■ TABLE 4. Prophylactic regimens for dental, oral, respiratory tract, or esophageal procedures

Situation	Agent	Regimen*
Standard general prophylaxis	Amoxicillin	Adults: 2.0 g; children: 50 mg/kg orally 1 h before procedure
Unable to take oral medications	Ampicillin	Adults: 2.0 g intramuscularly (IM) or intravenously (IV); children: 50 mg/kg IM or IV within 30 min before procedure
Allergic to penicillin	Clindamycin	Adults: 600 mg; Children: 20 mg/kg orally 1 h before procedure
	or	
	Cephalexin† or cefadroxil†	Adults: 2.0 g; children: 50 mg/kg orally 1 h before procedure
	or	
	Azithromycin or clarithromycin	Adults: 500 mg; children: 15 mg/kg orally 1 h before procedure
Allergic to penicillin and unable to take oral medications	Clindamycin	Adults: 600 mg; children: 20 mg/kg IV within 30 min before procedure
	or	
	Cefazolin†	Adults: 1.0 g; children: 25 mg/kg IM or IV within 30 min before procedure

*Total children's dose should not exceed adult dose.
†Cephalosporins should not be used in individuals with immediate-type hypersensitivity reaction (urticaria, angioedema, or anaphylaxis) to penicillins.
From Dajani AS, Taubart KA, Wilson W, et al.: Prevention of bacterial endocarditis recommendations by the American Heart Association. *JAMA* 277:1794–1801, 1997.

■ TABLE 5. Prophylactic regimens for genitourinary gastrointestinal (excluding esophageal) procedures

Situation	Agents*	Regimen†
High-risk patients	Ampicillin plus Gentamicin	Adults: ampicillin 2.0 g intramuscularly (IM) or intravenously (IV) plus gentamicin 1.5 mg/kg (not to exceed 120 mg) within 30 min of starting the procedure; 6 h later, ampicillin 1 g IM/IV or amoxicillin 1 g orally Children: ampicillin 50 mg/kg IM or IV (not to exceed 2.0 g) plus gentamicin 1.5 mg/kg IM/IV within 30 min of starting the procedure; 6 h later, ampicillin 25 mg/kg IM/IV or amoxicillin 25 mg/kg orally
High-risk patients allergic to ampicillin/amoxicillin	Vancomycin plus Gentamicin	Adults: vancomycin 1.0 g IV over 1-2 h plus gentamicin 1.5 mg/kg IV/IM (not to exceed 120 mg); complete injection/infusion within 30 min of starting the procedure Children: vancomycin 20 mg/kg IV over 1-2 h plus gentamicin 1.5 mg/kg IV/IM; complete injection/infusion within 30 min of starting the procedure
Moderate-risk patients	Amoxicillin or Ampicillin	Adults: amoxicillin 2.0 g orally 1 h before procedure, or ampicillin 2.0 g IM/IV within 30 min of starting the procedure Children: amoxicillin 50 mg/kg orally 1 h before procedure, or ampicillin 50 mg/kg IM/IV within 30 min of starting the procedure
Moderate-risk patients allergic to ampicillin/amoxicillin	Vancomycin	Adults: vancomycin 1.0 g IV over 1-2 h; complete infusion within 30 min of starting the procedure Children: vancomycin 20 mg/kg IV over 1-2 h; complete infusion within 30 min of starting the procedure

*Total children's dose should not exceed adult dose.
†No second dose of vancomycin or gentamicin is recommended.
From Dajani AS, Taubart KA, Wilson W, et al.: Prevention of bacterial endocarditis recommendations by the American Heart Association. *JAMA* 277:1794–1801, 1997.

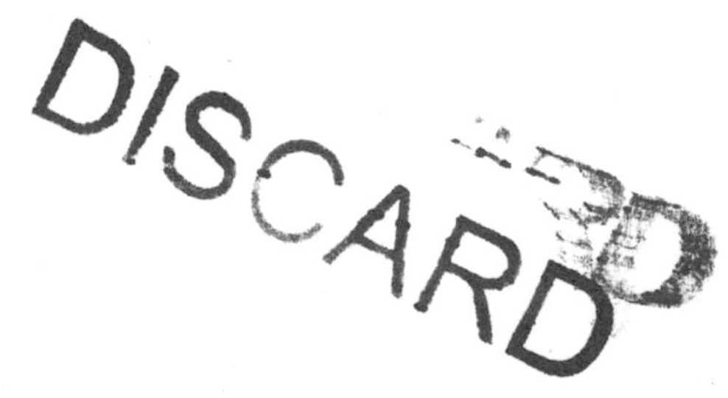
DISCARD

SMITH'S Anesthesia for Infants and Children

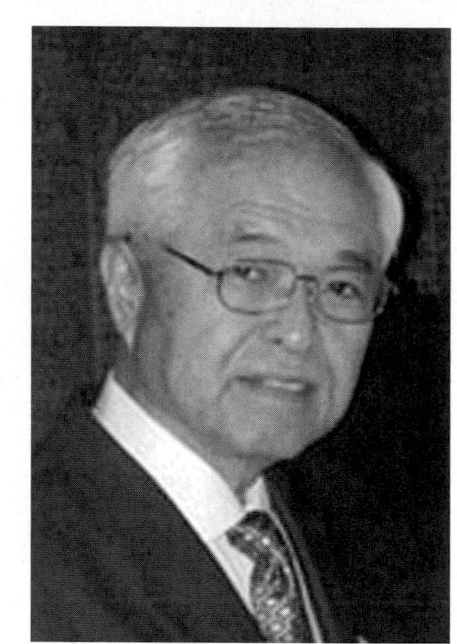
Etsuro K. Motoyama, M.D.

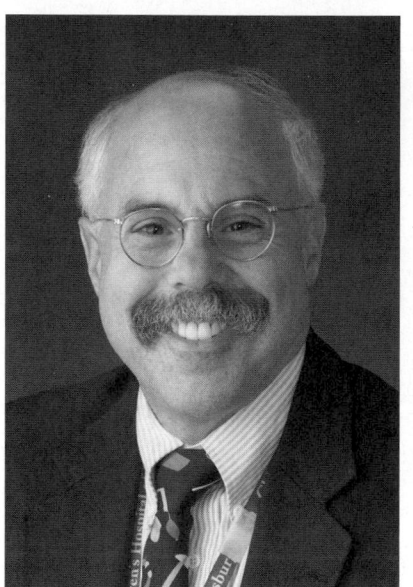
Peter J. Davis, M.D.

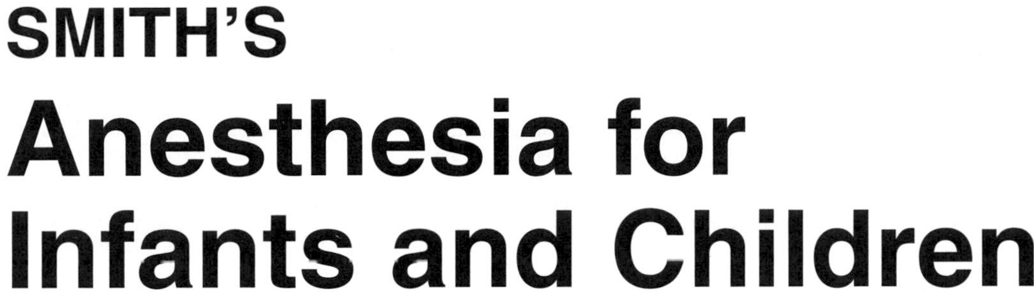

SMITH'S Anesthesia for Infants and Children

SEVENTH EDITION

Etsuro K. Motoyama, M.D.
Professor
Department of Anesthesiology
Department of Pediatrics (Pulmonology)
University of Pittsburgh School of Medicine
Attending Anesthesiologist and Pulmonologist
Director Pediatric Pulmonology Laboratory
Children's Hospital of Pittsburgh
Pittsburgh, Pennsylvania

Peter J. Davis, M.D.
Professor
Department of Anesthesiology
Department of Pediatrics
University of Pittsburgh School of Medicine
Anesthesiologist-in-Chief
Children's Hospital of Pittsburgh
Pittsburgh, Pennsylvania

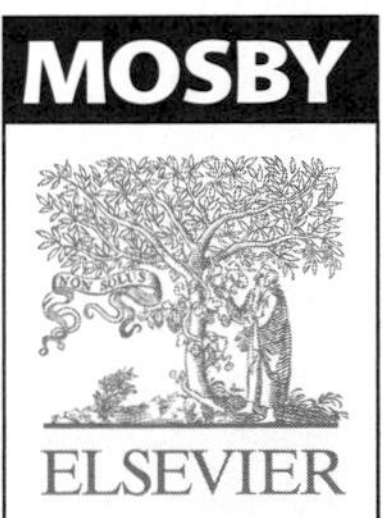

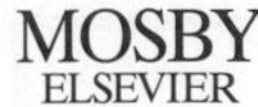

1600 John F. Kennedy Blvd.
Suite 1800
Philadelphia, PA 19103-2899

SMITH'S ANESTHESIA FOR INFANTS AND CHILDREN,
Seventh Edition
ISBN 978-0323-02647-5
ISBN 0-323-02647-8

Notice

Knowledge and best practice in the field are constantly changing. As new research and experience broaden our knowledge, changes in practice, treatment and drug therapy may become necessary or appropriate. Readers are advised to check the most current information provided (i) on procedures featured or (ii) by the manufaturer of each product to be administered, to verify the recommended dose or formula, the method and duration of administration, and contraindications. It is the responsibilty of the practitioner, relying on their own experience and knowledge of patient, to make diagnoses, to determine dosages and the best treatment for each individual patient, and to take all appropriate safety precautions. To the fullest extent of the law, neither the Publisher nor the Editors assume any liability for any injury and/or damage to persons or property arising out of or related to any use of the material contained in this book.

Cover design by Kaoru Kawasaki

Library of Congress Cataloging-in-Publication Data
Smith's anesthesia for infants and children / [edited by] Etsuro K. Motoyama, Peter J. Davis.-- 7th ed.
p. cm.
Includes bibliographical references and index.
ISBN 0-323-02647-8
1. Pediatric anesthesia. I. Title: Anesthesia for infants and children. II. Motoyama, Etsuro K. III. Davis, Peter, M.D.

RD139.S62 2006
617.9′6′083--dc22 2004065567

Publisher: Natasha Andjelkovic
Developmental Editor: Ann Ruzycka Anderson
Publishing Services Manager: Tina Rebane
Project Manager: Mary Anne Folcher
Designer: Karen O'Keefe Owens
Marketing Manager: Emily M. Christie

Printed in the United States of America.
Last digit is the print number: 9 8 7 6 5 4 3 2 1

To all the children we care for and from whom we learn every day

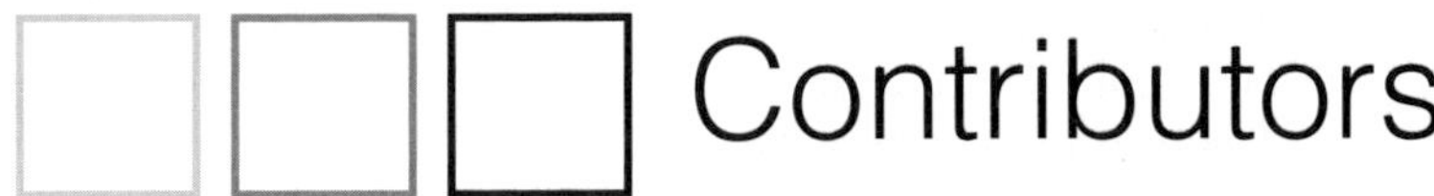

Contributors

Ann G. Bailey, M.D.
Professor of Anesthesiology and Pediatrics
University of North Carolina at Chapel Hill School of Medicine
Chapel Hill, North Carolina
Anesthesia for Pediatric Ophthalmic Surgery

Matthew B. Baker, M.D., Ph.D.
Chief Resident
Department of Anesthesiology
Vanderbilt University School of Medicine
Nashville, Tennessee
Anesthesia for Pediatric Plastic Surgery

Victor C. Baum, M.D.
Professor of Anesthesiology and Pediatrics
Executive Vice-Chair, Cardiac Anesthesia
Department of Anesthesiology
University of Virginia School of Medicine
Charlottesville, Virginia
Systemic Disorders in Infants and Children

David S. Beebe, M.D.
Professor
Department of Anesthesiology
University of Minnesota Medical School-Minneapolis
Fairview University Medical Center
Minneapolis, Minnesota
Anesthesia for Pediatric Organ Transplantation

Kumar G. Belani, M.D.
Professor of Anesthesiology and Pediatrics
University of Minnesota Medical School–Minneapolis
Minneapolis, Minnesota
Anesthesia for Pediatric Organ Transplantation

Richard A. Berkowitz, M.D.
Associate Professor
Department of Anesthesiolgy
University of Illinois at Chicago College of Medicine
Chicago, Illinois
Chairman and Medical Director
Department of Anesthesiology and Pain Medicine
Community Hospital
Munster, Indiana
Office-Based Pediatric Anesthesia

George B. Bikhazi, M.D.
Professor of Anesthesiology
University of Tennessee, Memphis, College of Medicine
St. Jude Children's Research Hospital
Memphis, Tennessee
Anesthesia for Neonates and Premature Infants

Bruno Bissonnette, M.D., F.R.C.P.C.
Professor of Anesthesiology
University of Toronto Faculty of Medicine
Director of Neuroanesthesiology
Department of Anaesthesia
Hospital for Sick Children
Toronto, Ontario
Thermoregulation: Physiology and Perioperative Disturbances

Barbara W. Brandom, M.D., M.P.H.
Professor of Anesthesiology
University of Pittsburgh School of Medicine
Attending Anesthesiologist
Department of Anesthesiology
Children's Hospital of Pittsburgh
Director, North American Malignant Hyperthermia Registry
Pittsburgh, Pennsylvania
Malignant Hyperthermia

Claire M. Brett, M.D.
Professor of Clinical Anesthesia and Pediatrics
University of California, San Francisco, School of Medicine
San Francisco, California
Anesthesia for Neonates and Premature Infants

Franklyn P. Cladis, M.D.
Assistant Professor of Anesthesiology
University of Pittsburgh School of Medicine
Childern's Hospital of Pittsburgh
Pittsburgh, Pennsylvania
Pediatric Drug Dosages
Index of Syndromes and Their Pediatric Anesthetic Implications

David E. Cohen, M.D.
Associate Professor of Anesthesiology and Pediatrics
Departments of Anesthesiology and Pediatrics
University of Pennsylvania School of Medicine
Perioperative Medical Director
Department of Anesthesiology and Critical Care Medicine
Children's Hospital of Philadelphia
Philadelphia, Pennsylvania
Pediatric Anesthesia Equipment and Monitoring

Ira T. Cohen, M.D.
Associate Professor of Anesthesiology and Pediatrics
George Washington University School of Medicine and Health Sciences
Attending Anesthesiologist
Children's National Medical Center
Washington, D.C.
Pediatric Intraoperative and Postoperative Management

D. Ryan Cook, M.D.
Professor of Anesthesiology
Duke University School of Medicine
Durham, North Carolina
Pharmacology of Pediatric Anesthesia

Peter J. Davis, M.D.
Professor
Department of Anesthesiology
Department of Pediatrics
University of Pittsburgh School of Medicine
Anesthesiologist-in-Chief
Children's Hospital of Pittsburgh
Pittsburgh, Pennsylvania
Special Characteristics of Pediatric Anesthesia
Thermoregulation: Physiology and Perioperative Disturbances
Pharmacology of Pediatric Anesthesia
Preoperative Preparation for Infants and Children
Anesthesia for Neonates and Premature Infants
Anesthesia for General Abdominal, Thoracic, Urologic, and Bariatric Surgery in Pediatric Patients
Perioperative Management of the Pediatric Trauma Patient
Systemic Disorders in Infants and Children

Jayant K. Deshpande, M.D., F.A.A.P.
Associate Professor of Pediatrics and Anesthesia
Vanderbilt University School of Medicine
Director, Division of Pediatric Critical Care and Anesthesia
Vanderbilt Children's Hospital
Nashville, Tennessee
Anesthesia for Pediatric Plastic Surgery

Karen B. Domino, M.D., M.P.H.
Professor of Anesthesiology
Adjunct Professor of Neurological Surgery
University of Washington School
Seattle, Washington
Anesthesia for Pediatric Neurosurgery

R. Blaine Easley, M.D.
Assistant Professor
Departments of Anesthesiology and Critical Care Medicine and Pediatrics
Johns Hopkins School of Medicine
Johns Hopkins Hospital
Baltimore, Maryland
Pediatric Cardiopulmonary Resuscitation

Demetrius Ellis, M.D.
Professor of Pediatrics
University of Pittsburgh School of Medicine
Director of Pediatric Nephrology
Children's Hospital of Pittsburgh
Pittsburgh, Pennsylvania
Regulation of Fluids and Electrolytes in Infants and Children

Gavin F. Fine, M.D., M.B.B.Ch.
Clinical Assistant Professor
University of Texas Southwestern Medical Center at Dallas Southwestern Medical School
Dallas, Texas
Attending Anesthesiologist
Cook's Children's Hospital
Fort Worth, Texas
Induction of Anesthesia and Maintenance of the Airway in Infants and Children

Carl G. Fischer, M.D.
Professor of Anesthesiology
University of Cincinnati College of Medicine
Anesthesiologist
Shriners Hospital for Children
Cincinnati, Ohio
Anesthesia for Children with Burns

Jeffrey L. Galinkin, M.D.
Associate Professor
University of Colorado School of Medicine
University of Colorado Health Science Center
Director of Research
Department of Anesthesia
Children's Hospital
Denver, Colorado
Anesthesia for Fetal Surgery

Salvatore R. Goodwin, M.D.
Associate Professor of Anesthesiology
Mayo Clinic Chairman
Department of Anesthesiology
Nemours Children's Clinic
Jacksonville, Florida
Systemic Disorders in Infants and Children

William J. Greeley, M.D.
Professor
Departments of Anesthesia and Pediatrics
University of Pennsylvania School of Medicine
Anesthesiologist-in-Chief
Children's Hospital of Philadelphia
Philadelphia, Pennsylvania
Anesthesia for Pediatric Cardiovascular Surgery

Brian J. Gronert, M.D.
Anesthesia Associates of New Mexico
Attending Anesthesiologist Presbyterian Hospital Albuquerque, New Mexico
Induction of Anesthesia and Maintenance of the Airway in Infants and Children

Steven C. Hall, M.D.
Anesthesiologist-in-Chief
Department of Pediatric Anesthesiology
Children's Memorial Hospital
Arthur C. King Professor of Anesthesiology
Northwestern University Medical School
Chicago, Illinois
Anesthesia for General Abdominal, Thoracic, Urologic, and Bariatric Surgery in Pediatric Patients

Gregory B. Hammer, M.D.
Professor of Anesthesiology and Pediatrics
Stanford University School of Medicine
Stanford University Hospital
Stanford, California
Anesthesia for General Abdominal, Thoracic, Urologic, and Bariatric Surgery in Pediatric Patients

Michael Winn Hauser, M.D.
Assistant Professor
University of North Carolina at Chapel Hill School of Medicine
Chapel Hill, North Carolina
Anesthesia for Pediatric Ophthalmic Surgery

Andrew Herlich, D.M.D., M.D.
Professor of Anesthesiology, Otolaryngology, and Pediatrics
Medical Director, Human Simulation Center
Temple University School of Medicine
Staff Anesthesiologist
Temple University Children's Medical Center and Shriners Hospital for Children of Philadelphia
Philadelphia, Pennsylvania
Anesthesia for Pediatric Dentistry

Robert S. Holzman, M.D.
Associate Professor of Anesthesia
Harvard Medical School
Children's Hospital
Boston, Massachusetts
Anesthesia and Sedation for Pediatric Procedures Outside the Operating Room

Richard J. Ing, M.B.B.Ch., F.C.A. (S.A.)
Department of Anesthesia
Duke University School of Medicine
Durham, North Carolina
Anesthesia for Pediatric Cardiovascular Surgery

Jodi Innocent, J.D.
Associate Counsel, Corporate Compliance and Privacy Officer
Children's Hospital of Pittsburgh
Pittsburgh, Pennsylvania
Medicolegal and Ethical Aspects of Pediatric Anesthesia

Zeev N. Kain, M.D., M.B.A.
Professor of Anesthesiology, Pediatrics, and Child Psychology
Executive Vice-Chair
Department of Anesthesiology
Yale University School of Medicine
Anesthesiologist-in-Chief
Yale–New Haven Children's Hospital
New Haven, Connecticut
Psychological Aspects of Pediatric Anesthesia

Kevin J. Kelly, M.D., D.D.S.
Associate Professor
Department of Plastic Surgery
Vanderbilt Medical Center
Medical Center South
Nashville, Tennessee
Anesthesia for Pediatric Plastic Surgery

Frank H. Kern, M.D., F.C.C.M.
Professor of Anesthesiology and Pediatrics
Chief of Pediatric Anesthesia and Critical Care Medicine
Duke University Medical Center
Durham, North Carolina
Anesthesia for Pediatric Cardiovascular Surgery

Elliot J. Krane, M.D.
Professor of Anesthesia and Pediatrics
Stanford University School of Medicine
Stanford, California
Chief, Pain Management
Lucile Salter Packard Children's Hospital at Stanford
Palo Alto, California
Preoperative Preparation for Infants and Children
Anesthesia for Pediatric Neurosurgery

Ira S. Landsman, M.D.
Associate Professor
Departments of Pediatrics and Anesthesiology
Vanderbilt University School of Medicine
Director, Division of Pediatric Anesthesiology
Vanderbilt Children's Hospital
Vanderbilt University Medical Center
Nashville, Tennessee
Anesthesia for Pediatric Otorhinolaryngologic Surgery

Jerrold Lerman, M.D., F.R.C.P.C., F.A.N.Z.C.A.
Clinical Professor of Anesthesia
Women and Children's Hospital of Buffalo, SUNY at Buffalo Strong Memorial Hospital
University of Rochester
Rochester, New York
Pharmacology of Pediatric Anesthesia

Ronald S. Litman, D.O.
Associate Professor of Anesthesiology and Pediatrics
University of Pennsylvania School of Medicine
Attending Anesthesiologist
Children's Hospital of Philadelphia
Philadelphia, Pennsylvania
Pediatric Anesthesia Equipment and Monitoring

Igor Luginbuehl, M.D.
Assistant Professor
Department of Anesthesiology
University of Toronto Faculty of Medicine
Staff Anesthesiologist
Hospital for Sick Children
Toronto, Ontario, Canada
Thermoregulation: Physiology and Perioperative Disturbances

Shobha Malviya, M.D.
Associate Professor of Anesthesiology
Section of Pediatric Anesthesiology
University of Michigan Medical School
C. S. Mott Children's Hospital
Ann Arbor, Michigan
Perioperative Management of the Pediatric Trauma Patient

Thomas J. Mancuso, M.D.
Assistant Professor of Anesthesia
Harvard Medical School
Director, Acute Pain Treatment Services
Children's Hospital
Boston, Massachusetts
Systemic Disorders in Infants and Children

Keira P. Mason, M.D.
Assistant Professor of Anesthesia (Radiology)
Harvard Medical School
Associate in Perioperative Anesthesia
Director of Radiology Anesthesia
Children's Hospital
Boston, Massachusetts
Anesthesia and Sedation for Pediatric Procedures Outside the Operating Room

Lynne Maxwell, M.D., F.A.A.P.
Associate Professor
Department of Anesthesia
University of Pennsylvania School of Medicine
Director, General Anesthesia Division
Department of Anesthesiology and Critical Care Medicine
Children's Hospital of Philadelphia
Philadelphia, Pennsylvania
Systemic Disorders in Infants and Children

John E. McCall, M.D.
Professor of Anesthesiology
University of Cincinnati College of Medicine
Director of Anesthesiology
Shriners Hospital for Children
Cincinnati, Ohio
Anesthesia for Children with Burns

Francis X. McGowan, Jr., M.D.
Professor of Anesthesiolgy
Harvard Medical School
Cardiac Anesthesia Service
Children's Hospital
Boston, Massachusetts
Anesthesia for Pediatric Organ Transplantation

Philip G. Morgan M.D.
Professor
Department of Anesthesiology, Genetics and Pharmacology
University Hospitals of Cleveland
Case Western Reserve University
Cleveland, Ohio
Systemic Disorders in Infants and Children

Etsuro K. Motoyama, M.D.
Professor
Department of Anesthesiology
Department of Pediatrics (Pulmonology)
University of Pittsburgh School of Medicine
Attending Anesthesiologist and Pulmonologist
Director, Pediatric Pulmonology Laboratory
Children's Hospital of Pittsburgh
Pittsburgh, Pennsylvania
Special Characteristics of Pediatric Anesthesia
Respiratory Physiology in Infants and Children
Induction of Anesthesia and Maintenance of the Airway in Infants and Children
Pediatric Intraoperative and Postoperative Management
Anesthesia for Fetal Surgery
Anesthesia for Pediatric Otorhinolaryngologic Surgery
Systemic Disorders in Infants and Children
Safety and Outcome in Pediatric Anesthesia

Bridget M. Philip, M.D.
Pediatric Anesthesia Fellow
Department of Anesthesia
Stanford University School of Medicine
Stanford, California
Attending Anesthesiologist
Santa Clara Valley Medical Center
San Jose, California
Anesthesia for Pediatric Neurosurgery

David M. Polaner, M.D., F.A.A.P.
Associate Professor of Anesthesiology
Department of Anesthesiology
University of Colorado School of Medicine
Attending Pediatric Anesthesiologist
Chief, Acute Pain Service
Children's Hospital
Denver, Colorado
Anesthesia for Pediatric Same-Day Surgical Procedures

Paul I. Reynolds, M.D.
Uma and Sujit Pandit Professor and Chief of Pediatric Anesthesiology
University of Michigan Medical School
University of Michigan Health System
Ann Arbor, Michigan
Perioperative Management of the Pediatric Trauma Patient

Kerri M. Robertson, M.D., F.R.C.P.(C.)
Associate Clinical Professor
Department of Anesthesiology
Duke University School of Medicine
Chief, Transplantation Services
Duke University Medical Center
Durham, North Carolina
Anesthesia for Pediatric Organ Transplantation

Mark A. Rockoff, M.D.
Professor of Anesthesiology
Harvard Medical School
Vice Chairman
Department of Anesthesiology
Children's Hospital
Boston, Massachusetts
History of Pediatric Anesthesia

Allison Kinder Ross, M.D.
Associate Professor of Anesthesiology
Duke University School of Medicine
Associate Chief, Division of Pediatric Anesthesia
Duke University Medical Center
Durham, North Carolina
Pediatric Regional Anesthesia

Lynn M. Rusy, M.D.
Associate Professor
Department of Anesthesia
Medical College of Wisconsin
Staff Anesthesiologist
Medical Acupuncturist
Children's Hospital of Wisconsin
Milwaukee, Wisconsin
Pain Management in Infants and Children

M. Ramez Salem, M.D.
Chairman
Department of Anesthesiology
Illinois Masonic Medical Center
Clinical Professor of Anesthesiology
University of Illinois College of Medicine
Attending Anesthesiologist
Shriners Hospital for Crippled Children
Chicago, Illinois
Blood Conservation in Children

Charles L. Schleien, M.D.
Professor of Pediatrics and Anesthesia
Director, Pediatric Intensive Care Unit
Columbia University Medical Center
New York, New York
Professor of Pediatrics and Anesthesiology
Coloumbia University College of Physicians and Surgeons
Medical Director, Pediatric Critical Care Medicine
Morgan Stanley Children's Hospitals-Presbyterian
New York, New York
Pediatric Cardiopulmonary Resuscitation

Uwe Schwarz, M.D.
Research Fellow
University of Pennsylvania School of Medicine
Children's Hospital of Philadelphia
Philadelphia, Pennsylvania
Anesthesia for Fetal Surgery

Robert J. Sclabassi, M.D., Ph.D.
Professor
Departments of Neurosurgery, Neuroscience, Electrical Engineering, and Biomedical Engineering
University of Pittsburgh School of Medicine
Attending Clinical Neurophysiologist
Department of Neurosurgery, Center for Clinical Neurophysiology
Children's Hospital of Pittsburgh, University of Pittsburgh Medical Center
Pittsburgh, Pennsylvania
Pediatric Anesthesia Equipment and Monitoring

Victor L. Scott, M.D.
Clinical Professor of Anesthesiology
University of Pittsburgh School of Medicine
Attending Anesthesiologist
Children's Hospital of Pittsburgh
Pittsburgh, Pennsylvania
Anesthesia for Pediatric Organ Transplantation

Donald H. Shaffner, M.D.
Associate Professor
Department of Anesthesiology and Critical Care Medicine
Johns Hopkins University School of Medicine
Johns Hopkins Hospital
Baltimore, Maryland
Pediatric Cardiopulmonary Resuscitation

Avinash C. Shukla, M.B.B.S., F.R.C.A.
Associate in Cardiac Anesthesia
Department of Anesthesia
Harvard Medical School
Children's Hospital
Boston, Massachusetts
Anesthesia for Pediatric Organ Transplantation

Robert M. Smith, M.D., F.R.A.R.C.S., Ireland (Hon.)
Clinical Professor of Anesthesia, Emeritus
Harvard Medical School
Chief of Anesthesia (1946–1980)
Children's Hospital
Boston Massachusetts
History of Pediatric Anesthesia

Oliver S. Soldes, M.D.
Clinical Assistant Professor
Section of Pediatric Surgery
University of Michigan Medical School
University of Michigan Health System
Ann Arbor, Michigan
Perioperative Management of the Pediatric Trauma Patient

Maureen A. Strafford, M.D.
Associate Professor of Anesthesiology and Pediatrics
Tufts University School of Medicine
Associate Anesthesiologist
Department of Anesthesiology
New England Medical Center Hospitals
Boston, Massachusetts
Cardiovascular Physiology in Infants and Children

Stevan P. Tofovic, M.D., D.Sc.
Assistant Professor
Medicine/Clinical Pharmacology
Center for Clinical Pharmacology
University of Pittsburgh School of Medicine
Pittsburgh, Pennsylvania
Pharmacology for Pediatric Anesthesia

Robert D. Valley, M.D.
Professor of Anesthesiology and Pediatrics
University of North Carolina at Chapel Hill School of Medicine
Director of Pediatric Anesthesia
North Carolina Children's Hospital
Chapel Hill, North Carolina
Anesthesia for Pediatric Ophthalmic Surgery

Jay A. Werkhaven, M.D.
Associate Professor
Department of Otolaryngology
Vanderbilt University School of Medicine
Nashville, Tennessee
Anesthesia for Pediatric Otorhinolaryngologic Surgery

Eva Vogeley, M.D., J.D., Mdiv.
Assistant Professor of Pediatrics
Division of Pediatric Emergency Medicine
University of Pittsburgh School of Medicine
Attending Physician
Children's Hospital of Pittsburgh
Pittsburgh, Pennsylvania
Medicolegal and Ethical Aspects of Pediatric Anesthesia

Steven J. Weisman, M.D.
Professor of Anesthesiology and Pediatrics
Medical College of Wisconsin
Medical Director, Jane B. Pettit Pain and Palliative Care Center
Associate Director, Pediatric Anesthesiology
Children's Hospital of Wisconsin
Milwaukee, Wisconsin
Pain Management in Infants and Children

Myron Yaster, M.D.
Richard J. Traystman Professor of Pediatric Anesthesiology, Critical Care Medicine, and Pediatric Pain Management
Department of Anesthesia and Critical Care Medicine
Johns Hopkins University School of Medicine
Attending Anesthesiologist
Johns Hopkins Hospital
Baltimore, Maryland
Anesthesia for Pediatric Orthopedic Surgery

Kelly K. Yeh, M.D.
Pediatric Anesthesia Fellow
Department of Anesthesia
Stanford University School of Medicine
Stanford, California
Pediatric Anesthesiologist
Department of Anesthesia
Santa Clara Valley Medical Center
San Jose, California
Anesthesia for Pediatric Neurosurgery

Steven E. Zgleszewski, M.D.
Instructor in Anesthesia
Harvard Medical School
Associate in Perioperative Anesthesia
Director, Endoscopy Unit Anesthesia Services
Children's Hospital
Boston, Massachusetts
Anesthesia and Sedation for Pediatric Procedures Outside the Operating Room

Aaron L. Zuckerberg, M.D.
Assistant Professor
Departments of Pediatrics Anesthesia and Critical Care Medicine
University of Maryland School of Medicine
Director, Pediatric Anesthesiology, Critical Care Medicine
Director, Children's Diagnostic Center
Sinai Hospital of Baltimore
Baltimore, Maryland
Anesthesia for Pediatric Orthopedic Surgery
Systemic Disorders in Infants and Children

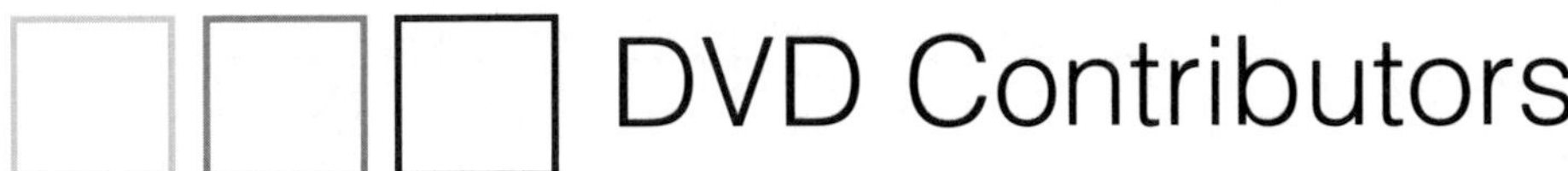

DVD Contributors

Cuneyt M. Alper, M.D.
Associate Professor of Otolaryngology
University of Pittsburgh School of Medicine
Department of Otolaryngology
Children's Hospital of Pittsburgh
Pittsburgh, Pennsylvania

Lawrence M. Borland, M.D.
Associate Professor of Anesthesiology
University of Pittsburgh School of Medicine
Department of Anesthesiology
Children's Hospital of Pittsburgh
Pittsburgh, Pennsylvania

James G. Cain, M.D.
Associate Professor of Anesthesiology
University of Pittsburgh School of Medicine
Department of Anesthesiology
Children's Hospital of Pittsburgh
Pittsburgh, Pennsylvania

Peter J. Davis, M.D.
Professor of Anesthesiology and Pediatrics
University of Pittsburgh School of Medicine
Anesthesiologist-in-Chief
Children's Hospital of Pittsburgh
Pittsburgh, Pennsylvania

William A. Devine
Senior Pathologists Assistant
Department of Pathology
Curator, Frank E. Sherman and Cora C. Lenox Heart Museum
Children's Hospital of Pittsburgh
Pittsburgh, Pennsylvania

Joseph E. Dohar, M.D.
Associate Professor of Otolaryngology
University of Pittsburgh School of Medicine
Department of Otolaryngology
Children's Hospital of Pittsburgh
Pittsburgh, Pennsylvania

Keith E. Georgeson, M.D.
Surgeon-in-Chief
The Children's Hospital of Alabama
Joseph M. Farely Chair of Pediatric Surgery
Director of the Division of Pediatric Surgery
Department of Surgery
University of Alabama School of Medicine
Birmingham, Alabama

Christopher M. Grande, M.D.
Visiting Clinical Professor of Anesthesiology
University of Pittsburgh School of Medicine
Pittsburgh, Pennsylvania

Gregory B. Hammer, M.D.
Professor of Anesthesiology and Pediatrics
Stanford University School of Medicine
Department of Anesthesia and Pain Management
Lucile Packard Children's Hospital
Stanford, California

Timothy D. Kane, M.D.
Assistant Professor of Surgery and Critical Care Medicine
University of Pittsburgh School of Medicine
Department of Pediatric Surgery
Children's Hospital of Pittsburgh
Pittsburgh, Pennsylvania

George V. Mazariegos, M.D
Associate Professor of Surgery
University of Pittsburgh School of Medicine
Director of Pediatric Transplant Program
Children's Hospital of Pittsburgh
Pittsburgh, Pennsylvania

Douglas A. Potoka, M.D
Assistant Professor of Surgery
University of Pittsburgh School of Medicine
Department of Pediatric Surgery
Children's Hospital of Pittsburgh
Pittsburgh, Pennsylvania

Paul I. Reynolds, M.D.
Clinical Associate Professor of Anesthesiology
Section Head, Pediatric Anesthesiology
Associate Chair, Department of Anesthesia
University of Michigan Health System
Ann Arbor, Michigan

Allison Kinder Ross, M.D
Clinical Associate Professor of Anesthesiology
Duke University Medical Center
Durham, North Carolina

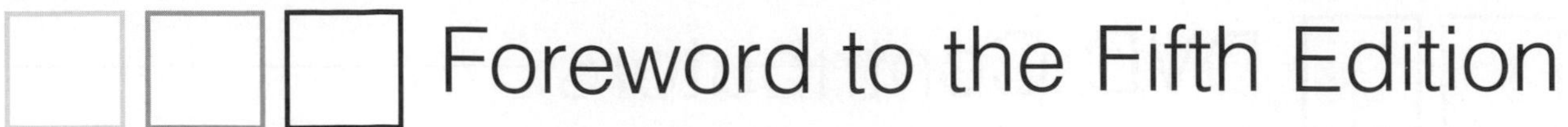

Foreword to the Fifth Edition

When the first edition of the book was published in 1959, the essentials of pediatric anesthesia were barely taking form. Teaching was limited to a few centers, literature was scanty, and research was virtually nonexistent. *Anesthesia for Infants and Children* was offered as a practical text presenting the fundamental differences in pediatric patients as related to older persons, with safety and simplicity as the main underlying principles.

During the following 20 years, pediatric anesthesia expanded along with the rapid development of pediatric surgery. Standards of clinical management became established and refined, training facilities were organized, and pediatric anesthesiology became a recognized and respected field of medicine. The three editions published during this period kept pace with the growing specialty while retaining the same general format as the first edition. In the fourth edition all but 6 of the 29 chapters were written by the principal author.

During the past 10 years clinical management has advanced to a highly developed science with unpredicted levels of accomplishment, educational programs have burgeoned, and the research approaches previously limited to older patients have been developed for even the smallest infants, resulting in a deluge of new and important information. The situation clearly demands a multiauthored text. I am delighted to pass the responsibility on to my former associate Etsuro K. Motoyama, who has authored an outstanding chapter on respiratory physiology in all earlier editions, and to his associate, Peter Davis. The chapters are written by experts in each area, adding much authority to the presentation. While benefiting greatly from scientific advances, our text still retains emphasis on the human approach to the whole patient.

I am greatly indebted to the editors and the collaborators for their painstaking efforts and for prolonging the existence of *Anesthesia for Infants and Children.*

Robert M. Smith, M.D.

Preface

Dr. Robert M. Smith's legacy is as a pioneer and a great educator in pediatric anesthesia. Long before the terminology became fashionable—before it even existed—Dr. Smith advocated patient monitoring and safety. In the 1950s, when pediatric anesthesia was still in its infancy, he made the use of the precordial stethoscope and the pediatric blood pressure cuff (Smith cuff) a standard of care. In 1959, he wrote a major comprehensive anesthesia textbook, *Anesthesia for Infants and Children,* which was specifically dedicated to the anesthetic management and the care of the children.

The first four editions of this book were written almost entirely by Dr. Smith himself. The scope of Dr. Smith's scholarship was reflected in the breadth of his firsthand clinical experience, his keen sense of observation, and his ability to apply scientific and technical developments in medicine and anesthesia to the field of pediatric anesthesia. In 1988, Dr. Smith became the first pediatric anesthesiologist to receive the Distinguished Service Award from the American Society of Anesthesiologists.

In 1980, with Dr. Smith's retirement from the Harvard Medical School faculty and the anesthesia directorship of Children's Hospital, Boston, the task of updating this classic textbook was bestowed upon the current editors. The fifth edition, published in 1990, was multiauthored and was reorganized to include new subjects of importance in the ever expanding field of anesthesiology and pediatric anesthesiology in particular. In the fifth edition, the editors tried to maintain Dr. Smith's compassion, philosophy, and emphasis on the personal approach to patients. To honor his pioneering work and leadership (and against Dr. Smith's initial strong resistance), the title of the fifth edition of the textbook was modified to read *Smith's Anesthesia for Infants and Children.*

In 1996, the sixth edition of the textbook was published. New developments with inhaled anesthetic agents (sevoflurane and desflurane), intravenous agents (propofol), neuromuscular blocking agents, and anesthetic adjuncts, coupled with changes in the approach to pediatric pain management and airway management, were highlights.

Today, the seventh edition further expands these areas of development. The roles of airway management, regional anesthesia, new local anesthetic agents, and innovative regional anesthetic techniques have been further developed. Newer intravenous anesthetic agents and adjuncts have also been included in this edition, while patient safety and compassion remain integral aspects of *Smith's Anesthesia for Infants and Children.* Extensive experience with the newer inhaled anesthetics has brought up hitherto unrecognized problems. In the case of sevoflurane, its breakdown products (i.e., compound A) in carbon dioxide absorbers and exothermic reactions led to the development of inert, calcium chloride-based absorbers. Consequently, sevoflurane anesthesia using a low-flow or even a closed-circle system is becoming a reality with lower cost and less environmental air pollution in the operating room. Development of an ultra-short-acting synthetic opioid (remifentanil) together with propofol has made the total intravenous anesthesia for young infants a reality. The assessment of anesthetic depth is aided by bispectral electroencephalographic index monitoring. Increased awareness and improvement in perioperative pain management over the last decade have led to the establishment of pain services by anesthesiologists. Though much has changed since Dr. Smith last edited the book, its underlying focus is still on patients and their families.

The seventh edition has been prepared with the same intention as the previous six editions: to give anesthesia care providers comprehensive coverage of the physiology, pharmacology, and clinical anesthetic management of infants and children of all ages. This edition remains organized into four sections. The first section, **Basic Principles in Pediatric Anesthesia,** has been updated by major revisions of the chapters on respiratory physiology, cardiovascular physiology, fluid and electrolyte regulation, thermal regulation, and pharmacology in infants and children. In the second section, **General Approach to Pediatric Anesthesia,** a new chapter on the psychological aspects of pediatric anesthesia has been created, reflecting anesthesiologists' increased awareness of the subject. New chapters on pain management and pediatric regional anesthesia have been added by new contributors. All other chapters in this section have been updated by the same group of contributors as in the sixth edition. The third section, **Clinical Management of Special Surgical Problems,** contains newly added chapters on anesthesia for fetal surgery, in response to the development of fetal surgical procedures, and office-based pediatric anesthesia. This section also contains newly reorganized chapters on anesthesia for general, thoracic, urologic, and bariatric surgery and for plastic surgery in infants and children. New chapters by new contributors are included on anesthesia for pediatric ophthalmic surgery, anesthesia for pediatric same-day surgical procedures, anesthesia for children with burns, and perioperative management of pediatric trauma patients. All other chapters in this section have been updated by the same group of contributors. The fourth section, **Associated Problems in Pediatric Anesthesia,** contains new chapters on pediatric cardiopulmonary resuscitation and ethical and medicolegal aspects of pediatric anesthesia. The remainder of the chapters went through major revisions and updates by the corresponding contributors. Of note, the chapter on the history of pediatric anesthesia has been updated by Dr. Mark A. Rockoff with direct consultation with Dr. Robert M. Smith—who, we are happy to report, still enjoys good health in his advancing age, at the time of this writing. The **Appendices** include an updated list of drugs and their dosages, normal growth curves, normal values for pulmonary function tests in children, and an expanded list of common and uncommon syndromes of clinical importance for pediatric anesthesiologists.

In keeping with the advancement in technology, this edition contains a DVD with video segments to provide visual and verbal descriptions to improve the understanding of some technically more demanding procedures. They include techniques of regional anesthesia, single-lung ventilation, and fiberoptic intubation. Video and still images of surgical procedures as well as the color images of syndromes of clinical importance for pediatric anesthesia are included. They are intended to help pediatric anesthesiologists for preoperative assessments and preparations.

In summary, considerable developments and progress in the practice of pediatric anesthesia over the last decade are reflected in this new edition. The emphasis on the safety and well-being of our young patients during the perianesthetic period remains unchanged.

Etsuro K. Motoyama, M.D.

Peter J. Davis, M.D.

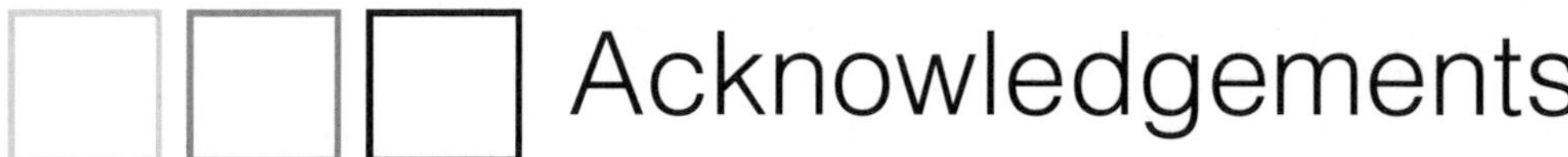

Acknowledgements

The project of revising a classic medical textbook presents many opportunities and challenges. The chance to review the many new developments that have emerged in pediatric anesthesia since the publication of the last edition of *Smith's Anesthesia for Infants and Children* in 1996 and to evaluate their effects on clinical practice have indeed been exciting. As always, we are deeply indebted to the extraordinary work done and commitment made by Dr. Robert M. Smith. Beginning shortly after World War II, Dr. Smith pioneered pediatric anesthesia in the United States. Between 1959 and 1980, he published the first four editions of his book, *Anesthesia for Infants and Children*. His work made this textbook a classic, establishing a quality and record of longevity. Editions 1st through 4th were written almost exclusively by Dr. Smith, with the exception of the chapter on respiratory physiology by E.K. Motoyama. Since the late 1980s, when Dr. Smith passed the book to the current editors, the subsequent 5th and 6th editions and now the new 7th edition have utilized the talents and expertise of many renowned pediatric anesthesiologists throughout North America. The 7th edition has been expanded further by the addition of new chapters and new contributors. The new edition has added DVD capabilities to further enhance the book's educational potential. These additions reflect the continual growth and complexity of the specialty of pediatric anesthesia.

Our ability to maintain this book's standard of excellence is not just a reflection of the many gifted contributors but is also a result of the level of support that we have received at work and at home. We wish to thank the staff members of the Department of Anesthesiology at the Children's Hospital of Pittsburgh and the University of Pittsburgh Medical Center for their support and tolerance.

Our special thanks go to David Chasey, Editorial Assistant, as well as Susan Danfelt and Patty Klein, Administrative Assistants, of the Department of Anesthesiology, Children's Hospital of Pittsburgh, for their many hours of diligent work on the book. We are appreciative of the photographic material supplied to us by various current and former members of the Children's Hospital of Pittsburgh staff. The credits for photography go to Dr. Brian Gronert; Ellen Kretchman, CRNA; David Wagner, CRNA (Anesthesiology); Drs. Charles Bluestone, Sylvan Stool, Robert Yellon (Otolaryngology), and Basil Zitelli (Pediatrics). The cover for this edition was created by Kaoru Kawasaki, graphic designer.

Our special thanks also go to Elsevier's Natasha Andjelkovic, Publisher; Ann Ruzycka Anderson, Senior Developmental Editor; and Mary Anne Folcher, Senior Project Manager, for their editorial assistance.

Finally, as with the previous two editions, we are deeply indebted to our family members, Yoko, Eugene, and Ray Motoyama and Katie, Evan, Julie, and Zava Davis, for remaining loyal, for being understanding, and for providing moral support throughout the lengthy and, at times, seemingly endless project.

Etsuro K. Motoyama, M.D.

Peter J. Davis, M.D.

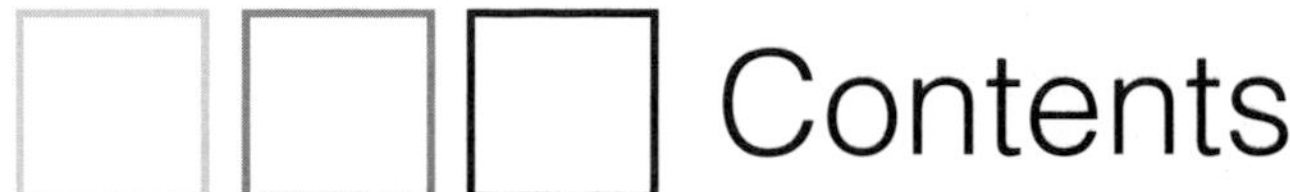

Contents

DVD Contents

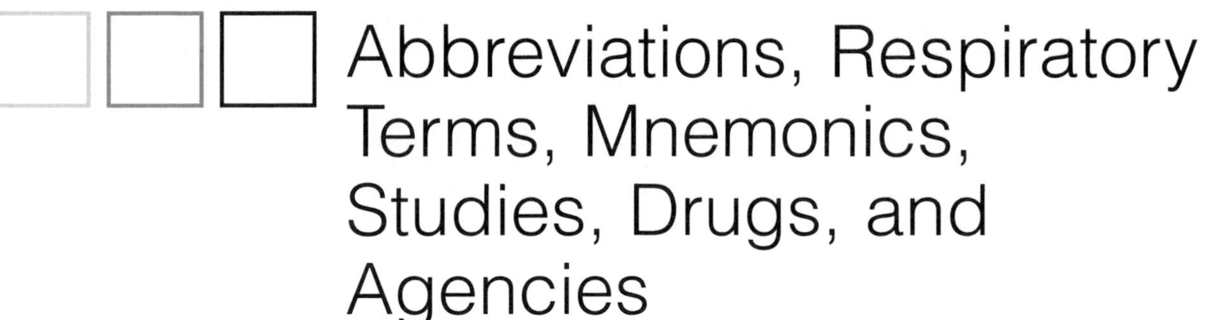

Abbreviations, Respiratory Terms, Mnemonics, Studies, Drugs, and Agencies

AAAAPSF: American Association for Accreditation of Ambulatory Plastic Surgery Facilities
AAASF: Association for Accreditation of Ambulatory Surgical Facilities
AAAHC: American Association for Ambulatory Health Care
AABB: American Association of Blood Banks
AAP: American Academy of Pediatrics
ABCs: airway, breathing, and circulation
ABL: allowable blood loss
ABMS: American Board of Medical Specialties
ABS: amniotic band syndrome
ACD: active compression–decompression
ACh: acetylcholine
ACE: alcohol, chloroform, and ether
ACE: angiotensin-converting enzyme
ACLS: advanced cardiac life support
ACT: activated coagulation (clotting) time
ADARPEF: French-Language Society of Pediatric Anesthesiologists
ADH: antidiuretic hormone
ADHR: autosomal dominant hypophosphatemic rickets
ADP: adenosine diphosphate
AED: automated external defibrillator
AGA: appropriate-for-gestational age
AHA: American Heart Association
AHCPR: Agency for Health Care Policy and Research
AIMS: Australian Incident Monitoring Study
ALG: antilymphocyte globulin
ALTE: apparent life-threatening event(s)
AMA: American Medical Association
AMC: arthrogryposis multiplex congenita
AMP: adenosine monophosphate
ANA: antinuclear antibody
ANH: acute isovolemic or normovolemic hemodilution
ANP: atrial natriuretic peptide
AP: action potential
APC: activated protein C
APSF: Anesthesia Patient Safety Foundation
aPTT: activated partial thromboplastin time
AQ: acoustic quantification
αAR: α-adrenergic receptor
ARDS: adult (acute) respiratory distress syndrome
ARF: acute renal failure
ASA: American Society of Anesthesiologists
ASC: ambulatory surgery center
ASD: atrial septal defect
ASPRS: American Society of Plastic and Reconstructive Surgery
ASTM: American Society for Testing and Materials
ATG: antithymocyte globulin
ATLS: advanced trauma life support (Advanced Trauma Life Support as course name)
ATN: acute tubular necrosis
ATP: adenosine triphosphate
AV: atrioventricular
AVM: arteriovenous malformation
AVP: L-arginine vasopressin
AVPU: Alert, responds to Voice, responds only to Pain, Unresponsive to stimuli
AVSD: atrioventricular septal defect
AVV: atrioventricular valve
BAEP: brainstem auditory evoked potential
Bi-PAP: bilevel positive airway pressure
BIS: bispectral index
BLS: basic life support
BMI: body mass index
BMP: bone morphogenetic protein
BP: blood pressure
BPD: bronchopulmonary dysplasia
BSA: body surface area
BSEP: brainstem somatosensory evoked potential
cAMP: cyclic adenosine monophosphate
CaO_2: arterial oxygen content
CaSR: Ca^{2+}-sensing receptor
CBF: cerebral blood flow
CBC: complete blood cell count
CCAM: congenital cystic adenomatoid malformation
CCD: cortical collecting duct
CCD: central core disease
CCL: cardiac cycle length
CCP: cerebral perfusion pressure
CDC: Centers for Disease Control and Prevention
CDH: congenital diaphragmatic hernia
CE: chloroform and ether
CEPOD: Confidential Enquiry into Perioperative Deaths
cGMP: cyclic guanosine monophosphate
CHAOS: congenital high airway obstruction syndrome
CHCT: caffeine-halothane contracture test
CHD: congenital heart disease
CHEOPS: Children's Hospital of Eastern Ontario Pain Scale
CI: cardiac index
CK: creatinine kinase
CL: compliance of lungs
CMAP: compound muscle action potential

$CMRO_2$: cerebral metabolic rate for oxygen
CMS: Centers for Medicare and Medicaid Services
CMV: cytomegalovirus
CNAP: compound nerve action potential
CNS: central nervous system
CO: cardiac output
COPD: chronic obstructive pulmonary disease
COPA: cuffed oropharyngeal airway
COPRA: Consolidated Omnibus Budget Reconciliation Act of 1986
COX: cyclooxygenase
CP: cerebral palsy
CPAP: continuous positive airway pressure
CPB: cardiopulmonary bypass
CPD: citrate-phosphate-dextrose
CPP: cerebral perfusion pressure
CPR: cardiopulmonary resuscitation
CP_{ss50}: steady-state plasma concentration associated with 50% neuromuscular blockade
CrCl: creatinine clearance
Cr-EDTA: ^{51}Cr-ethylenediaminetetra-acetic acid
CRIES: Crying Requires oxygen Increased vital signs Expression Sleep (scale)
CRNA: certified registered nurse anesthetist
CRNP: certified registered nurse practitioner
CRPS: complex regional pain syndrome
CRS: compliance of respiratory system
CSC: caffeine-specific concentration
CSF: cerebrospinal fluid
CT: computed tomography
CVA: cerebrovascular accident
CVL: central venous catheter (line)
$C\bar{v}O_2$: mixed venous oxygen content
CVP: central venous pressure
CVR: cerebrovascular resistance
CW: compliance of chest wall
CYPs: cytochrome P450 enzymes
DAG: diacylglycerol
DBS: double burst stimulation
DCA: dichloroacetate
DCD: donation after cardiac death
DDAVP: desmopressin (1-desamino-8-D-arginine vasopressin)
DDH: developmental dysplasia of the hip
DHCA: deep hypothermic circulatory arrest
DI: diabetes insipidus
DIC: disseminated intravascular coagulation
DLT: double-lumen tube
DMD: Duchenne's muscular dystrophy
DNR: do not resuscitate
2,3-DPG: 2,3-diphosphoglycerate
DPL: diagnostic peritoneal lavage
DRG: dorsal respiratory group of neurons
DTPA: gadolinium diethylenetriaminepenta-acetic acid
EACA: ε-aminocaproic acid
EAST: enzyme allergosorbent test
EBV: estimated blood volume
ECF: extracellular fluid
ECG: electrocardiogram, electrocardiography, electrocardiographic
ECMO: extracorporeal membrane oxygenation
ED_{50}m: median effective dose
EDP: end-diastolic pressure
EDRF: endothelium-derived relaxing factor
EDV: end-diastolic volume
EEG: electroencephalogram, electroencephalograph, electroencephalographic
EF: ejection fraction
EGD: esophagogastroduodenoscopy
EGF: epidermal growth factor
ELBW: extremely low birth weight
EMD: electromechanical dissociation
EMG: electromyogram, electromyography, electromyographic
EMLA (cream): eutectic mixture of local anesthetics, 2.5% lidocaine, and 2.5% prilocaine
EMTALA: Emergency Medical Treatment and Active Labor Act
ENaC: epithelial sodium specific channel
ENT: ear, nose, and throat
ERV: expiratory reserve volume
ESRD: end-stage renal disease
ESS: endoscopic sinus surgery
ESV: end-systolic volume
ESWS: end-systolic wall stress
ET: endotracheal
ETC: electron transport chain
ETT: endotracheal tube
EXIT: ex utero intrapartum therapy
f: respiratory frequency
FAST: focused abdominal sonogram for trauma
FDA: Food and Drug Administration
FEO_2: fraction of mixed expired oxygen
FES: fat embolism syndrome
FEV_1: forced expiratory volume at 1 second
FFA: free fatty acids
FFP: fresh frozen plasma
FGF: fibroblast growth factor
FHH: familial hypocalciuric hypercalcemia
FIO_2: fraction of inspired oxygen
FISH: fluorescent in situ hybridization
FOB: fiberoptic bronchoscope
FRC: functional residual capacity
FS-EMG: frequency sweep electromyogram
FSMB: Federation of State Medical Boards
FVC: forced vital capacity
Gaw: airway conductance (reciprocal of Raw)
GCS: Glasgow Coma Scale
GER: gastroesophageal reflux
GERD: gastroesophageal reflux disease
GFR: glomerular filtration rate
GH: growth hormone
GMP: guanosine monophosphate
GP: glycoprotein
GVHS: graft-versus-host disease
four Hs: Hypovolemia, Hypoxemia, Hypothermia, and Hyperkalemia
Hb: hemoglobin
HbA: hemoglobin A
HbA_2: hemoglobin A_2
HbF: fetal hemoglobin
HbS: hemoglobin S
HbSA: sickle cell trait
HbSC: sickle cell C disease
HbA_{1C}: glycosylated hemoglobin
Hct: hematocrit

HCV: hepatitis C virus
HES: hydroxyethyl starch
HFJV: high-frequency jet ventilation
HFO: high-frequency oscillatory ventilation
HFV: high-frequency ventilation
HHPR: hereditary hypophosphatemic rickets
HIPAA: Health Insurance Portability and Accountability Act of 1996
HLHS: hypoplastic left heart syndrome
HMD: hyaline membrane disease (IRDS)
HME: heat and moisture exchanger
HMWK: high-molecular-weight kininogen
HPA: hypothalamic-pituitary-adrenal (axis)
HPV: hypoxic pulmonary vasoconstriction
HR: heart rate
HR: hormonal resuscitation
HSR: heat storage rate
5-HT: 5-hydroxytryptamine (serotonin)
IAA: interrupted aortic arch
IASP: International Association for the Study of Pain
IC: inspiratory capacity
ICF: intracellular fluid
ICP: intracranial pressure
ICROP: International Classification of Retinopathy of Prematurity
ICU: intensive care unit
ID: internal (or inner) diameter
IFNγ: interferon γ
IL: interleukin
ILIH: ilioinguinal/iliohypogastric
INM: intraoperative neurophysiologic monitoring
INR: international normalized ratio
IOP: intraocular pressure
IP3: inositol triphosphate
IPPV: intermittent positive-pressure ventilation
IRB: institutional review board
IRDS: idiopathic (infantile) respiratory distress syndrome
IRV: inspiratory reserve volume
ISCs: irreversibly sickled cells
ITP: idiopathic thrombocytopenic purpura
ITV: inspiratory impedance threshold valve
IVC: inferior vena cava
IVRA: intravenous regional anesthesia
JCAHO: Joint Commission for the Accreditation of Healthcare Organizations
JET: junctional ectopic tachycardia
JRA: juvenile rheumatoid arthritis
KIU: kallikrein inactivator unit
KTP laser: potassium (kalium) titanyl phosphate laser
LA: left atrium, left atrial
LAGB: laparoscopic adjustable gastric banding
LBW: low birth weight
LD_{50}: median lethal dose
LEAN: lidocaine, epinephrine, atropine, and naloxone
LES: lower esophageal sphincter
LET: lidocaine/epinephrine/tetracaine
LFC: lateral femoral cutaneous (nerve)
LGA: large-for-gestational age
LHR: lung-to-head ratio
LIM: line-isolation monitor
LIP: lipoid interstitial pneumonia
LMA: laryngeal mask airway
LRI: lower respiratory tract infection
LTA_4: leukotriene A_4
LTB_4: leukotriene B_4
LTC_4: leukotriene C_4
LTD_4: leukotriene D_4
LV: left ventricle, left ventricular
LVAD: left ventricular assist device
LVOT: left ventricular outflow tract
MABL: maximum allowable blood loss
MAC: minimum alveolar concentration
MAP: mean arterial blood pressure
MAST: military antishock trousers
MBT: mean body temperature
MCHC: mean corpuscular hemoglobin content
MCV: mean corpuscular volume
MDI: metered-dose inhaler
MDMA: 3,4-methylenedioxymethamphetamine ("ecstasy")
MEFV: maximum expiratory flow-volume (curve)
MEN: multiple endocrine neoplasia (syndrome)
MEP: motor evoked potential
MFS: Marfan syndrome
MH: malignant hyperthermia
MHC: major histocompatibility
MHCPB: moderate hypothermic cardiopulmonary bypass
MHS: malignant hyperthermia susceptible
MIBG: *meta*-iodobenzylguanidine
MMC: myelomeningocele
MMEFR: maximum mid-expiratory flow rate (same as FEF_{25-75})
MMEP: myogenic motor evoked potential
MMF: mycophenolate mofetil
MMS: masseter muscle spasm
MMWT: Modified Maintenance of Wakefulness Test
MODS: multiple organ dysfunction syndrome
MPD: maximum permissible dose
MPP: myocardial perfusion pressure
MPS: mucopolysaccharidosis
MRA: magnetic resonance angiography
MRI: magnetic resonance imaging
MST: mean skin temperature
MSK: median nerve evoked potential
MUF: modified ultrafiltration
NAPA: *N*-acetyl procainamide
NCHS: National Center for Health Statistics
N-CPAP: nasal continuous positive airway pressure
NCQA: National Committee for Quality Assurance
Nd:YAG laser: neodymium:yttrium-aluminum-garnet laser
NEC: necrotizing enterocolitis
NFκB: nuclear factor-κB
NICO: noninvasive cardiac output
NIH: National Institutes of Health
NIPS: Neonatal Infant Pain Scale
NIRS: near infrared spectroscopy
NMDA: *N*-methyl-D-aspartate
NMEP: neurogenic motor evoked potential
NMJ: neuromuscular junction
NMS: neurolept malignant syndrome
NO: nitric oxide
NPSF: National Patient Safety Foundation
NPT2a: type IIa Na^+/P^- electrogenic cotransporter
NPTR: National Pediatric Trauma Registry
NSAID: nonsteroidal anti-inflammatory drug

OCR: oculocardiac reflex
OD: outer diameter
OER: oculoemetic reflex
OHRP: Office for Human Research Protections
OI: osteogenesis imperfecta
OIG: Office of the Inspector General
OLT: orthotopic liver transplantation
OPTN: Organ Procurement and Transplantation Network
ORR: oculorespiratory reflex
OSA: obstructive sleep apnea
OSAS: obstructive sleep apnea syndrome
OSHA: Occupational Safety and Health Administration
OTFC: oral transmucosal fentanyl citrate
P_{50}: arterial oxygen tension (PaO_2) at 50% hemoglobin saturation
PA: pulmonary artery
PA: alveolar pressure
Pa: arterial partial pressure of dissolved gas
PABD: preoperative autologous blood donation
PACAD: phased chest and abdominal compression–decompression
PACU: postanesthesia care unit
PAE: paradoxical air embolism
PAF: platelet-activating factor
PAH: *para*-aminohippuric acid
PAI: plasminogen activator inhibitor
Palv: alveolar pressure
PALS: pediatric advanced life support
$PaCO_2$: arterial carbon dioxide tension
Pao: airway opening pressure
PaO_2: arterial oxygen tension (or partial pressure)
PAPVC: partial anomalous pulmonary venous connection
PB: atmospheric pressure
PBF: pulmonary blood flow
PC: phosphatidylcholine
PCA: postconceptional age
PCA: patient-controlled analgesia
PCEA: patient-controlled epidural anesthesia
PCO_2: partial pressure of carbon dioxide
PCP: phencyclidine
PCWP: pulmonary capillary wedge pressure
PDA: patent ductus arteriosus
PDPH: postdural puncture headache
PE: phosphatidylethanolamine
PEA: pulseless electrical activity
PEEP: positive end-expiratory pressure
PEFR: peak expiratory flow rate
PEG: percutaneous endoscopic gastrostomy
PEmax: maximum expiratory pressure
PET: positron emission tomography
$PETCO_2$: end-tidal carbon dioxide tension
PFC: persistent fetal circulation
PFO: patent foramen ovale
PG: phosphatidylglycerol
PGE_1: prostaglandin E_1
PGE_2: prostaglandin E_2
PGF_{2a}: prostaglandin F_{2a}
PHBQ: Posthospitalization Behavior Questionnaire
pHi: intracellular pH
PICU: pediatric intensive care unit
PImax: maximum inspiratory pressure
PIP: peak inspiratory pressure
PIVKA: proteins induced in vitamin K's absence
PLA: perilaryngeal airway
PMCA: plasma membrane Ca^{2+}-ATPase
PNB: peripheral nerve block
PO_2: partial pressure of oxygen
POCA: Pediatric Perioperative Cardiac Arrests (Registry)
POG: Pediatric Oncology Group
PONV: postoperative nausea and vomiting
POPE: postobstructive pulmonary edema
PPHN: persistent pulmonary hypertension of the neonate (or newborn)
PPIA: parental presence during induction of anesthesia
Ppl: pleural pressure
PRA: plasma rennin activity
PRBCs: packed red blood cells
PRG: pontine respiratory group of neurons
PRIMACORP: Prophylactic Intravenous Use of Milrinone After Cardiac Operation in Pediatrics
PS: phosphatidylserine
PS: physical status (with ASA levels)
Pstl: static recoil pressure of the lungs
PT: prothrombin time
PTH: parathyroid hormone
PTHrP: parathyroid hormone–related peptide
PTLD: posttransplant lymphoproliferative disease
PTT: partial thromboplastin time
PV: pulmonary venous pressure
PVC: polyvinylchloride
PVC: premature ventricular contraction
PVO_2: venous oxygen tension
PVR: pulmonary vascular resistance
$\dot{Q}$: pulmonary blood flow
$\dot{Q}_{L\rightarrow R}$: left-to-right shunt
$\dot{Q}P/\dot{Q}S$: pulmonary-to-systemic blood flow ratio
QA: quality assurance
QI: quality improvement
R: resistance
ΔR: viscoelastic component of Rrs
RA: right atrium, right atrial
RAD: reactive airways disease
RAE tube: Ring-Adair-Elwyn endotracheal tube
RAR: rapidly adapting (irritant) receptor
RAST: radioallergosorbent test
Raw: airway resistance
RBC: red blood cell
RBF: renal blood flow
RCM: radiocontrast media
REM: rapid eye movement
RF: radiofrequency
rFVIIa: recombinant factor VIIa
RIA: radioimmunoassay
Rint: resistive component of Rrs
ROP: retinopathy of prematurity
ROSC: return of spontaneous circulation
RPF: renal plasma flow
Rrs: total resistance of the respiratory system
RSD: reflex sympathetic dystrophy
RSP: radial nerve evoked potential
RSV: respiratory syncytial virus
Rus: airway resistance of upstream segment
RV: residual volume
RV: right ventricle, right ventricular
RVOT: right ventricular outflow tract
RYR: ryanodine receptor
RYR1: type I ryanodine receptor

SaO_2: arterial SO_2
SAMBA: Society for Ambulatory Anesthesia
SAR: specific absorption rate
SAR: slowly adapting (pulmonary stretch) receptor
SBE: subacute bacterial endocarditis
SCD: sickle cell disease
SCFE: slipped capital femoral epiphysis
SCT: sacrococcygeal teratoma
SCV: simultaneous ventilation with compression
SEP: somatosensory evoked potential
SET: signal extraction technology
SFLP: selective fetoscopic laser photocoagulation
SGA: small-for-gestational-age
SIADH: syndrome of inappropriate secretion of antidiuretic hormone
SIC: systemic intravascular coagulation
SIDS: sudden infant death syndrome
SIRS: systemic inflammatory response syndrome
SLE: systemic lupus erythematosus
SLV: single-lung ventilation
SNGFR: single-nephron glomerular filtration rate
SO_2: oxygen saturation of hemoglobin
SOBA: Society for Office-Based Anesthesia
SPA: Society for Pediatric Anesthesia
SP-A (B, C, D): surfactant protein A (B, C, D)
SPECT: single-photon emission computed tomography
SpO_2: SO_2 measured with pulse oximetry
SR: sarcoplasmic reticulum
SSEP: somatosensory evoked potential
SSRI: selective serotonin reuptake inhibitor
SSRU: short-stay recovery unit
SV: stroke volume
SVC: superior vena cava
$S\bar{v}O_2$: mixed venous oxygen saturation
SVR: systemic vascular resistance
SVT: supraventricular tachycardia
T_3: triiodothyronine
T_4: thyroxine
four Ts: Tension pneumothorax, pericardial Tamponade, Thromboembolism to the lungs, and Toxins
TAC: tetracaine/Adrenalin (epinephrine)/cocaine
TAFI: thrombin-activatable fibrinolysis inhibitor
TA-GVHD: transfusion-associated graft-versus-host disease
TAPVC: total anomalous pulmonary venous connection
TAR syndrome: thrombocytopenia–absent radius syndrome
TBG: thyroid-binding globulin
TBI: total body irradiation
TBI: traumatic brain injury
TBSA: total body surface area
TBW: total body weight
TCA: tricyclic antidepressant
TCD: transcranial Doppler
^{99m}Tc: technetium-99m
Tc-DTPA: ^{99m}Tc-diethylenetriaminepenta-acetic acid
TE: expiratory time
TEE: transesophageal echocardiography
TEF: tracheoesophageal fistula
TEG: thromboelastography
TENS: transcutaneous electrical nerve stimulation
TF: tissue factor
TFPI: tissue factor pathway inhibitor
TGA: transposition of the great arteries
TGFβ: transforming growth factor-β
THAM: tromethamine, or tris-[hydroxymethyl]aminomethane
THC: tetrahydrocannabinol
TI: inspiratory time
TI/TTOT: respiratory duty cycle
TIVA: total intravenous anesthesia
TLC: total lung capacity
T_{mG}: maximal tubular glucose
TMJ: temporomandibular joint
TMP: transmembrane pressure
TNFα: tumor necrosis factor-α
TOF: train-of-four
TPA: tissue plasminogen activator
TPG: transpulmonary gradient
TPN: total parenteral nutrition
TRALI: transfusion-related acute lung injury
TRAP: twin reversed arterial perfusion sequence
TSP: tibial somatosensory evoked potential
TT: tracheal tube
TTF-1: thyroid-transcription factor-1
TTKG: transtubular potassium gradient
TTOT: total respiratory time (T_1 + TE)
TTTS: twin-twin transfusion syndrome
T-tubule: transverse tubule
TXA_2: thromboxane A_2
UCP: uncoupling protein
UGT: uridine 5′-diphosphate-glucuronosyltransferase
UMSS: University of Michigan Sedation Scale
UNOS: United Network of Organ Sharing
URI: upper respiratory tract infection
USP: ulnar nerve evoked potential
UW solution: University of Wisconsin solution
$\dot{V}A/\dot{Q}$: ventilation/pulmonary perfusion ratio
$\dot{V}E$: minute volume ($\dot{V} = VT \times f = VT/TI \times TI/TTOT$)
$\dot{V}max_{25}$: maximum expiratory flow at 25% FVC (FEF_{75} or MEF_{25})
$\dot{V}O_2$: oxygen consumption
VACTERL: vertebral, anal, cardiac, tracheal, esophageal, renal, and limb
VAD: ventricular assist device
VAE: venous air embolus
VATER: vertebral defects, imperforate anus, tracheoesophageal fistula, radial and renal dysplasia)
VAVD: vacuum-assist venous drainage
VC: vital capacity
V_{cf}: velocity of circumferential fiber shortening
VDR: vitamin D (calcitriol) receptor
VE: volume of expired gas (air)
VEP: visual evoked potential
VF: ventricular fibrillation
VI: volume of inspired air (mL/min)
VIP: vasoactive intestinal peptide
Viso$\dot{V}$: volume of isoflow
VLBW: very low birth weight
VMA: 3-methoxy-4-hydroxy-vanillyl-mandelic acid
VPB: ventricular premature beat
VRG: ventral respiratory group of neurons
VSD: ventricular septal defect
VSN: vagal nerve stimulation
VT/TI: mean inspiratory flow (neural drive)
VT: ventricular tachycardia
VT: tidal volume
vWF: von Willebrand factor
WHO: World Health Organization
XLH: X-linked hypophosphatemic rickets

Basic Principles

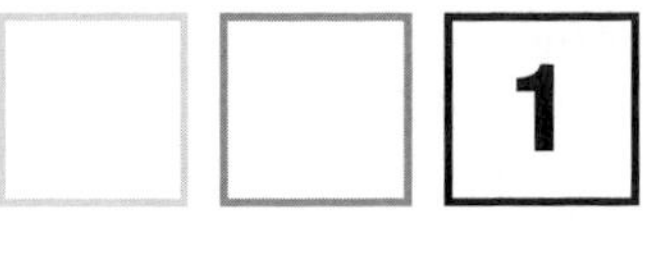

1 Special Characteristics of Pediatric Anesthesia

Etsuro K. Motoyama • Peter J. Davis

CHANGING CONCEPTS

In the 1940s and 1950s, the techniques of pediatric anesthesia, as well as the skills of those using and teaching them, evolved more as an art than as a science, as Dr. Robert Smith vividly and eloquently recollects through his firsthand experiences in his chapter on the history of pediatric anesthesia (see Chapter 35, History of Pediatric Anesthesia). The anesthetic agents and methods available were limited, as was the scientific knowledge of developmental differences in organ system function and anesthetic effect in infants and children. Monitoring in pediatric patients was limited to inspection of chest movement and occasional palpation of the pulse until the late 1940s, when Smith introduced the use of the precordial stethoscope for continuous auscultation of heartbeat and breath sounds (Smith, 1953, 1968). Until the mid-1960s, many anesthesiologists monitored only the heart rate in infants and small children during anesthesia and surgery. Electrocardiographic and blood pressure measurements were either too difficult or too extravagant and were thought to provide little or no useful information. Measurements of central venous pressure were thought to be inaccurate and too invasive even in major surgical procedures. The insertion of an indwelling urinary (Foley) catheter in infants was considered invasive and was resisted by surgeons.

The introduction of soft latex blood pressure cuffs suitable for newborn and older infants (Smith, 1968) encouraged the use of blood pressure monitoring in children (see Fig. 35–4). The "Smith cuff" remained the standard monitoring device in infants and children until the late 1970s, when it began to be replaced by automated blood pressure devices.

In the past two decades an explosion of new scientific knowledge in physiology and pharmacology in developing humans, as well as technologic advancements in perioperative monitoring, has markedly changed the concepts and techniques of pediatric anesthesia. At the same time the anesthesiologist's responsibilities have expanded well beyond the operating room and now cover the perioperative care of critically ill surgical and nonsurgical patients in intensive care settings. Resuscitative techniques, prolonged mechanical ventilatory support, and elaborate mechanical and physiologic instrumentation have become essential elements in anesthesiology. More recently, the roles of anesthesiologists have expanded to specialists in the management of acute and chronic pain beyond the perioperative period.

Significant developments in these areas over the past two decades include advances in perioperative monitoring techniques and standards; development and availability of new inhaled anesthetics, intravenous anesthetic and sedative-hypnotic agents, synthetic opioids, muscle relaxants, and other adjuvant drugs for both routine and complicated procedures; a better understanding of pain perception in neonates and advances in techniques of conduction analgesia as part of general anesthesia and perioperative pain management; parental presence during induction of anesthesia and in the postanesthesia care unit (PACU); and reevaluation of time-honored preoperative laboratory tests and fasting routines in ever-expanding, same-day (outpatient) surgery settings to improve efficiency and health care cost containment. (See Chapter 27, Anesthesia for Same-Day Procedures.)

RECENT DEVELOPMENTS IN PEDIATRIC ANESTHESIA

PERIOPERATIVE MONITORING TECHNIQUES AND STANDARDS

The introduction of pulse oximetry for routine clinical use since the early 1990s has been the single most important development in monitoring and patient safety, especially related to pediatric anesthesia, since the advent of the precordial stethoscope in the 1950s (Smith, 1956) (see Chapters 9, 10, 11, and 34, Anesthetic Equipment and Monitoring, Induction of Anesthesia, Intraoperative and Postoperative Management, and Safety and Outcome). Pulse oximetry is superior to clinical observation and other means of monitoring, such as capnography, for the detection of intraoperative hypoxemia (Coté et al., 1988, 1991). In addition, Spears and colleagues (1991) have indicated that experienced pediatric anesthesiologists may not have an "educated hand" or a "feel" adequate to detect changes in pulmonary compliance in infants. This report is particularly sobering for "old timers" who had always assumed that their clinical skills were sufficient to protect the safety of their young patients, without depending on monitors. Pulse oximetry has revealed that postoperative hypoxemia occurs commonly among otherwise healthy infants and children undergoing simple surgical procedures (Motoyama and Glazener, 1986).

Consequently, the use of supplemental oxygen in the PACU has become a part of routine postanesthetic care (see Chapter 11, Intraoperative and Postoperative Management).

Although pulse oximetry has greatly improved patient monitoring, there had been some limitations, namely motion artifact and inaccuracy in low-flow states and in children at levels of low oxygen saturation (e.g., cyanotic congenital heart disease). Advances have been made in the new generation of pulse oximetry (Masimo Signal Extraction Technology [SET]). This device minimizes the effect of motion artifact, improves accuracy, and has been shown to have advantages over the existing system in low-flow states, mild hypothermia, and moving patients (Malviya et al., 2000; Hay et al., 2002; Irita et al., 2003).

The standards for intraoperative patient monitoring proposed by the Harvard group (Eichhorn et al., 1986) and the American Society of Anesthesiologists (1986) (see Chapter 11, Intraoperative and Postoperative Management) strongly recommend the routine use of pulse oximetry and capnography or their equivalents. These standard monitoring procedures have been mandated by law in many state legislatures (New York State Hospital Code, 1988).

Depth of anesthesia can be difficult to assess in the pediatric patient. The bispectral index (BIS) monitor has been developed to objectively assess the depth of anesthesia continuously during general anesthesia. BIS monitor technology compresses electroencephalographic signals with use of a sophisticated algorithm into a digital readout ranging from 0 to 100 (Sebel et al., 1997). By comparing the reading with previously measured results in conscious, sedated, and anesthetized patients, a normogram for level of sedation has been generated. Studies in infants and children have confirmed the validity of this instrument and have demonstrated that more accurate titration of sedation and general anesthesia in children is achieved with the use of a BIS monitor (Denman et al., 2000; Bannister et al., 2001; Choudhry and Brenn, 2002; McCann et al., 2002). Although the BIS monitor has been used in adult patients to prevent awareness under general anesthesia (Sebel et al., 1997), its use for pediatric patients is expected to increase over the coming decade (also see Chapter 11, Intraoperative and Postoperative Management).

NEW VOLATILE ANESTHETICS

More than a decade after the release of isoflurane for clinical use, two volatile anesthetics, desflurane and sevoflurane, became available in the mid to late 1990s in most industrialized countries. Although these two agents are dissimilar in many ways, they share common physiochemical and pharmacologic characteristics: very low blood-gas partition coefficients (0.4 and 0.6, respectively), which are close to that of nitrous oxide and are only fractions of those of halothane and isoflurane; rapid induction of and emergence from surgical anesthesia; and hemodynamic stability (see Chapters 6, 10, and 11, Basic Pharmacokinetic Concepts, Induction of Anesthesia, and Intraoperative and Postoperative Management).

Although desflurane is not suitable for inhalation induction because of its pungent odor and airway irritability with frequent and often severe laryngospasms (Fisher and Zwass, 1992), sevoflurane appears to be an excellent anesthetic for inhalation induction with hemodynamic stability (Sarner et al., 1995). Indeed, in Japan, where sevoflurane has been in clinical use since 1993, and in most western European countries, where it was introduced much later than in the United States, halothane has been almost completely replaced by sevoflurane for pediatric anesthesia. Even in the United States, the clinical use of holothane has been limited almost exclusively for pediatric anesthesia over the last two decades and its future survival, commercially or otherwise, has become cloudy as of the spring of 2005. Although these newer, less-soluble inhaled agents allow for faster emergence from anesthesia, emergence excitation or delirium associated with their use has become a major concern to the pediatric anesthesiologists (Davis et al., 1994; Sarner et al., 1995; Lerman et al., 1996; Welborn et al., 1996; Cravero et al., 2000). However, issues of patient temperament, separation anxiety, postoperative pain, and hunger have clouded the etiology of the stormy emergence associated with these issues. Adjuncts, such as opioids, analgesics, serotonin antagonists, and α_1-adrenergic agonists, have been found to decrease the incidence of emergence agitation. In addition, risk factors such as patient age and type of surgery, in addition to the actual inhaled anesthetic agents, have also been identified as risk factors for emergence agitation (Aono et al., 1997, 1999; Davis et al., 1999; Galinkin et al., 2000; Cohen et al., 2001; Ko et al., 2001; Kulka et al., 2001; Voepel-Lewis et al., 2003).

INTRAVENOUS AGENTS

Propofol has increasingly been used in pediatric anesthesia as an induction agent, for intravenous sedation, or as the primary agent of a total intravenous technique (Martin et al., 1992). Propofol has the advantage of rapid emergence and causes less nausea and vomiting during the postoperative period, particularly in children with a high risk of vomiting, such as those who have undergone strabismus surgery (Wacha et al., 1991).

The eutectic mixture of local anesthetics (EMLA cream) for skin analgesia (Soliman et al., 1988) has become available since the 1990s and has made intravenous cannulation and intravenous induction of anesthesia less threatening for children.

The development of shorter-acting synthetic opioids and intermediate- and short-acting nondepolarizing muscle relaxants, as well as a better understanding of their pharmacokinetics and pharmacodynamics (see Chapter 6, Pharmacology of Pediatric Anesthesia), has increased the opportunities for pediatric anesthesiologists to provide safe and stable anesthesia with various approaches and less dependence on volatile anesthetics. For example, Anand and Hickey (1992) found that neonates undergoing cardiac surgery with a high-dose of sufentanil had a significantly better outcome than those who received morphine and halothane. Availability of shorter-acting opioids and muscle relaxants has also changed the approach to more routine pediatric procedures such as inguinal herniorrhaphy, tonsillectomy, and bronchoscopy for foreign body aspiration.

The most recent development has been the use of ultrashort-acting opioids in pediatric patients. Specifically, remifentanil, a μ agonist, is metabolized by nonspecific plasma and tissue esterases. The organ-independent elimination of remifentanil, coupled with its clearance rate, which is highest in neonates and infants compared with older children, makes its kinetic profile different from that of any other opioids (Davis et al., 1999; Ross et al., 2001). In addition, its ability to provide hemodynamic stability, coupled with its kinetic profile of rapid elimination and nonaccumulation, makes it an attractive anesthetic option for infants and children. Numerous clinical studies have described its use for pediatric anesthesia (Wee et al., 1999; Chiaretti et al., 2000; Davis et al., 2000, 2001; German et al., 2000; Dönmez et al., 2001; Galinkin et al., 2001; Keidan et al., 2001; Chambers et al., 2002; Friesen et al., 2003).

LARYNGEAL MASK AIRWAY

The laryngeal mask airway (LMA) (Brain, 1983), from the United Kingdom, has been used widely in pediatric anesthesia since the 1990s. Although it is not a substitute for the endotracheal tube, the LMA maintains upper airway patency in anesthetized patients who are breathing spontaneously (Keidan et al., 2000). It also serves as an emergency airway when the patient cannot be adequately ventilated with a conventional bag-and-mask system or when intubation is not successful. The LMA is also used as a conduit for endotracheal intubation with a fiberoptic bronchoscope (see Chapter 10, Induction of Anesthesia). The LMA may or may not be suitable for positive pressure ventilation because of air leaks and possible regurgitation of gastric contents, although a number of reports indicate its relative safety as long as the peak inspiratory pressure is limited to less than 10 to 15 cm H_2O (Barker et al., 1992; Devitt et al., 1994; Keidan et al., 2001). The LMA has been used in infants and children (Grevenik et al., 1990; Johnston et al., 1990; Mizushima et al., 1992; Wilson, 1993) (see Chapter 10).

In addition to LMA, other airway devices have been used in children that help decrease the need for tracheal intubation; the cuffed oropharyngeal airway (COPA) and the perilaryngeal airway (PLA) are newer airway devices that have been successfully used in children (see Chapter 9, Anesthetic Equipment and Monitoring and Chapter 27, Anesthesia for Same-Day Procedures).

INTRAOPERATIVE AND POSTOPERATIVE ANALGESIA IN NEONATES

It has long been thought that newborn infants do not appreciate pain the way older children and adults do and therefore do not require anesthetic or analgesic agents (Lippman et al., 1976). Later studies, however, have indicated that pain, such as that caused by circumcision without analgesia, is felt by the newborn infant and causes prolonged disruption of behavioral development (Dixon et al., 1984). In a landmark study, Anand and others (1987) reported that premature infants showed marked endocrine responses to surgically induced stress, as in the ligation of a patent ductus arteriosus. Pretreatment with fentanyl completely abolished these responses (Booker, 1988).

With this increased awareness has come new interest in the prevention and management of perioperative pain, particularly in neonates. Because of increased cardiovascular sensitivity to inhaled anesthetics and delayed elimination of opioids in the neonate and premature infant, conduction anesthesia is a suitable technique for those patients who are expected to be awake and breathing at the end of surgery and anesthesia. The development of remifentanil, an ultra short-acting opioid, has markedly improved the safety of general anesthesia for neonates and infants. (See Chapters 6 and 11, Pharmacology of Pediatric Anesthesia, and Intraoperative and Postoperative Management)

REGIONAL ANALGESIA IN INFANTS AND CHILDREN

Conduction analgesia has been used in infants and children since the beginning of the twentieth century, when open-drop ether and chloroform were the anesthetics of choice (Bainbridge, 1901). During the first half of the twentieth century, virtually all of the regional anesthetic techniques available for adults were applied to pediatric patients, mostly by surgeons. By the 1950s, however, when well-trained anesthesiologists were available and general anesthesia was considerably safer for children, the use of regional anesthesia went out of fashion and rapidly declined.

Since the mid-1980s there has been a resurgence of interest in regional anesthesia among pediatric anesthesiologists. One important reason is the difficulty of anesthetizing the increasing number of prematurely born infants who are being cared for in the newly organized neonatal intensive care units. These infants often have severe cardiopulmonary compromise and histories of apnea. Regional analgesia with or without supplemental inhalation or intravenous anesthesia has been used almost exclusively in these situations (Abajian et al., 1984).

As newer local anesthetic agents with less systemic toxicity become available, their role in the anesthetic/analgesic management of children is increasing. Studies of the use of levobupivacaine and ropivacaine have demonstrated safety and efficacy in children greater than that of bupivacaine, the standard regional anesthetic in the 1990s (Ivani et al., 1998, 2002, 2003; Hansen et al., 2000, 2001; Lönnqvist et al., 2000; McCann et al., 2001; Karmakar et al., 2002).

Pediatric anesthesiologists have been paying much closer attention to postoperative analgesia than they did even a few years ago as part of an overall anesthetic strategy. The pain management plan, either conduction analgesia or patient-controlled analgesia, is discussed with the surgeon and with the parents (and the child if he or she is old enough to understand) preoperatively. A single dose of local anesthetics through the caudal and epidural spaces is most often used for a variety of surgical procedures as part of general anesthesia and for postoperative analgesia. Insertion of an epidural catheter for continuous or repeated bolus injections of local anesthetics often with opioids and other adjunct drugs for postoperative analgesia has become a common practice in pediatric anesthesia. The addition of adjunct drugs, such as midazolam, neostigmine, tramadol, ketamine, and clonidine, to prolong the neuroaxial blockade from local anesthetic agents has become more popular even though the safety of these agents on the neuroaxis has not been determined (Ansermino et al., 2003; de Beer and Thomas, 2003) (see Chapters 13 and 14, Pain Management and Regional Anesthesia). By the beginning of the twenty-first century, pediatric pain service has been organized and practiced by pediatric anesthesiologists in most pediatric institutions, and the pain service rotation has become an integral part of the pediatric anesthesia fellowship training program.

SAME-DAY SURGERY—EFFICIENCY AND QUALITY OF CARE

Efficiency and health care cost-containment concerns, particularly in the United States, have resulted in an astonishing increase in same-day (outpatient) surgery in relatively healthy adult and pediatric patients. Most pediatric centers encourage children and families to participate in presurgical preparatory programs within a few weeks before scheduled surgery. On the day of surgery, all patients are seen by anesthesiologists and screened for acute illness and fasting status. Laboratory tests in healthy children are usually kept to a minimum. The necessity of a routine hemoglobin and hematocrit has been questioned, and these are mostly eliminated from practice (see Chapter 27, Anesthesia for Same-Day Procedures). The preoperative fasting requirement has been reevaluated and liberalized. In most institutions, clear fluid is now offered to infants and children up to 2 hours before admission to the same-day surgery unit. The safety of such a practice has been confirmed in the anesthesia literature (see Chapter 27, Anesthesia for Same-Day Procedures).

To reduce the anxiety of children and their parents, preoperative preparations of pediatric patients have undergone considerable changes since the 1990s. Premedication via the painful intramuscular injection, until the 1980s, has been replaced by transmucosal (oral, nasal, or rectal) midazolam, fentanyl, or ketamine and their combinations (see Chapters 8, 10, and 27, Preoperative Preparation, Induction of Anesthesia, and Anesthesia for Same-Day Procedures). Midazolam, given orally, has become the most popular and successful (Kain et al., 1997).

Since the 1990s, parental presence during the induction of anesthesia and in the PACU has become commonplace in most institutions to minimize separation anxiety. Both parents and anesthesiologists have had mostly positive responses to this approach, despite initial reservations and anxiety on the part of the anesthesiologists (Hannallah and Rosales, 1983). Some parents, however, are exceedingly anxious and may transmit this anxiety to their child (Bevan et al., 1990). Kain and others (1996, 1998, 2000, 2003a, 2003b, 2004) have shown that parental presence is as effective as a preanesthetic medication, and public awareness and consumer expectations place a high value on these family-centered care efforts. The value of parents being present for induction is a function of educating parents about their role in the process (see Chapter 7, Psychological Aspects).

Progress in biotechnology, medical knowledge, and postgraduate training in anesthesiology has produced remarkable advances in pediatric anesthesia in terms of patient safety and outcome and the patients' comfort perioperatively that would have been unthinkable even a few decades ago. These advances, however, were not achieved without cost—the increasing cost of health care in most industrialized nations. In the United States, health care reform is moving quickly by market force. Cost containment has become the major focus in the minds of practitioners, which, unfortunately, tends to impede further improvement in technology and the quality of anesthesia.

FUNDAMENTAL DIFFERENCES IN INFANTS AND CHILDREN

The reason for undertaking a special study of pediatric anesthesia is that children, especially infants younger than a few months, differ markedly from adolescents and adults. Many of the important differences, however, are not the most obvious. Although the most apparent contrast is size, it is the physiologic differences related to general metabolism and to immature function of the various organ systems (including the heart, lungs, kidneys, liver, blood, muscles, and central nervous system) that are of major importance to the anesthesiologist.

PSYCHOLOGICAL DIFFERENCES

For a child's normal psychological development, continual support of a nurturant family is indispensable at all stages of development; serious social and emotional deprivation (including separation from the parents during hospitalization), especially during the first 2 years of development, may cause temporary or even lasting damage to psychosocial development (Forman et al., 1987). A young child who is hospitalized for surgery is forced to cope with separation from parents, to adapt to a new environment and strange people, and to experience the pain and discomfort associated with anesthesia and surgery (see Chapter 7, Psychological Aspects).

The most intense fear of an infant or a young child is created by separation from the parents, often conceived as loss of love or abandonment. The sequence of reaction often observed is as follows: angry protest with panicky anxiety, depression and despair, and eventually apathy and detachment (Bowlby, 1973). Older children may be more concerned with painful procedures and the loss of self-control implicit with general anesthesia (Forman et al., 1987). Repeated hospitalizations for anesthesia and surgery may be associated with psychosocial disturbances in later childhood (Dombro, 1970). In children old enough to experience fear and apprehension during anesthesia and surgery, the emotional factor may be of greater concern than the physical condition; in fact, it may represent the greatest problem of the perioperative course (Smith, 1980) (see Chapter 7, Psychological Aspects).

All of these responses can and should be reduced or abolished through preventive measures to ease the child's adaptation to the hospitalization, anesthesia, and surgery. The anesthesiologist's role in this process is extremely important (see Chapters 7, 8, and 10, Psychological Aspects, Preopetrative Preparation, and Induction of Anesthesia). Description of the normal pattern of behavior that emerges during infancy and childhood is beyond the scope of this book. The reader is encouraged to consult standard pediatric textbooks.

DIFFERENCES IN RESPONSE TO PHARMACOLOGIC AGENTS

The extent of the differences among infants, children, and adults in response to the administration of drugs was not fully appreciated until fairly recently. Before the 1960s, the primary concern in pediatric pharmacology was to find a formula to convert adult dosages to pediatric ones. Application of a pharmacokinetic method in which mathematical and statistical analyses are used to relate drug dosage, pharmacologic effects, and time (Jusko, 1972) has been instrumental in the rapid development of pediatric pharmacology since the 1980s. During the first several months after birth, rapid development and growth of organ systems take place, altering the factors involved in uptake, distribution, metabolism, and elimination of anesthetics and related drugs. These changes appear responsible for developmental differences in the response to drugs. The pharmacology of anesthetics and adjuvant drugs and their different effects in neonates, infants, and children are discussed in detail in Chapter 6, Pharmacology of Pediatric Anesthesia.

ANATOMIC AND PHYSIOLOGIC DIFFERENCES

Body Size

As already stated, the most striking contrast between children and adults is size, but the degree of difference and the variation even within the pediatric age group are hard to appreciate. The contrast between an infant weighing 1 kg and an overgrown and obese adolescent weighing more than 100 kg appearing in succession in the same operating room is overwhelming. It makes considerable difference whether body weight, height, or body surface area is used as the basis for size comparison. As pointed out by Harris (1957), a normal newborn infant weighing 3 kg is

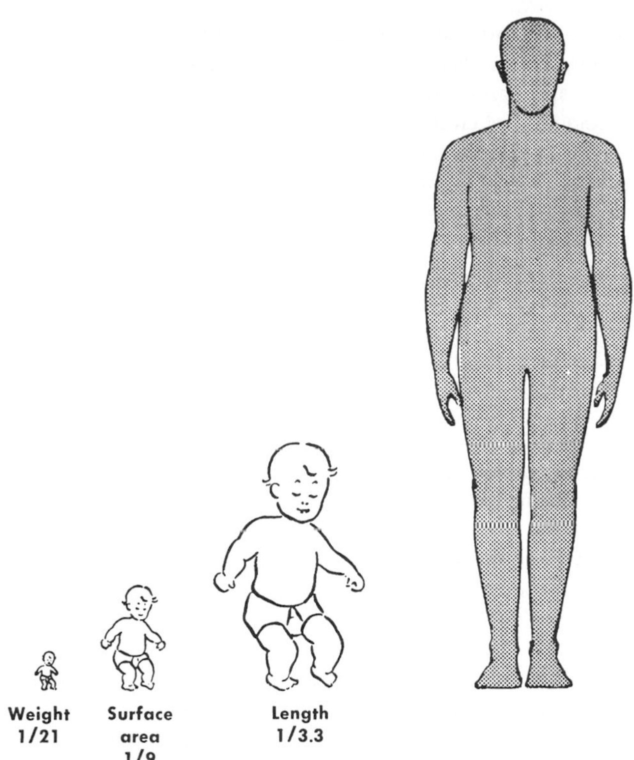

FIGURE 1–1. Proportions of newborn to adult with respect to weight, surface area, and length. (From Crawford JD, Terry ME, Rourke GM: *Pediatrics* 5:785, 1950.)

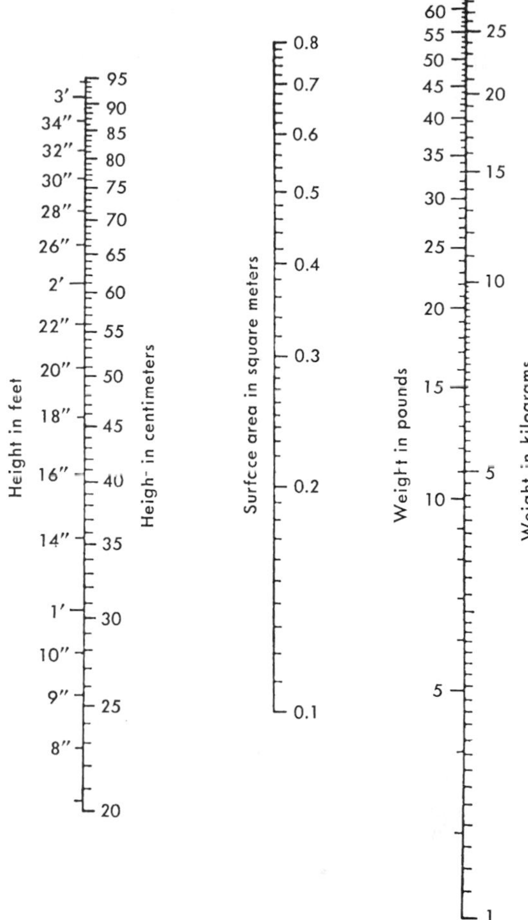

FIGURE 1–2. Body surface area nomogram for infants and young children. (Reprinted with permission of the publishers and The Commonwealth Fund, from Talbot NB, Sobel FH, McArthur JW, Crawford JD: *Functional Endocrinology From Birth Through Adolescence.* Cambridge, MA, 1952, Harvard University Press; copyright, 1952, by the Commonwealth Fund.)

$\frac{1}{3}$ the size of an adult in length but $\frac{1}{9}$ the adult size in body surface area and $\frac{1}{21}$ adult size in weight (Fig. 1–1). Of these body measurements, body surface area (BSA) is probably the most important because it closely parallels variations in basal metabolic rate measured in kilocalories per hour per square meter. For this reason, BSA is believed to be a better criterion than age or weight in judging basal fluid and nutritional requirements. For clinical use, however, BSA proves somewhat difficult to determine, although a nomogram such as that of Talbot and associates (1952) facilitates the procedure considerably (Fig. 1–2). For the anesthesiologist who carries a pocket calculator, the following formulas may be useful to derive BSA:

Formula of DuBois and Dubois (1916)

$$\text{BSA (m}^2) = 0.007184 \times \text{Height}^{0.725} \times \text{Weight}^{0.425}$$

Formula of Gehan and George (1970)

$$\text{BSA (m}^2) = 0.0235 \times \text{Height}^{0.42246} \times \text{Weight}^{0.51456}$$

At full-term birth, BSA averages 0.2 m^2, whereas in the adult it averages 1.75 m^2. A table of average height, weight, and BSA is presented for reference (Table 1–1). A simpler, crude estimate of BSA for children of average height and weight is given in Table 1–2. The formula BSA (m^2) = (0.02 × kg) + 0.40 is also reasonably accurate in children of normal physique weighing 21 to 40 kg (Vaughan and Litt, 1987).

The caloric need in relation to BSA of a full-term infant is about 30 kcal/m^2 per hour. It increases to about 50 kcal/m^2 per hour by 2 years of age and then decreases gradually to the adult level of 35 to 40 kcal/m^2 per hour.

Relative Size or Proportion

Less obvious than the difference in overall size is the difference in relative size of body structure in infants and children. This is particularly true with the head, which is large at birth (35 cm in circumference)—in fact, larger than chest circumference. Head circumference increases by 10 cm during the first year and an

TABLE 1–1. Relation of age, height, and weight to body surface area (BSA)*

Age (y)	Height (cm)	Weight (kg)	BSA (m^2)
Premature	40	1	0.1
Newborn	50	3	0.2
1	75	10	0.47
2	87	12	0.57
3	96	14	0.63
5	109	18	0.74
10	138	32	1.10
13	157	46	1.42
16 (Female)	163	50	1.59
16 (Male)	173	62	1.74

*Based on standard growth chart and the formula of DuBois and DuBois (1916): BSA (m^2) = 0.007184 × Height$^{0.725}$ × Weight$^{0.425}$.

■ **TABLE 1–2.** Approximation of body surface area (BSA) based on weight

Weight (kg)	Approximate BSA (m^2)
1 to 5	0.05 × kg + 0.05
6 to 10	0.04 × kg + 0.10
11 to 20	0.03 × kg + 0.20
21 to 40	0.02 × kg + 0.40

Modified from Vaughan VC III, Litt IF: Assessment of growth and development. In Behrman RE, Vaughn VC III (eds): *Nelson's Textbook of Pediatrics*, ed 13. Philadelphia, 1987, WB Saunders.

additional 2 to 3 cm during the second year, when it reaches three fourths the adult size.

At full-term birth, the infant has a short neck and a chin that often meets the chest at the level of the second rib; these infants are prone to upper airway obstruction during sleep. In infants with tracheostomy, the orifice is often buried under the chin unless the head is extended with a roll under the neck. In addition, infants are more prone to upper airway obstruction under anesthesia or sedation because upper airway muscles, which normally support the airway patency, are disproportionately sensitive to the depressant effect of anesthesia and sedation, resulting in pharyngeal airway collapse and obstruction (Ochiai et al., 1989) (see Chapter 2, Respiratory Physiology). The chest is relatively small in relation to the abdomen, which is protuberant with weak abdominal muscles (Fig. 1–3). Furthermore, the rib cage is cartilaginous and the thorax is too compliant to resist inward recoil of the lungs. In the awake state, the chest wall is maintained relatively rigid with sustained inspiratory muscle tension, which maintains the end-expiratory lung volume (functional residual capacity [FRC]). Under general anesthesia, however, the muscle tension is abolished and FRC collapses, resulting in airway closure, atelectasis, and venous admixture unless positive end-expiratory pressure (CPAP) or positive end-expiratory pressure (PEEP) is maintained.

Poor development of body support by bone and muscle, together with disproportion, creates problems in positioning the child for surgery. In the prone position, the shoulders are too small to provide adequate support despite attempts to build them up with rolls underneath both shoulders, thereby keeping the thorax and abdomen free for adequate ventilation. Occasionally, when the child must sit up for a craniotomy, special attention is needed to secure the head carefully, because the neck is a very weak stem for the heavy head. Structure and function of the thorax and airways, as well as respiratory physiology in infants and children, are detailed in Chapter 2.

Central and Autonomic Nervous Systems

The brain of the neonate is relatively large, weighing about $^1/_{10}$ of body weight compared with about $^1/_{50}$ in the adult. The brain grows rapidly; its weight doubles by 6 months of age and triples by 1 year. At birth, about one fourth of the neuronal cells are present. The development of cells in the cortex and brain stem is nearly complete by 1 year of age. Myelinization and elaboration of dendritic processes continue well into the third year. Incomplete myelinization is associated with primitive reflexes, such as the Moro and grasp reflexes, in the neonate; these are valuable in the assessment of neural development. Inadequate nutrition during this critical period of brain growth results in impaired neuronal function, as seen with inborn errors of metabolism.

At birth the spinal cord extends to the third lumbar vertebra. By the time the infant is 1 year old, the cord has assumed its permanent position, ending at the first lumbar vertebra (Gray, 1973).

In contrast to the central nervous system, the autonomic nervous system is relatively well developed in the newborn. The parasympathetic components of the cardiovascular system are fully functional at birth. The sympathetic components, however, are not fully developed until 4 to 6 months of age (Friedman, 1973). Baroreflexes to maintain blood pressure and heart rate, which involve medullary vasomotor centers (pressor and depressor areas), are functional at birth in awake newborn infants (Moss et al., 1968; Gootman, 1983). In anesthetized newborn animals, however, both pressor and depressor reflexes are diminished (Wear et al., 1982; Gallagher et al., 1987).

The laryngeal reflex is activated by the stimulation of receptors on the face, nose, and upper airways of the newborn. Reflex apnea,

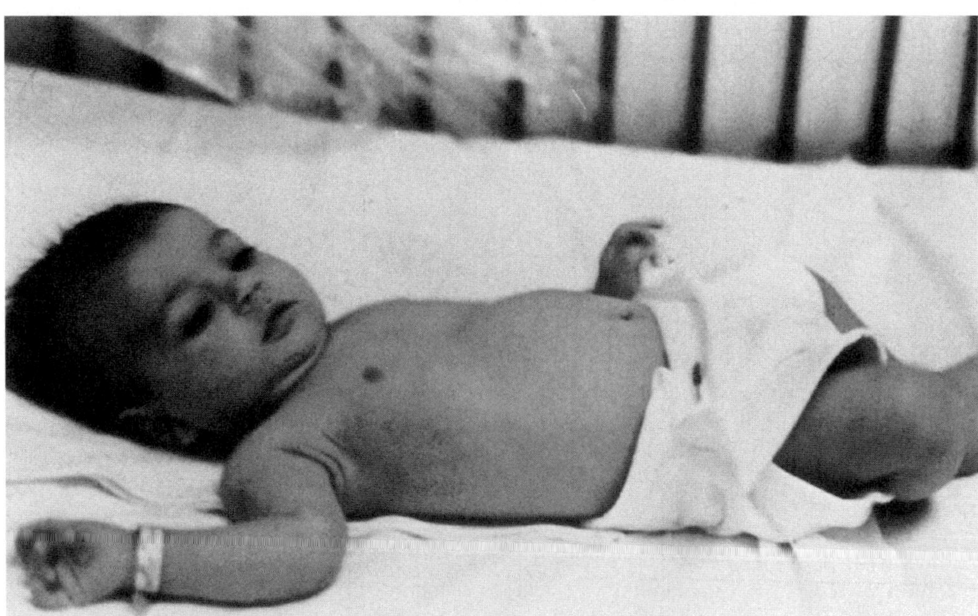

■ **FIGURE 1–3.** A normal infant has a large head, narrow shoulders and chest, and a large abdomen.

bradycardia, or laryngospasm may occur. Various mechanical and chemical stimuli, including water, foreign bodies, and noxious gases, can trigger this response. This protective response is so potent that it can cause death in the newborn (see Chapters 2 and 3, Respiratory Physiology and Cardiovascular Physiology).

Respiratory System

At full-term birth, the lungs are still in the stage of active development. The formation of adult-type alveoli begins at 36 weeks post conception but represents only a fraction of the terminal air sacs with thick septa at full-term birth. It takes more than several years for functional and morphologic development to be completed. Similarly, control of breathing during the first several weeks of extrauterine life differs notably from control in older children and adults. Of particular importance is the fact that hypoxemia depresses, rather than stimulates, respiration. The development of the respiratory system and its physiology are detailed in Chapter 2, Respiratory Physiology.

Cardiovascular System

During the first minutes after birth, the newborn infant must change his or her circulatory pattern dramatically from fetal to adult type to survive in the extrauterine environment. Even for several months after initial adaptation, the pulmonary vascular bed remains exceptionally reactive to hypoxia and acidosis. The heart remains extremely sensitive to volatile anesthetics during early infancy, whereas the central nervous system is relatively insensitive to these anesthetics. Cardiovascular physiology in infants and children is discussed in Chapter 3.

Fluid and Electrolyte Metabolism

Like the lungs, the kidneys are not fully mature at birth, although the formation of nephrons is complete by 36 weeks' gestation. Maturation continues for about 6 months after full-term birth. The glomerular filtration rate (GFR) is lower in the neonate because of the high renal vascular resistance associated with the relatively small surface area for filtration. Despite a low GFR and limited tubular function, the full term newborn can conserve sodium. Premature infants, however, experience prolonged glomerulotubular imbalance, resulting in sodium wastage and hyponatremia (Spitzer, 1982). On the other hand, both full-term and premature infants are limited in their ability to handle excessive sodium loads. Even following water deprivation, concentrating ability is limited at birth, especially in premature infants. After several days, neonates can produce dilute urine; however, diluting capacity does not mature fully until 3 to 5 weeks of life (Spitzer, 1978). The premature infant is prone to hyponatremia when sodium supplementation is inadequate or with overhydration. Furthermore, dehydration is detrimental in the neonate regardless of gestational age. The physiology of fluid and electrolyte balance is detailed in Chapter 4, Regulation of Body Fluids and Electrolytes.

Temperature Regulation

Temperature regulation is of particular interest and importance in pediatric anesthesia. There is a better understanding of the physiology of temperature regulation and the effect of anesthesia on the control mechanisms. General anesthesia is associated with mild to moderate hypothermia resulting from environmental exposure, anesthesia-induced central thermoregulatory inhibition, redistribution of body heat, and up to 30% reduction in metabolic heat production (Bissonette, 1991). Small infants have disproportionately large BSAs, and heat loss is exaggerated during anesthesia, particularly during the induction of anesthesia unless the heat loss is actively prevented. General anesthesia decreases but does not completely abolish thermoregulatory threshold temperature to hypothermia. Mild hypothermia can sometimes be beneficial intraoperatively, and profound hypothermia is effectively used during open heart surgery in infants to reduce oxygen consumption. Postoperative hypothermia, however, is detrimental because of marked increases in oxygen consumption, oxygen debt (dysoxia), and resultant metabolic acidosis. Regulation of body temperature is discussed in detail in Chapter 5, Thermoregulation: Physiology and Perioperative Disturbances.

■ SUMMARY

Pediatric anesthesia as a subspecialty has evolved because the needs of infants and young children are fundamentally different from those of adults. The pediatric anesthesiologist should be aware of the child's cardiovascular, respiratory, renal, neuromuscular, and central nervous system responses to various drugs, as well as to physical and chemical stimuli, such as changes in blood oxygen and carbon dioxide tensions, pH, and body temperature. Their responses are different both qualitatively and quantitatively from those of adults and among different pediatric age groups. More important, the pediatric anesthesiologist should always consider the child's emotional needs and create an environment that minimizes or abolishes fear and distress.

There have been many advances in the practice of anesthesia to improve the comfort of young patients since the sixth edition of this book was published in 1996. These advances include a relaxation of preoperative fluid restriction, more focused attention to the child's psychological needs with more extensive use of preoperative sedation via the transmucosal route, the wide use of topical analgesia with EMLA cream before intravenous catheterization, and more generalized acceptance of parental presence during anesthetic induction and in the recovery room. Furthermore, a more diverse anesthetic approach has evolved through the combined use of regional analgesia, together with the advent of newer and less soluble volatile anesthetics, intravenous anesthetics, and shorter-acting synthetic opioids and muscle relaxants. Finally, the scope of pediatric anesthesia is expanding as pediatric anesthesiologists assume the role of pain management specialists beyond the boundary of perioperative care.

REFERENCES

Abajina JC, Mellish RW, Browne AF, et al.: Spinal anesthesia for surgery in the high-risk infant. *Anesth Analg* 63:359–362, 1984.

American Society of Anesthesiologists: Standards for basic intraoperative monitoring. *ASA Newsletter* 50:12, 1986.

Anand KJS, Hickey PR: Halothane-morphine compared with high-dose sufentanil for anesthesia and postoperative analgesia in neonatal cardiac surgery. *N Engl J Med* 326:1, 1992.

Anand KJS, Sippell WG, Aynsley-Green A: Randomized trial of fentanyl anesthesia in preterm babies undergoing surgery. *Lancet* 1:243, 1987.

Ansermino M, Basu R, Vandebeek C, Montgomery C: Nonopioid additives to local anaesthetics for caudal blockade in children: A systematic review. *Paediatr Anaesth* 13:561–573, 2003.

Aono J, Mimiya K, Manube M: Preoperative anxiety is associated with high incidence of problematic behavior on emergence after halothane anesthesia in boys. *Acta Anaesthesiol Scand* 43:542–544, 1999.

Aono J, Ueda W, Mamiya K, et al.: Greater incidence of delirium during recovery from sevoflurane anesthesia in preschool boys. *Anesthesiology* 87:1298–1300, 1997.

Bainbridge WS: Report of 12 operations on infants and young children under spinal anesthesia. *Arch Pediatr* 18:510, 1901.

Bannister CF, Brosius KK, Sigl JC, Meyer BJ, Sebel PS: The effect of bispectral index monitoring on anesthetic use and recovery in children anesthetized with sevoflurane in nitrous oxide. *Anesth Analg* 92:877–881, 2001.

Barker P, Langton JA, Murphy PJ, Rowbotham DJ: Regurgitation of gastric contents during general anesthesia using the laryngeal mask airway. *Br J Anaesth* 69:314, 1992.

Bevan JC, Johnston C, Haig MJ, et al.: Preoperative parental anxiety predicts behavioural and emotional responses to induction of anesthesia. *Can J Anaesth* 37:177, 1990.

Bissonette B: Body temperature and anesthesia. *Anesth Clin N Am* 9:849, 1991.

Booker PD: Management of postoperative pain in infants and children. *Curr Opin Anesthesiol* 1:17, 1988.

Bowlby J: *Attachment and loss.* New York, 1973, Basic Books.

Brain AIJ: The laryngeal mask airway—A new concept in airway management. *Br J Anaesth* 55:801, 1983.

Chambers N, Lopez T, Thomas J, James MFM: Remifentanil and the tunneling phase of paediatric ventriculoperitoneal shunt insertion. A double-blind, randomized, prospective study. *Anaesthesia* 57:133–139, 2002.

Chiaretti A, Pietrini D, Piastra M, et al.: Safety and efficacy of remifentanil in craniosynostosis repair in children less than 1 year old. *Pediatr Neurosurg* 33:83–88, 2000.

Choudhry DK, Brenn BR: Bispectral index monitoring: a comparison between normal children and children with quadriplegic cerebral palsy. *Anesth Analg* 95:1582–1585, 2002.

Cohen IT, Hannallah RS, Hummer KA: The incidence of emergence agitation associated with desflurane anesthesia in children is reduced by fentanyl. *Anesth Analg* 93:88–91, 2001.

Coté CJ, Goldstein EA, Coté MA, et al.: A single-blind study of pulse oximetry in children. *Anesthesiology* 68:184, 1988.

Coté CJ, Rolf N, Liu LMP, Gousouzian NG: A single-blind study of pulse oximetry and capnography in children. *Anesthesiology* 74:984, 1991.

Cravero J, Surgenor S, Whalen K: Emergence agitation in paediatric patients after sevoflurane anaesthesia and no surgery: A comparison with halothane. *Paediatr Anaesth* 10:419–424, 2000.

Davis PJ, Cohen IT, McGowan FX Jr, Latta K: Recovery characteristics of desflurane vs. halothane for maintenance of anesthesia in pediatric ambulatory patients. *Anesthesiology* 80:293–302, 1994.

Davis PJ, Finkel J, Orr R, et al.: A randomized, double-blinded study of remifentanil versus fentanyl for tonsillectomy and adenoidectomy surgery in pediatric ambulatory surgical patients. *Anesth Analg* 90:863–871, 2000.

Davis PJ, Galinkin J, McGowan FX, et al.: A randomized multicenter study of remifentanil compared with halothane in neonates and infants undergoing pyloromyotomy. I. Emergence and recovery profiles. *Anesth Analg* 93: 1380–1386, 2001.

Davis PJ, Greenberg JA, Gendelman M, Fertal K: Recovery characteristics of sevoflurane and halothane in preschool aged children undergoing bilateral myringotomy and pressure equalization tube insertion. *Anesth Analg* 88:34–38, 1999.

Davis PJ, Wilson AS, Siewers RD, et al.: The effects of cardiopulmonary bypass on remifentanil kinetics in children undergoing atrial septal defect repair. *Anesth Analg* 89:904–908, 1999.

de Beer DA, Thomas ML: Caudal additives in children—Solutions or problems? *Br J Anaesth* 90:487–498, 2003.

Denman WT, Swanson EL, Rosow D, et al.: Pediatric evaluation of the bispectral index (BIS) monitor and correlation of BIS with end-tidal sevoflurane concentration in infants and children. *Anesth Analg* 90:872–877, 2000.

Devitt JH, Wenstone R, Noel AG, O'Donnell PO: The laryngeal mask airway and positive pressure ventilation. *Anesthesiology* 80:550, 1994.

Dixon S, Snyder J, Holve R, Bromberger P: Behavioral effects of circumcision with and without anesthesia. *J Dev Behav Pediatr* 5:246, 1984.

Dombro RH: The surgically ill child and his family. *Surg Clin North Am* 50:759, 1970.

Dönmez A, Kizilkan A, Berksun H, et al.: One center's experience with remifentanil infusions for pediatric cardiac catheterization. *J Cardiothoracic Vasc Anaesth* 15:736–739, 2001.

DuBois D, DuBois EF: A height-weight formula to estimate the surface area of man. *Proc Soc Exp Biol Med* 13:77, 1916.

Eichhorn SM, Cooper JB, Cullen DJ, et al.: Standards for patient monitoring during anesthesia at Harvard Medical School. *JAMA* 256:1017, 1986.

Fisher DM, Zwass MS: MAC of desflurane in 60% nitrous oxide in infants and children. *Anesthesiology* 76:354, 1992.

Forman MC, Kerschbaum WE, Hetznecker WH, Dunn JM: Psychosocial dimensions. In Behrman RE, Vaughan VC III, editors: *Nelson's textbook of pediatrics,* ed 13. Philadelphia, 1987, WB Saunders.

Friedman WF: The intrinsic physiologic properties of the developing heart. In Friedman WF, Lesch M, Sonnenblick EH, editors: *Neonatal heart disease.* New York, 1973, Grune & Stratton.

Friesen RH, Veit AS, Archibald DJ, Campanini RS: A comparison of remifentanil and fentanyl for fast track paediatric cardiac anaesthesia. *Paediatr Anaesth* 13:122–125, 2003.

Galinkin JL, Davis PJ, McGowan FX, et al.: A randomized multicenter study of remifentanil compared with halothane in neonates and infants undergoing pyloromyotomy: II. Perioperative breathing patterns in neonates and infants with pyloric stenosis. *Anesth Analg* 93:1387–1392, 2001.

Galinkin JL, Fazi LM, Cuy RM, et al.: Use of intranasal fentanyl in children undergoing myringotomy and tube placement during halothane and sevoflurane anesthesia. *Anesthesiology* 93:1378–1383, 2000.

Gallagher T, Lerman J, Volgyesi GA, et al.: Effects of halothane and isoflurane on the baroreceptor response in newborn swine. *Anesth Analg* 66:564, 1987.

Gehan EA, George SL: Estimation of human body surface area from height and weight. *Cancer Chemother Rep* 54(Pt 1):225, 1970.

German JW, Aneja R, Heard C, Dias M: Continuous remifentanil for pediatric neurosurgery patients. *Pediatr Neurosurg* 33:227–229, 2000.

Gootman PM: Neural regulation of cardiovascular function in the perinatal period. In Gootman N, Gootman PM, editors: *Perinatal cardiovascular function.* New York, 1983, Marcel Dekker.

Gray H: *Anatomy of the human body,* ed 29. Philadelphia, 1973, Lea & Febiger.

Grevenik CR, Ferguson C, White A: The laryngeal mask airway in pediatric radiology. *Anesthesiology* 72:474, 1990.

Hannallah RS, Rosales JK: Experience with parents' presence during anaesthesia induction in children. *Can Anaesth Soc J* 30:286, 1983.

Hansen TG, Ilett KF, Lim SI, et al.: Pharmacokinetics and clinical efficacy of long-term epidural ropivacaine infusion in children. *Br J Anaesth* 85:347–353, 2000.

Hansen TG, Ilett KF, Reid C, et al.: Caudal ropivacaine in infants. *Anesthesiology* 94:579–584, 2001.

Harris JS: Special pediatric problems in fluid and electrolyte therapy in surgery. *Ann N Y Acad Sci* 66:966, 1957.

Hay WW Jr, Rodden DJ, Collins SM et al.: Reliability of conventional and new pulse oximetry in neonatal patients. *J Perinatol* 22:360–366, 2002.

Irita K, Kai Y, Akiyoshi K et al.: Performance evaluation of a new pulse oximeter during mild hypothermic cardiopulmonary bypass. *Anesth Analg* 96:11–14, 2003.

Ivani G, DeNegri P, Conio A, et al.: Comparison of racemic bupivacaine, ropivacaine, and levobupivacaine for pediatric caudal anesthesia: Effects on postoperative analgesia and motor block. *Reg Anesth Pain Med* 27:157–161, 2002.

Ivani G, Lampugnani E, Torre M, et al.: Comparison of ropivacaine with bupivacaine for paediatric caudal block. *Br J Anaesth* 81:247–248, 1998.

Ivani G, Pasquale De Negri, Lönnqvist P, et al.: A comparison of three different concentrations of levobupivacaine for caudal block in children. *Anesth Analg* 97:368–371, 2003.

Johnston DF, Wrigley SR, Robb PJ, Jones HE: The laryngeal mask airway in paediatric anaesthesia. *Anaesthesia* 45:924, 1990.

Jusko WJ: Pharmacokinetic principles in pediatric problems. *Pediatr Clin North Am* 19:81, 1972.

Kain Z, Mayes L, Wang S, et al.: Parental presence and a sedative premedicant for children undergoing surgery: A hierarchical study. *Anesthesiology* 92:939–946, 2000.

Kain Z, Mayes L, Wang S, et al.: Parental presence during induction of anesthesia vs. sedative premedication: Which intervention is more effective? *Anesthesiology* 89:1147–1156, 1998.

Kain Z, Mayes LC, Bell C, et al.: Premedication in the United States: A status report. *Anesth Analg* 84:427–432, 1997.

Kain ZN, Caldwell-Andrews A, Wang S-M, et al.: Parental intervention choices for children undergoing repeated surgeries. *Anesth Analg* 96:970–975, 2003a.

Kain ZN, Caldwell-Andrews AA, Krivutza D, et al.: Trends in the practice of parental presence during induction of anesthesia and the use of preoperative sedative premedication in the United States, 1995-2002: Results of a followup national survey. *Anesth Analg* 2004.

Kain ZN, Caldwell-Andrews AA, Mayes LC, et al.: Parental presence during induction of anesthesia: Physiological effects on parents. *Anesthesiology* 98:58–64, 2003b.

Kain ZN, Mayes LC, Caramico LA, et al.: Parental presence during induction of anesthesia. A randomized controlled trial. *Anesthesiology* 84:1060–1067, 1996.

Karmakar MK, Aun CST, Wong ELY, et al.: Ropivacaine undergoes slower systemic absorption from the caudal epidural space in children than bupivacaine. *Anesth Analg* 94:259–265, 2002.

Keidan I, Berkenstadt H, Sidi A, Perel A: Propofol/remifentanil versus propofol alone for bone marrow aspiration in paediatric haemato-oncological patients. *Paediatr Anaesth* 11:297–301, 2001.

Keidan I, Berkenstadt H, Segal E, Perel A: Pressure versus volume-controlled ventilation with a laryngeal mask airway in paediatric patients. *Paediatr Anaesth* 11:691–694, 2001.

Ko Y-P, Huang C-J, Hung Y-C, et al.: Premedication with low-dose oral midazolam reduces the incidence and severity of emergence agitation in pediatric patients following sevoflurane anesthesia. *Acta Anaesthesiol Sin* 36:169–177, 2001.

Kulka PJ, Bressem M, Tryba M: Clonidine prevents sevoflurane-induced agitation in children. *Anesth Analg* 93:335–338, 2001.

Lerman J, Davis PJ, Welborn LG, et al.: Induction, recovery, and safety characteristics of sevoflurane I children undergoing ambulatory surgery: A comparison with halothane. *Anesthesiology* 84:1332–1340, 1996.

Lippmann M, Nelson J, Emmanouilides GC, et al.: Ligation of patent ductus arteriosus in premature infants. *Br J Anaesth* 48:365, 1976.

Lönnqvist PA, Westrin P, Laarsson BA, et al.: Ropivacaine pharmacokinetics after caudal block in 1- to 8-year-old children. *Br J Anaesth* 85:506–511, 2000.

Malviya S, Reynolds PI, Voepel-Lewis T, et al.: False alarms and sensitivity of conventional pulse oximetry versus the Masimo SET technology in the pediatric postanesthesia care unit. *Anesth Analg* 90:1336–1340, 2000.

Martin LD, Pasternak LR, Pudimar MA: Total intravenous anesthesia with propofol in pediatric patients outside the operating room. *Anesth Analg* 74:609, 1992.

McCann ME, Bacsik J, Davidson A, et al.: The correlation of bispectral index with end tidal sevoflurane concentration and haemodynamic parameters in preschoolers. *Paediatr Anaesth* 12:519–525, 2002.

McCann ME, Sethna NF, Mazoit JX, et al.: The pharmacokinetics of epidural ropivacaine in infants and young children. *Anesth Analg* 93:893–897, 2001.

Mizushima A, Wardall GJ, Simpson DL: The laryngeal mask airway in infants. *Anaesthesia* 47:849, 1992.

Moss AJ, Emmanouilides GC, Monset-Couchard M, Marcan B: Vascular responses to postural changes in normal newborn infants. *Pediatrics* 42:250, 1968.

Motoyama EK, Glazener CH: Hypoxemia after general anesthesia in children. *Anesth Analg* 65:267, 1986.

Murthy BVS, Pandya KS, Booker PD, et al.: Pharmacokinetics of tramadol in children after IV or caudal epidural administration. *Br J Anaesth* 84:346–349, 2000.

New York State Hospital Code, Section 405.13, 1988.

Ochiai R, Guthrie RD, Motoyama EK: Effects of varying concentrations of halothane on the activity of the genioglossus, intercostals, and diaphragm in cats: An electromyographic study. *Anesthesiology* 70:812–816, 1989.

Ross AK, Davis PJ, Dear G, et al.: Pharmacokinetics of remifentanil in anesthetized pediatric patients undergoing elective surgery or diagnostic procedures. *Anesth Analg* 93:1393–401, 2001.

Sarner JB, Levine M, David PJ, et al.: Clinical characteristics of sevoflurane in children: A comparison with halothane. *Anesthesiology* 82:38–46, 1995.

Sebel PS, Lang E, Rampil IJ, et al.: A multicenter study of bispectral electroencephalogram analysis for monitoring anesthetic effect. *Anesth Analg* 84: 891, 1997.

Smith RM: *Anesthesia for infants and children,* ed 3. St. Louis, 1968, The CV Mosby Co.

Smith RM: *Anesthesia for infants and children,* ed 4. St. Louis, 1980, The CV Mosby Co.

Smith RM: Anesthesia for pediatric surgery. In Gross RE, editor: *Surgery of infants and children.* Philadelphia, 1953, WB Saunders.

Smith RM: Some reasons for the high mortality in pediatric anesthesia. *N Y J Med* 56:2212, 1956.

Soliman IE, Broadman LM, Hannalah RS, McGill WA: Comparison of the analgesic effects of EMLA (eutectic mixture of local anesthetics) to intradermal lidocaine infiltration prior to venous cannulation in unpremedicated children. *Anesthesiology* 68:804, 1988.

Spears RS, Yeh A, Fisher DM, Zwass MS: The "Educated Hand." Can anesthesiologists assess changes in neonatal pulmonary compliance manually? *Anesthesiology* 75:693, 1991.

Spitzer A: Renal physiology and functional development. In Edelman CM Jr, editor: *Pediatric kidney disease.* Boston, 1978, Little, Brown and Co, p 25.

Spitzer A: The role of the kidney in sodium homeostasis during maturation. *Kidney Int* 21:539, 1982.

Talbot NG, Sobel EH, McArthur JW, Crawford JD: *Functional endocrinology from birth through adolescence.* Cambridge, MA, 1952, Harvard University Press.

Vaughan VC III, Litt IF: Assessment of growth and development. In Behrman BE, Vaughan VC ID, editors: *Nelson's textbook of pediatrics,* ed 13. Philadelphia, 1987, WB Saunders.

Voepel-Lewis T, Malviya S, Tait AR: A prospective cohort study of emergence agitation in the pediatric postanesthesia care unit. *Anesth Analg* 96:1625–1630, 2003.

Wacha MF, Simeon RM, White PF, Stevens JL: Effect of propofol on the incidence of postoperative vomiting after strabismus surgery in pediatric outpatients. *Anesthesiology* 75:204, 1991.

Wear R, Robinson S, Gregory GA: The effect of halothane on the baroresponse of adult and baby rabbits. *Anesthesiology* 56:188, 1982.

Wee LH, Moriarty A, Cranston A, Bagshaw O: Remifentanil infusion for major abdominal surgery in small infants. *Paediatr Anaesth* 9:415–418, 1999.

Welborn LG, Hannallah RS, Norden JM, et al.: Comparison of emergence and recovery characteristics of sevoflurane, desflurane, and halothane in pediatric ambulatory patients. *Anesth Analg* 83:917–920, 1996.

Wilson IG: The laryngeal mask airway in paediatric practice. *Br J Anaesth* 70:124, 1993.

Yelderman MF, New W: Evaluation of pulse oximetry. *Anesthesiology* 59:349, 1983.

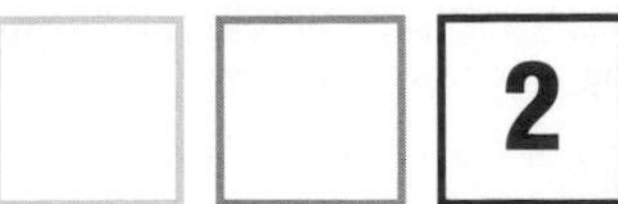

Respiratory Physiology in Infants and Children

Etsuro K. Motoyama

For an infant to survive in the extrauterine environment, the respiratory and circulatory systems must be developed sufficiently to withstand drastic changes at birth, from the fetal circulatory pattern with liquid-filled lungs to air breathing with transitional circulatory adaptation in a matter of a few minutes. The newborn infant must exercise an effective neuronal drive and respiratory muscles to displace the liquid filling the airway system and to introduce sufficient air against the surface force in order to establish sufficient alveolar surface for gas exchange. At the same time, pulmonary blood vessels must dilate to increase pulmonary blood flow and to establish adequate regional alveolar ventilation–pulmonary perfusion relationships for pulmonary gas exchange. The neonatal adaptation of lung mechanics and respiratory control takes several weeks to complete. Beyond this immediate neonatal period, the infant's lungs continue to mature at a rapid pace and postnatal development of the lungs and the thorax surrounding the lungs continues well beyond the first year of life. Respiratory function in infants and toddlers, especially during the first several months of age, as with cardiovascular system and hepatic function, is both qualitatively and quantitatively different from that in older children and adults.

This chapter reviews clinically important aspects of the development of the respiratory system and respiratory physiology in infants and children and their application to pediatric anesthesia. Such knowledge is indispensable for the proper care of infants and children before, during, and after general anesthesia and surgery, as well as for the care of those with respiratory insufficiency.

The respiratory system consists of the respiratory centers in the brainstem; the central and peripheral chemoreceptors; the phrenic, intercostal, hypoglossal (all efferent), and vagal (afferent) nerves; the thorax (including the thoracic cage; the muscles of the chest, abdomen, and diaphragm); the upper (extrathoracic) and lower (intrathoracic) airways; the lungs; and the pulmonary vascular system. The principal function of the respiratory system is to maintain the oxygen and carbon dioxide equilibrium in the body. The lungs also contribute importantly to the regulation of acid-base balance. The maintenance of body temperature (via loss of water through the lungs) is an additional but secondary function of the lungs. The lung is also an important organ of metabolism. A glossary of abbreviations used in this chapter is compiled in Box 2–1. An additional glossary of abbreviations specific to the mechanics of respiration is summarized in Box 2–2.

■ DEVELOPMENT OF THE RESPIRATORY SYSTEM

■ PRENATAL DEVELOPMENT OF THE LUNGS

The morphologic development of the human lung is seen as early as several weeks into the embryonic period and continues well into the first decade and beyond of postnatal life (Fig. 2–1). The fetal lungs begin to form within the first several weeks of the embryonic period, when the fetus is only 3 mm long. A groove appears in the ventral aspect of the foregut, creating a small pouch. The outgrowth of the endodermal cavity, with a mass of surrounding mesenchymal tissue, projects into the pleuroperitoneal cavity and forms lung buds. The future alveolar

BOX 2–1 Glossary of Abbreviations 1 (General Topics)

ALTE: Apparent life-threatening events (near-miss SIDS)
ARDS: Acute (adult) respiratory distress syndrome
cAMP: Cyclic adenosine monophosphate
CPAP: Continuous positive airway pressure
CSF: Cerebrospinal fluid
DPG: Diphosphoglycerate
DRG: Dorsal respiratory group neurons (versus VRG)
EGF: Epidermal growth factor
EMG: Electromyogram
ET: Endotracheal
ETT: Endotracheal tube
HMD: Hyaline membrane disease (IRDS)
HPV: Hypoxic pulmonary vasoconstriction
IRDS: Idiopathic (infantile) respiratory distress syndrome
Pa: Pulmonary arterial pressure
P_A: Alveolar pressure
Pao: Airway opening pressure
Palv: Alveolar pressure
P_V: Pulmonary venous pressure
P_{50}: Arterial oxygen tension (Pa_{O_2}) at 50% hemoglobin saturation
PC: Phosphatidylcholine
P_{CO_2}: Partial pressure of carbon dioxide
Pa_{O_2}: Arterial oxygen tension (or partial pressure)
P_{ETCO_2}: End-tidal carbon dioxide tension
PE: Phosphatidylethanolamine
PEEP: Positive end-expiratory pressure
PG: Phosphatidylglycerol
P_{O_2}: Partial pressure of oxygen
Pa_{O_2}: Arterial oxygen tension (or partial pressure)
P_{VO_2}: Venous oxygen tension
PPHN: Persistent pulmonary hypertension of the neonate
PRG: Pontine respiratory group of neurons
PS: Phosphatidylserine
$\dot{Q}$: Pulmonary blood flow
$\dot{Q}_P/\dot{Q}_S$: Pulmonary-to-systemic blood flow ratio
R: Resistance
Raw: Airway resistance
Rint: Resistive component of Rrs
Rrs: Total resistance of the respiratory system
ΔR: Viscoelastic component of Rrs
RARs: Rapidly adapting (irritant) receptors
REM: Rapid eye movement (sleep)
SARs: Slowly adapting (pulmonary stretch) receptors
SIDS: Sudden infant death syndrome
S_{O_2}: Oxygen saturation of hemoglobin
Sa_{O_2}: Arterial S_{O_2}
Sp_{O_2} Sa_{O_2}: As measured with a pulse oximeter
SP-A (B, C, D): Surfactant protein A (B, C, D)
TGFβ: Transforming growth factor-β
TNFα: Tumor necrosis factor-α
$\dot{V}_A/\dot{Q}$: Ventilation/pulmonary perfusion ratio
VRG: Ventral respiratory groups of neurons

membranes and mucous glands are derived from the endoderm, whereas the cartilage, muscle, elastic tissue, and lymph vessels originate from the mesenchymal elements surrounding the lung buds (Emery, 1969). During the pseudoglandular period, which extends until the seventeenth week of gestation, the budding of

BOX 2–2 Glossary of Abbreviations 2 (Respiratory Mechanics)

C_L: Compliance of lungs
Crs: Compliance of respiratory system
Cw: Compliance of chest wall
ERV: Expiratory reserve volume
f: Respiratory frequency
$FEV_{1.0}$: Forced expiratory volume at 1.0 second
FRC: Functional residual capacity
FVC: Forced vital capacity
Gaw: Airway conductance (reciprocal of Raw)
IC: Inspiratory capacity
IRV: Inspiratory reserve volume
MEFV: Maximum expiratory flow-volume (curve)
MMEFR: Maximum mid-expiratory flow rate (same as $FEF_{25\text{-}75}$)
PEFR: Peak expiratory flow rate
Pao: Airway opening pressure
Palv: Alveolar pressure
P_B: Atmospheric pressure
Ppl: Pleural pressure
Pstl: Static recoil pressure of the lungs
Raw: Airway resistance
Rrs: Resistance of respiratory system
Rus: Airway resistance of upstream segment
RV: Residual volume
T_I: Inspiratory time
T_I/T_{TOT}: Respiratory duty cycle
T_E: Expiratory time
T_{TOT}: Total respiratory time ($T_1 + T_E$)
TLC: Total lung capacity
V_T: Tidal volume
V_T/T_I: Mean inspiratory flow (neural drive)
VC: Vital capacity
Visov̇: Volume of isoflow
$\dot{V}_E$: Minute volume ($\dot{V} = V_T \times f = V_T/T_I \times T_I/T_{TOT}$)
$\dot{V}max_{25}$: Maximum expiratory flow at 25% FVC (FEF_{75} or MEF_{25})

the bronchi and lung growth rapidly takes place, forming a loose mass of connective tissue. The morphologic development of the human lung is illustrated in Figure 2–2.

By 16 weeks gestation, preacinar branching of the airways (down to the terminal bronchioli) is complete (Reid, 1967). A disturbance of the free expansion of the developing lung during this stage, as occurs with diaphragmatic hernia, results in hypoplasia of the airways and lung tissue (Areechon and Reid, 1963).

During the canalicular period, in mid-gestation, the future respiratory bronchioli develop as the relative amount of connective tissue diminishes. Capillaries grow adjacent to the respiratory bronchioli, and the whole lung becomes more vascular (Emery, 1969).

At about 24 weeks gestation, the lung enters the terminal sac (alveolar) period, which is characterized by the appearance of clusters of terminal air sacs, termed saccules, with flattened epithelium (Hislop and Reid, 1974). These saccules are large and irregular with thick septa and have few capillaries in comparison with the adult alveoli (Boyden, 1969). At about 26 to 28 weeks gestation, proliferation of the capillary network surrounding the terminal air spaces becomes sufficient for pulmonary gas exchange (Potter, 1961). These morphologic developments may occur earlier in some premature infants born at 24 to 25 weeks gestation who have survived with neonatal intensive care.

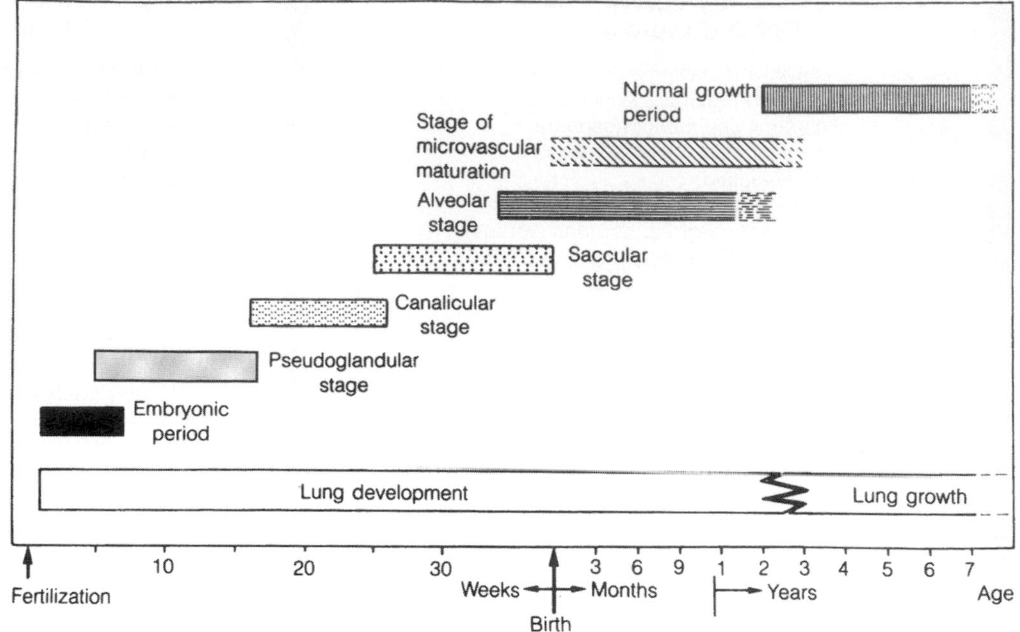

■ **FIGURE 2–1.** Stages of human lung development and their timing. Note the overlap between stages, particularly between the alveolar stage and the stage of microvascular maturation. Open-ended bars indicate uncertainty as to exact timing. (From Zeltner TB, Burri PH: *Respir Physiol* 67:269, 1987, with permission from Elsevier.)

Air space wall thickness decreases rapidly starting at 28 weeks gestation. From 28 weeks gestation to term, there is further lengthening of saccules with possible growth of additional generations of air spaces. Some species, such as the rat, have no mature alveoli at birth (Burri, 1974). Alveolar development from saccules begins in some human fetuses as early as 32 weeks gestation, but alveoli are not uniformly present until 36 weeks of gestation (Langston et al., 1984). Most alveolar formation, however, takes place during the first 12 to 18 months of postnatal life (Langston et al., 1984). Development of respiratory bronchioles by transformation of preexisting terminal airways does not take place until after birth (Langston et al., 1984).

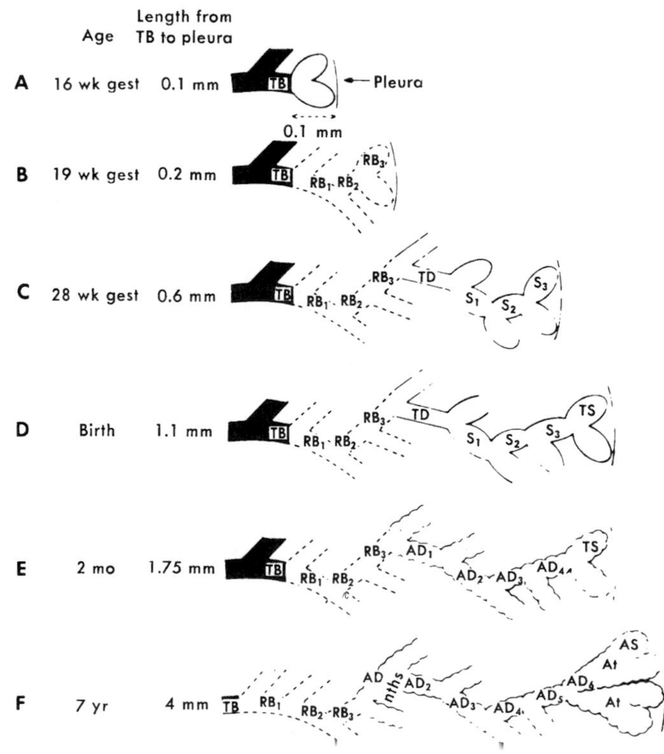

■ **FIGURE 2–2.** Development of the acinus in human lungs at various ages. TB, Terminal bronchiole; RB, respiratory bronchiole; TD, transitional duct; S, saccule; TS, terminal saccule; AD, alveolar duct; At, atrium; AS, alveolar sac. (From Hislop A, Reid L: *Thorax* 29:90, 1974.)

The fetal lung produces a large quantity of liquid, which expands the airways while the larynx is closed. This expansion helps to stimulate lung growth and development. The lung fluid is periodically expelled into the uterine cavity and contributes about one third of the total amniotic fluid. Prenatal ligation or occlusion of the trachea was tried in the 1990s with some success for the treatment of the fetus with congenital diaphragmatic hernia. This treatment causes the expansion of the fetal airways and results in an accelerated growth of the otherwise hypoplastic lung (see Chapter 15, Anesthesia for Fetal Surgery).

The type II pneumocytes, which produce pulmonary surfactant that forms the alveolar lining layer and stabilizes air spaces, appear at about 24 to 26 weeks gestation, but occasionally as early as 20 weeks (Spear et al., 1969; Lauweryns, 1970). Idiopathic (or infantile) respiratory distress syndrome (IRDS), also known as hyaline membrane disease (HMD), occurring in prematurely born infants, is caused by the immaturity of the lung, with its insufficient pulmonary surfactant production, and its inactivation by plasma proteins exudating onto the alveolar surface (see discussion under Surface Activity and Pulmonary Surfactant).

Experimental evidence from animals indicates that certain pharmacologic agents such as cortisol (deLemos et al., 1970; Motoyama et al., 1971) and thyroxin (Wu et al., 1973) administered to the mother or directly to the fetus accelerate the maturation of the lungs, resulting in the early appearance of type II pneumocytes and surfactant (Smith and Bogues, 1982; Rooney, 1985). In 1972, Liggins and Howie reported accelerated maturation of human fetal lungs after the administration of corticosteroids to mothers 24 to 48 hours before the delivery of premature babies. Despite initial concern that steroids are potentially toxic to other organs of the fetus, particularly to the development of the central nervous system, prenatal glucocorticoid therapy has been used widely since the 1980s to induce lung maturation and surfactant synthesis in mothers at risk of premature delivery (Avery, 1984, 1986).

NEONATAL RESPIRATORY ADAPTATION

Respiratory rhythmogenesis occurs in the fetus long before partition. The clamping of the umbilical cord and increasing arterial oxygen tensions with air breathing (but not transient hypoxia) initiate and maintain rhythmic breathing at birth.

To introduce air into the fluid-filled lungs at birth, the newborn infant must overcome large surface force with the first few breaths. Usually a negative pressure of 30 cm H_2O is necessary to introduce air into the fluid-filled lungs. In some normal full-term infants, even with sufficient surfactant, a force of as much as −70 cm H_2O or more must be exerted to overcome the surface force (Karlberg et al., 1962) (Fig. 2–3). Usually fluid is rapidly expelled via the upper airways. The residual fluid leaves the lungs through the pulmonary capillaries and lymphatic channels over the first few days of life, and changes in compliance parallel this time course. All changes are delayed in the prematurely born infant.

As the lungs expand with air, pulmonary vascular resistance decreases dramatically and pulmonary blood flow increases markedly, thus allowing gas exchange between alveolar air and pulmonary capillaries to occur. Changes in PO_2, PCO_2, and pH are largely responsible for this decrease in pulmonary vascular resistance (Cook et al., 1963). With the expansion of the lung, arterial oxygen tension (PaO_2) increases and reduces pulmonary vascular resistance dramatically. The resultant large increases in pulmonary blood flow and the increase in left atrial pressure with a decrease in right atrial pressure reverse the pressure gradient across the atria and functionally close the foramen ovale, a left-to-right one-way valve. With these adjustments, the cardiopulmonary system approaches adult levels of $\dot{V}A/\dot{Q}$ balance within a few days (Nelson et al., 1962, 1963). The process of expansion of the lungs during the first few hours of life and the resultant circulatory adaptation for establishing pulmonary gas exchange are greatly influenced by the adequacy of pulmonary surfactant. It should be remembered that these changes are delayed in immature newborns.

POSTNATAL DEVELOPMENT OF THE LUNGS AND THORAX

The development and growth of the lung and surrounding thorax continue with amazing speed during the first year of life. Although the formation of the airway system, all the way to the terminal bronchioles, is completed by the 16th week of gestation, alveolar formation begins only at about the 36th week. At birth, the number of terminal air sacs (most of which are saccules) is between 20 and 50 million, only one tenth that of adults. Most of the postnatal development of alveoli from primitive saccules occurs during the first year and is essentially completed by 18 months of age (Langston et al., 1984). The morphologic and physiologic development of the lungs, however, continues throughout the first decade of life (Mansell et al., 1972).

During the early postnatal period, the lung volume of infants is disproportionately small in relation to body size. In addition, because of higher metabolic rates in infants (oxygen consumption per unit body weight is twice as high as that of adults), the ventilatory requirement per unit of lung volume in infants is markedly increased. Infants have much less reserve of lung surface area for gas exchange. This is the primary reason why infants and young children become rapidly desaturated with hypoventilation or apnea of relatively short duration.

In the neonate, static (elastic) recoil pressure of the lung is very low (i.e., compliance, normalized for volume, is high), not dissimilar to that of geriatric or emphysematous lungs, because the elastic fibers do not develop until the postnatal period (whereas elastic fibers in geriatric lungs are not functional (Fagan, 1976; Mansel et al., 1972; Bryan and Wohl, 1986). In addition, the elastic recoil pressure of the infant's thorax (chest wall) is extremely low due to its compliant cartilaginous rib cage with poorly developed thoracic muscle mass, which does not add rigidity. These unique characteristics make infants more prone to lung collapse, especially under general anesthesia (see later). Throughout infancy and childhood, static recoil pressure of the lung steadily increases (compliance, normalized for volume, decreases) toward normal values for young adults (Zapletal et al., 1971; Motoyama, 1977).

The actual size of the airway from the larynx to the bronchioles in infants and children, of course, is much smaller than in adolescents and adults, and flow resistance in absolute terms is extremely high. When normalized for lung volume or body size, however, infants' airway size is much larger and airway resistance is much lower than in adults (Polgar, 1967; Motoyama, 1977; Stocks and Godfrey, 1977). Infants and toddlers, however, are more prone to severe obstruction of upper and lower airways because their absolute (not relative) airway diameters are much smaller than those in adults. As a consequence, relatively mild airway inflammation, edema, or secretions can lead to far greater degrees of airway obstruction like subglottic croup (laryngotracheobronchitis) or acute supraglottitis (epiglottitis) compared with adults.

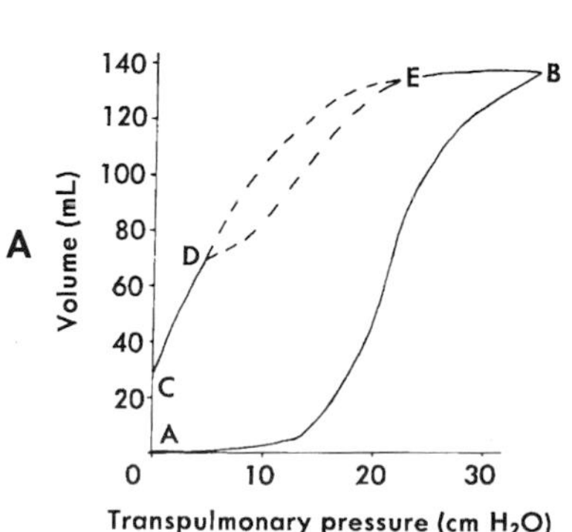

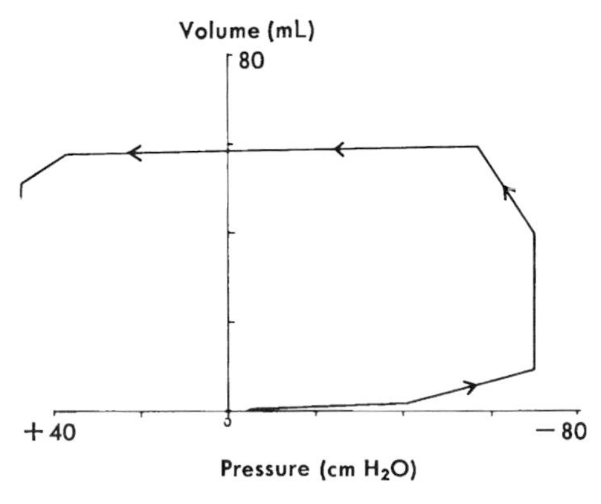

FIGURE 2–3. *(A)* Typical pressure-volume curve of expansion of a gas-free lung. (A, B) Initial expansion. In the example, approximately 30 cm H_2O pressure will be necessary to overcome surface forces. (C) Deflation to zero pressure with gas trapping. (D, E) Subsequent breaths with a further increase in FRC. *(B)* Pressure-volume relationships during the first breath of a newborn weighing 4.3 kg. Here, 60 to 70 cm H_2O negative pressure was necessary to overcome the surface forces. (From Karlberg P, Cherry RB, Escardo FE, Koch G: *Acta Paediatr Scand* 51:121, 1962.)

Further description on the development of the lungs and thorax and their effects on lung function, especially under general anesthesia, are described later in the chapter. Perinatal and postnatal adaptations of respiratory control are included in the following section on the control of breathing.

PRENATAL DEVELOPMENT OF BREATHING

Respiratory rhythmogenesis occurs long before parturition. Dawes and others (1970) were the first to demonstrate "breathing" activities with rhythmic diaphragmatic contractions in the fetal lamb. They found it to be episodic and highly variable in frequency. Boddy and Robinson (1971) recorded movement of the human fetal thorax with an ultrasound device and interpreted this as evidence of fetal breathing. Later studies (Patrick et al., 1980) have shown that in the last 10 weeks of pregnancy, fetal breathing is present approximately 30% of the time. The breathing rate in the fetus at 30 to 31 weeks gestation is higher (58/min) than that in the near-term fetus (47/min). A significant increase in fetal breathing movements occurs 2 to 3 hours after a maternal meal and is correlated with the increase in the maternal blood sugar level (Patrick et al., 1980).

Spontaneous breathing movements in the fetuses occur only during their active or rapid eye movement (REM) sleep and with low voltage electrocortical activity and appear to be independent of the usual chemical and nonchemical stimuli of postnatal breathing (Dawes et al., 1972; Jansen and Chernick, 1983). Later studies, however, have clearly shown that the fetus can respond to chemical stimuli known to modify breathing patterns postnatally (Dawes et al., 1982; Jansen et al., 1982; Rigatto et al., 1988; Rigatto, 1992). In contrast, hypoxemia in the fetus abolishes, rather than stimulates, breathing movements. This may be related to the fact that hypoxemia diminishes the incidence of REM sleep (Boddy et al., 1974). It appears that normally low Pa_{O_2} (19 to 23 mm Hg) in the fetus is a normal mechanism inhibiting breathing activities in utero (Rigatto, 1992). Severe hypoxemia induces gasping, which is independent of the peripheral chemoreceptors and apparently entirely independent of rhythmic fetal breathing (Jansen and Chernick, 1974).

The near-term fetus is relatively insensitive to Pa_{O_2} changes. Extreme hypercapnia ($Pa_{O_2} > 60$ mm Hg) in the fetal lamb, however, can induce rhythmical breathing movement that is preceded by a sudden activation of inspiratory muscle tone with expansion of the thorax and inward movement (inhalation) of amniotic fluid, as much as 30 to 40 mL/kg (an apparent increase in functional residual capacity [FRC]) (E. K. Motoyama, unpublished observation). When Pa_{O_2} was reduced, breathing activities ceased, followed by a reversal of the sequence of events noted above (i.e., relaxation of the thorax, decreased FRC as evidenced by outward flow of amniotic fluid) (Motoyama, 2001).

The inflation reflex of Hering-Breuer is present in the fetus. Distension of the lungs by saline infusion slows the frequency of breathing (Dawes et al., 1982). Transection of the vagi, however, does not change the breathing pattern (Dawes, 1974).

Maternal ingestion of alcoholic beverages abolishes human fetal breathing for up to 1 hour. Fetal breathing movement is also abolished by maternal cigarette smoking. These effects may be related to fetal hypoxemia resulting from changes in placental circulation (Jansen and Chernick, 1983).

It is unclear why the fetus must "breathe" in utero, when gas exchange is handled by the placental circulation. Dawes (1974) suggested that fetal breathing might represent "prenatal practice" to ensure that the respiratory system is well developed and ready at the moment of birth. Another reason may be that the stretching of the airways and lung parenchyma is an important stimulus for lung development; bilateral phrenic nerve sectioning in the fetal lamb results in hypoplasia of the lungs (Alcorn et al., 1980).

BOX 2–3 Mechanism of Continuous Neonatal Breathing

1. The onset of breathing activities occurs not at birth but in utero, as a part of normal fetal development.
2. The clamping of the umbilical cord initiates rhythmic breathing.
3. Relative "hyperoxia" with air breathing, compared with low fetal Pa_{O_2}, augments and maintains continuous and rhythmic breathing.
4. Continuous breathing is independent of the level of Pa_{CO_2}.
5. Breathing is unaffected by carotid denervation.
6. Hypoxia depresses or abolishes continuous breathing.

PERINATAL ADAPTATION OF BREATHING

During normal labor and vaginal delivery, the human fetus goes through a period of transient hypoxemia, hypercapnia, and acidemia. The traditional view of the mechanism of the onset of breathing at birth was that the transient fetal asphyxia stimulates the chemoreceptors and produces gasping followed by rhythmic breathing at birth. Subsequent observations have challenged this concept. First, in full-term fetal lambs, severe hypoxemia stimulates fetal gasping and ventilation even after denervation of the carotid and aortic chemoreceptors (Chernick et al., 1975). Second, total peripheral chemodenervation does not alter the pattern of fetal breathing or the initiation of continuous breathing at birth. Third, continuous breathing can be initiated and maintained by ventilating the fetal lamb through the endotracheal tube with 100% oxygen in utero and raising fetal Pa_{CO_2} (Baier et al., 1990). The occlusion of the umbilical cord also initiates the onset of rhythmic breathing, independent of Pa_{O_2} (Baier et al., 1990; Rigatto, 1992). The current concept regarding the mechanism of continuous neonatal breathing is summarized in Box 2–3.

Once the newborn has begun rhythmic breathing, ventilation is adjusted to achieve a lower Pa_{O_2} (Table 2–1) than is found in older children and adults. The reason for this difference is not

TABLE 2–1. Normal blood-gas values

	Pa_{O_2} (mm Hg)	Sa_{O_2} (%)	Pa_{CO_2} (mm Hg)	pH
Pregnant woman at term (artery)	88*	96	32	7.40
Umbilical vein	31	72*	42	7.35
Umbilical artery	19	38*	51	7.29
1 Hour of life (artery)	62	95	28	7.36
24 Hours of life (artery)	68	94	29	7.37
Child and adult (artery)	99	97	41	7.40

*Estimated values.

clear but most likely is related to a poor buffering capacity in the neonate and a ventilatory compensation for metabolic acidosis. The PaO_2 of the infant approximates the adult level within a few weeks after birth (Nelson, 1976).

Control of breathing in the neonate evolves gradually during the first month of extrauterine life and beyond and is different from that in older children and adults, especially in their response to hypoxemia and hyperoxia. The neonates' breathing patterns and responses to chemical stimuli are detailed later, following a general overview of the control of breathing.

■ CONTROL OF BREATHING

The mechanism that regulates and maintains pulmonary gas exchange is remarkably efficient. In a normal person, the level of arterial PCO_2 is maintained within a very narrow range, whereas oxygen demand and carbon dioxide production vary greatly during rest and exercise. This control is achieved by a precise matching of the level of ventilation to the output of carbon dioxide. Breathing is produced by the coordinated action of a number of inspiratory and expiratory muscles. Inspiration is produced principally by the contraction of the diaphragm, which creates negative intrathoracic pressure that draws air into the lungs. Expiration, on the other hand, is normally produced passively by the elastic recoil of the lungs and thorax. It may be increased actively by the contraction of abdominal and thoracic expiratory muscles during exercise. During the early phase of expiration, sustained contraction of the diaphragm with decreasing intensity (braking action) and the upper airway muscles activities impede and smoothen the rate of expiratory flow.

Rhythmic contraction of the respiratory muscles is governed by the respiratory centers in the brainstem and tightly regulated by feedback systems so as to match the level of ventilation to metabolic needs (Cherniack and Pack, 1988) (Fig. 2–4). These feedback mechanisms include central and peripheral chemoreceptors, stretch receptors in the airways and lung parenchyma via the vagal afferent, and segmental reflexes in the spinal cord provided by muscle spindles (Cherniack and Pack, 1988). The control of breathing comprises neural and chemical controls, which are closely interrelated.

■ NEURAL CONTROL OF BREATHING

Respiratory neurons in the medulla have inherent rhythmicity even when they are separated from the higher levels of the brainstem. In the cat, respiratory neurons are concentrated in two bilaterally symmetric areas in the medulla near the level of the obex. The dorsal respiratory group of neurons (DRG) is located in the dorsomedial medulla just ventrolateral to the nucleus tractus solitarius and contains predominantly inspiratory neurons. The ventral respiratory group (VRG) of neurons, located in the ventrolateral medulla, consists of both inspiratory and expiratory neurons (von Euler, 1986; Tabatabai and Behnia, 1995; Berger, 2000) (Fig. 2–5).

Dorsal Respiratory Group (DRG) of Neurons

The DRG is spatially associated with the tractus solitarius, which is the principal tract for the ninth and tenth cranial (glossopharyngeal and vagus) nerves. These nerves carry afferent fibers from the airways and lungs, heart, and peripheral arterial chemoreceptors. The DRG may constitute the initial intracranial site for processing some of these visceral sensory afferent inputs into a respiratory motor response (Berger, 2000).

On the basis of lung inflation, three types of neurons have been recognized in the DRG: type Iα (I stands for inspiratory), type Iβ, and pump (P) cells. Type Iα is inhibited by lung inflation (Cohen, 1981a). The axons of these neurons project to both the phrenic and the external (inspiratory) intercostal motoneurons of the spinal cord. Some type Iα neurons have medullary collaterals that terminate among the inspiratory and expiratory neurons of the ipsilateral VRG (Merrill, 1970).

The second type, Iβ, is excited by lung inflation and receives synaptic inputs from pulmonary stretch receptors. There is controversy as to whether Iβ axons project into the spinal cord respiratory neurons; the possible functional significance of such spinal projections is unknown. Both Iα and Iβ neurons receive excitatory inputs from the central pattern generator (or central inspiratory activity) for breathing, so that when lung inflation is terminated or the vagi in the neck are cut, the rhythmic firing activity of these neurons continues (Cohen, 198la, 1981b; Feldman and Speck, 1983).

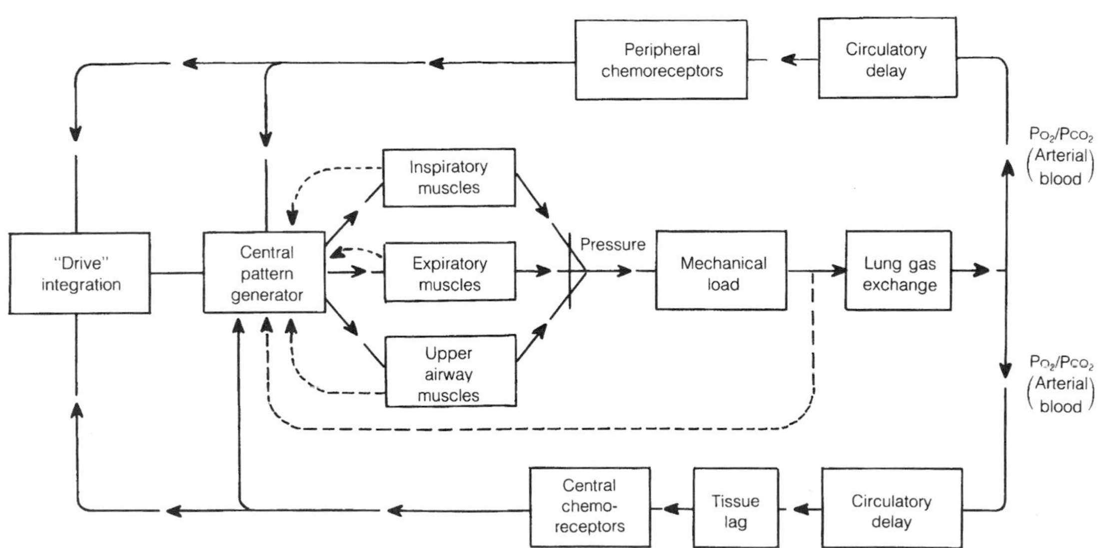

■ **FIGURE 2–4.** Block diagram of multi-input, multi-output system that controls ventilation. (From Cherniak NS, Pack AI: Control of ventilation. In Fishman AP, editor: *Pulmonary diseases and disorders,* ed 2. New York, 1988, McGraw-Hill Book Co.)

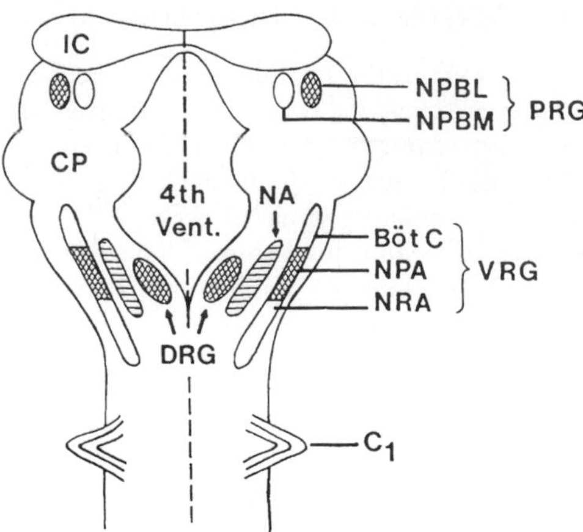

■ **FIGURE 2–5.** Schematic representation of the respiratory neurons on the dorsal surface of the brainstem. Crosshatched areas contain predominantly inspiratory neurons, blank areas contain predominantly expiratory neurons, and dashed areas contain both inspiratory and expiratory neurons. Böt C, Bötzinger complex; C_1, first cervical spinal nerve; CP, cerebellar peduncle; DRG, dorsal respiratory group; 4th Vent, fourth ventricle; IC, inferior colliculus; NA, nucleus ambiguus; NPA, nucleus para-ambigualis; NPBL, nucleus parabrachialis lateralis; NPBM, nucleus parabrachialis medialis; NRA, nucleus retroambigualis; PRG, pontine respiratory group; VRG, ventral respiratory group. (From Tabatabai M, Behnia R: Neurochemical regulation of respiration. In Collins VJ, editor: *Physiological and pharmacological basis of anesthesia.* Philadelphia, 1995, Williams & Wilkins.)

The third type of neurons in the DRG receives no input from the central pattern generator. The impulse of these neurons, called pump, or P cells, closely follows lung inflation during either spontaneous or controlled ventilation (Berger, 1977). The P cells are assumed to be relay neurons for visceral afferent inputs (Berger, 2000).

The excitation of Iβ neurons by lung inflation is associated with the shortening of inspiratory duration. The Iβ neurons appear to promote inspiration-to-expiration phase-switching by inhibiting Iα neurons. This network seems to be responsible for the Hering-Breuer reflex inhibition of inspiration by lung inflation (Cohen, 198la, 1981b; von Euler, 1986, 1991).

The DRG thus functions as an important primary and possibly secondary relay site for visceral sensory inputs via glossopharyngeal and vagal afferent fibers. Because many of the inspiratory neurons in the DRG project to the contralateral spinal cord and make excitatory connections with phrenic motoneurons, the DRG serves as a source of inspiratory drive to phrenic and possibly to external intercostal motoneurons (Berger, 2000).

Ventral Respiratory Group (VRG) of Neurons

The VRG extends from the rostral to the caudal end of the medulla and has three subdivisions (see Fig. 2–5). The Bötzinger complex, located in the most rostral part of the medulla in the vicinity of the retrofacial nucleus, contains mostly expiratory neurons (Lipski and Merrill, 1980; Merrill et al., 1983). These neurons send inhibitory signals to DRG and VRG neurons and project into the phrenic motoneurons of the spinal cord, causing its inhibition (Bianchi and Barillot, 1982; Merrill et al., 1983). The physiologic significance of these connections may be to ensure inspiratory neuronal silence during expiration (reciprocal inhibition) and to contribute to the "inspiratory off-switch" mechanism.

The nucleus ambiguus (NA) and nucleus para-ambigualis (NPA), lying side by side, occupy the middle portion of the VRG. Axons of the respiratory motoneurons originating from the NA project along with other vagal efferent fibers and innervate the laryngeal abductor (inspiratory) and adductor (expiratory) muscles via the recurrent laryngeal nerve (Barillot and Bianchi, 1971; Bastel and Lines, 1975). The NPA contains mainly inspiratory (Iγ) neurons, which respond to lung inflation in a manner similar to that of Iα neurons. The axons of these neurons project both to phrenic and external (inspiratory) intercostal motoneuron pools in the spinal cord. The nucleus retroambigualis (NRA) occupies the caudal part of the VRG and contains expiratory neurons whose axons project into the spinal motoneuron pools for the internal (expiratory) intercostal and abdominal muscles (Merrill, 1970; Miller et al., 1985).

The inspiratory neurons of the DRG send collateral fibers to the inspiratory neurons of the NPA in the VRG. These connections may provide the means for ipsilateral synchronization of the inspiratory activity between the neurons in the DRG and those in the VRG (Merrill, 1979, 1983). Furthermore, axon collaterals of the inspiratory neurons of the NPA on one side project to the inspiratory neurons of the contralateral NPA, and vice versa. These connections may be responsible for the bilateral synchronization of the medullary inspiratory motoneuron output, as evidenced by synchronous bilateral phrenic nerve activity (Merrill, 1979, 1983).

Pontine Respiratory Group of Neurons

In the dorsolateral portion of the rostral pons, both inspiratory and expiratory neurons have been found. Inspiratory neuronal activity is concentrated ventrolaterally in the region of the nucleus parabrachialis lateralis (NPBL). The expiratory activity is centered more medially in the vicinity of the nucleus parabrachialis medialis (NPBM) (Cohen, 1979; Mitchell and Berger, 1981) (see Fig. 2–5). The respiratory neurons of these nuclei are referred to as the pontine respiratory group (PRG) (Feldman, 1986), which was, and sometimes still is, called the pneumotaxic center, although the term is generally considered obsolete. There are reciprocal projections between the PRG neurons and the DRG and VRG neurons in the medulla. Electrical stimulation of the PRG produces rapid breathing with premature switching of respiratory phases (Cohen, 1971), whereas transaction of the brainstem at a level caudal to the PRG prolongs inspiratory time (Feldman and Gautier, 1976). Bilateral cervical vagotomies produce a similar pattern of slow breathing with prolonged inspiratory time; a combination of PRG lesions and bilateral vagotomy in the cat results in apneusis (apnea with sustained inspiration) or apneustic breathing (slow rhythmic respiration with marked increase end-inspiratory hold) (Feldman, 1986; Feldman and Gaultier, 1976). The PRG probably plays a secondary role in modifying the inspiratory off-switch mechanism (Gautier and Bertrand, 1975; von Euler and Trippenbach, 1975).

Respiratory Rhythm Generation

Rhythmic breathing in mammals can occur in the absence of feedback from peripheral receptors. Because transection of the brain rostral to the pons or high spinal transection has little effect on the respiratory pattern, respiratory rhythmogenesis apparently takes place in the brainstem. The PRG, DRG, and VRG have all been considered as possible sites of the central pattern generator, although its exact location is still unknown (Cohen, 1981b; von Euler, 1983, 1986). A study with an in vitro brainstem preparation of neonatal rats has indicated that respiratory rhythm is generated in the small area in the ventrolateral medulla just rostral to the Bötzinger complex (pre-Bötzinger complex), which contains pacemaker neurons (Smith et al., 1991).

The current consensus is that the pre-Bötzinger complex contains a group of neurons that is responsible for respiratory rhythmogenesis (Smith et al., 1991; Pierrefiche et al., 1998; Rekling and Feldman, 1998). Although the specific cellular mechanism responsible for rhythmogenesis is not known, two possible mechanisms have been proposed (Funk and Feldman, 1995; Ramirez and Richter, 1996). One hypothesis is that the pacemaker neurons possess intrinsic properties associated with various voltage- and time-dependent ion channels that are responsible for rhythm generation. Rhythmic activity in these neurons may depend on the presence of an input system that may be necessary to maintain the neuron's membrane potential in a range in which the voltage-dependent properties of the cell's ion channels result in rhythmic behavior. The network hypothesis is the alternative model in which the interaction between the neurons produces respiratory rhythmicity, such as reciprocal inhibition between inhibitory and excitatory neurons and recurrent excitation within any population of neurons (Berger, 2000). The output of this central pattern generator is influenced by various inputs from chemoreceptors (central and peripheral), mechanoreceptors (pulmonary receptors, muscle and joint receptors), thermoreceptors (central and peripheral), nociceptors, and higher central structures (such as the PRG). The function of these inputs is to modify the breathing pattern to meet and adjust to ever-changing metabolic and behavioral needs (Smith et al., 1991).

Airway and Pulmonary Receptors

The upper airways, trachea and bronchi, lungs, and chest wall have a number of sensory receptors sensitive to mechanical and chemical stimulation. These receptors affect ventilation as well as circulatory and other nonrespiratory functions.

Upper Airway Receptors

Stimulation of receptors in the nose can produce sneezing, apnea, changes in bronchomotor tone, and the diving reflex, which involves both the respiratory and the cardiovascular systems. Stimulation of the epipharynx causes the sniffing reflex, a short, strong inspiration to bring material (mucus, foreign body) in the epipharynx into the pharynx to be swallowed or expelled. The major role of receptors in the pharynx is associated with swallowing. It involves the inhibition of breathing, closure of the larynx, and coordinated contractions of pharyngeal muscles (Widdicombe, 1985; Nishino, 1993; Sant'Ambrogio et al., 1995).

The larynx has a rich innervation of receptors. The activation of these receptors can cause apnea, coughing, and changes in the ventilatory pattern (Widdicombe, 1981, 1985). These reflexes, which influence both the patency of the upper airway and the breathing pattern, are related to transmural pressure and/or airflow. Based on single-fiber action potential recordings from the superior laryngeal nerve in the spontaneously breathing dog preparation in which the upper airway is isolated from the lower airways, three types of receptors have been identified: pressure receptors (most common, about 65%), "drive" (or irritant) receptors (stimulated by upper airway muscle activities), and flow or cold receptors (Sant'Ambrogio et al., 1983; Fisher et al., 1985). The laryngeal flow receptors show inspiratory modulation with room air breathing but become silent when inspired air temperature is raised to body temperature and 100% humidity or saturation (Sant'Ambrogio et al., 1985). The activity of pressure receptors increases markedly with upper airway obstruction (Sant'Ambrogio et al., 1983).

Tracheobronchial and Pulmonary Receptors

Three major types of tracheobronchial and pulmonary receptors have been recognized: slowly adapting (pulmonary stretch) receptors, rapidly adapting (irritant or deflation) receptors, both of which lead to myelinated vagal afferent fibers, and unmyelinated C-fiber endings (J-receptors). Excellent reviews on pulmonary receptors have been published (Pack, 1981; Widdicombe, 1981; Sant'Ambrogio, 1982; Coleridge and Coleridge, 1984).

Slowly Adapting (Pulmonary Stretch) Receptors. Slowly adapting (pulmonary stretch) receptors (SARs) are mechanoreceptors that lie within the submucosal smooth muscles in the membranous posterior wall of the trachea and central airways (Bartlett et al., 1976). A small proportion of the receptors are located in the extrathoracic upper trachea (Berger, 2000). SARs are activated by the distension of the airways during lung inflation and inhibit inspiratory activity (Hering-Breuer inflation reflex), whereas they show little response to steady levels of lung inflation. The Hering-Breuer reflex also produces dilation of the upper airways from the larynx to the bronchi. Although SARs are predominantly mechanoreceptors, hypocapnia stimulates their discharge, and hypercapnia inhibits it (Pack, 1981). In addition, SARs are thought to be responsible for the accelerated heart rate and systemic vasoconstriction observed with moderate lung inflation (Widdicombe, 1974). These effects are abolished by bilateral vagotomy.

Studies by Clark and von Euler (1972) have demonstrated the importance of the inflation reflex in adjusting the pattern of ventilation in the cat and the human. In cats anesthetized with pentobarbital, inspiratory time decreases as tidal volume increases with hypercapnia, indicating the presence of the inflation reflex in the normal tidal volume range. Clark and von Euler demonstrated an inverse hyperbolic relationship between the tidal volume and inspiratory time. In the adult human, inspiratory time is independent of tidal volume until the latter increases to about twice the normal tidal volume, when the inflation reflex appears (Fig. 2–6). In the newborn, particularly the premature newborn, the inflation reflex is present in the eupneic range for a few months (Olinsky et al., 1974).

Apnea, frequently observed in adult patients at the end of surgery and anesthesia with the endotracheal tube cuff still inflated, may be related to the inflation reflex, since the trachea has a high concentration of stretch receptors (Bartlett et al., 1976; Sant'Ambrogio, 1982). Deflation of the cuff promptly restores rhythmic spontaneous ventilation.

Rapidly Adapting (Irritant) Receptors. Rapidly adapting (irritant) receptors (RARs) are located superficially within the airway epithelial cells, mostly in the region of the carina and the large bronchi (Pack, 1981; Sant'Ambrogio, 1982). RARs respond to both mechanical and chemical stimuli. In contrast to SARs, RARs adapt rapidly to large lung inflation, distortion, or deflation, thus possessing marked dynamic sensitivity (Pack, 1981). RARs are stimulated by cigarette smoke, ammonia, and other irritant gases including inhaled anesthetics, with significant interindividual variability (Sampson and Vidruk, 1975). RARs are stimulated more consistently by histamine (Vidruk et al., 1977) and prostaglandins (Coleridge et al., 1976; Sampson and Vidruk, 1977), suggesting their role in response to

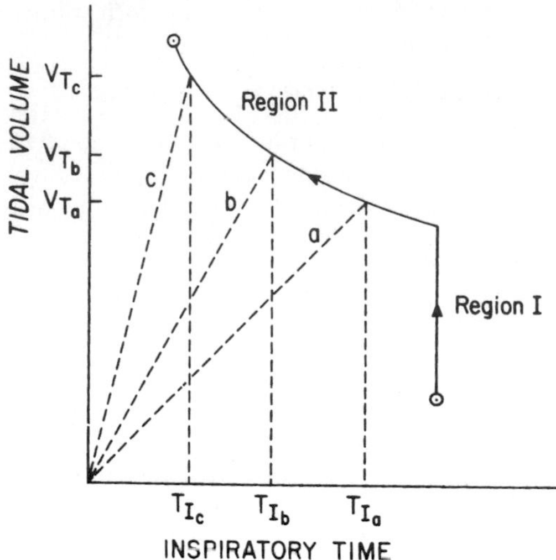

■ **FIGURE 2–6.** Relationship between tidal volume (VT) and inspiratory time (TI) as ventilation is increased in response to respiratory stimuli. Note that in region I, VT increases without changes in TI. Also shown as dashed lines are the VT trajectories for three different tidal volumes in region II. (From Berger AJ: Control of breathing. In Murray JF, Nadel JA: *Textbook of respiratory medicine.* Philadelphia, 1994, WB Saunders.)

pathologic states (Berger, 2000). The activation of RARs in the large airways may be responsible for various reflexes, including coughing, bronchoconstriction, and mucus secretion. Stimulation of RARs in the periphery of the lungs may produce hyperpnea. Because RARs are stimulated by deflation of the lungs to produce hyperpnea in animals, they are considered to play an important role in the Hering-Breuer deflation reflex (Sellick and Widdicombe, 1970). This reflex, if it exists in humans, may partly account for increased respiratory drive when the lung volume is abnormally decreased, as in premature infants with IRDS and in pneumothorax.

When vagal conduction is partially blocked by cold, inflation of the lung produces prolonged contraction of the diaphragm and deep inspiration instead of inspiratory inhibition. This reflex, the paradoxical reflex of Head, is most likely mediated by RARs. It may be related to the complementary cycle of respiration, or the sigh mechanism, that functions to reinflate and reaerate parts of the lungs that have collapsed because of increased surface force during quiet, shallow breathing (Mead and Collier, 1959). In the newborn, inflation of the lungs initiates gasping. This mechanism, which was considered to be analogous to the paradoxical reflex, may help to inflate unaerated portions of the newborn lung (Cross et al., 1960).

C-Fiber Endings. Most afferent axons arising from the lungs, heart, and other abdominal viscera are slow conducting (<2.5 m/sec), unmyelinated vagal fibers (C-fibers). Extensive studies by Paintal (1973) have suggested the presence of receptors supposedly located near the pulmonary or capillary wall (juxtapulmonary capillary or J-receptors) innervated by such C-fibers. C-fiber endings are stimulated by pulmonary congestion, pulmonary edema, pulmonary microemboli, and irritant gases such as anesthetics. Such stimulation causes apnea followed by rapid, shallow breathing, hypotension, and bradycardia. Stimulation of J-receptors also produces bronchoconstriction and increases mucus secretion. All these responses are abolished by bilateral vagotomy. In addition, stimulation of C-fiber endings can provoke severe reflex contraction of the laryngeal muscles, which may be partly responsible for the laryngospasm observed during induction of anesthesia with isoflurane or halothane.

In addition to receptors within the lung parenchyma (pulmonary C-fiber endings), there appear to be similar nonmyelinated nerve endings in the bronchial wall (bronchial C-fiber endings) (Coleridge and Coleridge, 1984). Both chemical and, to a lesser degree, mechanical stimuli excite these bronchial C-fiber endings. They are also stimulated by endogenous mediators of inflammation, including histamine, prostaglandins, serotonin, and bradykinin. Such stimulation may be a mechanism of C-fiber involvement in disease states such as pulmonary edema, pulmonary embolism, and asthma (Coleridge and Coleridge, 1984).

The inhalation of irritant gases or particles causes a sensation of tightness or distress in the chest, probably by activating pulmonary receptors. The pulmonary receptors may contribute to the sensation of dyspnea in lung congestion, atelectasis, and pulmonary edema. Bilateral vagal blockade in patients with lung disease abolished dyspneic sensation and increased breath-holding time (Noble et al., 1970).

Chest Wall Receptors

The chest wall muscles, including the diaphragm and the intercostal muscles, contain various types of receptors that can produce respiratory reflexes. This subject has been reviewed extensively (Newsom-Davis, 1974; Duron, 1981). The two types of receptors that have been most extensively studied are muscle spindles, which lie parallel to the extrafusal muscle fibers, and the Golgi tendon organs, which lie in series with the muscle fibers (Berger, 2000).

Muscle spindles are a type of slowly adapting mechanoreceptors that detect muscle stretch. As in other skeletal muscles, the muscle spindles of respiratory muscles are innervated by γ-motoneurons that excite intrafusal fibers of the spindle.

Intercostal muscles have a density of muscle spindles comparable to that of other skeletal muscles. The arrangement of muscle spindles is appropriate for the respiratory muscle load-compensation mechanism (Berger, 2000). By comparison with the intercostal muscles, the diaphragm has a very low density of muscle spindles and is poorly innervated by the γ-motoneurons. Reflex excitation of the diaphragm, however, can be achieved via proprioceptive excitation within the intercostal system (Decima and von Euler, 1969).

Golgi tendon organs are located at the point of insertion of the muscle fiber into its tendon and, like muscle spindles, are a slowly adapting mechanoreceptor. Activation of the Golgi tendon organs inhibits the homonymous motoneurons, possibly preventing the muscle from being overloaded (Berger, 2000). In the intercostal muscles, fewer Golgi tendon organs are present than muscle spindles, whereas the ratio is reversed in the diaphragm.

■ CHEMICAL CONTROL OF BREATHING

Regulation of alveolar ventilation and maintenance of normal arterial P_{CO_2}, pH, and P_{O_2} are the principal functions of the medullary and peripheral chemoreceptors (Leusen, 1972).

Central Chemoreceptors

The medullary, or central, chemoreceptors, located near the surface of the ventrolateral medulla, are anatomically separated from the medullary respiratory center (Fig. 2–7). They respond to changes in hydrogen ion concentration in the adjacent cerebrospinal fluid rather than to changes in arterial P_{CO_2} or pH

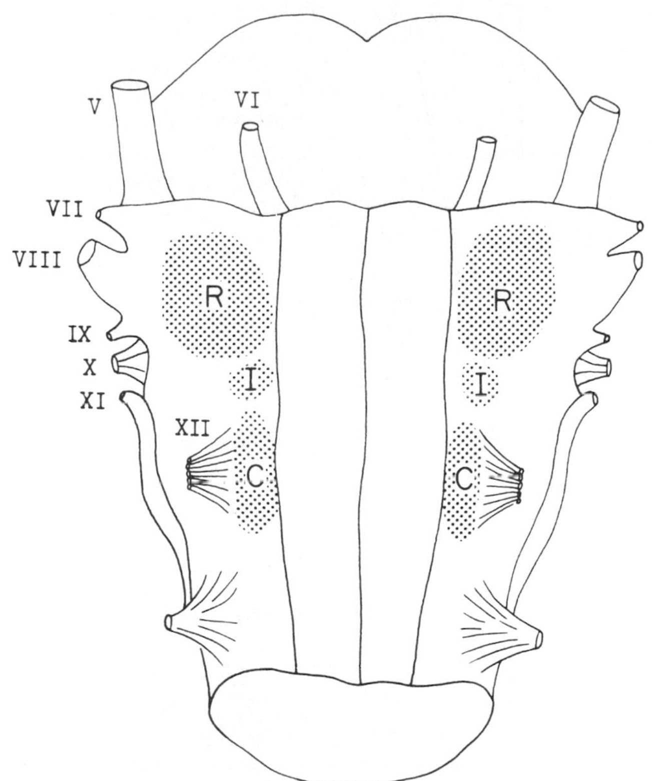

■ **FIGURE 2–7.** View of the ventral surface of the medulla shows the chemosensitive zones. The rostral (R) and caudal (C) zones are chemosensitive. The intermediate (I) zone is not chemosensitive but may have a function in the overall central chemosensory response. The roman numerals indicate the cranial nerves. (Reproduced with permission from Berger AJ, Hornbein TF: Control of respiration. In Patton HD, Fuchs AF, Hille B, et al., editors: *Textbook of physiology*, ed 21. Philadelphia, 1989, WB Saunders, pp 1026–1045.)

(Pappenheimer et al., 1965). Since carbon dioxide rapidly passes through the blood-brain barrier into the cerebrospinal fluid, which has poor buffering capacity, the medullary chemoreceptors are readily stimulated by respiratory acidemia. In contrast, ventilatory responses of the medullary chemoreceptors to acute metabolic acidemia and alkalemia are limited because changes in the hydrogen ion concentration in arterial blood are not rapidly transmitted to the cerebrospinal fluid. In chronic acid-base disturbances, the pH of cerebrospinal fluid (and presumably that of interstitial fluid) surrounding the medullary chemoreceptors is generally maintained close to the normal value of about 7.3 regardless of arterial pH (Mitchell et al., 1965). Under these circumstances, ventilation becomes more dependent on the hypoxic response of peripheral chemoreceptors.

Peripheral Chemoreceptors

Peripheral chemoreceptors, particularly the carotid bodies, located near the bifurcation of the common carotid artery, react rapidly to changes in PaO_2 and pH. Their contribution to the respiratory drive amounts to about 15% of resting ventilation (Severinghaus, 1972). The carotid body has three types of neural components: type I (glomus) cells, presumably the primary site of chemotransduction; type II (sheath) cells; and sensory nerve fibers (McDonald, 1981). Sensory nerve fibers originate from terminals in apposition to the glomus cells, travel via the carotid sinus nerve to join the glossopharyngeal nerve, and then enter the brainstem. The sheath cells envelop both the glomus cells and the sensory nerve terminals. A variety of neurochemicals have been found in the carotid body, including acetylcholine, dopamine, substance P, enkephalins, and vasoactive intestinal peptide. The exact functions of these cell types and the mechanisms of chemotransduction and the specific roles of these neurochemicals have not been well established (Berger, 2000).

The carotid bodies are perfused with extremely high levels of blood flow and respond rapidly to an oscillating PaO_2 rather than a constant PaO_2 at the same mean values (Dutton et al., 1964; Fenner et al., 1968). This mechanism may be partly responsible for hyperventilation during exercise.

The primary role of peripheral chemoreceptors is their response to changes in arterial PO_2. Moderate to severe hypoxemia (PaO_2 <60 mm Hg) results in a significant increase in ventilation in all age groups (Dripps and Comroe, 1947) except for newborn, particularly premature, infants, whose ventilation is decreased by hypoxemia (Rigatto et al., 1975). Peripheral chemoreceptors are also partly responsible for hyperventilation in hypotensive patients. Respiratory stimulation is absent in certain states of tissue hypoxia, such as moderate to severe anemia and carbon monoxide poisoning; despite a decrease in oxygen content, PaO_2 in the carotid bodies is maintained near normal levels, so that the chemoreceptors are not stimulated.

In acute hypoxemia, the ventilatory response via the peripheral chemoreceptors is partially opposed by hypocapnia, which depresses the medullary chemoreceptors. When a hypoxemic environment persists for a few days, for example, during an ascent to high altitude, ventilation increases further as cerebrospinal fluid bicarbonate decreases and pH returns toward normal (Severinghaus et al., 1963). However, later studies demonstrated that the return of cerebrospinal fluid pH toward normal is incomplete, and a secondary increase in ventilation precedes the decrease in pH, indicating that some other mechanisms are involved (Bureau and Bouverot, 1975; Foster et al., 1975). In chronic hypoxemia lasting for a number of years, the carotid bodies initially exhibit some adaptation to hypoxemia and then gradually lose their hypoxic response. In high altitude natives, the blunted response of carotid chemoreceptors to hypoxemia takes 10 to 15 years to develop and is sustained thereafter (Sorensen and Severinghaus, 1968; Lahiri et al., 1978). In cyanotic heart diseases, the hypoxic response is lost much sooner but returns after surgical correction of the right-to-left shunts (Edelman et al., 1970).

In patients who have chronic respiratory insufficiency with hypercapnia, hypoxemic stimulation of the peripheral chemoreceptors provides the primary impulse to the respiratory center. If these patients are given excessive levels of oxygen, the stimulus of hypoxemia is removed, and ventilation decreases or ceases. PCO_2 further increases, patients become comatose (carbon dioxide narcosis), and death may follow unless ventilation is supported. Rather than oxygen therapy, such patients need their effective ventilation increased artificially with or without added inspired oxygen.

Response to Carbon Dioxide

The graphic demonstration of relations between the alveolar or arterial PCO_2 and the minute ventilation ($\dot{V}E/PCO_2$) is commonly known as the CO_2 response curve (Fig. 2–8). This curve normally reflects the response of the chemoreceptors and respiratory center to carbon dioxide. The CO_2 response curve is a useful means for evaluation of the chemical control of breathing, provided that the mechanical properties of the respiratory system, including the neuromuscular transmission, respiratory muscles, thorax, and

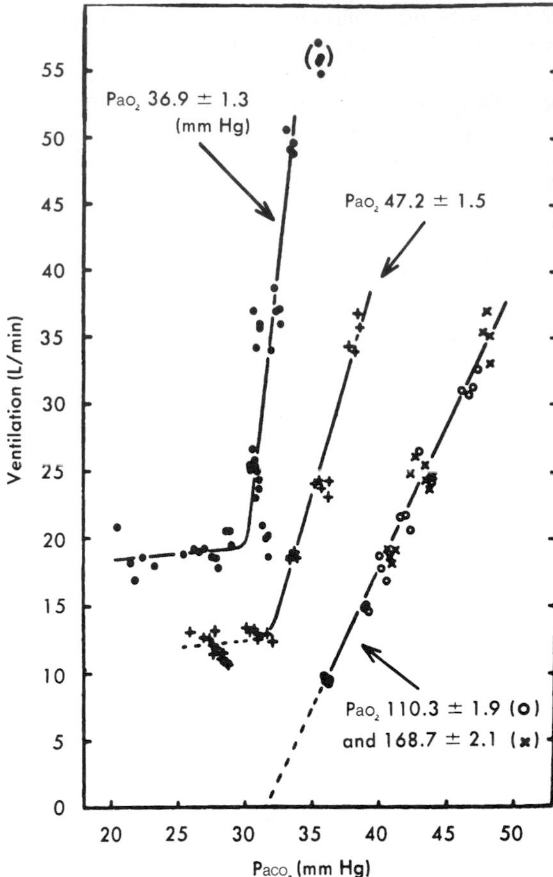

■ **FIGURE 2–8.** Effect of acute hypoxemia on the ventilatory response to steady-state PaO_2 in one subject. Inspired oxygen was adjusted in each experiment to keep PaO_2 constant at the level as indicated. (From Nielsen M, Smith H: *Acta Physiol Scand* 24:293, 1951.)

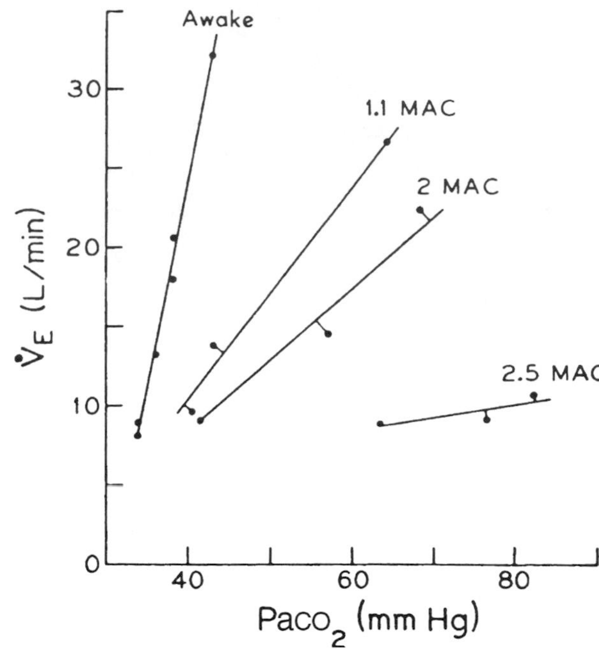

■ **FIGURE 2–9.** CO_2 response curve with halothane. Family of steady-state CO_2 response curves in one subject awake and at three levels of halothane anesthesia. Note progressive decrease in ventilatory response to PaO_2 with increasing anesthetic depth (MAC) (ventilatory response in awake state was measured in response to end-tidal PCO_2). (Courtesy Dr. Edwin S. Munson; data based on Munson ES, Larson CP Jr, Babad AA, et al.: *Anesthesiology* 27:716, 1966.)

lungs, are intact. In normal persons, ventilation increases more or less linearly as the inspired concentration of carbon dioxide increases up to 9% to 10%, above which ventilation starts to decrease (Dripps and Comroe, 1947). Under hypoxemic conditions the CO_2 response is potentiated, primarily via carotid body stimulation, resulting in a shift to the left of the CO_2 response curve (Nielsen and Smith, 1951) (see Fig. 2–8). On the other hand, anesthetics, opioids, and barbiturates in general depress the medullary chemoreceptors and, by decreasing the slope, shift the CO_2 response curve progressively to the right as the anesthetic concentration increases (Munson et al., 1966) (Fig. 2–9).

A shift to the right of the CO_2 response curve in an awake human may be caused by decreased chemoreceptor sensitivity to carbon dioxide, as seen in patients whose carotid bodies had been destroyed (Wade et al., 1970). It may also be caused by lung disease and resultant mechanical failure to increase ventilation despite intact neuronal response to carbon dioxide. In patients with various central nervous system dysfunctions, the CO_2 response may be partially or completely lost (Ondine's curse) (Severinghaus and Mitchell, 1962). In the awake state, these patients have chronic hypoventilation but can breathe on command. During sleep, they further hypoventilate or become apneic to the point of carbon dioxide narcosis and death unless mechanically ventilated or implanted with a phrenic pacemaker (Glenn et al., 1973).

It has been difficult to separate the neuronal component from the mechanical failure of the lungs and thorax, because the two factors often coexist in patients with chronic lung diseases (Guz et al., 1970). Whitelaw and others (1975) demonstrated that occlusion pressure at 0.1 second ($P_{0.1}$, or the negative mouth pressure generated by inspiratory effort against airway occlusion at FRC) correlates well with neuronal (phrenic) discharges but is uninfluenced by mechanical properties of the lungs and thorax. The occlusion pressure is a useful means for the clinical evaluation of the ventilatory drive.

As mentioned previously, hypoxemia potentiates the chemical drive and increases the slope of the CO_2 response curve ($\dot{V}E/PCO_2$). Such a change has been interpreted as "a synergistic (or multiplicative) effect" of the stimulus, whereas a parallel shift of the curve has been considered as "an additive effect." This analysis may be useful for descriptive purposes, but it is misleading. Because ventilation is the product of tidal volume and frequency ($\dot{V}E = VT \times f$), an additive effect on its components could result in a change in the slope of the CO_2 response curve. Obviously the response to carbon dioxide of tidal volume and frequency should be examined separately to understand the effect of various respiratory stimulants and depressants.

Milic-Emili and Grunstein (1975) proposed that ventilatory response to carbon dioxide be analyzed in terms of the mean inspiratory flow (VT/TI, where VT is tidal volume and TI is the inspiratory time) and in terms of the ratio of inspiratory time to total ventilatory cycle duration or respiratory duty cycle (TI/TTOT) (Fig. 2–10). Because the tidal volume is equal to VT/TI × TI and respiratory frequency *f* is 1/TTOT, ventilation can be expressed as follows:

$$\dot{V}E = VT \times f = VT/TI \times TI/TTOT$$

The advantage of analyzing the ventilatory response in this fashion is that VT/TI, is an index of inspiratory drive, which is independent of the timing element. The tidal volume, on the other hand, is time dependent, because it is (VT/TI) × TI. The second

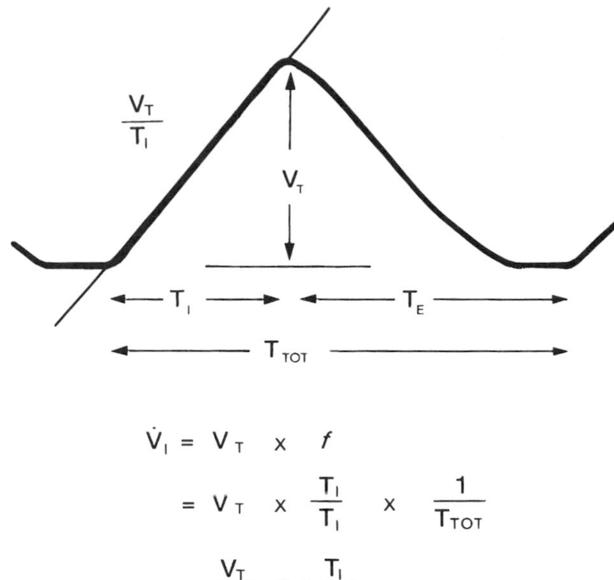

$$\dot{V}_I = V_T \times f$$

$$= V_T \times \frac{T_I}{T_I} \times \frac{1}{T_{TOT}}$$

$$= \frac{V_T}{T_I} \times \frac{T_I}{T_{TOT}}$$

■ **FIGURE 2–10.** Schematic drawing of tidal volume and timing components on time-volume axes. VT, Tidal volume; TI, inspiratory time; TE, expiratory time; TTOT, total time for respiratory cycle; *f*, respiratory frequency; VT/TI, mean inspiratory flow rate; TI/TTOT, respiratory duty cycle (see text).

parameter, TI/TTOT, is a dimensionless index of effective respiratory timing (respiratory duty cycle) that is determined by the vagal afferent or central inspiratory off-switch mechanism or by both (Bradley et al., 1975). From this equation, it is apparent that in respiratory disease or under anesthesia, changes in pulmonary ventilation may result from a change in VT/TI, TI/TTOT, or both. A reduction in TI/TTOT indicates that the relative duration of inspiration decreased or that expiration increased. Such a reduction in the TI/TTOT ratio may result from changes in central or peripheral mechanisms. In contrast, a reduction in VT/TI may indicate a decrease in the medullary inspiratory drive or neuromuscular transmission or an increase in inspiratory impedance (i.e., increased flow resistance, decreased compliance, or both). By relating the mouth occlusion pressure to VT/TI, it becomes clinically possible to determine whether changes in the mechanics of the respiratory system contribute to the reduction in VT/TI (Milic-Emili, 1977).

Analysis of inspiratory and expiratory durations provides useful information on the mechanism of anesthetic effects on ventilation. Figure 2–11 illustrates the effect of pentobarbital, which depresses minute ventilation, and diethyl ether, which "stimulates" ventilation in newborn rabbits. With both anesthetics the mean inspiratory flow (VT/TI) did not change, but VT decreased because TI was shortened. With pentobarbital, however, TE was prolonged disproportionately, and TI/TTOT and frequency decreased; consequently, minute ventilation was decreased. With ether, on the other hand, ventilation increased as the result of disproportionate decrease in TE and consequent increases in TI/TTOT and frequency (Milic-Emili, 1977).

CONTROL OF BREATHING IN NEONATES AND INFANTS

Response to Hypoxemia in Infants

During the first 2 to 3 weeks of age, both full-term and premature infants in a warm environment respond to hypoxemia (15% oxygen) with a transient increase in ventilation followed by sustained ventilatory depression (Brady and Ceruti, 1966; Rigatto and Brady, 1972a, 1972b; Rigatto et al., 1975a) (Fig. 2–12). In infants born at 32 to 37 weeks gestation, the initial period of transient hyperpnea is abolished in a cool environment, indicating the importance of maintaining a neutral thermal environment (Cross and Oppe, 1952; Ceruti, 1966; Perlstein et al., 1970). When 100% oxygen is given, a transient decrease in ventilation is followed by sustained hyperventilation. This ventilatory response to oxygen is similar to that of the fetus and is different from that of the adult, in whom a sustained decrease in ventilation is followed by little or no increase in ventilation (Dripps and Comroe, 1947). By 3 weeks after birth, hypoxemia induces sustained hyperventilation, as in older children and adults.

The biphasic depression in ventilation has been attributed to central depression rather than to depression of peripheral chemoreceptors (Albersheim et al., 1976). In newborn monkeys, however, tracheal occlusion pressure, an index of central neural drive, and diaphragmatic electromyographic output were increased above the control level during both the hyperpneic and the hypopneic phases in response to hypoxic gas mixture (LaFramboise et al., 1981; LaFramboise and Woodrum, 1985). These findings imply that the biphasic ventilatory response to hypoxemia results from changes in the mechanics of the respiratory system (thoracic stiffness or airway obstruction), rather than from neuronal depression, as has been assumed (Jansen and Chernick, 1983). Premature infants continue to show a biphasic response to hypoxemia even at 25 days after birth (Rigatto, 1986). Thus, in terms of a proper response to hypoxemic challenge, maturation of the respiratory system may be related to postconceptional rather than postnatal age.

Response to Carbon Dioxide in Infants

Newborn infants respond to hypercapnia by increasing ventilation but less so than do older infants. The slope of the CO_2 response curve increases appreciably with gestational age as well as with postnatal age, independent of postconceptional age (Rigatto et al., 1975a, 1975b, 1982; Frantz et al., 1976). This increase in slope

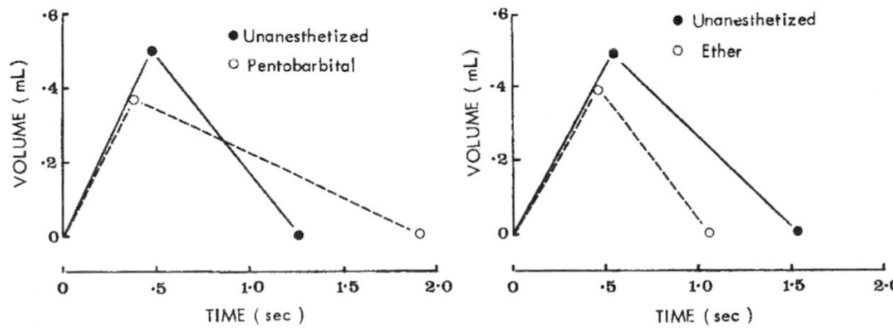

■ **FIGURE 2–11.** Schematic summary of changes in the average respiratory cycle in a group of newborn rabbits before and after sodium pentobarbital anesthesia *(left)* and before and during ether anesthesia *(right)*. Measurements obtained during spontaneous room air breathing. Zero on the time axis indicates onset of inspiration. Mean inspiratory flow is represented by the slope of the ascending limb of the spirograms.

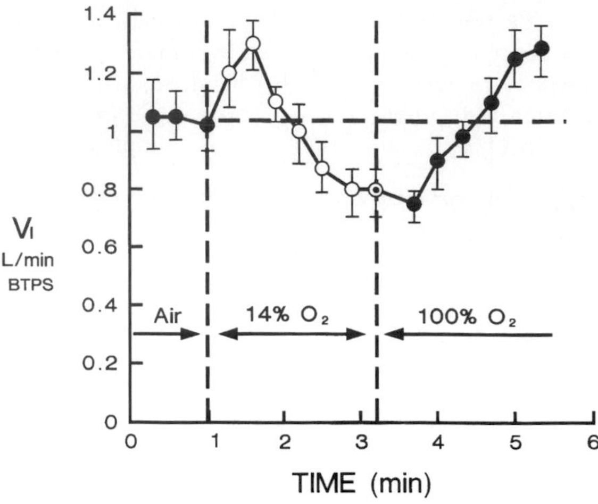

■ **FIGURE 2–12.** Effect on ventilation of 14% oxygen (hypoxia) from room air and then to 100% oxygen (hyperoxia) in three newborn infants. Ventilation (mean ± SEM) is plotted against time. During acute hypoxia there was a transient increase in ventilation followed by depression. Hyperoxia increased ventilation. (Modified from Lahiri S, Brody JS, Motoyama EK, Valasquez TM: Regulation of breathing in newborns. *J Appl Physiol* 44:673, 1978. Used with permission of the American Physiological Society.)

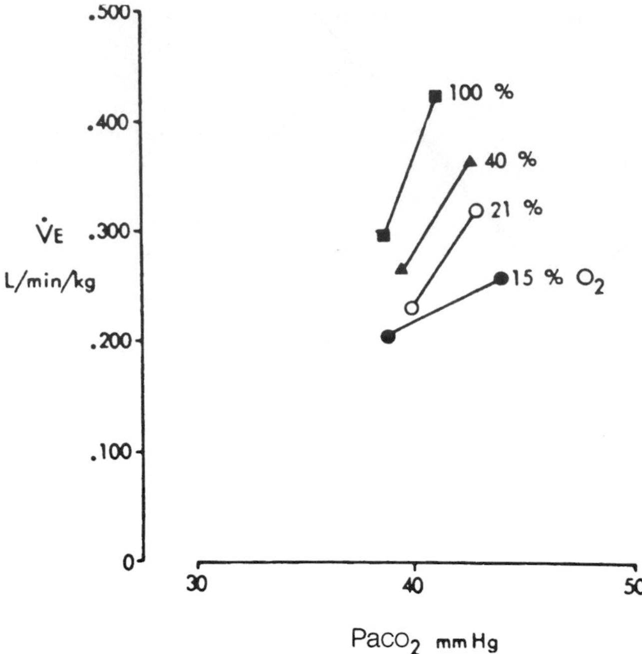

■ **FIGURE 2–13.** Mean steady-state CO_2 response curves at different inspired oxygen concentrations in eight preterm infants. The slope of the CO_2 response decreases with decreasing oxygen. (From Rigatto H, de la Torre Verduzco R, Cates DB: Effects of O_2 on the ventilatory response. *J Appl Physiol* 39:896, 1975. Used with permission of the American Physiological Society.)

may represent an increase in chemosensitivity, but it may also result from more effective mechanics of the respiratory system. In adults the CO_2 response curve both increases in slope and shifts to the left with the severity of hypoxemia (see Fig. 2–8). In contrast, in newborn infants breathing 15% oxygen, the CO_2 response curve decreases in slope and shifts to the right (Fig. 2–13). Inversely, hyperoxemia increases the slope and shifts the curve to the left (Rigatto et al., 1975).

Upper Airway Receptor Responses in the Neonatal Period

Newborn animals are particularly sensitive to the stimulation of the superior laryngeal nerve either directly or through the receptors (such as water in the larynx), which results in ventilatory depression or apnea. In anesthetized newborn puppies and kittens, negative pressure or airflow through the larynx isolated from the lower airways produced apnea or significant prolongation of inspiratory and expiratory time and a decrease in tidal volume, whereas similar stimulation caused little or no effect in 4- to 5-week-old puppies or in adult dogs and cats (Al-Shway and Mortola, 1982; Fisher et al., 1985).

In a similar preparation using puppies anesthetized with pentobarbital, water in the laryngeal lumen produced apnea, whereas phosphate buffer with sodium chloride and neutral pH did not. The principal stimulus for the apneic reflex was the absence or reduced concentrations of chloride ion (Boggs and Bartlett, 1982). In awake newborn piglets, direct electrical stimulation of the superior laryngeal nerve caused periodic breathing and apnea associated with marked decreases in respiratory frequency, hypoxemia, and hypercapnia with minimal cardiovascular effects. Breathing during superior laryngeal nerve stimulation was sustained by an arousal system (Donnelly and Haddad, 1986). The strong inhibitory responses elicited in newborn animals by various upper airway receptor stimulations have been attributed to the immaturity of the central nervous system (Lucier et al., 1979; Boggs and Bartlett, 1982).

Active (REM) Versus Quiet (Non-REM) Sleep

During the early postnatal period, full-term infants spend 50% of their sleep time in active or REM sleep compared with 20% REM sleep in adults (Stern et al., 1969; Rigatto et al., 1982). Wakefulness rarely occurs in neonates. Premature neonates stay in REM sleep most of the time, and quiet (non-REM) sleep is difficult to define before 32 weeks postconception (Rigatto, 1992). Neonates, particularly prematurely born neonates, therefore, breathe irregularly.

Neurologic and chemical control of breathing in infants is related to the state of sleep (Scher et al., 1992). During quiet sleep, breathing is regulated primarily by the medullary respiratory centers and breathing is regular with respect to timing as well as amplitude and is tightly linked to chemoreceptor input (Bryan and Wohl, 1986). During active (REM) sleep, however, breathing is controlled primarily by the behavioral system and is irregular with respect to timing and amplitude (Phillipson, 1984).

Periodic Breathing and Apnea

Periodic Breathing

Periodic breathing, in which breathing is interposed with repetitive short apneic spells lasting 5 to 10 seconds without hemoglobin desaturation or cyanosis, occurs frequently in neonates and young infants during wakefulness, active (REM) sleep, and quiet (non-REM) sleep (Rigatto et al., 1982a). Periodic breathing tends to be more regular in quiet sleep than in active sleep (Kalapezi et al., 1981) and has been observed more frequently during active sleep (Rigatto et al., 1982) or during quiet sleep (Kelly et al., 1985). Minute ventilation increases during REM sleep due to increases in respiratory frequency with little change in tidal volume (Kalapezi et al., 1981; Rigatto et al., 1982).

An addition of 2% to 4% carbon dioxide to the inspired gas mixture abolishes periodic breathing, probably by causing respiratory stimulation (Chernick et al., 1964). Nevertheless, the ventilatory response to hypercapnia seems to be diminished during periodic breathing (Rigatto and Brady, 1972a). The decreased hypercapnic response appears to result from changes in respiratory mechanics rather than from a reduction in chemosensitivity, because respiratory center output as determined by airway occlusion pressure is greater during REM sleep than during non-REM sleep.

The incidence of periodic breathing was reported to be 78% in full-term neonates (Kelly et al., 1985), whereas the incidence was much higher (93%) in preterm infants (mean postconceptional age, 37.5 weeks) (Glotzbach et al., 1989). The frequency of periodic breathing diminishes with increasing postconceptual age and decreases to 29% by 10 to 12 months of age (Fenner et al., 1973; Kelly et al., 1985).

Apnea of Prematurity and Hypoxia

Central apnea of infancy is defined as unexplained cessation of breathing for 15 seconds or longer or a shorter respiratory pause associated with bradycardia (heart rate <100), cyanosis, or pallor (Brooks, 1982). Apnea is common in preterm infants and may be related to an immature respiratory control mechanism (Jansen and Chernick, 1983). Most preterm infants with a birth weight of less than 2 kg have apneic spells at some time (Spitzer and Fox, 1984). Glotzbach and others (1989) reported a 55% incidence of central apnea in preterm infants, whereas it was rarely found in full-term infants (Kelly et al., 1985).

The report by the Collaborative Home Infant Monitoring Evaluation (CHIME) Study Group was based on the recordings of respiratory inductive plethysmography (Respitrace), electrocardiography (ECG), and pulse oximetry in normal infants and those with increased risk of sudden infant death syndrome (SIDS), and it involved a total of 1079 infants during the first 6 months after birth (Hunt et al., 1999; Ramanathan et al., 2001). This report has revealed evidence that the control of breathing and oxygenation during sleep in healthy term infants are not as precise as have been assumed. Normal infants, up to 2% to 3%, commonly have prolonged central, obstructive or mixed apnea lasting up to 30 seconds, which is associated with oxygen desaturation (Ramanathan et al., 2001). With a simple upper respiratory infection, prolonged obstructive sleep apneas were recorded in a few normal full-term infants but were present in 15% to 30% of preterm infants. The risk of having such episodes was 20 to 30 times higher among preterm infants than in full-term infants before 43 weeks postconception (Hunt et al., 1999). Healthy term infants had an average baseline Spo_2 of 98% throughout the recorded period. However, hypoxia (Spo_2 <90%, occasionally in 70%-to-80% range) occurred in 59% of these normal-term infants in 0.6% of recorded epochs (Hunt et al., 1999). Thus, levels of hypoxia previously considered pathologic are relatively common occurrences among normal infants.

Apparent life-threatening events (ALTE) is characterized by an episode of sudden onset characterized by color change (cyanosis or pallor), tone change (limpness or rarely stiffness), and apnea, which requires immediate resuscitation to revive the infant and restore normal breathing (National Institutes of Health Consensus Development Conference, 1987). The incidence of ALTE is as high as 3% and may occur in previously healthy infants. Overnight polysomnography (PSG) is particularly useful in the evaluation of infants with a history of unexplained apnea. Treatable etiology, however, was found only in about 30% of infants and, thus, normal PSG results are not necessarily diagnostic to rule out ALTE.

Postoperative Apnea

Life-threatening apnea has been reported postoperatively in prematurely born infants less than 41 weeks postconception, particularly in those with a history of apneic spells following simple surgical procedures, such as inguinal herniorrhaphy (Liu et al., 1983), and can occur up to 12 hours postoperatively (Steward, 1982). In another report, apnea was reported in 4 of 18 prematurely born infants who were 49 to 55 weeks postconception (Kurth et al., 1987). Malviya and others (1993) analyzed the relationship between the incidence of postoperative apnea and maturation. They reported a high incidence of postoperative apnea (26%) in infants less than 44 weeks postconception, whereas the incidence of apnea in those more than 44 weeks was only 3%.

Subsequently, Coté and others (1995) performed a meta-analysis of the data from previously published studies of postoperative apnea in ex-premature infants following inguinal hernia repairs. They concluded that postoperative apnea was strongly and inversely correlated to both gestational age as well as postconceptual age; was associated with previous history of apnea; and was associated with anemia (hematocrit <30) as a significant risk factor regardless of gestational or postconceptual age (see Chapter 11, Intraoperative and Postoperative Management).

Both theophylline and caffeine have been effective in reducing apneic spells in preterm infants (Aranda et al., 1979). Caffeine is especially useful for prematurely born infants during the postanesthetic period (Welborn et al., 1988). Xanthine derivatives are known to prevent muscle fatigue (Aubier et al., 1981), and their respiratory stimulation in the premature infant may occur via both central and peripheral mechanisms.

MAINTENANCE OF THE UPPER AIRWAY AND AIRWAY PROTECTIVE REFLEXES

Pharyngeal Airway

The pharyngeal airway, unlike the laryngeal airway, is not supported by a rigid bony or cartilaginous structure. Its wall consists of soft tissues and is surrounded by muscles for breathing and for swallowing. The pharyngeal airway is easily obstructed by the relaxation of the velopharynx (soft palate), posterior displacement of the mandible (and the base of the tongue) in the supine position during sleep, flexion of the neck, or external compression over the hyoid bone. The pharyngeal airway also is easily collapsed by negative pressure within the pharyngeal lumen created by inspiratory effort, especially when airway-maintaining muscles are depressed or paralyzed (Issa and Sullivan, 1984; Reed et al., 1985; Roberts et al., 1985). In neonates, with a relatively hypoplastic mandible, the oropharynx and the entrance to the larynx at the level of the aryepiglottic folds are the areas most easily collapsed (Reed et al., 1985).

Mechanical support to sustain the patency of the pharynx against the collapsing force of luminal negative pressure during inspiration is given by both the sustained muscle tension and cyclic contraction of the pharyngeal dilator muscles, acting synchronously with the contraction of the diaphragm. These include the genioglossus, geniohyoid, sternohyoid, sternothyroid, and thyrohyoid muscles (Bartlett et al., 1973; Pack et al., 1988; Thach, 1992) (Fig. 2–14). Similar phasic activities have been recorded in the scalene and sternomastoid muscles in humans (Onal et al., 1981; Drummond, 1987).

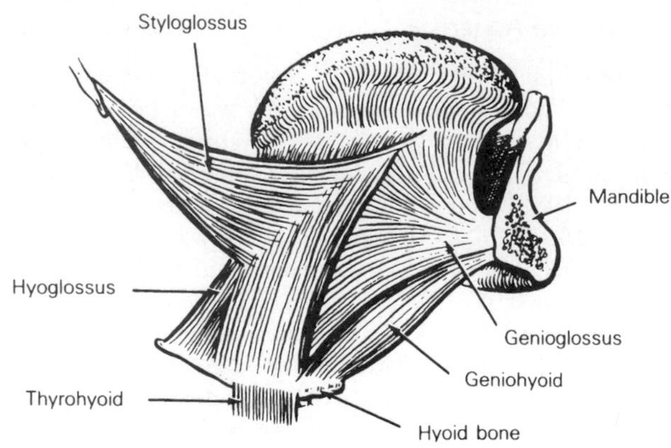

■ **FIGURE 2–14.** Lateral view of the musculature of the tongue and its relationship with a mandible and hyoid bone. (From Kuna ST, Remmers JE: Pathophysiology and mechanisms of sleep apnea. In Fletcher EC, editor: *Abnormalities of respiration during sleep.* Orlando, FL, 1986, Grune & Stratton.)

A model of pharyngeal airway maintenance proposed by Thach (1988) is shown in Figure 2–15. In this model, the suction force created in the pharyngeal lumen by the inspiratory activity of the diaphragm must be well balanced by the activities of upper airway–dilating muscles to maintain upper airway patency. Increased nasal and pharyngeal airway resistance exaggerates the suction force. In addition, once pharyngeal closure occurs, the mucosal adhesion force of the collapsed pharyngeal wall becomes an added force acting against the opening of pharyngeal air passages (Reed et al., 1985).

Several reflex mechanisms are present to maintain the balance between the dilating and collapsing forces in the pharynx. Chemoreceptor stimuli such as hypercapnia and hypoxemia stimulate the airway dilators preferentially over the stimulation of the diaphragm so as to maintain airway patency (Brouillette and Thach, 1980; Onal et al., 1981, 1982). Negative pressure in the nose, pharynx, or larynx activates the pharyngeal dilator muscles and simultaneously decreases the diaphragmatic activity (Mathew et al., 1982a, 1982b; Hwang et al., 1984; Thach, 1992) (Fig. 2–16). Such an airway pressure reflex is especially prominent in infants less than 1 year of age (Thach et al., 1989). Upper airway mechanoreceptors are located superficially in the airway mucosa and are easily blocked by topical anesthesia

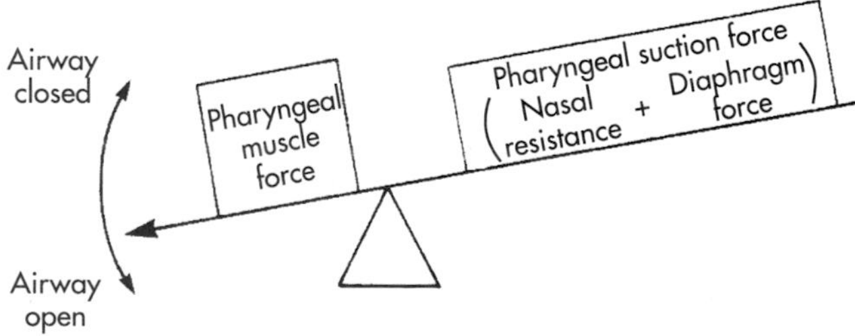

■ **FIGURE 2–15.** A schematic model of pharyngeal airway maintenance illustrating the balance of opposing forces that affect airway diameter. Airway constricting (suction force) and airway dilating forces (pharyngeal muscles) are shown on either side of the fulcrum. The balance of forces is dynamic; for example, a sudden increase in nasal resistance or diaphragm force during the course of an inspiration can result in airway closure in a fraction of a second. Change in neck posture shifts position of the fulcrum and thus can bias the balance toward airway closure or airway patency. (From Thach BT: Potential role of airway obstruction in SIDS. In Krous H, Culbertson H, editors: *Sudden infant death syndrome.* Baltimore, 1988, Johns Hopkins University Press.)

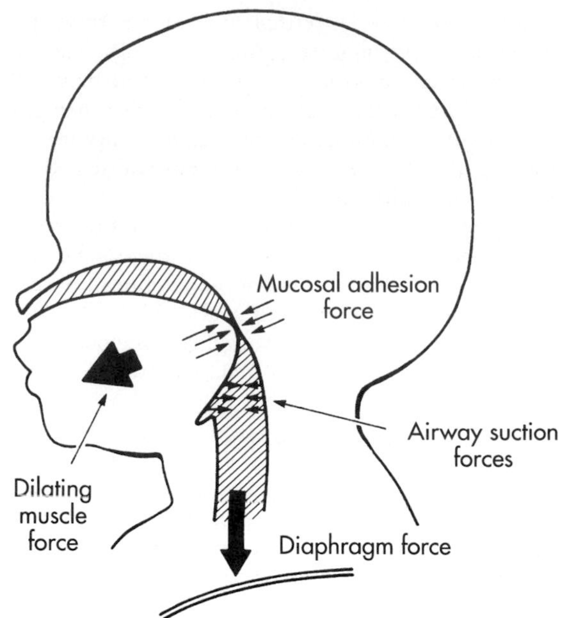

■ **FIGURE 2–16.** Schematic illustration of sequence of events showing one of the ways in which the upper airway pressure reflex operates to preserve pharyngeal airway patency. (From Thach BT: Neuromuscular control of the upper airway. In Beckerman RC, Brouillette RT, Hunt CE, editors: *Respiratory control disorders in infants and children.* Baltimore, 1992, Williams & Wilkins.)

(Mathew et al., 1982a, 1982b). Sleep, sedatives, and anesthesia depress upper airway muscles more than they do the diaphragm (Sauerland and Harper, 1976; Ochiai et al., 1989, 1992). The arousal from sleep shifts the balance toward pharyngeal dilation (Thach, 1992).

Laryngeal Airway

The larynx is composed of a group of cartilage, connecting ligaments, and muscles. It maintains the airway and functions as a valve to occlude and protect the lower airways from the alimentary tract. It is also an organ for phonation (Proctor, 1977a, 1977b, 1986; Fink and Demarest, 1978).

With the exception of the anterior nasal passages, the larynx at the subglottis is the narrowest portion of the entire airway system in all ages (Eckenhoff, 1951). The cricoid cartilage forms a complete ring, protecting the upper airway from compression. On the other hand, it is vulnerable to stenosis, because mucosal edema from infection can only expand inward, diminishing the lumen. In infants this edema may produce severe obstruction, whereas the same degree of swelling in adults may cause no more than mild discomfort. The mucosa covering the cricoid ring is also a frequent site of trauma and resulting edema from intubation with an oversized endotracheal tube in infants and young children (Koka et al., 1977). Ischemic mucosal edema may cause symptoms of upper airway obstruction (postintubation croup) and, if severe enough, subsequent fibrosis and subglottic stenosis.

The glottis widens slightly during tidal inspiration but narrows during expiration, thus increasing laryngeal airflow resistance (Bartlett et al., 1973). Laryngeal resistance is finely regulated in neonates and young infants to dynamically maintain end-expiratory lung volume (FRC) well above the small volume determined by the opposing elastic recoil forces of the thorax and the lungs, as discussed later (Harding, 1984; England and Stogren, 1986). In infants with IRDS, expiration is often associated with "grunting" caused by narrowing of the glottic aperture. This grunting maintains intrinsic PEEP during the expiratory phase and presumably reduces premature closure of airways and air spaces. In infants with IRDS, when grunting is eliminated by endotracheal intubation, respiratory gas exchange deteriorates unless continuous positive airway pressure (CPAP) is applied (Gregory et al., 1971).

Airway Protective Reflexes

Upper airway protective mechanisms involve both the pharynx and larynx and include sneezing, swallowing, coughing, and pharyngeal or laryngeal closure. Laryngospasm is a sustained tight closure of the vocal cords caused by the stimulation of the superior laryngeal nerve, a branch of the vagus, and contraction of the adductor muscles that persists beyond the removal of the stimulus. In puppies, it is elicited by repetitive stimulation of the superior laryngeal nerve with typical adductor afterdischarge activity. This response is not evoked by the stimulation of the recurrent laryngeal nerve (Suzuki and Sasaki, 1977). Hyperventilation and hypocapnia as well as light anesthesia increase the activity of adductor neurons, reduce the mean threshold of the adductor reflex, or increase upper airway resistance (Suzuki and Sasaki, 1977; Nishino et al., 1981). Hyperthermia and decreased lung volume also facilitate laryngospasm produced by stimulation of the superior laryngeal nerve (Sasaki, 1979; Haraguchi et al., 1983). Contrarily, hypoventilation and hypercapnia, positive intrathoracic pressure, and deep anesthesia depress excitatory adductor afterdischarge activity and increase the threshold of the reflex that precipitates laryngospasm (Suzuki and Sasaki, 1977; Ikari and Sasaki, 1980; Nishino et al., 1981). Hypoxia below an arterial PO_2 of 50 mm Hg also increases the threshold for laryngospasm (Ikari and Sasaki, 1980).

These findings are clinically relevant, suggesting a fail-safe mechanism by which asphyxia (hypoxia and hypercapnia) tends to prevent sustained laryngospasm. In healthy, awake adults, laryngospasm by itself is self-limiting and not a threat to life. On the other hand, in the presence of cardiopulmonary compromise, such as may occur during anesthesia (particularly in infants), laryngospasm may indeed become life threatening (Ikari and Sasaki, 1980). Increased depth of anesthesia increases the reflex threshold and diminishes excitatory adductor afterdischarge in puppies (Suzuki and Sasaki, 1977). This finding is in accord with the clinical experience of anesthesia practitioners—that laryngospasm occurs most readily under light anesthesia and that it can be broken by deepening anesthesia or awakening the patient. In puppies, positive intrathoracic pressure inhibits the glottic closure reflex and laryngospasm. This supports the clinical observation that during the emergence from anesthesia in infants and young children, maintenance of PEEP and inflation of the lungs at the time of extubation seem to reduce both the incidence and severity of laryngospasm (E. K. Motoyama, unpublished observation).

Infants are particularly vulnerable to laryngospasm. Animal studies suggest that during a discrete interval after birth and before complete neurologic maturation, there is a period of transient laryngeal hyperexcitability. This may relate to the transient reduction in central latency and a reduction in central inhibition of the vagal afferent. If these observations in puppies are applicable to human infants, they may explain the susceptibility of infants and young children to laryngospasm and have some causal relation in unexpected infant death such as SIDS (Sasaki, 1979).

Infants, particularly premature neonates, exhibit clinically important airway protective responses to fluid at the entrance to the larynx (Davies et al., 1988; Pickens et al., 1989). This response seems to trigger prolonged apnea in neonates and breath holding during inhalation induction of anesthesia in children. When a small quantity (<1 mL) of warm saline solution is dripped into the nasopharynx in a sleeping infant, it pools in the piriform fossa and then overflows into the interarytenoid space at the entrance to the larynx. This area is densely populated with various nerve endings, including a structure resembling a taste bud. The most common response to fluid accumulation is swallowing. The infant also develops central apnea with the glottis open or a closure of vocal cords; coughing is rare (Pickens et al., 1989). Apneic responses are more prominent with water than with saline solution (Davies et al., 1988).

These findings appear clinically important in pediatric anesthesia. During inhalation induction, pharyngeal reflexes (swallowing) are abolished, whereas laryngeal reflexes remain intact, as Guedel originally described in ether anesthesia (1937). Secretions would accumulate in the hypopharynx without swallowing and cause breath holding resulting from central apnea, a closure of the glottis, or both. Positive pressure ventilation using a mask and bag instead of suctioning the pharynx would push secretions farther down into the larynx, stimulate the superior laryngeal nerve, and trigger real laryngospasm.

ANESTHETIC EFFECTS ON CONTROL OF BREATHING

Effects of Anesthetic on Upper Airway Receptors

Inhalation induction of anesthesia is often associated with reflex responses such as coughing, breath holding, and laryngospasm. Volatile anesthetics stimulate upper airway receptors directly and affect ventilation. In dogs spontaneously breathing through tracheostomy under urethane-chloralose anesthesia, an exposure of isolated upper airways to halothane caused depression of respiratory-modulated mechanoreceptors or pressure receptors, whereas irritant receptors and flow (cold) receptors were consistently stimulated in a dose-dependent manner (Nishino et al., 1993). Responses to isoflurane and enflurane were less consistent. Laryngeal respiratory-modulated mechanoreceptors may be a part of a feedback mechanism that maintains the patency of upper airways; the depression of this feedback mechanism may play an important role in the collapse of upper airways during the induction of anesthesia. Furthermore, activation of irritant receptors by halothane and other volatile anesthetics may be responsible for laryngeal reflexes such as coughing, apnea, laryngospasm, and bronchoconstriction seen during inhalation induction of anesthesia (Nishino et al., 1993).

The same group of investigators showed that in young puppies (<2 weeks old), exposure of isolated upper airways to halothane (and to a lesser extent to isoflurane) as described previously resulted in a marked depression of ventilation (<40% of control) associated with decreases in both tidal volume and respiratory frequency (Sant'Ambrogio et al., 1993). Ventilatory effects caused by the exposure of isolated upper airways to volatile anesthetics were present but only mildly in 4-week-old puppies, whereas adult dogs were not affected. The superior laryngeal nerve section and topical anesthesia of the nasal cavity completely abolished the effects of halothane and isoflurane in the isolated upper airways of puppies (Sant'Ambrogio et al., 1993). Laryngeal receptor output in response to volatile anesthetics was not measured in this study. These findings in puppies appear to be clinically relevant because infants and young children often develop manifestations of upper airway reflexes during inhalation induction.

Effects of Anesthetics on Upper Airway Muscles

The genioglossus, geniohyoid, and other pharyngeal and laryngeal abductor muscles have phasic inspiratory activity synchronous with diaphragmatic contraction, in addition to their tonic activities that maintain upper airway patency in both animals and humans (Bartlett et al., 1973; Brouillette and Thach, 1979). The genioglossus and geniohyoid muscles increase the caliber of the pharynx by displacing the hyoid bone and the tongue anteriorly and are the most important muscles for the maintenance of oropharynx patency (see Fig. 2–14). They have both phasic inspiratory activity and tonic activity throughout the respiratory cycle in awake humans (Onal et al., 1981). These activities of the genioglossus muscle and presumably other pharyngeal and laryngeal abductor muscles are easily depressed by alcohol ingestion, sleep, and general anesthesia (Remmers et al., 1978; Nishino et al., 1984, 1985; Bartlett et al., 1990); their depression would result in upper airway obstruction (Brouillette and Thach, 1979).

Sensitivity to anesthetics differs among various inspiratory muscles and their neurons. In studies in cats with the use of electromyography, Ochiai, Guthrie, and Motoyama (1989) demonstrated that the phasic inspiratory activity of the genioglossus muscle was most sensitive to the depressant effect of halothane at a given concentration, whereas the diaphragm was most resistant; the sensitivity of inspiratory intercostal muscles was intermediate (Fig. 2–17). In addition, phasic genioglossus activity was more readily depressed in kittens than in adult cats. Phasic genioglossus activity was abolished with 1.5% halothane or more in all kittens studied, whereas the activity was diminished but present in most adult cats even at 2.5% (Ochiai, Guthrie, and Motoyama, 1992).

Early depression of the genioglossus muscle and other pharyngeal dilator muscles appears to be responsible for upper airway obstruction in infants and young children, especially during the induction of inhalation anesthesia. Because of the higher sensitivity to anesthetic depression, the upper airway muscles failed to increase the intensity of contraction to keep the pharynx patent while the diaphragm continues to contract vigorously, while the negative feedback mechanism to attenuate its contraction may be diminished or lost (Brouillett and Thach, 1979; Ochiai et al., 1989; Isono et al., 2002). Partial upper airway obstruction may occur more often in infants and young children than is clinically apparent during anesthesia by mask without an oral airway. Keidan and others (2000) found in infants and children breathing spontaneously under halothane anesthesia that the work of breathing (as an index of the degree of upper airway obstruction) significantly increased when breathing by mask without an oral airway than with an oral airway in place, even when partial upper airway obstruction was not clinically apparent. An addition of CPAP (5 to 6 cm H_2O) further improved airway patency as evidenced by significant decreases in the work of breathing (Keidan et al., 2000) (also see Chapter 10, Induction of Anesthesia).

Anesthetic Effects on Neural Control of Breathing

Most general anesthetics, opioids, and sedatives depress ventilation. They variably affect minute ventilation ($\dot{V}_E$ and its components (such as tidal volume [V_T], respiratory frequency [f], mean inspiratory flow [V_T/T_I], and respiratory duty cycle [T_I/T_{TOT}]). All inhaled anesthetics significantly depress

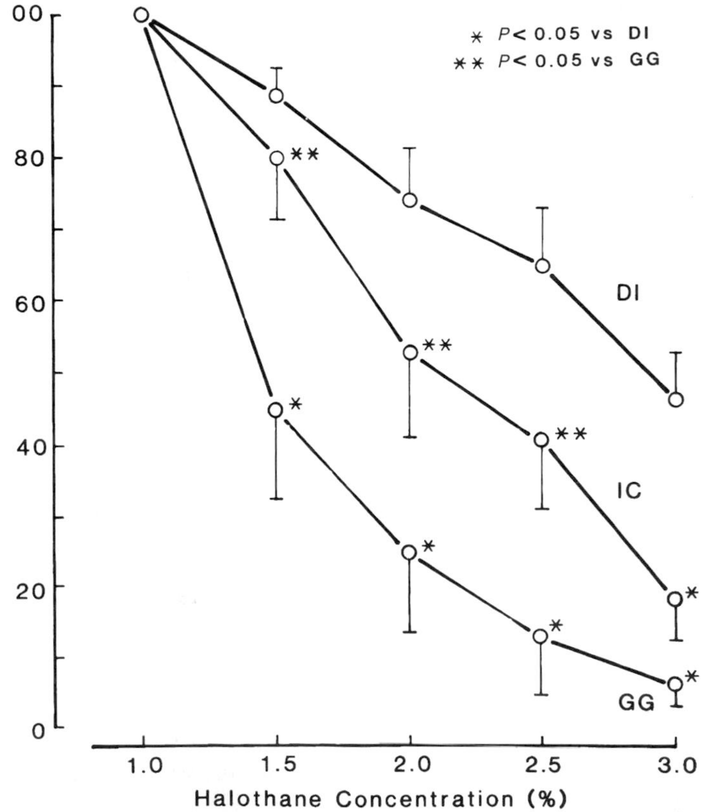

■ **FIGURE 2–17.** Decrease in phasic inspiratory muscle activity, expressed as peak height of moving time average (MTA), in percent change from control (1% halothane), during halothane anesthesia in adult cats. Values are mean ± SEM. $^*P < 0.05$ compared with the diaphragm (DI); $^{**}P < 0.05$ compared with the genioglossus muscle (GG). (From Ochiai R, Guthrie R, Motoyama EK: *Anesthesiology* 70:812, 1989.)

ventilation in a dose-dependent fashion (see Fig. 2–9). This subject has been extensively reviewed (Hickey and Severinghaus, 1981; Pavlin and Hornbein, 1986); information in human infants and children, however, remains limited.

Studies in adult human volunteers using the occlusion technique (Whitelaw, Derenne, Milic-Emili, 1975) and the timing component analysis (Milic-Emili and Grunstein, 1975) have indicated that the reduction in tidal volume with anesthetics results primarily from a reduction in the neural drive of ventilation (Derenne et al., 1976; Wahba, 1980). Inspiratory time tends to decrease but the respiratory duty cycle is relatively unaffected. In several studies in children 2 to 5 years of age, breathing was relatively well maintained at a light level of halothane (0.5 minimum alveolar concentration [MAC]) (Murat et al., 1985; Lindahl, Yates, Hatch, 1987; Benameur et al., 1993). In deeper, surgical levels of anesthesia (1.0 to 1.5 MAC), breathing was depressed in a dose-dependent manner and hypercapnia resulted. Decreased $\dot{V}_E$ was associated with reduced V_T and increased respiratory frequency. The neural respiratory drive was depressed as evidenced by reduced V_T/T_I, whereas the duty cycle (T_I/T_{TOT}) either tended to increase without changes in T_I (Lindahl, Yates, Hatch, 1987; Benameur et al., 1993) or decreased slightly (Murat et al., 1985). In infants less than 12 months of age, ventilatory depression was more pronounced and the duty cycle did not increase, partly because of high chest wall compliance and pronounced thoracic deformity (thoracoabdominal asynchrony) compared with older children (Benameur et al., 1993).

When an external load was imposed on the airway system of an awake individual, ventilation was maintained by increased inspiratory effort (Whitelaw, Derenne, Milic-Emili, 1975). This response was greatly diminished or abolished by the effect of general anesthetics (Nunn and Ezi-Ashi, 1966; Isaza et al., 1976), opioids (Kryger et al., 1976), and barbiturates (Savoy et al., 1982). In children under light halothane anesthesia (0.5 MAC), an addition of a resistive load initially decreased tidal volume. However, tidal volume returned to baseline within 5 minutes (Lindahl, Yates, Hatch, 1987).

Anesthetic Effects on Chemical Control of Breathing

In the dog, inhaled anesthetics diminish or abolish the ventilatory response to hypoxemia in a dose-dependent manner (Weiskopf et al., 1974; Hirshman et al., 1977). In human adult volunteers, the hypoxic ventilatory response was disproportionately depressed in light halothane anesthesia compared to the response to hypercapnia (Knill and Gelb, 1978). At 1.1 MAC of halothane, the hypoxic ventilatory response was completely abolished, whereas the hypercapnic response was about 40% of control in the awake state. Even at a subanesthetic or trace level (0.05 to 0.1 MAC), halothane, isoflurane, and enflurane attenuated the hypoxic ventilatory response to about 30% of control, whereas hypercapnic response was essentially intact (Knill and Gelb, 1979; Knill and Clement 1984). The site of the anesthetics' action appeared to be at the peripheral (carotid) chemoreceptors, because of the rapid response in humans (Knill and Clement 1984) as well as the direct measurement of neuronal chemoreceptor output in the cat (Davies, Edwards, Lahiri, 1982).

Subsequently, Temp and others (1992, 1994) challenged these findings by demonstrating that 0.1 MAC of isoflurane had no demonstrable ventilatory effect on hypoxia. On the other hand, Dahan and others (1994) confirmed the original findings by Knill and others (1978). The reason for the conflicting results appeared to be related to the contribution of visual and auditory inputs (Robotham, 1994). The study by Temp and others (1994) was conducted while the volunteers were watching television (open-eyed), whereas the volunteers in the study by Dahan and others (1994) were listening to soothing music with their eyes closed (but not asleep).

Pandit (2000) conducted a meta-analysis of 37 studies in 21 publications and analyzed the conflicting response to hypoxia under trace levels of anesthetics. Pandit's analysis supported the prediction by Robotham (1994) that the study condition has a major impact on the outcome of the study. Bandit concluded that the main factor for the difference in hypoxia response was the anesthetic agent used ($p < 0.002$). Additional factors included subject stimulation ($p < 0.014$) and agent–stimulation interaction ($p < 0.04$), whereas the rate of induction of hypoxia or the level of P_{CO_2} had no effect (Pandit, 2000).

The effect of subanesthetic concentrations of inhaled anesthetics on ventilation in infants and children has not been studied. However, high incidences of postoperative-hypoxemia in otherwise healthy infants and children without an apparent hypoxic ventilatory response in the postanesthetic period suggest that the hypoxic ventilatory drive in infants and children may be blunted with the presence of residual, subanesthetic levels of inhaled anesthetics (Motoyama and Glazener, 1986).

SUMMARY

The understanding of the control of breathing during the perinatal and early postnatal periods has increased significantly. In general, neural and chemical controls of breathing in older infants and children are similar to those in adolescents and adults. A major exception to this general statement is found in neonates and young infants, especially prematurely born infants less than 40 to 44 weeks postconception. In these infants, hypoxemia is a potent respiratory depressant, rather than a stimulant, either centrally or because of changes in respiratory mechanics. These infants often develop periodic breathing without apparent hypoxemia and occasionally central apnea with possible serious consequence, most likely because of immature respiratory control mechanisms.

LUNG VOLUMES

POSTNATAL DEVELOPMENT OF THE LUNGS

In the human fetus, alveolar formation does not begin until about 4 weeks before birth (Langston et al., 1984), although the airways, including the terminal bronchioles, are completely formed by 16 weeks' gestation (Reid, 1967). The full-term newborn infant has 20 to 50 million terminal airspaces, mostly primitive saccules from which alveoli later develop (Thurlbeck, 1975; Langston et al., 1984). During the early postnatal years, development and growth of the lungs continue at a rapid pace, particularly with respect to the development of new alveoli. By 12 to 18 months of age, the number of alveoli reaches the adult level of 300 million or more; subsequent lung development and growth are associated with increases in alveolar size as well as further structural development (Dunnill, 1962; Langston et al., 1984) (see Development of the Respiratory System).

During the early period of postnatal lung development, the lung volume of infants is disproportionately small in relation to body size. Furthermore, because the infant's metabolic rate, in

■ TABLE 2–2. Normal values for lung functions for persons of various ages

	AGE								
	1 wk	*1 yr*	*3 yr*	*5 yr*	*8 yr*	*12 yr*	*Male 15 yr*	*Male 21 yr*	*Female 21 yr*
Height (cm)	48	75	96	109	130	150	170	174	162
Weight (kg)	3.3	10	15	18	26	39	57	73	57
FRC (mL)	75*	(263)	(532)	660	1174	1855	2800	3030	2350
FRC/weight (mL/kg)	(25)	(26)	(37)	(36)	(46)	(48)	(49)	(42)	(41)
VC (mL)	100†	(475)	(910)	1100	1855	2830	4300	4620	3380
V_E (mL/min)	550	(1775)	(2460)	(2600)	(3240)	(4150)	5030	6000	5030
V_T (mL)	17	(78)	(112)	(130)	(180)	(260)	360	500	420
f (frequency)	30	(24)	(22)	(20)	(18)	16	14	12	12
V_A (mL/min)	385	(1245)	(1760)	(1800)	(2195)	(2790)	3070	4140	3530
V_D (mL)	75	21	37	49	75	105	141	150	126
C_l (mL/cm H_2O)	5	(16)	(32)	44	71	91	130	163	130
Peak flow rates (L/min)	10			136	231	325	437	457	365
R (cm H_2O/L per sec)	29‡	(13)	(10)	8	6	5	3	2	2
DLco (mL/mm Hg per min)§				11	15	20	27	28	24
Cardiac output (L/min)	(0.9)	1.9	2.7	3.2	4.4	5.7	(7.0)	(7.6)	(7.2)
Lung weight (g)	49	120	166	211	290	470	640	730	

Parentheses, interpolated values.
*Supine.
†Crying vital capacity.
‡Nose breathing.
§Single-breath technique.
Compiled from data in Cook CD, Cherry RB, O'Brien D, et al.: *J Clin Invest* 34:975, 1955; Cook CD, Sutherland JM, Segal S, et al.: *J Clin Invest* 36:440, 1957; Comroe JH Jr, et al.: *The lung.* Chicago, Year Book Medical Publishers, 1962; Bucci G, Cook CD, Barrie H: *J Pediatr* 58:820, 1961; Murray AB, Cook CD: *J Pediatr* 62:186, 1963; Cook CD, Hamann JF: *J Pediatr* 59:710, 1961; Long EC, Hull WE: *Pediatrics* 27:373, 1961; and Koch G: *Respir Physiol* 4:168, 1968.

relation to body weight, is nearly twice that of the adult, the ventilatory requirement per unit of lung volume in infants is greatly increased. Infants seem to have far less reserve in lung surface area for gas exchange. Furthermore, general anesthesia markedly reduces the end-expiratory lung volume (FRC or relaxation volume, Vr), especially in young infants, reducing their oxygen reserve severely (see later). Normal values for lung volumes and function in children of various ages are compiled in Table 2–2.

Total lung capacity (TLC) is the maximum lung volume allowed by the strength of the inspiratory muscles stretching the thorax and lungs. Subdivisions of TLC are shown schematically in Figure 2–18. Residual volume (RV) is the amount of air remaining in the lungs after maximum expiration and is approximately 25% of TLC in healthy children. FRC is determined by the balance between the outward stretch of the thorax and the inward recoil of the lungs (Fig. 2–19) and is normally roughly 50% of TLC in the upright posture in healthy children and young adults; it is about 40% in the supine position. The two opposing forces create an average negative average pleural pressure of approximately −5 cm H_2O in older children and adults. In the neonate the pleural pressure is only slightly negative or nearly atmospheric.

■ FUNCTIONAL RESIDUAL CAPACITY AND ITS DETERMINANTS

In infants, outward recoil of the thorax is exceedingly low and inward recoil of the lungs is only slightly lower than that of adults (Agostoni, 1959; Bryan and Wohl, 1986). Consequently, the FRC (or, more appropriately, Vr) of young infants at static conditions (such as apnea, under general anesthesia, or paralysis) decreases to 10% to 15% of TLC (Agostoni, 1959) (Fig. 2–20), a level incompatible with normal gas exchange because of airway closure, atelectasis, and ventilation/perfusion imbalance. In awake infants and young children, however, FRC is dynamically maintained by a number of mechanisms for preventing the collapse of the lungs, including a sustained inspiratory muscle tension to make the thorax stiffer (Box 2–4) (also see later, Elastic Properties). FRC in young infants, therefore, is dynamically determined; there is no fixed level of FRC.

In normal children and adolescents, lung volumes are related to body size, especially height. In most instances, the relative size of the lung compartment appears to be approximately constant from

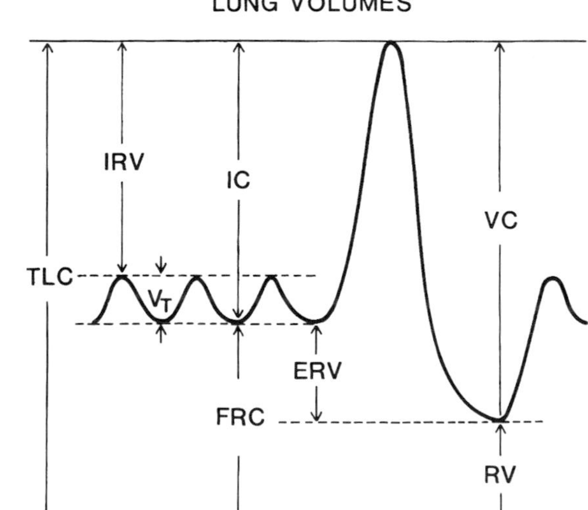

■ FIGURE 2–18. TLC and lung volume subdivisions. ERV, Expiratory reserve volume; FRC, functional residual capacity; IC, inspiratory capacity; IRV, inspiratory reserve volume; RV, residual volume; TLC, total lung capacity; VC, vital capacity; V_T, tidal volume. (From Motoyama EK: *Int Anesthesiol Clin* 26:6, 1988.)

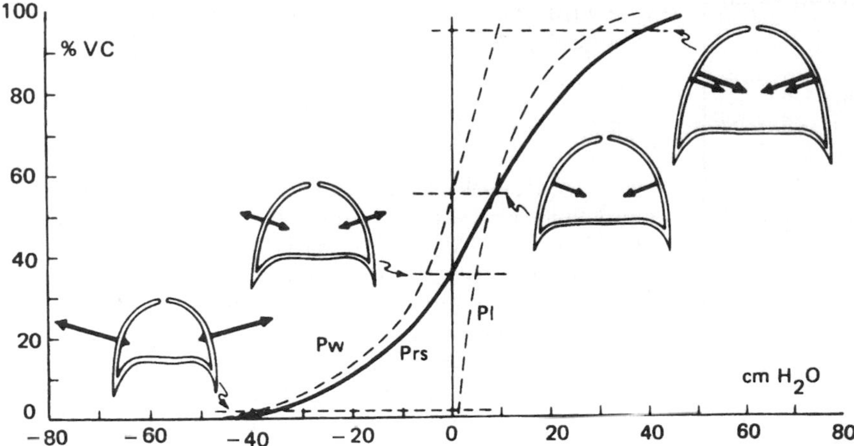

■ **FIGURE 2–19.** Static volume-pressure curves of the lung (Pl), chest wall (Pw), and respiratory system (Prs) during relaxation in the sitting position. The static forces of the lung and chest wall are pictured by the arrows in the side drawings. The dimensions of the arrows are not to scale; the volume corresponding to each drawing is indicated by the horizontal broken lines. (From Agostoni E, Mead J: Statics of the respiratory system. In Fenn WO, Rahn H, editors: *Handbook of physiology. Section 3. Respiration,* vol 1. Washington, DC, 1986, American Physiological Society. Used with permission of the American Physiological Society.)

school-aged children to young adults (see Table 2–2). A study in anesthetized and paralyzed infants and children (Thorsteinsson et al., 1994) indicates that TLC, as measured with a tracer gas washout technique, is relatively small in infants (≈60 mL/kg) when the lungs are inflated with relatively low inflation pressure (20 to 25 cm H_2O) (the recruitment of previously collapsed air space with this pressure might not have been complete). TLC in children older than 1.5 years of age (determined with inflation pressures of 35 to 40 cm H_2O) increases with growth until about 5 years of age (body weight, 20 kg), when it reaches that of older children and adolescents (90 mL/kg).

Negative pressure surrounding the lungs is the same, with respect to lung expansion, as positive pressure within the airways; thus, the net transpulmonary pressure represents the force expanding or contracting the lungs. In contrast, negative intrathoracic pressure has quite a different effect from positive airway pressure with respect to pulmonary circulation and the ventilation–pulmonary perfusion relationship.

Anesthesia, surgery, abdominal distention, and disease may all alter lung volumes. The patient in the prone or supine position has a smaller FRC than the patient standing or sitting because the abdominal contents shift. FRC is further decreased under general anesthesia with or without muscle relaxants (Westbrook et al., 1973). Such a decrease in FRC may result in the closure of small airways, uneven distribution of ventilation, ventilation–pulmonary perfusion imbalance, and hypoxemia. In certain conditions, such as respiratory distress syndrome of the newborn (IRDS), in which the lung resists expansion because of the high surface force, the FRC is further reduced. When the air passages are narrowed, as in asthma or cystic fibrosis, air trapping occurs on expiration, resulting in increased FRC.

The importance of the air remaining in the lungs at the end of normal expiration is often overlooked. This FRC serves as a buffer to minimize cyclic changes in PCO_2 and PO_2 of the blood during each breath. In addition, the fact that air normally remains in the lungs throughout the respiratory cycle means that relatively few alveoli collapse. Although alveolar collapse does not occur during normal breathing, unusually high pressures are needed to expand the lungs when they are liquid filled at birth, after open-chest surgery, or during general anesthesia without the maintenance of PEEP in infants. Transpulmonary pressure of 30 to 40 cm H_2O (and occasionally even more) is needed to reexpand the collapsed lungs. Thereafter, 5 to 6 cm H_2O of PEEP appears adequate to prevent airway closure and to maintain FRC.

■ MECHANICS OF BREATHING

To ventilate the lungs, the respiratory muscles must overcome certain opposing forces within the lungs themselves. These forces have both elastic and resistive properties. Although respiratory mechanics in adults have been studied extensively over the past four decades, most available information on infants and young children has emerged relatively recently, as reviewed by Bryan and Wohl (1986). More recently, new information on lung mechanics in infants was carefully scrutinized and compiled by researchers from North America, Europe, and Australia under

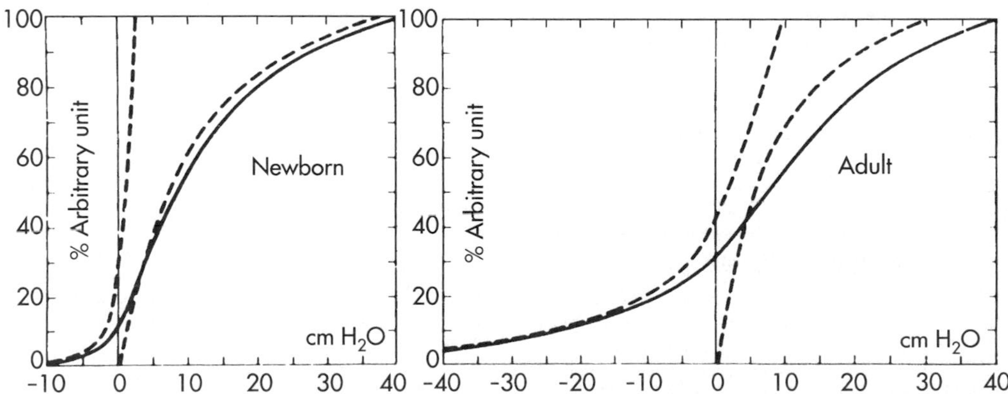

■ **FIGURE 2–20.** Static pressure-volume curve of lung *(right dashed line),* chest wall *(left dashed line),* and total respiratory system *(solid line)* in newborn and adult. (From Agostoni E: Volume-pressure relationships of the thorax. *J Appl Physiol* 14:909, 1959. Used with permission of the American Physiological Society.)

> **BOX 2–4 Maintenance of Functional Residual Capacity (FRC) in Young Infants**
>
> 1. Sustained tonic activities of inspiratory muscles throughout the respiratory cycle.
> 2. Breaking of expiration with continual but diminishing diaphragmatic activity.
> 3. Narrowing of the glottis during expiration.*
> 4. Inspiration starting in mid-expiration.*
> 5. High respiratory rate in relation to expiratory time constant.*
>
> All mechanisms of sustaining FRC are lost with anesthesia or muscle relaxant.

*Create intrinsic or auto-PEEP ($PEEP_i$).

the auspices of the American Thoracic Society (ATS) and the European Respiratory Society (ERS). A resulting position paper was published (ATS/ERS Joint Committee, 1993).

ELASTIC PROPERTIES

Compliance of the Lungs and Thorax

When the lungs are expanded by the contraction of inspiratory muscles or by positive pressure applied to the airways, elastic recoil of the lungs and thoracic structures surrounding the lungs counterreacts to reduce lung volume. This elastic force is fairly constant over the range of normal tidal volumes, but it increases at the extremes of deflation or inflation (Fig. 2–21). The elastic properties of the lungs or respiratory system (lungs and thorax) are measured and expressed as lung compliance (CL) or respiratory system compliance (Crs) in units of volume change per unit of pressure change. The following equation is derived:

$$CL = \frac{\Delta V}{\Delta P}$$

where ΔV is usually the tidal volume and ΔP is the change in transpulmonary pressure (the difference between the airway and pleural pressures [ΔP = Pao − Ppl]) for CL, and for Crs, ΔP is transrespiratory pressure (the difference between the airway pressure at end-inspiratory occlusion and atmospheric pressure [ΔP = Pao − PB]) necessary to produce the tidal volume. These measurements are made at points of no flow, that is, at the extremes of tidal volume when there is no flow-resistive component (static compliance). Lung compliance may vary with changes in the mid-position of tidal ventilation with no inherent alteration in the elastic characteristics of the lungs (see Fig. 2–21). The elastic properties of the lungs are described more accurately by measuring pressure-volume relationships over the entire range of TLC.

In normal persons, lung compliance measured during the respiratory cycle (i.e., the dynamic compliance during quiet breathing) is approximately the same as the static compliance. When there is airway obstruction, however, the ventilation of some lung units may be functionally decreased, resulting in decreased dynamic compliance, whereas the static compliance is relatively unaffected. This difference between static and dynamic compliance increases with increasing respiratory frequency (frequency dependence of compliance) and is a sign of airway obstruction (Woolcock et al., 1969).

Quiet, normal expiration occurs passively, resulting from the elastic recoil of the lungs and chest wall and involves little or no additional work. The situation in the infant or in the anesthetized and spontaneously breathing patient may be somewhat different because expiration may have an active phase, as discussed later. To consider volume-pressure relationships from another point of view, a normal tidal volume may be obtained using transpulmonary pressures of approximately 4 to 6 cm H_2O in persons of all sizes, provided that the lungs are normal and normally expanded initially and the airways are patent. The total transthoracopulmonary pressure needed to ventilate the lungs with positive pressure in a closed chest is, in the adult, approximately twice the required transpulmonary pressure during spontaneous breathing because the thoracic structures must also be expanded. The chest wall in the newborn is extremely compliant and therefore requires almost no force for expansion (see Fig. 2–20). The combined compliance of the chest wall and lungs, or the compliance of the total respiratory system (Crs), is expressed as follows:

$$\frac{1}{Crs} = \frac{1}{CL} + \frac{1}{Cw}$$

where Cl is lung compliance and Cw is chest wall compliance. The equation can be expressed in terms of elastance (E), an inverse of compliance (E = 1/C):

$$Ers = EL + Ew$$

where Ers is the elastance of the total respiratory system, EL is lung elastance, and Ew is chest wall elastance.

Lung compliance in normal humans of different sizes is, in general, directly proportional to lung size (see Table 2–2). The compliance is expressed per unit of lung volume (e.g., per FRC, VC, or TLC) for comparison (termed "specific compliance").

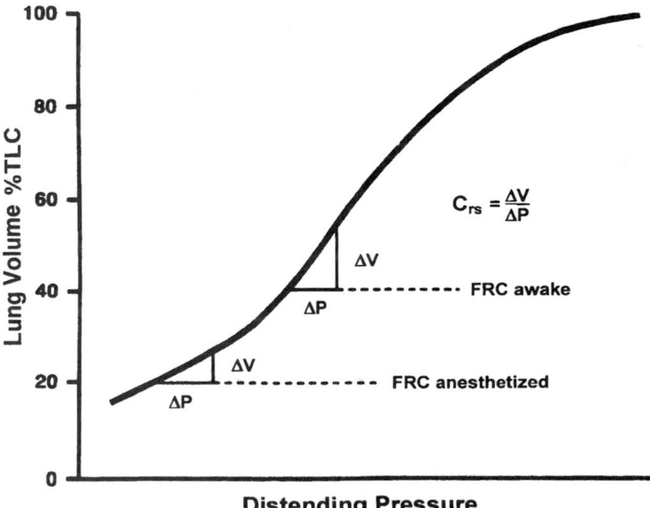

FIGURE 2–21. Schematic representation of the pressure-volume (P-V) curve and compliance of the respiratory system (CRS). At the midpoint of the P-V curve (indicated as FRC awake), the slope and compliance (CRS = ΔP/ΔV) is the highest. When FRC is decreased to the lower, flatter portion of the P-V curve under general anesthesia or paralysis (indicated as FRC anesthetized), CRS decreases even without changes in the mechanics of the lung or the respiratory system.

Developmental Changes in the Compliance of the Lungs and Thorax

After the initial period of neonatal adaptation, the compliance of the infant's lungs is extremely high (elastic recoil is low) (Motoyama, 1977), probably because of absent or poorly developed elastic fibers (Fagan, 1976, 1977) (Fig. 2–22). Oddly enough, their functional characteristics resemble those of geriatric, emphysematous lungs with pathologically high compliance caused by the loss of functioning elastic fibers (Fig. 2–23). Thus, at both extremes of human life, the lungs are prone to premature airway closure (Mansell et al., 1972). Elastic recoil pressure of the lungs at 60% TLC increases from about 1 cm H_2O in the newborn (Fagan, 1976, 1977) to 5 cm H_2O at 7 years of age and 9 cm H_2O at 16 years of age (Zapletal et al., 1987).

In infants the outward recoil of the chest wall is exceedingly small (Agostoni, 1959), because the rib cage is cartilaginous and horizontal and the respiratory muscles are not well developed, whereas the inward recoil of the lungs is only moderately decreased compared with that in adults (Gerhardt and Bancalari, 1980). Consequently, the static balance of these opposing forces would decrease FRC to a very low level (see Fig. 2–20). Such a reduction in FRC would make parenchymal airways unstable and subject them to collapse. In reality, however, dynamic FRC in spontaneously breathing infants is maintained at around 40% TLC, a value similar to that in adults in the supine position, because of a number of possible mechanisms or their combinations (Bryan and Wohl, 1986).

Maintenance of Functional Residual Capacity in Infants

Infants terminate the expiratory phase of the breathing cycle before lung volume reaches the relaxation volume (Vr), or true FRC, determined by the balance of opposing chest wall and lung elastic recoil (Kosch and Stark, 1979). This "premature" cessation of the expiratory phase, which results in intrinsic PEEP ($PEEP_i$) with higher FRC, probably results partly from the relatively long time constant of the respiratory system in infants in relation to their high respiratory rate (Olinsky et al., 1974). Additional mechanisms may help maintain dynamic FRC above the relaxation volume. Glottic closure, or laryngeal braking, during the expiratory phase of the breathing cycle is an important mechanism for the establishment of sufficient air space in the lungs during the early postnatal period (Fisher et al., 1982). Diaphragmatic braking, the diminishing diaphragmatic activity extending to the expiratory phase of breathing, is another important mechanism that extends expiratory time and maintains FRC.

Among all mechanisms that maintain FRC, tonic contractions of both the diaphragm and the intercostal muscles throughout the respiratory cycle in awake infants appear to be most important. This mechanism effectively stiffens the chest wall and maintains a higher end-expiratory lung volume (Muller et al., 1979). Henderson-Smart and Read (1979) have shown a 30% decrease in thoracic gas volume in sleeping infants changing from non-REM to REM sleep. This large reduction in dynamic FRC may result from loss of tonic activity of the respiratory muscles, loss of laryngeal braking, diaphragmatic braking, or all of these factors. All of these important mechanisms for maintaining FRC in infants (and to a lesser extent in older children) are lost with general anesthesia or muscle relaxants, causing marked reductions in FRC, airway closure and atelectasis (Serafini et al., 1999). The physiological mechanisms for maintaining FRC in young infants are listed in Box 2–4.

When is the FRC no longer determined dynamically but determined by the balance between the recoils of the thorax and the lungs to the opposing direction, as in adults? Colin and others (1989) have shown that, in infants and children during quiet, natural sleep, the transition from dynamically determined to relaxed end-expiratory volume or FRC takes place between 6 and 12 months of age. By 1 year of age the breathing pattern is predominantly that of relaxed end-expiratory volume, just as in older children and adults. These findings coincide with the upright posture and development of thoracic tissue and muscle strength in infants.

The breathing pattern of infants less than 6 months of age is predominantly abdominal (diaphragmatic) and the contribution of the rib cage (external intercostal muscles) to tidal volume is relatively small (20% to 40%), reflecting instability of the thorax or weakness of the intercostal muscles. After 9 months of age, the rib cage component of tidal volume increases to a level (50%) similar to that of older children and adolescents, reflecting the maturation of the thoracic structures (Hershenson et al., 1990). Furthermore, a study by Papastamelos and others (1995) has

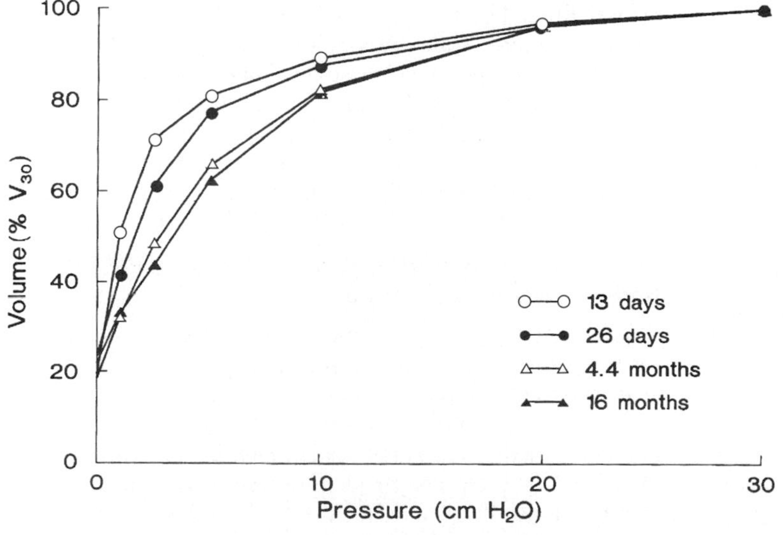

■ **FIGURE 2–22.** Pressure-volume curves obtained from excised lungs at autopsy. Data are grouped by postnatal ages as shown by symbols. It is evident that elastic recoil pressure (horizontal distance between nil distending pressure and the curve at a given distending volume) increases with postnatal development of the lungs. (Based on data from Fagan DG: *Thorax* 31:534, 1976, and 32:193, 1977.)

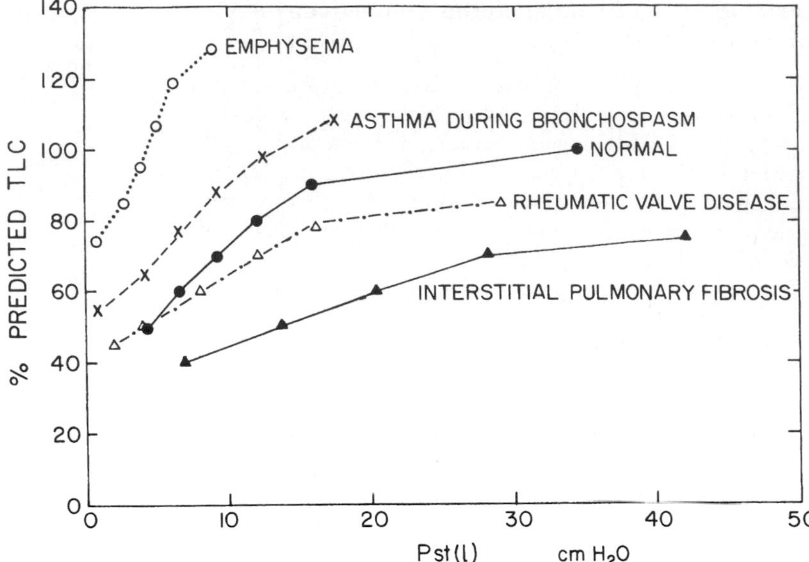

■ **FIGURE 2–23.** Static pressure-volume curves (deflation limbs) of the lungs in various conditions as indicated. (From Bates DV, editor: *Respiratory function in disease,* ed 3. Philadelphia, 1989, WB Saunders.)

shown that the stiffening of the chest wall continues throughout infancy and early childhood. By 12 months of age, however, chest wall compliance (which is extremely high in neonates) decreases and nearly equals lung compliance. The chest wall becomes stable and can resist the inward recoil of the lungs and maintain FRC passively. These relatively recent findings support the notion that the stability of the respiratory system is achieved by 1 year of age.

Effects of General Anesthesia on Functional Residual Capacity

General anesthesia with or without muscle relaxation results in a significant reduction of FRC in adult patients in the supine position soon after the induction of anesthesia (Rehder et al., 1971, 1974; Westbrook et al., 1973), whereas FRC is unchanged during anesthesia in the sitting position (Rehder et al., 1972). A decrease in FRC is associated with reductions in both lung and thoracic compliance, but the mechanism responsible for the reduction in FRC and the sequence of events that changes respiratory mechanics were not understood for many years.

In an excellent study, deTroyer and Bastenier-Geens (1979) showed that when a healthy volunteer was partially paralyzed with pancuronium, the outward recoil of the thorax decreased, whereas lung recoil (compliance) did not. This change altered the balance between the elastic recoil of the lung and thorax in opposite directions, and consequently FRC diminished. The compliance of the lungs decreased shortly thereafter, resulting from the reduced FRC and resultant airway closure. Based on their findings, deTroyer and Bastenier-Geens postulated that, in the awake state, inspiratory muscles have intrinsic tone that maintains the outward recoil and rigidity of the thorax. Anesthesia or paralysis would abolish this muscle tone, reducing thoracic compliance followed by a reduction in FRC, and eventually lung compliance in rapid succession (in a matter of a few minutes).

In healthy young adults, a reduction of FRC during general anesthesia is limited to between 9% and 25% from the awake control levels (Laws, 1968; Rehder et al., 1972; Westbrook et al., 1973; Hewlett et al., 1974; Juno et al., 1978). In older individuals, the average reduction in FRC is higher (30%), probably because of lower elastic recoil pressure and increased closing capacity (Bergman, 1963).

With the more compliant thoraces of infants and young children, general anesthesia and muscle relaxation would be expected to produce more profound reductions in FRC than in adolescents and adults. Henderson-Smart and Read (1979) have shown a 30% reduction in thoracic gas volume in infants changing the sleep pattern from quiet (non-REM) to active (REM) sleep. In children 6 to 18 years of age under general anesthesia and paralysis, Dobbinson and others (1973) found marked reductions in FRC (average reduction, 35%) from their own awake control values, as measured with a helium dilution technique. The average decrease in FRC among those younger than 12 years of age was 46%. Fletcher and others (1990) demonstrated that compliance of the respiratory system (Crs) in infants and children under general anesthesia decreased about 35%, a value comparable to the reduction reported in adults under similar conditions (Westbrook et al., 1973; Rehder and Marsh, 1986). This reduction in Crs occurred both during spontaneous breathing and during manual ventilation with low tidal volume after muscle relaxants were given. When tidal volume was doubled, however, Crs returned to preanesthetic control levels.

These findings are in accord with previous findings in adults (deTroyer and Bastenier-Geens, 1979; Hedenstierna and McCarthy, 1980) and support the notion that anesthesia reduces FRC. The finding that a larger tidal volume increases Crs toward control values also indicates that FRC decreases to the lower, flatter portion of the pressure-volume curve (see Fig. 2–21). Motoyama and others (1982a) reported moderate decreases in FRC (−46%) in children as measured with helium dilation and a marked decrease (−71%) in infants under halothane anesthesia and muscle paralysis, approaching the relaxation volume in the newborn infant reported by Agostoni (1959).

Effect of Positive End-Expiratory Pressure (PEEP) Under General Anesthesia

Thorsteinsson and others (1994) reported that the lung volume at FRC (or relaxation volume, Vr) was at a lower, flatter portion of the pressure-volume (P-V) curve in all infants and children studied. To restore FRC to the normal or steepest portion of the P-V curve of the respiratory system seen in the awake state, a PEEP of 5 to 6 cm H_2O had to be added to infants younger than 6 months of age and 12 cm H_2O in children.

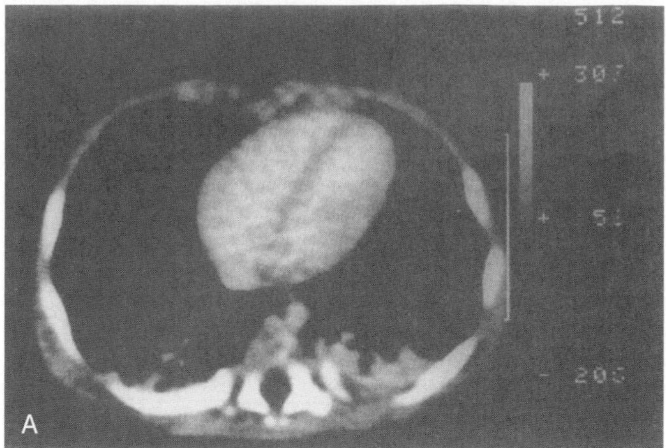

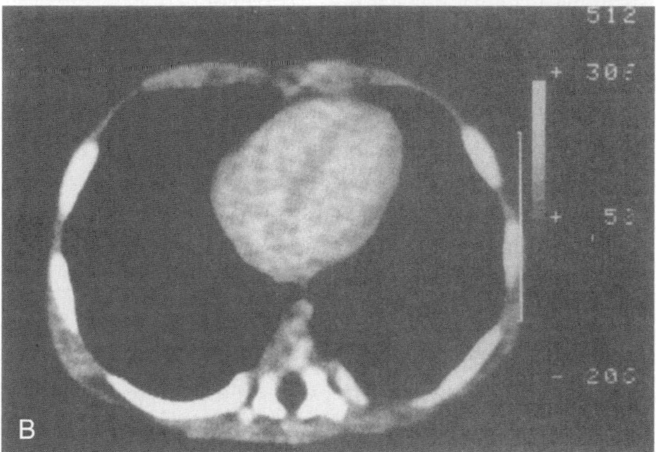

■ **FIGURE 2–24.** Computed tomography (CT) scan of the thorax during general endotracheal anesthesia. *(A)* Transverse CT scan of the thorax 5 minutes after the induction of anesthesia without PEEP. Note the appearance of atelectasis (density) in the dependent regions of both lungs. *(B)* Transverse CT scan of the thorax during anesthesia with a positive end-expiratory pressure (PEEP) of 5 cm H_2O, showing the complete disappearance of atelectasis in the dependent regions of both lungs. (From Serafini G, Cornara G, Cavalloro F, et al.: *Paediatr Anaesth* 9:225-228, 1999, with permission.)

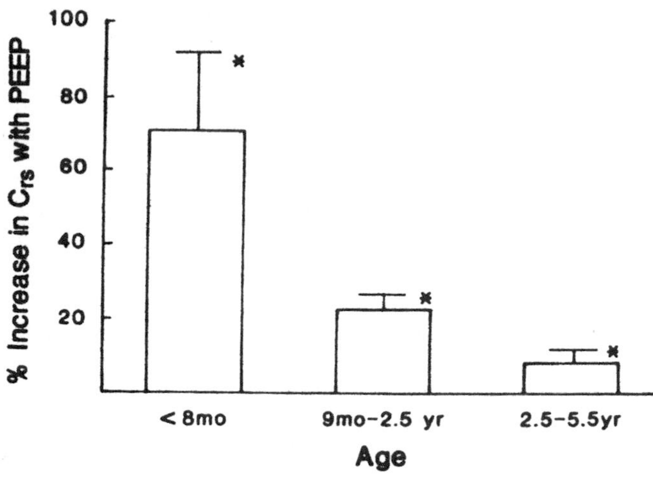

■ **FIGURE 2–25.** Compliance of the respiratory system (Crs) under general anesthesia in infants and children and the effect of PEEP. An addition of PEEP (5 to 6 cm H_2O) improves (restores) Crs significantly in all age groups studied. The beneficial effect of PEEP was most dramatic in infants younger than 8 months (see text). (From Motoyama EK: *Anesthesiology* 85:A1099, 1996.)

Increased density appearing on computed tomography (CT) scans in the dependent portion of the lung has been described in adult patients shortly after the induction of anesthesia and muscle relaxation. This increased density could be reduced or eliminated by adding PEEP (Brismar et al., 1996). Serafini and others (1999) were the first to report evidence of atelectasis in young children (1 to 3 years; mean age, 1.8 years) on CT scan in the dependent portion of the lungs shortly after the inhalation induction of anesthesia and intubation. These patients were given three deep inflations of the lungs (sighs) with 40% oxygen in nitrogen (air mix) and ventilated with 10 mL/kg of tidal volume. Atelectasis (density on the CT scan) appeared almost immediately when ventilated without PEEP (Fig. 2–24*A*). When the patients were ventilated for 5 minutes with an addition of PEEP (5 cm H_2O) with the same ventilator settings and end-tidal PCO_2, the density disappeared from the repeated CT scans in all 10 children studied, indicating the recruitment of atelectic lung segments (Fig. 2–24*B*) (Serafini et al., 1999).

As the stability of the thorax increases during the first year of life as stated earlier (Papastamelos et al., 1995), it is likely that the thorax would resist the lung collapse and atelectasis with increasing age. Motoyama (1996) examined this possibility by measuring respiratory system compliance (Crs) in infants and young children under 6 years of age undergoing halothane–nitrous oxide endotracheal anesthesia. These patients were ventilated either with or without PEEP (6 cm H_2O) for 15 minutes preceded by deep sighs. After a period of ventilation with PEEP, Crs was consistently higher after PEEP than without PEEP. There were significant age-related differences in the degree of increase in Crs after PEEP (6 cm H_2O) versus no PEEP (0 cm H_2O) (Fig. 2–25). The average increase of Crs with PEEP was greatest in infants less than 8 months of age (75% higher with PEEP versus without PEEP). In contrast, in older infants and toddlers (9 months to 2.5 years), an average increase in Crs with PEEP was 22%; in children (2.5 and 5.5 years), the increase was 9%, the level one would expect in adults. These results reflect greater reductions in FRC (or increases in atelectasis) in the younger age groups (Motoyama, 1996) (Fig. 2–25).

Persistent airway closure during general anesthesia would result in resorption atelectasis because alveolar gas (mostly oxygen and nitrous oxide) trapped below the occluded airways would be rapidly absorbed. Resultant pulmonary ventilation/perfusion imbalance and right-to-left shunting of blood in the lung may reduce arterial PO_2 in the postanesthetic recovery room. Such an effect would be expected to be more profound in infants. Motoyama and Glazener (1986) studied arterial oxygen saturation with a pulse oximeter (SpO_2) in otherwise healthy infants and children before and after general anesthesia for simple, relatively short surgical procedures (inguinal hernia repair, myringotomy tube insertions, etc.). On arrival at the postanesthetic care unit (PACU), the mean SpO_2 was 93% (estimated PaO_2, 66 mm Hg), significantly reduced from the preoperative value of 97%. In some children, SpO_2 decreased to the low 70s (estimated PaO_2 <40 mm Hg). These patients showed no sign of hypoxic ventilatory stimulation with normal cutaneous PCO_2 (Motoyama and Glazener, 1986).

A large percentage (20% to 40%) of otherwise healthy infants and children develop oxygen desaturation (SpO_2 ≤94%) during transport and on arrival at the PACU (Motoyama and Glazner, 1986; Pullertis et al., 1987; Patel et al., 1988). A later study of postoperative hypoxemia involving 1152 patients ranging from infants to adults has demonstrated that hemoglobin desaturation occurs sooner, is more pronounced, and lasts longer in infants than in children and in children than in adults (Xue et al., 1996).

All children, therefore, should be given oxygen by mask during the transport from the operating room and on arrival at the PACU until he or she can maintain satisfactory oxygen saturation by pulse oximeter without supplemental oxygen (see Chapter 11, Intraoperative and Postoperative Management).

Closing Volume and Closing Capacity

Besides the lungs and chest wall, the air passages themselves have a compliance that may be important. With deep inspiration the air passages of normal persons increase in size (interdependence of airways and lung volume), whereas on forced expiration they decrease to a point at which dynamic compression or airway closure with air trapping may take place. Closing volume is the lung volume above residual volume (RV) at which dependent lung zones (i.e., lower lung segments in the upright position) cease to ventilate, presumably because of the closure of small airways. Closing capacity is the sum of closing volume and RV. Whether this closure is anatomic or merely the result of dynamic compression and reduction in flow (see discussion of maximum expiratory flow-volume curves under Dynamic Properties) is controversial (Hughes et al., 1970; Hyatt et al., 1973). Because the patency of small airways depends in part on the elastic recoil of the lungs, closing capacity as a percentage of TLC is relatively high in young children (Mansell et al., 1972) and would be even higher, at least theoretically, in infants. Closing capacity increases with aging as well as with small airway disease, such as chronic bronchitis caused by smoking and emphysema in adults.

Lung compliance is reduced in most situations in which lung volume is decreased (e.g., the removal of lung tissue, atelectasis, intrapulmonary tumors), although it is normal when corrected for lung volumes. Compliance is also decreased when surface forces are increased (as in IRDS with increased surface force [or decreased surfactant]) or elastic recoil is abnormally increased (e.g., in interstitial pulmonary fibrosis).

Emphysema is associated with a loss of elastic recoil and therefore an abnormal increase in compliance. Chest wall compliance decreases with conditions such as scleroderma, kyphoscoliosis, and ankylosing spondylitis involving the thoracic structures.

DYNAMIC PROPERTIES

Breathing involves cyclic contractions of respiratory muscles and the generation of force, which must overcome resistive and elastic properties of the lung and chest wall. The resistive properties of the respiratory system include the resistance to airflow within the airways, the tissue viscoelastic resistance or the resistance of the lung and thoracic tissues themselves to deformation, and inertial resistance (inertance) resulting from the movement of gas molecules within the airways, especially at high velocities. In contrast to compliance (or elastance), which is measured at points of no flow, flow resistance is present only when the lung is in motion.

Airway Resistance

The pressure required to overcome frictional resistance and produce flow between the alveoli (Palv) and the airway opening (Pao) is proportional to flow rate. Airway resistance (Raw) is expressed as pressure gradient across the airways (P = Pao – Palv) per unit flow ($\dot{V}$):

$$Raw = P/\dot{V} \text{ (cm } H_2O\text{/L per sec)}$$

If the respiratory system is assumed to have a single compartment with a constant elastance or compliance (E = 1/C) and a constant resistance (R), the equation of forces acting on the respiratory system can be expressed as follows:

$$P = E\dot{V} + R\dot{V} + I\dot{V}$$

In tidal breathing, inertance (I) is very small and can be ignored. During normal tidal breathing, approximately 90% of the pressure gradient required is needed to overcome the elastic forces and the remaining 10% of the pressure is expended to counter the flow resistance (Sly and Hayden, 1998).

Flow resistance is related to the length (l), radius of the tube (r), and the viscosity of the gas (η) as follows:

$$R = \frac{8l\eta}{\pi r^4}$$

Assuming a laminar flow (as seen in small or peripheral airways), it is apparent from this equation (Poiseuille's law) that the most important factor affecting flow resistance is the change in the radius of the tube (airways), because resistance is inversely proportional to the fourth power of the radius. (When the flow is turbulent, as occurs in large airways, the flow resistance increases approximately with r^5.) Therefore, airway resistance in infants with smaller airway diameters is much higher, in absolute terms, than airway resistance in older children and adults. It might also be expected that inflammation or secretions in the airway system would result in exaggerated degrees of obstruction in infants compared with older persons (Fig. 2–26). One such example may be the severe and often life-threatening obstruction of upper airways seen only in infants and young children with acute supraglottitis (epiglottitis) and subglottic croup (laryngotracheobronchitis). In terms of body size, however, the caliber of airways in general is wider and airway resistance (specific resistance) lower in infants and children compared with adults (Motoyama, 1977; Stocks and Goddfrey, 1977).

In absolute terms, airway resistance (Raw) in the newborn is very high (19 to 28 cm H_2O/L per sec). It decreases to less than 2 cm H_2O/L per sec in the adolescent and the adult. In relative terms (as expressed per unit of lung volume, usually FRC), airway resistance is relatively low, or conductance (Gaw, the reciprocal of resistance) is very high, in the newborn. The specific conductance (sGaw = Gaw/FRC) decreases rapidly during the first year of life (Stocks and Godfrey, 1977, 1978), indicating a rapid increase in lung volume (alveolar formation) in relation to airway size. Between 6 and 18 years of age, Gaw increases

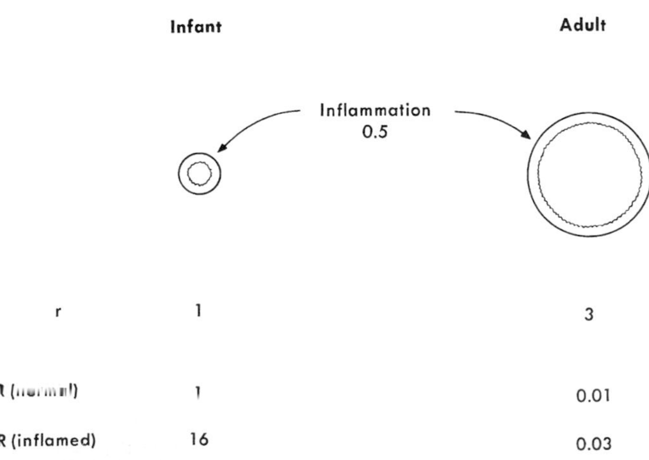

■ **FIGURE 2–26.** Effect of inflammation on airway resistance in infants and adults. r, Radius of an air passage; R, flow resistance.

linearly with increases in height; sGaw, however, stays fairly constant throughout this period at about 0.2 L/sec/cm H_2O (Zapletal et al., 1969, 1976, 1987).

Distribution of Airway Resistance

Rohrer's earlier work (1915) led to the belief that peripheral airways of small caliber were the major contributors to total airway resistance. However, the elegant morphometric studies of Weibel (1963) with inflated and fixed lungs proved that the total cross-sectional area of each generation of airways increases dramatically toward the periphery (Fig. 2–27). Indeed, about two thirds of the total airway resistance exists between the airway opening and the trachea, and most of the remaining resistance is in the large central airways. The airways smaller than a few millimeters in diameter (peripheral airways) contribute only about 10% of total resistance (Macklem and Mead, 1967).

These findings have important clinical implications. If the peripheral airways contribute little to the total airway resistance, disease processes involving small airways, such as emphysema in adults, cystic fibrosis in children, and bronchopulmonary dysplasia (BPD) in infants, will not be detectable by measurement of the total airway resistance. For instance, complete obstruction of one half of peripheral airways would increase the total airway resistance by only 10%, an increase within the usual variation in measurements. For this reason, the peripheral airways formerly were called the "quiet zone" of the lung (Mead, 1970). Apparently the measurement of total airway resistance is not a sensitive clinical test for detecting small airway obstruction.

Upper Airway Resistance

The airway system extends from the airway opening at the nares or the mouth to the alveolar duct at the periphery of the lung. Functionally, the airway system can be subdivided into the upper (extrathoracic) and lower (intrathoracic) airways. During quiet breathing, airflow resistance through the nasal passages accounts for approximately 65% of total airway resistance in adults (Ferris et al., 1964). This is more than twice the resistance during mouth breathing. For air warming, humidification, and particle filtration, it is important that one preferentially or instinctively breathes through the nose despite its higher resistance (Proctor, 1977a, 1977b). Stocks and Godfrey (1978) found nasal resistance comprised approximately 49% of the total airway resistance in European infants, whereas it was significantly less in infants of African origin (31%). Overall, upper airway resistance is approximately two thirds of the total airway resistance.

Except when crying, newborn infants are obligatory nose breathers. The cephalad position of the epiglottis and close approximation of the soft palate to the tongue and epiglottis in neonates may be a reason why mouth breathing is more difficult than nose breathing (Moss, 1965; Sasaki et al., 1977). When the nasal airway is occluded, some infants, especially during REM sleep, do not respond sufficiently to initiate adequate mouth breathing and obstructive apnea ensues. In infants, an insertion of a nasogastric tube significantly increases total resistance by as much as 50% and may compromise breathing (Stocks, 1980).

Lower Airway Resistance

Between the trachea and the alveolar duct are an average of 23 airway generations (Weibel, 1963) (see Fig. 2–27). As gas molecules move from the trachea toward the terminal airways during inspiration, the radius of the successive generations of airways becomes smaller and the flow resistance is expected to increase. In reality, however, the total cross-sectional area of the airway segments increases dramatically toward the periphery, although the diameter of successive single airways decreases. This is because the number of airways increases markedly and,

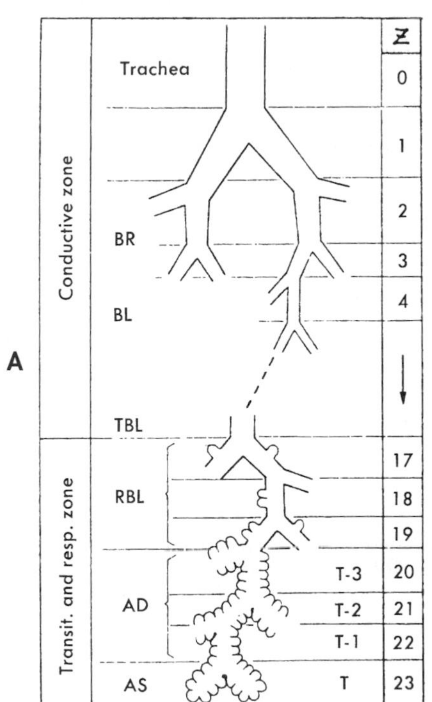

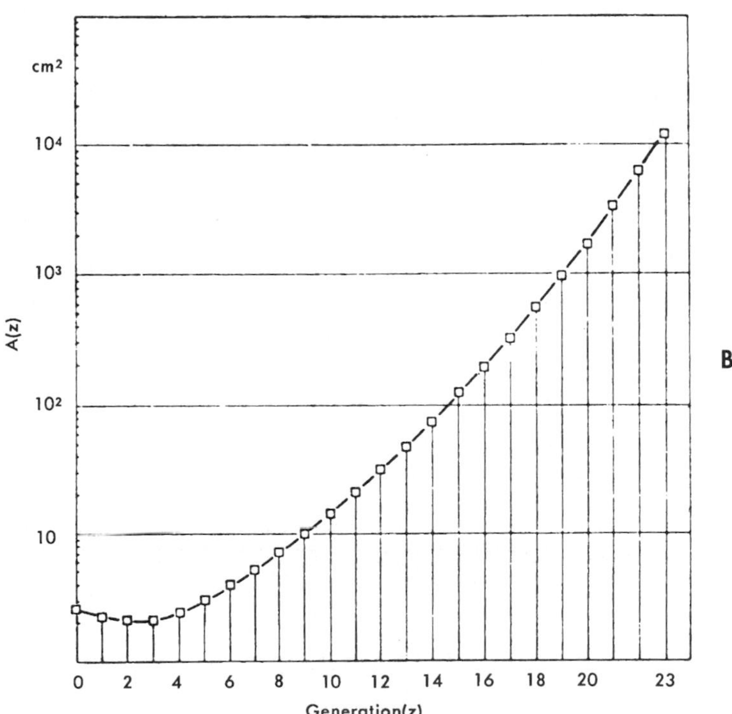

■ **FIGURE 2–27.** *(A)* Diagrammatic representation of the sequence of elements in the conductive, transitory, and respiratory zones of the airways. BR, Bronchi; BL, bronchioles; TBL, terminal bronchioles; RBL, respiratory bronchioles; AD, alveolar ducts; AS, alveolar sacs; z, order of generation of branching; T, terminal generation. *(B)* Total airway cross-sectional area, A(z), in each generation, z. (From Weibel ER: *Morphometry of the human lung.* New York, 1963, Academic Press.)

consequently, the flow resistance of airways decreases toward the periphery (Weibel, 1963) (see Fig. 2–27). Indeed, using a retrograde catheter technique, Macklem and Mead (1967) demonstrated that the peripheral airways, less than about 1 mm in diameter (around 14th generation), contribute less than 10% of the lower airway resistance (or 3% of the total airway resistance).

Tissue Viscoelastic Resistance

It had been assumed that airway (frictional) resistance represented the majority of total respiratory system resistance during breathing. The pressure needed to overcome tissue viscous resistance during inspiration was estimated to be about 35% in adults and 28% in children (Bryan and Wohl, 1986). Studies since the 1980s on mechanical ventilation, in both animals and humans, however, have indicated that viscoelastic resistance, or the energy required to counter the hysteresis or viscoelasticity of the lungs and thoracic tissues, contributes a significantly greater proportion of the total resistance than previously assumed (Milic-Emili et al., 1990). Furthermore, both airway resistance (Raw) and viscoelastic resistance (ΔR) have been found to be flow and volume dependent (i.e., both Raw and ΔR change with volume or flow changes) and to the opposite directions. Airway resistance (Raw) increases with increasing flow due to higher turbulence, whereas Raw decreases with increasing lung volume because airway caliber also increases with volume. The traditional view had been that the total resistance followed the same direction of flow resistance because it was thought to be the majority of total respiratory system resistance. Paradoxically, ΔR decreases with increasing flow, while the volume is kept constant; and, while the flow rate is kept constant, ΔR increases with increasing lung volume (D'Angelo et al., 1989) (Fig. 2–28). Furthermore, the direction of changes in total resistance followed that of ΔR, rather than that of Raw. Studies in anesthetized and ventilated children have shown the same flow and volume dependence of ΔR that exist in adults, that is, opposite of the direction of changes in Raw, although the total resistance did not necessarily follow the changes in ΔR (Kaditis et al., 1999a) (Fig. 2–29).

This new evidence on the behavior of viscoelastic resistance has important clinical implications. Traditionally, the patient with airway obstruction has been treated with large tidal volumes and a slow respiratory rate to allow complete exhalation to avoid intrinsic $PEEP_i$ (or auto-PEEP) and air trapping. With the new understanding, it makes more sense to breathe with a smaller VT and higher respiratory rate in order to minimize total respiratory system resistance and decrease work of breathing (Kaditis et al., 1999b).

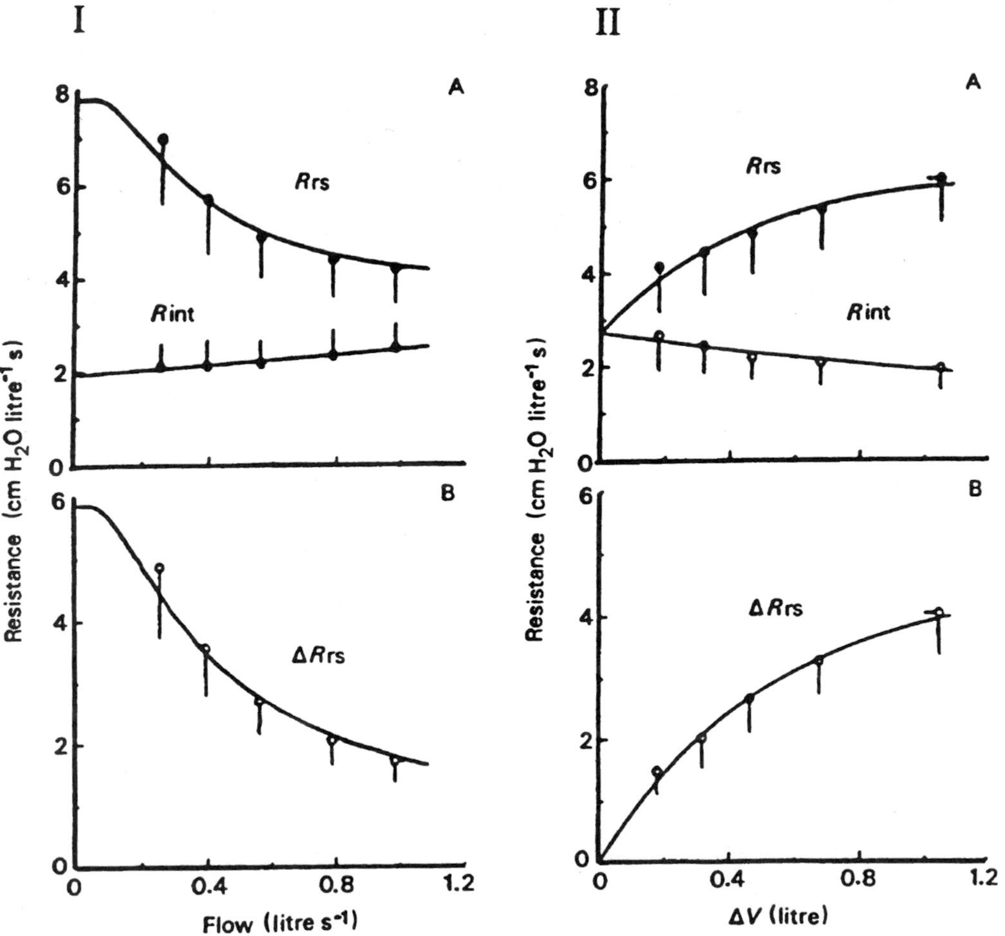

FIGURE 2–28. Flow and volume dependence of respiratory system resistance (Rrs) and its subdivisions, resistive component (Rint, mostly airway resistance Raw) and viscoelastic component (ΔRrs) (Rrs – Rint + ΔRrs). *(IA)* Average relationship of Rrs and Rint with increasing inspiratory flow on X-axis at a constant inspiratory volume (0.47 L) in 16 anesthetized and paralyzed adult subjects. *(IB)* Similar relationship between ΔRrs with variable inspiratory flow. *(IIA)* Average relationship of Rrs and Rint with variable inspiratory volume on X-axis at a constant inspiratory flow (0.56L/s) in the same subjects as IA. *(IIB)* Similar relationship in terms of ΔRrs. Bars, 1SD. (Modified from D'Angelo E, et al.: Respiratory mechanics in anesthetized paralyzed humans. *J Appl Physiol* 67:2556, 1989. Used with permission of the American Physiological Society.)

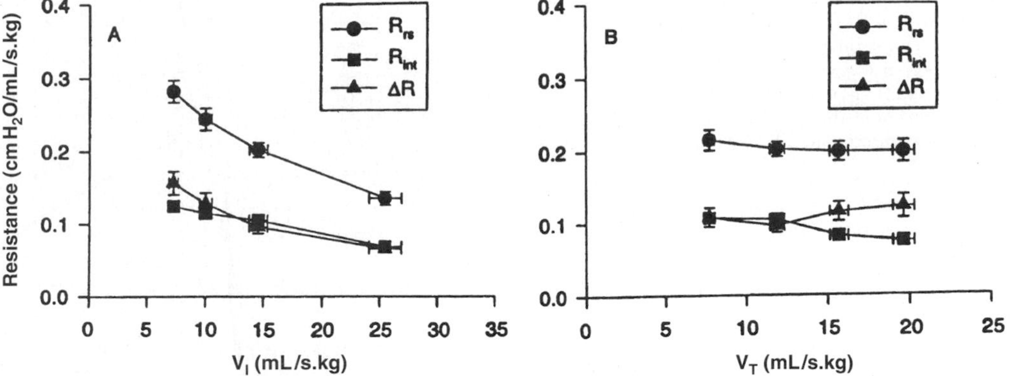

FIGURE 2–29. Flow and volume dependence of respiratory system resistance (Rrs) and its subdivisions, flow-resistive component (Rint or Raw) and viscoelastic component (ΔR) (Rrs = Rint + ΔR), in eight healthy children aged 2 to 5 years under general endotracheal anesthesia. *(A)* Average relationship of Rrs, Rint, and ΔR with increasing inspiratory flow on x-axis at a constant end-inspiratory volume (VT, 12 mL/kg). ΔR and Rrs decreased significantly with increasing flow as in adults (see Fig. 2–27). *(B)* Average relationship of Rrs, Rint, and ΔR with increasing volume on x-axis while flow was kept constant (15 mL/sec per kg) in the same subjects as in *A*. ΔR increased with increasing volume while Rint decreased with volume. Unlike in adults, there was no volume dependence of Rrs. Bars, 1 SEM; $\dot{V}$I, inspiratory flow; VT, tidal volume. (From Kaditis AG, Motoyama EK, Seki I, et al.: *Pediatr Res* 46:419–428, 1999.)

Time Constant of the Respiratory System

When the lung is allowed to empty passively from end-inspiration to FRC, the speed of lung deflation is determined by the product of respiratory system resistance and compliance (R × C or R/E), which is a unit of time (time constant, τ). If the respiratory system is considered as a single compartment with a constant resistance and compliance within the tidal volume range of breathing (which is a reasonable assumption in healthy individuals), then τ = RC.

Under these conditions, the volume-time profile can be represented by an exponential decay and at 1 time constant (1τ), tidal volume is reduced by 63%. It requires 3 × τ to nearly complete exhalation to FRC. In healthy children and adults, τ is 0.4 to 0.5 second; it is slightly shorter in neonates (0.2 to 0.3 second) (Bryan and Wohl, 1986). In patients with obstructive lung disease, such as bronchial asthma, τ is increased due to an increase in airway resistance; it is also increased markedly in patients breathing through an endotracheal tube under general anesthesia.

Maximum Expiratory Flow-Volume Curve and the Concept of Flow Limitation

During quiet breathing, pleural pressure remains subatmospheric, whereas during forced expiration, pleural pressure increases considerably above atmospheric pressure and, in turn, increases alveolar pressure. The resultant pressure gradient between the alveoli and the airway opening (atmospheric) produces the expiratory flow. In the periphery of the lungs this pressure within the airways is higher than the pleural pressure because of the elastic recoil of the lung. In comparison, in major intrathoracic airways the pressure within the lumen is near atmospheric and lower than the surrounding pleural pressure. At some point along the airways the pressure within the airway lumen should equal the pleural pressure surrounding the airway (equal pressure point [EPP]) (Mead et al., 1967). During forced expiration, the airway between EPP and the trachea is dynamically compressed, and the flow rates consequently become independent of effort (i.e., additional expiratory effort or pressure does not increase flow) (Fig. 2–30). Under these circumstances (dynamic flow limitation), the maximum expiratory flow rate ($\dot{V}$max) is determined by the flow resistance of the upstream segment (Rus) between the alveoli and the EPP and the elastic recoil pressure of the lung (Pstl), as follows (Mead et al., 1967):

$$\dot{V}max = \frac{Pstl}{Rus}$$

According to the wave-speed theory of expiratory flow limitation (Dawson and Elliot, 1977), compliance or collapsibility of lower airways around the EPP (choke point) is an additional determinant of $\dot{V}$max (Hyatt, 1986).

The maximum expiratory flow-volume (MEFV) curve obtained during forced expiration from TLC to RV relates instantaneous maximum expiratory flow rates ($\dot{V}$max) to corresponding lung volumes (Fig. 2–31). Clinically, the measurement of $\dot{V}$max is an extremely sensitive test for the detection of obstruction of the lower airways toward the periphery (silent zone) of the lungs because it eliminates the component of upper airway resistance

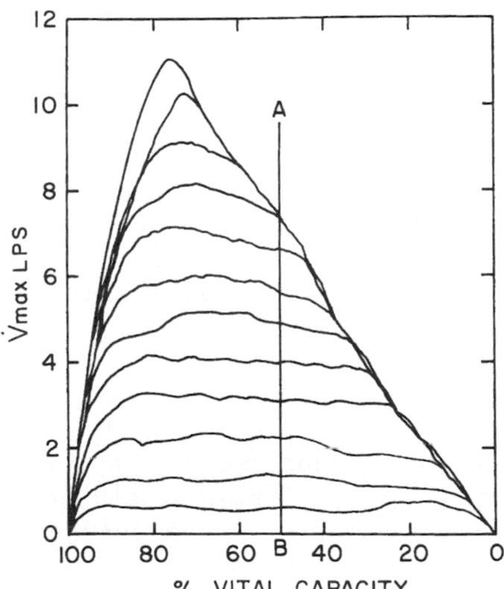

■ **FIGURE 2–30.** Flow-volume curves obtained when a subject performs a series of vital capacity expirations of graded effort, varying from a very slow breath out to one of maximal speed and effort. (From Bates DV, Macklem PT, Christie RV, editors: *Respiratory function in disease. An introduction to the integrated study of the lung.* Philadelphia, 1971, WB Saunders.)

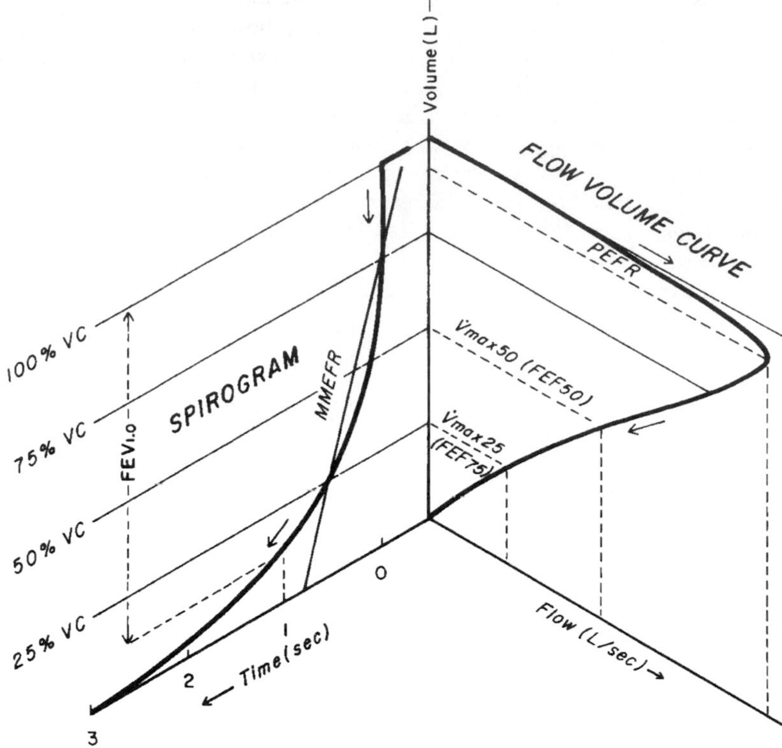

■ **FIGURE 2–31.** Maximum expiratory flow volume (MEFV) curve on volume-flow axis on the right is contrasted with spirometric tracing (spirogram) on volume-time axis on the left during a single forced vital capacity (VC) maneuver. $FEV_{1.0}$, Forced expiratory volume in 1 second; PEFR, peak expiratory flow rate; $\dot{V}max_{50}$, $\dot{V}max_{25}$, maximum expiratory flow at 50% and 25%, respectively, of forced VC. (From Motoyama EK: *Int Anesthesiol Clin* 26:6, 1988.)

between the mouth and EPP and is independent of the degree of effort or cooperation by the patient (Zapletal et al., 1971) (also see under Measurements of pulmonary function below).

Distribution of Flow Resistance

On the basis of physiologic measurements in lungs obtained at autopsy, Hogg and others (1970) reported that airway conductance of the peripheral airways in children less than 6 years of age was disproportionately low (i.e., resistance was high). They postulated that the diameter of small airways of the same generation was disproportionately smaller in infants than in older children and adults. Although this theory is consistent with the high incidence of severe lower airway disease in infants, it conflicts with later physiologic data obtained from healthy infants. Studies of MEFV curves in anesthetized infants and children (Motoyama, 1977), and more recently in sedated infants (Lambert et al., 2004), showed that at low lung volumes, the maximum expiratory flow ($\dot{V}max$) normalizes for lung volume and the conductance of the upstream segment is disproportionately high in infants and decreases with age (Motoyama, 1977), indicating that lower airway resistance toward the periphery of the lung parenchyma is relatively lower, rather than higher, in the early postnatal years (Fig. 2–32).

■ SUMMARY

Compliance of the respiratory system has both lung and chest wall components. During artificial ventilation of a healthy adult, about one half of the inspiratory pressure is required to expand the lungs and one half to expand the chest wall. In infants, the chest wall is extremely compliant and requires little pressure to expand. Accordingly, airway pressure during artificial ventilation should be reduced. In absolute terms, lung compliance increases with body or lung size. In relative terms, however, lung compliance is relatively high in infants and decreases with age, as elastic recoil pressure of the lungs increases. Most of the flow resistive force against breathing is exerted within the upper and large central airways; the small airways contribute only a fraction of total flow resistance. Flow resistance in absolute terms is largest when air passages are smallest; thus, infants are more

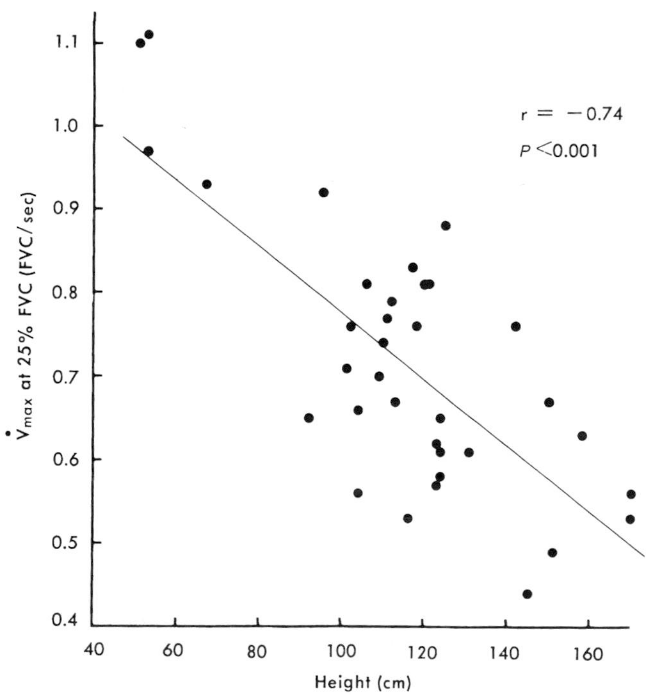

■ **FIGURE 2–32.** Maximum expiratory flow rate ($\dot{V}max$) at 25% forced vital capacity (FVC) from forced deflation flow-volume curves versus height in anesthetized boys and girls. $\dot{V}max_{25}$ is expressed in FVC units per second to normalize for lung size. FVC-adjusted $\dot{V}max_{25}$ is disproportionately higher in infants than in older children. (From Motoyama EK: *Pediatr Res* 11:220, 1977.)

prone to airway obstruction of the upper and lower airways. When lung volumes are taken into account, however, total airway resistance is relatively low during the newborn period and increases rapidly during the first year, as lung volume increases with alveolar formation. Resistance of smaller (parenchymal) airways appears to be relatively low at birth and increases with age. The contribution of viscoelastic resistance from the lung and thoracic tissue hysteresis has been found to be much larger than had been recognized in the past. Both flow-resistive and tissue viscoelastic resistance change with increasing flow and volume, but the directions of changes are opposite to each other. Forming a complex mechanism, the tonic activities of the pharyngeal and laryngeal dilator muscles protect the pharyngeal airway from collapse. During spontaneous breathing, the genioglossus and other upper airway muscles contract synchronously with the diaphragm and increase upper airway caliber. These muscles are easily depressed by sleep and anesthesia, causing upper airway obstruction both at the velopharynx and, to a lesser extent, at the base of the tongue, resulting in upper airway obstruction during anesthesia.

VENTILATION

Ventilation involves the movement of air in and out of the lungs. The diaphragm is the most important muscle for normal inspiration, although the intercostal and accessory respiratory muscles aid in a maximal inspiratory effort. Quiet expiration results from the elastic recoil of the lungs and chest wall and the relaxation of the diaphragm. The expiration of a newborn, even when resting or asleep, appears active rather than passive, as in the older child and adult. A similar active expiration has been observed in anesthetized patients (Freund et al., 1964), but the mechanism is unknown. Forced expiration is accomplished with the aid of the spinal flexors, the intercostal muscles, and especially the abdominal muscles.

Tidal volume (V_T) is the amount of air moved into or out of the lungs with each breath. Minute volume ($\dot{V}_E$) is the amount of air breathed in or out in a minute, or as follows:

$$\dot{V}_E = V_T \times f$$

The frequency (f) of quiet breathing decreases with increasing age. The exact basis for this change is unknown but may be related to the work of breathing. Humans seem to adjust their respiratory rate and tidal volume so that ventilatory needs are accomplished with a minimum of work (McIlroy et al., 1954). The relatively high rate in newborns (average, 34 breaths/min) as compared with adults (10 to 12 breaths/min) is consistent with this minimum work concept (Cook et al., 1957) (Fig. 2–33). Mead (1960), however, has presented data indicating that in the normal resting state, respiration is adjusted to require a minimum average force of the respiratory muscles. He postulated that the principal site of the sensory end of the control mechanism is in the lungs. In certain situations, the minimum work of breathing and minimum average force required would occur at the same frequency of respiration, but this would not invariably be true.

DEAD SPACE AND ALVEOLAR VENTILATION

Only part of the minute volume is effective in gas exchange—the alveolar ventilation ($\dot{V}_A$). The remainder merely ventilates the respiratory dead space. If the minute noneffective ventilation ($\dot{V}_E - \dot{V}_A$) is divided by the frequency, the physiologic respiratory dead space is calculated. In the normal person, the physiologic and anatomic dead spaces are approximately equal because alveolar dead space is negligible. Because the air passages are compliant structures, the size of the dead space correlates closely with the degree of lung expansion. When airway obstruction and emphysema are present, dead space increases. However, physiologic dead space is influenced more by the evenness of gas distribution within the lungs and by the perfusion of the alveoli. Thus,

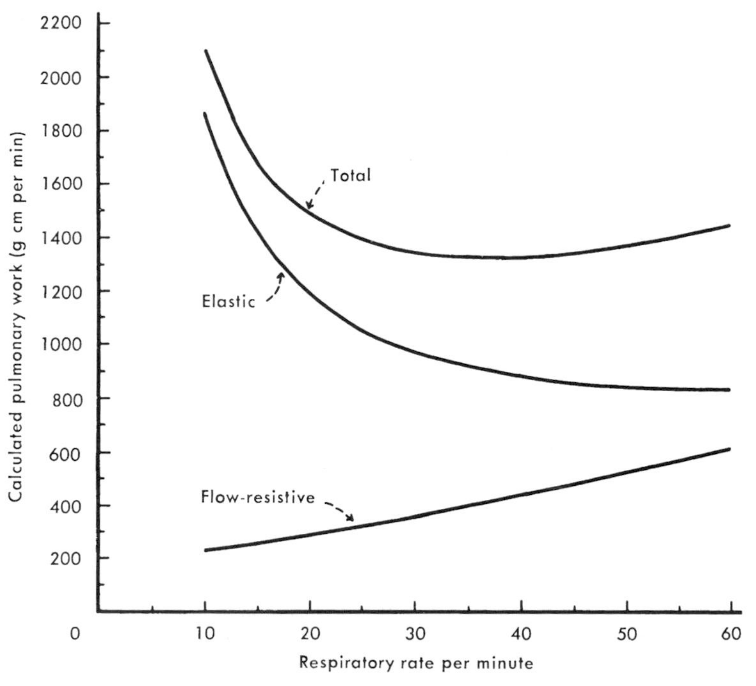

FIGURE 2–33. Calculated pulmonary work in newborns versus respiratory rate. The theoretical minimum work of respiration occurs at a rate of 37 breaths/min. Observed resting respiratory rates were 38 breaths/min. (From Cook CD, Sutherland JM, Segal S, et al.: *J Clin Invest* 36:440, 1957.)

when ventilation of the lungs is uneven (as in asthma or cystic fibrosis) or the blood supply to various areas of the lungs decreases (as with pulmonary emboli), the physiologic dead space increases.

Although the anatomic dead space represents an inefficient part of the respiratory tract with respect to gas exchange, it does have two important functions: warming and humidifying gas on inspiration. These functions are compromised by endotracheal intubation or tracheostomy.

In a normal person, dead space can be estimated as 1 mL/pound of body weight (Radford et al., 1954). In children and young adults, a more exact estimate may be obtained from its relation to body height (Hart et al., 1963).

The VD/VT ratio in normal lungs is approximately constant (0.3) from infancy to adulthood (see Table 2–2). An absolute increase in dead space, however, whether caused by respiratory abnormalities or external apparatus, is much more critical to the infant than to the adult because of the infant's small tidal volume and the relatively larger volume of dead space added.

Alveolar ventilation ($\dot{V}A$), or the minute effective ventilation, may be expressed in terms of the carbon dioxide in the peripheral arterial blood. Thus, the following equation is applicable:

$$\dot{V}A = \frac{(PB - 47) \times \dot{V}CO_2}{PaCO_2}$$

where $\dot{V}CO_2$ is the carbon dioxide production per minute, $PaCO_2$ is the arterial carbon dioxide tension, and PB − 47 is the barometric pressure minus water vapor tension at 37 °C.

The difference between minute volume and alveolar ventilation ($\dot{V}E - \dot{V}A$) is the wasted ventilation due to physiologic dead space. The concept of $\dot{V}A$ may be easier to understand if considered similar in some way to the renal clearance of a substance; in the lungs, carbon dioxide is the substance being cleared. If $\dot{V}CO_2$ remains constant when $\dot{V}A$ is halved, $PaCO_2$ will double. Measurement of $\dot{V}A$ provides a far better index of the efficacy of ventilation than measurement of $\dot{V}E$. $\dot{V}E$ may be very large, but if it is composed mostly of dead space or ineffective ventilation, $\dot{V}E$ may be inadequate and $PaCO_2$ may start to increase.

Physiologic dead space is calculated from the carbon dioxide tensions between arterial blood and mixed expired gas ($PECO_2$) and is often expressed as a fraction of the tidal volume:

$$\frac{VD}{VT} = \frac{(PaCO_2 - PECO_2)}{PaCO_2}$$

Alveolar ventilation is considerably higher per unit of lung volume in the normal infant than in the adult. This is expected because the oxygen consumption is also higher per unit of lung volume or body weight in the infant (Cook et al., 1955).

DISTRIBUTION OF VENTILATION

The distribution of ventilation is affected by a number of factors. At end-expiration with the mouth open and the larynx relaxed, alveolar pressure is zero, or atmospheric. The interpleural pressure is negative, and there is a vertical pressure gradient. The pressure surrounding the apex of the lung is more negative than that at the base. Accordingly, the transmural or distending pressure at the apex is greater and the regional FRC is larger than that at the base (Fig. 2–34*A*). At the end of tidal inspiration, a

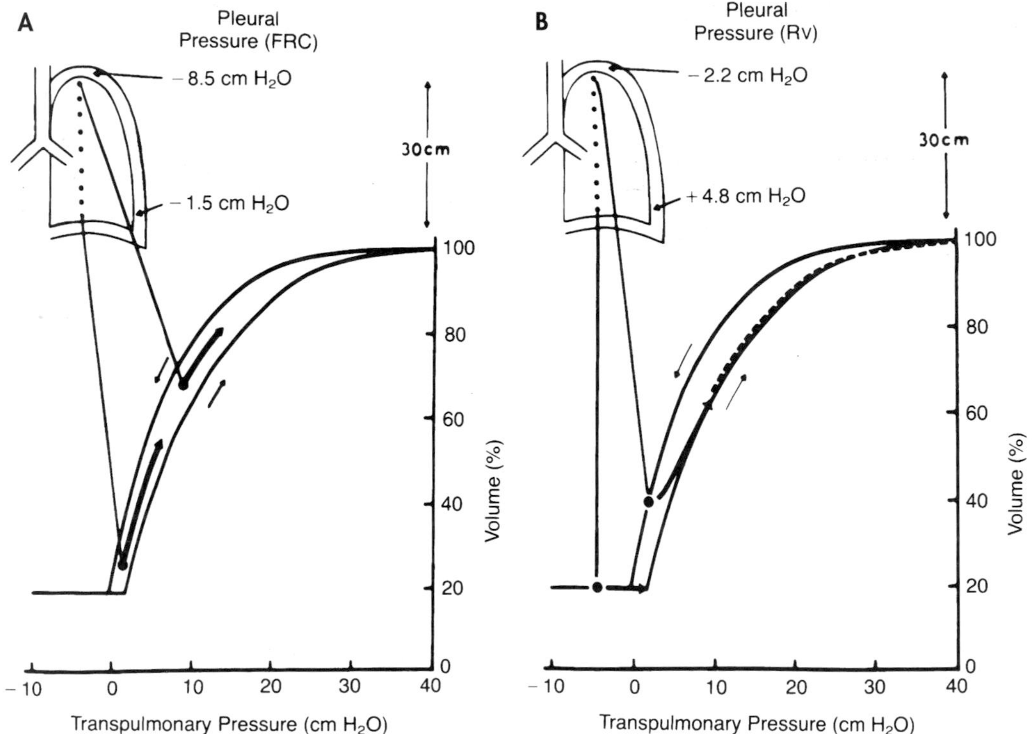

FIGURE 2–34 Effect of vertical gradient of pleural surface pressure on distribution of tidal ventilation. *(A)* At the beginning of lung inflation from functional residual capacity (FRC), lower regions are operating on a steeper part of the compliance curve of lungs than upper regions. Accordingly, during slow inspiration from FRC, ventilation is greater in lower lung regions *(arrows)*. *(B)* At residual volume (RV), pleural surface pressure at lung base is positive (+4.8 cm H_2O) and lower airways are closed. Consequently, at the beginning of slow inspiration from RV, lower lung regions are not ventilated and the uppermost part of the lung is preferentially ventilated *(arrows)*. (From Milic-Emili J: Pulmonary statics. In Widdicomb JG, editor: *Respiratory physiology, MTP International Review of Science. Series I, vol 2.* Borough Green, Kent, 1974, Butterworth.)

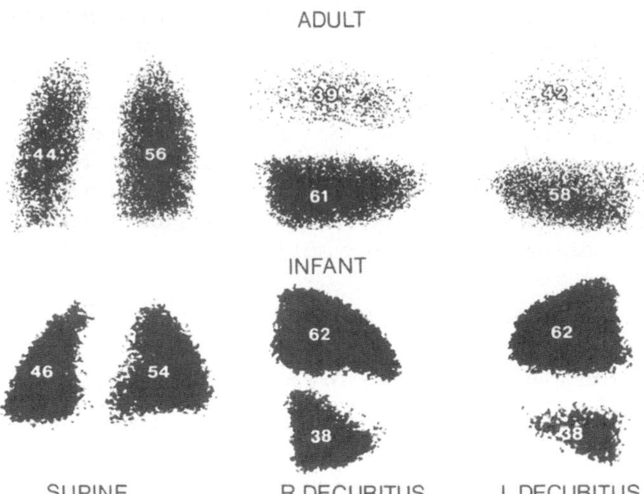

■ **FIGURE 2–35.** Posterior krypton 81m ventilation lung scan in a healthy 31-year-old man and in a 2-month-old girl. In the adult, ventilation is preferentially distributed to the dependent lung; in the infant, the reverse is seen, with ventilation greater in the uppermost lung. For all scans, the distribution of ventilation to each lung is expressed as a percentage of the total to both lungs. (From Heaf DP, Helms P, Gordon I, et al.: *N Engl J Med* 308:1505, 1983, with permission. Copyright © 1983. Massachusetts Medical Society. All rights reserved.)

greater proportion of the inspired air is distributed to the base because the regional FRC is at the steepest portion of the pressure-volume curve at the base. In a lateral decubitus position, the lower part of the lung receives a larger tidal volume than the upper part (Kaneko et al., 1966). In adults with unilateral lung disease, pulmonary gas exchange can be improved by positioning with the healthy lung down, or dependent (Remolina et al., 1981).

In infants with unilateral lung disease, however, the opposite seems to be the case. In the lateral decubitus position, oxygenation improves when the healthy lung is uppermost (Heaf et al., 1983; Davies et al., 1985). Furthermore, Heaf and others (1983) have shown, by means of a krypton-81m ventilation scan, that in infants and children up to 27 months of age, with or without radiologic evidence of lung disease, ventilation is preferentially increased in the uppermost part of the lung and diminished in the dependent lung (Fig. 2–35). This paradoxical distribution of ventilation in young children may be explained by premature airway closure (Davies et al., 1985). Because the infant's chest wall is extremely compliant the pleural pressure is near atmospheric. The condition resembles that of adults breathing at extremely low lung volumes (or near RV) (see Fig. 2–34*B*). Under these circumstances, airway closure occurs and, in the lateral decubitus position, ventilation preferentially shifts to the uppermost part of the lung (Milic-Emili et al., 1966). In paralyzed, mechanically ventilated adults, tidal ventilation is preferentially shifted to the uppermost part of the lung, presumably by a similar mechanism (i.e., reduction of FRC and airway closure) (Rehder et al., 1972).

Distortion of regional mechanical properties in the lungs results in far greater variations in the distribution of ventilation than is produced by gravitational forces. The product of regional flow resistance (R, expressed as pressure/flow in cm H_2O/mL/sec) and compliance (C, expressed as volume/pressure in mL/cm H_2O) determines the regional ventilation in the lungs. The product of resistance and compliance (RC) is a unit of time, termed the time constant (τ), as has been discussed earlier. In diseased lungs, as in asthma, bronchopulmonary dysplasia, and cystic fibrosis, the regional time constant becomes abnormal in affected areas, resulting in an uneven distribution of ventilation. The distribution of ventilation may be studied by measuring a nitrogen washout curve. The subject breathes 100% oxygen, and the decay of the alveolar nitrogen concentration is measured in successive expirations. Both in normal children and adults, nitrogen concentration is less than 2.5% after 7 minutes of oxygen breathing. This value is increased in patients with an uneven distribution of ventilation because the elimination of nitrogen from poorly ventilated areas is prolonged. In addition, radioactive xenon ventilation scans have been used to demonstrate macroscopic ventilatory abnormalities to aid in the interpretation of perfusion lung scans.

■ CLINICAL IMPLICATIONS

The anesthesiologist often controls a patient's ventilation manually or mechanically during general anesthesia because most anesthetic techniques cause spontaneous ventilation to decrease or cease. This is because most anesthetics are potent respiratory depressants and because the endotracheal tube and the anesthesia circuit add elastic and resistive loads to breathing. Because anesthesia generally causes a decrease in FRC, the uneven distribution of ventilation, and an increase in physiologic dead space, the tidal volume must be increased. The mechanical dead space and internal compliance of anesthetic equipment also must be taken into account for the proper estimation of a patient's ventilatory requirement. Physiologic dead space is further increased in patients with preexistent lung dysfunction. For these reasons, it is practical to start with a tidal volume of 10 to 15 mL/kg, or roughly 1.5 to 2.0 times that required in awake individuals.

The inspiratory-to-expiratory (I/E) ratio is set to 1:2, a duty cycle (TI/TTOT) of 0.33. Respiratory frequency should be 10 to 14/min in adolescents, 14 to 20/min in children, and 20 to 30/min in infants. Once the mechanical ventilation is established, it can be decreased and refined with the aid of capnographic monitoring. In patients with obstructive lung disease who have a prolonged respiratory system time constant, expiratory time is increased to allow sufficient time for passive lung deflation. Passive expiration is an exponential function and takes three times the time constant to return to FRC (Nunn, 1994). The addition of a low level of PEEP (5 to 7 cm H_2O) restores the volume (FRC) lost from the relaxation of inspiratory muscles and helps prevent airway closure.

■ SUMMARY

Ventilation comprises effective (alveolar) and dead space ventilation. In healthy subjects, ventilation in relation to body size is increased in early infancy and then remains fairly constant throughout childhood and adolescence. Changes in Pa_{O_2} reflect changes in alveolar ventilation; thus capnographic monitoring of end-tidal P_{CO_2} is useful for adjusting and maintaining appropriate alveolar ventilation. There is a vertical, hydrostatic gradient in negative pressure in the pleural space. Uneven distribution of ventilation exists both in health and in disease. The regional resting volume (FRC) is highest in the uppermost part of the lung, whereas the regional tidal volume is largest in the lowermost region of the lung in a spontaneously breathing subject. The opposite relationship exists in spontaneously breathing infants as well as in patients under anesthesia who are mechanically ventilated. In diseased lungs, uneven distribution of regional compliance (C), resistance (R), and a time constant (R × C) cause maldistribution of ventilation and increased physiologic dead space.

■ GAS DIFFUSION

The ultimate purpose of pulmonary ventilation is to allow the diffusion of oxygen through the alveolar epithelial lining, basement membrane, and capillary endothelial wall into the plasma and red cells and diffusion of carbon dioxide in the opposite direction. The distance for gases to diffuse between the alveolar space and the capillary lumen is extremely small, about 0.3 μm in humans (Weibel, 1973). Because these processes apparently follow the physical laws of diffusion, without any active participation by the lung tissue, pressure gradients must exist or gas exchange will not occur. On the other hand, if the gradient is increased by changes in gas tension either within the alveoli or in the blood, gas exchange is more rapid. Furthermore, since the blood PO_2 affects the blood PCO_2, changes in one moiety alter diffusion of the other. Carbon dioxide diffuses approximately 20 times faster than oxygen in a gas-liquid environment. Therefore, impairment of carbon dioxide diffusion does not become apparent in clinical situations until extremely severe disease is present.

The diffusing capacity of the lungs may be measured with a foreign gas, carbon monoxide, used in small concentrations (≤0.3%), or with various concentrations of inspired oxygen (Forster, 1957). The subjects of diffusion and diffusing capacity have been reviewed.

The diffusing capacity (DLCO) of carbon monoxide (CO) can be measured with a single breath technique by adding an inert gas to the inhaled gas mixture with a single alveolar gas sample (Ogilve et al., 1957). The DLCO test is not exactly a measure of diffusing capacity since "diffusing" implies that the uptake of CO is attributable to diffusion alone and "capacity" implies it is a maximal limit (Crapo et al., 2001). Indeed, the term "transfer factor" (TLCO) has become a standard term in most countries outside of North America (Forster, 1983; Cotes et al., 1993). The role of DLCO measurement in lung function testing is to provide information on the transport of gas from alveolar air to hemoglobin in pulmonary capillaries. More specifically, DLCO measures the uptake of CO from the lungs per minute per unit of CO driving pressure, as follows:

$$D_{LCO} = \frac{\dot{V}_{CO}}{(P_{ACO} - P_{cCO})}$$

where $\dot{V}_{CO}$ is uptake of CO (mL/min), P_{ACO} is alveolar partial pressure of CO, and P_{cCO} is average pulmonary capillary partial pressure of CO. Because the basic equation is flow/pressure change ($\dot{V}/\Delta P$), DLCO is a measure of conductance (G = 1/R).

Although the diffusion of gases within the lung is necessary for survival, comparatively few conditions occurring in children affect diffusion per se. Diffusing capacity is decreased in the "alveolar capillary block syndrome" (Bates, 1962). This decrease was considered to result primarily from increased thickness of the alveolocapillary membranes; but it is now believed that uneven distribution of ventilation with a resulting ventilation/perfusion imbalance is the more important cause of arterial oxygen desaturation (Finley et al., 1962). Diffusing capacity changes with hemoglobin concentrations; it increases as hemoglobin concentration increases. A correction factor has to be used according to the recommendation of American Thoracic Society guidelines (1995). Anemia, on the other hand, is associated with a decrease in diffusing capacity. This is partially explained by the decreased ability of blood to carry the inspired gases. Patients with congenital heart disease and left-to-right shunts frequently have an increased DLCO caused by increased blood volume and flow in the lungs (Bucci and Cook, 1961). Conversely, diffusing capacity may be reduced when the pulmonary blood flow is markedly decreased, as in pulmonic stenosis.

■ PULMONARY CIRCULATION

PERINATAL AND POSTNATAL ADAPTATION

In prenatal life, pulmonary vascular resistance is high and most of the right ventricular output runs parallel to the left ventricular output, bypassing the lungs and flowing into the descending aorta through the ductus arteriosus. With the onset of ventilation at birth, the pulmonary vascular resistance suddenly decreases and blood flow through the lungs increases, enabling the organism to exchange oxygen and carbon dioxide and sustain independent existence. The principal factors that control this vital adjustment in vascular resistance are chemical changes (i.e., changes in PO_2 and PCO_2 or pH) in the environment of the pulmonary vessels (Cook et al., 1963). An increase in PO_2 also produces constriction and subsequent closure of the ductus arteriosus. The pulmonary arterial pressure, which is slightly higher than the pressure in the ascending aorta in the fetus (Assali and Morris, 1964), suddenly decreases at birth and then continues to decrease, with a gradual decline in pulmonary vascular smooth muscle mass approaching the adult level within the first year of life (Rudolph, 1970). If the lungs do not expand adequately (as in RDS of the neonate) and PO_2 remains low, the pulmonary vascular resistance and pressure may remain high, and there may be prolonged patency of the ductus arteriosus and persistent right-to-left shunting of blood (Strang and MacLeish, 1961) (also see Chapter 3, Cardiovascular Physiology).

Under normal postnatal conditions, the systemic and pulmonary vascular beds are connected in series to form a continuous circuit. Although the systemic circulation has a high vascular resistance with a large pressure gradient between the arteries and veins, the pulmonary circulation presents a low resistance to flow.

Both hypoxemia and hypercapnia constrict the pulmonary vascular bed and increase resistance to flow. Chronic hypoxemia is associated with a pulmonary hypertension that returns to or toward normal when the hypoxemia is corrected (Goldring et al., 1964). Pulmonary hypertension that persists for months or years results in right-sided heart failure (cor pulmonale), which then further complicates the existing pulmonary insufficiency.

Under normal circumstances, the arterial blood from the left ventricle contains up to 5% unsaturated blood (venous admixture). This comes mainly from the bronchial circulation but also in part from blood in the pulmonary circulation bypassing the alveoli and from blood flowing through the thebesian veins. This physiologic venous admixture depresses the arterial PO_2 from approximately 102 to 97 mm Hg. In certain conditions, such as ventilation/perfusion imbalance (including decreased diffusing capacity), the amount of the venous admixture through the lungs increases sufficiently to cause significant arterial hypoxemia. Venous admixture also occurs because of intrapulmonary shunting as the result of atelectasis, pulmonary arteriovenous fistula, pulmonary hemangiomas, and increased collateral (bronchial) circulation, as in bronchiectasis. In addition, shunting may occur at the cardiac level when there is congenital heart disease with right-to-left shunting.

NITRIC OXIDE AND PULMONARY CIRCULATION

The vascular endothelial cells release various vasoactive factors that affect vascular tone. The endothelium-derived relaxing factor (EDRF), first described by Furchgott and Zawadski (1980), has been identified as nitric oxide (NO) (Ignaro et al., 1987; Palmer et al., 1987). NO is a unique endogenous regulatory molecule involved in a wide variety of biologic activities, including systemic and pulmonary vasodilation, neurotransmission, and immunomodulation (Welch and Loscalzo, 1994). Under physiologic conditions, nitric oxide is produced from the amino acid L-arginine catalyzed by constitutive nitric oxide synthase (cNOS) with a number of cofactors (NADPH, flavoproteins, tetrahydrobiopterin, reduced glutathione, and heme complex) and with the presence of ionized calcium and calmodulin. NO in the vascular endothelial cells diffuses into the adjacent vascular smooth muscle cells, stimulates guanylate cyclase activity, and increases cyclic guanylate monophosphate (cGMP), resulting in controlled smooth muscle relaxation and vasodilation (Furchgott and Vanhoutte, 1989; Moncada et al., 1989). In normal lungs, basal release of endothelium-derived NO contributes to the maintenance of low pulmonary vascular resistance (Celemajer et al., 1994; Stamler et al., 1994).

Certain cytokines and bacterial endotoxins induce a nitric oxide synthase isoform (inducible NOS [iNOS]) in macrophages, neutrophils, vascular and airway smooth muscles, and other cell types that normally do not produce cNOS. A massive release of NO by iNOS via activated macrophages and other cell types appears to be the primary cause of profound vasodilation and systemic hypotension in septic shock (Cohen, 1995).

NO is one of the principal industrial pollutants oxidized in the atmosphere to form highly toxic nitrogen dioxide (NO_2); NO_2, in turn, combines with water to form nitric acid (H_2NO_3), the cause of acid rain. Inhaled NO below the concentration of industrial safety standards (5 to 40 ppm) has been shown to be effective against experimental hypoxic pulmonary vasoconstriction and pulmonary hypertension by selectively dilating the vascular beds surrounding terminal air spaces that are ventilated (Frostell et al., 1993). Consequently, the ventilation/perfusion balance is improved and the venous admixture is decreased (Fratacci et al., 1991; Frostell et al., 1991; Pison et al., 1993). This selective pulmonary vasodilation results from the inactivation of nitric oxide by hemoglobin (Rimar and Gillis, 1993).

The use of inhaled NO appears safe in clinical settings because the exhaled concentration is extremely low and the production of toxic nitrogen dioxide is miniscule (Jacob et al., 1994). NO combines with hemoglobin and produces nitrosyl hemoglobin, but the level remains extremely low during continuous inhalation of NO (40 ppm) for 4 hours. The level of methemoglobin in blood is relatively low and remains stable during the same period, although the plasma levels of nitrite (NO_2) and nitrate (NO_3) increase with time (Jacob et al., 1994). Early clinical trials with inhaled NO in newborns with persistent pulmonary hypertension of neonates (PPHN) (Kinsella et al., 1992; Roberts et al., 1992), in newborns with congenital diaphragmatic hernia (Shah et al., 1994), in infants with congenital heart disease (Roberts et al., 1993; Wessel, 1993; Adatia and Wessel, 1994), and in those with adult respiratory distress syndrome (ARDS) (Rossaint et al., 1993; Bigatello et al., 1994; Puybasset et al., 1994) showed effectiveness but such treatment has not always been effective.

Studies have shown that various inhaled anesthetics attenuate endothelium-dependent relaxation of vascular ring preparations in vitro (Muldoon et al., 1988; Johns et al., 1992; Toda et al., 1992). The mechanism of this paradoxical phenomenon is not clear, but it may be related to the effect of anesthetics that reduces the intracellular influx of ionized calcium, a catalyst essential for NOS to form NO from L-arginine (Muldoon et al., 1988). Yoshida and Okabe (1992) postulated that the anesthetic sevoflurane increases oxygen free radicals, which, in turn, combine with NO and block its vasodilating effect because an addition of superoxide dismutase blocks the effect of anesthetics that antagonize endothelium-derived vasodilation.

DISTRIBUTION OF PULMONARY PERFUSION

As with regional ventilation, gravity results in a nonuniform distribution of pulmonary blood flow in normal lungs. West and others (1965) divided the characteristics of upright lung perfusion into three zones, later modified to four zones, of flow distribution (Hughes et al., 1968) (Fig. 2–36). Perfusion of lung tissue depends on the interrelation among three pressures: alveolar pressure (PA), pulmonary arterial pressure (Pa), and pulmonary venous pressure (Pv). Because pulmonary circulation normally is a low-pressure circuit, the pulmonary perfusion pressure varies from the top to the bottom of the lung, barely overcoming the hydrostatic pressure to reach the apex of the tall upright adult lung. Both pulmonary perfusion pressure and flow are relatively increased at the lung base (West, 1994).

In zone I, the apicalmost part, alveolar pressure is higher than both pulmonary arterial and venous pressures. Alveolar capillary

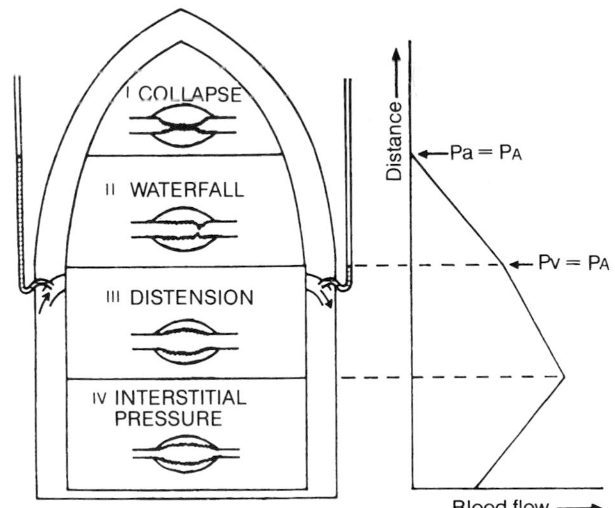

FIGURE 2–36. Four zones of lung perfusion. Zone I has no flow because alveolar pressure exceeds pulmonary arterial pressure, thereby collapsing alveolar vessels. Zone II is present when pulmonary arterial pressure exceeds alveolar pressure and both are greater than pulmonary venous pressure. This is termed the vascular waterfall, because flow is unaffected by downstream (pulmonary venous) pressure. Zone III is characterized by a constant driving force, the difference between pulmonary arterial and venous pressure. Both are greater than alveolar pressure. Flow increases throughout zone III, even though driving pressure is constant because the absolute pressures lower in the lung distend the vessels to a greater extent, thereby lowering resistance. Zone IV has less flow per unit lung volume, probably because of the increased parenchymal pressure surrounding pulmonary vessels. (From Hughes JMB, Glazier JB, Maloney JE, West JB: *Respir Physiol* 4:58, 1968. With permission from Elsevier.)

blood flow is absent in this zone or is only intermittently occurring with peak pulsatile pressure and flow. Ventilation in zone I is mostly wasted. Excessive PEEP increases zone I, thus increasing alveolar dead space, whereas increased pulmonary perfusion pressure, as occurs in exercise or hypoxemia, decreases or abolishes zone I.

In zone II (waterfall zone), as the vertical distance above the heart decreases (with alveolar pressure uniform throughout the lung), arterial pressure becomes higher than surrounding alveolar pressure while venous pressure remains lower than alveolar pressure. The driving pressure in this zone is the difference between arterial and alveolar pressures (Pa − PA), which determines blood flow regardless of venous or downstream pressure (waterfall phenomenon). The blood flow increases linearly as the driving pressure increases toward the base of the lung until pulmonary venous pressure equals alveolar pressure.

In zone III, both arterial and venous pressures are higher than alveolar pressure. The driving pressure for blood flow becomes the difference between arterial and venous pressures (Pa − PV) throughout this zone. Although the pressure gradient is the same throughout zone III, blood flow is greater toward the base, presumably because both arterial and venous pressures are greater and the pulmonary vascular bed is more distended. The relationships among arterial, venous, and alveolar pressures in zones I to III are summarized as follows:

Zone I: PA > Pa > PV
Zone II: Pa > PA > PV
Zone III: Pa > PV > PA

In zone IV, blood flow is progressively decreased toward the base of the lung, presumably because of increased interstitial pressure surrounding the extra-alveolar vessels. This zone increases in size with reduction in the lung volume toward RV (Hughes et al., 1968; West, 1994).

The vertical distance between the top and the bottom of the lung is decreased in the supine position, resulting in the disappearance of zone I. Zone II also decreases as pulmonary venous pressure becomes higher throughout the lung in the supine position. The effect of gravity in infants and small children, particularly in the supine position, would be small, although it has not been documented.

VENTILATION/PERFUSION RELATIONSHIPS

To achieve normal gas exchange in the lung the regional distribution of ventilation and pulmonary perfusion must be balanced. Without this balance, pulmonary gas exchange is impaired, even when the overall levels of ventilation and perfusion are adequate. The normal value for the ventilation/perfusion ($\dot{V}A/\dot{Q}P$ but usually $\dot{V}A/\dot{Q}$ is used instead) ratio is about 0.8. Studies with radioactive gases have shown that the elastic and resistive properties of various parts of the lung, as well as the pulmonary blood flow, are influenced by gravity. Both components of the $\dot{V}A/\dot{Q}$ ratio are affected by changes in a patient's position (West, 1965).

When the patient is in the upright position, blood flow and ventilation are both less in the apex than in the base of the lungs. Because the difference in blood flow between apex and base is relatively greater than that in ventilation, the $\dot{V}A/\dot{Q}$ ratio increases from the bottom to the top of the lungs, as shown in Figures 2–37 and 2–38. The apical regions (high $\dot{V}A/\dot{Q}$) have higher alveolar PO_2 and lower PCO_2 and PN_2, whereas the basal areas (low $\dot{V}A/\dot{Q}$) have lower PO_2 and higher PCO_2 and PN_2. Gravity has a greater effect on the $\dot{V}A/\dot{Q}$ ratio in hypotensive and hypovolemic patients and may be exaggerated with positive-pressure ventilation. In the supine position, similar differences exist between the anterior and posterior parts of the lung, but they are smaller. During exercise, pulmonary arterial pressure and blood flow, as well as ventilation, are increased and more evenly distributed. In infants and children the distribution of pulmonary blood flow is more uniform than in adults because the pulmonary arterial pressure is relatively high and the gravity effect in the lungs is less.

In diseased lungs, changes in the $\dot{V}A/\dot{Q}$ ratio occur as the result of uneven ventilation, or uneven perfusion, or both; for example, compression or occlusion of pulmonary vessels, reduced pulmonary vascular bed, or intrapulmonary-anatomic right-to-left shunting may contribute to nonuniform perfusion. In congenital heart diseases with increased pulmonary blood flow caused by left-to-right shunting, the $\dot{V}A/\dot{Q}$ ratio is decreased. When perfusion is diminished, as in tricuspid atresia or pulmonic stenosis with tetralogy of Fallot, $\dot{V}A/\dot{Q}$ is increased.

The lungs appear to have an intrinsic regulatory mechanism that, to a limited extent, preserves a normal $\dot{V}A/\dot{Q}$ ratio.

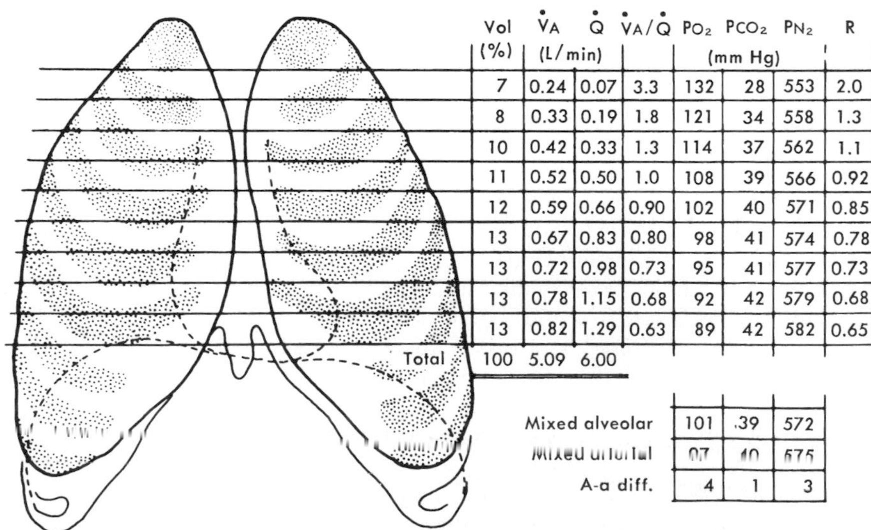

Vol (%)	$\dot{V}A$ (L/min)	$\dot{Q}$	$\dot{V}A/\dot{Q}$	PO_2 (mm Hg)	PCO_2	PN_2	R
7	0.24	0.07	3.3	132	28	553	2.0
8	0.33	0.19	1.8	121	34	558	1.3
10	0.42	0.33	1.3	114	37	562	1.1
11	0.52	0.50	1.0	108	39	566	0.92
12	0.59	0.66	0.90	102	40	571	0.85
13	0.67	0.83	0.80	98	41	574	0.78
13	0.72	0.98	0.73	95	41	577	0.73
13	0.78	1.15	0.68	92	42	579	0.68
13	0.82	1.29	0.63	89	42	582	0.65
Total 100	5.09	6.00					

	PO_2	PCO_2	PN_2
Mixed alveolar	101	39	572
Mixed arterial	[illegible]	40	575
A-a diff.	4	1	3

■ **FIGURE 2–37.** Effect of distribution of ventilation and perfusion on regional gas tensions in erect man. The lung is divided into nine horizontal slices, and the position of each slice is shown by its anterior rib markings. Vol, Relative lung volume; $\dot{V}A$, regional alveolar ventilation; $\dot{Q}$, regional perfusion; $\dot{V}A/\dot{Q}$, ventilation/perfusion ratio; R, respiratory exchange ratio. (From West JB: *J Appl Physiol* 17:893, 1962.)

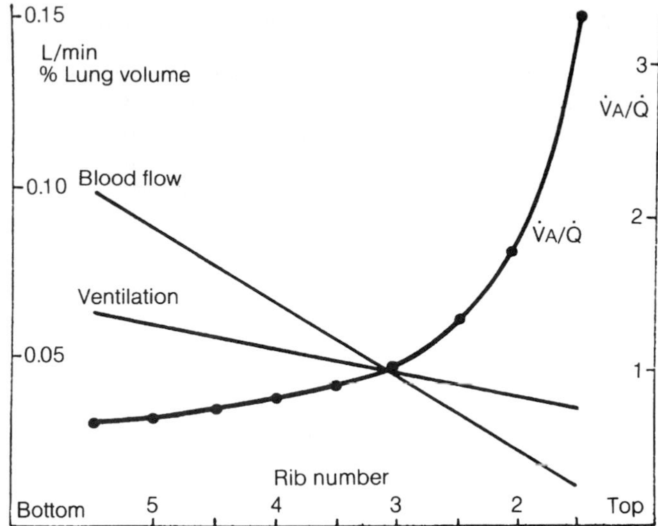

■ **FIGURE 2–38.** Effect of vertical height (expressed as the level of the anterior ends of the ribs) on ventilation and pulmonary blood flow (left ordinate) and the ventilation/perfusion ratio (right ordinate). (From West JB: *Ventilation/blood flow and gas exchange,* ed 2. Oxford, 1970, Blackwell Scientific Publications Ltd.)

In areas with a high $\dot{V}_A/\dot{Q}$ ratio, a low P_{CO_2} tends to constrict airways and dilate pulmonary vessels, and the opposite occurs in areas with a low $\dot{V}_A/\dot{Q}$ ratio. In the latter case, in addition to the effect of P_{CO_2}, hypoxic pulmonary vasoconstriction (HPV) decreases regional blood flow and helps to increase $\dot{V}_A/\dot{Q}$ ratios toward normal. The administration of drugs such as isoproterenol, nitroglycerin, theophylline, and sodium nitroprusside diminishes or abolishes HPV and increases intrapulmonary shunting (Goldzimer et al., 1974; Colley et al., 1979; Hill et al., 1979; Benumof, 1994). All inhaled anesthetics depress HPV in vitro (Sykes et al., 1972; Bjertnaes, 1978), contributing to an increase in venous admixture during general anesthesia. The effect of inhaled anesthetics on HPV, however, has not been conclusive in vivo (Marshall and Marshall, 1980, 1985; Pavlin and Su, 1994).

Wagner and others (1974) have developed a sophisticated quantitative method of studying the continuous spectrum of $\dot{V}_A/\dot{Q}$ mismatch. The technique is based on the pattern of elimination of multiple inert gases infused intravenously. At steady state after intravenous infusion of test gases dissolved in saline solution, arterial, mixed-venous, and expired gas samples are obtained, and minute ventilation and cardiac output are measured. The ratio of arterial to mixed venous concentration (retention) and the ratio of expired to mixed venous concentration (excretion) are computed for each gas, and retention-solubility and excretion-solubility curves are drawn by the computer. The ratio of the two curves represents the distribution of perfusion and ventilation on the spectrum of $\dot{V}_A/\dot{Q}$ ratios (West, 1974, 1994; Benumof, 1994) (Fig. 2–39).

Low $\dot{V}_A/\dot{Q}$ and Lung Collapse while Breathing Oxygen

In a lung unit with a low regional $\dot{V}_A/\dot{Q}$ ratio while breathing oxygen, collapse of the lung unit occurs, leading to atelectasis. As alveolar ventilation to the lung unit ($\dot{V}_A$) decreases, regional expiratory volume (V_E) decreases progressively in comparison to regional inspiratory volume (V_I) as it approaches the amount of

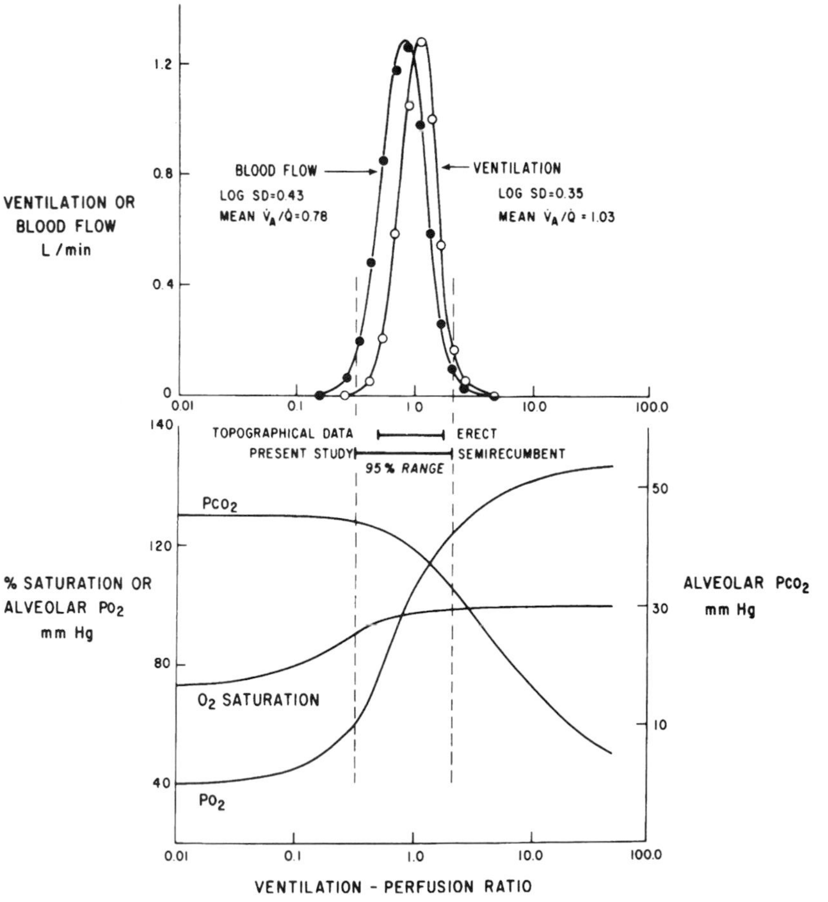

■ **FIGURE 2–39.** Upper graph shows the average distribution of ventilation/perfusion ratios in young semirecumbent normal subjects. The 95% range covers ventilation/perfusion from 0.3 to 2.1. The corresponding variations of P_{O_2}, P_{CO_2}, and oxygen saturation in the end-capillary blood can be seen in the lower panel. (From West JB: *Anesthesiology* 41:124, 1974.)

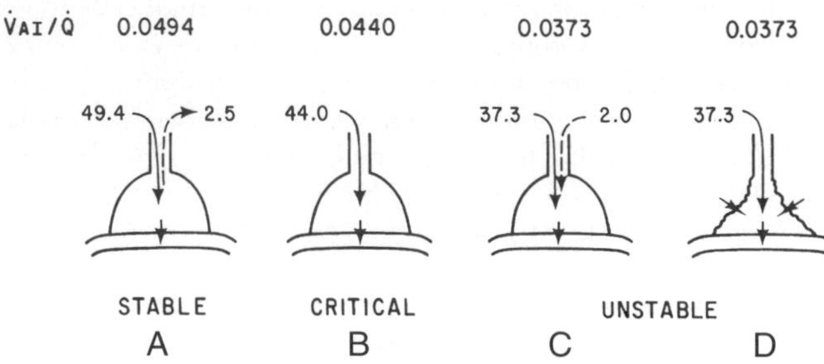

■ **FIGURE 2–40.** Schematic drawings to explain the development of shunts in lung units with low inspiratory $\dot{V}_A/\dot{Q}_S$ ($\dot{V}_{AI}/\dot{Q}$) caused by breathing high concentrations of oxygen. *A* (stable), There is a small expired alveolar ventilation ($\dot{V}_A$) and the unit is stable. *B* (critical), Inspired $\dot{V}_A$ is decreased slightly from *A* and expired $\dot{V}_A$ falls to zero. *C* (unstable), Inspired $\dot{V}_A$ is further reduced and gas enters in the lung unit during the expiratory phase. *D* (unstable), Reverse inspiration during expiratory phase is prevented and the unit gradually collapses. (From West JB: *Anesth Analg* 54:417, 1975.)

oxygen taken up by regional pulmonary blood flow ($\dot{Q}$). A point is reached at which the expired alveolar volume falls to zero (West, 1975). This situation occurs at the "critical" inspired $\dot{V}_A/\dot{Q}$. With inspired ratios less than the critical $\dot{V}_A/\dot{Q}$ value, the lung unit becomes unstable; oxygen may enter rather than leave the lung unit during the expiratory phase or the unit may gradually collapse (Briscoe et al., 1960) (Fig. 2–40). Figure 2–41 shows the calculated relationship between the critical inspired $\dot{V}_A/\dot{Q}$ ($\dot{V}_{AI}/\dot{Q}$) and the concentration of inspired oxygen (assuming mixed venous P_{O_2} of 40 mm Hg and P_{CO_2} of 45 mm Hg and no

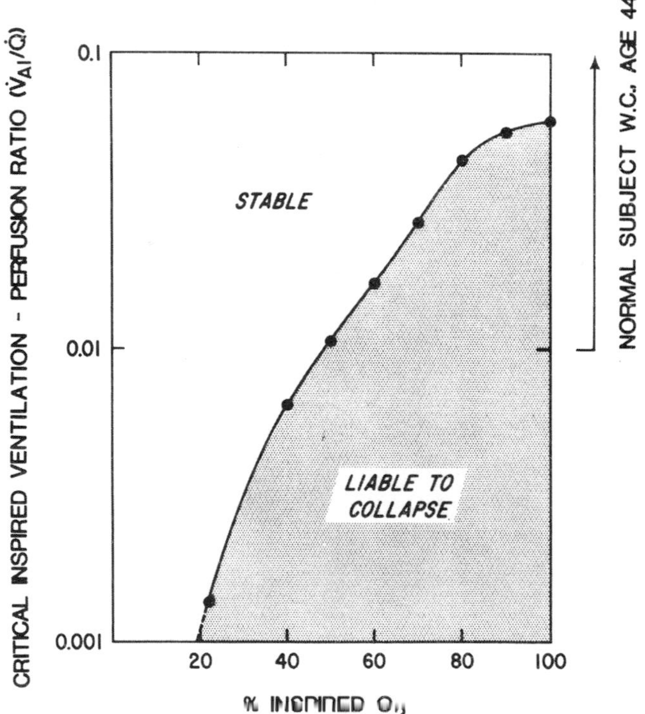

■ **FIGURE 2–41.** Relationship between inspired oxygen concentration and critical inspired $\dot{V}_A/\dot{Q}_S$, the value at which the expired ventilation of a given lung unit falls to zero. Lung units whose $\dot{V}_A/\dot{Q}_S$ is less than the critical value may be unstable and easily collapse. (From West JB: *Anesth Analg* 54:417, 1975.)

nitrogen exchange occurring across the whole lung) (Dantzker et al., 1975). From Figure 2–41, it can be seen that lung units with $\dot{V}_A/\dot{Q}$ < 0.01 become vulnerable when F_{IO_2} is increased above 0.5 while lung units with inspiratory $\dot{V}_{AI}/\dot{Q}$ of 0.1 are not at risk even with 100% oxygen (West, 1975). Although a $\dot{V}_A/\dot{Q}$ less than 0.1 is infrequent in normal awake children, lung units with a $\dot{V}_A/\dot{Q}$ less than 0.1 may occur in the diseased lung as well as in the normal lung under general anesthesia.

■ OXYGEN TRANSPORT

For normal metabolism, oxygen must be transported continuously to all body tissues. Changes in oxygen demand are met by the integrated response of three major functional components of the oxygen transport system: pulmonary ventilation, cardiac output, and blood hemoglobin concentration and characteristics. With acute oxygen demand, such as with severe exercise, high fever, or acute hypoxemia (<60 mm Hg), oxygen transport is increased mainly by increased cardiac output, while alveolar ventilation is increased to maintain proper levels of alveolar P_{O_2} and P_{CO_2}. Chronic hypoxemia increases erythropoietin production, thereby increasing erythrocyte production from the normal daily rate of approximately 1% of circulating red cell mass to about 2%. Thus increasing red cell mass in response to chronic hypoxemia is a slow process (Finch and Lenfant, 1972). Hemoglobin concentrations greater than the normal level (15 g/dL) raise viscosity and increase blood flow resistance until the plasma volume is also increased (Thorling and Erslev, 1968).

The amount of oxygen carried by the plasma depends on its solubility and is small (≈0.3 mL/dL per 100 mm Hg). Most oxygen molecules in blood combine reversibly with hemoglobin to form oxyhemoglobin. Each molecule of hemoglobin combines with four molecules of oxygen; 1 g of oxyhemoglobin combines with 1.34 mL of oxygen.

■ OXYGEN AFFINITY OF HEMOGLOBIN AND P_{50}

The oxygen-hemoglobin dissociation curve reflects the affinity of hemoglobin for oxygen (Fig. 2–42). As blood circulates through the normal lungs, oxygen tension increases from the mixed-venous P_{O_2} of around 40 mm Hg to pulmonary capillary P_{O_2} of above 100 mm Hg, and hemoglobin is saturated to about 97% in arterial blood. (Unfortunately, most pulse oximeters commercially available today are artificially modified to read 100% saturation in healthy subjects breathing room air rather than 97%; see later discussion.) The shape of the dissociation curve is such that further increases in P_{O_2} result in a very small increase in oxygen saturation (S_{O_2}) of hemoglobin.

As arterial blood circulates through the capillaries, tissues pick up oxygen, and both P_{O_2} and S_{O_2} decrease. The blood of normal adults has S_{O_2} of 50% when P_{O_2} is 27 mm Hg at 37°C and a pH of 7.4. The P_{50}, which is the P_{O_2} of whole blood at 50% S_{O_2}, indicates the affinity of hemoglobin for oxygen. An increase in blood pH increases the oxygen affinity of hemoglobin (Bohr effect). Similarly, a decrease in temperature increases oxygen affinity and shifts the oxygen-hemoglobin dissociation curve to the left; a decrease in pH or an increase in temperature has the opposite effect (Comroe, 1974) (see Fig. 2–42).

Benesch and Benesch (1967) and Chanutin and Curnish (1967) demonstrated that the oxygen affinity of a hemoglobin solution decreases by the addition of organic phosphates, in particular 2,3-diphosphoglycerate (2,3-DPG) and adenosine

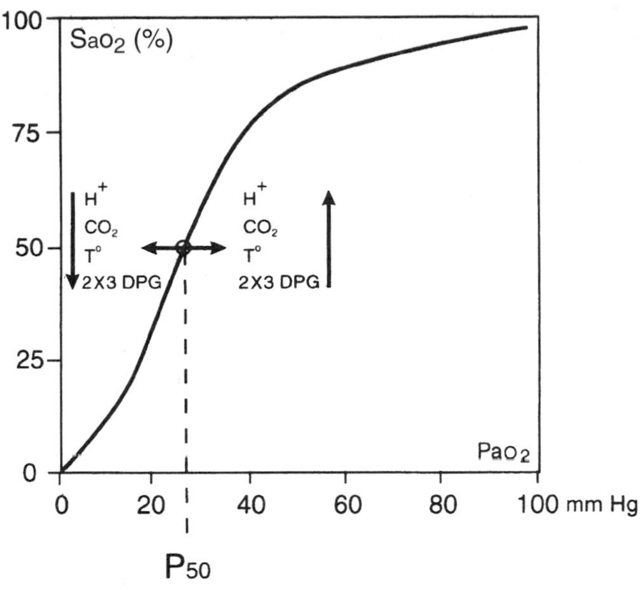

■ **FIGURE 2–42.** Schematic representation of oxygen dissociation curve and factors that affect blood oxygen affinity. Oxygen partial pressure at 50% oxygen saturation (P_{50}) is a convenient index of oxygen affinity. P_{50} of adult blood (at 37°C; pH, 7.40; PCO_2, 40 mm Hg) is roughly 27 mm Hg and is influenced by a number of factors. SaO_2, arterial oxygen saturation; PaO_2, arterial oxygen tension; H^+, hydrogen ion concentration; T°, blood temperature; 2,3 DPG, 2,3-diphosphoglycerate (see text).

triphosphate (ATP), which bind to deoxyhemoglobin but not to oxyhemoglobin. Human erythrocytes contain an extremely high concentration of 2,3-DPG, averaging about 4.5 mol/mL, compared with ATP (1 mol/mL) and other organic phosphates (Oski and Delivoria-Papadopoulos, 1970). Thus, an increase in red cell 2,3-DPG decreases the oxygen affinity of hemoglobin, increases P_{50} (shifts the dissociation curve to the right), and increases the unloading of oxygen at the tissue level. Increases in 2,3-DPG and P_{50} have been found in chronic hypoxemia.

In the newborn, blood oxygen affinity is extremely high and P_{50} is low (≈19 mm Hg) (Fig. 2–43) because fetal hemoglobin (HbF) reacts poorly with 2,3-DPG. Oxygen delivery at the tissue level is low despite high red blood cell mass and hemoglobin level. After birth, the total hemoglobin level decreases rapidly as the proportion of HbF diminishes, reaching its lowest level by 2 to 3 months of age (physiologic anemia of infancy) (Fig. 2–44). During the same early postnatal period, P_{50} increases rapidly (Oski and Delivoria-Papadopoulos, 1970); it exceeds the normal adult value by 3 months of age and remains high during the first decade of life (Oski, 1973a, 1973b) (Fig. 2–45). This high P_{50} is associated with a relatively low hemoglobin level (11 to 12 g/dL) and increased levels of ATP and 2,3-DPG, probably related to the process of general growth and development and high plasma levels of inorganic phosphate (Card and Brain, 1973). These observations engendered a hypothesis to explain why hemoglobin levels are lower in children than in adults (physiologic "anemia" of childhood). Because children have a lower oxygen affinity for hemoglobin, oxygen unloading at the tissue level is increased. Thus, a lower level of hemoglobin in infants and children is just as efficient, in terms of tissue oxygen delivery, as a higher hemoglobin level in adults (Oski, 1973a) (Table 2–3). Table 2–4 compares the hemoglobin concentrations at different ages in terms of equal tissue oxygen unloading (Motoyama et al., 1974).

Acceptable Hemoglobin Levels

These findings have important clinical implications for anesthesiologists. It was long assumed, until the 1980s, that children with a hemoglobin level of less than 10 g/dL were not acceptable for general anesthesia and surgery. This level of hemoglobin has been used arbitrarily without the knowledge of different oxygen affinity and tissue oxygen unloading at different ages. It appears from Table 2–4 that if a hemoglobin level of 10 g/dL is acceptable for an adult with a P_{50} of 27 mm Hg, 8.2 g/dL should theoretically be adequate for an infant more than 3 months of age with an average P_{50} of 30 mm Hg (without considering the high level of metabolism and oxygen consumption). In contrast, for a 2-month-old premature infant with a P_{50} of 24 mm Hg, a hemoglobin level of 10 g/dL is equivalent to only 6.8 g/dL in adults, and this may be inadequate to provide sufficient tissue oxygenation in patients with limited cardiac output or oxygen desaturation.

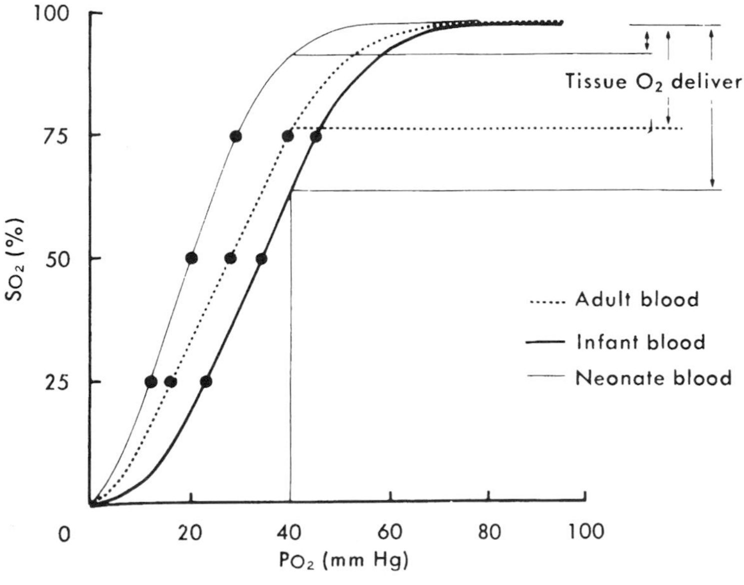

■ **FIGURE 2–43.** Schematic representation of oxygen-hemoglobin dissociation curves with different oxygen affinities. In infants older than 3 months with high P_{50} (30 mm Hg versus 27 mm Hg in adults), tissue oxygen delivery per gram of hemoglobin is increased. In neonates with a lower P_{50} (20 mm Hg) and a higher blood oxygen affinity, tissue oxygen unloading at the same tissue PO_2 is reduced.

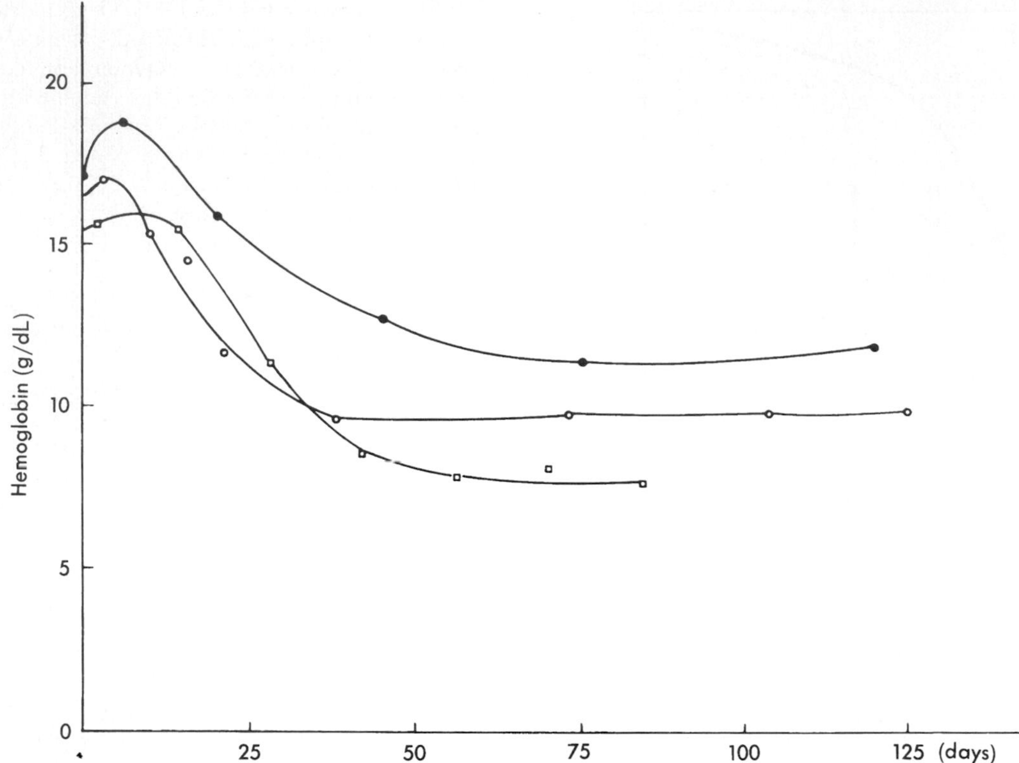

■ **FIGURE 2–44.** Hemoglobin concentration in infants of different degrees of maturation at birth. Filled circle, full-term infants; open circle, premature infants with birth weights of 1200 to 2350 g; open square, premature infants with birth weights less than 1200 g. (From Nathan DG, Oski FA: *Hematology of infancy and childhood,* ed 3. Philadelphia, 1987, WB Saunders.)

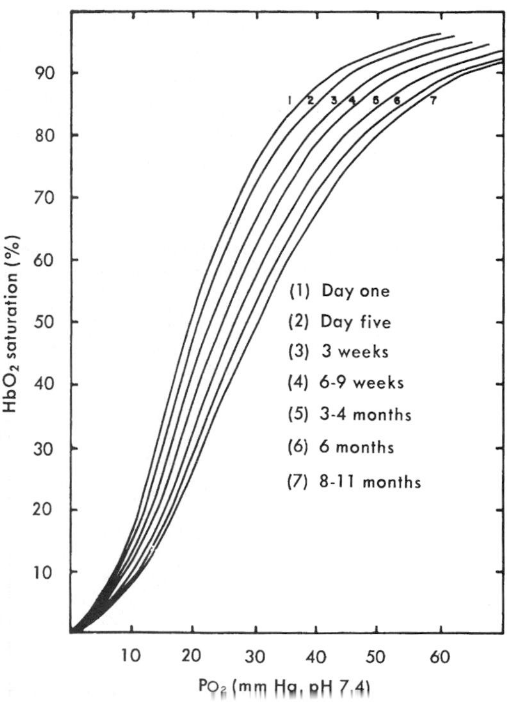

■ **FIGURE 2–45.** Oxyhemoglobin equilibrium curve of blood from normal term infants at different postnatal ages. The P_{50} on day 1 is 19.4 ± 1.8 mm Hg and has shifted to 30.3 ± 0.7 at age 11 months (normal adults = 27.0 ± 1.1 mm Hg). (From Oski FA: *Pediatrics* 51:494, 1973; copyright 1973 American Academy of Pediatrics.)

With the advent of human immunodeficiency virus (HIV) and acquired immunodeficiency syndrome (AIDS) and the resultant anxiety among the medical community and the lay public about homologous blood transfusion, the criteria for transfusion have changed significantly over the past two decades. At the consensus-developing conference by the National Institutes of Health and the Food and Drug Administration on perioperative red blood cell Transfusion (Consensus Conference, 1988), it was generally agreed that the available evidence does not support the "10/30" rule (that is, hemoglobin, 10 g/dL, or hematocrit, 30%), although the literature is remarkable for its lack of carefully controlled, randomized studies that would provide definitive conclusions. Other data suggest that cardiac output does not increase dramatically in healthy adult humans until the hemoglobin value decreases to approximately 7 g/dL.

It was also agreed that the decision to transfuse red blood cells in a specific patient should take into consideration the many factors that comprise clinical judgment. These factors include the duration of anemia, the intravascular volume, the extent of surgery, the probability of massive blood loss, and the presence of coexisting conditions, such as impaired cardiopulmonary function and inadequate cardiac output. A general consensus on acceptable perioperative levels of hemoglobin and hematocrit in infants and young children has not emerged. According to the data in Table 2–4, hemoglobin levels exceeding 8.2 g/dL (hematocrit, 25%) should be acceptable in children older than 3 months. Transfusion in otherwise healthy normovolemic infants with 8 g/dL of hemoglobin is hardly justifiable. On the other hand, postoperative hypoxemia is common even among healthy infants and children undergoing simple surgical procedures, such as inguinal hernia repair and myringotomies.

TABLE 2–3. Oxygen unloading changes with age

Age	P_{50} (mm Hg)	Percent Saturation at Venous Oxygen Tension of 40 mm Hg	Hemoglobin (g/100 mL)	Oxygen Unloaded* (mL/100 mL)
1 day	19.4	87	17.2	1.84
3 wk	22.7	80	13.0	2.61
6 to 9 wk	24.4	77	11.0	2.65
3 to 4 mo	26.5	73	10.5	3.10
6 mo	27.8	69	11.3	3.94
8 to 11 mo	30.0	65	11.8	4.74
5 to 8 yr	29.0†	67	12.6	4.73
9 to 12 yr	27.9†	69	13.4	4.67
Adult	27.0	71	15.0	4.92

*Assumes arterial oxygen saturation of 95%.
†From Oski FA: *J Pediatr* 83:353, 1973a.

These children with borderline hemoglobin levels must be given oxygen via mask and be monitored closely with a pulse oximeter in the recovery room (Motoyama and Glazener, 1986) (see Chapter 11, Intraoperative and Postoperative Management). The lowest safe limit of hemoglobin for infants less than 2 months of age has not been determined, although in sick infants it is desirable to maintain a hemoglobin level of 12 to 13 g/dL or a hematocrit of 40% (equivalent to 8 to 9 g/dL in adults) (also see Chapter 12, Blood Conservation).

There has been controversy about what constitutes abnormally low oxygen saturation in infants and children postoperatively and what is considered clinically unsafe. Mok and others (1986) reported that during the first week of life, oxygen saturation as monitored with pulse oximetry (SpO_2) was noticeably decreased, especially during active (REM) sleep (mean SpO_2, 92%) and during feeding (SpO_2, 91%). After 4 weeks of age, however, SpO_2 was more stable and was maintained at or above 94% during sleep. Thus, SpO_2 less than 94% can be considered as physiologically abnormal in infants beyond the first week of age. A study in preterm infants (mean gestational age, 33 weeks; postconceptional age, 37 weeks) has shown that median SpO_2 at the time of discharge was 99.5% and increased to 100% at follow-up 6 weeks later. The preterm infants had higher baseline saturation and no more incidence of desaturation than full-term infants of equivalent postconceptional ages (Poets et al., 1992). It is generally agreed that SpO_2 less than 95% in otherwise healthy infants and children is abnormal and that these patients require oxygen supplementation.

The routine use of pulse oximetry has dramatically improved the anesthesiologist's ability to monitor and properly maintain arterial oxygenation (Coté et al., 1988, 1991). This is especially true for premature infants, who are susceptible to oxygen toxicity and retinopathy of prematurity, even when breathing room air. In prematurely born infants weighing less than 1300 g, the incidence of retinopathy of prematurity increases markedly with exposure to 12 or more hours of PaO_2 exceeding 80 mm Hg (Flynn et al., 1992). Arterial oxygen saturation (SaO_2) must be adjusted properly so as to maintain PaO_2 in the normal neonatal range of 60 to 80 mm Hg (Orzalesi et al., 1967). As mentioned, oxygen affinity to hemoglobin is very high in the neonate and decreases rapidly during the first 3 to 6 months of life (Oski, 1973a, 1973b, 1981). Estimated PaO_2 should be adjusted according to age, as shown in Table 2–5. In the newborn, whose P_{50} is 18 to 20 mm Hg, the range of SaO_2 to maintain adequate PaO_2 (60 to 80 mm Hg) is 97% to 98%, whereas in the adult (P_{50}, 27), it is 91% to 96%. In the neonate, SaO_2 of 91% corresponds to PaO_2 of 41 mm Hg. Although the values in Table 2–5, based on Severinghaus's nomogram for the Bohr effect (Severinghaus, 1966), are only estimates, published data comparing arterial PO_2 and oxygen saturation seem to agree well with values in the nomogram (Ramanathan et al., 1987; Bucher et al., 1989).

Unfortunately, another factor compounding the confusion (and clinically too important to ignore) is that pulse oximeters by Nelcor (which are the most widely used in the United States) are artificially set to read 2% to 3% higher at the 90% to 95% range than actual arterial oxygen hemoglobin saturation (as measured by means of co-oximetry) and that Ohmeda pulse oximeters (which are more commonly used in Europe) tend to read somewhat lower than actual arterial oxygen saturation (Jennis and Peabody, 1987; Bucher et al., 1989). Unfortunately, the newer pulse oximeter (Masimo SET) with less motion artifact, which has increasingly been used in the United States and elsewhere, also artificially increased the reading by 2% to 3% higher to match the reading with the Nelcor pulse oximeter (see Chapter 10, Induction of Anesthesia). In view of these findings, the range of SpO_2 of 93% to 95%, corresponding to an estimated PaO_2 of 66 to 74 mm Hg in adults (but only 40 to 50 mm Hg in neonates), often recommended as desirable maintenance levels for neonates and premature infants in intraoperatively or in the intensive care settings, appears much too low for adequate tissue oxygenation. Furthermore, respiratory alkalosis, which may result from assisted or controlled ventilation, would shift the oxygen hemoglobin dissociation curve further to the left (P_{50}, even lower than it already is) and decrease PaO_2 and tissue oxygen delivery even further at this range of oxygen

TABLE 2–4. Hemoglobin requirements for equivalent tissue oxygen delivery

	P_{50} (mm Hg)	Hemoglobin for Equivalent O_2 Delivery (g/dL)						
Adult	27	7	8	9	10	11	12	13
Infant >3 mo	30	5.7	6.5	7.3	8.2	9.0	9.8	10.6
Neonate <2 mo	24	10.3	11.7	13.2	14.7	16.1	17.6	19.1

Calculated from data of Motoyama EK, Zigas CJ, Troll G: Functional basis of childhood anemia. *Am Soc Anesthesiol Abstr* 283–284, 1974.

■ **TABLE 2–5.** Estimated Po_2 at different P_{50} of hemoglobin*

	AGE				
	1 day	*2 wk*	*6 to 9 wk*	*6 mo to 6 yr*	*Adult*
P_{50} (mm Hg)†	19	22	24	29	27
So_2 (%)	**Estimated Po_2 (mm Hg) at neutral pH (7.40)**				
99	108	130	143	171	156
98	77	92	101	122	111
97	64	77	84	101	92
96	56	68	74	89	82
95	52	62	68	82	74
94	48	58	63	76	69
93	45	55	60	72	66
92	43	52	57	68	62
91	41	50	55	66	60
90	40	48	53	63	58
88	37	45	49	59	54
86	35	42	47	56	51
84	34	40	44	53	49
82	32	39	42	51	47
80	31	37	41	49	45
78	30	36	39	47	43
76	29	34	38	45	41
74	28	33	36	44	40
72	27	32	35	42	39
70	26	31	34	41	37

*Calculated from Severinghaus' (1966) assuming that the shift in oxygen dissociation curve of hemoglobin due to changes in its oxygen affinity at neutral pH (7.40) is the same as the shift due to the Bohr effect.

†Po_2 at which oxygen saturation of hemoglobin (So_2) is 50%.

saturation (see Fig. 2–42). In clinical practice, therefore, Spo_2 levels of 95% to 97% (corresponding Pao_2 of 50 to 70 mm Hg in neonates and 60 to 80 mm Hg in infants 1 to 2 months old) are recommended.

Some anesthetics affect the oxygen affinity of hemoglobin. The presence of cyclopropane (although it has not been used since the 1970s) significantly decreases oxygen affinity and increases P_{50} by 3 mm Hg without changes in the 2,3-DPG levels, whereas halothane has minimal effects (Orzalesi et al., 1971). Exposure to 50% nitrous oxide, on the other hand, has been reported to produce a marked reversible increase in oxygen affinity; P_{50} decreased from 26 to 18 mm Hg, a level similar to that of HbF (Fournier and Major, 1984). This finding contrasts with a report based on one patient by Prime (1951), who found no effect with 70% nitrous oxide, and with a study by Smith and others (1970), who reported a 3 mm Hg rightward shift of P_{50} with an unspecified concentration of nitrous oxide. The finding of Fournier and Major may be of considerable clinical importance. Nitrous oxide anesthesia combined with hyperventilation would markedly increase the oxygen affinity of hemoglobin and decrease oxygen unloading at the tissue level. This effect could be hazardous in neonates whose P_{50} is unusually low even without respiratory alkalosis or nitrous oxide.

■ SURFACE ACTIVITY AND PULMONARY SURFACTANT

The alveolar surfaces of human lungs are lined with surface active materials with unique properties that are responsible for the stability of air spaces. These materials, which contain specific phospholipids and proteins (discussed later), are collectively called pulmonary surfactant.

The relationship among pressure (P), surface tension (T), and radius (r) of a sphere, such as a soap bubble, is expressed by the Laplace equation, as follows:

$$P = \frac{2T}{r}$$

It can be seen from this equation that if surface tension (T) were constant, in a number of connected spheres the smallest sphere would have the highest pressure. Thus the smaller spheres would empty their gas contents into the larger ones. If this concept applied to lung units, the lungs would be unstable, with most units collapsing into several large ones, as seen in the lung of an infant with IRDS or HMD. Such instability does not exist in normal lungs. As Clements and others (1958) first demonstrated, saline extract of normal lungs has an extremely low surface tension (0 to 5 dynes/cm) during dynamic compression of the surface area and increased tension (30 to 50 dynes/cm) during expansion of the surface area. Their findings indicate that, in normal lungs, the surface tension decreases as the alveolar radius decreases and vice versa; the stability of the air spaces is maintained regardless of the size of each unit (Fig. 2–46).

The alveolar lining layer obtained from lung lavage contains approximately 10% lipoprotein and 90% phospholipid, of which surface-active dipalmiotylphosphatidylcholine is the major fraction. Phosphatidylglycerol was identified as the second major fraction (≈10%) of surface-active phospholipid (Rooney, Canavan, Motoyama, 1974). Other phospholipids include sphingomyelin (also surface active), phosphatidylethanolamine, and phosphatidylinositol (Rooney, 1985). Four surfactant-associated proteins have been isolated and characterized; their locations in specific chromosomes have been identified (Weaver and Whitsett, 1991). These substances are produced by type II alveolar epithelial cells (pneumocytes) stored in the osmiophilic lamellar inclusions within these cells, and are excreted into the air space to form tubular myelins and surface-active alveolar lining layers (Kikkawa, Motoyama, Cook, 1965) (Figs. 2–47, 2–48, and 2–49).

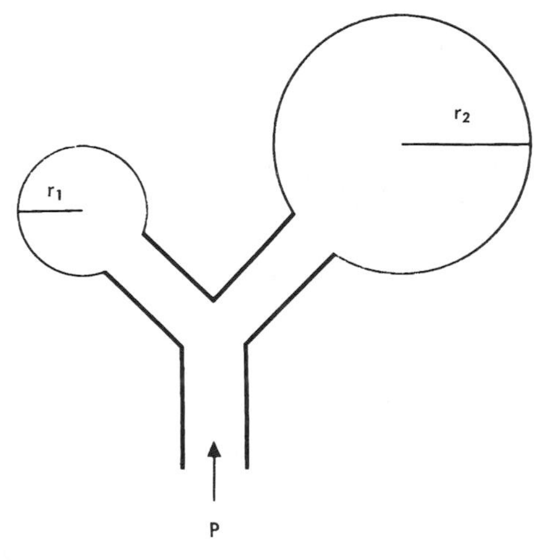

■ **FIGURE 2–46.** Schematic drawing of stable alveoli of different sizes (see text).

Surfactant protein-A (SP -A) is a 35-kDa hydrophilic protein and appears in the amniotic fluid by 28 weeks' gestation. Surfactant protein B and C (SP-B [8 kDa]; SP-C [3-5 kDa]) are hydrophobic and are bound to the phospholipid fraction. SP–A, SP-B, and SP-C are involved in the formation of myelin figures and are believed to enhance the rate of formation and the stability of surface monolayers at the air-liquid interface on the alveolar surface (deMello and Reid, 1995). In addition, SP-A increases the phagocytosis of alveolar macrophages and thus plays a role in host defense (van Iwaarden et al., 1990), whereas SP-B and SP-C have a direct immunosuppressive effect on lung lymphocytes (Ansfield and Benson, 1980). Surfactant also plays a role in the maintenance of alveolar fluid homeostasis by reducing transepithelial protein leakage (Hallman, 1984).

The production of phosphatidylcholine increases towards term, whereas that of sphingomyelin decreases. The ratio of these phospholipids (L/S ratio) in the amniotic fluid has been used as an index of fetal lung maturity (Kulovich, Hallman, Cluck, 1979).

Inadequacy or deficiency of the surfactant system is important in several clinical conditions. Historically, Avery and Mead (1959) showed that the minimum surface tension of lung extracts from premature infants dying of IRDS (or HMD) was unusually high when measured on the Wilhelmy balance. Surface-active phosphatidylcholine is markedly decreased or even absent in the alveolar linings in these lungs (Boughton, Gandy, Gardiner, 1970). These findings partially explain the atelectasis and low compliance in the lungs of infants with this syndrome.

Fujiwara and others first reported, with impressive results, the instillation in the trachea of bovine surfactant in premature infants born with surfactant deficiency (Fujiwara et al., 1980). Surfactant replacement therapy using human, bovine, or synthetic surfactant in premature infants with IRDS is now established as an important and essential form of therapy, reducing morbidity and mortality (Merritt et al., 1986; Lang et al., 1990; Hoekstra et al., 1991; Long et al., 1991; Holms, 1993). Surfactant replacement therapy has been extended to cover other clinical conditions with surfactant deficiency or inactivation not only in premature infants but also in full-term infants, children, and adults. These conditions include (1) neonates with persistent pulmonary hypertension (PPHN) in whom surfactant production by type II pneumocytes is depressed because of severe pulmonary hypoperfusion and hypoxia; (2) neonates with severe congenital diaphragmatic hernia (CDH) whose immature lungs are damaged by ventilator-induced lung injury and surfactant inactivation by plasma protein leak on the alveolar surface (see Chapter 16, Anesthesia for Neonates and Premature Infants); (3) meconium aspiration syndrome caused by pulmonary hypoperfusion, inflammation, and inactivation of

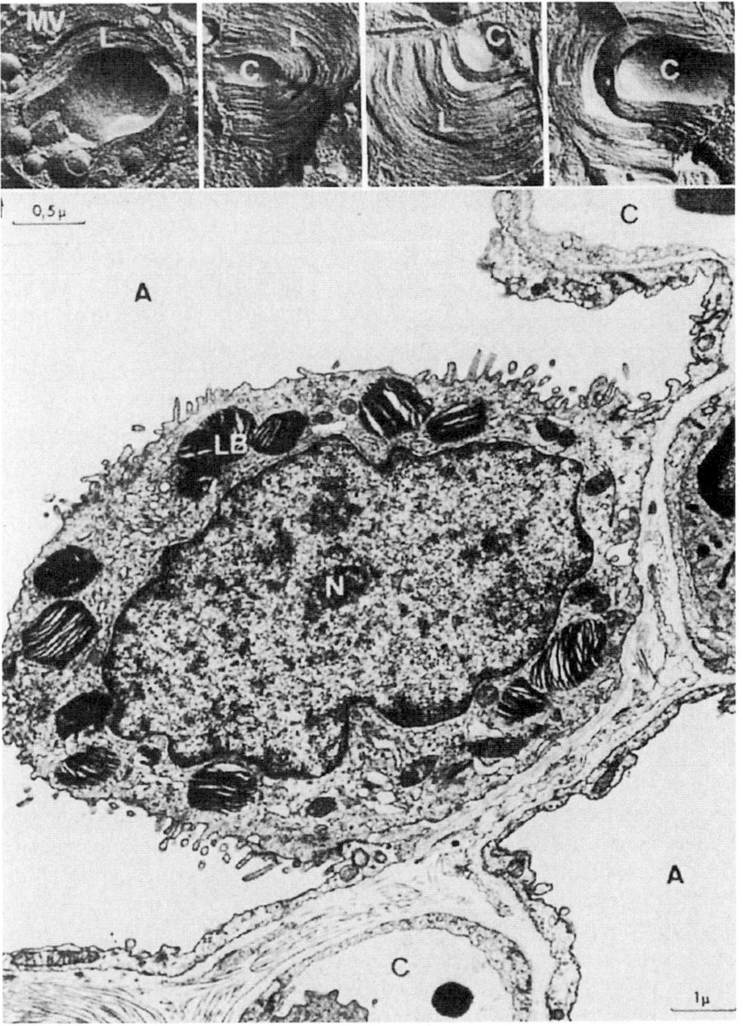

■ **FIGURE 2–47.** Granular pneumocyte (type II). Cytoplasm around the nucleus (N) contains many organelles, particularly osmophilic lamellar bodies (LB). A, Alveolar space; C, capillary space. Insets show lamellar bodies in freeze-etched preparation revealing form and existence of central core (C) around which lamellae (L) are stacked. (×22,400.) (From Weibel ER: *Physiol Rev* 53:419, 1973.)

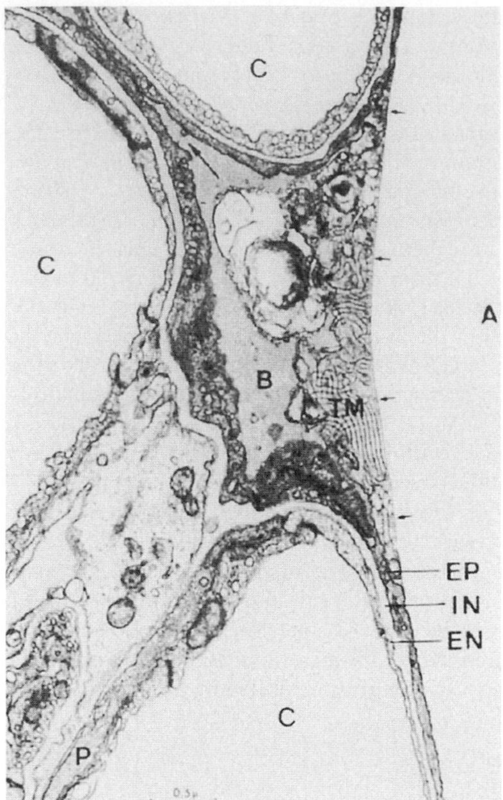

■ **FIGURE 2–48.** Perfusion-fixed rat lung showing three capillaries *(C)* and the extracellular lining layer toward the alveolus *(A)* composed of a base layer *(B)* and an osmophilic lining layer *(short arrows).* Base layer contains tubular myelin figures (TM) and extends into a cleft between capillaries closely opposed because of septal folding *(long arrow).* EP, Alveolar epithelial cell (type I); EN, capillary endothelial cell; IN, interstitium; P, pericyte (×23,000). (From Weibel ER: *Physiol Rev* 53:419, 1973.)

surfactant by protein leak; and (4) ARDS in children and adults (Jobe, 1993; Pramanik, Holtzman, Merritt, 1993).

■ CILIARY ACTIVITY

The tracheal and bronchial walls are lined with pseudo-stratified epithelium that consists of ciliated cells, nonciliated serous and brush cells, and abundant mucus-secreting goblet cells. The submucous contains numerous serous and mucous cell glands, which are major contributors of the mucus in the respiratory tract. Under normal circumstances both goblet cells and mucus-secreting glands diminish in number toward the periphery of the airway system. The mucosal surface is covered by a serous fluid layer, in which the cilia beat. Above this periciliary layer of serous fluid lie discontinuous flakes of mucus (rather than the continuous mucous blanket assumed previously), which are moved cephalad by the cilia (Jeffery and Reid, 1977) (Fig. 2–50).

The cilia in the respiratory tract play an important role in the removal of mucoid secretions, foreign particles, and cell debris and are an essential defense mechanism of the airway system. These cilia move in a synchronous, whip-like fashion at a rate of 600 to 1300 times/min. They can move particles toward the mouth at the rate of about 1.5 to 2 cm/min (Lichtiger, Landa, Hirsch, 1975).

Ciliary function is influenced by the thickness of the mucous layer and other factors that can occur with dehydration or infection. In tissue culture, some viral infections reduce ciliary motion as much as 50%, and repeated infections in vivo can destroy the cilia completely (Kilburn and Salzano, 1966). Inhalation of warm air with 50% humidity maintains normal ciliary activity, whereas breathing dry air for 3 hours results in a complete cessation of mucus movement. Ciliary activity can be restored by breathing warm, saturated air (Forbes, 1974; Hirsch et al., 1975). Breathing 100% oxygen and controlled positive-pressure ventilation also affect ciliary function (Wolfe, Ebert, Sabiston, 1972; Forbes, 1976; Forbes and Gamsu, 1979).

Inhaled anesthetics seem to decrease ciliary function in both animals and humans. Forbes and Horrigan (1977) observed a dose-related depression of ciliary activity during halothane and enflurane anesthesia. The same group of investigators found delayed mucus clearance during and 6 hours after discontinuation of halothane or diethyl ether anesthesia (Forbes and Gamsu, 1979). These findings suggest that inhaled anesthesia has adverse effects on mucociliary clearance, especially in patients with pulmonary disease. The effect of anesthetics on mucociliary clearance in infants and children has not been reported.

■ MEASUREMENTS OF PULMONARY FUNCTION IN INFANTS AND CHILDREN

Airway obstruction is often difficult to assess clinically, particularly in young infants. For instance, what appears to be stridor may not indicate obstruction of the upper or extrathoracic airways. Similarly, although wheezing commonly represents disorders of relatively large intrathoracic airways, such as bronchial asthma, other airway dysfunction, from the upper airways (such as stridors) to the lower airways (such as rhonchi from secretions) can be mistaken as wheezing.

The cause of abnormal breath sounds also include such airway abnormality as narrowing of the airway lumen by mucosal edema, compression, secretions, or foreign objects, and by hyperreactive airway smooth muscles. Stridor and wheezing may also be caused by increased collapsibility of airways, as seen in laryngotracheomalacia involving both the upper and lower (large central) airways. A careful evaluation of the medical history and physical examination are obviously essential and helpful but may be inadequate to determine the exact nature of the disorder.

Pulmonary function tests are most effective in evaluating the respiratory status of infants and children and in documenting the site(s), nature, and extent of airway dysfunction. In addition, pulmonary function tests allow objective and quantitative assessment of a reactive airway disease such as bronchial asthma and bronchopulmonary dysplasia and its response to bronchodilator therapy. For a detailed account of various measurements of pulmonary function in children and adolescents, the publications by Polgar and Promadhat (1971) and by Bates (1989) should be consulted.

The most frequent types of pulmonary disability may be classified under the general headings of (1) restrictive diseases and (2) obstructive diseases, although there is considerable overlap between the two groups. Restrictive disorders, whether intrapulmonary or extrapulmonary in origin, result in reduced lung volumes. Relatively common restrictive disorders in infants and children, from the anesthesiologist's point of view, include persistent PPHN and CDH in the newborn period, congestive heart failure (also obstructive), pulmonary fibrosis, kyphoscoliosis, obesity, and abdominal distention in older children.

In patients after surgery, especially those given muscle relaxants, the vital capacity (VC) is a practical guide to muscle strength. A VC of at least twice the tidal volume (15 mL/kg; normal range, 60 to 70 mL/kg) appears necessary to maintain adequate

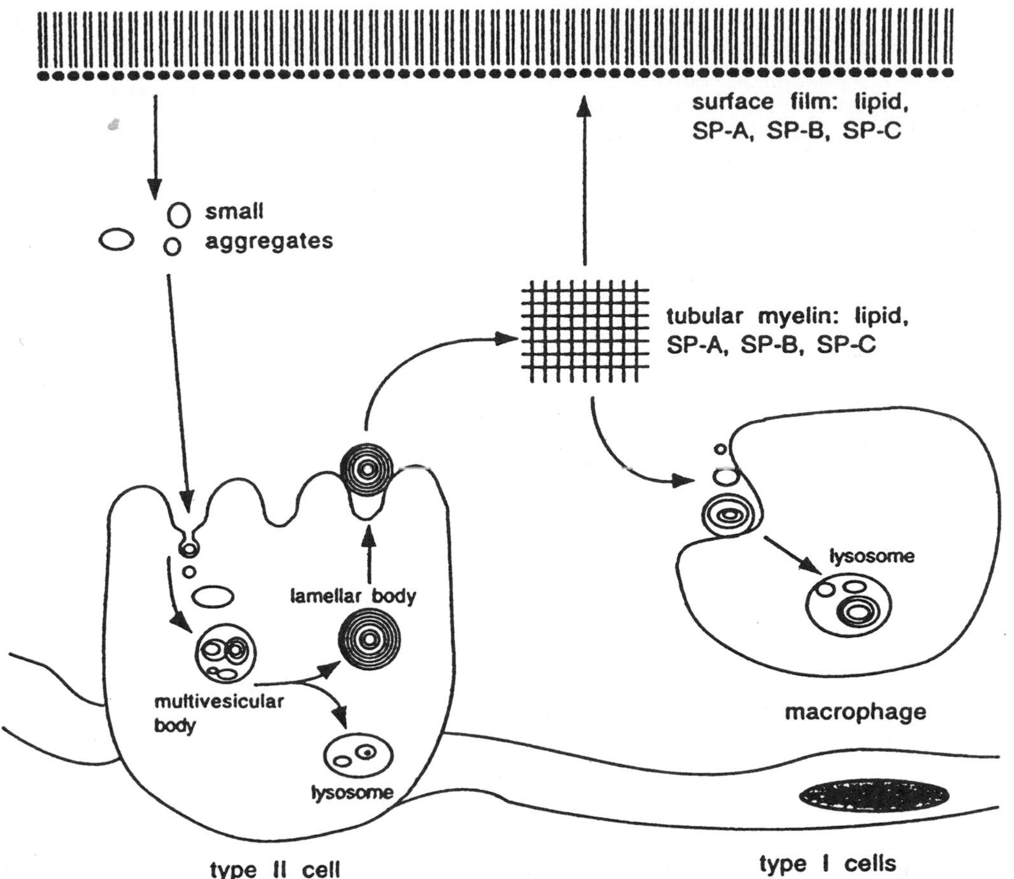

■ **FIGURE 2–49.** Life cycle of pulmonary surfactant. SP-A, SP-B, SP-C, and phospholipids are packaged in lamellar inclusion bodies and secreted by type II alveolar epithelial cells (pneumocytes) into the air space. Lamellar bodies unfold into tubular myelin, which gives rise to the phospholipid-surfactant protein film at the air-liquid interface. Used surfactant phospholipids are released from the film as small vesicles, which are taken up and recycled or degraded by type II cells. Alveolar macrophages also take up surfactant and degrade it. SP-A, SP-B, SP-C, surfactant proteins A, B, and C. (From Whitsett JA, Horowitz AD: Surfactant and associated proteins. In Fishman AP, editor: *Fishman's pulmonary diseases and disorders*, ed 3. New York, 1998, McGraw-Hill, with permission.)

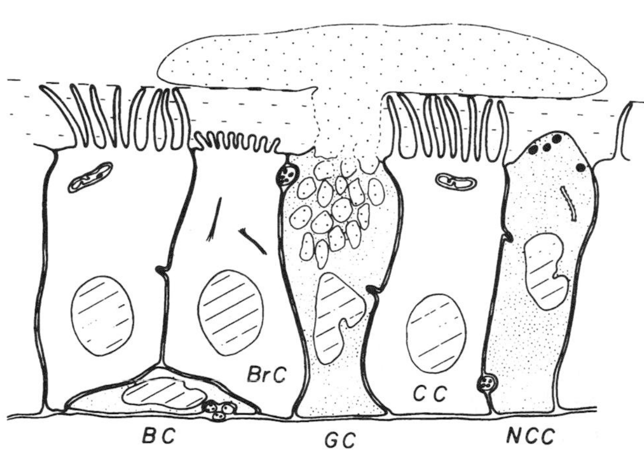

■ **FIGURE 2–50.** The ultrastructure of airway epithelium represented diagrammatically. Cilia beat in a fluid layer of low viscosity above which move flakes of mucus. Ciliated cells (CC), goblet cells (GC), nonciliated "serous" cells (NCC), brush cells (BrC), and basal cells (BC) are shown, as are nerves penetrating the epithelium. (Reprinted from Jeffery PK, Reid LM: The respiratory mucous membrane. In Brain JD, Procotor DF, Reid LM, editors: *Respiratory defense mechanisms.* New York, 1977, Marcel Dekker, p 198, by courtesy of Marcel Dekker, Inc.)

spontaneous ventilation. The measurement of peak inspiratory and expiratory pressures against airway occlusion at FRC provides additional information. A minimum of 30 cm H_2O is needed for effective coughing and adequate spontaneous breathing.

Obstructive pulmonary disorders may be classified into upper and lower airway diseases. Most of the severe upper airway diseases, such as acute epiglottitis and subglottic croup, occur in infancy and early childhood. Occasionally, however, upper airway obstruction can be seen in children with obstructive sleep apnea syndrome (OSAS) (see earlier) with chronic adenotonsillar hypertrophy as well as subglottic stenosis associated with prolonged intubation or tracheostomy. Vascular ring and vascular sling are rare but are associated with severe tracheobronchial (large central airway) obstruction.

The lower airway disorders commonly seen among children include bronchopulmonary dysplasia, cystic fibrosis, bronchial asthma, reactive airway disease associated with gastroesophageal reflux, and heart disease with left-to-right shunting and pulmonary hypertension.

STANDARD TESTS OF PULMONARY FUNCTION

Standard pulmonary function testing is largely limited to children older than 7 years who can understand and cooperate with the test procedures. In newborns, some physiologic indicators of pulmonary function can be measured using modifications of standard tests. The relatively recent introduction of tests that are applicable in infants and young children has considerably broadened the ability to assess their pulmonary dysfunction.

Zapletal and others (1987) compiled pulmonary function indices in children from the data he and his coworkers accumulated over the last two decades. Some of these normal values are reproduced in Appendix C.

Measurement of Lung Volumes

Total lung capacity (TLC) and its subdivisions (see Fig. 2–18 and the discussion of lung volumes) are measured either with spirometry and the gas dilution technique or with body plethysmography. FRC is commonly measured by the gas dilution technique with rebreathing of a known concentration of helium (10% He in O_2). TLC is obtained by adding inspiratory capacity (IC) and FRC. Residual volume (RV) is the difference between TLC and VC, the maximum amount of air one can breathe out from TLC. Forced vital capacity (FVC) is the VC obtained during maximum expiratory effort. Normally, FVC and VC in the same healthy person are nearly identical, but in patients with obstructive airway disease, airway closure worsens with effort and FVC may become considerably smaller than VC. VC per se is not a useful indicator for differential diagnosis because it decreases in both obstructive and restrictive lung disorders, such as atelectasis and pulmonary fibrosis. TLC, on the other hand, is decreased in restrictive disease but is increased by air trapping in obstructive disorders.

Gas dilution techniques underestimate TLC in obstructive lung disease because the test gas molecules (helium) do not sufficiently penetrate into trapped gas compartments. Under these circumstances, body plethysmography should be used to measure FRC more accurately. Measurement of FRC (or thoracic gas volume [TGV or VTG]) with body plethysmography is accomplished with a panting (or short, rapid breathing) maneuver against mouth occlusion. TGV is derived from simultaneous changes in lung volume (V) and airway pressure (P) using Boyle's law (P × V = k). When body plethysmography is not available, addition of a low level of end-expiratory positive airway pressure (EPAP) during helium rebreathing increases gas mixing, probably by preventing airway closure or by keeping the collateral channels open. The difference in calculated FRC with and without EPAP correlates well with the degree of air trapping in the lung (Motoyama et al., 1982). In obstructive lung disease, FRC and, in particular, RV, in relation to TLC (FRC/TLC, RV/TLC), are markedly increased.

Flow Function With Spirometry

In clinical pulmonary function laboratories, airway obstruction is usually assessed by the analysis of maximal forced expiration using a spirometer. The resultant volume change in relation to time is displayed on a kymograph (Fig. 2–51). Peak expiratory flow rate (PEFR) is by far the simplest of all expiratory flow measurements. PEFR is decreased most drastically by obstruction of the upper or large lower (central) airways, even when other indices of airway function are within normal limits. It is also decreased in patients with typical asthma, which primarily involves central airways, with severe peripheral airway disease such as cystic fibrosis, and with neuromuscular disorders. The measurement of PEFR is not a sensitive test for discriminating among various types of lung disease. Another major disadvantage of PEFR is that it varies with the degree of effort and cooperation, particularly in young children.

For many decades, the forced expiratory volume in 1 second ($FEV_{1.0}$) and maximum mid-expiratory flow rate (MMEFR or FEF_{25-75}) have been used extensively to evaluate airway function. These parameters are obtained from spirographic tracings made during an FVC maneuver from maximal inspiration (TLC) down to RV (see Fig. 2–51).

A reduction in $FEV_{1.0}$ correlates well with the clinical severity of lung disease, both in adults and in children. $FEV_{1.0}$ is expressed both in absolute terms and as a percentage of the value predicted on the basis of sex, age, and height. It is also expressed in relation to FVC ($FEV_{1.0}$/FVC). In obstructive lung disease, $FEV_{1.0}$ is decreased both in absolute terms and in relation to FVC because of prolonged expiration. On the other hand, in restrictive lung disease such as pulmonary fibrosis, in which airways are wide open, $FEV_{1.0}$ is decreased but $FEV_{1.0}$/FVC may be normal or even increased.

The MMEFR (FEF_{25-75}) is the average flow rate between 25% and 75% of FVC. Compared with $FEV_{1.0}$, MMEFR is a more sensitive index of airway disease involving smaller airways.

The major limitations of these indices of airway function are that they are variable depending on the patient's effort (effort dependent); they are also inadequate for identifying the site of obstruction (the upper versus lower airways, the central versus peripheral airways).

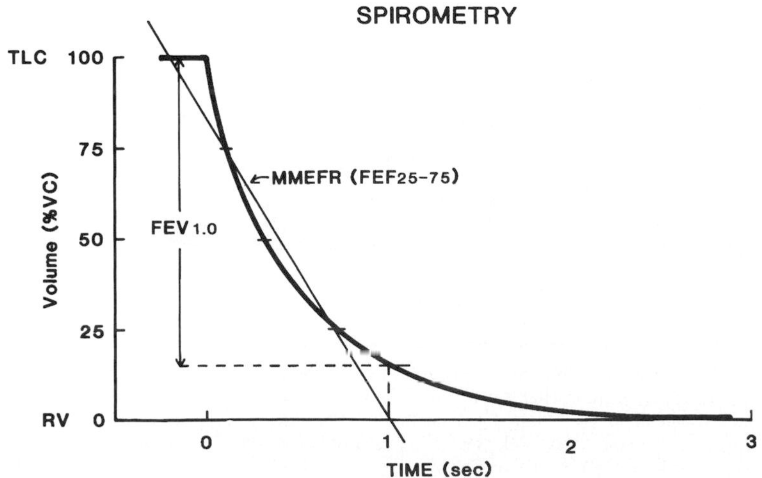

FIGURE 2–51. A spirometric tracing of forced vital capacity (FVC). $FEV_{1.0}$, forced expiratory volume in 1 second; MMEFR, maximum mid-expiratory flow rate, or FEF_{25-75}; RV, residual volume; TLC, total lung capacity. (See text.) (From Motoyama EK: Physiologic alterations in tracheostomy. In Myers EN, Stool SE, Johnson JT, editors: *Tracheotomy.* New York, 1985, Churchill Livingstone.)

Measurement of Airway Resistance

The standard technique for evaluating airway obstruction has been the measurement of airway resistance and forced expiratory flow. Airway resistance (Raw) is the most direct index of airway obstruction. It is, however, rarely used in clinical settings for several reasons: it requires a body plethysmograph, which is too costly, needs a trained pulmonology technician to perform it, and is too complicated for routine use. Furthermore, Raw is not a sensitive indicator of disease involving the lower airways, particularly small, peripheral airways, because the latter contribute only a fraction of total Raw, and abnormally high Raw does not indicate the site or location of airway disease.

Raw is influenced by the degree of lung inflation. As the lung volume increases, the airways expand and Raw falls. The airway conductance (Gaw), the reciprocal of resistance, changes linearly with lung volume in children (Zapletal et al., 1969).

Maximum Expiratory Flow-Volume Curves

Unlike other, conventional indices of airway function, which express volume change per unit of time (i.e., flow rates), maximum expiratory flow-volume (MEFV) curves relate maximum expiratory flow rates ($\dot{V}$max or MEF) to corresponding lung volumes during a FVC maneuver (see Fig. 2–30). As mentioned previously, the intrathoracic airways downstream (toward the mouth) from the equal pressure point (EPP) are subjected to dynamic compression during forced exhalation. As a result, the maximum expiratory flow rate ($\dot{V}$max, MEF, or FEF) at low lung volumes (i.e., <50% FVC) becomes independent of effort and is determined by the flow resistance of the upstream segment of airways between the alveoli and EPP (Rus) and by the static recoil pressure of the lung (Pstl):

$$\dot{V}\text{max} = \frac{\text{Pstl}}{\text{Rus}}$$

The measurement of $\dot{V}$max is a very sensitive test of lower airway obstruction because it eliminates the component of the upper and lower central airway resistance between the mouth and EPP, which may amount to as much as 80% to 90% of the total airway resistance. Another advantage of MEFV curve analysis over conventional spirometry is the effort independence of $\dot{V}$max, particularly in young children, whose effort may be submaximal or inconsistent. The normal values of $\dot{V}$max in children are shown in Appendix C.

Figure 2–52 is a schematic representation of MEFV curves from a patient with cystic fibrosis whose flow function is only mildly affected. PEFR is within normal limits, whereas values of $\dot{V}$max at 50% and 25% of FVC (FEF_{50} and FEF_{75}, respectively) are markedly reduced. With MEFV curves, lower airway disease can be further divided into central versus peripheral airway disorders by repeating MEFV curves with air (21% oxygen in nitrogen) versus a 20% oxygen–80% helium mixture.

In healthy persons the flow-limiting segment (EPP) is located in the central airways, usually within the first five generations of the tracheobronchial tree (Zapletal et al., 1969). Because the flow pattern here is turbulent and density dependent, air, with an average molecular weight of 29, has a lower flow rate than does the helium-oxygen mixture, with a much lighter average molecular weight of 9.6. In the case of peripheral airway obstruction, EPP moves upstream (peripherally) toward the area of obstruction, where the flow pattern is laminar and therefore viscosity dependent. The viscosity of helium is higher than that of nitrogen, so flow rates ($\dot{V}$max) in helium MEFV curves (He curve) at lower lung volumes become less than those in MEFV curves with air (air curve). In Figure 2–52, the He curve crosses the air curve at 30% of FVC (volume of isoflow [Viso$\dot{V}$]). Viso$\dot{V}$ of more than 20% of FVC is considered evidence of peripheral airway obstruction (Hutcheon et al., 1974). In children with mild to moderate asthma, both PEFR, an indicator of large airway function, and $\dot{V}max_{25}$, an indicator of lower airway function, are decreased because asthma involves constriction of both large and medium or even smaller airways (Fig. 2–53).

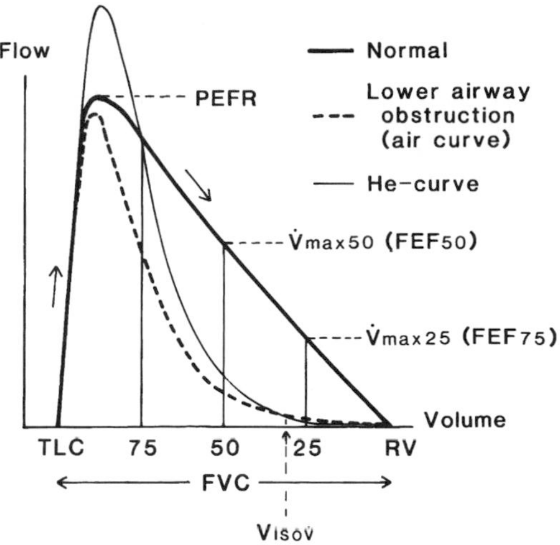

■ **FIGURE 2–52.** Maximum expiratory flow-volume (MEFV) curve of a 13-year-old boy with cystic fibrosis *(dotted line)* compared with predicted MEFV curve *(bold solid line)* breathing air. Note that peak expiratory flow rate (PEFR) is within normal limits, whereas maximum expiratory flows at 50% ($\dot{V}max_{50}$ or MEF_{50}) and at 25% ($\dot{V}max_{25}$ or MEF_{25}) are markedly reduced, indicating lower airway obstruction. The second MEFV curve *(thin solid line)* was obtained while he was breathing an 80% helium/20% oxygen mixture (He curve). The He curve crosses the air curve at 30% FVC (Viso$\dot{V}$), indicating peripheral airway disease. TLC, total lung capacity; RV, residual volume; FVC, forced vital capacity. (See text.) (From Motoyama EK: Physiologic alterations in tracheostomy. In Myers EN, Stool SE, Johnson JT, editors: *Tracheotomy.* New York, 1985, Churchill Livingstone.)

In contrast, in a typical case of mild cystic fibrosis with primary peripheral airway disease, $\dot{V}max_{25}$ is markedly reduced and PEFR is within normal limits (see Fig. 2–52). Figures 2–53 and 2–54 illustrate changes in flow and volume function in a 9-year-old boy with bronchial asthma. The control or baseline MEFV curve (curve 1 in Fig. 2–53) is markedly reduced from the predicted curve (curve 3, dotted line). His FVC is decreased because of air trapping and increases in RV. After an inhalation of nebulized bronchodilator, there is a marked increase in overall expiratory flow rates with decreased air trapping and a resultant increase in FVC (curve 2 in Fig. 2–54). TLC is decreased toward the predicted value.

EVALUATION OF UPPER AIRWAY FUNCTION

Upper airway obstruction is not uncommon in infants and young children because of anatomic factors such as a relatively large head, short neck, and small mandible in relation to tongue size. Also, the caliber of the upper airways is smaller in absolute terms than in older children and adults. Frequent causes of upper airway obstruction include, in descending order, obstructive sleep apnea (pharyngeal obstruction), laryngomalacia, vocal cord paralysis and dysfunction, laryngeal papillomas, and subglottic

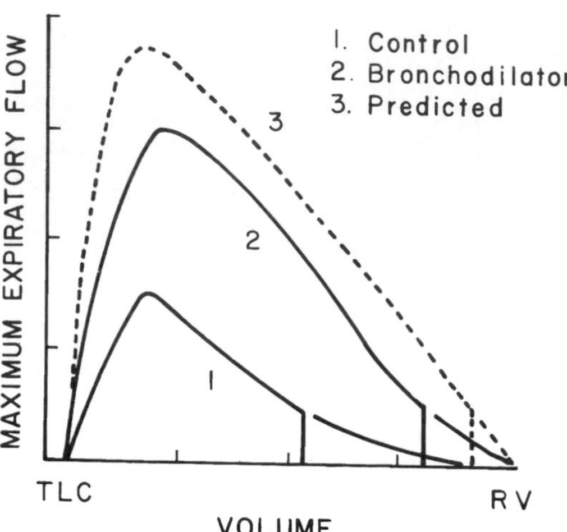

■ **FIGURE 2–53.** Maximum expiratory flow-volume (MEFV) curves of a 9-year-old boy with bronchial asthma before *(1)* and after *(2)* inhalation of nebulized bronchodilator compared with a predicted MEFV curve *(3)*. The volume between total lung capacity (TLC) and the vertical line for each MEFV curve is the forced expiratory volume in 1 sec ($FEV_{1.0}$). Note that peak expiratory flow rate (PEFR), $FEV_{1.0}$, and maximum expiratory flows ($\dot{V}max$ or MEF) at same volumes are all markedly diminished in the control curve. The bronchodilator produced a marked improvement in all flow parameters. (See text.) (From Motoyama EK: *Int Anesthesiol Clin* 26:6, 1988.)

stenosis of various causes. In addition, in older children, severe inspiratory obstruction may occur as the result of conversion reaction (Appelblatt and Baker, 1981). This condition may be mistakenly diagnosed as severe bronchial asthma. In some patients with bronchial asthma the primary site of airway obstruction is in the upper airways, with the clinical manifestation of coughing (Christopher et al., 1983).

The conventional pulmonary function tests already described are used primarily to detect impairment of lower, intrathoracic airway function and are inadequate for the evaluation of upper airway obstruction.

The intrathoracic airways narrow during forced expiration because of dynamic compression, whereas during forced inspiration they expand because of increases in surrounding negative pleural pressure. By contrast, the caliber of the extrathoracic trachea and larynx expands during forced expiration and narrows during forced inspiration, particularly when there is obstruction.

Functionally, obstructive airway lesions in the upper airways and large intrathoracic (central) airways can be classified into "variable" and "fixed" types of obstruction, based on the ability of the obstructed segment of the airways to alter its caliber in response to changes in transmural pressure. In variable extrathoracic airway obstruction, inspiratory flow is markedly reduced, whereas expiratory flow is relatively unchanged (Fig. 2–55*A*). The opposite is true with variable intrathoracic large airway obstruction (Fig. 2–55*B*). Large airway obstruction of a fixed type limits both inspiratory and expiratory flows nearly equally, because the changes in transmural pressure do not affect airway caliber (Fig. 2–55*C*). The measurement of maximum expiratory-inspiratory flow-volume curves is useful in diagnosing the location (extrathoracic versus intrathoracic) and the nature (variable versus fixed) of large airway obstruction (Kryger et al., 1976; Frenkiel et al., 1980). Figure 2–55*A* shows the maximum expiratory-inspiratory flow-volume curve of a 7-year-old girl with laryngeal papillomatosis, who, because of her "wheezing" (in reality, it was stridor) had previously been thought to have bronchial asthma. She had nearly normal MEFV curves with severe reductions in inspiratory flow. She did not respond to bronchodilators.

AIRWAY REACTIVITY

Because wheezing is often a manifestation of reactive airway disease, it is important to examine positive response to bronchodilators (hyperresponsiveness) or to stimuli that provoke bronchoconstriction. The most commonly used pulmonary function test for this purpose is the measurement of flow rates during forced expiration. Traditionally, $FEV_{1.0}$ and MMEFR have been used. More recently, however, the measurement of $\dot{V}max$ at 25% of 50% of FVC on MEFV curves has been shown to be most sensitive (Zapletal et al., 1971). Some healthy children (up to 15% of the general population) may respond to a bronchomotor challenge, but the degree of response is relatively small, usually less than 5% of the control value in $FEV_{1.0}$ and not more than 20% of the control value in MMEFR and $\dot{V}max$. When the response is beyond these ranges, hyperreactive

■ **FIGURE 2–54.** Bar graphs representing changes in total lung capacity (TLC) and its subdivisions in a 9-year-old boy with bronchial asthma before (control) and after bronchodilator use in relation to predicted values. Note the increase in TLC and residual volume (RV) and the reduction in vital capacity (VC) in the control period caused by air trapping. The RV/TLC and FRC/TLC ratios are abnormally increased. Bronchodilator use nearly abolished air trapping and restored VC. Compare these values with his flow function in Figure 2–50. IRV, inspiratory reserve volume; ERV, expiratory reserve volume; VT, tidal volume; IC, inspiratory capacity. (From Motoyama EK: *Int Anesthesiol Clin* 26:6, 1988.)

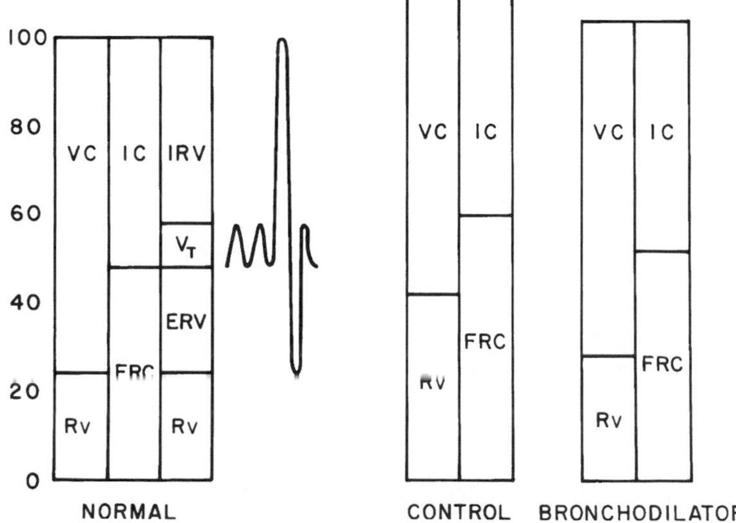

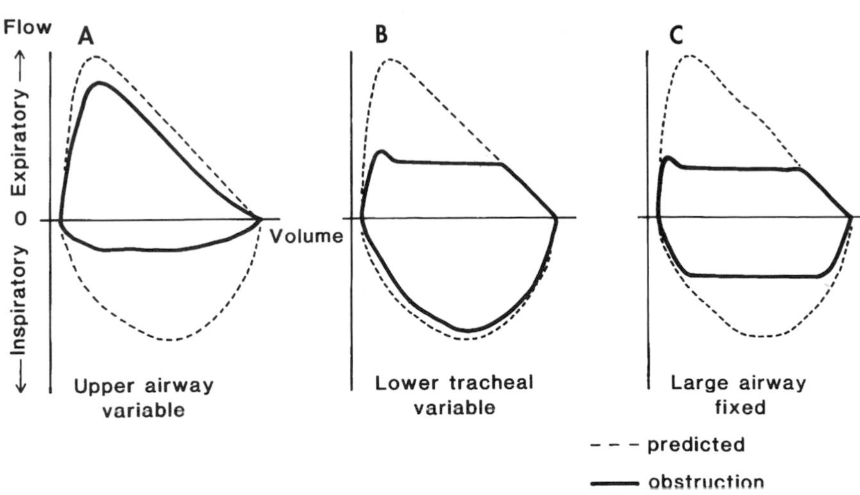

■ **FIGURE 2–55.** Schematic tracing of maximum expiratory-inspiratory flow-volume curves. *(A)* Variable upper airway obstruction due to papillomatosis of the larynx. *(B)* Variable central (intrathoracic) airway obstruction due to tracheomalacia. *(C)* Fixed-type obstruction due to tracheal stenosis. (From Motoyama EK: Physiologic alterations in tracheostomy. In Myers EN, Stool SE, Johnson JT, editors: *Tracheotomy.* New York, 1985, Churchill Livingstone.)

airway disease is suspected. In children, inhalation of aerosolized β_2-adrenergic agonists, such as albuterol (salbutamol) and metaproterenol, is used for bronchodilation. To provoke bronchoconstriction, exercise challenge has been used widely in children. The inhalation of bronchoconstrictors such as methacholine and histamine (Chatham et al., 1982), although a more definitive test, is used less frequently because of its discomfort in patients whose cooperation is less than optimal.

It has been recognized that exercise-induced bronchoconstriction results not from exercise per se but from reduction in tracheobronchial mucosal temperature caused by vigorous mouth breathing of dry air and resultant evaporative heat loss (McFadden et al., 1982). The exercise challenge test, therefore, has been replaced by cold air challenge with normocapnic hyperpnea with added carbon dioxide, which gives more consistent results (Deal et al., 1980). When MEFV curves are used to evaluate bronchial reactivity, expiratory flow rates ($\dot{V}max$) must be compared at the same lung volume before and after the challenge, which changes RV and, therefore, FVC. Because the absolute lung volume often is not available in clinical settings, $\dot{V}max$ (at 50% or 25% FVC) should be compared at the same volume below TLC, rather than at the volume above RV. The rationale for this practice is that TLC is altered relatively little (although affected by severe air trapping or its release) by comparison with large changes in RV.

PULMONARY FUNCTION TESTS IN INFANTS

Advances in neonatal intensive care and improved survival of prematurely born infants with variable degrees of chronic lung disease of prematurity since the 1980s prompted the focused interest and development of innovative techniques for pulmonary function testing in neonates, infants, and young children. A position paper was published by the International Committee on Infant Lung Mechanics based on critical evaluation of these techniques (American Thoracic Society/European Respiratory Society [ATS/ERS] Joint Committee, 1993). Guidelines for laboratory conditions, preparation of infants, sedation, and patient safety have also been published by the same group (Gaultier et al., 1995; Quanjer et al., 1995).

Measurements of Dynamic Respiratory Mechanics

Maximum or Partial Expiratory Flow-Volume Curves

Two techniques have been developed to produce flow-volume curves to evaluate lower airway function (ATS/ERS Joint Committee, 1993). Motoyama and others (1977, 1987) produced MEFV curves by "forced deflation" in infants and young children who were intubated and ventilated under sedation or general anesthesia and paralysis. With this technique, a moderate negative pressure is applied to the endotracheal tube at maximal inflation of the lung (TLC). While the lungs are rapidly deflated (within a few seconds), instantaneous expiratory flow and integrated volume signals produce an MEFV curve. $\dot{V}max$ is obtained at 25% and 10% of FEV. This forced deflation technique was found to be safe and reproducible and extremely sensitive for the evaluation of smaller airway function. The average normal value for $\dot{V}max_{25}$ (FEF_{75}) in full-term infants was 49 mL/kg per sec and $\dot{V}max_{25}$/FVC, an index of upstream conductance (or the caliber of airways toward the periphery) was 1.12, whereas in preterm infants without apparent lung disease $\dot{V}max_{25}$ was 95 mL/kg per sec and the $\dot{V}max_{25}$/FVC was 1.67. This indicates that in preterm infants, airway caliber in relation to lung volume is much larger than in full-term infants (Nakayama et al., 1991; ATS/ERS Joint Committee, 1993). A major drawback of this technique, however, is that its application is limited to the infants already intubated under general anesthesia or being cared for in the intensive care unit setting.

Another technique is the infant "squeeze" or "hugging" (thoracoabdominal compression) technique, originally reported by Adler and Wohl (1978) and later improved by Taussig and others (1982). In this technique a double-layer inflatable "jacket" is wrapped around the thorax and abdomen of a sedated infant. The inner compression bag is attached to a reservoir of compressed air, and the jacket is inflated rapidly at the end of spontaneous tidal inspiration. A partial flow-volume curve is produced, and $\dot{V}max$ at the end-tidal volume ($\dot{V}max_{FRC}$) is measured. Although the reproducibility of this test is somewhat limited, it has an advantage over the deflation technique in that it can be applied to infants who are not intubated. One major problem with this technique is that although it seems to work in infants with lower airway obstruction by producing flow limitation, the pressure and flow developed by external thoracoabdominal compression are insufficient to produce dynamic compression of the intrathoracic airways in healthy infants; no predicted normal values could be obtained (ATS/ERS Joint Committee, 1993).

Following the discussion at the mentioned ATS/ERS Joint Committee meetings, a modification of the "infant hugging" technique was developed. This technique, a raised volume thoracoabdominal compression technique, is accomplished by increasing the end-inspiratory volume initially to 20 cm H_2O and eventually to 30 cm H_2O by occluding the expiratory valve and "stacking" several tidal breathing while inspiratory flow is maintained (Feher et al., 1996; Goldstein et al., 2001). With this modified squeeze technique, expiratory flow limitation was achieved even in healthy infants (Lambert, Castile, Tepper, 2004). The advantage of this technique over the forced deflation technique is that infants can be studied with sedation alone, rather than under general endotracheal anesthesia or under sedation with muscle relaxation in ICU settings.

Measurements of Passive Respiratory Mechanics

The total respiratory system compliance (dynamic compliance) can be measured during the respiratory cycle by measuring the tidal volume and peak inspiratory pressure. In patients with airway dysfunction, however, dynamic compliance does not reflect the true (static) compliance. This problem is circumvented by a brief occlusion of the airway at end-inspiration. This approach is based on the principle that the active Hering-Breuer reflex in young infants causes a brief period of apnea during occlusion of the airway at lung volumes above FRC. The passive mechanical properties of the respiratory system can then be determined during this brief moment of respiratory muscle relaxation by removing the upper airway occlusion and allowing the lungs to deflate passively to FRC or relaxation volume (Zin, Pengelly, Milic-Emili, 1982; Mortola et al., 1982). The static compliance of the total respiratory system (Crs) is obtained by dividing the tidal volume by the relaxation pressure at the mouth during the occlusion and relaxation of the respiratory muscles, which reflects the elastic recoil of the respiratory system (LeSouef et al., 1984). In addition, by extrapolation from the plot of a flow-volume loop during passive deflation from airway occlusion, the resistance of the total respiratory system and the time constant can be obtained (LeSouef, England, Bryan, 1984). This technique can also be applied in intubated patients under general anesthesia or in intensive care unit settings, although the resistance of the endotracheal tube per se would be a major component of measured resistance.

According to published data compiled by the ATS/ERS Joint Committee (1993), dynamic lung compliance values for infants and both term and preterm infants range from 1.1 to 2.0 mL/kg per cm H_2O, whereas static compliance values range from 1.0 to 1.6 mL/kg per cm H_2O. Quasi-static compliance of the thorax (Cw) in preterm infants (6.4) exceeds that of term infants (4.2) (ATS/ERS Joint Committee, 1993). Compliance of the total respiratory system (Crs) between 1 and 12 months of age can be expressed as follows:

$Crs = 0.87 + 26.3 \times Height^3$ (Masters et al., 1987) or

$Crs = 0.88 \times Weight\ (kg)^{1.09}$ (Marchal and Crance, 1987)

Values for airway resistance (Raw) have been reported as

$Raw = 0.047 - 0.036 \times Height^3$ (Masters et al., 1987) or

$Raw = 5.36 \times Weight\ (kg)^{-0.75}$ (Marchal et al., 1988)

FRC is low in infants. As measured with the gas (helium) dilution method in infants sedated with chloral hydrate, the mean FRC was reported as 20.2 ± 4.7 mL/kg (SD; range, 20 to 24 mL/kg) up to 10 months of age, whereas FRC or VTG obtained by means of body plethysmography was higher: 23.8 ± 5.3 mL/kg (range, 29 to 34 mL/kg) (ATS/ERS Joint Committee, 1993; McCoy et al., 1996). The reason for the discrepancy between the two methods is unknown (ATS/ERS Joint Committee, 1993; Gappa et al., 1993; McCoy et al., 1996), but the magnitude of difference in FRC measured with gas dilution versus body plethysmograph (15% to 23%) was similar (McCoy et al., 1996). The values for boys and girls are similar in most studies. Table 2–6 shows the average values of respiratory rate and tidal volume in infants between birth and 12 months of age based on published data (ATS/ERS Joint Committee, 1993). The average respiratory rate is high at birth (47/min) and decreases rapidly with growth (26/min at 12 months). In contrast, average tidal volume is larger in infants (9 mL/kg) than in older children and adults (7 mL/kg) but is remarkably consistent between 3 and 12 months of age, whereas the respiratory rate changes markedly.

TABLE 2–6. Predicted values of respiratory rate and tidal volume in infants*

Age (mo)	Birth	3	6	9	12
Respiratory rate (/min)	47	38	33	29	26
Tidal volume (mL/kg)	7.4	9	9	9	9

*Weighted mean from published data.

Modified from ATS/ERS Joint Committee: Respiratory mechanics in infants: Physiologic evaluation in health and disease. *Am Rev Respir Dis* 147:474, 1993. Official Journal of the American Thoracic Society.

INDICATION FOR AND INTERPRETATION OF PULMONARY FUNCTION TESTS

Although pulmonary function tests usually do not help in diagnosing the exact location of a pathophysiologic process (for instance, left versus right lung), they do provide qualitative and quantitative assessment of the general type of disability (restrictive versus obstructive, upper versus lower airway, central versus peripheral airway), the extent of impairment, and the efficacy of various treatments, either medical or surgical.

Various indices of pulmonary function, as already described, are expressed in absolute terms as well as in percentage of the predicted normal values. Normal values are based usually on sex and height because height is better correlated with lung volumes and other ventilatory parameters than is body weight or age. More complicated multiple regression formulas include all these parameters. Ideally, each pulmonary function laboratory should establish normal values based on its own sample population, using the same instruments and techniques that are used to evaluate patients with pulmonary dysfunction as recommended by the ATS/ERS Joint Committee (1993). In reality, however, laboratories usually choose values from published data. Polgar and Promadhat (1971) compiled and compared all of the predicting formulas of pulmonary function in children published by 1969. Their data are still valid and useful today. Once the "normal" values are chosen, it is important to test a sample population of healthy children to make sure that the results fall within the predicted range of values.

For most pulmonary function indices the normal range (mean ± 2 SDs) is within 20% to 25% of the predicted values, with the exception of $\dot{V}max$ (MEF) values on MEFV curves, which range up to 40% of the mean. This does not necessarily indicate that patients with some pulmonary function indices outside of this range have lung disease. Serial pulmonary function tests in these patients are invaluable for a better understanding of the presence or absence of disease and its progression with time.

What particular test or combination of tests is most useful? In a child who wheezes, it is essential to investigate lower airway function, because wheezing is most often caused by reactive airway disease (bronchial asthma, bronchopulmonary dysplasia, etc.). Wheezing is usually caused by the narrowing of relatively large intrathoracic (lower) airways (i.e., tracheal and large bronchi) and occurs during expiration. It should be kept in mind that both stridors (mostly inspiratory), coming from narrowing of the extrathoracic (laryngopharyngeal) airways, and rhonchi (both inspiratory and expiratory), usually caused by rattling of secretions in the trachea or large bronchi, are often mistaken as wheezing.

If there is considerable lower airway dysfunction, lung volume should be measured to determine the extent of dysfunction and air trapping. Evaluation of bronchial hyperresponsiveness with a bronchodilator must also be done in these patients and, if it is present, the extent of reversibility should be evaluated. Upper airway function should be examined in patients with stridor and in those in whom lower airway dysfunction is absent or mild in relation to overall respiratory symptoms.

Which children should have pulmonary function tests preoperatively? All children with a history of severe neonatal respiratory disease, such as bronchopulmonary dysplasia or meconium aspiration, with severe bronchiolitis, and those who wheeze should have a consultation with a pulmonologist and have a baseline pulmonary function test performed to establish the nature of the lung dysfunction. These children often have lower airway obstruction and abnormal gas exchange with reactive airway disease (Motoyama, 1988). At the least, oxygen saturation should be measured in room air preoperatively as a guide for postoperative management. In addition, children with history of asthma, cystic fibrosis, or gastroesophageal reflux often have moderate to severe lung dysfunction, and they should be evaluated by a pulmonologist. Another condition requiring pulmonary function testing is scoliosis before surgical repair. Adolescents with scoliosis may have a moderate to severe restrictive defect, especially those with muscular dystrophy, and some of these patients cannot generate sufficient airway pressure for effective coughing or lung expansion postoperatively. These patients, as well as surgeons, should know what to expect postoperatively, and the anesthesiologist should make sure that an intensive care unit bed is reserved for postoperative care.

With advanced knowledge and new technology, the ability of a pulmonary function laboratory to evaluate and document pulmonary dysfunction has improved considerably. Standard pulmonary function testing is effective in identifying the site, nature, and extent of airway dysfunction, as well as changes in volume function in children. With new developments in the various noninvasive test methods, it is now possible in an increasing number of pediatric medical centers to evaluate lung function and the presence of reversible (reactive) airway disease in infants, even those in respiratory failure. Pulmonary function test results are helpful for planning the anesthetic approach and postoperative management of infants and children with known pulmonary dysfunction.

SUMMARY

It is apparent that respiration of pediatric patients, especially neonates and young infants, is considerably different from that of older children and adults. Respiratory control mechanisms are not fully developed until at least 42 to 44 weeks postconception, especially in terms of their response to hypoxia.

BOX 2–5 Infants Are Prone to Perioperative Hypoxemia

1. Immature respiratory control and irregular breathing
   Hypoxia does not stimulate, but rather depresses, ventilation.
   Trace anesthetics abolish hypoxic ventilatory response.
2. Infants have small FRC and high oxygen demand.
3. Anesthesia reduces FRC; airway closure and atelectasis result
   Prone to hypoxemia (Sp_{O_2} < 94%) in the PACU (20% to 40%).
4. Infants are prone to upper airway obstruction.
5. High oxygen affinity (low oxygen unloading) of fetal hemoglobin.

The lungs are immature at birth, even in full-term infants. Most alveolar formation and elastogenesis occurs postnatally during the first year of life. Thoracic structure is insufficient to support the negative pleural pressure generated during the respiratory cycle, at least until the infant develops the muscle strength for upright posture toward the end of the first year. Weakness of the thoracic structure is in part compensated by tonic contractions of the intercostal and accessory muscles. Anesthesia and muscle relaxation abolish this compensatory mechanism, and the end-expiratory lung volume (FRC) decreases to the point of airway closure, resulting in widespread alveolar collapse and atelectasis. Infants are prone to upper airway obstruction because of anatomic and physiologic differences, as discussed in this chapter. Anesthesia preferentially depresses tonic and phasic activities of the pharyngeal and other neck muscles, which normally resist the collapsing forces in the pharynx.

Fetal hemoglobin has high oxygen affinity and limits oxygen unloading at the tissue level. These factors, unique to young infants less than 3 months of age, result in decreases in oxygen delivery to the tissues that have much higher oxygen demands than those of adults. Thus, infants and young children are prone to perioperative hypoxemia and tissue hypoxia (Box 2–5).

REFERENCES

Adatia I, Wessel DL: Therapeutic use of inhaled nitric oxide. *Curr Opin Pediatr* 6:583, 1994.

Adler SM, Wohl MEB: Flow-volume relationship at low lung volumes in healthy term newborn infants. *Pediatrics* 61:636, 1978.

Agostoni E: Volume-pressure relationships of the thorax and lung in the newborn. *J Appl Physiol* 14:909, 1959.

Albersheim S, Boychuk R, Seshia MMK, et al.: Effects of CO_2 on immediate ventilatory response to O_2 in preterm infants. *J Appl Physiol* 41:609, 1976.

Alcorn D, Adamson DT, Maloney JE, et al.: Morphological effects of chronic bilateral phrenectomy or vagotomy in the fetal lamb lung. *J Anat* 130:683, 1980.

Al-Shway SE, Mortola JP: Respiratory effects of airflow through the upper airways in newborn kittens and puppies. *J Appl Physiol* 53:805, 1982.

American Thoracic Society: Single-breath carbon monoxide diffusing capacity (transfer factor). Recommendations for a standard technique—1995 Update. *Am J Respir Crit Care Med* 152:2185–2198, 1995.

American Thoracic Society/European Respiratory Society Joint Committee: Respiratory mechanics in infants: Physiologic evaluation in health and disease. *Am Rev Respir Dis* 147:474, 1993.

Ansfleld MJ, Benson BJ: Identification of the immunosuppressive components of canine pulmonary surface active material. *J Immunol* 125:1092, 1980.

Appelblatt NJ, Baker SR: Functional upper airway obstruction. *Arch Otolaryngol* 107:305, 1981.

Aranda JV, Trumen T: Methylxanthines in apnea of prematurity. *Clin Perinatal* 6:87, 1979.
Areechon W, Reid L: Hypoplasia of lung with congenital diaphragmatic hernia. *Br Med J* 1:230, 1963.
Assali NS, Morris JA: Maternal and fetal circulations and their interrelationships. *Obstet Gynecol Surv* 19:923, 1964.
ATS Assembly on Pediatrics and the ERS Paediatrics Assembly: ATS statement. Respiratory mechanics in infants: Physiologic evaluation in health and disease. *Am Rev Respir Dis* 147:474, 1993.
Aubier, DeTroyer A, Sampson M, et al.: Aminophylline improves diaphragmatic contractility. *N Engl J Med* 305:249, 1981.
Avery ME: The argument for prenatal administration of dexamethasone to prevent respiratory distress syndrome (editorial). *J Pediatr* 104:240, 1984.
Avery ME, Aylward G, Creasy R, et al.: Update on prenatal steroid for prevention of respiratory distress. Report of a conference, September 26–28, 1985. *Am J Obstet Gynecol* 155:2, 1986.
Avery ME, Mead J: Surface properties in relation to atelectasis and hyaline membrane disease. *Am J Dis Child* 97:517, 1959.
Baier RJ, Hasan SU, Gates DB, et al.: Effects of various concentrations of O_2 and umbilical cord occlusion on fetal breathing and behavior. *J Appl Physiol* 68:1597, 1990.
Barillot JC, Bianchi AL: Activité des motoneurons larynges pendant reflexes de Hering-Breuer. *J Physiol (Paris)* 63:783, 1971.
Bartlett D Jr, Jeffrey P, Sant'Ambrogio G, Wise JCM: Location of stretch receptors in the trachea and bronchi of the dog. *J Physiol (Lond)* 258:409, 1976.
Bartlett D Jr, Leiter JC, Hollowell E: Control and actions of the genio-glossus muscle. In Issa FG, Suratt PM, Remmers JE, editors: *Sleep and respiration.* New York, 1990, Wiley-Liss.
Bartlett D Jr, Remmers JE, Gautier H: Laryngeal regulation of respiratory airflow. *Respir Physiol* 18:194, 1973.
Bar-Yishay E, Shulman DL, Ecoffey C, Gaultier C: Functional residual capacity in healthy preschool children lying supine. *Am Rev Respir Dis* 135:954, 1987.
Bastel HL, Lines AJ: Neural mechanisms of sneeze. *Am J Physiol* 229:770, 1975.
Bates DV: Respiratory disorders associated with impairment of gas diffusion. *Annu Rev Med* 13:301, 1962.
Bates DV, editor: *Respiratory function in disease,* ed 3. Philadelphia, 1989, WB Saunders Co.
Bates DV, Macklem PT, Christie RV: *Respiratory Junction in disease,* ed 2. Philadelphia, 1971, WB Saunders.
Benameur M, Goldman MD, Ecoffey C, Gaultier C: Ventilation and thoracoabdominal asynchrony during halothane anesthesia in infants. *J Appl Physiol* 74:l591, l993.
Benesch R, Benesch RE: The effect of organic phosphates from the human erythrocytes on the allosteric properties of hemoglobin. *Biochem Biophys Res Commun* 26:162, 1967.
Benumof JL: Respiratory physiology and respiratory function during anesthesia. In Miller RD, editor: *Anesthesia,* ed 4. New York, 1994, Churchill Livingstone.
Berger AJ: Control of breathing. In Murray JF, Nadel JA, editors: *Textbook of respiratory medicine.* Philadelphia, 1988, WB Saunders.
Berger AJ: Control of breathing. In Murray JF, Nadel JA, editors: *Textbook of respiratory medicine.* Philadelphia, 2000, WB Saunders.
Berger AJ: Dorsal respiratory neurons in the medulla of cat: Spinal projections, responses to lung inflation and superior laryngeal nerve stimulation. *Brain Res* 135:231, 1977.
Berger AJ: Phrenic motoneurons in the cat: Subpopulations and nature of respiratory drive potentials. *J Neurophysiol* 42:76, 1979.
Bergman NA: Distribution of inspired gas during anesthesia and artificial ventilation. *J Appl Physiol* 18:1085, 1963.
Betts EK, Downes JJ, Schaffer DB, Johns R: Retrolental fibroplasia and oxygen administration during general anesthesia. *Anesthesiology* 47:518, 1977.
Bianchi AL, Bariollot JC: Respiratory neurons in the region of the retro-facial nucleus: Pontile, medullary, spinal and vagal projections. *Neuroscience Lett* 31:277, 1982.
Bigatello LM, Hurford WE, Kacmarek RM: Prolonged inhalation of low concentrations of nitric oxide in patients with severe adult respiratory distress syndrome. *Anesthesiology* 80:761, 1994.
Bjertnaes LJ: Hypoxia-induced pulmonary vasoconstriction in man: Inhibition due to diethyl ether and halothane anesthesia. *Acta Anaesthesiol Scand* 22:570, 1978.
Boddy K, Dawes GS, Fisher R, et al.: Fetal respiratory movements, electrocortical and cardiovascular responses to hypoxaemia and hypercapnia in sheep. *J Physiol (Lond)* 243:399, 1974.
Boddy K, Robinson JS: External method for detection of fetal breathing in utero. *Lancet* 2:1231, 1971.
Boggs DF, Bartlett D: Chemical specificity of a laryngeal apneic reflex in puppies. *J Appl Physiol* 53:455, 1982.
Boughton K, Gandy G, Gairdner D: Hyaline membrane disease. II. Lung lecithin. *Arch Dis Child* 45:311, 1970.
Boyden EA: The pattern of the terminal air spaces in a premature infant of 30-32 weeks that lived 19 1/4 hours. *Am J Anat* 126:31, 1969.
Bradley GW, von Euler C, Marttila I, Roos B: A model of the central and reflex inhibition of inspiration in the cat. *Biol Cybern* 19:105, 1975.
Brady JP, Ceruti E: Chemoreceptor reflexes in the newborn infant. Effects of varying degrees of hypoxia on heart rate and ventilation in a warm environment. *J Physiol (Lond)* 184:631, 1966.
Brody JS, Thurlbeck WM: Development, growth, and aging of the lung. In Geiger SR, Macklem PT, Mead J, Fishman AP, editors: *Handbook of physiology. Section 3. The respiratory system. Vol 3. Mechanics of breathing, part 1.* Bethesda, MD, 1986, American Physiological Society.
Brooks JG: Apnea of infancy and sudden infant death syndrome. *Am J Dis Child* 136:1012, 1982.
Brouillette RT, Thach BT: A neuromuscular mechanism maintaining extra-thoracic airway patency. *J Appl Physiol* 46:772, 1979.
Brouillette RT, Thach BT: Control of genioglossus muscle inspiratory activity. *J Appl Physiol* 49:801, 1980.
Bryan AC, Wohl ME: Respiratory mechanics in children. In Geiger SR, Macklem PT, Mead J, Fishman AP, editors: *Handbook of physiology. Section 3. The respiratory system. Vol 3. Mechanics of breathing, part 1.* Bethesda, MD, 1986, American Physiological Society.
Bucci G, Cook CD: Studies of respiratory physiology in children. VI. Lung diffusing capacity, diffusing capacity of the pulmonary membrane, and pulmonary capillary blood volume in congenital heart disease. *J Clin Invest* 40:1431, 1961.
Bucci G, Cook CD, Barrie H: *J Pediatr* 58:820, 1961.
Bucher HU, Fanconi S, Baeckert P, Duc G: Hyperoxemia in newborn infants: Detection by pulse oximetry. *Pediatrics* 84:226, 1989.
Bureau M, Bouverot P: Blood and CSF acid-base changes and rate of ventilatory acclimatization of awake dogs to 3,500 m. *Respir Physiol* 24:203, 1975.
Burri PH: The postnatal growth of the rat lung. III. Morphology. *Anat Rec* 178:711, 1974.
Card RT, Brain MC: The "anemia" of childhood; evidence for a physiologic response to hyperphosphatemia. *N Engl J Med* 288:388, 1973.
Celermajer DS, Dollery C, Burch M, Deanfield JE: Role of endothelium in the maintenance of low pulmonary vascular tone in normal children. *Circulation* 89:2035, 1994.
Ceruti E: Chemoreceptor reflexes in the newborn infant. Effect of cooling on the response to hypoxia. *Pediatrics* 37:556, 1966.
Chanutin A, Curnish RR: Effect of organic and inorganic phosphates on the oxygen equilibrium of human erythrocytes. *Arch Biochem* 121:96, 1967.
Chatham M, Bleecker ER, Norman P, et al.: A screening test for airway reactivity. An abbreviated methacholine inhalation challenge. *Chest* 82:15, 1982.
Cherniack NS, Pack AI: Control of ventilation. In Fishman AP, editor: *Pulmonary diseases and disorders,* ed 2. *Vol 1, part 2: Physiological principles.* New York, 1988, McGraw-Hill Book Co.
Chernick V, Faridy EE, Pagtakhan RD: Role of peripheral and central chemoreceptors in the initiation of fetal respiration. *J Appl Physiol* 38:407, 1975.
Chernick V, Heldrich F, Avery ME: Periodic breathing of premature infants. *J Pediatr* 64:330, 1964.
Christopher KL, Wood RP II, Eckert C, et al.: Vocal cord dysfunction presenting as asthma. *N Engl J Med* 308:1566, 1983.
Clark FJ, von Euler C: On the regulation of depth and rate of breathing. *J Physiol (Lond)* 222:267, 1972.
Clements JA, Brown ES, Johnson RP: Pulmonary surface tension and mucus lining of the lungs; some theoretical considerations. *J Appl Physiol* 12:262, 1958.
Cogswell JJ, Hull D, Milner AD, et al.: Lung function in childhood. III. Measurement of airflow resistance in healthy children. *Br J Dis Chest* 69:177, 1975.
Cohen J: Pathophysiology of sepsis: Role of nitric oxide and other mediators. *Curr Opin Anaesthesiol* 8:109, 1995.
Cohen MI: Central determinants of respiratory rhythm. *Anna Rev Physiol* 43:91, 1981b.
Cohen MI: How is respiratory rhythm generated? *Fed Proc* 40:2372, 1981a.
Cohen MI: Neurogenesis of respiratory rhythm in the mammal. *Physiol Rev* 59:1105, 1979.
Cohen MI: Switching of the respiratory phases and evoked phrenic responses produced by rostral pontine electrical stimulation. *J Physiol (Lond)* 217:133, 1971.
Coleridge HM, Coleridge JCG, Ginzel KH, et al.: Stimulation of "irritant" receptors and afferent C-fibers in the lungs by prostaglandins. *Nature* 264:451, 1976.

Coleridge JCG, Coleridge HMG: Afferent vagal C fibre innervation of the lungs and airways and its functional significance. *Rev Physiol Biochem Pharmacol* 99:1, 1984.

Colin AA, Wohl MEB, Mead J, et al.: Transition from dynamically maintained to relaxed end-expiratory volume in human infants. *J Appl Physiol* 67:2107. 1989.

Colley PS, Cheney FW Jr, Hlastala MP: Ventilation-perfusion and gas exchange effects of sodium nitroprusside in dogs with normal edematous lungs. *Anesthesiology* 30:489, 1979.

Comoe JH: *Physiology of respiration: An introductory text,* ed 2. Chicago, 1974, Year Book Medical Publishers.

Consensus Conference: Perioperative red blood cell transfusion. *JAMA* 260:2700, 1988.

Cook CD, Cherry RB, O'Brien D, et al.: Studies of respiratory physiology in the newborn infant. I. Observations on the normal premature and full-term infants. *J Clin Invest* 34:975, 1955.

Cook CD, Drinker PA, Jacobson HN, et al.: Control of pulmonary blood flow in the foetal and newly born lamb. *J Physial (Lond)* 169:10, 1963.

Cook CD, Sutherland JM, Segal S, et al.: Studies of respiratory physiology in the newborn infant. HI. Measurements of mechanics of respiration. *J Clin Invest* 36:440, 1957.

Coté CJ, Goldslein EA, Coté MA, et al.: A single-blind study of pulse oximetry in children. *Anesthesiology* 68:184, 1988.

Coté CJ, Rolf N, Liu LMP, Gousouzian NG: A single-blind study of pulse oximetry and capnography in children. *Anesthesiology* 74:984, 1991.

Coté CJ, Zaslavsky A, Downes JJ, et al.: Postoperative apnea in former preterm infants after inguinal herniorrhaphy. A combined analysis. *Anesthesiology* 82:809–822, 1995.

Cotes JE, Chinn DJ, Quanjer PH, et al.: Official statement of the European Respiratory Society: Standardization of the measurement of transfer factor (diffusing capacity). *Eur Respir J* 6:(suppl 16):41–52, 1993.

Crapo RO, Jensen RL, Wagner JS: Single breath carbon monoxide diffusing capacity. *Clin Chest Med* 22:637–649, 2001.

Cross KW, Klaus M, Tooley WH, Weisser K: The response of the newborn baby to inflation of the lungs. *J Physiol (Lond)* 151:551, 1960.

Cross KW, Oppe TE: The effect of inhalation of high and low concentrations of oxygen on the respiration of the premature infant. *J Physiol (Lond)* 117:38, 1952.

Dahan A, van den Elsen MJLW, Berkenbosch A, et al.: Effects of subanesthetic halothane on the ventilatory response to hypercapnia and acute hypoxia in healthy volunteers. *Anesthesiology* 80:727, 1994.

D'Angelo E, Calderini G, Torri FM et al: Respiratory mechanics in anesthetized paralyzed humans: Effects of flow, volume and time. *J Appl Physiol* 67:2556, 1989.

Davies AM, Koenig JS, Thach BT: Upper airway chemoreflex response to saline and water in preterm infants. *J Appl Physiol* 64:1412, 1988.

Davies H, Kitchman R, Gordon I, Helms P: Regional ventilation in infancy: Reversal of adult pattern. *N Engl J Med* 313:1626, 1985.

Davies RO, Edwards MW, Lahiri S: Halothane depresses the response of carotid body chemoreceptors to hypoxia and hypercarbia in the cat. *Anesthesiology* 57:153, 1982.

Dawes GS: Breathing before birth in animals and man. *N Engl J Med* 290:557, 1974.

Dawes GS, Fox HE, Leduc MB, et al.: Respiratory movements and paradoxical sleep in the fetal lamb. *J Physiol (Lond)* 210:47P, 1970.

Dawes GS, Fox HE, Leduc MB, et al.: Respiratory movements and rapid eye movement sleep in the fetal lamb. *J Physiol (Lond)* 2211:119, 1972.

Dawes GS, Gardner WN, Johnston BM, Walker DW: Effects of hypercapnia on tracheal pressure, diaphragm and intercostal electromyograms in unanesthetized fetal lambs. *J Physiol (Lond)* 326:461, 1982.

Dawson SV, Elliott EA: Wave-speed limitation on expiratory flow—A unifying concept. *J Appl Physiol* 43:498, 1977.

Deal EC, McFadden ER, Ingram RH, et al.: Airway responsiveness to cold air and hyperpnea in normal subjects and in those with hay fever and asthma. *Am Rev Respir Dis* 121:621, 1980.

Decima EE, von Euler C: Excitability of phrenic motoneurons to afferent input from lower intercostal nerves in the spinal cat. *Acta Physiol Scand* 75:580, 1969.

deLemos RA, Shermeta DW, Knelson JH, et al.: Acceleration of appearance of pulmonary surfactant in the fetal lamb by administration of corticosteroids. *Am Rev Respir Dis* 102:459, 1970.

deMello DE, Reid LM: Respiratory tract and lungs. In Reed GB, Claireaux AE, Cockburn F, editors: *Disease of the fetus and newborn,* ed 2. London, 1995, Chapman & Hall.

Derenne JP, Couture J, Iscoe S, et al.: Occlusion pressures in men rebreathing CO_2 under methoxyflurane anesthesia. *J Appl Physiol* 40:805, 1976.

deTroyer A, Bastenier-Geens J: Effect of neuromuscular blockade on respiratory mechanics in conscious man. *J Appl Physiol* 47:1162, 1979.

Dobbinson TL, Nisbet HIA, Pelton DA: Functional residual capacity (FRC) and compliance in anaesthetized paralysed children. Part I: In vitro tests with the helium dilution method of measuring FRC. *Can Anaesth Soc J* 20:310, 1973.

Don HF, Wahba M, Cuadrado L, Kelkar K: The effects of anesthesia and 100% oxygen on the functional residual capacity of the lungs. *Anesthesiology* 67:695, 1987.

Donnelly DF, Haddad GG: Respiratory changes induced by prolonged laryngeal stimulation in awake piglets. *J Appl Physiol* 61:1018, 1986.

Dripps RD, Comroe JH Jr: The respiratory and circulatory response of normal man to inhalation of 7.6 and 10.4 percent CO_2 with a comparison of the maximal ventilation produced by severe muscular exercise, inhalation of CO_2 and maximal voluntary hyperventilation. *Am J Physiol* 149:43, 1947.

Drummond GB: Reduction of tonic ribcage muscle activity by anesthesia with thiopental. *Anesthesiology* 67:695, 1987.

Dunnill MS: Postnatal growth of the lung. *Thorax* 17:329, 1962.

Duron B: Intercostal and diaphragmatic muscle endings and afferents. In Hornbein TF, editor: *Regulation of breathing,* part 1. New York, 1981, Marcel Dekker.

Dutton RE, Chernick V, Moses H, et al.: Ventilatory response to intermittent inspired carbon dioxide. *J Appl Physiol* 19:931, 1964.

Eckenhoff JE: Some anatomic considerations of the infant larynx influencing endotracheal anesthesia. *Anesthesiology* 12:401, 1951.

Edelman NH, Lahiri S, Brando L, et al.: The blunted ventilatory response to hypoxia in cyanotic congenital heart disease. *N Engl J Med* 282:405, 1970.

Emery JL: *The anatomy of the developing lung.* London, 1969, Heinemann Medical Books, Ltd.

England SJ, Stogren HAF: Influence of the upper airway on breathing pattern and expiratory time constant in dog pups. *Respir Physiol* 66:181, 1986.

Enhorning G, Shennan A, Possmayer F, et al.: Prevention of neonatal respiratory distress syndrome by tracheal instillation of surfactant: A randomized clinical trial. *Pediatrics* 76:145, 1985.

Fagan DG: Post-mortem studies of the semistatic volume-pressure characteristics of infants' lungs. *Thorax* 31:534, 1976.

Fagan DG: Shape changes in static V-P loops for children's lungs related to growth. *Thorax* 32:193, 1977.

Feher A, Castile R, Kisling J et al: Flow limitation in normal infants: A new method for forced expiratory maneuvers from raised lung volumes. *J Appl Physiol* 80:2019–2025, 1996.

Feldman JL: Neurophysiology of breathing in mammals. In Bloom FE, editor: *Handbook of physiology. Section I. Nervous system. Vol 4. Intrinsic regulatory systems of the brain.* Bethesda, MD, 1986, American Physiological Society.

Feldman JL, Gautier H: Interaction of pulmonary afferents and pneumotaxic center in control of respiratory pattern in cats. *J Neurophysiol* 39:31, 1976.

Feldman JL, Speck DF: Interaction among inspiratory neurons in dorsal and ventral respiratory groups in cat medulla. *J Neurophysiol* 49:472, 1983.

Fenner A, Jansson EH, Avery ME: Enhancement of the ventilatory response to carbon dioxide by tube breathing. *Respir Physiol* 4:91, 1968.

Fenner A, Schalk U, Hoenicke H, et al.: Periodic breathing in premature and neonatal babies: Incidence, breathing pattern, respiratory gas tensions, response to changes in the composition of ambient air. *Pediatr Res* 7:174, 1973.

Ferris BG, Mead J, Opie LH: Partitioning of respiratory flow resistance in man. *J Appl Physiol* 19:653, 1964.

Finch CA, Lenfant C: Oxygen transport in man, *N Engl J Med* 286:407, 1972.

Fink BR, Demarest RJ: *Laryngeal biomechanics.* Cambridge, MA, 1978, Harvard University Press.

Finley TN, Swenson EW, Comroe JH Jr: The cause of arterial hypoxemia at rest in patients with "alveolar-capillary block syndrome." *J Clin Invest* 41:618, 1962.

Fisher JT, Mathew OP, Sant'Ambrogio FB, Sant'Ambrogio G: Reflex effects and receptor responses to upper airway pressure and flow in developing puppies. *J Appl Physiol* 58:258, 1985.

Fisher JT, Mortola JP, Smith GS, et al.: Respiration in newborns: Development of the control of breathing. *Am Rev Respir Dis* 125:650, 1982.

Fletcher ME, Ewert M, Stack C, et al.: Influence of tidal volume on respiratory compliance in anesthetized infants and young children. *J Appl Physiol* 68:1127, 1990.

Flynn JT, Bancalari E, Snyder ES, et al.: A cohort study of transcutaneous oxygen tension and the incidence and severity of retinopathy of prematurity. *N Engl J Med* 326:1050, 1992.

Forbes AR: Temperature, humidity and mucous flow in the intubated trachea. *Br J Anaesth* 46:29, 1974.

Forbes AR: Halothane depresses mucociliary flow in the trachea. *Anesthesiology* 45:59, 1976.
Forbes AR, Gamsu G: Lung mucociliary clearance after anesthesia and spontaneous and controlled ventilation. *Am Rev Respir Dis* 120:857, 1979.
Forbes AR, Horrigan RW: Mucociliary flow in the trachea during anesthesia with enflurane, ether, nitrous oxide, and morphine. *Anesthesiology* 46:319, 1977.
Forster RE: Exchange of gases between alveolar air and pulmonary capillary blood; pulmonary diffusing capacity. *Physiol Rev* 37:391, 1957.
Forster RE II: The single breath carbon monoxide transfer test 25 years: A reappraisal 1. Physiological considerations. *Thorax* 38:1–5, 1983.
Foster HV, Dempsey JA, Chosy LW: Incomplete compensation of CSF (H^+) in man during acclimatization to high altitude (4,300 m). *J Appl Physiol* 38:1067, 1975.
Fournier L, Major D: The effect of nitrous oxide on the oxyhaemoglobin dissociation curve. *Can Anaesth Soc J* 31:173, 1984.
Frantz ID III, Adler SM, Thach BT, Taeusch HW Jr: Maturational effects on respiratory responses to carbon dioxide in premature infants. *J Appl Physiol* 41:634, 1976.
Fratacci MD, Frostell CG, Chen TY, et al.: Inhaled nitric oxide: A selective pulmonary vasodilator of heparin-protamine vasoconstriction in sheep. *Anesthesiology* 75:990, 1991.
Frenkiel S, Desmond K, Coates AL, et al.: Upper airway obstruction in children: The value of inspiratory-expiratory flow-volume curves. *J Otolaryngol* 9:7, 1980.
Freund F, Roos A, Dood RB: Expiratory activity of the abdominal muscles in man during general anesthesia. *J Appl Physiol* 19:963, 1964.
Frostell CG, Blomqvist H, Hedenstierna G, et al.: Inhaled nitric oxide selectively reverses human hypoxic pulmonary vasoconstriction without causing systemic vasodilation. *Anesthesiology* 78:427, 1993.
Frostell C, Fratacci MD, Wain JC, et al.: Inhaled nitric oxide: A selective pulmonary vasodilator reversing hypoxic pulmonary vasoconstriction. *Circulation* 83:2083, 1991.
Fujiwara T, Maeta H, Chida S, et al.: Artificial surfactant therapy in hyaline membrane disease. *Lancet* 1:55, 1980.
Funk GD, Feldman JL: Generation of respiratory rhythm and pattern in mammals: Insights from developmental studies. *Curr Opin Neurobiol* 5:778–785, 1995.
Furchgott RF, Vanhoutte PM: Endothelium-derived relaxing and contracting factors. *FASEB J* 3:2007, 1989.
Furchgott RF, Zawadzki JV: The obligatory role of endothelial cells in the relaxation of arterial smooth muscle by acetylcholine. *Nature* 288:373, 1980.
Gaultier C, Boule M, Allaire Y, et al.: Growth of lung volumes during the first three years of life. *Bull Eur Physiopathol Respir* 15:1103, 1979.
Gaultier C, Fletcher ME, Beardsmore C, et al.: Respiratory function measurement in infants: Measurement conditions. *Am J Respir Crit Care Med* 151:2058, 1995.
Gautier H, Bertrand F: Respiratory effects of pneumotaxic center lesions and subsequent vagotomy in chronic cats. *Respir Physiol* 23:71, 1975.
Gerhardt T, Bancalari E: Chest wall compliance in full term and premature infants. *Acta Paediatr Scand* 69:359, 1980.
Gerhardt T, Bancalari E: Components of effective elastance and their maturational changes in human newborns. *J Appl Physiol* 53:766, 1982.
Gerhardt T, Reifenberg L, Hehre D, et al.: Functional residual capacity in normal neonates and children up to 5 years of age determined by a N_2 washout method. *Pediatr Res* 20:668, 1986.
Glenn WWL, Holcomb WG, Hogan J, et al.: Diaphragm pacing by radiofrequency transmission in the treatment of chronic ventilatory insufficiency. *J Thorac Cardiovasc Surg* 66:505, 1973.
Glezen WP, Denny FW: Epidemiology of acute lower respiratory disease in children. *N Engl J Med* 288:498, 1973.
Glotzbach SF, Tansey PA, Baldwin RB, Ariagno RL: Periodic breathing in preterm infants: Influence of bronchopulmonary dysplasia and theophylline. *Pediatr Pulmonol* 7:78, 1989.
Goldberg MS, Milic-Emili J: Effect of sodium pentobarbital on respiratory control in newborn rabbits. *J Appl Physiol* 42:845, 1977.
Goldring RM, Fishman AP, Turino GM, et al.: Pulmonary hypertension and cor pulmonale in cystic fibrosis of the pancreas. *J Pediatr* 65:501, 1964.
Goldstein AB, Castile RG, Davis SD, et al.: Bronchodilator responsiveness in normal infants and young children. *Am J Respir Crit Care Med* 164:447–454, 2001.
Goldzimer EL, Konopka RG, Moser KM: Reversal of the perfusion defect in experimental canine labor pneumococcal pneumonia. *J Appl Physiol* 37:85, 1974.
Gregory GA, Kitterman JA, Phibbs RH, et al.: Treatment of the idiopathic respiratory-distress syndrome with continuous positive airway pressure. *N Engl J Med* 284:1333, 1971.
Guedel A: *Inhalation anesthesia.* New York, 1937, MacMillan Publishing Co.
Guz A, Noble MIM, Eisel JH, Trenchard D: The role of vagal inflation reflexes in man and other animals. In Porter R, editor: *Breathing: Hering-Breuer Centenary Symposium.* London, 1970, Churchill Livingstone.
Hallman M: Antenatal diagnosis of lung maturity. In Robertson B, van Golde LMG, Batenvurg JJ, editors: *Pulmonary surfactant.* Amsterdam, 1984, Elsevier.
Haraguchi S, Fung R, Sasaki CT: Effect of hyperthermia on the laryngeal closure reflex: Implications for the sudden infant death syndrome. *Ann Otol Rhinol Laryngol* 92:24, 1983.
Harding R: Function of the larynx in the fetus and newborn. *Annu Rev Physiol* 46:645, 1984.
Hart MC, Orzalesi MM, Cook CD: Relation between anatomic respiratory dead space and body size and lung volume. *J Appl Physiol* 18:519, 1963.
Heaf DP, Helms P, Gordon I, Turner HM: Postural effects on gas exchange in infants. *N Engl J Med* 308:1505, 1983.
Hedenstierna G, McCarthy GS: Airway closure and closing volume during mechanical ventilation. *Acta Anaesth Scand* 24:299, 1980.
Henderson-Smart DJ, Read DJC: Reduced lung volume during behavior active sleep in the newborn. *J Appl Physiol* 46:1081, 1979.
Hershenson MB, Colin AA, Wohl MEB, Start AR: Changes in contribution of the rib cage to tidal breathing during infancy. *Am Rev Respir Dis* 141:922, 1990.
Hewlett AM, Hulands GH, Nunn JF, Milledge JS: Functional residual capacity during anesthesia. III. Artificial ventilation. *Br J Anaesth* 46:495, 1974.
Hickey RF, Severinghaus JW: Regulation of breathing: Drug effect. In Hornbein TF, editor: *Lung biology in health and disease. Regulation of breathing.* New York, 1981, Dekker.
Hill AB, Chir B, Sykes MK, et al.: A hypoxic pulmonary vasoconstrictor response in dogs during and after infusion of sodium nitroprusside. *Anesthesiology* 50:484, 1979.
Hirsch JA, Tokayer JL, Robinson MJ, et al.: Effects of dry air and subsequent humidification on tracheal mucous velocity in dogs. *J Appl Physiol* 39:242, 1975.
Hirshman CA, McCullough RE, Cohen PJ, Weil JV: Depression of hypoxic ventilatory response by halothane, enflurane and isoflurane in dogs. *Br J Anaesth* 49:957, 1977.
Hislop A, Reid L: Development of the acinus in the human lung. *Thorax* 29:90, 1974.
Hoekstra RE, Jackson JC, Myers TF, et al.: Improved neonatal survival following multiple doses of bovine surfactant in very premature neonates at risk for respiratory distress syndrome. *Pediatrics* 88:10, 1991.
Hogg JC, Williams J, Richardson JB, et al.: Age as a factor in the distribution of lower airway conductance and in the pathologic anatomy of obstructive lung disease. *N Engl J Med* 282:1283, 1970.
Holms BA: Surfactant replacement therapy. New levels of understanding. *Am Rev Respir Dis* 148:834, 1993.
Hughes JMB, Glazier JB, Maloney JE, West JB: Effect of lung volume on the distribution of pulmonary blood flow in man. *Respir Physiol* 4:58, 1968.
Hughes JMB, Rosenzweig DY, Kivitz PB: Site of airway closure in excised dog lung: Histologic demonstration. *J Appl Physiol* 29:340, 1970.
Hutcheon M, Griffin P, Levison H, Zamel N: Volume of isoflow: A new test in detection of mild abnormalities of lung mechanics. *Am Rev Respir Dis* 110:458, 1974.
Hwang JC, St. John WM, Bartlett D: Afferent pathways for hypoglossal and phrenic responses to changes in upper airway pressure. *Resp Physiol* 55:341, 1984.
Hyatt RE: Forced expiration. In Geiger SR, Macklem PT, Mead J, Fishman AP, editors: *Handbook of physiology. Section 3. The respiratory system. Vol 3. Mechanics of breathing, part 1.* Bethesda, MD, 1986, American Physiological Society.
Hyatt RE, Okeson GC, Rodarte JR: Influence of expiratory flow limitation on the pattern of lung emptying in normal man. *J Appl Physiol* 35:411, 1973.
Ignarro LJ, Buga GM, Woods KS, et al.: Endothelium-derived relaxing factor produced and released from artery and vein is nitric oxide. *Proc Natl Acad Sci USA* 84:9265, 1987.
Ikari T, Sasaki CT: Glottic closure reflex: Control mechanisms. *Ann Otol Rhinol Laryngol* 89:220, 1980.
Isaza GD, Posner JD, Altose MD, et al.: Airway occlusion pressure in awake and anesthetized goats. *Respir Physiol* 27:87, 1976.
Isono S, Tanaka A, Nishino T: Lateral position decreases collapsibility of the passive pharynx in patients with obstructive sleep apnea. *Anesthesiology* 97:780, 2002.
Issa FQ, Sullivan CE: Upper airway closing pressures in obstructive sleep apnea. *J Appl Physiol* 57:520, 1984.
Jacob TD, Nakayama DK, Seki I, et al.: Hemodynamic effects and metabolic fate of inhaled nitric oxide in hypoxic piglets. *J Appl Physiol* 77:1794, 1994.

Jammes Y, Speck DF: Respiratory control by diaphragmatic and respiratory muscle afferents. In Dempsey JA, Pack AI, editors: Regulation of breathing. New York, Marcel Dekker, 1955, pp 543–582.

Jansen AH, Chernick V: Respiratory response to cyanide in fetal sheep after peripheral chemodenervation. *J Appl Physiol* 36:1, 1974.

Jansen AH, Chernick V: Development of respiratory control. *Physiol Rev* 63:437, 1983.

Jansen AH, Ioffe S, Russell BJ, Chernick V: Influence of sleep state on the response to hypercapnia in fetal lambs. *Respir Physiol* 48:125, 1982.

Jeffery PK, Reid LM: The respiratory mucous membrane. In Brain JD, Proctor DF, Reid LM. editors: *Respiratory defense mechanisms*. New York, 1977, Marcel Dekker.

Jennis MS, Peabody JL: Pulse oximetry: An alternative method for the assessment of oxygenation in newborn infants. *Pediatrics* 79:524, 1987.

Jobe AH: Pulmonary surfactant therapy. *N Engl J Med* 328(12):861, 1993.

Johns RA, Moscicki JC, DiFazio CA: Nitric oxide synthase inhibitor dose-dependently and reversibly reduces the threshold for halothane anesthesia. *Anesthesiology* 77:779, 1992.

Juno P, March HM, Knopp TJ, Render K: Closing capacity in awake and anesthetized-paralysed man. *J Appl Physiol* 44:238, 1978.

Kaditis AG, Motoyama EK, Seki I, et al: Flow and volume dependence of respiratory mechanics in anesthetized children. *Pediatr Res* 46:419, 1999a.

Kaditis AG, Venkataraman ST, Zin WA, et al: Partitioning of respiratory system resistance in children with respiratory insufficiency. *Am J Respir Crit Care Med* 159:389, 1999b.

Kaneko K, Milic-Emili J, Dolovich MB, et al.: Regional distribution of ventilation and perfusion as a function of body position. *J Appl Physiol* 21:767, 1966.

Karlberg P, Cherry RB, Escardo FE, Koch G: Respiratory studies in newborn infants. II. Pulmonary ventilation and mechanics of breathing in the first minutes of life, including the onset of respiration. *Acta Paediatr Scand* 51:121, 1962.

Keidan I, Fine GF, KagawaT, et al.: Work of breathing during spontaneous ventilation in anesthesized children: A comparative study among the face mask, laryngeal mask airway and endotracheal tube. *Anesth Analg* 91:1381–1388, 2000.

Kelly DL, Stellwagen LM, Kaitz E, Shannon DC: Apnea and periodic breathing in normal full-term infants during the first twelve months. *Pediatr Pulmonol* 1:215, 1985.

Kikkawa Y, Motoyama EK, Cook CD: Ultrastructure of lungs of lambs; the relation of osmiophilic inclusions and alveolar lining layer to fetal maturation and experimentally produced respiratory distress. *Am J Pathol* 47:877, 1965.

Kilburn KH, Salzano JV, editors: Symposium on structure, function and measurement of respiratory cilia. *Am Rev Respir Dis* 93:1, 1966.

Kinsella JP, Neish SR, Shaffer E, Abman SH: Low-dose inhalational nitric oxide in persistent pulmonary hypertension of the newborn. *Lancet* 340:819, 1992.

Knill RL, Clement JL: Site of selective action of halothane on the peripheral chemoreflex pathway in humans. *Anesthesiology* 61:121, 1984.

Knill RL, Gelb AW: Ventilatory response to hypoxia and hypercapnia during halothane sedation and anesthesia in man. *Anesthesiology* 49:244, 1978.

Koka BV, Jeon S, Andre JM, et al.: Post intubation croup in children. *Anesth Analg (Cleve)* 56:501, 1977.

Kosch PC, Stark AR: Determination and homeostasis of functional residual capacity (FRC) in infants. *Physiologist* 22:71, 1979.

Kryger M, Bode F, Antic R, Anthonisen N: Diagnosis of obstruction of upper and central airways, *Am J Med* 61:85, 1976.

Kryger MH, Jacob O, Dosman J, et al.: Effect of meperidine on occlusion pressure response to hypercapnia and hypoxia with and without external inspiratory resistance. *Am Rev Respir Dis* 114:133, 1976.

Kulovich MV, Hallman M, Cluck L: The lung profile. I. Normal pregnancy. *Am J Obstet Gynecol* 135:57, 1979.

Kuna ST, Remmers JE: Pathophysiology and mechanisms of sleep apnea. In Fletcher EC, editor: *Abnormalities of respiration during sleep*. Orlando, FL, 1986, Grune & Stratton.

Kurth CD, Spitzer AR, Broennle AM, Downes JJ: Postoperative apnea in preterm infants. *Anesthesiology* 66:483, 1987.

Lacourt G, Polgar G: Interaction between nasal and pulmonary resistance in newborn infants. *J Appl Physiol* 30:870, 1971.

LaFramboise WA, Standaert TA, Woodrum DE, Guthrie RD: Occlusion pressures during the ventilatory response to hypoxemia in the newborn monkey. *J Appl Physiol* 51:1169, 1981.

LaFramboise WA, Woodrum DE: Elevated diaphragm electromyogram during neonatal hypoxic ventilatory depression. *J Appl Physiol* 59:1040, 1985.

Lahiri S, Brody JS, Motoyama EK, Valasquez TM: Regulation of breathing in newborns in high altitude. *J Appl Physiol* 44:673, 1978.

Lahiri S, DeLaney RG: Stimulus interaction in the responses of carotid body chemoreceptor single afferent fibers. *Respir Physiol* 24:249, 1975.

Lambert RK, Castile RG, and Tepper RS: Model of forced expiratory flows and airway geometry in infants. *J Appl Physiol* 96:688–692, 2004.

Lang MJ, Hall RT, Reddy NS, et al.: A controlled trial of human surfactant replacement therapy for severe respiratory distress syndrome in very low birth weight infants. *J Pediatr* 116:295, 1990.

Langston C, Kida K, Reed M, Thurlbeck WM: Human lung growth in late gestation and in the neonate. *Am Rev Respir Dis* 129:607, 1984.

Lauweryns JM: "Hyaline membrane disease" in newborn infants: Macroscopic, radiographic and light and electron microscopic studies. *Hum Pathol* 1:175, 1970.

Laws AK: Effects of induction of anaesthesia and muscle paralysis on functional residual capacity of the lungs. *Can Anaesthesiol Soc J* 15:325, 1968.

LeSouef PN, England SJ, Bryan AC: Passive respiratory mechanics in newborns and children. *Am Rev Respir Dis* 129:552, 1984.

Leusen I: Regulation of cerebrospinal fluid composition with reference to breathing. *Physiol Rev* 52:1, 1972.

Levy AM, Tabakin BS, Hanson JS, Narkewicz RM: Hypertrophied adenoids causing pulmonary hypertension and severe congestive heart failure. *N Engl J Med* 277:506, 1967.

Lichtiger M, Landa JF, Hirsch JA: Velocity of tracheal mucus in anesthetized women undergoing gynecologic surgery. *Anesthesiology* 41:753, 1975.

Liggins GC, Howie RN: A controlled trial of antepartum glucocorticoid treatment for prevention of the respiratory distress syndrome in premature infants. *Pediatrics* 50:515, 1972.

Lindahl SGE, Yates AP, Hatch DJ: Respiratory depression in children at different end tidal halothane concentrations. *Anaesthesia* 42:1267, 1987.

Lipski J, Merrill EG: Electrophysiological demonstration of the projection from expiratory neurons in rostral medulla to contralateral dorsal respiratory group. *Brain Res* 197:521, 1980.

Litman RS, Keon TP: Postintubation croup in children. *Anesthesiology* 75:1122, 1991.

Liu LMP, Coté CJ, Goudsouzian NG, et al.: Life-threatening apnea in infants recovering from anesthesia. *Anesthesiology* 59:506, 1983.

Long SE, Duffin J: The medullary respiratory neurons: A review. *Can J Physiol Pharmacol* 62:161, 1984.

Long WA, Corbet A, Cotton R, et al.: A controlled trial of synthetic surfactant in infants weighing 1250 grams or more with the American Exosurf Neonatal Study Group I and the Canadian Exosurf Neonatal Study Group. *N Engl J Med* 325:1696, 1991.

Lucier GE, Storey AT, Sessle BJ: Effects of upper respiratory tract stimuli on neonatal respiration; reflex and single neuron analysis in the kitten. *Biol Neonate* 35:82, 1979.

Macklem PT, Mead J: Resistance of central and peripheral airways measured by a retrograde catheter. *J Appl Physiol* 22:395, 1967.

Mansell A, Bryan C, Levison H: Airway closure in children. *J Appl Physiol* 33:711, 1972.

Marcal F, Crance JP: Measurement of ventilatory system compliance in infants and young children. *Respir Physiol* 68:311, 1987.

Marcal F, Haouzi P, Gallina C, Crance JP: Measurement of ventilatory system resistance in infants and young children. *Respir Physiol* 73:201, 1988.

Marshall BE, Marshall C: Anesthesia and pulmonary circulation. In Covino BJ, Fozzard HA, Rehder K, Strichartz, editors: *Effects of anesthesia*. Bethesda, MD, 1985, American Physiological Society.

Marshall BE, Marshall C: Continuity of response to hypoxic pulmonary vasoconstriction. *J Appl Physiol* 49:189, 1980.

Masters IB, Seidenberg J, Hudson I, et al.: Longitudinal study of lung mechanics in normal infants. *Pediatr Pulmonol* 3:3, 1987.

Mathew OP, Abu-Osba YK, Thach BT: Genioglossus muscle responses to upper airway pressure changes: Afferent pathways. *J Appl Physiol* 52:445, 1982a.

Mathew OP, Abu-Osba YK, Thach BT: Influence of upper airway pressure changes on genioglossus muscle inspiratory activity. *J Appl Physiol* 52:438, 1982b.

McCoy KS, Castile RG, Allen ED et al: Functional residual capacity (FRC) measurements by plethysmography and helium dilution in normal infants. *Pediatr Pulmonol* 19:282–290, 1995.

McDonald DM: Peripheral chemoreceptors: Structure-function relationships of the carotid body. In Hornbein TF, editor: *Regulation of breathing, part 1*. New York, 1981, Marcel Dekker.

McFadden ER Jr, Denison DM, Waller JF, et al.: Direct recordings of the temperature in the tracheobronchial tree in normal man. *J Clin Invest* 69:700, 1982.

McIlroy MB, Marshall R, Christie RV: The work of breathing in normal subjects. *Clin Sci* 13:127, 1954.

Mead J: Control of respiratory frequency. *J Appl Physiol* 15:325, 1960.

Mead J: The lung's "quiet zone." *N Engl J Med* 28:1318, 1970.

Mead J, Collier C: Relation of volume history of lungs to respiratory mechanics in anesthetized dogs. *J Appl Physiol* 14:668, 1959.

Mead J, Turner JM, Macklem PT, Little JB: Significance of the relationship between lung recoil and maximum expiratory flow. *J Appl Physiol* 22:95, 1967.

Merrill EG: The lateral respiratory neurons of the medulla: Their association with nucleus ambiguus, nucleus retroambigualis, the spinal accessory nucleus and the spinal cord. *Brain Res* 24:11, 1970.

Merrill EG: Is there reciprocal inhibition between medullary inspiratory and expiratory neurons? In von Euler C, Lagercrantz H, editors: *Central nervous control mechanisms in breathing,* vol 32. New York, 1979, Pergamon Press.

Merrill EG, Lipski J, Kubin L: Origin of the expiratory inhibition of nucleus tractus solitarius inspiratory neurons. *Brain Res* 263:43, 1983.

Merritt TA, Hallman M, Bloom BT, et al.: Prophylactic treatment of very premature infants with human surfactant. *N Engl J Med* 315:785, 1986.

Milic-Emili J: Pulmonary statics. In Widdicomb JG, editor: *Respiratory physiology, MTP International Review of Science,* Series I, vol 2. Borough Green Kent, 1974, Butterworth.

Milic-Emili J: Recent advances in the evaluation of respiratory drive. *Int Anesthesiol Clin* 15:39, 1977.

Milic-Emili J, Grunstein MM: Drive and Timing components of ventilation. *Chest* 70(suppl):181, 1975.

Milic-Emili J, Henderson JAM, Dolovich MB, et al.: Regional distribution of gas in the lung. *J Appl Physiol* 21:749, 1966.

Milic-Emili J, Robatto FM, Gates JH: Respiratory mechanics in anaesthesia. *Br J Anaesth* 65:4, 1990.

Miller AD, Erure K, Suzuki I: Control of abdominal muscles by brain stem respiratory neurons in the cat. *J Neurophysiol* 54:155, 1985.

Miserocchi G, Mortola J, Sant'Ambrogio G: Localization of pulmonary stretch receptors in the airways of the dog. *J Physiol (Lond)* 235:775, 1973.

Mitchell RA: Cerebrospinal fluid and the regulation of respiration. In Caro CG, editor: *Advances in respiratory physiology.* Baltimore, 1966, Williams & Wilkins.

Mitchell RA, Berger AJ: Neurol regulation of respiration. In Hornbein TF, editor: *Regulation of breathing, part I.* New York, 1981, Marcel Dekker.

Mitchell RA, Carman CT, Severinghaus JW, et al.: Stability of cerebrospinal fluid pH in chronic acid-base disturbances in blood. *J Appl Physiol* 20:443, 1965.

Mok JY, McLaughlin FJ, Pintar M, et al.: Transcutaneous monitoring of oxygenation: What is normal? *J Pediatr* 108:365, 1986.

Moncada S, Palmer RMJ, Higgs EA: Biosynthesis of nitric oxide for L-arginine. A pathway for the regulation of cell function and communication. *Biochem Pharmacol* 38:1709, 1989.

Mortola JP, Fisher JT, Smith B, et al.: Dynamics of breathing in infants. *J Appl Physiol* 52:1209, 1982.

Moss ML: The veloepiglottic sphincter and obligate nose breathing in the neonate. *J Pediatr* 67:330, 1965.

Motoyama EK: Airway function tests in infants and children. *Int Anesthesiol Clin* 26:6, 1988.

Motoyama EK: Effects of positive end expiratory pressure (PEEP) on respiratory mechanics and oxygen saturation ($Sp{O_2}$) in infants and children under general anesthesia. *Anesthesiology* 85:A1099, 1996.

Motoyama EK: Physiologic alterations in tracheostomy. In Myers EN, Stool SE, Johnson JT, editors: *Tracheostomy.* New York, 1985, Churchill Livingstone.

Motoyama EK: Pulmonary mechanics during early postnatal years. *Pediatr Res* 11:220, 1977.

Motoyama EK: Respiratory physiology. In Bissonnette B, Dalens B, editors: *Pediatric Anesthesia: Principles and Practice*, New York, McGraw-Hill, 2001, pp 43-75.

Motoyama EK, Brinkmeyer SD, Mutich RL, Walczak SA: Reduced FRC in anesthetized infants: Effect of low PEEP. *Anesthesiology* 57:A418,1982a.

Motoyama EK, Fort MD, Klesh KW, et al.: Early onset of airway reactivity in premature infants with bronchopulmonary dysplasia. *Am Rev Respir Dis* 136:50, 1987.

Motoyama EK, Glazener CH: Hypoxemia after general anesthesia in children. *Anesth Analg* 65:267, 1986.

Motoyama EK, Hen J, Tamas L, Dolan FT: Spirometry with positive airway pressure: A simple method to evaluate obstructive lung disease in children. *Am Rev Respir Dis* 126:766, 1982.

Motoyama EK, Orzalesi MM, Kikkawa Y, et al.: Effect of cortisol on the development of fetal rabbit lungs. *Pediatrics* 48:547, 1971.

Motoyama EK, Zigas CJ, Troll G: Functional basis of childhood anemia [abstract]. *Am Soc Anesthesiology* 283, 1974.

Muldoon SM, Hart JL, Bowen KA, Freas W: Attenuation of endothelium-mediated vasodilation by halothane. *Anesthesiology* 68:31, 1988.

Muller N, Volgyesi G, Becker L, et al.: Diaphragmatic muscle tone. *J Appl Physiol* 47:279, 1979.

Munson ES, Larson CP, Babad AA, et al.: The effects of halothane, fluroxene and cyclopropane on ventilation: A comparative study in man. *Anesthesiology* 27:716, 1966.

Murat I, Delleur MM, Maggee K, Saint-Maurice C: Changes in ventilatory patterns during halothane anaesthesia in children. *Br J Anaesth* 57:569, 1985.

Nakayama DK, Mutich R, Motoyama EK: Pulmonary dysfunction in surgical conditions of the newborn infant. *Crit Care Med* 19:926, 1991.

Nathan DG, Oski FA: *Hematology of infancy and childhood,* ed 3. Philadelphia, 1987, WB Saunders.

Nelson NM: Respiration and circulation after birth. In Smith CA, Nelson NM, editors: *The physiology of the newborn infant,* ed 4. Springfield, IL, 1976, Charles C Thomas.

Nelson NM, Prod'hom LS, Cherry RB, et al.: Pulmonary function in the newborn infant. II. Perfusion-estimation by analysis of the arterial-alveolar carbon dioxide differences. *Pediatrics* 30:975, 1962.

Nelson NM, Prod'hom LS, Cherry RB, et al.: Pulmonary function in the newborn infant: The alveolar-arterial oxygen gradient. *J Appl Physiol* 18:534, 1963.

Newsom-Davis J: Control of the muscles of breathing. In Widdicombe JG, editor: *Respiratory physiology,* vol 2. Baltimore, 1974, University Park Press.

Nielsen M, Smith H: Studies on the regulation of respiration in acute hypoxia. *Acta Physiol Scand* 24:293, 1951.

Nishino T: Swallowing as a protective reflex for the upper respiratory tract. *Anesthesiology* 79:588, 1993.

Nishino T, Anderson JW, Sant'Ambrogio G: Effects of halothane, enflurane, and isoflurane on laryngeal receptors in dogs. *Respir Physiol* 91:247, 1993.

Nishino T, Kohchi T, Yonezawa T, Honda Y: Response of recurrent laryngeal, hypoglossal, and phrenic nerves to increasing depth of anesthesia with halothane or enflurane in vagotomized cats. *Anesthesiology* 63:404, 1985.

Nishino T, Shirahata M, Yonezawa T, Honda Y: Comparison of changes in the hypoglossal and the phrenic nerve activity in response to increasing depth of anesthesia in cats. *Anesthesiology* 60:19, 1984.

Nishino T, Yonezawa T, Honda Y: Modification of laryngospasm in response to changes in $Pa{O_2}$ in the cat. *Anesthesiology* 55:286, 1981.

Noble MIM, Eisele JH, Trenchard D, Guz A: Effect of selective peripheral nerve blocks on respiratory sensations. In Porter R, editor: *Breathing: Hering-Breuer Centenary Symposium.* London, 1970, Churchill Livingstone.

Nunn JF, Ezi-Ashi TI: The respiratory effects of resistance to breathe in anesthetized man. *Anesthesiology* 22:174, 1966.

Ochiai R, Guthrie R, Motoyama EK: Differential sensitivity of halothane anesthesia on the genioglossus, intercostals, and diaphragm in kittens. *Anesth Analg* 74:338, 1992.

Ochiai R, Guthrie RD, Motoyama EK: Effects of varying concentrations of halothane on the activity of the genioglossus, intercostals, and diaphragm in cats: An electromyographic study. *Anesthesiology* 70:812, 1989.

Ogilvie CM, Forster RE, Blakemore WS, et al: A standardized breath holding technique for the clinical measurement of the diffusing capacity of the lung for carbon monoxide. *J Clin Invest* 36:1–17, 1957.

Olinsky A, Bryan MH, Bryan AC: Influence of lung inflation on respiratory control in neonates. *J Appl Physiol* 36:426, 1974.

Onal E, Lopata M, O'Conner TD: Diaphragmatic and genioglossal electromyogram response to CO_2 rebreathing in humans. *J Appl Physiol* 49:638, 1981.

Onal E, Lopata M, O'Connor TD: Diaphragmatic and genioglossal electromyogram responses to chemical stimulation and loading. *J Appl Physiol* 53:1133, 1982.

Orzalesi MM, Cowan MJ, Motoyama EK: The in vitro effect of cyclopropane and halothane on the oxygen affinity of human blood [abstract]. *Am Soc Anesthesiol* 187, 1971.

Orzalesi MM, Mendicini M, Bucci G, et al.: Arterial oxygen studies in premature newborns with and without mild respiratory disorders. *Arch Dis Child* 42:174, 1967.

Oski FA: Designation of anemia on a functional basis. *J Pediatr* 83:353, 1973a.

Oski FA: The erythrocyte and its disorders. In Nathan DG, Oski FA, editors: *Hematology of infancy and childhood,* ed 2. Philadelphia, 1981, WB Saunders.

Oski FA: The unique fetal red cell and its function. *Pediatrics* 51:494, 1973b.

Oski FA, Delivoria-Papadopoulos M: The red cell, 2,3-diphosphoglycerate, and tissue oxygen release. *J Pediatr* 77:941, 1970.

Pack AI: Sensory inputs to the medulla. *Annu Rev Physiol* 43:73, 1981.

Pack AI, Kline LR, Hendricks JC, Morrison AR: Control of respiration during sleep. In Fishman AP, editor: *Pulmonary diseases and disorders,* ed 2. *Vol 1, part 2: Physiological principles.* New York, 1988, McGraw-Hill Book Co.

Paintal AS: Vagal sensory receptors and their reflex effects. *Physiol Rev* 53:159, 1973.

Palmer RMJ, Ferrige AG, Moncada S: Nitric oxide release accounts for the biologic activity of endothelium derived relaxing factor. *Nature* 327:524, 1987.

Papastamelos C, Panitch H, England S, Allen J: Developmental changes in chest wall compliance in infancy and early childhood. *J Appl Physiol* 78:179, 1995.

Pappenheimer JR., Fenci V, Heisey SR, Held D: Role of cerebral fluids in control of respiration as studied in unanesthetized goats. *Am J Physiol* 208:436, 1965.

Patel RI, Norden J, Hannallah RS: Oxygen administration prevents hypoxemia during postanesthetic transport in children. *Anesthesiology* 69:616, 1988.

Patrick J, Campbell K, Carmichael L, et al.: Patterns of human fetal breathing during the last 10 weeks of pregnancy. *Obstet Gynecol* 56:24, 1980.

Pavlin EG, Hornbein TF: Anesthesia and control of ventilation. In Fishman AP, Cherniack NS, Widdicombe JG, editors: *Handbook of physiology. Section 3. The respiratory system. Vol II. Control of breathing*. Bethesda, MD, 1986, American Physiological Society.

Pavlin EG, Su JY: Cardiopulmonary pharmacology. In Miller RD, editor: *Anesthesia*, ed 4. New York, 1994, Churchill Livingstone.

Perlstein PH, Edward NK, Sutherland JM: Apnea in premature infants and incubator-air-temperature changes. *N Engl J Med* 282:461, 1970.

Phillipson EA: Sleep disorders. In Murray JF, Nalel JA, editors: *Textbook of respiratory medicine*, 2nd ed. Philadelphia, 1994, WB Saunders.

Pickens DL, Schefft GL, Thach BT: Pharyngeal fluid clearance and aspiration preventive mechanisms in sleeping infants. *J Appl Physiol* 66:1164, 1989.

Pierrefiche O, Schwarzacher SW, Bischoff AM, et al: Blockade of synaptic inhibition within the pre-Boetzinger complex in the cat suppresses respiratory rhythm generation in vivo. *J Physiol Lond* 509:245–254, 1998.

Pison U, Lopez FA, Heidelmeyer CF, et al.: Inhaled nitric oxide reverses hypoxic pulmonary vasoconstriction without impairing gas exchange. *J Appl Physiol* 74:1287, 1993.

Pitts RF: Organization of the respiratory center. *Physiol Rev* 26:609, 1946.

Poets CF, Stebbens VA, Alexander JR, et al.: Arterial oxygen saturation in preterm infants at discharge from the hospital and six weeks later. *J Pediatr* 120:447, 1992.

Polgar G: Opposing forces to breathing in newborn infants. *Biol Neonate* 11:1, 1967.

Polgar G, Promadhat V: *Pulmonary function testing in children: Techniques and standards*. Philadelphia, 1971, WB Saunders.

Possmayer F: A proposed nomenclature for pulmonary surfactant-associated proteins. *Am Rev Respir Dis* 136:990, 1988.

Potter EL: *Pathology of the fetus and infant*. Chicago, 1961, Year Book Medical Publishers.

Pramanik AK, Holtzman RB, Merritt TA: Surfactant replacement therapy for pulmonary diseases. *Pediatr Clin North Am* 40:913, 1993.

Prime FJ: Oxygen dissociation curves of whole blood in the presence of anaesthetic gases. *Br J Anaesth* 23:171, 1951.

Proctor DF: The upper airways. I. Nasal physiology and defense of the lung. *Am Rev Respir Dis* 115:97, 1977a.

Proctor DF: The upper airways. II. The larynx and trachea. *Am Rev Respir Dis* 115:315, 1977b.

Proctor DF: Modifications of breathing for phonation. In Geiger SR, Macklem PT, Mead J, Fishman AP, editors: *Handbook of physiology. Section 3. The respiratory system. Vol 3. Mechanics of breathing, part 1*. Bethesda, MD, 1986. American Physiological Society.

Pullerits J, Burrows FA, Roy WL: Arterial desaturation in healthy children during transfer to the recovery room. *Can J Anaesth* 34:470, 1987.

Puybasset L, Stewart TE, Rouby JJ, et al.: Inhaled nitric oxide reverses the increase in pulmonary vascular resistance induced by permissive hypercapnia in patients with acute respiratory distress syndrome. *Anesthesiology* 80:1254, 1994.

Quanjer PH, Sly PD, Stocks J, et al: Respiratory function measurements in infants: symbols, abbreviations and units. *Am J Respir Crit Care Med* 151:2041–2057, 1995.

Radford EP Jr, Ferns BJ Jr, Kriet BC: Clinical use of nomogram to estimate proper ventilation during artificial respiration. *N Engl J Med* 251:877, 1954.

Ramanathan R, Durand M, Larrazabal C: Pulse oximetry in very low birth weight infants with acute and chronic lung disease. *Pediatrics* 79:612, 1987.

Ramirez JM, Richter DW: The neuronal mechanisms of respiratory rhythm generation. *Curr Opin Neurobiol* 6:817–825, 1996.

Reed R, Roberts JL, Thach BT: Factors influencing regional patency and configuration of the upper airway in human infants. *J Appl Physiol* 58:635, 1985.

Rehder K, Hatch DJ, Sessler AD, Fowler WS: The function of each lung of anesthetized and paralyzed man during mechanical ventilation. *Anesthesiology* 37:16, 1972.

Rehder K, Hatch DJ, Sessler AD, et al.: Effects of general anesthesia, muscle paralysis, and mechanical ventilation on pulmonary nitrogen clearance. *Anesthesiology* 35:591, 1971.

Rehder K, Mallow JE, Fibuch EE, et al.: Effects of isoflurane anesthesia and muscle paralysis on respiratory mechanics in normal man. *Anesthesiology* 41:477, 1974.

Rehder K, Marsh HM: Respiratory mechanics during anesthesia and mechanical ventilation. In Fishman A, Macklem PT, Mead J, editors: *Handbook of physiology. Section 3. The respiratory system. Vol 3. Mechanics of breathing*. Bethesda, MD, 1986, American Physiological Society.

Rehder K, Sittipong R, Sessler AD: The effect of thiopental-meperidine anesthesia with succinylcholine paralysis on functional residual capacity and dynamic lung compliance in normal sitting man. *Anesthesiology* 37:395, 1972.

Reid L: The embryology of the lung. In DeReuck AVS, Porter R, editors: *Development of the lung. Ciba Foundation Symposium*. London, 1967, Churchill Livingstone.

Rekling JC, Feldman JL: Pre-Boetzinger complex and pacemaker neurons: Hypothesized site and kernel for respiratory rhythm generation. *Annu Rev Physiol* 60:385–405, 1998.

Remmers JE, deGroot WJ, Sauerland EK, Anch AM: Pathogenesis of upper airway occlusion during sleep. *J Appl Physiol* 44:931, 1978.

Remolina C, Khan AU, Santiago TV, Edelman NH: Positional hypoxemia in unilateral lung disease. *N Engl J Med* 304:523, 1981.

Richard CC, Bachman L: Lung and chest wall compliance in apneic paralyzed infants. *J Clin Invest* 40:273, 1961.

Richter DW: Generation and maintenance of the respiratory rhythm. *J Exp Biol* 100:93, 1982.

Rigatto H: Apnea. In Thibeault DW, Gregory GA, editors: *Neonatal pulmonary care*. Norwalk, CT, 1986, Appleton-Century-Crofts.

Rigatto H: Maturation of breathing control in the fetus and newborn infant. In Beckerman RC, Brouillette RT, Hunt CE, editors: *Respiratory control disorders in infants and children*. Baltimore, 1992, Williams & Wilkins.

Rigatto H, Brady JP: Periodic breathing and apnea in preterm infants. II. Hypoxia as a primary event. *Pediatrics* 50:219, 1972a.

Rigatto H, Brady JP: Periodic breathing and apnea in preterm infants. I. Evidence for hypoventilation possibly due to central respiratory depression. *Pediatrics* 50:202, 1972b.

Rigatto H, Brady JP, Chir B, de la Tone Verduzco R: Chemoreceptor reflexes in preterm infants. II. The effect of gestational and postnatal age on the ventilatory response to inhaled carbon dioxide. *Pediatrics* 55:614, 1975a.

Rigatto H, Brady JP, de La Torre Verduzco R: Chemoreceptor reflexes in preterm infants. I. The effect of gestational and postnatal age on the ventilatory response to inhalation of 100% and 15% oxygen. *Pediatrics* 55:604, 1975b.

Rigatto H, Kalapesi Z, Leahy FN, et al.: Ventilatory response to 100% and 15% O_2 during wakefulness and sleep in preterm infants. *Early Hum Dev* 7:1, 1982.

Rigatto H, Lee D, Devi M, et al.: Effect of increasing arterial CO_2 on fetal breathing and behavior in sheep. *J Appl Physiol* 64:982, 1988.

Rimar S, Gillis CN: Selective pulmonary vasodilation by inhaled nitric oxide is due to hemoglobin inactivation. *Circulation* 88:2884, 1993.

Roberts JD, Lang P, Bigatello LM, et al.: Inhaled nitric oxide in congenital heart disease. *Circulation* 87:447, 1993.

Roberts JD, Polaner DM, Lang P, Zapol WM: Inhaled nitric oxide in persistent pulmonary hypertension of the newborn. *Lancet* 340:818, 1992.

Roberts JL, Reed WR, Mathew OP, et al.: Assessment of pharyngeal airway stability in normal and micrognathic infants. *J Appl Physiol* 58:290, 1985.

Robinson SL, Richardson CA, Willis MM, Gregory GA: Halothane anesthesia reduces pulmonary function in the newborn lamb. *Anesthesiology* 62:578, 1985.

Robotham JL: Do low-dose inhalation anesthetic agents alter ventilatory control? *Anesthesiology* 62:578, 1994.

Rohrer F: Der Stromungswiderstand in den menschlichen Atemwegen und der Einfluss der unregelmassigen Verzweigung des Bronchialsystems auf den Atmungsverlauf in verschiedenen Lungenbezirken. *Pflugers Arch* 162:225, 1915.

Rooney SA: The surfactant system and lung phospholipid biochemistry. *Am Rev Respir Dis* 131:439, 1985.

Rooney SA, Canavan PM, Motoyama EK: The identification of phosphatidyl glycerol in the rat, rabbit, monkey and human lung. *Biochem Biophys Acta* 360:56–67, 1974.

Rossaint R, Falke KJ, Lopez F, et al.: Inhaled nitric oxide for the adult respiratory distress syndrome. *N Engl J Med* 328:399, 1993.

Rudolph AM: The changes in the circulation after birth; their importance in congenital heart disease. *Circulation* 41:343, 1970.

Sampson SR, Vidruk EH: Chemical stimulation of rapidly adapting receptors in the airways. In Fitzgerald RS, Gautier H, Lahiri S, editors: *Thermoregulation of respiration during sleep and anesthesia*. New York, 1977, Plenum Press.

Sampson SR, Vidruk EH: Properties of "irritant" receptors in canine lung. *Respir Physiol* 25:9, 1975.

Sant'Ambrogio FB, Anderson JW, Nishino T, Sant'Ambrogio G: Effects of halothane and isoflurane in the upper airway of dogs during development. *Respir Physiol* 91:237, 1993.

Sant'Ambrogio G: Information arising from the tracheobronchial tree of mammals. *Physiol Rev* 62:531, 1982.

Sant'Ambrogio G, Mathew OP, Fisher JT, Sant'Ambrogio FB: Laryngeal receptors responding to transmural pressure, airflow and local muscle activity. *Respir Physiol* 54:317, 1983.

Sant'Ambrogio G, Mathew OP, Sant'Ambrogio FB, Fisher JT: Laryngeal cold receptors. *Respir Physiol* 59:35, 1985.

Sant'Ambrogio G, Tsubone H, Sant'Ambrogio FB: Sensory information from the upper airway: Role in the control of breathing. *Respir Physiol* 102:1–16, 1995.

Sasaki CT: Development of laryngeal function: Etiologic significance in the sudden infant death syndrome. *Laryngoscope* 89:1964, 1979.

Sasaki CT, Levine PA, Laitman JT, Crelin ES Jr: Postnatal descent of the epiglottis in man. *Arch Otolaryngol* 103:169, 1977.

Sauerland EK, Harper RM: The human tongue during sleep: Electromyographic activity of the genioglossus muscle. *Exp Neural* 51:160, 1976.

Savoy J, Arnup ME, Anthonisen NR: Response to external inspiratory resistive loading and bronchospasm in anesthetized dogs. *J Appl Physiol* 53:355, 1982.

Scher MS, Steppe DA, Dahl RE, et al.: Comparison of EEG sleep measures in healthy full-term and preterm infants at matching conceptional ages. *Sleep* 15:442–448, 1992.

Sellick H, Widdicombe JG: Vagal deflation and inflation reflexes mediated by lung irritant receptors. *J Exp Physiol* 55:153, 1970.

Serafini G, Cornara G, Cavalloro F, et al.: Pulmonary atelectasis during paediatric anaesthesia: CT scan evaluation and effects of positive end expiratory pressure (PEEP). *Paediatr Anaesth* 9:225–228, 1999.

Severinghaus JW: Blood gas calculator. *J Appl Physiol* 21:1108, 1966.

Severinghaus JW: Hypoxic respiratory drive and its loss during chronic hypoxia. *Clin Physiol* 2:57, 1972.

Severinghaus JW, Mitchell RA: "Ondine's curse": Failure of respiratory center automaticity while awake. *Clin Res* 10:122, 1962.

Severinghaus JW, Mitchell RA, Richardson BW, Singer MM: Respiratory control of high altitude suggesting active transport regulation of CSF pH. *J Appl Physiol* 18:1155, 1963.

Shah NS, Jacob TD, Exler R, et al.: Inhaled nitric oxide in congenital diaphragmatic hernia. *J Pediatr Surg* 29:1010, 1994.

Shannon DC, Kelly DH, O'Connor KG: Abnormal regulation of ventilation in infants: A risk for sudden infant death syndrome. *N Engl J Med* 297:747, 1977.

Sly PD, Hayden MJ: Applied clinical respiratory physiology. In Taussig LM, Landau LI (editors): *Pediatric respiratory medicine.* St. Louis, 1998, Mosby, p 95.

Smith BT, Bogues WG: Effects of drugs and hormones on lung maturation in experimental animal and man. *Pharmacol Ther* 9:51, 1982.

Smith JC, Ellenberger HH, Ballanyi K, et al.: Pre-Boetzinger complex: A brain stem region that may generate respiratory rhythm in mammals. *Science* 254:726–729, 1991.

Smith TC, Colton ET, Behar MG: Does anesthesia alter hemoglobin dissociation? *Anesthesiology* 32:5, 1970.

Sorensen SC, Severinghaus JW: Irreversible respiratory insensitivity to acute hypoxia in man born at high altitude. *J Appl Physiol* 25:217, 1968.

Spear GS, Vaeusorn O, Avery ME, et al.: Inclusions in terminal air spaces of fetal and neonatal human lung. *Biol Neonate* 14:344, 1969.

Spitzer AR, Fox WW: Infant apnea. *Clin Pediatr* 23:374, 1984.

Stamler JS, Loh E, Roddy MA, et al.: Nitric oxide regulates basal systemic and pulmonary vascular resistance in healthy humans. *Circulation* 89:2035, 1994.

Stark AR, Thach BT: Mechanisms of airway obstruction leading to apnea in newborn infants. *J Pediatr* 89:982, 1976.

Stern E, Parmelee AH, Akiyama Y, et al.: Sleep cycle characteristics in infants. *Pediatrics* 43:65, 1969.

Steward DJ: Preterm infants are more prone to complications following minor surgery than are term infants. *Anesthesiology* 56:304, 1982.

Stocks J: Effect of nasogastric tubes on nasal resistance during infancy. *Arch Dis Child* 55:17, 1980.

Stocks J, Godfrey S: Nasal resistance during infancy. *Respir Physiol* 34:233, 1978.

Stocks J, Godfrey S: Specific airway conductance in relation to postconceptional age during infancy. *J Appl Physiol* 43:144, 1977.

Stocks, J, Levy NM, Godfrey S: A new apparatus for the accurate measurement of airway resistance in infancy. *J Appl Physiol* 43:155, 1977.

Strang LB, MacLeish MH: Ventilatory failure and right-to-left shunt in newborn infants with respiratory distress. *Pediatrics* 28:17, 1961.

Suzuki M, Sasaki CT: Laryngeal spasm: A neurophysiologic redefinition. *Ann Otol Rhinol Laryngol* 86:150, 1977.

Swift PGF, Emery JL: Clinical observations in response to nasal occlusion in infancy. *Arch Dis Child* 48:947, 1973.

Sykes MK, Loh L, Seed RF, et al.: The effect of inhalational anaesthetics on hypoxic pulmonary vasoconstriction and pulmonary vascular resistance in the perfused lungs of the dog and cat. *Br J Anaesth* 44:776, 1972.

Tabatabai M, Behnia R: Neurochemical regulation of respiration. In Collins VJ, editor: *Physiological and pharmacological basis of anesthesia.* Philadelphia, 1995, Williams & Wilkins.

Tauesch HW Jr, Carson SH, Wang NS, Avery ME: Heroin induction of lung maturation and growth retardation in fetal rabbits. *J Pediatr* 82:869, 1973.

Taussig LM, Landau LI, Godfrey S, Arad I: Determinants of forced expiratory flows in newborn infants, *J Appl Physiol* 53:1220, 1982.

Temp JA, Henson LC, Ward DS: Does a subanesthetic concentration of isoflurane blunt the ventilatory response to hypoxia? *Anesthesiology* 77:1116, 1992.

Temp JA, Henson LC, Ward DS: Effect of subanesthetic minimum alveolar concentration of isoflurane on two tests of the hypoxic ventilatory response. *Anesthesiology* 80:739, 1994.

Thach BT: Sleep apnea in infancy and childhood. *Med Clin North Am* 69:1289, 1985.

Thach BT: Potential role of airway obstruction in SIDS. In Krous H, Culbertson H, editors: *Sudden infant death syndrome.* Baltimore, 1988, Johns Hopkins Press.

Thach BT: Neuromuscular control of the upper airway. In Beckerman RC, Brouillette RT, Hunt CE, editors: *Respiratory control disorders in infants and children.* Baltimore, 1992, Williams & Wilkins.

Thach BT, Menon PA, Schefft G: Effects of negative upper airway pressure on the pattern of breathing in sleeping infants. *J Appl Physiol* 66:1599, 1989.

Thorling EG, Erslev AJ: The "tissue" tension of oxygen and its relation to hematocrit and erythropoiesis. *Blood* 31:332, 1968.

Thorsteinsson A, Larsson A, Jonmarker C, Werner O: Pressure-volume relations of the respiratory system in healthy children. *Am J Respir Crit Care Med* 150:421, 1994.

Thurlbeck WM: Postnatal growth and development of the lung. *Am Rev Respir Dis* 111:803, 1975.

Toda H, Nakamura K, Hatano Y, et al.: Halothane and isoflurane inhibit endothelium-dependent relaxation elicited by acetylcholine. *Anesth Analg* 75:198, 1992.

van Iwaarden F, Welmers B, Verhoef J, et al.: Pulmonary surfactant protein A enhances the host-defense mechanism of rat alveolar macrophages. *Am J Respir Cell Mol Biol* 2:91, 1990.

Vidruk EH, Hahn HL, Nadel JA, Sampson SR: Mechanisms by which histamine stimulates rapidly adapting receptors in dog lungs. *J Appl Physiol* 43:397, 1977.

von Euler C: Brain stem mechanisms for generation and control of breathing pattern. In Cherniack NS, Widdicombe JG, editors: *Handbook of physiology. Section 3. The respiratory system. Vol 2. Control of breathing, part 1.* Bethesda, MD, 1986, American Physiology Society.

von Euler C: On the central pattern generator for the basic breathing rhythmicity. *J Appl Physiol* 55:1647, 1983.

von Euler C: Neural organization and rhythm generation. In Crystal RG, West JB: *The lung: Scientific foundations.* New York, 1991, Raven Press.

von Euler C, Trippenbach T: Cyclic excitability changes of the inspiratory "off switch" mechanism. *Acta Physiol Scand* 93:560, 1975.

Wade JG, Larson CP Jr, Hickey RF, et al.: Effect of carotid endarterectomy on carotid chemoreceptor and baroreceptor function in man. *N Engl J Med* 282:823, 1970.

Wahba WM: Analysis of ventilatory depression by enflurane during clinical anesthesia. *Anesth Analg* 59:103, 1980.

Wagner PD: Diffusion, diffusing capacity, and chemical reactions. In Fishman AP, editor: *Pulmonary diseases and disorders.* New York, 1988, McGraw-Hill Book Co.

Wagner PD, Saltzman HA, West JB: Measurement of continuous distributions of ventilation-perfusion ratios: Theory. *J Appl Physiol* 36:588, 1974.

Weaver T, Whitsett JA: Function and regulation of expression of pulmonary surfactant proteins. *Biochem J* 273:249, 1991.

Weibel ER: *Morphometry of the human lung.* New York, 1963, Academic Press.

Weibel ER: Morphological basis of alveolar-capillary gas exchange. *Physiol Rev* 53:419, 1973.

Weiskopf RB, Raymond LW, Severinghaus JW: Effects of halothane on canine respiratory response to hypoxia with and without hypercarbia. *Anesthesiology* 41:350, 1974.

Welborn LG, DeSoto H, Hannallah RS, et al.: The use of caffeine in the control of post-anesthetic apnea in former premature infants. *Anesthesiology* 68:796, 1988.

Welch G, Loscalzo J: Collective review: Nitric oxide and the cardiovascular system. *J Card Surg* 9:361, 1994.

Wessel DL: Inhaled nitric oxide for the treatment of pulmonary hypertension before and after cardiopulmonary bypass. *Crit Care Med* 21(suppl):S344, 1993.

West JB: Blood flow to the lung and gas exchange. *Anesthesiology* 41:124, 1974.

West JB: Topographical distribution of blood flow in the lung. In Fenn WO, Rahn H, editors: *Handbook of physiology. Vol 2. Section 3. Respiration.* Washington, DC, 1965, American Physiological Society.

West JB: *Ventilation/blood flow and gas exchange,* ed 2, Oxford, 1970, Blackwell Scientific Publications, Ltd.

West JB: Ventilation, blood flow, and gas exchange. In Murray JF, Nadel JA, editors: *Textbook of respiratory medicine,* ed 2. Philadelphia, 1994, WB Saunders.

Westbrook PR, Stubbs SE, Sessler AD, et al.: Effects of anesthesia and muscle paralysis on respiratory mechanics in normal man. *J Appl Physiol* 34:81, 1973.

Whitelaw WA, Derenne JP, Milic-Emili J: Occlusion pressure as a measure of respiratory center output in conscious man. *Respir Physiol* 23:181, 1975.

Whitsett JA, Horowitz AD: Surfactant and associated proteins. In Fishman AP, editor: *Fishman's pulmonary diseases and disorders,* ed 3. New York, 1998, McGraw-Hill, p 119.

Widdicombe JG: Nervous receptors in the respiratory tract and lungs. In Hornbein TF, editor: *Regulation of breathing, part 1.* New York, 1981, Marcel Dekker.

Widdicombe JG: Reflex control of breathing. In Widdicombe JG, editor: *Respiratory physiology. MTP International Review of Science, series 1, vol 2.* Borough Green, Kent, 1974, Butterworth.

Widdicombe JG: Reflexes from the upper respiratory tract. In Cherniak NS, Widdicombe JG, editors: *Handbook of physiology. Section 3. The respiratory system. Vol II. Control of breathing, Part 1.* Bethesda, MD, 1985, American Physiological Society.

Wohl MEB, Stigol LC, Mead J: Resistance of the total respiratory system in healthy infants and infants with bronchiolitis. *Pediatrics* 43:495, 1969.

Wolfe WG, Ebert PA, Sabiston DC: Effect of high oxygen tension on mucociliary function. *Surgery* 72:246, 1972.

Woolcock AJ, Vincent NJ, Macklem PT: Frequency dependence of compliance as a test for obstruction in small airways. *J Clin Invest* 48:1097, 1969.

Wu B, Kikkawa Y, Orzalesi MM, et al.: The effect of thyroxine on the maturation of fetal rabbit lungs. *Biol Neonate* 22:161, 1973.

Xue FS, Huang YG, Tong SY, et al: A comparative study of early postoperative hypoxemia in infants, children, and adults undergoing elective plastic surgery. *Anesth Analg* 83:709–715, 1996.

Yoshida K, Okabe E: Selective impairment of endothelium-dependent relaxation by sevoflurane: Oxygen free radicals participation. *Anesthesiology* 76:440, 1992.

Zapletal A, Motoyama EK, Gibson LE, Bouhuys A: Pulmonary mechanics in asthma and cystic fibrosis. *Pediatrics* 48:64, 1971.

Zapletal A, Motoyama EK, van de Woestijne KP, et al.: Maximum expiratory flow-volume curves and airway conductance in children and adolescents. *J Appl Physiol* 26:308, 1969.

Zapletal A, Paul T, Samanek M: Pulmonary elasticity in children and adolescents. *J Appl Physiol* 40:953, 1976.

Zapletal A, Samanek M, Paul T: *Lung function in children and adolescents: Methods, reference values.* New York, 1987, Karger.

Zeltner TB, Burri PH: The postnatal development and growth of the human lung. II. Morphology. *Respir Physiol* 67:269, 1987.

Zin WA, Pengelly LD, Milic-Emili J: Single-breath method for measurement of respiratory mechanics in anesthetized animals. *J Appl Physiol* 52:1266, 1982.

3 Cardiovascular Physiology in Infants and Children

Maureen A. Strafford

The clinical challenge of pediatric anesthesia is directly related to the ongoing development and maturation of multiple organs, especially the cardiopulmonary system, and the intricate interaction of anesthetic and surgical manipulation with these developing systems. Each child presents a challenge. Ironically, the dynamic nature of the cardiovascular system may make pediatric anesthesia appear confusing and complex to the anesthesiologist is inexperienced with children.

With respect to cardiovascular physiology, it is well recognized that the neonate is not just a small infant and that the infant differs from the older child and adolescent. To be safe and effective, an appropriate anesthetic plan must incorporate these vital differences. In addition, the anesthesiologist must be aware that when underlying congenital heart disease is present, cardiopulmonary development continues but may be adversely affected by the ongoing pathophysiology. The patient who undergoes surgical repair of congenital heart defects does not necessarily return to normal cardiac function despite an excellent surgical repair, because the preoperative cardiopulmonary effects of disease are often irreversible. Because cardiac function and pharmacologic responses are so closely tied to developmental changes, this discussion of cardiovascular physiology stresses the basic principles of cardiovascular physiology in the context of ongoing maturational changes. With a clear understanding of these developmental concepts, the anesthesiologist is able to formulate an intelligent and careful plan for a pediatric patient of any age, fully realizing the clinical challenge and rewards of caring for these children.

Maturation of the cardiovascular system is not complete at birth. Dynamic changes of the cardiovascular system occur throughout fetal development and continue into the neonatal period and infancy. The healthy school-aged child possesses a cardiovascular system that functions like that of a healthy young adult but continues to structurally mature as the child grows into adolescence. It is appropriate to begin with a discussion of fetal and neonatal circulation and the basic principles of cardiac function as an introduction to the pediatric cardiovascular system.

FETAL AND TRANSITIONAL CIRCULATION

The cardiovascular system exists to efficiently deliver oxygen and other metabolic nutrients to tissues throughout the body. The needs of the fetus differ from those of the neonate, as do the means of meeting those needs. In the fetus, gas exchange occurs at the placenta, a unique organ that receives blood flow from both the mother and the fetus. Because the lungs require only nutrient flow, not the entire cardiac output (CO) for respiratory exchange, fetal intracardiac and extracardiac shunts exist to minimize flow to the lungs while simultaneously maximizing the appropriate delivery of oxygen to all organ systems. At birth, the placenta is removed and the neonate must exchange gas in the lungs. Fetal shunts are no longer needed and must close to permit the efficient transition to a neonatal circulation. *Transitional circulation* describes the changes observed as the fetus adjusts to the circulatory changes after birth and establishes a neonatal circulation. The presence and persistence of the transitional circulation have important implications for the cardiac function of the neonate, whether the child is normal, is preterm, is critically ill, or has congenital heart disease.

Our understanding of the fetal, transitional, and neonatal cardiovascular circulations is derived from the pioneering research of Dawes and Rudolph in their fetal and neonatal lamb studies (Dawes, 1968; Rudolph, 1974a). Despite obvious species differences, these data have been extrapolated to the human species, and clinical experience continues to confirm their validity.

FETAL CIRCULATION

The chorionic villus is the functional unit of the placenta. Deoxygenated blood is pumped down the fetal descending aorta to the umbilical artery and then to the placenta. The umbilical artery branches and eventually gives rise to an intricate system of arterioles, capillaries, and venules in the intervillous spaces of the placenta, where oxygen and nutrient exchange occurs.

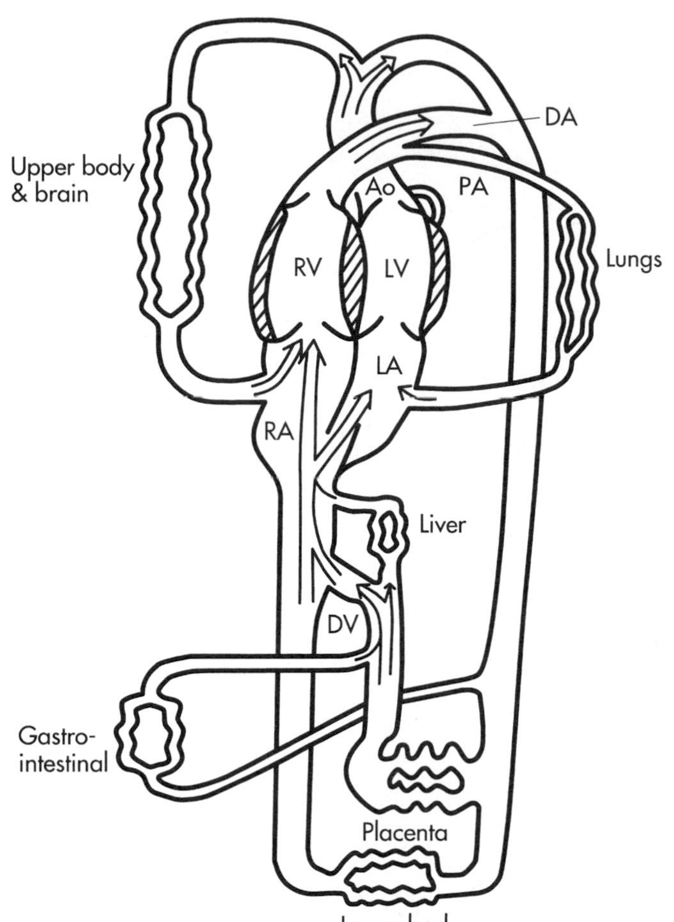

■ **FIGURE 3–1.** Fetal circulation. Ao, aorta; DA, ductus arteriosus; DV, ductus venosus; LA, left atrium; LV, left ventricle; PA, pulmonary artery; RA, right atrium; RV, right ventricle. (From Rudolph AM: Changes in the circulation after birth. In Rudolph AM, editor: *Congenital diseases of the heart.* Chicago, 1974, Year Book Medical.)

Oxygenated blood returns to the fetus via the umbilical vein for delivery to all organ systems. Not only do intracardiac and extracardiac shunts permit the lungs to be bypassed but also more highly oxygenated blood flow is delivered to organs with higher metabolic needs, such as the brain and heart (Fig. 3–1). A review of the anatomy and physiology of fetal circulation illustrates how the fetus with congenital heart disease, even with severe structural cardiac abnormalities, can survive in utero and exhibit clinical difficulties only when the transition from fetal to neonatal circulation is under way.

Because of the presence of shunts, fetal organs receive a mixed blood supply from either the right ventricle (RV) or the left ventricle (LV), often referred to as *parallel circulation.* In contrast, in adult circulation the RV and LV are in series (a *series circulation*), resulting in equal but separate outputs for each ventricle. The foramen ovale, ductus arteriosus, and ductus venosus are the fetal shunts needed for effective fetal circulation that must close after birth. Blood returning from the placenta in the umbilical vein has the highest oxygen content (Fig. 3–2*A*). The first shunt encountered is the ductus venosus, which shunts half of this richly oxygenated umbilical blood flow away from the liver, directly to the heart. Highly oxygenated ductus venosus blood mixes with inferior vena cava blood, but preferential streaming directs blood with more oxygen across the foramen ovale (an intracardiac shunt) into the left atrium (LA). As a result, highly oxygenated blood travels to the LV and is ejected into the aorta, thereby feeding the coronary arteries and arteries to the brain with the most oxygenated blood. Superior vena cava and hepatic venous blood flows to the RV directly, but because of the high resistance in the pulmonary vascular bed and relatively low systemic resistance due to the placental vasculature, right ventricular output is shunted away from the lungs via the ductus arteriosus to enter the descending aorta. The shunted blood entering the descending aorta returns to the placenta or perfuses the lower body. Only 5% to 10% of the combined ventricular output of both ventricles is circulated directly to the lungs.

Fetal CO is often described as combined ventricular output, meaning the sum of the output of both ventricles. However, each ventricle has a different afterload, against which it pumps. The RV ejects against the low-resistance ductus arteriosus, the low-resistance placenta, and the high-resistance lungs and lower body. The left ventricular afterload consists of the high resistance found in the brain, upper body, and aortic isthmus. The fetal RV has a slightly higher output because its afterload is significantly lower than that of the LV. The LV pumps into the much larger vascular bed of the brain, so in the end, the outputs of the RV and LV are almost equal. Studies by Rudolph (1974a, 1974b) suggested a ratio of RV to LV output equal to 2:1 in the fetal lamb. Echocardiographic evidence supports this concept of equal size and output as the ventricles develop in utero and have an RV/LV output ratio closer to 1.3:1 (St. John Sutton et al., 1984).

OXYGEN DELIVERY IN THE FETUS AND NEONATE

The cardiovascular system must efficiently deliver oxygen and other metabolic substrates to all tissues and organs. Nevertheless, the fetus functions and develops within a relatively hypoxemic environment and adequate oxygen delivery must depend on other compensatory mechanisms. Umbilical venous blood has an oxygen tension of about 35 mm Hg. The fetus has high concentrations (≈80% at term) of fetal hemoglobin (HbF), which binds oxygen much more efficiently than the adult form of hemoglobin (HbA). Oxygen competes with 2,3-diphosphoglycerate (2,3-DPG) for binding on the hemoglobin molecule. Levels of 2,3-DPG are lower in the fetus than in the adult. In addition, HbF has a low affinity for 2,3-DPG compared with HbA and therefore HbF preferentially binds oxygen. The P_{50} (oxygen tension at which 50% of the blood is saturated with oxygen) occurs at a lower PO_2 in the fetus as a result of HbF and its unique binding characteristics (see Fig. 2–45). Oxygen saturation of hemoglobin in umbilical venous blood is well maintained, often greater than 90%.

A review of fetal anatomy and physiology shows how a fetus with congenital heart disease may have little difficulty in utero. The fetal intracardiac and extracardiac shunts permit blood flow to the placenta and other vital organs despite the presence of severe underlying abnormalities. Hypoplastic left heart syndrome (HLHS), which is associated with severe hypoplasia of the LV, atresia of the mitral and aortic valve, and hypoplasia of the aortic arch, is incompatible with neonatal survival, but the fetus with HLHS has a viable circulation in utero. A neonate with HLHS has no way for blood to flow from the LA to the LV and therefore left atrial blood return is shunted completely via the foramen ovale to the RA, RV, and ductus arteriosus.

Retrograde flow from the ductus arteriosus perfuses the ascending aorta and coronary arteries. Intracardiac shunts, such

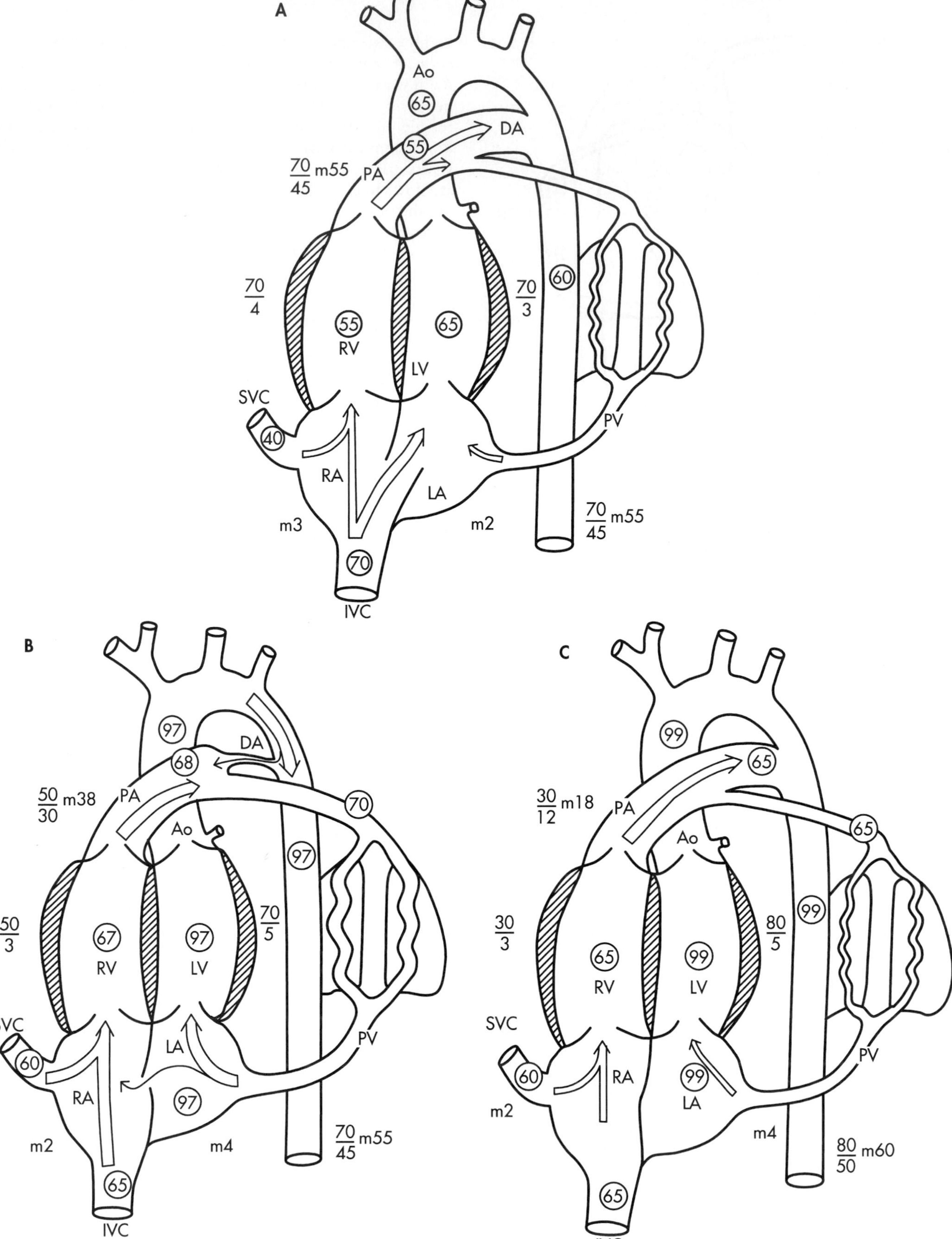

■ **FIGURE 3–2.** Hemodynamics of the fetus and neonate. Circled values represent oxygen saturation. Systolic, diastolic, and mean (m) pressures appear near their respective chambers and vessels. *(A)* Fetal circulation near term. *(B)* Transitional circulation less than 1 day after birth. *(C)* Neonatal circulation several days after birth. Ao, aorta; DA, ductus arteriosus; DV, ductus venosus; IVC, inferior vena cava; LA, left atrium; LV, left ventricle; PA, pulmonary artery; PV, pulmonary vein; RA, right atrium; RV, right ventricle; SVC, superior vena cava. (From Rudolph AM: Changes in the circulation after birth. In Rudolph AM, editor: *Congenital diseases of the heart.* Chicago, 1974a, Year Book Medical.)

as the foramen ovale and ductus arteriosus, remain essential to continued survival after birth in the neonate with HLHS. When the transition from fetal to neonatal circulation begins, with closure of the fetal shunts, the underlying congenital heart defect is unmasked, often because systemic blood flow (as in HLHS) depends on the presence of a ductus arteriosus, foramen ovale, or both. In contrast, dysrhythmias or conduction abnormalities, such as congenital complete heart block, often cause severe fetal problems such as hydrops and may contribute to fetal death. Cardiac function is limited in utero, and output is sensitive to changes in volume and heart rate (HR) changes (see later discussion). Because of these functional limitations, the fetus cannot tolerate bradycardia or persistent dysrhythmias in utero yet can survive severe structural abnormalities.

TRANSITIONAL CIRCULATION

At birth, various factors influence the change from a fetal circulation to the neonatal pattern (see Fig. 3–2*B*). When the placenta separates, with clamping of the umbilical vessels, and ventilation and pulmonary blood flow begin, profound effects are produced on fetal circulatory anatomy and physiology. As described, the circulation changes from a parallel to a series system, and intracardiac and extracardiac shunts close. The placenta ceases to function as the organ of respiration, and the lungs begin respiration in a gaseous rather than a liquid environment. The most dramatic changes at birth are related to changes in resistance throughout the circulatory system. The low-resistance placenta is excluded, as the umbilical cord vessels are clamped and systemic vascular resistance (SVR) increases. With the initiation of breathing, pulmonary vascular resistance (PVR) begins to decrease as pulmonary blood flow increases.

PVR falls dramatically at birth. More gradual decreases in PVR, pulmonary artery pressure, and pulmonary blood flow occur over the first few weeks of life (Fig. 3–3*A*). These more gradual declines reflect the *remodeling* of the pulmonary vascular musculature typical of this period. At birth, the increased pulmonary blood flow increases left atrial pressure, and the foramen ovale, a flaplike one-way valve, closes in response to these higher pressures relative to right atrial pressure. The foramen ovale can open in response to changing physiologic conditions. Fifty percent of children under age 5 and 25% of adults demonstrate probe patency of the foramen ovale (Scammon and Norris, 1918). Functional closure of the ductus arteriosus occurs with removal of the placenta and a consequent decrease in the levels of circulating prostaglandins.

In utero prostaglandins contribute to the patency of the ductus arteriosus, and the increasing oxygen tension after ventilation serves as a potent stimulus for ductal closure. Final anatomic closure results from thrombosis and fibrosis over the first few months of life, although the precise mechanisms of closure are not well elucidated (see Fig. 3–2*C*). Because these shunts are not anatomically closed immediately after birth, certain clinical conditions may contribute to either the persistence of or a return to a fetal circulation. Infants who are preterm or critically ill with a either medical (e.g., sepsis or meconium

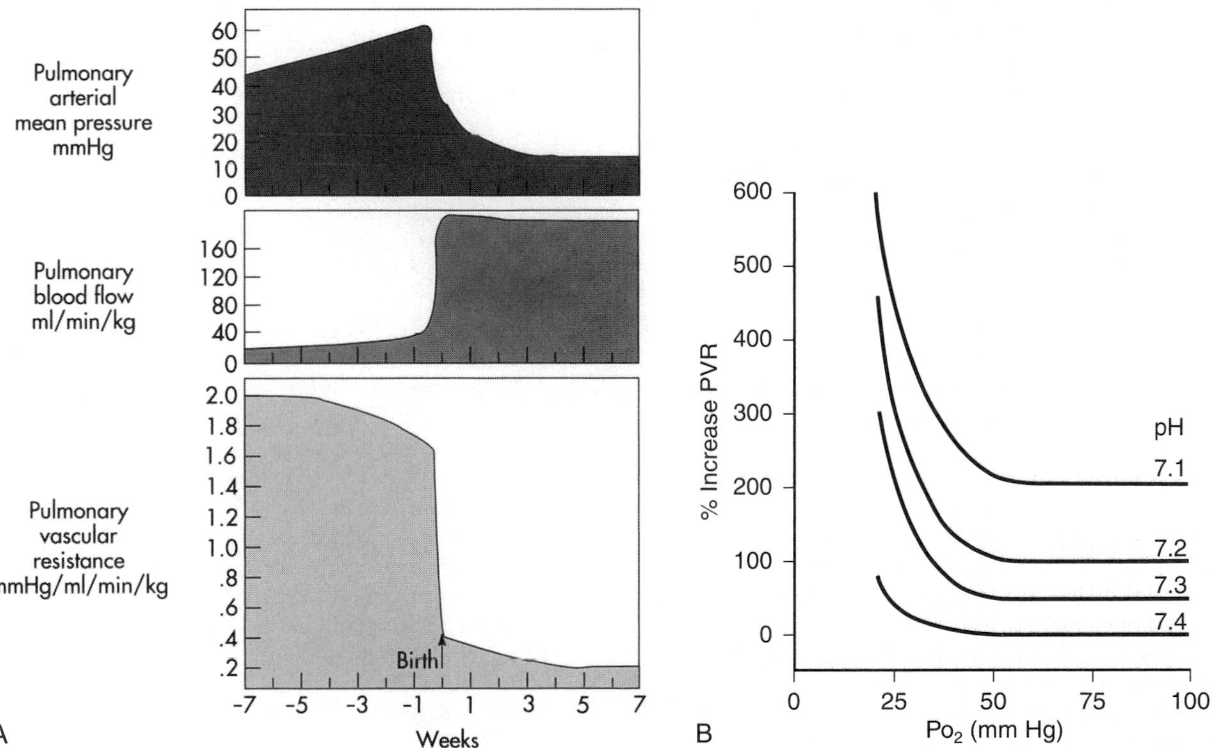

FIGURE 3–3. *(A)* Graphic representation of the changes in pulmonary artery pressure, pulmonary blood flow, and pulmonary vascular resistance that occur in the perinatal period. Pulmonary vascular resistance decreases during the latter part of gestation, mainly because of an increase in the number of pulmonary vessels associated with growth; it falls dramatically at birth because of the vasodilator effect of ventilating the lungs with air; a further decrease occurs as pulmonary vascular smooth muscle regresses. Pulmonary blood flow increases slightly during fetal growth and then increases dramatically after birth. Pulmonary arterial pressure falls rapidly immediately after birth and then more gradually to reach adult levels after 6 to 8 weeks. (From Rudolph AM: Changes in the circulation after birth. In Rudolph AM, editor: *Congenital diseases of the heart.* Chicago, 1974, Year Book Medical.) *(B)* Change in pulmonary vascular resistance (PVR) with changes in Po_2 and arterial pH. (From Rudolph AM, Yuan S: Response to the pulmonary circulation to hypoxia and H^+ ion concentration changes. *J Clin Invest* 45:399–411, 1966.)

aspiration) or surgical (e.g., tracheoesophageal fistula or omphalocele) crisis are at high risk for persistent fetal shunting. Hypoxemia and acidosis are two main factors known to reverse shunt patency. Neonates with these problems are at considerable risk for persistence of the fetal circulation (PFC), a clinical syndrome observed in neonates when fetal shunting persists beyond the normal transition period in the absence of structural congenital heart disease (Gersony et al., 1969). The presence of hypoxemia, acidosis, or both can be potent stimuli for maintaining high PVR in the neonate. Persistent fetal shunting (see Fig. 3–3*B*), PFC, or persistent pulmonary hypertension of the newborn (PPHN), illustrates the important interactions between pulmonary and cardiac development at the neonatal stage.

The process by which the vasoconstricted pulmonary vascular bed relaxes at birth is complex and not completely understood. The process most likely involves a cascade of humoral, vasoactive mediators that cause dynamic changes in PVR. PPHN can also result when there are structural abnormalities in the pulmonary vascular bed. For example, an intrauterine insult may result in maladaptation of the pulmonary vasculature, resulting in abnormal muscularization of normally nonmuscularized peripheral arteries and medial hypertrophy of the muscular arteries. At birth, this infant may present with signs or symptoms of PPHN. Some infants with severe meconium aspiration have been found to have these postmortem findings in the pulmonary vasculature, raising the possibility of a developmental insult resulting in these changes. The pathophysiology of neonatal pulmonary hypertension has been elucidated extensively in the past decades, but it is only since the 1990s that research has begun to explain the recovery process and its potential long-term effects on the pulmonary vasculature. In a well-studied animal model of chronic hypobaric hypoxia that reflects neonatal pulmonary hypertension in humans, the remodeling of the pulmonary arteries during recovery from pulmonary hypertension induced by neonatal hypoxia was studied (Hall et al., 2004). In neonatal pulmonary hypertension, the thickening of the pulmonary arteries is due to smooth muscle cell hyperplasia, hypertrophy, smooth muscle cell recruitment from the adventitia, and increased deposition of matrix proteins (Tulloh et al., 1997; Haworth and Hislop, 2003).

Recovery from neonatal pulmonary hypertension results in thinning of the elastic and muscular arteries, but the mechanisms of recovery are different in these two types of arteries and are age dependent. The study of recovery from abnormal fetal and neonatal cardiovascular physiology has also raised the challenging concept that abnormalities in this early period of life may have dramatic implications for adult cardiovascular risk. Both fetal hypoxia and fetal undernutrition may be linked to adult cardiovascular disease. In 1993, Barker and others (Barker, 1993; Barker and Fall, 1993) hypothesized that any alteration of the in utero environment that has the potential for alterations in fetal development may also irreversibly impair physiologic function, increasing susceptibility to disease in adulthood.

Jones and others (2004) demonstrated in the laboratory that perinatal exposure to chronic hypoxia had multiple and serious consequences in the adult, which included reduced body weight, right and left ventricular hypertrophy, reduced pulmonary arterial compliance, and alterations in pulmonary artery compliance.

While maladaptation of the pulmonary vasculature is one problem, maldevelopment of the pulmonary vasculature can also be seen in newborns. For example, infants with diaphragmatic hernia have underdevelopment of the lung parenchyma or pulmonary hypoplasia. These infants have a reduction in alveoli and pulmonary arterial vessels, but the arterial vessels present have an increased and abnormal muscularity and do not dilate normally after birth.

Figure 3–4 illustrates the normal arterial dilatation during transition from fetal to neonatal circulation. The initial change seen postnatally is preacinar dilatation. When there is underdevelopment of the lung, such as in diaphragmatic hernia, the vascular bed is hypoplastic and abnormally muscular and cannot dilate normally after birth. When the pulmonary vascular bed is maldeveloped, the vascular bed also has increased muscular development. Finally, if there is maladaptation, such as in neonates with medical or surgical emergencies or congenital heart disease, and resulting hypoxemia, acidosis, or both, normal dilatation does not occur. In these neonates, severe hypoxemia and circulatory compromise may occur and may first appear during the stress of surgery and anesthesia.

BASIC PRINCIPLES OF FETAL AND NEONATAL CARDIAC FUNCTION

Fetal circulatory anatomy has many clever design features, and the developing heart has significant functional limitations that continue into the neonatal period. In any discussion of cardiovascular physiology, several essential physiologic concepts must be understood: preload, afterload, contractility, SV, and CO. CO in both the fetus and the adult is directly proportional to HR, preload (ventricular distention), and contractility but is inversely related to afterload (combined resistances of blood, ventricular mass, and vascular beds).

An understanding of basic cardiac function is derived from studies examining the mechanical and contractile properties of isolated cardiac muscle fiber and the basic unit of contraction, the sarcomere. The heart is a muscle that lengthens and shortens against a load. It pumps blood from the low-pressure venous system to the high-pressure arterial vascular bed. How well the heart performs as a pump is measured by *cardiac output (CO),* or the volume of blood ejected per minute by the LV. *Stroke volume* is the volume of blood ejected during each contraction, and *CO* is the product of HR multiplied by SV. The SV, however, is determined by the loading conditions of the heart (preload and afterload) and the intrinsic contractility of the heart.

Intact heart function is influenced by multiple other factors, including geometry of fiber orientation, ventricular geometry, interdependence of right and left ventricular function, pericardial and pulmonary interactions, and the vascular beds and their various resistances. Finally, the immaturity of the fetal and neonatal circulatory system has important implications for cardiac function. This discussion focuses on these important concepts, with reviews of studies from isolated cardiac muscle and intact heart preparations and comparative studies that describe fetal, neonatal, and adult myocardial function. In this way, the potent effects of anesthetics on the circulatory system, especially at critical developmental stages such as the newborn period, can be better understood and anesthetic plans safely formulated.

PRELOAD

In cardiovascular physiology isolated muscle studies, a strip of isolated cardiac muscle is stretched and fixed at both ends in a physiologic solution (Fig. 3–5). An electrical stimulation is delivered, causing an isometric contraction. Because the muscle

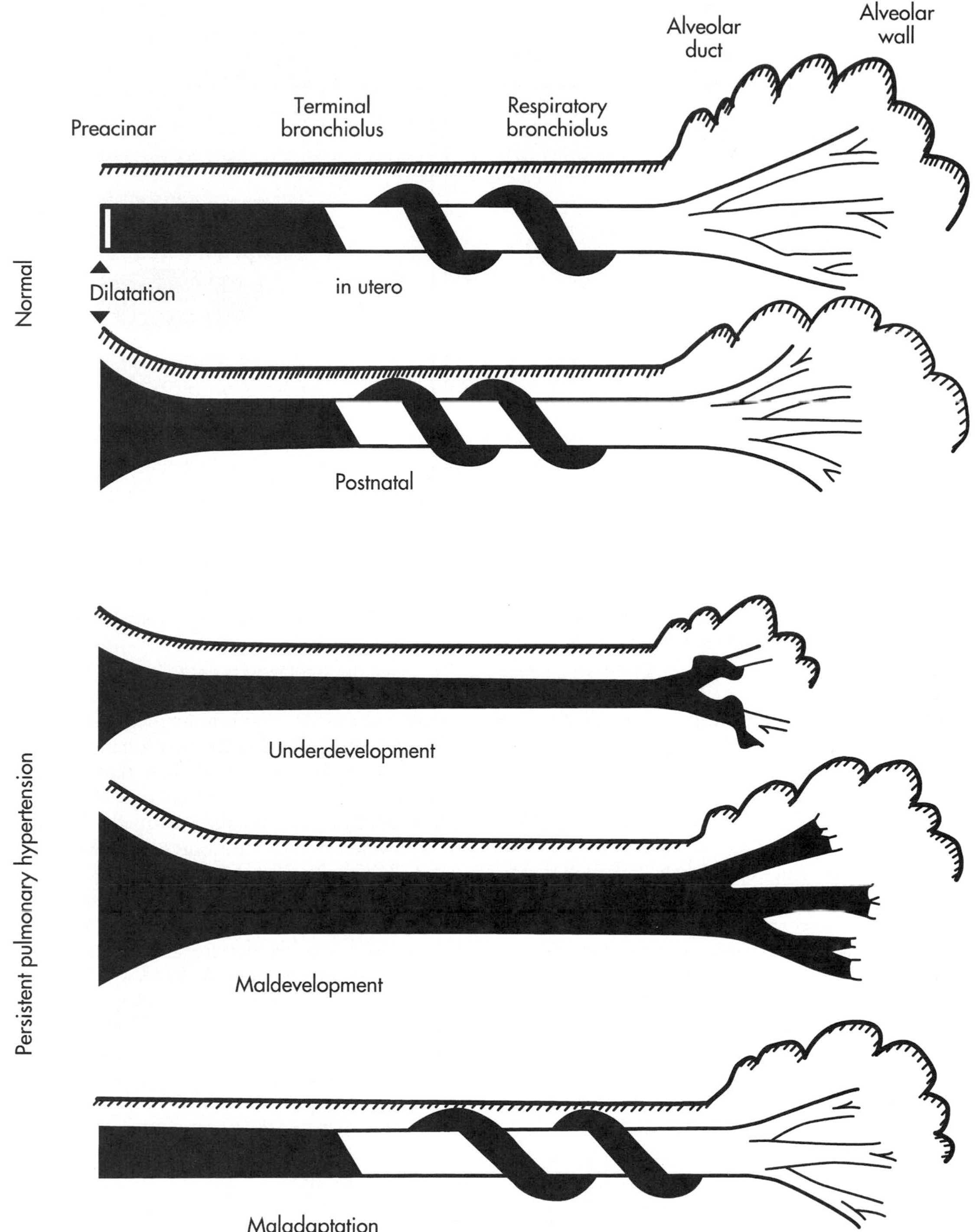

■ **FIGURE 3–4.** Schematic representation of normal arterial dilatation during transition from fetal to neonatal circulation. When the lung is underdeveloped, the vascular bed is abnormally muscular; when it is maladapted, it has not dilated appropriately at birth. (From Rabinovitch M: Pulmonary hypertension. In Adams FH, Emmanouilides GC, Riemenschnieder T, editors: *Moss' heart disease in infants, children, and adolescents,* 4th ed. Baltimore, 1989, Williams & Wilkins.)

is fixed on both ends, no fiber shortening occurs, but tension does increase. This tension varies directly with the amount of stretch put on the muscle before stimulation. The initial amount of stretch is defined as *preload.* Because different amounts of stretch can be applied to the muscle, different amounts of tension are developed. The point at which the maximal tension is developed is called L_{max}. The curve plotted using different stretch values (preload) against the tension developed is called the length–active tension curve (Fig. 3–6). As sarcomeres are stretched up to a finite length, the force of contraction (tension) increases. *Tension* is the force generated along a line. *Stress* is the force exerted across a cross-sectional area or surface. *Pressure* is the force generated within a cavity. When we apply the concept of preload to the intact heart, wall stress and intracavitary pressure

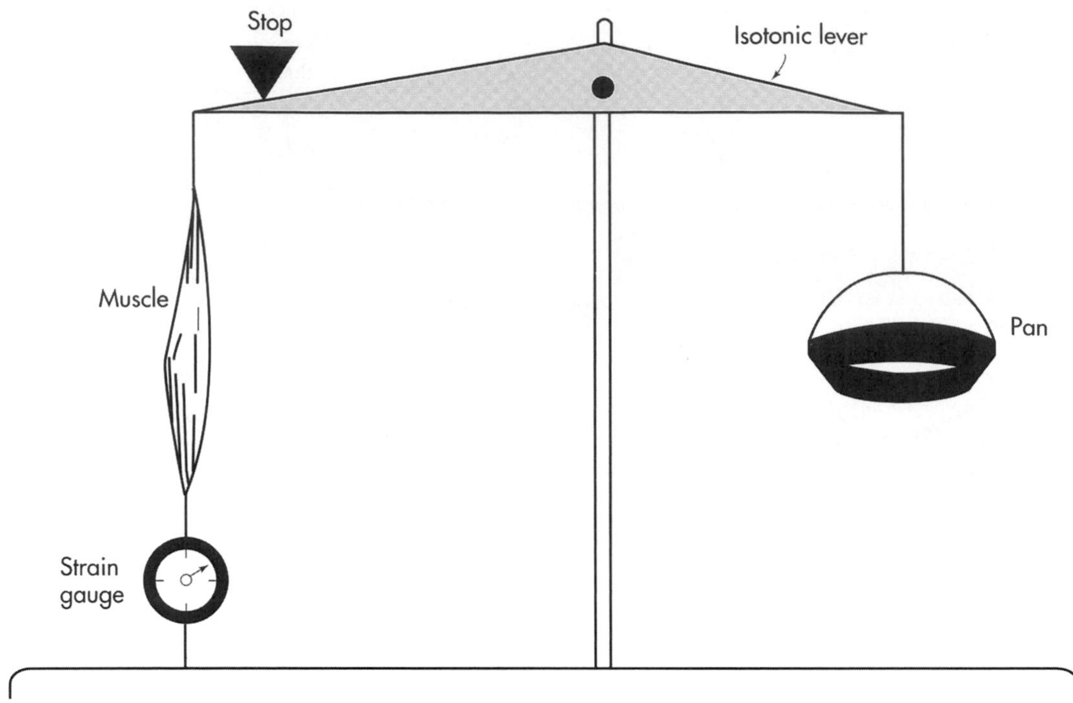

■ **FIGURE 3–5.** Study of length–tension relationships in isolated cardiac muscle strips. (From Braunwald E, Ross J, Sonnenblick EH: *Mechanisms of contraction of the normal and failing heart,* 2nd ed. Boston, 1976, Little, Brown.)

play important roles. Because the LV is conceptualized as a thick-walled cylinder, the law of La Place states that

$$\text{Wall stress} = \frac{(\text{P} \times \text{R})}{\text{h}} \tag{3.1}$$

where P is the pressure within the cylinder, R is the radius of curvature, and h is the thickness of the ventricular wall.

Despite the complex geometry of the LV, wall stress is considered uniform throughout. As a result, wall stress is said to increase as ventricular chamber volume increases even when intraventricular pressure is constant. In addition, if wall thickness increases (i.e., the total number of muscle fibers increases), the tension on any single muscle fiber is decreased, because it is distributed among more muscle fibers.

In the intact heart, preload is the diastolic wall stress resulting from a certain volume of blood distending the ventricle. The preload is the load present before contraction has started, at the end of diastole. The preload is a reflection of venous filling pressure that fills the RA or LA, which then fills the RV or LV during diastole. The relationship between end-diastolic volume (EDV) and developed pressure in the intact heart produces a curve similar to the length–tension curve defined in isolated muscle fiber preparations (Fig. 3–7). These curves appear similar to those shown in Figure 3–6 in isolated papillary muscle studies. Independent observations by Frank and Starling correlated the isolated muscle fiber results with intact heart observations (Frank, 1895; Starling, 1918). Frank's observations that the "length and tension changes in skeletal muscle correspond to changes in volume and pressure in the heart" and Starling's description that "the mechanical energy set free on passage from the resting to the contracted state is a function of the length of the muscle fiber" form the basis for the well-known Frank-Starling mechanism. When the preload increases, the LV distends during diastole and the SV rises according to Starling's law. This mechanism and the idealized ventricular function curves demonstrating the mechanism (Fig. 3–8) show that cardiac performance, represented by SV or CO, is related to preload, ventricular EDV, or pressure. In clinical practice, ventricular end-diastolic pressure (EDP) is often used as a measure of preload. However, compliance or "stiffness" of the ventricle after hypertrophy, scarring, or with aortic regurgitation may alter this response.

Why is preload important in regulating cardiac function? Preload acts as a functional reserve. Preload reserve, or the ability to increase SV with an increase in EDV, has important implications for the circulatory system during stress. Lee and others (1986) have shown a 9% increase in EDV coupled with a 13% increase in SV in resting dogs during volume loading. Cardiac muscle has a high degree of resting tension at all lengths, especially compared with skeletal muscle (Fig. 3–9). Because of the collagen network in which myocardial cells dwell in the intact heart, cardiac muscle operates on the ascending limb of the length–tension curve.

■ AFTERLOAD

Afterload has been studied in isolated muscle preparations as well as in the intact heart. In isolated muscle preparations, *afterload* is the weight or load that the contracting muscle must overcome to shorten. In single fiber studies, one end of the muscle strip is attached to a transducer while the other end is attached to an isotonic lever (Fig. 3–10). On the opposite end of the lever, a weight is attached, stretching the muscle to its resting length. At this point the resting tension or preload can be determined. Further stretch on the muscle is prevented by placing a stop where the muscle is attached to the lever. Then weight is added. After a stimulation, the muscle contracts until it develops sufficient tension to overcome the additional imposed weight.

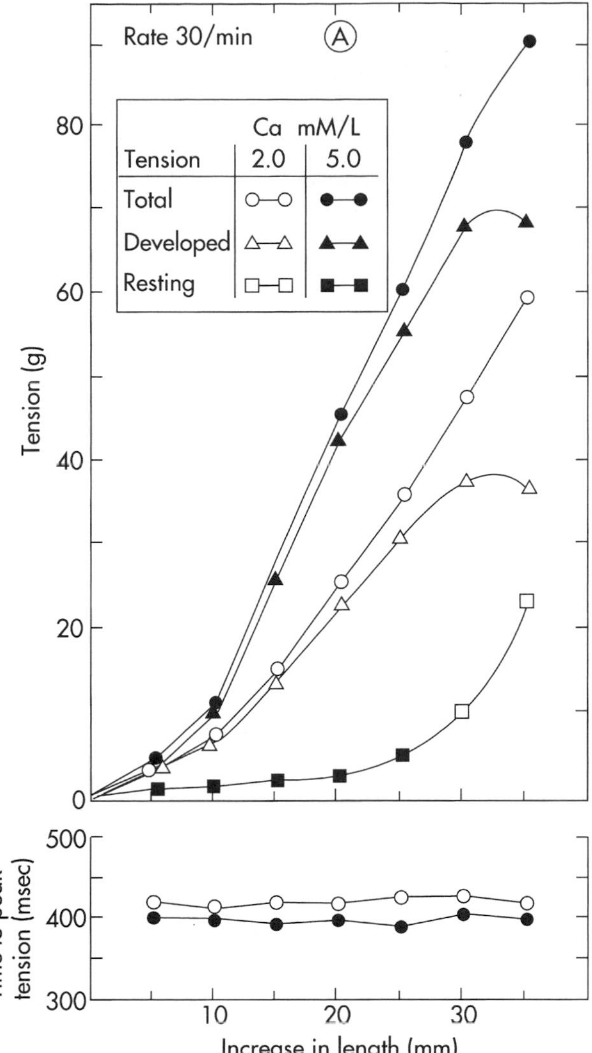

■ **FIGURE 3–6.** Length–active tension curve showing the relationship between length and tension in isolated cat papillary muscle. Note the effect of increased contractility due to increased calcium ion concentration. Neither the relation between muscle length and rising tension nor L_{max} is altered. However, developed tension at any given muscle length is increased at the higher calcium concentration. (From Braunwald E, Ross J, Sonnenblick EH: *Mechanisms of contraction of the normal and failing heart.* 2nd ed. Boston, 1976, Little, Brown.)

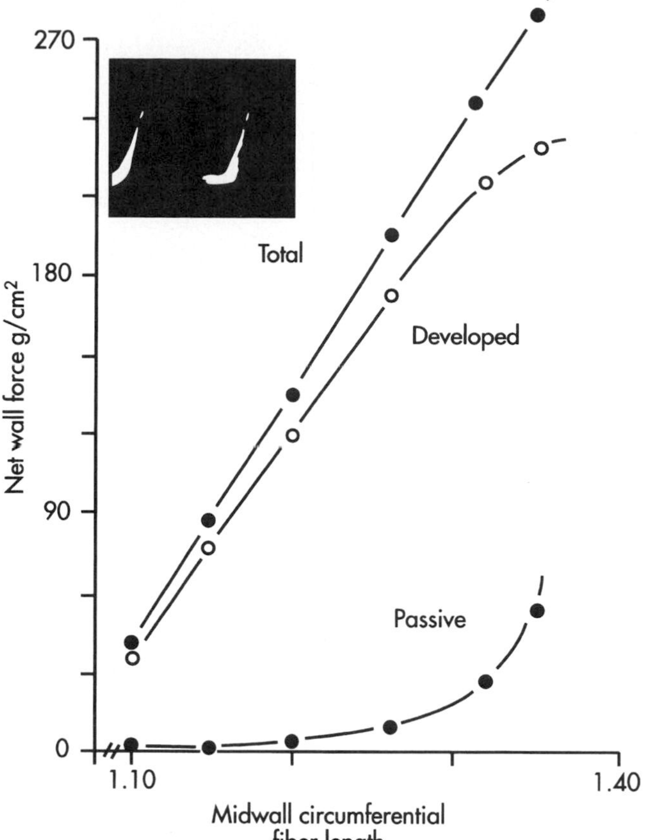

■ **FIGURE 3–7.** Relationship between midwall circumferential fiber length and maximal developed force obtained in the isovolumetrically beating left ventricle of the isolated canine heart. Note the similarity to Figure 3–6. (From Weber KT, Janicki JS: *Am J Cardiol* 40:740, 1977.)

This tension is the afterload. Preload in the intact heart is defined as the wall stress at the end of diastole, whereas afterload is the wall stress experienced by the intact heart during ventricular ejection. Because ventricular ejection is a dynamic event, afterload is more complicated conceptually.

Cardiac function is inversely related to afterload and directly related to preload. Afterload plays a critical role in cardiovascular regulation as summarized in Figure 3–11. In intact hearts, arterial pressure, resistance, or impedance is often used as a measure of afterload. As with preload, extrapolation from single-fiber studies to the intact heart is difficult because of asymmetric ventricular geometry and the process of ventricular ejection. Afterload is often related to vascular resistance even though resistance is a measure of the opposition to flow in a nonpulsatile system. Impedance is a more accurate measure of opposition to flow in a pulsatile system, but it is much more difficult to measure. Resistance is measured as the pressure difference across the circulation divided by mean aortic flow, or CO, as follows:

$$R = \frac{P}{Q} = 8\mu L/\pi r^4 \qquad (3.2)$$

where R is vascular resistance, P is mean pressure change across the arterial circuit, Q is mean flow or CO, μ is blood viscosity, L is length of the arterial system, and r is vessel radius.

Equating systolic arterial pressure with SVR is potentially erroneous, as Equation 3.2 demonstrates. Arterial blood pressure (BP) may remain constant in the face of opposite changes in CO and resistance, and profound changes in afterload would not be suspected.

Because the amount of blood ejected by the ventricle, the CO, is determined largely by afterload, changes in afterload affect performance in important ways. Increased afterload causes a reciprocal decline in the extent and velocity of fiber shortening and therefore the volume of blood ejected. However, this assumes the other determinants of output (HR, preload, contractility) are not changing. In addition, other factors, such as the neurohumoral control of vascular constriction, play important roles.

CONTRACTILITY

Contractility is a critical factor in cardiac performance. Multiple forces influence the contractile state of the myocardium, as

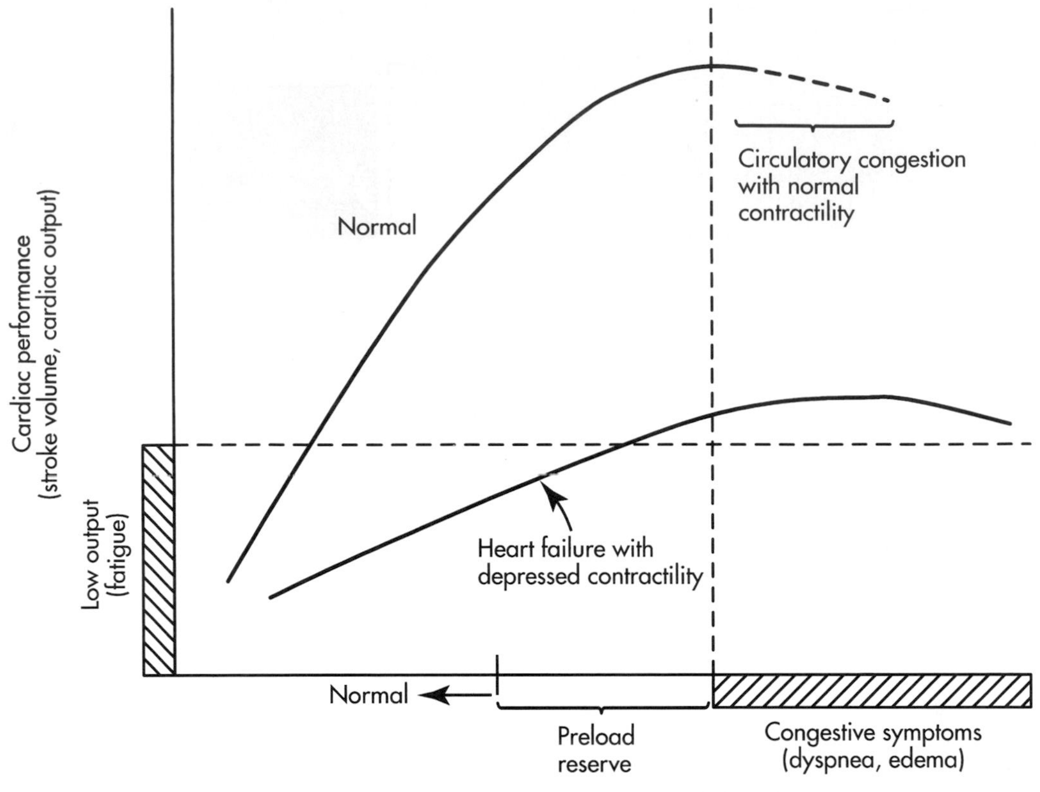

FIGURE 3–8. Frank-Starling mechanism. Cardiac performance, represented by stroke volume or cardiac output, is related to some estimation of preload, ventricular end-diastolic volume, or pressure. (From Friedman WF, George BL: Treatment of congestive heart failure by altering loading conditions of the heart. *J Pediatr* 106:697, 1985.)

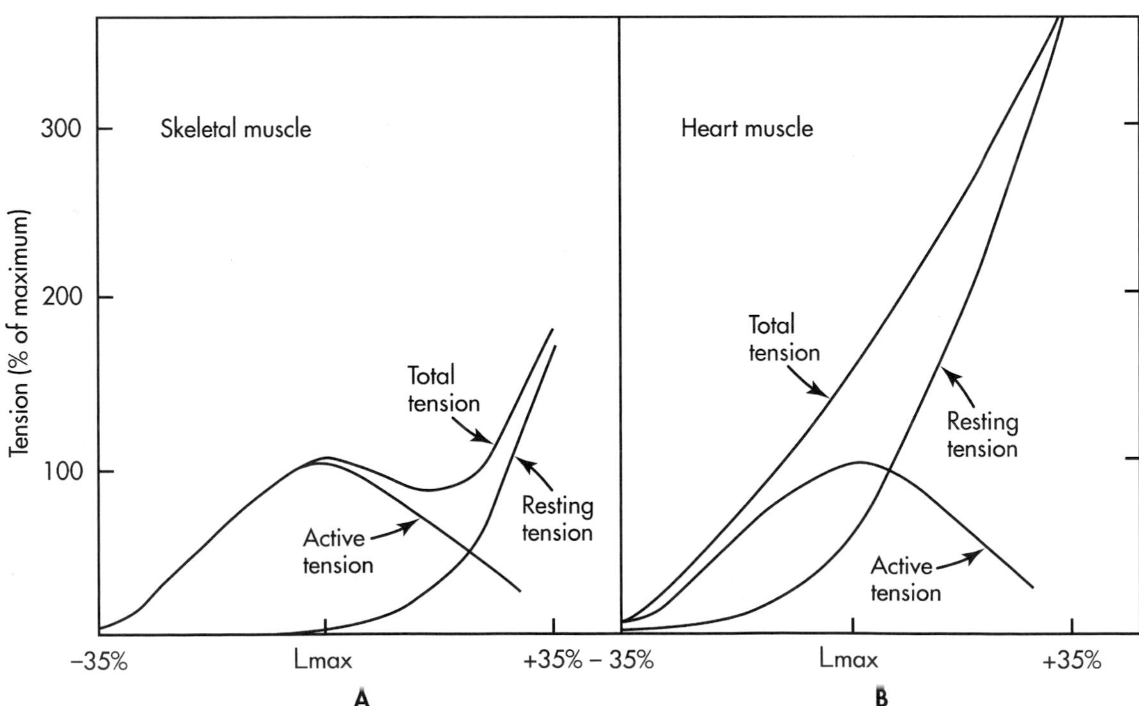

FIGURE 3–9. Comparison of total and active length–tension curves in skeletal *(A)* and cardiac *(B)* muscle allowed to contract under isometric conditions. Active tension, which is the tension developed during contraction, equals total tension after stimulation minus the tension recorded in the resting muscle before stimulation. Although the active length–tension curves are similar for the two muscle types, the resting tension in the cardiac muscle is much higher and, unlike skeletal muscle, is significant below L_{max}. (From Katz A: *Physiology of the heart.* New York, 1977, Raven Press.)

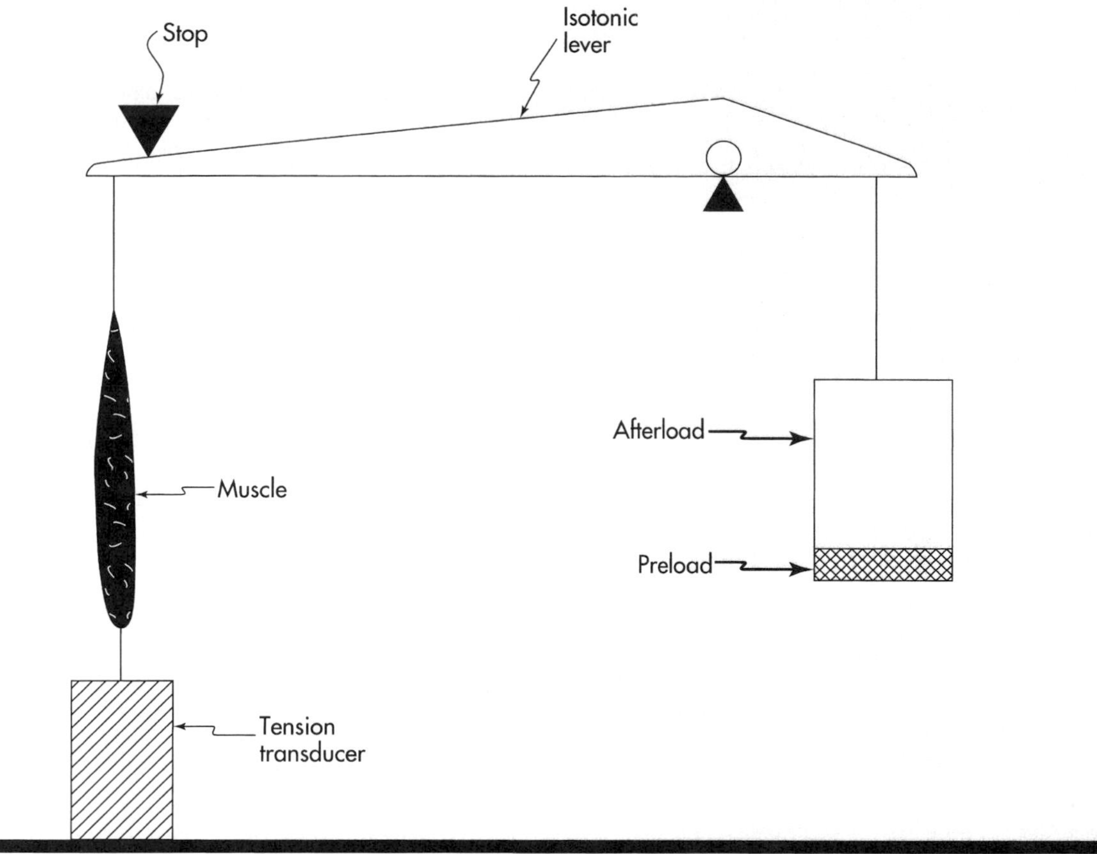

■ **FIGURE 3–10.** Diagrammatic representation of an isotonic lever system. (From Braunwald E, Ross J, Sonnenblick EH: *Mechanisms of contraction of the normal and failing heart.* 2nd ed. Boston, 1976, Little, Brown.)

summarized schematically in Figure 3–12. Isolated muscle studies show that if preload and afterload are held constant, the rate at which tension develops can nevertheless be increased in the presence of calcium or drugs such as norepinephrine (Fig. 3–13). With increased calcium, the intrinsic performance of the cardiac muscle is enhanced. However, contractility assessment is much more complex and difficult to measure in the intact heart. Because preload and afterload dynamically influence contractility, an assessment of contractility should be load independent. Obtaining a load-independent measurement remains controversial. The validity of contractility measurements must always be critically examined and understood, especially when the effects of anesthetics on cardiac function and contractility are described with echocardiographic measurements. This issue is reviewed in greater detail later.

INTERRELATIONSHIPS BETWEEN PRELOAD, AFTERLOAD, AND CONTRACTILITY

Realistic understanding of preload, afterload, and contractility and of how these factors affect cardiac performance must take into account the interrelationships between these forces in the

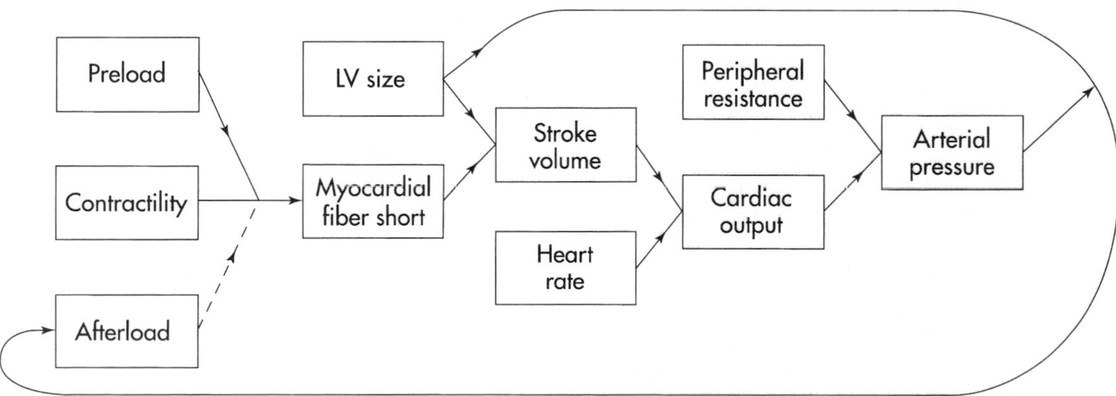

■ **FIGURE 3–11.** Interactions between the various components of cardiac activity. Solid lines indicate an increasing effect. Broken line represents a depressing effect. LV, left ventricle. (From Braunwald E: Regulation of the circulation. *N Engl J Med* 290:1124, 1974. © 1974 Massachusetts Medical Society. All rights reserved.)

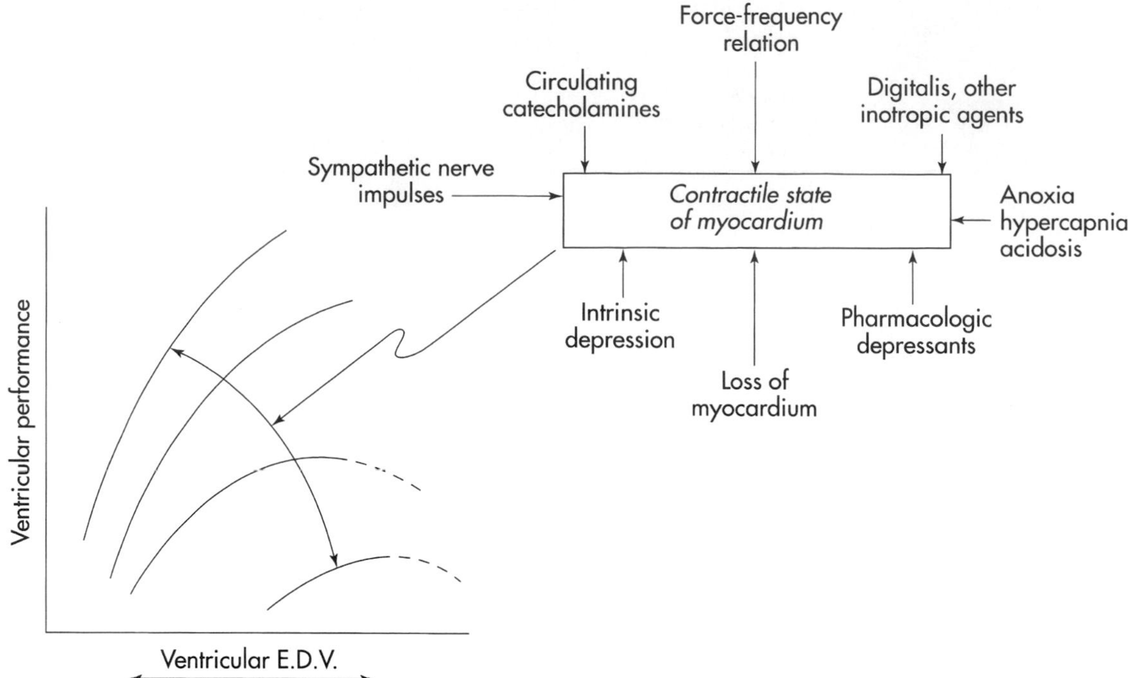

■ **FIGURE 3–12.** Major influences that elevate or depress the contractile state of the myocardium. *(Bottom left)* Effect of alterations in the contractile state of the myocardium on the level of ventricular performance at any given level of ventricular end-diastolic volume (E.D.V.). (From Braunwald E, Ross J, Sonnenblick EH: *Mechanisms of contraction of the normal and failing heart.* 2nd ed. Boston, 1976, Little, Brown.)

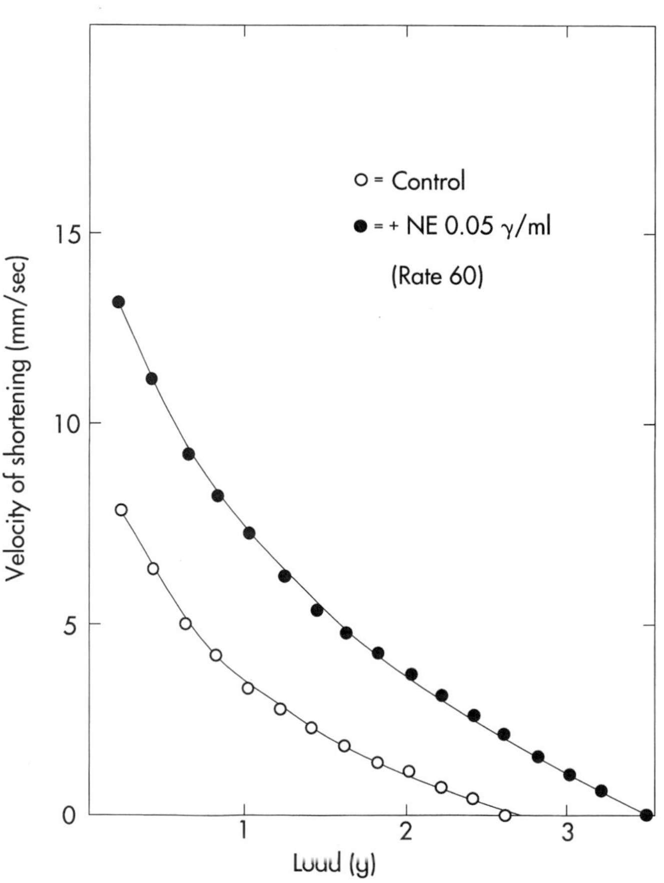

■ **FIGURE 3–13.** Effect of increased contractility due to norepinephrine (NE) administration on the force–velocity relation of the cat papillary muscle. (From Braunwald E, Ross J, Sonnenblick EH: *Mechanisms of contraction of the normal and failing heart.* 2nd ed. Boston, 1976, Little, Brown.)

intact heart. When the relationship of pressure and volume in the intact heart is schematically described, a pressure–volume loop is drawn. This loop demonstrates the phases of contraction and relaxation in the intact heart (Fig. 3–14). When a measurable pressure and volume are reached at point A, this is a determination of *preload.* The LV begins to contract and, as the pressure increases, the mitral valve closes. Before the aortic valve opens, there is the period of isovolumetric contraction. Once ventricular pressure exceeds aortic pressure, the aortic valve opens and ejection begins (point B = afterload). The distance between points B and C is a representation of SV. As the ventricle ejects, the force on the wall of the LV, or afterload, actually decreases. The law of La Place (wall stress = P × R/h) states that wall stress decreases as the ventricular chamber size decreases. Point C is reached when the muscle cannot shorten any farther; then the aortic valve closure occurs. The interval of point C to point D represents isovolumetric relaxation coincident with the sharp drop in ventricular pressure. Once ventricular pressure drops below left atrial pressure, the mitral valve opens and ventricular filling begins again, generating the preload for the next ejection.

These pressure–volume loops become extremely helpful in describing how changes in one determinant directly affect SV. When afterload and contractility are held constant, changes in preload are described in the following pressure–volume loop (Fig. 3–15). Points A, E, and F represent different ventricular EDVs or preloads. SV is increased ($SV_2 > SV_1$) with increasing preloads as described by the Frank-Starling mechanism.

If afterload is increased while preload and contractility remain the same, a different loop results (Fig. 3–16). Points A, B, and C represent increasing afterloads. SV decreases as afterload increases (SV A to F > SV B to E > SV C to D).

These loops serve to illustrate the relationships of preload, afterload, and contractility in the intact heart. However, preload

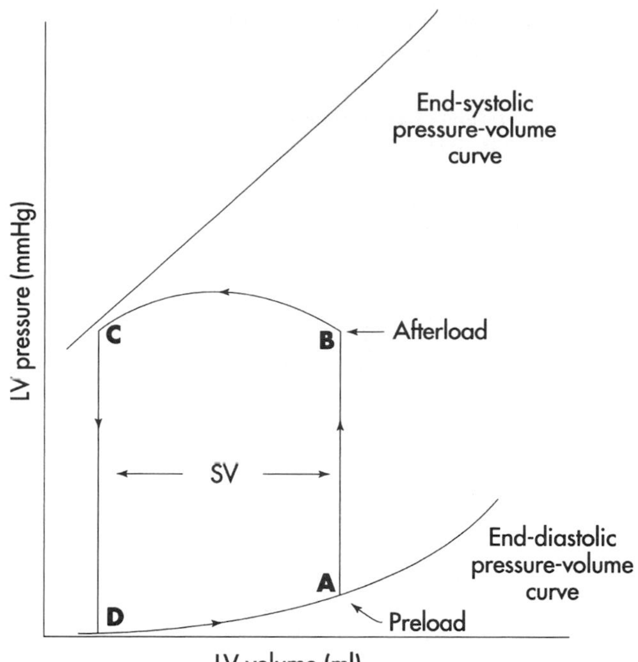

■ **FIGURE 3–14.** Schematic representation of the pressure–volume relation in the intact heart (see text for description). LV, left ventricular; SV, stroke volume. (From Braunwald E, Ross J, Sonnenblick EH: *Mechanisms of contraction of the normal and failing heart.* 2nd ed. Boston, 1976, Little, Brown.)

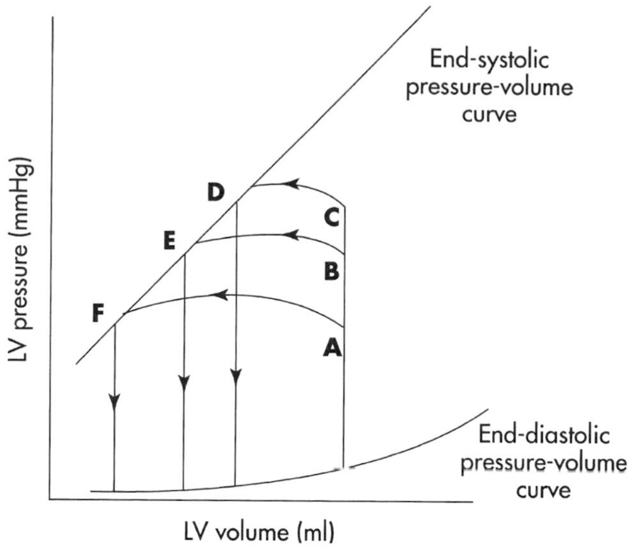

■ **FIGURE 3–16.** Schematic pressure–volume loops demonstrating the effect of increasing afterload on stroke volume during normal contraction when preload and contractility are held constant. As afterload is increased, stroke volume is diminished. The points D, E, and F at end ejection describe a line known as the end-systolic pressure–volume relation, the slope of which is used as a load-independent index of contractility. LV, left ventricular. (From Braunwald E, Ross J, Sonnenblick EH: *Mechanisms of contraction of the normal and failing heart.* 2nd ed. Boston, 1976, Little, Brown.)

and afterload do not always change independently, as described earlier (Fig. 3–17). Loop 1 schematically represents a normal EDV being reached and the subsequent ejection of a normal SV. When the heart must contract against an increased afterload, loop 2 is described and a decrease in SV is noted. However, the heart attempts to compensate for the decrease in SV by contracting at an increased EDV but with less afterload. The result is an SV very close to normal (loop 1).

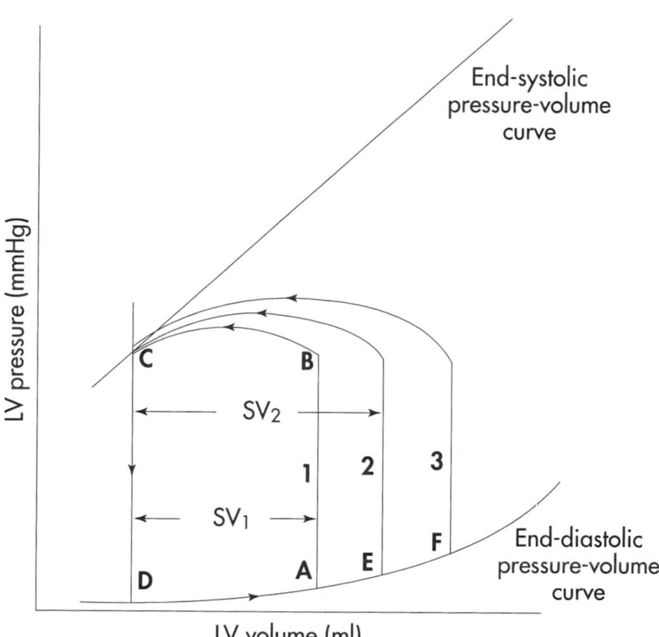

■ **FIGURE 3–15.** Schematic pressure–volume loops demonstrating the effect of increasing preload on stroke volume (SV) during normal contraction when afterload and contractility are held constant. LV, left ventricular. (From Braunwald E, Ross J, Sonnenblick EH: *Mechanisms of contraction of the normal and failing heart.* 2nd ed. Boston, 1976, Little, Brown.)

In each of these loops, a line is described known as the end-systolic pressure–volume curve. End-systolic volume (ESV) is linearly related to end-systolic ventricular pressure (Suga and Sagawa, 1974; Little et al., 1985). The slope of the end-systolic pressure–volume curve varies as a function of contractility but is independent of loading parameters. This relationship is not true when regional myocardial wall abnormalities exist. However, this curve has become an important basis for the noninvasive measurement of contractility in the intact heart. Borow and Grossman (1984) used M-mode echocardiography, noninvasive systemic arterial BP, and indirect carotid pulse recordings to study the changes in contractility in examining the end-systolic pressure–volume relationship. Figure 3–18 shows the effects of changing contractility where loop 1 normal represents normal contractility, loop 2 describes increased contractility, and loop 3 describes a condition in which contractility is decreased. A larger EDV in this depressed contractility state does not result in an increased SV, as would be expected in the normal heart. SV is restored with decreased contractility by lowering afterload (loop 5) or increasing preload (loop 4) even more than the preload increase described in loop 3.

■ EFFECT OF HEART RATE ON CARDIAC PERFORMANCE

Heart rate (HR) plays a major role in determining cardiac function for various reasons. HR affects preload by determining the length of time for ventricular filling. Because coronary and therefore myocardial blood supply occurs during diastole, HR directly affects subendocardial blood flow. If subendocardial flow

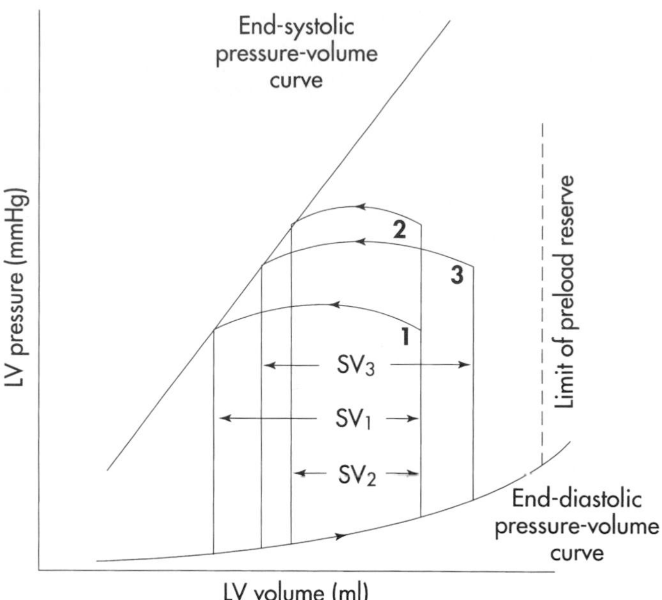

■ **FIGURE 3–17.** Response of the normal heart to an increase in afterload during function in the physiologic range of the pressure–volume relation (see text for full description). LV, left ventricular; SV, stroke volume. (From Strobeck JE and Sonnenblick EH: Myocardial contractile properties and ventricular performance. In Fozzard HA, et al., editors: *The heart and cardiovascular system.* New York, 1986, Raven Press.)

is compromised with shorter diastolic filling, ischemia may result. A downward spiral ensues because the ischemic, less-compliant heart resists optimal ventricular filling and preload decreases. Increased HR is critical during exercise to increase CO and meet increased metabolic needs. HR changes as a result of ongoing

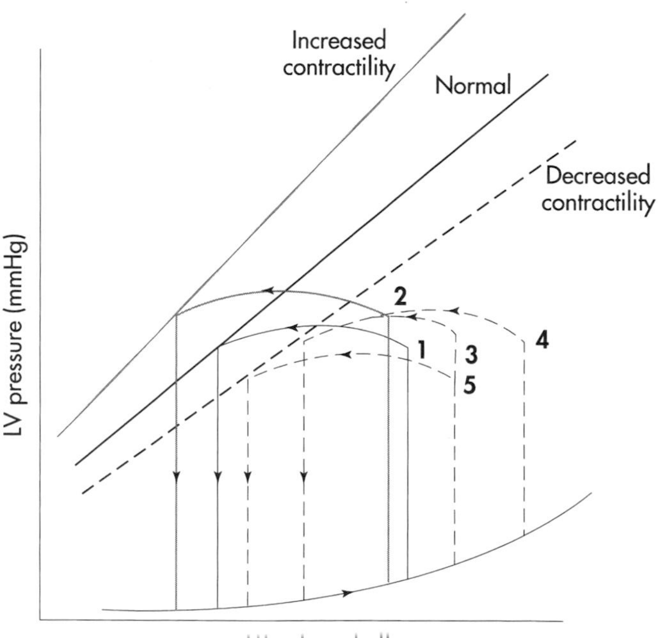

■ **FIGURE 3–18.** Effect of changing contractility on the left ventricular (LV) pressure–volume relation (see text for full description). (From Braunwald E, Ross J, Sonnenblick EH: *Mechanisms of contraction of the normal and failing heart.* 2nd ed. Boston, 1976, Little, Brown.)

multifactorial development; the effect of HR on cardiac function is discussed further in this context.

■ DEVELOPMENTAL ASPECTS OF MYOCARDIAL FUNCTION

Studies in fetal and neonatal lambs, as well as studies of isolated fetal and neonatal muscle fibers, have helped to define various maturational aspects related to cardiac function. The fetus is immature in the structure, function, and innervation of the heart. When the length–tension relationship is examined in the fetal and adult myocardium, the following findings have been described: (1) resting tension is higher in the fetus than in adult sheep and (2) the extent and velocity of shortening and developed tension differ between fetuses and adults (Figs 3–19 and 3–20). The higher percentage of noncontractile protein in fetal myocytes (60% versus 30% in the adult myocardium) (Rychik, 2004) may explain some of these findings. The fetal and newborn ventricle is less compliant, or "stiffer." As a result, the newborn responds poorly to volume loading and shows less ability to augment CO with changes in preload (Fig. 3–21). The increased negative effect of afterload on CO is exaggerated in fetal and newborn hearts. In addition, unlike in the adult, afterload reduction with drugs (such as nitroprusside) does not increase CO (Kuipers et al., 1984; Mirro et al., 1985).

Myocardial cellular replication differs in the fetus compared with that in the adult. Cardiomyocytes contain the contractile elements of the heart. Primitive mesodermal cells differentiate into cardiomyocytes and then receive a signal to exit the cell cycle at approximately the time of birth. It is these early fetal cardiomyocytes that have the potential to divide and increase in number (hyperplasia), in contrast to mature adult cardiomyocytes, which can only grow in size (hypertrophy). For example, the left ventricular myocyte increases in volume 30- to 40-fold during the neonatal to adolescent period (Rychik, 2004).

The fetal myocardium has different relaxation properties than that of the adult. Experimental animal studies in the fetus have demonstrated a difference in the process of rapid removal of calcium from troponin C, the mechanism responsible for myocardial relaxation (Mahoney, 1996). This may be due to diminished sarcoplasmic reticulum function and greater dependence on the sodium-calcium exchanger process to remove cytosolic calcium in the fetus (Artman, 1992). Finally, the energy source for myocardial cell metabolism differs. Long-chain fatty acids are the preferred fuel in adults; in the fetus and neonate, lactate is the primary agent metabolized (Fisher et al., 1981). In the fetus, this is due to a deficiency in the enzyme carnitine palmitoyl transferase-1, responsible for transporting long-chain fatty acids into the mitochondria.

Traditionally, the limitations in myocardial function in the fetus have been thought to be due to the fetal myocardial architecture. Grant and others (1992a, 1992b) and Grant and Walker (1996) proposed an interesting and plausible alternative theory: fetal SV is limited not by intrinsic properties of the fetal myocardium but by ventricular constraint due to extrinsic compression of the fetal heart. At birth, fetal SV doubles at the same time that ventricular constraint by tissues around the fetal heart is dramatically changed. The chest wall, the lungs, and the pericardium create limitations on fetal ventricular preload and are major determinants of fetal cardiac function. Expansion of the lungs and clearance of fetal lung liquid may be the major determinant of an increase in left ventricular preload and an

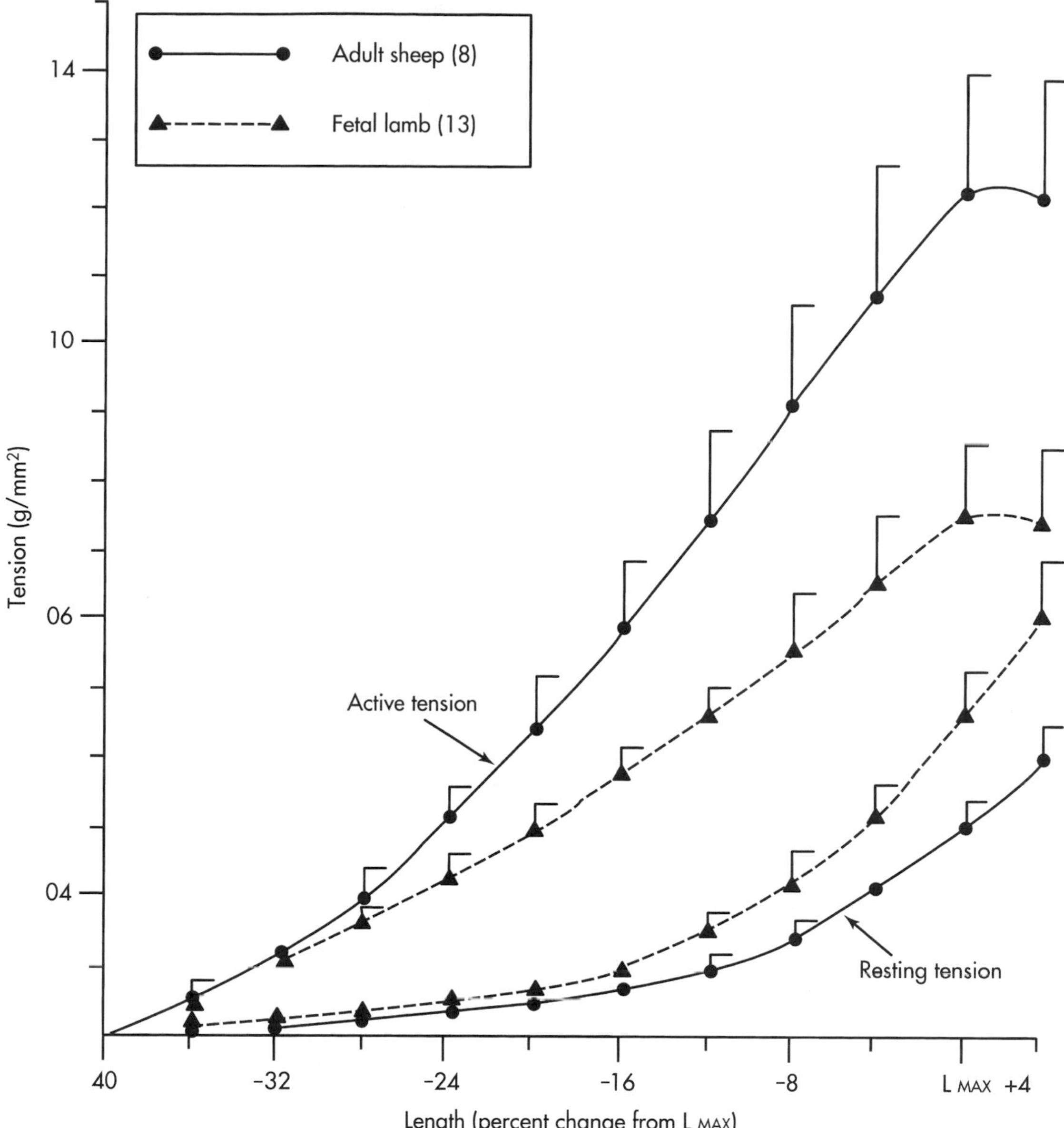

■ **FIGURE 3–19.** Length–tension relationships in fetal lambs and adult sheep demonstrating the lower resting tension and great active tension development in adult sheep. Fetal myocardium has a higher resting tension but less active tension development, indicating less compliance—a "stiffer" ventricle than in the adult. (From Friedman WF: The intrinsic properties of the developing heart. *Prog Cardiovasc Dis* 15:87, 1972.)

increase in SV seen in the newborn infant. Clinically, this theory is supported by observations in neonatal open chest surgery where closure of the chest wall has an often dramatic impact on cardiac function.

The neonatal heart has been shown experimentally to function with increased myocardial contractility (Geis et al., 1975; Riemenschneider et al., 1981; Rudolph et al., 1981). This may result from a number of factors, including increased β-stimulation after birth and the effects of thyroid hormone both prenatally and postnatally (Breall et al., 1984; Mahdavi et al., 1987) or the release of ventricular constraint as proposed by Grant (1999).

Because the newborn heart functions at high levels of preload, afterload, contractility, and HR, a resultant marked limitation in cardiac reserve occurs. Sudden and profound depression in CO is not unusual in neonates under certain adverse conditions, such as hypoxia or acidosis, or under the influence of anesthetics. Increased preload or afterload or depressed contractility is poorly tolerated by the newborn.

HR plays an important role in cardiac function. The limited ability of the fetal heart to increase SV results in marked changes in CO with changes in HR. For example, a 10% to 15% increase in CO is observed when HR increases from 160 to 240 beats per minute. Conversely, a 20% to 25% decrease in CO is observed when the HR falls to 120 beats per minute (Rudolph, 1987). The role of HR in regulating cardiac performance remains controversial. A study examining the role of HR (over a range of 130 to 175 beats per minute) and CO in fetuses demonstrated the relationship between cardiac cycle length and SV. As HR increases in fetal lambs, right and left ventricular output increases.

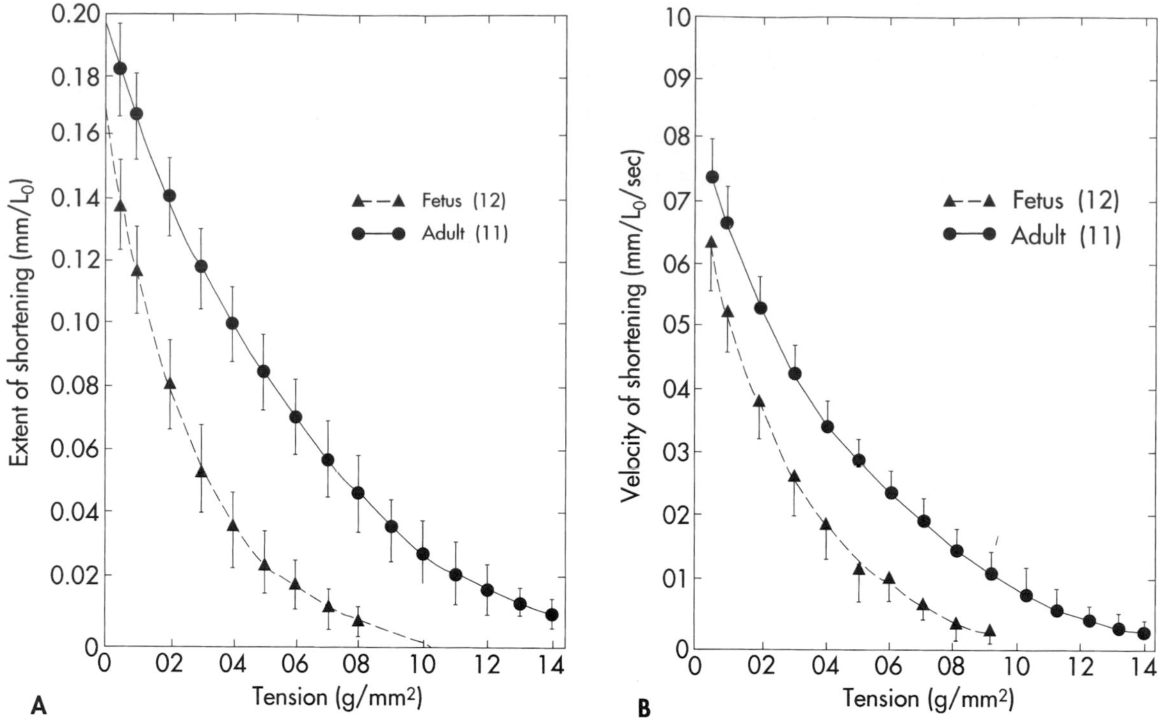

■ **FIGURE 3–20.** Relationships between *(A)* the extent of shortening and *(B)* the velocity of shortening and developed tension in fetal and adult cardiac muscle strips. (From Friedman WF: The intrinsic physiologic properties of the developing heart. *Prog Cardiovasc Dis* 15:87, 1972.)

At slower HRs, prolongation of diastole does not increase ventricular filling to the same degree as observed in the mature heart. This phenomenon is a reflection of the stiffness and ventricular interdependence of both ventricles in the fetus. In addition, observed decreases in SVs with increasing heart rate did not reveal changes in ventricular output (Fig. 3–22) (Kenny et al., 1987).

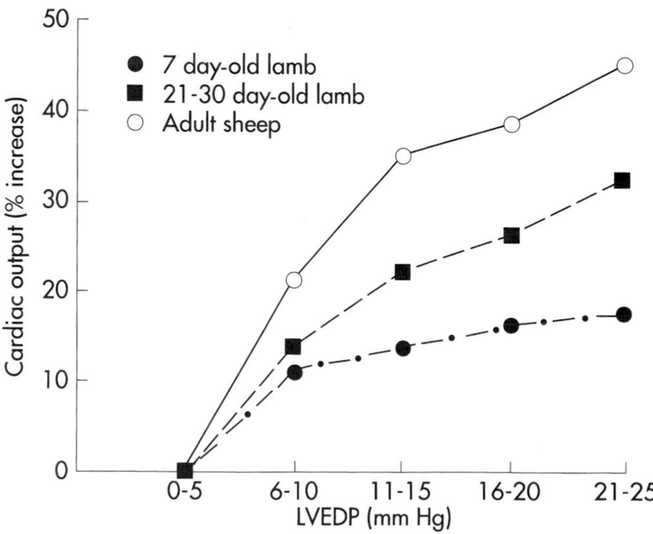

■ **FIGURE 3–21.** Response to volume loading in newborn lambs and adult sheep. At constant heart rate, limited cardiac reserve is demonstrated in the youngest lambs by a reduced ability to augment cardiac output at any filling pressure compared with the adult or older lambs. LVEDP, left ventricular end-diastolic pressure. (From Friedman WF, George BL: Treatment of congestive heart failure by altering loading conditions of the heart. *J Pediatr* 106:697, 1985.)

As fetal HR increases, the maximum diastolic cavity size diminishes but without any significant change in systolic function measured as left ventricular area shortening (Fig. 3–23). This figure shows a reduction in maximum diastolic cavity size with increasing HR but little or no change in systolic contractile function (as measured with fractional change in ventricular area). It appears that the Frank-Starling mechanism remains the major regulator of CO in the fetus. Clearly, the newborn is more sensitive to changes in HR, but this is probably because of the "stiffness," or decreased compliance, of the newborn myocardium. When sequential atrioventricular pacing is performed in newborn lambs and 1-month-old lambs, the contribution of atrial pacing is not as great as in the newborn, possibly because the atria are limited in the amount ejected into the stiffer newborn ventricle (Kaufman and Rudolph, 1988).

At birth and over the ensuing weeks and months of infant life, the cardiovascular system shows evidence of increasing functional reserves. With birth, left ventricular output increases as a result of increases in venous return and HR, as well as a result of increases in inotropic stimulation, removal of extracardiac restraints, and improvement of ventricular interaction. In the neonate, CO (indexed for body weight) falls gradually, dP/dt_{max} returns to fetal levels, and extrasystolic potentiation and the inotropic response to β-adrenergic receptor stimulation increase (Klopfenstein and Rudolph, 1978; Anderson et al., 1984). All of these changes result in an increase in functional reserve. Because of these reserves, the heart is better able to respond to stress. These concepts apply to the normal newborn. When congenital heart disease is present, dramatic changes in preload, afterload, and contractility may significantly impair cardiac performance and must be carefully considered.

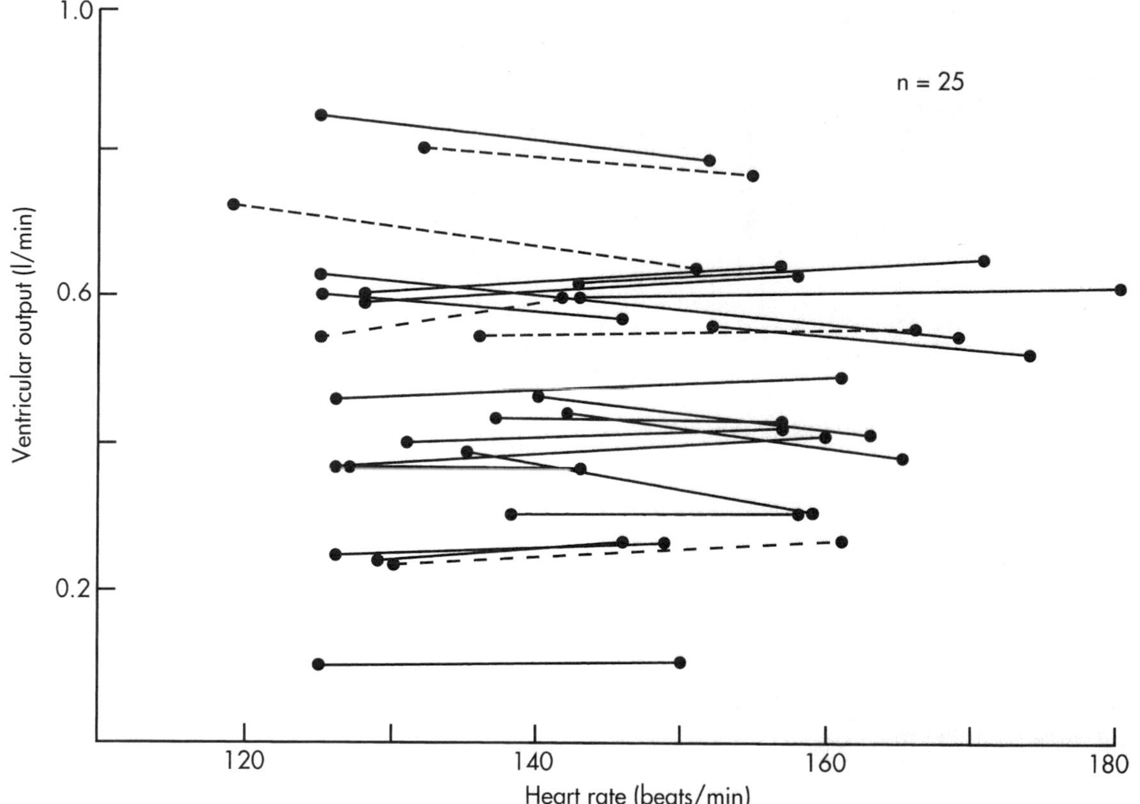

■ **FIGURE 3–22.** The relationship between right ventricular output (interrupted lines) and left ventricular output (solid lines) with varying heart rate in 25 human fetuses. (From Kenny J, et al.: Effects of heart rate on ventricular size, stroke volume and output in the normal human fetus: A prospective Doppler echocardiographic study. *Circulation* 76:52, 1987.)

DEVELOPMENTAL ELECTROPHYSIOLOGY

The electrophysiologic circuits of the fetus and neonate have been studied in chick and rat heart embryos, with limited data from human tissue. Resting membrane potential increases as development proceeds. Potassium permeability increases with development. In the neonatal heart, resting membrane potentials are higher compared with that in adults. Duration of the action potential increases during postnatal development, and atrioventricular conduction is more rapid in the newborn. Tissue refractory periods are significantly shorter in newborns and infants (Rosen et al., 1981). These laboratory findings support the ongoing maturation of sarcolemmal ionic channels, alterations in cell coupling, and structural changes in cell grouping. Clinically, both the neonate and infant can conduct rapid impulses from the atrium to the ventricle. Because of the shorter refractory periods, responses of the premature can be conducted at shorter coupling intervals (Box 3–1).

Cell membranes and cell metabolism develop and mature simultaneously with autonomic innervation of the heart. Parasympathetic innervation is noted very early in development. Sympathetic innervation may begin in the area of the sinoatrial node and proceed to the ventricular myocardium (Pappano, 1972; Pappano and Loeffelholz, 1974) but is definitely not complete at birth. Cardiac catecholamine levels are significantly less in the neonatal heart compared with the adult. Both α- and β-adrenergic receptors have been identified in cardiac myocytes. However, these receptors may respond quite differently with incomplete innervation.

Since the 1990s, it has become clear that cardiac development is complex and involves the induction of genes at certain times in development—an induction process that influences cardiac chamber formation, conduction path development, and function. The end result is that the early peristaltic tubular heart develops into a synchronously contracting four-chambered heart with predictable conduction paths (Moorman and Christoffels, 2003).

INTERACTION OF THE NERVOUS SYSTEM AND THE HEART

The nervous system plays a critical role in regulating cardiac function by ensuring adequate perfusion to all organ systems under various physiologic conditions. Fine-tuning of cardiac function is accomplished by the autonomic nervous system. A highly integrated and complex interaction occurs between the cardiovascular system, nervous system, and cardiovascular reflex arcs on cardiac function. Baroreceptor and chemoreceptor sensitivity may be protective reflexes in the fetus and are almost completely mature at birth. Arterial baroreceptors play a critical role in cardiovascular regulation. Baroreceptors are located in the aortic arch, at the carotid bifurcation, and send afferents to the vasomotor center in the medulla. In fetal lambs, denervation of these baroreceptors (Yardley, 1979) results in marked variability in arterial BP. Peripheral chemoreceptors are found in the aortic arch, carotid bodies, and main pulmonary artery. Dawes and Mott (1962) suggested that aortic chemoreceptors are important

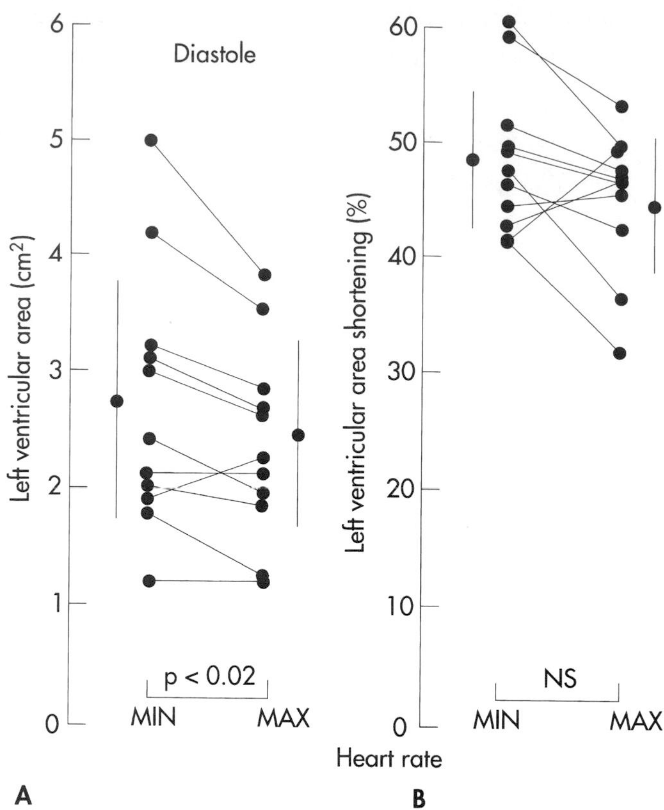

■ **FIGURE 3–23.** *(A)* Changes in left ventricular diastolic area with change in heart rate in 11 human fetuses. *(B)* Changes in the left ventricular area shortening with heart rate in the same 11 fetuses. (From Kenny J, et al.: Effects of heart rate on ventricular size, stroke volume and output in the normal human fetus: A prospective Doppler echocardiographic study. *Circulation* 76:52, 1987.)

for cardiovascular control, whereas carotid chemoreceptors regulate respiratory parameters. Peripheral autonomic regulation is important in cardiovascular homeostasis. Rudolph and Heymann (1973) suggested that basal sympathetic tone is present during early gestation and increases at birth, as evidenced clinically by gradually increasing arterial BP. In addition to direct innervation, circulating catecholamines play a role in cardiovascular control. These circulating catecholamines are derived from adrenal tissue and para-aortic chromaffin tissue and may exert effects directly even before the complete maturation of innervation.

Autonomic control of cardiovascular function is complex, differing under basal resting conditions compared with stressful stimulation. HR remains constant during most of fetal life and then decreases during the first 2 months of neonatal life. During this period, significant changes are occurring in sympathetic and parasympathetic innervation. Neither fetal vagotomy nor treatment with atropine or chemical sympathectomy alters fetal HR or BP (Woods et al., 1977; Assali et al., 1978; Zugaib et al., 1980; Tabsh et al., 1982). Immature autonomic neuronal or receptor development may contribute to differences described and verified by laboratory studies in fetuses and neonates. A lower level of neurotransmitters in fetal hearts compared with older hearts suggests a lack of mature innervation. In contrast, fetuses administered norepinephrine and isoproterenol show a hypersensitivity in comparison with adult responses, supporting the concept that the receptors are fully functional (Geis et al., 1975).

Baroreceptor reflexes are present and operative in early fetal life, but qualitative and quantitative differences exist in the neonate and adult. For example, norepinephrine infusions increase both HR and BP in the fetal lamb, whereas neonate and adult animals respond with bradycardia as BP is increased. The injection of veratridine into the RA of a mature fetus or neonate elicits the Bezold-Jarisch reflex, resulting in hypotension and bradycardia, just as in the adult. However, the younger fetus responds with tachycardia and hypertension (blocked by α- and β-blockade), suggesting sympathetic innervation is functional (Vappavouri et al., 1973; Assali et al., 1978).

Neonatal Cardiovascular Reflex Development

At birth, dramatic circulatory changes occur, accompanied by parasympathetic activity that regulates HR and pulmonary vascular reactivity, as well as a profound activation of the neurohumoral sympathoadrenal axis. Both norepinephrine and epinephrine are dramatically increased during vaginal delivery and directly affect HR, SVR, and BP. Infants delivered via cesarean section or prematurely show a diminished neurohumoral response, whereas infants stressed by hypoxia, acidosis, or both at birth show an exaggerated response (Faxelius et al., 1984). Diminished ventricular compliance with a simultaneous opening of vascular beds leads to a fall in circulating fluid volume and SVR. These observations may explain the normal decrease in BP seen soon after birth (Romero and Friedman, 1979). Many studies have examined the role of HR and its variability during maturation. The results of many studies suggest that HR develops as a function of postnatal age, whereas HR variability is a reflection of conceptional age. Around 6 months of age, differences between full-term and preterm infants with respect to HR variability and absolute HR disappear. HR declines gradually until adult levels are reached during adolescence (Church et al., 1967; Katona and Egbert, 1978; Katona et al., 1980; Mazza et al., 1980).

Childhood Cardiovascular Reflex Development

Studies examining the role of autonomic control are more limited in older children, but observed changes clearly vary with respect to age, gender, and race. Increased parasympathetic tone during rapid eye movement (REM) sleep has been observed in children with sleep dysrhythmias and sleep apnea (Guilleminault et al., 1981; Miller, 1982; McNicholas et al., 1983; Thach, 1985). Increased vagal tone has been described as a cause of syncope during exercise in some children. The values in older children and adolescents probably approach adult levels with respect to cardiovascular responses to exercise and Valsalva maneuver, although studies are definitely limited. The potent interaction between central respiratory and cardiovascular reflexes is an area of ongoing research in both children and adults.

Birth results in dramatic changes in the cardiovascular system that can be best summarized as an increase in left ventricular output, secondary to increases in venous return and HR, increases in inotropic stimuli, removal of extracardiac restraints, and improvement in ventricular interaction. During the neonatal period, CO (indexed for body weight) falls gradually, dP/dt_{max} returns to fetal levels, and postextrasystolic potentiation and the inotropic response to β-adrenergic receptor stimulation increase (Klopfenstein and Rudolph, 1978; Anderson et al., 1984). The end result is that the infant's heart is acquiring greater functional reserves. Ironically, it is this reserve that also permits many patients with congenital heart defects to survive the neonatal period.

Box 3–1 Diseases or Conditions Associated With Rhythm Disturbances

Sinus Tachycardia (Persistent)

Anemia
Infection
Hypoxia, acute
Hypotension, shock
Hyperthyroidism
Acute intermittent porphyria
Pheochromocytoma

Sinus Bradycardia (Persistent)

Hepatitis (jaundice)
Typhoid fever
Increased intracranial pressure
Cerebral hypoxia
Hypothyroidism
Drugs (morphine sulfate, digoxin, propranolol)
Hypothermia
Anorexia nervosa

Atrial Tachycardia

Infection
Trauma
Neoplasm
Cardiac catheterization
Anesthesia, surgery
Emotional stress
Thalassemia major
Digoxin toxicity

Atrial Flutter

Congenital thyrotoxicosis
Thalassemia major
Imipramine

Atrial Fibrillation

Hypokalemia
Thyrotoxicosis
Pseudoephedrine
Drugs
Tricyclic antidepressants

Ventricular Tachycardia

Anesthesia
Cardiac catheterization and surgery
Electrolyte imbalance
Cardiac neoplasm (primary or metastatic)
Subarachnoid hemorrhage
Drugs
Cardioauditory syndrome
Psychogenic
Tricyclic antidepressants

First-Degree Atrioventricular (AV) Block

Rheumatic fever
Diphtheria
Trichinosis
Familial

Second-Degree AV Block

Infection
Hypocalcemia
Hyperkalemia
Drugs and toxins
Familial
Brain abscess

Third-Degree AV Block

Infection
Diphtheria
Collagen disease
Hyperkalemia
Digitalis
Tricyclic antidepressants
Rheumatic fever

Congenital Arrhythmias

Congenital Malformation	*Arrhythmia*
Ventricular inversion with transposition of great arteries AV canal Secundum atrial septal defect Ebstein's anomaly Intrauterine cytomegalovirus infection	First-, second-, and third-degree AV block Preexcitation syndrome with supraventricular tachycardia, first-degree heart block Sinoatrial and AV nodal damage

Acquired Postoperative Arrhythmias

Intra-atrial repair of transposition of great arteries	Sick sinus syndrome, complete heart block, premature ventricular contractions, ventricular tachycardia and fibrillation, atrial flutter and fibrillation
Secundum atrial septal defect	Atrial flutter or fibrillation, first- and second-degree heart block, complete heart block

EFFECTS OF CONGENITAL HEART DISEASE ON CARDIOPULMONARY DEVELOPMENT

It is clear that cardiac and pulmonary development is intricately related in the normal fetus and neonate. In the presence of a congenital heart defect, this relationship has even more profound interactions. Despite the fact that pulmonary blood flow is minimal in the fetus, the presence of a congenital heart defect, which alters pulmonary hemodynamics, has important effects. For example, the presence of pulmonary atresia early in gestation (before the ninth week) results in the persistence of connections with primitive intersegmental arteries, which appear at birth as direct branches from the descending thoracic aorta. These abnormal vessels may be the only source of pulmonary blood flow—acting as mini-systemic artery-to-pulmonary artery collateral shunts in the neonatal period. If pulmonary stenosis or atresia occurs later in gestation, these bronchopulmonary collaterals are still noted. However, the pulmonary arteries are also hypoplastic and have a decrease in elastin in the media. This lack of elastin may explain the poor dilatation seen in pulmonary arteries even after a surgical shunt is placed in patients with pulmonary atresia (Rabinovitch et al., 1981; Rosenberg et al., 1987).

In patients with large left-to-right shunts, an increase in medial wall thickness and abnormal extension of muscle into peripheral pulmonary arteries is found. These patients may still exhibit evidence of severe pulmonary hypertension after surgical repair, because this anatomic substrate in the pulmonary vascular bed may take time to resolve postoperatively (Haworth and Reid, 1977).

The effects of increased volume and pressure—as seen in a large left-to-right shunt such as a ventricular septal defect—may have a toxic effect on the endothelial cell integrity in the pulmonary bed. Mechanical as well as humoral influences may cause a persistence of fetal muscularization throughout the pulmonary vascular bed, and if the shunt is not closed, the process results in irreversible pulmonary vascular obstructive disease.

Any patient who has undergone repair of a congenital heart defect may have residua of this abnormal physiology in the pulmonary vascular bed as well as within the cardiovascular system. Understanding of the dynamic nature of cardiopulmonary physiology in the fetus and neonate with congenital heart disease has resulted in a more aggressive attempt at early infant repair of defects so that the pulmonary vascular bed is spared the possibility of permanent changes. The fetal environment may indeed have long-lasting effects on adult cardiovascular health and disease and that, to be effective, cardiovascular disease prevention begins during the period of fetal development.

ASSESSMENT OF THE CARDIOVASCULAR SYSTEM

When a patient presents for anesthetic evaluation and management, the anesthesiologist must know about age-related differences in history, physical examination findings, routine laboratory results, and more sophisticated evaluations of cardiac function, such as electrocardiography, echocardiography, and cardiac catheterization. Age-related differences are not surprising in view of developmental cardiovascular physiology and are only briefly described. This discussion focuses on evaluation of the healthy child; evaluation of the child with congenital heart disease is discussed in greater detail in Chapter 17, Anesthesia for Cardiovascular Surgery. Routine cardiac catheterization is reviewed.

HISTORY AND PHYSICAL EXAMINATION

The well-being of a child is definitely reflected in his or her ability to "thrive," which includes the attainment of weight and height expectations during development. Obviously children vary in these parameters, and weight and height curves reflect the acceptable percentiles for children at different ages. In addition, acute and chronic illnesses may differentially affect these important parameters. Growth charts should be reviewed when obtaining a history in a young child. Weight may be the first parameter to show the negative effects of illness, followed by height and then head circumference measurements. In an adult, cardiac symptoms are often graded using established guidelines, such as those of the New York Heart Association. These guidelines often do not apply to pediatric patients. In the neonate and young infant, feeding difficulties, especially fatigue and tachypnea, are important symptoms of cardiac failure. The ability to maintain peer or sibling exercise levels is a less formal but helpful piece of historical information in children.

The healthy newborn may have a respiratory rate of 50 breaths per minute and a systolic BP of 55 mm Hg. These physical findings are obviously abnormal in a 3-year-old child. Tables 3–1 and 3–2 and Figures 3–24 and 3–25 outline normal values for respiratory rate, HR, and BP in healthy children of various ages. Table 3–3 defines normal values for more invasive evaluations of cardiac function, including hemodynamic and saturation data. Figure 3–26 summarizes the progression of changes in HR, CO, and SV over childhood.

The normal electrocardiogram and chest radiograph reflect changes in physiology as well as anatomic changes in chamber size and position. The normal neonatal chest radiograph and electrocardiogram would be read as abnormal in a teenager. The large thymic shadow on the neonatal chest radiograph may be misinterpreted as cardiomegaly. HR increases during the first 2 months of life and then decreases gradually over the ensuing years of early childhood. The progression from RV dominance at birth to LV dominance is reflected in the presence of increased right ventricular forces on the neonatal electrocardiogram. Detailed age-related electrocardiographic values are available for review to ensure proper electrocardiogram interpretation.

SPECIAL EVALUATION OF THE CARDIOVASCULAR SYSTEM

Cardiac Catheterization

Despite the dramatic contribution of echocardiography, especially two-dimensional echocardiography, in the diagnosis of congenital heart disease, cardiac catheterization laboratories are still active areas of investigation. In addition to diagnostic cardiac catheterization and angiocardiography, the catheterization laboratory is the site of major interventional procedures once delegated to the operating room, including dilatation of valvar stenosis, vascular stenoses, closure of patent ductus arteriosus, investigational closure of atrial and ventricular septal defects, complex electrophysiologic studies, ablation of abnormal foci of arrhythmias, and coil closure of collateral blood vessels. These complex procedures may be associated with hemodynamic instability, and the involvement of pediatric anesthesiologists in the sedation, monitoring, and, often, administration of general anesthesia has become increasingly important in the care of these patients.

TABLE 3–1. Normal values for respiratory rates in children

Age	Respiratory Rate (min)
Birth to 6 wk	45 to 60
6 wk to 2 yr	40
2 to 6 yr	30
6 to 10 yr	25
>10 yr	20

■ **TABLE 3–2.** Acceptable heart rates in children (beats/min)*

	Awake	Asleep	Exercise/Fever
Newborn	100 to 180	80 to 160	<220
1 wk to 3 mo	100 to 220	80 to 200	<220
3 mo to 2 yr	80 to 150	70 to 120	<200
2 to 10 yr	70 to 110	60 to 90	<200
>10 yr	55 to 90	50 to 90	<200

*From Adams FH, Emmanoulides GC, editors: *Moss' heart disease in infants, children, and adolescents*, 3rd ed. Baltimore, 1983, Williams & Wilkins.

Cardiac catheterization remains an important diagnostic tool in delineating anatomy and hemodynamics, especially preoperatively. Cardiac catheterization carries risk, especially in sick neonates and infants. Major complications occur in about 30% of high-risk infants, 14% of medium-risk infants, and 4% of low-risk infants (Cohn et al., 1985). In an 8-year survey of 6,101 children, the overall mortality rate within 48 hours of catheterization was 1.7%, ranging from 10.2% in the first week of life to 0.5% in patients older than 1 year. Approximately 1% of all interventional procedures result in death (Lock et al., 1992). Complications include arterial and venous complications, arrhythmias, myocardial perforation, hypoxia, acidosis, apnea, and air emboli. Despite the fact that the cardiac catheterization laboratory is not only the site for diagnosis but also the site for interventional treatment in younger and more critically ill infants, complication rates have improved.

Cassidy and others (1992) prospectively examined cardiac catheterization complications in a 3-year period (January 1986 through October 1988) and compared them with complications in the same laboratory in 1974. In their study, 1,037 catheterizations (885 diagnostic and 152 diagnostic/interventional procedures) were performed in 888 patients (age range, 1 day to 27 years; median age, 15.6 months). There were 15 major complications (1.4%), 70 minor complications (6.8%), and 30 incidents (2.9%). Two patients died as a result of the procedure, and two patients died as a result of pericatheterization clinical deterioration caused by the cardiac abnormality. The great majority of complications were successfully treated or were self-limited, and the patients had no residua. Of patients with 13 nonfatal major complications and 70 minor complications, residua were evident in 7 patients, and 3 without evident residua had the potential for sequelae (0.7% and 0.3% of catheterizations). A comparison of the diagnostic and balloon atrial septostomy cases in the present study with similar cases in the 1974 study shows that the incidence of major complications has decreased from 2.9% to 0.9%, minor complications and incidents have decreased from 11.7% to 7.9%, and pericatheterization deaths not attributable to catheterization have decreased from 2.8% to 0.2%.

Vitiello and others (1998) studied complications in 4,952 consecutive patients (age range, 1 day to 20 years; median age, 2.9 years) at The Hospital for Sick Children in Toronto. One or more complication occurred in 8.8% of the study patients (major complication in 102 patients and minor complication in 458 patients). Vascular complications were the most common adverse event (3.8% of procedures), and arrhythmic complications (n = 24) were the most common major complication. Death occurred in seven cases (0.14%) as a direct complication of the procedure and was more common in infants (n = 5). Medical management (including an increasing involvement of anesthesiology staff in monitoring, sedation, and anesthetic management), better patient selection, and stabilization before

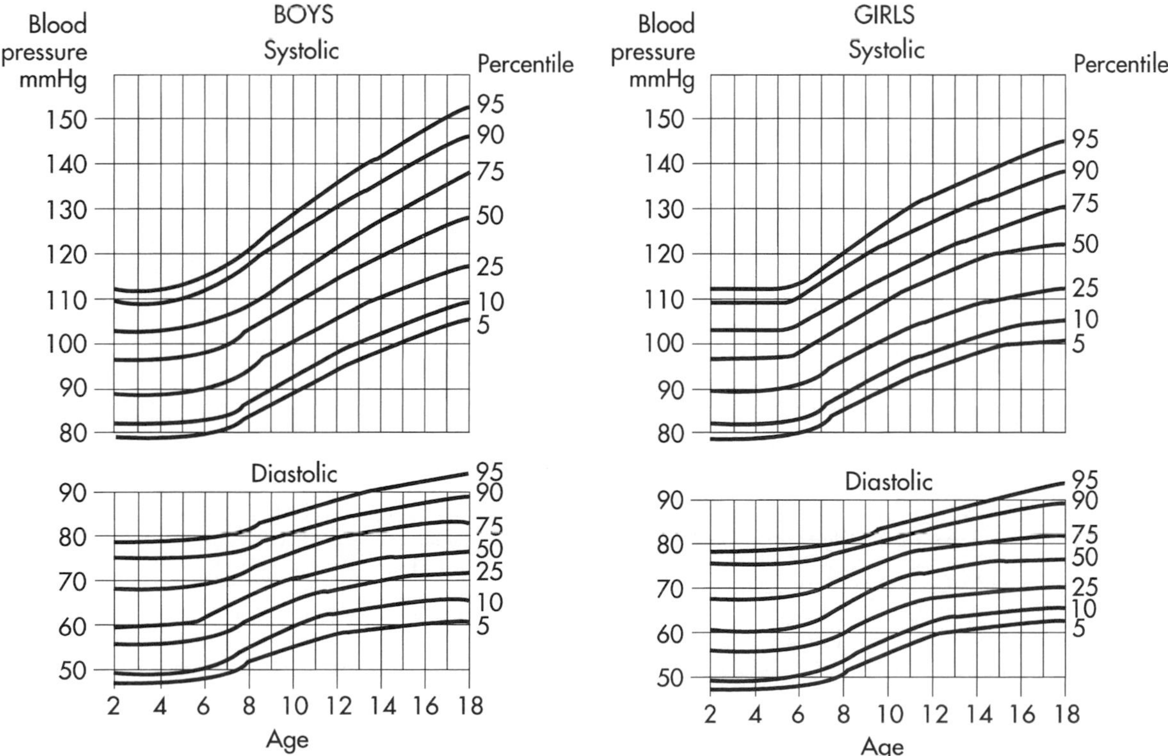

■ **FIGURE 3–24.** Normal values of resting blood pressure in boys and girls aged 2 to 18 years. (From Blumenthal S, et al.: *Pediatrics* 59:797, 1977.)

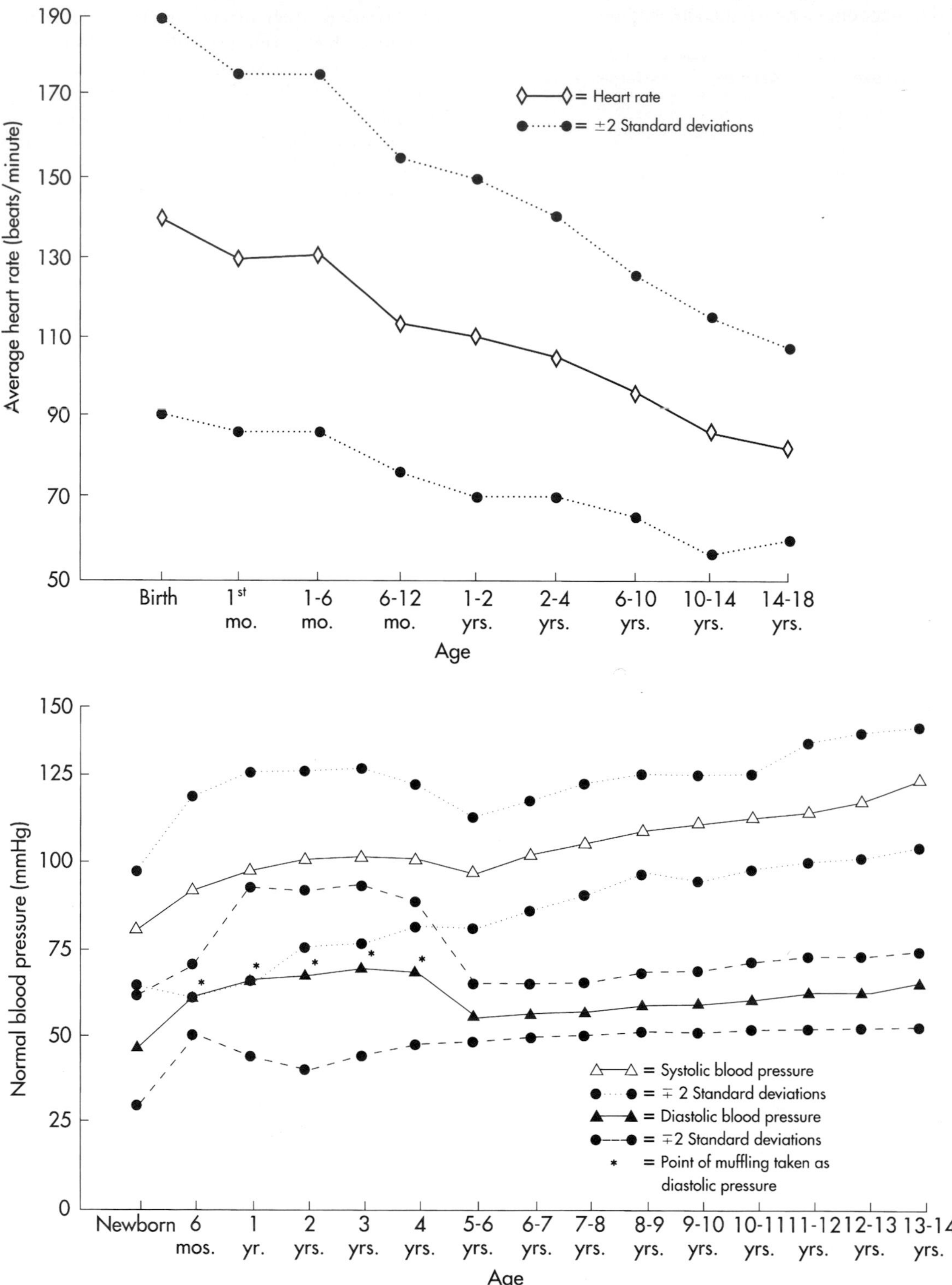

■ **FIGURE 3–25.** Variations in average heart rate and blood pressure with age. (From Moore RA: Anesthesia considerations for patients undergoing palliative or reoperative operations for congenital heart disease. In Swedlow DB, Russell RC, editors: *Cardiovascular problems in pediatric critical care.* New York, 1986, Churchill Livingstone.)

catheterization have all contributed to decreased complication rates in centers nationally.

Hemodynamic Evaluation

Cardiac catheterization includes the measurement of intracardiac pressures and oxygen saturation, gradients across valves, pulmonary and systemic blood flow, CO, quantity and direction of shunt flow, and resistance. In addition, the changes in these measurements are often assessed after the administration of drugs, oxygen, or both. Normal hemodynamic data in children beyond the neonatal period are given (Table 3–4); these data are obviously altered by structural or acquired heart disease.

■ TABLE 3–3. Normal values for invasive evaluations of cardiac function*

Location	Infants and Children	Newborns
Right atrium	a = 5 to 8 v = 2 to 6 M = 2 to 6	M = 0 to 4
Right ventricle	15 to 25/2 to 5	35 to 80/1 to 5
Pulmonary artery	15 to 25/8 to 12 M = 10 to 16	35 to 80/20 to 50 M = 25 to 60
Pulmonary wedge	a = 6 to 12 v = 8 to 15 M = 5 to 12	
Left atrium	a = 6 to 12 v = 8 to 15 M = 5 to 10	M = 3 to 6
Left ventricle	80 to 130/5 to 10	
Systemic artery	90 to 130/60 to 80 M = 70 to 95	65 to 80/45 to 60 M = 60 to 65

*Data from Rudolph AM: *Congenital disease of the heart*, Chicago, 1974, Year Book Medical Publishers. (a = a wave, v = v wave, M = mean.)

■ TABLE 3–4. Normal cardiovascular values beyond the neonatal and infancy period*

Location	Average	Range
Mean right atrial pressure (central venous pressure)	3	1 to 5 mm Hg
Right ventricular pressure		
Systolic	25	17 to 32 mm Hg
Diastolic	5	1 to 7 mm Hg
Pulmonary arterial pressure		
Systolic	25	9 to 19 mm Hg
Diastolic	10	17 to 32 mm Hg
Mean	15	4 to 13 mm Hg
Mean pulmonary artery wedge pressure	9	6 to 12 mm Hg
Mean left atrial pressure	8	2 to 12 mm Hg
Cardiac index	3.5	2.5 to 4.2 L/min per m^2
Stroke volume index	45 mL/m^2	
Oxygen consumption	140	110 to 150 L/min per m^2
Vascular resistance		
Pulmonary		1 to 3 hybrid units/m^2 80 to 240 dynes·s·cm^{-5}·m^{-2}
Systemic		10 to 20 hybrid units/m^2 800 to 1600 dynes·s·cm^{-5}·m^{-2}

*Data from Rudolph AM: *Congenital disease of the heart*, Chicago, 1974, Year Book Medical Publishers.

The difference in pressure between two sites in the cardiac system is called a *gradient* and can be measured as a mean gradient, a peak gradient, or an instantaneous gradient. Typically a gradient is measured during withdrawal of the pressure catheter across two locations. With severe stenosis, a minimal gradient may be described because flow is severely compromised. In addition to assessing a gradient, some measurement of flow must be made.

Oxygen Content and Saturation. *Oxygen saturation* is the percent of hemoglobin present as oxyhemoglobin; it is measured directly with oximetry. *Oxygen capacity* is the maximal amount of oxygen that can be bound to hemoglobin. This value is calculated by multiplying the patient's hemoglobin by 1.34 and is expressed in milliliters per 100 milliliters. *Oxygen content* is the total amount of oxygen present in blood and includes oxygen bound to oxyhemoglobin as well as oxygen dissolved in the plasma. Oxygen content is the product of the oxygen saturation value multiplied by 1.34 multiplied by 10, where 1.34 is the amount of O_2 that 1 g of hemoglobin carries when fully saturated. The number 10 converts 100 mL to liters. Dissolved oxygen is usually ignored because it is so small. However, when PO_2 is high, dissolved oxygen may be high and must be considered. Dissolved oxygen is equal to $PaO_2 \times 0.003$ mL/100 mL. Oxygen content and oxygen consumption ($\dot{V}O_2$) must be known to calculate systemic and pulmonary blood flow.

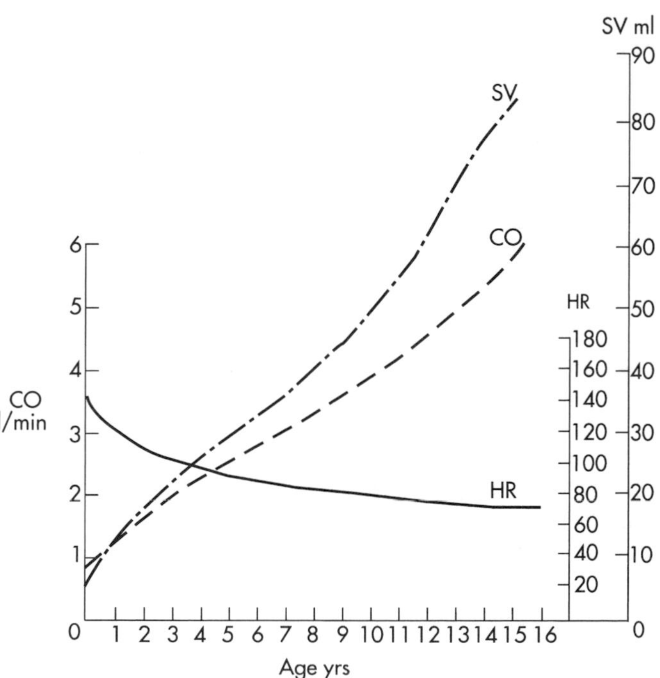

■ FIGURE 3–26. Changes in cardiac output *(CO)*, stroke volume *(SV)*, and heart rate *(HR)* with age. (From Rudolph AM, editor: *Congenital diseases of the heart*. Chicago, 1974, Year Book Medical.)

Pulmonary blood flow

$$\dot{Q}_P = \frac{\dot{V}O_2[\text{mL/min}]}{P\dot{V}O_2\ \text{content} - PaO_2\ \text{content}}$$

Systemic blood flow

$$\dot{Q}_S = \frac{\dot{V}O_2[\text{mL/min}]}{SaO_2\ \text{content} - M\dot{V}O_2\ \text{content}}$$

where $P\dot{V}O_2$ is the oxygen content in the pulmonary vein, PaO_2 is the oxygen content in the pulmonary artery, SaO_2 is the oxygen content in a systemic artery or aorta, and $M\dot{V}O_2$ is the oxygen content in a mixed venous sample.

The mixed venous oxygen content should be the same in the RA as in the pulmonary artery if no shunts are present. However, venous blood is poorly mixed in the RA where streaming and large variations in oxygen content are normally seen, as in coronary sinus return. Mixing on the left side of the heart is much more uniform. Saturation data become important in the detection and quantification of shunt flow.

Shunts. Shunts can be diagnosed with various techniques: angiocardiography, echocardiography, dye indicators such as radionucleotides and indocyanine green dye, and, more commonly, oxygen saturation data. Shunts can be left-to-right, right-to-left, or bidirectional. Using saturation data, quantity of shunt flow can be calculated.

Left-to-right shunts. When blood from the left side of the heart is shunted to the right side, pulmonary blood flow is increased and the saturation of mixed venous blood is increased by the presence of fully oxygenated left-sided blood. A series of samples is drawn in quick succession from each chamber of the right heart, including superior and inferior vena cava blood. An increase in blood saturation or "step-up" beyond a normally accepted variation indicates a left-to-right shunt. For example, a mid–right atrial saturation should be no higher than superior vena cava blood by 7% to 9%. Saturation step-up of 9% indicates a shunt at the atrial level. Because of streaming and poor mixing in the RA, calculation of shunt flow in shunts at the atrial level may be less accurate than at other levels. A step-up of greater than 6% between the RV and the pulmonary artery suggests a ventricular septal defect.

Right-to-left shunts. When desaturated right-sided blood is shunted into the left side of the heart, decreased saturation is observed, called a "step-down." Because left-sided saturations should be fully saturated except in the presence of pulmonary disease, a right-to-left shunt can be suspected whenever desaturation is seen in the left-sided saturation data. A decrease in saturation of more than 2% to 3% strongly suggests a right-to-left shunt.

Shunt magnitude. In addition to diagnosing the presence and direction of a shunt, the magnitude of the shunt must be determined. A left-to-right shunt increases the amount of pulmonary blood flow while decreasing the systemic blood flow. The quantity of left-to-right shunt can be calculated as follows:

$$\dot{Q}_{L\rightarrow R} = \dot{Q}_P - \dot{Q}_S \quad (3.3)$$

where $\dot{Q}_{L\rightarrow R}$ is left-to-right shunt and $\dot{Q}_P - \dot{Q}_S$ is pulmonary blood flow minus systemic blood flow.

Similarly, right-to-left shunts can be calculated as follows:

$$\dot{Q}_{R\rightarrow L} = \dot{Q}_S - \dot{Q}_P \quad (3.4)$$

In a discussion of shunts, the term $\dot{Q}_P/\dot{Q}_S$ is often used to describe the flow ratio between pulmonary and systemic flow. Combining these equations, shunt flow can be determined without obtaining oxygen consumption data, as follows:

$$\frac{\dot{Q}_P}{\dot{Q}_S} = \frac{\text{oxygen consumption}/\text{Spv}O_2 - \text{Spa}O_2}{\text{oxygen consumption}/\text{Sa}O_2 - S_vO_2}$$

$$\frac{\dot{Q}_P}{\dot{Q}_S} = \frac{\text{Sa}O_2 - S_vO_2}{\text{Spv}O_2 - \text{Spa}O_2} \quad (3.5)$$

For example, $\dot{Q}_P/\dot{Q}_S$ can be quickly calculated after reviewing available saturation data. If the superior vena cava saturation is 80, the pulmonary artery saturation is 95, and the systemic artery saturation is 100, then $\dot{Q}_P/\dot{Q}_S$ = (100 – 80)/100 – 95) = 20/5 = 4/1.

Mixed venous saturation data should always be obtained from the chamber most likely to represent complete admixture, which is usually the chamber proximal to the suspected shunt. For example, in a ventricular septal defect, the RA yields the best mixed venous sample, whereas the RV yields the best data in a patient with a suspected patent ductus arteriosus.

Measurement of Cardiac Output. CO is expressed in liters per minute and, when corrected for body surface area (L/min per m^2), is called *cardiac index* (CI). CO is calculated in the catheterization laboratory using indicator dye techniques. Thermodilution CO is calculated using cold saline solution as the indicator; with the Fick method, oxygen is used as the indicator. The Fick principle states that blood flow through an organ is proportional to the amount of an indicator (oxygen) that is added to or removed from the organ as the blood flows through it. When oxygen is the indicator, CO can be calculated and requires the measurement of oxygen consumption and oxygen content in arterial and venous blood.

Oxygen Consumption. Oxygen consumption ($\dot{V}O_2$) is calculated using the amount of oxygen in inspired and expired air as follows:

$$\dot{V}O_2 = V_I F_IO_2 - V_E F_EO_2 \quad (3.6)$$

where V_I is volume of inspired air (mL/min), F_IO_2 is fraction of inspired oxygen, V_E is volume of expired oxygen (mL/min), and F_EO_2 is fraction of mixed expired oxygen.

The volume of air collected in a Douglas bag is analyzed for oxygen, and carbon dioxide levels are compared with those in ambient air. Younger children and infants may make measurement of oxygen consumption technically challenging, although a hood analyzer can be used. Oxygen consumption may be estimated using HR and age as variables. In many calculations, oxygen consumption is assumed and values are obtained from published tables (Table 3–5).

Vascular Resistance. Vascular resistance (R) relates the mean pressure change (ΔP) across a circuit to the flow ($\dot{Q}$) across the circuit, as follows:

$$R = (\Delta P)/\dot{Q} \quad (3.7)$$

Poiseuille's Law relates flow to pressure, cross-sectional area, length, and viscosity of fluid and is defined by the following equation:

$$\dot{Q} = \pi(P_i - P_o)r^4(8hl) \quad (3.8)$$

where $\dot{Q}$ is flow of volume, $P_i - P_o$ is inflow pressure minus outflow pressure, r is the radius of the tube, h is viscosity of the fluid, and l is the length of the tube.

In this equation, l, h, and π are constant; therefore $\dot{Q}$ is directly proportional to the change in pressure multiplied by the fourth power of the radius (r^4) of the tube. If flow ($\dot{Q}$) remains constant, resistance increases when there is a large drop in pressure (ΔP) across a vascular bed. Poiseuille's Law assumes nonpulsatile laminar flow through rigid tubes, which is not completely

■ **TABLE 3–5.** Oxygen consumption table*

	HEART RATE (beats/min)												
Age	*50*	*60*	*70*	*80*	*90*	*100*	*110*	*120*	*130*	*140*	*150*	*160*	*170*
Male patients													
3				155	159	163	167	171	175	178	182	186	190
4			149	152	156	160	163	168	171	175	179	182	186
6		141	144	148	151	155	159	162	167	171	174	178	181
8		136	141	145	148	152	156	159	163	167	171	175	178
10	130	134	139	142	146	149	153	157	160	165	169	172	176
12	128	132	136	140	144	147	151	155	158	162	167	170	174
14	127	130	134	137	142	146	149	153	157	160	165	169	172
16	125	129	132	136	141	144	148	152	155	159	162	167	
18	124	127	131	135	139	143	147	150	154	157	161	166	
20	123	126	130	134	137	142	145	149	153	156	160	165	
25	120	124	127	131	135	139	143	147	150	154	157		
30	118	122	125	129	133	136	141	145	148	152	155		
35	116	120	124	127	131	135	139	143	147	150			
40	115	119	122	126	130	133	137	141	145	149			
Female patients													
3				150	153	157	161	165	169	172	176	180	183
4			141	145	149	152	156	159	163	168	171	175	179
6		130	134	137	142	146	149	153	156	160	165	168	172
8		125	129	133	136	141	144	148	152	155	159	163	167
10	118	122	125	129	133	136	141	144	148	152	155	159	163
12	115	119	122	126	130	133	137	141	145	149	152	156	160
14	112	116	120	123	127	131	134	133	143	146	150	153	157
16	109	114	118	121	125	128	132	136	140	144	148	151	
18	107	111	116	119	123	127	130	134	137	142	146	149	
20	106	109	114	118	121	125	128	132	136	140	144	148	
25	102	106	109	114	118	121	125	128	132	136	140		
30	99	103	106	110	115	118	122	125	129	133	136		
35	97	100	104	107	111	116	119	123	127	130			
50	94	98	102	105	109	112	117	121	124	128			

*From LaFarge CG, Miettinen OS: The estimation of oxygen consumption. *Cardiovas Res* 4:23, 1970.

analogous to the dynamic nature of the cardiovascular system. However, the calculation of resistance is helpful and the following equations are used.

$$\text{Systemic resistance} = \frac{\text{aortic mean pressure} - \text{right atrial mean pressure}}{\text{systemic blood flow}} \qquad (3.9)$$

$$\text{Pulmonary resistance} = \frac{\text{pulmonary artery mean pressure} - \text{left atrial mean pressure [or PCWP]}}{\text{pulmonary blood flow}} \qquad (3.10)$$

where PCWP is pulmonary capillary wedge pressure.

Resistance is measured in Woods units (mm Hg/L per minute) and is converted to metric units by multiplying by 80 and expressed as dynes/sec per cm^{-5}. Resistances are often indexed to body surface area by using CI, not CO. Normal PVR is less than 2 Woods units in older children but higher in neonates, a reflection of the anatomic and physiologic changes in cardiopulmonary maturation (Emmanouilides, 1964; Rudolph and Nadas, 1962). SVR is 10 to 15 Woods units in neonates and increases to 20 Woods units during infancy and then remains at that level (Rudolph, 1974a).

Interpretation of Cardiac Catheterization Data

Evaluation of a patient with congenital heart disease should include a careful review of the most recent catheterization data. In summary, the following information should be available for evaluation.

1. *Anatomic diagnosis:* This is confirmed with hemodynamic data, oxygen saturation data, angiocardiographic evaluation, or a combination.
2. *Hemodynamic data:* Important data include baseline oxygen saturation and routine intracardiac pressure measurements, valve gradients, shunt calculation (including the direction and quantity of shunt flow), systemic and pulmonary flow, and vascular resistance measurements.
3. *Response to sedation, anesthetic agents, or both:* This is the source of important information during a preanesthetic evaluation.
4. *Response to oxygen:* In patients with elevated PVR (usually with large left-to-right shunts), the response of pulmonary artery pressure, PVR, and shunting after the administration of oxygen is valuable information. Patients with "fixed" or irreversible vascular changes in the lung may not show the expected pulmonary vasodilatation with oxygen administration (i.e., a decrease in pulmonary artery pressure as well as an increase in the left-to-right shunt). These patients may not be candidates for surgical repair of intracardiac shunts in the face of irreversible pulmonary vascular obstructive disease.
5. *Effects of dysrhythmias on cardiac function:* The presence of intracardiac catheters often induces dysrhythmias, and the hemodynamic response to dysrhythmias or to treatment is valuable information for the anesthesiologist.

Echocardiography

Echocardiographic evaluation of the cardiovascular system has been a revolutionary advancement in the assessment of congenital heart disease and pediatric cardiac function. Many children with congenital heart disease may proceed to surgical repair without the need for additional invasive cardiac catheterization because of the precise anatomic information made available by two-dimensional echocardiography. Because infants and children have thin chests and excellent "echo windows," the size, location, orientation, and pattern of motion of all cardiac structures can be visualized in greater detail than in adults. Doppler ultrasound adds to the investigative capabilities of echocardiography, permitting assessment of blood flow to detect patterns, shunting, and valvular gradients. In addition, transesophageal echocardiography (TEE) has been used increasingly in congenital heart disease patients undergoing surgery as small probes have become available.

The evaluation of cardiac function and especially the effects of anesthetics on pediatric cardiac function cannot rely on the use of invasive monitors such as Swan-Ganz catheters, as used in many adult patients. Echocardiography has been extremely useful in children as a noninvasive monitor for cardiac function. Its applications and the limitations are reviewed here.

Echocardiography is the use of reflected ultrasound to create images of the heart and its structures. A pulse generator, timer, transducer and image processor, and display screen are the components of an echocardiographic machine. Electrical pulses are sent from the pulse generator to the transducer. The transducer emits a burst of sound energy and then acts as a receiver and detects the reflected sound. The sound energy reflected back is translated into an electrical impulse and then sent to an image processor.

M-mode echocardiography is the use of a thin beam of sound energy directed toward the heart. Only a small wedge of the heart is viewed with M-mode echocardiography, and, as a result, anatomic diagnosis is limited. However, temporal and spatial resolution of M-mode echocardiography permits the accurate measurement of changes in heart chamber or wall thickness size. As a result, M-mode is used to measure ventricular size and function (Fig. 3–27).

Two-dimensional echocardiography produces a cross-sectional view of the heart. The two-dimensional image results from a sound beam being directed through an arc, in contrast to the ice-pick view of the heart in M-mode. The diagnosis of anatomic abnormalities is superb with two-dimensional echocardiography, and this modality has supplanted cardiac catheterization in the diagnosis of many defects.

Doppler echocardiography uses continuous-wave Doppler and pulsed-wave Doppler. Continuous-wave Doppler is helpful in diagnosing stenotic lesions, atrioventricular valve regurgitation, and some shunt lesions. Pulsed-wave Doppler and Doppler color flow mapping are useful in the description of shunt lesions.

The value of intraoperative *transesophageal echocardiography (TEE)* has been evaluated at several centers (Ungerleider et al., 1989; Sutherland et al., 1989; Muhiudeen et al., 1992). Inaccurate preoperative diagnosis, inadequate surgical repair, or both are major reasons for difficulties in weaning from bypass in congenital heart disease patients. If a postbypass echocardiogram demonstrates good repair, the long-term outcome is shown to be good in 93% of patients in contrast to 55% when a postrepair study demonstrates a suboptimal repair (Ungerleider et al., 1990). In addition, assessment of ventricular function in the operating room carries predictive value for the postoperative period in general. Potential difficulties with TEE monitoring have been described and include the potential for airway obstruction and aortic compression, especially in small infants (Strafford et al., 1994).

A combined echo-Doppler technique can be a valuable monitor of continuous cardiovascular changes. Using a transesophageal echo-Doppler probe, changes in aortic blood flow were shown to agree with corresponding changes in CO measured intermittently with thermodilution CO. With the combined echo-Doppler technique, the Doppler beam can be properly positioned with M-mode echocardiography so that the aortic wall and aortic cross-sectional area are continuously measured (Odenstedt et al., 2001). Invasive monitoring during general anesthesia is not routine in healthy infants, and as a result, invasive evaluation of the use of anesthetic agents on cardiovascular function in healthy children is usually not justified. However, the measurement of continuous aortic blood flow with an esophageal echocardiographic probe has been used in infants as a less invasive tool for measurement (Gueugniaud et al., 1997). Aortic blood flow, preejection period, left ventricular ejection time, mean arterial blood pressure (MAP), HR, SV, and SVR can be obtained with this probe. A study in 12 healthy infants aged 8 to 26 months showed reliable measurements after easy positioning of the probe (Gueugniaud et al., 1998).

Automated real-time echocardiographic assessment or *acoustic quantification* is an advance in cardiac imaging. An automated left ventricular border detection system records beat-to-beat changes in left ventricular cavity area and fractional area change. This real-time assessment of left ventricular function became clinically available since the 1990s and has proved to be helpful in the quantification of left ventricular function (Cahalan et al., 1993). Normal values of left ventricular systolic and diastolic function were defined using acoustic quantification in a multicenter study (Spencer et al., 2003). This study examined adolescent and adult patients (aged 16 to 78 years). Of interest, the percentage of contribution to total left ventricular filling occurring during atrial filling nearly tripled during the six decades studied, from 13% in the youngest cohort to 36% in the eighth decade of life.

The smaller size of the LV in younger children was initially thought to predispose to greater measurement errors in younger children using acoustic quantification. However, the reliability and accuracy of automated border detection using acoustic quantification in children were determined by Rein and others (1998) and appears to be an acceptable method for estimating the cross-sectional area and fractional area change of the LV in children. Other, more objective evaluations of ventricular function have been developed. Tissue Doppler imaging uses Doppler color flow technology to evaluate myocardial velocity with the use of two-dimensional and M-mode echocardiography (Rychik, 1996; Miyatake et al., 1995). Tissue velocity Doppler has also been used in the assessment of atrial and ventricular electromechanical coupling and atrioventricular time intervals in children (Rein et al., 1998). The ability to simultaneously analyze mechanical events and electromechanical coupling in the atria and ventricles is very helpful in rhythm analysis. As a result tissue Doppler may have a role to play in rhythm diagnosis noninvasively when invasive electrophysiologic studies are difficult, such as for fetal arrhythmias. Color kinesis imaging is a visually enhanced mode of automated border detection in which sonographic backscatter analysis is used to color code blood and myocardium interfaces, which are then integrated over the cardiac cycle and analyzed to assess wall motion (Mor-Avi et al., 1997).

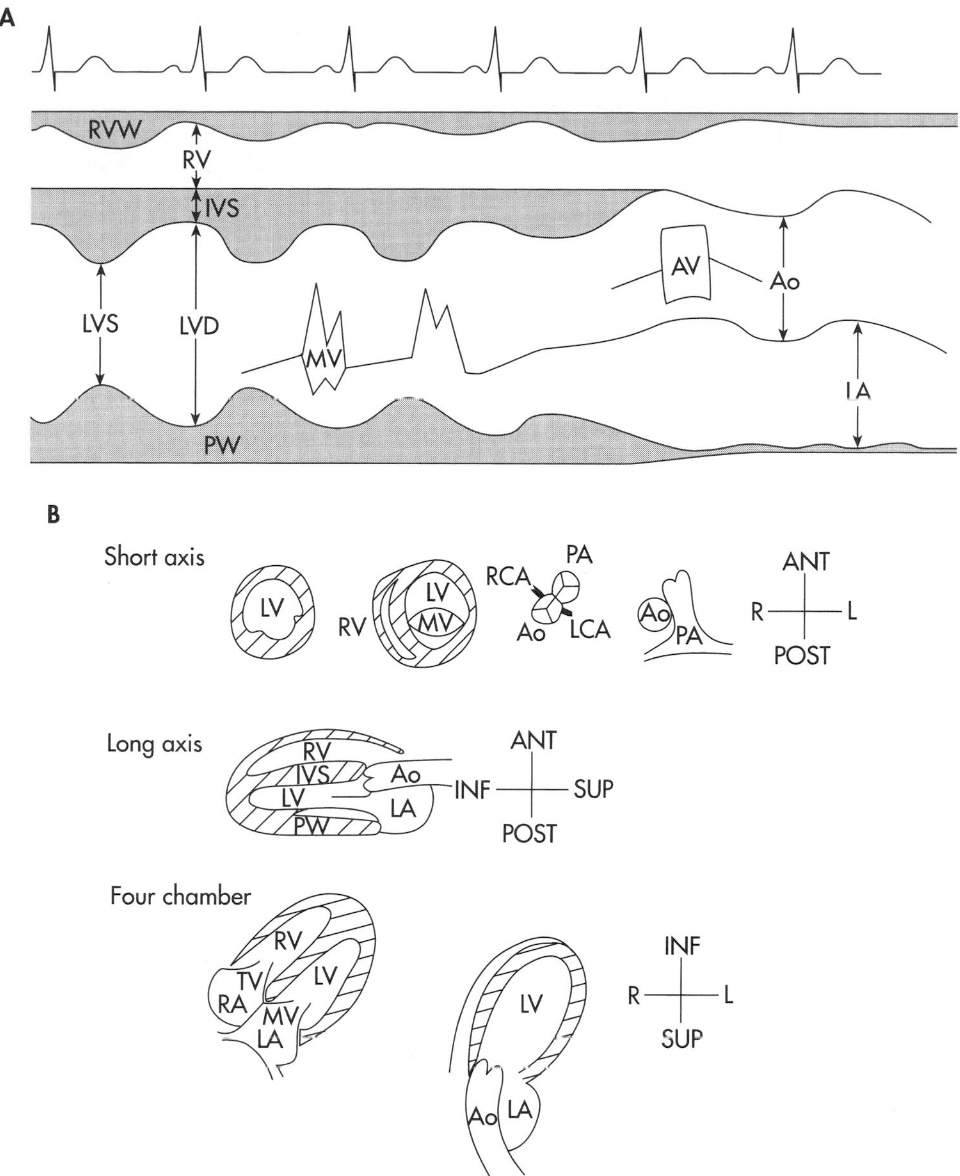

■ **FIGURE 3–27.** Schematic representation of M-mode *(A)* and two-dimensional *(B)* echocardiography. RVW, right ventricular wall; RV, right ventricle; IVS, intraventricular septum; LVS, left ventricular stress; LVD, left ventricular dimension; PW, posterior wall; MV, mitral valve; AV, atrial valve; Ao, aorta; LA, left atrium; LV, left ventricle; RV, right ventricle; RCA, right coronary artery; PA, pulmonary artery; LCA, left coronary artery; ANT, anterior; R, right; L, left; POST, posterior; SUP, superior; INF, inferior; TV, tricuspid valve; RA, right atrium; LA, left atrium. (From Cassell ES, Rogers MC, Zahka KG: Developmental physiology of the cardiovascular system. In Rogers MC, editor: *Textbook of pediatric intensive care.* Baltimore, 1987, Williams and Wilkins.)

Evaluation of Cardiac Function Using Echocardiography

The description of cardiac function earlier in the chapter defined the three major determinants of cardiac performance: preload, afterload, and contractility. In adults, thermodilution CO and pulmonary artery occlusion pressure have historically been used to assess cardiac function, although these methods also have limitations. Echocardiography has proved to be increasingly reliable in the noninvasive assessment of left ventricular function, especially in pediatric patients. For example, previous treatment with anthracylines, a group of chemotherapeutic drugs in use for childhood cancer, may enhance the myocardial depressive effect of anesthetics even in children and adolescents with normal resting cardiac function. Many of these cancer survivors have subtle cardiac abnormalities that are evident with exercise. The stress of anesthesia may also unmask these abnormalities. Huettemann and others (2004) noted that children who had undergone chemotherapy and were anesthetized with 1 MAC isoflurane along with 70:30% nitrous oxide/oxygen had significantly decreased cardiac function even though resting cardiac function was normal. This decrease in function with anesthesia was significantly different than that in the control group of children.

Preload. As defined earlier, preload is the stretching force put on a muscle fiber in the relaxed state. In the intact heart, the end-diastolic fiber length is equated with EDV and left ventricular EDV is generally assumed to be a measurement of preload. EDP is equated with EDV, which is probably a valid assumption when ventricular compliance is normal. However, measurement of ventricular preload using left ventricular EDP is probably less accurate in patients with mitral regurgitation, abnormal ventricular compliance, or both. Two-dimensional echocardiography can be used to measure left ventricular EDV directly. Although this method may be time consuming, the experienced echocardiographer can detect mild blood volume reductions by monitoring left ventricular short-axis changes with high sensitivity (80% to 95%) and specificity (80%). In the study by Reich and others (1993), TEE was used to accurately monitor cardiac filling changes in pediatric cardiac surgical patients.

Afterload. The clinical measurement of afterload (the stress imposed on the ventricular wall during systole) has been more difficult to obtain. SVR is often used as a measurement of afterload, but SVR is derived from the measurement of MAP, right atrial pressure, and CO, as follows:

$$SVR = \frac{MAP - \text{right atrial pressure}}{CO} \quad (3.11)$$

Each of these measurements has potential for error.

Left ventricular end-systolic wall stress (ESWS) is considered a better reflection of afterload because it includes both peripheral loading conditions and myocardial factors. The stress that the ventricle faces at the end of systole is probably the most accurate measurement of afterload. At the end of contraction, the force resisting further shortening determines when shortening ceases.

ESWS is the measurement of this force and is a clinically relevant measure of afterload. ESWS is the force per unit area within the ventricular wall and is determined by combining arterial pressure, phonocardiographic, and echocardiographic measurements (Colan et al., 1984). ESWS has found increased applicability as a possible factor influencing myocardial oxygen consumption, and multiple clinical studies in adults have examined this effect (O'Kelly et al., 1991; Goertz et al., 1993). On the other hand, wall stress may be a poorer reflection of afterload in children and young adults who have abnormal left ventricular geometry such as patients with valvar aortic stenosis, coarctation, and mitral and aortic regurgitation, as well as anthracycline-treated patients (Gentles and Colan, 2002).

Contractility. Contractility is a measurement of intrinsic properties of cardiac muscle that do not include afterload, preload, or both. The usual measures of ventricular performance described on echocardiographic data include shortening fraction and ejection fraction (EF) data, as follows:

$$EF = (SV/EDV) \times 100 \quad (3.12)$$

Normal values are between 65% and 80%, depending on the method used to measure systolic and diastolic volumes (Guttgesel et al., 1977). EFs do not change significantly with age but are affected by changes in preload and afterload. An increase in preload or a decrease in afterload increases the EF if there is no simultaneous change in contractility (Fisher et al., 1975; Sonnenblick and Stobeck, 1977), as seen here:

$$\text{Shortening fraction} = \frac{\text{diastolic diameter} - \text{systolic diameter}}{\text{diastolic diameter} \times 100} \quad (3.13)$$

Shortening fraction is similar to EF but shortening fraction does not rely on the calculation of ventricular volumes as does EF. A normal shortening fraction is 36%, with a range of 28% to 44% (Guttgesel et al., 1977).

The velocity of circumferential fiber shortening (V_{cf}) is a measurement of both the extent and the rapidity of ventricular fiber shortening, as follows:

$$V_{cf} = \frac{\text{left ventricular diastolic dimension} - \text{left ventricular systolic dimension}}{\text{left ventricular diastolic dimension} \times \text{left ventricular ejection time}} \quad (3.14)$$

The velocity of circumferential shortening is sensitive to changes in afterload but not to changes in preload. V_{cf} decreases with increasing afterload. In addition, V_{cf} increases with positive inotropic therapy, such as isoproterenol, and decreases with propranolol (Mahler, et al., 1975). HR also affects V_{cf}. The younger child with a normally higher HR has a different "normal" V_{cf} than do older children (Guttgesel et al., 1977). Normal V_{cf} for a child of a given age and HR can be calculated as follows:

$$V_{cf} = 1.075 + 0.005\,(HR) - 0.020\,(age) \quad (3.15)$$

Because of the influence of preload and afterload on these measurements, there are limitations to the use of shortening data. For example, children with chronic renal failure have depressed shortening fraction data on echocardiographic examination (Colan et al., 1987b). However, Colan and others have shown that these depressed shortening data were due entirely to altered load rather than abnormal contractility and were reversible with improved renal function. Studies on left ventricular mass and systolic performance in pediatric patients with chronic renal failure have shown that those on chronic dialysis do have increased left ventricular mass, left ventricular performance, and contractility at rest but decreased contractile reserve on exercise, which may portend the development over time of worsening systolic function (Mitsnefes et al., 2003). When athletes are studied, endurance athletes may show reduced shortening data, but again this is due to altered load and not reduced contractility (Colan et al., 1987a). Children with Duchenne's muscular dystrophy were studied before scoliosis repair. Percent of fiber shortening was depressed in these children. However, using the stress–velocity relationship, reduced systolic performance was due to excess afterload (elevated end-systolic stress) without significant reduction in contractility (normal stress–velocity relationship). This finding in Duchenne's patients can be explained by reviewing the pathologic results. The myocardium is characterized by fatty deposits and myocardial filament drop-out. The echocardiographic findings support reduced working muscle, but the remaining muscle fibers do have normal systolic function.

To return to our developmental assessment of cardiac function, infants and young children have been found to enhance systolic performance using shortening fraction data alone. When fractional shortening and velocity of shortening are examined in normal children, an age-related decline in performance is noted. However, much of this observed change is

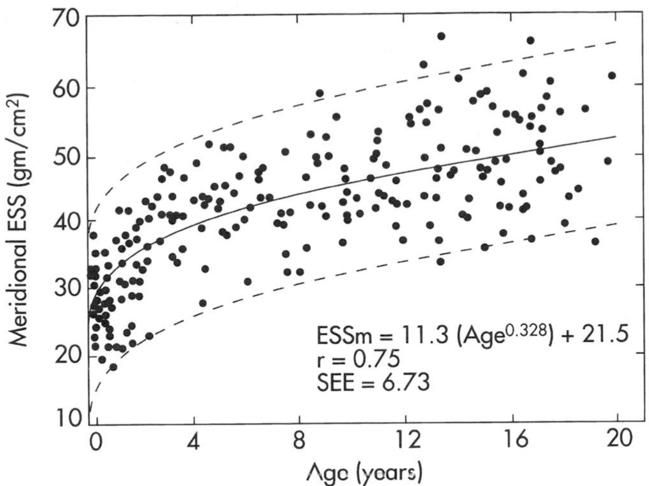

■ **FIGURE 3–28.** In normal subjects, there is a significant age-related rise in afterload. ESSm, mean end-systolic stress. (From Colan SD: Assessment of ventricular and myocardial performance. In Flyer DC, editor: *Nadas' pediatric cardiology.* Philadelphia, 1992, Hanley and Belfus.)

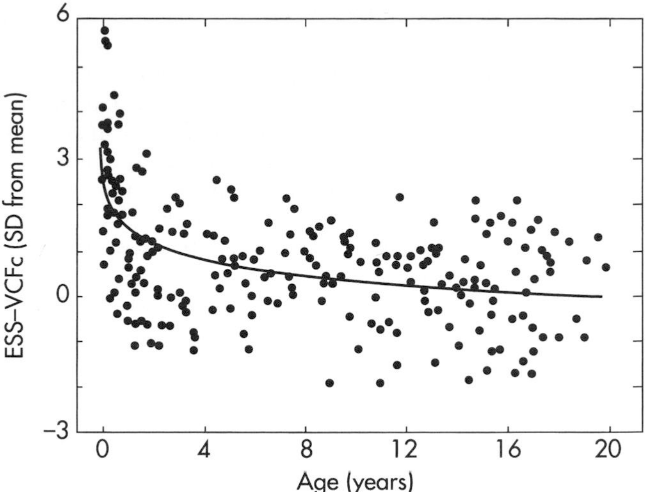

■ **FIGURE 3–30.** An inverse linear relationship exists between end-systolic stress (ESS) and velocity of shortening (VCFc) as demonstrated in this graphic representation of data from a large number of individuals. (From Colan SD: Assessment of ventricular and myocardial performance. In Flyer DC, editor: *Nadas' pediatric cardiology.* Philadelphia, 1992, Hanley and Belfus.)

due to increased afterload with age (Fig. 3–28) (Colan et al., 1989). When the stress–shortening relation is examined, contractility still decreases, mainly over the first 2 years of life (Fig. 3–29).

Research into defining a load-independent measure of contractility has been active. When the length of an isolated muscle strip is held constant, force and velocity are inversely correlated. In the intact heart, this relationship can be defined using arterial pressure and echocardiographic parameters. Colan and others (1984) used the relationship of left ventricular wall stress to the velocity of circumferential fiber-shortening corrected for HR (V_{cfc} [velocity of circumferential shortening corrected for HR]) as a measure of myocardial contractility (Fig. 3–30). Unlike EF and circumferential fiber shortening percentage, which are significantly affected by changes in preload, a change in V_{cfc} is

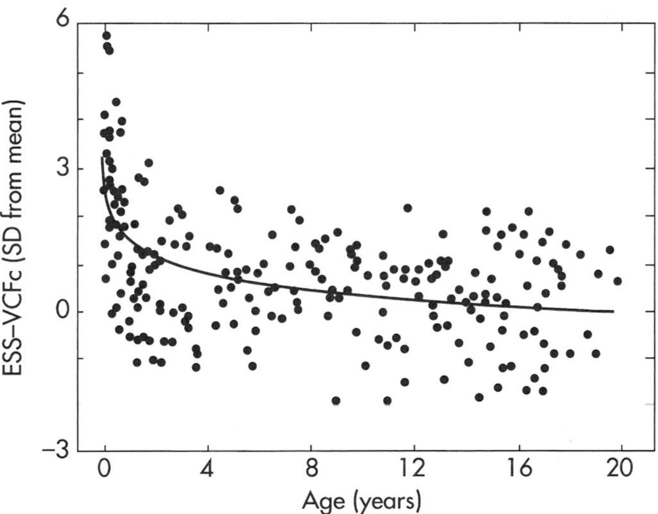

■ **FIGURE 3–29.** The stress-shortening relation falls with age with the most prominent effect in the first two years of life. This is consistent with age modulation of contractility. ESS, end-systolic stress; VCFc, velocity of shortening. (From Colan SD: Assessment of ventricular and myocardial performance. In Flyer DC, editor: *Nadas' pediatric cardiology.* Philadelphia, 1992, Hanley and Belfus.)

independent of preload. In fact, this relationship has been used in studies on the effects of anesthetics on myocardial contractility.

Another important relationship in examinations of contractility is the end-systolic pressure–volume relationship. Suga and others (1973) have shown that the relationship end-systolic pressure can be approximated by the following equation:

$$P_{es} = E_{max} \times (V_{es} - V_d)$$

where P_{es} is end-systolic arterial blood pressure, E_{max} is slope of end-systolic pressure–volume relationship, V_{es} is end-systolic volume, and V_d is the intercept of the end-systolic pressure–volume relationship line on the horizontal axis. They found that E_{max} is independent of preload and afterload and is an excellent indicator of contractility.

The wall stress–velocity and the end-systolic pressure–volume relationships are important parameters that can be measured noninvasively and add to our clinical understanding of an anesthetic agent's effects on cardiac function. These load-independent contractile indices should find increasing applicability in research describing the effects of anesthetics on pediatric cardiac function.

The echocardiographic assessment of cardiac function is important to review because the effects of anesthetics on cardiac function in children are often assessed using such noninvasive monitors. Clearly, conclusions regarding an anesthetic's effect on contractility must consider whether reliable indices have been studied, preferably load-independent indices. When the validity of echocardiographic measurements is understood, a conclusion regarding a drug's effect on cardiac function can be made more accurately.

■ EFFECTS OF ANESTHESIA ON THE CARDIOVASCULAR SYSTEM

The effects of anesthesia on the cardiovascular system must also be considered with a developmental framework. Studies examining the effects of different agents on cardiac function have helped to define age-related responses. Proper anesthetic management must carefully assess the risks of cardiac depression in different age groups and for different surgical procedures. A high-dose opioid technique may help maintain hemodynamic stability in a patient with congenital heart disease who is undergoing cardiac surgery but is an unacceptable technique if direct laryngoscopy and bronchoscopy or a short outpatient procedure is to be performed. The potent effects that anesthetics have on the respiratory system may also cause important interactions with normal cardiovascular function and must be considered, especially in neonates and infants or children with congenital heart disease. Finally, studies examining the cardiovascular effects of anesthetic agents in adults often rely on the availability of invasive monitors, such as pulmonary artery catheters and CO monitoring, which are inappropriate for or difficult to use in pediatric patients. Echocardiographic assessment of cardiac function has been used extensively to define in a more sophisticated and accurate way the effects of anesthesia on the cardiovascular system in children.

PREMEDICATION AND THE INDUCTION OF ANESTHESIA

A safe and effective anesthetic induction must consider psychological and developmental issues as well as the physiologic effects of the agents used. In addition to the use of effective sedative or hypnotic agents, careful preoperative education of parents and patient as well as parental presence during induction may provide for a smooth and safe induction. Since the 1990s, there has been a dramatic increase in the role of parental presence during induction and the use of premedication. Midazolam had become the most commonly used premedication (Kain et al., 2004) (see Chapters 6 and 7, Pharmacology of Pediatric Anesthesia, and Psychological Aspects). Induction techniques may vary, but the end result should be a calm patient with minimal hemodynamic stress, optimal airway control, and maintenance of cardiovascular stability.

Agents for Premedication and Induction

The importance of a smooth, calm induction in children has been recognized as an essential part of an effective anesthetic plan. Psychological benefits may seem obvious, but a smooth induction in a calm, cooperative, or sedated child may also minimize disturbances during induction secondary to increased airway secretions and agitation.

Cardiorespiratory effects of premedication in normal children were studied using three different oral, nasal, and rectal premedication regimens (Audenaert et al., 1995). Fifty-eight young children (average age, 2.7 years) were studied. Oral meperidine (3 mg/kg) with pentobarbital (4 mg/kg) decreased HR, MAP, CI, respiratory rate, and oxygen saturation. SV was maintained. Nasal ketamine (5 mg/kg) with midazolam (0.2 mg/kg) produced no significant cardiovascular or respiratory effects. Rectal methohexital (30 mg/kg) increased HR with a coincident decrease in SV but had no other positive or negative cardiac or respiratory effect.

Methohexital

Age-related differences have been described with the use of barbiturates. Animal studies suggest a lower LD_{50} for barbiturates in young animals (Carmichael, 1947; Domek et al., 1960). Differences in metabolism, including glucuronic acid conjugation and liver immaturity, may have potent effects on the pharmacologic aspects of this group of drugs in neonates and young infants.

Rectal methohexital is used as a premedication in young children. The effect of methohexital on cardiac function has been studied in children with normal cardiac function (Audenaert et al., 1992), using echocardiographic evaluations preoperatively and after rectal administration of 30 mg/kg of methohexital. HR increased and SV decreased, but BP and CI showed no significant changes. Shortening fraction and EF remained within normal parameters. Because baseline measurements were taken the day before surgery and blood levels of additional doses of methohexital were administered if sleep did not occur, the impact of fasting and different serum levels might have affected these results. However, rectally administered methohexital appears to have minimal cardiovascular side effects. Because respiratory depression must be considered a potential side effect of sedation with any barbiturate, the effects of airway compromise on cardiopulmonary interactions cannot be minimized, especially in young infants.

Midazolam and Diazepam

The benzodiazepines have been used widely for premedication and sedation via various routes. Midazolam has been shown to be effective as an induction agent while maintaining cardiovascular stability in adults (Gamble, 1981). Midazolam has found a significant place in premedication and sedation for procedures and intensive care unit sedation in children of all ages, and further research has elucidated its effects. The cardiovascular effects in postoperative cardiac surgery patients have been examined (Shekerdemian et al., 1997). Ten hemodynamically stable children, ventilated in the early postoperative period after cardiac surgery and receiving intravenous morphine infusions, were given an intravenous bolus followed by a continuous infusion of midazolam. Hemodynamic data were recorded before the bolus and 15 minutes and 1 hour later. A bolus of midazolam lowered the CO by 24.1%. Arterial BP, oxygen consumption, and mixed venous oxygen content decreased. There was a tendency for all variables subsequently to recover toward baseline values, within 1 hour, during a continuous infusion. An intravenous bolus of midazolam causes a decrease in CO. Continuous infusions may confer greater cardiovascular stability than intermittent boluses, especially in the compromised cardiac patient.

The standard dose of oral midazolam has been 0.5 to 1.0 mg/kg. The safety and efficacy of a higher oral dose, 1.5 mg/kg, compared with 0.5 and 1.0 mg/kg were studied in 193 children (aged 4 months to 2 years) undergoing cardiovascular surgery (Masue et al., 2003). Midazolam 1.5 mg/kg did not cause any statistically significant decrease in BP, HR, or SpO_2, although eight infants and children showed a 20% decrease in systolic BP and six infants and children showed a greater than 5% decrease in SpO_2. No "spelling attacks," seizure-like activity, apnea, or laryngospasm was observed in any infants and children during and after the medication.

Midazolam has also been found to be an important medication in the management of agitation and distress in the pediatric intensive care unit setting. Sedation in the intensive care unit may be needed for short interventions during difficult procedures or for continuous periods of assisted ventilation. Midazolam, with its characteristic of water solubility (unlike diazepam), short elimination half-life, and short duration of action, has been used with lorazepam to manage sedation in the pediatric intensive care unit. Abrupt cessation of therapy may result in withdrawal symptoms and must be anticipated and appropriate weaning schedules planned.

Midazolam has also been studied as an induction agent and compared with thiopentone and propofol (Jones et al., 1994). Thirty children undergoing circumcision were randomized to receive either thiopentone 4 mg/kg, propofol 2.5 mg/kg, or midazolam 0.5 mg/kg (n = 10 each) intravenously over 30 seconds for induction. There was no statistically significant hemodynamic difference between the three induction agents. Propofol caused a greater decrease in MAP compared with thiopentone at 1 minute ($P = .01$), and the MAP remained significantly lower than that with midazolam at 5 minutes. Of the three induction agents, thiopentone caused the least hemodynamic disturbance on induction.

MAINTENANCE OF ANESTHESIA

Inhalational Anesthesia

Halothane and Isoflurane

Inhalational anesthesia remains the most common method of anesthesia for pediatric patients. Unlike adult patients, halothane continued to hold a significant role in pediatric anesthesia. The introduction of sevoflurane since the 1990s has resulted in some change in choice of agents mainly because of sevoflurane's low blood-gas partition coefficient and low airway irritability, resulting in smooth conditions for rapid induction of anesthesia. It is well recognized that neonates and infants experience a higher incidence of bradycardia, hypotension, and cardiac arrest than older patients undergoing inhalational anesthesia (Nicodemus et al., 1969; Friesen and Lichtor, 1982; Diaz, 1985). Animal studies show a dose-related depression in cardiac function in young animals compared with adults for both halothane and isoflurane (Boudreaux et al., 1984; Murat et al., 1990). The depressant effects of halothane have been described in newborns and young infants. The hemodynamic effects of inhalational anesthesia were defined using basic parameters such as BP and HR, and echocardiographic assessment of cardiac function has refined these measurements.

Investigators using M-mode echocardiography have shown that halothane increases the preejection period (isovolumic contraction time), decreases the fraction of left ventricular shortening fraction, and increases the systolic time interval (preejection period/left ventricular ejection time). In contrast, isoflurane decreases the preejection period, maintains left ventricular shortening fraction, and shortens the systolic time interval. These M-mode measurements indicate a greater decrease in contractility associated with halothane compared with isoflurane (Wolf et al., 1986). However, a limitation in these M-mode results is the assumption that preload, afterload, HR, and cardiac conduction all remain constant.

The cardiac-depressant effects of halothane and isoflurane have also been examined using more definitive function parameters, such as pulsed Doppler and two-dimensional echocardiographic measurements as well as the addition of a fluid bolus challenge at three different anesthetic levels: 0.75, 1.0, and 1.25 MAC (Murray et al., 1987). Halothane and isoflurane both decreased mean BP. Halothane decreased HR at 1.25 MAC, whereas isoflurane increased HR at all levels. Cardiac index was decreased with both agents at 1.25 MAC. EFs decreased significantly with both agents at 1.0 and 1.25 MAC. After a fluid bolus of lactated Ringer's solution (15 mL/kg), EF and SV index increased significantly in the isoflurane group but decreased significantly in the halothane group, suggesting a diminished cardiovascular reserve in the halothane-anesthetized group. This response to fluid loading may have important implications in the clinical setting.

Continuous esophageal aortic blood flow echo-Doppler has been used in healthy infants and small children to examine the myocardial effects of isoflurane (Gueugniaud et al., 1998). Twenty-five healthy infants were studied; they had significant decreases in aortic blood flow and increased preejection period/left ventricular ejection time compared with control values 5 minutes after induction with halothane-fentanyl and atracurium. When isoflurane was discontinued, these changes were reversed. A 1% end-expired concentration of isoflurane caused no significant changes in HR but moderately decreased MAP.

The cardiovascular effects of sevoflurane, isoflurane, halothane, and fentanyl-midazolam have been studied in children with congenital heart disease (Rivenes et al., 2001). Fifty-four patients younger than 14 years who were scheduled to undergo congenital heart surgery were randomized to receive halothane, sevoflurane, isoflurane, or fentanyl-midazolam. Cardiovascular and echocardiographic data were recorded at baseline and at randomly ordered 1 and 1.5 MAC, or predicted equivalent fentanyl-midazolam plasma concentrations. Halothane caused a significant decrease in MAP, EF, and CI, preserving only HR at baseline levels. Fentanyl-midazolam in combination caused a significant decrease in CI secondary to a decrease in HR; contractility was maintained. Sevoflurane maintained CI and HR and had less profound hypotensive and negative inotropic effects than halothane. Isoflurane preserved both CI and EF, had less suppression of MAP than halothane, and increased HR.

The effect of adding nitrous oxide during halothane and isoflurane anesthesia has also been studied in infants (Murray et al., 1988). Baseline measurements were made in 19 healthy nonpremedicated infants (mean age, 12 months) with pulsed Doppler and two-dimensional echocardiography again at 1 MAC halothane or isoflurane and then at the addition of nitrous oxide. MAP, CI, SV, and EF decreased similarly and significantly at 1.0 MAC halothane and isoflurane. HR increased during isoflurane anesthesia but decreased during halothane anesthesia. The addition of nitrous oxide resulted in a decrease in HR, CI, and MAP compared with 1.0 MAC levels of halothane or isoflurane; however, SV and EF were not significantly changed from levels measured during 1.0 MAC halothane or isoflurane. The sympathetic stimulation seen in adults with nitrous oxide does not appear to be seen in infants and young children.

The role of HR in maintaining CO has also been examined in children undergoing inhalational anesthesia. Atropine, administered as a premedication or intraoperatively, has been shown to increase CO during halothane and nitrous oxide anesthesia (Barash et al., 1978; Friesen and Lichtor, 1982; Miller and Friesen, 1988). Using pulsed Doppler and two-dimensional echocardiographic measurements, the effect of atropine on infants and small children undergoing anesthesia with 1.5 MAC halothane or isoflurane was studied (Murray et al., 1989). Because this study examined hemodynamic effects at higher end-expired concentrations and for a longer period of time, halothane was shown to have greater decreases in EF and increases in left ventricular EDV compared with isoflurane.

The greater solubility of halothane compared with isoflurane would explain why evaluation of function parameters after only a short period of time might not reflect differences observed when higher myocardial levels have been attained after prolonged administration. Halothane and isoflurane had similar decreases in CO and SV. The use of atropine resulted in an increase in CO and SV in both groups but more significantly in the halothane group. Despite the greater increase in HR, halothane still produced greater increases in preload (left ventricular EDV) and decreases in EF than isoflurane. Atropine therefore increases CO by its effect on increasing HR but does not affect other cardiovascular effects of inhalational agents.

In summary, similar decreases in CO, SV, and EF are observed with equipotent concentrations of halothane and isoflurane. There is clearly a dose-related effect, with a 30% decrease noted at 1.5 MAC with both agents. HR is affected more by halothane than by isoflurane, but atropine may attenuate this effect. The accuracy of end-tidal measurements of inhalational agent concentrations may account for differences between agents described in other studies. Age has an important effect on MAC: as age decreases, MAC increases. Infants aged 1 to 6 months have a maximum MAC value, and this value decreases with age thereafter. Lerman and others (1983) have shown that the incidence of hypotension in neonates was similar to that in older infants when equipotent concentrations were inhaled.

The safety or therapeutic margin is a useful concept that defines the separation between MAC and a lethal concentration of an inhaled anesthetic, as follows:

$$\text{Therapeutic ratio} = \frac{\text{mean anesthetic heart concentration at cardiovascular failure}}{\text{mean anesthetic heart concentration at MAC}} \qquad (3.16)$$

Isoflurane has been shown to have a higher therapeutic ratio than halothane (Wolfson et al., 1973, 1978; Kissen et al., 1983). Animal studies show that young rats exhibit a 50% decrease in the therapeutic ratio for halothane compared with older animals (Cook et al., 1981). Isoflurane and halothane were found to have very similar therapeutic ratios in newborn animal studies (Schieber et al., 1986).

The cardiovascular effects of inhalational anesthetics are also modulated by baroreceptor responses. As the earlier discussion outlined, many of these reflexes may be limited or absent in very young infants and newborns. Gregory (1982) has shown that despite an increase in systemic blood flow after ligation of a patent ductus arteriosus in premature infants under halothane anesthesia, HR did not increase. In animal studies, halothane and nitrous oxide have been shown to diminish the baroreceptor reflexes in a concentration-dependent manner. Limitations in baroreceptor responsivity may explain the well-described clinical phenomenon of an increased incidence of hypotension and bradycardia in very young infants and newborns under halothane anesthesia. Murat and others (1989) studied eight neonates during the administration of 1 MAC isoflurane. No other anesthetic was administered. The pressor response was tested with the use of phenylephrine, and nitroglycerin was used to test the depressor response. At 1 MAC, MAP decreased about 30% and the mean pressor response decreased to 23% of control awake values. The depressor response decreased to 28% of control. These changes could be attributed to a significant resetting of HR itself. The sensitivity of the baroreceptor reflex was unchanged. This study demonstrated that the significant depression of baroreflex control of HR may impair the newborn's ability to compensate for changes in arterial pressure or to maintain an adequate CO with hypovolemia.

Sevoflurane is a volatile inhalational anesthetic with a low blood-tissue solubility and limited cardiorespiratory depression. It has often been described as an ideal inhalational agent because of its physical, pharmacodynamic, and pharmacokinetic properties.

Sevoflurane confers cardiovascular stability in children, especially compared with other agents such as desflurane and halothane. Sevoflurane produces less increase in HR than isoflurane (Frink et al., 1992) and less myocardial depression than halothane (Holzman et al., 1996). Sevoflurane has been safely used during spinal surgery to control hypotension (Tobias, 1998). At all concentrations in infants, sevoflurane caused less of a decrease in HR, myocardial contractility, and CO compared with halothane (Wodey et al., 1997). Arrhythmias are also less common in children undergoing ear, nose, and throat surgery (61% for halothane and 5% for sevoflurane [Johannesson et al., 1995]) and dental surgery (62% for halothane and 28% for sevoflurane [Paris et al., 1997]).

Lerman and others (1994) described the pharmacology of sevoflurane in infants and children. The MAC of sevoflurane in neonates is 3.3%; in infants (aged 1 to 6 months), 3.2%; and in older infants (aged 6 to 12 months) and children (aged 1 to 12 years), 2.5% (Lerman et al., 1994). In this study, systolic arterial pressure decreased significantly at 1 MAC before incision in all subjects except (1) children aged 1 to 3 years receiving 60% nitrous oxide and (2) children aged 5 to 12 years receiving sevoflurane with oxygen. Blood pressure returned to baseline after incision. HR was unchanged at 1 MAC in all patients except children older than 12 years, who had an increase in HR before incision. The cardiovascular effects of sevoflurane have been studied using transesophageal acoustic quantification (AQ). AQ is a computer-based automatic border detection method to describe echocardiographic images and real-time analysis of cardiac volume changes. AQ with TEE has the ability to detect small depressions in cardiac ejection performance in children undergoing sevoflurane anesthesia (aged 1.4 to 12 years). An increase in HR was balanced by a decrease in SVR (Tanaka et al., 1994).

The MAC and hemodynamic effects of halothane, isoflurane, and sevoflurane have been studied in newborn swine (Lerman et al., 1990). Compared with the awake HR, the mean HR decreased 35% at 1.5 MAC halothane, 19% at 1.5 MAC isoflurane, and 31% at 1.5 MAC sevoflurane. Compared with awake systolic arterial pressure, mean systolic pressure decreased 46% at 1.5 MAC halothane, 43% at 1.5 MAC isoflurane, and 36% at 1.5 MAC sevoflurane. Mean CI did not change significantly between awake and 1.5 MAC sevoflurane, whereas halothane and isoflurane caused significant changes (53% decrease at 1.5 MAC halothane and 43% decrease at 1.5 MAC isoflurane). At equipotent concentrations, halothane and isoflurane depressed hemodynamics to a greater extent than did sevoflurane.

Sevoflurane and halothane were also compared using echocardiographically derived indices of myocardial contractility during induction (Holzman et al., 1996). Left ventricular end-systolic meridian wall stress increased with halothane but remained unchanged with sevoflurane. SVR decreased from baseline to 1 MAC and 1.5 MAC with sevoflurane. Halothane depressed contractility as assessed by the stress–velocity index and stress–shortening index, whereas contractility remained within normal limits with sevoflurane. Total minute stress and normalized total mechanical energy expenditure, measures of myocardial oxygen consumption, did not change with either agent.

Infants may be a greater risk of hemodynamic compromise with inhalational anesthetics (Wodey et al., 1997). In a comparative hemodynamic study between halothane and sevoflurane in infants, sevoflurane showed less cardiac depression than did halothane. Sevoflurane did not alter HR or CI at all concentrations compared but did significantly decrease BP and SVR compared with awake values at all concentrations. Shortening fraction and rate-corrected velocity of circumferential fiber shortening decreased at 1.5 but not at 1 MAC. Myocardial contractility assessed by stress–velocity index and stress–shortening index decreased significantly but not to any abnormal value at all concentrations. Halothane caused a greater decrease in HR, shortening fraction, stress–shortening index, velocity of circumferential fiber shortening, stress–velocity index, and CI at all concentrations compared with sevoflurane.

The use of sevoflurane versus halothane in children has been studied with particular attention to electroencephalograms, clinical agitation, and autonomic cardiovascular activity (Constant et al., 1999). Sevoflurane induced a greater withdrawal of parasympathetic activity than halothane and a transient relative increase in sympathetic vascular tone at the time that the eyelash reflex was lost.

Induction with 8% sevoflurane in children has been studied (Wappler et al., 2003) and has been shown to be effective in creating ideal conditions, including hemodynamic stability, for endotracheal intubation without the use of muscle relaxants.

Desflurane has a lower blood-gas and tissue-blood partition coefficient than isoflurane. Rapid induction and emergence would thus be expected, although airway irritability is notable with desflurane and limits its use as an induction agent (Taylor and Lerman, 1992; Zwass et al., 1992). MAC and hemodynamic responses in neonates, infants, and children have been studied (Taylor and Lerman, 1991) and showed that the MAC of desflurane depends on age, but the age-related differences are much less than those observed with halothane and isoflurane. HR decreased an average of 16% before skin incision in infants aged 6 to 12 months and children aged 1 to 3 years and 3 to 5 years, but no significant change was observed in other age groups.

In a multicenter study examining induction and maintenance characteristics of anesthesia with nitrous oxide and desflurane in children, MAP of less than 80% of baseline was more common with halothane. However, HR and MAP of greater than 120% of baseline was more common with desflurane. Airway irritability, including laryngospasm, limited the use of desflurane as an induction agent (Zwass et al., 1992).

Nitrous Oxide

The effects of nitrous oxide on cardiovascular function have been studied in infants after surgical repair of congenital heart defects. Administration of nitrous oxide to infants with normal and elevated PVR revealed a 9% decrease in HR, a 12% decrease in MAP, and a 13% decrease in CI in both groups. The mild depressant effects of nitrous oxide on systemic hemodynamics are similar to those described in adults. However, reports of elevations in pulmonary artery pressure and PVR in adults were not observed in this group of infants (Hickey et al., 1986).

Nitrous oxide permits lower concentrations of other inhalational agents to maintain a similar depth of anesthesia. The cardiovascular effects of nitrous oxide during inhalational anesthesia with isoflurane and halothane have also been studied in infants and small children (Murray et al., 1988). Using two-dimensional and pulsed Doppler echocardiographic measurements, the effects of nitrous oxide were studied during halothane and isoflurane anesthesia. CO decreased significantly during both halothane and isoflurane anesthesia with and without nitrous oxide. The addition of nitrous oxide to halothane and isoflurane decreased HR and led to decreased CO. Unlike adults, infants and small children do not show the effects of sympathetic stimulation seen with nitrous oxide. The addition of nitrous oxide may have beneficial effects, such as rapid uptake and distribution because of its low solubility, minimal odor, and enhanced alveolar delivery of other inhalational agents. However, the addition of nitrous oxide does not appear to confer added cardiovascular protection from the depressant effects of inhalational agents. As investigative methods have become more sophisticated and accurate, especially the use of echocardiography, the cardiovascular effects of all anesthetic agents can be studied more accurately and direct the choice of safe anesthetics, especially in high-risk pediatric patients.

Opioids

Opioids, especially in high doses for cardiac surgery, have been widely used in children of all ages. Sufentanil, fentanyl, isoflurane, and halothane have been studied in pediatric patients undergoing cardiac surgery. Cardiovascular function was measured by echocardiography before induction, after induction, and after intubation. Left ventricular EF, systemic arterial pressure, and HR were recorded. Left ventricular EF decreased with each agent: sufentanil, 9%; fentanyl, 9%; isoflurane, 4%; and halothane, 8%. Left ventricular EF increased after intubation in all groups except the halothane group, in which left ventricular EF remained 13% below baseline (Glenski et al., 1988).

Pulmonary and systemic hemodynamic responses to 25 mcg/kg of fentanyl were examined in 12 infants after repair of congenital heart defects (Hickey et al., 1985a). No significant changes were found in HR, CI, mean pulmonary artery pressure, or PVR. There were small but statistically significant decreases in MAP and SVR. The use of high-dose opioid technique in neonates undergoing cardiac surgery has been shown to blunt the hormonal and metabolic responses to stress, which may affect postoperative morbidity and mortality (Anand and Hickey, 1992). High-dose opioid anesthesia may also affect the incidence of ventricular fibrillation in susceptible infants with HLHS who are undergoing cardiac surgery (Hansen and Hickey, 1986; Hickey and Hansen, 1991). Stress responses in the pulmonary circulation (during endotracheal suctioning for example) can have potent effects on cardiovascular stability. Fentanyl (25 mcg/kg) has been shown to blunt increases in mean pulmonary artery pressure and PVR (Hickey et al., 1985a, 1985b).

Sufentanil has been studied in children undergoing cardiac surgery. Fentanyl (50 to 75 mcg/kg) was compared with sufentanil at two doses of 5 and 10 mcg/kg. Hemodynamic responses were similar with each agent, and cardiovascular stability was maintained, lowering PVR and increasing oxygen saturations in cyanotic patients (Hickey and Hansen, 1984). Davis and others (1987) studied a high-dose sufentanil technique (15 mcg/kg) in pediatric cardiac surgery patients and described similar hemodynamic responses and the maintenance of cardiovascular stability.

Alfentanil has been examined in greater detail in adult patients, using high- and low-dose infusions. At low infusion rates (1.6 and 6.4 mcg/kg), no significant hemodynamic changes were noted. At higher rates (150 mcg/kg), HR, MAP, and SVR decreased and pulmonary capillary wedge pressure, PVR, and pulmonary artery pressure increased slightly (Kay and Stephenson, 1980; Kramer et al., 1983).

The cardiovascular effects on children of the administration of morphine, meperidine, methadone, and remifentanil have not been studied in children undergoing cardiac surgery in as much detail as have the effects of high-dose fentanyl and sufentanil. All opioids cause a shift to the right in ventilatory response. This potent effect on the respiratory system plays an important interactive role with the cardiac system and should be considered whenever opioids are used. The pharmacokinetics of various opioids in pediatric patients should be reviewed before use (see Chapter 6, Pharmacology for Pediatric Anesthesia).

Propofol

Propofol is a short-acting hypnotic with a rapid redistribution and metabolism. It has been used increasingly in short procedures or for sedation of limited duration. Although apnea can occur during induction, minimal respiratory depression has been observed after induction. Hannallah and others (1991) studied the ED_{50} and ED_{95} for loss of eyelash reflex and found the dose to be 1.3 and 2.0 mg/kg, respectively. Blood pressure decreased 20% in almost half (48%) of the children who received 1% to 3% halothane and propofol infusion.

Propofol has also been studied in children undergoing cardiac catheterization. In this study, children were randomly assigned to receive propofol or ketamine. Ketamine was given in an induction dose of 2 mg/kg IV followed by an infusion at 2 mg/kg per hour. The propofol group received 0.5-mg/kg boluses every 60 seconds titrated to an appropriate sedation level. An infusion of propofol was then started at an hourly infusion rate of three times the induction dose. The propofol group experienced significantly greater decreases in MAP (>20% from baseline). Several patients administered ketamine had episodes of increased HR and arterial pressure. There were significant desaturation effects in the propofol group. The slow titration of propofol used in this study is quite different from standard induction techniques using 2 to 2.5 mg/kg. The hemodynamic effects of a slower induction regimen may differ significantly (Lebovic et al., 1992).

In another study, 216 children were randomly allocated to receive one of six different doses of propofol, from 1.6 to 2.6 mg/kg in 0.2-mg/kg increments. MAP was reduced 15% after 1 minute and 30% after 5 minutes. HR decreased about 17% (Short and Aun, 1991). When thiopentone (5 mg/kg) and propofol (2.5 mg/kg) were compared as induction agents using echocardiographic measurements, MAP was significantly reduced in the propofol group, but the reduced CI did not differ between the two agents. Aun and others (1993) noted that the baroreflex-mediated increases in HR and SVR were less after propofol than after thiopentone. Hannallah and others (1994) studied hemodynamic changes during induction with four different induction/maintenance regimens—(1) propofol/propofol infusion, (2) propofol/halothane, (3) thiopentone/halothane, and (4) halothane/halothane—and noted no significant hemodynamic changes between the groups.

Pediatric anesthesiologists have found an increasing role in the sedation of pediatric patients undergoing cardiac catheterization. Hemodynamic stability is paramount for the patient's safety but also for the accuracy of hemodynamic measurements, which are essential for surgical and medical management decisions. Propofol has been studied in children with intracardiac shunts undergoing cardiac catheterization (Gozal et al., 2001). Mild systemic hypotension that has been described in pediatric patients with propofol may have deleterious effects on right-to-left intracardiac shunts. Fifteen children (aged 18 months to 9 years) underwent cardiac catheterization with sedation, without supplemental oxygen, using 1 mcg/kg of fentanyl followed by propofol bolus (1 to 2 mg/kg) and a continuous infusion (100 mcg/kg per minute). Hemodynamic data, including systemic venous and pulmonary artery and vein pressures and aortic saturation, were recorded; $\dot{Q}_P$ and $\dot{Q}_S$ were calculated. Despite lower pressures during propofol infusion, compared with those pressures measured after the discontinuation of propofol, the intracardiac shunt remained unchanged.

Ketamine

Ketamine is a nonbarbiturate cyclohexamine derivative that is classified as a dissociative anesthetic and has been widely used in children, especially patients with congenital heart disease (Singh et al., 2000; Jobeir et al., 2003; Kogan et al., 2003; Pees et al., 2003). It has been used extensively by pediatric cardiologists in pediatric cardiac catheterization laboratories for sedation. Morray and others (1984) studied the effects of intravenous ketamine (2 mg/kg) given during cardiac catheterization. No significant changes in arterial blood gases, pulmonary artery pressure, HR, or pulmonary-to-systemic arteriolar resistance ratios were found (Morray et al., 1984).

Propofol and ketamine were compared in three groups of children undergoing cardiac catheterization: (1) children without intracardiac shunts, (2) children with a left-to-right shunt, and (3) children with a right-to-left shunt. The children were premedicated with oral midazolam and then randomized to receive a continuous infusion of either propofol (100 to 200 mcg/kg per minute) or ketamine (50 to 75 mcg/kg per minute). Hemodynamic data, including systemic venous and pulmonary artery and vein pressures and aortic saturations, were recorded; $\dot{Q}_p$ and $\dot{Q}_s$ were calculated. The same set of data was recorded before discontinuation of infusions at the end of the procedure. All patients receiving propofol infusions had significant decreases in systemic MAP. In patients with cardiac shunts, propofol infusion significantly decreased SVR and increased systemic blood flow, whereas PVR and pulmonary blood flow did not change significantly. These changes resulted in decreased left-to-right shunting and increased right-to-left shunting; the pulmonary-to-systemic flow ratio decreased significantly. The ketamine-treated patients showed a significant increase in systemic MAP in all patient groups, but pulmonary MAP, SVR, and PVR was unchanged. Ketamine caused fewer effects on intracardiac shunting (Oklu et al., 2003).

Hickey and others (1985) studied children after cardiac surgery who had been administered intravenous ketamine (2 mg/kg). No significant changes in HR, systemic or pulmonary arterial mean pressures, CI, PVR, or SVR were noted after drug administration. Maintaining normal ventilation and normal PCO_2 plays an important role in assessing the effects of ketamine.

Wolfe and others (1991) and Berman and others (1990) studied the effects of ketamine in two high-altitude cities—Albuquerque and Denver—and found dramatic increases in pulmonary artery pressure and pulmonary arteriolar resistance with the administration of ketamine. Interpretation of these data must be evaluated in view of the contribution of the high altitude. Similarly, arterial blood gas data should be available when ketamine is administered during cardiac catheterization, because elevations in pulmonary artery pressure and resistance may result from hypercarbia during ketamine administration (Hickey et al., 1984). Apnea and excessive secretions are seen with ketamine and may contribute to hypoxia, hypercarbia, and the hemodynamic results described in various studies performed in catheterization laboratories. When adequate ventilation is maintained, the effect of ketamine on pulmonary resistance may be minimized in children.

Local Anesthetics

The use of local anesthetics for topical analgesia and anesthesia as well as for use in regional anesthetic techniques requires a clear understanding of pharmacokinetics, pharmacodynamics, and proper dosing. Because infants have low pseudocholinesterase levels, the metabolism of ester-type local anesthetics is decreased. The kinetics of intravenous lidocaine is similar in older infants, children, and adults, but a much longer elimination half-life is observed in children when this agent is delivered intrathecally. In an animal model of right-to-left intracardiac shunting, Bokesch and others (1987) showed higher plasma lidocaine levels in the systemic circulation. The absorption of lidocaine in the lung accounts for the potential toxicity of local anesthetics in patients with right-to-left shunts, and dosages should be adjusted accordingly.

Regional Anesthesia and Analgesia

The use of regional blocks in children of all ages has increased in popularity. Regional anesthesia and analgesia can be safe and effective. Both local anesthetics and opioids have been used in regional blockade. The hemodynamic response to sympathetic blockade by local anesthetics is age dependent, with children younger than 8 years old showing minimal hemodynamic changes with epidural or intrathecal administration of local anesthetics, even with high levels of blockade (Dohi et al., 1979). Children may have a different baseline sympathetic tone compared with adults, who typically respond to blockade with hypotension. In addition, children may have less venous pooling and smaller lower extremity–to–body surface area ratios. Doppler studies have shown minimal alterations in blood pressure and CO in young children (Payen et al., 1987). If a normal circulating blood volume is present, fluid loading, which is normally done in adults, is unnecessary in children. The effects of caudal extradural analgesia on pulmonary and systemic arterial pressure have been examined in children.

Kawamoto and others (1984) examined 27 children who had received a lidocaine caudal block, noting an insignificant change in pulmonary arterial pressure and aortic pressure in children with normal cardiac function. Aortic pressure did decrease significantly in children with cardiac disease. In addition, if pulmonary hypertension was present before blockade, pulmonary artery pressure increased significantly with a simultaneous decrease in aortic pressure. Serum levels of lidocaine were not toxic. Optimal postoperative pain management cannot be ignored because there is a profound interaction between cardiovascular stability and pain systems that has often been overlooked in the postoperative management of cardiac dysfunction (Randich and Maixner, 1984).

Pediatric caudal anesthesia has found a major place in pediatric anesthesia as well as in postoperative pain management. Although this technique has been widely applied, the cardiovascular effects were not well studied in children. Larousse and others (2002) used transesophageal Doppler, a noninvasive method, to examine the cardiovascular effects in healthy children. Ten children (aged 2 months to 5 years) who were scheduled for lower abdominal surgery were studied. General anesthesia was induced using sevoflurane and was followed by the insertion of a transesophageal Doppler probe. Caudal anesthesia was performed using 1 mL/kg of 0.25% bupivacaine with 1:200,000 epinephrine. Hemodynamic variables were collected before and after caudal anesthesia. No complications arose during insertion of the probe. The mean time between the two sets of measurements was 15 minutes. HR, MAP, and systolic and diastolic BPs were not modified by caudal anesthesia. Descending aortic blood flow increased significantly from 1.14 to 1.92 L/min (P = .0002). Aortic ejection volume increased from 8.5 to 14.5 mL (P = .0002). Aortic vascular resistances decreased from 6,279 to 3,901 dynes/sec per cm^{-5} (P = .005). Caudal anesthesia did not affect HR and MAP but induced a significant increase in descending aortic blood flow.

The hemodynamic and cardiovascular effects were studied of epidural anesthesia with plain bupivacaine 0.75 mL/kg in 13 nonpremedicated American Society of Anesthesiologists class 1 children using measurements of HR and BP and M-mode echocardiography. Using general anesthesia, M-mode echocardiographic evaluation of left ventricular function was performed in each patient at four points (after general anesthesia and 5, 10, and 25 minutes after epidural anesthesia). HR decreased significantly at 10 and 25 minutes, and MBP decreased at 5 and 10 minutes compared with point A. No other M-mode echocardiographic indices were changed at any point. Epidural anesthesia with 0.25% bupivacaine 0.75 mL/kg did not affect left ventricular function in young children (Tsuji et al., 1996).

The potent, even life-threatening, effects of local anesthetics when inadvertent intravascular injection occurs mandate that there be a reliable method of detecting intravascular injection. Epinephrine may induce tachycardia or hypertension, but this technique has produced false-positive and false-negative findings. Electrocardiographic changes as markers of intravascular injection of local anesthetics with epinephrine, during placement of epidural blocks in children, have been studied as a more reliable approach. During a 1-year period, all pediatric patients undergoing epidural anesthesia had an electrocardiogram rhythm strip recorded during test dose injection and analyzed for changes in rate, rhythm, and T-wave configuration. During the 1-year period, 742 pediatric epidural blocks and 644 caudal (284 without catheters), 97 lumbar, and 1 thoracic epidural anesthetic procedures were performed, with a satisfactory placement rate of 97.7%. Intravascular injection was detected in 42 (5.6%) epidural anesthetic procedures (3.8% and 6.7% of straight needle and catheter injections, respectively).

Detection was made by immediate aspiration of blood in 6 patients and by HR increases of greater than 10 beats per minute in 30 patients. Five patients had HR decreases suggesting a baroreceptor response. Five patients had HR increases of less than 10 beats per minute that were thought to be secondary to noxious stimuli. Of 30 patients with known intravascular injection and for whom electrocardiographic strips were available, 25 (83%) had T-wave amplitude increases of greater than 25%, and 29 (97%) had electrocardiographic changes in T-wave or rhythm in response to the epinephrine injection. There were no false-positive results. Epinephrine can be used effectively to test for intravascular injection, but slow, incremental dosing should be used as well. In children with cardiac disease who are undergoing cardiac surgery, the role of regional anesthesia has also found an important role, and its safety and efficacy are being verified in research since the 1990s (Dalens and Mazoit, 1998; Naguib et al.,

1998; Hammer et al., 2000; Holtby, 2002; Bosenberg, 2003; Rosen et al., 2002; Steven, 2000; Mazoit and Dalens, 2004).

EFFECTS OF CARDIOPULMONARY INTERACTIONS

CLINICAL CONSIDERATIONS AND NEW TREATMENT MODALITIES

The cardiovascular and respiratory systems interact dynamically at all stages of development. The delivery of oxygen to optimally meet the metabolic needs of all tissues and organs is the goal of both systems. In the neonatal period, evolving anatomic and physiologic changes in the pulmonary bed dramatically affect cardiovascular stability and the maturation from a fetal to a transitional and ultimately a neonatal circulatory pattern. Systemic and pulmonary venous return and the output of both ventricles are affected by cardiopulmonary interactions. Right ventricular preload derives from extrathoracic vessels, whereas right ventricular output is into intrathoracic vessels. On the other hand, left ventricular output is into extrathoracic vessels, and preload originates from intrathoracic vessels. This gives the RV the ability to augment left ventricular preload. Right ventricular preload cannot be similarly augmented. The ventricular septum responds dramatically to changes in both ventricles and can adversely affect left ventricular ejection when increased right ventricular afterload causes septal bowing into the left ventricular outflow tract. This can adversely affect myocardial function, especially in the neonate and young infant. Alterations in intrathoracic pressure have effects on myocardial wall tension. Modes of ventilation can have significant effects on preload, such as the use of positive pressure ventilation and peak end-expiratory pressure, both of which increase right atrial pressure and decrease preload. Increases in right ventricular pressure and right ventricular afterload are also observed (Pinsky, 1990). It is not surprising that patients with right ventricular dysfunction can decompensate with these changes.

How these modes of ventilation affect left ventricular function is less clear. A decrease in right ventricular preload should lead to a decreased volume of blood received by the LV. The increase in right ventricular afterload may adversely affect septal motion and dynamically contribute to left ventricular dysfunction. Ventilation affects PVR. PVR is high at very low or high lung volumes and lowest at functional residual capacity. These potent and dynamic interactions have important implications for respiratory management in patients with cardiac dysfunction and in the stressed neonate, in whom reversion to a fetal circulatory pattern is possible. Ventilatory manipulation is an important tool in minimizing high PVR and its subsequent negative effects on cardiac function. Right ventricular afterload and PVR can be decreased by ventilation with decreased intrathoracic pressures and increased respiratory rates, leading to respiratory alkalosis. High-frequency jet and oscillatory ventilation result in lower mean airway and intrathoracic pressures. High inspired oxygen concentrations are widely used to decrease PVR. Extracorporeal membrane oxygenation, surfactant replacement, and inhaled nitric oxide (NO) have been used to support a failing cardiorespiratory system. The clinical relevance of cardiorespiratory interactions, especially in the critically ill, artificially ventilated pediatric patient, was reviewed by Robotham (1987).

Nitric Oxide

During the past several decades, research on the control of vascular smooth muscle tone and the mediators of resting pulmonary vascular tone has contributed to a better understanding of pulmonary hypertension and its treatment. The synthesis and release of various vasoactive substances contribute to vasomotor tone. When this synthesis is impaired, vasomotor tone may be adversely affected. PFC (also called PPHN) or pulmonary hypertension in patients with severe congenital heart disease is the clinical manifestation of increased pulmonary vascular tone. Many vasoactive products are released by the pulmonary vasculature, including prostacyclin, endothelium-derived relaxant factor (EDRF), and vasoconstrictors such as endothelin. A change in blood flow or shear stress stimulates the release of prostacyclin or EDRF (Van Grondelle et al., 1986). In addition, the response of the endothelium to various pharmacologic agents, such as acetylcholine, may require an intact endothelium (Furchgott and Zawadzki, 1980).

NO has been identified as EDRF, and intensive research has demonstrated an important role for NO in the treatment of pulmonary hypertension among pediatric patients, especially during the perinatal period and after cardiopulmonary bypass. NO may be an important mediator in the development of transitional circulation of the newborn. NO directly activates soluble guanylate cyclase of vascular smooth muscle, thus increasing cyclic guanosine monophosphate and relaxing vascular smooth muscle. L-Arginine is the precursor for the formation of NO in vascular tissues. Davidson and Eldemerdash (1990) demonstrated that EDRF was present in the pulmonary and systemic arteries of newborn guinea pigs, and Roberts and others (1993) showed that inhaled NO was a selective vasodilator in hypoxic newborn lambs. NO has also been studied in PPHN in both low and high doses with a documented reversal in hypoxemia secondary to PPHN (Kinsella et al., 1992; Roberts et al., 1992). Inhalation of NO in these studies did not show any significant effect on systemic pressure. These clinical studies confirmed the laboratory findings that NO acts as a selective pulmonary vasodilator to reverse hypoxic pulmonary vasoconstriction in awake lambs. Lang and others (1992) studied congenital heart disease patients with pulmonary hypertension in the cardiac catheterization laboratory and postoperatively. Inhaled NO was shown to selectively reduce PVR in many patients and is useful for the diagnostic evaluation of severe congenital heart disease complicated by pulmonary hypertension.

Since the 1990s, NO has found wide application in pediatric medicine. A European consensus conference in 2004 reviewed the use of inhaled NO in neonates and children (Macrae et al., 2004). The cases of preterm neonates, children with cardiac disease, and children with acute lung injury and respiratory distress syndrome who were treated with NO were studied. With data from a Cochrane Review (Finer et al., 2000) on NO and expert consensus, certain recommendations were made regarding these groups. In preterm infants, there are three published, randomized controlled trials of NO therapy (The Franco-Belgium Collaborative NO Trial Group, 1999; Subhedar et al., 1997; Kinsella et al., 1999). The Cochrane Review concluded that sufficient data are lacking for evaluation of the possible effects of inhaled NO on periventricular hemorrhage and on long-term neurodevelopmental outcome. The European consensus group recommended that further use of NO in preterm infants be done within the format of controlled clinical trials or as a rescue therapy in life-threatening hypoxemia after all other modalities have failed.

In the clinical setting of acute lung injury and acute respiratory distress syndrome, many systemic disease processes are involved in patients of all ages. The use of NO to improve oxygenation by improving ventilation–perfusion mismatching has had increasing clinical application. Nevertheless, the transient improvement in oxygenation has not yet been proved to have an impact on mortality. Trials in children are very limited (Dobyns et al., 1999), and it appears that underlying disease and not respiratory failure alone may be a critical factor in outcome analysis.

NO in children with cardiac disease has found clinical use in those with pulmonary hypertension because of acquired or congenital heart disease. As a selective pulmonary vasodilator, NO has also been used to differentiate fixed and reactive pulmonary hypertension and therefore has found an important role in diagnostic cardiac procedures (Wessel et al., 1993; Adatia et al., 1995). Severe reactive pulmonary hypertension after cardiac bypass procedures has been treated with NO and in randomized controlled trials was shown to significantly reduce pulmonary hypertensive events (Day et al., 2000; Miller et al., 2000). NO has also been shown to improve the negative effects of elevated PVR after the Fontan operation and in those patients with right ventricular failure, but these observations have not been studied in randomized controlled trials. Because of the lack of extensive randomized controlled trial data, the routine prophylactic use of NO in postoperative congenital heart disease patients was not recommended by the consensus group. Continued research, especially more definitive randomized control trials, will define the place of NO in pediatric care.

The role of other pulmonary vasodilators is another area of research. Prostacyclin and its analogues (prostanoids) are potent vasodilators and possess antithrombotic and antiproliferative properties. All of these properties help to antagonize the pathologic changes that take place in the small pulmonary arteries of patients with pulmonary hypertension. Prostaglandins and phosphodiesterase inhibitors and endothelin receptor antagonists such as prostacyclin, treprostinil, beraprost, and iloprost may be combined to treat pulmonary hypertension, and these combination therapies may hold promise for future therapies (Olschewski et al., 2003).

■ SUMMARY

Anesthesiologists caring for children must have a clear and precise understanding of cardiovascular physiology, the developmental aspects of cardiac function, the effects of anesthetics, and the dynamic interactions of the cardiopulmonary systems. A safe and effective anesthetic plan can then be successfully formulated.

REFERENCES

Adatia I, Perry S, Landzberg M, et al.: Inhaled nitric oxide and hemodynamic evaluation of patients with pulmonary hypertension before transplantation. *J Am Coll Cardiol* 25:1656, 1995.

Anand KJS, Hickey PR: Halothane-morphine compared with high dose sufentanil for anesthesia and postoperative analgesia in neonatal cardiac surgery. *N Engl J Med* 326:1, 1992.

Anderson PAW, Glick K, Manring A, et al: Developmental changes in cardiac contractility in fetal and postnatal sheep: In vitro and in vivo. *Am J Physiol* 247:H371, 1984.

Artman M: Sarcolemmal sodium-calcium exchange activity and exchanger immunoreactivity in developing rabbit hearts. *Am J Physiol* 263:H1506–H1513, 1992.

Assali NS, et al.: Ontogenesis of the autonomic control of cardiovascular functions in the sheep. In Longo LD, Reneau DD, editors: *Fetal and newborn cardiovascular physiology,* vol 1: Developmental aspects. New York, 1978, Garland STPM Press, p 47.

Audenaert SM, Lock RL, Johnson GL, et al.: Cardiovascular effects of rectal methohexital in children. *J Clin Anesth* 4:116, 1992.

Audenaert SM, Montgomery CL, Thompson DE, Sutherland J: A prospective study of rectal methohexital: efficacy and side effects in 648 cases. *Anesth Analg* 81:957, 1995.

Aun CST, Sung RYT, O'Meara ME: Cardiovascular effects of IV induction in children: Comparison between propofol and thiopentone. *Br J Anaesth* 70:647, 1993.

Barash PG, Glanz S, Katz JD, et al.: Ventricular function in children during halothane anesthesia. *Anesthesiology* 49:79, 1978.

Barker DJ: The intrauterine origins of cardiovascular disease. *Acta Paediatr Suppl* 82(suppl 391):93–99; discussion 100, 1993.

Barker DJ, Fall CH: Fetal and infant origins of cardiovascular disease. *Arch Dis Child* 68:797–799, 1993.

Berman W, Fripp RR, Rubler M, et al.: Hemodynamic effects of ketamine in children undergoing cardiac catheterization. *Pediatr Cardiol* 11:72, 1990.

Bokesch PM, Castaneda AR, Ziemer G, et al.: The influence of a right-to-left shunt on lidocaine pharmacokinetics. *Anesthesiology* 67:739, 1987.

Borow KM, Grossman W: Clinical use of pressure-dimension and stress-shortening relations in systole and diastole. *Fed Proc* 43:2414–2417, 1984.

Bosenberg A: Neuraxial blockade and cardiac surgery in children. *Paediatr Anaesth* 13:559, 2003.

Boudreaux JP, Schieber RA, Cook DR: Hemodynamic effects of halothane in the newborn piglet. *Anesth Analg* 63:731, 1984.

Breall JA, Rudolph AM, Heymann MA: Role of thyroid hormone in postnatal circulatory and metabolic adjustments. *J Clin Invest* 73:1418, 1984.

Cahalan MK, Ionescu P, Melton HE, et al.: Automated real-time analysis of intraoperative transesophageal echocardiograms. *Anesthesiology* 78:477, 1993.

Carmichael EB: The median lethal dose (LD_{50}) of Pentothal sodium for both young and old guinea pigs and rats. *Anesthesiology* 8:589, 1947.

Cassidy SC, Schmidt KG, Van Hare GF, et al.: Complications of pediatric cardiac catheterization: a 3-year study. *J Am Coll Cardiol* 19:1285, 1992.

Church SC, Morgan BC, Oliver TK Jr, et al.: Cardiac arrhythmias in premature infants: An indication of autonomic immaturity? *J Pediatr* 71:542, 1967.

Cohn HE, Freed MD, Hellenbrand WF, et al.: Complications and mortality associated with cardiac catheterization in infants under one year: A prospective study. *Pediatr Cardiol* 6:123, 1985.

Colan SD, Borow KM, Neumann A: Left-ventricular end-systolic wall stress-velocity of fiber shortening relation: A load independent index of myocardial contractility. *J Am Coll Cardiol* 4:715, 1984.

Colan SD, Sanders SP, Borow K: Physiologic hypertrophy: Effects on left ventricular systolic mechanics in athletes. *J Am Coll Cardiol* 9:776, 1987a.

Colan SD, Sanders SP, Ingelfinger JR, et al.: Left ventricular mechanics and contractile state in children and young adults with end-stage renal disease: Effect of dialysis and renal transplantation. *J Am Coll Cardiol* 10:1085, 1987b.

Colan SD, Sanders SP, Parness IA, et al.: Evidence of enhanced contractility in normal infants compared to older children and adults [abstract]. *J Am Coll Cardiol* 13:135A, 1989.

Constant I, Dubois MC, Piat V, Moutard ML: Changes in electroencephalogram and autonomic cardiovascular activity during induction of anesthesia with sevoflurane compared with halothane in children. *Anesthesiology* 91:1604, 1999.

Cook DR, Brandom BW, Shiu G, et al.: The inspired median effective dose, brain concentration at anesthesia, and cardiovascular index for halothane in young rats. *Anesth Analg* 60:182, 1981.

Dalens BJ, Mazoit JX: Adverse effects of regional anesthesia in children. (Review). *Drug Saf* 19:251–268, 1998.

Davidson D, Eldemerdash A: Endothelium-derived relaxing factor: Presence in pulmonary and systemic arteries of the newborn guinea pig. *Pediatr Res* 27:128, 1990.

Davis PJ, Cook DR, Stiller RL, et al.: Pharmacodynamics and pharmacokinetics of high-dose sufentanil in infants and children undergoing cardiac surgery. *Anesth Analg* 66:203, 1987.

Dawes GS, Mott JC: The vascular tone of the foetal lung. *J Physiol* 164:465, 1962.

Dawes GS: *Fetal and neonatal physiology.* Chicago, 1968, Year Book Medical.

Day RW, Hawkins JA, McGough EC, et al.: Randomized controlled study of inhaled nitric oxide after operation for congenital heart disease. *Ann Thorac Surg* 69:1907, 2000.

Diaz JH: Halothane anesthesia in infancy: Identification and correlation of preoperative risk factors with intraoperative arterial hypotension and postoperative recovery. *J Pediatr Surg* 20:502, 1985.

Dobyns EL, Cornfield DN, Anas NG, et al.: Multicenter randomized controlled trial of the effects of inhaled nitric oxide therapy on gas exchange in children with acute hypoxemic respiratory failure. *J Pediatr* 134:406, 1999.

Dohi S, Naito H, Takasaki T: Age-related changes in blood pressure and duration of motor block in spinal anesthesia. *Anesthesiology* 50:319, 1979.

Domek NS, Barlow CF, Roth LJ, et al.: An octogenetic study of phenobarbital C-14 in cat brain. *J Pharmacol Exp Ther* 130:285, 1960.

Emmanouilides GC, Moss AJ, Duffie ER Jr, et al.: Pulmonary arterial pressure changes in human newborn infants from birth to three days of age. *J Pediatr* 65:327, 1964.

Faxelius G, Lagercrantz H, Yao A: Sympathoadrenal activity and peripheral blood flow after birth: Comparison in infants delivered vaginally and by cesarean section. *J Pediatr* 105:144, 1984.

Finer NN, Barrington KJ: Nitric oxide for respiratory failure in infants born at or near term. *Cochrane Database Syst Rev* 2:CD000399, 2000.

Fisher DJ, Heymann MA, Rudolph AM: Myocardial consumption of oxygen and carbohydrates in newborn sheep. *Pediatr Res* 15:843–846, 1981.

Fisher EA, DuBrow IW, Hastreiter AR: Comparison of ejection phase indices of left ventricular performance in infants and children. *Circulation* 52:916, 1975.

The Franco-Belgium Collaborative NO Trial Group: Early compared with delayed inhaled nitric oxide in moderately hypoxaemic neonates with respiratory failure: A randomized controlled trial. *Lancet* 354: 1066–1071, 1999.

Frank O: Zur Dynamik des Herzmuskels. *A Biol* 32:370, 1895 (translated by Chapman CB and Wasserman E: *Am Heart J* 58:282, 1959).

Friesen RH, Lichtor JL: Cardiovascular depression during halothane anesthesia in infants: A study of three induction techniques. *Anesth Analg*: 61:42, 1982.

Frink EJ Jr, Malan TP, Atlas M, et al.: Clinical comparison of sevoflurane and isoflurane in healthy patients. *Anesth Analg* 74:241, 1992.

Furchgott RF, Zawadzki JV: The obligatory role of endothelial cells in the relaxation of arterial smooth muscle. *Nature (Lond)* 288:373, 1980.

Gamble JA, Kawar P, Dundee JW, et al.: Evaluation of midazolam as an intravenous induction agent. *Anaesthesia* 36:868, 1981.

Geis WP, Tatooles CJ, Priola DV, et al.: Factors influencing neurohumoral control of the heart in the newborn dog. *Am J Physiol* 228:1685, 1975.

Gentles TL, Colan SD: Wall stress misrepresents afterload in children and young adults with abnormal left ventricular geometry. *J Appl Physio1* 92:1053, 2002.

Gersony WM, Duc GV, Sinclair JC: "PFC" syndrome (persistence of the fetal circulation). *Circulation* 40:111, 1969.

Glenski JA, Friesen RH, Berglund NL, et al.: Comparison of the hemodynamic and echocardiographic effects of sufentanil, fentanyl, isoflurane and halothane for pediatric cardiovascular surgery. *J Cardiothoracic Anesth* 2:147, 1988.

Goertz AW, Lindner KH, Seefelder C, et al.: Effect of phenylephrine bolus administration on global left ventricular function in patients with coronary artery disease and patients with valvular aortic stenosis. *Anesthesiology* 78:834, 1993.

Gozal D, Rein AJ, Nir A, Gozal Y: Propofol does not modify the hemodynamic status of children with intracardiac shunts undergoing cardiac catheterization. *Pediatr Cardio* 6:488, 2001.

Grant DA: Ventricular constraint in the fetus and newborn. *Can J Cardiol* 15:95, 1999.

Grant DA, Kondo CS, Maloney JE, et al.: Changes in pericardial pressure during the perinatal period. *Circulation* 86:1615, 1992a.

Grant DA, Maloney JE, Tyberg JV, et al.: Effects of external constraint on the fetal left ventricular function curve. *Am Heart J* 123:1601–1609, 1992b.

Grant DA, Walker AM: Pleural pressures limit fetal right ventricular output. *Circulation* 94:555–561, 1996.

Gregory GA: The baroresponses of preterm infants during halothane anesthesia. *Can Anaesth Soc J* 29:105, 1982.

Gueugniaud PY, Abisseror M, Moussa M, et al.: The hemodynamic effects of pneumoperitoneum during laparoscopic surgery in healthy infants: assessment by continuous esophageal aortic blood flow echo-Doppler. *Anesth Analg* 86:290, 1998.

Gueugniaud PY, Muchada R, Moussa M, et al.: Continuous oesophageal aortic blood flow echo-Doppler measurement during general anesthesia in infants. *Can J Anaesth* 44:745, 1997.

Guilleminault C, Briskin JG, Greenfield MS, et al.: The impact of autonomic nervous system dysfunction on breathing during sleep. *Sleep* 4:263, 1981.

Guttgesel HP, Paquet M, Duff DF, et al.: Evaluation of left ventricular size and function by echocardiography. Results in normal children. *Circulation* 56:457, 1977.

Hall SM, Hislop AA, Wu Z, et al.: Remodelling of the pulmonary arteries during recovery from pulmonary hypertension induced by neonatal hypoxia. *J Pathol* 203:575–583, 2004.

Hammer CB, Ngo K, Macario A: A retrospective examination of regional plus general anesthesia in children undergoing open heart surgery. *Anesth Analg* 90:1020, 2000.

Hannallah RS, Baker SB, Casey W, et al.: Propofol: Effective dose and induction characteristics in unpremedicated children. *Anesthesiology* 74:217, 1991.

Hannallah RS, Britton JT, Schafer PG, et al.: Propofol anaesthesia in paediatric ambulatory patients: A comparison with thiopentone and halothane. *Can J Anaesth* 41:12, 1994.

Hansen DD, Hickey PR: Anesthesia for hypoplastic left heart syndrome: Use of high-dose fentanyl in 30 neonates. *Anesth Analg* 65:127, 1986.

Haworth SG, Hislop AA: Lung development—the effects of chronic hypoxia [review]. *Semin Neonatol* 8:1–8, 2003.

Haworth SG, Reid L: Structural study of the pulmonary circulation in total anomalous pulmonary venous return in early infancy. *Br Heart J* 39:80, 1977.

Hickey PR, Hansen DD: Fentanyl and sufentanil-oxygen-pancuronium anesthesia for cardiac surgery in infants. *Anesth Analg* 63:117, 1984.

Hickey PR, Hansen DD: High-dose fentanyl reduces intraoperative ventricular fibrillation in neonates with hypoplastic left heart syndrome. *J Clin Anesth* 3:295, 1991.

Hickey PR, Hansen DD, Cramolini GM: Pulmanory and systemic hemodynamic responses to ketamine in infants with normal and elevated pulmonary vascular resistance. *Anesthesiology* 62:287, 1985.

Hickey PR, Hansen DD, Strafford M, et al.: Pulmonary and systemic responses to high dose fentanyl in infants. *Anesth Analg* 64:483, 1985a.

Hickey PR, Hansen DD, Strafford M, et al.: Pulmonary and systemic hemodynamic effects of nitrous oxide in infants with normal and elevated pulmonary vascular resistance. *Anesthesiology* 65:374, 1986.

Hickey PR, Hansen DD, Wessel DL, et al.: Blunting of stress responses in the pulmonary circulation of infants by fentanyl. *Anesth Analg* 64:1137, 1985b.

Holtby H: Con: regional anesthesia is not an important component of the anesthetic technique for pediatric patients undergoing cardiac surgical procedures. *J Cardiothorac Vasc Anesth* 16:379, 2002.

Holzman RS, Van der Velde ME, Kaus SJ, et al.: Sevoflurane depresses myocardial contractility less than halothane during induction of anesthesia in children. *Anesthesiology* 85:1260, 1996.

Huettemann E, Junker T, Chatzinikolaou KP, et al.: The influence of anthracycline therapy on cardiac function during anesthesia. *Anesth Analg* 98:941, 2004.

Jobeir A, Galal MO, Bulbul ZR, et al.: Use of low-dose ketamine and/or midazolam for pediatric cardiac catheterization. *Pediatr Cardiol* 24:236, 2003.

Johannesson GP, Floren M, Lindahl SG: Sevoflurane for ENT-surgery in chidren. A comparison with halothane. *Acta Anaesthesiol Scand* 39:546, 1995.

Jones RD, Visram AR, Chan MM, et al.: A comparison of three induction agents in paediatric anesthesia cardiovascular effects and recovery. *Anaesth Intensive Care* 22:545, 1994.

Jones RD, Morice AH, Emery CJ: Effects of perinatal exposure to hypoxia upon the pulmonary circulation of the adult rat. *Physiol Res* 53:11–17, 2004.

Kain ZN, Caldwell-Andrews AA, Krivutza DM, et al.: Trends in the practice of parental presence during induction of anesthesia and the use of preoperative sedative premedication in the United States, 1995-2002: results of a follow-up national survey. *Anesth Analg* 98:1252, 2004.

Katona PG, Egbert MS: Heart rate and respiratory rate differences between preterm and full term infants during quiet sleep: Possible implications for sudden infant death syndrome. *Pediatrics* 62:91, 1978.

Katona PG, Frasz A, Egbert J: Maturation of cardiac control in full term and pre-term infants during sleep. *Early Hum Dev* 4:145, 1980.

Kaufman TM, Rudolph AM: The effect of heart rate on the atrial contribution to stroke volume in newborn and one month old lambs. *Pediatr Res* 24:434A, 1988.

Kawamoto M, Takasaki M, Kawasaki H, et al.: Effects of caudal extradural analgesia on pulmonary and systemic arterial pressure in children. *Jpn J Anesthesiol* 33:520, 1984.

Kay B, Stephenson D: Alfentanil (R39209): Initial clinical experiences with a new narcotic analgesic. *Anaesthesia* 35:1197, 1980.

Kenny J, Plappert T, Doubliet P, et al.: Effects of heart rate on ventricular size, stroke volume and output in the normal human fetus: A prospective Doppler echocardiographic study. *Circulation* 76:52, 1987.

Kinsella JP, Neish SR, Shaffer E, et al.: Low-dose inhalational nitric oxide in persistent pulmonary hypertension of the newborn. *Lancet* 340:819, 1992.

Kinsella JP, Walsh WF, Bose CL, et al.: Inhaled nitric oxide in premature neonates with severe hypoxaemic respiratory failure: a randomized controlled trial. *Lancet* 354:1061, 1999.

Kissen I, Morgan PL, Smith LR: Comparison of isoflurane and halothane safety margins in rats. *Anesthesiology* 58:556, 1983.

Klopfenstein HS, Rudolph AM: Postnatal changes in the circulation and responses to volume loading in sheep. *Circ Res* 42:839 1978.

Kogan A, Efrat R, Katz J, Vidne BA: Propofol-ketamine mixture for anesthesia in pediatric patients undergoing cardiac catheterization. *J Cardiothorac Vasc Anesth* 17:691, 2003.

Kramer M, Kling D, Walter P, et al.: Alfentanil, a new short acting opioid: Haemodynamic and respiratory aspects. *Anaesthetist* 32:265, 1983.

Kuipers JRG, Sidi D, Heymann MA, et al.: Effects of nitroprusside on cardiac function, blood flow distribution and oxygen consumption in the conscious young lamb. *Pediatr Res* 118:618, 1984.

Lang P, Roberts JD, Bigatello LM, et al.: Inhaled nitric oxide: A selective vasodilator for the treatment of pulmonary artery hypertension in congenital heart disease. *Pediatr Res* 31:A104, 1992.

Larousse E, Asehnoune K, Dartayet B, et al.: The hemodynamic effects of pediatric caudal anesthesia assessed esophageal doppler. *Anesth Analg* 94:1165, 2002.

Lee JD, Tajimi T, Patritta J, et al.: Preload reserve and mechanisms of afterload mismatch in the normal conscious dog. *Am J Physiol* 250:H464, 1986.

Lerman J, Oyston JP, Gallagher TM, et al.: The minimum alveolar concentration (MAC) and hemodynamic effects of halothane, isoflurane, and sevoflurane in newborn swine. *Anesthesiology* 73:717, 1990.

Lerman J, Robinson S, Willis MM, et al.: Anesthetic requirements for halothane in young children 0-1 month and 1-6 months of age. *Anesthesiology* 59:421, 1983.

Lerman J, Sikich N, Kleinman S, et al.: The pharmacology of sevoflurane in infants and children. *Anesthesiology* 80:814, 1994.

Little WC, Freeman GL, O'Rourke RA. Simultaneous determination of left ventricular end-systolic pressure volume and pressure-dimension relationships in closed chest dogs. *Circulation* 71:1301, 1985.

Lock JL, Keane JF, Mandell VS, et al.: Cardiac catheterization. In Fyler DC, editor: *Nadas's pediatric cardiology.* St Louis, 1992, Mosby–Year Book, p 187.

Macrae DJ, Field D, Mercier JC, et al.: Inhalled nitric oxide therapy in neonates and children: reaching European consensus. *Intensive Care Med* 30:372, 2004.

Mahdavi V, Izumo S, Nadal-Ginard B: Developmental and hormonal regulation of sarcomeric myosin heavy chain gene family. *Circ Res* 60:804, 1987.

Mahler F, Ross J Jr, O'Rourke RA, Covell JW: Effects of changes in preload, afterload and inotropic state on ejection and isovolumic phase measures of contractility in the conscious dog. *Am J Cardiol* 35:626, 1975.

Mahoney L: Calcium homeostasis and control of contractility in the developing heart. *Semin Perinatol* 20:510–519, 1996.

Masue T, Shimonaka H, Fuako I, et al.: Oral high-dose midazolam premedication for infants and children undergoing cardiovascular sugery. *Paediatr Anaesth* 13:662, 2003.

Mazoit JX, Dalens BJ: Pharmacokinetics of local anaesthetics in infants and children. *Clin Pharmacokinet* 43:17, 2004.

Mazza NM, Epstein MA, Haddad GG, et al.: Relation of beat-to-beat variability to heart rate in normal sleeping infants. *Pediatr Res* 14:232, 1980.

McNicholas WT, Rutherford R, Grossman R, et al.: Abnormal respiratory pattern generation during sleep in patients with autonomic dysfunction. *Am Rev Respir Dis* 128:429, 1983.

Miller OI, Tang SF, Keech A, et al.: Inhaled nitric oxide and prevention of pulmonary hypertension after congenital heart surgery: a randomized double-blind study. *Lancet* 356:1464, 2000.

Miller RB, Friesen RH: Oral atropine premedication in infants attenuates cardiovascular depression during halothane anesthesia. *Anesth Analg* 67:180, 1988.

Miller WP: Cardiac arrhythmias and conduction disturbances in the sleep apnea syndrome. Prevalence and significance. *Am J Med* 73:31, 1982.

Mirro R, Milley JR, Holzman IR: The effects of sodium nitroprusside on blood flow and oxygen delivery to the organs of the hypoxemic newborn lamb. *Pediatr Res* 19:15, 1985.

Mitsnefes MM, Kimball TR, Witt SA, et al.: Left ventricular mass and systolic performance in pediatric patients with chronic renal failure. *Circulation* 107:864, 2003.

Miyatake K, Yamagishi M, Tanaka N, et al.: New method for evaluating left ventricular wall motion by color-coded tissue Doppler imaging: in vitro and in vivo studies. *J Am Coll Cardiol* 25:717, 1995.

Moorman AF, Christoffels VM: Cardiac chamber formation: Development, genes, and evolution. *Physiol Rev* 83:1223–1267, 2003.

Mor-Avi V, Vignon P, Koch R, et al.: Segmental analysis of color kinesis images: new method for quantification of the magnitude and timing of endocardial motion during left ventricular systole and distole. *Circulation* 95:2082, 1997.

Morray JP, Lynn AM, Stamm SJ, et al.: Hemodynamic effects of ketamine in children with congenital heart disease. *Anesth Analg* 63:895, 1984.

Muhiudeen IA, Roberson DA, Silverman MH, et al.: Intraoperative echocardiography for evaluation of congenital heart defects in infants and children. *Anesthesiology* 76:165, 1992.

Murat I, Hoerter J, Ventura-Claper R: Developmental changes in effects of halothane and isoflurane on contractile properties of rabbit cardiac skinned fibers. *Anesthesiology* 73:137, 1990.

Murat I, Lapeyre G, Saint-Maurice C: Isoflurane attenuates baroreflex control of heart rate in human neonates. *Anesthesiology* 70:395, 1989.

Murray D, Forbes R, Murphy K, et al.: Nitrous oxide: Cardiovascular effects in infants and small children during halothane and isoflurane anesthesia. *Anesth Analg* 67:1059, 1988.

Murray D, Vandewalker G, Matherne GP, et al.: Pulsed Doppler and two-dimensional echocardiography comparison of halothane and isoflurane on cardiac function in infants and small children. *Anesthesiology* 67:211, 1987.

Murray DJ, Forbes RB, Dillman JB, et al.: Haemodynamic effects of atropine during halothane or isoflurane anaesthesia in infants and small children. *Can J Anaesth* 36:295, 1989.

Murray DJ, Mehta MP, Forbes RB: The additive contribution of nitrous oxide to isoflurane MAC in infants and children. *Anesthesiology* 75:186, 1991.

Naguib M, Magboul MM, Samarkandi AH, Attia M: Adverse effects and drug interactions associated with local and regional anaesthesia. *Drug Saf* 18:221, 1998.

Nicodemus HF, Nassiri-Rahimi C, Bachman L, Smith TC: Median effective doses (ED50) of halothane in adults and children. *Anesthesiology* 31:344, 1969.

Odenstedt H, Aneman A, Oi Y, et al.: Descending aortic blood flow and cardiac output: a clinical and experimental study of continuous oesophageal echo-Doppler flowmetry. *Acta Anaesthesiol Scand* 45:180, 2001.

Oklu E, Bulutcu FS, Yalcin Y, et al.: Which anesthetic agent alters the hemodynamic status during pediatric catheterization? Comparison of propofol versus ketamine. *J Cardiothorac Vasc Anesth* 17:686, 2003.

Olschewski H, Rohde B, Behr J, et al.: Pharmacodynamics and pharmacokinetics of inhaled iloprost, aerosolized by three different devices, in severe pulmonary hypertension. *Chest* 124:1294, 2003.

O'Kelly BF, Tubau JF, Knight AA, et al.: Measurement of left ventricular contractility using transesophageal echocardiography in patients undergoing coronary artery bypass grafting. The Study of Perioperative Ischaemia (SPI) research group. *Am Heart J* 122:1041, 1991.

Pappano AJ: Ontogenic development of autonomic neuroeffector transmission and transmitter reactivity in embryonic and fetal hearts. *Pharmacol Rev* 29:3, 1972.

Pappano AJ, Loeffelholz K: Ontogenesis of adrenergic and cholinergic neuroeffector transmission in chick embryo heart. *J Pharmacol Exp Ther* 191:468, 1974.

Paris ST, Cafferkey M, Tarling M, et al.: Comparison of sevoflurane and halothane for outpatient dental anaesthesia in children. *Br J Anaesth* 79:280, 1997.

Payen D, Ecoffey C, Carli P, et al.: Pulsed Doppler ascending aortic, carotid, brachial and femoral artery blood flows during caudal anesthesia in infants. *Anesthesiology* 67:681, 1987.

Pees C, Haas NA, Ewert P, et al.: Comparison of analgesic/sedative effect of racemic ketamine and (+)-ketamine during cardiac catheterization in newborns and children. *Pediatr Cardiol* 24:424, 2003.

Pinsky MR: The effects of mechanical ventilation on the cardiovascular system. *Crit Care Clin* 6:663, 1990.

Rabinovitch M, Herrera-deLeon V, Castaneda AR, et al.: Growth and development of the pulmonary vascular bed in patients with tetralogy of Fallot with or without pulmonary atresia. *Circulation* 64:1234, 1981.

Randich A, Maixner W: Interactions between cardiovascular and pain regulatory systems. *Neurosci Behav Rev* 8:343, 1984.

Reich DL, Konstadt SN, Nejat M, et al.: Intraoperative transesophageal echocardiography for the detection of cardiac preload changes induced by transfusion and phlebotomy in pediatric patients. *Anesthesiology* 79:10, 1993.

Rein AJ, Tracey M, Colan SD, et al.: Automated left ventricular endocardial border detection using acoustic quantification in children. *Echocardiography* 15:111, 1998.

Riemenschneider TA, Brenner RA, Mason DT: Maturational changes in myocardial contractile state of newborn lambs. *Pediatr Res* 15:349, 1981.

Rivenes SM, Lewin MB, Stayer SA, et al.: Cardiovascular effects of sevoflurane, isoflurane, halothane, and fentanyl-midazolam in children with congenital heart disease: an echocardiographic study of myocardial contractility and hemodynamics. *Anesthesiology* 94:223, 2001.

Roberts JD, Chen TY, Kawai N, et al.: Inhaled nitric oxide reverses pulmonary vasoconstriction in the hypoxic and acidotic newborn lamb. *Circ Res* 72:246, 1993.

Roberts JD, Polaner DM, Lang P, et al.: Inhaled nitric oxide in persistent pulmonary hypertension of the newborn. *Lancet* 340:818, 1992.

Robotham JL: Cardiorespiratory interactions. In Rogers MC, editor: *Textbook of intensive care,* vol 1. Baltimore, 1987, Williams and Wilkins.

Robotham JL, Takata M, Berman M, et al.: Ejection fraction revisited. *Anesthesiology* 74:172, 1991.

Romero TE, Friedman WF: Limited left ventricular response to volume overload in the neonatal period: A comparative study with the adult animal. *Pediatr Res* 13:910, 1979.

Rosen DA, Rosen KR, Hammer GB: Pro: regional anesthesia is an important component of the anesthetic technique for pediatric patients undergoing cardiac surgical procedures. *J Cardiothorac Vasc Anesth* 16:374, 2002.
Rosen MR, Legato MJ, Weiss RM: Developmental changes in impulse conduction in the canine heart. *Am J Physiol* 240:H546, 1981.
Rosenberg HC, Williams WG, Trusler GA, et al.: Structural composition of central pulmonary artery shunts. *J Thorac Cardiovasc Surg* 94:498, 1987.
Rudolph AM: Cardiac catheterization and angiography. In Rudolph AM, editor: *Congenital diseases of the heart.* Chicago, 1974b, Year Book Medical.
Rudolph AM: Changes in the circulation after birth. In Rudolph AM, editor: *Congenital diseases of the heart.* Chicago, 1974a, Year Book Medical.
Rudolph AM: Fetal circulation and cardiovascular adjustments after birth. In Rudolph AM, editor: *Pediatrics.* East Norwalk, CT, 1987, Appleton and Lange.
Rudolph A, Nadas A: The pulmonary circulation and congenital heart disease. *N Engl J Med* 267:968, 1962.
Rudolph AM, Heymann MA: Circulation and breathing. Control of foetal circulation. In Bancroft JJ, editor: *Foetal and neonatal physiology.* Cambridge, 1973, Cambridge University Press, pp 89–111.
Rudolph AM, Itshovitz J, Heymann MA: Fetal cardiovascular responses to stress. *Semin Perinatol* 5:109, 1981.
Rychik J: Fetal cardiovascular physiology. *Pediatr Cardiol* 25:201, 2004.
Rychik J, Tian ZY: Quantitative assessment of myocardial tissue velocities in normal children with Doppler tissue imaging. *Am J Cardiol* 77:1254, 1996.
Scammon RE, Norris EH: On the time of obliteration of the fetal blood passages (foramen ovale, ductus arteriosus, ductus venosus). *Anat Rec* 15:165, 1918.
Schieber RA, Namnoum A, Sugden A, et al.: Hemodynamic effects of isoflurane in the newborn piglet: Comparison with halothane. *Anesth Analg* 65:633, 1986.
Shekerdemian L, Bush A, Redington A: Cardiovascular effects of intravenous midazolam after open heart surgey. *Arch Dis Child* 76:57, 1997.
Short SM, Aun CST: Haemodynamic effects of propofol in children. *Anaesthesia* 46:783, 1991.
Singh A, Girotra S, Mehta Y, et al.: Total intravenous anesthesia with ketamine for pediatric interventional cardiac procedures. *J Cardiothoracic Vasc Anesth* 14:36, 2000.
Sonnenblick EH, Stobeck JE: Derived indexes of ventricular and myocardial function. *N Engl J Med* 296:978, 1977.
Spencer KT, Mor-Avi V, Kirkpatrick J, et al.: Normal values of left ventricular systolic and diastolic function derived from signal-averaged acoustic quantification waveforms multicenter study. *J Am Soc Echocardiogr* 16:1244, 2003.
St. John Sutton MG, Raichlen JS, Reichek N, et al.: Quantitative assessment of right and left ventricular growth in the human fetal heart: A pathoanatomic study. *Circulation* 70:935, 1984.
Starling EH: *The Linacre lecture on the law of the heart.* London, 1918, Longmans, Green.
Steven JM, McGowan FX Jr.: Neuraxial blockade for pediatric cardiac surgery: lessons yet to be learned. *Anesth Analg* 90:1011, 2000.
Strafford M, Soliman D, Bokesch P, et al.: The risk of aortic compression from transesophageal echocardiographic probe in neonates and infants. *Anesthesiology* 81(suppl):A1219, 1994.
Subhedar NV, Shaw NJ: Changes in oxygenation and pulmonary haemodynamics in preterm infants treated with inhaled nitric oxide. *Arch Dis Child Fetal Neonatal Ed* 77:F191, 1997.
Suga H, Sagawa K: Instantaneous pressure-volume relationships and their ratio in the excised, supported canine left ventricle. *Circ Res* 35:117, 1974.
Suga H, Sagawa K, Shoukas AA: Load independence of the instantaneous pressure-volume ratio of the canine left ventricle and effects of epinephrine and heart rate on the ratio. *Circ Res* 32:314, 1973.
Sutherland GR, Balaji S, Monro JL: Potential value of intraoperative Doppler colour flow mapping in operations for complex intracardiac shunting. *Br Heart J* 62:467, 1989.
Tabsh K, Nuwayhid B, Murad S, et al.: Circulatory effects of chemical sympathectomy in fetal, neonatal, and adult sheep. *Am J Physiol* 243:H113, 1982.
Tanaka H, Takata M, Yamamoto S, et al.: Cardiovascular interaction during sevoflurane anesthesia in children assessed by transesophageal acoustic quantification. *Anesthesiology* 81:A132, 1994.
Taylor RH, Lerman J: Induction, maintenance and recovery characteristics of desflurane in infants and children. *Can J Anaesth* 39:6–13, 1992.
Taylor RH, Lerman J: Minimum alveolar concentration of desflurane and hemodynamic responses in neonates, infants, and children. *Anesthesiology* 75:975, 1991.
Thach BT: Sleep apnea in infancy and childhood. *Med Clin North Am* 69:1289, 1985.
Tobias JD: Sevoflurane for controlled hypotension during spinal surgery: preliminary experience in five adolescents. *Paediatr Anaesth* 8:167, 1998.
Tsuji MH, Horigome H, Yamashita M: Left ventricular functions are not impaired after lumbar epidural anaesthesia in your children. *Paediatr Anaesth* 6:405,1996.
Tulloh RM, Hislop AA, Boels PJ, et al.: Chronic hypoxia inhibits postnatal maturation of porcine intrapulmonary artery relaxation. *Am J Physiol* 272 (5 Pt 2):H2436–H2445, 1997.
Ungerleider RM, Greeley WJ, Kisslo J: Intraoperative echocardiography in congenital heart disease surgery: Preliminary report on a current study. *Am J Cardiol* 63(suppl 1):3F, 1989.
Ungerleider RM, Greeley WJ, Sheikh KH, et al.: Routine use of intraoperative epicardial echocardiography and Doppler color flow imaging to guide and evaluate repair of congenital heart defects. A prospective study. *J Thorac Cardiovasc* 100:297, 1990.
Van Grondelle AGS, Worthen GS, Ellis D, et al.: Altering hydrodynamic variables influences PGI_2 production by isolated lungs and endothelial cells. *J Appl Physiol* 52:705, 1986.
Vappavouri EK, Shinebourne EA, Williams RL, et al.: Development of cardiovascular responses to autonomic blockade in intact fetal and neonatal lambs. *Biol Neonate* 22:177, 1973.
Vitiello R, McCrindle BW, Nykanen D, et al.: Complications associated with pediatric cardiac catheterization. *J Am Coll Cardiol* 32:1433, 1998.
Wappler F, Frings DP, Scholz J, et al.: Inhalational induction of anaesthesia with 8% sevoflurane in children: conditions for endotracheal intubation and side-effects. *Eur J Anaesthesiol* 7:548, 2003.
Wessel DL, Adatia I, Giglia TM, et al.: Use of inhaled nitric oxide and acetylcholine in the evaluation of pulmonary hypertension and endothelial function after cardiopulmonary bypass. *Circulation* 88:2128, 1993.
Wessel DL, Adatia I, Thompson JE, Hickey PR: Delivery and monitoring of inhaled nitric oxide in patients with pulmonary hypertension. *Crit Care Med* 22:930, 1994.
Wodey E, Pladys P, Copin C, et al.: Comparative hemodynamic depression of sevoflurane versus halothane in infants: an echocardiographic study. *Anesthesiology* 87:795, 1997.
Wolf WJ, Neal NB, Peterson MD: The hemodynamic and cardiovascular effect of isoflurane and halothane in children. *Anesthesiology* 64:328, 1986.
Wolfe RR, Loehr JP, Schaffer MS, Wiggins JW Jr.: Hemodynamic effects of ketamine, hypoxia and hyperoxia in children with surgically treated congenital heart disease residing greater than or equal to 1,200 meters above sea level. *Am J Cardiol* 67:84,1991.
Wolfson B, Kielar CM, Lake C: Anesthetic index—a new approach. *Anesthesiology* 38:583, 1973.
Woods JR, Dandavino A, Murayama K, et al.: Autonomic control of cardiovascular functions during neonatal development and in adult sheep. *Circ Res* 40:401, 1977.
Yardley R: Baroreceptor regulation of blood pressure in unanesthetized fetal sheep. *Aust Paediatr J* 15:286, 1979.
Zugaib M, Forsythe AB, Nuwayhid B, et al.: Mechanisms of beat-to-beat variability in the heart rate of the neonatal lamb. *Am J Obstet Gynecol* 138:444, 1980.
Zwass MS, Fisher DM, Welborn LG, et al.: Induction and maintenance characteristics of anesthesia with desflurane and nitrous oxide in infants and children. *Anesthesiology* 76:373, 1992.

4 Regulation of Fluids and Electrolytes in Infants and Children

Demetrius Ellis

Concentrations of minerals and electrolytes in extracellular fluid (ECF) are maintained nearly constant despite large day-to-day variations in the dietary intake of salt and water. Such homeostasis is governed primarily by the kidneys through an array of intricate processes that may be influenced by intrarenal and extrarenal vasoactive substances and hormones. Although the basic tenants governing nephron function and homeostasis of body fluid composition have changed little over the past decade, major advances stemming from genetic research have greatly elucidated the structure and function of many renal tubular electrolyte transporters in both health and disease. A major objective of the present treatise is to enhance the understanding of electrolyte (and fluid) pathophysiology based on such newer information.

OVERVIEW OF ANATOMY AND PHYSIOLOGY

ANATOMY

The kidneys are retroperitoneal paired organs located on each side of the vertebral column. A normal adult kidney measures 11 to 12 cm in length, 5 to 7.5 cm in width, and 2.5 to 3.0 cm in thickness. In the adult male it weighs 125 to 170 g, and in the adult female, it weighs 115 to 155 g. Beneath its fibrous capsule lies the cortex, which contains the glomeruli, the convoluted proximal tubules, the distal tubules, and the early portions of the collecting tubules. The remainder of the tissue, the medulla, contains the pars recta, the loop of Henle, and the middle and distal portions of the collecting duct. The inner medulla borders the renal pelvis, where urine is received from the collecting ducts. The ducts and loops are arranged into cone-shaped bundles called pyramids, whose tips project into the renal pelvis and form papillae. The pelvis drains into the ureter, which in the adult human descends a distance of 28 to 34 cm to open into the fundus of the bladder. The walls of the pelvis and ureters contain smooth muscles that contract in a peristaltic manner to propel urine to the bladder.

RENAL BLOOD FLOW

Despite accounting for only 0.5% of body weight, the kidneys receive about 25% of the cardiac output with a blood flow of approximately 4 mL/min per g of kidney tissue. Renal plasma flow (RPF) in women is slightly lower than in men, even when normalized for body surface area, averaging 592 ± 153 mL/min per 1.73 m^2 and 654 ± 163 mL/min per 1.73 m^2, respectively (Smith, 1943). In children between the ages of 6 months and 1 year, normalized RPF is half that of adults but increases progressively to reach adult levels at about 3 years of age (McCrory, 1972). After the age of 30 years, renal blood flow (RBF) decreases progressively; by the age of 90 years, it is approximately half of the value present at 20 years (Davies et al., 1950). This generous supply provides not only for the basal metabolic needs of the kidneys but also for the high demands of ultrafiltration.

The basic arterial supply of the kidney is a single renal artery that divides into large anterior and posterior branches and subsequently into segmental or interlobar arteries. The latter form the arcuate and interlobular arteries. These blood vessels are end-arteries and therefore predisposed to tissue infarction in the presence of emboli. The arcuate arteries are short, large-caliber vessels supplying blood to the afferent arterioles of the glomeruli at a mean pressure of 45 mm Hg, which is higher than that found in most capillary beds. This high hydraulic pressure and large endothelial pore size lead to enhanced glomerular filtration (Brenner et al., 1978).

Glomerular capillaries have many anastomoses but recombine to form the efferent arteriole. The latter subdivide into an extensive peritubular capillary network. This arrangement allows solute and water to move between the tubular lumen and blood. These networks rejoin to form the venous channels by which blood exits the kidney.

Ninety percent of RBF goes to the cortex, which accounts for 75% of the renal weight, whereas the medulla and the rest of the kidney receive 25% of the RBF. Although cortical blood flow is 5 to 6 mL/g per min, outer medullary blood flow decreases to 1.3 to 2.3 mL/g per min, and the flow to the papilla is as low as 0.22 to 0.42 mL/g per min (Dorkin et al., 1991). The unevenness in the distribution of RBF between the cortex and the medulla is necessary to develop and maintain the medullary gradient of osmotically active solutes that drive the countercurrent exchange/multiplier, which is essential for the elaboration of concentrated urine. Outer medullary blood flow may preferentially supply Henle's loop, thereby accounting for the striking influence of loop diuretics in that region. Furthermore, papillary blood flow is far greater than the metabolic needs of the renal parenchyma and is well adapted to the countercurrent concentrating mechanism characteristic of this region.

RBF remains almost constant over a range of systolic blood pressures from 80 to 180 mm Hg, a phenomenon known as autoregulation. Consequently, glomerular filtration is also constant over this range of pressures (Selkurt et al., 1949) as a result of adaptations in the renal vascular resistance (Gertz et al., 1966). Because the changes in resistance that accompany graded reductions in renal perfusion pressure occur in both denervated and isolated perfused kidneys (Thurau, 1964), autoregulation appears not to depend on extrinsic neural or hormonal factors. According to the "myogenic hypothesis," first proposed by Bayliss (1902), the stimulus for vascular smooth muscle contraction in response to increasing intraluminal pressure is either the transmural pressure itself or the increase in the tension of the vascular wall. An increase in perfusion pressure, which initially distends the vascular wall, is followed by a contraction of the resistance vessels and a return of blood flow to basal levels.

There are only a few studies of autoregulation of RBF in developing animals. Aortic constriction in adult animals reduces renal perfusion by 30% but has minimal effects on RBF and glomerular filtration rate, compared with the significant changes observed in 4- to 5-week-old rats (Yared and Yoskioka, 1989). Furthermore, it has been demonstrated that autoregulation of RBF in young rats occurs at renal perfusion pressures between 70 and 100 mm Hg, compared with pressures of 100 to 130 mm Hg in the adult (Chevalier and Kaiser, 1985). A similar increase in the pressure set point for autoregulation has been found in dogs (Jose et al., 1975). It appears that autoregulation of RBF occurs in the very young and is sufficient to maintain blood flow constant over a wide range of perfusion pressures that are physiologically adequate for the age. No such human studies are available.

Several substances have been proposed to participate in the autoregulation of RBF, including vasoconstrictor and vasodilator prostaglandins (Herbacznska-Cedro and Vane, 1973), kinins (Maier et al., 1981), adenosine, vasopressin (Osswald et al., 1978), the renin-angiotensin-aldosterone system (Schnermann et al., 1984), endothelin, and endopeptidases. Nitric oxide (NO), previously known as endothelium-derived relaxing factor (EDRF), has also been shown to play an important role in regulating renal vascular tone, through its vasodilatory action. Bradykinin, thrombin, histamine, serotonin, and acetylcholine act on endothelial receptors to activate phospholipase C, which in turn results in the formation of inositol triphosphate and diacylglycerol, resulting in the release of intracellular calcium (Marsden and Brenner, 1991; Luscher et al., 1992). This, in turn, stimulates the synthesis of NO from L-arginine. Other factors that stimulate the formation of NO include hypoxia, calcium ionophores, and mechanical stimuli to the endothelium. NO increases RBF by decreasing efferent arteriolar vascular resistance, while glomerular filtration remains unchanged (Marsden and Brenner, 1991).

Because in the mature kidney autoregulation is lost at arterial pressures less than 80 mm Hg, the lower physiologic pressures prevailing in the newborn period may be expected to limit this important control mechanism. There is evidence both to support (Kleinman and Lubbe, 1972) and to refute (Jose et al., 1975) this conclusion.

RENAL PHYSIOLOGY

The glomerulus is a specialized capillary cluster arranged in loops that functions as a filtering unit. The capillary walls may be viewed as a basement membrane lined by a single layer of cells on either side. In contact with blood are endothelial cells, which contain many fenestrations, whereas podocytes, with their foot processes, line the other side of the basement membrane.

The route by which water and other solutes are filtered from the blood is not fully understood, but it appears that plasma ultrafiltrate traverses the large fenestrations of the glomerular capillary endothelium and penetrates the basement membrane and the slit pores located between the podocyte foot processes. Filtration of large molecules is greatly influenced by the size and charge of the specific molecule, as well as by the integrity and charge of the glomerular basement membrane. Abnormalities in various structural proteins of the slit pore diaphragm such as nephrin, podocin, and α-actinin may be responsible for several proteinuric disorders (Mundel and Shankland, 2002). In general, the endothelium and the lamina rara interna of the glomerular basement membrane slow the filtration of circulating polyanions such as albumin (Ryan and Karnovsky, 1976), and the lamina rara externa and the slit pores slow the filtration of cationic macromolecules such as lactoperoxidase (Graham and Kellermeyer, 1968). Neutral polymers such as ferritin are not filtered because of their large molecular size and shape (Farauhar et al., 1961). Molecules with a radius of 4.2 nm or more are excluded from the glomerular filtrate. In practical terms, red cells, white cells, platelets, and most proteins are restricted to the circulation.

GLOMERULAR FILTRATION

Among the main functions performed by the kidney is the process of glomerular filtration. The glomerulus is primarily responsible for the filtration of plasma. The glomerular filtration rate (GFR) is the product of the filtration rate in a single nephron and the number of such nephrons, which range from 0.7 to 1.4 million in each kidney (Keller et al., 2003). *Clearance,* which is defined as the volume of plasma cleared of a substance within a given time, provides only an estimate or approximation of GFR.

Although tubular reabsorption and tubular secretion may influence the blood level of numerous medications and endogenously produced substances such as urea, creatinine, and uric acid, the degree of elimination of such substances depends largely on GFR. Hence, in individuals with renal impairment, estimation or measurement of GFR is crucial in determining the dosage adjustment and choice of medications needed to achieve effectiveness while avoiding toxicity. GFR is also a major factor that affects electrolyte composition and volume of body fluids, as well as acid-base homeostasis.

Glomerular filtration is driven by hydrostatic pressure, which forces water and small solutes across the filtration barrier. In healthy individuals, changes in hydrostatic pressure rarely affect single-nephron GFR because autoregulatory mechanisms sustain or maintain a constant glomerular capillary pressure over a large range of systemic blood pressure (Robertson et al., 1972). Hydrostatic pressure is opposed by the oncotic pressure produced by plasma proteins and the hydrostatic pressure within Bowman's capsule. Mathematically, this relation can be expressed by the following equation:

$$\text{SNGFR} = K_f \times (\text{P} - \text{p}) = K_f \times \text{P}_{\text{UF}}$$

where SNGFR is the single-nephron glomerular filtration rate; K_f is the glomerular ultrafiltration coefficient; P and p are the average hydraulic and osmotic pressure differences, respectively; and P_{UF} is the net ultrafiltration pressure. As plasma water is filtered, the proteins within the capillaries become more concentrated, so oncotic pressure increases at the distal end of the glomerular capillary loop and the rate of filtration ceases at the efferent capillary (Blantz, 1977). Under normal conditions, about 20% of the plasma water that enters the glomerular capillary bed is filtered; this quantity is referred to as the filtration fraction.

Renal blood flow (RBF) has the greatest influence on GFR. Renal parenchymal disorders interfere with autoregulation of RBF such that GFR may fall even with low normal mean arterial blood pressure (MABP). Still more pronounced changes in GFR may occur with hypotension or hypertension, which may accelerate ischemic or hypertensive injury.

Clearance of a molecule may serve as an indicator of GFR only if the assayed molecule is biologically inert and freely permeable across the glomerular capillary, if it remains unchanged after filtration, and if it is neither reabsorbed nor secreted by the tubule. The exogenous filtration marker inulin (a fructose polymer) has all of these attributes and is the ideal, or "gold standard," for measuring GFR. However, inulin clearance measurement is rarely used clinically because it is an expensive and cumbersome method. Instead, measurement of an endogenous small molecule such as serum creatinine (molecular weight, 0.113 kDa), which is derived from muscle metabolism at a relatively constant rate and is freely filtered at the glomerulus, is a practical, rapid, and inexpensive means for estimating GFR, and thereby aiding clinical decisions. Thus, in the steady state, creatinine production and urinary creatinine excretion are equal even when GFR is reduced.

Serum creatinine concentrations vary by age and gender. In 1-year-old girls values are 0.35 ± 0.05 mg/dL (mean ± SD) and rise gradually to 0.7 ± 0.02 mg/dL (mean ± SD) by 17 years of age; boys have corresponding mean values that are 0.05 mg/dL higher until 15 years of age and 0.1 mg/dL higher subsequently (Schwartz et al., 1976). Expected creatinine excretion rates in 24-hour urine collections are often used to validate such collections. Values range from 8 to 14 mg/kg per day in neonates and up to 1 year of age, with an increase to about 22 ± 7 mg/kg per day (mean ± SD) in preadolescent children of either gender (Hellerstein et al., 2001). Subsequently, creatinine excretion in boys is 27 ± 3.4 mg/kg per day.

In healthy children with proportional height and weight, GFR can be estimated by creatinine clearance (CrCl) as calculated by the *Schwartz formula,* which does not rely on measurement of urinary creatinine or timed urine collections:

$$\text{CrCl (mL/min per 1.73 m}^2\text{)} = (\text{Height}/\text{P}_{\text{CR}}) \times k$$

where height is in centimeters, P_{CR} is the plasma creatinine concentration in mg/dL, and k is a constant proportion to muscle mass. The value of k is 0.45 in full-term newborns and until 1 year of age, 0.55 in children 2 years of age and older and in adolescent girls, and 0.70 in adolescent boys (Schwartz et al., 1987). Normal CrCl ranges from 90 to 143 mL/min per 1.73 m^2, with a mean of 120 mL/min per 1.73 m^2.

Although more cumbersome, calculation of CrCl based on values obtained in 12- or 24-hour urine collections provide a better estimate of GFR. Once the completeness of such collections is validated based on expected creatinine excretion, CrCl is calculated using the following formula:

$$\text{CrCl (mL/min/1.73 m}^2\text{)} = \frac{\text{U} \times \text{V} \times \text{SA m}^2}{\text{min} \times \text{P}_{\text{Cr}} \times 1.73\ \text{m}^2}$$

where U is the urinary concentration of creatinine in mg/dL, V is the total urine volume in mL, min is the time of collection in minutes, and P_{Cr} is the serum concentration of creatinine in mg/dL. To standardize the clearance of children of different sizes, the calculated result is multiplied by 1.73 m^2 (surface area of a standard man in meters squared) and divided by the surface area (SA) of the child (in meters squared).

In children with impaired renal function, GFR estimates based on creatinine methods may grossly overestimate the true GFR because tubular and gastrointestinal secretion of creatinine increases disproportionately and, hence, serum creatinine concentrations are less reflective of filtration at the glomerulus. For example, Schwartz formulas overestimate GFR by 10% ± 3% when GFR is greater than 50 mL/min per 1.73 m^2 but by 90% ± 15% when GFR is less than 50 mL/min per 1.73 m^2. Other limitations of creatinine-based GFR determinations stem from variation of analytical assays, reference values ranging from 0.1 to 0.6 mg/dL in children under 9 years of age, diurnal variation in serum creatinine levels due to high intake of cooked meat or intense exercise, influence of body mass index, and inaccurate urine collections all of which make comparisons of GFR difficult over time, especially in growing children (Levey et al., 1988). Use of cimetidine to block tubular secretion of creatinine prior to measuring CrCl in urine collections may improve such measurements (Hellerstein et al., 1998).

Measurement of cystatin-C, a 13-kDa serine proteinase produced at a constant rate by all nucleated cells, is purported to be a superior endogenous marker of filtration because cystatin-C is less susceptible to variation than is plasma creatinine. A meta-analysis compared the correlation between GFR measured by inulin

■ **TABLE 4–1.** Nonparametric 95% reference intervals for cystatin C in different age groups

Age Group	n	Reference Interval	90% CONFIDENCE LIMITS Lower Limit	Upper Limit	P*
Preterm infants	58	1.34 to 2.57	1.07 to 1.42	2.47 to 2.86	.000
Full-term infants	50	1.36 to 2.23	1.24 to 1.44	2.03 to 2.32	.000
>8 days to 1 yr	65	0.75 to 1.87	0.71 to 0.86	1.78 to 1.91	.000
>1 to 3 yr	72	0.68 to 1.60	0.65 to 0.79	1.39 to 1.67	.011
>3 to 16 yr	162	0.51 to 1.31	0.48 to 0.68	1.26 to 1.35	—

*Statistical significance versus the oldest group (including Bonferroni's correction factor 5).

Modified from Harmoinen A, Ylinen E, Ala-Houhala M, et al.: Reference intervals for cystatin C in pre- and full-term infants and children. *Pediatr Nephrol* 15:105–108, 2000, p 107, Table 1. (With kind permission of Springer Science and Business Media.)

clearance, radiolabeled methods, nonlabeled iothalamate or iohexol and either plasma creatinine, or cystatin-C concentrations measured nephelometrically (Dharnidharka et al., 2002). The correlation between GFR and cystatin-C was significantly higher compared with plasma creatinine (0.846 versus 0.742, $P < 0.001$). Thus, cystatin-C measurements are becoming increasingly popular in clinical practice and reference ranges have been generated in children up to 16 years of age (Bokenkamp et al., 1998; Finney et al., 2000; Harmoinen et al., 2000) (Table 4–1).

Studies in renal transplant donors and in individuals with various renal disorders have shown that plasma creatinine concentration changes minimally as GFR falls to about 50 mL/min per 1.73 m^2 (Shemesh, 1985) (Fig. 4–1). This compensation is largely due to hypertrophy and hyperfiltration of the remaining nephrons. When more than 50% of the nephrons cease to function and "renal reserve" is outstripped, serum creatinine may rise rapidly in a parabolic fashion (see Fig. 4–1). Thus, when a more accurate clinical assessment of GFR is desirable for research purposes, radiolabeled methods with an identity exceeding 97% give a better approximation of GFR relative to inulin clearance and may be more useful in aiding clinical decisions. In multicenter investigations conducted in the United States using a uniform method for GFR measurement, ^{125}I-iothalamate is frequently used because this isotope has low radiation exposure and long isotope half-life and can be assayed at a central laboratory (Bajaj et al., 1996). Otherwise, ^{99m}Tc-diethylenetriaminepenta-acetic acid (Tc-DTPA) is frequently used to estimate GFR for routine clinical purposes. In other countries, ^{51}Cr-ethylenediaminetetra-acetic acid (Cr-EDTA), which delivers a greater radiation dosage, is also popular as are nonlabeled iothalamate and iohexol methods.

Although GFR may fluctuate, the kidney retains the ability to regulate the rate of solute and water excretion according to changes in intake. This regulation is achieved by changes in tubular reabsorption rates—a phenomenon known as glomerular–tubular balance (Tucker and Blantz, 1977). The end result is preservation of ECF volume and chemical composition. Glomerular–tubular balance can be disturbed by several factors, including volume expansion, loop diuretics, and inappropriate secretion of antidiuretic hormone (ADH).

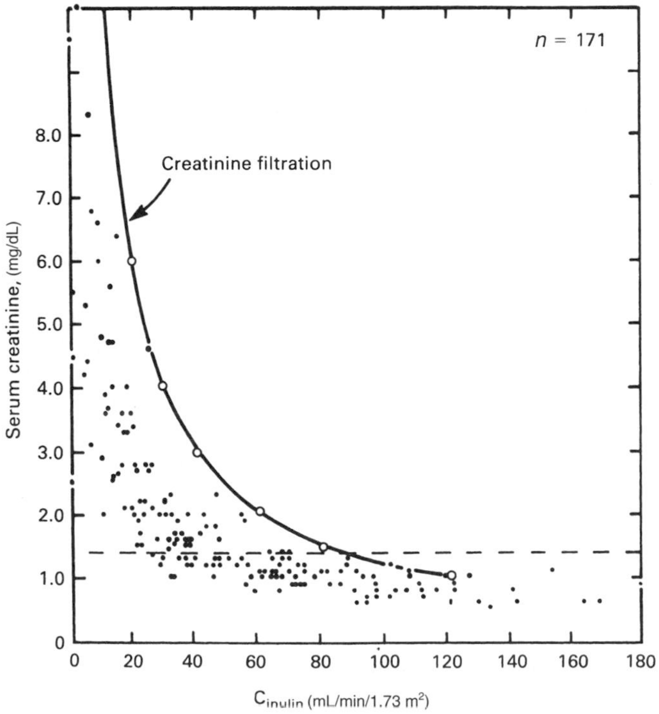

■ **FIGURE 4–1.** Relationship of serum creatinine to GFR. (From Shemesh O, Golbetz H, Kriss JP, et al.: Limitation of creatinine as a filtration marker in glomerulopathic patients. *Kidney Int* 28:830, 1985, Figure 1-3.)

■ OVERVIEW OF TUBULAR FUNCTION

The proximal tubule is the site of reabsorption of large quantities of solute and filtered fluid (Fig. 4–2). Many transporters subserving tubular electrolyte transport have been characterized at the genetic level, and various pathologic disorders have been elucidated (Epstein, 1999). Under physiologic conditions, the proximal convoluted tubule isotonically reabsorbs 50% to 60% of the glomerular filtrate (Berry and Rector, 1991). The initial portion of the proximal convoluted tubule reabsorbs most of the filtered glucose, amino acids, and bicarbonate. Glucose and amino acids are absorbed actively, whereby they are transported against their electrochemical gradient, coupled to sodium (Na^+). Active Na^+ transport at the peritubular membrane provides the driving force that ultimately is responsible for other transport processes. The system is driven by sodium, potassium (Na^+, K^+) (activated) adenosine triphosphatase (Na^+,K^+-ATPase) or Na^+ "pump," which requires the presence of potassium (K^+) in the peritubular fluid and is inhibited by ouabain. Micropuncture studies show that around 50% to 70% of the filtered Na^+ is reabsorbed in this segment, mostly by a process of active cotransport.

The major fraction of filtered bicarbonate (HCO_3^-) is absorbed early in the proximal convoluted tubule. Hydrogen (H^+) gains access to luminal fluid via an Na^+/H^+ electroneutral exchange mechanism and forms carbonic acid. The latter is dehydrated to H_2O and CO_2 under the influence of carbonic anhydrase. CO_2 diffuses into the cell, and HCO_3^- is re-formed and ultimately

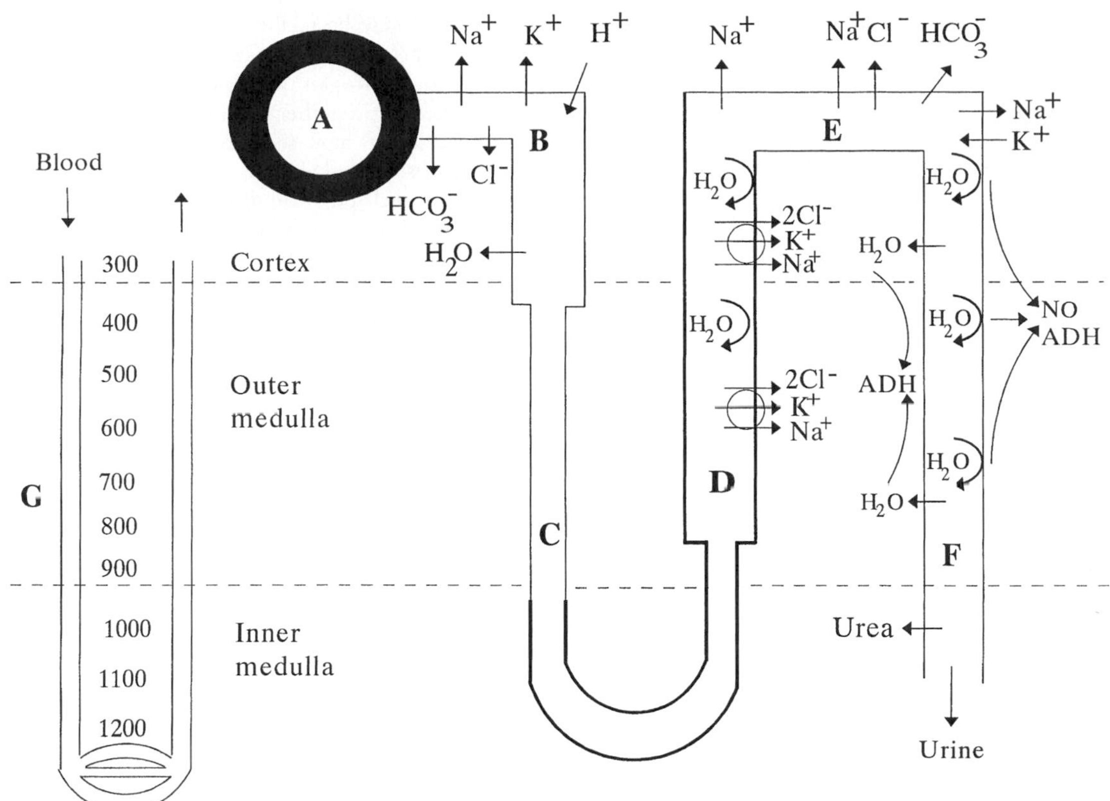

■ **FIGURE 4–2.** Sodium and water handling by the nephron. *A*, Glomerulus. *B*, Proximal tubule, the major site for the reabsorption of Na^+ (70%), Cl^-, K^+ (80%), HCO_3^- (80% to 90%), and water. The reabsorptive process is isomotic, regardless of whether the kidney is concentrating or diluting urine. *C*, Thin descending loop of Henle. *D*, Thick ascending loop of Henle. It is always impermeable to water. The medullary portion is important for the generation of free water. There is active Na^+, K^+, and Cl^- (20% to 25%) reabsorption, which is responsible for driving the countercurrent multiplier and creating increased medullary tonicity. The cortical thick ascending limb and the early distal tubule *(E)* are responsible for the reabsorption of the remaining HCO_3^-, to as well as 5% of the filtered Na^+ and Cl^-. These segments are impermeable to water and are unaffected by ADH. In the late distal tubule and the cortical collecting duct *(F)*, aldosterone action controls Na^+ and K^+ reabsorption and excretion. The medullary portion of the collecting duct is the major site for ADH-dependent water reabsorption. This segment is permeable to water in the presence of ADH. The vasa recta *(G)* is important in maintaining a concentrated medullary interstitium.

absorbed into the bloodstream. In general, the concentration of HCO_3^- is maintained at 26 mmol/L, which is slightly below the renal threshold of approximately 28 mmol/L (Pitts and Lotspeich, 1946).

The renal clearance of glucose is exceedingly low even after complete maturation of glomerular filtration. The amount filtered increases linearly as plasma glucose increases. Initially, all filtered glucose is reabsorbed until the renal threshold has been exceeded (at around 180 mg/dL), at which point filtered glucose appears in the urine. However, maximal tubular glucose (T_{mG}) reabsorption is attained at a filtrate glucose concentration of about 350 mg/mL (Pitts, 1974). The reabsorption of glucose in the proximal tubule occurs via a carrier-mediated, Na^+/glucose cotransport process across the apical membrane followed by passive facilitated diffusion and active Na^+ extrusion across the basolateral membrane.

Apart from Na^+, other solutes reabsorbed in the proximal tubule include K^+, Ca^{2+}, P^{2-}, Mg^{2+}, and amino acids. These are discussed in detail in other sections of this chapter.

The loop of Henle makes possible the formation of concentrated urine and contributes to the formation of dilute urine (Kokko, 1979). This dual function is achieved through the unique membrane properties of the loop, the postglomerular capillaries, and the hypertonicity of the interstitium. The proximity of the descending and ascending portions of loop allows it to function as a countercurrent multiplier, whereas the capillaries serve as countercurrent exchangers (see Fig. 4–2). The descending loop of Henle abstracts water from tubular fluid, increasing the intraluminal concentrations of NaCl and other solutes. However, the intraluminal osmolality remains in equilibrium with the interstitium, where 50% of the osmolality results from urea. In the thin ascending limb of the loop of Henle, there is passive efflux of NaCl and urea into the interstitium. The thick ascending limb of the loop of Henle, by being impermeable to water, contributes to the formation of dilute urine.

The final creation of hypotonic or hypertonic urine depends on the distal tubules and collecting ducts and their interaction with ADH. In the distal convoluted tubule, Na^+ reabsorption occurs against a steep gradient, largely under the influence of aldosterone. K^+ is secreted by the distal tubule in association with Na^+ reabsorption and H^+ secretion. Moreover, this segment of the nephron acidifies the urine and is the only site of new bicarbonate formation. At the end of the collecting duct, about 1% of the filtered water and about 0.5% of the filtered Na^+ appear in the final urine.

■ KIDNEY AND ANTIDIURETIC HORMONE

Antidiuretic hormone (ADH) plays a pivotal role in water homeostasis by acting on the most distal portion of the nephron.

ADH is a cyclic octapeptide that, along with its carrier protein, neurophysin, is synthesized in the supraoptic and paraventricular nuclei of the hypothalamus (Zimmerman and Defendini, 1977). The prohormone migrates along the nerve axons to the posterior pituitary gland, where it is stored as arginine vasopressin. It is released through exocytosis (Douglas, 1973).

Several variables affect ADH secretion. Physiologically, the most important factor is plasma osmolality. A very small rise in plasma osmolality is sufficient to trigger a response from the very sensitive osmoreceptors located in and around the hypothalamic nuclei leading to ADH secretion. Conversely, plasma ADH concentrations are less than 1 pg/mL at a physiologic plasma osmolality of less than 280 mOsm/kg water. The antidiuretic activity of ADH is maximal at plasma osmolality of greater than 295 mOsm/kg water, when plasma ADH exceeds 5 pg/mL (Robertson, 2001). Once plasma osmolality exceeds this limit—thus surpassing the capacity of the ADH system to affect maximal fluid retention—the organism depends on thirst to defend against dehydration. Intracerebral synthesis of angiotensin II largely mediates this thirst response along with the oropharyngeal reflex. Atrial natriuretic peptide (ANP) opposes the release of ADH and of angiotensin II. In summary, plasma osmolality and Na^+ are maintained within a narrow range. The upper limit of this range is determined by the sensitivity of the thirst mechanism located in the hypothalamus, whereas its lower range is affected by ADH release.

Nonosmolar factors also influence ADH secretion and may be key stimuli of ADH secretion in pathologic disorders leading to hypovolemia and hypotension. These changes are mediated by low pressure (located in the left atrium) and high-pressure (located in the carotid sinus) baroreceptors. Experimental studies suggest that this nonosmotic pathway of ADH release is less sensitive than the osmotic pathway and is triggered by a 5% to 10% fall in blood volume, whereas a 1% and 2% increase in ECF osmolality can trigger ADH release.

Nonhypovolemic conditions that stimulate ADH release often lead to diminished urine volume, hyponatremia, fractional excretion of uric acid greater than 10% and low serum uric acid level (<4 mg/dL), and urinary sodium greater than 20 mEq/L (Albanese et al., 2001). These conditions result in hyponatremia. Conversely, inhibitors of ADH release or primary or acquired nephropathies may lead to an inability to respond to ADH and to conserve water and are often accompanied by polyuria with Uosm less than 150 mOsm/kg, dehydration, and hypernatremia.

ADH has a major effect on the medullary thick ascending limb and thereby influences the countercurrent multiplier mechanism and urinary concentration. More directly, ADH binds to V_2 receptors in the basolateral membrane of the collecting duct leading to activation of adenylate cyclase and the formation of cyclic 3′,5′-adenosine monophosphate (cAMP) (Dorisa and Valtin, 1976; Schwartz et al., 1974). This results in insertion of aquaporin-2 water channels in apical membranes and in activation of apical Na^+ channels leading to water conservation (Andreoli 2001). These effects are counterbalanced by prostaglandin E_2 (PGE_2) and the calcium-sensing receptor in cells of the medullary thick ascending limb that mediate saluresis and diuresis.

Polyuric syndromes can be separated on the basis of urine osmolality and generally consist of water diuresis, solute diuresis, or a mixed water-solute diuresis with typical Uosm of less than 150 mOsm/kg, 300 to 500 mOsm/kg, and 150 to 300 mOsm/kg, respectively (Oster et al., 1997). The etiology of polyuria (Table 4–2) may be facilitated by obtaining a urinalysis, urine pH, and measurement of electrolytes, creatinine, osmolality, glucose, urea nitrogen, and bicarbonate, preferably in a timed urine collection together with the corresponding serum values. Such assessment may serve to prevent dehydration, acid-base disturbances, hypokalemia, or hypernatremia, which often accompany such polyuric disorders (Oster et al., 1997). Proper correction of acute hypernatremia is needed to prevent brain demyelination. Normal saline infusion may be the agent of choice in polyuric conditions associated with solute diuresis, whereas ADH and electrolyte-free fluid administration may be appropriate in cases of "pure" water diuresis. The recommended rate of correction of hypernatremia is about 10 mEq/L per 24 hours, amounting to a fall in plasma osmolality of about 20 mOsm/kg H_2O per day (Adrogue and Madias, 2000b).

RENIN-ANGIOTENSIN-ALDOSTERONE SYSTEM

The renin-angiotensin-aldosterone axis plays a key role in control of vascular tone, Na^+ and K^+ homeostasis, and, ultimately, circulatory volume and cardiovascular and renal function. Renin is an enzyme with a molecular weight of 40 kDa that is synthesized and stored in the juxtaglomerular apparatus surrounding the afferent arterioles of the glomeruli (Davis and Freeman, 1976). The primary stimuli for renal renin release are reductions in renal perfusion pressure, Na^+ restriction, and Na^+ loss as detected by the specialized macula densa cells located in the distal tubule. Mechanical (stretch of the afferent glomerular arterioles), neural (sympathetic nervous system), and hormonal (prostaglandin E_2 and prostacyclin) stimuli act in an integrated fashion to regulate the rate of renin secretion (Fig. 4–3).

Once released into the circulation, renin cleaves the leucine-valine bond of angiotensinogen, forming angiotensin I. Angiotensin-converting enzyme present in lung, as well as in kidney, large caliber vessels, and other tissues, cleaves the carboxyl terminal (histidine-leucine dipeptide) from angiotensin I to form the biologically active angiotensin II (Ng and Vane, 1967).

Angiotensin II has numerous important hemodynamic functions that are mediated largely by binding to angiotensin II T1 receptors in endothelial cells, tubular epithelial cells, and smooth muscle (Burnier and Brunner, 2000) (Box 4–1). It plays a key role in regulating blood volume and long-term blood pressure regulation through stimulation of several tubular transporters of Na^+ conversation largely located in the proximal tubule, as well as through its effects in enhancing aldosterone secretion and Na^+ reabsorption in the distal tubule. As a potent direct smooth muscle vasoconstrictor and as an enhancer of ADH and sympathetic nervous system activity, angiotensin II also participates in short-term blood pressure regulation in disorders associated with volume depletion or circulatory depression. Research has uncovered multiple nonhemodynamic functions largely mediated by binding to T1 receptors of angiotensin II, which are particularly important in the pathophysiology of progressive renal injury (Hall et al., 1999).

A rise in plasma aldosterone concentration stimulates urinary K^+ secretion, thus allowing maintenance of K^+ balance. Aldosterone also increases the excretion of ammonium (NH^{+4}) and magnesium (Mg^{2+}) and increases the absorption of Na^+ in the distal tubule, both by increasing the permeability of the apical membrane and by increasing the activity of Na^+, K^+-ATPase (Marver and Kokko, 1983). The net effect is to generate more negative potential in the lumen, a driving force for

■ **TABLE 4–2.** Studies done to evaluate polyuria

Abbreviation (Term)	Definition	Formula	Comment
C_{osm} (osmolal clearance)	Urine flow (volume/unit time) necessary to excrete the urinary solution isotonically (i.e., at osmolality of the plasma)	$\frac{(U_{osm})\,V}{P_{osm}}$	Classic clearance formula applied to solute
$C_{osm(E)}$ (electrolyte osmolal clearance)	Urine flow (volume/unit time) necessary to excrete urinary electrolytes at concentration of plasma Na	$\frac{(U_{[Na]}+U_{[K]})V}{P_{[Na]}}$	Assumes that contribution of $P_{[K]}$ is negligible compared with $P_{[Na]}$
$C_{osm(NE)}$ (nonelectrolyte osmolal clearance)	Urine flow (volume/unit time) necessary to excrete urinary nonelectrolytes isotonically (i.e., at osmolality of plasma)	$C_{osm}-C_{osm(E)}$	—
CH_2O (free water clearance)	Volume of urinary solute – free water excreted per unit time	$V-C_{osm}$	—
$CH_2O(E)$ (electrolyte – free water clearance	Volume of urinary electrolyte – free water excreted per unit time	$V-C_{osm(E)}$	$CH_2O(E)$, rather than CH_2O, influences $S_{[Na]}$
U_{TS} (urine total solute)	Measured total amount of urinary solute in 24 hr	(U_{osm}) (TV)	—
U_E (urine electrolyte solute)	Estimated total amount of urinary solute in 24 hr accounted for by electrolytes	(2) $(U_{[Na]}+U_{[K]})$ (TV)†	—
U_{NE} (urine nonelectrolyte solute)	Estimated total amount of urinary solute in 24 hr not accounted for by electrolytes	$U_{TS}-U_E$	—
UAG (urinary anion gap)	Difference (in milliequivalents per liter) between sum of urinary concentrations of Na and K, and that of Cl	$U_{[Na]}+U_{[K]}-U_{[Cl]}$	A large (positive) value usually implies a large concentration of anions other than Cl
PS (principal solute)	Principal urinary solute in millimoles per 24 hr	—	If PS is a monovalent ion such as Na^+ or Cl^-, PS is calculated as twice its total excretion
PS% (percent principal solute)	Contribution of principal solute to total solute excretion	$\frac{(100)\,(PS)}{(U_{osm})\,(TV)}$	The solute with the highest osmolal concentration in a 24-hr urine collection, expressed as a percentage of total solute excretion

*U_{osm} indicates urine osmolality; V, urine volume/unit time; P_{osm}, plasma osmolality; $U_{[Na]}$, urine sodium concentration; $U_{[K]}$, urine potassium concentration; $P_{[Na]}$, plasma sodium concentration; TV, total 24-hr urinary volume; and $U_{[Cl]}$, urine chloride concentration.
†U_E calculations assume that the corresponding anions are monovalent.
Modified from Oster JR, Singer I, Thatte L, et al.: The polyuria of solute diuresis. *Arch Intern Med* 157:721–729, 1997, p 722, Table 1.

increased K^+ secretion. In addition, aldosterone enhances reabsorption of sodium in the cortical collecting duct through activation of the epithelial sodium specific channel, ENaC (Greger, 2000). In performing these functions, aldosterone plays a key role in regulating fluid and electrolyte balance. Long-term aldosterone administration to healthy volunteers increases the extracellular fluid (ECF) volume. Clinical edema does not occur, however, because after several days the kidney "escapes" from the Na^+-retaining effect while maintaining the K^+-secretory effect (August et al., 1958).

KIDNEY AND ATRIAL NATRIURETIC PEPTIDE

Atrial natriuretic peptide (ANP) is secreted by atrial monocytes in response to local stretching of the atrial wall in cases of hypervolemia (e.g., congestive heart failure or renal failure) and ultimately results in reduction of intravascular volume and systemic blood pressure (Brenner et al., 1990). In the kidney, ANP acts in the medullary collecting duct to inhibit sodium reabsorption during ECF expansion. ANP induces hyperfiltration, natriuresis, and suppression of renin release and inhibits receptor-mediated aldosterone biosynthesis (Greger, 2000). In the cardiovascular system, it diminishes cardiac output and stroke volume and reduces peripheral vascular resistance. Some of these effects are mediated through the influence of ANP on vagal and sympathetic nerve activity.

BODY FLUID COMPARTMENTS

The internal environment of the body consists of fluids contained within compartments. Water accounts for 50% to 80% of the human body by weight. The variation in water content depends on tissue type: adipose tissue contains only 10% water, whereas muscle contains 75% water. Total body water (TBW) decreases with age, mainly as a result of loss of water in ECF. For clinical purposes, TBW is estimated at 60% of body weight in infants after 6 months of postnatal age, as well as in children and adolescents. This value is very inaccurate for low-birth-weight premature infants in whom TBW comprises as much as 80% of total body weight (Friis-Hansen, 1971; Kagan, 1972). In term infants under 6 months of age, TBW may be approximated as 75% of total body weight (Hill, 1990). Newer formulas that consider the height (cm) and weight (kg) but not the degree of

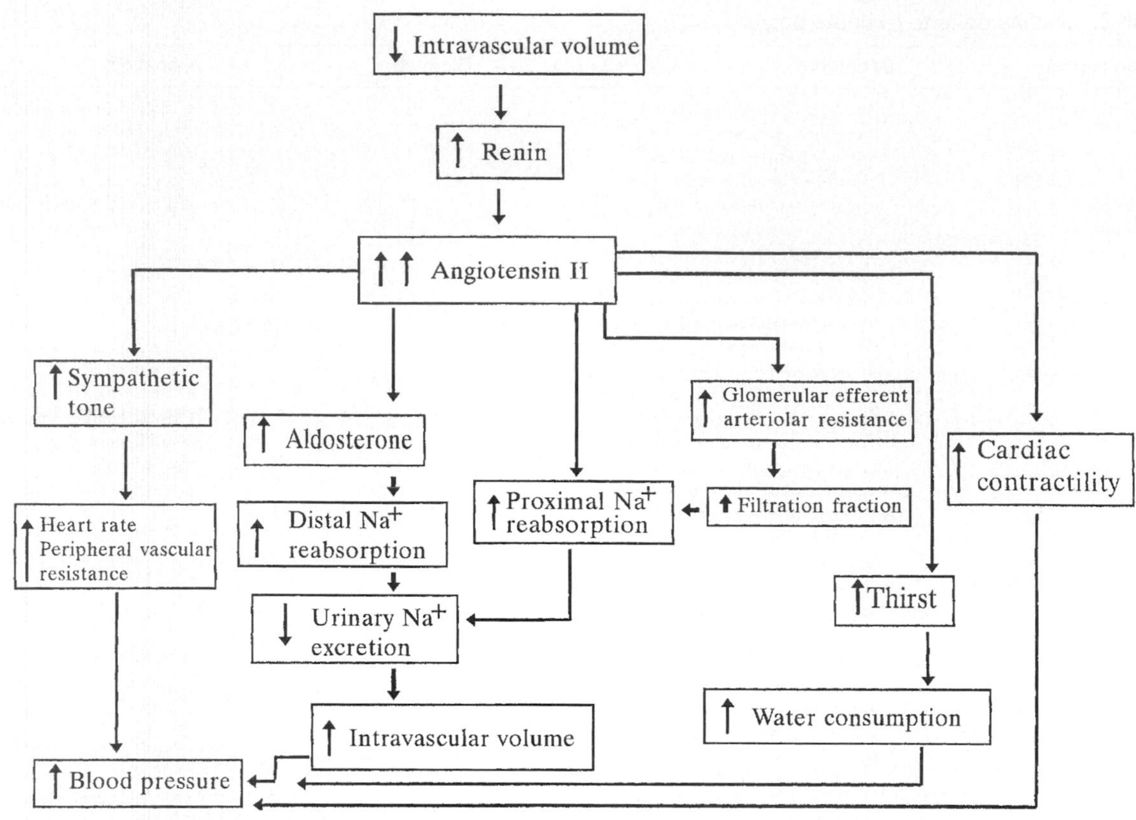

■ **FIGURE 4–3.** Effect of decreased intravascular volume on the renin-angiotensin-aldosterone system.

BOX 4–1 Effects of Angiotensin II Mediated via AT_1 and AT_2 Receptor Stimulation

AT_1 Receptor Stimulation

Vasoconstriction (preferentially coronary, renal, cerebral)
Sodium retention (angiotensin, aldosterone production)
Water retention (vasopressin release)
Renin suppression (negative feedback)
Myocyte and smooth muscle cell hypertrophy
Stimulation of vascular and myocardial fibrosis
Inotropic/contractile (cardiomyocytes)
Chronotropic/arrhythmogenic (cardiomyocytes)
Stimulation of plasminogen activator inhibitor-1
Stimulation of superoxide formation
Activation of sympathetic nervous system
Increased endothelin secretion

AT_2 Receptor Stimulation

Antiproliferation/inhibition of cell growth
Cell differentiation
Tissue repair
Apoptosis
Possible vasodilation
Kidney and urinary-tract development

Modified from Burnier M, Brunner HR: Angiotensin II receptor antagonists. *Lancet* 355:637–645, 2000, p 639, Panel 4. With permission from Elsevier.

adiposity or the child's surface area have improved the estimation of TBW particularly in healthy children between 3 months and 13 years of age (Fig. 4–4) (Mellits and Cheek, 1970; Morgenstern, 2002). TBW can be determined as follows:

$$0 \text{ to } 3 \text{ months: TBW} = 0.887 \times (\text{Wt})^{0.83}$$

$$\text{Children 4 to 13 years: TBW} = 0.0846 \times 0.95^{[\text{if female}]} \times (\text{Ht} \times \text{Wt})^{0.65}$$

$$\text{Children over 13 years: TBW} = 0.0758 \times 0.84^{[\text{if female}]} \times (\text{Ht} \times \text{Wt})^{0.69}$$

Intracellular Fluid

Intracellular fluid (ICF) represents about two thirds of the TBW, which is equivalent to 30% to 40% of total body weight. However, the proportion of ECF is much greater than that of ICF in preterm infants and reaches 60% of TBW at term. The membranes retaining this fluid allow the passive diffusion of water, whereas active transport mechanisms maintain an internal solute milieu different from that found outside the cells. K^+, P^{2-}, and Mg^{2+} are intracellular ions, and Na^+ and Cl^- are predominantly extracellular.

Extracellular Fluid

ECF accounts for about one third of TBW and is made up of two compartments: plasma and interstitial fluid. Plasma water represents 4% to 5% of body weight and 10% of TBW. It is the milieu in which blood cells, platelets, and proteins are suspended. Blood volume is usually estimated as a changing proportion,

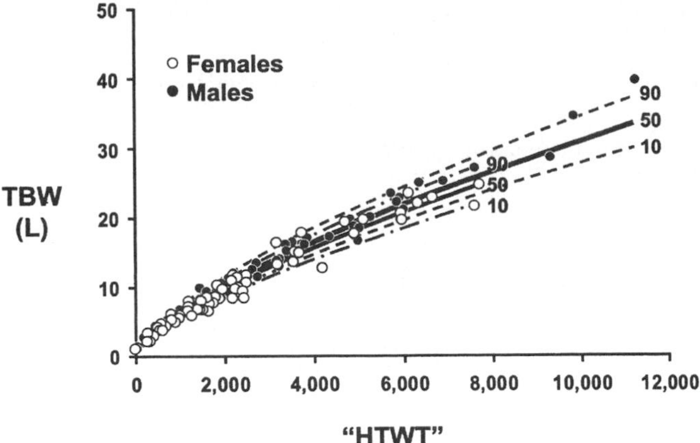

■ **FIGURE 4–4.** Total body water (TBW) plotted against the parameter (Ht × Wt) for children from 3 months to 13 years of age. The 10th, 50th, and 90th percentile curves, generated from the equations in the text, are shown. The curves for both males and females are presented. (From Morgenstern BZ, Mahoney DW, Warady BA: Estimating total body water in children on the basis of height and weight: A reevaluation of the formulas of Mellits and Cheek. *J Am Soc Nephrol* 13:1884–1888, 2002, p 186, Figure 2.)

with respect to body weight. When expressed as milliliters per kilogram of body weight, it decreases with age from 80 mL/kg at birth to 60 mL/kg in adulthood.

Interstitial Fluid

This accounts for 16% of body weight and has a solute composition almost identical to that of intravascular fluid except for a lower protein concentration. In general, the bulk distribution of ions and fluids between these two compartments is determined by the Donnan effect and Starling forces.

Transcellular Fluid

The transcellular fluid compartment (1% to 3% of body weight) is a specialized subdivision of the ECF compartment. Separated from blood by endothelium and epithelium, it represents fluid collections such as cerebrospinal fluid, aqueous and vitreous humors of the eye, synovial fluid, pleural fluid, and peritoneal fluid.

■ MATURATION OF RENAL FUNCTION

Although all nephrons of the mature kidney are formed by 36 weeks of gestation of normal intrauterine life, hyperplasia continues until the sixth postnatal month; thereafter, cell hypertrophy is responsible for increase in renal size. Growth in the size of the kidney tends to be directly proportional to increase in height (Schultz et al., 1962).

While the fetal kidney receives 3% to 7% of cardiac output (Rudolph et al., 1971), RBF increases gradually after birth. RBF, as measured by *para*-aminohippuric acid (PAH) clearance (C_{PAH}), correlates with gestational age. For example, C_{PAH} is 10 mL/min per m^2 at 28 weeks of gestation and 35 mL/min per m^2 at 35 weeks of gestation (Fawer et al., 1979). C_{PAH} corrected for body surface area doubles by 2 weeks of age and reaches adult levels at 2 years. Furthermore, changes in RBF are associated with considerable increases in the relative RBF to the outer cortex where most glomeruli are located (Olbing et al., 1973).

Selected renal functions measured at different ages are summarized in Table 4–3. The GFR in the full-term newborn infant averages 40.6 ± 14.8 mL/min per 1.73 m^2 and increases to 65.8 ± 24.8 mL/min per 1.73 m^2 by the end of the second postnatal week (Schwartz et al., 1987). GFR reaches adult levels after 2 years of age. Premature newborns have a lower GFR that increases more slowly than that in full-term infants. The low GFR at birth is attributed to the low systemic arterial blood pressure, high renal vascular resistance, and low ultrafiltration pressure together with decreased capillary surface area for filtration.

Despite a low GFR, full-term infants are able to conserve Na^+ (Spitzer, 1982). This is explained by the existence of glomerulotubular balance such that as GFR and the filtered load of Na^+ increase, so does the ability of the proximal tubule to reabsorb Na^+. In contrast, premies have a prolonged glomerulotubular imbalance so that GFR is high relative to tubular capacity to reabsorb Na^+. The glomerulotubular imbalance is caused by structural immaturity of the proximal convoluted tubule and the incomplete development of the transport system responsible for conserving Na^+. This, together with poor response of the distal tubule to mineralocorticoids in premies, results in Na^+ wastage and susceptibility to hyponatremia.

The tubular mechanisms involved in the excretion of organic acids are poorly developed in neonates. The tubular transport of PAH, which is a weak acid, is around 16 ± 5 mg/min per 1.73 m^2 in full-term infants and about half this value in premature babies. It increases with age and reaches adult rates ranging from 55 to 104 mg/min per 1.73 m^2 by 12 to 18 months (Spitzer, 1978). PAH excretion is limited by a number of factors, including low GFR, immaturity of the systems providing energy for transport, and low number of transporter molecules. This is further accentuated by a low extraction ratio for PAH and other organic acids caused by the predominance of juxtamedullary circulation in the immature kidney (Calcagno and Rubin, 1963),

■ **TABLE 4–3.** Maturation of renal function with age

Measurement	Premature Newborn	Full-term Newborn	1 to 2 Weeks	6 Months to 1 Year	1 to 3 Years	Adult
GFR (mL/min per 1.73 m^2)	14 ± 3	40.6 ± 14.8	65.8 ± 24.8	77 ± 14	96 ± 22	Male: 125 ± 15 Female: 110 ± 15
RBF (mL/min per 1.73 m^2)	40 ± 6	88 ± 4	220 ± 40	352 ± 73	540 ± 118	620 ± 92
Tm_{PAH} (mg/min per 1.73 m^2)	10 ± 2	16 ± 5	38 ± 8	51 ± 20	66 ± 19	79 ± 12
Maximal concentration ability (mOsm/kg)	480	700	900	1200	1400	1400
Serum creatinine (mg/dL)	1.3	1.1	0.4	0.2	0.4	0.8 to 1.5
Tm_P/GFR (mg/dL)	—	7.39 ± 0.37	—	5.58 ± 0.28	5.71 ± 0.28	3.55 ± 19
Fractional excretion of sodium (%)	2% to 6%	<1	<1	<1	<1	<1
Tm_G (mg/min per 1.73 m^2)	—	—	71 ± 20	—	—	339 ± 51

Tm_G, tubular maximum for reabsorption of glucose; GFR, glomerular filtration rate; RBF, renal blood flow; Tm_{PAH}, tubular maximum for para-aminohippuric acid; Tm_P, tubular maximum for phosphorus.

a phenomenon that allows increased shunting of blood through the vasa recta and exclusion of postglomerular blood from the proximal tubular excretory surface.

Concentrating ability is low at birth, especially in premature infants. After water deprivation in the full-term newborn, urine concentrates to only 600 to 700 mOsm/kg, or 50% to 60% of maximum adult levels. Healthy children 0.5 to 3 years of age given 20 mcg of desmopressin intranasally demonstrate a gradual rise in urinary concentration starting from a mean value of 525 mOsmol/kg and reach a mean maximum plateau of 825 mOsm/kg (Marild et al., 1992). The major cause for the reduced concentration of urine in the neonate is the hypotonicity of the renal medulla (Aperia and Zetterstrom, 1982). Several mechanisms that contribute to interstitial hypertonicity are not well developed, including urea accumulation in the medulla (Trimble, 1970), length of the loop of Henle and the collecting ducts within the medulla (Edwards, 1981), and Na^+ reabsorption in the ascending, water-impermeable loop (Horster, 1978). In addition, the collecting duct cells in immature kidneys may be less sensitive to ADH than those of mature nephrons (Schlondorff et al., 1978).

A water-loaded infant can excrete dilute urine with osmolality as low as 50 mOsm/kg. In the first 24 hours of life, however, the infant may be unable to increase water excretion to approximate water intake (Aperia and Zetterstrom, 1982). The diluting capacity becomes mature by 3 to 5 weeks of postnatal life.

TABLE 4–4. Average fluid need of low-birth-weight infants (mL/kg per 24 hr) during first week of life*

Age (days)	Component	Body weight (gm) 751 to 1000	1001 to 1250	1251 to 1500	1501 to 2000
1	IWL†	65	55	40	30
	Urine‡	20	20	30	30
	Stool	0	0	0	0
	Total	85	75	70	60
2 to 3	IWL	65	55	40	30
	Urine	40	40	40	40
	Stool	0	0	0	5
	Total	105	95	80	75
4 to 7	IWL	65	55	40	30
	Urine	60	60	60	60
	Stool	5	5	5	5
	Total	130	120	105	95

*Allowances for increased metabolic rate (cold stress, increased activity) are not included; these infants are in an incubator and naked.

†Insensible water loss.

‡Volume required to achieve a urine osmolarity of 250 mOsm/kg of renal solute load during the first day (no sodium and protein added), 10 mOsm/kg per day on the second and third days, and 15 mOsm/kg per day on the fourth to seventh days.

FLUID AND ELECTROLYTE NEEDS IN HEALTHY INFANTS AND CHILDREN

The normal need for fluids varies markedly in low-birth-weight and full-term neonates, as well as during infancy and later childhood. This variability in fluid needs is caused by differences in the rate of caloric expenditure and growth, the ratio of evaporative surface area to body weight, the degree of renal functional maturation and reserve, and the amount of total body water (TBW) at different ages. For instance, compared with older children and adults, infants have greater fluid needs because of higher rates of metabolism and growth; a surface area-to-weight ratio that is about three times greater, resulting in higher insensible fluid loss; and greater urinary excretion of solutes combined with lower tubular concentrating ability, which increases obligatory fluid loss. On the other hand, as previously noted, low-birth-weight and full-term neonates have a greater percentage of TBW compared with older children and adults (Friis-Hensen, 1971; Kagan et al., 1972). This increase in TBW results mainly from expansion of the ECF compartment, which at birth may comprise as much as 50% of the TBW. During the first 3 postnatal days, when this "extra fluid" is eliminated by the kidneys, full-term neonates require less fluid intake (Silverman, 1961; Oh, 1980; Winters, 1982).

The needs of low-birth-weight infants are more variable (Table 4–4) and may be markedly altered by relatively minor changes in ambient temperature or by phototherapy (Fanaroff et al., 1972; Oh and Karecki, 1972; Wu and Hodgman, 1974). In contrast to more mature infants, the immature skin in very low-birth-weight infants (<1500 g) allows disproportionate evaporative heat loss relative to basal metabolic rate (Levine et al., 1929; Levinson et al., 1966). This greater evaporative heat loss, together with a large body surface area, accounts for the much greater insensible fluid needs in infants with very low birth weight.

PARENTERAL AND ORAL FLUIDS AND ELECTROLYTES

Except for the first 3 postnatal days when full-term neonates require only 40 to 60 mL/kg fluid per day, in general, 100 mL of water is needed for each 100 kcal expended. Notably, an additional 15 mL of water is generated endogenously for each 100 kcal used (water of oxidation), which is also available for body functions. In premies, fluid intake may be gradually increased to 150 mL/kg per day, while 100 to 125 mL/kg per day generally suffices for infants weighing less than 10 kg. The fluid requirement decreases to 50 mL/kg per day for those weighing 11 to 20 kg and to 20 mL/kg per day for those with body weight above 20 kg. These fluid volumes are sufficient to allow excretion of dietary solute load, as well as to replace insensible fluid loss through the skin, lungs, and intestines (Winters, 1982) (Table 4–5). It should be noted that energy expenditure and, therefore, fluid intake may be significantly increased with stress (Holliday et al., 1994) (Table 4–6).

The high fractional excretion of Na^+ (FE_{Na^+}) in premature infants can lead to negative Na^+ balance, hyponatremia, neurologic disturbances, and poor growth unless an Na^+ intake of 3 to 5 mmol/kg per day is given; in full-term infants and older children, 2 to 3 mmol/kg per day is sufficient (Drukker et al., 1980). Premature infants have a lower renal threshold for bicarbonate. In addition, several functional and anatomic factors combine to limit tubular excretion of weak organic acids (Avner et al., 1990). Consequently, premature infants may need small supplements of base. Sodium bicarbonate at 1 to 2 mmol/kg per day is generally recommended for the very small premature infant. Clinically important disturbances in acid-base status are unusual in full-term neonates unless they consume excessive amounts of protein.

TABLE 4–5. Normal losses and maintenance requirements for fluid, electrolytes, and dextrose in infants and children

H_2O = 100 to 125 mL/100 kcal Expended		
Components:	Insensible loss (mL)	45
	Sweat (mL)	0 to 25
	Urine (mL)	50 to 75
	Stool (mL)	5 to 10
	Food oxidation (mL)	12
Na^+ = 2.5 mmol/100 kcal Expended		
Components:	Body growth	
	Sweat	Variable
	Urine	Variable
	Stool	Variable
K^+ = 2.5 mmol/100 kcal Expended		
Components:	As for Na^+	
Cl^- = 5 mmol/100 kcal Expended		
Components:	As for Na^+	
Dextrose = 25 g/100 kcal Expended		
Components:	Basal metabolic rate	
	Growth and tissue repair	
	Physical activity	
Maintenance Solution (per liter of water)		
Dextrose (g)		50
Na^+ (mmol)		25
K^+ (mmol)		25
Cl^- (mmol)		50

Adapted from Winters RW: *Principles of pediatric fluid therapy,* ed 2. Boston, 1982, Little, Brown.

DEHYDRATION IN INFANTS AND CHILDREN

Because premature infants and mature neonates have a greater TBW–to–body weight ratio than do older infants and children, they tolerate a greater degree of dehydration before manifesting clinical symptoms. A 10% fluid deficit in such patients may produce symptoms consistent with moderate dehydration, whereas a similar deficit in adults will produce severe symptoms. However, dehydration can occur very quickly in infants because disorders such as vomiting or diarrhea very rapidly produce deficits of 50 to 100 mL/kg. Dehydration can also develop in healthy premature infants if insensible water losses are underestimated and are not adequately replaced. This situation may result from use of an open radiant warmer without appropriate plastic shields; forced convection in nonhumidified incubators; skin immaturity, resulting in greater transcutaneous evaporative fluid loss; use of phototherapy, causing insensible fluid loss; hyperthermia; or tachypnea. In older infants and children, gastrointestinal disorders are the major causes of dehydration.

TABLE 4–6. Method to predict metabolic rates during critical illness

AVERAGE HOSPITAL ENERGY REQUIREMENTS		INCREASES IN ENERGY EXPENDITURE WITH STRESS	
Body Weight(kg)	*kcal/kg per day*		
0 to 10	100	Fever	12% per°C
10 to 20	1000 + 50/kg	Cardiac failure	>37°C
>20	1500 + 20/kg	Major surgery	15% to 25%
		Burns	20% to 30%
		Severe sepsis	Up to 100%
			40% to 50%

Modified from Holliday MA: Fluid and nutrition support. In Holliday MA, Barratt TM, Avner ED, editors: *Pediatric nephrology,* ed 3. Williams and Wilkins, 1994, Baltimore, p 301, Table 14B.5.

ASSESSMENT OF DEHYDRATION

Assessment of the extent and type of dehydration is important for formulating a therapeutic strategy. Table 4–7 provides guidelines for the clinical assessment of the severity of dehydration in children (Ellis and Avner, 1985). Laboratory measurements should include hematocrit, blood gases, glucose, calcium, blood urea nitrogen, and albumin, as well as serum and urinary creatinine, osmolality, and electrolytes. A urinalysis should be done to detect cellular elements and to measure specific gravity. Urinary osmolality and specific gravity are of minimal value in assessing dehydration in premature infants with tubular immaturity and in infants with reduced urinary concentrating ability caused by low protein intake. In general, however, such data, together with a careful medical history, physical examination, and assessment of fluid input and loss, aid in the diagnosis of dehydration and guide adjustment of the amount and composition of fluid administration during various phases of therapy.

TREATMENT OF DEHYDRATION

Severely dehydrated infants and children should be cared for in the intensive care unit with constant monitoring of central venous pressure and serial measurements of the initial laboratory studies. Box 4–2 shows a stepwise approach to the treatment of isotonic, hypotonic, and hypertonic dehydration (Ellis and Avner, 1985). Particular attention should be given to hypernatremic dehydration and brain injury. The initial measures for fluid resuscitation are to stabilize the vital signs by administering crystalloid or colloid solutions and to correct severe acid-base imbalance, hypoglycemia, and other metabolic disturbances. The objective of subsequent measures is to assess further the kind of dehydration and to plan a time course for administration of the appropriate fluid volume and chemical composition needed to correct previous deficits and to replace ongoing losses.

The composition of selected parenteral and oral rehydration solutions are shown in Tables 4–8 and 4–9. In most infants and children receiving parenteral solutions for brief periods, the normal fluid and electrolyte needs can be easily satisfied. The caloric needs, however, are not readily met. It is customary to provide 5% dextrose in parenteral solutions. While this concentration provides only a fraction of the optimal number of calories (20% of total kilocalories needed by infants less than 1 year of age), it is sufficient to prevent ketosis. In less mature neonates, higher infusion rates of 5% dextrose generally suffice to maintain blood glucose concentrations between 50 to 90 mg/dL (Roy and Sinclair, 1975; Winters, 1982).

Provided that infants and children are less than 10% dehydrated and have minimal electrolyte abnormalities, good level of consciousness, adequate bowel sounds, and absence of signs of hypovolemia, oral rehydration may be used to replace deficits and maintain fluid volume. Commercially available preparations such as Pedialyte RS (Ross) with a Na^+ content of 45 mmol/L may be used. In children with diarrhea in developing countries, the World Health Organization (WHO) has recommended

■ **TABLE 4–7.** Clinical and laboratory assessment of the severity of dehydration in children*

Signs and Symptoms	Mild Dehydration	Moderate Dehydration	Severe Dehydration
Weight loss (%)	5	10	15
Fluid deficit (mL/kg)	50	100	150
Vital signs			
Pulse	Normal	Increased; weak	Greatly increased; feeble
Blood pressure	Normal	Normal to low	Reduced and orthostatic
Respiration	Normal	Deep	Deep and rapid
General appearance			
Infants	Thirsty, restless, alert	Thirsty, restless, or lethargic, but arousable	Drowsy to comatose; limp, cold, sweaty; gray color
Older children	Thirsty, restless, alert	Thirsty, alert, postural hypotension	Usually comatose; apprehensive, cyanotic, cold
Skin turgor†	Normal	Decreased	Greatly decreased
Anterior fontanel	Normal	Sunken	Markedly depressed
Eyes	Normal	Sunken	Markedly sunken
Mucous membranes	Moist	Dry	Very dry
Urine			
Flow (mL/kg per hr)	<2	<1	<0.5
Specific gravity	1.020	1.020-1.030	>1.030

*When hypernatremia is present, the severity of dehydration may be clinically underestimated because of the relative preservation of extracellular fluid volume (ECFV) at the expense of intracellular fluid volume (ICFV). In such states, neurologic symptoms (lethargy alternating with hyperexcitability, progressing to focal or generalized seizures) may predominate.

†With hypernatremia, the skin may have a thick, "doughy" consistency or a soft, velvety texture.

the use of an inexpensive and effective oral rehydration solution consisting of 90 mmol/L Na^+ and 111 mmol/L of glucose (total osmolarity, 311 mOsmol/L). However, glucose-based solutions with a lower osmolality may further optimize fluid and glucose-sodium coupled absorption in the small intestine (Hahn et al., 2001).

■ PERIOPERATIVE PARENTERAL GUIDELINES OF FLUIDS AND ELECTROLYTES

The optimal perioperative fluid volume and composition requirements in infants and children have not been adequately investigated. The formulas provided by Berry (1986) (Table 4–10) are widely used to determine the hourly rates of intraoperative fluid volume administration, which consists of four major components:

1. Maintenance fluid established by Holliday and Segar (1957) based on calorie expenditure at different ages.
2. Estimated volume deficit incurred during preoperative fasting or gastrointestinal or by other fluid deficits; one third of such deficits may be replaced during the first hour of surgery while the remaining volume may be spread over the duration of the surgery.
3. Severity of surgical and nonsurgical trauma. This may comprise the largest volume of fluid loss or fluid redistribution, which derives largely from the ECF compartment.
4. Blood losses and fluids needed to support systemic blood pressure.

A key goal of perioperative fluid management is to maintain an adequate intravascular volume without the development of hyponatremia. Perioperative patients are at risk for developing hyponatremia because of multiple factors, including prehydration with hypotonic fluid, and nausea, pain, and stress associated with surgery, that may lead to nonhypovolemic stimulation of ADH release during and after surgery (i.e., inappropriate secretion of ADH; Burrows et al., 1983; Arieff, 1998). The limited ability of such individuals to excrete a large water load may be influenced by any preexisting edema-forming disorder, obstructive uropathy, or the use of thiazide diuretics or other drugs such as narcotics and antiemetics. However, hypotonic fluid infusion is the single most important cause of acute hyponatremia developing in the intraoperative period. Acute hyponatremia results in increased water content in neurons (brain edema) without a change in solute content. This may cause subclinical symptoms such as headache, nausea, vomiting, or muscle weakness in any age group. Younger children are more susceptible to more severe hyponatremic encephalopathy due to a larger brain-to-skull ratio (Moritz and Ayus, 2002). Unless there is a free water deficit, isotonic fluid infusion is recommended during the perioperative period. The need for potassium, calcium, chloride, and bicarbonate (or lactate or citrate, which may be converted to bicarbonate in individuals without hepatic failure) is more controversial. Such components are contained in lactated Ringer's solution, which is nearly isonatremic (Na^+ = 130 mEq/L) and isotonic but also contains K^+ (4 mEq/L), Ca^{2+} (0.9 mmol/L), Cl^- (109 mEq/L), and lactate (27.7 mmol/L).

The amount of dextrose commonly used is 5% (equals 5000 mg/dL or 278 mmol/L). Although this is more than 50 times more concentrated than normal plasma glucose concentration (90 to 100 mg/dL or ≈5 mmol/L), the energy delivery based on the volume of fluid given to an infant weighing 10 kg amounts to 50 kcal for the first hour of surgery. Such energy supply is particularly important in preventing hypoglycemia in premature and full-term neonates who have greater energy requirements than older children, but may lead to hyperglycemia in 0.5% to 2% of pediatric patients. This disorder may be less common in children receiving regional anesthesia, which reduces the hyperglycemic effects of surgery per se. Although such transient hyperglycemia is purported to have various potential deleterious consequences, these have not been well substantiated. A review suggests that a solution of lactated Ringer's with 1% dextrose is sufficient to prevent both hypoglycemia and hyperglycemia (Berleur et al., 2003) in most children excluding premature and term neonates. This practice, however, is not yet widely used.

BOX 4–2 Stepwise Approach to Fluid Therapy in Infants and Young Children With Moderate (100 mL/kg) to Severe (150 mL/kg) Dehydration*

Phase I (0 to 4 hr)

1. Assess vital signs and body weight, approximate fluid deficit, and begin fluid balance sheet.
2. Obtain blood for immediate chemical and acid-base analysis and, if possible, obtain a urine sample for chemical and microscopic determinations.
3. Regardless of the type of dehydration (see below), begin immediately with 0.9% NaCl at 20 to 30 mL/kg given over 1 hr or faster, depending on the severity of circulatory compromise. If the major cause of dehydration is diarrhea, a mixture of 0.45% NaCl and 0.45% $NaHCO_3$ is preferred as the initial hydrating solution. If shock is present, administer 5% salt-poor albumin (10 mL/kg).
4. Stabilize vital signs by repeating step 3 if needed, and continue fluid administration at 10 mL/kg per hr until urine output is established.
5. On the basis of serum electrolyte values, determine the type of dehydration. Also, make a more precise assessment of the total fluid deficit and proceed to phase II.

Phase II (4 hr to 2 days)

1. Repeat phase I, steps 1 and 2.
2. Isotonic dehydration (serum $[Na^+]$ = 130 to 150 mmol/L).
   a. Replace 60% to 70% of the remaining fluid deficit over the next 24 hr using a solution containing 0.45% NaCl with 20 mmol/L KCl and 50 g/L dextrose; add 20 mmol $NaHCO_3$/L if serum pH is <7.25. Replace maintenance fluid plus continued fluid loss using the same solution.
   b. Replace remainder of fluid deficit over subsequent 24 hr, in addition to maintenance fluid and ongoing fluid loss, with solution containing 0.2% NaCl with 20 mmol KCl and 50 g/L dextrose.
   c. Additional dextrose, K^+, or HCO_3^- may be needed and is added according to serial serum measurements.
3. Hypotonic dehydration (serum $[Na^+]$ < 130 mmol/L).
   a. Estimate Na^+ deficit as follows: $[Na^+]$ deficit (mmol) = (135 – Serum $[Na^+]$) × Total body water (L). Replace 60% of fluid deficit over the next 24 hr using a similar choice of solution as in phase I, step 3, plus 5% to 10% dextrose. If serum $[Na^+]$ is <120 mmol/L or symptoms of water intoxication are present, give 12 mL/kg of 3% saline solution over 1 hr. During this period, replace maintenance fluid and ongoing fluid loss with the solution noted in phase II, step 2b.
   b. Same as for phase II, step 2b.
   c. Same as for phase II, step 2c.
4. Hypertonic dehydration (serum $(Na^+]$ > 150 mmol/L).
   a. Add fluid deficit, 48 hr of maintenance water, and estimate of continued fluid loss to determine total volume of fluid to be administered initially at a constant rate over 48 hr.
   b. Use a solution containing 0.2% NaCl with 40 mmol KCl/L and 25 g/L dextrose.
   c. Add 20 mmol lactate or acetate if plasma pH is <7.25. (Do not use $NaHCO_3$, since calcium may need to be added to the fluid.)
   d. If serum calcium level is <8.5 mg/dL, add 1 g calcium gluconate to every 500 mL of administered fluid. Additional calcium is administered as required by serial serum values or clinical symptoms of hypocalcemia. Discontinue when serum calcium level is ≥9.0 mg/dL.
   e. If serum $[Na^+]$ is decreasing at 0.50 mmol/L per hr, decrease rate of administration by 30% to 50%. If serum $[Na^+]$ is decreasing at <0.25 mmol/L per hr, increase rate of fluid administration by 30% to 50%.

Phase III (3 to 6 days)

1. Same as for phase I, steps 1 and 2.
2. Replace any residual fluid or solute deficits over the next 2 to 4 days using the solution described in phase II, step 2b.
3. For severe hypertonic dehydration (serum $[Na^+]$ >175 mmol/L), phase II therapy is continued for 3 to 4 days and subsequently may be switched to phase III therapy, step 2, when serum $[Na^+]$ is <145 mmol/L.

*For mild dehydration (50 mL/kg), requiring parenteral fluid therapy, start therapy with phase II.

PERIOPERATIVE FLUID MANAGEMENT OF PREMATURE AND TERM NEONATES

Guidelines for the intraoperative fluid and electrolyte management of premature and term neonates are largely based on available knowledge of renal physiology rather than on data obtained from clinical investigation. The physiology of the healthy neonate is influenced by the short tubular length and is characterized by immature reabsorption mechanisms, an activated renin-angiotensin-aldosterone system, and low circulating ADH concentrations (Avner et al., 1990; El-Dahr and Chevalier, 1990). Thus, healthy preterm neonates weighing less than 1300 g, or of less than 32 weeks' gestation, have fractional excretion rates of Na^+ (FE_{Na^+}) that range from 8.2% to 2.1% from 28 to 32 weeks' gestation, with further gradual decrease to less than 1% at term (Arant, 1978; Delgado et al., 2003); such rates may increase to 15% with stress. The high FE_{Na^+} in preterm infants is ascribed to decreased Na^+ reabsorption in the proximal tubule together with hyporesponsiveness of the distal tubule to aldosterone (Sulyok et al., 1979). When combined with a negative Na^+ balance due to inadequate Na^+ supplementation as well as decreased sensitivity of the collecting duct to ADH, up to one third of such infants develop significant hyponatremia (Na^+ < 130 mEq/L), often manifesting with neurologic

■ **TABLE 4–8.** Composition of frequently used parenteral fluids

Liquid	CHO (g/100 mL)	Prot.* (g/100 mL)	Cal/L	Na^+ (mEq/L)	K^+ (mEq/L)	Cl^- (mEq/L)	HCO_3^-† (mEq/L)	Ca^{2+} (mg/dL)	P‡ (mg/dL)
D_5W	5	—	170	—	—	—	—	—	—
$D_{10}W$	10	—	340	—	—	—	—	—	—
Normal saline (0.9% NaCl)	—	—	—	154	—	154	—	—	—
½ Normal saline (0.45% NaCl)	—	—	—	77	—	77	—	—	—
D_5 (0.2% NaCl)	5	—	170	34	—	34	—	—	—
3% Saline	—	—	—	513	—	513	—	—	—
8.4% Sodium bicarbonate (1 mEq/mL)	—	—	—	1000	—	—	1000	—	—
Ringer's	0 to 10	—	0 to 340	147	4	155.5	—	4.5	—
Ringer's lactate	0 to 10	—	0 to 340	130	4	109	28	3	—
Amino acid 8.5% (Travasol)	—	8.5	340	3	—	34	52	—	—
Plasmanate	—	5	200	110	2	50	29	—	—
Albumin 25% (Salt poor)	—	25	1000	150 to 160	—	<120	—	—	—
Intralipid	2.25	—	1100	2.5	0.5	4.0	—	—	0.8

*Protein or amino acid equivalent.
†Bicarbonate or equivalent (citrate, acetate, lactate).
‡Approximate values: actual values may vary somewhat in various localities depending on electrolyte composition of water supply used to reconstitute solution. Values are approximate—may vary from lot to lot.
Modified from DeYoung L, Patterson J, Johns Hopkins Hospital, Children's Medical and Surgical Center: *The Harriet Lane handbook: A manual for pediatric house officers*, ed 14. Mosby, 1996, p 234, Table 11.18.

disturbances during the first 6 weeks of life (Roy and Sinclair, 1975).

Both premature and term neonates have a limited capacity to excrete K^+, possibly because of distal tubular insensitivity to aldosterone. Hence, baseline reference plasma K^+ concentrations range from 3.9 to 5.9 mEq/L. Moreover, both preterm and term neonates are capable of producing maximally dilute urine while concentrating capacity is limited. Yet, hyponatremia may develop after administration of large volumes of hypotonic fluids because fluid excretion may be limited mainly because of low GFR. Stress may cause profound reduction in GFR in premature and term neonates through release of various extrarenal vasoactive and hormonal substances that modify the response of "immature kidneys," thereby further disturbing fluid and electrolyte homeostasis. The higher body content of water and the higher metabolic rate, as well as a propensity to metabolic acidosis and hypocalcemia in premature newborns, are other important factors in deciding the volume and composition of intraoperative fluids.

Such considerations support the avoidance of boluses of hypotonic fluids while keeping in mind the lower age- and size-appropriate circulatory pressures that may serve as the goal of fluid management. In the absence of the expected physiologic fluid loss, which may range from 5% to 15% of body weight during the first 3 days of postnatal life, fluid volume during this time period may be limited to 60 mL/kg per day while blood pressure support may be sustained with small infusions (5 mL/kg) of 5% albumin or other blood products as needed. Beyond 3 days of life, maintenance fluid volume is gradually increased to 150 mL/kg per day. Deficits beyond the expected physiologic losses and ongoing losses and allowance for surgical

■ **TABLE 4–9.** Comparison of oral rehydration solutions and "clear fluids"

Product	Na^+	K^+	Cl^-	Base	CHO, g/L	Glucose/Na^+ Ratio	Osmolality
World Health Organization ORS	90	20	80	30	20	1.2	310
Pedialyte	45	20	35	30	25	3.1	250
Rehydralyte	75	20	65	30	25	1.6	305
Infalyte	50	25	45	10	30	—	200
Cereal-based ORT	90	20	80	30	50	—	175
Gatorade	23	3	17	3	46	11.1	330
Cola	2	2	0.1	13	120	—	750
Ginger ale	3	3	1	4	90	—	540
Apple juice	3	3	28	0	120	—	730
Chicken broth	250	8	250	0	0	—	450
Tea	0	5	0	0	0	—	5

ORS, oral rehydration solution.
Na^+, K^+, Cl^-, and base levels are measured in mmol/L.
Modified from Meyers A: Fluid and electrolyte therapy for children. *Curr Opin Pediatr* 6:303–309, 1994, p 305, Table 1.

TABLE 4–10. Guidelines for fluids for newborn and children during the perioperative period*

Age (yr)	Hydrating Solution During First Hour (mL/kg)	Hydrating Solution During Following Hours
Neonates		Maintenance fluid: 4 mL/kg per hr 5% to 10% dextrose in 0.75 normal saline plus 20 mEq sodium bicarbonate/L Trauma: 6 to 10 mL/kg per hr for intra-abdominal or 4 to 7 mL/kg per hr for intrathoracic surgery replaced with Ringer's lactate
<3	25	Maintenance fluid: 4 mL/kg per hr 5% Dextrose in normal saline
3 to 4	20	Maintenance and trauma: basic hourly fluid 4 mL/kg 5% Dextrose in normal saline + If mild trauma 2 mL/kg = 6 mL/kg per hr
>4	15	+ If moderate trauma 4 mL/kg = 8 mL/kg per hr + If maximal trauma 6 mL/kg = 10 mL/kg per hr

Modified from Berry FA: Practical aspects of fluid and electrolyte therapy. In Berry FA, editor: *Anesthetic Management of Difficult and Routine Pediatric Patients.* New York, 1986, Churchill Livingstone, pp 107–135.

*Plus blood replacement with blood or 3:1 volume replacement with crystalloid. Replace blood loss in excess of 20 mL/kg with equal volume of packed red blood cells.

trauma may be replaced by a similar fluid composition, but the volume replacement may be more gradual or less rapid than outlined for older infants and children (see Table 4–10). Na^+ bicarbonate and calcium may be supplemented, while K^+ should be limited. Also, a higher glucose concentration is generally desirable in premature infants. My preferred fluid composition is 0.75 normal saline with 20 mEq sodium bicarbonate/L (total Na^+ = 135 mmol/L) in 5% to 10% dextrose, as well as 20 mEq/L KCl if plasma K^+ falls below 3.5 mEq/L. Close attention to change in body weight and urine output and serial measurements of plasma electrolytes are essential in guiding the perioperative fluid management of the sick premature and full-term neonate.

FLUID MANAGEMENT OF CHILDREN UNDERGOING RENAL TRANSPLANTATION

The key goal of intraoperative management is to expand the circulatory volume and to maintain systemic blood pressure between the 90th and 95th percentile for age gender and height percentile (Update on the 1987 Task Force Report on High Blood Pressure in Children and Adolescents, 1996), so as to allow for adequate perfusion of the renal allograft. An adult kidney may sequester up to 250 mL of blood, and in infants, nearly 50% of the cardiac output may be directed toward perfusion of the allograft. To ensure adequate perfusion of the allograft the anesthesiologist actually needs to maximize the circulatory volume of the recipient, mainly with crystalloid or packed cytomegalovirus-safe, leukocyte-poor red blood cells if hemoglobin is below 9 g/dL, while closely monitoring the central venous pressure (CVP) and systemic MABP during vessel anastomosis. Near the completion of the vascular anastomoses, 20% mannitol (0.5 to 1.0 g/kg) and intravenous furosemide, 1 mg/kg, may be given before the cross-clamps are released. Before cross-clamp release, CVP should be maintained at 8 to 12 cm H_2O, and the systolic blood pressure and MABP above 120 mm and 70 mm Hg, respectively. If the MABP is inadequate to achieve good renal perfusion of the adult kidney, a constant dopamine infusion of up to 5 mcg/kg per min may be started. Intraoperative blood gases may be monitored frequently, because clamping of the aorta and accumulation of lactic acid can result in metabolic acidosis and vasoconstriction. The critical goal is to obtain immediate allograft function; hypotension after cross-clamp release in an infant with inadequate circulatory volume and an underperfused allograft is a potential catastrophe.

Intravenous furosemide (1 to 2 mg/kg per dose), 25% salt-poor albumin (0.5 g/kg per dose), 20% mannitol (0.3 to 0.5 g/kg per dose), or 0.9 normal saline solution (10 mL/kg bolus) may be given to help promote urine output in the immediate postoperative period.

The volume and composition of intravenous fluid administered during the first 48 postoperative hours are essential to ensure continued renal function. The urine output frequently exceeds 5 mL/kg per hr. Thus, insensible losses are quantitatively less important. In children with such high urine output, we routinely reduce the concentration of dextrose to 1% to prevent hyperglycemia, which may compound osmotic diuresis due to high preoperative blood urea nitrogen concentrations. Urine output is replaced on a milliliter-for-milliliter basis. In infants and children with body weight below 30 kg, the CVP should be maintained in the range of 5 to 10 cm H_2O and MABP greater than 70 mm Hg. Our preferred fluid solution during the first 24–48 hours consists of 1% dextrose, 0.45 mEq/L NaCl solution, and 10 to 20 mEq sodium bicarbonate per liter. During the first 24 to 36 hours, additional fluid boluses of 10 mL/kg of normal saline or a 5% albumin solution may be given if CVP falls below 5 cm H_2O with the goal of maintaining a urine output above certain arbitrary limits (5, 4, and 3 mL/kg per hr for body weight <10 kg, <20 kg, and <30 kg, respectively). In conjunction with such fluid boluses, we also administer intravenous furosemide (1 mg/kg) because renal allografts tend to be diuretic dependent in the early perioperative setting.

Serum electrolytes (Na^+, K^+, Cl^-, HCO_3^-, Ca^{2+}, P^{2-}, Mg^{2+}) may be monitored at 8- to 12-hour intervals during the first 2 postoperative days. Potassium chloride is given separately as needed when the plasma K^+ falls below 3.5 mEq/L. In infants and young children, close monitoring of fluid balance and cardiovascular examination are essential to prevent electrolyte imbalance and fluid overload, which may result in severe hypertension or pulmonary edema, or, in reduction of intravascular volume and acute tubular necrosis (ATN). A bladder catheter inserted intraoperatively is necessary for accurate measurement of urine volume. Unless there are specific urologic indications, the catheter is removed after 4 to 5 days.

Immediate measures must be undertaken to improve postoperative oliguria. Besides the most easily correctable causes of oliguria such as hypovolemia or a malfunctioning catheter, other potential causes include vascular bleeding or occlusion, ATN due to prolonged cold ischemia storage, hyperacute rejection, or urinary extravasation or obstruction. In patients with oxalosis, precipitation of calcium oxalate crystals in the graft may cause acute allograft failure. Children with delayed graft function, congestive heart failure, or marked electrolyte abnormalities may require removal of fluid by hemodialysis or peritoneal dialysis. Fluid removal should be performed cautiously to avoid allograft hypoperfusion.

DISORDERS OF SODIUM METABOLISM

Among the many kidney functions, sodium homeostasis via multiple or redundant systems is paramount (Greger, 2000). About 75% of the filtered Na^+ is reabsorbed in the proximal tubule by the luminal Na^+/H^+ exchanger and by the basolateral Na^+,K^+-ATPase. Such reabsorption is increased by the action of angiotensin II, which preferentially constricts the efferent arteriole, thereby increasing filtration fraction and limiting fluid reentry into the peritubular capillaries. Dopamine has an opposing effect in this tubule segment causing natriuresis. About 20% of NaCl reabsorption occurs in the ascending loop of Henle via the electroneutral $Na^+/K^+/2Cl^-$ transporter (NKCC2), leading to formation of dilute urine. Vasopressin and loop diuretics inhibit such reabsorption. In the distal tubule, Na^+ is reabsorbed by a thiazide-sensitive Na^+/Cl^- cotransporter. In the connecting tubule and in the cortical collecting duct, Na^+ is reabsorbed by the sodium-specific amiloride-sensitive epithelial sodium channel (ENaC). ENaC is activated by aldosterone. In the medullary collecting duct, Na^+ reabsorption is under the influence of ANP.

Much experimental evidence suggests that regulation of ECF volume and maintenance of systemic blood pressure prevail over Na^+ homeostasis; plasma Na^+ concentration and plasma osmolality are secondary regulators (Bricker, 1982; Rees et al., 1984; Gennari, 1998; Kumar and Berl, 1998; Scheinman et al., 1999). Thus, in the strict sense, virtually all of the conditions associated with hyponatremia are primarily disorders of ADH excess with an impaired ability to excrete free water. Disturbances in serum Na^+ concentration may be associated with hypervolemia, normovolemia, or hypovolemia.

HYPONATREMIA (Plasma Na^+ <135 mmol/L)

In infants and children, hyponatremia occurs much more frequently than hypernatremia. Although premature and full-term infants are capable of producing hypotonic urine, large hypotonic fluid loads cannot be excreted, especially during the first 6 weeks of postnatal life. This is most evident during the first week of life, when only 10% to 50%, rather than 80%, of an intravenous challenge of 5% dextrose in water is excreted within 4 hours. The major factor limiting the response to a fluid challenge, especially in preterm infants during the first 5 weeks of postnatal life, is the physiologically low GFR and low urinary flow rate (Svenningsen and Aronson, 1974; Leake et al., 1976). Moreover, high urinary Na^+ excretion and negative Na^+ balance may contribute to the hyponatremia found in about one third of low-birth-weight premature infants (Engelke et al., 1978). This Na^+ wasting has been attributed to deficient proximal and distal tubular reabsorption of Na^+ in such infants (Sulyok et al., 1979).

A positive water balance, rather than Na^+ wasting, has also been implicated in the hyponatremia of healthy premature infants (Rees et al., 1984; Sulyok et al., 1985). Low serum albumin concentrations and reduced plasma oncotic pressure may also lead to fluid retention and "late hyponatremia" in preterm infants (Menon et al., 1986). Thus, independent of the specific pathologic process, preterm infants are at high risk of developing hyponatremia. Therefore, electrolytes should be monitored frequently during the first 4 to 6 weeks of life, especially in infants of less than 34 weeks gestation. Other causes of hyponatremia in neonates are shown in Table 4–11. In older infants and children, hyponatremia may occur with dehydration, edema-forming states, and syndrome of inappropriate secretion of antidiuretic hormone (SIADH). Such conditions may be differentiated clinically at the bedside. In addition, the simple laboratory studies described in the section on dehydration may reveal urinary hypotonicity, suggesting water intoxication, or dilutional hyponatremia associated with renal failure.

Surgery and anesthesia stimulate ADH release. This may persist for 2 or more days and may result in acute hypotonic hyponatremia, particularly when hypotonic fluids are also administered. Even isotonic fluid administration may not prevent hyponatremia due to ADH release, because such individuals often excrete urine with sodium and potassium concentrations higher than plasma. This is partly because of high ANP concentrations that may coexist in this setting. The syndrome of SIADH is discussed separately.

Several causes of hyponatremia require special emphasis. Pseudohyponatremia is associated with normal plasma osmolality and occurs in the setting of severe hyperlipidemia, hyperproteinemia, or disorders in which solutes other than sodium such as glucose, mannitol, or sorbitol result in high plasma osmolality. Administration of thiazide diuretics to individuals with cardiac failure may impair distal tubular dilution of urine and the ability to excrete a water load. Finally, large amounts of hypotonic fluid intake during prolonged exercise can cause acute symptomatic hyponatremia and noncardiogenic pulmonary edema, particularly under high ambient temperatures when sweat sodium and chloride are high or when nonsteroidal anti-inflammatory agents are administered.

In hyponatremic patients who require parenteral fluids, the decision to correct the plasma Na^+ level may be based both on clinical symptoms and signs and on the rapidity with which the disorder developed. Children are especially prone to neurologic symptoms (Laureno and Karp, 1997; Lauriat and Berk, 1997; Albanese et al., 2001). In clinical practice, the most important prophylactic measure for preventing hyponatremia is to avoid the infusion of hypotonic fluids. Common symptoms and signs of hyponatremia include headache, fatigue, nausea, and vomiting; seizures and respiratory arrest are more severe and sometimes delayed manifestations. Guidelines for replacing such sodium deficits may be based on the following formula:

$$Na^+ \text{ deficit (mmol)} = \text{TBW} \times (\text{Desired} - \text{Actual plasma } Na^+)$$

For example, the amount of 3% saline solution needed to raise the plasma Na^+ to 125 mmol/L in a 10-kg infant with a plasma Na^+ concentration of 115 mmol/L (assuming that TBW is 65% of body weight) may be calculated as follows:

$$\text{TBW} = 0.65 \text{ TBW} \times 10 \text{ kg} = 6.5 \text{ L}$$

$$Na^+ \text{ deficit} = 6.5 \text{ L } (125 \text{ mmol/L} - 115 \text{ mmol/L}) = 65 \text{ mmol}$$

■ **TABLE 4–11.** Causes of hyponatremia

Neonates	Infants and Children
Drugs	
Prolonged use of diuretics in mother or infant Oxytocin for labor Dopamine >5 mcg/kg per min Prostaglandin infusion Excessive administration of electrolyte-free solutions	Diuretics (thiazides, osmotic diuretics) Arginine vasopressin Carbamazepine Vincristine Theophylline Cyclophosphamide Morphine Estrogen Barbiturates Nonsteroidal anti-inflammatory agents Mannitol Hypotonic 1.5% glycine irrigant Ecstasy Selective serotonin reuptake inhibitors All conditions listed for neonates
Endocrine Disorders	
Pseudohypoaldosteronism Adrenogenital syndrome Adrenal insufficiency problems Hypothyroidism SIADH due to asphyxia	Hyperglycemia Myxedema Glucocorticoid deficiency Decreased atrial natriuretic peptide Diabetes/ketonuria All conditions listed for neonates
Renal Disorders	
Dysplasia Multicystic kidneys Obstructive uropathy Polycystic kidney disease Renal tubular acidosis Acute or chronic renal failure	Nephrotic syndrome Acute or chronic renal failure Medullary cystic kidneys Nephronophthisis Chronic pyelonephritis Drug-induced tubulointerstitial nephritis Hypokalemic nephropathy Metabolic alkalosis Bicarbonaturia Postobstructive diuresis All conditions listed for neonates
Gastrointestinal Disorders	
Dilute formulas	Pancreatitis Cirrhosis Vomiting Diarrhea Ileus Bowel edema Protein-losing enteropathy Colonoscopy
Central Nervous System Disorders	
	SIADH Cerebral salt wasting Reset osmostat
Miscellaneous	
Negative Na^+ balance caused by high FE_{Na^+} in infants ≤34 weeks gestation Hypoalbuminemia and decreased oncotic pressure Osmotic diuresis caused by hyperalimentation and low Tm_G Ketonuria Congestive heart failure Hydrops fetalis Congenital nephrotic syndrome Surgery Infection Pulmonary disorders	Congestive heart failure "Third-space" from burns, peritonitis, or severe muscle injury Water intoxication (psychogenic polydipsia, dilute formulas) Physical and emotional stress Cystic fibrosis Pain Postoperative Porphyria Rickettsial disease Fresh-water drowning Pseudohyponatremia in patients with hypoproteinemia, hyperglycemia, or hyperlipidemia Prolonged exercise

CNS, central nervous system; FENa+, excreted fraction of filtered sodium; SIADH, syndrome of inappropriate antidiuretic hormone; TmG, tubular maximum for glucose reabsorption.

In asymptomatic children, the Na^+ deficit of 65 mmol may be replaced by 422 mL of normal saline (154 mmol/L) given over 24 hours; symptomatic children may receive 127 mL of 3% saline solution (513 mmol/L) given at a rate of about 5 mL/kg per hr, that is, 2.5 mmol/kg per hr.

With chronic hyponatremia (over 48 hours in duration), adaptive increases in neuronal osmolytes (glutamine, taurine, phosphocreatinine, myoinositol) diminish cellular uptake of water, hence preventing brain edema (Gullans and Verbalis, 1993). Thus, in contrast to acute hyponatremia, in which brain edema combined with noncardiogenic pulmonary edema and hypoxia can disrupt neuronal function, such events are uncommon with chronic hyponatremia. Edema-forming disorders such as nephrosis, liver failure, or congestive heart failure are frequently associated with chronic hyponatremia in children. Although physiologic mechanisms stimulate both sodium and fluid retention aimed at preventing hypovolemia, hypovolemic stimuli for ADH release result in free fluid retention and hyponatremia. Treatment includes the possible correction of the primary disorder, the elimination of diuretics and other offending agents, and limitation of electrolyte–free water intake. Because most individuals with chronic hyponatremia are asymptomatic, and because slow recovery of brain osmolytes coupled with iatrogenic correction of chronic hyponatremia can result in fatal or serious pontine and extrapontine myelinolysis, the rate of correction of serum sodium should be slow (about 0.3 mEq/L per hr) (Ayus, 1987; Adrogue and Madias, 2000a).

Syndrome of Inappropriate Secretion of Antidiuretic Hormone

Syndrome of inappropriate secretion of antidiuretic hormone (SIADH) is a diagnosis by exclusion. It is a hypo-osmolar, saline-resistant form of hyponatremia that occurs in the absence of dehydration, hypoadrenalism, renal failure, hypothyroidism, or myxedema. The nonhypovolemic and nonhypotonic release of ADH impairs the ability of the kidneys to excrete free water.

The main causes of SIADH in infants and children are shown in Box 4–3. Hyponatremia due to SIADH is uncommon in premature and full-term infants before 4 to 6 weeks of postnatal life because of factors that limit the urinary concentrating ability to values below 600 mOsm/kg. These factors include a low dietary solute intake, low circulating levels of ADH, and tubular hyporesponsiveness to endogenous ADH (Svenningsen and Aronson, 1974; Godard et al., 1979). Because of these circumstances, it is indeed difficult to establish the diagnosis of SIADH in such infants. In children with bacterial meningitis, ADH may be directly released through leaky, inflamed vessels, with secondary alterations in the blood-brain barrier. Despite the hyponatremia, mean plasma ADH levels are relatively high rather than suppressed (3.3 U/mL versus 1 U/mL) in such children, and SIADH develops in about 50% (Kaplan and Feigin, 1978).

The diagnosis of SIADH should be suspected in any child with asphyxia, meningitis, brain tumor, trauma, surgery, or pulmonary disease who does not appear dehydrated but has hyponatremia, hypochloremia, persistent natriuresis, decreased plasma osmolality (<270 mOsm/kg), and urine that is not maximally dilute (>100 mOsm/kg). The blood urea nitrogen (BUN) and plasma uric acid levels are frequently reduced.

Na^+ excretion in SIADH may vary depending on the extent of ECF expansion, which may raise the GFR and suppress aldosterone release. In addition, intravascular volume expansion stimulates the secretion of ANP, which enhances the renal excretion of Na^+. Moreover, Na^+ excretion will match or exceed Na^+ intake.

BOX 4–3 Disorders Associated With Syndrome of Inappropriate Secretion of Antidiuretic Hormone

Central Nervous System Disorders

Asphyxia in newborns (intraventricular hemorrhage in neonates, mask ventilation)
Encephalitis
Meningitis (viral, bacterial, tuberculous)
Cerebrovascular accident (stroke)
Postpituitary surgery
Brain tumors
Brain abscesses
Hydrocephalus
Head trauma
Guillain-Barré syndrome
Lupus cerebritis

Pulmonary Disorders

Atelectasis or pneumothorax in newborns
Positive pressure ventilation
Pneumothorax
Hyaline membrane disease
Pneumonia (viral, bacterial)
Abscess
Tuberculosis
Aspergillosis
Positive-airway pressure breathing
Ligation of patent ductus arteriosus

Medications

Vincristine
Cyclophosphamide
Carbamazepine
Selected serotonin reuptake inhibitors

The initial treatment of children with SIADH with a few or no symptoms may consist of restricting fluid intake to between one half and two thirds of the maintenance rate, or 800 to 1000 mL/m^2 per day. For severely symptomatic children, 3% saline may be given at a rate of 2.5 mmol/kg per hr, or 5 mL/kg per hr to maintain serum Na^+ concentrations at or above 125 mmol/L. In patients with urinary osmolality greater than 500 mOsm/kg, an alternative method for faster correction of severe hyponatremia is to use loop diuretics to inhibit reabsorption of free water while replacing measured urinary Na^+ losses. In young children, such treatment must be monitored especially closely to prevent volume contraction, hypokalemia, or acid-base imbalance. Furosemide at a dose of 1 mg/kg may be given intravenously one or two times daily. Other therapies used to manage adults with SIADH, such as osmotically active agents, dimethyl chlortetracycline, and lithium carbonate, are generally not used in children with this condition. V_{1a} and V_2 receptor blockers are newer agents that may soon become available and may be more effective in managing this disorder (Palm et al., 2001).

HYPERNATREMIA (Plasma Na^+ >145 mmol/L)

The causes of hypernatremia in infants and children are listed in Table 4-12. Hypernatremia commonly results from excessive water loss and inadequate water intake and occurs most frequently in individuals who are unable to communicate or satisfy their own thirst by accessing water. Thus, infants and debilitated

TABLE 4–12. Causes of hypernatremia

Hypernatremia Caused by Pure Water Loss
Inadequate water replacement of mucocutaneous fluid losses, especially in low-birth-weight infants or young children with fever and lack of access to water; phototherapy; or use of radiant warmers.
Central diabetes insipidus (low plasma ADH concentration)
Congenital thalamic/pituitary disorders
Acquired: trauma or tumor involving the thalamic/pituitary areas
Nephrogenic diabetes insipidus with failure of thirst response (high plasma ADH concentration)
Congenital distal tubular and collecting duct unresponsiveness to ADH
Biochemical: hypercalcemia, hypokalemia
Dietary: severe protein malnutrition or marked restriction in NaCl intake
Drug-induced: lithium carbonate, demeclocycline, amphotericin B
Anesthetic-induced: methoxyflurane
Hyperventilation

Hypernatremia Caused by Water Loss in Excess of Sodium Loss
Lactation failure (breast feeding)
Overdressing of neonates and infants
Neonates receiving phototherapy or kept in incubators without normothermal control
Diarrhea or colitis
Vomiting
Profuse sweating
Hyperosmolar nonketotic coma
Hypertonic dialysis
Renal disorders with partial diabetes insipidus or limited concentrating ability, including chronic renal failure, polycystic kidney disease, medullary cystic disease, pyelonephritis, obstructive uropathy, amyloidosis, and sickle cell nephropathy
High protein intake with high urea appearance rate
Diuretics: mannitol, furosemide

Hypernatremia Caused by Sodium Excess
Excess NaCl intake secondary to improper preparation of oral formulas or electrolyte solutions
Excessive administration of $NaHCO_3$
Ingestion of NaCl tablets, sea water, or near-drowning in sea water
Inadequate free fluid relative to NaCl intake because of defective thirst mechanism or unconsciousness
Cushing's syndrome or excessive administration of glucocorticoids
Hyperaldosteronism or excessive administration of mineralocorticoids.

individuals of any age are particularly susceptible to this disorder. A primary lack of thirst sensation is a very rare cause of this disorder in children. The condition has been caused by improper mixing of formulas and is also increasingly reported with inadequate breastfeeding (Manganaro et al., 2001; Oddie et al., 2001). It is also increasingly recognized as a complication in hospitalized very ill individuals with edema in association with renal failure, heart failure, hypotension, or liver failure resulting in impaired sodium excretion and sodium overload (Kahn, 1999; Adrogue and Madias, 2000). Administration of isotonic saline given to maintain systemic blood pressure together with associated hyperglycemia may promote hypernatremia in these settings. Also, the deliberate use of hypertonic saline for the treatment of brain edema has occasionally resulted in severe hypernatremia (Peterson et al., 2000).

Premature infants and full-term neonates are also prone to hypernatremia because, in addition to an inability to excrete a water load, they are unable to excrete a large solute load (Aperia et al., 1975a, 1975b, 1977). The renal response to an Na^+ load improves gradually, so that by the end of the first year of life, Na^+ excretion reaches maximal levels of 16 mmol/hr per 1.73 m^2 (Aperia et al., 1975b). The limited ability to excrete an Na^+ load appears to result from a reduced GFR and tubular inability to significantly increase the fractional excretion of Na^+ (FE_{Na^+}) because of the effect of aldosterone in increasing distal tubular Na^+ reabsorption.

Signs and symptoms associated with hypernatremia in infants include muscle weakness, hyperpnea, apnea, bradycardia, restlessness, a high-pitched cry, lethargy, insomnia or coma, and muscular hypertonicity (Finberg and Harrison, 1955). Older children may exhibit thirst, lethargy, confusion, muscle irritability, rhabdomyolysis, respiratory arrest, seizures, or coma. Tachycardia and hypotension are symptoms of hypovolemia, which is an ominous sign suggestive of extreme dehydration. Because of hypertonicity, fluid shift from the intracellular compartment may result in brain shrinkage, subarachnoid hemorrhage, and permanent brain injury when chronic adaptive solute gain fails to maintain cell volume. Even with such correction, the ensuing neuronal hyperosmolality may predispose to cerebral edema and serious neurologic consequences when rehydration with hypotonic fluid is used aggressively.

The initial laboratory investigation of hypernatremia is similar to that noted in the section on dehydration. In the absence of dehydration, the treatment of hypernatremia depends largely on the underlying disorder. The judicious administration of insulin and avoidance of colloids may be needed in patients with hyperosmolar nonketotic hyperglycemic coma. On the other hand, the administration of free water, together with appropriate replacement of arginine vasopressin, is useful for treatment of central diabetes insipidus. Surgery may be used to treat several endocrinopathies, whereas thiazides and a diet low in osmotic activity may be of benefit in nephrogenic diabetes insipidus.

In children with acute hypernatremia due to pure water loss such as those with nephrogenic diabetes insipidus, a hypotonic fluid may be given at a rate that will decrease plasma osmolality by no more than 2 mOsmol/kg per hour calculated using the following formula:

$$\text{Current TBW} = 65\% \text{ of body weight (kg)}$$

$$\text{Former TBW} = \frac{\text{Current Na}^+ \times \text{Current TBW}}{\text{Desired Na}^+}$$

$$\text{Water deficit (L)} = \text{Former TBW} - \text{Current TBW}$$

For example, to calculate the water deficit in a 10-kg infant with diabetes insipidus, a current serum Na^+ concentration of 160 mmol/L, and a desired plasma Na^+ concentration of 140 mmol/L, the following applies:

$$\text{Current TBW} = 0.65 \times 10 \text{ kg} = 6.5 \text{ L}$$

$$\text{Former TBW} = \frac{160 \text{ mmol/L} \times 6.5\text{L}}{140 \text{ mmol/L}} = 7.43 \text{ L}$$

$$\text{Water deficit} = 7.43 \text{ L} - 6.5 \text{ L} = 0.93 \text{ L}$$

In children with hypotonic sodium loss, this fluid deficit, together with ongoing fluid losses occurring during the time of replacing such deficits, may be infused as $^1/_8$ or $^1/_4$ saline with 1% to 2% dextrose.

With chronic hypernatremia, correction of plasma osmolality may occur at a rate of less than 1 mOsmol/kg per hr, or a reduction in serum sodium of less than 0.5 mEq/L. Hypotonic fluids given at a low rate are the most suitable for this purpose. In individuals with accidental sodium loading, furosemide, combined with adequate replacement of urine volume with 5% dextrose in water, is usually effective unless renal failure is present, in which case dialysis may be of benefit.

Hypernatremic Dehydration

This disorder is relatively common in premature infants of less than 27 weeks gestation (Baumgart, 1982; Baumgart et al., 1982). Its typical presentation, however, is in infants less than 12 months of age, with diarrhea being the usual predisposing cause. Such infants have inadequate access to free water, increased insensible water loss, proportionally greater water loss than Na^+ loss from the gastrointestinal tract, and, at times, a positive solute balance from the improper use of electrolyte solutions used to manage the diarrhea (Paneth, 1980). Patients with hypertonic dehydration often do not have dehydration of the interstitial fluid compartment and thus may not manifest the poor skin turgor, dryness of mucous membranes, and postural changes in pulse and blood pressure often associated with isotonic or hypotonic dehydration. Muscular hypertonicity may result in nuchal rigidity. Other potential complications include brain hemorrhage and edema following rehydration because of fluid shifting into the brain. Because of impaired insulin secretion initial serum glucose concentrations often exceed 130 mg/dL in 50% and 200 mg/dL in 25% of children with hypernatremia. Hence, the amount of dextrose administered to such individuals may be limited or insulin may be given to prevent further hyperglycemia, osmotic diuresis, and hypernatremia. Hypocalcemia also occurs in 10% to 20% of patients with hypertonic dehydration. The management of this disorder is outlined in Box 4–2.

■ DISORDERS OF POTASSIUM METABOLISM

Potassium (K^+) is the principal cation in the intracellular fluid (ICF), ranging in concentration from 140 to 160 mmol/L; the normal K^+ concentration in ECF varies between 3.5 and 5.5 mmol/L (same as 3.5 and 5.5 mEq/L). The low proportion of ECF K^+ to ICF K^+ is necessary to maintain transmembrane electrical potential, which is essential for proper function of muscle and neural tissue (Suki, 1976).

■ POTASSIUM HOMEOSTASIS

Total body K^+ content correlates with body weight and height and depends on muscle mass (Pierson et al., 1974; Patrick, 1977). In a healthy 20-year-old adult, total body K^+ approximates 58 mmol/kg, a value that decreases progressively with age as muscle mass decreases and body fat increases. In children, total body K^+ is 38 mmol/kg or less (Pierson et al., 1974). More than 90% of body K^+ is intracellular, and most of that is in muscle tissue. Of the extracellular K^+, only 1.4% is contained within the ECF, whereas the remaining 8.6% is contained in the bone matrix.

The daily need for K^+ is about 2 mmol/100 kcal of expended energy. The daily intake from a standard Western diet is estimated to be 0.75 to 1.5 mmol/kg body weight. Typically, approximately 90% of the K^+ ingested each day is eliminated in the urine. Less than 15% is eliminated in the stool while a negligible amount is lost through the skin. The amount of K^+ eliminated in stool increases, however, with a significant degree of renal failure (Hayes et al., 1967), reaching 34% of dietary intake at a GFR of less than 5 mL/min per 1.73 m^2.

The renal tubular mechanisms involved in K^+ homeostasis have been extensively reviewed (Halperin and Kamel, 1998). Nearly 85% of the filtered K^+ is reabsorbed in the proximal tubule and the ascending thick limb of the loop of Henle. The amount of K^+ in the final urine depends on the amount of intake and on the tubular secretion of K^+.

Two key hormones lower ECF K^+ acutely through redistribution in various tissues. Insulin causes Na^+ to enter and H^+ to exit cells through the electroneutral Na^+/H^+ exchanger, and epinephrine (and β_2-adrenergic agonists) activates the Na^+,K^+-ATPase, which exports three Na^+ ions for each two K^+ ions that enter the cell. Although epinephrine possesses both α- and β-adrenergic properties, it first causes a hyperkalemic response (during the first 1 to 3 minutes) and then a sustained decrease in plasma K^+ concentration through trapping of K^+ in cells by maintenance of an intracellular net negative charge that is essential in determining the electronegative resting membrane potential. By contrast, α-adrenergic agonists raise plasma K^+ concentration by modifying muscle K^+ uptake (Rosa et al., 1980).

Chronic K^+ homeostasis is largely regulated by secretion of K^+ by principal cells that predominate in the renal cortical collecting duct and are located in smaller numbers in the connecting tubule. The main mechanisms of K^+ secretion are depicted in Figure 4–5. Secretion is aided by (1) the plasma aldosterone level that is stimulated by angiotensin II and by high plasma K^+ concentrations. Aldosterone activates the epithelial Na^+ channel (ENaC). This results in Na^+ reabsorption and development of an electronegative lumen voltage that favors K^+ secretion. An ATP-sensitive ROMK channel aids the efflux of K^+ into the tubular lumen. Many primary adrenal disorders or renal disorders associated with high circulating levels of renin and angiotensin II may lead to secondary stimulation of aldosterone and result in hypokalemia. (2) The peritubular fluid K^+ concentration directly stimulates Na^+/K^+-ATPase and may be the most important mediator of K^+ secretion. (3) High urinary flow rates are associated. (4) Hypomagnesemia, possibly through inactivation of the Na^+/K^+-ATPase pump; (5) higher pH in the lumen of the cortical collecting duct; and (6) reabsorption of bicarbonate and Na^+

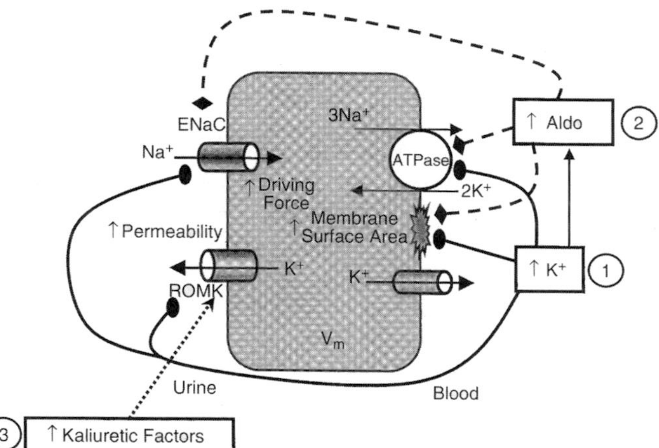

■ **FIGURE 4–5.** Major factors that regulate K^+ secretion in principal cells. Sodium is reabsorbed across the luminal membrane through ENaC Na^+ channels, with the resultant cellular depolarization increasing the electrical driving force for K^+ secretion through ROMK K^+ channels. (1) Elevation of peritubular [K^+] (*circular arrowheads*) increases the density of luminal ENaC and ROMK channels, which promote both K^+ secretion by increasing the electrical driving force and K^+ permeability, respectively. Increases in peritubular [K^+] also activate the Na^+,K^+-ATPase pump in the basolateral membrane and stimulate aldosterone release. (2) Aldosterone (*diamond arrowheads*) increases the density of ENaC (but not ROMK) channels and activates the Na^+,K^+-ATPase pump, both of which increase the driving force for K^+ secretion. The surface area of the BLM containing the Na^+, K^+-ATPase pump undergoes amplification during prolonged exposure to either increased peritubular [K^+] or aldosterone. (3) Kaliuretic factors, including K^+ itself, have been proposed to somehow directly increase K^+ secretion. For example, high luminal [K^+] may directly increase the activity of ROMK channels. (From Gennari FJ, Segal AS: Hyperkalemia: An adaptive response in chronic renal insufficiency. *Kidney Int* 62:1–9, 2002, p 4, Figure 3.)

influence the electronegativity in the lumen of the cortical collecting duct.

Understanding of such mechanisms provides physiologic explanations for plasma K^+ alterations and for therapeutic rationale. An example is the individual with hypovolemia and hyperkalemia. The kidney guards against extracellular volume contraction by raising angiotensin II levels. The latter increases bicarbonate reabsorption in the proximal and distal tubules such that the cortical collecting duct lumen becomes less electronegative and favors NaCl retention but reduced K^+ secretion despite elevated aldosterone levels. In this clinical setting low urinary flow rate also contributes to hyperkalemia. This is in contrast to euvolemic or hypervolemic individuals, in whom a high plasma K^+ concentration inhibits proximal tubular bicarbonate reabsorption while it directly stimulates aldosterone release, thereby promoting K^+ secretion (along with Cl^- and HCO_3^-) in the cortical collecting duct. In this setting Na^+ is reabsorbed through the important effect of aldosterone in activating the specific epithelial Na^+ channel (ENaC) at the apical membrane of principal cells (Halperin and Kamel, 1998). When ENaC is blocked by trimethoprim, amiloride, or triamterene, kaliuresis is inhibited.

HYPOKALEMIA (Plasma K^+ <3.5 mmol/L or <3.5 mEq/L)

Although hypokalemia usually implies total body K^+ depletion, it can also be caused by transcellular shifts of K^+ without extrarenal losses. Several classifications of hypokalemia have been devised depending on whether the condition is acute or chronic, with or without K^+ shift, renal or extrarenal. One classification is shown in Box 4–4. Because the etiology of renal K^+ wasting is extensive, it may be facilitated by further subclassification on the basis of systemic blood pressure (Box 4–5).

Hypokalemia Without Potassium Depletion

Pseudohypokalemia can result by increased uptake of K^+ when large numbers of leukemic cells (white blood cell count of 100,000 to 250,000 mm^3) are allowed to stand at room temperature (Adams et al., 1981). This confounding effect is eliminated by rapid separation of plasma or by cold storage of blood samples at 4°C.

Hypokalemia caused by intracellular shift of K^+ is particularly common in metabolic or in respiratory alkalosis, and approximates a 0.6-mmol/L fall for every 0.1-unit increase in blood pH (Kim and Brown, 1968; Adrogue and Madias, 1981). Endogenous or exogenous β-adrenergic agonists such as albuterol, dopamine, dobutamine, and theophylline mediate transcellular shifts of K^+ (see earlier discussion). Barium poisoning (Roza and Berman, 1971) or toluene intoxication resulting from the inhalation of paint or glue vapors (Streicher et al., 1981) can produce hypokalemia by trapping K^+ within the cells. Insulin administration activates the Na^+,K^+-ATPase, resulting in active K^+ uptake and hypokalemia. This is frequently encountered during the treatment of diabetic ketoacidosis.

Hypokalemic periodic paralysis is a rare autosomal dominant disorder characterized by recurrent episodes of flaccid paralysis of the trunk and limbs lasting 6 to 24 hours. Paralysis may be accompanied by cardiac arrhythmias, which may be provoked by high carbohydrate intake, exertion, and a high Na^+ diet (Griggs et al., 1970). This condition is more common in the Asian population and is characterized by low urinary K^+ excretion, low transtubular potassium gradient (TTKG), and no acid-base disturbances

BOX 4–4 Causes of Hypokalemia

Hypokalemia Without Potassium Depletion

Spurious

High white blood cell count

Transcellular Shifts

Metabolic alkalosis
Insulin excess
β-Adrenergic agonists
Barium intoxication
Toluene intoxication
Hypokalemic periodic paralysis
Delirium tremens

Hypokalemia With Potassium Depletion

Nutritional

Inadequate nutritional intake
Chloride-deficient infant formula

Extrarenal Causes

Copious perspiration (cystic fibrosis)
Gastrointestinal losses/malabsorption
Chronic diarrhea
Vomiting
Gastrointestinal fistulas
Ostomy/short gut syndrome
Ureterosigmoidostomy
Rectal villous adenoma
Geophagia
Laxative abuse
Full-thickness burns

Renal Causes

Renal tubular acidosis (RTA, types I and II)
Fanconi syndrome
Carbonic anhydrase inhibitors
Correction phase of metabolic alkalosis

Chloride Depletion

Vomiting/gastric drainage with metabolic alkalosis
Congenital chloride diarrhea
Cystic fibrosis
Diuretics (thiazide, loop, osmotic)
Cisplatin

Potassium Wasting

Bartter's syndrome
Gitelman's syndrome
Liddle's syndrome
Renal artery stenosis (high renin and aldosterone release)
Mineralocorticoid excess (Cushing's syndrome, hyperaldosteronism, prolonged use of glucocorticoids, licorice ingestion, 17α- or 11β-hydroxylase deficiency)
Pyelonephritis and other interstitial nephritides
Magnesium depletion
Postobstructive diuresis
Diuretic phase of acute tubular necrosis
Antibiotics (carbenicillin, penicillins, amphotericin B, aminoglycosides, cidofovir)

BOX 4–5 Renal Wasting of Potassium in Relation to Systemic Blood Pressure

Renal Wasting of K^+ Associated With Normal Blood Pressure

High Renin, High Aldosterone

Renal tubular acidosis
Bartter's syndrome
Gitelman's syndrome
Magnesium-losing tubulopathy
Calcium-losing tubulopathy
Osmotic diuresis (hyperglycemia)
Covert diuretic abuse
Prolonged emesis or nasogastric suction
Drugs (penicillins, amphotericin B, aminoglycosides, cisplatin, ifosfamide)

Renal Wasting of K^+ Associated With Hypertension

Low Renin, High Aldosterone

Aldosterone-producing adenoma
Idiopathic hyperaldosteronism
Dexamethasone-suppressible hyperaldosteronism
Adrenocortical carcinoma

Low Renin, Low Aldosterone

17α-Hydroxylase deficiency
11β-Hydroxylase deficiency
11β-Hydroxysteroid dehydrogenase deficiency, licorice ingestion
Liddle's syndrome

High Renin, High Aldosterone

Malignant hypertension
Renal artery stenosis
Renin-secreting tumor (Wilms, nephroblastomatosis)
Chronic renal disease

Gill JR, Santos F, Chan JCM: Disorders of potassium metabolism. In Chan JCM, Gill JR, editors: *Kidney electrolyte disorders*. New York, 1990, Churchill Livingstone, Table 4-6, p 157.

(Lin et al., 2001). Dietary restriction of salt and carbohydrates together with spironolactone may help prevent such attacks. Intravenous K^+ infusion should be avoided as rebound hyperkalemia can occur. Potassium-sparing diuretics and the ingestion of foods rich in K^+ are of limited benefit in treating or in preventing the disorder. Notably, affected individuals are susceptible to malignant hyperthermia with administration of general anesthesia.

Potassium Depletion

K^+ depletion accounts for most cases of hypokalemia. Three basic disturbances can affect total body K^+ balance and result in cellular depletion: poor nutritional intake, extrarenal loss of K^+, and renal loss of K^+.

Nutritional Causes

A deficient diet alone seldom causes symptomatic hypokalemia because K^+ is ubiquitous in foodstuffs. In adults, a reduction in K^+ intake to less than 10 mmol/day for 7 to 10 days will cause a relative total body K^+ deficit of 250 to 300 mmol, or a decrement of 7% to 8% (Wormersley and Darragh, 1955). Occasionally K^+ depletion occurs in hospitalized patients maintained on K^+-free intravenous fluids. In these instances, the kidney responds by appropriately decreasing K^+ excretion, although it cannot produce K^+-free urine.

Extrarenal Causes

Diarrhea, vomiting, and abuse of laxatives result in hypokalemia via a complex process. In addition to K^+ loss in vomiting and stool, these conditions cause intravascular volume contraction, secondary hyperaldosteronism, and enhanced urinary excretion of K^+. In children, diarrhea is often accompanied by hyperchloremic metabolic acidosis (Welfare et al., 2002), whereas laxative abuse is associated with normal acid-base status or mild metabolic alkalosis.

Copious perspiration from intense physical exertion in a hot environment causes K^+ depletion (Knochel et al., 1972). This condition is characterized by normal plasma K^+ concentration with total body K^+ depletion and a high rate of urinary K^+ excretion. Loss of K^+ via sweat and secondary hyperaldosteronism explains the depletion state and the urinary loss; the sustained normal plasma K^+ level, however, is not adequately explained. The human colon responds to aldosterone in a similar fashion resulting in an increase in the renal collecting duct transepithelial potential difference followed by an increase in Na^+,K^+-ATPase activity (Thompson and Edmonds, 1971). Glucocorticoids are kaliuretic, and evidence suggests that their effect is independent of any action on the mineralocorticoid receptor (Bia et al., 1982). Furthermore, glucocorticoids appear to cause an increase in K^+ and a decrease in Na^+ stool concentration associated with increased Na^+,K^+-ATPase activity (Charney et al., 1975).

Renal Causes

Renal wastage of K^+ occurs by several different yet interrelated mechanisms. First, an increased Na^+/K^+ exchange may occur in the distal tubule in conditions associated with increased circulating mineralocorticoid or glucocorticoid concentrations resulting in circulatory volume expansion and suppression of plasma renin and aldosterone levels. Hypokalemia often occurs in Conn's syndrome (Ganguly and Donohue, 1983). It also occurs in 30% of patients with adrenal hyperplasia (Cushing's syndrome) (Prunty et al., 1963). The ingestion of certain foods and use of glucocorticoids or other drugs possessing mineralocorticoid activity can also result in hypokalemia. Licorice, for example, contains large amounts of glycyrrhizic acid, which impairs adrenal 11β-hydroxysteroid dehydrogenase action. This impairs the degradation of endogenous glucocorticoids, resulting in a mineralocorticoid-like response (Brem, 2001).

Second, increased delivery of Na^+ to the distal tubule, which occurs in various proximal tubulopathies, including proximal renal tubular acidosis and Fanconi's syndrome, may enhance K^+ secretion. Similarly, thiazides and loop diuretics increase the delivery of Na^+ to the distal nephron, thus promoting K^+ excretion (Kassirer and Harrington, 1977). This effect by diuretics is augmented by concomitant Cl^- depletion (Kassirer and Harrington, 1977) and by contraction alkalosis (Seldin and Rector, 1972).

Third, large concentrations of nonabsorbable anions in the distal tubules, such as penicillins, increase the electronegativity of tubular fluid and induce kaliuresis and hydrogen ion secretion (Lipner et al., 1975). Carbenicillin is particularly notorious for causing hypokalemia because it is secreted actively in the proximal tubule, and high concentrations of the anion are delivered to the distal nephron (Stapleton et al., 1976).

Fourth, kaliuresis may occur secondary to direct damage to the renal epithelium. Conditions such as pyelonephritis and other interstitial nephritides may be associated with hypokalemia. Similarly, antibiotics such as amphotericin B, polymyxin, and outdated tetracycline can lead to K^+ depletion through their direct toxic effects on the renal tubules (Chesney, 1976). Aminoglycosides result in magnesium as well as K^+ wasting, probably because of a change in the permeability of the renal epithelium to these cations (Humes et al., 1982). Experimentally, hypokalemia tends to occur within the first 7 days of aminoglycoside administration and often occurs in the absence of overt acute tubular necrosis and renal failure. This tubular defect and the risk of hypokalemia usually resolve within 1 to 2 weeks after discontinuation of the drug.

Fifth, several genetic disorders are known to cause K^+ depletion. Box 4–5 characterizes such disorders of hypokalemia based on the presence or absence of hypertension. Hypertensive disorders may be associated with high peripheral renin activity (renovascular disorders comprise the majority of such causes in children) or low renin states that are associated with either increased plasma mineralocorticoid or glucocorticoid levels or with more direct activation of the principal cell amiloride-sensitive Na^+ channel (ENaC) in the cortical collecting duct resulting in salt retention, chronic volume expansion, renin and aldosterone suppression (hence "pseudoaldosteronism"), and hypertension as exemplified in Liddle's syndrome. In the latter disorder, treatment consisting of blockade of the mineralocorticoid receptor with spironolactone, or of the aldosterone receptor by amiloride, is less effective than the combination of triamterene and a low-salt diet.

Manifestations of Potassium Depletion

Hypokalemia results in multiple biochemical and neurophysiologic disturbances (Weiner and Wingo, 1997) (Box 4–6). Chronic hypokalemia and moderate degrees of acute K^+ depletion (5% to 10% of total body K^+) are generally well tolerated. More profound deficits result in clinical manifestations independent of the underlying cause of hypokalemia.

Biochemical consequences of hypokalemia include impairment in insulin release (Rowe et al., 1980) and insulin end-organ sensitivity, thereby increasing the risk of hyperglycemia or precipitation of frank diabetes mellitus. Metabolic alkalosis results from direct stimulation of proximal tubular bicarbonate reabsorption and ammonia genesis by increased proton secretion via H^+,K^+-ATPase located in the collecting duct and by decreasing citrate excretion. Inadequate ADH response and increased synthesis of angiotensin II in the central nervous system may cause polyuria. Hypokalemia may raise plasma ammonia levels in patients with reduced hepatic function. Also, chronic renal K^+ wasting may predispose to formation of renal cysts and interstitial fibrosis (Torres, 1990).

Many of the symptoms of acute hypokalemia relate to disturbed neuromuscular functions. Skeletal muscle weakness due to cell hyperpolarization is the earliest manifestation of K^+ depletion. Plasma K^+ concentrations below 3.0 mEq/L lower the resting cell membrane potential and thereby increase the voltage needed to reach the threshold and initiate an action potential (Fig. 4–6). The symptoms include restless leg syndrome, fatigue, muscle cramps, paralysis, and rhabdomyolysis. Frank muscle necrosis may occur with serum K^+ concentrations below

BOX 4–6 Pathophysiologic Consequences of Hypokalemia

Neuromuscular

Peripheral nerves (paresthesias)
Skeletal muscle (fatigue, weakness, cramps, flaccid paralysis, rhabdomyolysis, myoglobinuria)
Smooth muscle (paralytic ileus, increased vascular pressor resistance)

Renal

Concentration defect (polyuria, nocturia)
Sodium retention
Increased ammonia production, enhanced bicarbonate reabsorption
Reduced renal blood flow, decreased GFR
Predisposition to urinary tract infection
Interstitial fibrosis
Cyst formation

Metabolic

Metabolic alkalosis
Impaired hepatic glycogen storage
Impaired protein metabolism
Insulin resistance
Increased plasma ammonia
Growth retardation

Hormonal

Impaired growth hormone release
Impaired insulin secretion
Decreased aldosterone secretion
Increased renin release
Increased synthesis of prostaglandins

Gill JR, Santos F, Chan JCM: Disorders of potassium metabolism. In Chan JCM, Gill JR, editors: *Kidney electrolyte disorders.* New York, 1990, Churchill Livingstone, Table 4-7, p 158.

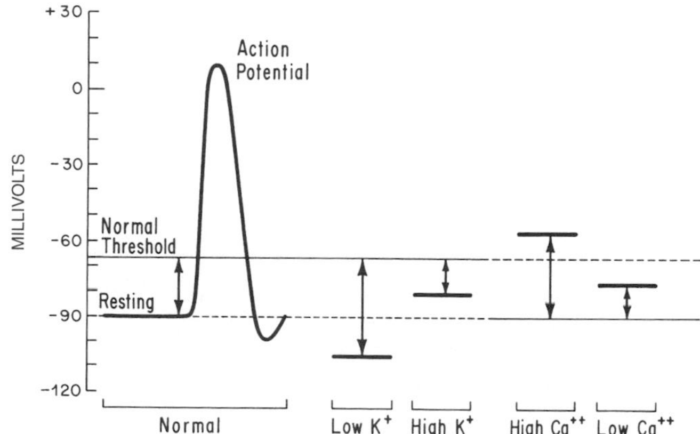

■ **FIGURE 4–6.** Typical action potential profile. Normal threshold is influenced by Ca^{2+} concentrations, whereas K^+ concentrations affect the resting potential. (From Leaf A, Cotran RS: *Renal pathophysiology*, ed 2. New York, 1980, Oxford University Press, p 119, Figure 1.2.)

2.0 mEq/L (Knochel, 1982). Cardiac manifestations of hypokalemia include abnormalities in rhythm as a result of slowed repolarization (Helfant, 1986). The presence of electrocardiographic changes helps to exclude spurious hypokalemia and may aid the decision to manage the hypokalemia urgently (Fig. 4–6). Abnormalities include depression of the ST segment, lower T-wave voltage, and appearance of U waves. Patients receiving cardiac glycosides are especially at risk of developing such abnormalities. Hypokalemia also impairs the cardiovascular responses to norepinephrine and angiotensin II.

K^+ depletion may lead to several functional and structural abnormalities in the kidney, including reduced RBF and GFR, renal hypertrophy, tubuloepithelial dilation, vacuolization, and sclerosis (Relman and Schwartz, 1956). Functionally, patients develop urinary acidification and concentration defects and polyuria.

Diagnosis of Hypokalemia

When hypokalemia is diagnosed, the underlying pathophysiologic cause may not be apparent. Measurement of urinary K^+ levels may be helpful. A urinary concentration less than 10 mEq/L suggests nearly maximal conservation and usually implies extrarenal loss of K^+. Urinary K^+ concentrations exceeding 30 mEq/L suggest the kidney is a likely route for the depletion. In patients maintained on diuretics, the caveat is that within hours of discontinuation of these agents, the kidney responds by conserving K^+.

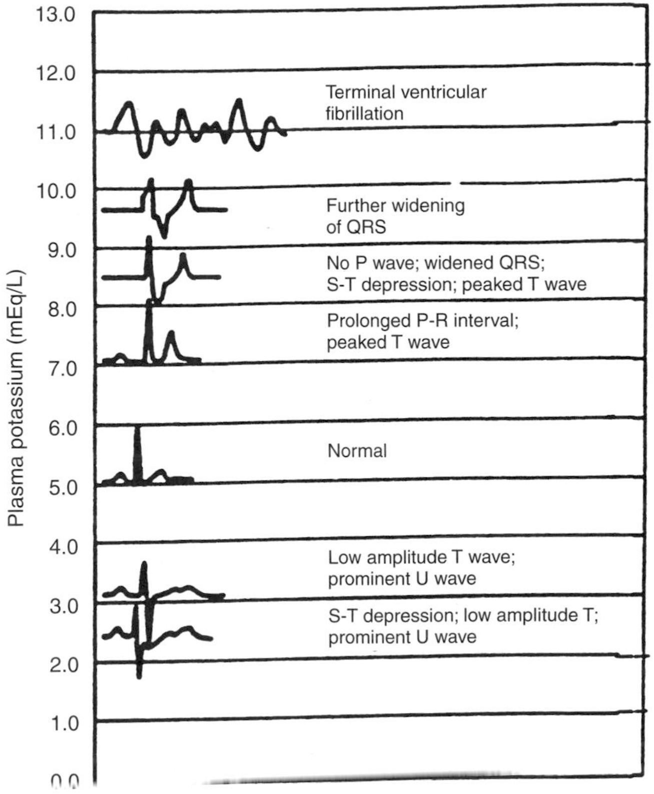

■ **FIGURE 4–7.** The relationship between plasma potassium concentration and electrocardiographic changes. (From Winters RW: *The body fluids in pediatrics.* Boston, 1973, Little, Brown, p 134, Figure 10.1.)

Treatment of Hypokalemia

The treatment of hypokalemia requires extreme caution, as the magnitude of loss is difficult to measure clinically. In the absence of cellular shifts, the percent of total body K^+ deficit may be grossly estimated from the plasma concentration and intracellular K^+ content (0.40 × body weight × 145 mEq/L) as follows:

Plasma K^+ 2.6 to 3.5 mEq/L = 5% to 10%

Plasma K^+ 1.8 to 2.5 mEq/L = 10% to 20%

Plasma K^+ <1.8 mEq/L = >20%

The concurrence of hypokalemia and metabolic acidosis suggests an even greater K^+ depletion. In such children the correction of the acidosis should follow, rather than precede, the correction of hypokalemia. Guidelines for potassium supplementation in dietary or medication forms are available for adults but not for children (Cohn, 2000). Such supplements should be given with close monitoring of blood levels, particularly when combined with potassium-sparing diuretics such as amiloride and spironolactone. Providing details of managing children with specific disorders associated with chronic hypokalemia is beyond the scope of this chapter. Supplemental K^+ at a dosage of 3 to 5 mEq/kg per day (plus maintenance amounts) may be given orally as the chloride salt, because most disorders are associated with chloride depletion. Several liquid and salt preparations are available. Microencapsulated salt preparations are associated with a lower rate of gastrointestinal bleeding and hemorrhage. In patients with combined K^+ and phosphate depletion, the phosphate salt is recommended. Magnesium correction may help improve the hypokalemia, especially in refractory states such as Gitellman syndrome (Whang et al., 1992). High K^+-containing foods are useful in individuals managed with laxatives and diuretics.

Intravenous K^+ repletion is often desirable for the management of acute hyperkalemia, particularly when neuromuscular or electrocardiographic alterations are clinically evident.Concentrations as high as 40 mEq/L may be given peripherally. Higher concentrations should be administered in large veins to prevent phlebitis. Concentrations exceeding 60 mEq/L generally are not recommended. In special clinical situations, higher K^+ concentrations may be delivered in limited fluid volumes by diluting 20 mEq of KCl in 100 mL in a Soluset with a microdip and infusing it at a rate not to exceed 0.5 mEq/kg per hr (maximum, 30 to 40 mEq/hr). Such higher infusion rates, although reserved for life-threatening situations, can be given perioperatively in hypokalemic children with close cardiac monitoring and frequent measurement of plasma K^+ concentrations.

■ HYPERKALEMIA (Plasma K^+ >5.5 mEq/L in Infants and Children, or >6 mmol/L in Neonates)

Conditions causing hyperkalemia are listed in Box 4–7. Hyperkalemia may result from a surprisingly small increase in total body K^+ or may result rapidly from transcellular shift. Normally, the kidney provides the crucial defense against slight elevations in serum K^+ level. Thus, with a few exceptions, hyperkalemia occurs with high frequency in conditions characterized by decreased urine flow rates or marked reduction in GFR. In the absence of renal insufficiency, drugs are responsible for most cases of hyperkalemia. Several agents may cause hyperkalemia by

BOX 4–7 Causes of Hyperkalemia

Pseudohyperkalemia

Ischemic blood drawing
Hemolysis
Thrombocytosis (>1,000,000/mm^3)
Leukocytosis (>500,000/mm^3)
Familial "leaky red blood cell"
Infectious mononucleosis

Transcellular Shifts

Metabolic acidosis
Hyperglycemia with insulin insufficiency
Extracellular hypertonicity
Tissue damage: trauma, exercise, burns, rhabdomyolysis, asphyxia, catabolic states, sepsis, rojection of transplanted orqans (such as liver, kidney)
Drugs (see Table 4–13)
Familial hyperkalemic periodic paralysis

Increased Potassium Load

Dietary excess, oral or intravenous K^+ supplementation
Use of aged bank blood/hemolysis
Geophagia
High doses of K^+-containing medications (such as potassium penicillin)

Decreased Renal Excretion of Potassium

Acute renal failure
Chronic renal failure
Low-birth-weight infants
Spitzer-Weinstein syndrome
Drugs (see Table 4–13)
Hyporeninemic hypoaldosteronism
Type I and type II pseudohypoaldosteronism
Addison's disease (hypoaldosteronism)
Obstructive uropathy
Impaired steroidogenesis (congenital adrenal hyperplasia, mitochondrial disorders, Smith-Lemli-Opitz syndrome)

increasing the K^+ load, by facilitating transcellular K^+ efflux, or by impairing renal excretion of K^+ (Perazella, 2000) (Table 4–13).

Transcellular Shift

Among conditions associated with altered K^+ distribution across cell membranes is poorly controlled insulin-dependent diabetes mellitus. The mechanism is twofold: hyperglycemia causes hypertonicity with resultant extrusion of K^+ from cells, whereas insulin deficiency does not promote K^+ entry into the cells (Ammon et al., 1978). These effects are independent of aldosterone response and level of renal function.

Cellular damage from rhabdomyolysis, burns, tissue necrosis, or fulminant rejection of a grafted organ may release large quantities of K^+ into the extracellular space. In patients with normal renal function, most of the excess K^+ is easily excreted. In those with large tumor lysis after induction of chemotherapy (Araseneau et al., 1973) or those with renal impairment, however, hyperkalemia may occur.

During metabolic acidosis, part of the hydrogen ion load is buffered within cells in exchange for K^+. It has been noted that

■ TABLE 4–13. Medications that can cause hyperkalemia and their mechanism of action

Medication	Mechanism
Increased Potassium Input	
Potassium supplements and salt substitutes	Potassium ingestion
Nutritional and herbal supplements	Potassium ingestion
Stored packed red blood cells	Potassium infusion
Penicillin G potassium	Potassium ingestion
Transcellular Potassium Shifts	
β-Blockers	Decrease β_2-driven potassium uptake
Intravenous amino acids (lysine, arginine, and ε-aminocaproic acid)	Release of potassium from cells
Succinylcholine	Depolarize cell membranes
Digoxin intoxication	Decrease Na^+,K^+-ATPase activity
Impaired Renal Excretion	
Potassium-sparing diuretics	
Spironolactone	Aldosterone antagonism
Triamterene	Block Na^+ channels in principal cells
Amiloride	Block Na^+ channels in principal cells
Nonsteroidal anti-inflammatory drugs	Decrease aldosterone synthesis
	Decrease renal blood flow and glomerular filtration rate
ACE Inhibitors and Angiotensin II Receptor Blockers	Decrease aldosterone synthesis
	Decrease renal blood flow and glomerular filtration rate
Trimethoprim and pentamidine	Block Na^+ channels in principal cells
Cyclosporine and tacrolimus	Decrease aldosterone synthesis
	Decrease Na^+,K^+-ATPase activity
	Decrease K^+ channel activity
Heparin	Decrease aldosterone synthesis

ACE, angiotensin-converting enzyme.
Modified from Perazella MA: Drug-induced hyperkalemia: Old culprits and new offenders. *Am J Med* 109:307–314, 2000, p 308, Table 2.

for every 0.1-U decrease in blood pH, serum K^+ changes by 0.6 mEq/L. Changes in plasma HCO_3^- concentration per se may influence K^+ concentration independent of changes in pH. Clinically, serum K^+ can be decreased with bicarbonate administration in the absence of metabolic acidosis (Fraley and Adler, 1977).

Pseudohyperkalemia

Ischemic blood drawing is a very common cause of pseudohyperkalemia, especially in infants and young children undergoing blood sampling by lancing and squeezing the finger or heel or because of hemolysis from prolonged application of tourniquets. Several conditions cause false elevations in plasma K^+ concentrations, including thrombocytosis (Ingram and Seki, 1962), leukocytosis (Chumbley, 1970), hemolysis, and sampling of ischemic blood. In general, immediate determination of K^+ in plasma instead of in serum minimizes the release of K^+ from the cellular components and avoids the development of pseudohyperkalemia.

High Potassium Intake

An oral intake of as little as 50 mmol of K^+ (<2% of normal body K^+ content) by an adult can cause a transient increase in plasma K^+ of 0.5 to 1.0 mmol/L. From 70% to 90% of this load is sequestered intracellularly within 15 to 30 minutes and ultimately excreted in the urine. Thus, when renal function is normal, large amounts of K^+ may be ingested without adverse sequelae. However, the intravenous administration of K^+ at a rate higher than 0.5 mmol/kg per hr may result in life-threatening hyperkalemia. In patients with renal insufficiency, hyperkalemia may occur due to increased excretory burden associated with large doses of potassium penicillin (10^6 U contain 1.7 mEq K^+), juices with high K^+ content, overuse of salt substitutes (1 g contains 10 to 13 mEq of K^+), and the administration of banked stored blood (1 L contains 15 to 20 mEq of K^+) (Bostic and Duvernoy, 1972).

Decreased Potassium Excretory Capacity

Regardless of the underlying cause, impaired renal function predisposes to K^+ retention and hyperkalemia. However, hyperkalemia is uncommon even in advanced renal failure unless endogenous or exogenous loads are excessive. Nonoliguric individuals with impaired GFR can excrete ordinary dietary intakes of K^+ until GFR decreases to as low as 5 mL/min per 1.73 m^2 (Gonick et al., 1971). An increase in K^+ secretion per nephron, as well as increased colonic secretion (van Ypersele de Strihou, 1977), helps to prevent hyperkalemia in severe renal failure. If hyperkalemia occurs with a GFR above 10% of normal, other causes should be sought, such as worsening metabolic acidosis, increased catabolism, cell injury, hemorrhage, or use of potassium-sparing diuretics.

The most common clinical setting in which hyperkalemia occurs is acute oliguric renal failure of any etiology. In addition to the decreased excretory capacity, an increased K^+ burden is imposed by an increased catabolic rate. The daily increase in K^+ concentration averages 0.3 to 0.5 mmol/L in oliguric acute renal failure under optimal conditions of nutrition, whereas the increase exceeds 0.7 mmol/L in patients with trauma, a high rate of catabolism, or both (Schrier, 1979).

Hyporeninemic hypoaldosteronism accounts for more than 50% of adults or older children with unexplained hyperkalemia accompanying adequate, albeit decreased, GFR (Schambelan et al., 1980). Most patients have a component of chronic interstitial renal disease, and more than half have diabetes mellitus.

Obstructive uropathy may be associated with a defect in K^+ excretion associated with a mild hyperchloremic acidosis, decreased fractional excretion of K^+, and mild hyperkalemia (Battle et al., 1981) because of end-organ resistance to the action of aldosterone or because of hypoaldosteronism per se.

Many drugs or drug combinations can cause hyperkalemia, particularly when KCl supplements are coadministered (Perazella, 2000) (see Table 4–13). For example, a potassium-sparing diuretic and an angiotensin-converting enzyme inhibitor can result in life-threatening hyperkalemia-induced arrhythmia, especially in diabetics with renal insufficiency or other high-risk groups. The mechanisms may involve (1) direct suppression of renin release by β-blockers or by prostaglandin synthetase inhibitors leading to secondary hypoaldosteronism, (2) lowering aldosterone synthesis by angiotensin-converting enzyme inhibitors, or (3) inhibition of Na^+,K^+-ATPase and other transporters in principal cells by digitalis, trimethoprim, cyclosporine, or tacrolimus. Succinylcholine increases plasma K^+ concentration by increasing the permeability of muscle membranes during depolarization (Gronert and Theye, 1975).

Adrenal destruction due to hemorrhage, tumor, infection, autoimmune polyglandular syndrome, or adrenoleukodystrophy can cause an Addison-like presentation with fatigue, muscle weakness, hypotension, and hyponatremia. Congenital disorders associated with reduced steroidogenesis may have a similar clinical presentation (Ten et al., 2001; Bonny and Rosier, 2002). Hereditary disorders with similar sodium wasting and hyperkalemia, but with increased, rather than low, plasma renin and aldosterone levels, include the autosomal dominant (self-limited) and autosomal recessive (permanent) forms of pseudohypoaldosteronism I. In these disorders, a defective mineralocorticoid receptor is responsible for hyponatremia, hyperkalemia, and metabolic acidosis (Ten et al., 2001; Bonny and Rosier, 2002). In contrast, pseudohypoaldosteronism Type II (Gordon syndrome) is a sporadic or autosomal dominant condition associated with hypertension, suppressed plasma renin activity, normal plasma aldosterone concentration, and mild hyperchloremic acidosis that respond well to thiazide diuretic (Milford, 1999).

Manifestations of Hyperkalemia

The clinical manifestations of hyperkalemia relate to interference with the electrophysiologic activities of muscle. Under the influence of hyperkalemia, the ratio of intracellular to extracellular K^+ is decreased, resulting in delayed depolarization, hastened repolarization, and slow conduction velocity (Knochel, 1982). The most important effect involves the heart. Diagnostic electrocardiographic alterations include tenting or symmetric peaking of the T wave in the precordial leads and depression of the ST wave (Fig. 4–7). In severe hyperkalemia, there is widening of the QRS complex, lengthening of the PR interval, first-degree or second-degree heart block, disappearance of the P wave, and, finally, atrial standstill. Ventricular fibrillation or asystole follows the development of a sinusoid wave. Although the magnitudes of hyperkalemia and of cardiotoxicity correlate well, arrhythmias may develop with even mild hyperkalemia when other metabolic abnormalities such as hyponatremia, acidosis, or calcium disorders coexist.

Hyperkalemia affects electrical activities in noncardiac muscle as well. Such manifestations as paresthesias, weakness, and flaccid paralysis that spare the head and trunk are not rare.

Clinical Evaluation of Dyskalemia

The initial step involves a clinical assessment of circulatory volume (Halperin and Kamel, 1998; Rodriguez-Soriano, 1990). Assuming that Na^+ and fluid conservation mechanisms are intact, the next step is to assess if the excretion of K^+ is appropriate compared with expected values in healthy children (Rodriguez-Soriano, 1990). If K^+ excretion is abnormal, urinary flow rate and K^+ excretion rate are measured separately. The flow rate in the terminal portion of the cortical collecting duct (CCD) is proportional to the osmolar particles in urine, which consist primarily of urea derived from protein metabolism, with Na^+ and Cl^- contributing to a lesser extent. This is derived as follows:

$$\text{Flow rate in CCD} = (U_{osm} \times U_{vol}) \div P_{osm}$$

where U refers to urine and P refers to plasma. Under the influence of ADH, a minimum flow rate in the CCD is 1 L for each 300 mOsmol excreted, which is approximately the osmolality of plasma. Thus, a lesser osmolality in the CCD would result in a lower flow rate and reduced net K^+ secretion.

If the flow rate in the CCD is adequate, then the ability of principal cells to secrete K^+ depends largely on the appropriate activity and secretion of K^+ by ENaC and ROMK channels (see Fig. 4–5). This is assessed by measurement of urinary chloride excretion and by estimation of the transtubular $[K^+]$ gradient, or, TTKG:

$$TTKG = ([K^+]_U) \div (U_{osm}/P_{osm}) \div [K^+]_P$$

This equation provides an estimate of the K^+ concentration in the CCD relative to plasma K^+ concentration after correcting for further water reabsorption past the CCD, in the medullary collecting duct, under the influence of ADH. TTKG values under 4.9 in infants or under 4.1 in children indicate a reduced ability to secrete K^+ due to hypoaldosteronism or pseudohypoaldosteronism and prompt further investigation of renal and adrenal disorders (Rodriguez-Soriano, 1990). Such evaluation may consist of venous blood gas, electrolyte measurement of gastric fluids, urinary nitrogen, plasma renin, aldosterone, cortisol and corticosterone concentrations, and, possibly, identification of mutated genes.

Treatment of Hyperkalemia

The strategy of managing hyperkalemia (Box 4–8) depends on the plasma K^+ concentration, renal function, and cardiac manifestations. Mild to moderate hyperkalemia without major electrocardiographic changes responds to a simultaneous decrease in K^+ intake and increase in Na^+ intake. In certain instances, loop diuretics may be used to increase K^+ excretion.

The fastest means of reversing cardiotoxicity is to antagonize the membrane effects of high plasma K^+ concentration. Calcium decreases the threshold potential of excitable tissue, thus restoring the normal difference between threshold and transmembrane potentials (see Fig. 4–6).

Calcium gluconate, infused intravenously at 100 to 200 mg/kg per dose, is an effective initial measure even in the absence of hypocalcemia.

If the clinical setting permits administration of a high fluid volume rate, a solution consisting of glucose and insulin added to 0.9 N NaCl is the most effective means for lowering plasma K^+ concentration (10% glucose solution, with insulin added at a ratio of 1 unit per 4 or 5 g of glucose). In children with metabolic acidosis, K^+ can be driven intracellularly by intravenous $NaHCO_3$ given at 1 to 2 mEq/kg per dose. Both treatment measures decrease plasma K^+ levels within minutes and are effective regardless of acid-base or insulin status. Hyperventilation (with resultant hypocapnia and respiratory alkalosis) abruptly increases the urinary excretion of K^+. Its effect, however, is not sustained beyond 24 hours (Gennari, 2002).

Sodium polystyrene sulfonate (Kayexalate), a cation exchange resin, can be administered at a dose of 1 g/kg, in sorbitol for oral use, or in mineral oil for rectal instillation. This dosage may be repeated every 2 to 4 hours. Typically, plasma K^+ concentration decreases by 1 mEq/L per dose. The onset of action for the oral route is 1 to 4 hours, whereas an enema removes K^+ within 30 to 60 minutes. In patients with renal failure, repeated administration of Kayexalate may impose a high Na^+ load with resultant hypertension and edema.

Dialysis may be useful in the treatment of hyperkalemia, especially in patients with renal failure. Hemodialysis can remove 1 mEq K^+/kg per hour. The duration of this effect depends on the rate of ongoing endogenous release of K^+. Peritoneal dialysis is less efficient than hemodialysis, but it can be performed more safely in small infants and children.

BOX 4–8 Treatment of Hyperkalemia

Treatment of Mild Hyperkalemia

- Decrease dietary K^+ burden
- Discontinue K^+-containing medications or K^+-sparing diuretics
- Eliminate conditions that favor hyperkalemia (acidosis, sodium restriction)

Treatment of Moderate to Severe Hyperkalemia

To Reverse Membrane Effects

- Calcium gluconate, 100 to 200 mg/kg per dose

To Produce Transcellular Shifts

- Sodium bicarbonate, 1 to 2 mmol/kg per dose
- Glucose, 0.3 to 0.5 g/kg as 10% glucose solution with insulin, 1 U per 4 to 5 g glucose IV
- Albuterol by nebulizer
- Hyperventilation

To Remove Potassium

- Kayexalate, 1 g/kg per dose PO or enema
- Furosemide (Lasix), 1 mg/kg per dose IV
- Dialysis (hemodialysis or peritoneal dialysis)
- Hemofiltration (continuous arteriovenous hemofiltration or continuous venovenous hemofiltration with or without dialysis)

■ DIURETIC THERAPY

Pharmacologic agents that promote diuresis represent a major advance in the treatment of edema and hypertension. The principal therapeutic purpose of these agents is to induce a negative Na^+ and fluid balance. The increase in urine output merely reflects the linkage of salt and water transport in the kidney: solute reabsorption limits the osmotic reabsorption of water, and "diuresis" ensues.

■ CLASSIFICATION OF DIURETICS AND SITE OF ACTION

In this section diuretics are classified according to the site of action in the nephron. This system is oversimplified, because several agents have pharmacologic effects that are not localized to a single tubular site (Table 4–14).

Proximal Tubule Diuretics

Mannitol

This is a nonmetabolizable sugar that is osmotically active. Mannitol is freely filtered at the glomerulus, but it is poorly reabsorbed and, hence, it obligates the renal excretion of water (Warren and Blantz, 1981). It limits water reabsorption in segments of the nephron that are freely permeable to water, namely, the proximal tubule, the descending limb of Henle's loop, and the collecting tubule. This results in a decreased gradient for NaCl reabsorption in the late proximal and distal

■ **TABLE 4–14.** Site, mechanism, duration of action, and dose of diuretics

			ACTION (hr)				
Site of Action	**Diuretic**	**Mechanism of Action***	*Onset*	*Peak*	*Duration*	**Dose (mg/kg per day)**	**Potency**
Proximal tubule	Acetazolamide (Diamox)	Carbonic anhydrase inhibitor	1 to 2	2	4 to 6	5 to 7	Mild
	Mannitol	Osmotic diuretic	1 to 2	2	Variable	0.5 to 1.0 g/kg per dose	Moderate
Ascending loop of Henle	Fursemide (Lasix)	Inhibition of chloride reabsorption	0.5 to 1	2 to 4	6 to 8	2 to 6 (oral) 1 to 6 (IV)	Very potent
	Bumetanide (Bumex)		0.25 to 0.5	0.45	5 to 8	0.08 to 0.6 (oral) 0.04 to 0.4 (IV)	Very potent
	Ethacrynic acid (Edecrin)		0.5 to 1	2 to 4	6 to 8	1 to 2	Very potent
Distal convoluted tubule (early)	Hydrochlorothiazide (Hydrodiuril)	Inhibition of sodium reabsorption	1 to 2	4 to 6	12 to 24	2 to 3.5	Moderate
	Chlorothiazide (Diuril)		1 to 2	4 to 6	12 to 24	20 to 40	Moderate
	Metolazone† (Zaroxolyn)		2	6	24 to 36	0.5 to 5.0 mg/day	Moderate to potent
Distal convoluted tubule (late) and collecting duct	Spironolactone (Aldactone)	Competitive inhibitor of aldosterone	8 to 24	24 to 48	48 to 72	1 to 2	Mild
	Triamterene (Dyrenium)	Direct effect by reducing electrical potential between cell and lumen	2 to 4	6 to 8	19 to 24	3	Mild

*See text for details of mechanisms of action.

†Metolazone acts at the proximal tubule (as a carbonic anhydrase inhibitor) and hence can be used in patients with renal failure, unlike the other thiazides. It is only available in oral form.

tubule, which, together with a mannitol-induced washout of the hypertonic medullary interstitium brought about by increased blood flow, potentiates natriuresis. The magnitude of the natriuresis depends on the pretreatment intravascular volume status and on RBF.

Mannitol has limited use when GFR is severely compromised and may aggravate congestive heart failure or other conditions in which intravascular volume is often increased.

In nonedematous oliguric conditions, mannitol may be used to increase water excretion in preference to natriuresis. It is also useful in the prophylaxis of acute renal failure due to its ability to expand the extracellular volume, increase tubular fluid flow, redistribute blood to hypoxic inner cortical and outer medullary regions, and scavenge free radicals (Warren and Blantz, 1981). The rationale for using mannitol in oliguric acute renal failure is to convert the condition into a nonoliguric one, thereby permitting easier management of fluids, nutritional support, and electrolytes. In addition, mannitol has been reported to decrease the incidence of acute renal failure in cardiopulmonary bypass surgery (Rigden et al., 1984), myoglobinuria (Eneas et al., 1979), transfusion of mismatched blood (Byrne, 1966), and contrast nephropathy (in patients with chronic renal failure) (Anto et al., 1981). The usual dose is 0.5 g/kg given intravenously as a 12.5% solution. A good response is usually observed within 2 hours and consists of a urine output of at least three times the volume injected (10 to 12 mL/kg). In oliguric conditions, however, loop diuretics may be used initially because these may be effective without risking further intravascular volume expansion.

Because osmotic diuretics such as mannitol reduce TBW and intracellular volume, they help to decrease intracranial pressure in neurosurgical conditions associated with brain edema and to decrease intraocular pressure in ophthalmologic procedures. They also ameliorate symptoms associated with dialysis-related disequilibrium syndrome (Arieff, 1982).

Acetazolamide (Diamox)

This carbonic anhydrase inhibitor causes sodium bicarbonate diuresis and a reduction in total body bicarbonate stores. Its effectiveness is limited by the development of hyperchloremic metabolic acidosis. The bicarbonaturia induces phosphaturia (Beck and Goldberg, 1973), whereas the metabolic acidosis increases calcium excretion (Lemman et al., 1967). Both factors are responsible for renal stone formation and nephrocalcinosis during prolonged use of acetazolamide. It can cause severe K^+ wasting, especially during the acute bicarbonaturic phase.

Therapeutically, acetazolamide may be effective in the chronic treatment of glaucoma (Maren, 1987), in alkalinization of the urine (Conger and Falk, 1977), in the treatment of acute mountain sickness (Greene et al., 1981), to stimulate ventilation in central sleep apnea (White et al., 1982), to reduce endolymph formation in Meniere's disease (Brookes et al., 1982), and in the treatment of refractory hydrocephalus (Vogh, 1980).

Loop Diuretics

These agents are rapidly absorbed from the gastrointestinal tract and are excreted by glomerular filtration and by tubular secretion (Rane et al., 1978). Diuretic response is usually very rapid after intravenous administration and greatly exceeds that produced by most other diuretic agents.

Loop diuretics inhibit the $Na^+/K^+/2Cl^-$ (NKCC2) electroneutral cotransport system in the luminal membrane of both the medullary and the cortical segments of the ascending limb of Henle's loop, where 20% of the filtered Na^+ and Cl^- are reabsorbed (Burg et al., 1973). They also inhibit NaCl transport at the level of the proximal and distal tubules (Imbs et al., 1987) and are known to possess weak carbonic anhydrase inhibitory properties (Radtke et al., 1972). Loop diuretics tend to increase RBF without increasing GFR, especially after intravenous administration.

Increased RBF is associated with a redistribution of blood flow from the medulla to the cortex and within the cortex (Higashio et al., 1978). The hemodynamic effects appear to involve the renin-angiotensin system and vasodilatory prostaglandins (Gerger, 1983). These hemodynamic effects have not been linked to the diuretic response, however, and tend to be short-lived.

By markedly increasing the movement of solute in the distal segments of the nephron, loop diuretics induce potent diuresis and natriuresis. The large Na^+ load presented to the distal tubule is associated with increased K^+ and H^+ ion secretion. Thus, hypokalemia and metabolic alkalosis may ensue. The hypercalciuric action of loop diuretics makes them suitable agents for treatment of hypercalcemia (Dirks, 1979), but their use in newborns with chronic respiratory disorders has been implicated in the development of nephrocalcinosis (Schell-Feith et al., 2000).

In addition to inducing rapid diuresis, loop diuretics appear to improve cardiac function before the onset of diuresis by increasing venous capacitance (Dikshit et al., 1973). These drugs are also effective in the treatment of refractory edema as long as interstitial fluid can be mobilized without compromising intravascular volume. Because furosemide, ethacrynic acid, and bumetanide are effective with GFR as low as 10 mL/min per 1.73 m^2, they are useful for management of edema in patients with chronic renal failure. Despite the obvious benefits of high-dose furosemide in certain experimental models of acute renal failure (deTorrente et al., 1978), its use in humans for conversion of oliguric acute renal failure to a nonoliguric state is controversial (Brown et al., 1981). All loop diuretics are ototoxic when given in large dosages to patients with severe renal failure (Gallagher and Jones, 1979). Unique to the loop diuretics, ototoxicity has been ascribed to drug-induced changes in the electrolyte composition of endolymph.

Finally, furosemide must be used cautiously in infants with hyperbilirubinemia because it is highly protein bound (Prandota and Pruitt, 1975) and thus capable of displacing bilirubin from albumin (Wenneberg et al., 1977). This phenomenon usually occurs with repeated dosages exceeding 1 mg/kg (Aranda et al., 1978).

Distal Convoluted Tubule Diuretics

The diuretic action of thiazides depends on the direct inhibition of the Na^+/Cl^- cotransporter in the distal convoluted tubule (Kunau et al., 1975), which is accompanied by enhanced excretion of K^+ and hypokalemia. By increasing Na^+ delivery to the cortical collecting duct, thiazides induce a kaliuresis that rivals that of loop diuretics, whereas the natriuresis of furosemide is 5 to 10 times greater than that produced by thiazides.

Apart from their use in managing edema and hypertension, thiazides have also been used successfully for treatment of hypercalciuria because they augment the reabsorption of calcium in the distal tubule (Sutton, 1986). Thiazides can also reduce polyuria and polydipsia in nephrogenic diabetes insipidus (Shirley et al., 1982). Such beneficial effect probably results from plasma volume depletion with an attendant decrease in GFR, which promotes NaCl and obligatory fluid reabsorption in the proximal tubule. This effect of thiazides is augmented by dietary salt restriction. Finally, thiazides are useful in the treatment of proximal renal tubular acidosis, characterized by marked bicarbonaturia. Depletion of intravascular volume is necessary to increase proximal bicarbonate reabsorption, an effect that is also promoted by restricting dietary Na^+ (Donckerwolke et al., 1970).

Combined therapy with thiazides and loop diuretics can be used to manage refractory edema due to cirrhosis, nephrotic syndrome, or severe cardiac dysfunction. Synergy occurs when these classes of diuretics are administered together. NaCl delivery out of the proximal tubule is increased, whereas Na^+ reabsorption is inhibited in the loop of Henle and distal tubule. Thus, the resulting diuretic action is greater than that achieved with either agent alone (Ghose and Gupta, 1981). Similarly, metolazone, a thiazide-like diuretic, is particularly useful in the management of edema accompanying congestive heart failure and renal disorders including nephrotic syndrome and states of decreased renal function. While other thiazides lose their diuretic effectiveness at a CrCl of about 30 to 40 mL/min, metolazone retains its effectiveness, especially when used in conjunction with loop diuretics. This is attributed to its action on the proximal tubule in addition to its action on the distal diluting tubular segments. A limiting factor to the use of metolazone is its availability in tablet form, which may preclude its use in patients whose gastrointestinal tract cannot be used. In such instances, chlorothiazide may be used intravenously in conjunction with loop diuretics.

Adverse effects of thiazides include hypokalemia, metabolic alkalosis, carbohydrate intolerance (Hoskins and Jackson, 1978), hyperuricemia (Manuel and Steele, 1974), hyponatremia in the presence of severe restriction of dietary Na^+, and hypercalcemia (Popovtzer et al., 1975). In general, the hypercalcemia resolves within a few days.

Late Distal Tubule Diuretic

These diuretics are primarily K^+-sparing diuretics. Because of their distal site of action, they are not potent when used alone. Their major use is as adjuncts to thiazide or loop diuretics. Spironolactone competitively antagonizes aldosterone (Corvol et al., 1981), whereas triamterene and amiloride inhibit the epithelial Na^+ channel (ENaC) in the cortical collecting duct and thereby limit kaliuresis (Stoner et al., 1974). In addition, triamterene may depress the GFR through its effect on urinary prostaglandin E_2 excretion (Favre et al., 1982). In general, these agents should be used cautiously in children with renal failure because of the danger of hyperkalemia. Furthermore, concurrent use of K^+-sparing diuretics and K^+ supplements is hazardous.

■ ANESTHETIC AGENTS AND THE KIDNEY

Inhalational and intravenous anesthetics and many intravenous and oral analgesics and sedatives may influence renal function through their hemodynamic, cardiovascular, autonomic, and neuroendocrine effects. The trauma of surgery and possible accompanying dehydration per se are more likely, however, to result in renal dysfunction through elevations in plasma renin, aldosterone, and ADH that accompany surgery. These perturbations are reduced by morphine or halothane anesthesia (Philbin et al., 1978). Prolonged release of ADH associated with surgical stress and use of anesthetics, combined with high infusions of hypotonic fluids, may result in hyponatremia. Moreover, well-hydrated patients may not experience reductions in glomerular filtration (Philbin et al., 1981) and may actually experience increases in RBF with subsequent increases in urine output and sodium excretion (Bastron et al., 1981).

More direct nephrotoxic acute renal failure was common before discontinued use of the fluorinated anesthetic methoxyflurane (Pezzi et al., 1966; Halpren et al., 1973). Inhaled anesthetics in current use, such as sevoflurane and halothane, result in lesser amounts of metabolic byproducts composed of inorganic fluoride, as well as oxalic acid, and hence, renal dysfunction is rare with these agents. Fluoride, in particular, may decrease ATP availability and thereby impair the action of the Na^+,K^+-ATPase in the loop of Henle and in the collecting duct. This may result in a salt-losing, vasopressin-resistant high urine output renal dysfunction (Whitford and Taves, 1973). Conversely, a preexisting reduction in GFR may prolong the pharmacologic half-life of many agents that have significant renal elimination, such as morphine, and thereby exacerbate their hemodynamic and other systemic adverse effects. Moreover, because of short tubular length and enzymatically immature secretory mechanisms, proximal tubular secretion of propofol metabolites and of other substances may be limited in infants under 6 months of age. Awareness of the previously discussed developmental differences in GFR and tubular function in preterm and term neonates and early infancy is essential to determine the choice and dosage modification of many such agents.

DISORDERS OF DIVALENT ION METABOLISM

CALCIUM

Calcium plays many vital physiologic roles, not the least of which is to maintain the health of bones. It is essential for the stability of cellular membranes and regular neuromuscular excitation–contraction coupling, blood coagulation, and transport and secretory functions of the cell. Furthermore, Ca^{2+} acts as a "second messenger" in the signal transduction of extracellular hormones and other substances that affect numerous cellular functions.

Calcium Homeostasis

A typical adult diet contains about 800 mg of elemental Ca^{2+}, of which only 20%, or about 4 mmol (160 mg), is absorbed principally in the duodenum and jejunum. This net Ca^{2+} absorption is closely matched by renal excretion such that all but 4 mmol of the 270 mmol of Ca^{2+} filtered by the kidneys is excreted in the urine. This contrasts with a net Ca^{2+} absorption of 40% to 45% in infants and as high as 80% in low-birth-weight infants and breastfed babies (Liu et al., 1989; Matkovic et al., 1992). Normal daily bone turnover in adults accounts for 14 mmol of Ca^{2+} and comprises only a small proportion of the bone reservoir consisting of about 20 moles, or 800 g.

Plasma Ca^{2+} is maintained at a concentration of 9 to 10.5 mg/dL (2.2 to 2.4 mmol/L) as total calcium, with approximately 40% of this value comprising the protein-bound nonfiltratable fraction, and 10% is chelated. Ionized calcium accounts for 47% of the total circulating Ca^{2+} and ranges from 4 to 5 mg/dL (1.0 to 1.25 mmol/L) (Moore, 1970).

The extent of protein binding per deciliter of plasma is approximately 0.8 mg of Ca^{2+} for every 1 g of albumin and 0.16 mg for each 1 g of globulin. Furthermore, a threefold increase in serum phosphate or sulfate concentration results in a 10% decrease in serum Ca^{2+} concentration. In addition, the binding of Ca^{2+} to albumin is pH-dependent between pH 7 and 9. An acute increase or decrease in the pH by 0.1 U results in an increase or a decrease, respectively, of protein bound Ca^{2+} of 0.2 mg/dL (0.05 mmol/L). Thus, infusion of blood products, rapid correction of metabolic acidosis by infusion of sodium bicarbonate, or acute alkalosis caused by hyperventilation in the presence of hypocalcemia may precipitate tetany and/or seizures because of increased binding of Ca^{2+} to albumin. Calcium homeostasis is complex and occurs at three main levels, often involving similar calcitropic hormones, receptors, and transporters.

In the small intestine, Ca^{2+} is absorbed via two mechanisms: (1) a nonsaturable passive paracellular pathway such that a high Ca^{2+} intake results in higher Ca^{2+} absorption, and (2) an active energy-dependent intracellular pathway that predominates when calcium intake is low. This latter mechanism is highly influenced by 1,25-dihydroxyvitamin D_3 [1,25$(OH)_2D_3$ or calcitriol], which stimulates the synthesis and/or activity of enterocyte apical Ca^{2+} transporters known as CaT1 and ECaC. Calcium crosses the cytoplasm bound to calbindin-D_{9K} and then is extruded against an electrochemical gradient at the basolateral side by plasma membrane Ca^{2+}-ATPase (PMCA). Disorders leading to hypersensitivity or increased synthesis of 1,25$(OH)_2D_3$ can result in increased intestinal absorption and hypercalciuria. Lactose stimulates calcium absorption even in the absence of vitamin D via an effect that may involve 25-hydroxylase (Lester et al., 1982). This may explain the higher plasma Ca^{2+} levels seen in infants. The efficiency of intestinal Ca^{2+} absorption depends on needs, age, sex, dietary intake, pregnancy, and vitamin D status.

The kidneys play a major role in Ca^{2+} homeostasis. The mechanisms of renal transport have been reviewed extensively by Suki and Rouse (1991), Bushinsky (2001), and Frick and Bushinsky (2003) and are reviewed here briefly. Only the fraction of Ca^{2+} not bound to protein is filtered, accounting for 60% of the plasma concentration. About 70% of the filtered Ca^{2+} is reabsorbed in the proximal convoluted tubule through a paracellular pathway involving solvent drag of salt and water (convection). It is then returned to the circulation from the interstitium. About 20% of the filtered Ca^{2+} is reabsorbed in the thick ascending limb of Henle's loop via both paracellular and transcellular processes. Paracellin is the major protein component of the paracellular tight junction. Similar to the pathway of magnesium reabsorption (Fig. 4–8*A* and *B*), the Ca^{2+}-sensing receptor (CaSR) detects small changes in interstitial Ca^{2+} concentrations and regulates the apical ROMK channel, thereby producing a lumen-positive voltage that drives Ca^{2+} through the tight junctions. In this tubular segment mutations in paracellin, NKCC2 transporter, ROMK, or CaSR, or inhibition of the NKCC2 transporter by loop diuretics, can result in significant hypercalciuria, nephrocalcinosis, and osteopenia. The distal convoluted tubule reabsorbs 8% of the filtered calcium mainly via an active transcellular transport. This mechanism is similar to that found in enterocytes except for intracellular calcium transport occurring through binding to calbindin-D_{28K} and extrusion mainly by a Na^+/Ca^{2+} exchanger and less by PMCA. This mechanism is influenced by parathyroid hormone (PTH) and perhaps by other calcitropic hormones.

Bone reabsorption and formation also contribute to calcium homeostasis. The mechanisms by which osteoclasts and osteoblasts affect these processes are less well understood, but several hormonal regulators and transport processes are thought to resemble those found in intestine and kidney.

PTH is a major regulator of serum Ca^{2+} homeostasis. PTH acts via cAMP to increase proximal tubular Ca^{2+} excretion while it increases reabsorption in the distal and collecting ducts, so that the net effect is conservation of Ca^{2+} (Suki and Rouse, 1991). PTH also resorbs Ca^{2+} from the vast skeletal reservoir of Ca^{2+} and increases intestinal Ca^{2+} absorption by stimulating

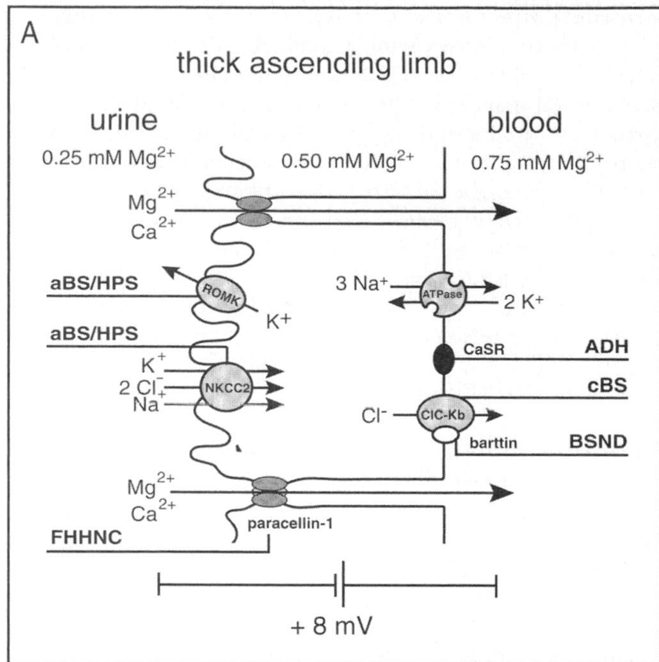

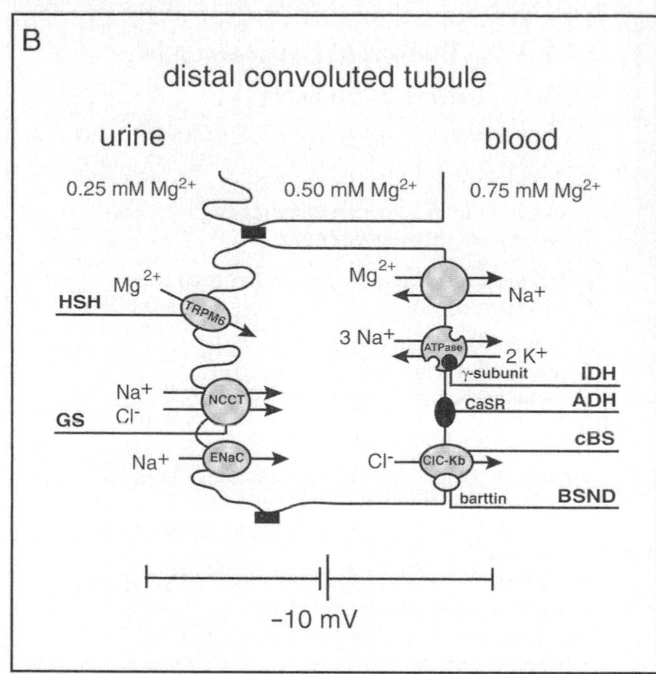

■ **FIGURE 4–8.** *(A)* Magnesium reabsorption in the thick ascending limb of the loop of Henle. Driving force for the paracellular reabsorption of magnesium and calcium is the lumen-positive electrochemical gradient generated by the transcellular reabsorption of NaCl. *(B)* Magnesium reabsorption in the distal convoluted tubule. In this segment, magnesium is reabsorbed by an active transcellular pathway involving an apical entry step probably via a magnesium permeable ion channel and a basolateral exchange mechanism, presumably an Na^+/Mg^{2+} exchanger. The molecular identity of this exchanger is still unknown. See text for details. ADH, autosomal dominant hypocalcemia. (From Konrad M, Weber S: Recent advances in molecular genetics of hereditary magnesium-losing disorders. *J Am Soc Nephrol* 14:249–260, 2003, p 251, Figure 4-3 *[A]* and *[B]*.)

1α-hydroxylase and calcitriol synthesis by proximal tubular epithelium, thereby guarding against hypocalcemia. High plasma phosphorus concentrations directly stimulate PTH release. This causes phosphaturia and raises serum Ca^{2+} concentration by the body's tendency to maintain a constant $Ca^{2+} \times P^{2-}$ product. Conversely, preterm infants fed diets low in phosphorus develop hypophosphatemia and are susceptible to hypercalcemia through direct stimulation of calcitriol synthesis.

Calcitriol is another major independent homeostatic factor. It increases intestinal absorption of Ca^{2+}, and, in concert with PTH, it stimulates osteoclast-mediated resorption of bone. High serum calcium concentrations, on the other hand, interact with the parathyroid cell Ca^{2+}-sensing receptors to inhibit PTH secretion. High calcitriol levels also exert a negative feedback role on PTH secretion.

Other endogenous or exogenous substances play a lesser role in Ca^{2+} homeostasis. A hypercalcemic substance produced in several malignant or paraneoplastic syndromes is known as PTH-related peptide (PTHrP). The N-terminal of PTHrP functions like PTH and often contributes to humoral or tumoral hypercalcemia. Increased synthesis of other hypercalcemic cytokines such as interleukins-1,-6, and -11, as well as tumor necrosis factor-α and prostaglandins, may also be released in various malignancies (Mundy and Guise, 1997). Macrophages may be an important source of such factors that act synergistically to produce significant osteolysis. Glucocorticoids lower calcium levels by reducing its intestinal absorption. Excessive thyroid hormone accelerates bone turnover, and calcitonin lowers serum calcium by increasing its excretion at the medullary portion of the thick ascending limb of the loop of Henle while inhibiting bone turnover. Immobilization may raise serum calcium levels by lowering the inflow of calcium into bone hydroxyapatite. Hypervitaminosis D, or a combination of vitamin A administration and decreased vitamin A catabolism in individuals with reduced renal function, may cause hypercalcemia by stimulating intestinal absorption.

Hypocalcemia (Plasma Ionized Calcium <1.0 mmol/L, or Total Calcium <7.0, 8.0, and 8.8 mg/dL, or <1.7, 2.0, and 2.2 mmol/L in Preterm, Term Newborns, and Children, Respectively)

The causes of hypocalcemia in neonates and children are listed in Box 4–9, and the biochemical features of these disorders are shown (Umpaichitra et al., 2001) (Table 4–15). "Early neonatal hypocalcemia" develops within the first 48 hours after birth in about 33% of infants less than 37 weeks gestation, in 50% of infants of insulin-dependent diabetic mothers, and in 30% of infants with neonatal asphyxia. In this disorder, there appears to be a significant correlation between gestational age and serum calcium levels. Plasma PTH concentrations are usually normal. Hence, the mechanism for the hypocalcemia may involve decreased calcium intake associated with increased P^{2-} loading (Tsang et al., 1973) and possibly resistance to the action of PTH (Linarelli et al., 1972). Elevated calcitonin levels have been recently suggested as a cause of early hypocalcemia, particularly in neonatal asphyxia (Venkataraman et al., 1987).

In term infants, hypocalcemia may occur 5 to 7 days after birth, often associated with the ingestion of cow's milk (Root and Harrison, 1976). Maternal vitamin D status may also play an important role in late neonatal hypocalcemia (Cockburn et al., 1980). Nutritional deficiency of vitamin D, inadequate photoconversion of vitamin D, and decreased calcium intake are currently uncommon causes of hypocalcemia and rickets in infants. In the neonate with micrognathia, hypertelorism,

BOX 4–9 Causes of Hypocalcemia*

Early Neonatal Hypocalcemia

Preterm (related to decreased PTH secretion)
Neonates with asphyxia (limitation of calcium intake)
Infants of diabetic mothers (related to maternal urinary magnesium loss because of glycosuria leading to hypomagnesemia)

Late Neonatal Hypocalcemia (End of the First Week of Life)

Dietary phosphate loading
Hypoparathyroidism
Hypomagnesemia

Childhood Hypocalcemia

Vitamin D–related: Vitamin D–deficient rickets, vitamin D–dependent rickets type I (1β-hydroxylase deficiency), and type II (end-organ resistance to calcitriol)
Parathyroid hormone–related: Hypoparathyroidism, pseudohypoparathyroidism type I and type II
Calcium/phosphorus–related: Malabsorption, hyperphosphatemia
Organ-related: Hepatic rickets, acute pancreatitis, renal osteodystrophy
Miscellaneous: Drugs, such as calcitonin, phosphate, and bisphosphonates; magnesium deficiency; calcium-sensing receptor defect

*Causes at different ages at onset can overlap.
Modified from Umpaichitra V, Bastian W, Castells S: *Clin Pediatr (Phila)* 40:306, 2001, Table 1.

fishmouth, low-set posteriorly rotated ears, and cardiac disease, one must consider branchial dysembryogenesis, or DiGeorge anomaly. In this disorder, there is aplasia or hypoplasia of the parathyroid glands in association with diverse genetic deletions that can be detected by fluorescent in situ hybridization (FISH) DNA probes (Hong, 1998).

In children, autoimmune disorders that are either isolated or associated with other polyglandular syndromes comprise the majority of causes of acquired hypoparathyroidism and are often diagnosed by detection of specific autoantibodies directed against various endocrine tissues. Pseudohypoparathyroidism is associated with mutations in the PTH receptor, which is a G protein–coupled receptor. Circulating PTH levels are high, but there is PTH resistance in bone and kidney or in the kidney alone (Farfel et al., 1999). In the first subtype (Ia), the phenotype consists of hereditary osteodystrophy (Albright's), short fingers, short stature, mental retardation, and subcutaneous calcifications, whereas in subtype Ib, the phenotype is normal. Pseudohypoparathyroidism type II is caused by disturbances in the pathway past the PTH receptor. Plasma PTH levels are also increased in this disorder.

Hypocalcemia is a frequent complication of hypomagnesemia. Three mechanisms have been suggested: resistance to the action of PTH (Estep et al., 1969); subnormal secretion of PTH (Suh et al., 1973); and defective Ca^{2+}/Mg^{2+} exchange in bone (Chase and Slatopolsky, 1974). Correction of hypomagnesemia has been shown to restore calcium homeostasis.

Hepatic disorders that interfere with vitamin D and other fat-soluble vitamin absorption and conversion to 25-vitamin D_3, or calcidiol, can cause hypocalcemia particularly in debilitated or immobilized individuals. In children with renal failure due to a variety of chronic renal disorders, impaired conversion of calcitriol by proximal tubular α-hydroxylase to the active calcitriol form, along with phosphate retention, impaired intestinal absorption of Ca^{2+}, and high circulating PTH concentrations that impair osteoclastic activity, all combine to cause hypocalcemia (Slatopolski and Delmez, 1992). Mutations in 1α-hydroxylase lead to vitamin D–resistant rickets, an autosomal dominant disorder presenting at 4 to 12 months of age with low serum Ca^{2+} but normal 25-vitamin D_3 levels. If calcitriol levels are normal, hypocalcemia can be the result of mutations in the vitamin (calcitriol) D receptor (VDR), which is also an autosomal dominant, vitamin D–resistant condition presenting at 3 to 12 months with rickets and alopecia (Levine and Carpenter, 1999).

Manifestations of Hypocalcemia

Many of the symptoms associated with hypocalcemia are attributed to increased neuromuscular excitability. These symptoms include numbness and tingling of the hands, toes, and lips; irritability, anxiety, and depression; prolonged QT interval; cardiac arrhythmias; and congestive heart failure. In the neonatal period, jitteriness, twitching, and seizures are more common. The seizures may be generalized or focal and usually are short-lived but repetitive, with very little postictal depression.

TABLE 4–15. Causes of hypocalcemia and their biochemical profile clues

	SERUM						URINE	
Causes of Hypocalcemia	*Ca*	*P*	*PTH*	*Alk Phos*	*25OHD$_3$*	*1,25(OH) 2D$_3$*	*Mg*	*Ca*
Vitamin D–deficient rickets	↓, ↔	↔,↓	↑	↑	↓	*	↔	↓
Vitamin D–dependent rickets type I	↓	↓, ↔	↑	↑	↔	↓	↔	↓
Vitamin D–dependent rickets type II	↓	↓, ↔	↑	↑	↔	↑	↔	↓
Hypoparathyroidism	↓	↑	↓	↔	↔	↔, ↓	↔	↓
Pseudohypoparathyroidism	↓	↑	↑	↔	↔	↔, ↓	↔	↓
Rickets of prematurity	↔, ↓	↔, ↓	↑	↑	↔	↔, ↓	↔	?
Renal osteodystrophy	↓	↑	↑	↑	↔	↓	↔, ↑	↓
Calcium-sensing receptor defect	↓	↑, ↔	**	↔	↔	↔, ↓	↔	↑
Mg deficiency	↓	↔	**	↔	↔	↓	↓	↑

Ca, calcium; P, phosphorus; PTH, parathyroid hormone; Alk Phos, alkaline phosphatase; Mg, magnesium; ↔, normal; ↓, decrease; ↑, increase; ?, difficult to interpret owing to different degree of renal immaturity in preterm infants; *, decrease or normal or increase; **, decrease or normal or slight increase (relatively low for degree of hypocalcemia).
Modified from Umpaichitra V, Bastian W, Castells S: Hypocalcemia in children: Pathogenesis and management. *Clin Pediatr* 40:305–312, 2001, p 307, Table 2.

Chvostek's and Trousseau's signs and a high-pitched cry are useful indications, especially in the older infant and child. Infants may have cyanosis, vomiting, or feeding intolerance, whereas older children may present with laryngospasm. With prolonged hypocalcemia, cataracts can develop because of the increased intake of Na^+ and water by the lens (Ireland et al., 1968).

Treatment of Hypocalcemia

If hypocalcemia is not life threatening, it is preferable to administer a calcium-containing solution amounting to 15 mg of elemental calcium/kg body weight infused over a period of 4 to 6 hours. For clinical emergencies (seizures, tetany), 10% calcium gluconate is infused, preferably in a large vein or central venous catheter, to provide an elemental Ca^{2+} dosage of 2 to 4 mg/kg body weight in newborns and 2 to 3 mg/kg body weight in children, given over 5 to 10 minutes under constant electrocardiographic monitoring. Subsequently 25 to 50 mg of intravenous elemental Ca^{2+}/kg body weight per day may be used until hypocalcemia resolves. If hypomagnesemia is also present, 50% magnesium sulfate (48 mg elemental Mg^{2+}/mL) at a dosage of 6 mg of elemental Mg^{2+}/kg body weight may be infused over 1 hour.

Hypoparathyroidism requires the use of calcitriol at an initial dosage of 0.01 mcg/kg body weight daily to maintain plasma Ca^{2+} concentrations between 8.5 and 9.0 mg/dL. Monitoring of plasma levels and urinary Ca^{2+} excretion may limit the risk of hypercalcemia, hypercalciuria, and nephrocalcinosis (evident on renal ultrasound). In vitamin D–dependent rickets type I, the dose of calcitriol is 10 to 15 ng/kg per day combined with elemental calcium of 500 to 1000 mg/day. Children with vitamin D–deficient rickets may receive vitamin D (ergocalciferol or Drisdol, 8000 units/mL = 0.2 mg/mL) at 2000 to 10,000 IU/day orally for 4 to 8 weeks, or a single oral megadose of 200,000 to 600,000 IU (Stosstherapy), which is safe and more effective, particularly when compliance is in question. Oral or intravenous calcitriol may be used in pseudohypoparathyroidism or in children with chronic renal failure to increase intestinal absorption Ca^{2+} and suppress PTH secretion.

Hypercalcemia (Plasma Ionized Calcium >1.35 mmol/L or >5.4 mg/dL, or Total Calcium >10.5 mg/dL, or 2.6 mmol/L)

It is important to exclude pseudohypercalcemia as a cause of hypercalcemia in individuals with essential thrombocytosis after clotting of phlebotomized blood. The causes of hypercalcemia vary by age (Box 4–10) (Rodd and Goodyer, 1999; Ziegler, 2001). Although hypercalcemia is uncommon in newborns, the most common cause is iatrogenic resulting from excessive administration of calcium salts. Other causes in this age group include idiopathic infantile hypercalcemia, which is usually mild; more severe hypercalcemia occurs in Williams syndrome. Primary neonatal hyperparathyroidism is a very rare disorder caused by homozygous inheritance of mutations in the Ca^{2+}-sensing receptor that result in familial hypocalciuric hypercalcemia (FHH). Although these patients' heterozygous parents are often asymptomatic, the condition may be life-threatening in the offspring due to plasma calcium of 15 to 30 mg/dL, unexplained anemia, hepatosplenomegaly, and nephrocalcinosis. Primary hyperparathyroidism is extremely rare in childhood but may occur in the multiple endocrine adenoma syndrome, in which hypercalcemia, hypercalciuria, and nephrolithiasis relate to elevated levels of $1,25(OH)_2D_3$ (Broadus et al., 1980).

BOX 4–10 **Causes of Hypercalcemia**

Neonates

Iatrogenic (calcium salts)
Idiopathic infantile hypercalcemia
Williams syndrome
Vitamin D
- Vitamin D intoxication
- Subcutaneous fat necrosis

Parathyroid related
- Hyperparathyroidism
  - Neonatal severe hyperparathyroidism
  - Secondary hyperparathyroidism
- Familial hypocalciuric hypercalcemia
- PTHrP (humoral hypercalcemia) tumor related
- PTH receptor mutation—Jansen's metaphyseal chondrodysplasia

Miscellaneous
- Hypophosphatasia
- Hypophosphatemia
- Vitamin A intoxication
- Blue-diaper syndrome
- Thiazide diuretics

Children

Primary hyperparathyroidism
"Tertiary hyperparathyroidism"
Ectopic secretion of PTH by tumors
Neoplasms (bony metastases)
Neoplastic production of $1,25(OH)_2D_3$
Phosphate depletion with hypophosphatemia
Sarcoidosis, tuberculosis, and other granulomatous disorders
Immobilization
Milk-alkali syndrome
Medications (thiazide diuretics, theophylline, lithium, salicylate intoxication, vitamin D or vitamin A intoxication)
Thyrotoxicosis
Exsiccosis
AIDS
Multiple fractures
Acute renal failure

PTH, parathyroid hormone; PTHrP, parathyroid hormone–related protein

Diagnostic Studies

Diagnostic studies to consider in newborns and in children with hypocalcemia or hypercalcemia are shown (Box 4–11) (Rodd and Goodyer, 1999). In general, PTHrP and calcitrophic cytokines need not be measured unless plasma PTH levels are normal or suppressed and the cause of hypercalcemia is cryptic. If PTHrP is measured, the blood tube should contain a proteinase inhibitor.

Manifestations of Hypercalcemia

Newborns and infants with hypercalcemia present with nonspecific symptoms such as failure to thrive because of anorexia and vomiting. Irritability, lethargy, hypotonia, and seizures are common with more severe hypercalcemia. Bradycardia, a short QT interval, and hypertension are other findings. In older children, nausea, vomiting, constipation, and vague central nervous system symptoms of headaches and fatigue may be apparent.

BOX 4–11 Evaluation of Infants With Persistent Hypercalcemia

Blood—Total and ionized calcium, pH, phosphorus, alkaline phosphatase, creatinine, intact PTH, 25-hydroxyvitamin D, 1,25-dihydroxyvitamin D
Urine—Calcium/creatinine ratio, tubular reabsorption of phosphate
Renal ultrasonography
Other tests that can be performed, if the above do not yield a diagnosis
- PTHrP
- Vitamin A
- Parents' serum calcium and urine calcium
- Long bone X-rays

From Rodd C, Goodyer P: Hypercalcemia of the newborn: etiology, evaluation, and management. *Pediatr Nephrol* 13:542–547, 1999, p 545, Table 2.

Renal function may be markedly decreased because of diminished RBF due to vasoconstriction induced by hypercalcemia and by circulatory volume depletion due to acquired nephrogenic diabetes insipidus. Nephrocalcinosis, nephrolithiasis, hematuria, and sterile pyuria may occur secondary to hypercalciuria. An inability to concentrate the urine because of resistance to the action of ADH may result in polyuria, polydipsia, and dehydration. Hypokalemia may occur secondary to diuresis. The development of rapid and severe hypercalcemia (>17 mg/dL) can result in dehydration, azotemia, coma, and death.

Management of Hypercalcemia

The first step in the management of acute hypercalcemia is to discontinue all of the sources of calcium and vitamin D. In neonates, a formula with low calcium and vitamin D content may be used (Calci-loXD; Ross Laboratories) along with immediate provision of hydration consisting of normal saline at 20 mL/kg body weight per hr for 4 hours. Excretion of calcium may be further promoted by intravenous furosemide at a dosage of 0.5 to 1.0 mg/kg body weight given every 6 hours with frequent monitoring of plasma ionized Ca^{2+}, Na^+, K^+, Cl^-, and Mg^{2+} concentrations. Supplementation with such ions is essential. Thiazides are anticalciuric and are contraindicated. Calcitonin given at 4 to 8 IU/kg body weight subcutaneously every 6 hours is particularly useful if there is concurrent renal insufficiency. Methylprednisolone at 1 mg/kg body weight per 24 hr may be useful in this setting. Biphosphonates inhibit macrophage and osteoclast activity and are increasingly used to treat hypercalcemia but also to prevent osteoporosis, osteopathy, or calcinosis. Pamidronate at a single dose of 0.5 mg/kg intravenously (may be repeated daily as needed for 3 days) is the agent of choice in tumoral hypercalcemia, vitamin D intoxication, resistant hypercalcemia, or in newborns with subcutaneous fat necrosis and elevated plasma $1,25(OH)_2D_3$ concentrations. Etidronate at an oral dosage of 5 mg/kg per dose given twice daily along with sodium supplementation at 3 mmol/kg per day is also effective for managing chronic disorders. In severe hypercalcemia or when oliguria or renal insufficiency is present, dialysis with a low calcium dialysate concentration (1.25 mmol/L) is recommended. In cases of severe neonatal hyperparathyroidism due to homozygous FHH or other forms of primary hyperparathyroidism, expeditious parathyroidectomy may be lifesaving.

MAGNESIUM

Magnesium is the fourth most abundant cation in the body, and it is largely located intracellularly. Its principal role is to stabilize electrically excitable membranes. Magnesium is also an important co-factor of numerous important enzymes, including adenosine triphosphatase (Na^+,K^+-ATPase) (Gums, 1987), alkaline phosphatase, and adenylate cyclase and is essential in oxidative phosphorylation, protein synthesis, and DNA metabolism.

Magnesium Homeostasis

Normal plasma magnesium levels range from 1.7 to 2.5 mg/dL or 0.7 to 1.0 mmol/L. In general, plasma levels of Mg^{2+} correlate well with tissue levels; such correlation is poor, however, in circumstances such as renal failure or hepatic cirrhosis (Cohen and Kitzes, 1982).

Despite being very abundant in the body, defense against hypomagnesemia is limited by (1) an inappropriately low parathyroid secretion when plasma levels are below 1.0 mg/dL, (2) PTH resistance at the skeletal level, and (3) decreased calcitriol levels predisposing to combined hypocalcemia (Agus, 1999). Hypomagnesemia is very common in hospitalized individuals, particularly when nutritional intake is low for 3 or more days.

An average Western diet provides 400 mg of Mg^{2+} (16 mmol) per day, of which 30% to 50% is absorbed in the jejunum and ileum (Brannan et al., 1976). Intestinal absorption can increase to 80% in the presence of mild hypomagnesemia (plasma Mg^{2+} <1.2 mg/dL, <1.0 mEq/L, or <0.5 mmol/L). In the blood, 30% of Mg^{2+} is bound to proteins and is not filtered at the glomerulus. Of the filtered Mg^{2+}, about 3% is excreted in the urine.

Once filtered, Mg^{2+} is reabsorbed in the proximal tubule (15% to 20%), in the thick ascending limb of the loop of Henle (65% to 76%), and in the distal convoluted tubule (5% to 10%). As with Ca^{2+}, the bulk of Mg^{2+} reabsorption occurs in the thick ascending limb of Henle's loop via a passive paracellular mechanism that is facilitated by the positive transepithelial voltage generated by apical Na^+ entry and diffusion of K^+ into the lumen generated by the interplay of the apical NKCC2 cotransporter, the basolateral Na^+,K^+-ATPase, and the return of K^+ into the tubular lumen via the action of ROMK (Konrad and Weber, 2003) (see Fig. 4–8*A*). The resultant change in luminal charge affects the configuration of structural proteins, especially that of paracellin-1 (also known as "claudin 16") present in tight junctions. Mutations in paracellin-1 become manifest in early childhood with often familial hypomagnesemia, hypercalciuria, hematuria and nephrocalcinosis leading to polyuria, and progressive decline in GFR such that one third of these children develop renal failure by age 15 years (Weber et al., 2001).

Interference with NKCC2 cotransport by loop diuretics diminishes the luminal voltage and leads to Mg^{2+} wasting, hypomagnesemia, and hypocalcemia. Metabolic acidosis, K^+ depletion, and hypophosphatemia may cause magnesuria by affecting the transepithelial voltage. In contrast, Mg^{2+} transport in the distal convoluted tubule is active and transcellular (see Fig. 4–8*B*). Specific, but not well-characterized, Mg^{2+} channels transport Mg^{2+} in and out of the cells in this region and are influenced by multiple agents, including the Mg^{2+}-sparing diuretics amiloride and chlorothiazide (Cole and Quamme, 2000; Konrad and Weber 2003). Mutations in these channels or in the Ca^{2+}/Mg^{2+}–sensing receptor (CaSR), which inhibits Na^+, Ca^{2+}, and Mg^{2+} absorption at the basolateral membrane (DiStefano et al., 1997), are responsible for several inherited disorders (Box 4–12), which

BOX 4–12 Inherited Disorders of Renal Magnesium Handling

Primary Inherited Disorders of Renal Magnesium Handling

Hypomagnesemia with secondary hypocalcemia (HSH)
Infantile isolated hypomagnesemia with autosomal dominant inheritance (IDH)
Infantile primary hypomagnesemia with autosomal recessive inheritance

Other Inherited Disorders

Idiopathic hypermagnesuria
Congenital hypomagnesemia not yet classified

Hypomagnesemia Associated With Hypercalciuria and Nephrocalcinosis

Familial hypomagnesemia with hypercalciuria and nephrocalcinosis (FHHNC)

Inherited Disorders Associated With Abnormal Extracellular Mg^{2+}/Ca^{2+} Sensing

Autosomal dominant hypoparathyroidism
Familial hypocalciuric hypercalcemia and neonatal severe hyperparathyroidism (FHH)

Hypomagnesemia Associated With Abnormal Renal NaCl Transport

Gitelman's syndrome (GH)
Bartter's syndrome
 Classic form (cBS)
 Antenatal form with hyperprostaglandin E (aBS/HPS)
 With sensorineural hearing loss (BSND)

Cole D, Quamme GA: Inherited disorders of renal magnesium handling. *J Am Soc Nephrol* 11:1937–1947, 2000, p 1940, Table 2. (With kind permission of Springer Science and Business Media.)

often present in infancy and childhood with symptoms related to hypomagnesemia.

Etiology and Manifestations of Dysmagnesemia

Hypomagnesemia (Plasma Concentration <1.7 mg/dL, or <0.7 mmol/L)

Hypomagnesemia is far more common and more clinically relevant than hypermagnesemia (>2.5 mg/dL, or >1.0 mmol/L). Genetic disorders resulting in renal Mg^{2+} wasting are highlighted in Box 4–12, and nonheritable or acquired causes of hypomagnesemia and its clinical manifestations are shown in Box 4–13 (Elin, 1988). Pediatric transplant recipients maintained on cyclosporine or tacrolimus are particularly susceptible to hypomagnesemia. This disorder is associated with an increase in the fractional excretion of Mg^{2+} (Barton et al., 1987). Experimental studies demonstrate that cyclosporine leads to a decrease in the serum magnesium concentration, associated with renal Mg^{2+} wasting and Mg^{2+} shift into tissue compartments with no effect on intestinal absorption of Mg^{2+} (Barton, 1989).

Because of the type of clinical conditions leading to hypomagnesemia and because hypomagnesemia per se may contribute to refractory hypokalemia and hypocalcemia, it is common to find concurrent hypokalemia, hypocalcemia, and metabolic alkalosis. Symptoms may be exclusively attributed to hypomagnesemia only after excluding these other electrolyte disturbances. Patients with renal wasting of magnesium present with nephrocalcinosis, nephrolithiasis, and decreased GFR. Neurologic symptoms resemble those of hypocalcemia and may include personality changes, tremors, seizures, and carpopedal spasm.

Hypermagnesemia

Hypermagnesemia occurs frequently in individuals with acute renal failure who also consume a high level of dietary Mg^{2+} or because of cellular efflux in association with acute ketoacidosis or pheochromocytoma crisis. Although individuals with plasma Mg^{2+} concentrations below 10 mg/dL are usually asymptomatic, hypermagnesemia may cause central nervous system depression, decreased deep-tendon reflexes, muscle weakness, respiratory muscle paralysis, hypotension, bradycardia, heart block, and other arrhythmias.

Etiology and Management of Dysmagnesemia

Diagnosis of Dysmagnesemia

In individuals with normal renal function and absence of renal Mg^{2+} wasting, a fractional excretion of Mg^{2+} ($FE_{Mg^{2+}}$) below 0.5% indicates low dietary intake or gastrointestinal losses of Mg^{2+}, whereas an $FE_{Mg^{2+}}$ over 2% suggests renal Mg^{2+} wasting.

$$FE_{Mg^{2+}} = \frac{U_{Mg^{2+}} \times Pcr}{(0.7 \times P_{Mg^{2+}}) \times Ucr} \times 100$$

where $U_{Mg^{2+}}$ and $P_{Mg^{2+}}$ and Ucr and Pcr are the urinary and plasma concentrations of Mg^{2+} and creatinine, respectively. In this equation, plasma Mg^{2+} concentration is multiplied by 0.7 because only 70% of plasma Mg^{2+} is free. This implies that administration of albumin or blood products may further lower the ionized form of Mg^{2+} and precipitate symptoms. In individuals with low normal plasma Mg^{2+} concentrations, total body Mg^{2+} depletion may be confirmed by an Mg^{2+} excretion in a 24-hour urine collection amounting to less than 80% after an intravenous or intramuscular load of 2.4 mg/kg of lean body mass (this may be administered over 4 hours as the chloride or the sulfate solution in 5% dextrose in water or normal saline) (Gullestad et al., 1994).

Management of Dysmagnesemia

The first step is to discontinue offending medications and to attempt to correct the primary etiology of hypomagnesemia (Box 4–15). In individuals with tetany or cardiac arrhythmias, intravenous Mg^{2+} may be infused slowly to avoid hypotension. The usual dosage is 0.2 mEq/kg (0.1 mmol/kg, or, 2.4 mg/kg) every 4 to 6 hours until blood levels exceed 1.0 mg/dL (0.4 mmol/L, or 0.8 mEq/L). The intravenous or intramuscular administration of 25 to 50 mg/kg body weight of magnesium sulfate solution, or 0.2 to 0.4 mEq/kg body weight of elemental Mg^{2+}, is also preferred in symptomatic individuals with normomagnesemia who exhibit refractory hypokalemia or hypocalcemia. Amiloride may be used to reduce renal Mg^{2+} wasting by stimulating reabsorption in the cortical collecting duct. Because Mg^{2+} has a low renal tubular threshold (1.3 to 1.7 mEq/L), intravenous infusions or large single oral loads of Mg^{2+} are quickly excreted in the urine. Thus, smaller, more frequent doses or use of oral sustained-release preparations, such as Slow-Mag or Mag-Tab SR, are more effective. Symptomatic hypermagnesemia

BOX 4–13 Causes of Hypomagnesemia

Gastrointestinal

Chronic diarrhea
Bowel bypass or resection
Congenital inflammatory bowel disease
Malabsorption syndromes
Tropical sprue
Gluten enteropathy
Laxative abuse
Pancreatitis
Specific magnesium malabsorption
Prolonged nasogastric suctioning
Caloric malnutrition

Renal Excretion

Gitelman's syndrome
Acute renal failure
Renal tubular acidosis
Chronic pyelonephritis
Postobstructive diuresis
Primary renal tubular magnesium wasting
Drug induced
- Acetazolamide
- Alcohol
- Aminoglycosides
- Amphotericin B
- Bumetanide
- Capreomycin
- Carbenicillin
- Chlorthalidone
- Cisplatin
- Cyclosporine
- Digoxin
- Ethacrynic acid
- Furosemide
- Mannitol
- Methotrexate
- Osmotic agents
- Pentamidine
- Tacrolimus
- Theophylline
- Thiazides
- Torsemide
- Viomycin

Nutritional Deficiencies

Malnutrition or eating disorders
Magnesium-free parenteral feedings
Long-term alcohol abuse

Endocrine Disorders

- Hyperaldosteronism
- Hypocalcemia
- Hyperparathyroidism
- Hyperthyroidism
- Diabetes mellitus
- Ketoacidosis
  - Diabetic
  - Alcoholic

Hypoparathyroidism
Syndrome of inappropriate secretion of antidiuretic hormone
Excessive lactation

Redistribution

Insulin treatment for diabetic ketoacidosis
High-catecholamine states
Major trauma or stress
Hungry-bone syndrome

Multiple Mechanisms

Chronic alcoholism
Alcohol withdrawal
Major burns
Liquid-protein diet
Acute porphyria

Neonates

Gestational diabetes
Gestational hyperparathyroidism
Gestational hypoparathyroidism
Exchange transfusion (citrate)

Modified from Elin RJ: Magnesium metabolism in health and disease. *Dis Mon* 34:161–218, 1988, Table 1.

may be acutely managed by dialysis using a dialysate Mg^{2+} concentration of 0.2 mmol/L, as well as calcium infusion or anticholinesterase administration.

PHOSPHORUS

Most total body P^{2-} exists in the form of the inorganic phosphate, but it also exists in an organic intracellular form, where it is the major anion. Phosphorus is an integral component of intracellular nucleic acids and cell membrane phospholipids and is involved in phosphorylation of proteins and lipids. Severe hypophosphatemia (<1 mg/mL) may have profound effects on all body functions through its effect in limiting 2,3-diphosphoglycerate and oxygen dissociation from hemoglobin and by reducing phosphate available for synthesis of high energy bonds in the form of adenosine triphosphate (ATP), which is involved in virtually all energy-requiring processes (Knochel, 1977). Phosphorus, along with Ca^{2+}, is a major constituent of bone.

Phosphorus Homeostasis

Approximately 85% of the total body P^{2-} is in bone (hydroxyapatite, octacalcium phosphate, and amorphous calcium phosphate) (Raisz, 1977) and teeth, while 15% is a constituent of carbohydrate, lipid, and protein in soft tissues and 0.1% is in the ECF.

Serum P^{2-} concentration is maintained between 3.0 and 8.5 mg/dL, depending on age (Parfit and Kleerekoper, 1980). It is highest in infants (4.5 to 8.5 mg/dL) and is relatively high in children (3.7 to 5.9 mg/dL), presumably because of increased concentrations of growth hormone and reduced levels of gonadal hormones until the completion of adolescence.

BOX 4–14 Clinical and Laboratory Manifestations of Hypomagnesemia

Neuromuscular	Central Nervous System
Weakness	Personality change
Tremors	Depression
Muscle fasciculation	Agitation
Positive Chvostek's sign	Psychosis
Positive Trousseau's sign	Nystagmus
Dysphagia	Seizure
Cardiac	**Metabolic**
Arrhythmias (torsades de pointes)	Hypokalemia
ECG changes	Hypocalcemia

Modified from Elin RJ: Magnesium metabolism in health and disease. *Dis Mon* 34:161–218, 1988, Table 4.

About 50% to 60% of dietary P^{2-} is absorbed in the small intestine, especially in the duodenum and jejunum, via an active vitamin D-dependent process which is Na^+-dependent (Harrison and Harrison, 1961), and by passive diffusional flux through paracellular pathways. The absorption of P^{2-} depends on the availability of adequate glucose, Na^+, P^{2-}, and Ca^{2+}. Absorption is decreased by the ingestion of antacids such as aluminum hydroxide, which binds phosphorus in the gut and thereby inhibits gastrointestinal absorption.

At least 90% of plasma P^{2-} appears in the glomerular ultrafiltrate. Most of the filtered P^{2-} is reabsorbed in the proximal tubule. The process is active and Na^+-dependent, and it occurs against an electrochemical gradient (Suki and Rouse, 1991). The amount of P^{2-} in the urine closely parallels the amount absorbed by the intestine. Normally the kidney excretes 10% to 20% of the filtered P^{2-}, suggesting that the maximal capacity of the tubules to reabsorb P^{2-}, or Tmp, is met or exceeded. Saline expansion causes phosphaturia, which can be blocked by total parathyroidectomy. In the absence of PTH, the reabsorption of P^{2-} by the pars recta and the distal nephron is complete and accounts for the hyperphosphatemia in hypoparathyroidism (Knox et al., 1977).

The urinary excretion of P^{2-} depends on the oral intake of P^{2-} (high intake causing increased excretion), the oral intake of Ca^{2+} (high intake causing hypophosphaturia), the presence of catabolism (high catabolic rates causing hyperphosphatemia and hyperphosphaturia), acid-base status (chronic metabolic acidosis decreasing the tubular reabsorption of P^{2-} by decreasing the Vmax of Na^+/P^{2-} cotransport in the brush border membrane of the proximal tubule) (Kempson, 1982), and the levels of PTH and calcitriol. Severe respiratory alkalosis stimulates glycolysis and carbohydrate phosphorylation resulting in secondary intracellular shift of phosphate. Untreated diabetes causes hypophosphatemia through volume expansion, osmotic diuresis, or ketonuria and also through extracellular shift after insulin administration.

BOX 4–15 Treatment of Magnesium Depletion

The following guidelines are suggested for treatment of magnesium deficiency regardless of etiology:

1. It is important to know that the kidneys are producing urine and that the BUN (blood urea nitrogen) and/or creatinine is normal. Magnesium may be needed and may be administered even in an instance of renal insufficiency, but the treatment must be monitored by frequent serum or plasma level assays.
2. On the first day of therapy, at least 1 mEq mg/kg per day should be given parenterally. Subsequently, at least 0.5 mEq mg/kg per day should be given for 3 to 5 days. If parenteral fluid therapy continues, at least 0.2 mEq/kg per day should be given.
3. Give the above in intravenous infusions if such infusions are being given anyway; otherwise, intramuscular administration is satisfactory.
4. The following schedule for an average adult is safe and effective. (1) *Intramuscular route:* [ampules of 1 g $MgSO_4(H_2O)_7$, 50% solution = 8.13 mEq Mg^{2+}] Day 1: 2.0 g (16.3 mEq) every 4 hours for six doses. Days 2 to 5: 1.0 g (9.1 mEq) every 6 hours. (2) *Intravenous route* (same ampules) Day 1: 6 g (41 mEq) in each liter of fluid and at least 2 L of 83 mEq. Days 2 to 5: A total of 6 g (49 mEq) distributed equally in total fluids of the day.
   If the patient's condition requires continued intravenous infusions, 2 g of $MgSO_4$ should be given daily in the infusion as long as infusions are necessary. When a patient who has a reason to have magnesium deficiency is convulsing, 2.0 g of $MgSO_4$ solution may be administered intravenously in a 10-minute period. For symptomatic infants and children, such doses may be 0.025 g $MgSO_4$/kg, or 0.2 to 0.3 mEq/kg per dose of elemental mg^{2+}, in 10 minutes.
5. Oral preparations

Magnesium oxide	(Uro-Mg) 50 mEq magnesium per g of salt
	(Mag-Ox) 50 mEq magnesium per g of salt
Magnesium chloride	(Slo-Mag) 9.75 mEq magnesium per g of salt
Magnesium lactate	(MagTab) 7.6 mEq magnesium per g of salt

- Note: 50% solution of $MgSO_4$ = 500 mg/mL (1 g/2 mL), or 49.3 mg elemental Mg^{2+}/mL, or 98.6 mg elemental Mg^{2+}/2 mL. Given an atomic gram weight of 24.3 and a valence of 2 for Mg^{2+}, 98.6 mg = 4.058 mmol or 8.13 mEq elemental Mg^{2+}/g salt.
- Example. A 10-kg infant with seizures, hypomagnesemia, and an adequate serum calcium level may receive 2.0 mEq elemental Mg^{2+} (0.2 mEq/kg • 10 kg). This may be accomplished by diluting 0.5 mL of the 50% $MgSO_4$ in 9.5 mL of dextrose and infusing over 2 to 10 minutes.

Adapted from Flink EB, et al.: Magnesium deficiency and magnesium toxicity in man. In Prasad AS, Oberleas D, editors: *Trace elements in human health and disease.* New York, 1976, Academic Press, p 13.

Phosphate transport at the proximal tubule is the main means for regulating total body phosphate balance. The latter process is largely mediated by a type IIa Na^+/P^{2-} electrogenic cotransporter (NPT2a) in the proximal tubule (Murer et al., 2000; Kronenberg, 2002; Tenenhouse and Murer, 2003). An increase or a decrease in the number of NPT2a in the brush border cell membrane is associated with either an increase or a decrease in P^{2-} reabsorption. Modulators of NPT2a endocytosis, internalization, recycling, and lysosomal degradation include PTH, fibroblast growth factor (FGF-23), and several proteins that interact with this phosphate transporter. High levels of PTH or FGF-23 increase NPT2a endocytosis and breakdown and cause phosphaturia. Reduction in dietary phosphate lowers PTH levels while concurrently promoting insertion of NPT2a at the apical membrane thereby promoting phosphate reabsorption (Fig. 4–9).

Human disorders of phosphate transport may relate to aberrations in these phosphate-regulating genes. Certain tumors can cause oncogenic hypophosphatemic osteomalacia (OHO) by stimulating mRNA encoding for FGF-23, while activating mutations of FGF-23 can cause autosomal dominant hypophosphatemic rickets (ADHR). Another phosphate-regulating gene is named *PHEX* (Phosphate-regulating gene with Homology to Endopeptidases on the X chromosome). Many mutations in this gene, which is largely expressed in osteoblasts, osteoclasts, and odontoblasts, lead to decreased degradation of FGF-23, which may be the key defect in X-linked hypophosphatemic rickets (XLH). However, the mechanism by which PHEX dysfunction leads to renal phosphate wasting is unclear (Kronenberg, 2002).

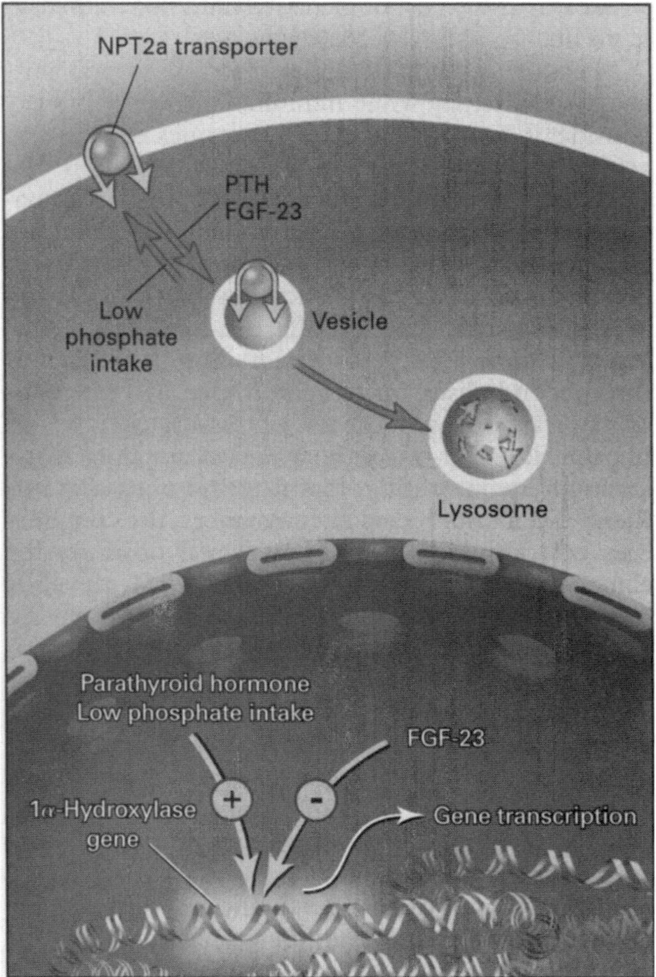

■ **FIGURE 4–9.** Regulation of the NPT2a sodium-phosphate cotransporter and synthesis of 1,25-dihydroxyvitamin D_3 in the renal proximal tubule. Parathyroid hormone (PTH) and fibroblast growth factor 23 (FGF-23) both lead to rapid internalization and subsequent lysosomal destruction of NPT2a. A low-phosphate diet causes the insertion of NPT2a into the plasma membrane. PTH and a low-phosphate diet both stimulate production of 25-hydroxyvitamin D 1α-hydroxylase messenger RNA (mRNA), whereas FGF-23 lowers mRNA levels. (From Kronenberg HM: NPT2a—The key to phosphate homeostasis. *N Engl J Med* 347:1022–1024, 2002, p 1022, Figure 1. Copyright © 1974 Massachusetts Medical Society. All rights reserved)

Regulation of phosphate shifts in and out of bone is principally mediated by PTH and calcitriol synthesized mainly by proximal tubular epithelial cells. Several plasma proteins prevent precipitation of calcium phosphate in vessels and soft tissues, whereas alkaline phosphatase aids deposition of such minerals in bone. Other hormones that may affect the renal handling of P^{2-} include vasopressin, thyroxin, glucagon, insulin, and glucocorticoids (Ritz et al., 1980). The antiphosphaturic action of growth hormone is believed to occur via mechanisms involving increased reabsorption of Na^+, release of insulin, or increased synthesis of $1,25(OH)_2D_3$.

Hypophosphatemia stimulates calcitriol synthesis. The adaptive increases in plasma calcitriol concentrations on bone and intestine raise serum phosphate levels and cause hypercalciuria. This is evident in hereditary hypophosphatemic rickets (HHPR) but not in the disorders involving excessive amounts or activating mutations of FGF-23 (XLH, ADHR, or OHO) in which calcitriol expression is suppressed. The transporter abnormality in HHPR remains elusive.

Hypophosphatemia (Plasma Concentration <2.5 mg/dL)

The etiologies of hypophosphatemia are summarized in Box 4–16. Because it is found in most foods, particularly in dairy products, and because intestinal absorption is efficient and minimally regulated, phosphorus depletion is rare except in patients with hyperparathyroidism. Hypophosphatemia usually coexists with total body P^{2-} depletion, which is defined precisely as P^{2-} content in lean muscle below 0.28 mol/g dry weight. One may occur without the other, however, particularly when the decrease in serum P^{2-} results from intracellular shifts (Popovtzer and Knochel, 1986).

Clinical manifestations of hypophosphatemia are quite diverse and may be due to the underlying disorder (e.g., pseudofractures and osteopenia in chronic hypoparathyroidism) or because of hypoxic effects on any and all body processes resulting in hemolysis, rhabdomyolysis, respiratory muscle paralysis, myocardial failure, encephalopathy, or neuropsychiatric symptoms and in secondary disturbances in renal tubular bicarbonate, magnesium, calcium, and glucose reabsorption. Plasma Ca^{2+} concentration may increase due to stimulation of calcitriol and from mobilization of bone Ca^{2+} due to reduction in the blood $Ca^{2+} \times P^{2-}$product. Glucose intolerance may occur with severe P^{2-} depletion (Marshall et al., 1978). Osteomalacia, rickets, hypercalcemia, hypercalciuria, and distal tubular acidification defects (Kurtz and Hsu, 1978) are known to occur in chronic hypophosphatemia of any cause. Chronic administration of antacids (e.g., calcium carbonate or aluminum hydroxide) combined with inadequate P^{2-} intake may result in severe hypophosphatemia. In addition to acting as P^{2-} binders, antacids can induce net P^{2-} secretion in the gut and create a negative P^{2-} balance.

BOX 4–16 **Causes of Hypophosphatemia**

Excessive Renal Losses as Primary Cause

Drugs: Cyclosporine, tacrolimus, diuretics, salicylates, carbonic anhydrase inhibitors
Primary hypophosphatemic rickets
Hereditary hypophosphatemic rickets with hypercalciuria
Postobstructive diuresis
Renal tubular acidosis
Postrenal transplantation
Fanconi syndrome
Recovery from acute tubular necrosis
Potassium deficiency
Oncogenic osteomalacia or rickets
Vitamin D deficiency and dependency (also related to decreased intestinal absorption)
Volume expansion or osmotic diuresis (hyperglycemia)

Negative Intestinal Balance as Primary Cause

Breastfed premature infants
Term infants fed with low phosphate source
Use of phosphate-binding antacids
Decreased dietary intake (rare) especially with dialysis and phosphate binders
Vomiting or gastric suction
Glucocorticoids

Acute Flux of Plasma Phosphate to Intracellular and Skeletal Pools*

Nutritional recovery, usually TPN associated
Therapy of diabetic ketoacidosis
Salicylate intoxication
Alkalosis (especially respiratory)
Androgen therapy
Burn therapy
Hungry-bone phenomenon
Increased tumor burden (uptake by tumor cells)

*The serum phosphate is maintained but total body pools are depressed. In many of these conditions, recovery results in restoration of intracellular phosphate, precipitating acute hypophosphatemia.

Many genetic disorders causing hypophosphatemia are characterized by an abnormal response to PTH, alteration in the structure and function of renal tubular transporters, or defective regulatory proteins within the proximal tubular epithelium. Several of these disorders are inherited and are associated with other metabolic disturbances such as aminoaciduria, glucosuria, hypocalcemia, rickets, and growth failure.

Hypophosphatemia is commonly seen after successful renal transplantation. Contributory factors include the persistence of preexisting parathyroid hyperplasia, volume expansion and osmotic diuresis in the immediate postoperative period, glucocorticoid administration (which increases the renal excretion of P^{2-} and inhibits the gastrointestinal absorption of this ion), ingestion of antacids (which also function as phosphate binders), and an inherent renal tubular defect for P^{2-} reabsorption that is independent of all other hormonal and metabolic factors (Parfit et al., 1986).

Moderate hypophosphatemia (plasma concentrations of 1.0 to 2.5 mg/dL) generally results in few symptoms and can be managed with oral rather than intravenous phosphate salts. Whenever possible, this may be accomplished through dietary supplements. One quart of milk provides about 1 g of elemental phosphorus (≈32 mmol). The dosage of oral salt supplements ranges from 1.0 to 3.0 mmol/kg per day, with the larger dosages given to infants. Children with hypophosphatemia after renal transplantation may temporarily require phosphate replacement with Neutra-Phos and calcitriol supplements. This drug combination is also effective in the management of children with hypophosphatemic rickets.

Symptomatic children, those with profound hypophosphatemia (plasma concentration <1.0 mg/dL), or children requiring parenteral nutrition may be managed with intravenous phosphate at about 50% of the oral dosage. The choice of the preparation, including sodium phosphate or potassium phosphate, of either oral or intravenous phosphate preparations (see Table 4–13), depends on plasma K^+ concentrations and level of renal function.

Hyperphosphatemia

The pathogenesis of hyperphosphatemia is related to redistribution of P^{2-} from the intracellular compartment, P^{2-} overdose, or decreased renal clearance of P^{2-} (Box 4–17). Symptoms result from the reciprocal decrease in serum calcium. Convulsions, cardiac arrhythmias, laryngospasm, and tetany may reflect hypocalcemia. Also, hyperphosphatemia can produce, contribute to, or be associated with acute renal failure. Conditions such as crush injury, tumor lysis syndrome, rhabdomyolysis, and hemolysis are often associated with oliguria and acute renal failure. The most serious side effect of hyperphosphatemia relates to calcium-phosphorus precipitation in the form of hydroxyapatite

BOX 4–17 **Causes of Hyperphosphatemia**

Decreased Glomerular Filtration Rate

Acute and chronic renal failure

Increased Tubular Reabsorption of Phosphate

Parathyroid Dysfunction

Hypoparathyroidism (transient hypoparathyroidism of infancy, pseudohypoparathyroidism; transient parathyroid resistance of infancy)

Other Endocrine Causes

Hyperthyroidism, tumoral calcinosis, growth hormone excess; juvenile hypogonadism
High ambient temperature

Increased Phosphate Loads

Exogenous Loads

Enemas and laxatives; vitamin D intoxication; parenteral phosphate; blood transfusions; white phosphorus burns; phosphorus-rich cow's milk

Endogenous Loads

Cellular shift in diabetic ketoacidosis; lactic acidosis; tissue hypoxia; rhabdomyolysis; cytotoxic therapy of neoplasms; hemolysis; malignant hyperthermia

Miscellaneous

Familial intermittent hyperphosphatemia

crystals in nonosseous tissue including the cornea, lungs, kidneys, pancreas, blood vessels, and brain.

■ SUMMARY

Elucidation of nephron transporters and their interacting substrates has greatly enhanced our understanding of fluid and electrolyte regulation in children and in adults. However, unlike in adults, anatomic, metabolic, and physiologic differences stemming from the evolving aspects of development ranging from prematurity to adolescence result in a spectrum of responses of the nephron to perturbations in fluid and electrolyte balance. This treatise provides guidelines for fluid and electrolyte management based on an understanding of renal function and tubular transporter physiology in health and disease and during various periods of childhood.

REFERENCES

Acker CG, Johnson JP, Palevsky PM, et al.: Hyperkalemia in hospitalized patients. *Arch Intern Med* 158:917–924, 1998.

Adams PC, Woodhouse KW, Adela M: Exaggerated hypokalemia in acute myeloid leukemia. *Br Med J* 282:1034, 1981.

Adrogue HJ, Madias NE: Changes in plasma potassium concentration during acute acid-base disturbances. *Am J Med* 71:456, 1981.

Adrogue HJ, Madias NE: Hypernatremia. *N Engl J Med* 342:1493–1499, 2000b.

Adrogue HJ, Madias NE: Hyponatremia. *N Engl J Med* 342:1581–1589, 2000a.

Agus ZS: Hypomagnesemia. *J Am Soc Nephrol* 10:1616–1622, 1999.

Albanese A, Hindmarsh P, Stanhope R: Management of hyponatraemia in patients with acute cerebral insults. *Arch Dis Child* 85:246–251, 2001.

Ammon RA, May WS, Nightingale SD: Glucose-induced hyperkalemia with normal aldosterone levels. *Ann Intern Med* 89:349, 1978.

Andreoli TE: The polyuric hypertonic syndrome. *Nephrol Dial Transplant* 16(suppl 6):10–12, 2001.

Anto HR, Chou SY, Poroush JG, et al.: Infusion intravenous pyelography and renal function: Effects of hypertonic mannitol in patients with chronic renal insufficiency. *Arch Intern Med* 131:1652, 1981.

Aperia A, Broberger O, Herin P, et al.: A comparative study of the response to an oral NaCl and $NaHCO_3$ load in newborn preterm and full term infants. *Pediatr Res* 11:1109, 1977.

Aperia A, Broberger O, Thodenius J, et al.: Development of renal control of salt and fluid homeostasis during the first year of life. *Acta Paediatr Scand* 64:393, 1975b.

Aperia A, Broberger O, Thodenius J, et al.: Renal control of sodium and fluid balance in newborn infants during intravenous maintenance therapy. *Acta Paediatr Scand* 64:725, 1975a.

Aperia A, Zetterstrom R: Renal control of fluid homeostasis in the newborn infant. *Clin Perinatal* 9:523, 1982.

Aranda JV, Perez J, Sitar DS: Pharmacokinetic disposition and protein binding of furosemide in newborn infants. *Pediatr Pharmacol Ther* 93:507, 1978.

Arant BS Jr: Developmental patterns of renal functional maturation compared in the human neonate. *J Pediatr* 92:705–712, 1978.

Araseneau JC, Bagley CL, Anderson T, et al.: Hyperkalemia, a sequel of the chemotherapy of Burkitt's lymphoma. *Lancet* 1:10, 1973.

Arieff A, Llach F, Massry SG: Neurological manifestations and morbidity of hyponatremia: Correlation with brain water and electrolytes, *Medicine* 55:121, 1976.

Arieff AI: Dialysis disequilibrium syndrome: Current concepts on pathogenesis. In Schriener GE, Winchester JF, editors: *Controversies in nephrology,* vol 4. Washington, DC, 1982, Georgetown University Press, p 367.

Arieff AI: Postoperative hyponatremic encephalopathy following elective surgery in children. *Pediatr Anaesth* 8:1–4, 1998.

August JT, Nelson D, Thorn G: Response of normal subjects to large amounts of aldosterone. *J Clin Invest* 37:1549, 1958.

Avner ED, Ellis D, Ichikawa L, et al.: Normal neonates and the maturational development of homeostatic mechanisms. In Ichikawa I, editor: *Pediatric textbook of fluids and electrolytes.* Baltimore, 1990, Williams & Wilkins, pp 107–118.

Ayus JC, Krothapalli RK, Arieff AI: Treatment of symptomatic hyponatremia and its relation to brain damage. *N Engl J Med* 317:1190-1195, 1987.

Bajaj G, Alexander SR, Browne R, et al.: ^{125}Iodine-iothalamate clearance in children. A simple method to measure glomerular filtration. *Pediatr Nephrol* 10:25–28, 1996.

Barton CH, Vaziri ND, Martin DC, et al.: Hypomagnesemia and renal magnesium wasting in renal transplant recipients receiving cyclosporine. *Am J Med* 83:693, 1987.

Barton CH, Vaziri ND, Mina-Araghi S, et al.: Effects of cyclosporine on magnesium metabolism in rats. *J Lab Clin Med* 114:232, 1989.

Bastron RD, Pyne JL, Inagaki M: Halothane-induced renal vasodilatation. *Anesthesiology* 50:126, 1981.

Battle DC, Arruda JAL, Kurtzman NA: Hyperkalemic distal tubular acidosis associated with obstructive uropathy. *N Engl J Med* 304:373, 1981.

Baumgart S, Langman CB, Sosulski R, et al.: Fluid, electrolyte, and glucose maintenance in the very low birth-weight infant. *Clin Pediatr* 21:199, 1982.

Baumgart S: Radiant energy and insensible water loss in the premature newborn infant under a radiant warmer. *Clin Perinatal* 8:483, 1982.

Bayliss WM: On the local reactions of the arterial wall to changes in internal pressure. *J Physiol (Lond)* 28:220, 1902.

Beck LM, Goldberg M: Effects of acetazolamide and parathyroidectomy on renal transport of sodium, calcium and phosphate. *Am J Physiol* 224:1136, 1973.

Berleur MP, Dahan A, Murat I, et al.: Perioperative infusions in paediatric patients: Rationale for using Ringer-lactate solution with low dextrose concentration. *J Clin Pharm Ther* 28:31–40, 2003.

Berry CA, Rector FC Jr: Renal transport of glucose, amino acids, sodium, chloride and water. In Brenner BM, Rector FC Jr, editors: *The kidney.* Philadelphia, 1991, WB Saunders, p 245.

Bia MJ, Tyler K, DeFronzo RA: The effect of dexamethasone on renal electrolyte excretion in the adrenalectomized rat. *Endocrinology* 111:882, 1982.

Blantz RC: Dynamics of glomerular ultrafiltration in the rat. *Fed Proc* 36:2602, 1977.

Bockenhauer D: Ion channels in disease. *Curr Opin Pediatr* 13:142–149, 2001.

Bokenkamp A, Domanetzki M, Zinck R, et al.: Cystatin C—a new marker of glomerular filtration rate in children independent of age and height. *Pediatrics* 101:875–881, 1998.

Bonioli E, Bellini C: Therapy for hereditary nephrogenic diabetes insipidus. *J Pediatr* 119:331–332, 1991.

Bonny O, Rossier BC: Disturbances of Na/K balance: Pseudohypoaldosteronism revisited. *J Am Soc Nephrol* 13:2399–2414, 2002.

Bostic O, Duvernoy WFC: Hyperkalemic cardiac arrest during transfusion of stored blood. *J Endocrinol* 5:407, 1972.

Brannan PG, Vergne-Marini P, Pak CYC, et al.: Magnesium absorption in the human small intestine. *J Clin Invest* 57:1421–1418, 1976.

Brem AS: Insights into glucocorticoid-associated hypertension. *Am J Kidney Dis* 37:1–10, 2001.

Brenner BM, Ballermann BJ, Gunning ME, et al.: The diverse biological actions of atrial peptides. *Physiol Rev* 70:665, 1990.

Brenner BM, Beeuwkes R III: The renal circulations. *Hosp Pract* 13:35, 1978.

Bricker NS: Sodium homeostasis in chronic renal disease. *Kidney Int* 21:886, 1982.

Broadus AE, Horst RL, Lang R: The importance of circulating 1,25-dihydroxy vitamin D in the pathogenesis of hypercalciuria and renal stone formation in primary hyperparathyroidism. *N Engl J Med* 302:421, 1980.

Brookes GB, Hodge RA, Booth JB, et al.: The immediate effects of acetazolamide in Meniere's disease. *J Laryngol Otol* 96:57, 1982.

Brown CB, Ogg CS, Cameron JS: High dose furosemide in acute renal failure: A controlled trial. *Clin Nephrol* 13:90, 1981.

Burg M, Stoner L, Cardinal J, et al.: Furosemide effect on isolated perfused tubules. *Am J Physiol* 225:119, 1973.

Burrows FA, Shutack JG, Crone RK: Inappropriate secretion of antidiuretic hormone in a post-surgical pediatric population. *Crit Care Med* 11:527–531, 1983.

Bushinsky DA, Monk RD: Calcium. *Lancet* 352:306–311, 1998.

Bushinsky DA: Disorders of calcium and phosphorous homeostasis. In Greenberg A, editor: *Primer on kidney diseases,* ed 3. San Diego, 2001, Academic Press, pp 107–115.

Byme JJ: Shock. *N Engl J Med* 275:659, 1966.

Calcagno PL, Rubin MI: Renal extraction of para-aminohippurate in infants and children. *J Clin Invest* 42:1632, 1963.

Charney AN, Kinsey MD, Myers L, et al.: NaK-activated adenosine triphosphatase and intestinal electrolyte transport. *J Clin Invest* 56:653, 1975.

Chase LR, Slatopolsky E: Secretion and metabolic efficacy of parathyroid hormone in patients with severe hypomagnesemia. *J Clin Endocrinol Metab* 38:363, 1974.

Chesney RW: Drug-induced hypokalemia. *Am J Dis Child* 130:1055, 1976.

Chevalier RL, Kaiser DL: Effects of acute uninephrectomy and age on renal blood flow autoregulation in the rat. *Am J Physiol* 249(5 Pt 2):F672–F679, 1985.

Chumbley LC: Pseudohyperkalemia in acute myelocytic leukemia. *JAMA* 211:1007, 1970.

Cockburn F, Belton NR, Purvis RJ, et al.: Maternal vitamin D intake and mineral metabolism in mothers and their newborn infants. *Br Med J* 28:11, 1980.

Cohen L, Kitzes R: Relationship of bone and plasma magnesium in magnesium-deficient cirrhosis patients. *Isr J Med Sci* 18:679, 1982.

Cohn JN, Kowey PR, Whelton PK, et al.: New guidelines for potassium replacement in clinical practice: A contemporary review by the National Council on Potassium in Clinical Practice. *Arch Intern Med* 160:2429–2436, 2000.

Conger JF, Falk SA: Intrarenal dynamics in the pathogenesis and prevention of acute urate nephropathy. *J Clin Invest* 59:786, 1977.

Corvol P, Claire M, Oblin ME, et al.: Mechanism of the antimineralocorticoid effect of spironolactones. *Kidney Int* 20:1, 1981.

Davies DF, Shock NW: Age changes in glomerular filtration rate, effective renal plasma flow, and tubular excretory capacity in adult males. *J Clin Invest* 29:496, 1950.

Davis JO, Freeman RH: Mechanisms regulating renin release. *Physiol Rev* 56:1, 1976.

Delgado MM, Rohatgi R, Khan S, et al.: Sodium and potassium clearances by the maturing kidney: Clinical-molecular correlates. *Pediatr Nephrol* 18:759–767, 2003.

deTorrente A, Miller PD, Cronin RE, et al.: Effects of furosemide and acetylcholine in norepinephrine-induced acute renal failure. *Am J Physiol* 235: 131, 1978.

Dharnidharka VR, Kwon C, Stevens G: Serum cystatin C is superior to serum creatinine as a marker of kidney function: A meta-analysis. *Am J Kidney Dis* 40:221–226, 2002.

Di Stefano A, Desfleurs E, Simeone S, et al.: Ca^{2+} and Mg^{2+} sensor in the thick ascending limb of the loop of Henle. *Kidney Blood Press Res* 20:190–193, 1997.

Dikshit K, Vyden JK, Forrester JS, et al.: Renal and extrarenal hemodynamic effects of furosemide in congestive heart failure after acute myocardial infarction. *N Engl J Med* 288:1087, 1973.

Dirks JH: Mechanism of action and clinical use of diuretics. *Hosp Pract* 14:99, 1979.

Donckerwolcke RA, Vanstekelenburg J, Tilddburg J, et al.: Therapy of bicarbonate losing tubular renal acidosis. *Arch Dis Child* 45:774, 1970.

Dorisa TP, Valtin H: Cellular actions of vasopressin in the mammalian kidney. *Kidney Int* 10:46, 1976.

Dorkin LD, Brenner BM: The renal circulations. In Brenner BM, Rector FC Jr, editors: *The kidney.* Philadelphia, 1991, WB Saunders, p 164.

Douglas WW: How do neurons secrete peptides? Exocytosis and its consequences, including "synaptic vesicle" formation in the hypothalamo-neurohypophyseal system. *Prog Brain Res* 39:21, 1973.

Drukker A, Goldsmith DI, Spitzer A, et al.: The renin-angiotensin system in newborn dogs. Developmental patterns and response to acute saline loading. *Pediatr Res* 14:304, 1980.

Edwards BR: Postnatal development of urinary concentrating ability in rats: Changes in renal anatomy and neurohypophyseal hormones. In Spitzer A, editor: *The kidney during development.* Paris, 1981, Masson, p 233.

El-Dahr SS, Chevalier RL: Special needs of the newborn infant in fluid therapy. *Pediatr Clin North Am* 37:323–336, 1990.

Ellis D, Avner ED: Fluid and electrolyte disorders in pediatric patients. In Puschett JB, editor: *Disorders of fluid and electrolyte balance.* New York, 1985, Churchill Livingstone, p 217.

Eneas JF, Schoenfeld PY, Humphreys MH: The effect of infusion of mannitol-sodium bicarbonate on the clinical course of myoglobinuria. *Arch Intern Med* 139:801, 1979.

Engelke SC, Shah BL Vasan U, et al.: Sodium balance in very low birth weight infants. *J Pediatr* 93:837, 1978.

Epstein FH: Genetic disorders of renal electrolyte transport. *N Engl J Med* 340:1177–1187, 1999.

Epstein FH: Renal excretion of sodium and the concept of a volume receptor. *Yale J Biol Med* 29:282, 1957.

Estep H, Shaw WA, Watlington C, et al.: Hypocalcemia due to hypomagnesemia and reversible parathyroid hormone unresponsiveness. *J Clin Endocrinol Metab* 29:842, 1969.

Fanaroff AA, Wald M, Gruber HS, et al.: Insensible water loss in low birth weight infants. *Pediatrics* 50:236, 1972.

Farauhar MG, Wissig SL, Palade GE: Glomerular permeability. I. Ferritin transfer across the normal glomerular capillary wall. *J Exp Med* 113:47, 1961.

Farfel Z, Bourne HR, Iiri T: The expanding spectrum of G protein disease. *N Engl J Med* 340:1012–1120, 1999.

Favre L, Glasson P, Valloton MB: Reversible acute renal failure from combined triamterene and indomethacin. *Ann Intern Med* 96:317, 1982.

Fawer CL, Torrado A, Guignard JP: Maturation of renal function in full-term and premature neonates. *Helv Pediatr Acta* 34:11, 1979.

Felsenfeld AJ, Gutman RA, Drezner M, et al.: Hypophosphatemia in long-term renal transplant recipients; effects on bone histology and 1,25-dihydroxycholecalciferol. *Miner Electrolyte Metab* 12:233, 1986.

Finberg L, Harrison HE: Hypernatremia in infants: An evaluation of the clinical and biochemical findings accompanying this state. *Pediatrics* 16:1–14, 1955.

Finney H, Newman DJ, Thakkar H, et al.: Reference ranges for plasma cystatin C and creatinine measurements in premature infants, neonates and older children. *Arch Dis Child* 82:71–75, 2000.

Fraley DS, Adler S: Correction of hyperkalemia by bicarbonate despite constant blood pH. *Kidney Int* 12:354, 1977.

Frick KK, Bushinsky DA: Molecular mechanisms of primary hypercalciuria. *J Am Soc Nephrol* 14:1082 1095, 2003.

Friis-Hensen B: Body composition during growth. In vivo measurements and biochemical data correlated to differential anatomical growth. *Pediatrics* 47:264, 1971.

Gallagher KL, Jones JK: Furosemide-induced ototoxicity. *Ann Intern Med* 91:744, 1979.

Ganguly A, Donohue JP: Primary aldosteronism: Pathophysiology, diagnosis and treatment. *J Urol* 129:241, 1983.

Gennari FJ: Hypo-hypernatraemia: disorders of water balance. In Davidson AM, Camerom JS, Grunfeld JP, et al., editors: *Oxford textbook of clinical nephrology, vol 1*, ed 2. Oxford, England, 1998, Oxford University Press, pp 175–200.

Gennari FJ: Hypokalemia. *N Engl J Med* 339:451–458, 1998.

Gennari FJ, Segal AS: Hyperkalemia: An adaptive response in chronic renal insufficiency. *Kidney Intl* 62:1–9, 2002.

Gerger JG: Role of prostaglandins in the hemodynamic and tubular effects of furosemide. *Fed Proc* 42:1707, 1983.

Gertz KH, Mangos JA, Braum G, et al.: Pressures in the glomerular capillaries of the rat kidney in relation to arterial blood pressure. *Pflugers Arch* 288:369, 1966.

Ghose RR, Gupta SK: Synergistic action of metal ozone with "loop" diuretics. *Br Med J* 282:1432, 1981.

Godard C, Geering JM, Geering K, and others: Plasma renin activity related to sodium balance, renal function, and urinary vasopressin in the newborn infant. *Pediatr Res* 13:742, 1979.

Gonick HC, Kleeman CR, Rubini ME, et al.: Functional impairment in chronic renal disease. III. Studies of potassium excretion. *Am J Med Sci* 261:281, 1971.

Graham RC, Kellermeyer RW: Bovine lactoperoxidase as a cytochemical protein tracer for electron microscopy. *J Histochem Cytochem* 16:275, 1968.

Greene MK, Kerr AM, McIntosh IB, et al.: Acetazolamide in prevention of acute mountain sickness: A double-blind controlled crossover study. *Br Med J* 283:811, 1981.

Greger R: Ion transport mechanisms in thick ascending limb of Henle's loop of mammalian nephron. *Physiol Rev* 65:760, 1985.

Greger R: Physiology of renal sodium transport. *Am J Med Sci* 319:51–62, 2000.

Griggs RC, Engel WK, Resnick JS: Acetazolamide treatment of hypokalemic periodic paralysis. Prevention of attacks and improvement of persistent weakness. *Ann Intern Med* 73:39, 1970.

Gronert GA, Theye RA: Pathophysiology of succinylcholine induced hyperkalemia. *Anesthesiology* 43:89, 1975.

Guay-Woodford LM: Bartter syndrome: Unraveling the pathophysiologic enigma. *Am J Med* 105:151–161, 1998.

Gullans SR, Verbalis JG: Control of brain volume during hyperosmolar and hypo-osmolar conditions. *Annu Rev Med* 44:289, 1993.

Gullestad L, Midtvedt K, Dolva, et al.: The magnesium loading test: Reference values in healthy subjects. *Scand J Clin Lab Invest* 54:23–31, 1994.

Gums JG: Clinical significance of magnesium: A review. *Drug Int Clin Pharmacol* 21:240–246, 1987.

Hahn S, Kim Y, Garner P: Reduced osmolarity oral rehydration solution for treating dehydration due to diarrhea in children: Systematic review. *Br Med J* 323:81–85, 2001.

Hall JE, Brands MW, Henegar JR: Angiotensin II and long-term arterial pressure regulation: the overriding dominance of the kidney. *J Am Soc Nephrol* 10(suppl 12):S258–S265, 1999.

Halperin ML, Bichet DG, Oh MS: Integrative physiology of basal water permeability in the distal nephron: Implications for the syndrome of inappropriate secretion of antidiuretic hormone. *Clin Nephrol* 56:339–345, 2001.

Halperin ML, Kamel KS: Potassium. *Lancet* 352:135–140, 1998.

Halpren BA, Kempson RC, Coplon NS: Interstitial fibrosis and chronic renal failure following methoxyflurane anesthesia. *JAMA* 223:1239, 1973.

Harrison HE, Harrison HC: Intestinal transport of phosphate: Action of vitamin D, calcium and potassium. *Am J Physiol* 201:2001, 1961.

Hayes CP Jr, McLeod ME, Robinson RR: An extrarenal mechanism for the maintenance of potassium balance in severe chronic renal failure. *Trans Assoc Am Physicians* 50:207, 1967.

Helfant RH: Hypokalemia and arrhythmias. *Am J Med* 80(suppl 4A):13, 1986.

Hellerstein S, Berenbom M, Alon US, et al.: Creatinine clearance following cimetidine for estimation of glomerular filtration rate. *Pediatr Nephrol* 12:49–54, 1998.

Hellerstein S, Simon SD, Berenbom M, et al.: Creatinine excretion rates for renal clearance studies. *Pediatr Nephrol* 16:637–643, 2001.

Hendricks SA, Lippe B, Kaplan SA, et al.: Differential diagnosis of diabetes insipidus: Use of DDAVP to terminate the seven-hour water deprivation test. *J Pediatr* 98:244–246, 1981.

Herbacznska-Cedro K, Vane JR: Contribution of intrarenal generation of prostaglandins in autoregulation of renal blood flow in the dog. *Circ Res* 33:428, 1973.

Higashio T, Abe Y, Yamamoto K: Renal effects of bumetanide. *J Pharmacol Exp Ther* 207:212, 1978.

Hill LL: Body composition, normal electrolyte concentrations, and maintenance of normal volume, tonicity, and acid-base metabolism. *Pediatr Clin North Am* 37:241, 1990.

Holliday MA, Segar WE: The maintenance need for water in parenteral fluid therapy. *Pediatrics* 19:823–832, 1957.

Hong R: The Di-George anomaly (catch 22, DiGeorge/velocardiofacial syndrome). *Semin Hematol* 35:282–290, 1998.

Horster M: Principles of nephron differentiation. *Am J Physiol* 235:F387, 1978.

Hoskins B, Jackson CM: The mechanism of chlorothiazide-induced carbohydrate intolerance. *J Pharmacol Exp Ther* 206:423, 1978.

Humes HD, Weinberg JM, Knauss TC: Clinical and pathophysiologic aspects of aminoglycoside nephrotoxicity. *Am J Kidney Dis* 2:5, 1982.

Imbs JL, Schmidt M, Giesen-Crouse E: Pharmacology of loop diuretics: State of the art. *Adv Nephrol* 16:137, 1987.

Ingram RH Jr, Seki M: Pseudohyperkalemia with thrombocytosis. *N Engl J Med* 267:895, 1962.

Ireland AW, Hornbrook JW, Neale FC, et al.: The crystalline lens in chronic surgical hypoparathyroidism. *Arch Intern Med* 122:406, 1968.

Jones G, Strugnell SA, DeLuca HF: Current understanding of the molecular actions of vitamin *D. Physiol Rev* 78:1193–1231, 1998.

Jose PA, Slotkoff LM, Montgomery S, et al.: Autoregulation of renal blood flow in the puppy. *Am J Physiol* 229:983, 1975.

Kagan BM, Stanincova V, Felix NS, et al.: Body composition of premature infants: Relation to nutrition. *Am J Clin Nutr* 25:1153, 1972.

Kahn T: Hypernatremia with edema. *Arch Intern Med* 159:93–98, 1999.

Kaloyanides GJ, DiBona GF: Effect of an angiotensin II antagonist on autoregulation in the isolated dog kidney. *Am J Physiol* 230:1073, 1976.

Kaplan SL, Feigin RD: The syndrome of inappropriate secretion of antidiuretic hormone in children with bacterial meningitis. *J Pediatr* 92:758, 1978.

Kassirer JP, Harrington JT: Diuretics and potassium metabolism: Reassessment of the need, effectiveness and safety of potassium therapy. *Kidney Int* 11:505, 1977.

Keller G, Zimmer G, Mall G, et al.: Nephron number in patients with primary hypertension. *N Engl J Med* 348:101–108, 2003.

Kelly J: Disorders of sodium balance. *Lancet* 352:1146–1147, 1998.

Kempson SA: Effect of metabolic acidosis on renal brush border membrane adaptation to low phosphorus diet. *Kidney Int* 22:225–233, 1982.

Kim WG, Brown EB Jr: Potassium transfer with constant extracellular pH. *J Lab Clin Med* 71:678–685, 1968.

Kleinman LI, Lubbe RJ: Factors affecting the maturation of glomerular filtration rate and renal plasma flow in the newborn dog. *J Physiol* 223:395–409, 1972.

Knochel JP, Dotin LN, Hamburger RJ: Pathophysiology of intense physical conditioning in a hot climate. *J Clin Invest* 51:242, 1972.

Knochel JP: Neuromuscular manifestations of electrolyte disorders. *Am J Med* 72:521, 1982.

Knochel JP: The pathophysiology and clinical characteristics of severe hypophosphatemia. *Arch Intern Med* 137:203, 1977.

Knoers N, Monnen LAH: Amiloride-hydrochlorothiazide versus indomethacin-hydrochlorothiazide in the treatment of nephrogenic diabetes insipidus. *J Pediatr* 117:499–502, 1990.

Knoers N, Monnens LAH: Nephrogenic diabetes insipidus: Clinical symptoms, pathogenesis, genetics and treatment. *Pediatr Nephrol* 6:476–482, 1992.

Knox FG, Osswald H, Marchand GR, et al.: Phosphate transport along the tubule. *Am J Physiol* 233:F261, 1977.

Kokko JP: Renal concentrating and diluting mechanisms. *Hosp Pract* 14:110, 1979.

Kumar S, Berl T: Sodium. *Lancet* 352:220–228, 1998.

Kunau RT Jr, Walter DR, Webb HL: Clarification of action of chlorothiazide in the rat nephron. *J Clin Invest* 56:401, 1975.

Kurnik BRC, Hruska KA: Effects of 1,25-dihydroxycholecalciferol on phosphate transport in vitamin D-deprived rats. *Am J Physiol* 247:F177–F182, 1984.

Kurnik BRC, Hruska KA: Mechanism of stimulation of renal phosphate transport by 1,25-dihydroxycholecalciferol. *Biochem Biophys Acta* 817:42–50, 1985.

Kurtz E, Hsu CH: Impaired distal nephron acidification in chronically phosphate deprived rats. *Pflugers Arch* 377:229, 1978.

Laureno R, Karp BI: Myelinolysis after correction of hyponatremia. *Ann Intern Med* 126:57–62, 1997.

Lauriat S, Berl T: The hyponatremic patient: Practical focus on therapy. *J Am Soc Nephrol* 8:1599–1607, 1997.

Leake RD, Zabauddin S, Trygstad CW, et al.: The effects of large volume intravenous infusion on neonatal renal function. *J Pediatr* 89:968, 1976.

Lemman J Jr, Litzow JR, Lennon JR: Studies of the mechanism by which metabolic acidosis augments urinary calcium excretion in man. *J Clin Invest* 46:1318, 1967.

Lester GE, Vander Wiel CJ, Gray TK, et al.: Vitamin D deficiency in rats with normal serum calcium concentrations. *Proc Natl Acad Sci USA* 79:4791, 1982.

Levey AS, Greene T, Schluchter MD, et al.: Glomerular filtration rate measurements in clinical trials. *J Am Soc Nephrol* 4:1159–1171, 1993.

Levey AS, Perrone RD, Madias NE: Serum creatinine and renal function. *Annu Rev Med* 39:465–490, 1988.

Levine BS, Carpenter TO: Evaluation and treatment of heritable forms of rickets. *Endocrinologist* 9:358–365, 1999.

Levine SZ, Wilson JR, Kelly M: The insensible perspiration on infancy and childhood. I. Its constancy in infants under various physiologic factors. *Am J Dis Child* 37:791, 1929.

Levinson H, Linsao L, Swyer PR, et al.: A comparison of infra-red and convective heating for newborn infants. *Lancet* 2:1346, 1966.

Lin SH, Lin YF, Halperin ML: Hypokalemia and paralysis. *QJM* 94:133–139, 2001.

Lineralli LG, Bobik J, Bobik C: Newborn urinary cyclic AMP and developmental renal responsiveness to parathyroid hormone. *Pediatrics* 50:14, 1972.

Lipner HI, Rusany R, Dasgupta M, et al.: The behavior of carbenicillin as a nonabsorbable anion. *J Lab Clin Med* 86:183, 1975.

Liu Y-M, Neal P, Ernst J, et al.: Absorption of calcium and magnesium from fortified human milk by very low birth weight infants. *Pediatr Res* 25:496, 1989.

Luscher TF, Boulanger CM, Dohi Y, et al.: Endothelium-derived contracting factors. *Hypertension* 19:117, 1992.

Maier M, Starlinger M, Wagner M, et al.: The effect of hemorrhagic hypoperfusion on urinary kallikrein excretion, renin activity and renal cortical blood flow in the pig. *Circ Res* 48:386, 1981.

Manganaro R, Mami C, Marrone T, et al.: Incidence of dehydration and hypernatremia in exclusively breast-fed infants. *J Pediatr* 139:673–675, 2001.

Manuel MA, Steele TH: Changes in renal urate handling after prolonged thiazide administration. *Am J Med* 57:741, 1974.

Maren TH: Carbonic anhydrase: General perspective and advances in glaucoma research. *Drug Dev Res* 10:255, 1987.

Marild S, Jodal U, Jonasson G, et al.: Reference values for maximal renal concentrating capacity in children by the desmopressin test. *Pediatr Nephrol* 6:254–257, 1992.

Marsden PA, Brenner BM: Nitric oxide and endothelins: Novel autocrine/paracrine regulators of the circulation. *Semin Nephrol* 11:169, 1991.

Marshall WP, Banasiak MF, Kalkhoff RK: Effects of phosphate deprivation on carbohydrate metabolism. *Harm Metab Res* 10:369, 1978.

Marver D, Kokko JP: Renal target sites and the mechanism of action of aldosterone. *Miner Electrolyte Metab* 9:1, 1983.

Matkovic V, Heaney RP: Calcium balance during human growth: Evidence for threshold behavior. *Am J Clin Nutr* 55:992, 1992.

McCrory WW: *Developmental nephrology.* Cambridge, MA, 1972, Harvard University Press.

Mellits ED, Cheek DB: The assessment of body water and fatness from infancy to adulthood. *Monogr Soc Res Child Dev* 35:12–26, 1970.

Menon RK, Fouseca V, Dandoya P: Late hyponatremia in preterm infants. *J Pediatr* 108:487, 1986.

Milford DV: Investigation of hypertension and the recognition of monogenic hypertension. *Arch Dis Child* 81:452–455, 1999.

Moore EW: Ionized calcium in normal serum, ultrafiltrates, and whole blood determined by ion-exchange electrodes. *J Clin Invest* 49:318, 1970.

Moritz M, Ayus JC: Disorders of water metabolism in children: Hyponatremia and hypernatremia. *Pediatr Rev* 23:371–380, 2002.

Mundel P, Shankland SJ: Podocyte biology and response to injury. *J Am Soc Nephrol* 13:3005–3015, 2002.

Mundy GR, Guise TA: Hypercalcemia of malignancy. *Am J Med* 103:134–135, 1997.

Murer H, Hernando N. Forster I, Biber J: Proximal tubular phosphate reabsorption: Molecular mechanisms. *Physiol Rev* 80:1373–1409, 2000.

Narins RG: Hyponatraemia—review of a controversial case. *Nephrol Dial Transplant* 16(suppl 6):36–37, 2001.

Ng KKF, Vane JR: Conversion of angiotensin I to angiotensin II. *Nature* 216:762, 1967.

Nussberger J, Waeber B, Brunner HR: Clinical pharmacology of ACE inhibition. *Cardiology* 76(suppl 2):11–22, 1990.

Oddie S, Richmond S, Coulthard M: Hypernatraemic dehydration and breast feeding: A population study. *Arch Dis Child* 85:318–320, 2001.

Oh W, Karecki H: The effects of radiant warmer on insensible water loss in newborn infants. *Am J Dis Child* 124:230, 1972.

Oh W: Fluid and electrolyte therapy in low birth weight infants. *Pediatr Rev* 1:313, 1980.

Olbing J, Blaufox MD, Aschinberg LC, et al.: Postnatal changes in glomerular blood flow distribution in puppies. *J Clin Invest* 52:2885, 1973.

Osswald H, Spielman WS, Knox FG: Mechanism of adenosine-mediated decreases in glomerular filtration rate in dogs. *Circ Res* 43:465, 1978.

Palm C, Reimann D, Gross P: The role of V_2 vasopressin antagonists in hyponatremia. *Cardiovasc Res* 51:403–408, 2001.

Paneth N: Hypernatremic dehydration of infancy. *Am J Dis Child* 134:785, 1980.

Parfit AM, Kleerekoper M, Cruz C: Reduced phosphate reabsorption unrelated to parathyroid hormone after renal transplantation: Implications for the pathogenesis of hyperparathyroidism in chronic renal failure. *Miner Electrol Metab* 12:356, 1986.

Parfitt AM, Kleerekoper M: Clinical disorders of calcium, phosphorus and magnesium metabolism. In Maxwell MH, Kleeman CR, editors: *Clinical disorders of fluid and electrolyte metabolism.* New York, 1980, McGraw-Hill Book, p 947.

Patrick J: Assessment of body potassium stores. *Kidney Int* 11:476, 1977.

Peterson B, Khanna S, Fisher B, et al.: Prolonged hypernatremia controls elevated intracranial pressure in head-injured pediatric patients. *Crit Care Med* 28:1136–1143, 2000.

Pezzi PJ, Frobese AS, Greenberg SR: Methoxyflurane and renal toxicity. *Lancet* I:73, 1966.

Philbin DM, Coggins CH: Plasma antidiuretic hormone levels in cardiac surgical patients during morphine and halothane anesthesia. *Anesthesiology* 49:95, 1978.

Philbin DM, Levine FH, Kono K, et al.: Attenuation of the stress response to cardiopulmonary bypass by the addition of pulsatile flow. *Circulation* 64:808, 1981.

Pierson RN Jr, Lin DHY, Phillips RA: Total body potassium in health: Effects of age, sex, height, and fat. *Am J Physiol* 226:206, 1974.

Pitts RF, Lotspeich WD: Bicarbonate and the renal regulation of acid-base balance. *Am J Physiol* 147:136, 1946.

Pitts RF: Tubular disorders. In Pitts RF, editor: *Physiology of the kidney and body fluids.* Chicago, 1974, Year Book Medical Publishers, p 71.

Popovtzer MM, Knochel JP: Disorders of calcium, phosphorus, vitamin D and parathyroid hormone activity. In Schrier RW, editor: *Renal and electrolyte disorders.* Boston, 1986, Little, Brown & Co, p 251.

Popovtzer MM, Subryan VL, Alfrey AC, et al.: The acute effect of chlorothiazide on serum-ionized calcium. Evidence for a parathyroid hormone-dependent mechanism. *J Clin Invest* 55:1295, 1975.

Prandota J, Pruitt AW: Furosemide binding to human albumin and plasma of nephrotic syndrome. *Clin Pharmacol Ther* 17:159, 1975.

Prie D, Huart V, Bakouh N et al.: Nephrolithiasis and osteoporosis associated with hypophosphatemia caused by mutations in the type 2a sodium-phosphate cotransporter. *N Engl J Med* 347:983–991, 2002.

Prunty FTG, Brooks RV, Dupre J, et al.: Adrenocortical hyperfunction and potassium metabolism with "non-endocrine" tumors and Cushing's syndrome. *J Clin Endocrinol Metab* 23:737, 1963.

Radtke HW, Rumrich G, Kinne-Saffran E, et al.: Dual actions of acetazolamide and furosemide on proximal volume absorption in the rat kidney. *Kidney Int* 1:100, 1972.

Raisz LG: Bone metabolism and calcium regulation. In Avioli LV, Karne SM, editors: *Metabolic bone disease, vol 1.* New York, 1977, Academic Press, p 1.

Rane A, Villeneuve JP, Stone WJ, et al.: Plasma binding and disposition of furosemide in the nephrotic syndrome and in uremia. *Clin Pharmacol Ther* 24:199, 1978.

Rao TLK, Shanmugam M: Succinylcholine administration—another contraindication? *Anesth Analg* 58:61, 1979.

Rees L, Shaw JCL, Brook CGD, et al.: Hyponatremia in the first week of life in preterm infants. *Arch Dis Child* 59:423, 1984.

Reimann D, Gross P: Chronic, diagnosis-resistant hypokalaemia. *Nephrol Dial Transplant* 14:2957–2961, 1999.

Relman AS, Schwartz WB: The nephropathy of potassium depletion, *N Engl J Med* 255:195, 1956.

Rigden SP, Dillon MJ, Kind PR, et al.: The beneficial effect of mannitol on postoperative renal function in children undergoing cardiopulmonary bypass surgery. *Clin Nephrol* 21:148, 1984.

Ritz E, Kreusser W, Bommer J: Effects of hormones other than parathyroid hormones on renal handling of phosphate. In Massry SG, Fleisch H, editors: *The renal handling of phosphate.* New York, 1980, Plenum Press, p 137.

Robertson CR, Deen WM, Troy JL, et al.: Dynamics of glomerular ultrafiltration in the rat. III. Hemodynamics and autoregulation. *Am J Physiol* 223:1191, 1972.

Robertson G: Antidiuretic hormone: Normal and disordered functions. *Endocrinol Metab Clin North Am* 30:671–694, 2001.

Robertson GL: Thirst and vasopressin function in normal and disordered states of water balance. *J Lab Clin Med* 101:351, 1983.

Rodd C, Goodyer P: Hypercalcemia of the newborn: etiology, evaluation, and management. *Pediatr Nephrol* 13:542–547, 1999.

Rodriguez-Soriano J, Ubetagoyena M, Vallo A: Transtubular potassium concentration gradient: A useful test to estimate renal aldosterone bio-activity in infants and children. *Pediatr Nephrol* 4:105–110, 1990.

Rodriguez-Soriano J, Vallo A: Renal tubular hyperkalaemia in childhood. *Pediatr Nephrol* 2:498–509, 1988.

Root AW, Harrison HE: Recent advances in calcium metabolism. *J Pediatr* 88:1, 1976.

Rosa RM, Silva P, Young JB, et al.: Adrenergic modulation of extra-renal potassium disposal. *N Engl J Med* 302:431, 1980.

Rowe JW, Tobin JD, Rosa RM, et al.: Effect of experimental potassium deficiency on glucose and insulin metabolism. *Metabolism* 29:498, 1980.

Roy RN, Sinclair JC: Hydration of the low birth weight infants. *Clin Perinatal* 2:393, 1975.

Roza O, Berman LB: The pathophysiology of barium: Hypokalemic and cardiovascular effects. *J Pharmacol Exp Ther* 177:433, 1971.

Rudolph AM, Heymann MA, Teramo AW, et al.: Studies on the circulation of the previable human fetus. *Pediatr Res* 5:452, 1971.

Ryan GB, Karnovsky MJ: Distribution of endogenous albumin in rat glomerulus. Role of hemodynamic factors in glomerular barrier function. *Kidney Int* 9:36, 1976.

Schambelan M, Sebastian A, Biglieri EG: Prevalence, pathogenesis, and functional significance of aldosterone deficiency in hyperkalemia patients with chronic renal insufficiency. *Kidney Int* 17:89, 1980.

Scheinman SJ, Guay-Woodford LM, Thakker RV, et al.: Genetic disorders of renal electrolyte transport. *N Engl J Med* 340:1177–1187, 1999.

Schell-Feith EA, Kist-van Holthe JE, Conneman N, et al.: Etiology of nephrocalcinosis in preterm neonates: Association of nutritional intake and urinary parameters. *Kidney Int* 58:2102–2110, 2000.

Schiffrin EL: Vascular and cardiac benefits of angiotensin receptor blockers. *Am J Med* 113:409–418, 2002.

Schlondorff D, Wever H, Trizna W: Vasopressin responsiveness of renal adenylate cyclase in newborn rats and rabbits. *Am J Physiol* 234:F16–F21, 1978.

Schnermann J, Briggs JP, Weber PC: Tubulo-glomerular feedback, prostaglandins, and angiotensin in the autoregulation of glomerular filtration rate. *Kidney Int* 25:53, 1984.

Schrier RW: Acute renal failure. *Kidney Int* 15:205, 1979.

Schultz DM, Giordano DA, Schultz DH: Weights of organs of fetuses and infants. *Arch Pathol* 74:244, 1962.

Schwartz GL, Brion LP, Spitzer A: The use of plasma creatinine concentration for estimating glomerular filtration in infants, children and adolescents. *Pediatr Clin North Am* 34:571, 1987.

Schwartz IL, Shlatz LI, Kinne-Saffran E: Target cell polarity and membrane phosphorylation in relation to the mechanism of action of antidiuretic hormone. *Proc Natl Acad Sci USA* 71:2695, 1974.

Seldin DW, Rector FC Jr: The generation and maintenance of metabolic alkalosis. *Kidney Int* 1:306, 1972.

Selkurt EE, Hall PW, Spencer MP: Influence of graded arterial pressure decrement on renal clearance of creatinine, *p*-amino-hippurate and sodium. *Am J Physiol* 159:369, 1949.

Shaer AJ: Inherited primary renal tubular hypokalemic alkalosis: A review of Gitelman and Bartter syndromes. *Am J Med Sci* 322:316–332, 2001.

Shipley RE, Study RS: Changes in renal blood flow, extraction of insulin, glomerular filtration rate, tissue pressure and urine flow with acute alterations of renal artery blood pressure. *Am J Physiol* 167:676, 1951.

Shirley DG, Walter SJ, Laycock JF: The anti-diuretic effects of chronic hydrochlorothiazide treatment in rats with diabetes insipidus: Renal mechanism. *Clin Sci* 63:533, 1982.

Shoemaker LR: Expanding role of biphosphonate therapy in children. *J Pediatr* 134:264–267, 1999.

Silverman WA: *Dunham's premature infants,* ed. New York, 1961, Paul B Hoeber, p 531.

Slatopolsky E, Delmez J: Bone disease in chronic renal failure and after renal transplantation. In Coe FL, Favus MJ, editors: *Disorders of bone and mineral metabolism.* New York, 1992, Raven Press, p 905.

Smith HW: *Lectures on the kidney.* Lawrence, KS, 1943, University Extension Division of University of Kansas, p 97.

Spitzer A: Renal physiology and functional development. In Edelman CM Jr, editor: *Pediatric kidney disease.* Boston, 1978, Little, Brown & Co, p 25.

Spitzer A: The role of the kidney in sodium homeostasis during maturation. *Kidney Int* 21:539, 1982.

Stapleton FB, Nelson B, Vats TS, et al.: Hypokalemia associated with antibiotic treatment. *Am J Dis Child* 130:1104, 1976.

Stein JH: The pathogenetic spectrum of Banter's syndrome. *Kidney Int* 28:85, 1985.

Stoner LC, Brug MB, Orloff J: Ion transport in cortical collecting tubule: Effect of amiloride. *Am J Physiol* 227:453, 1974.

Streicher HZ, Gabow PA, Moss AH, et al.: Syndromes of toluene sniffing in adults. *Ann Intern Med* 94:758, 1981.

Suh SM, Tashjian AH Jr, Matsuo N: Pathogenesis of hypocalcemia in primary hypomagnesemia: Normal end-organ responsiveness to parathyroid hormone, impaired parathyroid gland function. *J Clin Invest* 51:531, 1973.

Suki WN, Rouse D: Renal transport of calcium, magnesium, and phosphorus. In Brenner BM, Rector FC Jr, editors: *The kidney.* Philadelphia, 1991, WB Saunders, pp 340–423.

Suki WN: Disposition and regulation of body potassium: An overview. *Am J Med Sci* 272:31, 1976.

Sulyok E, Kovacs L, Lichardus B, et al.: Late hyponatremia in premature infants: Role of aldosterone and arginine vasopressin. *J Pediatr* 106:990, 1985.

Sulyok E, Varga F, Gyory E, et al.: Postnatal development of renal sodium handling in premature infants. *J Pediatr* 95:787–792, 1979.

Sutton RA: Calcium disorders. In Dirks JH, Sutton RA, editors: *Diuretics: Physiology, pharmacology and clinical use.* Philadelphia, 1986, WB Saunders, p 259.

Svenningsen NW, Aronson AS: Postnatal development of renal concentrating capacity as estimated by DDAVP-test in normal and asphyxiated neonates. *Biol Neonate* 25:230, 1974.

Ten S, New M, Maclaren N: Addison's disease. *J Clin Endocrinol Metabl* 86:2909–2922, 2001.

Tenenhouse HS, Murer H: Disorders of renal tubular phosphate transport. *J Am Soc Nephrol* 14:240–247, 2003.

The ADHR Consortium: Autosomal dominant hypophosphatemic rickets is associated with mutations in FGF23. *Nat Genet* 26:345–348, 2000.

Thompson BD, Edmonds CJ: Comparison of effects of profound aldosterone administration on rat colon and renal electrolyte excretion. *J Endocrinol* 50:163, 1971.

Thurau K: Renal hemodynamics. *Am J Med* 36:698, 1964.

Torres VE, Young WF, Offord KP, Hattery RR: Association of hypokalemia, aldosteronism and renal cysts. *N Engl J Med* 322:345–351, 1990.

Trimble ME: Renal response to solute loading in infant rats: Relation to anatomical development. *Am J Physiol* 219:1089, 1970.

Tsang RC, Light IJ, Sutherland JM, et al.: Possible pathogenic factors in neonatal hypocalcemia of prematurity. *J Pediatr* 82:423, 1973.

Tucker BJ, Blantz RC: An analysis of the determinants of nephron filtration rate. *Am J Physiol* 232:447, 1977.

Update on the 1987 Task Force Report on High Blood Pressure in Children and Adolescents: A work group report from the National High Blood Pressure Education Program. *Pediatrics* 98:649–658, 1996.

van Ypersele de Strihou C: Potassium homeostasis in renal failure. *Kidney Int* 11:49, 1977.

Venkataraman PS, Tsang RC, Chen IW, et al.: Pathogenesis of early neonatal hypocalcemia: Studies of serum calcium, gastrin, and plasma glucagon. *J Pediatr* 110:599, 1987.

Vogh DP: The relation of choroid plexus carbonic anhydrase activity to cerebrospinal fluid formation: Study of three inhibitors in cat with extrapolation to man. *J Pharmacol Exp Ther* 213:321, 1980.

Warren SE, Blantz RC: Mannitol. *Arch Intern Med* 141:493, 1981.

Weber S, Schneider L, Peters M, et al.: Novel paracellin-1 mutations in 25 families with familial hypomagnesemia with hypercalciuria and nephrocalcinosis. *J Am Soc Nephrol* 12:1872–1881, 2001.

Weiner DI, Wingo CS: Hypokalemia—consequences, causes and correction. *J Am Soc Nephrol* 7:1179–1188, 1997.

Welfare W, Sasi P, English M: Challenges in managing profound hypokalemia. *Br Med J* 324:269–270, 2002.

Wenneberg RP, Rasmussen LF, Ahlfors CE: Displacement of bilirubin from human albumin by three diuretics. *J Pediatr* 90:647, 1977.

Whang R, Whang DD, Ryan MP: Refractory potassium depletion: A consequence of magnesium deficiency. *Arch Intern Med* 152:40–45, 1992.

White DP, Zwillich CW, Pickett CK, et al.: Central sleep apnea: Improvement with acetazolamide therapy. *Arch Intern Med* 142:1816, 1982.

Whitford GM, Taves DR: Fluoride-induced diuresis: Renal-tissue solute concentrations, functional, hemodynamic and histologic correlates in the rat. *Anesthesiology* 39:416, 1973.

Winters RW: *Principles of pediatric fluid therapy,* ed 2. Boston, 1982, Little, Brown & Co.

Wormersley RA, Darragh JH: Potassium and sodium restriction in the normal human. *J Clin Invest* 34:456, 1955.

Wu PYK, Hodgman JE: Insensible water loss in preterm infants: Changes with postnatal development and nonionizing radiant energy. *Pediatrics* 54:704, 1974.

Yared A, Yoskioka A: Autoregulation of glomerular filtration in the young. *Semin Nephrol* 9:94, 1989.

Zelikovic I: Molecular pathophysiology of tubular transport disorders. *Pediatr Nephrol* 16:919–935, 2001.

Ziegler R: Hypercalcemic crisis. *J Am Soc Nephrol* 12:S3–S9, 2001.

Zimmerman EA, Defendini R: Hypothalamic pathways containing oxytocin, vasopressin, and associated neurophysins. In Moses AM, Share L, editors: *Neurohypophysis: International Congress on the Neurohypophysis.* Basel, 1977, S Karger.

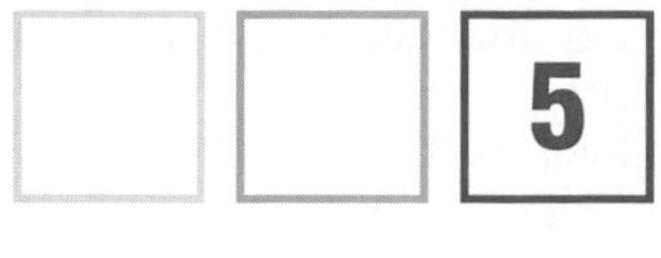

5 Thermoregulation: Physiology and Perioperative Disturbances

Igor Luginbuehl • Bruno Bissonnette • Peter J. Davis

One of many physiologic adaptations required for human survival is the ability to establish and maintain a constant core body temperature. The significance of thermal regulation for neonates was appreciated as early as the 1900s when Budin noted a significant difference in the mortality rate among infants with different body temperatures (1907). Other investigators have confirmed the importance of thermal stability in the adaptive process and further elucidated the mechanisms by which infants and children behave as homeotherms (Silverman and Blanc, 1957; Cross et al., 1958; Silverman et al., 1958; Bruck, 1961). By definition, a *homeothermic organism* maintains a constant core temperature despite changes in the ambient temperature. Only a few other physiologic parameters are as vigorously and effectively controlled as the central temperature. The central body temperature in humans refers to the temperature of the vessel-rich group organs (brain, heart, lungs, liver, and kidneys) and under normal circumstances is maintained within ±0.2°C of its set point of 37.0°C. This so-called interthreshold range defines the limits, within which no thermoregulatory effector responses are triggered and the human organism in fact behaves in a poikilothermic manner. The musculoskeletal system makes up the major part of the peripheral compartment, which can be seen as a dynamic buffer in the thermoregulatory system, whereas the skin represents the shell compartment, which acts as a barrier to the environment.

Although temperature control is subjected to a circadian rhythm, which starts in the first months of life, nocturnal oscillations in infants (Brown et al., 1992) and a monthly rhythm in fertile women (due to a higher set point temperature in the luteal phase of the menstrual cycle) (Hardy, 1961) are found. The control within these rhythms is very tight, however, and accomplished by a delicate and effective system that balances heat production and heat loss. Despite this effective regulatory system, the ability of the organism to dissipate or generate heat by regulating skin blood flow, sweat production, minute ventilation, and metabolism is often overwhelmed by external factors. Anesthesia and surgery have a powerful effect on this sophisticated thermoregulatory system, and minor changes in body temperature may result in cellular and tissue dysfunction, explaining the need not only for a regulation within so narrow limits but also for perioperative temperature monitoring.

Accidental hypothermia is a frequent occurrence in patients of any age undergoing anesthesia and surgery. Hence, it is unfortunately often accepted as a consequence of the surgical procedure. This common occurrence led Pickering to comment that "The most effective means of cooling a man is to give him an anesthetic" (1958).

This chapter discusses the principles of thermoregulation in infants and children and the relative merits of different anatomic sites of temperature monitoring. In addition, we review the influence of anesthetic agents on the child's thermoregulatory system, the physiologic consequences of hypothermia and hyperthermia, and the techniques to prevent perioperative hypothermia.

TEMPERATURE MONITORING

The unit for temperature in the Système Internationale is Kelvin (K), where 0 K = –273.15°C. Most countries measure temperature in Celsius degrees and a few measure in Fahrenheit degrees. The following formulas can be used to convert them from one unit into the other:

$$°\text{Celsius} = [(°\text{Fahrenheit} - 32)5]/9 \quad (5.1)$$

$$°\text{Fahrenheit} = (9 \cdot °\text{Celsius}/5) + 32 \quad (5.2)$$

To detect perioperative changes in temperature, an appropriate measurement of temperature is mandatory. Guidelines of the American Society of Anesthesiologists require that one method for measuring body temperature during anesthesia be available.

Mercury-in-glass thermometers were standard in earlier times; currently, the most common thermometers are thermocouples and thermistors. A thermocouple consists of two different metals, often copper and constantan (a copper-nickel-manganese-iron alloy). The principle is based on the Seebeck effect, which states a small current is produced at any junction of two different metals from the thermoelectric series. The magnitude of this voltage is temperature dependent and therefore can be used for temperature measuring.

An exponential change in electrical resistance with temperature is the principle of the thermistor type of thermometer, which is a semiconductor resistor that consists of a tiny piece of metal (copper, nickel, manganese, or cobalt). The change in resistance is used to measure temperature. Both thermocouple and thermistor probes are inexpensive and sufficiently accurate for clinical purposes.

Temperature-sensitive liquid crystals have been used to measure skin temperature. Although these devices are easy and convenient to handle, they generally do not meet the accuracy criteria for clinical use, because they can be influenced by changes in body temperature and skin blood flow (Leon et al., 1990; MacKenzie and Asbury, 1994). Simply adding a constant correcting value (e.g., 2.2°C) to an arbitrary skin temperature such as the forehead is highly unlikely to provide a reliable estimate of central temperature (Burgess et al., 1978; Leon et al., 1990).

Body temperature varies widely throughout the body. On the one hand, core tissues tend to maintain a constant temperature due to high perfusion. On the other hand, peripheral tissues have much lower and less uniform temperatures (Colin et al., 1971), which may differ several degrees within a short distance from each other.

Core temperature is difficult to define. Benzinger suggested that core temperature is the temperature of the hypothalamus and that tympanic membrane probes reliably indicate core temperature (1969). No physiologic evidence suggests that hypothalamic temperature precisely represents central temperature, however. Core temperature is the most important thermoregulatory controller and therefore of most clinical interest. Core temperature–measuring sites available for clinical use are tympanic membrane, nasopharynx, distal esophagus, pulmonary artery, and, with some limitations, bladder and rectum. These sites usually provide equal readings in awake and anesthetized humans undergoing noncardiac surgery (Cork et al., 1983). Different monitoring sites under certain conditions may represent different temperatures. The physiologic and clinical significance of such differences may vary.

Body temperature can be monitored at numerous anatomic sites. The precision and accuracy of measurements at these sites have been studied (Cork et al., 1983; Bissonnette et al., 1989a), and each site has its advantages and disadvantages. The site of temperature monitoring should reflect core temperature and be associated with none or only minimal morbidity.

Skin temperature offers little as a reflection of core temperature (Lacoumenta and Hall, 1984; Bissonnette et al., 1989a). Skin temperature varies depending on the site of monitoring. A number of investigators have suggested monitoring between 4 and 15 sites, using both weighted and unweighted formulas to accurately describe mean skin temperature (Ramanathan, 1964; Colin et al., 1971; Shanks, 1975; Puhakka et al., 1994). To be of clinical value, skin temperature must accurately reflect central temperature in the perioperative setting such as mild hypothermia and malignant hyperthermia. It is unlikely that skin temperature correlates well with central temperature during the early phase of malignant hyperthermia, because the circulating catecholamine concentrations may be up to 20 times higher than normal and significantly affect skin perfusion (Sessler, 1986; Sessler and Moayeri, 1990).

Tympanic membrane temperature has been suggested to be the most ideal temperature-monitoring site. To reflect tympanic temperature, it is not necessary for the temperature probe to be in contact with the tympanic membrane, as long as the external auditory canal is sealed by the probe, thereby allowing the air column trapped between the probe and the tympanic membrane to reach a steady state. In the initial postoperative period in infants and children after cardiac reconstructive surgery, tympanic temperature does not correlate well with brain temperature (Bissonnette et al., 2000) and therefore does not provide an accurate estimate of central body temperature (Muma et al., 1991). Because of the difficulty associated with obtaining appropriate-sized thermistors and reports of tympanic membrane perforation, its clinical use has been discouraged.

Nasopharyngeal temperature probes can accurately reflect core temperature if placed properly (i.e., placing the tip of the temperature probe in the posterior nasopharynx close to the soft palate). This should provide a good estimate of the hypothalamic temperature. If used in combination with uncuffed tubes with a moderate to large air leak, the resulting airflow may lead to inaccurate reading. Slight and self-limiting bleeding from the nose is not uncommon (especially in children with large adenoids), and its preclusion in mask anesthesia has limited its routine use. In contrast, oral temperature is considered less adequate (Cork et al., 1983) and therefore is not recommended as an accurate intraoperative temperature-monitoring site.

Esophageal temperature probes are often combined with an esophageal stethoscope, which makes this site particularly attractive in the pediatric population. In infants and children, and in cachetic patients, the thermal insulation is minimal between the tracheobronchial tree and the esophagus. The respiratory gas flow, therefore, may result in erroneous temperature readings (Bissonnette et al., 1989a), especially when the respiratory gas flow is high and its temperature differs significantly from the body temperature. Furthermore, central temperature is measured only if the tip of the probe is placed in the distal third of the esophagus at the point where the heart sounds are the loudest (Bissonnette et al., 1989a; Stoen and Sessler, 1990). In patients with endotracheal intubation, esophageal temperature is more reliable than rectal temperature and more practical than tympanic temperature.

Axillary temperature probes are notoriously unreliable guides to core temperature, because they are frequently malpositioned. It is not only the most commonly used but also the most convenient site for temperature monitoring. Axillary temperature has been reported to be as accurate in measuring central temperature as tympanic membrane, esophageal, and rectal temperature sites (Bissonnette et al., 1989a) but only when the tip of the thermometer is carefully placed over the axillary artery and the arm is closely adducted (Bissonnette et al., 1989a). Infusing cool solutions at high flow rates in small children on the ipsilateral side of the thermometer may result in falsely low temperature readings.

Rectal temperature monitoring bears the problems of probe insulation by feces, exposure of the probe to cooler blood returning from the legs, the influence of an open abdominal cavity during laparotomy, or bladder irrigations with either cold or warm solutions. Nonetheless, with these restrictions kept in mind, the rectal site can provide central temperature reading (Bissonnette et al., 1989a), and the minimal morbidity associated with its use and its ease of insertion confer major advantages. Relative contraindications for the use of a rectal probe are patients with inflammatory bowel disease, neutropenia, or thrombocytopenia and patients whose bowel or bladder is to be irrigated.

Bladder temperature is considered to be one of the most accurate sites for measuring core temperature. It has been demonstrated to be identical to pulmonary artery temperature as long as urinary output is high (Horrow and Rosenberg, 1988). When urinary output is normal or less than normal, this site becomes inaccurate to represent central temperature. A pulmonary artery catheter with a distal-tip thermistor can accurately reflect pulmonary blood temperature, but due to its invasive nature, its use is limited to special situations, namely, in critically ill children.

The site or sites of temperature monitoring generally are a function of the operative procedure. For cardiac surgery patients, in whom temperatures from different body sites convey useful information, temperature is usually measured at multiple sites (e.g., rectum, bladder, esophagus, nasopharynx, tympanic membrane).

In the pediatric patient who does not have an endotracheal tube and is undergoing a short operative procedure, either rectal or axillary temperature monitoring can be used. If the child has an endotracheal tube in place, another option includes the use of a distal esophageal temperature probe.

PHYSIOLOGY OF THERMAL REGULATION

Survival from body temperatures as low as 13.7°C has been reported (Gilbert et al., 2000), whereas death resulting from protein denaturation occurs within 7°C from normality at approximately 44°C. Compared with each other, the tolerance to cold is more than three times higher than that to heat, which explains why the system to dissipate heat has to be much more effective than the cold defense system.

The thermoregulatory system is similar to other physiologic control systems in the sense that the brain uses negative feedback mechanisms to keep variations from normal values as minimal as possible (Shanks, 1975). The principal site of temperature regulation is the hypothalamus, which integrates afferent signals from temperature-sensitive cells found in most tissues, including other parts of the brain, spinal cord, central core tissues, respiratory tract, gastrointestinal tract, and the skin surface (Fig. 5–1). The processing of thermoregulatory information occurs in three stages:

1. Afferent thermal sensing
2. Central regulation
3. Efferent response

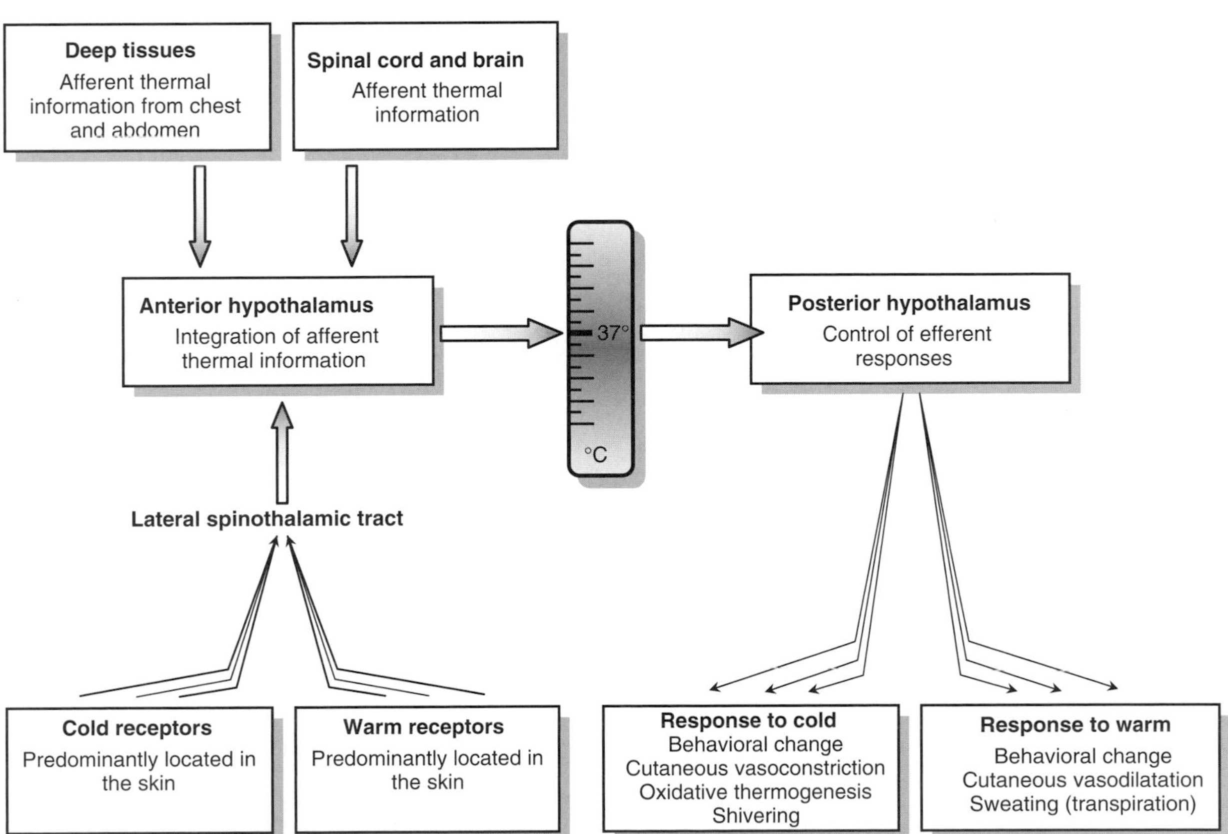

FIGURE 5–1. Illustration of the thermoregulatory pathways with afferent information from the body being integrated in the anterior hypothalamus and triggering of efferent responses in the posterior hypothalamus.

AFFERENT THERMAL SENSING

In the periphery, anatomically distinct warm and cold receptors sense the ambient temperature. The skin contains about 10 times more cold than warm receptors, acknowledging the important function of the skin in the detection of cold (Poulos, 1981). Thermosensitive receptors are also found in close proximity to the great vessels, the viscera, and the abdominal wall and in the brain and the spinal cord. Each receptor type transmits the information through an afferent nerve conduction pathway. Although they originate from anatomically different nerve fibers, the speed of transmission is influenced by the intensity of the stimulus rather than the type of nerve fiber. It is well established that the rate of the change in skin temperature alters its apparent importance. Rapid changes contribute about five times as much to the central regulatory system as comparable slow changes (Wyss et al., 1975). In patients not undergoing cardiopulmonary bypass, the rate of change in core temperature does not appear to substantially influence the magnitude of the provoked regulatory responses. The thermal information from cold-sensitive receptors, which have their maximal discharge rate of impulses at a temperature of 25° to 30°C, is transmitted to the preoptic area of the hypothalamus by A delta fibers.

The thermal information gathered by peripheral warm receptors, which have their maximal discharge rate at 45° to 50°C (Pierau and Wurster, 1981), is carried by unmyelinated C fibers. These C fibers also detect and convey pain sensations, which explains why intense heat cannot be distinguished from severe pain (Pierau and Wurster, 1981; Poulos, 1981). Although most ascending thermal information travels along the spinothalamic tracts in the anterolateral spinal cord, no single spinal tract is solely responsible for conveying thermal information (Hellon, 1981).

CENTRAL REGULATION

The anterior hypothalamus is responsible for the integration of the afferent thermal information, whereas the posterior hypothalamus controls the descending pathways to the effectors. Thermal inputs from skin surface, spinal cord, and deep body tissues are integrated in the preoptic area of the anterior hypothalamus and compared with the threshold temperatures for heat and cold. The hypothalamus then carefully regulates mechanisms for heat generation and dissipation to maintain body temperature within the narrow limits of its set point (interthreshold range).

The preoptic area of the hypothalamus contains cold- and heat-sensitive neurons, with the latter predominating by 4:1 (Boulant and Bignall, 1973). This area also receives and processes nonthermic afferent information, which seems to be important in controlling the adaptive mechanisms and the behavior of the organism (Hori and Katafuchi, 1998).

Local heat sensation results in increased discharge rate from these heat-sensitive neurons and leads to the activation of heat loss mechanisms. Conversely, cold-sensitive neurons in the hypothalamus respond with increased discharge rates to cooling of the preoptic area of the hypothalamus (Boulant and Hardy, 1974; Boulant and Demieville, 1977). Thermosensitive neurons also exist in the posterior hypothalamus, the reticular formation, the medulla, the lower brainstem, and the spinal cord, although their function remains to be fully elucidated (Guieu and Hardy, 1970; Simon, 1974; Cabanac, 1975; Dickenson, 1977).

It seems that under normal conditions, the contribution of the central thermoreceptors to thermal regulation is limited by the marked predominance of the input of peripheral receptors (Downey et al., 1964). These central receptors take over thermoregulation if the sensory input from peripheral sensors is disrupted (e.g., central neuraxial anesthesia or spinal cord transsection), but they are less efficient compared with peripheral thermoreceptors (Downey et al., 1967).

The threshold represents the central temperature for which a particular regulatory effector becomes active (Box 5–1). When the integrated input from all sources exceeds the upper or falls below the lower threshold, efferent responses are initiated from the hypothalamus to maintain normal body temperature. The slope of the response intensity plotted against the difference between the thermal input temperature and the threshold temperature is called the *gain* of that response (i.e., the intensity of the response).

The difference between the lowest temperature at which warm responses are triggered and the highest temperature at which cold responses are triggered indicates the thermal sensitivity of the system. As previously stated, the interthreshold range is the temperature range over which no regulatory responses occur (although the brain presumably detects these temperature changes). It changes from approximately 0.4°C in the awake state to approximately 3.5°C during anesthesia. Compared with normal human body temperature (37.0 ± 0.2°C), the interthreshold range is wider in the hypothermic state than in the hyperthermic state. This physiologic system acts as an "all-or-none" phenomenon. The mechanism by which the body determines the absolute threshold temperatures is not known, but it appears that the thresholds are influenced by several factors such as sodium, calcium, thyroid hormones, tryptophan, general anesthetics and other drugs, circadian rhythm, exercise, pyrogens, food intake, and cold and warm adaptation. Central regulation is fully functional in infancy but may be impaired in the premature,

BOX 5–1 Definition of Temperature Regulation Terms

Threshold temperature	Central temperature that elicits a regulating effect, e.g., vasoconstriction, vasodilatation, shivering, sweating, nonshivering thermogenesis
Interthreshold range	Temperature range over which no regulatory response occurs
Gain	Intensity of regulatory response
Mean body temperature	Physiologically weighted average temperature from various tissues
Nonshivering thermogenesis	Heat production (above basal metabolism) not associated with muscle activity
Shivering thermogenesis	Heat production through voluntary muscle activity
Dietary thermogenesis	Heat production through metabolism of nutrients

elderly, or extremely ill patient. It is now known that regulatory responses are based on mean body temperature.

EFFERENT RESPONSE

Mean body temperature (MBT) is a physiologically weighted average temperature that reflects the thermoregulatory importance of various tissues but in particular that of the central compartment. In unanesthetized subjects, the MBT can be calculated as follows:

$$\text{MBT} = 0.85(\text{central T}) + 0.15(\text{skin T}) \quad (5.3)$$

where T denotes temperature measured in °C or as follows (several different formulas exist: Ramanathan, 1964; Colin et al., 1971; Shanks, 1975; Puhakka et al., 1994):

$$\text{MBT} = 0.66 \text{ rectal T} + 0.34 \text{ MSK} \quad (5.4)$$

where MSK reflects the mean skin temperature (in °C), which then equals

$$\text{MSK} = 0.3(\text{chest T} + \text{arm T}) + 0.2(\text{thigh T} + \text{calf T}) \quad (5.5)$$

From that it follows:

$$\text{MBT} = 0.66 \text{ rectal T} + 0.34[0.3(\text{chest T} + \text{forearm T}) + 0.2(\text{thigh T} + \text{calf T})] \quad (5.6)$$

Although skin temperature is the most important parameter in triggering behavioral changes, for the thermoregulatory autonomic response, the thermal input from the skin contributes only about 20% (Cheung and Mekjavic, 1995; Lenhardt et al., 1999). The main part of this autonomic response depends on the afferent information from the central core (Jessen and Mayer, 1971; Simon, 1974; Jessen and Feistkorn, 1984), which includes the brain (parts other than the hypothalamus), the spinal cord, and deep abdominal and thoracic tissues, with each of them contributing about 20% to the central thermoregulatory control (Jessen and Mayer, 1971; Mercer and Jessen, 1978).

Although the most commonly described thermoregulatory model is a set point system in which hypothalamic temperatures above or below a predetermined level trigger warm or cold defenses, respectively, temperature regulation may also be described by a system of thresholds and gains for each particular thermoregulatory response. Efferent responses (behavioral changes, cutaneous vasoconstriction or vasodilatation, nonshivering thermogenesis, shivering, and sweating) appear to be mediated according to the central interpretation of the afferent input.

The thermal steady state is actively defended when the hypothalamus responds to thermal changes, that is, temperatures exceeding the interthreshold range. Thus, thermal deviations from the threshold temperature initiate efferent responses that either increase metabolic heat production (nonshivering thermogenesis and shivering) and decrease environmental heat loss (active vasoconstriction and behavioral changes), or increase heat loss (active vasodilatation, sweating, and behavioral maneuvers). These thermoregulatory effectors work by adjusting their own threshold and gain according to the physiologic needs, and they do so by selecting the order of responses and by regulating the intensities.

Behavioral responses to environmental temperatures outside the thermoneutral range (approximately 28°C for an unclothed adult) are quantitatively the most important thermoregulatory effectors in humans (e.g., heating the home, looking for shelter, putting on a jacket, etc.) and are much more efficient than all of the autonomic responses combined. Cutaneous vasoconstriction is not only the first thermoregulatory response to hypothermia, but also the most consistent one. Total digital skin blood flow can be categorized into a nutritional (capillaries) and a thermoregulatory (arteriovenous shunts) component. Cold-mediated decreases in cutaneous blood flow are most pronounced (down to 1% of the normal blood flow in an environment with neutral temperature) in arteriovenous shunts of the hands, feet, ears, lips, and nose (Grant and Bland, 1931; Hillman et al., 1982). These shunts are typically 100 μm in diameter, which means that one can divert 10,000 times as much blood as a capillary with a 10-μm diameter under otherwise unchanged conditions (i.e., same length and pressure gradient). Shunt flow is primarily regulated by norepinephrine (released from presynaptic adrenergic terminals), which binds to peripheral α_2-receptors that are sensitized by local cooling and inhibited by temperatures equal to or higher than 35°C (Sessler and Ponte, 1982). Flow decreases not only in the arteriovenous shunts but also in the far more numerous capillaries (Coffman and Cohen, 1971). Despite the impressive decrease in cutaneous perfusion secondary to thermoregulatory vasoconstriction, the resulting reduction of heat loss from the hands and feet decrease by 50%, but only by 17% from the trunk, resulting in an overall heat loss reduction of only 25% (Sessler et al., 1991).

In contrast, warm exposure initially results in sweating, which results in the triggering of massive precapillary vasodilatation with marked increase in skin blood flow. This allows for huge amounts of heat to be transported to the skin, which then dissipate to the environment, mainly by evaporation due to preconditioning by sweat. Voluntary muscle activity, nonshivering thermogenesis, and shivering are efferent mechanisms, which lead to heat generation.

THERMAL REGULATION IN THE NEWBORN

Premature infants or infants small for gestational age, but also full-term neonates, have an exceptionally large skin surface area compared with their body mass (normal ratio: term neonate, 1; adult, about 0.40) and an increased thermal conductance (thin layer of subcutaneous fat). Furthermore, evaporative heat loss is increased due to a reduced keratin content in the infant's skin. Therefore, neonates lose proportionately more heat through skin than do adults in a similar environment. In contrast to the adult, the capabilities and the functional range of the neonate's thermoregulatory system are significantly limited and easily overwhelmed by environmental factors. The lower temperature limit of thermal regulation in adults is 0°C, whereas that in newborns is 22°C. The combination of increased heat loss and a diminished efficacy of the thermoregulatory response with a reduced ability to generate heat makes these infants prone to hypothermia. The same anatomic properties that are responsible for the increased risk of hypothermia also allow for three to four times faster rewarming in infants and children compared with adults (Szmuk et al., 2001).

The *neutral temperature* is defined as the ambient temperature, at which the oxygen demand (as a reflection of metabolic heat production) is minimal and temperature regulation is achieved through nonevaporative physical processes alone. For unclothed adults, the neutral temperature is about 28°C; for neonates, 32°C; and for preterm infants, 34°C (see later). In a thermoneutral environment, the cutaneous arteriovenous shunts are open and skin blood flow is maximal.

In general, the maintenance of the core temperature in a cool environment results in an increased oxygen consumption and metabolic acidosis. It was demonstrated long ago that in full-term neonates, oxygen consumption does not correlate with rectal temperature but rather increases directly with the skin surface–to–environment temperature gradient (Adamson et al., 1965). Oxygen consumption was minimal at gradients of 2° to 4°C. Thus, at environmental temperatures of 32° to 34°C and abdominal skin temperature of 36°C, the resting newborn infant is in a state of minimal oxygen consumption (i.e., the neutral thermal state). Normal rectal temperature, therefore, does not imply a state of minimal oxygen consumption in this age group (Fig. 5–2).

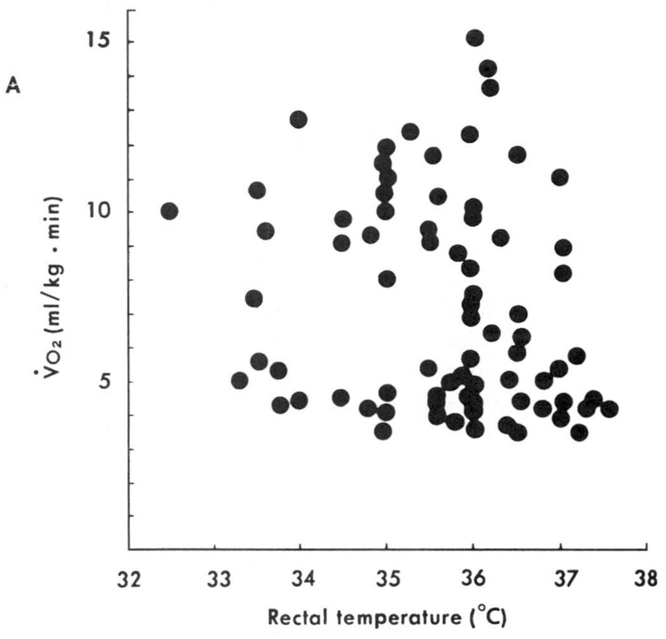

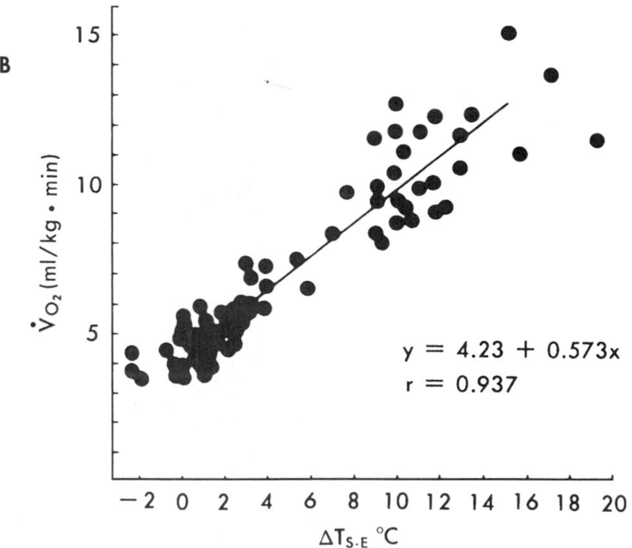

■ **FIGURE 5–2.** *A,* Relation of oxygen consumption ($\dot{V}O_2$) to rectal temperature. Note complete lack of correlation. *B,* Relation between oxygen consumption and temperature gradient between skin temperature and environment ($\Delta T_{S\text{-}E}$) in full-term human newborns with varying deep body and skin temperatures. (From Adamson KJ Jr, Gandy GM, James LS: The influence of thermal factors upon oxygen consumption of the newborn human infant. *J Pediatr* 66:495, 1965.)

Of particular concern in view of thermoregulation in the newborn is the head, which comprises up to 20% of the total skin surface area and shows the highest regional heat flux ability (Anttonen et al., 1995). In addition, the thin skull bone and the usually sparse scalp hair in combination with the close proximity to the well-perfused brain (core temperature) further favor heat loss from the head. Facial cooling may increase oxygen requirements by up to 23% in the term infant and up to 36% in the premature infant (Sinclair, 1972), thereby demonstrating the effectiveness of protecting the infant from heat loss by covering the head.

Thermoregulatory vasoconstriction and vasodilatation most likely establish during the first day of life (Lyons et al., 1996) and can occur in both the premature and the full-term infant (Bruck, 1961). With vasoconstriction, cutaneous blood flow decreases and the effect of tissue insulation increases, which results in an overall reduction in conductive and convective heat losses.

Heat dissipation in the premature or small-for-gestational-age infant represents the extreme of thermal regulation in the neonate. Small size and decreased insulation tissue result in increased volume index and thermal transfer coefficients, thereby challenging the thermoregulating capacity of these infants. These disadvantages narrow the temperature range for thermoregulatory stability. In small-for-gestational-age infants, a slightly lower skin surface area–to–volume ratio and an increased motor tone offer some protection compared with the premature infant in regard to heat loss or transfer. In addition to the physical limitations of heat conservation in infants and children, surgery can further increase heat loss and fluid requirements by exposing the visceral surfaces of the abdomen and thorax, thereby exacerbating evaporative heat and water losses.

■ HEAT LOSS MECHANISMS

For an organism to be homeothermic, it must be able both to dissipate and to produce heat. Controlled heat loss is fundamental in homeotherms and is accomplished in two stages (Swyer, 1973), both governed by the physical laws of conduction, radiation, convection, and evaporation (Box 5–2). The second law of thermodynamic states that heat transfer is only possible from a warmer to a cooler object, never from a cooler to a warmer object. This means that the warmer object (in the operating room setting, this is almost exclusively the patient) is used to warm up the surrounding cooler objects (operating room walls, tables, etc.). Although most anesthesiologists consider heat loss to be a nuisance, we have to keep in mind that without any heat loss to the environment (i.e., perfect insulation), the body of an awake adult at rest (assuming a metabolic rate of 75 W) would warm up by at least 1°C per hour! (Keep in mind that during

BOX 5–2 **Mechanisms (by Percent) of Heat Loss in Neutral Thermal Environments**

Radiation	39%
Convection	34%
Evaporation	24%
Conduction	3%

exercise, the metabolic heat generation can increase 10-fold.) This can be calculated with the following formula:

$$HSR = m\kappa \, dT_B/dt \tag{5.7}$$

where HSR is the heat storage rate (W), m is the body mass (kg), κ is the specific heat coefficient of the human body ($3.5 \cdot 10^3$ J/°C) (Burton, 1935), dT_B is the change in body temperature (°C), and dt is the time interval (seconds).

The first stage of heat loss is transfer of heat from the body core (central compartment) to the periphery and the skin surface, which is referred to as the concept of internal redistribution of heat. The second stage is dissipation of heat from the skin surface to the environment. Physiologic manipulations of regional blood flow and changes in the thermal conductance properties of the insulation tissue can influence both gradients. Most studies of thermal regulation in infants and children have quantified the relative contributions of radiation, convection, evaporation, and conduction to heat loss. A study in newborns in an environment at neutral temperature found radiation, convection, evaporation, and conduction to account for 39%, 34%, 24%, and 3%, respectively, of total heat loss (Hey, 1973). Changes in the environment (e.g., the operating room) can alter not only the magnitude of heat loss but also the relative contribution of each of these four physical components. Figure 5–3 gives an overview of the heat loss mechanisms involved in the operating room setting.

CONDUCTION

Conduction is heat transfer between two surfaces in direct contact. The amount of heat transferred (C) depends on the temperature difference between two objects in contact ($T_1 - T_2$), the surface area in contact (A), and the conductive heat transfer coefficient h_k of the materials. It can be calculated as follows:

$$C = h_k \, A \, (T_1 - T_2) \tag{5.8}$$

The coefficient h_k is a property of the material or interface between objects that determines the rate of heat transfer per unit area per unit temperature difference ($W/m^2 \cdot °C$). It seems convenient to think of conductance as the inverse of resistance. During surgery, relatively little heat is lost to the environment via conduction, because patients are well insulated from surrounding objects (Allen, 1987). Conduction is also represented in the energy needed to warm cool irrigation solutions and intravenous fluids, which have the potential to significantly reduce body temperature. Care should also be taken to ensure that the patient's skin is not in contact with metallic surfaces. (In addition, contact with metallic surfaces during surgery must be avoided to prevent skin burns from electrocautery.) The physiologic factors controlling conductive heat loss in newborns are cutaneous blood flow and the thickness of the subcutaneous tissue (insulation).

RADIATION

Radiant heat loss is the transfer of heat between two objects of different temperature but not in contact with each other (e.g., radiation is the mechanism by which the sun warms the earth). The emitted radiation carries energy from the warmer to the cooler object, therefore causing the warmer object to cool and the cooler object to warm. This heat transfer occurs in the

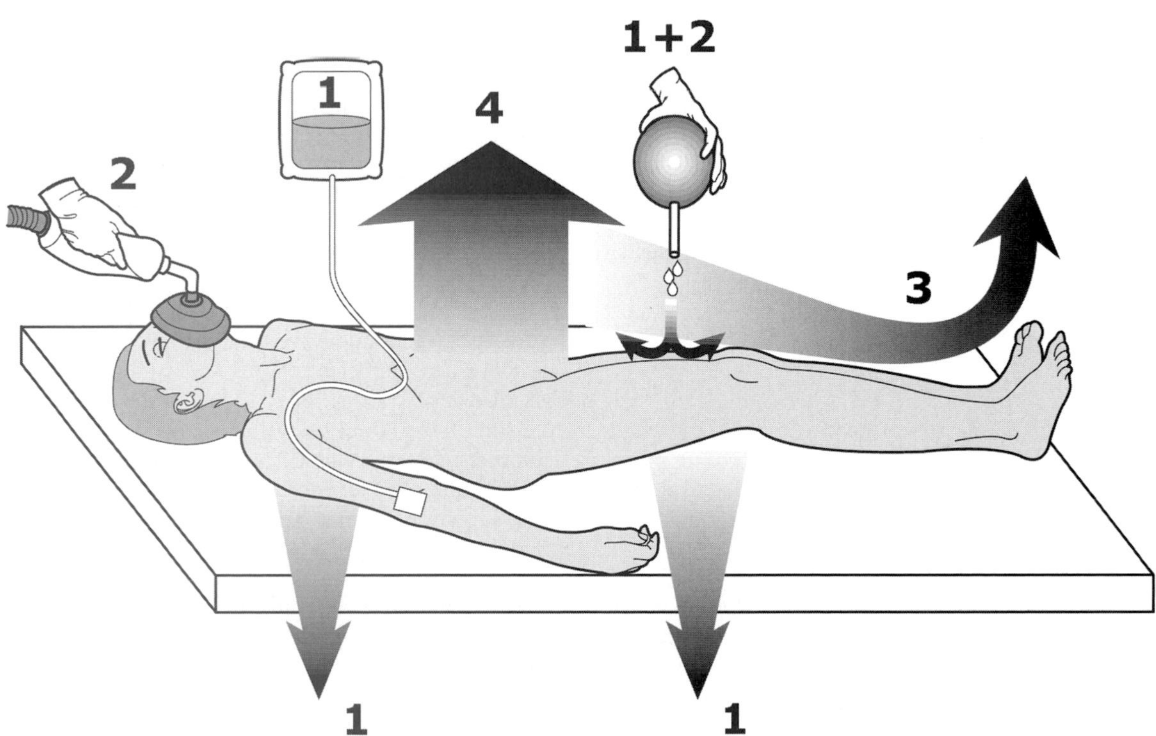

FIGURE 5–3. Schematic illustration of the mechanisms contributing to perioperative hypothermia: (1) conduction, (2) evaporation, (3) convection, and (4) radiation. (Modified from Gurtner C, Paul O, Bissonnette B: Temperature regulation: physiology and pharmacology. In Bissonnette B, Daleus B, editors: *Pediatric anesthesia. Principles and Practice*. New York, 2002, McGraw-Hill, p173.)

infrared light spectrum. Heat exchange by radiation depends on the difference of the fourth power of the absolute temperatures of the two objects:

$$R = e\sigma A\,(T_{sk}^4 - T_r^4) \tag{5.9}$$

where R is heat transfer by radiation (W), e is the emissivity (a material property with a value between 0 and 1), σ is the Stefan Boltzmann constant ($5.67 \cdot 10^{-8}$ J/sec · m² · K^4), A denotes the surface area of the object (m²), T_{sk} is the skin temperature, and T_r is the temperature of the second object (both temperature values in K).

To calculate radiation heat exchange for clinical purposes, where T_{sk} and T_r are close to each other, it is acceptable to use a first-power relationship as follows:

$$R = h_r A\,(T_{sk} - T_r) \tag{5.10}$$

where h_r denotes the radiation coefficient. The value of h_r depends on the temperatures of the two surfaces and such surface characteristics as emittance and reflectance (reflected in the emissivity value). It is obvious that heat transfer by radiation principally depends on the temperature of the two surfaces concerned but is unaffected by air movement or the distance between the surfaces. It can take place across a vacuum (Allen, 1987).

As previously stated, newborns and infants have a large surface area–to–volume ratio, thus radiant heat loss is proportionally greater the smaller the infant. In both the awake and the anesthetized infant, radiation is the major factor for heat loss under normal conditions. The human body is an excellent emitter of energy at wavelengths relevant for heat transfer, and the probability of photon reflection in the standard operating room is near zero. Radiant heat loss in the operating room is therefore a function of the difference between the patient's body temperature and the objects in the room, such as the walls and solid objects. Radiant heat loss is diminished by increasing the ambient temperature of the room, thereby reducing the temperature gradient between the patient and the operating room walls and its content. As long as a temperature gradient exists, the patient continues to warm up walls and solid objects by exchanging radiant energy. At a room temperature of 22°C, about 70% of the total heat loss is due to radiation (Hardy et al., 1941). A single-layer covering dramatically reduces the losses by convection and radiation; thus, a thin shirt (e.g., a silk blouse providing negligible insulation) results in considerably increased thermal comfort.

CONVECTION

Convective heat loss is the transfer of heat to moving molecules such as air and liquid. The thin air layer adjacent to the skin is warmed by conduction from the body. Although changes in body posture and minute ventilation may affect convective heat loss, convection plays only a minor role in heat loss. In the case of a naked individual exposed to air, the rate and direction of convective heat exchange depend on the airflow velocity and the temperature difference between the air and the skin surface. The situation is more complicated in a clothed individual. Convective heat transfer may be calculated as follows:

$$Q = h_q A\,(T_{sk} - T_a) \tag{5.11}$$

where Q is the heat exchange by convection (W), A is the surface area (m²), h_q is the convective heat transfer coefficient (W/m² · °C), T_{sk} is the mean skin temperature (°C), and T_a is the ambient temperature (°C). The convective heat exchange coefficient is not a constant and depends on the rate of air movement, the shape of the body, and the medium. It may be calculated from $h_c = 8.3\ V^{0.5}$ (W/m² · °C), where V is the air movement (m/sec) (Allen, 1987). Thus, convective heat losses increase in proportion to the temperature difference between the body surface and the surrounding fluid (liquid or gas) and the square root of the flow velocity of the fluid (liquid or gas) in contact with the patient. Convective losses are experienced outdoors as the "wind chill factor."

EVAPORATION

Evaporative heat loss occurs through the skin and the respiratory system. Under conditions of thermal neutrality, evaporation accounts for 10% to 20% of heat loss. Physical factors that govern evaporative heat loss include relative humidity of the ambient air, velocity of airflow, and lung minute ventilation. The driving force for evaporation is the vapor pressure difference between the body surface and the environment. Evaporative losses include several components: (1) sweat (sensible water loss), (2) insensible water loss from the skin, respiratory tract, and open surgical wounds, and (3) evaporation of liquids applied to the skin such as antibacterial solutions. The evaporation of water from a surface is an energy-dependent process, energy that is absorbed from the surface during transition from the liquid to the gaseous state. This energy is called the *latent heat of vaporization,* and in the case of sweat, it has a value of 2.5×10^6 J/kg. This figure emphasizes the extraordinary power of the human sweating mechanism as a means of dissipating heat, especially when it is considered that an adult in good physical condition can produce up to 2 liters of sweat per hour. In an environment where the air temperature is equal to or higher than the skin temperature, sweating is the only mechanism available for the dissipation of heat from metabolic production. In this situation, anything that limits evaporation, such as high ambient humidity or impermeable clothing, easily leads to heat storage and a potentially fatal rise in body temperature.

Evaporative heat loss depends on the water vapor pressure gradient between the skin surface and the ambient air and may be calculated from the following:

$$E = h_e A_{wet}\,(P_{sk} - P_a) \tag{5.12}$$

where E is the evaporative heat loss (W); h_e is the evaporative heat transfer coefficient (W/m² · kPa), P_{sk} is the water vapor pressure at the skin surface, and P_a is the ambient water vapor pressure (both pressure values in kPa). The coefficient for evaporative heat exchange (h_e) incorporates the latent heat of vaporization of water and the paramount effect of air movement on evaporation. For practical purposes, h_e may be calculated from $h_e = 124\ V^{0.5}$ (W/m² · kPa), where V is the airflow velocity (m/sec). Similar to convection, the important point to note is that evaporation is determined by the vapor pressure gradient between the exposed body surface and the ambient air and the rate of airflow across the surface (Allen, 1987).

Physiologic factors that affect evaporative losses relate to the infant's ability to sweat and to increase the minute ventilation. Although the physical characteristics of the newborn predispose him or her to heat loss, it has been demonstrated that neonates are capable of sweating in a warm environment (Bruck, 1961).

Full-term neonates begin to sweat when rectal temperature is between 37.5° and 37.9°C and ambient temperature exceeds 35°C. Although the onset of sweat production in infants small for gestational age is slower than in full-term infants, the maximum rates of sweat production are comparable (Sulyok et al., 1973). Premature infants with a gestational age of less than 30 weeks show no response because their sweat glands are not yet fully developed.

A small amount of heat is lost when dry inspired respiratory gases are humidified by water evaporating from the tracheobronchial epithelium. In adults, respiratory losses account for only 5% to 10% of total heat loss during anesthesia and surgery (Bickler and Sessler, 1990), and total insensible loss accounts for approximately 25% of the total heat dissipated. Because minute ventilation on a per-kilogram basis is significantly higher in infants and children than in adults, respiratory losses represent about one third of the total heat loss. Heat loss from the respiratory tract increases if one breathes cool, dry gas as opposed to warm, moisturized gas (Bissonnette et al., 1989a, 1989b).

Heat loss from evaporation inside a large surgical incision may equal all other sources of intraoperative heat loss combined (Roe, 1971). Because of increased evaporative heat loss, hypothermia is also more likely to occur if the skin of the patient is wet or in contact with wet drapes.

HEAT GENERATION

The ability to produce heat by increasing the metabolic rate and oxygen consumption is the other component of thermal regulation in the homeotherm (Hull and Smales, 1978). Although three of the physical mechanisms that lead to heat loss (i.e., conduction, radiation, and convection) can theoretically also be used to passively warm up a patient, the body has the ability to actively produce heat. Heat generation is achieved via four mechanisms:

1. Voluntary muscle activity
2. Nonshivering thermogenesis
3. Involuntary muscle activity (shivering)
4. Dietary thermogenesis

The behavioral aspect of heat production (voluntary muscle activity) is absent in the perioperative period and therefore its role in heat production is not discussed further. Of the two remaining mechanisms for heat production, nonshivering thermogenesis is the major component in the newborn, whereas shivering thermogenesis is the main mechanism for heat production in the adult. The contribution of nonshivering thermogenesis in adults is debatable (Jessen, 1980a).

Although the time course and relation between nonshivering thermogenesis and shivering thermogenesis in infants have been described (Hull and Smales, 1978), the exact time sequence and factors involved in the developmental aspects of switching on and off the nonshivering thermogenesis mechanism remain to be elucidated. It seems that the importance of nonshivering thermogenesis is rapidly decreasing after the first year of life, while at the same time shivering thermogenesis is becoming more and more effective.

NONSHIVERING THERMOGENESIS

Nonshivering thermogenesis is defined as an increase in metabolic heat production (above the basal metabolism) not associated with muscle activity. It occurs mainly through metabolism of brown fat, but to a lesser degree also in skeletal muscle, liver, brain, and white fat.

Brown fat differentiates in the human fetus at 26 to 30 weeks of gestational age. It comprises only 2% to 6% of the infant's total body weight and is located in six main areas: between the scapulae, in small masses around blood vessels in the neck, in large deposits in the axilla, in medium-size masses in the mediastinum, around the internal mammary vessels in the mediastinum, and around the adrenal glands or kidneys.

Brown fat is a highly specialized tissue whose brown color is secondary to the abundant content of mitochondria in the cytoplasm of its multinucleated cells. These mitochondria appear to be densely packed with cristae and have an increased content of respiratory chain components (Himms-Hagen, 1976). They are unique in their ability to uncouple oxidative phosphorylation, resulting in heat production instead of generating adenosine triphosphate. This uncoupling is mediated by the presence of the uncoupling protein (UCP), also termed thermogenin, which is located in the inner mitochondrial membrane.

Brown fat is highly vascularized and has a rich innervation, which appears to be primarily β-sympathetic in origin and responsible for the uncoupling of oxidative phosphorylation (Karlberg et al., 1962, 1965). Cold stress increases sympathetic nerve system activity and norepinephrine production, leading to increased lipase activity in the brown fat tissue (Schiff et al., 1966). As a consequence, hydroxylation of triglycerides and release of free fatty acids occur. These free fatty acids appear to act on the UCP and thereby to increase the protein conductance across the mitochondrial membrane. In addition to norepinephrine, glucocorticoids and thyroxin have been implicated as factors triggering nonshivering thermogenesis (Gale, 1973; Jessen, 1980b, 1980c). The heat produced by nonshivering thermogenesis is mainly a byproduct of fatty acid metabolism, but to a minor degree it can also be a product of glucose metabolism. The activation of brown fat metabolism results in an increased proportion of the cardiac output being diverted through the brown fat. This proportion may reach as much as 25% of the cardiac output, thereby facilitating the direct warming of the blood.

Pharmacologic inhibition of nonshivering thermogenesis is possible with ganglionic and β-receptor blockade (Silverman et al., 1964), inhalational anesthetics (Ohlson et al., 1994), and surgically by sympathectomy (Stern et al., 1965). The inhibition of nonshivering thermogenesis by inhalational anesthetics begins as early as 5 minutes after turning on the vapor and starts to wean off within approximately 15 minutes after discontinuation of the anesthetic (Ohlson et al., 1994). Nonshivering thermogenesis is also inhibited in infants anesthetized with fentanyl and propofol (Plattner et al., 1997).

Nonshivering thermogenesis seems to be quite variable in adults but most often does not appear to be functional or relevant (van Marken Lichtenbelt and Daanen, 2003). This is supported by the fact that oxygen consumption does not increase significantly when patients are vasoconstricted (Mestyan et al., 1964; Dawkins and Scopes, 1965; Sessler et al., 1988). It seems that adults have the potential to regenerate brown fat tissue under certain pathologic conditions, such as high and sustained sympathetic stimulation (pheochromocytoma), Chagas disease, hibernoma (benign brown fat tumor), and marked cold acclimatization (Lean et al., 1986; Garruti and Ricquier, 1992; Vybiral et al., 2000).

In contrast, prematures, full-term neonates, and infants are able to double their metabolic heat production during cold exposure (Mestyan et al., 1964; Dawkins and Scopes, 1965; Hey and Katz, 1969). Clinically significant nonshivering thermogenesis is possible within hours after birth (Oya et al., 1997) and may persist up to the age of 2 years. Although it is the main source of thermoregulatory heat production in infants, it should be kept in mind that its effect is limited and does not compensate for the decreased ability of newborns and infants to effectively reduce heat loss through cutaneous vasoconstriction or to increase heat production through shivering.

During general anesthesia in children, nonshivering thermogenesis is not triggered by core hypothermia or cold exposure and therefore does not seem to be functional (Plattner et al., 1997). Halothane anesthesia has been shown to block nonshivering thermogenesis in children (Ohlson et al., 1994, 1997; Dicker et al., 1995). It has been demonstrated in animal studies that pharmacologic inhibition of nonshivering thermogenesis by β-blockade does not prevent shivering thermogenesis (Bruck and Wunnenberg, 1965). In the animals studied, shivering did not fully compensate for the lack of heat produced by nonshivering thermogenesis. The magnitude of nonshivering thermogenesis in animals varies among species, but it appears that in newborn versus adult animals and in cold-adapted versus warm-adapted animals, nonshivering thermogenesis is significant (Himms-Hagen, 1976).

SHIVERING THERMOGENESIS

Although there appears to be some developmental sequence in human thermal regulation to the onset of shivering thermogenesis, the precise mechanisms and/or factors that govern this development are unclear. With increasing age, shivering thermogenesis assumes a more prominent role in thermoregulation. It has been demonstrated that shivering occurs only after all of the other mechanisms, such as behavioral responses, nonshivering thermogenesis (both ineffective under anesthesia), and maximal vasoconstriction, have failed to maintain body temperature within the interthreshold range (Hemingway, 1963; Hemingway and Price, 1968). Until recently, newborns and infants were considered not to be able to shiver, presumably because of the general immaturity of the musculoskeletal system on the one hand and the limited muscle mass on the other hand, which would render muscle activity ineffective in cold defense. A few reports exist about shivering in neonates with shivering occurring at rectal temperatures of 35.0° to 35.3°C (Brück, 1992; Petrikovsky et al., 1997). It is debatable whether this shivering was indeed thermoregulatory in origin or whether drugs and other factors (all mothers received an intrapartum amnioinfusion) were to blame. In general, neonates do not shiver, and if they do, it is of minor importance in thermoregulation.

Shivering can briefly result in an up to sixfold increase in metabolic heat production (Giesbrecht et al., 1994), but only a twofold increase is sustained (Horvath et al., 1956). Shivering is characterized by involuntary, irregular muscular activity that begins in the muscles of the upper body. The basal frequency of the shivering tremor in the electromyogram is typically around 200 Hz (Israel and Pozos, 1989). Superimposed slow tremor spasms also occur, producing a "waxing and waning" electromyographic pattern at a rate of two to eight cycles per minute (Stuart et al., 1966; Sessler et al., 1991).

The impulses from cold receptors impinge at the motor center for shivering, which is located in the dorsomedial part of the posterior hypothalamus adjacent to the wall of the third ventricle. Under warm conditions, this center is inhibited by impulses from the heat-sensitive area in the preoptic region of the anterior hypothalamus; however, a predominance of cold impulses from the skin and the spinal cord activates the shivering center, which results in stimulation of the anterior motor neurons of the spinal cord. Initially, this results in an increased skeletal muscle tone throughout the body. These signals do not cause the actual shivering. Only when this tone is raised over a certain level does shivering become visible (Guyton, 2000).

Because of this increased muscle activity, oxygen consumption ($\dot{V}O_2$) and CO_2 production proportionally increase by up to 400% to 600% for a short period of time (Horvath et al., 1956; Benzinger, 1969; Ciofolo et al., 1989; Just et al., 1992; Giesbrecht et al., 1994).

In healthy patients, this increase in $\dot{V}O_2$ is met by an increase in cardiac output without any hemodynamic compromise. In patients with already limited hemodynamic and coronary reserves, this increase in $\dot{V}O_2$ can lead to a decreased mixed venous oxygen content that, under a less-than-perfect ventilation/perfusion ratio, may result in a decreased arterial oxygen content and, consequently, decreased tissue oxygen delivery. An inverse correlation has been shown between intraoperative temperature and postoperative $\dot{V}O_2$ (Roe et al., 1966), as well as between different anesthetics (see "Thermoregulation and General Anesthesia") and postoperative $\dot{V}O_2$. Shivering not only is an unpleasant experience for the patient in the postoperative period but it can also increase intraocular and intracranial pressure (Mahajan et al., 1987; Rosa et al., 1995).

The incidence of postoperative shivering is inversely related to the core temperature; shivering was also found in patients kept strictly normothermic during anesthesia with isoflurane or desflurane, indicating that a substantial fraction of shivering is nonthermoregulatory (Horn et al., 1998) with pain being a potential trigger (Horn et al., 1999). Inhibition of shivering with meperidine in unanesthetized, actively cooled volunteers results in a more than threefold higher and more than fourfold prolonged core temperature afterdrop and a 37% decreased rewarming rate compared with the shivering control group (Giesbrecht et al., 1997).

DIETARY THERMOGENESIS

Stimulation of energy expenditure and thermogenesis by certain nutrients (i.e., proteins and amino acids) is well known. Despite muscle paralysis and decreased metabolism during general anesthesia, the infusion of small amounts of amino acids resulted in an up to fivefold increased heat generation during anesthesia compared with awake adults (Sellden et al., 1994). Using preoperative and intraoperative amino acid infusions, the same researchers were able to prove this advantage clinically in achieving a core temperature of 36.5 ± 0.1°C at the end of surgery, whereas the temperature dropped to 35.7 ± 0.1°C in the control group (Sellden and Lindahl, 1999). Similar findings have been reported for preoperative amino acid infusion in patients undergoing spinal anesthesia (Kasai et al., 2003). Although effective, the exact mechanism behind this form of thermogenesis has not been fully elucidated. It seems that stimulation of cellular amino acid oxidation is crucial. Furthermore, protein synthesis and breakdown in extrasplanchnic tissues, requiring extra synthesis of ATP, could be a contributing factor as well. It has been concluded that about half of the heat generated in association with amino acid infusion is splanchnic in origin and that blood flow in extrasplanchnic (but not splanchnic) tissues is increased significantly, reflected by an increase in cardiac output of almost 20% (Brundin and Wahren, 1994). Except for a different time course, the average whole body thermic effect of intravenous amino acid administration was not different from the one seen with oral protein ingestion.

■ EFFECT OF ANESTHESIA ON THERMOREGULATION

■ THERMOREGULATION AND GENERAL ANESTHESIA

Anesthetics may interfere with thermal regulation at both peripheral and central receptor sites. In adults, general anesthesia has been shown to decrease the thermoregulatory threshold temperature triggering a response to hypothermia on average by approximately 2.5°C and increases the threshold temperature initiating a response to hyperthermia to a lesser degree (approximately 1.3°C) (Sessler et al., 1988a and b) (Boxes 5–3 and 5–4). This anesthesia-induced expansion of the interthreshold range (Fig. 5–4) results in a wider temperature range over which active thermoregulatory responses are absent. Within this range, patients are poikilothermic, and body temperature is changing passively in proportion to the difference between metabolic heat production and heat loss to the environment. Vasoconstriction and nonshivering thermogenesis are the only thermoregulatory responses available to anesthetized, paralyzed, hypothermic infants and children. Patients with mild hypothermia during surgery (e.g., a central body temperature of about 34.5°C) demonstrate profound peripheral vasoconstriction, which can easily be verified using skin surface temperature gradients (e.g., forearm versus fingertip skin temperature), laser Doppler flowmeter, volume plethysmography, or other techniques (Stuart et al., 1966; Sessler et al., 1988a and b).

Under anesthesia, the maximal intensity of peripheral vasoconstriction is similar to that in awake volunteers, indicating that the gain of the response is preserved, although at a markedly lowered threshold. The only exemption seems to be desflurane, which lowers not only the threshold temperature for vasoconstriction but also the gain (Kurz et al., 1995). The temperature at which vasoconstriction and nonshivering thermogenesis occur identifies the corresponding lower thermoregulatory threshold for the anesthetic agent at any given concentration or dose.

For halothane administered in a concentration of 1.0% in oxygen to healthy adults undergoing donor nephrectomy, the thermoregulatory threshold is 34.4 ± 0.2°C (Sessler et al., 1988a). In infants and children anesthetized with 0.6% halothane and a caudal epidural block with bupivacaine, the threshold for vasoconstriction was 35.7°C (Bissonnette and Sessler, 1992). Of note is that in children weighing more than 30 kg, the central temperature continued to drop after the vasoconstriction threshold had been reached, whereas in children and infants below 30 kg, the central temperature remained constant or even slightly increased. These data show that thermoregulatory defense in infants and smaller children is more effective than in older children and adults.

> **BOX 5–3 General Effects of Anesthetics on Thermoregulation**
>
> 1. Lower hypothermia threshold
> 2. Increase hyperthermia threshold
> 3. Widen interthreshold range
> 4. No effect on gain response (except for desflurane)

> **BOX 5–4 Specific Effects of Anesthetics on Thermoregulation**
>
> 1. Opioids reduce threshold for vasoconstriction and shivering as a linear function of dose.
> 2. Propofol reduces threshold for vasoconstriction and shivering as a linear function of dose.
> 3. Volatile anesthetics produce nonlinear inhibition, the threshold being proportionally greater at higher end-tidal concentrations.
> 4. Volatile anesthetics at comparable minimum alveolar concentration values produce similar amounts of inhibition.
> 5. N_2O decreases vasoconstriction threshold less than other volatile agents.

The administration of subanesthetic concentrations of nitrous oxide (10% to 25% in a normoxic mixture) to healthy adult volunteers resulted in a significant and dose-independent reduction of shivering thermogenesis (Cheung and Mekjavic, 1995). In a concentration of 0.6 (63%) minimum alveolar concentration (MAC), nitrous oxide resulted in a calculated reduction of the vasoconstriction threshold to 35.7 ± 0.6°C (Goto et al., 1999). Overall, nitrous oxide decreased the vasoconstriction threshold less than equipotent concentrations of the volatile anesthetic agents sevoflurane and isoflurane.

In a small study in adults anesthetized with isoflurane, the decrease in the thermoregulatory threshold for vasoconstriction was found to be inversely correlated to the isoflurane concentration, and the threshold temperature decreased by approximately 3°C/% end-tidal isoflurane concentration (Stoen and Sessler, 1990). In a more recent study, the same group found that the dose dependence was not linear, with isoflurane reducing the threshold temperature disproportionately at higher anesthetic concentrations (Xiong et al., 1996). In adults anesthetized with 0.7% isoflurane, the shivering temperature threshold was decreased as was the maximum intensity of shivering. The gain of shivering increased significantly and was associated with a clonic muscular activity that was not a component of regular shivering (Ikeda et al., 1998).

Inhaled Anesthetic Agents

The vasoconstriction threshold in infants and children anesthetized with isoflurane differs only slightly from that in adults (Bissonnette and Sessler, 1990). The thermoregulatory threshold for vasoconstriction in pediatric patients anesthetized with 1 MAC halothane in 70% nitrous oxide is higher (35.8 ± 0.5°C) (Bissonnette and Sessler, 1992) than reported in an adult study (34.4°C) (Sessler et al., 1988a). In the adult study, the patients were anesthetized without nitrous oxide and the administered halothane concentration (1.3 MAC) was significantly greater

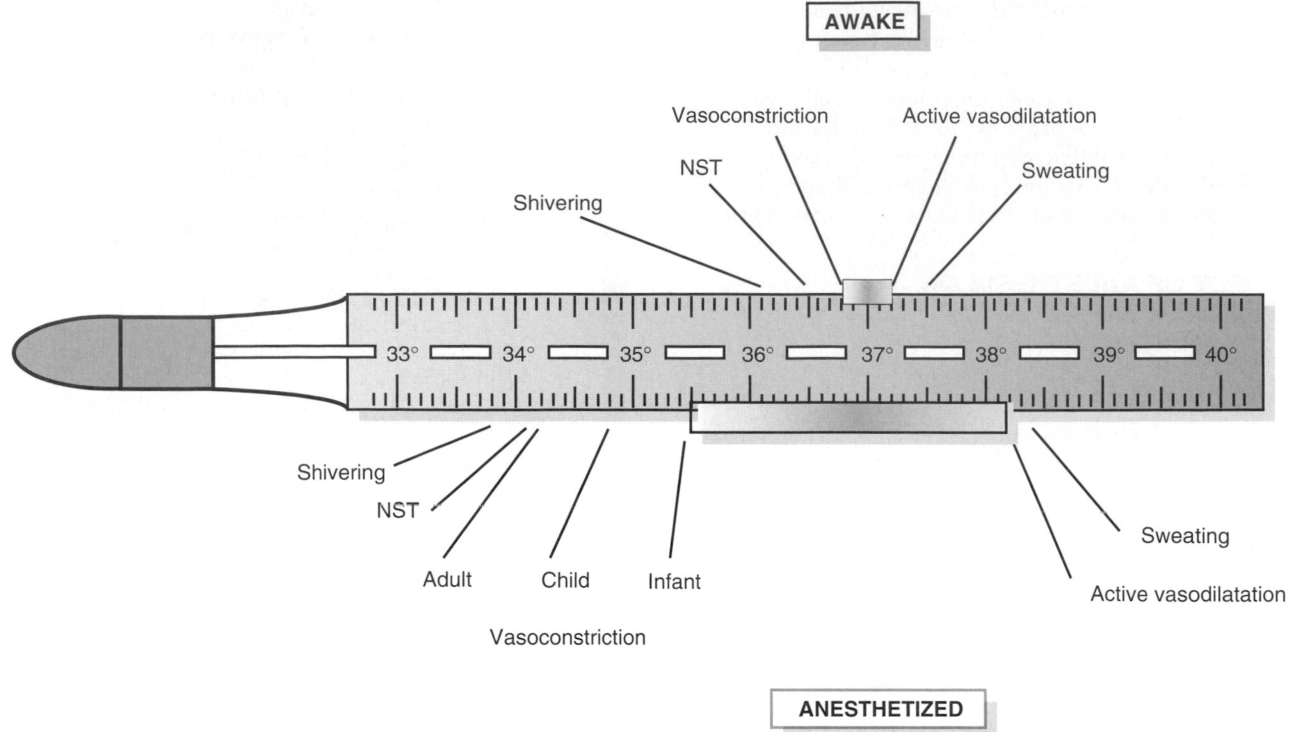

■ **FIGURE 5–4.** Schematic illustration of the thermoregulatory thresholds and gains in awake and anesthetized adults, children, and infants. The vertical height/depth of the lines represents the maximal intensity of each effector response, whereas the slope (negative values for anesthetized patients in this graph) represents the gain of the response. The horizontal axis corresponds to the core temperature. The threshold is defined as the core temperature triggering a response. The sensitivity of the thermoregulatory system is the range between the first cold response (vasoconstriction) and the first warm response (sweating) and is called interthreshold range. NST, nonshivering thermogenesis.

than the halothane concentration used in the pediatric study (1.0 MAC). In a separate study, Nebbia and others (1996) noted a similar thermoregulatory threshold (35.8 ± 0.3°C) in pediatric patients who were anesthetized with a caudal epidural block with bupivacaine and 1 MAC halothane in oxygen.

Thermoregulatory inhibition under general anesthesia with equipotent doses of halothane is therefore likely to affect adults and children similarly. The high surface area–to–mass ratio in infants, which allows for a rapid loss of heat to the environment, is largely offset by a high intrinsic metabolic rate. Environmental heat loss is further reduced by a well-developed thermoregulatory vasoconstriction (Bissonnette and Sessler, 1990). Although there was a trend toward increased threshold temperatures in smaller infants and children anesthetized with similar (age-corrected) concentrations of isoflurane, differences between the groups were not statistically significant and spanned only about 0.3°C. This indicates that inhibition of thermoregulatory vasoconstriction is similar in anesthetized infants and children and relatively independent of the body weight (Bissonnette and Sessler, 1990). This relatively constant degree of thermoregulatory inhibition in infants and children of different ages is in marked contrast to the age-related changes in MAC of isoflurane. In infants 1 to 6 months of age, the MAC for isoflurane is approximately 1.5 times higher than the MAC for adults. Because of the physical and physiognomic properties of infants and children, the speed of cooling is higher than in adults.

Sevoflurane was found to be similar to isoflurane in regard to decreasing the thermoregulatory threshold for vasoconstriction, although at a slower rate (Ozaki et al., 1997; Saito, 1997). Desflurane has been shown to increase the sweating threshold temperature in a concentration-dependent, linear way. The threshold temperatures for vasoconstriction and shivering at 0.8 MAC were in the same range as expected for other volatile anesthetics; however, at 0.5 MAC, the vasoconstrictive threshold was reduced less. Thus, for desflurane there may be a nonlinear concentration-response relationship (Annadata et al., 1995). Desflurane also decreases the gain of thermoregulatory vasoconstriction (Kurz et al., 1995).

Enflurane is an interesting inhalational agent with respect to thermoregulatory effects. In healthy adult volunteers anesthetized with 1.3% enflurane (equivalent to approximately 0.77 MAC), the thermoregulatory threshold for vasoconstriction was found to be 35.1 ± 0.6°C without any stimulation and 35.5 ± 0.8°C during painful electrical stimulation, demonstrating a slight, although clinically insignificant, effect of nociception in offsetting the anesthesia-induced thermoregulatory inhibition (Washington et al., 1992). Caudal or lumbar epidural blockade is useful in eliminating this effect during abdominal and peripheral surgical procedures. Thermoregulatory studies with enflurane in the pediatric population are hampered by the lack of enflurane MAC studies for this age group. In pediatric patients aged 1 to 12 years, 1.67% enflurane (equals 1 MAC in adults, which is estimated to be the equivalent of 0.75 to 1.0 MAC for the population studied) with caudal bupivacaine caused a profound depression of the thermoregulatory threshold temperature for vasoconstriction. Most patients in this study failed to achieve vasoconstriction despite reaching mean temperatures of 33.9 ± 0.9°C (Nebbia et al., 1996). These researchers therefore concluded that the risk of hypothermia is significantly higher compared with isoflurane or halothane.

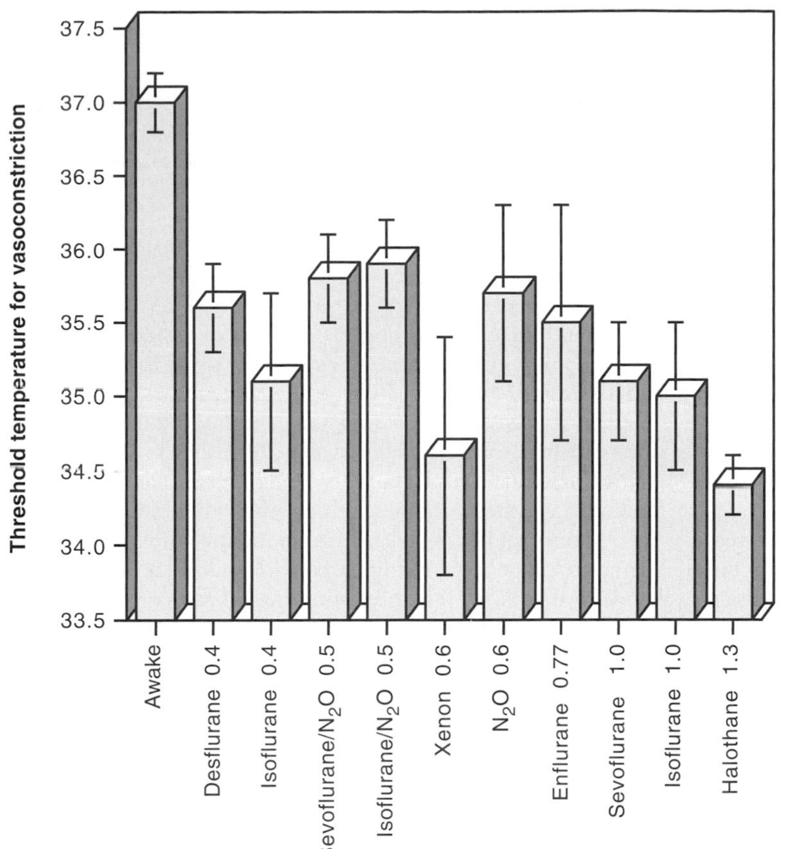

■ **FIGURE 5–5.** Threshold temperature (in °C) for thermoregulatory vasoconstriction in adults at different concentrations of inhalational anesthetics alone or in combination with nitrous oxide. The x-axis denotes the minimum alveolar concentration (MAC) equivalents of the different inhalational anesthetics. (Data compiled from Sessler and Ponte, 1982; Washington et al., 1992; Kurz et al., 1995; Ozaki et al., 1995; Annadata et al., 1995; Goto et al., 1999.)

The effects of different inhalational anesthetics on the threshold for thermoregulatory vasoconstriction are summarized in Figure 5–5. Furthermore, hypothermia can affect not only the physical characteristics of inhalational anesthetics but also the pharmacokinetics and pharmacodynamics of intravenous agents. For inhalational agents, hypothermia lowers the MAC (for isoflurane there is a linear decrease of 5.1%/°C) and increases the tissue solubility (Vitez et al., 1974; Eger and Johnson, 1987; Antognini, 1993; Antognini et al., 1994; Liu et al., 2001). Thus, for any inspired concentration of an inhalational agent in a hypothermic patient, an increased amount of the anesthetic agent is delivered to the tissues when in fact the anesthetic requirements are decreased. The pharmacokinetics of barbiturates (Kadar et al., 1982) and narcotics are also affected by hypothermia (Koren et al., 1987).

Intravenous Agents

The effect of opioids on thermoregulation remained unclear until recently. Alfentanil has been demonstrated to significantly reduce the thermoregulatory threshold temperature for vasoconstriction. This reduction appears to be linear and in proportion to the plasma drug concentration (Kurz et al., 1995). Meperidine (pethidine) and sufentanil linearly reduce the shivering threshold temperature (Alfonsi et al., 1998). This side effect can be used to treat postoperative shivering. Neither meperidine nor alfentanil reduces the gain and the maximum shivering intensity (Ikeda et al., 1998). Tramadol slightly decreases the threshold temperature for sweating, whereas the thresholds for vasoconstriction and shivering decrease linearly with the tramadol plasma concentration. Overall, with a doubling of the interthreshold range, its effects on thermoregulation can be considered mild (De Witte et al., 1998).

A comparison between the temperature effects in children anesthetized with either ketamine or halothane showed that halothane decreases rectal temperature more than ketamine and that children with the highest surface area–to–body weight ratio had the greatest decrease in body temperature regardless of the agent used (Engelman and Lockhart, 1972). In adults, ketamine causes less thermoregulatory suppression than other anesthetic agents (Hunter et al., 1981).

In the case of propofol, a small study in adult volunteers showed a significant and linear decrease in the threshold temperatures for vasoconstriction and shivering, whereas the sweating threshold temperature increased only slightly (Leslie et al., 1994; Matsukawa et al., 1995). Furthermore, the induction of anesthesia with a single bolus dose of propofol (2.5 mg/kg) in adults and maintenance of anesthesia with sevoflurane in 60% nitrous oxide resulted in lower core temperatures (35.5 ± 0.3°C) compared with patients where sevoflurane and nitrous oxide only were used for induction and maintenance of anesthesia (36.2 ± 0.2°C) (Ikeda et al., 1999). This led to the suggestion that the brief propofol-induced vasodilatation is sufficient to facilitate the core-to-peripheral redistribution of body heat resulting in nonrecoverable heat loss to the environment.

Midazolam only slightly decreases the threshold temperature for sweating, but more so for vasoconstriction with a tripling of the interthreshold range, which is quite similar to the results found for central neuraxial nerve blockade (Kurz et al., 1995).

These results contrast with the findings for volatile anesthetics, propofol or opioids, where the interthreshold range increases by a factor of 10 to 15 (Kurz et al., 1995).

A bolus dose of clonidine followed by an infusion results in a dose-independent increase in the threshold temperature for sweating, but the gain remains unchanged (Delaunay et al., 1996). Its use for premedication neither affects redistribution hypothermia nor worsens hypothermia during general anesthesia (Bernard et al., 1998). Atropine not only blocks sympathetic cholinergic-mediated sweating but also increases the threshold temperatures for sweating and therefore may lead to hyperthermia in children (Fraser, 1978).

THERMOREGULATION AND REGIONAL ANESTHESIA

During regional anesthesia, central thermoregulation remains intact and therefore provides some protection against hypothermia. Anesthetic interference with regional thermal sensation (afferent and efferent pathways) with inhibition of cutaneous vasoconstriction and shivering in the anesthetized area, internal redistribution of body heat, and increased heat loss to the environment may contribute to intraoperative hypothermia. In many aspects, the factors causing intraoperative hypothermia under neuraxial anesthesia are similar to those under general anesthesia. Like during general anesthesia, redistribution of body heat from core to peripheral compartments accounts for 89% of the initial (first hour) drop in core temperature. In the subsequent 2 hours, redistribution contributed 62% to the core temperature decrease (Matsukawa et al., 1995a, 1995b). The extent of this redistribution, and thus also the decrease in core temperature, depends on inhibition of peripheral vasoconstriction rather than on centrally mediated effects. Neuraxial anesthesia usually affects a major part of the body mass; hence, the decrease in core temperature can be quite pronounced. Heat production during regional anesthesia is only minimally decreased (Hynson et al., 1991).

In contrast to general anesthesia, patients under central neuraxial anesthesia may fail to reach an equilibrium state where heat loss and heat generation are equal, because peripheral vasoconstriction is completely inhibited by neuraxial blockade. In addition, extensive regional anesthesia may alter or even block the thermal input to the hypothalamus from a major part of the body (the information from the more active cold sensors at a normal leg skin temperature of about 33°C seems not to reach the hypothalamus, which could potentially be interpreted as relative leg warming), with the number of dermatomes blocked being directly proportional to the inhibition of central thermoregulation (Ozaki et al., 1994; Leslie and Sessler, 1996; Frank et al., 2000). Heat loss may therefore be an ongoing issue until sympathetic function and consequently vasoconstriction have been restored. Under these circumstances, hypothermia may become even more severe than under general anesthesia. Although peripheral vessels not affected by regional anesthesia are maximally vasoconstricted, a further drop in core temperature may not be prevented, because the body mass cephalad to the block is usually much smaller.

Once the patient's core temperature reaches the shivering threshold, shivering is initiated; however, neuraxial blockade reduces the gain of shivering by more than 60%, mainly due to a failure of the upper body muscles to compensate for lower body paralysis (Kim et al., 1998). It is unlikely that the thermoregulatory changes seen under regional anesthesia are influenced by systemic absorption of local anesthetics, because a study aiming to generate equal plasma drug concentrations without regional anesthesia failed to reproduce these effects (Glosten et al., 1991).

Compared with general anesthesia, the administration of a regional anesthetic technique reduces the risk of hypothermia, especially during surgery in which a small incision is made and the patient is kept well insulated. In contrast, with large surgical incisions, hypothermia can be profound and even more severe than with general anesthesia, and recovery to normal body temperature may be prolonged (Cattaneo et al., 2000).

In adults, threshold temperatures for sweating, vasoconstriction, and shivering during spinal anesthesia and epidural anesthesia seem to be comparable with a doubling of the interthreshold range (Ozaki et al., 1994). It has been demonstrated in adults that the combination of general anesthesia with epidural anesthesia further reduces the threshold temperature for thermoregulatory vasoconstriction and thus significantly aggravates hypothermia compared with general anesthesia alone (Joris et al., 1994). It is interesting that in this context, diabetic patients with autonomic neuropathy showed lower core temperatures and delayed thermoregulatory vasoconstriction during general anesthesia than diabetic patients without autonomic dysfunction (Kitamura et al., 2000).

In contrast to the thermoregulatory effects of regional anesthesia in adults, the presence of a caudal block in children anesthetized with halothane has been shown not to significantly affect the threshold temperature for vasoconstriction in children (35.7°C without versus 35.9°C with caudal block) (Bissonnette and Sessler, 1992). A survey revealed that only a third of clinicians is monitoring temperature during regional anesthesia (Frank et al., 1999). From the aforementioned, it is obvious that temperature should also be monitored in these patients, as significant hypothermia is common, which otherwise remains undetected and therefore also untreated.

ANESTHESIA AND HYPOTHERMIA

General anesthesia decreases the temperature threshold at which the body initiates a thermoregulatory response to cold stress. Mild intraoperative hypothermia (1° to 3°C below normal) is common and results from a combination of events:

1. An approximately 30% reduction in metabolic heat generation during anesthesia (Brismar, 1982)
2. Increased environmental exposure
3. Anesthetic-induced central inhibition of thermoregulation (Sessler and Ponte, 1982; Sessler, 1991)
4. Redistribution of heat within the body (Hynson et al., 1991)

Hypothermia has a typical profile during general anesthesia and usually develops in three phases (Fig. 5–6).

1. Internal redistribution of heat
2. Thermal imbalance
3. Thermal steady state (plateau or rewarming)

INTERNAL REDISTRIBUTION

To simplify the understanding of the internal redistribution concept, it is useful to divide the human body into three compartments: central, peripheral, and skin (or "shell"). The core

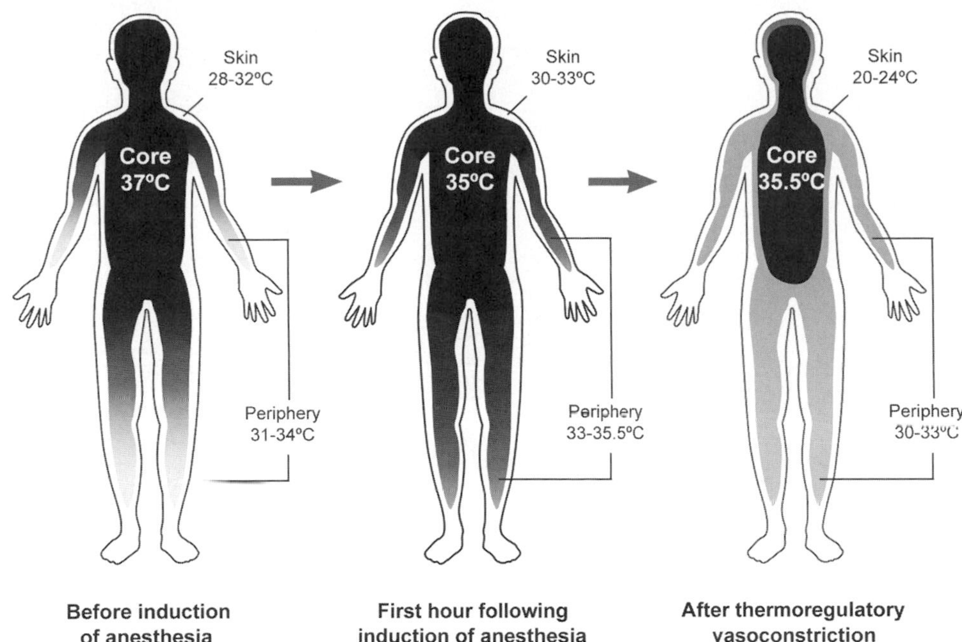

■ **FIGURE 5–6.** The body of a child demonstrating the dynamic changes within the three temperature compartments before induction of anesthesia, during the first hour of anesthesia, and after thermoregulatory vasoconstriction. In the awake human, temperature and size of the compartments are well preserved and considered normal. Following induction of anesthesia, the internal redistribution of heat results in a rapid decrease in core temperature and an increase in peripheral temperature, together resulting in enlargement of the central and shrinkage of the peripheral compartments. The drop in central temperature is mainly caused by the distribution of its heat to a larger volume and actual heat loss is minimal at this stage. Once thermoregulatory vasoconstriction has been initiated (after about 3 hours of anesthesia), the central compartment is shrinking in favor of the peripheral compartment. The raise in central temperature is now due to generated heat being contained in a smaller volume.

temperature represents the central compartment temperature. The vessel-rich group organs are part of this central compartment and represent about 10% of the body weight in adults but up to 22% in neonates, and they receive about 75% of the cardiac output. At rest, the central compartment in an awake adult accounts for approximately 66% of the body mass and extends to about 71% during general anesthesia (Deakin, 1998).

The peripheral compartment comprises the remaining part of the body mass and acts as a dynamic buffer to accommodate any changes in core temperature by vasodilatation or vasoconstriction. Its estimated buffer capacity of more than 600 kJ allows the body to maintain a constant core temperature with a minimal amount of energy spent for thermoregulation despite absorption or dissipation of significant amounts of heat.

The skin compartment (or "shell") is almost virtual and represents the barrier between the previous two compartments and the environment. After induction of anesthesia, the peripheral vasodilatation causes an increase in the size of the central compartment, forcing it to redistribute its heat within a larger volume. Furthermore, the decrease in metabolic heat production caused by anesthesia reduces the amount of energy available to compensate for the enlargement of this compartment. The concept of internal redistribution of heat therefore consists not of heat loss to the environment but of a measurable decrease in central temperature and an increase in the peripheral and skin compartment temperatures due to redistribution of heat.

With induction of anesthesia, the central core temperature starts to decrease rapidly by approximately 0.5° to 1.5°C during the first 30 to 45 minutes of anesthesia (Fig. 5–7). Although this process results in reduced core temperature, the total body heat decreases only slightly. Heat is—as the name implies—mainly redistributed and not dissipated. This redistribution of heat accounts for 81% of the core temperature decrease in the first hour of anesthesia, whereas the remainder is the result of the anesthesia-induced reduction in metabolism and increased heat loss. For the subsequent 2 hours of anesthesia, the impact of redistribution on total heat loss decreases to approximately 43% (Matsukawa et al., 1995). Accordingly, by using a vasoconstrictor such as phenylephrine, the magnitude of hypothermia caused by redistribution can be decreased (Ikeda et al., 1999).

The internal redistribution results in shrinkage of the peripheral and enlargement of the central compartment, which explains not only the decreased core temperature (the same amount of heat is now distributed to a larger volume) but also the increased temperature in the peripheral and skin compartments. This is reflected by a more than fourfold increase in the perfusion of forearms and particularly legs after induction of anesthesia, and a forearm–fingertip or calf–toe temperature gradient that may exceed 8°C (Matsukawa et al., 1995).

■ THERMAL IMBALANCE

This is the result of a combination of reduced heat production and increased heat loss to the environment. During this second phase, which lasts about 2 to 3 hours, the heat loss to the environment leads to an approximately linear decrease in mean body temperature (typically 0.5 to 1.0°C/hr). Anesthesia contributes to the decreased heat production by limiting muscular activity, reducing the metabolic rate, and eliminating the work of breathing (Stoen and Sessler, 1990; Washington et al., 1992). Heat loss to the environment is a function of the temperature difference

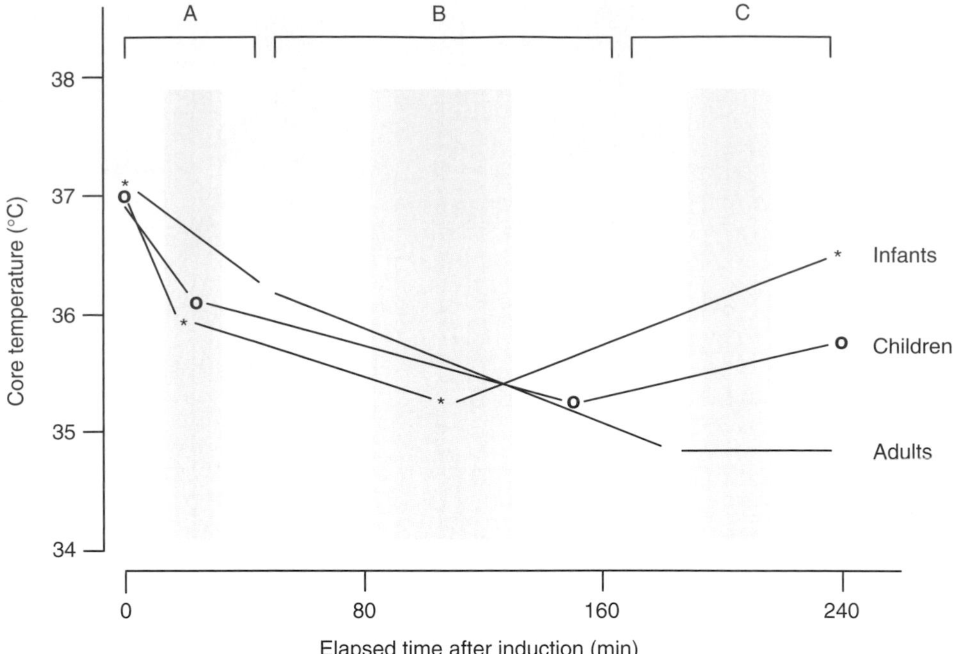

■ **FIGURE 5–7.** This graph represents the three phases typical for the course of hypothermia during general anesthesia. *A* represents the internal redistribution of heat; *B,* the phase with ongoing net loss of heat to the environment; and *C,* the thermal steady state, which in children and infants is in fact a rewarming phase. The slope of each phase varies as a function of the age group. (Modified from Bissonnette B: Thermoregulation and paediatric anaesthesia. *Curr Opin Anaesthesia* 6:537, 1993.)

between body surface and ambient structures (concept of patient warming up the environment). Heat loss, therefore, decreases passively as patients become more hypothermic. Radiation, convection, evaporation, and conduction all contribute to heat loss from the patient to the environment during anesthesia and surgery.

THERMAL STEADY STATE (PLATEAU OR REWARMING)

The third phase of the hypothermic response to anesthesia consists of a thermal steady state, where metabolic heat production equals heat dissipation to the environment and the core temperature therefore remains constant. This plateau occurs between 34.5° and 35.5°C. Thus, the patient must increase the heat production, decrease the heat loss, or both to prevent further hypothermia.

A study in adults undergoing isoflurane anesthesia showed that the effect of cutaneous vasoconstriction reduces heat loss by a maximum of 25%, which is relatively small compared with the fall in metabolic rate and the increase in evaporative heat losses from the surgical incision (Sessler et al., 1992). It is presumed that this happens because heat loss to the environment is determined principally by the capillary blood flow in large areas of the skin covering the limbs and the trunk. These capillaries cannot constrict as effectively as the arteriovenous shunts but markedly outnumber the arteriovenous shunts. Thus, it is possible that vasoconstriction contributes to the thermal plateau by reestablishing the temperature gradient between the central and the peripheral compartments and thereby preventing metabolic heat from being transported to the periphery, from where it would dissipate. The metabolic heat produced in the body core is distributed to a now smaller central compartment, allowing the temperature of this compartment to be maintained at a constant level.

To reinforce this theory of compartment size, it should be noted that the use of a limb tourniquet during surgical procedures influences the thermoregulatory response in children and adults (Bloch et al., 1992; Estebe et al., 1996). The tourniquet-induced hyperthermia is most likely due to reduction in the size of the peripheral compartment and the containment of metabolic heat within the central thermal compartment. Accordingly, the core temperature drops after deflation of the tourniquet (Estebe et al., 1996; Sanders et al., 1996; Akata et al., 1998). Despite a now constant core temperature, total body heat content is diminishing as heat loss to the environment continues.

In contrast to that in adults, the third phase in infants and children is a rewarming rather than a plateau phase (see Fig. 5–7). As mentioned earlier, general anesthesia decreases heat production by inhibiting muscular activity and nonshivering thermogenesis and by reducing metabolic rate production. Thus, the only possible explanation for this rewarming phase must be the occurrence of marked vasoconstriction within the peripheral and central compartments, leading to shrinkage of the central compartment. Thus, the amount of metabolic heat produced is distributed within a smaller central compartment volume, resulting in raised core temperature. Furthermore, this is also associated with a simultaneous increase in oxygen consumption, CO_2 production, and systemic norepinephrine levels, which have been observed in infants anesthetized with isoflurane and paralyzed with vecuronium (B. Bissonnette, unpublished data).

Infants differ from adults in that intraoperative thermoregulatory responses are sufficiently effective to significantly increase the core temperature despite constant ambient temperatures. A clinical study in children undergoing general anesthesia for surgery found a twofold increase in $\dot{V}O_2$ during mild hypothermia (Ryan, 1982). With either active or passive rewarming, significant physiologic stress is imposed on the infant. Passive surface rewarming (with the use of warm blankets, bundling, or other measures) turns off the skin cold receptors. If the normal core temperature is not reached or maintained with passive surface rewarming, hypothermia may result in hypoventilation or even apnea, relative anesthetic overdose (reduced MAC at lower temperatures), and finally metabolic acidosis (Fig. 5–8). The increased oxygen demand to

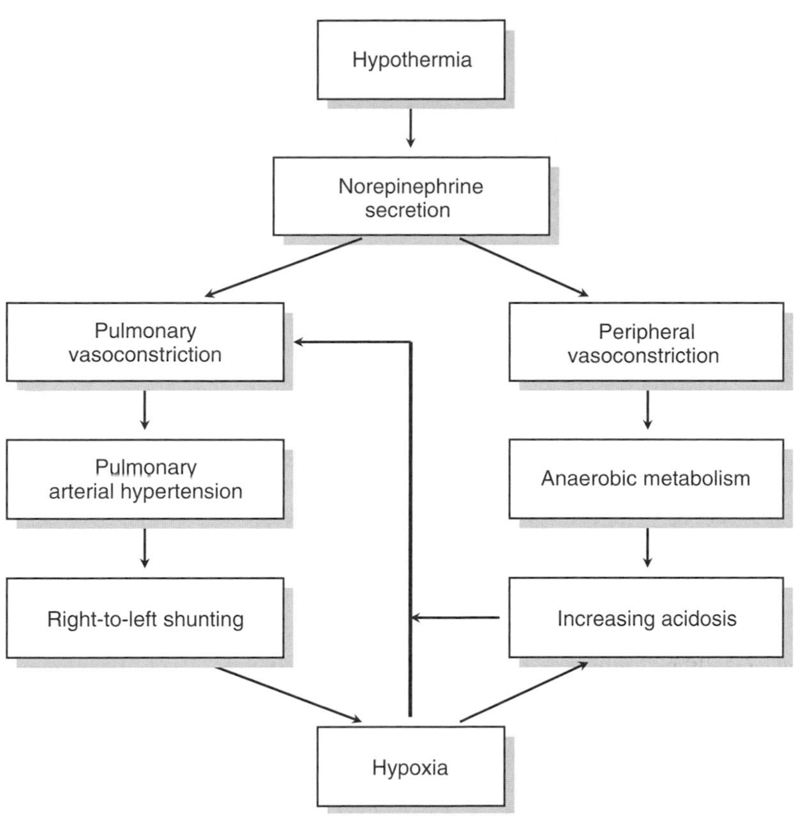

■ **FIGURE 5–8.** Vicious cycle resulting from hypothermia in neonates. (Modified from Klaus M, Faranoff A: *Care of the high-risk neonate.* Philadelphia, 1986, WB Saunders.)

maintain the normal core temperature in the anesthetized infant may create or exacerbate a preexisting cardiopulmonary insufficiency. The release of norepinephrine to trigger vasoconstriction may contribute to the development of acidosis and hypoxia, thereby increasing right-to-left pulmonary shunting. Sustained pulmonary artery hypertension and right-to-left pulmonary shunting may lead to the formation of a vicious cycle.

In adult patients, a correlation of intraoperative hypothermia with an early increase in postoperative $\dot{V}O_2$ has been demonstrated (Roe et al., 1966). In addition, this study evaluated the effects of various anesthetic agents on postoperative $\dot{V}O_2$. Although halothane anesthesia in adults was associated with the largest increase in $\dot{V}O_2$, no anesthetic agent or combination of agents in pediatric patients has been shown to clearly offer more protection from the adverse effects of hypothermia. It has been demonstrated in adults that although anesthetics can modify the thermoregulatory response to hypothermia, anesthetized patients are not poikilothermic (Sessler et al., 1987).

■ ANESTHESIA AND HYPERTHERMIA

Similar to hypothermia, hyperthermia triggers important physiologic thermoregulatory responses using threshold and gains. The threshold represents the central temperature for which a particular regulatory effector becomes active, whereas the gain quantifies the intensity of the response (see Fig. 5–4). The effector mechanisms during hyperthermia are well preserved during anesthesia when central temperature increases. Regarding controlled hyperthermia (i.e., increased central temperature), it has been demonstrated that the efferent responses seen in awake individuals were also preserved in anesthetized subjects (Lopez et al., 1993). The efferent response threshold was shifted to higher temperatures, thereby creating an expansion of the interthreshold range, which corresponds to the difference between the normal central temperature and the first efferent response triggered by the hypothalamus. In a healthy, awake person, the variability of the system (interthreshold range) is only 0.4°C. Within this range, it is said that the individual is poikilothermic; that is, the change in central temperature does not trigger any thermoregulatory effector responses. The interesting observation in regard to the interthreshold range resides in the difference between the shift observed in hypothermia and the shift in hyperthermia.

The poikilothermic range to the hypothermic side in the anesthetized patient may be expanded up to 2.5° to 3.5°C. Clinical studies in human volunteers have suggested that the threshold for active vasodilatation and sweating was only 1.0° to 1.4°C higher in anesthetized than in awake individuals (Lopez et al., 1993). This observation suggests that the human physiology responds more aggressively to the threats of hyperthermia than it does for hypothermia. Thus, the speculative explanation is that hyperthermia is far more dangerous than a comparable degree of hypothermia (Lopez et al., 1993).

The efferent responses during hyperthermic stress in anesthesia are limited to two mechanisms: active vasodilatation and sweating. The vasodilatation triggered in response to warm stress is not simply the absence of vasoconstriction but rather an active and effective vasodilatation resulting in increased dissipation of heat (Detry et al., 1972; Rübsamen and Hales, 1984). It has been demonstrated that the effect of hyperthermia on the peripheral vasculature causes a significant increase in blood flow (Tankersley et al., 1991; Matsukawa et al., 1995). The observation of active cutaneous vasodilatation in infants under anesthesia, although difficult to quantify (skin flushing), suggests that the thermoregulatory response to hyperthermia may be preserved.

Sweating represents an increase in evaporative cutaneous heat loss during episodes of heat stress. The relatively high heat of vaporization of sweat ($2.5 \cdot 10^6$ J/kg) makes sweating an extremely effective process. It allows an up to fivefold increase in heat loss to the environment, making it proportionally more effective than all of the defense mechanisms against cold combined (Fusi et al., 1989).

A study in adult volunteers showed that sweating remains functional during isoflurane anesthesia (Sessler, 1991). It has also been demonstrated that men sweat more than women. In infants and children who weigh less than 15 kg, scientific evidence suggests that sweating under anesthesia in this age group is less effective than in older children and adults (B. Bissonnette, unpublished data).

The benefits provided by induced hyperthermia may be desirable during peripheral microvascular surgery when an increase in regional blood flow is important. The physiologic relationship between maximal vasodilatation and sweating is not fully understood, and the possibility that maximal vascular dilatation may not occur until the central temperature increases even further remains possible. One of the clinical limitations of the use of induced hyperthermia in increasing cutaneous blood flow is the efficiency of the sweating mechanism. Despite active transfer of about 50 W across the patient's skin via convection and radiation (Sessler, 1993), it was possible to show that the central temperature remains relatively constant or even decreases. Although shivering can easily double the heat production, sweating can result in the dissipation of more than 10 times the amount of normal basal heat production (Guyton, 2000).

PREVENTION OF HYPOTHERMIA

Heat loss in an infant can occur for a variety of reasons. Exposure of body cavities to low environmental temperatures and humidity, infusion of cold fluids, and ventilation with cold and dry gases, in combination with the infant's physical characteristics of the large body surface area–to–volume ratio and the minimal insulating tissue layer, all increase the potential for an infant or a child to become hypothermic during anesthesia. Nevertheless, hypothermia must not be viewed as an inevitable consequence of surgery. Although hypothermia may be protective in a small subgroup of patients with certain ischemic conditions (Illievich et al., 1994), for the majority of our patients the adverse effects outweigh the benefits and inadvertent core hypothermia must be avoided.

A study in 200 adult patients scheduled for colorectal surgery showed that patients who were allowed to become hypothermic (34.7 ± 0.6°C) during the procedure showed a more than threefold higher rate of surgical wound infection than did the group who was actively warmed to keep the body normothermic (36.6 ± 0.5°C) (Kurz et al., 1996). Furthermore, the times to suture removal and discharge from hospital in the hypothermia group were prolonged by 1 and 2.6 days, respectively. It has been suggested by these and other researchers (Jonsson et al., 1991) that the vasoconstriction triggered by hypothermia may result in a decreased partial pressure of oxygen in the tissues, which leads to increased wound infection and, finally, delayed wound healing, even in the absence of an infection (Fig. 5–9). A shorter hospital stay for normothermic versus hypothermic

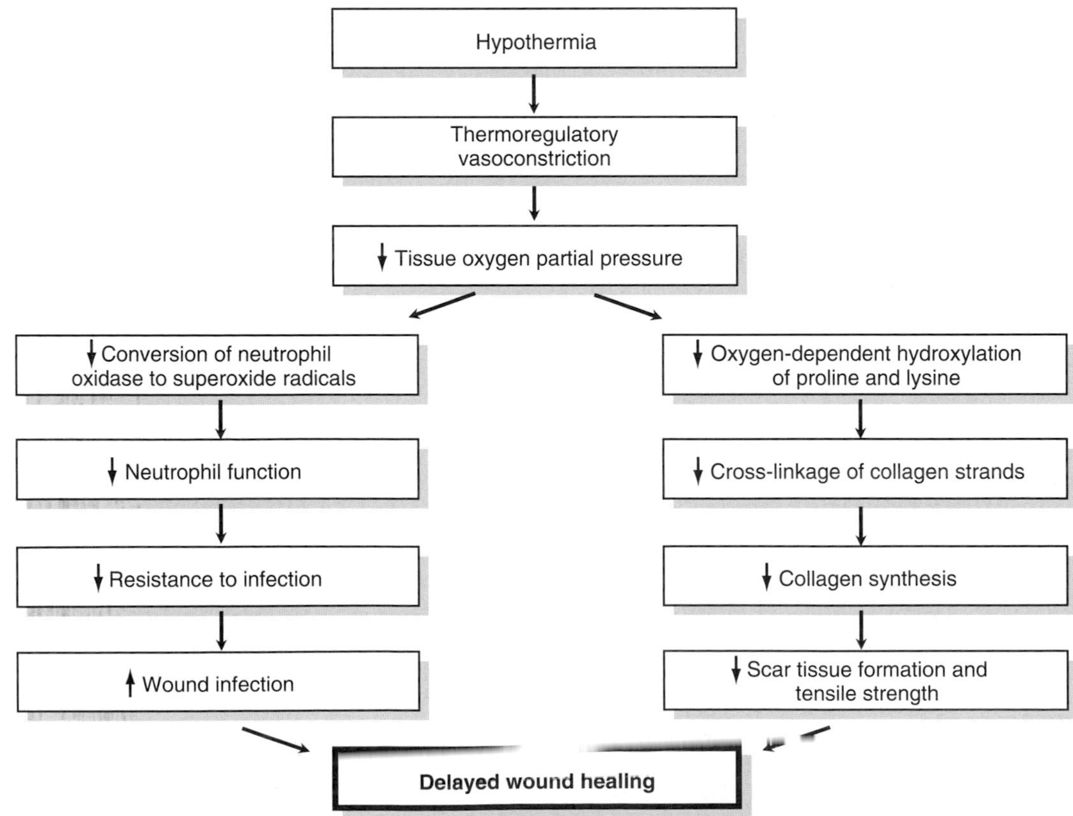

FIGURE 5–9. Hypothermia and its consequences on immune function and wound healing (↓ represents a decrease; ↑, an increase in the corresponding response).

patients has also been reported by others (Sellden and Lindahl, 1999). In addition, hypothermia per se has been shown to reduce chemotaxis and phagocytosis of granulocytes, natural killer cell cytotoxicity, migration of macrophages, and synthesis of immunoglobulins and thereby directly affect the immune response (Leijh et al., 1979; van Oss et al., 1980; Wenisch et al., 1996; Beilin et al., 1998).

Hypothermia significantly delays the reactions of the coagulation cascade (most likely due to a direct effect on the activity of the coagulation factors) with prolongation of prothrombin time and partial thromboplastin time (Rohrer and Natale, 1992). An inhibition of platelet function with prolonged bleeding time was found during hypothermia, secondary to inhibited upregulation of platelet surface protein GMP-140 and downregulation of the glycoprotein GP Ib-IX complex, reduced platelet aggregation, and thromboxane B_2 (the stable metabolite of thromboxane A_2) generation (Michelson et al., 1994). This platelet dysfunction is fully reversible with rewarming. Thromboelastography confirms these findings with a prolongation of the reaction and coagulation times as well as a reduction in the clot formation rate (Douning et al., 1995). It is therefore not surprising that blood loss in patients undergoing hip arthroplasty was found to be significantly higher in the hypothermia group (core temperature, 35 ± 0.5°C) than in the normothermia group (core temperature, 36.6 ± 0.4°C) (Schmied et al., 1996). Similar results have been confirmed by other researchers (Bock et al., 1998).

A significantly greater incidence of myocardial ischemia and PaO_2 values below 80 mm Hg has been reported in hypothermic patients (defined by sublingual temperature measured on arrival to the recovery room) compared with normothermic patients during the first 24 hours after lower extremity vascular surgery with either epidural or general anesthesia (Frank et al., 1993). Although these data are most likely not of relevance to most pediatric patients due to the absence of coronary heart disease, they nevertheless demonstrate the widespread and potential impact of hypothermia on the body in surgical patients.

Hypothermia affects drug metabolism and results in diminished metabolism and prolonged action. Although in adults intraoperative hypothermia resulted in delayed recovery from anesthesia compared with normothermic patients (Lenhardt et al., 1997), no such differences could be demonstrated in children (Bissonnette and Sessler, 1993). Studies on the effects of hypothermia and muscle relaxants have demonstrated that hypothermia decreases the requirements for nondepolarizing muscle relaxants, due to an increased sensitivity of the neuromuscular junction and to diminished biliary (indicating a reduced affinity for the drug substrate to microsomal enzymes) and renal elimination of the drug (Ham et al., 1978; Miller et al., 1978). The same has been confirmed for other medications (McAllister and Tan, 1980).

Even in the absence of similar studies for the pediatric population, there are no reasons to believe that the results would be significantly different from those in adults. Avoiding hypothermia in the infant and child is therefore crucial and requires not only an understanding of thermal physiology but also meticulous attention to detail in anesthetic care. The following recommendations are intended to help minimize intraoperative heat loss.

OPERATING ROOM TEMPERATURE

Because evaporative heat losses from the respiratory tract account for only about 5% to 10% of total heat loss during anesthesia, it is obvious that keeping the operating room temperature at an optimal level is crucial in the prevention of hypothermia. The major source of heat loss in the anesthetized patient is radiation. As mentioned previously, radiant heat loss is a function of the temperature difference between that of the patient and that of the environment. The effectiveness of controlling ambient operating room temperature in regulating the temperature of newborns during surgery has been demonstrated (Bennett et al., 1977). In adults, 21°C is reported as the critical ambient temperature for maintaining normal (36° to 37.5°C) nasopharyngeal or esophageal temperatures (Morris and Wilkey, 1970; Morris, 1971a, 1971b). Operating room temperatures of 27° and 29°C are recommended for full-term and premature newborns, respectively. It is essential that every operating room be equipped with an individual thermistor control unit so that the temperature in each operating room can be controlled individually to meet the needs of each child.

RADIANT HEATERS

Radiant heaters are used during induction of anesthesia and insertion of catheters, until the patient is prepared and draped. Prolonged use of radiant heaters may result in increased insensible water losses. Also, if radiant heaters are too close to the patient, they can cause skin burns.

REFLECTING BLANKETS

The use of reflective blankets in adults has produced conflicting results, and data on their use in infants and children are sparse. In adults, it has been reported that normothermia can be maintained with reflective blankets if 60% or more of the patient's body surface area is covered (Bourke et al., 1984). Although wrapping infants in reflective blankets to cover 60% of the body surface area may be cumbersome or impossible, we recommend that uninvolved skin areas be covered. Of particular concern in this regard is the head, which comprises up to 20% of the total skin surface area in a neonate and shows the highest regional heat flux ability (Anttonen et al., 1995). Facial cooling increases oxygen requirements by 23% in the term infant and by 36% in the premature infant (Sinclair, 1972). The practice of covering the head with a plastic bag easily and significantly reduces radiant, convective, and evaporative heat loss. Passive insulators are commonly used to prevent cutaneous heat loss. Insulating covers may be chosen on the basis of cost and convenience. Most likely, the percentage of skin surface area covered is more important than the choice of insulating material or the skin region covered (Sessler et al., 1991) (Fig. 5–10).

SKIN-WARMING DEVICES

The use of skin surface–warming devices in adults before the induction of anesthesia reduces the magnitude of the hypothermic response resulting from internal redistribution of heat (Glosten et al., 1991). Aggressive skin surface warming induces peripheral vasodilatation and favorably increases the temperature of the peripheral compartment to values approaching those of the central compartment. The net result is an increased mean body temperature, because skin surface warming reduces the amount of energy transferred from the central to the peripheral compartment after induction of anesthesia. A variety of passive

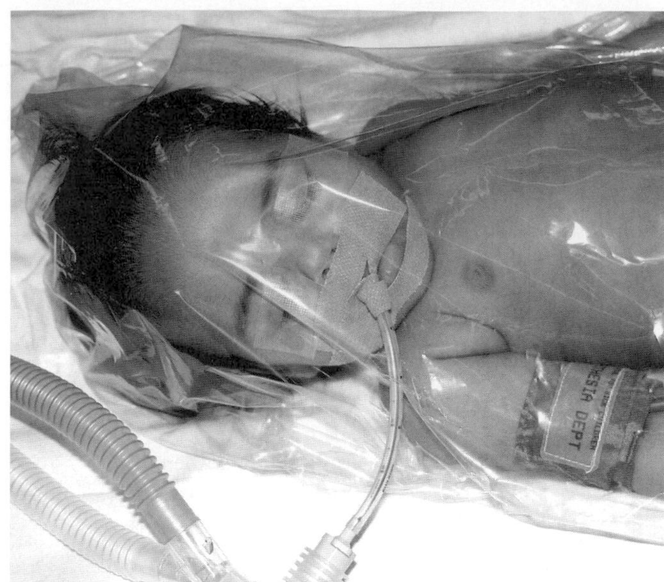

■ **FIGURE 5–10.** Because the head of an infant constitutes a large fraction of its body size, covering the infant's head and uninvolved areas of the child's body with plastic wrap can greatly affect evaporative heat loss.

and active skin surface warmers are available, including circulating hot water blankets (Stephen et al., 1960; Vale and Lunn, 1969), infrared radiant heaters (Morris, 1971; Goldblat and Miller, 1972), and convective forced-air heaters, which blow warm air through a disposable blanket to raise the effective ambient temperature immediately surrounding the patient (Sessler and Moayeri, 1990; Steele et al., 1996). A new system simulating water immersion with use of a special garment and feedback algorithms analyzed by computer to achieve a preset body temperature is available and seems to perform well and safe in children (Nesher et al., 2001). Of all these devices, convective forced-air warmers are by far the most effective. They not only can maintain a certain body temperature but also can rewarm a hypothermic patient (Sessler and Moayeri, 1990; Kurz et al., 1993; Ciufo et al., 1995; Karayan et al., 1996).

WARMING MATTRESSES

The use of warming mattresses reduces conductive heat loss. Warming mattresses set at 40°C and covered with two layers of cotton blankets have been demonstrated to effectively conserve heat (Goudsouzian et al., 1973). This measure was especially significant for infants with a surface area of less than 0.5 m^2. In older children and adults, only a small proportion of the skin surface area is in contact with the heating mattress, which makes it generally ineffective.

WARMING FLUIDS

It is well known that the rapid infusion of chilled (1° to 6°C) intravenous fluids can be used effectively to induce hypothermia. The administration of 1 L of an ice-cold infusion in an adult is expected to drop core temperature by approximately 1.7°C, but values of up to 3°C are possible (Baumgardner et al., 1999; Rajek et al., 2000). Intravenous fluids and blood products should thus be warmed before administration. It is particularly important to warm fluids in instances of rapid or massive fluid administration. In addition, attention should be paid to the length and the type of the infusion tubing, because significant heat loss of the infusate during transit from the warming device to the intravenous cannula may occur (Faries et al., 1991; Bissonnette and Paut, 2002). Although a study demonstrated that conservative fluid management (1 mL/kg per hour of crystalloids warmed to 37°C) in patients aged 1 to 3 years resulted in less core hypothermia compared with the control group that received aggressive fluid replacement (10 mL/kg per hour) (Ezri et al., 2003), this should not preclude pediatric patients from receiving appropriate fluid resuscitation.

Because both the peritoneal and thoracic cavities are large heat-exchanging areas, solutions for intraoperative lavage should always be warmed to body temperature. Although desirable from a thermoregulatory point of view, preparation solutions should not be warmed, because heat can cause a chemical breakdown of the iodine solution and thereby inactivate its antimicrobic properties.

HUMIDIFIED AND HEATED GASES

To minimize convective and evaporative heat losses via the respiratory tract, inspiratory gases should be heated and humidified. Airway humidification in intubated patients prevents tracheal damage from dry inspired gases (Chalon et al., 1979), increases tracheal mucus flow (Forbes, 1974), and minimizes respiratory heat losses (Berry et al., 1973; Tollofsrud et al., 1984). Heat and humidity can be added actively to inspired gases by evaporative or ultrasonic heated humidifiers or passively by heat and moisture exchanging filters ("artificial noses") (Newton, 1975; Chalon et al., 1984; Bissonnette et al., 1989). Furthermore, there is considerable evidence that a relative humidity of at least 50% maintains normal ciliary function in the respiratory tract and helps prevent bronchospasm (Chalon et al., 1972; Forbes, 1974; Mercke, 1975). Humidification to 50% is easily obtained with heat and moisture exchanging filters and is mandatory for long procedures. In adults, heating and humidifying of gases to 37°C and 100% relative humidity not only effectively maintains normothermia but also reverses hypothermia during general surgery (Pflug et al., 1978; Stone et al., 1981).

Because of the higher minute ventilation per kilogram of body weight in pediatric patients, airway humidification is even more effective in maintaining normothermia than in adults (Bissonnette and Sessler, 1989; Bissonnette et al., 1989). In newborns, heat loss during general anesthesia is significantly reduced when heated, humidified gases are used instead of dry anesthetic gases (Fonkalsrud et al., 1980). Although high-temperature humidification can decrease intraoperative evaporative heat loss, it may result in tracheal burns. Because there may be a large temperature gradient between the humidifier and the endotracheal tube, it is important to measure airway temperature as close to the airway as possible. This has the advantage of preventing heated gases from accidentally burning the trachea while providing the warmest possible inspiratory gas. On the other hand, it results in decreased intraoperative heat loss. If these devices are used, it is recommended to heat inspiratory gases to normal body temperature only. Although heat and moisture exchanging filters are less effective than active humidifiers (especially in the first hour after the induction of anesthesia), they seem to provide a reasonable alternative (Bissonnette et al., 1989b).

Additional advantages of the use of heat and moisture exchangers in small infants include the absent danger of airway burns and risk of overhumidification with the consequences of overhydration, and the reduced risk of breathing circuit disconnection (Smith and Allen, 1986; Shroff and Skerman, 1988). A heat-moisture exchanger falsely increases the esophageal temperature by about 0.35°C above tympanic temperature or mean body temperature (Bissonnette et al., 1989a).

The addition of an artificial nose with a dead space of approximately 1 mL introduces trivial airway resistance and can be safely used even in the smallest infants (Jones et al., 1988). Differences in the efficiency among heat and moisture exchangers are negligible (Baumgarten, 1985; Bickler and Sessler, 1990).

TRANSPORTATION

Care in the transportation of an infant cannot be overemphasized. All intraoperative efforts at maintaining intraoperative thermal stability can be lost during even a brief transport to either the post–anesthetic care room or the intensive care unit. It is therefore essential that the incubator be warmed before transport both to and from the operating room. Older infants and children should at least be covered with a warmed blanket during transport.

SUMMARY

Because of their small size with increased body surface area–to–body weight ratio and increased thermal conductance, infants and young children are at significant risk for thermal instability. This risk is even more pronounced for premature and small-for-gestational-age infants. Although unanesthetized infants are able to maintain homeothermic functions, they can do so only within a narrow range of ambient temperatures. In undergoing general anesthesia for surgery, the combination of exposure to the operating room with its usually low ambient temperature and high airflow and the use of cold infusions and dry anesthetic gases can easily overwhelm the thermal homeostatic mechanisms and, in certain instances, result in potentially serious complications. A better understanding of the physiology of the temperature-regulation system during anesthesia has improved the recognition, prevention, and management of these perioperative disturbances. The identification of the hypothermia and hyperthermia patterns in relation to the severity and the duration of the anesthetic procedure has contributed to this improvement. Furthermore, the knowledge of the different effects of each anesthetic agent on the thermoregulatory mechanism undoubtedly proves useful in providing a safe anesthesia.

REFERENCES

Adamson KJ Jr, Gandy GM, James LS: The influence of thermal factors upon oxygen consumption of the newborn human infant. *J Pediatr* 66:495, 1965.

Akata T, Kanna T, Izumi K, et al.: Changes in body temperature following deflation of limb pneumatic tourniquet. *J Clin Anesth* 10:17, 1998.

Alfonsi P, Sessler DI, Du Manoir B, et al.: The effects of meperidine and sufentanil on the shivering threshold in postoperative patients. *Anesthesiology* 89:43, 1998.

Allen JA: The thermal environment and human heat exchange. In Ernsting J, King P, editors: *Aviation medicine*. London, 1987, Butterworths, p 219.

Annadata R, Sessler DI, Tayefeh F, et al.: Desflurane slightly increases the sweating threshold but produces marked, nonlinear decreases in the vasoconstriction and shivering thresholds. *Anesthesiology* 83:1205, 1995.

Antognini JF: Hypothermia eliminates isoflurane requirements at 20 degrees C. *Anesthesiology* 78:1152, 1993.

Antognini JF, Lewis BK, Reitan JA: Hypothermia minimally decreases nitrous oxide anesthetic requirements. *Anesth Analg* 79:980, 1994.

Anttonen H, Puhakka K, Niskanen J, et al.: Cutaneous heat loss in children during anaesthesia. *Br J Anaesth* 74:306, 1995.

Baumgardner JE, Baranov D, Smith DS, et al.: The effectiveness of rapidly infused intravenous fluids for inducing moderate hypothermia in neurosurgical patients. *Anesth Analg* 89:163, 1999.

Baumgarten RK: Humidifiers are unjustified in adult anesthesia. *Anesth Analg* 64:1224, 1985.

Beilin B, Shavit Y, Razumovsky J, et al.: Effects of mild perioperative hypothermia on cellular immune responses. *Anesthesiology* 89:1133, 1998.

Bennett EJ, Patel KP, Grundy EM: Neonatal temperature and surgery. *Anesthesiology* 46:303, 1977.

Benzinger M: Tympanic thermometry in surgery and anesthesia. *JAMA* 209:1207, 1969.

Benzinger TH: Heat regulation: homeostasis of central temperature in man. *Physiol Rev* 49:671, 1969.

Bernard JM, Fulgencio JP, Delaunay L, et al.: Clonidine does not impair redistribution hypothermia after the induction of anesthesia. *Anesth Analg* 87:168, 1998.

Berry FA Jr, Hughes-Davies DI, DiFazio CA: A system for minimizing respiratory heat loss in infants during operation. *Anesth Analg* 52:170, 1973.

Bickler PE, Sessler DI: Efficiency of airway heat and moisture exchangers in anesthetized humans. *Anesth Analg* 71:415, 1990.

Bissonnette B, Holtby HM, Davis AJ, et al.: Cerebral hyperthermia in children after cardiopulmonary bypass. *Anesthesiology* 93:611, 2000.

Bissonnette B, Paut O: Active warming of saline or blood is ineffective when standard infusion tubing is used: an experimental study. *Can J Anaesth* 49:270, 2002.

Bissonnette B, Sessler DI: Mild hypothermia does not impair postanesthetic recovery in infants and children. *Anesth Analg* 76:168, 1993.

Bissonnette B, Sessler DI: Passive or active inspired gas humidification increases thermal steady-state temperatures in anesthetized infants. *Anesth Analg* 69:783, 1989.

Bissonnette B, Sessler DI: The thermoregulatory threshold in infants and children anesthetized with isoflurane and caudal bupivacaine. *Anesthesiology* 73:1114, 1990.

Bissonnette B, Sessler DI: Thermoregulatory thresholds for vasoconstriction in pediatric patients anesthetized with halothane or halothane and caudal bupivacaine. *Anesthesiology* 76:387, 1992.

Bissonnette B, Sessler DI, LaFlamme P: Intraoperative temperature monitoring sites in infants and children and the effect of inspired gas warming on esophageal temperature. *Anesth Analg* 69:192, 1989a.

Bissonnette B, Sessler DI, LaFlamme P: Passive and active inspired gas humidification in infants and children. *Anesthesiology* 71:350, 1989b.

Bloch EC, Ginsberg B, Binner RA Jr, et al.: Limb tourniquets and central temperature in anesthetized children. *Anesth Analg* 74:486, 1992.

Bock M, Muller J, Bach A, et al.: Effects of preinduction and intraoperative warming during major laparotomy. *Br J Anaesth* 80:159, 1998.

Boulant JA, Bignall KE: Hypothalamic neuronal responses to peripheral and deep-body temperatures. *Am J Physiol* 225:1371, 1973.

Boulant JA, Demieville HN: Responses of thermosensitive preoptic and septal neurons to hippocampal and brain stem stimulation. *J Neurophysiol* 40:1356, 1977.

Boulant JA, Hardy JD: The effect of spinal and skin temperatures on the firing rate and thermosensitivity of preoptic neurones. *J Physiol* 240:639, 1974.

Bourke DL, Wurm H, Rosenberg M, et al.: Intraoperative heat conservation using a reflective blanket. *Anesthesiology* 60:151, 1984.

Brismar B, Hedenstierna G, Lundh R, et al.: Oxygen uptake, plasma catecholamines and cardiac output during neurolept-nitrous oxide and halothane anaesthesias. *Acta Anaesthesiol Scand* 26:541, 1982.

Brown PJ, Dove RA, Tuffnell CS, et al.: Oscillations of body temperature at night. *Arch Dis Child* 67:1255, 1992.

Bruck K: Temperature regulation in the newborn infant. *Biol Neonate* 3:65, 1961.

Brück K: Neonatal thermal regulation. In Polin RA, Fox WW, editors: *Fetal and neonatal physiology*. Philadelphia, 1992, WB Saunders, p 493.

Bruck K, Wunnenberg B: The influence of ambient temperature in the process of replacement of non-shivering thermogenesis during postnatal development. *Fed Proc* 25:1332, 1965.

Brundin T, Wahren J: Effects of i.v. amino acids on human splanchnic and whole body oxygen consumption, blood flow, and blood temperatures. *Am J Physiol* 266:E396, 1994.

Budin P: *The nursling.* London, 1907, Caxton Publishing Co.

Burgess GE 3rd, Cooper JR, Marino RJ, et al.: Continuous monitoring of skin temperature using a liquid-crystal thermometer during anesthesia. *South Med J* 71:516, 1978.

Burton AC: Human calorimetry: The average temperature of the tissues of the body. *J Nutr* 9:261, 1935.

Cabanac M: Temperature regulation. *Annu Rev Physiol* 37:415, 1975.

Cattaneo CG, Frank SM, Hesel TW, et al.: The accuracy and precision of body temperature monitoring methods during regional and general anesthesia. *Anesth Analg* 90:938, 2000.

Chalon J, Loew DA, Malebranche J: Effects of dry anesthetic gases on tracheobronchial ciliated epithelium. *Anesthesiology* 37:338, 1972.

Chalon J, Markham JP, Ali MM, et al.: The Pall Ultipor breathing circuit filter—an efficient heat and moisture exchanger. *Anesth Analg* 63:566, 1984.

Chalon J, Patel C, Ali M, et al.: Humidity and the anesthetized patient. *Anesthesiology* 50:195, 1979.

Cheung SS, Mekjavic IB: Human temperature regulation during subanesthetic levels of nitrous oxide-induced narcosis. *J Appl Physiol* 78:2301, 1995.

Ciofolo MJ, Clergue F, Devilliers C, et al.: Changes in ventilation, oxygen uptake, and carbon dioxide output during recovery from isoflurane anesthesia. *Anesthesiology* 70:737, 1989.

Ciufo D, Dice S, Coles C: Rewarming hypothermic postanesthesia patients: a comparison between a water coil warming blanket and a forced-air warming blanket. *J Post Anesth Nurs* 10:155, 1995.

Coffman JD, Cohen AS: Total and capillary fingertip blood flow in Raynaud's phenomenon. *N Engl J Med* 285:259, 1971.

Colin J, Timbal J, Houdas Y, et al.: Computation of mean body temperature from rectal and skin temperatures. *J Appl Physiol* 31:484, 1971.

Cork RC, Vaughan RW, Humphrey LS: Precision and accuracy of intraoperative temperature monitoring. *Anesth Analg* 62:211, 1983.

Cross K, Tizard J, Trythall D: Gaseous metabolism of newborn infant breathing 15% oxygen. *Acta Paediatr* 47:217, 1958.

Dawkins MJ, Scopes JW: Non-shivering thermogenesis and brown adipose tissue in the human new-born infant. *Nature* 206:201, 1965.

De Witte JL, Kim JS, Sessler DI, et al.: Tramadol reduces the sweating, vasoconstriction, and shivering thresholds. *Anesth Analg* 87:173, 1998.

Deakin CD: Changes in core temperature compartment size on induction of general anaesthesia. *Br J Anaesth* 81:861, 1998.

Delaunay L, Herail T, Sessler DI, et al.: Clonidine increases the sweating threshold, but does not reduce the gain of sweating. *Anesth Analg* 83:844, 1996.

Detry JM, Brengelmann GL, Rowell LB, et al.: Skin and muscle components of forearm blood flow in directly heated resting man. *J Appl Physiol* 32:506, 1972.

Dickenson AH: Specific responses of rat raphe neurones to skin temperature. *J Physiol* 273:277, 1977.

Dicker A, Ohlson KB, Johnson L, et al.: Halothane selectively inhibits nonshivering thermogenesis. Possible implications for thermoregulation during anesthesia of infants. *Anesthesiology* 82:491, 1995.

Douning LK, Ramsay MA, Swygert TH, et al.: Temperature corrected thromboelastography in hypothermic patients. *Anesth Analg* 81:608, 1995.

Downey J, Mottram R, Pickering G: The location by regional cooling of central temperature receptors in the conscious rabbit. *J Physiol (Lond)* 170:415, 1964.

Downey JA, Chiodi HP, Darling RC: Central temperature regulation in the spinal man. *J Appl Physiol* 22:91, 1967.

Eger EI 2nd, Johnson BH: MAC of I-653 in rats, including a test of the effect of body temperature and anesthetic duration. *Anesth Analg* 66:974, 1987.

Engelman DR, Lockhart CH: Comparisons between temperature effects of ketamine and halothane anesthesia in children. *Anesth Analg* 51:98, 1972.

Estebe JP, Le Naoures A, Malledant Y, et al.: Use of a pneumatic tourniquet induces changes in central temperature. *Br J Anaesth* 77:786, 1996.

Ezri T, Szmuk P, Weisenberg M, et al.: The effects of hydration on core temperature in pediatric surgical patients. *Anesthesiology* 98:838, 2003.

Faries G, Johnston C, Pruitt KM, et al.: Temperature relationship to distance and flow rate of warmed i.v. fluids. *Ann Emerg Med* 20:1198, 1991.

Fonkalsrud EW, Calmes S, Barcliff LT, et al.: Reduction of operative heat loss and pulmonary secretions in neonates by use of heated and humidified anesthetic gases. *J Thorac Cardiovasc Surg* 80:718, 1980.

Forbes AR: Temperature, humidity and mucus flow in the intubated trachea. *Br J Anaesth* 46:29, 1974.

Frank SM, Beattie C, Christopherson R, et al.: Unintentional hypothermia is associated with postoperative myocardial ischemia. The Perioperative Ischemia Randomized Anesthesia Trial Study Group. *Anesthesiology* 78:468, 1993.

Frank SM, El-Rahmany HK, Cattaneo CG, et al.: Predictors of hypothermia during spinal anesthesia. *Anesthesiology* 92:1330, 2000.

Frank SM, Nguyen JM, Garcia CM, et al.: Temperature monitoring practices during regional anesthesia. *Anesth Analg* 88:373, 1999.

Fraser JG: Iatrogenic benign hyperthermia in children. *Anesthesiology* 48:375, 1978.

Fusi L, Steer PJ, Maresh MJ, et al.: Maternal pyrexia associated with the use of epidural analgesia in labour. *Lancet* 1:1250, 1989.

Gale CC: Neuroendocrine aspects of thermoregulation. *Annu Rev Physiol* 35:391, 1973.

Garruti G, Ricquier D: Analysis of uncoupling protein and its mRNA in adipose tissue deposits of adult humans. *Int J Obes Relat Metab Disord* 16:383, 1992.

Giesbrecht GG, Goheen MS, Johnston CE, et al.: Inhibition of shivering increases core temperature afterdrop and attenuates rewarming in hypothermic humans. *J Appl Physiol* 83:1630, 1997.

Giesbrecht GG, Sessler DI, Mekjavic IB, et al.: Treatment of mild immersion hypothermia by direct body-to-body contact. *J Appl Physiol* 76:2373, 1994.

Gilbert M, Busund R, Skagseth A, et al.: Resuscitation from accidental hypothermia of 13.7 degrees C with circulatory arrest. *Lancet* 355:375, 2000.

Glosten B, Sessler DI, Ostman LG, et al.: Intravenous lidocaine does not cause shivering-like tremor or alter thermoregulation. *Reg Anesth* 16:218, 1991.

Goldblat A, Miller R: Prevention of incidental hypothermia in neurosurgical patients. *Anesth Analg* 51:536, 1972.

Goto T, Matsukawa T, Sessler DI, et al.: Thermoregulatory thresholds for vasoconstriction in patients anesthetized with various 1-minimum alveolar concentration combinations of xenon, nitrous oxide, and isoflurane. *Anesthesiology* 91:626, 1999.

Goudsouzian NG, Morris RH, Ryan JF: The effects of a warming blanket on the maintenance of body temperatures in anesthetized infants and children. *Anesthesiology* 39:351, 1973.

Grant RJ, Bland E: Observations on arteriovenous anastomoses in human skin and in bird's foot with special reference to the reaction to cold. *Heart* 15:385, 1931.

Guieu JD, Hardy JD: Effects of heating and cooling of the spinal cord on preoptic unit activity. *J Appl Physiol* 29:675, 1970.

Gurtner C, Paut O, Bissonnette B: Temperature regulation: physiology and pharmacology. In Bissonnette B, Dalens B, editors: *Pediatric anesthesia. Principles and practice.* New York, 2002, McGraw-Hill, p 173.

Guyton AC: Body temperature, temperature regulation and fever. In Guyton AC, Hall JE, editors: *Textbook of medical physiology*, 10th ed. Philadelphia, 2000, WB Saunders, p 822.

Ham J, Miller RD, Benet LZ, et al.: Pharmacokinetics and pharmacodynamics of d-tubocurarine during hypothermia in the cat. *Anesthesiology* 49:324, 1978.

Hardy JD: Physiology of temperature regulation. *Physiol Rev* 41:521, 1961.

Hardy JD, Milhorat A, DuBois A: Basal metabolism and heat loss of young women at temperatures from 22 degrees C to 35 degrees C. *J Nutr* 21:38, 1941.

Hellon RF: Neurophysiology of temperature regulation: problems and perspectives. *Fed Proc* 40:2804, 1981.

Hemingway A: Shivering. *Physiol Rev* 43:397, 1963.

Hemingway A, Price WM: The autonomic nervous system and regulation of body temperature. *Anesthesiology* 29:693, 1968.

Hey EN: Physiological principles involved in the care of the pre-term human infant. In Austin CR, editor: *The mammalian fetus in vitro.* London, 1973, Chapman and Hall, p 251.

Hey EN, Katz G: Temporary loss of a metabolic response to cold stress in infants of low birthweight. *Arch Dis Child* 44:323, 1969.

Hillman PE, Scott NR, van Tienhoven A: Vasomotion in chicken foot: dual innervation of arteriovenous anastomoses. *Am J Physiol* 242: R582, 1982.

Himms-Hagen J: Cellular thermogenesis. *Annu Rev Physiol* 38:315, 1976.

Hori T, Katafuchi T: Cell biology and the functions of thermosensitive neurons in the brain. *Prog Brain Res* 115:9, 1998.

Horn EP, Schroeder F, Wilhelm S, et al.: Postoperative pain facilitates nonthermoregulatory tremor. *Anesthesiology* 91:979, 1999.

Horn EP, Sessler DI, Standl T, et al.: Non-thermoregulatory shivering in patients recovering from isoflurane or desflurane anesthesia. *Anesthesiology* 89:878, 1998.

Horrow JC, Rosenberg H: Does urinary catheter temperature reflect core temperature during cardiac surgery? *Anesthesiology* 69:986, 1988.

Horvath S, Spurr G, Hutt B, et al.: Metabolic cost of shivering. *J Appl Physiol* 8:595, 1956.

Hull D, Smales O: Heat production in the newborn. In Sinclair J, editor: *Temperature regulation and energy metabolism in the newborn.* New York, 1978, Grune & Stratton, p 129.

Hunter WS, Holmes KR, Elizondo RS: Thermal balance in ketamine-anesthetized rhesus monkey Macaca mulatta. *Am J Physiol* 241:R301, 1981.

Hynson JM, Sessler DI, Glosten B, et al.: Thermal balance and tremor patterns during epidural anesthesia. *Anesthesiology* 74:680, 1991.

Ikeda T, Kim JS, Sessler DI, et al.: Isoflurane alters shivering patterns and reduces maximum shivering intensity. *Anesthesiology* 88:866, 1998.

Ikeda T, Ozaki M, Sessler DI, et al.: Intraoperative phenylephrine infusion decreases the magnitude of redistribution hypothermia. *Anesth Analg* 89:462, 1999.

Ikeda T, Sessler DI, Kikura M, et al.: Less core hypothermia when anesthesia is induced with inhaled sevoflurane than with intravenous propofol. *Anesth Analg* 88:921, 1999.

Ikeda T, Sessler DI, Tayefeh F, et al.: Meperidine and alfentanil do not reduce the gain or maximum intensity of shivering. Anesthesiology 88:858, 1998.

Illievich UM, Zornow MH, Choi KT, et al.: Effects of hypothermia or anesthetics on hippocampal glutamate and glycine concentrations after repeated transient global cerebral ischemia. *Anesthesiology* 80:177, 1994.

Israel DJ, Pozos RS: Synchronized slow-amplitude modulations in the electromyograms of shivering muscles. *J Appl Physiol* 66:2358, 1989.

Jessen C, Feistkorn G: Some characteristics of core temperature signals in the conscious goat. *Am J Physiol* 247:R456, 1984.

Jessen C, Mayer ET: Spinal cord and hypothalamus as core sensors of temperature in the conscious dog. I. Equivalence of responses. *Pflugers Arch* 324:189, 1971.

Jessen K: An assessment of human regulatory nonshivering thermogenesis. *Acta Anaesthesiol Scand* 24:138, 1980a.

Jessen K: The cortisol fluctuations in plasma in relation to human regulatory nonshivering thermogenesis. *Acta Anaesthesiol Scand* 24:151, 1980b.

Jessen K: The relation between thyroid function and human regulatory non-shivering thermogenesis. *Acta Anaesthesiol Scand* 24:144, 1980c.

Jones B, Ozaki G, Benumof J, et al.: Airway resistance caused by a pediatric heat and moisture exchanger. *Anesthesiology* 69:A786, 1988.

Jonsson K, Jensen JA, Goodson WH 3rd, et al.: Tissue oxygenation, anemia, and perfusion in relation to wound healing in surgical patients. *Ann Surg* 214:605, 1991.

Joris J, Ozaki M, Sessler DI, et al.: Epidural anesthesia impairs both central and peripheral thermoregulatory control during general anesthesia. *Anesthesiology* 80:268, 1994.

Just B, Delva E, Camus Y, et al.: Oxygen uptake during recovery following naloxone. Relationship with intraoperative heat loss. *Anesthesiology* 76:60, 1992.

Kadar D, Tang BK, Conn AW: The fate of phenobarbitone in children in hypothermia and at normal body temperature. *Can Anaesth Soc J* 29:16, 1982.

Karayan J, Thomas D, Lacoste L, et al.: Delayed forced air warming prevents hypothermia during abdominal aortic surgery. *Br J Anaesth* 76:459, 1996.

Karlberg P, Moore R, Oliver TJ: The thermogenic response of the newborn infant to noradrenaline. *Acta Paediatr* 51:284, 1962.

Karlberg P, Moore R, Oliver TJ: Thermogenic and cardiovascular response of the newborn baby to noradrenaline. *Acta Paediatr* 54:225, 1965.

Kasai T, Nakajima Y, Matsukawa T, et al.: Effect of preoperative amino acid infusion on thermoregulatory response during spinal anaesthesia. *Br J Anaesth* 90:58, 2003.

Kim JS, Ikeda T, Sessler DI, et al.: Epidural anesthesia reduces the gain and maximum intensity of shivering. *Anesthesiology* 88:851, 1998.

Kitamura A, Hoshino T, Kon T, et al.: Patients with diabetic neuropathy are at risk of a greater intraoperative reduction in core temperature. *Anesthesiology* 92:1311, 2000.

Klaus M, Faranoff A: *Care of the high-risk neonate*. Philadelphia, 1986, WB Saunders.

Koren G, Barker C, Goresky G, et al.: The influence of hypothermia on the disposition of fentanyl—human and animal studies. *Eur J Clin Pharmacol* 32:373, 1987.

Kurz A, Go JC, Sessler DI, et al.: Alfentanil slightly increases the sweating threshold and markedly reduces the vasoconstriction and shivering thresholds. *Anesthesiology* 83:293, 1995.

Kurz A, Kurz M, Poeschl G, et al.: Forced-air warming maintains intraoperative normothermia better than circulating-water mattresses. *Anesth Analg* 77:89, 1993.

Kurz A, Sessler DI, Annadata R, et al.: Midazolam minimally impairs thermoregulatory control. *Anesth Analg* 81:393, 1995.

Kurz A, Sessler DI, Lenhardt R: Perioperative normothermia to reduce the incidence of surgical-wound infection and shorten hospitalization. Study of Wound Infection and Temperature Group. *N Engl J Med* 334:1209, 1996.

Kurz A, Sessler DI, Narzt E, et al.: Morphometric influences on intraoperative core temperature changes. *Anesth Analg* 80:562, 1995.

Kurz A, Xiong J, Sessler DI, et al.: Desflurane reduces the gain of thermoregulatory arteriovenous shunt vasoconstriction in humans. *Anesthesiology* 83:1212, 1995.

Lacoumenta S, Hall GM: Liquid crystal thermometry during anaesthesia. *Anaesthesia* 39:54, 1984.

Lean ME, James WP, Jennings G, et al.: Brown adipose tissue in patients with phaeochromocytoma. *Int J Obes* 10:219, 1986.

Leijh PC, van den Barselaar MT, van Zwet TL, et al.: Kinetics of phagocytosis of Staphylococcus aureus and Escherichia coli by human granulocytes. *Immunology* 37:453, 1979.

Lenhardt R, Greif R, Sessler DI, et al.: Relative contribution of skin and core temperatures to vasoconstriction and shivering thresholds during isoflurane anesthesia. *Anesthesiology* 91:422, 1999.

Lenhardt R, Marker E, Goll V, et al.: Mild intraoperative hypothermia prolongs postanesthetic recovery. *Anesthesiology* 87:1318, 1997.

Leon JE, Bissonnette B, Lerman J: Liquid crystalline temperature monitoring: does it estimate core temperature in anaesthetized paediatric patients? *Can J Anaesth* 37: S98, 1990.

Leslie K, Sessler DI: Reduction in the shivering threshold is proportional to spinal block height. *Anesthesiology* 84:1327, 1996.

Leslie K, Sessler DI, Bjorksten AR, et al.: Propofol causes a dose-dependent decrease in the thermoregulatory threshold for vasoconstriction but has little effect on sweating. *Anesthesiology* 81:353, 1994.

Liu M, Hu X, Liu J: The effect of hypothermia on isoflurane MAC in children. *Anesthesiology* 94:429, 2001.

Lopez M, Ozaki M, Sessler DI, et al.: Physiologic responses to hyperthermia during epidural anesthesia and combined epidural/enflurane anesthesia in women. *Anesthesiology* 78:1046, 1993.

Lyons B, Taylor A, Power C, et al.: Postanaesthetic shivering in children. *Anaesthesia* 51:442, 1996.

MacKenzie R, Asbury AJ: Clinical evaluation of liquid crystal skin thermometers. *Br J Anaesth* 72:246, 1994.

Mahajan RP, Grover VK, Sharma SL, et al.: Intraocular pressure changes during muscular hyperactivity after general anesthesia. *Anesthesiology* 66:419, 1987.

Matsukawa T, Kurz A, Sessler DI, et al.: Propofol linearly reduces the vasoconstriction and shivering thresholds. *Anesthesiology* 82:1169, 1995.

Matsukawa T, Sessler DI, Christensen R, et al.: Heat flow and distribution during epidural anesthesia. *Anesthesiology* 83:961, 1995.

Matsukawa T, Sessler DI, Sessler AM, et al.: Heat flow and distribution during induction of general anesthesia. *Anesthesiology* 82:662, 1995.

McAllister RG Jr, Tan TG: Effect of hypothermia on drug metabolism. In vitro studies with propranolol and verapamil. *Pharmacology* 20:95, 1980.

Mercer JB, Jessen C: Central thermosensitivity in conscious goats: hypothalamus and spinal cord versus residual inner body. *Pflugers Arch* 374:179, 1978.

Mercke U: The influence of varying air humidity on mucociliary activity. *Acta Otolaryngol* 79:133, 1975.

Mestyan J, Jarai I, Bata G, et al.: The significance of facial skin temperature in the chemical heat regulation of premature infants. *Biol Neonat* 7:243, 1964.

Michelson AD, MacGregor H, Barnard MR, et al.: Reversible inhibition of human platelet activation by hypothermia in vivo and in vitro. *Thromb Haemost* 71:633, 1994.

Miller RD, Agoston S, van der Pol F, et al.: Hypothermia and the pharmacokinetics and pharmacodynamics of pancuronium in the cat. *J Pharmacol Exp Ther* 207:532, 1978.

Morris RH: Influence of ambient temperature on patient temperature during intraabdominal surgery. *Ann Surg* 173:230, 1971a.

Morris RH: Operating room temperature and the anesthetized, paralyzed patient. *Arch Surg* 102:95, 1971b.

Morris RH, Wilkey BR: The effects of ambient temperature on patient temperature during surgery not involving body cavities. *Anesthesiology* 32:102, 1970.

Muma BK, Treloar DJ, Wurmlinger K, et al.: Comparison of rectal, axillary, and tympanic membrane temperatures in infants and young children. *Ann Emerg Med* 20:41, 1991.

Nebbia SP, Bissonnette B, Sessler DI: Enflurane decreases the threshold for vasoconstriction more than isoflurane or halothane. *Anesth Analg* 83:595, 1996.

Nesher N, Wolf T, Uretzky G, et al.: A novel thermoregulatory system maintains perioperative normothermia in children undergoing elective surgery. *Paediatr Anaesth* 11:555, 2001.

Newton DE: Proceedings: The effect of anaesthetic gas humidification on body temperature. *Br J Anaesth* 47:1026, 1975.

Ohlson KB, Lindahl SG, Cannon B, et al.: Analysis of the cellular mechanism for halothane inhibition of brown adipose tissue thermogenesis. *Ann N Y Acad Sci* 813:718, 1997.

Ohlson KB, Mohell N, Cannon B, et al.: Thermogenesis in brown adipocytes is inhibited by volatile anesthetic agents. A factor contributing to hypothermia in infants? *Anesthesiology* 81:176, 1994.

Oya A, Asakura H, Koshino T, et al.: Thermographic demonstration of non-shivering thermogenesis in human newborns after birth: its relation to umbilical gases. *J Perinat Med* 25:447, 1997.

Ozaki M, Kurz A, Sessler DI, et al.: Thermoregulatory thresholds during epidural and spinal anesthesia. *Anesthesiology* 81:282, 1994.

Ozaki M, Sessler DI, Suzuki H, et al.: Nitrous oxide decreases the threshold for vasoconstriction less than sevoflurane or isoflurane. *Anesth Analg* 80:1212, 1995.

Ozaki M, Sessler DI, Suzuki H, et al.: The threshold for thermoregulatory vasoconstriction during nitrous oxide/sevoflurane anesthesia is lower in elderly than in young patients. *Ann N Y Acad Sci* 813:789, 1997.

Petrikovsky B, Silverstein M, Schneider EP: Neonatal shivering and hypothermia after intrapartum amnioinfusion. *Lancet* 350:1366, 1997.

Pflug AE, Aasheim GM, Foster C, et al.: Prevention of post-anaesthesia shivering. *Can Anaesth Soc J* 25:43, 1978.

Pickering G: Regulation of body temperature in health and disease. *Lancet* 1:59, 1958.

Pierau FK, Wurster RD: Primary afferent input from cutaneous thermoreceptors. *Fed Proc* 40:2819, 1981.

Plattner O, Semsroth M, Sessler DI, et al.: Lack of nonshivering thermogenesis in infants anesthetized with fentanyl and propofol. *Anesthesiology* 86:772, 1997.

Poulos DA: Central processing of cutaneous temperature information. *Fed Proc* 40:2825, 1981.

Puhakka K, Anttonen H, Niskanen J, et al.: Calculation of mean skin temperature and changes in body heat content during paediatric anaesthesia. *Br J Anaesth* 72:548, 1994.

Rajek A, Greif R, Sessler DI, et al.: Core cooling by central venous infusion of ice-cold (4 degrees C and 20 degrees C) fluid: isolation of core and peripheral thermal compartments. *Anesthesiology* 93:629, 2000.

Ramanathan NL: A new weighting system for mean surface temperature of the human body. *J Appl Physiol* 19:531, 1964.

Roe CF: Effect of bowel exposure on body temperature during surgical operations. *Am J Surg* 122:13, 1971.

Roe CF, Santulli TV, Blair CS: Heat loss in infants during general anesthesia and operations. *J Pediatr Surg* 1:266, 1966.

Rohrer MJ, Natale AM: Effect of hypothermia on the coagulation cascade. *Crit Care Med* 20:1402, 1992.

Rosa G, Pinto G, Orsi P, et al.: Control of post anaesthetic shivering with nefopam hydrochloride in mildly hypothermic patients after neurosurgery. *Acta Anaesthesiol Scand* 39:90, 1995.

Rübsamen K, Hales JR: Role of arteriovenous anastomoses in determining heat transfer across the hindleg skin of sheep. In Hales JR, editor: *Thermal physiology.* New York, 1984, Raven Press, p 259.

Ryan JF: Altered temperature regulation section two: unintentional hypothermia. In Cooperman L, Orkin F, editors: *Complications in anesthesiology.* Philadelphia, 1982, JB Lippincott, p 284.

Saito T: A comparison of the body temperature during sevoflurane anesthesia and isoflurane anesthesia. *Ann N Y Acad Sci* 813:786, 1997.

Sanders BJ, D'Alessio JG, Jernigan JR: Intraoperative hypothermia associated with lower extremity tourniquet deflation. *J Clin Anesth* 8:504, 1996.

Schiff D, Stern L, Ledue J: Chemical thermogenesis in newborn infants. Catecholamine excretion and the plasma non-esterified fatty acid-response to cold exposure. *Pediatrics* 37:577, 1966.

Schmied H, Kurz A, Sessler DI, et al.: Mild hypothermia increases blood loss and transfusion requirements during total hip arthroplasty. *Lancet* 347:289, 1996.

Sellden E, Brundin T, Wahren J: Augmented thermic effect of amino acids under general anaesthesia: a mechanism useful for prevention of anaesthesia-induced hypothermia. *Clin Sci (Lond)* 86:611, 1994.

Sellden E, Lindahl SG: Amino acid-induced thermogenesis reduces hypothermia during anesthesia and shortens hospital stay. *Anesth Analg* 89:1551, 1999.

Sessler DI: Central thermoregulatory inhibition by general anesthesia. *Anesthesiology* 75:557, 1991.

Sessler DI: Malignant hyperthermia. *J Pediatr* 109:9, 1986.

Sessler DI: Perianesthetic thermoregulation and heat balance in humans. *FASEB J* 7:638, 1993.

Sessler DI: Sweating threshold during isoflurane anesthesia in humans. *Anesth Analg* 73:300, 1991.

Sessler DI, McGuire J, Hynson J, et al.: Thermoregulatory vasoconstriction during isoflurane anesthesia minimally decreases cutaneous heat loss. *Anesthesiology* 76:670, 1992.

Sessler DI, McGuire J, Moayeri A, et al.: Isoflurane-induced vasodilation minimally increases cutaneous heat loss. *Anesthesiology* 74:226, 1991.

Sessler DI, McGuire J, Sessler AM: Perioperative thermal insulation. *Anesthesiology* 74:875, 1991.

Sessler DI, Moayeri A: Skin-surface warming: heat flux and central temperature. *Anesthesiology* 73:218, 1990.

Sessler DI, Olofsson CI, Rubinstein EH, et al.: The thermoregulatory threshold in humans during halothane anesthesia. *Anesthesiology* 68:836, 1988a.

Sessler DI, Olofsson CI, Rubinstein EH: The thermoregulatory threshold in humans during nitrous oxide-fentanyl anesthesia. *Anesthesiology* 69:357, 1988b.

Sessler DI, Ponte J: Disparity between thermal comfort and psychological thermoregulatory responses during epidural anesthesia. *Anesthesiology* 71:A682, 1982.

Sessler DI, Rubinstein EH, Eger EI 2nd: Core temperature changes during N_2O fentanyl and halothane/O_2 anesthesia. *Anesthesiology* 67:137, 1987.

Sessler DI, Rubinstein EH, Moayeri A: Physiologic responses to mild perianesthetic hypothermia in humans. *Anesthesiology* 75:594, 1991.

Shanks CA: Heat balance during surgery involving body cavities. *Anaesth Intensive Care* 3:114, 1975.

Shanks CA: Mean skin temperature during anaesthesia: an assessment of formulae in the supine surgical patient. *Br J Anaesth* 47:871, 1975.

Shroff PK, Skerman JH: Humidifier malfunction—a cause of anesthesia circuit occlusion. *Anesth Analg* 67:710, 1988.

Silverman W, Blanc W: Effects of humidity on survival of newly born premature infants. *Pediatrics* 22:876, 1957.

Silverman W, Fertig J, Bergen A: Influence of thermal environent upon survival of newly born premature infants. *Pediatrics 22*:876, 1958.

Silverman W, Zamelis A, Sinclair J, et al.: Warm nape of the newborn. *Pediatrics* 33:984, 1964.

Simon E: Temperature regulation: the spinal cord as a site of extrahypothalamic thermoregulatory functions. *Rev Physiol Biochem Pharmacol* 1, 1974.

Sinclair JC: Thermal control in premature infants. *Annu Rev Med* 23:129, 1972.

Sinclair JG: The effects of meperidine and morphine in rabbits pretreated with phenelzine. *Toxicol Appl Pharmacol* 22:231, 1972.

Smith HS, Allen R: Another hazard of heated water humidifiers. *Anaesthesia* 41:215, 1986.

Steele MT, Nelson MJ, Sessler DI, et al.: Forced air speeds rewarming in accidental hypothermia. *Ann Emerg Med* 27:479, 1996.

Stephen CR, Dent S, Hall K: Body temperature regulation during anesthesia in infants and children. *JAMA* 174:1579, 1960.

Stern L, Lees MH, Leduc J: Environmental temperature, oxygen consumption, and catecholamine excretion in newborn infants. *Pediatrics* 36:367, 1965.

Stoen R, Sessler DI: The thermoregulatory threshold is inversely proportional to isoflurane concentration. *Anesthesiology* 72:822, 1990.

Stone DR, Downs JB, Paul WL, et al.: Adult body temperature and heated humidification of anesthetic gases during general anesthesia. *Anesth Analg* 60:736, 1981.

Stuart D, Ott K, Ishikawa K, et al.: The rhythm of shivering. 3. Central contributions. *Am J Phys Med* 45:91, 1966.

Sulyok E, Jequier E, Prod'hom LS: Thermal balance of the newborn infant in a heat-gaining environment. *Pediatr Res* 7:888, 1973.

Swyer P: Heat loss after birth. In Sinclair JC, editor: *Temperature regulation and energy metabolism in the newborn.* New York, 1973, Grune & Stratton, p 91.

Szmuk P, Rabb MF, Baumgartner JE, et al.: Body morphology and the speed of cutaneous rewarming. *Anesthesiology* 95:18, 2001.

Tankersley CG, Smolander J, Kenney WL, et al.: Sweating and skin blood flow during exercise: effects of age and maximal oxygen uptake. *J Appl Physiol* 71:236, 1991.

Tollofsrud SG, Gundersen Y, Andersen R: Peroperative hypothermia. *Acta Anaesthesiol Scand* 28:511, 1984.

Vale RJ, Lunn HF: Heat balance in anaesthetized surgical patients. *Proc R Soc Med* 62:1017, 1969.

van Marken Lichtenbelt WD, Daanen HA: Cold-induced metabolism. *Curr Opin Clin Nutr Metab Care* 6:469, 2003.

van Oss CJ, Absolom DR, Moore LL, et al.: Effect of temperature on the chemotaxis, phagocytic engulfment, digestion and O_2 consumption of human polymorphonuclear leukocytes. *J Reticuloendothel Soc* 27:561, 1980.

Vitez TS, White PF, Eger EI 2nd: Effects of hypothermia on halothane MAC and isoflurane MAC in the rat. *Anesthesiology* 41:80, 1974.

Vybiral S, Lesna I, Jansky L, et al.: Thermoregulation in winter swimmers and physiological significance of human catecholamine thermogenesis. *Exp Physiol* 85:321, 2000.

Washington DE, Sessler DI, McGuire J, et al.: Painful stimulation minimally increases the thermoregulatory threshold for vasoconstriction during enflurane anesthesia in humans. *Anesthesiology* 77:286, 1992.

Wenisch C, Narzt E, Sessler DI, et al.: Mild intraoperative hypothermia reduces production of reactive oxygen intermediates by polymorphonuclear leukocytes. *Anesth Analg* 82:810, 1996.

Wyss CR, Brengelmann GL, Johnson JM, et al.: Altered control of skin blood flow at high skin and core temperatures. *J Appl Physiol* 38:839, 1975.

Xiong J, Kurz A, Sessler DI, et al.: Isoflurane produces marked and nonlinear decreases in the vasoconstriction and shivering thresholds. *Anesthesiology* 85:240, 1996.

6 Pharmacology of Pediatric Anesthesia

Peter J. Davis • Jerrold Lerman • Stevan P. Tofovic • D. Ryan Cook

DEVELOPMENTAL PHARMACOLOGY

Pharmacokinetics and pharmacodynamics in the pediatric population are significantly different from those in adults. As recognized by Dr. Abraham Jacobi more than a century ago, children should not be regarded as "little adults." He wrote that, "Pediatrics does not deal with miniature men and women, with reduced doses and the same class of disease in smaller bodies" but rather "has its own independent range and horizon" (Kearns et al., 2003; Halpern, 1988). The physical growth and major physiologic changes that occur during the child's maturation (i.e., from preterm newborn to adolescence) may substantially affect drug disposition (Table 6–1). However, the pharmacologic maturation and rapid changes in factors that govern the drug absorption, distribution, redistribution, metabolism, and excretion occur mainly during the first 12 months of life. The factors that influence different phases of drug disposition, their differences in various pediatric age groups, and basic pharmacokinetic concepts for intravenously administered drugs important for pediatric anesthesia are presented in this chapter.

TABLE 6–1. Changes in organ weights with age (percentage of body weight)

Organ System	Fetus	Full-Term Newborn	Adult
Skeletal muscle	25.0	25.0	40.0
Skin	13.0	4.0	6.0
Skeleton	22.0	18.0	14.0
Heart	0.6	0.5	0.4
Liver	4.0	5.0	2.0
Kidneys	0.7	1.0	0.5
Brain	13.0	12.0	2.0

Reproduced with permission from Widdowson EM: *Scientific foundations of paediatrics*, ed 2. Baltimore, 1982, University Park Press.

Distribution of drugs is the process by which a drug leaves the bloodstream and enters the extracellular fluids (ECFs) and tissues. The rate and extent of distribution of a drug are determined by body composition, permeability of tissue membranes for drugs, cardiac output and regional blood flow, and relative distribution of the drug between tissue and blood. The latter is dependent on the binding of the drug in blood and tissues, the lipid solubility of the drug, and, for ionizable drugs, the pK_a and the pH of the environment.

Body composition (i.e., body water and fat content) undergoes dramatic changes during the maturation process (Table 6–2). Because drug distribution between ECF and fat tissue depends on its lipid–water partition coefficient, the changes in body composition affect drug disposition in the pediatric population. The fetus has high total body water, which at birth accounts for about 75% of the body weight in the full-term newborn infant and 80% in the preterm newborn. The total body water decreases during the first year of life to about 60% of body

TABLE 6–2. Body composition during growth

Body Compartment	Premature Infant (1.5 kg)	Full-Term Infant (3.5 kg)	Adult (70 kg)
Total body water (% body weight)	83	73	60
Extracellular fluid (% body weight)	62	44	20
Blood volume (mL/kg)	60	85-105	70
Intracellular water (% body weight)	25	33	40
Muscle mass (% body weight)	15	20	50
Fat (% body weight)	3	12	18

From Cook DR, Marcy JH: Neonatal anesthesia. Pasadena, CA, 1988, Appleton Davies.

weight and remains at that level until puberty (Friis-Hansen, 1961). Importantly, there is a dramatic shift in ECF content versus intracellular fluid (ICF) content during the first year of life. The newborn infants have a much higher ECF volume, which in premature infants constitutes 50%, and in full-term, 45%, of body weight. The postnatal diuresis induces an immediate decrease in ECF volume and by 1 year of age, the ratio of ECF volume (20% to 25%) to ICF volume (35% to 40%) approaches adult levels. In contrast to water content, the fat content gradually increases with maturation, from 3% in premature infants and 12% in full-term newborns, to 30% at 1 year of age and about 18% in the average adult. These changes result in a relatively higher volume of distribution of water-soluble drugs and a relatively smaller volume of distribution of liposoluble drugs in neonates and infants. The volume of distribution of water-soluble gentamicin is 0.5 to 1.2 L/kg in neonates and infants compared with 0.2 to 0.3 L/kg in adults (Echeverria et al., 1975), and in neonates the volume of distribution of sulfisoxazole is twice as large as that in adults (Morselli, 1976). Also, the volume of distribution of liposoluble drugs such as diazepam and flunitrazepam has been reported to be smaller in infants than in adults (Treluyer et al., 1997). Table 6–3 gives developmental estimates of gas and tissue volumes and tissue blood flow derived from physiologic studies and autopsies of normal tissue (Altman and Dittmer, 1971; Widdowson, 1974; Guignard et al., 1975; Smith and Nelson, 1976).

The *membrane permeability* changes during the maturation period. It is particularly high in immature neonates, and the penetration of drugs into the central nervous system (CNS) should be considered in preterm infants. In full-term infants, the myelinization (which counteracts drug passage) continues, and due to the immature blood–brain barrier, the distribution of drugs into the CNS should be expected. In infants, administration of first-generation histamine type 1 receptor (H_1) antagonists was reported to be associated with marked central adverse effects, suggesting significant CNS distribution of these lipophilic drugs (Yokoyoma et al., 1993; Simons et al., 1996). The CNS permeability decreases as a function of age, as evidenced by decreased brain/plasma ratio of anticonvulsant agents in infants compared with that in neonates (Benedetti and Baltes, 2003).

Plasma protein binding is another factor that determines drug distribution and elimination. Pharmacologic response may also be altered, because it is the free (unbound) fraction of drug that is available at the site of action (receptor) and is pharmacologically active. In general, acidic drugs mainly bind to albumin, whereas basic drugs bind to α_1-acid glycoprotein and, to a lesser extent, to globulins and lipoproteins. The clinical pharmacokinetic profile of weak acid drugs that significantly (>90%) bind to albumin may be affected by changes in binding affinity/capacity and the amount of circulating albumin. In neonates, the reduced amount of total plasma protein (including the albumin), the presence of fetal albumin that has reduced binding affinity for weak acids, and the increased concentrations of endogenous substances (i.e., bilirubin and free fatty acids) that reduce binding capacity of albumin may contribute to a higher free-unbound fraction of highly protein-bound drugs (phenytoin, valproic acid, salicylates) (Ehrnebo et al., 1971; Kurz et al., 1977; Wallace, 1977).

Basic drugs, including propranolol, lidocaine, imipramine, and carbamazepine, bind with high affinity to α_1-acid glycoprotein. The plasma levels of this high-affinity, low-capacity globulin range from 40 to 100 mg/L, and because plasma levels are relatively low, it may be saturated over the therapeutic plasma concentration range of the binding drug. This protein behaves as an acute-phase reactant, and plasma levels of α_1-acid glycoprotein are increased during acute myocardial infarction, burns, cancer, inflammatory disease, surgery, and trauma. This increase in protein level may lead to increased binding of basic drugs. In contrast, severe liver disease, including cirrhosis and nephrotic syndrome, leads to decreased plasma levels of α_1-acid glycoprotein and increased free-unbound fraction of basic drugs. The concentrations of α_1-acid glycoprotein are low at birth but reach adult levels over the first year of life. It has been reported that the free-unbound (i.e., pharmacologically active) fraction of sufentanil decreases with age (i.e., 20% in neonates, 12% in infants, and 8% in children and adults). It seems that the lower α_1-acid glycoprotein levels in neonates and infants are responsible for the decrease in protein binding of sufentanil in these age groups compared with adults (Meistelman et al., 1990).

TABLE 6–3. Age-related estimates of gas and tissue volumes and blood flow

	GAS AND TISSUE VOLUME (mL/kg)		TISSUE BLOOD FLOW (% CO)	
Tissue Volume	*Adult*	*Infant*	*Adult*	*Infant*
Tidal volume (V_T)	7	7	—	—
Functional residual capacity (FRC)	40	25	—	—
Blood volume	70	90	—	—
Brain	21	90	14.3	34
Heart	4	4.5	4.3	3
Abdominal viscera	57	70	28.6	25
Kidney	6	10	25.7	18
Muscle	425	180	11.4	10
Fat	150	100	5.7	5
Poorly perfused tissue	270	270	10.0	5

From Cook DR, Marcy JH: Neonatal anesthesia. Pasadena, CA, 1988, Appleton Davies.

PHARMACOKINETIC PARAMETERS

Volume of distribution is one of the basic pharmacokinetic parameters, and it describes disposition of the drug in the body. It is defined as a space in the body where the drug is uniformly distributed. It is an important pharmacokinetic parameter that relates the amount of the drug in the body (A_B) to the concentration of drug in plasma (C_p) or other measured fluid:

$$V_d = A_B / C_p \tag{6.1}$$

This volume does not necessarily correlate with any anatomic space or physiologic volume in the body. It is defined as a fluid of volume that would be required to contain all of the drug in the body at the same C_p as the measured one. This theoretical or fictitious space is also called the *apparent* volume of distribution. Tissue binding increases the volume of distribution, whereas binding to plasma proteins reduces the volume of distribution (Fig. 6–1). Water-soluble drugs have a relatively smaller volume of distribution, whereas lipophilic drugs have a larger volume of distribution. A volume of distribution greater than the total body water volume (>40 L) suggests extensive tissue binding of drug. For example, due to high binding for myocardial Na^+,K^+-ATPase, digoxin concentrations in the adult heart are 50 times higher than concentrations in plasma, and volume of distribution in adults is up to 700 L (6 to 10 L/kg). In the pediatric

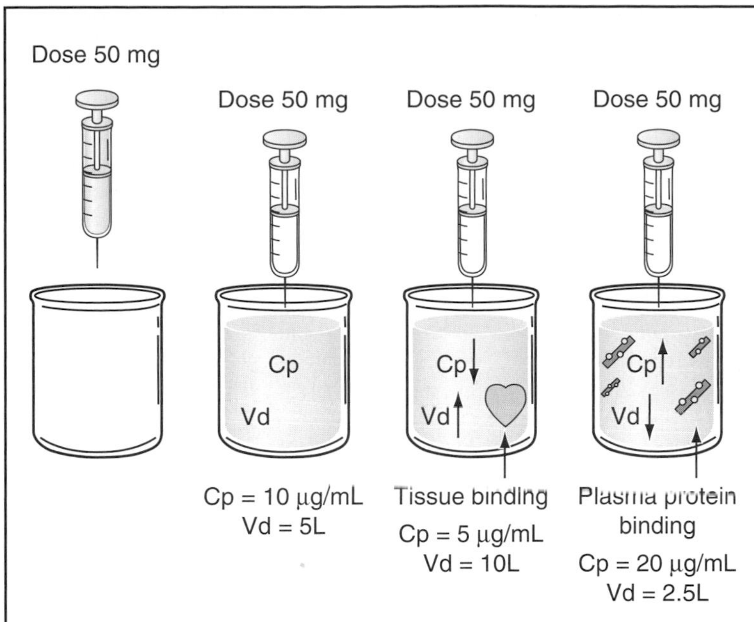

■ **FIGURE 6–1.** Apparent volume of distribution. The real volume of the beaker is 5 L (V_d = 50 mg/10 mcg/mL = 5 L). However, based on measured concentrations in fluid, and calculated according Eq. 1, the volume of distribution (V_d) may vary (i.e., apparent volume). It depends on significant tissue or plasma protein binding. Significant tissue binding (i.e., significant digoxin binding to myocardial Na^+,K^+-ATPase) increases V_d (V_d = 10 L; see the text for explanation). Because routinely measured fluid concentration includes both free-unbound and plasma protein bound drug, the increased protein binding reduces V_d (V_d = 2.5 L).

population there is an even greater binding affinity for myocardial Na^+,K^+-ATPase, and neonates (10 L/kg) and infants and toddlers (16 L/kg) have a larger volume of distribution digoxin than do adults.

This fictitious volume helps clinicians to estimate the loading dose of a drug that would be required to achieve a desired C_p. For drugs administered intravenously, the loading dose (L_D or A_B from Eq. 6.1) would depend on volume of distribution:

$$L_D = V_d \times C_p \qquad (6.2)$$

Clearance (CL) is the intrinsic ability of the body to eliminate the drug. Clearance is not an indicator of the amount of drug eliminated but rather represents the theoretical volume of biologic fluid (blood or plasma) that is completely cleared of drug per unit of time (mL/min; L/hr). The amount of drug removed depends on the plasma concentration of the drug and clearance. At the steady state, when the rate of administration (R_A) is equal to the rate of elimination, CL can be considered as the proportionality constant that defines the rate of administration (or maintenance dose) for given steady-state plasma concentrations (C_{ss}) to be maintained.

$$R_A = CL \times C_{ss} \qquad (6.3)$$

The drugs are eliminated or cleared unchanged by the kidney, metabolized in the liver or other organs, or both. The total systemic clearance represents the sum of all of these separate clearances.

$$CL_{systemic} = CL_{renal} + CL_{hepatic} + CL_{other} \qquad (6.4)$$

■ HEPATIC CLEARANCE

The principal determinants of hepatic clearance (CL_H) are the metabolizing and excretory capacity (intrinsic clearance, CL_{int}), hepatic blood flow (Q_H), and plasma protein binding (i.e., fraction of unbound drug in the plasma [f_u]) of the liver.

The relation of these factors is defined by the following equation:

$$CL_H = (Q_H \cdot f_u \cdot CL_{int})/(Q_H + f_u \cdot CL_{int}) \qquad (6.5)$$

The CL_{int} can be referred to as the extraction ratio (E), which is equal to the differences in arterial blood concentration presented to the liver (C_A) and concentration of drug in the venous blood leaving the liver (C_V), divided by the arterial blood drug concentration:

$$E = (C_A - C_V)/C_A \qquad (6.6)$$

For drugs that exhibit a high (i.e., lidocaine, propofol, ketamine, fentanyl, sufentanil) or intermediate (methohexital, midazolam, alfentanil) hepatic extraction ratio, hepatic clearance depends mainly on hepatic blood flow. The elimination of drugs with low hepatic extraction ratios (diazepam) depends on enzymatic activity of the liver and is independent of hepatic blood flow (Fig. 6–2). Hepatic blood flow is decreased in patients with congestive heart failure, volume depletion, hypocapnia, circulatory shock, and β-adrenergic blockade. Based on similar systemic clearance values for lidocaine in infants and adults, it seems not that hepatic blood flow is a limiting factor for drug metabolism in infants but rather that the immature metabolizing enzyme systems and inefficient excretory function are major limiting factors for hepatic clearance of drugs in infants (*infra vide*). Protein binding may also alter drug clearance. In contrast to highly extracted drugs where protein binding does not influence clearance, for drugs with low extraction ratios, protein binding inversely affects the clearance. That is, increased protein binding results in reduced clearance, whereas decreased protein binding and subsequent increase in free-unbound fraction augment the hepatic clearance of the drug.

Regarding *drug metabolism,* hepatic biotransformation is a main route of elimination for many drugs. In general, hepatic metabolism increases the hydrophilicity of drugs and allows their renal elimination and termination of their pharmacologic

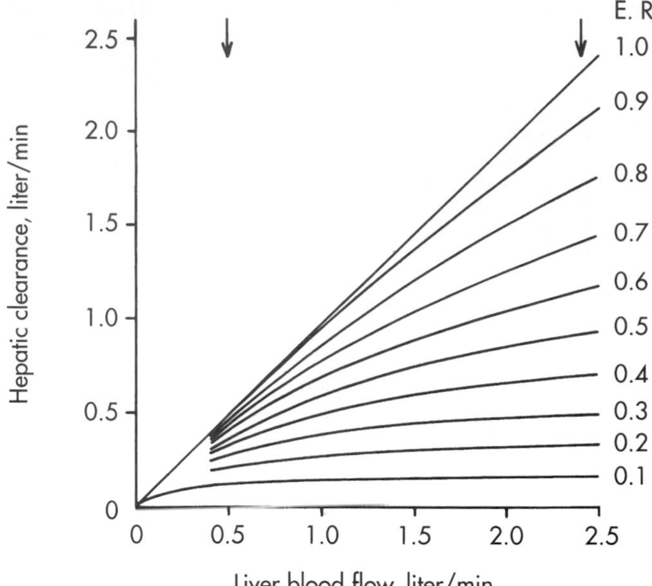

■ **FIGURE 6–2.** Effect of increasing liver blood flow on the hepatic clearance of drugs with varying extraction ratios. Each curve represents a drug whose extraction ratio (E.R.) at 1.5 L/min is shown above that flow. For drugs with a low extraction ratio, increase in liver blood flow within the physiologic range (indicated by *arrow*) produces very little change in hepatic clearance. For a drug with a high E.R., however, increases in liver blood flow produce an almost proportional increase in hepatic clearance. (With permission from Wilkinson GR, Shank DG: *Clin Pharmacol Ther* 18:377, 1975.)

and toxicologic activity. Drug metabolism that takes place in the liver involves various pathways that are generally categorized as phase I and phase II reactions (Table 6–4). Although the phase I and phase II reactions are well characterized in adults, there is limited information on the ontogeny of these important metabolic pathways.

The *phase I reactions* (oxidation, reduction, and hydrolysis) that result in addition, formation, or uncovering of a functional group on the drug molecule are mediated mainly by cytochrome P450 enzymes (CYPs). The CYP enzymes are a superfamily of heme-containing enzymes that catalyze the oxidative metabolism of a variety of exogenous and endogenous compounds, including many lipophilic drugs. At least 12 CYP gene families have been identified in humans. Based on amino acid sequence similarities, CYPs are divided into families when the amino acid sequence possesses more than 40% homology (denoted by Arabic number) and grouped into subfamilies (>55% homology; designated by letter). Individual enzymes (labeled by Arabic letter) may have up to 97% homology between the sequences. Only families 1 through 4 play an important role in drug metabolism. In general, CYP enzymes have broad substrate specificity for both exogenous and endogenous compounds. However, some CYPs have narrow substrate specificity with little overlapping activity. The presence of constitutive and inducible forms and documented genetic polymorphism for several CYPs may affect the metabolic clearance and have significant clinical ramification (Leeder and Kearns, 1997; Rane, 1999). Oxidation is the phase I reaction most deficient in neonates, whereas reduction is less affected and hydroxylation is almost equally effective as in adults. Parturition triggers the dramatic development of CYP enzymes.

The fetal liver and liver in infants exhibit significant differences in CYP mRNA and protein level and enzyme activity compared with adults. CYP1A2, the only member of the CYP1A subfamily present in the liver, is responsible for metabolism of caffeine and theophylline, two methylxanthines used frequently in pediatrics. The CYP1A2 is practically absent in the fetal liver and has very low activity in neonates, with 85% of a caffeine dose being excreted unchanged by the kidney in neonates (Cazeneuve et al., 1994). It reaches adult levels by the age of 4 to 6 months (Besunder et al., 1988; Cazeneuve et al., 1994; Hakkola et al., 1994; Yang et al., 1995; Leeder, 2001). The metabolism of caffeine in neonates primarily depends on CYP3A4 and not, as in the case of infants and adults, on CYP1A2 activity (Cazeneuve et al., 1994). The CYP3A subfamily (CYP3A4, CYP3A5, and CYP3A7) is the most important group of CYPs in regard to hepatic drug metabolism. The CYP3A4 isoform is the major isoenzyme (30% to 40% of the total CYP content) present in the adult liver and in the intestinal wall, where it markedly participates in the first-pass metabolism of midazolam (Thummel et al., 1996). In addition to midazolam, it metabolizes important drugs for pediatric anesthesiology

■ **TABLE 6–4.** Pathways in drug metabolism

Reaction	Examples
Phase I	
Oxidation Reactions	Thiopental, methohexital
Aliphatic hydroxylation	Pentazocine, meperidine, glutethimide, doxapram, ketamine, chlorpromazine
Aromatic	Lidocaine, bupivacaine, mepivacaine, meperidine, glutethimide, fentanyl, propranolol
Expoxidation	Phenytoin
O-Dealkylation	Pancuronium, vecuronium, codeine, phenacetin, methoxyflurane
N-Dealkylation	Morphine, meperidine, fentanyl, diazepam, amide local anesthetics, ketamine, codeine, atropine, methadone
N-Oxidation	Meperidine, normeperidine, morphine, tetracaine
S-Oxidation	Chlorpromazine
Oxidative deamination	Amphetamine, epinephrine
Desulfuration	Thiopental
Dehalogenation	Halogenated anesthetics
Dehydrogenation	Ethanol
Reduction Reactions	
Axoreduction	Fazadinium
Nitroreduction	Nitrazepam, dantrolene
Carbonyl reduction	Prednisolone
Alcohol dehydrogenation	Ethanol, chloral hydrate
Hydrolysis Reactions	
Ester hydrolysis	Ester local anesthetics, succinylcholine, acetylsalicyclic acid, propanidid
	Amide local anesthetics
Phase II: Conjugation Reactions	
Glucuronamide	Oxazepam, lorazepam, morphine, nalorphine, codeine, fentanyl, naloxone
Sulfate	Paracetamol, morphine, isoproterenol, cimetidine
Methylation	Norepinephrine
Acetylation	Procainamide
Amino acid	Salicyclic acid
Mercapturic acid	Sulfobromophthalein
Glutathione	Paracetamol

Adapted from Tucker GT: *Br J Anaesth* 51:603, 1979.

such as alfentanil, fentanyl, lidocaine, diazepam, and methadone. The CYP3A5, which is 83% homologous with CYP3A4, is less expressed in the liver but is the main CYP3A in the kidney and has similar substrate specificity to CYP3A4 (Yang et al., 1994). The CYP3A7 is 90% homologous to CYP3A4 and is a major highly active isoform present in fetal liver, with maximal activity in the early neonatal period and with progressive, and almost complete, loss of the activity within the first months after birth (Leeder and Kearns, 1997; Leeder, 2001). Only a few substrates have been studied with respect to the CYP3A7 activity, and it has minor contribution in metabolism of midazolam, carbamazepine, and cisapride (Thummel et al., 1996; de Wildt et al., 1999). CYP2D6 is another important isoenzyme involved in the metabolism of up to 25% of drugs (antidepressants, antipsychotics, antiarrhythmics, β-blockers, and opioids). This includes the metabolism of codeine and tramadol, which are converted by CYP2D6 to their respective pharmacologically active entities, morphine and *O*-desmethyl tramadol. In vitro studies suggest limited fetus CYP2D6 activity that reaches 20% of adult activity by 1 month of age (Treluyer et al., 1991). Both CYP2C19 (diazepam) and CYP2C9 (fluoxetine, phenytoin, torsemide) are absent in the fetal liver, and they reach the activity seen in adults by 6 months of age.

Phase II reactions catalyze the conjugation (glucuronidation, sulfation, glutathione conjugation) of a water-soluble endogenous molecule to the drug compound and further enhance the water solubility of drugs and their renal or biliary excretion. Glucuronidation, glutathione conjugation, and acetylation are deficient in the neonate, whereas sulfate conjugation is an effective pathway at birth (Cappiello et al., 1991). Uridine 5′-diphosphate-glucuronosyltransferase (UGT) catalyzes the conjugation of glucuronic acid to their substrates. Like the CYPs, the UGTs are a gene superfamily of enzymes that, according to the sequence homologues, are divided into two families (UGT1A and UGT2B) with more than 18 different enzymes. The conjugation of bilirubin (UGT1A1) is practically undetectable in the fetal liver but increases immediately after birth and reaches adult levels by the age of 6 to 9 months. The glucuronidation of morphine (a UGT2B7 substrate) in the fetal liver in vitro is 10% to 20% of that in the adult liver (Anderson et al., 1997). Clinical studies suggest deficient morphine glucuronidation in young infants with adult values reached by 6 to 30 months of age, depending on the method used to calculate clearance (clearance corrected by body weight or body surface area) (Choonara et al., 1989; Balistreri, 1983).

RENAL CLEARANCE

The kidney is the most important organ for elimination of drugs, and renal clearance contributes to the elimination of a significant number of water-soluble drugs and their metabolites. Glomerular filtration rate (CL_{GFR}), tubular secretion ($CL_{tub\text{-}sec}$), and tubular reabsorption ($CL_{tub\text{-}abs}$) mainly govern renal clearance. Their relationship is defined by the following equation:

$$CL = CL_{GFR} + CL_{tub\text{-}sec} - CL_{tub\text{-}abs} \quad (6.7)$$

The renal clearance mechanisms are also subject to maturational changes, with each renal clearance process exhibiting a different rate and pattern of development. Changes in renal clearance of digoxin (which includes glomerular filtration and tubular excretion) from 0.6 L/hr per 1.73 m^2 and 2.0 L/hr per 1.73 m^2 in premature and full-term infants, respectively, to 5.3 L/hr per 1.73 m^2 and 8.7 L/hr per 1.73 m^2 in 3-month-old infants and 18-month-old children, respectively, are representative of renal growth and maturation processes (Halkin et al., 1978; Ng et al., 1981).

The nephrogenesis that begins in the eighth week of gestation is completed by 36 weeks of age. At that time, for the full complement of nephrons, GFR is only 5% of the adult values (Haycock, 1998). Measurements of renal plasma flow (para-aminohippuric acid) and GFR (inulin or mannitol) that are normalized for the body surface area indicate that adult values are reached between 6 and 12 months of age (Rubin et al., 1949; Heilbron et al., 1991). Notably, if clearance numbers are related to body weight, the adult values for plasma flow and GFR are reached much earlier (i.e., within weeks to a month). Both anatomic and functional immaturity of renal tubules is present at birth and both passive reabsorption and active secretion are diminished. The maturation of renal tubular function has a more protracted time course and reaches the adult renal tubular function values by 12 to 18 months of age (Alcorn and McNamara, 2002). The reduced GFR in the perinatal period seems to be due to the active vasoconstriction of the renal microvasculature, and diminished renal blood flow accounts mainly for the differences in GFR between full-term infants and adults. The low GFR at birth seems to protect the immature proximal tubules from an overload of electrolytes and other solutes. Parturition triggers dramatic increase in renal blood flow, with a 10-fold increase of para-aminohippuric acid clearance in the first year of life. For most drugs eliminated predominantly by the kidney, there is prolonged half-life in the first 1 to 3 weeks of life, with a significantly shorter half-life by 4 weeks and adult values for $t_{1/2}$ reached by 6 months of age.

NONLINEAR PHARMACOKINETICS

For some drugs, an increase in dose is not followed by proportional increase in steady-state plasma concentrations (C_{ss}) and area-under-the-plasma-concentration curve (AUC). Instead, the C_{ss} and AUC increase more than expected. The explanation for this nonlinear pharmacokinetics is that enzymes responsible for metabolism and elimination of the drug may be saturated. The nonlinear pharmacokinetics, also called *Michaelis-Menten kinetics*, occur when the maximum rate of metabolism (Vmax) for the drug is approached. The Michaelis-Menten–type pharmacokinetics describe the rate of production of molecules (drug metabolites) produced by *enzymatic* chemical reactions. Enzymes can perform up to several million *catalytic* reactions per second. To determine the maximum rate of an enzymatic reaction, the *substrate* (plasma drug) concentration should be increased until a constant rate of product (drug metabolite) formation is achieved. This is the *maximum velocity* (V_{max}) of the enzyme, and at this point the active sites of the enzymes are saturated with drug and a constant *amount* of drug begins to be eliminated per unit of time ("zero-order" kinetics). Because the substrate (drug plasma) concentration at V_{max} cannot be measured exactly, the metabolism of drug can be characterized by Michaelis-Menten constant (K_m), i.e., the drug plasma concentration at which the rate of metabolism is half of its maximum ($K_m = V_{max}/2$). For practical purposes, the K_m is the plasma concentration at which, when the dose is increased, the nonproportional increase in C_{ss} and AUC start to occur.

For most of drugs that are metabolized by hepatic enzymes and eliminated by the liver, the K_m is above the required therapeutic range and they follow linear kinetics. However, when the therapeutic range is above the K_m, nonlinear kinetics occurs. For example, the average K_m and therapeutic range for phenytoin are 4 mg/L and 10 to 20 mg/L, respectively, and many patients on phenytoin experience nonlinear pharmacokinetics.

The nonlinear pharmacokinetics may also be seen in low-clearance drugs for which elimination is significantly influenced by the binding of the drug to plasma proteins. In this scenario, after increasing the dose of drug, a less-than-expected increase in C_{ss} and AUC occurs. This would suggest that the plasma protein binding sites have been saturated and that the free fraction of low-clearance drug has increased. The latter would result with increased clearance and a less-than-expected increase C_{ss} occurs. However, if measured, the free fraction of the low-clearance drug increases proportionally. Both valproic acid and disopyramide follow this type of nonlinear pharmacokinetics (Bowdle et al., 1980; Lima et al., 1991).

■ COMPARTMENT MODELS

For many drugs, after intravenous administration, the process of distribution throughout plasma and tissues occurs rapidly and simultaneously, and the whole body could be thought of as a single compartment. In this single-compartment model, after bolus intravenous administration of the drug, there is a monoexponential decrease in plasma concentration. The latter is due to the elimination process that allows a constant *portion* of the drug (not amount) in the body to be eliminated per unit of time. In this case, the drug follows the *first-order kinetic*. The first order elimination of a drug from the body or plasma (C_p) is defined as follows:

$$A_B = A_B^0 \times e^{-K\text{dt}} \text{ or } C_p = C_p^0 \times e^{-K\text{dt}} \quad (6.8)$$

A_B^0 is the initial amount in the body and C_p^0 plasma concentration immediately after the bolus; t is the time since bolus and K_d is the rate constant of elimination. The $e^{-K\text{dt}}$ represents the fraction of the A_B^0 remaining at time t. The drug elimination rate constant (K_d) is an index of the body's capacity to remove the drug. The elimination rate constant K_d is the fraction of the total amount of drug in the body that is removed per unit of time. It is a function of clearance and volume of distribution:

$$K_d = CL/V_d \quad (6.9)$$

The elimination rate constant (K_d) can be also thought of as the fraction of the volume of distribution that is effectively cleared of drug per unit of time. Because the drug plasma concentration diminishes monoexponentially, a graph plot of the logarithm of the plasma concentrations versus time yields a straight line. The elimination rate constant defines the slope of this curve (Fig. 6–3), and two plasma concentrations measured during the decay or elimination phase can be used to calculate the K_d:

$$K_d = \ln C_{p1} - \ln C_{p2}/(t_2 - t_1) \quad (6.10)$$

The elimination rate constant is often expressed in terms of a time required for half of the total amount of drug in the body to be eliminated, or the plasma concentrations to decrease by one half, that is, by the half-life of the drug ($t_{1/2}$). If plasma concentrations drop by 50% and $C_{p1} = 2\,C_{p2}$, then in Eq. 5, $t_2 - t_1 = t_{1/2}$ and

$$K_d = \ln 2/t_{1/2} \quad (6.11)$$

$$t_{1/2} = 0.693/K_d \quad (6.12)$$

The half-life, like K_d, is dependent on volume of distribution and clearance, and this relationship is shown in Eq. 13.

$$t_{1/2} = (0.693 \times V_d)/CL \quad (6.13)$$

The half-life is a variable that determines (1) the time needed ($5 \times t_{1/2}$) to reach plasma steady-state concentrations of the drug after initiation of an infusion, (2) the time needed to reach new steady-state concentrations after increasing or decreasing the infusion rate, (3) the time needed for drug to disappear from plasma after the infusion is stopped, and (4) the time it takes for all drug from the body to be eliminated after cessation of the drug infusion (Fig. 6–4). The short half-life is an obvious advantage for drugs given by intravenous infusion: it allows for drug effects to be easily and dynamically titrated; a relatively shorter time is required for steady-state concentrations to be achieved; and if toxicity occurs, it is easier to handle. For drugs used by intermittent administration (oral or parenteral), a short half-life is a disadvantage because multiple doses are needed; it is difficult to keep the plasma concentration within the therapeutic window; and a missed dose could drop plasma concentrations below the minimal therapeutic level. It should be emphasized that V_d and CL may change independent of one another and alter the half-life in the same or opposite directions. For the given clearance, drugs with smaller V_d have a shorter $t_{1/2}$ and a faster recovery after the infusion of an anesthetic agent. Reduced clearance, with no changes in volume of distribution, increases the half-life and recovery time after intravenous infusion.

Most of the drugs used in anesthesia do not follow the simple, one-compartment pharmacokinetics but rather behave like a two- or even three-compartment model. Distribution of anesthetic drugs into and out of peripheral tissues determines the pharmacokinetic profile and the time course of the anesthetic drug effect. For the two-compartment model, the central

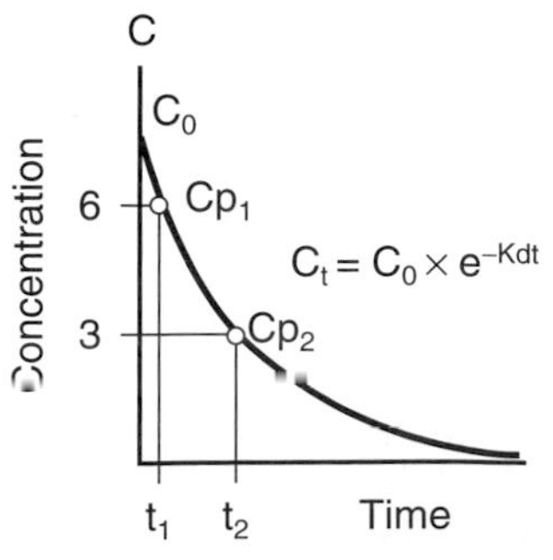

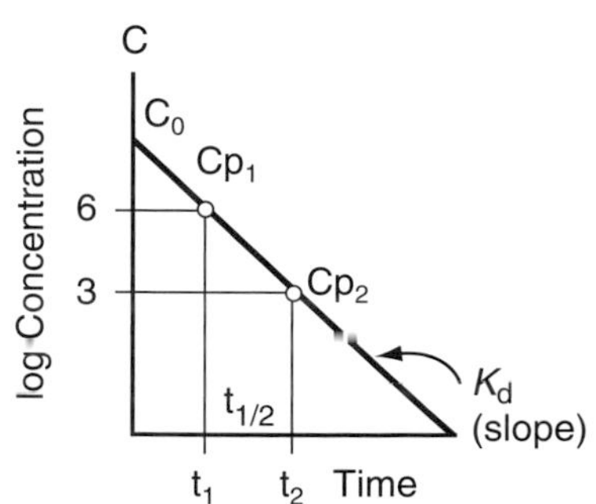

■ **FIGURE 6–3.** Single-compartment model. The initial plasma (body) drug concentration (C_p^0) produced by single loading dose diminishes monoexponentially *(left)*. The semilogarithmic graph of concentration versus time yields a straight line *(right)*.

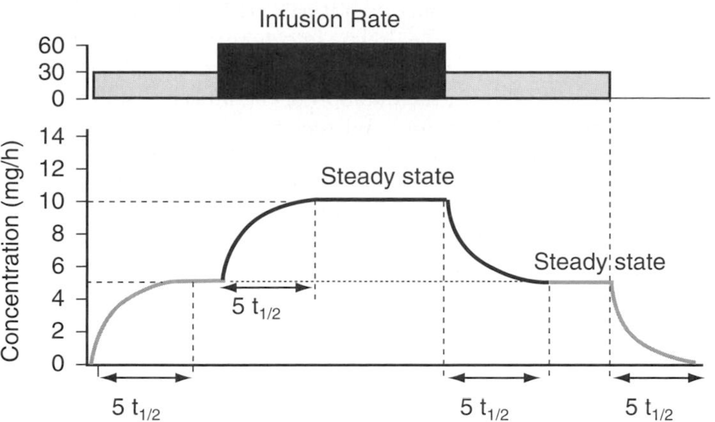

■ **FIGURE 6–4.** Changes in plasma concentration and steady-state level after intravenous infusion are in the function of half-life.

compartment includes the blood and organs or tissues that have high blood flow and can be thought of as a rapidly equilibrating volume. The second compartment has a volume (V_t) that equilibrates at a much slower pace. After bolus administration of a drug that follows the two-compartment model, two distinct phases can be distinguished—distribution phase and terminal elimination—and the decay of plasma concentration over time is defined by the biexponential equation (Fig. 6–5). Changes in plasma and the site of action concentrations would depend on drug elimination and on the equilibrium between central and peripheral tissue compartments.

For many anesthetic drugs, even three phases can be distinguished after intravenous bolus administration. This three-compartment model is composed of the central compartment and two additional compartments that include the respective rapid and slow equilibrating tissues and organs (Fig. 6–6). Likewise, the three-compartment model is characterized by the triexponential plasma concentration equation, three volumes of distribution, and five rate constants of distribution and terminal elimination (K_{12}, K_{21}, K_{13}, K_{31}, and K_{10}).

After an intravenous bolus, the anesthetic/hypnotic drug dilutes almost immediately, within the single circulation time, into the central compartment (i.e., in the bloodstream and in the highly perfused organs such as brain and spinal cord). The central volume of distribution can be used to calculate the loading dose. Subsequently, there is a redistribution of drug out from the CNS back into the blood and to the peripheral compartments with rapid equilibrium (muscles viscera; $V_{d\,rapid}$). Finally, the drug diffuses into poorly perfused tissues (fat) that slowly equilibrate with the central compartment. The initial redistribution, rather than metabolic clearance, determines the termination of the effect of single boluses of parenteral anesthetics. If prolonged anesthesia is required, the maintenance infusion rate should compensate not only for the drug clearance but initially also for the transient loss of anesthetic by redistribution to the peripheral compartments that are governed by "intercompartmental clearance" and elimination rate constants (K_{12}, K_{21}, K_{13}, and K_{31}).

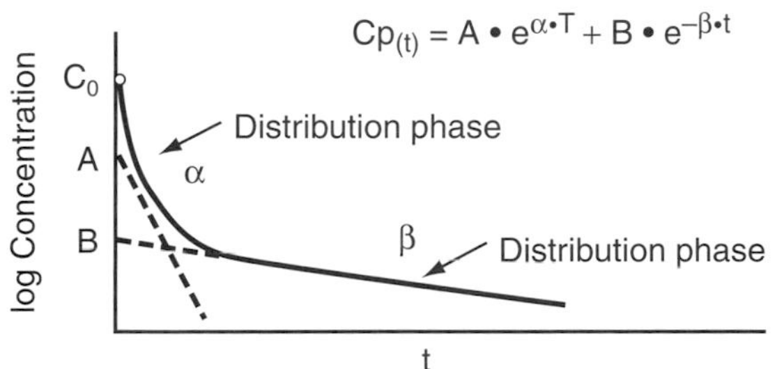

■ **FIGURE 6–5.** Two-compartment model. For many drugs, after an intravenous bolus, there is no "instantaneous" and even distribution of the drug throughout the body (as in the one-compartment model). Drugs distribute with different paces between the initial/central (V_c) compartment (i.e., circulation and well-perfused organs, including the brain) and the tissue/peripheral compartment (V_t). The changes in plasma concentrations follow the biexponential decay.

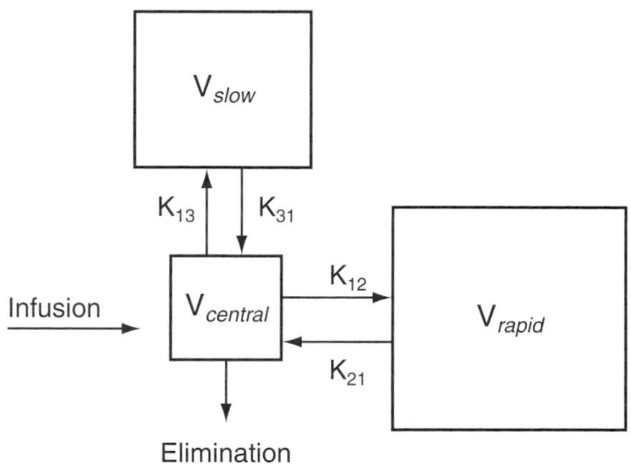

■ **FIGURE 6–6.** Three-compartment model. After intravenous administration, for many anesthetic drugs three phases in distribution can be distinguished. After immediate distribution into central compartment (i.e., bloodstream and highly perfused organs), there is redistribution of drugs (i.e., from the brain) back into circulation (K_{21}) and to peripheral tissue with rapid equilibrium (K_{12}). Drug also diffuses at very slow pace into and out from the poorly perfused tissues (K_{13}, K_{31}). The triexponential decay describes the changes in plasma concentrations.

■ OFFSET OF DRUG EFFECT AND CONTEXT-SENSITIVE HALF-TIME CONCEPT

Traditionally, clearance, volume of distribution, and half-life are standard pharmacokinetic parameters used to characterize the drug offset of action. As presented earlier, they are derived from one- and two-compartment models or, through the use of computer simulation programs, from multicompartment models. These pharmacokinetic parameters can be relatively easy to apply to calculate the infusion rate and predict the offset of action of water-soluble drugs with small V_d and relatively "simple pattern of disposition" (i.e., muscle relaxants).

For the anesthesiologist, pharmacokinetic factors are frequently used for the routine selection and use of various intravenous anesthetic agents. Drugs with short elimination half-lives are frequently selected for brief procedures, whereas drugs with longer half-lives are selected for lengthier procedures. Drugs with small volumes of distribution tend to decrease the time required for recovery after intravenous infusion, and agents with decreased plasma clearances may increase the time for recovery. In general, formulas for the calculation of continuous infusions incorporate knowledge of these pharmacokinetics. For bolus administration of drug, the volume of distribution and the desired plasma concentration are needed. Table 6–5 lists plasma concentrations in adults for some of the opioids. The bolus dose is calculated as the product of the volume of distribution (V_d) and the desired plasma concentration (C_p):

$$\text{Bolus dose} = V_d \times C_p \qquad (6.14)$$

The maintenance infusion rate (MIR) is calculated as the product of the desired plasma concentration (C_p) and the clearance (CL):

$$\text{MIR} = \text{CL} \times C_p \qquad (6.15)$$

Although these formulas work well, Shafer and Varvel (1991) and Hughes and others (1992) have demonstrated the complex interactions that occur with prolonged infusions, especially in drugs that are lipid soluble.

The offset of drug effect depends on reduction of the plasma concentrations and the withdrawal of drug from the site of action, that is, for anesthetic from the receptor site in the CNS. If steady state is achieved and all compartments are saturated, then the half-life of elimination phase, which is a function of the first-order processes of elimination, would correlate with decrease in the site-of-action drug concentrations and with the offset of drug action. However, after infusion of a highly lipophilic anesthetic agent, when steady state is not achieved and not all compartments are saturated, the decline in concentrations (i.e., the offset of action and recovery from anesthesia) depends on complex interaction between the duration of the infusion and initial distribution, redistribution, and metabolic/elimination first-order processes. The classic descriptors of a drug's pharmacokinetics and offset of action (terminal half-time) are of little help to anesthesiologists in predicting the offset of action and recovery from anesthesia for the intravenous anesthetic drugs. Fortunately, with the help of pharmacokinetic/pharmacodynamic simulation models, new predictors of offset of drug effect have evolved (Shafer and Varvel, 1991; Huges et al., 1992; Youngs and Shafer, 1994).

Using a pharmacokinetic/pharmacodynamic model and basic pharmacokinetics profile of commonly used synthetic opioid analogs, Shafer and Varel (1991) were the first to construct the offset of action (recovery) curves as a function of the duration of infusion for fentanyl, alfentanil, and sufentanil (Fig. 6–7). Huges and others (1992) introduced the term "context-sensitive half-time" (*context* refers to the duration of infusion) as a time required for a drug concentration to decrease to half of its value after drug infusion of a given duration. Of importance is that for any given drug, its context-sensitive half-time varies with the duration of the drug infusion. Thus, a 2-hour context-sensitive half-time is a time required for the plasma or effects site concentrations to decrease by 50% after termination of a 2-hour infusion. Because for most intravenous anesthetic drugs the 50% fall in concentration is not sufficient for recovery from anesthesia, other decrement times have been introduced (Youngs and Shafer, 1994). For example, 1-hour 80% and 3-hour 90% decrement times describe the time needed for concentrations to decrease by 80% and 90% after the cessation of the 1- and 3-hour infusions, respectively.

After a short intravenous infusion (>10 to 15 minutes), fentanyl and other synthetic opioid analogs have similar context-sensitive half-times (see Fig. 6–7). However, after prolonged infusion (>1 hour), there is a marked difference among four synthetic opioid analogs (fentanyl, sufentanil, alfentanil, and remifentanil), and these differences do not correlate with their classic pharmacokinetic parameters (Table 6–6). In contrast to its older congeners, remifentanil has a short and steady context-sensitive half-life of 3 minutes, which does not change with the increasing duration of infusion (Egan et al., 1996). This contrasts with alfentanil, with a context-sensitive half-time that increases to 1 hour after a 4-hour infusion (Ebling et al., 1990; Scholz et al., 1996). This difference is due to the unique pharmacokinetic profile of remifentanil. It is a highly liposoluble (volume of distribution at steady state [Vd_{ss}], 30 L) opioid analog that undergoes widespread metabolism (deesterification), including metabolism in the circulation. Unlike other opioids, the termination of action of remifentanil does not depend on redistribution but rather on extremely rapid metabolic clearance. Kapila and others (1995) demonstrated that the context-sensitive half-times of remifentanil (3 minutes) and alfentanil (50 to 55 minutes) derived from computer modeling are similar to measured context-sensitive half-times (3.2 and 47 minutes for remifentanil and alfentanil, respectively), and both correlate with measured pharmacodynamic offset (recovery of minute ventilation). The latter confirms the value and clinical applicability of this new pharmacokinetic/pharmacodynamic parameter in predicting the offset of anesthetic drugs.

The context-sensitive half-time curves provide a better, clinically more relevant comparison of the pharmacokinetic profiles

■ TABLE 6–5. Opioid concentrations that ablate responsiveness to intraoperative noxious stimuli and permit adequate ventilation on emergence*

	Fentanyl	Alfentanil	Sufentanil
Induction and intubation			
Thiopental	3 to 5	250 to 400	0.4 to 0.6
O_2/N_2O only	8 to 10	400 to 750	0.8 to 1.2
Maintenance			
N_2O/potent vapor	1.5 to 4	100 to 300	0.25 to 0.5
O_2/N_2O only	1.5 to 10	100 to 750	0.25 to 1.0
O_2 only	15 to 60	1000 to 4000	10 to 60
Adequate ventilation on emergence	1.5	125	0.25

*Opioid concentration given in ng/mL.

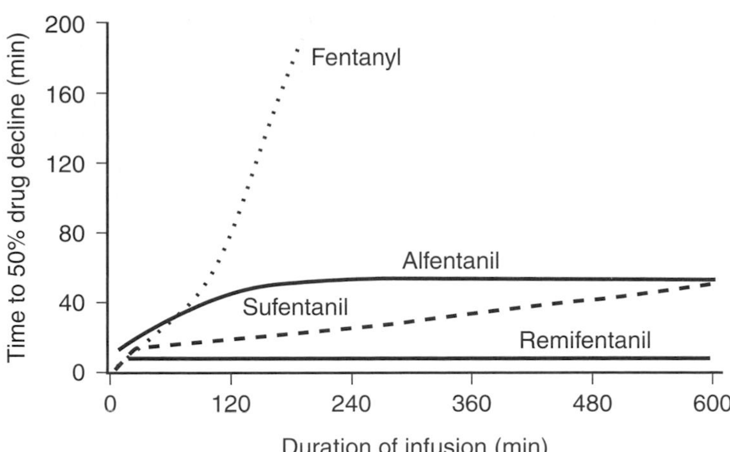

■ **FIGURE 6–7.** Context-sensitive half-time: the time required for drug concentration to decrease by half of its value (Y axis) after cessation of infusion of given duration (X axis) for fentanyl and its congeners, sufentanil, alfentanil, and remifentanil (see the text for explanation). (Adapted from Shafer SL, Varvel MD: Pharmacokinetics, pharmacodynamics and rational opioid selection. *Anesthesiology* 74:53, 1991; and Egan TD: *Clin Pharmacokinet* 29:80, 1995.)

of anesthetic drugs than the traditional pharmacokinetic parameters (Fig. 6–8). After a single intravenous dose, commonly used anesthetic/hypnotic drugs have a short duration of action. However, after prolonged infusions, the context-sensitive half-times and duration of action increase. For some drugs (propofol, ketamine), this increase is modest, whereas for others (diazepam, thiopental), it is quite dramatic. In the case of midazolam, the rapid increase in its context-sensitive half-time with prolonged duration of infusion occurs in the presence of a relatively short elimination half-life ($t_{1/2}\beta$), and this is most likely due to the low clearance of midazolam.

The data regarding the context-sensitive half-times and other decrement times of anesthetic agents in the pediatric population are limited, at best. In children aged 3 to 11 years, longer context-sensitive half-times than in adults were reported for propofol. After a 1-hour infusion in children and adults, the context-sensitive half-times for propofol are 10.4 and 6.6 minutes, respectively, and after a 4-hour infusion, they are 19.6 and 9.5 minutes, respectively (McFarlan et al., 1999). This is probably due to the altered compartment volumes and may lead to slower recovery from a propofol infusion in children than in adults (Short et al., 1994). In contrast, the shorter context-sensitive half-time of fentanyl was determined in pediatric population (2 to 11 years old) compared with published data in adults (Ginsberg et al., 1996; Reves et al., 1994).

■ INTRAVENOUS DRUGS

■ SEDATIVE-HYPNOTIC AGENTS

A variety of sedative-hypnotic agents can be used for premedication or induction of anesthesia. Most commonly these agents are administered intravenously, but oral, rectal, or intramuscular routes are occasionally used.

On a milligram-per-kilogram basis, barbiturates are more lethal to newborns than to more mature animals (Carmichael, 1938, 1947; Weatherall, 1960; Goldenthal, 1971). The sleeping times of newborn animals are markedly prolonged at sublethal doses given on an equal milligram-per-kilogram basis (Weatherall, 1960). Greater penetration of the blood–brain barrier by barbiturates has been found in neonates as opposed to older animals (Domek et al., 1960).

Neonates have a decreased ability to metabolize barbiturates (Mirkin, 1975). The longer-acting barbiturates, which are in part excreted unmetabolized in the urine, would be expected to have prolonged or elevated blood levels (Knauer et al., 1973; Boreus et al., 1975). Glucuronic acid conjugation of barbiturates develops rapidly and increases 30-fold during the first 3 weeks of life (Brown et al., 1958).

Short-acting barbiturates (e.g., methohexital, thiamylal, and thiopental) can be used to induce anesthesia in infants and children. These agents produce rapid induction of hypnosis with minimal relaxation or analgesia. The pharmacokinetics of short-acting barbiturates in infants, children, and adults were studied extensively by Brodie (1952), Dundee and Barron (1962), Mark (1963), Saidman and Eger (1966), and Lindsay and Shepherd (1969). Because of the child's proportionately greater amount of vessel-rich tissue, the uptake of short-acting barbiturates should be more rapid (Eger, 1974), the effect more quickly achieved, and metabolism, excretion, and recovery more prompt unless retarded by supplementary agents.

Thiopental

Thiopental is a commonly administered intravenous induction agent. Hiccoughs, sneezing, and other irregularities are rarely seen on induction, and there is no excitement or extrapyramidal activity. Cerebrospinal fluid pressure is reduced, making the

■ **TABLE 6–6.** Pharmacokinetic parameters of synthetic opioids after single intravenous bolus administration

	Volume of Distribution (Vd_{ss}; L/kg)	Elimination Half-Life ($t_{1/2}\alpha$; min)	Distribution Half-Life ($t_{1/2}\beta$; min)	Total Body Clearance (mL/min per kg)	Context-Sensitive Half-Time (3-hr infusion)
Fentanyl	4	2 to 3	220 to 300	10 to 20	100
Sufentanil	1.7	1.4	160	10 to 15	30
Alfentanil	0.75	0.6 to 12	90 to 120	8	50
Remifentanil	0.3 to 0.4	1 to 1.5	6 to 14	50	3

Data from Egan et al., 1996; Ebling et al., 1990; and Scholz et al., 1996.

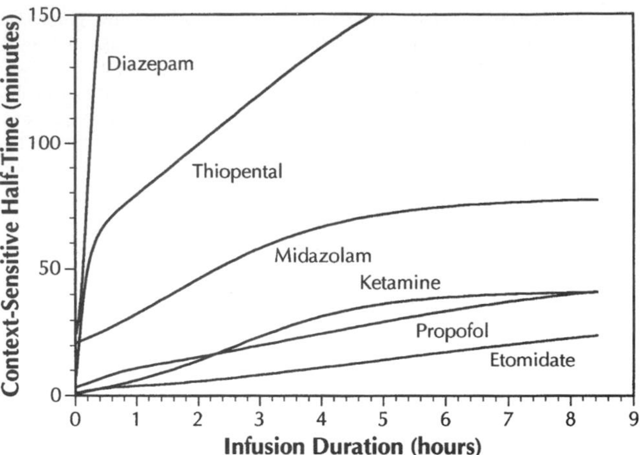

■ **FIGURE 6–8.** Context-sensitive half-time for commonly used general anesthetics. (From Reves JG, Glass PSA, Lubarsky DA: Non-barbiturate intravenous anesthetics. In Miller RD, editor: *Anesthesia,* 5th ed. New York, 2000, Churchill Livingstone, p 228, Fig. 9-5.)

agent useful for diagnostic and operative neurologic procedures (Dawson et al., 1971), and intraocular pressure also is decreased. Awakening is quiet, occasionally interrupted by shivering (Smith et al., 1955), and associated with a low incidence of nausea. Porphyria, seldom encountered in the United States, is a specific contraindication to barbiturates (Dundee and Barron, 1962). Thiopental requirements for induction of anesthesia reveal an inverse relation with age. Jonmarker and others (1987) reported that the ED_{50} of thiopental in infants is significantly greater (7 mg/kg) than that in adults (4 mg/kg) (Jonmarker et al., 1987) (Fig. 6–9). Westrin and others (1989) determined the dose of thiopental needed for satisfactory induction of 10 healthy, nonpremedicated neonates, 0 to 14 days old, and 20 infants, 1 to 6 months old. In this study the ED_{50} for thiopental induction was 3.4 ± 0.2 mg/kg in neonates and 6.3 ± 0.7 mg/kg in infants aged 1 to 6 months. In an in vitro study in which the free fraction of thiopental was measured in the serum of neonates and adult volunteers, Kingston and others (1990) noted that neonates had a free drug fraction 1.5× to 2×

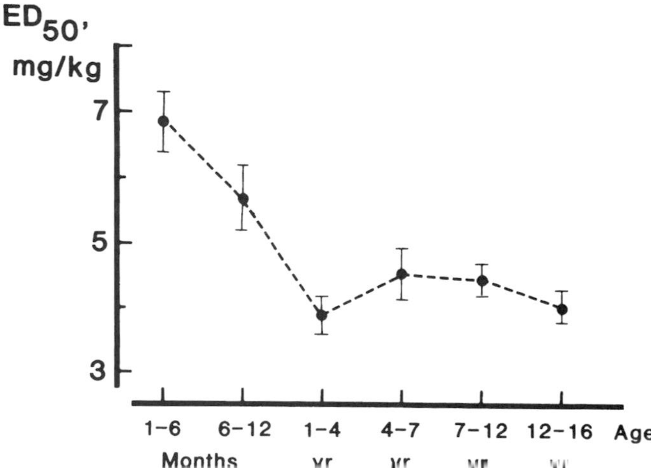

■ **FIGURE 6–9.** Estimated ED_{50} ± SE for thiopental in the various age groups. (With permission from Jonmarker C, Westrin P, Larsson S, et al.: *Anesthesiology* 67:104, 1987.)

greater than that of adults. The increased free fraction of thiopental may explain the decreased induction dose required by the neonate. Sorbo and others (1984) studied the pharmacokinetics of thiopental in 24 surgical patients aged 5 months to 13 years. The volume of distribution of the central compartment ranged from 0.3 to 0.4 L/kg. The Vd_{ss} was approximately 2.0 L/kg and did not differ statistically from values previously measured in adults. The elimination half-time and clearance of thiopental in these infants and children were 6.1 ± 3.3 hours and 6.6 ± 2.2 mL/kg per minute, respectively. These values were significantly different from the values of 12.0 ± 6.0 hours and 3.1 ± 0.5 mL/kg per minute, respectively, observed in adults.

Methohexital

Methohexital, a methylated oxybarbiturate, is more potent than thiopental by a ratio of about 3:1 (Clarke et al., 1968), is more rapidly eliminated, and produces more undesirable side effects. Greater speed of recovery provides its principal indication, especially for outpatient care or for situations where very brief effect is wanted, as for cardioversion or electroconvulsive therapy. The incidence of involuntary muscular movement, hiccough, and respiratory irregularity during induction is definitely greater with methohexital than with thiopental. Although methohexital has been used via the intramuscular or rectal route without tissue damage (Miller et al., 1961), some studies suggest that the high concentration of rectal methohexital can cause mucosal damage. Administration of 10% methohexital to rats via the rectal route produces minor, self-limiting lesions in the rectal mucosa (Hinkle and Weinlander, 1989). The recommended dose for intravenous use is 1 to 2 mg/kg, and in children younger than 5 years, 25 to 30 mg/kg can be administered rectally.

In a study of 85 children, Khalil and others (1990) compared 25 mg/kg of rectal methohexital in a 10% and a 1% concentration. In this study, 1% was associated with a better success rate, faster onset time, high plasma concentration, and longer recovery time than the 10% concentration. In addition, Khalil and others noted that the length of the rectal catheter had no effect on the pharmacodynamics of the drug. A 10% solution of methohexital at a dose of 25 mg/kg usually produced sleep in 6 to 10 minutes (Goresky and Steward, 1979), which coincided with peak serum levels (Letty et al., 1985).

Forbes and others (1989a) reported on the plasma concentrations of 60 children after doses of 15, 20, 25, or 30 mg/kg of rectal methohexital (Fig. 6–10). The dose of 30 mg/kg resulted in significantly higher plasma concentrations for up to 20 minutes. In addition, in a separate study of 12 patients who were premedicated with 25 mg/kg of 2% rectal methohexital, Forbes and others (1989b), using pulsed Doppler and two-dimensional echocardiography, noted a significant increase in heart rate but no change in cardiac index, stroke volume, ejection fraction, or blood pressure.

Audenaert and others (1995) prospectively reviewed the effects of rectal methohexital in 648 patients. They noted that after a 30 mg/kg dose of 10% methohexital, children fell asleep 85% of the time. Sleep occurred usually in 6 minutes. Sleep was less likely to occur in patients with myelomeningocele or in patients on phenobarbital or Dilantin (phenytoin) therapy. Side effects of defecation after administration occurred in 10% of patients and hiccups occurred in 13% (Audenaert et al., 1995). The intravenous dose for induction using methohexital dissolved in a rapid emulsion was determined by Westrin (1992). Westrin noted that the dose (adjusted by body weight) needed

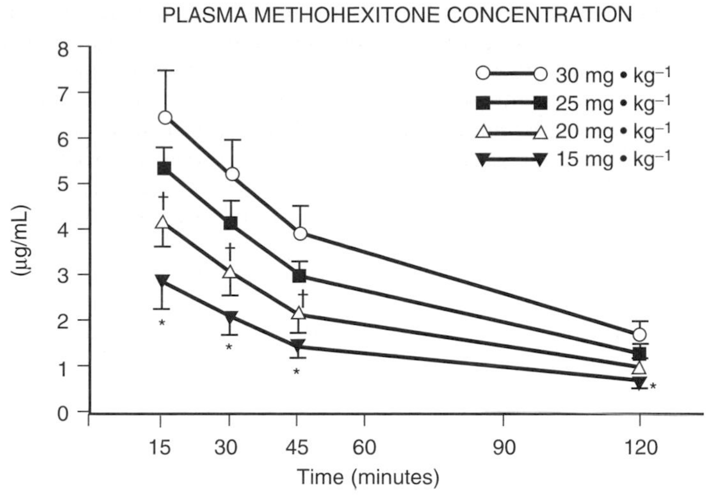

■ **FIGURE 6–10.** Plasma methohexitone concentrations following rectal administration of methohexitone 15 mg/kg, 20 mg/kg, 25 mg/kg, or 30 mg/kg. Mean ± SEM. *P < 0.05 15 mg/kg versus 30 mg/kg; †P < 0.05 20 mg/kg versus 30 mg/kg. (Redrawn from Forbes RB, Murray DJ, Dillman JB, et al.: *Can J Anaesth* 36:160–164, 1989.)

for induction in infants younger than 5 months was almost twice that for older children (Fig. 6–11).

Beskow and others (1995) compared intravenous induction of methohexital (3 mg/kg) and thiopental (7.3 mg/kg) in 41 infants aged 1 month to 1 year. In this study of short surgical procedures, recovery as measured by spontaneous eye opening after methohexital was significantly shorter than for thiopental.

Benzodiazepines and Antagonists

Diazepam

Diazepam produces relatively pleasant sedation or hypnosis with few side effects and prompt recovery. Its action is due to depression of the amygdala of the limbic system and spinal internuncial neurons. It is a specific treatment of seizure disorders in children

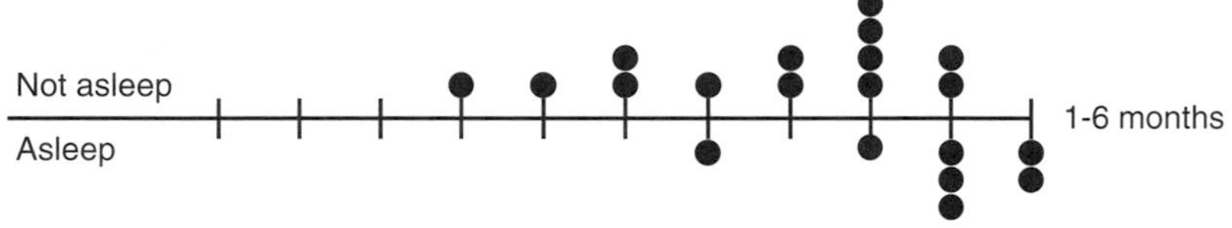

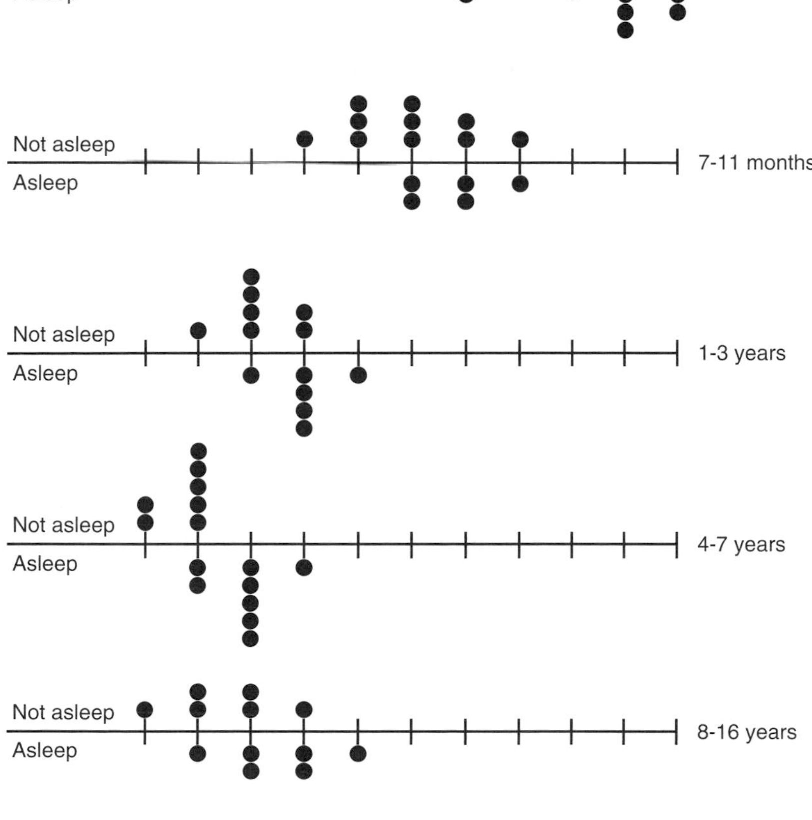

■ **FIGURE 6–11.** Results of injection of different doses of methohexital. Each filled circle represents one patient. The position of the circle below or above the line indicates whether induction was classified as satisfactory or not satisfactory. (Redrawn from Westrin P: *Anesthesiology* 76:917–921, 1992.)

(Lombroso, 1966; Carter and Gold, 1977). Intravenous administration of 0.2 to 0.3 mg/kg usually induces hypnosis, but the requirement varies widely. Diazepam appears to cause less cardiac depression than do barbiturates (Muenster et al., 1967; Abel and Reis, 1971).

Diazepam is metabolized by the CYP-linked mono-oxygenase system. In adults, the metabolite (desmethyldiazepam) is eliminated slower ($t_{1/2}$ = 150 hours) than the parent compound ($t_{1/2}$ = 20 to 30 hours) (Meberg, 1978).

The plasma half-life of diazepam and the nature of the diazepam metabolites formed vary with maturity (Morselli et al., 1974). The premature infant and the mature infant at term eliminate diazepam at a slower rate than do older infants, children, and adults. In premature infants, a demethylated derivative of diazepam, *N*-demethyldiazepam, could not be measured in plasma until 4 hours after injection, in comparison to older infants and children, in whom, *N*-demethyldiazepam was measured in the plasma by 1 hour and had peaked by 24 hours. In adults, 71% of diazepam or its metabolites was excreted in the urine, and about 10% was excreted in the feces. As an oral premedicant or intravenous induction agent, the recommended dose of diazepam is 0.1 to 0.2 mg/kg.

Midazolam

Midazolam is a water-soluble, short-acting benzodiazepine. Its chemical configuration confers a pH-dependent ring phenomenon. At pH 4, the diazepine ring opens, and a highly stable water-soluble compound results. At physiologic pH values, the ring closes and thereby increases the drug lipophilic activity. Cardiovascular stability, transient mild respiratory depression, minimal venous irritation, retrograde amnesia, and short duration of action are reasons why midazolam has replaced diazepam.

Midazolam is metabolized in the liver; less than 1% is excreted unchanged in the urine. Midazolam undergoes extensive metabolism (CYP3A4, CYP3A5, CYP3A7) to a major hydroxylated form, 1-OH-midazolam. The protein binding of midazolam is extensive, with a free fraction of only 3% to 6%. Midazolam has an intermediate rate of absorption (0.5 to 1.5 hours) and a bioavailability of 30% to 50%. The terminal elimination phase ranges from 1 to 4 hours (Smith et al., 1981).

In children, the pharmacokinetics of midazolam were reported. Payne and others (1989) noted that in healthy children administered 0.15 mg/kg intravenously, the volume of distribution at steady state, the elimination half-life, and the clearance were 1.29 L/kg, 70 minutes, and 9.1 mL/kg per minute, respectively. Jones and others (1993) have also reported on the kinetics of intravenous midazolam (0.5 mg/kg) in 12 healthy Chinese children and noted that the kinetics were consistent with a three-compartment model with a volume of distribution of 1.9 L/kg, $t_{1/2}\beta$ of 107 minutes, and a clearance of 15.4 mL/kg per minute. However, because the drug exhibits dose-related changes in clearance (Salonen et al., 1987), comparisons between studies become difficult. The kinetics of midazolam have also been determined after intramuscular, rectal, and oral administration. Payne and others (1989) noted that times for peak serum concentrations after intramuscular, rectal, and oral administration were 15, 30, and 53 minutes, respectively, whereas the drug clearance and bioavailability via these three different routes were 10.4, 50.8, and 33.4 mL/kg per minute and 87%, 18%, and 27%, respectively.

In a study involving pediatric patients aged 6 months to 16 years, Reed and others (2001) characterized the pharmacokinetic profile of both oral and intravenous midazolam using noncompartment models. After oral administration, midazolam absorption was rapid with adolescents absorbing the drug at half that seen with children younger than 12 years. In young children, the volumes of distribution were larger; the largest volume of distribution was observed in children, whereas adolescents had a slower clearance and longer half-life after intravenous administration. There was little effect of age on volume of distribution or clearance and the half-life was slightly shorter in children (Reed et al., 2001).

The pharmacokinetics of rectally administered midazolam in children were reported by Saint-Maurice and others (1986). In this study of 16 children administered 0.3 mg/kg, the terminal half-life and clearance were 106 minutes and 42.5 mL/kg per minute, respectively. Differences in the plasma clearance rates between pharmacokinetic studies involving rectal, oral, and intramuscular forms of administration were probably related to changes in drug bioavailability. Decreases in bioavailability increase the apparent drug clearance.

Commercially prepared solutions for oral midazolam are available. Literature on the pharmacokinetics and pharmacodynamics of oral midazolam has been hindered by the fact that studies have used different vehicles for administering the drug. Different vehicles affect drug absorption and, consequently, onset time and drug bioavailability (Brosius and Bannister, 2003). In addition, concurrent antacid use and grapefruit juice may increase the onset time and drug bioavailability (Lammers et al., 2002; Goho, 2001) of midazolam.

Population studies involving the pharmacokinetics of midazolam in neonates have been reported. Using NONMEM and a two-compartment model, 531 midazolam concentrations from 187 infants were analyzed. The clearance and the central volume were noted to be 70 ± 13 mL/kg per hour and 591 ± 65 mL/kg, respectively. Of interest was that the clearance was 1.6× higher in neonates with a gestational age of more than 39 weeks than in neonates of less than 39 weeks (Burtin et al., 1994).

The pharmacokinetics of midazolam in premature infants after both oral and intravenous administration were described by de Wildt and others (2002, 2001). In premature infants, 24 to 34 weeks' gestational age and 3 to 11 days of age, de Wildt and others noted the apparent volume of distribution, clearance, and half-life were 1.1 L/kg, 1.8 mL/kg per minute, and 6.3 hours, respectively, after a single 0.1-mg/kg bolus dose. In addition, the metabolite 1-OH midazolam was markedly reduced compared with reports in older children. Also of note was that in those infants exposed to indomethacin, midazolam clearance was increased (de Wildt et al., 2001) (Fig. 6–12).

In a separate study of preterm infants who were administered oral midazolam, de Wildt and others (2002) noted that midazolam clearance was markedly decreased and the bioavailability was 0.4. The decrease in clearance was thought to mirror the pattern of CYP3A4 intestinal and hepatic activity (de Wildt et al., 2002). The kinetics of midazolam are affected by the use of extracorporeal membrane oxygenation (ECMO); Mulla and others (2003) noted that the volume of distribution and half-life of midazolam are significantly increased in neonates requiring ECMO.

The cardiovascular and respiratory effects of midazolam have been reported in adults. Midazolam decreases systolic and diastolic blood pressures by 5% to 10%, decreases systemic vascular resistance by 15% to 30%, and increases heart rate by 20%. Right- and left-sided filling pressures are usually unaffected. Reeves and others (1979) observed that 0.2 mg/kg midazolam was a safe agent for induction of anesthesia in patients with

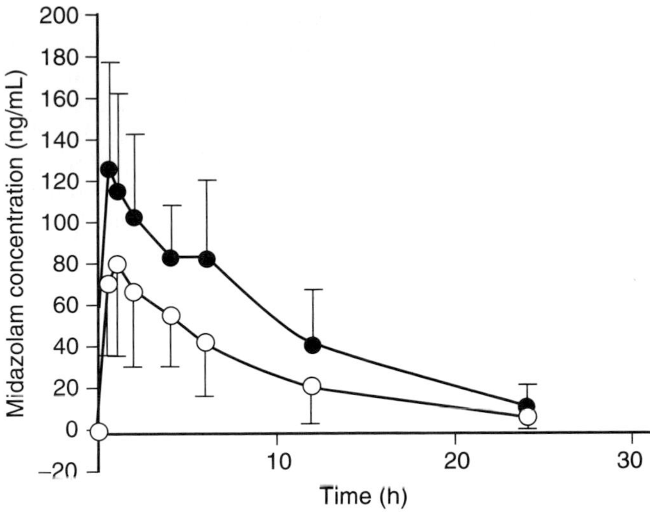

■ **FIGURE 6–12.** Effect of postnatal indomethacin exposure on midazolam disposition in preterm infants. Midazolam concentration versus time curve after a single intravenous dose (0.1 mg/kg) to preterm infants with (n = 11, open circles) and without (n = 13, solid circles) postnatal indomethacin exposure. Each dot represents mean ± SD concentration at each time point. (Redrawn from de Wildt SN, Kearns GL, Hop WCJ, et al.: *Clin Pharmacol Ther* 70:525–531, 2001.)

compromised myocardial function. In healthy patients (Lebowitz et al., 1982), no significant difference was found in the hemodynamic effects of induction doses of 0.25 mg/kg midazolam and 4 mg/kg thiopental.

Respiratory depression is frequently associated with midazolam administration, and this respiratory depression is poorly related to dose, not reversed by naloxone, and independent of the rate of administration of the drug (Forster et al., 1983; Alexander and Gross, 1988; Alexander et al., 1992).

As an intravenous induction agent in children, midazolam in doses as high as 0.6 mg/kg was not as reliable as thiopental (Salonen et al., 1987). The most common pediatric use for intravenous midazolam other than as an anesthetic adjunct has been its use as a sedative for intensive care patients. Rosen and Rosen (1991) demonstrated the usefulness of continuous midazolam in critically ill pediatric patients. In their retrospective report of patients sedated for 4 to 72 hours who received a slow intravenous bolus (0.25 mg/kg) followed by a continuous infusion at 0.4 to 4.0 mg/kg per minute, they noted that all of their patients were adequately sedated, their patients' oxygen consumption was significantly reduced, and enteral feedings were successful in all of those in whom it was attempted. However, others have noted reversible neurologic abnormalities associated with prolonged intravenous midazolam infusions (Engstrom and Cohen, 1989; Sury et al., 1989; Bergman et al., 1991).

Even with the extensive experience of intravenous midazolam in adult patients and volunteers, most of the pediatric experience with midazolam is derived from its use as a preanesthetic medication delivered via the intramuscular, oral, rectal, intranasal, and sublingual routes of administration. More than 85% of anesthesiologists responding to a survey of premedication practices indicated that they prescribe midazolam (Kain et al., 1997). In children, midazolam has been shown to produce tranquil and calm sedation, reduce separation anxiety, facilitate induction of anesthesia, and enhance antegrade amnesia (Twersky et al., 1993). Kain and others (2000) have shown that 0.5 mg/kg of oral midazolam can produce significant anterograde amnesia at 10 and 20 minutes, and anxiolysis as early as 15 minutes after administration.

Numerous studies have documented the efficacy of orally administered midazolam (Feld et al., 1990; Weldon et al., 1992; Levine et al., 1993b). The appropriate dose appears to range between 0.5 and 1.0 mg/kg. Its time of onset ranges from 15 to 30 minutes. Oral midazolam can also be safely administered to children with cyanotic heart disease without affecting oxygen saturation (Levine et al., 1993a). Serious side effects of midazolam are uncommon. However, potential postoperative behavior problems (fearfulness, nightmares, food rejection) were observed in children premedicated with oral (0.5 mg/kg) midazolam (McGraw, 1993). In addition, McMillan and others (1992) have noted loss of balance, dysphoria, and blurred vision in some patients receiving 0.75 and 1.0 mg/kg orally. Hiccups have been associated with midazolam administration via the rectal, nasal, and oral routes (Marhöfer et al., 1999). The major disadvantage of oral midazolam is its bitter taste; it has to be administered in a flavored syrup or drink; however, a commercially available liquid preparation is now available.

Oral midazolam has been associated with prolonged recovery times in some children (Viitanen and others (1999), but studies by Brosius and Bannister (2001, 2002) using bispectral index and measured end-tidal gases refute this.

In a multicenter study involving 455 children, Coté and others (2002) reported on the effectiveness of commercially prepared midazolam syrup. In this study, oral midazolam was effective for sedation and anxiolysis at a dose as low as 0.25 mg/kg. Doses as high as 1.0 mg/kg had minimal effect on respiration and oxygen saturation (Fig. 6–13).

Rectal administration of midazolam has been successfully used to sedate patients. Saint Maurice and others (1986) have shown that after a dose of 0.3 mg/kg, a maximum plasma concentration of 100 ng/mL was achieved with levels of sedation as judged by mask acceptance, with patient cooperation being satisfactory in all 16 patients. Coventry and others (1991), in

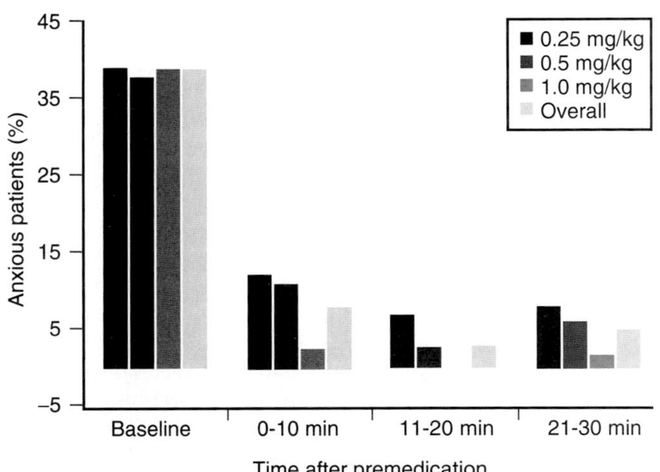

■ **FIGURE 6–13.** Percentage of patients exhibiting anxiety from baseline to time after oral midazolam. There was a positive association between dose and onset of anxiolysis ($P = 0.01$); a larger proportion of children achieved satisfactory anxiolysis within 10 minutes at the higher doses. (Redrawn from Coté CJ, Cohen IT, Suresh S, et al.: *Anesth Analg* 94:374, 2002.)

a double-blind study of pediatric patients requiring sedation for computed tomography evaluations, noted that 0.3 and 0.6 mg/kg of rectal midazolam was ineffective in providing satisfactory sedation. Spear and others (1991) noted that the optimum dose of rectal midazolam was 1.0 mg/kg and that doses of 0.3 mg/kg resulted in patient struggling during anesthesia induction.

Nasal and sublingual transmucosal routes of administration have also been used for midazolam preanesthesia medications. Wilton and others (1988) and Davis and others (1995a) demonstrated the usefulness of preanesthetic sedation of preschool children with 0.2 to 0.3 mg/kg of intranasal midazolam. Walbergh and others (1991) determined plasma concentrations after administration of 0.1 mg/kg of intranasal midazolam. In these patients, peak plasma concentrations of midazolam occurred within 10 minutes after its administration, with peak plasma concentrations ranging from 43 to 106 ng/mL. In this study, plasma midazolam concentrations exceeded threshold sedation values for adults (40 ng/kg) as early as 3 minutes after its nasal administration and exceeded this level for as long as 30 minutes. Because intranasal midazolam can irritate the nasal mucosa, its use is limited by the volume of drug to be administered. The sublingual mucosa has a rich vascular supply and drugs are absorbed systemically, thereby eliminating hepatic first-pass metabolism. Karl and others (1993), in a comparative study of intranasal and sublingual midazolam administration, demonstrated the two routes to be equally effective but that the sublingual route of administration had better patient acceptance.

Pandit and others (2001) demonstrated that when aliquots of midazolam dissolved in strawberry syrup were placed on the anterosuperior aspect of the child's tongue, 0.2 mg of midazolam was effective in 95% of patients for parental separation. When midazolam was administered sublingually, Khalil and others (1998) noted that in children aged 12 to 129 months who received either placebo or one of three doses of midazolam, none of the children receiving placebo, 28% of those receiving 0.25 mg/kg, 52% of those receiving 0.5 mg/kg, and 64% of those receiving 0.75 mg/kg of midazolam showed satisfactory sedation (drowsy) 15 minutes after drug administration. Children receiving the two higher doses of midazolam (0.5 and 0.75 mg/kg) accepted mask induction willingly, whereas the group receiving 0.25 mg/kg resembled the placebo group.

Flumazenil

Flumazenil blocks the effects of benzodiazepines on the GABAergic inhibition pathway in the CNS. Flumazenil does not have much agonist activity of its own and does not appear to reverse the effects of opioids. Flumazenil has a short duration of action. Its plasma half-life is between 0.7 and 1.3 hours. It is metabolized and cleared by the liver and excreted in the urine (Rocari et al., 1986). Adverse effects of flumazenil include nausea, vomiting, blurred vision, sweating, anxiety, and emotional lability. Serious adverse events include seizures and cardiac dysrhythmias; these serious events have been associated with patients physically dependent on benzodiazepines, patients with epilepsy, and patients having taken multiple drug ingestions or overdoses. Clinical trials in adults suggest a use of flumazenil in reversing the effects of conscious sedation, general anesthesia in benzodiazepine overdose, and hepatic encephalopathy.

Use of midazolam in pediatric patients has been related to clinical situations requiring benzodiazepine reversal in anesthesia and for the treatment of benzodiazepine overdose (Roald and Dohl, 1989; Jones et al., 1991). Doses of flumazenil varied between 0.005 and 0.1 mg/kg, with 0.01 mg/kg being the most frequently used dose. In a study of 107 children undergoing procedural sedation, Shannon and others (1997) noted that a mean dose of 0.017 mg/kg of flumazenil was used to reverse a mean midazolam dose of 0.18 mg/kg (Shannon et al., 1997). Because of its short half-life relative to the half-life of most benzodiazepines, resedation is a frequent finding after flumazenil use. Consequently, repeat administrations and careful patient observations are necessary (Jones, et al., 1993).

Nonbarbiturate Nonbenzodiazepines

Etomidate

Etomidate is a potent, short-acting, nonbarbiturate sedative-hypnotic agent without analgesic properties. It produces a central depressant effect through γ-aminobutyric acid (GABA) mimetic action. Administered intravenously, it has been used for induction and maintenance of anesthesia as well as for prolonged sedation in critically ill patients. Little information is available about etomidate in infants and small children.

Etomidate is metabolized in the liver. Only 2% of the drug appears unchanged in the urine. Etomidate causes little change in cardiovascular function in either healthy or compromised patients (Guldner et al., 2003). In a study of children with ASDs undergoing cardiac catheterizaion, Sarkar and others (2005) noted that induction doses of intravenous etomidate had no significant effect on the hemodynamics or on the shunt fraction ($\dot{Q}p{:}\dot{Q}s$). Myoclonic movements that are not associated with ipileptiform electroencephalographic activity (Ghonheim and Yamanda, 1977) occur in 30% to 75% of patients after induction with etomidate.

Etomidate has both anticonvulsant and proconvulsant qualities. In patients with known seizure disorders, etomidate can produce epileptiform activity (Ebrahim et al., 1986; Modica et al., 1990). The major side effect regarding etomidate is it can suppress adrenal steroid synthesis and increase mortality (Ledinham and Watt, 1983). Etomidate blocks adrenal steroid synthesis through inhibition of two mitochondrial enzymes dependent on CYP: cholesterol side-chain cleavage enzyme and 11β-hydroxylase (Wagner et al., 1984). The inhibition of steroid synthesis occurs with both prolonged continuous infusions and with single induction doses (Wagner and White, 1984; Longnecker, 1984). In 30 children undergoing cardiopulmonary bypass, Donmez and others (1998) in a randomized prospective study noted that when etomidate (0.3 mg/kg) was used as an induction agent, it significantly suppressed the increased cortisol levels associated with the stress response of surgery and cardiopulmonary bypass. For induction of anesthesia, the recommended intravenous dose is 0.3 to 0.4 mg/kg.

Propofol

Propofol is an alkyl phenol that is formulated in 10% soybean oil, 2.25% glycerol, and 12% purified egg phosphatide. This form of reconstitution is used because of anaphylactic reactions that occurred when propofol was reconstituted with Cremophor EL. The rapid redistribution and metabolism of propofol result in a short duration of action and allow for the drug to be administered via repeated injections or continuous infusions with minimal accumulation. Kinetic studies in both adults and children reveal a drug with a large steady state, a slow elimination half-life, and a rapid clearance. In radiolabeled isotope studies, 88% of the radioactivity is excreted in the urine, 2% is excreted in the feces, and the remainder is excreted as 1- and 4-glucuronides and 4-sulfate conjugates. In patients with hepatic and renal impairment, no statistically significant alterations occur in the pharmacokinetics. Because the clearance of the drug exceeds the capacity of the liver blood supply, extrahepatic sites of metabolism appear to be involved with the clearance of propofol. These extrahepatic sites of metabolism were suggested in studies of patients undergoing liver transplantation where metabolic products of propofol metabolism were produced when propofol was administered only during the anhepatic phase of the operation. The effect of fentanyl on propofol clearance is not clear. In studies by Cockshott and others (1987), fentanyl decreased propofol clearance, whereas in other studies, no effect was noted (Saint Maurice et al., 1989; Gill et al., 1990).

Another important aspect of propofol pharmacokinetics is that the drug can limit its own clearance. Propofol is eliminated by hepatic conjugation to inactive metabolites, which are excreted by the kidneys. A 2-mg/kg bolus dose of propofol for the induction of anesthesia can reduce blood flow to the liver by 14%. Bolus doses of propofol may cause a small but persistent change in blood flow to the liver, resulting in decreased clearance and higher-than-predicted plasma concentrations.

The pharmacokinetics of propofol in children were described by numerous investigators (Saint-Maurice et al., 1989; Jones et al., 1990; Marsh et al., 1991; Kataria et al., 1994; Knibbe et al., 2002; Zuppa et al., 2003). In computer-controlled infusions of propofol in children younger than 10 years, Marsh and others (1991) noted the volume of the central compartment to be 0.34 L/kg and the clearance of the drug to be 34.3 mL/kg per minute. Kataria and others (1994), using three different pharmacokinetic modeling approaches, analyzed the kinetics of single-bolus and continuous infusions of propofol in children. In all three models, the pharmacokinetics were well described by a three-compartment model with a central compartment of 0.52 L/kg and a clearance of 34 mL/kg per minute.

The pharmacokinetics of propofol were studied in a small number of children after cardiac surgery. When propofol was used to provide sedation for 6 hours, Knibbe and others (2002), using population kinetics, reported propofol to have a two-compartment model with a clearance of 35 mL/kg per minute and a central compartment of 0.78 L/kg. In addition, the authors suggested that children may have a lower pharmacodynamic sensitivity to propofol in that higher plasma concentrations were needed to maintain sedation.

The pharmacodynamics of propofol have been well described and reviewed (Glass, 1993). Because of the pharmacokinetic properties of propofol, infusions allow for more rapid decreases in plasma concentrations (Shafer, 1993) (Fig. 6–14) and allow for faster patient recoveries from anesthesia (Mirakhur, 1988; Borgeat et al., 1990; Watcha et al., 1991; Larsson et al., 1992; Lebovic et al., 1992; Nightingale and Lewis, 1992; Reimer et al., 1993).

In general, with induction doses of propofol, blood pressure decreases, as does systemic vascular resistance. Changes in heart rate are variable, and cardiac output decreases slightly. In studies evaluating propofol requirements for induction of anesthesia in children, Manschot and others (1992) noted that in children aged 3 to 15 years receiving 5 mg/kg of alfentanil to reduce the pain of propofol injection, age-related differences in propofol requirements were demonstrated. In children aged 10 to 15 years, 1.5 mg/kg of propofol was sufficient to induce sleep, whereas in children aged 3 to 9 years, a dose of 2.5 mg/kg was needed.

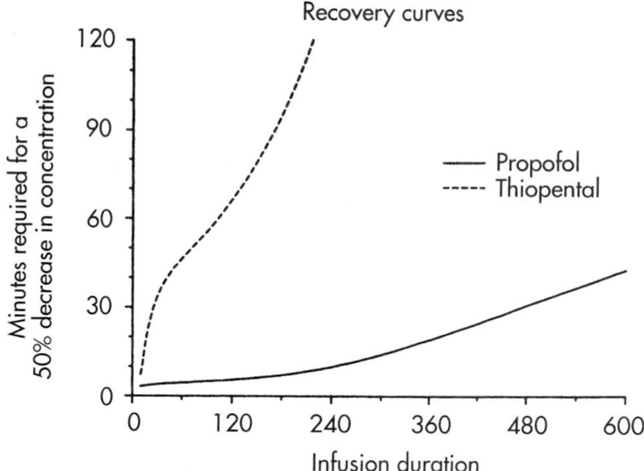

■ **FIGURE 6–14.** Curves showing time required for a 50% decrease in propofol and thiopental concentration after discontinuation of a continuous infusion. (With permission from Shafer SL: *J Clin Anesth* 5:145, 1993.)

In a study by Hannallah and others (1991) in which alfentanil was not administered, the ED_{50} and ED_{95} for loss of eyelash reflex were 1.3 and 2.0 mg/kg, whereas the ED_{50} and ED_{95} for induction of anesthesia were 1.5 and 2.3 mg/kg, respectively. Westrin (1991), in a study of infants aged 1 to 6 months and children aged 10 to 16 years, noted that the ED_{50} of propofol was 3.0 mg/kg for infants and 2.4 mg/kg for the older children. In all three of these studies, propofol was administered over 10 to 30 seconds. However, as with most hypnotic agents, propofol also demonstrates a rate-dependent induction. Stokes and Hutton (1991) demonstrated that with the use of slower infusion rates, induction time for anesthesia increases but smaller doses could be used.

In patients with congenital heart disease, Gozal and others (2001) demonstrated that despite lower systemic and pulmonary pressures, propofol did not modify the characteristics of the patient's underlying intracardiac shunts.

In normal children aged 1 to 6 years, Karsli and others (2002), using transcranial Doppler, noted that propofol decreases cerebral blood flow velocity and that there is a relationship between cerebral blood flow velocity and propofol dosing. In addition, Wilson-Smith and others (2003) noted that in healthy children administered propofol for their elective surgery, the effects of nitrous oxide on cerebral blood flow velocity were preserved.

In addition to its anesthetic action, propofol appears to have antiemetic properties. In adult patients, Borgeat and others (1992) demonstrated that 10 mg of propofol administered in the recovery room was effective in reducing the incidence of nausea and vomiting. In pediatric patients, Watcha and others (1991) noted that in patients undergoing strabismus surgery, propofol alone effectively decreases the incidence of postoperative emesis compared with a similar group of patients anesthetized with halothane and nitrous oxide and supplemented with prophylactic droperidol 23% versus 50%. However, in patients who received propofol and nitrous oxide, Watcha and others (1991) noted that the incidence of emesis increased significantly (60%). Weil and others (1993) also noted the antiemetic effect in pediatric strabismus patients anesthetized with propofol and nitrous oxide compared with patients anesthetized with halothane and nitrous oxide. This antiemetic effect of propofol was even more pronounced in patients who received no opioids. Reimer and others (1993) noted no difference in the incidence of emesis between pediatric patients undergoing strabismus repair anesthetized with halothane and nitrous oxide and those receiving propofol in oxygen or propofol with nitrous oxide. Differences between studies with regard to the antiemetic effect of propofol may be a function of the basic design of each study. Variations in premedications, opioid administration, and postoperative fluid intake may be factors that make comparisons of the studies difficult.

The antiemetic effects of propofol have also been demonstrated in pediatric patients undergoing short ear, nose, and throat surgical procedures (Borgeat et al., 1990) and ambulatory surgical procedures (Martin et al., 1993).

In patients undergoing radiofrequency ablation, a procedure that is associated with emesis as frequently as 60%, Erb and others (2002) noted that propofol-based anesthesia was associated with a markedly decreased incidence of nausea (21%) and emesis (6%) compared with a rate of nausea and vomiting of 63% and 55%, respectively, in children anesthetized with isoflurane.

Side effects from propofol include tolerance to the drug, pain on injection, spontaneous excitatory movements, and anaphylactic reactions. Tolerance has been reported in a pediatric patient undergoing numerous exposures for radiation therapy (Deer and Rich, 1992). Pain on injection is a common problem with propofol administration and may be related to the size of the vein in which it is administered. Westrin (1991) noted that pain on injection occurred more frequently in the infants (50%) than in the older children (18%). The addition of 5 mg/kg of alfentanil, 1% xylocaine (1 mg), or 0.1 mg/kg xylocaine can markedly attenuate the pain on injection (Valtonen et al., 1989; Manschot et al., 1992). The addition of thiopental (Cox, 2002) and the use of inhaled nitrous oxide (Beh et al., 2002) also have been shown to attenuate the pain on injection.

Involuntary motor movements have been associated with propofol (Reynolds and Koh, 1993), and these spontaneous movement disorders appear to occur in the absence of epileptic form activity on electroencephalography (Borgeat et al., 1993). Anaphylactic reactions have also been reported. Initial studies with propofol using 10% Cremophor EL as a solubilizing agent had reported instances of anaphylactic reactions (Briggs et al., 1982). Laxenaire and others (1992) have reported on 14 patients with life-threatening reactions within minutes after receiving propofol in its current preparation. In some patients, these anaphylaxis reactions occurred during the patient's first exposure to propofol.

Because of its lipid base, propofol has been associated with bacterial growth and patient infection if strict aseptic techniques during handling are not observed. Because of patient safety concerns, 0.005% EDTA or metabisulfite was added to the formulation by different manufacturers. In a study comparing propofol with and without EDTA, Cohen and others (2001) noted no differences in clinical profiles between the two drugs and noted that both formulations lower ionized calcium without any apparent clinical effect.

Ketamine

Ketamine is a racemic nonbarbiturate cyclohexamine derivative that produces dissociation of the cortex from the limbic system. Ketamine appears to block afferent impulses in the diencephalon and associated pathways of the cortex, sparing the reticular formation of the brain stem. This may be the mechanism of its action. It may also act on the brain stem (Domino et al., 1965). There frequently is electroencephalographic seizure activity, particularly in the limbic system and cortex, without clinical manifestations (Schwartz et al., 1974). Clinically ketamine anesthetic produces effective analgesia, but patients may keep their eyes open. Many reflexes are preserved. Preservation of gag reflex, laryngeal irritability, and continued muscle tension occur. Two mg/kg produces a highly predictable response in children. On a milligram-per-kilogram basis, the amount of ketamine required to prevent gross movements is four times greater in infants younger than 6 months than in 6-year-old children (Lockhart and Nelson, 1974).

TABLE 6–7. Pharmacokinetics of ketamine: effect of age

Age	$t_{1/2}\beta$ (min)	Vd_{ss} (L/kg)	CL (mL/min per kg)
<3 mo	184.7	3.46	12.9
4 to 12 mo	65.1	3.03	35.0
4 yr	31.6	1.18	25.1
Adult	107.3	0.75	20.0

$t_{1/2}\beta$, Elimination half-life; Vd_{ss}, volume of distribution at steady state; CL, clearance.

Modified from Lake CL: *Pediatric anesthesia.* East Norwalk, CT, 1988, Appleton & Lange.

White and others (1980) compared both the L- and D-isomers of ketamine in adult surgical patients with respect to the efficacy and side effects of these isomers. In this study they noted that the *d*-isomer produced the most satisfactory anesthetic state and the lowest incidence of negative emergence reactions, whereas the *l*-isomer produced the least satisfactory anesthesia and the highest incidence of emergence reactions.

The pharmacokinetics of ketamine in patients of different ages were determined (Table 6–7). In infants younger than 3 months, the volume of distribution was similar to that in older infants but the elimination half-life was prolonged. Clearance was reduced in the younger infants; reduced metabolism and renal excretion in the young infant are the likely causes. Ketamine is metabolized in the liver, and its major metabolite is norketamine. Norketamine has about 30% of the clinical activity of ketamine.

In the "anesthetic" state associated with ketamine, respiration and blood pressure are usually well maintained. The use of ketamine in infants, particularly at the high doses required for lack of movement, has been associated with respiratory depression and apnea (Eng et al., 1975). Generalized extensor spasm with opisthotonos also has been seen in infants (Radney and Badola, 1973). In addition, acute increases in pulmonary artery pressure have occasionally occurred in infants with congenital heart disease during ketamine anesthesia for cardiac catheterization. Studies suggest that pulmonary vascular resistance is not changed by ketamine in infants with either normal or elevated pulmonary vascular resistance as long as the airway and ventilation are maintained (Hickey et al., 1984; Murray et al., 1984).

The mechanism of cardiorespiratory stimulation has not been entirely clarified. Dowdy and Kaya (1968), Traber and others (1970), and other groups have shown that there is a direct negative inotropic action on denervated heart. In the presence of intact sympathetic and autonomic nervous systems, however, a pressor effect causes increased blood pressure, heart rate, and cardiac output, a response present at all ages. This serves as a most valuable adjunct in management of poor-risk patients but is a contraindication in the presence of hypertension or tachycardia. In their investigation of ketamine, Dowdy and Kaya (1968) also found evidence of antiarrhythmic activity.

Ketamine increases cerebrospinal fluid pressure significantly for 5 to 15 minutes (Gardner et al., 1971; Lockhart and Jenkins, 1972), but as shown by Dawson and others (1971), the increase may be held within acceptable limits by pretreatment with thiopental. Elevation of intraocular pressure also occurs after ketamine administration. In a group of 15 children, Yoshikawa and Murai (1971) noted an average increase of 30% that was maximum within 15 minutes after administration of ketamine and evident for approximately 30 minutes. In addition to the elevation of intraocular pressure, nystagmus movements limit its usefulness in eye surgery.

With the present concern over toxicity of anesthetic agents, ketamine has the advantage of a clean record with no known toxic effects on liver, kidney, or other organ systems. The major drawback to ketamine administration is the high incidence of hallucinations and bad dreams. In adults, this occurs in 30% to 50% of patients, and in prepubescent children, the incidence is noted at 5% to 10%. Hallucinations were uncommon in children, but the awakening phase may entail considerable excitement (Wilson et al., 1970).

Ketamine can be administered orally, and part of its effect is secondary to its metabolic norketamine. Gutstein and colleagues compared oral premedication with ketamine at either 3 or 6 mg/kg. With 3 mg, 73% of the children were sedated within 30 minutes. At the 6 mg/kg dose, 100% of the patients were sedated and 67% tolerated intravenous cannulation. Onset times for the 3- and 6-mg/kg dose groups were 19.6 and 11.2 minutes, respectively (Gutstein et al., 1992).

OPIOIDS

To avoid the major adverse hemodynamic effects caused by potent inhalation anesthetic agents, the use of narcotic anesthesia has reemerged. Relative potencies of the various narcotics are listed in Table 6–8. Initially, meperidine (0.5 to 1.0 mg/kg) and morphine (0.05 to 0.1 mg/kg) were used to reinforce nitrous oxide anesthesia in the neonate. However, concerns regarding the toxicity and increased sensitivity of neonates to narcotics were raised. Way and others (1965) have demonstrated that morphine depresses newborn respiration more than does meperidine and that these decreases in respiration occur at a dose one third (on a milligram-per-kilogram basis) of that administered to adults. In laboratory animals, narcotics are more toxic to newborn animals than to older animals (Goldenthal, 1971). For morphine and dihydromorphine, the blood–brain barrier is more permeable in newborn animals than in older animals. The brain concentration of morphine several hours after injection was two to four times greater in brains of younger rats despite equal blood concentration. This finding may be related to greater perfusion, to greater permeability, or to both in the newborn. Such developmentally increased permeability is not seen with meperidine (Kupferberg and Way, 1963); this is not surprising because the lipid solubility of meperidine is quite high.

TABLE 6–8. Comparative narcotic potencies

Drug	Potency
Morphine	1
Meperidine	0.1
Alfentanil	40
Fentanyl	150
Sufentanil	1500

Studies involving opiate receptor–binding sites in rats have suggested that changes in receptor ontogeny also may be responsible for the respiratory depressant and analgesic effects observed in newborns. Zhang and others (1981) have shown that both low-affinity and high-affinity opiate receptors are present in rats. Low-affinity receptors are associated with respiratory depression, whereas high-affinity receptors are associated with analgesia. In the rat model, low-affinity receptors are present in large numbers at birth, and the number remains constant to 18 days of life. By contrast, high-affinity receptors are scarce at birth and do not reach significant proportions (50% of the adult value) until 15 days of life. Respiratory depression in infants may be a function not only of the lipophilicity of opioids but also of the maturational changes in the opiate receptor pool. In addition to age-related changes in opioid receptor pools, genetic factors may affect the OPRMJ opioid receptor. Single nucleotide polymorphisms, resulting in a single amino acid change, can have effects on opioid side effects and analgesia (Matthes et al., 1996; Klepstad et al., 2004; Romberg et al., 2004, 2005).

Clinical studies on opioid sensitivity have been conflicting. Early reports by Kupferberg and Way suggested neonates had more respiratory depression after opioid administration than did adults. However, Lynn and others (1993) evaluated the respiratory depressant effects of intravenous morphine infusions in 30 patients aged 2 to 570 days and noted no evidence of a relationship of any given morphine concentration with respiratory depression and age.

Nichols and others (1993) studied the extent and duration of respiratory depression after intrathecal administration of 0.02 mg/kg of morphine to 10 patients aged 4 months to 15 years. Although intrathecal morphine depresses ventilation for at least 18 hours, there was no relationship of age and ventilatory depression.

Age-related sensitivities have also been studied after intravenous fentanyl administration. Hertzka and others (1989) determined that fentanyl-induced ventilatory depression as assessed by skin surface PCO_2 and ventilatory patterns was not greater in infants older than 3 months than in children or adults. In addition to age sensitivities, Zhou and others (1993) demonstrated ethnic differences in the disposition and effects of morphine.

Morphine

The pharmacology of morphine has been studied in both adults and children. In adults, morphine is 30% to 35% protein bound, while in neonates, it is 18% to 22% bound (Bhat et al., 1990). Morphine is a drug with a high hepatic extraction coefficient; consequently, morphine clearance is determined by hepatic blood flow. Increases in hepatic blood flow can further increase morphine clearance, whereas decreases in hepatic blood flow can lower drug clearance. Morphine is inactivated by *N*-demethylation and glucuronidation. The two major metabolic products are morphine 6-glucuronide and morphine 3-glucuronide, which are mainly excreted by the kidney. In adults, sulfate metabolism accounts for 5% to 10% of the drug metabolism. Although in neonates the enzymes for glucuronide metabolism are immature and the role of sulfation in morphine metabolism may be more pronounced, Choonara and others (1989) demonstrated that in the neonate sulfation contributes little to morphine metabolism.

As with other drugs, morphine appears to undergo age-related changes in its pharmacokinetic profile (Table 6–9). The presence

■ **TABLE 6–9.** Morphine age-related pharmacokinetics

Reference	Age	No. of Patients	V_d (L/kg)	CL (mL/kg per min)	$t_{1/2}\beta$ (min)
Dahlstrom et al. (1979)	1 to 7 yr	8	1.13	6.17	183
Dahlstrom et al. (1979)	7 to 15 yr	8	1.36	6.71	202
Lynn and Slattery (1987)	2 to 4 days	7	3.3	6.3	408
Lynn and Slattery (1987)	17 to 65 days	4	5.15	23.8	234
Barret et al. (1991)	1 to 37 days	26	2.7	3.6	534

V_d, Volume of distribution; CL, clearance; $t_{1/2}\beta$, elimination half-life.

of age-related changes in the neonatal period appears somewhat controversial. Bhat and others (1990) studied the pharmacokinetics in 20 newborn infants less than 5 days of age after a single bolus administration of intravenous morphine. In this study, they concluded that with increasing gestational age, drug clearance increases by 0.9 mL/kg per minute per week gestation and that with increasing gestational age, both distribution and elimination half-life also decreased. Compared with term infants, Bhat and others noted that infants less than 30 weeks' gestation had a longer elimination half-life (50 versus 19 minutes) and slower clearances (3.4 versus 15 mL/kg per minute). However, Chay and others (1992) reported no difference in the pharmacokinetics of continuous morphine infusions in preterm and term infants. There was no reported correlation of gestational age or conceptual age with drug clearance or elimination half-life. In addition, these investigators noted that a plasma concentration of 125 ng/mL was necessary to provide adequate sedation in 50% of the neonates. These values are quite high compared with analgesic values of 12 ng/mL needed after cardiac surgery (Lynn et al., 1984).

In addition to age, morphine pharmacokinetics can be influenced by disease. Patients with renal failure were reported to be sensitive to narcotic intoxication after morphine administration. Chauvin and others (1987b) studied the pharmacokinetics of morphine in adult patients with renal insufficiency. For morphine, they found that patients with chronic renal failure have similar rates of clearance and half-lives but significantly smaller steady-state volumes of distribution compared with age- and weight-matched control patients. Although chronic renal failure did not alter the elimination of unchanged morphine, metabolites of morphine accumulated at higher plasma levels for longer periods of time in the patients with chronic renal failure (Chauvin et al., 1987b). In studies of patients with renal failure, Osbourne and others (1993) noted that morphine metabolism is impaired and that the metabolites of morphine (morphine 3-glucuronide and morphine 6-glucuronide) accumulate in the plasma (Fig. 6–15). Hanna and others (1993) have also demonstrated abnormal kinetics of morphine metabolites in patients with renal failure. Patients with renal failure had a prolonged elimination half-life and decreased clearance in the pharmacokinetic profile of morphine 6-glucuronide. In patients with renal impairment, the increased opioid sensitivity may be a function of decreased morphine metabolism coupled with impaired clearance of the metabolites.

In patients with liver disease, the effects of disease can be unpredictable. Patwardhan and others (1981) described the effects of liver disease on morphine kinetics in adult patients with cirrhosis and healthy adult volunteers. Compared with healthy subjects, patients with moderate-to-severe cirrhosis had a normal elimination and disposition of morphine but a prolonged elimination half-life and decreased clearance of indocyanine. Because morphine is a highly extracted drug and its clearance depends on hepatic blood flow, the investigators postulated that morphine has extrahepatic sites of metabolism in the gastrointestinal tract and kidneys.

In a limited study of 21 children aged 6 months to 10 years who underwent cardiopulmonary bypass for repair of their underlying heart defects, Dagan and others (1993) noted that morphine clearance in the postbypass period for patients requiring inotropic support was 50% less than that reported for other children.

In addition to intravenous infusions, intraspinal axis administration of opioids has been studied. In adults, Nordberg and others (1984) noted that after 0.5 mg of intrathecally (L2-4) administered morphine, the cerebrospinal fluid kinetics revealed a terminal half-life of 175 minutes, volume of cerebrospinal fluid distribution of 0.88 mL/kg, and a clearance of 2.8 mL/kg per minute. In pediatric patients undergoing craniofacial surgical repairs, Nichols and others (1993) noted that the cerebrospinal fluid concentrations at 6, 12, and 18 hours after 0.02 mg/kg intrathecal administration were 2860, 640, and 220 mg/mL, respectively.

In children, Attia and others (1986) demonstrated that the pharmacokinetics of epidural morphine were similar to values reported in adults. After a 50-mg/kg epidural bolus, the volume of distribution was 7.9 L/kg, the elimination half-life was 74 minutes, and the clearance was 28 mL/kg per minute. In addition to morphine pharmacokinetics, Attia and others noted that the onset and duration of analgesia were 30 minutes and 19 hours, respectively, and that respiratory depression as evidenced by changes in the slope of the ventilatory response to CO_2 was impaired for 22 hours after epidural administration.

Fentanyl

Fentanyl is a synthetic opiate with a clinical potency 50× to 100× that of morphine. It is metabolized by dealkylation, hydroxylation, and amide hydrolysis to inactive metabolites. It has a high hepatic extraction coefficient and a high pulmonary uptake (Roerig et al., 1987). In adults, Heberer noted that cirrhosis had no effect on fentanyl kinetics. Fentanyl has relatively minimal hemodynamic effects and is used both as an adjunct to nitrous oxide anesthesia and as a sole anesthetic agent. Bradycardia and chest wall rigidity are potential features of high-dose fentanyl anesthesia. The cardiovascular effects of fentanyl at doses of 30 to 75 mcg/kg fentanyl (with pancuronium) are minimal (Hickey et al., 1984). Modest decreases in mean arterial pressure and systemic vascular resistance index were noted by Hickey and others (1985).

In neonates, Murat and others (1988) have shown that although baroreceptor control of heart rate is present, fentanyl anesthesia (10 mcg/kg) can significantly depress the baroreceptor response to both hypotension and hypertension. Respiratory depression is probably concentration related as well. In adult comparative studies of opioid-induced respiratory depression with sufentanil and fentanyl administration, Bailey and others (1990) noted that ventilatory depression (both magnitude and

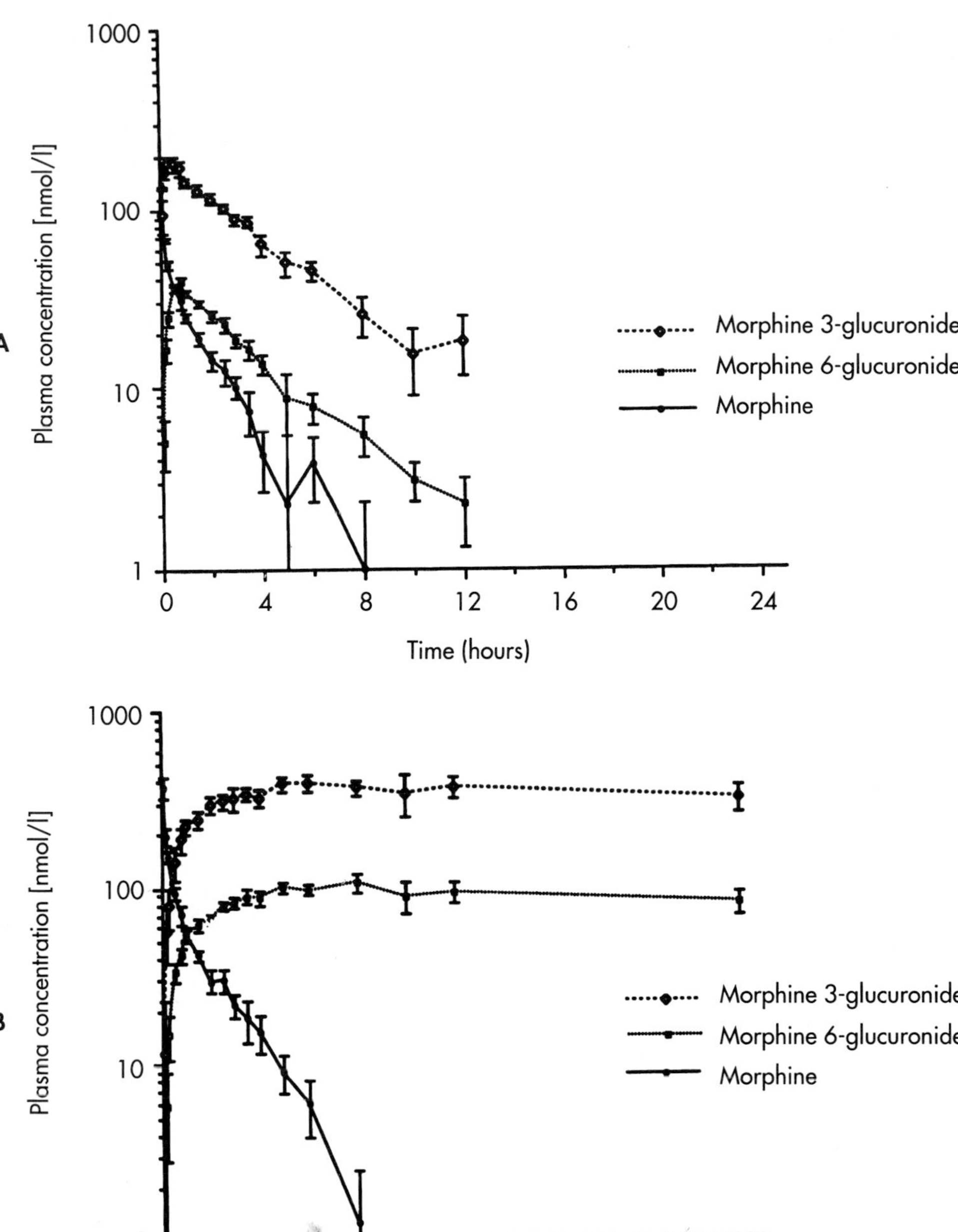

■ **FIGURE 6–15.** *(A)* Morphine and metabolite levels in normal volunteers (mean ± SEM; data correction to 10 mg/70 kg). *(B)* Pharmacokinetics of morphine and morphine glucuronides in patients with kidney failure. (With permission from Osborne R, Joel S, Grebenik K: *Clin Pharmacol Ther* 54:158, 1993.)

duration) was less after sufentanil administration. In addition, although the two drugs have similar half-lives, analgesia lasted longer after sufentanil administration.

The dose of fentanyl needed to ensure satisfactory anesthesia for infants varies with the surgical stress. Hickey and Retzack (1993) have shown that in a pediatric patient with reactive pulmonary vasculature, 25 mcg/kg of fentanyl was needed to prevent an acute episode of right ventricular failure secondary to pulmonary hypertension in the patient who was undergoing upper airway instrumentation and manipulation. Ellis and Steward (1990) have shown that in children undergoing hypothermic cardiopulmonary bypass or profound hypothermia with circulatory arrest anesthetized with fentanyl, a dose of at least 50 mcg/kg of fentanyl was needed to blunt the hyperglycemic response to hypothermia and circulatory arrest. Yaster (1987) noted that in neonates anesthetized with fentanyl, metocurine, and oxygen who were undergoing a wide variety of surgical procedures, fentanyl (10 to 12.5 mcg/kg) provided reliable hemodynamic stability for 75 minutes (Yaster, 1987).

In a study of children aged 6 months to 6 years undergoing cardiac surgery with cardiopulmonary bypass, Pirat and others (2002) compared three groups of patients. One group received intravenous fentanyl, the second group received intrathecal fentanyl, and the third group received both intravenous and intrathecal fentanyl. In this study, intrathecal fentanyl offered no advantage over intravenous fentanyl with regard to hemodynamic stability or suppression of the biochemical stress response. However, the combination of intrathecal and intravenous fentanyl was associated with better hemodynamic stability in the prebypass period compared with either group alone.

Duncan and others (2000) reported a dose-ranging study of 40 pediatric patients undergoing cardiac surgery using one of five intravenous fentanyl doses: 2, 25, 50, 100, and 150 mcg/kg. In this study, patients in the 2 mcg/kg group had significant rises in prebypass glucose, prebypass and postbypass cortisol, and prebypass and postbypass norepinephrine. No significant rise occurred in glucose, cortisol, and catecholamines in any of the higher dosage groups. Patients in the 2 mcg/kg group had significantly higher mean systolic blood pressure and heart rate. Higher doses of fentanyl (100 and 150 mcg/kg) offered little advantage over 50 mcg/kg.

Age-related differences in the kinetics and sensitivity to fentanyl and changes in kinetics associated with pathophysiologic conditions and types of surgery create variability and make generalizations difficult (Johnson et al., 1984; Collins et al., 1985; Koehntop et al., 1986; Singleton et al., 1987; Koren, et al., 1984). In the neonate, fentanyl clearance seems comparable to that of the older child or adult, whereas in the premature infant, fentanyl clearance is markedly reduced. In premature infants, fentanyl half-life was reported as 6 to 32 hours (Collins et al., 1985). In infants and children, fentanyl plasma concentrations were less than those in adults after similarly administered intravenous doses (milligrams per kilogram) (Singleton et al., 1987) (Fig. 6–16). These marked variations in kinetics reflect age differences and perhaps differences in anesthetic, dose, and duration of sampling.

Fentanyl pharmacokinetics after continuous infusions for less than 24 hours in critically ill children have demonstrated increased steady-state volume of distribution (15.2 L/kg), prolonged terminal elimination half-life (24 hours), and normal clearances (Katz and Kelly, 1993). The pharmacokinetics after 48 hours of continuous fentanyl infusion in newborns were reported in 12 neonates. In these infants (mean gestational age, 32 weeks; mean weight, 1.88 kg; mean postnatal age, 6 ± 9 days), the volume of distribution was noted as 17 ± 9 L/kg, total body clearance was 1154 mL/kg per hour, and the half-life was 9.5 ± 2.6 hours (Santeiro et al., 1997). In addition, the relatively high total body clearance was noted to correlate with postnatal age, suggesting that hepatic blood flow increases with age. Gauntlett and others (1988) found that fentanyl clearance increased with postnatal age, with most of the increase occurring by 2 weeks of age.

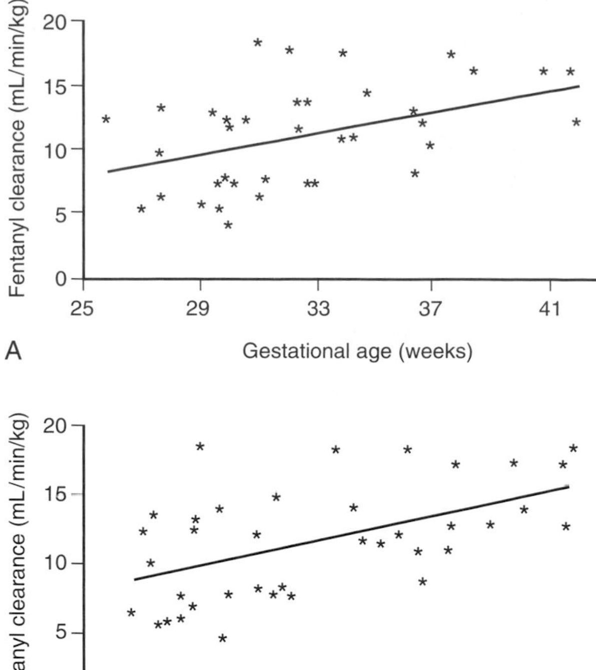

■ **FIGURE 6–17.** Plasma clearance of fentanyl correlates with gestational age and birth weight. (Redrawn with permission from Saarenmaa E, Neuvonen P, Fellman V: Gestational age and birth weight effects on plasma clearance of fentanyl in newborn infants. *J Pediatr* 136:767–770, 2000.)

In a study of nonsurgical neonates, Saarenmaa and others (2000) studied the fentanyl clearance in the first few days of life of 38 infants who were at 26 to 42 weeks gestation and had birth weights of 835 to 3550 g. This study reported a correlation of fentanyl clearances with gestational age and birth weight (Fig. 6–17).

Prolonged fentanyl infusions, however, were associated with tolerance. In neonates sedated with fentanyl via continuous

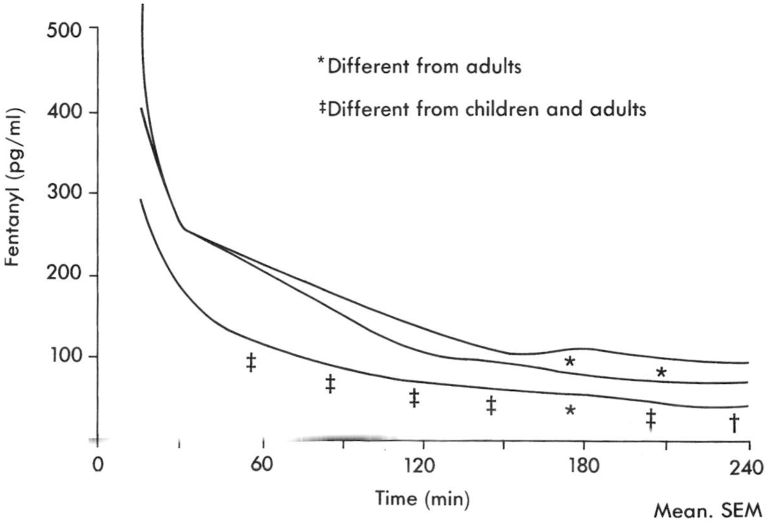

■ **FIGURE 6–16.** Fentanyl concentration-versus-time curves for adults *(top curve),* children *(middle curve),* and infants *(bottom curve).* (With permission from Singleton MA, Rosen JI, Fisher DM: *Can Anaesth Soc J* 34:152, 1987.)

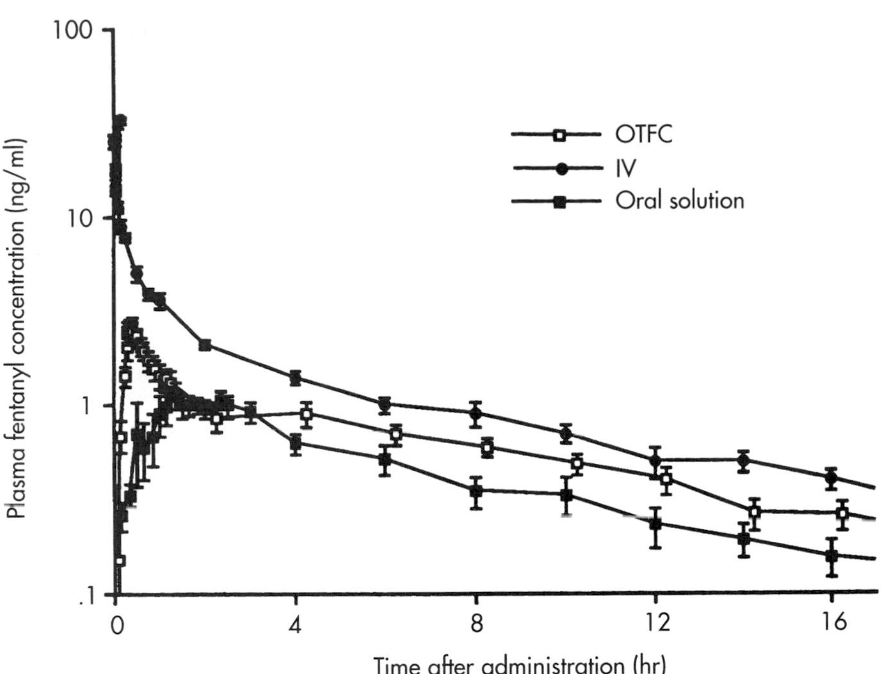

■ **FIGURE 6–18.** Plasma concentrations of fentanyl following oral transmucosal (OTFC), intravenous (IV), and oral administration. (With permission from Streisand JB, Varvel JR, Stanski DR: *Anesthesiology* 75:226, 1991.)

infusion while undergoing ECMO, Arnold and others (1991) noted that the daily infusion rates and plasma concentrations required to keep the infant sedated increased over time. Although prolonged continuous infusions of fentanyl may increase the volume of distribution, prolong the elimination half-life of the drug, and consequently prolong recovery on discontinuation, the development of tolerance may minimize this pharmacologic consequence.

In addition to intravenous administration, fentanyl has been administered transmucosally as a means of providing sedation to children. The pharmacokinetics and bioavailability of oral transmucosal fentanyl citrate (OTFC) were studied by Streisand and others (1991) using adult volunteers studied on three separate occasions (Fig. 6–18). Plasma levels of fentanyl were determined after either the intravenous, transmucosal, or gastrointestinal (oral) route of administration. Regardless of the mode of administration, the terminal elimination half-life was similar in all three groups (425 to 469 minutes). Compared with the oral group, peak plasma concentrations of fentanyl occurred earlier (22 versus 101 minutes) and were higher (30 versus 1.6 ng/mL) in the OTFC groups. The bioavailability of OTFC was 50% compared with 30% in the oral group. This difference in the bioavailability probably relates to the first-pass (hepatic extraction) effect observed with orally administered drugs (Streisand et al., 1991).

Intranasal administration of fentanyl has also been used to provide postoperative analgesia for pediatric patients (Galinkin et al., 2000; Manjushree et al., 2002). After 2 mcg/kg of intranasal fentanyl, Galinkin and others noted the mean fentanyl concentrations at 10 and 34 minutes were 0.8 and 0.6 ng/mL, respectively. In a study comparing intranasal fentanyl with intravenous fentanyl, Manjushree and others noted that onset time to analgesia after 1 mcg/kg of fentanyl was slower (13 minutes) for the intranasal route than for the intravenous route of administration (8 minutes).

Sufentanil

With the supposition that increase in potency is associated with increased opiate effects and decreased nonspecific cardiovascular effects, other fentanyl congeners have been developed. Sufentanil, a potent synthetic opioid, is an N-4 substituted derivative of fentanyl. It is a highly lipophilic compound that is distributed rapidly and extensively to all tissues. Sufentanil is approximately 5 to 10 times more potent than fentanyl and has an extremely high margin of safety. The major pathways for sufentanil metabolism involve *O*-demethylation and *N*-dealkylation; minimal amounts are excreted unchanged in urine. Desmethyl sufentanil, the major metabolite of sufentanil, possess about 10% the activity of the potent compound.

Pharmacokinetic and pharmacodynamic studies of sufentanil were conducted in infants, children, and adults. In adults, compared with fentanyl, the smaller volume of distribution (2.48 L/kg) and high clearance rate (11.3 mL/kg per minute) of sufentanil contribute to its short terminal elimination half-life (149 minutes). Meuldermans and others (1982) demonstrated that sufentanil is more protein bound (92%) than fentanyl (84%) and that pH affects protein binding. Decreasing pH from 7.4 to 7.0 increased protein binding by 28%; conversely, increasing pH from 7.4 to 7.8 decreased protein binding by 28%.

Clinical studies assessing the hemodynamic and endocrine stress response of sufentanil have been done in adults undergoing cardiopulmonary bypass (deLange et al., 1982; Sebel and Bovill, 1982). Sufentanil appears to block some of the stress responses to cardiac surgery. Stress-induced increases in antidiuretic hormone (ADH) and growth hormone (GH) appear to be blocked before, during, and after cardiopulmonary bypass, whereas the catecholamines (norepinephrine, epinephrine, and dopamine) show a large surge during the bypass and postbypass periods (deLange et al., 1982; Bovill et al., 1983). In a double-blind study, Rosow and others (1984) found the drugs, fentanyl and sufentanil, to be comparable with regard to hemodynamic stability.

■ **TABLE 6–10.** Hemodynamics during sufentanil anesthesia in infants and children undergoing open-heart surgery

Variable	Baseline	1 min	5 min	Incision	Sternotomy
Heart rate	140 ± 14	129 ± 25	118 ± 23*	116 ± 20*	123 ± 32
Systolic blood pressure	101 ± 9	86 ± 15*	74 ± 11*	99 ± 15	106 ± 13
Diastolic blood pressure	65 ± 10	48 ± 9*	46 ± 12*	65 ± 14	67 ± 13

Values are mean ± SD.
*$P<.01$ compared with baseline.
Reprinted with permission from the International Anesthesia Research Society from Davis PJ, Cook DR, Stiller RL, Davin-Robinson KA: Pharmacodynamics and pharmacokinetics of high-dose sufentanil in infants and children undergoing cardiac surgery. *Anesth Analg* 66:203, 1987.

The pharmacokinetic and pharmacodynamic effects of sufentanil in children were studied. Hickey and others (1984) compared the hemodynamic response of 5 and 10 mcg/kg of sufentanil to 50 to 75 mcg/kg of fentanyl in patients with complex congenital heart disease. Although heart rate and blood pressure changed slightly, they noted marked improvement in the patient's oxygenation with both fentanyl and sufentanil. They concluded that both sufentanil and fentanyl were safe anesthetics in high doses and that both agents favorably decreased pulmonary vascular resistance and thereby increased pulmonary blood flow and systemic oxygenation in patients with cyanotic heart disease. Davis and others (1987) examined both the pharmacodynamics and pharmacokinetics of high-dose sufentanil (15 mcg/kg) and oxygen in infants and children undergoing cardiac surgery. Sufentanil provided marked hemodynamic stability after an infusion and during the stress periods of incision and sternotomy (Table 6–10). The hemodynamic responses to sufentanil were similar to those noted by Hickey and others (1984) but differed from the increases in blood pressure and heart rate occurring after intubation, sternotomy, and incision observed in older children having repair of their congenital heart defect (Moore et al., 1985).

Greeley and others (1987) investigated age-related changes in the pharmacokinetics of sufentanil in pediatric patients undergoing cardiothoracic surgery. They noted that sufentanil best fit a three-compartment model and that neonates had significantly smaller clearance rates, larger volumes of distribution at steady state, and longer elimination half-lives than infants, children, and adolescents (Table 6–11). The developmental pharmacokinetic changes of improved clearance and elimination for sufentanil were further substantiated in another report in which infants were studied within the first 8 days of life and then again at 3 to 4 weeks of age (Greeley and de Bruijn, 1988).

Guay and others (1992) studied the pharmacokinetics of sufentanil in 20 healthy pediatric patients aged 2 to 8 years. After intravenous administration of 1 to 3 mcg/kg of sufentanil, the elimination half-life was 97 minutes, the volume of distribution at steady state was 2.9 L/kg, and the plasma clearance was 30.5. It is unclear whether the doubling of the plasma clearance value in healthy children was a function of the study design or the patient's underlying disease.

In addition to its use as an anesthetic agent, sufentanil has been used as a preanesthetic medication in children. Pharmacokinetic studies in adults after intravenous and intranasal administration show that the area under the curve from 0 to 120 minutes after intranasal dosing was 78% of that after intravenous injection (Helmers et al., 1989). By 30 minutes after drug administration, plasma sufentanil concentrations were identical for the two routes of administration.

The role of the kidney in sufentanil elimination and metabolism has not been well defined. The effects of renal failure in sufentanil kinetics were assessed in adolescent patients with chronic renal failure (Davis et al., 1988). Although there was no statistical difference in apparent volume of distribution, elimination, and clearance between patients with renal failure and control patients, patients with renal failure demonstrated more variability in clearance and half-life (Table 6–12). In patients with renal failure, sufentanil must be administered carefully on the basis of responses elicited in individual patients.

The pharmacodynamics of sufentanil were also evaluated in neurosurgical patients. The effects of opioids on intracranial pressure (ICP) and cerebral perfusion pressure have been controversial. In intubated patients with severe head injuries (Glasgow Coma Scale GCS < 8), sufentanil administration was associated

■ **TABLE 6–11.** Age-related pharmacokinetic values for sufentanil

Age	N	$t_{1/2}\alpha$ (min)	$t_{1/2}\beta$ (min)	CL (mL/kg per min)	Vd_{ss} (L/kg)
Neonates (0 to 8 days)	3	20.5	635	4.2	2.7
Neonates (20 to 28 days)	3	8.8	217	17.3	3.4
0 to 1 mo	9	23.4	737	6.7	4.15
1 mo to 2 yr	7	15.8	214	18.1	3.09
2 to 12 yr	7	19.6	140	16.9	2.73
12 to 16 yr	5	20.4	209	13.1	2.75

$t_{1/2}\alpha$, Distribution phase half-life; $t_{1/2}\beta$, elimination phase half-life; CL, clearance; Vd_{ss}, volume of distribution at steady state.
Reprinted with permission from the International Anesthesia Research Society from Greeley WJ, de Bruijn NP: Sufentanil pharmacokinetics in pediatric cardiovascular patients. *Anesth Analg* 67:86, 1988.

■ **TABLE 6–12.** Pharmacokinetics of sufentanil in adolescent patients with chronic renal failure (group 1) and in patients without renal disease (group 2)

Group	Vd_{180} (L/kg)	$t_{1/2}\alpha$ (min)	$t_{1/2}\beta_{180}$	CL (mL/kg per min)
1	1.65 ± 0.6	2.85 ± 1.7	89.7 ± 15.7	16.4 ± 6.1
2	1.28 ± 0.62	2.5 ± 0.73	76.0 ± 32.8	12.8 ± 12.0

Values are mean ± SD. Vd_{180}, Volume of distribution at 180 min; $t_{1/2}\alpha$, distribution phase half-life; $t_{1/2}\beta_{180}$, elimination phase half-life at 180 min; CL, clearance.
Reprinted with permission from the International Anesthesia Research Society from Davis PJ, Stiller RL, Cook DR, et al: Effects of cholestatic hepatic disease and chronic renal failure on alfentanil pharmacokinetics in children. *Anesth Analg* 67:268, 1988.

with an increase in ICP, a decrease in mean arterial blood pressure, and a decrease in cerebral perfusion pressure (Albanese et al., 1993). The effects of sufentanil in the EEG of premature infants was reported by Nguyen and others (2003). Bolus injection and continuous infusion increased EEG discontinuity, decreased burst suppression, and increased interburst intervals.

In adult patients undergoing nonintracranial neurosurgical procedures, Trindle and others (1993) noted that cerebral blood flow velocity (as assessed by transcranial Doppler) increased after sufentanil infusion. This increase in velocity was similar for equipotent doses of fentanyl (Trindle et al., 1993).

In a study of adult head trauma patients, Scholz and others (1994) noted that sufentanil bolus (2 mcg/kg), combined with a sufentanil continuous infusion (150 mcg/hr) and midazolam continuous infusion (9.0 mg/hr), resulted in a decrease in both ICP and mean arterial pressure. Perfusion pressure was noted to be stable.

Alfentanil

Alfentanil, a potent, short-acting analog of fentanyl, is rapidly distributed to the brain and central organs and then rapidly redistributed to more remote sites. It is about one fourth as potent as fentanyl and has one third the duration of action. Following a single bolus injection, the drug's decreased volume of distribution results in a significantly shorter elimination half-life. Its low lipid solubility allows less penetration of the blood–brain barrier. The concentration in brain tissue is markedly less than that in plasma. The duration of narcotic effect appears to be governed by redistribution and elimination. The redistribution principle operates in a small single-dose infusion, whereas elimination determines the effect of a large single bolus, a multiple small-bolus infusion, or a continuous infusion. Alfentanil is metabolized in the liver by oxidative *N*-dealkylation and *O*-demethylation in the CYP3A4 system (Yun et al., 1992). The pharmacologically inactive metabolites are excreted in the urine (Camu et al., 1982), with the major metabolite being noralfentanil. Alfentanil metabolism is catalyzed by CYP3A3/4 and CYP3A5 (Klees et al., 2005). Interindividual differences in the expression of this cytochrome and its susceptibility to inducers and inhibitors may account for the clinical variability in alfentanil kinetics and dynamics (Kharasch and Thummel, 1993). Although gender differences in CYP activity can affect drug metabolism, Kharasch and others (1997), in a study of young women, could find no differences in alfentanil clearance on different days of the menstrual cycle. Differences in CYP activity can markedly influence the pharmacokinetics of alfentanil, specifically its context-sensitive half-time. Using normal, low, and high CYP3A4 activity, Kharasch and others (1997b) have postulated through computer simulations that alfentanil can behave similarly to remifentanil (high CYP3A4 activity) or fentanyl (*low* CYP3A4 activity) (Fig. 6–19).

Protein binding has a significant influence on the pharmacokinetics of alfentanil. Alfentanil is 88% to 95% protein bound in the plasma and is independent of concentration and blood pH. The plasma protein most responsible for binding of alfentanil is α_1-acid glycoprotein. In adults, changes in the binding and in the pharmacokinetics of alfentanil occur during and after cardiopulmonary bypass (Hug, 1984). Disease states including end-stage kidney or liver failure can alter protein binding of opioids in children. Davis and others (1989b) studied the effects of liver disease and kidney disease on the binding characteristics of alfentanil. Compared with the healthy children, patients with

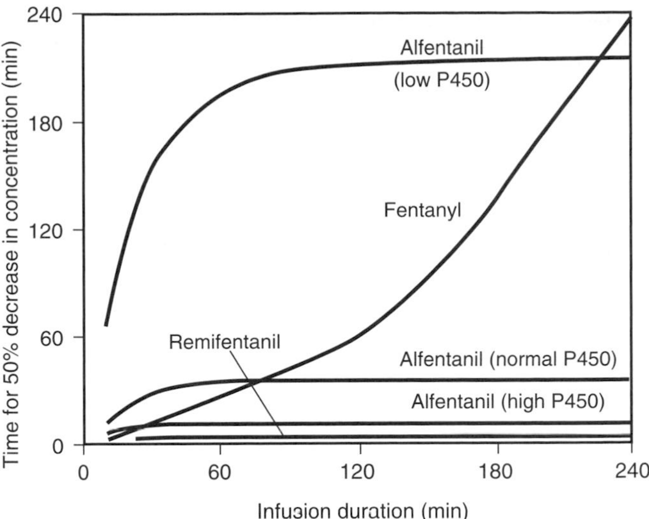

■ **FIGURE 6–19.** Effect of P450 3A4 activity on the time required for a 50% decrease in alfentanil venous plasma concentration after targeted infusions of variable durations. Half-times for fentanyl and remifentanil in normal participants were calculated using reported kinetic parameters. (Redrawn from Kharasch E, Russell M, Mautz D, et al.: The role of cytochrome P450 3A4 in alfentanil clearance: implications for interindividual variability in disposition and perioperative drug interactions. *Anesthesiology* 87:36–50, 1997.)

kidney disease had a significant decrease in protein binding (89.2 ± 5.4% versus 93.1 ± 3.2%), an increase in α_1-acid glycoprotein concentration (108.8 ± 44.3 versus 71.8 ± 30.7 mg/dL), and no change in albumin concentration (3910 ± 754 versus 4555 ± 524 mg/dL), whereas patients with liver disease had a significant decrease in protein binding (85.9 ± 6.2% versus 93.1 ± 3.2%), no change in α_1-acid glycoprotein concentration (65.8 ± 31.8 versus 71.8 ± 30.7 mg/dL), and a decrease in albumin concentration (3045 ± 1255 versus 4555 ± 524 mg/dL). Alfentanil binding has been studied in adult burn patients and noted to be increased from 90% to 94% protein bound (Macfie et al., 1992). Because alfentanil is highly protein bound, even small changes in the drug's free fraction could have marked pharmacodynamic effects in patients with kidney or liver failure.

The pharmacokinetics of alfentanil have been studied in both adults and children, but limited information is available for children of different ages. The limited, age-related, developmental pharmacokinetic data for alfentanil are presented in Table 6–13. In a study by Meistelman and others (1987), children aged 5 ± 1.1 years had a significantly smaller volume of distribution and shorter elimination half-life but similar clearance values compared with young adult patients aged 31 ± 4 years. Gorskey and others (1987) noted no difference in volume of distribution, elimination half-life, or clearance in infants aged 3 to 12 months compared with children aged 1 to 14 years. Roure and others (1987), on the other hand, noted that children aged 33 ± 18 months had faster clearance rates and elimination half-lives but similar volumes of distribution compared with those of adults. As Maitre and others (1987) noted in population studies of alfentanil pharmacokinetics in adults, differences in the pharmacokinetic profiles among the pediatric studies may be related to the large interpatient variability of alfentanil. Davis and others (1989a) have studied the pharmacokinetics of a single bolus of alfentanil in newborn premature infants and older children. In their study, newborn premature infants had considerably longer elimination half-lives (525 ± 305 versus 60 ± 11 minutes),

TABLE 6–13. Alfentanil age-related pharmacokinetics

Reference	Age	No. of Patients	V_d (L/kg)	CL (mL/min per kg)	$t_{1/2}\beta$ (min)
Meistelman et al. (1987)	4 to 8 yr	8	0.163	4.7	40
Meistelman et al. (1987)	25 to 40 yr	5	0.457	4.2	97
Goresky et al. (1987)	4 to 12 mo	5	0.500	8.3	76
Goresky et al. (1987)	1 to 14 yr	8	0.416	7.7	84
Davis et al. (1989a)	1 to 3 days (premature, 26 to 35 wk)	5	0.840	1.35	455
Killian et al. (1990)	1 to 3 days (term)	5	0.820	1.7	328

V_d, Volume of distribution; CL, clearance; $t_{1/2}\beta$, elimination half-life.

slower clearance rates (2.2 ± 2.4 versus 5.6 ± 2.4 mL/kg per minute), and larger volumes of distribution (1.0 ± 0.39 versus 0.48 ± 0.19 L/kg) than those observed in the older children (Fig. 6–20).

In a report on the influence of gestational age on the pharmacokinetics of alfentanil in neonates, Killian and others (1990) noted no change in alfentanil kinetics between preterm and term infants. Wiest and others (1991) studied the kinetics of alfentanil in neonates after a loading dose and variable continuous infusion route. Noncompartmental analysis revealed a clearance rate of 3.24 mL/kg per minute, a volume of distribution of 0.54 L/kg, and an elimination half-life of 4.1 hours. However, they noted an effect of alfentanil plasma concentration and plasma clearance.

The effects of renal failure and cirrhosis on alfentanil kinetics were studied in adult and in pediatric patients. Chauvin and others (1987a) have studied the pharmacokinetics of alfentanil in adult patients with chronic renal failure. The clearance and half-life values for alfentanil were similar in patients with renal failure and in control patients, but the steady-state volumes of distribution of alfentanil were significantly greater in patients with renal disease than in control patients. However, when the kinetic values for alfentanil were corrected for protein binding, the steady-state volumes of distribution and rates of clearance of unbound drug were similar in both groups of patients.

The effects of cirrhosis on alfentanil pharmacokinetics in adults were demonstrated by Ferrier and others (1985). Cirrhotic patients have lower total plasma clearance (1.60 versus 3.06 mL/kg per minute) and prolonged terminal elimination half-life (219 versus 97 minutes) but similar volume of distribution (0.390 versus 0.355 L/kg) compared with control patients.

By contrast to the studies in adults, the pharmacokinetics of alfentanil in children with cholestatic liver disease or end-stage kidney disease who are about to undergo either liver or kidney transplantation appear to be unaffected by the disease process (Davis et al., 1989b). Whether this difference is related to age or to the underlying pathophysiology of the disease states remains unanswered.

As do other narcotics, alfentanil produces a shift to the right in the ventilatory response curve. Although this shift is dose dependent, the ventilatory depressant effects dissipate by 30 to 50 minutes after the dose is given (Kay and Pleuvry, 1980; Kay and Stephenson, 1980).

Goldberg and others (1992) noted that in healthy adult patients, prolonged alfentanil administration sometimes resulted in arterial oxygen desaturation and depression of the hypercapneic respiratory drive even though the patients were easily arousable. Muscle rigidity can occur with rapid-acting opiates such as fentanyl, sufentanil, and alfentanil. Pokela and others (1992) have reported that rigidity occurs in neonates after alfentanil administration.

The cardiovascular effects of alfentanil were assessed during both low- and high-dose infusions (Kay and Pleuvry, 1980; Kay and Stephenson, 1980). At doses of 150 mcg/kg, heart rate, mean arterial pressure, and systemic vascular resistance were noted to decrease. Pulmonary capillary wedge pressure, pulmonary vascular resistance, right atrial pressure, and pulmonary artery pressure increased slightly (Kramer et al., 1983).

The neuroendocrine stress response with alfentanil has been studied in adults. Alfentanil incompletely suppresses the stress response. High-dose alfentanil can blunt the GH, ADH, and cortisol response to bypass. Epinephrine and norepinephrine concentrations are increased with the onset of bypass (Stanley, et al., 1983; deLange, et al., 1982).

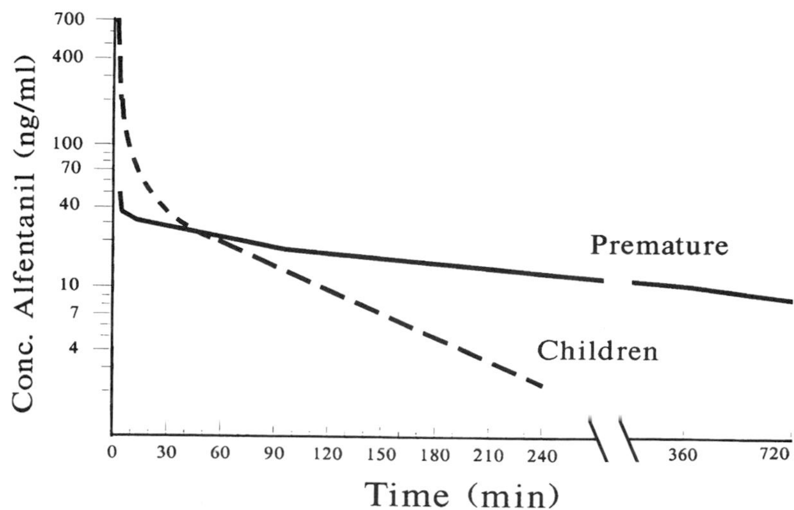

FIGURE 6–20. Alfentanil concentration-versus-time curves in newborn premature infants and older children. Both groups received 25 mcg/kg of alfentanil. (With permission from Davis PJ, Killian A, Stiller RL, et al.: *Dev Pharmacol Ther* 13:21, 1989.)

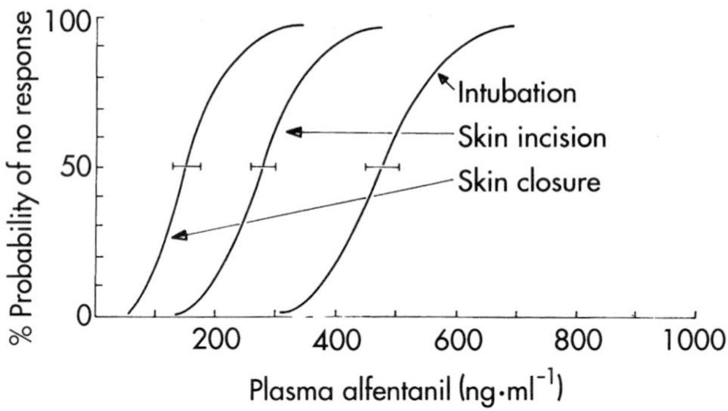

■ **FIGURE 6–21.** Relationship between the alfentanil plasma concentrations (with 66% nitrous oxide) and their effects for three specific events of short duration (intubation, skin incision, and skin closure). (With permission from Ausems ME, Hug C, Stanski DR, et al.: *Anesthesiology* 65:362, 1986.)

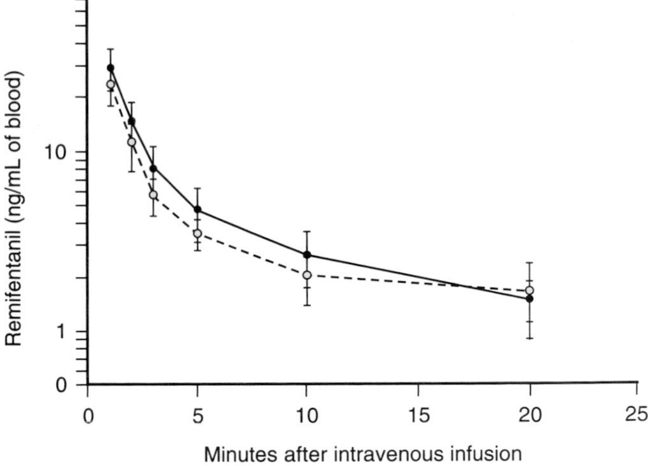

■ **FIGURE 6–22.** Prebypass *(filled circles)* and postbypass *(open circles)* pharmacokinetic decay curves of remifentanil were constructed from the average concentrations of the 12 patients. (Redrawn with permission from Davis PJ, Wilson AS, Siewers RD, et al.: The effects of cardiopulmonary bypass on remifentanil kinetics in children undergoing atrial septal defect repair. *Anesth Analg* 89:904–908, 1999.)

In children, Meretoja and Rautiainen (1990) noted that in children aged 1 month to 2 years, oral flunitrazepam premedication and alfentanil bolus of 20 mcg/kg followed by a continuous infusion of 0.5 mcg/kg per minute provided adequate sedation for patients spontaneously breathing room air who were undergoing cardiac catheterization. In these patients, hemodynamic variables changed less than 11%.

In adults, Ausems and Hug (1986) have defined the Cp_{50} values of alfentanil for various surgical and anesthetic stimulations (Fig. 6–21). Using these adult Cp_{50} plasma values, initial bolus and infusion rates can be estimated for children.

Remifentanil

Remifentanil is the hydrochloride salt of 3-[4-methoxycarbonyl]-4-[(1-oxopropyl) phenylamino]-1-piperidine] propanoic acid, methyl ester. Because of its ester linkage, remifentanil is susceptible to metabolism by blood and tissue esterases. Its primary metabolic pathway is through deesterification to form a carboxylic acid metabolite, which is only one-300th to one-1000th the potency of the parent compound. In adult studies, the pharmacokinetic profile of remifentanil is best described by a biexponential decay curve, with a small volume of distribution (0.39 L/kg), a rapid distribution phase (0.94 minute), and an extremely short elimination half-life (10 minutes) (Egan et al., 1993; Glass et al., 1993; Westmoreland et al., 1993).

In addition, computer simulations show that the duration of remifentanil infusion has no effect on the time to decrease the plasma or effect site concentration by 50%. The $t_{1/2}$ keo, or half-time for equilibration between plasma and the effect compartment, is 1.3 minutes. Thus, the context-sensitive half-time is a flat line.

For opioids, which undergo organ elimination, the neonatal profile of opioids demonstrates prolonged clearances, large volume of distributions, and markedly prolonged half-lives. However, in neonates remifentanil has a rapid clearance, a large volume of distribution, and a half-life that does not change with age. In an age-related study of remifentanil pharmacokinetics, Ross and others (2001) noted that the volume of distribution was largest in the infants younger than 2 months (mean, 452 mL/kg) and decreased to mean values of 223 to 308 mL/kg in the older patients. There was a more rapid clearance in the infants younger than 2 months (90 mL/kg per minute) and infants aged 2 months to 2 years (92 mL/kg per minute) than in the other groups (mean, 46 to 76 mL/kg per minute). The half-life was similar in all age groups, with mean values of 3.4 to 5.7 minutes. Because the redistribution phase and elimination half-life are so rapid, a bolus injection prior to a continuous infusion of remifentanil is unnecessary.

Another unique feature of remifentanil kinetics in children is that its pharmacokinetic profile is unchanged by cardiopulmonary bypass. For opioids, which undergo organ elimination, cardiopulmonary bypass prolongs drug clearance, increases volume of distribution, and increases half-life. The pharmacokinetic profile of remifentanil appears to be unaffected by cardiopulmonary bypass (Davis et al., 1999) (Fig. 6–22).

The pharmacodynamics of remifentanil were studied in children and infants. Multiple case reports of remifentanil use in neonates and infants suggest its usefulness (Wee and Stokes, 1999; Chiaretti et al., 2000; German et al., 2000; Dönmez et al., 2001; Foubert et al., 2002). In a multicenter trial of infants younger than 2 months who were undergoing pyloromyotomy, Galinkin and others (2001) and Davis and others (2001) noted that remifentanil provides stable hemodynamic conditions and that new onset of postoperative apnea, as detected by pneumograms, did not occur with remifentanil.

In older children, pharmacodynamic studies suggest that the short duration of remifentanil can be used to promote faster emergence times (Davis et al., 1997, 2000). As with other opioids, the issue of tolerance is a concern with remifentanil. Acute tolerance to remifentanil has been suggested in the nonblinded studies of Guignard and others (2000) and Vinik and others (1998) but not in the studies of Gustorff and others (2002) and Schraag and others (1999). The incidence of postoperative nausea and vomiting appears similar to the incidence seen with other opioids (Eltzschig et al., 2002).

Methadone

Methadone is a synthetic narcotic analgesic. It is a racemic mixture with the L-isomer 10 to 50 times more potent than the D-isomer. Methadone has an oral bioavailability of 80% with a range of 41% to 99%. It is 60% to 90% protein bound, and α_1-acid glycoprotein is the main determinant of the free factor of methadone. After an intravenous dose in adults, the pharmacokinetic profile fits a two-compartment model with a distribution half-life of 6 minutes and an elimination half-life of 35 hours (Gourlay et al., 1982). Findings of the pharmacokinetics of methadone in children suggest that it has a large volume of distribution (7.1 L/kg), a high plasma clearance (5.4 mL/kg per minute), and a long half-life (19.2 hours) (Berde et al., 1991).

Although methadone is metabolized in the liver, little information is available with respect to its p*K* profile in end-stage liver or kidney failure. Urinary pH is another important determinant of the elimination half-life of methadone. Acidifying the urine markedly decreases the half-life of methadone and increases its renal clearance (Bellward et al., 1977).

Clinical use in children is somewhat limited. Berde and others (1991), in a randomized, double-blind study of morphine and methadone, noted that the children receiving methadone had significantly less opioid requirements and better pain scores in the postoperative period than did children receiving equipotent doses of morphine. Recommended doses of perioperative methadone include a loading dose of 0.1 to 0.2 mg/kg with 0.05 mg/kg supplemental dose every 4 to 12 hours.

LOCAL ANESTHETICS

Local anesthetics are divided into two types: esters (tetracaine, chlorprocaine, procaine) and amides (lidocaine, bupivacaine, ropivacaine, and levobupivacaine). The ester compounds are metabolized by plasma cholinesterase, and the amide class of drugs undergoes hepatic biotransformation and clearance. Local anesthetic agents work by blocking voltage-gated sodium channels.

Local toxicity involves the spinal cord and peripheral nerves and usually occurs at the site of injection. General or systemic toxicity involves either the central nervous system or the heart. In general, there is a direct relationship between local anesthetic potency and systemic toxicity, and, in general, central nervous system toxicity occurs at lower plasma concentrations than for cardiac toxicity. The systemic effects of local anesthetics are a function of dose rapidity of injection and site of injection. Highly vascular areas are prone to local anesthetic uptake and, consequently, toxicity. The order of site absorption from highest to lowest is intercostal, intratracheal > caudal, epidural > brachial plexus > subcutaneous.

The amide local anesthetics are bound to serum proteins. Alpha$_1$-acid glycoprotein is the major binding protein. The free drug fraction for lidocaine ranges from 30% to 40%, and for both ropivacaine and bupivacaine it ranges from 4% to 7%. Metabolism of amides is by the liver's cytochrome P450 system. CYP3A4 metabolizes bupivacaine while CYP1A2 is mostly involved with ropivacaine's metabolism. Lidocaine has a high hepatic extraction ratio, and its clearance is dependent on hepatic blood flow. In addition, the metabolic product of lidocaine metabolism (ME6X) may inhibit the intrinsic enzyme involved with its degradation. Lidocaine has a longer elimination half-life and larger volume of distribution in children than in adults after either intratracheal or caudal anesthsia (Eyres et al., 1978; Ecoffey et al., 1984). Bokesch and others (1985) demonstrated higher plasma lidocaine levels in the systemic circulation in animals with right-to-left shunts.

Bupivacaine

Bupivacaine and ropivacaine have a low hepatic extraction ratio. Thus, protein binding and CYP enzyme activity effect drug clearance (Lonnqvist et al., 2000). Bupivacaine is a racemic mixture of equiosmolar amounts of R-(+)–bupivacaine and S–(-)–bupivacaine. Drug clearance is low at birth and increases throughout the first year of life. Pharmacokinetic studies have demonstrated age-related differences between infants and children (Ecoffey et al., 1985; Desparmet et al., 1987; Mazoit et al., 1988; Mazoit and Dalens, 2004; Eyres et al., 1983). Extrapolation of pharmacokinetic data after single-bolus bupivacaine administration for infants and children suggests that for continuous caudal/epidural infusions, rates of 0.2 to 0.4 mg/kg per hour for infants and 0.2 to 0.75 mg/kg per hour for children would provide efficacious and safe plasma concentrations (McCloskey et al., 1992) (Table 6–14).

TABLE 6–14. Pharmacokinetics of bolus caudal-epidural bupivacaine in infants and children

	C_{max} (mcg/mL)	$t_{1/2}\beta$ (hr)	V_d (L/kg)	CL (mL/min per kg)
Infants* (2.5 mg/kg)	0.97 ± 0.42	7.7 ± 2.4	3.9 ± 2.0	7.1 ± 3.2
Children† (2.5 mg/kg)	1.25 ± 0.09	4.6 ± 0.5	2.7 ± 0.2	10.0 ± 0.7

C_{max}, Maximal serum concentration; $t_{1/2}\beta$, elimination half-life; V_d, volume of distribution; CL, clearance.
*Expressed as value ± SD (Mazoit et al., 1988).
†Expressed as value ± SEM (Ecoffey et al., 1985).

Ropivacaine

Ropivacaine is a long-acting amide, local anesthetic agent with fewer cardiac and CNS toxicities. It is thought to provide a greater separation of sensory and motor effects. Compared with bupivacaine, Karmakar and others (2002) have shown that after 2.0 mg/kg of either caudal ropivacaine or bupivacaine, ropivacaine undergoes slower systemic absorption from the caudal space but with comparable peak venous plasma concentrations. In comparative studies of caudal blocks with ropivacaine and bupivacaine, Khalil and others (1999) and Ivani and others (1998) noted that for children the quality and duration of postoperative pain relief, motor and sensory effects, and time to first micturition were similar.

In infants and children, the pharmacokinetics of ropivacaine have been reported after caudal, epidural, and ilioinguinal blocks (Hansen, 2000, 2001; Lönnqvist et al., 2000; Wulf et al., 2000; Dalens, 2001). Hansen and others (2001) have shown that infants 0 to 3 months of age have higher to medium maximum free ropivacaine concentrations than infants 3 to 12 months of age, and for both these groups of infants the free drug concentrations were within the concentrations reported for adults. However, Wulf and others (2000) noted that in infants less than one year of age and toddlers 1 to 5 years of age, infants had higher peak plasma concentrations than toddlers, with the peak concentration occurring at 60 minutes in both groups. In a dosing study of children 4 to 12 years of age, Bosenberg and others (2001) noted that single shot caudals in doses of 1 to 3 mg/kg resulted in peak plasma levels of free ropivacaine that increased proportionately to the increase in dose.

McCann and others (2001) reported on the pharmacokinetics of epidural ropivacaine (1.7 mg/kg) in infants and young children. In this study, they noted that ropivacaine has a biphasic absorption. As with bupivacaine, ropivacaine shows age-related clearance changes with infants having slower clearance than children, but in both groups the peak plasma concentrations were well below the maximum tolerated venous concentration (2100 mcg/mL for adults).

The pharmacodynamics of ropivacaine after caudal blocks have been shown to be similar to bupivacaine with regard to onset time, efficacy, duration of analgesia, and incidence of motor block. Local anesthetic supplements can also affect ther duration of action. Ropivacaine's duration of action can be prolonged with neostigmine, clonidine, or ketamine supplementation (Da Conceicao et al., 1998; Ivani et al., 1998, 1999-2000; Khalil et al., 1999; Morton, 2000; Turan et al., 2003).

Levobupivacaine

Levobupivacaine is one of the enantiomers of bupivacaine. Information regarding its use in children is less than with the other local anesthetics (Locatelli et al., 2005; DeNegri et al., 2004; Chalkiadis et al., 2004; Kokki et al., 2004; Lerman et al., 2003; Ivani et al., 2003; Gunter et al., 1999; Ivani et al., 2005).

In studies of children 1 to 7 years of age, Ivani and others (2002) noted that caudal bupivacaine, levobupivacaine, and ropivacaine were thought to be clinically comparable. Locatelli and others (2005) reported that caudal bupivacaine was associated with more motor block and longer analgesic block. In pediatric patients with continuous infusions of epidurals, DeNegri and others (2004) noted that ropivacaine and levobupivacaine were associated with less motor block than bupivacaine.

In a dose-response study by Ivani and others (2003) in children undergoing caudal block for subumbilical surgical procedures, three concentrations (0.125%, 0.20%, and 0.25%) of levobupivacaine were compared. A dose-response relationship was observed with median duration of postoperative analgesia and with motor blockade (Fig. 6-23). Based on these relationships, they noted the optimal concentration to be 0.2% (Ivani, 2003). More information on local anesthetics is given in Chapter 14, Regional Anesthesia.

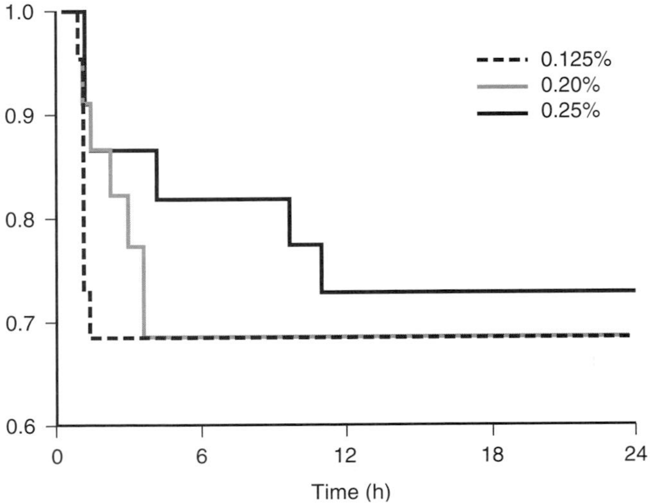

FIGURE 6–23. Fraction of patients without a need for supplemental analgesia in relation to various concentrations of levobupivacaine. (Redrawn with permission from Ivani G, Pasquale De Negri, et al.: A comparison of three different concentrations of levobupivacaine for caudal block in children. *Anesth Analg* 97:368–371, 2003.)

COMMONLY ADMINISTERED ANESTHETIC ADJUNCTS

Atropine

Strong cholinergic stimulation such as occurs from halothane and succinylcholine can produce profound bradycardia and reduce cardiac output in infants. The primary purpose of atropine in pediatric anesthesia is to protect against cholinergic stimulation; its secondary purpose is to inhibit the production of secretions.

If atropine is administered intravenously in incremental doses, more atropine on weight basis is needed to accelerate the heart rate in children younger than 2 years; however, acceleration uniformly occurs with 14.3 mcg/kg (Dauchot and Gravenstein, 1971). Infants need higher doses of atropine to increase heart rate compared with adults (Palmisano et al., 1991). The onset of the chronotopic effects of atropine appears to be related to the underlying heart rate at the time of administration of atropine. Children with slower heart rates have longer onset times than do children with faster heart rates (Zimmerman and Steward, 1986). Although atropine can increase heart rate and cardiac output, it does not appear to change the neuromuscular blocking onset time of atracurium (Simhi et al., 1997). A dose of 30 mg/kg appears to be vagolytic in infants, children, and adults. This dose provides adequate protection against a cholinergic challenge. In a study of 20 healthy children aged 1 to 36 months undergoing elective surgery, McAuliffe and others (1997) noted that 20 mcg/kg intravenously caused a variable increase in heart rate and cardiac output in anesthetized children. In 40 children, 2 to 6 years of age, intratracheal atropine (20 mcg/kg) produced only a modest increase in heart rate after 5 minutes (Jorgensen et al., 1997). However, 50 mcg/kg increased heart rate rapidly (Howard et al., 1990). The site of injection has a role in the onset time of atropine effect. In a randomized study of children 1 to 10 years of age anesthetized with nitrous oxide, oxygen, and halothane, Sullivan and others (1997) noted that a subglossal injection resulted in a faster onset time than either a deltoid or vastus lateralis intramuscular injection.

In all age groups, 5 to 10 mcg/kg atropine minimally decreases salivation (Gaviotaki and Smith, 1962). Children with Down syndrome may have an increased sensitivity to atropine; the pupils dilate in response to atropine, and large increases in heart rate occur after repeated doses of atropine (Berg et al., 1960; Priest, 1960; Harris and Goodman, 1968). In retrospective study by Kobel and others (1982), however, patients with Down syndrome were no more sensitive to intravenous atropine than were other patients.

Ketorolac

Ketorolac is a nonsteroidal anti-inflammatory drug (NSAID). The analgesic properties of NSAIDs are thought to be related to their ability to attenuate the hyperalgesic state caused by prostaglandins as opposed to producing analgesia directly. Ketorolac may act both peripherally and centrally. Ketorolac is an enantiomeric compound. The pharmacokinetics of ketorolac were described after single and continuous infusion (Olkkola et al., 1991; Hamunen et al., 1999; Kauffman et al., 1999; Dsida et al., 2002; Kokki et al.; 2002; Gillis et al., 1997).

In a study of 43 pediatric surgical patients, Dsida and others (2002) noted no age-related differences in the pharmacokinetics, and the kinetic profile was similar to that reported for adults. In a pharmacokinetic study of the stereoisomers of ketorolac in children, Kauffman and others (1999) noted that concentrations of the (*S*)-(-)-enantiomer were lower than those of the (*R*)-(+)-enantiomer and that the (*S*)-(-)-enantiomer had a shorter half-life, greater clearance, and larger volume of distribution. These differences in the enantiomer kinetic profile appear similar for children, adolescents, and adults (Hamunen et al., 1999) (Fig. 6–24). In addition to its analgesic properties, ketorolac may have antiemetic properties (Munro et al., 1994), and in children undergoing ureteral reimplantation procedures, ketorolac can decrease the incidence and severity of postoperative bladder spasms (Park et al., 2000).

Tramadol

Tramadol is a centrally acting agent with two distinct mechanisms of action: opioid and nonopioid. Tramadol acts as an opioid agonist. Tramadol also acts on monoamine systems to inhibit the reuptake of norepinephrine and serotonin. Tramadol is structurally related to codeine. It is metabolized by liver CYP2D6; about 0.8% of the white population is deficient in this enzyme. Its metabolite, *O*-demethyl metabolic intermediate has some analgesic effect. Tramadol is a stereoisomer. The (+)-stereoisomer form provides similar analgesia as the racemic form. The bioavailability of tramadol in adults is 68%, and it is 20% protein bound. In 14 children aged 1 to 12 years, the intravenous tramadol pharmacokinetic profile demonstrated a volume of distribution, clearance, and half-life of 3.1 L/kg, 6.1 mL/kg per minute, and 6.4 hours, respectively. In the same study, the kinetics of tramadol after caudal administration revealed a volume of distribution, clearance, and half-life of 2.06 L/kg, 6.6 mL/kg per minute, and 3.7 hours, respectively. Of note was that the ratio of caudal and intravenous AUC was 0.83, suggesting there is extensive systemic absorption of caudal tramadol (Murthy et al., 2000) (Fig. 6–25).

The clinical efficacy of tramadol has been reviewed in adults and children by Scott and Perry (2000); in summary, the overall efficacy of tramadol is comparable to equianalgesic doses of parenteral opioids. In children, tramadol has been administered orally, intravenously, intramuscularly, and caudally. Its major advantage is its lack of respiratory depression after its administration (Scott and Perry, 2000; Ozcengiz et al., 2001; Viitanen and Annila, 2001; Finkel et al., 2002; Engelhardt et al., 2003; Rose et al., 2003).

5-HT_3 Receptor Antagonists

Ondansetron is a 5-hydroxytryptamine$_3$ (serotonin) (5-HT_3) receptor antagonist. The mechanism of action, although not totally elucidated, appears to block the effects of serotonin on 5-HT_3 receptors on vagal afferents. Ondansetron is well absorbed orally and has an oral bioavailability of 60%. Ondansetron is metabolized in the liver by the CYPIA2, CYP2D6, and CYP3A4 (Gregory et al., 1998; Sweetland et al., 1992). After oral administration, peak plasma levels occur in 1 to 2 hours. In adults after oral, intramuscular, or intravenous administration, the volume of distribution and half-life are 140 L/kg and 3.5 hours. In children, the half-life ranged from 2.5 to 3.0 hours, the volume of distribution ranged from 1.9 to 2.4 L/kg, and the clearance ranged from 6.6 to 15.6 mL/kg per minute (Bryson et al., 1991; Spahr-Schopfer et al., 1995). The major clinical use in anesthesia has been for prophylaxis and treatment of postoperative nausea and vomiting. Both large-scale studies and meta-analyses noted ondansetron to be a superior prophylactic drug compared with placebo, droperidol, and

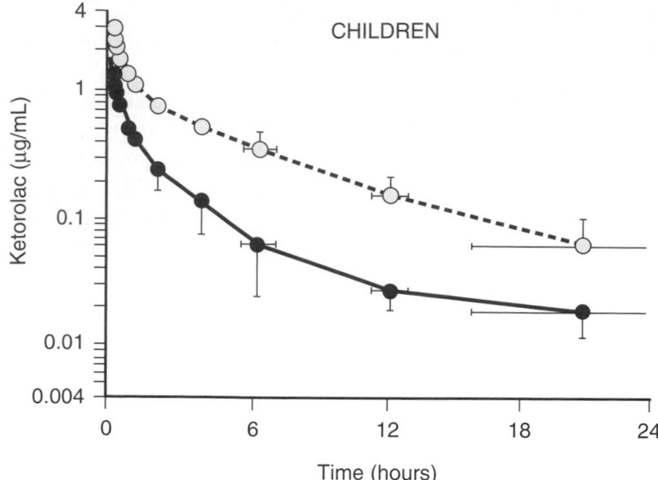

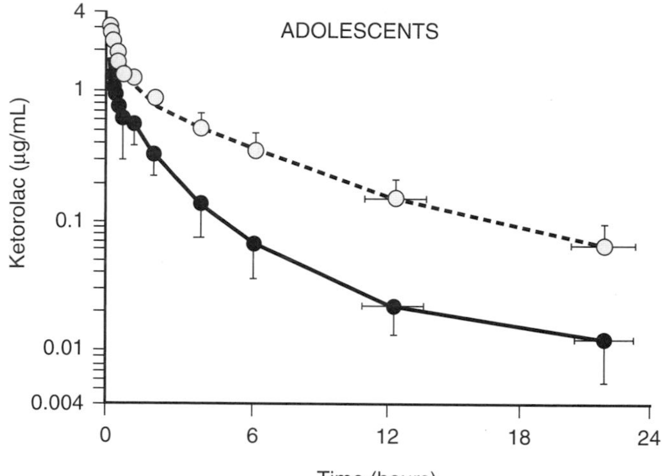

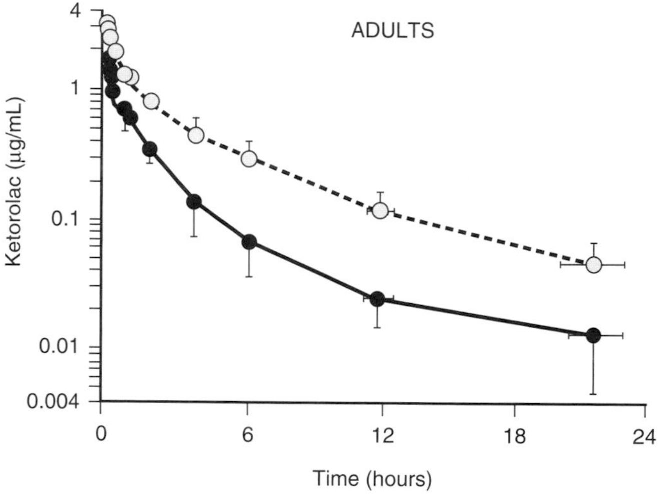

FIGURE 6–24. Concentrations (mean ± SD) of (*S*)-ketorolac *(filled circles)* and (*R*)-ketorolac *(shaded circles)* in plasma following intravenous administration of 0.5 mg/kg of racemic ketorolac tromethamine to 18 children, 28 adolescents, and 18 adults. (Redrawn with permission from Hamunen K, Maunuksela EL, Sarvela J, et al.: Stereoselective pharmacokinetics of ketorolac in children, adolescents and adults. *Acta Anaesthesiol Scand* 43:1041–1046, 1999.)

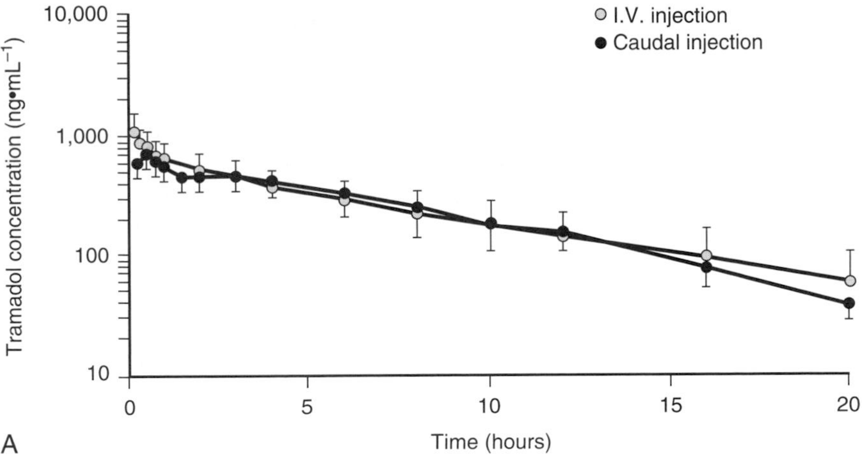

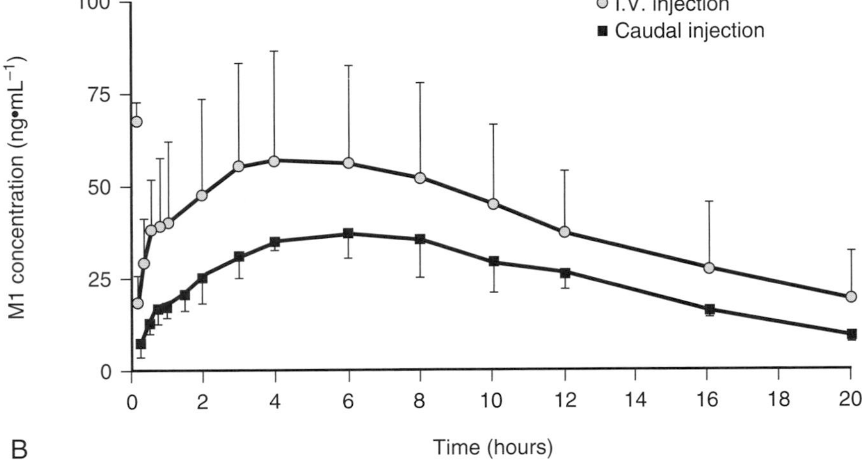

■ **FIGURE 6–25.** *(A)* Mean (SD) serum concentrations of total tramadol after intravenous (IV) or caudal injection of tramadol 2 mg/kg. *(B)* Mean (SD) serum concentrations of *O*-dimethyl tramadol (M1) after IV or caudal injection of tramadol 2 mg/kg. (Redrawn from Murthy BVS, Pandya KS, Booker PD, et al.: Pharmacokinetics of tramadol in children after IV or caudal epidural administration. *Br J Anaesth* 84:346–349, 2000.)

metaclopramide (Patel et al., 1997; Domino et al., 1999; Lim et al., 1999). The addition of dexamethasone to prophylactic ondansetron further increases the antiemetic efficacy of the drugs (Splinter et al., 1998). When used for treatment of postoperative nausea and vomiting, ondansetron (0.1 mg/kg, maximum 4.0 mg) appears to be superior to placebo (Khalil et al., 1996; Culy et al., 2001).

Granisetron, with an elimination half-life of 9 to 12 hours, has been reported to be effective at a dose of 40 mcg/kg when administered either orally or intravenously (Fujii et al., 1998, 1999a, 1999b, 2001; Fujii and Tanaka, 1999, 2001, 2002).

Tropisetron is another 5-HT$_3$ receptor antagonist whose half-life is two to three times longer than that of ondansetron. In studies of children, doses ranging from 0.1 to 0.2 mg/kg were found to be effective for postoperative nausea and vomiting (Ang et al., 1998; Holt et al., 2000; Jensen et al., 2000).

Dolasetron, a highly potent and selective 5-HT$_3$ receptor antagonist, appears to provide prophylactic antiemetic efficiency similar to that of ondansetron (Sukhani et al., 2002; Olutoye et al., 2003). Dolasetron appears to have an active metabolite that has a half-life of about 8 hours. In a pharmacokinetic study of 30 children, the kinetics of the metabolite were similar after both intravenous and oral administration. The volume of distribution, clearance, and half-life were 5.2 L/kg, 22.1 mL/kg per minute, and 5.7 hours, respectively. Bioavailability has been estimated at 59% (Lerman et al., 1996).

Dexmedetomidine

Alpha$_2$-adrenoreceptor agonists are being used increasingly in anesthesia and critical care because they not only decrease sympathetic tone and attenuate the stress responses to anesthesia and surgery, but also cause sedation and analgesia. They are used as adjuvants during regional anesthesia. Clonidine, which was initially introduced as an antihypertensive, is the most commonly used alpha$_2$ agonist by anesthesiologists. Dexmedetomidine is the most recent agent in this group, approved by the FDA in 1999 for use in humans for analgesia and sedation. It is used to sedate ICU patients. In addition to its sedative properties, dexmedetomidine also acts synergistically with other sedative drugs to lower the overall analgesic and sedative doses of the other agents. Although clonidine, another alpha$_2$-adrenoreceptor agonist, has been used in pediatric patients to promote sedation and reduce anesthetic requirements, dexmedetomidine differs from clonidine in that dexmedetomidine possesses selective alpha$_2$-adrenoreceptor activity, especially for the 2A subtype of this receptor. Dexmedetomidine is 8 to 10 times more specific than clonidine. This selectivity, coupled with its pharmacokinetic profile, allows the drug to be administered as a continuous infusion with a relatively quick onset and offset of action.

The hemodynamic effects of dexmedetomidine are similar to clonidine and vary depending on the dose rate and route of administration (Dyck et al., 1993; Ebert et al., 2000). Its use in pediatric anesthesia has been limited, but its ability to provide sedation for pediatric patients has been reported in case reports and small series (Tobias et al., 1997; Serlin, 2004; Finkel and Elretai, 2004; Tobias et al., 2003; Ard et al., 2003; Dyck et al., 1993; Ebert et al., 2000; DeRuiter and Crawford, 2001; Meretoja et al., 1995). Ibacache and others (2003) have noted that as an adjunct to sevoflurane, a single-dose of dexmedetomidine (0.3 μg/kg) markedly attenuated the incidence of sevoflurane-associated emergence agitation.

INHALATION ANESTHETICS

Sevoflurane, isoflurane, and nitrous oxide are the most widely used inhalational anesthetics in the practice of pediatric anesthesia. During the 1990s, sevoflurane displaced halothane as the pediatric induction agent of choice. Where economic issues prevail, halothane continues to dominate the pediatric anesthetic practice. Desflurane has not established itself as a widely used maintenance/emergence agent in children, although this role is under review.

NITROUS OXIDE

Nitrous oxide reduces the anesthetic requirements for the more potent inhalational anesthetics, speeds uptake of the more potent agents, and serves to dilute the inspired oxygen concentration. Nitrous oxide expands gas-containing spaces because it is 34× more soluble in blood (blood/gas partition coefficient, 0.47) than nitrogen (blood gas partition coefficient, 0.014). Assuming a trivial quantity of nitrogen diffuses out of the space while ventilating the lungs with nitrous oxide, then the maximum multiple expansion of the original space that can occur is as follows (Eger, 1974):

$$\text{Multiple} = 100/(100 - \%\ \text{nitrous oxide}) \qquad (6.16)$$

Using this equation, if 75% nitrous oxide is inspired, then the space volume may expand up to threefold. The rate at which the space expands varies with the site: a pneumothorax may double in size in 12 minutes, whereas a small bowel obstruction may double in 120 minutes (Eger, 1974). This 10-fold difference in the rate of expansion is determined in part by the reduction in (mural) blood flow to the bowel as the gas volume within the lumen expands. The same limitation of blood flow does not occur with a pneumothorax. Other cavities that may expand in the presence of nitrous oxide include the middle ear, gas within the ocular globe, and CNS air from a pneumoencephalogram. In situations where oxygenation (either inspired oxygen concentration or tissue oxygenation) must be maximized, the use of nitrous oxide, particularly in concentrations in excess of 50%, must be judiciously reviewed. The potency of nitrous oxide is affected by barometric pressure, being less effective at high altitude than at sea level or below.

Once believed to be entirely nontoxic, nitrous oxide has aroused increasing suspicion of cellular and atmospheric toxicity on several counts. Lymphocyte depression, miscarriage (first trimester), cancer, defects in spermatogenesis, apoptosis, and others have raised concerns about health risks after prolonged exposure (Brodsky et al., 1984; Rowland et al., 1995; Jevtovic-Todorovic et al., 2003). The half-life of nitrous oxide, an oxygen-free radical scavenger, in the troposphere is approximately 150 years compared with the half-lives of the polyhalogenated inhalational anesthetics, which are 5 to 10 years. Although less than 5% of the nitrous oxide released into the atmosphere originates from medical sources, limiting the waste of nitrous oxide through the use of low fresh gas flows and smoke stack scrubbers curbs the depletion of the ozone layer.

Potent inhalational anesthetics are sevoflurane, isoflurane, halothane, and desflurane. Sevoflurane and isoflurane have become

TABLE 6–15. The pharmacology, solubility, and minimum alveolar concentration (MAC) of five potent inhalational anesthetics

	Halothane	Isoflurane	Sevoflurane	Desflurane
Pharmacology				
Chemical structure	F—C(F)(F)—C(H)(Cl)—Br	H—C(F)(F)—O—C(Cl)(H)—C(F)(F)—F	F—C(H)(F)—O—C(CF_3)(CF_3)—H	H—C(F)(F)—O—C(F)(H)—C(F)(F)—F
Molecular weight	197.4	184.5	200.1	168
Boiling point (°C)	50.2	48.5	58.6	23.5
Vapor pressure (mm Hg)	244	240	185	664
Odor	Mild, pleasant	Etheral	Pleasant	Etheral
Metabolized (%)	15-25	0.2	5	0.02
Solubility				
$\lambda_{b/g}$ adults	2.4	1.4	0.66	0.42
$\lambda_{b/g}$ neonates	2.1	1.2	0.66	—
$\lambda_{fat/b}$ adults	51	45	48	27
MAC				
MAC_{adults}	0.75	1.2	2.05	7.0
$MAC_{neonates}$	0.87	1.60	3.3	9.2

b/g, blood/gas; fat/b, fat/blood.

Note that the boiling point of desflurane is close to room temperature and that the solubilities of the anesthetics in blood and fat decrease from left to right across the table, whereas MAC increases from left to right.

With permission from Lerman J: *Anesth Clin North Am* 9:764, 1991.

the dominant maintenance anesthetics in children, displacing halothane because of their "forgiving" qualities; that is, they are less soluble in blood and tissues than is halothane. The pharmacology of available inhalational anesthetics is summarized in Table 6–15.

SEVOFLURANE

Sevoflurane is a polyfluorinated methyl isopropyl ether anesthetic that is the first ether anesthetic to be widely used for induction of anesthesia in children. Its low blood solubility, half that of isoflurane, speeds the equilibration of alveolar and inspired anesthetic partial pressures (Fig. 6–26). However, the tissue/blood solubilities of sevoflurane and isoflurane in the vessel-rich group (brain, heart, liver, kidneys, and endocrine glands), muscle, and fat groups are indistinguishable. Because the wash-in of inhalational anesthetics is increased by use of the overpressure technique, these physicochemical differences affect the wash-in of the anesthetics to a lesser extent than they do the rate of washout and the rate of emergence from anesthesia. In terms of the pharmacokinetics of inhaled anesthetics, changes in alveolar ventilation and cardiac output affect the wash-in of more-soluble anesthetics (halothane and methoxyflurane) more than that of the less-soluble anesthetic agents (sevoflurane and desflurane) (Eger, 1974). In contrast, increases in the right-to-left shunt (as in an intrapulmonary or intracardiac shunt) affect the wash-in of the less-soluble anesthetics (sevoflurane) compared with the more-soluble anesthetics (halothane and methoxyflurane) (Lerman, 2002). Because of the low blood and tissue solubilities of sevoflurane, its elimination in infants and children is rapid.

Sevoflurane is a far less potent anesthetic than isoflurane and halothane, as reflected by the minimum alveolar concentration (MAC) of sevoflurane. The MAC of sevoflurane is twice that of isoflurane and three times that of halothane (Lerman et al., 1994). The relationship between age (in the pediatric range) and the MAC of sevoflurane differs from the relationships for isoflurane and halothane in two respects: first, the MAC of sevoflurane does not increase steadily as age decreases, and second, the contribution of nitrous oxide to the MAC of sevoflurane in children is less than that of halothane. MAC of sevoflurane in neonates and infants younger than 6 months (3.2%) and in infants older than 6 months and children up to 12 years (2.5%) is constant. Why the MAC of sevoflurane does not increase as age decreases as it does with the other inhalational anesthetics is unclear. Although nitrous oxide reduces the MAC of inhalational anesthetics in proportion to its concentration, the same does not hold true for sevoflurane in children. In the case of sevoflurane in children aged 1 to 3 years, nitrous oxide (inspired concentration, 60%) decreases the MAC of sevoflurane by only 25%. The explanation for the blunted effect of nitrous oxide on the MAC of sevoflurane in children also remains unclear.

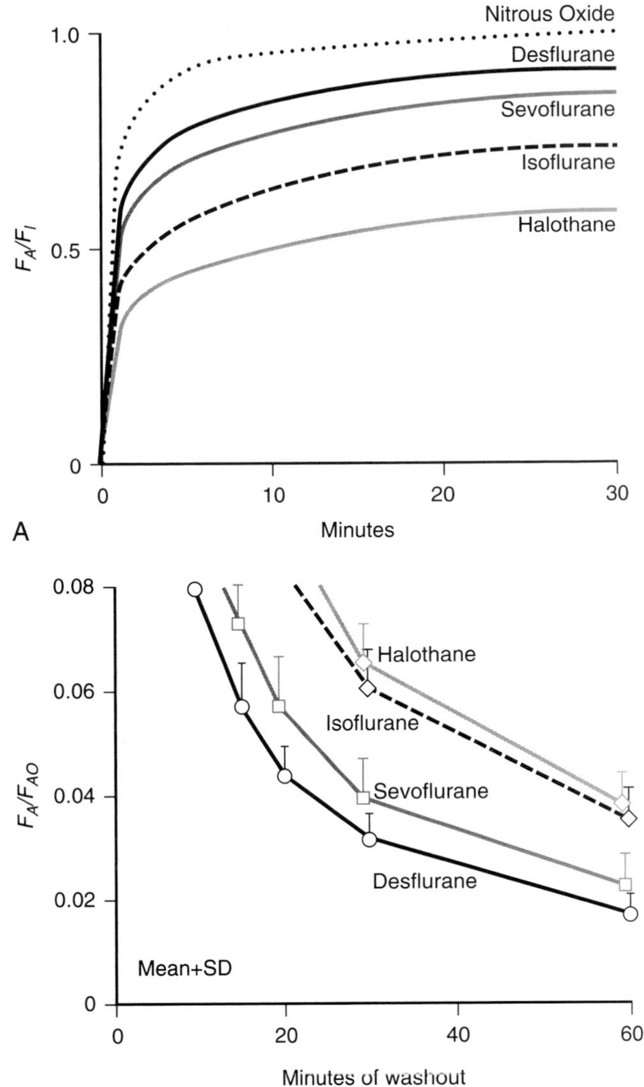

FIGURE 6–26. *(A)* In unstimulated human volunteers, the increase in the alveolar concentration (F_A) toward the inspired concentration (F_I) is more rapid with the least soluble potent inhaled anesthetic (desflurane) and slowest with the most soluble potent inhaled anesthetic (halothane). Only nitrous oxide has a more rapid increase in F_A/F_I than desflurane. Nitrous oxide enjoys a still more rapid increase because of its low solubility in blood and tissues, and because of the employment of a greater inspired concentration (i.e., its rise is influenced by the concentration effect). *(B)* Elimination, as defined by the decrease in alveolar concentration relative to the last alveolar concentration found during anesthesia (F_{AO}), is most rapid with desflurane, less rapid with sevoflurane, and slowest with isoflurane and halothane. Despite its greater solubility, the decrease with halothane is as rapid as the decrease with isoflurane because halothane is metabolized and thus is cleared from the body by both lungs and liver, whereas isoflurane is cleared only by the lungs.

Sevoflurane is unique among the currently used ether anesthetics in that in nonpremedicated children, it is well tolerated when administered for induction of anesthesia, even without nitrous oxide. The incidences of breath holding, coughing, laryngospasm, and desaturation during induction of anesthesia with sevoflurane and halothane are infrequent and similar with the two anesthetics (Black et al., 1996; Lerman et al., 1996). However, induction of anesthesia with sevoflurane is not always uneventful. Although exceedingly rare, electroencephalographic and epileptiform activities were reported during inhalational inductions with sevoflurane in children (Komatsu et al., 1994; Vakkuri et al., 2001; Jaaskelainen et al., 2003). Investigations failed to identify a cause for these episodes (Constant et al., 1999). Rare instances of twitching of the face or limb usually dissipate rapidly as the depth of anesthesia is increased. If the inspired concentration of sevoflurane is increased slowly (i.e., in 0.5% to 1% increments every few breaths), a protracted excitement phase may ensue during the induction. This can be obviated by increasing the inspired concentration of sevoflurane very quickly, without inducing airway reflex responses.

Administering 60% to 70% nitrous oxide for approximately 1 minute and then adding 8% (inspired concentration) sevoflurane to the nitrous oxide makes the induction rapid and smooth. Recall of the odor of sevoflurane is rare, and excitement during the induction of anesthesia is minimal. Other techniques for rapid induction of anesthesia in children with sevoflurane have included a single breath (vital capacity) induction with 8% sevoflurane, which is 40% more rapid than a single breath induction with 5% halothane (Agnor et al., 1998). Whichever technique is used to induce anesthesia, clinicians continue to be surprised by anesthetized children who withdrew on attempted cannulation of a vein. This results not from a flaw in the anesthetic, sevoflurane, but rather in the combination of its pharmacology and delivery. Compared with halothane, the modestly increased maximum vaporizer concentration of sevoflurane is overshadowed by the 250% greater MAC. This limits the alveolar concentration that can be achieved in the first few minutes of anesthesia. This may reduce the probability of circulatory depression during induction of anesthesia with sevoflurane, but it also prevents clinicians from inducing a deep level of anesthesia quickly and thereby preventing a response to stimulation.

Like halothane, sevoflurane is a potent respiratory depressant. At concentrations greater than 1.5 MAC, sevoflurane is a more potent respiratory depressant than halothane. Indeed, apnea may occur in the nonstimulated child breathing 8% inspired sevoflurane. Premedication with midazolam or other medications may potentiate the respiratory depression with sevoflurane. After an inhalational induction with sevoflurane, spontaneous ventilation usually resumes after a brief period of apnea or manual ventilation of the lungs and a reduction in the inspired concentration of sevoflurane. Sevoflurane maintains cardiovascular homeostasis in infants and children. At 1 MAC sevoflurane, heart rate is usually maintained in infants and children even when they are not pretreated with atropine (Lerman et al., 1994), although rare instances of a slowing of the heart rate have been reported, particularly at concentrations exceeding 1 MAC. Systolic pressure is usually reduced 20% to 25% from awake values. These responses to 1 MAC sevoflurane are similar to those after other inhalational anesthetics. Arrhythmias during sevoflurane anesthesia are infrequent; the incidence of arrhythmias during sevoflurane anesthesia after exogenous epinephrine is similar to that during isoflurane anesthesia. In infants and children with congenital heart disease undergoing cardiac surgery, hypotension and desaturation in cyanotic children after sevoflurane anesthesia occurred less frequently than they did after halothane anesthesia (Russell et al., 2001). In parallel with the rapid elimination of sevoflurane, the recovery profile for sevoflurane is rapid compared with that for halothane. Transient agitation and involuntary movements during emergence from anesthesia have been reported. Emergence agitation occurs primarily in preschool age children, lasts 10 to 20 minutes, and is often self-limiting. Although agitation has been attributed to pain, pain as the sole explanation was dispelled when agitation was noted in children after lower abdominal surgery with a working caudal block in situ and after sevoflurane for magnetic resonance imaging procedures, where no pain occurs (Aono et al., 1997; Cravero et al., 2000). One of the most difficult problems has been defining emergence agitation, which could not previously be assessed with any scale or measurement (Sikich and Lerman, 2004). It is important to note that emergence agitation is not unique to sevoflurane; it also occurs after other anesthetic agents, including isoflurane and desflurane.

Sevoflurane is degraded both in vivo (to inorganic fluoride and hexafluoroisopropanol) and in vitro (via alkaline hydrolysis in the presence of soda lime or Baralyme [barium hydroxide lime] to five compounds: A to E [Hanaki et al., 1987; Morio et al., 1992]). In vivo, sevoflurane is metabolized by microsomal CYP IIE1 isozyme in both the liver and kidney (Kharasch et al., 1995a, 1995b). The peak plasma concentration of inorganic fluoride is proportional to the duration of exposure to sevoflurane in children. However, there have been no instances of sevoflurane-induced nephrotoxicity after several million anesthetic procedures. Two plausible explanations for the absence of nephrotoxicity are the rapid elimination of sevoflurane and the small extent of intrarenal metabolism of sevoflurane, the putative source of inorganic fluoride–induced nephrotoxicity (Kharasch et al., 1995a). In vitro, sevoflurane is both absorbed and degraded in the presence of soda lime and Baralyme, yielding only compound A in significant concentrations; up to 20 to 40 ppm in closed circuits in humans (Liu et al., 1991). Alkaline hydrolysis of sevoflurane is enhanced by high temperatures, decreased water content in the absorbent, increased inspired concentration of sevoflurane, and new absorbent. In infants and children, compound A concentrations during sevoflurane anesthesia in a closed circuit increase in parallel with increasing in age (Frink et al., 1996). In concentrations up to 100 ppm for 3 hours, compound A causes histopathologic changes in the kidneys of rats (Gonsowski et al., 1994a, 1994b), although no evidence of histopathologic or pathophysiologic renal changes have been reported in humans. In the presence of desiccated soda lime and Baralyme, sevoflurane is degraded to only an extremely small extent to carbon monoxide (Fang et al., 1995; Wissing et al., 2001). When both potassium hydroxide and sodium hydroxide are eliminated from the absorbent (i.e., Amsorb), sevoflurane produces only minute concentrations of carbon monoxide (Murray et al., 1999; Versichelen et al., 2001). The combination of high-dose sevoflurane with desiccated Baralyme has resulted in instances of extreme heat and fire within the absorbent canister.

DESFLURANE

Desflurane is a potent polyfluorinated methyl ethyl ether anesthetic available for use in infants and children. The single substitution of a fluorine atom for a chlorine atom on the carbon atom of isoflurane dramatically changes the physicochemical properties of this anesthetic (see Table 6–15). Blood/gas and tissue/blood solubilities are only fractions of those of halothane and isoflurane (Yasuda et al., 1989). As a result, the wash-in of desflurane is the fastest of all of the available potent inhalational anesthetics (see Fig. 6–26). As in the case of sevoflurane, changes in alveolar ventilation and cardiac output exert small effects on the pharmacokinetics of this anesthetic, whereas changes in right-to-left shunting exert a large effect (Eger, 1974; Lerman, 2002). Just as the wash-in of desflurane is extremely fast, so, too, the washout of desflurane is extremely rapid. Of the potent inhalational anesthetics, the elimination of desflurane is most rapid (Yasuda, 1991) (see Fig. 6–26).

The MAC of desflurane in infants and children is least in neonates, increasing throughout infancy and reaching a zenith of 9.9% in infants aged 6 to 12 months. MAC decreases thereafter with increasing age through adolescence (Taylor and

Lerman, 1991). Nitrous oxide (60%) decreases the MAC of desflurane by only 26% in children (Fisher and Zwass, 1992), an effect similar to that of sevoflurane.

Inhalational inductions with desflurane are not recommended because upper airway reflexes are frequently triggered (50% incidence of breath holding, 40% incidence of laryngospasm) (Taylor and Lerman, 1992; Zwass et al., 1992). If anesthesia is induced by either the intravenous or inhalational route, desflurane may be used to maintain anesthesia (Taylor and Lerman, 1992; Zwass et al., 1992). Like sevoflurane, desflurane maintains cardiovascular homeostasis at 1 MAC (Taylor and Lerman, 1991). At this concentration, heart rate and systolic blood pressure are depressed 20% to 25% compared with awake values (Taylor and Lerman, 1991). Arrhythmias and bradycardia are uncommon with this anesthetic.

The rate of recovery after desflurane anesthesia parallels the extremely rapid washout of this anesthetic (Taylor and Lerman, 1992; Davis et al., 1994). Early experience with the rapid recovery after discontinuation of desflurane resulted in the precipitous onset of excruciating surgical pain. A strategy to prevent pain on emergence must be considered and the intervention instituted before discontinuation of this anesthetic.

Desflurane resists metabolism both in vivo (0.02%) (Smiley et al., 1991) and in vitro (in the presence of soda lime and Baralyme). In vivo, insignificant blood concentrations of inorganic fluoride are produced after desflurane anesthesia. However, in vitro degradation of desflurane may be problematic. If the carbon dioxide absorbent becomes desiccated and is incubated with desflurane, then desflurane may react with the constituents to release carbon monoxide into the inspired limb of the breathing circuit (Fang et al., 1995; Wissing et al., 2001). Other ether anesthetics, including isoflurane and enflurane, all difluoromethyl ethyl ether anesthetics (including desflurane), undergo a similar path of degradation to carbon monoxide in the presence of desiccated absorbent, albeit to a lesser extent than desflurane (Baxter et al., 1998). Absorbent becomes desiccated by circulating fresh gas through an absorbent canister for a prolonged period of time without a reservoir bag in place. In some anesthetic machines, this continuous fresh gas flow desiccates the absorbent by flowing retrograde through the canister, exiting where the reservoir bag usually is attached. Without the ability to detect carbon monoxide in the breathing circuit, contamination of the breathing circuit with carbon monoxide might present a serious risk to patients, particularly those anesthetized after the anesthetic machine has not been used for a prolonged period (i.e., Monday mornings). To preclude this complication, the fresh gas flow should be discontinued when the anesthetic machine is not in use, the reservoir bag should never be removed from the canister, and, most important, the anesthetic machine should be turned off when not in use. If one suspects that the absorbent has been desiccated, the absorbent must be replaced before any anesthetic is administered. There are no guidelines for rehumidifying desiccated absorbents. Not all absorbents produce carbon monoxide when they are exposed to the desflurane. Those absorbents that lack both potassium hydroxide and sodium hydroxide (i.e., Amsorb) do not produce carbon monoxide.

With a boiling point close to room temperature, a heated pressurized vaporizer was developed to deliver a predictable concentration of desflurane. This vaporizer requires electrical current to maintain a predictable temperature and pressure that are independent of ambient conditions.

ISOFLURANE

The pharmacology of isoflurane is very similar to that of desflurane with a few exceptions. As mentioned, the chemical structure of isoflurane is identical to that of desflurane except that isoflurane has a chlorine atom instead of a fluoride atom on the carbon atom (see Table 6–15). Because isoflurane is more soluble in blood and tissues than desflurane, the wash-in and washout of isoflurane are slower than those of desflurane (see Fig. 6–26) (Yasuda et al., 1991). The MAC of isoflurane is intermediate between those of halothane and sevoflurane, as described previously (see Table 6–15) (Cameron et al., 1984).

Like desflurane, isoflurane triggers airway reflex responses during inhalational inductions and is not suited for this purpose. Although numerous attempts were made to ameliorate the airway responses to an inhalational induction, clinicians abandoned the notion of using it for this purpose. Isoflurane is used similarly to desflurane for the maintenance phase of anesthesia.

Once anesthesia is induced, whether the airway is instrumented or not, children and adults breathe isoflurane without difficulty. Similarly, they emerge from isoflurane anesthesia without difficulty.

Isoflurane, like desflurane, does not depress the circulation in children. In fact, heart rate often increases during isoflurane anesthesia and blood pressure is well maintained. Unlike in the adult, rapid increases in the inspired concentration of isoflurane do not trigger a central sympathetic (tachycardia and hypertension) response that requires intervention with an opioid or other agent.

The in vivo metabolism of isoflurane, 0.2%, yields very small concentrations of inorganic fluoride in the blood without significant intrarenal production. Nephrotoxicity after isoflurane anesthesia is not a substantive risk. However, in the presence of desiccated soda lime and Baralyme, isoflurane can produce carbon monoxide, as discussed earlier.

HALOTHANE

Halothane has been the standard of practice against which all other inhalational anesthetics were compared until the introduction of sevoflurane. Halothane is the only nonether anesthetic that is used today, being an alkane in structure. The wash-in of halothane is the slowest of the currently used anesthetic agents because it is the most soluble (see Table 6–15). This means that the time to equilibration of inspired and alveolar (or brain) partial pressures of halothane is the greatest of the anesthetics. Although this may be viewed as a safety factor, the potency of halothane is the greatest of the anesthetic agents. These two factors, together with the ability to deliver a maximum inspired concentration of 5% halothane with all vaporizers, resulted in numerous episodes of cardiorespiratory instability that included hypotension and bradycardia/arrhythmias. In particular, concern was expressed in the 1980s about the ability of neonates to tolerate halothane anesthesia because of the hemodynamic consequences. Based on our current understanding of the pharmacology of halothane, several conclusions may be made about the past experience with this anesthetic in pediatric anesthesia:

1. The MAC for halothane in neonates is less than that in older infants.
2. Halothane depresses both the circulation and respiration in infants and children.

3. With the design of the vaporizer and given the potency of halothane, it is easier to overdose children with halothane than with other anesthetic agents.

Halothane is metabolized approximately 15% to 20% in humans. Immunologic responses including hepatitis have been documented after repeat halothane anesthesia even in children (Kenna et al., 1989). With the declining use of this agent in clinical practice, it is unlikely to pose a serious threat to children.

UPTAKE AND DISTRIBUTION

The uptake and distribution of inhaled anesthetics are more rapid in infants and small children than in adults (Salanitre and Rackow, 1969; Steward and Creighton, 1978; Gallagher and Black, 1985). Studies have shown inspired and expired partial pressures of nitrous oxide equilibrate in infants in 25 minutes, in children in 30 minutes, and in adults in 60 minutes (Salanitre and Rackow, 1969). However, the differences in uptake between children and adults are magnified as the solubility of the agents increases. In the case of halothane, the wash-in in infants and children is more rapid than it is in adults (Fig. 6–27).

Four factors explain the more rapid wash-in of alveolar to inspired anesthetic partial pressures in children compared with adults:

1. Increased alveolar ventilation–to–functional residual capacity (FRC) ratio
2. Increased cardiac output
3. Decreased blood/gas partition coefficient (Lerman et al., 1984)
4. Decreased tissue/blood partition coefficients (Lerman et al., 1986)

The alveolar ventilation–to–FRC ratio in infants (5:1) is about threefold greater than it is in adults (1.5:1). Because the time to achieve 63% equilibration of alveolar to inspired anesthetic partial pressures (one time constant) is the ratio of the volume to the flow through the volume, the greater the ratio of alveolar ventilation to FRC, the faster is the time to equilibration. This effect is more pronounced for soluble anesthetics than it is for less-soluble anesthetics.

Although an increased cardiac output should delay the equilibration of alveolar to inspired anesthetic partial pressures (Eger, 1974), an increased cardiac output in infants actually speeds the equilibration of partial pressures. This paradoxical effect may be attributed to the vessel-rich group (VRG) (brain, heart, liver, kidneys, and endocrine glands) representing 18% of body weight in infants compared with 8% in adults. This effect is compounded by the limited muscle and fat mass in the infant. An increased cardiac output distributed primarily to the VRG in infants speeds the equilibration of anesthetic partial pressures in the VRG.

The lower solubilities of inhalational anesthetics in blood and tissues in neonates and infants (Lerman et al., 1984, 1986) compared with those in adults speed the equilibration of alveolar to inspired anesthetic partial pressures. The time constant for equilibration of inspired and alveolar anesthetic partial pressures in tissues is similar to that for the lungs, but this equation includes the tissue solubility, as follows:

$$\text{Time constant} = (\text{Organ volume} \times \text{tissue/blood solubility})/\text{organ blood flow} \quad (6.17)$$

Hence, if the tissue/blood solubility in infants is one half that in adults, then the time constant is reduced by one half and the time to 95% equilibration (four time constants) is one half that in adults. This effect is augmented by the reduced mass of the neonatal myocardium compared with that of the adult (Fig. 6–28).

Effect of Shunting

Intracardiac and intrapulmonary shunts can affect the uptake of inhalational anesthetics (Stoelting and Longnecker, 1972; Tanner et al., 1985; Huntington et al., 1999). A right-to-left shunt slows the uptake of anesthetic as the partial pressure in arterial blood increases more slowly. The effect of the shunt is

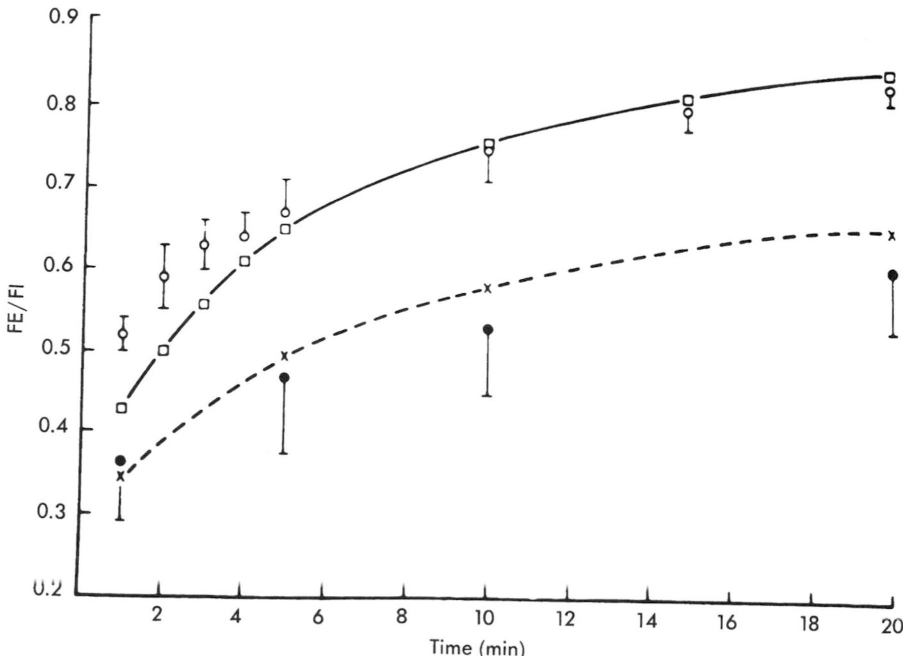

FIGURE 6–27. The observed ratio of expired to inspired halothane (FE/FI) in infants demonstrates their more rapid uptake of halothane compared with adults. |—O—|, Infant observed (mean ± SD); —□—, infant predicted; |—●—|, adult observed (mean ± SD); x– – –x, adult predicted. (Observed data from adults from Sechzer PH, Linde HW, Dripps RD, et al.: *Anesthesiology* 24:779, 1963; Eger EI II, Bahlman SH, Munson ES: *Anesthesiology* 35:365, 1971a. Predicted curves generated from a computerized model. Reprinted with permission from the International Anesthesia Research Society from Brandom BW, Brandom RB, Cook DR: *Anesth Analg* 62:404, 1983.)

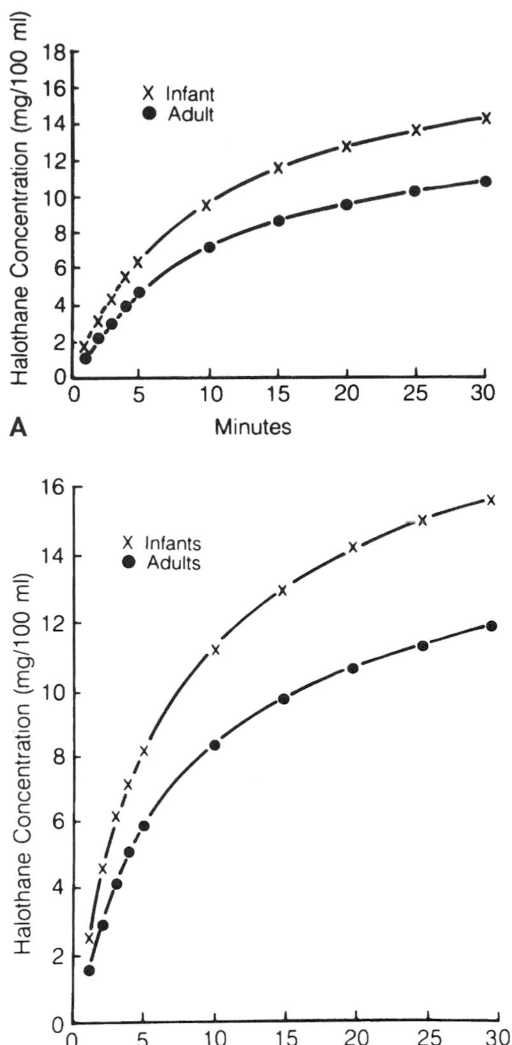

■ **FIGURE 6–28.** *(A)* Predicted concentration of halothane in the brain. Values were derived from a computerized model of anesthetic uptake and distribution. *(B)* Predicted concentration of halothane in the heart. (Reprinted with permission from the International Anesthesia Research Society from Brandom BW, Brandom RB, Cook DR: *Anesth Analg* 62:404, 1983.)

more pronounced with less soluble anesthetics than it is with more soluble anesthetics (Lerman, 2002) (Fig. 6–29). Induction of anesthesia is protracted in the presence of an insoluble anesthetic with a right-to-left shunt. Evidence suggests that when anesthetizing children with congenital heart disease, sevoflurane may better preserve cardiovascular homeostasis than halothane (Russell et al., 2001). Care must be taken to avoid an inadvertent overdose of a soluble inhaled anesthetic as removal of the anesthetic in the presence of a right-to-left shunt may be prolonged. The effect of a left-to-right shunt depends on the magnitude of the shunt and on whether there is a coincidental right-to-left shunt. A large (>80%) left-to-right shunt increases the rate of uptake of anesthetic from the FRC to the arterial blood: smaller shunts (<50%) have a negligible effect on uptake.

Anesthetic Requirements and Minimum Alveolar Concentration

The MACs for various inhalation anesthetics generally are inversely related to age (Gregory et al., 1969; Lerman et al., 1983; LeDez and Lerman, 1987; Taylor and Lerman, 1991; Lerman et al., 1994). Anesthetic requirement is usually quantified by the MAC, at which 50% of the subjects move in response to a surgical stimulus. Alternatively, the MAC for an individual subject can be estimated as an intermediate concentration between a concentration associated with movement and one associated with no movement. To prevent a sympathetic response to a surgical stimulus, the end-tidal concentration must exceed the MAC by 30%.

In the first months of life, the relationship between age and MAC is complex. The neurologic connections are intact beginning about 24 weeks' gestation. Gregory and others (1983) noted that MAC in lambs increased during gestation and in the first few hours of postnatal life. Several plausible explanations have been proposed to explain the age-related change in MAC, including change in progesterone levels, endorphin levels, and enkephalin levels; however, none of these have been substantiated.

Equally perplexing is the change in MAC with age in humans. In this case, MAC increases throughout gestation from 24 weeks' gestation, reaching a peak during infancy (LeDez and Lerman, 1987). For isoflurane and halothane, MAC reaches its zenith in infants aged 1 to 6 months (Lerman et al., 1983; Cameron et al., 1984). For desflurane, MAC reaches its zenith in infants aged 6 to 12 months (Taylor and Lerman, 1991). In the case of sevoflurane, MAC does not peak in infancy but rather is constant in neonates and infants younger than 6 months (Lerman et al., 1994). After reaching its peak, MAC decreases with increasing age to adulthood.

Although MAC additivity has been widely accepted, two exceptions were reported in children. The contribution of the MAC of nitrous oxide to the MAC of sevoflurane and desflurane in children appear to be less than additive. In both of these instances, 60% nitrous oxide reduced the MAC values of these two anesthetics in children by only 26% (Fisher and Zwass, 1992; Lerman et al., 1994). The explanation for this attenuated effect remains unclear.

Frei and others (1997) reported that the MAC of halothane in cognitively challenged children was reduced. In particular, they noted a 25% decrease in the MAC in those challenged children who were not receiving seizure medication and a further 15% reduction in the MAC if they had been taking seizure medication. Although the cognitively challenged children had a heterogeneous group of disorders, this is the first evidence of a reduced anesthetic requirement in these children.

Respiration

All inhalational anesthetics depress respiration in a dose-dependent manner. In general, tidal volume and the response to carbon dioxide decrease and respiratory rate increases as the anesthetic concentration increases. These effects are most pronounced in the neonate and young infant because the mechanics of respiratory effort are compromised due to the child's immature chest wall (bones) and lungs (lack of elastin). In the case of sevoflurane, the extent of respiratory depression is similar to that of halothane up to 1.4 MAC, but thereafter respiratory depression may be greater with sevoflurane. It is important to note that compared with halothane, sevoflurane decreases intercostal muscle tone to a lesser extent. If hypopnea or apnea should occur during sevoflurane or desflurane anesthesia, it is important to recognize that their low solubilities in blood and tissues should facilitate a rapid reduction in anesthetic concentration and resolution of the respiratory depression.

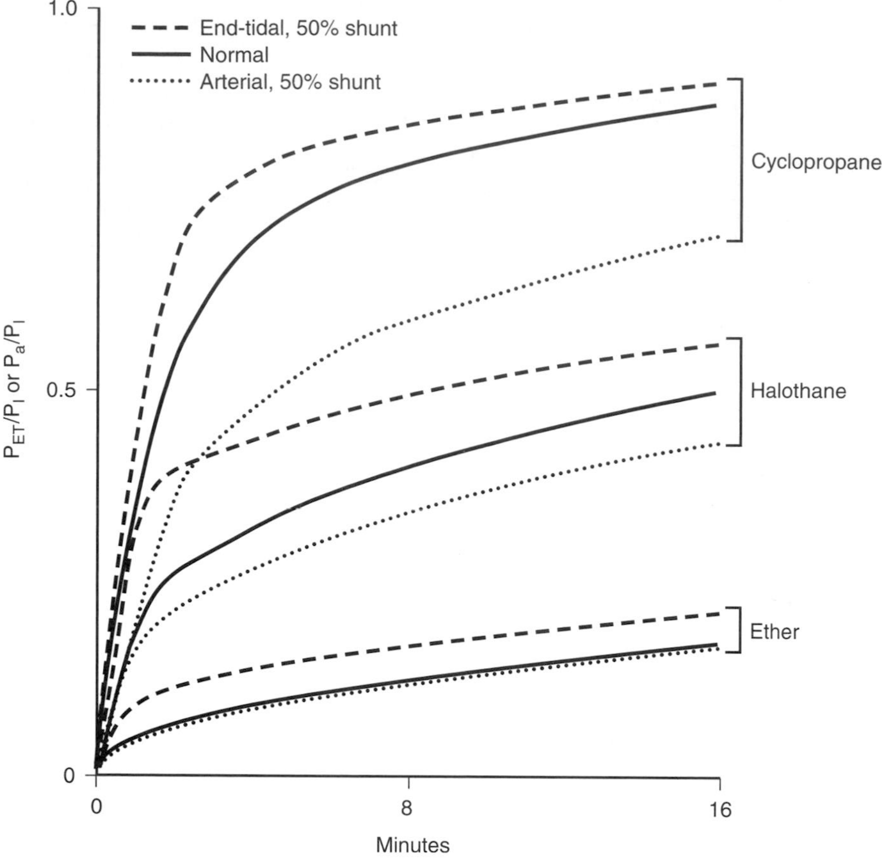

■ **FIGURE 6–29.** When no ventilation–perfusion abnormalities exist, the alveolar (P_A or P_{ET}) and arterial a) anesthetic partial pressures rise together *(solid lines)* toward the inspired partial pressure P_a). When 50% of the cardiac output is shunted through the lungs, the rate of rise of the end-tidal partial pressure *(dashed lines)* is accelerated, whereas the rate of rise of the arterial partial pressure *(dotted lines)* is retarded. The greatest retardation is found with the least soluble anesthetic, cyclopropane. (Redrawn from Eger EI II: *Anesthetic uptake and action.* Baltimore, 1974, Williams & Wilkins. ©1974, El Eger II, MD.)

Circulation

The incidence of bradycardia, hypotension, and cardiac arrest during induction of anesthesia is greater in infants and children than in adults (Leigh and Belton, 1960; Rackow et al., 1961; Keenan and Boyan, 1985; Cohen et al., 1990). This has been attributed in part to the administration of excessive concentrations of inhalational anesthetics to neonates (Lerman et al., 1983) and to an increased sensitivity of the myocardium in neonates to inhalational anesthetics. Inhalational anesthetics depress contractility of the myocardium in neonatal rats and rabbits compared with adult animals (Rao et al., 1986; Krane and Su, 1987; Murat et al., 1990; Palmisano et al., 1994). This may result from structural or functional differences, or both, in the myocardium of neonates and adults. In particular, there is a paucity of contractile elements and decreased sarcoplasmic reticulum in neonatal myocardium. The latter increases the neonate's dependency on the influx of extracellular calcium to support contractility. Current evidence suggests that inhalational anesthetics decrease the calcium flux by their actions on the calcium channels themselves, Na^+–Ca^{2+} exchange pumps, and the sarcoplasmic reticulum (Baum and Palmisano, 1997). Further evidence now suggests that inhalational anesthetics may attenuate contractility of ventricular myocytes via voltage-dependent L-type calcium channels (which release large amounts of calcium from the sarcoplasmic reticulum) (Baum and Wetzel, 1994). This may explain why neonates are more sensitive to the cardiodepressant effects of inhalational anesthetics than are adults. To clearly define the issue of age-related cardiovascular sensitivity, it is necessary to measure simultaneously the determinants of cardiac output in anesthetized subjects (or animals) at known end-tidal concentrations of anesthetic and at known MAC multiples. In addition, it is necessary to define the sensitivity of cardiovascular "protective" reflexes (baroreceptor reflexes) at MAC multiples of the anesthetic. Direct measurement of cardiac output, contractility, preload, and afterload involves invasive techniques, although the application of an indirect measurement of these variables using noninvasive techniques such as echocardiography has provided some evidence of age-related effects of inhalational anesthetics in humans in early infancy. This, together with neonatal animal data, has clarified these effects in this age group.

The cardiovascular effects of 1.0 and 1.5 MAC halothane and isoflurane were compared in healthy neonates and infants with the use of two-dimensional echocardiography (Murray et al., 1992). Depression of the cardiovascular system was dose dependent and similar with both anesthetics (>30% decrease in ejection fraction and stroke volume at 1.5 MAC) in the two age groups. Atropine (0.02 mg/kg) increased heart rate and cardiac output up to 20% at 1.5 MAC for both anesthetics in both age groups (Barash et al., 1978). In a previous study that included infants and children between 9 days and 32 months old, 15 mL/kg lactated Ringer's solution decreased the stroke volume index at 1.25 MAC halothane, whereas it increased the stroke volume index with isoflurane (Murray et al., 1987). Interpretation of the latter study is difficult in view of the large age range of the infants studied.

Halothane depresses cardiovascular function in direct proportion to the depth of anesthesia (MacGregor et al., 1958; Reynolds, 1962; Barash et al., 1978). This depression results from direct myocardial depression, dromotropic (cardiac slowing), and a reduction in peripheral resistance (Goldberg, 1968;

Skovsted et al., 1969; Eger et al., 1970, 1971). This cardiovascular depression can be attenuated by the use of atropine (Barash et al., 1978; Murray et al., 1992).

Isoflurane has a direct negative inotropic effect on myocardium and causes a marked reduction in peripheral resistance. It is considered to have a less depressant effect than halothane on the cardiovascular system, however, because cardiac output is more adequately sustained during hypotension by a compensatory increase in heart rate. In normal adults, both drugs cause reduced blood pressure with increasing depth of agent when used without supplementation, with the hypotension with halothane being greater.

Sevoflurane and desflurane confer similar cardiodepressant activity as isoflurane at equipotent concentrations. At approximately 1 MAC sevoflurane and desflurane, heart rate and blood pressure are similarly reduced in neonates, infants, and children as they are with isoflurane.

Metabolism

Inhalational anesthetics are metabolized to varying degrees in vivo. The extent of metabolism in adults is as follows: methoxyflurane (50%) > halothane (15% to 25%) > sevoflurane (5%) > enflurane (2.4%) > isoflurane (0.2%) > desflurane (0.02%). Metabolism of inhalational anesthetics in vivo in neonates is less than that in adults. This may be attributed to several factors, including reduced activity of the hepatic microsomal enzyme activities, reduced fat stores, and more rapid elimination of inhalational anesthetics in neonates compared with adults. Halothane and, more recently, enflurane have been suspected of causing liver dysfunction. Several cases of postoperative liver failure have been attributed to "halothane hepatitis" in children (Kenna et al., 1989). The exact mechanism that leads to this response remains unclear, although some have speculated that it may be caused by a specific metabolite of halothane. This putative toxic substance may be produced when the reductive pathway for halothane biotransformation in the liver microsomes is active as, for example, when hepatic blood flow is impaired and liver enzyme induction has occurred. Because the reductive metabolic pathways in the liver are poorly developed in infants and children, this may account for the very low incidence of halothane hepatitis in children. Perioperative liver dysfunction has been associated with the use of halothane, isoflurane, enflurane, and desflurane (Carrigan et al., 1987; Martin et al., 1995). Transient hepatic dysfunction has been reported after administration of halothane and sevoflurane in children (Kenna et al., 1989; Ogawa et al., 1991; Watanabe et al., 1993).

In vivo metabolism of inhalational anesthetics to inorganic fluoride has been discussed for each anesthetic. Similarly, the propensity of these anesthetics to undergo in vitro degradation to compound A in the case of sevoflurane and carbon monoxide in the cases of desflurane, isoflurane, and enflurane has also been discussed.

Malignant Hyperthermia

All inhalational anesthetics can trigger malignant hyperthermia (MH) reactions. However, whether the probability of triggering a reaction or the severity of a reaction, were it to occur, differs among these anesthetics is less clear. For example, the relative capability of these anesthetics to augment a caffeine-induced contracture in vitro follows the order of halothane > enflurane > isoflurane > methoxyflurane. The onset of an MH reaction in susceptible swine differs among the anesthetics: halothane > isoflurane > desflurane (Wedel et al., 1993). MH is discussed in further detail in Chapter 31, Malignant Hyperthermia.

NEUROMUSCULAR BLOCKING AGENTS

Neuromuscular blocking agents are frequently used to facilitate endotracheal intubation, to provide surgical relaxation, and to facilitate controlled mechanical ventilation in both the operating room and the intensive care unit (ICU). Neuromuscular blocking agents have no sedative, hypnotic, or analgesic side effects, but they may indirectly decrease metabolic demand, prevent shivering, decrease nonsynchronous ventilation, decrease ICP, and improve chest wall compliance. The purposes of this section are to review (1) the growth and development of the neuromuscular junction and (2) the age-related pharmacologic characteristics of neuromuscular blocking agents.

NEUROMUSCULAR SYSTEM

Throughout infancy, the neuromuscular junction matures physically and biochemically, the contractile properties of skeletal muscle change, and the amount of muscle in proportion to body weight increases; as a result, the neuromuscular junction is variably sensitive to relaxants. In addition, there are changes in the apparent volume of distribution of relaxants, their redistribution and excretion (clearance), and possibly their rate of metabolism. These factors influence the dose-response relationship of relaxants (i.e., ED_{50} and ED_{95}) and the duration of neuromuscular blockade. The ED_{95}, which is the mean dose that produces a maximal effect of 95% twitch suppression or neuromuscular blockade, of a neuromuscular blocking agent can be viewed conceptually as proportional to both the volume of distribution (the bucket size) and the concentration of the blocker at its effect site. Both factors have major age-related differences. Although the concentration of drug at the neuromuscular junction in vivo is inaccessible, the drug concentration in plasma that produces 95% twitch suppression at steady-state conditions (C_{ss95}) provides a means of comparing drug potencies and the factors that affect them. The volume of distribution of neuromuscular blocking agents is highly correlated with (but not equal to) the ECF volume. The ECF of the volume of the infant is significantly greater than that of the older child and adult on a weight basis. ECF volume and surface area, by contrast, bear a nearly constant relationship throughout life (6 to 8 L/m^2). Major organ failure, upregulation of acetylcholine (ACh) receptors, poor nutrition, electrolyte and acid-base abnormalities, hypothermia drug interactions, and muscle atrophy can also profoundly influence both the kinetics and dynamics of relaxants (Fiamengo and Savarese, 1991; Klessig et al., 1992; Magorian and Lynam, 1992; Martyn et al., 1992; Rupp, 1987; Viby-Mogensen, 1993; Fleming, 1994; Watling and Dasta, 1994; Elliot and Bion, 1995; Kim et al., 1995; Lee, 1995; Miller, 1995).

Neuromuscular Junction and Neuromuscular Transmission

The general anatomy, age-related physiology, and pharmacology of the neuromuscular junction have been well defined (Meakin et al., 1992; Wareham et al., 1994; Calakos and Scheller, 1996; Prince and Since, 1998; Sanes and Lichtman, 1999). The neuromuscular system is incompletely developed at birth. The conduction velocity of motor nerves increases throughout gestation as nerve fibers are myelinated. The myotubules connect to mature

TABLE 6–16. Development of skeletal muscle fibers

Age	Development
4 wk	Mesenchymal cells become syncytial; myoblasts become myotube.
5 wk	Syncytial myotube grows in length.
9 wk	Primitive muscle fibers with myofilaments appear.
5 mo	More myofilaments appear and grow in length.
Birth	Nuclei are centralized.
Adult	Muscle fibers become thicker and longer; myofilaments multiply; myofilaments differentiate into actin and myosin; nuclei move more peripherally; myofilaments aggregate into bundles and form myofibrils; muscle fibers grow still thicker and longer; nuclei have shifted peripherally; muscle fibers are thick and mature; alternating actin and myosin myofilaments aggregate into longitudinal bundles.

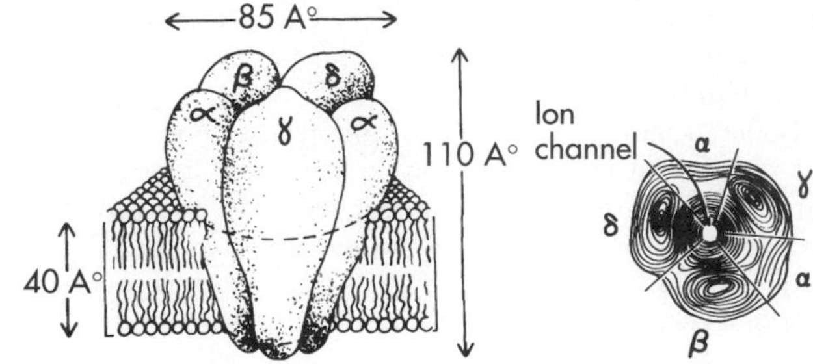

FIGURE 6–30. Structure of the nicotinic acetylcholine receptor and a description of the requirements to activate and competitively antagonize receptor function. The five subunits (2α, β, γ, and δ with apparent molecular masses of 40, 50, 60, and 65 kDa, respectively), which are partly homologous in sequence, are arranged to form the perimeter of an internal cavity, which is believed to be the ion channel. Each of the subunits has an extracellular and a cytoplasmic exposure, with the bulk of the peptide chain existing on the extracellular side. The α subunits each carry a recognition site for agonists and competitive antagonists. (With permission from Taylor P: Are neuromuscular blocking agents more efficacious in pairs? *Anesthesiology* 63:1, 1985.)

muscle fibers in the latter part of intrauterine life and in the first several weeks after birth (Table 6–16). Some slow-contracting muscle (e.g., intrinsic muscles of the hand) is progressively converted to fast-contracting muscle, with a concomitant change in the force–velocity relationship. Both the diaphragm and the intercostal muscles increase their percentage of slow muscle fibers in the first months of life. Synaptic transmission is relatively slow at birth but, more important, the rate at which ACh is released during repeated nerve stimulation is limited in the infant. The margin of safety for neurotransmissions is smaller in infants than in adults. Age-related changes in the ACh receptor may also contribute to the reduced margin of safety of neurotransmission. See Box 6–1.

Acetylcholine Receptors

Prejunctional, postjunctional, and extrajunctional ACh receptors are involved with neuromuscular transmission. The postjunctional ACh receptor is organized into five subprotein units, forming a rosette with a central pit at the mouth of the ion channel, a so-called doughnut hole (Fig. 6–30). Each rosette is made up of two α_1 units and a β_1, ε, and δ unit. These subunits are arranged in a specific order (counterclockwise α_1*–ε–α_1–δ–β_1). The α* subunit has a higher affinity binding site for *d*-tubocurarine. The binding sites for ACh and neuromuscular blocking drugs are at the α_1/δ interface (Blount and Merlie, 1989; Gu et al., 1990; Pederson and Cohen, 1990). Fetal ACh receptor subtypes differ in the structure of one subunit from the adult subtype (i.e., a γ subunit is present in the fetal ACh receptor instead of the ε subunit present in the adult ACh receptor). One presumes that neonates have a mix of both adult and fetal receptors, but at term the adult subtypes are more common. Functional differences exist between these two forms of ACh receptors (Table 6–17; Fig. 6–31). These differences appear to contribute to the sensitivity of fetal ACh muscle receptors to nondepolarizing and depolarizing neuromuscular blocking drugs. Some uncertainty exists concerning these observations (Martyn et al., 1992; Yost and Dodson, 1993; Paul et al., 2002).

Prejunctional receptors (α_3 subunits) modulate both ACh mobilization and release. They have different binding characteristics and possibly different channel characteristics than the postjunctional receptors (Bowman, 1980). Antagonism of the prejunctional receptor results in diminished release of ACh from neurons stimulated at high frequency. These prejunctional receptors increase ACh mobilization to readily releasable stores and provide feedback control during high-frequency stimulation. The ontogeny of α_3 subunits is not known.

BOX 6–1 Characteristics of neonatal neuromuscular junction

- Acetylcholine receptors change in function and distribution.
- Slow twitch fibers (type I increase severalfold in first 6 months).
- Infants younger than 2 months have lower train-of-four ratio.
- Infants younger than 2 months have increased fade.
- Differences more pronounced in premature infants than in term infants.

TABLE 6–17. Distinguishing features of mature and fetal receptors

Mature Receptors	Fetal Receptors*
ε Subunit	γ Subunit
Localized to end-plate region	Junctional and extrajunctional sites
Metabolically stable (half-life 2 wk)	Metabolically unstable (half-life ≈24 hr)
Larger single-channel conductance	Smaller single-channel conductance
Shorter mean open time	Twofold to 10-fold longer mean open time
Agonists depolarize less easily	Agonists depolarize more easily
Competitive agents block more easily	Competitive agents block less easily†

*Immature junctional receptors have the same characteristics as upregulated extrajunctional receptors.

Data from Martyn JA, White DA, Gronert GA, et al.: *Anesthesiology* 76:822, 1992.

†Recent data conflict with this statement (M. Paul, C. H. Kindler, R. M. Fokt, et al.: 2002).

Fetal receptors are more sensitive to pancuronium, vecuronium, mivacurium, and rocuronium but not to *d*-tubocurarine or gallamine.

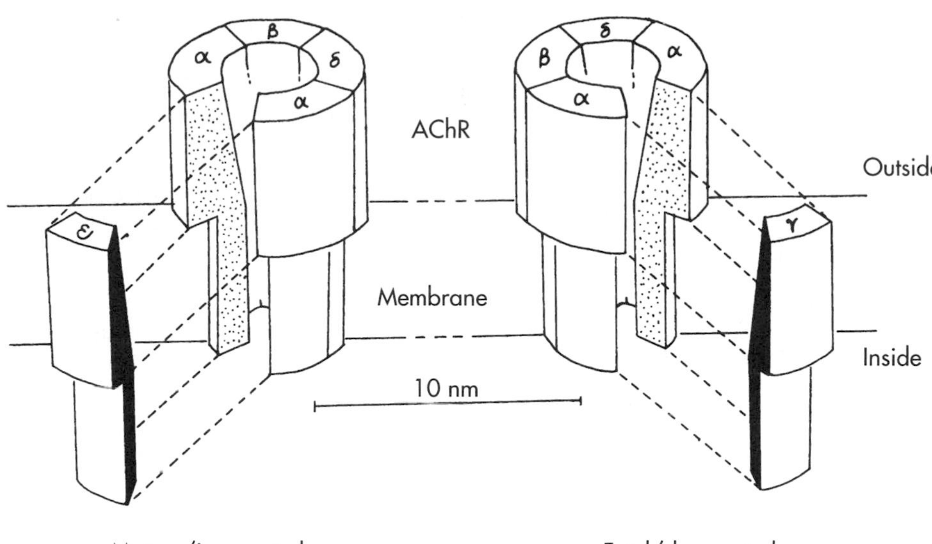

■ **FIGURE 6–31.** Acetylcholine receptor (AChR) channels with the subunits (α, β, ε, and δ or α, β, γ, and δ) arranged around the central cation channel. Binding of acetylcholine to the two α subunits induces the conformational change that converts the channel from closed to open, although the mean channel open times differ between the two types of AChRs depicted here. (With permission from Martyn JAJ, White DA, Gronert GA, et al.: *Anesthesiology* 76:822, 1992.)

A limited number of extrajunctional ACh receptors (i.e., fetal or upregulated receptors) are also loosely incorporated in the muscle membrane of older infants, children, or adults. Nerve activity inhibits the biosynthesis of ACh receptors at extrajunctional sites. Neurologic motor defects, direct muscle trauma, thermal injury, disease atrophy, sepsis, and prolonged use of relaxants can markedly increase the number of normal ACh receptors and, more important, the number of extrajunctional ACh receptors (i.e., upregulation of receptors) (Martyn et al., 1992).

Neuromuscular Transmission

The issues of ACh transfer, release, or reformation in the nerve terminal have been well reviewed (Lee, 1987; Naguib et al., 2002). Mobilization of ACh during tetanic stimulation may be limited in the neonate and particularly in the premature infant. Unanesthetized newborns appear to have less neuromuscular reserve during tetanic stimulation than do adults. In neonates, there is no fade of twitch height with repeated stimulation at rates of 1 to 2 Hz; at 20 Hz, however, there is significant fade. Premature infants may show posttetanic exhaustion for 15 to 20 minutes. Goudsouzian (1980) noted slower contraction times of the thumb after slow and rapid rates of stimulation in term infants (aged 1 to 10 days, anesthetized with halothane) than in older children. The percentage of fade at 20, 50, or 100 Hz did not differ between the infants and the older children, but the tetanic stimulus was applied for only 5 seconds. The *train-of-four (TOF) ratio* (the ratio of the amplitude of the fourth evoked response to the amplitude of the first response in the same train), the degree of posttetanic facilitation, and the tetanus/twitch ratio increase with age. Crumrine and Yodlowski (1981) noted a decrease in the amplitude of the frequency sweep electromyogram (FS-EMG) at frequencies of 50 to 100 Hz in infants younger than 12 weeks (Fig. 6–32). The FS-EMG is a recording of the action potential from an electrical stimulus rate that increases exponentially from one pulse per second to 100 Hz during a stimulation period of 10 seconds. The exponential increase in frequency allows assessment of neuromuscular transmission at tetanic rates without inducing fatigue. In older infants and children, Crumrine and Yodlowski found little or no decrement in the FS-EMG at the high frequencies of stimulation.

■ TYPES OF NEUROMUSCULAR BLOCKING AGENTS: SUCCINYLCHOLINE

Succinylcholine, the only depolarizing relaxant that is used, produces two different types of blockade: phase 1 and phase 2 (Fig. 6–33). During phase 1, succinylcholine binds to ACh receptors, causing membrane ionic channels to open in the same fashion as does ACh. The molecules remain bound to the receptor for an extended period and cause the membrane to remain depolarized and unable to trigger any further muscle action potentials. With prolonged exposure, a succinylcholine-induced blockade begins to assume the characteristics of a nondepolarizing blockade. This is referred to as phase 2, desensitization, or

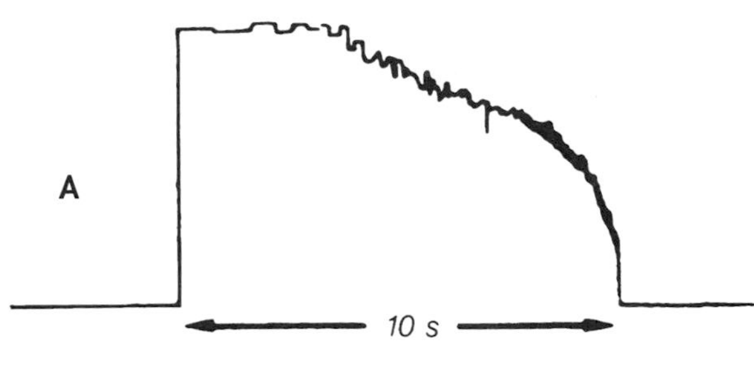

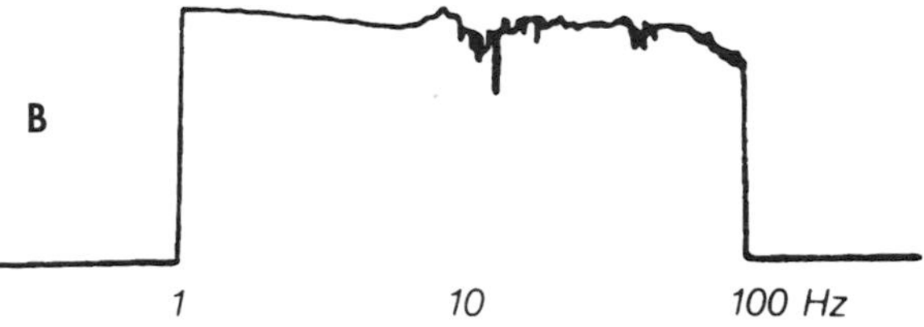

■ **FIGURE 6–32.** Tracings of the frequency sweep electromyographic (FS-EMG) responses from the tibialis anterior muscles of a 1-day-old infant *(A)* and a 4-month-old infant *(B)* premedicated with methohexital. (From Crumrine RS, Yodlowski EH: *Anesthesiology* 54:29, 1981.)

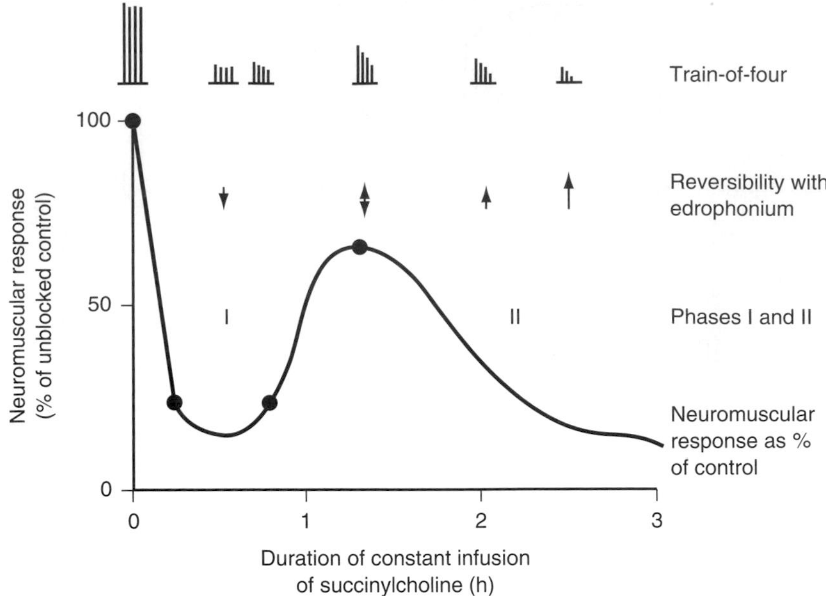

■ **FIGURE 6–33.** During continuous infusion of succinylcholine chloride, a phase I block—characterized by reduced neuromuscular response, little fade of train-of-four (TOF), and increased blockade with edrophonium—is seen initially. During phase II, there is a fade on TOF, increasing reversibility of the block by edrophonium, and accumulation of the slowly recovering residual block.

dual blockade (Sutherland et al., 1980; Donati and Bevan, 1983; Goudsouzian and Liu, 1984; Lee, 1986). Nondepolarizing agents competitively bind to the α units of the ACh receptor and may also physically block the ion channel in the motor end-plate. Channel blockade can also occur.

Dose-Response Relationships

Several multiples of the ED_{95} (e.g., 2× ED_{95})—the so-called intubating dose—are usually administered to ensure adequate neuromuscular blockade and to minimize the time to maximum neuromuscular blockade (the onset time) (Kopman et al., 2001). Table 6–18 gives the relative potencies and duration of effect of various neuromuscular blocking agents in infants and children. By current convention, *onset* is defined as the time to maximum effect, and *duration* is defined as the time for return to 25% neuromuscular transmission after a 2× ED_{95} dose (Bedford, 1995). In general, the ED_{95} of relaxants was determined on the intrinsic muscles of the hand (e.g., adductor pollicis muscle of the thumb) under steady-state anesthetic conditions.

The response to neuromuscular blocking agents and the time to achieve a given degree of blockade (i.e., degree of neuromuscular blockade) vary somewhat with the nerve motor unit being monitored (Law and Cook, 1990). When neuromuscular blocking drugs are used to facilitate tracheal intubation, the goal is to produce relaxation of laryngeal, jaw, abdominal, and intercostal muscles. Diaphragmatic relaxation is of less concern during intubation, but ideally, coughing, bucking, or pushing are not wanted (Table 6–19). The laryngeal adductors are less sensitive than the adductor pollicis to nondepolarizing relaxants, and that response is similar in intensity and time course to the orbicularis oculi (Fig. 6–34). This means that thumb twitch may cease before relaxation of the vocal cords; the opposite is true for succinylcholine (Donati et al., 1991; Meistelman et al., 1991, 1992; Ungureanu et al., 1993; Iwasaki et al., 1994a, 1994b; Plaud et al., 1996). Alternatively, small priming doses of the nondepolarizing relaxant (<ED_{5-10}) can be given to partially

■ **TABLE 6–18.** Time course of neuromuscular blockade with various drugs*

Drug	Dose (mg/kg)	Time to Complete Neuromuscular Blockade (min)	Recovery Time to T_{25} (min)
Succinylcholine	2.0	1.0	4
Mivacurium	0.3	1.5	6
Rocuronium	0.6	1.3	27
Atracurium	0.5	1.5	33
Vecuronium	0.1	1.3	24
Pancuronium	0.4	0.7	75
Doxacurium	0.1	2.5	NA
cis-Atracurium	0.05	5.3	51

*Drug dose (~2× ED_{95}) represents so-called intubating dose.
Adapted from Gronert BJ, Brandom BW: *Pediatr Clin North Am* 41:73–92, 1994.
In general, maintenance dose (one-fourth that in table) is given when one palpable twitch is present with train-of-four monitoring.

■ **TABLE 6–19.** Degrees of neuromuscular blockade

Neuromuscular Blockade (%)	Clinical Relaxation	Ventilation
0	None; train-of-four >0.70; tetanus sustained at 50 Hz	Normal; vital capacity normal; inspiratory force >50 cm H_2O
25	Poor; head lift inadequate; leg flexion inadequate	Slightly to moderately diminished vital capacity
50	Fair	Moderately to markedly diminished vital capacity; tidal volume may be adequate
75	Good	Tidal volume diminished
90	Good	Tidal volume inadequate
95	Very good—adequate for tracheal intubation under light anesthesia	Some diaphragmatic motion possible
100	Excellent; very good for tracheal intubation	Apnea

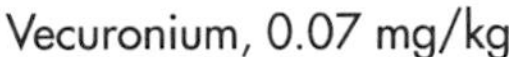

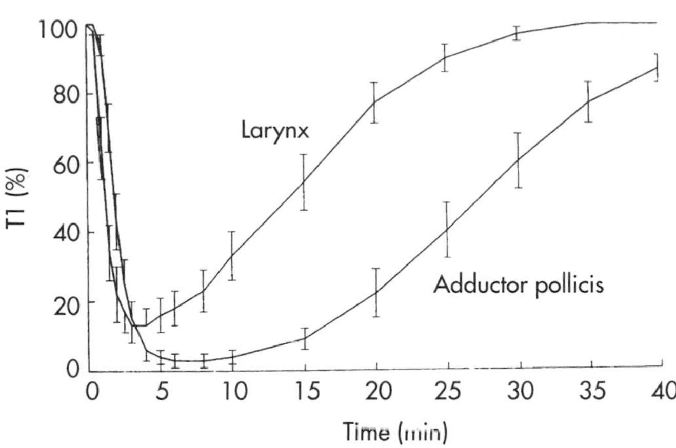

■ **FIGURE 6–34.** First twitch height (T1) against time for vocal cords and adductor pollicis, after vecuronium 0.07 mg/kg. Bars indicate SEM. (With permission from Donati F, Meistelman C, Plaud B: *Anesthesiology* 74:833, 1991.)

occupy the receptor (Kopman et al., 2001). Larger, top-up doses (total dose, 2× ED_{95}) given several minutes later seem to accelerate the onset time. This approach avoids potential cardiovascular changes from even higher multiples of the ED_{95} (i.e., 6× to 8× ED_{95}) and still provides rapid onset time of neuromuscular blockade.

As neuromuscular transmission recovers to 25% of control twitch height (T_{25}), the patient may require an additional top-up dose of relaxant (Fig. 6–35). Published T_{10} or T_{25} indexes of recovery provide some prediction of the expected duration of effect, but monitoring of neuromuscular transmission is preferable. Traditional long-acting relaxants such as pancuronium or intermediate ones such as atracurium, vecuronium, or rocuronium provide about 0.5 to 1 hour of clinical relaxation (1× to 1.5× ED_{95}).

Intermittent administration of neuromuscular blocking agents for prolonged periods may be inconvenient, and administration via infusion appears to be a practical alternative. The goal of such infusion techniques is to maintain a constant plasma concentration of relaxant and a constant degree of neuromuscular blockade. The steady-state infusion rate (I_{ss}) is proportional to the required plasma concentration (C_{ss95}) and clearance rate and, thus, the removal rate (R_{ss}).

$$I_{ss} = R_{ss} = \text{clearance} \times C_{ss95} \quad (6.18)$$

■ **TABLE 6–20.** Comparison of neuromuscular blocking agents by infusion

	Loading Dose (mcg/kg)	Infusion Rate (mcg/kg per min)	\$/mg	\$/HR
Pancuronium	50 to 100	0.5 to 1.0	0.42	4.70
Vecuronium	80 to 100	1.0 to 1.5	0.96	2.77
Pipecuronium	40 to 80	0.2 to 0.3	0.44	30.15
Atracurium	200 to 500	5 to 8	1.06	16.32
Doxacurium	25 to 50	0.2 to 0.35	4.06	20.20
Mivacurium	250 to 300	10 to 15	0.92	77.15
Succinylcholine	2000	5.0	0.005	0.86

*Based on 70-kg adult.
Modified from Fleming NW: *Semin Anesth* 13:255, 1994.

Although traditional long-acting agents (e.g., pancuronium) have been used via infusion, there are drawbacks such as recurrent cardiovascular effects and accumulation. It may be more prudent to infuse agents with an intermediate duration (e.g., atracurium, *cis*-atracurium, rocuronium, or vecuronium) for prolonged periods. Short-acting agents (e.g., mivacurium) may be even more preferable. Shorter-acting agents may allow more rapid recovery of neuromuscular transmission and are more easily titrated but are clearly more expensive (Table 6–20). Monitoring of neuromuscular blockade with a nerve–muscle stimulator or clinical indicators diminishes the likelihood of prolonged neuromuscular blockade. Additional boluses of relaxant should not be administered until there is reappearance of a single twitch in the TOF-evoked response. Infusion rates can be adjusted to maintain a perceptible single twitch or a level that just abolishes the twitch.

Characteristics of Specific Agents

The sensitivity of the postjunctional cholinergic receptor to neuromuscular blocking agents may vary with age. When allowance is made for differences in the volume of distribution, infants appear as sensitive to succinylcholine as adults but more sensitive to nondepolarizing relaxants.

Succinylcholine

Succinylcholine, a rapid-acting and ultrashort-duration depolarizing muscle relaxant, is useful when given as a bolus to facilitate endotracheal intubation. The onset times (i.e., time to maximum neuromuscular blockade) at so-called intubating doses are listed in Table 6–21. Succinylcholine is metabolized by

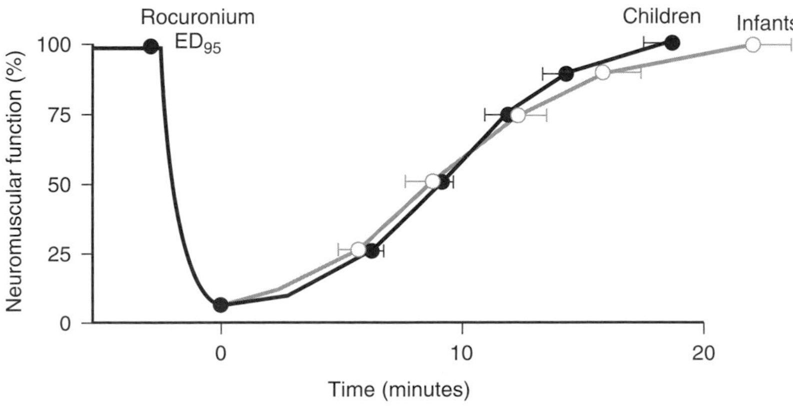

■ **FIGURE 6–35.** Spontaneous recovery of neuromuscular function after a dose of rocuronium (1× ED_{95}) in children and infants.

■ **TABLE 6–21.** Variation in onset time at different epochs for various relaxants

	RESPONDERS (%)			
Onset Time (sec)	*Succinylcholine*	*Rapacuronium**	*Rocuronium*	*Mivacurium*
<30	0	0	0	0
31 to 60	90	62	50	27
61 to 90	10	19	25	45
91 to 120	0	14	17	9
121 to 150	0	0	0	9
151 to 180	0	0	8	9
>180	0	5	0	0

Data from various studies by the author.
Onset times from 2× ED_{95}.
*Not commercially available.

butyrylcholinesterase. Markedly prolonged neuromuscular blockade can result from atypical or abnormally low enzyme concentrations.

Butyrylcholinesterase activity is reduced in neonates, but there is little change in butyrylcholinesterase activity between 3 months and 12 years of age (B. Gronert, B. W. Brandom, D. R. Cook, unpublished data).

When differences in volume of distribution and concentration of anesthesia are taken into account, infants and small children (<2 years old) appear relatively resistant to succinylcholine, have a faster clearance, and have a shorter onset time (at equal multiples of the ED_{95}) than do older children and adults. Most of the side effects of succinylcholine were described within years of its introduction: dysrhythmias, increased intraocular pressure, prolonged apnea, injured muscle membranes with associated hyperkalemia, association with masseter spasm and malignant hyperthermia, and death. Infants and small children have a high incidence of such complications. Intractable, unexpected cardiac arrest (ventricular fibrillation or asystole) associated with a 40% to 50% mortality has been reported after the use of succinylcholine in children with undiagnosed Duchenne's muscular dystrophy. In these patients, succinylcholine may cause rhabdomyolysis and massive hyperkalemia (Tang et al., 1992; Hopkins, 1995; Gronert, 2001). This series of case reports created a small firestorm that culminated in the Food and Drug Administration issuing a "box" warning against the elective use of succinylcholine.

Age-Related Responses

Neonates and infants require about twice as much succinylcholine on a weight basis as do older children or adults to depress respiration or neuromuscular transmission or to produce apnea. In infants, 1 mg/kg succinylcholine produces neuroblockade about equal to that produced by 0.5 mg/kg in children aged 6 to 8 years (Cook and Fischer, 1975). At these equipotent doses, there is no statistically significant difference between the times to recover to 50% and 90% (T_{90}) neuromuscular transmission in the two groups. Complete neuromuscular blockade develops in children given 1 mg/kg of succinylcholine. Cook and Fischer (1975) estimated the ED_{95} of succinylcholine to be 2.2 mg/kg. Estimates of the ED_{95} of succinylcholine were made in additional age groups by Meakin and others (1989) (Table 6-22, Fig. 6-36). Neonates and infants may require 2 to 3 mg/kg and children may require 1 to 2 mg/kg of succinylcholine to achieve comparable intubation conditions seen in adults who are given

■ **TABLE 6–22.** Calculated ED_{50} and ED_{95} for succinylcholine as a function of age

Age Group	ED_{50} (mcg/kg)	ED_{95} (mcg/kg)	ED_{50} (mcg/m²)	ED_{95} (mcg/m²)
Neonates	250	625	3952	9881
Infants	317	729	6277	14,436
Children	184	423	4416	10,154
Adults	—	290	—	11,940

Data from Meakin G, McKiernan EP, Morris P, et al.: Dose-response curves for suxamethonium in neonates, infants and children. *Br J Anaesth* 62:655, 1989.

1 to 1.5 mg/kg of succinylcholine. In view of the marked variability in neuromuscular block produced by small doses of succinylcholine, it would seem advisable to select doses at the upper end of these ranges. Spontaneous recovery from succinylcholine-induced apnea may not occur sufficiently quickly to prevent hemoglobin desaturation in patients whose ventilation is not assisted (Heir et al., 2001).

Goudsouzian and Liu (1984) found that a threefold higher infusion rate of succinylcholine (milligrams per kilogram per hour) was needed to maintain a 90% twitch depression in young infants compared with older infants or children. A slightly larger dose of succinylcholine was needed in infants than in the other age groups to achieve phase II block. Differences in butyrylcholinesterase activity, receptor sensitivity, or volume of distribution may explain these age-related differences in succinylcholine requirements. The neonate has about one half the butyrylcholinesterase activity of the older child or adult; it is unlikely that augmented butyrylcholinesterase activity is responsible for the infant's resistance to succinylcholine. When succinylcholine was given on a surface area basis (40 mg/m²), no difference existed between infants and adults in the times to recover to 10%, 50%, or 90% neuromuscular

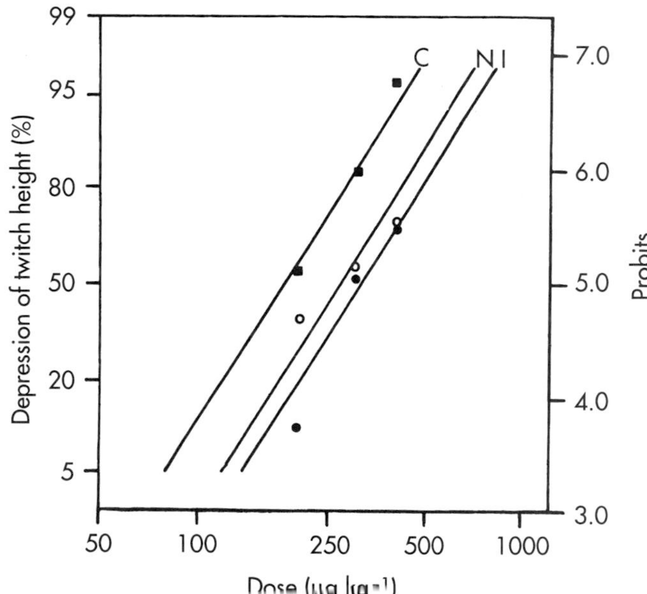

■ **FIGURE 6–36.** Log dose-probit response regression lines for succinylcholine for neonates (N), infants (I), and children (C). Points along the lines represent mean responses from subgroups of five patients. (With permission from Meankin G, McKiernan EP, Morris P, et al.: *Br J Anaesth* 62:655, 1989.)

transmission; this dose of succinylcholine produced complete neuromuscular blockade in all patients. A linear relationship occurs between the log dose on a milligram-per-meter squared basis and the maximum intensity of neuromuscular blockade for infants, children, and adults. They also observed a linear relationship between the logarithm of the dose on a milligram-per-meter squared basis and either 50% or 90% recovery time for infants and children as a combined group. Similar findings were noted by others (see Table 6–22). Because of the small molecular size of succinylcholine, it is rapidly distributed throughout the ECF. The blood volume and ECF volume of the infant are significantly greater than those of the child and adult on a weight basis. On a weight basis (milligram per kilogram), twice as much succinylcholine is needed in infants as in adults to produce a given degree of neuromuscular blockade.

Because ECF volume and surface area bear a nearly constant relationship throughout life, it is not surprising that there is a good correlation between succinylcholine dose (micrograms per meter squared) and response throughout life. The data of Goudsouzian and Liu (1984) suggest that relative resistance to succinylcholine persists in some infants even when the dose is transformed to micrograms per meter squared per minute. These data suggest that the ACh receptor matures with age, or that butyryl cholinesterase activity is high in infants. Indeed, butyryl cholinesterase activity is quite high in infants compared with adults.

Side Effects

Succinylcholine can have profound cardiovascular effects; increase intraocular, intragastric, and intracranial pressures; and be associated with hyperkalemia, myoglobinemia, and malignant hyperthermia.

Dysrhythmias. Succinylcholine exerts variable and seemingly paradoxical effects on the cardiovascular system. Typically, intravenous succinylcholine produces initial bradycardia and hypotension, followed after 15 to 30 seconds by tachycardia and hypertension. In the infant and small child, profound sustained sinus bradycardia (rates of 50 to 60 beats/min) commonly is observed; rarely, asystole occurs. Nodal rhythm and ventricular ectopic beats are seen in about 80% of children given a single intravenous injection of succinylcholine; such dysrhythmias are rarely seen after an intramuscular injection of succinylcholine. The incidence of bradycardia and other dysrhythmias is higher after a second dose of succinylcholine.

Atropine (0.1 mg) appears to offer adequate protection against these bradyarrhythmias in all age groups of infants and children. (In infants, vagolytic doses of 0.03 mg/kg are required for protection; in older children, adequate protection is provided by doses of 0.005 mg/kg.)

Pulmonary Edema and Pulmonary Hemorrhage. Cook and others (1981) have described several young infants in whom fulminant pulmonary edema developed only minutes after intramuscular injection of succinylcholine (4 mg/kg). The edema responded to ventilation with continuous positive airway pressure.

Intragastric Pressure. Succinylcholine may increase intragastric pressure. The increase in intragastric pressure is directly related to the intensity of muscle fasciculations. In adults, pressures as high as 40 cm H_2O have been recorded after violent fasciculations. When the intragastric pressure exceeds 20 cm H_2O, the cardioesophageal valve ("sphincter") mechanism may become incompetent; regurgitation and aspiration may occur. Because of limited muscle mass, the infant or small child, in contrast to the adult, seldom has strong fasciculations. Salem and others (1972) observed only a 4 cm H_2O increase in intragastric pressure after intravenous administration of succinylcholine in infants; in some patients, the intragastric pressure decreased.

Intraocular Pressure. Intravenous or intramuscular administration of succinylcholine increases intraocular pressure in infants and adults. Although dilation of choroidal vessels by succinylcholine is a contributory factor, the increase in intraocular pressure is primarily the result of contraction of extraocular muscles. Typically after intravenous succinylcholine administration, the intraocular pressure begins to increase within 60 seconds, peaks at 2 to 3 minutes, and then returns to control levels 5 to 7 minutes after injection. A succinylcholine-induced increase in intraocular pressure in the presence of a penetrating wound of the eye can result in extrusion of vitreous humor through the site of injury and possibly loss of vision. The transient increase in intraocular pressure may be misinterpreted and lead to unnecessary surgery in a patient with glaucoma if tonometry is performed within 5 to 7 minutes of the injection of succinylcholine.

Increased Intracranial Pressure. Minton and others (1986) suggested that succinylcholine per se may increase ICP. Increases in ICP after the administration of succinylcholine are produced by cerebral metabolic stimulation and increases in cerebral blood flow. These effects are attenuated by prior administration of a non-depolarizing agent and by treatment with thiopental or lidocaine.

Hyperkalemia and Myoglobinemia. In normal patients, succinylcholine increases plasma levels of potassium by 0.3 to 0.5 mEq/L. Alarming levels of potassium, as high as 11 mEq/L, along with cardiovascular collapse, were frequently reported with succinylcholine in a variety of conditions, including burns, massive trauma, stroke, spinal cord injury, and muscle diseases (Delphin et al., 1987; Rosenberg and Gronert, 1992; Schow et al., 2002). The common denominator appears to be either massive tissue destruction or CNS injury with muscle wasting. Strong fasciculations are not necessary to produce hyperkalemia in susceptible patients. There are no data to suggest that the infant is any less vulnerable than the adult to massive potassium flux from the listed conditions (Henning and Bush, 1982; Dierdorf et al., 1984). A seemingly high incidence of myoglobinemia occurs after succinylcholine (1 mg/kg) in prepubertal patients, especially those anesthetized with halothane. Myoglobinemia rarely results from succinylcholine administration in adults. Plasma levels of creatine phosphokinase, an indicator of muscle injury, have been shown to be significantly increased after succinylcholine administration in children. Myoglobinemia and increased plasma levels of creatine phosphokinase occurred without strong fasciculations. The tendency of muscle in children to release myoglobin after depolarization with succinylcholine is not readily explained. Such changes seem to be rare in infants.

Masseter Spasm, Trismus, and Malignant Hyperthermia. Most clinicians are well aware of the association of succinylcholine with malignant hyperthermia (MH). Typically, MH develops as a profound rigidity or violent fasciculations, a rapid increase in temperature, an increase in pulse rate, and an increase in end-tidal carbon dioxide tension. These are the classic signs, but occasionally the only manifestation of MH is trismus (Flewellen and Nelson, 1984; Schwartz et al., 1984). The rigid jaw can be forced open but only with considerable difficulty. Only about half of the patients in whom trismus follows administration of succinylcholine have a predisposition to MH (Flewellen and Nelson, 1984). Resting tension or stiffness in the masseter muscle increases in a dose-related manner as succinylcholine blocks neuromuscular function (DeCook and Goudsouzian, 1980; Plumley et al., 1990; Sadler et al., 1990; Van Der Spek et al., 1989, 1988). These changes can make laryngoscopy difficult. Perhaps masseter spasm is an extreme case of the apparently normal dose-related increase in resting tension observed in some studies. A more complete evaluation of the force required to open the mouth is necessary to clarify this issue. Perhaps masseter spasm is not only quantitatively different from the changes in resting tension but also qualitatively different. If so, the identifying features of masseter spasm have yet to be described in sufficient detail to allow differentiation of masseter spasm from an extreme instance of the normal increase in resting tension of the masseter after the administration of succinylcholine. It is not possible to define susceptibility to MH solely on the basis of trismus. Creatine phosphokinase measurement and muscle biopsy may be of some help, but most centers are reluctant to perform major muscle biopsies in children younger than 8 to 10 years. The diagnosis is extraordinarily difficult to make on clinical grounds alone. See Chapter 31, Malignant Hyperthermia.

Decreasing Use

Rumors of the total withdrawal from use of succinylcholine have become more common in the past several years. Many have suggested that succinylcholine be eliminated from clinical use; others have demanded that succinylcholine be eliminated altogether. Both the "box" warning against the elective use of succinylcholine and increased availability of alternative agents have contributed to the markedly diminished use of this agent (Cook, 2000). Many of the profound cardiovascular complications of succinylcholine were described within 5 to 15 years of its introduction: the hazards of the use of succinylcholine in patients with neural injuries, neuromuscular disease, burns, and massive trauma were established; and the hazards of succinylcholine as a "triggering" agent for myotonia, masseter spasm, and MH were established. Despite these hazards, succinylcholine remained popular to facilitate endotracheal intubation because there was no reasonable alternative. The clinical introduction of the new short-acting and intermediate-acting relaxants and the development of the so-called *priming principle* and other clinical strategies to minimize the onset time of relaxants have minimized the need for succinylcholine. Priming or administration of 8× to 10× the ED_{95} of a relaxant can be used to accelerate the onset of neuromuscular blockade. Infants and small children rarely demonstrate histamine release after relaxants are administered; thus large top-up doses can be used after the priming dose or initial megadoses of relaxants. Such uses convert atracurium, *cis*-atracurium, rocuronium, and vecuronium from intermediate-acting to long-acting relaxants.

NONDEPOLARIZING NEUROMUSCULAR BLOCKING DRUGS

Nondepolarizing neuromuscular blocking agents can be categorized by the time to maximum blockade (onset time) and by the clinical duration of effect (i.e., time to return of neuromuscular transmission to 25% of control) after a 2× ED_{95} dose during a standard anesthetic technique (Bedford, 1995) (Table 6–23).

TABLE 6–23. Definitions of adjectives describing nondepolarizing neuromuscular blocking agents

	TIME (min)	
Adjective	*Minimum*	*Maximum*
Onset		
Ultrarapid	Not needed	<1
Rapid	1	2
Intermediate	2	4
Slow	4	Not needed
Duration		
Ultrashort	Not needed	8
Short	8	20
Intermediate	20	50
Long-acting	>50	Not needed

From Bedford RF: *Anesthesiology* 82:33A, 1995.

There is a clear trend to use short-duration and intermediate-duration relaxants rather than long-acting relaxants for most surgical patients. There also is a thought that more rapid-acting relaxants are preferable to those of longer onset. In general, at equal multiples of the ED_{95}, the less potent agents have more rapid onset times than the more potent agents (i.e., rocuronium has a more rapid onset time than vecuronium). The coefficient of variation in onset time for various relaxants is listed in Table 6–24. Long-acting relaxants are probably reserved for long surgical procedures and procedures in which postoperative ventilation is anticipated.

There are four routes of elimination of nondepolarizing muscle relaxants: renal excretion; hepatic uptake, storage and excretion; biotransformation (including Hofmann elimination); and tissue binding (Table 6–25). Nondepolarizing muscle relaxants filter freely through the glomerulus, and the renal clearance of these drugs does not exceed the GFRe (1 to 2 mL/kg per minute). The degree of metabolism that nondepolarizing muscle relaxants undergo varies widely. Hofmann elimination and ester hydrolysis are largely responsible for the breakdown of atracurium and *cis*-atracurium; butyrylcholinesterase is primarily associated with the metabolism of mivacurium. Hepatic biodegradation has been demonstrated for steroidal relaxants (Savage et al., 1980; Bencini et al., 1983). A small fraction (20% to 30%) of pancuronium undergoes metabolism. The metabolism of vecuronium is significant (Savage et al., 1980; Marshall et al., 1983). Spontaneous deacetylation occurs in the liver, and the byproducts are 3-hydroxy and 17-hydroxy derivatives. The metabolism of steroidal relaxants is not mediated by CYP systems but by nonspecific esterases (personal observations).

TABLE 6–24. Coefficient of variation in onset time of intubating doses of relaxants in infants and children*

	COEFFICIENT OF VARIATION (%)	
Drug	*Infants*	*Children*
Atracurium	45.9	46.5
Vecuronium	40.0	58.3
Mivacurium	53.3	42.8
Succinylcholine	36.4	22.2
cis-Atracurium	NA	53.5

*Intubating dose = 2× ED_{95}.

TABLE 6–25. Elimination routes of muscle relaxants

Agent	Hepatobiliary Metabolism in Plasma	Uptake and Metabolism	Renal Excretion
Mivacurium	XX	—	—
Atracurium	XX	—	—
cis-Atracurium	XX	—	—
Vecuronium	—	XX	X
Rocuronium	—	XX	X
Pancuronium	—	XX	X
Pipecuronium	—	XX	X
Doxacurium	—	—	XX

XX, major route; X, alternative route.

TABLE 6–26. Pharmacokinetic parameters for the three isomers of mivacurium in children

	trans-trans	*cis-trans*	*cis-cis*
AUC (ng/mL per min)	4032 ± 1095	1768 ± 569*	1502 ± 414*
MRT (min)	2.2 ± 1.1	1.5 ± 1.0	7.7 ± 2.4*†
V_d (mL/kg)	85.1 ± 53.5	83.9 ± 67.8	83.9 ± 15.7
CL (mL/min per kg)	38.5 ± 10.9	56.3 ± 17.9*	11.6 ± 4.0*†
$t_{1/2}\beta$ (min)	1.2 ± 0.2	0.8 ± 0.2	4.5 ± 1.6*†

AUC, area-under-the-plasma-concentration curve; MRT, mean residence time; V_d, volume of distribution; CL, clearance; $t_{1/2}\beta$, elimination half-life.
Analysis of variance with Student-Newman-Keuls test.
*Different from *trans-trans*.
†Different from *cis-trans*.
Unpublished data of the author.

The 3-OH metabolites of both vecuronium and pancuronium are roughly one half to equally potent at the neuromuscular junction as the parent compounds. The 17-OH and 3,17-OH metabolites are far less active (Marshall et al., 1983).

Short-Acting Agents

Mivacurium

Mivacurium, a nondepolarizing muscle relaxant with a short duration of action, is metabolized by butyrylcholinesterase, which clearly influences the duration of action (Beaufort et al., 1998; Ostergaard et al., 2000; Gatke et al., 2001). Mivacurium is a mixture of three optical isomers. The two active isomers of mivacurium (*trans-trans* and *cis-trans*) have a short half-life and rapid clearance because of rapid enzymatic hydrolysis. The *cis-cis* isomer has minimal neuromuscular blocking effects but is slowly hydrolyzed (Cook et al., 1992a, 1992b; Head-Rapson et al., 1994; Lien et al., 1994). The ED_{95} of mivacurium during halothane anesthesia in infants and children is 85 and 89 mcg/kg, respectively (Woelfel et al., 1993; Meretoja et al., 1994). Mivacurium is metabolized by butyrylcholinesterase more slowly than is succinylcholine. In infants, mivacurium produces complete neuromuscular blockade as quickly as succinylcholine, but at that time the intubating conditions were less desirable after mivacurium (i.e., a higher incidence of coughing and diaphragmatic movement) (Gronert et al., 1995). In children, mivacurium produces complete neuromuscular blockade more slowly than does succinylcholine. During halothane anesthesia increasing the dose of mivacurium from 0.2 mg/kg to 0.3 mg/kg does not shorten the time to complete paralysis after mivacurium administration (1.5 minutes) (Gronert and Brandom, 1994). After administration of 0.3 mg/kg of mivacurium during halothane anesthesia, hypotension or cutaneous flushing was not observed in children. Mivacurium can induce histamine release when large bolus doses (e.g., 0.4 mg/kg) are administered rapidly. The most common manifestation of histamine release is transient cutaneous flushing and mild decreases in blood pressure. Recovery to T_{25} was faster in infants (6.3 minutes) compared with children (10 minutes). Increasing the dose of mivacurium given to children from 0.2 to 0.3 mg/kg did not significantly prolong the time to spontaneous recovery of neuromuscular function to 25% of baseline (Gronert et al., 1995). Mivacurium (0.3 mg/kg) has little or no effect on lung mechanics (flow–volume loops) (Fine et al., 2002).

It is remarkable that the duration of action of mivacurium is so short in children. Mivacurium is one of the few neuromuscular blocking agents that are cleared in the plasma rather than by the kidneys or liver. This may be the reason why infants recover from this drug at least as rapidly as do children and why children recover more rapidly than do adults. There have been several studies of the kinetics of mivacurium in infants and children (Ostergaard et al., 2002; Markakis et al., 1998; Meretoja, et al., 1994) (Table 6–26). The volume of distribution of mivacurium is seemingly greater in the infant than in the child, and the clearance in infants and children is faster than that of the adult. These conclusions are indirectly supported by the observations that the infusion rate of mivacurium to maintain constant neuromuscular block (≈95% twitch depression) is about twice as great in infants and children as in adults (Markakis et al., 1998). An advantage of mivacurium is that it can be given via infusion for hours without accumulation or prolongation of recovery once the infusion is stopped (Brandom et al., 1990; Goudsouzian et al., 1994).

In adults with renal or hepatic failure and subsequently reduced butyrylcholinesterase activity, the duration of mivacurium-induced neuromuscular blockade is increased by renal and hepatic failure. Similar studies in children have not been performed. In adults given 0.15 mg/kg, the duration of block was approximately three times normal in those with liver failure (Cook et al., 1992; Head-Rapson et al., 1994, 1995; Levy, 1994). There was a significant nonlinear, negative correlation between butyrylcholinesterase and time to spontaneous recovery of neuromuscular function to 25% of baseline in these patients.

Intermediate-Acting Agents

Atracurium

Atracurium, a muscle relaxant of intermediate duration, is metabolized by nonspecific esters and spontaneously decomposed by Hofmann degradation. Both processes are sensitive to pH and temperature. Under physiologic conditions, the breakdown of atracurium is mainly by ester hydrolysis; Hofmann elimination plays a minor role. Deficient or abnormal butyryl cholinesterases have little or no effect on atracurium degradation. The effects of both age and potent inhaled anesthetics on the dose-response relationships of atracurium in infants, children, and adolescents have been studied (Brandom et al., 1985; Goudsouzian et al., 1983, 1985; Stiller et al., 1985a, 1985b; Meretoja, et al., 1994). On the basis of weight (micrograms per kilogram), the ED_{95} for atracurium was similar in infants aged 1 to 6 months and in adolescents, whereas children had a higher dose requirement. On the basis of surface area (micrograms per meter squared), the

■ **TABLE 6–27.** Age-related pharmacokinetics of atracurium

Variable	Children	Infants
$t_{1/2}\alpha$ (min)	2.1 ± 0.56	1.04 ± 0.34*
$t_{1/2}\beta$ (min)	19.1 ± 4.5	13.6 ± 1.4*
V_d (mL/kg)	139.0 ± 23.48	176.6 ± 22.2*
CL (mL/kg per min)	5.1 ± 0.56	9.0 ± 1.65*

Values are mean ± SEM. $t_{1/2}\alpha$, half-life of the distribution phase; $t_{1/2}\beta$, elimination half-life; V_d, volume of distribution; CL, clearance.
*$P < 0.5$ in infants compared with values in children.
From Cook DR, Marcy JH: *Neonatal anesthesia.* Pasadena, CA, 1988, Appleton Davies.

ED_{95} for atracurium was similar in children and adolescents, and the ED_{95} (milligrams per meter squared) for atracurium in infants was much lower. At equipotent doses (1× ED_{95}), the duration of effect (time from injection to 95% recovery) was 23 minutes in infants and 29 minutes in children and adolescents, compared with 44 minutes in adults. The time from injection to T_{25} (i.e., 25% neuromuscular transmission) was 10 minutes in infants, 15 minutes in children and adolescents, and 16 minutes in adults. At T_{25}, supplemental doses are needed to maintain relaxation for surgery. At higher multiples of the ED_{95}, the duration of effect is longer, but the times from T_5 to T_{25} are the same. The shorter duration of effect in the infant may represent a difference in pharmacokinetics. The pharmacokinetics of atracurium differ among infants, children, and adults. The volume of distribution is larger, clearance is more rapid, and the elimination half-life is seemingly shorter in infants than in children or adults (Table 6–27).

Brandom and others (1985) used a continuous infusion of dilute atracurium (200 mcg/mL) after a bolus infusion to maintain neuromuscular blockade at 95 ± 5%. To maintain this degree of steady-state blockade, 8 to 10 mcg/kg per minute was required with nitrous oxide, thiopental, and narcotic anesthesia after an initial bolus. No accumulation was seen with prolonged infusion; recovery of neuromuscular transmission was prompt. The recovery of neuromuscular transmission from the same degree of blockade was similar if potent anesthetics were used (i.e., halothane). With these data the removal of atracurium can be estimated. At steady state, the infusion rate (I_{ss}) equals the removal rate (R_{ss}) of atracurium. Removal is directly related to the clearance and the $C_{ss}95$. In children, during so-called balanced anesthesia, $C_{ss}95$ is about 2 mcg/mL. Atracurium infusion requirements in children during nitrous oxide and narcotic anesthesia can be compared with those noted in several age groups of adults during similar anesthetic administrations. d'Hollander and others (1983) noted that in patients aged 16 to 85 years, the steady-state atracurium infusion rate averaged 14.4 mg/kg per hour; this corresponds to 240 mg/m² per minute. This value is similar to the 226 mg/m² per minute rate we noted. Atracurium does not depend on the kidney or the liver for elimination because it is biodegraded by Hofmann elimination and ester hydrolysis. However, the parent compound and its metabolites are normally found in bile and urine (Neill and Chapple, 1983). Because atracurium does not depend on the kidney for excretion, its elimination half-life and duration of action are not prolonged in patients with renal failure (Hunter et al., 1982; Ward and Neill, 1983; Fahey et al., 1984) (Table 6–28). Fahey and others (1984) found no change in the kinetics or the duration of action and rate of recovery from atracurium in these patients. Hunter and others (1982) also found no difference in duration of action.

The *cis*-atracurium is a mixture of 10 optical and geometric isomers (Welch et al., 1995). The R-R[1] optical isomer in the *cis-cis* configuration, *cis*-atracurium, is about 1.5× more potent than atracurium and does not liberate histamine at very high doses (Tobias et al., 2001). Seemingly *cis*-atracurium is primarily degraded by Hofmann elimination, pH-dependent chemical degradation, with the initial formation of laudanosine and a monoquaternary acrylate. Plasma esterases hydrolyze the monoquaternary acrylate to a monoquaternary alcohol; further Hofmann elimination can form another molecule of laudanosine. Renal failure or liver disease has minimal effect on the pharmacodynamics of *cis*-atracurium (Prielipp et al., 1995; DeWolf et al., 1996). Because *cis*-atracurium is more potent than atracurium, less laudanosine accumulates in patients after a bolus of prolonged infusion. Dhonneur and others (2001) infused *cis*-atracurium for 0.5 to 8 days in patients with adult respiratory distress syndrome. Clearance of *cis*-atracurium was little different from that seen in normal patients, and laudanosine plasma concentrations were less than 1200 ng/mL. Reich and others (2002) infused *cis*-atracurium in infants after congenital heart surgery. The clearance of *cis*-atracurium was quite high and the duration of residual blockade was low. Laudanosine plasma concentrations were less than 2000 ng/mL.

DeRuiter and Crawford (2001) have noted that *cis*-atracurium is equipotent in infants and children. During nitrous oxide-narcotic thiopentone administration, the ED_{50} and ED_{95} values for infants (29 ± 3 μg/kg and 43 ± 9 μg/kg, respectively) were similar for children (29 ± 2 μg/kg and 47 ± 7 μg/kg) (DeRuiter and Crawford, 2001).

Using halothane anesthesia, Meretoja noted that the rate of recovery following a dose of 1 to 2× the ED_{95} was rapid with a recovery index of 9 to 11 minutes and a time from 5% to 95% recovery of 25 to 30 minutes. In a separate study of infants and children anesthetized with nitrous oxide and opioids,

■ **TABLE 6–28.** Pharmacokinetic parameters in normal and organ failure patients

	NORMAL PATIENTS			HEPATIC PATIENTS			RENAL FAILURE PATIENTS		
Drug	*Vd_{SS} (L/kg)*	*$t_{1/2}\beta$ (hr)*	*CL (mL/kg per min)*	*Vd_{SS} (L/kg)*	*$t_{1/2}\beta$ (hr)*	*CL (mL/kg per min)*	*Vd_{SS} (L/kg)*	*$t_{1/2}\beta$ (hr)*	*CL (mL/kg per min)*
d-Tubocurarine	0.3 to 0.5	2 to 5.8	1 to 2.7	NA	NA	NA	0.25	2.2	1.5
Pancuronium	0.14 to 0.4	1.7 to 2.4	1 to 2	0.21 to 0.42	3.4 to 5.1	0.6 to 1.5	0.29	4.3	0.9
Vecuronium	0.18 to 0.26	0.5 to 1.3	3	0.23	1.2	2.7	0.19	0.8	5.3
Atracurium	0.18	0.33	5 to 6	0.16	0.35	5.2	0.22	0.4	5.3
Rocuronium	0.20	1.5	3.7 to 5	0.25	2.5	2.6	0.20	1	2.5
cis-Atracurium	0.16	—	5.7	0.20	—	6.6	—	—	—

■ **TABLE 6–29.** Age-related potency and time course for vecuronium

	POTENCY			TIME COURSE (70 mcg/kg)	
Age Group	*ED_{50} (mcg/kg)*	*ED_{95} (mcg/kg)*	*ED_{95} (multiple)*	*Onset Time (min)*	*Duration (min)*
Infants	16.5	27.7	2.5	4.5 ± 0.6	73 ± 27
Children	19.0	45.5	1.5	2.4 ± 1.4	35 ± 6
Adults	15.0	33.8	2	2.9 ± 0.2	53 ± 21

Values are mean ± SD. ED_{50}, effective dose for 50% twitch depression; ED_{95}, estimated dose needed to produce 95% neuromuscular blockade.
From Cook DR, Marcy JH: *Neonatal anesthesia.* Pasadena, CA, 1988, Appleton Davies.

Taivainen and others (2000) noted that following 0.1 mg/kg of *cis*-atracurium, the mean (SD) onset time of maximum blockade was more rapid in infants (2.0 ± 0.8 min) than in children (3.0 ± 1.2 min). The clinical duration of action of *cis*-atracurium (recovery of evoked response to 25% of control) was significantly longer in infants (43.3 ± 6.2 min) than in children (36.0 ± 5.4 min). Once neuromuscular function started to recover, the rate was similar in both age groups. It appears that liver disease and renal failure do not alter *cis*-atracurium's pharmacologic profile.

Laudanosine is the major end-product of atracurium or *cis*-atracurium degradation (Stiller et al., 1985; Eddleston et al., 1989). The byproducts of atracurium metabolism have no neuromuscular blocking effect, and they are excreted by the liver and the kidney (Neill and Chapple, 1983; Parker et al., 1988). Laudanosine accumulates in patients with liver or renal failure, and its serum concentration remains elevated for a prolonged period (Fahey et al., 1985). In large doses, laudanosine has been shown to cause CNS stimulation in dogs and rabbits but not in cats (Babel, 1989; Ingram et al., 1986). It also increases the MAC of halothane in rabbits (Shi et al., 1985), and in dogs it causes electroencephalographic changes of arousal during halothane anesthesia (Lanier et al., 1985).

Adverse effects observed with laudanosine accumulation may be partially attributed to an interaction with neuronal nicotinic receptors (e.g., $\alpha_4\beta_2$ and $\alpha_3\beta_4$ receptors) (Chiodini et al., 2001). The clinical importance of laudanosine in patients with renal failure, particularly after repeated doses of atracurium, has not been determined. Atracurium has been infused in patients for 22 to 106 hours, however, without adverse effect (Parker et al., 1988).

Vecuronium

The ED_{95} for vecuronium is somewhat higher in children than in infants and adults (d'Hollander et al., 1982; Fisher and Miller, 1983). At equipotent doses (2× ED_{95}) of vecuronium, the duration of effect (time from injection to 90% recovery) was longest in infants (73 minutes) compared with that in children (35 minutes) and adults (53 minutes). Thus vecuronium does not have intermediate duration in infants. An infusion rate of 2.4 mcg/kg per minute (60 mg/m^2 per minute) vecuronium is generally required to maintain approximately 95% neuromuscular blockade in children during narcotic and nitrous oxide anesthesia. These infusion rates are several times higher than those noted by d'Hollander and others (1982) in adults (aged 18 to 85 years). Young adults required 0.9 mcg/kg per minute (45 mcg/m^2 per minute) to maintain 95% neuromuscular blockade. Children recover more rapidly from vecuronium infusion than do adults. Several groups have noted long-term vecuronium infusion requirements in adults with multiple organ failure in the ICU (Segredo et al., 1992). Infusion rates of about 1.6 mcg/kg per minute are required, and the degree of block may gradually increase, a sign of accumulation. Increasing vecuronium infusion requirements, by contrast, may be seen during very prolonged infusions (i.e., lasting 3 to 14 days). These increased requirements could not be clearly associated with various pathophysiologic states, concurrent drug administration, or biochemical abnormalities. Proliferation of extrajunctional cholinergic receptors resulting from prolonged nondepolarizing blockade has also been offered as an explanation.

Fisher and others (1983) determined the pharmacodynamics and pharmacokinetics of vecuronium in infants and children (Tables 6–29 and 6–30). The volume of distribution and the mean residence time were greater in infants than in children. Clearance was similar in the two groups; the C_{ss50} was lower in infants than in children. The combination of a large volume of distribution in infants and fixed clearance results in a longer mean residence time. After a single dose of relaxant, recovery of neuromuscular transmission depends on both distribution and elimination. The combination of a longer mean residence time and a lower sensitivity for vecuronium explains the prolongation of neuromuscular blockade in infants. Little or no 3-OH vecuronium is seemingly formed after a single dose of vecuronium (0.1 to 0.2 mg/kg).

Lebrault and others (1985) studied the pharmacokinetics and pharmacodynamics of vecuronium in patients with cirrhosis compared with normal subjects. The volume of distribution in patients with cirrhosis was normal, but the clearance was reduced by roughly 50%. The time interval between the administration of vecuronium and 50% recovery of twitch height was 130 minutes in patients with cirrhosis versus 62 minutes in normal subjects. The time to recovery from 25% to 75% of control twitch height was 68 minutes in patients with cirrhosis versus 21 minutes in normal subjects. Plasma concentration of vecuronium at 50% twitch recovery (CP_{50}) was similar in both groups. This similarity suggests that patients with cirrhosis have normal sensitivity to vecuronium. Despite the prolonged

■ **TABLE 6–30.** Pharmacokinetics and pharmacodynamics of vecuronium

Age Group	$t_{1/2}\beta$ (min)	CL (mL/kg per min)	Vd_{ss} (mL/kg)	Cp_{ss50} (ng/mL)
Infants	64.7 ± 30.2	5.6 ± 1.0	357 ± 70	57.3 ± 17.7
Children	41.0 ± 15.1	5.9 ± 24	204 ± 116	109.8 ± 28.1
Adults	70.7 ± 20.4	5.2 ± 0.7	269 ± 42	93.7 ± 33.5

Values are mean ± SD. $t_{1/2}\beta$, elimination half-life; CL, clearance; Vd_{ss}, volume of distribution at steady state; Cp_{ss50}, steady-state plasma concentration associated with 50% neuromuscular blockade.
From Cook DR, Marcy JH: *Neonatal anesthesia.* Pasadena, CA, 1988, Appleton Davies.

duration of action of vecuronium in cirrhotic patients, it was still shorter than that of pancuronium in patients free of liver disease.

Vecuronium is only slightly dependent on renal elimination (10% to 30%), and its elimination should be minimally affected by renal failure. Although some found no change in volume of distribution, clearance, elimination half-life, or recovery time with vecuronium in patients with renal failure, subsequent studies demonstrated that the duration of neuromuscular blockade was longer in patients with renal failure than in those with normal renal function (Lynam et al., 1988). This increased duration of effect may be related to both a decreased plasma clearance and a prolonged elimination half-life of vecuronium in the renal failure group. Similarly, Bencini and others (1983) found a 50% decrease in clearance, an increase in volume of distribution, and a 50% increase in elimination half-life. The duration of action was not reported. Metabolites of vecuronium were not measured in these studies. Reich and others (2002) infused vecuronium in infants after congenital heart surgery. The clearance of vecuronium was low, significant amounts of 3-OH vecuronium were noted, and return of neuromuscular transmission was quite slow.

Rocuronium

Rocuronium (ORG-9426) is a nondepolarizing, steroidal neuromuscular blocking drug similar to vecuronium but with one-eighth to one-tenth the potency. It is similar in many ways to vecuronium, but the lesser potency of rocuronium produces a more rapid onset of paralysis in comparison with equipotent doses of other drugs (i.e., equal multiples of the ED_{95}) (Kopman, 1989). Bolus administration of 0.6 mg/kg of rocuronium, twice the ED_{95}, is associated with a transient increase in heart rate of about 15 beats/min (O'Kelly et al., 1994). Bolus intravenous administration of 0.6 mg/kg of rocuronium produces complete neuromuscular blockade (at the adductor pollicis) in infants and children in 50 and 80 seconds, respectively (Woelfel et al., 1992). Increasing the dose to 0.8 mg/kg in children shortens this time to an average of 30 seconds (O'Kelly et al., 1994). The time to recovery of neuromuscular function to T_{25} after a dose of 0.6 mg/kg is almost twice as long in infants younger than 10 months compared with children aged 1 to 5 years (45.1 versus 26.7 minutes, respectively). This age-related difference is similar to that observed with vecuronium (Meretoja, 1989). Its rapid onset of action with minimal tachycardia and intermediate duration of action makes it an attractive neuromuscular blocking drug for use in pediatric patients. The role of rocuronium in ICU patients is unclear. Hepatic uptake and biliary excretion are the dominant mechanisms for its clearance; hepatobiliary clearance is about 75% and renal clearance is about 9% (Khuenl-Brady et al., 1990). The effects of rocuronium are prolonged in patients with renal disease (Cooper et al., 1993). Little or no metabolism of rocuronium takes place (i.e., about 3%).

Long-Acting Agents

d-Tubocurarine

Although *d*-tubocurarine is no longer commercially available, studies of its dose-response relationships and kinetics were the prototypes for future studies with other nondepolarizing relaxants and have helped provide key concepts (Goudsouzian et al., 1981, 1984, Cook, 1981; Fisher et al., 1982). The volume of distribution for *d*-tubocurarine is quite high in the newborn infant compared with that in the older child or adult, but plasma clearance of *d*-tubocurarine does not differ with age. The volume of distribution for *d*-tubocurarine appears relatively constant on a liter-per-meter squared basis (estimated by author). Adults and children require about 7 to 8 mg/m^2 of *d*-tubocurarine, 6- to 9-month-old infants require about 5 to 6 mg/m^2, and neonates require only about 4 mg/m^2. These differences suggest that the neonate and, to a lesser degree, the infant are quite sensitive to *d*-tubocurarine if compensation is made for the wide variation in volumes of distribution. More important, the steady-state plasma concentration associated with 50% neuromuscular blockade (C_{ss50}) was age related; C_{ss50} in neonates was about one third that noted for adults. The largest variability in elimination half-lives and volumes of distribution was seen in the data from neonates.

Pancuronium

Pancuronium, a steroidal bisquaternary muscle relaxant, has been used frequently for infants and children because of its rather predictable neuromuscular blocking action and associated cardiovascular stimulating properties. The dose-response relationships for pancuronium were determined in infants and children by Goudsouzian and others (1981) and by Blinn and others (1992). Older children require a higher dose on a weight basis (micrograms per kilogram) than do infants and small children (Table 6–31).

Within 24 hours after administration of pancuronium, Duvaldestin and others (1982) recovered 67% of the drug in the urine in the form of the parent compound and its metabolites. In other studies, about 25% of the injected pancuronium appeared in the urine in the form of the 3-OH metabolite and less than 5% each appeared in the form of the 17-OH and 3,17-dehydroxy metabolites. Approximately 11% of the pancuronium was excreted in the bile as the parent compound and its metabolites.

Pancuronium has been studied extensively in patients with hepatic dysfunction or renal dysfunction (Duvaldestin et al., 1982; Lavine and Hindein, 1983) (see Table 6–28). The studies demonstrate that different types of liver disease have different effects on the disposition of muscle relaxants. Studies show prolonged elimination half-life and delayed recovery from pancuronium in patients with cholestasis. Duvaldestin and others (1982) studied the pharmacokinetics of pancuronium in patients with cirrhosis and found a prolonged distribution half-life, an almost twofold increase in elimination half-life, and a 20% decrease in clearance. These effects are related primarily to an increase in ECF and in volume of distribution (see Table 6–28). On the basis of these observations, one would predict that, in cirrhotic patients, resistance and increased sensitivity to pancuronium exist at the same time. On one hand, the onset time

TABLE 6–31. Cumulative dose-response relationship of pancuronium

Age	ED_{50} (mg/kg; mg/m^2)	ED_{95} (mg/kg; mg/m^2)
3 to 6 mo	24 ± 7; 448 ± 136	45 ± 7; 849 ± 151
7 to 12 mo	30 ± 5; 602 ± 90	52 ± 9; 1050 ± 175
1 to 3 yr	34 ± 9*; 753 ± 198	62 ± 18*; 1394 ± 401
4 to 6 yr	29 ± 8; 1022 ± 524*	62 ± 13*; 2136 ± 855*

*Statistically significant difference from the 3- to 6-month age group (analysis of variance).

Data from Blinn A, Woefel SK, Cook DR, et al.: 1992.

of pancuronium would be prolonged because of an increase in the volume of distribution, suggesting resistance to the drug; on the other hand, recovery would be delayed because of the prolonged elimination half-life, suggesting increased sensitivity.

If pancuronium is given to a patient in renal failure, it may cause prolonged paralysis. The clearance of pancuronium is reduced by one half to two thirds, whereas the volume of distribution is only minimally affected (see Table 6–28). The metabolites accumulate in renal failure because they normally depend on renal excretion. The metabolites, especially 3-hydroxy pancuronium, have some neuromuscular blocking activity, and they further prolong paralysis. A twofold to fourfold increase in elimination half-life results.

Pipecuronium

Pipecuronium, an analog of pancuronium, is free of cardiovascular side effects. It is a long-acting neuromuscular blocking drug with duration of action similar to pancuronium. After administration of an ED_{95} dose, complete recovery of neuromuscular function occurs in approximately 1 hour in children. The ED_{95} of pipecuronium in children is 80 mcg/kg during nitrous oxide/fentanyl anesthesia (Pittet et al., 1989) and 50 mcg/kg during nitrous oxide/halothane anesthesia (Sarner et al., 1990). The ED_{95} of pipecuronium in infants is only about 35 mcg/kg during nitrous oxide/halothane anesthesia, but spontaneous recovery is not prolonged in infants relative to older patients after a dose titrated to produce close to maximal effect (i.e., not overdose) (Pittet et al., 1989). Prolonged recovery is to be expected when multiples of the ED_{95} are administered.

Pipecuronium is largely excreted by the kidneys. In adults with renal failure, mean duration of neuromuscular blockade after one dose of 70 mcg/kg was similar to that in patients with normal renal function, but there was more variability in duration of action in the renal failure group (Caldwell et al., 1989). Prolonged neuromuscular blockade in an adult with renal failure has been reported (Caballero and Johnson, 1992). It is to be expected that a dose of pipecuronium administered to facilitate rapid endotracheal intubation in children with no renal function lasts at least several hours. Pipecuronium is not easily removed through peritoneal dialysis.

Doxacurium

Doxacurium has a duration of action similar to that of pancuronium. Unlike pancuronium, doxacurium has minimal cardiovascular side effects. In children, Sarner and others (1988) noted that the ED_{50} and ED_{95} of doxacurium in children during halothane/nitrous oxide/oxygen anesthesia are 14.8 mcg/kg and 27.3 mcg/kg, respectively. These values are comparable to the requirements seen in adults administered nitrous oxide/oxygen narcotic anesthesia. In addition, at equipotent doses of doxacurium, the investigators noted age-related differences with respect to the time of recovery of neuromuscular transmission to T_{25} and time of onset to maximal blockade; the children anesthetized with halothane had a shorter onset time to maximal block and shorter recovery times compared with adults anesthetized with nitrous oxide/oxygen and narcotic. Doxacurium is eliminated largely unchanged in the urine (Dresner et al., 1990). At equal doses of doxacurium, patients with hepatic failure achieve a lesser and more variable degree of neuromuscular blockade than do normal patients; the onset time and clinical duration tended to be longer in patients with hepatic failure (Cook et al., 1991).

Selection of Nondepolarizing Relaxant

At appropriate doses, all nondepolarizing relaxants produce neuromuscular blockade; at equipotent doses, each relaxant produces the same degree of relaxation as any other. Potency is important not only to the drug concentration in the vial but perhaps also to the disparity between neuromuscular blocking effects and autonomic side effects. In addition, onset time is markedly reduced with relaxants with high ED_{95} values, a mass effect. Potent inhaled anesthetic agents may decrease the onset time of neuromuscular blocking agents (i.e., mivacurium) and duration in a concentration-dependent manner (Jalkanen and Meretoja, 1997). However, this has not been studied in a systematic fashion for a variety of relaxants. In selecting one relaxant over another, one should consider its onset time, duration of effect, side effects, and routes of elimination (renal, liver, or spontaneous). In addition, one should consider how the age or the pathologic condition of the patient may have an influence on the kinetics of the relaxant. The side effects of the nondepolarizing relaxants are primarily cardiovascular; these cardiovascular effects are related to the magnitude of histamine release, ganglionic blockade, and vagolysis. In addition, the cardiovascular effects appear to be age related. In infants and children, minimal cardiovascular effects are seen after administration of atracurium or vecuronium at several multiples of the ED_{95} (Brandom et al., 1983, 1984; Fisher and Miller, 1983; Goudsouzian et al., 1983). In adults, atracurium at 3× ED_{95} causes slightly less histamine release than 2× ED_{95} of metocurine and less than half as much histamine release as the ED_{95} of *d*-tubocurarine (Tullock et al., 1990). Vecuronium (at any multiple of ED_{95}) is not associated with histamine release (Tullock et al., 1990). Infants and children appear to be less susceptible than adults to histamine release after administration of relaxants. In a small series of infants, 5× ED_{95} of atracurium did not elicit flushing or alter heart rate or blood pressure (Brandom et al., 1984; Goudsouzian et al., 1985). However, local signs of histamine release after direct intravenous injection of atracurium in infants and children have been described; rarely, flushing with or without mild hypotension is seen at high multiples of the ED_{95} (Nightingale and Bush, 1983). At high doses, *d*-tubocurarine may cause hypotension and histamine release in children. The different pattern of tryptase release by the various types of relaxants suggests different mechanisms of mast cell activation (Koppert et al., 2001). Bronchospasm may be related to histamine release or release of leukotrienes. Some relaxants may block prejunctional muscarinic receptors in the airway.

At 2× ED_{95}, increases in heart rate are seen with pancuronium and rocuronium in children; in contrast, both have minimal effect on heart rate in infants. Because the infant responds with bradycardia to a variety of stimuli (hypoxia, tracheal intubation), the "potential" vagolytic effects of pancuronium or rocuronium may be desired side effects.

Priming Principle

The priming principle, or the judicious use of a subparalyzing dose of a nondepolarizing muscle relaxant several minutes before an intubating dose is given, has been used in attempts to achieve a shorter onset time of neuromuscular blocking agents for endotracheal intubation. The priming principle is based on the concept that neuromuscular junction has a large margin of safety. When 75% to 80% of the receptors are blocked, seemingly normal neuromuscular transmission still occurs. Consequently, the pharmacodynamic effects of neuromuscular blocking agents are seen when the remaining 20% to 25% of unoccupied ACh receptors bind the drug. Because the initial dose is subtherapeutic and binds to less than 75% of the available receptors, no apparent pharmacologic or clinical effect is observed. When the second dose or intubating dose is administered, it interacts with the remainder of the unoccupied receptors. Because the second dose exerts its effect on the remaining 25% of the receptor pool, the pharmacologic effect (i.e., onset of a clinical neuromuscular block) occurs faster. Certain cautions need to be emphasized when using the priming principle: (1) the time interval between the initial dose and the second intubating dose needs to be of sufficient length such that the initial dose has time to occupy the receptors and (2) the dose-response curve for any given muscle relaxant has significant patient variability. For some patients, the initial dose may not be sufficient and the intubating dose does not have a rapid onset time. Conversely, for other patients, the initial dose may be too much and consequently those patients may be unable to protect their airways.

Synergism (supra-additivity) has been demonstrated between some neuromuscular blocking drugs of different molecular structures (Satwicz and Martyn, 1984; Naguib, 1994; Rautoma et al., 1995a, 1995b; Erkola et al., 1996; Naguib et al., 1997, 1998). For example, in children the amount of an equipotent combination of atracurium and vecuronium that produces 95% block is only 60% of the amount of either atracurium or vecuronium administered alone that would produce the same effect (Meretoja et al., 1993). When ED_{50} (the dose expected to cause 50% neuromuscular block) of pancuronium was given simultaneously with one half of an ED_{50} dose of mivacurium, 97% depression of neuromuscular function occurred (Meretoja et al., 1993). When children receive a long-acting muscle relaxant (pancuronium) followed by a short-acting muscle relaxant (mivacurium) (Brandom et al., 1993), the duration of neuromuscular blockade is prolonged beyond what would be expected with mivacurium alone (Fig. 6–37).

Modes of Evaluation of Neuromuscular Transmission

Restoration of complete skeletal muscle strength is essential to ensure that patients are able to sustain adequate ventilation, to

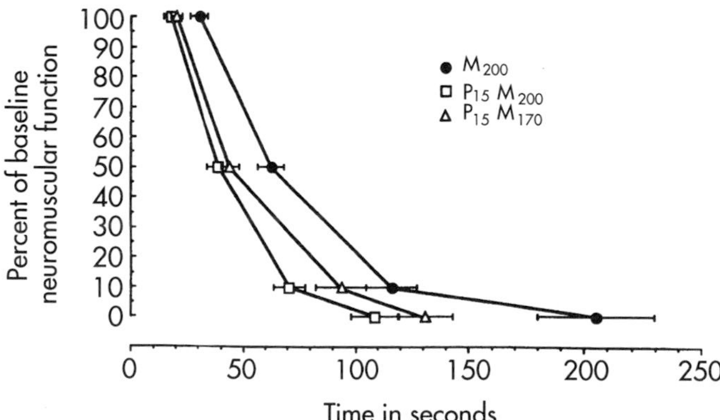

■ **FIGURE 6–37.** Onset of paralysis induced either by 200 mcg/kg of mivacurium preceded by saline solution (M_{200}) or 15 mcg/kg of pancuronium ($P_{15}M_{200}$), or by 170 mcg/kg of mivacurium preceded by 15 mcg/kg of pancuronium ($P_{15}M_{170}$). A small dose of pancuronium did shorten the onset significantly. (With permission from Brandom BW, Meretoja OA, Taivaninen T, et al: *Anesth Analg* 76:998, 1993.)

cough, and to maintain a patent airway after chronic administration of relaxants. Peripheral nerve stimulation (usually the ulnar nerve) adequately measures recovery from nondepolarizing neuromuscular blockade. Peripheral nerve stimulation (e.g., TOF, double burst or tetanic stimulation) is often used in preference to tests of ventilation. Nerve stimulators used for neuromuscular monitoring in the ICU may need to deliver at least 100 mA to generate supramaximal stimulation (Harper et al., 2001). TOF stimulation has been established as the pattern of stimulation for clinical monitoring of neuromuscular blockade. This stimulation mode allows for convenient and reliable tactile evaluation of moderate degrees of nondepolarizing blockade without undue discomfort accompanying tetanic bursts (i.e., 50 to 100 Hz for 5 seconds). However, several studies suggest that these rigorous criteria for adequacy of neuromuscular transmission are indeed needed. The rationale for this approach is the following: first, the diaphragm recovers from the effects of nondepolarizing neuromuscular blocking drugs more rapidly than does the adductor pollicis; and second, at a TOF ratio of 0.9, vital capacity returns to normal (>15 to 20 mL/kg), pharyngeal muscle strengthens with recovery of swallowing, diplopia disappears, and maximum inspiratory and expiratory force are only slightly depressed (−50 cm H_2O). Intense neuromuscular blockade of the peripheral muscles is indicated by disappearance of the response to TOF and single-twitch stimulation (Pavlin et al., 1989). It is possible, however, to quantify part of this period of no response by applying tetanic stimulation (50 Hz for 5 seconds), followed by 1-Hz stimulation and observing the posttetanic single-twitch response (posttetanic count). The posttetanic count is highly correlated with recovery from intense blockade caused by relaxants and with antagonism less than or equal to the neuromuscular blockade.

During recovery of neuromuscular transmission, it is difficult, however, to estimate the TOF ratio with sufficient certainty to exclude residual paralysis (Viby-Mogensen et al., 1985). In this situation it may be more reliable to ascertain the ability to sustain tetanus (50 Hz) for 5 seconds or to evaluate double burst stimulation (DBS). DBS is a new pattern of stimulation that was developed to reveal residual neuromuscular blockade (Drenck et al., 1989). DBS consists of two short tetanic bursts separated by 750 milliseconds. A DBS with three impulses (200-microsecond square-wave impulses) in each of two tetanic bursts of 50 Hz (DBS 3.3) is most suitable for clinical work. Fade in the response results from residual neuromuscular blockade as is seen with TOF stimulation. However, DBS is more sensitive than TOF in the manual detection of residual neuromuscular blockade. Absence of fade in response to DBS 3.3 normally excludes severe residual neuromuscular blockade but does not necessarily indicate adequate clinical recovery. Sustained tetanus (50 Hz) correlates with a TOF ratio of at least 0.85 (Kopman et al., 2001; Dahaba et al., 2002).

Myoneuropathies (Critical Illness Polyneuropathy)

Unexpectedly prolonged duration of paralysis after the administration of muscle relaxants to ICU patients has seemingly reached epidemic proportions (Segredo et al., 1992; Tobias et al., 1995). Individual patients with so-called ICU neuromuscular syndrome have had a variety of relaxants administered for variable times, have had a variety of underlying critical diseases and coexisting conditions, and have had a spectrum of muscle weakness. Unfortunately, there is considerable overlap by this syndrome, disuse atrophy, polyneuropathy of critical illness, and steroid myopathy. Multiorgan dysfunction, corticosteroid administration, prolonged immobilization, and female sex have been suggested as key risk factors. Some cases appear to represent a pharmacologic overdose (i.e., pharmacokinetic category), but other cases seemingly represent specific pathology of the neuromuscular structures (Lee, 1995; Watling and Dasta, 1994; De Jonghe et al., 2002). The pathology includes marked atrophy of type I and type II muscle fibers, destruction of muscle, relatively little inflammation, and relatively intact motor and sensory nerves (Lee, 1995). This syndrome may be related in part to synergistic dysfunctional upregulation of ACh receptors from both a critical illness and the administration of muscle relaxants (Lee, 1995). It has been suggested that reducing the amount of relaxants used (i.e., dose over time) by monitoring neuromuscular transmission may decrease the risk of prolonged paralysis (Fine et al., 2001). Lee suggests that periodic interruption of relaxant administration, pharmacodynamic studies, and neurologic and electrophysiologic studies may be useful in the early detection of this complication. Prolonged neuromuscular blockade in infants and small children may interfere with normal growth and development of muscle and result in moderate to severe residual weakness for months. Immobilization-induced atrophy may not be reversible in developing muscle. Recovery of muscle function thus may be more likely in older infants and children, in whom neuromuscular development has already progressed to a fair degree, than in newborns and especially premature newborns immobilized shortly after birth (Shear, 1981).

Reversal of Neuromuscular Blockade

Because of the increased potential for respiratory inadequacy from residual neuromuscular blockade in infants, most anesthesiologists routinely antagonize nondepolarizing relaxants. The rule has been always to reverse neuromuscular blockade. Large doses of neostigmine (70 mcg/kg) are usually used. In infants, as in adults, neurotransmission returns promptly if few receptors are blocked at the time of reversal. Proper choice of relaxant and careful timing and titration of the dose of relaxant usually ensure that some motor tone is present by the time antagonism is attempted. Certain antibiotics, hypotension, hypothermia, acidosis, or hypocalcemia can prolong or potentiate neuromuscular blockade from nondepolarizing relaxants. Hypothermia, deep sedation, or narcosis per se can also lead to respiratory depression in infants.

The use of intermediate-acting relaxants forces one to reexamine the dictum to "always reverse blockade." Clearly, the margin of safety of relaxants is increased by using objective criteria to judge the adequacy of neuromuscular transmission. As stated in the preceding section, these criteria include a TOF ratio greater than 0.9, the ability to sustain tetanus at 50 Hz, a vital capacity of 15 to 20 mL/kg, the ability to flex the arms and legs, and an inspiratory force greater than 50 cm H_2O. If the infant or child can meet several of these criteria without reversal, no reversal is needed. When there is doubt, however, a drug should be given to antagonize blockade.

Fisher and others (1983, 1984) examined the dose of neostigmine and edrophonium required in infants, children, and adults to reverse a 90% blockade from a continuous *d*-tubocurarine infusion. In infants and children, 15 mcg/kg of neostigmine produced a 50% antagonism of the *d*-tubocurarine blockade; in adults, 23 mcg/kg was required. It was claimed that the duration of antagonism was equal in all three groups, although the elimination half-life was clearly shorter in infants. A larger dose than that seemingly recommended would give a higher sustained blood concentration; whether this is of pharmacologic benefit in the absence of a continuous infusion or relaxant is doubtful. The dissociation between the elimination half-life and the duration of antagonism may result from the carbamylation of cholinesterase by neostigmine. In infants, 145 mcg/kg of edrophonium produced a 50% antagonism of the *d*-tubocurarine blockade; in children, 233 mcg/kg was required; and in adults, 128 mcg/kg was required. The volume of distribution of edrophonium was similar in all age groups. The elimination half-life of edrophonium was shorter in infants than in children or adults; hence, clearance was more rapid in infants. Because the molecular interaction between edrophonium and cholinesterase is readily reversible, Fisher and others (1983, 1984) suggest that the shorter elimination half-life for edrophonium might limit its value in pediatric patients. This is doubtful.

Meakin and others (1983) compared the rate of recovery from pancuronium-induced neuromuscular blockade after various doses of neostigmine (0.036 or 0.07 mg/kg) or edrophonium (0.7 or 1.43 mg/kg) in infants and children. In the first 5 minutes, recovery of neuromuscular transmission was more rapid after edrophonium than after neostigmine in all age groups; recovery was more rapid in infants and children than in adults. By 10 minutes, there was no difference in neuromuscular transmission achieved in infants and children with either reversal agent (at either dose); adults had lower neuromuscular transmission at the lower dose (0.036 mg/kg) of neostigmine. If speed of initial recovery is a critical issue, edrophonium is better than neostigmine, and a high dose of neostigmine is better than a low dose. At 30 minutes after injection of either reversal agent (at any dose), there was no difference between neuromuscular transmission among age groups.

SUMMARY

To provide appropriate anesthesia care for pediatric surgical patients, the anesthesiologist should have not only an appreciation of the pathophysiology of the child's disease but also a firm understanding of how developmental changes affect the pharmacology of anesthetic agents. As the child's cardiac output becomes less rate dependent, hemodynamic stability occurs with inhalational anesthetics. For the infant, anesthetics that decrease heart rate and myocardial contractility can have a profound cardiovascular effect. Because infants' baroreceptors are less mature, compensatory mechanisms for the inhalational anesthetics cannot compensate. In addition to inhalational anesthetics, intravenous agents are also offered by pharmacokinetic parameters; that is, volume distribution, clearance, and elimination half-life also develop. Consequently, drug dosages need to be individualized. The anesthetic management of the infant and child requires a careful approach; knowledge of pharmacologic and physiologic development is essential for optimum patient management.

REFERENCES

Abel RM, Reis RL: Intravenous diazepam for sedation following cardiac operations: Clinical and hemodynamic assessments. *Anesth Analg (Cleve)* 50:244, 1971.

Agnor RC, Sikich N, Lerman J: Single breath vial capacity rapid inhalation induction in children: 8% Sevoflurane versus 5% halothane. *Anesthesiology* 89:379, 1998.

Albanese J, Durbec O, Viviand X: Sufentanil increases intracranial pressure in patients with head trauma. *Anesthesiology* 79:493, 1993.

Alcorn J, McNamara PJ: Ontogeny of hepatic and renal systemic clearance pathways in infants. Part I. *Clin Pharmacokinet* 41:959–998, 2002.

Alexander CM, Gross JB: Sedative doses of midazolam depress hypoxic ventilatory responses in humans. *Anesth Analg* 67:377, 1988.

Alexander CM, Teller LE, Gross JB: Slow injection does not prevent midazolam-induced ventilatory depression. *Anesth Analg* 74:260, 1992.

Anderson BJ, McKee AD, Holford NH: Size, myths and the clinical pharmacokinetics of analgesia in paediatric patients. *Clin Pharmacokinet* 33:313–327, 1997.

Ang C, Habre W, Sims C: Tropisetron reduces vomiting after tonsillectomy in children. *Br J Anaesth* 80:761–763, 1998.

Aono J, Ueda W, Mamiya K, et al.: Greater incidence of delirium during recovery from sevoflurane anesthesia in preschool boys. *Anesthesiology* 87:1298, 1997.

Ard J, Doyle W, Bekker A: Awake craniotomy with dexmedetomidine in pediatric patients. *J Neurosurg Anesthesiol* 15:263, 2003.

Arnold JH, Truog RD, Scavone JM: Changes in the pharmacodynamic response to fentanyl in neonates during continuous infusion. *J Pediatr* 119:639, 1991.

Attia J, Ecoffey C, Sandouk P: Epidural morphine in children: Pharmacokinetics and CO_2 sensitivity. *Anesthesiology* 65:590, 1986.

Audenaert SM, Montgomery CL, Thompson DE, et al: A prospective study of rectal methohexital: Efficacy and side effects in 648 cases. *Anesth Analg* 81:957–961, 1995.

Ausems ME, Hug C Jr, Stanski DR, et al.: Plasma concentrations of alfentanil required to supplement nitrous oxide anesthesia for general surgery. *Anesthesiology* 65:362, 1986.

Babel A: Etude comparative de la laudanosine et de la papaverine au point de vue pharmacodynamique. *Rev Med Suisse Romande* 19:657, 1989.

Bailey PL, Stresand JB, East KA: Differences in magnitude and duration of opioid-induced respiratory depression and analgesia with fentanyl and sufentanil. *Anesth Analg* 77:708, 1990.

Balistreri WF: Immaturity of hepatic excretory function and the ontogeny of bile acid metabolism. *J Pediatr Gastroenterol Nutr* 2(Suppl 1):S207–S214, 1983.

Barash PG, Glanzz S, Katz JD, et al.: Ventricular function in children during halothane anesthesia: An echocardiographic evaluation. *Anesthesiology* 49:79, 1978.

Baum VC, Plamisano BW: The immature heart and anesthesia. *Anesthesiology* 87:1529, 1997.

Baum VC, Wetzel GT: Sodium-calcium exchange in neonatal myocardium: Reversible inhibition by halothane. *Anesth Analg* 78:1105, 1994.

Baxter PJ, Garten K, Kharasch ED: Mechanistic aspects of carbon monoxide formation from volatile anesthetics. *Anesthesiology* 89:929–941, 1998.

Beaufort TM, Nigrovic V, Proost JH, et al.: Inhibition of the enzymic degradation of suxamethonium and mivacurium increases the onset time of submaximal neuromuscular block. *Anesthesiology* 89:707–714, 1998.

Bedford RF: The FDA protects the public by regulating the manufacture of anesthetic agents and the production devices used in anesthetic practice. *Anesthesiology* 82:33A, 1995.

Beh T, Splinter W, Kim J: In children, nitrous oxide decreases pain on injection of propofol mixed with lidocaine. *Can J Anesth* 49:1061–1063, 2002.

Bellward GD, Warren PM, Howald W, et al.: Methadone maintenance: Effect of urinary pH on renal clearance in chronic high and low doses. *Clin Pharmacol Ther* 22:92, 1977.

Bencini A, et al.: Clinical pharmacokinetics of vecuronium. In Agoston S, et al. (eds): *Clinical experiences with Norcuron (Org NC 45 vecuronium bromide).* Amsterdam, 1983, Excerpta Medica.

Benedetti SM, Baltes EL: Drug metabolism and disposition in children. *Fundam Clin Pharmacol* 17:281–299, 2003.

Berde CB, Beyer JE, Bournaki M-C, et al.: Comparison of morphine and methadone for prevention of postoperative pain in 3- to 7-year-old children. *J Pediatr* 119:136–141, 1991.

Berg JM, Brandon MWG, Kirwan BH: Atropine in mongolism. *Cancer* 2:441, 1960.

Bergman I, Steeves M, Burckart G: Reversible neurologic abnormalities associated with prolonged intravenous midazolam and fentanyl administration. *J Pediatr* 119:644, 1991.

Beskow A, Werner O, Westrin P: Faster recovery after anesthesia in infants after intravenous induction with methohexital instead of thiopental. *Anesthesiology* 83:976–979, 1995.

Besunder JB, Reef MD, Blumer JL: Principles of drug biodisposition in the neonate. A critical evaluation of the pharmacokinetic-pharmacodynamic interface. *Clin Pharmacokinet* 14:189–216, 1988.

Bhat R, Chari G, Golati A: Pharmacokinetics of a single dose of morphine in preterm infants during the first week of life. *J Pediatr* 117:477, 1990.

Black A: A comparison of the induction characteristics of sevoflurane and halothane in children. *Anaesthesia* 51:539, 1996.

Blinn A, Woelfel SK, Cook DR, et al.: Pancuronium dose-response revisited. *Paediatr Anesth* 2:133, 1992.

Blount P, Merlie JP: Molecular basis of the two nonequivalent ligand binding sites of the muscle nicotinic acetylcholine receptor. *Neuron* 3:349, 1989.

Bokesch PM, Ziemer G, Castaneda AR, et al.: Arterial lidocaine concentrations in intracardiac right-to-left shunts. *Anesthesiology* 63:468, 1985.

Boreus LO, Jalling B, Kallberg N: Clinical pharmacology of phenobarbital in the neonatal period. In Morselli PL, Garatini S, Sereni F (eds): *Basic and therapeutic aspects of perinatal pharmacology.* New York, 1975, Raven Press, p 331.

Borgeat A, Popovic V, Meier D: Comparison of propofol and thiopental/halothane for short-duration ENT surgical procedures in children. *Anesth Analg* 71:511, 1990.

Borgeat A, Wilder-Smith OHG, Despland PA: Spontaneous excitatory movements during recovery from propofol anaesthesia in an infant: EEG evaluation. *Br J Anaesth* 70:459, 1993.

Borgeat A, Wilder-Smith OHG, Saiah M, et al.: Subhypnotic doses of propofol possess direct antiemetic properties. *Anesth Analg* 74:539, 1992.

Bosenberg AT, Thomas J, Lopez T, et al.: Plasma concentrations of ropivacaine following a single-shot caudal block of 1, 2 or 3 mg/kg in children. *Acta Anaesthesiol Scand* 45:1276–1280, 2001.

Bovill J, Sebel P, Fiolet J, et al.: The influence of sufentanil on endocrine and metabolic responses to cardiac surgery. *Anesth Analg* 62:391, 1983.

Bowdle TA, Patel IH, Levy RH, et al.: Valproic acid dosage and plasma protein binding and clearance. *Clin Pharmacol Ther* 28:486–492, 1980.

Bowman WC: Prejunctional and postjunctional cholinoreceptors at the neuromuscular junction. *Anesth Analg* 59:935, 1980.

Brandom BW, Cook DR, Woelfel SK, et al.: Atracurium infusion in children during fentanyl, halothane, and isoflurane anesthesia. *Anesth Analg* 64:471, 1985.

Brandom BW, Meretoja OA, Taivainen T, et al.: Accelerated onset and delayed recovery of neuromuscular block induced by mivacurium preceded by pancuronium in children. *Anesth Analg* 76:998, 1993.

Brandom BW, Rudd GD, Cook DR: Clinical pharmacology of atracurium in pediatric patients. *Br J Anaesth* 55:117S, 1983.

Brandom BW, Sarner JB, Woelfel SK, et al.: Mivacurium infusion requirements in pediatric surgical patients during nitrous oxide-halothane and during nitrous oxide-narcotic anesthesia. *Anesth Analg* 71:16, 1990.

Brandom BW, Woelfel SK, Cook DR, et al.: Clinical pharmacology of atracurium in infants. *Anesth Analg* 63:309, 1984.

Briggs LP, Clarke RSJ, Watkins J: An adverse reaction to the administration of disoprofol (Diprivan). *Anaesthesia* 37:1099, 1982.

Brodie BB: Physiological disposition and chemical fate of thiobarbiturates in the body. *Fed Proc* 11:632, 1952.

Brodsky JB, Baden JM, Serra M, et al.: Nitrous oxide inactivates methionine synthetase activity in rat testis. *Anesthesiology* 61:66–68, 1984.

Brosius KK, Bannister CF: Effect of oral midazolam premedication on the awakening concentration of sevoflurane, recovery times and bispectral index in children. *Paediatr Anaesth* 11:585–590, 2001.

Brosius KK, Bannister CF: Midazolam premedication in children: A comparison of two oral dosage formulations on sedation score and plasma midazolam levels. *Anesth Analg* 96:392–395, 2003.

Brosius KK, Bannister CF: Oral midazolam premedication in preadolescents and adolescents. *Anesth Analg* 94:31–36, 2002.

Brown AK, Zwelzin WW, Burnett HH: Studies on the neonatal development of the glucuronide conjugating system. *J Clin Invest* 37:332, 1958.

Bryson JC, Pritchard JF, Shurin S, et al.: Efficacy, pharmacokinetics (PK), and safety of ondansetron (OND) in pediatric chemotherapy patients [abstract]. *Clin Pharmacol Ther* 49:161, 1991.

Burtin P, Jacqz-Aigrain E, Girard P, et al.: Population pharmacokinetics of midazolam in neonates. *Clin Pharmacol Ther* 56:615, 1994.

Caballero PA, Johnson RE: Long-lasting neuromuscular blockade from pipecuronium. *Anesthesiology* 76:154, 1992.

Calakos N, Scheller RH: Synaptic vesicle biogenesis, docking, and fusion: A molecular description. *Physiol Rev* 76:1–29, 1996.

Caldwell JE, Canfell PC, Castagnoli KP, et al.: The influence of renal failure on the pharmacokinetics and duration of action of pipecuronium bromide in patients anesthetized with halothane and nitrous oxide. *Anesthesiology* 70:7, 1989.

Cameron CB, Robinson S, Gregory GA: The minimum anesthetic concentrations of isoflurane in children. *Anesth Analg* 63:418, 1984.

Camu F, Gepts E, Rucquoi M, et al.: Pharmacokinetics of alfentanil (R39709) in man. *Anesth Analg* 61:657, 1982.

Cappiello M, Giuliani L, Rane A, et al.: Dopamine sulphotransferase is better developed than p-nitrophenol sulphotransferase in the human fetus. *Dev Pharmacol Ther* 16:83–88, 1991.

Carmichael EB: The median lethal dose (LD_{50}) of pentothal sodium for both young and old guinea pigs and rats. *Anesthesiology* 8:589, 1947.

Carrigan TW, Straughen WJ: A report of hepatic necrosis and death following isoflurane anesthesia. *Anesthesiology* 67:581, 1987.

Carter S, Gold AP: Status epilepticus. In Smith CA (ed): *The critically ill child.* 2nd ed. Philadelphia, 1977, WB Saunders.

Cazeneuve C, Pons G, Rey E, et al.: Biotransformation of caffeine in human liver microsomes from foetuses, neonates, infants and adults. *Br J Clin Pharmacol* 37:405–412, 1994.

Chalkiadis GA, Eyers RI, Cranswick N, et al.: Pharmacokinetics of levobupivacaine 0.25% following caudal administration in children under 2 years of age. *Br J Anaesth* 92:218-22, 2004.

Chauvin M, Lebrault C, Levron JC, et al.: Pharmacokinetics of alfentanil in chronic renal failure. *Anesth Analg* 66:53, 1987a.

Chauvin M, Sandouk P, Schermann JM, et al.: Morphine pharmacokinetics in renal failure. *Anesthesiology* 66:327, 1987b.

Chay PCW, Duffy BJ, Walker JS: Pharmacokinetic-pharmacodynamic relationships of morphine in neonates. *Clin Pharmacol Ther* 51:334, 1992.

Chiaretti A, Pietrini D, et al.: Safety and efficacy of remifentanil in craniosynostosis repair in children less than 1 year old. *Pediatr Neurosurg* 33:83–88, 2000.

Chiodini F, Charpantier E, Muller D, et al.: Blockade and activation of the human neuronal nicotinic acetylcholine receptors by atracurium and laudanosine. *Anesthesiology* 94:643–651, 2001.

Choonara IA, McKay P, Hain R, et al.: Morphine metabolism in children. *Br J Clin Pharmacol* 28:599–604, 1989.

Clarke RS, Dundee JW, Barron DW, et al.: Clinical studies of induction agents. XXVI. The relative potencies of thiopentone, methohexitone and propanidid. *Br J Anaesth* 40:593, 1968.

Cockshott ID, Briggs IP, Douglas EJ, et al.: Studies using single bolus injection. *Br J Anaesth* 59:1103, 1987.

Cohen MM, Cameron CB, Duncan PG: Pediatric anesthesia morbidity and mortality in the perioperative period. *Anesth Analg* 70:160, 1990.

Cohen IT, Hannallah RS, Goodale DB: The clinical and biochemical effects of propofol infusion with and without EDTA for maintenance anesthesia in healthy children undergoing ambulatory surgery. *Anesth Analg* 93:106–111, 2001.

Collins G, Koren G, Crean P, et al.: Fentanyl pharmacokinetics and hemodynamic effects in preterm infants ligation of patent ductus arteriosus. *Anesth Analg* 64:1078, 1985.

Constant I, Dubois MC, Piat V, et al.: Changes in electroencephalogram and autonomic cardiovascular activity during induction of anesthesia with sevoflurane compared with halothane in children. *Anesthesiology* 91:1604, 1999.

Cook DR: Can succinylcholine be abandoned? *Anesth Analg* 90:S24–S28, 2000.

Cook DR: Sensitivity of the newborn to tubocurarine. *Br J Anaesth* 53:320, 1981.

Cook DR, Chakravorti S, Brandom BW, et al.: Effects of neostigmine, edrophonium and succinylcholine on the in vitro metabolism of mivacurium: Clinical correlates. *Anesthesiology* 77:A948, 1992a.

Cook DR, Fischer CG: Neuromuscular blocking effects of succinylcholine in infants and children. *Anesthesiology* 42:662–665, 1975.

Cook DR, Freeman JA, Lai AA, et al.: Pharmacokinetics of mivacurium in normal patients and in those with hepatic or renal failure. *Br J Anaesth* 69:580, 1992b.

Cook DR, Freeman JA, Lai AA, et al.: Pharmacokinetics and pharmacodynamics of doxacurium in normal patients and in those with hepatic or renal failure. *Anesth Analg* 72:145, 1991.

Cook DR, Westman HR, Rosenfeld L, et al.: Pulmonary edema in infants: Possible association with intramuscular succinylcholine. *Anesth Analg* 60:220, 1981.

Cooper RA, Maddineni VR, Mirakhur RK, et al.: Time course of neuromuscular effects and pharmacokinetics of rocuronium bromide (ORG 9426) during isoflurane anesthesia in patients with and without renal failure. *Br J Anaesth* 71:222, 1993.

Coté CJ, Cohen IT, Suresh S, et al.: A comparison of three doses of a commercially prepared oral midazolam syrup in children. *Anesth Analg* 94:37–43, 2002.

Coventry DM, Martin CS, Burke AM: Sedation for paediatric computerized tomography—a double-blind assessment of rectal midazolam. *Eur J Anaesth* 8:29, 1991.

Cox RG: Are children just little adults when it comes to propofol injection pain? *Can J Anesth* 49:1016–1020, 2002.

Cravero J, Surgenor S, Whalen K: Emergence agitation in paediatric patients after sevoflurane anaesthesia and no surgery: A comparison with halothane. *Paediatr Anaesth* 10:419–424, 2000.

Crumrine RS, Yodlowski EH: Assessment of neuromuscular function in infants. *Anesthesiology* 54:29, 1981.

Culy CR, Bhana N, Plosker GL: Ondansetron. A review of its use as an antiemetic in children. *Paediatr Drugs* 3:441–479, 2001.

DaConceicao MJ, Coelho L: Caudal anaesthesia with 0.375% ropivacaine or 0.375% bupivacaine in paediatric patients. *Br J Anaesth* 80:507, 1998.

Dagan O, Klein J, Bohn D, et al.: Morphine pharmacokinetics in children following cardiac surgery: Effects of disease and inotropic support. *J Cardiothorac Vasc Anesth* 7:396–398, 1993.

Dahaba AA, von Klobucar F, Rehak PH, et al.: The neuromuscular transmission module versus the relaxometer mechanomyograph for neuromuscular block monitoring. *Anesth Analg* 94:591–596, 2002.

Dalens B, Ecoffey C, Joly A, et al.: Pharmacokinetics and analgestic effect of ropivacaine following illioinguinal/iliohypogastric nerve block in children. *Pediatr Anaesth* 11:415, 2001.

Dauchot P, Gravenstein JS: Effects of atropine on the electrocardiogram in different age groups. *Clin Pharmacol Ther* 12:274, 1971.

Davis PJ, Cohen RT, McGowan FX Jr, et al.: Recovery characteristics of desflurane versus halothane for maintenance of anesthesia in pediatric ambulatory patients. *Anesthesiology* 80:298, 1994.

Davis PJ, Cook DR, Stiller RL, et al.: Pharmacodynamics and pharmacokinetics of high-dose sufentanil in infants and children undergoing cardiac surgery. *Anesth Analg* 66:203, 1987.

Davis PJ, Finkel JC, Orr RJ, et al.: A randomized, double-blinded study of remifentanil versus fentanyl for tonsillectomy and adenoidectomy surgery in pediatric ambulatory surgical patients. *Anesth Analg* 90:863–871, 2000.

Davis PJ, Galinkin J, McGowan FX, et al.: A randomized multicenter study of remifentanil compared with halothane in neonates and infants undergoing pyloromyotomy. I. Emergence and recovery profiles. *Anesth Analg* 93:1380–1386, 2001.

Davis PJ, Lerman J, Suresh S, et al.: A randomized multicenter study of remifentanil compared with alfentanil, isoflurane, or propofol in anesthetized pediatric patients undergoing elective strabismus surgery. *Anesth Analg* 84:982–989, 1997.

Davis PJ, Killian A, Stiller RL, et al.: Pharmacokinetics of alfentanil in newly born premature infants and older children. *Dev Pharmacol Ther* 13:21, 1989a.

Davis PJ, Stiller RL, Cook DR, et al.: Effects of cholestatic hepatic disease and chronic renal failure on alfentanil pharmacokinetics in children. *Anesth Analg* 68:568, 1989b.

Davis PJ, Stiller RL, Cook DR, et al.: Pharmacokinetics of sufentanil in adolescent patients with chronic renal failure. *Anesth Analg* 67:268, 1988.

Davis PJ, Stiller RL, McGowan FX, Jr: Decreased protein binding of alfentanil in plasma from children with kidney or liver failure. *Paediatr Anaesth* 3:19, 1993.

Davis PJ, Stiller RL, McGowan FX Jr, et al.: Preanesthetic medication with intranasal midazolam for brief surgical procedures: Effect on recovery and hospital discharge times. *Anesthesiology* 82:2, 1995.

Davis PJ, Wilson AS, Siewers RD, et al.: The effects of cardiopulmonary bypass on remifentanil kinetics in children undergoing atrial septal defect repair. *Anesth Analg* 89:904–908, 1999.

Dawson B, Michenfelder JD, Theye RA: Effects of ketamine on canine cerebral blood flow and metabolism: Modification by prior administration of thiopental. *Anesth Analg (Cleve)* 50:443, 1971.

De Ruiter J, Crawford MW: Does-response relationship and infusion requirement of cisatracurium besylate in infants and children during nitrous oxide-narcotic anesthesia. *Anesthesiology* 94:790–2, 2001.

de Wildt SN, Kearns GL, Hop WCJ, et al.: Pharmacokinetics and metabolism of oral midazolam in preterm infants. *Br J Clin Pharmacol* 53:390–392, 2002.

de Wildt SN, Kearns GL, Hop WCJ, et al.: Pharmacokinetics and metabolism of intravenous midazolam in preterm infants. *Clin Pharmacol Ther* 70:525–531, 2001.

de Wildt SN, Kearns GL, Leeder JS, et al.: Cytochrome P4503A: Ontogeny and drug disposition. *Clin Pharmacokinet* 37:486–505, 1999.

DeCook TH, Goudsouzian NG: Tachyphylaxis and phase II block development during infusion of succinylcholine in children. *Anesth Analg* 59:639, 1980.

Deer TR, Rich GF: Propofol tolerance in a pediatric patient. *Anesthesiology* 77:828, 1992.

DeJonghe B, Sharshar T, Lefaucheur JP, et al.: Paresis acquired in the intensive care unit. *JAMA* 288:2859–2867, 2002.

deLange S, Boscoe M, Stanley T, et al.: Comparison of sufentanil-oxygen and fentanyl-oxygen for coronary artery surgery. *Anesthesiology* 56:112, 1982.

Delphin E, Jackson D, Rothstein P: Use of succinylcholine during elective pediatric anesthesia should be reevaluated. *Anesth Analg* 66:1190, 1987.

DeNegri P, Ivani G, Tirri T, et al.: A comparison of epidural bupivacaine, levobupivacaine, and ropivacaine on postoperative analgesia and motor blockade. *Anesth Analg* 99:45–8, 2004.

Desparmet J, Meistelman C, Barre J, et al.: Continuous epidural infusion of bupivacaine for postoperative pain relief in children. *Anesthesiology* 67:108, 1987.

DeWolf AM, Freeman JA, Scott VL, et al.: Pharmacokinetics and pharmacodynamics of cisatracurium in patients with end-stage liver disease undergoing liver transplantation. *Br J Anesth* 76:624, 1996.

d'Hollander A, Massaux F, Nevelsteen M, et al.: Age-dependent dose-response relationship of ORG NC45 in anesthetized patients. *Br J Anaesth* 54:653, 1982.

d'Hollander AA, Luyckx C, Barvais L, et al.: Clinical evaluation of atracurium besylate requirement for a stable muscle relaxation during surgery: Lack of age-related effects. *Anesthesiology* 59:237, 1983.

Dhonneur G, Cerf C, Lagneau F, et al.: The pharmacokinetics of cisatracurium in patients with acute respiratory distress syndrome. *Anesth Analg* 93:400–404, 2001.

Dierdorf SF, McNiece WL, Wolfe TM, et al.: Effect of thiopental and succinylcholine on serum potassium concentrations in children. *Anesth Analg* 63:1136, 1984.

Doenicke A, Lorenz W, Beigl R, et al.: Histamine release after intravenous application of short-acting hypnotics. *Br J Anesth* 45:1097, 1973.

Domek NS, Batlow CF, Roth LJ: An ontogenetic study of phenobarbital C-14 in cat brain. *J Pharmacol Exp Ther* 130:285, 1960.

Domino KB, Anderson EA, Polissar NL, et al.: Comparative efficacy and safety of ondansetron, droperidol, and metoclopramide for preventing postoperative nausea and vomiting: A meta-analysis. *Anesth Analg* 88:1370–1379, 1999.

Domino EF, Chodoff P, Corssen G: Pharmacologic effects of CI-581, a new dissociative anesthetic, in man. *Clin Pharmacol Ther* 6:279, 1965.

Donati F, Bevan DR: Long-term succinylcholine infusion during isoflurane. *Anesthesiology* 58:6, 1983.

Donati F, Meistelman C, Plaud B: Vecuronium neuromuscular blockaded at the adductor muscles of the larynx and adductor pollicies. *Anesthesiology* 74:833–837, 1991.

Dönmez A, Kaya H, Haberal A, et al.: The effect of etomidate induction on plasma cortisol levels in children undergoing cardiac surgery. *J Cardiothorac Vasc Anesth* 12:182–185, 1998.

Dönmez A, Kizilkan A, Berksun H, et al.: One center's experience with remifentanil infusions for pediatric cardiac catheterization. *J Cardiothorac Vasc Anesth* 15:736–739, 2001.

Dowdy EG, Kaya K: Studies of mechanism of cardiovascular responses to CI-581. *Anesthesiology* 29:931, 1968.

Drenck NE, Ueda N, Olsen NV, et al.: Manual evaluation of residual curarization using double burst stimulation: A comparison with train-of-four. *Anesthesiology* 70:578, 1989.

Dresner DL, Basta SJ, Ali HA, et al.: Pharmacokinetics and pharmacodynamics of doxacurium in young and elderly patients during isoflurane anesthesia. *Anesth Analg* 71:498, 1990.

Dsida RM, Wheeler M, Birmingham PK, et al.: Age-stratified pharmacokinetics of ketorolac tromethamine in pediatric surgical patients. *Anesth Analg* 94:266–270, 2002.

Duncan HP, Cloote PM, Weir I, et al.: Reducing stress responses in the pre-bypass phase of open heart surgery in infants and young children: A comparison of different fentanyl doses. *Br J Anaesth* 84:556–564, 2000.

Dundee JW, Barron DW: The barbiturates. *Br J Anaesth* 34:240, 1962.

Duvaldestin P, Saada J, Berger JL, et al.: Pharmacokinetics, pharmacodynamics, and dose-response relationships of pancuronium in control and elderly subjects. *Anesthesiology* 56:36, 1982.

Dyck JB, Maze M, Haack C, et al.: The pharmocokinetics and hemodynamic effects of intravenous and intramuscular dexmedetomidine hydrochloride in adult human volunteers. *Anesthesiology* 78:813–20, 1993.

Ebert TJ, Hall JE, Barney JA, et al.: The effects of increasing plasma concentrations of dexmedetomidine in humans. *Anesthesiology* 93:382–94, 2000.

Ebling WF, Lee EN, Stanski DR: Understanding pharmacokinetics and pharmacodynamics through computer simulation: I. The comparative clinical profiles of fentanyl and alfentanil. *Anesthesiology* 72:650–658, 1990.

Ebrahim ZY, DeBoer GE, Luders H, et al.: Effect of etomidate on the electroencephalogram of patients with epilepsy. *Anesth Analg* 65:1004–6, 1986.

Echeverria P, Siber GR, Paisley J, et al.: Age-dependent dose response to gentamicin. *Pediatrics* 87:805–808, 1975.

Ecoffey C, Desparmet J, Berdeaux A, et al.: Bupivacaine in children: Pharmacokinetics following caudal anesthesia. *Anesthesiology* 63:447, 1985.

Ecoffey C, Desparmet J, Berdeaux A, et al.: Pharmacokinetics of lignocaine in children following caudal anesthesia. *Br J Anaesth* 56:1399, 1984.

Eddleston JM, Harper NJ, Pollard BJ, et al.: Concentrations of atracurium and laudanosine in cerebrospinal fluid during intracranial surgery. *Br J Anaesth* 63:525, 1989.

Egan TD, Lemmens HJM, Fiset P: The pharmacokinetics of the new short-acting opioid remifentanil (GI87084B) in healthy adult male volunteers. *Anesthesiology* 79:881, 1993.

Egan TD, Minto CF, Hermann DJ, et al.: Remifentanil versus alfentanil: Comparative pharmacokinetics and pharmacodynamics in healthy adult male volunteers. *Anesthesiology* 84:821–833, 1996.

Eger EI II: *Anesthetic uptake and action*. Baltimore, 1974, Williams & Wilkins.

Eger EI II, Smith NT, Cullen DJ, et al.: A comparison of cardiovascular effects of halothane, fluroxene, ether and cyclopropane in man. *Anesthesiology* 34:325, 1971.

Eger EI II, Smith NT, Stoeling RK, et al.: Cardiovascular effects of halothane in man. *Anesthesiology* 32:396, 1970.

Ehrnebo M, Agurell S, Jalling B, et al.: Age differences in drug binding by plasma proteins: Studies on human foetuses, neonates and adults. *J Eur Clin Pharmacol* 3:189–193, 1971.

Elliot JM, Bion JF: The use of neuromuscular blocking drugs in intensive care practice. *Acta Anaesthesiol Scand* 39:70, 1995.

Ellis DJ, Steward DJ: Fentanyl dosage is associated with reduced blood glucose in pediatric patients with hypothermic cardiopulmonary bypass. *Anesthesiology* 72:812, 1990.

Eltzschig HK, Schroeder TH, Eissler BJ, et al.: The effect of remifentanil or fentanyl on postoperative vomiting and pain in children undergoing strabismus surgery. *Anesth Analg* 94:1173–1177, 2002.

Eng M, Bonica JJ, Akamatsu TJ, et al.: Respiratory depression in newborn monkeys at cesarean section following ketamine administration. *Br J Anaesth* 47:917, 1975.

Engelhardt T, Steel E, Johnston G, et al.: Tramadol for pain relief in children undergoing tonsillectomy: A comparison with morphine. *Paediatr Anaesth* 13:249–252, 2003.

Engstron RH, Cohen SE: A complication associated with the use of midazolam [letter]. *Anesthesiology* 70:719, 1989.

Erb TO, Hall JM, Ing RJ, et al.: Postoperative nausea and vomiting in children and adolescents undergoing radiofrequency catheter ablation: A randomized comparison of propofol- and isoflurane-based anesthetics. *Anesth Analg* 95:1577–1581, 2002.

Erkola O, Rautoma P, Meretoja OA: Mivacurium when preceded by pancuronium becomes a long-acting muscle relaxant [comment]. *Anesthesiology* 84:562–565, 1996.

Eyres RL, Bishop W, Brinn TCK: Plasma bupivacaine concentrations in children during caudal epidural analgesia. *Anesth Intensive Care* 11:20, 1983.

Eyres RL, Kidd J, Oppenheim R, et al.: Local anaesthestic plasma levels in children. *Anaesth Intensive Care* 6:243, 1978.

Fahey MR, Rupp SM, Canfell C, et al.: The effect of renal failure on laudanosine excretion in man. *Br J Anaesth* 57:1049, 1985.

Fahey MR, Rupp SM, Fisher DM, et al.: The pharmacokinetics and pharmacodynamics of atracurium in patients with and without renal failure. *Anesthesiology* 61:699, 1984.

Fang ZX, Eger EI 2nd, Laster MJ, et al.: Carbon monoxide production from degradation of desflurane, enflurane, isoflurane, halothane and sevoflurane by soda lime and Baralyme. *Anesth Analg* 80:1187, 1995.

Feld LH, Negus JB, White PF: Oral midazolam preanesthetic medication in pediatric outpatients. *Anesthesiology* 73:831, 1990.

Ferrier C, Marty J, Bouffard Y, et al.: Alfentanil pharmacokinetics in patients with cirrhosis. *Anesthesiology* 62:480, 1985.

Fiamengo SA, Savarese JJ: Use of muscle relaxants in intensive care units. *Crit Care Med* 19:1457, 1991.

Fine GF, Brandom BW, Yellon RF: Unmasked residual neuromuscular block after administration of vecuronium for days. *Anesth Analg* 93:345–347, 2001.

Fine GF, Motoyama EK, Brandom BW, et al.: The effect on lung mechanics in anesthetized children with rapacuronium: A comparative study with mivacurium. *Anesth Analg* 95:56–61, 2002.

Finkel JC, Elrefai A: The use of dexmedetomidine to facilitate opioids and benzodiazepine detoxification in an infant. *Anesth Analg* 98:1658–9, 2004.

Finkel JC, Rose JB, Schmitz ML, et al.: An evaluation of the efficacy and tolerability of oral tramadol hydrochloride tablets for the treatment of postsurgical pain in children. *Anesth Analg* 94:1469–1473, 2002.

Fisher DM, Cronnelly R, Miller RD, et al.: The neuromuscular pharmacology of neostigmine in infants and children. *Anesthesiology* 59:220, 1983.

Fisher DM, Cronnelly R, Sharma M, et al.: Clinical pharmacology of edrophonium in infants. *Anesthesiology* 61:428, 1984.

Fisher DM, Miller RD: Neuromuscular effects of vecuronium (ORG NC45) in infants and children during N_2O-halothane anesthesia. *Anesthesiology* 58:519, 1983.

Fisher DM, O'Keeffe C, Stanski DR, et al.: Pharmacokinetics and pharmacodynamics of d-tubocurarine in infants, children, and adults. *Anesthesiology* 57:203, 1982.

Fisher DM, Zwass MS: MAC of desflurane in 60% nitrous oxide in infants and children. *Anesthesiology* 76:354, 1992.

Fleming NW: Neuromuscular blocking drugs in the intensive care unit: Indications, protocols, and complications. *Semin Anesth* 13:255, 1994.

Flewellen EH, Nelson TE: Halothane-succinylcholine induced masseter spasm: Indicative of malignant hyperthermia susceptibility. *Anesth Analg* 63:693, 1984.

Forbes RB, Murray DJ, Dillman JB, et al.: Pharmacokinetics of two percent rectal methohexitone in children. *Can J Anaesth* 36:160–164, 1989a.

Forbes RB, Murray DJ, Dull KL, et al.: Haemodynamic effects of rectal methohexitone for induction of anaesthesia in children. *Can J Anaesth* 36:526–529, 1989b.

Forster A, Morel D, Bachmann M: Respiratory depressant effects of different doses of midazolam and lack of reversal with naloxone—a double-blind randomized study. *Anesth Analg* 62:920, 1983.

Foubert L, Reyntjens K, De Wolf D, et al.: Remifentanil infusion for cardiac catheterization in children with congenital heart disease. *Acta Anesthiol Scand* 46:355–360, 2002.

Frei FJ, Haemmerle MH, Brunner R, et al.: Minimum alveolar concentration for halothane in children with cerebral palsy and severe mental retardation. *Anaesthesia* 52:1056, 1997.

Friis-Hansen B: Body water compartments in children: Changes during growth and related changes in body composition. *Pediatrics* 28:169–181, 1961.

Frink EJ Jr, Green WB Jr, Brown EA, et al.: Compound A concentrations during sevoflurane anesthesia in children. *Anesthesiology* 84:566, 1996.

Fujii Y, Saitoh Y, Kobayashi N: Prevention of vomiting after tonsillectomy in children: Granisetron versus ramosetron. *Laryngoscope* 111:255–258, 2001.

Fujii Y, Saitoh Y, Tanaka H, et al.: Preoperative oral antiemetics for reducing postoperative vomiting after tonsillectomy in children: Granisetron versus perphenazine. *Anesth Analg* 88:1298–1301, 1999a.

Fujii Y, Saitoh Y, Tanaka H, et al.: Prevention of postoperative vomiting with granisetron in paediatric patients with and without a history of motion sickness. *Paediatr Anaesth* 9:527–530, 1999b.

Fujii Y, Tanaka H: Comparison of granisetron, droperidol, and metoclopramide for prevention of postoperative vomiting in children with a history of motion sickness undergoing tonsillectomy. *J Pediatr Surg* 36:460–462, 2001.

Fujii Y, Tanaka H: Granisetron reduces postoperative vomiting in children: A dose-ranging study. *Eur J Anesthesiol* 16:62–65, 1999.

Fujii Y, Tanaka H: Preoperative oral granisetron for the prevention of vomiting following paediatric surgery. *Paediatr Anaesth* 12:267–271, 2002.

Fujii Y, Toyooka H, Tanaka H: A granisetron-droperidol combination prevents postoperative vomiting in children. *Anesth Analg* 87:761–765, 1998.

Galinkin JL, Davis PJ, McGowan FX, et al.: A randomized multicenter study of remifentanil compared with halothane in neonates and infants undergoing pyloromyotomy. II. Perioperative breathing patterns in neonates and infants with pyloric stenosis. *Anesth Analg* 93:1387–1392, 2001.

Galinkin JL, Fazi LM, Cuy RM, et al.: Use of intranasal fentanyl in children undergoing myringotomy and tube placement during halothane and sevoflurane anesthesia. *Anesthesiology* 93:1378–1383, 2000.

Gallagher TW, Black GW: Uptake of volatile anaesthetics in children. *Anaesthesia* 40:1073, 1985.

Gardner AE, Olson BE, Lichtiger M: Cerebrospinal fluid pressure during dissociative anesthesia with ketamine. *Anesthesiology* 35:226, 1971.

Gatke MR, Ostergaard D, Bundgaard JR, et al.: Response to mivacurium in a patient compound heterozygous for a novel and a known silent mutation in the butyrylcholinesterase gene: Genotyping by sequencing. *Anesthesiology* 95:600–606, 2001.

Gauntlett IS, Fisher DM, Hertzka RE, et al.: Pharmacokinetics of fentanyl in neonatal humans and lambs: Effects of age. *Anesthesiology* 69:683–687, 1988.

Gaviotaki A, Smith RM: Use of atropine in pediatric anesthesia. *Int Anesthesiol Clin* 1:97, 1962.

German JW, Aneja R, Heard C, et al.: Continuous remifentanil for pediatric neurosurgery patients. *Pediatr Neurosurg* 33:227–229, 2000.

Ghonheim M, Yamanda T: Etomidate: A clinical and electroencephalographic comparison with thiopental. *Anesth Analg* 56:479, 1977.

Gill SS, Wright EM, Reilly CS: Pharmacokinetic interaction of propofol and fentanyl: Single bolus injection study. *Br J Anaesth* 65:760, 1990.

Gillis JC, Brogden RN: Ketorolac. A reappraisal of its pharmacodynamic and pharmacokinetic properties and therapeutic use in pain management. *Drugs* 53:139–188, 1997.

Ginsberg B, Scott H, Glass PSA, et al.: Pharmacokinetic model-driven infusion of fentanyl in children. *Anesthesiology* 85:1268–1275, 1996.

Glass PSA, Hardman D, Kamiyama Y: Preliminary pharmacokinetics and pharmacodynamics of an ultra-short-acting opioid: Remifentanil (GI87084B). *Anesth Analg* 77:1031, 1993.

Goho C: Oral midazolam-grapefruit juice drug interaction. *Pediatr Dent* 23:365–366, 2001.

Goldberg AH: Effects of halothane on force-velocity, length-tension, and stress-strain curves of isolated heart muscle. *Anesthesiology* 29:192, 1968.

Goldberg ME, Torjman M, Bartkowski RR: Time-course of respiratory depression after an alfentanil infusion-based anesthetic. *Anesth Analg* 75:965, 1992.

Goldenthal EI: A compilation of LD50 values in newborn and adult animals. *Toxicol Appl Pharmacol* 18:185, 1971.

Gonsowski CT, Laster MJ, Eger EI II, et al.: Toxicity of compound A in rats: Effect of a 3-hour administration. *Anesthesiology* 80:556, 1994a.

Gonsowski CT, Laster MJ, Eger EI II, et al.: Toxicity of compound A in rats. *Anesthesiology* 80:566, 1994b.

Goresky GV, Koren G, Sabourin MA, et al.: The pharmacokinetics of alfentanil in children undergoing surgery. *Anesthesiology* 67:654, 1987.

Goresky GV, Steward DJ: Rectal methohexitone for induction of anaesthesia in children. *Can Anaesth Soc J* 26:213, 1979.

Goudsouzian N, Chakravorti S, Denman W, et al.: Lack of accumulation of the cis-cis isomer of mivacurium in patients with low butyryl cholinesterase activity. *Anesthesiology* 81:1060, 1994.

Goudsouzian N, Liu LM, Gionfriddo M, et al.: Neuromuscular effect of atracurium in infants and children. *Anesthesiology* 62:75, 1985.

Goudsouzian NG, Liu LM, Cote CJ, et al.: Safety and efficacy of atracurium in adolescents and children anesthetized with halothane. *Anesthesiology* 59:459, 1983.

Goudsouzian NG, Liu LMP, Cote CJ: Comparison of equipotent doses of non-depolarizing muscle relaxants in children. *Anesth Analg* 60:862, 1981.

Goudsouzian NG, Liu LMP: The neuromuscular response of infants to a continuous infusion of succinylcholine. *Anesthesiology* 60:97, 1984.

Goudsouzian NG, Martyn JJA, Liu LMP: The dose response effect of long-acting non-depolarizing neuromuscular blocking agents in children. *Can J Anaesth* 3:246, 1984.

Goudsouzian NG: Maturation of neuromuscular transmission in the infant. *Br J Anaesth* 52:205, 1980.

Gourlay GK, Wilson PR, Glynn CJ: Pharmacodynamics and pharmacokinetics of methadone during the perioperative period. *Anesthesiology* 57:458, 1982.

Gozal D, Rein AJJT, Nir A, et al.: Propofol does not modify the hemodynamic status of children with intracardiac shunts undergoing cardiac catheterization. *Pediatr Cardiol* 22:488–490, 2001.

Greeley WJ, de Bruijn NP: Changes in sufentanil pharmacokinetics within the neonatal period. *Anesth Analg* 67:86, 1988.

Greeley WJ, de Bruijn NP, Davis DP: Sufentanil pharmacokinetics in pediatric cardiovascular patients. *Anesth Analg* 66:1067, 1987.

Gregory GA, Eger EI II, Munson ES: The relationship between age and halothane requirement in man. *Anesthesiology* 30:488, 1969.

Gregory GA, Wade JG, Beihl DR, et al.: Fetal anesthetic requirement (MAC) for halothane. *Anesth Analg* 62:9–14, 1983.

Gregory RE, Ettinger DS: 5-HT3 receptor antagonists for the prevention of chemotherapy-induced nausea and vomiting: A comparison of their pharmacology and clinical efficacy. *Drugs* 55:173–189, 1998.

Gronert BJ, Brandom BW: Neuromuscular blocking drugs in infants and children. *Pediatr Clin North Am* 41:73, 1994.

Gronert BJ, Woelfel SK, Cook DR: Comparison of the neuromuscular effects of mivacurium and succinylcholine in infants and children. *Acta Anaesthesiol Scand* 39:35, 1995.

Gronert GA: Mortality greater with rhabdomyolysis than receptor upregulation. *Anesthesiology* 94:523–529, 2001.

Gu Y, Franco A Jr, Gardner PD, et al.: Properties of embryonic and adult muscle acetylcholine receptors transiently expressed in COS cells. *Neuron* 5:147, 1990.

Guay J, Gaudreault P, Tang A: Pharmacokinetics of sufentanil in normal children. *Can J Anaesth* 39:14, 1992.

Guignard B, Bossard AE, Coste C, et al.: Acute opioid tolerance: Intraoperative remifentanil increases postoperative pain and morphine requirement. *Anesthesiology* 93:409–417, 2000.

Guignard JP, Torrado A, Cunha OD, et al.: Glomerular filtration rate in the first three weeks of life. *J Pediatr* 87:268, 1975.

Guldner G, Schultz J, Sexton P, et al.: Etomidate for rapid-sequence intubation in young children: hemodynamic effects and adverse events. *Acad Emerg Med* 10:134–9, 2003.

Gunter JB, Gregg T, Varughese AM, et al.: Levobupivacaine for ilioinguinal/iliohypogastric nerve block in children. *Anesth Analg* 89:647–649, 1999.

Gustorff B, Nahlik G, Hoerauf KH, et al.: The absence of acute tolerance during remifentanil infusion in volunteers. *Anesth Analg* 94:1223–1228, 2002.

Gutstein HB, Johnson KL, Heard MB, et al.: Oral ketamine preanesthetic medication in children. *Anesthesiology* 76:28–33, 1992.

Hakkola J, Pasanen M, Purkunen R, et al.: Expression of xenobiotic-metabolizing cytochrome P450 forms in human adult and fetal liver. *Biochem Pharmacol* 48:59–64, 1994.

Halkin H, Radomsky M, Millman P, et al.: Steady state serum concentrations and renal clearance of digoxin in neonates, infants and children. *Eur J Clin Pharmacol* 13:113–117, 1978.

Halpern SA: *American pediatrics: The social dynamic of professionalism, 1880-1980.* Berkeley, 1988, University of California Press.

Hamunen K, Maunuksela EL, Sarvela J, et al.: Stereoselective pharmacokinetics of ketorolac in children, adolescents and adults. *Acta Anaesthesiol Scand* 43:1041–1046, 1999.

Hamza J, Ecoffey C, Gross JB: Ventilatory response to CO_2 following intravenous ketamine in children. *Anesthesiology* 70:422–25, 1989.

Hanaki C, Fujii K, Morio M, et al.: Decomposition of sevoflurane by soda lime. *Hiroshima J Med Sci* 36:61, 1987.

Hanna MH, D'Costa F, Peat SJ: Morphine-6-glucuronide disposition in renal impairment. *Br J Anaesth* 70:511, 1993.

Hannallah RS, Baker SB, Casey W: Propofol: Effective dose and induction characteristics in unpremedicated children. *Anesthesiology* 74:217, 1991.

Hansen TG, Ilett KF, Lim SI, et al.: Pharmacokinetics and clinical efficacy of long-term epidural ropivacaine infusion in children. *Br J Anaesth* 85:347–353, 2000.

Hansen TG, Ilett KF, Reid C, et al.: Caudal ropivacaine in infants. *Anesthesiology* 94:579–584, 2001.

Harper NJ, Greer R, Conway D: Neuromuscular monitoring in intensive care patients: Milliamperage requirements for supramaximal stimulation. *Br J Anaesth* 87:625–627, 2001.

Harris WS, Goodman PM: Hyperactivity to atropine in Down's syndrome. *N Engl J Med* 279:407, 1968.

Haycock GB: Development of glomerular filtration and tubular sodium reabsorption in the human fetus and newborn. *Br J Urol* 81(Suppl 2):33–38, 1998.

Head-Rapson AG, Devlin JC, Parker CJ, et al.: Pharmacokinetics and pharmacodynamics of the three isomers of mivacurium in health, in end-stage renal failure and in patients with impaired renal function. *Br J Anaesth* 75:31–36, 1995.

Head-Rapson AG, Devlin JC, Parker CJ, et al.: Pharmacokinetics of the three isomers of mivacurium and pharmacodynamics of the chiral mixture in hepatic cirrhosis. *Br J Anaesth* 73:613–618, 1994.

Heilbron DC, Holliday MA, al-Dahwi A, et al.: Expressing glomerular filtration rate in children. *Pediatr Nephrol* 5:5–11, 1991.

Heir T, Feiner JR, Lin J, et al.: Hemoglobin desaturation after succinylcholine-induced apnea. *Anesthesia* 94:754–759, 2001.

Helmers JH, Noorduin H, Van Peer A: Comparison of intravenous and intranasal sufentanil absorption and sedation. *Can J Anaesth* 36:494, 1989.

Henning RD, Bush GH: Plasma potassium after halothane suxamethonium induction in children. *Anaesthesia* 37:802, 1982.

Hertzka RE, Gauntlett IS, Fisher DM: Fentanyl-induced ventilatory depression: Effects of age. *Anesthesiology* 70:213, 1989.

Hickey PR, Hansen DD, Cramolini GM: Pulmonary and systemic hemodynamic responses to ketamine in infants with normal and elevated pulmonary vascular resistance. *Anesthesiology* 61:A438, 1984.

Hickey PR, Hansen DD, Wessel DL: Pulmonary and systemic hemodynamic responses to fentanyl in infants. *Anesth Analg* 64:483, 1985.

Hickey PR, Retzack SM: Acute right ventricular failure after pulmonary hypertensive responses to airway instrumentation: Effect of fentanyl dose. *Anesthesiology* 78:372, 1993.

Hinkle AJ, Weinlander CM: The effects of 10% methohexital on the rectal mucosa in mice. *Anesthesiology* 71:550, 1989.

Holt R, Rask P, Coulthard KP, et al.: Tropisetron plus dexamethasone is more effective than tropisetron alone for the prevention of postoperative nausea and vomiting in children undergoing tonsillectomy. *Paediatr Anaesth* 10:181–188, 2000.

Hopkins PM: Use of suxamethonium in children. *Br J Anaesth* 75:675–677, 1995.

Howard RF, Bingham RM: Endotracheal compared with intravenous administration of atropine. *Arch Dis Childhood* 65:449–50, 1990.

Hug C: *Alfentanil: Pharmacology and uses in anaesthesia.* Auckland, New Zealand, 1984, Adis Press.

Huges MA, Glass PS, Jacobs JR: Context-sensitive half-time in multi-compartment pharmacokinetic models for intravenous anesthetic drugs. *Anesthesiology* 76:334–341, 1992.

Hunter JM, Jones RS, Utting JE: Use of atracurium in patients with no renal function. *Br J Anaesth* 54:1251, 1982.

Huntington JH, Malviya S, Voepel-Lewis T, et al.: The effect of right-to-left intracardiac shunt on the rate of rise of arterial and end-tidal halothane in children. *Anesth Analg* 88:759–762, 1999.

Ibacache ME, Munoz HR, Brandes V, Morales AL: Single-dose dexmedetomidine reduces agitation after sevoflurane anesthesia in children. *Anesth Analg* 98:60, 2004.

Ingram MD, et al.: Cardiovascular and electroencephalographic effects of laudanosine in "nephrectomized" cats. *Br J Anaesth* 58:14S, 1986.

Ivani G, DeNegri P, Conio A, et al.: Comparison of racemic bupivacaine, ropivacaine, and levobupivacaine for pediatric caudal anesthesia: Effects on postoperative analgesia and motor block. *Reg Anesth Pain Med* 27:157–161, 2002.

Ivani G, DeNegri P, Conio A, et al.: Ropivacaine-clonidine combination for caudal blockade in children. *Acta Anaesth Scand* 44:446, 2000.

Ivani G, DeNegri P, Lonngvist PA, et al.: Caudal anesthesia for minor pediatric surgery: a prospective randomized comparison of ropivacaine 0.2% vs levobupivacaine 0.2%. *Paediatr Anaesth* 15:491, 2005.

Ivani G, DeNegri P, Lonqvist PA, et al.: A comparison of three different concentrations of levobupivacaine for caudal block in children. *Anesth Analg* 97:368–71, 2003.

Ivani G, Lampugnani E, DeNegri P, et al.: Ropivacaine vs bupivacaine in major surgery in infants. *Can J Anaesth* 46:467, 1999.

Ivani G, Lampugnani E, Torre M, et al.: Comparison of ropivacaine with bupivacaine for paediatric caudal block. *Br J Anaesth* 81:247–248, 1998.

Iwasaki H, Igarashi M, Namiki A, et al.: Differential neuromuscular effects of vecuronium on the adductor and abductor laryngeal muscles and tibialis anterior muscle in dogs. *Br J Anaesth* 72:321–323, 1994a.

Iwasaki H, Igarashi M, Omote K, et al.: Vecuronium neuromuscular blockade at the cricothyroid and posterior cricoarytenoid muscles of the larynx and at the adductor pollices muscle in humans. *J Clin Anesth* 6:14–17, 1994b.

Jaaskelainen SK, Kaisti K, Suni L, et al.: Sevoflurane is epileptogenic in healthy subjects at surgical levels of anesthesia. *Neurology* 61:1073–1078, 2003.

Jalkanen L, Meretoja OA: The influence of the duration of isoflurane anesthesia on neuromuscular effects of mivacurium. *Acta Anesthesiol Scand* 41:248–251, 1997.

Jalkanen L, Meretoja OA, Taivainen T, et al.: Synergism between atracurium and mivacurium compared with that between vecuronium and mivacurium [comment]. *Anesth Analg* 79:998–1002, 1994.

Jensen AB, Christiansen DB, Coulthard K, et al.: Tropisetron reduces postoperative vomiting in children undergoing tonsillectomy. *Paediatr Anaesth* 10:69–75, 2000.

Jevtovic-Todorovic V, Beals J, Benshoff N, et al.: Prolonged exposure to inhalational anesthetic nitrous oxide kills neurons in adult rat brain. *Neuroscience* 122:609–616, 2003.

Johnson KL, Erickson JP, Holley FO, et al.: Fentanyl pharmacokinetics in the pediatric population. *Anesthesiology* 61:A441, 1984.

Jones RDM, Chan K, Andrew LJ: Pharmacokinetics of propofol in children. *Br J Anaesth* 65:661, 1990.

Jones RDM, Chan K, Roulson CJ: Pharmacokinetics of flumazenil and midazolam. *Br J Anaesth* 70:286, 1993.

Jones RDM, Lawson AD, Andrew LJ: Antagonism of the hypnotic side effects of midazolam in children: A randomized double-blind study of placebo and flumazenil administered after midazolam-induced anesthesia. *Br J Anaesth* 66:660, 1991.

Jonmarker C, Westrin P, Larsson S, et al.: Thiopental requirements for induction of anesthesia in children. *Anesthesiology* 67:104, 1987.

Jorgensen BG, Ostergaard D: Tracheal administration of atropine in children–effect on heart rate. *Paed Anaesth* 7:461–63, 1997.

Kain ZN, Hofstadter MB, Mayes L, et al.: Midazolam: Effects on amnesia and anxiety in children. *Anesthesiology* 93:676–684, 2000.

Kain ZN, Mayes LC, Bell C, et al.: Premedication in the United States: A status report. *Anesth Analg* 84:427–432, 1997.

Kapila A, Glass PS, Jacobs JR, et al.: Measured context-sensitive half-times of remifentanil and alfentanil. *Anesthesiology* 83:968–975, 1995.

Karl HW, Rosenberger JL, Larach MG: Transmucosal administration of midazolam for premedication of pediatric patients: Comparison of nasal and sublingual routes. *Anesthesiology* 78:885, 1993.

Karmakar MK, Aun CST, Wong ELY, et al.: Ropivacaine undergoes slower systemic absorption from the caudal epidural space in children than bupivacaine. *Anesth Analg* 94:259–265, 2002.

Karsli C, Luginbuehl I, Farrar M, et al.: Propofol decreases cerebral blood flow velocity in anesthetized children. *Can J Anesth* 49:830–834, 2002.

Kataria BK, Ved SA, Nicodemus HF: The pharmacokinetics of propofol in children using three different data analysis approaches. *Anesthesiology* 80:104, 1994.

Katz R, Kelly HW: Pharmacokinetics of continuous infusions of fentanyl in critically ill children. *Crit Care Med* 21:995, 1993.

Kauffman RE, Lieh-Lai MW, Uy HG, et al.: Enantiomer-selective pharmacokinetics and metabolism of ketorolac in children. *Clin Pharmacol Ther* 65:382–388, 1999.

Kay B, Pleuvry B: Human volunteer studies of alfentanil (R39209), a new short-acting narcotic analgesic. *Anaesthesia* 35:952, 1980.

Kay B, Stephenson D: Alfentanil (R34209) initial clinical experience with a new narcotic analgesic. *Anaesthesia* 35:1182, 1980.

Kearns GL, Abdel-Rahman SM, Alander SW, et al.: Drug therapy: Developmental pharmacology: Drug disposition, action, and therapy in infants and children. *N Engl J Med* 349:1157–1167, 2003.

Keenan RL, Boyan CP: Cardiac arrest due to anesthesia. *JAMA* 253:2372, 1985.

Kenna JG, Neuberger J, Mieli-Vergani G, et al.: Halothane hepatitis in children. *Br Med J* 294:1209, 1989.

Khalil S, Campos C, Farag AM, et al.: Caudal block in children. *Anesthesiology* 91:1279–1284, 1999.

Khalil S, Philbrook L, Rabb M, et al.: Sublingual midazolam premedication in children: A dose response study. *Paediatr Anaesth* 8:461–465, 1998.

Khalil S, Rodarte A, Wildon BC, et al.: Intravenous ondansetron in established postoperative emesis in children. S3A-381 Study Group. *Anesthesiology* 85:270–276, 1996.

Khalil SN, Florence FB, Van den Nieuwenhuyzen MCO, et al.: Rectal methohexital: Concentration and length of the rectal catheters. *Anesth Analg* 70:645–649, 1990.

Kharasch E, Russell M, Mautz D, et al.: The role of cytochrome P450 3A4 in alfentanil clearance: Implications for interindividual variability in disposition and perioperative drug interactions. *Anesthesiology* 87:36–50, 1997b.

Kharasch ED, Armstrong AS, Gunn K, et al.: Clinical sevoflurane metabolism and disposition: II. The role of cytochrome P450 2E1 in fluoride and hexafluoroisopropanol formation. *Anesthesiology* 82:1379, 1995a.

Kharasch ED, Hankins DC, Thummel KE: Human kidney methoxyflurane and sevoflurane metabolism: Intrarenal fluoride production as a possible mechanism of methoxyflurane nephrotoxicity. *Anesthesiology* 82:689, 1995b.

Kharasch ED, Russell M, Garton K, et al.: Assessment of cytochrome P450 3A4 activity during the menstrual cycle using alfentanil as a noninvasive probe. *Anesthesiology* 87:26–35, 1997.

Kharasch ED, Thummel KE: Human alfentanil metabolism by cytochrome P450 3A3/4. An explanation for the interindividual variability in alfentanil clearance? *Anesth Analg* 76:1033–1039, 1993.

Khuenl-Brady K, Castagnoli KP, Canfell C, et al.: The neuromuscular blocking effects and pharmacokinetics of ORG 9426 and ORG 9616 in the cat. *Anesthesiology* 72:669–674, 1990.

Killian A, Davis PJ, Stiller RL: Influence of gestational age on pharmacokinetics of alfentanil in neonates. *Dev Pharmacol Ther* 15:82, 1990.

Kim C, Hirose M, Martyn JAJ: d-Tubocurarine accentuates the burn-induced upregulation of nicotinic acetylcholine receptors at the muscle membrane. *Anesthesiology* 83:309–315, 1995.

Kingston HGG, Kendrick A, Sommer KM: Binding of thiopental in neonatal serum. *Anesthesiology* 72:428, 1990.

Klees TM, Sheffels P, Thummel KE, Kharasch ED: Pharmacogenetic determinants of human liver microsomal alfentanil metabolism and the role of cytochrome P450 3A5. *Anesthesiology* 102(3):550–6, 2005.

Klepstad P, Rakvag TT, Kaasa S, et al.: The 118A>G polymorphism in the human microopioid receptor gene may increase morphine requirements in patients with pain caused by malignant disease. *Acta Anaesthesiol Scand* 48:1232, 2004.

Klessig HT, Geiger HJ, Murray MJ, et al.: A national survey on the practice patterns of anesthesiologist intensivists in the use of muscle relaxants. *Crit Care Med* 20:1341, 1992.

Knauer B, Draffen GA, WIlliams FM: Elimination kinetics of amobarbital in mothers and their newborn infants. *Clin Pharmacol Ther* 14:442, 1973.

Knibbe CAJ, Melenhorst-de Jong G, Mestrom M, et al.: Pharmacokinetics and effects of propofol 6% for short-term sedation in paediatric patients following cardiac surgery. *Br J Clin Pharmacol* 54:415–422, 2002.

Kobel M, Creighton RE, Steward DJ: Anaesthetic considerations in Down's syndrome: Experience with 100 patients and a review of the literature. *Can Anaesth Soc J* 29:593, 1982.

Koehntop DE, Rodman JH, Brundage DM, et al.: Pharmacokinetics of fentanyl in neonates. *Anesth Analg* 65:227, 1986.

Kokki H, Ylonen P, Heikkinen M, Reinikainen M: Levobupivacaine for pediatric spinal anesthesia. *Anesth Analg* 98:64–7, 2004.

Kokki H, Karvinen M, Jekunen A: Pharmacokinetics of a 24-hour intravenous ketoprofen infusion in children. *Acta Anaesthesiol Scand* 46:194–198, 2002.

Komatsu H, et al.: Electrical seizures during sevoflurane anesthesia in two pediatric patients with epilepsy. *Anesthesiology* 81:1535, 1994.

Kopman A: Pancuronium, gallamine, and d-tubocurarine compared: Is speed of onset inversely related to drug potency? *Anesthesiology* 70:915, 1989.

Kopman AF, Khan NA, Neuman GG: Precurarization and priming: A theoretical analysis of safety and timing. *Anesth Analg* 93:1253–1256, 2001.

Kopman AF, Klewicka MM, Neuman GG: Reexamined: The recommended endotracheal intubating dose for nondepolarizing neuromuscular blockers of rapid onset. *Anesth Analg* 93:954–959, 2001.

Kopman AF, Kumar S, Klewicka MM, et al.: The staircase phenomenon: Implications for monitoring of neuromuscular transmission. *Anesthesiology* 95:403–407, 2001.

Koppert W, Blunk JA, Petersen LJ: Different patterns of mast cell activation by muscle relaxants in human skin. *Anesthesiology* 95:659–667, 2001.

Koren G, Goresky G, Crean P: Pediatric fentanyl dosing based on pharmacokinetics during cardiac surgery. *Anesth Analg* 63:577, 1984.

Kramer M, Kling D, Walter P, et al.: Alfentanil: A new short acting opioid: Haemodynamic and respiratory aspects. *Anaesthetist* 32:265, 1983.

Krane EJ, Su JY: Comparison of the effects of halothane on newborn and adult rabbit myocardium. *Anesth Analg* 66:1240, 1987.

Kupferberg HI, Way EL: Pharmacologic basis for the increased sensitivity of the newborn rat to morphine. *J Pharmacol Exp Ther* 141:105, 1963.

Kurz H, Michels H, Stickel HH: Differences in the binding of drugs to plasma proteins from newborn to adult man. *Eur J Clin Pharmacol* 11:469–472, 1977.

Lammers CR, Rosner JL, Crockett DE, et al.: Oral midazolam with an antacid may increase the speed of onset of sedation in children prior to general anaesthesia. *Paediatr Anaesth* 12:26–28, 2002.

Lanier WL, Milde JH, Michenfelder JD: The cerebral effects of pancuronium and atracurium in halothane-anesthetized dogs. *Anesthesiology* 63:589, 1985.

Larsson S, Asgeirsson B, Magnusson J: Propofol-fentanyl anesthesia compared with thiopental-halothane with special reference to recovery and vomiting after pediatric strabismus surgery. *Acta Anaesthesiol Scand* 36:182, 1992.

Lavine LM, Hindein BI: Hemodialysis as treatment for prolonged neuromuscular blockade in anephric patients. *Anesthesiology* 59:264, 1983.

Law SC, Cook DR: Monitoring the neuromuscular junction. In Lake CL (ed): *Clinical monitoring.* Philadelphia, 1990, WB Saunders, pp 719–755.

Laxenaire M-C, Mata-Bermejo E, Moneret-Vautrin DA: Life-threatening anaphylactoid reactions to propofol (Diprivan®). *Anesthesiology* 77:275, 1992.

Lebovic S, Reich DL, Steinberg LG: Comparison of propofol versus ketamine for anesthesia in pediatric patients undergoing cardiac catheterization. *Anesth Analg* 74:490, 1992.

Lebowitz P, Cote E, Daniels A, et al.: Comparative cardiovascular effects of midazolam and thiopental in healthy patients. *Anesth Analg* 61:77, 1982.

Lebrault C, Berger JL, D'Hollander AA, et al.: Pharmacokinetics and pharmacodynamics of vecuronium (*ORG NC45*) in patients with cirrhosis. *Anesthesiology* 62:601–605, 1985.

LeDez KM, Lerman J: The minimum alveolar concentration (MAC) of isoflurane in preterm neonates. *Anesthesiology* 67:301, 1987.

Ledingham I, Watt I: Influence of sedation on mortality in critically ill multiple trauma patients. *Lancet* 1:1270, 1983.

Lee C: Intensive care unit neuromuscular syndrome? *Anesthesiology* 83:237, 1995.

Lee C: Self antagonism: Possible mechanism of tachyphylaxis in suxamethonium-induced neuromuscular block in man. *Br J Anaesth* 48:1097, 1986.

Lee C: Structure, conformation, and action of neuromuscular blocking drugs. *Br J Anaesth* 5:755–769, 1987.

Leeder JS: Pharmacogenetics and pharmacogenomics. *Pediatr Clin North Am* 48:765–781, 2001.

Leeder JS, Kearns GL.: Pharmacogenetics in pediatrics. Implications for practice. *Pediatr Clin North Am* 44:55–77, 1997.

Leigh MD, Belton MK: *Pediatric anesthesiology.* 2nd ed. New York, 1960, Macmillan.

Lerman J: Induction, recovery and safety characteristics of sevoflurane in children undergoing ambulatory surgery: A comparison with halothane. *Anesthesiology* 84:1332, 1996.

Lerman J: Inhalational agents. In: Bissonnette B, Dalens BJ, editors: Pediatric anesthesia: Principles and practice. New York, 2002, McGraw-Hill Professional, Chapter 13.

Lerman J: Pharmacokinetics of inhalational anesthetic agents. In Bowdle TA, Horita A, Kharasch ED (eds): *The pharmacologic basis of anesthesiology.* New York, 1994, Churchill Livingstone.

Lerman J, Gregory GA, Eger EI II: Age and the solubility of volatile anesthetics in blood. *Anesthesiology* 61:139, 1984.

Lerman J, Nolan J, Eyers R, et al.: Efficacy, Safety, and pharmacokinetics of levobupivacaine with and without fentanyl after continuous epidural infusion in children: a multicenter trial. *Anesthesiology* 99:1166–74, 2003.

Lerman J, Robinson S, Willis MM, et al.: Anesthetic requirements for halothane in young children 0-1 month and 1-6 months of age. *Anesthesiology* 59:421, 1983.

Lerman J, Schmitt BI, Willis MM, et al.: Effect of age on the solubility of volative anesthetics in human tissues. *Anesthesiology* 65:63, 1986.

Lerman J, Sikich N, Kleinman S, et al.: The pharmacology of sevoflurane in infants and children. *Anesthesiology* 80:814, 1994.

Lerman J, Sims C, Sikich N, et al.: Pharmacokinetics of the active metabolite (MDL 74,156) of dolasetron mesylate after oral or intravenous administration to anesthetized children. *Clin Pharmacol Ther* 60:485–492, 1996.

Letty MP, Gaudreault P, Friedman PA: Methohexital plasma concentrations in the child following rectal administration. *Anesthesiology* 62:567, 1985.

Levine MF, Hartley EJ, Macpherson BA: Oral midazolam premedication for children with congenital cyanotic heart disease undergoing cardiac surgery. *Can J Anaesth* 40:934, 1993a.

Levine MF, Spahr-Schopfer I, Hartley E: Oral midazolam premedication in children. *Can J Anaesth* 40:726, 1993b.

Levy G: Effect of hepatic cirrhosis on the pharmacodynamics and pharmacokinetics of mivacurium in humans. *Pharmaceut Res* 11:772–773, 1994.

Lien CA, Schmith VD, Embree PB, et al.: The pharmacokinetics and pharmacodynamics of the stereoisomers of mivacurium in patients receiving nitrous oxide/opioid/barbiturate anesthesia. *Anesthesiology* 80:1296, 1994.

Lim L-Y, Dear KBG, Heller RF: A systematic review of the antiemetic efficacy of prophylactic ondansetron compared with droperidol and with metoclopramide in children. *Clin Res Regul Aff* 16:59–70, 1999.

Lima JJ, Boudonlans H, Blanford M: Concentration dependence of disopyramide binding to plasma protein and its influence kinetics and dynamics. *J Pharmacol Exp Ther* 219:741–747, 1991.

Lindsay WA, Shepherd J: Plasma levels of thiopentone after premedication with rectal suppositories in young children. *Br J Anaesth* 41:977, 1969.

Liu J, Laster MJ, Eger EI 2nd, et al.: Absorption and degradation of sevoflurane and isoflurane in a conventional anesthetic circuit. *Anesth Analg* 72:785, 1991.

Locatelli B, Ingelmo P, Sonzogni V, et al.: Randomized, double-blind, phase III, controlled trial comparing levobupivacaine 0.25%, ropivacaine 0.25% and bupivacaine 0.25% by the caudal route in children. *Br J Anaesth* 94:366–71, 2005.

Lockhart CH, Jenkins JJ: Ketamine-induced apnea in patients with increased intracranial pressure. *Anesthesiology* 37:92, 1972.

Lockhart CH, Nelson WL: The relationship of ketamine requirements to age in pediatric patients. *Anesthesiology* 40:507, 1974.

Lombroso CT: Treatment of status epilepticus with diazepam. *Neurology* 16:629, 1966.

Longnecker DR: Stress free: To be or not to be? *Anesthesiology* 61:643, 1984.

Lönnqvist PA, Westrin P, Larsson BA, et al.: Ropivacaine pharmacokinetics after caudal block in 1-8 year old children. *Br J Anaesth* 85:506–511, 2000.

Lynam DP, Cronnelly R, Castagnoli KP, et al.: The pharmacodynamics and pharmacokinetics of vecuronium in patients anesthetized with isoflurane with normal renal function or with renal failure. *Anesthesiology* 69:227, 1988.

Lynn AM, Nespeca MK, Opheim KE: Respiratory effects of intravenous morphine infusions in neonates, infants, and children after cardiac surgery. *Anesth Analg* 77:695, 1993.

Lynn AM, Opheim KE, Tyler DC: Morphine infusion after pediatric cardiac surgery. *Crit Care Med* 12:863, 1984.

Macfie AG, Magides AD, Reilly CS: Disposition of alfentanil in burn patients. *Br J Anaesth* 69:447, 1992.

Magorian T, Lynam DP: Clinical use of muscle relaxants in patients with hepatic disease. In Rupp SM (ed): *Problems in anaesthesia: Neuromuscular relaxants.* Philadelphia, 1992, JB Lippincott.

Maitre PO, Vozeh S, Heykants J, et al.: Population pharmacokinetics of alfentanil. *Anesthesiology* 66:3, 1987.

Manjushree R, Lahiri A, Ghosh BR, et al.: Intranasal fentanyl provides adequate postoperative analgesia in pediatric patients. *Can J Anaesth* 49:190–193, 2002.

Manschot HJ, Meuring AEE, Axt P: Propofol requirements for induction of anesthesia in children of different age groups. *Anesth Analg* 75:876, 1992.

Marhofer P, Glaser C, Krenn CG, et al.: Incidence and therapy of midazolam induced hiccups in paediatric anaesthesia. *Paediatr Anaesth* 9:295–298, 1999.

Mark LC. Thiobarbiturates. In Papper EM, Kitz RJ (eds): *Uptake and distribution of anesthetic agents.* New York, 1963, McGraw-Hill.

Markakis DA, Lau M, Brown R, et al.: The pharmacokinetics and steady state pharmacodynamics of mivacurium in children. *Anesthesiology* 88:978–983, 1998.

Marsh B, White M, Morton N: Pharmacokinetic model driven infusion of propofol in children. *Br J Anaesth* 67:41, 1991.

Martin JL, Plevak DJ, Flannery KD, et al.: Hepatotoxicity after desflurane anesthesia. *Anesthesiology* 83:1125, 1995.

Martin TM, Nicolson SC, Bargas MS: Propofol anesthesia reduces emesis and airway obstruction in pediatric outpatients. *Anesth Analg* 76:144, 1993.

Martyn JAJ, White DA, Gronert GA, et al.: Up-and-down regulation of skeletal muscle acetylcholine receptors. *Anesthesiology* 76:822–843, 1992.

Matthes HW, Maldonado R, Simonin F, et al.: Loss of morphine-induced analgesia, reward effect and withdrawal symptoms in mice lacking the mu-opioid-receptor gene. *Nature* 383:819, 1996.

Mazoit JX, Denson DD, Samil K: Pharmacokinetics of bupivacaine following caudal anesthesia in infants. *Anesthesiology* 68:387, 1988.

Mazoit JX, Dalens BJ: Pharmacokinetics of local anaesthetics in infants and children. *Clin Pharmacokinet* 43:17–32, 2004.

McAuliffe G, Bissonnette B, Cavallé-Garrido T, et al.: Heart rate and cardiac output after atropine in anaesthetized infants and children. *Can J Anaesth* 44:154–159, 1997.

McCann ME, Sethna NF, Mazoit JX, et al.: The pharmacokinetics of epidural ropivacaine in infants and young children. *Anesth Analg* 93:893–897, 2001.

McCloskey JJ, Haun SE, Deshpande JK: Bupivacaine toxicity secondary to continuous caudal epidural infusion in children. *Anesth Analg* 75:287, 1992.

McFarlan CS, Anderson BJ, Timothy SG: The use of propofol infusion in pediatric anesthesia: A practical guide. *Pediatr Anaesth* 9:209–216, 1999.

McGraw T: Oral midazolam and postoperative behaviour in children. *Can J Anaesth* 40:682, 1993.

McGregor M, Davenport HT, Jegier W, et al.: The cardiovascular effects of halothane in normal children. *Br J Anaesth* 30:398, 1958.

McMillan CO, Spahr-Schopfer IA, Sikich N: Premedication of children with oral midazolam. *Can J Anaesth* 39:545, 1992.

Meakin G, McKiernan EP, Morris P, et al.: Dose-response curves for suxamethonium in neonates, infants and children. *Br J Anaesth* 62:655, 1989.

Meakin G, Morton RH, Wareham AC: Age-dependent variation in response to tubocurarine in the isolated rat diaphragm. *Br J Anaesth* 68:161–163, 1992.

Meakin G, Sweet PT, Bevan JC, et al.: Neostigmine and edrophonium as antagonists of pancuronium in infants and children. *Anesthesiology* 59:316, 1983.

Meberg A, Langslet A, Bredesen JE, et al.: Plasma concentration of diazepam and N-desmethyldiazepam in children after a single rectal or intramuscular dose of diazepam. *Eur J Clin Pharmacol* 14:273–276, 1978.

Meistelman C, Plaud B, Donati F: Neuromuscular effects of succinylcholine on the vocal cords and adductor pollicis muscles. *Anesth Analg* 73:278–282, 1991.

Meistelman C, Plaud B, Donati F: Rocuronium (ORG 9426) neuromuscular blockade at the adductor muscles of the larynx and adductor pollicies in humans. *Can J Anesth* 39:665–669, 1992.

Meistelman C, Benhamou D, Barre J, et al.: Effects of age on plasma protein binding of sufentanil. *Anesthesiology* 72:470–473, 1990.

Meistelman C, Saint-Maurice C, Lepaul M, et al.: A comparison of alfentanil pharmacokinetics in children and adults. *Anesthesiology* 66:13, 1987.

Meretoja OA, Rautiainen P: Alfentanil and fentanyl sedation in infants and small children during cardiac catheterization. *Can J Anaesth* 37:624, 1990.

Meretoja OA, Brandom BW, Taivainen T, et al.: Synergism between atracurium and vecuronium in children. *Br J Anaesth* 71:440–442, 1993.

Meretoja OA, Taivainen T, Jalkanen L, et al.: Synergism between atracurium and vecuronium in infants and children during nitrous oxide-oxygen-alfentanil anaesthesia. *Br J Anaesth* 73:605–607, 1994.

Meretoja OA, Taivainen T, Wirtavuori K: Pharmacodynamics of mivacurium in infants. *Br J Anaesth* 73:490, 1994.

Meretoja OA: Is vecuronium a long-acting neuromuscular blocking agent in neonates and infants? *Br J Anaesth* 62:184, 1989.

Meretoja OA, Taivainen T, Wirtavuori K: Pharmacodynamic effects of 51 W89, an isomer of atracurium, in children during halothane anaesthesia. *Br J Anaesth* 74:6–11, 1995.

Meuldermans W, Hurkmans R, Heykants J: Plasma protein binding and distribution of fentanyl, sufentanil and lofentanil in blood. *Arch Int Pharmacol Ther* 25:4, 1982.

Miller JR, Stoelting VK, Dann MW: A preliminary report on the use of intramuscular methohexital sodium (Brevital) for pediatric anesthesia. *Anesth Analg (Cleve)* 40:573, 1961.

Miller RD: Use of neuromuscular blocking drugs in intensive care unit patients. *Anesth Analg* 81:1–2, 1995.

Minton MD, Grosslight K, Stirt JA, et al.: Increases in intracranial pressure from succinylcholine: Prevention by prior nondepolarizing blockade. *Anesthesiology* 65:165, 1986.

Mirakhur RK: Induction characteristics of propofol in children. *Anaesthesia* 43:593, 1988.

Mirkin BL: Developmental pharmacology. *Anesthesiology* 43:156, 1975.

Modica PA, Pempelhoff R, White PF: Pro-and anticonvulsant effects of anesthetics (Part II). *Anesth Analg* 70:433–44, 1990.

Moore RA, Yang SS, McNicholas KW, et al.: Hemodynamic and aesthetic effects of sufentanil as the sole anesthetic for pediatric cardiovascular surgery. *Anesthesiology* 62:725, 1985.

Morio M, Fugii K, Satoh N, et al.: Reaction of sevoflurane and its degradation products with soda lime. *Anesthesiology* 77:1155, 1992.

Morselli PL, et al.: Drug interactions in the human fetus and in the newborn infant. In Morselli PL, Cohen SN (eds): *Drug interactions.* New York, 1974, Raven Press, p 320.

Morselli PL: Clinical pharmacokinetics in neonates. *Clin Pharmacokinet* 1:81–98, 1976.

Morton NS: Editorial. II. Ropivacaine in children. *Br J Anaesth* 85:344–346, 2000.

Muenster JJ, et al.: Comparison between diazepam and sodium thiopental during D.C. countershock. *JAMA* 199:758, 1967.

Mulla H, McCormack P, Lawson G, et al.: Pharmacokinetics of midazolam in neonates undergoing extracorporeal membrane oxygenation. *Anesthesiology* 99:275, 2003.

Munro HM, Riegger LQ, Reynolds PI, et al.: Comparison of the analgesic and emetic properties of ketorolac and morphine for paediatric outpatient strabismus surgery. *Br J Anaesth* 71:624–628, 1994.

Murat I, Levron J-C, Berg A: Effects of fentanyl on baroreceptor reflex control of heart rate in newborn infants. *Anesthesiology* 68:717, 1988.

Murat I, Hoerter J, Ventura-Clapier R: Developmental changes in effects of halothane and isoflurane on contractile properties of rabbit cardiac skinned fibers. *Anesthesiology* 73:137, 1990.

Murray D, Vandewalker G, Matherne GP, et al.: Pulsed Doppler and two-dimensional echocardiography: Comparison of halothane and isoflurane on cardiac function in infants and small children. *Anesthesiology* 67:211, 1987.

Murray DJ, Forbes RB, Mahoney LT: Comparative hemodynamic depression of halothane versus isoflurane in neonates and infants: An echocardiographic study. *Anesth Analg* 74:329, 1992.

Murray JM, Renfrew CW, Bedi A, et al.: Amsorb: A new carbon dioxide absorbent for use in anesthetic breathing systems. *Anesthesiology* 91:1342, 1999.

Murray JP, et al.: Hemodynamic effects of ketamine in children with congenital heart disease. *Anesth Analg* 63:895, 1984.

Murthy BVS, Pandya KS, Booker PD, et al.: Pharmacokinetics of tramadol in children after IV or caudal epidural administration. *Br J Anaesth* 84:346–349, 2000.

Naguib M, Flood P, McArdle JJ, et al.: Advances in neurobiology of the neuromuscular junction. *Anesthesiology* 96:202–231, 2002.

Naguib M, Samarkandi AH, Ammar A, et al.: Comparative clinical pharmacology of rocuronium, cis-atracurium, and their combination. *Anesthesiology* 89:1116–1124, 1998.

Naguib M, Samarkandi AH, Ammar A, et al.: Comparison of suxamethonium and different combinations of rocuronium and mivacurium for rapid tracheal intubation in children. *Br J Anaesth* 79:450–455, 1997.

Naguib M: Neuromuscular effects of rocuronium bromide and mivacurium chloride administered alone and in combination. *Anesthesiology* 91:388–395, 1994.

Neill EAM, Chapple DJ: Metabolic studies in the cat with atracurium: neuromuscular blocking agent designed for non-enzymatic inactivation at physiological pH. *Xenobiotica* 12:203, 1983.

Ng PK, Cote J, Schiff D, et al.: Renal clearance of digoxin in premature neonates. *Res Commun Chem Pathol Pharmacol* 34:207–216, 1981.

Nguyen TTS, Vecchierini MF, Debillon T, Pereon Y: Effects of sufentanil on electroencephalogram in very and extremely peterm neonates. *Pediatrics* 11:123–8, 2003.

Nichols DG, Yaster M, Lynn AM: Disposition and respiratory effects of intrathecal morphine in children. *Anesthesiology* 79:733, 1993.

Nightingale DA, Bush GH: Atracurium in paediatric anesthesia. *Br J Anaesth* 55:115S, 1983.

Nightingale JJ, Lewis IH: Recovery from day-case anesthesia. *Br J Anaesth* 68:356, 1992.

Nordberg G, Hedner T, Mellstrand T: Pharmacokinetic aspects of intrathecal morphine analgesia. *Anesthesiology* 60:448, 1984.

Ogawa M, et al.: Drug-induced hepatitis following sevoflurane anesthesia in a child. *Masui* 40:1952, 1991.

O'Kelly B, Fiset P, Meistelman C, et al.: Pharmacokinetics of rocuronium in pediatric patients. *Eur J Anesth Suppl* 9:57–58, 1994.

Olkkola KT, Maunuksela EL: The pharmacokinetics of postoperative intravenous ketorolac tromethamine in children. *Br J Clin Pharmac* 31:182–184, 1991.

Olutoye O, Jantzen EC, Alexis R, et al.: A comparison of the costs and efficacy of ondansetron and dolasetron in the prophylaxis of postoperative vomiting in pediatric patients undergoing ambulatory surgery. *Anesth Analg* 97:390–396, 2003.

Osbourne R, Joel S, Grebenik K: The pharmacokinetics of morphine and morphine glucuronides in kidney failure. *Clin Pharmacol Ther* 54:158, 1993.

Ostergaard D, Gatke MR, Rasmussen BH, et al.: The pharmacodynamics and pharmacokinetics of mivacurium in children. *Acta Anaesthesiol Scand* 46:512–518, 2002.

Ostergaard D, Rasmussen SN, Vib-Mogensen J, et al.: The influence of drug-induced low butyryl cholinesterase activity on the pharmacokinetics and pharmacodynamics of mivacurium. *Anesthesiology* 92:1581–1587, 2000.

Ozcengiz D, Gunduz M, Ozbek H, et al.: Comparison of caudal morphine and tramadol for postoperative pain control in children undergoing inguinal herniorrhaphy. *Paediatr Anaesth* 11:459–464, 2001.

Palmisano BW, Mehner RW, Stowe DF, et al.: Direct myocardial effects of halothane and isoflurane. *Anesthesiology* 81:718, 1994.

Palmisano BW, Setlock MA, Brown MP, et al.: Dose-response for atropine and heart rate in infants and children anesthetized with halothane and nitrous oxide. *Anesthesiology* 75:238–42, 1991.

Pandit UA, Collier PJ, Malviya S, et al.: Oral transmucosal midazolam premedication for preschool children. *Can J Anesth* 48:191–195, 2001.

Park JM, Houck CS, Sethna NF, et al.: Ketorolac suppresses postoperative bladder spasms after pediatric ureteral reimplantation. *Anesth Analg* 91:11–15, 2000.

Parker CJR, Jones JE, Hunter JM: Disposition of atracurium and its metabolite, laudanosine, in patients in renal and respiratory failure in an ITU. *Br J Anaesth* 61:531, 1988.

Patel RI, Davis PJ, Orr RJ, et al.: Single-dose ondansetron prevents postoperative vomiting in pediatric outpatients. *Anesth Analg* 85:538–545, 1997.

Patwardhan RV, et al.: Normal metabolism of morphine in cirrhosis. *Gastroenterology* 81:1006, 1981.

Paul M, Folt DM, Kindler CH, et al.: Characterization of the interactions between volatile anesthetics and neuromuscular blockers at the muscle nicotinic acetylcholine receptor. *Anesth Analg* 95:362–367, 2002.

Paul M, Kindler CH, Fokt RM et al.: The potency of new muscle relaxants on recombinant muscle-type acetylcholine receptors. *Anesth Analg* 94:597–603, 2002.

Pavlin EG, Halle RH, Schaene R: Recovery of airway protection compared with ventilation in humans after paralysis with curare. *Anesthesiology* 70:381, 1989.

Payne K, et al.: The pharmacokinetics of midazolam in paediatric patients. *Eur J Clin Pharmacol* 37:267, 1989.

Pedersen SE, Cohen JB: d-Tubocurarine binding sites are located at alpha-gamma and alpha-delta subunit interfaces of the nicotinic acetylcholine receptor. *Proc Natl Acad Sci USA* 87:2785, 1990.

Pirat A, Akpek E, Arslan G: Intrathecal versus IV fentanyl in pediatric cardiac anesthesia. *Anesth Analg* 95:1207–1214, 2002.

Pittet JF, Tassonyi E, Morel DR, et al.: Pipecuronium-induced neuromuscular blockade during nitrous oxide-fentanyl, isoflurane, and halothane anesthesia in adults and children. *Anesthesiology* 71:210, 1989.

Plaud B, Debaine B, Lequean F, et al.: Mivarcurium neuromuscular block at the adductor muscles of the larynx and adductor pollicis in humans. *Anesthesiology* 85:77–81, 1996.

Plumley MH, Bevan JC, Saddler JM, et al.: Dose-related effects of succinylcholine on the adductor pollicis and masseter muscles in children. *Can J Anaesth* 37:15, 1990.

Pokela M-L, Ryhanen PT, Koivisto ME: Alfentanil-induced rigidity in newborn infants. *Anesth Analg* 75:252, 1992.

Prielipp RC, Coursin DB, Scuderi PE, et al.: Comparison of the infusion requirements and recovery profiles of vecuronium and cisatracurium 51W89 in intensive care unit patients. *Crit Care Trauma* 81:3, 1995.

Priest JH: Atropine response of the eyes to mongolism. *Am J Dis Child* 100:869, 1960.

Prince RJ, Since SM: The ligand binding domains of the nicotinic acetylcholine receptor. In Barrantes FJ (ed): *The nicotinic acetylcholine receptor: Current views and future trends.* Berlin/New York, 1998, Springer-Verlag.

Rackow H, Salinitre E, Green LT: Frequency of cardiac arrest associated with anesthesia in infants and children. *Pediatrics* 28:697, 1961.

Radney PA, Badola RP: Generalized extensor spasm in infants following ketamine anesthesia. *Anesthesiology* 39:459, 1973.

Rane A: Phenotyping of drug metabolism in infants and children: Potentials and problems. *Pediatrics* 104: 640–645, 1999.

Rao CC, et al.: Increased sensitivity of the isometric contraction of the neonatal isolated rat atria to halothane, isoflurane, and enflurane. *Anesthesiology* 64:13, 1986.

Rautoma P, Erkola O, Meretoja OA: Potency and maintenance requirement of atracurium and vecuronium given alone or together. *Acta Anaesthesiol Scand* 39:220–223, 1995a.

Rautoma P, Erkola O, Meretoja OA: Synergism between mivacurium and pancuronium in adults. *Acta Anaesthesiol Scand* 39:733–737, 1995b.

Reed MD, Rodarte A, Blumer JL, et al.: The single-dose pharmacokinetics of midazolam and its primary metabolite in pediatric patients after oral and intravenous administration. *J Clin Pharmacol* 41:1359–1369, 2001.

Reeves J, Samuelson P, Lewis S: Midazolam maleate induction in patients with ischemic heart disease: Hemodynamic observation. *Can Anaesth Soc J* 26:402, 1979.

Reimer EJ, Montgomery CJ, Bevan JC: Propofol anaesthesia reduces early postoperative emesis after paediatric strabismus surgery. *Can J Anaesth* 40:927, 1993.

Reich DL, Hollinger I, Harrington DJ, et al.: Pharmacokinetic comparison of cisatracurium and vecuronium infusions in neonates and infants following congenital heart surgery. *Anesthesiology* October 2002.

Reves JG, Glass PSA, Lubarsky DA: Non-barbiturate intravenous anesthetics. In Miller RD (ed): *Anesthesia.* 5th ed. New York, 2000, Churchill Livingstone, pp 228–272.

Reynolds LM, Koh JL: Prolonged spontaneous movement following emergence from propofol/nitrous oxide anesthesia. *Anesth Analg* 76:192, 1993.

Reynolds RN: Halothane in pediatric anesthesia. *Int Anesthesiol Clin* 1:209, 1962.

Roald OK, Dohl V: Flunitrazepam intoxication in a child successfully treated with the benzodiazepine antagonist flumazenil. *Crit Care Med* 17:1355, 1989.

Rocari G, Ziegler WH, Guentert TW: Pharmacokinetics of the new benzodiazepine antagonist Ro 15-788 in man following intravenous and oral administration. *Br J Clin Pharmacol* 22:421, 1986.

Roerig DL, Kotrly KJ, Vucins EJ: First pass uptake of fentanyl, meperidine, and morphine in the human lung. *Anesthesiology* 67:466, 1987.

Romberg R, Olofsen E, Sarton E, et al.: Pharmacokinetic-pharmacodynamic modeling of morphine-6-glucuronide-induced analgesia in healthy volunteers: Absence of sex differences. *Anesthesiology* 100:120, 2004.

Romberg RR, Olofsen E, Bijl H, et al.: Polymorphism of mu-opioid receptor gene (OPRM1:c.118A>G) does not protect against opioid-induced respiratory depression despite reduced analgesic response. *Anesthesiology* 102:522, 2005.

Rose JB, Finkel JC, Arquedas-Mohs A, et al.: Oral tramadol for the treatment of pain of 7-30 days' duration in children. *Anesth Analg* 96:78–81, 2003.

Rosen DA, Rosen KR: Midazolam for sedation in the pediatric intensive care unit. *Intens Care Med* 17 Suppl 1:515, 1991.

Rosenberg H, Gronert GA: Intractable cardiac arrest in children given succinylcholine. *Anesthesiology* 77:1054, 1992.

Rosow C, Philbin D, Moss J, et al.: Sufentanil vs. fentanyl: I Suppression of hemodynamic responses. *Anesthesiology* 59:A323, 1983.

Rosow CE, Philbin DM, Keegan CR, Moss J: Hemodynamics and histamine release during induction with sufentanil or fentanyl. *Anesthesiology* 60:489, 1984.

Ross AK, Davis PJ, et al.: Pharmacokinetics of remifentanil in anesthetized pediatric patients undergoing elective surgery or diagnostic procedures. *Anesth Analg* 93:1392–1401, 2001.

Roure P, Jean N, Leclerc A-C, et al.: Pharmacokinetics of alfentanil in children undergoing surgery. *Br J Anaesth* 59:1437, 1987.

Rowland AS, Baird DD, Shore DL, et al.: Nitrous oxide and spontaneous abortion in female dental assistants. *Am J Epidemiol* 141:531–538, 1995.

Rubin M, Bruck E, Rapoport M: Maturation of renal function in childhood: Clearance studies. *J Clin Invest* 28:1144–1162, 1949.

Rupp SM: Muscle relaxants and the patient with renal and/or hepatic failure. In Azar I (ed): *Muscle relaxants.* New York: Dekker, 1987.

Russell IA, Miller Hance WC, Gregory G, et al.: The safety and efficacy of sevoflurane anesthesia in infants and children with congenital heart disease. *Anesth Analg* 92:1152–1158, 2001.

Saarenmaa E, Neuvonen P, Fellman V: Gestational age and birth weight effects on plasma clearance of fentanyl in newborn infants. *J Pediatr* 136:767–770, 2000.

Sadler JM, et al.: Jaw tension after succinylcholine in children undergoing strabismus surgery. *Can J Anaesth* 37:21, 1990.

Saidman LJ, Eger EI II: The effect of thiopental metabolism on duration of anesthesia. *Anesthesiology* 27:118, 1966.

Saint-Maurice C, et al.: Pharmacokinetics of propofol in young children after a single dose. *Br J Anaesth* 63:667, 1989.

Saint-Maurice C, et al.: The pharmacokinetics of rectal midazolam for premedication in children. *Anesthesiology* 65:536, 1986.

Salanitre E, Rackow H: The pulmonary exchange of nitrous oxide and halothane in infants and children. *Anesthesiology* 30:388, 1969.

Salem MR, Wong AY, Lin YH,: The effect of suxamethonium on the intragastric pressure in infants and children. *Br J Anaesth* 44:166, 1972.

Salonen M, Kanto J, Iisalo E: Midazolam as an induction agent in children. *Anesth Analg* 66:625, 1987.

Sanes JR, Lichtman JW: Development of vertebrate neuromuscular junction. *Annu Rev Neurosci* 22:389–442, 1999.

Santeiro ML, Christie J, Stromquist C, et al.: Pharmacokinetics of continuous infusion fentanyl in newborns. *J Perinatol* 17:135–139, 1997.

Sarkar M, Laussen PC, Zurakowski D, et al.: Hemodynamic responses of etomidate on induction of anesthesia in pediatric patients. *Anesth Analg* 2005 (in press).

Sarner JB, Brandom BW, Cook DR, et al.: Clinical pharmacology of doxacurium chloride (BW A938U) in children. *Anesth Analg* 67:303–306, 1988.

Sarner JB, Brandom BW, Dong ML, et al.: Clinical pharmacology of pipecuronium in infants and children during halothane anesthesia. *Anesth Analg* 71:362, 1990.

Satwicz PR, Martyn JA, Szyfelbein SF, et al.: Potentiation of neuromuscular blockade using a combination of pancuronium and dimethyltubocurarine. Studies in children following acute burn injury or during reconstructive surgery. *Br J Anaesth* 56:479–484, 1984.

Savage DS, Sleigh T, Carlyle I: The emergence of ORG NC 45 from the pancuronium series. *Br J Anaesth* 52:3S, 1980.

Scholz J, Bause H, Schulz M, et al.: Pharmacokinetics and effects on intracranial pressure of sufentanil in head trauma patients. *Br J Clin Pharmacol* 38:369–372, 1994.

Scholz J, Steinfath M, Shultz M: Clinical pharmacokinetics of alfentanil, fentanyl and sufentanil. An update. *Clin Pharmacokinet* 31:275– 292, 1996.

Schow AJ, Lubarsky DA, Olson RP, et al.: Can succinylcholine be used safely in hyperkalemic patients? *Anesth Analg* 95:119–122, 2002.

Schraag S, Checketts MR, Kenny GN: Lack of rapid development of opioid tolerance during alfentanil and remifentanil infusions for postoperative pain. *Anesth Analg* 89:753–757, 1999.

Schwartz L, Rockoff MA, Koka BV: Masseter spasm with anesthesia: incidence and implications. *Anesthesiology* 61:772, 1984.

Schwartz MS, et al.: Effects of ketamine on the electroencephalograph. *Anaesthesia* 29:135, 1974.

Scott LJ, Perry CM: Tramadol. A review of its use in perioperative pain. *Drugs* 60:139–176, 2000.

Sebel P, Bovill J: Cardiovascular effects of sufentanil anesthesia. *Anesth Analg* 61:115, 1982.

Segredo V, Caldwell JE, Matthay MA, et al.: Persistent paralysis in critically ill patients after long-term administration of vecuronium. *N Engl J Med* 327:524, 1992.

Serlin S: Dexmedetomidine in pediatrics: controlled studies needed. *Anesth Analg* 98:1814, 2004.

Shafer SL: Advances in propofol pharmacokinetics and pharmacodynamics. *J Clin Anesth* 5:14S, 1993.

Shafer SL, Varvel JR: Pharmacokinetics, pharmacodynamics and rational opioid selection. *Anesthesiology* 74:53–63, 1991.

Shannon M, Albers G, Burkhart K: Safety and efficacy of flumazenil in the reversal of benzodiazepine-induced conscious sedation. The Flumazenil Pediatric Study Group. *J Pediatr* 131:582–586, 1997.

Shear CR: Effects of disuse on growing and adult chick skeletal muscle. *J Cell Sci* 48:35, 1981.

Shi WZ, Fahey MR, Fisher DM, et al.: Laudanozine (a metabolite of atracurium) increases the minimum alveolar concentration of halothane in rabbits. *Anesthesiology* 63:584, 1985.

Short TC, Aun CS, Tan P: A prospective evaluation of pharmacokinetic model controlled infusion of propofol in pediatric patients. *Br J Anesth* 72:302–306, 1994.

Sikich N, Lerman J: Development and psychometric evaluation of the pediatric anesthesia emergence delirium scale. *Anesthesiology* 100:1138–1145, 2004.

Simhi E, Brandom BW, Lloyd ME, Woelfel SK: Administration of atropine and onset of neuromuscular block produced by atracurium in infants. *Paediatr Anaesth* 7:375–8, 1997.

Simons FE, Fraser TG, Reggin JD, et al.: Adverse central nervous system effects of older antihistamines in children. *Pediatr Allergy Immunol* 7:22–27, 1996.

Singleton MA, Rosen JI, Fisher DM: Plasma concentrations of fentanyl in infants, children and adults. *Can J Anaesth* 34:152, 1987.

Skovsted P, Price ML, Price HL: The effects of halothane on arterial pressure, preganglionic sympathetic activity and barostatic reflexes. *Anesthesiology* 31:507, 1969.

Smiley RM, Ornstein E, Pantuck EJ, et al.: Metabolism of desflurane and isoflurane to fluoride ion in surgical patients. *Can J Anaesth* 38:965, 1991.

Smith CA, Nelson NM: *The physiology of the newborn infant*, ed 4. Springfield, IL, 1976, Charles C Thomas, Publisher, p179.

Smith M, Eadie M, Brophy T: The pharmacokinetics of midazolam in man. *Eur J Clin Pharmacol* 19:271, 1981.

Smith RM, Bachman L, Bougas T: Shivering following thiopental sodium and other anesthetic agents. *Anesthesiology* 16:655, 1955.

Sorbo RM, Hudson RJ, Loomis JC: The pharmacokinetics of thiopental in pediatric surgical patients. *Anesthesiology* 61:666, 1984.

Spahr-Schopfer IA, Lerman J, Sikich N, et al.: Pharmacokinetics of intravenous ondansetron in healthy children undergoing ear, nose and throat surgery. *Clin Pharmacol Ther* 58:316–321, 1995.

Spear RM, Yaster M, Berkowitz ID: Preinduction of anesthesia in children with rectally administered midazolam. *Anesthesiology* 74:670, 1991.

Splinter WM, Rhine EJ: Low-dose ondansetron with dexamethasone more effectively decreases vomiting after strabismus surgery in children than does high-dose ondansetron. *Anesthesiology* 88:72–75, 1998.

Stanley T, Pace N, Liu W, et al.: Alfentanil-N_2O vs fentanyl-N_2O balanced anesthesia: Comparison of plasma hormonal changes, early postoperative respiratory function and speed of postoperative recovery. *Anesth Analg* 62:285, 1983.

Steward DJ, Creighton RE: The uptake and excretion of nitrous oxide in the newborn. *Can Anaesth Soc J* 25:215, 1978.

Stiller RL, Brandom BW, Cook DR: Determination of atracurium by high-performance liquid chromatography. *Anesth Analg* 64:58, 1985a.

Stiller RL, Cook DR, Chakravorti S: In vitro degradation of atracurium in human plasma. *Br J Anaesth* 57:1085, 1985b.

Stoelting RK, Longnecker DE: The effect of right-to-left shunt on the rate of increase of arterial anesthetic concentration. *Anesthesiology* 36:352, 1972.

Stokes DN, Hutton P: Rate-dependent induction phenomena with propofol: Implications for the relative potency of intravenous anesthetics. *Anesth Analg* 72:578, 1991.

Streisand JB, Varvel JR, Stanski DR: Absorption and bioavailability of oral transmucosal fentanyl citrate. *Anesthesiology* 72:223, 1991.

Sukhani R, Pappas AL, Lurie J, et al.: Ondansetron and dolasetron provide equivalent postoperative vomiting control after ambulatory tonsillectomy in dexamethasone-pretreated children. *Anesth Analg* 95:1230–1235, 2002.

Sullivan KJ, Berman LS, Koska J, et al.: Intramuscular atropine sulfate in children: Comparison of injection sites. *Anesth Analg* 84:54–58, 1997.

Sury MRJ, Billingham I, Russell GN: Acute benzodiazepine withdrawal syndromes after midazolam infusions in children (letter). *Crit Care Med* 17:301, 1989.

Sutherland GA, Bevan JC, Bevan DR: Neuromuscular blockade in infants following intramuscular succinylcholine in two or five percent solution. *Can J Anaesth* 30:342, 1980.

Sweetland J, Lettis S, Fowler PA, et al.: Duration of the inhibitory effect of intravenous ondansetron on intradermal 5-HT-induced flare. *Br J Clin Pharmacol* 33:565P, 1992.

Taivainen T, Meakin GH, Meretoja OA, et al.: The safety and efficacy of cisatracurium 0.15 mg.kg(-1) during nitrous oxide-opioid anaesthesia in infants and children. *Anaesthesia* 55:1047, 2000.

Tang TT, Oechler HW, Siker D, et al.: Anesthesia-induced rhabdomyolysis in infants with unsuspected Duchenne dystrophy. *Acta Paediatr* 81:716–719, 1992.

Tanner GE, Angers DG, Barash PG, et al.: Effect of left-to-right, mixed left-to-right, and right-to-left shunts on inhalational anesthetic induction in children: a computer model. *Anesth Analg* 64:101, 1985.

Taylor P: Are neuromuscular blocking agents more efficacious in pairs? *Anesthesiology* 63:1, 1985.

Taylor RH, Lerman J: Induction and recovery characteristics for desflurane in children. *Can J Anaesth* 39:6, 1992.

Taylor RH, Lerman J: Minimum alveolar concentration (MAC) of desflurane and hemodynamic responses in neonates, infants and children. *Anesthesiology* 75:975, 1991.

Thummel KE, O'Shea D, Paine MF, et al.: Oral first-pass elimination of midazolam involves both gastrointestinal and hepatic CYP3A-mediated metabolism. *Clin Pharmacol Ther* 59:491–502, 1996.

Tobias JD, Berkenbosch JW: Sedation during mechanical ventilation in infants and children: Dexmedetomidine versus midazolam. *South Med J* 97(5):451–5, 1997.

Tobias JD, Berkenbosch JW, Russo P: Additional experience with dexmedetomidine in pediatric patients. *South Med J* 96:871–5, 2003.

Tobias JD, Johnson JO, Sprague K, et al.: Effects of rapacuronium on respiratory function during general anesthesia. *Anesthesiology* 95:908–912, 2001.

Tobias JD, Lynch A, McDuffee A, et al.: Pancuronium infusion for neuromuscular block in children in the pediatric intensive care unit. *Anesth Analg* 81:13, 1995.

Traber DL, Wilson RD, Priano LL: Blockade of the hypertensive response to ketamine. *Anesth Analg (Cleve)* 49:420, 1970.

Treluyer JM, Jacqz-Aigrain E, Alvarez F, et al.: Expression of CYP2D6 in developing human liver. *Eur J Biochem* 202:583–588, 1991.

Trindle MR, Dodson BA, Rampil IJ: Effects of fentanyl versus sufentanil in equianesthetic doses on middle cerebral artery blood flow velocity. *Anesthesiology* 78:454, 1993.

Tullock WC, Diana P, Cook DR, et al.: Neuromuscular and cardiovascular effects of high-dose vecuronium. *Anesth Analg* 70:80–90, 1990.

Turan A, Memis D, Basaran UN, et al.: Caudal ropivacaine and neostigmine in pediatric surgery. *Anesthesiology* 98:719–722, 2003.

Twersky RS, Hartung J, Berger BJ: Midazolam enhances anterograde but not retrograde amnesia in pediatric patients. *Anesthesiology* 78:51, 1993.

Urgureanu D, Meistelman C, Frossard J, et al.: The arbicularis oculi and the adductor pollicis muscles as monitors of atracurium block of laryngeal muscles. *Anesth Analg* 77:775–779, 1993.

Vakkuri A, Yli-Hankala A, Sarkela M, et al.: Sevoflurane mask induction of anaesthesia is associated with epileptiform EEG in children. *Acta Anaesthesiol Scand* 45:805–811, 2001.

Valtonen M, Iisalo E, Kanto J: Propofol as an induction agent in children: Pain on injection and pharmacokinetics. *Acta Anaesthesiol Scand* 33:152, 1989.

Van der Spek AF, Fang WB, Ashton-Miller JA, et al.: Increased masticatory muscle stiffness during limb muscle flaccidity associated with succinylcholine administration. *Anesthesiology* 69:11, 1988.

Van der Spek AF, Reynolds PI, Ashton-Miller JA, et al.: Differing effect of agonist and antagonist muscle relaxants on cat jaw muscles. *Anesth Analg* 69:76, 1989.

Versichelen LFM, Bouche M-PLA, Georges R, et al.: Only carbon dioxide absorbents free of both NaOH and KOH do not generate compound A during in vitro closed-system sevoflurane evaluation of five absorbents. *Anesthesiology* 95:750–755, 2001.

Viby-Mogensen J, Jensen NH, Engbaek J, et al.: Tactile and visual evaluation of the response to train-of-four stimulation. *Anesthesiology* 63:440, 1985.

Viby-Mogensen J: Monitoring neuromuscular function in the intensive care unit. *Intensive Care Med* 19(Suppl):S74, 1993.

Viitanen H, Annila P: Analgesic efficacy of tramadol 2 mg kg-1 for paediatric day-case adenoidectomy. *Br J Anaesth* 86:572–575, 2001.

Viitanen H, Annila P, Viitanen M, et al.: Premedication with midazolam delays recovery after ambulatory sevoflurane anesthesia in children. *Anesth Analg* 89:75–79, 1999.

Vinik HR, Kissin I: Rapid development of tolerance to analgesia during remifentanil infusion in humans. *Anesth Analg* 86:1307–1311, 1998.

Wagner R, White P, Kan P, et al.: Inhibition of adrenal steroidogenesis by the anesthetic etomidate. *N Engl J Med* 310:1415, 1984.

Wagner R, White P: Etomidate inhibits adrenocortical function in surgical patients. *Anesthesiology* 61:647, 1984.

Walbergh FJ, Wills RJ, Eckhert J: Plasma concentrations of midazolam in children following intranasal administration. *Anesthesiology* 74:233, 1991.

Wallace S: Altered plasma albumin in the newborn infant. *Br J Clin Pharmacol* 4: 83–85, 1977.

Ward S, Neil EAM: Pharmacokinetics of atracurium in acute hepatic failure (with acute renal failure). *Br J Anaesth* 55:1169, 1983.

Wareham AC, Morton RH, Meakin GH: Low quantal content of the endplate potential reduces safety factor for neuromuscular transmission in the diaphragm of the newborn rat. *Br J Anaesth* 72:205–209, 1994.

Watanabe K, Hatakenaka S, Ikemune K, et al.: A case of suspected liver dysfunction induced by sevoflurane anesthesia. *Masui* 42:902, 1993.

Watcha MF, Simeon RM, White PF: Effect of propofol on the incidence of postoperative vomiting after strabismus surgery in pediatric outpatients. *Anesthesiology* 75:204, 1991.

Watling SM, Dasta JF: Prolonged paralysis in intensive care unit patients after the use of neuromuscular blocking agents: A review of the literature. *Crit Care Med* 22:884, 1994.

Way WL, Costley EC, Way EL: Respiratory sensitivity of the newborn infant to meperidine and morphine. *Clin Pharmacol Ther* 6:454, 1965.

Weatherall JA: Anaesthesia in newborn animals. *Br J Pharmacol* 15:454, 1960.

Wedel DJ, Gammel SA, Milde JH, et al.: Delayed onset of malignant hyperthermia induced by isoflurane and desflurane compared with halothane in susceptible swine. *Anesthesiology* 78:1138, 1993.

Wee L, Stokes MA: Bladder extrophy in a neonate at risk of transient myasthenia gravis: A role for remifentanil and epidural analgesia. *Br J Anaesth* 82:774–776, 1999.

Weil PM, Munro HM, Reynolds PI: Propofol infusion and the incidence of emesis in pediatric outpatient strabismus surgery. *Anesth Analg* 76:760, 1993.

Welch RM, Brown A, Ravitch J, et al.: The in vitro degradation of cisatracurium, the R, cis-R′-isomer of atracurium, in human and rat plasma. *Clin Pharmacol Ther* 58:132, 1995.

Weldon BC, Watcha MF, White PF: Oral midazolam in children: Effect of time and adjunctive therapy. *Anesth Analg* 75:51, 1992.
Westmoreland CL, Hoke JF, Sebel PS: Pharmacokinetics of remifentanil (GI87084B) and its major metabolite (GI90291) in patients undergoing elective inpatient surgery. *Anesthesiology* 9:893, 1993.
Westrin P: The induction dose of propofol in infants 1-6 months of age and in children 16 years of age. *Anesthesiology* 74:455, 1991.
Westrin P: Methohexital dissolved in lipid emulsion for intravenous induction of anesthesia in infants and children. *Anesthesiology* 76:917–921, 1992.
Westrin P, Jonmarker C, Werner O: Thiopental requirements for induction of anesthesia in neonates and infants one to six months of age. *Anesthesiology* 71:344, 1989.
White PF, Ham J, Way WL, Trevor AJ: Pharmacology of ketamine isomers in surgical patients. *Anesthesiology* 52:231, 1980.
Widdowson EM: Changes in body proportions and composite during growth. In Davis JA, Dobbing J, editors: *Scientific foundations of pediatrics*. Philadelphia, 1974, WB Saunders Co, p 153.
Wiest DB, Oyning BL, Garner SS: The disposition of alfentanil in neonates with respiratory distress. *Pharmacotherapy* 11:308, 1991.
Wilson RD, Traber DL, Evans BL: Correlation of psychologic and physiologic observations from children undergoing repeated ketamine anesthesia. *Anesth Analg (Cleve)* 48:995, 1970.
Wilson-Smith E, Karsli C, Luginbuehl IA, et al.: The effect of nitrous oxide on cerebral blood flow velocity in children anesthetized with propofol. *Acta Anaesthesiol Scand* 47:307–311, 2003.
Wilton NCT, Leigh J, Rosen DR: Preanesthetic sedation of preschool children using intranasal midazolam. *Anesthesiology* 69:972, 1988.
Wissing H, Kuhn I, Warnken U, et al.: Carbon monoxide production from desflurane, enflurane, halothane, isoflurane and sevoflurane in dry soda lime. *Anesthesiology* 95:1205–1212, 2001.
Woelfel SK, Brandom BW, Cook DR, et al.: Effects of bolus administration of ORG-9426 in children during nitrous oxide-halothane anesthesia. *Anesthesiology* 76:939, 1992.
Woelfel SK, Brandom BW, McGowan FX, et al.: Clinical pharmacology of mivacurium in pediatric patients less than two years old during nitrous oxide-halothane anesthesia. *Anesth Analg* 77:713, 1993.
Wulf H, Peters C, Behnke H: The pharmacokinetics of caudal ropivacaine 0.2 in children. *Anaesthesia* 55:575–560, 2000.
Yang HY, Lee QP, Rettie AR, et al.: Functional cytochrome P4503A isoforms in human embryonic tissues: Expression during organogenesis. *Mol Pharmacol* 46:922–928, 1994.
Yang HYL, Namkung MJ, Juchau MR: Expression of functional cytochrome P4501A1 in human embryonic hepatic tissues during organogenesis. *Biochem Pharmacol* 49:717–726, 1995.
Yaster M: The dose response of fentanyl in neonatal anesthesia. *Anesthesiology* 66:433, 1987.
Yasuda N, Lockhart SH, Eger II, et al.: Kinetics of desflurane, isoflurane, and halothane in humans. *Anesthesiology* 74:489,1991.
Yasuda N, Targ AG, Eger EI II: Solubility of I–653, sevoflurane, isoflurane, and halothane in human tissues. *Anesth Analg* 69;370, 1989.
Yokoyama H, Iinuma K, Yanai K, et al.: Proconvulsant effect of ketotifen, a histamine H_1-antagonist, confirmed by the use of d-chlorpheniramine with monitoring electroencephalography. *Methods Fundam Exp Clin Pharmacol* 15:183–188, 1993.
Yoshikawa K, Murai Y: The effect of ketamine on intraocular pressure in children. *Anesth Analg (Cleve)* 50:199, 1971.
Yost CS, Dodson BA: Inhibition of the nicotinic acetylcholine receptor by barbiturates and by procaine: Do they act at different sites? *Cell Mol Neurobiol* 13:159, 1993.
Youngs EJ, Shafer SL: Pharmacokinetic parameters relevant to recovery from opioids. *Anesthesiology* 81:833–842, 1994.
Yun C-H, Wood M, Wood AJJ, et al.: Identification of the pharmacogenetic determinants of alfentanil metabolism: Cytochrome P-450 3A4. *Anesthesiology* 77:467, 1992.
Zhang AZ, Pasternak GW: Ontogeny of opioid pharmacology and receptors. High and low affinity site differences. *Eur J Pharmacol* 73:29, 1981.
Zhou HH, Sheller JR, Nu H, et al.: Ethnic differences in response to morphine. *Clin Pharmacol Ther* 54:507, 1993.
Zimmerman G, Steward DJ: Bradycardia delays the onset of action of intravenous atropine in infants. *Anesthesiology* 65:320, 1986.
Zuppa AF, Helfaer MA, Adamson PC: Propofol pharmacokinetics. *Pediatr Crit Care Med* 4:124–125, 2003.
Zwass MS, Fisher DM, Welborn LG, et al.: Induction and maintenance characteristics of anesthesia with desflurane and nitrous oxide in infants and children. *Anesthesiology* 76:373, 1992.

II

GENERAL APPROACH

7 Psychological Aspects of Pediatric Anesthesia

Zeev N. Kain

Surgery and anesthesia induce considerable emotional stress on both parents and children. Because the consequences of this stress occur in the immediate postoperative period (Aono et al., 1999; Holm-Knudsen et al., 1998; Kain and Mayes, 1996) and may remain long after the hospital experience has passed (Chapman et al., 1956; Kain et al., 1999a, 1999b), it is one of the tasks of the pediatric anesthesiologist to ensure the psychologic as well as the physiologic well-being of patients. To minimize the emotional stress of anesthesia and surgery, the anesthesiologist must understand the psychological developmental milestones of childhood and anticipate situations that the child may find threatening. The latter can often be accomplished with a careful and thoughtful preoperative visit and by administering preoperative sedation when a comforting person alone is inadequate. During the preoperative visit to the patient, the anesthesiologist can optimally evaluate the levels of anxiety of both parent(s) and child, while assessing the child's medical condition. In this chapter, the psychological facets of hospitalization and surgery for children and the psychological and medical preparation of pediatric patients for anesthesia and surgery are discussed. A summary of premedications used for children undergoing anesthesia is included.

PSYCHOLOGICAL PREPARATION FOR ANESTHESIA AND SURGERY

More than 4 million children undergo surgery in the United States each year, and it is estimated that 50% to 75% of these children experience significant fear and anxiety before their operation (Corman et al., 1958; Vernon et al., 1965; Melamed and Siegel, 1975; Beeby and Hughes, 1980; Kain et al., 1996c). Based on behavioral and physiological measures of anxiety, induction of anesthesia in children has been identified as the most stressful point during the entire preoperative period (Kain and Mayes, 1996). Appropriate understanding and management of fear and anxiety before surgery are important because they can lead to both psychological and physiologic adverse outcomes. Increased child anxiety before surgery has been linked to outcomes such as parent satisfaction, perioperative neuroendocrine response, and postoperative, clinical, and psychological recovery (Kain et al., 2002a). As an indicator of the importance of preoperative anxiety, a panel of 72 anesthesiologists ranked various anesthesia low-morbidity clinical outcomes based on importance and frequency (Macario et al., 1999). The three clinical outcomes with the highest combined score were incisional pain, nausea and vomiting, and preoperative anxiety. Thus, it is important to understand the psychological issues involved when a child undergoes surgery.

INCIDENCE AND DEFINITION

Although the exact prevalence of preoperative anxiety in children is difficult to assess because of issues related to measurement and developmental variations, it is estimated that up to 75% of children are reported to exhibit significant psychological and/or physiologic manifestations of anxiety during the preoperative period (Corman et al., 1958; Vernon et al., 1965; Melamed and Siegel, 1975; Beeby and Hughes, 1980; Kain et al., 1996c). That is, every year up to 3 million children in the United States exhibit significant fear and anxiety before undergoing surgery.

Preoperative anxiety is operationally defined as a subjective feeling of tension, apprehension, nervousness, worry, and vigilance associated with increased autonomic nervous system activity (Burton, 1984; Kain and Mayes, 1996). Children are threatened by anticipated parental separation, pain or discomfort, loss of control, uncertainty about "going to sleep," and masked strangers working in a technical, sterile, non–child-focused environment. Younger children are more concerned about separation from parents, and older children are more anxious about the anesthetic and surgical processes. The stress and anxiety experienced by children during induction of anesthesia represent an interaction between child-related factors and environmental conditions in the operating room. Child-related factors include age and developmental maturity, previous experience with medical procedures and illness, individual capacity for affect regulation and trait anxiety, and parental trait anxiety (Lumley et al., 1990; Lumley et al., 1993; Kain et al., 1996c).

Operating room–related environment factors include factors such as interactions with the medical staff, intensity of lights, level of noise produced by the staff and instrument preparation, and number of medical personnel who interact with the child. Children may look scared and/or agitated, breathe deeply, tremble, stop talking or playing, and/or start to cry. Other children may become nauseous, wet themselves, have increased motor tone, and/or attempt to escape from the operating room personnel (Burton, 1984; Kain and Mayes, 1996). These behaviors, which are likely to prolong the induction of anesthesia, give children a sense of control over the situation and therefore diminish the sense of helplessness.

IDENTIFICATION OF CHILDREN AT RISK

The first step in psychologically preparing children to undergo surgery is the identification of those children who are at a particularly high risk to develop extreme anxiety and fear before surgery. This is particularly important in an environment that is sensitive to operational hospital and operating room costs. To date, studies looking into risk factors that affect the behavioral responses of children during the preoperative period have identified several categories: age, temperament and developmental stage of the child, trait (baseline) and state (situational) anxiety of the parent, various demographic characteristics of the child and parent, and quality of previous experience of the child with medical procedures.

Young children, between the ages of 1 and 5 years, are reported to be at the highest risk for developing significant anxiety before anesthesia and surgery (Brophy and Erickson, 1990; Lumley et al., 1993; Vetter, 1993; Kain et al., 1996a, 1996c). At this age, children are particularly vulnerable because they are both young enough to be dependent on their parents and old enough to recognize the parent's absence. Additional factors enhancing the vulnerability of this age group include degree of inexperience in social contact, ability to communicate and benefit from psychological preparation, and ability to relieve anxiety through play (Hyson, 1983). Although the younger child may not have the cognitive ability to anticipate potential dangers or painful situations during induction of anesthesia, the older child (older than 6 years) may anticipate pain and fear "going to sleep" (Sparrow et al., 1984). Older children may also rely on a number of coping strategies, including verbal questioning and cognitive mastery (e.g., learning about heart monitors or about what surgeons do), to mediate their anxiety.

Children who have high trait anxiety and who have experienced in the past poor-quality medical encounters are at a particularly high risk to develop high anxiety during the preoperative period (Kain et al., 1996a, 1996c). Interestingly, a child who presents for repeated surgical procedures may respond in *either* higher-than-expected preoperative anxiety levels or lower-than-expected preoperative anxiety levels. Based on a conditioned learning model, the preoperative situation presents unconditioned fear stimuli that occur repeatedly over short intervals. Thus, children's previous surgical and medical histories may either exacerbate or attenuate fear conditioning, and the quality of the previous medical experience (e.g., how distressing it was to the child) is more crucial than its occurrence (Box 7-1).

> **BOX 7–1 Risk Factors for Preoperative Anxiety**
>
> **Child Related**
>
> Young age (1 to 5 years)
> Poor previous experience with medical procedures and illness
> Children with shy and inhibited temperament
> Lack of developmental maturity and social adaptability
> High cognitive levels
> Not enrolled in daycare
>
> **Parent Related**
>
> High trait and state anxiety
> Divorced parents
> Parents who had multiple surgical procedures
>
> **Environment Related**
>
> Sensory overload
> Conflicting messages
> Operating

Several investigations indicate that children who have a shy and inhibited temperament present with higher levels of fear and anxiety on the day of surgery compared with other children (Melamed and Ridley-Johnson, 1988; Kain et al., 1996c, 2001). Conversely, children who have a more socially adaptive temperament are less anxious in the perioperative settings (Kain et al., 2001a). Temperament in a child refers to individual patterns of behavior and has been compared with personality traits in adults (Buss et al., 1973; Buss and Plomin, 1975). Kagan et al. (1987) reported that temperament characteristics can be used to predict how a child responds emotionally in a stressful situation; for example, children who are "shy" or "inhibited" tend to become more anxious in novel settings, as suggested by the adrenocortical response and elevated heart rate.

A child's anxiety before surgery is strongly affected by the state and trait anxiety of the parent (Kain et al., 1996c, 2001a). Parental anxiety mediates the child's response to stressful situations through two pathways (Kain and Mayes, 1996). First, while parents may act as stress reducers for their children, parents who are themselves more anxious in a given situation are less available to respond to their child's needs. Indeed, in these cases, the child's distress may further compound parental anxiety, thus rendering the parent increasingly less able to respond effectively. The second pathway of the effect of parental anxiety on a child's response reflects the genetics of parental disposition to being overanxious. It was described that mothers who were more anxious in the surgical setting had children who were also more anxious and that these mothers were less able to respond in these situations (Kagan et al., 1987).

Divorced parents, parents with lower educational levels, and parents of children who were not enrolled in a daycare setting rate themselves as significantly more anxious preoperatively (Kain et al., 1996a, 1996c). Finally, parents of children who are less than 1 year old, parents who themselves underwent multiple admissions, and parents of children who underwent multiple admissions all report being more anxious (Litman et al., 1996; Shirley et al., 1998). Preoperative anxiety in young children undergoing surgery can be managed with behavioral or pharmacologic (preoperative sedative medication) interventions, or both (Fig. 7–1).

PSYCHOLOGICAL PREPARATION PROGRAMS

The concept of psychological preparation of children and parents who undergo surgery was introduced almost 50 years ago (Mellish, 1969; Robinson and Kobayashi, 1991). Earlier programs provided the child with information regarding the surgical and anesthetic procedures and sought to develop a rapport between the medical staff and the child (Melamed and Siegel, 1975; Melamed et al., 1976, 1978). In the 1970s, modeling preparation programs were introduced to multiple hospitals in the United States. These modeling programs included the use of illustrated books, video programs, and puppet shows (Melamed and Siegel, 1975; Melamed et al., 1976, 1978). The theory behind

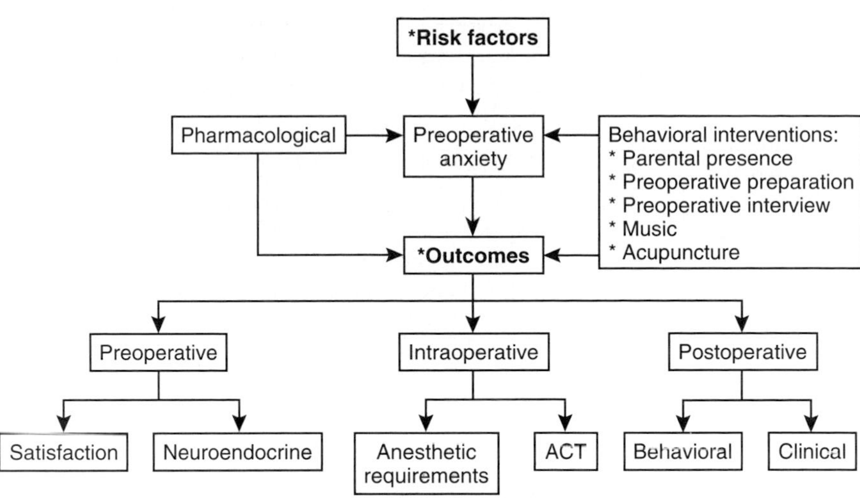

■ **FIGURE 7–1.** Operational view of preoperative anxiety in children. ACT, anesthesia control time.

these programs was that children would be prepared for the surgical experience by observing other children who underwent similar procedures. During the 1990s, the idea of family-centered care was introduced to medicine in general and to the area of preoperative preparation in particular (Melamed, 1993). Coupled with the development of the child-life discipline and teaching of coping skills, these concepts dominate the preparation programs in current use. Child-life specialists are individuals who facilitate the child's coping and the perioperative adjustment of children and parents by providing play experiences using modeling techniques (AAP statement, 1993). Child-life specialists incorporate descriptions of the perioperative sensations children experience and provide opportunities to examine, rehearse, and "play" with perioperative equipment to be used in their care. Child-life specialists also aim to establish supportive relationships with children and parents and to teach relaxation skills and present information to the child and parent about the anesthetic and surgical procedures (AAP statement, 1993).

The frequency at which preparation programs aimed at children undergoing surgery are being used has changed over the past decades. Although these programs were scarce in the 1970s and 1980s, they became quite popular in the 1990s. In fact, in 1996 about 80% of all major acute care children's hospitals in the United States offered such programs to children and their parents (O'Byrne et al., 1997). Unfortunately, the number of comprehensive preparation programs has been reported to decrease over the past few years; this new trend is likely the result of new economical constraints in the perioperative environment.

The type of preparation programs used varies significantly among the various children's hospitals in the United States (O'Byrne et al., 1997). About 89% of children's hospitals are reported to provide narrative preparation, 87% provide operating room tours, 86% provide play therapy, and 84% provide printed material (O'Byrne et al., 1997). More comprehensive preparation such as child-life preparation is provided at about 50% of children's hospitals, and relaxation is taught at about 40% of the hospitals (O'Byrne et al., 1997). Interestingly, a panel of experts indicated their consensus regarding the effectiveness of psychological preparation programs before surgery (O'Byrne et al., 1997). On a scale of 1 (least effective) to 9 (most effective), child life was ranked the most effective, followed by play therapy, operating room tour, and printed material (O'Byrne et al., 1997).

Although the effectiveness of preparation programs in reduction of anxiety in the holding area is well established, their effectiveness for reducing anxiety during the induction process is questionable (Kain et al., 1996a, 1998a). Methodologic flaws such as the absence of an appropriate outcome instrument and small sample size hinder many of the studies that report reduced child's anxiety. In fact, a study that included a validated outcome measure has clearly documented that while a comprehensive psychological preparation program (i.e., child life) is effective in reduction of anxiety in the holding area, it was *not* effective during the induction of anesthesia or in the recovery room period (Kain et al., 1998a). It is likely that the extreme anxiety experienced during induction of anesthesia inhibits processing and implementing of the content of the preoperative preparation program by children.

Considerations in Choosing a Preparation Program

It is vital to realize that psychological preparation programs have to be tailored based on the individual needs of each child. That is, a preparation program that is appropriate for a 3-year-old is not appropriate for a 12-year-old. Thus, once the type of the preparation has been chosen (e.g., child life versus a tour of the operating room), the preparation has to be individualized based on developmental considerations of the child.

Timing of the preparation in relation to the day of surgery is a significant factor. That is, children 6 years and older benefit most if they participate in the program more than 5 to 7 days before surgery and benefit the least if the program is given 1 day before surgery (Melamed et al., 1976; Robinson and Kobayashi, 1991; Kain et al., 1996a). This longer interval between the preparation and surgery is needed for the older children to have adequate time to process new information provided to them during the preparation process (Melamed et al., 1983; Kain et al., 1996a, 1998a). Typically, older children prepared 1 week ahead of surgery show an immediate increase in the anxiety during the preparation period with a gradual decrease until the time of surgery (Melamed et al., 1983). Interestingly, there may be a *negative* effect of a preparation program on younger children. This may be a result of the inability of children younger than 3 years to separate fantasy from reality (Melamed et al., 1976; Robinson and Kobayashi, 1991). From ages 3 to 6 years, children experience increased ability to separate fantasy from reality, and by the age of 6, this distinction of fantasy versus reality is typically completed (Piaget, 1955).

Designing a preparation program for children who were previously hospitalized is a particular challenge. Information about what occurs on the day of surgery does not provide new information for these children. Studies have documented that simple modeling and play programs are *not* beneficial for these children and may actually sensitize these children (Melamed et al., 1983; Faust and Melamed, 1984). Alternative psychological programs, such as extensive individualized coping skills training, combined with actual practice, is more helpful for these children (Melamed et al., 1983; Kain et al., 1996a). These alternative programs should be based on the particular experience the child had during the previous surgeries.

Parental Issues

Clearly, preoperative preparation should be directed to parents as well as to children. Multiple studies have reported that parents typically become very anxious when their child undergoes surgery (Pinto and Hollandsworth, 1989; Kain et al., 1996a, 1996c; Litman et al., 1996; Shirley et al., 1998; Cassady et al., 1999), and parental anxiety was identified as a significant risk factor for increased preoperative anxiety in children (Pinto and Hollandsworth, 1989; Kain et al., 1996a; Litman et al., 1996; Cassady et al., 1999). Parents experience preoperative anxiety for reasons such as separation and bodily harm to their children, guilt, and financial stresses (Cassady et al., 1999). Indeed, many parents are more anxious regarding their children's health than their own (Kain et al., 1997d). Mothers are more prone to preoperative anxiety than are fathers (Litman et al., 1996; Shirley et al., 1998). Compared with fathers, mothers are known to be more anxious preoperatively when their child is less than 1 year old or when coping with their child's first surgical experience (Litman et al., 1996). Previous research has also documented that women are significantly more concerned with risks and side effects in general, although men specifically articulate a fear of death twice as often as do women.

Parents who undergo a preoperative preparation program or who have viewed a preoperative videotape featuring factual information about anesthesia display reduced preoperative anxiety on the day of surgery (Table 7–1) (Pinto and Hollandsworth, 1989; Kain et al., 1996a; Cassady et al., 1999) but not during the anesthetic induction, in the recovery room, and at 2 weeks postoperatively (Kain et al., 1998a). Presently, the use of videotapes is receiving increasing attention as a supplementary educational modality for parents (Karl et al., 1990; Cassady et al., 1999) because they are informative, perhaps anxiolytic, and cost effective in certain settings (Pinto and Hollandsworth, 1989; Cassady and Kain, 2000).

Future of Preparation Programs

The need for preoperative preparation programs that are cost sensitive created a void that will inevitably be filled technologically. The future will be characterized by the development and implementation of computerized multimedia displays and interactive technology. The latter offers particular appeal, because its multimodal capability can provide specific interventions for individuals with a wide range of medical problems and coping styles. The capacity, programmability, and rapid response of current interactive technology are suitable for such tasks, but the cost remains high. In the future, it is the hope that all children and their parents will be able to realize the benefits of specialized, technologically advanced educational systems programmed to meet their individual and cultural needs and coping styles.

PARENTAL PRESENCE

Parental presence during the induction of anesthesia has been suggested as an alternative to sedative premedication. Although there is general agreement about the desirability of parents visiting during their child's hospitalization, their presence during invasive medical procedures, such as induction of anesthesia, remains very controversial (Lerman, 2000; Kain, 2001). Potential benefits from parental presence include reducing the need for preoperative sedatives and reducing the child's anxiety and distress on separation to the operating room. Increased child compliance and reduced child anxiety during induction of anesthesia have been suggested to be benefits as well. Common objections to this practice include delays in operating room schedules, crowded operating rooms, and a possible adverse reaction of the parent during the induction process.

A large-scale nationwide survey indicated that there is a large variability in hospital policy in the United States toward parental presence in operating rooms. Thirty-two percent of the hospitals allow parental presence, 11% encourage parental presence, 23% have no formal hospital policy, and 26% do not allow it (Kain et al., 2004b).

The same survey reported that only 10% of anesthesiologists have parents present during induction of anesthesia in more than 75% of cases and that 27% of anesthesiologists have parents

TABLE 7–1. Use of preoperative video for increased parental education and decreased parental anxiety

	EXPERIMENTAL GROUP		CONTROL GROUP		*P* Value
Measure	*Prevideo*	*Postvideo*	*Prevideo*	*Postvideo*	
SALT (% correct)	75.2 ± 1.8	84.9 ± 2.3	73.4 ± 1.4	75.4 ± 1.9	<.0220
STAI State Anxiety	40.5 ± 1.7	36.0 ± 1.4	39.2 ± 1.5	37.7 ± 1.2	<.0310
APAIS Total	22.0 ± 1.2	17.0 ± 0.9	22.0 ± 0.8	21.6 ± 0.7	<.0001
APAIS Anxiety	12.7 ± 0.8	9.0 ± 0.6	12.6 ± 0.6	12.2 ± 0.5	<.0001
APAIS Need for Information	9.3 ± 0.7	8.0 ± 0.3	9.4 ± 0.6	9.3 ± 0.6	<.0001

Values are given as mean ± SEM.

SALT, Standard Anesthesia Learning Test; STAI State Anxiety, State-Trait Anxiety Inventory (State Anxiety); APAIS, Amsterdam Preoperative Anxiety and Information Scale.

Group × time interaction obtained by repeated-measures analyses of variance.

From Cassady JF Jr, Wysocki TT, Miller KM, and others: Use of a preanesthetic video for facilitation of parental education and anxiolysis before pediatric ambulatory surgery. *Anesth Analg* 88:246–250, 1999.

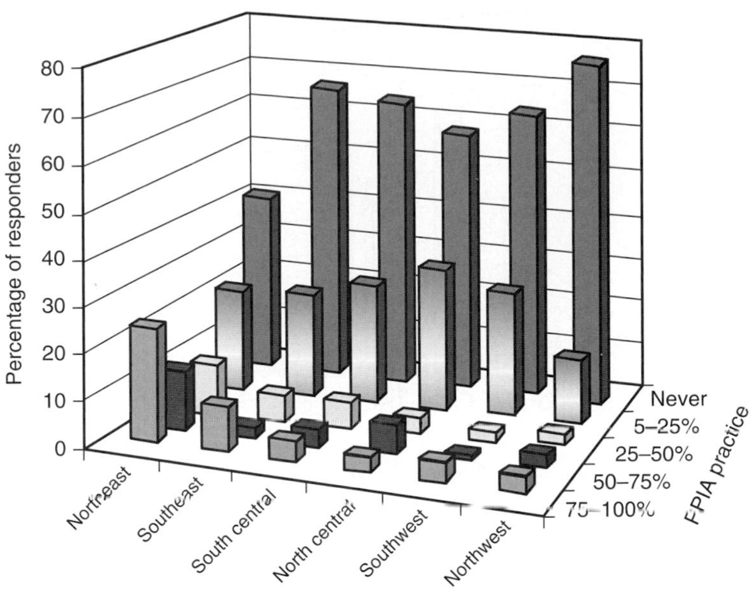

■ **FIGURE 7–2.** Practice of parental presence during induction of anesthesia as a function of geographic areas in the United States. PPIA, parental presence during induction of anesthesia. (Kain ZN, Caldwell-Andrews AA, Krivutza DM, Weinberg ME, Wang SM, Gaal D: Trends in the practice of parental presence during induction of anesthesia and the use of preoperative sedative premedication in the United States, 1995–2002: results of a follow-up national survey. *Anesth Analg* 98:1252–9, 2004.)

present during induction in less than 25% of cases. About 50% of all anesthesiologists never have parents present during induction (Kain et al., 2004b). The reported prevalence of parental presence varies widely among the different geographic locations in the United States.

Parental presence during induction of anesthesia was practiced most often in the northeast region and least often in the south central region of the United States (Fig. 7–2). Interestingly, the findings in this survey (Kain et al., 2004b) are very much different from the findings in a nationwide survey conducted in 1995 (Kain et al., 1997c). Overall, there is an increase in the frequency of parental presence from 1995 to 2002, and the number of anesthesiologists who *never* allow parental presence dropped in every geographic region (Kain et al., 1997c, 2004b). These findings may represent a new trend in this practice in the United States (Fig. 7–3).

Parental Perspectives

A number of surveys have indicated that most parents prefer to be present during the induction of anesthesia regardless of the child's age (Braude et al., 1990; Ryder and Spargo, 1991). Further, a majority of parents believe that they are of some help to their child and to the anesthesiologist during the induction process (Ryder and Spargo, 1991). A study indicates that over 80% of parents chose to be present in the operating room when returning for a second operation regardless of whether they were

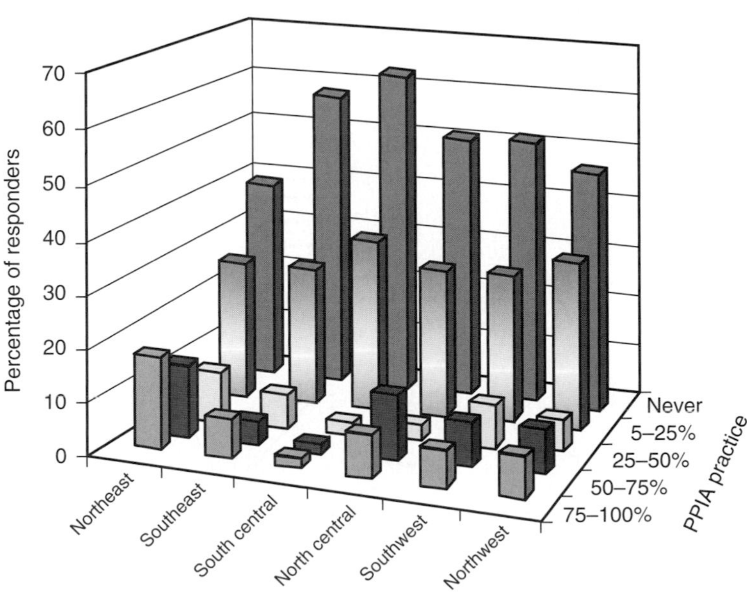

■ **FIGURE 7–3.** Practice of parental presence during induction of anesthesia as a function of geographic areas in the United States. PPIA, parental presence during induction of anesthesia. (Kain ZN, Caldwell-Andrews AA, Krivutza DM, Weinberg ME, Wang SM, Gaal D: Trends in the practice of parental presence during induction of anesthesia and the use of preoperative sedative premedication in the United States, 1995–2002: results of a follow-up national survey. *Anesth Analg* 98:1252–9, 2004.)

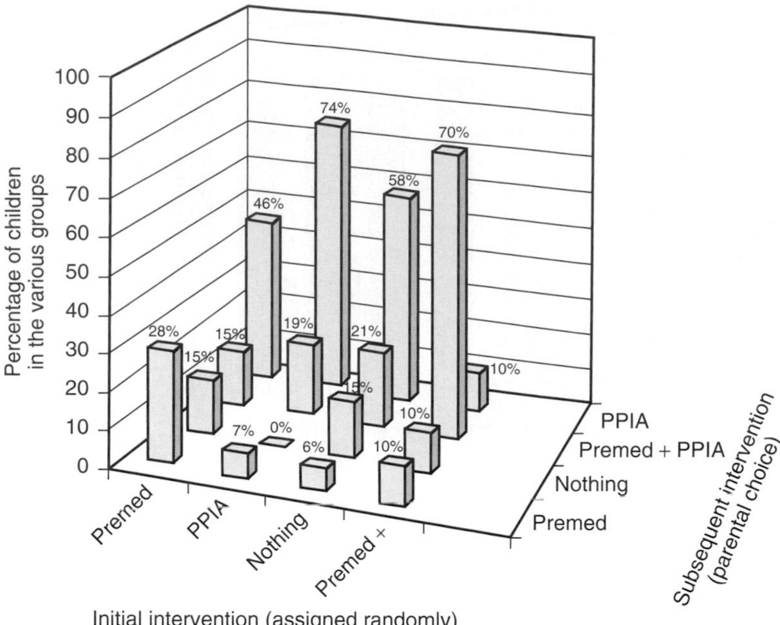

■ **FIGURE 7–4.** Data regarding the parental intervention choice in the subsequent surgery as a function of the initial surgery. For example, 28% of the parents who were assigned to the premedication group in the initial intervention chose to be in the premedication group in the subsequent surgery. PPIA, parental presence during induction of anesthesia. (Kain ZN, Caldwell-Andrews AA, Wang SM, Krivutza DM, Weinberg ME, Mayes LC: Parental intervention choices for children undergoing repeated surgeries. *Anesth Analg* 96:970–5, 2003.)

present in the operating room in the first operation (Kain et al., 2003b). This preference for parental presence during induction shown by parents who had experience with other interventions, including preoperative midazolam, is similar to the preference for parental presence shown by parents of children undergoing surgery for the first time (Kain et al., 2003b) (Fig. 7–4). It is no surprise, therefore, that parental presence during the induction of anesthesia is associated with increased parental satisfaction regarding not only the separation process from their child but also with the overall functioning of the hospital (Kain et al., 2000).

Many parents report increased anxiety when present during induction of anesthesia (Vessey et al., 1994). An investigation found, however, that anxiety following induction of anesthesia among parents who were present during induction did *not* differ significantly from anxiety among parents who were not present during the induction process (Kain et al., 2003a). This finding is in agreement with previous randomized controlled trials that have examined this issue (Bevan et al., 1990; Kain et al., 1996b, 1998b, 2000).

Parental physiologic responses during induction of anesthesia have been examined as well (Kain et al., 2003a). It was found that parental heart rate and skin conductance levels significantly increase as the parents walk to the operating room. Interestingly, once the induction begins, parental heart rate decreases, only to peak again once the parents have to leave the operating room. This second peak in heart rate is in agreement with previous data that indicate the most upsetting factors are seeing the child go limp during induction and then having to leave the child (Vessey et al., 1994). Parental blood pressure following induction of anesthesia was not elevated and examination of parental Holter data revealed no rhythm abnormalities and no electrocardiographic changes indicating ischemia (Kain et al., 2003a) (Fig. 7–5).

There have been isolated reports of parental presence resulting in disruptive behavior, and even removal of a child from the operating room by a grandmother (Schofield and White, 1989; Bowie, 1993). In contrast, a 4-year experience with 3,086 children in a free-standing ambulatory surgery center found that no

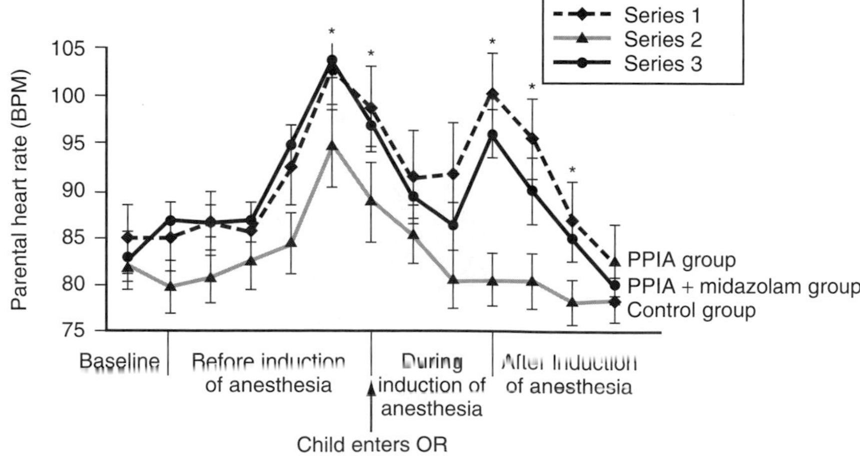

■ **FIGURE 7–5.** Changes in parental heart rate (HR) from baseline measurement until after induction of anesthesia. Data are reported as mean (SE). *Time points at which differences between groups are statistically significant ($P < .05$). OR, operating room; PPIA, parental presence during induction of anesthesia. (Kain ZN, Caldwell-Andrews AA, Mayes LC, Wang SM, Krivutza DM, LoDolce ME: Parental presence during induction of anesthesia: physiological effects on parents. *Anesthesiology* 98:58–64, 2003.)

parent needed to be escorted from the operating room (Gauderer et al., 1989).

Experimental Studies Involving Parental Presence

Early studies involving parental presence during induction of anesthesia indicated that the presence of a parent might lower the anxiety of the child (Schulman et al., 1967; Hannallah and Rosales, 1983). These studies, however, were nonrandomized, did not control for confounding variables, and lacked appropriate outcome measurement tools. It is important to note that measurement of a child's anxiety during induction of anesthesia is a complex issue that necessitates the use of a validated and reliable instrument of a child's anxiety. Such an instrument, the Yale Preoperative Anxiety Scale, was developed and validated a number of years ago (Kain et al., 1995, 1997b). Later studies that used appropriate sample size, eliminated confounding variables, and used appropriate end points and assessment instruments concluded that parental presence does *not* result in decreased child's anxiety during the induction process (Hickmott et al., 1989; Bevan et al., 1990; Kain et al., 1996b, 1998b, 2000; Kain, 2001). Further, parental presence during induction of anesthesia was also compared with the use of oral midazolam (0.5 mg/kg) administered 30 minutes before surgery (Kain et al., 1998b). The investigations concluded that the use of oral midazolam is significantly more effective than parental presence in terms of both reduced child's anxiety and increased child's compliance (Kain et al., 1998b) (Fig. 7–6).

On critical examination of this area, however, one realizes that the basic concepts underlying parental presence during induction of anesthesia–related research have not changed during the past two decades and that the present body of research simply deals with the question of whether parents should be present during induction of anesthesia. Research interests should shift toward an emphasis on what parents actually *do* during induction of anesthesia rather than simply on their presence. A preliminary publication reports the development of an intervention that consists of an informational and modeling video, instructed graduated exposure and shaping exercises, coached distraction techniques, supportive telephone coaching, and adherence checks (Kain et al., 2002b). This informative modeling intervention is directed at parents of children undergoing surgery and is quite extensive. Results show that children and parents who underwent the extensive parental preparation program were significantly less anxious than were children whose parents were present during induction of anesthesia and who did not receive the preparation program. More data regarding this preparation program are needed.

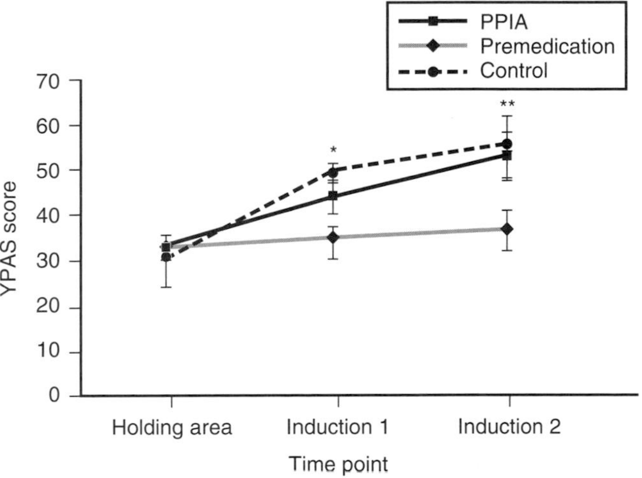

■ **FIGURE 7–6.** Anxiety of child across the perioperative period. Induction 1, entrance to the operating room; Induction 2, introduction of the anesthesia mask to the child. Premedication group was significantly less anxious compared with the parental presence and control groups at induction 1 (*) and induction 2 (**). PPIA, parental presence during induction of anesthesia; YPAS, Yale Preoperative Anxiety Scale. (Kain ZN, Mayes LC, Wang SM, Caramico LA, Hofstadter MB: Parental presence during induction of anesthesia versus sedative premedication: which intervention is more effective? *Anesthesiology* 89:1147–1156, 1998.)

Satisfaction Issues

Previously, the medical community held the view that the only "real" outcomes are those that have an immediate and direct impact on patient morbidity and mortality. This view has changed dramatically, and issues such as patient satisfaction and quality of life are considered by many as equally important as morbidity (Ford et al., 1997). This new development is echoed in review articles in the anesthesia literature that suggest that patient satisfaction should serve as an important end point and indicator of overall quality of anesthesia care (Fung and Cohen, 1998).

Typically, parents are not aware of any of the events that take place inside an operating room. To parents, the most important thing is their child's safety. However, with anesthetic mortality rates approaching 1:100,000, safety is expected. In contrast, parents evaluate an anesthesiologist, in part, based on the separation experience with their child. That is, if their child is taken to the operating room upset and crying, their satisfaction and impression of the anesthesiologist and the surgery center may be poor.

A study evaluated parental satisfaction as a function of their presence during induction of anesthesia. The study also evaluated the effectiveness of parental presence when used in conjunction with oral midazolam (0.5 mg/kg) (Kain et al., 2000). The study has demonstrated that while parental presence did *not* provide added value in terms of reduced child's anxiety or increased child's compliance, it did improve parental satisfaction with both the separation process and the entire perioperative process (Kain et al., 2000). Thus, although experimental studies fail to demonstrate the effectiveness of parental presence with regard to anxiety reduction or increased compliance, parental satisfaction seems to improve if the parents are present during the induction of anesthesia.

Medicolegal Issues

The practicing anesthesiologist should also be aware of legal issues associated with parental presence during induction of anesthesia—that is, what additional risks the anesthesiologist is incurring because of the presence of a parent in the operating room. The legal literature is not clear with this issue. Of note, however, is a decision made by the Illinois Supreme Court with regard to parental presence during an invasive procedure. In its verdict the Illinois Supreme Court stated that a hospital that *allows* a nonpatient to accompany a patient during treatment does not have a duty to protect the nonpatient from fainting (Lewyn, 1993). If medical personnel invite the nonpatient to be present during the treatment, however, the hospital has a legal responsibility toward the nonpatient. Thus, there is an important distinction between *allowing* parental presence and *inviting* parental presence. As a response to such possible litigation, a number of hospitals require parents to sign a separate consent form when they express the wish to be present during induction of anesthesia. A nationwide survey indicated, however, that at the current time only 5% of all hospitals in the United States indicate that they routinely obtain a separate written consent for parental presence during induction of anesthesia (Kain et al., 2004b).

BEHAVIORAL INTERVENTIONS

Music

Music has well-established psychological effects, including the induction and modification of moods and emotions (Baeck, 2002; Kain et al., 2002a; Lipe, 2002). Kane, in 1914, is reported to be one of the first individuals to provide intraoperative music to distract patients from "the horror of surgery" (Kane, 1914). It was not until about 1960, however, that a group of dentists reported that between 65% and 90% of their patients needed little or no anesthesia for dental extractions with routine use of music during dental surgery (Gardner and Licklider, 1959; Gardner et al., 1960). Music has gained popularity as a part of complementary medicine directed at patients undergoing medical and surgical procedures (Wang et al., 2002a, 2002b, 2003).

The role of music as a therapeutic modality for the treatment of preoperative anxiety in adult patients has been evaluated in several studies. Although a number of studies conducted in this area were hindered by multiple methodologic flaws, the anxiolytic effects of perioperative music are well documented in adults (Standley, 1986; Miluck-Kolasa et al., 1996; Thompson and Kam, 1995; Wang et al., 2002a). As indicated earlier, the anxiety experienced by a child during the induction period is related to personality factors as well as to operating room factors such as bright lights and high noise levels. Several studies that have assessed noise levels in the operating room concluded that while overall sound levels are not excessive, loud intermittent noises up to 108 dB are present intermittently (Hodge and Thompson, 1990; Nott and West, 2003). Cohen classified noises as just audible (10 dB), very quiet (50 dB, comparable to light traffic at 30 miles/hr), moderately loud (70 dB, comparable to a dishwasher), very loud (90 dB, comparable to a food blender), and uncomfortably loud (130 dB, comparable to a rock-and-roll band) (Cohen, 1970). Interestingly, a sudden noise with a level as little as 30 dB above the background noise (e.g., an SpO_2 alarm) might cause an immediate startle response, which is associated with an activation of the sympathetic system and an anxiolytic response (Falk and Woods, 1973). A study introduced an intervention that consisted of dimmed operating room lights (200 Lx) and soft background music (Bach's "Air on a G String" [50 to 60 dB]), and only the attending anesthesiologist was allowed to interact with the child during induction (Kain et al., 2001b) (Fig. 7–7).

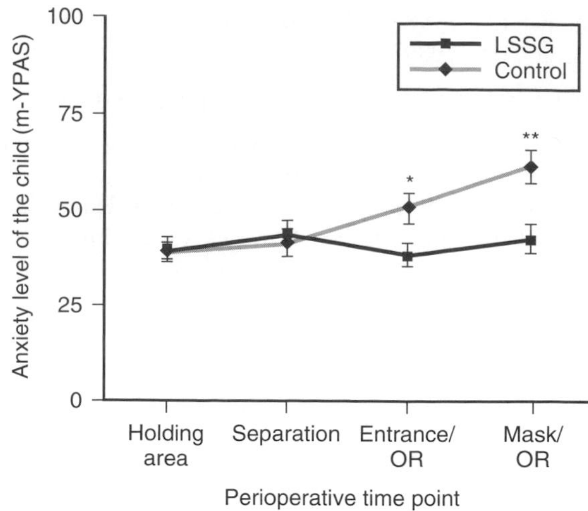

FIGURE 7–7. Levels of anxiety manifested by children during the perioperative period. Anxiety was assessed by the m-PAS (modified Yale Preoperative Anxiety Scale). Observed anxiety differed significantly between the two groups [$F(1,67) = 6.3$, $P = .014$]. LSSG, low sensory stimulation group; OR, operating room. $^{*}P = .03$; $^{**}P = .003$. (Kain ZN, Wang SM, Mayes LC, Krivutza DM, Teague BA: Sensory stimuli and anxiety in children undergoing surgery: a randomized, controlled trial. *Anesth Analg* 92:897–903, 2001.)

The number of medical personnel interacting with the child is of particular importance as it is not infrequent that the surgeon, the circulating nurse, the anesthesia resident, and the anesthesia attending are all trying to help the child through the induction process. This may result in conflicting messages and increased anxiety of the child. The study found that this combination of music, dim light, and only the attending anesthesiologist interacting with the child was effective and those children who received this intervention exhibited significantly less anxiety during induction of anesthesia (Kain et al., 2002b).

To date, most reported studies of music therapy in the medical literature describe interventions that consist of patients passively listening to music. Interestingly, results from a meta-analytical review appear to indicate that studies using live-participation music therapy, although significantly fewer in number, showed overall higher effect sizes compared with engagement of the patient. Earlier studies that examined live-participation music therapy with children undergoing surgery concluded that this type of music therapy resulted in reduced anxiety in children undergoing surgery (Chetta, 1981; Robb et al., 1995). These studies, however, were limited because of a small sample size and a lack of reliable and valid outcome anxiety measures. A more recent trial that used an appropriate sample size and a reliable outcome measure instrument indicated some complexities related to this issue (Kain et al., 2004a). The study found that at separation and on entrance to the operating room, only children who received music therapy from one of the therapists involved in the study were significantly less anxious than the control group. This anxiolytic effect was present only in the holding area and at separation but not during induction of anesthesia. Thus, one should conclude that the provision of live-participation music therapy is quite expensive, and considering the results of the more recent study, one can seriously doubt if this modality should be routinely used to reduce preoperative anxiety in all children undergoing surgery.

Acupuncture

Acupuncture originated in China between the years 2000 and 100 B.C.E. (Hsu, 1996). Despite slow progression of scientific evidence, acupuncture and related techniques have become very popular in the western medical culture over the last few decades.

Several studies have examined whether acupuncture is an effective treatment modality for preoperative anxiety. Wang and Kain (2001a, 2001b) found that both healthy volunteers and adult patients undergoing routine outpatient surgery report lower levels of state anxiety after auricular acupuncture provided in specific points. This effect started as early as 30 minutes after insertion of the acupuncture needles. The use of acupuncture as a treatment for parental anxiety was examined as well.

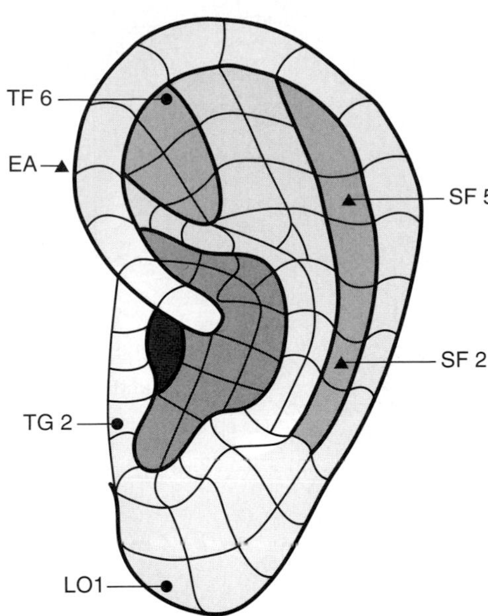

● Intervention group
TF6 - Triangular fossa zone 6, hypertension
TG2 - Tragus zone 2, valium (tranquilizer point)
LO1 - Lobe zone 1, master cerebral
▲ Control group
SF2 - Scaphoid fossa zone 2 wrist
SF5 - Scaphoid fossa zone 5 shoulder
Extraneous point

■ **FIGURE 7–8.** Auricular acupuncture points that are used to treat parental anxiety. (Wang SM, Maranets I, Weinberg ME, Caldwell-Andrews AA, Kain ZN: Parental auricular acupuncture as an adjunct for parental presence during induction of anesthesia. *Anesthesiology* 100:1399–404, 2004.)

Wang and Kain randomized mothers of children who were scheduled for surgery to an acupuncture intervention group or a sham acupuncture control group (Fig. 7–8). The intervention was performed at least 30 minutes before the child's induction of anesthesia and all mothers were present during induction of anesthesia.

The investigators found that after induction, maternal anxiety in the acupuncture group was significantly lower *and* children whose mothers received the acupuncture intervention were significantly less anxious on entrance to the operating room (Wang et al., 2004). Thus, auricular acupuncture may have various uses in the pediatric perioperative environment.

Preoperative Interview

There is no question that anesthesiologists have the ability to either increase or decrease the anxiety of patients; one should consider the preoperative interview as a psychological intervention that is administered routinely to parents and children (Egbert et al., 1963; Kain et al., 2002a). The anxiety-moderating effect of anesthesiologists is dependent on multiple variables such as environmental stimuli and the coping style of the parent. That is, while overall, patients undergoing surgery ask for all relevant information to be provided to them (Kain et al., 1997a, 1997d), some patients and parents have an information-seeking coping style, and others have an information-avoiding coping style (Miller, 1995). The challenge for the anesthesiologist is to identify the individual coping style of a parent without the benefit of using structured psychological instruments during the preoperative visit.

The impact of information given in the preoperative settings on the anxiety of patients was examined. Miller and Mangan (1983) found that adult patients who were given extensive information preoperatively were more anxious and uncomfortable. In contrast, no increase in preoperative anxiety was demonstrated in a study that involved English and Scottish men undergoing elective herniorrhaphy who were presented with detailed risk information (Kerrigan et al., 1993). Similarly, a study that involved parents of children undergoing surgery found that the provision of detailed anesthetic information in the setting of a randomized controlled trial did not increase the anxiety of the parents (Kain et al., 1997d). Thus, the practicing anesthesiologist should be aware of these data and provide information in the perioperative settings as dictated by the settings and the needs of the parents and the children.

■ BEHAVIORAL OUTCOMES OF PREOPERATIVE ANXIETY IN CHILDREN

■ POSTOPERATIVE BEHAVIORAL CHANGES

Epidemiology

In 1945, Levy (1945) described 25 cases of children who developed significant fear of physicians after tonsillectomy. Vernon et al. (1966) developed a structured parental instrument (Posthospitalization Behavior Questionnaire [PHBQ]) that addressed the issue of postoperative behavioral changes in children. Earlier studies that used the PHBQ reported that up to 88% of all children undergoing anesthesia and surgery develop new-onset postoperative behavioral changes (Vernon et al., 1966; Peterson and Shigetomi, 1982; Thompson and Vernon, 1993). More recent studies conducted in the United States and Europe documented that up to 54% of young children undergoing outpatient surgery experience general anxiety, nighttime crying, enuresis, separation anxiety, and temper tantrums at 2 weeks postoperatively (Kain et al., 1996c; Kotiniemi et al., 1996, 1997a; Kain, 2000) (Fig. 7–9).

Nightmares and waking up crying are particularly common problems after surgery in children, and the incidence of these behaviors is as high as 20% at 2 weeks postoperatively (Kain et al., 1996c). The effect of outpatient surgery on postoperative sleep patterns was also addressed in a study that used actigraphy, which is an objective measure that aims to quantify sleep (Kain et al., 2002d). The study found that 47% of all children developed postoperative sleeping problems as assessed by either actigraphy or the PHBQ (Kain et al., 2002d). Fourteen percent of children experienced a decrease of at least 1 SD in percentage sleep as assessed by actigraphy (Kain et al., 2002d) (Fig. 7–10).

Considering the dramatic changes that have occurred with health care delivery, this relatively high incidence of postoperative behavioral changes is surprising (Kain, 2000). That is, one would expect a lower incidence considering that these were studies that were conducted with *outpatients*. It is important to appreciate, however, that because of economical issues, outpatient surgery is being performed with children with high levels of medical acuity. These children underwent *inpatient* surgery just a few years ago; it may be that efforts to improve the psychological climate of hospitals may have been neutralized by other variables.

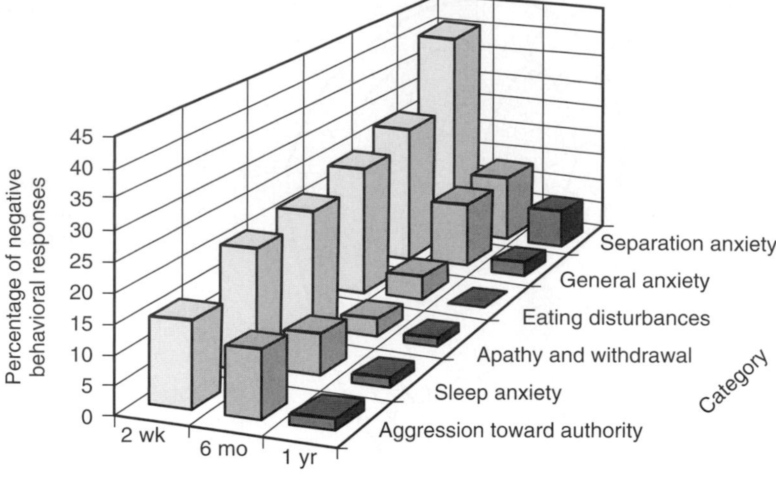

■ **FIGURE 7–9.** The incidence of postoperative behavioral changes as a function of time after surgery. (Kain ZN, Mayes LC, O'Connor TZ, Cicchetti DV: Preoperative anxiety in children. Predictors and outcomes. *Arch Pediatr Adolesc Med* 150:1238–45, 1996.)

Predictors

Several studies report that young age is a significant risk factor for the development of postoperative behavioral changes. In 1945, Levy noted a marked reduction in the emotional reaction following surgery after the age of 3 years, when the incidence of the new-onset behaviors dropped from 50% to 10%. More recent investigations confirm this observation and report that these postoperative behavioral changes are most common in ages 1 to 4 years (Vernon et al., 1965; Kain et al., 1996c). At this age, children are particularly vulnerable because of issues such as separation anxiety, degree of inexperience in social contact, ability to communicate and benefit from psychological preparation, and ability to relieve anxiety through play (Kain, 2000).

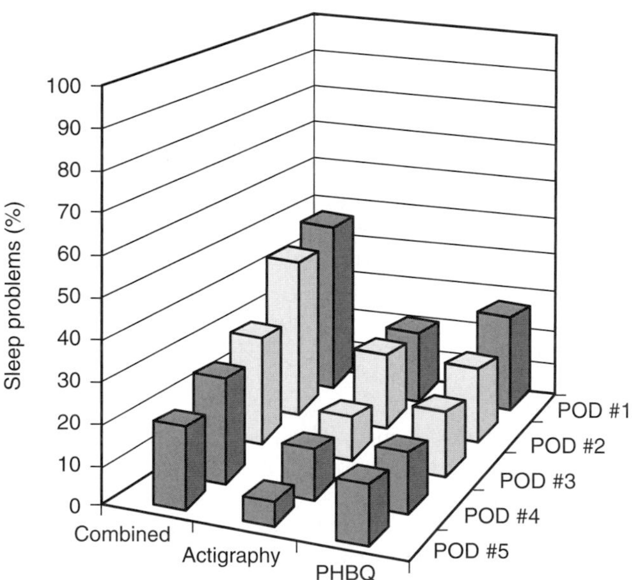

■ **FIGURE 7–10.** Postoperative sleeping disturbances during the first 5 postoperative nights, as determined either by actigraphy *or* the Posthospitalization Behavior Questionnaire (PHBQ). (Kain ZN, Mayes LC, Caldwell-Andrews AA, Alexander GM, Krivutza D, Teague BA, Wang SM: Sleeping characteristics of children undergoing outpatient elective surgery. *Anesthesiology* 97:1093–101, 2002.)

Increased anxieties of the child and of the parent in the holding area and during induction of anesthesia are both good predictors for later emergence of maladaptive postoperative behaviors (Eckenhoff, 1958; Kain et al., 1996c, 1999a; Lumley et al., 1993). Meyers and Muravchick (1977) compared postoperative behavioral responses in a group of children who underwent a "steal induction" versus a group of children who underwent an "awake" induction. One month after discharge of the children from the hospital, the investigators reported that the rate of behavioral changes was 88% in the awake group and 58% in the steal group. Kain et al. (1999a) confirmed these previous findings and observed that extreme anxiety during induction of anesthesia and forcing the child to the table ('brutane anesthesia') is associated with a significantly increased occurrence of postoperative negative behavioral changes.

Several reports indicate that these behavioral changes are significantly more common among children undergoing tonsillectomy and genitourinary surgery (Manley, 1982; Kain et al., 1996c). Finally, positive behavioral changes have also been reported after surgery, particularly in children with chronic conditions (e.g., recurrent otitis media) that have been improved by the surgery (Kain et al., 1996c; Kotiniemi et al., 1996).

The issue of anesthetic techniques (intravenous versus mask) has not been demonstrated to be a significant predictor of the incidence of postoperative maladaptive behavioral changes (Kotiniemi and Ryhanen, 1996). Although a history of previous surgery predicted increased incidence of postoperative maladaptive behavior in one study (Lumley et al., 1993), other studies did not confirm this finding (Kain et al., 1996c; Kotiniemi et al., 1997b). It is likely that the quality of surgical experiences is an important predictor, not simply the history of surgery. Quality of past medical experience as a predictor of future anxiety of the child has been reported in studies exploring the issue of preoperative anxiety (Kain et al., 1996c).

Interventions

Preparation Programs

The impact of preparation programs on the incidence of postoperative behavioral changes is not clear. Vernon and Thompson (1993) completed a meta-analysis of published studies that evaluated the effects of preoperative behavioral preparation programs on postoperative behavior. The meta-analysis concluded that on the average, children who received preoperative interventions tended to have less postoperative maladaptive behavioral changes than did control subjects. In contrast, Kain et al. (1998a) compared several types of preoperative preparation programs in children and found no effect of preoperative preparation on the incidence of postoperative behavioral changes.

Parental Presence

The impact of parental presence during induction of anesthesia on the incidence of postoperative behavioral changes was evaluated (Kain et al., 1996b). To date, all studies concluded that the presence of a parent during induction does *not* have an impact on the issue of postoperative behavioral changes (Kain et al., 1996b; Kain, 2000).

Sedatives

Investigations that looked into the association between preoperative sedative premedication and postoperative behavioral changes report contradictory findings. Two investigations report some beneficial effects of premedication on postoperative behavior (Padfield et al., 1986; Payne et al., 1992), but others report no effect (Parnis et al., 1992). Furthermore, an investigation found a higher incidence of negative postoperative behavioral changes in children who were premedicated (McGraw and Kendrick, 1998). These contradictory results may be explained by the methodologic complexity of this issue. Confounding variables such as age of child, surgical procedure, postoperative pain, and recent stressful major life events must be considered. An investigation by Kain and others (1999b) addressed all of these methodologic issues and screened all children for recent stressful life events. The investigators found that a significantly smaller number of children who were premedicated with oral midazolam before surgery presented with negative behavioral changes on postoperative days 1 through 7 (Fig. 7–11). Postoperative behaviors that were most improved included apathy and withdrawal, separation anxiety, and eating disturbances. At postoperative week 2, however, there were no significant differences between the placebo and midazolam groups. Thus, it can be concluded that in addition to its significant beneficial preoperative effects, sedative premedication improves immediate postoperative behavioral outcomes in young children undergoing general anesthesia and outpatient surgery.

CLINICAL OUTCOMES

Five decades ago, Janis (1958) proposed that moderate levels of preoperative anxiety in adult patients were associated with good postoperative behavioral recovery and that low and high levels of preoperative anxiety were associated with poor behavioral recovery. Although Janis' theory is intriguing, his studies were based on descriptive data from nonrandom, limited samples and retrospective reports of questionable validity. Subsequent studies have been critical of Janis' methodology and have reported a linear rather than a curvilinear relationship between anxiety level and postoperative behavioral recovery (Johnson et al., 1971; Johnston, 1980; Johnston and Carpenter, 1980; Newman, 1984; Pick et al., 1994). That is, low levels of preoperative anxiety are associated with good postoperative behavioral recovery, while high levels of preoperative anxiety are associated with poor postoperative recovery. To date, the adult literature indicates that intensity of pain, analgesic requirements, postsurgical complications, length of hospital stay, poor patient satisfaction, and blood cortisol levels have all been reported to be associated with high levels of preoperative anxiety (Devine, 1992; Johnston and Vogele, 1993; Contrada et al., 1994; Kiecolt-Glaser et al., 1998).

Many reviews of this research have appeared that, although critical of the methodology of a large number of studies, concluded that high preoperative anxiety is associated with impaired postoperative recovery (Mathews and Ridgeway, 1984; Mumford et al., 1982; Rogers and Reich, 1986; Anderson, 1987; Suls and Wan, 1989; Johnston and Wallace, 1990; Kincey and Saltmore, 1990; Devine, 1992; Johnston and Vogele, 1993; Contrada et al., 1994; Kiecolt-Glaser et al., 1998).

The fact that low preoperative anxiety is predictive of good postoperative outcome underlies many interventions in which the aim is to reduce preoperative anxiety. As with the cohort studies described earlier, preparation studies have used diverse postoperative outcome measures, including pain, analgesic

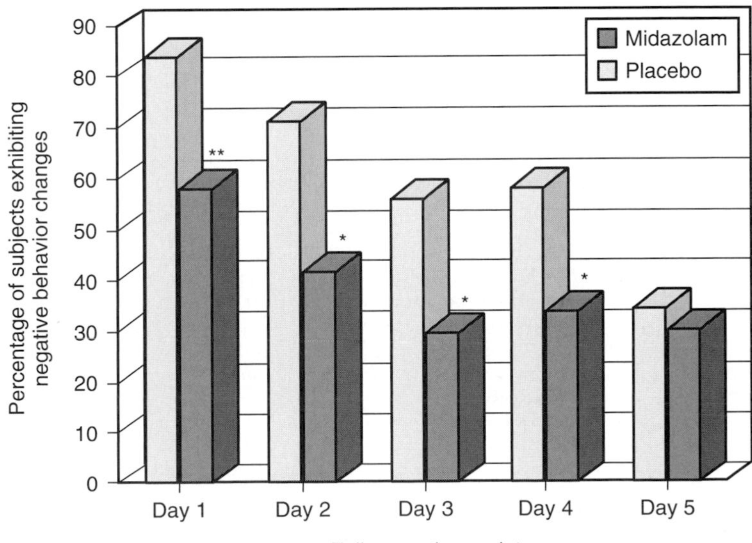

FIGURE 7–11. The effect of oral midazolam on the incidence of postoperative behavioral outcomes. (Kain ZN, Mayes LC, Wang SM, Hofstader MB: Postoperative behavioral outcomes in children: effects of sedative premedication. *Anesthesiology* 90:758–65, 1999.)

requirements, length of hospital stays, patient satisfaction, cortisol levels, blood pressure, heart rate, and behavioral indices of recovery (Mumford et al., 1982; Andersen and Masur, 1983; Mathews and Ridgeway, 1984; Anderson, 1987; Johnston and Vogele, 1993). Reviews of this research concluded that psychologically prepared adult patients have improved postoperative recovery (Mumford et al., 1982; Suls and Wan, 1989; Johnston and Wallace, 1990; Devine, 1992; Johnston and Vogele, 1993; Contrada et al., 1994; Kiecolt-Glaser et al., 1998).

In contrast to the adult literature, there is a paucity of peer-reviewed, published outcome data regarding the question of whether heightened preoperative anxiety impairs postoperative recovery in children undergoing surgery. A large-scale study assessed this question with convergent clinical, neuroendocrinologic, and behavioral measures and found that increased preoperative anxiety in children is associated with impaired postoperative behavioral and clinical recovery. Analysis of the data indicated that children who were more anxious preoperatively showed poorer immediate clinical recovery (Kain et al., 2002c). The study also found a significant relationship between preoperative anxiety and postoperative pain and postoperative behavioral recovery. That is, children who were more anxious preoperatively were in more pain postoperatively and had a higher incidence of postoperative behavioral changes.

SUMMARY

The perioperative period may be very stressful for the young child undergoing surgery. The fear and anxiety during this period are associated not only with immediate hardship to parents and children but also with outcomes such parental satisfaction and the postoperative behavioral and clinical recovery. Here, we described a variety of behavioral interventions that can and should be used for the management of anxiety during this time period. Although some interventions such as preparation programs are well established, others, such as parental presence, music, and acupuncture, are still under development. The individual clinician should have the knowledge of the risk factors, management, and outcome of this important clinical phenomenon.

REFERENCES

American Academy of Pediatrics Committee on Hospital Care: Child life programs. *Pediatrics* 91:671–3, 1993.

Andersen KO, Masur FT: Psychological preparation for invasive medical and dental procedures. *J Behav Med* 6:17–40, 1983.

Anderson E: Preoperative preparation for cardiac surgery facilitates recovery, reduces psychological distress, and reduces the incidence of acute postoperative hypertension. *J Consult Clin Psychol* 55:513–520, 1987.

Aono J, Mamiya K, Manabe M: Preoperative anxiety is associated with a high incidence of problematic behavior on emergence after halothane anesthesia in boys. *Acta Anaesthesiol Scand* 43:542–544, 1999.

Baeck E: The neural networks of music. *Eur J Neurol* 56:449–454, 2002.

Beeby DG, Hughes JOM: Behaviour of unsedated children in the anaesthetic room. *Br J Anaesth* 52:279–281, 1980.

Bevan JC, Johnston C, Haig MJ, et al.: Preoperative parental anxiety predicts behavioral and emotional responses to induction of anesthesia in children. *Can J Anaesth* 37:177–182, 1990.

Bowie JR: Parents in the operating room. *Anesthesiology* 78:1192–1193, 1993.

Braude N, Ridley SA, Summer E: Parents and paediatric anaesthesia: A prospective survey of parental attitudes to their presence at induction. *Ann R Coll Surg Engl* 72:41–44, 1990.

Brophy CJ, Erickson MT: Children's self-statements and adjustment to elective outpatient surgery. *J Dev Behav Pediatr* 11:13–6, 1990.

Burton L: Anxiety relating to illness and treatment. In Verma V, editor: *Anxiety in children*. New York, 1984, Methuen Croom Helm.

Buss A, Plomin R: *A temperament theory of personality development*. New York, 1975, Wiley-Interscience Publications.

Buss A, Plomin R, Willevuan L: The inheritance of temperament. *J Pers* 41:513–524, 1973.

Cassady J, Kain Z: Preoperative preparation for parents of pediatric surgery patients. *Curr Anesthesiol Rep* 1:10–17, 2000.

Cassady JF Jr, Wysocki TT, Miller KM, et al.: Use of a preanesthetic video for facilitation of parental education and anxiolysis before pediatric ambulatory surgery. *Anesth Analg* 88:246–250, 1999.

Chapman AH, Loeb DG, Gibbons MJ: Psychiatric aspects of hospitalizing children. *Arch Paediatr* 73:77, 1956.

Chetta HD: The effect of music and desensitization on preoperative anxiety in children. *J Music Ther* 18:74–87, 1981.

Cohen A: Environmental noise problems in broad perspective. In *Proceedings of Symposium on Environmental Noise—Its Human and Economic Effects*. Chicago, 1970, Chicago Hearing Society.

Contrada RJ, Leventhal EA, Anderson JR: Psychological preparation for surgery: Marshalling individual and social resources to optimize self-regulation. In Maes S, Leventhal H, Johnston M, editors: *International review of health psychology*, vol 3. Hoboken, NJ, 1994, Wiley.

Corman H, Hornick E, Kritchman M, et al.: Emotional reactions of surgical patients to hospitalization, anesthesia and surgery. *Am J Surg* 96:646–653, 1958.

Devine E: Effects of psychoeducational care for adult surgical patients: A meta-analysis of 191 studies. *Patient Educ Counsel* 19:129–142, 1992.

Eckenhoff JE: Relationship of anesthesia to postoperative personality changes in children. *Am J Dis Child* 86:587–591, 1958.

Egbert L, Battit G, Turndorf H, et al.: The value of the preoperative visit by an anesthetist. *JAMA* 185:553–555, 1963.

Falk SA, Woods NF: Hospital noise—Levels and potential health hazards. *N Engl J Med* 289:774–781, 1973.

Faust J, Melamed B: Influence of arousal, previous experience, and age on surgery preparation of same day of surgery and in-hospital pediatric patients. *J Consult Clin Psychol* 52:359–365, 1984.

Ford RC, Bach SA, Fottler MD: Methods of measuring patient satisfaction in health care organizations. *Health Care Manage Rev* 22:74–89, 1997.

Fung D, Cohen MM: Measuring patient satisfaction with anesthesia care: A review of current methodology. *Anesth Analg* 87:1089–1098, 1998.

Gardner WJ, Licklider JCR: Auditory analgesia in dental operations. *J Am Dent Assoc* 59:1144–1149, 1959.

Gardner WJ, Licklider JCR, et al.: Suppression of pain by sound. *Science* 132:32–33, 1960.

Gauderer MW, Lorig JL, Eastwood DW: Is there a place for parents in the operating room? *J Pediatr Surg* 24:705–706, 1989.

Hannallah RS, Rosales JK: Experience with parents' presence during anaesthesia induction in children. *Can Anaesth Soc J* 30:286–289, 1983.

Hickmott KC, Shaw EA, Goodyer I, et al.: Anaesthetic induction in children: The effect of maternal presence on mood and subsequent behaviour. *Eur J Anaesthesiol* 6:145–155, 1989.

Hodge B, Thompson JF: Noise pollution in the operating theatre. *Lancet* 335:891–894, 1990.

Holm-Knudsen RJ, Carlin JB, McKenzie IM: Distress at induction of anaesthesia in children. A survey of incidence, associated factors and recovery characteristics. *Paediatr Anaesth* 8:383–392, 1998.

Hsu D: Acupuncture: A review. *Reg Anesth* 21:361–370, 1996.

Hyson M: Going to the doctor: A developmental study of stress and coping. *J Child Psychol Psychiatr* 24, 1983.

Janis IL: *Psychological stress: Psychoanalytic and behavioral studies of surgical patients*. New York, 1958, Wiley.

Johnson JE, Leventhal H, Dabbs JM Jr: Contribution of emotional and instrumental response processes in adaptation to surgery. *J Pers Soc Psychol* 20:55–64, 1971.

Johnston M: Anxiety in surgical patients. *Psychol Med* 10:145–152, 1980.

Johnston M, Carpenter L: Relationship between pre-operative anxiety and post-operative state. *Psychol Med* 10:361–367, 1980.

Johnston M, Vogele C: Benefits of psychological preparation for surgery: A meta-analysis. *Ann Behav Med* 15:245–256, 1993.

Johnston M, Wallace L: *Stress and medical procedures*. Oxford, England, 1990, Oxford University Press.

Kagan J, Reznick JS, Snidman N: The physiology and psychology of behavioral inhibition in children. *Child Dev* 58:1459–1473, 1987.

Kain Z: Parental presence and premedication revisited. *Curr Opin Anesth* 14:331–337, 2001.

Kain Z: Postoperative maladaptive behavioral changes in children: Incidence, risks factors and interventions. *Acta Anaesth Scand* 51:217–226, 2000.

Kain Z, Andrews-Caldwal A, Wang S: Psychological preparation of the pediatric surgical patient. *Anesth Clin North Am* 20:29–44, 2002a.

Kain Z, Caldwell-Andrews A, Blount R, et al.: Parental presence during induction of anesthesia: The development of a new intervention. *Anesthesiology* 96:A1242, 2002b.

Kain Z, Caramico L, Mayes L, et al.: Preoperative preparation programs in children: A comparative study. *Anesth Analg* 87:1249–1255, 1998a.

Kain Z, Hernandez Conte A, Kosarusavadi B, et al.: Desire for information in adults patients: A cross sectional study. *J Clin Anesth* 9:467–472, 1997a.

Kain Z, Mayes L: Anxiety in children during the perioperative period. In Borestein M, Genevro J, editors: *Child development and behavioral pediatrics*. Mahwah, NJ, 1996, Lawrence Erlbaum Associates.

Kain Z, Mayes L, Caramico L, et al.: Distress during induction of anesthesia *and* postoperative behavioral outcomes. *Anesth Analg* 88:1042–1047, 1999a.

Kain Z, Mayes L, Caramico L, et al.: Postoperative behavioral outcomes in children: Effects of sedative premedication. *Anesthesiology* 90:758–765, 1999b.

Kain Z, Mayes L, Caramico L, et al.: Social adaptability and other personality characteristics as predictors for children's reactions to surgery. *J Clin Anesth* 12:549–554, 2001a.

Kain Z, Mayes L, Cicchetti D, et al.: Measurement tool for pre-operative anxiety in children: The Yale Preoperative Anxiety Scale. *Child Neuropsychol* 1:203–210, 1995.

Kain Z, Mayes L, Cicchetti D, et al.: The Yale Preoperative Anxiety Scale: How does it compare to a gold standard? *Anesth Analg* 85:783–788, 1997b.

Kain Z, Mayes L, Wang S, et al.: Parental presence during induction of anesthesia *vs.* sedative premedication: Which intervention is more effective? *Anesthesiology* 89:1147–1156, 1998b.

Kain Z, Mayes L, Wang S, et al.: Parental presence and a sedative premedicant for children undergoing surgery: A hierarchical study. *Anesthesiology* 92:939–946, 2000.

Kain Z, Mayes LC, Bell C, et al.: Premedication in the United States: A status report. *Anesth Analg* 84:427–432, 1997c.

Kain Z, Wang SM, Caramico LA, et al.: Parental desire for perioperative information and informed consent: A two-phase study. *Anesth Analg* 84:299–306, 1997d.

Kain ZN, Caldwell-Andrews AA, Krivutza DM, et al.: Interactive music therapy as a treatment for preoperative anxiety in children: A randomized controlled trial. *Anesth Analg* 98:1260–1266, 2004a.

Kain ZN, Caldwell-Andrews AA, Krivutza D, et al.: Trends in the practice of parental presence during induction of anesthesia and the use of preoperative sedative premedication in the United States, 1995-2002: Results of a follow-up national survey. *Anesth Analg* 2004b.

Kain ZN, Caldwell-Andrews AA, LoDolce ME, et al.: The perioperative behavioral stress response in children. *Anesthesiology* 96:A1242, 2002c.

Kain ZN, Caldwell-Andrews AA, Mayes LC, et al.: Parental presence during induction of anesthesia: Physiological effects on parents. *Anesthesiology* 98:58–64, 2003a.

Kain ZN, Caldwell-Andrews AA, Wang S-M, et al.: Parental intervention choices for children undergoing repeated surgeries. *Anesth Analg* 96:970–975, 2003b.

Kain ZN, Mayes LC, Alexander GM, et al.: Sleeping characteristics of children undergoing outpatient elective surgery. *Anesthesiology* 96:1093–1101, 2002d.

Kain ZN, Mayes LC, Caramico LA: Preoperative preparation in children: A cross-sectional study. *J Clin Anesth* 8:508–514, 1996a.

Kain ZN, Mayes LC, Caramico LA, et al.: Parental presence during induction of anesthesia. A randomized controlled trial. *Anesthesiology* 84:1060–1067, 1996b.

Kain ZN, Mayes LC, O'Connor TZ, et al.: Preoperative anxiety in children. Predictors and outcomes. *Arch Pediatr Adolesc Med* 150:1238–1245, 1996c.

Kain ZN, Mayes LC, Wang SM, et al.: Parental presence and a sedative premedicant for children undergoing surgery: A hierarchical study. *Anesthesiology* 92:939–946, 2000.

Kain ZN, Rimar S, Barash PG: Cocaine abuse in the parturient and effects on the fetus and neonate. *Anesth Analg* 77:835–845, 1993.

Kane E: The phonograph in the operating room. *JAMA* 62:1829, 1914.

Karl HW, Pauza KJ, Heyneman N, et al.: Preanesthetic preparation of pediatric outpatients: The role of a videotape for parents. *J Clin Anesth* 2:172–177, 1990.

Kerrigan DD, Thevasagayam RS, Woods TO, et al.: Who's afraid of informed consent? *BMJ* 306:298–300, 1993.

Kiecolt-Glaser JK, Page G, Marucha P, et al.: Psychological influences on surgical recovery. *Am Psychol* 53:1209–1218, 1998.

Kincey J, Saltmore S: Surgical treatments. In Johnston M, Wallace L, editors: *Stress and medical procedures*. Oxford, England, 1990, Oxford University Press.

Kotiniemi L, Ryhanen P: Behavioural changes and children's memories after intravenous, inhalation and rectal induction of anaesthesia. *Paediatr Anaesth* 6:201–207, 1996.

Kotiniemi LH, Ryhanen PT, Moilanen IK: Behavioural changes in children following day-case surgery: A 4-week follow-up of 551 children. *Anaesthesia* 52:970–976, 1997a.

Kotiniemi LH, Ryhanen PT, Moilanen IK: Behavioural changes following routine ENT operations in two-to-ten-year-old children. *Paediatr Anaesth* 6:45–49, 1996.

Kotiniemi LH, Ryhanen PT, Valanne J, et al.: Postoperative symptoms at home following day-case surgery in children: A multicentre survey of 551 children. *Anaesthesia* 52:963–969, 1997b.

Lerman J: Anxiolysis—By the parent or for the parent? *Anesthesiology* 92:925, 2000.

Levy D: Psychic trauma of operations in children. *Am J Dis Child* 69:7–25, 1945.

Lewyn MJ: Should parents be present while their children receive anesthesia? *Anesth Malpract Protect* May:56–57, 1993.

Lipe A: Beyond therapy: Music, spirituality, and health in human experience: A review of literature. *J Music Therapy* 39:209–240, 2002.

Litman R, Berger A, Chhibber A: An evaluation of preoperative anxiety in a population of parents of infants and children undergoing ambulatory surgery. *Paediatr Anaesth* 6:443–447, 1996.

Lumley M, Abeles L, Melamed B, et al.: Coping outcomes in children undergoing stressful medical procedures: The role of child-environment variables. *Behav Assess* 12:223–238, 1990.

Lumley MA, Melamed BG, Abeles LA: Predicting children's presurgical anxiety and subsequent behavior changes. *J Pediatr Psychol* 18:481–497, 1993.

Macario A, Weinger M, Truong P, et al.: Which clinical anesthesia outcomes are both common and important to avoid? The perspective of a panel of expert anesthesiologists. *Anesth Analg* 88:1085–91, 1999.

Manley C: Elective genital surgery at one year of age: Psychological and surgical considerations. *Surg Clin North Am* 62:941–953, 1982.

Mathews A, Ridgeway V: Psychological preparation for surgery. In Steptoe A, Mathews A, editors: *Health care and human behaviour*. London, 1984, Academic Press.

McGraw T, Kendrick A: Oral midazolam premedication and postoperative behavior in children. *Paediatr Anaesth* 8:117–121, 1998.

Melamed B, Meyer R, Gee C, et al.: The influence of time and type of preparation on children's adjustment to hospitalization. *J Pediatr Psychol* 1:31–37, 1976.

Melamed BG: Putting the family back in the child. *Behav Res Ther* 31:239–247, 1993.

Melamed BG, Dearborn M, Hermecz DA: Necessary considerations for surgery preparation: Age and previous experience. *Psychosom Med* 45:517–525, 1983.

Melamed BG, Ridley-Johnson R: Psychological preparation of families for hospitalization. *Dev Behav Pediatr* 9:96–102, 1988.

Melamed BG, Siegel LJ: Reduction of anxiety in children facing hospitalization and surgery by use of filmed modeling. *J Consult Clin Psychol* 43:511–521, 1975.

Melamed BG, Yurcheson R, Fleece EL, et al.: Effects of film modeling on the reduction of anxiety-related behaviors in individuals varying in level of previous experience in the stress situation. *J Consult Clin Psychol* 46:1357–1367, 1978.

Mellish RWP: Preparation of a child for hospitalization and surgery. *Pediatr Clin North Am* 16:543–553, 1969.

Meyers EF, Muravchick S: Anesthesia induction technics in pediatric patients: A controlled study of behavioral consequences. *Anesth Analg* 56:538–542, 1977.

Miller S, Mangan C: Interacting effects of information and coping style in adapting to gynecologic stress: Should the doctor tell all? *J Pers Soc Psychol* 45:223–226, 1983.

Miller SM: Monitoring versus blunting styles of coping with cancer influence the information patients want and need about their disease. Implications for cancer screening and management. *Cancer* 76:167–177, 1995.

Miluck-Kolasa B, Matejek M, Stupnicki R: The effects of music listening on changes in selected physiological parameters in adult presurgical patients. *J Music Ther* 33:208–218, 1996.

Mumford E, Schlesinger HJ, Glass GV: The effects of psychological intervention on recovery from surgery and heart attacks: An analysis of the literature. *Am J Pub Health* 72:141–151, 1982.

Newman S: Anxiety, hospitalization, and surgery. In Fitzpatrick R, Hinton J, Newman S, et al., editors: *The experience of illness*. London, 1984, Tavistock Publications.

Nott M, West P: Orthopaedic theatre noise: A potential hazard to patients. *Anaesthesia* 58:784–787, 2003.

O'Byrne K, Peterson L, Saldana L: Survey of pediatric hospitals' preparation programs: Evidence of the impact of health psychology research. *Health Psychol* 16:147–154, 1997.

Padfield NL, Twohig M, Fraser ACL: Tempazepam and trimeprazine compared with placebo as premedication in children. *Br J Anaesth* 58:487–493, 1986.

Parnis SJ, Foate JA, van-der-Walt JH, et al.: Oral midazolam is an effective premedication for children having day-stay anaesthesia. *Anaesth Intensive Care* 20:9–14, 1992.

Payne KA, Coetzee AR, Mattheyse FJ, et al.: Behavioural changes in children following minor surgery—Is premedication beneficial? *Acta Anaesthesiol Belg* 43:173–179, 1992.

Peterson L, Shigetomi C: One-year follow-up of elective surgery child patients receiving preoperative preparation. *J Pediatr Psychol* 7:43–48, 1982.

Piaget J: *The language and thought of the child.* New York, 1955, Meridian Books.

Pick B, Molloy A, Hinds C, et al.: Post-operative fatigue following coronary artery bypass surgery: Relationship to emotional state and to the catecholamine response to surgery. *J Psychosom Res* 38:599–607, 1994.

Pinto RP, Hollandsworth JG Jr: Using videotape modeling to prepare children psychologically for surgery: Influence of parents and costs versus benefits of providing preparation services. *Health Psychol* 8:79–95, 1989.

Robb SL, Nichols RJ, Rutan RL, et al.: The effects of music assisted relaxation on preoperative anxiety. *Music Ther* 32:2–21, 1995.

Robinson PJ, Kobayashi K: Development and evaluation of a presurgical preparation program. *J Pediatr Psychol* 16:193–212, 1991.

Rogers M, Reich P: Psychological intervention with surgical patients: Evaluation outcome. In Fava G, Guggenheim FG, Lipowski ZJ, et al., editors: *Psychological aspects of surgery*, vol 15. Basel, 1986, Karger.

Ryder I, Spargo P: Parents in the anesthetic room: A questionnaire survey of parents' reactions. *Anaesthesia* 46:977–979, 1991.

Schofield NM, White JB: Interrelations among children, parents, premedication, and anaesthetists in paediatric day stay surgery. *BMJ* 299:1371–1375, 1989.

Schulman JL, Foley JM, Vernon DT, et al.: A study of the effect of the mother's presence during anesthesia induction. *Pediatrics* 39:111–114, 1967.

Shirley P, Thompson N, Kenward M, et al.: Parental anxiety before elective surgery in children. *Anaesthesia* 53:956–959, 1998.

Sparrow SS, Balla DA, Cicchetti DV: *Manual for the Vineland Adaptive Behavior Scales.* Circle Pines, 1984, American Guidance Services.

Standley JM: Music research in medical/dental treatment: Meta-analysis and clinical applications. *J Music Ther* 23:56–122, 1986.

Suls J, Wan CK: Effects of sensory and procedural information on coping with stressful medical procedures and pain: A meta-analysis. *J Consult Clin Psychol* 57:372–379, 1989.

Thompson JF, Kam PC: Music in the operating theatre [editorial]. *Br J Surg* 82:1586–1587, 1995.

Thompson R, Vernon D: Research on children's behavior after hospitalization: A review and synthesis. *Dev Behav Pediatr* 14:28–35, 1993.

Vernon D, Foley J, Sipowicz R, et al.: *The psychological responses of children to hospitalization and illness.* Springfield, IL, 1965, Thomas Books.

Vernon D, Thompson R: Research on the effect of experimental interventions on children's behavior after hospitalization: A review and synthesis. *Dev Behav Pediatr* 14:36–44, 1993.

Vernon DT, Schulman JL, Foley JM: Changes in children's behavior after hospitalization. *Am J Dis Child* 111:581–593, 1966.

Vessey JA, Bogetz MS, Caserza CL, et al.: Parental upset associated with participation in induction of anaesthesia in children. *Can J Anaesth* 41:276–280, 1994.

Vetter T: The epidemiology and selective identification of children at risk for preoperative anxiety reactions. *Anesth Analg* 77:96–99, 1993.

Wang S, Caldwell-Andrews A, Kain Z: The use of complementary and alternative medicines by surgical patients: A follow-up survey study. *Anesth Analg* 97:1010–1015, 2003.

Wang S, Kain Z: Acupuncture as a treatment for preoperative anxiety. *Anesth Analg* 2001a.

Wang S, Kain Z: Auricular acupuncture: A potential treatment for anxiety. *Anesth Analg* 92:548–553, 2001b.

Wang S, Kulkarni L, Dolev J, et al.: Music and preoperative anxiety: A randomized controlled study. *Anesth Analg* 94:1489–1494, 2002a.

Wang S, Maranets I, Weinberg M, et al.: Parental auricular acupuncture as an adjunct for parental presence during induction of anesthesia. *Anesthesiology* 2004.

Wang S, Peloquin C, Kain Z: Attitudes of patients undergoing surgery toward alternative medical treatment. *J Altern Complement Med* 8:351–356, 2002b.

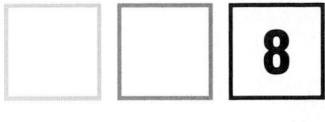

8 Preoperative Preparation for Infants and Children

Elliot J. Krane • Peter J. Davis

In addition to appreciating the emotional stresses that affect both the child and parent, the anesthesiologist must have a sound understanding of the child's medical disease and anticipated surgical procedure. The preoperative meeting with the patient and his or her parents is not only a responsibility of the anesthesiologist but also an important opportunity to learn facts that could otherwise be missed. It is a chance to win the confidence of the patient and the gratitude of the parents, if they are present. The anesthesiologist should conduct the preoperative visit wearing the operating room scrub attire and hat (Fig. 8–1), so that when the child comes to the operating room and is met by the anesthesiologist, the face and garb are familiar.

A careful preoperative examination of the child and the child's medical record enables the anesthesiologist to assess the general state of health and to identify the presence of chronic, acute, or intercurrent diseases, as well as to recognize previous anesthetic problems (Black, 1999). From this knowledge, appropriate subspecialty consultation can be sought, the operative medical condition can be optimized for the surgery, and the anesthetic plans can be made. In addition to monitoring practices and anesthetic techniques, anesthetic plans should include provisions for the patient's postoperative care, particularly an analgesic plan. It is the general goal of the preanesthetic visit to anticipate potential complications before they occur, to avert them when possible, and, in so doing, to minimize the risks to the health of the child. The risk of anesthesia is assessed during the preoperative visit, and the child's parents should be informed of the plans for anesthesia and monitoring and apprised of the anticipated risk.

■ PREANESTHETIC VISIT

The preanesthetic visit should begin with a careful review of the medical record; particular attention is paid to previous anesthetic agents and problems encountered, the successful and unsuccessful techniques used in the past for airway management, and any history of cardiorespiratory diseases or airway anomalies. A history of medical or environmental allergies should be elicited, including questions specifically directed toward evaluating the presence of allergy to latex in children at risk, notably those with meningomyelocele or urogenital anomalies; those who undergo bladder self-catheterization; or those whose medical histories indicate frequent latex exposure in the past (Beal, 1992; Levy, 1992; Sussman, 1992; Yassin et al., 1992; Meeropol et al., 1993). Results of laboratory tests should be reviewed, focusing on hematologic evaluations, renal function, and electrolyte profiles, as well as blood gas analysis and pulmonary function tests when appropriate.

The anesthesiologist must be aware of the child's current drug therapy and how it may interact with the anesthetic. The perioperative administration of bronchodilators, cancer chemotherapeutic agents, or anticholinesterases has significant implications for anesthesia (Schein and Winoker, 1975; Selvin, 1981; Drummond, 1984). Corticosteroid administration for patients who are receiving chronic corticosteroid therapy and for patients who have received steroids in the past must be addressed (see Chapter 32, Systemic Disorders). Current drug therapy must also include questions regarding the use of herbal medications. Potential complications in the perioperative period have been attributed to the use of complementary medicines. Table 8–1 summarizes the most commonly used herbal remedies (Ang-lee et al., 2001).

Many unusual syndromes occur in childhood, and they often have multisystem involvement; consequently, they have an important impact on anesthetic management. An important caveat in pediatric medicine is that when one congenital anomaly exists, there is a significant likelihood of anomalies involving other organs. For example, infants with tracheoesophageal fistulas have an increased frequency of congenital heart disease,

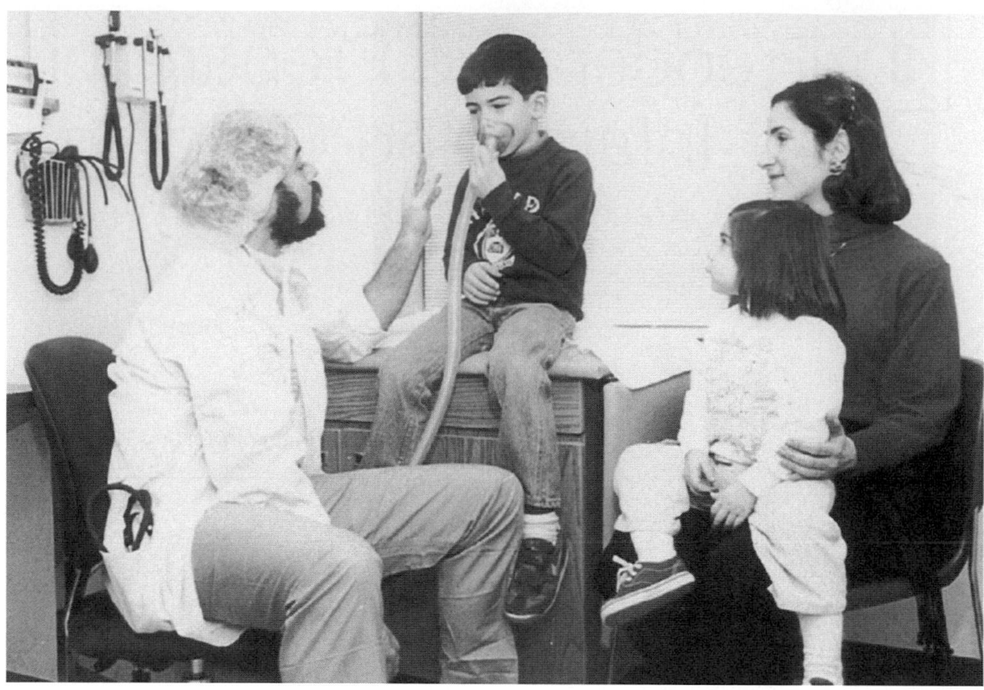

■ **FIGURE 8–1.** An instructive approach to the anesthesia induction can be taken during the preoperative visit, enabling the anesthesiologist to gain the child's trust and confidence.

and some forms of radial dysplasia may be associated with thrombocytopenia or atrial septal defects. The topic of congenital anomalies was extensively discussed in a review by Lynn (1985). Table 8–2 describes the anesthetic implications of positive findings derived from the medical history and review of systems. The remainder of this section is a review of pediatric diseases that may be important to the anesthesiologist. Information regarding these problems may be forthcoming from the child's medical history, the physical examination, or both.

■ PHYSICAL EXAMINATION

The extent of the physical examination that the anesthesiologist performs depends on the circumstances. If a small infant scheduled for a minor operation has been crying all afternoon and has finally dropped off to sleep, one can observe from the bedside the child's general nutritional state, skin color, character of respiration, and presence or absence of nasal discharge. Although the surgeon's or pediatrician's notes are helpful, they should not be a substitute for the anesthesiologist's independent examination.

Certain general principles are applied to the preoperative evaluation. In examining a child, one should look for somewhat different signs than in examining an adult. Between the ages of 4 and 8 years, children must be examined for loose primary teeth. Finding an empty dental socket after an operation is not disturbing if one knows that the child lost the tooth before admission. There is always the danger of the recent onset of an

■ **TABLE 8–1.** Pharmacologic effects and potential perioperative complications of eight commonly used herbal remedies

Name of Herb	Common Uses	Potential Perioperative Complications
Echinacea, purple cone flower root	Prophylaxis and treatment of viral, bacterial, and fungal infections	Reduced effectiveness of immunosuppressants; potential for wound infection; may cause hepatotoxicity when used with other hepatotoxic drugs
Ephedra, ma-huang	Diet aid	Dose-dependent increase in heart rate and blood pressure; arrhythmias with halothane; tachyphylaxis with intraoperative ephedrine
Garlic, ajo	Antihypertensive, lipid-lowering agent, anti–thrombus forming	May potentiate other platelet inhibitors; perioperative bleeding
Ginkgo, maidenhair; fossil tree	Circulatory stimulant; used to treat Alzheimer's disease, peripheral vascular disease, and erectile dysfunction	May potentiate other platelet inhibitors; perioperative bleeding
Ginseng	To protect the body against stress and restore homeostasis	Perioperative bleeding; potential for hypoglycemia
Kavakava, pepper	Anxiolytic	Potentiates sedative effects of anesthetic agents; possible withdrawal syndrome after sudden abstinence; Kavakava-induced hepatotoxicity
St. John's wort, goatweek, amber, hardhay	Treatment for depression and anxiety	Decreased effectiveness of cyclosporin, alfentanil, midazolam, lidocaine, calcium channel blockers, and digoxin
Valerian, vandal root, all heal	Anxiolytic and sleep aid	Potentiates sedative effects of anesthetic agents; withdrawal-type syndrome with sudden abstinence

From Skinner CM, Rangasami J: Preoperative use of herbal medicines: A patient survey. *Br J Anaesth* 89:792–795, 2002.

■ TABLE 8–2. Medical history and review of systems: Anesthetic implications

System	History	Potential Anesthetic Implication
Central nervous and neuromuscular systems	Seizure	Medications: drug interactions, inadequate anticonvulsant therapy, drug-induced hepatopathology
	Head trauma	Elevated intracranial pressure
		Anemia
	Hydrocephalus	Elevated intracranial pressure
	Central nervous system tumor	Elevated intracranial pressure
		Chemotherapeutic drug interactions
		History of steroid use
	Developmental delay	Bulbar dysfunction
		Risk of aspiration
	Neuromuscular disease	Altered response to relaxants
	Muscle disease	Risk of malignant hyperthermia
Cardiovascular system	Heart murmur	Risk of right-to-left air embolism of intravenous air bubbles
		Need for SBE prophylaxis
	Cyanotic heart defect	Right-to-left cardiac shunt
		Risk of right-to-left air embolism of intravenous air bubbles
		Hemoconcentration
		Need for SBE prophylaxis
	History of squatting	Teratology of Fallot
	Diaphoresis with feeding or crying	Congestive heart failure
	Hypertension	Coarctation of the aorta, renal disease, or pheochromacytoma
Respiratory system	Prematurity	Increased risk of postoperative apnea
	Bronchopulmonary dysplasia	Lower airway obstruction
		Reactive airway disease
		Subglottic stenosis
		Pulmonary hypertension
	Respiratory infection, cough	Reactive airways and bronchospasm
		Medication history
	Croup	Subglottic stenosis or anomaly
	Snoring	Obstructive sleep apnea
		Perioperative airway obstruction
	Asthma	β-Agonist or theophylline therapy
		History of steroid use
	Cystic fibrosis	Drug interactions
		Pulmonary toilet
		Pulmonary dysfunction and VQ mismatch
		Reactive airway disease
Gastrointestinal/hepatic systems	Vomiting, diarrhea	Electrolyte abnormality
		Dehydration
		Risk of aspiration
	Growth failure	Low glycogen reserves/risk of hypoglycemia
		Anemia
	Gastroesophageal reflux	Risk of aspiration
		Reactive airway disease
		Anemia
	Jaundice	Altered drug metabolism
		Risk of hypoglycemia
	Liver transplant recipient	Altered drug metabolism
		Immunosuppression
Renal system	Frequency, nocturia	Occult diabetes mellitus
		Electrolyte disturbance
		Urinary sepsis
	Renal failure/dialysis	Electrolyte disturbance
		Hypervolemia or hypovolemia
		Anemia
		Medication history
	Kidney transplant recipient	Immunosuppression
Endocrine system	Diabetes	Insulin requirement
		Intraoperative hyperglycemia or hypoglycemia
	Steroid therapy	Adrenocorticoid suppression
Genitourinary system	Pregnancy	Teratogenic effects
		Risk of spontaneous abortion
Hematologic system	Anemia	Transfusion requirement
		Occult sickle cell disease
	Bruising, history of bleeding	Coagulopathy
	Sickle cell disease	Anemia
		Need for hydration
		Limb tourniquet use
	Human immunodeficiency virus infection	Susceptibility to infection
		Infectious risk to medical personnel
Dental system	Loose primary teeth	Risk of aspiration of avulsed tooth

SBE, subacute bacterial endocarditis; VQ, ventilation perfusion.

Modified with permission from Coté CJ, Todres ID, Ryan JF: Preoperative evaluation of pediatric patients. In Ryan JF, Todres ID, Coté CJ, Goudsouzian N, editors: *A practice of anesthesia for infants and children.* New York, 1986, Grune & Stratton. (With permission from Elsevier.)

upper respiratory tract infection with cough, rhinitis, and pharyngitis. If an infant has a runny nose, it may be hard to determine whether it is due to an infection or simply the result of crying. Enlarged cervical nodes and otitis media occur frequently with respiratory tract infections.

Partial airway obstruction may result from infection, anatomic anomalies, or tumors. The exact diagnosis should be made before anesthesia is started. Unilateral nasal discharge is unusual and suggests a foreign body (or, rarely, choanal atresia).

When a child is scheduled for procedures such as repair of lacerations, removal of a tumor, or excision of a nevus, the anesthesiologist should personally observe the location and size of the lesion. A tumor may be the size of a pea or a melon, and a nevus may be a spot on a child's elbow or cover half a limb. The anesthesia cannot be planned intelligently without knowledge of these points.

REVIEW OF BODY SYSTEMS

CENTRAL NERVOUS SYSTEM

Disorders of the neuromuscular system only rarely escape notice during the history and review of systems; the purpose of the central nervous system (CNS) examination is primarily to assess the severity of the abnormality and the implications for anesthetic care.

Trauma is the most frequent cause of death in children, and most fatal trauma involves injury to the CNS. Head injuries frequently result in an altered level of consciousness, cerebral edema, and elevated intracranial pressure. Tumors of the brain are the most common solid tumors of childhood and usually occur in the posterior fossa. They generally increase intracranial pressure as a mass effect and often obstruct cerebrospinal fluid pathways, resulting in hydrocephalus. The anesthetic care of children with elevated intracranial pressure is discussed in Chapter 18, Anesthesia for Neurosurgery.

Serum levels of certain anticonvulsant drugs should be measured or should have been measured before elective surgery in children with chronic seizure disorders to ensure therapeutic levels. Most anticonvulsants have a long plasma half-life; missing one dose in the perioperative period does not significantly diminish the serum level. Of the commonly used anticonvulsants, only phenobarbital and phenytoin may be given intravenously in the perioperative period. Other frequently administered anticonvulsants, however, such as sodium valproate and carbamazepine, are available only as oral medications. If a prolonged period without oral intake is anticipated (such as after abdominal surgery), a neurologist should be consulted concerning possible alternative drug therapy.

Conditions such as a development delay and spastic cerebral palsy have important implications for anesthesia. In such children, the response to opioids and anesthetic agents is less predictable than that with healthy children. Many patients with cerebral palsy or mental retardation have difficulty managing oral secretions, and gastroesophageal reflux is particularly common in these children. They are at a greater risk of aspirating oral or gastric contents during induction. Cerebral palsy in later years frequently produces restrictive lung disease resulting from deformities of the spine and thoracic cage and from uncoordinated respiratory muscle function.

Neuromuscular diseases, such as congenital myotonia, muscular dystrophy, and the various forms of myositis, contraindicate the use of succinylcholine (see Chapter 32, Systemic Disorders). In myotonia, succinylcholine produces a sustained contracture of skeletal muscle, which may impede the ability to maintain a patent airway and ventilate the lungs. In other myopathies, such as clinically active dermatomyositis, succinylcholine may produce life-threatening hyperkalemia.

Several case reports noted cardiac arrest and rhabdomyolysis after the administration of halothane and succinylcholine or succinylcholine alone to children with Duchenne's muscular dystrophy (Genever, 1971; Miller et al., 1978; Seay et al., 1978; Brownell et al., 1983; Kelfer et al., 1983). As a result, the suggestion has been made that the incidence of malignant hyperthermia (MH) may be elevated in Duchenne's muscular dystrophy (Miller et al., 1978; Brownell et al., 1983). In these cases, the diagnosis of malignant hyperthermia was based on muscle biopsy and caffeine or halothane contracture test results (Brownell et al., 1983; Kelfer et al., 1983; Rosenberg and Heiman-Patterson, 1983). Although not all children with Duchenne's muscular dystrophy are susceptible, Rosenberg and Heiman-Patterson (1983) recommend that precautions against malignant hyperthermia be taken in all patients with this disorder.

CARDIOVASCULAR SYSTEM

Evaluation of the cardiovascular system is critical to the delivery of safe anesthesia. The physical examination infrequently reveals an unexpected CNS lesion, but a careful history and auscultation of the child's chest more frequently demonstrate a congenital cardiac lesion unknown to the parents or the child's surgeon.

The history and systems review yield information regarding known cardiac anomalies of an acquired disease, cyanotic defects, or the presence of congestive heart failure. Symptoms of congestive heart failure may be insidious. In an infant, whose level of activity is of course not high, the symptoms of congestive heart failure or cyanosis are most likely limited to those few periods of physical exertion, such as feeding and crying, and the only symptoms of congestive heart failure may be pallor and diaphoresis, which are subtle findings. Parents should be asked about diaphoresis during nursing or sucking. Resting tachypnea and failure to thrive also are consequences of more advanced degrees of congestive heart failure, which may be the result of ventricular volume overload (most commonly, a ventricular septal defect, patent ductus arteriosus, or anomalous pulmonary venous return), either right- or left-sided outflow obstruction, or pulmonary hypertension.

Preoperative evaluation of a patient with a known or suspected physiologically significant heart defect should include thorough history and physical examination, an electrocardiogram (ECG) and echocardiogram, determination of hematocrit, a baseline oxygen saturation value (SpO_2), a chest radiograph, and definitive knowledge of the type of cardiac lesion, its degree of severity, and its physiologic effect on cardiac efficiency and oxygen delivery. These patients should be examined meticulously and should not be accepted for anesthesia until they are in the best possible physical condition. For children with compromising lesions or those requiring cardiac medication, it is advisable to consult the cardiologist shortly before surgery.

The presence of polycythemia should be ascertained in children with cyanotic heart disease; a hematocrit greater than 65% may be reduced by red blood cell pheresis or isovolemic hemodilution. Dehydration must be avoided, preferably through the use of controlled intravenous hydration beginning the night

BOX 8–1 Pediatric Syndromes Associated With Cardiac Conditions

Syndromes Associated With Congenital Heart Disease

Apert's syndrome
Aspenia syndrome (Ivemark's syndrome)
Conradi's syndrome
DiGeorge syndrome
Down syndrome (trisomy 21)
Edwards' syndrome (trisomy 18)
Ellis-van Creveld syndrome
Goldenhar's syndrome
Holt-Oram syndrome
I-cell disease
Laurence-Moon-Biedl syndrome
LEOPARD syndrome (multiple lentigines syndrome)
Marfan syndrome
Meckel's syndrome
Noonan's syndrome
Patau's syndrome (trisomy 13)
Polysplenia
Rubinstein's syndrome
Sebaceous nevi syndrome
TAR syndrome (thrombocytopenia–absent radius syndrome)
VACTERL (vertebral, anal, cardiac, tracheal, esophageal, renal, and limb) association
VATER (vertebral defects, imperforate anus, tracheoesophageal fistula, radial and renal dysplasia) association
Williams syndrome

Syndromes Associated With Cardiomyopathy

Cretinism
Duchenne's muscular dystrophy
Farber's disease
Friedreich's ataxia
Hunter's syndrome
Hurler's syndrome
Maroteaux-Lamy syndrome
Myotonic dystrophy
McArdle's disease
Pompe's disease
Stevens-Johnson syndrome

Syndromes Associated With Autonomic Dysfunction or Arrhythmias

Albright's osteodystrophy
Guillain-Barré syndrome
Jervell and Lange-Nielsen syndrome
Riley-Day syndrome
Shy-Drager syndrome
Short QT syndrome
Sipple's syndrome
Wolff-Parkinson-White syndrome

Syndromes Associated With Thromboses or Ischemic Heart Disease

Ehlers-Danlos syndrome
Fabry's disease
Grönblad-Strandberg syndrome
Homocystinuria
Progeria
Tangier disease
Werner's syndrome

before surgery or by following the NPO guidelines and ensuring adequate oral intake of clear liquids up until 2 hours before surgery.

Particular care must be taken to rule out the existence of any infection, especially in the throat, ears, skin, or genitourinary tract. Bacteremia and infections of the teeth or gums should be controlled with appropriate antibiotics. The preoperative appearance of fever or rhinitis or a significant preoperative exposure to a source of infection should be considered a possible indication for postponement of the operation.

Asymptomatic cardiac murmurs occasionally have implications for anesthesia. If they represent small ventricular septal defects or mild valvular disease, bacterial endocarditis prophylaxis is indicated for procedures that may result in bacteremia, such as dental surgery, gastrointestinal or urogenital endoscopy, and nasotracheal intubation (see inside cover). Atrial septal defects contraindicate the use of the sitting position for suboccipital craniotomies, to minimize the risk of paradoxical air embolism (Fischler, 1992), and may make intraoperative transesophageal echocardiography desirable in certain cases that have been associated with venous air embolism (e.g., posterior spine fusions, liver transplantation), to detect the movement of air from the pulmonary to the systemic circulation. If the anesthesiologist detects a previously undescribed murmur in these circumstances, a consultation with the cardiologist is indicated to further delineate the nature of the lesion. Many congenital anomalies and syndromes are associated with cardiac defects or other cardiovascular problems; Box 8–1 provides an outline of these conditions.

RESPIRATORY SYSTEM

Chapter 2, Respiratory Physiology, describes the anatomic and physiologic differences between the pediatric and adult respiratory systems. The differences in dimension and function predispose the child to perioperative airway obstruction, which mandates a critical preoperative evaluation of the airway. The upper airway of the child may be further compromised by many entities, including tonsillar or adenoidal hypertrophy or both; craniofacial anomalies such as Crouzon's disease, Apert's syndrome, hemifacial microsomia, Goldenhar's syndrome, Treacher Collins syndrome, or Pierre Robin syndrome; lingular hypertrophy, common in Down syndrome (trisomy 21), Beckwith's syndrome, and the various forms of mucopolysaccharidosis (Hurler's syndrome and Hunter's syndrome being the most common); isolated airway anomalies such as cleft palate, laryngeal web or cleft, laryngomalacia, or subglottic stenosis; or tumors, such as hemangiomas and lymphangiomas, which may occur anywhere along the airway.

Acute upper respiratory tract infections provide a frequent dilemma for the anesthesiologist (Tait and Malviya, 2005). In the best of all worlds, no child would be anesthetized electively during an acute respiratory illness. Although not all have identified acute respiratory illness as a cause of perioperative complications in children (Elwood et al., 2003), there is compelling evidence that the occurrence of both intraoperative and postoperative hypoxemia and other airway complications is increased in children with upper respiratory tract infection (DeSoto et al., 1988; Cohen and Cameron, 1991; Kinouchi et al., 1992; Levy et al., 1992; Rolf and Coté, 1992; Parnis et al., 2001; Bordet et al., 2002) and that the incidence of bronchospasm is increased in the presence of upper respiratory infections in children who are intubated (Rolf and Coté, 1992). In a prospective study, Tait and others (2001) noted that endotracheal intubation, a history of prematurity, reactive airway disease, parental smoking, airway surgery, and nasal congestion were risk factors associated with respiratory complications in infants and children with an upper respiratory infection who were undergoing anesthesia. Furthermore, the child with an acute respiratory disease exposes other patients and health care workers to their contagion, which may not be a trivial concern when these individuals are immunocompromised.

Other considerations, however, must be taken into account in the decision to postpone surgery. For example, the small additional risk to the child must be weighed against the expense and effort the family has made to come to the hospital, often from a distant locale and at the cost of lost income. Some children, particularly many seen for otolaryngologic surgery, appear to never be free from respiratory infections during much of the year. Postponement of surgery may not be practical in these circumstances. Indeed, one study indicates myringotomy is therapeutic in these children and is not associated with an incidence of increased postoperative pulmonary complications (Tait and Knight, 1987).

The presence of acute disease of the lower airways, however, should delay elective surgery. The presence of fever, cough, and an abnormal auscultatory examination is reason for radiographic evaluation and possibly cancellation of scheduled surgery. Patients with viral lower respiratory tract infection, such as influenza, develop airway hyperreactivity that is indistinguishable from bronchial asthma and can last as long as 6 to 7 weeks from onset.

Chronic diseases of the lower respiratory tract occur in both children and adults. Asthma and cystic fibrosis are the most common chronic pulmonary diseases of childhood. A careful history and physical examination usually suffice in the preoperative evaluation of these diseases. If preoperative impairment is severe, however, or if the planned surgery is extensive, formal pulmonology consultation and pulmonary function testing may provide the anesthesiologist with information that can be used to provide optimal postoperative care. Children with asthma are frequently medicated with β_2-adrenergic agents and inhaled corticosteroids. Other first-line drugs include cromolyn sodium and leukotriene receptor antagonists; sometimes theophylline preparations are administered. The serum concentration of theophylline should be measured preoperatively to ensure a therapeutic level (10 to 20 mcg/mL), and the anesthesiologist should be aware of potential interactions among theophylline, β_2-adrenergic drugs, and halothane (although infrequently used). Asthmatic children who receive corticosteroids should also receive perioperative therapy with stress doses of corticosteroids if steroid therapy has been recent, for those children who have required systemic steroids in the past, a short course of steroids beginning 1 to 2 days before the day of surgery may be beneficial (see Chapter 32, Systemic Disorders).

Severe kyphoscoliosis frequently leads to significant restrictive lung disease. The cause of the kyphoscoliosis should be assessed because it frequently results from neuromuscular disease such as cerebral palsy or muscular dystrophy. Preoperative pulmonary function testing also predicts which children will need admission to the intensive care unit with or without mechanical ventilation postoperatively (see Chapter 21, Anesthesia for Orthopedic Surgery).

A growing population, now frequently seen in the operating room, consists of infants who have graduated from neonatal intensive care. The formerly premature infant is often left with residual chronic obstructive pulmonary disease, called bronchopulmonary dysplasia, the consequence of both oxygen toxicity and ventilator-induced lung injury to immature lungs. Children with bronchopulmonary dysplasia exhibit a combination of fibrotic changes in the lung parenchyma and reactive small airways disease with or without wheezing and air trapping. The latter may respond to steroids and bronchodilators to varying degrees. More advanced bronchopulmonary dysplasia is associated with chronic hypoxia, carbon dioxide retention, pulmonary hypertension, and ultimately cor pulmonale (Berman et al., 1982).

As in the adult with chronic pulmonary disease, elective surgery is best delayed until preoperative cardiopulmonary function has been optimized. Children with severe bronchopulmonary dysplasia are usually treated with diuretics to reduce extravascular lung water; abnormal serum electrolyte levels are common preoperatively. Adequate arterial saturation must be ensured at all times, which reduces pulmonary hypertension, and perioperative bronchodilator therapy should be given. Alterations in anesthetic care include judicious, if any, use of nitrous oxide, to avoid aggravation of pulmonary gas trapping; very careful fluid therapy and restriction of sodium load; and continuation of bronchodilator therapy. Postoperative mechanical ventilation may be required in this population.

Life-threatening apnea and bradycardia may occur after general anesthesia, most commonly in the formerly premature infant who is still less than 45 or as old as 60 weeks of postconceptional age (the sum of gestational age and the postnatal age) (Liu et al., 1980; Kurth et al., 1986; Wellborn et al., 1986). Hospital admission and respiratory monitoring are necessary for infants at risk, even after brief general anesthesia. Risk factors for postoperative apnea in formerly premature infants include a history of mechanical ventilation, a history of apnea and bradycardia, and anemia at the time of surgery (Kurth and LeBard, 1991; Wellborn et al., 1991; Spear, 1992; Malviya et al., 1993; Coté et al., 1995). In a meta-analysis of eight studies, Coté and others (1995) reported that the postconceptual age required to reduce the risk of postoperative apnea to 1% was 54 weeks for infants born at 35 weeks' gestation and 56 weeks for infants born before 32 weeks' gestation.

Congenital diseases of the lungs are usually recognized and surgically corrected in the newborn period. These conditions and their anesthetic management are discussed in Chapter 32, Systemic Disorders.

GASTROINTESTINAL SYSTEM

The primary concern of the anesthesiologist is to assess the integrity of the gastroesophageal sphincter, the emptiness of the stomach, and, hence, the risk of aspiration on induction of or emergence from anesthesia. Gastroesophageal reflux occurs as an isolated entity in some otherwise normal infants. Parents describe frequent spitting up after meals, and there may be a history of frequent lower respiratory tract infections, small airways disease, wheezing, or esophagitis, which point to the diagnosis. Gastroesophageal reflux is very common in the developmentally delayed child. After repair of tracheoesophageal fistulas, abnormalities of esophageal motility and decreased competence of the gastroesophageal sphincter are often present, increasing the risk of vomiting and aspiration on induction of anesthesia. Children who fall into these categories should be considered to have a "full stomach."

RENAL SYSTEM

Renal failure is infrequent in childhood. Chronic renal failure is typically managed with either peritoneal dialysis or, in the older child, hemodialysis. The evaluation of the child with preoperative renal disease includes serial measurements of blood pressure to assess the adequacy of antihypertensive therapy, careful determination of vascular volume, and measurement of serum levels of electrolytes, urea nitrogen, creatinine, phosphate, calcium, and magnesium, as well as hematocrit. Electrolyte levels should be within a reasonably normal range; if significant derangement exists, additional electrolyte therapy or dialysis should be performed before elective surgery. The acceptable lower limit of hematocrit is generally considered to be about 20% with chronic renal failure. Such an assumption of adaptation, however, is controversial because the blood levels of 2,3-diphosphoglycerate in these children are not necessarily increased, depending on the chronicity of anemia or recent history of dialysis.

Milder degrees of renal dysfunction may also affect anesthetic care. In small children with mild or moderate underlying renal disease, clinically significant hypervolemia may occur without compensation by augmented urine output, and an excessive sodium or free water load further deranges the serum electrolyte level. Particular caution is important in the management of fluids in children, and central venous pressure monitoring is required during major surgery in which significant blood loss or fluid shifts are anticipated (see Chapter 4, Regulation of Body Fluids and Electrolytes).

HEMATOLOGIC SYSTEM

Underlying disorders of the hematologic system are infrequent. The systems review should include an inquiry into unusual bleeding in the family's or child's medical history to explore possible genetic coagulopathies. A report of excessive bleeding from a circumcision or tonsillectomy should raise the possibility of thrombocytopenia, von Willebrand's disease, or one of the inherited factor deficiencies and is a reason to measure platelet count, bleeding time, and coagulation times (see Chapter 32, Systemic Disorders).

Sickle cell anemia typically produces no symptoms in early childhood, so a systems review is unlikely to detect its presence. For this reason, children of African heritage should be screened for sickle cell disease before surgery. A positive result should be followed by a hemoglobin electrophoresis to confirm the diagnosis or to define other hemoglobinopathies. The anesthetic plan may then be altered to ensure preoperative and postoperative hydration and to provide a high concentration of inspired oxygen. The use of a tourniquet during orthopedic surgery is contraindicated when sickle cell disease or trait is present, to prevent ischemia and subsequent sickling in the operated limb. This has become controversial, however.

In a report by the Preoperative Transfusion in Sickle Cell Disease Study Group, aggressive treatment (transfusion to a hemoglobin S level of less than 30%) was compared with a more conservative management regimen (hemoglobin maintained at 10 g/dL). The conservative approach was equally as effective as the aggressive approach in preventing serious complications but associated with half the number of transfusion-associated complications (Vichinsky et al., 1995). A hematologic consultation should be sought when diagnosis is made (see Chapter 32, Systemic Disorders).

CHILD WITH PHYSICAL OR MENTAL HANDICAPS

The most important principle in dealing with all types of physically and/or mentally handicapped children is to be considerate. In any situation involving the care of handicapped patients, it is appropriate to show appreciation of the position of the families and the dedication and deprivation they endure with remarkably little complaint. It is frequently inspiring to learn about their ability to cope with misfortune.

BRAIN DAMAGE

Children surviving severe hypoxic or traumatic brain damage and those with postinfectious encephalopathy may undergo various surgical procedures. Preoperative evaluation should include determination of the type and degree of original neurologic lesion and the patient's present neurologic status. Patients with severe neurologic lesions may depend on implanted ventriculoperitoneal shunts, and shunt patency should be ensured before the administration of anesthesia. Signs and symptoms of a blocked shunt include an abnormally low or high heart rate or blood pressure, headache, vomiting, irritability, and drowsiness. At some point in the child's past, pulmonary management may have required tracheostomy, which, if still present, may simplify induction of anesthesia, but if the patient was decannulated in the past, the upper airway may have been rendered stenotic.

Because of difficulty in swallowing, these patients often aspirate secretions, and atelectasis or pneumonia may develop. Consequently, a chest radiograph may be indicated to determine the presence and degree of ventilatory compromise. The same patients frequently have gastrostomy tubes for feeding, which should be identified, drained before the induction of anesthesia, and left open throughout the operative period to prevent gastric distension.

Old injuries, strictures, flexions, deformities, and scars should be noted, with careful description of the signs of recent injuries, pressure sores, or self-inflicted scratches and marks that might otherwise be attributed to anesthetic care. During anesthesia, added care is taken to protect all parts of the body from abnormal pressure and positioning.

CEREBRAL PALSY

Special consideration is needed when caring for patients with the diagnosis of cerebral palsy or spastic diplegia or quadriplegia (Nolan et al., 2000). Inexperienced personnel frequently make the serious mistake of assuming that patients with spastic diplegia or quadriplegia are mentally retarded, which may not be true. *Cerebral palsy* is a general term applied to several different forms of neuromuscular disability (Stiles, 1981), arising from various anatomic lesions of the brain, and not always involving mental retardation. The treatment of patients with cerebral palsy should include careful assessment of their level of intelligence. When in doubt, as with all patients who have difficulty communicating, one should assume that they can both hear and understand what is said.

MENTAL RETARDATION AND PSYCHOLOGICAL DISORDERS

The term *mental retardation* is one of the broadest in medicine, encompassing about 30 different forms (Thorn et al., 1977). Simple familial retardation, Down syndrome, autism, and phenylketonuria are well-known forms; information on more obscure forms may be found in special texts, such as that of Katz and Steward (1987). Familial mental retardation bears no specific outward stigmata, and anesthesia is adapted to the child's level of consciousness and cooperation. Down syndrome is frequently associated with congenital heart defects as well as other congenital defects. It is also frequently associated with blunting of the styloid process of the second cervical vertebra, which combined with the ligamental laxity of the syndrome allows atlanto-occipital subluxation or dislocation on marked flexion of the head and neck, resulting in spinal cord injury (Moore et al., 1987; Williams et al., 1987) (see Chapter 32, Systemic Disorders).

Autistic children are difficult to deal with and frequently are wildly resistant to any intervention. These patients may appear to be remarkably alert, in contrast to most mentally retarded patients, but they also appear to be locked within themselves. The management of the autistic child must be individualized to the dynamics particular to each child's circumstances (Rainey et al., 1998; van der Walt et al., 2001). As for other mentally retarded children, the presence of a parent at induction often has a soothing effect. Premedication with oral midazolam is often effective to sedate these children and to improve cooperation.

HYPERACTIVITY AND LACK OF COOPERATION

Hyperactive, aggressive, resistant, and uncooperative children offer challenging situations to the anesthesiologist. Such conditions are seen in pure behavioral syndromes without retardation, as well as in various forms of neurologic disease or posthypoxic lesions.

The history is carefully reviewed to determine the extent of the hyperactivity and factors that affect the behavior. Parents or attendants are questioned as to which approaches have succeeded in the past and which have not. Trial-and-error methods are not advisable. Oral premedication with benzodiazepines may be helpful. Intramuscular ketamine (2 to 4 mg/kg) may be used as a last resort.

DRUG-ABUSING CHILD AND ADOLESCENT

Drugs such as cocaine, marijuana, and lysergic acid diethylamide (LSD) have been of increasing social and medical concern. Abuse of illicit drugs is unfortunately not limited to adults. In 1993, about one of three (35.5%) high school seniors in the United States had used marijuana in their lifetime (Fig. 8–2) (Johnston et al., 1994). A survey of schoolchildren in Great Britain showed that 15.8% of boys have been offered the drug Ecstasy and that 5.7% have taken it (Milroy, 1999). A survey among college students in Great Britain indicated that the most frequently used drugs are marijuana (59%), amphetamines (19%), cocaine (18%), and LSD (18%) (Christophersen, 2000). Because drug abuse may result in increased morbidity and mortality, a thorough understanding of the consequences of drug abuse is essential for the practicing anesthesiologist.

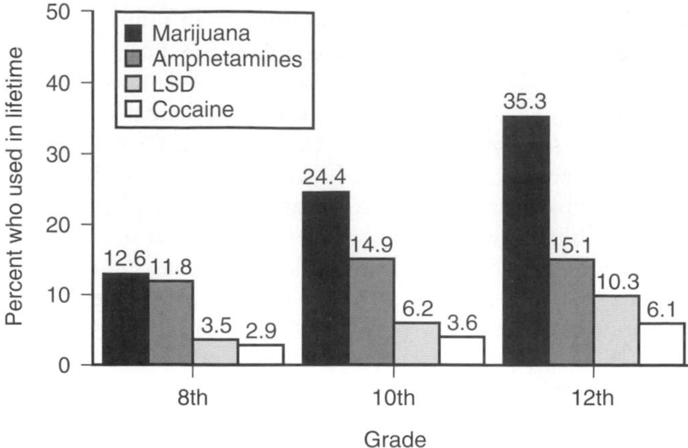

FIGURE 8–2. Percentage of high school seniors in the United States who had used marijuana in their lifetime.

COCAINE

Cocaine is an alkaloid derived from the leaves of the South American shrub *Erythroxylon coca*; it is prepared by dissolving the alkaloid base to form a water-soluble salt (cocaine hydrochloride), which can be marketed as crystals or granules (Fleming et al., 1990). Cocaine can be abused via every possible route, including oral, nasal, intravenous, and rectal. The hydrochloride form can be chemically altered to the base form, which is then concentrated by extraction in ether or baking soda (Perez-Reyes et al., 1982; Fleming et al., 1990). The residue from this method is a form of cocaine base commonly called "crack" (based on the cracking sounds it makes when heated) (Fleming et al., 1990; Julien, 1994). High levels of cocaine may persist for 6 hours after nasal administration (Inaba et al., 1978). The metabolism of cocaine occurs primarily through plasma and hepatic cholinesterase, and patients with pseudocholinesterase deficiency are at increased risk for cocaine toxicity. Less than 5% of ingested cocaine is excreted unchanged in the urine (Inaba et al., 1978). Ecgonine methyl ester and benzoylecgonine constitute over 80% of cocaine metabolites and are detected in the urine for 14 to 60 hours after cocaine use.

Medical Complications

Myocardial ischemia and infarction have been described among young cocaine users with no other known cardiac risk factors (Box 8–2) (Mittleman et al., 1999; Feldman et al., 2000). The pathophysiologic basis for cocaine-related cardiac effects is not clear, and multiple mechanisms have been postulated, including increase in myocardial oxygen demand, accelerated atherosclerosis, thrombus formation, coronary vasospasm and vasoconstriction, and abnormally enhanced platelet aggregation (Pitts et al., 1997).

BOX 8–2 Medical Complications of Cocaine Abuse

Cardiac

Myocardial ischemia/infarction
Arrhythmias
Cardiomyopathy
Myocardial depression

Neurologic

Seizures
Cerebral infarctions
Subarachnoid hemorrhage
Intracerebral bleed

Obstetric

Preterm labor
Premature rupture of membranes
Abruptio placentae
Precipitate delivery
Sudden infant death syndrome

Pediatric

Prematurity
Congenital anomalies
Neurobehavioral abnormalities
Partial ankyloglossia
Necrotizing enterocolitis

Pulmonary

Cocaine-induced asthma
Hypersensitivity pneumonitis
Chronic cough
Pulmonary edema
Pneumothorax
Pulmonary hemorrhage

Endothelin-1, a potent vasoconstrictor, is released by cocaine and may play a significant role in vasospastic angina, acute myocardial infarction, and sudden cardiac death (Wilbert-Lampen et al., 1998). Cocaine abuse has also been associated with ventricular hypertrophy, myocardial depression, and cardiomyopathy (Ghuran and Nolan, 2000). Dysrhythmias associated with cocaine use include sinus tachycardia, ventricular premature contractions, ventricular tachycardia/fibrillation, and asystole (Mouhaffel et al., 1995). Dilated cardiomyopathy, myocarditis, and congestive heart failure have also been reported secondary to cocaine use (Kloner et al., 1992; Mouhaffel et al., 1995). In addition, there is an increased incidence of hemorrhagic cerebrovascular accidents in patients who abuse cocaine (Brust, 1993).

Cocaine-related pulmonary effects occur primarily in patients who smoke crack; these include cocaine-induced asthma, hypersensitivity pneumonitis, chronic cough, pulmonary edema, and pneumopericardium (Albrecht et al., 2000). The prevalence of cocaine abuse in the obstetric population reportedly ranges from 7.5% to 45% (Kain et al., 1993). Acute cocaine use during the third trimester may result in abruptio placenta and premature labor. In the newborn, meconium staining, multiple congenital anomalies, and increased incidence of sudden infant death syndrome have been reported (Kain et al., 1993). Short- and long-term neurobehavioral problems have also been described.

Anesthetic Management

Identification of the cocaine user during the preoperative assessment presents a special challenge to the anesthesiologist, as self-reporting of drug abuse is notoriously unreliable. The nasal mucosa should be carefully observed for ulceration signs. All extremities should be examined for sclerosis of peripheral veins and needle marks from intravenous injections. Recent cocaine injection sites may also have a characteristic look of multiple ecchymoses. Auscultation over the lungs is important to exclude cocaine-induced asthma, and a careful cardiovascular and neurologic examination is necessary (Fleming et al., 1990; Kain and Rosenbaum, 1994).

Preoperative laboratory tests include complete blood cell count, with a platelet count, to rule out thrombocytopenia; ECG to identify signs of rhythm disturbance or myocardial ischemia; chest radiography to rule out any pulmonary or cardiac involvement; and abdominal radiography—cocaine and heroin addicts may present with pseudo-obstruction.

Cocaine-induced thrombocytopenia has been reported among parturients, and until the incidence of cocaine-induced thrombocytopenia is defined through prospective studies, a platelet count should be obtained before instituting a regional anesthetic. Ester local anesthetics, which undergo metabolism by plasma cholinesterase, may compete with cocaine, resulting in decreased metabolism of both drugs.

Induction and Maintenance of Anesthesia

Of concern is that (1) ketamine should be used with extreme caution in these patients because it can markedly potentiate the cardiovascular toxicity of cocaine; (2) because both cocaine and succinylcholine undergo metabolism by plasma cholinesterase, the use of succinylcholine may result in prolonged paralysis; (3) an increased anesthetic requirement for volatile anesthetics may be present in the acutely intoxicated patient; and (4) the temperature rise and sympathomimetic effects associated with cocaine can mimic malignant hyperthermia (MH), and it may be difficult to differentiate between the two.

Acutely Intoxicated Patient

General stabilization and hemodynamic control should precede induction of anesthesia. Propranolol was used successfully in the past to treat the β-adrenergic cardiac effects of cocaine (Fleming et al., 1990). Propranolol may worsen coronary vasoconstriction and should not be used if the patient presents with chest pain. Labetalol, hydralazine, and esmolol have been documented to adequately control cocaine-induced hypertension (Hollander, 1995). Intravenous nitroglycerin, which was shown to reverse both cocaine-induced hypertension and coronary vasoconstriction, may be the preferable drug. Further, Brogan and others (1991) reported that sublingual nitroglycerin, in a dose sufficient to reduce the mean arterial pressure by 10% to 15%, reverses cocaine-induced coronary artery vasoconstriction.

Clinical experience and experimental evidence support the use of benzodiazepines as a first-line treatment for cocaine-intoxicated patients (Hollander, 1995). In addition to anxiolytic effects, benzodiazepines may lower blood pressure and heart rate, thereby decreasing myocardial oxygen consumption. Benzodiazepines are recommended for patients who present with cocaine-associated chest pain and cardiac ischemic changes and for patients who present with convulsions. Also, although there are no clinical data to support the use of acetylsalicylic acid (aspirin) in patients with cocaine-associated ischemia, there is experimental evidence to support the use of this drug (Rezkalla et al., 1993).

AMPHETAMINE-RELATED DESIGNER DRUGS

The term *designer drugs* includes compounds that have been chemically altered from federally controlled substances to produce special effects and to bypass legal regulation. The largest group consists of the methylenedioxy derivatives of amphetamine and methamphetamine. Amphetamine designer drugs produce indirect sympathetic activation by releasing norepinephrine, dopamine, and serotonin from terminals in the central and autonomic central nervous system (Albertson et al., 1999; Christophersen, 2000). The best known and most widely used designer drug is 3,4-methylenedioxymethamphetamine (MDMA ["Ecstasy"]), which resembles chemically a combination of amphetamine and mescaline (Milroy, 1999). The drug can be ingested orally, injected, smoked, or snorted. The onset of action is directly related to the route of administration, and for an oral dose, onset usually occurs in 20 to 45 minutes and generally lasts up to 6 hours (Milroy, 1999). Ecstasy is metabolized by the liver and excreted by the kidney. Ecstasy was first produced in 1914 by Merck as an appetite suppressant, but it never became commercially successful (Shulgin, 1986). It resurfaced in the 1950s as a method of lowering inhibitions in patients undergoing psychoanalysis (Shulgin, 1986). Recreational use of MDMA began to surface in the early to mid-1980s in Great Britain and later in the United States. Most MDMA use occurs during "raves" (dance parties attended by thousands in abandoned warehouses) (Boot et al., 2000).

Most people who use Ecstasy experience no complications, but a number of deaths have occurred as a result of hyperthermia or idiosyncratic reactions to the drug. The most commonly seen reaction to severe or toxic ingestion of MDMA is a syndrome of altered mental status, tachycardia, tachypnea, profuse sweating, and hyperthermia (Henry, 2000). This constellation of symptoms closely resembles that caused by acute amphetamine overdose, which is not surprising given the chemical similarity of MDMA. Severe reported complications from MDMA ingestion include hyperthermia, rhabdomyolysis, renal failure, cardiovascular collapse, disseminated intravascular coagulation, hepatic failure, hyponatremia, urinary retention, cerebral infarct, and cerebral hemorrhage (Hall, 1997a; Milroy, 1999; Ghuran and Nolan, 2000; Henry, 2000; Reneman et al., 2000). Liver damage was recognized among the first deaths in the United Kingdom (Henry, 2000) and seems to be a function of hyperthermia and resulting shock and disseminated intravascular coagulopathy.

The usual presentation of cases of acute toxicity includes hyperthermia, muscle rigidity, and rise in creatinine kinase (CK) (Hall, 1997b). These patients may deteriorate toward multiple-organ failure, requiring intensive cardiovascular and respiratory support. These patients should be treated with active cooling and dantrolene given over 72 hours (Dar and McBrien, 1996). MDMA-induced hyperthermia results from augmentation of central serotonin function by stimulation of neuronal serotonin release (Dar and McBrien, 1996). Interestingly, Rittoo and Rittoo suggest that serum MDMA concentrations be measured in the admission blood sample of young adults who develop hyperthermia during general anesthesia (Rittoo and Rittoo, 1992). They also raise the question of whether patients who develop hyperthermia after Ecstasy use are at higher risk for the development of severe hyperthermia after general anesthesia.

Management is aimed at controlling symptoms. Benzodiazepines are suggested for agitation or seizures and dopamine or norepinephrine for hypotension unresponsive to fluid challenges. Also suggested are phentolamine or nitroprusside for hypertension, lidocaine for ventricular dysrhythmias, and aggressive cooling and possibly the use of dantrolene (Milroy, 1999; Ghuran and Nolan, 2000; Henry, 2000). In addition, the use of bicarbonate for rhabdomyolysis and correction of electrolyte abnormalities may be needed in the management of these patients.

MARIJUANA ABUSE

Marijuana is the most commonly used illegal drug. The hemp plant *Cannabis sativa*, from which marijuana grows throughout the world, flourishes in most temperate and tropical regions. Marijuana is commonly ingested by smoking, which increases the bioavailability of the primary psychoactive constituent, tetrahydrocannabinol (THC) (Musty et al., 1995; Hall and Solowij, 1998). Inhalation of marijuana smoke produces euphoria, signs of increased sympathetic nervous system activity, and decreased parasympathetic nervous system activity (Schwartz, 1987). At high doses, however, sympathetic activity is inhibited and parasympathetic activity is increased, leading to bradycardia and hypotension. Reversible ECG abnormalities have been reported, as well as an increase in supraventricular and ventricular ectopic activity (Ghuran and Nolan, 2000). The clinical relevance of this finding is unclear.

Pharmacologic effects of inhaled marijuana occur within minutes but rarely persist longer than 2 to 3 hours. The likelihood that an acutely intoxicated patient would present to the operating room is small. Severe tachycardia should be controlled preoperatively with labetalol or esmolol. Animal studies demonstrated decreased dose requirements for volatile anesthetics, barbiturates, and ketamine after intravenous injection of THC. Possible intraoperative complications include bronchospasm secondary to airway irritability by the marijuana smoke, although marijuana is a bronchodilator.

PHENCYCLIDINE AND LYSERGIC ACID DIETHYLAMIDE ABUSE

Phencyclidine (PCP) was developed in 1956, and it was briefly used as an anesthetic in humans before being abandoned because of the high incidence of bizarre and serious psychiatric reactions, including agitation, excitement, delirium, disorientation, and hallucinatory phenomenon (Abraham et al., 1996). If taken orally, the effects of PCP develop in 1 to 2 hours and last from 8 to 12 hours. The mechanisms of action of both PCP and LSD are quite complex and include agonist, partial agonist, and antagonist effects at various serotonin, dopaminergic, and adrenergic receptors (Abraham et al., 1996). No data exist that examines PCP and its effect on patients undergoing general anesthesia, but anesthesiologists should be familiar with the management of issues related to PCP, because this product is a structural analogue of ketamine (Jansen, 1993).

The CNS effects of LSD begin approximately 15 to 30 minutes after intake and last about 6 to 12 hours (Abraham et al., 1996). The psychological effects related to LSD are intense and include alterations in mood and emotion, euphoria, dysphoria, and visual hallucinations (Abraham and Aldridge, 1993).

LSD abuse is associated with only a mild sympathetic discharge that does not resemble that of cocaine, Ecstasy, or amphetamines (Ghuran and Nolan, 2000). These patients may also present with severe attacks of anxiety and panic. Anesthesia and surgery may precipitate these uncontrollable panic responses; diazepam or midazolam may be useful for the management of such responses. Postoperative hallucinations in patients undergoing general anesthesia have been reported as well (Morris and Magee, 1995).

PREOPERATIVE PREGNANCY TESTING

Although the pregnancy rates for teenagers continue to fall, reaching record lows for the United States in 2002, teen pregnancy remains a significant public health concern and poses a dilemma for pediatric anesthesiologists. The birth rate for the youngest teenagers is about 0.7 birth per 1000 females aged 10 to 14 years and about 44 per 1000 for girls aged 15 to 19 years (Martin et al., 2003). At least 5% of girls are or have been pregnant by the time they reach their 19th birthday, and a significant percentage of girls who present for elective or emergent surgery in their teen years have unsuspected or unrecognized pregnancies. General anesthesia and surgery in this population place them at risk for spontaneous abortions and the fetus at risk to exposure to known teratogenic substances during both the anesthetic and the perioperative period, after which the patient is no longer under the control of the anesthesiologist. It is this knowledge that leads many departments of anesthesiology to have a policy of routinely screening postmenarchal girls for pregnancy.

On the other hand, routine pregnancy screening opens a Pandora's box of legal, ethical, and practical concerns. Some of the issues are as follows:

- If an unsuspected (and, chances are, unwanted) pregnancy is discovered, the disclosure of this upsetting information to the patient and her family is a challenging task best done by a physician well acquainted with the family. The likelihood is that the anesthesiologist, and often the surgeon, have little personal knowledge of the patient and the family. How to best disclose test results, and then ensure appropriate high-risk obstetrical care, must be prospectively determined before embarking on a testing program.
- Complicating test result disclosure further is the fact that in the United States, it is illegal to share confidential medical information with a third party without the consent of the patient. If a preoperative screening pregnancy test is positive, it is necessary to share the result with the patient, who may well be a child, but it remains illegal to share the test result with a parent without the consent of the patient. This creates a challenging logistical problem for the anesthesiologist.
- The fact that there is a teenage pregnancy may imply the prior commitment of a criminal offense against the child, such as statutory rape or incest. Because of mandatory reporting requirements when child abuse is suspected, there may be criminal legal overtones to a positive pregnancy test that the anesthesiologist must address.
- Finally, although the recognition of an unsuspected teen pregnancy may be a theoretically advantageous accomplishment before elective anesthesia, the fact is that within a hospital there are many more potentially injurious events that can occur to a fetus, including exposure to ionizing radiation, teratogenic antibiotics, antineoplastic agents, etc. A pregnancy screening program makes more sense if instituted on a hospital-wide basis rather than strictly within a preoperative screening program. Hospital-wide institution of such a program relieves the anesthesiologist of the burden of test result disclosure and institution of appropriate social services.

PREOPERATIVE ORDERS

After the medical history and physical examination have been completed, preoperative orders are written.

For preoperative fasting ("NPO orders," Box 8–3), the anesthesiologist must consider the patient's age, size, and general medical condition as well as the scheduled time of surgery, if that is known. The younger the child, the smaller are the glycogen stores, and the more likely is the occurrence of hypoglycemia with prolonged intervals of fasting. For this reason, fasting time is reduced in the infant and young child. In general, solid food and milk products are prohibited within 8 and 6 hours, respectively, before surgery (generally after midnight), breast milk is prohibited within 4 hours of surgery, and clear liquids are prohibited within 2 hours of surgery. Liquids such as apple or grape juice, flat cola, and sugar water may be encouraged up to 2 hours before the induction of anesthesia. Ample experience has shown that shortened fasting times are safe, diminish preoperative anxiety and agitation, and may reduce the volume of gastric contents (Coté, 1990; Miller et al., 1990; Schreiner et al., 1990; Emerson et al., 1998; Ferrari et al., 1999). When surgery is to be delayed beyond the anticipated time, it is important that small infants, generally younger than 12 to 18 months, are offered clear fluids or given intravenous fluids to prevent significant dehydration or hypovolemia.

Regardless of the amount of time for which the patient fasts, there remains a defined population of children who are at an increased risk for regurgitation and aspiration of stomach contents. This group of children includes patients who have not fasted the requisite length of time and have sustained a severe injury during this period and children with esophageal dysmotility, incompetent gastroesophageal sphincters (gastroesophageal reflux diseases), delayed gastric emptying times, and abdominal pathology associated with ileus, vomiting, and electrolyte disorders. In addition, children with medical disorders associated with fluid and electrolyte abnormalities (such as diabetic ketoacidosis) are at risk for regurgitation and aspiration secondary to delayed gastric emptying.

BOX 8–3 Fasting (NPO) Guidelines for Elective Surgery in Infants and Children

Substance	Minimum Hours of Fasting
Solid food	8
Commercial formula	6
Milk or milk products	6
Citrus juices	6
Breast milk	4
Clear liquids	2

In these children at risk for aspiration, appropriate medical evaluation is important and preanesthetic medication with a nonparticulate antacid (e.g., Bicitra [sodium citrate/citric acid] 0.5 mL/kg), metoclopramide (0.1 mg/kg), and/or H_2-blocking agents (e.g., ranitidine 2.5 mg/kg) may be considered.

PREANESTHETIC MEDICATIONS

Preoperative anxiety not only is an unpleasant experience for the patient but also makes the induction and recovery from anesthesia more complicated (Aono et al., 1999). In addition to allaying the anxieties of surgery, separation, pain, and body disfigurement, premedication should allow a smoother and safer induction of anesthesia. The issue of which child should be premedicated and what agent should be used must be considered according to the specific needs of each child (Coté, 1999; McCann and Kain, 2001).

Which is the best agent to use for premedication? The sheer volume of articles on the subject in the literature attests to the lack of an ideal agent or combination of agents as premedication for children. Most preoperative medication is dictated by tradition. As Beecher (1959) remarked more than 40 years ago, "Empirical procedures firmly entrenched in habits of good doctors seem to have a vigor and life, not to say an immortality of their own."

The remainder of this chapter offers a discussion on the various premedications according to their drug classification. In selecting premedication, three important factors must be remembered:

1. A child's major fear concerning hospitalization is pain from needles and injections. Often hospitalization is synonymous with needles. Many children remember the premedication injection more than they do the pain associated with the operative procedure. Thus, in selecting a premedication agent, any form other than intramuscular is preferred.
2. Children who undergo frequent hospitalizations need as much or more preoperative medication during preparation than do patients undergoing surgery for the first time. Previous hospital experiences have formed the basis of their fears, so questions directed at determining their past experiences are invaluable. The previous anesthetic record should be reviewed, with careful attention given to the premedication agent and its effect.
3. The effects of premedications in children vary. Some children may be sedated, others may be excited and restless. In addition, to obtain a given level of sedation, some children may need half the recommended dose, others may need twice the recommended dose. The dosages in Table 8–3 are intended to serve only as useful guidelines.

Anticholinergic Agents

Anticholinergic agents are at present uncommonly used, although in years past they were often administered to prevent unwanted autonomic vagal reflexes or bradycardia associated with airway instrumentation, nasopharyngeal stimulation, and anesthetic drugs, particularly halothane. In addition, these compounds were administered to block the excessive secretions formerly encountered on induction of anesthesia when diethyl ether was commonly administered. There are few indications for routine premedication with an anticholinergic agent, and fewer still that cannot wait until the patient has had anesthesia induced and intravenous access established, allowing intravenous administration of the agent. Like all anesthetic agents, use of anticholinergic agents, whether as premedication or as a vagolytic agent during surgery, should be governed by the same considerations as any anesthetic agent. Side effects (temperature elevation, flushing, dry mouth, and CNS irritability) can be significant.

TABLE 8–3. Guidelines for commonly used preanesthesia medications in children

	ROUTE OF ADMINISTRATION			
Medication	*Oral*	*Intravenous*	*Transmucosal*	*Rectal*
Midazolam (mg/kg)	0.25 to 1	0.1	0.2 to 0.3 (nasal)	
Morphine (mg/kg)		0.05 to 0.1		
Fentanyl (mcg/kg)		0.5 to 1	10 to 15 (oral)	
Methohexital (mg/kg)				20 to 30
Ketamine (mg/kg)	5 to 10	1		5 to 10

Although atropine is the most commonly used agent, scopolamine and glycopyrrolate may also be used to premedicate children. Atropine, in doses of 0.02 mg/kg (0.03 mg/kg in infants), is an extremely effective vagolytic agent.

Oral atropine has been shown to be effective in preventing the adverse cardiovascular changes during induction of anesthesia (Miller and Friesen, 1987). Although injection is avoided with the use of oral atropine, the timing of its use relative to the operative procedure still must be anticipated.

Glycopyrrolate is a quaternary ammonium complex that does not cross the blood-brain barrier. As a result, it has a minimal CNS effect. It causes less tachycardia than atropine, but it is as effective as atropine at half the dose (0.01 mg/kg) as a vagolytic and antisialagogue. Studies in children have shown that glycopyrrolate reduced gastric fluid volume and altered its pH (Brock-Utne et al., 1978; Stoelting, 1978).

Opioids

Most pediatric anesthesiologists prefer not to use opioid premedication in infants younger than 6 months (Kupferberg and Way, 1963; Way et al., 1965). Opioid premedication can result in unpleasant dysphoria and an increased incidence of preoperative and postoperative vomiting. Opioids can be administered via oral, rectal, intravenous, intramuscular, and transmucosal routes. Interest in the use of opioids as preanesthetic medications has focused on the intranasal (Henderson et al., 1988) and oral transmucosal (Leiman et al., 1987; Nelson et al., 1989) forms of administration. The advantage of the latter technique is that the dose of premedication can be titrated to effect. Oral transmucosal fentanyl (OTFC) appears to have a relatively short onset time without adversely increasing gastric pH, but it does slightly increase gastric volume (Stanley et al., 1989) and delays the time that children require to tolerate postoperative fluids (Ashburn et al., 1990).

Pharmacokinetic studies have demonstrated that OTFC is absorbed through the buccal mucosa (Streisand et al., 1991). In volunteers administered an oral drink of both fentanyl and OTFC, OTFC produced higher and earlier peak plasma concentrations as well as increased bioavailability (50% versus 30%).

In blinded studies in children in which OTFC (15 to 20 mcg/kg) was compared with placebo, OTFC was superior to placebo in allowing children to separate from parents and undergo inhalation induction of anesthesia (Moore et al., 2000) but was associated with considerable untoward side effects, including nausea and vomiting, oversedation, and oxygen desaturation (Nelson et al., 1989; Streisand et al., 1989; Ashburn et al., 1990; Goldstein-Dresner et al., 1991; Moore et al., 2000). The postoperative nausea and vomiting are not attenuated by intraoperative intravenous droperidol (50 mcg/kg) (Freisen and Lockhart, 1992). The optimum dose as a preanesthetic medication appears to be 10 to 15 mcg/kg, whereas the dose for breakthrough cancer pain and postoperative analgesia may be higher (Ashburn et al., 1989, 1993). Because of the high incidence of reported side effects, as well as the need for continuous pulse oximetry while this drug is administered, OTFC as a preoperative sedative in children has not gained widespread use or popularity.

Hypnotics

Midazolam (Versed) is a water-soluble benzodiazepine with a more rapid onset time and a shorter duration of action than diazepam (Valium). Its water solubility allows better absorption after intramuscular injection and eliminates the venous irritant properties associated with diazepam (Ghoneim and Korttila, 1977). Midazolam's peak plasma concentration occurs 45 minutes after intramuscular injection, but its anxiolytic effects occur in 5 to 60 minutes. Its duration of action is usually 2 hours, with a range of 1 to 6 hours (Reves et al., 1985).

Now approved as a premedication for children, and marketed as an oral preparation, midazolam has become the most commonly administered premedication before routine surgery in virtually every pediatric center. A national survey of over 5000 anesthesiologists has indicated that midazolam is the preoperative sedative of choice in more than 90% of all routine cases in children (Kain et al., 1997). The experience with midazolam is extensive and demonstrates the drug to be highly effective in alleviating anxiety, increasing cooperation (Payne et al., 1991a; Parnis et al., 1992; Gillerman et al., 1996), and diminishing antegrade recall without affecting retrograde memory (Twersky et al., 1993; McCann and Kain, 2001). Premedication with midazolam is safe and free of side effects and does not prolong recovery times (Payne et al., 1991b; Sievers et al., 1991; McMillan et al., 1992; Weldon et al., 1992; Davis et al., 1995; Viitanen et al., 1999; Brosius and Bannister, 2002). Finally, midazolam premedication smoothes the postoperative recovery of children and diminishes the incidence of delirium (Ko et al., 2001).

Nasal midazolam has also been reported to be highly effective in reducing anxiety in children within 10 to 12 minutes of administration (Griffith et al., 1998). Furthermore, Davis and others (1995) demonstrated that nasal midazolam (0.2 to 0.3 mg/kg) administered to patients undergoing myringotomies led to reduced preoperative anxiety and did not prolong recovery time and hospital discharge time. A drawback of nasal midazolam, however, is that more than 50% of children cry on administration because it irritates the nasal passages. Midazolam can also be administered sublingually (0.2 to 0.3 mg/kg), but it may be difficult to prevent small children from either swallowing the midazolam or spitting it out immediately (Karl et al., 1993). Occasionally, younger children who refuse to take oral or nasal midazolam are more inclined to accept the midazolam rectally (McCann and Kain, 2001). Midazolam administered rectally in doses of 0.5 to 1.0 mg/kg was reported to effectively reduce the anxiety of children before induction of anesthesia, although about 20% of the children who receive rectal midazolam develop hiccups (Marhofer et al., 1999).

Flunitrazepam is a benzodiazepine 10 times more potent than diazepam. Its hypnotic and amnesic effects predominate over its sedative, anxiolytic, muscle-relaxing, and anticonvulsant effects. Flunitrazepam is relatively insoluble and has slow times of onset and recovery. Studies of this drug in children are limited, but it appears to be an effective pediatric premedication (Richardson and Manford, 1979).

As with other benzodiazepines, flunitrazepam can be administered as a rectal premedication. In a double-blind, placebo-controlled study, 0.04 mg/kg of rectal flunitrazepam provided better sedation and mask acceptance scores without prolonging recovery from anesthesia (Esteve and Saint-Maurice, 1990).

Triazolam (Halcion) is another benzodiazepine used as a preanesthetic medication. It has a short half-life, reaches peak serum concentrations in 1 to 2 hours, and has no active metabolites (Pakes et al., 1981). Baughman and others (1989) noted that in healthy adult surgical patients, 0.5 mg of triazolam provided better anxiolysis, sedation, and amnesia than placebo but similar anxiolysis and sedation as oral diazepam (15 mg). Its use in pediatric anesthesia is not well established. In children requiring dental procedures, 0.02 mg/kg of triazolam was noted to be as effective as 40 mg/kg of chloral hydrate compared with 25 mg of hydroxyzine (Meyer et al., 1990).

Ketamine

In high doses (4 to 12 mg/kg), intramuscular ketamine has been frequently used to induce and maintain anesthesia in children (Wyant, 1971). Hannallah and Patel (1989) demonstrated that at low doses (2 mg/kg), intramuscular ketamine can facilitate inhalation induction of anesthesia. In this study of uncooperative children undergoing tympanostomy tube insertion, low-dose intramuscular ketamine was very effective in completing a mask induction with halothane in a shorter time than in cooperative children who did not need premedication. Although the induction time was shorter in the group receiving ketamine, ketamine did prolong the hospital discharge times.

As an alternative to intramuscular administration, rectal, nasal transmucosal, and oral routes of ketamine administration have been reported. Rectal administration of ketamine has been reported in children undergoing a wide variety of surgical procedures. Van der Bijl and others (1991) compared rectal administration of midazolam (0.3 mg/kg) with rectal administration of ketamine (5 mg/kg). Thirty minutes after the administration of either drug, good anxiolysis, cooperation, and sedation were achieved. In doses of 8 to 10 mg/kg, Saint-Maurice and others (1979) noted that the interval from rectal administration to loss of verbal contact and acceptance of the facemask was 7 and 9 minutes, respectively.

Nasal transmucosal ketamine has also been shown to be an effective means of premedicating children. Weksler and others (1993) demonstrated that 6.0 mg/kg of nasal ketamine 20 to 40 minutes before surgery achieved satisfactory sedation in 78% of the patients.

Oral ketamine has been used as a preoperative anesthetic medication in healthy children undergoing routine surgical procedures and in children undergoing corrective surgery for congenital heart defects (Stewart et al., 1990). Gutstein and others (1992), in a double-blind, prospective study, evaluated placebo and oral ketamine at both 3.0 and 6.0 mg/kg doses as a preanesthetic medication in children. At some time during the study, 100% of the children administered 6.0 mg/kg were sedated as opposed to 73% of the children administered 3.0 mg/kg. In both groups of children who received ketamine, the onset of sedation occurred in 12 minutes, and in the 6.0 mg/kg group, 67% of patients were sufficiently sedated to have an intravenous cannula inserted. Similarly, Funk and others (2000) reported that the combination of oral midazolam and oral ketamine had a 90% success rate of satisfactory anxiolysis compared with less than 75% with either drug alone. Postanesthesia care unit discharge time of children who received orally administered ketamine is reported not to be prolonged compared with orally administered midazolam, provided that duration of surgery is longer than 30 minutes (Funk et al., 2000). Oral ketamine has also been found to be an effective premedication in alleviating the distress of invasive procedures in pediatric oncology patients (Tobias et al., 1992).

α_2-ADRENORECEPTOR AGONISTS

The role of α_2-adrenoreceptor agonists is continuing to be developed. In adults, α_2-adrenoreceptor agonists have been shown to provide perioperative sedation, postoperative analgesia, improved perioperative hemodynamic stability, and reduced anesthetic requirements (Ghignone et al., 1987; Wright et al., 1990; Carabine et al., 1991). In children, less is known about the role of α_2-adrenoreceptor agonists. The MAC-sparing effect of premedication with 1 to 10 mcg/kg of oral clonidine has been demonstrated (Nishina et al., 1996, 1997; Inomata et al., 2002). In a double-blind, randomized study, Mikawa and others (1993) demonstrated that in children, oral clonidine could produce sedation in a dose-dependent manner, and that at a dose of 4 mcg/kg, clonidine provided satisfactory sedation and better quality of child/parent separation and facemask acceptance than did standard (0.4 mg/kg) oral diazepam premedication. Fazi and others (2001) showed that oral clonidine was generally inferior to oral midazolam; although clonidine 4 mcg/kg was associated with faster awakening than midazolam 0.5 mg/kg. After clonidine premedication, children were more distressed and agitated during inhalation induction and had higher pain scores and greater analgesic requirement in the postoperative period.

Oral clonidine produces several desirable aspects of a premedication agent, notably sedation and analgesia, but the necessity to administer it 60 minutes before induction renders it an impractical drug to use for this purpose in most practices. In children, peak plasma concentration is at 60 to 90 minutes for orally administered clonidine and 50 minutes for rectally administered clonidine (Nishina et al., 1999).

SUMMARY

The pediatric anesthesiologist not only must recognize developmental differences in anatomy and physiology but also must understand and deal effectively with the emotional reactions and needs of children at various ages. Although premedication agents often alleviate the anxieties of anesthesia and surgery, these pharmacologic adjuncts cannot substitute for a thorough and thoughtful preoperative visit and discussion with the patient and family.

REFERENCES

Abraham H, Aldridge A: Adverse consequences of lysergic acid diethylamide. *Addiction* 88:1327–1334, 1993.

Abraham H, Aldridge A, Gogia P: The psychopharmacology of hallucinogens. *Neuropsycopharma* 14:285–298, 1996.

Albertson TE, Derlet RW, Van Hoozen BE: Methamphetamine and the expanding complications of amphetamines. *West J Med* 170:214–219, 1999.

Albrecht CA, Jafri A, Linville L, et al.: Cocaine-induced pneumopericardium. *Circulation* 102:2792–2794, 2000.

American Academy of Pediatrics Committee on Hospital Care: Child life programs. *Pediatrics* 91:671–673, 1993.

Ang-lee MK, Moss J, Yuan CS: Herbal medicines and perioperative care. *JAMA* 286:208, 2001.

Arthur DS, McNichol LR: Local anaesthetic techniques in paediatric surgery. *Br J Anaesth* 58:760, 1986.

Ashburn MA, Fine PG, Stanley TH: Oral transmucosal fentanyl citrate for the treatment of breakthrough cancer pain: A case report. *Anesthesiology* 71:615, 1989.

Ashburn MA, Lind GH, Gillie MN, et al.: Oral transmucosal fentanyl citrate (OTFC) for the treatment of postoperative pain. *Anesth Analg* 76:377, 1993.

Ashburn MA, Streisand JB, Tarver SD, et al.: Oral transmucosal fentanyl citrate for premedication in paediatric outpatients. *Can J Anaesth* 37:857, 1990.

Baughman VL, Becker GL, Ryan CM, et al.: Effectiveness of triazolam, diazepam, and placebo as preanesthetic medications. *Anesthesiology* 71:196, 1989.

Beal JA: Latex allergy risk management considerations. *Implant Soc* 3:5, 1992.

Beecher H: *Measurement of subjective responses—a quantitative effect of drugs.* New York, 1959, Oxford University Press.

Bellew M, Atkinson KR, Dixon G, et al.: The introduction of a paediatric anaesthesia information leaflet: An audit of its impact on parental anxiety and satisfaction. *Paediatr Anaesth* 12:124–130, 2002.

Berman W, Yabek SM, Dillon T: Evaluation of infants with bronchopulmonary dysplasia using cardiac catheterization. *Pediatrics* 55:783, 1982.

Bhatt-Mehta V, Rosen DA: Management of acute pain in children. *Clin Pharm* 10:667, 1991.

Black AE: Medical assessment of the paediatric patient. *Br J Anaesth* 83:3–15, 1999.

Boot BP, McGregor IS, Hall W: MDMA (Ecstasy) neurotoxicity: Assessing and communicating the risks. *Lancet* 355:1818–1821, 2000.

Bordet F, Allaouchiche B, Lansiaux S, et al.: Risk factors for airway complications during general anaesthesia in paediatric patients. *Paediatr Anaesth* 12:762–769, 2002.

Brock-Utne JG, Rubin J, Wilman S, et al.: The effect of glycopyrrolate (Robinul) on the lower esophageal sphincter. *Can Anaesth Soc J* 25:14, 1978.

Brogan WC 3rd, Lange RA, Kim AS, et al.: Alleviation of cocaine-induced coronary vasoconstriction by nitroglycerin. *J Am Coll Cardiol* 18:581–586, 1991.

Brosius KK, Bannister CF: Oral midazolam premedication in preadolescents and adolescents. *Anesth Analg* 94:31–36, 2002.

Brownell AKW, Paasuke RT, Elash A, et al.: Malignant hyperthermia in Duchenne muscular dystrophy. *Anesthesiology* 58:180, 1983.

Brust JC: Clinical, radiological, and pathological aspects of cerebrovascular disease associated with drug abuse. *Stroke* 24(Suppl I):I-129–I-133; discussion I-134–I-135, 1993.

Carabine UA, Wright PMC, Moore J: Preanesthetic medication with clonidine: A dose-response study. *Br J Anaesth* 67:79, 1991.

Christophersen AS: Amphetamine designer drugs—an overview and epidemiology. *Toxicol Lett* 112/113:127–131, 2000.

Cohen MM, Cameron CB: Should you cancel the operation when a child has an upper respiratory tract infection? *Anesth Analg* 72:282, 1991.

Coté CJ: NPO after midnight for children—a reappraisal. *Anesthesiology* 72;589, 1990.

Coté CJ, Todres ID, Ryan JF: Preoperative evaluation of pediatric patients. In Ryan JF, Todres ID, Coté CJ, Goudsouzian N, editors: *A practice of anesthesia for infants and children.* New York, 1986, Grune & Stratton, p 27.

Coté CJ, Zaslavsky A, Downes JJ, et al.: Postoperative apnea in former preterm infants after inguinal herniorrhaphy: A combined analysis. *Anesthesiology* 82:809–822, 1995.

Coté CJ. Preoperative preparation and premedication. *Br J Anaesth* 83:16–28, 1999.

Dalens B, Tanguy A, Haberer JP: Lumbar epidural anesthesia for operative and postoperative pain relief in infants and young children. *Anesth Analg* 65:1069, 1986.

Dar KJ, McBrien ME: MDMA induced hyperthermia: Report of a fatality and review of current therapy. *Intensive Care Med* 22:995–996, 1996.

Davis P, Tome J, McGowan F, et al.: Preanesthetic medication with intranasal midazolam for brief surgical procedures. *Anesthesiology* 82:2–5, 1995.

Davis PJ, et al.: Preanesthetic medication with intranasal midazolam for brief pediatric surgical procedures: Effect on recovery and hospital discharge times. *Anesthesiology* 82:2–5, 1995.

DeSoto H, Patel RI, Soliman IE, et al.: Changes in oxygen saturation following general anesthesia in children with upper respiratory infection and symptoms undergoing otolaryngological procedures. *Anesthesiology* 68:276, 1988.

Drummond JC: Of venous air embolism, aminophylline, and volatile agents. *Anesthesiology* 60:389, 1984.

Elwood T, Morris W, Martin LD, et al.: Bronchodilator premedication does not decrease respiratory adverse events in pediatric general anesthesia. *Can J Anaesth* 50:277–284, 2003.

Emerson BM, Wrigley SR, Newton M: Pre-operative fasting for paediatric anaesthesia. A survey of current practice. *Anaesthesia* 53:326–330, 1998.

Esteve C, Saint-Maurice C: Rectal flunitrazepam as premedication in preschool children. A double-blind, randomized study. *Acta Anaesthesiol Scand* 34:662, 1990.

Fazi L, Jantzen EC, Rose JB, et al.: A comparison of oral clonidine and oral midazolam as preanesthetic medications in the pediatric tonsillectomy patient. *Anesth Analg* 92:56–61, 2001.

Feldman JA, Fish SS, Beshansky JR, et al.: Acute cardiac ischemia in patients with cocaine-associated complaints: Results of a multicenter trial. *Ann Emerg Med* 36:469–476, 2000.

Ferrari LR, Rooney FM, Rockoff MA: Preoperative fasting practices in pediatrics. *Anesthesiology* 90:978–980, 1999.

Fishchler M: Patent foramen ovale and sitting position. *Anesthesiology* 76:46, 1992.

Fleming JA, Byck R, Barash PG: Pharmacology and therapeutic applications of cocaine. *Anesthesiology* 73:518–531, 1990.

Funk W, Jakob W, Reidl T, et al.: Oral preanaesthetic medication for children: Double-blind randomized study of a combination of midazolam and ketamine vs midazolam or ketamine alone. *Br J Anaesth* 84:335–340, 2000.

Gauderer MW, Lorig JL, Eastwood DW: Is there a place for parents in the operating room? *J Pediatr Surg* 24:705–706, 1989.

Genever EE: Suxamethonium-induced cardiac arrest in unsuspected pseudohypertrophic muscular dystrophy: Case report. *Br J Anesth* 43:984, 1971.

Ghignone M, Calvillo O, Quintin L: Anesthesia and hypertension: The effects of clonidine on perioperative hemodynamics and isoflurane requirements. *Anesthesiology* 67:3, 1987.

Ghoneim MM, Korttila K: Pharmacokinetics of intravenous anaesthetics: Implications for clinical use. *Clin Pharmacokinet* 2:344, 1977.

Ghuran A, Nolan J: Recreational drug misuse: Issues for the cardiologist. *Heart* 83:627–633, 2000.

Gillerman RG, Hinkle AJ, Green HM, et al.: Parental presence plus oral midazolam decreases frequency of 5% halothane inductions in children. *J Clin Anesth* 8:480–485, 1996.

Griffith N, Howell S, Mason D: Intranasal midazolam for premedication of children undergoing day-case anaesthesia: Comparison of two delivery systems with assessment of intra-observer variability. *Br J Anaesth* 81:65–69, 1998.

Gutstein HB, Johnson KL, Heard MB, et al.: Oral ketamine preanesthetic medication in children. *Anesthesiology* 76:28, 1992.

Hall AP: "Ecstasy" and the anaesthetist. *Br J Anaesth* 79:697–698, 1997a.

Hall AP: Ecstasy: Creatinine kinase. *Anaesth Intens Care* 25:586–587, 1997b.

Hall W, Solowij N: Adverse effects of cannabis. *Lancet* 352:1611–1616, 1998.

Hannallah R, Patel RI: Low-dose intramuscular ketamine for anesthesia pre-induction in young children undergoing brief outpatient procedures. *Anesthesiology* 70:598, 1989.

Henderson JM, Brodsky DA, Fisher DM, et al.: Pre-induction of anesthesia in pediatric patients with nasally administered sufentanil. *Anesthesiology* 68:671, 1988.

Henry J: Metabolic consequences of drug misuse. *Br J Anaesth* 85:136–142, 2000.

Hollander JE: The management of cocaine-associated myocardial ischemia. *N Engl J Med* 333:1267–1272, 1995.

Inaba T, Stewart DJ, Kalow W: Metabolism of cocaine in man. *Clin Pharmacol Ther* 23:547–552, 1978.

Inomata S, Kihara S, Miyabe M, et al.: The hypnotic and analgesic effects of oral clonidine during sevoflurane anesthesia in children: A dose-response study. *Anesth Analg* 94:1479–1483, table of contents, 2002.

Jansen K: Non-medical use of ketamine. *BMJ* 306:601–602, 1993.

Johnston L, O'Malley P, Bachman J: *National survey results on drug use from the monitoring the future study, 1975-1993. Volume I: Secondary school students.* Rockville, MD, National Institute on Drug Abuse, 1994, DHHS Publication No. [NIH] 94-0000.

Julien R: *Psychostimulants: Cocaine and amphetamines*, ed 7. New York, 1994, W.H. Freeman.

Kain Z: Parental presence and premedication revisited. *Curr Opin Anesth* 14:331–337, 2001.

Kain Z, Mayes LC, Bell C, et al.: Premedication in the United States: A status report. *Anesth Analg* 84:427–432, 1997.

Kain Z, Rosenbaum H: Physiology and management of cocaine exposure preceding emergency anesthesia and surgery. *Curr Opin Anesthesiol* 7:293–298, 1994.

Kain ZN, Mayes LC, Caramico LA, et al.: Parental presence during induction of anesthesia. A randomized controlled trial. *Anesthesiology* 84:1060–1067, 1996.

Kain ZN, Rimar S, Barash PG: Cocaine abuse in the parturient and effects on the fetus and neonate. *Anesth Analg* 77:835–845, 1993.

Kam PC, Voss TJ, Gold PD, et al.: Behaviour of children associated with parental participation during induction of general anaesthesia. *J Paediatr Child Health* 34:29–31, 1998.

Karl HW, Rosenberger JL, Larach MG, et al.: Transmucosal administration of midazolam for premedication of pediatric patients. Comparison of the nasal and sublingual routes. *Anesthesiology* 78:885–891, 1993.

Katz J, Steward DJ, editors: *Anesthesia and uncommon pediatric diseases*, Philadelphia, PA, 1987, WB Saunders.

Kelfer HM, Singer WD, Reynolds RN: Malignant hyperthermia in a child with Duchenne muscular dystrophy. *Pediatrics* 71:118, 1983.

Kinouchi K, Tanigami H, Tashiro C, et al.: Duration of apnea in anesthetized infants and children required for desaturation of hemoglobin to 95%. The influence of upper respiratory infection. *Anesthesiology* 77:1105, 1992.

Kloner RA, Hale S, Alker K, et al.: The effects of acute and chronic cocaine use on the heart. *Circulation* 85:407–419, 1992.

Ko YP, Huang CJ, Hung YC, et al.: Premedication with low-dose oral midazolam reduces the incidence and severity of emergence agitation in pediatric patients following sevoflurane anesthesia. *Acta Anaesthesiol Sin* 39:169–177, 2001.

Koinig H: Preparing parents for their child's surgery: Preoperative parental information and education. *Paediatr Anaesth* 12:107–109, 2002.

Korsch BM: The child and the operating room. *Anesthesiology* 43:251, 1975.

Kotiniemi LH, Ryhanen PT, Moilanen IK: Behavioural changes following routine ENT operations in two-to-ten-year-old children. *Paediatr Anaesth* 6:45–49, 1996.

Krane EJ, Jacobson LE, Lynn AM, et al.: Caudal morphine for postoperative analgesia in children. *Anesth Analg* 66:647, 1987.

Kupferberg HJ, Way EL: Pharmacologic basis for the increased sensitivity of the newborn rat to morphine. *J Pharmacol Exp Ther* 141:105, 1963.

Kurth CD, LeBard SE: Association of postoperative apnea, airway obstruction and hypoxemia in former premature infants. *Anesthesiology* 75:22, 1991.

Kurth CD, Spitzer AR, Broennie AM, et al.: Postoperative apnea in preterm infants. *Anesthesiology* 66:483, 1986.

Leigh JM, Walker J, Janaganathan P: Effect of preoperative anaesthetic visit on anxiety. *Br J Med* 2:987, 1977.

Leiman BC, Walford A, Rawal N, et al.: The effects of oral transmucosal fentanyl citrate premedication on gastric volume and acidity in children. *Anesthesiology* 87:A489, 1987.

Levy DA, Charpin D, Pecquet C, et al.: Allergy to latex. *Allergy* 47:579, 1992.

Levy L, Pandit UA, Randel GI, et al.: Upper respiratory tract infections and general anaesthesia in children. Perioperative complications and oxygen saturation. *Anaesthesia* 47:678, 1992.

Liu LMP, Coté CJ, Goudsouzian NG, et al.: Life-threatening apnea in infants recovering from anesthesia. *Anesthesiology* 59:283, 1980.

Lockhart CH: *Preoperative preparation of the child for hospitalization, anesthesia, and surgery.* Annual Refresher Course Lectures, American Society of Anesthesiologists, Philadelphia, No. 125, 1984, Lippincott.

Lynn AM: Unusual conditions in paediatric anaesthesia. *Clin Anaesth* 3:379, 1985.

Malviya S, Swartz J, Lerman J: Are all preterm infants younger than 60 weeks post conceptual age at risk for postanesthetic apnea? *Anesthesiology* 78:1076, 1993.

Marhofer P, Glaser C, Krenn CG, et al.: Incidence of therapy of midazolam induced hiccups in paediatric anaesthesia. *Paediatr Anaesth* 9:295–298, 1999.

Martin JA, Hamilton BE, Sutton PD, et al.: *Births: Final data for 2002. National vital statistics reports.* Hyattsville, MD, 2003, National Center for Health Statistics, publication 52(10).

Mather L, Mackie J: The incidence of postoperative pain in children. *Pain* 15:271, 1983.

McCann M, Kain ZN: Management of preoperative anxiety in children: An update. *Anesth Analg* 93:98–105, 2001.

McMillan CO, Spahr Schopfer IA, Sikich N, et al.: Premedication of children with oral midazolam. *Can J Anaesth* 39:545, 1992.

Meeropol E, Frost J, Pugh L, et al.: Latex allergy in children with myelodysplasia: A survey of Shriners hospitals. *J Pediatr Orthop* 13:1, 1993.

Meyer ML, Mourino AP, Farringtron FH: Comparison of triazolam to a chloral hydrate/hydroxyzine combination in the sedation of pediatric dental patients. *Pediatr Dent* 12:283, 1990.

Mikawa K, Mackawa N, Nishina K, et al.: Efficacy of oral clonidine premedications in children. *Anesthesiology* 79:926, 1993.

Miller BR, Friesen RH: Oral atropine premedication in infants. *Anesthesiology* 67:A491, 1987.

Miller BR, Tharp JA, Isaacs WB: Gastric residual volume in infants and children following a 3-hour fast. *J Clin Anesth* 2:301, 1990.

Miller ED Jr, Sanders DB, Rowlington JC, et al.: Anesthesia-induced rhabdomyolysis in a patient with Duchenne's muscular dystrophy. *Anesthesiology* 48:146, 1978.

Milroy CM: Ten years of "ecstasy." *J R Soc Med* 92:68–71, 1999.

Miluk-Kolasa B, Obminski Z, Stupnicki R, et al.: Effects of music treatment on salivary cortisol in patients exposed to pre-surgical stress. *Exp Clin Endocrinol* 102:118–120, 1994.

Mittleman MA, Mintzer D, Maclure M, et al.: Triggering of myocardial infarction by cocaine. *Circulation* 99:2737–2741, 1999.

Moore PA, Cuddy MA, Magera JA, et al.: Oral transmucosal fentanyl pretreatment for outpatient general anesthesia. *Anesth Prog* 47:29–34, 2000.

Moore RA, McNicholas KW, Warren SP: Atlantoaxial subluxation with symptomatic spinal cord compression in a child with Down's syndrome. *Anesth Analg* 66:89, 1987.

Morris G, Magee P: Anaesthesia and past use of LSD. *Can J Anaesth* 42:177, 1995.

Mouhaffel AH, Madu EC, Satmary WA, et al.: Cardiovascular complications of cocaine. *Chest* 107:1426–1434, 1995.

Musty R, Reggio P, Consroe P: A review of recent advances in cannabinoid research and the 1994 International Symposium on Cannabis and the Cannabinoids. *Life Sci* 56:1933–1940, 1995.

Nelson PS, Streisand JB, Mulder SM, et al.: Comparison of oral transmucosal fentanyl citrate and an oral solution of meperidine, diazepam, and atropine for premedication in children. *Anesthesiology* 70:616, 1989.

NIH Consensus Development Panel on Acupuncture: Acupuncture. *JAMA* 280:1518–1524, 1998.

Nishina K, Mikawa K, Shiga M, et al.: Clonidine in paediatric anaesthesia. *Paediatr Anaesth* 9:187–202, 1999.

Nishina K, Mikawa K, Maekawa N, et al.: The efficacy of clonidine for reducing perioperative haemodynamic changes and volatile anaesthetic requirements in children. *Acta Anaesthesiol Scand* 40:746–751, 1996.

Nishina K, Mikawa K, Shiga M, et al.: Oral clonidine premedication reduces minimum alveolar concentration of sevoflurane for tracheal intubation in children. *Anesthesiology* 87:1324–1327, 1997.

Nolan J, Chalkiadis GA, Low J, et al.: Anaesthesia and pain management in cerebral palsy. *Anaesthesia* 55:32–41, 2000.

Pakes GE, Brogden RN, Heel RC, et al.: Triazolam: A review of its pharmacological properties and therapeutic efficacy in patients with insomnia. *Drugs* 22:81, 1981.

Parnis SJ, Barker DS, van der Walt JH: Clinical predictors of anaesthetic complications in children with respiratory tract infections. *Paediatr Anaesth* 11:29–40, 2001.

Parnis SJ, Foate JA, van der Walt JH, et al.: Oral midazolam is an effective premedication for children having day-stay anaesthesia. *Anaesth Intensive Care* 20:9–14, 1992.

Payne KA, Coetzee AR, Mattheyse FJ: Midazolam and amnesia in pediatric premedication. *Acta Anaesthesiol Belg* 42:101, 1991a.

Payne KA, Coetzee AR, Mattheyse FJ, et al.: Oral midazolam in paediatric premedication. *S Afr Med J* 79:372, 1991b.

Perez-Reyes M, Di Guiseppi S, Ondrusek G, et al.: Free-base cocaine smoking. *Clin Pharmacol Ther* 32:459–465, 1982.

Pitts W, Lange R, Cigarroa J, et al.: Cocaine-induced myocardial ischemia and infarction: Physiology, pathology, recognition, and management. *Prog Cardiovasc Dis* 40:65–76, 1997.

Rainey L, van der Walt JH: The anaesthetic management of autistic children. *Anaesth Intensive Care* 26:682–686, 1998.

Reneman L, Habraken JB, Majoie CB, et al.: MDMA ("Ecstasy") and its association with cerebrovascular accidents: Preliminary findings. *AJNR Am J Neuroradiol* 21:1001–1007, 2000.

Reves JG, Fragen RJ, Vinik HR, et al.: Midazolam: Pharmacology and uses. *Anesthesiology* 62:310, 1985.

Rezkalla SH, Mazza JJ, Kloner RA, et al.: Effects of cocaine on human platelets in healthy subjects. *Am J Cardiol* 72:243–246, 1993.

Richardson F, Manford M: Comparison of flunitrazepam and diazepam for oral premedication in older children. *Br J Anaesth* 51:313, 1979.

Rittoo DB, Rittoo D: Complications of "ecstasy" misuse. *Lancet* 340:725–726, 1992.

Rolf N, Coté CJ: Frequency and severity of desaturation events during general anesthesia in children with and without upper respiratory infections. *J Clin Anesth* 4:200, 1992.

Rosenberg H, Heiman-Patterson T: Duchenne's muscular dystrophy and malignant hyperthermia: another warning [letter]. *Anesthesiology* 59:362, 1983.

Saint-Maurice C, Laguenie G, Couturier C, et al.: Rectal ketamine in paediatric anaesthesia. *Br J Anaesth* 51:573, 1979.

Saint-Maurice C, Meistelman C, Rey E, et al.: The pharmacokinetics of rectal midazolam for premedication in children. *Anesthesiology* 65:536, 1986.

Schechter NL: Status of pediatric pain control. *Pediatrics* 77:11, 1986.

Schein PS, Winoker SH: Immunosuppressive and cytotoxic chemotherapy: Long-term complications. *Ann Intern Med* 82:84, 1975.

Schreiner MS, Triebwasser A, Keon TP: Ingestion of liquids compared with perioperative fasting in pediatric outpatients. *Anesthesiology* 72:593, 1990.

Schwartz R: Marijuana: An overview. *Pediatr Clin North Am* 34:305–317, 1987.

Seay AR, Ziter FA, Thompson JA: Cardiac arrest during induction of anesthesia in Duchenne muscular dystrophy. *J Pediatr* 93:88, 1978.

Selvin BL: Cancer chemotherapy: Implications for the anesthesiologist. *Anesth Analg* 60:425, 1981.

Shulgin A: The background and chemistry of MDMA. *J Psychoactive Drugs* 18:291–304, 1986.

Sievers TD, Yee JD, Foley ME, et al.: Midazolam for conscious sedation during pediatric oncology procedures: Safety and recovery parameters. *Pediatrics* 88:172, 1991.

Skinner CM, Rangasami J: Preoperative use of herbal medicines: A patient survey. *Br J Anaesth* 89:792–795, 2002.

Spear RM: Anesthesia for premature and term infants: Perioperative implications. *J Pediatr* 120:165, 1992.

Stanley TH, Leiman BC, Rawal N, et al.: The effects of oral transmucosal and gastric volume and acidity in children. *Anesth Analg* 69:328, 1989.

Steward DJ: Psychological preparation and premedication. In Gregory GA, editor: *Pediatric anesthesia*. New York, 1983, Churchill Livingstone.

Stewart KG, Rowbottom SJ, Aiken AW, et al.: Oral ketamine premedication for paediatric cardiac surgery—a comparison with intramuscular morphine (both after oral trimeprazine). *Anaesth Intensive Care* 18:11, 1990.

Stiles CM: Anesthesia for the mentally retarded patient. *Orthop Clin North Am* 12:45, 1981.

Stoelting RK: Responses to atropine, glycopyrrolate, and Riopan on gastric fluid pH and volume in adult patients. *Anesthesiology* 18:367, 1978.

Streisand JB, Varvel JR, Stanski DR, et al.: Absorption and bioavailability of oral transmucosal fentanyl citrate. *Anesthesiology* 75:223, 1991.

Sussman GL: Latex allergy: Its importance in clinical practice. *Allergy Proc* 13:67, 1992.

Tait AR, Knight PR: The effects of general anesthesia on upper respiratory tract infections in children. *Anesthesiology* 67:930, 1987.

Tait AR, Malviya S, Voepel-Lewis T, et al.: Risk factors for perioperative adverse respiratory events in children with upper respiratory tract infections. *Anesthesiology* 95:299–306, 2001.

Tait AR, Malviya S: Anesthesia for the child with an upper respiratory tract infection: Still a dilemma? *Anesthesiol Analg* 100:59–65, 2005.

Thorn GW, Adams RD, Braunwaid E, et al.: *Harrison's principles of internal medicine*, ed 8. New York, 1977, McGraw-Hill Book Co.

Tobias JD, Phipps S, Smith B, et al.: Oral ketamine premedication to alleviate the distress of invasive procedures in pediatric oncology patients. *Pediatrics* 90:537, 1992.

Twersky RS, Hartung J, Berger BJ, et al.: Midazolam enhances antegrade but not retrograde amnesia in pediatric patients. *Anesthesiology* 78:51, 1993.

Van der Bijl P, Roelofse JA, Stander IA: Rectal ketamine and midazolam for premedication in pediatric dentistry. *J Oral Maxillofac Surg* 49:1050, 1991.

van der Walt JH, Moran C: An audit of perioperative management of autistic children. *Paediatr Anaesth* 11:401–408, 2001.

Vernon DTA, Bailey WC: The use of motion pictures in the psychological preparation of children for induction of anesthesia. *Anesthesiology* 40:68, 1974.

Vichinsky EP, Haberkern CM, Neumayr L, et al.: The Preoperative Transfusion in Sickle Cell Disease Study Group: A comparison of conservative and aggressive transfusion regimens in the perioperative management of sickle cell disease. *N Engl J Med* 333:206–213, 1995.

Viitanen H, Annila P, Viitanen M, et al.: Midazolam premedication delays recovery from propofol-induced sevoflurane anesthesia in children 1-3 yr. *Can J Anaesth* 46:766–771, 1999.

Visintainer MA, Wolfer JA: Psychological preparation for surgical pediatric patients: The effect on children's and parent's stress responses and adjustment. *Pediatrics* 56:187, 1975.

Way WL, Costley EC, Way EL: Respiratory sensitivity of the newborn infant to meperidine and morphine. *Clin Pharmacol Ther* 6:454, 1965.

Weksler N, Ovadia L, Muati G, et al.: Nasal ketamine for paediatric premedication. *Can J Anaesth* 40:119, 1993.

Weldon BC, Watcha MF, White PF: Oral midazolam in children: Effect of time and adjunctive therapy. *Anesth Analg* 75:51, 1992.

Wellborn LG, Hannallah RS, Luban NL, et al.: Anemia and postoperative apnea in former preterm infants. *Anesthesiology* 74:1003, 1991.

Wellborn LG, Ramirez N, Oh TH, et al.: Postanesthetic apnea and periodic breathing in infants. *Anesthesiology* 65:658, 1986.

Wilbert-Lampen U, Seliger C, Zilker T, et al.: Cocaine increases the endothelial release of immunoreactive endothelin and its concentrations in human plasma and urine: Reversal by coincubation with sigma-receptor antagonists. *Circulation* 98:385–390, 1998.

Williams JO, Somerville GM, Miner ME, et al.: Atlanto-axial subluxation and trisomy-21: Another perioperative complication. *Anesthesiology* 67:253, 1987.

Wright PMC, Carabine UA, McClune S, et al.: Preanesthetic medication with clonidine. *Br J Anaesth* 65:628, 1990.

Wyant GM: Intramuscular ketalar (CI-581) in paediatric anaesthesia. *Can Anaesth Soc J* 18:72, 1971.

Yassin MS, Sanyurah S, Lierl MB, et al.: Evaluation of latex allergy in patients with meningomyelocele. *Ann Allergy* 69:207, 1992.

Yaster M, Deshpande JK, Maxwell LG: The pharmacologic management of pain in children. *Compre Ther* 15:14, 1989.

Zuwala R, Barber KR: Reducing anxiety in parents before and during pediatric anesthesia induction. *AANA J* 69:21–25, 2001.

9 Pediatric Anesthesia Equipment and Monitoring

Ronald S. Litman • David E. Cohen • Robert J. Sclabassi

Confronted with the task of caring for the tiny neonate or the large adolescent while providing optimal conditions for simple or complex surgical procedures, the pediatric anesthesiologist requires a wide variety of equipment and monitors often specifically adapted or developed for the pediatric patient. Specific modifications and adaptations of complex monitoring technology enhance the moment-to-moment surveillance of the anesthetized child, supplementing the anesthesiologist's direct observation of the patient. National and local standards reinforce this need for specially adapted electronic surveillance even in the simplest of anesthetic procedures and in the healthiest of children. This chapter focuses on the types of equipment and monitoring devices that are used in pediatric anesthesia.

■ LATEX ALLERGY

With an increasing frequency, anaphylactic reactions to latex (natural rubber) have produced catastrophic problems for the pediatric anesthesiologist (Slater et al., 1990; Holzman, 1993; Hepner and Castells, 2003). Children with myelodysplasia, congenital urologic abnormalities, or cerebral palsy with ventriculoperitoneal shunts are at the greatest risk for intraoperative reactions (Kelly et al., 1991; Dormans et al., 1994, 1997). This may be related to repeated exposure to rubber products during surgery or other procedures. The U.S. Food and Drug Administration has recommended that all patients should be questioned for latex hypersensitivity (1991). Even with a negative history for sensitivity to latex products, anaphylactic reactions have occurred, especially in the high-risk groups noted (Gold et al., 1991). Prophylactic management of children with known hypersensitivity or those at high risk may minimize both the incidence and severity of possible reactions (Dormans et al., 1994). The benefit of this type of management is unknown and there are numerous reports of failure of premedication to prevent allergic reactions to latex (Kwittken et al., 1992). Minimizing exposure to latex in the operating room is vitally important to both patients and workers. The use of a latex-safe protocol without premedication has been used successfully (Holzman, 1997; Berry et al., 2001). Unfortunately, latex is ubiquitous in anesthetic and surgical equipment.

Substitution of latex-containing products and devices with latex-free devices minimizes exposure to the patient. The Food and Drug Administration has mandated that medical devices with natural rubber latex be identified on product and package labeling (Hubbard, 1997). Careful examination of the components of each device or disposable product in the operating room complex is needed to identify problematic products. When substitute products are not available, efforts need to be made to shield or minimize contact between these devices and the child at risk.

■ ANESTHESIA MACHINES

Although much of the equipment discussed in this chapter is designed specifically for pediatric use, no anesthesia machines are dedicated exclusively to pediatric applications. There are certain characteristics that should be sought in an anesthesia machine to be used in pediatric patients.

Measures should be taken to eliminate the risk of unintentional administration of an hypoxic gas mixture. The American Society for Testing and Materials (ASTM) (F-1850-00, 2005) specifies that all machines be designed to deliver a preset oxygen concentration at any flow and oxygen gas pressure. Because these safety mechanisms can fail, an oxygen analyzer should be maintained in-line as specified in the *Standards for Basic Anesthetic Monitoring* of the American Society of Anesthesiologists (ASA) (2003; Box 9-1).

When fragile hemodynamics or the patient's condition (e.g., necrotizing enterocolitis) precludes the use of nitrous oxide, compressed air should be available to reduce the inspired oxygen concentration (F_{IO_2}). Another example is the premature infant at risk for retinopathy of prematurity (ROP). Clinical studies implicate arterial oxygen tension as one of several variables linked to ROP in the most vulnerable population of preterm infants (<1300 grams) whose retinas are immature (Flynn et al., 1992). The contribution of brief periods of intraoperative hyperoxemia to the development of ROP remains unknown; oxygen concentrations greater than necessary should be avoided in this vulnerable population. Compressed air is usually required during airway laser surgery to reduce the concentration of inhaled gas mixtures that support combustion (i.e., nitrous oxide, oxygen). Specially adapted anesthesia machines capable of delivering inspired carbon dioxide to achieve hypercarbia or increased inspired nitrogen to produce hypoxia may be indicated in the care of the neonate with specific types of congenital heart disease (Tabbutt et al., 2001).

Another feature of an anesthesia machine that is useful in pediatric anesthesia is the ability to accommodate special pediatric circuits (e.g., Mapleson). This represents more than a convenience, as it avoids the inherent dangers of "modifying" vital equipment to meet the needs of these circuits. A well-designed pediatric breathing circuit reduces the risk of incorrect assembly by those who use these circuits infrequently.

■ ANESTHESIA MACHINE VENTILATORS

An anesthesia machine ventilator appropriate for infants and small children should be capable of accurately delivering a range of small tidal volumes and high ventilatory rates. Newer anesthesia machines have ventilators that can precisely deliver small volumes at high rates (e.g., NAD 6000; North American Dräger, Telford, PA) (Stayer et al., 2000). The standard ventilators used in pediatric intensive care units can be adapted for use in the operating room (e.g., Siemens Servo 900C; Siemens-Elema AB, Sweden). The added cost and complexity of this approach may be warranted only in children with preexisting pulmonary disease.

■ HUMIDIFIERS

In the human respiratory tract, inspired gases are warmed and brought to 100% relative humidity (44 mg H_2O/L at 37°C). The caloric expenditure of humidification consumes approximately five times the energy required to heat the inspired gases (Rashad and Benson, 1967); this may amount to 20% of the basal metabolic rate of an infant.

Benefits of heating and humidifying anesthetic gases include prevention of intraoperative hypothermia, decreased atelectasis, improved mucociliary clearance, and reduced impairment of ciliary function caused by inhalation of dry anesthetic gases. Partial humidification of gas in the anesthesia breathing circuit takes place within the carbon dioxide absorber, which uses an exothermic reaction that may raise the water vapor content to as much as 29 mg/L. Further humidification is accomplished by reducing the amount of fresh gas flow, thereby increasing rebreathing of humidified gases, and using a heat and moisture exchanger (HME) ("artificial nose"), which uses a fine mesh to cause condensation of exhaled water vapor. The latter may increase the resistance to breathing for some infants and children, although these changes are usually tolerable. HMEs increase airway humidification and preserve temperature in anesthetized children at a lower cost than active humidification systems (Bissonnette and Sessler, 1989). They require 80 minutes to achieve optimal saturation of the membrane, during which time they are less efficient. Specially designed HMEs filter out infectious pathogens and minimize the risk of cross-infection between patients (Wilkes et al., 2000).

Active humidification is the most efficient means by which to heat and humidify inspired gases (Bissonnette and Sessler, 1989). A servo-controlled, shielded heated wire in the fresh gas line helps to prevent cooling and condensation of the water as it passes through the inspiratory limb. The temperature should be

BOX 9–1 **Standards for Basic Anesthetic Monitoring**
(Approved by House of Delegates on October 21, 1986, and last affirmed on October 15, 2003)

Standard I

Qualified anesthesia personnel shall be present in the room throughout the conduct of all general anesthetics, regional anesthetics and monitored anesthesia care.

Objective

Because of the rapid changes in patient status during anesthesia, qualified anesthesia personnel shall be continuously present to monitor the patient and provide anesthesia care. In the event there is a direct known hazard, e.g., radiation, to the anesthesia personnel which might require intermittent remote observation of the patient, some provision for monitoring the patient must be made. In the event that an emergency requires the temporary absence of the person primarily responsible for the anesthetic, the best judgment of the anesthesiologist is exercised in comparing the emergency with the anesthetized patient's condition and in the selection of the person left responsible for the anesthetic during the temporary absence.

Standard II

During all anesthetics, the patient's oxygenation, ventilation, circulation and temperature shall be continually evaluated.

Oxygenation

Objective

To ensure adequate oxygen concentration in the inspired gas and the blood during all anesthetics.

Methods

1. *Inspired gas:* During every administration of general anesthesia using an anesthesia machine, the concentration of oxygen in the patient breathing system shall be measured by an oxygen analyzer with a low oxygen concentration limit alarm in use.*
2. *Blood oxygenation:* During all anesthetics, a quantitative method of assessing oxygenation such as pulse oximetry shall be employed.* Adequate illumination and exposure of the patient are necessary to assess color.*

Ventilation

Objective

To ensure adequate ventilation of the patient during all anesthetics.

Methods

1. Every patient receiving general anesthesia shall have the adequacy of ventilation continually evaluated. Qualitative clinical signs such as chest excursion, observation of the reservoir breathing bag and auscultation of breath sounds are useful. Continual monitoring for the presence of expired carbon dioxide shall be performed unless invalidated by the nature of the patient, procedure or equipment. Quantitative monitoring of the volume of expired gas is strongly encouraged.*
2. When an endotracheal tube or laryngeal mask is inserted, its correct positioning must be verified by clinical assessment and by identification of carbon dioxide in the expired gas. Continual end-tidal carbon dioxide analysis, in use from the time of endotracheal tube/laryngeal mask placement, until extubation/removal or initiating transfer to a postoperative care location, shall be performed using a quantitative method such as capnography, capnometry or mass spectroscopy.*
3. When ventilation is controlled by a mechanical ventilator, there shall be in continuous use a device that is capable of detecting disconnection of components of the breathing system. The device must give an audible signal when its alarm threshold is exceeded.
4. During regional anesthesia and monitored anesthesia care, the adequacy of ventilation shall be evaluated, at least, by continual observation of qualitative clinical signs.

Circulation

Objective

To ensure the adequacy of the patient's circulatory function during all anesthetics.

Methods

1. Every patient receiving anesthesia shall have the electrocardiogram continuously displayed from the beginning of anesthesia until preparing to leave the anesthetizing location.*
2. Every patient receiving anesthesia shall have arterial blood pressure and heart rate determined and evaluated at least every five minutes.*
3. Every patient receiving general anesthesia shall have, in addition to the above, circulatory function continually evaluated by at least one of the following: palpation of a pulse, auscultation of heart sounds, monitoring of a tracing of intra-arterial pressure, ultrasound peripheral pulse monitoring, or pulse plethysmography or oximetry.

BOX 9–1 **Standards for Basic Anesthetic Monitoring** (Continued)

Body temperature

Objective

To aid in the maintenance of appropriate body temperature during all anesthetics.

Methods

Every patient receiving anesthesia shall have temperature monitored when clinically significant changes in body temperature are intended, anticipated or suspected.

These standards apply to all anesthesia care although, in emergency circumstances, appropriate life support measures take precedence. These standards may be exceeded at any time based on the judgment of the responsible anesthesiologist. They are intended to encourage quality patient care, but observing them cannot guarantee any specific patient outcome. They are subject to revision from time to time, as warranted by the evolution of technology and practice. They apply to all general anesthetics, regional anesthetics and monitored anesthesia care. This set of standards addresses only the issue of basic anesthetic monitoring, which is one component of anesthesia care. In certain rare or unusual circumstances, 1) some of these methods of monitoring may be clinically impractical, and 2) appropriate use of the described monitoring methods may fail to detect untoward clinical developments. Brief interruptions of continual† monitoring may be unavoidable. *Under extenuating circumstances, the responsible anesthesiologist may waive the requirements marked with an asterisk (*); it is recommended that when this is done, it should be so stated (including the reasons) in a note in the patient's medical record.* These standards are not intended for application to the care of the obstetrical patient in labor or in the conduct of pain management.

†Note that "continual" is defined as "repeated regularly and frequently in steady rapid succession" whereas "continuous" means "prolonged without any interruption at any time."

regulated by a probe near the patient connection, because overheating of the inspired gases can produce injury to the airway (Klein and Graves, 1974). Active humidifiers may also increase the compression volume of the breathing circuit (Coté et al., 1983); thus, compensatory increases in the tidal volume during controlled ventilation may be necessary.

ANESTHESIA BREATHING SYSTEMS

Since Philip Ayre's landmark article (1937) began the modern era of breathing systems for pediatric anesthesia, this has been a topic of controversy. Using Magill's technique of endotracheal anesthesia for the repair of cleft lip and palate in infants, Ayre noted adverse results. Breathing through a "closed" system, these infants often developed "rapid, 'sighing' respirations" and "ashy pallor and sweating." They exhibited a "dark, congested oozing at the site of operation." Postoperatively, the infants were "in varying degrees of shock: some ... for days." The contribution of hypotension or hypovolemia to this picture remains unknown, because blood pressure was not measured and blood loss was difficult to quantify by Ayre's account.

Ayre noted dramatic clinical improvement when he adopted an open T-piece breathing system. The T-piece, an extremely simple device, consists of an inspiratory limb, a connection to the patient, and an expiratory limb. It has no unidirectional or overflow valves, nor any breathing bag. The expiratory limb serves as a reservoir for fresh gas, a means of monitoring the infant's respirations, and, if the distal end is intermittently occluded, a means of providing positive pressure ventilation. If the volume of the expiratory limb is one third of the tidal volume, rebreathing can be virtually eliminated during spontaneous ventilation with a fresh gas flow that is twice the minute ventilation (Ayre, 1956). Ayre attributed the salutary effect of the T-piece to marked reductions in resistance to gas flow and rebreathing.

NONREBREATHING AND PARTIAL REBREATHING SYSTEMS

Despite its apparent benefits, the T-piece is far from ideal. The major flaws are its release of anesthetic gases into the operating room and its inability to provide assisted or controlled ventilation. A series of modifications followed. Jackson-Rees first proposed the addition of a breathing bag to the expiratory limb (Jackson-Rees, 1950). Another system, the Magill attachment, which predated Ayre's publication, introduced fresh gas distal to a breathing bag and an overflow valve near the patient connection. These and other variations were brought together under a single classification scheme proposed by Mapleson (1954) in which each system was distinguished on the basis of the location of its fresh gas inflow and overflow valves relative to the patient connection (Fig. 9–1).

The Mapleson systems share the benefit of reduced resistance to breathing by virtue of the absence of unidirectional valves and canisters; the elimination of these components results in various degrees of rebreathing. Rebreathing is not necessarily bad, as it serves to conserve heat, humidity, and anesthetic gases. Yet in the absence of a mechanism by which to monitor the accumulation of carbon dioxide, the consequences of hypercarbia and respiratory acidosis probably outweigh these benefits.

Each system has very different rebreathing characteristics depending on the location of the fresh gas inflow and overflow valves, the fresh gas flow rate, the respiratory rate (i.e., expiratory time) and tidal volume, carbon dioxide production, and the mode of ventilation (i.e., spontaneous or controlled). The following sections describe the Mapleson A (Magill attachment) and D systems. The B and C systems are virtually never used today. The Mapleson E system is the T-piece described earlier.

MAPLESON A SYSTEM

The Mapleson A system results in virtually no rebreathing during spontaneous ventilation when the fresh gas flow is more than 75% of the minute ventilation; it requires a large fresh gas flow to eliminate rebreathing during controlled ventilation (Waters and Mapleson, 1961; Kain and Nunn, 1967) (Fig. 9–2). This design is also impractical in the operating room because the proximal location of the overflow valve makes it cumbersome for scavenging waste gases, difficult to adjust during head and neck surgery, and potentially dangerous, as the heavy valve could dislodge a small endotracheal tube.

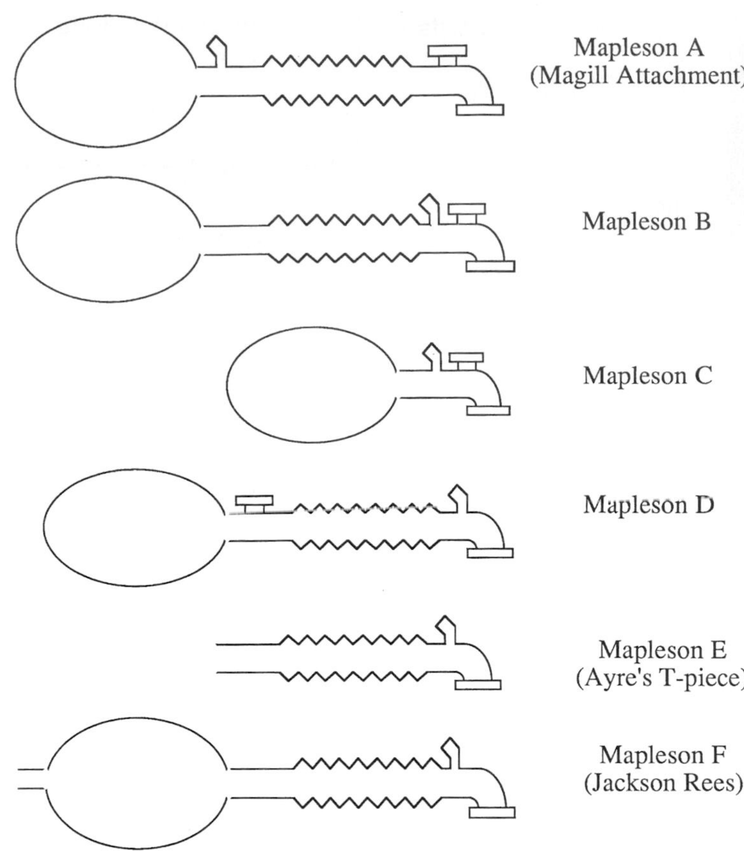

FIGURE 9–1. The Mapleson circuits. Each circuit is classified on the basis of the relative position of the fresh gas inlet, overflow valve, corrugated tubing, and reservoir bag in relation to the patient connection. (Adapted from Mapleson WW: The elimination of rebreathing in various semi-closed anaesthetic systems. *Br J Anaesth* 26:323, 1954.)

MAPLESON D SYSTEM

The Mapleson D system is characterized by a proximal fresh gas inflow and a distal overflow valve. It is a modification of the T-piece in which a breathing bag and an overflow valve have been added to the distal expiratory limb. Although it requires slightly more fresh gas flow to eliminate rebreathing during spontaneous ventilation than the Mapleson A system, it is the most economical during controlled ventilation (Waters and Mapleson, 1961). On balance, considering both spontaneous and controlled ventilation, the Mapleson D requires the lowest fresh gas flow rates among all Mapleson circuits. This system has become the most widely used of the Mapleson circuits for pediatric anesthesia.

The precise flow dynamics in the Mapleson D system is a subject of controversy that has resulted in a variety of complex recommendations (Mapleson, 1954; Waters and Mapleson, 1961; Nightingale et al., 1965; Bain and Spoerel, 1973; Rose et al., 1978; Spoerel et al., 1978; Rose and Froese, 1979). To eliminate rebreathing, higher fresh gas flows are needed during spontaneous ventilation than during controlled ventilation. With spontaneous

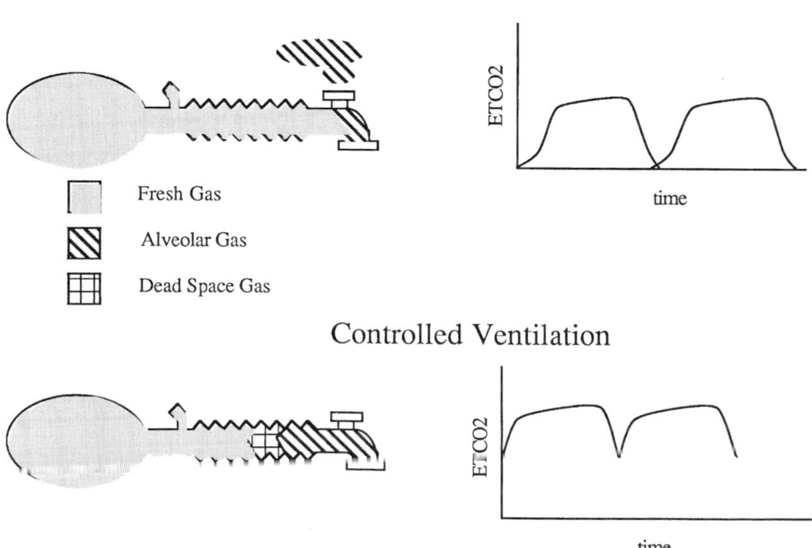

FIGURE 9–2. Rebreathing characteristics of the Mapleson A circuit. During spontaneous ventilation, the overflow valve is open and exhaled gases are discharged. There is virtually no rebreathing as long as fresh gas flow is more than 75% of the minute ventilation. With controlled ventilation, the valve is closed and rebreathing is significant.

ventilation, rebreathing is virtually eliminated by provision of fresh gas flow equal to the mean inspiratory flow rate (Mapleson, 1954; Rose et al., 1978). If one assumes an inspiratory/expiratory ratio of 1:1 to 1:2, the mean inspiratory flow rate is two to three times the minute ventilation. Although Spoerel and others (1979) have demonstrated that a normal $PaCO_2$ can be maintained during spontaneous ventilation at fresh gas flows as low as 100 mL/kg per minute, an increased minute ventilation (and hence, more respiratory work) is required to compensate for rebreathed carbon dioxide.

The recommendations for fresh gas flow during controlled ventilation are complex and varied (Waters and Mapleson, 1961; Nightingale et al., 1965; Bain and Spoerel, 1973). This reflects the importance of several factors that were summarized by Rose and Froese (1979) (Fig. 9–3). When a high fresh gas flow (>100 mL/kg per minute) is used, the P_ACO_2 is governed by minute ventilation (ventilation limited). At low fresh gas flow (<90 mL/kg per minute), P_ACO_2 is independent of minute ventilation, varying instead as a function of the amount of rebreathing, which is governed by the fresh gas flow rate (flow limited).

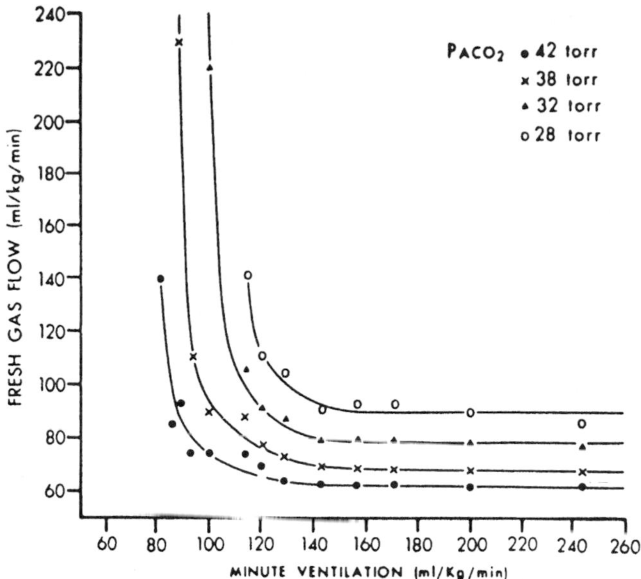

■ **FIGURE 9–3.** Mapleson D, controlled ventilation. Illustrates factors in determining alveolar PCO_2 during controlled ventilation with Mapleson D. At low fresh gas flow (FGF) (<90 mL/kg per minute), $PaCO_2$ changes only with FGF ("flow-limited") regardless of ventilation. At higher FGF (>100 mL/kg per minute), $PaCO_2$ changes as a result of changes in delivered minute ventilation ("ventilation-limited"). (From Froese AB: *ASA annual refresher course,* 1978.)

Additional important factors that govern the magnitude of rebreathing include carbon dioxide production, respiratory rate, and respiratory waveform characteristics (inspiratory flow, inspiratory and expiratory times, and expiratory pause) (Rose and Froese, 1979). Adjustments to the ventilatory pattern that allow the fresh gas flow to constitute a larger proportion of the inspired gas (e.g., slow inspiratory time, low inspiratory flow) or that enable exhaled gases to be more completely washed out (e.g., long expiratory pause, slow rate) reduce the amount of rebreathing. If one were using a Mapleson D circuit with controlled ventilation and low fresh gas flow (flow limited), an attempt to reduce the $PaCO_2$ by increasing the respiratory rate would reduce the expiratory pause and thus promote rebreathing (Fig. 9–4). In this situation, the increased ventilation is offset by increased $FICO_2$, resulting in no net change in $PaCO_2$. To wash out the exhaled gas at this higher respiratory rate and take advantage of the increased minute ventilation, the fresh gas

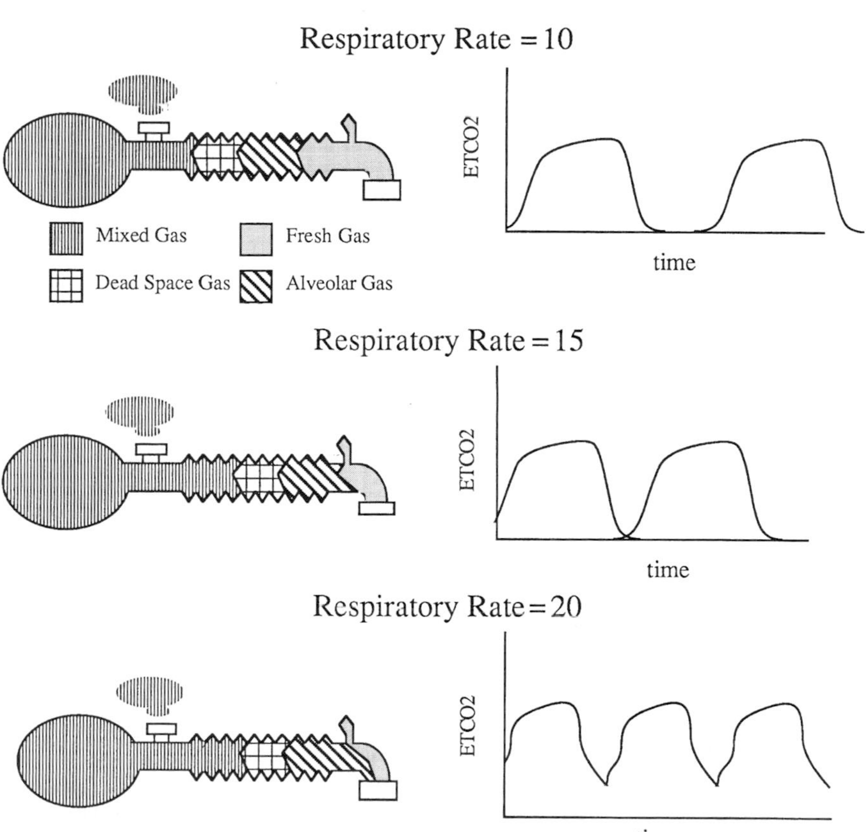

■ **FIGURE 9–4.** Fresh gas flow–limited controlled ventilation using a Mapleson D circuit. Note that higher respiratory rate reduces the washout of exhaled gases. Rebreathing occurs so that there is no net reduction in end-tidal carbon dioxide ($ETCO_2$). Fresh gas flow must be increased to wash out exhaled gases and lower the $ETCO_2$.

flow must be increased. These fresh gas flow and ventilatory recommendations are predicated on a normal metabolic rate and hence normal carbon dioxide production (Bain and Spoerel, 1977; Nightingale and Lambert, 1978). Conditions that increase carbon dioxide production (e.g., fever, catabolic state, malignant hyperthermia) must be met with a proportional increase in fresh gas flow or ventilation.

Bain Modification of Mapleson D

The Bain modification of the Mapleson D circuit incorporates the fresh gas supply within the expiratory limb in a coaxial arrangement (Bain and Spoerel, 1972) (Fig. 9–5). This circuit is light and streamlined with only a single hose to the patient. It also provides some countercurrent warming of the inspired gases and effective scavenging of expired gases. Its major disadvantage lies in the inability to directly inspect the integrity of the inspiratory limb. Pethick (1975) described an indirect test of the Bain inspiratory limb integrity in which the oxygen flush is passed through the circuit for several seconds. If the inspiratory limb is intact, the rapid flow of gas through it exerts a Venturi effect on the expiratory limb, resulting in a slight negative pressure and collapse of the breathing bag. With a leak from the inspiratory limb into the expiratory limb, the pressure in the latter rises, tending to inflate the reservoir bag. The rebreathing characteristics of the Bain circuit are essentially identical to those of any other Mapleson D. The major reasons that proponents have advocated the use of these Bain circuits for pediatric anesthesia are their relatively lower resistance to breathing and the simplicity with which a heating circuit may be added.

The primary sources of resistance in an anesthesia delivery system are (1) the endotracheal tube, (2) the valves, and (3) the carbon dioxide absorber. With modern equipment, the endotracheal tube represents a major source of resistance in the neonate (Cave and Fletcher, 1968; Brown and Hustead, 1969). Lightweight, large-diameter, modern disc valves exert resistance in two ways. There is a minimum, flow-independent resistance necessary to displace the valve, usually much less than 1 cm H_2O (Hunt, 1955). A much higher resistance may be required when the expiratory valve is wet. At high gas flows (>30 L/min), the valves also become a source of turbulent resistance proportional to the flow through them. Carbon dioxide canisters are also a source of turbulence. Their resistance is inversely proportional to the length of the path the gas must take through the resistor. Modern absorbers are short and wide to minimize this path of resistance.

At approximately a half-century after Ayre introduced the T-piece, the extent to which his work applies remains unclear.

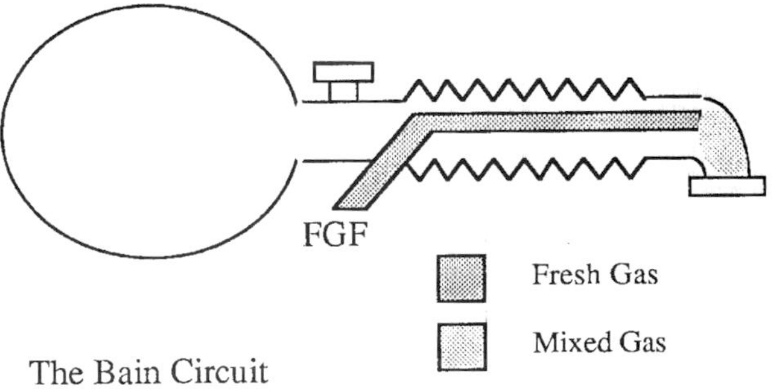

■ FIGURE 9–5. The Bain circuit. The Bain modification of the Mapleson D circuit provides a low profile circuit and allows simple connection to the patient's airway.

If the infants he described were victims of rebreathed carbon dioxide in those days before the carbon dioxide absorber came into common use, it would seem that infants are more likely to be faced with rebreathing in the Mapleson circuits than in the modern circle system. Perhaps Ayre's infants were subjected to the significant resistance imposed by the valves of that era. Although the neonate has a lower proportion of fatigue-resistant fibers in the diaphragm (Muller et al., 1979), infants as small as those 2 weeks old have been shown to be able to compensate for increases in resistance of 200% without changes in blood gases, at least for relatively short periods of time (Graff, 1966). The benefits of the Mapleson systems must be weighed against their inherent problems on an individual basis. One must also factor in the added risks of a practitioner who uses Mapleson circuits infrequently and is unfamiliar with their characteristics or who may have to make substantial alterations to an anesthesia machine to accommodate them. Even if one uses a circle system for most children, it is important to understand the flow requirements of this circuit, as it continues to be used very commonly in intensive care units and for transport of critically ill patients.

■ CIRCLE SYSTEMS

The circle system is standard equipment on anesthesia machines designed to meet the standards specified in ASTM 1850-00 (2005). When functioning properly, it enables lower fresh gas flows than the Mapleson D; a circle system conserves heat, humidity, and anesthetic agent. It also minimizes environmental pollution. Compared with the resistance of an endotracheal tube, the additional resistance imposed by the addition of unidirectional valves and a carbon dioxide canister seems trivial. Because the ratio of the patient's tidal volume to the total circuit volume is small in young children, changes in the anesthetic concentration can take some time to reach equilibrium unless higher fresh gas flows are used. One must be vigilant for the manifestations of stuck (resistance) or floating (rebreathing) unidirectional valves, because both have harmful consequences in small children.

Special circle breathing systems have been designed for infants and children. They incorporate the same components as the standard adult circuits but have been modified to minimize dead space and resistance to breathing. Most incorporate short, narrow-caliber hoses and Y connections and smaller carbon dioxide absorbers.

Although these circuits have been shown to minimize dead space and the resistance work of breathing, they have not gained wide acceptance. They require significant modifications of standard equipment and thus are inconvenient. Unlike the adult circle system and Mapleson circuits, these circuits have not been marketed in modern, disposable materials that readily adapt to standard anesthesia machines.

■ ANESTHESIA FACEMASKS

The most appropriate anesthesia facemask for a child spans vertically from the bridge of the nose to just below the lower lip, without compressing the nasal passages (Fig. 9–6). It should contain the least volume inside (i.e., dead space) possible. The pediatric facemask should be constructed as a clear (non–latex-containing) plastic that allows recognition of cyanosis, the condensation of exhaled gas, and the presence of excess secretions or vomitus.

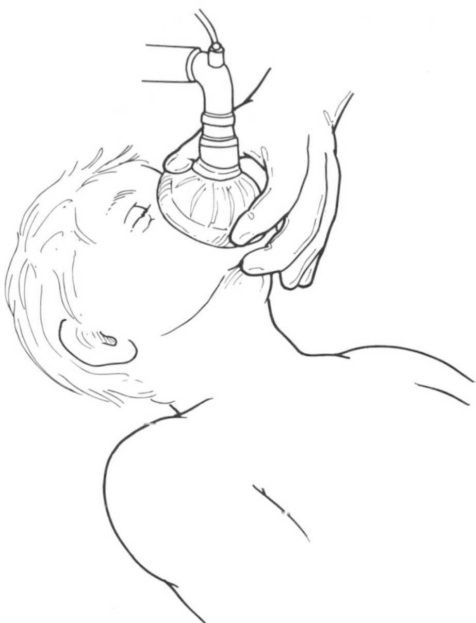

■ **FIGURE 9–6.** The most effective mask ventilation technique for infants and young children is for the anesthesiologist to hold the mask over the mouth and nose with the thumb and forefinger, while the middle finger is placed on the bony portion of the mandible. (From Litman RS: Pediatric airway management. In: Litman RS, ed: *Pediatric anesthesia, The requisites.* St. Louis, 2004, Mosby.)

A constant challenge in pediatric anesthesia, especially for small infants, is to find a facemask that conforms to the shape of the infant's face without a significant leak. During positive pressure ventilation, the anesthesia practitioner often must twist or torque the facemask, without applying undue pressure against the child's face, to reduce the amount of air that escapes from within the mask. To achieve these purposes, a variety of facemasks have been used in the pediatric population.

The most common anesthesia facemask in use today is the plastic disposable type that contains an adjustable pneumatic cushion that, when inflated or deflated with air, can be altered to conform to the shape of the child's face. A variety of different manufacturers produce this type of facemask (Fig. 9–7). An alternative variety for use in pediatric patients is the Rendell-Baker-Soucek mask, which remains in use in many centers (Fig. 9–7). This mask is available in malleable rubber or non–latex-containing silicone and allows an effective seal on the child's face while minimizing internal dead space. It was originally designed on the basis of anatomic molds of a large number of children (Rendell-Baker and Soucek, 1962).

■ ORAL AND NASAL AIRWAYS

Oral and nasal pharyngeal airway devices are used in pediatric anesthesia to improve patency of the upper airway and to facilitate delivery of oxygen or anesthetic gases to the lungs. Minimum requirements for these devices are noted in ASTM F1573-95 (Subcommittee F29.12 on Airways, 2000). The Guedel-type oral airway is probably the airway most commonly used in pediatric patients. It contains a central lumen for the

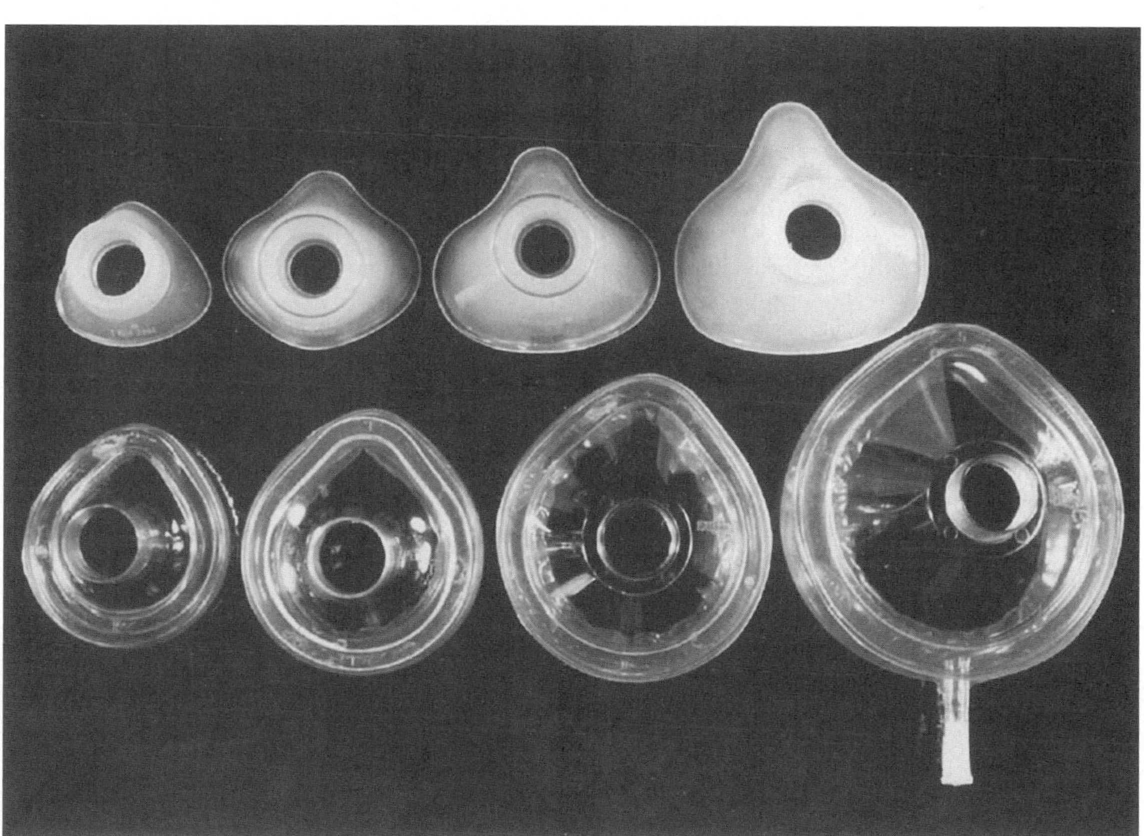

■ **FIGURE 9–7.** Pediatric facemasks. Various mask sizes are available for the wide range of pediatric patients. *Top row,* Four different Rendell-Baker-Soucek masks (Willy Rusch, Kernen, Germany). *Bottom row,* Disposable bubble masks (Vital Signs, Totowa, NJ).

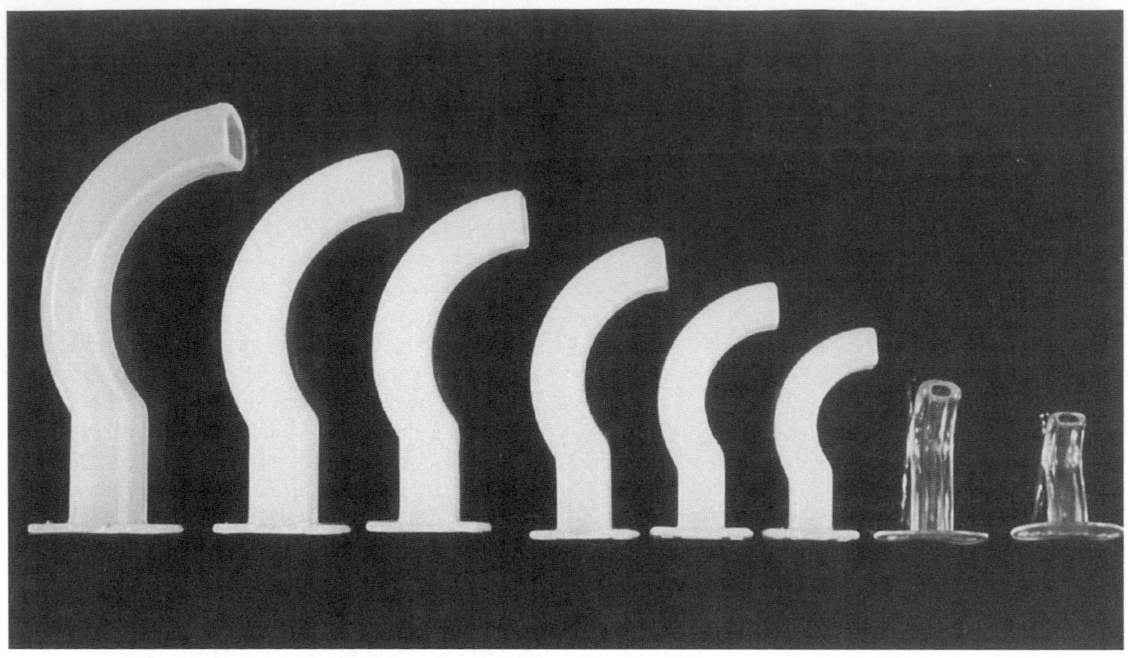

■ **FIGURE 9–8.** Oral airways for the entire spectrum of pediatric patients from infancy through adolescence.

passage of airflow and for suctioning of the posterior pharynx (Fig. 9–8). The oral airway device is primarily used when manual airway-opening techniques have failed to alleviate upper airway obstruction, which is usually caused by tonsillar or adenoidal hypertrophy, or normal pharyngeal tissue obstruction, as often occurs in small infants (see Chapter 2, Respiratory Physiology).

Oral airways are usually manufactured from plastic or polyethylene and are latex free. They are sized depending on the total length of the device (50 to 80 mm, flange to tip, for most children) or based on an arbitrary scale designated by the manufacturer. The appropriate size is determined by placing the airway adjacent to the child's face to approximate its position in the oral cavity (Fig. 9–9). When appropriately placed, its distal end snugly curves around the back of the tongue, without the proximal end protruding out of the mouth. Too small an oral airway pushes the posterior portion of the tongue against the posterior pharyngeal wall, and too large an oral airway may itself cause upper airway obstruction at the laryngeal inlet by compressing or distorting the epiglottis.

The oral airway device should be inserted in its normal orientation position with the aid of a tongue depressor. In older children, insertion may be accomplished with the distal tip oriented cephalad, and then turned 180 degrees when the tip has reached the posterior aspect of the palate. In younger children, this maneuver may push the tongue posteriorly and exacerbate airway obstruction.

Complications of oral airway use in children are not infrequent and usually occur during emergence. Lip or tooth damage is possible; a loose tooth may become dislodged and lost in the oral cavity, where it may accidentally travel into the bronchopulmonary tree. Compression of oral structures by the oral airway may result in transient postoperative numbness.

The nasal airway device is made from soft latex-free rubber to allow easy insertion through the nasal passage and into the nasal or oropharynx. It can be bathed in warm or cold water to decrease or increase its stiffness, respectively. Some nasal airways contain an enlarged flange at the proximal end to prevent unintentional advancement into the nasal cavity. Others contain an adjustable ring to secure against the outside of the nasal opening (Fig. 9–10). Nasal airways are available in sizes 12 F to 36 F (outer diameter). If required, a stiffer nasal airway can be fashioned out of a standard endotracheal tube by cutting it off at the appropriate length. An anesthesia breathing circuit can be connected to any type of nasal airway using an appropriately sized endotracheal tube adaptor (Fig. 9–11).

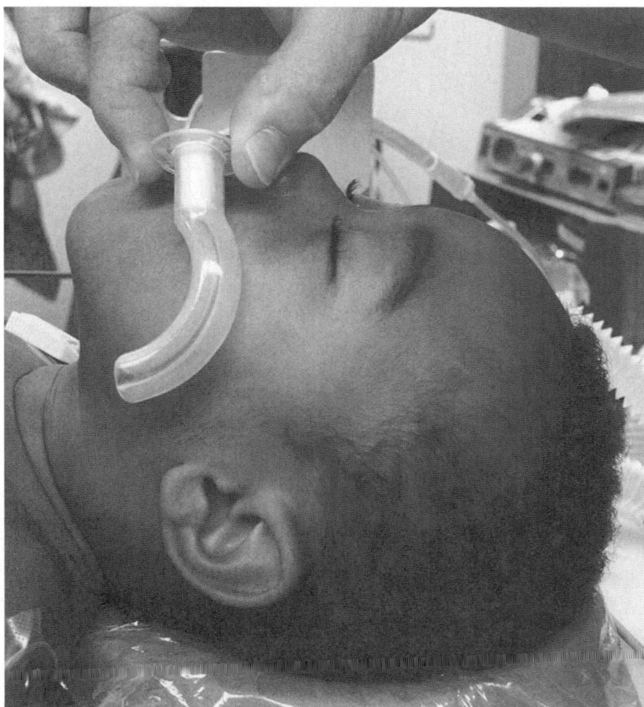

■ **FIGURE 9–9.** The appropriate-size oral airway device is chosen by placing it adjacent to the face to approximate its position in the oral cavity.

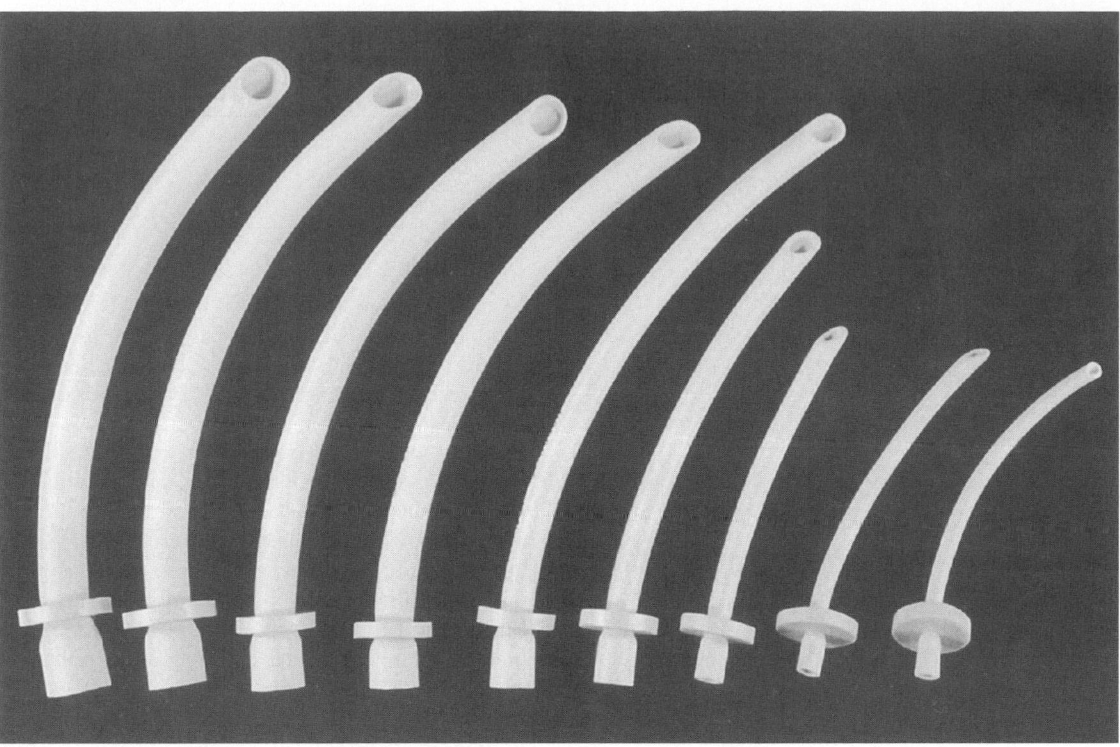

■ **FIGURE 9–10.** A large selection of nasal airways is needed for pediatric patients. Those pictured (Willy Rusch, Kernen, Germany) can be adjusted for length by moving the circular disc along the tube.

Before insertion, the nasal cavities should be inspected to ensure the absence of significant septal deviation or other causes of narrowing (e.g., polyp) that obstruct passage of the nasal airway. To avoid trauma and bleeding of the delicate nasal mucosa, the nasal airway should be lubricated and gently inserted in a posterocaudad direction along the floor of the nasal cavity. A topical vasoconstrictor, such as 0.05% oxymetazoline, can be applied to the nasal mucosa before nasal airway insertion to shrink nasal mucosal tissue and reduce bleeding. The proper diameter of the nasal airway is determined by approximating the circular diameter of the nasal opening. The proper length of the nasal airway is estimated by measuring the distance from the nares to the tragus of the ear. When appropriately placed, its distal tip should lie at the level of the angle of the mandible, between the posterior aspect of the tongue and above the tip of the epiglottis.

The most common complication from nasal airway insertion is trauma to the nasal or pharyngeal mucosa that results in minor bleeding. Adenoidal tissue may be disrupted and may bleed into the oropharynx. Occasionally, a friable vessel is encountered in the nasal mucosa and bleeding is brisk. A lesser known, although not rare, complication is the insertion of the nasal airway device into a false passage beneath the posterior wall mucosa of the nasal and oral pharynx. This is not usually accompanied by bleeding and may be caused by a patent bursa of Thornwaldt (James et al., 1968). Nasal airways should not be inserted in children with a coagulopathy, neutropenia, or suspicion of a traumatic basilar skull fracture.

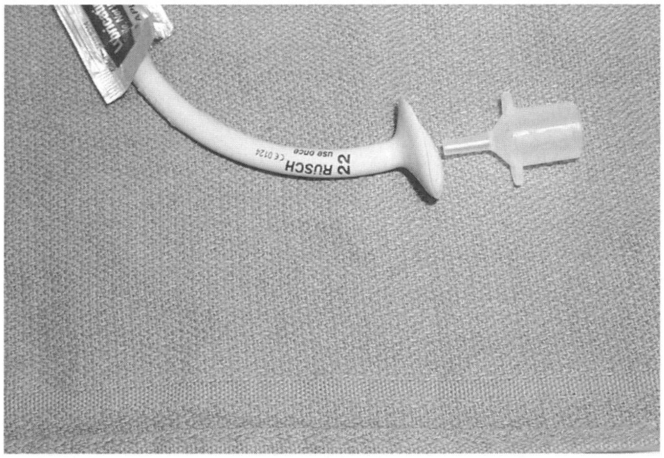

■ **FIGURE 9–11.** The nasal airway can easily be connected to a standard 15-mm endotracheal tube adaptor for connection into an anesthesia breathing circuit.

■ CUFFED OROPHARYNGEAL AIRWAY

The cuffed oropharyngeal airway (COPA) is essentially a Guedel airway manufactured with a 15-mm anesthesia breathing circuit connector on the proximal end and an inflatable cuff on the distal end (Fig. 9–12). It has an integrated bite block, which is color coded for size and to help with proper positioning. The device is inserted in a similar manner to that of an oral airway; once inserted, the cuff is inflated (with 20 to 40 mL air) to provide a low-pressure seal in the hypopharynx to facilitate spontaneous or controlled ventilation. Once inserted, the COPA can be secured in place using an accompanying head strap that attaches to the posts on the tooth/lip guard. The COPA is intended as a single-use device.

The principal indication of the COPA is to aid airway management by replacing the use of an anesthesia facemask, freeing up the hands of the anesthesia practitioner (Robbins and Connelly, 2000; Sammartino and Ferro, 2002). It is primarily

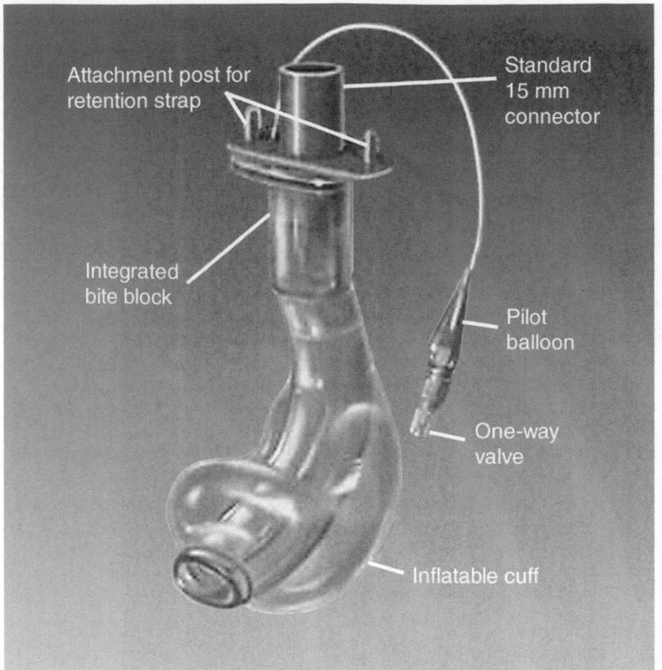

■ **FIGURE 9–12.** The cuffed oropharyngeal airway (COPA) is essentially a Guedel airway manufactured with a 15-mm anesthesia breathing circuit connector on the proximal end and an inflatable cuff on the distal end.

intended for use in anesthetized patients who are breathing spontaneously, but it also can be used with controlled ventilation in some patients.

The COPA is available in four sizes (Table 9–1). The smallest (size 8) is appropriate for most school-aged children. When held adjacent to the patient's head, the appropriately sized COPA should rest with the bite block just above the teeth and the distal tip at the angle of the mandible. This is usually one size larger than the corresponding appropriately sized oral airway. Before insertion, the distal end of the device is lubricated and

■ **TABLE 9–1.** Characteristics of the cuffed oropharyngeal airway

Size	Color	Amount of Air Needed to Inflate Cuff (mL)
8	Green	25
9	Yellow	30
10	Red	35
11	Light green	40

the cuff is tested for leaks. When sized correctly, the COPA "locks into place" behind the base of the tongue. If the proper size has been chosen, the colored bite block should "transition" at the teeth. Once inserted, the COPA is fastened to the head strap, a jaw-thrust/chin-lift maneuver is performed, and the cuff is inflated with the proper amount of air (see Table 9–1).

On occasion, manual airway adjustments may be required to enhance the proper functioning of the COPA; these include increased or decreased head tilt, turning the head to one side, supporting the shoulders, gentle chin lift, or application of continuous positive airway pressure (CPAP) up to 10 cm H_2O (Bussolin and Busoni, 2002). The COPA can be removed at any time, preferably with the cuff remaining inflated to facilitate removal of oral secretions.

When compared with the laryngeal mask airway (LMA) in children, the use of a COPA resulted in a greater number of subsequent airway maneuvers or a switch to another airway method to establish ventilation (Mamaya, 2002). Its use was also associated with less airway response with cuff inflation and decreased requirement for assisted ventilation compared with the LMA.

■ LARYNGEAL MASK AIRWAY

The LMA has become an accepted standard device for airway management in pediatric patients (Lopez-Gil et al., 1996). It consists of a rigid tube with a standard 15-mm connector at the most proximal end and a fenestrated, elliptical cuff cavity at the distal end (Brain, 1983; Brain et al., 1985) (Fig. 9–13).

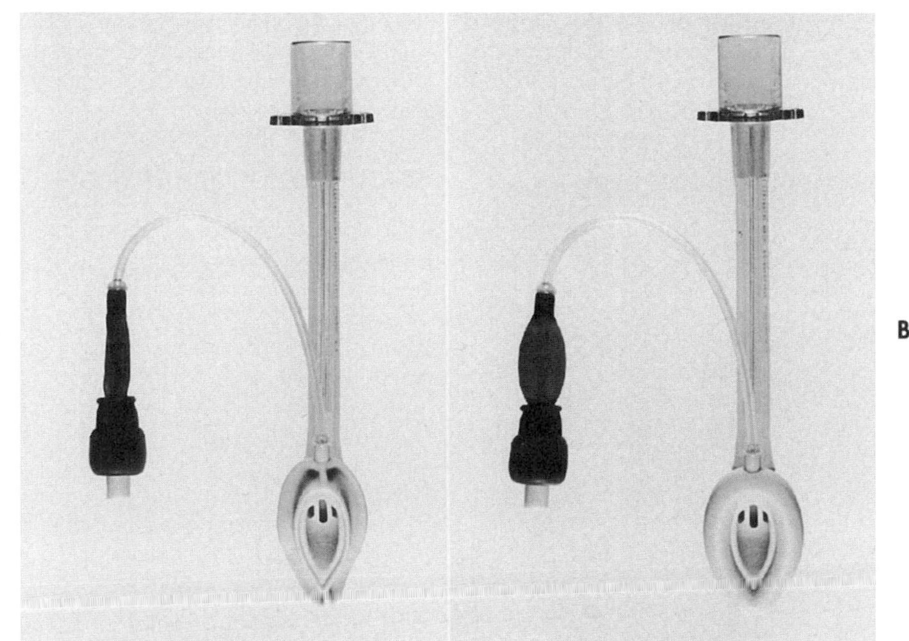

■ **FIGURE 9–13.** A laryngeal mask airway, *(A)* deflated and *(B)* inflated.

■ **TABLE 9–2.** Laryngeal mask airway size characteristics

Laryngeal Mask Airway Size	Approximate Weight (kg)	Cuff Volume (mL)
1	<5	2 to 5
1.5	5 to 10	3 to 8
2	10 to 20	5 to 10
2.5	20 to 30	10 to 15
3	30 to 50	15 to 20
4	50 to 70	≤30
5	70 to 100	≤40
6	>100	≤50

When placed properly, the distal cuff overlies the laryngeal inlet, and the fenestrations prevent the epiglottis from obstructing the lumen. Once inflated through a pilot tube, the cuff creates a seal in the pharynx that permits both spontaneous and controlled ventilation without a large gas leak when the peak pressure is below 15 cm H_2O (Epstein and Halmi, 1994). A black line runs longitudinally along the posterior curvature to permit orientation of the tube after placement. A variety of LMA sizes are available to accommodate all pediatric age groups (Table 9–2). Newer, disposable models are available in all pediatric sizes (Portex, Keene, NH). Several larger reusable sizes are made with a port that allows passage of an orogastric tube to facilitate gastric emptying (ProSeal; LMA North America, Inc., San Diego, CA).

The LMA is used in pediatric anesthesia as a routine airflow conduit during general anesthesia, as a tool with which to facilitate endotracheal intubation in difficult-to-intubate children, and as an airway rescue device for the difficult-to-ventilate child. The LMA is recommended as a component of the ASA difficult airway algorithm to facilitate ventilation when bag-mask ventilation or endotracheal intubation is unsuccessful in adults (ASA Task Force on Management of the Difficult Airway, 1993; Benumof, 1996).

When the LMA was first introduced in the 1980s, its use as an elective airway device was reserved for procedures that were amenable to facemask anesthesia (Grebenik et al., 1990; Johnston et al., 1990; Mason and Bingham, 1990; Watcha et al., 1994). Except for the emergency rescue situation, the LMA was considered a substitute for an anesthesia facemask but not for an endotracheal tube. As practitioners have become more comfortable with its use, the LMA has become a useful alternative to an endotracheal tube in certain nonemergent cases, such as tonsillectomy or strabismus repair. An LMA that is specially designed with a wire-reinforced shaft is available for use during procedures that would otherwise require an oral RAE endotracheal tube, named after its inventors, Ring, Adair, and Elwyn (1975) (Mallinckrodt, Inc., St. Louis, MO) (Webster et al., 1993). In most children, positive pressure ventilation can be accomplished via an LMA, but peak inspiratory pressures greater than approximately 15 cm H_2O are associated with a leak around the distal cuff into the esophagus, subsequent gastric insufflation, and possible regurgitation and aspiration (Fawcett et al., 1991; Gursoy et al., 1996).

A variety of methods of LMA placement in children are possible. The manufacturer recommends that the mask be advanced across the hard palate with the cuff fully deflated, distal aperture facing anteriorly, and head in the classic "sniffing" position. The index finger of the right hand helps guide the LMA over the surface of the tongue. A water-based lubricant smeared onto the posterior surface of the LMA may decrease the resistance to insertion. On meeting the characteristic resistance of the upper esophageal sphincter, the cuff is inflated through the pilot tube. With cuff inflation, the tube usually moves outward a short distance as the tube centers itself over the laryngeal inlet.

The LMA can also be inserted with the cuff partially inflated or with the aperture facing posterior and then turned 180 degrees once in the larynx (Chow et al., 1991; McNicol, 1991; O'Neill et al., 1994; Nakayama et al., 2002). There are no advantages to one particular insertion method, but one method may be easier than another in any particular child. Additional maneuvers that may facilitate ease of insertion include increasing head extension, pushing the tongue forward with a jaw-thrust maneuver, inserting the LMA slightly laterally to avoid the uvula, or using a laryngoscope to lift the tongue anteriorly (Brain, 1989; van Heerden and Kirrage, 1989; Cass, 1991). Nevertheless, in some children, insertion is difficult and associated with pharyngeal bleeding (Marjot, 1991). The LMA is usually placed in an anesthetized child; insertion in a conscious or sedated child (after use of topical analgesia) is occasionally necessary when one desires to gain control of the child's airway in a potentially difficult-to-ventilate situation (Denny et al., 1990; Markakis et al., 1992).

When inserted correctly, the distal end of the LMA cuff rests in the proximal end of the esophagus, the proximal portion of the LMA cuff pushes the epiglottis anteriorly, and the grille lies over the laryngeal inlet (Goudsouzian et al., 1992) (Fig. 9–14). The relatively cephalad location of the pediatric larynx does not lend itself to ideal LMA placement. Fiberoptic bronchoscopy and magnetic resonance imaging (MRI) studies in pediatric patients demonstrate a high incidence of malpositioning of the LMA after placement in children (Keidan et al., 2000). In general, the smaller the size of the LMA, the higher the incidence of malposition, usually with the epiglottis contained within the grille of the LMA (Rowbottom et al., 1991; Mizushima et al., 1992; Dubreuil et al., 1993). Studies have revealed that even in the presence of this malpositioning, ventilation is not usually impaired (Mason and Bingham, 1990; Rowbottom et al., 1991). Ventilation may become impaired more easily in children subsequent to seemingly minor movements of the child or LMA.

LMA use with spontaneously ventilating patients results in fewer episodes of arterial oxygen desaturation than does standard mask ventilation (Johnston et al., 1990; Watcha et al., 1994). In addition, the work of breathing through an LMA is less than the work of breathing through a standard facemask

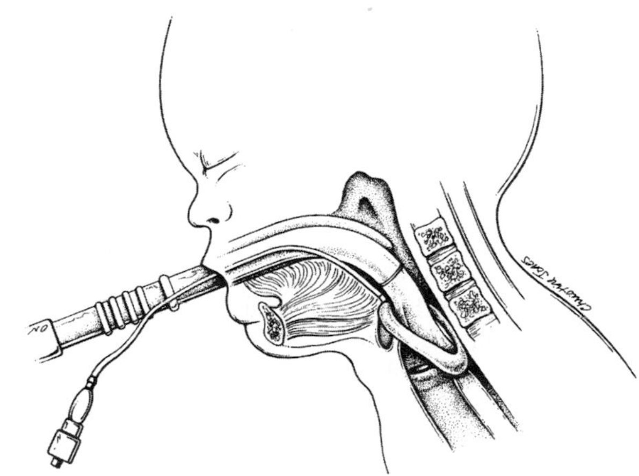

■ **FIGURE 9–14.** When properly inserted, the distal outlet of the laryngeal mask airway is situated over the laryngeal inlet.

TABLE 9–3. Pediatric-sized laryngeal mask airways and compatible endotracheal tubes*

Laryngeal Mask Airway Size	Maximum Lubricated Uncuffed Standard Endotracheal Tube Inner Diameter (mm)	Maximum Lubricated Cuffed Standard Endotracheal Tube Inner Diameter (mm)	Maximum Flexible Bronchoscope Size†
1	3.5	3.0	2.7
1.5	4.0	4.0	3.0
2	5.0	4.5	3.5
2.5	6.0‡	5.0	4.0
3	—	6.0	5.0
4	—	6.0	5.0
5	—	7.0†	5.0
6	—	7.0†	5.0

*Based on experiments performed by the author.
†As per LMA North America.
‡Largest available uncuffed endotracheal tube available at The Children's Hospital of Philadelphia.
With permission from Litman RS: The difficult pediatric airway. In Litman RS, editor: *Pediatric anesthesia: The requisites*, St. Louis, 2004, Mosby.

(Keidan et al., 2000). Unlike a facemask, the LMA can be secured to the face with tape in the manner of a tracheal tube, thereby freeing the anesthesiologist to attend to other care responsibilities such as drug and fluid administration or record-keeping.

Compared with tracheal intubation, the LMA produces less sympathetic stimulation, despite a lighter plane of anesthesia, and is associated with fewer postoperative sore throats than tracheal intubation (Alexander and Leach, 1989; Hickey et al., 1990; Wilkins et al., 1992). Compared with an endotracheal tube, the LMA is associated with less laryngeal stimulation and a decreased incidence of airway complications in children with upper respiratory tract infections (Tait et al., 1998).

The cardiovascular response produced with LMA insertion is not as pronounced or prolonged as that observed with tracheal intubation (Hickey et al., 1990; Wilson et al., 1992). Changes in intraocular pressure are similarly blunted (Lamb et al., 1992; Watcha et al., 1992). Accurate intraocular pressure measurements may be obtained during LMA use in children.

For the pediatric anesthesiologist, the LMA has significantly improved the care of children with congenital facial anomalies, such as Robin's syndrome or Treacher Collins syndrome, who in the past would have been difficult to ventilate and intubate (Beveridge, 1989; Ebata et al., 1991; Hansen et al., 1995; Stocks et al., 2002; Bucx et al., 2003; Gandini and Brimacombe, 2003). Initial reports of successful LMA placement in these children while conscious led to the widespread use of the device after the induction of general anesthesia. It is unusual that the LMA cannot provide adequate ventilation in an anesthetized child with a congenital facial anomaly. Once inserted, the LMA has also been used to facilitate endotracheal intubation using flexible fiberoptic bronchoscopy (Heard et al., 1996). This technique is limited by the small size of the LMA relative to the size of the flexible bronchoscope and endotracheal tube (Table 9–3). Blind intubation of the trachea with an endotracheal tube or an intubating guide that subsequently serves as a stylet can often be accomplished without fiberoptic visualization because the apertures of the LMA and larynx are usually closely approximated (Chadd et al., 1992; Kihara et al., 2000). This blind technique is problematic in small children, in whom the approximation of aperture and larynx is perfect in only 27% of patients (Dubreuil et al., 1993).

A specially designed LMA (Fastrach; The Laryngeal Mask Company, Henley-on-Thames, UK) is available in larger sizes to facilitate intubation in individuals with difficult airways (Brimacombe, 1997; Ferson et al., 2001) (Fig. 9–15). The Fastrach is shorter than the standard LMA and has a rigid handle to allow easy manipulation and a different distal aperture to allow easier elevation of the epiglottis when passing an endotracheal tube.

Because of its inability to adequately seal off the trachea, the LMA is not indicated for use in children at risk for pulmonary aspiration of gastric contents. The extent of protection provided by the LMA against regurgitation of stomach contents into the trachea or aspiration of oral contents is unclear. In adults without significant risk for reflux or aspiration, there was a 25% incidence of regurgitation of methylene blue into the laryngeal mask (Barker et al., 1992). No tracheal soiling was noted. Nevertheless, multiple cases of aspiration of gastric contents have been reported in conjunction with LMA use (Cyna, 1990; Wilkinson, 1990; Maroof et al., 1993). Aspiration of stomach contents may result from high intragastric pressure, a decrease in lower esophageal sphincter tone, or inclusion of the esophageal opening within the rim of the LMA cuff. In contrast, the study of Williams and Bailey (1993) suggests that the LMA may offer protection from aspiration of oral contents. In this study of

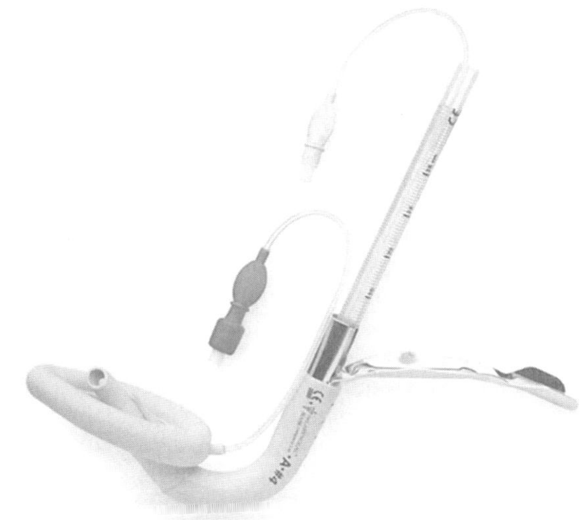

FIGURE 9–15. Laryngeal mask airway Fasttrach is designed to facilitate intubation in individuals with difficult airways (Fastrach, Henley-on-Thomes, UK).

patients undergoing adenotonsillectomy, fiberoptic inspection of the laryngeal trachea after surgery did not reveal any blood (Williams and Bailey, 1993).

During emergence from general anesthesia, the LMA can be removed at any time; compared with adults, children demonstrate more problems (7% to 13%), including laryngospasm, coughing, biting on the tube, or breath holding, when the LMA remains until the child has recovered his or her protective reflexes (Mason and Bingham, 1990; McGinn, 1993; Laffon, 1994; O'Neill et al., 1994). Removal with the cuff inflated facilitates removal of blood or secretions that have collected above the cuff. If one chooses to wait until the child is strong and awake before removing the LMA, a soft bite block should be inserted between the patient's teeth to prevent compression of the lumen of the LMA, which, as a result of a completely obstructed airway, may result in negative pressure pulmonary edema. During the excitement phase of emergence, removal of the LMA is associated with a lower incidence of airway complications compared with removal of an endotracheal tube. Nevertheless, airway complications during emergence are least when the LMA is removed before the child regains airway reflexes and full consciousness. Rapid removal of the LMA may cause displacement of loose teeth.

PERILARYNGEAL AIRWAY

The perilaryngeal airway (PLA) (CobraPLA; Engineered Medical Systems, Inc., Indianapolis, IN) is an addition to the supply of laryngeal masklike devices that aid in airway management. The PLA consists of a distal softened tip that has slotted openings for ventilation and is designed to be positioned in the hypopharynx overlying the laryngeal inlet (Fig. 9–16). It is secured in place by a more proximal cuff, and it contains a proximal 15-mm connector that attaches to the anesthesia breathing circuit.

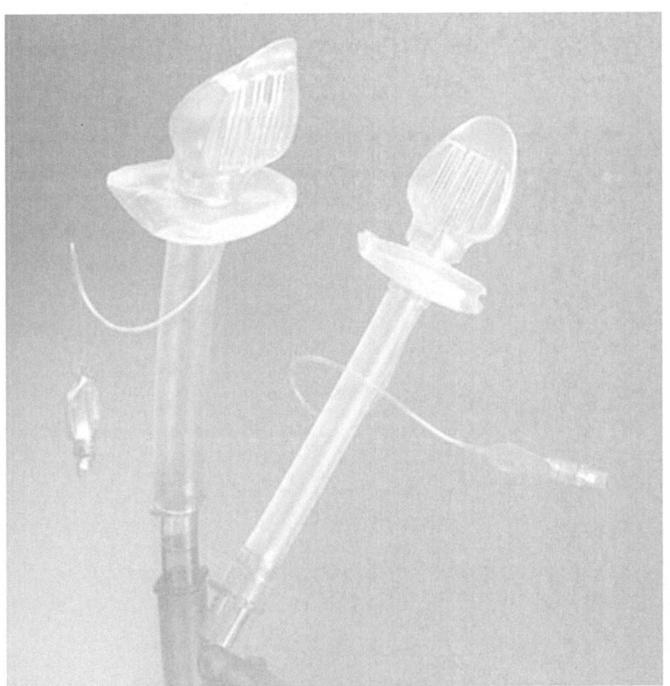

FIGURE 9–16. Perilaryngeal airway consists of a distal softened tip that contains slotted openings for ventilation, a more proximal cuff to secure the airway, and a proximal 15-mm connector that attaches to the anesthesia breathing circuit. (Reproduced with permission of Engineered Medical Systems, Inc., Indianapolis, IN.)

TABLE 9–4. Classification of the Cobra perilaryngeal airway

	PERILARYNGEAL AIRWAY CHARACTERISTICS			
Perilaryngeal Airway Size	*Patient Size*	*Weight (kg)*	*Internal Diameter (mm)*	*Cuff Volume (mL)*
0.5	Neonatal	>2.5	5	<8
1	Infant	>5	6	<10
1.5	Child	>10	6	<25
2	Child	>15	10.5	<40
3	Child/small adult	>35	10.5	<65
4	Adult	>70	12.5	<70
5	Large adult	>100	12.5	<85
6	Large adult	>130	12.5	<85

Reproduced with permission from Engineered Medical Systems, Inc., Indianapolis, IN.

The PLA is available in eight different sizes, of which five are suitable for pediatric age and weight ranges (Table 9–4). It is suitable for use during spontaneous or controlled ventilation, and the larger sizes can accommodate an appropriately sized fiberoptic bronchoscope and endotracheal tube for difficult intubations.

The PLA is inserted in a similar manner to the LMA. A preliminary study in adults demonstrated that the PLA frequently requires readjustment up or down to effect adequate ventilation once inserted (Agro et al., 2003). There are no published studies on efficacy or complications with the use of this device in children.

LARYNGEAL TUBE

The Laryngeal Tube (VBM Medical Inc., Noblesville, IN) is another supraglottic ventilatory device that is used for airway management assistance. It has been described as a single-lumen, shortened Combitube. It consists of an oval ventilation aperture placed between two distal low-pressure cuffs (Fig. 9–17), and it is inserted in a similar manner as the LMA. The distal (esophageal) balloon is designed to seal the airway distally and

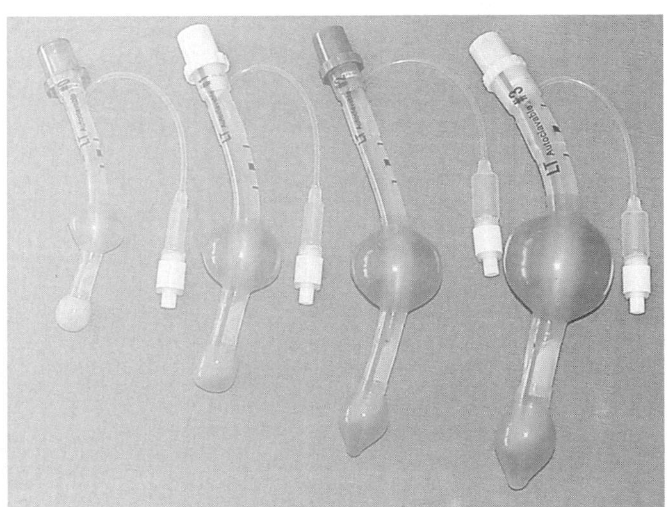

FIGURE 9–17. The laryngeal tube consists of an oval ventilation aperture placed between two distal low-pressure cuffs. The distal (esophageal) balloon is designed to seal the airway distally and protect against regurgitation. (Reproduced with permission of VBM Medical Inc., Noblesville, IN.)

protect against regurgitation. The proximal (oropharyngeal) balloon is designed to seal off the pharynx above the ventilation port. The two balloons are inflated sequentially via a unique connector at a pressure of 60 cm H_2O by using a manometer. There are six sizes that encompass all age ranges.

Like the LMA and PLA, the laryngeal tube is designed as an alternative to the anesthesia facemask and as a potential tool for providing ventilation in patients with a difficult airway. It can be used during spontaneous or controlled ventilation. In adult studies, the rate of successful placement exceeds 90% (Cook et al., 2003), but pediatric trials have not been performed.

■ ENDOTRACHEAL TUBES

In evaluating endotracheal tubes for use in infants and children, one must consider their influence on dead space, resistance to breathing, and tracheal or laryngeal injury. Endotracheal intubation reduces the dead space of the natural extrathoracic airway (Glauser et al., 1961) but can have a dramatic negative impact on the resistance to breathing. Resistance to laminar flow through a tube is governed by Hagen-Poiseuille Law, which dictates that resistance is proportional to the length of the tube and inversely proportional to the fourth power of the radius. Thus, small changes in the lumen of a tube can dramatically increase the resistance to flow through it. Assuming that flow is laminar and that all other variables are constant, one can predict that a reduction in internal diameter (ID) from 7.5 to 7.0 mm increases resistance 24%, whereas a reduction from 3.5 to 3.0 mm increases resistance by nearly 50%. Because luminal changes between the endotracheal tube and the adapter promote turbulent flow, measured differences are even more exaggerated. The resistance to breathing through the natural airway of a neonate is greater than that through a 3.5-mm-ID endotracheal tube but significantly less than that through a 2.5-mm-ID endotracheal tube (Polgar and Kong, 1965). A small amount of secretions or debris can increase resistance substantially, yet these accumulations are difficult to avoid in small-lumen tubes. The use of 2.5-mm-ID endotracheal tubes should be restricted to situations in which no other tube fits.

Resistance to breathing is governed by the ID of a tube, but the potential for laryngeal or tracheal mucosal injury is related to the outer diameter (OD). Mild trauma to the airway producing as little as 1-mm mucosal edema can result in significant narrowing of the infant's airway. As little as 25 mm Hg pressure on the lateral wall of the trachea causes local ischemia and mucosal injury in adults (Ching et al., 1974) and presumably in children as well.

Endotracheal tubes are made of nonreactive polyvinylchloride (PVC). Biologically inert materials reduce the risk of airway inflammatory reactions. PVC tubes are flammable and cannot be used in airway laser surgery. One must substitute a tube that is either nonflammable (e.g., metal) or laser resistant (e.g., red rubber tube wrapped with aluminum foil or manufactured with special surface treatments) (see Chapter 23, Anesthesia for Pediatric Otorhinolaryngologic Surgery). These special tubes should have labeling indicating they are intended for use in laser surgery (Subcommittee F29.18 on Operating Room Fire Safety, 1995). Patients with difficult airways or tracheal abnormalities often require a spiral wire-embedded silicone, or "anode" tube (Fig. 9–18). This tube has the flexibility to assume virtually any position, while the wire coil embedded in its wall preserves the lumen. Extreme caution must be taken with anode tubes, because their flexibility makes accidental extubation more likely.

There are a variety of endotracheal tubes for special needs. An RAE tube has a preformed contour that facilitates access to the surgical field (Fig. 9–19). Oral RAE tubes were initially developed for cleft palate surgery. The proximal end of the oral RAE tube rests over the middle of the mandible, whereas the proximal end of a nasal RAE tube rests on the forehead (Fig. 9–20). These preformed tracheal tubes can be used for any type of head or neck surgery in which the operating room table is turned away from the anesthesiologist and the head is maintained in a neutral position. The greatest disadvantage of preformed tubes

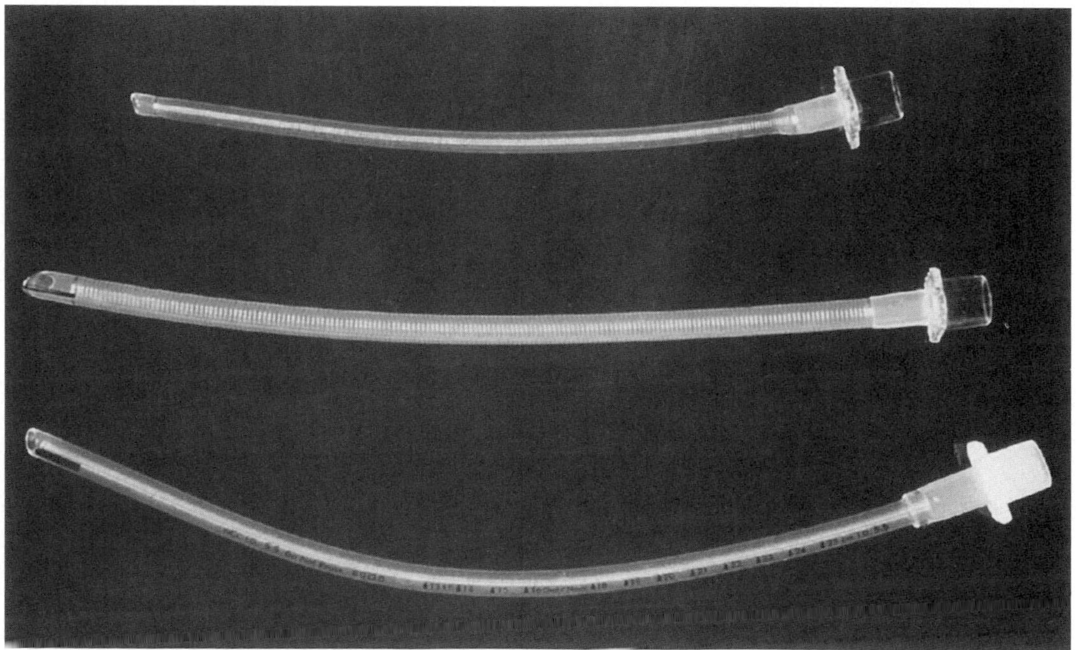

■ **FIGURE 9–18.** The flexibility of the anode tube and its ability to maintain a patent lumen with extremes in position make this endotracheal tube useful in surgery of the face and the airway. This is only a representative sample of the sizes of anode tubes that are available.

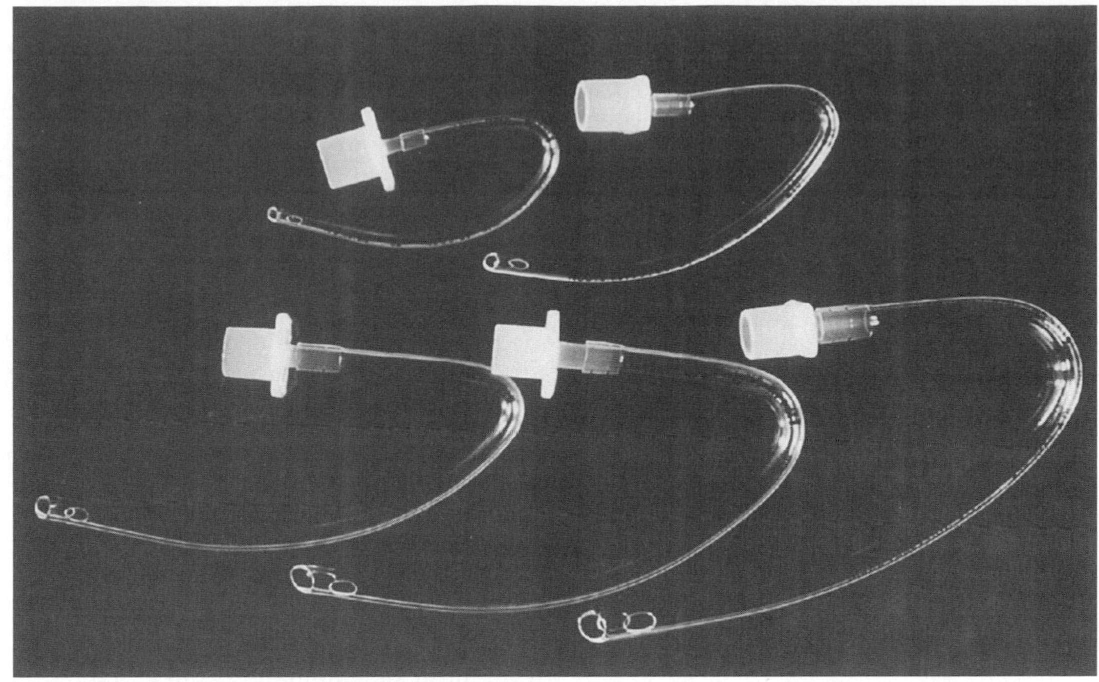

■ **FIGURE 9–19.** Oral RAE tubes. Preformed oral RAE tubes are made in a variety of sizes. They are especially useful in facial surgery. (From: Litman RS: Pediatric airway management. In: Litman RS, ed: *Pediatric anesthesia: The requisites.* St. Louis, 2004, Mosby.)

is that the flexion point is fixed. The length may be inappropriate, especially in patients whose cricoid diameter is unusually large or small, increasing the risk of endobronchial intubation or accidental extubation, respectively. Similarly, in a patient with a laryngeal or proximal tracheal stenosis, a standard endotracheal tube of a caliber small enough to be admitted to the airway may be too short. Tubes of small caliber with extra length are commercially available for this purpose.

Double-Lumen Endotracheal Tubes

A double-lumen endotracheal tube is commonly used to attain lung separation in adults. Its advantages include rapid and easy separation of the lungs, access to both lungs to facilitate suctioning, the ability to rapidly switch to two-lung ventilation if needed, and the ability to administer CPAP or oxygen insufflation to the operative lung, when necessary. The smallest commercially available double-lumen endotracheal tube is size 28 F, which precludes its placement in children weighing less than 30 to 35 kg or younger than 8 to 10 years (Table 9-5). With this smallest double-lumen endotracheal tube, bronchoscopic confirmation of its appropriate location within the trachea and bronchus requires use of an ultrathin flexible bronchoscope.

ENDOTRACHEAL TUBES FOR ONE-LUNG VENTILATION

Because of mechanical difficulties of one-lung ventilation in small children, pediatric surgeons historically have used retractors and surgical packs to improve surgical exposure during thoracic surgery.

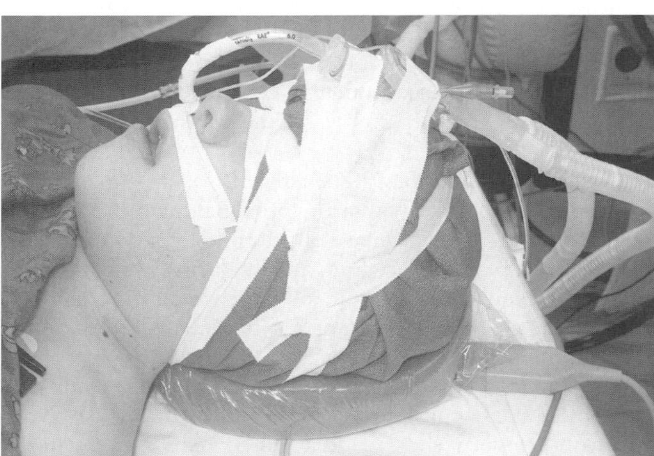

■ **FIGURE 9–20.** The nasal RAE tube is preformed to sit on the forehead for procedures in the oral cavity or neck. (From Litman RS: Pediatric airway management. In: Litman RS, ed: *Pediatric anesthesia: The requisites.* St. Louis, 2004, Mosby.)

■ **TABLE 9–5.** Comparison of tracheal tube dimensions used for one-lung ventilation

Tracheal Tube	Tracheal Lumen (mm)	Bronchial Lumen (mm)	Outside Diameter (mm)
Broncho-Cath*			
28 F (L)	4.5	4.5	9.8
35 F (L)	6.0	6.0	12.1
37 F (L)	6.5	6.5	13.2
39 F (L)	7.0	7.0	14.3
41 F (L)	7.4	7.4	15.4
Univent†	6.0		11.0
Standard*			
7.0	7.0		9.5
9.0	9.0		11.1
10.0	10.0		13.2

*Nellcor, Pleasanton, CA.
†Fuji Systems, Inc., Tokyo, Japan.

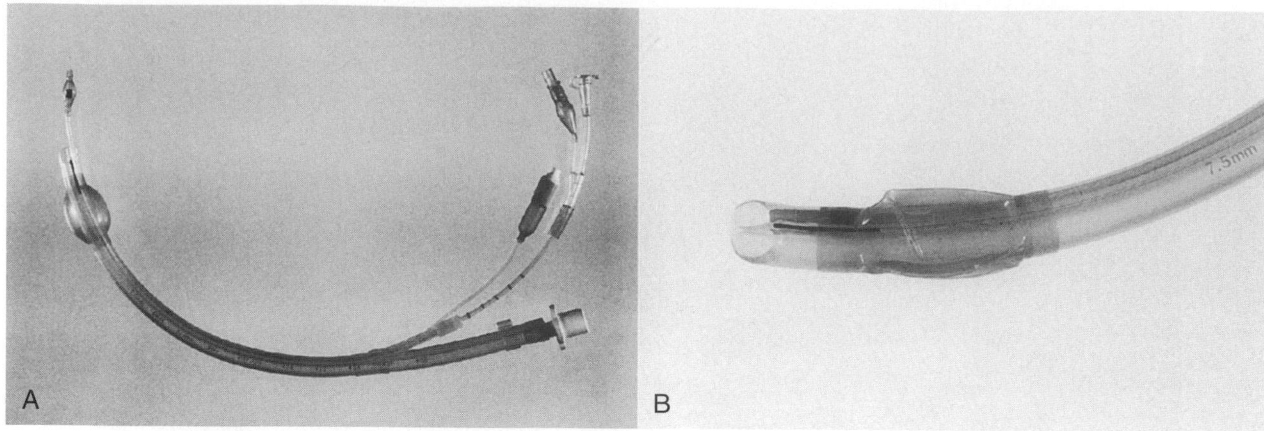

■ **FIGURE 9–21.** *(A)* Univent tube. A bronchial blocker is incorporated into this tracheal tube to allow for isolation of one of the lungs during an anesthetic. It can be withdrawn and ventilation can be continued in the postoperative period without the need to change to a single-lumen tube. *(B)* The blocker in its retracted state.

With the popularity of thoracoscopic surgical techniques in the pediatric population, there is an increasing need to provide one-lung ventilation to facilitate surgical exposure (Rowe et al., 1994; Tobias, 1999; Hammer, 2001). The pediatric anesthesiologist has a number of choices with which to provide one-lung ventilation.

UNIVENT ENDOTRACHEAL TUBE

The Univent endotracheal tube (Fuji Systems Corporation, Tokyo, Japan) is a single-lumen endotracheal tube with a moveable bronchial blocker built into its side wall (Kamaya and Krishna, 1985; MacGillivray, 1988; Hammer, 1998) (Fig. 9–21). The bronchial blocker contains a low-pressure high-volume cuff and has a central channel used to suction the blocked lung and to insufflate oxygen. The Univent tube is inserted into the trachea like a standard tracheal tube with the bronchial blocker withdrawn into the main tube. The bronchial blocker can then be advanced into the main stem bronchus of the operative lung under bronchoscopic guidance. Rotation of the tracheal tube determines the direction that the blocker takes as it is advanced. Inflation of the endobronchial cuff on the balloon tip catheter enables isolation of the operative lung. At the end of the procedure, the blocker tube can be withdrawn into the main tube, permitting postoperative ventilation without the need to change to a separate single-lumen tube.

Advantages of the Univent tube include ease of placement and the ability to easily change from one-lung ventilation to two-lung ventilation. In addition, unlike the standard double-lumen endotracheal tube, the bronchial blocker can be pulled back into its channel with the Univent tube left in place for postoperative ventilation. The Univent tube is available in sizes 3.5- (uncuffed), 4.5-, 6.0-, 6.5-, 7.5-, 8.0-, 8.5-, and 9.0-mm ID. The OD is larger than that of a conventional endotracheal tube of the same ID (Table 9–5). The IDs of the 3.5- and 4.0-mm Univent tubes limit the passage of a standard pediatric bronchoscope with an OD of 3.5 mm or greater, thereby requiring an ultrathin pediatric bronchoscope to visualize the bronchial blocker.

SELECTIVE ENDOBRONCHIAL INTUBATION

In infants and young children whose small size precludes placement of a double-lumen endotracheal tube or Univent tube, there are two additional options for one-lung ventilation: selective endobronchial intubation with a standard endotracheal tube or placement of a separate "bronchial blocker."

Endobronchial Intubation With a Standard Endotracheal Tube

An endotracheal tube can be inserted into either main bronchus with the use of bronchoscopic guidance. In children older than 2 years, a cuffed endotracheal tube maintains an effective seal of the lung while maintaining the tube in a proximal position within the main bronchus. The major disadvantage of selective endobronchial intubation is that it is not possible to quickly change from one-lung ventilation to two-lung ventilation because it requires repositioning the endotracheal tube from the bronchus into the trachea and vice versa. Furthermore, with unintentional movement of the endotracheal tube and minimal cephalad displacement, selective intubation may be lost because of bronchial extubation.

Bronchial Blocker Devices

A bronchial blocker device consists of a small balloon that is purposefully inflated within the proximal portion of the main bronchus to isolate one of the lungs under bronchoscopic guidance. Several different devices can be used as bronchial blockers, including a Fogarty embolectomy catheter and the Arndt (Cook Critical Care, Bloomington, IN) endobronchial blocker (Fig. 9–22). These devices contain a central channel that allows suctioning (for lung deflation) and the application of oxygen and CPAP.

A Fogarty embolectomy catheter contains a balloon at the distalmost end to place within the proximal main bronchus to isolate the lung. A disadvantage of the embolectomy catheter is that the tip can be displaced proximally during the course of a surgical procedure, especially if the patient's position changes. Total airway obstruction can result if the inflated balloon slips back into the trachea.

The Arndt Endobronchial Blocker is a bronchial blocker with an inflatable cuff and a central lumen, through which a wire with a looped end has been passed (Arndt et al., 1999; Hammer et al., 2002) (see Fig. 9–22). The bronchial blocker is passed through a specialized adapter that is placed at the proximal end of the endotracheal tube. This adapter contains four ports: (1) a connection to the endotracheal tube, (2) a standard

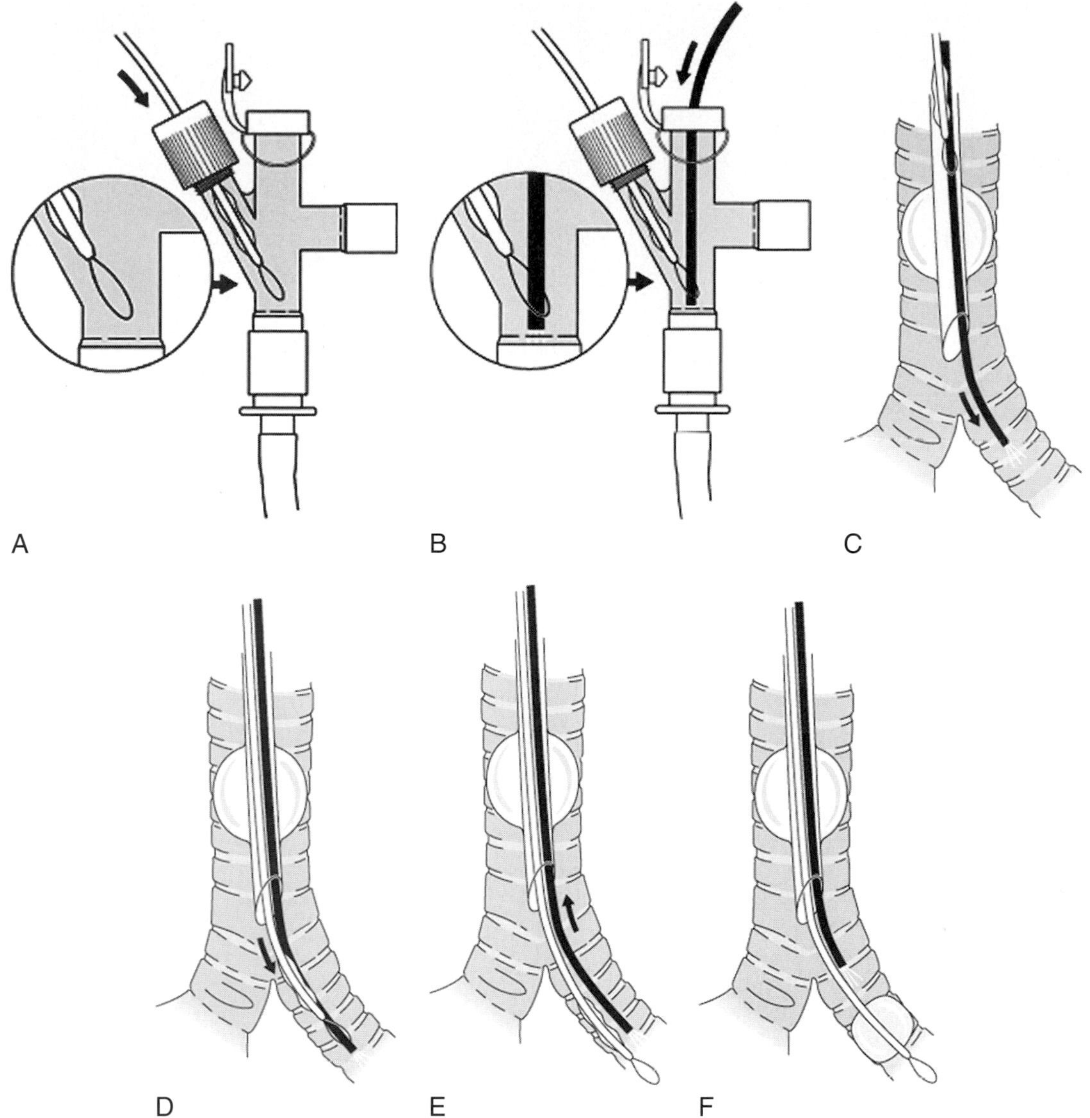

■ **FIGURE 9–22.** The Arndt bronchial blocker is inserted under fiberoptic guidance. *(A)* With a special multi-port adapter that is attached to the tracheal tube, the blocker is inserted through a side port into the main body of the connector. Ventilation with 100% oxygen is enabled through a second side port. *(B)* A flexible bronchoscope is inserted through the remaining port engaging the wire loop at the end of the bronchial blocker. *(C)* The bronchoscope is advanced into the bronchus to be isolated. *(D)* The blocker is advanced into the bronchus sliding down the bronchoscope. *(E)* The bronchoscope is withdrawn leaving the blocker in place. *(F)* The blocker's balloon is inflated and placement is verified using the bronchoscope before it is withdrawn completely. (Drawings courtesy of Cook, Inc., Bloomington, IN.)

15-mm adaptor for the anesthesia circuit, (3) a port for the bronchial blocker with a self-sealing diaphragm that can be tightened around the bronchial blocker to hold it in place, and (4) a port for the flexible bronchoscope. The bronchial blocker is passed through the port and placed at the entrance of the endotracheal tube. The bronchoscope is passed through the port and then through the wire loop at the end of the bronchial blocker. The bronchoscope and bronchial blocker are passed under direct vision as a single unit into the main bronchus of the operative side. The bronchoscope is withdrawn into the trachea, and the balloon is inflated under direct visualization. When correct placement has been confirmed, the wire loop is removed from the central channel. Once the wire guide is removed from the channel, it cannot be replaced. The Arndt blocker is currently available in 3 sizes (5 F, 7 F, and 9 F) with the 9 F recommended for endotracheal tubes of 7.5 mm and above, 7 F for endotracheal tubes of 6.0 to 7.0 mm, and 5 F for endotracheal tubes of 4.5 to 5.5 mm.

■ TRACHEOSTOMY TUBES

The three most common indications for tracheostomy in children are (1) prolonged mechanical ventilation (>50%), (2) upper airway obstruction (40%), and (3) pulmonary toilet (10%) (Wetmore et al., 1999). Within each category are congenital, traumatic, metabolic, infectious, and neoplastic conditions that require tracheostomy. Although the underlying medical conditions may be numerous, the most common diagnoses in pediatric tracheostomy patients are bronchopulmonary dysplasia and neurologic disorders.

The ideal tracheostomy tube should be made of a material that causes minimal tissue reactivity, can be easily cleaned and

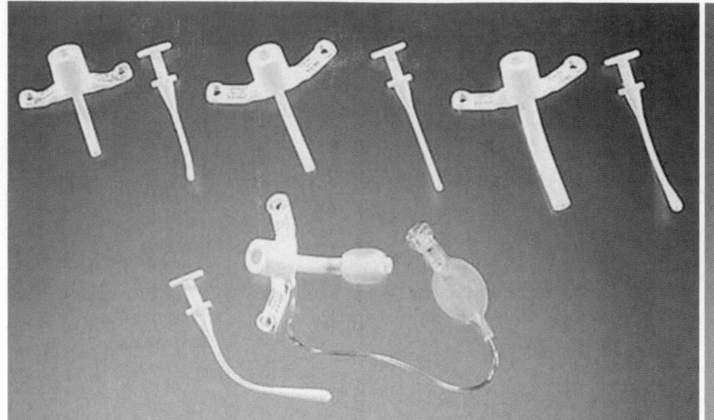
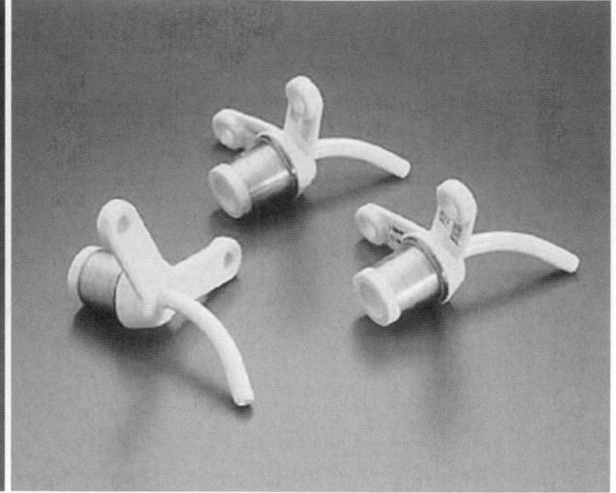

■ **FIGURE 9–23.** Representative models of pediatric tracheostomy tubes include Shiley *(left)* and Bivona *(right)*.

maintained, and is available in a variety of shapes, diameters, and lengths (Fig. 9–23). The tube needs to be rigid enough to prevent kinking or collapse, yet soft enough to be comfortable for the patient. Early tracheostomy tubes were made of stainless steel or silver (Downes and Schreiner, 1985). These tubes had the advantages of causing minimal tissue reaction and avoiding tracheal collapse. Their rigidity caused significant discomfort to the patient because of injury to the tracheal mucosa. Most manufacturers use silicone tubes that have minimal tissue reactivity and conform to the structure of the airway. The ideal tube also contains an inner cannula that can be removed and cleaned. Modern tracheostomy tubes have a 15-mm male connector for the attachment of standard respiratory equipment. To improve the patient's comfort and ease of care, a low-profile swivel is commonly added to the tracheostomy tube (Schreiner, 1986). This allows unrestricted neck movement and easy care through a suction port. Tracheostomy tubes for infants are uncuffed; in larger children and adolescents, cuffed tracheostomy tubes are preferred.

The appropriate tracheostomy tube is selected on the basis of the ID and OD and the length. The OD determines the size of the tube that may be inserted, whereas the ID determines the actual airway size. The diameter of the tube should be large enough to allow adequate air exchange, easy suctioning, and clearance of secretions. If the indication for tracheostomy is assisted ventilation, the size of the tube should be adjusted to prevent excessive air leak. Predictors of the appropriate tube size include the child's age and the size of a preexisting endotracheal tube. A tube that is too large compromises the capillary blood flow in the tracheal wall, which may result in mucosal ischemia, ulceration, and development of fibrous stenosis. Overinflation of a cuffed tracheostomy tube for a prolonged period of time may produce similar injuries. This complication may be avoided by selecting the proper size of tracheostomy tube (Table 9–6) and adjusting the cuff pressure to less than 20 cm H_2O. The choice of the tube size is also influenced by visualization of the size of the tracheal lumen.

The length of the tube is important, especially in neonates and infants. A tube that is too short may result in accidental decannulation or the development of a false passage. If a tube is too long, the tip may abrade the carina or become situated in the right main bronchus. Some plastic tubes may be cut to the desired length as necessary. Extra-long custom-made tubes

■ **TABLE 9–6.** Tracheostomy tube dimensions

Model	Inner Diameter (mm)	Outer Diameter (mm)	Overall Length (mm)
Shiley*			
Shiley Neonatal			
3.0	3.0	4.5	30
3.5	3.5	5.2	32
4.0	4.0	5.9	34
4.5	4.5	6.5	36
Shiley Pediatric			
3.0	3.0	4.5	39
3.5	3.5	5.2	40
4.0	4.0	5.9	41
4.5	4.5	6.5	42
5.0	5.0	7.1	44
5.5	5.5	7.7	46
Shiley Pediatric Long			
5.0	5.0	7.1	50
5.5	5.5	7.7	52
6.0	6.0	8.3	54
6.5	6.5	9.0	56
Shiley Cuffed Pediatric			
4.0	4.0	5.9	41
4.5	4.5	6.5	42
5.0	5.0	7.1	44
5.5	5.5	7.7	46
Shiley Cuffed Pediatric Long			
5.0	5.0	7.1	50
5.5	5.5	7.7	52
6.0	6.0	8.3	54
6.5	6.5	9.0	56
Bivona†			
Standard Neonatal Uncuffed			
60N025	2.5	4.0	30
60N030	3.0	4.7	32
60N035	3.5	5.3	34
60N040	4.0	6.0	36
60N045	4.5	6.5	36
Neonatal FlexTend Plus‡			
60NFP25	2.5	4.0	30
60NFP30	3.0	4.7	32
60NFP35	3.5	5.3	34
60NFP40	4.0	6.0	36

TABLE 9–6. Tracheostomy tube dimensions (Continued)

Model	Inner Diameter (mm)	Outer Diameter (mm)	Overall Length (mm)
Bivona† (Continued)			
Standard Pediatric Uncuffed			
60P025	2.5	4.0	38
60P030	3.0	4.7	39
60P035	3.5	5.3	40
60P040	4.0	6.0	41
60P045	4.5	6.7	42
60P050	5.0	7.3	44
60P055	5.5	8.0	46
Standard Pediatric FlexTend Plus‡			
60PFS25	2.5	4.0	38
60PFS30	3.0	4.7	39
60PFS35	3.5	5.3	40
60PFS40	4.0	6.0	41
60PFS45	4.5	6.7	42
60PFS50	5.0	7.3	44
60PFS55	5.5	8.0	46
Extra Long Pediatric FlexTend Plus‡			
60PFS35	3.5	5.3	40
60PFS40	4.0	6.0	44
60PFS45	4.5	6.7	48
60PFS50	5.0	7.3	50
60PFS55	5.5	8.0	52
Neonatal Cuffed§			
N025	2.5	4.0	30
N030	3.0	4.7	32
N035	3.5	5.3	34
N040	4.0	6.0	36
Pediatric Cuffed§			
P025	2.5	4.0	38
P030	3.0	4.7	39
P035	3.5	5.3	40
P040	4.0	6.0	41
P045	4.5	6.7	42
P050	5.0	7.3	44
P055	5.5	8.0	46
Adjustable and Extra Length¶			
60HA25	2.5	4.0	55
60HA30	3.0	4.7	60
60HA35	3.5	5.3	65
60HA40	4.0	6.0	70
60HA45	4.5	6.7	75
60HA50	5.0	7.3	80
60HA55	5.5	8.0	85
550050	5.0	7.7	50
550055	5.5	8.3	52
550060	6.0	8.3	55

*Shiley is manufactured by Mallinckrodt Inc., St. Louis, MO.

†Bivona is manufactured by Portex, Keene, NH.

‡FlexTend tubes feature a flexible, kink-resistant proximal extension that allows easier access and enables distal connections away from the infant's chin, neck, and chest.

§Bivona cuffed tubes are available in three different models: Fome-Cuf tubes (85 series) include a SidePort AutoControl Adapter that synchronizes cuff and ventilator pressure. A complete seal is possible for patients with high peak end-expiratory pressure or high inspiratory pressure needs. Aire-Cuf tubes (65 series) feature a traditional air-filled cuff. TTS cuffs (67 series) feature an uncuffed tube profile when the cuff is deflated but provide the protection of a cuff when it is inflated.

¶Adjustable Hyperflex (HA series) is an instantly customizable, soft, flexible, kink-resistant, silicone tube with an adjustable neck flange. The flexible shaft adapts to the unique contours of each patient's anatomy. The Adjustable Hyperflex tube is primarily used as a measuring device and temporizing measure until the child can receive a permanent tube with a fixed neck flange. The 550 series is made of polyvinylchloride that softens at body temperature. It features a long tube shaft and a traditional anatomic curve.

may be helpful in unusual situations, such as tracheomalacia or tracheal stenosis, to span the diseased area.

LARYNGOSCOPES

A variety of pediatric-sized laryngoscope blades are available (Table 9–7). The laryngoscope has three basic parts: a handle, a blade, and a light. The blade consists of a spatula, a flange, and a tip. Blades differ in length, width, and curvature. Laryngoscopes can be purchased with incandescent or fiberoptic light sources. Those with fiberoptic light sources provide extremely bright, highly focused light that occasionally can be obscured by the tongue and soft tissue. Standards for each component are specified by ASTM standard F-1195-99 (ASTM, 2005). Selection of a particular laryngoscope is usually based on personal preference and experience, the size of the child, and the peculiarities of a specific airway problem.

Generally, the straight Miller blade is used in children (Miller, 1941). This blade allows the cephalad aspect of the larynx to be exposed more easily, because the base of the tongue can be lifted out of the line of sight, and the protruding epiglottis can be retracted with the tip. Wide blades and large-flange blades, like the Robertshaw, the Flagg, and the Wis-Hipple, allow the wide tongue of the small child to be flattened during laryngoscopy (Flagg, 1928; Robertshaw, 1962) (Fig. 9–24). The 1.5 Wis-Hipple blade is especially useful in the toddler (Fig. 9–25). For older children and young adults, longer straight blades (e.g., Miller 2) or curved blades (e.g., the Macintosh) allow the anesthesiologist to achieve good exposure and avoid prominent dentition (Macintosh, 1943).

During laryngoscopy, neonates may rapidly develop hypoxemia secondary to apnea, decreased functional residual capacity, and increased oxygen consumption (Gibbons, 1986). The Oxyscope is a modified Miller blade that allows insufflation of oxygen into the pharynx and decreases the rapidity with which hypoxemia occurs during laryngoscopy (Todres and Crone, 1981) (Fig. 9–26).

DEVICES AND TECHNIQUES FOR A DIFFICULT INTUBATION

Children with micrognathia, such as those with Goldenhar's syndrome, Pierre Robin sequence, or Treacher Collins syndrome, are often difficult to intubate with standard laryngoscopy equipment. A number of different devices have been designed to facilitate endotracheal intubation in these types of children; these include the Bullard laryngoscope, the lighted stylet, and the fiberoptic flexible bronchoscope.

TABLE 9–7. Laryngoscope blade types and sizes

Age	BLADE TYPE AND SIZE		
	Miller	*Wis-Hippel*	*Macintosh*
Premature neonate	0	—	—
Term neonate	0 to 1	—	—
1 to 12 mo	1	1	—
1 to 2 yr	1	1.5	2
2 to 6 yr	2	—	2
6 to 12 yr	2	—	3

Modified from Coté CJ: A practice of anesthesia for infants and children. Philadelphia, 2001, WB Saunders.

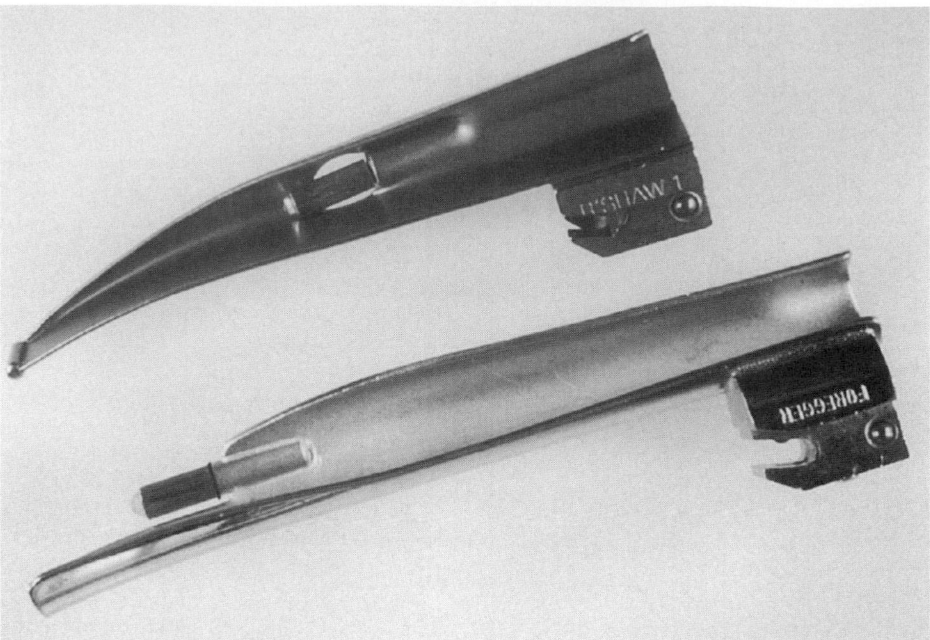

■ **FIGURE 9–24.** Robertshaw blade *(top)* and Flagg blade *(bottom)*.

Bullard Laryngoscope

The Bullard laryngoscope (ACMI, Stamford, CT) uses a fiberoptic telescope attached to a rigid curved blade to enhance glottic visualization (Borland and Casselbrant, 1990; Brown et al., 1993; Shulman et al., 1997; Shulman and Connelly, 2000) (Fig. 9–27). It is available in two pediatric sizes. Tube placement can be performed using a mechanical device on the scope to position the tube or by directing the tube along the side of the laryngoscope using the telescope. Use of the device by novices is often awkward, but experienced users tout its ease of use. Comparison trials of the Bullard scope with other methods to secure the difficult pediatric airway have not been performed.

Lighted Stylet

The lighted stylet ("light wand") consists of a semirigid stylet with a bright light at the distalmost end (Fiberoptic Intubation Stilette; Anesthesia Medical Specialties, Santa Fe Springs, CA; and Trachlight; Laerdal Medical, Armonk, NJ) (Fig. 9–28). The lighted stylet is prepared by inserting it inside a standard

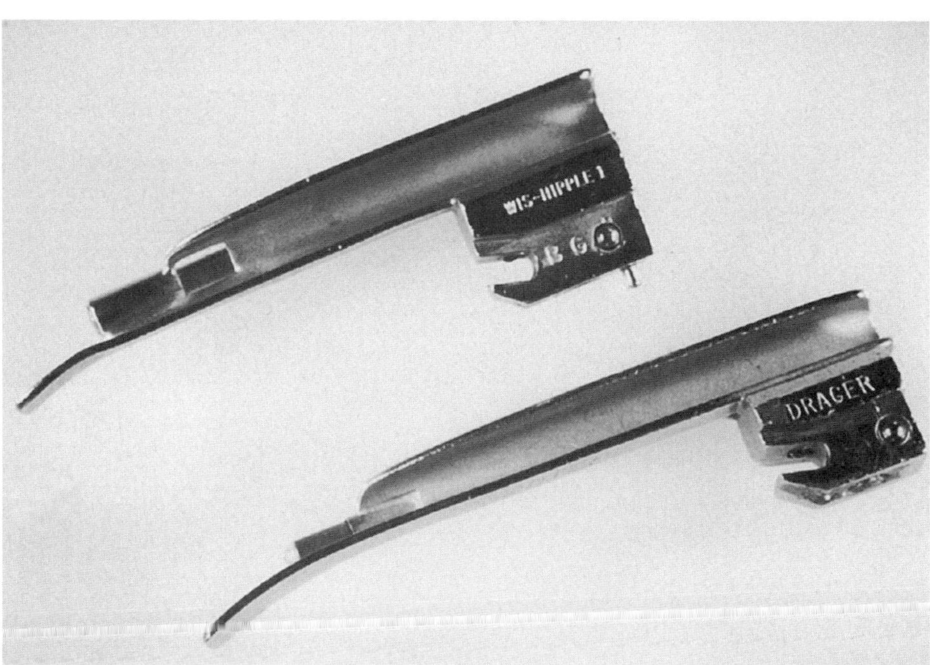

■ **FIGURE 9–25.** Two sizes of the Wis-Hipple blade are available.

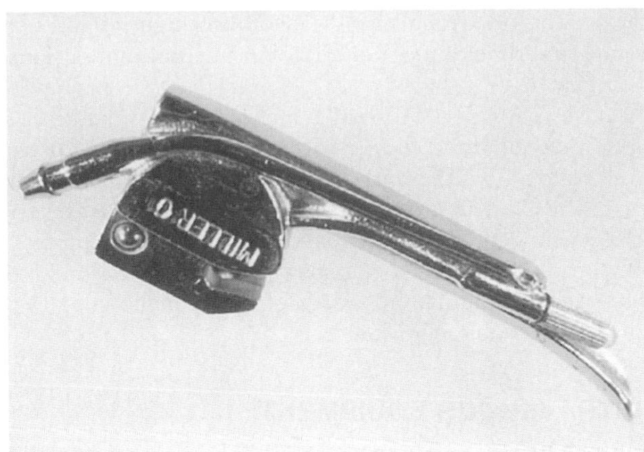

■ **FIGURE 9–26.** Oxyscope. This is a Miller O blade that is specially fitted; 2 to 3 L/min of oxygen is connected to the cannula on the left side of the blade, as shown. The oxygen is then directed by the lumen of this cannula into the trachea.

endotracheal tube, which is then blindly inserted into the pharynx. In a darkened room, the transmitted light is used to guide accurate glottic location, and the endotracheal tube is slid off the lighted stylet and into the trachea. It is useful when the child has an anatomically normal larynx that is difficult to visualize with direct methods. This may occur with micrognathia (Krucylak and Schreiner, 1992), temporomandibular joint disorders (or any condition that limits mandibular mobility), cervical spine instability, or facial trauma. It is particularly suited to children with limited neck and mandible mobility, but it is not useful in cases of fixed upper or lower airway obstructive pathology or in the presence of a foreign body.

Innovative solutions to the size limitations have been overcome, and the lighted stylet can be used with endotracheal tubes as small as 2.5-mm ID (Davis et al., 2000). A "home-grown" version lightwand for small infants and neonates has been created, with a 20-gauge fiberoptic illuminating lightpipe (Storz Ophthalmics Inc., St. Louis, MO) attached to any standard fiberoptic light source (Fig. 9–29*A* to *C*).

Flexible Fiberoptic Bronchoscopy

Fiberoptic bronchoscopes with flexible tips have been used successfully both in infants and in children whose intubation would otherwise have been difficult or impossible. With the child sedated or anesthetized and breathing spontaneously, a fiberoptic bronchoscope that has been passed through an endotracheal tube is inserted through the mouth or nose to visualize the larynx. The endotracheal tube is slid off the bronchoscope after its entrance into the trachea. In the past, the major limitation of this technique was the inability of large adult bronchoscopes to fit through small pediatric endotracheal tubes. This problem has been solved by the availability of new, smaller ultrathin fiberoptic laryngoscopes (Fan et al., 1986; de Blic et al., 1991; Roth et al., 1994) (Table 9–8). Anesthesiologists have become more adept at manipulating the ultrathin bronchoscope, which may be used inside a 2.5- or 3.0-mm-ID endotracheal tube (depending on the manufacturer). In addition, the optical aspects of the equipment have improved with these smaller fiberscopes to allow better screen resolution.

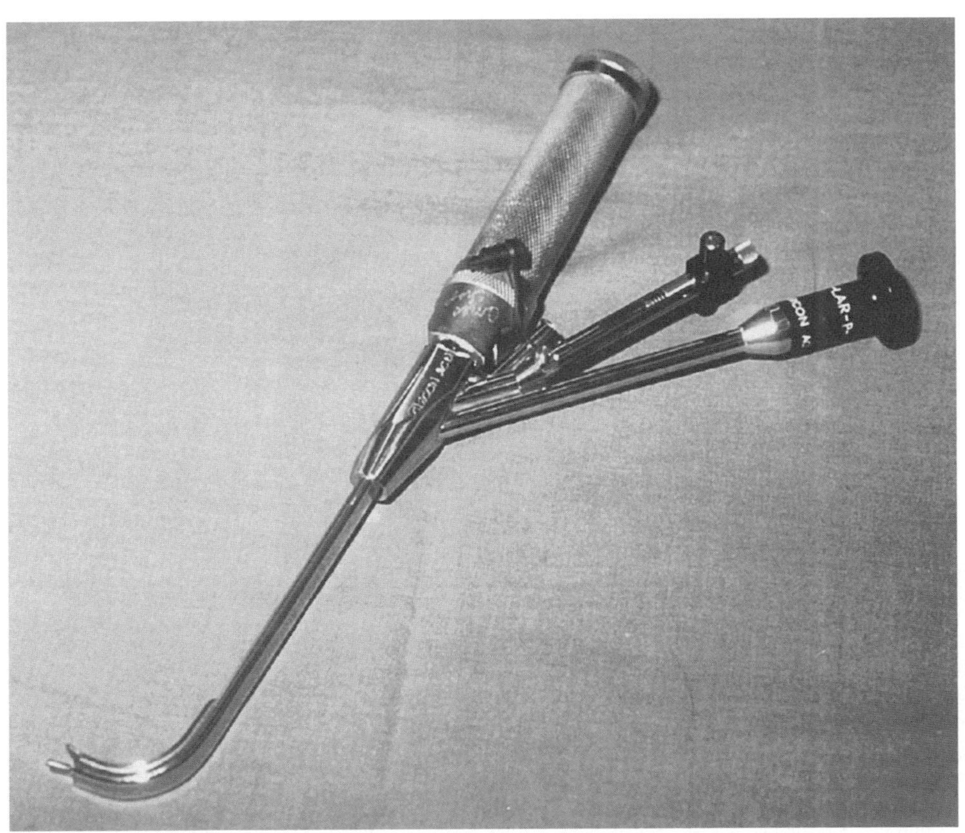

■ **FIGURE 9–27.** The Bullard laryngoscope allows a view of the larynx in children with limited ability to open the mouth and whose larynx is positioned relatively anterior (cephalad).

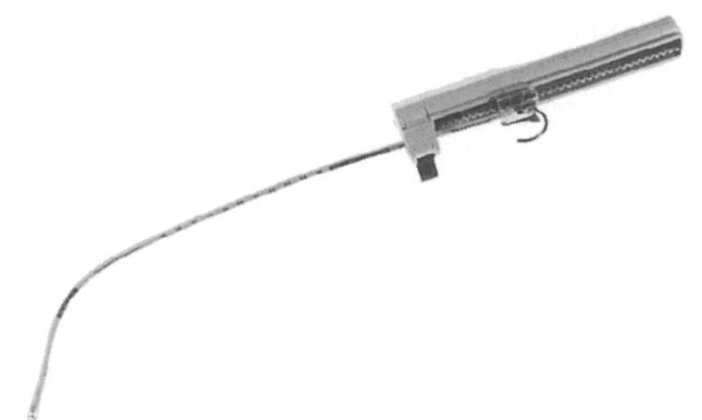

■ **FIGURE 9–28.** Using a lighted stylet, the endotracheal tube can be guided into the trachea with the use of the surface anatomy of the child and projection of the lighted stylet tip. (From Litman RS: Pediatric airway management. In: Litman RS, ed: *Pediatric anesthesia: The requisites*. St. Louis, 2004, Mosby.)

These ultrathin bronchoscopes may or may not be manufactured with suction ports; secretions and blood are more likely to obscure the view in smaller children. Some ultrathin bronchoscopes contain a suction port, but it is too narrow to allow effective suctioning of secretions. Furthermore, oxygen insufflation should not be performed via this port in small children because of the possibilities of generating dangerously high intrabronchial pressures and development of a tension pneumothorax (Iannoli and Litman, 2002).

Apneic ventilation is usually ineffective in small children because of their limited time to oxyhemoglobin desaturation. This is caused by the markedly reduced functional residual capacity (FRC) in anesthetized small children and their relatively high oxygen consumption. Ventilation can be accomplished during bronchoscopy by the use of a special anesthesia mask that incorporates a conduit for passage of the bronchoscope (VBM Medical Inc., Noblesville, IN).

■ INTRAVENOUS EQUIPMENT

■ CATHETERS

Intravenous catheters appropriate for the smallest premature infant and the largest adolescent patient are made by a wide variety of companies. The appropriate catheter is usually dictated by the patient's size, expected fluid requirements, and the operator's preference. In general, a 22- or 24-gauge catheter suffices in the small infant. Patients with significant fluid requirements, such as neonates undergoing gastroschisis repair,

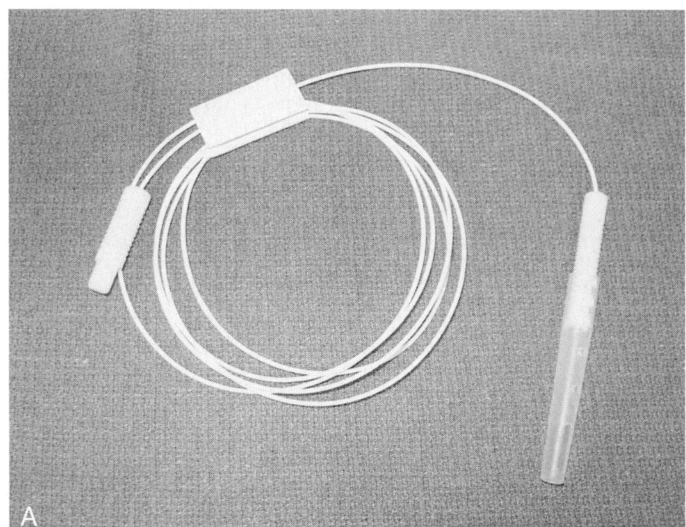

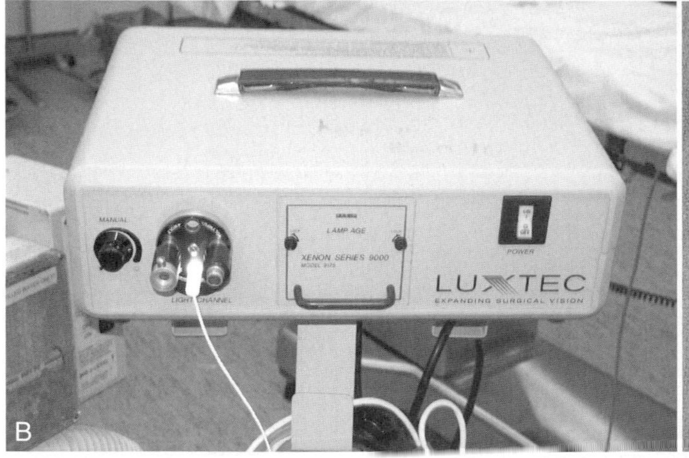

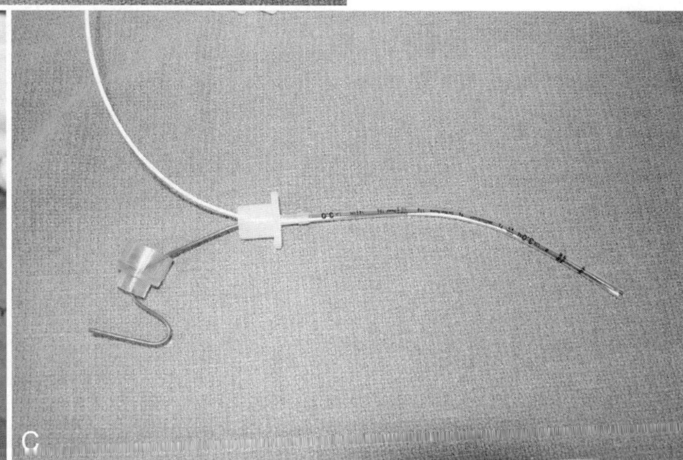

■ **FIGURE 9–29.** *(A)* A thin fiberoptic bundle is used as a lightwand. *(B)* The fiberoptic bundle can be attached to any commercially available light source with adjustable light intensity. *(C)* The fiberoptic bundle is inserted alongside a thin pliable stylet into an endotracheal tube. (From Litman RS: The difficult pediatric airway. In: Litman RS, ed: *Pediatric anesthesia: The requisites*. St. Louis, 2004, Mosby.)

TABLE 9–8. Pediatric fiberoptic bronchoscopes

Manufacturer	Model No.	Outer Diameter (mm)	Suction Channel Diameter (mm)	Working Length (cm)	Field of View (°)	Angulation Up (°)	Angulation Down (°)
Fujinon, Wayne, NJ	BRO-YP2	4.8	2.0	57.5	90	160	100
Olympus, Melville, NY	LF-P	2.2	None	60	75	120	120
Olympus	BF-N20	2.2	None	55	75	160	90
Pentax, Golden, CO	FI-7P	2.4	None	60	95	130	130
Storz, Culver City, CA	BN 11301	5.0	2.3	65	110	160	160
Storz	BD 11302	3.7	1.5	65	80	120	120

may need two or three intravenous catheters. In older children, a 22- or 20-gauge catheter usually suffices. Butterfly needles inserted into tiny veins are not adequate for infusions during surgery because they are easily dislodged. They are convenient for performing rapid intravenous induction in a young child or an anxious adolescent. Pain can be minimized when using a 25- or 27-gauge butterfly needle.

In accordance with Poiseuille's relationship, the resistance to flow through an intravenous catheter is related most significantly to the radius of the lumen, but the length of the catheter and the viscosity of the fluid also have an impact (Table 9–9). Although small differences exist between comparable catheters of various manufacturers (Hodge and Fleisher, 1985; Rosen and Rosen, 1986), major flow reductions occur when they are lengthened to enable central venous cannulation. Viscosity of the infused fluid (e.g., blood versus crystalloid) imposes significant resistance changes only when small (<20 gauge) or long (>3 inches) catheters are used (Hodge and Fleisher, 1985; Rothen et al., 1992). For example, an 18-gauge catheter lengthened to 8 inches to enable central venous placement exhibits the flow characteristics of a short 24-gauge catheter.

With the widespread concern of the danger of accidental needlestick injuries, many medical centers have replaced standard intravenous and butterfly catheters with those that provide retractable needles and less danger of a needlestick after intravenous catheter insertion. A number of studies have determined that needleless intravenous catheters reduce the rate of needlestick injuries by up to 60% (Orenstein et al., 1995; Lawrence et al., 1997). Consequently, in 2001 the U.S. Occupational Safety and Health Administration (OSHA) authored the Needlestick Safety and Prevention Act (H.R. 5178), which stipulates that the 1991 Bloodborne Pathogens Standard (29 CFR 1910.1030) be revised to strengthen the requirements related to the use of safety-engineered sharp devices (*Federal Register* on January 18, 2001). The Needlestick Safety and Prevention Act provides a legislative mandate that health care facility employers provide employees with safety-engineered sharp devices.

TABLE 9–9. Catheter sizes and their flow rates

Catheter Size (gauge)	Length (inches)	MEAN FLOW RATE RANGE (mL/min) *Crystalloid (gravity)*	*Crystalloid (pressure)*	*Blood (pressure)*
24	0.75	14 to 15	42 to 47	20 to 30
22	1	24 to 26	65 to 77	44 to 50
20	1.25 to 2	38 to 42	103 to 126	69 to 81
18	1.25 to 2	55 to 62	164 to 214	150 to 164
16	2	75 to 81	248 to 280	216 to 286
14	2	92 to 93	301 to 319	334 to 410
20	8	5	16	3
18	8	13	51	22
16	8	31	97	35

Data summarized from Hodge D III, Fleisher G: Pediatric catheter flow rates. *Am J Emerg Med* 3:403, 1985.

INFUSION SETS

Intravenous infusion sets must also be tailored to the patient and the planned surgical procedure. Microdrip infusion sets (60 drops/mL) allow the anesthesiologist to more accurately deliver small volumes of infusate to the small child compared with the standard 15 drops/mL infusion set. For an older child (older than approximately 10 years), the standard adult infusion set is adequate. The addition of extension tubes to all pediatric infusion sets permits the intravenous catheter to be placed in any available extremity and allows a small child to be moved down on the operating table for better surgical access. Insertion of multiple stopcocks in the infusion tubing allows precise volumes of blood or colloid to be administered. The blood set is attached to the stopcock closest to the patient, and a syringe is placed proximally. The stopcocks are opened to allow blood to flow into the syringe and then adjusted to allow an accurate volume of blood to be infused from the syringe into the patient. Before their use, all infusion sets should be "de-bubbled" to prevent air entrainment into the circulation, a task especially important in a small premature infant, who is likely to have a patent foramen ovale or ductus arteriosus, or in a child with a known intracardiac defect. To decrease the incidence of accidental needlestick injuries, all manufacturers now offer injection ports throughout the length of the tubing that are accessible with needleless Luer-Loc ports. These ports can easily inject air that is trapped in the injection ports.

WARMING DEVICES

Heat conservation is critical in the care of the newborn infant. A decrease of 2°C in the environmental temperature is sufficient to double the oxygen consumption of a full-term infant (Hill and Rahimtulla, 1965). To meet this increase in oxygen consumption, the neonate must double its minute ventilation. For a critically ill premature infant who is unable to mount this increase in ventilation, an oxygen debt and progressive lactic acidosis ensue (see Chapter 5, Thermoregulation: Physiology and Perioperative Disturbances). The rate of heat loss in newborn infants is four times that in adults because of a higher surface area–to–body weight ratio, increased curvature of body surfaces, and decreased insulation from skin and subcutaneous fat (Adamsons and Towell, 1965). Special efforts must be made to maintain body temperature during anesthesia, especially in small infants, in operative procedures with large insensible losses, and with rapid fluid administration.

Heated water-filled mattresses are routinely used to prevent conductive heat loss from the infant to the operating room table and to transfer heat to the infant (see Chapter 5, Thermoregulation: Physiology and Perioperative Disturbances). The safe temperature range is narrow—below 35°C, infants may lose heat to the mattress, and above 38°C, there is the possibility of overheating and burns. In children who weigh less than 0.5 m^2 (≈10 kg), circulating water warming blankets have been shown to conserve heat (Goudsouzian et al., 1973). Circulating water warming blankets placed under the patient have no significant effect on temperature conservation in larger children and adults, although they do make the operating room table more comfortable. This difference in warming blanket effectiveness relative to the patient's size probably reflects the proportionally larger surface area in contact with the blanket in the smaller infant than in the larger child or adult. Placing the circulating water blanket over the patient is more effective than having the child lie on the warming device (Sessler and Moayeri, 1990). Inappropriate use of warming blankets can result in overheating and burns (Crino and Nagel, 1968). Burns can be minimized by placing one or two sheets between the patient and the water filled blanket; each additional sheet reduces heat transfer by 20%. To decrease further the risk of burns, the warming blanket should have a maximum temperature of 42°C and an automatic shutoff if this temperature is exceeded or if the patient's temperature exceeds a preset value. In addition, the machine should display both the patient's temperature and the water temperature so that periodic visual comparison can act as a further safety monitor. Excess surgical preparation solution should not be allowed to pool over the blanket because skin irritation can occur, especially under pressure points. The cause of this irritation is not known.

FORCED WARM AIR DEVICE

The flow of warm air across a child's skin produced by a forced air warming blanket prevents heat loss to the environment and may even effectively warm patients via radiant shielding and convection. Of all devices, these are one of the most effective and should be used in all cases where hypothermia is a possibility (Sessler et al., 1991; Camus et al., 1993; Kurz et al., 1993). Forced air systems inject warm air through a connecting hose into a quiltlike blanket that has small holes on one surface. Warm air escaping through these holes provides conductive and convective warming to the patient. Different size blankets permit maximum coverage of specific body areas over a range of patient sizes. The most effective units direct flow toward areas with major blood vessels like the chest, axilla, abdomen, and groin, where convective heating is most effective (Giesbrecht et al., 1994). Like overhead radiant warmers and circulating water blankets, forced air systems can produce burns and overheating when used inappropriately (Truell et al., 2000). Maximum air temperatures on these devices are designed to minimize the risk of burns. Ensuring that the tube carrying the warm air to the blanket does not touch the patient also decreases the likelihood of thermal injury. Furthermore, directing warm air from the hose without the blanket ("free-hosing") has been associated with patient burns.

WRAPPING AND DRAPING WITH PLASTIC SHEETS

Because of their large surface area, infants have significant evaporative and radiant heat loss. Wrapping and draping the patient with special blankets are also effective in decreasing heat loss during prolonged surgery, especially when forced air devices are impractical. Radiant heat loss can be decreased with the use of Webril cotton wrapping (Kendall Corporation, Boston, MA) covered with plastic bags over exposed extremities. For small infants with relatively large heads, cranial heat loss can be decreased up to 73% by wrapping the head in an insulated hat or plastic bag. This is significant in neonates, because their brain is responsible for 44% of their total heat production (Rowe et al., 1983). The use of reflective blankets, made from the material used in outdoor survival apparel (e.g., space blankets), is also effective in reducing heat loss (Bourke et al., 1984). Cutaneous heat loss is proportional to the surface area of the patient, making the percentage of skin surface covered far more important than the region of the body covered or the type of material used for passive insulation (Sessler et al., 1991).

HUMIDIFICATION OF INSPIRED GASES

Humidification of inspired gases, as noted previously, is an important technique for conserving heat in anesthetized patients. Because 12% to 14% of body heat is lost through the respiratory tract, the use of warm, humidified gases decreases the potential heat drain in addition to preventing damage to the ciliated cells of the tracheobronchial tree caused by dry gases (Clarke et al., 1954). The humidifier should be servo-controlled, shutting off when the preset temperature equals the patient's airway temperature, so that airway burns are avoided. Maximum temperature limits, causing automatic shutoff, should also be an integral aspect of the humidifier. Heat and moisture exchangers (e.g., Humid-Vent) can provide 80% inspired humidity when 80 minutes of use is allowed to saturate the hygroscopic membrane (Bissonnette and Sessler, 1989; Bissonnette et al., 1989b).

MONITORING

Most studies that have determined the rate of cardiac arrests due to anesthesia have found a three- to fivefold greater risk among children compared with adults (Graff et al., 1964; Keenan and Boyan, 1985). In children younger than 1 year, the incidence increases to 9.2 to 17 per 10,000 anesthetics, or 10 times the adult incidence (Olsson and Hallen, 1988; Cohen et al., 1990). Factors contributing to cardiac arrests in anesthetized children are likely to be related to the cardiovascular or respiratory system (Salem et al., 1975). The incidence of other serious complications is also greater for infants than for adults in the operating room (Tiret et al., 1988) and postanesthesia care unit (PACU) (Cohen et al., 1990). These data indicate that children represent a high-risk population and should be monitored with particular attention to cardiovascular and respiratory variables.

Guidelines for the intraoperative monitoring of patients under anesthesia have been published by the ASA (2003) (see Box 9–1). These standards mandate the continuous presence of a anesthesiologist or a nurse anesthetist throughout the conduct of anesthesia and require continuous monitoring of oxygenation, electrocardiography, and adequacy of ventilation and circulation. The minimum standard for monitoring oxygenation includes an oxygen analyzer in the anesthesia breathing circuit, sufficient illumination to evaluate the patient's color, and a quantitative method such as pulse oximetry, except under extenuating circumstances. Tracheal intubation must be verified by physical examination and qualitative detection of carbon dioxide in the exhaled gas. Regardless of whether endotracheal intubation has been performed, continuous capnography is required unless it becomes invalidated by the nature of the patient, procedure, or equipment. Furthermore, quantitative monitoring of the volume of expired gas is strongly encouraged. The ASA also recommends monitoring of ventilation using observation of chest excursion and the reservoir breathing bag, as well as auscultation of breath sounds. When ventilation is controlled by a mechanical ventilator, there shall be in continuous use a device that is capable of detecting disconnection of components of the breathing system, and the device must give an audible signal when its alarm threshold is exceeded.

ASA monitoring standards for circulation mandate that every patient receiving anesthesia shall have continuous ECG and determination of arterial blood pressure and heart rate at least every 5 minutes. In addition to these, every patient shall have circulatory function continually evaluated with use of at least one of the following methods: palpation of a pulse, auscultation of heart sounds, monitoring of an intra-arterial pressure tracing, ultrasound peripheral pulse monitoring, or pulse plethysmography or oximetry. Finally, a method by which the temperature can be measured should be readily available during general anesthesia, and patients should have their temperature monitored when clinically significant changes in body temperature are intended, anticipated, or suspected.

Many of these provisions have been extended to the PACU. In standards adopted by the ASA in 1988 and updated in 1994, PACU monitoring should emphasize oxygenation, ventilation, circulation, and temperature assessment with specific capability for quantitative determination of systemic oxygenation by pulse oximetry or its equivalent. Equipment should be readily available to enable the practitioner to meet these standards in all pediatric patients.

The anesthesiologist is the ultimate monitor. Devices that provide electronic surveillance should not distract the anesthesiologist from direct monitoring using observation, auscultation, and palpation. In healthy pediatric patients, under certain circumstances, it may be appropriate to induce anesthesia while using these senses alone. This enables smooth "steal" inductions, in which the patient enters the operating room asleep and does not awaken during the induction of general anesthesia. It also allows the practitioner to enlist the cooperation of a child who might otherwise become increasingly anxious and less cooperative if the induction were delayed or altered by the application of monitors. When anesthetizing an infant (i.e., <1 year old) or a critically ill child, the benefit of delaying the application of monitors must be weighed against the risks of not having them in place during induction of general anesthesia.

PHYSICAL EXAMINATION

Observation

The anesthesiologist can gain a tremendous amount of information from observation alone. Anesthetic depth can be inferred from the rate and pattern of respiration, and airway obstruction can be detected by chest wall retractions or "seesaw" paradoxical motion. The skin and mucous membranes should be continually assessed to confirm adequate oxygenation, because a pulse oximeter reading may significantly lag behind other indices of hypoxemia when placed on an extremity (Reynolds et al., 1993), or it may not detect a pulse at all during intense vasoconstriction. In rare circumstances, pulse oximetry falsely indicates normal saturations during hypoxic conditions (Costarino et al., 1987).

Capillary refill can provide valuable information about the intravascular volume and cardiac output of an euthermic patient. A child with cool, mottled, poorly perfused extremities should be examined closely for additional evidence of hypovolemia or reduced cardiac output even if the systemic arterial pressure remains normal. Progression of this mottled appearance onto the trunk indicates the extreme vasoconstriction that may herald imminent cardiovascular collapse.

Auscultation

Continuous auscultation of heart and lung sounds by means of a precordial stethoscope is useful during all phases of general anesthesia, as well as during transport of the child between hospital locations. A precordial stethoscope allows the anesthesiologist to immediately detect changes in the rate and character of heart and breath sounds and is often the first warning of a physiologic alteration (e.g., right main bronchial intubation, wheezing, etc.). Crisp heart tones are produced by the flow of blood through a briskly contracting heart. Myocardial depression initially results in a muffled and then a distant quality to the heart tones. Careful auscultation may reveal arrhythmias or murmurs such as the "mill wheel" murmur that results from a venous air embolus. During the administration of halothane, the character of the heart sounds is often used to judge the depth of anesthesia. During ligation of a patent ductus arteriosus (PDA), auscultation with an esophageal stethoscope can help the surgeon identify the correct structure, because clamping the ductus results in disappearance of the murmur.

In selecting and placing a precordial or an esophageal stethoscope, one should consider the nature of the planned surgery, the proposed anesthetic, and any underlying patient condition that may affect auscultation. Breath sounds and heart tones are best heard when a precordial stethoscope is positioned near the left sternal border between the second and fourth interspaces (above the nipple line). An esophageal stethoscope is reserved for patients whose anesthetic management includes endotracheal intubation and in whom a precordial stethoscope either provides inadequate information or violates the surgical field. The proper method for accurate placement of the esophageal stethoscope is to listen while simultaneously advancing the device and placing it at the level where the heart and lung sounds are maximal. In small infants, unintentional placement of the esophageal stethoscope into the stomach can occur easily.

Esophageal stethoscopes are contraindicated in patients with esophageal atresia or in those who have a disease process involving the proximal portion of the esophagus. They confer a rigid feel to the esophagus, which might be mistaken for the trachea (Schwartz and Downes, 1977). As a result, the esophageal stethoscope is relatively contraindicated in neck dissections where the trachea is a critical landmark, such as tracheostomy.

ELECTROCARDIOGRAPHY

In pediatric anesthesia, the electrocardiogram (ECG) is most useful for tracking the heart rate and diagnosing intraoperative rate-related arrhythmias, of which the two most common are bradycardia and supraventricular tachycardia (SVT). The ECG is much less prone to movement-related artifact than is the original pulse oximeter; new pulse oximeter devices have eliminated most motion artifacts. In small infants, hypoxemia-related bradycardia may occur before the pulse oximeter reveals oxyhemoglobin desaturation. Conversely, resolution of hypoxemia is heralded by the transition from bradycardia to normal sinus rhythm. Premature ventricular contractions (PVCs) are commonly observed when halothane is used as the general anesthetic agent, especially during periods of hypercapnia and/or catecholamine release. The precordial stethoscope as a single monitor provides a much better indication of cardiac contractility and thus the overall hemodynamic status.

Electrolyte abnormalities may also be uncovered through the use of the ECG. Hyperkalemia produces the characteristically prominent T waves. Hypocalcemia, which may occur during rapid administration of citrated blood products, prolongs the QT interval. Because ischemic changes in normal pediatric patients are rare and lead II provides a good view of atrial activity for arrhythmia diagnosis, the latter is recommended for the routine intraoperative electrocardiographic monitoring of pediatric patients.

In children, the normal heart rate varies with age (Table 9–10). The normal heart rate of the newborn ranges from 120 to 160 beats per minute, although lower rates (e.g., 70) are frequently observed during sleep, and higher rates (>200) are common during anxiety or pain. Heart rates tend to decrease with age and in parallel with decreases in oxygen consumption. In addition, many children have a noticeable variation in heart rate with respiration (i.e., sinus arrhythmia).

SYSTEMIC ARTERIAL PRESSURE

Noninvasive Measurement

Blood pressure is easily measured noninvasively in children and small infants using oscillotonometry. In children, oscillometric measurements of systolic arterial pressure (Bruner et al., 1981; Friesen and Lichtor, 1981) and mean arterial pressure (Kimble et al., 1981) usually correlate well with the Riva Rocci mercury column method as well as with direct arterial pressure measurement but tend to underestimate the diastolic component. During routine uncomplicated cases, measurement of blood pressure should be performed every 3 to 5 minutes while the child is anesthetized—determinations that are too frequent can result in limb ischemia. The blood pressure cuff is most commonly placed on the upper arm but can be placed on the forearm, thigh, or calf. There is inconsistent correlation of measurements obtained between the upper and lower limbs.

The width of the blood pressure cuff should cover approximately two thirds the total length of the upper arm (or other extremity portion to which it is applied). A cuff that is too small or too narrow incompletely occludes the artery, resulting in the premature return of detectable flow and hence falsely increasing the pressure measurement (Park et al., 1976; Kimble et al., 1981). The error can be as great as 30 mm Hg. A cuff that is too wide may dampen the arterial wave and result in a falsely low pressure, but the magnitude of this error is small (Kimble et al., 1981). Blood pressure increases gradually throughout childhood (Figs. 9–30 and 9–31) and is dependent on the height of the child such that taller children demonstrate a higher blood pressure (Table 9–11). Blood pressure ranges in premature infants have been defined (Table 9–12) and vary depending on the health status of the infant and mother.

Direct Measurement

Direct measurement of blood pressure via an arterial catheter is indicated when there is a need for precise beat-to-beat blood pressure monitoring or for frequent determination of arterial blood gas values. This patient population may include children

TABLE 9–10. Normal resting heart rates of infants and children

Age	HEART RATE (beats/min) Mean	Range (±2 SDs)
0 to 24 hr	119	94 to 145
1 to 7 days	133	100 to 175
8 to 30 days	163	115 to 190
1 to 3 mo	152	124 to 190
3 to 12 mo	140	111 to 179
1 to 3 yr	126	98 to 163
3 to 5 yr	98	65 to 132
5 to 8 yr	96	70 to 115
8 to 16 yr	77	55 to 105

Modified from Liebman J, Plonsey R, Gilette PC, editors: *Pediatric electrocardiography.* Baltimore, MD, 1982, Williams & Wilkins.

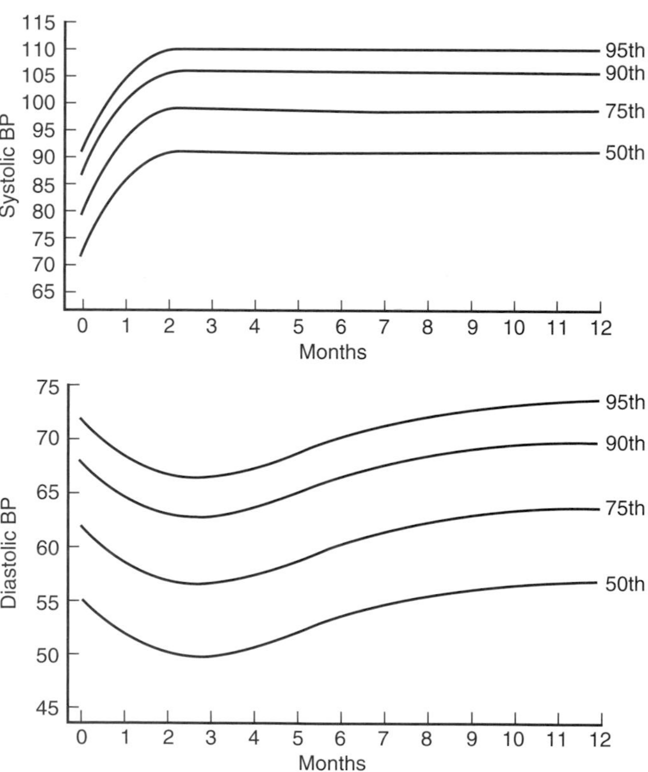

FIGURE 9–30. Age-specific percentiles of blood pressure measurements in boys, from birth to 12 months of age. Values for girls are slightly lower. (From National Heart, Lung, and Blood Institute: *Report of the Second Task Force on Blood Pressure Control in Children.* Bethesda, MD, 1987, The Institute. Reproduced by permission of *Pediatrics,* Vol. 79, p. 1. Copyright 1987.)

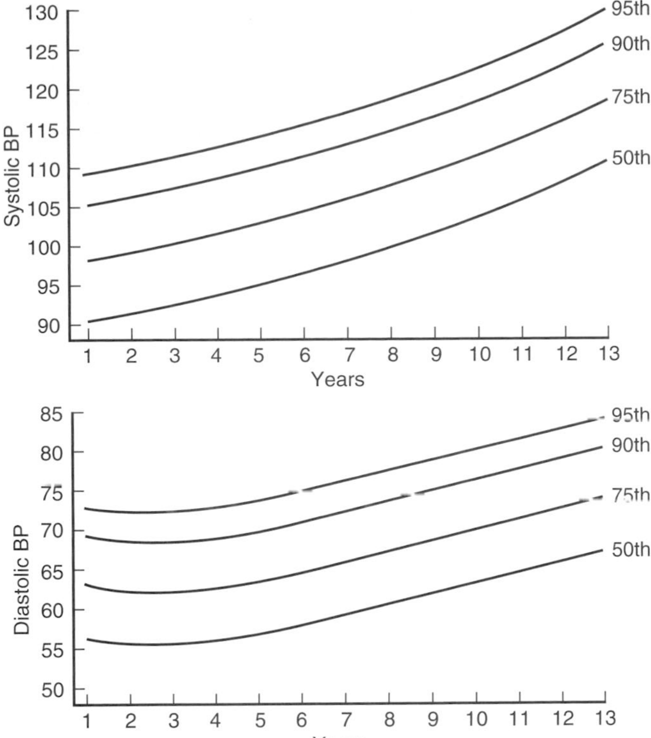

FIGURE 9–31. Age-specific percentiles for blood pressure measurements in boys, 1-13 years of age. Values for girls are slightly lower. (From National Heart, Lung, and Blood Institute, Bethesda, MD: *Report of the second task force on blood pressure control in children*, 1987. Reproduced by permission of *Pediatrics*. Vol. 79, p. 1. Copyright 1987.)

who are expected to develop unstable hemodynamics or those undergoing a surgical procedure that could result in profound hemodynamic alterations related to blood loss (i.e., total loss >50% estimated blood volume [EBV] or acute loss >10% EBV), fluid shifts (i.e., third space losses >50% EBV), deliberate hypotension, or nonpulsatile blood flow (e.g., cardiopulmonary bypass). The respiratory indications for direct arterial monitoring include significant abnormalities in gas exchange due to either preexisting disease or the procedure (e.g., thoracotomy). Rarely, direct arterial monitoring is necessary because of the

TABLE 9–12. Blood pressure ranges in healthy premature infants (birth weight between 501 and 2000 g)

	SYSTOLIC BLOOD PRESSURE (mm Hg)		DIASTOLIC BLOOD PRESSURE (mm Hg)	
Age (days)	*Minimum*	*Maximum*	*Minimum*	*Maximum*
1	48 ± 9	63 ± 12	25 ± 7	35 ± 10
2	54 ± 10	63 ± 10	30 ± 0	39 ± 8
3	53 ± 9	67 ± 10	31 ± 8	43 ± 8
4	57 ± 10	71 ± 11	32 ± 8	45 ± 10
5	56 ± 9	72 ± 14	33 ± 9	47 ± 12
6	57 ± 9	71 ± 11	32 ± 7	47 ± 10

Values are mean ± standard deviation.
From Hegyi T, Anwar M, Carbone MT, et al.: Blood pressure ranges in premature infants: II. The first week of life. *Pediatrics* 97:336–342, 1996.

inability to measure systemic arterial pressure by any indirect technique.

There are no absolute contraindications to placing an arterial catheter, but a risk-benefit analysis should be performed in patients with a hypercoagulable state or bleeding disorder. The radial artery is a favored site for arterial cannulation because the vessel is superficial and easily accessible. Other anatomic sites frequently used are the ulnar, dorsalis pedis, posterior tibial, and femoral arteries. The axillary artery has gained favor because of increased collateral blood flow compared with the brachial or femoral artery (Lawless and Orr, 1989; Cantwell et al., 1990; Greenwald et al., 1990; Piotrowski and Kawczynski, 1995). In general, the brachial artery should be avoided because of the risk of median nerve damage and poor collateral flow around the elbow. Umbilical vessels provide an alternate site via which the aorta and inferior vena cava may be cannulated in neonates. In determining a site, one needs to consider the history of that vessel (i.e., whether it has been cannulated before), its collateral flow, the experience of the person inserting the catheter, and special physiologic issues (e.g., whether it arises on aortic root proximal to the ductus arteriosus) or surgical issues (e.g., whether it arises from a vessel likely to be clamped or sacrificed during the procedure). Cannulation of vessels with good collateral flow, such as the arch vessels of the wrist or foot, may reduce the risk of ischemic tissue damage distal to the catheter.

TABLE 9–11. Systemic arterial pressure

Age	Systolic Pressure (mm Hg) (±95% confidence limits)	Diastolic Pressure (mm Hg) (±95% confidence limits)	Mean Pressure (mm Hg) (±95% confidence limits)
Newborn (kg)*			
1	47 (9)	27 (10)	35 (7)
2	54 (9)	32 (10)	40 (7)
3	62 (9)	37 (10)	45 (7)
4	69 (9)	42 (10)	50 (7)
6 wk–9 yr†			
Boys	93 (18)	59 (18)	
Girls	96 (24)	62 (22)	
10–19 yr†			
Boys	108 (20)	67 (18)	
Girls	105 (20)	64 (22)	

*Adapted from Versmold HT, et al.: Aortic blood pressure during the first 12 hours of life in infants with birth weight 610 to 4,220 grams. *Pediatrics* 67:607, 1981.
†Adapted from Adams FH, Landaw EM: What are healthy blood pressures for children? *Pediatrics* 68:268, 1981.

As the largest superficial vessel, the femoral artery can be cannulated most predictably in situations where intense peripheral vasoconstriction may accompany low cardiac output and blood pressure. In less dire circumstances, the selection of a vessel may reflect a variety of anatomic and physiologic characteristics exhibited by certain vessels. The pedal vessels exhibit pressure wave amplification that results in pressure determinations exceeding aortic values by as much as 30% (Park et al., 1983).

After palpation and localization of the artery with the nondominant hand, one can cannulate the selected artery either by inserting the catheter directly into the artery using a catheter-over-needle device or by using the Seldinger technique. The Seldinger technique involves entering the vessel with a needle, placing a guidewire through the needle after the vessel is entered, removing the needle, and then placing the catheter over the wire into the vessel. A 22-gauge catheter is appropriate for peripheral artery cannulation in infants and children younger than 5 years, whereas a 20-gauge catheter may be substituted in older children. Aseptic technique should always be followed when placing an arterial line. When cannulating a peripheral artery, it is helpful to immobilize the extremity with a board.

A Doppler flow transducer is occasionally useful to locate an artery that is difficult to palpate. Surgical cutdown may be the preferred option in patients in whom percutaneous placement is likely to be difficult or has failed. Indwelling arterial catheters are associated with several possible complications. Proximal emboli, distal ischemia, arterial thrombosis, and infection are common to all sites. Thrombosis of the radial artery is generally temporary, although it is more likely to persist after a cutdown (Miyasaka et al., 1976). Although small flush volumes (0.3 mL) in radial arterial catheters can be detected in the aortic arch vessels, cerebral infarcts have not been reported (Edmonds et al., 1980). The tip of an umbilical artery catheter should be placed in either a high (above the diaphragm) or a low (below L-3) position to avoid direct flushing into the renal arteries. Despite these precautions, as many as 10% of neonates exhibit hypertension as a late complication attributed to umbilical artery catheterization (Bauer et al., 1975; Plumer et al., 1976; Horgan et al., 1987). Minor complications of umbilical artery monitoring include vasospasm of the lower extremity vessels, which are more common with low tip placement. Major complications (e.g., necrotizing enterocolitis, renal artery thrombosis) occur independent of location (Mokrohisky et al., 1978; Umbilical Artery Catheter Trial Study Group, 1992). The rarity of clinical complications is remarkable given an incidence of aortic thrombosis on removal of umbilical artery catheters that approaches 95% in some series (Neal et al., 1972), although most series define the incidence at 12% to 31% of neonates (Symansky and Fox, 1972; Horgan et al., 1987; Seibert et al., 1987).

CENTRAL VENOUS PRESSURE

There are four relative indications for central venous catheterization: inadequate peripheral venous access, central venous pressure monitoring, infusion of hyperosmolar or sclerosing substances, and a planned operative procedure with a high risk of hemodynamically significant venous air embolism. There is no absolute indication for central venous pressure monitoring in pediatrics. Unlike direct systemic arterial pressures, central venous pressure itself rarely provides the sole basis for therapeutic action. It does, however, provide useful information that, taken together with other data, helps to form a management plan. The procedures in which this monitoring deserves consideration include large estimated blood loss or fluid shifts (>50% EBV), deliberate hypotension, cardiac surgery with cardiopulmonary bypass, situations in which the usual signs of hypovolemia are likely to be misleading (e.g., renal failure, congestive heart failure), and procedures with expected moderate blood loss or fluid shifts. The normal values for central venous pressure in children are similar to those in adults (mean, 2 to 6 mm Hg).

Every insertion site that has been used in adults can be used in children. Access to the central circulation can be achieved from the internal and external jugular, subclavian, basilar, umbilical, and femoral veins. The site selected depends on the experience of the operator and the indication for the catheter. If venous access is the only requirement, one might elect to use visible veins (e.g., basilar, external jugular) or those with a lower risk of complications (e.g., femoral). Situations that require true intrathoracic central venous placement also require placement of the catheter into the internal jugular vein or subclavian vein. The umbilical vein can be used in neonates for volume resuscitation, but the high frequency with which these catheters enter the branch portal veins introduces a significant risk of permanent liver injury if sclerosing or hyperosmolar solutions are infused. Because a catheter tip can erode through the wall of the right atrium, care must be taken to avoid intracardiac tip placement. The catheter should be advanced only until the orifice lies in the intrathoracic great vessels, and its position should be confirmed radiographically.

Catheters of various sizes (2.5 to 10 F), lengths, and composition are available for pediatric applications (Cook Critical Care, Bloomington, IN, and other companies). Selection is based on the size of the patient (Andropoulos et al., 2001) and the purpose of the catheter. The composition of the catheter depends on its intended use. Teflon is fairly resistant to thrombus formation, but concerns about perforation by catheters have prompted the development of softer catheter materials, especially for long-term use (e.g., Silastic and polyurethane). The catheters are generally inserted via a Seldinger technique using landmarks that are similar to those used in adults.

There are no absolute contraindications to placing a central venous catheter, but each site has potential risks. All sites share the common complications of infection (site cellulitis, bacteremia), venous thrombosis with potential emboli, air embolism, catheter malfunction (occlusion, dislodgment, or fractures), dysrhythmias (when the catheter tip is in the heart), and bleeding. Universal precautions and sterile technique should be used when placing a central venous catheter. The risks involved in cannulating the internal jugular vein include carotid artery puncture, Horner's syndrome, pneumothorax, and injury to the thoracic duct when the left internal jugular vein is cannulated. The high approach to the internal jugular vein, at the midpoint of the sternocleidomastoid muscle, results in comparable success with fewer complications than lower approaches (Coté et al., 1979). Two-dimensional ultrasound scanning improves localization of the internal jugular vein and increases the success rate of central venous cannulation in adults and children (Verghese et al., 2002; Hind et al., 2003) (Fig. 9–32). Using this device, Alderson and others (1993) reported an 18% prevalence of anatomic variations in children younger than 6 years that would preclude or significantly hinder the successful cannulation of the internal jugular vein using anatomic landmarks alone.

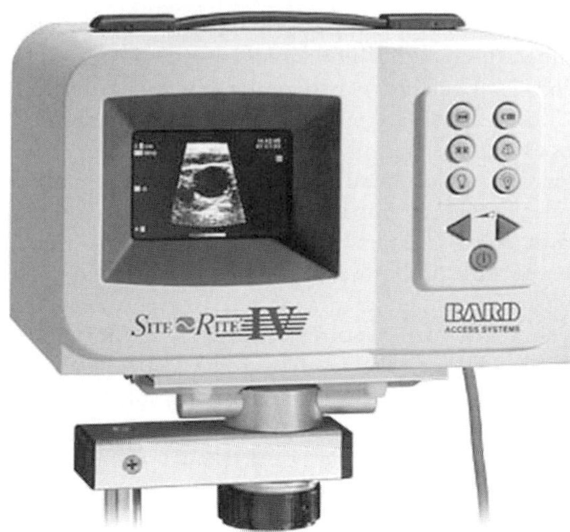

■ FIGURE 9–32. The Site-Rite (Bard Access Systems, Pittsburgh, PA) is an ultrasound device that is used to localize the anatomic position and relationship of large vessels and to facilitate central venous access. (Reproduced with permission.)

PULMONARY ARTERY CATHETERS

Since its introduction in 1970, indications for the use of the flow-directed balloon-tipped pulmonary artery catheter (Swan-Ganz) in pediatric patients have been slow to evolve. While the validity and value of the data that these catheters generate remain controversial in pediatrics, the technical difficulties and complications associated with their use are significant. Pulmonary artery pressure measurement can help guide therapy in children with elevated or volatile pulmonary vascular resistance, but the interpretation of the flow data they generate is hindered by several factors. First, the desired cardiac output varies according to age, disease state, and other elements of management that alter metabolic demand in complex ways, thereby introducing significant uncertainty in assigning a target value. Second, the prevalence of intracardiac communications that permit shunting of blood causes discrepancies in pulmonary and systemic blood flow that may vary continuously and are difficult to quantify. Finally, despite several studies demonstrating reasonable accuracy when thermodilution is compared with other methods of flow determination, such as the Fick equation (Freed and Keane, 1978) and dye dilution (Colgan and Stewart, 1977), the precision of these determinations in small infants is low and has a 25% intersample variability. In patients with congenital heart malformations, for example, measurement errors are introduced by shunting and complex anatomy, and the risks of improper placement of the flow-directed pulmonary artery catheter are increased. Alternatively, directly placed pulmonary artery catheters can provide the necessary information regarding pulmonary vascular resistance and residual left-to-right shunts, whereas left atrial catheters reflect filling and diastolic function of the left ventricle after cardiac surgery.

There are situations in which pulmonary artery catheters can provide useful information. In children who have severe coexisting pulmonary and circulatory failure, pulmonary artery catheters can help to quantify the hemodynamic impact of extreme respiratory support measures and guide complex fluid and pharmacologic regimens. They may also be useful in patients with underlying pulmonary hypertension or poorly compensated left ventricular dysfunction who undergo acute surgical stress (e.g., arteriovenous malformation clipping or aortic cross-clamping). Given the uncertainty regarding optimal systemic flow in a given child, mixed venous oxygen saturation may serve as a better indication of global perfusion. In the absence of left-to-right shunts, this sample is best obtained from the pulmonary artery.

Pulmonary artery catheters can be difficult to insert, especially in infants or in children with low cardiac output. They may be placed in any vein used for access to the central venous system, but the most reliable veins are the right internal jugular and the femoral. In infants and children smaller than 15 kg, it is technically difficult to place an introducer sheath in the neck vessels; the femoral veins are preferable. Multilumen catheters capable of thermodilution are available in two sizes, 5 and 7 F, with four options for the right atrium–pulmonary artery interluminal distance. Catheter recommendations are based on age (Table 9–13). The proper placement of these catheters can take a long time, and thus the assistance of fluoroscopy is recommended in infants and children less than 30 kg and in larger children who have a low cardiac output.

The risks of balloon-tipped pulmonary artery catheters are numerous and include the risks of central venous catheter placement discussed previously, as well as the complications seen in adult patients with pulmonary artery catheters: infection, air emboli, thrombus, pulmonary artery rupture, acute right bundle branch block, and intracardiac knots. There are also complications that are more common with children: misleading information, paradoxical systemic emboli, disruption of an intracardiac repair, and high-grade right ventricular outflow tract obstruction because of the relatively large balloon diameter. The presence of intracardiac and extracardiac malformations may result in an aberrant catheter course leading to incorrect data as well as an increased risk of systemic emboli.

Cardiac output can be estimated in children through indicator dilution (e.g., thermodilution or dye dilution) and noninvasive techniques. Doppler determinations of aortic blood velocity can be used to quantify systemic flow if the angle of the incident ultrasound beam and the cross-sectional area of the aorta are reliably determined (Alverson et al., 1982). Transthoracic and transesophageal evaluations of Doppler cardiac output in children have proved to be less promising (Notterman et al., 1989; Muhiudeen et al., 1991). Thoracic bioimpedance, a method that estimates stroke volume on the basis of changes in thoracic impedance, has been applied to children as small as 3.6 kg. Although some correlation exists between bioimpedance and indicator dilution methods, reproducibility is poor (O'Connell et al., 1991). Further details and the complexities encountered in the measurement of cardiac output in children are beyond the scope of this chapter but have been reviewed previously (Tibby and Murdoch, 2002).

■ TABLE 9–13. Guidelines for multilumen pulmonary artery catheters in infants and children

Age (yr)	Size (F)	CVP – Pulmonary Artery Port Distance (cm)
Newborn to 3	5	10
3 to 8	5	15
8 to 14	7	20
>14	7	30

CVP, central venous pressure.

A noninvasive cardiac output (NICO) monitor has been developed that determines cardiac output via the Fick principle for rebreathed carbon dioxide (Respironics; Novametrix Medical Systems Inc., Wallingford, CT) (Capek and Roy, 1988). The NICO monitor has been clinically validated in adults and is approved by the Food and Drug Administration for use, but it requires tidal volumes of 200 mL or greater (Guzzi et al., 2003; Watt et al., 2004). Unpublished studies in children have demonstrated a similar validation compared with thermodilution (personal communication, Richard J. Levy, M.D., 2004) and represents a possible future method for NICO determination.

TRANSESOPHAGEAL ECHOCARDIOGRAPHY

Transesophageal echocardiography (TEE) provides anatomic and physiologic information in small infants and children (Phoon et al., 1999; Kavanaugh-McHugh et al., 2000). Because of its esophageal position, it affords a unique perspective when the transthoracic approach is either unavailable (e.g., during cardiac surgery) or not helpful. For small infants, transesophageal probes with decreased size (9 mm) are available with "omniplane" imaging, in which, once the transducer is directed at a specific site of interest, the imaging plane can be rotated 180 degrees. As the technical resolution of TEE probes has improved, posterior cardiac structures such as the pulmonary veins, left atrium, mitral valve, and left ventricular outflow tract are often better visualized from the esophagus. The wide spectrum of anatomic variability with congenital heart malformations and the judgment necessary to make physiologic determinations under the varying functional and loading conditions typical in the operating room require extensive experience (Hsu et al., 1991; Muhiudeen et al., 1992). Unlike many anesthesia practices devoted to acquired heart disease, TEE investigations in children with congenital malformations are usually performed in conjunction with pediatric cardiologists.

TEMPERATURE

Temperature monitoring is vital during pediatric anesthesia as children may exhibit hypothermia or hyperthermia, both of which can have profound physiologic consequences (see Chapter 5, Thermoregulation: Physiology and Perioperative Disturbances). As discussed previously in this chapter, temperature maintenance in the operating room is difficult for the infant and the small child; hypothermia is common in this group. Although axillary temperature measurements are easier to obtain, core temperature measurement using rectal or esophageal probes better reflects the magnitude of hypothermia and should be used routinely, particularly in small children.

The site selected for temperature monitoring depends on one's objectives. Rectal temperature provides a good index of core temperature but lags behind temperature monitors in more vascularized locations (e.g., esophagus, nasopharynx), especially during rapid core cooling, as occurs during institution of cardiopulmonary bypass. Esophageal temperature is influenced by the great vessels and thus rapidly reflects changes in core temperature if the probe is in the middle or distal portion of the esophagus. Probes in the proximal portion of the esophagus may be influenced by the inspired gas temperature in the trachea (Bissonnette et al., 1989a). These probes should be used only in patients who have undergone endotracheal intubation. Nasopharyngeal temperature probes more accurately reflect the temperature of the blood perfusing the brain (Hindman et al., 1992). Usually, a small probe inserted a distance equal to that between the ala nasi and the tragus of the ear reaches the mucosa of the nasopharynx. Tympanic membrane probes also accurately reflect brain temperature. In early studies, thermocouples provided tympanic membrane temperature. Because they must make contact with the tympanic membrane, the insertion of these probes was noxious and traumatic to children, resulting in a small incidence of bleeding and even tympanic rupture. Axillary temperature is usually 1°C lower than core temperature. Axillary probes should be placed over the axillary artery with the arm tightly adducted. Skin surface temperature varies from core temperature by an unpredictable and often substantial amount as a function of changes in skin perfusion. Algorithms used by manufacturers of liquid crystal skin thermography sensors tend to overestimate core temperature in anesthetized children (Leon et al., 1990).

URINE OUTPUT

Urine output often reflects intravascular volume status and cardiac output. Proper assessment of urine output requires recognition of the physiologic mechanisms that exert an affect on urine flow in children. During the first week of life, the glomerular filtration rate and renal plasma flow are only 25% of normal adult values (Arant, 1978). The neonatal kidney is limited in its ability to concentrate the urine (Simpson and Stephenson, 1993). By the end of the first week of life, the kidney begins to reach absorption thresholds for sodium and glucose that approach adult levels.

Normal newborns produce between 0.5 and 4 mL urine/kg per hour in the first 3 hours of life (Strauss et al., 1981). Urine flow, which initially ranges from 15 to 60 mL/kg per day, reaches as much as 120 mL/kg per day by the end of the first week of life, with 90% of neonates producing 0.5 to 5 mL/kg per hour (Douglas, 1972; Guignard, 1982). In the neonate less than 1 week old, urine flow alone is not a sensitive index of changes in cardiac output or intravascular volume. The limited capacity of the neonatal kidney to compensate for diminished or excessive intravascular volume demands more precise management of blood and fluid replacement in these infants.

Beyond the neonatal period, a urine flow of 0.5 to 1 mL/kg per hour usually indicates adequate renal perfusion and function. When the systemic arterial pressure exceeds a critical opening pressure for the afferent arteriole of the glomerulus (approximately 75 mm Hg systolic pressure in the adult), urine flow is directly proportional to circulating blood volume. Urine flow may be subject to several modulating factors in the operating room: the hormonal response to anesthesia and surgery, previous diuretic therapy, preexistent renal disease, hypothermia, deliberate hypotension, and the nonpulsatile flow of cardiopulmonary bypass. When these modulating factors are likely to have a significant impact on urine flow, alternative measures for estimating circulating blood volume must be used.

Intraoperative monitoring of urine output is indicated in procedures in which large shifts in fluid, blood, or hemodynamics are anticipated, including blood loss greater than 20% of the EBV, third space replacement exceeding 50% of the EBV, cardiopulmonary bypass, neurosurgery, deliberate hypotension, planned use of diuretics, or planned hemodilution. Silastic Foley

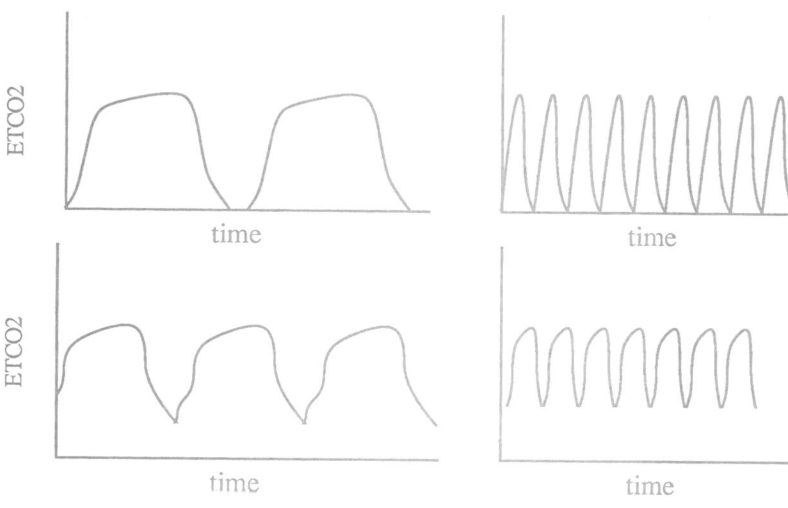

■ **FIGURE 9–33.** Common capnographic diagnoses—rebreathing. *Top tracings*, normal capnographs with the graph on the right compressed over a longer time. Note plateau suggesting valid end-tidal carbon dioxide data and the return to baseline between breaths; there is no rebreathing. Lower curves illustrate rebreathing, as there is no return to baseline. This can occur with inadequate fresh gas flow or floating unidirectional valves. The small initial deflection before exhalation ("pre-exhalation hump") can occasionally be seen. It represents the inhalation late in the inspiratory phase of more concentrated exhaled gas from the previous exhalation.

catheters are available in sizes small enough (6 F) for full-term neonates. Alternatively, a small feeding tube can be used in premature infants and in those with a small urethra. In infants, urinary bladder catheters should be connected to a urinometer capable of measuring small volumes or to a vented 10- to 20-mL syringe.

NONINVASIVE RESPIRATORY GAS MONITORING

Carbon Dioxide

Capnometry is the instantaneous measurement of carbon dioxide in the breathing circuit; capnography depicts this information in a continuous graphic display by which both the quality and the quantity of ventilation can be evaluated (Figs. 9–33 to 9–36).

Before 1998, capnography was considered a standard monitor by the ASA for the purpose of confirming the initial placement and continuous presence of an endotracheal tube. This section of the ASA monitoring standards was updated in 1998 and states that capnography should be used to confirm adequate ventilation during general anesthesia with or without an endotracheal tube (during laryngeal mask airway, facemask, or natural airway anesthesia). Specifically, these guidelines state:

Continual monitoring for the presence of expired carbon dioxide shall be performed unless invalidated by the nature of the patient, procedure or equipment . . . . Continual end-tidal carbon dioxide analysis, in use from the time of endotracheal tube/laryngeal mask placement, until extubation/removal or initiating transfer to a postoperative care location, shall be performed using a quantitative method such as capnography, capnometry or mass spectroscopy (ASA, 2003).

Most capnometers use the principle of infrared light absorption by sampling circuit gas in either a mainstream or a sidestream fashion. Sidestream analyzers aspirate a sample from the circuit and transport it via a long, narrow-bore tube to a distant analyzing chamber. Advantages include a lightweight airway adapter and the remote location of the delicate components of the analyzing chamber. Disadvantages of sidestream systems include potential occlusion of the sampling tube, distortion or dilution of the exhaled gas wave during aspiration and transport to the analyzing chamber, and the delay necessary to transport and analyze the sample. Innovations in capnography technology have allowed a sampling rate as low as 30 mL/min ("microstream technology").

Mainstream analyzers use a sample chamber placed directly into the circuit. They have the advantage of providing virtually instantaneous analysis by avoiding transport of the sample. Such a system necessitates the addition of a delicate and bulky sensor to the proximal airway connection, where it might easily serve as a fixation point to dislodge a small tracheal tube. Solid-state innovations have dramatically reduced the weight of the mainstream sensors, but they remain significantly more hazardous when added to the circuits of neonates and small infants. Although early mainstream sample chambers added as much as

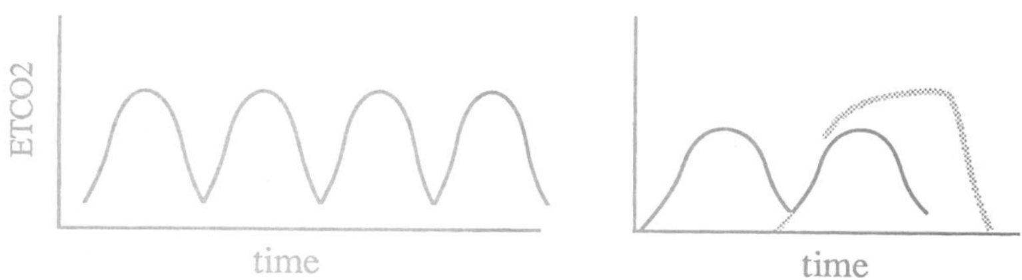

■ **FIGURE 9–34.** Common capnographic diagnoses—poor sampling. *Left*, poor sampling as evidenced by absence of a plateau phase. One would not be able to make this diagnosis with a capnometer that is incapable of real-time graphics. This is typical of small neonates whose small exhaled volumes are washed out by fresh gas flow. The speckled curve to the right projects the full exhaled breath if fresh gas flow were diverted. Note that the plateau would be higher than the actual curve by an unpredictable amount. The digital information derived from a curve like that on the left is useless.

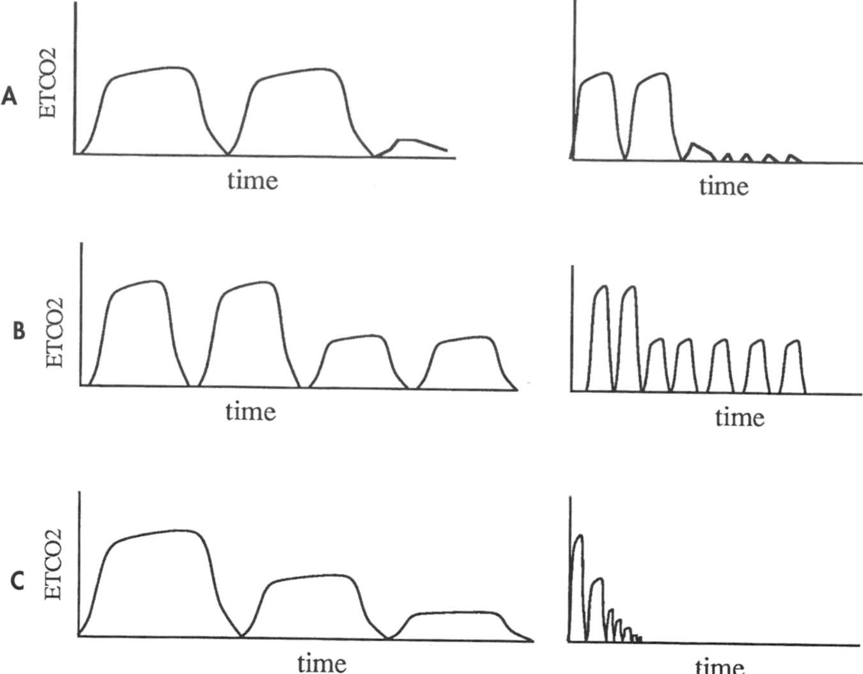

■ **FIGURE 9–35.** Common capnographic diagnoses—reduction in P_{ETCO_2}. There are many reasons for sudden reduction in the P_{ETCO_2}, some of which result in characteristic capnographic patterns. *(A)* Abrupt reduction to zero or nearly zero typically indicates mechanical disruption, disconnection, accidental extubation, or plugged sampling line. *(B)* Sudden reduction to a lower P_{ETCO_2} while preserving plateau and characteristics of a good trace indicates sudden increase in dead space ventilation as occurs with a pulmonary embolus (either thrombus or air). *(C)* Exponential reduction to zero (carbon dioxide washout curve) is characteristic of no pulmonary blood flow and thus either massive embolus or cardiac arrest.

17 mL of dead space to the circuit, currently available models reduced this volume to 2 mL or less.

Capnography in pediatric anesthesia is used to confirm placement of an endotracheal tube in the correct tracheal position and to continuously assess the adequacy of ventilation. Capnography also provides information about the respiratory rate, breathing pattern, endotracheal tube patency, and, indirectly, degree of neuromuscular blockade. Capnography can assist with the diagnosis of metabolic and cardiovascular events and can provide an early warning of a faulty anesthesia delivery system. In pediatric patients, an abnormal increase in end-tidal carbon dioxide (P_{ETCO_2}) most commonly signifies hypoventilation but, rarely, also indicates the presence of increased carbon dioxide production as occurs with temperature elevation or as an early sign of malignant hyperthermia. Conversely, an abnormally low P_{ETCO_2} may indicate an increase in dead space or suggest a state of low pulmonary perfusion. Sudden absence of the capnographic tracing indicates a breathing circuit disconnection, and the abnormal presence of inspired carbon dioxide signifies the presence of a faulty unidirectional valve, an exhausted carbon dioxide absorber, or, when a semiopen circuit is being used, rebreathing secondary to an insufficient fresh gas flow.

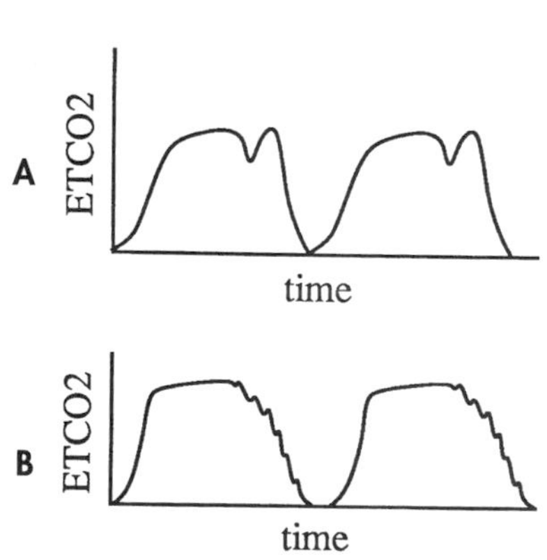

■ **FIGURE 9–36.** Common capnographic diagnoses—irregular tracings. Irregularities in the curve are common especially at the end of exhalation when exhaled gas flow is lowest. *(A)* Diaphragmatic activity indicating spontaneous respiratory effort, usually the result of dissipating neuromuscular blockade. *(B)* Cardiac oscillations: fluctuations in intrathoracic gas volume as a result of cardiac activity, usually a benign finding.

The capnographic tracing of small infants is often characterized by the lack of an apparent alveolar plateau. This is usually a result of a higher respiratory rate, an excessively high sampling flow for the volume of carbon dioxide produced, excessive dead space in the breathing circuit, or an excessive leak around an uncuffed endotracheal tube.

The degree to which P_{ETCO_2} reflects Pa_{CO_2} is subject to many variables, some technical and others physiologic. The technical issues of primary importance in the accurate measurement of mean alveolar carbon dioxide tension include the volume and flow rate of exhaled gas, the aspirating flow rate (for sidestream analyzers), the fresh gas flow rate, the type of breathing circuit, and the circuit location of the sampling chamber (mainstream analyzers) or lumen of the aspirating tubing (sidestream analyzers). These variables are of particular importance in the small neonate whose small exhaled volumes at low flow rates are often diluted by high fresh gas flows or aspirating gas flows (Badgwell et al., 1987, 1993; Rich et al., 1990; Spahr-Schopfer et al., 1993). Badgwell and others (1987) demonstrated exponential increases in the discrepancy between P_{ETCO_2} and Pa_{CO_2} values with progressive reduction in patients with weight of

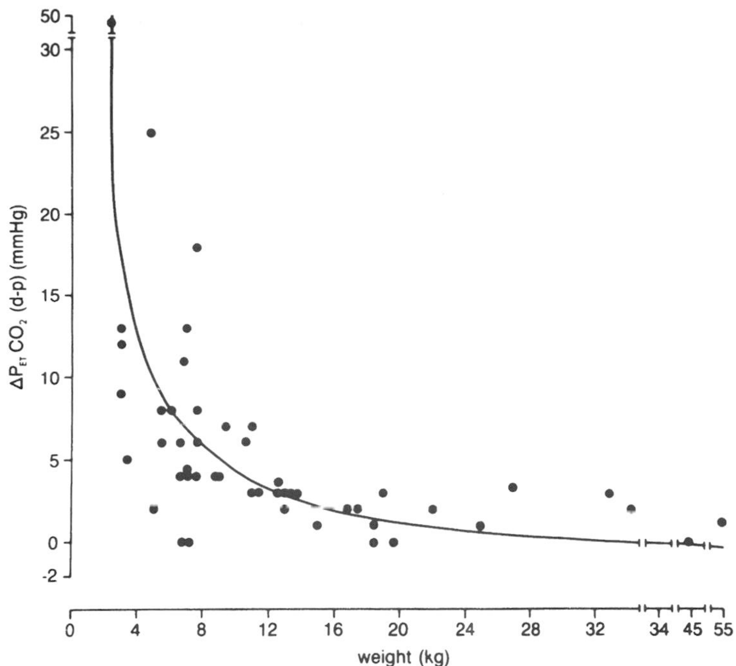

■ **FIGURE 9–37.** Gradient between end-tidal carbon dioxide (ET_{CO_2}) determinations made in the proximal and distal ends of a tracheal tube. Exponential increases in the gradient suggest substantial potential inaccuracy in proximal ET_{CO_2} determinations for children under 12 kg. (From Badgwell JM, McLeod ME, Lerman J, et al.: End-tidal PCO_2 measurements sampled at the distal and proximal ends of the endotracheal tube in infants and children. *Anesth Analg* 66:959, 1987.)

less than 12 kg (Fig. 9–37). The coaxial distal sampling tube that they advocated dramatically improved the correlation.

The physiologic variable that introduces the most significant error in $PETCO_2$ is dead space ventilation (Swedlow, 1986). Apart from children with severe pulmonary pathology or acute events such as pulmonary embolus, the most prevalent pediatric population in whom substantial dead space ventilation occurs are those with cyanotic congenital heart disease, particularly right-to-left shunts (Burrows, 1989; Fletcher, 1991).

Other Gases

The ability to measure other respiratory and anesthetic gases can provide important information about cardiopulmonary physiology. Confirming the elimination of nitrogen is useful in determining adequate preoxygenation, whereas its presence during anesthesia may reveal a leak in the delivery system or, in combination with a sudden decrease in end-tidal carbon dioxide, a venous air embolism. The measurement of anesthetic gases and vapors serves to illustrate the uptake and elimination of these agents and to confirm the purity and the accuracy of the tanks and vaporizers used to administer them. The quantity of residual inhaled anesthetic agent has obvious importance in the evaluation of prolonged emergence from anesthesia.

The techniques enabling multigas analysis that have found clinical application are based on properties such as ionized mass separation (mass spectrometry), ultraviolet and infrared light absorption, and absorption into lipophilic substances. A variety of manufacturers produce devices that quantify respiratory and anesthetic gases in the same unit as the capnograph; their complete description is beyond the scope of this chapter.

■ MONITORING OXYGEN AND CARBON DIOXIDE

Because of the high oxygen consumption and small functional residual capacity of infants and small children, they are more likely to become hypoxemic during general anesthesia than adults. Careful tracking of arterial oxygenation is vitally important. Noninvasive monitors of oxygenation are ubiquitous in the perioperative setting because of technological advances that have improved their reliability and because of standards that require their application not only in the operating room but also in the PACU and sedation room. These devices are of two basic types: those that measure cutaneous (transcutaneous) oxygen tension and others that evaluate arterial oxygen saturation (pulse oximeters).

■ CUTANEOUS OXYGEN TENSION

In 1972, a miniature Clark polarographic oxygen electrode, similar to those used in in vitro blood gas analysis, became available for application to the skin. When a probe heats the skin to 42° to 44°C, the cutaneous oxygen tension (PsO_2) approaches arterial oxygen tension because the skin blood flow and permeability to oxygen are increased (Barker and Tremper, 1985). The correlation may be better in neonates because their epidermis is less keratinized and their cutaneous capillary bed is denser. In fact, skin heating alters oxygen dissociation and may even result in a PsO_2 value that is higher than the PaO_2 value (Lubbers, 1981). In older children and adults, as the keratinized layer thickens, the diffusion gradient for oxygen becomes more significant. In practice, transcutaneous gas monitors are subject to the effects of these and myriad other nonlinear variables that influence skin perfusion, such as hypotension, hypothermia, and pharmacologic agents. They are the only noninvasive monitors that can provide information regarding significant hyperoxemia (Monaco et al., 1982; Rafferty et al., 1982; Barker and Tremper, 1985). The correlation, especially outside the physiologic range of PaO_2, is variable depending on the individual conditions, and the data produced may differ from that provided by the PsO_2 by a substantial yet unpredictable amount (American Academy of Pediatrics, 1989). Such results led Barker and Tremper (1985) to propose a more reasonable role for this monitor in determining peripheral tissue oxygen delivery (perfusion) rather than arterial oxygenation.

From a practical standpoint, the monitor is cumbersome. It requires calibration, a warm-up time of 10 to 20 minutes, and meticulous skin preparation and probe placement. It is sensitive to electrosurgical interference and mechanical manipulation. The technical demands of this monitor have limited its current use to special applications, such as detection of hyperoxemia in premature infants. A frequent side effect of transcutaneous monitoring is the occurrence of first- and second-degree burns.

CUTANEOUS CARBON DIOXIDE TENSION

Cutaneous carbon dioxide tension ($Psco_2$) measurement using a variant of the Severinghaus electrode is also available (Nosovitch et al., 2002). Although $Psco_2$ is always higher than $Paco_2$ as a result of tissue carbon dioxide production and the increased metabolism caused by a heating sensor, these monitors accurately follow trends in arterial carbon dioxide tension. The predictable gradient from arterial to cutaneous carbon dioxide tensions enables the monitors to calculate the gradient and display a "corrected" value. These devices are less altered by changes in skin temperature and perfusion than are cutaneous oxygen analyzers. The reasonably good correlation of end-tidal and arterial carbon dioxide tensions in all but extremely small subjects has limited the interest in cutaneous carbon dioxide tension monitoring in the operating room to very rare situations.

PULSE OXIMETRY

Pulse oximetry provides an estimate of the oxyhemoglobin saturation. The pulse oximeter uses plethysmography to determine the systolic portion of the cardiac cycle. During systole, there is a greater volume of blood in a pulsatile arterial vascular bed. This vascular bed is positioned between a sensor that contains a two-wavelength (660 and 940 nm) light-emitting diode and a photodiode receptor. Less light is transmitted in systole than in diastole because of the increased volume of the arterial bed. Sophisticated algorithms based on the amount of light absorbed differentiate systole from diastole. Oxygenated and deoxygenated blood absorb different quantities of light, proportional to their concentrations or the percent saturation according to the Beer-Lambert law. Once systole is identified through plethysmography, the arterial saturation during this period is determined by using the ratio of light absorption at the two different wavelengths through this vascular bed. The ratio is matched to data acquired over a range of experimentally determined saturations and ratios of light absorption stored in the instrument's memory to determine the arterial saturation. Using the ratio of light absorption at two different wavelengths makes unnecessary individual calibration and zeroing to adjust to the size of the patient or skin pigment. Within the 80% to 100% saturation range, arterial saturation values determined by this method correlated well with in vitro measurements (New, 1985).

Based on the algorithm used to determine systole and the time-averaging process used over several cardiac cycles, different pulse oximeters have slightly different responses to a variety of clinical situations. Because the device must identify the pulse-added absorption, it may confuse motion of the extremity to which the sensor is attached with pulsating motion and abort the display of saturation data or, worse, display inaccurate data. Decreased peripheral perfusion that is caused by decreased temperature or low cardiac output, a pulseless state, also makes determination of the pulse interval difficult, causing loss of data during critical episodes. Because the machine identifies the pulse as systole, high venous pressure causing venous pulse waves, as in secondary severe tricuspid regurgitation, elevated intrathoracic pressure, or obstructed venous return, can also create false readings (New, 1985).

Pulse oximetry was widely introduced into pediatric practice in the United States in the 1980s (Salyer, 2003). It serves as an early warning signal of impending or actual hypoxemia, often before the onset of cyanosis, and frequently reminds anesthesiologists of the alarming rapidity with which infants develop hypoxemia. Continuous use pulse oximetry is included in the Basic Monitoring Standards of the ASA (2003).

There are no outcome studies that demonstrate proved benefit from the use of pulse oximetry (Moller et al., 1993; Pedersen et al., 2001). Anesthesiologist-blinded studies have demonstrated that the use of pulse oximetry facilitates earlier recognition and fewer episodes of hypoxemia (Coté et al., 1988, 1991). Pulse oximetry has evolved into a standard monitor during pediatric anesthesia and has never been subjected to rigorous outcome studies with a true control group (an anesthetic without a pulse oximeter) (Cohen et al., 1988).

There are a number of well-described limitations of pulse oximetry, in which values are dependent on ambient lighting conditions, motion, peripheral circulation to the extremity, and abnormal hemoglobins, among other factors.

Although the pulse oximeter is a continuous monitor, it does not instantaneously reflect the arterial saturation or the degree of desaturation. When fully saturated, a substantial decrease in Pao_2 can occur without a change in Sao_2. Reynolds (1993) detected desaturation in children 30 seconds earlier in probes placed centrally (facial) than in those placed on an extremity (Reynolds et al., 1993). By the time the value indicated by a peripheral sensor had decreased 5%, the value indicated by a central sensor was 30% to 40% lower. The precise mechanism for this discrepancy remains unknown, although Severinghaus and Naifeh (1987) postulated that it reflects peripheral blood transit, capillary composition, and oxygen utilization.

Pulse oximeters are designed to warn practitioners when the arterial saturation decreases below normal, not to serve as quantitative devices in hypoxemic patients. Compared with measured arterial saturation in children with cyanotic congenital heart disease, most pulse oximeters exhibit a progressively positive bias typically reaching 5% to 15% at an Sao_2 of 60%, in addition to a significant reduction in precision (±8% to 10%) (Gidding, 1992; Schmitt et al., 1993) (Fig. 9–38).

Interference with the expected spectrophotometric absorption pattern also causes errors in measurement. Low hemoglobin, less than 5 g/dL, and abnormal hemoglobin species, like methemoglobin or carboxyhemoglobin, cause inaccurate saturation estimates by the pulse oximeter (New, 1985; Barker and Tremper, 1987; Barker et al., 1989; Watcha et al., 1989). In contrast, abnormal hemoglobin molecules, like fetal hemoglobin, apparently have little effect on the saturation measurement (Jennis and Peabody, 1987). Intravenous dyes, like methylene blue and indocyanine green, affect the expected light absorption and produce spurious information (Sidi et al., 1987). Aberrant radiation, like the electromagnetic energy from the electrocautery, infrared heat lamps, or operating room lights, also causes incorrect

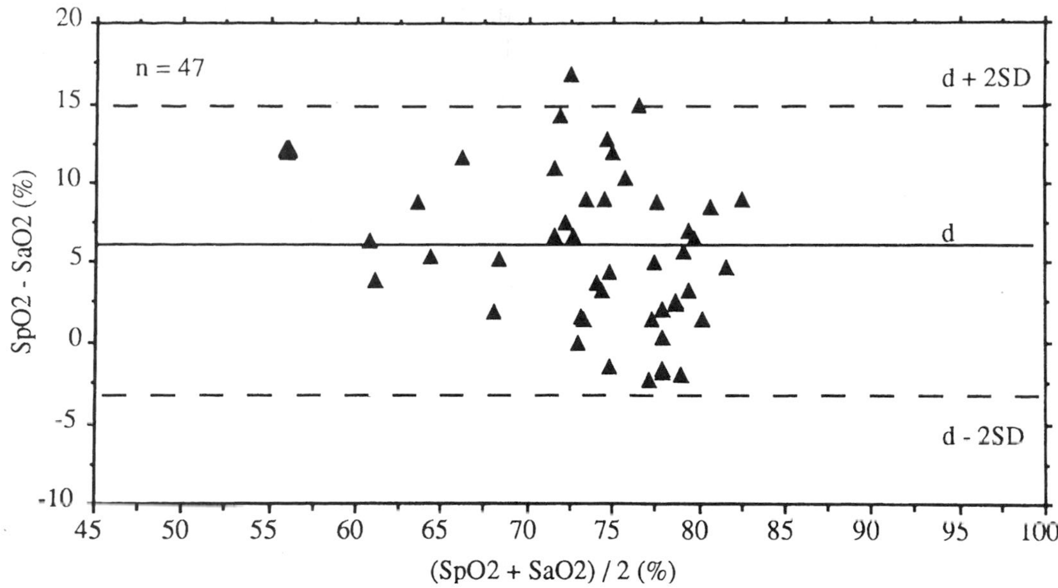

■ **FIGURE 9–38.** Accuracy and precision of pulse oximetry (Nellcor N-100) in chronically hypoxemic children with congenital heart malformations. Data comparing pulse oximetry (Spo_2) with co-oximetry (Sao_2) reflect a 5.8% mean positive bias for Spo_2 with wide discrepancies between the two techniques (±2 SDs = −3.8% to +15.4%). (From Schmitt HJ, Schuetz WH, Proeschel PA, et al.: Accuracy of pulse oximetry in children with cyanotic congenital heart disease. *J Cardiothorac Vasc Anesth* 7:61, 1993.)

saturation determination (Brooks et al., 1984; Costarino et al., 1987; Hanowell et al., 1987).

Innovative pulse oximetry technologies using signal extraction technology (SET) have claimed improved performance during extremity motion and states of poor perfusion (Masimo Corporation, Mission Viejo, CA) (Anonymous, 2000; Goldman et al., 2000). Studies comparing SET with conventional pulse oximetry during pediatric anesthesia have demonstrated superior performance with SET (Malviya et al., 2000). Its application in the perioperative setting has not been universally adopted.

BISPECTRAL INDEX

In 1996, the Food and Drug Administration approved the use of the bispectral index (BIS) monitor (Aspect Medical Systems, Nattick, MA), an electroencephalogram (EEG)-based device that is used to predict the relative level of hypnosis, or unconsciousness, in anesthetized patients (Rosow and Manberg, 1998). With use of a patch that affixes to the patient's forehead, the BIS monitor integrates various EEG descriptors into a single dimensionless, empirically calibrated number ranging from 0 to 100, where 0 represents electrical silence and 100 represents full wakefulness. A state of unconsciousness consistent with BIS values less than 60 usually ensures a lack of intraoperative recall (Glass et al., 1997). In adults, titration of anesthetics to a targeted BIS value between 40 and 60 results in the administration of smaller doses of anesthetics and earlier awakening (Gan et al., 1997). Preliminary data in adults suggest that routine BIS monitoring is associated with reduced intraoperative awareness during high-risk surgical procedures (e.g., microlaryngeal surgery, cesarean section, cardiac bypass, etc.) (Myles et al., 2003).

In anesthetized children, BIS values are inversely proportional to the end-tidal concentration of sevoflurane (Denman et al., 2000; Davidson et al., 2001; Degoute et al., 2001). This association weakens in infants younger than 1 year. In adolescents undergoing scoliosis surgery, BIS can predict voluntary patient movement in response to commands during the intraoperative wake-up test (McCann et al., 2002). BIS values during sevoflurane anesthesia appear to be proportionately less in children with quadriplegic cerebral palsy and mental retardation (Choudhry and Brenn, 2002).

BIS monitoring in children aged 3 to 18 years who are undergoing tonsillectomy and adenoidectomy is associated with reduced recovery times; in the same study, BIS monitoring did not affect recovery times in children younger than 3 years who were undergoing hernia repair (Bannister et al., 2001).

Because of age-related differences in brain maturation and synapse formation throughout childhood, BIS monitoring may not be as useful an intraoperative monitor as for adults (Watcha, 2001). Future studies are expected to further delineate the use of BIS in the pediatric population.

NEUROPHYSIOLOGIC MONITORING

It has long been appreciated that the patient's physiologic status is dynamic and that rapid and life-threatening changes may occur during surgery. The comparative ability to evaluate the functional status of the nervous system by either clinical means or the commonly used physiologic monitoring tools that are available to the anesthesiologists is limited. Routine monitoring may reflect stress on the central nervous system (CNS), yet changes in heart rate related to both brainstem and vagal stimulation provide only a nonspecific, insensitive view of global function. Intraoperative neurophysiologic monitoring adds another dimension as well as specificity to assessment of the status of the patient during surgery and anesthesia.

Neurophysiologic techniques provide important and reliable alternative tools for assessment of function of the pediatric CNS (Taylor, 1993). These techniques provide objective measures of the functioning of the CNS and can serve to document and localize deterioration in neuronal function. Intraoperatively, continuous monitoring of the area of the CNS that is at risk from surgical and anesthetic manipulation provides immediate insight into the effects of these operative interventions. Rather than waiting to evaluate the neurologic examination in the postoperative period of a child at risk for intraoperative diminution of neurologic function, continuous neurophysiologic monitoring provides an immediate view of the integrity of the CNS, permitting intraoperative changes in operative and anesthetic technique to minimize or correct the deleterious effects of the intraoperative manipulation. Advantages of these methods are that the results are objective and quantifiable, the site of the lesion can be identified, clinically latent or evolving lesions can be frequently demonstrated, and distinctions can often be made between disease entities. These techniques have a role to play both in the diagnostic investigation of pediatric CNS function and in the developing field of intraoperative assessment of CNS function.

It is imperative that the measures used are both specific to the neural tissue being manipulated and sensitive to changes in the functioning of the neural tissue produced by the surgical manipulations. Monitoring of the electrical activity dependent on the functioning of the brainstem (brainstem auditory evoked potentials [BAEPs] and brainstem somatosensory evoked potentials [BSEPs]), the cortex (the EEG, somatosensory evoked potentials [SEPs], and visual evoked potentials [VEPs]), the spinal cord (SEPs and motor evoked potentials [MEPs] and electromyograms [EMGs]), the various cranial nerves (EMGs), and peripheral nerves (compound action potentials and EMGs) provides a multidimensional assessment of the integrity of the neural structures at risk. In addition, many of these measures provide information not only about function itself but also about variables that directly or indirectly affect function, such as blood flow, hypoxia, and hypotension. The goal of intraoperative neurophysiologic monitoring is to provide information to the surgeon and anesthesiologist to allow them to modify their operative strategy before inducing additional deficits in the functioning of the CNS.

PERIOPERATIVE ASSESSMENT

An important aspect necessary for successful intraoperative monitoring is the planning and execution of surgical procedures in such a way that the neurophysiologists are in close communication with all other members of the surgical team, including surgeons, anesthesiologists, and radiologists. This preoperative and intraoperative communication among members of the surgical team ensures that the appropriate neurophysiologic measures are used during the procedure, that the anesthesiologist is prepared to switch anesthetic technique in support of the requirements imposed by the monitoring techniques, and that the significance of observed changes is appreciated by all members of the operative team. The surgeon needs to understand the level of information that the neurophysiologist can provide as the operative procedure is evolving, and the anesthesiologist needs to understand the effects of the pharmacologic manipulations on the monitoring tools available to the neurophysiologist. In addition, preoperative and postoperative neurophysiologic studies to determine and to reaffirm baseline responses increase understanding of the significance of intraoperative findings.

TECHNICAL METHODOLOGY

The recording of high-quality neurophysiologic data is dependent on the appropriate use of technology. In particular, attention must be paid to the electrode properties, the amplifiers, and the equipment used to acquire and display the data.

ELECTRODES

The bioelectrical activity at the scalp and the surface of the body is sensed using metal electrodes and transferred through conducting leads to recording amplifiers. Disk electrodes are typically used in the diagnostic laboratory, whereas subdermal needle electrodes are used in the operating room. Both disk and needle electrodes may also be used as stimulating electrodes as well as recording electrodes.

SIGNAL AMPLIFICATION

Techniques of data acquisition and handling before analysis are of considerable importance in the operating room environment. Functions such as signal scaling, bias levels, prefiltering, artifact removal, and analog-to-digital conversion must be optimized by trained individuals using specialized equipment. For example, evoked potentials are typically a fraction of the size of the spontaneous brain activity appearing in the background EEG and about one-thousandth the size of the other physiologic and extraneous potentials with which they are intermixed. The most effective method for extracting the signal of interest from the noise, after amplifying the signal with differential amplifiers, is to use signal averaging, which is in effect a cross-correlation between a point-process defined by the occurrence of the stimuli and the recorded evoked activity (i.e., an optimal filter) (Lee, 1960). In averaging, the signal component at each point is coherent and adds directly, whereas the background and noise components tend to be statistically independent and summate in a more-or-less root-mean-square fashion. The resultant recording highlights the signal of interest and deemphasizes the background and noise components.

STIMULATORS

Evoked SEPs are usually produced by electrical stimulators that produce a shock through the skin. MEPs are produced by either electrical or magnetic stimulators. Electrical activation of the motor cerebral cortex or brainstem can be performed transcranially. Electroencephalographic scalp electrodes or electrode plates placed adjacent to the scalp or hard palette can be used to stimulate the cortex. Transcranial magnetic stimulation involves the generation of a rapidly changing magnetic field that induces an electric current in nearby conductors. The magnetic field induced by transcranial magnetic stimulation passes through the scalp and skull and induces an electric current in underlying cerebral tissues. Auditory stimulation is obtained using one of several techniques, depending on the surgical procedure involved and thus on whether the auricle is retracted, as well as other considerations. Miniature open-air high-fidelity earphones (commonly used with personal tape players or radios) that rest in the concha of the ear or a tubal insert earphone (3A; EAR Tone, Indianapolis, IN). The tubal insert is attractive by virtue of distancing the transducer from the recording electrode (producing reduced stimulus artifact) and ease of support. For stimulation of the visual system, a fiberoptic system, which is positioned directly under the eye but not on the globe, is designed to be mounted on the flash stimulator driven by a Grass-Telefactor photic stimulator. With any of the stimulators, precise synchronization with the monitoring and averaging process must occur.

■ ANESTHETIC TECHNIQUES

It is well known that the type of anesthesia and the patient's blood pressure, cerebral blood flow, body temperature, hematocrit, and blood gas tensions all affect the functioning of the patient's CNS and thus intraoperatively observed neurophysiologic measures (Grundy, 1983; McPherson, 1994). The neurophysiologist must communicate with the anesthesiologist concerning the anesthetic plan before the start of the procedure to ensure that no conflicts exist over the required anesthetic and neurophysiologic monitoring. Both neurophysiologist and anesthesiologist must understand the needs of each other and develop a plan for the monitoring and anesthesia that allows both individuals to provide care that is appropriate for the specific patient. The halogenated hydrocarbon inhalation agents tend to significantly reduce the amplitude of somatosensory evoked responses (Salzman et al., 1986). The best SEPs are often recorded with use of a narcotic relaxant technique, consisting of an opioid, nitrous oxide (<65%), and a muscle relaxant. Boluses of medications produce more disruption of signals than do constant infusions. Regardless of how medications are delivered, the anesthesiologist must inform the neurophysiologist of medication administration, changes in patient temperature or blood pressure, or any other change in the patient's condition.

In many situations, the use of halogenated hydrocarbon inhalation agents is desired to help control blood pressure. Once baseline responses have been obtained and compared with the preoperative responses, many children can maintain their responses to an isoflurane level of approximately 0.3 MAC (minimum alveolar concentration), whereas many adults can maintain their responses to 0.5 MAC. This is highly variable and strongly dependent on the patient and his or her individual reaction to the inhalation agent. A slow increase in isoflurane until either the blood pressure is controlled or the responses significantly deteriorate usually leads to satisfactory results; it should be noted that there are a small number of patients who cannot maintain their somatosensory evoked potentials (SEPs) with any inhalation agent on board. Propofol, etomidate, and ketamine also appear to maintain SEPs at anesthetic concentrations and may be particularly useful when signals are expected to be difficult to obtain (Schubert et al., 1990; Kalkman et al., 1991; Taniguchi et al., 1992; McPherson, 1994).

■ NEUROPHYSIOLOGIC MEASURES

Neurophysiologic measures that are routinely used provide a functional map of much of the entire neuroaxis. These include the EEG, an unstimulated measure of cortical function suitable for providing information concerning the degree of cortical activation related to either metabolic process (e.g., hypoxia) or to pharmacologic manipulation (e.g., pentobarbital-induced burst suppression to protect the patient's cortical function) (Niedermeyer and Lopes da Silva, 1987); SEPs and VEPs, which provide additional measures of cortical function specific to certain pathways and vasculature; BAEPs and BSEPs, which provide information about the functioning of the brainstem, again specific to certain pathways (Regan, 1989); and EMGs, produced either by muscles innervated by the various cranial nerves, which provide information about both the cranial nerves themselves and their underlying brainstem nuclei (Kamura, 1983), or by somatic muscles providing information about spinal cord or peripheral nerve function.

■ MATURATIONAL EFFECTS

The functional assessment of the pediatric CNS presents difficult and unique problems compared with that of the more mature adult CNS. The pediatric CNS differs from the adult CNS in that it is maturing over the first several years of life; that is, the neural tissue, the myelin coating of the axonal processes, and the vascular supply to the CNS all show significant changes. These developmental anatomic changes are reflected in maturational functional changes as measured by both ascending SEP and descending MEP activity, VEPs, and BAEPs (Starr et al., 1977; Cracco et al., 1979; Guthkelch et al., 1982). There are a number of factors that contribute to the maturational changes of evoked potentials, and the use of age- and size-matched normal controls is essential. For intraoperative monitoring purposes, infants act as their own controls. Central and peripheral myelination is believed to be completed by 5 years of age, and from then until maturity the dominant factor affecting SEP latency is height (Yakovlev and Lecours, 1967; Gilmore et al., 1985) (Fig. 9–39).

■ GENERAL PROCEDURES

Neurophysiologic recording during pediatric operations can rapidly become quite complex. It is not unusual to monitor several different neurophysiologic variables simultaneously, such as EEGs, BAEPs, BSEPs, SEPs, and EMGs relating to several cranial nerves. This requires a well-organized and theoretically parsimonious approach to monitoring.

The positioning of recording electrodes should be chosen in relation to the expected distribution of the responses to be recorded. Many laboratories place scalp electrodes at sites determined with use of the international 10-20 system (Jasper, 1958). This system, originally devised for EEG recordings, specifies the position of 21 evenly spaced locations on the scalp. Recording electrodes are placed symmetrically to provide for control recordings from the side contralateral to the surgery, even when electrodes may not be positioned in the standard recording sites.

All recordings are usually performed using subdermal needle electrodes. Electrodes that are not in the operative field but are on the scalp and are not accessible during surgery are either sutured or stapled in place. Electrodes on the face, which are placed to record electromyographic activity, are taped in place. Electrodes in the operative field are placed by the surgeons using sterile technique, usually early in the procedure.

Baseline responses are obtained before draping the patient and compared with the preoperative evaluation. Significant differences must be accounted for, because signal deterioration may be caused by the effects of inadequate patient positioning.

■ ELECTROENCEPHALOGRAPHY

The functioning of the cerebral cortex is extremely sensitive to changes in arterial oxygenation and insufficient cerebral blood

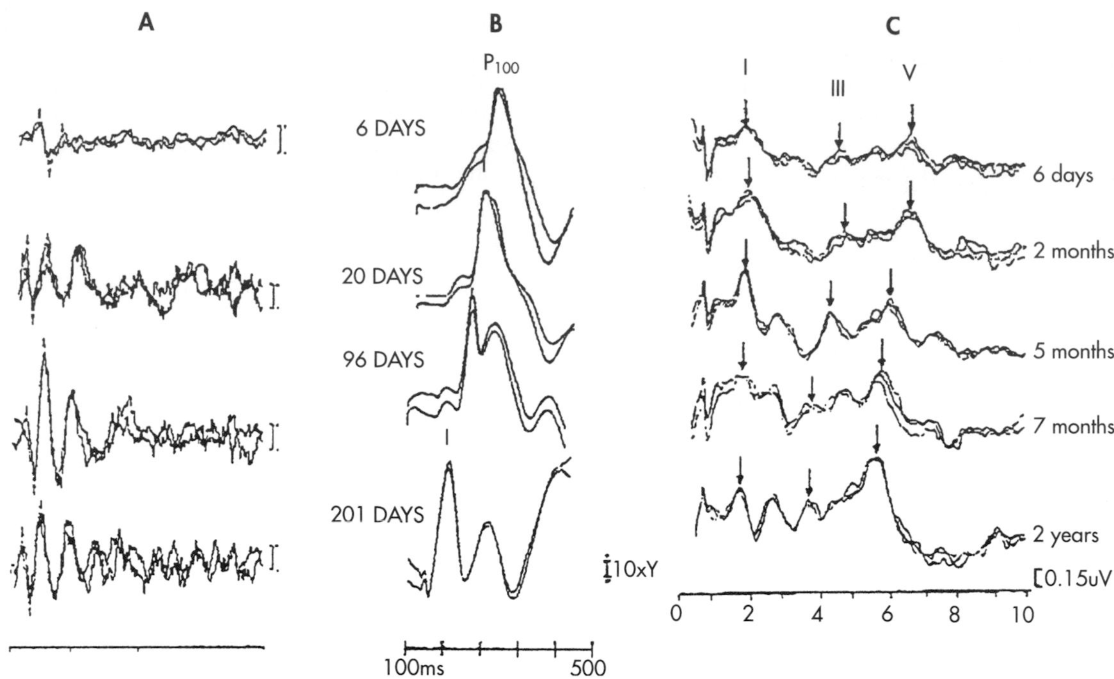

■ **FIGURE 9–39.** Maturational changes in cortical somatosensory evoked potentials to median nerve stimulation *(A)*, visual evoked potentials to flash stimulation *(B)*, and brainstem auditory evoked potentials to click stimulation *(C)*, in early infancy. Note the decreasing latency (the time measured from the initiation of the stimulus to the point of maximum amplitude of signal) and enhancing morphology for the identified waves in all three modalities.

flow or an inadequate partial pressure of oxygen; this sensitivity is rapidly reflected in the EEG (Meyer and Marx, 1972). Oxidative metabolism supplies the energy for maintenance of the membrane potential of nerve cells, and the EEG is directly dependent on the transmembrane potentials of neurons; it reflects disturbances of cerebral metabolism such as hypoxia. Some factors that may contribute to ischemic events in surgical patients are decreased oxygen-carrying capacity due to hypovolemia or decreased cerebral perfusion pressure due to factors associated with decreased systemic arterial pressure, increased intracranial pressure, and mechanical obstruction of cerebral vessels (Freye, 1990).

Two channels of continuous EEG monitoring is thought to be adequate, because the problems are not related to precise focality but rather are of global or hemispheric importance. The EEG can be observed both as the ongoing unprocessed signal and in a Fourier transformed representation. The electroencephalographic appearances of any ischemic or hypoxic events are similar, and differentiation between the various putative causative factors is made by being particularly attentive to the clinical situation; for example, blood pressure, ECG, oxygen saturation, administered drugs, and surgical manipulations may all have an observable effect. Other concurrent factors that may alter the EEG are changes in the depth of anesthesia, temperature changes, and changes in carbon dioxide content. These factors may be recognized by their relatively slow onset, lasting for several minutes, in contrast to the changes of ischemia, which generally occur within seconds. There are situations where the EEG may be acutely depressed on injection of an anesthetic that rapidly passes the blood-brain barrier. Such situations may be found with the use of high-dose opioid anesthesia, in which fentanyl induces an immediate and marked reduction in fast-frequency activity in the EEG, with an increase in low-frequency, high-amplitude activity in the delta range (Freye, 1990).

A simple but useful summary of possible changes is that decreased frequency with increased amplitude (Van der Drift, 1972) implies an ischemic event to the cortex; widespread frequency slowing and decreased amplitude usually imply brainstem ischemia (Roger et al., 1954); ischemic events affecting the thalamus and the internal capsule produce unremarkable changes in the EEG (Van der Drift, 1972) but possible significant changes in the SEPs.

■ SOMATOSENSORY AND MOTOR EVOKED POTENTIALS

The neurophysiologic measures of value in assessing the spinal cord consist of SEPs, produced by stimulating various peripheral nerves, and MEPs, which may be observed as either compound muscle or nerve action potentials and which may be produced by either transcranial or spinal cord stimulation. It is currently advantageous to think of the SEPs as characterizing the ascending activity in the spinal cord and of the MEPs as characterizing the descending activity in the spinal cord. This distinction, although not particularly important with respect to the sensory activity, is potentially extremely important with respect to the descending activity, because important questions remain as to what pathways are being stimulated (Rose et al., 1994).

■ SOMATOSENSORY EVOKED POTENTIALS (ASCENDING ACTIVITY)

SEPs are dependent on the stimulation of the large afferent fibers of peripheral nerves. Following stimulation of peripheral nerves in the arms or the legs, SEPs can be reproducibly recorded over the spine and scalp. In the spinal cord, the SEPs are conducted primarily through the dorsal columns.

SEPs are a sequence of potentials generated in the peripheral nerves, dorsal horn nuclei, dorsal column pathways, and dorsal column nuclei of the spinal cord; the medial lemniscal pathways of the brainstem; and the thalamus, thalamocortical, parietal region of the brain after the application of a transient electrical stimulus to a peripheral nerve (Sclabassi et al., 1993). When recorded from electrodes on the surface of the body, the potentials of interest are very small, ranging in size from 2 to 5 μV, and occur in approximately the first 100 milliseconds after the application of a stimulus (often referred to as early and middle latency potentials). Evoked potentials are typically a fraction of the size of the spontaneous brain activity appearing in the background EEG and about one-thousandth the size of the other physiologic and extraneous potentials with which they are intermixed. Unwanted activity (noise) originates with both the signal recorded from the subject and electrical devices in the immediate neighborhood of the recording equipment. The aim of evoked potential recording is to ensure a large, clear response with the least possible noise contamination (i.e., the best signal-to-noise ratio possible); the elimination of these unwanted signal components is essential. Evoked potentials are described in terms of latency and amplitude. *Latency* is the time measured from the application of a stimulus to the point of maximum amplitude of the evoked potential. Some types of SEP have more than one peak and the time between peaks is the *interpeak latency*. The *amplitude* is the voltage difference between two peaks of opposite polarity or a reference potential. Measurement of latencies, amplitudes, and interpeak latencies characterize SEP recordings. Changes in these measurements during an anesthetic and surgical procedure may represent injury to the neural tissue between the stimulus generator and the recording electrode.

In all cases, the stimuli are electrical impulses applied transcutaneously, at a rate of 0.7 to 5.3 Hz, depending on the robustness of the response, which is typically a function of the patient's age and pathology. Typically, responses to 128 stimuli are averaged; in many cases, as few as 12 responses may be averaged, providing near real-time updating of the responses.

All types of SEPs are used for intraoperative monitoring, primarily during spinal surgery. Potentials can be recorded after stimulation of the median nerve at the wrist, the common peroneal nerve, the posterior tibial nerve, and the dorsal nerve of the penis and the clitoris. Multiple types of responses from different stimuli and different sources often are simultaneously recorded, allowing the entire neuroaxis to be monitored. Monitoring multiple upper and lower extremity responses simultaneously during spinal surgery allows cord injury to be distinguished from global problems or localized monitoring difficulty.

MEDIAN, ULNAR, AND RADIAL NERVE POTENTIALS

The median (MSPs), ulnar (USPs), and radial (RSPs) nerve evoked potentials are all useful in assessing the brachial plexus, upper spinal cord, brainstem, and telencephalon. One important distinction is that the USPs provide information regarding level C-8 and above, whereas the MSPs provide information about level C-7 and above (Fig. 9–40). At Erb's point, the response consists of an apparently triphasic (positive-negative-positive) nerve action potential, reflecting the passage of the mixed nerve volley through the brachial plexus. This component is usually labeled N11 for the large negative going component. At the cervical C-7 recording site, the main component is a negative peak occurring at 14-millisecond latency, N14, with an associated complex structure. It has been postulated that these waves are generated in the dorsal roots, dorsal horn, posterior columns, and structures of the lower brainstem. During spinal fusions, monitoring of the brachial plexus may also alert the anesthesiologist to poor positioning of the arms.

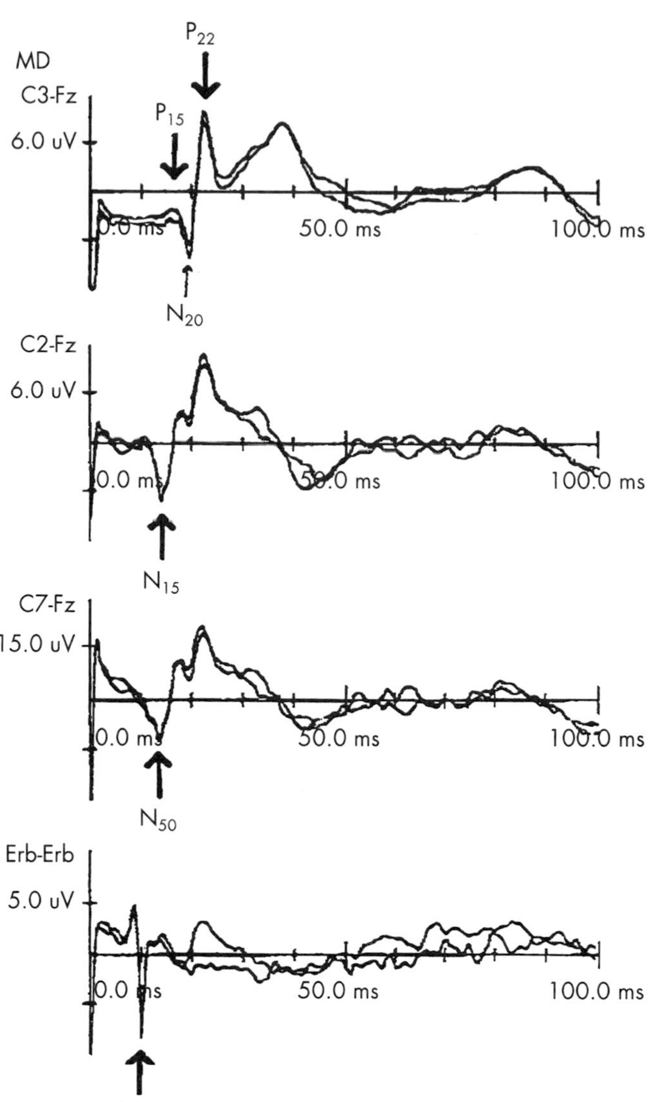

FIGURE 9–40. Median nerve potentials produced by right median nerve (MD) stimulation. Data are recorded from Erb's point *(bottom)*, cervical C-7, C-2, and cranial C-3 and all referenced to Fz. Note the increase in latency of large negative depression noted by the N11 wave at Erb's point and N14, N15, and N20 at the other respective electrode locations as the recording electrode becomes more distant from the stimulator.

COMMON PERONEAL AND TIBIAL NERVE POTENTIALS

In the lower limb, nerves used to elicit cortical SEPs include the tibial, peroneal, sural, saphenous, and others. Spinal potentials are most consistently obtained through stimulation of the tibial nerve at the medial malleolus or peroneal nerve in the popliteal fossa.

SEPs recorded over the spine reflect the afferent volley traversing the dorsal columns. These responses can be recorded from electrodes attached to the skin over the spine, and they progressively increase in latency at more rostral recording locations. Spinal SEPs are relatively easy to obtain in children, with the amplitude and definition of the waves decreasing with increasing age such that by the mid-teenage years, these responses are more difficult to obtain, as is the case with adults. More rostral recording locations reflect potentials arising in multiple ascending pathways, including the dorsal and dorsolateral columns, which lie primarily ipsilateral to the side of stimulation.

DERMATOMAL RESPONSES

A disadvantage of SEPs produced by stimulation of large nerve trunks is that input to the spinal cord usually occurs over more than one level. This problem can be addressed by delivering the stimulus to a small cutaneous nerve that is believed to derive from a single dorsal root or to the "signature area" of a particular dermatome. Significant disagreement exists concerning the cutaneous distributions of dermatomes, and care should be taken to stimulate the commonly accepted receptive fields of a root.

Pudendal nerve responses are a special type of dermatomal responses that are particularly useful, especially in patients with spina bifida. The pudendal nerve carries sensory fibers from the penis, urethra, anus, and pelvic floor muscles and supplies motor innervation to the bulbocavernosus and pelvic floor muscles, the external urethral sphincter, and the external anal sphincter. Cortical responses to electrical stimulation of the dorsal nerve of the penis, the urethra, and the urinary bladder have all been described (Badr et al., 1982; Haldeman et al., 1982). Pudendal nerve responses are of similar morphology to the tibial nerve SEP (TSP) and are best recorded from the same area of the scalp (Fig. 9–41).

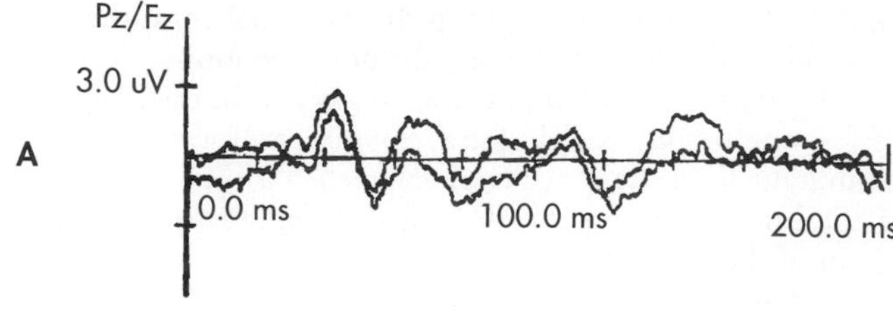

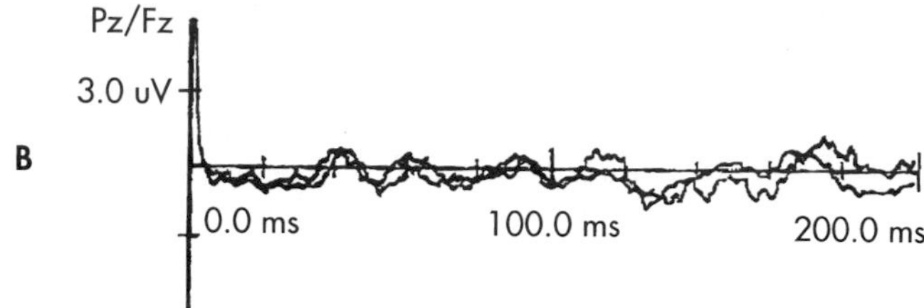

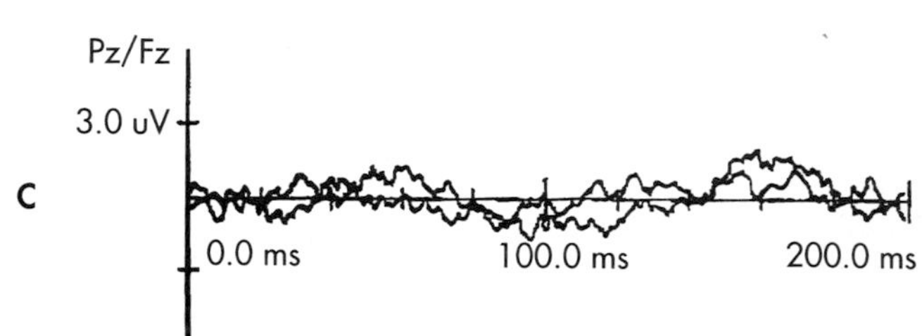

FIGURE 9–41. Pudendal nerve responses obtained from a male tethered cord patient with symptoms referable to the pudendal nerve. All responses are recorded from Pz referenced to Fz. *A* was obtained by stimulating the right branch of the dorsal nerve of the penis, whereas *B* was obtained by stimulating the left. Note the significant reduction in amplitude in response to the left-sided stimulation. *C* represents control data recorded during every procedure.

MOTOR EVOKED POTENTIALS

Because SEPs reflect function in the dorsal columns of the spinal cord, SEPs do not directly assess the integrity of descending spinal motor tracts. It is possible to have focal damage to the motor areas in the spinal cord in which the SEPs remain normal. Accordingly, there have occasionally been misleading results when using SEPs alone for intraoperative monitoring and diagnosis (Lesser et al., 1986), but this is rare. MEPs, which may be either evoked EMGs or compound action potentials, can be used to test the integrity of the motor pathways through either electrical or magnetic stimulation (Merton and Morton, 1980; Barker et al., 1985). MEPs can be obtained via stimulation of the motor areas of the brain or spinal cord through the intact skin, direct stimulation of exposed neuronal tissue, or direct root stimulation (e.g., during the release of a tethered cord) and recording of a stimulus-related response either as a compound muscle action potential (CMAP) or as an efferent compound nerve action potential (CNAP) (Fig. 9–42).

Transcranial and electrical surface stimulation may be used to elicit motor responses. There is no general consensus about the location of recording electrodes, outside of specific muscle groups for evoked CMAPs or over the obvious peripheral nerves for evoked CNAPs, nor is there a general consensus concerning which class of these activities is more advantageous to record. CNAPs allow the patient to have neuromuscular blockade agents.

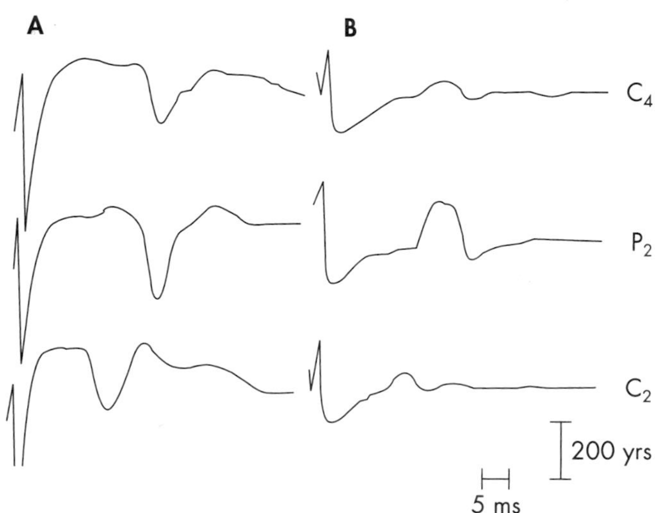

FIGURE 9–42. Compound muscle action potentials *(A)* and compound muscle action potentials *(B)* produced by transcranial simulation at C4, Pz, and C2, using a magnetic stimulator. The compound muscle action potentials are recorded from the abductor pollicis brevis, whereas the compound nerve action potentials were recorded from the left median nerve at the wrist.

COMBINED ASCENDING AND DESCENDING ACTIVITY

Intraoperative monitoring of CNAPs and posterior TSPs is used to provide a simultaneous measure of the ascending and descending activities in the spinal cord. Through this approach, sequential stimulation is performed of the left tibial nerve, the right tibial nerve, and the spinal cord through the spinous processes. Recording electrodes positioned on the scalp record the bilateral SEPs from the tibial nerve stimuli as well as the afferent activity induced in the spinal area via direct spinal stimulation. Recording electrodes in the popliteal fossa allow the afferent stimulus compound action potentials to be observed, and then the descending compound action potentials produced by the spinal cord stimulation. This combined technique aids in localizing spinal cord dysfunction during surgery by continuously evaluating the adequacy of both the sensory and motor components of spinal cord neural activity.

AUDITORY BRAINSTEM RESPONSES

Monitoring of the function of cranial nerve VIII through the use of BAEPs assists in preserving hearing, locating cranial nerve VIII, or determining whether the overall function of the brainstem is altered. BAEPs are also sensitive to the retraction on the frontal poles, most likely due to force transmission to the brainstem.

The classic BAEP consists of a minimum of five and a maximum of seven peaks. All occur with 10 milliseconds of a brief click or tone presentation. Wave I is generated in the auditory portion of nerve VIII. Wave II is generated bilaterally at or in the proximity of the cochlear nucleus. Wave III is generated bilaterally from the lower pons near the superior olive and trapezoid body. Waves IV and V are probably generated in the upper pons or lower midbrain, near the lateral lemniscus or possibly near the inferior colliculus.

Waves I through V are relatively resistant to sedative medication and general anesthetics; these responses place no constraints on the anesthesiologist. They are sensitive to temperature changes, with absolute and interpeak latencies increasing by approximately .20 milliseconds. The latency of wave V is the primary concern in intraoperative monitoring of the BAEPs, because this is the most robust and easily identifiable of the waves in this response.

VISUAL SYSTEM

VEPs are used to aid in determining the functional integrity of the visual system, primarily in the region of the optic nerves, chiasm, and optic radiations. The recorded activity is generated either at the retina (electroretinogram) or at the cortex.

Stimulation of the visual system using a bright flash is not recommended for diagnostic purposes due to intersubject variability (Ciganek, 1961), except in selected situations; in the operating room this is a very helpful and effective technique (Fig. 9–43).

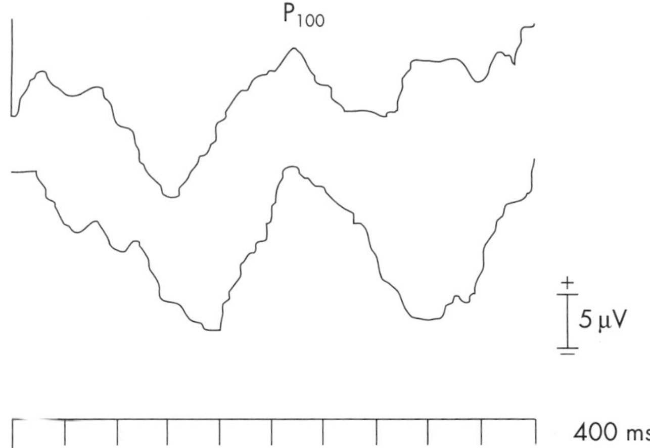

FIGURE 9–43. Intraoperative visual evoked potentials (VEPs), obtained between midline occipital and vertex electrodes, to flash stimuli. Results were obtained from a 10-month-old girl who was being operated on for a chiasmal glioma, which was 90% removed. *Top trace,* preresection response; *bottom trace,* postresection response. The responses were abnormal but unchanged during the procedure.

ELECTROMYOGRAPHY

The EMG is electrical activity produced in muscle fibers below the skin; it has a frequency content ranging from 1 to 150 Hz. Three different types of electrodes are used to record the EMGs: fine wire electrodes, which have the highest impedance and the narrowest field of view; subdermal needles, which have an intermediate impedance and a larger field of view; and disk surface electrodes, which have the lowest impedance and the largest field of view (*field of view* means the integrated level of electrical activity). The recording techniques are essentially the same for all cranial nerves and all muscle groups. Subdermal platinum needle electrodes are used in bipolar recording configurations; that is, all recordings are made between a pair of electrodes inserted into the same muscle group. Bipolar recordings are used to minimize confusion regarding which cranial nerve or branch of a cranial nerve is producing the observed EMG. The electrodes are normally placed before the start of the procedure; occasionally electrodes are placed in a sterile field by the surgeons.

These signals are listened to continuously for evaluation of nerve function both by the neurophysiologists and by the surgeons. Four categories of EMG activity are observed: (1) no activity, which in an intact nerve is the best situation but which may also be the case in a nerve that has been sharply dissected; (2) irritation activity, which sounds like soft intermittent flutter and is consistent with working near the nerve; (3) injury activity, which sounds like a continuous, nonaccelerating tapping and which can be an indicator of permanent injury to the cranial nerve; and (4) a "killed-end" response, which sounds like an accelerating firing pattern and is an unequivocal indicator of nerve injury. It is important to note that a sharply cut nerve may produce only a brief burst of activity; monitoring cannot be expected to replace extreme caution when working near the cranial nerves.

EVALUATION OF CRANIAL NERVE FUNCTION

Cranial nerve function is monitored continuously during surgery for two reasons: first, to establish the location and orientation of the cranial nerves in the operative field; and second, to preserve functioning in the cranial nerves and their related brainstem nuclei (Sclabassi et al., 1993). The major observed variables are the EMGs from the appropriate muscle group innervated by the cranial nerves of interest. In general, the cranial nerves ipsilateral to the operative side are monitored; when appropriate, bilateral activity is monitored.

In addition to monitoring the ongoing EMG activity related to the various cranial nerves, the various cranial nerves may also be electrically stimulated. This is usually done to determine the location of the nerve in the operative field, because many times the nerve is enveloped by tumor and may not be directly observable, or to determine the functional integrity of the nerve (Daube and Harper, 1989). The most common example of this procedure is the direct stimulation of nerve VII. The return path for the stimulating current is provided by a metal electrode inserted into the adjacent muscle mass. In some situations, where very precise localization of the nerve is required, bipolar stimulating electrodes are used. The great majority of the time, the question being asked is, Is the nerve there?

ELECTROMYOGRAMS IN TETHERED CORD RELEASES AND SELECTIVE RHYZOTOMIES

The EMG is a useful indicator of the integrity of descending activity in the spinal cord. The EMG is either spontaneous, such as anal sphincter activity produced by irritation of the S3-5 roots during an untethering procedure involving the lower portion of the cauda equina, or evoked of the type produced in either stimulation of nerve roots when attempting to identify the cauda equina or selective rhyzotomy for the treatment of spasticity. Anesthetic management involves the avoiding of neuromuscular blockade during this type of evaluation.

The commonly accepted principal goal of intraoperative monitoring is to prevent morbidity, and at a certain level this is true; the more fundamental goal of intraoperative monitoring is to provide the operative team with information that allows them to accomplish the desired operative objective with as optimal an anesthetic and surgical strategy as possible, while having a clear idea of what morbidity is being induced along the way. This latter goal is particularly important in cases where the degree of difficulty is high and it is virtually impossible to prevent morbidity.

Stringent time constraints exist in intraoperative monitoring of neurophysiologic function, and damage to the CNS may occur rapidly, over seconds. This constraint has inspired the development of methods for extracting and analyzing evoked potential, EMG, and EEG waveforms rapidly and efficiently. A corollary of the increased sensitivity required to decrease the monitoring time is a higher rate of individually false-positive measures. These are usually rapidly identified as such and produce no disruption in the flow of the case. Intraoperative monitoring requires rapid interpretations to be made of complex data, recorded in less-than-optimal conditions. It does no good to inform the surgeon 10 minutes after the fact that a significant change has occurred. Successful intraoperative monitoring of the pediatric CNS requires the acquisition of as many appropriate neurophysiologic variables simultaneously as possible. In addition, the correct interpretation of these responses is greatly aided by the ability to display the history of all of the acquired data in such a way as to facilitate a comparison of all of the data. This includes the baseline values acquired both at the beginning of the procedure and from the preoperative studies.

SUMMARY

The anesthesiologist caring for infants and children has a wide array of equipment and monitors available. The exact configuration of equipment and monitors necessary depends primarily on the patient's illness, the experience of the anesthesiologist, and the proposed surgery. With the increasing complexity of anesthesia equipment and monitors, the anesthesiologist needs to understand thoroughly the operation and limitations of each device. Last, the anesthesiologist should never rely too heavily on the monitoring equipment and abandon the direct, close, personal surveillance of each patient during anesthesia and surgery.

REFERENCES

Adamsons K, Towell ME: Thermal homeostasis in the fetus and newborn. *Anesthesiology* 26:531, 1965.

Agro F, Barzoi G, Carassiti M, et al.: Getting the tube in the oesophagus and oxygen in the trachea: Preliminary results with the new supraglottic device (Cobra) in 28 anaesthetised patients. *Anaesthesia* 58:920, 2003.

Alderson PJ, Burrows FA, Stemp LI, et al.: Use of ultrasound to evaluate internal jugular vein anatomy and to facilitate central venous cannulation in paediatric patients. *Br J Anaesth* 70:145, 1993.

Alexander CA, Leach AB: Incidence of sore throats with the laryngeal mask. *Anaesthesia* 44:791, 1989.

Alverson DC, Eldridge M, Dillon T, et al.: Noninvasive pulsed Doppler determination of cardiac output in neonates and children. *J Pediatr* 101:46, 1982.

American Academy of Pediatrics Task Force on Transcutaneous Oxygen Monitors: Report of consensus meeting, December 5 to 6, 1986. *Pediatrics* 83:122, 1989.

American Society for Testing and Materials (ASTM): Standard Specification for Particular Requirements for Anesthesia Workstations and their Components. ASTM, West Conshohocken, PA. (F-1195-99, 2005).

American Society for Testing and Materials (ASTM): Standard Specification for Particular Requirements for Anesthesia Workstations and their Components. ASTM, West Conshohocken, PA. (F-1850-00, 2005).

American Society of Anesthesiologists Task Force on Management of the Difficult Airway: Practice guidelines for management of the difficult airway. *Anesthesiology* 78:597, 1993.

American Society of Anesthesiologists: Standards for basic anesthesia monitoring. 10-15-2003, Park Ridge, IL.

Andropoulos DB, Bent ST, Skjonsby B, et al.: The optimal length of insertion of central venous catheters for pediatric patients. *Anesth Analg* 93:883, 2001.

Anonymous: Next-generation pulse oximetry. Focusing on Masimo's signal extraction technology. *Health Devices* 29:349, 2000.

Arant BS Jr: Developmental patterns of renal functional maturation compared in the human neonate. *J Pediatr* 92:705, 1978.

Arndt GA, DeLessio ST, Kranner PW, et al.: One-lung ventilation when intubation is difficult—presentation of a new endobronchial blocker. *Acta Anaesthesiol Scand* 43:356, 1999.

Ayre P: Endotracheal anesthesia for babies with special references to hare-lip and cleft palate operations. *Anesthesia Analg* 16:330, 1937.

Ayre P: The T piece technique. *Br J Anesth* 28:520, 1956.

Badgwell JM, Kleinman SE, Heavner JE: Respiratory frequency and artifact affect the capnographic baseline in infants. *Anesth Analg* 77:708, 1993.

Badgwell JM, McLeod ME, Lerman J, et al.: End-tidal PCO_2 measurements sampled at the distal and proximal ends of the endotracheal tube in infants and children. *Anesth Analg* 66:959, 1987.

Badr G, Carlsson CA, Fall M, et al.: Cortical evoked potentials following stimulation of the urinary bladder in man. *Electroencephalogr Clin Neurophysiol* 54:494, 1982.

Bain JA, Spoerel WE: A streamlined anaesthetic system. *Can Anaesth Soc J* 19:426, 1972.

Bain JA, Spoerel WE: Carbon dioxide output and elimination in children under anaesthesia. *Can Anaesth Soc J* 24:533, 1977.

Bain JA, Spoerel WE: Flow requirements for a modified Mapleson D system during controlled ventilation. *Can Anaesth Soc J* 20:629, 1973.

Bannister CF, Brosius KK, Sigl JC, et al.: The effect of bispectral index monitoring on anesthetic use and recovery in children anesthetized with sevoflurane in nitrous oxide. *Anesth Analg* 92:877, 2001.

Barker AT, Jalinous R, Freeston IL: Noninvasive magnetic stimulation of the human motor cortex. *Lancet* 2:1106, 1985.

Barker P, Langton JA, Murphy PJ, et al.: Regurgitation of gastric contents during general anaesthesia using the laryngeal mask airway. *Br J Anaesth* 69:314, 1992.

Barker SJ, Tremper KK, Hyatt J; Effects of methemoglobinemia on pulse oximetry and mixed venous oximetry. *Anesthesiology* 70:112, 1989.

Barker SJ, Tremper KK: The effect of carbon monoxide inhalation on pulse oximetry and transcutaneous PO_2. *Anesthesiology* 66:677, 1987.

Barker SJ, Tremper KK: Transcutaneous oxygen tension: A physiological variable for monitoring oxygenation. *J Clin Monit* 1:130, 1985.

Bauer SB, Feldman SM, Gellis SS, et al.: Neonatal hypertension. A complication of umbilical-artery catheterization. *N Engl J Med* 293:1032, 1975.

Benumof JL: Laryngeal mask airway and the ASA difficult airway algorithm. *Anesthesiology* 84:686, 1996.

Berry AJ, Katz JD, Brown RH, et al.: *Latex allergy: Considerations for anesthesiologists.* Committee on Occupational Health of Operating Room Personnel, American Society of Anesthesiologists, 2001, Park Ridge, IL.

Beveridge ME: Laryngeal mask anaesthesia for repair of cleft palate. *Anaesthesia* 44:656, 1989.

Bissonnette B, Sessler DI: Passive or active inspired gas humidification increases thermal steady-state temperatures in anesthetized infants. *Anesth Analg* 69:783, 1989.

Bissonnette B, Sessler DI, LaFlamme P: Intraoperative temperature monitoring sites in infants and children and the effect of inspired gas warming on esophageal temperature. *Anesth Analg* 69:192, 1989a.

Bissonnette B, Sessler DI, LaFlamme P: Passive and active inspired gas humidification in infants and children. *Anesthesiology* 71:350, 1989b.

Borland LM, Casselbrant M: The Bullard laryngoscope. A new indirect oral laryngoscope (pediatric version). *Anesth Analg* 70:105, 1990.

Bourke DL, Wurm H, Rosenberg M, et al.: Intraoperative heat conservation using a reflective blanket. *Anesthesiology* 60:151, 1984.

Brain AI: Further developments of the laryngeal mask. *Anaesthesia* 44:530, 1989.

Brain AIJ, McGhee TD, McAteer EJ, et al.: Laryngeal mask airway—development and preliminary trials of a new type of airway. *Anaesthesia* 40:356, 1985.

Brain AIJ: Laryngeal mask—a new concept in airway management. *Br J Anaesth* 55:801, 1983.

Brimacombe JR: Difficult airway management with the intubating laryngeal mask. *Anesth Analg* 85:1173, 1997.

Brooks TD, Paulus DA, Winkle WE: Infrared heat lamps interfere with pulse oximeters. *Anesthesiology* 61:630, 1984.

Brown ES, Hustead RF: Resistance of pediatric breathing systems. *Anesth Analg* 48:842, 1969.

Brown RE Jr, Vollers JM, Rader GR, et al.: Nasotracheal intubation in a child with Treacher Collins syndrome using the Bullard intubating laryngoscope. *J Clin Anesth* 5:492, 1993.

Bruner JM, Krenis LJ, Kunsman JM, et al.: Comparison of direct and indirect measuring arterial blood pressure. *Med Instrum* 15:11, 1981.

Bucx MJ, Grolman W, Kruisinga FH, et al.: The prolonged use of the laryngeal mask airway in a neonate with airway obstruction and Treacher Collins syndrome. *Paediatr Anaesth* 13:530, 2003.

Burrows FA: Physiologic dead space, venous admixture, and the arterial to end-tidal carbon dioxide difference in infants and children undergoing cardiac surgery. *Anesthesiology* 70:219, 1989.

Bussolin L, Busoni P: The use of the cuffed oropharyngeal airway in paediatric patients. *Paediatr Anaesth* 12:43, 2002.

Camus Y, Delva E, Just B, et al.: Leg warming minimizes core hypothermia during abdominal surgery. *Anesth Analg* 77:995, 1993.

Cantwell GP, Holzman BH, and Caceres MJ: Percutaneous catheterization of the axillary artery in the pediatric patient [published erratum appears in *Crit Care Med* 19:746, 1991]. *Crit Care Med* 18:880, 1990.

Capek JM, Roy RJ: Noninvasive measurement of cardiac output using partial CO_2 rebreathing. *IEEE Trans Biomed Eng* 35:653, 1988.

Cass L: Inserting the laryngeal mask. *Anaesth Intensive Care* 19:615, 1991.

Cave P, Fletcher G: Resistance of nasotracheal tubes used in infants. *Anesthesiology* 29:588, 1968.

Chadd GD, Crane DL, Phillips RM, et al.: Extubation and reintubation guided by the laryngeal mask airway in a child with the Pierre-Robin syndrome. *Anesthesiology* 76:640, 1992.

Ching NP, Ayres SM, Spina RC, et al.: Endotracheal damage during continuous ventilatory support. *Ann Surg* 179:123, 1974.

Choudhry DK, Brenn BR: Bispectral index monitoring: A comparison between normal children and children with quadriplegic cerebral palsy. *Anesth Analg* 95:1582, 2002.

Chow BFM, Lewis M, Jones SEF: Laryngeal mask airway in children: Insertion technique. *Anaesthesia* 46:590, 1991.

Ciganek L: The EEG response to light stimulus in man. *Electroenceph Clin Neurophysiol* 13:165–172, 1961.

Clarke RE, Orkin LR, Rovenstine EA: Body temperature studies in anesthetized man: Effect of environmental temperature, humidity, and anesthesia systems. *JAMA* 154:311, 1954.

Cohen DE, Downes JJ, Raphaely RC: What difference does pulse oximetry make? *Anesthesiology* 68:181, 1988.

Cohen MM, Cameron CB, Duncan PG: Pediatric anesthesia morbidity and mortality in the perioperative period. *Anesth Analg* 70:160, 1990.

Colgan FJ, Stewart S: An assessment of cardiac output by thermodilution in infants and children following cardiac surgery. *Crit Care Med* 5:220, 1977.

Cook TM, McCormick B, Asai T: Randomized comparison of laryngeal tube with classic laryngeal mask airway for anaesthesia with controlled ventilation. *Br J Anaesth* 91:373, 2003.

Costarino AT, Davis DA, Keon TP: Falsely normal saturation reading with the pulse oximeter. *Anesthesiology* 67:830, 1987.

Coté CJ, Goldstein EA, Coté MA, et al.: A single-blind study of pulse oximetry in children. *Anesthesiology* 68:184, 1988.

Coté CJ, Jobes DR, Schwartz AJ, et al.: Two approaches to cannulation of a child's internal jugular vein. *Anesthesiology* 50:371, 1979.

Coté CJ, Petkau AJ, Ryan JF, et al.: Wasted ventilation measured in vitro with eight anesthetic circuits with and without inline humidification. *Anesthesiology* 59:442, 1983.

Coté CJ, Rolf N, Liu LMP, et al.: Single-blind study of combined pulse oximetry and capnography in children. *Anesthesiology* 74:980, 1991.

Cracco JB, Cracco RQ, Stolove R: Spinal evoked potentials in man: A maturational study. *Electroencephalogr Clin Neurophysiol* 46:58, 1979.

Crino MH, Nagel EL: Thermal burns caused by warming blankets in the operating room. *Anesthesiology* 29:149, 1968.

Cyna AM, MacLeod SM: The laryngeal mask: cautionary tales. *Anaesthesia* 45:167, 1990.

Daube JR, Harper CM: Surgical monitoring of cranial and peripheral nerves. In Desmedt JE, editor: *Neuromonitoring in surgery.* Amsterdam, 1989, Elsevier.

Davidson AJ, McCann M, Devavaram P, et al.: The differences in the bispectral index between infants and children during emergence from anesthesia after circumcision surgery. *Anesth Analg* 93:326, 2001.

Davis L, Cook-Sather SD, Schreiner MS: Lighted stylet tracheal intubation: A review. *Anesth Analg* 90:745, 2000.

de Blic J, Delacourt C, Scheinmann P: Ultrathin flexible bronchoscopy in neonatal intensive care units. *Arch Dis Child* 66:1383, 1991.

Degoute CS, Macabeo C, Dubreuil C, et al.: EEG bispectral index and hypnotic component of anaesthesia induced by sevoflurane: Comparison between children and adults. *Br J Anaesth* 86:209, 2001.

Denman WT, Swanson EL, Rosow D, et al.: Pediatric evaluation of the bispectral index (BIS) monitor and correlation of BIS with end-tidal sevoflurane concentration in infants and children. *Anesth Analg* 90:872, 2000.

Denny NM, Desilva KD, Webber PA: Laryngeal mask airway for emergency tracheostomy in a neonate. *Anaesthesia* 45:895, 1990.

Dormans JP, Templeton JJ, Edmonds C, et al.: Intraoperative anaphylaxis due to exposure to latex (natural rubber) in children. *J Bone Joint Surg Am* 76:1688, 1994.

Dormans JP, Templeton J, Schreiner MS, et al.: Intraoperative latex anaphylaxis in children: classification and prophylaxis of patients at risk. *J Pediatr Orthop* 17:622, 1997.

Douglas M: Urinary flow rates and urea excretion in newborn infants. *Biol Neonate* 21:321, 1972.

Downes JJ, Schreiner MS: Tracheostomy tubes and attachments in infants and children. *Int Anesthesiol Clin* 23:37, 1985.

Dubreuil M, Laffon M, Plaud B, et al.: Complications and fiberoptic assessment of size 1 laryngeal mask airway. *Anesth Analg* 76:527, 1993.

Ebata T, Nishiki S, Masuda A, et al.: Anaesthesia for Treacher Collins syndrome using a laryngeal mask airway. *Can J Anaesth* 38:1043, 1991.

Edmonds JF, Barker GA, Conn AW: Current concepts in cardiovascular monitoring in children. *Crit Care Med* 8:548, 1980.

Epstein RH, Halmi BH: Oxygen leakage around the laryngeal mask airway during laser treatment of port-wine stains in children. *Anesth Analg* 78:486, 1994.

Fan LL, Sparks LM, Dulinski JP: Applications of an ultrathin flexible bronchoscope for neonatal and pediatric airway problems. *Chest* 89:673, 1986.

Fawcett WJ, Ravilia A, Radford P: Laryngeal mask airway in children. *Can J Anaesth* 38:685, 1991.

Ferson DZ, Rosenblatt WH, Johansen MJ, et al.: Use of the intubating LMA-Fastrach in 254 patients with difficult-to-manage airways. *Anesthesiology* 95:1175, 2001.

Flagg P: Exposure and illumination of the pharynx and larynx by the general practitioner. A new laryngoscope designed to simplify the technique. *Arch Laryngol* 8:716, 1928.

Fletcher R: The relationship between the arterial to end-tidal PCO_2 difference and hemoglobin saturation in patients with congenital heart disease. *Anesthesiology* 75:210, 1991.

Flynn JT, Bancalari E, Snyder ES, et al.: Cohort study of transcutaneous oxygen tension and the incidence and severity of retinopathy of prematurity. *N Engl J Med* 326:1050, 1992.

Food and Drug Administration: Allergic reactions to latex-containing medical devices. *FDA Med Bull* 2: 1991.

Freed MD, Keane JF: Cardiac output measured by thermodilution in infants and children. *J Pediatr* 92:39, 1978.

Freye E: *Cerebral monitoring in the operating room and the intensive care unit.* Boston, 1990, Kluwer Academic Publishers.

Friesen RH, Lichtor JL: Indirect measurement of blood pressure in neonates and infants utilizing an automatic noninvasive oscillometric monitor. *Anesth Analg* 60:742, 1981.

Gan TJ, Glass PS, Windsor A, et al.: Bispectral index monitoring allows faster emergence and improved recovery from propofol, alfentanil, and nitrous oxide anesthesia. *Anesthesiology* 87:808, 1997.

Gandini D, Brimacombe J: Laryngeal mask airway for ventilatory support over a 4-day period in a neonate with Pierre Robin sequence. *Paediatr Anaesth* 13:181, 2003.

Gibbons PA, Swedlow DB: Changes in oxygen saturation during elective tracheal intubation in infants [abstract]. *Anesth Analg* 65:S58, 1986.

Gidding SS: Pulse oximetry in cyanotic congenital heart disease. *Am J Cardiol* 70:391, 1992.

Giesbrecht GG, Ducharme MB, McGuire JP: Comparison of forced-air patient warming systems for perioperative use. *Anesthesiology* 80:671, 1994.

Gilmore RL, Bass NH, Wright EA, et al.: Developmental assessment of spinal cord and cortical evoked potentials after tibial nerve stimulation: Effects of age and stature on normative data during childhood. *Electroencephalogr Clin Neurophysiol* 62:241, 1985.

Glass PS, Bloom M, Kearse L, et al.: Bispectral analysis measures sedation and memory effects of propofol, midazolam, isoflurane, and alfentanil in healthy volunteers. *Anesthesiology* 86:836, 1997.

Glauser EM, Cook CD, Bougas TP: Pressure-flow characteristics and dead spaces of endotracheal tubes used in infants. *Anesthesiology* 22:339, 1961.

Gold M, Swartz JS, Braude BM, et al.: Intraoperative anaphylaxis: An association with latex sensitivity. *J Allergy Clin Immunol* 87:662, 1991.

Goldman JM, Petterson MT, Kopotic RJ, et al.: Masimo signal extraction pulse oximetry. *J Clin Monit Comput* 16:475, 2000.

Goudsouzian NG, Denman W, Cleveland R, et al.: Radiologic localization of the laryngeal mask airway in children. *Anesthesiology* 77:1085, 1992.

Goudsouzian NG, Morris RH, Ryan JF: The effects of a warming blanket on the maintenance of body temperatures in anesthetized infants and children. *Anesthesiology* 39:351, 1973.

Graff TD, Phillips OC, Benson DW, et al.: Baltimore Anesthesia Study Committee: Factors in pediatric anesthesia mortality. *Anesth Analg* 43:407, 1964.

Graff TD, Sewall K, Lim HS, et al.: The ventilatory response of infants to airway resistance. *Anesthesiology* 27:168, 1966.

Grebenik CR, Ferguson C, White A: Laryngeal mask airway in pediatric radiotherapy. *Anesthesiology* 72:474, 1990.

Greenwald BM, Notterman DA, DeBruin WJ, et al.: Percutaneous axillary artery catheterization in critically ill infants and children. *J Pediatr* 117:442, 1990.

Grundy BL, Nash CL, Brown RH: Arterial pressure manipulation alters spinal cord function during the correction of scoliosis. *Anesthesiology* 54:249, 1981.

Guignard JP: Renal function in the newborn infant. *Pediatr Clin North Am* 29:777, 1982.

Gursoy F, Algren JT, Skjonsby BS: Positive pressure ventilation with the laryngeal mask airway in children. *Pediatr Anaesth* 82:33, 1996.

Guthkelch AN, Sclabassi RJ, Vries JK: Changes in the visual evoked potentials of hydrocephalic children. *Neurosurgery* 11:599, 1982.

Guzzi L, Jaffe M, Orr J: Clinical evaluation of a new noninvasive method of cardiac output measurement: Preliminary results in CABG patients [abstract]. *Anesthesiology* 89:A543, 2003.

Haldeman S, Bradley WE, Bhatia NN, et al.: Cortical evoked potentials on stimulation of the pudendal nerve in women. *Urology* 21:590, 1983.

Hammer G, Brodsky JB, Redpath JH, et al.: The Univent tube for single-lung ventilation in paediatric patients. *Pediatr Anaesth* 8:55, 1998.

Hammer G, Harrison TK, Vricella LA, et al.: Single lung ventilation in children using a new paediatric bronchial blocker. *Pediatr Anaesth* 12:69, 2002.

Hammer GB: Pediatric thoracic anesthesia. *Anesth Analg* 92:1449, 2001.

Hanowell L, Eisele JH Jr, Downs D: Ambient light affects pulse oximeters. *Anesthesiology* 67:864, 1987.

Hansen TG, Joensen H, Henneberg SW, et al.: Laryngeal mask airway guided tracheal intubation in a neonate with the Pierre Robin syndrome. *Acta Anaesthesiol Scand* 39:129, 1995.

Heard CMB, Caldicott LD, Fletcher JE, et al.: Fiberoptic-guided endotracheal intubation via the laryngeal mask airway in pediatric patients: A report of a series of cases. *Anesth Analg* 82:1287, 1996.

Hepner DL, Castells MC: Latex allergy: An update. *Anesth Analg* 96:1219, 2003.

Hickey S, Cameron AE, Asbury AJ: Cardiovascular response to insertion of Brain's laryngeal mask. *Anaesthesia* 45:629, 1990.

Hill JR, Rahimtulla KA: Heat balance and the metabolic rate of new-born babies in relation to environmental temperature; and the effect of age and of weight on basal metabolic rate. *J Physiol* 180:239, 1965.

Hind D, Calvert N, McWilliams R, et al.: Ultrasonic locating devices for central venous cannulation: Meta-analysis. *BMJ* 327:361, 2003.

Hindman BJ, Dexter F, Cutkomp J, et al.: Brain blood flow and metabolism do not decrease at stable brain temperature during cardiopulmonary bypass in rabbits. *Anesthesiology* 77:342, 1992.

Hodge D III, Fleisher G: Pediatric catheter flow rates. *Am J Emerg Med* 3:403, 1985.

Holzman RS: Latex allergy: An emerging operating room problem. *Anesth Analg* 76:635, 1993.

Holzman RS: Clinical management of latex-allergic children. *Anesth Analg* 85:529, 1997.

Horgan MJ, Bartoletti A, Polansky S, et al.: Effect of heparin infusates in umbilical arterial catheters on frequency of thrombotic complications. *J Pediatr* 111:774, 1987.

Hsu YH, Santulli T Jr, Wong AL, et al.: Impact of intraoperative echocardiography on surgical management of congenital heart disease. *Am J Cardiol* 67:1279, 1991.

Hubbard W: Natural rubber-containing medical devices; user labeling. *Federal Register* 62:51021, 1997.

Hunt KH: Resistance in respiratory valves and canisters. *Anesthesiology* 16:190, 1955.

Iannoli ED, Litman RS: Tension pneumothorax during flexible fiberoptic bronchoscopy in a newborn. *Anesth Analg* 94:512, 2002.

Jackson-Rees GJ: Anesthesia in the newborn. *Br Med J* 2:1419, 1950.

James AE, Macmillan AS, Momose KJ: Thornwaldt's cyst. *Br J Radiol* 41:902, 1968.

Jasper HH: Report of Committee on Methods of Clinical Examination in EEG: The Ten-Twenty System of the International Federation. *Electroenceph Clin Neurophysiol* 10:371–375, 1958.

Jennis MS, Peabody JL: Pulse oximetry: An alternative method for the assessment of oxygenation in newborn infants. *Pediatrics* 79:524, 1987.

Johnston DF, Wrigley SR, Robb PJ, et al.: Laryngeal mask airway in paediatric anaesthesia. *Anaesthesia* 45:924, 1990.

Kain ML, Nunn JF: Fresh gas flow and rebreathing in the Magill circuit with spontaneous respiration. *Proc R Soc Med* 60:749, 1967.

Kalkman CJ, ten Brink SA, Been HD, et al.: Variability of somatosensory cortical evoked potentials during spinal surgery: Effects of anesthetic technique and high-pass filtering. *Spine* 16:924, 1991.

Kamaya H, Krishna PR: New endotracheal tube (Univent tube) for selective blockade of one lung. *Anesthesiology* 63:342, 1985.

Kamura J: *Electrodiagnosis in diseases of nerve and muscle.* Philadelphia, 1983, FA Davis.

Kavanaugh-McHugh A, Tobias JD, Doyle T, et al.: Transesophageal echocardiography in pediatric congenital heart disease. *Cardiol Rev* 8:288, 2000.

Keenan RL, Boyan P: Cardiac arrest due to anesthesia—a study of incidence and causes. *JAMA* 253:2373, 1985.

Keidan I, Fine GF, Kagawa T, et al.: Work of breathing during spontaneous ventilation in anesthetized children: A comparative study among the face mask, laryngeal mask airway and endotracheal tube. *Anesth Analg* 91:1381, 2000.

Kelly K, Setlock M, Davis JP: Anaphylactic reactions during general anesthesia among pediatric patients—United States, January 1990-January 1991. *Morb Mortal Wkly Rep* 40:437, 1991.

Kihara S, Watanabe S, Taguchi N, et al.: A comparison of blind and lightwand-guided tracheal intubation through the intubating laryngeal mask. *Anaesthesia* 55:427, 2000.

Kimble KJ, Darnall RA Jr, Yelderman M, et al.: An automated oscillometric technique for estimating mean arterial pressure in critically ill newborns. *Anesthesiology* 54:423, 1981.

Klein EF Jr, Graves SA: "Hot pot" tracheitis. *Chest* 65:225, 1974.

Krucylak CP, Schreiner MS: Orotracheal intubation of an infant with hemifacial microsomia using a modified lighted stylet. *Anesthesiology* 77:826, 1992.

Kurz A, Kurz M, Poeschl G, et al.: Forced-air warming maintains intraoperative normothermia better than circulating-water mattresses. *Anesth Analg* 77:89, 1993.

Kwittken P, Becker J, Oyefara B, et al.: Latex hypersensitivity reactions despite prophylaxis. *Allergy Proc* 13:123, 1992.

Laffon M, Plaud B, Dubousset A, et al.: Removal of laryngeal mask airway, airway complications in children, anesthetized versus awake. *Paediatr Anaesth* 3:35, 1994.

Lamb K, James MF, Janicki PK: The laryngeal mask airway for intraocular surgery: Effects on intraocular pressure and stress responses. *Br J Anaesth* 69:143, 1992.

Lawless S, Orr R: Axillary arterial monitoring of pediatric patients. *Pediatrics* 84:273, 1989.

Lawrence LW, Delclos GL, Felknor SA, et al.: The effectiveness of a needleless intravenous connection system: An assessment by injury rate and user satisfaction. *Infect Control Hosp Epidemiol* 18:175, 1997.

Lee YW: *Statistical theory of communication*. New York, 1960, Wiley.

Leon JE, Bissonnette B, Lerman J: Liquid crystalline temperature monitoring: Does it estimate core temperature in anaesthetized paediatric patients? *Can J Anaesth* 37:S98, 1990.

Lesser RP, Raudzens P, Luders H, et al.: Postoperative neurological deficits may occur despite unchanged intraoperative somatosensory evoked potentials. *Ann Neurol* 19:22, 1986.

Lopez-Gil M, Brimacombe J, Alvarez M: Safety and efficacy of the laryngeal mask airway. *Anaesthesia* 51:969, 1996.

Lubbers DW: Theoretical basis of the transcutaneous blood gas measurements. *Crit Care Med* 9:721, 1981.

MacGillivray RG: Evaluation of a new tracheal tube with a movable bronchus blocker. *Anaesthesia* 43:687, 1988.

Macintosh RR: A new laryngoscope. *Lancet* 1:205, 1943.

Malviya S, Reynolds PI, Voepel-Lewis T, et al.: False alarms and sensitivity of conventional pulse oximetry versus the Masimo SET technology in the pediatric postanesthesia care unit. *Anesth Analg* 90:1336, 2000.

Mamaya B: Airway management in spontaneously breathing anaesthetized children: Comparison of the laryngeal mask airway with the cuffed oropharyngeal airway. *Paediatr Anaesth* 12:411, 2002.

Mapleson WW: The elimination of rebreathing in various semi-closed anaesthetic systems. *Br J Anaesth* 26:323, 1954.

Marjot R: Trauma to the posterior pharyngeal wall caused by a laryngeal mask airway. *Anaesthesia* 46:589, 1991.

Markakis DA, Sayson SC, Schreiner MS: Insertion of the laryngeal mask airway in awake infants with the Robin sequence. *Anesth Analg* 75:822, 1992.

Maroof M, Khan RM, Siddique MS: Intraoperative aspiration pneumonitis and the laryngeal mask airway. *Anesth Analg* 77:409, 1993.

Mason DG, Bingham RM: The laryngeal mask airway in children. *Anaesthesia* 45:760, 1990.

McCann ME, Brustowicz RM, Bacsik J, et al.: The bispectral index and explicit recall during the intraoperative wake-up test for scoliosis surgery. *Anesth Analg* 94:1474, 2002.

McGinn G, Haynes S, Morton N: An evaluation of the laryngeal mask airway during routine pediatric anesthesia. *Pediatr Anesth* 3:23, 1993.

McNicol LR: Insertion of laryngeal mask airway in children [letter]. *Anaesthesia* 46:330, 1991.

McPherson RW: General anesthetic considerations in intraoperative monitoring: Effects of anesthetic agents and neuromuscular blockade on evoked potentials, EEG and cerebral blood flow. In Loftus CM, Traynelis VC, editors: *Intraoperative monitoring techniques in neurosurgery*. New York, 1994, McGraw-Hill.

Merton PA, Morton HB: Stimulation of the cerebral cortex in the intact human subject. *Nature* 285:227, 1980.

Meyer JS, Marx PW: The pathogenesis of EEG changes during cerebral anoxia. In Van der Drift JHA, editor: *Cardiac and vascular diseases. Handbook of electroencephalography and clinical neurophysiology*. Amsterdam, 1972, Elsevier.

Miller RA: A new laryngoscope. *Anesthesiology* 2:317, 1941.

Miyasaka K, Edmonds JF, Conn AW: Complications of radial artery lines in the paediatric patient. *Can Anaesth Soc J* 23:9, 1976.

Mizushima A, Wardall GJ, Simpson DL: The laryngeal mask airway in infants. *Anaesthesia* 47:849, 1992.

Mokrohisky ST, Levine RL, Blumhagen JD, et al.: Low positioning of umbilical-artery catheters increases associated complications in newborn infants. *N Engl J Med* 299:561, 1978.

Moller JT, Johannessen NW, Espersen K, et al.: Randomized evaluation of pulse oximetry in 20,802 patients: II. Perioperative events and postoperative complications. *Anesthesiology* 78:445, 1993a.

Moller JT, Pedersen T, Rasmussen LS, et al.: Randomized evaluation of pulse oximetry in 20,802 patients: I. Design, demography, pulse oximetry failure rate, and overall complication rate. *Anesthesiology* 78:436, 1993b.

Monaco F, Nickerson BG, McQuitty JC: Continuous transcutaneous oxygen and carbon dioxide monitoring in the pediatric ICU. *Crit Care Med* 10:765, 1982.

Muhiudeen IA, Kuecherer HF, Lee E, et al.: Intraoperative estimation of cardiac output by transesophageal pulsed Doppler echocardiography. *Anesthesiology* 74:9, 1991.

Muhiudeen IA, Roberson DA, Silverman NH, et al.: Intraoperative echocardiography for evaluation of congenital heart defects in infants and children. *Anesthesiology* 76:165, 1992.

Muller N, Gulston G, Cade D, et al.: Diaphragmatic muscle fatigue in the newborn. *J Appl Physiol* 46:688, 1979.

Myles PS, Symons JA, Leslie K: Anaesthetists' attitudes towards awareness and depth-of-anaesthesia monitoring. *Anaesthesia* 58:11, 2003.

Nakayama S, Osaka Y, Yamashita M: The rotational technique with a partially inflated laryngeal mask airway improves the ease of insertion in children. *Paediatr Anaesth* 12:416, 2002.

Neal WA, Reynolds JW, Jarvis CW, et al.: Umbilical artery catheterization: Demonstration of arterial thrombosis by aortography. *Pediatrics* 50:6, 1972.

New W Jr: Pulse oximetry. *J Clin Monit* 1:126, 1985.

Niedermeyer E, Lopes da Silva F: *Electroencephalography*, 3rd ed. Baltimore, 1993, Williams & Wilkins.

Nightingale DA, Richards CC, Glass A: An evaluation of rebreathing in a modified T-piece system during controlled ventilation of anaesthetized children. *Br J Anaesth* 37:762, 1965.

Nightingale DA, Lambert TF: Carbon dioxide output in anaesthetised children. *Anaesthesia* 33:594, 1978.

Nosovitch MA, Johnson JO, Tobias JD: Noninvasive intraoperative monitoring of carbon dioxide in children: End tidal versus transcutaneous techniques. *Paediatr Anaesth* 12:48, 2002.

Notterman DA, Castello FV, Steinberg C, et al.: A comparison of thermodilution and pulsed Doppler cardiac output measurement in critically ill children. *J Pediatr* 115:554, 1989.

O'Connell AJ, Tibballs J, Coulthard M: Improving agreement between thoracic bioimpedance and dye dilution cardiac output estimation in children. *Anaesth Intensive Care* 19:434, 1991.

Olsson GL, Hallen B: Cardiac arrest during anaesthesia. A computer-aided study in 250,543 anaesthetics. *Acta Anaesthesiol Scand* 32:653, 1988.

O'Neill B, Templeton JJ, Caramico L, and Schreiner MS: The laryngeal mask airway in pediatric patients: Factors affecting ease of use during insertion and emergence. *Anesth Analg* 78:659, 1994.

Orenstein R, Reynolds L, Karabaic M, et al.: Do protective devices prevent needlestick injuries among health care workers? *Am J Infect Control* 23:344, 1995.

Park MK, Kawabori I, Guntheroth WG: Need for an improved standard for blood pressure cuff size. The size should be related to the diameter of the arm. *Clin Pediatr* 15:784, 1976.

Park MK, Robotham JL, German VF: Systolic pressure amplification in pedal arteries in children. *Crit Care Med* 11:286, 1983.

Pedersen T, Pedersen P, Moller AM: Pulse oximetry for perioperative monitoring. *Cochrane Database Syst Rev* CD002013, 2001.

Pethick SL: Letter to the editor. *Can Anaesthet Soc J* 22:115, 1975.

Phoon CK, Divekar A, Rutkowski M: Pediatric echocardiography: Applications and limitations. *Curr Probl Pediatr* 29:157, 1999.

Piotrowski A, Kawczynski P: Cannulation of the axillary artery in critically ill newborn infants. *Eur J Pediatr* 154:57, 1995.

Plumer LB, Kaplan GW, Mendoza SA: Hypertension in infants—a complication of umbilical arterial catheterization. *J Pediatr* 89:802, 1976.

Polgar G, Kong GP: The nasal resistance of newborn infants. *J Pediatr* 67:557, 1965.

Rafferty TD, Marrero O, Nardi D, et al.: Transcutaneous PO_2 as a trend indicator of arterial PO_2 in normal anesthetized adults. *Anesth Analg* 61:252, 1982.

Rashad KF, Benson DW: Role of humidity in prevention of hypothermia in infants and children. *Anesth Analg* 46:712, 1967.

Regan D: *Human brain electrophysiology: Evoked potentials and evoked magnetic fields in science and medicine*. East Norwalk, CT, 1989, Appleton & Lange.

Rendell-Baker L, Soucek DH: New pediatric face masks and anaesthetic equipment. *Br Med J* 5293:1690, 1962.

Reynolds LM, Nicolson SC, Steven JM, et al.: Influence of sensor site location on pulse oximetry kinetics in children. *Anesth Analg* 76:751, 1993.

Rich GF, Sullivan MP, Adams M: Is distal sampling of end-tidal CO_2 necessary in small subjects? *Anesthesiology* 73:265, 1990.

Ring WH, Adair JC, Elwyn RA: A new pediatric endotracheal tube. *Anesth Analg* 54:273, 1975.

Robbins L, Connelly NR: An evaluation of the cuffed oropharyngeal airway for elective pediatric anesthesia. *J Clin Anesth* 12:555, 2000.

Robertshaw FL: A new laryngoscope for infants and children. *Lancet* 2:1034, 1962.

Rose DK, Byrick RJ, Froese AB: Carbon dioxide elimination during spontaneous ventilation with a modified Mapleson D system: Studies in a lung model. *Can Anaesth Soc J* 25:353, 1978.

Rose DK, Froese AB: The regulation of $PaCO_2$ during controlled ventilation of children with a T-piece. *Can Anaesth Soc J* 26:104, 1979.

Rose RD: Role of afferent activation in cervically evoked motor responses. Proceedings of The American Society of Neurophysiological Monitoring, Chicago, May 1994.

Rosen KR, Rosen DA: Comparative flow rates for small bore peripheral intravenous catheters. *Pediatr Emerg Care* 2:153, 1986.

Rosow C, Manberg P: Bispectral index monitoring. *Anesthesiol Clin North Am* 2:89, 1998.

Roth AG, Wheeler M, Stevenson GW, et al.: Comparison of a rigid laryngoscope with the ultrathin fibreoptic laryngoscope for tracheal intubation in infants. *Can J Anaesth* 41:1069, 1994.

Rothen HU, Lauber R, Mosimann M: An evaluation of the rapid infusion system. *Anaesthesia* 47:597, 1992.

Rowbottom SJ, Simpson DL, Grubb D: Laryngeal mask airway in children—a fibreoptic assessment of positioning. *Anaesthesia* 46:489, 1991.

Rowe MI, Weinberg G, Andrews W: Reduction of neonatal heat loss by an insulated head cover. *J Pediatr Surg* 18:909, 1983.

Rowe R, Andropoulos D, Heard M, et al.: Anesthetic management of pediatric patients undergoing thoracoscopy. *J Cardiothorac Vasc Anesth* 8:563, 1994.

Salem MR, Bennett EJ, Schweiss JF, et al.: Cardiac arrest related to anesthesia. *JAMA* 233:238, 1975.

Salyer JW: Neonatal and pediatric pulse oximetry. *Respir Care* 48:386, 2003.

Salzman SK, Beckman AL, Marks HG, et al.: Effects of halothane on intraoperative scalp-recorded somatosensory-evoked potentials posterior tibial nerve stimulation in man. *Electroencephalogr Clin Neurophysiol* 65:36, 1986.

Sammartino M, Ferro G: Cuffed oropharyngeal airway: An option during paediatric ophthalmic surgery. *Paediatr Anaesth* 12:559, 2002.

Schmitt HJ, Schuetz WH, Proeschel PA, et al.: Accuracy of pulse oximetry in children with cyanotic congenital heart disease. *J Cardiothorac Vasc Anesth* 7:61, 1993.

Schreiner MS: Swivel-connector system for pediatric tracheostomy: An improvement. *Respir Care* 31:109, 1986.

Schubert A, Licina M, Lineberry PJ: The effect of ketamine on human somatosensory evoked potentials and its modification by nitrous oxide. *Anesthesiology* 72:33, 1990.

Schwartz AJ, Downes JJ: Hazards of a simple monitoring device, the esophageal stethoscope. *Anesthesiology* 47:64, 1977.

Sclabassi RJ, Kalia K, Sekhar L, et al.: Assessing brainstem function. In Haines SJ, Heros RC, editors: *Surgery of the brainstem. Neurosurg Clin North Am* 4:3, 415, 1993.

Seibert JJ, Taylor BJ, Williamson SL, et al.: Sonographic detection of neonatal umbilical-artery thrombosis: Clinical correlation. *AJR Am J Roentgenol* 148:965, 1987.

Sessler DI, McGuire J, Sessler AM: Perioperative thermal insulation. *Anesthesiology* 74:875, 1991.

Sessler DI, Moayeri A: Skin-surface warming: Heat flux and central temperature. *Anesthesiology* 73:218, 1990.

Severinghaus JW, Naifeh KH: Accuracy of response of six pulse oximeters to profound hypoxia. *Anesthesiology* 67:551, 1987.

Shulman B, Connelly NR: The adult Bullard laryngoscope as an alternative to the Wis-Hipple 1(1/2) in paediatric patients. *Paediatr Anaesth* 10:41, 2000.

Shulman GB, Connelly NR, Gibson C: The adult Bullard laryngoscope in paediatric patients. *Can J Anaesth* 44:969, 1997.

Sidi A, Rush W, Gravenstein N, et al.: Pulse oximetry fails to accurately detect low levels of arterial hemoglobin oxygen saturation in dogs. *J Clin Monit* 3:257, 1987.

Simpson J, Stephenson T: Regulation of extracellular fluid volume in neonates. *Early Hum Dev* 34:179, 1993.

Slater JE, Mostello LA, Shaer C, et al.: Type I hypersensitivity to rubber. *Ann Allergy* 65:411, 1990.

Spahr-Schopfer IA, Bissonnette B, et al.: Capnometry and the paediatric laryngeal mask airway. *Can J Anaesth* 40:1038, 1993.

Spoerel WE, Aitken RR, Bain JA: Spontaneous respiration with the Bain breathing circuit. *Can Anaesth Soc J* 25:30, 1978.

Standard Specification for Particular Requirements for Anesthesia Workstations and their Components. ASTM, West Conshohocken, PA.

Starr A, Amlie RN, Martin WH, et al.: Development of auditory function in newborn infants revealed by auditory brainstem potentials. *Pediatrics* 60:831, 1977.

Stayer SA, Bent ST, Campos CJ, et al.: Comparison of NAD 6000 and servo 900C ventilators in an infant lung model. *Anesth Analg* 90:315, 2000.

Stocks RM, Egerman R, Thompson JW, et al.: Airway management of the severely retrognathic child: Use of the laryngeal mask airway. *Ear Nose Throat J* 81:223, 2002.

Strauss J, Daniel SS, James LS: Postnatal adjustment in renal function. *Pediatrics* 68:802, 1981.

Subcommittee F29.18 on Operating Room Fire Safety: Standard specification for labeling and marking of cuffed and uncuffed tracheal tubes and related treatments intended for use during laser surgery. In ASTM Committee F29 on Anesthesia and Respiratory Equipment, editor: *Annual book of ASTM standards.* West Conshohocken, PA, 1995, ASTM International.

Swedlow DB: Capnometry and capnography, the anesthesia disaster early warning system. *Semin Anesth* 5:194, 1986.

Symansky MR, Fox HA: Umbilical vessel catheterization: Indications, management, and evaluation of the technique. *J Pediatr* 80:820, 1972.

Tabbutt S, Ramamoorthy C, Montenegro LM, et al.: Impact of inspired gas mixtures on preoperative infants with hypoplastic left heart syndrome during controlled ventilation. *Circulation* 104(Suppl II):I-159–I-164, 2001.

Tait AR, Pandit UA, Voepel-Lewis T, et al.: Use of the laryngeal mask airway in children with upper respiratory tract infections: A comparison with endotracheal intubation. *Anesth Analg* 86:706, 1998.

Taniguchi M, Nadstawek J, Pechstein U, et al.: Total intravenous anesthesia for improvement of intraoperative monitoring of somatosensory evoked potentials during aneurysm surgery. *Neurosurgery* 31:89, 1992.

Taylor MJ: Evoked potentials in paediatrics. In Halliday AM, editor: *Evoked potentials in clinical testing.* Edinburgh, 1993, Churchill Livingstone.

Tibby SM, Murdoch IA: Measurement of cardiac output and tissue perfusion. *Curr Opin Pediatr* 14:303, 2002.

Tiret L, Nivoche Y, Hatton F, et al.: Complications related to anaesthesia in infants and children. A prospective survey of 40,240 anaesthetics. *Br J Anaesth* 61:263, 1988.

Tobias JD: Anaesthetic implications of thoracoscopic surgery in children. *Paediatr Anaesth* 9:103, 1999.

Todres ID, Crone RK: Experience with a modified laryngoscope in sick infants. *Crit Care Med* 9:544, 1981.

Truell KD, Bakerman PR, Teodori MF, et al.: Third-degree burns due to intraoperative use of a Bair Hugger warming device. *Ann Thorac Surg* 69:1933, 2000.

Umbilical Artery Catheter Trial Study Group: Relationship of intraventricular hemorrhage or death with the level of umbilical artery catheter placement: A multicenter randomized clinical trial. *Pediatrics* 90:881, 1992.

Van der Drift JHA: The EEG in cerebrovascular disease. In Vinken PJ and Bruyn GW, editors: *Handbook of clinical neurology.* Amsterdam, 1972, Elsevier.

van Heerden PV, Kirrage D: Large tonsils and the laryngeal mask airway. *Anaesthesia* 44:703, 1989.

Verghese ST, Nath A, Zenger D, et al.: The effects of the simulated Valsalva maneuver, liver compression, and/or Trendelenburg position on the cross-sectional area of the internal jugular vein in infants and young children. *Anesth Analg* 94:250, 2002.

Watcha MF, Connor MT, Hing AV: Pulse oximetry in methemoglobinemia. *Am J Dis Child* 143:845, 1989.

Watcha MF, Garner FT, White PF, et al.: Laryngeal mask airway vs face mask and Guedel airway during pediatric myringotomy. *Arch Otolaryngol Head Neck Surg* 120:877, 1994.

Watcha MF, White PF, Tychsen L, et al.: Comparative effects of laryngeal mask airway and endotracheal tube insertion on intraocular pressure in children. *Anesth Analg* 75:355–360, 1992.

Watcha MF: Investigations of the bispectral index monitor in pediatric anesthesia: First things first. *Anesth Analg* 92:805, 2001.

Waters DJ, Mapleson WW: Rebreathing during controlled respiration with various semiclosed anesthetic systems. *Br J Anaesth* 33:374, 1961.

Watt RC, Loeb RG, Orr J: Comparison of a new noninvasive cardiac output technique with invasive bolus and continuous thermodilution [abstract]. *Anesthesiology* 89:A536, 2004.

Webster AC, Morley-Forster PK, Dain S, et al.: Anaesthesia for adenotonsillectomy: A comparison between tracheal intubation and armoured laryngeal mask airway. *Can J Anaesth* 40:1171, 1993.

Wetmore RF, Marsh RR, Thompson ME, et al.: Pediatric tracheostomy: A changing procedure? *Ann Otol Rhinol Laryngol* 108:695, 1999.

Wilkes AR, Benbough JE, Speight SE, et al.: The bacterial and viral filtration performance of breathing system filters. *Anaesthesia* 55:458, 2000.

Wilkins CJ, Cramp PGW, Staples J, et al.: Comparison of the anesthetic requirement for tolerance of laryngeal mask airway and endotracheal tube. *Anesth Analg* 75:794, 1992.

Wilkinson PA: The larygeal mask: cautionary tales. *Anaesthesia* 45:167, 1990.

Williams PJ, Bailey PM: Comparison of the reinforced laryngeal mask airway and tracheal intubation for adenotonsillectomy. *Br J Anaesth* 70:30, 1993.

Wilson IG, Fell D, Robinson SL, et al.: Cardiovascular responses to insertion of the laryngeal mask. *Anaesthesia* 47:300, 1992.

Yakovlev PI, Lecours AR: The myelogenetic cycles of regional maturation in the brain. In Minkowski A, editor: *Regional development of the brain in early life.* Oxford, 1967, Blackwell.

10 Induction of Anesthesia and Maintenance of the Airway in Infants and Children

Etsuro K. Motoyama • Brian J. Gronert • Gavin F. Fine

INDUCTION OF GENERAL ANESTHESIA

The induction of anesthesia is the most crucial and stressful period of general anesthesia for the young patient as well as for the anesthesiologist. The consequences of this stressful experience by a child become apparent in the immediate postanesthetic period and may persist for weeks or even longer (Kain and Mayers, 1996; Kotiniemi et al., 1997; Kain et al., 1999; McCann and Kain, 2001). Regrettably, anesthesia is often induced with too little consideration for the child's anxiety, despite better awareness by anesthesiologists of preoperative stress experienced by the young patient and improved psychological preparations since the 1980s (see Chapter 7, Psychological Aspects). This discrepancy continues in part because the anesthesiologist is preoccupied with the technical aspects of anesthetic induction and is naturally focused on the maintenance of cardiorespiratory stability, particularly when dealing with a poor-risk child, and pays too little attention to the child's psychological needs. In addition, in the era of managed care in the United States and elsewhere and with the economical pressure for efficiency and quick turnover between surgical cases, it has become increasingly difficult for the pediatric anesthesiologist to spend sufficient time with young patients and his or her parents preoperatively to get to know each other and earn the child's confidence. No matter how healthy the child or how minor the procedure, the experience of being placed on an operating table and forcefully put to sleep (a.k.a. "gorilla induction" or "brutaine") can be a terrifying and never-to-be-forgotten horror. Consequently, children who must return for repeated anesthesia and surgery could be emotionally disturbed (Dombro, 1970), although the adverse effects of the anesthetic experience are not easy to separate from the overall effects of hospitalization (Myers and Muravchick, 1977). It is the responsibility of the pediatric anesthesiologist to understand the emotional needs of young patients and to provide the optimal psychological preparation before and during the induction of anesthesia.

PSYCHOLOGICAL CONSIDERATION

The psychological environment for hospitalized children has improved substantially since the 1980s, with organized preoperative hospital tours, audiovisual programs, and playrooms with trained child life specialists, who are trained to facilitate the child's coping with the perioperative environment and stress by providing play experiences using modeling techniques, particularly in the preoperative waiting area (Melamed and Ridley-Johnson, 1988; Melamed, 1993). By the mid-1990s most major children's hospitals in the United States had developed the child life program for children and their parents (O'Bryrne et al., 1997). Unfortunately, while effective preparation programs to reduce the child's anxiety in the preoperative holding area are well established, progress in the effectiveness of reducing anxiety during the process of anesthetic induction has been limited (Kain et al., 1996, 1998).

Stress and anxiety manifested in children before and during anesthetic induction result from the interaction between the child's personal predisposition (age, maturity, personality, and his or her past experiences in the hospital environment) and the environmental factors (unfamiliar environment, exposure to many strangers, the noise level, intensity of lights in the operating room, etc.). The child may look scared (e.g., clinging to his or her mother), may try to ignore or escape from the anesthesiologist, or may start to cry. During the preoperative examination, it is extremely important to identify the child who is likely to develop extreme fear and anxiety before the induction of anesthesia (see Chapter 7, Psychological Aspects). Premedication with sedatives has been shown to be most effective, especially for those who are at high risk of developing extreme anxiety and distress, although some parents are reluctant to allow or even refuse premeditation altogether, against the anesthesiologist's advice.

MEDICAL CONSIDERATIONS

Infants and children with preexisting medical conditions should be carefully examined, and, when a decision is made to go ahead with induction with known medical problems, appropriate measures, including medications, should be taken before or shortly after anesthetic induction. This issue has been detailed elsewhere (Chapter 8, Preoperative Preparation; Chapter 27, Anesthesia for Same-Day Procedures; and Chapter 32, Systemic Disorders). Some basic preparations before anesthetic induction are listed next.

Upper Respiratory Tract Infections

Upper respiratory tract infection (URI) is by far the most common problem the pediatric anesthesiologist has to deal with before the induction of anesthesia, especially in the same-day surgery setting. Although a recent history or the presence of URI per se may not necessarily increase the risk of long-term outcome beyond the immediate postoperative period, URI or lower respiratory tract infection and inflammation does increase the irritability and secretion of the respiratory tract and may increase the incidence of laryngospasm, bronchospasm, and perioperative hypoxemia (DeSoto et al., 1988; Cohen and Cameron, 1991; Coté, 2001; Bordet et al., 2002; Elwood et al., 2003). Risk factors for respiratory complications include endotracheal intubation, history of prematurity (even in older children), reactive airway disease and passive smoking, nasal congestion and copious secretions, and airway surgery (Tait et al., 2001).

It is also important to note that with viral lower respiratory infection clinically limited to upper airway symptoms, airway reactivity and hyperresponsiveness indistinguishable from bronchial asthma often develop, even in patients without a history of asthma (de Kluijver et al., 2002). Increased airway reactivity with viral respiratory infection lasts as long as 6 to 8 weeks (Empey et al., 1976). Special consideration should be made to provide a warmed humidified gas mixture during the induction and maintenance of anesthesia, because anesthetic dry gas mixture irritates already inflamed upper airways and may trigger coughs, laryngospasm, or bronchospasm. Prophylactic bronchodilator treatment should be given, as indicated, before the induction of anesthesia and/or before the emergence from anesthesia and extubation.

For children with a history of reactive airway disease, one has to make sure that each patient has received optimal treatment before reaching the operating room. Careful history taking is the single most important element of the preoperative evaluation of children with reactive airway disease. If a child has had symptoms of URI with episodes of wheezing requiring bronchodilator treatment in the previous weeks, the anesthesiologist should consider postponing elective surgery for at least 4 to 6 weeks after an episode of symptomatic asthma, although this is often not practical. The history of the child's steroid requirement over the past several months is important for determining if he or she should be given stress-dose steroid coverage (see Chapter 32, Systemic Disorders).

For patients with recent episodes of wheezing and bronchodilator treatment but requiring surgery, preinduction treatment with a β_2-agonist with or without corticosteroids is recommended to minimize respiratory complications, especially laryngospasm and bronchospasm. A study in adult patients with reactive airway disease showed significant decreases in bronchospasm after tracheal intubation (Silvanus et al., 2004).

The patient's history, physical examination, and laboratory tests are all helpful for determining if the patient's condition is adequately managed. A child with active wheezing at a preoperative physical examination, especially wheezing with symptoms of upper or lower respiratory infection, should not be operated on unless it is a dire emergency (see Chapter 32, Systemic Disorders).

Children With Congenital Heart Disease

Many children with congenital heart lesions will require antibiotic prophylaxis preoperatively for the prevention of bacterial endocarditis. Recommendations by the American Heart Association (AHA) are listed in the inside cover of this publication (Dajani et al., 1997). The recommendations can also be downloaded from the AHA website at http://www.americanheart.org. The consensus statement for the AHA subacute bacterial endocarditis (SEB) prophylaxis has been formulated by the writing group within AHA and has been reviewed by outside experts. It consists of five tables that are periodically updated:

- Table 1: Cardiac conditions associated with endocarditis
- Table 2: Dental procedures and endocarditis prophylaxis
- Table 3: Other procedures and endocarditis prophylaxis
- Table 4: Prophylactic regimens for dental, oral, respiratory tract, or esophageal procedures
- Table 5: Prophylactic regimens for genitourinary/gastrointestinal (excluding esophageal) procedures

Amoxicillin, 50 mg/kg (with an addition of gentamicin, 1.5 mg/kg for genitourinary or gastrointestinal procedures), given intravenously or intramuscularly 30 minutes before the procedure, has been the standard prophylaxis. Alternative antibiotics for those who are allergic to penicillin are also listed (clindamycin, cephalexin, azithromycin, vancomycin, etc.).

For optimal effect, the intravenous antibiotics should be administered 30 minutes prior to the start of the surgical or endoscopic procedures. This procedure, however, can be problematic for infants and young children without an access to an intravenous route preoperatively, especially in same-day surgery settings. In case the preoperative establishment of intravenous access under sedation is not practical for any reason, it is often the practice in many centers to start the infusion of antibiotics during or right after inhalation induction of general anesthesia and intravenous access is established. The patient may be positioned and prepared for surgery, but the skin incision should be delayed at least for 20 minutes after the infusion of an antibiotic. In case preoperative antimicrobial prophylaxis was missed for any reason, an animal study indicates that the prophylaxis given within 2 hours (but not after 4 hours) following the procedure will still provide effective prophylaxis (Dajani et al.,

1997; Berney and Francioli, 1990), although, for obvious reasons, no clinical studies have confirmed this finding.

Latex Allergy

Since the first report of intraoperative anaphylactic reaction due to latex allergy in the anesthesiology literature in 1989 (Gerber et al., 1989), latex allergy has increased at an alarming pace in the latter part of the twentieth century (Murat, 2000) and is detailed elsewhere in this publication (Chapter 32, Systemic Disorders). Allergy to latex is the main cause of intraoperative anaphylaxis in children, whereas in adults, allergy to muscle relaxants is the main cause (Murat, 1993). Children with congenital urogenital abnormalities, myelomeningocele, and hydrocephalus with ventriculoperitoneal shunts are among the high-risk groups (Dormans et al., 1994, 1997). Repeated exposure to latex-containing products in the neonatal period and early childhood is the apparent cause of the development of a latex allergy. High-risk groups of children have been well defined (Kwittken et al., 1995; Porri et al., 1997; Cremer et al., 1998). Fortunately, over the past decade, latex-containing products, including adhesive tapes, blood pressure cuffs, tourniquets, and surgical gloves, have largely been replaced by latex-free products in the United States and other industrialized countries. It has become much simpler to provide a latex-free environment for children with high risks during the early postnatal years. Anesthesiologists should remain vigilant, however, to protect their patients from inadvertent exposures to latex, especially with latex gloves used by the surgeons. The U.S. Food and Drug Administration (1991) recommended that all patients should be questioned preoperatively for latex hypersensitivity.

PREOPERATIVE FASTING

The purpose of preoperative fasting is to allow sufficient time for gastric emptying of ingested food and liquid and, thus, to minimize the risk of aspiration of gastric contents into the lungs during anesthesia. For the preparation of infants and children for general anesthesia and surgery, it is extremely important to properly instruct the family in regard to preoperative food and fluid intake.

To decrease the incidence of aspiration, it was routine practice prior to the 1990s to keep all children NPO after midnight before surgery. This practice ignored both the differences in the rate of gastric emptying between ingested solid food and clear liquids and the differences in the scheduled times of surgery (Welborn, 1993). A number of studies in the 1990s demonstrated that clear liquids with or without added sugar are rapidly cleared from the stomach and that the gastric fluid pH and volume are independent of the duration of fasting beyond 2 hours, provided that only clear liquids are given on the day of surgery (Schreiner, 1990; Splinter and Schaefer, 1990; Litman et al., 1994). The liberalization of guidelines for preoperative fluid administration in the 1990s offers the benefit of improved patient comfort. It also means that fewer infants and children demonstrate signs of hypoglycemia or dehydration at the time of anesthetic induction (Welborn et al., 1993). Over the last decade, most pediatric hospitals have altered and shortened the fasting period of clear liquids to 2 hours prior to induction of anesthesia for all ages (Ferrari et al., 1999).

In 1999, Ferrari and coworkers reported the results of a survey of current practice of preoperative fasting in pediatric institutions in the United State and Canada. Of 51 institutions surveyed, 44 responded. The survey revealed that a "2-4-6-8 rule" represents the majority of institutions providing pediatric care in North America (Ferrari et al., 1999). This rule restricts clear fluids for 2 hours. Infants less than 6 months of age on breast milk require 4 hours of fasting. Older infants over 6 months of age on milk or infant formula should be fasted for 6 hours; milk or infant formula should be considered as solid food because the fat is the main determinant delaying gastric emptying (Litman et al., 1994). Children on solid food, including toast, cereal, and juice with pulp, such as orange juice, are usually fasted for 8 hours (or NPO after midnight) prior to induction of anesthesia.

PREMEDICATION

The use of premedication is most effective for reducing preoperative anxiety for young patients and their parents. Preanesthetic medication is described in detail in Chapter 8 (Preoperative Preparation) and is discussed only briefly here. There has been progress in the effectiveness of premedication and preoperative sedation during the past 10 years. With the advent of newer anesthetic agents, especially sevoflurane for inhalation induction, the nature of premedication has also evolved. With less secretions and fewer cardiorespiratory side effects with sevoflurane compared with halothane, anticholinergic agents (atropine, glycopyrrolate) are rarely required before induction, perhaps with the exception of neonates and preterm infants. Furthermore, with few exceptions (such as intramuscular ketamine in agitated, uncontrollable children), intramuscular premedication is all but eliminated from routine pediatric anesthesia practice.

Hypnotics

The most common drug for premedication has been midazolam, a water-soluble benzodiazepine, in fruit-flavored syrup to mask its bitter taste (0.3 to 0.5 mg/kg given orally). It is effective within 10 to 15 minutes (Kain et al., 2000). Even lesser doses of oral midazolam (0.25 mg/kg) have been reported to be effective, although it may take slightly longer than the larger dose to produce effective sedation (Coté et al., 2002). Midazolam has also been used less frequently via the nasal (0.2 to 0.3 mg/kg) or rectal (0.3 mg/kg) routes but with their own disadvantages. In 10 to 15 minutes of oral medication administration, most children become calm, euphoric, or drowsy and are unsteady walking, and they must be held carefully or placed in bed. There is minimal separation anxiety when taken away from parents toward the induction area. Prolonged recovery time with midazolam premedication had been a concern, especially for infants and children for same-day surgery, but the time of discharge from the hospital is not increased (Bevan et al., 1997, Viitanen et al., 1999).

Opioids

Opioid premedication is infrequently used in healthy children because of potential respiratory depression, especially in young infants less than 6 months of age. Oral transmucosal fentanyl citrate (OTFC) has the advantage of self-titration and has a relatively rapid onset without increases in gastric pH (Nelson et al., 1989; Stanley et al., 1989). However, it causes more preoperative and postoperative side effects such as pruritus, vomiting, and hypoxemia (Goldstein-Dresner et al., 1991; Ashburn et al., 1990, 1993) (see Chapter 8, Preoperative Preparation).

Ketamine

Intramuscular injection of ketamine in a relatively low dose (2 to 3 mg/kg, undiluted) is effective in uncooperative, combatant children as the last resort to avoid inhalation induction by force or for the insertion of an intravenous catheter. Ketamine may be combined with glycopyrrolate to reduce secretions. Hannallah and Patel (1989) reported that inhalation induction with halothane in uncooperative children with intramuscular ketamine took even less time than induction with cooperative children without premedication. Ketamine has also been given via the oral, nasal transmucosal, or rectal routes. Ketamine solution (6 mg/kg) diluted with fruit-flavored syrup and given orally produced effective sedation in 12 minutes (Stewart et al., 1990; Gutstein et al., 1992). Ketamine mixed with midazolam was reported to produce a better anxiolysis than either drug alone (Funk et al., 2000). Nasal transmucosal ketamine has also produced effective sedation (Weksler et al., 1993).

Clonidine

An α_2-adrenergic receptor agonist, clonidine has been shown to produce perioperative sedation and reduce the anesthetic requirement and postoperative analgesia (Ghinone et al., 1987). Clonidine has been used for premedication in children over the past decade, although it is most frequently used as an adjunct to caudal and epidural blocks ((Mikawa et al., 1993; Nishina and Mikawa, 2002). Oral clonidine (4 mcg/kg) provides satisfactory anxiolysis and sedation (Nishina et al., 1999). A study compared the efficacy of premedication between clonidine (4 mcg/kg orally, given 60 minutes before induction) and midazolam (0.4 mg/kg rectally, given 30 minutes before induction) by means of clinical observation, and bispectral index (BIS). During rapid sevoflurane induction (8% in 50% N_2O in O_2), both agitation requiring restraint and hemodynamic responses were significantly less and shorter in duration with clonidine premedication than with midazolam premedication (Constant et al., 2004). A major limitation of oral clonidine as a premedicant, especially in the same-day surgery setting, is that it must be given at least 60 minutes prior to induction.

A mail survey of randomly selected practicing anesthesiologists in the United States in 2002 (27% response, n = 1362) showed that a significantly larger proportion of young children undergoing surgery were reported to receive sedative premedication compared with a previous survey in 1995 (50% versus 30%, $P = 0.001$) and that midazolam was the predominant, if not exclusive, sedative for premedication (Kain et al., 2004).

PREANESTHETIC PREPARATIONS

It is essential for the anesthesiologist to try to gain the patient's confidence in the preoperative waiting area, especially when the child is not properly premedicated. Dressed in a strange operating room outfit and standing tall over the frightened child is not the way to initiate contact with a young patient. The anesthesiologist should sit close to the child or even down on the floor to be at the child's eye level before starting communication with the child. If a line of communication has been found through a child's toy, pet, or favorite television program, then focusing attention on this may help to gain the child's confidence and divert or reduce fear and anxiety. The game of "peek-a-boo" in infants and young children may calm them and even bring a smile to their faces. Infants less than 6 months of age may be less subject to anxiety and need gentle handling and a reassuring voice long before words can be understood. During the brief stay in the preanesthetic waiting area, a child is encouraged to be engaged in play, with a toy or a video game with or without the presence of parents (Fig. 10–1*A*); an infant can also be held in arms for comfort (Fig. 10–1*B*).

Most unpremedicated children can be well managed in this friendly environment. The anesthesia mask may be given to the child to play with in the waiting area before induction. Provide a sense of self-control by letting the child choose his or her favorite flavor (bubble gum, cherry, strawberry, etc.) to be added to the mask. The additional support of pacifiers, toys, and music

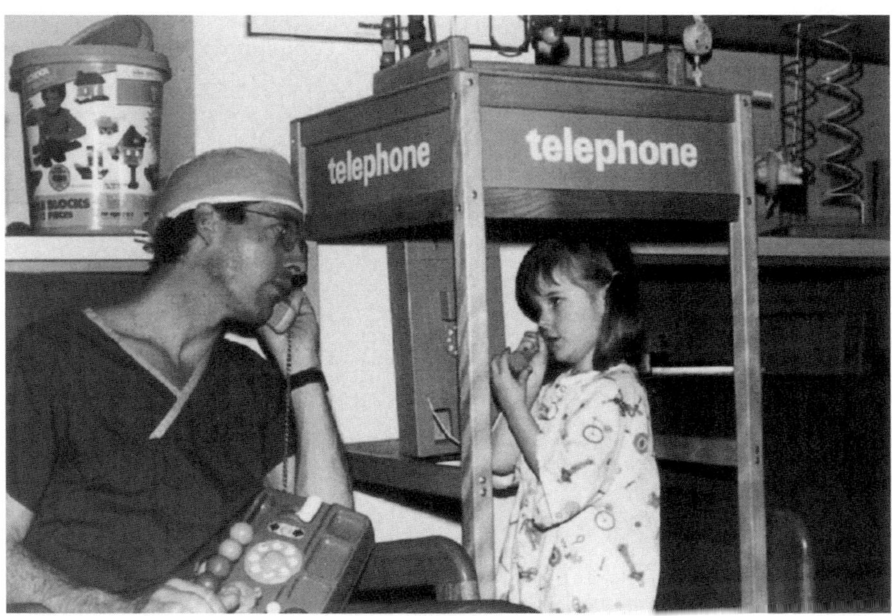

A

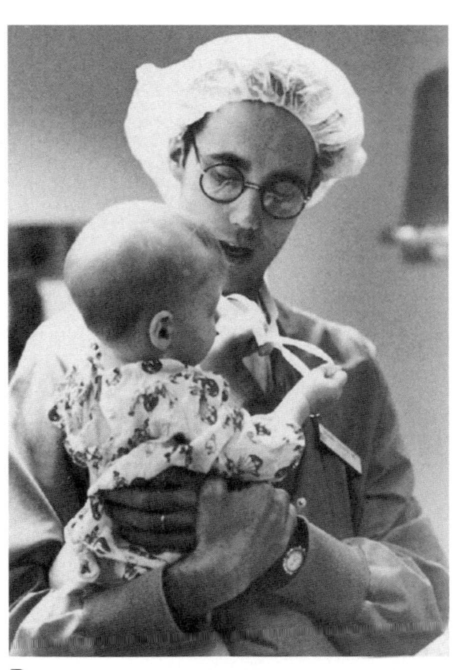

B

■ **FIGURE 10–1.** The preoperative waiting (play) area provides a last opportunity for the anesthesiologist to improve his or her communication with the child in a relaxed atmosphere. (Photograph by Frank A. Leavens, Pittsburgh, PA.)

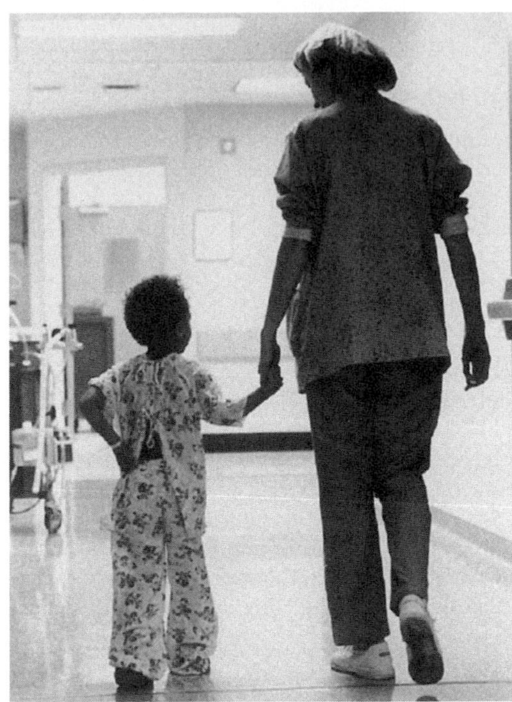

■ **FIGURE 10–2.** Some children prefer to walk from the play area to the operating room with the anesthesiologist. (Photograph by Frank A. Leavens, Pittsburgh, PA.)

boxes often is helpful. Children should keep the object of their choice brought from home, particularly a "security blanket," during the induction of anesthesia. The short trip from waiting area to operating or induction room can be extremely important. The child is moved back onto a stretcher from the play area and wheeled to the operating room, or held in the arms of the anesthesiologist, taking the security blanket and/or best-loved toys with him or her. Some older unpremedicated children prefer to walk along with the anesthesiologist (Fig. 10–2). If the child proves actively resistant at this stage, he or she may be convinced by a parental presence at induction (see later), but if this also fails, then further sedation may be administered.

Sedation at this point can be in the form of intranasal midazolam, 0.2 to 0.3 mg/kg, undiluted (5 mg/mL) to minimize the volume (Wilton et al., 1988). Mixing with 1% to 2% lidocaine decreases the stinging discomfort to the nasal mucosa. For a larger combative child, intramuscular ketamine (2 to 3 mg/kg) can be used effectively as the last resort (see earlier). In the case of an older resistant child for an elective procedure, consideration should also be given to postponing the procedure until the child is properly prepared. One is rarely justified in bringing a screaming and resisting child into an operating room.

Parental Presence During Induction

A parental presence is desirable because it may reduce the need for preoperative sedatives and decrease the level of preoperative anxiety, especially upon separation to the operating room (Berry, 1986) (see Chapter 7, Psychological Aspects). A parental presence results in a significant decrease in the number of very upset children during induction in unpremedicated children (Hannallah and Rosales, 1983). The disadvantages of a parental presence in the operating room include delays in the operative schedule, crowding of limited operating room space, and possible adverse effects on the parent during the induction process, especially if something goes wrong during induction.

If a separate induction room equipped with all the essential monitors and an anesthesia machine is not available, a parent, masked and gowned, may be allowed to enter the operating room and sit on a stool right next to the operating table, holding the child's hands during the induction. The induction process should be explained in layman's terms to the parent and he or she should be prewarned of possible excitement and upper airway obstruction ("loud snoring") as part of a possible occurrence during induction. And the parents should be assured that they need not be concerned. The parent should be escorted out of the operating room by an operating room nurse as soon as the child loses consciousness.

In a 2002 national survey via mail with questionnaires sent to randomly selected anesthesiologists in the United States, Kain and others (2004) found that the practice of having a parental presence during induction of anesthesia (PPIA) has increased significantly, compared with a similar survey in 1995, and that regional differences in this practice have decreased. Overall, 10% of respondents allow parental presence during induction in more than 75% of the time, whereas 27% reported PPIA in less than 25% of all cases. Approximately 50% of all respondents never allowed parental presence during induction of anesthesia when anesthetizing children (Kain et al., 2004). The frequency of practicing PPIA in the United States, however, remains far less than that in the United Kingdom.

Preparation for Induction

Before the induction of anesthesia, the temperature of the operating room should be properly adjusted and warming devices (warming blanket, radiant heat lamp) should be turned on, particularly for young infants (Box 10–1). The anesthetic and monitoring equipment must be properly set up and ready before the child enters the room. The preinduction checklist should include gas pressures of accessory oxygen and nitrous oxide cylinders, gas tightness of the anesthesia circuit, and the necessary small equipment and supplies. These include a properly sized face mask, oral and nasal airways, a tongue depressor, three sizes of endotracheal tubes (the expected size plus one size larger and one size smaller), and a stylet; all must be available regardless of whether endotracheal intubation is planned. A laryngeal mask airway (LMA) appropriate for the patient's age should also be available if it is to be used. A suction apparatus with a Yankauer tonsil suction tip or a 14F oral suction catheter must be turned on, and additional sterile endotracheal suction catheters (6F to 10F, depending on the patient's age) and nasogastric tubes (10F to 18F) must be available. Adhesive tape, torn and ready for use, and a padded or foam rubber head ring or a small pillow should also be at hand.

Monitoring devices such as an in-flow oxygen analyzer, an automatic blood pressure measuring apparatus, an electrocardiograph (ECG), a pulse oximeter, an anesthetic gas monitor, and capnographic equipment should be turned on. In addition to intravenous drugs that are to be used in anesthetic management, atropine and succinylcholine should always be drawn into syringes and clearly labeled just in case of severe laryngospasm.

Monitoring During Induction

Because vital signs can vary markedly during the induction of anesthesia, it is important to attach a basic monitoring device to the patient before induction. Most children will accept a

BOX 10–1 Preanesthetic Preparation

Operating Room Preparation

Warm operating room
Turn on warming devices (e.g., warming blanket, intravenous line warmer, radiant light heat source)

Anesthesia Equipment

Anesthesia machine checkout
Monitoring equipment (pulse oximeter, capnograph, anesthetic gas monitor) turned on and checked
Precordial stethoscope with double-stick adhesive
Proper-size blood pressure cuff, pulse oximeter probe, temperature probe
Proper-size facemask
Oral and nasal airways
Tongue depressor
Laryngeal mask airway (LMA) if planned
Laryngoscope handle and at least two blades
Three sizes of endotracheal tubes
Stylet
Suction turned on with Yankauer suction tip or suction catheter
Adhesive tape torn and ready for use
Intravenous fluid bag connected to appropriate tubings and injection ports
Intravenous catheters

Drugs

Intravenous drugs drawn up

- Propofal and/or thiopental
- Atropine, succinylcholine, nondepolarizing muscle relaxant
- Reversal drugs (neostigmine, edrophonium, glycopyrrolate)
- Opioids (morphine, fentanyl, or remifentanil on infusion pump)

precordial stethoscope when it is warmed properly and quietly applied, and a pulse oximeter probe on a fingertip or a toe. If the child is anxious, it is unwise to further upset him or her by placing ECG leads and a blood pressure cuff before induction. They can be applied soon after the patient loses consciousness. On the other hand, particularly in a small and sick infant, it is important to place all of the monitors before induction and to obtain a baseline blood pressure measurement, which may be unexpectedly low. After the induction, the same blood pressure could be mistaken as a sign of anesthesia-induced hypotension and trigger unnecessary treatment such as fluid resuscitation or vasoactive drugs. Monitoring the child continuously with a pulse oximeter and capnograph is extremely important and is part of the American Society of Anesthesiologists (ASA) monitoring standards for patient safety (1986).

METHODS OF INDUCTION

There are a number of techniques for safely inducing general anesthesia in children. The particular technique chosen varies with the age of the child, underlying illness, surgical procedure, and the skill and preference of the anesthesiologist. The induction techniques vary from inhalational, intravenous, and intramuscular, to rectal administration of anesthetics, although the latter is rarely used today.

Inhalation Induction

Inhalation induction by mask is the most commonly used technique in pediatric anesthesia in the United States because it can be achieved relatively easily and rapidly in most children and is less objectionable to most children than the insertion of an intravenous catheter. The pediatric anesthesiologist must be flexible and able to suit the child's need by varying his or her method of induction.

If a child has dozed off while awaiting induction or is well sedated with premedication, anesthesia can be induced by the "steal technique," with the child on the stretcher as originally described by Guedel in 1921 (Calverley, 1986). This can be achieved by blowing a high flow of 70% nitrous oxide in oxygen into the anesthesia mask while it is held closely over the face, without touching the skin at first, and then placed gently on the face for a few minutes while increasing the concentration of sevoflurane up to 2 MAC (minimum anesthetic concentration) before the child is moved to the operating table. Minimal monitoring is used to avoid awakening the child, but adequate monitoring must be established as soon as the patient is sufficiently asleep to tolerate this without causing excitement phase reflexes. Monitoring devices, particularly a precordial stethoscope and a pulse oximeter probe, should be attached as soon as possible before transferring the child to the operating table.

Once in the operating room, the average child is cooperative but may be frightened by noisy personnel and strange sights. The conversation and communication between the child and the anesthesiologist should not be interrupted throughout the transition from the preanesthetic holding area through the transport and onto the operating table. The child needs repeated reassurance that he or she is doing fine and that no one is going to hurt him or her. An assistant (an operating room nurse, nurse anesthetist, attending anesthesiologist, etc.) should help position the child on the operating table and stand by. It is usually best if the anesthesiologist alone does the talking; and the talking should be continual. Surgeons and nurses are reminded to be quiet immediately before and during the induction or are asked to stay out of the operating room if they need to carry on a conversation.

The procedure should be smooth and continuous and unbroken by the last-minute preparation of equipment. The two most important pieces of monitoring equipment during an inhalation induction are a precordial stethoscope and a pulse oximeter. The stethoscope should be positioned over the left sternal border at the second to fourth intercostal space (not below the nipple line) with a double stick adhesive so that both the breath and heart sounds will be heard clearly (Fig. 10–3). A layer of blanket or a pajama top over the stethoscope and ECG pads will help divert the child's attention away from the strange objects on the chest wall.

Frequently a small child is content to sit up and play but has no intention of lying down on the operating table. In such cases, it is much better to proceed with induction with the child sitting up near the upper edge of the operating table and his or her back leaning against the anesthesiologist's chest or the child on the anesthesiologist's lap (Fig. 10–4).

Some children may object strenuously to both the sight and smell of the mask, even before the gas flow is started. Varied approaches may be used to temper these emotional reactions. Fruit-scented lipsticks have been successful in hiding the smell of inhaled anesthetics from a reluctant child. Bubble gum flavor seems to be the favorite scent of most children. A regular

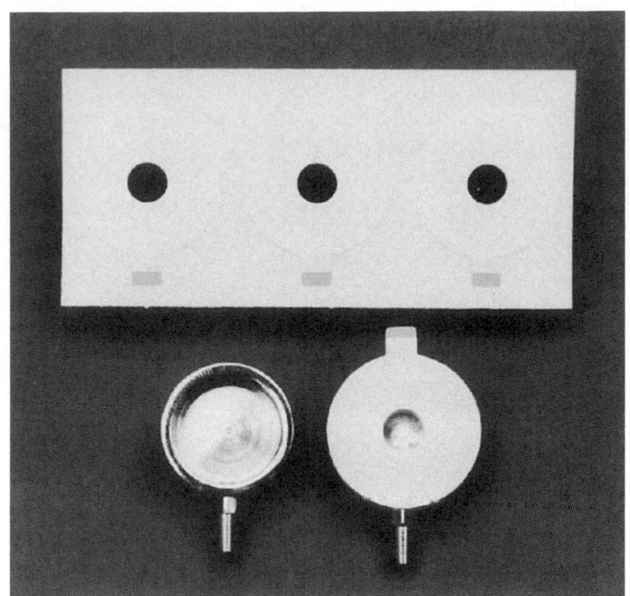

■ **FIGURE 10–3.** Precordial stethoscopes with double-stick adhesive. (Courtesy 3M Company, St. Paul, MN.)

disposable clear plastic mask with an inflatable cuff around the rim is acceptable to children. One should never begin the induction by putting a mask on the child's face abruptly and without warning. The mask, detached from the anesthesia circuit and scented with a fruit flavor of choice, should be shown to the child, even if he or she has seen it previously. Let your assistant (nurse or attending anesthesiologist) or the parent (most often the mother), if he or she is present at the bedside, try the mask first and let approve the sweet flavor before applying it to the child's face to assure the child that it is harmless. The anesthetic circuit is then connected and started with N_2O and O_2 (2:1).

At the outset, the child may be responsive, apprehensive, resistant, or alert; the approach must be suited to the child's mood. It is best to rely on the establishment of communication and especially on the building of self-confidence. One can pretend to need a child's help by having him or her hold the mask on his or her face by himself or herself (Fig. 10–5). If the child objects to the smell of the inhaled anesthetic, he or she should be told to breathe through the mouth because this reduces the smell. A child's imagination may be used to alleviate anxiety. Unlike adult patients, it is not useful to ask a child to take a deep breath because he or she may not respond to the command or may become apneic after deep breaths and disrupt smooth induction with a steady increase in inhaled anesthetic concentrations. One does not stimulate a quiet child by asking questions and prodding him or her awake. It is better to discourage activity by suggesting more and more soporific themes. Some degree of hypnosis is involved in most inhalation inductions.

As the child goes to sleep, he or she may close the eyes and not move but may lose consciousness slowly and continue to hear very accurately, especially when halothane is used for induction. Apprehension may increase as the child becomes dizzy and disoriented and may feel that he or she is floating off in space, completely helpless and abandoned. To prevent these sensations, the anesthesiologist must be sure to maintain contact with the child, continually reassuring him or her by touching him or her lightly. The assistant stands quietly beside the patient. Most children, and many teenagers and adults, appreciate having a hand to hold as they begin to lose control of things.

It is extremely important to know the signs of early induction and to check them before disturbing the child. The first sign of anesthetic induction usually is the appearance of nystagmus; then the eyes usually close, respiration becomes slower, regular, and deeper, then shallower and more rapid, and the child becomes still. For some time after that the child may be only half asleep and responds to verbal command. Until he or she no longer reacts to one's voice and the eyelash reflex in gone, nothing should be done to move or stimulate the patient, unless airway obstruction or a similar need arises. Nurses and surgeons should know not to touch the patient without getting a nod to go ahead from the anesthesiologist. As soon as anesthesia is induced and the patient can tolerate moderately painful stimuli, an intravenous infusion can be started. An intravenous dose of atropine (0.01 to 0.02 mg/kg) may be given to infants to prevent bradycardia and hypotension caused by inhaled anesthetics, especially with halothane.

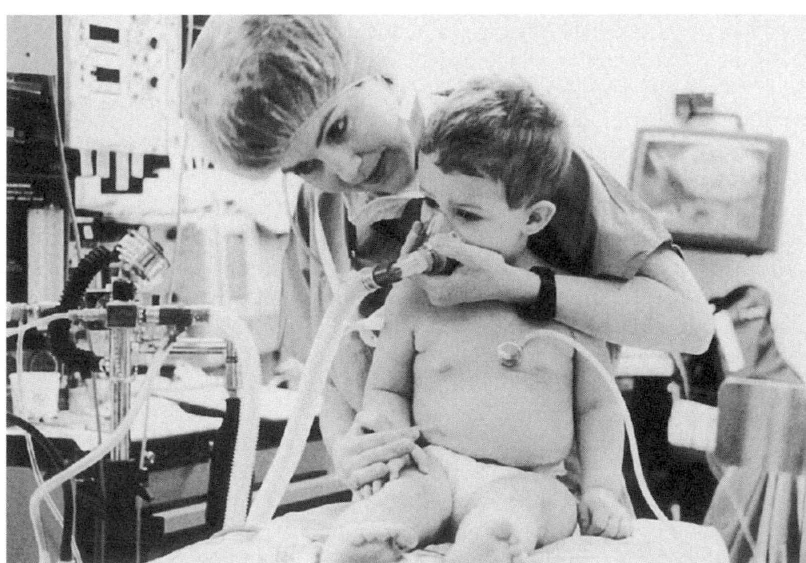

■ **FIGURE 10–4.** Children who refuse to lie down on the operating table often have little objection to a "sitting up" induction with minimal monitoring, usually with a precordial stethoscope and a pulse oximeter probe.

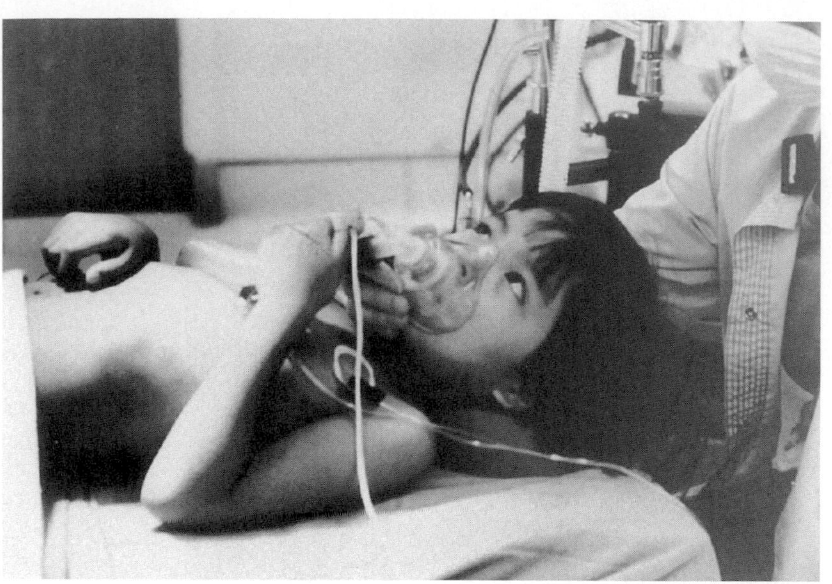

■ **FIGURE 10–5.** The child may hold the mask himself.

An effective and safe method of inhalation induction for children is to run a high flow of nitrous oxide and oxygen, 2:1, over the mouth and nose as one slowly lowers the mask onto the face as oxygen saturation (usually 100%) is continuously monitored. The patient will get the full effect of nitrous oxide within 1 to 2 minutes, as evidenced by the appearance of nystagmus and a regular and slower respiratory pattern of breathing. Then sevoflurane is added. Except for young infants less than 3 to 6 months of age, the concentration of sevoflurane can be increased rapidly to 6% to 8% in otherwise healthy patients without causing significant hypotension or bradycardia. DuBois and others (1999) compare the three techniques of sevoflurane induction: incremental increases in sevoflurane (2%, 4%, 6%, and 8%) in 100% oxygen, a high concentration of sevoflurane (8%) in O_2, and a high concentration of sevoflurane in the 1:1 mixture of N_2O and O_2. There were minimal differences among the three approaches. An addition of N_2O with a high concentration of sevoflurane decreased the time to eyelash reflex and tended to decrease the incidence of excitement during the induction.

Halothane is a potent, relatively nonirritant, volatile anesthetic with a sweet odor that was introduced for clinical use in 1956 in the United Kingdom (1958 in the United States). It soon displaced all existing volatile agents for pediatric use (Wark, 1997). Fulminant hepatitis associated with halothane anesthesia (halothane hepatitis) eventually eliminated its use in adults, and it was replaced by isoflurane in the early 1980s. Until recently, halothane enjoyed the role of the sole agent for inhalation induction, mostly because there was no alternative to halothane and the incidence of halothane hepatitis in children has been reported to be relatively low, estimated as less than 1:80,000 to 1:500,000; it has not been a major concern for clinical use (Wark, 2001).

When halothane is used for induction, the concentration must be increased by 0.5% increments every 2 or 3 breathes. Concentrations of 3.5% to 4.0% halothane are considered proper limits for induction and should be reduced to 1.0% to 1.5% once anesthesia is established. For practitioners who are not familiar with halothane, inhalation induction with halothane should be discouraged, especially for infants, without proper supervision, because, in comparison with sevoflurane, halothane causes more myocardial depression, hypotension, and arrhythmias (Holzman et al., 1996; Blayney et al., 1999). The Pediatric Perioperative Cardiac Arrest (POCA) Registry reports that cardiac arrest related to medication is the most common cause (37% of total), of which 66% were associated with halothane (versus 4% with sevoflurane) (Morray et al., 2000).

Soon after the approval of sevoflurane for clinical use in the mid 1990s in North America and in Europe (since 1993 in Japan), it rapidly replaced halothane as the primary (if not the sole) inhalation induction agent. Sevoflurane has a low blood-gas partition coefficient of 0.6 (Wallin et al., 1975) and is well tolerated by infants and children for inhalation induction (Naito et al., 1991; Sarner et al., 1995). Children anesthetized with sevoflurane exhibited more rapid emergence and a significantly shorter postoperative recovery time compared with those receiving halothane (Naito et al., 1991).

There are several potential problems with the clinical use of sevoflurane: its degradation in CO_2 absorbers (Morio et al., 1992), the production of carbon monoxide and excessive heat, and biodegradation to inorganic fluoride ion (Frink et al., 1992).

Metabolism of sevoflurane in vivo produces inorganic fluoride, the level of which may be proportional to the concentration and duration of exposure to sevoflurane (MAC hour). There have been no reports of renal toxicity with sevoflurane, although serum fluoride concentrations in excess of 50 μmol/L have been reported in adults (Frink et al., 1992). It has been suggested that sevoflurane exposures up to 15 MAC hours are safe in adults (Sarner et al., 1995).

A breakdown product, fluoromethyl-2-2-difluoro-1-(trifluoromethyl) vinyl ether (compound A), is formed by the reaction of sevoflurane with CO_2 absorber (there is more breakdown with barium hydroxide lime [Baralyme] than with sodium hydroxide base [soda lime]). The formation of compound A increases with decreasing gas flow, with increasing sevoflurane concentrations, with increasing CO_2 production and temperature, and with the drying of the absorbent (Biebuyck and Eger, 1994; Steffey et al., 1997; Meakin, 1999). However, the degradation of sevoflurane to compound A in CO_2 absorbents is not a clinical issue if a minimum of 2 L/min fresh gas flow is maintained for a circle system or, alternatively, Mapleson D circuits (such as Bain circuit) are used on the anesthesia machine and the biotransformation does not seem to be associated with renal toxicity (Frink et al., 1996; Mazze and Jamison, 1997).

The degradation of sevoflurane with the presence of CO_2 absorbents has led to several new products that absorb CO_2 but without reacting with sevoflurane (Lerman, 2004). Amsorb and Dragersorb-Free are such "inert" CO_2 absorbers (Kharasch et al., 2002; Kobayashi et al., 2003). The degradation of inhaled anesthetics is virtually eliminated by excluding the sodium and potassium bases from these products. Amsorb contains only calcium hydroxide (Kharasch et al., 2002; Kobayashi et al., 2003). With the advent of the new class of CO_2 absorbers, it is likely that low-flow sevoflurane anesthesia with semiclosed or even closed circle ventilation will become a reality in the near future (Peters et al., 1998; Meakin, 1999).

Another problem with sevoflurane is its exothermic reaction with desiccated CO_2 absorber, especially with barium hydroxide lime (Baralyme), producing carbon monoxide (CO) and/or excessive heat. The reaction with desflurane produces more CO, whereas sevoflurane is associated with the most heat production compared with all other inhaled anesthetics (Wissing et al., 2001). Excessive overheating and melting of CO_2 canisters and spontaneous ignition and explosions within anesthesia circle systems have been reported. These accidents were associated with a combined use of sevoflurane and desiccated Baralyme (resulting from high fresh gas flow) (Castro et al., 2004; Wu et al., 2004); the data also included a case report of a serious injury (acute respiratory distress syndrome [ARDS]) to the patient (Fatheree and Leighton, 2004). In order to prevent excessive dehydration or desiccation of CO_2 absorbents, it is recommended that the common practice of running oxygen through the anesthesia circuit overnight and weekend be discontinued, especially in the remote and infrequently used anesthetizing locations (Woehlck, 2004). Routine monitoring of CO_2 canister temperature using a skin temperature probe may be an easy addition to the circle system for detecting the overheating of CO_2 absorbent during sevoflurane anesthesia (Woehlck, 2004). The new class of calcium hydroxide-based CO_2 absorbents appears to be safe against exothermic reactions in part because calcium hydroxide is hydrophilic and prevents excessive dehydration.

Whether there still is a place for halothane in pediatric anesthesia has been actively debated in the literature (Wark, 1997, 2001; Holzki and Kretz, 1999; Murat, 1998, 2001b). The relatively high blood-gas partition coefficient of halothane and its slower emergence and analgesic effects in comparison to sevoflurane could be advantages for certain cases for different reasons (e.g., bronchoscopy, myringotomy) (see Chapter 11, Intraoperative and Postoperative Management). In addition, sevoflurane is 20 times more expensive than halothane, one major reason why halothane is still used for the maintenance of pediatric anesthesia in the cost-conscious managed care environments of the United States and Australia (Wark, 2001). With the advent of a new class of "inert" CO_2 absorbents that do not degrade inhaled anesthetics (see earlier), low-flow circle absorber techniques in the future would decrease the cost of sevoflurane anesthesia. Sevoflurane, even with the advantage of a low blood-gas solubility coefficient, is not the ideal inhaled anesthetic, having its own drawbacks, like postoperative agitation that especially occurs after short surgical procedures. In addition, there have been reports of QT prolongation associated with sevoflurane anesthesia (Kleinsasser et al., 2001; Maier et al., 2002). Yet, with the cardiovascular stability and the lack of airway irritation that sevoflurane provides, the risk/benefit ratio of sevoflurane is much better than that of halothane (Murat, 2001b) (also see Chapter 6, Pharmacology).

Desflurane is not recommended for inhalation induction due to a high incidence of coughing not altered by premedication (58%) and frequent and severe laryngospasm (49%) with significant hemoglobin desaturation (Zwass et al., 1992).

Maintenance of the Upper Airway During Induction

The pharyngeal airway is composed of collapsible soft tissues surrounded by bony structures (the mandible anteriorly and spinal column posteriorly). In the awake state, the pharyngeal airway is kept open by tonic and phasic contractions of pharyngeal dilator muscles contracting synchronously with contractions of the diaphragm with inspiration (see Chapter 2, Respiratory Physiology). During induction of anesthesia, airway obstruction frequently occurs as the pharyngeal and laryngeal muscles are preferentially relaxed (Nishino et al., 1984; Ochiai et al., 1989). In order to maintain the airway patent, the neck must be extended, the jaw thrust forward in a sniffing position, and the mouth open in case of nasal obstruction (the triple airway maneuver), with a moderate continuous positive airway pressure (CPAP; 10 to 15 cm H_2O). It is therefore essential to establish an airtight system with the bag and mask and maintain CPAP to resist the collapsing force of relaxed upper airway structures (Motoyama, 1997; Hammer et al., 2001) until the patient is sufficiently anesthetized to tolerate the insertion of an oral airway without developing laryngospasm (Guedel's Stage 3, including the loss of intercostal muscle activities) (see Chapter 2, Respiratory Physiology). Once the steady state of surgical anesthesia is achieved, CPAP of 5 to 10 cm H_2O appears sufficient to maintain upper airway patency in spontaneously breathing children (Reber et al., 2001).

Major causes of airway obstruction during induction of anesthesia are (1) preexistent nasal obstruction when the mouth is closed by the anesthesiologist; (2) obstruction of the oropharynx and/or nasopharynx (velopharynx) by the relaxation of upper airway dilator muscles, and resultant collapse of velopharynx and/or posterior displacement of the tongue (Ochiai et al., 1989; Motoyama, 1997; Hammer et al., 2001); and (3) laryngospasm. Insertion of an oropharyngeal or nasopharyngeal airway usually solves the first and second problems, provided that the anesthesia is sufficiently deep to prevent pharyngeal reflex. During sevoflurane anesthesia, an oropharyngeal airway is tolerated relatively early during induction compared with halothane. Laryngospasm is common with isoflurane anesthesia and more frequent and severe with desflurane anesthesia (Zwass et al., 1992). A nasopharyngeal airway is better tolerated even when the anesthesia is too light for insertion of an oropharyngeal airway; it should be well lubricated and inserted very gently to prevent mucosal injury and epistaxis.

The oropharyngeal airway should be large enough to extend the tip behind the base of the tongue. The proper length can be estimated by holding the airway over the side of the child's face; the tip should be at or near the angle of the mandible. In children, the oral airway should always be inserted with the aid of a tongue depressor to pull the tongue forward. One should avoid the method of inserting the airway upside down to get it past the front teeth and then swinging it around into place. This practice, although used commonly and successfully in adult patients, tends to push the tongue posteriorly and obstruct the pharyngeal airway, particularly in infants; it also easily twists out loose front teeth in children (Smith, 1980a).

If the insertion of an airway does not relieve the obstruction, the patient may have laryngospasm due to mucosal irritation often initiated by the aspiration of saliva; the presence of oral airways may make matters worse. If the vocal cords are tightly closed, the use of continuous high pressure, pushing the secretions down into the larynx, simply intensifies the spasm and may also inflate the stomach, further interfering with pulmonary gas exchange and increasing the chance of regurgitation and aspiration of gastric contents. A normal child can tolerate a few moments of laryngospasm. By using 100% oxygen and a high intermittent positive pressure (40 to 60 mm Hg), one can usually squeeze enough oxygen through the child's glottis to avoid serious hypoxemia. One successful approach is to maintain moderate continuous positive pressure with an air-tight mask and to add a firm, intermittent squeeze to the bag synchronous with the end of each "expiratory" phase (or the "bearing-down" phase of the laryngospasm cycle) when the glottis relaxes momentarily, with or without evidence of inspiratory effort against the closed glottis. However, if the child begins to show bradycardia with rapid oxygen desaturation, one should not delay any longer and should administer succinylcholine (2 mg/kg) and atropine (0.02 mg/kg) intravenously or 5 mg/kg of succinylcholine intramuscularly (Liu et al., 1981; Hannallah et al., 1986) and reestablish the airway patency without delay, with or without tracheal intubation.

Intravenous Induction

In children, as well as in adults, induction via the intravenous route has the advantage of speed plus elimination of the mask and its unpleasant odors. The major disadvantage is the child's exaggerated fear of the needle and the difficulty of venipuncture. EMLA (eutectic mixture of local anesthetics 2.5% lidocaine and 2.5% prilocaine) cream seems to help alleviate this problem (Ehrenstrom et al., 1982; Maunuksela and Korpela, 1986; Freeman et al., 1993). Children under 6 to 7 years of age, however, have shown less overall benefit than older children in the use of EMLA for venous cannulation. This is probably due to the fact that the young child still sees the intravenous needle and fears that the cannulation will be painful. EMLA cream must be applied at least 1 hour prior to intravenous cannulation to provide sufficient dermal analgesia compared with placebo. The EMLA cream is placed on intact skin over a promising vein with an occlusive dressing applied over the cream. Two potential sites of venous cannulation should be prepared with EMLA cream, usually on opposite hands. EMLA sometimes causes vasoconstriction and makes the insertion of a cannula more difficult. Removing the EMLA patch 10 to 15 minutes before venipuncture and warming the site causes vasodilation and eases the cannulation. EMLA should not be used in infants under 12 months of age with glucose-6-phosphate deficiency or other children more susceptible to methemoglobinemia (Frayling et al., 1990). Children 8 to 10 years of age and older may prefer an intravenous induction to a mask, often because they have some fear of the mask from a previous unpleasant experience.

The dorsum of the hand, the radial vein, and the saphenous and other veins of the foot are examined as preferential sites for venipuncture. The volar aspect of the wrist has small visible veins that are inviting but are difficult to maintain in an awake child unless the wrist is immobilized and fixed in an extended position beforehand. Furthermore, venipuncture here is extremely painful. Likewise, venipuncture on the scalp is exceptionally painful and should be done only when peripheral veins appropriate for venipuncture are not found elsewhere.

To avoid frightening a child, one should hold the needle out of sight, avoid use of the word "needle," and divert attention. If EMLA cream has been applied, the occlusive dressing is removed and the cream is wiped off. The skin should be allowed to dry after wiping with alcohol lest the venipuncture be unnecessarily painful. The assistant should hold the extremity gently but firmly to avoid jerky movement. In order to fixate the veins in the dorsum of the hand, the skin is pulled down toward the fingers. If EMLA has not been used, intradermal injection of approximately 0.1 mL of 1% lidocaine is made with a 25-gauge (or smaller) needle, particularly when larger than a 20-gauge catheter is used. One should give a warning like "here comes a little pinch" and command "take a deep breath" at the time of inserting a needle to divert attention. Subsequent intravenous insertion of a larger needle through the skin wheal is painless and more often successful.

Unless excessive fluid and blood losses are anticipated, a 22-gauge catheter in young children and a 20-gauge catheter in older children undergoing an elective surgical procedure are sufficient for the need for fluid replacement. For a small infant, a 24-gauge catheter usually is sufficient for fluid replacement, and a 22-gauge catheter can be used for blood transfusion. Before the infusion of propofol or sodium thiopental, the anesthesiologist should make sure that there is a free flow of intravenous fluid in order to avoid an inadvertent, painful subcutaneous infusion.

The patient is oxygenated just before the induction of anesthesia. If the child objects to a facemask, oxygen can be delivered by holding the right-angle connector, without the mask, between the fingers of a cupped hand and insufflating oxygen without touching the patient's face. The effect of oxygen insufflation should be immediately apparent as the pulse oximeter reading rises from the high 90's to 100%.

Propofol

An intravenous induction dose of propofol in healthy unpremedicated children 3 to 12 years of age with a smooth transition to inhalation anesthesia (ED_{95}) usually requires 2.5 to 3.0 mg/kg (Manschot et al., 1992). Children younger than 2 years required a significantly larger dose (2.6 to 3.4 mg/kg) (Aun et al., 1992), whereas older children needed less (Manschot et al., 1992). Induction with propofol in children causes significant decreases in blood pressure and heart rate, similar to those observed after thiopental (Mirakhur, 1988; Hannallah et al., 1991; Manschot et al., 1992). Propofol has antiemetic properties and causes less laryngospasm than thiopental (Borgeat et al., 1990). Propofol, however, has some undesirable properties, such as pain on injection, allergic reactions, and rapid microbial growth (Eyres, 2004). The pain on injection is troublesome and often causes erythema near the site of injection (Manschot et al., 1992). Pain is less frequent if a large antecubital vein is used or lidocaine is administered into the intravenous catheter prior to the injection of propofol (Hannallah et al., 1991). Alternatively, a mixture of 9 mL of propofol (1%) with 1 mL (25 mg) of thiopental reduces injection pain considerably (Fine GF, personal communication). The duration of propofol anesthesia is largely due to its redistribution rather than to metabolism and elimination from the body. Because larger induction doses are needed in infants and children, the recovery time from propofol is more prolonged in children than in adults (McFarlan et al., 1999; Eyres, 2004).

Thiopental

An intravenous dose of thiopental in healthy children is 5 to 6 mg/kg (Coté et al., 1981). In infants 1 to 6 months of age, the median effective dose (ED_{50}) is reported to be 6.8 mg/kg; in infants less than 2 weeks of age, it is 3.4 mg/kg (Jonmarker et al., 1987). In a well-premedicated child or when the intravenous injection of opioids (such as 1 to 2 mcg/kg of fentanyl or 0.1 mg/kg of morphine) is given as basal anesthesia preceding thiopental, 2 to 4 mg/kg of thiopental usually is sufficient for a modified inhalation induction with nitrous oxide and sevoflurane or halothane.

A reasonable and safer approach to intravenous induction and intubation, particularly in infants, is a "modified inhalation induction" in which the child is given a sedative intravenous dose of opioids (e.g., fentanyl 1 to 2 mcg/kg) or benzodiazepine (e.g., midazolam 0.1 to 0.2 mg/kg, unless the patient is already well premedicated), followed by propofol or thiopental. As soon as the patient loses consciousness, mask induction is initiated with 2 to 3 MAC of an inhaled anesthetic (sevoflurane or halothane) until anesthesia is induced and ventilation is assisted or controlled.

Ketamine

Ketamine may be chosen for intravenous induction in specific situations, especially in high-risk patients with cardiovascular instability. Ketamine increases airway secretions; atropine (0.01 to 0.02 mg/kg) or glycopyrrolate, half the dose of atropine, should be given to counteract this effect. In these patients, one should try to maintain the airway through the careful positioning of the head rather than with insertion of an oral airway, to avoid laryngospasm. With a dose of 2 mg/kg, a child usually assumes a catatonic condition and is "asleep" within 1 to 2 minutes.

Intramuscular Induction

Low-dose intramuscular ketamine (2 to 3 mg/kg) is also useful to facilitate inhaled induction of anesthesia in those children who are uncooperative (Hannallah and Patel, 1989). Although it is preferable to avoid intramuscular injections, children who are unhappy despite parents being present and do not permit oral or transmucosal premedication are better served with an expeditious ketamine intramuscular injection. Inhalation induction or the insertion of intravenous cannula is easily performed 2 to 3 minutes after intramuscular ketamine.

Rectal Administration of Anesthetic

For the anxious child who is deathly afraid of a mask as well as a needle stick, inducing anesthesia via the rectum is probably the least disturbing method. This method is particularly appropriate when the parents are present during induction. Thiopental sodium and methohexital sodium have been used successfully for rectal administration. Both agents induce drowsiness and sleep rapidly and effectively (see Chapter 6, Pharmacology). For practical purposes, the standard 2.5% intravenous solution often is most convenient, although 5% and 10% solutions are also used. The usual dose of thiopental for children who have had no other sedation is 30 to 40 mg/kg (Kaufman, 1973). If thiopental is given as a supplement to previous but inadequate sedation, 20 mg/kg is advised.

Methohexital is reputed to produce more rapid induction than thiopental, but this is of little clinical significance when it is given rectally. Rectal methohexital should always be regarded as an agent to induce anesthesia rather than as a premedication. Airway irritability and hiccoughs, frequently observed during intravenous use, do not usually occur with rectal administration. Hypersensitivity reactions to methohexital have been reported but are rare (Driggs and O'Day, 1972; Wyatt and Watkin, 1975; Liu et al., 1984). Apnea after rectal methohexital has been reported in children with meningomyeloceles and should be used with caution in these children (Yemen et al., 1991).

With either thiopental or methohexital, the exact dose of thiopental and an additional 5 mL or so of air is aspirated in a 10- to 20-mL syringe, depending on the age of the child. The syringe is then connected to a 8F to 12F feeding tube, which is lubricated with surgical lubricant. The child is placed on the stretcher or held by the mother in the lateral or supine position with hips and knees flexed. The catheter filled to the tip with the barbiturate solution is inserted rectally. The syringe containing the medication and air is held vertically and the contents injected with a single gentle downward push of the plunger into the rectum. The syringe and the catheter should be removed as a unit. With this technique, the solution is pulsed by air and the catheter should be clear of solution when it is removed. Children often feel as though they need to have a bowel movement after the drug is administered (Berry, 1986). The buttocks must be held together firmly with the hands to avoid the loss or evacuation of the barbiturate solution. It is effective in 95% of children within 5 to 10 minutes; waiting longer than 10 minutes will not increase the incidence of success. Without additional sedative/hypnotics, the child awakens in about 20 to 60 minutes.

Induction by rectal thiopental is suitable for administration in the child's bed or the child held by a parent. It is useful for resistant children, especially the developmentally delayed or those who, for any reason, comprehend poorly. Rectal induction is less desirable in children older than 4 years or with a weight greater than 20 kg because it becomes an issue of the volume of drug to be instilled, as well as it being somewhat socially unacceptable. Because of the rapid onset and profound sedation, an anesthesiologist should remain with the child from the time of its administration until the end of surgery and anesthesia. This adds considerably to total anesthesia time and is a major deterrent to the widespread use of rectal methohexital. Midazolam has also been used rectally (Spear et al., 1991). A dose of 1.0 mg/kg (0.2% solution or, if volume exceeded 10 mL, undiluted 0.5% is used) is effective for preinduction of anesthesia and does not delay discharge from the postanesthesia care unit. It produces enough sedation for easy acceptance of the anesthesia mask, although loss of consciousness does not occur.

Combinations of rectally administered midazolam (0.5 mg/kg), ketamine (3 mg/kg), and atropine (0.02 mg/kg) are effective in facilitating separation of children aged 8 months to 7 years from their parents or intravenous cannulation (Beebe et al., 1992). The addition of ketamine to midazolam caused more children to be asleep when separating from parents.

Indications for Altered Induction Techniques

Many patients in the pediatric age group have various pathophysiologic conditions requiring special methods of anesthetic induction. Those with obstructive respiratory disorders at different airway levels, including "tonsil bleeders"; those with cardiac or renal disorders, increased intracranial pressure, open eye injury, or a full stomach; and those with many other conditions involve special considerations. Each of these situations is discussed in a section in different chapters devoted to the field involved.

■ LARYNGEAL MASK AIRWAY

The laryngeal mask airway (LMA) is a device that is being used increasingly since the early 1990s, both in children and in adults for general anesthesia where mask ventilation is appropriate but the procedure is long enough that endotracheal intubation would be used. The original LMA is constructed of reusable soft medical-grade silicone rubber. It does not contain latex and will withstand repeated autoclaving. Disposable LMAs are available and are made of soft plastic. There are six sizes of LMA (Table 10–1, Fig. 10–6), with the appropriate size based on the patient's weight. Studies by Voyagis and others (1996) and Loh and others (2002), however, have suggested that larger than previously suggested sizes may be needed for young children of between 10 and 20 kg body weight. For older adolescents, the gender should also be considered, with size 5 for males and size 4 for females (Voyagis et al., 1996). Flexible LMAs are also available in all six sizes and are advantageous for certain types of procedures, such as tonsillectomy. The Fastrach LMAs for blind oral intubation are available only in three large sizes (3, 4, and 5).

The LMA ProSeal is a new LMA with a rear cuff and a drainage tube that allows the insertion of a gastric tube and the evacuation of gastric gas and liquid. Pediatric-size LMA ProSeals (sizes 1.5 and up) without a rear cuff have become available. Insertion of a ProSeal LMA is as easy as insertion of the classic LMA (Shimbori et al., 2004). Before use, the LMA cuff is checked for leaks by inflating air into the cuff, as done with cuffed endotracheal tubes.

There are several methods of LMA insertion. The classic insertion, as originally described by Brain (1983), is to aspirate the air from the cuff of the LMA, making sure that the cuff deflates flat by placing it on a flat surface as it is deflated. The LMA is inserted blindly into the pharynx, forming a low-pressure seal around the laryngeal inlet in a spontaneously breathing patient (Haynes and Morton, 1993; Pennant and White, 1993). The sniffing position is recommended for insertion of the LMA, as with endotracheal intubations. With the patient's mouth open, the distal aperture of the LMA facing anteriorly, the tip of the cuff is slid down as it is firmly and continuously pressed against the hard palate using the index finger of the right hand to guide the tube over the back of the tongue. The tube is then advanced in one smooth movement until a characteristic resistance is felt as the upper esophageal sphincter is engaged (Pennant and White, 1993). The reverse technique has also become a common practice: inserting the LMA with the aperture facing the palate and, when the resistance is felt, the tube is then rotated 180 degrees to cover the laryngeal inlet. There is no statistical difference between the two methods regarding successful insertion (Soh and Ng, 2001), and when one method is not working, it may be possible to change to the other. Alternatively, insertion of the LMA partially inflated in children requires less time and is associated with a higher success rate (O'Neill et al., 1994).

Once the LMA has been inserted, it is then inflated with 5 to 30 mL of air (depending on the size as recommended (see Table 10–1). A slight and outward movement of the LMA usually follows this maneuver by 1 to 2 cm. Any further movement is usually indicative of incorrect placement and the LMA should be deflated, removed, and reinserted. After the LMA is positioned in the midline, stabilized with bite blocks in both sides of the LMA, and taped across the upper lip (as with the endotracheal tube), the 15-mm proximal connector is attached to the anesthesia circuit and the patient may breath either spontaneously or through controlled ventilation with a low peak pressure (<15 cm H_2O).

When correctly placed, a seal pressure of 20 cm H_2O is usually adequate and may predict correct placement. Inagawa and others (2002), however, found little correlation between seal and positioning of the LMA. Several studies have looked into the placement of the LMA both fiberoptically (Rowbottom et al., 1991; Dubreuil et al., 1993) and radiologically (Goudsouzian et al., 1992) and found that clinically functioning LMAs were not necessarily in the correct position. Keidan and others (2000), however, reported a significant correlation between the inspiratory work of breathing and percent of airway obliteration by the epiglottis examined fiberoptically through the LMA. Movement of the head from the neutral position may easily dislodge the LMA and could have a profound effect on the LMA position and the ability to ventilate the patient (Okuda et al., 2001). When general anesthesia under a caudal block and spontaneous breathing is planned for urogenital or other procedures, the anesthesiologist should induce the patient via mask and bag, insert an oral airway, and turn the patient to the lateral position to perform the caudal block; the patient is then turned back to the supine position, the stomach is emptied, and the LMA is inserted in order to avoid its dislodgment.

The LMA is more difficult to use in children than in adults and is associated with a higher incidence of misplacement (Rowbottom et al., 1991; Dubreuil et al., 1992). The smaller the child, the more difficult is the placement of the LMA in the

■ **TABLE 10–1.** Laryngeal mask airway sizes*

Mask Size	Patient Weight (kg)	Internal Diameter (cm)	Length (cm)	Maximum Cuff Volume Air (mL)	Largest ETT† (ID, mm)
1	<5	5.25	11.5	4	3.5
1.5	5 to 10	6.1	13.5	7	4.0
2	10 to 20	7.0	15.5	10	4.5
2½	20 to 30	8.4	17.5	14	5.0
3	30 to 50	10	22	20	6.0 Cuffed
4	50 to 70	10	22	30	6.5 Cuffed
5	Adult, 70 to 100	11.5	23.5	40	7.0 Cuffed
6	Large adult >100	11.5	23.5	50	7.0 Cuffed

*From LMA™ Instructional Manual, Revised 2003, LMA North America, Inc., San Diego, CA. (Courtesy of LMA North America, Inc.)
†ETT, endotracheal tube. This is the largest ETT that will pass inside the LMA™ for endotracheal intubation after the LMA™ is properly placed.

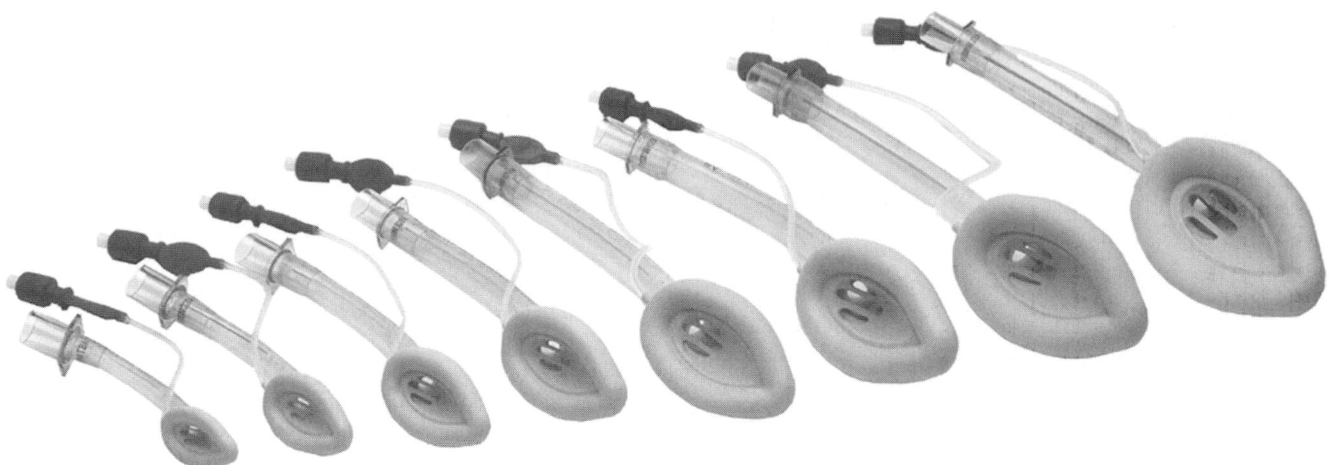

■ **FIGURE 10–6.** The original laryngeal mask airways (LMA Classic). From the top to bottom: sizes 1, 1.5, 2.0, 2.5, 3, 4, 5, and 6. (Courtesy of LMA North America, Inc, San Diego, CA, with permission.)

correct position (Park et al., 2001). This is due to the fact that pediatric LMAs are miniaturized adult-sized LMAs and have a smaller margin of error in positioning the device; it thus can be more easily dislodged.

Problems of LMA insertion are often related to inadequate depth of anesthesia. The LMA may be inserted immediately after an adequate dose of an intravenous induction agent (Allsop et al., 1995) or administration of a volatile anesthetic agent, although the depth of anesthesia for LMA insertion is less than that required for endotracheal intubation (Aantaa et al., 2001). The depth of anesthesia for placing an LMA, however, is greater than when an oral airway is placed. Complications relating to poor positioning are airway obstruction, higher ventilatory pressures in patients on intermittent positive pressure ventilation or controlled ventilation, larger inspiratory leakage, more gastric insufflation, and other related complications that occur more frequently with younger than with older children. A study by Verghese and Brimacombe (1996) has shown the LMA to be safe and effective with a less-than-0.15% complication rate. The LMA is relatively contraindicated in patients who are obese or at risk for aspiration.

The LMA has been used in both conventional and nonconventional ways. Properly inserted LMA with the cuff inflated provides a low-pressure seal around the larynx, enabling positive pressure ventilation. The new LMA with the suction channel (LMA ProSeal) has a definite advantage over the classic LMA for positive pressure ventilation because the pediatric ProSeal LMA allows the passage of a 10F suction catheter more than 90% of the time (Shimbori et al., 2004) and, at the same cuff inflation pressure, air leak pressure around the cuff is much higher than with the classic LMA (30 versus 20 cm H_2O) (Gaitini et al., 2004). Both pressure-controlled and volume-controlled ventilation have been used without the major problems of inflating the stomach. However, one is able to ventilate the patient more effectively with lower pressures using the pressure control mode (Keidan et al., 2001). In patients with marked craniofacial abnormalities whose vocal cords cannot be visualized with conventional laryngoscopy for intubation, the LMA has a unique advantage and may be inserted with the patient awake, allowing for spontaneous inhalation induction and airway maintenance (Markakis et al., 1992; Carenzi et al., 2001).

■ ENDOTRACHEAL INTUBATION

The indications for endotracheal intubation in children are similar to those in adults, with small, but important, differences, particularly in infants. These differences are due to the altered respiratory mechanics in infants and children compared with adults and to the fact that infants are more prone to upper airway obstruction and gastric distention with positive-pressure ventilation under general anesthesia. Potential disadvantages of endotracheal intubation include increased airway resistance when the patient is breathing spontaneously; trauma of intubation to larynx and subglottis; possible laryngospasm during both intubation and extubation; damaged or dislodged teeth; and laceration of soft tissues and hemorrhage, especially with nasotracheal intubation, esophageal intubation, and endobronchial intubation.

■ INDICATIONS FOR ENDOTRACHEAL INTUBATION

In general, intubation is indicated in most infants less than 6 months of age. The benefit of preventing potential difficulties in maintaining upper airway patency and the likelihood of distending the stomach by anesthetic gases with manual ventilation outweigh the potential complications of carefully executed intubation.

In infants and children between 6 and 12 months of age undergoing simple elective surgical procedures such as inguinal herniorrhaphy, intubation is optional, depending on the experience and choice of the anesthesiologist and the patency of upper airways under general anesthesia. Orthopedic or plastic procedures in children involving the extremities and lasting longer than 1 to 2 hours may be a relative indication for intubation for the purpose of safety, but more often in such cases it is used for the anesthesiologist's convenience.

Elective procedures in children older than 1 year that seldom justify intubation include short orthopedic procedures (wire removal, cast change), perineal and urologic procedures (inguinal hernia repairs, circumcision, cystoscopy), minor surgery on body or limbs, extraction of three or four deciduous teeth, probing and irrigation of lacrimal ducts, and myringotomy and tube insertion.

Needless to say, endotracheal intubation is as mandatory in children as in adults for intrathoracic, upper abdominal, and head and neck surgery and for laparoscopic procedures, as well as for procedures requiring prone, lateral, and sitting positions. In addition, intubation is necessary in patients with a full stomach or intestinal obstruction.

■ EQUIPMENT

■ LARYNGOSCOPES AND BLADES

Laryngoscope handles of standard length are suitable for pediatric use, although those of smaller diameter are easier to manipulate and are recommended, particularly for infants and small children. In the evaluation of laryngoscope blades, the length is of obvious importance, but additional features to note are the width and shape of the tip, the bore, and the curvature.

The use of a straight blade requires slightly more relaxation than use of a curved blade, but a straight blade gives better exposure in children. The curved tip of the Phillips blade makes it possible to retract the epiglottis, as with a Macintosh blade, without actually picking it up and lifting it directly (Fig. 10–7). In infants, the wider bore of the Wis-Hipple and Flagg blades enables one to see and to pass a tube more easily than does the flattened aperture of the Miller blade. For older children, the flatter, No. 2 Miller blade becomes more advantageous, because it is less likely to chip large new incisors. The blade designed by Phillips and Duerkson (1973), with a more pronounced terminal curve, has been particularly useful in a situation where the exposure of the larynx is more difficult (Fig. 10–8).

The Macintosh curved blade allows more room to pass the bulky cuffed endotracheal tube but may require a stylet unless the tube is properly curved. The small curved blade (No. 2 Macintosh) occasionally is useful in special situations, as in a small child with an ankylosed jaw or contractures of the neck secondary to burns.

The light bulb deserves special attention. For small patients, it is important to have the bulb near the tip of the blade. One finds considerable variation in this feature (see Fig. 10–8). If the bulb is far recessed from the tip, such as in the No. 1 Miller blade, the soft tissues of the infant's pharynx close around it and obstruct the light.

When testing a laryngoscope, one should be sure that the light is bright and of high intensity. A dim yellow light of low intensity denotes a failing battery and may prove inadequate. It is also important to confirm proper electrical conduction between the laryngoscope handle and blade by engaging the blade in position and observing a steady bright light before its use. It is advisable to have laryngoscope blades of several different shapes and sizes available before beginning induction and intubation.

The newer fiberoptic laryngoscopes have certain advantages. A high-intensity bulb housed in the handle, not on the blade itself, emits cool, high-intensity light through the glass fiber rod, eliminating the usual electrical problems associated with ordinary laryngoscopes. The blade is easier to clean; there is no bulb to change. One possible disadvantage may be that the sight of laryngeal structures can be blocked by the glare of bright, focused light reflecting from intervening soft tissues when exposure is inadequate.

■ FLEXIBLE (FIBEROPTIC) BRONCHOSCOPE

Technological advances in flexible fiberoptic bronchoscopy enable one to intubate patients with difficult airways (Patil et al., 1983) (see Chapter 9, Anesthetic Equipment and Monitoring). The smallest fiberoptic bronchoscope with flexible control of the tip has an outer diameter (OD) of 1.8 mm (Olympus Corporation of America, New Hyde Park, NY) and can easily accommodate an endotracheal tube 2.5 mm in inner diameter (ID) without the connector (Fig. 10–9) (Finer et al., 1992). The smallest bronchoscope with a suction channel that can be used to instill topical anesthetic or to insufflate oxygen has an OD of 2.8 mm (ID = 1.2 mm) and accommodates an endotracheal

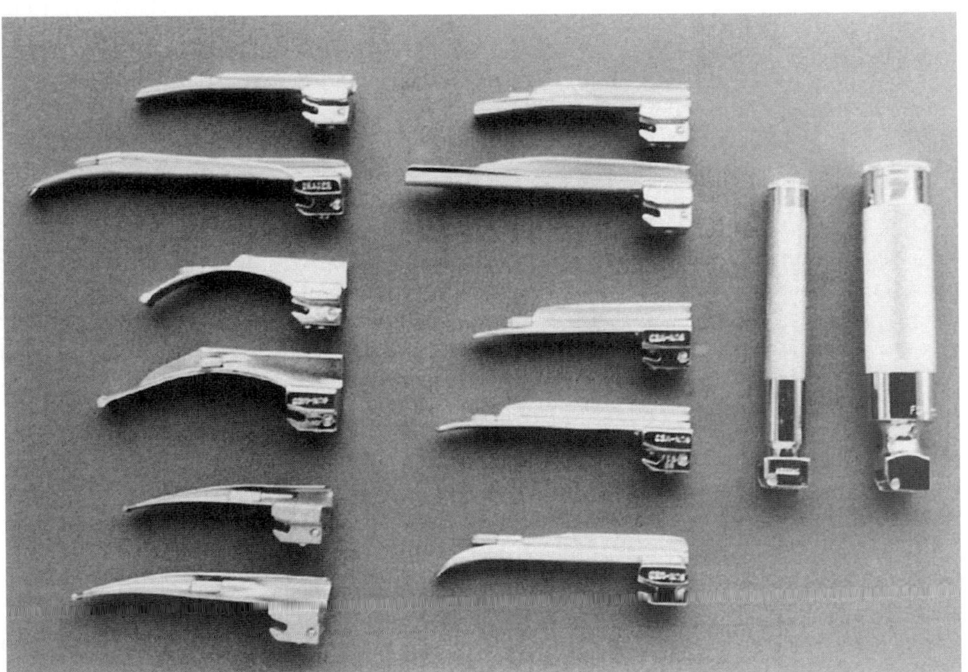

■ **FIGURE 10–7.** Standard laryngoscope blades commonly used in pediatric anesthesia. Left (top to bottom), Miller 1 and 2, Macintosh 1 and 2, Bradshaw 1 and 2. Center, Flagg 1 and 2, Wis-Hipple 1 and 1.5, and Phillips 1. Right, Pediatric and standard laryngoscope handles.

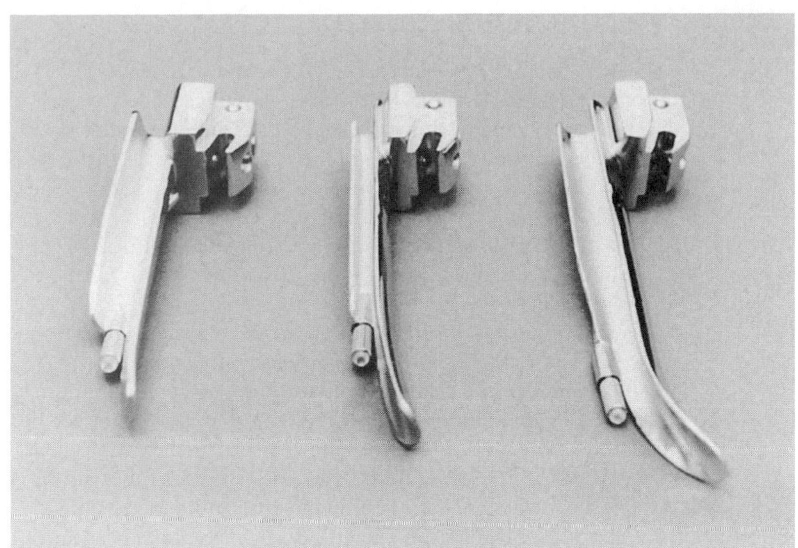

■ **FIGURE 10–8.** Infant laryngoscope blades with different curvatures and light bulb positions (left to right): Wis-Hipple 1, Miller 1, and Phillips 1.

tube with an ID of 3.5 mm. With advanced digital camera technology, the quality of video images has improved markedly. A major disadvantage of this instrument and technology, however, is that its proper use requires considerable practice and experience. In addition, the optic fibers are extremely delicate and are easily broken, leaving black dots on the image; and the instrument is too expensive for casual use.

BULLARD LARYNGOSCOPE

The Bullard laryngoscope, a fiberoptic and mirror combination instrument, deserves mention (Fig. 10–10) (also see Chapter 9, Anesthesia Equipment and Monitoring). The Bullard laryngoscope can be attached to a regular laryngoscope handle, it facilitates indirect oral laryngoscopy and endotracheal intubation with minimal practice; and it is particularly useful for difficult airways (Borland, 1988). To insert the Bullard laryngoscope, the mouth is opened manually and the blade is inserted while the shaft of the scope (and the laryngoscope handle) is kept horizontally (Fig. 10–10*A*). The laryngoscope handle is then rotated from the horizontal to vertical position so that the tip of the blade can be slid around the tongue (Fig. 10–10*B* and *C*). The blade is then elevated beyond the epiglottis and lies against the dorsal surface of the tongue (Fig. 10–10*C*) (Borland, 1988). It can also be attached to a video camera, and the enlarged image can be viewed on a video screen by multiple observers.

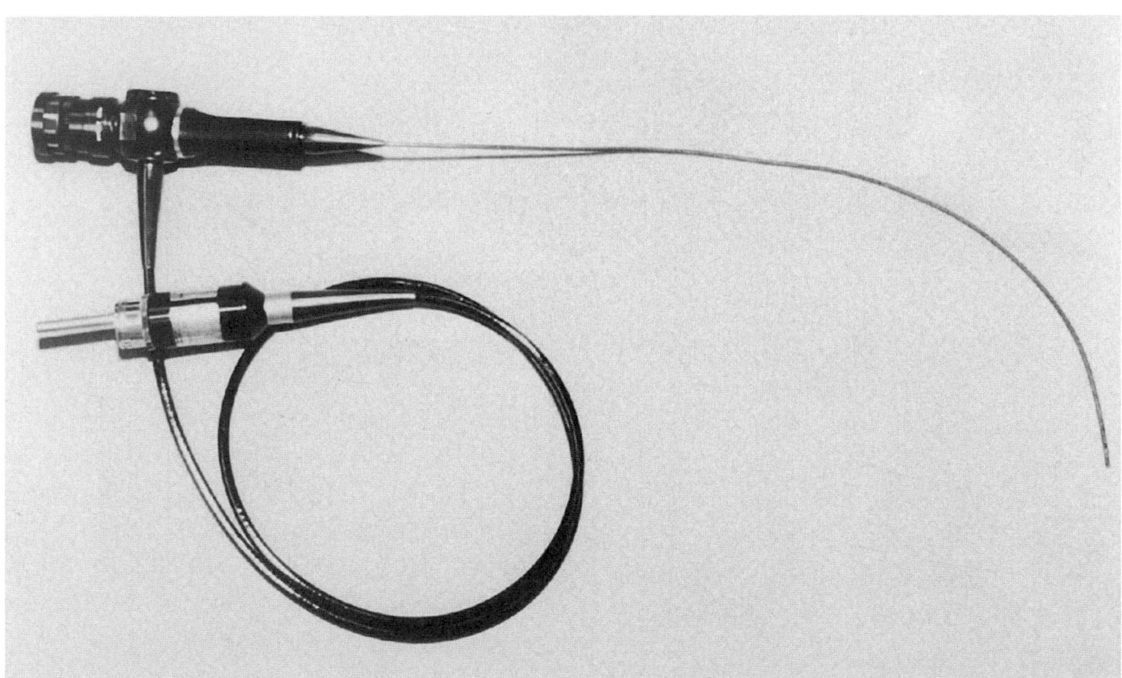

■ **FIGURE 10–9.** A small Olympus pediatric fiberoptic bronchoscope (2.7 mm OD) with a flexible tip accommodates a 3-mm ID Shiley nasal tube (right) for intubation.

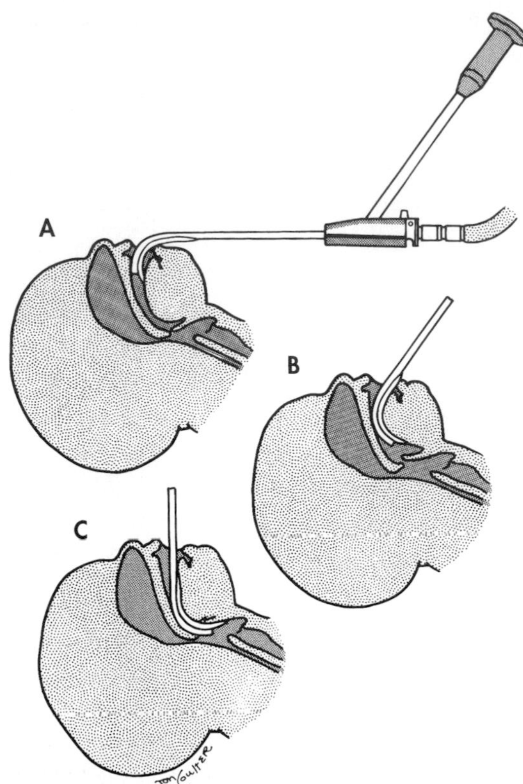

■ **FIGURE 10–10.** Sequence of placement of Bullard laryngoscope (lateral view). The mouth is opened manually, and the laryngoscope handle is rotated from the horizontal to vertical position, so that the blade can be slid around the tongue (*A* and *B*). The blade is then elevated to lie against the tongue's dorsal surface (*C*). (From Borland LM: *Int Anesthesiol Clin* 26:27, 1988.)

ENDOTRACHEAL TUBES

Since the early 1980s, disposable, sterile endotracheal tubes have been used in the United States and elsewhere. They are made of biologically inert, implant-tested (bearing the mark Z-79) polyvinyl chloride (PCV) in order to prevent chemical irritation to the upper airways. These disposable tubes are packaged with a suitable plastic, thin-walled adapter that minimally affects the internal diameter of the tube. PCV tubes are flammable and should not be used for laser surgery involving the airways. Under these circumstances, one should use nonflammable or laser resistant tubes specifically manufactured for this purpose (see Chapter 23, Anesthesia for Otorhinolaryngology Surgery).

Most endotracheal tubes for infants and small children today have length markers from the tip, printed at 1-cm intervals, to aid the anesthesiologist in securing the tube at the proper depth (Fig. 10–11). The Magill-type oral endotracheal tubes are relatively short and are exclusively for oral intubation, although endobronchial intubation can still occur if the tube is advanced indiscriminately, particularly in infants and young children. The tube has a black band or bold black line around the wall 2.0 to 5.0 cm from the tip (the distance varies according to the size as well as by the manufacturer) that should be situated at the vocal cords when the tube is at the proper depth in infants and children of normal anatomy. Variations in the depth mark among different manufacturers are considerable (Goel and Lim, 2003; Wallace and Bell, 2004), and reliance upon these markers (especially the black band) is potentially hazardous with endobronchial intubation or accidental extubation (Munro et al., 1995; Molendijk, 2001). Sound clinical judgment is essential for optimal tube placement, especially with premature infants and those with abnormal facial and airway anatomy.

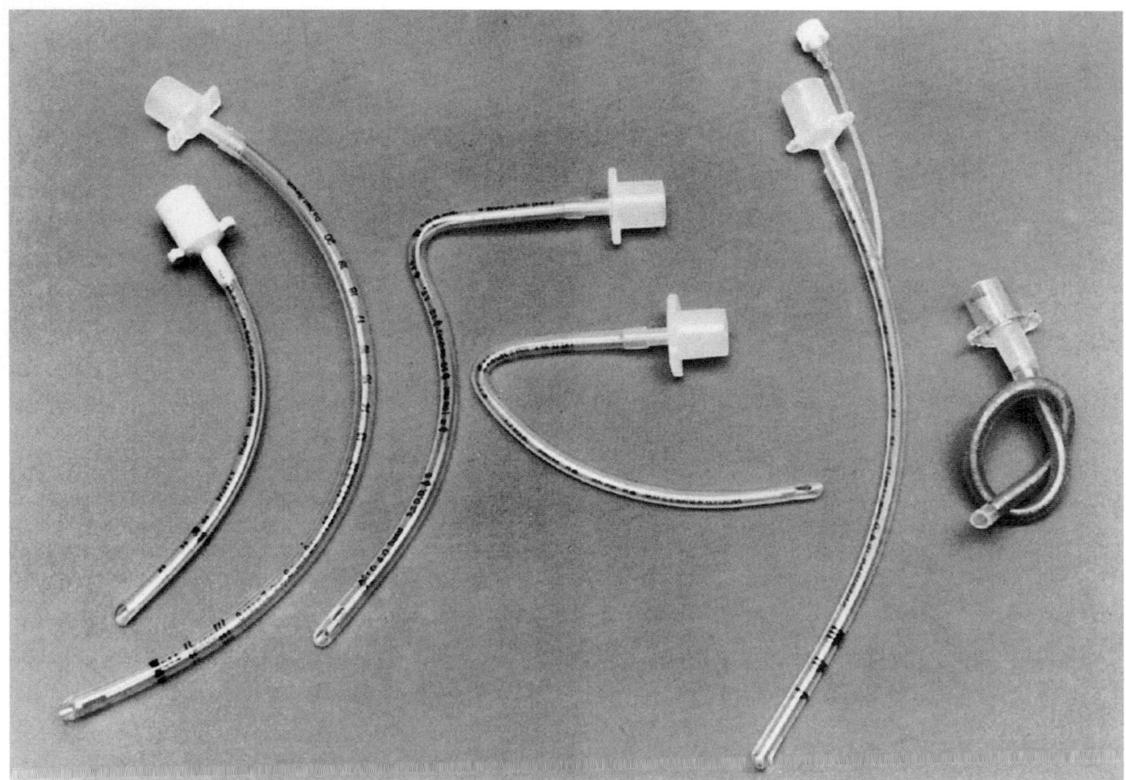

■ **FIGURE 10–11.** Endotracheal tubes used in pediatric anesthesia (left to right): Magill oral tube, Shiley nasal tube, nasal and oral RAE tubes, Sheridan tube with a gas sampling port, and armored tube tied in knot.

The Shiley nasotracheal tube (see Fig. 10–11) is a soft, flexible tube used primarily for nasal intubation. It can be cut to suit individual needs and preferences and can be used orally or through a tracheostomy stoma under special circumstances. This and many other tubes have single, double, and triple circumferential line markers about 1 cm apart, starting 2.0 to 2.5 cm from the tip. The distance of the middle (double) line from the tip usually is the proper depth for the glottis.

Armored or anode endotracheal tubes (see Fig. 10–11), consisting of thin silicon rubber (Silastic) reinforced by coiled wire, have the advantage of tolerating extreme flexion without kinking. In limited situations they prove valuable. Although Silastic anode tubes have improved considerably from older versions made of latex, their wall is still much thicker than that of the PVC tube, and there is a tendency for the tip of the tube to flip out of the trachea even when the tube is properly secured at the mouth (Cohen and Dilon, 1972). For this reason some pediatric anesthesiologists prefer Magill or preformed, acute-angled (RAE) tubes for neurosurgical procedures, reserving the anode tube for exceptional surgical procedures about the face.

The preformed, acute angle oral and nasal endotracheal tubes developed by Ring, Adair, and Elwyn in 1975 (RAE tubes) (see Fig. 10–11) are particularly useful for oral surgery as well as for certain neurosurgical procedures. There are other preformed orotracheal tubes not commonly used in the United States (Lindholm, 1973; Morgan and Steward, 1982b).

The oral RAE tube is bent sharply at the lower incisors and can be fixed over the mandibular midline for surgery involving the oral cavity, such as adenotonsillectomy or cleft palate repair. The nasal RAE tubes are about 1 inch longer, and the preformed acute bend is opposite to that of the oral RAE tube. The bend is directed over the patient's forehead yet eliminates pressure on the naris. A potential problem of this otherwise excellent innovation is that the length of the oral RAE tube to the acute angle, particularly in smaller oral RAE tubes, is slightly too long in some children, so that one must be careful to avoid endobronchial intubation. The uncuffed nasal RAE tubes (Mallinckrodt), on the other hand, tend to be a little too short and may cause accidental extubation, whereas the cuffed nasal RAE tubes of the same internal diameters are about 1 inch longer than the uncuffed nasal RAE tube.

Cuffed Endotracheal Tubes

Until the mid-1990s, the routine use of cuffed endotracheal tubes was not recommended in children younger that 8 to 10 years (Fisher, 1989; Coté and Todres, 1993; Wood, 1986), although the recommended age for cuffed tubes varied among the authors of pediatric textbooks (Uejima, 1989). Literature, however, suggests that the recommendation for the use of uncuffed endotracheal tubes in children may be outdated (Khine et al., 1997; Fine et al., 2000; James, 2001; Fine and Borland, 2004).

The use of uncuffed tubes had been an important consideration through the 1960s, when most young patients breathed spontaneously under diethyl ether anesthesia. The primary reason for not using a cuffed endotracheal tube had been that one must choose a cuffed tube one or two sizes (0.5 to 1.0 mm ID) smaller than the uncuffed tube to accommodate the bulk of the cuff through the subglottis, the narrowest portion of the upper airway (Eckenhoff, 1951). An endotracheal tube with a smaller diameter would markedly increase flow resistance (as much as fourth power of the diameter) and result in increases in work of breathing (see Chapter 2, Respiratory Physiology).

Another major argument against cuffed endotracheal tubes had been based on early experiences relating to laryngeal damage caused by overinflated, high-pressure/low-volume cuffed tubes for prolonged periods of time (Hawkins, 1977; Honig, 1979). Laryngeal damage should not occur from inflated endotracheal cuffs of limited duration intraoperatively if care is taken to make sure that the cuff is properly placed in the mid trachea, rather than straddling in the larynx (James, 2001). Okuyama and others (1995) determined the proper positioning of the cuff in small children by palpating the cuff externally between the cricoid and sternal notch. There were no complications attributable to the use of small (3.5 to 5.0 mm ID) cuffed tubes in children (Okuyama et al., 1995). Studies using low pressure-high volume cuffs have shown no difference in the rate of complications between cuffed and uncuffed endotracheal tubes in terms of long-term complications, such as subglottic stenosis (Deakers et al., 1994).

Care must be taken not to inflate the cuff greater than 25 cm H_2O to remain below the capillary perfusion pressure (20 to 25 mm Hg) of the laryngotracheal mucosa and to avoid pressure-induced mucosal ischemia and scarring (Tonnenson et al., 1981; Seegobin et al., 1984; James, 2001). During general anesthesia, nitrous oxide increases cuff pressure in a time-dependent fashion (Mehta, 1981); as high as six times the initial pressure can be reached and could cause laryngeal and tracheal mucosal ischemia (Patel et al., 1984). Alternatively, Patel and others (1984) recommend using saline, instead of air, to inflate the cuff. Inflating the cuff with the same gas mixture of nitrous oxide and oxygen should also protect the cuff from hyperinflation. In 174 children under general anesthesia with nitrous oxide using cuffed tubes inflated with room air, the cuff pressure was noted to increase variably, with increased cuff pressure occurring in 39% of cases. Numerous gas removals were required to maintain the cuff pressure less than 25 cm H_2O, especially during the first hour of anesthesia, independent of the tube sizes (Felten et al., 2003). For prolonged endotracheal anesthetics with nitrous oxide, a manometer should be attached to the cuff to monitor cuff pressures and prevent mucosal injury to the upper airways.

With a cuffed endotracheal tube, there is rarely a need for repeated laryngoscopic procedures because an endotracheal tube 0.5 to 1.0 mm (ID) smaller than the uncuffed tube is always selected and the leak around the tube is sealed by inflating the cuff (to 20 to 25 cm H_2O), thus avoiding multiple intubation attempts, important risk factors for trauma to the larynx and trachea (Khine et al., 1997). Choosing the correctly sized uncuffed endotracheal tube based on formulas tends to be extremely difficult (King et al., 1993). Additionally, the leak test (listening for leakage of air around the endotracheal tube) is unreliable, with large interobserver variations (Schwartz et al., 1993). Choosing cuffed endotracheal tubes solves all of these problems.

Finally, the use of cuffed endotracheal tubes is more economical than using uncuffed tubes. With cuffed tubes, a lower fresh gas flow can be used. Maintenance of inhalation anesthesia with low gas flow is not possible with uncuffed tubes with large leaks, and consumption of anesthetic agents increases as fresh gas flow is increased. Khine and others (1997) have shown that increased gas leak around the tube into the operating room environment importantly contributes to air pollution of the operating room, increasing anesthetic gases above the safe levels recommended by the National Institute of Occupational Safety and Health (NIOSH) (1997) (see www.osha.gov). Increased pollution of the operating room with anesthetic gases (particularly nitrous oxide) has been causatively linked to an increased incidence of miscarriages among female anesthesia providers exposed to anesthesia (Rowland et al., 1992, 1995).

In 1995, Okuyama and others in Japan reported a routine use of cuffed endotracheal tubes in small children without complications associated with this practice. At Hopital d'enfants Armand Trousseau in Paris, all children requiring mechanical ventilation intraoperatively have been intubated with cuffed endotracheal tubes since 1997 (Murat, 2001a). Of 3434 children under 8 years of age, 904 were infants (<1 year old). Of 55 respiratory complications reported, none were attributable to intubation and no subglottic stenosis was reported. The atmospheric level of nitrous oxide measured at the level of the anesthesia provider decreased from 48.1 ppm to 0.3 ppm after the institution wide adoption of the cuffed tube and closed circle system (Murat, 2001a).

One potential problem of using cuffed pediatric endotracheal tubes may be the inconsistency of existing cuffed tubes produced by different manufacturers, in terms of outer diameter for the same size (ID) tubes, different depth markings, and cuff length. There is the potential of cuffs inflating within the larynx or endobronchial intubation even when the cuff is properly positioned in the mid trachea (Weiss et al., 2004).

Stylets

Intubation in normal children rarely calls for the use of a stylet, particularly as a straight laryngoscope blade is used routinely. A stylet is likely to complicate the procedure, because its extraction after passage of the tube sometimes is difficult (it should be lubricated when used), inviting laryngospasm and hypoxia. The presence of a stiff, pointed object always adds potential trauma. A stylet, however, may help when patients have anatomic abnormalities and they should be kept available. The stylet of silicone-coated soft wire, manufactured for this use, is preferable; three different sizes are usually available to accommodate various tube sizes. Except for the most difficult intubation, the tip of a stylet should be recessed at least 1.5 to 2 cm from the tip of the endotracheal tube to keep the tip of the tube flexible and less traumatic, and the tube should be stoppered by a silicon rubber cork, or the stylet should be bent at the endotracheal tube adaptor to prevent accidental forward displacement of the stylet.

Guidelines for Endotracheal Tube Size and Depth

Various methods have been devised for choosing the correct diameter of endotracheal tubes in infants and children. Several formulas have been suggested and proved to be useful. These formulas should be used only as a general guide, however, because of the great variations in laryngeal size in relation to age, weight, or body length, revealed in data obtained at postmortem dissection (Engel, 1962; Butz, 1968), in living subjects using graduated bougies (Chodoff and Helrich, 1967; Keep and Manford, 1974; Mostafa, 1976), and by radiographic examination (Wittenborg et al., 1967). The formula most frequently used is that of Cole (1957):

$$\text{Tube size (French)} = \text{age (yr)} + 17$$

Or its modification (Morgan and Steward, 1982):

$$\text{Tube size (mm ID)} = [\text{age (yr)} + 16]/4$$

Both versions are applicable in children older than 2 years.

Penlington's formula (1974) is based on analysis of the data of Keep and Manford (1974) and gives a tube size similar to that derived with the Cole formula.

For children less than $6^1/_2$ years of age:

$$\text{Tube size (mm ID)} = \text{age (yr)}/3 + 3.5$$

For children $6^1/_2$ years and older:

$$\text{Tube size (mm ID)} = \text{age (yr)}/4 + 4.5$$

Another clinically useful yet scientifically untested method used by some anesthesiologists is to compare the outer diameter of the tube with that of the child's small (fifth) finger. Again, these formulas are useful as general guides, but the airway size varies greatly from one child to the next, necessitating a leak test after every intubation to confirm that the tube size is adequate. The leak test is accomplished by gently squeezing the anesthesia bag or by closing the pop-off valve of the anesthesia circuit and letting the airway pressure rise slowly; the airway pressure at which audible gas leak occurs around the tube is detected with a stethoscope. The leak pressure should be between 15 and 25 cm H_2O. When a cuffed endotracheal tube is used, the selection of the tube size is less important, because an endotracheal tube one or two sizes (0.5 to 1.0 mm ID) smaller than the uncuffed tube normally used is selected and the gas leak around the tube is accommodated by inflating the cuff.

In the classic retrospective study by Koka and others (1977), postoperative laryngotracheitis (postintubation croup) was associated with excessive endotracheal tube size (no leak at 40 cm H_2O) more than any other factor. Furthermore, the use of an oversized tube has a greater effect on the incidence of postintubation croup in children with a history of infectious or postintubation croup compared with those without a similar history (Lee et al., 1980). Khalil and others (1998) did not find a similar correlation between the leakage of airway gas mixture around the tube and the incidence of postoperative croup among 159 healthy outpatient children undergoing strabismus correction. They, however, did find a positive correlation between the duration of surgery (>2 hours) and the incidence and severity of postoperative croup. This difference in the postintubation croup may be related in part to the difference in the materials of the endotracheal tube—sterile, implant-tested tubes versus the older-type tubes used in the earlier study, which were not sterilized. Indeed, Litman and Keon (1991) found far less incidence of postintubation croup (0.1%) among 5589 healthy children compared with the incidence of 1% among the 7875 children reported in the original study by Koka and others (1977). Nevertheless, oversized endotracheal tubes are clearly associated with subglottic injury, and the air leakage around the endotracheal tube should be kept between 15 and 25 cm H_2O for both cuffed and uncuffed tubes to prevent ischemia of mucosa around the endotracheal tube. This also ensures adequate tidal ventilation.

A report with an editorial in *Anesthesiology* has raised renewed awareness of laryngeal trauma from routine endotracheal intubation. Tanaka and others (2003) studied laryngeal resistance under general anesthesia in adult patients before and after clinically atraumatic intubations lasting 1 to 4 hours. After extubation they found that airway resistance (pressure drop across the larynx) increased significantly from preintubation values, whereas there was no change in laryngeal resistance postoperatively in the control group of patients anesthetized with LMA. Furthermore, flexible laryngoscopy revealed considerable laryngeal swelling and narrowing of the vocal cord angle only in the postextubation group (Tanaka et al., 2003). This study raises a great deal of concern about safety, regarding whether routine endotracheal intubation is as safe as one assumes (or wishes)

TABLE 10–2. Endotracheal tube size*

Age	Weight (kg)	ID (mm)	Length (OT) (cm)	Length (NT) (cm)	Suction Catheter (F)
Premie	0.7 to 1.0	2.5	7 to 8	9	5
Premie	1.0 to 2.5	3.0	8 to 9	9 to 10	5
Newborn	2.5 to 3.5	3.5	9 to 10	11 to 12	6
3 mo	3.5 to 5.0	3.5	10 to 11	12	6
3 to 9 mo	5.0 to 8.0	3.5 to 4.0	11 to 12	13 to 14	6
9 to 18 mo	8.0 to 11.0	4.0 to 4.5	12 to 13	14 to 15	8
1.5 to 3 yr	11.0 to 15.0	4.5 to 5.0	12 to 14	16 to 17	8
4 to 5 yr	15.0 to 18.0	5.0 to 5.5	14 to 16	18 to 19	10
6 to 7 yr	19.0 to 23.0	5.5 to 6.0	16 to 18	19 to 20	10
8 to 10 yr	24.0 to 30.0	6.0 to 6.5	20 to 22	21 to 23	10
10 to 11 yr	30.0 to 35.0	6.0 to 6.5†	20 to 22	22 to 24	12
12 to 13 yr	35.0 to 40.0	6.5 to 7.0*	20 to 22	23 to 25	12
14 to 16 yr	45.0 to 55.0	7.0 to 7.5*	20 to 22	24 to 25	12

ID, inner diameter; OT, orotracheal tube; NT, nasotracheal tube; F, French size (number is approximately equal to ID × 4).

*The endotracheal tube should fit so as to allow full normal expansion of both lungs with positive airway pressure but to permit a gas leak about the tube at 20 to 25 cm H_2O.

†Cuffed tube.

Data modified from Smith RM: *Anesthesia for infants and children.* CV Mosby, 1980, St. Louis; Davenport HT: *Paediatric anaesthesia.* Year Book Medical Publishers, 1973, Chicago.

(Maktabi et al., 2003). This concern is especially valid with pediatric anesthesiologists, because the effect of upper airway swelling on airway resistance would be far greater in infants and young children with smaller airways sized in absolute terms (see Chapter 2, Respiratory Physiology).

Table 10–2 is a general guide for the choice of tube diameter related to age, as recommended by Smith (1980b) and Davenport (1973), with modifications. One takes the endotracheal tube size indicated as most suitable as indicated in the table, as well as the next larger and next smaller sizes. Of these three, one should be the correct size. The tube diameters listed should allow some leakage around the tube at 20 to 25 cm H_2O of airway pressure if the size is adequate yet not excessive.

Should the child be reintubated if there is no gas leakage around the endotracheal tube (>30 cm H_2O) after the initial intubation? A practical guideline would be to consider changing the tube to the next smaller (i.e., 0.5 mm less ID) size, if the surgical procedure is expected to take longer than 2 hours (Khalil et al., 1998). If the passage of the endotracheal tube was smooth without resistance and the case is expected to be relatively short (i.e., <1 hour), the tube may be kept in place, considering the fact that each attempt for intubation would add an additional chance of causing more mucosal damage to the larynx (Tanaka et al., 2003). In either case, the patient should be pretreated with dexamethasone (0.4 to 0.5 mg/kg) to prevent mucosal swelling and postoperative croup. If one plans to use a cuffed endotracheal tube, the tube size should be 0.5 to 1.0 mm ID smaller than the uncuffed tube, to accommodate the easy passage of the cuff through the subglottic space.

Endotracheal Tube Length

Much concern has also been shown for establishing the proper lengths for oral and nasal endotracheal tubes at different ages (Shellinger, 1964; Fearson and Whalen, 1967; Coldiron, 1968; Mattila et al., 1971; Morgan and Steward, 1982a, 1982b). In most full-term newborn infants, the proper distance is 9 to 10 cm at the incisor; it is considerably less in the premature infant. At 1 year of age, the length increases to about 12 cm (Davenport, 1973), and at 3 years, it increases to 14 cm (Morgan and Steward, 1982b). Beyond this age, Morgan and Steward (1982a) found remarkably good correlations between airway length (incisors to midarea of trachea) and age, height, or weight. Their formula, based on regression equations for age (>3 years), can be approximated by the following simplified formula:

$$\text{Airway length (cm)} = \text{age (yr)}/2 + 13$$

which closely resembles that of Cole (1957) (age/2 + 12). Airway length also can be estimated by the following equations by Morgan and Steward (1982a):

$$\text{Airway length (cm)} = \text{height (cm)}/10 + 5 = \text{weight (kg)}/5 + 12$$

As with tube diameter, however, the variations prove too great to allow a reliance on any predetermined reference scale. The correct length, therefore, must be determined individually at the time of intubation. The tip of the endotracheal tube should be advanced under direct vision, not more than 2.5 cm in newborn infants, because the distance between the glottis and the carina is only 4 to 5 cm and is even shorter in premature neonates (Fearson and Whalen, 1967). In older children, a cuffed endotracheal tube is advanced not more than 1 cm beyond the upper end of the cuff, to disappear through the glottis. The desired length of a nasotracheal tube may be considered to be 20% more than that of an orotracheal tube for practical use (Smith, 1980b).

Yates and others (1987) derived a simple formula for estimating the nasotracheal tube length in infants and children, based on the tube size S (ID) chosen by the formula of Morgan and Steward (1982b):

$$S = [\text{age (yr)} + 16]/4)$$

The length of the nasotracheal tube (L) is:

$$L = (2.8 \times S) + 2.7 \ (r = 0.99)$$

The practical formula is simplified as follows:

$$L = (3 \times S) + 2$$

Table 10–3 is a comparison of the estimated nasotracheal tube length with this formula and two previously published formulas (Rees, 1966; Steward, 1979).

■ **TABLE 10–3.** Recommended nasotracheal tube dimensions

		TUBE LENGTH (L) (cm)		
Age (yr)	***Tube Size (S) (ID, mm)***	***Yates et al. (1987)***	***Rees (1966)***	***Steward (1979)***
0 to 3 mo	2.5 to 3.0	9.5 to 11.0	11.8	13.5
4 to 7 mo	3.5 to 4.0	12.5 to 14.0	13.6	
1	4.0	14.0	14.5	15.0
2	4.5	15.5	15.2	16.0
3	4.5 to 5.0	15.5 to 17.0	15.6	
4	5.0	17.0	16.5	17.0
5	5.0 to 5.5	17.0 to 18.5	16.8	
6	5.5	18.5	17.1	19.0
7	5.5 to 6.0	18.5 to 20.0	17.8	
8	6.0	20.0	18.3	21.0
9	6.0 to 6.5	20.0 to 21.5	18.8	
10	6.5	21.0	19.1	22.0
11	6.5 to 7.0	21.5 to 23.0	19.1	
12	7.0	23.0		22.0

■ TECHNIQUES FOR ENDOTRACHEAL INTUBATION

■ ORAL INTUBATION UNDER GENERAL ANESTHESIA AND MUSCLE RELAXANTS

Once anesthesia has been induced and an intravenous route established, an intravenous bolus of atropine (0.01 to 0.02 mg/kg) is recommended for neonates and young infants, especially when the patient is bradycardic (<100/min) or hypotensive, because compliance of ventricles is low and cardiac output is rate dependent in this age group (see Chapter 3, Cardiovascular Physiology). Until recently, atropine or glycopyrrolate (half the dose of atropine) was given routinely to children for halothane induction to prevent bradycardia and hypotension. With sevoflurane induction, the use of vagolytic agents is optional in older infants and children because, with careful induction, marked myocardial depression and bradycardia are not commonly encountered. If the procedure dictates muscle relaxation, a nondepolarizing muscle relaxant is usually administered next, to facilitate endotracheal intubation. Intermediate-acting nondepolarizing relaxants, such as cisatracurium (0.2 mg/kg) and vecuronium (0.1 mg/kg), are most commonly used for endotracheal intubation (Brandom et al., 1984; Meakin et al., 1988; Meretoja, 1989; Sloan et al., 1991; Kenaan et al., 2000; Taivanien et al., 2000). Intubating doses of muscle relaxants are shown in Table 10–4.

Intravenous succinylcholine, the only depolarizing muscle relaxant in use, has the fastest onset of action and shortest duration of action of all muscle relaxants (Brandom et al., 1989; Gronert et al., 1993a, 1993b) and is especially useful in patients with a full stomach, in whom a rapid sequence induction with propofol or thiopental is required. The *routine* use of succinylcholine in children under 10 years of age is not recommended, due to the small chance that the child may have an unrecognized muscle disease (e.g., Duchenne's) that may result in hyperkalemia and cardiac arrest (Delphin et al., 1987; Rosenberg and Gronert, 1992). Under these circumstances, as many as 60% of afflicted children could not be resuscitated. This finding is coupled with the fact that there are many good alternative nondepolarizing muscle relaxants to succinylcholine, even for short pediatric surgical cases. However, in infants and children with a full stomach requiring emergency surgery, succinylcholine provides the fastest onset of muscle relaxation and spontaneous recovery.

■ **TABLE 10–4.** Intravenous doses of muscle relaxants for intubation

Drug	**Dose (mg/kg)**
Succinylcholine	
Infants	3.0 (Meakin et al., 1989)
Children	2.0
Adolescents/adults	1.0
Pancuronium	0.1 to 0.15 (Cunliffe et al., 1986)
Vecuronium	0.1 to 0.15 (Meretoja, 1989)
Cisatracurium	0.15 to 0.2 (Taivanien et al., 2000)
Mivacurium	0.2 to 0.3 (Gronert et al., 1994)
Rocuronium	0.6 to 0.8 (O'Kelly et al., 1991)

Rocuronium and vecuronium, nondepolarizing muscle relaxants, offer a possible alternative to succinylcholine for rapid sequence intubation. Bolus intravenous administration of 0.6 mg/kg of rocuronium produces complete neuromuscular blockade of the adductor pollicis in infants and children in an average of 49 and 80 seconds, respectively (Woelfel et al., 1994). Increasing the dose to 0.8 mg/kg in children shortens this time to an average of 28 seconds (O'Kelly et al., 1991). Spontaneous recovery of T1 (the first of the train-of-four twitches) to 25% of control requires 26.7 minutes and 45.1 minutes in infants and children, respectively, with 0.6 mg/kg of rocuronium. If the dose of vecuronium in children is increased from 0.1 mg/kg to 0.4 mg/kg, the time to paralysis of the thumb (to 95% depression of twitch response) shortens from an average of 83 seconds to 39 seconds (Sloan et al., 1991). With this increased dose of vecuronium, however, the duration of action of vecuronium approaches that of pancuronium.

When the patient is adequately anesthetized, the anesthetic concentration is reduced to a maintenance level, nitrous oxide is turned off, and the patient is preoxygenated with increased ventilation briefly with 100% oxygen in preparation for endotracheal intubation. Alternatively, in most children a 50% nitrous oxide–oxygen mixture may be used safely before intubation while oxygen saturation of hemoglobin is monitored continuously with a pulse oximeter. The time for achieving FIO_2 of greater than 0.9, after nitrous oxide is turned off and 100% oxygen is

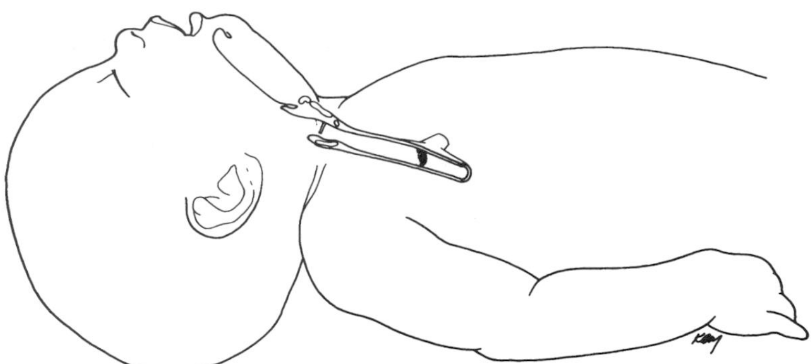

■ **FIGURE 10–12.** Anatomic drawing of neonatal airway with actual relations of the larynx, trachea, and supporting cartilages.

turned on, was reported to be less than 60 seconds (mean, 36 seconds) in spontaneously breathing infants. In older children, the time for achieving FIO_2 of greater than 0.9 was within an average of 40 to 70 seconds (Morrison et al., 1998). The time for achieving FIO_2 sufficient for intubation would be substantially shorter were the patient manually hyperventilated. Intubation normally is relatively easy to perform in children, but it may prove rather difficult in young infants.

The anatomic drawing in Figure 10–12 illustrates the dimensional relations of the glottis, trachea, and supporting cartilages with the head of an infant properly positioned for laryngoscopy and intubation. The large tongue relative to small mandible, large head, and short neck is obvious, as is the high (cephalad) location of the epiglottis. In infants at or younger than 4 months, the epiglottis is at or above the level of the first cervical vertebra overlapping with the soft palate (Fig. 10–13) (Sasaki et al., 1977). By 6 months of age, the epiglottis has moved down to the level of the third cervical vertebra and separated from the soft palate (Fig. 10–14) (Sasaki et al., 1977), probably making oral breathing more feasible. Unlike in adults, the epiglottis in infants and young children is hard and narrow, folded into an omega or "U" shape (Fig. 10–15, see also Color Plate on the DVD), and is often difficult to lift with the tip of a laryngoscope blade. Until adolescence, the shape of a child's larynx is that of an inverted cone, with the circular cricoid cartilage at its narrowest (lowest) point; the shape of the adult larynx is more cylindrical (Eckenhoff, 1951; Coté and Todres, 1993).

Before intubation is attempted, the anesthesiologist is seated comfortably or standing at the proper height in relation to the operating table, with eye level about 1 foot above the patient's head. This positioning provides the proper angle and distance for visualization. The child's neck is moderately extended beyond a neutral position or "sniffing" position to align the oral, pharyngeal, and laryngeal axes (Stoelting, 1986). A soft head ring may be used to help stabilize the head. In infants, it is not necessary to elevate the head by placing pads under the occiput to align the upper airway axes because the infant's head is disproportionately large.

For laryngoscopy a straight blade is most commonly used. The mask is lifted and the oral airway, if used, is removed. The blade held by the left hand is moistened and inserted through the right corner of the mouth while the head is held in the extended position by the right hand. Opening the mouth by crossing or scissoring the right index finger and the thumb at the right corner of the mouth, the technique commonly practiced

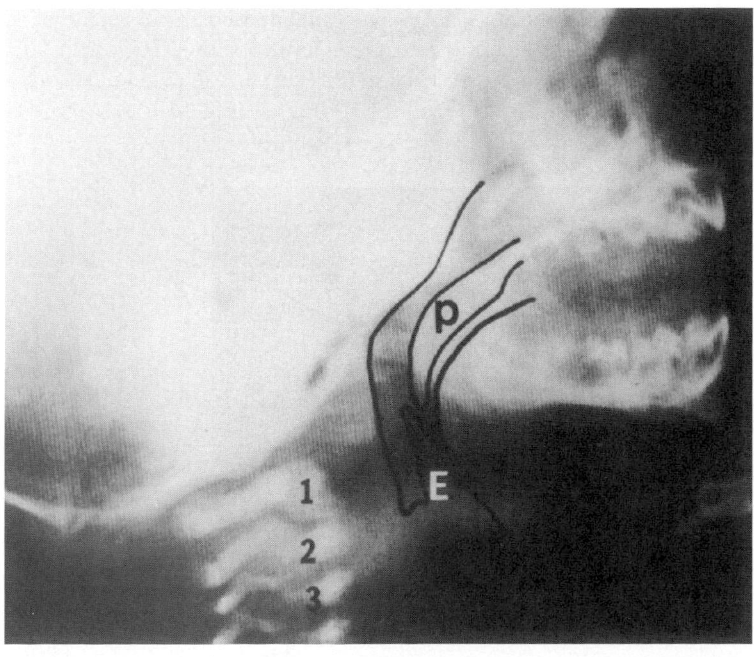

■ **FIGURE 10–13.** Lateral neck radiograph in the neonatal period indicates epiglottis at level of first cervical vertebra. Epiglottis (E) engages posterior surface of soft palate (P) during tidal respiration. (From Sasaki CT, Levine PA, Laitman JT, et al.: *Arch Otolaryngol* 103:169, 1977. Copyright 1977, American Medical Association.)

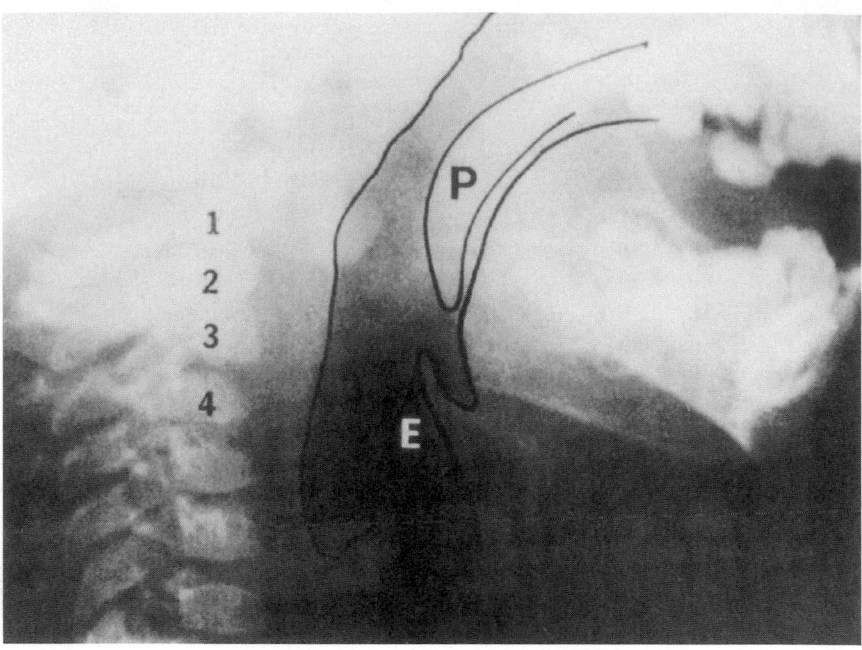

■ **FIGURE 10–14.** Lateral neck radiograph at age 18 months. Epiglottis (E) remains at level of third cervical vertebra. P, soft palate. (From Sasaki CT, Levine PA, Laitman JT, et al.: *Arch Otolaryngol* 103:169, 1977. Copyright 1977, American Medical Association.)

for the adult patient, should not be used in infants and young children because the small mouth opening prevents the practitioner from properly inserting the laryngoscope blade at the right corner of the mouth and swinging the tongue to the left.

The laryngoscope blade is now moved gently toward the midline to displace the tongue to the left. It is then advanced further toward the epiglottis at about a 45-degree angle to the horizontal plane, and the laryngoscope handle is gently lifted forward and upward along its axis. The larynx is now exposed, and the posterior portion of the vocal cords should be visible below or behind the epiglottis.

In an anesthetized, relaxed child, the blade should barely touch the upper teeth and lip. Needless to say, one should never use the upper teeth as a lever to pivot the laryngoscope blade; such a motion would easily result in the damage to or loss of teeth and bleeding. One should also be careful not to pinch the upper or lower lip between the teeth and the laryngoscope blade.

In older children, the distal end of the straight blade is further advanced beneath the lower (laryngeal) surface of the epiglottis, and the laryngoscope handle is lifted upward along the axis of the handle to achieve full exposure of the glottis. In infants, however, because the epiglottis is hard and omega shaped (see Fig. 10–15), it may be difficult to pick up with the blade. In this situation, the straight blade is simply advanced into the pharyngeal base of the epiglottis or the vallecula, and the laryngoscope handle is lifted upward and slightly forward, as with a Macintosh blade, to expose the glottis. A straight blade with a curved tip, such as a No. 1 Phillips blade, is especially useful under these circumstances.

The endotracheal tube, held lightly with the right thumb and index finger and supported by the middle finger, is inserted along the right side of the blade but not through the straight part of the blade, so as to maintain an unobstructed view as the tip of the tube slips through the glottic opening. The tube is further advanced to the black marker on the tube or about 2.5 cm

A

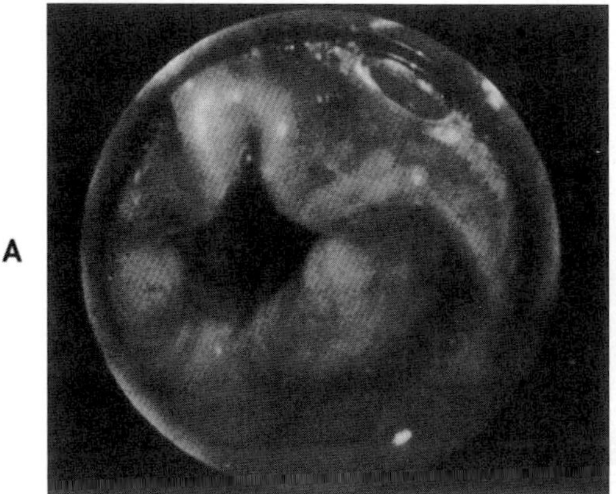

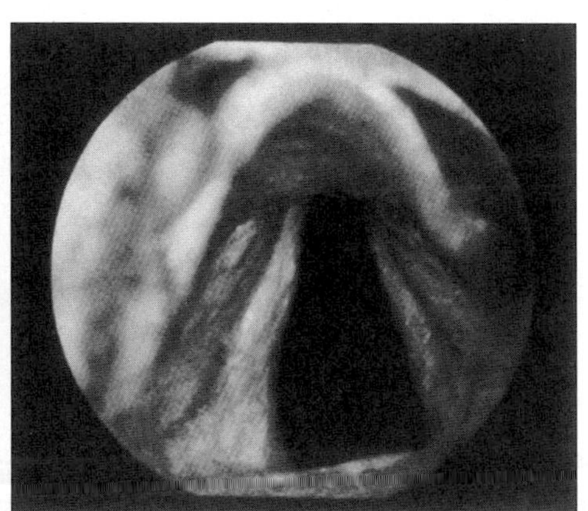

B

■ **FIGURE 10–15.** A, Infant glottis. B, Adult glottis. Note the soft, edematous appearance of infant tissue and folded, omega (Ω) or "U" shape of the infant glottis (see Color Plates on the DVD) (Courtesy Dr. Hollinger, Chicago.)

(more in older children) from the tip, halfway between the glottis and the carina in newborn infants. When a cuffed endotracheal tube is used, one should make sure that the upper end of the cuff disappears out of sight and the tube advanced an additional centimeter or two. One eye should be kept on the glottis throughout the process of intubation. The tube is then held tightly against the child's upper teeth or lip as the laryngoscope blade is withdrawn gently and a distance number, or any symbol on the tube wall at the lip, is noted as the proper depth marker.

If the tube meets resistance at the cords, the fingers holding the tube should rotate the tip of the tube slightly and gently. If resistance beyond the vocal cords cannot be cleared by this maneuver, the tube should be withdrawn, remembering that the narrowest diameter of the upper airway system is at the cricoid cartilage rather than at the glottis (Eckenhoff, 1951). After reoxygenation, laryngoscopy is repeated with a smaller endotracheal tube.

Correct positioning of the endotracheal tube is confirmed by symmetric ventilatory movements of both hemithoraces with manual positive pressure ventilation, by equal and satisfactory breath sounds bilaterally in the upper aspect of the chest, and by the presence of an end-tidal carbon dioxide waveform on a capnograph. It is important to listen to the right upper aspect of the chest because ventilation of the right upper lobe is most vulnerable in cases of endobronchial intubation, especially if the tube is without a Murphy eye. Occasionally, the right upper lobe originates from an anomalous tracheal bronchus above the carina, which is easily blocked if the tip of the tube is close to the carina (Vredevoe et al., 1981). Once the correct position has been verified, and the depth marker on the tube that is aligned with the lip or incisors has been reconfirmed, the endotracheal tube is fixed with adhesive tape.

Induction of anesthesia and intubation may be achieved by means of intravenous atropine, propofol or thiopental, and succinylcholine, followed by intubation, fixation of the tube, and establishment of controlled ventilation with high concentrations of inhalation anesthesia in healthy, well-prepared children and adolescents, as in healthy adults. This technique is not suitable in infants and young children, however, because their cardiovascular system is exceptionally sensitive to a sudden increase in anesthetic concentration after the administration of propofol or thiopental. In the presence of airway problems, such as in patients with upper airway obstruction or difficult anatomy, one should never induce apnea with muscle relaxants unless it is certain that manual ventilation can be maintained.

INTUBATION UNDER GENERAL ANESTHESIA ALONE

In infants and children with intact cardiovascular function, endotracheal intubation can be accomplished safely under deep inhalation anesthesia without muscle relaxants. Once anesthesia has been induced by mask with a volatile anesthetic and intravenous access is established, the patient is deepened with a high concentration of sevoflurane (6% to 8%) in oxygen with controlled ventilation for a few minutes while the heart rate and tone are continuously monitored through a precordial stethoscope and blood pressure watched to avoid excessive myocardial depression. Intravenous atropine may be given as indicated. After the child has become motionless and apneic, with fixed pupils, vocal cords are sprayed with 1% to 2% lidocaine (1 mg/kg) under direct vision with a laryngoscope. Lidocaine spray can be accomplished with a metal or plastic atomizer tip attached to a 3-mL syringe. Alternatively, a 20- or 22-gauge plastic intravenous catheter with the needle removed can be used for the same purpose if an appropriate atomizer is not readily available. The child's lungs are manually ventilated for an additional 6 to 12 breaths with sevoflurane in oxygen to give enough time for topical anesthetic to take effect before laryngoscopy and endotracheal intubation. With this technique, laryngospasm is avoided even when the patient becomes too light or if intubation is not swiftly accomplished. Alternatively, a dose of intravenous propofol (1 to 2 mg/kg) is given once the patient is sufficiently deepened for laryngoscopy and intubation. In most children undergoing relatively short surgical procedures requiring endotracheal tubes for airway protection, such as adenotonsillectomies, endotracheal intubation can be achieved without muscle relaxants, the potential side effects of these drugs thus being avoided.

The depth of anesthesia is often difficult to judge. The most reliable signs of adequate depth for intubation are centrally fixed pupils, flaccidity of arms and hands, jaw relaxation, apnea, and blood pressure lower than the preinduction level. Because infants and young children have relatively high MAC and increased myocardial sensitivity to inhaled anesthetics, intubation under deep inhaled anesthetics should be performed with the utmost care, with continuous attention to the quality of heart tone, by means of a precordial stethoscope, in addition to standard monitoring. In healthy children, 1 to 12 years old, deep sevoflurane provides satisfactory anesthetic induction and intubating conditions and more rapid emergence than provided by halothane (Sarner et al., 1995). Heart rate and systolic blood pressure were better maintained during the anesthetic induction period with sevoflurane than with halothane.

Position, Size, and Fixation of Endotracheal Tube

Numerous complications are caused by the incorrect placement of endotracheal tubes and their dislodgment after intubation. Accidental intubation of the esophagus may occur and may be difficult to immediately recognize. For this reason, auscultation with a stethoscope over both sides of the chest and confirmation of CO_2 waveforms with capnography are essential. Endobronchial intubation is a relatively common occurrence. As stated earlier, the endotracheal tube should be advanced under direct vision just beyond the vocal cords, that is, 2 to 2.5 cm in newborn infants and not more than 3 to 4 cm in older children. Unfortunately, this approach is not always possible, especially when unusual anatomy makes it difficult to visualize the larynx. Alternatively, the endotracheal tube may be advanced until the breath sounds in one lung (usually left side) start to diminish; the tube is then pulled back by 2 to 4 cm and taped securely.

After intubating the child, the anesthesiologist should keep the patient's head in the intended position for surgery when confirming breath sounds because flexion and extension of the head can cause considerable movement of the tube (Bosman and Foster, 1977). Continuous auscultation with a precordial stethoscope over the left sternal border is a reliable method for detecting endobronchial intubation (Smith, 1975). In this situation auscultation is better than pulse oximeter because breath sounds diminish or disappear over the left chest long before oxygen desaturation is noticed on pulse oximetry. When intubation is intended for prolonged ventilatory support, as in the intensive care unit, radiographic confirmation of its position is essential at the outset and at subsequent intervals as indicated.

To securely fix the endotracheal tube, common cloth-backed adhesive tape usually serves well. Both the tube and skin surface over and under the lips should be clean and dry. Nearly every pediatric anesthesiologist has his or her own "right" way of taping the endotracheal tube. One method is to use two strips of 1-inch-wide tape that are long enough to extend halfway to the ear on each side of the mouth. Each tape is split halfway longitudinally. The intact half of the first tape is applied to the right cheek. The upper half of the split strip is taped across the mouth between the nose and upper lip to the left cheek, while the lower half of the strip is wrapped spirally toward the proximal end of the tube, which is usually situated at the right corner of the mouth. The second tape is again applied on the right cheek. The lower half of the split strip is taped across the mouth below the lower lip toward the left cheek, while the upper half of the strip is wrapped spirally around the endotracheal tube as with the first tape. Tincture of benzoin seldom is needed for the average procedure in children, although it should be used before prolonged procedures, particularly for craniotomies and posterior spinal fusions, in which the patient is in the prone position or the endotracheal tube is out of sight or reach of the anesthesiologist.

When the maintenance of patent airway is difficult, requiring oropharyngeal airway during the induction of anesthesia, the airway should be reinserted before extubation at the conclusion of surgery and anesthesia to make sure that an adequate airway is maintained during emergence from anesthesia after extubation. During the maintenance of anesthesia, a soft bite block commonly made of rolled and taped 4 × 4-inch gauze sponges suffices to keep the patient from clamping down on the tube. If the head is moved either laterally or vertically, the anesthesiologist should hold both the head and tube together so that there is no change in relative position. If the child's body is to be moved or the operating table turned, the tube is disconnected from the anesthesia breathing apparatus until the new position has been reestablished.

NASOTRACHEAL INTUBATION

Nasotracheal intubation is indicated for a number of surgical procedures involving the mouth and face. In addition, nasal tubes are preferred when patients are expected to require postoperative ventilatory care, because the nasal tube can be fixed more securely, is less irritating to the patient, and cannot be bitten. Nasal intubation is more difficult and time consuming to perform compared with oral intubation and can start profuse hemorrhage from the nose or pharynx. Furthermore, pieces of adenoidal tissues can be torn away, and these and other scrapings may be carried into the trachea, increasing the danger of lower airway obstruction and pulmonary infection (Berry et al., 1973).

Before starting anesthesia, one should check the patency of the nares by having the child breathe through the nose with the mouth closed while each nostril is blocked in turn (Block and Brechner, 1973). Frequently, air moves better through one nostril than the other, making it the better one to use for intubation. The application of a nasal decongestant (such as 0.05% oxymetazoline) is recommended to vasoconstrict the nasal mucosa and to minimize hemorrhage, especially when the turbinate appears swollen. If phenylephrine (0.25%) is used instead, the dose should be limited to 20 mcg/kg to prevent possible systemic side effects.

In preadolescent children, one may expect to use uncuffed nasotracheal tubes of the same size that is required for oral intubation (Yates et al., 1987). Older children may require a nasal tube that is two or three sizes (1.0 to 1.5 mm OD) smaller with a cuff. The length of a nasal tube at the nostril should be approximately 20% longer than that of an oral tube at the incisors (see Table 10–3).

Nasal intubation may be expected to take longer and thus requires a well-established depth of anesthesia and/or muscle relaxation. In addition to the use of a lubricant on the endotracheal tube and a nasal decongestant, a topical spray of a local anesthetic (1% to 4% lidocaine) applied to the nostrils, pharynx, and glottis reduces the chance of inducing laryngeal responses in patients who are not given muscle relaxants. One must be careful, however, not to overdose the child with local anesthetic (one squeeze of the atomizer equals approximately 0.1 mL, or 4 mg of lidocaine, if a 4% solution is used), because topical anesthetics are absorbed rapidly from the mucosal surface. In addition, if the atomizer is not held upright during spraying, a large unknown quantity of local anesthetic can be deposited inadvertently on the mucosal surface and can cause a circulatory catastrophe. It is therefore imperative to preset the total dose of lidocaine (not more than 5 to 6 mg/kg) in an atomizer or a disposable cannula-syringe set (LTA set; Abbott Laboratories, North Chicago, Ill.). Alternatively, intravenous lidocaine (1.5 mg/kg) may be used. With rapid onset of action, it seems to be as effective as topical anesthesia in the adult (Hamill et al., 1981).

When the child is suitably prepared, the head is slightly elevated and the neck extended as with oral intubation. A well-lubricated nasotracheal tube is inserted through a nostril and advanced gently as the remaining body of the tube is pushing down against the upper rim of the nostril. If the tip of the tube is pointed straight downward or toward the base of the skull, as frequently happens when inserted by the inexperienced, the tube would gouge its way through the turbinate, causing bleeding. When properly directed, the tube may meet mild resistance, which may be overcome by pulling the tube back slightly and rotating it before it is again gently advanced. If one encounters a solid obstruction, the attempt should be halted, the tube withdrawn, and the opposite naris tried.

As noted previously, there is a definite danger of shearing off adenoidal tissues in children, with bothersome bleeding and the additional risk that pieces of adenoid may either be carried into the trachea or remain as obstructing plugs in the tube. To prevent this from occurring, a suction catheter can be inserted through the endotracheal tube with its tip protruding beyond the tip of the tube, thus acting as a probe as the tube is advanced. The nasotracheal tube that is hung up in the nasopharynx can also be redirected safely by inserting a gloved finger through the mouth (provided the child is well anesthetized or paralyzed) and gently lifting the tip of the tube off the posterior pharyngeal wall as it is advanced.

When the tube has reached the pharynx, the child can be ventilated manually through the tube as a nasopharyngeal airway by connecting the anesthesia circuit to it while the opposite nostril and the mouth are occluded by the left hand. With this maneuver, the patient can be adequately ventilated without removing and reinserting the nasotracheal tube through the nasopharynx, especially when intubation is difficult or prolonged.

A laryngoscope is then passed to visualize the tube and glottis. It may be possible to maneuver the glottis into position by flexing

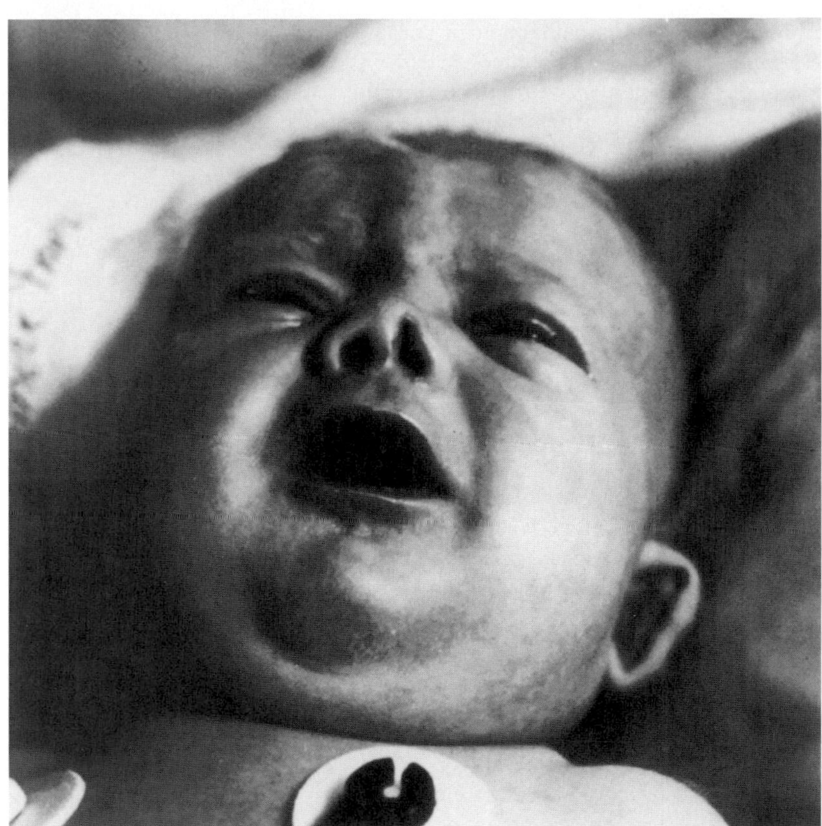

■ **FIGURE 10–16.** Nasal ulceration caused by pressure of nasotracheal tube during critical neonatal illness.

or extending the neck and inserting the tube under direct vision. If the tube is too straight, the neck should be extended. If the tube is too sharply curved, the head must be lifted and the neck flexed. Frequently, the Magill forceps are needed to direct the tube into the glottic opening, with an assistant ready to advance the tube when it is properly positioned. If the tube is too straight, its tip is grasped with the Magill forceps and redirected downward or posteriorly as the assistant advances the tube. If a cuffed endotracheal tube is being used, it is imperative to position the Magill forceps either proximal or distal to the cuff when directing the endotracheal tube advancement, because grasping the cuff portion of the tube often damages the cuff.

In taping the nasotracheal tube in place, it is extremely important to avoid creating pressure of the tube against the edge of the nostril. This could easily traumatize the soft tissue and, if prolonged, would produce ulceration followed by nasal scarring and obvious facial distortion (Fig. 10–16). The tube should be taped so that the entire upper rim of the nostril is visible and can be observed throughout the surgery and during postoperative intensive care, should this be necessary.

Blind nasotracheal intubation in children, particularly in infants, is rather difficult and is not recommended because the glottis is situated more cephalad and the tubes are less adaptable, increasing the likelihood of trauma and hemorrhage. With the advent of ultrathin fiberoptic bronchoscopy, allowing atraumatic intubation in infants and small children with difficult airways (Patil et al., 1983), there is no justification for blind nasotracheal intubation (Berry, 1984, 1986).

■ INTUBATION IN A CHILD WITH A FULL STOMACH

Overview

One of the most dangerous and challenging situations in anesthetizing all age groups is the patient whose stomach is filled with solid food or distended by intestinal obstruction. Mendelson (1946) reported 66 cases of fulminating chemical pneumonitis (Mendelson syndrome) occurring in pregnant women following pulmonary aspiration of gastric contents during obstetric anesthesia. The report drew attention to the danger of a full stomach and aspiration during general anesthesia, although the incidence of aspiration in this report was relatively low and only two patients died of causes not directly associated with anesthesia. Additional early studies, however, reported high morbidity and mortality, especially among infants and children associated with gastric aspiration (Smith, 1956; Graff et al., 1964).

These reports of high mortality associated with perioperative aspiration alerted the emerging specialty of anesthesiology to the problem and have resulted in numerous experimental and clinical studies during the ensuing half century, attempting to minimize the risk of perianesthetic gastric aspiration and its associated complications. Prophylaxes of gastric aspiration included rapid sequence intubation with a cuffed endotracheal tube; cricoid pressure (Sellick, 1961); attempts to reduce gastric acidity with sodium citrate (Henderson et al., 1987) and H_2 blockers (Goudsouzian et al., 1981; Goudsouzian and Young, 1987); and attempts to reduce gastric fluid volume with glycopyrrolate (Salem et al., 1976) and metoclopramide (Lerman et al., 1988).

A large-scale epidemiologic study from Sweden in the mid-1980s involving more than 185,000 general anesthetics revealed quite a different story. Although the radiographic evidence of pneumonia (or atelectasis) was confirmed in 47% of cases, the mortality rate in children was relatively low (0.2:10,000). The incidence of aspiration of gastric contents in children, however, was significantly higher than that in the adult population (8.6 versus 4.5:10,000) (Olsson et al., 1986). Risk factors for perianesthetic aspiration included the skill and experience of anesthetists; a number of coexisting diseases and ASA physical status (PS) 3 to 5; emergency surgery, especially at night; and neurologic or esophagogastric abnormality (Olsson et al., 1986). Other high-risk categories included children with intestinal obstruction, increased intracranial pressure, and increased abdominal pressure and obesity. Incidence of gastric aspiration was even lower in studies from the French-speaking countries (1.0:10,000) (Tiret et al., 1988) and from Norway (2.9:10,000) (Mellin-Olsen et al., 1988) in the 1980s.

The first study from the United States came from Children's Hospital of Pittsburgh and reported an incidence of aspiration of gastric contents of 4.9:10,000 based on 50,880 anesthetic procedures (Borland et al., 1998). In this institution, pulmonary aspiration of gastric contents was treated aggressively with flexible bronchoscopy and removal of solid food particles, if any were present, followed by reexpansion of the lungs and the maintenance of CPAP. Twenty-nine percent of these children were kept intubated in the postanesthetic care unit (PACU) and only 23% of these patients stayed overnight. None of these children developed clinically significant pneumonia, and there were no deaths (Borland et al., 1998). Similarly, a study from the Mayo Clinic reported the incidence of aspiration being low (3.8:10,000) and similar to that of adults (3.1:10,000) with no serious respiratory morbidity and no associated deaths (Warner et al., 1999). These epidemiologic studies suggest that the incidence of gastric aspiration and associated morbidity and mortality in both adults and children has declined considerably. The risk of aspiration, however, remains higher in infants and children than in adults (Olsson et al., 1986; Tiret et al., 1988; Weaver, 1993).

Based on these findings of reduced incidence, morbidity, and mortality associated with aspiration of gastric contents in children, the routine use of preoperative antacid or H_2 blocker may not be justified (Weaver, 1993; Borland et al., 1998). In children, the majority of gastric aspiration occurs during inhalation induction without muscle relaxants (Warner et al., 1999) or during intravenous induction (Borland et al., 1998). About 30% of aspiration took place during emergence and extubation.

These reports are encouraging and are no doubt the results of improved training in pediatric anesthesia and sophisticated and vigilant clinical practice. One should be aware, however, that a combination of factors makes infants and young children potentially more susceptible to regurgitation and aspiration. These factors include excessive swallowing of air during crying, strenuous diaphragmatic breathing, possible relaxation of the gastroesophageal sphincter, a shorter esophagus and smaller hydrostatic pressure gradient between the stomach and larynx in the sitting position, and, most important, the tendency in infants and children for upper airway obstruction (Salem et al., 1973). Furthermore, in pediatric anesthesia, patients are less adaptable to alternatives such as local and regional anesthesia and intubation while awake. Children also give less reliable information about when, what, and how much they have ingested (Splinter et al., 1990). When gastric pH and residual volume have been measured in fasted normal children, nearly all have gastric pH less than 2.5 as well as a residual volume greater than 0.4 mL/kg (Coté et al., 1982).

Preparation and Management

Although there has been some disagreement about the right approach to take for this problem, the following essential safety factors are generally accepted for the management of children with a full stomach:

1. Avoidance or delay of general anesthesia, if possible; consideration of regional block with minimal sedation
2. Careful preparation if anesthesia is required
3. Preanesthetic relief of gastric distention, if present
4. Rapid and smooth induction and cricoid pressure until intubation is completed successfully

Delaying anesthesia is an important consideration, although it is well known that food may lie in the stomach undigested for many hours or even overnight when an accident occurs shortly after a meal or when the patient is in pain. The anesthetic management of children considered at high risk for aspiration is controversial. If the surgical procedure is emergent, H_2 receptor antagonists (Goudsouzian et al., 1981) (e.g., cimetidine, ranitidine), nonparticulate antacids (Taylor and Pryse-Davies, 1966) (e.g., sodium citrate), or agents to stimulate gastric emptying (e.g., metoclopramide) are effective in decreasing the pH of gastric fluid, or gastric volume. A reduction in gastric fluid pH or volume, however, does not prevent aspiration of gastric contents per se, which can still be life threatening.

In healthy children without known causes of delayed gastric emptying, "preoperative fasting" guidelines have been liberalized. Drinking clear liquids up to 2 hours prior to induction of anesthesia for elective surgical procedures does not substantially affect the volume of gastric fluid contents or the percentage of patients with a gastric fluid pH less than 2.5 (Schreiner et al., 1990; Nicolson et al., 1992). In addition, parents report less difficulty adhering to the preoperative feeding instructions, rated their children as less irritable, and rated the overall preoperative experience more positively (Schreiner et al., 1990). While human milk has been shown to leave the stomach more rapidly than formula in both preterm and full-term infants (Cavall, 1979, 1981), there is controversy as to whether this should be considered a clear liquid preoperative. A clear glucose-containing fluid should be used for feeding infants 2 to 3 hours before an elective surgical procedure (see Chapter 8, Preoperative Preparation).

In addition to a full complement of airways, endotracheal tubes, laryngoscope and blades, emergency drugs, the usual monitoring devices, and two strong, functioning suction devices, also readily at hand should be several suction catheters small enough to pass easily through the endotracheal tube, larger suction catheters (14F) to clear the mouth and pharynx, rigid "tonsil" (Yankauer) suction tips, and large-bore nasogastric tubes. In addition, a large uncuffed endotracheal tube without the plastic connector and fitted with an adapter to the suction apparatus is useful for removal of solid vomitus from the mouth and pharynx should copious vomiting with solid food occur during induction or emergence from anesthesia. A bite block is useful for preventing the jaws from clamping together. Equipment for rigid bronchoscopy and tracheotomy should also be readily available.

Premedication may be given to alleviate fear and anxiety in the holding area or in the operating room before induction. Intravenous midazolam (0.05 to 0.1 mg/kg) in divided doses usually works well for this purpose. A dose of atropine (0.01 to 0.02 mg/kg) should be given in anticipation of administering succinylcholine. If gastric distention is present or suspected, the stomach should be decompressed before induction using a large-bore nasogastric tube, nasally or orally, although this is uncomfortable and may upset the child even with intravenous sedation.

The most common technique for induction and intubation in a healthy or hemodynamically stable child with a full stomach is a rapid sequence induction with intravenous propofol (3 to 4 mg/kg) or thiopental (4 to 6 mg/kg) followed by succinylcholine (1 to 2 mg/kg), while cricoid pressure is applied (Sellick, 1961) to prevent regurgitation (Salem et al., 1972b). Atropine (0.01 to 0.02 mg/kg) should always be given prior to induction with succinylcholine. In older children, fasciculations and the incidence of postoperative myalgias can be decreased by pretreatment with approximately 10% of the paralyzing dose of a nondepolarizing muscle relaxant. Salem and others (1972a), however, found in infants and children that succinylcholine caused much less fasciculation and actually decreased mean gastric pressure slightly. Alternatively, a modified rapid-sequence intubation can be achieved within 60 seconds with higher doses of vecuronium (0.4 mg/kg) or rocuronium (1.0 mg/kg), but the duration of neuromuscular blockade is prolonged (O'Kelly et al., 1991; Sloan et al., 1991). If a combination of thiopental and rocuronium is planned, thiopental must be cleared from the intravenous tubing before rocuronium is infused so as to avoid precipitation in the tubing. Rocuronium may be associated with some tachycardia (O'Kelly et al., 1991).

The Sellick maneuver has been shown to be effective in both adult and pediatric patients (Salem et al., 1972b). By obliterating the esophageal lumen, it prevents regurgitated material from reaching the pharynx (Sellick, 1961; Salem et al., 1972b). Before induction, an assistant palpates the cricoid ring lightly between the thumb and the middle finger; then, after the patient has lost consciousness, the pressure is steadily increased using the index finger while the neck is kept extended (Salem et al., 1973). The pressure necessary for preventing gastric reflux is reported to be 30 to 40 Newtons (equivalent to 3 to 4 kg of force), which creates the pressure of about 50 cm H_2O in the upper esophagus (Vanner et al., 1992). Moynihan and others (1993) showed that the appropriate application of cricoid pressure in infants and young children was effective for preventing gastric insufflation during mask ventilation up to 40 cm H_2O peak airway pressure (Landsman, 2004). The Sellick maneuver also effectively seals the esophagus in the presence of a nasogastric tube. Nevertheless, removal of the nasogastric tube before intubation is recommended (Salem et al., 1973). This provides a much better mask fit and glottic exposure to facilitate endotracheal intubation.

The efficacy of cricoid pressure to prevent gastric regurgitation has been questioned (Brock-Utne, 2002); some clinicians believe the technique is ineffective and even unnecessary (Brimacombe and Berry, 1997). Surveys among pediatric anesthetists in the United Kingdom indicate that cricoid pressure is used in only 40% to 50% of patients with a full stomach (Stoddart et al., 1994; Engelhardt et al., 2001). Even when cricoid pressure is used, it is not certain whether and how often the maneuver is applied appropriately, that is, with the correct position and pressure in clinical settings (Landsman, 2004).

A study by Smith and others (2003) further casts doubt about the efficacy of cricoid pressure for preventing gastric regurgitation. They studied the anatomical relationship between the upper esophagus and the cricoid cartilage in anesthetized spontaneously breathing adult volunteers in a supine position with the use of magnetic resonance imaging (MRI), with and without cricoid pressure. The study revealed that the esophagus was situated lateral to the cricoid cartilage in more than 50% of the patients without cricoid pressure; with cricoid pressure, the esophagus was laterally displaced more than 90% of the time. Cricoid pressure distorts the anatomy of the upper airways and makes laryngoscopy more difficult (Mac et al., 2000); the pressure must be eased to improve the exposure of the larynx. Cricoid pressure is also associated with decreases in upper and lower esophageal sphincter tones (Vanner et al., 1992; Tournadre et al., 1997). From the foregoing discussion, it appears rather difficult to apply cricoid pressure correctly to prevent gastric regurgitation. Nevertheless, properly applied cricoid pressure facilitates intubation with rapid sequence induction and mask ventilation. The safe and effective use of this maneuver requires a knowledge of neck anatomy and proper training or experience to know the appropriate technique and pressure to be applied (Landsman, 2004).

The head-up tilt position has been proposed for reducing the danger of regurgitation in adults (Snow and Nunn, 1959) as well as in children (Gregory, 1994), with the belief that the gastric pressure would be less than the hydrostatic pressure reaching the larynx. Gastric pressure in infants, however, can reach 18 cm H_2O or more, much higher than the hydrostatic distance of the head-up tilt position in infants (7 to 8 cm) or even in adults (18 cm). The head-up tilt is of little value in preventing material from reaching the laryngeal level in pediatric patients (Salem et al., 1973). Indeed, Roe (1962) showed that vomiting could easily overcome a head-up tilt, which would then increase the hazard of aspiration. On the other hand, the head-down position was proposed for reducing the danger of aspiration, because gastric contents would find their way into the oropharynx rather than flow against gravity into the larynx in case of regurgitation (Inkster, 1963). It is obvious, however, that a head-down tilt also would increase the hazard of regurgitation. Consequently, most anesthesiologists believe that it is best for the patient to be level during induction with the head turned well to the side to enable secretions to flow into the cheek and escape.

Aspiration of Gastric Contents

Despite the best efforts of the anesthesiologist, aspiration of secretions, blood, or vomitus unfortunately occurs occasionally and may cause airway obstruction, bronchospasm, and/or hypoxia. Although aspiration occurs most commonly during the induction of anesthesia, it can also occur during maintenance of or emergence from anesthesia (Borland et al., 1998). The first sign of aspiration is often laryngospasm with oxygen desaturation. Laryngospasm tends to be intense and sustained, especially if the patient is lightly anesthetized and not paralyzed. Localized rhonchi or rales on auscultation, especially over the lower dependent lung fields, after an episode of vomiting and laryngospasm, are the classic signs of aspiration. A definite diagnosis, however, is often difficult at the time of incidence, unless foodstuff or bile-stained liquid is recovered by tracheal suction or by flexible bronchoscopy through the endotracheal tube. A chest radiograph may or may not show changes for some time after aspiration. When in doubt, it is best to assume the worst, notify the surgeon and postpone the planned surgery if nonemergent, and start treatment without delay. Continuous monitoring with a pulse oximeter, along with a precordial stethoscope, is most useful for the evaluation and care of a patient after suspected pulmonary aspiration.

The management of pulmonary aspiration in children is essentially the same as in adults, as reviewed by Gibbs and Modell (1990). The treatment should be aimed at restoring pulmonary function and gas exchange as soon as possible. After a minor incidence or questionable aspiration, the child may be observed and given supplemental oxygen via mask if satisfactory oxygen saturation (>96% in room air) and ventilation can be maintained. Otherwise, the trachea should be intubated and the patient given general anesthesia or additional sedation and muscle relaxants as indicated. The trachea and major bronchi may be examined with a small fiberoptic bronchoscope and any solid food particles, if present, removed, while ventilation is continued without interruption (Borland et al., 1998). Aspirated food particles may be found in the midtrachea, between the tracheal wall and endotracheal tube, whereas the lower trachea and carina are free of aspirated material. In these circumstances, the endotracheal tube may be gently moved cephalad as the anesthesiologist suctions the aspirated particles and the trachea is reintubated; this procedure can be repeated to clear the trachea of food particles successfully without resorting to rigid bronchoscopy.

Lungs should be gently inflated fully to total lung capacity (i.e., end-inspiratory pressure of 40 cm H_2O) and kept inflated for several seconds. This (vital capacity) maneuver is repeated several times; then continuous positive end-expiratory pressure (PEEP) is instituted and kept at the level that maintains the optimal oxygenation or compliance without interfering with circulation (Suter et al., 1975). Inspiratory oxygen concentration is gradually lowered and kept at the lowest level necessary to maintain adequate oxygen saturation. With this aggressive management of gastric regurgitation and aspiration, Borland and others (1998) reported excellent outcome without serious pulmonary outcome among more than 50,000 pediatric general anesthetic procedures.

Pulmonary lavage with a bicarbonate solution is not helpful because mucosal damage by acidic gastric juice occurs within 20 seconds (Hamelberg and Bosomworth, 1964; Gibbs and Modell, 1990) and may even be harmful by spreading vomitus farther down the tracheobronchial tree. Corticosteroid therapy is not recommended because it does not reduce the inflammatory process of aspiration pneumonitis and may interfere with healing (Wynne et al., 1979). Antibiotics should not be used unless there is a known pathogen because they are not only ineffective but also their routine use would select out drug-resistant organisms.

INTUBATION IN AN AWAKE INFANT

Intubation can be performed quickly and safely in an awake infant by a skillful pediatric anesthesiologist. Even in the hands of the inexperienced, this method may be relatively safe, as it is widely practiced by medical and paramedical personnel in neonatal intensive care settings. Nevertheless, it is rather cruel to the helpless, struggling infant, who can respond to noxious stimuli (Anand and Hickey, 1987), and it may cause trauma to the mouth, larynx, and pharynx. Thus, its use has been declining over the years and should be limited to infants with severe airway obstruction (such as lymphangioma of the tongue) and intestinal obstruction (as in meconium ileus), and perhaps to very young, nonresistant infants (premature and newborns <1 week of age). When the infant is strong enough to resist vigorously, this approach should not be used.

Because intubation in an awake infant often provokes strong vagal stimulation and bradycardia, a vagolytic dose of atropine (0.03 mg/kg) is administered via the intravenous route shortly before the attempted intubation. If the condition permits, intravenous lidocaine (1.5 mg/kg) or a small dose of fentanyl (1 to 2 mcg/kg) may be considered. In addition, to reduce the infant's discomfort, it may help to expose the pharynx and apply topical anesthesia with 1 or 2 atomizer bursts of 1% to 2% lidocaine directed toward the base of the tongue and vocal cords. Oxygen is given for 1 additional minute while the anesthetic takes effect.

The patient should be monitored with an electrocardiograph, precordial stethoscope, and pulse oximeter and should be preoxygenated for 1 to 2 minutes, or until 100% saturation is observed on the pulse oximeter monitor, before intubation is attempted. An assistant, the key person for successful intubation, holds down the infant's shoulders and chest on the table and immobilizes the head in the "sniffing position." The use of a modified Miller 0 blade with a port for oxygen running 1 to 3 L/min (Oxyscope; Foregger, Smithtown, NY) (Fig. 10–17) or its further modification (Diaz, 1984) improves oxygenation during intubation in the awake neonate and is highly recommended (Todres and Crone, 1981). The anesthesiologist chooses the most likely endotracheal tube size (usually 3.0 mm ID for a newborn infant weighing 2 to 4 kg) lightly coated with lubricant and keeps it in his or her right hand until the time for insertion, to avoid having to grope for the tube on the table after the glottis is exposed. The anesthesiologist dips the blade of the laryngoscope into warm water and then inserts the tip over the right edge of the infant's mouth, gently opening the mouth and sweeping the tongue to the left. The tips of the blade and tube are advanced side by side to bring the glottis into view, so that the infant continues to breathe. If the infant chokes or stops breathing, or pulse oximeter reading drops below 95%, the laryngoscope is withdrawn just enough to let the infant breathe briefly with oxygen insufflation, until saturation returns to 100% (or the highest level previously achieved for a given patient). When possible, the blade should not be completely withdrawn from the mouth, for then the entire process must be started again. The blade is advanced again, keeping the pressure on the tongue upward without touching the upper jaw with the blade. If the glottis appears too far "anterior," the left little finger is used to apply a gentle pressure over the larynx to position and hold the glottis precisely as needed (Fig. 10–18).

At this point, the anesthesiologist waits with the tips of the blade and tube, side by side, within a centimeter above the glottis. As the infant takes the next deep breath, the glottic aperture widens momentarily, and the tube is advanced swiftly about 2 cm beyond the cords. The tube must be held firmly until its position is confirmed by visible motion of the chest, capnographic tracing, and auscultation. Then the tube is taped in place, and general anesthesia with intravenous injections of propofol, fentanyl, and a nondepolarizing muscle relaxant with or without an inhalation anesthetic follows immediately as cardiorespiratory stability is monitored continuously.

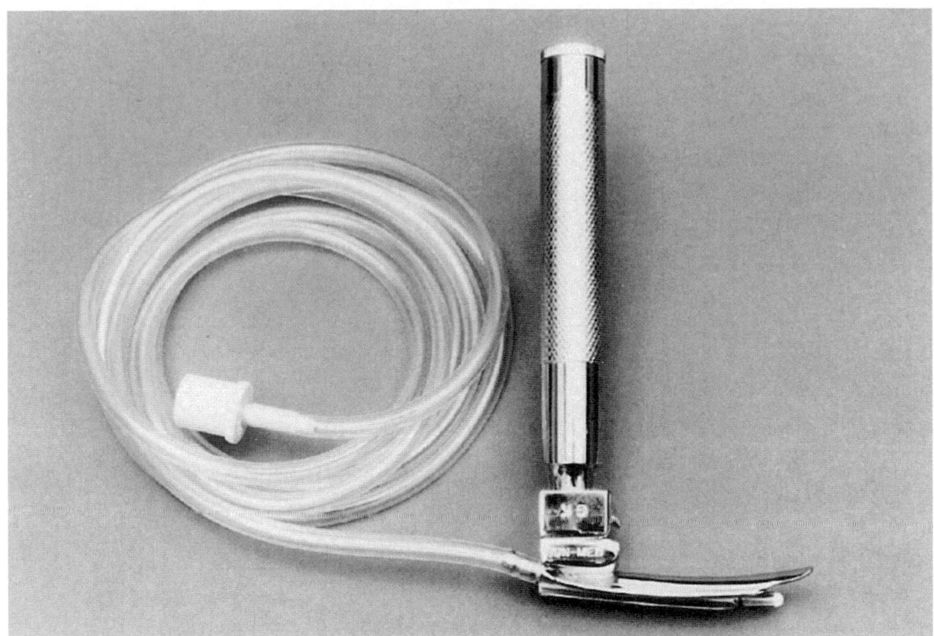

■ **FIGURE 10–17.** Oxyscope (modified Miller 0 blade with oxygen delivery channel) with pediatric laryngoscope handle for intubation of the awake infant.

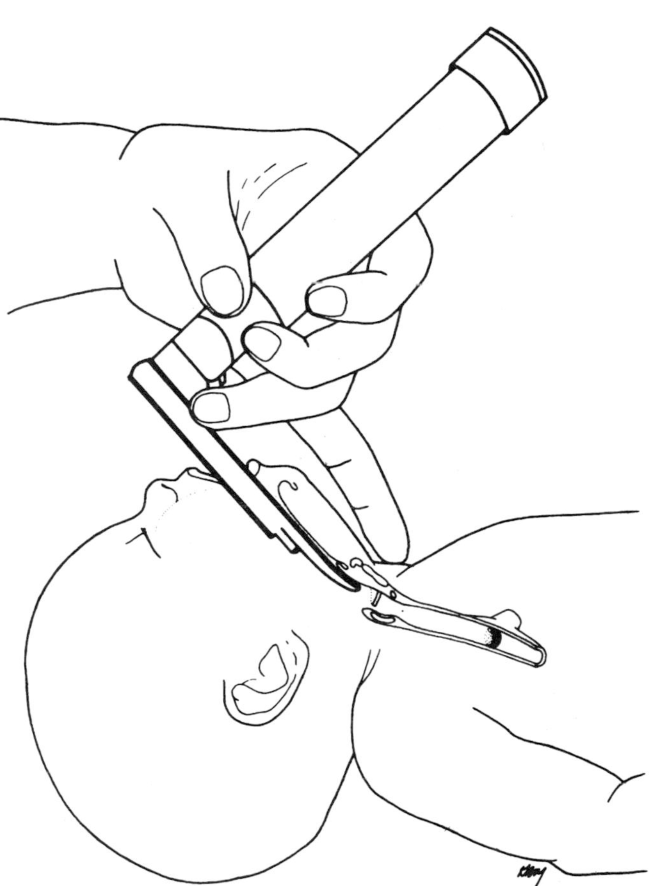

■ **FIGURE 10–18.** A diagram of intubating an infant showing the anesthesiologist's use of the left fifth finger to bring glottis into position and immobilize it before intubation.

■ DIFFICULT AIRWAY AND INTUBATION TECHNIQUES

In infants and children, a wide variety of difficult airways occur that can be extremely challenging as well as nerve-racking for the pediatric anesthesiologist. Some conditions, such as Pierre Robin association (syndrome) and large hemangioma of the tongue, are obvious and are likely to exhibit airway obstruction, whereas other conditions, such as Hurler's and Hunter's syndromes (mucopolysaccharidosis) and ankylosis of the jaw, usually are not associated with airway difficulty when the patient is awake and may escape recognition before the induction of anesthesia.

Nothing could be worse for the pediatric anesthesiologist than encountering severe airway obstruction after induction of anesthesia and paralysis in a child who could not be ventilated and whose jaw is found to be ankylosed. The best approach to the difficult airway problem is not to be caught by surprise. Careful history taking and physical examinations and making a rational plan (and alternative plans in case the first approach fails) to the problem are essential to prevent such a catastrophe.

A history of difficult intubation, particularly with the cancellation of planned surgery, should not be taken lightly, whether it is documented in the hospital record or at a different institution or recounted by a parent. One should always assume that the anesthesiologist previously involved was experienced and competent. Infants and young children with a history of prolonged intubation or of recurrent or severe croup are likely to have airway difficulties during the perioperative period.

The difficult airway algorithm for adult patients has been developed and recommended by the American Society of Anesthesiologists' Task Force on Airway Management (Caplan et al., 1993) and has been updated with an addition of LMA in the algorithm (Benumof, 1996). A difficult airway algorithm for children has been proposed (Fig. 10–19) (Wheeler, 1998).

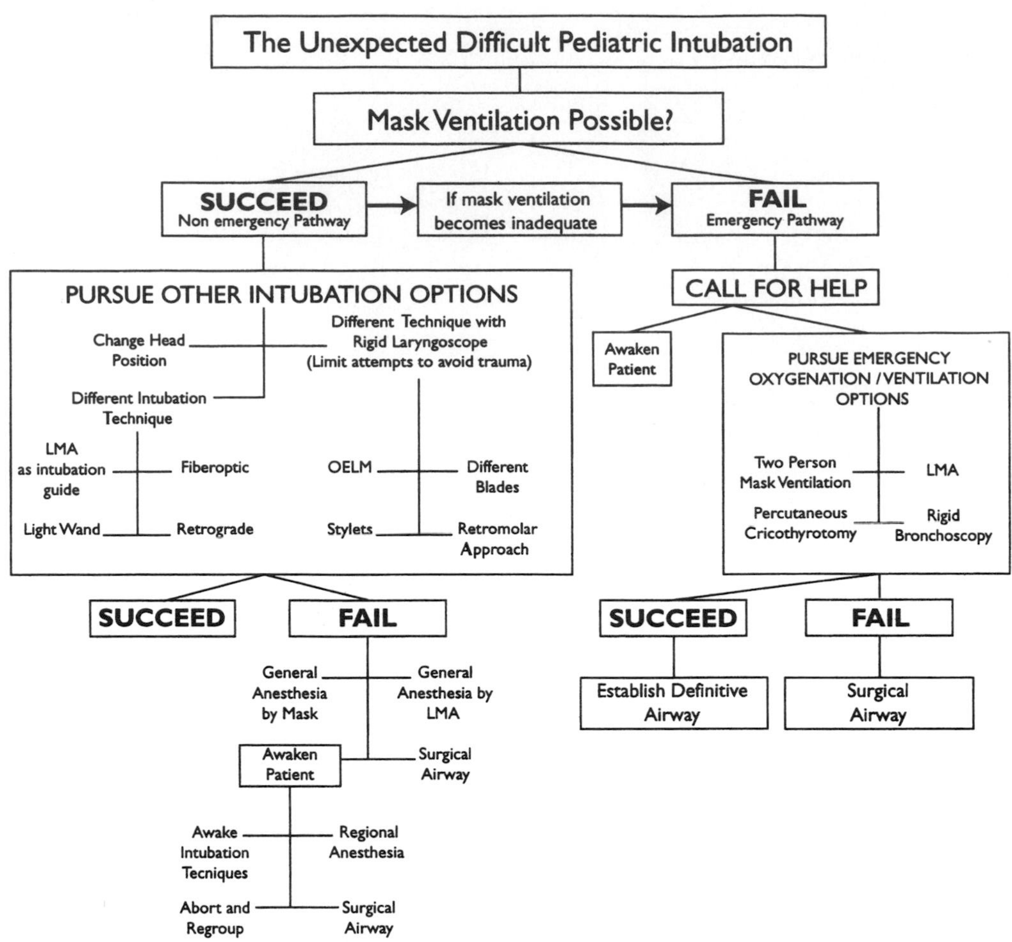

■ **FIGURE 10–19.** A difficult airway algorithm for the unexpected difficult airway in pediatric patients. LMA, laryngeal mask airway; OELM, optimal external laryngeal manipulation. (From Wheeler M: Management strategies for the difficult pediatric airway. *Anesth Clin North Am* 16:759, 1998, Figure 1.)

During the preoperative visit, it is important to ask the child to open the mouth wide and to extend the neck, to rule out ankylosis of the jaw and cervical spine. An unstable cervical spine, congenital (Down's syndrome) or acquired, is noted. A high arched palate with a narrow mouth is often associated with difficult exposure of the larynx. One should examine the size and shape of the mandible in relation to that of the tongue. The distance between the lower edge of the mandible and the thyroid notch in the adult is about 6.5 cm and that between the mandible and the hyoid cartilage is 3 cm. The distance in the newborn is about one-half that in the adult (Berry, 1986). A reduction in submandibular space (micrognathia) leaves too little room to displace the tongue and surrounding soft tissues for laryngoscopy and often is associated with difficult exposure and intubation (Patil et al., 1983; Berry, 1986). The classification of difficult airway by the exposure of the larynx (Grades 1 to 4) proposed by Mallampati and others (1985) can be useful in older and cooperative children but is not helpful in younger or frightened children who are not willing or capable of opening the mouth for examination.

If the child is already having difficulty breathing, the ventilation and degree of obstruction should be observed carefully. In case of acute upper airway obstruction such as supraglottitis, one should refrain from examining the pharynx, because immediate and severe airway occlusion may develop if the pharynx is manipulated. Other factors to be examined include the state of stomach emptying, adequacy of oxygen-carrying capacity, and presence of complicating lesions. Box 10–2 lists the diversity of conditions in which difficult airway and intubation problems may be encountered in pediatric anesthesia. The difficulties involved are quite varied, with the most hazardous being a child presenting with upper airway obstruction and/or in a critical hypoxic state, as with acute supraglottitis, when therapy must be immediate and involves great risk.

Several generalities apply to many situations. To avoid trouble, one must be prepared for trouble. General anesthesia in children with airway problems should be administered only by an experienced anesthesiologist (or under his or her close supervision) and should be performed in the area where personnel and equipment are available for bronchoscopy, tracheostomy, and resuscitation. The anesthesiologist should go into the procedure with a definite strategy, one best suited for the particular circumstances (Plan A), and with alternative courses of action in mind (Plans B and C) in case the intubation is not successful with Plan A. Parents, surgeons, and nurses should be forewarned of the possibility of prolonged time, the risk of manipulative trauma and the possible need for tracheostomy (with the consent signed), and the possible postponement of the planned surgery (Plan D).

BOX 10–2 Difficult Airways in Pediatric Anesthesia

Congenital Anomalies

Encephalocele
Double cleft lip and palate
Micrognathia, Pierre Robin syndrome (sequence)
Macroglossia (Beckwith-Wiedman syndrome, Down syndrome)
Craniofacial deformity (Crouzon's disease, Apert's syndrome)
Mandibular dysplasia, microsomia (Treacher Collins syndrome, Goldenhar's syndrome)
Mucopolysaccharidosis I, II (Hurler's syndrome, Hunter's syndrome)

Tumors

Cystic hygroma
Hemangioma of tongue, pharynx
Teratoma

Infection

Retropharyngeal abscess
Acute supraglottitis (epiglottitis)
Laryngotracheobronchitis (subglottic croup)
Ludwig's angina
Adenotonsillitis, abscess, hypertrophy (obstructive sleep apnea)

Musculoskeletal Problems

Ankylosis of jaw, cervical spine
Unstable or dislocated cervical vertebrae (Down syndrome, trauma)
Wired teeth, jaw
Cervical cord tumor
Halo traction apparatus

Trauma

Facial fractures, lacerations
Burns of mouth, airway
Foreign body aspiration

When difficult intubation is anticipated, a difficult airway cart (stocked with added equipment necessary for difficult airway management) should be wheeled into the induction area. The difficult airway cart should include different types of laryngoscope blades; endotracheal tubes of various sizes, curves, and length (oral and nasal); stylets; forceps; bite blocks; local anesthesia equipment; Bullard laryngoscopes; lighted stylets; and apparatus for retrograde intubation (Box 10–3). In addition, a setup for fiberoptic bronchoscopy, rigid bronchoscopy, as well as equipment for tracheostomy and resuscitation should be on hand.

Premedication may be varied to suit the situation but, in general, should be given intravenously and be carefully titrated in a monitored situation. Atropine (0.01 to 0.02 mg/kg) or glycopyrrolate (0.005 to 0.01 mg/kg) is indicated for most situations for both vagolytic and antimuscarinic effects. No sedative should be given to the infant with upper airway obstruction who is to be intubated while awake or to the child with supraglottitis

BOX 10–3 Equipment Included in the Difficult Airway Cart

Oral and nasal airways and lubricant
Intubating oral airways for fiberoptic bronchoscopic intubation
Airway endoscopy (Frei) mask
Laryngoscope handles, blades (various types and sizes)
Bullard laryngoscope
Endotracheal tubes and stylets
Laryngeal mask airway (all sizes)
Intubation (Frei) masks (all sizes)
Tracheal tube exchangers
Lighted stylets (with light source)
Retrograde intubation kits
Cricothyrotomy kit
Saunders jet ventilation stylets (with equipment available)
Additional equipment at hand with the difficult airway cart

- Manual (Saunders) or high-frequency jet ventilator
- Fiberoptic bronchoscopy setup including a video monitor
- Rigid bronchoscopy setup
- Tracheostomy setup

or subglottic croup (laryngotracheobronchitis). However, children who have airway problems but who are not in acute distress, such as those with facial deformities, may be given small divided doses of propofol to facilitate inhalation induction. With few exceptions, the presence of airway obstruction contraindicates the use of ketamine (see later). Muscle relaxants should not be used, at least until the airway is secured or an endotracheal tube is placed. When difficult intubation is anticipated, an intravenous dose of corticosteroid (dexamethasone 0.4 mg/kg) should be given as prophylaxis against edema formation (Biller et al., 1970).

Sevoflurane with oxygen without nitrous oxide is most commonly used for inhalation induction. As the upper airway muscles start to relax with general anesthesia, especially with sevoflurane, one frequently encounters progressive airway obstruction. A combination of the head extension, the jaw thrust, and (especially if the nasal airway is compromised) the mouth kept open (the triple airway maneuver) should be used during induction. A well-lubricated nasopharyngeal airway often is helpful when the patient is too lightly anesthetized to accept an oral airway. It is advisable to use a nasal decongestant (0.05% oxymetazoline or 0.25% phenylephrine) before induction to prevent nasal bleeding, which could seriously compromise difficult intubation. A moderate (10 to 15 cm H_2O) level of CPAP is also helpful for maintaining upper airway patency as described previously. If adequate ventilation can be maintained manually, ventilation may be gradually taken over and controlled while anesthesia is deepened. Sevoflurane may be switched to halothane or propofol infusion at this point to provide a steady level of anesthesia and allow the anesthesiologist more time for laryngoscopy. Intubation may be attempted after the use of topical lidocaine. Muscle relaxants should be avoided, so that in the event the patient cannot be intubated, mask ventilation or spontaneous ventilation can be maintained.

Alternatively, the patient with a potential difficult airway may be managed with intravenous induction. Propofol with divided doses, combined with topical anesthesia with lidocaine spray, may be used for intubation attempted while the patient is spontaneously breathing. Ketamine should be avoided for intubating patients with difficult airway because it maintains or exaggerates pharyngeal and laryngeal reflexes (Green, 1990). It also stimulates salivation and airway secretions, even with pretreatment by atropine or glycopyrrolate. The risk of cough and laryngospasm may be increased (Faithful and Haider, 1971; Cook et al., 1996). Anecdotal accounts exist of severe laryngospasm with attempted intubation with ketamine. Such reports, however, have been scarce in the literature (Sussman, 1974; Lassiter, 1982). Ketamine has been used successfully, however, as a bronchodilator for patients with status asthmaticus (Strube and Hallam, 1986; L'Hommedieu and Arens, 1987); for the treatment of bronchospasm during mechanical ventilation (Hemmingsen et al., 1994); and as an anesthetic in symptomatic and asymptomatic asthmatic patients (Corssen et al., 1972). Furthermore, studies report the successful use of ketamine comparable with propofol and topical lidocaine for emergency procedures involving the insertion for laryngeal mask airway, with relatively low incidence of coughs (2%) and laryngospasms (1.5%) (Gloor et al., 2001; Bahk et al., 2002).

Dexmedetomidine, an α_2-adrenergic receptor agonist, has been used for its sedative and analgesic effects and as an adjunct to general anesthetics with circulatory stability in both adult and pediatric patients (Tobias and Berkenbosch, 2002; Ard et al., 2003; Jorden et al., 2004). With an intravenous dose of 0.5 to 1.0 mcg/kg given slowly for induction followed by continuous infusion of dexmedetomidine (0.5 to 1.25 mcg/kg per hr), spontaneous breathing is well maintained. Ramsey and Luterman (2004) has reported the use of high-dose dexmedetomidine (10 mcg/kg per hr) as a total intravenous anesthetic in three adult patients with difficult airways while spontaneous breathing was well maintained in room air with satisfactory hemoglobin saturation on pulse oximetry. The patients tolerated fiberoptic bronchoscopy with the addition of topical lidocaine. Only one patient required a chin lift to maintain airway patency. End-tidal PCO_2 was measured in one patient and was well within normal limits. In addition, dexmedetomidine is a potent bronchodilator antagonizing histamine challenge in the dog (Groeben et al., 2004). Dexmedetomidine in lower clinical doses decreases systemic blood pressure, presumably due to central sympatholytic effect. At higher plasma levels, however, it may increase both pulmonary and systemic blood pressures due to peripheral α_2-adrenergic receptor–mediated vasoconstriction (Ebert and Maze, 2004). Although at the time of this writing the literature on the clinical experience with dexmedetomidine has been limited, procedural sedation or even total intravenous anesthesia with dexmedetomidine with or without topical lidocaine appears to provide an excellent condition for fiberoptic intubation while spontaneous breathing is well maintained (Grant et al., 2004).

During attempts at intubating the patient with difficult airway, it is mandatory to monitor oxygen saturation by means of pulse oximetry with an audible pulse signal to warn of developing hypoxia. Attempts at intubation must be interrupted for frequent and sufficient periods of oxygenation and stabilization. During attempted intubation, one must not persist with a maneuver that is unsuccessful; every attempt increases the chance of injury. One should instead try various instruments, techniques, and approaches. For a difficult exposure, the infant Phillips blade with its sharply curved tip often is helpful. Mandibular advancement with both hands by an assistant may improve the exposure of the larynx with laryngoscopy, especially for inexperienced physicians (Tamura et al., 2004).

When the problem of exposure is due to a large tongue combined with micrognathia, a paraglossal approach using a straight blade may be helpful for laryngeal exposure (Henderson, 1997). With this approach, the head is slightly tilted to the left and the laryngoscope blade is inserted from the right corner of the mouth over the molars while the assistant retracts the right corner of the mouth with a small retractor and the tongue is pulled out to the opposite corner of the mouth with forceps (M. B. Borland, personal communication).

The Bullard laryngoscope is superior to conventional laryngoscopes for the exposure of difficult airways with limited mouth opening, micrognathia, and/or macroglossia, although this instrument, as with most other tools, requires prior experience (Borland, 1988). The use of this instrument has been described earlier in this chapter (see Fig. 10–10) (also see Chapter 9, Anesthetic Equipment and Monitoring).

INTUBATION USING A FLEXIBLE FIBEROPTIC BRONCHOSCOPE

In experienced hands, endotracheal intubation with a flexible fiberoptic bronchoscope is usually successful, with minimal or no injury to the patient, even with the most difficult airway (Ovassapian et al., 1983) (see DVD). The nasotracheal route is preferred with this technique, particularly in infants and children, because it is less traumatic and considerably easier than the oral approach for visualizing the glottis (Wood, 1985, 1988).

The safest and most common approach for all ages is to have the patient well sedated and breathing spontaneously. A topical decongestant (0.05% oxymetazoline or 0.25% phenylephrine) should be given to prevent nasal bleeding, which would interfere with viewing through the fiberscope. A nasotracheal tube, one or two sizes smaller than that appropriate for the patient, with the connector removed, is threaded over the scope retrograde and is held at the upper end of the scope until it is ready to be lowered down into the trachea. A low-flow oxygen (<1 L/min) source may be attached to the suction port during flexible laryngoscopy to improve the patient's oxygenation during the procedure.

The tip of the flexible bronchoscope is introduced through the nostril and advanced through the center of the air passages without touching the nasal mucosa, toward the choana. It is then advanced into the nasopharynx by adjusting the vertically flexible tip with the lever situated near the eyepiece with the right thumb and by holding and rolling a portion of the scope above the nostril between the left thumb and index finger. The tip of the scope is farther advanced without touching the pharyngeal wall. Once the glottis is visualized, the bronchoscopist gives topical anesthesia by spraying the vocal cords and tracheal mucosa by pushing 1 mL of 2% lidocaine and air in a vertically held 5-mL non–Luer-Loc syringe through the suction port.

As the patient inhales and the glottic aperture widens, the tip of the fiberscope is swiftly advanced into the midtrachea. The tracheal rings, the carina, and the bronchial lumens beyond are now visible through the scope. The tip of the bronchoscope is steadied with the right hand of the operator with its tip in the mid trachea; the lubricated tip of the nasotracheal tube is slid down with the left thumb and index finger over the flexible scope through the nasal cavity and past the vocal cords into the mid trachea while the bronchoscope is held steadily without being advanced too far past the carina as the nasotracheal tube is advanced. The tip of the endotracheal tube is visualized above the carina through the scope as it is pulled back 1 to 2 cm to the mid trachea, and the tube is held firmly at the nostril, as the scope is completely withdrawn. Satisfactory and equal breath sounds on both sides of the chest are confirmed, and then the patient is anesthetized rapidly by intravenous injection of propofol or thiopental, an opioid, and a muscle relaxant of choice, with or without inhalation anesthesia as indicated.

Alternatively, fiberoptic intubation can be performed under general anesthesia. The patient may be anesthetized with sevoflurane and oxygen, switched over to propofol infusion with spontaneous breathing, as with rigid bronchoscopy, while intubation is attempted with a flexible bronchoscope as described earlier. In this case, however, extreme caution should be exercised and adequate topical anesthesia is used to prevent laryngospasm.

Fiberoptic bronchoscopy may also be performed orally on a patient whose ventilation is controlled under sevoflurane or halothane anesthesia with or without neuromuscular blockade. It is mandatory, however, to have a special intubation oral airway for bronchoscopic intubation. Its cross section is "C" shaped so that it can be removed once the tip of the bronchoscope is advanced into the tracheal lumen before the endotracheal tube is advanced over the bronchoscope (IMD Inc., Park City, UT). However, there are only three sizes available (infant, child, and adult), and these are often inadequate. When exposure of the oropharynx is difficult due to either relative macroglossia or micrognathia, it is helpful to have an assistant (a surgeon or an anesthesiologist) pull the tongue outward and downward over the lower incisors with a pair of forceps, towel clips, or a suture through the tongue to improve visualization.

Intubation With a Flexible Bronchoscope and an Endoscopy (Frei) Mask

Frei and others (1995) constructed a special endoscopy mask from a disposable clear plastic facemask. The original connector in the center of the mask was cut out to leave a large hole (40 mm in diameter) and was covered with a distensible silicon rubber (Silastic) membrane with a small hole off-center to accommodate a pediatric fiberoptic bronchoscope. An additional hole (10 mm in diameter) was cut over the lateral aspect of the mask, an airtight silicone rubber adapter was connected to a flexible extension tube, and a 15-mm adapter was inserted to serve as a connector to the anesthesia breathing circuit (Fig. 10–20). A flexible, pediatric fiberoptic bronchoscope can be threaded through the tiny hole in the Silastic diaphragm and an uncuffed endotracheal tube (up to 7 mm ID) can be slid over the scope into the trachea, while the patient can be ventilated manually and continually uninterrupted with manual intermittent positive pressure ventilation (Fig. 10–21). The same endoscopy mask can be used for either nasal or oral intubation by simply adjusting the position of the small hole in the Silastic diaphragm up or down, respectively. Frei and others reported nearly 100% success in fiberoptic intubation without hypoxemia (SpO_2 <95%) or significant trauma or complications (Frei and Ummerhofer, 1996; Erb et al., 1997).

Intubation With a Flexible Bronchoscope and Laryngeal Mask Airway

The LMA has been exceptionally useful as an emergency airway in the patients whose lungs cannot be ventilated adequately with the conventional mask and bag and who cannot be intubated (Benumof, 1992). Under these circumstances, an LMA in place can be used to ventilate the patient and as a conduit to place a flexible bronchoscope and facilitate endotracheal intubation in children (Maekawa et al., 1991; Theroux et al., 1995; Walker et al., 1997), as well as in the neonate (Tom et al., 1995). Using a long endotracheal tube, the LMA can be left in place after intubation facilitated by a flexible bronchoscope. If the LMA must be removed for any reason, an endotracheal tube exchanger, made of a long, stiff plastic catheter, exists for this purpose (Cook Airway Exchange Catheter; Cook Critical Care, Bloomington, IN). The endotracheal tube exchanger is inserted into the endotracheal tube before removing the LMA so that the

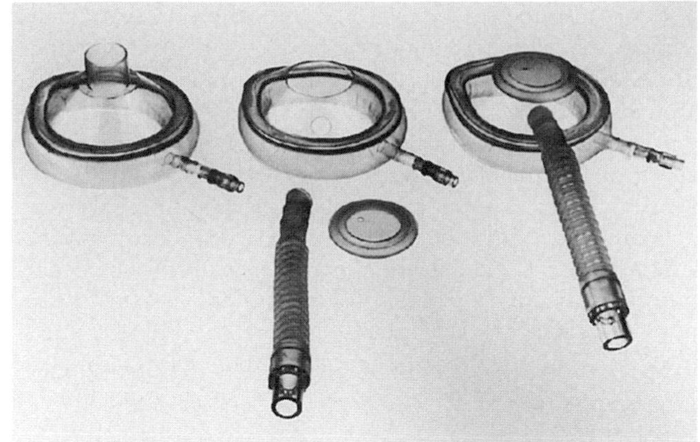

■ **FIGURE 10–20.** The airway endoscopy mask assembly (Frei mask) for fiberoptic bronchoscopic intubation. (Courtesy Dr. Franz Frei, Basel, Switzerland.)

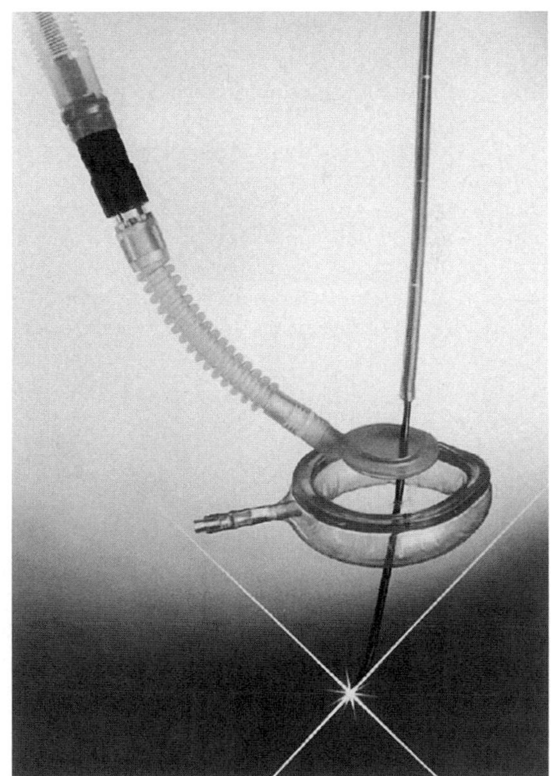

■ **FIGURE 10–21.** A fiberoptic bronchoscope with an overriding endotracheal tube penetrating through an airway endoscopy mask. (Courtesy Dr. Franz Frei, Basel, Switzerland.)

endotracheal tube can be reinserted over the tube exchanger in case it is inadvertently pulled out with the LMA (Thomas and Parry, 2001; Jöhr and Berger, 2004). Oxygen can be insufflated through the tube exchanger while the tube is being exchanged. The smallest tube exchanger accommodates an endotracheal tube with a 3-mm ID.

Alternatively, two endotracheal tubes are connected back to back, are loaded onto the flexible bronchoscope, and advanced into the trachea as described earlier. The flexible bronchoscope is withdrawn first and then the LMA is withdrawn. The proximal endotracheal tube is then detached; the tracheal tube connector is attached to the distal endotracheal tube before it is reconnected to the anesthesia circuit to resume assisted or controlled manual ventilation.

INTUBATION WITH A LIGHTED STYLET

Stylets with a light at the tip (lighted stylets or light-wands) have been used successfully in patients for both oral and nasal intubations (Ellis et al., 1986; Fox et al., 1987). Lighted stylets are advantageous for intubation in patients with difficult anatomy because the endotracheal tube can be guided by observing the movement of light under the skin. Fiberoptic lighted stylets consist of a reusable fiberoptic light guide, the distal portion of which is coated with annealed surgical stainless steel and covered with a sterile, disposable sheath. The fiberoptic light guide connects to most light sources for fiberoptic or rigid bronchoscopy. The lighted stylet is inserted through a properly sized endotracheal tube, making sure that the end does not protrude out of the tip of the endotracheal tube. Intubation with a lighted stylet is performed orally in an anesthetized patient with or without muscle paralysis. The stylet and endotracheal tube are sharply curved at the tip and are inserted into the mouth so that the end of the styletted tube is pointing in the midline toward the glottis.

In a darkened operating room, the light of the stylet can be seen through the skin over the anterior neck, especially in young children with fewer tissues for the light to penetrate through, and the styletted tube is manipulated so that the light is visible as the operator attempts to pass the tube down the trachea. When the styletted endotracheal tube is successfully introduced into the trachea beyond the larynx, the stylet is withdrawn as the endotracheal tube is advanced farther. Proper placement of the endotracheal tube must be confirmed by auscultation of both lung fields, chest movement, and the presence of end-tidal carbon dioxide waveforms on the capnograph. The lighted stylet appears to have a place in pediatric anesthesia as an additional device and technique for difficult intubation.

INTUBATION WITH THE RETROGRADE TECHNIQUE

Endotracheal intubation can be accomplished using a retrograde guide through the cricothyroid membrane. This technique is not without the risks of airway obstruction and hemorrhage and other complications, and it should not be used casually (Smith et al., 1975). In addition, in infants and young children less than 2 to 3 years, there is a potential for damage to the immature cartilages in the larynx, resulting in laryngeal obstruction and impairment in speech development (Berry, 1986). Furthermore, with the availability of ultrathin, flexible, fiberoptic bronchoscopes and lighted stylets, as described earlier, the indications and justification for the retrograde technique have diminished considerably.

Retrograde intubation may be accomplished with the patient under sedation or under either inhalation or intravenous anesthesia and spontaneously breathing. The patient is premedicated with atropine to prevent vagal stimulation and to reduce secretions. In addition, a topical anesthetic is atomized in the pharynx and larynx to prevent laryngospasm. The neck is extended by placing pads under the shoulders. The cricothyroid membrane (very narrow in infants) is palpated and a local anesthetic (1% lidocaine) is injected intradermally. The needle is then advanced into the tracheal lumen, as confirmed by the aspiration of air into the syringe, and a transtracheal block is performed. A 20-gauge needle attached to a saline-filled syringe is introduced through the skin wheal and the cricothyroid membrane (Powell and Ozdil, 1967). After confirming the intratracheal position with air aspiration into the syringe, a flexible-tip guide wire, used for central venous cannulation, is threaded cephalad via the needle through the larynx and is retrieved in the oropharynx with a Magill forceps (Borland et al., 1981).

In case of nasotracheal intubation, a rubber catheter is passed through the naris into the oropharynx and is tied with the guide wire and retrieved through the nasal cavity. A well-lubricated endotracheal tube is then threaded over the guide wire while tension is maintained on the guide wire from both ends (Borland et al., 1981).

Complications in Pediatric Patients with Difficult Airway

Complications from intubation attempts in patients with difficult airway can increase the risk of injury to the upper airways. The upper airways are lined with the mucosa supported by a rigid framework of cartilages, bone, and muscles. These structures with a relatively rigid external skeleton are predisposed to acute and chronic injuries from attempted intubation (Loh and Irish, 2002).

Acute nasal mucosal injuries can occur as a result of nasotracheal intubation. The use of an inappropriately large tube for the nasal passages is the most common factor, particularly when the nasal mucosa is not adequately decongested and the tube is not sufficiently lubricated. A deviated nasal septum, nasal polyps, and enlarged adenoidal tissues can predispose the patient for nasal and nasopharyngeal injuries. The failure to direct the tip of the nasotracheal tube anteriorly at the site of the nasopharynx can lead to deep mucosal injury. Softening of the nasotracheal tube by immersion in warm water before intubation can reduce epistaxis and mucosal injury (Kim et al., 2000).

Dental injury with partial or complete dental fracture and root avulsion may result during intubation with a difficult exposure of the larynx. When dental injuries occur, it is imperative to recover the loose tooth immediately to prevent aspiration. A dental consultation is required, especially when the permanent teeth are involved (see Chapter 24, Anesthesia for Dentistry).

Mucosal laceration can occur at the lips, the tongue, and the pharyngeal mucosa as the result of trauma caused by a laryngoscope blade, by an endotracheal tube, and during fiberoptic bronchoscopy when the endotracheal tube is advanced inappropriately. Most lacerations are superficial, however, and heal without surgical intervention. The contributing factors to laryngotracheal mucosal injuries are similar to those of pharyngeal mucosa with difficult airways; and bleeding often complicates the exposure and the process of securing airway access. Most injuries are superficial but may require consultation with a laryngologist (Weymuller, 1992; Loh and Irish, 2002).

SUMMARY

Preparations for the induction of anesthesia in infants and children differ considerably from those for adult patients. Equipment and techniques must be adjusted to accommodate a wide range of sizes in patients, from a premature infant weighing less than 1 kg to an obese teenager weighing well over 100 kg. Psychological preparation for anesthesia induction is as important as clinical readiness. The approach must be adjusted according to the maturity of the child and his or her psychological needs and at times to the psychological needs of the parents as well. A variety of newer and safer drugs and techniques have become available for the preparation and induction of anesthesia for pediatric patients. The characteristics and uses of standard, as well as newer anesthetic and adjuvant agents, are discussed. Indications and techniques of endotracheal intubation and the use of LMAs are discussed in detail, although their indications vary, depending on different surgical procedures and durations as well as the use of regional anesthetic techniques, as detailed in subsequent chapters for specific surgical procedures. With the advent of newer anesthetic and adjuvant agents, standard induction agents have evolved from halothane to sevoflurane and from thiopental to propofol for inhalation and intravenous inductions, respectively. Standard and various approaches to the management of the difficult airway are also covered, including the use of fiberoptic bronchoscopy alone or together with the intubation mask or LMA. In addition, a technique of fiberoptic intubation in infants and children can be viewed with the audiovisual program attached to this chapter.

REFERENCES

Aantaa R, Takala R, Muittair P: Sevoflurane EC_{50} and EC_{95} values for laryngeal mask insertion and tracheal intubation in children. *Br J Anaesth* 86:213–216, 2001.

Allsop E, Innes P, Jackson M, et al.: Dose of propofol required to insert the laryngeal mask airway in children. *Paediatr Anaesth* 5:47–51, 1995.

American Society of Anesthesiologists: Standards for basic intraoperative monitoring. *ASA Newsletter* 50:12, 1986.

Anand KJS, Hickey PR: Pain and its effects in the human neonate and fetus. *N Engl J Med* 317:1321, 1987.

Ard J, Doyle W, Bekker A: Awake craniotomy with dexmedetomidine in pediatric patients. *J Neurosurg Anesthesiol* 15:263–266, 2003.

Ashburn MA, Lind GH, Gillie MN, et al.: Oral transmucosal fentanyl citrate (OTFC) for the treatment of postoperative pain. *Anes Analg* 76:377-381, 1993.

Ashburn MA, Straisand JB, Tarver SD, et al.: Oral transmucosal fentanyl citrate for premedication in paediatric outpatients. *Can J Anaesth* 37:857–866, 1990.

Aun CS, Short SM, Leung DH, et al.: Induction dose-response of propofol in unpremedicated children. *Br J Anaesth* 68:64–67, 1992.

Bahk JH, Sung J, Jang IJ: A comparison of ketamine and lidocaine spray with propofol for the insertion of laryngeal mask airway in children: a double-blinded randomized trial. *Anesth Analg* 95:1586–1589, 2002.

Barash PG, Glanz S, Katz JD, et al.: Ventricular function in children during halothane anesthesia: An echocardiographic evaluation. *Anesthesiology* 49:79, 1978.

Beebe DS, Belani KG, Chang P, et al.: Effectiveness of preoperative sedation with rectal midazolam, ketamine, or their combination in young children. *Anesth Analg* 75:880, 1992.

Benumof JL: Laryngeal mask airway. Indications and contraindications. *Anesthesiology* 77:843–846, 1992.

Benumof JL: The laryngeal mask airway and the ASA difficult airway algorithm. *Anesthesiology* 84:689–699, 1996.

Berney P, Francioli P: Successful prophylaxis of experimental streptococcal endocarditis with single-dose amoxicillin administered after bacterial challenge. *J Infect Dis* 161:281–285, 1990.

Berry FA, Blankenbaker WL, Ball CG: A comparison of bacteremia occurring with nasotracheal and orotracheal intubation. *Anesth Analg* 52:873, 1973.

Berry FA: Anesthesia for the child with a difficult airway. In Berry FA, editor: *Anesthetic management of difficult and routine pediatric patients.* New York, 1986, Churchill Livingstone.

Berry FA: General philosophy of patient preparation, premedication, and induction of anesthesia; and inhalation anesthetic agents. In Berry FA, editor: *Anesthetic management of difficult and routine pediatric patients.* New York, 1986, Churchill Livingstone, pp 13–55.

Berry FA: The use of a stylet in blind nasotracheal intubation. *Anesthesiology* 61:469, 1984.

Beven JC, Veall GR, Macnab AJ, et al.: Midazolam premedication delays recovery after propofol without modifying involuntary movements. *Anesth Analg* 85:50–54, 1997.

Biebuyck JF, Eger EI II: New inhaled anesthetic. *Anesthesiology* 80:906–922, 1994.

Biller HF, Harvey JB, Bone R, et al: Laryngeal edema: An experimental study. *Trans Am Laryngeal Assoc* 91:68, 1970.

Blayney MR, Malins AF, Cooper GM: Cardiac arrhythmias in children during outpatient anaesthesia for dentistry: a prospective randomized trial. *Lancet* 354:1864–1867, 1999.

Block C, Brechner KL: Unusual problems in airway management II. *Anesth Analg* 50:114, 1973.

Bordet F, Allaouchiche B, Lansiaux S, et al.: Risk factors for airway complications during general anesthesia in paediatric patients. *Paediatr Anaesth* 12:762–769, 2002.

Bordet F, Allaouchiche B, Lansiaux S, et al.: Risk Factors for airway complications during general anaesthesia in paediatric patients. *Paediatr Anaesth* 12:762–769, 2001.

Borgeat A, Popovic V, Meier D: Comparison of propofol and thiopental/halothane for short-duration ENT surgical procedures in children. *Anesth Analg* 71:511, 1990.

Borland LM, Saitz EW, Woelfel SK: Evaluation of pediatric anesthesia care. Presented at the Section on Anesthesiology, American Academy of Pediatrics, March 1989 (abstract 23 and personal communication).

Borland LM, Sereika SM, Woelfel SK, et al.: Pulmonary aspiration in pediatric patients during general anesthesia: Incidence and outcome. *J Clin Anesth* 10:95–1102, 1998.

Borland LM, Swan DM, Leff S: Difficult endotracheal intubation: A new approach to the retrograde technique. *Anesthesiology* 55:577, 1981.

Borland LM: Establishing the pediatric airway. *Int Anesthesiol Clin* 26:27, 1988.

Bosman YK, Foster PA: Endotracheal intubation and head positions in infants. *S Afr Med J* 52:71, 1977.

Brain AIJ: The laryngeal mask airway – a new concept in airway management. *Br J Anaesth* 55:801, 1983.

Brandom BW, Woelfel SK, Cook DR, et al.: Clinical pharmacology of atracurium in infants. *Anesth Analg* 63:309, 1984.

Brandom BW, Woelfel SK, Cook DR, et al.: Comparison of mivacurium and suxamethonium administered by bolus and infusion. *Br J Anaesth* 62:488, 1989.

Brimacombe JR, Berry A: The incidence of aspiration associated with the laryngeal mask airway: A meta analysis of published literature. *J Clin Anesth* 7:297–305, 1995.

Brimacombe JR, Berry AM: Cricoid pressure. *Can J Anaesth* 44:414–425, 1997.

Brock-Utne JG: Is cricoid pressure necessary? [Editorial] *Paediatar Anaesth* 12:1–4, 2002.

Browning DH, Graves SA: Incidence of aspiration with endotracheal tubes in children. *J Pediatr* 102:582, 1983.

Butz RO Jr: Length and cross-section growth patterns in the human trachea. *Pediatrics* 42:336, 1968.

Calverly RK: A magnificent heritage: The history of pediatric anesthesia. In Berry FA, editor: *Anesthetic management of difficult and routine pediatric patients.* New York, 1986, Churchill Livingstone.

Caplan R, Benumof JL, Berry FA, et al.: A practice guideline for management of the difficult airway: A report by the ASA Task Force on Management of the Difficult Airway. *Anesthesiology* 78:596–602, 1993.

Carenzi B, Corso RM, Stellino V, et al.: Airway management in an infant with congenital centrofacial dysgenesia. *Br J Anaesth* 87:726–728, 2001.

Castro BA, Freedman LA, Craig WL, et al: Explosion within an anesthesia machine: Baralyme®, high fresh gas flows and sevoflurane concentration. *Anesthesiology* 101:537–539, 2004.

Cavall B: Gastric emptying in infants fed human milk or infants formula. *Acta Paediatr Scand* 70:639, 1981.

Cavall B: Gastric emptying in preterm infants. *Acta Paediatr Scand* 68:725, 1979.

Chodoff P, Helrich M: Factors affecting pediatric endotracheal tube size: A statistical analysis. *Anesthesiology* 28:779, 1967.

Cohen DD, Dillon JB: Hazards of armored endotracheal tubes. *Anesth Analg* 51:856, 1972.

Cohen MM, Cameron CB: Should you cancel the operation when a child has an upper respiratory tract infection? *Anesth Analg* 72:282, 1991.

Coldiron JS: Estimation of nasotracheal tube length in neonates. *Pediatrics* 41:823, 1968.

Cole F: Pediatric formulas for the anesthesiologist. *Am J Dis Child* 94:472, 1957.

Constant I, Leport Y, Richard P, et al: Agitation and changes of Bispectral Index™ and electroencephalographic-derived variables during sevoflurane induction in children: Clonidine premedication reduces agitation compared with midazolam. *Br J Anaesth* 92:504, 2004.

Cook DR, Davis PJ, Lerman J: Pharmacology of pediatric anesthesia. In Motoyama EK, Davis PJ (editors): *Smith's anesthesia for infants and children*, 6th edition. St. Louis, 1996, Mosby, pp 159–209.

Corssen G, Guiterrez J, Reves JG, Huber FC Jr: Ketamine in the anesthetic management of asthmatic patients. *Anesth Analg* 51:588–595, 1972.

Coté C: The upper respiratory tract infection (URI) dilemma: Fear of a complication or litigation? *Anesthesiology* 95:283–285, 2001.

Coté CJ, Goudsouzian NG, Liu LM, et al.: The dose response of intravenous thiopental for the induction of general anesthesia in unpremedicated children. *Anesthesiology* 55:703, 1981.

Coté CJ, Goudsouzian NG, Liu LMP, et al.: Assessment of risk factors related to the acid aspiration syndrome in pediatric patients—gastric pH and residual volume. *Anesthesiology* 56:70, 1982.

Coté CJ, Todres ID: The pediatric airway. In Ryan JF, Todres ID, Coté CJ, Goudsouzian N, editors: *A practice of anesthesia for infants and children*, ed 2. Orlando, 1993, Grune and Stratton.

Coté CJ, Cohen IT, Suresh S, et al.: A comparison of three doses of a comercially prepared oral midazolam syrup in children. *Anesth Analg* 94:37–43, 2002.

Cremer R, Kleine-Diepenbruch U, Hoppe A, Blaker F: Latex allergy in spina bifida patients - prevention by primary prophylaxis. *Allergy* 53:709–711, 1998.

Cunliffe M, Lucero VM, McLeod ME, et al.: Neuromuscular blockade for rapid tracheal intubation in children: Comparison of succinylcholine and pancuronium. *Can Anaesth Soc J* 33:760, 1986.

Dajani AS, Taubert KA, Wilson W, et al.: Prevention of bacterial endocarditis: Recommendation by the American Heart Association. *JAMA* 277:1794–1801, 1997.

Davenport HT, editor: *Paediatric anaesthesia,* ed 2. Chicago, 1973, Year Book Publishers, p 70.

Davenport HT, Werry JS: The effect of general anaesthesia, surgery, and hospitalization upon the behavior of children. *Am J Orthopsychiatr* 40:806, 1970.

De Kluijver J, Grunberg K, Sont JK, et al.: Rhinovirus infection in nonasthmatic subjects: Effect on intrapulmonary airways. *Eur Respir J* 20:274–279, 2002.

Deakers TW, Reynolds G: Cuffed endotracheal tubes in pediatric intensive care. *J Pediatr* 125:57–62, 1994.

Delphin E, Jackson D, Rothstein P: Use of succinylcholine during elective pediatric anesthesia should be reevaluated. *Anesth Analg* 66:1190, 1987.

DeSoto H, Patel RI, Soliman IE, et al.: Changes in oxygen saturation following general anesthesia in children with upper respiratory infection and symptoms undergoing otolaryngological procedures. *Anesthesiology* 68:276, 1988.

Diaz JH: Further modifications of the Miller blade for difficult pediatric laryngoscopy. *Anesthesiology* 60:612, 1984.

Dombro RH: The surgically ill child and his family. *Surg Clin North Am* 50:759, 1970.

Dormans JP, Templeton J, Edmonds C, et al.: Intraoperative anaphylaxis due to exposure to latex (natural rubber) in children. *J Bone Joint Surg* 76:1688, 1994.

Dormans JP, Templeton J, Schreiner MS, et al.: Intraoperative latex anaphylaxis in children: classification and prophylaxis of patients at risk. *J Pediatr Orthop* 17:622, 1997.

Driggs RL, O'Day RA: Acute allergic reaction associated with methohexital anesthesia: Report of six cases. *J Oral Surg* 30:906, 1972.

DuBois M-C, Piat V, Constant I, et al.: Comparison of three techniques for induction of anaesthesia with sevoflurane in children. *Paediatr Anaesth* 9:19–23, 1999.

Dubreuil M, Laffon M, Plaud B, et al.: Complications and fiberoptic assessment of size 1 laryngeal mask airway. *Anesth Analg* 76:527–529, 1993.

Dubreuil M, Laffon M, Plaud B, et al.: Incidence of complications with size 1 laryngeal mask. *Anesthesiology* 77:A1174, 1992.

Ebert T, Maze M: Dexmedetomidine: Another arrow of the clinician's quiver. *Anesthesiology* 101, 2004.

Eckenhoff JE: Some anatomic considerations of the infant larynx influencing endotracheal anesthesia. *Anesthesiology* 12:401–410, 1951.

Ehrenstrom Reiz GME, Reiz SLA: EMLA: A eutectic mixture of local anaesthetics for topical anaesthesia. *Acta Anaesthesiol Scand* 26:596, 1982.

Ellis DG, Jakymec A, Kaplan RM, et al.: Guided orotracheal intubation in the operating room using a lighted stylet: A comparison with direct laryngoscopic technique. *Anesthesiology* 64:823, 1986.

Elwood T, Morris W, Martin LD, et al.: Bronchodilator premedication does not decrease respiratory adverse events in pediatric general anesthesia. *Can J Anaesth* 50:277–284, 2003.

Empey DW, Laitinen LA, Jacobs L: Mechanism of bronchial hyperreactivity in normal subjects after upper respiratory infections. *Am Rev Respir Dis* 113:131–139, 1976.

Engel S: *The child's lung*, ed 2. London, 1962, Edward Arnold, Publishers.

Engelhardt T, Strachan L, Johnston G: Aspiration and regurgitation prophylaxis in paediatric anaesthesia. *Paediatr Anaesth* 11:147–150, 2001.

Erb T, Marsch SC, Hampl KF, et al.: Teaching the use of fiberoptic intubation for children older than two years of age. *Anesth Analg* 85: 1037–41, 1997.

Eyres R: Update on TIVA. *Pediatr Anesth* 14:374–379, 2004.

Faithful NS, Haider R: Ketamine for cardiac catheterization. *Anaesthesia* 26:318–323, 1971.

Fatheree RS, Leighton BL: Acute respiratory distress syndrome after an exothermic Baralyme®-sevoflurane reaction. *Anesthesiology* 101:531–3, 2004.

FDA: Allergic reactions to latex-containing medical devices. *FDA Med Bull* 2:1991.

Fearson B, Whalen JS: Tracheal dimensions in the living infant. *Ann Otol Rhinol Laryngol* 76:964, 1967.

Feld LH, Negus JB, White PF: Oral midazolam preanesthetic medication in pediatric outpatients. *Anesthesiology* 73:831, 1990.

Felton M-L, Schmautz E, Delaporte-Cerceau S, et al.: Endotracheal tube cuff pressure is unpredictable in children. *Anesth Analg* 97:1612–6, 2003.

Ferrari LR, Rooney FM, Rockoff MA: Preoperative fasting practices in pediatrics. *Anesthesiology* 90:978–989, 1999.

Fine GF, Borland LM: The future of the cuffed endotracheal tube. *Pediatr Anesth* 14:38–42, 2004.

Fine GF, Fertal K, Motoyama EK: The effectiveness of controlled ventilation using uncuffed versus uncuffed endotracheal tubes in children. *Anesthesiology* 93:A1276, 2000.

Finer NN, Muzyka D: Flexible endoscopic intubation of the neonate. *Pediatr Pulmonol* 12:48, 1992.

Fisher DM: Anesthesia equipment for pediatrics. In Gregory GA, editor: *Pediatric anesthesia.* New York, 1989, Churchill Livingstone, pp 464–465.

Flick RP, Schears GJ, Warner MA: Aspiration in pediatric anesthesia: Is there a higher incidence compared with adults? *Curr Opin Anesthesiol* 15:323–327, 2002.

Forbes RB, Dull DL, Murray DJ, et al.: Cardiovascular effects of rectal methohexital in children. *Anesthesiology* 69:A752, 1988a.

Forbes RB, Gail E, Vandewalker GE: Comparison of two and ten percent rectal methohexitone for induction of anaesthesia in children. *Can J Anaesth* 35:345, 1988b.

Fox DJ, Castro T Jr, Rastrelli AJ: Comparison of intubation technique in the awake patient: The Flexi-lum surgical light (lightwand) versus blind nasal approach. *Anesthesiology* 66:69, 1987.

Frayling IM, Addison GM, Chattergee K, et al.: Methaeglobinaemia in children treated with prilocaine-lignocaine cream. *Br Med J* 301:153, 1990.

Freeman JA, Doyle E, Tee IM, et al.: Topical anaesthesia of the skin: A review. *Paediatr Anaesth* 3:129, 1993.

Frei FJ, Ummenhofer W: Difficult intubation in paediatrics. *Paediatr Anaesth* 6:251–263, 1996.

Frei FJ, Wengen DF, Rutishauser M, et al.: The airway endoscopic mask: Useful device for fiberoptic evaluation and intubation of the paediatric airway. *Paediatr Anaesth* 5:319–324, 1995.

Frink EJ Jr, Green WB Jr, Brown EA, et al.: Compound A concentrations during sevoflurane anesthesia in children. *Anesthesiology* 84:566–571, 1996.

Frink EJ, Ghantous J, Malan TP, et al.: Plasma inorganic fluoride with sevoflurane anesthesia: Correlation with indices of hepatic and renal function. *Anesth Analg* 74:231, 1992.

Funk W, Jakob W, Reidl T, et al.: Oral preanaesthetic medication for children: Double-blind randomized study of a combination of midazolam and ketamine vs midazolam or ketamine alone. *Br J Anaesth* 84:335–340, 2000.

Gaitini LA, Vaida SJ, Somri M, et al.: Randomized and prospective study comparing the ProSeal and the classic laryngeal mask airway in anesthetized, paralyzed children. *Anesthesiology* 101:A515, 2004.

Gibbs CP, Modell JH: Aspiration pneumonitis. In Miller RD, editor: *Anesthesia*, ed 3. New York, 1990, Churchill Livingstone.

Ghinone N, Quintin L, Duke PC, et al.: Effects of clonidine on narcotic requirements and hemodynamic response during induction of fentanyl anesthesia and endotracheal intubation. *Anesthesiology* 64:36–42, 1986.

Gloor A, Diller C, Gerber A: Ketamine for short ambulatory procedures in children: an audit. *Paediatr Anaesth* 11:533–539, 2001.

Goel S, Lim SL: The intubation depth marker: The confusion of the black line. *Paediatr Anaesth* 13:579–583, 2003.

Goldstein-Dresner MC, Davis PJ, Kretchman EK, et al.: Double-blind comparison of oral transmucosal fentanyl citrate with oral meperidine, diazepam, and atropine as preanesthetic medication in children with congenital heart disease. *Anesthesiology* 74:28, 1991.

Goodwin SR, Graves SA, Haberkern CM: Aspiration in intubated premature infants. *Pediatrics* 75:85, 1985.

Goresky GV, Steward DJ: Rectal methohexitone for induction of anaesthesia in children. *Can Anaesth Soc J* 26:213, 1979.

Goudsouzain NG, Denman W, Cleveland R, et al.: Radiologic localization of the laryngeal mask airway in children. *Anesthesiology* 77:1085–1089, 1992.

Goudsouzian NC, Young ET: The efficacy of ranitidine in children. *Acta Anaesthesiol Scand* 31:387–390, 1987.

Goudsouzian NG, Cote CJ, Liu LMP, et al.: The dose-response effect of oral cimetidine of gastric pH and volume in children. *Anesthesiology* 55:533, 1981.

Graff TD, Phillips OC, Benson DW, Kelley E: Baltimore Anesthesia Study Committee: Factors in pediatric anesthesia mortality. *Anesth Analg* 43:407, 1964.

Grant SA, Breslin DS, MacLeod DB, et al.: Dexmedetomidine infusion for sedation during fiberoptic intubation: A report of three cases. *J Clin Anesth* 16:124–126, 2004.

Green SM, Johnson NE: Ketamine sedation for pediatric procedures: Review and implications. *Ann Emerg Med* 19:(Part 2)1033–46, 1990.

Gregory GA: Induction of anesthesia. In Gregory GA, editor: *Pediatric anesthesia.* New York, 1989, Churchill Livingstone, pp 539–560.

Groeben H, Mitzner W, Brown RH: Effects of the α2-adrenoreceptor agonist dexmedetomidine on bronchoconstriction in dogs. *Anesthesiology* 100:359–363, 2004.

Gronert BJ, Woelfel SK, Cook DR: Comparison of equipotent intubating doses of mivacurium and succinylcholine in infants 2-12 months old. *Anesthesiology* 79:A932, 1993a.

Gronert BJ, Woelfel SK, Cook DR: Comparison of high equipotent doses of mivacurium and succinylcholine in children 2-12 years old. *Anesthesiology* 79:A966, 1993b.

Gronert BJ, Woelfel SK, Cook DR: Comparison of neuromuscular effects of mivacurium and succinylcholine in infants and children. *Acta Anaesth Scand* 1994.

Gutstein HB, Johnson KL, Heard MB, et al.: Oral ketamine preanesthetic medication in children. *Anesthesiology* 76:28, 1992.

Hamelberg W, Bosomworth PP: Aspiration pneumonitis: Experimental studies and clinical observations. *Anesth Analg* 43:669–677, 1964.

Hamill JF, Bedford RF, Weaver DC, et al.: Lidocaine before endotracheal intubation: Intravenous or laryngotracheal? *Anesthesiology* 55:578, 1981.

Hammer J, Reber A, Trachsel D, et al.: Effect of jaw-thrust and continuous positive airway pressure on tidal breathing in deeply sedated infants. *J Pediatr* 138:826–830, 2001.

Hannallah RS, Baker SB, Casey W, et al.: Propofol: Effective dose and induction characteristics in unpremedicated children. *Anesthesiology* 74:217, 1991.

Hannallah RS, Oh TH, McGill WA, et al.: Changes in heart rate and rhythm after intramuscular succinylcholine with or without atropine in anesthetized children. *Anesth Analg* 65:1329, 1986.

Hannallah RS, Patel RI: Low-dose intramuscular ketamine for anesthesia pre-induction in young children undergoing brief outpatient procedures. *Anesthesiology* 70:598, 1989.

Hannallah RS, Rosales JK: Experience with parents' presence during anaesthesia induction in children. *Can Anaesth Soc J* 30:286, 1983.

Hawkins DB: Glottic and subglottic stenosis from endotracheal intubation. *Laryngoscope* 87:339–346, 1977.

Hay WW, Brockway JM, Eyzaguirre M: Neonatal pulse oximetry: Accuracy and reliability. *Pediatrics* 83:717, 1989.

Haynes SR, Morton NS: The laryngeal mask airway: A review of its use in paediatric anaesthesia. *Paediatr Anaesth* 3:65, 1993.

Hemmingsen C, Nielsen PK, Odorico J: Ketamine in the treatment of bronchospasm during mechanical ventilation. *Am J Emerg Med* 12:417–420, 1994.

Henderson JJ: The use of paraglossal straight blade laryngoscopy in difficult tracheal intubation. *Anaesthesia* 52:522–560, 1997.

Henderson JM, Spence DG, Clarke WN: Sodium citrate in paediatric patients. *Can J Anaesth* 34:560–562, 1987.

Holaday DA, Smith FR: Clinical characteristics and biotransformation of sevoflurane in healthy human volunteers. *Anesthesiology* 54:100, 1981.

Holzki J, Kretz FJ: Changing aspects of sevoflurane in paediatric anaesthesia 1975-99. *Paediatr Anaesth* 9:283, 1999.

Holzman RS: Morbidity and mortality in pediatric anesthesia. *Pediatr Clin North Am* 41:239, 1994.

Honig EG: Persistent tracheal dilatation: Onset after brief mechanical ventilation with a "soft-cuff" endotracheal tube. *South Med J* 72:487–490, 1979.

Inagawa G, Okuda K, Takaaki M, et al.: Higher airway seal does not imply adequate positioning of laryngeal mask airways in paediatric patients. *Paediatr Anaesth* 12:322–326, 2002.

Inkster JS: The induction of anaesthesia in patients likely to vomit with special reference to intestinal obstruction. *Br J Anaesth* 35:160, 1963.

James I: Cuffed tubes in children. *Paediatr Anaesth* 11:259–263, 2001.

Jöhr M, Berger TM: Fiberoptic intubation through the laryngeal mask airway (LMA) as a standardized procedure. *Pediatr Anesth* 14:614, 2004.

Jonmarker C, Westrin P, Larsson S, et al.: Thiopental requirements for induction of anesthesia in children. *Anesthesiology* 67:104, 1987.

Jordan WS, Graves CL, Elwyn RA: New therapy for post-intubation laryngeal edema and tracheitis in children. *JAMA* 212:585, 1970.

Jorden VS, Pousman RM, Sanford MM, et al.: Dexmedetomidine overdose in the perioperative setting. *Ann Pharmacother* 38:803–807, 2004.

Kain ZN, Caldwell-Andrews AA, Krivutza D, et al.: Trends in the practice of parental presence during induction of anesthesia and the use of preoperative sedative premedication in the United States, 1995-2002: Results of a follow-up national survey. *Anesth Analg* 98:1252–1259, 2004.

Kain ZN, Caramico L, Mayes L, et al.: Preoperative preparation programs in children: A comparative study. *Anesth Analg* 87:1249–1255, 1998.

Kain ZN, Mayes L: Anxiety in children during the perioperative period. In Borestein M, Genevro J (editors): *Child development and behavioral pediatrics.* Mahwah, NJ, 1996, Lawrence Erlbaum Associates.

Kain Z, Mayes L, Caramico L, et al.: Distress during induction of anesthesia and postoperative behavioral outcomes. *Anesth Analg* 88:1042–1047, 1999.

Kain Z, Mayes L, Wang S, et al.: Parental presence and a sedative premedicant for children undergoing surgery: A hierarchial study. *Anesthesiology* 92:939–946, 2000.

Kallar SK, Everett LL: Potential risks and preventive measures for pulmonary aspiration: new concepts in preoperative fasting guidelines. *Anesth Analg* 77:171, 1993.

Kaufman L: Anaesthesia for the older child. In Gray TC, Nunn JF, editors: *General anesthesia*, ed 3. Borough Green, Kent, 1973, Butterworth & Co.

Keep PJ, Manford ML: Endotracheal tubes for children. *Anaesthesia* 29:181, 1974.

Keidan I, Erkenstadt H, Segal E, et al.: Pressure versus volume-controlled ventilation with a laryngeal mask airway in paediatric patients. *Paediatr Anaesth* 11:691–694, 2001.

Keidan I, Fine GF, Kagawa T, et al.: Work of breathing during spontaneous ventilation in anesthetized children: A comparative study among the face mask, laryngeal mask airway and endotracheal tube. *Anesth Analg* 91:1381–1388, 2000.

Kellehar JF: Pulse oximetry. *J Clin Monit* 5:37, 1989.

Kenaan CA, Estacio RL, Bikhazi GB: Pharmacodynamics and intubation conditions of cisatracurium in children. *J Clin Anesth* 12:173–176, 2000.

Khalil SN, Mankarious R, Campos C, et al.: Absence or presence of a leak around tracheal tube may not affect postoperative croup in children. *Paediatr Anaesth* 8:393–396, 1998.

Kharasch ED, Powers KM, Artru AA: Comparison of Amsorb, soda lime and Baralyme degradation of volatile anesthetics and formation of carbon monoxide and compound A in swine in vivo. *Anesthesiology* 96:173–182, 2002.

Khine HH, Corddry DH, Kettrick RG, et al.: Comparison of cuffed and uncuffed endotracheal tubes in young children during general anesthesia. *Anesthesiology* 86:627–631, 1997.

Kim YC, Lee SH, Noh GL, et al.: Thermosoftening of the nasotracheal tube before intubation can reduce epistaxis and nasal damage. *Anesth Analg* 91: 698–701, 2000.

King BR, Baker MD, Braitman LE, et al.: Endotracheal tube selection in children: A comparison of four methods. *Ann Emerg Med* 22:530–534, 1993.

Kleinsasser A, Loekinger A, Lindner KH, et al.: Reversing sevoflurane associated Q-Tc prolongation by changing to propofol. *Anaesthesia* 56:248–250, 2001.

Kobayashi S, Bito H, Obara Y, et al.: Compound A concentration in the circle absorber system during low-flow sevoflurane anesthesia: Comparison of Dragersorb Free, Amsorb, and Sodasorb II. *J Clin Anesth* 15:33–37, 2003.

Koka BV, Jeon S, Andre JM, et al.: Postintubation croup in children. *Anesth Analg* 56:501, 1977.

Kotoniemi LH, Ryhanen PT, Moilanen IK: Behavioral changes in children following day-case surgery. A 4-week follow-up of 551 children. *Anaesthesia* 52:970–976, 1997.

Kwittken PL, Sweinberg SK, Campbell DE, et al.: Latex hypersensitivity in children: Clinical presentation and detection of latex-specific immunoglobulin E. *Pediatrics* 95:693–699, 1995.

Laishley RS, O'Callhaghan AC, Lerman J: Effects of dose and concentration of rectal methohexitone for induction of anaesthesia in children. *Can Anaesth Soc J* 33:427, 1986.

Landsman I: Cricoid pressure: Indications and complications. *Pediatr Anesth* 14:43–47, 2004.

Lassiter HA: Epiglottitis: Laryngospasm at intubation. *J Kans Med Soc* 83:9–10, 1982.

Lee KW, Templeton JJ, Douglas R: Tracheal tube size and postoperative croup in children. *Anesthesiology* 53:S325.

Lerman J, Christenson SK, Farrow-Gillespie AC: Effects of metoclopramide and ranitidine on gastric fluid volume and pH in children. *Can J Anaesth* 35:142–143, 1988.

Lerman J: Inhalational anesthetics. *Pediatr Anesth* 14:380–383, 2004.

Leske JS: Effects of intraoperative progress reports on anxiety of elective surgical patients' family members. *Clin Nursing Res* 1:266, 1992.

L'Hommedieu CS, Arens JJ: The use of ketamine for the emergency intubation of patients with status asthmaticus. *Ann Emerg Med* 16:568–571, 1987.

Lindholm CE: Experience with a new endotracheal tube. *Acta Otolaryngol* 75:389–390, 1973.

Litman RS, Keon TP: Postintubation croup in children [letter]. *Anesthesiology* 75:1122–1123, 1991.

Litman RS, Wu CL, Quinlivan JK: Gastric volume and pH in infants fed clear liquids and breast milk prior to surgery. *Anesth Analg* 79:482–485, 1994.

Liu LMP, Goudsouzian NG, Liu PL: Rectal methohexital premedication in children, a dose-comparison study. *Anesthesiology* 53:343, 1980.

Liu LMP, Liu PL, Moss J: Severe histamine-mediated reaction to rectally administered methohexital. *Anesthesiology* 61:95, 1984.

Liu MPL, DeCook TH, Goudsouzian NG, et al.: Dose response to intramuscular succinylcholine in children. *Anesthesiology* 55:599, 1981.

Loh KS, Irish JC: Traumatic complications of intubation and other airway management procedures. *Anesthesiol Clin North Am* 20:953–969, 2002.

Mac G, Palmer JH, Ball DR: The effect of cricoid pressure on the cricoid cartilage and vocal cords: An endoscopic study in anaesthetized patients. *Anaesthesia* 55:263–268, 2000.

MacFarlan CS, Anderson BJ, Short TG: The use of propofol infusions in paediatric anaesthesia: A practical guide. *Paediatr Anaesth* 9:209–216, 1999.

Maekawa N, Mikawa K, Tanaka O, et al.: The laryngeal mask airway may be useful device for fiberoptic airway endoscopy in pediatric anesthesia. *Anesthesiology* 75:169–170, 1999.

Maier S, Klingsasser A, Keller C, et al.: QT prolongation under sevoflurane in infants. *Paediatr Anaesth* 12:826, 2002.

Maktabi MA, Smith RB, Todd MM: Is routine endotracheal intubation as safe as we think or wish? *Anesthesiology* 99:247–248, 2003.

Mallampati SR, Gatt SP, Gugino LD, et al.: A clinical sign to predict difficult tracheal intubation: A prospective study. *Can Anaesth Soc J* 32:429–434, 1985.

Manschot HJ, Meursing AE, Axt P, et al.: Propofol requirement for induction of anaesthesia in children of different age groups. *Anesth Analg* 75:876–879, 1992.

Markakis D, Sayson SC, Schreiner MS: Insertion of the laryngeal mask airway in awake infants with the Robin sequence. *Anesth Analg* 75:822–824, 1992.

Mattila M, Heikel PE, Suutarinen T, et al.: Estimation of a suitable nasotracheal length for infants and children. *Acta Anaesthesiol Scand* 15:239, 1971.

Maunuksela E-L, Korpela R: Double-blind evaluation of lignocaine-prilocaine cream (EMLA) in children: Effect on the pain associated with venous cannulation. *Br J Anaesth* 58:1242, 1986.

Mazze RI, Jamison RL: Low-flow (1 l/minutes) sevoflurane: Is it safe? *Anesthesiology* 86:1225–1227, 1997.

McCann ME, Kain ZN: The management of preoperative anxiety in children: An update. *Anesth Analg* 93:98–105, 2001.

McFarlan CS, Anderson BJ, Short TG: The use of propofol infusions in paediatric anaesthesia: a practical guide. *Paediatr Anaesth* 9:209–216, 1999.

Meakin G, McKeirnan EP, Morris P, et al.: Dose-response curves for suxamethonium in neonates, infants, and children. *Br J Anaesth* 62:655, 1989.

Meakin G, Shaw EA, Baker RD, et al.: Comparison of atracurium-induced neuromuscular blockade in neonates, infants and children. *Br J Anaesth* 60:171, 1988.

Meakin GH: Low-flow anaesthesia in infants and children. *Br J Anaesth* 83:50–57, 1999.

Mehta S: Effects of nitrous oxide and oxygen on tracheal tube cuff gas volumes. *Br J Anaesth* 53:1227, 1981.

Melamed BG: Putting the family back in the child. *Behav Res Ther* 31:239–247, 1993.

Melamed BG, Ridley-Johnson R: Psychological preparation of families for hospitalization. *Dev Behav Pediatr* 9:96–102, 1988.

Mellin-Olsen J, Fasting S, Gisvold SE: Routine preoperative gastric emptying is seldom indicated. A study of 85,594 anaesthetics with special focus on aspiration pneumonia. *Acta Anaesthesiol Scand* 40:1184–1188, 1996.

Mendelson CL: Aspiration of stomach contents into lungs during obstetric anesthesia. *Am J Obstet Gynecol* 52:191–205, 1946.

Meretoja O: Is vecuronium a long-acting neuromuscular blocking agent in neonates and infants? *Br J Anaesth* 62:184, 1989.

Mikawa K, Maekawa N, Nishina K, et al.: Efficacy of oral clonidine premedication in children. *Anesthesiology* 79:926–931, 1993.

Miller JR, Stoelting VK, Darin MW: A preliminary report on the use of intramuscular methohexital sodium (Brevital) for pediatric anesthesia. *Anesth Analg* 54:64, 1973.

Mirakhur RK: Induction characteristics of propofol in children: Comparison with thiopentone. *Anaesthesia* 43:593, 1988.

Molendijk H: Use of the black area on the tubetip for rapid estimation of insertional depth of endotracheal tubes in neonates: a potential hazard. *Arch Dis Child Fetal Neonatal Ed* 85:F77, 2001.

Morgan GAR, Steward DJ: A pre-formed paediatric orotracheal tube design based on anatomical measurements. *Can Anaesth Soc J* 29:9–11, 1982b.

Morgan GAR, Steward DJ: Linear airway dimensions in children: Including those with cleft palate. *Can Anaesth Soc J* 29:1–8, 1982a.

Morio M, Fujii K, Satoh N, et al.: Reaction of sevoflurane and its degradation products with soda lime. *Anesthesiology* 77:1155, 1992.

Morray JP, Geiduscheck JM, Ramamoorthy C, et al.: Anesthesia-related cardiac arrest in children: Initial findings of the Pediatric Perioperaive Cardiac Arrest (POCA) registry. *Anesthesiology* 93:6–14, 2000.

Morrison JE, Collier E, Friesen RH, et al.: Preoxygenation before laryngoscopy in children: How long is enough? *Paediatr Anaesth* 8:293–298, 1998.

Mostafa SM: Variation in subglottis size in children. *Proc R Soc Med* 69:793, 1976.

Motoyama EK, Cohen IT: Continuous positive airway pressure (CPAP) improves airway patency and ventilation during inhalation induction in children. *Anesthesiology* 77:A1198, 1992.

Motoyama EK: Inspiratory muscle incoordination and upper airway obstruction during inhalation anesthesia. *Int Anesthesiol Clin* 35:45–47, 1997.

Moynihan RJ, Brock-Ute JG, Archer JH, et al.: The effect of cricoid pressure on preventing gastric insufflation in infants and children. *Anesthesiology* 78:652–656, 1993.

Munro HM, Ghurye MR, Thomas VL: Potential hazard due to differing markings of paediatric tracheal tubes. *Paediatr Anaesth* 5:339–342, 1995.

Murat I: Anaphylactic reactions during paediatric anaesthesia: Results of the survey of the French Society of Paediatric Anaesthetists (ADARPEF) 1991-1992. *Paediatr Anaesth* 3:339–343, 1993.

Murat I: Cuffed tubes in children: A 3-year experience in a single institution. *Paediatr Anaesth* 11:748–749, 2001a.

Murat I: Halothane: The last word? *Paediatr Anaesth* 11:249, 2001b.

Murat I: Is there still a place for halothane in paediatric anaesthesia? *Paediatr Anaesth* 8:183, 1998.

Murat I: Latex allergy: Where are we? *Paediatr Anaesth* 10:577–579, 2000.

Murray DJ, Forbes RB, Dull DL, et al.: Does atropine improve myocardial performance during halothane and isoflurane anesthesia in infants? *Anesthesiology* 69:A751, 1988.

Murray JP, Geidushek JM, Ramamoorthy C, et al.: Anesthesia-related cardiac arrest in children. *Anesthesiology* 93:6–14, 2000.

Myer EF, Muravchick S: Anaesthesia induction technics in paediatric patients: A controlled study of behavioral consequences. *Anesth Analg* 56:538, 1977.

Naito Y, Tamai S, Shingu K, et al.: Comparison between sevoflurane and halothane for paediatric ambulatory anaesthesia. *Br J Anaesth* 67:387, 1991.

Nelson PS, Streisand JB, Mulder SM, et al.: Comparison of oral transmucosal fentanyl citrate and an oral solution of meperidine, diazepam and atropine for premedication in children. *Anesthesiology* 70:616–621, 1989.

Nicolson SC, Dorsey AT, Schreiner MS: Shortened preanesthetic fasting interval in pediatric cardiac surgical patients. *Anesth Analg* 74:694, 1992.

NIOSH: *Anesthetic gases: Guidelines for workplace exposures.* Washington, DC, 1997, U.S. Department of Labor, Occupational Safety and Health Administration.

Nishida T, Nishimura M, Kagawa K, et al.: The effects of dexmedetomidine on the ventilatory response to hypercapnia in rabbits. *Intensive Care Med* 28:969–975, 2002.

Nishina K, Mikawa K, Shiga M, et al.: Clonidine in paediatric anaesthesia. *Paediatr Anaesth* 9:187–202, 1999.

Nishina K, Mikawa K: Clonidine in paediatric anaesthesia. *Curr Opin Anaesthesiol* 15:309–316, 2002.

Nishino T, Shirahata M, Yonezawa T, et al.: Comparison of changes in the hypoglossal and the phrenic nerve activity in response to increasing depth of anesthesia in cats. *Anesthesiology* 60:19, 1984.

Norton ML, de Vos P: New endotracheal tube for laser surgery of the larynx. *Ann Otol Rhinol Laryngol* 87:554, 1978.

O'Byrne K, Peterson L, Salada L: Survey of pediatric hospitals' preparation programs: Evidence of the impact of health psychology research. *Health Psychol* 16:147–154, 1997.

Ochiai R, Guthrie RD, Motoyama EK: Effects of varying concentrations of halothane on the activity of the genioglossus, intercostals and diaphragm in cats: an electromyographic study. *Anesthesiology* 70:812–816, 1989.

Ochiai R, Gutherie RD, Motoyama EK: Differential sensitivity to halothane anesthesia of the genioglossus intercostals and diaphragm in kittens. *Anesth Analg* 74:338, 1992.

O'Kelly B, Frossard J, Meistelman C, et al.: Neuromuscular blockade following ORG 9426 in children during N_2O-halothane anesthesia. *Anesthesiology* 76:A787, 1991.

Okuda K, Inagawa G, Miwa T, et al.: Influence of head and neck position on cuff position and oropharyngeal sealing pressure with the laryngeal mask airway in children. *Br J Anaesth* 86:122–124, 2001.

Okuyama M, Imai M, et al.: Finding appropriate tube position by the cuff palpation method in children. *Masui* 44:845–848, 1995.

Olsson GL, Hallen B, Hambraeus-Jonzon K: Aspiration during anaesthesia: A computer-aided study of 185,358 anaesthetics. *Acta Anaesthesiol Scand* 30:84, 1986.

O'Neill B, Templeton JJ, Caramic L, et al.: The laryngeal mask airway in pediatric patients: factors affecting ease of use during insertion and emergence. *Anesth Analg* 78:659, 1994.

Ovassapian A, Yelich SJ, Dykes MHM, et al.: Fiberoptic nasotracheal intubation—incidence and causes of failure. *Anesth Analg* 62:692, 1983.

Park C, Bahk JH, Ahn WS, et al.: The laryngeal mask airway in infants and children. *Can J Anaesth* 48:413–417, 2001.

Patel RI, Oh TH, Chandra R, et al.: Tracheal tube cuff pressure. Changes during nitrous oxide anaesthesia following inflation of cuffs with air and saline. *Anaesthesia* 39:862, 1984.

Patil VU, Stehling LC, Zauder HL: *Fiberoptic endoscopy in anesthesia.* Chicago, 1983, Year-Book Medical Publishers.

Penlington GN: Endotracheal tube sizes for children. *Br J Anaesth* 29:494, 1974.

Pennant JH, White PF: The laryngeal mask airway. *Anesthesiology* 79:144–163, 1993.

Peters JWB, Bezstarosti-van Eeden J, Erdmann W, et al.: Safety and efficacy of semi-closed circle ventilation in small infants. *Paedatr Anaesth* 8:299–304, 1998.

Phillips OC, Duerkson RL: Endotracheal intubation: A new blade for direct laryngoscopy. *Anesth Analg* 52:691, 1973.

Porri F, Prada M, Lemiere C, et al.: Association between latex sensitization and repeated latex exposure in children. *Anesthesiology* 86:599–602, 1997.

Powell WF, Ozdil T: A translaryngeal guide for tracheal intubation. *Anesth Analg* 46:231, 1967.

Ramsey MAE, Luterman DL: Dexmedetomidine as a total intravenous anesthetic agent. *Anesthesiology* 101:787–790, 2004.

Reber A, Paganoni R, Frei FJ: Effect of common airway manoeuvres on upper airway dimension and clinical signs in anaesthetized, spontaneously breathing children. *Br J Anaesth* 86:217–222, 2001.

Rees GJ, Owen Thomas JB: A technique of pulmonary ventilation with a nasotracheal tube. *Br J Anaesth* 38:901, 1996.

Rendall-Baker L, Roberts RB: Hazards of ethylene oxide sterilization. *Anesthesiology* 30:179, 1962.

Roe RB: The effect of suxamethonium on intragastric pressure. *Anaesthesia* 17:179, 1962.

Rosenberg H, Gronert GA: Intractable cardiac arrest in children given succinylcholine. *Anesthesiology* 77:1054, 1992.

Rowbottom SJ, Simpson DL, Grub D: Forum: The laryngeal mask airway in children—a fibreoptic assessment of positioning. *Anaesthesia* 46:489–491, 1991.

Rowland ASA, Baird DD, Shore DL, et al.: Nitrous oxide and spontaneous abortion among female dental assistants. *Am J Epidemiol* 141:531–538, 1995.

Rowland ASA, Baird DD, Weinberg CR, et al.: Reduced fertility among women employed as dental assistants exposed to high levels of nitrous oxide. *N Engl J Med* 327:993–997, 1992

Ruffle JM, Snider MT, Rosenberger JL, et al.: Rapid induction of halothane anaesthesia in man. *Br J Anaesth* 57:607, 1985.

Salem MR, Wong AY, Collins VJ: The pediatric patient with a full stomach. *Anesthesiology* 39:435, 1973.

Salem MR, Wong AY, Fozzoti GF: Efficacy of cricoid pressure in preventing aspiration of gastric contents in paediatric patients. *Br J Anaesth* 44:401, 1972a.

Salem MR, Wong AY, Lin YH: The effect of suxamethonium on the intragastric pressure in infants and children. *Br J Anaesth* 44:166, 1972b.

Salem MR: Anesthetic management of patients with a "full stomach." A critical review. *Anesth Analg* 49:47, 1970.

Sarner JB, Levine M, Davis PJ, et al.: Clinical characteristics of sevoflurane in children: A comparison with halothane. *Anesthesiology* 82:38–46, 1995.

Sasaki CT, Levine PA, Laitman JT, et al.: Postnatal descent of the epiglottis in man. *Arch Otolaryngol* 103:169, 1977.

Schreiner MS, Triebwasser A, Keon TP: Ingestion of liquids compared with preoperative fasting in pediatric outpatients. *Anesthesiology* 72:593–597, 1990.

Schwartz RE, Stayer SA, et al.: Tracheal tube leak test—is there inter-observer agreement? *Can J Anaesth* 40:1049–1052, 1993.

Seegobin RD, Hasselt GL: Endotracheal tube cuff pressure and tracheal mucosal blood flow: Endoscopic study of effects of four volume cuffs. *BMJ* 288:965–968, 1994.

Sellick BA: Cricoid pressure to control the regurgitation of stomach contents during the induction of anaesthesia. *Lancet* 2:204, 1961.

Shellinger RR: The length of the airway to the bifurcation of the trachea. *Anesthesiology* 25:169, 1964.

Shimbori H, Ono K, Miwa T, et al.: Comparison of the LMA-ProSeal and LMA-Classic in children. *Br J Anaesth* 93:523–531, 2004.

Silvanus M-T, Groeben H, Peters J: Corticosteroids and inhaled salbutamol in patients with reversible airway obstruction markedly decrease the incidence of bronchospasm after tracheal intubation. *Anesthesiology* 100:1047–1048, 2004.

Sloan MH, Lerman J, Bissonnette B: Pharmacodynamics of high-dose vecuronium in children during balanced anesthesia. *Anesthesiology* 74:656, 1991.

Smith KJ, Dobranowski J, Yip G, et al.: Cricoid pressure displaces the esophagus: An observational study using magnetic resonance imaging. *Anesthesiology* 99:60–64, 2003.

Smith RM, Schaer WB, Pfaeffle H: Percutaneous transtracheal ventilation for anaesthesia and resuscitation: A review and report of complications. *Can Anaesth Soc J* 22:607, 1975.

Smith RM: *Anesthesia for infants and children,* Chapter 7: Technics of the induction of anesthesia. St. Louis, 1980a, CV Mosby, p 152.

Smith RM: *Anesthesia for infants and children,* Chapter 8: Endotracheal intubation. St. Louis, 1980b, CV Mosby, p 164.

Smith RM: Indications for endotracheal anesthesia in pediatric anesthesia. *Anesth Analg* 33:107, 1954.

Smith RM: Some reasons for the high mortality in pediatric anesthesia. *N Y State J Med* 56:2212, 1956.

Smith RM: The pediatric anesthetist. *Anesthesiology* 43:144, 1975.

Smith RM: The prevention of tracheitis in children following endotracheal anesthesia. *Anesth Analg* 32:102, 1953.

Snow RG, Nunn JF: Induction of anaesthesia in the footdown position for patients with a full stomach. *Br J Anaesth* 31:493, 1959.

Soh CR, Ng AS: Laryngeal mask airway insertion in paediatric anaesthesia: Comparison between the reverse and standard techniques. *Anaesth Intensive Care* 29:515–519, 2001.

Sosis MB: Which is the safest endotracheal tube for use with the CO2 laser? *J Clin Anesth* 4:217, 1992.

Southhall DP, Bignall S, Stebbens VA, et al.: Pulse oximeter and transcutaneous arterial oxygen measurements in neonatal and paediatric intensive care. *Arch Dis Child* 62:882, 1987.

Spear RM, Yaster M, Berkowitz ID, et al.: Preinduction of anesthesia in children with rectally administered midazolam. *Anesthesiology* 74:670, 1991.

Splinter WM, Schaefer JD: Unlimited clear fluid ingestion two hours before surgery in children does not affect volume or pH of stomach contents. *Anaesth Intensive Care* 18:522–526, 1990.

Splinter WM, Stewart JA, Muir JG: Large volumes of apple juice preoperatively do not affect gastric pH and volume in children. *Can J Anaesth* 37:36, 1990.

Stanley TH, Leiman BC, Rawal N, et al.: The effects of oral transmucosal fentanyl citrate premedication on preoperative behavioral responses and gastric volume and acidity in children. *Anesth Analg* 69:328–335, 1989.

Steffey EP, Lasteer MJ, Ionescu P, et al.: Dehydration of Baralyme® increases the concentration of compound A resulting from sevoflurane degradation in a standard anesthetic circuit. *Anesth Analg* 85:892–898, 1997.

Steward DJ: *Manual of paediatric anaesthesia.* New York, 1979, Churchill Livingstone, p 39.

Stewart KG, Rowbottom SJ, Aiken AW, et al.: Oral ketamine premedication for paediatric cardiac surgery—a comparison with intramuscular morphine (both after oral trimeprazine). *Anaesth Intens Care* 18:11, 1990.

Stoddart PA, Brennen L, Hatch DJ, et al.: Postal survey of paediatric practice and training among consultant anaesthetists in the UK. *Br J Anaesth* 73:559–563, 1994.

Stoelting RK: Endotracheal intubation. In Miller RD, editor: *Anesthesia*, ed 2. New York, 1986, Churchill Livingstone, pp 523–552.

Strube PJ, Hallam PL: Ketamine by continuous infusion in status asthmaticus. *Anaesthesia* 41:1017–1019, 1986.

Strum DP, Eger EI: Partition coefficient for sevoflurane in human blood, saline, and olive oil. *Anesth Analg* 66:654, 1987.

Sussman DR: A comparative evaluation of ketamine anesthesia in children and adults. *Anesthesiology* 40:459–464, 1974.

Suter PM, Fairly HB, Isenberg MD: Optimum end-expiratory airway pressure in patients with acute pulmonary failure. *N Engl J Med* 292:284, 1975.

Tait AR, Malviya S, Voepel-Lewis T, et al.: Risk factors for perioperative adverse respiratory events in children with upper respiratory tract infections. *Anesthesiology* 95:299–306, 2001.

Taivanien T, Meakin GH, Meretoja OA, et al.: The safety and efficacy of cisatracurium 0.15 mg.kg^{-1} during nitrous oxide opioid anesthesia in infants and children. *Anaesthesia* 55:1047–1051, 2000.

Tamura M, Ishikawa T, Kato R, et al.: Mandibular advancement improves the laryngeal view during direct laryngoscopy performed by inexperienced physicians. *Anesthesiology* 100:598–601, 2004.

Tanaka A, Isono S, Ishikawa T, et al.: Laryngeal resistance before and after minor surgery. *Anesthesiology* 99:252, 2003.

Taylor G, Pryse-Davies J: The prophylactic use of antacids in the prevention of the acid-pulmonary-aspiration syndrome (Mendelson's syndrome). *Lancet* 1:288, 1966.

Theroux MC, Kettrick RG, Khine HH: Laryngeal mask airway and fiberoptic endoscopy in an infant with Schwartz-Jampel syndrome. *Anesthesiology* 82:605, 1995.

Thomas PB, Parry MG: The difficult paediatric airways: A new method of intubation using the laryngeal mask airway, Cook airway exchange catheter and tracheal intubation fiberscope. *Paediatr Anaesth* 11:618–621, 2001.

Tiret L, Nivoche Y, Hatton F, et al.: Complications related to anaesthesia in infants and children. A prospective survey of 40240 anaesthetics. *Br J Anaesth* 61:263–269, 1988.

Tisza VB, Angoff KA: A play program for hospitalized children: The role of the play-room teacher. *Pediatrics* 28:841, 1961.

Tobias JD, Berkenbosch JW: Initial experience with dexmedetomidine in paediatric-aged patients. *Paediatr Anaesth* 12:171–175, 2002.

Todres ID, Crone RK: Experience in modified laryngoscope in sick infants. *Crit Care Med* 9:544, 1981.

Tom GH, Henning J, Steen WH, et al.: Laryngeal mask airway guided trachea: Intubation in a neonate with the Pierre Robin syndrome. *Acta Anesthesiol Scand* 39:129–131, 1995.

Tonnenson AS, Vereen L, Aren JF: Endotracheal tube cuff residual volume and lateral wall pressure in a model trachea. *Anesthesiology* 55:680–683, 1981.

Tournadre JP, Chassard D, Berrada KR, et al.: Cricoid cartilage pressure decreases lower esophageal sphincter tone. *Anesthesiology* 86:7–9, 1997.

Uejima T: Cuffed endotracheal tubes in pediatric patients. *Anesth Analg* 68:413, 1989,

Vanner RG, O'Dwyer JP, Pryle BJ, et al.: Upper oesophageal sphincter pressure and the effect of cricoid pressure. *Anaesthesia* 47:95–100, 1992.

Verghese C, Brimacombe JR: Survey of laryngeal mask airway usage in 11910 patients: Safety and efficacy for conventional and non-conventional usage. *Anesth Analg* 82:129–133, 1996.

Viitanen H, Annila P, Viitanen M, et al.: Midazolam premedication delays recovery from propofol-induced sevoflurane anesthesia in children 1-3 yr. *Can J Anaesth* 46:766–771, 1999.

Voyagis GS, Batzioulis PG, Secha-Doussaitou PG: Selection of the proper size of the laryngeal mask airway in adults. *Anesth Analg* 83:663–664, 1996.

Vredevoe LA, Bretcher T, Moy P: Obstruction of anomalous tracheal bronchus with endotracheal intubation. *Anesthesiology* 55:581, 1981.

Vulcan BM, Nikulich-Barrett M: The effect of selected information on mothers' anxiety levels during their children's hospitalizations. *J Pediatr Nursing* 3:97, 1988.

Walker RWM, Aklen DL, Rothera MR: A fiberoptic intubation technique for children with mucopolysaccharidoses using the laryngeal mask airway. *Paediatr Anaesth* 7:421–426, 1997.

Wallace CJ, Bell GT: Tracheal tube markings. *Pediatr Anesth* 14:283–285, 2004.

Wallin RF, Regan BM, Napoli MD, et al.: Sevoflurane: A new inhalational anesthetic agent. *Anesth Analg* 54:758, 1975.

Wark H: Halothane: The last word? *Paediatr Anaesth* 11:249, 2001.

Wark H: Is there still a place for halothane in paediatric anaesthesia? *Paediatr Anaesth* 7:359, 1997.

Warner MA, Warner ME: Warner DO, et al.: Perioperative pulmonary aspiration in infants and children. *Anesthesiology* 90:66–71, 1999.

Weaver MK: Perioperative pulmonary aspiration in children: A review. *Paediatr Anaesth* 3:333–338, 1993.

Weiss M, Dullenkopf A, Gysin C, et al.: Shortcomings of cuffed paediatric tracheal tubes. *Br J Anaesth* 92:78–88, 2004.

Weksler N, Ovadia L, Muati G, et al.: Nasal ketamine for paediatric premedication. *Can J Anaesth* 40:119, 1993.

Welborn LG, Norden JM, Seiden N, et al.: Effect of minimizing preoperative fasting on perioperative blood glucose homeostasis in children. *Paediatr Anaesth* 3:167–171, 1993.

Weymuller EA: Prevention and management of intubation injury of the larynx and trachea. *Am J Otolaryngol* 13:139–144, 1992.

Wheeler M: Management strategies for the difficult pediatric airway. *Anesthesiol Clin North Am* 16:743–761, 1998.

Wilton NCT, Leigh J, Rosen DR, et al.: Preanesthetic sedation of preschool children using intranasal midazolam. *Anesthesiology* 69:972, 1988.

Wissing H, Kuhn I, Warnken R, et al.: Carbon monoxide production from desflurane, enflurane, halothane, isoflurane and sevoflurane with dry soda lime. *Anesthesiology* 95:1205–1212, 2001.

Wittenborg MH, Gyepes MT, Crocker D: Tracheal dynamics in infants with respiratory distress, stridor, and collapsing trachea. *Radiology* 88:653, 1967.

Woehlck HJ: Sleeping with uncertainty: Anesthesia and desiccated absorbent. *Anesthesiology* 101:276–278, 2004.

Woelfel SK, Brandom BW, McGowan FX, et al.: Neuromuscular effects of 600 mcg/kg of rocuronium in infants during nitrous oxide-halothane anaesthesia. *Paediatr Anaesth* 4:173, 1994.

Wood RE: Clinical applications of ultrathin flexible bronchoscopes. *Pediatr Pul* 1:244, 1985.

Wood RE: Endoscopy of the airway in infants and children. *J Pediatr* 112:1, 1988.

Wood RE: Pediatric bronchoscopy, bronchography, and laryngoscopy. In Berry FA, editor: *Anesthetic management of difficult and routine pediatric patients.* New York, 1986, Churchill Livingstone.

Wu J, Previte JP, Adler E, et al.: Spontaneous ignition, explosion, and fire with sevoflurane and barium hydroxide lime. *Anesthesiology* 101:534–537, 2004.

Wyatt R, Watkin J: Reaction to methohexitone. *Br J Anaesth* 47:1119, 1975.

Wynne JW, Reynolds JC, Hood I, et al.: Steroid therapy for pneumonitis induced in rabbits by aspiration of food-stuff. *Anesthesiology* 51:11, 1979.

Yates AP, Harris AJ, Hatch DJ: Estimation of nasotracheal tube length in infants and children. *Br J Anaesth* 59:524–526, 1987.

Yemen TA: Pediatric induction rooms: Clinical applications. *Anesthesiology* 71:A1166, 1989.

Yemen TA, Pullerits J, Stillman R, et al.: Rectal methohexital causing apnea in two patients with meningomyeloceles. *Anesthesiology* 74:1139, 1991.

Zwass MS, Fisher DM, Welborn LG, et al.: Induction and maintenance characteristics of anesthesia with desflurane and nitrous oxide in infants and children. *Anesthesiology* 76:373, 1992.

11 Pediatric Intraoperative and Postoperative Management

Ira T. Cohen • Etsuro K. Motoyama

The anesthetic plan should be designed as a continuous process that cares for the patient from preinduction to discharge, anticipating the patient's intraoperative requirements and postoperative recovery. Each step in the continuum is interrelated and interdependent. All factors, including the patient's age, medical history, surgical procedure, and discharge disposition, must be considered in selecting drugs and techniques to ensure safe induction, a stable intraoperative course, and comfortable, rapid recovery.

Once anesthesia is induced, the anesthesiologist is responsible for maintaining a state of analgesia, amnesia, adequate muscle relaxation, and autonomic nervous system stability, while communicating with the surgeon closely and providing the optimum working conditions for surgical procedures. To achieve this goal, the anesthesiologist chooses appropriate anesthetics and adjuvant drugs and carefully and continually monitors anesthetic depth, oxygenation, ventilation, cardiovascular function, fluid balance, body temperature, and glucose and electrolyte levels. For critically ill patients or those undergoing major or prolonged procedures, more extensive and invasive monitoring may be required. The pediatric anesthesiologist must use appropriate positioning and protective measures with soft pads to avoid soft tissue injury. Management of all factors, from the choice of pharmacologic agents to the use of regional anesthetic adjuncts to the adjustment of ambient temperature, is the role of the pediatric anesthesiologist.

Postoperatively, the pediatric anesthesiologist should plan a relatively swift awakening to ensure adequate airway maintenance, protective reflexes, and hemodynamic stability while avoiding emergence delirium, agitation, and pain. A rapid return to the preoperative level of consciousness, although ideal for ambulatory and short-stay patients, may be frightening and disorienting to a child who is not prepared to awaken in a new and unfamiliar environment among strangers. Pain, however slight, magnifies these responses dramatically. Nonambulatory and critically ill patients may not need a rapid emergence and can benefit from an extended period of sedation and analgesia. If they are being transferred directly to an intensive care unit (ICU), continuous monitoring is indicated. Once the patient is in the postanesthetic care unit (PACU or recovery room) or ICU, the anesthesiologist must assess airway patency, cardiovascular status, body temperature, and level of discomfort. Nausea, vomiting, and pain should be assessed and treated appropriately.

INTRAOPERATIVE MANAGEMENT

EARLY POSTINDUCTION PERIOD

Airway Protection

After anesthetic induction, securing the pediatric airway, maintaining patency, and reducing the risk of aspiration are crucial. Healthy, supine children over the age of 1 year who are having elective surgical procedures not involving the head and neck can safely be breathed spontaneously or by assisted breathing through a face mask. Suctioning of gastric contents, avoiding insufflation of gas into the stomach, and maintaining an appropriate level of anesthesia decrease the risk of regurgitation and pulmonary aspiration. Typically a handheld mask is adequate for short cases while the head is positioned in a sniffing position to maintain upper airway patency. Both the insertion of an oral airway and moderate levels of continuous positive airway pressure (CPAP) improve the upper airway patency and reduce inspiratory work of breathing (Keidan et al., 2000) (see Chapter 10, Induction of Anesthesia). Head straps are usually not necessary. If the use of straps is chosen, however, the anesthesiologist must be extremely careful not to press too tight on the face because soft tissues and neurovascular structures are more easily damaged in pediatric patients.

The advent of the laryngeal mask airway (LMA) has added an important alternative for managing the pediatric airway (Brain, 1983). LMAs offer the advantage of securing the airway without the need for additional manipulation, head straps, or instrumentation; an addition of a low CPAP further improves the patency of the pharyngeal airway and is recommended (Keidan et al., 2000). Ranging in sizes of 1 to 4 with half-sizes between 1 and 2 and 2 and 3, LMAs can be used in most pediatric patients over 6 months of age (Haynes and Morton, 1993; Pennant and White, 1993). These devices are designed for insertion into the pharynx by sliding over the tongue, imitating the swallowing motion. At times, inserting the LMA upside down and then rotating the devices 180 degrees is necessary for placement (Nakayama et al., 2002). After inflation of the cuff, one must check the position and fit of the mask over the larynx by confirming airway patency. Securing the LMA to prevent inadvertent displacement is essential (see Chapter 10, Induction of Anesthesia).

For infants, especially those younger than 6 months, endotracheal (ET) intubation is indicated because upper airway obstruction occurs commonly and is often unrecognized. In addition, vigorous manual ventilation with a mask by inexperienced hands tends to inflate the stomach with anesthetic gases, resulting in compression of the lower lungs and an increase in the dangers of regurgitation and aspiration of gastric secretions. Between 7 and 12 months of age, ET intubation is optional, although it is still recommended unless one is well experienced in the management of infant airways.

After intubation, the ET tube should be properly secured with adhesive tapes. For patients who are to be turned or have extensive movement of the head before or during the surgical procedures, the ET tube and adhesive tape should be secured to the face with the aid of adherent adjuncts, such as tincture of benzoin. In all patients, the corrugated delivery tubing of the anesthesia breathing circuit should be anchored securely near the ET tube connection to prevent to-and-fro movement with positive pressure ventilation, a major source of laryngeal injury. Most nonrebreathing circuits are relatively heavy and bulky, placing tension on the ET tube. Immobilizing the circuit with an anesthesia circuit stabilizing device (Fig. 11–1) or a drape sheet folded to about 1 foot wide and then rolled from both ends and held together by an elastic band can prevent laryngeal injury and accidental extubation (Fig. 11–2).

The stomach should be evacuated by using a lubricated suction catheter after the patient is well anesthetized. Usually a 12F catheter passes easily through the mouth in children younger than 6 years; in older children and adolescents, a regular nasogastric tube (12F to 18F) with side holes seems easier to insert, either orally or nasally.

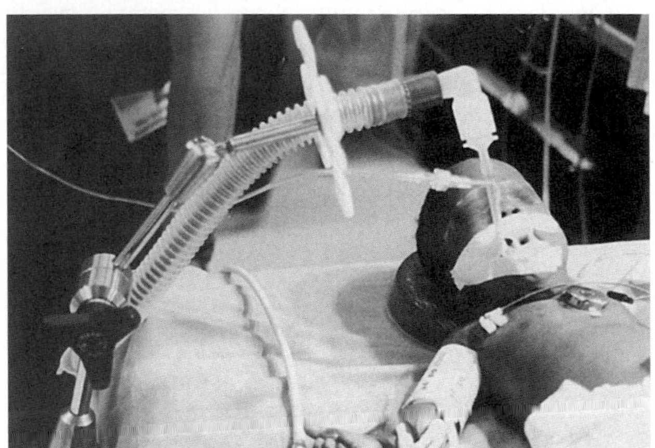

■ **FIGURE 11–1.** Circuit immobilized with an anesthesia circuit stabilizing device.

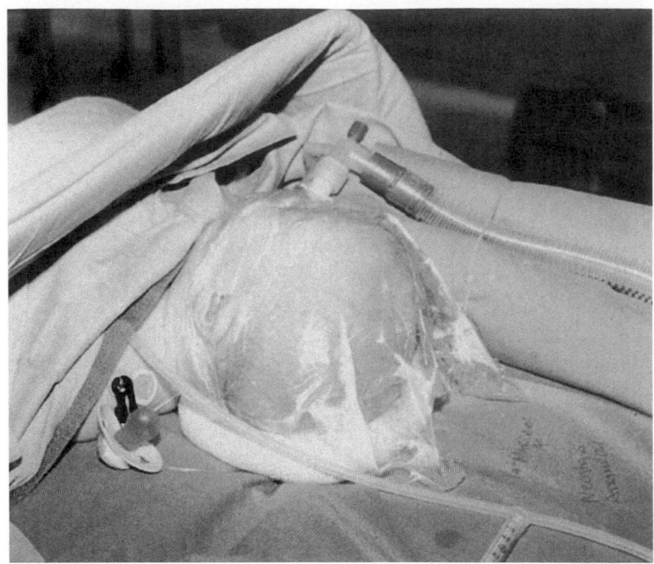

■ **FIGURE 11–2.** A rolled drape sheet held together by a rubber band ("jelly roll") provides a convenient stabilizer for a nonbreathing anesthesia delivery tube.

If auscultation of the chest after intubation indicates the presence of secretions in the tracheobronchial lumen, the anesthesia apparatus is briefly disconnected, and an appropriate suction catheter with a proximal side vent is passed through the ET tube for tracheobronchial toilette. The patient is ventilated with a high inspired concentration of oxygen and air without nitrous oxide before and after ET suction to prevent hypoxemia. Sometimes the air leakage around the ET tube with positive airway pressure is mistaken for rhonchi caused by increased airway secretions. Gentle pressure applied by the thumb and index finger over the intubated trachea, just above the sternal notch (resembling the Sellick maneuver but lower and with less pressure), minimizes air leak and noise and helps to identify the presence of airway secretions. The duration of apnea during ET suctioning should be kept to a minimum, especially in infants, since Pa_{CO_2} in apneic infants increases at a rate of 9 to 11 mm Hg/min (Motoyama et al., 2001). Furthermore, the suction catheter should be sufficiently small in relation to the ET tube to leave enough space between the two to avoid the direct application of high negative pressure to the airway system and inadvertent collapse of the lungs.

Protection of the Eyes

General anesthesia eliminates protective eyelid and corneal reflexes and decreases tear production with the eyelids partially open (Krupin et al., 1977). To prevent injury and desiccation, the eyelid should be completely closed and carefully sealed with hypoallergenic clear tape (Batra and Bali, 1977). Taping partially opened eyes can result in corneal abrasion from the tape adhesive itself. The eye tape should be placed horizontally, not diagonally, to ensure a complete seal. Orkin and Cooperman (1983) suggest placing artificial tears in the eyes before taping. Petroleum-based ophthalmic ointment may also protect against abrasions but is more irritating than water-soluble artificial tears (Boggild-Madsen and Schmidt, 1981), although Cucchiarra and Black (1988) were not able to demonstrate a significant difference with its use. Eye irritation and resultant mucosal edema can be severe when halothane (presumably other inhaled anesthetics as well) is used, probably because the anesthetic is absorbed into the ointment through the capillaries (Boggild-Madsen et al., 1981). Ointments also cause blurring of vision and should be avoided in ambulatory patients. In addition, these ointments support combustion and should never be used during laser surgery.

Intravenous Catheters

In children undergoing elective surgery, intravenous access is commonly established after an inhalation induction. These catheters should be large enough to allow the delivery of necessary fluids as indicated by the patient's medical status and surgical procedure. Unless excessive fluid or blood loss is anticipated, a 20-gauge catheter for children and a 22- to 24-gauge catheter for infants and small children fulfill the need for routine elective procedures. It is an error to use small-gauge catheters in infants and children merely because of their size. This is especially true for patients who come to the operating room with previously placed catheters that are typically small in size and may be inappropriate for major surgical procedures. If adequate percutaneous sites are not available, use of a central venous catheter or surgical cut-downs may be indicated.

In response to the growing concern in the medical community regarding percutaneous injury and exposure to blood-borne pathogens, needleless intravenous systems and self-sheathing needles and catheters have been developed and are now mandated in the United States and other countries. Limitations and complications secondary to the use of these catheters have been reported (Asai et al., 2002; Coté et al., 2003). The technical problems encountered with these self-sheathing catheters are of particular concern in preterm and young infants.

Securing the intravenous insertion site is particularly important in children because they often emerge in an uncooperative and agitated state. The extremity in which the catheter is inserted should be taped to a cushioned board with a loop of intravenous tubing to prevent accidental removal of the catheter. If a scalp vein is used, caution is advised. Inadvertent subcutaneous injection of certain drugs, such as thiopental or calcium, can cause tissue destruction and sloughing of the scalp.

Positioning

The relative lack of subcutaneous adipose tissue, poorly developed musculature, and more superficially located neurovascular structures place infants and children at greater risk for injuries caused by incorrect positioning. Cushioning with a sponge rubber cushion ("egg crating") or cotton towels to soften the otherwise hard surface of the operating room table can prevent pressure injuries, especially during procedures that require a long period of time. The patient must be prevented from lying on any monitoring cords, cables, or tubing, with particular attention to areas such as the distal humerus and femur where superficial nerves are at increased risk for injury. Extra precautions should be taken when placing infants and children in special positions, such as the prone, lateral, and lithotomy positions. Incorrectly sized rolls and straps can do more harm than good if they press or pull on delicate structures. Infants typically have large abdomens and require ample elevation of the pelvis and shoulders when prone. An infant's underdeveloped muscles and more elastic tendons and ligaments allow for greater flexibility and abnormal positioning of the extremities. As in adults, upper extremities should not be extended more than 90 degrees, hips should not be hyperextended, and bony prominences should not be allowed to press against each other. Head rings and horseshoe devices must be appropriately sized for the patient's head, preventing pressure on the globes or ears. Occasional turning of the patient's head is necessary during long surgical procedures to ensure the protection of soft tissues.

VENTILATION

Partial Rebreathing Versus Circle Systems

To maintain alveolar ventilation in infants and small children, partial rebreathing or nonrebreathing Mapleson D- or F-type circuits (such as the Bain or Jackson-Rees systems) are most commonly used and are desirable because of their relatively light weight, lower flow resistance, and easy access to heated humidifiers, although adult circle systems with lightweight pediatric circuits are increasingly used for convenience. The adult circle system should be used with caution for young infants because it does not provide adequate humidity, especially when fresh CO_2 absorbers are added to the circuit. Relative humidity of at least 50% at body temperature is necessary to maintain normal ciliary activity in the trachea and bronchi (Forbes, 1974; Mercke, 1975). A low dead space heat and moisture exchanging filter (artificial nose) should be used at the anesthesia circuit—ET tube junction to maintain humidity, although the artificial nose is far less effective than the heated humidifier, particularly during the first hour after induction of anesthesia (Bissonnette et al., 1989). Adequate humidification of inspired gas mixtures also decreases heat loss and increases thermal stability (Bissonnette and Sessler, 1989) (see Chapter 5, Thermoregulation: Physiology and Perioperative Disturbances). Adult circle systems may also add extra airway resistance to breathing, especially when the inspiratory valve is wet and sticky; circuit compliance may diminish the accuracy of measured tidal volume, although in vitro experiments using an infant lung model did not report major problems (Stevenson et al., 1998, 1999a, b).

In older children, an adult circle system can be used satisfactorily with a smaller anesthesia bag (0.5 to 3 L capacity) and pediatric corrugated tubing. The infant circle systems, although once popular, have become obsolete because of their lack of a built-in scavenging system and the availability of disposable coaxial circuits and effective, easy-to-use humidifiers. The advantages and disadvantages of pediatric anesthesia circuits are discussed in Chapter 9 (Anesthesia Equipment and Monitoring).

Fresh Gas Flow

There has been controversy as to what fresh gas flow rate is needed for the Mapleson D or F (Jackson Rees) systems to maintain adequate alveolar ventilation in different pediatric age groups. For adults with moderately increased artificial ventilation, Bain and Spoerel (1973) found that a fresh gas flow of 70 mL/kg was sufficient to maintain eucapnia. In a later study, Bain and Spoerel (1977) proposed a minimum flow of 3.5 L/min for children weighing 10 to 35 kg and 2 L/min for infants weighing 10 kg or less.

Using a Mapleson D circuit, Nightingale (1965) demonstrated that, with adequate controlled ventilation, a fresh gas flow of 220 mL/kg (50% to 100% of minute ventilation depending on age) was adequate to maintain eucapnia or mild hypocapnia in all children studied (aged 5 months to 10 years). Although end-tidal carbon dioxide with this fixed fresh gas flow decreased significantly with increasing age, the gas flow rate was not adjusted for age.

Rayburn and Graves (1978) ventilated children at three times the calculated minute ventilation with a Mapleson D system and found that, on the basis of body surface area (BSA), a fresh gas flow of 2500 mL/m^2 per min was needed to maintain eucapnia (2900 to 3000 mL/m^2 per min for mild hypocapnia). Their data imply that the fresh gas flow needed to maintain eucapnia in a newborn weighing 3 kg (BSA, 0.2 m^2) would be 170 mL/kg per min; for a typical 10-year-old child (weight, 30 kg; BSA, 1 m^2), it would be 80 mL/kg per min.

Rose and Froese (1979) studied the factors determining $Pa{CO_2}$ during controlled ventilation with either a Bain circuit or an Ayre T-piece in a lung model and substantiated their findings with data obtained in children under general anesthesia. They found that, at a fixed minute ventilation, assuming constant carbon dioxide production, $Pa{CO_2}$ varied inversely with fresh gas flow until it reached a plateau as the circuit became completely nonrebreathing. When the fresh gas flow was kept constant, $Pa{CO_2}$ decreased with increasing ventilation, but it reached a plateau at high levels of minute ventilation, apparently because of increased carbon dioxide rebreathing. The formulas by Rose and Froese (1979) for the fresh gas flow needed to achieve $Pa{CO_2}$ of 37 mm Hg are as follows:

10 to 30 kg: 1000 mL + 100 mL/kg
>30 kg: 2000 mL + 50 mL/kg

For optimum predictability, the minute ventilation should be set at 1.5 to 2.0 times the fresh gas flow. Most of these studies, however, included only small numbers of children and no young infants.

Badgwell and others (1987a) reported that a fresh gas flow of approximately 270 mL/kg per min in infants weighing less than 10 kg and 240 mL/kg per min in children weighing 10 to 20 kg was needed to maintain mild hypocapnia (end-tidal $P{CO_2}$, 38 mm Hg). These flow rates were not significantly different.

The variation in the fresh gas flow rates recommended by a number of investigators for pediatric partial rebreathing circuits is considerable. Such discrepancies are related to a number of factors, including the difference in minute ventilation used, variations in metabolic rate resulting from anesthetic technique and depth, measurement of arterial versus end-tidal $P{CO_2}$, site and method of end-tidal gas sampling, and differences in experimental design. Table 11–1 compares fresh gas flow rates needed to maintain mild hypocapnia as calculated from the data of various investigators.

In clinical practice, the fresh gas flow is adjusted to 200 mL/kg with a minimum flow of 3 to 4 L/min after the induction of anesthesia, while ventilation is usually maintained manually. Once a steady state of general anesthesia and controlled ventilation is established, the fresh gas flow rate is fine-tuned with the aid of end-tidal $P{CO_2}$ readings on a capnograph. To maintain mild hypocapnia with the use of a partial rebreathing system with recommended gas flow rates, the patient's minute ventilation must be increased considerably. Note that the end-tidal gas concentrations do not necessarily represent alveolar concentrations and that an end-tidal–to–arterial $P{CO_2}$ difference of 5 mm Hg or more exists in anesthetized patients (Nunn and Hill, 1960; Rayburn and Graves, 1978). End-tidal $P{CO_2}$ measurements are not reliable unless there is a plateau on the capnographic waveform (see Fig. 9–33 in Chapter 9, Anesthesia Equipment and Monitoring). Indeed, Badgwell and others (1986, 1987a) have shown that when a Mapleson D system is used, reliable end-tidal $P{CO_2}$ measurements cannot be obtained in children less than 8 kg in body weight unless the end-tidal gas is sampled at the tip of the ET tube (Badgwell et al., 1987b). Alternatively, the accurate end-tidal or alveolar $P{CO_2}$ can be obtained by temporarily turning off completely the fresh gas flow, having the pop-off valve closed, and having the child rebreathed by manual ventilation for five or six breaths or until the end-tidal CO_2 waveform reaches a plateau.

■ TABLE 11–1. Fresh gas flow rate for Mapleson D system*

	Newborn	1 Year	10 Years
Weight (kg)	3.0	10	30
Body surface area	0.2	0.5	1.0
Fresh gas flow (mL/kg per min)			
Nightingale and others (1965)	220	220	220
Rayburn and Graves (1978)	200	150	100
Rose and Froese (1979)	—	200	133
Badgwell and others (1987a, 1987b)	270	230	—

*Minute ventilation moderately increased to maintain mild hypocapnia.

For sevoflurane using adult circle systems with a conventional CO_2 absorber, a minimum fresh gas flow of 2 L/min is recommended to minimize the accumulation of a sevoflurane degradation product, fluoromethyl-2-2-difluoro-1-(trifluoromethyl)vinyl ether (Compound A). More breakdown occurs with barium hydroxide (Baralyme) than with soda lime; the breakdown increases with decreasing gas flow, increasing sevoflurane concentrations, CO_2 production, temperature, and the drying of the absorbent (Biebuyck and Eger, 1994; Meakin, 1999).

Several new CO_2 absorbers, which do not react with sevoflurane, have been developed (Lerman, 2004). The new products, such as Amsorb and Dragersorb-Free, have eliminated the problem of sevoflurane degradation by replacing CO_2 absorbers containing sodium, barium, and potassium bases with calcium hydroxide (Kharasch et al., 2002; Kobayashi, 2003). When this new class of CO_2 absorbers becomes available, it is likely that low-flow sevoflurane anesthesia with semiclosed or closed circle ventilation will become a reality in the very near future, with considerable cost savings (Peters et al., 1998; Meakin, 1999).

For controlled ventilation in infants and children without major respiratory dysfunction, the ventilator can be set initially at a tidal volume of 10 mL/kg or peak pressure of 16 to 18 cm H_2O. The respiratory rates between 20/min for infants and 12/min for older children are sufficient as long as one maintains adequate positive end-expiratory pressure (PEEP) between 5 and 6 cm H_2O, although much higher respiratory rates have been recommended for young infants (Peters et al., 1998). The PEEP of at least 5 cm H_2O is necessary to prevent airway closure and atelectasis in anesthetized infants and young children (Thorsteinsson et al., 1994; Motoyama, 1996; Serafini et al., 1999). A lower level of PEEP (3 cm H_2O), often used in the past for pediatric patients under general anesthesia or in intensive care settings, is inadequate to counteract the reduction in functional residual capacity (FRC) and prevent atelectasis under general anesthesia or paralysis (Motoyama, 1996) (see Chapter 2, Respiratory Physiology). Once the steady state of ventilation is established, tidal volume and respiratory rate can be fine-tuned to adjust end-tidal $P{CO_2}$ between 35 and 40 mm Hg.

Ventilators

Traditionally, anesthesia machines were equipped with only a volume-control mode system. For decades, the advantages of pressure-controlled or pressure-limited ventilation in premature infants, neonates, and patients with pulmonary pathology have been recognized. Badgwell and others (1996) described varying success in infants using volume control-mode ventilators with large compression volumes and compliant breathing systems. Tobin and others (1998) reported on a pressure-limited ventilation system on the Narkomed 2B (North America Draeger) anesthesia machines using infant lung models. This group's findings (Stevenson et al., 1999a, 1999b) support the use of this system with adult circuits in infants with pulmonary disease when the appropriate level of peak inspiratory pressure is selected. Ventilation was comparable to free-standing NICU ventilators (Servo 3000 and Babylog 8000). Intraoperative ventilation of children has been reviewed in detail (Marraro, 1998).

MONITORING

In children, close, fastidious observation of the patient's clinical signs is crucial. Physiologic changes can be both subtle and sudden in this age group, and their rapid detection is of paramount importance. Monitoring devices alone are not sufficient in caring for these patients. Changes in chest movement and symmetry, breath sounds, heart tones, skin color, capillary refill, and muscle tone can be perceived only with a precordial stethoscope and careful and continuous clinical observation. Although Spears and others (1991) found that manual ventilation may not provide an anesthesiologist with information as precise as once thought, it still allows for earlier detection of changes in respiratory system compliance resulting from ET tube obstruction caused by kinking or anesthesia circuit disconnection.

Routine monitoring devices include a precordial or esophageal stethoscope, pulse oximeter, capnograph, electrocardiogram, automated blood pressure–measuring device, and temperature probe. Of particular importance is the use of the precordial stethoscope, which is indispensable for continuous monitoring of heart and breath sounds (Smith, 1980), and the use of the pulse oximeter, which allows for rapid detection of oxygen desaturation (Coté et al., 1988). For surgical procedures lasting longer than 3 hours or those in which a major shift in fluid balance is anticipated, an indwelling urinary (Foley) catheter and monitoring urinary output provide useful information in assessing the state of hydration and adequacy of circulatory blood volume. Invasive monitors such as arterial, central venous, and pulmonary artery catheters are indicated only when the benefits of their use exceed the risks.

Standards of Intraoperative Monitoring

To reduce anesthesia-related catastrophes, minimum standards for intraoperative monitoring were initially proposed by the Harvard teaching hospitals in 1986 (Einhorn et al., 1986) and were adopted and amended as guidelines by the American Society of Anesthesiologists (ASA) (1986, 1999, 2004; http://www.asahq.org/publicationsAndServices/stantards/02.pdf#2). These standards are realistic, rather than idealistic, and must be attainable by average practicing anesthesiologists. The monitoring standards must be technologically attainable and affordable in terms of personnel and utilization (that is, not dependent on state-of-the-art technology). It should be noted that the fundamental focus of the standards is on behavior rather than on technology (Eichhorn, 1988a). For example, the ASA standards mandate the "continual" (means intermittent versus continuous) monitoring of ventilation. Initially, a list of methods to achieve this goal was given, including qualitative clinical signs such as chest excursion and observation of the reservoir breathing bag or breath sounds by means of a precordial stethoscope, as well as the use of capnography (see Chapter 9, Anesthesia Equipment and Monitoring). The updated guidelines, which now state that "continual monitoring for the presence of expired carbon dioxide shall be performed unless invalidated by the nature of the patient, procedure, or equipment" (ASA, 1999), still leave monitoring practices to the discretion of the practitioner.

The ASA standards specifically mandate that oxygenation, ventilation, circulation, and body temperature be evaluated "continually" (meaning frequently at regular intervals, as opposed to "continuously," as stated in Harvard's standards). For each component, the clear objectives, to ensure adequacy and specific methods, are stated. There is a strong emphasis on combining clinical evaluation and technological methods. Although no specific methodology or instrumentation is mandated for monitoring these components, ASA standards strongly encourage quantitative methods, such as pulse oximetry and capnography, over qualitative clinical assessment with inspection and auscultation for monitoring cardiopulmonary functions. These recommendations are meant to be minimal requirements and are expected to be routinely exceeded (Eichhorn, 1988b). Since the late 1980s, the use of a pulse oximeter and capnography in all patients has become a part of standard anesthesia practice in the United States. Indeed, the routine use of pulse oximetry and capnography has been mandated by law in a number of states (New York State Hospital Code, 1988). Although the benefit of government-imposed regulation of anesthetic practice is debatable, these standards should be observed by practicing anesthesiologists to further the desirable goal of minimizing unfortunate anesthesia-related mishaps (see Chapter 34, Safety and Outcome). The potential medicolegal consequences of ignoring these standards are also an incentive for compliance (Eichhorn, 1988a). Standard monitoring and supplemental measures recommended in pediatric anesthesia are shown in Box 11–1.

Clinical Observation

To evaluate various factors that determine the child's condition, the anesthesiologist should rely on continuous clinical observation in addition to information provided by various monitoring devices. In pediatric anesthesia, it is mandatory to be fully aware of surgical progress at all times; consequently, the anesthesiologist should remain standing or positioned so that the whole patient is in view throughout the procedure.

Even with the modern technology of noninvasive monitoring, such as pulse oximetry or infrared capnography, it is indispensable to have continual clinical assessment of information and interpretation with experience. Perhaps with the exception of pulse oximetry, this continual clinical assessment is often more valuable than what is provided by monitors. The anesthesiologist should observe, both visually as well as with a precordial stethoscope, the rate and depth of ventilation, whether assisted or controlled—that it is without obstruction, with equal expansion of both sides of the chest, and with good compliance and normal color of the skin and blood.

Stridor indicates a narrowing of the extrathoracic airways, most commonly at the glottis. Expiratory stridor usually denotes light anesthesia with tightening of the vocal cords, whereas inspiratory stridor indicates narrowing caused either by flaccid soft tissue being sucked together with inspiration during deep anesthesia or by impending laryngospasm.

BOX 11–1 Standard Monitors and Supplementary Measurements in Pediatric Anesthesia

Standard Monitors

Physiology

Clinical observation by qualified anesthesiologist
Oxygenation: pulse oximeter
Ventilation: stethoscope, capnograph, gas flow meter
Circulation: stethoscope, blood pressure cuff
Electrocardiograph
Temperature probe: rectal, esophageal, or axillary
Anesthetic depth: BIS monitor

Safety

Oxygen analyzer with low concentration alarm
Ventilator with low pressure and disconnect alarm

Supplemental Measurements

Continual

Fluids given
Urine output (catheterization and urinometer)
Blood loss
Direct arterial pressure
Central venous pressure
Pulmonary arterial pressure and wedge pressure
Cardiac output (noninvasive or invasive)
Electroencephalogram
Somatosensory-evoked potentials

Intermittent

Train-of-four twitch response on nerve stimulator
Arterial blood gas tensions, pH hematocrit
Serum levels of Na^+, K^+, Ca^{2+}, glucose
Colloid oncotic pressure
Coagulation profile

Manual ventilation of the patient, as opposed to mechanical ventilation, is encouraged, at least intermittently or whenever possible, because the hand on the anesthesia bag is an additional and an excellent monitor for detection of changes in the patient's dynamic compliance and respiratory resistance resulting from air leaks in the anesthesia circuit, airway obstruction of various origins, or movement of the diaphragm.

Normal cardiovascular function is evident in suitable heart tone and rate, rhythm, pulse volume, vascular tone, capillary refill, and skin color. Blood loss can be quantified reasonably well by visual estimation of bleeding in the surgical field and on drapes, pulse rate and volume, color of the conjunctivas, the counting and weighing of blood-soaked sponges, and measuring the volume of blood in suction bottles. With continuous monitoring with a precordial or an esophageal stethoscope, changes in the heart tone can readily be heard even before a reduction in the systemic blood pressure as indicated by automated blood pressure measurements by cuff.

The amended guidelines from the ASA (1999) state that "every patient receiving anesthesia shall have temperature monitored when clinically significant changes in body temperature are intended, anticipated or suspected." The standards for monitoring temperature should be applied more strictly in the pediatric patient, especially infants, because of their greater susceptibility to temperature change. Temperature should be monitored directly, but heating and cooling of the skin often can be sensed by touch. This helps to detect a faulty thermistor probe, avoiding initiation of treatment for false hypothermia or hyperthermia. Neuromuscular tone in infants (without relaxants) is easily assessed by just sensing changes in respiratory compliance while manually compressing the anesthesia bag or passively extending the child's flexed arm or fingers.

Depth of anesthesia can be difficult to assess in the pediatric patient. Bispectral index analysis (BIS) monitoring measures the effects of anesthetic agents on electroencephalography (see later). Extensively validated in adults and children, BIS monitoring can effectively estimate the level of sedation/anesthesia (Denman et al., 2000; Bannister et al., 2001; Choudhry and Brenn, 2002; McCann et al., 2002). In addition, central nervous system responses, such as pupillary responses and lid reflexes and autonomic responses such as sweating, vasomotion, and vagal activity, are informative and easily recognizable by clinical observation. Again, clinical observation, if properly used, provides a great deal of information that cannot be obtained by electronic monitors.

Monitoring Apparatus

Perioperative monitoring of patients receiving general anesthesia can be subdivided into physiologic monitoring and safety (accident prevention) monitoring. Both types are included in the ASA basic standards discussed previously. Safety monitoring is primarily the monitoring of the anesthesia delivery system, but this often overlaps with physiologic monitoring. Monitoring can also be classified as noninvasive or invasive. Most noninvasive monitors are mandated by the ASA standards as described earlier. These and some additional noninvasive monitors are considered mandatory for all pediatric procedures; others are indicated for special situations or procedures. Invasive monitors should be used only if they give truly essential information without exposing the child to undue risk (Smith, 1980). Various monitoring devices, together with their mechanism of action and clinical use, are detailed in Chapter 9, Anesthetic Equipment and Monitoring. In the current chapter, additional brief comments are made only on the most essential monitors, namely, the stethoscope, pulse oximeter, and anesthesia record.

Stethoscope

The use of a precordial stethoscope as an intraoperative monitoring device was first advocated by Smith in the late 1940s (Smith, 1953). It was gradually recognized and its use expanded in the United States and abroad over the next two decades (Ploss, 1955; Smith, 1962, 1978; Bosomworth et al., 1963; Domette, 1963, 1973; Bethune, 1965; Patterson, 1966). By the 1970s, the precordial (or esophageal) stethoscope was established as the most important monitoring device in pediatric anesthesia, essential for all procedures involving general anesthesia (Smith, 1980).

Several types of stethoscope heads without a diaphragm are available for adult and pediatric patients. The most convenient and popular have double-sided adhesive tape (see Fig. 10–3 in Chapter 10, Induction of Anesthesia). Before the stethoscope is fixed to a child's chest, the site should be determined by where both heart tones and breath sounds can be heard most distinctly. This usually is near the left sternal border at the nipple line (the fourth intercostal space), bordering the heart and major airways (Smith, 1980). Alternatively, the stethoscope may be placed over the third or second interspace at the left sternal border or over the second interspace at the right sternal border (to transmit pulmonic valve sounds). Auscultation of heart and breath sounds is satisfactory at these alternative sites in all ages but especially in muscular or obese adolescents. A disposable, soft, compressible foam rubber earpiece, attached to lightweight tubing, is commercially available as a convenient connector to the precordial stethoscope head, although, because of the small diameter of the tubing, the heart and breath sounds are often excessively attenuated. A large-bore silicone rubber tubing, attached to a custom-molded earpiece, gives more satisfactory results.

An esophageal stethoscope is valuable when children are placed in the prone position or when the precordium cannot be used because of surgery or injury. Esophageal stethoscopes are available commercially in sizes 12F, 18F, and 24F, which are suitable for most infants and children.

Pulse Oximeter

The pulse oximeter, which became available clinically in the mid 1980s, measures the arterial oxygen saturation of hemoglobin continuously and noninvasively. Within 5 years, it was widely accepted as an essential (if not mandatory) monitoring device for clinical anesthesia. Its probe, usually affixed to a fingertip or a toe, senses changes in light absorption of two wavelengths (saturated and unsaturated hemoglobin) that occur synchronously with arterial pulsation. Thus, the oxygen saturation detected by this device (Spo_2) represents arterial, rather than capillary, hemoglobin saturation on a beat-to-beat basis without previous heating or arteriorization (Yelderman and New, 1983; Motoyama and Glazener, 1986). The pulse oximeter accurately reflects Sao_2 in all age groups with various hematocrit values, including premature infants with fetal hemoglobin, over the range of 60% to 100% Sao_2 (Deckardt and Steward, 1984).

Pulse oximetry is the most important advancement in perioperative monitoring in pediatric anesthesia, since the precordial stethoscope was introduced by Smith more than 50 years ago (Smith, 1953). Coté and others (1988) found that the use of a pulse oximeter significantly reduced the occurrence of major hypoxic events during general anesthesia and surgery in children. The pulse oximeter detected hypoxemia before its signs and symptoms were apparent. Not surprisingly, hypoxemic events occurred more frequently in children younger than 2 years of age and in those with ASA physical status 3 or 4. A greater number of children not monitored by the pulse oximeter (not visible for the anesthesiologists administering anesthesia) experienced borderline hypoxemia (Spo_2 <90%, estimated Pao_2 <58 to 60 mm Hg) while breathing room air at the end of anesthesia than those with the monitor visible to the anesthesiologist. In a subsequent single-blind study of combined pulse oximetry and capnography in children, Coté and others (1991) showed that, of all major hypoxemic events, nearly 70% were first discovered with the pulse oximeter, 22% by the anesthesiologist (clinical signs), and only 8% with the capnograph. Thus, compared with changes in clinical signs and capnography, pulse oximetry provides by far the most sensitive warning of developing hypoxemia in anesthetized children.

The limitations of pulse oximetry have been noted. Accuracy of measurement is greatest in the range of 90% to 100%. Schmitt and others (1993) observed that accuracy was compromised in children with cyanotic congenital heart disease. Advances have been made in pulse oximetry by Masimo Signal Extraction Technology (SET). This device minimizes the effect of motion artifact, improves accuracy, and has been shown to have advantages over the existing systems, especially when used in neonates and with low-flow states, mild hypothermia, and in moving patients (Malviya et al., 2000; Hay et al., 2002; Irita et al., 2003).

Anesthesiologists should be aware that the most commonly used pulse oximetry system in the United States and elsewhere is artificially modified to read Spo_2, 2% to 3% higher than real values and, consequently, gives a false sense of security regarding patients' oxygenation (see Chapter 2, Respiratory Physiology). The reason for the built-in "deception" is not clear (it probably is for the convenience of reading Spo_2 of 100% in room air in the healthy individual). In reality, true oxygen saturation of hemoglobin at Po_2 of 100 mm Hg is 97% to 98% (arterial Po_2 of 130 to 150 mm Hg is necessary for 100% hemoglobin saturation). Unfortunately, the newer pulse oximetry system has also adopted the practice of raising Spo_2 readings by 2% to 3% above the true pulse oximetry reading, presumably in response to consumer demands and to avoid discrepancies between the two pulse oximeter systems. It is not clear if these pulse oximeters read falsely higher values at lower oxygen saturation where the accuracy of pulse oximeter diminishes markedly.

Bispectral Index

Bispectral analysis, comparing paired wave activity, quantifies the level of synchronization in an electroencephalogram, along with the traditional measurements of amplitude and frequency. BIS monitors compress electroencephalographic signals by a sophisticated algorithm into a digital readout ranging from 0 to 100. By comparing the reading with previously measured results in conscious, sedated, and anesthetized patients, a normogram for level of sedation has been generated. Studies in infants and children have confirmed the validity of this instrument and have demonstrated that more accurate titration of general anesthesia in children is achieved with the use of a BIS monitor (Denman et al., 2000; Bannister et al., 2001; Choudhry and Brenn, 2002; McCann et al., 2002). Davidson and others (2001) did not find the usual BIS–MAC relationship in children less than 1 year old. Attempts to refine this technology by interpreting high-frequency electroencephalographic data are in the initial phase.

Anesthesia Record

The anesthesia record or chart is extremely valuable as a data sheet during anesthesia, as a source of information for anesthetic management at a later date, and as a legal document (see Chapter 36, Medicolegal and Ethical Aspects). It should be considered an essential part of monitoring for the anesthesiologist, particularly when caring for infants and children. The record should contain all the important information obtained preoperatively:

- Patient's systemic disease or condition and ASA physical status (PS)
- Hemoglobin and hematocrit, when applicable
- Time of the last food and liquid intake
- Preanesthetic state of anxiety, if any
- Premedication, time and its effect
- Calculated fluid deficit, estimated blood volume, and allowable blood loss
- Completed preinduction and postinduction checklists

The chart should be properly documented and signed by the trainee as well as by the attending anesthesiologist legally responsible for administering anesthetic.

After induction a brief description of induction and intubation should be recorded, noting the drugs given, the size of the ET tube, whether cuffed or uncuffed, and verification of proper air leak around the ET tube. Subsequently, gas flow rates, maintenance concentrations and doses of anesthetic and adjuvant drugs, blood pressure, pulse, respiratory rate, temperature, oxygen saturation readings from the pulse oximeter, and end-tidal P_{CO_2} should be entered at frequent intervals.

With advances in computer technology, attempts have been made to elaborate the anesthesia record into a fully automated data entry system (Stanley and Reves, 1994). Computerized systems seem to increase efficiency by automatically entering cardiorespiratory and other data from various monitors into the anesthesia record and improving the accuracy and security of records. A number of automated charting systems have become commercially available but have not been widely used in clinical practice. Studying data collected from automated anesthesia records, Sanborn and others (1996) found that electronic scanning recorded a higher incidence of intraoperative incidents than those reported voluntarily. Lubarsky and others (1997) applied data collected toward management practice and cost containment. In review, Dorman and Fackler (2000) state that available automated anesthesia information systems are primitive, focusing only on the charting process. They believe that until these systems can be integrated with the care process, they will be of no true benefit. Others have reported improvements in patient safety and care with automated systems (Junger et al., 2001; Merry et al., 2001).

TEMPERATURE MAINTENANCE

Control of thermal regulation requires special consideration in infants and small children because of their relative lack of subcutaneous adipose tissue and increased BSA in relation to body weight. Vasodilation, exposure to the cold operating room environment, insensible heat losses, and infusion of cold intravenous fluid often result in loss of heat and resultant hypothermia (Smith, 1969). The mechanisms of thermoregulation in infants and children are discussed in detail in Chapter 5 (Thermoregulation: Physiology and Perioperative Disturbances).

To prevent excessive heat losses, a heated humidifier in the anesthetic circuit should always be turned on to humidify anesthetic gas mixtures (with 0% humidity) to prevent evaporative heat loss, damage to the ciliated airway epithelia, and postoperative pulmonary complications (Chalon et al., 1979). A warming mattress on the operating table is helpful for infants weighing less than 10 kg (Goudsouzian et al., 1973). Additional measures for heat conservation, such as increasing room temperature, use of a radiant warming lamp, use of a forced air warmer, and wrapping the child's head and other exposed areas with plastic sheet, should be practiced as needed to maintain normal body temperature. Kurz and others (1993) found in both adults and children that forced-air warming maintains intraoperative normothermia better than circulating-water mattresses. Intravenous fluids should be prewarmed with a fluid warmer, especially in infants and young children. Conversely, prolonged periods in a warmed environment with plastic drapes and wraps can sometimes cause hyperthermia. To reduce elevated temperature, reversing the measures of heat conservation is often sufficient.

Accurate and close monitoring of body temperature is essential for keeping pediatric patients in the normothermic range. Rectal or esophageal thermistor probes reliably measure core and peripheral temperature. Axillary probes, which are more easily placed, record temperatures 0.7° to 1.0°C less than core readings and are more appropriate for older children undergoing surgery without expected major hemodynamic changes. For the best results with this method, the sensing tip should be located as near the axillary artery as possible by taping the probe to the lateral chest wall and then adducting the arm down close to the body. The safe range for a child's core temperature is approximately 35.5° to 37.5°C (96° to 100°F). To minimize temperature changes under general anesthesia, action should be taken as soon as or before the temperature deviates from this narrow range (see Chapter 5, Thermoregulation: Physiology and Perioperative Disturbances).

FLUID MAINTENANCE

Regulation of fluids and electrolytes is detailed in Chapter 4 (Regulation of Body Fluids and Electrolytes). Intraoperative fluid and glucose management in children was reviewed (Leelanukrom and Cunliffe, 2000). The maintenance fluid requirement is most commonly based on the energy needs proposed by Holliday and Segar (1957). The basal caloric needs of infants and children dictate their fluid requirement. Infants weighing up to 10 kg use 100 kcal/kg per day; those weighing 10 to 20 kg require 1000 kcal plus 50 kcal/kg above 10 kg; and those weighing more than 20 kg need 1500 kcal plus 20 kcal/kg above 20 kg. For every 100 kcal consumed, these authors estimate that 67 mL of water is needed for solute excretion, plus an average of 50 mL/100 kcal is associated with insensible loss, while 17 mL/100 kcal is produced by oxidation. Thus, an infant needs 100 mL (67 + 50 − 17 = 100) of water per 100 kcal of caloric expenditure. On the basis of 1 mL of fluid per 1 kcal of caloric requirement, the fluid requirements in infants and children can be approximated as follows:

Body Weight Fluid Requirement

0 to 10 kg: 4 mL/kg per hr
10 to 20 kg: 40 mL + 2 mL/kg per hr above 10 kg
>20 kg: 60 mL + I mL/kg per hr above 20 kg

Alternatively, Oh (1980) proposed a modification of this formula as follows:

Body Weight Fluid Requirement

0 to 10 kg: 4 mL/kg per hr
10 to 20 kg: 20 mL + (2 × kg) mL per hr
>20 kg: 40 + kg × mL per hr

An increase or decrease in metabolic rate changes the fluid requirement. For each 1°C increase in body temperature, an 8% to 10% increase in fluid requirement occurs. For every 100 calories of energy expenditure or 100 mL of water, a child needs 3 mmol of sodium, 2 mmol of potassium, 5 mmol of chloride, and 5 g of dextrose. Usually 5% dextrose in ¼ or ½ normal saline solution (0.2% or 0.45% NaCl) suffices; potassium is not replaced routinely because of the hazard of accidental rapid infusion.

Pediatric patients are usually kept fasting (NPO status) for 2 hours for clear fluids and 4 to 8 hours for solid food, depending on the age (and sometimes much longer by default) before induction of anesthesia for elective surgery (see Preoperative Fasting Guidelines in Chapter 10, Induction of Anesthesia). With the exception of simple, same-day surgery procedures of short duration, half of the estimated fluid deficit, plus the hourly maintenance fluid requirement, should be given during the first hour of anesthesia, with a balanced salt solution such as lactated

Ringer's solution; one quarter of the fluid deficit plus the hourly maintenance fluid is infused during the second and third hours of anesthesia and surgery, along with the hourly maintenance fluid and the replacement of any third-space fluid loss (Furman et al., 1975). While the fluid deficit should be replaced by a balanced salt solution not containing glucose, 5% dextrose in 0.2% or 0.45% NaCl may be used for the hourly fluid maintenance. Infants and occasionally healthy children who have fasted for a prolonged period become hypoglycemic during general anesthesia and surgery without apparent clinical symptoms (Welborn et al., 1986). The intraoperative monitoring of blood glucose levels is recommended in infants and toddlers who have not received glucose supplementation for prolonged periods.

The intraoperative use of glucose supplementation has been reevaluated (Seiber et al., 1987). Administration of fluid containing 5% dextrose invariably produces hyperglycemia and causes osmotic diuresis. Hyperglycemia may worsen neurologic outcome in cerebral ischemia (Lanier et al., 1987). On the other hand, hypoglycemia is known to cause cerebral ischemia and brain damage, particularly in infants, and is difficult to detect during general anesthesia unless the blood glucose level is determined directly.

Welborn and others (1986, 1987) reassessed the need for intravenous glucose in otherwise healthy children undergoing outpatient surgery for minor procedures with minimal blood loss. They found that children who were given 5% dextrose in lactated Ringer's solution consistently developed hyperglycemia, whereas those given 2.5% dextrose in lactated Ringer's solution maintained a normal blood glucose level. At the infusion rate given, children who had intravenous fluid containing less than 2.5% dextrose did not meet the glucose maintenance requirement of 5 mg/kg per min. On the basis of these studies, these authors recommended the use of 2.5% dextrose rather than the 5% glucose solution (given routinely back in the 1980s) for healthy children undergoing minor surgical procedures.

A urethral catheter allows continual monitoring of urine output and the state of hydration and blood volume during major surgical procedures or with injuries that involve large loss of blood and fluid. Urethral catheterization is usually recommended in surgical procedures lasting for 3 hours or longer. In newborn and small infants, it is safest to use a soft 6F or 8F infant feeding tube. This avoids the retention balloon, which may contribute to bladder irritability and spasm. Even in premature infants weighing less than 1 kg, the feeding tube, when connected to a small syringe, provides an accurate measure of urine output and the state of hydration. In older infants and children, urine output can be read ultrasonically on a minute-to-minute basis with a urinometer (Lilly et al., 1980). Urine output of more than 0.5 mL/kg per hr should be maintained to avoid damage to the renal tubules (see Chapter 4, Regulation of Body Fluids and Electrolytes). Foley catheters sizes 8F to 10F made of nonreactive silicone rubber are generally used in the 6-month- to 6-year-old age group (Litvak et al., 1976). Although urethral catheterization can be achieved safely for intraoperative monitoring, the risk of complications increases with longer periods of drainage, so every effort is made to shorten its duration (Kaplan and Brock, 1983).

BLOOD LOSS AND BLOOD COMPONENT THERAPY

Accurate and continuous monitoring of blood loss and accurate assessment of acceptable blood loss and its timely replacement are essential in pediatric patients. Seemingly small losses in infants can cause significant changes in hemoglobin concentration and hemodynamic stability. Careful assessment of blood loss by weighing blood-soaked sponges, tallying blood and fluid losses using calibrated miniaturized suction bottles, and making a visual estimation of blood lost on surgical drapes allow determination of the extent of total blood loss. Factors that determine allowable blood losses include the patient's estimated blood volume, which is age dependent, preoperative and intraoperative hematocrit, cardiopulmonary and general medical conditions to provide adequate oxygen transport, and risk versus benefit of the transfusion. Estimated blood volumes in pediatric patients of different ages are listed in Table 11–2.

TABLE 11–2. Estimates of circulating blood volume

Patient	Blood Volume (mL/kg)
Premature newborn	90 to 100
Full-term newborn	80 to 90
3 mo to 1 yr	75 to 80
3 to 6 yr	70 to 75
>6 yr	65 to 70

As mentioned earlier, estimated blood volume and maximal allowable blood loss should be computed before the induction of anesthesia. There have been several methods proposed to estimate allowable blood loss based on blood volume, body weight, and hematocrit using a simple proportion, an approximation of circulating red blood cell (RBC) mass, and a logarithmic function (Bourke and Smith, 1974; Kallos and Smith, 1974; Furman et al., 1975). The results from these equations are compatible. The following simple formula can be used to estimate allowable blood loss (ABL):

$$ABL = EBV \times [H_O - H_L]/[H_A]$$

where EBV is the estimated blood volume, H_O is the original hematocrit, H_L is the lowest acceptable hematocrit, and H_A is the average hematocrit (that is, $[H_O + H_L]/2$) (Bennett, 1975). The estimated blood volume can be determined by the patient's age using Table 11–2. For example, in an 8-kg, 10-month-old infant whose original hematocrit (H_O) is 35% and blood volume is approximately 80 mL/kg, EBV is 80 × 8, or 640 mL. Allowing the lowest hematocrit (H_L) to fall to 25% yields an ABL of 640 × (35 − 25)/(35 + 25)/2, or 213 mL.

Whether a crystalloid or a colloid solution should be used to replace blood volume as the hematocrit is allowed to decrease has been debated. If a colloid solution (albumin, plasma protein, fresh frozen plasma) is used, blood loss is replaced milliliter for milliliter. If a crystalloid solution is used, two to three times the volume of the blood loss is replaced because the intravascular volume cannot be sustained with crystalloid solutions (Shires et al., 1961, 1964). In most cases the replacement of ABL with crystalloid alone is safe and effective, provided the patient is healthy otherwise. The replacement of blood loss with colloid solutions may be more physiologic but is much more expensive and exhibits no clear-cut evidence of superiority over crystalloid replacement. With excessive blood loss and large volumes of crystalloid replacement, however, hypoproteinemia would result. Furman and others (1975) recommend that continuing blood loss be replaced with an equal volume of lactated Ringer's solution until the serum total protein concentration decreases to 5 g/dL. Then blood volume is maintained with 5% albumin until the ABL has occurred.

Until the early 1980s, 10 g/dL of hemoglobin was used as a guideline for the minimal adequate level for elective anesthesia and surgery. This guideline began long before the physiologic effects of organic phosphates and the different oxygen affinities of fetal and adult hemoglobins were discovered (see Chapter 2, Respiratory Physiology). With the exception of patients in the early neonatal period (with high oxygen affinity of fetal hemoglobin and decreased oxygen unloading at tissue levels) and those with cyanotic cardiopulmonary disease, it is evident that 10 g/dL of hemoglobin is not a prerequisite in healthy, normovolemic patients for elective surgery.

A study on acute normovolemic hemodilution in animals indicated that hemoglobin values of 6 to 7 g/dL may be acceptable (Stehling and Zander, 1991). In another study of acute normovolemic hemodilution in dogs at hematocrit levels below 20%, hemodynamic stability was maintained with colloid solution but crystalloids caused massive whole body edema and hemodynamic instability (Brinkmeyer, Safar, and Motoyama, 1983). Furthermore, Dong and others (1986) demonstrated that normovolemic hemodilution to a hematocrit of 15% for 1 hour was associated with depression of evoked brain activities (somatosensory evoked potentials); the combination of hemodilution with hypotension resulted in either death or permanent brain damage.

Based on these limited findings, the best recommendation to date appears to be that of the National Institutes of Health Consensus Conference on Perioperative Red Cell Transfusion (1988): Healthy patients with hemoglobin values of 10 g/dL or greater rarely require transfusion, whereas those with values less than 7 g/dL frequently require transfusion. Thus, to keep operative hemorrhage and blood volume under control in a situation such as spinal fusion, hemoglobin may be decreased temporarily to as low as (but not below) 7 g/dL (hematocrit 20%), with proper monitoring of blood pressure, arterial and mixed venous PO_2, etc. The hemoglobin level should be increased (i.e., to 8 g/dL with a hematocrit of ≥25%) postoperatively when the patient needs more oxygen uptake for increased metabolic needs.

When the estimated blood loss approaches or exceeds the ABL, transfusion, most commonly with packed RBCs, becomes necessary. The hematocrit of packed RBCs varies between 60% and 80% and can be adjusted according to the need of the physician administering the blood. If the packed RBCs have a hematocrit of 75% and the patient's hematocrit is to be maintained at 30%, the volume of packed RBCs needed to replace the blood loss beyond ABL can be calculated as follows:

$$\text{Packed RBCs (ml)} = \frac{[\text{Blood loss} - \text{ABL}] \times \text{Desired hematocrit (30\%)}}{\text{Hematocrit of packed RBCs (75\%)}}$$

Using the example given earlier of the 8-kg infant and a total blood loss of 270 mL, or about 60 mL above ABL, the volume of packed RBCs needed would be as follows:

$$\text{Packed RBCs (mL)} = 60 \times 30/75 = 24 \text{ mL}$$

When the blood loss exceeds one blood volume (massive blood loss), labile clotting factors are significantly diminished. In patients with massive blood loss, packed RBCs are often given with 1 to 2 volumes of normal saline solution to achieve desired hematocrit, reduce viscosity, and facilitate transfusion. In patients with clinical signs of nonsurgical bleeding or abnormal activated clotting time, fresh frozen plasma (FFP) is given in place of crystalloid solution, with equal volumes of packed RBCs. The management of blood component therapy and massive blood loss is detailed elsewhere (Chapter 12, Blood Conservation).

PHARMACOLOGIC AGENTS

INHALED ANESTHETICS

A majority of general anesthetics administered to pediatric patients still involves the use of inhaled anesthetics. The pharmacokinetics and pharmacodynamics of inhaled anesthetics are detailed in Chapter 6 (Pharmacology of Pediatric Anesthesia). Nitrous oxide is commonly used for the initiation of mask induction and as an adjunct agent during inhalation and intravenous anesthetics, although its use has been decreasing considerably.

Since its introduction in North America in 1995, sevoflurane has replaced halothane as the preferred agent for inhalation induction and is commonly used in relatively simple and short procedures. The bronchodilating action and longer, smoother emergence of halothane offer advantages over the less-soluble agent when managing patients with reactive or difficult airways. Isoflurane, desflurane, and sevoflurane provide better cardiovascular stability with less or minimal biodegradation in the liver and are preferred for most other procedures. Each of these agents, however, has properties that may limit their use in certain patients and situations. Their effect on induction and emergence should be of particular consideration. Physical and pharmacologic characteristics of volatile anesthetics are shown in Table 11–3.

Nitrous Oxide

Nitrous oxide has been the most widely used anesthetic in adults and children because of its inoffensive odor; low solubility, which results in rapid uptake and distribution (blood-gas partition coefficient of 0.47); hypnotic and analgesic action; and relatively

TABLE 11–3. Characteristics of volatile anesthetics

	Molecular Weight (Da)	Boiling Point (°C)	Vapor Pressure at 20°C (mm Hg)	Blood Gas Partition Coefficient	MAC (%)		
					Infant (1 to 6 mo)	*Child (3 to 10 yr)*	*Adult*
Halothane	197.4	50.2	244	2.3	1.1	0.9	0.7
Enflurane	184.5	56.5	172	1.9	—	—	1.6
Isoflurane	184.5	48.5	239	1.4	1.7	1.6	1.2
Desflurane	168.0	23.5	664	0.4	9.4	8.0	6.0
Sevoflurane	200.1	58.5	160	0.6	3.3	2.5	2.0

MAC, Minimum alveolar concentration.

Adapted in part from Jones RM: Desflurane and sevoflurane; inhalation anesthetics for this decade? *Br J Anaesth* 65:527, 1990.

minimal depressant effects (Smith, 1971). Nitrous oxide requires a concentration greater than 100% to achieve 1 MAC, making its use as a sole anesthetic agent impossible at normal atmospheric pressures (Hornbien et al., 1982). Its use with volatile agents reduces the risk of untoward effects and the duration of emergence by lowering their MAC requirements. When intravenous anesthetics are used, nitrous oxide potentiates the analgesic effect of opioids and the amnesic actions of hypnotics.

In several situations, however, its use demands special consideration. In adults with moderate pulmonary hypertension, nitrous oxide increased pulmonary artery and pulmonary capillary wedge pressures (Schulte-Sasse et al., 1982). In healthy infants, however, Hickey and others (1986) observed no increase in pulmonary artery pressure or vascular resistance. Mild but significant decreases in heart rate, systemic blood pressure, and cardiac index were seen. These effects of nitrous oxide on systemic hemodynamics may be clinically insignificant in healthy infants but may affect the hemodynamic stability of sick infants, particularly those with pulmonary hypertension. Furthermore, the presence of nitrous oxide in blood may increase the oxygen affinity of hemoglobin, decreasing the P_{50} by as much as 8 mm Hg and thereby reducing the oxygen-unloading capacity of blood at the tissue level (Fournier and Major, 1984).

Of greater concern is the accumulation of nitrous oxide in a closed, gas-containing space such as an obstructed loop of bowel or a pneumothorax. In situations where maximal oxygen delivery is essential, as in bronchoscopy, massive blood loss, severe anemia, shock, and compromised cerebrospinal blood flow, the use of high concentrations of nitrous oxide is not recommended. Other possible undesirable side effects include risk to operating room personnel, inhibition of methionine synthetase, and teratogenic effects, as demonstrated in experimental animals.

The role of nitrous oxide in causing postoperative nausea and vomiting (PONV) has been reexamined since Watcha and others (1991) reported an increased incidence when it was used with propofol. Crawford and others (1998) confirmed this finding. A meta-analysis by Sneyd and others (1998), however, found that nitrous oxide had no effect on the incidence of PONV when propofol was compared with inhalation agents for the maintenance of general anesthesia. In children, no difference was seen in the incidence of PONV with or without nitrous oxide when general anesthesia was administered with sevoflurane (Bortone et al., 2002) or desflurane (Kuhn et al., 1999). This evidence supports avoiding the use of nitrous oxide to reduce the incidence of PONV only when propofol is the primary anesthetic agent.

Sevoflurane

Sevoflurane is an excellent induction agent in infants and children because of its relatively pleasant aroma, minimal airway irritation, and rapid induction time. Systolic blood pressure and heart rate are unchanged during the induction with nitrous oxide–sevoflurane anesthesia compared with nitrous oxide–halothane anesthesia, and hemodynamic stability is retained during the maintenance of anesthesia (Sarner et al., 1995). Concentrations can be increased rapidly to 8% during induction in healthy ASA I/II children without laryngospasm or hypotension (Baum et al., 1997).

Sevoflurane is a fluorinated methyl isopropyl ether with a blood-gas partition coefficient of 0.60 to 0.69 (Strum and Eger, 1987). One MAC of sevoflurane is 3.3% in neonates and infants 1 to 6 months of age (Lerman et al., 1994), 2.5% in younger children (Katoh and Ikeda, 1992), and 2.0% in older children and adults (Scheller et al., 1988; Inomata et al., 1994). The biotransformation of sevoflurane in humans is about 3%, roughly one fifth that of halothane (Holaday and Smith, 1981) and significantly greater than that of desflurane and isoflurane (see Chapter 6, Pharmacology of Pediatric Anesthesia).

Sevoflurane has minimal effect on hemodynamic parameters. Wodey and others (1997), using echocardiographic studies, found that sevoflurane at 1 and 1.5 MAC did not alter the heart rate or cardiac index. They did find a significant change from baseline when measuring blood pressure and vascular resistance but no abnormal values when assessing myocardial contractility. Unlike halothane, sevoflurane does not sensitize the myocardium to epinephrine (Hayashi et al., 1987).

Sevoflurane has been observed to profoundly depress ventilation (Doi and Ikeda, 1988). In comparison to halothane, minute ventilation and respiratory frequency were significantly lower in infants on 1 MAC of sevoflurane, although end-tidal P_{CO_2} values were only moderately increased (Brown et al., 1998). The bronchodilatory effect of sevoflurane appears to be similar to that of halothane (Hashimoto et al., 1996; Rooke et al., 1997). Neurologic effects of sevoflurane include decreasing cerebral blood flow compared with halothane (Monkhoff et al., 2001) and eliciting epileptiform electroencephalographs in adults and children (Yli-Hnankala et al., 1999; Vakkuri et al., 2001).

Metabolism of sevoflurane in vivo produces inorganic fluoride, the level of which may be proportional to the concentration and duration of exposure to sevoflurane (MAC-hour). There have been no reports of renal toxicity with sevoflurane, although serum fluoride concentrations in excess of 50 μmol/L have been reported in adults (Frink et al., 1992). It has been suggested that sevoflurane exposures up to 15 MAC-hours are safe in adults (Sarner et al., 1995). Sevoflurane is not stable in soda lime, and the rate of degradation (especially accumulation of Compound A) increases with increasing sevoflurane concentrations, decreasing fresh gas flow, and increasing temperature (Strum et al., 1987); this degradation may not be of clinical significance with a semiclosed anesthesia breathing circuit with moderate to high flows (i.e., >2 L/min of fresh gas flow). Ebert and others (1998) reported no sign of renal or hepatic toxicity in healthy volunteers exposed to 3% sevoflurane for 8 hours. In addition, as described previously, a new class of CO_2 absorbers, which do not react with sevoflurane, may solve the problem of sevoflurane breakdown in the near future (Karasch et al., 2002; Kobayashi et al., 2003; Lerman, 2004).

Another infrequent but potentially catastrophic problem with sevoflurane is its extreme exothermal reaction with desiccated CO_2 absorbers, especially with Baralyme, producing spontaneous ignition, fire, and even explosion, and the production of carbon monoxide, first reported in Europe (Baum et al., 1998) and more recently in the United States (Olympio and Morell, 2003; Castro et al., 2004; Wu et al., 2004).

Degradation of sevoflurane increases as the water content of the CO_2 absorber with strong monovalent base contents (KOH and NaOH) decreases. Complete desiccation occurs within several days of constant flow of dry gas at room temperature, such as oxygen flowing through the canister over the weekend (Woehlck et al., 2001; Wu et al., 2004). Fatheree and Leigon (2004) reported an unfortunate case of a patient developing acute respiratory distress syndrome (ARDS) and tracheobronchial burn with increased carboxyhemoglobin (29%) in arterial blood following an exposure to an apparent exothermic reaction (without explosion) between sevoflurane and Baralyme.

Wu and others (2004), in reporting an explosion in an unused, unattended anesthesia machine in which oxygen and sevoflurane were left running, identified several areas where CO_2 absorbent desiccation may be of concern. These areas include infrequently used anesthesia machines at off-site locations and in the operating rooms where high fresh gas flows relative to body size are used (such as myringotomies and tube insertions) and for bronchoscopy (Wu et al., 2004).

After an incidence of explosion during sevoflurane anesthesia for rigid bronchoscopy, Castro and others changed CO_2 absorbers from KOH- and NaOH-based Baralyme to soda lime (less carbon monoxide production than Baralyme) or $Ca(OH)_2$-based Amsorb (Castro et al., 2004; Fatheree and Leighton, 2004). In an editorial in *Anesthesiology* that accompanied these case reports, Woehlck (2004) recommended the monitoring of canister temperature intraoperatively using a skin temperature probe, which is readily available in the operating room. Alternatively, one should consider using a Mapleson D (Bain or Jackson-Rees) circuit with a humidifier, which totally circumvents the problems related to the use of adult circle systems with CO_2 absorbers, especially for infants and small children who are too small to produce enough exhaled CO_2 to humidify adult circle systems.

There have been case reports of hepatitis possibly associated with the administration of sevoflurane in Japan, with the estimated incidence of less than 1:250,000. These reports included three children between the ages of 1 to 18 months, all of whom recovered from hepatic dysfunction, although several deaths were reported among adult patients. Hepatic microsomal induction and its potential for hepatotoxicity may be no greater than those associated with isoflurane (Stoelting et al., 1987). Clinical case reports have noted malignant hyperthermia occurring with sevoflurane anesthesia in both adults and children and with or without the use of succinylcholine for intubation (Otsuka et al., 1991; Ochiai et al., 1992; Maeda et al., 1997; Kinouchi et al., 2001).

Postanesthetic emergence and the time for attaining discharge criteria are significantly shorter with sevoflurane than with halothane, consequently requiring the administration of postoperative analgesics sooner (Naito et al., 1991; Sarner et al., 1995). Approximately 40% to 50% of children experience emergence agitation depending on anesthetic technique and diagnostic criteria. Severe agitation often necessitates the use of sedatives and prolonging the recovery time (Greenspun et al., 1994). Intraoperative use of analgesics without delaying emergence and recovery has met varying success in minimizing this untoward response (Davis et al., 1999; Cohen et al., 2001).

Halothane

Although abandoned in Japan (within 6 months after introduction of sevoflurane in clinical use) and in most of Europe, halothane still offers some advantages over other agents, including excellent airway conditions and low cost. The relative lack of airway response (secretion, spasm) is a favorable characteristic of halothane, and, together with its bronchodilatory effect, halothane had been the drug of choice for inhaled anesthetics in the presence of airway pathology such as bronchopulmonary dysplasia or bronchial asthma. Pharyngeal reflexes are obtunded sufficiently by halothane to allow the use of an oral airway relatively early in induction. Its longer duration of action makes it a useful agent during procedures that require spontaneous respiration and instrumentation of the airway.

The MAC of halothane varies during infancy and childhood. It is highest in infants 1 to 6 months of age at 1.1%, measures 0.97% for children 1 to 2 years of age, and progressively decreases with increasing age until reaching adult values at around 10 years of age (Gregory et al., 1969; Nicodemus et al., 1969). A subsequent study showed that the MAC of halothane in neonates (0.87%) is much lower than that in older infants (Lerman et al., 1983).

As with other potent inhaled anesthetics, halothane depresses the neural respiratory drive and increases P_{CO_2} progressively with increasing depth of anesthesia in children (Graff et al., 1964; Wren et al., 1987). Spontaneous breathing under light halothane anesthesia increases alveolar dead space and wasted ventilation (Hulse et al., 1984). It is not unusual to find the end-tidal P_{CO_2} increased to 60 mm Hg and beyond in infants and children breathing spontaneously under halothane anesthesia. Although infants and children seem to tolerate mild to moderate hypercapnia, the extent of stress response to severe hypercapnia and respiratory acidosis in anesthetized infants and children is not known. It is therefore recommended that ventilation be assisted in infants and children as needed to keep end-tidal P_{CO_2} below 60 cm H_2O, especially to avoid myocardial irritability (see later).

Halothane depresses stroke volume, cardiac output, and mean arterial blood pressure in proportion to the depth of anesthesia (Eger et al., 1970, 1971), primarily because of a direct negative inotropic effect on the myocardium (Goldberg, 1968). Barash and others (1978) found that a halothane concentration greater than 2% can result in severe cardiac depression. This effect can be attenuated or even reversed by intravenous atropine (0.02 mg/kg).

Cardiac arrhythmias, particularly premature ventricular contractions, are much more likely to occur with halothane than with isoflurane (Rodrigo et al., 1986). Children, however, appear to tolerate epinephrine better than adults (Melgrave, 1970; Wallbank, 1970). While the hazard of arrhythmias with epinephrine may be less in children than in adults, a smaller dose of epinephrine (up to 5 mcg/kg in less than 10 minutes) during halothane anesthesia is recommended as a precautionary measure. It is also important to maintain adequate alveolar ventilation to reduce the effects of hypercapnia and resultant increases in endogenous catecholamines on the myocardium (Joas and Stevens, 1971).

Halothane, like other volatile anesthetics, causes cerebral vasodilation, increases cerebral blood flow and volume (Wollman et al., 1964; Todd and Drummond, 1984), and, at high concentrations, abolishes autoregulation of cerebral blood flow in response to changes in arterial blood pressure (Miletich et al., 1976). At concentrations greater than 1%, these agents increase intracranial pressure (DiGiovanni et al., 1974). Such effects present a definite danger in patients with increased intracranial pressure. Use of an opioid and a muscle relaxant technique with mild hypocapnia is the method of choice in these patients.

Hepatitis secondary to exposure to halothane is rare in children. A few documented accounts exist of fatal posthalothane hepatic necrosis in pediatric patients (Walton, 1986; Kenna et al., 1987). Retrospective studies have identified only a few cases of possible halothane-related hepatitis in children—1:82,000 halothane anesthesia procedures in one study (Wark, 1983) and 1:>200,000 cases in the other (Warner et al., 1984). In contrast, the estimated incidence in adults is between 1:6000 and 1:35,000 cases

(Summary of the National Halothane Study, 1966; Inman and Mushin, 1978; Brown, 1985). Thus, although children cannot be assumed to be immune to acute halothane hepatic necrosis, the incidence is extremely rare.

Isoflurane

Isoflurane is a stable, colorless liquid requiring no stabilizing agent. Isoflurane undergoes minimal biotransformation in vivo (Holaday et al., 1975). It has an unpleasant, pungent odor and often causes cough and laryngospasm during inhalation induction when the concentration is increased too rapidly. Its blood-gas partition coefficient (1.4) is lower than that of halothane (2.4) but much higher than that of desflurane (0.42) and sevoflurane (0.66). As with halothane, the MAC of isoflurane is age dependent, ranging from 1.3% in preterm infants (LeDez and Lerman, 1987) to 1.7% in infants 6 to 12 months of age and decreasing to 1.6% in children 1 to 5 years of age, compared with 1.2% in adults (Cameron et al., 1984). Clinically, emergence from isoflurane anesthesia in children is similar to that from halothane despite the lower solubility of isoflurane. This apparent discrepancy between solubility and clinical effect may be related to different extents of biotransformation of these agents, which may affect their alveolar concentration and their washout during emergence (Eger, 1984).

Isoflurane depresses ventilation progressively with increasing concentration but more so than does halothane at equipotent concentrations in adults as well as in children. The depression of minute ventilation and respiratory frequency with isoflurane in children is more than that with halothane, but the degree of tidal volume depression and hypercapnia is similar (Wren et al., 1987). Because of its potent ventilatory depressant effect, isoflurane anesthesia requires controlled ventilation.

During isoflurane anesthesia, as with other volatile agents, systemic arterial blood pressure decreases progressively with increasing anesthetic depth. In contrast to halothane, however, clinical concentrations of isoflurane maintain cardiac output; hypotension is caused primarily by a reduction in peripheral vascular resistance (Wolf et al., 1986). With minimal negative inotropic effect and decreased myocardial oxygen consumption, isoflurane may have a wider margin of safety than halothane. Isoflurane increases heart rate but does not precipitate arrhythmias. In adults, when exogenous epinephrine is used for subcutaneous hemostasis during isoflurane anesthesia, three times the dose that precipitates arrhythmias with halothane anesthesia is well tolerated.

Isoflurane causes more potentiation of pancuronium than does halothane (Miller et al., 1972). Vecuronium is less affected by the choice of inhalation anesthetic (Miller et al., 1984). The dose of nondepolarizing muscle relaxants should be adjusted accordingly.

Desflurane

Desflurane, a polyfluorinated methyl ethyl ether, has a blood-gas solubility coefficient (0.42) similar to that of nitrous oxide (0.47) (Yasuda et al., 1989). As with other inhaled anesthetics, the MAC of desflurane is age dependent. Taylor and Lerman (1991) report that MAC in neonates is 9.2%, in infants 1 to 6 months of age is 9.4%, in infants 6 to 12 months of age is 9.9%, and then progressively decreases to 8.0% in older children. These differences are similar to those reported for halothane and isoflurane but smaller in magnitude. Desflurane appears to be similar to isoflurane in terms of negligible biodegradation, absence of myocardial sensitization to epinephrine, and effect on electroencephalography. Because of its lower boiling point (23.5°C), desflurane requires a heated pressurized vaporizer.

Desflurane has a strong pungent odor and is highly irritating to the airways (Rampil et al., 1991; van Hemelrijck et al., 1991). Among infants and children undergoing inhalation induction with desflurane without premedication, severe laryngospasm occurred in 73% of patients (Fisher and Zwass, 1992). Zwass and others (1992) concluded that desflurane should be limited in its use as an anesthetic for maintenance.

Desflurane causes dose-related respiratory depression, with the major effect being a reduction in tidal volume and minute ventilation, whereas the respiratory rate is increased (Lockhart et al., 1991). Behforouz and others (1998) documented similar results in children when concentrations were greater than 1 MAC. The blunted ventilatory response to carbon dioxide is dose dependent and is qualitatively similar to that with isoflurane. Desflurane does not appear to have similar bronchodilating properties as halothane or sevoflurane (Goff et al., 2000).

The cardiovascular effects of desflurane have been extensively studied in healthy adult volunteers (Cahalan et al., 1991; Weiskopf et al., 1991a, 1991b). During steady-state anesthesia, desflurane provides a high degree of cardiovascular stability, although it markedly decreases systemic vascular resistance, leading to a significant decrease in systemic blood pressure without changes in cardiac output. Heart rate increases with desflurane in a dose-dependent manner. The myocardial depressant effect of desflurane is mild. In children, cardiovascular stability is well maintained if anesthesia is induced by sevoflurane, halothane, or intravenous agents. Bradycardia and arrhythmias are uncommon. At 1 MAC, heart rate and systolic blood pressure are decreased by 20% to 25% from awake controls (Taylor and Lerman, 1991).

Because of its low blood-gas partition coefficient, desflurane should allow for a more rapid emergence and recovery than halothane, isoflurane, or even sevoflurane. Indeed, in two studies in adults, emergence from desflurane anesthesia was significantly faster than emergence from sevoflurane, especially after prolonged anesthesia (Eger et al., 1998). The time to eye opening and orientation following anesthesia and the time to being ready for discharge were significantly shorter in the desflurane group (Mahmoud et al., 2001). The use of desflurane in pediatric patients, however, is complicated by a high incidence (50% to 80%) of emergence agitation, often characterized by violent thrashing and inconsolability. This necessitates the use of sedation with opioids and/or hypnotic medications (Davis et al., 1994). Moderate doses of fentanyl (average, 2.8 mcg/kg) have been successful in reducing the incidence of emergence agitation in pediatric patients, but postoperative vomiting incidence was high (75%) in this study (Cohen et al., 2001). On the other hand, the original multicenter study of desflurane in children reported a significantly lower incidence of PONV in children induced with halothane who were switched over to desflurane than those with halothane alone (10% versus 26%) (Zwass et al., 1992).

INTRAVENOUS AGENTS

There has been an increased use of intravenous anesthesia in infants and children as a result of an improved understanding of pediatric pharmacokinetics and the introduction of new shorter-acting agents, such as propofol and remifentanil. In general, neonates and infants have larger volumes of distribution and decreased rates of elimination. The density of receptors, blood-brain barrier permeability, and pharmacodynamic effects of various drugs also vary greatly during the early postnatal period. These differences are discussed in greater detail in Chapter 6 (Pharmacology of Pediatric Anesthesia). In general, the newer opioids with shorter durations, as well as hypnotic and anesthetic agents, have all been shown to be safe and effective in infants and children. Their increased use has changed pediatric anesthetic practice from a classic single-agent inhalation anesthetic to a vast array of possible techniques that can be specifically tailored to the patient's needs.

Total intravenous anesthesia (TIVA) offers both advantages (rapid recovery, cleaner environment, and portability) and disadvantages (awareness, vagal reflexes, movement, and need for supplemental analgesia) for the pediatric patient. The cost of TIVA compared with an inhalation technique, which is an important consideration, is difficult to assess. Often, in the pediatric age group, an inhalation induction precedes TIVA, which negates some of its advantages. Of the available agents, propofol has been the most widely adopted.

Propofol is a short-acting intravenous anesthetic with high lipid solubility and a short elimination half-life, can be used as an induction agent as well as a maintenance anesthetic when given as a continuous infusion. Propofol is increasingly the agent of choice for general anesthesia and sedation in and outside of the operating room settings. Often, it is the sole anesthetic agent used in magnetic resonance imaging (MRI), endoscopy, bronchoscopy, and "painful procedure" suites (Keengwe et al., 1999; Elitsur et al., 2000; Jayabose et al., 2001).

Hannallah and others (1994) demonstrated that children have higher dose requirements than adults. With a background of 60% nitrous oxide, pediatric patients require a dose of approximately 250 to 300 mcg/kg per min to prevent movement in response to surgical stimulation, and a dose of approximately 150 to 200 mcg/kg per min to stabilize the hemodynamic indices of those who received muscle relaxants. The higher dose requirement in children may be secondary to a 50% increase in the volume of distribution (Marsh et al., 1991) and a shorter elimination half-life (Valtonen et al., 1989). A shorter recovery period and decreased incidence of PONV have been described in children receiving propofol infusions compared with those receiving halothane anesthetics (Marsh et al., 1991; Watcha et al., 1991; Hannallah et al., 1994). Watcha and others (1991) found the incidence of nausea and vomiting to be even lower when nitrous oxide was not administered. Emergence times are reduced in infants and children when propofol is used as the induction agent for short procedures. Schrum and others (1994) found this to be especially true of infants aged 1 to 6 months. Cohen and others (2003) found in patients aged 2 to 36 months that propofol at 200 mcg/kg with analgesic supplementation had the same hemodynamic, recovery, and antiemetic profile as sevoflurane. Emergence delirium has not been described as occurring after the use of propofol in children.

Similar to adults, hypotension and bradycardia are associated with the use of propofol. These responses are accentuated by the concurrent use of opioids and attenuated with the use of an anticholinergic drug, such as atropine. Pain during injection, possible allergic reactions, and the need for intravenous access are additional problems related to propofol use, especially in children who have distinct fear and dislike of a needle stick. These disadvantages can usually be easily overcome by choosing inhalation induction or using a small dose of thiopental or lidocaine before or mixed with propofol to abolish or minimize pain at the injection site. Propofol is an excellent agent for the maintenance of anesthesia that permits rapid recovery not associated with agitation and disorientation on emergence and decreased PONV.

ADJUVANT AGENTS

There are numerous agents available to the pediatric anesthesiologist that can be incorporated into the maintenance anesthetic for both intraoperative and postoperative effects. Opioids and other analgesics are discussed in detail in Chapter 6 (Pharmacology of Pediatric Anesthesia). Reducing the amount of inhaled agent required during the anesthetic, a smooth, calm emergence, a comfortable patient, and appreciative family are just some of the benefits. Much discussion has been addressed to the issue of preemptive analgesia. Although, theoretically, preventing the reception and/or transmission of noxious stimuli in an organism should reduce the overall experience, the timing of analgesics, blocks, and paraxial opioids (i.e., presurgical versus postsurgical) has not been shown to effect acute postoperative pain measurements. Moiniche and others (2002) performed an extensive review of the available literature and found no benefit to pretreating patients undergoing surgical procedures. Studies in children that examined preemptive analgesia using axillary blocks (Altintas et al., 2000) or new-generation nonsteroidal anti-inflammatory drugs (NSAIDs) (Kokki and Salomen, 2002) for tonsillectomy also failed to show any difference in postoperative scores or analgesic requirements. Preemptive analgesia, however, may play an important role in preventing chronic pain syndromes.

Opioids

Opioids and their synthetic analogs have been widely used for infants and children as adjuncts to inhaled anesthetics, as the primary or major anesthetic component for "balanced anesthesia" techniques, or as analgesics for postoperative pain. Morphine, fentanyl, and, more recently, remifentanil are the opioids most commonly used in pediatric anesthesia. The dosage used varies a great deal, depending on the purpose and plan for postoperative management (spontaneous breathing versus mechanical ventilation) (Table 11–4).

TABLE 11–4. Intravenous dosage of opioids in children

Drug	As Major Anesthetic	As Adjunct	As Postoperative Analgesic
Morphine	2 to 3 mg/kg	0.05 to 0.1 mg/kg per hr	0.05 to 0.1 mg/kg
Fentanyl	50 to 100 mcg/kg	1 to 3 mcg/kg per hr	1 to 2 mcg/kg
Sufentanil	10 to 15 mcg/kg	0.1 to 0.3 mcg/kg per hr	—
Alfentanil	150 to 200 mcg/kg	1 to 3 mcg/kg per min	—
Remifentanil	0.2 to 1.0 mcg/kg per min	0.1 to 0.4 mcg/kg per min	—
Hydromorphone	5 to 10 mcg/kg	3 to 5 mcg/kg per hr	3 to 5 mcg/kg

Morphine is a long-acting, hydrophilic analgesic that initially appeared to be unsafe in infants. Kupferberg and Way (1963) and Way and others (1965) demonstrated increased sensitivity to morphine in neonatal rats and humans, respectively. An increased permeability of the infant blood-brain barrier, which was suggested by both groups, is supported by evidence cited by Cook and Marcy (1988). Lynn and Slattery (1987) described lower clearance and longer elimination half-life in neonates. Because of greater drug availability to the central nervous system and longer pharmacologic half-life, morphine dosing in the newborn should be reduced in amount and given at increased intervals. Morphine can be used safely in older infants and children who have pharmacokinetics similar to those of adults. In high doses, morphine can cause hypotension as a result of bradycardia, vasodilation, and histamine release as well as hypertension (Conahan et al., 1973; Moss and Roscow, 1983). Urticaria (frequent) and bronchospasm (rare) are also described. As with other opioids, morphine may cause nausea and vomiting postoperatively. Because of its longer duration of action and euphoric effect, however, morphine is commonly used for inpatients who require postoperative analgesia and sedation.

Hydromorphone is a hydrogenated ketone derivative of morphine that is 7 to 10 times more potent. Hydrophilic in nature, its time to onset and duration of action are shorter than those of morphine. In addition, it manifests less sedation, nausea, and vomiting but is still capable of inducing pronounced respiratory depression. Both morphine and hydromorphone are widely used in patient controlled and epidural analgesia.

Meperidine is about one tenth as potent as morphine. It does not have the same marked increased narcotic effect in the newborn as morphine (Way et al., 1965). In newborn animals, the plasma half-life of meperidine is about twice that of the adult, but because it is lipophilic, its active plasma level may not differ in infants (Mirkin, 1970). In older infants and children, meperidine offers the same advantages as morphine. Histamine release is also associated with its use. Relatively small doses of meperidine ($\leq$0.5 mg/kg) continue to be a reliable treatment of postanesthesia shivering (Macintyre et al., 1987; Tsai and Chu, 2001).

Fentanyl is a lipophilic synthetic opioid with a relatively short duration of action, 1 to 2 hours, but a plasma half-life similar to that of morphine. It is about 100 times as potent as morphine. From 20 to 50 mcg/kg is suggested for general anesthesia in neonates and infants for cardiac surgery, but there is great variability found in kinetic studies. Koehntop and others (1986) measured decreased elimination times and increased volumes of distribution in neonates, whereas Singleton and others (1987) described values similar to those in older infants and children. Hertzka and others (1989) demonstrated, in infants older than 3 months, no increased risk of respiratory depression, but Koehntop and others (1986) found the need for postoperative ventilatory support in some neonates and evidence of rebound in fentanyl serum levels. Fentanyl appears to be safe in infants and children as a primary anesthetic agent and as a supplementary analgesic during an inhalation anesthetic. Pharmacokinetic studies of fentanyl in neonates have demonstrated a highly variable volume of distribution, rate of clearance, and half-life. Because the effect is less predictable in neonates and premature infants, postoperative ventilatory support should be considered.

Two common side effects of high-dose fentanyl are bradycardia and chest wall rigidity. Bradycardia is typically beneficial in adults, because they rarely experience hemodynamic changes with these doses, even with poor ventricular function (Stanley and Webster, 1978). However, bradycardia is undesirable in infants, who are unable to accommodate the increased preload by increasing stroke volume. Vagolytic agents or muscle relaxants that cause tachycardia should be administered concurrently. Muscle relaxants also reduce the difficulty of mask-bag ventilation experienced with chest wall rigidity. If mask-bag ventilation is planned, then fentanyl doses should be limited to 2 to 3 mcg/kg.

Fentanyl is ideal for patients needing short-term anesthesia and analgesia. It is useful for patients who require rapid recovery to baseline ventilatory function and respiratory drive, such as patients having same-day surgery, neurosurgical procedures, and airway instrumentation. Unless administered as a continuous infusion, fentanyl is not the drug of choice for patients requiring extended periods of analgesia.

Sufentanil is about 1000 times as potent as morphine and has an elimination half-life of approximately half that of fentanyl. The neonatal pharmacokinetics profile is similar to that of fentanyl (Davis et al., 1987a, 1987b). Bradycardia is not as prevalent and can be minimized with muscle relaxants that cause tachycardia (Hickey and Hansen, 1984).

Alfentanil is about 25 to 100 times as potent as morphine, with a small volume of distribution and an elimination half-life about one third that of fentanyl. Davis and others (1989) found that in neonates, alfentanil, like fentanyl, has a prolonged elimination time and increased volume of distribution that markedly prolong its pharmacologic half-life. Alfentanil has great patient-to-patient variability, and its effect can be difficult to predict. Alfentanil is associated with a high incidence of PONV.

Remifentanil is an ultrashort-acting opioid with an elimination half-life about one sixth that of fentanyl (Egan et al., 1993; Westmoreland et al., 1993). Davis and others (2000) describe an infusion at 0.25 mcg/kg per min as being effective for general anesthesia for children undergoing adenotonsillectomy. Rapid emergence and the need for supplementary postoperative analgesia were also noted. Ross and others (2001) found a consistent pharmacokinetic profile of remifentanil in the pediatric population. Infants had the largest volume of distribution and the most rapid clearance, but the elimination half-life (3.4 to 5.7 minutes) was the same for all age groups. Pinsker and Carrol (1999) found in children undergoing dental restoration a low incidence of PONV in those patients anesthetized with remifentanil. When used for general anesthesia in premature and full-term infants undergoing pyloromyotomy, remifentanil provided safe and stable intraoperative and postoperative conditions (Davis et al., 2001). No new-onset postoperative apnea was reported. Remifentanil, with predictable pharmacokinetic and hemodynamic effects, is extremely well suited for intraoperative anesthesia and analgesia in infants and children but typically requires analgesic supplementation for emergence and recovery.

Methadone is a long-acting synthetic opioid with an elimination half-life of about 35 hours. It is equipotent to morphine when given intravenously. It can be administered as part of a general anesthetic for prolonged surgical procedures (such as anteroposterior spinal fusions) and when protracted postoperative pain relief is anticipated.

Nonsteroidal Anti-inflammatory Drugs

NSAIDs have no known role in the maintenance of anesthesia but may be used intraoperatively to decrease postoperative pain and discomfort. Intraoperative treatment with ketorolac has been shown to be effective in decreasing postoperative pain and the incidence of nausea and vomiting associated with opioid use (Watcha et al., 1992; Cohen et al., 1993; Munro et al., 1994). Unfortunately, ketorolac's interference with platelet function has been reported to increase the risk of bleeding, especially in surgeries with an increased risk of bleeding, such as tonsillectomy (Gunter et al., 1995; Splinter et al., 1996). Ketorolac should also be avoided in patients with compromised renal and hepatic function.

Cyclooxygenase-2 (COX-2) inhibitors offer the advantage of having minimal to no effect on renal, gastrointestinal, and platelet function. By selectively blocking prostaglandin production in response to inflammation, this group of drugs is more selective in treating pain. In a review, parecoxib (40 mg PO) was found to be more effective than placebo for pain after laparoscopic cholecystectomy in adults (Joshi et al., 2004). Rofecoxib (50 mg PO) was also found to be effective for postoperative pain relief after outpatient inguinal herniorrhaphy in adults (Ma et al., 2004). Romsing and Moiniche (2004) reported significant decreases in postoperative pain in 33 studies, including 62 comparisons of four COX-2 inhibitors with placebo. However, rofecoxib, a COX-2 inhibitor, given orally, did not decrease the postoperative use of opioids compared with placebo in children following adenotonsillectomies, although there was no increase in postoperative bleeding (Sheeran et al., 2004). An intravenous formulation, parecoxib, is available and a preinduction dose of 40 mg intravenously was reported to be more effective compared with placebo (Gan et al., 2004; Joshi et al., 2004) but not as effective as ketorolac (30 mg IV) after laparoscopic procedures in adult patients (Ng et al., 2004). The use of COX-2 inhibitors is being re-evaluated at the time of this writing due to increased mortalities reported among long-term users, in high doses (Lenzer, 2005).

Acetaminophen has for many years been given per rectum intraoperatively to supplement opioid analgesia. Birmingham and others (1997, 2001) demonstrated that doses of 40 mg/kg and an onset time of 2 hours were necessary to achieve antipyretic levels with this mode. They also reported marked interpatient variability. It should be noted that these one-time doses are at near toxic levels and subsequent doses should be modified.

Hypnotics and Sedatives

Benzodiazepines, commonly used for premedication and preinduction medication, can be used intraoperatively to ensure amnesia during "balanced anesthetics" and to prevent emergence delirium. Diazepam has a slower elimination time in neonates (Morselli et al., 1974) and greater blood-brain barrier penetration in newborn rodents (Marcucci et al., 1973). The shorter serum half-life of midazolam makes it better suited for intraoperative use. Davis and others (1995b) found that intranasal midazolam premedication did not prolong recovery from ultrashort procedures, such as bilateral myringotomies.

Antiemetics

The introduction of a serotonin receptor (5-HT_3) antagonist has markedly improved the anesthesiologist's ability to decrease the incidence of and treat PONV (Litman, Wu, and Catanzaro, 1994; Patel et al., 1997; Khalil et al., 1996). *Ondansetron*, compared with droperidol (the most effective antiemetic at that time), was shown to be equally effective with a minimum of side effects causing no delay in emergence or discharge (Davis et al., 1995a; Splinter et al., 1995). The half-life of ondansetron in infants and children under 2 years of age is 50% greater than in adults, so this age group should not require repeat dosing in the PACU. Other 5-HT_3 antagonists, granisetron and tropisetron, have been shown to be equally efficacious (Fuji et al., 1996; Ang et al., 1998).

Broadman and others (1990) found *metoclopramide* (0.15 mg/kg) to be an effective antiemetic in a similar group of pediatric patients. Its effects may be both central, where it antagonizes dopamine receptors, and peripheral, where it increases gastroesophageal sphincter tone and gastric emptying (Taylor, 1985). Other agents with demonstrated effectiveness include *dimenhydrinate* at 0.5 mg/kg (Kranke et al., 2002) or *perphenazine* at 70 mcg/kg (Splinter et al., 1998).

Dexamethasone has also been shown to be effective in reducing the incidence of vomiting in children recovering from tonsillectomy (Splinter and Roberts, 1996; Pappas et al., 1998). In addition, dexamethasone appears to decrease postoperative pain in this patient population (Elhakim et al., 2003). In a meta-analysis of antiemetic studies, Henzi and others (2000) found that dexamethasone is effective for a prolonged period of time. They concluded that the best available treatment for patients at increased risk for PONV is a combination of a 5-HT_3 antagonist and dexamethasone.

Muscle Relaxants

Muscle relaxants are discussed in greater detail in Chapter 6 (Pharmacology of Pediatric Anesthesia). The following overview briefly discusses the advantages and disadvantages of the different agents available. Table 11–5 summarizes recommended doses, duration, and sites of metabolism.

Succinylcholine is a depolarizing, fast- and short-acting muscle relaxant that offers important advantages but has important disadvantages compared with other available muscle relaxants. Succinylcholine is still the only muscle relaxant that dependably creates muscle relaxation for intubation conditions within 1 minute. It is also the only relaxant available approved for intramuscular use. Meakin and others (1989) recommend that 3 mg/kg in infants and 2 mg/kg in children intravenously

TABLE 11–5. Intravenous doses of muscle relaxants in children

	MAINTENANCE			ED_{95} (mg/kg)	
Drug	*Intubation (mg/kg)*	*Bolus (mg/kg)*	*Continuous Infusion (mcg/kg/m)*	*Infants*	*Children*
Mivacurium	0.2 to 0.3	0.1	10 to 20	0.1	0.1
Cisatracurium	0.15	0.1	1 to 5	0.05	0.05
Vecuronium	0.05 to 0.1	0.025	1	0.024	0.026
Rocuronium	0.8 to 1.0	0.3 to 0.5	15	0.2	0.3
Pancuronium	0.1	0.5	—	0.05	0.05
Pipecuronium	0.1	—	—	0.035	0.05

dependably produce the profound degree of paralysis needed for ET intubation. Atropine (0.02 mg/kg) should always be infused before the use of succinylcholine to prevent bradyarrhythmias. Liu and others (1981) recommend a dose of 4 mg/kg for intramuscular use for an onset time of 30 seconds to relieve laryngospasm and 3 to 4 minutes to achieve intubating conditions. Serious complications of succinylcholine include hyperkalemia in patients with neuromuscular disorders and burns, dysrhythmias, muscle rigidity, masseter spasm, postoperative myalgias, and triggering of malignant hyperthermia in susceptible patients. Due to these serious complications, the use of succinylcholine in children should be limited to emergency situations.

Mivacurium is a short-acting nondepolarizing muscle relaxant with a structure similar to that of *d*-tubocurarine and with a fairly rapid onset of action (Sarner et al., 1989). It is metabolized by plasma cholinesterase but more slowly than is succinylcholine. If needed, its neuromuscular effects can be satisfactorily antagonized by edrophonium or neostigmine. Histamine release and patient-to-patient variability can be seen with its use, particularly in pediatric patients (Gronert et al., 1993a, 1993b; Gronert and Brandom, 1994). Brandom and others (1998) described intubating conditions to be acceptable 90 seconds after a dose of 0.3 mg/kg. Infants were found to require a higher rate than adults for mivacurium infusion secondary to greater clearance (Marakakis et al., 1998).

Vecuronium is an intermediate-acting steroidal nondepolarizing muscle relaxant similar to pancuronium in structure. The vagolytic response and hemodynamic alterations do not occur with its use. Vecuronium in children has a higher ED_{95} than in infants and adults (Meretoja et al., 1988). At an equipotent dose ($2 \times ED_{95}$), the duration of its effect is much more prolonged in infants (73 minutes) compared with in children (35 minutes) or adults (53 minutes) (Meretoja, 1989). Because its duration of action is similar to that of pancuronium in infants, vecuronium cannot be considered as an intermediate-acting muscle relaxant for this age group.

Rocuronium is an intermediate-acting steroidal nondepolarizing agent similar in structure to vecuronium but with about one-tenth the potency. It produces a more rapid onset of paralysis than other nondepolarizing muscle relaxants. Woelfel and others (1992) described, at a dose of 0.6 mg/kg, that onset of maximal block was 1.3 (± 0.2) minutes in children 1 to 5 years of age and the time to recovery (T_{25}) was 26.7 ± 1.9 minutes. Increases in heart rate have been reported with its use. Meretoja and others (1995) found that the ED_{95} of rocuronium in infants was considerably less than that in adults and children but that the recovery times were similar in all age groups. In lightly anesthetized patients, intravenous injection is associated with pain and tachycardia (Shevchenko Y et al., 1999).

Cisatracurium, an intermediate nondepolarizing agent, is one of the 10 optical and geometric isomers (1R-isomer) of atracurium with four times the potency but a slower onset of action (Wastila et al., 1996; Brandom et al., 1998). Taivainen and others (2000) found at a dose of 0.15 mg/kg that onset of maximal block was 2 ± 0.8 and 3 ± 1.2 minutes in infants and children, respectively. Time to recovery (T_{25}) was longer in infants (43.3 ± 6.2 minutes) than in older children (36.0 ± 5.4 minutes). *cis*-Atracurium under goes hydrolysis at body temperature and physiologic pH (Hoffmann elimination), but this accounts for about only 23% of its elimination. Histamine is not an issue with this isomer, and hemodynamic stability is reported with its use.

Pancuronium is a long-acting steroidal nondepolarizing agent and is about 5 to 10 times more potent than *d*-tubocurarine with a comparative duration of action. Pancuronium causes tachycardia by blocking vagal activity at the ganglionic level and by releasing norepinephrine. The tachycardia may be advantageous in pediatric patients, who often demonstrate decreased heart rates and blood pressures caused by inhaled agents or synthetic opioids. Pancuronium is in part metabolized in the liver and the kidney excretes the rest; its effect is prolonged in patients with hepatic or renal failure.

Pipecuronium is an analogue of pancuronium with minimal or no cardiovascular effects. The duration of neuromuscular action is similar to that of pancuronium. The effective dose (ED_{95}) of pipecuronium in children with nitrous oxide–halothane anesthesia is 50 mcg/kg, and the dose during nitrous oxide–fentanyl anesthesia is 80 mcg/kg. The ED_{95} in infants under nitrous oxide–halothane anesthesia is only 35 mcg/kg (Pittet et al., 1989; Sarner et al., 1990). Pipecuronium is largely excreted by the kidneys.

REGIONAL ANESTHESIA

The reintroduction and adaptation of regional anesthetic techniques in the 1980s have helped advance pediatric pain management. The caudal approach is the simplest and most popular, but other methods, including peripheral nerve blocks, epidural anesthesia, and neuroaxial opioid use, have also become common practice. As in adults, the treatment course can be extended with the placement of catheters. Extensive experience with these methods intraoperatively and postoperatively has shown their efficacy and safety. The various regional analgesia techniques and the choice and dosage of local anesthetics and opioids for regional analgesia are detailed in Chapter 13 (Pain Management in Infants and Children). The volumes (and doses) of local anesthetics recommended for various regional blocks are summarized in Table 11–6.

Caudal Anesthesia

Caudal blocks are most often used as an adjunct to general anesthesia and for postoperative analgesia for surgical procedures involving the lower abdomen, pelvis, or lower extremities. The combination of inhalation anesthesia and regional block allows the anesthesiologist to lower anesthetic concentrations and facilitate postoperative emergence from general anesthesia. The caudal block is easily performed with minimal associated complications, such as dural puncture and intravascular injection (Dalens and

TABLE 11–6. Volumes of local anesthetic solutions for peripheral nerve blocks and regional anesthesia in children

Block	Volume (mL/kg)
Axillary	0.2 to 0.5*
Interscalene	0.33*
Sciatic	0.15 to 0.2*
Femoral	0.5*
Intravenous	0.5 to 10†
Caudal	0.5 to 1.0‡
Intrapleural (infusion)	0.5 (per hr)§

*Broadman and Rice, 1988.
†Yaster and Maxwell, 1989.
‡Armitage, 1979.
§McIlvaine and others, 1989.

Hasnaoui, 1989). Anatomical features that contribute to these occurrences are the caudal position of the dural sac in infants (S3), the high degree of vascularity of the region, and the development of the sacral fat pad in school-aged children. Awareness of these factors should reduce the risk of untoward events.

A caudal block in infants and children is most often performed after the induction of general anesthesia. After the airway is secured with an ET tube or the insertion of an oral airway, the child is turned to a lateral decubitus position and the sacral hiatus is identified, cleaned, and prepared. (If LMA is chosen for airway maintenance, it is safer to wait until the caudal block is completed, the patient turned back to the supine position, and the stomach emptied with a gastric tube before LMA is inserted. This is because LMA in infants and children tends to dislodge with the changes in the neck or body position.) A short beveled needle (22 gauge) is inserted through the sacrococcygeal ligament and advanced into the caudal space. Although different needle types and sizes are recommended (Broadman and Rice, 1988; Yaster and Maxwell, 1989), the only difference in outcome observed is that shorter needles result in fewer inadvertent intrathecal and intravascular injections. The syringe is withdrawn before injecting to make sure that an intravascular or intrathecal space is not inadvertently entered. Tobias (2001) reviewed the available literature on the efficacy of test doses, with epinephrine-containing solutions, for detecting the signs and symptoms of intravascular injection and concluded that they may be of limited benefit depending on anesthetic technique and previous use of anticholinergic medications.

Bupivacaine is the most widely used local anesthetic because of its relative safety and longer duration of action. Takasaki and colleagues (1977) recommended a volume of 0.056 mL/kg per segment, whereas Armitage (1979) uses 0.5 mL/kg for a sacral or saddle block and 1.0 mL/kg for an upper abdominal blockade. The optimal concentration of bupivacaine is one that provides adequate analgesia without producing postoperative motor blockade of the lower extremities (Wolf et al., 1990). Both 0.125% and 0.175% of bupivacaine have been shown to be appropriate concentrations, whereas 0.25% bupivacaine may occasionally produce a motor blockade in the lower extremities (Gunter et al., 1991). The (*S*)-isomer of bupivacaine, *levo*-bupivacaine, which has less cardiac toxicity with similar local anesthetic properties, may afford some benefit in at risk patients (Ivani et al., 2002).

Ropivacaine, a congener of bupivacaine with less toxicity and, at concentrations of 0.2%, with a lower incidence of motor block (Khalil, 1999), is gaining wider use. In infants, the incidence of cardiac arrhythmias, systemic absorption, and serum-free fraction are all lower compared with bupivacaine (Hansen et al., 2001; Karmakar et al., 2002). Hansen and others (2000) described a similar safety profile when ropivacaine was used in epidural infusions. These properties make ropivacaine the drug of choice when anticipating prolonged exposure in neonates or in patients with impaired metabolisms.

Other medications with analgesic properties, injected into the caudal space with and without local anesthetics, have been shown to be efficacious. Opioids, clonidine, and ketamine have been used with varying success and are discussed in greater detail in Chapters 13 and 14 (Pain Management and Pediatric Regional Anesthesia).

Urinary retention and the masking of essential diagnostic symptoms of surgical complications have been cited as postoperative concerns. Urinary retention occurs in approximately 10% of patients and is typically short lived (Yaster and Maxwell, 1989). Postoperative emptying of the urinary bladder along with parental education and reassurance should minimize this problem. A report describing an unrecognized compartment syndrome in a patient who received epidural anesthesia for an orthopedic procedure has raised concerns (Strecker et al., 1986). It was thought that the absence of pain prolonged the time to diagnosis. The administration of caudal anesthesia must be selective, but, more important, careful postoperative monitoring and nursing care should minimize the incidence of such complications.

Field and Nerve Blocks

Other regional and field block techniques have also been used as adjuncts to general anesthesia and to manage postoperative pain. Compared with caudal anesthesia, ilioinguinal-hypogastric nerve block, wound infiltration, local anesthesia "splash," dorsal penile nerve block, and subcutaneous ring block have all been shown to be equally effective for the chosen surgical procedure (Yeoman et al., 1983; Cross and Barrett, 1987; Hannallah et al., 1987; Fell et al., 1988; Casey et al., 1990). These techniques are applicable to orchiopexy, herniorrhaphy, hypospadias repair, and circumcision.

Peripheral nerve blocks can also supply analgesia for the upper and lower extremities. Axillary, interscalene, sciatic, and femoral nerve blocks have all been described. Recommended volumes appear in Table 11–6. The blocks can often be easily performed in young children, who tend to have better defined anatomy and landmarks. In older children, the use of a nerve stimulator can be helpful (Bosenberg et al., 2002). Toxic doses of local anesthetics can be avoided by using diluted solutions and solutions containing epinephrine (Berde, 1989). Head and face nerve blocks can also reduce the need for opioid analgesia and so reduce the incidence of nausea and vomiting (Suresh et al., 2002).

Epidural Anesthesia

Epidural block, by either a single injection, repeated injections, or continuous infusion via catheter, has been described in children (Dalens et al., 1986; Desparmet et al., 1987: Tusi et al., 2002). Bupivacaine (0.125% to 0.25%) and ropivacaine (0.2%) are recommended for both methods. A continuous infusion through a lumbar catheter at a rate of 0.3 mL/kg per hr maintains an analgesic level between T10 and L1. Although traditionally described from the lumbar approach, epidural analgesia can also be performed in children at the thoracic level (Bosenberg et al., 1988). Needle placement at these locations tends to be technically more challenging, with an increased risk of complications in small infants. Because of these difficulties, thoracic epidural blocks should be performed only by anesthesiologists who are experienced in their use and reserved for children undergoing a surgical procedure in the thoracic area or upper abdominal area that is associated with considerable postoperative pain (see Chapter 14, Regional Anesthesia).

Caudal catheters can be inserted with relative ease and minimal risk, similar to single-injection techniques previously described. A Touhy needle is inserted into the caudal space, and an appropriately sized catheter is advanced through it. The catheters are frequently styletted to facilitate direct advancement to higher levels with decreased risk of accidental placement in the nerve root sheath. The relatively short and straight path found in infants also minimizes complications. More rostral positioning of the catheter allows for improved postoperative pain management for upper abdominal procedures and thoracotomies.

Epidural Opioids

As described in adults, extremely effective analgesia can be achieved by injecting opioids into the epidural space (Jensen, 1981; Shapiro et al., 1984; Attia et al., 1986; Rosen and Rosen, 1989). Activation of opioid receptors in the dorsal horn of the spinal cord produces regional analgesia without the discomfort or danger of sympathetic, sensory, or motor blockade. Respiratory depression is a major complication requiring careful dosing and observation. Other side effects, including pruritus, nausea, vomiting, and urinary retention, can be prevented by using smaller doses of opioids, and are relatively easily managed by a small dose (0.5 to 1.0 mcg/kg) of naloxone. Nalbuphine 50 mcg/kg or 60 mcg/kg per hr has been shown to be effective in treating epidural morphine side effects without attenuating analgesia (Wang et al., 1998).

Various techniques, opioids, and opioid-local anesthetic combinations have been described. Preservative-free morphine (30 to 70 mcg/kg caudally and 50 mcg/kg epidurally) has resulted in effective and safe analgesia in children after various surgical procedures (Jensen, 1981; Krane et al., 1989; Rosen and Rosen, 1989; Rash et al., 1990; Wolf et al., 1990; Irving et al., 1993). Morphine's hydrophilic nature reduces its absorption from the epidural space, resulting in delayed onset of effect, decreased systemic uptake, rostral spread, and prolonged duration of action. The delayed onset (20 to 40 minutes) and duration of analgesia (mean range of 15 to 20 hours) in children are similar to those in adults, although the plasma half-life is shorter in children (Attia et al., 1986; Rash et al., 1990). Adequate monitoring of respiratory rate and depth and level of sedation is essential because serious respiratory depression has been reported in children with a higher dose (100 mcg/kg) of caudal morphine (Krane, 1988). Even at a recommended lower dose (50 mcg/kg) without clinical respiratory depression or apnea, ventilatory response to carbon dioxide is reported to be depressed throughout the duration of analgesia, independent of plasma morphine levels (Attia et al., 1986).

In contrast to morphine, fentanyl, sufentanil, and hydromorphone are lipophilic and have a more rapid onset, greater systemic absorption, shorter duration of action, and limited epidural redistribution (Dalens et al., 1986; Benlabed et al., 1987). These drugs are appropriate for rapid treatment of pain and are better suited for continuous infusions. Alone or in combination with diluted local anesthetics, their site of action is limited to the general location of the catheter tip placement.

Subarachnoid Opioids

Subarachnoid injection of morphine has also been studied (Dalens and Tanguy, 1988). The efficacy, side effects, and duration of analgesia with this technique are similar to those of epidural instillation with doses of 10 to 20 mcg/kg (Krechel and Helikson, 1993). Respiratory depression may be more severe. Intrathecal opioids are often restricted to intraoperative and postoperative management of patients undergoing extremely painful surgical procedures, such as scoliosis repair and open heart surgery. Delayed respiratory depression may occur, necessitating monitoring and observation in a more closely staffed setting (Jones et al., 1984; Nichols et al., 1993).

EMERGENCE AND EXTUBATION

EMERGENCE

Emergence from anesthesia begins as soon as the anesthesiologist stops the administration of anesthetic agents. In current practice, general anesthesia is often produced with a combination of inhaled or intravenous anesthetics, muscle relaxants, intravenous opioids and/or hypnotics, and, sometimes, regional nerve blocks. The presence of diverse agents makes the process of emergence more complex than after the use of a single agent. To facilitate prompt awakening and tracheal extubation, the anesthesiologist must anticipate, with reasonable accuracy, the conclusion of the surgical procedure. This allows for appropriate tapering of the concentration of inhaled anesthetics and decreasing or withholding intravenous agents, including muscle relaxants, before the procedure ends.

Normal recovery from anesthesia begins in the operating room with the reestablishment of adequate spontaneous breathing and extubation of the trachea. Discontinuation of the volatile agent, increasing the oxygen–nitrous oxide, oxygen, or oxygen-air mixture fresh gas flow, and moderately increasing the rate of manually controlled ventilation increase the pulmonary venous-to-alveolar concentration gradient of an inhaled anesthetic and facilitate the elimination of residual inhaled anesthetic, whereas excessive hyperventilation causes cerebral vasoconstriction and impedes the elimination of anesthetic from the brain. Furthermore, excessive hyperventilation depletes the carbon dioxide stores in the body tissues, delaying the onset of spontaneous breathing.

The less-soluble volatile anesthetics, such as desflurane and sevoflurane, may produce more rapid emergence, as discussed earlier, but with careful anticipation and appropriate timing, all patients anesthetized with various agents and techniques should emerge when planned. The timing for the discontinuation of intravenous medications must be determined by considering each agent's pharmacokinetics. Infants have longer elimination half-lives for many agents and thus require earlier termination of agents. Nitrous oxide (or, alternatively, sevoflurane or desflurane) is often continued during this period, to smooth the emergence from general anesthesia to wakefulness. Because of its low solubility and pleasant, minimal odor, nitrous oxide is an ideal transitional agent.

A smooth emergence is achieved by anticipating the patient's response to the pain caused by the surgical procedure and the disorientation caused by the anesthetic agents or the sudden wakefulness. The analgesic action of opioids and regional anesthesia and the sedative effects of opioids and hypnotics may help reduce agitation on emergence. If patient status or surgical procedure did not allow for the intraoperative use of these agents, they should be considered before emergence.

As the anesthetics are curtailed, the anesthesiologist observes the rate and pattern of spontaneous breathing. A rapid respiratory rate may be seen during stage 2 (the excitement phase) or in a patient with inadequate analgesia. Synchronous contraction of the intercostal muscles and diaphragm (that is, the upper part of the chest expands, as opposed to sinking paradoxically, during inspiration) is important because the intercostal muscles are more sensitive to inhaled anesthetics (Tusiewicz et al., 1977; Nishino et al., 1984, 1985; Ochiai et al., 1989). Paradoxical movement of the thorax and abdomen (thoracoabdominal asynchrony) may indicate incomplete recovery from general anesthesia or residual paralysis. The paradoxical breathing pattern may also indicate partial or complete upper airway obstruction as a result of relaxation of the upper airway muscles, which are most sensitive to the depressant effect of anesthetics and sedatives, especially in young infants (Ochiai et al., 1989, 1992). Careful and continuous auscultation with a precordial stethoscope is extremely important during the period of emergence.

Recovery From Neuromuscular Blockade

Recovery from neuromuscular relaxation can be monitored by means of peripheral nerve stimulation. As newer intermediate-acting and short-acting nondepolarizing muscle relaxants have become available, anesthetic management is more easily controlled, especially for simple pediatric surgical procedures such as inguinal herniorrhaphy and tonsillectomy. The degree of neuromuscular blockade may change relatively quickly when short-acting or intermediate-acting muscle relaxants are used and can be monitored closely by observing the train-of-four and double burst nerve stimulations. If repeat dosing is needed, the drug dose is titrated to maintain twitch height at 10% to 25% of the control height, or one to two twitches on the train-of-four monitor.

Neuromuscular blockade is reversed with intravenous atropine (0.02 mg/kg) followed by neostigmine (0.06 mg/kg). In infants, a higher dose of atropine (0.03 mg/kg) is recommended to prevent bradycardia and hypersecretion. Glycopyrrolate (0.1 mg/kg) is as effective as atropine and may produce a more stable heart rate (Cozanitis et al., 1980; Warran et al., 1981). Edrophonium (0.5 to 1.0 mg/kg) is faster acting (with shorter duration of action) and is as effective as neostigmine, but reversal with either drug is faster in children and infants than in adults (Meakin et al., 1983). Recovery of the train-of-four (TOF) ratio over 0.70 had long been considered adequate recovery of neuromuscular function (Ali and Kitz, 1973; Ali et al., 1975). This ratio is based on the observation that the diaphragm is more resistant to nondepolarizing muscle relaxants than skeletal muscles in adults (Wymore and Eisele, 1978; Pansard et al., 1987) and in infants and children (Laycock et al., 1988). In a more recent study, however, healthy young adult volunteers experienced considerable muscle weakness (diplopia, grip strength, and head lift) with TOF ratios between 0.70 and 0.90 after mivacurium infusion (Kopman et al., 1997). These authors concluded that "adequate" recovery of neuromuscular function, especially in the same-day surgery settings, requires the return of the TOF value to at least over 0.90 and ideally to unity. A minimum of at least two strong twitches on the TOF monitor should be confirmed before the reversal with neostigmine (and a minimum of three strong twitches for edrophonium reversal) to ensure that adequate reversal of neuromuscular blockade can be achieved (B. Brandom, personal communication).

The criteria for adequate clinical recovery from nondepolarizing neuromuscular blockade in adults (Ali and Miller, 1986) must be modified for use in infants and young children because of their inability to respond to verbal commands. Before tracheal extubation, the child should be able to do the following:

- Maintain adequate, nonparadoxical breathing
- Generate a negative inspiratory pressure against airway occlusion greater than 30 cm H_2O
- Sustain tetanic contraction at 50 Hz and strong double-burst contractions
- Sustain hip flexion with leg elevation for 10 seconds
- Lift the head and/or cough forcefully

When the child is awake, he or she should be able to perform the following:

- Grimace using eyebrows and/or forehead
- Spontaneously open the eyes
- Perform purposeful movement, such as reaching for the ET tube

The anesthesiologist must make the final judgment on the adequacy of neuromuscular function and the readiness for tracheal extubation. Timing of extubation is based on careful clinical observation rather than solely on monitoring with a nerve stimulator or other instruments. Before the trachea is extubated, the child must be breathing normally and adequately, without paradoxical movements. In addition to inadequate neuromuscular function, paradoxical breathing can also suggest other complications, such as airway obstruction, pneumothorax, or phrenic nerve injury.

EXTUBATION OF THE TRACHEA

Emptying of the Stomach

At the conclusion of surgery, while the child is still under general anesthesia, a suction catheter, lubricated with a surgical lubricant (or dipped in water), is gently passed into the stomach to remove gastric contents that accumulated or remained after suction at the beginning of the procedure. This practice reduces the risk of vomiting and aspiration during emergence. Gastric suctioning is especially important in patients thought to have a full stomach or an increased risk for gastroesophageal reflux. This practice is also indicated for patients who were mask ventilated during the procedure because it is helpful in removing any gases inadvertently introduced into the stomach with positive pressure ventilation. When the stomach contents are evacuated, the decrease in intra-abdominal pressure allows greater expansion of the lungs with manual expansions of the lungs, decreasing atelectasis at the base of the lungs and increasing the patient's functional residual capacity toward normal levels. For all patients, mucosal injury and bleeding from suctioning should be avoided. These preventable tissue injuries are usually sustained by forcing a dry catheter or by withdrawing the catheter with the suction generator attached.

Monitoring During Extubation

Once all anesthetics have been discontinued, muscle relaxation has been reversed, and vital signs are stabilized, the nerve stimulator, temperature probe, and blood pressure cuff may be removed. A precordial stethoscope should be applied, replacing an esophageal stethoscope if the latter was used intraoperatively. Electrocardiography should be continued at least until the trachea has been extubated, rhythmic breathing reestablished, and a stable sinus rhythm confirmed. Arterial saturation and heart rate should be continuously monitored by pulse oximetry throughout this period. Children are more likely to desaturate during emergence from anesthesia (Motoyama et al., 1987), and pulse oximetry is a more sensitive indicator of hypoxia than are clinical signs and symptoms or capnography (Coté et al., 1988, 1991).

Timing of Extubation

Extubation of the trachea must be performed with special care to avoid complications, such as laryngospasm or aspiration of gastric contents. Both of these complications can rapidly lead to severe hypoxia, cardiac depression, and significant patient compromise. Suzuki and Sasaki (1977) confirmed the age-old clinical impression by demonstrating in puppies that laryngospasm (defined as sustained adductor neural discharge after the cessation of a noxious stimulus) is worse during "light" general anesthesia than during wakefulness or deep anesthesia. The safest approach is to extubate the patient when he or she is either awake or well anesthetized.

One method of extubating older infants and children takes place while they are still anesthetized with sufficient inhaled or intravenous anesthetics (a minimum of 2 MACs by briefly increasing sevoflurane or desflurane concentration) to avoid coughing or laryngospasm. This technique (the deep extubation) is especially useful for patients with a history of reactive airway disease, such as asthma or bronchopulmonary dysplasia. Before considering this method, however, the anesthesiologist should know that the patient's airway had been well maintained by mask ventilation during induction of anesthesia. A prophylactic bronchodilator treatment (such as albuterol with a metered-dose inhaler) should be given to patients with a history of reactive airway disease (see later). An oropharyngeal airway should be placed to avoid upper airway obstruction caused by the collapse of velopharynx or the tongue falling back against the posterior pharyngeal wall after extubation (see Chapter 2, Respiratory Physiology). If airway patency was satisfactory before intubation, the return to spontaneous breathing is not a prerequisite for extubation in deeply anesthetized patients. Deep extubation can be performed safely when using sevoflurane or desflurane and awakening the patient expediently shortly after extubation (Valley et al., 2003). Airway problems may be more frequent with desflurane, and maintaining a higher concentration at extubation is recommended (Cranfield and Bromely, 1997).

The child suspected of having a full stomach should be awake and have complete return of protective laryngeal reflexes before extubation. Other conditions that require awakening before extubation include wiring of the jaw or a surgical intervention with a danger of airway obstruction. In such patients without a full stomach, intravenous lidocaine (1.0 to 1.5 mg/kg), given 2 to 3 minutes before extubation, helps decrease laryngeal responses to the ET tube. However, intravenous lidocaine tends to sedate and prolong the recovery from anesthesia, particularly in infants. A child with a history of reactive airway disease may also be safely extubated awake after pretreatment with a nebulized bronchodilator, such as albuterol. The patient is given two puffs of bronchodilator in a metered-dose inhaler into a mixing chamber, inserted between the anesthesia circuit and ET tube, followed immediately by slow and deep inspiration by gently squeezing the anesthesia bag to a static end-inspiratory pressure (>30 cm H_2O) for several seconds. This maneuver is repeated once more to conclude the pretreatment.

Before awake extubation, young children, particularly infants in the early months, may respond to laryngeal stimulation by breath-holding, bronchospasm, chest wall rigidity, marked cyanosis, and oxygen desaturation. The oxygen saturation on a pulse oximeter often drops suddenly to 70% or lower and continues to nose-dive even when both lungs are well ventilated manually with 100% oxygen. This phenomenon is impressive and frightening for a pediatric anesthesiologist; it resembles the cyanotic spells that occur in infants with tetralogy of Fallot. It has been observed mostly in young infants but occasionally in children up to 4 years of age (E. K. Motoyama, unpublished observation). In one case report, echocardiography showed a transient right-to-left shunt through a reopened foramen ovale (Moorthy et al., 1987), presumably as the result of a sudden increase in pulmonary vascular resistance, right ventricular afterload, and a shift in the right–to–left atrial pressure gradient and shunt. Fortunately, these episodes are self-limiting, provided that alveolar ventilation is maintained. Older children show less tendency toward sudden desaturation, but greater laryngeal response and irritation that produce forceful "bucking" (coughing with an ET tube in place) when extubation is delayed. This may lead to a greater incidence of postintubation croup (Koka et al., 1977). Thus, older children should be extubated as soon as protective reflexes return.

Technique of Extubation

Removal of the ET tube must be carried out with as much attention to detail as was needed for its insertion. As the child awakens, any stimulation may cause tightening of the jaw, occlusion of the teeth on the ET tube, and compromise of the airway. Severe or complete occlusion of the ET tube or the upper airways associated with marked inspiratory effort and intrathoracic negative pressure can result in postobstructive pulmonary edema (POPE) and hypoxemia (Galvis et al., 1980; Sofer et al., 1984). These children require supplemental oxygen, diuretics, and possible reintubation to provide continuous positive airway pressure (see later). This condition usually is resolved within 24 to 48 hours. Placement of an oral airway or a bite block before awakening can greatly reduce the risk of this occurring. Soft bite blocks made of rolled gauze and tape can reduce the incidence of soft tissue damage to the gums, palate, and lips associated with plastic airways. Oropharyngeal airways are preferred in patients whose airway patency was less than satisfactory during anesthetic induction. An oral airway does not stimulate laryngeal reflexes in most patients as long as it is inserted when the patient is still anesthetized and is left undisturbed. The oropharynx is then suctioned and, if indicated, the ET tube is suctioned of any secretions by passing a sterile suction catheter that takes up no more than half the internal diameter of the ET tube, to avoid the strong negative pressure collapsing the alveolar gas.

Until recently, it has been a standard practice before extubation to "preoxygenate" the patient with increased flow of 100% oxygen for several minutes, to wash out residual anesthetics and nitrous oxide, and to replace them with oxygen. Studies, however, have convincingly demonstrated that the age-old practice of preoxygenation must be modified and that the patient must be breathed with an oxygen-air mixture, rather than 100% oxygen, before extubation to minimize airway closure and atelectasis.

The reason for this maneuver is based on the fact that general anesthesia always produces significant reductions in resting lung volume (FRC), due to relaxation of the thoracic inspiratory muscles, especially in infants and young children (see Chapter 2, Respiratory Physiology). Reductions in FRC, in turn, result in small airway closure and considerable atelectasis, as oxygen and nitrous oxide in the trapped airways are absorbed into the pulmonary circulation (Serafini et al., 1999; Benoit et al., 2002). To eliminate the atelectasis developed during general anesthesia, the lungs must be reinflated with several vital capacity maneuvers (sustained airway pressure of 40 cm H_2O for several seconds) with a 30% to 70% oxygen and air mixture and an additional PEEP of 5 cm H_2O immediately thereafter, in both adults and children (Benoit et al., 2002; Lindahl and Mure, 2002; Tusman et al., 2003). Administering 100% oxygen before extubation worsens the gas exchange and increases atelectasis, even when the lungs have been sighed with vital capacity maneuvers (Loeckinger et al., 2002).

Based on these findings, it is now recommended, instead of the traditional preoxygenation with 100% oxygen, that the patient be ventilated with an oxygen and air mixture between the ratio of 1:1 and 2:1 (FIO_2, 0.6 to 0.73), to wash out residual anesthetics and nitrous oxide, and that the lungs be gently inflated by a sustained peak pressure between 30 and 40 cm H_2O for 3 to 5 seconds. This maneuver should be repeated several times to reexpand the lungs and eliminate atelectasis, and then PEEP of 5 to 6 cm H_2O be added thereafter to sustain FRC before extubation. Before extubation, the lungs are inflated synchronously with the child's inspiration by gently squeezing the anesthesia bag. The bag is then held momentarily at end-inspiration with a positive pressure of 15 to 20 cm H_2O to maintain a high lung volume as the ET tube is gently pulled out. This last maneuver serves three functions: (1) it inflates the lungs with an oxygen-rich gas mixture and provides an increased oxygen reservoir that may be needed if breath-holding or laryngospasm occurs (Motoyama et al., 1987); (2) the positive pressure (or stretching the airway walls) decreases the incidence and intensity of laryngospasm (Suzuki and Sasaki, 1977; Sasaki, 1979); and (3) the patient's first response after extubation will be a forceful exhalation or coughing, expelling any secretions trapped between the ET tube and the laryngeal wall, thus minimizing the laryngeal reflex to secretions and laryngospasm.

The initial moments after extubation are critical. The larynx is suctioned quickly to remove the secretions brought up from the upper trachea by the ET tube and then a facemask is applied to reestablish the breathing circuit and CPAP. The patency of the airway is maintained by lifting the mandible forward (the jaw-thrust position) and administering an oxygen mixture by a facemask. Unless laryngospasm develops, spontaneous ventilation resumes promptly. If laryngospasm does occur, oxygen can be forced past the vocal cords using a bag and mask in most patients, if a proper approach is used. Even during severe laryngospasm, there often is a pattern of rhythmicity in the child's respiratory movement. This is characterized by a period of stiffness or bearing down ("expiratory" phase), followed by a transient period of relative relaxation of the larynx ("inspiratory" phase). To oxygenate the child in laryngospasm, the anesthesiologist applies a tightly fitting facemask and maintains no more than 20 cm H_2O of CPAP. He or she then watches the patient's breathing pattern very closely and, during the brief moment of laryngeal relaxation, gives a firm squeeze on the anesthesia bag. In most cases, this maneuver delivers enough oxygen through the vocal cords to avoid severe hypoxemia and cardiac depression until laryngospasm resolves. Indiscriminate use of high positive pressure, regardless of the pattern or phase of laryngospasm, often makes matters worse.

Laryngospasm often results from overstimulation of the laryngeal reflexes by regurgitation or retained secretions. Under these circumstances the pharynx and larynx must be cleared of secretions swiftly, even during laryngospasm, to prevent further stimulation of the superior laryngeal nerve. Throughout laryngospasm, oxygen saturation, heart rate, and heart rhythm are continuously monitored with a pulse oximeter, precordial stethoscope, and electrocardiograph.

In the most severe episodes of laryngospasm, when all maneuvers seem ineffective, intravenous atropine (0.02 mg/kg) and succinylcholine (2 to 3 mg/kg) can be given for immediate relief. If an intravenous route is not available, succinylcholine (4 to 5 mg/kg) can be given as a sublingual injection for rapid results (Smith, 1980).

Once alveolar ventilation is reestablished, the patient is carefully examined for gastric distension, airway secretions, foreign body aspiration, and pneumothorax. Even if the stomach was suctioned previously, the child may still retch and vomit enough to cause laryngospasm and aspiration. Suction equipment must be immediately available and used with care and efficiency. If vomiting occurs, it is often sufficient to turn the child's head to the side to allow secretions to fall into the cheek for removal or to roll the child on to the side. Tipping of the head of the table is not necessarily helpful.

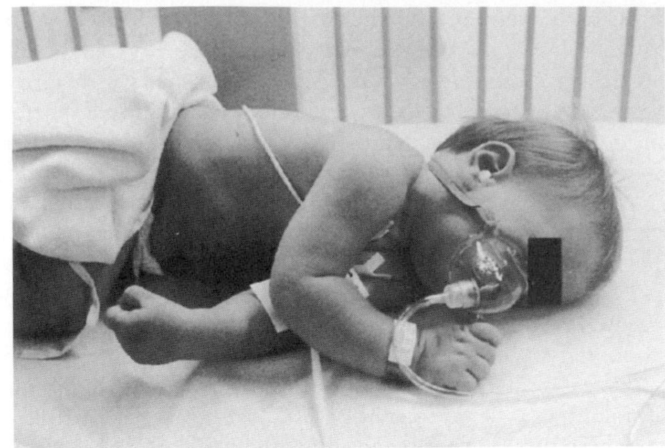

■ **FIGURE 11–3.** The infant is transported to the PACU in the lateral position.

TRANSPORT TO THE POSTANESTHETIC CARE UNIT

When ventilation is satisfactory, the patient is transported to the postanesthetic care unit (PACU, or recovery room) in the lateral position with supplemental oxygen via mask, keeping the airway clear of the tongue and secretions and protecting against aspiration (Fig. 11–3). During transport to the PACU, the guardrails should be up and the safety straps securely fastened. If the patient were to become agitated during transport, this simple restraint could prevent serious injury. Patients should be covered with warmed blankets to reduce heat loss during transport. Monitoring during transport should include clinical observation of chest movement, color, and gas exchange in awake and active patients and heart and breath sounds with a precordial stethoscope in sleeping patients. A portable pulse oximeter should be used during the transport for the patients with cardiorespiratory problems.

Smith (1959) advocated the lateral position for transport nearly half a century ago, based on his clinical experience. A study by Isono and others in 2002, using flexible laryngoscopy, clearly corroborated the assertion by Smith that the lateral head position best maintains the upper airway patency by decreasing the collapsibility of the pharynx. By holding the chin up and extending the neck, the anesthesiologist can further ensure a patent airway and feel the warm breaths, indicating gas exchange.

The newer (Masimo SET) pulse oximeter can be used as a convenient transport monitor, as its monitoring head is battery operated and it can easily be detached from the main monitoring console and placed onto the stretcher without being disconnected from the patient or the sensor. More extensive monitoring, including continuous pulse oximetry, electrocardiography, and invasive blood pressure measurements, should be maintained for critically ill patients or those undergoing extensive surgical procedures and who are being transported to the intensive care unit. These patients, whether intubated or not, must have a self-inflating resuscitation bag or a Mapleson D circuit connected to an oxygen cylinder with a flow rate set to maintain adequate alveolar ventilation and oxygenation. Appropriately sized ET tubes, a laryngoscope, and medications for intubation and resuscitation should also accompany the patient.

POSTANESTHETIC RECOVERY

The postanesthetic recovery period is a time of high risk for pediatric patients.

A large percentage (20-40%) of otherwise healthy infants and children develop oxygen desaturation ($Spo_2 \leq 94\%$) during transport and upon arrival at the PACU (Motoyama and Glazner, 1986; Pullertis et al., 1987; Patel et al., 1988). Oxygen desaturation occurs sooner, is more pronounced, and has a longer duration in infants than in children and in children than in adults (Xue et al., 1996). All children, therefore, should be given oxygen supplementation during their transport from the operating room and upon arrival at the PACU, until he/she can maintain satisfactory oxygen saturation by pulse oximeter without supplemental oxygen.

One should also be aware that the Nelcor pulse oximeter is artificially preset to read Spo_2, 2% to 3%, higher than real values and, consequently, gives a false sense of security about the patient's oxygenation (see previous discussion).

The cause of postoperative hypoxemia is most likely due to atelectasis secondary to a reduction in FRC and resultant small airway closure under general anesthesia, as mentioned above (Motoyama and Glazener, 1986; also see Chapter 2). Children are more likely than adults to have airway problems, with an occurrence rate of 4% to 5% (Cohen et al., 1990). Upper airway obstruction, postextubation croup, and apnea account for the majority of untoward events. Nearly 50% of all perioperative cardiac arrests caused by respiratory problems occurred during the recovery period (Salem et al., 1975). Dysrhythmias and hypotension occur less frequently in children than adults but require quick and appropriate treatment when they do occur. Nausea, vomiting, temperature instability, and postoperative pain also require prompt and effective treatment to ensure patient comfort and efficient discharge timing.

RECOVERY IN THE POSTANESTHETIC CARE UNIT (PACU)

The PACU should be situated adjacent to the operating rooms to facilitate rapid and safe patient transport and to allow the anesthesiologist ready access in case of an emergency. The number of beds depends on hospital size, caseload, and average length of stay. Each bed space should have an oxygen supply with humidification, a self-inflating resuscitation bag, suction apparatus, pulse oximeter, electrocardiographic monitor, and automated blood pressure apparatus. Other supplies and frequently used medications should be readily available (Box 11–2). In addition, the PACU should be equipped to handle any emergency that may arise when caring for infants and children (Boxes 11–3 and 11–4). The number of nursing personnel required depends on case type and load. Pediatric patients typically require closer observation, and 1:1 or 1:2 nurse-to-patient care ratio is recommended.

Additional features needed for PACUs are an isolation room for either infectious or immunosuppressed patients and the ability to function as a critical care unit with additional mechanical ventilatory and invasive monitoring capabilities. Ready access to portable radiography service and equipment and personnel for measuring blood gas tensions, pH, hemoglobin, and electrolyte analysis is important.

Initial Care

On arrival at the PACU, the anesthesiologist confirms the patency of the patient's airway, assesses the adequacy of ventilation, and ensures the supply of humidified oxygen. The anesthesiologist records the heart rate, respiratory rate, blood pressure, Spo_2, and temperature, which are reported by the nurse. The anesthesiologist then gives a report to the nurse concerning the child's condition, special problems related to any underlying illnesses, the events of surgery, anesthetic technique, and medications given. The anesthesiologist should remain at the bedside until the child is in a reasonably stable condition and is well attended. PACU staff must be competent in recognizing and initiating the treatment of commonly encountered problems, including inadequate ventilation, agitation, pain, vomiting, temperature instability, and delayed awakening. Before leaving the PACU, the anesthesiologist writes a summary note in the chart and verifies that suitable postoperative orders have been written or entered into the computer.

Awakening Responses

With most currently used general anesthetic techniques, awakening occurs within a few minutes of the conclusion of surgery. Many children wake up quietly, without excitement, nausea, vomiting, or other obvious disturbances, when an opioid-based technique (Chinyanga et al., 1984) or propofol infusion (Hannallah et al., 1994) is used. Unfortunately, no one technique guarantees a smooth emergence, and agitation may occur in the early recovery period (Downs and Nicodemus, 1969). Agitation may be caused by numerous factors, including emergence delirium from anesthetic agents, especially with a newer inhaled anesthetic with low blood-gas solubility (sevoflurane or desflurane); pain; metabolic disturbances (hypothermia, hyperthermia, hypoglycemia, hyponatremia); neurologic disturbances;

BOX 11–2 Bedside Equipment and Supplies in PACU

- Oxygen, flow meter, humidifier, facemask, and tent
- Resuscitation bag with oxygen and anesthesia masks
- Oral and nasal airways and lidocaine jelly
- Suction apparatus, catheters, and tonsil suction tips
- Nasogastric tubes and lubricant
- Cups and water for clearing suction catheter
- Blood pressure manometer and cuffs
- Thermometer
- Intravenous fluids, tubing, and three-way and T-connectors
- Intravenous catheters, syringes, alcohol, and povidone-iodine (Betadine) wipes
- Adhesive tape and tincture of benzoin

BOX 11–3 Emergency Cart Equipment and Supplies in PACU

- Cardiac defibrillator
- Two laryngoscope handles and a variety of blades
- Endotracheal tubes (2.5- to 7.5-mm inner diameter), stylets, tape, benzoin, and syringes for cuff
- Resuscitation bags, oral airways, and bite blocks
- Cutdown and tracheostomy sets
- Sterile gloves, drapes, gowns, towels, and masks
- Intravenous solutions, tubing, catheters, and syringes
- Central venous catheter sets
- Foley catheter
- Bedboard for cardiopulmonary resuscitation

BOX 11–4 PACU Emergency Cart Medications

α-Adrenergic agonist (phenylephrine)
Aminophylline
Antihypertensives (sodium nitropruside, labetalol)
Atropine
β-Adrenergic blocker (propranolol)
Calcium chloride
Catecholamines (epinephrine, norepinephrine, dopamine, dobutamine, isoproterenol)
Dextrose (50%)
Diuretics (furosemide, mannitol)
Heparin
Lidocaine (intravenous)
Naloxone
Phenytoin (Dilantin)
Racemic epinephrine and nebulizer
Steroids (cortisol, dexamethasone, methylprednisolone)
Succinylcholine

a behavioral response to sudden awakening in a strange environment; separation anxiety; airway obstruction with resultant hypoventilation and hypoxia; and combinations of these factors.

As discussed at the beginning of this chapter, a pediatric anesthesiologist should plan the general anesthetic approach to minimize or avoid many of these factors. Emergence delirium should be avoided with an opioid or benzodiazepine. Pain can be prevented in these patients by judicious use of analgesics or regional techniques intraoperatively. Monitoring and maintenance of metabolic homeostasis are essential aspects of all general anesthetics. Any disturbances should be quickly recognized and treated swiftly and appropriately. Adequate preoperative preparation for the recovery period can help minimize postoperative anxiety in children developmentally capable of understanding (Peterson and Toler, 1986).

Alternative measures, other than the use of pharmacologic agents, can often be effective in calming the awakening pediatric patient. Some patients simply need reassurance or the comfort of being touched or held to alleviate anxiety. Parental presence has been shown to reduce the incidence of fear, crying, anger, and clinging during hospitalization (Fiorentini, 1993; Fina et al., 1997; Patel et al., 2001). Both parents and PACU staff have reported beneficial results from parental involvement. Once the infant or child has documented stable vital signs, a parent should be present.

Last but not least, the importance of detecting airway obstruction, inadequate ventilation, hypercarbia, and/or hypoxemia as causes of agitation cannot be overemphasized. Misdiagnosis can lead to inappropriate use of opioids and sedatives. Delayed and erroneous treatment of these problems can have serious consequences, including respiratory and cardiac arrests. The etiology and treatment of these phenomena are discussed next.

COMMON PROBLEMS IN THE POSTANESTHETIC CARE UNIT

Airway Obstruction

Although patients should be able to maintain airway patency before leaving the operating room, it is not uncommon for an infant or a child to have obstruction after the stimulation of extubation and transportation has subsided. The anesthesiologist must be acutely aware of any changes in the breathing pattern at this time because hypoventilation can lead to a reaccumulation of volatile agents in the alveoli that can further blunt the respiratory drive. Hypercarbia may result in dysrhythmias and hypertension, and hypoxemia in infants may lead to further suppression of breathing (Knill and Gelb, 1978; Knill and Clement, 1984; Motoyama and Glazner, 1986). Neck extension, mouth opening, and jaw lift alone or together may be enough to correct the problem. Nasopharyngeal airways, if necessary, are better tolerated than oropharyngeal airway in this setting. If obstruction continues, reassessment of anesthetic and neuromuscular blockade reversal should be conducted and possible reintubation may be considered.

Other causes of respiratory distress may be present in a way similar to upper airway obstruction. Pneumothorax, silent aspiration, and pulmonary edema should be considered and investigated if the patient continues to exhibit respiratory compromise.

Apnea of Prematurity

Apnea may be central (no respiratory effort), obstructive (respiratory effort without gas flow), or mixed (both central and obstructive) (Rigatto, 1986). Clinically, apnea is defined as cessation of breathing for longer than 15 seconds or for less than 15 seconds associated with bradycardia, cyanosis, or pallor (Nelson et al., 1978; Thatch, 1985). Repetitive pauses of breathing, lasting 5 to 10 seconds and not associated with other changes in infants, are termed periodic breathing. These abnormal respiratory patterns, which are observed commonly in neonates and preterm infants (Rigatto, 1986), can appear or worsen in preterm infants after exposure to anesthetic agents. This is particularly true for prematurely born infants with a previous history of apnea (Liu et al., 1983) and those younger than 44 weeks postconceptional age (PCA) after simple surgical procedures such as inguinal herniorrhaphy (Gregory and Steward, 1983). It had been recommended that former preterm infants less than 44 to 46 weeks PCA should be carefully observed postoperatively for at least 18 to 24 hours (Gregory and Steward, 1983; Liu et al., 1983).

Kurth and others (1987), meanwhile, reported prolonged apneic spells among preterm infants up to 55 weeks PCA in 18 of 49 occasions (37%) following inguinal herniorrhaphy as well as laparotomies and ventriculoperitoneal shunts. They proposed that all ex-premature infants less than 60 weeks PCA (adding 2 SDs to their data) were at high risk for postoperative apnea and should be monitored continuously for at least 12 hours. Malviya and others (1993) subsequently reported that the incidence of postoperative apnea following inguinal herniorrhaphy in ex-premature infants is different depending on their PCA. They reported a high incidence of postoperative apnea (26%) in infants less than 44 weeks PCA, whereas the incidence of apnea in those more than 44 weeks PCA was only 3%.

Subsequently, Coté and others (1995) performed a meta-analysis of the data from eight previously published studies of postoperative apnea involving 384 ex-premature infants following inguinal hernia repairs. In this report, they found that postoperative apnea was (1) strongly and inversely correlated to both gestational age and PCA; (2) associated with a previous history of apnea; (3) not associated with small-for-gestational age infants; they were somewhat protected from postoperative apnea; and (4) associated with anemia (hematocrit <30) as a significant risk factor, regardless of gestational age or PCA. Coté and others (1995) concluded that the probability of developing apnea in nonanemic infants free of the history of apnea is not insignificant (<5% with 95% confidence limits) until PCA was 48 weeks and gestational age of 35 weeks. The risk of apnea is not less than 1% until PCA was 54 to 56 weeks with gestational age of 32 weeks. They further concluded that older infants with apnea in the PACU and those with anemia should be admitted and monitored overnight (Coté et al., 1995). Because of these findings, it is generally recommended that preterm infants less than 44 to 46 weeks PCA be admitted for monitoring following general anesthesia (Gregory and Steward, 1983; Coté et al., 1995). Welborn and others (1988) found caffeine (10 mg/kg) to be effective in treating apnea in premature infants undergoing elective surgery. These patients, however, are still routinely admitted for observation and treatment.

Obstructive Sleep Apnea

Another group of patients predisposed to postoperative apnea consists of those with chronic obstructive sleep apnea syndrome (OSAS). OSAS is a disorder of breathing during sleep that is characterized by prolonged partial upper airway obstruction with or without intermittent complete obstruction and cessation of airflow that disrupts normal sleep time breathing and normal sleep patterns (American Thoracic Society, 1996). Although OSAS in adults is common among obese middle-aged men and women, it is commonly associated with enlarged tonsils and adenoids in children (Young et al., 1993). Surgical removal of enlarged adenoids and tonsils often markedly improves upper airway patency (Schechter et al., 2002). OSAS also occurs in children with a narrowing of upper airways secondary to craniofacial abnormalities, muscular dystrophy, cerebral palsy, and Down syndrome (trisomy 21), which may worsen during the postoperative period (Clark, 1980; Marcus, 2001). Some children with OSAS but without adenotonsillar hypertrophy may have abnormal neural control of upper airway muscles (Marcus et al., 1994). The risk of postobstructive pulmonary edema is expected to be high in patients with OSAS (see later).

Hypoxemia

Supplemental oxygen should be administered to all children on arrival in the PACU. Pulmonary gas exchange deteriorates during general anesthesia primarily because of a reduction of FRC and resultant airway closure and atelectasis (Westbrook et al., 1973; Motoyama and Glazener, 1986; Motoyama, 1996; Serafini et al., 1999). Infants and children, being even more susceptible to reductions in FRC and to atelectasis, demonstrate frequent (28% to 43%) and marked oxygen desaturations (SpO_2 ≤94%, estimated PaO_2 <67 mm Hg) if allowed to breathe room air immediately after general anesthesia (Motoyama and Glazner, 1986). Infants, especially those younger than 6 months (Kataria et al., 1988; Xue et al., 1996) and those with upper respiratory infection (DeSoto et al., 1988), are at increased risk. Humidified oxygen should be delivered by “blow-by” or with a funnel-shaped facemask (face tent). Termination of oxygen therapy is determined by normal and stable pulse oximeter readings at or above preoperative levels with the patient breathing room air. Clinical signs of wakefulness and a high score on the modified Aldrete scale have been shown to be unreliable indicators (Soliman et al., 1988).

Postobstructive Pulmonary Edema

Pulmonary edema developing shortly after the relief of upper airway obstruction is known as postobstructive pulmonary edema (POPE). POPE was first described in 1977 following difficult intubation in children (Travis et al., 1977). Subsequently, POPE was described following the relief of laryngospasm both in infants and children (Galvis et al., 1980; Sofer et al., 1984). The first sign of POPE may occur immediately after the relief of upper airway obstruction. They are characterized by rales, wheezing, and hemoglobin desaturation with the appearance of copious, frothy, pink (pulmonary edema) fluid pouring out of the trachea. Although POPE can occur in patients without a history of intrinsic pulmonary or cardiac disease, patients with acute or chronic upper airway obstruction are more vulnerable to POPE. These conditions in children may include subglottic croup, acute supraglottitis, OSAS, laryngomalacia, tracheomalacia, craniofacial dysmorphology and soft tissue obstruction of different etiologies (Tami et al., 1986; Oudjhane et al., 1992).

Among a number of factors associated with the development of pulmonary edema, increased interstitial negative pressure by forced inspiratory effort against the closed glottis (Mueller maneuver), which would increase transudation of fluid from pulmonary capillaries to interstitial space, and altered capillary permeability, due to acute hypoxia, may be the likely causative factors of POPE (Stalcup and Mellins, 1977; Smith-Erichsen and Bo, 1979; Palvin et al., 1981).

Once upper airway obstruction is cleared, the patient with POPE should receive CPAP by mask (5 to 10 cm H_2O) with a high concentration of oxygen with an air mix to maintain oxygen saturation by pulse oximeter. Diuretics should be considered along with intravenous fluid restriction. If hypoxemia (SpO_2 <95%) persists the patient may require ET intubation and ventilation with a moderate PEEP (10 cm H_2O) under sedation, often with morphine or other opioids, until pulmonary edema is dissolved. In most cases of POPE, pulmonary wedge pressure remains within normal range and pulmonary arterial pressure is also normal or only slightly increased (Willms and Shure, 1988).

Postintubation Croup

The incidence of postintubation croup was reported to be about 1% (Koka et al., 1977). The most common cause is a tight-fitting ET tube without an air leak at 30 to 40 cm H_2O with positive airway pressure (Koka et al., 1977). Patients less than 4 years of age seem to be more susceptible to croup, probably because of their small laryngeal lumen, which is more readily obstructed with mucosal edema. Other factors associated with postintubation croup may include traumatic or repeated intubation, “bucking” or coughing with the ET tube in place, changing the head position (Koka et al., 1977), duration of surgery, and neck surgery. An increased incidence is also seen in children with trisomy 21 (Sherry, 1983). Additional factors that may contribute to the incidence of postintubation croup include the use of analgesic jelly for lubricating the ET tube (Loeser et al., 1980), insufficient intraoperative anesthetic gas humidification, and the presence of upper respiratory infection.

The incidence of postintubation croup seems to have decreased with or without a leak around the ET tube at or above 20 to 25 cm H_2O positive airway pressure (Khalil et al., 1998). Whether this trend is due to less irritating ET tube material (implant tested versus red rubber ET tubes), more liberal use of corticosteroids for laryngeal surgery or other factors needs to be explored. In addition, the trend of using the cuffed ET tube in infants and young children (Khine et al., 1997; Fine et al., 2000; Fine and Borland, 2004) would theoretically reduce the incidence

■ TABLE 11–7. Croup score

Criteria	SCORE 0	1	2	3
Stridor	None	Only with agitation	Mild at rest	Severe at rest
Retractions	None	Mild	Moderate	Severe
Air entry	Normal	Mild decrease	Moderate decrease	Severe decrease
Color	Normal	N/A	N/A	Cyanotic
Level of consciousness	Normal	Restless when disturbed	Restless when undisturbed	Lethargic

Total Score	Degree	Management
≤4	Mild	Outpatient; given mist therapy
5 to 6	Mild to moderate	Outpatient if child improves in emergency room after mist, is greater than 6 months old, and has a reliable family
7 to 8	Moderate	Admitted; given racemic epinephrine
>8	Severe	Admitted; given racemic epinephrine, oxygen, and intensive care therapy

From Downes JJ and Raphaely RC: Pediatric intensive care. *Anesthesiol* 43:238, 1975.

of postintubation croup, by choosing an ET tube that is one to two sizes (0.5 to 1.0 mm OD) smaller to accommodate the cuff and thereby avoid having the ET tube tightly fitting the subglottis and decreasing attempts for reintubation due to a tube that is either too tight or too small in diameter (with excessive gas leakage around the tube). At Hopital d'Enfants Armand Trousseau in Paris, all children requiring mechanical ventilation intraoperatively have been intubated exclusively with cuffed ET tubes since 1997 (Murat, 2001). Of more than 15,000 children intubated with cuffed ET tubes in the 4-year period, there were no increases in respiratory complications. In a prospective study between 2000 and 2001, 55 respiratory complications were reported in the recovery room out of 3434 children less than 8 years of age but none of them were attributable to ET intubation (Murat, 2001).

The croup scoring system by Downs and Raphaely (1975) objectively quantifies the severity of the condition and its use can be helpful in treatment decisions (Table 11–7). Cool humidified mist administered after extubation may be helpful in mild cases of croup. Racemic epinephrine (0.5 mL of 2.25% solution), diluted in 3 to 5 mL of normal saline solution and administered by nebulizer for 5 to 10 minutes, assists patients with progressively worsening symptoms and stridor by producing mucosal vasoconstriction, resulting in a shrinking of swollen airway mucosa. Jordan and others (1970) found that only the L-isomer of epinephrine is pharmacologically active, so the reduced incidence of dysrhythmias may be a dilutional effect. The "rebound effect" and reoccurrence of symptoms are well described and necessitate observing the patient up to 4 hours after treatment.

The efficacy of corticosteroids on postintubation croup has been controversial (Koren et al., 1983; Kuusela and Vesikari, 1988). However, Anene and others (1996), in a prospective, double-blind, placebo-controlled study, found that dexamethasone is effective in reducing the incidence of postintubation croup in children intubated for longer than 48 hours.

Cardiovascular Instability

Cardiac rhythm disturbances and blood pressure fluctuations tend to be less problematic in infants and children recovering from general anesthesia than in adults (Fogliani et al., 1982). Electrocardiographic monitoring is not routinely performed in pediatric PACUs because abnormalities, such as ST-segment and T-wave changes, are extremely rare. Bradycardia is typically a response to medications such as neuromuscular blockade reversing agents or fentanyl, or a normal variant that should be treated only if associated with hypotension. Tachycardia may be secondary to hypovolemia, inadequately treated pain, or anticholinergic medications. Careful assessment and appropriate therapy should be instituted to correct volume deficit or the need for analgesia. Hypertension may also reflect inadequate analgesia, an anticholinergic effect, or excessive hydration, or it may be an artifact caused by the use of an inappropriately small blood pressure cuff. Hypotension is more unusual and is most often caused by hypovolemia secondary to inadequate fluid replacement or ongoing blood loss. Appropriate fluid resuscitation should be instituted.

Nausea and Vomiting

Postoperative nausea and vomiting (PONV) is a relatively frequent and unpleasant complication of anesthesia in infants and children and a major cause of delayed discharge from the PACU or unscheduled admission for same-day or outpatient surgery patients (Patel and Hannallah, 1988). Although rarely life threatening in the PACU, vomiting has the potential for causing aspiration, hypovolemia, and/or hypernatremia. The average incidence of postoperative vomiting in children above 3 years of age has been reported to be 40% or greater (Lerman, 1992). The risk of PONV is higher after certain types of surgery, such as strabismus repair, adenotonsillectomy, and orchiopexy. Other factors affecting the incidence of nausea and vomiting can include age, gender, history of motion sickness, anesthetic techniques (inhaled anesthetics, nitrous oxide versus intravenous anesthetic with propofol), inadequate analgesia, gastric distention, and the skill of the anesthesiologist. Intraoperative use of opioids without antiemetics may also precipitate postoperative vomiting. Early ambulation and offering clear liquids, in an attempt to meet the discharge criteria in the short-stay surgery settings, may precipitate vomiting, particularly in susceptible patients (Schreiner et al., 1992).

For PONV prophylaxis, intravenous serotonin ($5\text{-}HT_3$) receptor antagonist, such as ondansetron (0.1 to 0.15 mg/kg) and granisetron (0.04 mg/kg) given intraoperatively 30 minutes before the emergence, has been shown to be highly effective in preventing PONV with rare side effects (Patel et al., 1997; Fujii et al., 2002). A small dose of dexamethasone (0.2 to 0.5 mg/kg), with or without ondansetron, is also effective (Aouad et al., 2001). Gan and others (2003) published guidelines for preventing and treating PONV and recommend prophylaxis only in patients with moderate to high risk. In untreated or pretreated patients who develop PONV in the PACU, a repeated dose of ondansetron or granisetron should be considered. For those patients for whom prophylaxis fails, antiemetic drugs that work via other mechanisms, such as dexamethasone (0.5 mg/kg) (Aouad et al., 2001), diphenhydramine (0.5 mg/kg) (Kranke et al., 2002), or perphenazine (70 mcg/kg) (Splinter et al., 1998), are suggested.

Temperature Instability

Even with the most careful attention to maintaining normothermia, patients frequently arrive in the PACU with lowered body temperature. Usually covering the patient with warm blankets is sufficient, but radiant warming lamps and conductive warming blankets should be used in extreme cases. Hyperthermia that develops in the PACU may indicate the onset of an infectious process and should be watched closely. Malignant hyperthermia may be seen initially during the postanesthetic period. If malignant hyperthermia is suspected, appropriate investigation and therapy should be instituted without delay (see Chapters 6 and 31, Pharmacology of Pediatric Anesthesia and Malignant Hyperthermia).

Emergence Agitation

The increased use of short-acting opioids, sedatives, and regional techniques has significantly reduced the incidence of this problem. With the introduction of desflurane and sevoflurane, however, emergence delirium and agitation have reappeared, particularly in children (Davis et al., 1994; Aono et al., 1997; Walker et al., 1997; Grundmann et al., 1998). Because it is not feasible to fully evaluate a young child's psychological state during emergence, the term delirium is often replaced with the descriptive terms agitation or excitation. Proposed theoretical explanations for this occurrence have included increased pain sensation, rapid emergence to a strange environment, variable recovery resulting in a dissociative state, and a yet-to-be-defined psychomotor side effect.

Inadequately treated pain has been proposed to be a major contributor to this phenomenon. Studies, though, have demonstrated a high incidence of emergence agitation in presumably pain-free patients; those who received desflurane for genitourinary surgery with adequate caudal blocks and those who received sevoflurane for noninvasive procedures and magnetic resonance imaging (Wells et al., 1999; Uezono et al., 2000). Davis and others (1999) demonstrated that in children undergoing bilateral myringotomies and tube insertions with a brief exposure to sevoflurane, incidence of emergence agitation was minimal when analgesia was achieved with ketorolac (0.5 mg/kg). Finkel and others (2001) reported similar results using intranasal fentanyl 0.1 mcg/kg. Cohen and others (2001) found in children undergoing adenodectomy that an intraoperative dose of fentanyl (2.5 mcg/kg) was effective in reducing the incidence of emergence agitation but that pain scores were similar between treated and control groups. Postoperative analgesics and sedatives have also been shown to be effective but prolong recovery and time to discharge from the PACU.

Pain and Discomfort

All pediatric patients, including neonates and premature infants, experience pain if untreated (see Chapter 13, Pain Management in Infants and Children). Differentiating between pain, anxiety, and other causes of stress in this age group is still an unresolved challenge. Each age group and each patient has a different behavioral manifestation and communication ability regarding pain. The selection of the appropriate pain assessment tool, from the multitude available, is crucial. Many of these tools are not designed for patients recovering from surgery and general anesthesia. Disorientation, fear, and regression may alter communication and behavior, causing misinterpretation. Some pain scales have a limited application in the clinical setting.

As with pain assessment, selection of a pain management technique must be individualized for the patient, the surgical procedure, and the hospital setting. Selection must also be made with a good understanding of each technique's advantages and shortcomings. For these techniques to be successful, conscientious postoperative care must be given.

Pain Measurement and Assessment

Most techniques measure the intensity of pain by assigning incremental values. The most common technique, self-reporting, depends on verbal, cognitive, and developmental skills. Adapting adult patient surveying tools such as the McGill Pain Questionnaire (Melzack, 1975), researchers have developed scales using verbal description and graphic rating. Such tools are modified for age, culture, and cognitive ability (McGrath et al., 1985; Varni et al., 1987). Word lists and questioning techniques have been developed (Abu-Saad et al., 1990; Wilkie et al., 1990).

Graphic or symbolic representations of pain intensity also require modification. The visual analog pain scale, initially developed for adult pain measurement, is typically a 10-cm horizontal line defined by "no pain" on the left end and "severe pain" on the right. In older children and adolescents, this instrument has been used with success (Abu-Saad, 1984; McGrath et al., 1985). In younger children, replacing the definers with different words, such as "no hurt"/"most hurt," numbers, or happy/sad faces has also been tested (Broadman et al., 1988; Savedra and Tesler, 1989). For younger children, with preoperational reasoning, less abstract quantitative measurements, including counting poker chips (Hester, 1979), selecting color scales (Eland and Anderson, 1977), and marking graduate thermometers (Jeans and Johnston, 1985), are more easily understood and used. Further variations include a progression of happy to crying faces either illustrated, as in McGrath's Facial Affective Scale (McGrath et al., 1985), or photographed, as in Beyer's Oucher Scale (Beyer and Aradine, 1988). Numerical values are assigned in each of these methods for progressive levels of pain intensity.

In infants and preverbal children, observational pain scales must be implemented. For the evaluation of postoperative pain, the Children's Hospital of Eastern Ontario Pain Scale (CHEOPS) (McGrath et al., 1985) and the Objective Pain Scale (Hannallah et al., 1987) grade behavioral manifestations of pain. The CHEOPS assesses six categories: cry, facial expression, verbal response, torso position, leg activity, and arm movement in relationship to the surgical wound. The Objective Pain Scale contains physiologic and behavioral changes associated with pain. These scales were designed for research purposes and are specific for age. Neonatal and premature infant pain scales have been created and verified; these include the Neonatal Infant Pain Scale (NIPS), the CRIES (Crying Requires oxygen Increased vital signs Expression Sleep) scale, and the Premature Infant Pain Profile.

Physiologic alterations, such as changes in heart rate, blood pressure, respiration, transcutaneous oxygen saturation, and sweating caused by pain, can be observed and easily measured (Holve et al., 1983; Williamson and Williamson, 1983; Owens and Todt, 1984). Using changes in vital signs removes the subjectivity of behavioral pain scoring methods, but these parameters may reflect change for reasons other than pain. To assess pain accurately in children, location, duration, frequency, historical precedent, and present setting must be assessed, as well as intensity of pain. In addition, the child's developmental level, coping style, and motivation must be considered. In older children and adolescents, verbal responses are the most accurate. The Vami/Thompson Questionnaire and The Children's Comprehensive Pain Questionnaire, as well as less-structured interview techniques, can elicit accurate and detailed descriptions of pain (McGrath and Unruh, 1987). How the questions are phrased, who asks them, and what the child expects all affect the response.

Observational pain assessment techniques are also fraught with variability. Studies have demonstrated that scoring by parents, nurses, and physicians can be unreliable when assessing pain by cry, behavior, and constructed pain scales (Wasz-Hocket et al., 1985; Beyer et al., 1990; Favaloro and Toozel, 1990; Watt-Watson et al., 1990). As with older children, previous experience, emotional and medical status, and clinician interaction can affect the response.

Because no single technique or approach is ideal, medical personnel assessing pain in children must be well versed and flexible. Verbal, graphic, behavioral, and physiologic measures have been examined and tested, but further work on psychology and emotional interplay is needed. Although cognitive development is well understood, a hospitalized child often regresses, and expected and previously observed abilities may be lost. Much progress has been made in acknowledging that infants and children experience pain, but a great deal of work is still needed to fully reveal the degree and manner of their experience.

Pain Management

The intraoperative use of opioids and regional anesthesia for preventing postoperative pain has been discussed. Even with the best planning, patients may still experience pain in the PACU. Although most pain and discomfort originate from surgical incision and tissue irritation, other causes, including tight bandages or casts, distended bladders, and corneal abrasions, should not be overlooked. Each of these problems requires immediate attention from the appropriate medical personnel. Foley catheters and nasogastric tubes may also be causes for distress. Preoperatively, patients should be prepared to expect these catheters, which will reduce anxiety during recovery.

Treatment of pain in the PACU depends on the patient's medical condition, the surgical procedure, and discharge disposition. Oral acetaminophen (10 to 15 mg/kg) is useful in patients without intravenous access who have had minor surgical procedures. Rectal acetaminophen (30 to 40 mg/kg) may take up to 2 hours to achieve a therapeutic level and so is not effective for treating acute pain in the PACU. NSAIDs can play an important role in pain management for patients with compromised airways and respiratory function and can serve as adjuncts to opioid techniques, including neuraxial and patient-controlled analgesia use. Ketorolac should be avoided in patients with an increased risk for bleeding and those post bone-grafting procedures.

Morphine (0.025 to 0.05 mg/kg) or fentanyl (0.5 to 1.0 mcg/kg), given in incremental doses, can be used to achieve an analgesic state in patients recovering from a general anesthetic. If hospital admission overnight or longer is planned, then morphine use is preferable because of its longer duration of action. For patients undergoing extensive surgical procedures with moderate to severe pain anticipated, continuous infusion of an opioid should be considered. Hendrickson and others (1990) demonstrated better analgesia and greater patient satisfaction with continuous infusion compared with intermittent dosing. Continuous infusion can create consistent analgesic blood levels of morphine and remove the need for children to communicate their pain (Berde, 1989; Esmail et al., 1999).

Patient-controlled analgesia (PCA) allows the patient to self-administer small incremental doses of a local anesthetic and an opioid. PCA has been extensively studied in children, and studies support its efficacy and safety (Gaukroger et al., 1989; Lawrie et al., 1990; Tyler, 1990; Berde et al., 1991). In younger children and infants, nurse-assisted PCA is a useful alternative (Monitto et al., 2000). It is most effective if patients are selected, evaluated, and instructed before surgery. Side effects of opioid use, including nausea, vomiting, pruritus, and urinary retention, should be anticipated and treated when they occur.

Placement of indwelling catheters in the epidural space, body cavities, and nerve sheaths allows for continued use of local anesthetics and opioids for several days after surgery. In older children, patient-controlled epidural anesthesia (PCEA) has been shown to be safe and effective (Birmingham et al., 2003). Careful dosing and monitoring for side effects, including oversedation, respiratory arrest, and toxicity of local anesthetics, are essential. The advantages, limitations, and possible dangers of these techniques are discussed more fully elsewhere (see Chapter 13, Pain Management in Infants and Children and Chapter 14, Pediatric Regional Anesthesia).

DISCHARGE FROM THE POSTANESTHETIC CARE UNIT

With more rapid recovery from general anesthesia and a greater variety of surgical cases being scheduled on an outpatient basis, strict time criteria for discharge from the PACU are becoming less useful. The Modified Aldrete Score (Soliman et al., 1988) (Table 11–8) examines the following five criteria: motor activity, respiration, blood pressure, consciousness, and color. The Simplified Postanesthetic Recovery Score (Steward, 1975) assesses three criteria: consciousness, airway, and movement. Both scores can be helpful as guidelines in determining when a patient is ready for discharge. Inclusion of oxygen saturation by pulse oximetry is indicated. Before a child can be safely discharged from the PACU, a careful examination should be conducted to ensure safety on the patient floor, with its reduced nursing care and observation. The following criteria must be met:

1. The child is fully awake or easily aroused when called.
2. The airway is maintained and protective reflexes are present.
3. Oxygen saturation is maintained above 95% on room air or stable at the preoperative level with or without oxygen.
4. Hypothermia is absent, and hyperthermia is controlled.
5. Pain and nausea/vomiting are controlled.
6. There is no active bleeding.
7. Vital signs are stable.

■ **TABLE 11–8.** The Aldrete score

Able to move 4 extremities voluntarily or on command	2	
Able to move 2 extremities voluntarily or on command	1	Activity
Unable to move extremities voluntarily or on command	0	
Able to breathe deeply and cough freely	2	
Dyspnea or limited breathing	1	Respiration
Apneic	0	
BP ±20% of preanesthetic level	2	
BP ±20–49% of preanesthetic level	1	Circulation
BP ±50% of preanesthetic level	0	
Fully awake	2	
Arousable on calling	1	Consciousness
Not responding	0	
Able to maintain O_2 saturation > 92% on room air	2	
Needs O_2 inhalation to maintain O_2 saturation > 90%	1	O_2 Saturation
O_2 saturation < 90% even with O_2 supplement	0	

Modified from Aldrete JA, Kroulik D: A post-anesthetic recovery score. *Anesth Analg* 9:924–928, 1970. In Aldrete JA: The post-anesthesia recovery score revisited (Letters to the editor). *J Clin Anesth* 7:89, 1995.

From the PACU, patients can be admitted to a short-stay recovery unit or to a hospital ward. Regardless of the patient's disposition, the anesthesiologist is responsible for the follow-up, to ensure that no anesthetic complications occur and to continue treatment for those patients receiving special pain management techniques. For ambulatory patients, a single visit is usually all that is needed, whereas for patients with complicated medical conditions and/or extensive surgery, visits should continue until the patient is stable. Postanesthetic notes should be written in the patient's chart to communicate any findings or suggestions that may assist in the patient's recovery.

■ SHORT-STAY RECOVERY UNIT

Patients undergoing outpatient procedures continue to recover in an ambulatory or a short-stay recovery unit (SSRU) (also see Chapter 27, Anesthesia for Pediatric Same-Day Surgical Procedures). Complications seen in the PACU can also occur here. The most frequent causes for unplanned hospital admission from the SSRU are vomiting, croup, fever, and family request (Patel and Hannallah, 1988).

Patel and Rice (1991) set forth the following criteria for discharge to home:

- Vital signs are stable.
- Intact gag reflex, swallowing, and cough allow for oral intake.
- Ambulation or movements are appropriate for developmental level. (Patients who received regional analgesia must demonstrate returning motor function.)
- Nausea and vomiting should be minimal, allowing for retaining of ingested fluids.
- No signs of respiratory distress such as stridor retractions, nasal flaring, "barking" cough, wheezing, cyanosis, or dyspnea.
- Patient is oriented to person, place, and time as appropriate for age.

Voiding is not necessary, but if present, it is helpful to assess fluid status and residual regional anesthesia.

When discharged to home, the patient's family should be instructed concerning fluid intake, pain control, nausea and vomiting, and any special directives concerning the surgical procedure. In addition, a telephone number where someone will be available 24 hours a day should be supplied.

■ SUMMARY

Maintenance of anesthesia, emergence, and postoperative care are parts of the continuous perioperative care of a patient. With improved technology in intraoperative monitoring under the guidelines for standards of monitoring and vigilance, anesthetic management of infants and children has become much safer in recent years. Yet the understanding of the young patient's special needs in terms of equipment, fluid requirement, airway management, and altered pharmacokinetics is essential. Newer anesthetic agents and adjuvant drugs, together with progress in regional analgesic techniques in infants and children, allow pediatric anesthesiologists to combine conduction analgesia with various general anesthetics for prompt and smooth emergence with appropriate postoperative analgesia. The great variety in patient age, size, and physiology necessitates planning and execution of postoperative management to be patient specific.

REFERENCES

Abu-Saad H: Assessing children's responses to pain. *Pain* 19:163, 1984.

Abu-Saad HH, Droonen E, Jialfens R: On the development of a multidimensional Dutch pain assessment tool for children. *Pain* 43:249, 1990.

Aldrete LA, Kroulik D: A post anesthetic recovery score. *Anesth Analg* 49:924, 1970.

Ali HH, Kitz RJ: Evaluation of recovery from non-depolarizing neuromuscular block using a digital neuromuscular transmission analyzer-preliminary report. *Anesth Analg* 52:740, 1973.

Ali HH, Miller RD: Monitoring of neuromuscular function. In Miller RD, editor: *Anesthesia,* ed 2. New York, 1986, Churchill Livingstone, p 871.

Ali HH, Wilson RS, Savarese JJ, Kitz RJ: The effect of tubocurarine on indirectly elicited train-of-four muscle response and respiratory measurements in humans. *Br J Anaesth* 47:570–574, 1975.

Altintas F, Bozkurt P, Ipek N, et al.: The efficacy of pre- versus postsurgical axillary block on postoperative pain in paediatric patients. *Paediatr Anaesth* 10:23–28, 2000.

American Society of Anesthesiologists: Standards for basic intraoperative monitoring. *ASA Newsletter* 50:12, 1986.

American Society of Anesthesiologists: Standards for Basic Anesthetic Monitoring http://www.asahq.org/publicationsAndServices/standards/02.pdf#2

American Thoracic Society: Standards and indications for cardiopulmonary sleep studies in children. *Am J Respir Crit Care Med* 153:866–878, 1996.

Anene O, Meert KL, Uy H, et al.: Dexamethasone for the prevention of postextubation airway obstruction: A prospective, randomized, double-blind, placebo-controlled trial. *Crit Care Med* 24:1666–1669, 1996.

Ang C, Habre W, Sims C: Tropisetron reduces vomiting after tonsillectomy in children. *Br J Anaesth* 80:761–763, 1998.

Aono J, Ueda W, Mamiya K, et al.: Greater incidence of delirium during recovery from sevoflurane anesthesia in preschool boys. *Anesthesiology* 87:1298–1300, 1997.

Aouad MT, Siddik SS, Rizk LB, et al.: The effect of dexamethasone on postoperative vomiting after tonsillectomy. *Anesth Analg* 92:636–640, 2001.

Armitage EN: Caudal block in children. *Anaesthesia* 34:396, 1979.

Asai T, Hidaka I, Kawashima A, et al.: Efficacy of catheter needles with safeguard mechanisms. *Anaesthesia* 57:572–577, 2002.

Attia J, Ecoffey C, Sandouk P, et al.: Epidural morphine in children: Pharmacokinetics and CO_2 sensitivity. *Anesthesiology* 65:590, 1986.

Badgwell JM, Heaver JE, May WS, et al.: End tidal P_{CO_2} monitoring in infants and children ventilated with either a partial rebreathing or a non-rebreathing circuit. *Anesthesiology* 66:405, 1987a.

Badgwell JM, McLeod ME, Lerman J, Creighton RE: End tidal P_{CO_2} measurements sampled at the distal and proximal ends of the endotracheal tube in infants and children. *Anesth Analg* 66:959, 1987b.

Badgwell JM, Wolf AR, Morton WD, et al.: Fresh gas flow requirements based on end-tidal P_{CO_2} measurements in infants and children during anesthesia and controlled ventilation. *Anesthesiology* 65:A419, 1986.

Badgwell M, Swan J, Foster AC: Volume-controlled ventilation is made possible in infants by using compliant breathing circuits with large compression volume. *Anesth Analg* 82:719–723, 1996.

Bain JA, Spoerel WE: Carbon dioxide output and elimination in children under anesthesia. *Can Anaesth Soc J* 24:533, 1977.

Bain JA, Spoerel WE: Flow requirements for a modified Mapleson D system during controlled ventilation. *Can Anaesth Soc J* 20:629, 1973.

Bannister CF, Brosius KK, Sigl JC, et al.: The effect of bispectral index monitoring on anesthetic use and recovery in children anesthetized with sevoflurane in nitrous oxide. *Anesth Analg* 92:877–881, 2001.

Barash PG, Glanz S, Katz JD, et al.: Ventricular function in children during halothane anesthesia: An echocardiographic evaluation. *Anesthesiology* 49:79, 1978.

Batra YK, Bali MI: Corneal abrasion during general anesthesia. *Anesth Analg* 56:363, 1977.

Baum VC, Yemen TA, Baum LD: Immediate 8% sevoflurane induction in children: A comparison with incremental sevoflurane and incremental halothane. *Anesth Analg* 85:313–316, 1997.

Baum J, Sitte T, Strauss JM, et al.: Die Reaktion von Sevofluran mit trockenem Atemkalk-überlegungen anlässlich eines aktuellen Zweischenfalls. *Anaesth Intensivmed* 39:11–16, 1998.

Behforouz N, Dubousset AM, Jamali S, et al.: Respiratory effects of desflurane anesthesia on spontaneous ventilation in infants and children. *Anesth Analg* 87:1052–1055, 1998.

Benlabed M, Ecoffey C, Levron JC, et al.: Analgesia and ventilation response to CO, following epidural sufentanil in children. *Anesthesiology* 67:948, 1987.

Bennett EJ: Fluid balance in the newborn. *Anesthesiology* 43:210, 1975.

Benoit Z, Wicky S, Fischer J-F, et al.: The effect of increased F_{IO_2} before tracheal extubation on postoperative atelectasis. *Anesth Analg* 95:1477, 2002.

Berde CB, L4ehn BM, Yee JD, et al.: Patient-controlled analgesia in children and adolescents: A randomized, prospective comparison with intramuscular administration of morphine for postoperative analgesia. *J Pediatr* 118:460, 1991.

Berde CB: Pediatric postoperative pain management. *Pediatr Clin North Am* 36:921, 1989.

Bethune RW: Precordial electrocardiograph stethoscope. *Anesthesiology* 26:228, 1965.

Beyer J, Aradine C: The convergent and discriminant validity of a self report measure of pain intensity for children. *Child Health Care* 16:274, 1988.

Beyer JE, McGraw PJ, Berde CB: Discordance between self-report and behavioral pain measures in children aged 3-7 years after surgery. *J Pain Sympt Manage* 5:350, 1990.

Biebuyck JF, Eger EI 2nd: New inhaled anesthetics. *Anesthesiology* 80:906–922, 1994.

Birmingham PK, Tobin MJ, Fisher DM, et al.: Initial and subsequent dosing of rectal acetaminophen in children: A 24-hour pharmacokinetic study of new dose recommendations. *Anesthesiology* 94:385–389, 2001.

Birmingham PK, Tobin MJ, Henthorn TK, et al.: Twenty-four-hour pharmacokinetics of rectal acetaminophen in children: an old drug with new recommendations. *Anesthesiology* 87:244–252,1997.

Birmingham PK, Wheeler M, Suresh S, et al.: Patient-controlled epidural analgesia in children: Can they do it? *Anesth Analg* 96:686–691, 2003.

Bissonnette B, Sessler DI: Passive or active inspired gas humidification increases thermal steady-state temperatures in anesthetized infants. *Anesth Analg* 69:784, 1989.

Bissonnette B, Sessler DI, Laflamme P: Intraoperative temperature monitoring sites in infants and children. *Anesth Analg* 76:168, 1989.

Boggild-Madsen NB, Bundgarrd-Nielsen P, Hammer U, Jakobsen B: Comparison of eye protection with methylcellulose and paraffin ointments during general anaesthesia. *Can Anaesth Soc J* 28:575, 1981.

Boggild-Madsen NB, Schmidt P: Protection of the eyes with ophthalmic ointments during general anesthesia. *Acta Ophthalmol* 59:422, 1981.

Booker PD: Management of postoperative pain in infants and children. *Curr Opin Anaesth* 1:17, 1988.

Bortone L, Picetti E, Mergoni M: Anaesthesia with sevoflurane in children: Nitrous oxide does not increase postoperative vomiting. *Paediatr Anaesth* 12:775–779, 2002.

Bosenberg AT, Bland BAR, Schulte-Steinberg O, et al.: Thoracic epidural anesthesia via caudal route in infants. *Anesthesiology* 69:265, 1988.

Bosenberg AT, Raw R, Boezaart A: Surface mapping of peripheral nerves in children with a nerve stimulator. *Paediatr Anaesth* 12:398–403, 2002.

Bosomworth PP, Dietsch JD, Hamelberg W: The effects of controlled hemorrhage on heart sounds. *Anesth Analg (Cleve)* 42:131, 1963.

Bourke DL, Smith TC: Estimating allowable hemodilution. *Anesthesiology* 41:609, 1974.

Brain AIJ: The laryngeal mask airway—a new concept in airway management. *Br J Anaesth* 55:801, 1983.

Brandom BW, Meretoja OA, Simhi E, et al.: Age related variability in the effects of mivacurium in paediatric surgical patients. *Can J Anaesth* 45:410–416, 1998.

Brandom BW, Woelfel SK, Ference A, et al.: Effects of cisatracurium in children during halothane-nitrous oxide anesthesia. *J Clin Anesth* 10:195, 1998.

Brinkmeyer L, Safar P, Motoyama EK: Superiority of colloid over electrolyte solution for severe normovolemic hemodilution (NVHD) in concurrent treatment of hemorrhage. *Disaster Med* 1:171, 1983.

Broadman LM, Cerruzi W, Patane PS, et al.: Metoclopramide reduces the incidence of vomiting following strabismus surgery in children. *Anesthesiology* 72:245, 1990.

Broadman LM, Higgins TT, Hannallah RS, et al.: Intraoperative subarachnoid morphine for postoperative pain control following Harrington Rod instrumentation in children. *Can J Anaesth* 34:S96, 1987.

Broadman LM, Rice L, Hannallah R: Evaluation of an objective pain scale for infants and children. *Reg Anaesth* 13:45, 1988.

Brown BR Jr.: Halothane hepatitis revisited. *N Engl J Med* 313:1347, 1985.

Brown K, Aun C, Stocks J, et al.: A comparison of the respiratory effects of sevoflurane and halothane in infants and young children. *Anesthesiology* 89:86–92, 1998.

Cahalan MK, Weiskopt RB, Eger E, et al.: Hemodynamic effects of desflurane/nitrous oxide anesthesia in volunteers. *Anesth Analg* 73:157, 1991.

Cameron CB, Robinson S, Gregory GA: The minimum alveolar concentration of isoflurane in children. *Anesth Analg* 63:418, 1984.

Casey WF, Rice IJ, Hannallah RS, et al.: A comparison between bupivacaine instillation versus ilioinguinal/iliohypogastric nerve block for postoperative analgesia following inguinal herniorrhaphy in children. *Anesthesiology* 72:637, 1990.

Castro BA, Freedman LA, Craig WL, et al.: Explosion within an anesthesia machine: Baralyme, high fresh gas flow and sevoflurane concentration. *Anesthesiology* 101:537–539, 2004.

Chalon J, Patel C, Ali M, et al.: Humidity and the anesthetized patient. *Anesthesiology* 50:195, 1979.

Chinyanga HM, Vandenberghe H, MacLeod S, Soldin S: Assessment of immediate postanaesthetic recovery in young children following intravenous morphine infusions, halothane and isoflurane. *Can Anaesth Soc J* 31:28, 1984.

Choudhry DK, Brenn BR: Bispectral index monitoring: A comparison between normal children and children with quadriplegic cerebral palsy. *Anesth Analg* 95:1582–1585, 2002.

Clark RW: Sleep-induced ventilatory dysfunction in Down's syndrome. *Arch Intern Med* 140:45, 1980.

Cohen MM, Cameron CB, Duncan PG: Pediatric anesthesia morbidity and mortality in the perioperative period. *Anesth Analg* 70:160, 1990.

Cohen IT, Finkel JC, Hannallah RS, et al.: Clinical and biochemical effects of propofol versus sevoflurane in healthy infants and young children. *Paediatr Anaesth* 14:135–142, 2004.

Cohen IT, Finkel JC, Hannallah RS, et al.: Effects of fentanyl on the emergence characteristics following desflurane or sevoflurane anesthesia in children. *Anesth Analg* 94:1178–1181, 2002.

Cohen IT, Hannallah RS, Hummer KA: The incidence of emergence agitation associated with desflurane anesthesia in children is reduced by fentanyl. *Anesth Analg* 93:88–91, 2001.

Cohen IT, Latta K, Wiener E, et al.: A study of ketorolac for intraoperative and postoperative analgesia for herniorrhaphy in children. *Anesth Analg* 76:S50, 1993.

Conahan TJ, Ominsky AJ, Wollman H, et al.: A prospective random comparison of halothane and morphine for open heart anesthesia: One year's experience. *Anesthesiology* 38:523, 1973.

Cook DR, Marcy JH: Pediatric anesthesia pharmacology. In Cook DR, Marcy JH, editors: *Neonatal anesthesia.* Pasadena, CA, 1988, Appleton Davies, pp 87–125.

Coté CJ, Goldstein EA, Coté MA, et al.: A single-blind study of pulse oximetry in children. *Anesthesiology* 68:184, 1988.

Coté CJ, Rolf N, Liu LMP, Goudsouzian NG: A single-blind study of pulse oximetry and capnography in children. *Anesthesiology* 74:984, 1991.

Coté Cl, Zaslavsky A, Downes JJ, et al.: Postoperative apnea in former preterm infants after inguinal herniorrhaphy. A combined analysis. *Anesthesiology* 82:809, 1995.

Coté CJ, Roth AG, Wheeler M, et al.: Traditional versus new needle retractable i.v. catheters in children: Are they really safer, and whom are they protecting? *Anesth Analg* 96:387–391, 2003.

Cozanitis DA, Dundee JW, Merrett JD, et al.: Evaluation of glycopyrrolate and atropine as adjuncts to reversal of non-depolarizing neuromuscular blocking agents in a "true-to-life" situation. *Br J Anaesth* 52:85, 1980.

Cranfield KA, Bromley LM: Minimum alveolar concentration of desflurane for tracheal extubation in deeply anaesthetized, unpremedicated children. *Br J Anaesth* 78:370–371, 1997.

Crawford MW, Lerman J, Sloan MH, et al.: Recovery characteristics of propofol anaesthesia, with and without nitrous oxide: A comparison with halothane/nitrous oxide anaesthesia in children. *Paediatr Anaesth* 8:49–54, 1998.

Cross GD, Barrett RF: Comparison of two regional techniques for postoperative analgesia in children following herniotomy and orchidopexy. *Anaesthesia* 42:845, 1987.

Cucchiara RF, Black S: Corneal abrasions during surgery. *Anesthesiology* 69:978, 1988.

Dalens B, Hasnaoui A: Caudal anesthesia in pediatric surgery: Success rate and adverse effects in 750 consecutive patients. *Anesth Analg* 68:83, 1989.

Dalens B, Tanguy A, Haberer JP: Lumbar epidural anesthesia for operative and postoperative pain relief in infants and young children. *Anesth Analg* 65:1069, 1986.

Dalens B, Tanguy A: Intrathecal morphine for spinal fusion in children. *Spine* 13:494, 1988.

Davidson AJ, McCann ME, Devavaram P, et al.: The differences in the bispectral index between infants and children during emergence from anesthesia after circumcision surgery. *Anesth Analg* 93:326–330, 2001.

Davis PJ, Cohen IT, McGowan FX, Latta K: Recovery characteristics of desflurane versus halothane for maintenance of anesthesia in pediatric ambulatory patients. *Anesthesiology* 80:298, 1994.

Davis PJ, Cook DR, Stiller RL, et al.: Pharmacodynamics and pharmacokinetics of high-dose sufentanil in infants and children. *Anesth Analg* 66:203, 1987a.

Davis PJ, Cook DR, Stiller RL, Robinson KA: Pharmacodynamic and pharmacokinetics of high-dose sufentanil in infants and children undergoing cardiac surgery. *Anesth Analg* 66:203, 1987b.

Davis PJ, Finkel JC, Orr RJ, et al.: A randomized, double-blinded study of remifentanil versus fentanyl for tonsillectomy and adenoidectomy surgery in pediatric ambulatory surgical patients. *Anesth Analg* 90:863–871, 2000.

Davis PJ, Galinkin J, McGowan FX, et al.: A randomized multicenter study of remifentanil compared with halothane in neonates and infants undergoing pyloromyotomy. I. Emergence and recovery profiles. *Anesth Analg* 93:1380–1386, 2001.

Davis PJ, Greenberg JA, Gendelman M, Fertal K: Recovery characteristics of sevoflurane and halothane in preschool-aged children undergoing bilateral myringotomy and pressure equalization tube insertion. *Anesth Analg* 88:34–38, 1999.

Davis PJ, Killian A, Stiller RL, et al.: Pharmacokinetics of alfentanil in newborn premature infants and older children. *Dev Pharmacol Ther* 13:21, 1989.

Davis PJ, Lerman J, Suresh S, et al.: A randomized multicenter study of remifentanil compared with alfentanil, isoflurane, or propofol in anesthetized pediatric patients undergoing elective strabismus surgery. *Anesth Analg* 84: 982, 1997.

Davis PJ, McGowan FX Jr, Landsman I, et al.: Effect of antiemetic therapy on recovery and hospital discharge time. A double-blind assessment of ondansetron, droperidol, and placebo in pediatric patients undergoing ambulatory surgery. *Anesthesiology* 83:956–960, 1995a.

Davis PJ, Tome JA, McGowan FX, et al.: Preanesthesic medication with intranasal midazolam for very brief pediatric surgical procedures: Effect on recovery and hospital discharge times. *Anesthesiology* 82:2, 1995b.

Deckardt R, Steward DJ: Noninvasive arterial hemoglobin oxygen saturation versus transcutaneous oxygen tension monitoring in the preterm infant. *Crit Care Med* 12:935, 1984.

Denman WT, Swanson EL, Rosow D, et al.: Pediatric evaluation of the bispectral index (BIS) monitor and correlation of BIS with end-tidal sevoflurane concentration in infants and children. *Anesth Analg* 90:872–877, 2000.

DeSoto H, Patel RI, Soliman IE, Hannallah RS: Changes in oxygen saturation following general anesthesia in children with upper respiratory infection signs and symptoms undergoing otolaryngological procedures. *Anesthesiology* 68:276, 1988.

Desparmet J, Meistelman C, Barr J, Saint-Maurice C: Continuous epidural infusion of bupivacaine for postoperative pain relief in children. *Anesthesiology* 67:108, 1987.

DiGiovanni AJ, Goodnick J, Neign JL, et al.: The effect of halothane anesthesia on intracranial pressure in the presence of intracranial hypertension. *Anesth Analg* 53:823, 1974.

Doi M, Ikeda K: Respiratory effects of sevoflurane. *Anesth Analg* 66:241, 1987.

Domette WHL: The stethoscope: The anesthesiologist's best friend. *Anesth Analg (Cleve)* 42:171, 1963.

Domette WS: Monitoring in anesthesia, the signal to be monitored. *Clin Anesth* 9:19, 1973.

Dong W, Bledsoe SW, Chadwick HS, et al.: Electrical correlates of brain injury resulting from severe hypotension and hemodilution in monkeys. *Anesthesiology* 65:617, 1986.

Dorman T, Fackler J: Automated information systems in anesthesiology. *Int Anesthesiol Clin* 38:105–113, 2000.

Downs JJ, Nicodemus H: Preparation for and recovery from anesthesia. *Pediatr Clin North Am* 16:601, 1969.

Downs JJ, Raphaely RC: Pediatric intensive care. *Anesthesiology* 43:238, 1975.

Ebert TJ, Frink EJ Jr, Kharasch ED: Absence of biochemical evidence for renal and hepatic dysfunction after 8 hours of 1.25 minimum alveolar concentration sevoflurane anesthesia in volunteers. *Anesthesiology* 88:601–610, 1998.

Eckenhoff JE, Kneale DH, Dripps RD: The incidence and etiology of postanesthetic excitement. *Anesthesiology* 22:667, 1961.

Egan TD, Lemmens HJM, Fiset P, et al.: The pharmacokinetics of the new short-acting opioid remifentanil (GI87084B) in health adult male volunteers. *Anesthesiology* 78:882, 1993.

Eger EI, Smith NT, Stoelting RK, et al.: Cardiovascular effects of halothane in man. *Anesthesiology* 32:396, 1970.

Eger EI, Smith NT, Cullen DJ, et al.: A comparison of cardiovascular effects of halothane, fluroxene, ether and cyclopropane in man: A resume. *Anesthesiology* 34:25, 1971.

Eger EI: Current controversies concerning enflurane and isoflurane. American Society of Anesthesiologists Annual Refresher Course Lectures 402, 1984.

Eger EI, Gong D, Koblin DD, et al.: The effect of anesthetic duration on kinetic and recovery characteristics of desflurane versus sevoflurane, and on the kinetic characteristics of compound A, in volunteers. *Anesth Analg* 86:414, 1998.

Eichhorn JH: Are there standards for intraoperative monitoring? In Stoelting RK, Barash PG, Gallagher JF, editors: *Advances in anesthesia,* vol 5. Chicago, 1988a, Year Book Medical Publishers.

Eichhorn JH: Monitoring standards for clinical practice. *Int Anesth Res Soc Rev Course Lect* 113, 1988b.

Eichhorn JH, Cooper JB, Cullen DJ, et al.: Standards for patient monitoring during anesthesia at Harvard Medical School. *JAMA* 256:1017–1020, 1986.

Eikermann M, Hunkemoller I, Peine L, et al.: Optimal rocuronium dose for intubation during inhalation induction with sevoflurane in children. *Br J Anaesth* 8:277–278, 2002.

Eland JM, Anderson JE: The experiences of pain in children. In Jacob AK, editor: *Pain: A source book for nurses and other health professionals.* Boston, 1977, Little Brown & Co, p 453.

Elhakim M, Ali NM, Rashed I, et al.: Dexamethasone reduces postoperative vomiting and pain after pediatric tonsillectomy. *Can J Anaesth* 50:392–397, 2003.

Eliaschar I, Lavie P, Halperin E, et al.: Sleep apneic episodes as indications for adenotonsillectomy. *Arch Otolaryngol* 106:492, 1980.

Elitsur Y, Blankenship P, Lawrence Z: Propofol sedation for endoscopic procedures in children. *Endoscopy* 32:788–791, 2000.

Esmail Z, Monotgomery C, Courtrn C, et al.: Efficacy and complications of morphine infusions in postoperative paediatric patients. *Paediatr Anaesth* 9:321–327, 1999.

Fatheree RS, Leighton BL: Acute respiratory distress syndrome after an exothermic Baralyme®-sevoflurane reaction. *Anesthesiology* 101:531–533, 2004.

Favaloro R, Touzel B: A comparison of adolescents' and nurses' postoperative pain ratings and perceptions. *Pediatr Nurs* 16:414, 1990.

Fell D, Derrington MC, Taylor E, et al.: Paediatric postoperative analgesia. A comparison between caudal block and wound infiltration of local anaesthetic. *Anaesthesia* 43:107, 1988.

Ferrari LD, Donlon JV: Metoclopramide reduces the incidence of vomiting after tonsillectomy in children. *Anesth Analg* 75:351, 1992.

Fina DK, Lopas LJ, Stagnone JH, et al.: Parent participation in the postanesthesia care unit: fourteen years of progress at one hospital. *J Perianesth Nurs* 12:152–162, 1997.

Fine GF, Fertal M, Motoyama EK: The effectiveness of controlled ventilation using cuffed vs. uncuffed endotracheal tubes (ETT) in infants. *Anesthesiology* 93:A1251, 2000.

Fine GF, Borland LM: The future of the cuffed endotracheal tube. *Pediatr Anesth* 14:38–42, 2004.

Finkel JC, Cohen IT, Hannallah RS, et al.: The effect of intranasal fentanyl on the emergence characteristics after sevoflurane anesthesia in children undergoing surgery for bilateral myringotomy tube placement. *Anesth Analg* 92:1164–1168, 2001.

Fiorentini SE: Evaluation of a new program: Pediatric parental visitation in the postanesthesia care unit. *J Postanesth Nurs* 8:249–256, 1993.

Fisher DM, Zwass MS: MAC of desflurane in 60% N_2O in infants and children. *Anesthesiology* 76:354, 1992.

Fogliani J, Didier G, Domenget JF, Dahan R: Clinical surveillance of wakening from anesthesia following 1006 regular operations. *Can Anesthesiol* 30:1003, 1982.

Forbes AR: Temperature, humidity and mucus flow in the intubated trachea. *Br J Anaesth* 46:29, 1974.

Fournier L, Major D: The effect of nitrous oxide on the oxyhaemoglobin dissociation curve. *Can Anaesth Soc J* 31:173, 1984.

Friedman M, Baim H, Stobnicki M, et al.: Laryngeal injuries secondary to nasogastric tubes. *Ann Otol* 90:469, 1981.

Frink EJ, Malan P, Morgan SE, et al.: Quantification of the degradation products of sevoflurane in two CO2 absorbents during low-flow anesthesia in surgical patients. *Anesthesiology* 77:1064, 1992.

Fujii Y, Tanaka H, Ito M: Treatment of vomiting after paediatric strabismus surgery with granisetron, droperidol, and metoclopramide. *Ophthalmologica* 216:359–362, 2002.

Fujii Y, Toyooka H, Tanaka H: Antiemetic efficacy of granisetron and metoclopramide in children undergoing ophthalmic or ENT surgery. *Can J Anaesth* 43:1095–1099, 1996.

Furman EB, Roman DG, Lemmer LAS, et al.: Specific therapy in water, electrolyte and blood volume replacement during pediatric surgery. *Anesthesiology* 42:187, 1975.

Galvis AG, Stool SE, Bluestone CD: Pulmonary edema following relief of acute upper airway obstruction. *Ann Otol Rhinol Laryngol* 89:124–128, 1980.

Gan TJ, Joshi GP, Zhao SZ, et al.: Presurgical intravenous parecoxib sodium and follow-up oral valdecoxib for pain management after laparoscopic cholecystectomy surgery reduces opioid requirements and opioid-related adverse effects. *Acta Anaesthesiol Scand* 48:1194–1207, 2004.

Gan TJ, Meyer T, Apfel CC, et al.: Consensus guidelines for managing postoperative nausea and vomiting. *Anesth Analg* 97:62–71, 2003.

Gaukroger PB, Tomkins DP, van der Walt JH: Patient-controlled analgesia in children. *Anaesth Intensive Care* 17:264, 1989.

Goff MJ, Arain SR, Ficke DJ, et al.: Absence of bronchodilation during desflurane anesthesia: A comparison to sevoflurane and thiopental. *Anesthesiology* 93:404–408, 2000.

Goldberg AH: Effects of halothane on force-velocity, length-tension, and stress-strain curves of isolated heart muscle. *Anesthesiology* 29:192, 1968.

Goudsouzian NG, Liu LMP, Coté CJ: Comparison of equipotent doses of nondepolarizing muscle relaxants in children. *Anesth Analg* 60:862, 1981.

Goudsouzian NG, Martyn JJA, Lou LMP: The dose-response effect of long-acting nondepolarizing neuromuscular blocking agents in children. *Can Anaesth Soc J* 3:246, 1984.

Goudsouzian NG, Morris RH, Ryan JF: The effects of a warming blanket on the maintenance of body temperature in anesthetized infants and children. *Anesthesiology* 39:351, 1973.

Graff TD, Holzman RS, Benson DW: Acid-base balance in infants during halothane anesthesia with the use of an adult circle-absorption system. *Anesth Analg* 43:583, 1964.

Greene LT: Physostigmine treatment of anticholinergic-drug depression in postoperative patients. *Anesth Analg* 50:222, 1971.

Greenspun JC, Hannallah RS, Welborn LG, Norden J: Comparison of sevoflurane and halothane in pediatric ENT surgery. *Anesth Analg* 78:S140, 1994.

Gregory GA, Eger EI II, Munson EW: The relationship between age and halothane requirement in man. *Anesthesiology* 30:488, 1969.

Gregory GA, Steward DJ: Life-threatening perioperative apnea in the ex-"premie." *Anesthesiology* 59:495, 1983.

Gronert B, Woelfel S, Cook DR: Comparison of equipotent doses of mivacurium and succinylcholine in children 2-12 years old. *Anesthesiology* 79:A966, 1993a.

Gronert B, Woelfel S, Cook DR: Comparison of equipotent intubating doses of mivacurium and succinylcholine in infants 2-12 months old. *Anesthesiology* 79:A932, 1993b.

Gronert BJ, Brandom BW: Neuromuscular blocking drugs in infants and children. *Pediatr Clin North Am* 41:73, 1994.

Gunter JB, Dunn CM, Bennie JB, et al.: Optimum concentration of bupivacaine for combined caudal-general anesthesia in children. *Anesthesiology* 75:57, 1991.

Gunter JB, Varughese AM, Harrington JF, et al. Recovery and complications after tonsillectomy in children: A comparison of ketorolac and morphine. *Anesth Analg* 81:1136–1141, 1995.

Grundmann U, Uth M, Eichner A, et al.: Total intravenous anaesthesia with propofol and remifentanil in paediatric patients: A comparison with a desflurane-nitrous oxide inhalation anaesthesia. *Acta Anaesthesiol Scand* 42:845, 1998.

Hannallah RS, Britton JT, Schafer PG, et al.: Propofol anaesthesia in paediatric ambulatory patients: A comparison with thiopentone and halothane. *Can J Anaesth* 41:12, 1994.

Hannallah RS, Broadman LM, Belman AB, et al.: Comparison of caudal and ilioinguinal/iliohypogastric nerve blocks for control of postorchiopexy pain in pediatric ambulatory surgery. *Anesthesiology* 66:832, 1987.

Hansen TG, Ilett KF, Lim SI, et al.: Pharmacokinetics and clinical efficacy of long-term epidural ropivacaine infusion in children. *Br J Anaesth* 85:347–353, 2000.

Hansen TG, Ilett KF, Reid C, et al.: Caudal ropivacaine in infants: Population pharmacokinetics and plasma concentrations. *Anesthesiology* 94:579–584, 2001.

Harxison GG, Bull AB, Schmidt HJ: Temperature changes in children during general anaesthesia. *Br J Anaesth* 32:60, 1960.

Hashimoto Y, Hirota K, Ohtomo N, et al.: In vivo direct measurement of the bronchodilating effect of sevoflurane using a superfine fiberoptic bronchoscope: comparison with enflurane and halothane. *J Cardiothorac Vasc Anesth* 10:213–216, 1996.

Hay WW Jr, Rodden DJ, Collins SM, et al.: Reliability of conventional and new pulse oximetry in neonatal patients. *J Perinatol* 22:360–366, 2002.

Hayashi Y, Sumikawa K, Tashiro C, et al.: Arrhythmogenic plasma levels of epinephrine during sevoflurane, isoflurane and enflurane anesthesia in the dog. *Anesthesiology* 67:A57, 1987.

Haynes SR, Morton NS: The laryngeal mask airway: A review of its use in paediatric anaesthesia. *Paediatr Anaesth* 3:65, 1993.

Hendrickson M, Myre L, Johnson DG, et al.: Postoperative analgesia in children: A prospective study of intermittent intramuscular injection versus continuous intravenous infusion of morphine. *J Pediatr Surg* 25:185, 1990.

Henzi I, Walder B, Tramer MR: Dexamethasone for the prevention of postoperative nausea and vomiting: A quantitative systematic review. *Anesth Analg* 90:186–194, 2000.

Hertzka RE, Fisher DM, Gauntlett IS, Spellman M: Are infants sensitive to respiratory depression from fentanyl? *Anesthesiology* 67:A512, 1987.

Hertzka RE, Gauntlett IS, Fisher DM, et al.: Fentanyl-induced ventilatory depression: Effect of age. *Anesthesiology* 70:213, 1989.

Hester NK: The preoperational child's reaction to immunization. *Nurs Res* 28:250, 1979.

Hickey PR, Hansen DD, Strafford M, et al.: Pulmonary and systemic hemodynamic effects of nitrous oxide in infants with normal and elevated pulmonary vascular resistance. *Anesthesiology* 65:374, 1986.

Hickey RR, Hansen DD: Fentanyl- and sufentanil-oxygen-pancuronium anesthesia for cardiac surgery in infants. *Anesth Analg* 63:117, 1984.

Holaday DA, Fiserova-Bergerova VF, Latto IP, Zumbiel MA: Resistance of isoflurane to biotransformation in man. *Anesthesiology* 43:325, 1975.

Holaday DA, Smith FR: Clinical characteristics and biotransformation of sevoflurane in healthy human volunteers. *Anesthesiology* 54:100, 1981.

Holliday MA, Segar WE: The maintenance need for water in parenteral fluid therapy. *Pediatrics* 19:823, 1957.

Holve DL, Bromberger P, Grovement HD, et al.: Regional anesthesia during newborn circumcision. *Clin Pediatr* 22:813, 1983.

Hornbein TF, Eger EI, II, Winter PM, et al.: The minimum alveolar concentration of nitrous oxide in man. *Anes Analg* 61:553–556, 1982.

Hulse MG, Lindahl SG, Hatch DJ: Comparison of ventilation and gas exchange in anaesthetized infants and children during spontaneous and artifical ventilation. *Br J Anaesth* 56:131–135, 1984.

Inman WHW, Mushin WW: Jaundice after repeated exposure to halothane: A further analysis of reports to the Committee on Safety of Medicine. *Br Med J* 11:1455, 1978.

Inomata S, Watanabe S, Taguchi M, et al.: End-tidal sevoflurane concentration for tracheal intubation and minimum alveolar concentration in pediatric patients. *Anesthesiology* 80:93, 1994.

Isono S, Tanaka A, Nishino T: Lateral position decreases collapsibility of the passive pharynx in patients with obstructive sleep apnea. *Anesthesiology* 97:780, 2002.

Irita K, Kai Y, Akiyoshi K, et al.: Performance evaluation of a new pulse oximeter during mild hypothermic cardiopulmonary bypass. *Anesth Analg* 96:11–14, 2003.

Irving GA, Butt AD, Van der Veen B: A comparison of caudal morphine given pre- or post-surgery for postoperative analgesia in children. *Paediatr Anaesth* 3:217, 1993.

Ivani G, DeNegri P, Conio A, et al.: Comparison of racemic bupivacaine, ropivacaine, and levo-bupivacaine for pediatric caudal anesthesia: Effects on postoperative analgesia and motor block. *Reg Anesth Pain Med* 27:157–161, 2002.

Jayabose S, Levendoglu-Tugal O, Giamelli J, et al.: Intravenous anesthesia with propofol for painful procedures in children with cancer. *J Pediatr Hematol Oncol* 23:290–293, 2001.

Jeans ME, Johnston CC: Pain in children: Assessment and management. In Lipton M, editor: *Persistent pain: Modern methods of treatment.* London, 1985, Grune & Stratton, p III.

Jensen BH: Caudal block for postoperative pain relief in children after genital operations. A comparison between bupivacaine and morphine. *Acta Anaesthesiol Scand* 25:373, 1981.

Joas TA, Stevens WC: Comparison of the arrhythmic doses of epinephrine during Forane, halothane, and fluroxene anesthesia in dogs. *Anesthesiology* 35:48, 1971.

Jones RM: Desflurane and sevoflurane: Inhalation anesthetics for this decade? *Br J Anaesth* 65:527, 1990.

Jones SE, Beasley JM, Macfarlane DW, et al.: Intrathecal morphine for postoperative pain relief in children. *Br J Anaesth* 56:137, 1984.

Jordan WS, Graves CL, Elwyn RA: New therapy for post-intubation laryngeal edema and tracheitis in children. *JAMA* 212:585, 1970.

Jordan WS: Laryngotracheobronchitis: Evaluation of new therapeutic approaches. *Rocky Mountain Med J* 63:69, 1966.

Joshi GP, Viscusi ER, Minkowitz H, et al.: Effective treatment of laparoscopic pain with intravenous followed by oral COX-2 specific inhibitor. *Anesth Analg* 98:336–342, 2004.

Junger A, Hartmann B, Benson M, et al.: The use of an anesthesia information management system for prediction of antiemetic rescue treatment at the postanesthesia care unit. *Anesth Analg* 92:1203–1209, 2001.

Kallos T, Smith. TC: Replacement of intraoperative blood loss. *Anesthesiology* 41:239, 1974.

Kaplan GW, Brock WA: Urethral strictures in children. *J Urol* 129:1200, 1983.

Karmakar MK, Aun CS, Wong EL, et al.: Ropivacaine undergoes slower systemic absorption from the caudal epidural space in children than bupivacaine. *Anesth Analg* 94:259–265, 2002.

Kataria BK, Hamik EV, Mitchard R, et al.: Postoperative arterial oxygen saturation in the pediatric population during transportation. *Anesth Analg* 67:280, 1988.

Katoh T, Ikleda K: Minimum alveolar concentration of sevoflurane in children. *Br J Anaesth* 68:134, 1992.

Kenna JG, Neuberger J, Mieli-Vergani G, et al.: Halothane hepatitis in children (review). *Br Med J (Clin Res)* 294:1209, 1987.

Keengwe IN, Hegde S, Dearlove O, et al.: Structured sedation program for magnetic resonance imaging examination in children. *Anaesthesia* 54:1069–1072, 1999.

Keidan I, Fine G, Kagawa T, et al.: Work of breathing during spontaneous ventilation in anesthetized children: A comparative study among the face mask, laryngeal mask airway and endotracheal tube. *Anes Analg* 91:1381–1388, 2000.

Khalil S, Campos C, Farag A, et al.: Caudal block in children: Ropivacaine compared with bupivacaine. *Anesthesiology* 91:1279–84, 1999.

Khalil SN, Mankanous R, Campos C, et al.: Absence of presence of a leak around tracheal tube may not affect postoperative croup in children. *Paediatr Anaesth* 8:393–396, 1998.

Khalil S, Rodarte A, Weldon BC, et al.: Intravenous ondansetron in established postoperative emesis in children. S3A-381 Study Group. *Anesthesiology* 85:270–276, 1996.

Kharasch ED, Powers KM, Artru AA: Comparison of Amsorb, soda lime and Baralyme degradation of volatile anesthetics and formation of carbon monoxide and compound A in swine in vivo. *Anesthesiology* 96:173–182, 2002.

Khine HH, Corddry DH, Kettrick RG, et al.: Comparison of cuffed and uncuffed endotracheal tubes in young children during general anesthesia. *Anesthesiology* 86:627–631, 1977.

Kinouchi K, Okawa M, Fukumitsu K, et al.: Two pediatric cases of malignant hyperthermia caused by sevoflurane. *Masui* 50:1232–1235, 2001.

Knill RI, Gelb AW: Ventilatory response to hypoxia and hypercapnia during halothane sedation and anesthesia in man. *Anesthesiology* 49:244, 1978.

Knill RL, Clement JL: Site of selective action of halothane on the peripheral chemoreflex pathway in humans. *Anesthesiology* 61:121, 1984.

Kobayashi S, Bito H, Obara Y, et al.: Compound A concentration in the circle absorber system during low-flow sevoflurane anesthesia: Comparison of Dragersorb Free, Amsorb, and Sodasorb II. *J Clin Anesth* 15:33–37, 2003.

Koehntop DE, Rodman IH, Brundage DM, et al.: Pharmacokinetics of fentanyl in neonates. *Anesth Analg* 65:227, 1986.

Koka BV, Jeon IS, Andre JM, et al.: Postintubation croup in children. *Anesth Analg* 56:501, 1977.

Kokki H, Salonen A: Comparison of pre- and postoperative administration of ketoprofen for analgesia after tonsillectomy in children. *Paediatr Anaesth* 12:162–167, 2002.

Kopman AF, Yee PS, Neuman GG: Relationship of the train-of-four fade ratio to clinical signs and symptoms of residual paralysis in awake volunteers. *Anesthesiology* 86:765–771, 1997.

Koren G, Frand M, Barzilay Z, et al.: Corticosteroid treatment of laryngotracheitis vs spasmodic croup in children. *Am J Dis Child* 137:941, 1983.

Krane EJ, Tyler DC, Jacobson LE: The dose response of caudal morphine children. *Anesthesiology* 71:48, 1989.

Krane EJ: Delayed respiratory depression in a child after caudal epidural morphine, *Anesth Analg* 67:79, 1988.

Kranke P, Mortin AM, Roewer N, et al.: H. Dimenhydrinate for prophylaxis of postoperative nausea and vomiting: a meta-analysis of randomized controlled trials. *Acta Anaesthesiol Scand* 46:238–244, 2002.

Krechel SW, Helikson MA: Intrathecal morphine for pain control in term infants for esophageal atresia/tracheoesophageal fistula repair. *Paediatr Anaesth* 3:243, 1993.

Krupin T, Cross DA, Becker B: Decreased basal tear production associated with general anesthesia. *Arch Ophthalmol* 95:107, 1977.

Kuhn I, Scheifler G, Wissing H: Incidence of nausea and vomiting in children after strabismus surgery following desflurane anaesthesia. *Paediatr Anaesth* 9:521–526, 1999.

Kupferberg J, Way EL: Pharmacologic basis for the increased sensitivity of the newborn rat to morphine. *J Pharmacol Exp Ther* 141:105, 1963.

Kurth CD, Spitzer AK, Broennle AM, Downes JJ: Postoperative apnea in preterm infants. *Anesthesiology* 66:483, 1987.

Kurz A, Kurz M, Poeschl G, et al.: Forced-air warming maintains intraoperative normothermia better than circulating-water mattresses. *Anesth Analg* 77:89–95, 1993.

Kuusela A, Vesikari T: A randomized double-blind, placebo-controlled trial of dexamethasone and racemic epinephrine in the treatment of croup. *Acta Paediatr Scand* 77:99, 1988.

Lanier WL, Strangland KJ, Scheithauer BW, et al: The effects of dextrose infusion and head position on neurologic outcome after complete cerebral ischemia in primates: Examination of a model. *Anesthesiology* 66:39, 1987.

Lawrence J, Alcock D, Kay J, et al.: The development of a tool to assess neonatal pain. *J Pain Sympt Manage* 6:AI59, 1991.

Lawrie SC, Forbes DW, Akhtar TM, et al.: Patient-controlled analgesia in children. *Anaesthesia* 46:1074, 1990.

Laycock JRD, Baxter MK, Bevan JC, et al.: The potency of pancuronium at the adductor pollicis and diaphragm in infants and children. *Anesthesiology* 68:908, 1988.

LeDez KM, Lerman J: The minimum alveolar concentration (MAC) of isoflurane in preterm neonates. *Anesthesiology* 67:301, 1987.

Leelanukrom R, Cunliffe M: Intraoperative fluid and glucose management in children. *Paediatr Anaesth* 10:353, 2000.

Lenzer J: FDA advisers warn: COX2 inhibitors increase risk of heart attack and stroke. *Br Med J* 330.:440, 2005.

Lerman J, Robinson S, Willis MM, Gregory GA: Anesthetic requirements for halothane in young children 0-1 month and 1-6 months of age. *Anesthesiology* 59:421, 1983.

Lerman J, Sikich N, Kleinman S: The pharmacology of sevoflurane in infants and children. *Anesthesiology* 80:814, 1994.

Lerman J: Inhalational anesthetics. *Pediatr Anesth* 14:380–383, 2004.

Lerman J: Surgical and patient factors involved in postoperative nausea and vomiting. *Br J Anaesh* 69:24–32,1992.

Lilly JK, Boland JP, Zekan S: Urinary bladder temperature monitoring: A new index of body core temperature. *Crit Care Med* 8:742, 1980.

Lindahl SG, Mure M: Dosing oxygen: A tricky matter or a piece of cake? *Anesth Analg* 95:1472, 2002.

Litman RS, Wu LL, Catanzaro FA: Ondansetron decreases emesis after tonsillectomy in children in tonsillectomies. *Anesth Analg* 78:478, 1994.

Litvak AS, Morris JA Jr, McRoberts JW: Normal size of the urethral meatus in boys. *J Urol* 115:736, 1976.

Liu LMP, Coté CJ, Goudsouzian NG, et al.: Life-threatening apnea in infants recovering from anesthesia. *Anesthesiology* 59:506, 1983.

Liu LMP, DeCook TH, Goudsouzian NG, et al.: Dose response to intramuscular succinylcholine in children. *Anesthesiology* 55:599, 1981.

Lockhart SH, Rampil U, Yasuda N, et al.: Depression of ventilation by desflurane in humans. *Anesthesiology* 74:484, 1991.

Loeckinger A, Kleinsasser A, Keller C, et al.: Administration of oxygen before tracheal extubation worsens gas exchange after general anesthesia in a pig model. *Anesth Analg* 95:1472, 2002.

Loeser EA, Stanley TH, Jordan W, Machin R: Postoperative sore throat: Influence of tracheal tube lubrication versus cuff design. *Can Anaesth Soc J* 27:156, 1980.

Lubarsky DA, Sanderson IC, Gilbert WC, et al.: Using an anesthesia information management system as a cost containment tool. Description and validation. *Anesthesiology* 86:1161–1169, 1997.

Lynn AM, Slattery JT: Morphine pharmacokinetics in early infancy. *Anesthesiology* 66:136, 1987.

Ma H, Tang J, White PF, Zaentz A, et al.: Perioperative rofecoxib improves early recovery after outpatient herniorrhaphy. *Anesth Analg* 98:970–975, 2004.

Macintyre PE, Pavlin EG, Dwersteg JF: Effect of meperidine on oxygen consumption, carbon dioxide production, and respiratory gas exchange in postanesthesia shivering. *Anesth Analg* 66:751–755, 1987.

Maeda H, Iranami H, Hatano Y: Delayed recovery from muscle weakness due to malignant hyperthermia during sevoflurane anesthesia. *Anesthesiology* 87:425–426, 1997.

Mahmoud NA, Rose DJA, Laurence AS: Desflurane or sevoflurane for gynaecological day: Case anaesthesia with spontaneous respiration? *Anaesthesia* 56:171, 2001.

Malan TP Jr, Marsh G, Hakki SI, et al.: Parecoxib sodium, a parenteral cyclooxygenase 2 selective inhibitor, improves morphine analgesia and is opioid-sparing following total hip arthroplasty. *Anesthesiology* 98:950–956, 2003.

Malviya S, Swarz J, Lerman J: Are all preterm infants younger than 60 weeks postconceptual age at risk of postanesthetic apnea? *Anesthesiology* 78:1076, 1993.

Malviya S, Reynolds PI, Voepel-Lewis T, et al.: False alarms and sensitivity of conventional pulse oximetry versus the Masimo SET technology in the pediatric postanesthesia care unit. *Anesth Analg* 90:1336–1340, 2000.

Mangat D, Orr WC, Smith RO: Sleep apnea, hypersomnolence, and upper airway obstruction secondary to adenotonsillar enlargement. *Arch Otolaryngol* 103:383, 1977.

Marcucci F, Mussini E, Airoldi L, et al.: Diazepam metabolism and anticonvulsant activity in newbom animals. *Biochem Pharmacol* 22:3051, 1973.

Marcus CL: Sleep-disordered breathing in children. *Am J Respir Crit Care Med* 164:16–30, 2001.

Marcus CL, McColley SA, Carroll JL, et al.: Upper airway collapsibility in children with obstructive sleep apnea syndrome. *J Appl Physiol* 77:918, 1994.

Marcy JH, editor: *Neonatal anesthesia.* Pasadena, CA, 1988, Appleton Davies, pp 87–125.

Markakis DA, Lau M, Brown R, et al.: The pharmacokinetics and steady state pharmacodynamics of mivacurium in children. *Anesthesiology* 88:978–983, 1998.

Marraro G: Intraoperative ventilation. *Paediatr Anaesth* 8: 373, 1998.

Marsh B, White M, Morton N, et al.: Pharmacokinetic model driven infusion of propofol in children. *Br J Anaesth* 67:41–48, 1991.

Marshall BE, Longnecker DE: General anesthetics. In Gilman AG, Goodman LS, Rall TW, et al., editors: *Pharmacological basis of therapeutics*, ed 8. New York, 1990, Pergamon Press, pp 285–310.

McCann ME, Bacsik J, Davidson A, et al.: The correlation of bispectral index with end tidal sevoflurane concentration and haemodynamic parameters in preschoolers. *Paediatr Anaesth* 12:519–525, 2002.

McGrath JA, Johnson G, Goodman JT, et al.: The CHEOPS: A behavioral scale to measure postoperative pain in children. In Fields HL, Dubner R, Ceveto F, editors: *Advances in pain research and therapy.* New York, 1985, Raven Press, p 395.

McGrath PA, DeVeber LH, Heam MJ: Multidimensional pain assessment in children. *Adv Pain Res Therapy* 9:387, 1985.

McGrath PJ, Unruh AM: *Pain in children and adolescents.* New York, 1987, Elsevier Science.

Mcllvaine WB: Perioperative pain management in children: A review. *J Pain Sympt Manage* 4:215, 1989.

Meakin GH: Low-flow anaesthesia in infants and children. *Br J Anaesth* 83:50–57, 1999.

Meakin G, McKieman EP, Morris P, et al.: Dose-response curves for suxamethonium in neonates, infants, and children. *Br J Anaesth* 62:655, 1989.

Meakin G, Sweet PT, Bevan JC, et al.: Neostigmine and edrophonium as antagonists of pancuronium in infants and children. *Anesthesiology* 59:316, 1983.

Melgrave AP: The use of epinephrine in the presence of halothane in children. *Can Anaesth Soc J* 17:256, 1970.

Melzack R: The McGill Pain Questionnaire: Major properties and scoring methods. *Pain* 1:277, 1975.

Mercke U: The influence of varying air humidity on mucociliary activity. *Acta Otolaryngol* 79:133, 1975.

Meretoja OA, Taivainen T, Erkola O, et al.: Dose-response and time-course of effect of rocuronium bromide in paediatric patients. *Eur J Anaesthesiol* 11:19–22, 1995.

Meretoja OA, Wirtavuori K, Neuvonen PJ: Age-dependence of the dose response curve of vecuronium in pediatric patients during balanced anesthesia. *Anesth Analg* 67:21, 1988.

Meretoja OA: Is vecuronium a long-acting neuromuscular blocking agent in neonates and infants? *Br J Anaesth* 62:184, 1989.

Merry AF, Webster CS, Mathew DJ: A new, safety-oriented, integrated drug administration and automated anesthesia record system. *Anesth Analg* 93:385–390, 2001.

Miletich DJ, Ivankovich AD, Albrecht R-F, et al.: Absence of autoregulation of cerebral blood flow during halothane and enflurane anesthesia. *Anesth Analg* 55:100, 1976.

Miller RD, Rupp SM, Fisher DM, et al.: Clinical pharmacology of vecuronium and atracurium. *Anesthesiology* 61:444, 1984.

Miller RD, Way WL, Dolan WM, et al.: The dependence of pancuronium and d-tubocurarine induced neuromuscular blockades on alveolar concentrations of halothane and Forane. *Anesthesiology* 37:573, 1972.

Mirkin BL: Developmental pharmacology. *Annu Rev Pharmacol Toxicol* 10:255, 1970.

Moiniche S, Kehlet H, Dahl JB: A qualitative and quantitative systematic review of preemptive analgesia for postoperative pain relief: The role of timing of analgesia. *Anesthesiology* 96:725–741, 2002.

Monitto CL, Greenberg RS, Kost-Byerly S, et al.: The safety and efficacy of parent-/nurse-controlled analgesia in patients less than six years of age. *Anesth Analg* 91:573–579, 2000.

Monkhoff M, Schwarz U, Gerber A, et al.: The effects of sevoflurane and halothane anesthesia on cerebral blood flow velocity in children. *Anesth Analg* 92:891–896, 2001.

Moorthy SS, Dietdorf SF, Krishna G, et al.: Transient hypoxemia from a transient right-to-left shunt in a child during emergence from anesthesia. *Anesthesiology* 66:234, 1987.

Morselli PL, Mandelli M, Tognoni G, et al.: Drug interactions in the human fetus and in the newborn infant. In Morselli PL, Cohen SN, editors: *Drug interactions.* New York, 1974, Raven Press, p 320.

Moss J, Rosow CE: Histamine release by narcotics and muscle relaxants in humans. *Anesthesiology* 59:330, 1983.

Motoyama EK: Effect of positive end expiratory pressure (PEEP) on respiratory mechanics and oxygen saturation (Spo_2) in infants and children under general anesthesia. *Anesthesiology* 85:A1099, 1996.

Motoyama EK, Borland L, Mutich R: The time course of hemoglobin desaturation during the immediate post anesthetic period in children. *Anesthesiology* 67:508, 1987.

Motoyama EK, Fine GF, Jacobson KH, et al.: Accelerated increases in end-tidal CO_2 ($P_{ET}CO_2$) in anesthetized infants and children during rebreathing. *Anesthesiology* 94:A1276, 2001.

Motoyama EK, Glazener CH: Hypoxemia after general anesthesia in children. *Anesth Analg* 65:267, 1986.

Munroe HM, Riegger LQ, Reynolds PI, Wilton NC, Lewis IH: Comparison of the analgesic and emetic properties of ketorolac and morphine for paediatric outpatient strabismus surgery. *Br J Anaesth* 72:624–628, 1994.

Murat I: Cuffed tubes in children: A 3-year experience in a single institution. *Paediatr Anaesth* 11:745–750, 2001.

Mushin WW, Rosen M, Jones EV: Post-halothane jaundice in relation to previous administration of halothane. *Br Med J* 3:18, 1971.

Naito Y, Tamai S, Shingu K, et al.: Comparison between sevoflurane and halothane for pediatric ambulatory anaesthesia. *Br J Anaesth* 67:387, 1991.

Nakayama S, Osaka Y, Yamashita M: The rotational technique with a partially inflated laryngeal mask airway improves the ease of insertion in children. *Paediatr Anaesth* 12:416–419, 2002.

Nelson NM, Members of Task Force on Prolonged Apnea: Reports of the Task Force on Prolonged Apnea of the American Academy of Pediatrics. *Pediatrics* 61:651, 1978.

Neuberger J, Williams R: Halothane anaesthesia and liver damage. *Br Med J* 289:1136, 1984.

New York State Hospital Code, Section 405.13, endorsed by the New York State Hospital Review and Planning Council, June 9, 1988; approved by the Commissioner of the New York State Department of Health for January 1, 1989, implementation. New York, 1994, Churchill Livingstone.

Ng A, Temple A, Smith G, et al.: Early analgesic effects of parecoxib versus ketorolac following laparoscopic sterilization: a randamized controlled trial. *Br J Anaesth* 92:846–849, 2004.

Nichols CG, Yaster M, Lynn AM, et al.: Disposition and respiratory effects of intrathecal morphine in children. *Anesthesiology* 79:733, 1993.

Nicodemus HF, Nassiri-Rahimi C, Bachman L, Smith TC: Median effective doses (ED50) of halothane in adults and children. *Anesthesiology* 31:347, 1969.

Nightingale DA, Richards CC, Glass A: An evaluation of rebreathing in a modified T-piece system during controlled ventilation of anaesthetized children. *Br J Anaesth* 37:762, 1965.

NIH Consensus Conference: Perioperative red cell transfusion. *JAMA* 260:2700, 1988.

Nishino T, Kohchi T, Yonezawa T, Honda Y: Response of recurrent laryngeal hypoglossal, and phrenic nerves to increasing depth of anesthesia with halothane or enflurane in vagotomized cats. *Anesthesiology* 63:404, 1985.

Nishino T, Shirahata M, Yonezawa T, Honda Y: Comparison of changes in the hypoglossal and the phrenic nerve activity in response to increasing depth of anesthesia in cats. *Anesthesiology* 60:19, 1984.

Nunn JF, Hill DW: Respiratory dead space and arterial to end-tidal CO2 tension difference in anaesthetised man. *J Appl Physiol* 15:583, 1960.

Ochiai R, Guthrie RD, Motoyama EK: Differential sensitivity to halothane anesthesia of the genioglossus intercostals and diaphragm in kittens. *Anesth Analg* 74:338, 1992.

Ochiai R, Guthrie RD, Motoyama EK: Effects of varying concentrations of halothane on the activity of the genioglossus, intercostals, and diaphragm in cats: An electrographic study. *Anesthesiology* 70:812, 1989.

Ochiai R, Toyoda Y, Nishio I, et al.: Possible association of malignant hyperthermia with sevoflurane anesthesia. *Anesth Analg* 74:616, 1992.

Oh TH: Formulas for calculating fluid maintenance requirements. *Anesthesiology* 53:351, 1980.

Olympio MA, Morell RC: Canister fires become a hot safety concern. *Anesth Patient Safety Found Newsletter* 18:45–64, 2003.

Orkin FK, Cooperman LH: *Complications in anesthesiology.* Philadelphia, 1983, JB Lippincott.

Otsuka H, Komura Y, Mayumi T, et al.: Malignant hyperthermia during sevoflurane anesthesia in a child with central core disease. *Anesthesiology* 75:699, 1991.

Oudjhane K, Bowen A, Oh KS, et al.: Pulmonary edema complicating upper airway obstruction in infants and children. *Can Assoc Radiol J* 43:278–282, 1992.

Owens ME, Todt EH: Pain in infancy: Neonatal reaction to a heel lance. *Pain* 20:77, 1984.

Palvin DJ, Nersley ML, Cheney FW: Increased pulmonary vascular permeability as a cause of re-expansion pulmonary oedema. *Am Rev Respir Dis* 124: 422–427, 1981.

Pansard JL, Chauvin M, Lebrault C, et al.: Effect of an intubating dose of succinylcholine and atracurium on the diaphragm and the adductor pollicis muscle in humans. *Anesthesiology* 67:326, 1987.

Pappas AL, Sukhani R, Hotaling AJ, et al.: The effect of preoperative dexamethasone on the immediate and delayed postoperative morbidity in children undergoing adenotonsillectomy. *Anesth Analg* 87:57–61, 1998.

Patel RI, Davis PJ, Orr RJ, et al.: Single-dose ondansetron prevents postoperative vomiting in pediatric outpatients. *Anesth Analg* 85:538–545, 1997.

Patel RI, Hannallah RS: Anesthetic complications following pediatric ambulatory surgery: A 3-year study. *Anesthesiology* 69:1009, 1988.

Patel RI, Norden J, Hannallah RS: Oxygen administration prevents hypoxemia during postanesthetic transport in children. *Anesthesiology* 69:616, 1988.

Patel RI, Rice LJ: Special considerations in the recovery room of children from anesthesia. *Int Anesthesiol Clin* 29:55, 1991.

Patel RI, Verghese ST, Hannallah RS, et al.: Fast-tracking children after ambulatory surgery. *Anesth Analg* 92:918–922, 2001.

Patterson JF: Stethoscope monitoring during anesthesia. *Anesth Analg* 45:572, 1966.

Pennant JH, White PF: The laryngeal mask airway. *Anesthesiology* 79:144, 1993.

Peters JWB, Bezstarosti-van Eeden J, Erdmann W, Meursing AEE: Safety and efficacy of semi-closed circle ventilation in small infants. *Paediatr Anaesth* 8:299, 1998.

Peterson L, Toler SM: An information seeking disposition in child surgery patients. *Health Psychol* 5:343, 1986.

Pinsker MC, Carroll NV: Quality of emergence from anesthesia and incidence of vomiting with remifentanil in a pediatric population. *Anesth Analg* 89:71–74, 1999.

Pittet JF, Tassonyi E, Morel DR, et al.: Pipecuronium-induced neuromuscular blockade during nitrous oxide-fentanyl, isoflurane, and halothane anesthesia in adults and children. *Anesthesiology* 71:210, 1989.

Ploss RE: A simple constant monitor system. *Anesthesiology* 16:466, 1955.

Pullerits J, Burrows FA, Roy WL: Arterial desaturation in healthy children during transfer to the recovery room. *Can J Anaesth* 34:470, 1987.

Rampil IJ, Lockhart SH, Zwass MS, et al.: Clinical characteristics of desflurane in surgical patients: Minimum alveolar concentration. *Anesthesiology* 74:429, 1991.

Rash DK, Webster DE, Pollard TG, et al.: Lumber and thoracic epidural analgesia via the caudal approach for postoperative pain relief in infants and children. *Can J Anaesth* 37:359, 1990.

Rayburn RL, Graves SA: A new concept in controlled ventilation of children with the Bain anesthesia circuit. *Anesthesiology* 48:250, 1978.

Rehder K, Mallow JE, Fibush EE, et al.: Effects of isoflurane anesthesia and muscle paralysis on respiratory mechanics in normal man. *Anesthesiology* 41:477, 1974.

Rigatto H: Apnea. In Thibeault DW, Gregory GA, editors: *Neonatal pulmonary care.* Norwalk, CT, 1986, Appleton-Century-Crofts, p 641.

Rodrigo MRC, Moles TM, Lee PK: Comparison of the incidence and nature of cardiac arrhythmias occurring during isoflurane and halothane anaesthesia. *Br J Anaesth* 58:394, 1986.

Romsing J, Moiniche S: A systematic review of COX-2 inhibitors compared with traditional NSAIDs, or different COX-2 inhibitors for post-operative pain. *Acta Anaesthesiol Scand* 48:525–546, 2004.

Rooke GA, Choi JH, Bishop MJ: The effect of isoflurane, halothane, sevoflurane, and thiopental/nitrous oxide on respiratory system resistance after tracheal intubation. *Anesthesiology* 86:1294–1299, 1997.

Rose DK, Froese AB: The regulation of $PaCO_2$ during controlled ventilation of children with a T-piece. *Can Anaesth Soc J* 26:104, 1979.

Rosen KR, Rosen DA: Caudal epidural morphine for control of pain following open heart surgery in children. *Anesthesiology* 70:418, 1989.

Ross AK, Davis PJ, Dear G, et al.: Pharmacokinetics of remifentanil in anesthetized pediatric patients undergoing elective surgery or diagnostic procedures. *Anesth Analg* 93:1393–1401, 2001.

Rubin AH, Eliaschar I, Joachim Z, et al.: Effects of nasal surgery and tonsillectomy on sleep apnea. *Bull Eur Physiopathol Respir* 19:612, 1983.

Salem RM, Bennett EJ, Schweiss JF, et al.: Cardiac arrest related to anesthesia: Contributing factors in infants and children. *JAMA* 233:238, 1975.

Sanborn KV, Castro J, Kuroda M, Thys DM: Detection of intraoperative incidents by electronic scanning of computerized anesthesia records. Comparison with voluntary reporting. *Anesthesiology* 85:977–987, 1996.

Sarner BJ, Brandom BW, Woelfel SK, et al.: Clinical pharmacology of mivacurium chloride in children during nitrous oxide-halothane and nitrous oxide-narcotic anesthesia. *Anesth Analg* 68:116, 1989.

Sarner JB, Brandom BW, Dong ML, et al.: Clinical Pharmacology of pipercuronium in infants and children during halothane anesthesia. *Anesth Analg* 71:362, 1990.

Sarner JB, Levine M, Davis PJ, et al.: Clinical characteristics of sevoflurane in children: A comparison with halothane. *Anesthesiology* 82:38, 1995.

Sasaki CT: Development of laryngeal function: Etiologic significance in the sudden infant death syndrome. *Laryngoscope* 89:1964, 1979.

Savedra MC, Tesler MD: Assessing children's and adolescents' pain. *Pediatrician* 16:24–29, 1989.

Schechter MS: Section on Pediatric Pulmonology, Subcommittee on Obstructive Sleep Apnea Syndrome. Technical report: Diagnosis and management of childhood obstructive sleep apnea syndrome. *Pediatrics* 109:e69, 2002.

Scheller MS, Tateishi A, Drummond JC, Zomow MH: The effect of sevoflurane on cerebral blood flow, cerebral metabolic rate for oxygen, intracranial pressure, and the electroencephalogram are similar to those of isoflurane in the rabbit. *Anesthesiology* 68:548, 1988.

Schmitt HJ, Schuetz WH, Proeschel PA, Jaklin C: Accuracy of pulse oximetry in children with cyanotic congenital heart disease. *J Cardiothorac Vasc Anesth* 7:61–65, 1993.

Schreiner MS, Nicolson SC, Martin T, et al.: Should children drink before discharge from day surgery? *Anesthesiology* 76:528, 1992.

Schrum SF, Hannallah RS, Verghese PM, et al.: Comparison of propofol and thiopental for rapid anesthesia induction in infants. *Anesth Analg* 78:482, 1994.

Schulte-Sasse U, Hess W, Tamow J: Pulmonary vascular responses to nitrous oxide in patients with normal and high pulmonary resistance. *Anesthesiology* 57:9, 1982.

Seiber FE, Smith DS, Traysman RJ, et al.: Glucose: A reevaluation of its intraoperative use. *Anesthesiology* 67:72, 1987.

Serafini G, Cornara G, Cavalloro F, et al.: Pulmonary atelectasis during paediatric anaesthesia CT scan evaluation and effect of positive end expiratory pressure (PEEP). *Paediatr Anaesth* 9:225, 1999.

Shapiro LA, Jedeikin RJ, Shalev D, et al.: Epidural morphine analgesia in children. *Anesthesiology* 61:210, 1984.

Sheeran PW, Rose JB, Fazi LM, et al.: Rofecoxib administration to paediatric patients undergoing adenotonsillectomy. *Paediatr Anaesth* 14:579–583, 2004.

Sherry KM: Post-extubation stridor in Down's syndrome. *Br J Anaesth* 55:53, 1983.

Shevchenko Y, Jocson JC, McRae VA, et al.: The use of lidocaine for preventing the withdrawal associated with the injection of rocuronium in children and adolescents. *Anesth Analg* 88:746–748, 1999.

Shires T, Coin D, Carrico J, et al.: Fluid therapy in hemorrhagic shock. *Arch Surg* 88:688, 1964.

Shires T, Williams J, Brown F: Acute changes in extracellular fluids associated with major surgical procedures. *Ann Surg* 154:803, 1961.

Singleton MA, Rosen JL, Fisher DM: Plasma concentrations of fentanyl in infants, children and adults. *Can Anaesth Soc J* 34:152, 1987.

Smith RM: Anesthesia for pediatric surgery. In Gross RE, editor: *Surgery of infants and children.* Philadelphia, 1953, WB Saunders Co.

Smith RM: Signs of depth and danger. *Int Anesthesiol Clin* 1:153, 1962.

Smith RM: *Pediatric anesthesia for infants and children,* ed 4. St Louis, 1980, CV Mosby.

Smith RM: Pediatric anesthesia in perspective: Sixteenth Annual Baxter Travenol Lecture. *Anesth Analg* 57:634, 1978.

Smith RM: Temperature monitoring and regulation. *Pediatr Clin North Am* 16:643, 1969.

Smith WD: Pharmacology of nitrous oxide. *Int Anesthesiol Clin* 9:91, 1971.

Smith-Erickson N, Bo G: Airway closure and fluid filtration in the lung. *Br J Anesth* 51:475, 1979.

Sneyd JR, Carr A, Byrom WD, Bilski AJ: A meta-analysis of nausea and vomiting following maintenance of anaesthesia with propofol or inhalational agents. *Eur J Anaesthesiol* 15:433–445,1998.

Sofer S, Bar-Ziv 1, Schafer SM: Pulmonary edema following relief of upper airway obstruction. *Chest* 86:401, 1984.

Soliman IE, Patel RI, Ehrenpreis MB, Hannallah RS: Recovery scores do not correlate with postoperative hypoxemia in children. *Anesth Analg* 67:53, 1988.

Spears RS Jr, Yeh A, Fisher DM, Zwass MS: The "educated hand." *Anesthesiology* 75:693, 1991.

Splinter WM, Rhine EJ, Roberts DW, et al.: Ondansetron is a better prophylactic antiemetic than droperidol for tonsillectomy in children. *Can J Anaesth* 42:848–851, 1995.

Splinter WM, Rhine EJ, Roberts DW, et al.: Preoperative ketorolac increases bleeding after tonsillectomy in children. *Can J Anaesth* 43:560–563, 1996.

Splinter WM, Roberts DJ: Dexamethasone decreases vomiting by children after tonsillectomy. *Anesth Analg* 83:913–916, 1996.

Splinter WM, Rhine EJ: Prophylaxis for vomiting by children after tonsillectomy: Ondansetron compared with perphenazine. *Br J Anaesth* 80:155–158, 1998.

Stalcup SA, Mellins RB: Mechanical forces producing pulmonary edema in acute asthma. *N Engl J Med* 297:592–596, 1997.

Stanley TE III, Reves JG: Cardiovascular monitoring. In Miller RD, editor: *Anesthesia,* ed 4. New York, 1994, Churchill-Livingstone, p 1161.

Stanley TH, Webster LR: Anesthetic requirements and cardiovascular effects of fentanyl-oxygen and fentanyl-diazepam-oxygen anesthesia in man. *Anesth Analg* 57:411, 1978.

Stehling L, Zander HL: Acute normovolemic hemodilution. *Transfusion* 31:857, 1991.

Stevenson GW, Tobin MJ, Horn BJ, et al.: The effect of circuit compliance on delivered ventilation with use of an adult circle system for time cycled volume controlled ventilation using an infant lung model. *Paediatr Anaesth* 8:139, 1998.

Stevenson GW, Tobin M, Horn B, et al.: An adult system versus a Bain system: Comparative ability to deliver minute ventilation to an infant lung model with pressure-limited ventilation. *Anesth Analg* 88:527–530, 1999a.

Stevenson GW, Horn B, Tobin M, et al.: Pressure-limited ventilation of infants with low-compliance lungs: The efficacy of an adult circle system versus two free-standing intensive care unit ventilator systems using an in vitro model. *Anesth Analg* 89:638, 1996b.

Steward DJ: A simplified scoring system for the postoperative recovery room. *Can Anaesth Soc J* 22:111, 1975.

Stoelting RK, Blitt CD, Cohen PJ, Merin RG: Hepatic dysfunction after isoflurane anesthesia. *Anesth Analg* 66:147, 1987.

Strecker WB, Wood MB, Bierber EJ: Compartment syndrome mask by epidural anesthesia for postoperative pain. *J Bone Joint Surg* 68:1447, 1986.

Strobl KP, Chemiack NS, Gothe B: Physiologic basis of therapy for sleep apnea. *Am Rev Respir Dis* 134:791, 1986.

Strum CP, Eger EI, Johnson BH, et al.: Toxicity of sevoflurane in rats. *Anesth Analg* 66:769, 1987.

Strum DP, Eger EI: Partition coefficients for sevoflurane; in human blood, saline, and olive oil. *Anesth Analg* 66:654, 1987.

Summary of the National Halothane Study: A study of the possible association between halothane anesthesia and postoperative hepatic necrosis. *JAMA* 197:775, 1966.

Suresh S, Barcelona SL, Young NM, et al.: Postoperative pain relief in children undergoing tympanomastoid surgery: Is a regional block better than opioids? *Anesth Analg* 94:859–862, 2002.

Suzuki M, Sasaki CT: Laryngeal spasm: A neurophysiologic redefinition. *Ann Otol Rhinol Laryngol* 86:150, 1977.

Taivainen T, Meakin GH, Meretoja OA, et al.: The safety and efficacy of cisatracurium 0.15 mg.kg(–1) during nitrous oxide-opioid anaesthesia in infants and children. *Anaesthesia* 55:1047–1051, 2000.

Takasaki M, Dohi S, Kawabata Y, et al.: Dosage of lidocaine for caudal analgesia in infants and children. *Anesthesiology* 47:527, 1977.

Tami TA, Chu F, Wildes TO, et al.: Pulmonary edema and acute upper airway obstruction. *Laryngoscope* 96:506–509, 1986.

Taylor P: Cholinergic agonists. In Gilman AG, Goodman LS, Rail TW, Murad F, editors: *The pharmacological basis of therapeutics,* ed 7. New York, 1985, Macmillan Publishing Co, p 108.

Taylor RH, Lerman J: Minimum alveolar concentration of desflurane and hemodynamic responses in neonates, infants and children. *Anesthesiology* 75:975, 1991.

Thatch BT: Sleep apnea in infancy and childhood. *Med Clin North Am* 69:1289, 1985.

Thorsteinsson A, Larsson A, Jonmarker C, Werner O: Pressure-volume relations of the respiratory system in healthy children. *Am J Respir Crit Care Med* 150:421, 1994.

Tobias JD: Caudal epidural block: A review of test dosing and recognition of systemic injection in children. *Anesth Analg* 93:1156–1161, 2001.

Tobin MJ, Stevenson GW, Horn BJ, et al.: A comparison of three modes of ventilation with the use of an adult circle system in an infant lung model. *Anesth Analg* 87:766–771, 1998.

Todd MM, Drummond JC: A comparison of the cerebrovascular and metabolic effects of halothane and isoflurane in the cat. *Anesthesiology* 66:720, 1984.

Travis KW, Todres ID, Shannon DC: Pulmonary edema associated with croup and epiglottitis. *Pediatrics* 59:695–698, 1977.

Tsai YC, Chu KS: A comparison of tramadol, amitriptyline, and meperidine for postepidural anesthetic shivering in parturients. *Anesth Analg* 93:1288–1292, 2001.

Tunnessen WW Jr, Feinstein AR: The steroid-croup controversy: An analytic review of methodologic problems. *J Pediatr* 96:751, 1980.

Tusi BC, Seal R, Koller J: Thoracic epidural catheter placement via the caudal approach in infants by using electrocardiographic guidance. *Anesth Anal* 95:326–330, 2002.

Tusiewicz K, Bryan AC, Froese AB: Contribution of changing rib cage diaphragm interactions to the ventilatory depression of halothane anesthesia. *Anesthesiology* 47:327, 1977.

Tusman G, Bohm SH, Tempra A, et al.: Effects of recruitment maneuver on atelectasis in anesthetized children. *Anesthesiology* 98:14, 2003.

Tyler DC: Patient-controlled analgesia in adolescents. *J Adolesc Health Care* 11:154, 1990.

Uezono S, Goto T, Terui K, et al.: Emergence agitation after sevoflurane versus propofol in pediatric patients. *Anesth Analg* 91:563–566, 2000.

Ummenhofer W, Frei FJ, Urwyler A, et al.: Effects of ondansetron in the prevention of postoperative nausea and vomiting in children. *Anesthesiology* 81:804, 1994.

Vakkuri A, Yli-Hankala A, Sarkela M, et al.: Sevoflurane mask induction of anaesthesia is associated with epileptiform EEG in children. *Acta Anaesthesiol Scand* 45:805, 2001.

Valley RD, Freid EB, Bailey AG, et al.: Tracheal extubation of deeply anesthetized pediatric patients: A comparison of desflurane and sevoflurane. *Anesth Analg* 96:1320–1324, 2003.

Valtonen M, Lissalo E, Kanto J, Rosenberg P: Propofol as an induction agent in children: Pain on injection and pharmacokinetics. *Acta Anaesthesiol Scand* 33:152, 1989.

Van Hemelrijck J, Smith I, White PF. Use of desflurane for outpatient anesthesia: A comparison with propofol and nitrous oxide. *Anesthesiology* 75:197, 1991.

Varni JW, Thompson KL, Hanson V: The Varni/Thompson Pediatric Pain Questionnaire. 1. Chronic musculoskeletal pain in juvenile rheumatoid arthritis. *Pain* 28:27, 1987.

Wallbank WA: Cardiac effects of halothane and adrenaline in hare-lip and cleft-palate surgery. *Br J Anaesth* 42:548, 1970.

Walker SM, Haugen RD, Richards A: A comparison of sevoflurane with halothane for paediatric day case surgery. *Anaesth Intens Care* 25:643–649, 1997.

Walton B: Halothane hepatitis in children. *Anaesthesia* 41:575, 1986.

Wang JJ, Ho ST, Tzeng JI: Comparison of intravenous nalbuphine infusion versus naloxone in the prevention of epidural morphine-related side effects. *Reg Anesth Pain Med* 3:479–484, 1998.

Wark HJ: Post-operative jaundice in children. The influence of halothane. *Anaesthesia* 38:237, 1983.

Warner LO, Beach TP, Garvin JP, Warner EJ: Halothane and children: The first quarter century. *Anesth Analg* 63:838, 1984.

Warran P, Radford P, Manford ML: Glycopyrrolate in children. *Br J Anaesth* 53:1273, 1981.

Wastila WB, Maehe RB, Turner GL, et al.: Comparative pharmacology of cisatracurium (51W89), atracurium and five isomers in cats. *Anesthesiology* 85:169, 1996.

Wasz-Hocket O, Michelsson K, Lind J: Twenty-five years of Scandinavian cry research. In Lester BM, Bookydsis CFZ, editors: *Infant crying: Theoretical and research perspectives.* New York, 1985, Plenum Press, p 83.

Watcha M, Jones M, Barry M, et al.: Comparison of ketorolac and morphine as adjuncts during pediatric surgery. *Anesthesiology* 76:368, 1992.

Watcha MF, Bras PJ, Cieslak GD, Pennant JH: The dose-response relationship of ondansetron in preventing postoperative emesis in pediatric patients undergoing ambulatory surgery. *Anesthesiology* 82:47, 1995.

Watcha MF, Simeon RM, White PF, Stevens JL: Effect of propofol on the incidence of postoperative vomiting after strabismus surgery in pediatric outpatients. *Anesthesiology* 75:204, 1991.

Watt-Watson IH, Evemden C, Lawson C: Parents' perception of their child's acute pain experience. *J Pediatr Nurs* 5:344, 1990.

Way WL, Costley EC, Way EL: Respiratory sensitivity of the newborn infant to meperidine and morphine. *Clin Pharmacol Ther* 6:454, 1965.

Weiskopf RB, Cahalan MK, Eger EI II, et al.: Cardiovascular actions of desflurane in normocarbic volunteers. *Anesth Analg* 73:143, 1991.

Weiskopf RB, Cahalan MK, Lonescu PB, et al.: Cardiovascular actions of desflurane with and without nitrous oxide during spontaneous ventilation in humans. *Anesth Analg* 73:165, 1991.

Weiskopf RB, Eger EI II, Lonescu P, et al.: Desflurane does not produce hepatic or renal injury in human volunteers. *Anesth Analg* 74:570, 1992.

Welborn LG, deSoto H, Hannallah RS, et al.: The use of caffeine in the control of post-anesthetic apnea in former premature infants. *Anesthesiology* 68:796, 1988.

Welborn LG, Hannallah RS, Norden JM, et al.: Comparison of emergence and recovery characteristics of sevoflurane, desflurane, and halothane in pediatric ambulatory patients. *Anesth Analg* 83:917–920, 1996.

Welborn LG, Hannallah RS, McGill WA, et al.: Glucose concentration for routine intravenous infusion in pediatric outpatient surgery. *Anesthesiology* 67:427, 1987.

Welborn LG, McGill WA, Hannallah RS, et al.: Perioperative blood glucose concentrations in pediatric outpatients. *Anesthesiology* 65:543, 1986.

Wells LT, Rasch DK: Emergence "delirium" after sevoflurane anesthesia: A paranoid delusion? *Anesth Analg* 88:1308–1310, 1999.

Westbrook PR, Stubbs SE, Sessler AD, et al.: Effects of anesthesia and muscle paralysis on respiratory mechanics in normal man. *J Appl Physiol* 34:81, 1973.

Westmoreland CL, Hoke JF, Sebel PS, et al.: Pharmacokinetics of remifentanil (GI87084B) and its major metabolite (GI90291) in patients undergoing elective inpatient surgery. *Anesthesiology* 78:893, 1993.

Wilkie DJ, Hokemer WL, Tesler MD, et al.: Measuring pain quality: Validity and reliability of children's and adolescents' pain language. *Pain* 41:151, 1990.

Williamson PS, Williamson ML: Physiological stress reduction by a local anesthetic during newborn circumcision. *Pediatrics* 71:36, 1983.

Willms D, Shure D: Pulmonary edema due to upper airway obstruction in adults. *Chest* 94:1090–1092, 1998.

Wodey E, Pladys P, Copin C, et al.: Comparative hemodynamic depression of sevoflurane versus halothane in infants: an echocardiographic study. *Anesthesiology* 87:795–800, 1997.

Woelfel SK, Brandom BW, Cook DR, Sarner JB: Effects of bolus administration of ORG-9426 in children during nitrous oxide-halothane anesthesia. *Anesthesiology* 76:939–942, 1992.

Woehlck HJ: Sleep with uncertainty: Anesthesia and desiccated absorbent. *Anesthesiology* 101:276–278, 2004.

Wolf AR, Hughes D, Wade A, et al.: Postoperative analgesia after paediatric orchiopexy: Evaluation of a bupivacaine-morphine mixture. *Br J Anaesth* 64:430, 1990.

Wolf AR, Valley RD, Fear DW, et al.: Bupivacaine for caudal analgesia in infants and children: The optimal effective concentration. *Anesthesiology* 69:102, 1988.

Wolf WJ, Neal MB, Paterson MD: The hemodynamic and cardiovascular effects of isoflurane and halothane anesthesia in children. *Anesthesiology* 64:328–333, 1986.

Wollman H, Alexander SC, Cohen PJ, et al.: Cerebral circulation of man during halothane anesthesia. *Anesthesiology* 25:180, 1964.

Wren WS, Allen P, Synnott A, et al.: Effects of halothane, isoflurane and enflurane on ventilation in children. *Br J Anaesth* 59:399, 1987.

Wu J, Previte JP, Adler E, et al.: Spontaneous ignition, explosion and fire with sevoflurane and barium hydroxide lime. *Anesthesiology* 101:534–537, 2004.

Wymore ML, Eisele JH: Differential effects of d-tubocurarine on inspiratory muscles and two peripheral muscle groups in anesthetized man. *Anesthesiology* 48:360, 1978.

Xue FS, Huang YG, Tong SY, et al.: A comparative study of early postoperative hypoxemia in infants, children and adults undergoing elective surgery. *Anesth Analg* 83:709–715, 1996.

Yaster M, Maxwell LG: Pediatric regional anesthesia. *Anesthesiology* 70:324, 1989.

Yasuda N, Targ AG, Eger EI H: Solubility of desflurane, sevoflurane, isoflurane and haloflurane in human tissues. *Anesth Analg* 69:370, 1989.

Yelderman MF, New W: Evaluation of pulse oximetry. *Anesthesiology* 59:349, 1983.

Yeoman PM, Cooke R, Hain WR: Penile block for circumcision? A comparison with caudal block. *Anaesthesia* 38:862, 1983.

Yli-Hankala A, Vakkuri A, Sarkela M, et al.: Epileptiform electroencephalogram during mask induction of anesthesia with sevoflurane. *Anesthesiology* 91:1596–1603, 1999.

Young T, Palta M, Dempsy J, et al.: The occurrence of sleep-disordered breathing among middle-aged adults. *N Engl J Med* 328:1230, 1993.

Zwass MS, Fisher DM, Welborn LG, et al.: Induction and maintenance characteristics of anesthesia with desflurane and nitrous oxide in infants and children. *Anesthesiology* 76:373, 1992.

12 Blood Conservation in Infants and Children

M. Ramez Salem

Merriam-Webster's Collegiate Dictionary defines *conservation* as "a careful preservation and protection of something; especially: planned management of a natural resource to prevent... destruction..." This definition is essential as applied to blood conservation. Efforts to conserve this natural human resource during operative procedures have assumed escalating importance in recent years. The increased demands for blood and blood products for major surgery; the risks and complications of allogenic blood transfusion; the fear of transfusion-transmitted diseases, especially acquired immunodeficiency syndrome; and the progress made in techniques have all contributed to the development of blood conservation strategies, which have been extended to pediatric surgery. Anesthesiologists should be familiar with the principles and practices of blood conservation. The techniques used to conserve blood in pediatric operative procedures may be classified as (1) adoption of appropriate transfusion guidelines, (2) techniques to reduce blood loss, (3) autologous blood transfusion, (4) combination of techniques, and (5) oxygen therapeutics (Box 12–1).

■ ADOPTION OF TRANSFUSION GUIDELINES WITH LOWER PERIOPERATIVE HEMOGLOBIN LEVELS

Transfusion practices vary widely despite similar patient and surgical variables, suggesting that attention is being paid more to certain arbitrary criteria for transfusion than to the patients' actual needs. To improve transfusion practices, the American Society of Anesthesiologists Task Force on Blood Component Therapy (1994) concluded that (1) transfusion is rarely indicated when the hemoglobin concentration is greater than 10 g/dL and is almost always indicated when it is less than 6 g/dL; (2) the determination of whether intermediate hemoglobin concentrations (6 to 10 g/dL) justify or require red blood cell transfusion should be based on the patient's risk of developing complications of inadequate oxygenation; (3) the use of a single hemoglobin "trigger" for all patients, and other approaches that fail to consider all important physiological and surgical factors affecting oxygenation, is not recommended; (4) where appropriate, preoperative autologous blood donation (PABD), acute normovolemic hemodilution (ANH), intraoperative and postoperative cell recovery, and measures to decrease blood loss (deliberate hypotension and pharmacologic agents) should be used; and (5) the indications for transfusion of autologous red blood cells may be more liberal than for allogenic red blood cells because of lower risks associated with the former.

Transfusion decisions based on hemoglobin measurements alone are associated with some degree of imprecision and can be misleading because of concomitant administration of fluids. Aspects of oxygen delivery and utilization should be considered when deciding to transfuse a patient; these include blood volume, cardiac output, PaO_2, myocardial ischemia, probability of massive blood loss, and factors causing increased oxygen requirements, such as pain, shivering, sepsis, or increased physical activity postoperatively. The decision to transfuse should depend on clinical assessment, aided by hemodynamic profile and indices of oxygen use (mixed venous partial pressure of oxygen [$P\bar{v}O_2$] and oxygen extraction ratio), if available. Severe chronic anemia (<7 g/dL) is typically characterized by an increase in erythrocyte 2,3 diphosphoglycerate (2,3-DPG), causing a rightward shift of the oxyhemoglobin dissociation curve that benefits oxygen delivery to the tissues (although 2,3-DPG may or may not

BOX 12–1 Blood Conservation Strategies in Pediatric Surgery

Adoption of Appropriate Transfusion Guidelines

Reduction in Blood Loss

Preoperative assessment and preparation
Anesthetic and surgical technique
Positioning
Infiltration with vasoconstrictors
Tourniquets
Prevention and treatment of hypothermia
Minimizing blood sampling for laboratory testing
Deliberate hypotension
Pharmacologic enhancement of hemostatic activity

Autologous Blood Transfusion

Preoperative autologous blood donation
Blood salvage procedures
Acute normovolemic hemodilution

Combination of Techniques

Oxygen Therapeutics

increase in patients with renal failure). This time-dependent adaptation is not a feature of acute anemia. Consequently, lower hemoglobin levels are tolerated better in chronic than in acute anemia. When anesthetizing patients with low hemoglobin levels, high PaO_2, adequate cardiac output, and adequate intravascular volume are essential, whereas factors associated with increased oxygen consumption (e.g., inadequate muscular relaxation, shivering) or leftward shifting of the oxyhemoglobin dissociation curve (e.g., hypocapnia, alkalosis, hypothermia) should be avoided (see Chapter 2, Respiratory Physiology).

Institutions should be committed to enforce the appropriateness of allogenic transfusions. Empiric or "shotgun" therapy approaches to transfusions can no longer be justified. A quality assessment program to study, monitor, and improve transfusion practices should be implemented, and appropriate blood conservation measures may be introduced. Physician education should be an integral part of the success of such a program.

The etiology of anemia is traditionally considered under three general pathophysiologic categories: (1) decreased production of red blood cells, (2) increased destruction of red blood cells, and (3) blood loss. In infants, this classic approach to anemia is complicated by hemoglobin concentration and oxygen affinity that undergoes physiologic changes during the first few months of life. Although anemia in infants has been defined as a "reduction in hemoglobin concentration," a more meaningful definition would be "a decrease in the level of hemoglobin content of a unit volume of blood below the level previously established as normal for age and sex."

PHYSIOLOGIC ANEMIA OF INFANCY

The mean hemoglobin concentration in cord blood at full-term birth is 16.8 g/dL, with 95% of all values falling between 13.7 and 20.1 g/dL. Based on these data, cord hemoglobin levels of less than 13 g/dL are considered abnormal (Blanchette and Zapursky, 1984). At birth, blood is rapidly transferred from the placenta to the infant, with 25% of the placental transfusion occurring within 15 seconds of birth and 50% occurring by the end of the first minute.

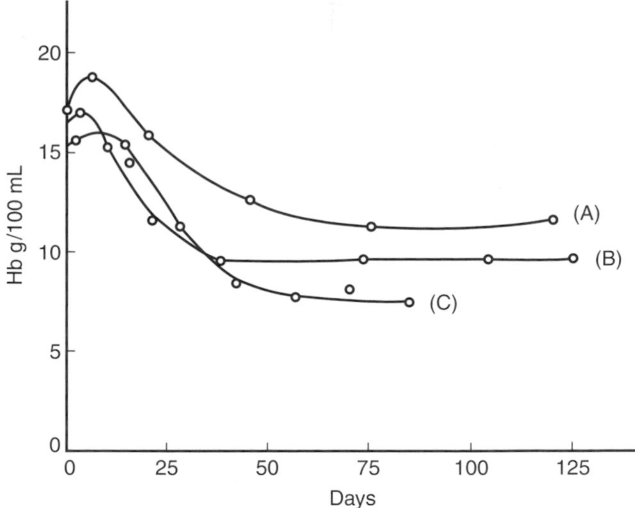

■ **FIGURE 12–1.** Hemoglobin (Hb) concentration in infants of different degrees of maturation at birth. *A*, Full-term infants. *B*, Premature infants with birth weights of 1200 to 2350 g. *C*, Premature infants with birth weights less than 1200 g. (From Nathan DG, Oski FA: *Hematology of infancy and childhood*, 3rd ed. Philadelphia, 1987, WB Saunders, p 29, with permission.)

After birth there is a transient increase in hemoglobin concentration as plasma moves extravascularly to compensate for the placental transfusion and an increase in circulating red blood cell volume that occurs at the time of delivery (Fig. 12–1) (Nathan and Oski, 1987). Thereafter, the hemoglobin level decreases rapidly as the proportion of hemoglobin F (HbF) diminishes, reaching a level between 10.5 and 11.5 g/dL in term infants by age 8 to 12 weeks and 7 to 10 g/dL in premature infants by age 6 weeks (Stockman and Oski, 1978). The high hemoglobin and reticulocyte values seen in cord blood reflect an erythropoietic response to the hypoxemic intrauterine environment. In response to the increase in arterial oxygen content after birth, erythropoietin levels decrease markedly, and there are corresponding falls in reticulocyte levels and marrow erythroid activity. Consequently, hematopoiesis virtually ceases after birth. The decrease in erythropoietin production after birth is the major cause of the physiologic anemia of infancy (Nathan and Oski, 1987). Coupled with the shortened red blood cell survival in term (80 to 100 days) and premature (60 to 80 days) infants, progressive fall in hemoglobin concentration occurs during the first 1 to 3 months of life (the life span of normal red blood cells in adults is approximately 120 days). When the hemoglobin concentration falls to a level low enough to affect tissue oxygen delivery, erythropoietin production is stimulated, active marrow erythropoiesis resumes, a reticulocytosis occurs, and the hemoglobin concentration increases. In newborns with congenital cyanotic heart disease, hypoxemia continues to stimulate active erythropoiesis and the postnatal fall in hemoglobin concentration rarely occurs.

OXYGEN UNLOADING IN THE NEWBORN, INFANT, AND CHILD

The umbilical venous blood in the mother has an oxygen content of approximately 13.5 vol% and oxygen saturation of 65%, but in the fetal side of the placenta, oxygen content is about 17 vol% and more than 80% saturated. The difference is caused by a beneficial leftward shift in the fetal oxyhemoglobin dissociation curve. HbF has a relatively low affinity for and a low concentration of 2,3-DPG compared with adult hemoglobin (hemoglobin-A [HbA]). Because both oxygen and 2,3-DPG compete for binding to hemoglobin, the reduced availability of 2,3-DPG causes oxygen to bind more tightly to HbF than to HbA. Before 34 weeks of gestational age, in the human fetus, hemoglobin consists of about 90% of HbF and 10% of HbA. At birth, the concentration of HbF is about 80%; thereafter, HbF decreases and HbA increases rapidly. The switchover is normally completed by 6 months of age (see Chapter 2, Respiratory Physiology). At birth, P_{50} (the Po_2 at which hemoglobin is 50% saturated with oxygen) is only 18 to 20 mm Hg compared with 27 mm Hg in the adult. During the first 3 months of life, there is a rapid increase in red blood cell HbA and 2,3-DPG, which results in increases in P_{50} (shifting of the curve to the right) as well as tissue oxygen unloading. At about 10 weeks of age, the increase in P_{50} reaches the adult level of 27 mm Hg. The oxyhemoglobin dissociation curve shifts farther to the right, and a level as high as 30 mm Hg may be reached by 6 to 11 months of age. Thereafter, P_{50} remains elevated during childhood and gradually decreases (shifting of the curve to the left), reaching the adult level of approximately 27 mm Hg during the first decade of life (Fig. 12–2). This is accompanied by a gradual decrease in 2,3-DPG levels toward the adult level by 10 years of age (Motoyama, 1990).

In the fetus, oxygen unloading occurs across the steep portion of the oxyhemoglobin dissociation curve (Fig. 12–3) (Smith and Nelson, 1976). The leftward shifting of the HbF curve makes it steeper than the HbA curve, and therefore HbF unloads oxygen to the fetal tissues better than does HbA. After birth, however, the presence of HbF puts the newborn at a disadvantage, because it reduces the amount of oxygen that would be otherwise unloaded to the tissues. The decline in hemoglobin levels after birth and the rapid increase in P_{50} seem to be related to the process of general growth and high plasma levels of inorganic phosphate. Normal children have plasma inorganic phosphate levels that are 50% above the normal adult range. This produces major alterations in red blood cell metabolism and leads to raised levels of red blood cell adenosine triphosphate (ATP) and 2,3-DPG, with a resultant increase in P_{50}. These observations engendered a hypothesis to explain why hemoglobin levels are lower in children than in adults: because infants (older than 3 months) and children have a lower oxygen affinity for hemoglobin (high P_{50}) than younger infants, oxygen unloading at the tissue level is increased. Thus, a lower level of hemoglobin in these infants and children is just as efficient, in terms of tissue oxygen delivery, as a higher hemoglobin level in adults (see Chapter 2, Respiratory Physiology).

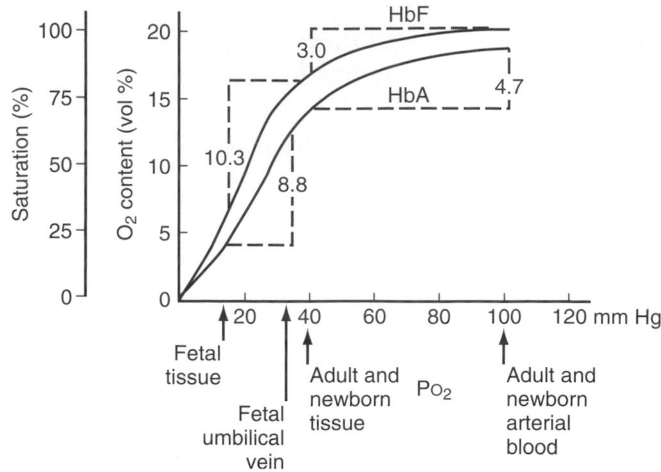

■ **FIGURE 12–3.** Oxygen unloading capacities of fetal and adult hemoglobin before and after birth. In the fetus, fetal hemoglobin (HbF) has 15% greater oxygen unloading capacity to the tissues than does adult hemoglobin (HbA). In the newborn, HbF has 36% less oxygen unloading capacity than HbA. (Modified from Smith CA, Nelson NM: *The physiology of the newborn infant.* Springfield, IL, 1976, Charles C Thomas, with permission.)

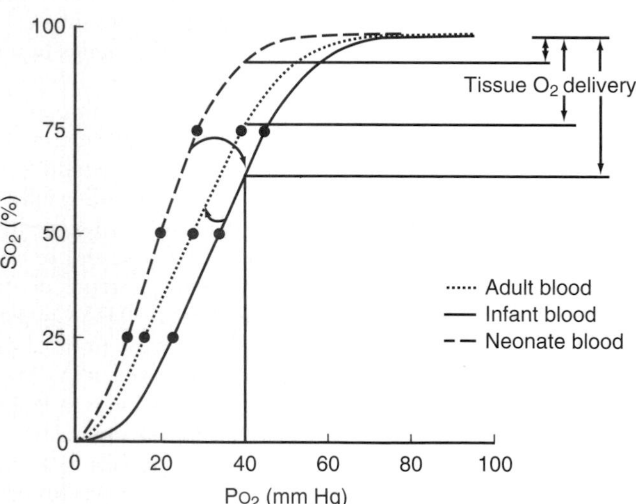

■ **FIGURE 12–2.** Schematic representation of oxyhemoglobin dissociation curves with different oxygen affinities. In infants older than 3 months with high P_{50} (30 mm Hg versus 27 mm Hg in adults), tissue oxygen delivery per gram of hemoglobin is increased. In neonates with a lower P_{50} (20 mm Hg) and a higher oxygen affinity, tissue oxygen unloading at the same tissue Po_2 is reduced. *Top arrow,* Direction of rightward shifting of the oxyhemoglobin dissociation curve (and P_{50}) after birth. By 10 weeks of age, the adult position of the curve is reached. Rightward shifting continues and maximum shifting is observed at 6 to 11 months of age. *Lower arrow,* Leftward shifting of the curve (and P_{50}) back to the adult level, which is usually completed by approximately 10 years of age. (From Motoyama EK: Respiratory physiology in infants and children. In Motoyama EK, Davis PJ, editors: *Smith's anesthesia for infants and children,* 5th ed. St Louis, 1990, CV Mosby, pp 11–76, with permission.)

It is evident that the hemoglobin concentration per se, in physiologic as well as other types of anemia, is neither an adequate descriptor of the severity of anemia nor reflective of the adaptive factors that preserve oxygen delivery to the tissues. This led Oski (1973) to introduce the concept of "designation of anemia on a functional basis." Motoyama (1990) compared hemoglobin requirements for equivalent tissue oxygen delivery (Table 12–1). Functionally, in terms of oxygen unloading capacity, a 10 g/dL hemoglobin level in an adult is equivalent to a level of 8.2 g/dL in infants older than 3 months, whereas a level of 10 g/dL of hemoglobin in preterm infants and in infants younger than 2 months is only as good as a level of 5 to 6 g/dL of hemoglobin in infants older than 3 months and children.

Value of Routine Preoperative Hemoglobin Measurements

The value of routine preoperative hemoglobin determinations in pediatric outpatients has been questioned. In a Canadian study (Hackmann, Steward and Sheps, 1991), several interesting

TABLE 12–1. Hemoglobin requirement for equivalent tissue oxygen delivery

	P_{50} (mm Hg)				Hemoglobin for Equivalent O_2 Delivery (g/dL)			
Adult	27	7	8	9	10	11	12	13
Infant (>3 mo)	30	5.7	6.5	7.3	8.2	9.0	9.8	10.6
Neonate (<2 mo)	24	10.3	11.7	13.2	14.7	16.1	17.6	19.1

From Motoyama EK: Respiratory physiology in infants and children. In Motoyama EK, Davis PJ, editors: Anesthesia of infants and children, 6th ed. St. Louis, Mosby, pp 11–67.

findings emerged, as follows. (1) The prevalence of anemia in their population was remarkably low (0.29%). (2) Anesthesiologists could not reliably predict preoperative anemia in patients presenting for outpatient surgery. (3) In the presence of mild anemia, anesthesia was safely conducted. (4) In view of the costs and patient discomfort, it was concluded that routine preoperative hemoglobin measurements may not be required. In centers where the patient population came from a lower socioeconomic background, the prevalence of anemia may be much higher and more severe than that reported within populations with a higher socioeconomic background.

ANEMIA OF PREMATURITY

In preterm infants, the hemoglobin concentration may fall steeply after birth and often reaches 8 g/dL or lower. Anemia of prematurity is attributed mainly to the abrupt increase in oxygen delivery after birth. It is characterized by diminished erythropoietin response (inappropriately low serum concentration of erythropoietin) to decreased oxygen delivery (Stockman et al., 1984). Other factors may contribute to the occurrence of anemia of prematurity, including (1) diagnostic sampling; (2) more rapid destruction of fetal cells and hemodilution due to rapid growth between 30 and 40 weeks' postconception; and (3) nutritional factors, including iron, vitamin E, and folic acid deficiencies, with iron deficiency being the most important.

Iron reserves at birth are quantitatively a direct function of birth weight; the smaller the preterm infant, the greater is the risk of developing iron deficiency. At birth, the majority of body iron is in the hemoglobin fraction. During the postnatal period, iron released from the destruction of red blood cells is either stored or used for tissue growth, with practically zero excretion. Because of the diminished iron stores and the need for expansion of the red blood cell mass with rapid tissue growth, iron deficiency anemia is a common etiology of the late anemia of prematurity. This late anemia occurs at a time when storage iron has been completely utilized in new red blood cell formation and coincides with a doubling of birth weight. In term infants, this occurs by the third to sixth month after birth, whereas in preterm infants, it may occur as soon as 1 to 2 months. It is believed that iron deficiency plays no role in the early or physiologic anemia of prematurity. Other conditions, including infection, renal disease, malignancy, and nutritional deficiencies, may prevent the hematopoietic response to iron and worsen the anemia.

The current opinion is that the addition of iron should be deferred in premature infants until supplementation is really necessary. The reasons are twofold. First, the administration of iron can aggravate the anemia of prematurity. This has been attributed to iron acting as a catalyst in the nonenzymatic autooxidation of unsaturated fatty acids and can, in the absence of antioxidants, result in red blood cell lipase peroxidation. Second, large doses of iron may stimulate the proliferation of microorganisms and affect the host's resistance to infection.

Iron supplementation should be provided to preterm infants to prevent the "late anemia" of prematurity. A prudent decision would be to delay iron supplementation until the time of the doubling of birth weight. However, it may be given earlier if the infant has been made iron deficient iatrogenically. Supplementation should start no later than 4 months of age in term infants and no later than 2 months of age in preterm infants. The recommended dosage is 1 mg/kg per day for term infants and 2 mg/kg per day for preterm infants.

Prophylaxis

The severity of anemia in preterm infants may be limited by (1) optimization of placental transfusion at birth, (2) minimal blood loss, (3) adequate nutritional uptake, (4) clinical and laboratory monitoring, and (5) recombinant human erythropoietin therapy.

Recombinant Human Erythropoietin Therapy

Stimulation of the infant's own erythropoiesis could maintain red blood cell volume and oxygen delivery, thus decreasing the need for transfusion and minimizing the complications associated with anemia. Like the anemia of end-stage renal disease, the anemia of prematurity is associated with a specific deficiency of erythropoietin in which erythroid progenitors remain highly sensitive to erythropoietin. Preterm infants may require relatively larger doses of erythropoietin than adults (in excess of 250 mcg/kg given twice weekly) to stimulate erythropoiesis.

BLOOD TRANSFUSION THERAPY

Two expressions have been used as a guide to transfuse critically ill infants (Holland et al., 1987).

1. *Available oxygen.* This uses the difference in oxygen content between arterial blood based on a measured PaO_2 and an assumed $P\bar{v}O_2$ of 20 mm Hg. When the available oxygen is calculated from infants of less than 32 weeks' gestational age, a value of less than 7 mL/dL is often associated with clinical signs of anemia, some of which respond to transfusion.
2. *Infants' $P\bar{v}O_2$ (or central venous PO_2).* Studies confirmed that, of all variables examined, $P\bar{v}O_2$ correlated best with plasma erythropoietin levels (Stockman et al., 1984). Thus the decline in $P\bar{v}O_2$ would seem to be the most sensitive indicator of the presence of anemia, as its value represents the integration of all the variables that determine oxygen supply and demand (Fig. 12–4). When $P\bar{v}O_2$ is between 35 and 38 mm Hg (normal, ≥38 mm Hg), 41% of erythropoietin

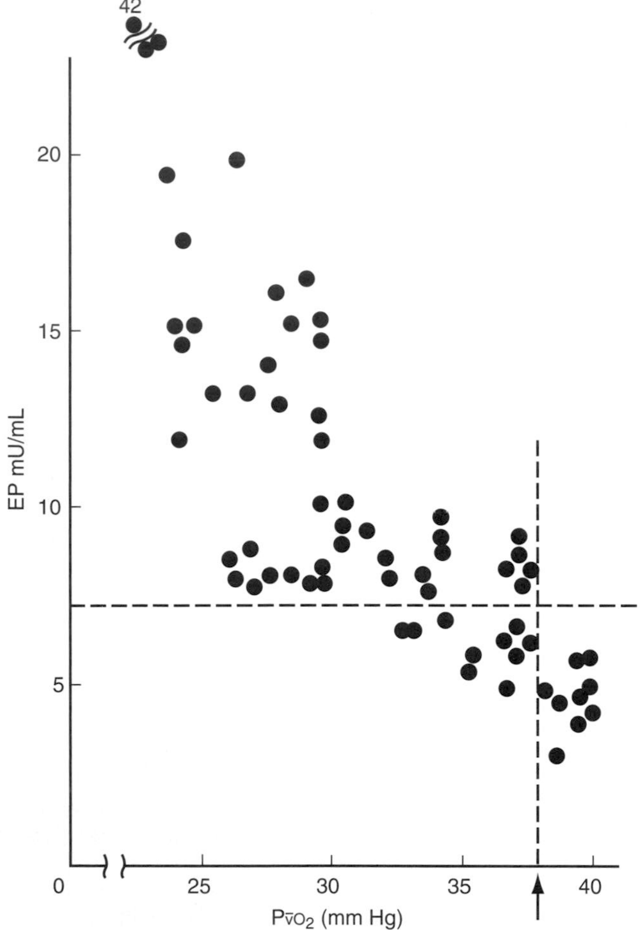

FIGURE 12–4. Changes in plasma erythropoietin (EP) concentrations in response to declines in central venous oxygen tension in preterm neonates. *Arrow,* Position of 38 mm Hg, which for the purposes of this figure is the lower limit of normal $P\bar{v}O_2$. *Horizontal dashed line,* Upper limit of normal for erythropoietin, taking $P\bar{v}O_2 \geq 38$ as normal. (From Stockman JA III, Graeber JE, Clark DA, et al.: Anemia of prematurity: Determinants of the erythropoietin response. *J Pediatr* 105:786, 1984, with permission.)

levels are above the normal range; for values between 30 and 35 mm Hg, 79% of erythropoietin levels are increased; and at $P\bar{v}O_2$ values less than 30 mm Hg, erythropoietin levels are uniformly above the normal range.

GUIDELINES FOR PERIOPERATIVE MANAGEMENT OF INFANTS AND CHILDREN WITH ANEMIA

1. In infants older than 3 months, hemoglobin levels of 8 g/dL or higher may be acceptable.
2. In infants younger than 2 months (or in preterm infants, 50 to 52 weeks' postconceptual age), a hemoglobin level of 9.5 to 10 g/dL is probably the absolute minimum.
3. In infants in their first week of life, infants weighing less than 1500 g, and infants with cardiac or pulmonary disease, a preoperative hemoglobin level of 12 g/dL or higher is advisable.
4. If the hemoglobin levels are lower than these recommended levels and the operation is purely elective, the operation may be postponed for 1 month or longer (if the risk of postponing surgery is small), especially if the anemia is associated with apneic episodes (Welborn et al., 1991). The anemia should be evaluated, and supplemental iron therapy may be given during this time.
5. If surgery cannot be postponed, anesthesia agent may then be administered with extreme care.
6. The decision to transfuse intraoperatively should take into consideration the many factors that comprise clinical judgment, including blood volume estimates, preoperative hemoglobin or hematocrit, previous blood transfusion (replacement of HbF in preterm infants), duration of anemia, general condition of the patient, ability to provide adequate tissue oxygenation (cardiopulmonary function and cardiac output), extent of surgical procedure, probability of massive blood loss, and risks versus benefits of transfusion.

GUIDELINES FOR TRANSFUSION OF CRITICALLY ILL INFANTS

Although precise indications for blood transfusion in critically ill infants cannot be given, a decline in available oxygen or central venous PO_2 is the most sensitive indicator of the severity of anemia and is very useful in deciding when to transfuse. The following guidelines may be useful.

1. A cumulative record of blood losses should be kept on all critically ill infants admitted to neonatal units. An infant sufficiently ill to require frequent blood sampling may have such blood losses replaced, especially when 10% of the estimated blood volume has been exceeded. For the infant with low PaO_2, there is a lower threshold for early replacement of blood withdrawn.
2. Infants during the first week of life who weigh less than 1500 g should have a hemoglobin value greater than 12 g/dL. In the presence of cardiac or pulmonary disease resulting in a lower PaO_2, the infant hemoglobin level may be maintained in the range of 16 to 17 g/dL.
3. At several weeks of age, when the clinical status of the preterm infant may have been stabilized, transfusion may or may not be needed at the nadir of the anemia. (a) Infants without compromised cardiopulmonary function and in whom no unusual metabolic needs exist are unlikely to be aided by transfusions when the hemoglobin level is greater than 10 or 11 g/dL. (b) Infants who had been previously transfused with HbA are usually able to tolerate lower levels of hemoglobin because of improved tissue oxygen delivery. (c) Premature infants at the nadir of their anemia when hemoglobin levels may be as low as 7 to 8 g/dL should not receive supplemental red blood cell transfusions unless they manifest clinical signs of tissue hypoxemia.
4. Other indications for blood transfusion in critically ill infants include improving oxygen delivery in infants with respiratory distress syndrome and stabilizing cardiac dynamics in some forms of acyanotic congenital heart disease. In infants with respiratory distress syndrome, if PaO_2 is greater than 50 mm Hg, transfusion of blood containing HbA improves oxygen delivery.

The most common blood component used is packed red blood cells, which have a hematocrit value between 70% and 80%. An average of 1 mL/kg packed red blood cells raises the hematocrit value by 1.5%.

■ REDUCTION IN BLOOD LOSS

■ PREOPERATIVE ASSESSMENT AND PREPARATION

The importance of preoperative assessment of anemia and hemostasis cannot be overemphasized. Preoperative anemia should be thoroughly evaluated and, if time permits, appropriately treated. Patients, patients' families, or both should be questioned about history of bleeding after previous surgery; family history; severe renal, liver, and other systemic diseases; and history of medications in the past 2 weeks (nonsteroidal anti-inflammatory drugs). The clinical assessment then determines the need for further testing to investigate possible disturbances of hemostasis.

■ SURGICAL AND ANESTHETIC TECHNIQUES

Although blood loss can be controlled by meticulous and expeditious surgical techniques, anesthesiologists should be aware of the anesthetic factors that may increase bleeding. This includes light anesthesia, intraoperative hypertension, systemic or regional increase in venous pressure, hyperdynamic circulation (increased cardiac output), and hypercapnia. Thus the anesthetic technique should be planned and executed to avoid increased blood loss.

During light anesthesia, bleeding may increase because of increases in skin and muscle blood flow. The redistribution of cardiac output during anesthesia has been recognized for years and has been reconfirmed during isoflurane anesthesia (Gelman et al., 1984). Coughing, bucking, increased airway resistance, airway obstruction, venous obstruction, inadequate muscular relaxation, positive end-expiratory pressure (PEEP), improper positioning, fluid overload, and congestive heart failure can cause an increase in central venous pressure and increased venous oozing.

Hypercapnia may increase bleeding by augmenting cardiac output and increasing blood pressure. To avoid hypercapnia, it is essential that the anesthesiologist (1) understand the basics of anesthetic equipment, including monitoring devices; (2) detect an abnormal arterial carbon dioxide tension ($PaCO_2$); (3) recognize potential causes of hypercapnia; and (4) correct these problems (Salem, 1987). Because clinical signs are unreliable in detecting hypercapnia (Cullen and Eger, 1974; Don, 1983; Nunn, 1993), it is essential that ventilation be monitored during anesthesia.

■ POSITIONING

Much of the physiology of posture can be learned from the giraffe (Warren, 1974). Because the head of this animal is far above its heart, the task of supplying it with oxygenated blood calls for a remarkably high blood pressure. At heart level, its blood pressure is much higher than in normal humans, approximately 260/160 mm Hg. Nevertheless, the pressure at which the brain is perfused is the same in the giraffe, humans, and most other animals (Warren, 1974; Salem, 1978) (Fig. 12–5).

In a normal subject, in the supine position the arterial (and venous) pressures are the same in various parts of the body. Moving from the supine to the erect position results in considerable changes in arterial pressures. Parts above the heart are perfused at lower pressures, whereas parts below the heart are perfused at higher pressures. Similar changes occur in the veins. In the standing position, the venous pressure is near zero above the heart and is subatmospheric in the cerebral sinuses where venous

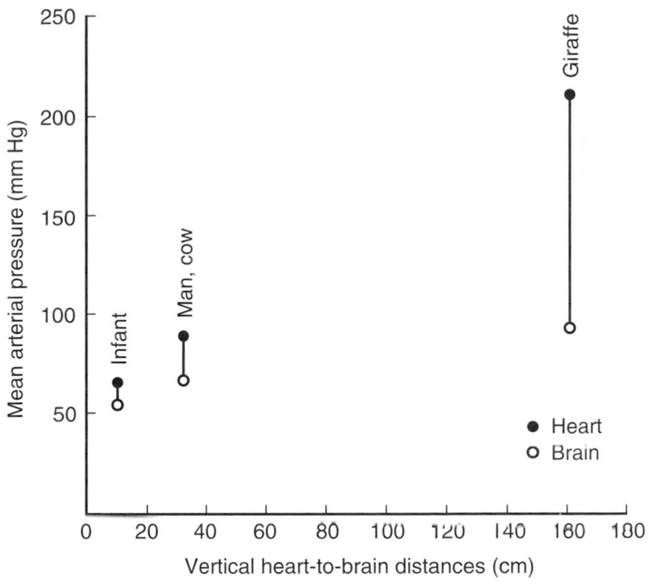

■ **FIGURE 12–5.** Mean arterial pressures at the heart and brain levels in various animals and man. While there is an appreciable difference between mean arterial pressure in the giraffe and in man at the level of the heart, the pressure perfusing the brain is the same in both species. (From Feldman Z, Narayan RK: Intracranial pressure monitoring: Techniques and pitfalls. In Cooper PR, editor. *Head injury*. Baltimore, 1993, Williams & Wilkins.)

collapse is prevented (Hainsworth, 1985). Below the heart level, the venous pressure progressively increases, reaching its highest levels in the feet. Vertical tilting produces a gradient of about 2 mm Hg for each inch of vertical height above which the arterial pressure is recorded, and it produces similar increases below the level of the heart. In the adult patient of average height (68 inches), the difference between arterial pressure at the head and that at the feet could be as great as 120 mm Hg. Because of their smaller stature, gravitational effects in arterial and venous pressures are less in children (and even much less in infants) than in adults. When head-up tilting is used during surgery, pressure gradients should be taken into consideration. Either an estimate of the pressure gradient is calculated at the heart and head (brain), or the transducer (in the case of arterial cannulation) is positioned parallel to the site where the perfusion pressure is measured.

With vertical tilting, twice as much blood can accumulate in the legs, and even larger volumes can be accommodated in the abdomen. Tilting also increases the capillary pressure in dependent parts, and, if the tilt is prolonged, increased filtration results in tissue edema, ultimately reducing blood volume. The converse is seen in elevated parts when tissue fluid is effectively reabsorbed.

In awake individuals, tilting initiates increased sympathetic and baroreceptor reflex activity, which leads to an increased production of catecholamines and plasma renin activity, in turn inducing the formation of angiotensin II with aldosterone release and sodium and water retention. These mechanisms result in constriction of the capacitance vessels, thus enhancing the venous return, whereas constriction of the resistance vessels (arterioles) minimizes the decrease in arterial pressure. The effects of these mechanisms become evident 15 to 30 minutes after tilting. In the normal subject, little change occurs in arterial pressure at the heart level during tilting or standing, although heart rate may increase. Anesthetics, ganglionic, and β-adrenergic–blocking drugs interfere with these compensatory mechanisms. Consequently, head-up tilt in the anesthetized patient favors arterial hypotension. Hypotension also tends to occur with the use of muscle relaxants and controlled ventilation.

Although tilting is less effective in infants and children compared with adults, the combination of decreased arterial and venous pressure above the heart and peripheral venous pooling below the heart makes tilting useful in reducing bleeding in pediatric head and neck procedures. It can also be used postoperatively to reduce swelling and edema. Added benefit may be derived in reducing postoperative laryngeal and upper airway edema after airway manipulations, instrumentation, and intubation.

If the prone position is used, as in scoliosis surgery, meticulous attention should be given to positioning so that adverse effects are avoided. The vertebral venous system provides channels into which blood may be diverted from the lower parts of the body if the inferior vena cava is partially or completely obstructed. Any rise in abdominal pressure (increased muscle tone, external pressure on the abdomen, gastric inflation, coughing, bucking, airway obstruction, and increased airway pressure) tends to increase inferior vena cava pressure and causes blood to be diverted into the vertebral venous plexuses, resulting in increased oozing during surgery. Complete relaxation of the diaphragm and the abdominal musculature decreases the intra-abdominal pressure as well as the inferior vena cava pressure and therefore is desirable to reduce bleeding (Relton, 1975).

Probably no modification has greater impact on minimizing blood loss during scoliosis correction than the use of specially designed frames (Relton and Hall, 1967; Relton, 1975; Schwentker, 1978). When the patient is positioned on the frame, the abdomen is free of pressure, and the pressure on the inferior vena cava is minimized (Fig. 12–6). Also, by avoiding abdominal pressure, the functional residual capacity can be maintained at a near-normal level, helping to prevent atelectasis and hypoxemia.

INFILTRATION WITH VASOCONSTRICTORS

A commonly used method of reducing bleeding involves local infiltration of the skin and subcutaneous tissues with a solution containing a vasoconstrictor drug, usually epinephrine. An undesirable side effect of epinephrine is cardiac arrhythmias. Certain anesthetics such as halothane sensitize the myocardium to epinephrine. The dose of epinephrine needed to produce arrhythmias is lower in halothane-anesthetized patients than in those who are awake. Johnston and associates (1976) determined the median effective dose (ED_{50}) of epinephrine in adult patients; this variable was defined by the appearance of three premature ventricular contractions at any time during or immediately after the subcutaneous injection of epinephrine. The ED_{50} for epinephrine and halothane was 2.1 mcg/kg; for halothane-lidocaine-epinephrine, it was 3.7 mcg/kg. The ED_{50} for enflurane was 10.9 mcg/kg, whereas for isoflurane it was 6.7 mcg/kg (Fig. 12–7). Accordingly, for subcutaneous infiltration in adults the maximum doses of epinephrine recommended as unlikely to produce arrhythmias with halothane and isoflurane are 1, 3, and 5.5 mcg/kg, respectively. The "arrhythmogenic" dose of epinephrine during sevoflurane anesthesia seems to be similar to that during isoflurane anesthesia (Navarro et al., 1994). Thiopental lowers the arrhythmogenic threshold when administered with any of the inhalation anesthetics (Atlee and Roberts, 1986; Hayashi et al., 1988).

Children seem to have a higher arrhythmogenic threshold for epinephrine than do adults. Ueda and associates (1983) found that a mean epinephrine dose of 7.8 mcg/kg given with lidocaine was safe during halothane anesthesia for closure of the cleft palate. Karl and others (1983) found that no arrhythmias occurred during various pediatric operations using cutaneous infiltration of 1:100,000 epinephrine (2 to 15 mcg/kg), with a wide range of halothane concentrations. They concluded that at least 10 mcg/kg of subcutaneous epinephrine could be used safely with a normal or lower-than-normal $Pa{CO_2}$. Furthermore, adding lidocaine to the epinephrine solution increases the margin of safety. If a large volume is required, as in scoliosis correction, a 1:500,000 solution may be used.

Infiltration with epinephrine solution to reduce bleeding is used in various minor and major pediatric surgical procedures. One drawback of epinephrine infiltration is that it may produce swelling and distortion of the tissues if an excessive volume is injected. This may interfere with a "precise" repair in certain plastic surgery operations. Close monitoring to detect arrhythmias is essential during and after epinephrine infiltration.

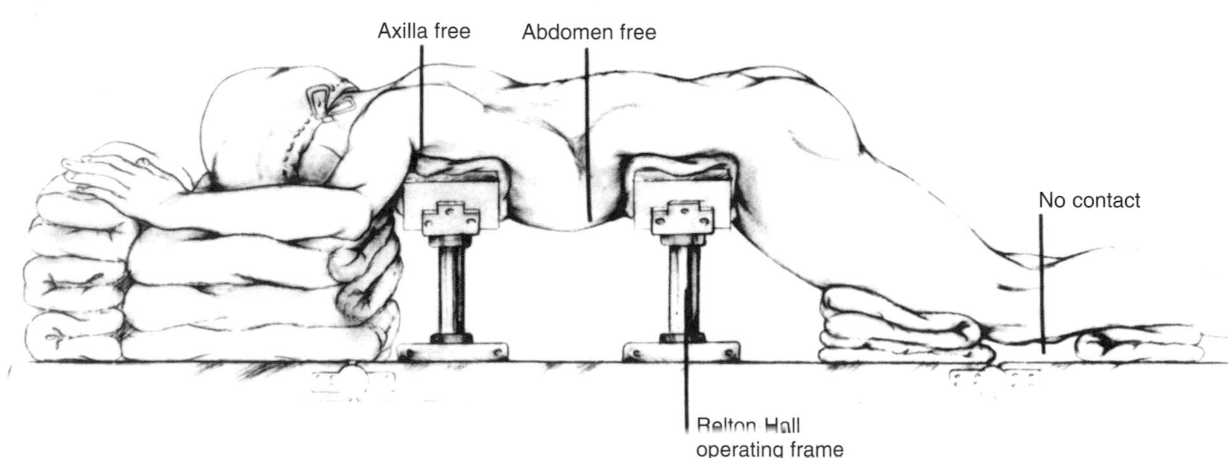

FIGURE 12–6. Position of patient on Relton-Hall frame. (From Schwenker EP: Posterior fusion of the spine for scoliosis. *Surg Rounds* 1:12, 1978, with permission.)

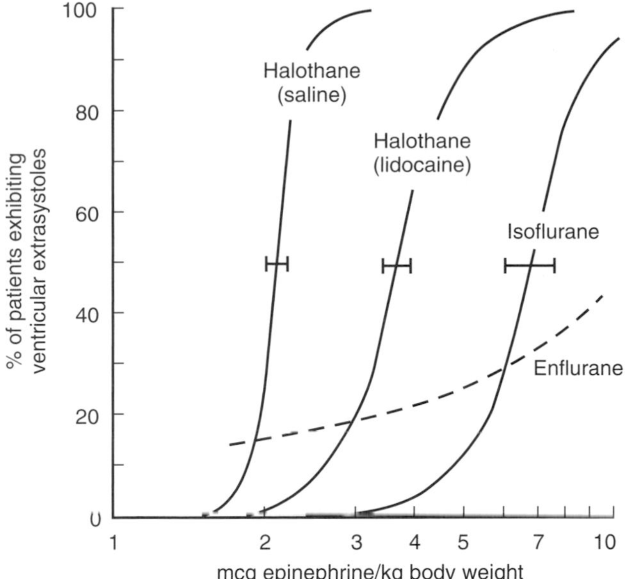

■ **FIGURE 12–7.** Submucosal doses of epinephrine produce PVCs in patients during 1.25 MAC inhalation anesthesia. Notice that the enflurane curve is flat. (Modified from Johnston RR, Eger EI, Wilson C: A comparative interaction of epinephrine with enflurane, isoflurane, and halothane in man. *Anesth Analg* 55:516, 1976, with permission.)

TOURNIQUETS

The use of pneumatic tourniquets after exsanguination of the upper and lower extremity decreases blood loss and permits a bloodless operative field. The tourniquet is placed over the arm, thigh, or leg (depending on the site of surgery) over cotton padding. After the limb is raised, an Esmarch bandage is applied tightly to exsanguinate that portion of the limb distal to the tourniquet. The tourniquet is then inflated to a pressure 100 mm Hg above systolic pressure for a lower extremity and 50 mm Hg above systolic pressure for an upper extremity. The size of the cuff is important; the width should be greater than half the limb's diameter. The main concerns associated with the use of tourniquets include hemodynamic, metabolic, and respiratory changes as a result of inflation and deflation; tourniquet pain; and potential injury to nerves and muscles if inflation is prolonged.

After tourniquet inflation, progressive decreases in venous pH and PO_2 and increases in venous PCO_2, lactate, intracellular enzymes, and potassium occur. Creatine phosphate and nicotinamide adenine dinucleotide stores decrease in muscles within 30 to 50 minutes. When the tourniquet is deflated, products of anaerobic metabolism enter the circulation, causing a transient state of reactive hyperemia and a mixed respiratory and metabolic acidosis. Mixed venous oxygen saturation ($S\bar{v}O_2$) may fall 20% in 1 minute. The accumulated acid metabolites are buffered by plasma bicarbonate, resulting in the release of CO_2 and increase in $PaCO_2$ (and $PETCO_2$).

Time for clearance of the accumulated metabolites after tourniquet deflation depends on duration of inflation, levels of metabolites before deflation, the extremity exsanguinated (upper versus lower and one versus both), efficacy of the buffering capacity, patient's circulatory status, ventilation, and the patient's response to the extra load of metabolites. The time to maximal increase in $PETCO_2$ is 1.5 to 2.5 minutes (Bourke et al., 1989). The maximum increase in $PETCO_2$ is approximately 3 mm Hg after the release of an upper extremity tourniquet and about 9 mm Hg after the release of a lower extremity tourniquet (Dickson et al., 1990).

Because of the higher metabolic rate in infants and children, it was assumed that tourniquet hemostasis might result in a greater accumulation of ischemic metabolites and that physiologic compensation might not be adequate. Lynn and associates (1986) found that children tolerated tourniquet release with fewer hemodynamic changes than have been reported in adults. A slight decrease in systolic blood pressure (8 to 10 mm Hg), lasting less than 10 minutes with no change in heart rate, was noted. The potassium levels increased slightly with tourniquet deflation but remained within the normal range. The respiratory acidosis was quickly compensated, but the metabolic acidosis persisted for longer than 10 minutes after tourniquet release. Large increases in lactate were seen with long inflation times (more than 75 minutes) and when bilateral tourniquets were used. The greatest decrease in arterial pH was seen when bilateral tourniquets were deflated simultaneously.

The following measures are recommended to minimize the systemic and metabolic consequences after tourniquet release: (1) attempt to limit inflation times to less than 75 minutes; (2) monitor $PETCO_2$ closely before and after the release of tourniquet; (3) if controlled ventilation is used, minute ventilation should be increased by 50% just before and for 5 minutes after tourniquet deflation; and (4) if a Mapleson D circuit is used, an increase in fresh gas flow may be needed to maintain $PETCO_2$ at a near-normal level after tourniquet deflation. These measures are of great importance with long tourniquet inflation times (>75 minutes) and when bilateral tourniquets are deflated simultaneously or within 30 minutes of each other.

A progressive increase in temperature in anesthetized infants and children (0.4° to 1.6°C) can occur during prolonged leg tourniquet inflation (90 minutes), and a greater increase (1.1° to 2.3°C) can occur with bilateral leg tourniquets (Mostello et al., 1991; Bloch et al., 1992). This slight hyperthermia may be related to a decrease in the effective heat loss from the skin and an altered distribution of heat within the body. Thus, during prolonged leg tourniquet inflation, attention should be given to the patient's temperature.

The use of tourniquets in patients with sickle cell disease has been discouraged for fear that it may lead to circulatory stasis, acidosis, and hypoxemia, the triad known to induce sickling. Clinical experience in a limited number of patients with sickle cell disease suggests that tourniquets are not associated with harmful effects, provided oxygenation and mild hyperventilation are maintained (Adu-Gyamfi et al., 1993). These patients should not be denied the benefits of tourniquets when indicated, but the usual precautions for tourniquet use should be adhered to.

A dull aching pain may occur 45 minutes after tourniquet inflation in awake children undergoing limb surgery, despite a successful regional anesthetic. The pain becomes unbearable with time but subsides immediately after tourniquet deflation. Attempts to relieve upper extremity tourniquet pain by stellate ganglion block, intercostobrachial nerve block, or intravenous opioids are usually ineffective. Tourniquet pain has been correlated with the sensory level, type of regional anesthetic technique, the local anesthetic, and the dose administered. Prophylaxis includes a high level of spinal or epidural anesthesia (for the lower extremity) and the addition of an opioid to the local anesthetic used for neural blockade. Therapy includes general anesthesia or tourniquet deflation.

Prolonged ischemia results in mitochondrial swelling, myelin degeneration, depletion of glycogen storage, Z-line lysis, and tissue edema. Thromboxane is released with disruption of endothelial integrity. Within 30 minutes of inflation, nerve conduction ceases, reflecting ischemia or direct extrinsic pressure on the nerves by the tourniquet. Paralysis after tourniquet use, although very rare, is a known complication. Direct pressure caused by the cuff is probably the main cause of nerve lesions, although ischemic injury may also play a part. Tourniquet paralysis nearly always resolves spontaneously, although recovery can be slow. If prolonged inflation (>90 minutes) is required, the tourniquet should be deflated periodically every 75 to 90 minutes to minimize the risk of postoperative neurapraxis.

To minimize the risk of complications from excessive inflation pressures, the use of wider tourniquet cuffs and minimal inflation pressures has been suggested. It has also been suggested that with the use of a hypotensive technique, it is possible to decrease the applied tourniquet inflation pressure to 110 to 140 mm Hg, while maintaining a bloodless surgical field (Tuncali et al., 2003). This technique may lead to reduction of complications due to excessive tourniquet inflation.

PREVENTION AND TREATMENT OF HYPOTHERMIA

During hypothermia, platelet dysfunction, impaired coagulation, and enhanced fibrinolytic activity can occur. Valeri and associates (1992) showed that local skin hypothermia produces an increased bleeding time and a marked reduction in thromboxane B_2 level at the bleeding site. Conversely, local rewarming produces an increase in shed blood thromboxane B_2 level. This hemostatic defect has been attributed to the involvement of platelet glycoprotein receptor (glycoprotein Ib and granule membrane protein 140) alteration. The enzymatic reaction of the coagulation cascade is strongly inhibited by hypothermia, as demonstrated by the dramatic prolongation of prothrombin time and activated partial thromboplastin time (Rohrer and Natale, 1992). The contribution of hypothermia to the hemolytic diathesis may be overlooked, because coagulation testing is performed at 37°C rather than at the patient's actual body temperature.

Although a few studies suggested that the indices of platelet activation during cardiopulmonary bypass vary similarly in hypothermic and normothermic patients (Mazer et al., 1995), the evidence is overwhelming that hypothermia contributes to increased bleeding (Rohrer and Natalie, 1992; Valeri et al., 1992; Yau et al., 1992). When bleeding without an obvious surgical cause is encountered in a hypothermic patient, rewarming may simply correct the hypothermia-induced coagulopathy. Operating under normothermic conditions may also decrease bleeding and the use of blood products and antifibrinolytics (Rohrer and Natale, 1992).

MINIMIZING BLOOD SAMPLING FOR LABORATORY TESTING

Laboratory testing is an often-overlooked source of blood loss in critically ill patients. Despite the use of micromethods, cumulative blood loss through sampling for laboratory measurements can have a great impact on hemoglobin levels. Much of the transfusion requirement in sick premature infants is a direct consequence of blood removed for laboratory use. The removal of 1 mL of blood from a 1-kg infant is equivalent to removing 70 mL of blood from an average adult. Various approaches to minimizing iatrogenic blood loss are presented in Box 12–2.

BOX 12–2 Techniques to Minimize Iatrogenic Blood Loss

Avoidance of Unnecessary Phlebotomy

Heightening staff awareness of iatrogenic blood loss
Charting cumulative diagnostic blood loss
Ordering tests according to need rather than by rigid protocol
Reliance on noninvasive (Sao_2 and $ETco_2$) or continuous "in-line" arterial and mixed venous blood gas/saturation monitors
Multiple tests from a single phlebotomy (Batch ordering)

Limiting Sample Volume

Modifying laboratory procedures regarding sample volume
Use of pediatric blood collection tubes
Use of analyzers requiring smaller samples (microsamples)
Use of whole blood stat laboratory and bedside ("point of care" technology) analyzers

Decreasing Blood Waste

Use of small dead space tubing sets
Reinfusion of dead space (discard) volume

PHARMACOLOGIC ENHANCEMENT OF HEMOSTATIC ACTIVITY

Studies continue to define the role of antifibrinolytics, desmopressin, and aprotinin for modulating hemostasis in surgical patients, especially during cardiopulmonary bypass.

Desmopressin

Desmopressin (DDAVP) is an analogue of the natural hormone vasopressin. Deamination of cysteine in position 1 allows for an increase in the antidiuretic, or V_2, effect. Through its V_2 effects, DDAVP causes endothelial cells to release von Willebrand factor, tissue-type plasminogen activator, and certain prostaglandins. An increase in the release of von Willebrand factor accounts for the hemostatic activity of DDAVP by promoting platelet adhesion to the vascular endothelium. A single dose of 10 mcg/m^2 of DDAVP after the induction of anesthesia could reduce intraoperative bleeding by 30% in patients undergoing spinal fusion with normotensive anesthesia (Kobrinsky et al., 1987); however, some have found that it does not reduce bleeding in patients without a known bleeding diathesis (Guay et al., 1992). The differences in these findings may be attributed to the side effects of DDAVP, including the release of tissue-type plasminogen activator, producing fibrinolysis and its vasodilator effect, which tend to offset the beneficial release of von Willebrand factor. It is also possible that bleeding in certain operations on bony tissues is particularly difficult to control and may not be readily influenced by substances that modify hemostasis, because blood vessels in bone are noncollapsible structures and consequently remain open when the bone is cut. Although randomized trials have shown no benefit from DDAVP on transfusion requirements when used nonselectively, this drug has been associated with reduction in allogenic transfusion in patients receiving aspirin before cardiac surgery and in patients with documented depression of platelet function after cardiopulmonary bypass (Mongan and Hosking, 1992; Dilthey et al., 1993).

Aprotinin

Aprotinin, a proteinase inhibitor, has been reported to decrease blood loss during cardiac and orthopedic surgery and liver transplantation (Van Oeveren et al., 1987; Alajmo et al., 1989; Dietrich et al., 1990; Havel et al., 1991; Janssens et al., 1994). Several mechanisms have been proposed to explain the observed decrease in blood loss with high-dose aprotinin:

1. It inhibits the fibrinolytic activity both via direct inhibition of plasmin and via inhibition of the kinin-kallikrein system. Decreased production of bradykinin reduces the release of tissue plasminogen activator, resulting in decreased formation of plasmin.
2. It has a protective effect on platelet function.
3. It partially inhibits the intrinsic coagulation pathway with preservation of the extrinsic system.

Although the exact hemostatic mechanisms of aprotinin are under investigation and remain to be elucidated, its inhibition of the intrinsic coagulation pathway has been confirmed.

In patients undergoing hip replacement, high-dose aprotinin (2 million kallikrein inactivator units [KIU] followed by an infusion of 500,000 KIU per hour until the end of surgery) resulted in a decrease in blood loss of approximately 25%, allowing almost 50% reduction in transfusion (Janssens et al., 1994). No adverse effects of aprotinin on renal or hepatic function have been reported, and the incidence of deep venous thrombosis was not increased. Aprotinin treatment alone is insufficient to avoid transfusion in most patients. However, when combined with other blood conservation measures, blood transfusions are substantially decreased or virtually eliminated in certain operations. Although aprotinin is expensive, the economic benefit of reducing the requirement for blood transfusion may justify the cost.

DELIBERATE HYPOTENSION

HISTORICAL BACKGROUND

The concept of intentional reduction of the blood pressure to decrease blood loss and thereby decrease the need for allogenic blood transfusion and improve operative conditions for intracranial surgery was first proposed by Cushing in 1917. Gardner (1946) reported on the deliberate decrease in blood pressure in neurosurgical procedures by arteriotomy. The blood removed was kept in heparinized bottles and reinfused at the end of the procedure. The many complications ("irreversible shock," tissue hypoxemia, acidosis, and overheparinization) indicated that the boundaries of physiologic trespass were broken down, and the technique was abandoned. Griffiths and Gillies (1948) advocated the use of high spinal analgesia to induce hypotension and to produce relatively bloodless conditions for certain operations. The major advancement with normovolemic hypotension was achieved when ganglionic blockade was combined with foot-down tilt. Enderby (1950) described the new method as "controlled circulation with hypotensive drugs and posture to reduce bleeding in surgery." The enthusiastic initial reception was followed by reports of unexplained morbidity and mortality (Hampton and Little, 1953).

After initial investigations of the use of hexamethonium (C_6), one of the series of polymethylene bistrimethyl ammonium salts, attention was drawn to pentolinium, which proved to be superior to other drugs. The knowledge that triethylsulfonium salts, like the quaternary and bisquarternary ammonium ions, possess ganglionic blocking activity culminated in the synthesis of trimethaphan (also known as trimetaphan) (Magill et al., 1953). Because it was short acting, trimethaphan offered a new dimension in the control of blood pressure through continuous infusion. Its short action has been surpassed only by sodium nitroprusside, which was introduced into clinical practice in 1962 by Moraca and associates.

The effects of controlled ventilation and *d*-tubocurarine on blood pressure had become apparent by 1952. The introduction of halothane achieved a remarkable breakthrough and allowed an easier and more gentle induction of hypotension with and without ganglionic blockade (Enderby, 1960). This milestone in vascular control was responsible for a great improvement in safety (Enderby, 1985a). β-Adrenergic–blocking drugs were introduced to treat and prevent tachycardia (Hellewell and Potts, 1966; Salem and Ivankovich, 1970). The discovery that labetalol given intravenously was effective in the treatment of severe hypertension prompted its use in hypotensive anesthesia (Scott et al., 1978). Nitroglycerin was introduced as a hypotensive drug by Fahmy in 1978.

The use of controlled hypotension in pediatric surgery was first reported by Anderson and McKissock in 1953. In 1974, Salem and his associates reported on the use of deliberate hypotension in 137 pediatric patients and concluded that the technique offered definite advantages and played a major role in the success of certain surgical procedures. Thereafter, deliberate hypotension became widely used in various pediatric surgical procedures, including scoliosis surgery, primary excision in burned children, vascular surgery, and neurosurgery (McNeill et al., 1974; Szyfelbein and Ryan, 1974; Diaz and Lockhart, 1979). Advances in understanding of the physiology and pharmacology of deliberate hypotension, as well as in the application of the newer monitoring techniques, have all contributed to the evolution and safety of the technique.

TECHNIQUES FOR INDUCING HYPOTENSION

Hypotensive drugs have been used in modern anesthetic practice to achieve one or more of the following goals (Salem, 1978): (1) reduction in blood loss, (2) facilitation of vessel surgery, and (3) improvement of myocardial performance by reducing the preload and afterload.

Many drugs and techniques have been described for the induction of hypotension (Adams, 1975; Salem, 1978; Green, 1985). Most of them rely on a combination of physiologic and pharmacologic means for inducing hypotension.

Two basic hypotensive anesthetic techniques currently in use are (1) the conventional technique and (2) deep anesthesia, with or without head-up tilt and PEEP (Box 12–3).

Conventional Technique

Hypotension is to be induced only when a steady state of light anesthesia is ensured and airway patency is secured with tracheal intubation. A reliable intravenous catheter and basic monitoring, including accurate blood pressure measurements, should be established before hypotension is initiated. Light anesthesia may be achieved with either an opioid–nitrous oxide–oxygen mixture

BOX 12–3 Techniques of Induced Hypotension

Requirements Before Inducing Hypotension

Stable clinical state
Secure airway (tracheal intubation)
Reliable intravenous catheters, basic monitoring
Means of accurate blood pressure measurements
Light anesthesia: inhalation anesthetic (with or without relaxants), or nitrous oxide, propofol, opioid, relaxant
Controlled ventilation

Conventional Technique

Steps of inducing gradual hypotension:

1. Intravenous administration of a vasodilator or a ganglionic blocker; a β-adrenergic–blocking drug may be given before the hypotensive drug
2. Tilting (if feasible)
3. Gradual increase of inhalation anesthetic (rarely used)
4. PEEP (very rarely needed)

Alternative Technique

Deep anesthesia (halothane or isoflurane) with tilting, PEEP, or both (very rarely needed or used)

supplemented with a muscle relaxant or with a volatile anesthetic, while ventilation is controlled. With the patient in the horizontal position, hypotension is then induced gradually with the aid of a hypotensive drug (a comparison of five hypotensive drugs is shown in Table 12–2). The drug is administered at least 10 minutes before surgery commences if hypotension is required before the incision is made. If surgery is to be performed with the patient in the prone position, hypotension is induced after the patient is carefully positioned and proper placement of the tracheal tube is verified. It is preferable to give a β-adrenergic–blocking drug before the hypotensive drug is administered. The time of the onset of hypotension depends on the drug given (see Table 12–2).

After the effect of the drug (or drugs) is assessed, the patient is then tilted (head-up or foot-down). In some patients a hypotensive response may not be evident in the horizontal position, but subsequent tilting results in a decrease in the arterial pressure as a result of peripheral venous pooling. The patient should not be tilted too quickly. Cerebral autoregulation requires several minutes (Salem, 1975; Patel, 1981). Head-up tilt may not be feasible in some operations (hip and back surgery). However, some degree of peripheral pooling may be obtained by lowering the legs while maintaining the operative site horizontally. A further decrease in arterial pressure can be obtained by a gradual increase in the concentration of the volatile anesthetic. This is particularly useful when tilting is not possible.

Deep Anesthesia With or Without Tilting and PEEP

Some anesthesiologists prefer to initiate hypotension by deepening the anesthetic level or relying on posture to maintain the hypotensive state without the use of hypotensive drugs (Thompson et al., 1978; Diaz and Lockhart, 1979). Dose-related depression of cardiovascular function by inhalational anesthetics has been well documented. The extent of this depression varies among anesthetics (Calverley et al., 1978; Merin, 1981). In healthy individuals, both halothane and enflurane have minimal effects on the systemic vascular resistance, and reduced arterial pressure is secondary to a dose-dependent decrease in left ventricular function. Isoflurane decreases the arterial pressure by decreasing the systemic vascular resistance, whereas the cardiac output is well preserved even at twice the minimum alveolar concentration (MAC) because of the associated decrease in afterload (Lam and Gelb, 1983; Van Aken and Cottrell, 1986). The intravascular volume status contributes to the decrease in cardiac output during isoflurane anesthesia. Halothane has little effect on heart rate, whereas enflurane produces a dose-related increase in heart rate. Isoflurane also increases heart rate, although the increase is not dose related. The effects of sevoflurane and desflurane seem to be similar to those of isoflurane (Pagel et al., 1994). Because of the impairment of the myocardial contractile function, the use of volatile anesthetics as the sole means of inducing hypotension is not recommended (Prys-Roberts et al., 1974). With high concentrations of volatile anesthetics, blood pressure control may be difficult, and the return of blood pressure to a normal level may be sluggish when the anesthetic is discontinued.

As a result of the decreased cerebrovascular resistance, halothane increases cerebral blood flow in a dose-dependent manner. Intracranial pressure may also increase as a result of increased intracranial blood volume. Cerebral autoregulation is lost with increasing anesthetic concentration. Isoflurane (up to 1 MAC) produces a concentration-related depression of cerebral metabolism, whereas the physiologic relationships between flow and pressure and between flow and metabolism are preserved (Van Aken and Van Hemelrijck, 1993). With higher concentrations, the vasodilator effect predominates; autoregulation is impaired and cerebral blood flow increases (Van Aken and Cottrell, 1986; Madsen et al., 1987). Higher concentrations also interfere with the somatosensory evoked potential (SSEP) monitoring (see Chapter 9, Anesthetic Equipment and Monitoring). Even low concentrations of isoflurane can provoke increases in intracranial pressure in patients with reduced intracranial compliance, and cerebral edema may occur, especially if blood pressure increases (Grosslight et al., 1985). Isoflurane-induced hypotension increases both brain edema and neurologic deficits in dogs with cryogenic brain lesions in contrast to dogs given labetalol (Bendo et al., 1993). A hypotensive technique based on a combination of α- and β-adrenergic receptor–blocking drugs with light isoflurane attenuates the undesirable effects of isoflurane when used as the sole hypotensive drug (Toivonen et al., 1992). Because intracranial pressure increases before the dura is open and cerebral edema may develop, inhalational anesthetics should not be used as the sole means of inducing hypotension in patients with intracranial lesions (Van Aken and Van Hemelrijck, 1993).

Positive End-Expiratory Pressure

Increased mean airway pressure has been used to fine-tune hypotension to the desired level (Salem, 1978; Green, 1985). For example, systolic pressure can be decreased rapidly from 80 to 70 mm Hg by adding PEEP (10 cm H_2O), and this change can be quickly reversed by discontinuing PEEP. PEEP, however, may have the following undesirable effects:

1. It exerts its hypotensive effect by restricting venous return (preload) and thereby reducing cardiac output.
2. It tends to increase intracranial (Shapiro and Marshall, 1978; Luce et al., 1982) and intraocular pressures (Nimmagadda et al., 1991).

TABLE 12–2. Comparison of five hypotensive drugs

Characteristic	Trimethaphan Camphorsulfonate	Sodium Nitroprusside	Nitroglycerin	Labetalol	Esmolol
Onset of action	Rapid onset, usually rapid recovery	Rapid onset, very rapid recovery	Rapid onset, moderately slower recovery	Gradual onset, slower recovery	Rapid onset, rapid recovery
Duration	Short acting; may be prolonged with halothane and propranolol	Evanescent action; prolonged with cyanide toxicity	Short acting	Long acting	Very short acting
Method of administration	IV drip (0.2% in D_5W solution)	IV drip (0.01% solution)	IV drip (0.01% in D_5W or 0.9% NaCl)	IV injection, repeated increments	IV drip followed by constant infusion
Mode of action	Ganglionic blockade, direct effect, α-adrenergic blockade, histamine release?	Direct effect (resistance and capacitance vessels)	Direct effect, capacitance vessels predominantly	α- and β-Adrenoceptor antagonist	β_1-Selective adrenoceptor antagonist
Tachycardia	Occurs in children (less likely in adults)	Very common	May occur in children (unlikely in adults)	None, usually slight bradycardia	None, usually slight bradycardia
Cardiac output	May remain unchanged, increase, or decrease, depending on posture (venous pooling), changes in heart rate, preload and afterload, anesthetics, other myocardium-depressant drugs, ventilation, intravascular volume status			Slight decrease	Slight decrease
Blood-brain barrier	Minimal or no derangement	Pronounced dysfunction	Probably same as sodium nitroprusside	Probably none	Probably none
Metabolism	Unclear, inhibits plasma cholinesterase but not metabolized by it	Metabolized to cyanide and thiocyanate	Degraded rapidly in the liver	Degraded in the liver	Rapidly metabolized by esterases in cytosol of red blood cells, not by plasma cholinesterases
Stability	Unstable; kept refrigerated	Available as powder, unstable when reconstituted, protect from light, use within 12 h	Stable; colorless, absorbed by plastics, use high-density polyethylene drip set	Stable	Stable
Dose	Total IV dose should not exceed 10 mg/kg	Initial dose 0.5 to 1.5 mcg/kg/min, dose usually <8 mcg/kg/min Total dose not to exceed 1.5 mg/kg in 4 hr	10-20 mcg/kg/min	0.2 to 0.4 mg/kg followed by increments of 0.1 to 0.2 mg/kg	500 mcg/kg/min loading dose plus 300 mcg/kg/min constant infusion
Histamine release	Histamine release related to administration rate	Unknown	Unknown	Unknown	Unknown
Neuromuscular function	A weak nondepolarizing effect in large doses	Probably no effect	A weak nondepolarizing effect	Probably no effect	Slight prolongation of succinylcholine-induced neuromuscular blockade
Rebound hypertension	Does not occur	Occurs in absence of β-blockade	Does not occur	Does not occur	Does not occur
Intracranial pressure	Variable, but may decrease	Increases in early stages, less with hypocapnia	Increases, greater than with trimethaphan	Does not increase	Does not increase

3. Cerebral venous pressure tends to increase, thus reducing perfusion pressure gradient to the brain. Some patients developed critically low jugular bulb oxygen tension, indicating a substantial decrease in cerebral blood flow (Eckenhoff et al., 1963b).
4. Maintaining high alveolar pressure in normal lungs causes increased resting lung volume and physiologic dead space (Eckenhoff et al., 1963a).
5. Excessive PEEP may diminish urine flow (Berry, 1981).
6. In vertebral surgery, PEEP may increase the inferior vena cava pressure, resulting in a diversion of blood into the vertebral venous plexuses and increased bleeding (Relton, 1975).

MODE OF ACTION OF HYPOTENSIVE DRUGS

Normovolemic hypotension can be produced by either a reduction in cardiac output or a decrease in systemic vascular resistance. Drugs with different modes of action have been used alone or in combination with anesthetics or with other drugs to induce hypotension. These drugs may be classified as (1) ganglionic-blocking drugs (e.g., pentolinium, trimethaphan); (2) nitrovasodilators (e.g., sodium nitroprusside and nitroglycerin); (3) α-adrenergic receptor–blocking drugs (e.g., phentolamine, urapidil, nicergoline); (4) β-adrenergic receptor–blocking drugs (e.g., propranolol, esmolol); (5) drugs with combined α- and β-adrenergic receptor–blocking drugs (e.g., labetalol); (6) calcium channel–blocking drugs (e.g., verapamil, nicardipine); and (7) other vasodilators (e.g., hydralazine, adenosine, prostaglandin E_1, fenoldopam).

Vasodilator drugs act primarily on the peripheral circulation. The smaller precapillary arterioles contain relatively large amounts of smooth muscle and thus are the major determinants of resistance. Because systemic vascular resistance is inversely related to arteriolar caliber by approximately the fourth power of the radius, relatively small changes in intraluminal radius have profound effects on systemic vascular resistance (Longnecker, 1985).

Ganglionic-Blocking Drugs

Ganglionic-blocking drugs may compete with acetylcholine for the nicotinic receptors on the postjunctional membrane at the autonomic ganglia. Because most organs are reciprocally innervated by sympathetic and parasympathetic nerves, the overall effect of autonomic blockade depends on the predominance of one or the other system at the end organ. The arterioles and venules of the skin and splanchnic viscera have predominantly sympathetic vasoconstrictor innervation, and ganglionic blockade produces peripheral vasodilation, increased venous capacitance, and hypotension. In contrast, the iris, ciliary muscle, gastrointestinal tract, urinary bladder, and sweat glands are all under predominantly parasympathetic control. Ganglionic blockade thus produces mydriasis, cycloplegia, constipation, urinary retention, and abolition of sweating. Because of these side effects, ganglionic-blocking drugs are no longer used for the treatment of hypertension. However, these side effects are of no consequence after intravenous use during anesthesia (except mydriasis and cycloplegia, which can be misinterpreted in the postoperative neurologic assessment of patients in the early postoperative period).

The hypotensive action of trimethaphan has been attributed to ganglionic blockade, a direct effect on vascular smooth muscle, β-adrenergic blockade, and histamine release (Taylor, 1985). Although histamine release occurs in humans, especially after bolus injections of trimethaphan, it does not play an important role in the hypotensive effect of the drug (Fahmy and Soter, 1985).

Nitrovasodilators

Nitric oxide is produced in cardiac and vascular endothelial cells from the amino acid L-arginine in a reaction requiring the constitutive enzyme nitric oxide synthase (Palmer et al., 1987; Rees et al., 1989a, 1989b; Moncada et al., 1991). Nitric oxide production is stimulated by increases in intracellular calcium, in response to the interaction of a chemical agent in the blood, such as bradykinin or acetylcholine, with its specific membrane receptor or by increases in shear stress. It diffuses into the underlying vascular smooth muscle, where it stimulates production of cyclic guanosine monophosphate, thus causing vascular relaxation. The vasodilating effects of sodium nitroprusside and nitroglycerin, so-called nitrovasodilators, have been explained by their ability to provide exogenous nitric oxide (Kruszyna et al., 1987). Inhaled nitric oxide has been used as a treatment for pulmonary hypertension (Rich et al., 1994).

Sodium nitroprusside exerts its hypotensive action primarily by decreasing systemic vascular resistance, while the venous effect is minimal, so that cardiac output is maintained. In contrast, nitroglycerin has little effect on arteriolar resistance vessels but exhibits relatively pronounced effects on the venous capacitance vessels, resulting in decreased venous return, decreased ventricular filling pressures, and ultimately reduced cardiac output (Longnecker, 1985).

β-Adrenergic–Blocking Drugs

Treatment with a β-adrenergic–blocking drug prevents the increase in heart rate, cardiac output, plasma renin activity, and catecholamine levels and prevents rebound hypertension after cessation of sodium nitroprusside infusion. Furthermore, the dose requirements of sodium nitroprusside are decreased by approximately 40%.

Propranolol given slowly in small increments up to 60 mcg/kg before or after the administration of a hypotensive drug is effective in preventing the rise in heart rate and in facilitating the control of blood pressure (Salem et al., 1974). It is preferable to give propranolol before rather than after the onset of tachycardia, when a much larger dose may be needed. In this dose range, the action of propranolol is almost exclusively ascribed to blockade of the β-adrenergic receptors. Being a nonselective β-adrenergic–blocking drug, propranolol blocks both β_1- (predominantly the heart) and β_2- (predominantly blood vessels and bronchial smooth muscles) receptors. Increased airway resistance in normal subjects and the occurrence of bronchospasm in asthmatics after the use of propranolol led to the development of more selective β_1-adrenergic–blocking drugs. The currently available β-adrenergic–blocking drugs that can be used as adjuvants to hypotensive anesthesia are listed in Table 12–3. Some clinicians have found esmolol-induced hypotension to be more effective than sodium nitroprusside in producing better operative conditions (Blau et al., 1992; Boezaart et al., 1995). Because these drugs can produce severe myocardial depression (especially with anesthetics), these drugs should be used mostly as adjuvants rather than as the sole hypotensive drug (Edmondson et al., 1989). The advantages of esmolol are its rapid onset, titration of action, short duration, and cardioselectivity (Sum et al., 1983; Menkhaus et al., 1985). The drug may be given in a loading dosage of 500 mcg/kg per minute for 2 to 4 minutes and continued via constant infusion at a rate of 300 mcg/kg per minute.

Labetalol

Labetalol acts as a competitive antagonist at both α_1- and β-adrenergic receptors. Its pharmacologic properties include selective blockade of α_1-adrenergic receptors, blockade of β_1- and β_2-adrenergic receptors, partial agonist activity at β_2-receptors, and inhibition of neural uptake of norepinephrine (cocaine-like effect) (Hoffman and Lefkowski, 1990). The potency of labetalol for β-adrenergic blockade is 5-fold to 10-fold that for α-adrenergic blockade. Ten milligrams of labetalol is the equivalent of 2 mg of propranolol at β_1-receptors, 0.75 mg of propranolol at β_2-receptors, and 2 mg of phentolamine (a pure α_1-antagonist) at α-receptors (Scott et al., 1978; Green, 1985; Fahmy et al., 1989; Goldberg et al., 1990). After the administration of labetalol, blood pressure decreases gradually over a 5- to 10-minute period. The hypotensive effect of labetalol is less pronounced when given with intravenous rather than inhalation anesthetics, and therefore the desired level of hypotension cannot always be achieved. Because its elimination half-life is rather

TABLE 12–3. Dose, cardioselectivity, and elimination half-life of currently available β-adrenergic–blocking drugs

Drug	Dose	Cardioselectivity (β_1)	Elimination Half-life
Propranolol	0.06 mg/kg	0	4 hr
Practolol	0.15 mg/kg	+	10 hr
Metoprolol	0.15 mg/kg	+	3 to 4 hr
Esmolol	Loading dose 0.5 mg/kg per minute, followed by 300 mcg/kg per minute (constant infusion)	+	10 min
Labetalol	0.2 to 0.4 mg/kg depending on background anesthetic, additional increments until desired effect	0 (Has α-, β_1-, and β_2-adrenergic–blocking properties)	3.5 to 4.5 hr

long (3 to 6 hours), it may be the preferred hypotensive drug when prolonged hypotension is required. In contrast, its prolonged action may mask the adrenergic response to acute blood loss in the early postoperative period. Labetalol is usually given in an initial dose of 0.2 to 0.4 mg/kg. Incremental doses (half the initial dose) may be repeated after 5 to 10 minutes until the desired hypotension is achieved. It has advantages over sodium nitroprusside, including absence of tachycardia, no increase in cardiac output, no rebound hypertension, no increase in intrapulmonary shunt ($\dot{Q}s/\dot{Q}t$), and no increase in intracranial pressure even in the presence of a reduced intracranial compliance (Van Aken et al., 1982).

Calcium Channel–Blocking Drugs

Nicardipine and verapamil exert their hypotensive effects primarily by decreasing systemic vascular resistance. Because verapamil also produces myocardial depression and delays atrioventricular conduction, it is not recommended for inducing hypotension. Nicardipine has been successfully used as a hypotensive drug during anesthesia. It vasodilates the peripheral, coronary, and cerebral vessels while maintaining the cardiac output without producing tachycardia. Careful titration of nicardipine infusion (10 to 250 mcg/kg per hour) is mandatory because of "increasing effect" over time and because nicardipine-induced hypotension may be resistant to conventional treatment (Flamm et al., 1988; Bernard et al., 1992; Van Aken and Hemelrijck, 1993). Because of these potential problems, calcium channel–blocking drugs are not recommended for use as hypotensive drugs in pediatric patients.

Adenosine

Adenosine, a metabolic end-product of ATP, is an endogenous vasodilator that has been implicated in local regulation of several vascular beds, including the heart and brain. Although ATP has been used as a hypotensive drug, its effect has been attributed to the arterial adenosine concentration (Sollevi et al., 1984). Intravenous infusion of adenosine causes arterial hypotension that is rapidly achieved, easily controlled, short lasting, and not accompanied by rebound hypertension when the infusion is discontinued (Lagerkranser et al., 1984; Sollevi et al., 1984; Crystal et al., 1988). The hypotensive effect of adenosine results entirely from a sharp decrease in systemic vascular resistance with minimal effect on the venous vascular bed because of the rapid degradation of adenosine or the decreased sensitivity of the venous vascular bed for adenosine. Because it increases the coronary blood flow and decreases the afterload, adenosine favorably influences the myocardial oxygen supply/demand balance. However, patients with coronary artery disease may develop signs of myocardial ischemia during adenosine-induced hypotension. Increased cardiac output has been noted. Although decreased heart rate occurs (probably because of direct depressive effect on the sinoatrial node) in dogs, this has not been consistent in humans. Adenosine inhibits renin release in the kidney and therefore prevents the activation of the renin-angiotensin system. β-Adrenergic–blocking drugs are not usually needed to control the heart rate. Adenosine-induced hypotension is not associated with cardiovascular, hematologic, central nervous system, renal, or hepatic toxicity. However, adenosine dilates cerebral vessels, increases intracranial pressure, and impairs autoregulation (Lagerkranser et al., 1984; Van Aken et al., 1984). Other potential adverse features of adenosine include its paradoxical ability to cause renal vasoconstriction and heart block (Lagerkranser et al., 1984; Crystal et al., 1988). Adenosine has not been approved for use as a hypotensive drug in the United States.

Prostaglandin E_1

Prostaglandin E_1 (PGE_1) has a potent vasodilator effect on the pulmonary and systemic vascular beds. Despite its vasodilator properties, PGE_1 infusion causes slight hypotension in conscious humans because of the concomitant increase in cardiac output secondary to its positive inotropic effect and the reflex increase in heart rate (Carlson et al., 1969). PGE_1 infusion (100 to 150 ng/kg per minute) has been successfully and safely used to induce hypotension during inhalation anesthesia. Resistance was encountered in 2 of 14 patients (Goto et al., 1982). Blood pressure returns to within 15% of normal 15 minutes after the infusion is stopped.

Increase in plasma renin activity occurs during PGE_1 infusion, presumably due to the fall in pressure rather than a direct effect on the kidney. PGE_1 also causes increases in renal blood flow, urine flow, and sodium excretion (Goto et al., 1982). Although an inhibitory effect on both platelet aggregation and thrombus formation has been described, PGE_1 in clinical doses has no discernible effect on platelet aggregation (Goto and Fujita, 1980). Use of PGE_1 as a hypotensive drug is not currently recommended pending further investigation.

Fenoldopam

Fenoldopam is a pure dopamine$_1$ receptor antagonist with selective coronary, renal, mesenteric, and peripheral arteriolar vasodilator action. Mild reflex tachycardia usually occurs with its use. The maximal response is usually achieved in 10 to 20 minutes. Fenoldopam is given via a continuous infusion (0.1 to 0.6 mcg/kg per minute). Unlike other hypotensive drugs, fenoldopam has renal vasodilatation and natriuretic actions that maintain or increase urine flow during hypotension. These properties may constitute a renal protective effect (Aronson et al., 1990).

HEMODYNAMIC EFFECTS OF HYPOTENSIVE DRUGS

Resistance to Hypotensive Drugs

After the introduction of hypotensive drugs into anesthetic practice, the problem of failure to achieve or maintain hypotension was soon observed. This phenomenon was assumed to be due to tachyphylaxis, that is, a diminished response despite continued administration of the drug. However, resistance to hypotensive drugs is almost always associated with tachycardia. This is more frequently seen in children than in adults (Salem et al., 1974). Resistance to hypotension is not a unique feature of one drug but has been reported with all ganglionic-blocking drugs, β-adrenergic–blocking drugs, and other direct-acting drugs, including sodium nitroprusside, nitroglycerin, and phentolamine.

Several mechanisms have been postulated to explain tachycardia or resistance to hypotension, or both (Box 12–4). The relative importance of these mechanisms may differ with the various hypotensive drugs. Sodium nitroprusside–induced hypotension is associated with increases in heart rate and cardiac output, activation of the renin-angiotensin system, and release of catecholamines (Khambatta et al., 1981; Knight et al., 1983; Fahmy et al., 1984). In contrast, ganglionic blockade results in less of an increase in circulating catecholamines and no activation of the renin-angiotensin axis (Knight et al., 1980, 1983). The increase in heart rate with the use of ganglionic-blocking drugs is probably the result of parasympathetic blockade, which may be more prominent in children because of their increased vagal tone (Salem et al., 1978; Yaster et al., 1986). In response to the initial decrease of pressure, reflex tachycardia, mediated through the baroreceptors, occurs with almost all hypotensive drugs. Because the cardiac output in children is rate dependent, increased heart rate results in an increase in cardiac output and counteracts the decrease in blood pressure. As a result of sympathetic activation, renin is released from the juxtaglomerular apparatus in the kidney. This acts on an α_2-globulin from the liver to produce the decapeptide angiotensin I, which is converted in the lungs to the octapeptide angiotensin II, a potent vasoconstrictor.

Stimulation of the sympathetic and the renin-angiotensin systems may adversely affect the operative course during induced hypotension. Even when hypotension is established, the increased cardiac output can cause bleeding. Rebound hypertension may occur after abrupt termination of the sodium nitroprusside infusion. This is related to the increase in systemic vascular resistance because of the unopposed activation of the sympathetic and renin-angiotensin systems. The consequences of rebound hypertension include wound bleeding, hematoma formation, cerebral edema, cerebrovascular accidents, disrupted cerebral autoregulation, increased myocardial oxygen demand, and pulmonary edema. The varying sensitivities of vessels to catecholamines in different organs may cause major changes in the distribution of blood flow among the various organs, as well as a redistribution of blood flow within organs. Evidence suggests that very high circulating catecholamine and angiotensin II levels have deleterious effects on myocardial and renal tubular cells and may adversely affect arterial and capillary function (McDonald et al., 1969; Giese, 1973; Gavras et al., 1975).

The key to successful hypotension is control of the heart rate. The techniques advocated to prevent resistance to hypotensive drugs are shown in Box 12–5. The simplest effective means is the judicious use of a β-adrenergic–blocking drug. Other alternatives include pretreatment with saralasin, an angiotensin II competitive antagonist, and captopril (clonidine), an oral angiotensin-converting enzyme inhibitor (Delaney and Miller, 1980; Fahmy and Gavras, 1985). Pretreatment with captopril results in lower dosage requirements and prevents rebound hypertension. A 10:1 mixture of trimethaphan (250 mg) and sodium nitroprusside (25 mg) in a solution of 5% dextrose in water has been advocated (Wildsmith et al., 1983; Fahmy, 1985a). The mixture produces hypotension with smaller doses of sodium nitroprusside and trimethaphan than when either drug is used separately (synergistic effect). When the mixture is

BOX 12–5 Techniques to Prevent Resistance to Hypotensive Drugs

Halothane (inactivates the baroreceptor response)
Avoiding fluid overload
Omitting belladonna drugs (or decreasing dosage)
Preoperative sedation and intravenous opioids
Use of a β-adrenergic–blocking drug
Pretreatment with angiotensin II competitive antagonist
Pretreatment with angiotensin-converting enzyme inhibitor
Combining hypotensive drugs
Premedication with clonidine

BOX 12–4 Theories Postulated to Explain Tachycardia and Resistance to Hypotension

1. Parasympathetic blockade causing tachycardia (ganglionic blockade)
2. Reflex tachycardia mediated through the baroreceptors in response to the initial fall in pressure (probably all hypotensive drugs)
3. Stimulation of the sympathetic and renin-angiotensin systems leading to increased plasma renin activity and angiotensin II and catecholamine levels (direct-acting drugs, especially sodium nitroprusside)
4. Constrictive effect of sympathetic blockade on the α-adrenoceptive blood vessels leading to rise in blood pressure
5. Inappropriate (excessive) fluid therapy before and during hypotension (causing expansion of blood volume and difficulty in controlling pressure)

used, the dose of sodium nitroprusside is approximately one third to one fifth the amount required when sodium nitroprusside is used alone and blood pressure returns gradually without rebound hypertension.

Clonidine, an α_2-adrenoceptor agonist, has been shown to reduce the requirement of isoflurane (by 60%) and sodium nitroprusside (by 45%) and to substantially reduce the need for labetalol during induced hypotension (Woodcock et al., 1988). Through its central effect at sites within the medulla and hypothalamus, clonidine effectively blocks the increased central adrenergic activity concomitant with the use of hypotensive drugs. Other actions include inhibition of renin release in the kidney and a reduction in vasopressin release. The recommended dose is 4 to 8 mcg/kg to be given orally 2 hours before surgery. The main disadvantage associated with premedication with clonidine is a slightly prolonged recovery from anesthesia (Maroof et al., 1994). Clonidine can also be given intravenously in a dose of 2 to 3 mcg/kg as an adjuvant for controlling blood pressure. In addition to the intraoperative hypotensive effect, the analgesic and sedative effects of the drug can last well into the postoperative period.

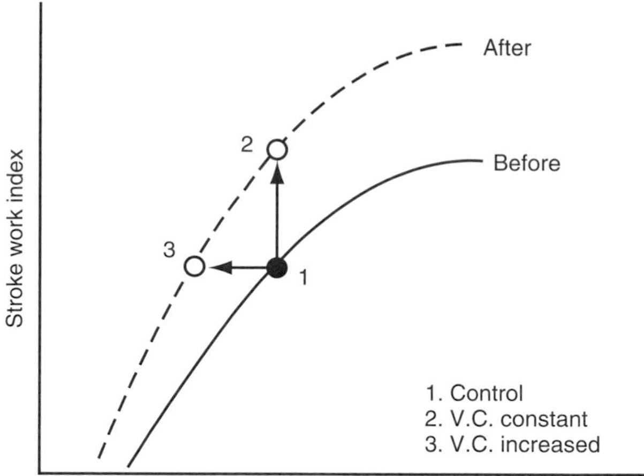

FIGURE 12–8. Effect of a vasodilator on the Frank-Starling relation. Decreased afterload shifts the curve (*solid line*) to the left (*dashed line*). If transmural pressure (preload) remains constant, cardiac output increases; if the decrease in afterload is also associated with decreased preload (transmural pressure), cardiac output remains constant. VC, venous compliance. (From Fahmy NR, Laver MB: Hemodynamic response to ganglionic blockade with pentolinium during N_2O-halothane anesthesia in man. *Anesthesiology* 44:6, 1976, with permission.)

Effects on Cardiac Output and Regional Blood Flows

The cardiovascular effects of hypotensive drugs may be modified by many factors: the anesthetic and other drugs given, position of the patient, degree of hypotension, intrathoracic pressure, acid-base status, circulating blood volume, age, and change in preload and afterload.

Cardiac Output

Vasodilators alter the cardiac output through changes in stroke volume and heart rate. They decrease afterload by lowering arterial impedance and reduce preload by increasing venous compliance. Depending on the ventricular function as defined by the Frank-Starling mechanism and the relative effect of the drug on the preload and afterload, stroke volume may rise, remain constant, or even decline (Fahmy and Laver, 1976). A decrease in afterload shifts the curve to the left (Fig. 12–8). If preload remains constant, stroke volume increases. If the decrease in afterload is associated with a decrease in preload, stroke volume probably remains constant. A decrease in preload without a decrease in afterload probably results in decreased stroke volume.

Changes in cardiac output during deliberate hypotension are a function of heart rate. Changes in heart rate depend mainly on the predominant autonomic tone existing at the time of hypotension. For example, if vagal tone is predominant, heart rate increases via the baroreceptor pathway, as in the case of children. Halothane blunts this reflex increase in heart rate during hypotension by "resetting the baroreceptors," depressing vasomotor centers, and depressing sinoatrial node activity.

In anesthetized humans with normal cardiac function, sodium nitroprusside–induced hypotension is associated with either increased or unchanged cardiac output. In contrast, nitroglycerin, because of its effect on venous capacitance and venous pressure, decreases ventricular filling pressure and ultimately reduces cardiac output (Fahmy, 1978; Gerson et al., 1982; Longnecker, 1985). Hypotension secondary to ganglionic blockade has variable effects on cardiac output.

Coronary Circulation

The driving pressure for coronary blood flow is aortic diastolic pressure. During deliberate hypotension, reduced myocardial work secondary to decreased afterload reduces the requirement for coronary blood flow. A decrease in the heart rate × systolic pressure product (an index of myocardial oxygen demand) has been observed during deliberate hypotension in adults and children (Fahmy and Laver, 1976; Salem et al., 1978). Unless hypotension is severe, locally mediated changes in vasomotor tone ensure that coronary blood flow remains adequate during deliberate hypotension. This may explain the lack of electrocardiographic evidence of myocardial ischemia during induced hypotension in children (Salem et al., 1974).

Cerebral Circulation

The physiologic response to a change in arterial pressure is a compensatory change in cerebral vascular resistance, that is, autoregulation. In the healthy unanesthetized human, cerebral blood flow remains virtually constant as long as mean systemic blood pressure remains between 50 and 150 mm Hg. Below or above these levels, flow becomes pressure dependent. Cerebral autoregulation is compromised in disease states, by anesthetics, and following head trauma (Strunin, 1975). Because the normal blood pressure in infants and children is lower than that of adults, the blood pressure limits established for adults may not be appropriate for pediatric patients. In general, lower blood pressures are needed to achieve a dry operative field in pediatric patients and the cerebral perfusion pressure–cerebral blood flow relation is likely shifted to the left in infants and young children (Rogers et al., 1980). Chronic hypertension blunts the cerebral autoregulatory response to reduced perfusion pressure (Strandgaard, 1976) (see Chapter 18, Neurosurgery).

Anesthetics might afford some protection against cerebral metabolic deficits during severe hypotension (Newberg et al., 1983; Newberg and Michenfelder, 1983). With reduction in cerebral blood flow, widening of the arteriovenous oxygen difference occurs, resulting in no change in cerebral oxygen consumption. In normotensive individuals, cerebral blood flow changes linearly with changes in $PaCO_2$. At $PaCO_2$ between 20 and 70 mm Hg, a 1 mm Hg change in Pa_{CO_2} produces a corresponding 2.6% change in cerebral blood flow. With progressive hypotension, this relationship becomes progressively flatter, so that at a mean arterial blood pressure below 50 mm Hg, cerebral blood flow does not change in response to variations in Pa_{CO_2} (Harper and Glass, 1965). However, findings in humans indicate that cerebral vascular response to CO_2 continues at moderate levels of induced hypotension (Salem et al., 1970; Eckenhoff et al., 1963a). Therefore, unless indicated, hypocapnia should be avoided during deliberate hypotension (Levin et al., 1980).

Sodium nitroprusside can abolish cerebral autoregulation and increase cerebral blood flow in both awake and anesthetized patients (Ivankovich et al., 1976). Increases in intracranial pressure are mostly seen during the early stages of sodium nitroprusside infusion and may vary widely from patient to patient (Stullken and Sokoll, 1975; Turner et al., 1977; Cottrell et al., 1978a). Hypocapnia tends to attenuate sodium nitroprusside–induced increases in intracranial pressure. Similar increases in intracranial pressure have been reported during nitroglycerin-induced hypotension (Rogers et al., 1979). In contrast, trimethaphan does not usually result in increased intracranial pressure except when intracranial compression is severe.

Spinal Cord Blood Flow

With the popularity of deliberate hypotension for the operative correction of scoliosis, there has been concern that hypotension may decrease spinal cord blood flow and predispose to spinal cord injury, particularly during instrumentation (Grundy et al., 1981; Jacobs et al., 1982). The spinal cord exhibits well-functioning autoregulation between mean pressures of 50 and 150 mm Hg. Autoregulation allows normal spinal cord metabolism in the face of decreased arterial blood pressure. However, hypotension and direct pressure on the spinal cord can combine to impair spinal cord function. In anesthetized cats, neither spinal cord compression nor reduction of aortic pressure (by clamping the thoracic aorta) altered spinal cord function when applied separately (Brodkey et al., 1972). When both were applied simultaneously, spinal cord function, as evidenced by changes in somatosensory evoked potentials, was reversibly altered. Hypotension aggravated the effects of compression, whereas intentional hypertension reversed these effects.

Changes in somatosensory evoked potentials at normotension have also been observed in patients undergoing spinal distraction but have resolved with slight increases of blood pressure. Ponte (1974) reported that in two patients in whom paraplegia developed after hypercorrection of scoliosis, partial recovery of neurologic function occurred when blood was infused to correct hypovolemic hypotension. These reports did not document demonstrable deleterious effects of well-conducted normovolemic hypotension on spinal cord function during scoliosis correction. However, they emphasize that (1) hemorrhagic hypotension could result in a severe reduction in spinal cord blood flow and alteration of spinal cord function; (2) spinal distraction (even without hypotension) may result in altered spinal cord function; (3) changes in somatosensory evoked potentials noted during hypotension may return to normal after increases in blood pressure; and (4) monitoring spinal cord function is essential whenever the spinal cord is potentially at risk for injury or interruption of its blood supply (Grundy et al., 1981). Details for monitoring spinal cord function are addressed in Chapter 18, Anesthesia for Neurosurgery, and Chapter 21, Anesthesia for Orthopedic Surgery.

Renal Circulation

Studies in humans show that trimethaphan- and sodium nitroprusside–induced hypotension have similar effects on the kidney (Behnia et al., 1978, 1982). The findings suggest that renal medullary tissue oxygenation, an index of tissue viability, remains adequate despite a significant reduction in creatinine clearance during the hypotensive period. Renal blood flow is normally autoregulated over a range of changes in mean arterial pressure (80 to 180 mm Hg). This capability is attenuated during anesthesia (Strunin, 1975). Below 60 mm Hg, renal blood flow may decrease to the point where urine flow ceases. Provided that induced hypotension does not decrease the renal blood flow below the critical value for the kidney, it is unlikely that renal damage ensues. Because glomerular filtration rate also is not autoregulated during anesthesia, monitoring the urine output may be useful, especially during prolonged hypotension. Other important factors affecting renal blood flow and urine flow during anesthesia include sympathetic stimulation, exogenous or endogenous catecholamines, renin-angiotensin system, antidiuretic hormone levels, and hypercapnia.

Hepatic and Other Regional Blood Flows

A 40% decrease in arterial pressure by sodium nitroprusside results in a decrease in portal pressure (44%) and portal blood flow (25%) and in an increase in hepatic arterial blood flow (13%) (Gelman and Ernst, 1978). Sodium nitroprusside decreases portal sinusoidal resistance, does not interfere with the ability of the liver to increase hepatic arterial blood flow (in conditions of insufficient portal circulation), and does not lead to hepatic hypoxia.

Dry Operative Field and Deliberate Hypotension

Controversy surrounds the relative importance of arterial pressure and cardiac output (or blood flow at the operative site) in producing a dry operative field. Some authors maintain that a reduction in cardiac output is essential to reduce bleeding and that even when blood pressure is low, bleeding is not necessarily reduced unless there is a concomitant fall in cardiac output (Enderby, 1985b). Salem and associates (1978) observed that the onset of a dry operative field during induction of hypotension in the supine position in children was not accomplished unless cardiac output was reduced by 35%. Knight and associates (1980) found a positive correlation between blood loss and left ventricular stroke work index during hypotensive anesthesia for surgical correction of scoliosis. Other investigators reported that blood pressure was the important factor determining blood loss. Amaranath and associates (1975) found correlations between systolic blood pressure and blood loss. Sivarajan and associates (1980) concluded that operative blood loss during induced hypotension is determined by mean arterial pressure, not cardiac output. Their study, however, was conducted on patients undergoing mandibular osteotomies placed in a head-up tilt. This may have resulted in pooling of blood in the dependent areas so that blood flow at the operative site was decreased.

A relatively dry operative field and improved operative conditions are not automatically achieved at a predetermined hypotensive level. The skillful anesthesiologist should ascertain that hypotensive anesthesia has achieved its objective and that improved operative conditions have, in fact, ensued. A lower level of blood pressure or other hemodynamic adjustments (e.g., control of heart rate, positioning) may be needed to improve the operative field.

In orthopedic procedures, where bleeding is mostly of venous origin, blood loss is less with nitroglycerin than with sodium nitroprusside at comparable levels of hypotension (Fahmy, 1978). Lower venous pressure associated with nitroglycerin may be partly responsible for the decreased blood loss. These findings have not yet been confirmed in children (Yaster et al., 1986). The requirement of a relatively bloodless field in children depends on decreased cardiac output, decreased blood flow at the operative site, or both. In contrast, when hypotension is used to facilitate surgery on large vessels, the reduction in vessel tension and not necessarily the decrease in blood flow is required. A hypotensive technique that does not decrease cardiac output may be preferred in these situations.

Both sodium nitroprusside and nitroglycerin infusions lead to prolonged bleeding times in a dose-dependent manner. When the dose of sodium nitroprusside exceeds 3 mcg/kg per minute, a dose-related inhibition of platelet aggregation occurs (Hines and Barash, 1989). The prolonged bleeding time with nitroglycerin seems to result from vasodilation and increased venous capacitance rather than inhibition of platelet aggregation (Lichtenthal et al., 1985). In contrast, trimethaphan has no effect on platelet function (Hines, 1990).

SAFETY FACTORS OF INDUCED HYPOTENSION IN CHILDREN

Onset and Degree of Hypotension

Hypotension should be induced slowly over 10 to 15 minutes. Time is needed for the cerebral, coronary, and renal vasculature to dilate in the face of decreased pressure so as to maintain adequate perfusion. If the blood pressure decreases too rapidly, a sharp decrease in mixed venous oxygen saturation ($S\bar{v}O_2$) and content ($C\bar{v}O_2$) may occur, reflecting inadequate tissue oxygenation (Salem, 1979) (Fig. 12–9). Cardiac arrest and other complications during the induction of hypotension have been related to a rapid decrease in pressure.

Because of individual variations, blood pressure should not be decreased to a "predetermined" level. The desired level of hypotension depends on the age, condition, position of the patient, and on the surgical requirement. In young children, a systolic pressure of 55 or 60 mm Hg in the supine position may be necessary to achieve a relatively bloodless field. The anesthesiologist should look for warning signs, including an excessively dry operative field and dark venous blood, which are indicators to increase the blood pressure (Salem et al., 1971). $P\bar{v}O_2$ (or central venous or jugular venous PO_2) below 30 mm Hg indicates tissue hypoxia, and the blood pressure should be increased. Unusually high $P\bar{v}O_2$ may be an early sign of cyanide toxicity (if sodium nitroprusside is used). If the blood pressure drifts too low, attempts should be made to raise it by decreasing the degree of head-up tilt, slowing the infusion of the hypotensive drug, lightening the level of anesthesia, and speeding up the intravenous fluids. Vasopressors are best avoided unless uncontrollable hypotension occurs.

Maintenance of Near-Normal $PaCO_2$ and Acid-Base Balance

Unless hypocapnia is required to reduce the intracranial pressure, a near-normal $PaCO_2$ should be maintained. Hypocapnia decreases cardiac output; decreases coronary, cerebral, and spinal cord blood flows; may alter drug action (by altering blood pH); decreases both ionized calcium and serum potassium concentrations; causes leftward shift of the oxyhemoglobin dissociation curve; may increase the oxygen consumption; and may inhibit hypoxic pulmonary vasoconstriction (HPV). If adequate oxygenation and a near-normal $PaCO_2$ are maintained, metabolic acidosis is not a feature of well-managed hypotensive technique.

The redistribution of pulmonary blood during induced hypotension may lead to alteration in alveolar ventilation and perfusion ratios. Eckenhoff and associates (1963b) demonstrated that the alveolar dead space may increase to as much as 80% of the tidal volume in the hypotensive adult patient in the head-up position and with an increased airway pressure. Further studies showed that the increase in alveolar dead space is less than previously thought (Askrog et al., 1964). Data from infants

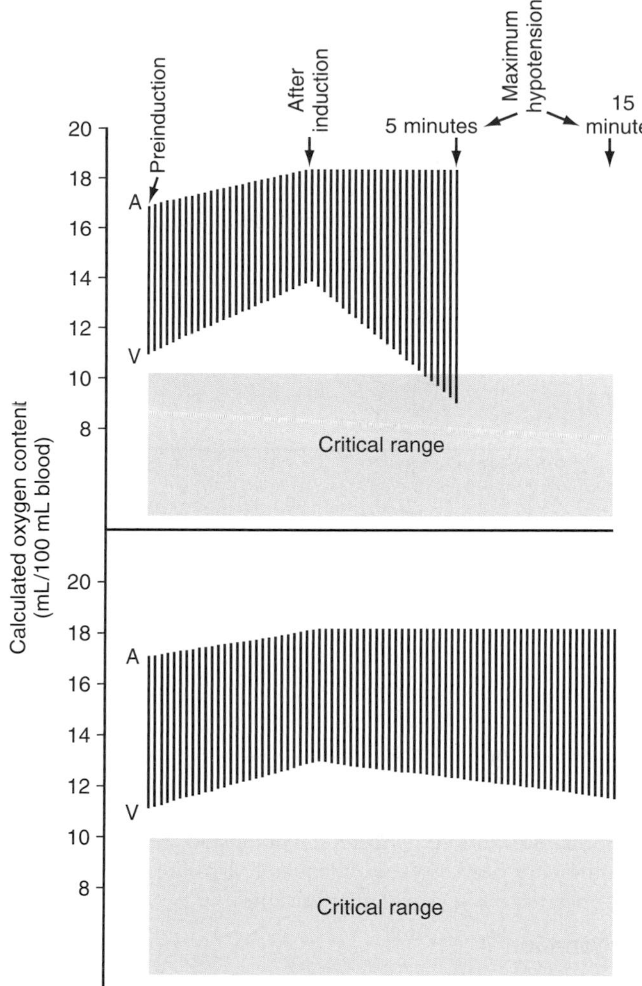

■ **FIGURE 12–9.** Effect of speed of onset of hypotension on central venous oxygen content. *Top*, Changes in arterial and venous oxygen content when maximum hypotension was achieved in 5 minutes in six patients. The venous oxygen content fell within the critical range, indicating a state of circulatory inadequacy. *Bottom*, In six other patients, hypotension was induced slowly (15 minutes). No remarkable increase in arteriovenous oxygen content difference occurred, and venous oxygen content was above the critical range. (Modified from Salem MR: Deliberate hypotension is a safe and accepted anesthetic technique. In Eckenhoff JE, editor: *Controversy in anesthesiology.* Philadelphia, 1975, WB Saunders, p 95.)

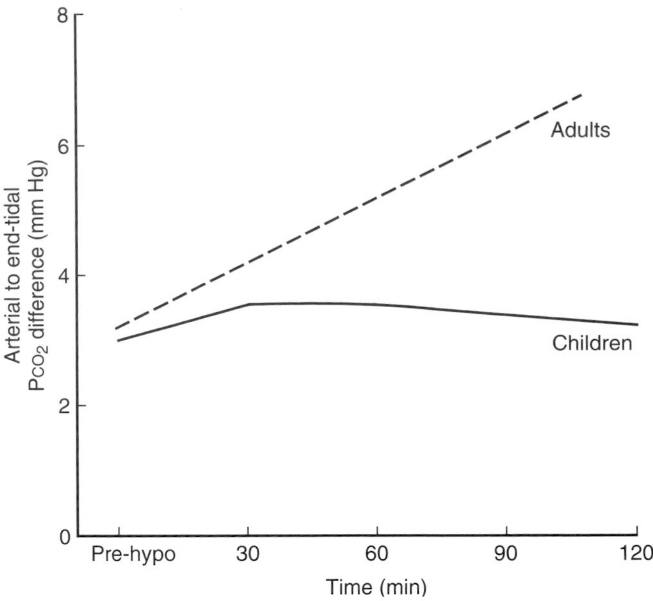

■ **FIGURE 12–10.** Arterial-to-end-tidal P_{CO_2} difference during deliberate hypotension in adults (from Askrog et al., 1964) and in children. (Reprinted with permission from the International Anesthesia Research Society from Salem MR, Wong AY, Bennett EJ: Deliberate hypotension in infants and children. *Anesth Analg* 53:975, 1974, with permission).

and children suggest that the alveolar dead space does not increase during controlled hypotension even with the head-up tilt (Salem et al., 1974) (Fig. 12–10). Others found that sodium nitroprusside–induced deliberate hypotension caused no change in pulmonary dead space in adequately hydrated patients who were operated on in the prone position.

Oxygenation

An increased difference between alveolar-to-arterial oxygen tensions ($A-aD_{O_2}$) is observed during induced hypotension (Stone et al., 1976; Casthely et al., 1982). This may be explained by (1) increased $\dot{Q}s/\dot{Q}t$ and (2) decreased cardiac output.

Increased $\dot{Q}s/\dot{Q}t$

Changes in functional residual capacity and closing volume during anesthesia and surgery contribute to airway closure, trapping of gas distal to the closure, and alveolar collapse. This local alveolar hypoxia is normally offset (to a degree) by reflex HPV that directs blood from hypoxic areas of the lung to adequately ventilated alveoli. Blunting or inhibition of this reflex may occur with pulmonary hypertension, inhalation anesthetics, and vasodilators (Benumof and Wahrenbrock, 1975). Although the inhibition of HPV occurs with all vasodilators, it is greater with sodium nitroprusside than with nitroglycerin. Inhibition of HPV is associated with a decrease in pulmonary vascular resistance and pulmonary artery pressure and results in increased $\dot{Q}s/\dot{Q}t$.

Decreased Cardiac Output

Decreased cardiac output is accompanied by increased extraction of oxygen by the tissues resulting in decreased $P\bar{v}_{O_2}$ and $C\bar{v}_{O_2}$ (Kelman et al., 1967; Philbin et al., 1970). Any portion of blood with decreased $C\bar{v}_{O_2}$ that passes through hypoventilated or nonventilated areas (low $\dot{V}_A/\dot{Q}_P$) contributes to a greater decrease in Pa_{O_2}. A decrease in cardiac output during deliberate hypotension can result in a decrease in Pa_{O_2}, significant only in the presence of regional atelectasis (Cheney and Colley, 1980).

A high F_{IO_2} (>0.9) during deliberate hypotension tends to compensate for the venous admixture contributed by ventilation–perfusion imbalance and is recommended. High F_{IO_2} is also desirable in children because of their increased oxygen demands. Robinson (1967) showed that the lactate-to-pyruvate ratio does not increase during profound hypotension when the Pa_{O_2} is kept above 300 mm Hg. Jugular bulb oxygen tension rises significantly when F_{IO_2} is altered from 0.4 to 1.0 during hypotensive anesthesia, although the oxygen delivery would have increased only slightly with an F_{IO_2} of 1.0 (Salem et al., 1970). These findings stress the importance of using high F_{IO_2}, monitoring oxygenation, and avoiding profound decreases in cardiac output.

Monitoring

In addition to routine monitoring (electrocardiography, pulse oximetry, capnography), accurate recording of the blood pressure is essential during induced hypotension. Although various methods have been used, direct measurement via arterial cannulation allows continuous blood pressure measurements and arterial blood sampling. A variety of automated noninvasive devices may be used as a backup system for direct arterial pressure measurement. Central venous access permits measurement of central venous blood gases, a fairly accurate estimation of mixed venous blood gases.

Cyanide Toxicity

Sodium nitroprusside has the molecular formula $Na_2[Fe(CN)_5NO]\cdot 2H_2O$. Although cyanide ($CN^-$) released from the sodium nitroprusside molecule is transformed mostly into relatively nontoxic products, CN^- can be toxic and sufficient amounts can cause death (Tinker and Michenfelder, 1976; Michenfelder, 1977; Verner, 1985) (Fig. 12–11). There are four pathways for the disposal of this free CN^-.

Binding to Cytochrome Oxidase

Cyanide binds to mitochondrial cytochrome oxidase, inhibiting oxidative phosphorylation. The subsequent anaerobic metabolism leads to acidosis. This binding to cytochrome oxidase is reversible in vitro, but reversibility probably does not contribute to short-term survival in humans.

Conversion to Thiocyanate

Transformation of CN^- into thiocyanate is the major metabolic pathway for CN^- in humans. It occurs in the liver and kidney, is catalyzed by the enzyme rhodanese, and requires B_{12a} as a cofactor. Added thiosulfate speeds the reaction, which is slowly reversible.

Conversion of B_{12a} to Cyanocobalamin

In the presence of adequate hydroxocobalamin, CN^- becomes cyanocobalamin. This is probably not an important pathway in normal humans, but hydroxocobalamin has been suggested for prophylaxis.

Conversion to Cyanmethemoglobin

One of every five CN^- ions is normally converted to cyanmethemoglobin. When exposed to light, sodium nitroprusside is rapidly converted to unstable ionic aquapentoferrocyanate, a substance that readily releases free CN^-. Sodium nitroprusside solutions should be protected from photolytic decomposition

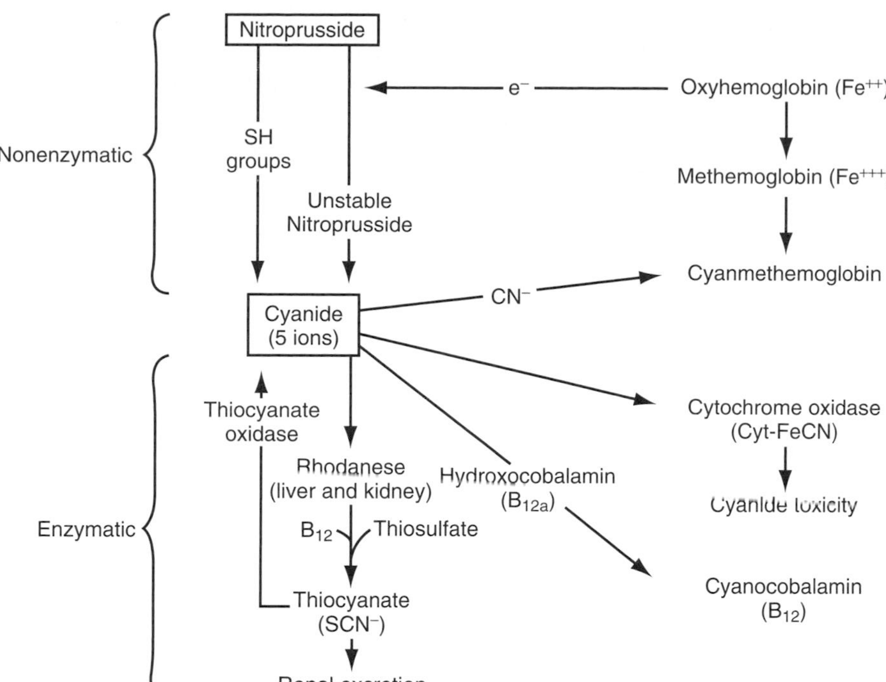

■ **FIGURE 12–11.** Metabolism of sodium nitroprusside. (Modified from Tinker JH, Michenfelder JD: Sodium nitroprusside: Pharmacology, toxicology and therapeutics. *Anesthesiology* 45:340, 1976, with permission.)

during infusion (Verner, 1985). Although it has been recommended that sodium nitroprusside solution be discarded 4 hours after reconstitution, evidence substantiates its safety for 24 hours if properly protected from light (Ikeda et al., 1987).

The mechanism for CN^- intoxication with sodium nitroprusside overdose is interference with aerobic metabolism, which is the major pathway of high-energy phosphate production (Tinker and Michenfelder, 1976; Michenfelder and Tinker, 1977). Free CN^- inhibits the reoxidation of reduced cytochrome oxidase by oxygen, and, by crossing cell and mitochondrial membranes, CN^- rapidly inhibits the electron transport system. The consequences of CN^- intoxication are decreased oxygen utilization, decreased CO_2 production via inhibition of the Krebs' cycle, and increased production of anaerobic metabolites. Metabolic acidosis and deterioration in the central nervous and cardiovascular systems ensue. The combination of tissue hypoxia with normal or elevated $P\bar{v}O_2$ levels is the hallmark of cytotoxic hypoxia produced by CN^- (Michenfelder, 1977).

Detection of Cyanide Toxicity

In the awake patient, the manifestations of cyanide toxicity are fatigue, nausea, vomiting, headache, anorexia, tremors, angina-like syndrome, disorientation, psychotic behavior, muscle spasms, rigidity, convulsions, and cardiovascular collapse. Prolonged intravenous sodium nitroprusside infusion may result in hypothyroidism due to the antithyroid action of thiocyanate (Palmer and Lasseter, 1975). The clinical manifestations of CN^- intoxication during anesthesia are shown in Box 12–6 (Jack, 1974; Merrifield and Blundell, 1974; Davies et al., 1975).

In children and adolescents three abnormal responses have been recognized that suggest impending CN^- intoxication: (1) a requirement for high doses of sodium nitroprusside (>10 mcg/kg per minute); (2) tachyphylaxis, which is apparent in 30 to 60 minutes after the start of the infusion; and (3) definite resistance becoming apparent within 5 to 10 minutes after the start of the infusion. The incidence of these abnormal responses may be as high as 30% (Greiss et al., 1976). Tachyphylaxis may or may not be associated with concurrent metabolic acidosis (Cottrell et al., 1978c). The severity of acidosis is usually proportional to the CN^- level. The progressive hypotension may be responsive to discontinuing the sodium nitroprusside infusion, administering fluid and blood products, or infusing vasopressors. Cardiovascular collapse may ensue and may not respond to cardiopulmonary resuscitation, but a dramatic response may be observed after the administration of sodium thiosulfate.

Early laboratory recognition of CN^- intoxication poses difficulties because of the absence of specific tests. The lethal blood CN^- level in humans is approximately 500 mcg/dL, whereas lethal blood thiocyanate levels have been reported to be as low as 340 mcg/dL, but this varies with the rate of CN^- release as well as the total dose. Measurement of blood levels of CN^- or thiocyanate does not reflect the magnitude of CN^- released. Consequently, nonspecific tests are relied upon as indicators of CN^- toxicity. The most sensitive metabolic indicators of CN^- toxicity are blood pH, blood lactate (or lactate/pyruvate), $P\bar{v}O_2$ or $S\bar{v}O_2$, sagittal sinus PO_2 (reflecting cerebral tissue oxygen tension),

BOX 12–6 Clinical Manifestations of Cyanide Toxicity

Metabolic acidemia
Progressive hypotension with narrow pulse pressure
Refractory hypotension unresponsive to fluids and vasopressors but responsive to thiosulfate
Cardiovascular collapse
Bright venous blood
Increased $S\bar{v}O_2$ and $P\bar{v}O_2$

cerebral oxygen consumption, and brain lactate (or lactate/pyruvate) (Michenfelder, 1977). Of these, arterial pH and gas tensions, as well as $P\bar{v}O_2$ or jugular venous PO_2, are easily obtained and should be measured when CN^- intoxication is suspected. "Bright" venous blood during sodium nitroprusside infusion should alert the anesthesiologist to the possibility of early CN^- intoxication.

Prevention of Cyanide Toxicity

Cyanide intoxication associated with the use of sodium nitroprusside is a preventable complication. The total projected dose should not exceed 1.5 mg/kg for short exposures or 0.5 mg/kg per hour for prolonged exposures. Infusion rates exceeding 10 mcg/kg per minute should not be allowed. The rate of sodium nitroprusside infusion should be adjusted to 0.5 to 1 mcg/kg per minute via use of a microdrop or infusion pump, and the infusion rate may be gradually increased as needed. A satisfactory response can be obtained well below the recommended maximum of 10 mcg/kg per minute. The patient's response to the infusion should be ascertained constantly, especially in the first 30 minutes. Frequent (half-hourly) arterial acid-base determinations are recommended during sodium nitroprusside infusion. In addition, CN^- antidote therapy should be available. If either a constant response to high doses of sodium nitroprusside (>10 mcg/kg per minute) or a tachyphylactic response is noted, a β-adrenergic–blocking drug should be administered and the inhaled anesthetic concentration increased. A quick response is usually noted after these measures are instituted, and a rapid decline in the dose requirement usually follows. If resistance is detected (within 5 to 10 minutes), the infusion should be abandoned and a different hypotensive drug given.

Treatment of Cyanide Toxicity

The rational approach in the treatment of CN^- toxicity is to prevent the CN^- from binding to cytochrome oxidase. Sodium thiosulfate can afford complete protection against CN^- and complete detoxification if three times more thiosulfate than CN^- is present. In experimental animals, thiosulfate resulted in no noticeable adverse hemodynamic or respiratory effects. Thiosulfate ensures the plentiful supply of sulfhydryl radicals needed to form thiocyanate from CN^-. Because thiosulfate is rapidly eliminated by the kidneys, a high level of plasma thiosulfate is best maintained by constant infusion. A bolus injection of 30 mg/kg followed by a continuous infusion of 60 mg/kg per hour appears to be the most effective and safest prophylactic antidote against CN^- toxicity and also prevents CN^--induced circulatory failure (Ivankovich et al., 1980). Being an osmotic diuretic, thiosulfate can ultimately decrease the plasma volume.

Hydroxocobalamin (vitamin B_{12a}) has been advocated as a treatment for cyanide intoxication (Posner et al., 1976; Cottrell et al., 1978b). It prevents the increase in the CN^- concentration in erythrocytes when given prophylactically with large doses of sodium nitroprusside. Problems associated with the use of vitamin B_{12a} include requirement of a large dose, lack of cardiovascular stability, scarcity, expense, solubility, and proper storage of the powder. The recommended dose is a 50-mg/kg bolus, plus 100 mg/kg per hour. In addition to these specific antidotes, correction of acidosis and fluid replacement are important in the management of CN^- intoxication. If the patient is bleeding, blood transfusion may help to "exchange the blood volume" and thus eliminate CN^- (Vesey et al., 1975).

BOX 12–7 Contraindications to Deliberate Hypotension

Inexperience
Infants (except when there is a definite indication)
Significant reduction in oxygen delivery
Systemic diseases compromising major organ function
Renal, cerebral, or coronary artery stenosis
Children with cardiac shunts
Patients with sickle cell disease
Uncorrected polycythemia
Ganglionic blockers in patients with narrow-angle glaucoma

CONTRAINDICATIONS TO INDUCED HYPOTENSION

At one time, almost all systemic diseases were considered absolute contraindications to induced hypotension (Box 12-7). With this stringent rule, many patients were denied the benefits of the technique. Many heretofore absolute contraindications are now regarded as relative. Because most of the complications associated with deliberate hypotension are related to inexperience and unfamiliarity with the technique, the technique should not be attempted by inexperienced practitioners. Anesthesiologists and surgeons should be familiar with the pharmacology of hypotensive drugs and the physiologic effects of hypotension. Teamwork and cooperation are of great importance in the care of patients who undergo hypotension.

Age is not a contraindication to induced hypotension. Except in infants, in whom blood pressure may be difficult to measure accurately, the technique need not be withheld (Salem, 1978). Significant reduction in oxygen delivery to the tissues, as in anemia, low fixed cardiac output, severe lung disease, and the presence of severe acute cardiac, cerebral, or renal disease or any combination of these factors, may contraindicate the use of induced hypotension. In the presence of renal artery stenosis, hypotension can cause further decrease in perfusion pressure to the kidney. In children with cardiac shunts, reduction of systemic vascular resistance may increase right-to-left shunting and cause hypoxemia. In patients with sickle cell disease, a decrease in $P\bar{v}O_2$ (<30 mm Hg) due to decreased cardiac output can trigger a crisis. Uncorrected polycythemia is an additional contraindication, because it may increase sludging and thrombosis.

Diabetes is not a contraindication to induced hypotension if blood sugar levels are controlled perioperatively. β-Adrenergic blockade, through its actions on carbohydrate metabolism, may lower the blood sugar level although not seriously with the small doses given. The pupillary dilation caused by trimethaphan is short lived but may be misinterpreted as cerebral ischemia in the immediate postoperative period.

AUTOLOGOUS BLOOD TRANSFUSION

PREOPERATIVE AUTOLOGOUS BLOOD DONATION

Although preoperative autologous blood donation (PABD) was practiced in the 1960s, it did not gain wide acceptance until the 1980s. By 1990, as much as 5% of all blood collected for transfusion was intended for use by the patient-donor from whom it was collected (Surgenor et al., 1990). In some centers, up to 80% of the blood needed for certain surgical procedures has been met by PABD. Contributing to growth in PABD programs were (1) concerns about litigation for blood borne infection; (2) patient fears and concerns about human immunodeficiency virus (HIV) infection; and (3), in some states, hastily conceived legislation. The California Statute CB-37, the Paul Gann Blood Safety Act (1990), requires that in addition to the risks and benefits of blood transfusion, alternatives to allogenic blood must be presented to patients.

Preoperative autologous blood may be donated by patients who are likely to require transfusion during or after surgery. The ideal patient for PABD is one who (1) is healthy enough to undergo elective surgery; (2) is likely to need a transfusion during or after surgery; (3) has 2 or more weeks before surgery; and (4) has a hemoglobin level above 11 g/dL (hematocrit >33%). Some centers accept patients with slightly lower hemoglobin values, especially when there is a strong need for PABD.

Autologous transfusion is ideally suited for children and adolescents because isoimmunization during youth can complicate future transfusion needs. Children weighing less than 50 kg can safely donate blood, although the volume drawn at each donation is reduced in proportion to body weight. Withdrawal of amounts equal to 10% of their estimated blood volume is usually well tolerated. Although PABD has been extended to children as young as 4 years, technical problems and lack of cooperation make young children unlikely candidates for autologous blood donation.

The American Association of Blood Banks (AABB) standards recommend a minimum 4-day interval between phlebotomies and at least 3 days between the last phlebotomy and surgery (Widman, 1991). These minimum intervals are required to allow for synthesis and mobilization of proteins and the return of plasma volume to normal. The commonly used schedule, however, is one donation per week. This permits preoperative acquisition of up to four donations with conventional storage techniques (blood stored as liquid at 1° to 6°C). The shelf-life of red blood cells stored in the liquid state can be prolonged to 42 days when additive solutions such as Adsol (Fenwal Laboratoris, Roundlake, IL) are used. With this longer shelf-life, a weekly donation results in the collection of sufficient amounts of blood before surgery for most patients.

The total volume of blood that the patient can donate preoperatively may be increased by (1) iron therapy and (2) recombinant human erythropoietin therapy to increase the rate of endogenous red blood cell production (Goodnough et al., 1989). Although weekly donations stimulate erythropoiesis, with iron therapy the marrow can double or triple production, and this response can be maintained over several weeks, even with repeated phlebotomies. In patients undergoing weekly phlebotomy without added iron, the hematocrit decreases from 44% to 33% over an 8-week period. In patients who receive iron, it decreases from 44% to 38% during the same period. Because of the side effects of parenteral iron administration, the oral route is preferred. The recommended dose is 5 mg/kg two to three times daily with meals. It is preferable to begin iron therapy 1 month before the first donation and continue therapy for several months after the last donation (Widman, 1991).

The ability of recombinant human erythropoietin therapy to enhance the procurement of autologous blood is now unquestioned. Goodnough and associates (1989) demonstrated that the red blood cell volume donated by the patients who received erythropoietin was 41% greater than the volume donated by the patients who received placebo (961 versus 683 mL). Side effects (hypertension, thrombotic events) observed for long-term treatment in patients with end-stage renal disease are uncommon in surgical patients (Goodnough et al., 1997).

Various regimens for the administration of recombinant erythropoietin have been suggested. Initially, 600 U/kg IV was recommended at each visit for blood collection (twice weekly). This required repeated visits to the blood bank. Kulier and associates (1993) advocated a single weekly dose of erythropoietin (400 U/kg) given subcutaneously once a week starting 4 weeks before surgery. They found that this simple protocol provided a constant and efficient stimulus for erythropoiesis and adequately compensated for the hemoglobin decrease after the weekly donation. To maximize the response, oral iron supplementation is also implemented (Goodnough et al., 1997).

The efficacy of PABD in reducing allogenic blood exposure is well established (Thomas et al., 1996). Nevertheless, some drawbacks exist, including patient inconvenience, delay of the operative procedure, cost efficiency, and the occurrence of adverse reactions. Transient vasovagal reactions vary between 1.5% and 5.5% but could be higher among first-time donors (13%) and females (Stehling, 1990). Donors younger than 17 years, those who weigh less than 45 kg, and those who have experienced reactions during earlier donations are most likely to have a reaction. These reactions consist of light-headedness as a result of transient hypotension and bradycardia; 10% of these patients lose consciousness. Intravenous replacement with crystalloids and monitoring cardiovascular function during blood donation may decrease the incidence of these reactions.

Contraindications to PABD are bacteremia, decrease in oxygen delivery (low cardiac output, severe anemia, and hypoxemia), and very young age of the patient. Clinical judgment is essential when there are relative contraindications or concerns that patients may not tolerate phlebotomies. Establishing an intravenous catheter for infusion of isotonic saline or lactated Ringer's solution (one to two times the volume of blood removed) and close monitoring may be advisable in these patients. Despite the wide acceptance of PABD, controversial issues regarding the extent of testing, disposition of infectious blood, and crossover into the allogenic blood supply remain unresolved (Silvergleid, 1991).

Extent of Testing

Arguments in favor of minimal or no testing of blood intended for autologous blood use include cost savings and simplified bookkeeping. Complete testing, however, makes crossover into the allogenic blood supply possible. Unfortunately, a positive infectious disease test may create a conflict between the patient's right to privacy and the hospital team's right to take additional precautions (Silvergleid, 1991).

Release of Potentially Infectious Units

The rationale for not releasing a potentially infectious unit is to protect health care workers and to prevent the transmission of disease should the blood be unintentionally transfused to the wrong patient.

Crossover Into the Allogenic Blood Supply

Because of logistic problems and concerns about safety, only 15% of centers currently transfer unused autologous blood to the allogenic blood supply. The high cost and the improved safety of allogenic blood account for the low cost-effectiveness of PABD reported recently (Tretiak et al., 1996; Etchason et al., 1995).

BLOOD SALVAGE PROCEDURES

The salvage and reinfusion of blood during the perioperative period represents the most common form of autologous blood transfusion. Used in conjunction with other techniques in a comprehensive blood conservation program, blood salvage is frequently used during pediatric surgical procedures where moderate blood loss is foreseen. Salvaged blood is a source of immediately available, type-specific, compatible blood without the risks of disease transmission or isoimmunization. The use of salvaged blood greatly reduces or abolishes the incidences of febrile, allergic, graft-versus-host, and hemolytic transfusion reactions. Because salvaged blood usually does not require handling, transport, typing, compatibility, or disease testing, technical errors are virtually eliminated. Salvaged blood is normothermic, and thus hypothermia and the necessity of a blood warmer are avoided. Other advantages may also include psychologic benefit to recipient and parents and avoidance of modification of any immunosuppressive effects of transfusion.

Indications for Blood Salvage

Blood salvage procedures are currently used for some surgical procedures in children, such as orthopedic correction of spinal deformities, correction of congenital cardiac defects, and orthotopic liver transplantation. An indication for the use of blood salvage in children (>10 kg) includes an anticipated blood loss of 20% or more of their estimated blood volume or a procedure in which greater than 10% of patients are transfused with more than one unit (Williamson and Taswell, 1991; Zauder, 1991; Simpson et al., 1993).

Blood salvage in infants and small children (<10 kg) is rarely feasible or indicated, because current pediatric blood salvage technology would require a minimum anticipated blood loss equal to 1 to 1.5 times their estimated blood volume. With allogenic blood transfusion unavoidable in these patients, many of the advantages of autologous transfusion are negated. These patients are probably best served through the use of minimal (single) blood donor exposure—that is, the use of mini (50 or 100 mL) blood packs derived from a single donor (Salem and Podraza, 1992).

Blood Salvage Techniques

Clinicians have often raised concerns about possible physical and biochemical alterations of blood following extravasation, collection and processing, and reinfusion that might render salvaged blood inferior to banked blood. That salvaged blood differs significantly from allogenic banked blood or from circulating blood is undisputed (Table 12–4). The diverse circumstances under which shed blood is salvaged and the various techniques that are used result in salvaged blood products with differing characteristics. Blood salvage in the pediatric patient

TABLE 12–4. Hematologic comparison of bank and salvaged blood

Index Factor	Processed Salvaged Blood*	Unprocessed Salvaged Blood*	Bank Blood	Normal Blood
Hemoglobin (g/dL)	17.9	6.3 ± 1.1	16.0 ± 3.5	12 to 17†
Hematocrit (%)		17.0 ± 3.3	46.5 ± 10.5	37 to 50†
Red blood cells (/mm³ × 10⁶)		2.0 ± 0.4	5.0 ± 1.1	4.8 to 5.8†
Leukocytes (/mm³ × 10³)	1.1	3.4 ± 1.3	5.3 ± 2.3	7.0
Platelets (/mm³ × 10³)	64	384 ± 141	Inactivated	250 to 350
Free hemoglobin (mg/dL)	123	1000 ± 625	13.3 ± 10.8	<2.5
Screen filtration pressure (mm Hg)	200	170		
pH	7.72 ± 0.18		6.63 ± 0.06	7.33 to 7.43
P_{CO_2} (mm Hg)		8.5 ± 4.0	158 ± 68	38 to 50
P_{O_2} (mm Hg)		160 ± 17	50 ± 25	60 to 108
Sodium (mmol/L)	147 ± 2.4	136 ± 5	162 ± 6	135 to 148
Potassium (mmol/L)	1.6 ± 1.5	6.8 ± 1.9	12.6 ± 4.6	3.5 to 5.3
Chloride (mmol/L)	134 ± 3.3	123 ± 5	76 ± 9	98 to 106
CO_2 (mmol/L)	5.4 ± 1.6	6 ± 1	11 ± 2	19 to 26
Calcium (ionized) (mmol/L)	2.3 ± 0.5	1.25 ± 0.2	2.25 ± 0.1	2.1 to 2.7
SGOT (units)	9 ± 5	128 ± 74	14 ± 4	6 to 21
SGPT (units)	15 ± 9	14 ± 6	11 ± 5	7 to 14
Lactate dehydrogenase (units)	214 ± 103	1605 ± 718	299 ± 146	85 to 190
Creatine phosphokinase (units)	1073 ± 983	96 ± 27	10 to 65	
Direct bilirubin (mg/dL)		0.4 ± 0.1	0.06 ± 0.02	0 to 0.2
Total bilirubin (mg/dL)	0.11 ± 0.07	0.7 ± 0.2	0.41 ± 0.13	0.2 to 1.0

Modified Bentley ATS100 used for blood salvage.

†Range includes both male and female adults.

Processed salvage data modified from Yawn DH: Properties of salvaged blood. In Taswell HF, Pineda AA, editors: *Autologous transfusion and hemotherapy.* Boston, 1991, Blackwell Scientific Publishers, with permission. Filtration data modified from Aaron RK, Beazley RM, Riggle GC: Hematologic integrity after intraoperative allotransfusion. *Arch Surg* 108:831, 1974. Normal data from Fiereck EA: Appendix. In Tietz NW, editor: *Fundamentals of clinical chemistry*, 2nd ed. Philadelphia, 1976, WB Saunders, pp 1177–1227, with permission.

can be accomplished by three different techniques: (1) filtration by a canister device, (2) cell processing by centrifugation and cell washing, and (3) hemoconcentration via hemofiltration.

Filtration

Blood salvage by filtration is based on the tenet that the mere extravasation of blood does not render that blood unfit for reinfusion, provided that coagulation, contamination, and significant hemolysis are prevented. Shed blood is altered only by filtration and the addition of anticoagulant, if required. Various filtration systems that are currently available differ slightly depending on the route of administration of anticoagulant, intraoperative or postoperative use, portability, and direct-versus-indirect reinfusion.

Blood is collected in a reservoir that is either divided into two chambers separated by a coarse mesh filter (170 μm) or a single chamber with the filter incorporated into the inlet (Fig. 12–12). A regulated vacuum source is connected to the reservoir, and negative pressure should not exceed −150 mm Hg (and usually kept between −30 and −50 mm Hg) to prevent damage to formed blood elements during aspiration. Defoaming material inside the reservoir chamber or present as a coating on the coarse filter prevents foaming. In the nonheparinized patient, anticoagulant must either be added to the reservoir or mixed with shed blood near the tip of a specially designed dual-channel suction tubing/wand assembly. Heparinized saline, citrate-phosphate-dextrose, and acid-citrate-dextrose formulas have all been used. Citrate anticoagulants are particularly advantageous in filtration systems because of their negligible systemic effects (provided citrated blood is not reinfused too rapidly or in excessive volumes). Anticoagulant requirements may vary depending on the location and extent of bleeding, with citrated solutions used in a ratio of 1 part anticoagulant to 7 parts blood. In the heparinized patient, heparin in a concentration of 20,000 to 40,000 U/L is usually effective (Zauder, 1991). After collection and coarse filtration, salvaged blood can be reinfused directly to the patient. Reinfusion through a microaggregate filter (10 to 50 μm) is recommended by most filtration system manufacturers, although data in favor of the use of these filters are not convincing. If blood cannot be immediately reinfused, it can be stored in the reservoir for up to 6 hours at 20° to 24°C, according to the AABB guidelines (1993). Blood salvaged by filtration can also be transported to the blood bank for processing (centrifugation and washing) (Pineda and Valbonesi, 1990).

The principal advantages of blood salvage by filtration are the simplicity of filter design, ease of operation, and portability. Setup and operation do not require specialized training, nor is a dedicated operator normally necessary. Other than a vacuum source and an anticoagulant solution, the disposable units are entirely self-contained. The collection reservoir can usually follow the patient from operating room to postanesthesia care or intensive care units to minimize costs and maximize salvage yield (Blevins et al., 1993; Davis et al., 1993). Because no blood processing (beyond filtration) is required, shed blood drawn into the collection chamber is immediately available for reinfusion. The cost of blood salvage by filtration is generally lower than that associated with cell processing.

Postoperative anemia is a common occurrence after autotransfusion with filtration devices, particularly when salvaged blood is the sole or primary source of replacement red blood cells. Blood salvaged by filtration typically has a low hemoglobin value, ranging between 6 and 9 g/dL (Yawn, 1991). However, the red blood cells that are salvaged have a relatively normal half-life, higher concentrations of 2,3-DPG and adenosine triphosphate (ATP) than banked blood, and normal P_{50} and pH. Salvaged red blood cells are more resistant to osmotic lysis, because the most frail red blood cells lyse during collection and filtration (Ray et al., 1986; Williamson and Taswell, 1991).

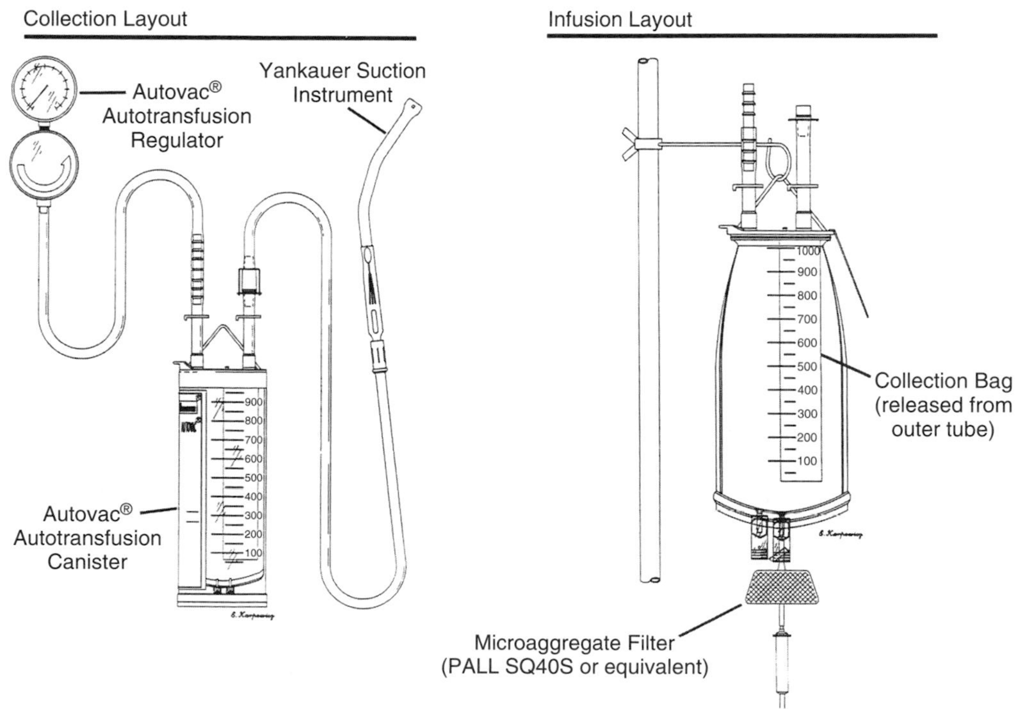

■ **FIGURE 12–12.** Schematic diagram of a filtration system. (Courtesy of Boehringer Laboratories, Inc., Norristown, PA.)

Platelets, leukocytes, and coagulation factors are often reduced in salvaged blood. The concentration of these components in unprocessed salvaged blood depends on their concentration in the patient's blood, loss in salvage apparatus, and dilution with anticoagulant, tissue fluids, and irrigation solutions (Yawn, 1991). Those platelets present in salvaged blood are considered dysfunctional, having shown signs of activation (Wilson et al., 1988; Yawn, 1991; Kongsgaard et al., 1993).

The concentration of coagulation factors and the clotting competency of salvaged blood are specifically determined by the location and circumstances of collection. Blood salvaged from the mediastinum, pleural space, and peritoneal cavity has undergone extensive coagulation and clot lysis and is virtually devoid of fibrinogen. Fibrinogen may be significantly higher in blood salvaged from systemically anticoagulated patients. Fibrin degradation products are markedly increased in filtered blood. Although signs of clinical bleeding should be monitored and the need for fresh frozen plasma and platelet concentrates considered, component replacement is rarely necessary (Yawn, 1991; Kongsgaard et al., 1993).

As a result of hemolysis, shed blood also can contain high concentrations of free plasma hemoglobin and cellular debris. Under normal circumstances the reticuloendothelial system can remove free plasma hemoglobin in concentrations up to 120 mg/dL. Levels exceeding 1600 mg/dL have been measured in salvaged blood. The filtration technique is not effective for free plasma hemoglobin or cell debris. Regardless of the toxic level, adequate hydration, avoidance of hypotension and acidosis, and maintenance of urinary output with appropriate use of diuretics or dopamine have been shown to prevent this complication.

Cell Processing

Blood salvaging is most commonly accomplished by cell processing. Shed blood is aspirated from the surgical field, mixed with an anticoagulant, and stored in a cardiotomy reservoir. When a sufficient amount of blood has collected, it is pumped into a spinning (5000 rpm) centrifuge bowl, which separates blood components on the basis of density. As the bowl fills, higher-density red blood cells continually displace other constituents of blood, which spill over into a waste container. When the bowl is filled with red blood cells, a wash cycle rinses away all residual contaminants and anticoagulants, suspending the red blood cells to any desired hematocrit (usually 50% to 70%) in normal saline solution (Stehling and Zauder, 1991) (Fig. 12–13). The trauma imposed by suction, centrifugation, washing, and reinfusion appears to have negligible effects on red blood cell survival (Ray et al., 1986). For optimal results and safety, a trained operator whose only responsibility is to "recycle shed blood" should operate these sophisticated systems (AABB, 1993).

The characteristics of salvaged blood following processing (centrifugation and washing) differ significantly from those of nonprocessed blood (see Table 12–4). Centrifugation virtually eliminates all the plasma constituents of blood. Washing significantly reduces any residual contaminants, including anticoagulant, free plasma hemoglobin and potassium, fibrin-degradation products and D-dimer fragments, products of platelet activation and lysis, products of complement activation, cellular and tissue debris, and microaggregates. The resulting product is similar to packed red blood cells but suspended in normal saline solution rather than plasma.

Unlike filtration systems, the hematocrit of the infusate following cell processing is unrelated to that of the shed blood. The hematocrit of processed red blood cells depends on the flow rate of salvaged blood into the centrifuge bowl and the rotational speed of the centrifuge and can be further adjusted by varying the volume of saline solution used for resuspension. If negative pressure in the recovery system is low, hemolysis during harvest and processing is between 2% and 10% of all salvageable red blood cells.

Because platelets and plasma constituents, including coagulation factors and plasma proteins, are totally eliminated during processing of salvaged blood, patients transfused with large volumes of processed red blood cells may show a slight reduction of coagulation factors, dilution of platelets, and prolonged

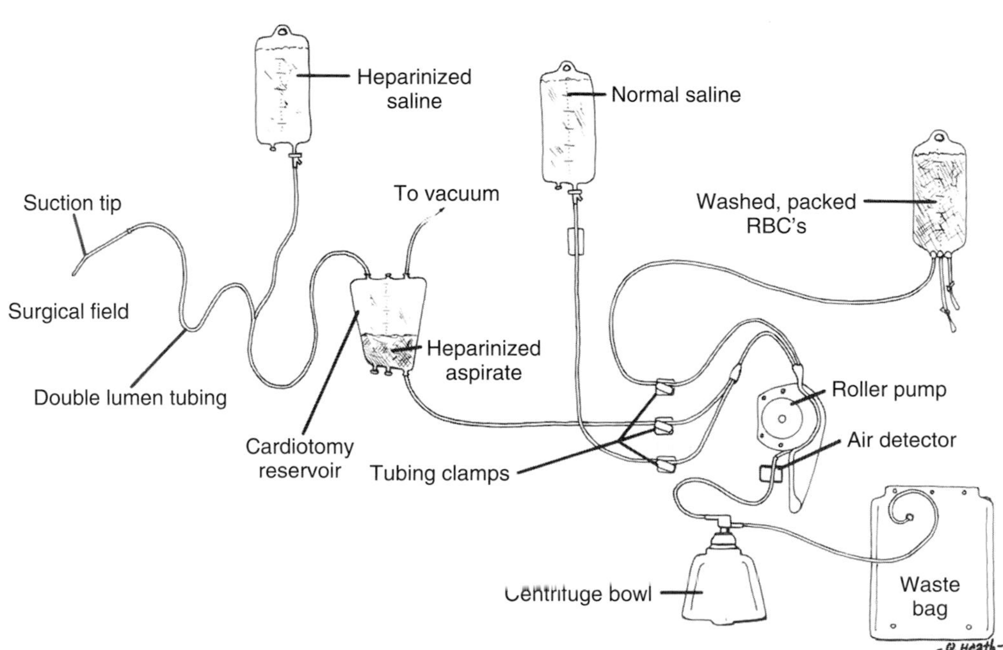

■ **FIGURE 12–13.** Schematic diagram of a cell-processing system.

prothrombin, activated partial thromboplastin, thrombin, and bleeding times (Otteson and Frøysaker, 1982). Massive autotransfusions of processed blood (usually several blood volumes) often require fresh frozen plasma administration. Various formulas for the replacement of plasma constituents and platelets have been advanced based on the volume of autotransfusion. However, coagulopathy often cannot be predicted based on such formulas. Because coagulopathy can result from the dilution of coagulation factors, fibrinogen, and platelets or a consumption process (disseminated intravascular coagulation), in vitro hemostatic laboratory testing is important in differentiating dilutional from consumptional coagulopathies.

Hemoconcentration

The hemofilter has been used as an adjunct to the extracorporeal circuit during cardiopulmonary bypass in children to facilitate collection of red blood cells (Tuman et al., 1988, Naik et al., 1991). The hemofilter is either a hollow fiber filter or a parallel plate with designated membrane pore size. Hemoconcentration is based on a process that imitates physiologic glomerular filtration by applying a hydrostatic pressure gradient across a porous membrane. This efficient method of removing excess circulating blood volume can be achieved without significant alteration in serum electrolyte concentrations or acid-base status. The technique of hemoconcentration is a convective process with plasma and dissolved solutes filtering at the same rate, limited only by the pore size of the device. Transmembrane pressure (gradient) is the driving force, and is calculated by the following formula:

$$TMP = \frac{P_A + P_V}{2} + |P_N|$$

where TMP is transmembrane pressure (mm Hg), P_A is arterial (inlet) pressure (mm Hg), P_V is venous (outlet) pressure (mm Hg), and P_N is absolute value of the suction applied on the ultrafiltrate outlet (mm Hg).

To avoid red blood cell lysis, the transmembrane pressure should remain below 600 mm Hg. Ultrafiltrate flux is determined by several factors, including properties of the membrane, pump flow rate, transmembrane pressure, hematocrit, and plasma protein concentration. Membrane pore size varies among manufacturers (16,000 to 60,000 Da). Depending on pore size, heparin with a molecular weight of less than 20,000 Da can be removed. Anticoagulation status should be closely monitored during intraoperative use and for postbypass concentration of residual oxygenator blood. The hemoconcentrator can be used in a similar manner as a cell processor in conjunction with cardiopulmonary bypass for cardiac (Naik et al., 1991; Friesen et al., 1993) or liver transplantation surgery (Tuman et al., 1988), as well as for nonbypass procedures (Solem et al., 1987).

Under normal circumstances, the management of excess hemodilution during extracorporeal circulation is accomplished by pharmacologically induced diuresis. However, certain situations arise when diuresis is impractical or too inefficient. In such situations, the control of plasma water volume during cardiopulmonary bypass can be achieved through hemofiltration much more effectively than through cell processing. By allowing more precise control of blood volume, the hemoconcentrator enables the use of greater hemodilution during cardiopulmonary bypass (Naik et al., 1991).

The main advantage of hemoconcentration over cell processing by centrifugation and washing appears to be the ability to hemoconcentrate blood to any desired hematocrit with preservation of valuable plasma constituents. Better platelet and fibrinogen preservation might avoid coagulopathy associated with the autotransfusion of large amounts of salvaged blood. Electrolytes, which pass through the hemofilter, remain relatively normal, and plasma proteins, which cannot, are concentrated (Solem et al., 1987). Other advantages of the hemoconcentrator are speed, lower cost, and single-pass hemofiltration at rates of 500 mL/min.

Postoperative Blood Salvage

The volume of blood lost after surgery can be significant, but this blood is salvageable by either filtration or cell-processing apparatus. Situated between a vacuum source and the wound drains, a reservoir with an internal 150- to 170-μm filter collects sanguineous wound drainage. This blood may be continuously reinfused, allowed to collect for a period of time (not longer than 6 hours) before reinfusion without processing through a fine filter (10 to 50 μm), or processed and reinfused. Anticoagulation is usually not required because this blood is totally defibrinogenated through extensive contact with wound surfaces (Yawn, 1991). The reinfusion of volumes up to 15% of the estimated blood volume has been shown to be safe (Kongsgaard et al., 1993).

Complications and Contraindications

The potential complications of blood salvaging are mostly related to the infusion of salvaged blood. Salvaged blood may be hemoglobinemic, thrombocytopenic, leukopenic, hypofibrinogenemic, and depleted or diluted of coagulation factors and plasma proteins. Furthermore, the state of those red blood cells, platelets, and leukocytes present has also been questioned. Because neither filtration nor cell processing can remove all contaminants, some soluble or insoluble foreign substances may be transfused to the patient. Cell washing has been shown to significantly reduce (by ≥80%) bacterial cell counts in enteric-contaminated blood. Finally, the concentrations and metabolisms of perioperatively administered drugs are unpredictable following the reinfusion of shed blood.

Various contraindications to the use of blood salvage have been suggested (Box 12–8). Extravasated blood older than 6 hours or excessively hemolyzed blood should not be reinfused. Although cell processing can eliminate most contaminants, shed blood in contact with bowel contents or malignant cells or that

BOX 12–8 Potential Contraindications of Blood Salvage

- Extravasated blood over 6 hours old
- Suspected or confirmed enteric contamination
- Suspected or confirmed malignant cell contamination
- Sickle cell anemia patients
- Hemolyzed blood
- Some Jehovah's Witness patients
- In the presence of certain hemostatic substances
- In the presence of some wound sterilizing substances
- Surgical excision of pheochromocytoma tumors
- Patients with positive viral antigen markers

aspirated from an infected wound site should not be reinfused except with life-threatening hemorrhage. The collection of shed blood should be interrupted following the application of thrombin, microfibrillar collagen hemostat (Avitene), methylmethacrylate, and irrigation with wound-sterilizing solutions (e.g., Betadine) or antibiotic solutions not meant for parenteral use (Stehling and Zauder, 1991; Williamson and Taswell, 1991; AABB, 1993).

The safety of blood salvaging in infants and children with sickle cell disease remains unclear. Although sickle cell disease has been described as a contraindication for the use of blood salvage, the scant literature that is available is inconclusive. In infancy, precautions are probably unnecessary, because erythrocytes with high concentrations of HbF molecules appear to be resistant to sickling. However, as HbF concentrations decline, sickle cell disease may begin to manifest itself (Karayalcin, 1979; Esseltine et al., 1988). Further studies are required before sickle cell patients are categorically denied the benefits of this important technique.

ACUTE NORMOVOLEMIC HEMODILUTION

Acute isovolemic or normovolemic hemodilution (ANH) entails the withdrawal of a calculated volume of the patient's blood and the simultaneous replacement with a cell-free substitute to maintain a near-normal blood volume. This intentional decrease in hemoglobin concentration (dilutional anemia) is accomplished sometime after anesthetic induction but before the critical phases of surgery are started. The patient's own fresh blood is reinfused near the end of the surgical procedure after the major blood loss has ceased. The rationale for the use of ANH as a method for blood conservation is that if intraoperative blood loss is relatively constant, the loss of blood constituents, especially red blood cells, would be reduced if the blood were diluted. The term *normovolemic* is commonly used although there are no simple means of predicting the accuracy of the *normovolemic status* and thus slight hypervolemia or hypovolemia cannot be excluded. Although no standard nomenclature for the degree of hemodilution has been established, a decrease in hematocrit from the normal value of 40% to between 25% and 35% is referred to as moderate or limited hemodilution, whereas a hematocrit below 20% has been referred to as profound or extreme hemodilution.

Although hemodilution was recognized as early as 1882 by Kronecker, who demonstrated that the acute dilution of blood to a hematocrit of 15% was compatible with survival, it was not until the 1960s that intentional hemodilution was used as a method of blood conservation during surgery. Since then, its use has been extended to various surgical procedures, including pediatric surgery (Lawson et al., 1974; Laver et al., 1975; Viviani et al., 1978; Watzek et al., 1980; Wong et al., 1980; Fahmy, 1985b).

ANH can alter oxygen transport via its influences on arterial oxygen–carrying capacity and the rheological properties of blood. This important rheological consequence of hemodilution warrants a discussion of some principles of blood viscosity.

Hemorheology of Hemodilution

The viscosity of a liquid is a measure of its internal friction. *Viscosity* may be defined as the resistance to flow that depends on the intermolecular forces operating within the liquid. The term *internal friction* emphasizes that as a fluid moves within a tube, laminae in the fluid slip on one another and move at different speeds. This results in a velocity gradient in a direction perpendicular to the wall of the tube, termed the *shear rate*.

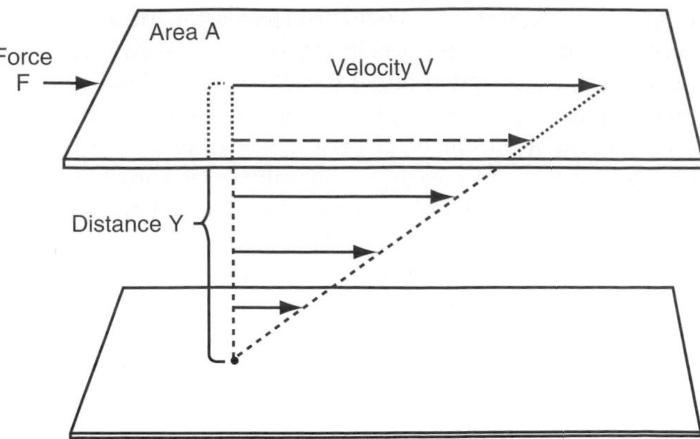

FIGURE 12–14. Relation between shear stress and shear rate when a fluid is sheared between two parallel plates. See text for details. (From Fahmy NR: Techniques for deliberate hypotension: Haemodilution and hypotension. In Enderby GEH, editor: *Hypotensive anaesthesia.* Edinburgh, 1985b, Churchill Livingstone, with permission.)

In the circulation, shear rate bears a positive correlation to blood flow.

In an experiment, a liquid is confined between two closely spaced parallel plates (analogous to playing cards) (Fig. 12–14). The area of each plate is A, and the distance between the plates is Y. If a tangential force is applied along one plate, while the other is kept stationary, the plate moves in the direction of the force and a velocity gradient develops in the fluid. For a given fluid, the velocity gradient (or shear rate) varies with the force applied (F) per plate surface area (or shear stress). The force required to displace one plate relative to its neighbor divided by the surface area of the plate is defined as shear stress (dynes/cm^2). The distance that the plate is displaced horizontally per unit time relative to its neighbor is known as the shear rate, which is expressed in units of distance per unit time divided by the thickness of the plate. The shear stress required to achieve a given shear rate varies with the viscosity of the fluid. Hence,

$$\text{Viscosity} = \frac{\text{Shear stress}}{\text{Shear rate}}$$

The units of viscosity are expressed in dynes/sec per cm^2, or *poise*. The relation between shear stress and shear rate is the basis for comparing viscosities of different fluids and for studying the effect of hemodilution on whole blood viscosity (Messmer and Sunder-Plassman, 1974; Messmer, 1975).

Factors affecting whole blood viscosity include (1) shear rate (rate of flow), (2) red blood cell deformability, (3) plasma proteins, (4) red blood cell aggregation, (5) hematocrit, (6) temperature, and (7) size of vessel.

A Newtonian fluid is characterized by constant viscosity during changes in shear rate. Plasma and saline solution are typical Newtonian fluids; the shear rates increase linearly with increasing shear stress and thus the viscosity remains unaltered. Because blood is a suspension of cells in plasma, it does not exhibit strict Newtonian behavior. Blood behaves like a non-Newtonian fluid when moving slowly and like a Newtonian fluid when flowing rapidly. The viscosity of whole blood increases sharply at low flow rates (as in postcapillary venules) but remains constant at high and moderate rates of blood flow (as in arteries and arterioles). This results from the increased tendency of red blood cells to concentrate in the center of the stream (axial streaming) and from the increased red blood cell deformation occurring at high flow rates (the tendency of red blood cells to assume ellipsoid patterns with their longitudinal axis aligned in the direction of the flow). Plasma proteins, specifically fibrinogen and γ-globulins, exert pronounced effects on red blood cell aggregation. When normal red blood cells are suspended in a medium with the same fluid viscosity as plasma but without the long plasma proteins required for cell bridging, shear-dependent behavior is decreased markedly.

Hematocrit directly influences blood viscosity. The higher the hematocrit, the more friction exists between the layers of blood, resulting in increased viscosity. An increase in hematocrit from 40% to 60% is associated with an approximate doubling of the viscosity, whereas a decrease from 40% to 20% results in an approximate 50% decrease in viscosity (Messmer, 1975) (Fig. 12–15). The most dramatic decrease in blood viscosity during hemodilution is seen in the postcapillary venules, when the hematocrit decreases from the normal level to approximately 25%. Further decrease in hematocrit is not accompanied by further reduction in viscosity (Fig. 12–16).

Temperature bears an inverse relation to blood viscosity. The decrease in hematocrit required to maintain constant blood viscosity during hypothermia is shown (Fig. 12–17). At 20°C, a reduction in hematocrit from 45% to 25% is needed to restore viscosity to the same value measured at 37°C. After circulatory arrest, however, the shear stress required to reinitiate flow and break up the red blood cell aggregates is likely to be high. Additional rheologic benefit may be gained by a further decrease in hematocrit.

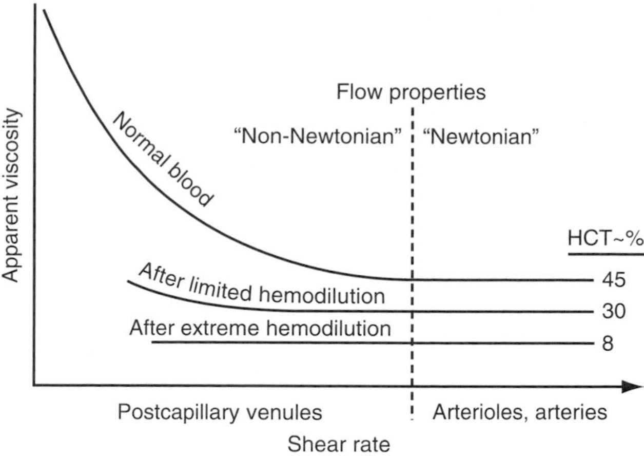

■ **FIGURE 12–16.** Schematic representation of the effect of hemodilution on whole blood viscosity as related to changes in shear rate in vivo in different vascular compartments. The most pronounced decrease in blood viscosity, and hence resistance to flow, should occur within the postcapillary venules when the hematocrit (HCT) is decreased from its control level (45%) to approximately 30%, that is, limited hemodilution. Further decreases in hematocrit (extreme hemodilution) will reduce viscosity remarkably less. (Modified from Messmer K, Sunder-Plassman L: Hemodilution. *Prog Surg* 13:208, 1974.)

The tendency for increased hematocrit to increase blood viscosity is attenuated when blood flows through tubes of capillary diameter. This is because red blood cells are normally very deformable, and with a diameter similar to that of the capillary, they can squeeze through the vessel lumen in single file with

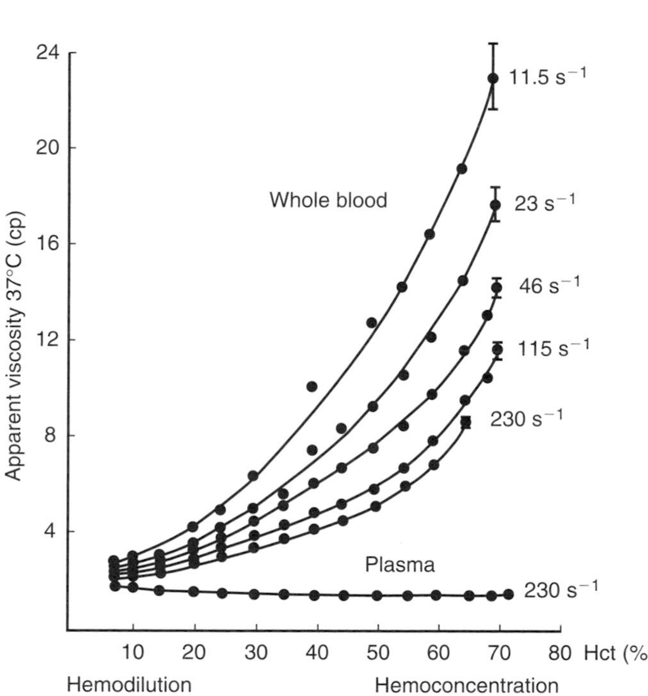

■ **FIGURE 12–15.** Viscosity of whole blood at various hematocrit values, determined at various shear rates (from 11.5 to 230 per second). Hematocrit was varied by the addition of dextran and packed red blood cells. The viscosity of plasma is also shown for comparison. Note that whole blood viscosity increases with hematocrit and that the increments in viscosity are greatest at the lower shear rates. (From Messmer K, Sunder-Plassman L: Hemodilution. *Prog Surg* 13:208, 1974.)

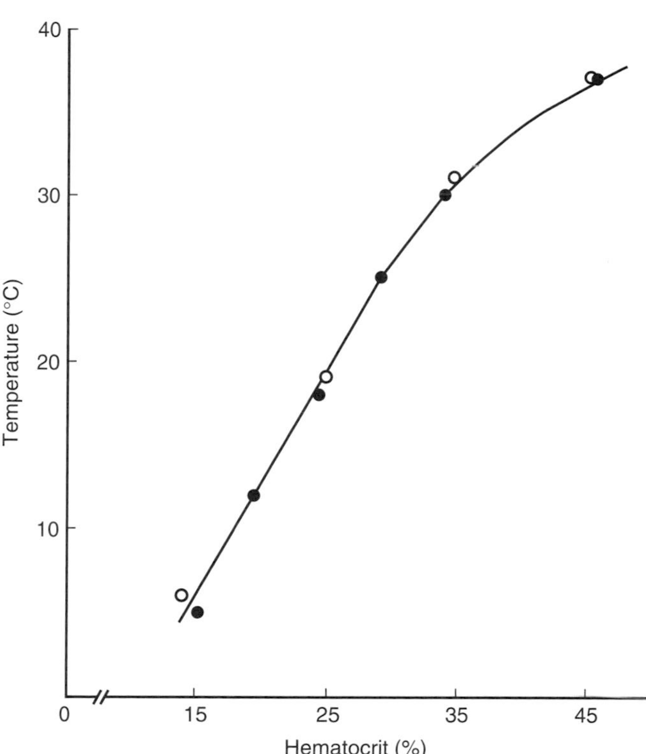

■ **FIGURE 12–17.** Illustration of decrease in hematocrit in two patients that must accompany a reduction in body temperature if viscosity is to remain constant. The measurements were made at a low shear rate with an initial hematocrit at 37°C of 45%. Data were obtained with whole blood from two normal adults. (Modified from Larson L: *Changes in flow properties in human blood* [thesis]. Bozeman MT, 1973, Montana State University.)

minimal extra force required. The rate at which red blood cells pass through the capillary has little influence on blood viscosity.

Physiologic Responses to Acute Normovolemic Hemodilution

The cardiovascular responses during ANH depend on the degree of hemodilution, the circulating blood volume, the nature of the diluent, and the efficacy of compensatory physiologic mechanisms.

Systemic Responses

The decrease in hemoglobin concentration during ANH leads to a proportional decrease in arterial oxygen content (CaO_2). Physiological mechanisms available to compensate for this decrease in CaO_2 are (1) increased cardiac output and (2) increased oxygen extraction ratio.

An increase in cardiac output is the main compensatory mechanism during moderate ANH. The increases in cardiac output are primarily due to an augmented stroke volume, although an increased heart rate may assume an important role when basal heart rate is low. The increases in stroke volume are attributable to (1) enhanced myocardial contractility involving activation of the cardiac sympathetic nerves and β-adrenergic receptors, (2) reduction in impedance to left ventricular ejection as a result of decreases in blood viscosity and peripheral vascular resistance, and (3) increased venous return because of reduced peripheral vascular resistance.

The systemic oxygen delivery, the product of cardiac output and $C\bar{v}O_2$, is reasonably well maintained as long as hematocrit is not reduced below 25% (Fig. 12–18). When oxygen delivery decreases during extreme ANH, oxygen consumption can be maintained if mixed venous oxygen content ($C\bar{v}O_2$) falls more than $C\bar{v}O_2$; that is, if oxygen extraction ratio increases resulting in reductions in mixed venous oxygen saturation ($S\bar{v}O_2$). Increases in oxygen extraction ratio from the normal value of 25% to 50% or higher have been demonstrated during extreme ANH.

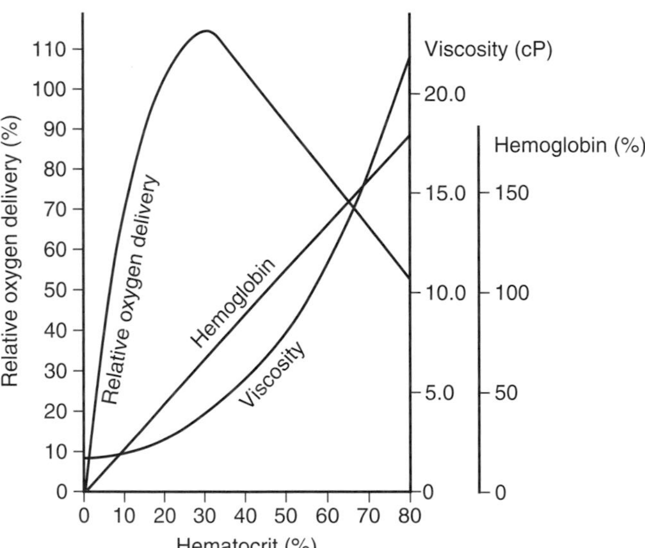

■ **FIGURE 12–18.** Relationship between hematocrit value and theoretical relative oxygen delivery of blood. Values were calculated from the whole blood viscosity assuming that a hematocrit value of 45% corresponds with a hemoglobin value of 100% and that the velocity of flow is inversely proportional to the viscosity of blood. (Modified from Hint H: The pharmacology of dextran and clinical background of the clinical use of Rheomacrodex. *Acta Anaesthesiol Belg* 19:119, 1968, with permission.)

Such increases in oxygen extraction ratio have been shown to coincide with the onset of cardiac lactate production and cardiac dysfunction. Based on this finding, it has been proposed that an oxygen extraction ratio of 50% may serve as a "trigger" for blood transfusion in severely hemodiluted patients.

In chronic anemia, a rightward shift of the oxyhemoglobin dissociation curve may facilitate unloading of oxygen at tissue. This mechanism, which apparently is due to an increased 2,3-DPG concentration within the red blood cells, appears to have no important role during ANH.

Regional Responses

Heart. During ANH, the heart is the principal organ at risk. This is due to (1) an augmented contractile demand, (2) a low baseline coronary venous PO_2 resulting in a limited oxygen extraction reserve, and (3) the tendency for subendocardial ischemia in the left ventricular wall, when tachycardia, aortic hypotension, or both occur in the presence of a dilated coronary vasculature.

In normal hearts, blood flow to both the left and right ventricular myocardium increases in proportion to the decreases in hematocrit during ANH (Fig. 12–19). As long as hematocrit is not reduced below a critical value (approximately 10%), the increases in myocardial blood flow are transmurally uniform and sufficient to maintain myocardial oxygen consumption and oxygen delivery. The adequacy of myocardial oxygen delivery is indicated by the unchanged PO_2 of coronary venous blood (a reflection of PO_2 within the myocardium) and well-preserved myocardial lactate extraction and uptake (Fig. 12–20), as well as by stability of indices of cardiac performance, including aortic pressure, left atrial pressure, and left ventricular contractility. Although a reduction in blood viscosity has been shown to contribute to the decreased coronary vascular resistance during ANH, significantly diminished reactive hyperemic responses imply that coronary vasodilation via metabolic mechanisms (presumably in response to reduced CaO_2) plays a prominent role (Fig. 12–21). Hearts with stenotic coronary arteries (resulting in diminished vasodilator reserve) are less tolerant of ANH; that is, they exhibit signs of global cardiac dysfunction at a higher hematocrit.

Other Organs. ANH has been shown to increase blood flow throughout the central nervous system, to both normal tissue and to areas with impaired autoregulation. The findings of unimpaired electroencephalographic activity, lack of anaerobic metabolism, and well-maintained cerebral oxygen consumption suggest that, on a global basis, cerebral oxygenation is adequate during moderate ANH.

Studies showed that the renal blood flow may increase or decrease during ANH. Although the hepatic arterial and portal vein blood flow may increase during ANH, there is increased hepatic oxygen extraction. In general, blood flow in the splanchnic organs and kidney changes minimally during ANH, resulting in decreases in regional oxygen delivery. These findings suggest that in these organs, the favorable influence of reduced viscosity on blood flow is antagonized by vasoconstriction, which is presumably mediated by the sympathetic vasoconstrictor nerves. The selective peripheral vasoconstriction during ANH serves two important functions: (1) it combines with an increased cardiac output to support aortic pressure and (2) it ensures that the increased cardiac output is preferentially distributed to the vital organs, namely, the heart and brain.

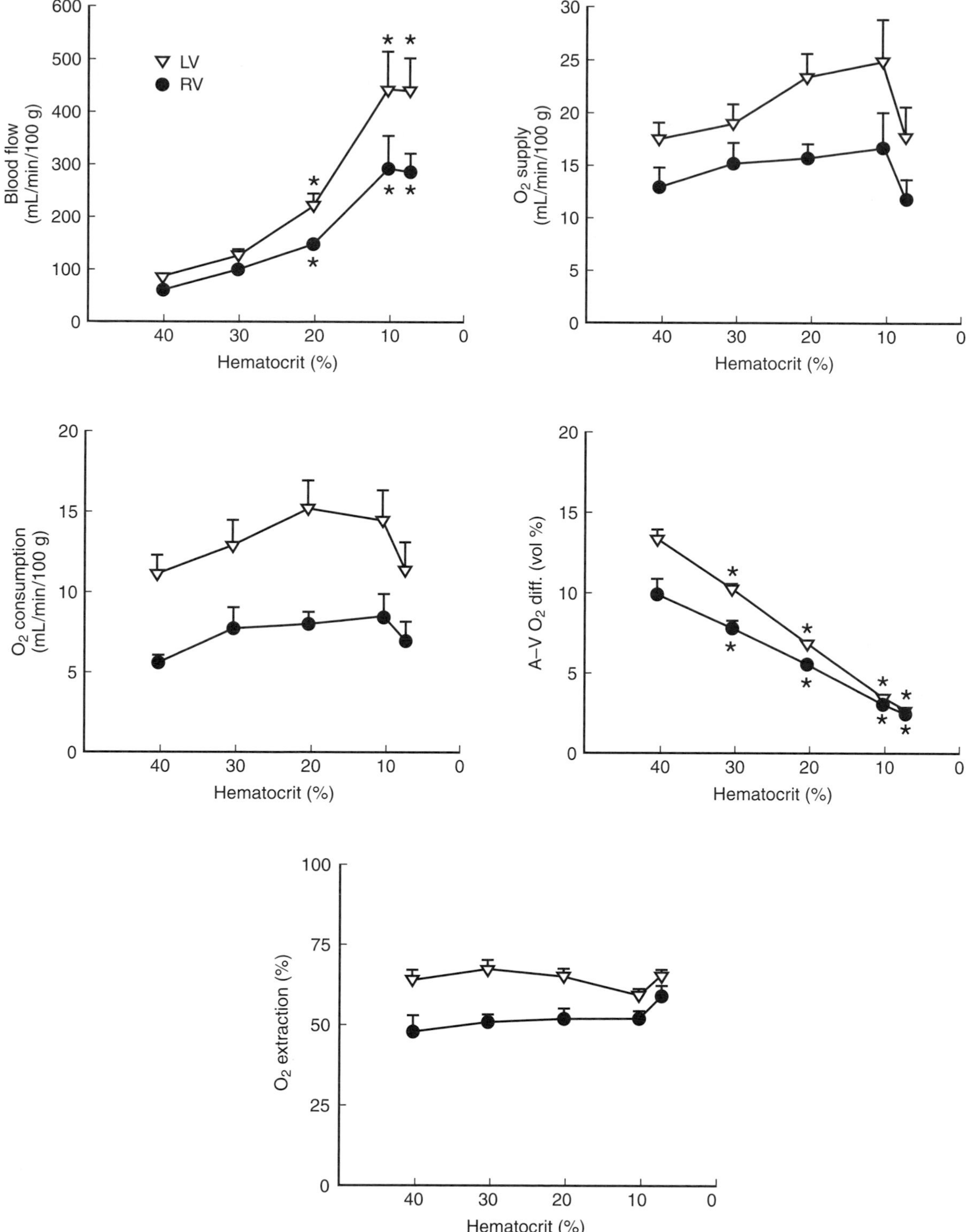

■ **FIGURE 12–19.** Comparison of effect of graded hemodilution on parameters of O_2 delivery and uptake in the right and left ventricles (RV and LV, respectively) in anesthetized dogs. A-V O_2 diff, arteriovenous O_2 difference. *$P < .05$, from value at hematocrit of 40%. (From Crystal GJ, Kim S-J, Salem MR: Right and left ventricular O_2 uptake during hemodilution and β-adrenergic stimulation. *Am J Physiol* 265:H1769–H1777, 1993, with permission.)

The effect of hemodilution on pulmonary gas exchange is controversial. In one study, blood gas levels did not change significantly among 47 patients in whom normovolemic hemodilution was conducted before anesthetic induction (Fahmy, 1985b). On the other hand, during hemodilution, the intrapulmonary shunt ($\dot{Q}s/\dot{Q}t$) may increase or decrease, depending on the ventilation–perfusion relationship. When the $\dot{V}/\dot{Q}$ ratios are low, atelectatic areas may have increased perfusion because of hemodilution despite HPV. As a result, a large $\dot{Q}s/\dot{Q}t$ (between 6% and 15%) may be found. When $\dot{V}/\dot{Q}$ ratio is normal, $\dot{Q}s/\dot{Q}t$ may actually decrease.

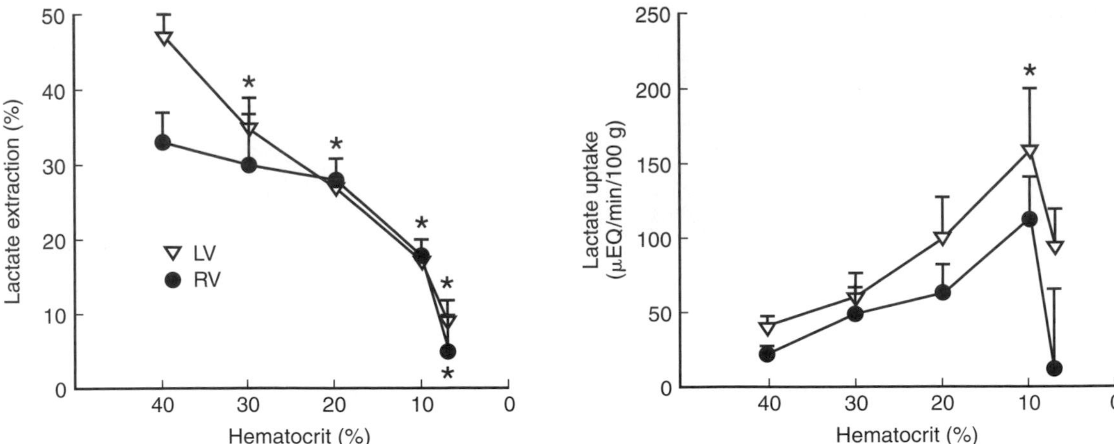

FIGURE 12–20. Comparison of effect of graded hemodilution on right ventricular (RV) and left ventricular (LV) lactate extraction and uptake in anesthetized dogs (*P<.05 from value at hematocrit of 40%). (From Crystal GJ, Kim S-J, Salem MR: Right and left ventricular O_2 uptake during hemodilution and β-adrenergic stimulation. *Am J Physiol* 265:H1769–H1777, 1993, with permission.)

Effects on Coagulation

Theoretically, ANH can influence coagulation, bleeding, or both via three mechanisms: (1) the increase in blood flow can increase oozing; (2) the diluent used can adversely influence coagulation; and (3) dilution of fibrinogen, platelets, and other coagulation factors concomitant with ANH can also impair coagulation. Tuman and others (1987) showed that progressive hemodilution does not result in hypocoagulability as measured by thromboelastography. In fact, the coagulation appears to be stimulated during progressive blood loss. It is likely that surgical stress and tissue trauma (with release of tissue thromboplastin and elevations in catecholamine levels) offset any hypocoagulable tendency resulting from hemodilution and loss of coagulation factors. These offsetting factors are probably responsible for the observed increase in coagulability. Other studies showed that as the hematocrit decreases from 39% to 25%, there are proportionate decreases in fibrinogen, platelets, and factors V and VIII; blood coagulation is not significantly impaired as long as the hematocrit is above 20%.

The slight prolongation of prothrombin time and partial thromboplastin time observed during ANH is not associated with any discernible increase in surgical bleeding or blood loss. Although Kramer and others (1979) found a 30% decrease in platelets and a 50% decrease in fibrinogen levels at a hematocrit of 25% during ANH for major vascular procedures, the values returned to normal levels by the end of the first postoperative day. Because the patient's own fresh blood is reinfused after most of the surgical bleeding has ceased when ANH is terminated, coagulation may be improved and the need for allogenic blood and blood products, including plasma and platelets, is reduced.

Choice of Replacement Fluid

ANH can be tolerated only with adequate circulating blood volume. Crystalloids, colloids, and combinations of both have been used as diluents during hemodilution. Lactated Ringer's solution is the most common crystalloid given. A number of colloids have been used, including albumin (5% solution), dextran (5% dextran solution with a molecular weight of 70,000 Da),

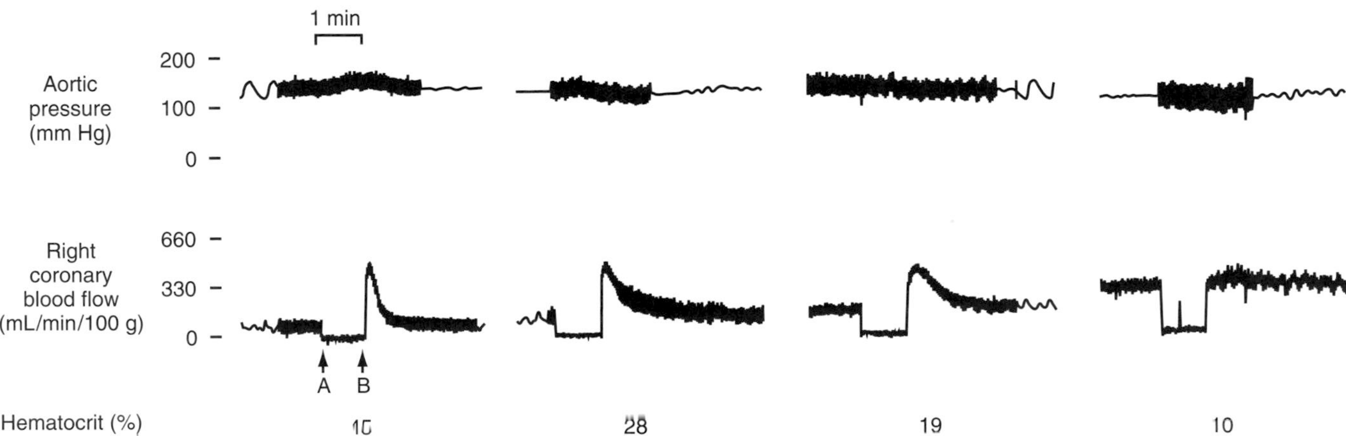

FIGURE 12–21. Original tracings demonstrating effect of graded hemodilution on reactive hyperemia after 60-second occlusion of right coronary artery of an anesthetized dog. At *A*, right coronary artery was occluded; at *B*, occlusion was released. (From Crystal GJ, Kim S-J, Salem MR: Right and left ventricular O_2 uptake during hemodilution and β-adrenergic stimulation. *Am J Physiol* 265:H1769–H1777, 1993, with permission.)

■ TABLE 12–5. Crystalloid versus colloid as the replacement fluid for hemodilution

	Crystalloid	Colloid
Volume required	3 times volume of shed blood	1 to 2 times volume of shed blood
Plasma volume	80% leaves intravascular compartment in 2 hr	Retained longer in the circulation—a better plasma volume expander
Water balance	Positive water balance, more peripheral edema, responds to diuretics	Less peripheral edema
Colloidal osmotic pressure	Reduced, probably not important	Maintained
Postoperative hematocrit	Higher hematocrit	Lower hematocrit
Coagulation defect	None	May occur with excessive colloid therapy (dextrans)
Cost	Inexpensive	Expensive

and hydroxyethyl starch (hetastarch). Dextran-40 (molecular weight = 40,000 Da) has the advantage of retarding rouleaux formation and sludging, but it may result in allergic reactions and coagulation defects. The maximum recommended doses for dextran-40 and dextran-70 are 2 and 1 g/kg, respectively (Arfors and Bergquist, 1975). When colloids are administered, there is a minimal risk of anaphylaxis and blood coagulation may be compromised, especially if a larger volume of hydroxyethyl starch is given (Egli et al., 1997). The advantages and disadvantages of crystalloids and colloids are compared in Table 12–5.

When crystalloids are given as the sole replacement fluid, to maintain normovolemia they should be administered in a volume three times that of the blood withdrawn. Less volume is required when colloids are used as the sole diluents. Crystalloids traverse the capillary endothelium so that, within 2 hours, 80% of the administered volume is in the extravascular space (Gammage, 1987). In contrast, colloids are retained longer in the circulation, thereby maintaining the colloid osmotic pressure and plasma volume for several hours. Consequently, albumin and other colloids produce slightly lower hematocrits intraoperatively and postoperatively than does lactated Ringer's solution (Hallowell et al., 1978). Crystalloids dilute serum proteins and lead to a reduction in colloid osmotic pressure, the importance of which is still controversial. Diuresis follows the administration of crystalloids, and there usually is a rapid response to furosemide.

Although peripheral edema may occur after crystalloid therapy, pulmonary edema rarely ensues (Brinkmeyer et al., 1983). When the lungs are normal, pulmonary edema is usually prevented by intrinsic compensatory factors, including the plasma–interstitial oncotic gradient, the high lymphatic capacity of the lung, the physicochemical characteristics of the interstitial space, the integrity of the microvascular membrane, and a low vascular hydrostatic driving pressure. These factors appear to be less effective in patients with underlying cardiopulmonary disease, thus promoting the development of pulmonary edema. If administered in the presence of capillary leak, albumin may cross the pulmonary capillary endothelium, pulling water with it and increasing pulmonary interstitial water. It must be emphasized that any fluid can be administered in excess to produce pulmonary edema. Probably the amount of the fluid administered and the vigilance in monitoring the hemodynamic variables are more important than the choice of fluid.

Clinical Management of Acute Normovolemic Hemodilution

Patients who are to undergo operations in which major blood losses are expected (more than one third of their blood volume) may be considered candidates for ANH. The technique has been extended to pediatric cardiac surgery, spinal surgery for scoliosis, and operations for malignant disease (Wilms tumor, neuroblastoma, teratomas, retroperitoneal ganglioneuroma, liver tumors, and pancreatic tumors). Although age is not considered an absolute contraindication to the use of ANH and has been used in patients weighing 5 kg (Schaller et al., 1983), the use of ANH in small children should be limited to experienced clinicians.

The parents or responsible guardians should be fully informed as to the rationale and methods of hemodilution before surgery. Risks of massive intraoperative blood loss and transfusion of allogenic blood should be explained. A realistic assessment of the benefit-to-risk ratio of the technique must be presented. Accurate preoperative assessment of the cardiovascular, respiratory, and other systems is essential. A history of drug therapy is important, and steps should be taken to correct any coagulation disorders present. Unless their use is necessary, salicylates (such as indomethacin) and other cyclooxygenase inhibitors should be discontinued 1 or 2 weeks before surgery.

After anesthetic induction and tracheal intubation, an arterial cannula is inserted for blood sampling and arterial blood pressure monitoring. Additional large-bore peripheral intravenous catheters may be placed. A central venous (or a pulmonary artery) catheter may be placed, if indicated. Other monitors should include use of a precordial or an esophageal (or both) stethoscope, electrocardiography, pulse oximetry, capnography, and an esophageal or rectal temperature probe. An indwelling catheter is inserted in the urinary bladder to permit urine volume measurements.

Anesthesia is maintained with an inhalational anesthetic and oxygen. Opioids or combinations of inhaled anesthetics and opioids may also be used. Muscular relaxation is maintained with appropriate monitoring of the neuromuscular function. Ventilation is adjusted to maintain $Pa{CO_2}$ between 30 and 40 mm Hg. Arterial pH, blood gas tensions, and hematocrit are measured every 30 minutes during and after hemodilution and during the critical stages of surgery. If central or pulmonary artery catheters are placed, measurements of central venous or mixed venous blood gas tensions may yield valuable information.

After a steady state of anesthesia is achieved, ANH is started. Using a strictly sterile technique, the predetermined volume of blood (Box 12–9) is withdrawn from either the arterial or the central venous catheter and collected into one or more 250-mL citrate-phosphate-dextrose (CPD) blood donor bags. If an adult bag is used in an adolescent, the bag should contain no less than 300 mL and no more than 450 mL to ensure proper blood-to-anticoagulant ratio. The collection of blood from a central venous line is facilitated by placing the bag lower than the patient level. If a peripheral vein is used, withdrawal of blood can be enhanced by cycling the cuff of a noninvasive blood pressure monitor at 2- or 3-minute intervals. The use of kits that contain two blood bags, a Y-type connector set with a Luer-Loc

BOX 12–9 Calculation of Volume of Blood Removed for Hemodilution

1. $ERCV_T = [HcT \times V \times \text{bodyweight (kg)}]/100$
   where $ERCV_T$ = estimated total red cell volume (mL) and V = estimated blood volume per kilogram of body weight:
   - 90 mL/kg (neonates)
   - 90 mL/kg (infants and children)
   - 65 to 75 mL/kg (teenagers)
2. $ERCV_{20} = 0.2 \times V \times \text{bodyweight (kg)}$
   where $ERCV_{20}$ = estimated red blood cell volume at HcT 20%.*
3. $RCW = ERCV_T - ERCV_{20}$
   where RCW = red blood cell volume to be withdrawn.
4. $WBW = 3 \times RCW$
   where WBW = whole blood volume to be withdrawn.†

*Hematocrit of 20% is chosen because it is commonly used.

†The average hematocrit value of the blood withdrawn is assumed to be 33% and thus the total volume withdrawn is three times the red blood cell volume to be withdrawn.

From Schaller RT Jr, Schaller J, Morgan A, et al.: Hemodilution anesthesia: a valuable aid to major cancer surgery in children. *Am J Surg* 146:79, 1983, with permission of Excerpta Medica, Inc.

adapter, and a blood recipient identification band simplifies the procedure. The collected blood should be mixed with the anticoagulant in the blood bag, and care should be taken to exclude air bubbles. The volume of blood in the CPD bags is determined by weighing the bags (1 mL = 1 g). As blood is being withdrawn, two to three times this amount of lactated Ringer's solution (or an appropriate amount of other diluents) is infused simultaneously. The lactated Ringer's solution should be warmed before its administration to prevent a decrease in the patient's temperature. The blood bags are numbered sequentially, labeled, and kept at room temperature for up to 6 hours to preserve platelet function. If it is expected that the blood will not be transfused within this period, the blood bags should be kept in a small cooler containing wet ice or arrangements should be made with the blood bank for storage up to 24 hours. Although surgery may be started earlier, phases of surgery during which large blood loss tends to occur should not be allowed until ANH is completed. This usually takes about 30 minutes.

A decision should be made regarding the lowest acceptable hematocrit. Unless hypothermia is used, the lowest safe acceptable hematocrit is 20% in normal healthy children. A higher hematocrit may be chosen depending on the condition of the patient and the anticipated blood loss. Measurements of hematocrit must be accurate during ANH, and it is preferable to do more than one measurement per sample. Heel sticks are unreliable and should not be used for measurements of hematocrit during hemodilution. Conventional laboratory hematocrit measurements, including the microcentrifuge technique or the Coulter method, are accurate during ANH. In contrast, hematocrit values derived by the conductivity of whole blood used in portable compact devices provide artificially low readings in situations where plasma has been replaced by crystalloids.

During the operative procedure, blood loss is initially replaced with an equal volume of lactated Ringer's solution. Third-space losses during surgery are compensated for by additional volumes of lactated Ringer's solution. If the hematocrit decreases below the desired level, allogenic packed red blood cells may be infused to maintain the hematocrit at an acceptable level. The temptation to reinfuse the patient's own blood should be resisted until blood loss has ceased.

The autologous blood is reinfused after most of the blood loss has ceased. Reinfusion is started with the latest collected blood bag. The first obtained blood bag, which is rich in red blood cells, platelets, and coagulation factors, is administered last. The autologous blood is infused through a 170-μm filter, rather than through a 40-μm filter, to avoid trapping of platelets. Fresh autologous blood flows easily through the filter compared with allogenic blood, and the filter remains remarkably free from debris. The hematocrit should be returned to 28% to 30% after surgery. The remaining autologous blood may be refrigerated and can be used within 24 hours.

Furosemide (0.5 to 1 mg/kg) may be administered to promote diuresis and the rapid excretion of excess crystalloids. Large urine volumes with high electrolyte content are expected over the next several hours after ANH is reversed, especially if crystalloids have been given as the sole diluent. Additional doses of furosemide may be needed over the next 2 hours. Blood electrolyte levels may be measured so that hypokalemia resulting from diuresis can be corrected. Postoperatively, the patients should be cared for in an intensive care environment.

Acute Normovolemic Hemodilution and Cardiopulmonary Bypass

ANH before the institution of cardiopulmonary bypass provides a source of autologous blood rich in hemoglobin, platelets, and coagulation factors, for reinfusion after the cessation of cardiopulmonary bypass, and it mitigates the increase in viscosity that accompanies hypothermia. During hypothermic cardiopulmonary bypass to 20°C, a decrease in hematocrit from 45% to 25% is necessary to restore viscosity to the same level observed at 37°C (see Fig. 12–17). After hypothermic circulatory arrest, the shear stress required to reinitiate flow and to break up red blood cell aggregates is likely to be high. An additional rheologic benefit may be given by further decrease in hematocrit.

Although blood can be withdrawn after induction of anesthesia or during the early stage of surgery in patients with normal cardiac function, it is usually done after heparinization and cannulation immediately before instituting cardiopulmonary bypass. The blood is withdrawn from the tubing to the oxygenator or before the blood passes through the roller pump. Alterations in the pump flow rate can be used to compensate for hemodynamic instabilities associated with blood removal. On initiation of cardiopulmonary bypass with a crystalloid (or crystalloid-colloid) prime, a further and sometimes profound hemodilution results depending on the patient's hemoglobin level before bypass.

Current Status of Acute Normovolemic Hemodilution

Prospective, randomized clinical trials showed that the use of ANH reduces allogenic red blood cell transfusion requirements. Some found that ANH decreases allogenic blood use by 25% to 60%, whereas others reported that more than 90% of patients did not require allogenic blood when ANH is combined with other strategies such as PABD or intraoperative blood salvage (Spahn and Casutt, 2000; Matot et al., 2002). The use of ANH was also found to be an independent factor reducing allogenic red blood cell transfusion in addition to maintaining normothermia and the use of cell salvage (Schmied et al., 1998). Although the effect of moderate ANH in reducing blood loss is not as great as deliberate hypotension, evidence suggests that the combination of both techniques leads to marked reduction in blood loss and in the need for allogenic blood (Fahmy, 1985b). Despite these enthusiastic reports, concerns have been raised as to the efficacy of ANH as a blood conservation measure. Large well-controlled, randomized studies with clearly defined transfusion triggers have been recommended (Spahn and Casutt, 2000).

It is apparent that moderate ANH used as the sole method may contribute only modestly to blood conservation. The efficacy may vary greatly and is certainly enhanced if a lower posthemodilution hematocrit level, in the range from 28% to 20%, is targeted. Although a hematocrit level of 20% has been recommended as the lowest acceptable hematocrit, profound ANH has been advocated in a few centers, especially when combined with hypothermia or when avoiding allogenic blood transfusion is vital. Fontana and others (1995) showed that healthy patients undergoing scoliosis surgery can be safely hemodiluted to an average hemoglobin of 3 g/dL without signs of global hypoxia or impairment of global cardiac performance. However, that study was limited to children/adolescents with normal cardiac function and performed under very controlled conditions. The use of extreme ANH is not recommended unless it is performed in specialized centers.

ANH offers unique advantages. It can be used in situations where PABD is not planned because of urgency of the operative procedure or scheduling conflicts and whenever blood salvage cannot be performed because of unavailability of technical personnel or lack of equipment. Unlike PABD or blood salvage, ANH is performed by the anesthesiologist and therefore may not require the presence of blood bank technicians or perfusionists. The cost of ANH is approximately one third of the cost of PABD. Finally, ANH is the only practical means of providing fresh autologous whole blood for transfusion.

Despite its simplicity and safety, ANH should not be undertaken in certain situations. Inexperience of the team is an absolute contraindication to the use of ANH. The presence of a coexisting disease that may potentially jeopardize tissue oxygen delivery, especially to the heart or brain, is also a contraindication. ANH should not be performed in anemic patients (hemoglobin <11 g/dL) and also should not be used if the anticipated compensatory increase in cardiac output is neither possible nor desirable. The technique is contraindicated in patients with pulmonary disease resulting in impaired arterial oxygenation. Patients with renal disease may not be suitable candidates for ANH because of inability to excrete large amounts of crystalloids. The success of ANH depends on a cooperative effort between surgeon, anesthesiologist, nurses and laboratory personnel, and on good communication between them.

It seems that in the future ANH will continue to be practiced either as the sole blood conservation measure or in combination with other strategies to maximize its efficacy. It may totally replace PABD (Goodnough et al., 1997). It may also be used in conjunction with preoperative erythropoietin therapy and with oxygen-carrying blood substitutes (Spahn and Cassut, 2000). Because the compensatory increase in cardiac output may be insufficient in itself to restore the oxygen extraction reserve, it has been hypothesized (and confirmed in an animal study) that augmentation of the cardiac output pharmacologically could reverse the increase in oxygen extraction ratio, restore the margin of safety for tissue oxygenation, and extend the limit to which hematocrit can be reduced safely during ANH (Crystal and Salem, 2002). The safety of this approach has not yet been confirmed in humans.

COMBINED TECHNIQUES

COMBINED HEMODILUTION AND DELIBERATE HYPOTENSION

Because deliberate hypotension can decrease blood loss and because ANH minimizes the need for allogenic blood transfusion, a combination of the techniques has been proposed (Fahmy, 1985a). This combined technique has been used primarily for major orthopedic procedures. When hemodilution and hypotension were combined, allogenic blood replacement was decreased by about 80% of the blood replacement required during normotensive anesthesia compared with 45% when hypotension was used alone (Fahmy, 1985a). Observations with the combined use of both techniques indicate that cardiac output tends to decrease after ANH, when the blood pressure decreases below 60 mm Hg. Because decreases in blood pressure can be achieved easily in hemodiluted patients, the dose of hypotensive drugs should be decreased accordingly.

Animal studies of the regional hemodynamic responses to the combination of hemodilution and controlled hypotension reveal that maintenance of oxygen delivery to critical tissue beds may be at risk (Plewes and Farhi, 1985; Crystal et al., 1988). These animal studies emphasize the importance of preoperative evaluation of patients, vigilance, experience, use of high FIO_2, and continuous monitoring of the arterial pressure, blood gases, blood loss, body temperature, and urine output when hypotension and hemodilution are combined (Fahmy, 1985a).

HEMODILUTION, HYPOTENSION, AND HYPOTHERMIA

The technique of combined ANH, hypotension, and hypothermia was stimulated by the need to carry out major surgical operations (usually associated with massive blood loss) in patients of the Jehovah's Witness faith who refuse to receive blood or blood products (Laver et al., 1975; Lilleaasen et al., 1978; Schaller et al., 1983; Singler, 1989). The rationale of this technique is that because the increased cardiac output may not be sufficient to maintain an adequate oxygen delivery during profound ANH, the protective effects of cooling are used, that is, decreased tissue oxygen requirement and increased fraction of dissolved oxygen in the blood. Anesthetics also decrease the tissue oxygen demand. Moderate hypotension decreases both blood losses and myocardial oxygen demand.

During air breathing at normothermia, the dissolved oxygen in the blood represents 0.3 mL/dL. This value rises to 1.3 to 1.5 mL/dL in normal patients during 100% oxygen administration. This represents about 7% of the CaO_2 and 30% of the total oxygen extraction in patients with a normal hemoglobin level at normal temperature (Singler, 1989). As temperature and plasma protein content fall during ANH combined with hypothermia, the fraction of dissolved oxygen increases. With hypothermia to 30° to 31°C and an FIO_2 of 1.0, the amount of dissolved oxygen increases to 2 mL/dL; during ANH a hemoglobin of 5 g/dL represents 23% of the total oxygen content (8.7 mL/dL). This dissolved oxygen accounts for more than half of the metabolic

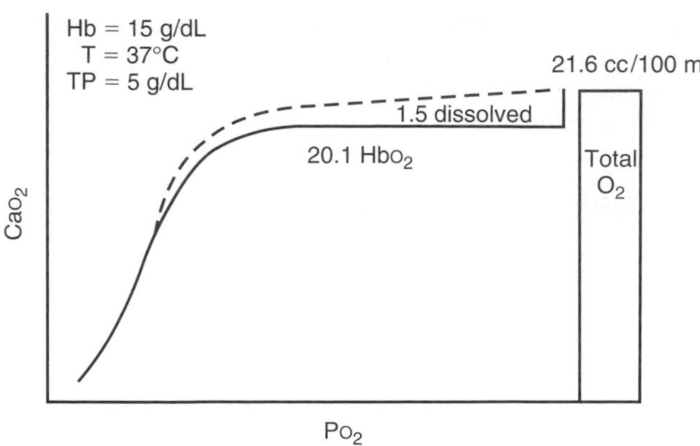

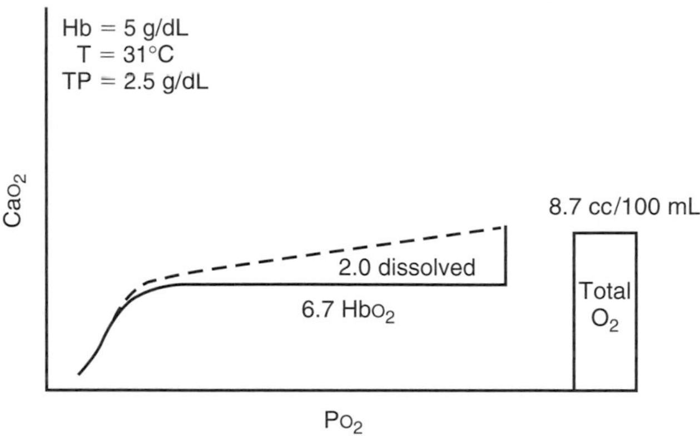

■ **FIGURE 12–22.** Curves plotting total arterial oxygen content (CaO_2) against PO_2 during the awake normal state and during hemodilution. The increase in dissolved oxygen during hemodilution represents approximately 30% of total CaO_2. See text for details. (From Singler RC: Special techniques: Deliberate hypotension, hypothermia, and acute normovolemic hemodilution. In Gregory GA, editor: *Pediatric anesthesia.* New York, 1989, Churchill Livingstone, with permission.)

requirements (Fig. 12–22). When oxygen consumption decreases by 40% as a result of anesthesia and cooling to 31°C, $S\bar{v}O_2$ does not change during a reduction in hemoglobin concentration from 15 g/dL to 5 g/dL. When this technique is used properly, the combined effect of increased dissolved oxygen in the blood, increased blood flow, decreased systemic vascular resistance, and decreased oxygen requirements offsets the effect of decreased hemoglobin concentration and results in maintenance of adequate tissue perfusion and adequate oxygen extraction. Because this technique of hemodilution, hypotension, and hypothermia requires extensive experience, it should be used only by experienced clinicians in very specialized centers.

■ OXYGEN THERAPEUTICS

The search for a blood substitute that could be stored at room temperature and administered on the battlefield without the need for cross-matching began more than 70 years ago. With time, the focus gradually shifted from the search for a "blood substitute" to the development of "oxygen therapeutics" (Wahr, 2003). There are three types of "oxygen therapeutic" agents: (1) hemoglobin-based solutions, (2) perfluorochemical solutions, and (3) allosteric modifiers of hemoglobin.

■ HEMOGLOBIN-BASED OXYGEN CARRIERS

Removal of hemoglobin, the oxygen-carrying moiety, from red blood cells initially seemed to offer the following advantages: purification, elimination of ABO incompatibility by removal of the antigens on the red blood cell surface, and extension of the shelf-life to several months or even years. Because hemoglobin is an inherently unstable molecule once it is removed from the red blood cell, the normal tetramer dissociates resulting in dimers easily filtered by the kidney. In addition, the loss of 2,3-DPG markedly reduces the P_{50}. Furthermore, free hemoglobin in the plasma is rapidly engulfed by the reticuloendothelial system, resulting in an intravascular half-life of 24 to 36 hours (Wahr, 2003). In the current generation of solutions, many of the problems have been resolved through chemical or genetic manipulations. The hemoglobin molecules under development are tetramers or large polymers, have a P_{50} of 28 to 37 mm Hg, have hemoglobin concentrations of 10 to 14 g/dL, and are free of antigens and pathogens. Formation of methemoglobin is still a problem, although the maximal amount of methemoglobin remains less than 10% (Sprung et al., 2002).

The hemoglobin in these solutions is derived from several sources—outdated human volunteer donations, cattle (a potential source of nearly 1 million units per day), and recombinant technology using *Escherichia coli* (Wahr, 2003). Regardless of the source, they share common problems: short intravascular half-life, some degree of vasoconstriction particularly in the pulmonary circulation, and interference with spectrophotometric laboratory measurements. The pulmonary vasoconstriction is probably related to the role of hemoglobin in nitric oxide equilibration (Wahr, 2003). Nitric oxide is produced by the vascular endothelium and diffuses both to the smooth muscles, where it exerts its vasodilating effect, and into the vascular lumen, where it is scavenged by hemoglobin inside the red blood cells. Free hemoglobin scavenges nitric oxide much more avidly than does red blood cell hemoglobin, resulting in vasoconstriction. Free hemoglobin in the plasma absorbs light and interferes with spectrophotometric measurements.

■ PERFLUOROCHEMICAL SOLUTIONS

Perfluorocarbons are inert substances that have high solubility for all gases, including oxygen and carbon dioxide. Because these liquids are completely immiscible in water, intravenous administration causes a fatal lipid embolus. However, a microemulsion of a perfluorocarbon in normal saline was used to perform exchange transfusion in a rat, which survived breathing 100% oxygen with a hematocrit of zero (Clark and Gollan, 1966).

Fluosol is the only "blood substitute" to have been approved by the U.S. Food and Drug Administration. Because of low demand and major disadvantages, namely low concentration (10%), a short intravascular half-life (Tremper et al., 1982; Gould et al., 1986), and instability of the emulsion, commercial production was stopped in the late 1990s. Perfluoroctyl bromide (Oxygent; Alliance Pharmaceuticals, San Diego, CA), a second-generation perfluorocarbon emulsion, has been produced, which contains 90% perflubron (C8F17) by weight or 45% by volume. It is emulsified with lecithin and stable at room temperature for longer than 6 years (Henry et al., 1994).

Perfluorocarbons are not metabolized but rather are cleared by the reticuloendothelial system and eventually are exhaled as vapor. A bloodless animal could survive with a "fluorocrit" of 10%, 20%, and 50% with PaO_2 values of 800, 650, and 250 mm Hg, respectively. Because the emulsion is cleared within 24 to 36 hours and because repeat dosing results in hepatosplenomegaly in animals, long-term survival would be problematic. There seems to be a dose-related effect on the platelet count, which decreases by 15% to 25% at 2 to 4 days after administration (Leese et al., 2000). With a maximum dose of 3 g/kg, no bleeding abnormalities have been noted in humans (Wahr, 2003).

ALLOSTERIC MODIFIERS

Two antilipidemic drugs (clofibrate and benzofibrate) were found to decrease the affinity of hemoglobin for oxygen, thereby enhancing oxygen release to tissues (Poyart et al., 1994; Perutz and Poyart, 1983). This in vitro "allosteric" effect of these drugs is inhibited by in vivo serum albumin. Effort to synthesize drugs that would affect allosteric modifications of hemoglobin in vivo culminated in development of a compound known as RSR13 (Abraham et al., 1992; Randad et al., 1991). Studies showed dose-dependent rightward shift of the oxyhemoglobin dissociation curve (Wahr et al., 2001). A right shift in P_{50} of 10 mm Hg was achieved at doses of 75 and 100 mg/kg. The only marked side effect reported is a transient increase in the serum creatinine level of three patients who received RSR13. The rightward shift of the oxyhemoglobin dissociation curve is a double-edged sword; although it enhances the release of oxygen to the tissue, SaO_2 decreases if FIO_2 is not increased.

CURRENT STATUS OF OXYGEN THERAPEUTICS

Unforeseen adverse side effects have kept commercially available oxygen therapeutics tantalizingly "just out of reach." However, there are indications that clinical use is very near for a number of these products. Transfusion alternatives eventually become commercially available—the question is "when" rather than "if." After successful use in adults, the use of oxygen therapeutics will ultimately be extended to the pediatric population.

SUMMARY

A variety of simple and special blood conservation procedures are currently available and applicable to pediatric patients. The anesthesiologist should be familiar with the principles and practices of various blood conservation strategies. A "flawless" anesthetic technique and proper positioning are essential so as to avoid increased blood loss during surgery. Infiltration with vasoconstrictors is a simple technique that can be used in many minor and major surgical procedures. The use of pneumatic tourniquets after exsanguination of the upper and lower extremity permits a bloodless operative field.

Advances in knowledge of the physiology of acute normovolemic hemodilution have expanded the application of the technique to a variety of surgical procedures and may in the future replace preoperative autologous blood donation. Similarly, refinements in perioperative blood salvage techniques have led to their use in certain pediatric surgical procedures.

Various hypotensive drugs and techniques are available, but the power to initiate hypotension resides entirely with the anesthesiologist who can, by skillful use of gravity, controlled ventilation, and choice of appropriate drugs, maintain the desired level of blood pressure. Factors that may improve the safety of the technique include careful selection of patients, maintenance of airway patency, avoidance of hypercapnia and hypocapnia, use of high FIO_2, gradual onset of hypotension aiming at a level consistent with the patient's condition, proper monitoring, and adequate postoperative care. Some pertinent points should be borne in mind when hypotensive anesthesia is used for pediatric patients. (1) Children respond to some hypotensive drugs with tachycardia. (2) The incidence of failed hypotension may be relatively high unless the heart rate is controlled. (3) Because of the child's smaller stature, tilting may not produce as great a pressure gradient and peripheral venous pooling. (4) The physiologic dead space does not increase in infants and children. (5) Lower arterial pressure may be necessary to achieve the desired bloodless field. (6) Cyanide toxicity is a preventable complication.

There has been an increased tendency to combine blood conservation measures so as to markedly reduce or virtually eliminate allogenic blood transfusion. However, these combined techniques demand the utmost in skill, training, and experience. Great advances have been made in the use of oxygen-carrying blood substitutes, as well as drugs that enhance hemostatic activity, and these approaches are expected to be in common use in the near future.

REFERENCES

American Association of Blood Banks: *Guidelines for blood salvage and reinfusion in surgery and trauma.* Bethesda, MD, 1993.

Abraham DJ, Wireko RC, Randad RS, et al.: Allosteric modifiers of hemoglobin: 2-[4-[[(3,5-disubstituted anilino)carbonyl]methyl]phenoxy]-2-methylpropionic acid derivatives that lower the oxygen affinity of hemoglobin in red cell suspensions, in whole blood, and in vivo in rats. *Biochemistry* 31:9141, 1992.

Adams AP: Techniques of vascular control for deliberate hypotension during surgery. *Br J Anaesth* 47:777, 1975.

Adu-Gyamfi Y, Sankarankutty M, Marwa S: Use of a tourniquet in patients with sickle-cell disease. *Can J Anaesth* 40:24, 1993.

Alajmo F, Calamai G, Perna AM, et al.: High-dose aprotinin: Hemostatic effects in open heart operations. *Ann Thorac Surg* 48:536, 1989.

Amaranath L, Cascorbi HF, Singh-Amaranath AV, et al.: Relation of anesthesia to total hip replacement and control of operative blood loss. *Anesth Analg* 54:641, 1975.

Anderson S, McKissock W: Controlled hypotension with Arfonad in neurosurgery with special reference to vascular lesions. *Lancet* 2:754, 1953.

Arfors KE, Bergquist D: Microvascular haemostatic plug formation in the rabbit mesentery. *Bibl Haematol* 41:84, 1975.

Aronson S, Goldberg LI, Roth S, et al.: Preservation of renal blood flow during hypotension induced with fenoldopam in dogs. *Can J Anaesth* 37:380, 1990.

Askrog VF, Pender JW, Eckenhoff JE: Changes in physiological dead space during deliberate hypotension. *Anesthesiology* 25:774, 1964.

Atlee JL, Roberts FL: Thiopental and epinephrine-induced dysrhythmias in dogs anesthetized with enflurane and isoflurane. *Anesth Analg* 65:437, 1986.

Behnia R, Martin A, Koushanpour E, et al.: Trimethaphan-induced hypotension: Effect on renal function. *Can Anaesth Soc J* 29:581, 1982.

Behnia R, Raymon F, Cheng SE, et al.: Metabolism of sodium nitroprusside in dogs awake and anesthetized with halothane. *Anesthesiology* 48:260, 1978.

Bendo AA, Kozlowski PB, Capuano C, et al.: Cerebral edema formation in dogs following hypotension induced with isoflurane and labetalol. *Acta Anaesthesiol Belg* 44:103–9, 1993.

Benumof JL, Wahrenbrock EA: Blunted hypoxic pulmonary constriction by increased lung vascular pressure. *J Appl Physiol* 38:846, 1975.

Bernard J-M, Passuti N, Pinaud M: Long-term hypotensive technique with nicardipine and nitroprusside during isoflurane anesthesia for spinal surgery. *Anesth Analg* 75:179, 1992.

Berry AJ: Respiration support and renal function. *Anesthesiology* 55:655, 1981.

Biro GP: Large venous compliance in carboxyhemoglobinemia and hemodilutional anemia. *Can J Physiol Pharmacol* 64:556, 1986.

Blanchette VS, Zipursky A: Assessment of anemia in newborn infants. *Clin Perinatol* 11:489, 1984.

Blau WS, Kafer ER, Anderson JA: Esmolol is more effective than sodium nitroprusside in reducing blood loss during orthognathic surgery. *Anesth Analg* 75:172, 1992.

Blevins FT, Shaw B, Valeri CR, et al.: Reinfusion of shed blood after orthopaedic procedures in children and adolescents. *J Bone Joint Surg [Am]* 75:363, 1993.

Bloch EC, Ginsberg B, Binner RA Jr, et al.: Limb tourniquets and central temperature in anesthetized children. *Anesth Analg* 74:486, 1992.

Boezaart AP, van der Merwe I, Coetzee A: Comparison of sodium nitroprusside- and esmolol-induced controlled hypotension for functional endoscopic sinus surgery. *Can J Anaesth* 42:373, 1995.

Bourke DL, Silberberg MS, Ortega R, et al.: Respiratory responses associated with release of intraoperative tourniquets. *Anesth Analg* 69:541, 1989.

Brinkmeyer S, Safar P, Motoyama EK: Superiority of colloid over electrolyte solution for severe normovolemic hemodilution (NVHD) in concurrent treatment of hemorrhage. *Disaster Med* 1:171, 1983.

Brodkey JS, Richards DE, Blasingame JP, et al.: Reversible spinal cord trauma in cats: Additive effects of direct pressure and ischemia. *J Neurosurg* 37:591, 1972.

California statute SB-37. Paul Gann Blood Safety Act, January 1, 1990.

Calverley RK, Smith NT, Jones CW, et al.: Ventilatory and cardiovascular effects of enflurane anesthesia during spontaneous ventilation in man. *Anesthesiology* 57:610, 1978.

Carlson LA, Ekelund LG, Orö L: Circulatory and respiratory effects of different doses of prostaglandin E_1 in man. *Acta Physiol Scand* 75:161, 1969.

Casthely PA, Lear S, Cottrell JE, et al.: Intrapulmonary shunting during induced hypotension. *Anesth Analg* 61:231, 1982.

Cheney FW, Colley PS: The effect of cardiac output on arterial blood oxygenation. *Anesthesiology* 52:496, 1980.

Clark L Jr, Gollan F. Survival of mammals breathing organic liquids equilibrated with oxygen at atmospheric temperature. *Science* 152:1755, 1966.

Cottrell JE, Patel K, Turndorf H, et al.: Intracranial pressure changes induced by sodium nitroprusside in patients with intracranial mass lesions. *J Neurosurg* 48:329, 1978a.

Cottrell JE, Casthely P, Brodie JD, et al.: Prevention of nitroprusside-induced cyanide toxicity with hydroxocobalamin. *N Engl J Med* 298:809, 1978b.

Cottrell JE, Patel K, Cathely P, et al.: Nitroprusside tachyphylaxis without β acidosis. *Anesthesiology* 9:141, 1978c.

Crystal GJ, Kim S-J, Salem MR: Right and left ventricular O_2 uptake during hemodilution and β-adrenergic stimulation. *Am J Physiol* 265:H1769–H1777, 1993.

Crystal GJ, Rooney MW, Salem MR: Regional hemodynamics and oxygen supply during isovolemic hemodilution alone and in combination with adenosine-induced controlled hypotension. *Anesth Analg* 67:211, 1988.

Crystal GJ, Salem MR: Acute normovolemic hemodilution. In Salem MR, editor: *Blood conservation in the surgical patient.* Baltimore, MD, 1996, Williams & Wilkins, pp 168–188.

Crystal GJ, Salem MR: Beta-adrenergic stimulation restores oxygen extraction reserve during acute normovolemic hemodilution. *Anesth Analg* 95:851, 2002.

Cullen DJ, Eger EI II: Cardiovascular effects of carbon dioxide in man. *Anesthesiology* 41:345, 1974.

Davies DW, Greiss L, Kadar D, et al.: Sodium nitroprusside in children: Observations on metabolism during normal and abnormal responses. *Can Anaesth Soc J* 22:553, 1975.

Davis RJ, Agnew DK, Shealy CR, et al.: Erythrocyte viability in postoperative autotransfusion. *J Pediatr Orthop* 13:781, 1993.

Delaney TJ, Miller ED Jr: Rebound hypertension after sodium nitroprusside prevented by saralasin in rats. *Anesthesiology* 52:154, 1980.

Diaz JH, Lockhart CH: Hypotensive anaesthesia for craniectomy in infancy. *Br J Anaesth* 51:233, 1979.

Dickson M, White M, Kinney W, et al.: Extremity tourniquet deflation increases end-tidal PCO2. *Anesth Analg* 70:457, 1990.

Dietrich W, Spannagl M, Jochum M, et al.: Influence of high-dose aprotinin treatment on blood loss and coagulation patterns in patients undergoing myocardial revascularization. *Anesthesiology* 73:1119, 1990.

Dilthey G, Dietrich W, Spannagl M, Richter J: Influence of desmopressin acetate on homologous blood requirements in cardiac surgical patients pretreated with aspirin. *J Cardiothorac Vasc Anesth* 7:425, 1993.

Don H: Hypoxemia and hypercapnia during and after anesthesia. In Orkin FK, Cooperman LH, editors: *Complications in anesthesiology.* Philadelphia, 1983, Lippincott, pp 183–207.

Eckenhoff JE, Enderby GEH, Larson A, et al.: Pulmonary gas exchange during deliberate hypotension. *Br J Anaesth* 35:750, 1963a.

Eckenhoff JE, Enderby GEH, Larson A, et al.: Human cerebral circulation during deliberate hypotension and head-up tilt. *J Appl Physiol* 18:1130, 1963b.

Edmondson R, Del Valle O, Shah N, et al.: Esmolol for potentiation of nitroprusside-induced hypotension: Impact on the cardiovascular, adrenergic, and renin-angiotensin systems in man. *Anesth Analg* 69:202, 1989.

Egli GA, Zollinger A, Seifert B, et al.: Effect of progressive haemodilution with hydroxyethyl starch, gelatin and albumin on blood coagulation: An in vitro thromboelastography study. *Br J Anaesth* 78:684, 1997.

Enderby GEH: Controlled hypotension with hypotensive drugs and posture to reduce bleeding surgery. Preliminary results with pentamethonium iodide. *Lancet* 1:1145, 1950.

Enderby GEH: Halothane and hypotension. *Anaesthesia* 15:25, 1960.

Enderby GEH: Historical review of the practice of deliberate hypotension. In Enderby GEH, editor: *Hypotensive anaesthesia.* New York, 1985a, Churchill-Livingstone, pp 75–91.

Enderby GEH: Blood pressure and bleeding. In Enderby GEH, editor: *Hypotensive anaesthesia.* New York, 1985b, Churchill-Livingstone, pp 92–98.

Esseltine DW, Baxter MRN, Bevan JC: Sickle cell states and the anaesthetist. *Can J Anaesth* 35:385, 1988.

Etchason J, Petz L, Keeler E, et al.: The cost effectiveness of preoperative blood donations. *N Engl J Med* 332:719, 1995.

Fahmy NR: Nitroglycerine as a hypotensive drug during general anesthesia. *Anesthesiology* 49:17, 1978.

Fahmy NR: Nitroprusside vs a nitroprusside-trimethaphan mixture for induced hypotension: Hemodynamic effects and cyanide release. *Clin Pharmacol Ther* 37:264, 1985a.

Fahmy NR: Techniques for deliberate hypotension: Haemodilution and hypotension. In Enderby GEH, editor: *Hypotensive anaesthesia.* New York, 1985b, Churchill-Livingstone, pp 164–183.

Fahmy NR, Bottros MR, Charchafieh J, et al.: A randomized comparison of labetalol and nitroprusside for induced hypotension. *J Clin Anesth* 1:409, 1989.

Fahmy NR, Gavras HP: Impact of captopril on hemodynamic and hormonal effects of nitroprusside. *J Cardiovasc Pharmacol* 7:869, 1985.

Fahmy NR, Laver MB: Hemodynamic response to ganglionic blockade with pentolinium during N_2O-halothane anesthesia in man. *Anesthesiology* 44:6, 1976.

Fahmy NR, Mihelakos PT, Battit GE, et al.: Propranolol prevents hemodynamic and humoral events after abrupt withdrawal of nitroprusside. *Clin Pharmacol Ther* 36:470, 1984.

Fahmy NR, Soter NA: Effects of trimethaphan on arterial blood histamine and systemic hemodynamics in humans. *Anesthesiology* 62:562, 1985.

Flamm ES, Adams HP Jr, Beck DW, et al.: Dose-escalation study of intravenous nicardipine in patients with aneurysmal subarachnoid hemorrhage. *J Neurosurg* 68:393, 1988.

Fontana JL, Welborn L, Mogan PD, et al.: Oxygen consumption and cardiovascular function in children during profound intraoperative normovolemic hemodilution. *Anesth Analg* 80:219, 1995.

Friesen RH, Tornabene MA, Coleman SP: Blood conservation during pediatric cardiac surgery: Ultrafiltration of the extracorporeal circuit volume after cardiopulmonary bypass. *Anesth Analg* 77:702, 1993.

Gammage G: Crystalloid versus colloid: Is colloid worth the cost? In Kirby RR, Brown DL, editors: Anesthesia for trauma. *Int Anesthesiol Clin* 25:37–60, 1987.

Gardner WJ: The control of bleeding during operation by induced hypotension. *JAMA* 132:572, 1946.

Gavras H, Kremer D, Brown JJ, et al.: Angiotensin and norepinephrine induced myocardial lesions: Experimental and clinical studies in rabbits and man. *Am Heart J* 89:321, 1975.

Gelman S, Ernst EA: Hepatic circulation during sodium nitroprusside infusion in the dog. *Anesthesiology* 49:182, 1978.

Gelman S, Fowler K, Smith L: Regional blood flow during isoflurane and halothane anesthesia. *Anesth Analg* 63:557, 1984.

Gerson JI, Allen FB, Seltzer JL, et al.: Arterial and venous dilation by nitroprusside and nitroglycerin: Is there a difference? *Anesth Analg* 61:256, 1982.

Giese J: Renin, angiotensin, hypertensive vascular damage: A review. *Am J Med* 55:315–320, 1973.

Goldberg ME, McNulty SE, Azad SS, et al.: A comparison of labetalol and nitroprusside for inducing hypotension during major surgery. *Anesth Analg* 70:537, 1990.

Goodnough LT, Rudnick S, Price TH, et al.: Increased preoperative collection of autologous blood with recombinant erythropoietin therapy. *N Engl J Med* 321:1163, 1989.

Goodnough LT, Despotis GJ, Parvin CA: Erythropoietin therapy in patients undergoing cardiac operations. *Ann Thorac Surg* 64:1579, 1997.

Goodnough LT, Monk TG, Brecher ME: Acute normovolemic hemodilution should replace the preoperative donation of autologous blood as a method of autologous-blood procurement. *Transfusion* 38:396, 1997.

Goto F, Fujita T: Prostaglandins and circulation. *Circ Control* 1:139, 1980.

Goto F, Otani E, Dato S, et al.: Prostaglandin E_1 as a hypotensive drug during general anesthesia. *Anaesthesia* 37:530, 1982.

Gould SA, Rosen AL, Sehgal LR, et al.: Fluosol-DA as a red cell substitute in acute anemia. *N Engl J Med* 314:1653, 1986.
Green DW: Techniques for deliberate hypotension: Pharmacological blockade. In Enderby, GEH, editor: *Hypotensive anaesthesia.* New York, 1985, Churchill-Livingstone, pp 109–133.
Greiss L, Tremblay NAG, Davies DW: The toxicity of sodium nitroprusside. *Can Anaesth Soc J* 23:480, 1976.
Griffiths HWC, Gillies J: Thoracolumbar splanchnicectomy and sympathectomy: Anaesthetic procedure. *Anaesthesia* 3:134, 1948.
Grosslight K, Forster R, Calahan AR, et al.: Isoflurane for neuro-anesthesia. Risk factors for increases in intracranial pressure. *Anesthesiology* 63:533, 1985.
Grundy BL, Nash CL Jr, Brown RH: Arterial pressure manipulation alters spinal cord function during correction of scoliosis. *Anesthesiology* 54:249, 1981.
Guay J, Reinberg C, Poitras B, et al.: A trial of desmopressin to reduce blood loss in patients undergoing spinal fusion for idiopathic scoliosis. *Anesth Analg* 75:405, 1992.
Hackmann T, Steward DJ, Sheps SB: Anemia in pediatric day-surgery patients: Prevalence and detection. *Anesthesiology* 75:27, 1991.
Hainsworth R: Arterial blood pressure. In Enderby GEH, editor: *Hypotensive anaesthesia.* London, 1985, Churchill Livingstone, pp 3–29.
Hallowell P, Bland JHL, Dalton BC, et al.: The effect of hemodilution with albumen or Ringer's lactate on water balance and blood use in open-heart surgery. *Ann Thorac Surg* 25:22, 1978.
Hampton LJ, Little DM: Complications associated with the use of "controlled hypotension" in anesthesia. *Arch Surg* 67:549, 1953.
Harper AM, Glass HI: Effects of alterations in the arterial carbon dioxide tension on the blood flow through the cerebral cortex at normal and low arterial blood pressures. *J Neurol Neurosurg Psychiatry* 28:449, 1965.
Havel M, Teufelsbauer H, Knöbl P, et al.: Effect of intraoperative aprotinin administration on postoperative bleeding in patients undergoing cardiopulmonary bypass operation. *J Thorac Cardiovasc Surg* 101:968, 1991.
Hayashi Y, Sumikawa K, Tashiro C, et al.: Arrhythmogenic threshold of epinephrine during sevoflurane, enflurane, and isoflurane anesthesia in dogs. *Anesthesiology* 69:145, 1988.
Hellewell J, Potts MW: Propranolol during controlled hypotension. *Br J Anaesth* 38:794, 1966.
Henry CJ, Brewer W Jr, Henderson RA, et al.: Pharmacokinetics and tolerance of weekly Oxygent CA infusions in the dog. *Artif Cells Blood Substit Immobil Biotechnol* 22:1155, 1994.
Hines R: Preservation of platelet function during trimethaphan infusion. *Anesthesiology* 72:834, 1990.
Hines R, Barash PG: Infusion of sodium nitroprusside induces platelet dysfunction. *Anesthesiology* 70:611, 1989.
Hoffman BB, Lefkowitz RJ: Adrenergic receptor antagonists; In Goodman Gilman A, Rall TW, Nies AS, Taylor P, editors: *Goodman and Gilman's the pharmacological basis of therapeutics,* 8th ed. New York, 1990, McGraw-Hill.
Holland BM, Jones JG, Wardrop CAJ. Lessons from the anemia of prematurity. *Hematol/Oncol Clin N Am* 1:355, 1987.
Ikeda S, Schweiss JF, Frank PA, et al.: In vitro cyanide release from sodium nitroprusside. *Anesthesiology* 66:381, 1987.
Ivankovich AD, Braverman B, Kanuru RP, et al.: Cyanide antidotes and methods of their administration in dogs. *Anesthesiology* 52:210, 1980.
Ivankovich AD, Miletich DJ, Albrecht RF, et al.: Sodium nitroprusside and cerebral blood flow in the anesthetized and unanesthetized goat. *Anesthesiology* 44:21, 1976.
Jack RD: Toxicity of sodium nitroprusside. *Br J Anaesth* 46:952, 1974.
Jacobs HK, Lieponis JV, Bunch WH, et al.: The influence of halothane and nitroprusside on canine spinal cord hemodynamics. *Spine* 7:35, 1982.
Janssens M, Joris J, David JL, et al.: High-dose aprotinin reduces blood loss in patients undergoing total hip replacement surgery. *Anesthesiology* 80:23, 1994.
Johnston RR, Eger EI II, Wilson C: A comparative interaction of epinephrine with enflurane, isoflurane, and halothane in man. *Anesth Analg* 55:709, 1976.
Karl HW, Swedlow DB, Lee KW, et al.: Epinephrine-halothane interactions in children. *Anesthesiology* 58:142, 1983.
Karayalcin G: Sickle cell anemia in the neonatal period. *South Med J* 72:492, 1979.
Kelman GR, Nunn JF, Prys-Roberts C, et al.: The influence of cardiac output on arterial oxygenation. *Br J Anaesth* 39:450, 1967.
Khambatta HJ, Stone JG, Kahn E: Propranolol alters renin release during nitroprusside induced hypotension and prevents hypertension on discontinuation of nitroprusside. *Anesth Analg* 60:569, 1981.
Knight PR, Lane GA, Hensinger RN, et al.: Catecholamine and renin-angiotensin response during hypotensive anesthesia induced by sodium nitroprusside or trimethaphan camsylate. *Anesthesiology* 59:248, 1983.
Knight PR, Lane GA, Nicholls MG, et al.: Hormonal and hemodynamic changes induced by pentolinium and propranolol during surgical correction of scoliosis. *Anesthesiology* 53:127, 1980.
Kobrinsky NL, Letts RM, Patel LR, et al.: 1-Deamino-8-D-arginine vasopressin (desmopressin) decreases operative blood loss in patients having Harrington rod spinal fusion surgery. *Ann Intern Med* 107:446, 1987.
Kongsgaard UE, Hovig T, Brosstad F, et al.: Platelets in shed mediastinal blood used for postoperative autotransfusion. *Acta Anaesthesiol Scand* 37:265, 1993.
Kramer AH, Hertzer NR, Beven EG: Intraoperative hemodilution during elective vascular reconstruction. *Surg Gynecol Obstet* 149:831, 1979.
Kruszyna H, Kruszyna R, Smith RP, et al.: Red blood cells generate nitric oxide from directly acting, nitrogenous vasodilators. *Toxicol Appl Pharmacol* 91:429, 1987.
Kulier AH, Gombotz H, Fuchs G, et al.: Subcutaneous recombinant human erythropoietin and autologous blood donation before coronary artery bypass surgery. *Anesth Analg* 76:102, 1993.
Lagerkranser M, Irestedt L, Sollevi A, et al.: Central and splanchnic hemodynamics in the dog during controlled hypotension with adenosine. *Anesthesiology* 60:547, 1984.
Lam AM, Gelb AW: Cardiovascular effects of isoflurane-induced hypotension for cerebral aneurysm surgery. *Anesth Analg* 62:742, 1983.
Laver MB, Buckley MJ, Austen WG: Extreme haemodilution with profound hypothermia and circulatory arrest. *Bibl Haematol* 41:225, 1975.
Lawson NW, Ochsner JL, Mills NL, et al.: The use of hemodilution and fresh autologous blood in open-heart surgery. *Anesth Analg* 53:672, 1974.
Leese PT, Noveck RJ, Shorr JS, et al.: Randomized safety studies of intravenous perflubron emulsion. I. Effects on coagulation function. *Anesth Analg* 91:804, 2000.
Levin RM, Zadigian ME, Hall SC: The combined effect of hyperventilation and hypotension on cerebral oxygenation in anaesthetized dogs. *Can Anaesth Soc J* 27:264, 1980.
Levy PS, Kim SJ, Eckel PK, et al.: Limit to cardiac compensation during acute isovolemic hemodilution: Influence of coronary stenosis. *Am J Physiol* 265:H340, 1993.
Lichtenthal PR, Rossi EC, Louis G, et al.: Dose-related prolongation of the bleeding time by intravenous nitroglycerin. *Anesth Analg* 64:30, 1985.
Lilleaason P, Frøysaker T, Stokke O: Cardiac surgery in extreme haemodilution without donor blood, blood products or artificial macromolecules. *Scand J Thorac Cardiovasc Surg* 12:249, 1978.
Longnecker DE: The microvascular response to hypotensive drugs. In Enderby GEH, editor, *Hypotensive anaesthesia.* London, 1985, Churchill Livingstone, pp 54–65.
Luce JM, Huseby JS, Kirk W, et al.: Mechanisms by which positive end expiratory pressure increases cerebrospinal fluid pressure in dogs. *J Appl Physiol* 52:231, 1982.
Lynn AM, Fischer T, Brandford HG, et al. Systemic responses to tourniquet release in children. *Anesth Analg* 65:865, 1986.
Madsen JB, Cold GE, Hansen ES, et al.: Cerebral blood flow and metabolism during isoflurane-induced hypotension in patients subjected to surgery for cerebral aneurysms. *Br J Anaesth* 59:1204, 1987.
Magill IW, Scurr CF, Wyman JB: Controlled hypotension by a thiophanium derivative. *Lancet* I:219, 1953.
Maroof M, Khan RM, Bhatti TH: Clonidine premedication for induced hypotension with total intravenous anaesthesia for middle ear microsurgery. *Can J Anaesth* 41:164, 1994.
Matot I, Scheinin O, Jurim O, Eid A: Effectiveness of acute normovolemic hemodilution to minimize allogeneic blood transfusion in major liver resection. *Anesthesiology* 97:794, 2002.
Mazer CD, Hornstein A, Freedman J: Platelet activation in warm and cold heart surgery. *Ann Thorac Surg* 59:1481, 1995.
McDonald FD, Thiel G, Wilson DR, et al.: The prevention of acute renal failure in the rat by long-term saline loading: A possible role of the renin-angiotensin axis. *Proc Soc Exp Biol Med* 131:610, 1969.
McNeil TW, DeWald RL, Kuo KN, et al.: Controlled hypotensive anesthesia in scoliosis surgery. *J Bone Joint Surg [Am]* 56:1167, 1974.
Menkhaus PG, Reves JG, Kissin I, et al.: Cardiovascular effects of esmolol in anesthetized humans. *Anesth Analg* 64:327, 1985.
Merin RG: Are the myocardial, functional, and metabolic effects of isoflurane really different from those of halothane and enflurane? *Anesthesiology* 55:398, 1981.
Merriam-Webster's collegiate dictionary, 11th ed. Springfield, MA, 2003, Merriam-Webster, Inc.
Merrifield AJ, Blundell MD: Toxicity of sodium nitroprusside [letter]. *Br J Anaesth* 1974; 46:324.
Messmer K: Hemodilution. *Surg Clin N Am* 55:659, 1975.
Messmer K, Sunder-Plassmann L: Hemodilution. *Prog Surg* 13:208, 1974.
Michenfelder JD: Cyanide release from sodium nitroprusside in the dog. *Anesthesiology* 46:196, 1977.

Michenfelder JD, Tinker JH: Cyanide toxicity and thiosulfate protection during chronic administration of sodium nitroprusside in the dog: Correlation with a human case. *Anesthesiology* 47:441, 1977.

Moncada S, Palmer RM, Higgs EA: Nitric oxide: Physiology, pathophysiology, and pharmacology. *Pharmacol Rev* 43:109, 1991.

Mongan PD, Hosking M: The role of desmopressin acetate in patients undergoing coronary artery bypass surgery. *Anesthesiology* 77:38, 1992.

Moraca PP, Elmars MB, Hale DE, et al.: Clinical evaluation of sodium nitroprusside as a hypotensive agent. *Anesthesiology* 23:193, 1962.

Mostello LA, Casey WF, McGill WA: Does the use of a surgical tourniquet induce fever in infants? *Anesth Analg* 72:S191, 1991.

Motoyama EK: Respiratory physiology in infants and children. In Motoyama EK, Davis PJ, editors: *Smith's anesthesia for infants and children*, 5th ed. St Louis, 1990, Mosby–Year Book.

Naik SK, Knight A, Elliott MJ: A successful modification of ultrafiltration for cardiopulmonary bypass in children. *Perfusion* 6:41, 1991.

Nathan DG, Oski FA: *Hematology of infancy and childhood,* 3rd ed. Philadelphia, 1987, WB Saunders.

Navarro R, Weiskopf RB, Moore MA, et al.: Humans anesthetized with sevoflurane or isoflurane have similar arrhythmic response to epinephrine. *Anesthesiology* 80:545, 1994.

Newberg LA, Michenfelder JD: Cerebral protection by isoflurane during hypoxemia or ischemia. *Anesthesiology* 59:29, 1983.

Newberg LA, Milde JH, Michenfelder JD: The cerebral metabolic effects of isoflurane at and above concentrations that suppress cortical electrical activity. *Anesthesiology* 59:23, 1983.

Nimmagadda U, Joseph NJ, Salem MR, et al.: Positive end-expiratory pressure increases intraocular pressure. *Crit Care Med* 19:796, 1991.

Nunn JF: *Applied respiratory physiology*, 4th ed. Boston, 1993, Butterworth.

Oski FA: Designation of anemia on a functional basis. *J Pediatr* 83:353, 1973.

Ottesen S, Frøysaker T: Use of the haemonetic cell saver for autotransfusion in cardiovascular surgery. *Scand J Thorac Cardiovasc Surg* 16:263, 1982.

Pagel PS, Kersten JR, Hettrick DA, et al.: Negative inotropic and lusitropic actions of sevoflurane in chronically instrumented dogs. *Anesth Analg* 78:S332, 1994.

Palmer RF, Lassiter KC: Sodium nitroprusside. *N Engl J Med* 292:294, 1975.

Palmer RM, Ferrige AG, Moncada S: Nitric oxide release accounts for the biological activity of endothelium-derived relaxing factor. *Nature* 327:524, 1987.

Patel H: Experience with the cerebral function monitor during deliberate hypotension. *Br J Anaesth* 53:639, 1981.

Perutz MF, Poyart C. Bezafibrate lowers oxygen affinity of haemoglobin. *Lancet* 2:881, 1983.

Philbin DM, Sullivan SF, Bowman FO, et al.: Postoperative hypoxemia: Contribution of the cardiac output. *Anesthesiology* 32:136, 1970.

Pineda A, Valbonesi M: Intraoperative blood salvage. *Clin Haematol* 3:385, 1990.

Plewes JL, Farhi LE: Cardiovascular responses to hemodilution and controlled hypotension in the dog. *Anesthesiology* 62:149, 1985.

Ponte A: Postoperative paraplegia due to hypercorrection of scoliosis and drop of blood pressure. *J Bone Joint Surg [Am]* 56:444, 1974.

Posner MA, Tobey RE, McElroy H: Hydroxocobalamin therapy of cyanide intoxication in guinea pigs. *Anesthesiology* 44:157, 1976.

Poyart C, Marden MC, Kister J: Bezafibrate derivatives as potent effectors of hemoglobin. *Methods Enzymol* 232:496, 1994.

Prys-Roberts C, Lloyd JW, Fisher A, et al.: Deliberate profound hypotension induced with halothane. Studies of haemodynamics and pulmonary gas exchange. *Br J Anaesth* 46:105, 1974.

Randad RS, Mahran MA, Mehanna AS, et al.: Allosteric modifiers of hemoglobin. *J Med Chem* 34:752, 1991.

Ray JM, Flynn JC, Bierman AH: Erythrocyte survival following intraoperative autotransfusion in spinal surgery. An in vivo comparative study and 5 year update. *Spine* 11:879, 1986.

Rees DD, Palmer RM, Hodson HF, et al.: A specific inhibitor of nitric oxide formation from L-arginine attenuates endothelium-dependent relaxation. *Br J Pharmacol* 96:418, 1989a.

Rees DD, Palmer RMJ, Moncada S: Role of endothelium-derived nitric oxide in regulation of blood pressure. *Proc Natl Acad Sci USA* 86:3375, 1989b.

Relton JES: Anesthesia in the original correction of scoliosis. In Riseborough EJ, Herndon JH, editors: *Scoliosis and other deformities of the axial skeleton.* Boston, 1975, Little, Brown and Co, pp 309–316.

Relton JES, Hall JE: An operation frame for spinal fusion. A new apparatus designed to reduce haemorrhage during operation. *J Bone Joint Surg [Br]* 49:327, 1967.

Rich GF, Lowson SM, Johns RA, et al.: Inhaled nitric oxide selectivity decreases pulmonary vascular resistance without impairing oxygenation during one-lung ventilation in patients undergoing cardiac surgery. *Anesthesiology* 80:57, 1994.

Robinson JS: Hypotension without hypoxia. In Stetson JB, editor: Metabolism. *Int Anesthesiol Clin* 5:467–480, 1967.

Rogers MC, Hamburger C, Owen K, et al.: Intracranial pressure in the cat during nitroglycerin-induced hypotension. *Anesthesiology* 51:227, 1979.

Rogers MC, Nugent SK, Traystman RJ: Control of cerebral circulation in the neonate and infant. *Crit Care Med* 8:570, 1980.

Rohrer MJ, Natale AM: Effect of hypothermia on the coagulation cascade. *Crit Care Med* 20:1402, 1992.

Salem MR: Deliberate hypotension is a safe and accepted anesthetic technique. In Eckenhoff JE, editor: *Controversy in anesthesiology.* Philadelphia, 1975, WB Saunders, pp 95–104.

Salem MR: Therapeutic uses of ganglionic blocking drugs. In Ivankovich AD, editor: Nitroprusside and other short-acting hypotensive agents. *Int Anesthesiol Clin* 16:171–200, 1978.

Salem MR: Hypercapnia, hypocapnia, and hypoxemia. *Semin Anesth* 6:202, 1987.

Salem MR, Ivankovich AD: The place of beta adrenergic blocking drugs in the deliberate induction of hypotension. *Anesth Analg* 49:427, 1970.

Salem MR, Ivankovich AD, Shaker MH: Safety factors in deliberately induced hypotension. *Middle East J Anesthesiol* 3:107, 1971.

Salem MR, Kim Y, Shaker MH: The effect of alteration of inspired oxygen concentration on jugular-bulb oxygen tension during deliberate hypotension. *Anesthesiology* 33:358, 1970.

Salem MR, Podraza AG: Blood conservation and massive transfusion. *Semin Anesth* 11:339, 1992.

Salem MR, Toyama T, Wong AY, et al.: Haemodynamic responses to induced arterial hypotension in children. *Br J Anaesth* 50:489, 1978.

Salem MR, Wong AY, Bennett EJ, et al.: Deliberate hypotension in infants and children. *Anesth Analg* 53:975, 1974.

Schaller RT Jr, Schaller J, Morgan A, et al.: Hemodilution anesthesia: A valuable aid to major cancer surgery in children. *Am J Surg* 146:79, 1983.

Schmied H, Schiferer A, Sessler DI, Meznik C: The effects of red-cell scavenging, hemodilution, and active warming on allogenic blood requirements in patients undergoing hip or knee arthroplasty. *Anesth Analg* 86:387, 1998.

Schwentker EP: Posterior fusion of the spine for scoliosis. *Surg Rounds* 1:12, 1978.

Scott DB, Buckley FP, Littlewood DG, et al.: Circulatory effects of labetalol during halothane anaesthesia. *Anaesthesia* 33:145, 1978.

Shapiro HM, Marshall LF: Intracranial pressure responses to PEEP in head-injured patients. *J Trauma* 18:254, 1978.

Silvergleid AJ: Preoperative autologous donation: What have we learned? *Transfusion* 31:99, 1991.

Simpson MB, Georgopolulos G, Eilert RE: Intraoperative blood salvage in children and young adults undergoing spinal surgery with predeposited autologous blood: Efficacy and cost effectiveness. *J Pediatr Orthop* 13:777, 1993.

Singler RC: Special techniques. Deliberate hypotension, hypothermia, and acute normovolemic hemodilution. In Gregory GA, editor: *Pediatric anesthesia.* New York, 1989, Churchill Livingstone, pp 553–577.

Sivarajan M, Amory DW, Everett GB, et al.: Blood pressure, not cardiac output, determines blood loss during induced hypotension. *Anesth Analg* 59:203, 1980.

Smith CA, Nelson NM: *The physiology of the newborn infant.* Springfield, IL, 1976, Charles C Thomas.

Solem JO, Tengborn L, Steen S, et al.: Cell saver versus hemofilter for concentration of oxygenator blood after cardiopulmonary bypass. *Thorac Cardiovasc Surg* 35:42, 1987.

Sollevi A, Lagerkranser M, Irestedt L, et al.: Controlled hypotension with adenosine in cerebral aneurysm surgery. *Anesthesiology* 61:400, 1984.

Spahn DR, Casutt M: Eliminating blood transfusions. *Anesthesiology* 93:242, 2000.

Sprung J, Kindscher JD, Wahr JA, et al.: The use of bovine hemoglobin glutamer-250 (Hemopure) in surgical patients: Results of a multicenter, randomized, single-blinded trial. *Anesth Analg* 94:799, 2002.

Stehling LC: Autologous transfusion. *Int Anesthesiol Clin* 28:190, 1990.

Stehling LC, Zauder HL: Autologous blood salvage procedures. *Biotechnology* 19:47, 1991.

Stockman JA, Graeber JE, Clark DA, et al.: Anemia of prematurity: Determinants of the erythropoietin response. *J Pediatr* 105:786, 1984.

Stockman JA, Oski FA: Physiological anemia of infancy and the anemia of prematurity. *Clin Haematol* 7:3, 1978.

Stone JG, Khambatta HJ, Matteo RS: Pulmonary shunting during anesthesia with deliberate hypotension. *Anesthesiology* 45:508, 1976.

Strandgaard S: Autoregulation of cerebral blood flow in hypertensive patients. *Circulation* 53:720, 1976.

Strunin L: Organ perfusion during controlled hypotension. *Br J Anaesth* 47:793, 1975.

Stullken EH, Sokoll MD: Intracranial pressure changes during hypotension and subsequent vasopressor therapy in anesthetized cats. *Anesthesiology* 42:425, 1975.

Sum CY, Yacobi A, Katzinel R, et al.: Kinetics of esmolol, an ultra-short-acting beta blocker, and of its major metabolite. *Clin Pharmacol Ther* 34:427, 1983.

Surgenor DM, Wallace EL, Hao SH, Chapman RH: Collection and transfusion of blood in the United States, 1982–1988. *N Eng J Med* 322:1666–1668, 1990.

Szyfelbein SK, Ryan JF: Use of controlled hypotension for primary surgical excision in an extensively burned child. *Anesthesiology* 41:501, 1974.

Taylor P: Ganglionic stimulating and blocking drugs. In Gilman AG, Goodman LS, Rall TW, Murad F, editors, *The pharmacological basis of therapeutics,* 7th ed. New York, 1985, Macmillan Publishing, p 215.

Thomas MJ, Gillon J, Desmond MJ: Consensus conference on autologous transfusion: Preoperative autologous donation. *Transfusion* 36:633, 1996.

Thompson GE, Miller RD, Stevens WC, et al.: Hypotensive anesthesia for total hip arthroplasty: A study of blood loss and organ function (brain, heart, liver, and kidney). *Anesthesiology* 48:91, 1978.

Tinker JH, Michenfelder JD: Sodium nitroprusside: Pharmacology, toxicology and therapeutics. *Anesthesiology* 45:340, 1976.

Toivonen J, Virtanen H, Kaukinen S: Labetalol attenuates the negative effects of deliberate hypotension induced by isoflurane. *Acta Anesthesiol Scand* 36:84, 1992.

Tremper KK, Freedman AE, Levine EM: The preoperative treatment of severely anemic patients with perfluorochemical emulsion oxygen transporting fluid, Fluosol-DA. *N Engl J Med* 307:277, 1982.

Tretiak R, Laupacis A, Rivière M, et al.: Cost of allogenic and autologous blood transfusion in Canada. *Can Med Assoc J* 154:1501, 1996.

Tuman KJ, Spiess BD, McCarthy RJ, Ivankovich AD: Effect of progressive blood loss and coagulation as measured by thromboelastography. *Anesth Analg* 66:856–963, 1987.

Tuman KJ, Spiess BD, McCarthy RJ, et al.: Effects of continuous arteriovenous hemofiltration on cardiopulmonary abnormalities during anesthesia for orthotopic liver transplantation. *Anesth Analg* 67:363, 1988.

Tuncali B, Karci A, Kadir A, et al.: Controlled hypotension and minimal inflation pressure: A new approach for pneumatid tourniquet application in upper limb surgery. *Anesth Analg* 97:1529, 2003

Turner JM, Powell D, Gibson RM, et al.: Intracranial pressure changes in neurosurgical patients during hypotension induced with sodium nitroprusside or trimetaphan. *Br J Anaesth* 49:419, 1977.

Valeri CR, Khabbaz K, Khuri SF: Effect of skin temperature on platelet function in patients undergoing extracorporeal bypass. *J Thorac Cardiovasc Surg* 104:108, 1992.

Van Aken H, Cottrell JE: Hypotensive anesthesia and its effect on the cardiovascular system. In Altura BM, Halevey S, editors: *Cardiovascular actions of anesthetics and drugs used in anesthesia,* vol 2, 5th ed. Basel, 1986, Karger, pp 260–279.

Van Aken H, Van Hemelrijck J: *Deliberate hypotension.* 1993 Review Course Lectures, International Anesthesia Research Society, Cleveland, Ohio.

Van Aken H, Puchstein C, Schweppe ML, et al.: Effect of labetalol on intracranial pressure in dogs with and without intracranial hypertension. *Acta Anaesth Scand* 26:615, 1982.

Van Aken H, Puchstein C, Anger C, et al.: Changes in intracranial pressure and compliance during adenosine triphosphate-induced hypotension in dogs. *Anesth Analg* 63:381, 1984.

Van Oeveren W, Jansen NJG, Bidstrup BP, et al.: Effects of aprotinin on haemostatic mechanisms during cardiopulmonary bypass. *Ann Thorac Surg* 44:640, 1987.

Verner IR: Techniques for deliberate hypotension: Direct acting vasodilators. In Enderby GEH, editor: *Hypotensive anaesthesia.* London, 1985, Churchill Livingstone, pp 138–163.

Vesey CJ, Cole PV, Simpson PJ: Sodium nitroprusside in anaesthesia. *Br Med J* 3:229, 1975.

Viviani GR, Sadler JTS, Ingham GK: Autotransfusions in scoliosis surgery. *Clin Orthop Related Res* 135:74, 1978.

Wahr JL: Clinical potential of blood substitutes or oxygen therapeutics during cardiac surgery. *Anesthesiol Clin N Am* 21:553, 2003.

Wahr JL, Gerber M, Venitz J, et al.: Allosteric modification of oxygen delivery by hemoglobin. *Anesth Analg* 92:615, 2001.

Warren JV: The physiology of the giraffe. *Sci Am* 231:96, 1974.

Watzek G, Watzek C, Draxler V, et al.: Experience with 'isovolaemic' haemodilution in extensive surgery for oro-facial tumours. *J Oral Maxillofac Surg* 8:131, 1980.

Welborn LG, Hannallah RS, Luban NLC, et al.: Anemia and postoperative apnea in former preterm infants. *Anesthesiology* 74:1003, 1991.

Widman FK: *Standards for blood banks and transfusion services,* 14th ed. Arlington, VA, 1991, American Association of Blood Banks.

Wildsmith JA, Sinclair CJ, Thorn J, et al.: Haemodynamic effects of induced hypotension with a nitroprusside-trimethaphan mixture. *Br J Anaesth* 55:381, 1983.

Williamson KR, Taswell HF: Intraoperative blood salvage. In Taswell HF, Pineda AA, editors: *Autologous transfusion and hemotherapy.* Boston, 1991, Blackwell Scientific, pp 122–154.

Wilson AJ, Cuddigan BJ, Wyatt AP: Early experience of intraoperative autotransfusion. *J R Soc Med* 81:389, 1988.

Wong KC, Webster LR, Coleman SS, et al.: Hemodilution and induced hypotension for insertion of a Harrington rod in a Jehovah's Witness patient. *Clin Orthop Relat Res* 152:237, 1980.

Woodcock TE, Millard RK, Dixon J, et al.: Clonidine premedication for isoflurane-induced hypotension. *Br J Anaesth* 60:388, 1988.

Yaster M, Simmons RJ, Tolo VT, et al.: A comparison of nitroglycerin and nitroprusside for inducing hypotension in children: A double-blind study. *Anesthesiology* 65:175, 1986.

Yau TM Carson S, Weisel RD, et al.: The effect of warm heart surgery on postoperative bleeding. *J Thorac Cardiovasc Surg* 103:1155, 1992.

Yawn DH: Properties of salvaged blood. In Taswell HF, Pineda AA, editors: *Autologous transfusion and hemotherapy,* Boston, 1991, Blackwell Scientific, pp 194–206.

Zauder HL: Intraoperative and postoperative blood salvage devices. In Stehling LC, editor: *Perioperative autologous transfusion.* Arlington, VA, 1991, American Association of Blood Banks, pp 25–36.

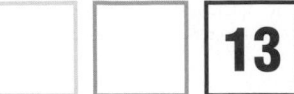

Pain Management in Infants and Children

Steven J. Weisman • Lynn M. Rusy

The International Association for the Study of Pain defines *pain* as "an unpleasant sensory and emotional experience associated with actual or potential tissue damage, or described in terms of such damage" (Merskey and Bogduk, 1994). In children, even the definition of pain has been debated (Anand and Craig, 1996). Pain is a complex constellation of unpleasant sensory, perceptual, and emotional experiences and certain associated autonomic, psychological, emotional, and behavioral responses. In many newborns or infants, as well as others who have mental retardation, are comatose, are severely demented, or are verbally handicapped, pain cannot be described in such self-report terms. In fact, pain experienced by infants and children often goes unrecognized, even neglected, because of the operational definition of *pain* that requires self-report (Walco et al., 1994; Anand and Craig, 1996). Untreated pain in children, as the result of vaccinations and blood draws, surgery, headaches, or repeated painful procedures, can have long-term effects (McGrath and Unruh, 1987).

Pain management is an essential component of care provided by pediatric anesthesiologists. Most obvious, of course, is the integration of a pain management plan into the overall perioperative plan. In addition, since the 1990s, many pediatric anesthesiologists have become the pain management experts in their institutions. This is particularly true in many of the freestanding children's hospitals that do not have ready access to more mature and developed adult pain management services. This chapter outlines developmental issues in pain management, measurement of pain in children, pharmacologic ways to treat pain (including opioid infusions, patient-controlled analgesia [PCA], epidural anesthesia, single-shot caudal blocks), behavioral pain management, physical modalities for pain management (transcutaneous electrical nerve stimulation [TENS] units), and alternative techniques (acupuncture) now being used in children to manage pain. A glossary of terms used in this chapter is given in Box 13–1.

■ UNDERTREATMENT OF PAIN IN CHILDREN

For many years, it has been recognized that pediatric patients are more likely to have pain treated less aggressively than are their adult counterparts (Eland, 1974; Asprey, 1994; Ferrell et al., 1995; Bildner and Krechel, 1996; Twycross et al., 1999; Sahler et al., 2000). Unfortunately, one can argue that this has led to a considerable amount of unnecessary suffering on the part of these patients. In addition, this may have contributed to a collective sense of guilt on the part of the health care provider teams that results in rationalization for policies and procedures that lead to undertreatment (Craig et al., 1996). Children have consistently been offered and/or received fewer, smaller, and less frequent doses of opioid analgesics (McCaffery and Hart, 1976; Perry and Heidrich, 1982; Beyer et al., 1983; Mather and Mackie, 1983; Sriwatanakul et al., 1983; Schechter and Allen, 1986).

BOX 13–1 Abbreviations in Pain Management

AHCPR : Agency for Health Care Policy and Research
COX : Cyclooxygenase
JCAHO : Joint Commission for the Accreditation of Healthcare Organizations
LET : Lidocaine/epinephrine/tetracaine
PCA : Patient-controlled analgesia
RAP : Recurrent abdominal pain
SSRIs : Selective serotonin reuptake inhibitors
TAC : Tetracaine/Adrenalin/cocaine
TCAs : Tricyclic antidepressants
TENS : Transcutaneous electrical nerve stimulation

■ **TABLE 13–1.** Survey of major pediatric textbooks

Textbook/Editor(s)/Publisher	Year of Publication	Edition	Total No. of Pages in Text Management*	No. of Chapters on Pain	No. of Pages on Pain Management*
Oski's pediatrics: Principles and practice/McMillan, DeAngelis, Feigin, Warshaw/Lippincott Williams and Wilkins	1999	3	2,848	1	2
Primary pediatric care/Hoekelman/Mosby	2001	4	2,199	5	34
Gellis and Kagan's current pediatric therapy/Burg, Ingelfinger, Polin, Gershon/Saunders	2002	17	1,280	1	9
Current pediatric diagnosis and treatment/Hay, Hayward, Levin, Sondheimer/McGraw-Hill/Appleton & Lange	2002	16	1,320	None	4
Rudolph's pediatrics/Rudolph, Rudolph, Hostetter, Lister, Siegel/McGraw-Hill Professional	2002	21	2,688	2	11
Saunders manual of pediatric practice/Finberg, Kleinman/W.B. Saunders	2002	2	1,214	None	0
Nelson textbook of pediatrics edition: Text with continually updated online reference/Behrman/W.B. Saunders	2004	17	2,618	1	8
Totals			14,167	10	68

*Chapters dedicated to pain management were identified. Total number of pages of text present in either these chapters or other sections of the book were calculated.

Most health care professionals, even many in surgical specialties, do not receive formal training in pain management (Taylor and Harris, 1997; Sloan et al., 1998; Ferrell et al., 2000; Fins and Nilson, 2000; Sahler et al., 2000; Jubelirer et al., 2001). In addition, even pediatricians lack relatively easy access to information about pain management. For example, a survey of major textbooks in pediatrics shows the minimal amount of pain management information that is available (Table 13–1). Despite the fact that more than 80% of children who present for nonroutine care have pain as a chief complaint, these 13,811 pages of pediatric text contain only 68 pages that address pain management. Many students complete medical school with only 1 to 2 hours of analgesic pharmacology lectures incorporated into their initial pharmacology course. In addition, although most practitioners involved in the care of children are well aware of the benefits of cognitive-behavioral interventions for pain or procedure management, few ever receive formal training to help incorporate these techniques into daily practice (Eland, 1974; Asprey, 1994). Johnston and others (1992) surveyed 150 hospitalized children and found that more than 87% reported having had pain within 24 hours and, of these, 19% reported their usual pain intensity as being in the severe range. Only 38% of the children received analgesic medication during the preceding 24 hours. Broome and others (1996) reported the results of a survey of pain management in pediatric residency training programs. Sixty percent of the respondents were aware of institutional standards of care or protocols for pain management, but only one fourth reported that the standards were followed 80% or more of the time. In another survey of hospitalized children, Cummings and others (1996) reported on patient or parent interviews that were conducted in 200 patients. They reported the intensity and source of the worst, usual, and current pain during the past 24 hours and the help received for pain. Forty-nine percent of the children had clinically significant levels of worst pain. Twenty-one percent had clinically significant levels of usual pain. The causes of pain included disease, surgery, and intravenous catheters. Children received significantly less medication than was prescribed, regardless of the reported pain level. In addition, many children identified "no one" as being helpful in relieving their pain.

Since 1990, many different national and international standards for pain management have been released. Although there have been individual examples of intensive local efforts to implement some of these guidelines, in general, the guidelines have not been adopted as practice guidelines. McMillan and others (2000) surveyed nurses at two large veterans hospitals and found that even 7 years after the initial Agency for Health Care Policy and Research (AHCPR) guideline was released, nurses continued to have major knowledge deficits about the physiology and pharmacology of pain. The majority of nurses did not agree that patients and their families should have the most control over analgesic scheduling and that a constant level of analgesic should be maintained in the blood. In fact, 82% indicated that around-the-clock analgesics increase the risk for sedation and respiratory depression. Dalton and others (1999) developed a comprehensive program to implement the AHCPR 1992 acute pain management guideline in 6 community hospitals. They were able to demonstrate improved pain assessment and documentation, as well as improved practice in the adopting hospitals.

In 1999, in the United States, the Joint Commission for the Accreditation of Healthcare Organizations (JCAHO) incorporated comprehensive standards of pain management into all of its clinical care manuals. The ripple effects from this are quite evident in the medical, nursing, and administrative communities of all health care organizations. Organizations are beginning to report improvement in assessment and management of pain as well as improvements in satisfaction by patients and their families (Phillips, 2000; Blank et al., 2001; Manworren, 2001; Ruzicka and Daniels, 2001; Starck et al., 2001; Goodman, 2003; O'Connor, 2003).

Fortunately, pediatric anesthesiologists have become proponents for the improvement of pain management in children. Many children's hospitals have developed acute, chronic, or combined programs for the management of pain in children (Shapiro et al., 1991; Miller, 1996; Harmer and Davies, 1998; Rawal, 1999). In this capacity, pediatric anesthesiologists must remain on the forefront of knowledgeable and safe use of a variety of pain interventions for infants and children.

■ NEUROPHYSIOLOGY OF PAIN

A variety of chemical, thermal, or mechanical insults can result in the sensation of pain. A mosaic of pain receptors or nociceptors in the body tissues ultimately project to pain centers in the brain. The somatosensory system is subserved by different groups of afferent fibers differentiated by their anatomy, rate of transmission, and sensory modality transmitted. The fibers relay pain information to the dorsal horn of the spinal cord and then on to the brain. These fibers include rapidly conducting, small-diameter C-fibers and thinly myelinated A-δ fibers. The majority of nociceptive input to the central nervous system is carried by C-fibers.

The dorsal horn is organized into fairly discreet lamellae. The primary afferent first-order synapses (nociceptive-specific neurons) are usually located in layers 1, 2, and 5 of the dorsal horn. Signals are then relayed rostrally to the thalamus and the cortex. In addition, afferent impulses are carried to the brainstem, limbic system, and hypothalamus to mediate many of the autonomic and affective component responses to noxious stimuli. Deeper in the dorsal horn are located wide dynamic range neurons (class 2 neurons) that appear to be important in the development of hyperalgesia, or wind-up. These synapses in lamella 5 process signals from hair movement and weak mechanical stimuli. However, they also respond vigorously to a variety of other tissue-damaging stimuli. These neurons may be responsible for firing in pain syndromes that are not associated with obvious tissue damage as well. Reviews of the mechanisms of pain transduction, processing, and modulation have been published by Woolf and colleagues (Costigan and Woolf, 2000, 2002; Woolf and Max, 2001).

■ NEURODEVELOPMENT AND NOCICEPTION

Until recently, physicians also lacked a clear understanding of the normal development of nociception in young or premature infants (Schechter and Allen, 1986; Anand and Hickey, 1987; Anand, 1998). Their nervous system is immature, and it has been shown that there is incomplete myelination of the nerve tracts bearing afferent impulses. Pain perception does begin before birth, and potent analgesics alter the stress response to surgery, even in premature infants. The landmark article published by Anand and Hickey in 1987 clearly addressed the issue that newborns and infants do in fact experience pain. In addition, the same investigators demonstrated that infants undergoing cardiac procedures do much better clinically if treated appropriately for pain (Anand and Hickey, 1992). Infants received either high-dose opioid (sufentanil) intraoperatively and postoperatively or halothane for surgery and morphine on an as-needed basis in the cardiac intensive care unit. Plasma levels of epinephrine, norepinephrine, glucagon, corticosterone, 11-deoxycorticosterone, and 11-deoxycortisol were significantly elevated in the halothane group up to 24 hours after surgery. They clearly demonstrated that the group that received the sufentanil had greater hemodynamic stability, required less postoperative ventilatory support, and had improved clinical outcome as measured by these markers. The reduced hormonal response and improved clinical outcome following surgery led to the conclusion that neonates do experience pain and that this pain needs to be controlled (Rogers, 1992).

This has also led to speculation that the fetus is capable of experiencing clinically meaningful pain. The anatomic requirements for pain are in place before birth (Anand and Hickey, 1987). Fitzgerald (1994) reviewed the biologic development of the fetus and showed that at 7.5 weeks, there are reflex responses to somatic stimuli. Touching the perioral region results in bending the head away from the stimulus, and repeated stimulation of the limbs at 10 weeks results in hyperexcitability, interpreted as evidence for a functional pain system, even in the very young fetus (Fitzgerald, 1994). Studies observing the muscle response of young infants using electromyography demonstrate a graded response reflective of the stimulus intensity (Andrews and Fitzgerald, 1999, 2000).

It is important to understand that pain due to surgical procedures not only results in an immediate nociceptive response but also results in changes in the nociceptive activation pathways that lead to hypersensitivity, hyperalgesia, and allodynia. Infants exposed to repeated heel lancing develop hypersensitivity so that mechanical sensory reflex thresholds are reduced on the affected side compared with the nonlanced control side (Fitzgerald et al., 1988, 1989). Neonatal rats that are studied after repeated needle sticks develop prolonged thermal hyperalgesia (Anand et al., 1999). In other rodent models, newborns demonstrate relatively large nociceptive receptor fields (Yi and Barr, 1995) and immature descending inhibitory systems (Fitzgerald and Koltzenburg, 1986). Actual neural remodeling in the spinal cord has been demonstrated by Ruda and others (2000) in a rat model of chronic inflammation. There was increased sprouting of primary sensory fibers as well as caudal extension in the spinal cord. In addition, there was hyperexcitability in dorsal horn neurons connecting to these fibers, plus abnormal and increased pain behaviors seen later in the adult animals.

■ ASSESSMENT OF PAIN

Children have a more intense physical and emotional reaction to painful procedures than do adults. In the 1800s, Darwin wrote about matching facial expressions to emotions, with pain being one of those he recognized (Grunau and Craig, 1987). In 1986, Johnston and Strada (1986) found that facial expressions are useful markers for pain in infants up to 6 months of age. They found facial expressions to be less well developed in premature babies and a high-pitched cry to be a better marker of pain. Grunau and others (1990) developed the Neonatal Facial Coding System to quantify facial actions in newborns exposed to brief painful stimuli. Various investigators have developed composite observational pain measurement tools to assist in the assessment of pain in the preverbal or nonverbal pediatric populations. Because of neurodevelopmental differences, tools have been refined to accommodate measurement in the premature infant; examples of these tools are given in Tables 13–2 through 13–5.

Wong and Baker (1988) described the original, and possibly most popularized, FACES pain scale for children aged 3 years or older (Fig. 13–1). Bieri and others (1990) investigated the use of facial expressions as a way of rating subtle behaviors. They adapted children's drawings to derive a cartoon scale with more anthropomorphically realistic faces (Fig. 13–2). This scale was revised and validated to correspond to a 0- to 10-point verbal analog scale (Hicks et al., 2001).

Numeric self-report measures are widely accepted for use in children older than 6 to 8 years (Maunuksela et al., 1987; Vetter and Heiner, 1996). Although the visual analog scale (10-cm line that is anchored as "no pain" to "worst possible pain" at each end) is often considered the gold standard of pain assessment, in children the verbal analog scale (pain rated from 0 [no pain] to 10 [most pain possible]) may be more reliable (Briggs and Closs, 1999).

Pain assessment in the cognitively impaired child has been a challenge and a barrier to effective pain treatment. As many as

■ **TABLE 13–2.** Behavioral and composite pain assessment scales

Measure	Target Age	Indicators	Comments	References
Premature Infant Pain Profile (PIPP)	Preterm and full-term neonates	Gestational age, behavioral state, heart rate, oxygen saturation, brow bulge, eye squeeze, nasolabial furrow	Developed with procedural pain model (heel lance); 0-to-21 scoring	Stevens et al., 1996; Ballantyne et al., 1999
Neonatal Infant Pain Scale (NIPS)	Preterm and full-term infants	Facial expression, cry, breathing pattern, arms, legs, state of arousal	Developed with procedural pain model (heel lance); also validated for preterm infants; 0-to-7 scoring	Lawrence et al., 1993; Johnston et al., 1999
CRIES (*c*rying *r*equires O_2 saturation, *i*ncreased vital signs, *e*xpression, and *s*leeplessness)	Full-term neonates	Crying, O_2 saturation, heart rate, blood pressure, expression, sleeplessness	Developed with postoperative pain model; 0-to-10 scoring	Krechel and Bildner, 1995
FLACC (*f*ace, *l*egs, *a*ctivity, *c*rying, *c*onsolability)	2 mo to 7 yr	Facial expression, crying, legs, activity state, consolability	Developed with postoperative pain model; 0-to-10 scoring	Merkel et al., 1997
Children's Hospital of Eastern Ontario Pain Scale (CHEOPS)	1 to 7 yr	Cry, facial expression, verbalization, torso position, touch (affected area), legs	Developed with postoperative pain model but tested in procedural pain as well; 4-to-13 scoring	McGrath et al., 1985
COMFORT Score	All ages	Alertness, calmness/agitation, respiratory response, physical movements, heart rate, blood pressure, muscle tone, facial tension	Developed for use in critical care setting (intubated patient); 0-to-40 scoring	Ambuel et al., 1992

10% of children who are cared for in major pediatric centers have mental retardation, autism, metabolic disorders, neurotrauma, or significant other communication disorders. Breau and others (1999, 2002) identified common pain problems likely to occur in these children, such as gastroesophageal reflux, muscle spasm, and constipation. In addition, the same group of investigators developed a tool to measure pain in these at-risk children, the Non-Communicating Pain Behavior Check List (Breau et al., 2002).

Individual institutions have developed their own algorithm for a series of pain assessment tools to span the developmental continuum. It is imperative for caretakers to incorporate the

■ **TABLE 13–3.** Children's Hospital of Eastern Ontario Pain Scale (CHEOPS)

Item	Behavior	Score	Definition
Cry	No cry	1	Child is not crying.
	Moaning	2	Child is moaning or quietly vocalizing, silent cry.
	Crying	2	Child is crying but the cry is gentle or whimpering.
	Scream	3	Child is in a full-lunged cry; sobbing: may be scored with complaint or without complaint.
Facial	Composed	1	Neutral facial expression
	Grimace	2	Score only if definite negative facial expression.
	Smiling	0	Score only if definite negative facial expression.
Child Verbal	None	1	Child is not talking.
	Other complaints	1	Child complains but not about pain, e.g., "I want to see my mommy," or "I am thirsty."
	Pain complaints	2	Child complains about pain.
	Both complaints	2	Child complains about pain and about other things, e.g., "It hurts; I want my mommy."
	Positive	0	Child makes any positive statement or talks about other things without complaint.
Torso	Neutral	1	Body (not limbs) is at rest; torso is inactive.
	Shifting	2	Body is in motion in a shifting or serpentine fashion.
	Tense	2	Body is arched or rigid.
	Shivering	2	Body is shuddering or shaking involuntarily.
	Upright	2	Child is vertical or in upright position.
	Restrained	2	Body is restrained.
Touch	Not touching	1	Child is not touching or grabbing at wound.
	Reach	2	Child is reaching for but not touching wound.
	Touch	2	Child is gently touching wound or wound area.
	Grab	2	Child is grabbing vigorously at wound.
	Restrained	2	Child's arms are restrained.
Legs	Neutral	1	Legs may be in any position but are relaxed; includes gentle swimming or serpentine-like movements.
	Squirming/kicking	2	Definitive uneasy or restless movements in the legs and/or striking out with foot or feet.
	Drawn up/tensed	2	Legs tensed and/or pulled up tightly to body and kept there.
	Standing	2	Standing, crouching, or kneeling
	Restrained	2	Child's legs are being held down.

From McGrath P, Johnson G, et al.: CHEOPS: A behavioral scale for rating postoperative pain in children. In Fields H, editor: *Advances in pain research and therapy.* New York, 1985, Raven Press, pp 395–402.

TABLE 13–4. FLACC (Face, Legs, Activity, Crying, Consolability) Scale

Category	SCORING 0	1	2
Face	No particular expression or smile	Occasional grimace or frown, withdrawn, disinterested	Frequent to constant quivering chin, clenched jaw.
Legs	Normal position or relaxed	Uneasy, restless, tense	Kicking, or legs drawn up
Activity	Lying quietly, normal position, moves easily	Squirming, shifting back and forth, tense	Arched, rigid or jerking
Cry	No cry (awake or asleep)	Moans or whimpers; occasional complaint	Crying steadily, screams or sobs, frequent complaints
Consolability	Content, relaxed	Reassured by occasional touching, hugging, or being talked to, distractible	Difficult to console or comfort

From Merkel SI, Voepel-Lewis T, et al.: The FLACC: A behavioral scale for scoring postoperative pain in young children. *Pediatr Nurs* 23:293–297, 1997.

various ages or developmentally appropriate tools into their language of pain assessment and management.

PHARMACOLOGIC APPROACHES TO PAIN MANAGEMENT

The management of pediatric pain can be accomplished using a multimodal approach in which pharmacologic techniques and nonpharmacologic approaches complement one another. The nonpharmacologic approaches include relaxation training, cognitive-behavioral techniques, biofeedback, physical therapy, occupational therapy, TENS, acupuncture, and progressive muscle relaxation training. We first discuss pharmacologic approaches and, later in the chapter, discuss in greater detail nonpharmacologic ways to manage pain. Unfortunately, nonpharmacologic methods for pain management continue to be underused in children. An in-depth discussion of this topic is, obviously, beyond the scope of this chapter; the reader is referred to an excellent monograph by Lynnda Dahlquist (1999).

NONSTEROIDAL ANTI-INFLAMMATORY DRUGS

Acetaminophen (paracetamol) is an antipyretic and weak analgesic that blocks prostaglandin synthesis centrally, reduces substance P–induced hyperalgesia, and modulates spinal cord hyperalgesic nitric oxide production (Bjorkman et al., 1994; Bjorkman, 1995). It is a weak analgesic indicated for mild pain or as an adjunct for the treatment of moderate or severe pain. Although it produces dose-dependent responses, it is limited by a ceiling effect, above which dose increases do not produce further analgesia (Skoglund et al., 1991; Hahn et al., 2003). Acetaminophen is safe to use in neonates, especially because it is primarily metabolized in the liver. Because neonates have immature hepatic function, they are less likely to produce toxic metabolites (Lesko and Mitchell, 1999; van Lingen et al., 1999a, 1999b; Anderson et al., 2002). Oral doses of 10 to 15 mg/kg, although antipyretic, are not analgesic until doses of 20 to 35 mg/kg are used (Anderson and Holford, 1997; Anderson et al., 1999). In fact, there is evidence that rectal doses of 40 to 45 mg/kg are needed to achieve effective plasma concentrations (Korpela et al., 1999).

Nonsteroidal anti-inflammatory drugs (NSAIDs) inhibit peripheral cyclooxygenase (COX) and decrease prostaglandin production and are more potent analgesics than acetaminophen (Malmberg and Yaksh, 1992; Yaksh and Malmberg, 1993; Yaksh et al., 1998). NSAID pharmacology has advanced so that agents have been developed that target the different isozymes of COX. COX-1 is constitutive, whereas COX-2 is induced after trauma and inflammation (Mitchell et al., 1993; Everts et al., 2000). Commonly used NSAIDs actively inhibit both COX enzymes (Table 13–6). A newer series of agents have become available that target primarily the COX-2 isozyme. None of these agents have received approval for use in children. However, several reports of the successful perioperative use of celecoxib (Celebrex) and rofecoxib (Vioxx) have been published (Cummins et al., 2000; Pickering et al., 2002; Stempak et al., 2002; Joshi et al., 2003; Kerr et al., 2003). These are helpful in mild postoperative pain problems, such as ear tube insertions, inguinal hernia repairs, and other minor surgical procedures.

These publications target the opioid-sparing effect of the COX-2 inhibitors in children, as has been clearly documented with several older-generation NSAIDs. Diclofenac and ketorolac have been most extensively studied in this setting (Nordbladh et al., 1991; Maunuksela et al., 1992; Watcha et al., 1992; Sutters et al., 1995; Nishina et al., 2000; Park et al., 2000; Oztekin et al., 2002). Ketorolac remains the only parenteral NSAID used in the perioperative setting. Several injectable COX-2 inhibitors are in development. Because all cells, except red cells, produce prostanoids via the COX pathway, the COX agents have significant toxic effects. Use is limited by gastropathy,

TABLE 13–5. Self-report measures pain assessment scales

Measure	Target	Age	Indicators/ Comments	References
FACES	>3 yr	Cartoon drawings of faces from smiling to crying with tears	Some cultural variability; 0-to-5 or 0-to-10 scoring	Littmer and LePage, 1988; Wong and Baker 1988
Bieri–Modified	>3 yr	Line drawings of faces from neutral to crying	Validated for 6–8 yr; 0-to-6 (original) scoring; 0-to-5 or -10 (modified) scoring	Bieri et al., 1990; Hicks et al., 2001
Oucher	>3 yr	Photographs of child from neutral to crying	Available in versions for whites, Hispanics, and blacks; 0-to-100 scoring	Beyer et al., 1992

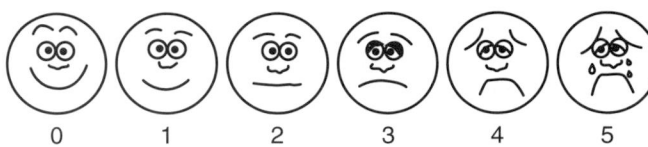

■ **FIGURE 13–1.** Wong-Baker FACES scale. Scored from 0 to 5; it can also be scored from 0 to 10. Wong and Baker (1988) described the original, and possibly most popularized, FACES pain scale for children aged 3 years or older. (From Wong DL, Hockenberry–Eaton M, Wilson DJ, et al.: *Wong's essentials of pediatric nursing,* 8th ed. St. Louis, Mosby, 2001, p 1301.)

inhibition of platelet function, and marked reduction in renal blood flow. The COX-2 inhibitors have marked less gastrointestinal toxicity, as well as no hemostatic effects, but they are still able to induce significant renal toxicity. No data are available on potential cardiovascular toxicity of COX-2 inhibitors in children.

■ **TABLE 13–6.** Nonsteroidal anti-inflammatory drugs (NSAIDs)

Drug	Age Group	Dose (mg/kg)	Interval
Acetaminophen	Preterm Term	Load: 20; 15(PO), 20 (PR)	q12h
	>3 mo	Load: 20 to 30; 20 (PO)	q8h
		Load: 20 (PO); 15 (PO)	q4h
		40 (PR), 20 (PR)	q6h
Diclofenac	>1 yr	1 (PO)	q8h
Ibuprofen	>6 mo	10 to 15 (PO)	q6h
Ketorolac	>6 mo	0.25 to 0.5 (IM, IV)	q6h
Naproxen	>6 mo	5 to 10 (PO)	q8-12h
Celecoxib	>1 yr	1.5 to 3 (PO)	q12h

Note: In the perioperative setting, or in other medical settings where hypovolemia may occur, extreme caution is advised when using NSAIDs (except acetaminophen).

■ OPIOIDS

A review of opioid pharmacology can be found in Chapter 6, Basic Pharmacokinetic Concepts. Opioids are one of the foundations of analgesia in a balanced anesthetic, as well as the basis of analgesia for patients with moderate to severe pain. Opioids are used as part of a "balanced" or multimodal analgesic plan (Table 13–7). Such a plan will incorporate an NSAID, if possible, and/or use of local anesthetics. In addition, careful attention must be paid to the specific neurodevelopmental pharmacology of these drugs, because it affects the distribution and clearance of all the opioid analgesics.

Morphine and Fentanyl

Premature and term newborns show reduced clearance of morphine and prolonged elimination half-life (Lynn and Slattery, 1987). In opioid naïve young infants, doses that are one fourth to one half of those normally recommended should be used. By 3 to 6 months of age, morphine pharmacokinetics resembles that in older children and adults (McRorie et al., 1992; Lynn et al., 1998). Fentanyl has a prolonged elimination half-life and diminished clearance in premature infants and newborns (Singleton et al., 1987). The same authors report that in infants older than 3 months, clearance is actually double that in older children and adults. Because fentanyl clearance is dependent on hepatic blood flow, it must be used with caution in infants who have increased intra-abdominal pressure, particularly during and after surgery (Yaster, 1987; Yaster et al., 1988). Small infants, younger than 6 months, who are receiving opioid analgesics must be carefully monitored with pulse oximetry in a setting that provides adequate supervision, if respiratory compromise were to occur.

In many clinical settings, use of continuous opioid infusions may be preferable to the use of intermittent dosing. In general, continuous therapy is used in children who are too young to take advantage of PCA systems. In neonates, because of lowered morphine clearance, continuous infusion should be initiated cautiously, even at dosages as low as 5 mcg/kg per hour (Hartley et al., 1993). Infants between 1 and 3 months of age have been successfully managed with morphine infusions of 10 to 30 mcg/kg per hour (Bray, 1983; Bray et al., 1986, 1996). Lynn and others (1984) have shown that after a loading dose of 25 to 75 mcg/kg, infusions of 15 to 25 mcg/kg per hour provide adequate postoperative analgesia.

Alternatively, continuous fentanyl infusions are widely used in both pediatric and newborn intensive care units. Loading doses are usually in the 1 to 4 mcg/kg range followed by infusions of 2 to 4 mcg/kg per hour. Fentanyl affords some degree of cardiovascular stability compared with morphine in the very critically ill infant (Collins et al., 1985; Yaster et al., 1987, 1994).

Success in the use of continuous opioid therapy is often dependent on successful management of side effects or effective dose adjustment in children who continue to have pain. Nausea, vomiting, pruritus, urinary retention, dysphoria, constipation, and somnolence must all be treated promptly (Table 13–8). Inadequate analgesia will be difficult to treat if adjustments are only made to the rate of infusion. If the overall assessment is that the child is having significant pain at the current infusion rate, a bolus dose of approximately 50% of the standard dose for age should be administered and followed by a rate increase of 10% to 20%.

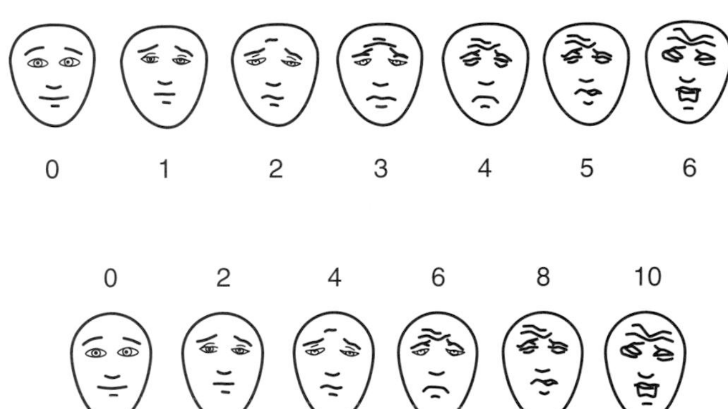

■ **FIGURE 13–2.** Bieri faces scales. *(Top)* Original panel. *(Bottom)* Revised scale corresponding to a 0-to-10 metric. Bieri and others (1990) investigated the use of facial expressions as a way of rating subtle behaviors. They adapted children's drawings to derive a cartoon scale with more anthropomorphically realistic faces. This scale was recently revised and validated to correspond to a 0- to 10-point verbal analog scale. (From Hicks CL, Baeyer CL, Spaffard PA, et al.: The faces pain scale-revised: Toward a common metric in pediatric pain measurement. *Pain* 93:173–183, 2001. Copyright © 2001, with permission from the International Association for the Study of Pain.)

Hydromorphone

Hydromorphone is a phenanthrene derivative of morphine. It is approximately five times more potent than morphine, is nearly as water soluble, and has a similar elimination half-life. Hydromorphone is metabolized to hydromorphone-3-glucuronide, dihydromorphone, and dihydroisomorphine. Its pharmacokinetic profile appears to be similar in children and

■ **TABLE 13–7.** Opioid analgesics (μ-agonists)

Drug	Equipotent IV Dose (mg/kg)	IV:PO Equivalence	IV Dose (mg/kg)	PO Dose (mg/kg)	Interval (Minimum)	Comments
Codeine	1	1:1.5	NA	0.5-1.0	q3h	Usually prescribed with acetaminophen; limited analgesia in patients deficient in P450 2D6 isozyme
Fentanyl	0.001	1:10	0.001 to 0.002	Transmucosal: 200-mcg unit smallest available; titrate to effective dose	q1h (IV)	Chest wall rigidity associated with doses >0.005 mg/kg; also available as transdermal system (12.5 to 100 mcg/hr delivery) for chronic pain neuraxial
Hydromorphone	0.02	1:5	0.015 to 0.02	0.1	q3h	May cause less itching and nausea; no active metabolites; good in renal failure; neuraxial
Meperidine	1.0	1:4	1.0	4	q3h	Avoid monoamine oxidase inhibitors; normeperidine (metabolite) causes seizures; only short-term use
Methadone	0.1	1:2	0.1 to 0.2 (load)	0.1 to 0.2	q12h	Very long-acting
Morphine	0.1	1:3	0.1	0.3	q3h	Histamine release; several slow-release oral forms available (MS Contin; Kadian; Avinza, Oramorph SR); neuraxial
Oxycodone	0.2			0.1 to 0.2	q3h	Little nausea or itch; slow-release oral form available (OxyContin); available in combination with acetaminophen or ibuprofen

adults (Babul et al., 1995). There is still some controversy over the clinically relevant side effect profile of hydromorphone. Several authors contend that hydromorphone results in less pruritus and less respiratory depression compared with morphine (Chaplan et al., 1992; Goodarzi, 1999). Both of these studies examined epidural administration and use equianalgesic conversions well above the 5:1 ratio commonly accepted in children (Collins et al., 1996). Other investigators have found very similar side effects with hydromorphone compared with morphine (Collins, 1996; Halpern et al., 1996; Rapp et al., 1996; Miller et al., 1999). Nonetheless, hydromorphone is an excellent alternative to morphine when one desires opioid rotation in the very tolerant patient, when there are unacceptable morphine side effects, and in patients with significant renal impairment.

■ **TABLE 13–8.** Medications commonly used to treat opioid side effects

Side Effect	Treatment
Pruritus	Diphenhydramine (0.5 mg/kg per dose q6h PRN) **or** Naloxone gtt (0.5 to 2 mcg/kg per hour) **or** Nalmefene (0.25 to 0.5 mcg/kg per dose *scheduled* q8h)
Nausea/vomiting	Ondansetron (0.15 mg/kg per dose q6h PRN to a maximum of 4 mg/dose) **or** Narcan gtt (0.5 to 2 mcg/kg per hour) **or** Nalmefene (0.25 to 0.5 mcg/kg per dose *scheduled* q8h)
Somnolence	Methylphenidate (0.1 mg/kg per dose); consider slow-release preparations
Urinary retention	Naloxone gtt (0.5 to 2 mcg/kg per hour) **or** Nalmefene (0.25 to 0.5 mcg/kg per dose *scheduled* q8h) May require placement of continuous indwelling catheter

Note: Often symptoms can be managed with a reduction in opioid dosing by 20% to 25%. However, this may reduce analgesia and adjunctive therapy should be considered.

Although hydromorphone metabolites can accumulate in patients with renal impairment, they do not appear to be associated with the respiratory depressive effects seen with morphine metabolites in these patients (Babul et al., 1995). Hydromorphone does not appear to have significantly active water-soluble metabolites (Bruera et al., 1996; Collins et al., 1996).

Methadone

Methadone is also a μ-agonist, but it has an extremely long elimination half-life of 19 hours in children (Berde et al., 1991). It behaves similarly to a slow-release preparation because of this property. It can be administered intravenously or orally. Berde and colleagues (Berde et al., 1989; Shannon and Berde, 1989) described a convenient and effective technique for the management of postoperative pain using methadone. Patients receive a load of 0.1 to 0.2 mg/kg, usually during the surgery. Postoperative pain management is accomplished by the as-needed administration of doses of 0.03 to 0.08 mg/kg every 4 to 12 hours.

Another important role for methadone is in weaning opioid-tolerant patients (Tobias et al., 1990; Anand and Arnold, 1994). Different techniques have been proposed for conversion of morphine to oral methadone equivalents. Siddappa and others (2003) recommend administering methadone as 2.5 times the total daily fentanyl dose each day. Berens and Meyer (Meyer and Berens, 2001; Berens and Meyer, 2002) calculate the 24-hour morphine requirement and then administer one sixth of that amount as methadone every 12 hours. In addition, Berens and Meyer suggest, in preliminary data, that opioid-tolerant patients can be successfully weaned over as brief a period as 5 days.

Codeine

Codeine is a commonly prescribed oral opioid analgesic that is often used for mild to moderate pain. Oral codeine has reasonable oral bioavailability and undergoes hepatic metabolism via O-demethylation to morphine. Interestingly, this conversion relies on the cytochrome P-450 2D6 isozyme, which is absent or diminished in 5% to 10% of certain ethnic populations (Leeder, 2001, 2003). These individuals have a markedly diminished or absent analgesic response to codeine. This, plus the well-known profile of codeine that includes nausea, vomiting, and constipation, has led many clinicians to switch to either hydrocodone or oxycodone as first-line oral opioid analgesics. Codeine and hydrocodone offer some additional ease in prescribing in that both agents are listed as schedule III opioids, whereas all of the other available agents are listed as schedule II by the Drug Enforcement Agency of the United States. All of these oral opioid analgesics are often used in fixed combination with acetaminophen or ibuprofen. Particularly with the former, attention must be paid to the total daily acetaminophen dose to avoid hepatotoxic levels.

Tramadol

Tramadol is a synthetic analog of codeine that was first introduced in Europe in the late 1970s (Cossmann et al., 1997). It did not receive approval in the United States until 1995, even though it had been extensively used and studied elsewhere. It appears to be a unique analgesic that works via both μ-receptor–mediated activity and inhibition of serotonin and norepinephrine reuptake (Lee et al., 1993; Dayer et al., 1994; Goeringer et al., 1997). It has excellent oral bioavailability (75%); however, it is metabolized by the cytochrome P-450 hepatic pathways, resulting in potentially significant drug interactions, such as with the tricyclic antidepressants (TCAs). Tramadol has been associated with seizures, especially in patients already on drugs that inhibit hepatic metabolism (Tobias, 1997; Jick et al., 1998; Gardner et al., 2000; Gasse et al., 2000). Tramadol (100 mg) compares favorably, in adults, to hydrocodone/acetaminophen (5 mg/325 mg) (Turturro et al., 1998). Investigators have evaluated the use of tramadol as an adjunct to caudal analgesia (Baraka et al., 1993; Delilkan and Vijayan, 1993; Motsch et al., 1997; Prosser et al., 1997; Russell, 1998; Batra et al., 1999; Gunduz et al., 2001; Ozcengiz et al., 2001; Senel et al., 2001). Finkel and others (2002) and Rose and others (2003) reported on the use of tramadol (1 to 2 mg/kg per dose every 6 hours) for acute and subacute postoperative pain management.

Oxycodone

Oxycodone is a semisynthetic phenanthrene-derivative opioid that is being used more frequently because of the issues touched on earlier regarding codeine. Oxycodone is extensively metabolized to noroxycodone (major) and oxymorphone (minor) and their glucuronide conjugates in the liver (Weinstein and Gaylord, 1979; Ishida et al., 1982). Although oxymorphone metabolism is mediated by cytochrome P-450 2D6, blockade of this pathway by concomitant medications or genetic variation has not yet been shown to be of clinical significance with controlled-release oxycodone. Oxycodone has excellent oral bioavailability (≈60%). It is available as liquid, tablets, and then in various fixed combinations with acetaminophen, ibuprofen, or aspirin. It is also available in a slow-release form, OxyContin. Although its use in children is off-label, it would appear that it is being used in many situations. Czarnecki and others (2004), for example, describe its use as an oral analgesic for the management of postoperative pain after spinal fusion. Interestingly, these authors report an OxyContin/intravenous morphine conversion ratio of 1:1. The manufacturer suggests that this ratio be 3:1, from adult studies.

OTHER DRUGS

Clonidine is an α_2-agonist that has been available for some time for the treatment of hypertension, attention deficit disorder, migraine prophylaxis (Sillanpaa, 1977; Sills et al., 1982), and Tourette's syndrome. It has undergone investigation as an analgesic, particularly for neuraxial use (Eisenach et al., 1996). This agent shows promise as part of an analgesic regimen for postoperative and cancer pain. It is associated with hypotension, bradycardia, and somnolence, but it avoids respiratory depression, pruritus, and urinary retention, commonly associated with opioids. It has been given orally, before surgery, and been shown to reduce postoperative analgesic requirements (Mikawa et al., 1995, 1996; Broadman et al., 1997; Goyagi et al., 1999). Clonidine is now commonly added to local anesthetics for epidural or caudal block (Jamali et al., 1994; Ivani et al., 1996, 2000; Luz et al., 1999). Epidural doses of 1 to 2 mcg/kg appear safe and not only prolong the duration of analgesia from epidural blockade but can also significantly reduce the need to use opioids. Caution must be taken when using clonidine in neonates or young infants who may be more susceptible to the development of apnea (Bouchut et al., 2001). Clonidine can also be used as a preoperative sedative that also reduces postoperative analgesic requirements (Mikawa et al., 1996; Broadman et al., 1997; Reimer et al., 1998; Goyagi et al., 1999; Nishina et al., 2000; Fazi et al., 2001). Doses of 3 to 5 mcg/kg (PO) appear effective. Some clinicians also apply transdermal clonidine for continued analgesia in the postoperative period (0.1 mg/24 hr for patients <40 kg and 0.2 mg/day if >40 kg).

Ketamine is a phencyclidine derivative agent with amnestic, sedative, and analgesic properties. It has been used as a general anesthetic as well as an adjunct for postoperative analgesia (Cook et al., 1995; De Negri et al., 2000; Dix et al., 2003), chronic pain management (Stubhaug and Breivik, 1997; Fine, 1999), and procedural sedation (Green et al., 1990; Tobias et al., 1992; Parker et al., 1997; Lawrence and Wright, 1998; Kennedy and Luhmann, 2001). Interestingly, ketamine has been shown to have significant *N*-methyl-D-aspartate (NMDA) receptor antagonism activity (Stubhaug and Breivik, 1997; Stubhaug et al., 1997). Activation of this pathway is thought to play an important role in the development of hyperalgesia and spinal cord windup. In addition, ketamine exerts local anesthetic properties when administered intrathecally. Although it is not yet available in the United States in a suitable neuraxial preparation, its use as an additive to caudal and epidural analgesia has been reported from Europe (De Negri et al., 2000; Koinig et al., 2000; Zenz and Zenner, 2000).

Tricyclic antidepressants have consistently provided analgesia in a variety of chronic pain conditions including neuropathic pain (McQuay et al., 1996; Sindrup and Jensen, 1999; Orza et al., 2000), migraine (Saeed et al., 1992; Silberstein et al., 2003), and abdominal pain (Rajagopalan et al., 1998; Hyams, 1999; Hyams et al., 2002). It is thought that these agents are analgesic by inhibiting serotonin and norepinephrine uptake, resulting in facilitating inhibitory neurotransmitter activity at the level of the spinal cord. Because of anticholinergic side effects, most TCAs must be slowly titrated to an effective dose. It is prudent to initiate therapy with either amitriptyline or nortriptyline at 0.2 mg/kg and over 1 to 2 weeks target trial doses of 0.5 to 1.0 mg/kg per day. If sleep disturbance is a part of the pain syndrome, amitriptyline, given 1 to 2 hours before bed, can help facilitate better sleep. Alternatively, nortriptyline can be used at similar doses, because amitriptyline is metabolized to nortriptyline in vivo. Because these drugs can prolong the QTc interval with resultant tachyarrhythmias in patients with predisposing prolonged QTc syndrome, baseline electrocardiography is indicated.

■ **TABLE 13–9.** Tricyclic antidepressants and anticonvulsants for pain management

Drug	Dose	Dose Interval	Comments
Amitriptyline	*Initial:* 0.2 mg/kg per day *Target:* 0.5 to 1.0 mg/kg per day	Once each night; 1 to 2 hr before bed.	Sedating; constipating; dry mouth; monitor electrocardiogram; may need to monitor plasma levels
Nortriptyline	See Amitriptyline	See Amitriptyline	Less sedating and fewer anticholinergic effects
Carbamazepine	*Initial:* 5 to 10 mg/kg per day *Target:* 15 to 30 mg/kg per day	Divide into 2 or 3 doses.	Blood dyscrasias; must follow plasma levels
Gabapentin	*Initial:* 5 mg/kg per day *Target:* 15 to 30 mg/kg per day	Divide into three doses.	Initial sedation; may affect memory
Sodium valproate	*Initial:* 10 mg/kg per day	Divide into three doses.	Blood dyscrasias; hepatotoxicity; monitor plasma levels, complete blood cell count, liver function tests

In addition, if selective serotonin reuptake inhibitors (SSRIs) are also being used, periodic measurement of TCA levels is also warranted (Table 13–9).

Anticonvulsant treatment for chronic pain management has become the mainstay of neuropathic pain disorders (McQuay, 1988; Galer, 1995; Backonja, 2000; Wallace, 2001). In addition, there is considerable support for their use in migraine prophylaxis (Rapoff et al., 1988; Baumel, 1994; Grazzi et al., 1998; Silberstein et al., 2000). Phenytoin, carbamazepine, sodium valproate, and gabapentin are the most commonly used agents. Carbamazepine was the most widely studied and best supported antiepileptic agent for use in neuropathic pain (Backonja, 2000; Wiffen et al., 2000; Harke et al., 2001). Gabapentin, which has a much more acceptable side effect profile, has been gathering more attention (Wetzel and Connelly, 1997; Attal et al., 1998; Backonja et al., 1998; Fudin and Audette, 2000; Nicholson, 2000; Rusy et al., 2001). Unfortunately, virtually all of these studies have been completed in adults and are yet to be replicated in children (see Table 13–9).

■ ACUTE PAIN MANAGEMENT

Postoperative pain management should begin with preoperative teaching and preparation. Because as many as 70% of pediatric procedures are completed as same-day surgery, a true preoperative visit is often not possible. Nonetheless, a thorough discussion of how pain is going to be managed postoperatively is crucial to both the patient and parent and should take place before surgery. Recovery room nurses can then further instruct the patient and family to reinforce the preoperative teaching. Nonpharmacologic techniques discussed later commonly reduce anxiety and pain and may even reduce the need for opioids or other analgesics. Pharmacologic techniques include nonopioid medications (acetaminophen, NSAIDs, clonidine, and tramadol), opioids, and local anesthetics. A potentially beneficial principle to adhere to for acute postoperative pain management is that local anesthetics should be part of the initial pain management plan. This can be accomplished by using a peripheral regional anesthetic technique, a central neuraxial block, or local infiltration of the surgical site either before or after the procedure.

■ TOPICAL ANESTHESIA

Painless topical anesthesia has become possible since the introduction of EMLA (eutectic mixture of local anesthetics, 2.5% lidocaine, and 2.5% prilocaine) cream in the 1980s. Application to skin for 60 minutes with an occlusive dressing leads to effective cutaneous anesthesia (Ehrenstrom-Reiz and Reiz, 1982; Hallen and Uppfeldt, 1982; Maunuksela and Korpela, 1986). EMLA has been studied for use in multiple situations that require trauma to the skin, including venipuncture, intravenous catheter placement, circumcision, port access, shunt access, lumbar puncture, bone marrow aspiration, laceration repair, and even myringotomy (Cooper et al., 1987; Soliman et al., 1988; Halperin et al., 1989; Miser et al., 1994; Calamandrei et al., 1996; Taddio et al., 1997; Zempsky and Karasic, 1997). Other topical creams have subsequently been approved for use that include a 4% liposomal lidocaine mixture or 4% tetracaine gel (Ametop Gel). Both are reported to have quicker onset than EMLA and to cause less local vasoconstriction, which sometimes can obscure veins with EMLA (Doyle et al., 1993; Choy et al., 1999; Friedman et al., 1999; Chen and Cunningham, 2001; Eichenfield et al., 2002).

Cutaneous anesthesia can also be achieved using careful intradermal infiltration with local anesthetics. Obviously, most pediatric patients prefer not to undergo a needle puncture procedure. However, if one incorporates the use of buffered lidocaine with a 30-gauge needle, this procedure can be done virtually without discomfort (McKay et al., 1987; Christoph et al., 1988; Bartfield et al., 1990). Good cutaneous anesthesia can also be achieved in open skin wounds (lacerations) using a fixed combination of either tetracaine/Adrenalin (epinephrine)/cocaine (TAC) or lidocaine/epinephrine/tetracaine (LET) (Blackburn et al., 1995; Ernst et al., 1995, 1997; Schilling et al., 1995; Liebelt, 1997; Adler et al., 1998; Resch et al., 1998; Singer and Stark, 2000). TAC, however, has been associated with seizures, especially in young children who have lacerations in more vascular areas, such as the face or scalp (Fitzmaurice et al., 1990).

Several other relatively noninvasive systems have been developed to effect the delivery of lidocaine into the dermis without using a needle-based technique. Numby Stuff (Iomed, Salt Lake City, UT) uses iontophoretic delivery of lidocaine with epinephrine using an impregnated electrode, current generator, and a return pad. It provides dense cutaneous analgesia in about 8 minutes (Zempsky et al., 1998; Schultz et al., 2001). Another interesting delivery system, the Epiture Easytouch (Norwood Abbey, Victoria, Australia), uses a single-pulse Er:YAG laser to remove the stratum corneum layer of skin. One then applies 4% liposomal lidocaine cream and cutaneous analgesia is achieved in 5 minutes (Baron et al., 2003). Both of these techniques are limited by the relatively high cost of each individual application.

■ PATIENT-CONTROLLED ANALGESIA

PCA is a common and effective method of analgesia for postsurgical pain management in children, adolescents, and adults (Berde and Sethna, 2002). The rationale for PCA analgesia is that the usual doses of as-needed (PRN) medication can lead to episodes or cycles of pain, followed by rescue dosing that causes excessive sedation and other opioid side effects. More frequent, smaller doses of opioids, which can be self-administered by the patient, lead to better analgesic titration with fewer side effects. The child's control over his or her own analgesia has considerable psychological benefits and allows him or her to anticipate increased activity, such as physical therapy or pulmonary toilet maneuvers (McKenzie et al., 1997). A controlled opioid delivery system also eliminates the need for the nurses to sign out controlled substances and the need to administer the medication (Kho and Thomas, 1994; Chan et al., 1995; Colwell and Morris, 1995). PCA is safe and effective in children as young as 5 years (Berde et al., 1991) and compares well with continuous morphine infusions in the older child (Bray et al., 1996). There have been occasional reports of children as young as 2 using PCA devices effectively (Rusy et al., 1997). PCA technology can be safely used in children younger than 5 years, using a basal infusion with parents or nurses delivering the bolus doses (Monitto et al., 2000). Characteristics of maturity, computer dexterity, family and nursing support, and patient familiarity with the hospital environment can be good predictors of successful use of PCA at such a young age. Adaptable PCA control buttons are helpful for the patient with cerebral palsy, who can understand the concept of PCA but may not have the manual dexterity to use the typical small button to activate the machine.

Parent- and nurse-controlled analgesia is another way to use PCA technology, when the patient is incapable of delivering doses, due to either immaturity, developmental delay, or medical condition. This technique often uses a higher level of basal infusion with a longer lockout time for individual doses (Lloyd-Thomas, 1995; Monitto et al., 2000). Instruction and strictly set guidelines are needed when parents are activating the PCA, as they are often emotionally involved in the care of the patient and need to understand safety features of the PCA. This technique has been used successfully for many years with specific attention to the rule that no bolus doses may be administered if the child is asleep or drowsy. This attempts to recapitulate the intrinsic safety features of self-administered PCA. This approach is considered to be a safe and well-accepted form of analgesia (Monitto et al., 2000).

It is important to initiate PCA in the recovery room or the emergency department to avoid the potential long delay in obtaining the PCA device by the floor nurse, obtaining the proper medication, and then programming the device (Table 13–10). Typical starting doses of morphine are 0.01 to 0.02 mg/kg, every 6 to 10 minutes, with an hourly maximal dose of 0.1 to 0.15 mg/kg. A low-dose background infusion of 0.004 mg/kg per hour was reported as useful, in the first 24 hours, and shown to improve sleep patterns without increasing the adverse effects seen with higher background infusions in children (Doyle et al., 1993). Others advocate basal infusions that are somewhat more generous (0.01 to 0.02 mg/kg per hour) (Berde et al., 1991). In studies comparing three methods of administering morphine—intramuscularly, PCA alone, and PCA plus low-dose basal (Berde et al., 1991)—it was noted that the best analgesia and greatest patient satisfaction occurred with PCA and with low-dose basal infusion. Other opioids can be used in instances where there is morphine sensitivity or intolerance. Hydromorphone, meperidine, and fentanyl can be administered with PCA (Yaster et al., 1997) (see Table 13–10).

An exciting new PCA system has been described for postoperative pain control in adults. This system uses a credit card–sized iontophoretic delivery system that uses fixed-dose fentanyl (Gupta et al., 1998). Two separate trials have been reported in adults that demonstrate excellent tolerability, side effects, and analgesia with this system (Chelly et al., 2004; Viscusi et al., 2004). The technique does not require intravenous access and analgesia is achieved rapidly, due to the excellent skin penetration of iontophoretic fentanyl.

CONTINUOUS INTRAVENOUS OPIOIDS

Continuous infusion of opioids is a means of managing postoperative pain in infants and young children unable to use a PCA device. Morphine dosages of 0.02 to 0.03 mg/kg per hour can provide consistent levels of analgesia with minimal respiratory depression (Bray, 1983; Bray et al., 1986; Bosenberg, 1988). Bray and others (Bray et al., 1996; Bray et al., 1996; Lynn et al., 2000) have also demonstrated analgesic efficacy similar to PCA in various pediatric populations. This technique may be the preferred method of morphine delivery in the hospitalized child with moderate or severe pain.

EPIDURAL ANALGESIA

Epidural analgesia is another way to approach acute postoperative pain management in the pediatric patient (Table 13–11). Pulmonary function may be enhanced with effective epidural analgesia after upper abdominal surgery and thoracic procedures in pediatric patients (Tyler, 1989). Murrell and others (1993) reported that in neonates undergoing primary abdominal procedures, prolonged postoperative ventilation could be avoided by combining general anesthesia with epidural analgesia. Epidural analgesia is associated with a lower incidence of postoperative respiratory depression and cardiovascular complications compared with intravenous opioids (Wolf et al., 1993). Continuous lumbar epidural analgesia has been reported to decrease the incidence of bladder spasm in patients undergoing

TABLE 13–10. Patient-controlled analgesia (PCA) doses

	PCA Dose (mg/kg per dose)	PCA Hourly Maximum (mg/kg)	Basal Rate (mg/kg per hour)	Registered Nurse–Administered Additional Bolus (mg/kg) for Pain (Above Basal/Doses Administered)
Morphine	0.01 to 0.03	0.1	0.01 to 0.03	0.05 to 0.1
Hydromorphone	0.002 to 0.006	0.02	0.002 to 0.006	0.01 to 0.02
Fentanyl	0.0005 to 0.002 (0.5 to 2 mcg/kg per dose)	0.0035 to 0.005 (3.5 to 5 mcg/kg per hour)	0.001–0.004 (1 to 4 mcg/kg per hour)	0.001 to 0.002 (1 to 2 mcg/kg)

*Load with 0.5 to 1 time hourly max if no opioid in >2 hours. Lockout: 6 to 10 min for patient; 8 to 12 min for parent/registered nurse. Consider setting the PCA dose equal to the hourly basal rate. Adjust up for pain by increments of 10% to 20% in both doses.

For patients not well controlled, consider adding a basal, increasing dose or basal by 10% to 20% after an additional bolus is given.

■ **TABLE 13–11.** Doses of epidural analgesics

				AFTER EPIDURAL DISCONTINUED, MAY...				
Solution	**Epidural Loading Doses**	**Epidural Infusion (mL/kg per hour)**	**PCEA Dose (mcg/kg/ dose)**	*Onset (min)*	*Duration (hr)*	*Discontinue Monitors (hr)*	*Discontinue Foley (hr)*	*Give IV or PO Analgesics*
Infants younger than 6 mo or patients at risk for respiratory depression								
Morphine 10 mcg/mL + 1/16% bupivacaine	10 to 30 mcg/kg + 0.3 to 0.5 mL/kg (0.25%)	0.1 to 0.3	NA	20 to 30	6 to 12	4	4	As soon as patient experiences discomfort
Hydromorphone 3 mcg/mL + 1/16% bupivacaine	1 to 3 mcg/kg + 0.3 to 0.5 mL/kg (0.25%)	0.1 to 0.3	NA	15	4 to 6	4	4	As soon as patient experiences discomfort
Fentanyl 1 mcg/mL + 1/16% bupivacaine	0.5 to 1 mcg/kg + 0.3 to 0.5 mL/kg (0.25%)	0.1 to 0.2 (neonates; < 6 mo; tip at site)	NA	10	2 to 3	4	4	As soon as patient experiences discomfort
Morphine 20 mcg/mL + 1/16% bupivacaine	25 to 50 mcg/kg + 0.5 to 1 mL/kg (0.25%)	0.1 to 0.3	1/6 to 1/4 hourly rate	20	6 to 12	12	4	As soon as patient experiences discomfort
Hydromorphone 5 to 10 mcg/mL + 1/16% bupivacaine	5 to 10 mcg/kg + 0.5 to 1 mL/kg (0.25%)	0.1 to 0.3	1/6 to 1/4 hourly rate	15	4 to 6	4	2 to 4	As soon as patient experiences discomfort
Fentanyl 2 mcg/mL + 1/16% bupivacaine	1 to 2 mcg/kg + 0.5 to 1 mL/kg (0.25%)	0.1 to 0.3	1/6 to 1/4 hourly rate	10	2 to 3	0 to 2	0 to 2	As soon as patient experiences discomfort

Note: Maximum dosage for bupivacaine is 0.2 mg/kg per hour in newborns (0.4 mg/kg per hour in older infants and children).

Thoracic epidural doses should be at the lower end of these ranges (0.1 to 0.15 mL/kg per hour maximum).

Morphine dose is usually between 3 and 5 mcg/kg per hour; may be increased if patient is not overly sedated.

Ropivacaine may be substituted for bupivacaine. Consider loading with 0.2% and using 0.1% for infusions.

Clonidine may be added to any of these solutions. Consider using 1 mcg/mL and reducing the opioid dose by 50%. Also consider loading with 1 mcg/kg and reducing the original opioid load by 50%. AVOID CLONIDINE IN NEONATES (APNEA).

For patients who are not well controlled, consider a bolus equal to the volume of 1 hour basal infusion and then increase the rate by 20%. If there is a question of whether the epidural is working, test with 3 to 5 mg/kg lidocaine (0.5% to 1%). If there is no block, D/C epidural and change pain therapy.

Avoid testing with bupivacaine (0.25%) as inadvertent intravascular administration can lead to cardiovascular collapse.

ureteral reimplantation surgery (Park et al., 2000). McNeely and others (1997) studied high-risk pediatric patients undergoing gastric fundoplication procedures and showed that the complication rate was decreased in those receiving epidural versus intravenous opioid techniques. Patients in the epidural group were discharged earlier from the intensive care unit and the hospital (McNeely et al., 1997).

Single-shot caudal analgesia with bupivacaine is very safe, can last as long as 6 to 8 hours, and has been effectively used for outpatient procedures such as inguinal hernia repair and orchidopexy (McGown, 1982; Broadman et al., 1987; Dalens and Hasnaoui, 1989) (see Chapter 14, Regional Anesthesia). Others have also reported substituting ropivacaine, which may provide less risk of cardiovascular compromise from inadvertent vascular injection (Ivani et al., 1998; Khalil et al., 1999; Luz et al., 2000). The addition of epidural opioids provides longer-lasting analgesia but adds the potential for respiratory depression. Consequently, patients receiving caudal or epidural opioids should be monitored in the hospital (Krane, 1988; Krane et al., 1989; Karl et al., 1996).

The epidural space can be approached at any level: caudal, lumbar, or thoracic. Most children can have the epidural space accessed with 18- or 20-gauge Touhy or Crawford needles and a saline technique for loss of resistance (see Chapter 14, Regional Anesthesia). Air should be avoided in children to avoid the risk of air embolus, if a patent foramen ovale, a ventricular septal defect, or an atrial septal defect is present (Williams et al., 1991). In addition, in small infants, epidural catheters can be threaded from the caudal space to even thoracic levels (Bosenberg et al., 1988; Gunter and Eng, 1992). Tucker and Mather (1975) demonstrated that the epidural fat of infants has a spongy gelatinous quality with distinct spaces found between fat lobules. The location of the catheter tip is best placed at the dermatome where the surgery is to occur. This can be accomplished by approaching the epidural space at the level of the surgical incision. Alternatively, a radiopaque catheter can be used so that the location can be checked by radiograph. If the catheter is not plainly visible, water-soluble dye can be used to identify the catheter and the exact location of the tip. Tsui and others (Tsui et al., 1998, 1999; Goobie et al., 2003) described a novel technique to determine catheter tip location of caudally advanced epidural catheters. This technique uses a low current nerve stimulator to detect muscle twitches as the catheter is advanced to its final destination.

Epidural catheters inserted below the first or second lumbar vertebra offer the safety feature of being below the termination of the spinal cord. However, the delivery of the epidural solution several dermatomes well below a thoracic surgical procedure may result in inadequate analgesia. Caudle and others (1993) showed that patients with thoracic epidural catheters placed for thoracic or upper abdominal procedures had better pain relief than did patients with lower catheters. Because of the potential difficulties of placing catheters in awake, young pediatric patients, it has been the standard of care for many years among pediatric anesthesiologists to place epidural catheters in anesthetized patients (Krane et al., 1998). Giaufré and others (1996) preformed the largest prospective study evaluating the morbidity of regional anesthesia in anesthetized children. There were 24,409 regional blocks performed in patients between 3 and 12 years of age: 15,013 were caudal blocks, 5215 were nerve blocks, 506 were spine blocks, and 135 were thoracic epidurals. Local infiltration accounted for all of the other blocks. There were 23 complications, 4 total spinal blocks, 6 intravascular injections with convulsions in 2 and cardiac arrhythmias in 2, and 2 transient paresthesias. More than half of the complications may have been influenced by the patient's alertness during performance of the block and none of the sequelae were long term (see Chapter 14, Regional Anesthesia).

To minimize the side effects of epidural analgesia, a combination of local anesthetic and opioids is used to permit using a lower dose of each agent. Morphine, fentanyl, and hydromorphone are frequently combined with 0.0625% to 0.1% bupivacaine. Standardized concentrations of these mixtures allow the pharmacy to have premixed bags readily available. Epidural infusions can be set up as epidural PCA, in which the patient or registered nurse can administer additional doses for breakthrough pain (McDonald and Cooper, 2001; Molik et al., 2001; Lin, 2002; Birmingham et al., 2003; Hansen et al., 2004). All patients are administered epidural bupivacaine, with the opioid of choice, at the start of the operation with consideration of a repeat dose, if an appropriate amount of time has elapsed. In general, fentanyl can be reloaded every 4 hours, whereas redosing of morphine or hydromorphone depends on the amount initially administered and the elapsed time. In general, redosing is not needed for procedures that take less than 6 to 8 hours. Bupivacaine can be redosed every 1 to 2 hours, using about half of the initial loading dose, so that a denser block can be maintained intraoperatively.

When the catheter tip is close to the dermatome of surgery, fentanyl is the opioid of choice. When the tip is farther from the site of the operation, such as a lumbar catheter in a patient who underwent a thoracotomy, more water-soluble opioids, such as morphine and hydromorphone, are chosen to have the desired spread. The morphine load is usually 30 to 50 mcg/kg, hydromorphone is 3 to 5 mcg/kg, and fentanyl is 0.5 to 2 mcg/kg. Infusion rates of the bupivacaine must be kept below 0.2 mg/kg per hour in the neonate and infant under 4 to 6 months of age and below 0.4 to 0.75 mg/kg per hour in the child over 2 years of age to avoid toxicity and cardiovascular instability (McCloskey et al., 1992; Wood et al., 1994; Luz et al., 1996, 1998). Adjuvant NSAIDs (ketorolac, etc.) can also be safely used with epidural analgesia.

Contraindications to placement of an epidural catheter include intrinsic coagulopathy or use of anticoagulants, sepsis, and infection in the skin at the site of insertion. Relative contraindications might include neurologic disease such as multiple sclerosis. Infection from epidural catheters for postsurgical pain management in pediatric patients is rare (Strafford et al., 1995; McNeely et al., 1997). However, it may occur when epidural catheters are tunneled in terminally ill patients for long-term pain management and needs to be aggressively monitored and treated if diagnosed (DuPen et al., 1987).

CHRONIC PAIN MANAGEMENT

Chronic pain has become a significant problem in the pediatric population, conservatively estimated to affect 10% to 15% of the population (Goodman and McGrath, 1991). Signs of sympathetic nervous system arousal rarely accompany chronic pain, in contrast to acute pain. The lack of objective signs may prompt the inexperienced clinician to say the patient "does not look like he or she is in pain" (American Pain Society, 2003). Signals of facial grimacing, limping, and tachycardia may be absent in the chronic pain patient. There is no neurophysiologic or chemical test that can measure pain; the clinician must accept the patient's report of pain. The International Association for the Study of Pain (IASP) classifies chronic pain as less than 1 month, 1 to 6 months, and greater than 6 months (Merskey and Bogduk, 1994). Formerly, chronic pain was defined as having pain for longer than 6 months, but it is now recognized that chronic pain can be evident much earlier.

> **BOX 13–2 Pediatric Chronic Pain**
>
> Headache
> Chronic abdominal pain, functional abdominal pain
> Irritable bowel syndrome
> Crohn's disease, ulcerative colitis
> "Growing pains"
> Myofascial pain
> Fibromyalgia
> Juvenile rheumatoid arthritis
> Sports injuries
> Complex regional pain syndrome
> Phantom limb pain
> Sickle cell anemia
> Cancer
> Cerebral palsy
> Arthritis

Patients with chronic pain can include children with headaches, myofascial pain, chronic abdominal pain, complex regional pain syndrome, cancer pain, phantom limb pain, cerebral palsy, arthritis, and sickle cell anemia (Box 13–2). These patients have significant alterations in their lifestyles; often have poor school attendance and social withdrawal. The entire family is affected significantly by the pain condition. Most child health specialists have limited experience in treating patients with chronic pain, and pediatric textbooks offer little guidance. Some patients move from one physician to the next, even to different cities or states, and almost all have undergone extensive medical testing that has been costly and often revealed little or no insight into what the problem may be.

Chronic pain can be differentiated from acute pain in that acute pain signals a specific nociceptive event and is self-limited. Chronic pain may start out as an acute event but continues beyond the normal time expected for recovery. Chronic pain in children is a result of a dynamic integration of biologic processes with contributing psychological factors, sociocultural factors, and developmental and family dynamics. To evaluate and treat chronic childhood pain effectively and efficiently, a multidisciplinary approach is most successful, incorporating physicians with nurses, psychologists, psychiatrists, physical therapists, social workers, and occupational therapists. The mind–body dualism must be abandoned. To continue to think that pain is associated with a single physical cause can result in the physician investigating the patient with repeated invasive testing, laboratory tests, and procedures and lead to overprescription of medications. One needs to acknowledge the patient's multidimensional experience of pain and treat it from the various angles to which each participant in the multidisciplinary team can contribute.

ORGANIZATION OF THE MULTIDISCIPLINARY PAIN TEAM

The evaluation of a patient with chronic pain should begin with a complete history, where all members of the multidisciplinary team participate (Box 13–3). Factors to investigate include the pain itself; the time frame for the painful condition; the descriptors of the pain, such as *sharp, dull, burning, throbbing,* or *pounding*; and what helps or exacerbates the pain. One should find out how it has affected the patient's activities of daily living such as sleep, exercise, nutrition, family relations, and school attendance. It is important to determine what, if any, therapies have afforded some degree of relief. Assessment should include what the family perceives as causing the pain and how they have responded to it. Family history of chronic pain problems should be investigated. One should review whether alternative forms of pain therapies have been tried. The review of systems should pay special attention to possible symptoms of depression. Social history of how the pain problem has affected the family structure, including who lives at home, how the patient is doing in school, and the parents' vocations and work status, should be clarified. Recent stressors should be identified, including a death in the family, parental separation or divorce, or a move. Frequently, the chronic pain patient has missed a considerable amount of school and extracurricular activities.

All members of the team may interview the family and patient together to obtain the medical and pain history (see Box 13–3). The psychologist or therapist then interviews the parents alone while the physician is performing the physical evaluation in collaboration with the advanced practice nurse and physical or occupational therapist. The psychologist then meets briefly and alone with the patient. The members of the team gather and formulate a plan of treatment. The plan is then presented to the family and patient with the entire team present. A written summary of the plan is given to the family during this exit session. It includes, as appropriate, a combination of pharmacologic, physical, and occupational therapy interventions; massage therapy; acupuncture; cognitive-behavioral pain strategies including meditation, deep relaxation, guided imagery techniques, and mindfulness meditation; and individual and/or family counseling. Patients are also counseled on how nutrition, sleep habits, and exercise can play a role in their pain condition.

BOX 13–3 Recommended Staff for Multidisciplinary Pain Management Center

Pain specialist physician
Pediatric psychologist
Consulting psychiatrist
Advanced practice nurses
Pediatric physical/occupational therapist
Social worker
Administrative assistants

Major goals are established to improve psychological functioning (decreased school absences); psychological support for the entire family and communication with both the patient's school and physician can occur. When elimination of pain is likely not to occur with a simple intervention, efforts focus on modulating the pain to tolerable levels, allowing there to be return to school (even if part time) and return to participation in activities with friends and family. The time course of such an intake evaluation is about 90 minutes, and most patients are then seen over a period of 1 to 6 months to accomplish these goals.

HEADACHE

As many as 20% of children younger than 5 years have headache as a common chronic pain complaint (Sillanpaa et al., 1991). In another report, 10% to 20% of children younger than 10 years complained of headache (Carlsson, 1996). At puberty, migraine headaches become common with 10% to 27% of adolescent girls and 4% to 20% of adolescent boys reporting them (Abu-Arafeh and Russell, 1993). Approximately 60% of children who have migraines continue to have migraines as adults (Bille, 1997). Tension-type headache is also a highly prevalent condition that can be quite disabling (Schwartz et al., 1998).

Evaluation of the patient is performed as described earlier and includes a detailed neurologic evaluation. Virtually every headache patient seen in a chronic pain clinic has had prior neuroimaging with, most commonly, magnetic resonance imaging (MRI), to rule out brain tumors, vascular anomalies, and other structural abnormalities. Ophthalmological, dental, and sinus conditions, especially potential infections, should not be overlooked. Burton and others (1997) reviewed the etiology of headaches in children presenting to an emergency department. Thirty-nine percent had headache associated with a viral illness; an equal number (16%) had sinusitis and migraine. In addition, temporomandibular joint dysfunction can result in recurrent bitemporal headaches (Reik and Hale, 1981).

Treatment approaches include medications for both preventative and abortive therapy, including NSAIDs, acetaminophen, TCAs, SSRIs, ergotamines, β-adrenergic blockers, or triptans. The occasional use of opioids to abort a refractory headache may be indicated. One of the most important components of any chronic headache treatment program is cognitive-behavioral therapy; this may include biofeedback (Gauthier et al., 1981; Saeed et al., 1992; Silberstein, 2000), relaxation techniques, cognitive reframing, and a variety of standard psychotherapeutic interventions (Reid and McGrath, 1996; Grazzi et al., 1998). Simple home-based therapy with minimal therapist contact can be effective in headache management (Rowan and Andrasik, 1996). A complete review of this topic is presented in recent reviews of the subject by Larsson (1999) and McGrath and Hillier (2001).

CHRONIC ABDOMINAL PAIN

Recurrent abdominal pain was defined many years ago as pain occurring at least once per month for 3 consecutive months (Apley and Naish, 1958). The pain is usually periumbilical, lasting 1 to 3 hours, and may be associated with pallor, vomiting, sweating, and nausea. Sleep patterns may be disturbed. Although it is important for physicians to exclude organic illness, almost all studies have found that only 10% of children with recurrent abdominal pain have recognizable organic illness accounting for the pain complaints (Apley and Naish, 1958;

Saavedra and Perman, 1989). Organic causes include ulcer, lactose intolerance, ulcerative colitis, infection (*Helicobacter pylori*), and Crohn's disease. Once organic causes are excluded, it is important to communicate to the family that even though an organic cause cannot be found, the treating medical personnel believe the pain is real and attempts must be made to manage it. There is some evidence that these patients may have forms of irritable bowel syndrome with associated visceral hyperalgesia (Di Lorenzo et al., 2001; Alaradi and Barkin, 2002). Animal models have confirmed that in a variety of stimulus models, abnormal responses to colonic or rectal stimulation can be elicited (Kamp et al., 2003; Palecek and Willis, 2003; Gaudreau and Plourde, 2004; Miranda et al., 2004). These animals demonstrate central sensitization, possibly mediated by NMDA receptor activity. These studies, plus several others in adult patients with irritable bowel syndrome (Delvaux, 2002; Hunt and Tougas, 2002; Verne and Price, 2002; Verne et al., 2003), lend support to the notion that even without clear-cut pathologic findings, patients can have persistent abdominal pain syndromes. Again, a multidisciplinary approach is taken, incorporating medications (COX-2 inhibitor, NSAIDs, TCAs, tramadol, or SSRIs); behavioral approaches to manage stress and anxiety; sleep hygiene, biofeedback training, and encouragement of return to normal activities. There is some evidence that these patients respond to amitriptyline (Jailwala et al., 2000; Huertas-Ceballos et al., 2002a, 2002b). The reader is referred to recent reviews on this subject by Walker (1999) and Hyams and others (1999, 2002).

MYOFASCIAL PAIN/FIBROMYALGIA

Myofascial pain or fibromyalgia is characterized by widespread pain, multiple tender points on physical examination, fatigue, sleep difficulties, abdominal pain, headaches, and mood disturbance and is estimated to occur in 1% to 6% of the juvenile population (Kashikar-Zuck et al., 2002). In 1985, Yunus and Masi (1985) described the juvenile primary fibromyalgia syndrome (Table 13–12). Malleson and others (1992) reported that, using these diagnostic criteria, a significant percentage of children showed no improvement in symptoms when followed for more than 2 years. Current management includes improving sleep hygiene, regular physical activity (aerobic exercise), cognitive-behavioral strategies, and low-dose TCAs to improve both pain and sleep disturbance (Breau et al., 1999). Acupuncture is another form of therapy that, on a regular basis, can be very beneficial in controlling muscle tender points (Sprott et al., 1998).

COMPLEX REGIONAL PAIN SYNDROME (CRPS TYPE I; FORMERLY KNOWN AS REFLEX SYMPATHETIC DYSTROPHY [RSD])

Complex regional pain syndrome (CRPS) refers to a syndrome of persistent neuropathic pain associated with nondermatomal autonomic dysfunction. It often is seen after minor injury, and patients have findings that include temperature and color changes, allodynia, edema, cyanosis, eventual trophic changes of the skin, and osteoporotic changes, if left untreated. The current IASP diagnostic criteria (published by Stanton-Hicks et al. [1995]) include (1) at least two neuropathic pain descriptors (burning, dysesthesias, paresthesias, mechanical allodynia, and hyperalgesia to cold) and (2) at least two physical signs of autonomic dysfunction (cyanosis, mottling, hyperhidrosis, >3°C lower temperature in affected limb, edema).

The cause of pain is not completely understood but is thought to be related to abnormal discharges in sympathetic afferent nerves along with nociceptive effects produced by the incidental trauma. Sensitivity of nerve receptors, spontaneous neuronal ectopy, and psychological components of the pain are always present. Ruggeri and others (1982) published data to show that CRPS in children is benign and responds to physical therapy. Others suggest that a subset of patients continue to have severe pain and disability (Greipp and Thomas, 1987). Wilder and others (1992) published a report of 70 patients, who were predominately female, who had involvement of the lower extremity disease. Conservative treatment, including physical therapy, transcutaneous electrical nerve stimulation (TENS), TCAs, cognitive-behavioral therapies, and relaxation therapies, was used with some success. Two thirds of the patients in this series responded to sympathetic blockade. In a 2002 study by Lee and others, reduced pain and improved functioning were reported after a 6-week course of intensive physical therapy and cognitive-behavioral therapies without the need for sympathetic blockade. This approach does not incorporate any invasive regional nerve blockade but instead used neuromodulating drug therapy (TCAs with gabapentin or other antiepileptic agents) with intensive physical therapy, administered on a 3-day-per-week regimen up to even twice a day. In patients who were unable to tolerate this degree of physical therapy, anesthesia-monitored deep sedation with propofol has been used to allow manipulation of the affected extremity or extremities. Psychotherapy that includes a focus on cognitive-behavioral interventions plus intensive decatastrophizing of the illness is also used in the treatment of patients with CRPS. In addition, intensive family

TABLE 13–12. Juvenile primary fibromyalgia syndrome

Major Criteria	Minor Criteria
1. General musculoskeletal aching at 3 or more sites for 3 or more months in the absence of any underlying condition	1. Subjective soft tissue swelling
2. Normal laboratory tests	2. Pain modulated by physical activities
3. Severe pain in 5 of 18 bilateral tender point sites with palpation of less than 4-kg force: occiput; low cervical area; trapezius; supraspinatus; second rib; lateral epicondyle; gluteal, upper outer quadrant of buttock; greater trochanter; knee	3. Pain modulated by weather factors
	4. Pain modulated by anxiety/stress
	5. Irritable bowel syndrome
	6. Chronic anxiety or tension
	7. Fatigue
	8. Poor sleep
	9. Numbness
	10. Chronic headaches
Diagnosis is based on ALL 3 major criteria plus 3 of 10 minor criteria OR 1 and 2 plus 4 of 18 tender points and 5 of 10 minor criteria.	

Modified from Yunus MB, Masi AT: Juvenile primary fibromyalgia syndrome. A clinical study of thirty-three patients and matched normal controls. *Arthritis Rheum* 28:138–145, 1985. (Copyright © 1985. Reprinted with permission of Wiley-hiss, Inc., a subsidiary of John Wiley & Sons, Inc.)

psychotherapy may be needed to restore intrafamily relationships that interfere with recovery. Except for a small proportion of patients who respond quickly to over-the-counter pain medications and increased physical activity of the involved extremity, CRPS type I is a disease that is best managed at a pediatric pain management center.

SICKLE CELL ANEMIA

Sickle cell anemia is an inherited hemoglobinopathy that results in recurrent acute and chronic pain due to red cell sickling and obstruction of the microvasculature with subsequent embolism and inflammation. Painful vaso-occlusive episodes occur in the hands and feet, extremity long bones, chest, and abdomen, leading to frequent hospitalizations for intensive pain management with intravenous opioids. The recognition of pervasive undertreatment or inappropriate treatment prompted the American Pain Society to develop guidelines for pain treatment (1999). Chronic pain in sickle cell anemia can be associated with bony changes such as avascular necrosis of the femoral heads, vertebral collapse, and chronic, recurrent leg ulcerations (Esseltine et al., 1988). The superimposition of unpredictable acute pain crises on top of chronic pain compounds the chronic pain assessment of these patients. It is imperative to complete a thorough evaluation of all the biologic and psychological aspects of the individual and his or her family and support system. Emotional support, possible chronic transfusions, hydroxyurea (to stimulate fetal hemoglobin production), and the selective administration of NSAIDs or TCAs, with liberal use of short- and long-acting opioids, can help the patient who has sickle cell crises.

Patients with sickle cell anemia often have used opioids for pain control and may even be managed on chronic, long-acting opioid medications, such as MS Contin (morphine sulfate), OxyContin (oxycodone), or methadone. They may have a high tolerance to opioid analgesics. In general, children with vaso-occlusive episodes consume more than twice as much morphine as children with postoperative pain (Shapiro et al., 1993). Pseudo-addiction has been reported in patients with sickle cell disease (Kirsh et al., 2002; Elander et al., 2004). In these patients, underprescription of adequate doses and amounts of analgesics leads to the expression of behaviors that are interpreted as drug seeking. A variety of sociocultural factors contribute to this syndrome of gross undertreatment of sickle cell pain.

Regional anesthesia may be a good choice to help manage a sickle cell crisis in the lower extremity or pelvis, including priapism. It may also be quite beneficial in the management of the acute chest syndrome. Epidural anesthesia with local anesthetics administered alone or in combination with fentanyl has been shown to effectively treat sickle cell vaso-occlusive crisis unresponsive to conventional methods with fewer side effects such as sedation or respiratory depression (Yaster et al., 1994; Labat et al., 2001).

CANCER

Cancer is the second leading cause of death in children after trauma. Almost all children who have cancer experience pain during the course of diagnosis, treatment, and end of life (Miser et al., 1987). Children with cancer may have pain that can be classified into four broad categories; cancer-related pain (bone pain, neuropathic pain, somatic pain, terminal care); treatment-related pain from chemotherapy, radiation, infection, and phantom limb pain; procedure-related pain; and pain unrelated to the cancer (preexisting pain such as headache, trauma, or other medical problems such as appendicitis). Children who survive cancer rate the pain from procedures and treatment as worse than pain related to the cancer itself (Fowler-Kerry, 1990). In fact, in a survey of Swedish children with cancer, Ljungman and others (1999) found that almost 50% of reported pain was from treatment, 40% was from procedures, and only 10% was from the disease itself. For almost 15 years, cancer pain treatment has been guided by the World Health Organization *Analgesic Ladder* (1990). Mild pain can be treated with nonopioids first, with it kept in mind that these agents have a ceiling effect and side effects that include inhibition of platelet function, gastritis, and decreased renal blood flow. Moderate pain can be treated with an oral opioid plus the nonopioid. Severe pain can be managed with potent intravenous opioids. As it was originally proposed, the "ladder" suggests a progression of therapy that escalates as the patient fails the lowest rungs (Ljungman et al., 1996, 1999). However, a more appropriate conceptualization of the ladder demands selecting the analgesic agent that seems best matched to the severity of the patient's pain. In addition, some pain in cancer can be opioid resistant, such as spinal cord or nerve root compression from an intraspinal Ewing's sarcoma. In this case, the prompt addition of adjuvant analgesics such as the TCAs or gabapentin is indicated, even though these agents were not part of the original schema. Unless the individual has unusual, intermittent pain episodes, a regimen of around-the-clock, long-acting opioids (sustained-release morphine or methadone) should be chosen, with a short-acting, immediate-release agent available for breakthrough pain (immediate-release morphine or oxycodone). Patients unable to tolerate the oral administration of opioids can be managed with intravenous drugs, with either as-needed dosing, continuous infusions, or PCA.

Because patients with progressive malignancy may need chronic opioid therapy, it is important to titrate doses as needed. Fortunately, the opioid analgesics do not demonstrate an analgesic ceiling effect; it is not uncommon to encounter situations where massive doses of opioids are required to continue analgesia (Collins et al., 1995; Sirkia et al., 1998). The majority of children can be successfully managed using oral or intravenous therapy, even through the end of life (Ljungman et al., 1996). Although most children remain comfortable with moderate dosing, a subgroup of patients may require drastic escalation of dosing (Collins et al., 1995). This is especially true in patients with solid tumors that have metastasized to nerves, the spine, or the central nervous system.

Under rare circumstances, terminally ill children with cancer may benefit from invasive neuraxial therapy delivered via an implanted intraspinal or epidural catheter (Collins, 1996; Ljungman et al., 1996). Other invasive approaches to drug delivery, such as celiac plexus blockade (Rykowski and Hilgier, 2000) or even neurosurgical ablations (Cherny, 2000), are even less commonly used.

The key to the success of opioid pain management for cancer pain is incorporation of a careful plan for the management of side effects. Constipation is common, and regular stool softeners or laxatives are needed; enemas must usually be avoided in cancer patients due to the risk in causing perirectal infection by introducing bacteria into the bloodstream. Small doses of stimulants (methylphenidate, amphetamines, modafinil, or atomoxetine) may help combat sedation. Antihistamines and antiemetics are often also needed on an as-needed basis. Neuropathic pain secondary to metastasis or chemotherapeutic agents (e.g., vincristine) is common in these children and often requires management with

TCAs, gabapentin, or TENS units (Foley, 1995; Breitbart, 1998; Wiffen et al., 2000).

ALTERNATIVE FORMS OF PAIN MANAGEMENT

Traditionally, health care practitioners have approached pain management in children on an "either/or" basis—that is, pharmacologic interventions or "alternative" approaches. A multidisciplinary approach that combines several different modalities is best. Cognitive-behavioral approaches such as relaxation techniques, breathing exercises, TENS, biofeedback, and even acupuncture can augment any of the pharmacologic interventions (Rusy and Weisman, 2000).

COGNITIVE-BEHAVIORAL INTERVENTIONS

Children are highly responsive to pain-reducing strategies that involve their imagination and sense of play. Children younger than 6 years can be distracted by blowing bubbles, playing with pop-up toys, or looking through a kaleidoscope (Zeltzer and Lebaron, 1982). Older children engage well in external or abstract interventions, such as guided imagery, counting, and breathing techniques (Zeltzer and Lebaron, 1982; Kuttner, 1988; LeBaron et al., 1988; Chen et al., 2000). Preschoolers can imagine a superhero who can "turn off the pain switch" (Kachoyeanos and Friedhoff, 1993). Zeltzer and Lebaron (1982) compared hypnotic and nonhypnotic techniques for reducing pain associated with bone marrow aspirations and lumbar punctures in children with cancer; hypnosis was found to be significantly better in reducing procedural distress. A potential physiologic explanation of the effectiveness of hypnosis in reducing pain is that hypnosis inhibits transmission of pain signals from peripheral fibers at the level of the dorsal horn (Crawford et al., 1998). Alternatively, hypnosis may work by causing amnesia of the events surrounding the hypnotic trance.

Progressive muscle relaxation is designed to help children recognize and reduce tension associated with pain, decrease anxiety, and decrease discomfort. Learning to decrease body tension is an acquired skill, and relaxation training requires initial instruction and then frequent practice to be successful. An occupational therapist or a psychologist often teaches these skills. Biofeedback uses alpha-electroencephalography, muscle electromyography, skin temperature, and temporal pulse feedback to provide immediate information to allow a child to observe and modify the level of tension in the body (Andrasik and Attanasio, 1985; Williamson et al., 1988; Labbe and Ward, 1990; Finley and Jones, 1992; Labbe, 1995; Blanchard et al., 1997). These techniques can be very effective for the management of headache (Andrasik et al., 1983; Daly et al., 1983; Druckro and Cantwell-Simmons, 1989; Engel and Rapoff, 1990; Labbe, 1995; Bussone et al., 1998), procedure pain (Broome, 1984), and chronic abdominal pain (Masek et al., 1984; Banez and Steffen, 2001; Weydert et al., 2003).

TRANSCUTANEOUS ELECTRICAL NERVE STIMULATION

TENS can be an additive technique for pain management (Long, 1978; Avellanosa and West, 1982; Meyler et al., 1994). A TENS unit generates a nonpainful stimulus at peripheral nerves and appears to facilitate the closing of the gate for transmission of pain. TENS may stimulate the body to produce endorphins, that then act as natural painkillers (Chapman and Benedetti, 1977; Mannheimer and Carlsson, 1979; Hughes et al., 1984; O'Brien et al., 1984; Facchinetti et al., 1986). In fact, several investigators have demonstrated that opioid antagonists can reverse the effect of TENS (Chapman and Benedetti, 1977; Mannheimer and Carlsson, 1979). TENS is useful in management of many pain problems, including acute pain after chest surgery (Cotter, 1983), fibromyalgia (Stone and Wharton, 1997), chronic knee pain (Jensen et al., 1986; Meyler et al., 1994; Ng et al., 2003; Breit and Van Der Wall, 2004), and cancer pain (Avellanosa and West, 1982).

ACUPUNCTURE

Acupuncture is among the most commonly used forms of complementary medicine for various pain problems. Acupuncture may provide analgesia through a mechanism similar to TENS. Stimulation of small pain fibers may inhibit spinal transmission of other pain signals (Wang et al., 1992). Similarly, there is emerging evidence that through stimulation of the acupuncture energy channels, intrinsic opioid pathways are activated, causing profound analgesia (He et al., 1985; He, 1987; Kho et al., 1993; Pintov et al., 1997). The National Institutes of Health found promising results in the use of acupuncture for the treatment of tennis elbow, myofascial pain, dental pain, stroke rehabilitation, and postoperative or chemotherapeutic nausea (1998). Zeltzer and others (2002) conducted a phase I investigation examining the acceptability of using acupuncture for chronic pediatric pain management and found significant improvement in pain measures. A retrospective case study on pediatric pain patients' experience with acupuncture revealed that 67% of children aged 5 to 18 years (median age, 16 years) rated their experience as positive or pleasant, and 70% of patients thought that the acupuncture helped the pain associated with headaches, endometriosis, or CRPS (Kemper et al., 2000). Lin and others (2002) found that acupuncture significantly reduced pediatric pain associated with headaches, limb pain, chest pain, and abdominal pain when used in a multimodal approach to pain. Acupuncture is an exciting "new" technology that seems well tolerated by children, despite their general needle phobia, and now there is preliminary evidence of effectiveness for our young patients.

SUMMARY

We have the tools to clearly understand the neurophysiology of pain transmission in children and ways to measure the amount of pain that a child is experiencing. Pain should be managed using a broad range of demonstrated tools that include pharmacologic, regional anesthetic, behavioral, and alternative therapies. Acute and chronic pain can be best handled when they are approached in a multidisciplinary fashion. Pediatric anesthesiologists can be active members of hospital-based acute pain services, as well as members of teams evaluating children with chronic pain. Ideally, centers will build multidisciplinary pain teams where physicians, nurses, physical therapists, and psychologists can assess pain and incorporate the various forms of therapy that were discussed in this chapter.

REFERENCES

Abu-Arafeh IA, Russell G: Epidemiology of headache and migraine in children. *Dev Med Child Neurol* 35:370–371, 1993.

Adler AJ, Dubinisky I, Eisen J: Does the use of topical lidocaine, epinephrine, and tetracaine solution provide sufficient anesthesia for laceration repair? *Acad Emerg Med* 5:108–112, 1998.

Alaradi O, Barkin JS: Irritable bowel syndrome: Update on pathogenesis and management. *Med Princ Pract* 11:2–17, 2002.

Ambuel B, Hamlett KW, Mars CM: Assessing distress in pediatric intensive care environments: The COMFORT Scale. *J Pediatr Psychol* 17:95–109, 1992.

American Pain Society: *Guideline for the management of acute and chronic pain in sickle cell disease.* Glenview, IL, 1999, American Pain Society, p 98.

American Pain Society: *Principles of analgesic use in the treatment of acute pain and cancer pain.* Glenview, IL, 2003, American Pain Society.

Anand KJ, Coskun V, Thrivikraman KV, et al.: Long-term behavioral effects of repetitive pain in neonatal rat pups. *Physiol Behav* 66:627–637, 1999.

Anand KJ, Craig KD: New perspectives on the definition of pain. *Pain* 67:3–6, 1996; discussion 209–211, 1996.

Anand KJ, Hickey PR: Pain and its effects in the human neonate and fetus. *N Engl J Med* 317:1321–1329, 1987.

Anand KJ: Neonatal analgesia and anesthesia. Introduction. *Semin Perinatol* 22:347–349, 1998.

Anand KJS, Arnold JH: Opioid tolerance and dependence in infants and children. *Crit Care Med* 22:334–342, 1994.

Anand KJS, Hickey PR: Halothane-morphine compared with high-dose sufentanil for anesthesia and postoperative analgesia in neonatal cardiac surgery. *N Engl J Med* 326:1–9, 1992.

Anderson BJ, Holford NH, Woollard GA, et al.: Perioperative pharmacodynamics of acetaminophen analgesia in children. *Anesthesiology* 90:411–421, 1999.

Anderson BJ, Holford NH: Rectal paracetamol dosing regimens: Determination by computer simulation. *Paediatr Anaesth* 7:451–455, 1997.

Anderson BJ, van Lingen RA, Hansen TG, et al.: Acetaminophen developmental pharmacokinetics in premature neonates and infants: A pooled population analysis. *Anesthesiology* 96:1336–1345, 2002.

Andrasik F, Blanchard EB, Edlund SR, et al.: EMG biofeedback treatment of a child with muscle contraction headache. *Am J Clin Biofeedback* 6:96–102, 1983.

Andrasik F, Attanasio V: Biofeedback in pediatrics: Current status and appraisal. *Adv Dev Behav Pediatr* 6:241–286, 1985.

Andrews K, Fitzgerald M: Cutaneous flexion reflex in human neonates: A quantitative study of threshold and stimulus-response characteristics after single and repeated stimuli. *Dev Med Child Neurol* 41:696–703, 1999.

Andrews K, Fitzgerald M: Flexion reflex responses in biceps femoris and tibialis anterior in human neonates. *Early Hum Dev* 57:105–110, 2000.

Apley J, Naish N: Recurrent abdominal pains: A field survey of 1,000 school children. *Arch Dis Child* 33:165–170, 1958.

Asprey JR: Postoperative analgesic prescription and administration in a pediatric population. *J Pediatr Nurs* 9:150–157, 1994.

Attal N, Brasseur L, Parker F, et al.: Effects of gabapentin on the different components of peripheral and central neuropathic pain syndromes: A pilot study. *Eur Neurol* 40:191–200, 1998.

Avellanosa AM, West CR: Experience with transcutaneous electrical nerve stimulation for relief of intractable pain in cancer patients. *J Med* 13:203–213, 1982.

Babul N, Darke AC, Hagen N: Hydromorphone metabolite accumulation in renal failure. *J Pain Symptom Manage* 10:184–186 1995.

Babul N, Darke AC, Hain R: Hydromorphone and metabolite pharmacokinetics in children. *J Pain Symptom Manage* 10:335–337, 1995.

Backonja M, Beydoun A, Edwards KR, et al.: Gabapentin for the symptomatic treatment of painful neuropathy in patients with diabetes mellitus: A randomized controlled trial. *JAMA* 280:1831–1836, 1998.

Backonja MM: Anticonvulsants (antineuropathics) for neuropathic pain syndromes. *Clin J Pain* 16(2 Suppl):S67–S72, 2000.

Ballantyne M, Stevens B, McAllister M, et al.: Validation of the premature infant pain profile in the clinical setting. *Clin J Pain* 15:297–303, 1999.

Banez GA, Steffen RM: Treatment of recurrent abdominal pain: Components analysis of four treatment protocols. *Clin Pediatr (Phila)* 40:470–471, 2001.

Baraka A, Jabbour S, Ghabash M, et al.: A comparison of epidural tramadol and epidural morphine for postoperative analgesia. *Can J Anaesth* 40:308–313, 1993.

Baron ED, Harris L, Redpath WS, et al.: Laser-assisted penetration of topical anesthetic in adults. *Arch Dermatol* 139:1288–1290, 2003.

Bartfield JM, Gennis P, Barbera J, et al.: Buffered versus plain lidocaine as a local anesthetic for simple laceration repair. *Ann Emerg Med* 19:1387–1389, 1990.

Batra YK, Prasad MK, Arya VK, et al.: Comparison of caudal tramadol vs bupivacaine for post-operative analgesia in children undergoing hypospadias surgery. *Int J Clin Pharmacol Ther* 37:238–242, 1999.

Baumel B: Migraine: A pharmacologic review with newer options and delivery modalities. *Neurology* 44(5 Suppl 3):S13–S17, 1994.

Berde CB: Pediatric postoperative pain management. *Pediatr Clin North Am* 36:921–940, 1989.

Berde CB, Beyer JE, Bournaki MC, et al.: Comparison of morphine and methadone for prevention of postoperative pain in 3- to 7-year-old children. *J Pediatr* 119:136–141, 1991.

Berde CB, Lehn BM, Yee JD, et al.: Patient-controlled analgesia in children and adolescents: A randomized, prospective comparison with intramuscular morphine for postoperative analgesia. *J Pediatr* 118:460–466, 1991.

Berde CB, Sethna NF: Analgesics for the treatment of pain in children. *N Engl J Med* 347:1094–1103, 2002.

Berens RJ, Meyer MT: Comparison of 5 versus 10 days of methadone wean in pediatric critical care patients. *Anesthesiology* 96:A1297, 2002.

Beyer JE, DeGood DE, Ashley LC, et al.: Patterns of postoperative analgesic use with adults and children following cardiac surgery. *Pain* 17:71–81, 1983.

Beyer JE, Denyes MJ, Villarruel AM: The creation, validation, and continuing development of the Oucher: A measure of pain intensity in children. *J Pediatr Nurs* 7:335–346, 1992.

Bieri, D, Reeve RA, Champion GD, et al.: The Faces Pain Scale for the self-assessment of the severity of pain experienced by children: Development, initial validation, and preliminary investigation for ratio scale properties. *Pain* 41:139–150, 1990.

Bildner J, Krechel SW: Increasing staff nurse awareness of postoperative pain management in the NICU. *Neonatal Netw* 15:11–16, 1996.

Bille B: A 40-year follow-up of school children with migraine. *Cephalalgia* 17:488–491, 1997; discussion 487, 1997.

Birmingham PK, Wheeler M, Suresh S, et al.: Patient-controlled epidural analgesia in children: Can they do it? *Anesth Analg* 96:686–691, 2003, table of contents.

Bjorkman R: Central antinociceptive effects of non-steroidal anti-inflammatory drugs and paracetamol. Experimental studies in the rat. *Acta Anaesthesiol Scand Suppl* 103:1–44, 1995.

Bjorkman R, Hallman KM, Hedner J, et al.: Acetaminophen blocks spinal hyperalgesia induced by NMDA and substance P. *Pain* 57:259–264, 1994.

Blackburn PA, Butler KH, Hughes MJ, et al.: Comparison of tetracaine-adrenaline-cocaine (TAC) with topical lidocaine-epinephrine (TLE): Efficacy and cost. *Am J Emerg Med* 13:315–317, 1995.

Blanchard EB, Peters ML, Hermann C, et al.: Direction of temperature control in the thermal biofeedback treatment of vascular headache. *Appl Psychophysiol Biofeedback* 22:227–245, 1997.

Blank FS, Mader TJ, Wolfe J, et al.: Adequacy of pain assessment and pain relief and correlation of patient satisfaction in 68 ED fast-track patients. *J Emerg Nurs* 27:327–334, 2001.

Bosenberg AT: Continuous morphine infusion for postoperative pain in children. *S Afr Med J* 73:136–137, 1988.

Bosenberg AT, Bland BA, Schülte-Steinberg O, et al.: Thoracic epidural anesthesia via the caudal route in infants. *Anesthesiology* 69:265–269, 1988.

Bouchut JC, Dubois R, Godard J: Clonidine in preterm-infant caudal anesthesia may be responsible for postoperative apnea. *Reg Anesth Pain Med* 26:83–85, 2001.

Bray RJ: Postoperative analgesia provided by morphine infusion in children. *Anaesthesia* 38:1075–1078, 1983.

Bray RJ, Beeton C, Hinton W, et al.: Plasma morphine levels produced by continuous infusion in children. *Anaesthesia* 41:753–755, 1986.

Bray RJ, Woodhams AM, Vallis CJ, et al.: A double-blind comparison of morphine infusion and patient controlled analgesia in children. *Paediatr Anaesth* 6:121–127, 1996.

Bray RJ, Woodhams AM, Vallis CJ, et al.: Morphine consumption and respiratory depression in children receiving postoperative analgesia from continuous morphine infusion or patient controlled analgesia. *Paediatr Anaesth* 6:129–134, 1996.

Breau LM, Finley GA, McGrath PJ, et al.: Validation of the Non-communicating Children's Pain Checklist-Postoperative Version. *Anesthesiology* 96:528–535, 2002.

Breau LM, McGrath PJ, Ju LH: Review of juvenile primary fibromyalgia and chronic fatigue syndrome. *J Dev Behav Pediatr* 20:278–288, 1999.

Breit R, Van Der Wall H: Transcutaneous electrical nerve stimulation for post-operative pain relief after total knee arthroplasty. *J Arthroplasty* 19:45–48, 2004.

Breitbart W: Psychotropic adjuvant analgesics for pain in cancer and AIDS. *Psychooncology* 7:333–345, 1998.

Briggs M, Closs JS: A descriptive study of the use of visual analogue scales and verbal rating scales for the assessment of postoperative pain in orthopedic patients. *J Pain Symptom Manage* 18:438–446, 1999.

Broadman LM, Hannallah RS, Norden JM, et al.: Kiddie caudals: Experience with 1154 consecutive cases without complications. *Anesth Analg* 66:S18, 1987.

Broadman LM, Rice LJ, Hannallah RS: Oral clonidine and postoperative pain. *Anesth Analg* 84:229, 1997.

Broome AK: Psychological approaches to chronic pain. *Nurs Times* 80:36–39, 1984.

Broome ME, Richtsmeier A, Maikler V, et al.: Pediatric pain practices: A national survey of health professionals. *J Pain Symptom Manage* 11:312–320, 1996.

Bruera E, Pereira J, Watanabe S, et al.: Opioid rotation in patients with cancer pain. A retrospective comparison of dose ratios between methadone, hydromorphone, and morphine. *Cancer* 78:852–857, 1996.

Burton LJ, Quinn B, Pratt-Cheney JL, et al.: Headache etiology in a pediatric emergency department. *Pediatr Emerg Care* 13:1–4, 1997.

Bussone G, Grazzi L, D'Amico D, et al.: Biofeedback-assisted relaxation training for young adolescents with tension-type headache: A controlled study. *Cephalalgia* 18:463–467, 1998.

Calamandrei M, Messeri A, Busoni P, et al.: Comparison of two application techniques of EMLA and pain assessment in pediatric oncology patients. *Reg Anesth* 21:557–560, 1996.

Carlsson J: Prevalence of headache in schoolchildren: Relation to family and school factors. *Acta Paediatr* 85:692–696, 1996.

Caudle CL, Freid EB, Bailey AG, et al.: Epidural fentanyl infusion with patient-controlled epidural analgesia for postoperative analgesia in children. *J Pediatr Surg* 28:554 559, 1993.

Chan VW, Chung F, McQuestion M, et al.: Impact of patient-controlled analgesia on required nursing time and duration of postoperative recovery. *Reg Anesth* 20:506–514, 1995.

Chaplan SR, Duncan SR, Brodsky JB, et al.: Morphine and hydromorphone epidural analgesia. A prospective, randomized comparison. *Anesthesiology* 77:1090–1094, 1992.

Chapman CR, Benedetti C: Analgesia following transcutaneous electrical stimulation and its partial reversal by a narcotic antagonist. *Life Sci* 21:1645–1648, 1977.

Chelly JE, Grass J, Houseman TW, et al.: The safety and efficacy of a fentanyl patient-controlled transdermal system for acute postoperative analgesia: A multicenter, placebo-controlled trial. *Anesth Analg* 98:427–433, 2004.

Chen BK, Cunningham BB: Topical anesthetics in children: Agents and techniques that equally comfort patients, parents, and clinicians. *Curr Opin Pediatr* 13:324–330, 2001.

Chen E, Joseph MH, Zeltzer LK: Behavioral and cognitive interventions in the treatment of pain in children. *Pediatr Clin North Am* 47:513–525, 2000.

Cherny NI: The management of cancer pain. *CA Cancer J Clin* 50:70–116, 2000; quiz 117–120, 2000.

Choy L, Collier J, Watson AR: Comparison of lignocaine-prilocaine cream and amethocaine gel for local analgesia before venepuncture in children. *Acta Paediatr* 88:961–964, 1999.

Christoph RA, Buchanan L, Begalla K, et al.: Pain reduction in local anesthetic administration through pH buffering. *Ann Emerg Med* 17:177–181, 1988.

Collins C, Koren G, Crean P, et al.: Fentanyl pharmacokinetics and hemodynamic effects in preterm infants during ligation of patent ductus arteriosus. *Anesth Analg* 64:1078–1080, 1985.

Collins J, Grier H, Kinney H, et al.: Control of severe pain in children with terminal malignancy. *J Pediatr* 126:653–657, 1995.

Collins JJ, Geake J, Grier HE, et al.: Patient-controlled analgesia for mucositis pain in children: A three-period crossover study comparing morphine and hydromorphone. *J Pediatr* 129:722–728, 1996.

Collins JJ, Grier HE, Kinney HC, et al.: Control of severe pain in children with terminal malignancy. *J Pediatr* 126:653–657, 1995.

Collins JJ, Grier HE, Sethna NF, et al.: Regional anesthesia for pain associated with terminal pediatric malignancy. *Pain* 65:63–69, 1996.

Colwell CW Jr, Morris BA: Patient-controlled analgesia compared with intramuscular injection of analgesics for the management of pain after an orthopaedic procedure. *J Bone Joint Surg Am* 77:726–733, 1995.

Cook B, Grubb DJ, Aldridge LA, et al.: Comparison of the effects of adrenaline, clonidine and ketamine on the duration of caudal analgesia produced by bupivacaine in children. *Br J Anaesth* 75:698–701, 1995.

Cooper CM, Gerrish SP, Hardwick M, et al.: EMLA cream reduces the pain of venipuncture in children. *Eur J Anaesthesiol* 4:441–448, 1987.

Cossmann M, Kohnen C, Langford R, et al.: [Tolerance and safety of tramadol use. Results of international studies and data from drug surveillance]. *Drugs* 53(Suppl 2):50–62, 1997.

Costigan M, Woolf CJ: No DREAM, no pain. Closing the spinal gate. *Cell* 108:297–300, 2002.

Costigan M, Woolf CJ: Pain: Molecular mechanisms. *J Pain* 1(3 Suppl):35–44, 2000.

Cotter DJ: Overview of transcutaneous electrical nerve stimulation for treatment of acute postoperative pain. *Med Instrum* 17:289–292, 1983.

Craig KD, Lilley CM, Gilbert CA: Social barriers to optimal pain management in infants and children. *Clin J Pain* 12:232–242, 1996.

Crawford HJ, Knebel T, Vendemia JMC: The nature of hypnotic analgesia: Neurophysiological foundation and evidence. *Contemp Hypnosis* 15:22–33, 1998.

Cummings EA, Reid GJ, Finley GA, et al.: Prevalence and source of pain in pediatric inpatients. *Pain* 68:25–31, 1996.

Cummins R, Wagner-Weiner L, Paller A: Pseudoporphyria induced by celecoxib in a patient with juvenile rheumatoid arthritis. *J Rheumatol* 27:2938–2940, 2000.

Czarnecki ML, Jandrisevits MD, Theiler SC, et al.: Controlled-release oxycodone for the management of pediatric postoperative pain. *J Pain Symptom Manage* 27:379–386, 2004.

Dahlquist LM: *Pediatric pain management*. New York, 1999, Plenum Press.

Dalens B, Hasnaoui A: Caudal anesthesia in pediatric surgery: Success rate and adverse effects of 750 consecutive patients. *Anesth Analg* 68:83–89, 1989.

Dalton JA, Blau W, Lindley C, et al.: Changing acute pain management to improve patient outcomes: An educational approach. *J Pain Symptom Manage* 17:277–287, 1999.

Daly EJ, Donn PA, Galliher MJ, et al.: Biofeedback applications to migraine and tension headaches: A double-blinded outcome study. *Biofeedback Self Regul* 8:135–152, 1983.

Dayer P, Collart L, Desmueles J: The pharmacology of tramadol. *Drugs* 47(Suppl 1):3–7, 1994.

De Negri P, Visconti C, Ivani G, et al.: Caudal additives to ropivacaine in children: Preservative free S-ketamine versus clonidine. *Paediatr Anaesth* 10:704–705, 2000.

Delilkan AE, Vijayan R: Epidural tramadol for postoperative pain relief. *Anaesthesia* 48:328–331, 1993.

Delvaux M: Role of visceral sensitivity in the pathophysiology of irritable bowel syndrome. *Gut* 51(Suppl 1):i67–i71, 2002.

Di Lorenzo C, Youssef NN, Sigurdsson L, et al.: Visceral hyperalgesia in children with functional abdominal pain. *J Pediatr* 139:838–84, 2001.

Dix P, Martindale S, Stoddart PA: Double-blind randomized placebo-controlled trial of the effect of ketamine on postoperative morphine consumption in children following appendicectomy. *Paediatr Anaesth* 13:422–426, 2003.

Doyle E, Freeman J, Im NT, et al.: An evaluation of a new self-adhesive patch preparation of amethocaine for topical anaesthesia prior to venous cannulation in children. *Anaesthesia* 48:1050–1052, 1993.

Doyle E, Robinson D, Morton NS: Patient-controlled analgesia with low dose background infusions after lower abdominal surgery in children. *Br J Anaesth* 71:818–822, 1993.

Druckro PN, Cantwell-Simmons E: A review of studies evaluation biofeedback and relaxation training in the management of pediatric headache. *Headache* 29:428–43, 1989.

DuPen SL, Peterson DG, Bogosian AC, et al.: A new permanent exteriorized epidural catheter for narcotic self-administration to control cancer pain. *Cancer* 59:986–993, 1987.

Ehrenstrom-Reiz GME, Reiz SLA: EMLA—A eutectic mixture of local anaesthetics for topical anaesthesia. *Acta Anaesthesiol Scand* 26:596–598, 1982.

Eichenfield LF, Funk A, Fallon-Friedlander S, et al.: A clinical study to evaluate the efficacy of ELA-Max (4% liposomal lidocaine) as compared with eutectic mixture of local anesthetics cream for pain reduction of venipuncture in children. *Pediatrics* 109:1093–1099, 2002.

Eisenach JC, De Kock M, Klimscha W: Alpha-adrenergic agonists for regional anesthesia. A clinical review of clonidine: 1984-1995 *Anesthesiology* 85:655–674, 1996.

Eland JM: Children's communication of pain. *Educational Psychology*. Iowa City, 1974, University of Iowa.

Elander J, Lusher J, Bevan D, et al.: Understanding the causes of problematic pain management in sickle cell disease: Evidence that pseudoaddiction plays a more important role than genuine analgesic dependence. *J Pain Symptom Manage* 27:156–169, 2004.

Engel JM, Rapoff MA: Biofeedback-assisted relaxation training for adult and pediatric headache disorders. *Occup Therapy J Res* 10:283–299, 1990.

Ernst AA, Marvez E, Nick TG, et al.: Lidocaine adrenaline tetracaine gel versus tetracaine adrenaline cocaine gel for topical anesthesia in linear scalp and facial lacerations in children aged 5 to 17 years. *Pediatrics* 95:255–258, 1995.

Ernst AA, Marvez-Valls E, Nick TG, et al.: Topical lidocaine adrenaline tetracaine (LAT gel) versus injectable buffered lidocaine for local anesthesia in laceration repair. *West J Med* 167:79–81, 1997.

Esseltine DW, Baxter MR, Bevan JC: Sickle cell states and the anaesthetist. *Can J Anaesth* 35:385–403, 1988.

Everts B, Wahrborg P, Hedner T: COX-2-specific inhibitors—the emergence of a new class of analgesic and anti-inflammatory drugs. *Clin Rheumatol* 19:331–343, 2000.

Facchinetti F, Sforza G, Amidei M, et al.: Central and peripheral beta-endorphin response to transcutaneous electrical nerve stimulation. *NIDA Res Monogr* 75:555–558, 1986.

Fazi L, Jantzen EC, Rose JB, et al.: A comparison of oral clonidine and oral midazolam as preanesthetic medications in the pediatric tonsillectomy patient. *Anesth Analg* 92:56–61, 2001.

Ferrell B, Virani R, Grant M, et al.: Analysis of pain content in nursing textbooks. *J Pain Symptom Manage* 19:216–228, 2000.

Ferrell BR, Dean GE, Grant M, et al.: An institutional commitment to pain management. *J Clin Oncol* 13:2158–2165, 1995.

Fine PG: Low-dose ketamine in the management of opioid nonresponsive terminal cancer pain. *J Pain Symptom Manage* 17:296–300, 1999.

Finkel JC, Rose JB, Schmitz ML, et al.: An evaluation of the efficacy and tolerability of oral tramadol hydrochloride tablets for the treatment of postsurgical pain in children. *Anesth Analg* 94:1469–1473, 2002.

Finley WW, Jones LC: Biofeedback with children. In *Handbook of clinical child psychology*. Wiley Series on Personality. New York, 1992, John Wiley & Sons, pp 809–827.

Fins JJ, Nilson EG: An approach to educating residents about palliative care and clinical ethics. *Acad Med* 75:662–625, 2000.

Fitzgerald M: Neurobiology of fetal and neonatal pain. In Wall PD, Melzack R, editors: *Textbook of pain*. Edinburgh, 1994, Churchill Livingstone, pp 153–163.

Fitzgerald M, Millard C, McIntosh N: Cutaneous hypersensitivity following peripheral tissue damage in newborn infants and its reversal with topical anaesthesia. *Pain* 39:31–36, 1989.

Fitzgerald M, Koltzenburg M: The functional development of descending inhibitory pathways in the dorsolateral funiculus of the newborn rat spinal cord. *Brain Res* 389:261–270, 1986.

Fitzgerald M, Millard C, MacIntosh N: Hyperalgesia in premature infants. *Lancet* 1(8580):292, 1988.

Fitzmaurice LS, Wasserman GS, Knapp JF, et al.: TAC use and absorption of cocaine in a pediatric emergency department. *Ann Emerg Med* 19:515–518, 1990.

Foley KM: Misconceptions and controversies regarding the use of opioids in cancer pain. *Anticancer Drugs* 6(Suppl 3):4–13, 1995.

Fowler-Kerry S: Adolescent oncology survivors' recollection of pain. In Tyler D, Krane E, editors: *Advances in pain research and therapy: Pediatric pain*. New York, 1990, Raven Press, pp 365–371.

Friedman PM, Fogelman JP, Nouri K, et al.: Comparative study of the efficacy of four topical anesthetics. *Dermatol Surg* 25:950–954, 1999.

Fudin J, Audette CM: Gabapentin vs amitriptyline for the treatment of peripheral neuropathy. *Arch Intern Med* 160:1040–1041, 2000.

Galer BS: Neuropathic pain of peripheral origin: Advances in pharmacologic treatment. *Neurology* 45(12 Suppl 9):S17–S25, 1995; discussion S35–S36, 1995.

Gardner JS, Blough D, Drinkard CR, et al.: Tramadol and seizures: A surveillance study in a managed care population. *Pharmacotherapy* 20:1423–1431, 2000.

Gasse C, Derby L, Vasilakis-Scaramozza C, et al.: Incidence of first-time idiopathic seizures in users of tramadol. *Pharmacotherapy* 20:629–634, 2000.

Gaudreau GA, Plourde V: Involvement of N-methyl-d-aspartate (NMDA) receptors in a rat model of visceral hypersensitivity. *Behav Brain Res* 150:185–189, 2004.

Gauthier J, Bois R, Allaire D, et al.: Evaluation of skin temperature biofeedback training at two different sites for migraine. *J Behav Med* 4:407–419, 1981.

Giaufré E, Dalens B, Gombert A: Epidemiology and morbidity of regional anesthesia in children: A one-year prospective survey of the French-Language Society of Pediatric Anesthesiologists. *Anesth Analg* 83:904–912, 1996.

Goeringer KE, Logan BK, Christian GD: Identification of tramadol and its metabolites in blood from drug-related deaths and drug-impaired drivers. *J Anal Toxicol* 21:529–537, 1997.

Goobie SM, Montgomery CJ, Basu R, et al.: Confirmation of direct epidural catheter placement using nerve stimulation in pediatric anesthesia. *Anesth Analg* 97:984–988, 2003.

Goodarzi M: Comparison of epidural morphine, hydromorphone and fentanyl for postoperative pain control in children undergoing orthopaedic surgery. *Paediatr Anaesth* 9:419–422, 1999.

Goodman GR: Outcomes measurement in pain management: Issues of disease complexity and uncertain outcomes. *J Nurs Care Qual* 18:105–111, 2003; quiz 112–113, 2003.

Goodman JE, McGrath PJ: The epidemiology of pain in children and adolescents: A review. *Pain* 46:247–264, 1991.

Goyagi T, Tanaka M, Nishikawa T: Oral clonidine premedication enhances postoperative analgesia by epidural morphine. *Anesth Analg* 89:1487–1491, 1999.

Grazzi L, D'Amico D, Leone M, et al.: Pharmacological and behavioral treatment of pediatric migraine and tension type headache. *Ital J Neurol Sci* 19:59–64, 1998.

Green SM, Nakamura R, Johnson NE: Ketamine sedation for pediatric procedures: Part 1, A prospective series. *Ann Emerg Med* 19:1024–1032, 1990.

Greipp ME, Thomas AF: Reflex sympathetic dystrophy syndrome: A nursing challenge. *Orthop Nurs* 6:32–36, 72, 1987.

Grunau RV, Craig KD: Pain expression in neonates: Facial action and cry. *Pain* 28:395–410, 1987.

Grunau RV, Johnston CC, Craig KD: Neonatal facial and cry responses to invasive and non-invasive procedures. *Pain* 42:295–305, 1990.

Gunduz M, Ozcengiz D, Ozbek H, et al.: A comparison of single dose caudal tramadol, tramadol plus bupivacaine and bupivacaine administration for postoperative analgesia in children. *Paediatr Anaesth* 11:323–326, 2001.

Gunter JB, Eng C: Thoracic epidural anesthesia via the caudal approach in children. *Anesthesiology* 76:935–938, 1992.

Gupta SK, Bernstein KJ, Noorduin H, et al.: Fentanyl delivery from an electrotransport system: Delivery is a function of total current, not duration of current. *J Clin Pharmacol* 38:951–958, 1998.

Hahn TW, Mogensen T, Lund C, et al.: Analgesic effect of i.v. paracetamol: Possible ceiling effect of paracetamol in postoperative pain. *Acta Anaesthesiol Scand* 47:138–145, 2003.

Hallen B, Uppfeldt A: Does lidocaine-prilocaine cream permit painfree insertion of IV catheters in children? *Anesthesiology* 57:340–342, 1982.

Halperin DL, Koren G, Attias D, et al.: Topical skin anesthesia for venous, subcutaneous drug reservoir and lumbar punctures in children. *Pediatrics* 84:281–284, 1989.

Halpern SH, Arellano R, Preston R, et al.: Epidural morphine vs hydromorphone in post-caesarean section patients. *Can J Anaesth* 43:595–598, 1996.

Hansen TG, Henneberg SW, Walther-Larsen S, et al.: Caudal bupivacaine supplemented with caudal or intravenous clonidine in children undergoing hypospadias repair: A double-blind study. *Br J Anaesth* 92:223–227, 2004.

Harke H, Gretenkort P, Ladleif HU, et al.: The response of neuropathic pain and pain in complex regional pain syndrome I to carbamazepine and sustained-release morphine in patients pretreated with spinal cord stimulation: A double-blinded randomized study. *Anesth Analg* 92:488–495, 2001.

Harmer M, Davies KA: The effect of education, assessment and a standardised prescription on postoperative pain management. The value of clinical audit in the establishment of acute pain services. *Anaesthesia* 53:424–430, 1998.

Hartley R, Green M, Quinn M, et al.: Pharmacokinetics of morphine infusion in premature neonates. *Arch Dis Child* 69(1 Spec No):55–58, 1993.

He LF, Lu RL, Zhuang SY, et al.: Possible involvement of opioid peptides of caudate nucleus in acupuncture analgesia. *Pain* 23:83–93, 1985.

He LF: Involvement of endogenous opioid peptides in acupuncture analgesia. *Pain* 31:99–121, 1987.

Hicks CL, von Baeyer CL, Spafford PA, et al.: The Faces Pain Scale-Revised: Toward a common metric in pediatric pain measurement. *Pain* 93:173–183, 2001.

Huertas-Ceballos A, Macarthur C, Logan S: Dietary interventions for recurrent abdominal pain (RAP) in childhood. *Cochrane Database Syst Rev* CD003019, 2002a.

Huertas-Ceballos A, Macarthur C, Logan S: Pharmacological interventions for recurrent abdominal pain (RAP) in childhood. *Cochrane Database Syst Rev* CD003017, 2002b.

Hughes GS Jr, Lichstein PR, Whitlock D, et al.: Response of plasma beta-endorphins to transcutaneous electrical nerve stimulation in healthy subjects. *Phys Ther* 64:1062–1066, 1984.

Hunt RH, Tougas G: Evolving concepts in functional gastrointestinal disorders: Promising directions for novel pharmaceutical treatments. *Best Pract Res Clin Gastroenterol* 16:869–883, 2002.

Hyams J, Colletti R, Faure C, et al.: Functional gastrointestinal disorders: Working Group Report of the First World Congress of Pediatric Gastroenterology, Hepatology, and Nutrition. *J Pediatr Gastroenterol Nutr* 35(Suppl 2):S110–S117, 2002.

Hyams JS: Functional gastrointestinal disorders. *Curr Opin Pediatr* 11:375–378, 1999.

Ishida T, Oguri K, Yoshimura H: Determination of oxycodone metabolites in urines and feces of several mammalian species. *J Pharmacobiodyn* 5:521–525, 1982.

Ivani G, De Negri P, Conio A, et al.: Ropivacaine-clonidine combination for caudal blockade in children. *Acta Anaesthesiol Scand* 44:446–469, 2000.

Ivani G, Lampugnani E, Torre M, et al.: Comparison of ropivacaine with bupivacaine for paediatric caudal block. *Br J Anaesth* 81:247–248, 1998.

Ivani G, Mattioli G, Rega M, et al.: Clonidine-mepivacaine mixture vs plain mepivacaine in paediatric surgery. *Paediatr Anaesth* 6:111–114, 1996.

Jailwala J, Imperiale TF, Kroenke K: Pharmacologic treatment of the irritable bowel syndrome: A systematic review of randomized, controlled trials. *Ann Intern Med* 133:136–147, 2000.

Jamali S, Monin S, Begon C, et al.: Clonidine in pediatric caudal anesthesia. *Anesth Analg* 78:663–636, 1994.

Jensen JE, Etheridge GL, Hazelrigg G: Effectiveness of transcutaneous electrical neural stimulation in the treatment of pain. Recommendations for use in the treatment of sports injuries. *Sports Med* 3:79–88, 1986.

Jick H, Derby LE, Vasilakis C, et al.: The risk of seizures associated with tramadol. *Pharmacotherapy* 18:607–611, 1998.

Johnston CC, Abbott FV, Gray-Donald K, et al.: A survey of pain in hospitalized patients aged 4-14 years. *Clin J Pain* 8:154–163, 1992.

Johnston CC, Sherrard A, Stevens B, et al.: Do cry features reflect pain intensity in preterm neonates? A preliminary study. *Biol Neonate* 76:120–124, 1999.

Johnston CC, Strada ME: Acute pain response in infants: A multidimensional description. *Pain* 24:373–382, 1986.

Joshi W, Connelly NR, Reuben SS, et al.: An evaluation of the safety and efficacy of administering rofecoxib for postoperative pain management. *Anesth Analg* 97:35–38, 2003.

Jubelirer SJ, Welch C, Babar Z, et al.: Competencies and concerns in end-of-life care for medical students and residents. *W V Med J* 97:118–121, 2001.

Kachoyeanos MK, Friedhoff M: Cognitive and behavioral strategies to reduce children's pain. *MCN Am J Matern Child Nurs* 18:14–19, 1993.

Kamp EH, Jones RC 3rd, Tillman SR, et al.: Quantitative assessment and characterization of visceral nociception and hyperalgesia in mice. *Am J Physiol Gastrointest Liver Physiol* 284:G434–G444, 2003.

Karl HW, Tyler DC, Krane EJ: Respiratory depression after low-dose caudal morphine. *Can J Anaesth* 43:1065–1067, 1996.

Kashikar-Zuck S, Vaught MH, Goldschneider KR, et al.: Depression, coping, and functional disability in juvenile primary fibromyalgia syndrome. *J Pain* 3:412–419, 2002.

Kemper KJ, Sarah R, Silver-Highfield E, et al.: On pins and needles? Pediatric pain patients' experience with acupuncture. *Pediatrics* 105(4 Pt 2):941–947, 2000.

Kennedy RM, Luhmann JD: Pharmacological management of pain and anxiety during emergency procedures in children. *Paediatr Drugs* 3:337–354, 2001.

Kerr SJ, Mant A, Horn FE, et al.: Lessons from early large-scale adoption of celecoxib and rofecoxib by Australian general practitioners. *Med J Aust* 179:403–407, 2003.

Khalil S, Campos C, Farag AM, et al.: Caudal block in children: Ropivacaine compared with bupivacaine. *Anesthesiology* 91:1279–1284, 1999.

Kho HG, Kloppenborg PW, van Egmond J: Effects of acupuncture and transcutaneous stimulation analgesia on plasma hormone levels during and after major abdominal surgery. *Eur J Anaesthesiol* 10:197–208, 1993.

Kho P, Thomas VJ: Patient-controlled analgesia (PCA): Does time saved by PCA improve patient satisfaction with nursing care? *J Adv Nurs* 20:61–70, 1994.

Kirsh KL, Whitcomb LA, Donaghy K, et al.: Abuse and addiction issues in medically ill patients with pain: Attempts at clarification of terms and empirical study. *Clin J Pain* 18(4 Suppl):S52–S60, 2002.

Koinig H, Marhofer P, Krenn CG, et al.: Analgesic effects of caudal and intramuscular S(+)-ketamine in children. *Anesthesiology* 93:976–980, 2000.

Korpela R, Korvenoja P, Meretoja OA: Morphine-sparing effect of acetaminophen in pediatric day-case surgery. *Anesthesiology* 91:442–427, 1999.

Krane EJ, Dalens BJ, Murat I, et al.: The safety of epidurals placed during general anesthesia. *Reg Anesth Pain Med* 23:433–438, 1998.

Krane EJ, Tyler DC, Jacobson LE: The dose response of caudal morphine in children. *Anesthesiology* 71:48–52, 1989.

Krane EJ: Delayed respiratory depression in a child after caudal epidural morphine. *Anesth Analg* 67:79–82, 1988.

Krechel SW, Bildner J: CRIES: A new neonatal postoperative pain measurement score. Initial testing of validity and reliability. *Paediatr Anaesth* 5:53–61, 1995.

Kuttner L, LePage T: Face scales for the assessment of pediatric pain: A critical review. *Canad J Behave Sci* 21:198–209, 1988.

Kuttner L: Favorite stories: A hypnotic pain-reduction technique for children in acute pain. *Am J Clin Hypn* 30:289–295, 1988.

Labat F, Dubousset AM, Baujard C, et al.: Epidural analgesia in a child with sickle cell disease complicated by acute abdominal pain and priapism. *Br J Anaesth* 87:935–936, 2001.

Labbe EE: Treatment of childhood migraine with autogenic training and skin temperature biofeedback: A component analysis. *Headache* 35:10–13, 1995.

Labbe EE, Ward CH: Electromyographic biofeedback with mental imagery and home practice in the treatment of children with muscle-contraction headache. *J Dev Behav Pediatr* 11:65–68, 1990.

Larsson B: Recurrent headaches in children and adolescents. In McGrath PJ, Finley GA, editors: *Chronic and recurrent pain in children and adolescents.* Seattle, 1999, IASP Press, pp 115–140.

Lawrence J, Alcock D, McGrath P, et al.: The development of a tool to assess neonatal pain. *Neonat Network* 12:59–66, 1993.

Lawrence LM, Wright SW: Sedation of pediatric patients for minor laceration repair: Effect on length of emergency department stay and patient charges. *Pediatr Emerg Care* 14:393–395, 1998.

LeBaron S, Zeltzer LK, Fanurik D: Imaginative involvement and hypnotizability in childhood. *Int J Clin Exp Hypn* 36:284–295, 1988.

Lee BH, Scharff L, Sethna NF, et al.: Physical therapy and cognitive-behavioral treatment for complex regional pain syndromes. *J Pediatr* 141:135–140, 2002.

Lee CR, McTavish D, Sorkin EM: Tramadol. A preliminary review of its pharmacodynamic and pharmacokinetic properties, and therapeutic potential in a cute and chronic pain states. *Drugs* 46:313–340, 1993.

Leeder JS: Developmental and pediatric pharmacogenomics. *Pharmacogenomics* 4:331–341, 2003.

Leeder JS: Pharmacogenetics and pharmacogenomics. *Pediatr Clin North Am* 48:765–781, 2001.

Lesko SM, Mitchell AA: The safety of acetaminophen and ibuprofen among children younger than two years old. *Pediatrics* 104:e39, 1999.

Liebelt EL: Current concepts in laceration repair. *Curr Opin Pediatr* 9:459–464, 1997.

Lin YC, Bioteau AB, Lee AC: Acupuncture for the management of pediatric pain: A pilot study. *Med Acupuncture* 14:45–46, 2002.

Lin YC: Patient controlled analgesia (PCA), nurse controlled analgesia (NCA), or epidural controlled analgesia (ECA). *Anaesthesia* 57:518, 2002.

Ljungman G, Gordh T, Sorensen S, et al.: Pain in paediatric oncology: Interviews with children, adolescents and their parents. *Acta Paediatr* 88:623–630, 1999.

Ljungman G, Kreuger A, Gordh T, et al.: Treatment of pain in pediatric oncology: A Swedish nationwide survey. *Pain* 68:385–394, 1996.

Lloyd-Thomas A: Assessment and control of pain in children. *Anaesthesia* 50:753–755, 1995.

Long DM: Electrical stimulation of the nervous system for pain control. *Electroencephalogr Clin Neurophysiol Suppl* 34:343–348, 1978.

Luz G, Innerhofer P, Bachmann B, et al.: Bupivacaine plasma concentrations during continuous epidural anesthesia in infants and children. *Anesth Analg* 82:231–234, 1996.

Luz G, Innerhofer P, Haussler B, et al.: Comparison of ropivacaine 0.1% and 0.2% with bupivacaine 0.2% for single-shot caudal anaesthesia in children. *Paediatr Anaesth* 10:499–504, 2000.

Luz G, Innerhofer P, Oswald E, et al.: Comparison of clonidine 1 microgram kg-1 with morphine 30 micrograms kg-1 for post-operative caudal analgesia in children. *Eur J Anaesthesiol* 16:42–46, 1999.

Luz G, Wieser C, Innerhofer P, et al.: Free and total bupivacaine plasma concentrations after continuous epidural anaesthesia in infants and children. *Paediatr Anaesth* 8:473–478, 1998.

Lynn A, Nespeca MK, Bratton SL, et al.: Clearance of morphine in postoperative infants during intravenous infusion: The influence of age and surgery. *Anesth Analg* 86:958–963, 1998.

Lynn AM, Nespeca MK, Bratton SL, et al.: Intravenous morphine in postoperative infants: Intermittent bolus dosing versus targeted continuous infusions. *Pain* 88:89–95, 2000.

Lynn AM, Opheim KE, Tyler DC: Morphine infusion after pediatric cardiac surgery. *Crit Care Med* 12:863–866, 1984.

Lynn AM, Slattery JT: Morphine pharmacokinetics in early infancy. *Anesthesiology* 66:136–139, 1987.

Malleson PN, al-Matar M, Petty RE: Idiopathic musculoskeletal pain syndromes in children. *J Rheumatol* 19:1786–1789, 1992.

Malmberg AB, Yaksh TL: Hyperalgesia mediated by spinal glutamate or substance P receptor blocked by spinal cyclooxygenase inhibition. *Science* 257:1276–1279, 1992.

Mannheimer C, Carlsson CA: The analgesic effect of transcutaneous electrical nerve stimulation (TNS) in patients with rheumatoid arthritis. A comparative study of different pulse patterns. *Pain* 6:329–334, 1979.

Manworren RC: Development and testing of the Pediatric Nurses' Knowledge and Attitudes Survey Regarding Pain. *Pediatr Nurs* 27:151–158, 2001.

Masek BJ, Russo DC, Varni JW: Behavioral approaches to the management of chronic pain in children. *Pediatr Clin North Am* 31:1113–1131, 1984.

Mather L, Mackie J: The incidence of postoperative pain in children. *Pain* 15:271–282, 1983.

Maunuksela EL, Kokki H, Bullingham RES: Comparison of intravenous ketorolac with morphine for postoperative pain in children. *Clin Pharmacol Ther* 52:436–443, 1992.

Maunuksela E, Korpela R: Double-blind evaluation of lignocaine-prilocaine cream (EMLA) in children. *Br J Anaesth* 58:1242–1245, 1986.

Maunuksela EL, Olkkola KT, Korpela R: Measurement of pain in children with self-reporting and behavioral assessment. *Clin Pharmacol Ther* 42:137–141, 1987.

McCaffery M, Hart LL: Undertreatment of acute pain with narcotics. *Am J Nurs* 76:1586–1591, 1976.

McCloskey JJ, Haun SE, Deshpande JK: Bupivacaine toxicity secondary to continuous caudal epidural infusion in children. *Anesth Analg* 75:287–290, 1992.

McDonald AJ, Cooper MG: Patient-controlled analgesia: An appropriate method of pain control in children. *Paediatr Drugs* 3:273–284, 2001.

McGown RG: Caudal analgesia in children: Five hundred cases for procedures below the diaphragm. *Anaesthesia* 37:806–810, 1982.

McGrath P, Johnson G, Goodman J: CHEOPS: A behavioral scale for rating postoperative pain in children. In Fields H, editor: *Advances in pain research and therapy*. New York, 1985, Raven Press, pp 395–402.

McGrath PA, Hillier LM: *The child with headache: Diagnosis and treatment.* Seattle, 2001, IASP Press.

McGrath PJ, Unruh AM: *Pain in children and adolescents*. Amsterdam, 1987, Elsevier.

McKay W, Morris R, Mushlin P: Sodium bicarbonate attenuates pain on skin infiltration with lidocaine, with and without epinephrine. *Anesth Analg* 66:572–574, 1987.

McKenzie IM, Gaukroger PB, Ragg PG, et al.: *Manual of acute pain management in children*. New York, 1997, Churchill Livingstone.

McMillan SC, Tittle M, Hagan S, et al.: Knowledge and attitudes of nurses in veterans hospitals about pain management in patients with cancer. *Oncol Nurs Forum* 27:1415–1423, 2000.

McNeely JK, Farber NE, Rusy LM, et al.: Epidural analgesia improves outcome following pediatric fundoplication. A retrospective analysis. *Reg Anesth* 22:16–23, 1997.

McNeely JK, Trentadue NC, Rusy LM, et al.: Culture of bacteria from lumbar and caudal epidural catheters used for postoperative analgesia in children. *Reg Anesth* 22:428–431, 1997.

McQuay HJ, Tramer M, Nye BA, et al.: A systematic review of antidepressants in neuropathic pain. *Pain* 68:217–227, 1996.

McQuay HJ: Pharmacological treatment of neuralgic and neuropathic pain. *Cancer Surv* 7:141–159, 1988.

McRorie TI, Lynn AM, Nespeca MK, et al.: The maturation of morphine clearance and metabolism. *Am J Dis Child* 146:972–976, 1992.

Merkel SI, Voepel-Lewis T, Shayevitz JR, et al.: The FLACC: A behavioral scale for scoring postoperative pain in young children. *Pediatr Nurs* 23:293–297, 1997.

Merskey H, Bogduk N, editors: *Classification of chronic pain, IASP Task Force on Taxonomy*. Seattle, 1994, IASP Press.

Meyer MM, Berens RJ: Efficacy of an enteral 10-day methadone wean to prevent opioid withdrawal in fentanyl-tolerant pediatric intensive care unit patients. *Pediatr Crit Care Med* 2:329–333, 2001.

Meyler WJ, de Jongste MJ, Rolf CA: Clinical evaluation of pain treatment with electrostimulation: A study on TENS in patients with different pain syndromes. *Clin J Pain* 10:22–27, 1994.

Mikawa K, Nishina K, Maekawa N, et al.: Oral clonidine premedication reduces vomiting in children after strabismus surgery. *Can J Anaesth* 42:977–981, 1995.

Mikawa K, Nishina K, Maekawa N, et al.: Oral clonidine premedication reduces postoperative pain in children. *Anesth Analg* 82:225–230, 1996.

Miller BR: *Establishing a pediatric acute pain service.* Pediatric Anesthesiology 1996, Tampa, FL, 1996, Society for Pediatric Anesthesia.

Miller MG, McCarthy N, O'Boyle CA, et al.: Continuous subcutaneous infusion of morphine vs. hydromorphone: A controlled trial. *J Pain Symptom Manage* 18:9–16, 1999.

Miranda A, Peles S, Rudolph C, et al.: Altered visceral sensation in response to somatic pain in the rat. *Gastroenterology* 126:1082–1089, 2004.

Miser A, Dothage J, Wesley R, et al.: The prevalence of pain in a pediatric and young adult cancer population. *Pain* 29:73–83, 1987.

Miser AW, Goh S, Dose AM, et al.: Trial of a topically administered local anesthetic (EMLA cream) for pain relief during central venous port access in children with cancer. *J Pain Symptom Manage* 9:259–264, 1994.

Mitchell JA, Akarasereenont P, Thiemermann C, et al.: Selectivity of nonsteroidal antiinflammatory drugs as inhibitors of constitutive and inducible cyclooxygenase. *Proc Natl Acad Sci U S A* 90:11693–11697, 1993.

Molik KA, Engum SA, Rescorla FJ, et al.: Pectus excavatum repair: Experience with standard and minimal invasive techniques. *J Pediatr Surg* 36:324–328, 2001.

Monitto CL, Greenberg RS, Kost-Byerly S, et al.: The safety and efficacy of parent-/nurse-controlled analgesia in patients less than six years of age. *Anesth Analg* 91:573–579, 2000.

Motsch J, Bottiger BW, Bach A, et al.: Caudal clonidine and bupivacaine for combined epidural and general anaesthesia in children. *Acta Anaesthesiol Scand* 41:877–883, 1997.

Murrell D, Gibson PR, Cohen RC: Continuous epidural analgesia in newborn infants undergoing major surgery. *J Pediatr Surg* 28:548–552, 1993; discussion 552–553, 1993.

National Institutes of Health: NIH Consensus Conference. Acupuncture. *JAMA* 280:1518–1524, 1998.

Ng MM, Leung MC, Poon DM: The effects of electro-acupuncture and transcutaneous electrical nerve stimulation on patients with painful osteoarthritic knees: A randomized controlled trial with follow-up evaluation. *J Altern Complement Med* 9:641–649, 2003.

Nicholson B: Gabapentin use in neuropathic pain syndromes. *Acta Neurol Scand* 101:359–371, 2000.

Nishina K, Mikawa K, Shiga M, et al.: Diclofenac and flurbiprofen with or without clonidine for postoperative analgesia in children undergoing elective ophthalmological surgery. *Paediatr Anaesth* 10:645–651, 2000.

Nordbladh I, Ohlander B, Bjorkman R: Analgesia in tonsillectomy: A double-blind study on pre and post-operative treatment with diclofenac. *Clin Otolaryngol* 16:554–558, 1991.

O'Brien WJ, Rutan FM, Sanborn C, et al.: Effect of transcutaneous electrical nerve stimulation on human blood beta-endorphin levels. *Phys Ther* 64:1367–1374, 1984.

O'Connor M: Pain management: Improving documentation of assessment and intensity. *J Healthc Qual* 25:17–21, 2003; quiz 22, 2003.

Orza F, Boswell MV, Rosenberg SK: Neuropathic pain: Review of mechanisms and pharmacologic management. *NeuroRehabilitation* 14:15–23, 2000.

Ozcengiz D, Gunduz M, Ozbek H, et al.: Comparison of caudal morphine and tramadol for postoperative pain control in children undergoing inguinal herniorrhaphy. *Paediatr Anaesth* 11:459–464, 2001.

Oztekin S, Hepaguslar H, Kar AA, et al.: Preemptive diclofenac reduces morphine use after remifentanil-based anaesthesia for tonsillectomy. *Paediatr Anaesth* 12:694–699, 2002.

Palecek J, Willis WD: The dorsal column pathway facilitates visceromotor responses to colorectal distention after colon inflammation in rats. *Pain* 104:501–507, 2003.

Park JM, Houck CS, Sethna NF, et al.: Ketorolac suppresses postoperative bladder spasms after pediatric ureteral reimplantation. *Anesth Analg* 91:11–15, 2000.

Parker RI, Mahan RA, Giugliano D, et al.: Efficacy and safety of intravenous midazolam and ketamine as sedation for therapeutic and diagnostic procedures in children. *Pediatrics* 99:427–431, 1997.

Perry S, Heidrich G: Management of pain during debridement: A survey of U.S. burn units. *Pain* 13:267–280, 1982.

Phillips DM: JCAHO pain management standards are unveiled. Joint Commission on Accreditation of Healthcare Organizations. *JAMA* 284:428–429, 2000.

Pickering AE, Bridge HS, Nolan J, et al.: Double-blind, placebo-controlled analgesic study of ibuprofen or rofecoxib in combination with paracetamol for tonsillectomy in children. *Br J Anaesth* 88:72–77, 2002.

Pintov S, Lahat E, Alstein M, et al.: Acupuncture and the opioid system: Implications in management of migraine. *Pediatr Neurol* 17:129–133, 1997.

Prosser DP, Davis A, Booker PD, et al.: Caudal tramadol for postoperative analgesia in pediatric hypospadias surgery. *Br J Anaesth* 79:293–296, 1997.

Rajagopalan M, Kurian G, John J: Symptom relief with amitriptyline in the irritable bowel syndrome. *J Gastroenterol Hepatol* 13:738–741, 1998.

Rapoff M, Walsh D, Engel JM: Assessment and management of chronic pediatric headaches. Special Issue: Pain in children. *Iss Compr Pediatr Nursing* 11:159–178, 1988.

Rapp SE, Egan KJ, Ross BK, et al.: A multidimensional comparison of morphine and hydromorphone patient-controlled analgesia. *Anesth Analg* 82:1043–1048, 1996.

Rawal N: 10 Years of acute pain services—achievements and challenges. *Reg Anesth Pain Med* 24:68–73, 1999.

Reid GJ, McGrath PJ: Psychological treatments for migraine. *Biomed Pharmacother* 50:58–63, 1996.

Reik L Jr, Hale M: The temporomandibular joint pain-dysfunction syndrome: A frequent cause of headache. *Headache* 21:151–156, 1981.

Reimer EJ, Dunn GS, Montgomery CJ, et al.: The effectiveness of clonidine as an analgesic in paediatric adenotonsillectomy. *Can J Anaesth* 45:1162–1167, 1998.

Resch K, Schilling C, Borchert BD, et al.: Topical anesthesia for pediatric lacerations: A randomized trial of lidocaine-epinephrine-tetracaine solution versus gel. *Ann Emerg Med* 32:693–697, 1998.

Rogers MC: Do the right thing. Pain relief in infants and children. *N Engl J Med* 326:55–56, 1992.

Rose JB, Finkel JC, Arquedas-Mohs A, et al.: Oral tramadol for the treatment of pain of 7-30 days' duration in children. *Anesth Analg* 96:78–81, 2003.
Rowan AB, et al.: Efficacy and cost-effectiveness of minimal therapist contact treatments of chronic headaches: A review. *Behav Therapy* 27:207–234, 1996.
Ruda MA, Ling QD, Hohmann AG, et al.: Altered nociceptive neuronal circuits after neonatal peripheral inflammation. *Science* 289:628–631, 2000.
Ruggeri SB, Athreya BH, Doughty R, et al.: Reflex sympathetic dystrophy in children. *Clin Orthop* 163:225–230, 1982.
Russell W: Caudal tramadol for postoperative analgesia in hypospadias surgery. *Br J Anaesth* 80:408–409, 1998.
Rusy LM, Olsen DJ, Farber NE: Successful use of patient-controlled analgesia in pediatric patients 2 and 3 years old: Two case reports. *Am J Anesthesiol* 14:212–214, 1997.
Rusy LM, Troshynski TJ, Weisman SJ: Gabapentin in phantom limb pain management in children and young adults: Report of seven cases. *J Pain Symptom Manage* 21:78–82, 2001.
Rusy LM, Weisman SJ: Complementary therapies for acute pediatric pain management. *Pediatr Clin North Am* 47:589–599, 2000.
Ruzicka DL, Daniels D: Implementing a pain management service at an Army Medical Center. *Milit Med* 166:146–151, 2001.
Rykowski JJ, Hilgier M: Efficacy of neurolytic celiac plexus block in varying locations of pancreatic cancer: Influence on pain relief. *Anesthesiology* 92:347–354, 2000.
Saavedra JM, Perman JA: Current concepts in lactose malabsorption and intolerance. *Annu Rev Nutr* 9:475–502, 1989.
Saeed MA, Pumariega AJ, Ciniripini PM: Psychopharmacological management of migraine in children and adolescents. *J Child Adolesc Psychopharm* 2:199–211, 1992.
Sahler O, Frager G, Levetown M, et al.: Medical education about end-of-life care in the pediatric setting: Principles, challenges, and opportunities. *Pediatrics* 105:575–584, 2000.
Schechter NL, Allen D: Physicians' attitudes toward pain in children. *J Dev Behav Pediatr* 7:350–354, 1986.
Schilling CG, Bank DE, Borchert BA, et al.: Tetracaine, epinephrine (adrenalin), and cocaine (TAC) versus lidocaine, epinephrine, and tetracaine (LET) for anesthesia of lacerations in children. *Ann Emerg Med* 25:203–208, 1995.
Schultz AA, Strout TD, Jordan P, et al.: Safety, tolerability, and efficacy of dermal anesthesia by lidocaine iontophoresis in emergency department pediatric patients. *Acad Emerg Med* 8:429–430, 2001.
Schwartz BS, Stewart WF, Simon D, et al.: Epidemiology of tension-type headache. *JAMA* 279:381–383, 1998.
Senel AC, Akyol A, Dohman D, et al.: Caudal bupivacaine-tramadol combination for postoperative analgesia in pediatric herniorrhaphy. *Acta Anaesthesiol Scand* 45:786–789, 2001.
Shannon M, Berde CB: Pharmacologic management of pain in children and adolescents. *Pediatr Clin North Am* 36:855–871, 1989.
Shapiro BS, Cohen DE, Covelman KW, et al.: Experience of an interdisciplinary pediatric pain service. *Pediatrics* 88:1226–1232, 1991.
Shapiro BS, Cohen DE, Howe CJ: Patient-controlled analgesia for sickle-cell-related pain. *J Pain Symptom Manage* 8:22–28, 1993.
Siddappa R, Fletcher JE, Heard AM, et al.: Methadone dosage for prevention of opioid withdrawal in children. *Paediatr Anaesth* 13:805–810, 2003.
Silberstein SD, Goadsby PJ, Lipton RB: Management of migraine: An algorithmic approach. *Neurology* 55(9 Suppl 2):S46–S52, 2000.
Silberstein SD, Winner PK, Chmiel JJ: Migraine preventive medication reduces resource utilization. *Headache* 43:171–178, 2003.
Silberstein SD: Practice parameter: Evidence-based guidelines for migraine headache (an evidence-based review): Report of the Quality Standards Subcommittee of the American Academy of Neurology. *Neurology* 55:754–762, 2000.
Sillanpaa M, Piekkala P, Kero P: Prevalence of headache at preschool age in an unselected child population. *Cephalalgia* 11:239–242, 1991.
Sillanpaa M: Clonidine prophylaxis of childhood migraine and other vascular headache. A double blind study of 57 children. *Headache* 17:28–31, 1977.
Sills M, Congdon P, Forsythe I: Clonidine and childhood migraine: A pilot and double-blind study. *Dev Med Child Neurol* 24:837–841, 1982.
Sindrup SH, Jensen TS: Efficacy of pharmacological treatments of neuropathic pain: An update and effect related to mechanism of drug action. *Pain* 83:389–400, 1999.
Singer AJ, Stark MJ: Pretreatment of lacerations with lidocaine, epinephrine, and tetracaine at triage: A randomized double-blind trial. *Acad Emerg Med* 7:751–756, 2000.
Singleton MA, Rosen JI, Fisher DM: Plasma concentrations of fentanyl in infants, children, and adults. *Can J Anaesth* 34:152–155, 1987.
Sirkia K, Hovi L, Pouttu J, et al.: Pain medication during terminal care of children with cancer. *J Pain Symptom Manage* 15:220–226, 1998.
Skoglund LA, Skjelbred P, Fyllingen G: Analgesic efficacy of acetaminophen 1000 mg, acetaminophen 2000 mg, and the combination of acetaminophen 1000 mg and codeine phosphate 60 mg versus placebo in acute postoperative pain. *Pharmacotherapy* 11:364–369, 1991.
Sloan PA, Montgomery C, Musick D: Medical student knowledge of morphine for the management of cancer pain. *J Pain Symptom Manage* 15:359–364, 1998.
Soliman IE, Broadman LM, Hannallah RS, et al.: Comparison of the analgesic effects of EMLA (eutectic mixture of local anesthetics) to intradermal lidocaine infiltration prior to venous cannulation in unpremedicated children. *Anesthesiology* 68:804–806, 1988.
Sprott H, Franke S, Kluge H, et al.: Pain treatment of fibromyalgia by acupuncture. *Rheumatol Int* 18:35–36, 1998.
Sriwatanakul K, Weis OF, Alloza JL, et al.: Analysis of narcotic analgesic usage in the treatment of postoperative pain. *JAMA* 250:926–929, 1983.
Stanton-Hicks M, Janig W, Hassenbusch S, et al.: Reflex sympathetic dystrophy: Changing concepts and taxonomy. *Pain* 63:127–133, 1995.
Starck PL, Sherwood GD, Adams-McNeill J, et al.: Identifying and addressing medical errors in pain mismanagement. *Jt Comm J Qual Improv* 27:191–199, 2001.
Stempak D, Gammon J, Klein J, et al.: Single-dose and steady-state pharmacokinetics of celecoxib in children. *Clin Pharmacol Ther* 72:490–497, 2002.
Stevens B, Johnston C, Petryshen P, et al.: Premature Infant Pain Profile: Development and initial validation. *Clin J Pain* 12:13–22, 1996.
Stone RG, Wharton RB: Simultaneous multiple-modality therapy for tension headaches and neck pain. *Biomed Instrum Technol* 31:259–262, 1997.
Strafford MA, Wilder RT, Berde CB: The risk of infection from epidural analgesia in children: A review of 1620 cases. *Anesth Analg* 80:234–238, 1995.
Stubhaug A, Breivik H, Eide PK, et al.: Mapping of punctuate hyperalgesia around a surgical incision demonstrates that ketamine is a powerful suppressor of central sensitization to pain following surgery. *Acta Anaesthesiol Scand* 41:1124–1132, 1997.
Stubhaug A, Breivik H: Long-term treatment of chronic neuropathic pain with the NMDA (N-methyl-D-aspartate) receptor antagonist ketamine. *Acta Anaesthesiol Scand* 41:329–331, 1997.
Sutters KA, Levine JD, Dibble S, et al.: Analgesic efficacy and safety of single-dose intramuscular ketorolac for postoperative pain management in children following tonsillectomy. *Pain* 61:145–153, 1995.
Taddio A, Stevens B, Craig K, et al.: Efficacy and safety of lidocaine-prilocaine cream for pain during circumcision. *N Engl J Med* 336:1197–1201, 1997.
Taylor I, Harris R: Education in pain management. *Int Anesthesiol Clin* 35:197–206, 1997.
Tobias JD, Phipps S, Smith B, et al.: Oral ketamine premedication to alleviate the distress of invasive procedures in pediatric oncology patients. *Pediatrics* 90:537–541, 1992.
Tobias JD, Schleien CL, Haun SE: Methadone as treatment for iatrogenic narcotic dependency in pediatric intensive care units. *Crit Care Med* 18:1292–1293, 1990.
Tobias JD: Seizure after overdose of tramadol. *South Med J* 90:826–827, 1997.
Tsui BC, Gupta S, Finucane B: Confirmation of epidural catheter placement using nerve stimulation. *Can J Anaesth* 45:640–644, 1998.
Tsui BC, Gupta S, Finucane B: Detection of subarachnoid and intravascular epidural catheter placement. *Can J Anaesth* 46:675–678, 1999.
Tucker GT, Mather LE: Pharmacology of local anaesthetic agents. Pharmacokinetics of local anaesthetic agents. *Br J Anaesth* 47(Suppl):213–224, 1975.
Turturro MA, Paris PM, Larkin GL: Tramadol versus hydrocodone-acetaminophen in acute musculoskeletal pain: A randomized, double-blind clinical trial. *Ann Emerg Med* 32:139–143, 1998.
Twycross A, Mayfield C, Savory J: Pain management for children with special needs: A neglected area? *Paediatr Nurs* 11:43–45, 1999.
Tyler DC: Respiratory effects of pain in a child after thoracotomy. *Anesthesiology* 70:873–874, 1989.
van Lingen RA, et al.: Multiple-dose pharmacokinetics of rectally administered acetaminophen in term infants. *Clin Pharmacol Ther* 66:509–515, 1999a.
van Lingen RA, et al.: Pharmacokinetics and metabolism of rectally administered paracetamol in preterm neonates. *Arch Dis Child Fetal Neonatal Ed* 80:F59–F63, 1999b.
Verne GN, et al.: Central representation of visceral and cutaneous hypersensitivity in the irritable bowel syndrome. *Pain* 103:99–110, 2003.
Verne GN, Price DD: Irritable bowel syndrome as a common precipitant of central sensitization. *Curr Rheumatol Rep* 4:322–328, 2002.
Vetter TR, Heiner EJ: Discordance between patient self-reported visual analog scale pain scores and observed pain-related behavior in older children after surgery. *J Clin Anesth* 8:371–375, 1996.

Viscusi ER, Reynolds L, Chung F, et al.: Patient-controlled transdermal fentanyl hydrochloride vs intravenous morphine pump for postoperative pain: A randomized controlled trial. *JAMA* 291:1333–13341, 2004.

Walco GA, Cassidy RC, Schechter NL: Pain, hurt, and harm. The ethics of pain control in infants and children. *N Engl J Med* 331:541–544, 1994.

Walker LS: The evolution of research on recurrent abdominal pain: History, assumptions, and a conceptual model. In McGrath PJ, Finley GA, editors: *Chronic and recurrent pain in children and adolescents.* Seattle, WA, 1999, IASP Press, pp 141–172.

Wallace MS: Pharmacologic treatment of neuropathic pain. *Curr Pain Headache Rep* 5:138–150, 2001.

Wang JQ, Mao L, Han JS: Comparison of the antinociceptive effects induced by electroacupuncture and transcutaneous electrical nerve stimulation in the rat. *Int J Neurosci* 65:117–129, 1992.

Watcha MF, Jones B, Lagueruela RG, et al.: Comparison of ketorolac and morphine as adjuvants during pediatric surgery. *Anesthesiology* 76:368–372, 1992.

Weinstein SH, Gaylord JC: Determination of oxycodone in plasma and identification of a major metabolite. *J Pharm Sci* 68:527–528, 1979.

Wetzel CH, Connelly JF: Use of gabapentin in pain management. *Ann Pharmacother* 31:1082–1083, 1997.

Weydert JA, Ball TM, Davis MF: Systematic review of treatments for recurrent abdominal pain. *Pediatrics* 111:e1–e11, 2003.

Wiffen P, Collins S, McQuay H, et al.: Anticonvulsant drugs for acute and chronic pain. *Cochrane Database Syst Rev* CD001133, 2000.

Wilder RT, Berde CB, Wolohan M, et al.: Reflex sympathetic dystrophy in children. Clinical characteristics and follow-up of seventy patients. *J Bone Joint Surg Am* 74:910–919, 1992.

Williams EL, Templehoff R, Modica PA, et al.: Sudden cardiac arrest during epidural anesthesia: Venous air embolism? *Anesthesiology* 74:1171, 1991.

Williamson DA, McKenzie SJ, Goreczny AJ: Biofeedback. In Witt JC, et al., editors: *Handbook of behavior therapy in education.* New York, 1988, Plenum Press, pp 547–565.

Wolf AR, Eyres RL, Laussen PC, et al.: Effect of extradural analgesia on stress responses to abdominal surgery in infants. *Br J Anaesth* 70:654–660, 1993.

Wong DL, Baker CM: Pain in children: Comparison of assessment scales. *Pediatr Nurs* 14:9–17, 1988.

Wood CE, Goresky GV, Klassen KA, et al.: Complications of continuous epidural infusions for postoperative analgesia in children. *Can J Anaesth* 41:613–620, 1994.

Woolf CJ, Max MB: Mechanism-based pain diagnosis: Issues for analgesic drug development. *Anesthesiology* 95:241–249, 2001.

World Health Organization: *Cancer pain relief and palliative care. Report of a WHO expert committee.* Geneva, Switzerland, 1990, World Health Organization.

World Health Organization: *Cancer pain relief and palliative care in children.* Geneva, Switzerland, 1998, World Health Organization.

Yaksh TL, Dirig DM, Malmberg AB: Mechanism of action of nonsteroidal anti-inflammatory drugs. *Cancer Invest* 16:509–527, 1998.

Yaksh TL, Malmberg AB: Spinal actions of NSAIDs in blocking spinally mediated hyperalgesia: The role of cyclooxygenase products. *Agents Actions Suppl* 41:89–100, 1993.

Yaster M, Buck JR, Dudgeon DL, et al.: Hemodynamic effects of primary closure of omphalocele/gastroschisis in human newborns. *Anesthesiology* 69:84–88, 1988.

Yaster M, Koehler RC, Traystman RJ: Effects of fentanyl on peripheral and cerebral hemodynamics in neonatal lambs. *Anesthesiology* 66:524–530, 1987.

Yaster M, Koehler RC, Traystman RJ: Interaction of fentanyl and nitrous oxide on peripheral and cerebral hemodynamics in newborn lambs. *Anesthesiology* 80:364–371, 1994.

Yaster M, Krane E, Kaplan R, et al.: *Pediatric pain management and sedation handbook.* St. Louis, 1997, Mosby–Year Book.

Yaster M, Tobin JR, Billett C, et al.: Epidural analgesia in the management of severe vaso-occlusive sickle cell crisis. *Pediatrics* 93:310–315, 1994.

Yaster M: The dose response of fentanyl in neonatal anesthesia. *Anesthesiology* 66:433–435, 1987.

Yi DK, Barr GA: The induction of Fos-like immunoreactivity by noxious thermal, mechanical and chemical stimuli in the lumbar spinal cord of infant rats. *Pain* 60:257–265, 1995.

Yunus MB, Masi AT: Juvenile primary fibromyalgia syndrome. A clinical study of thirty-three patients and matched normal controls. *Arthritis Rheum* 28:138–145, 1985.

Zeltzer L, Lebaron S: Hypnosis and nonhypnotic techniques for reduction of pain and anxiety during painful procedures in children and adolescents with cancer. *J Pediatr* 101:1032–1035, 1982.

Zeltzer LK, Tsao JC, Stelling C, et al.: A phase I study on the feasibility and acceptability of an acupuncture/hypnosis intervention for chronic pediatric pain. *J Pain Symptom Manage* 24:437–446, 2002.

Zempsky WT, Anand KJ, Sullivan KM, et al.: Lidocaine iontophoresis for topical anesthesia before intravenous line placement in children. *J Pediatr* 132:1061–1063, 1998.

Zempsky WT, Karasic RB: EMLA versus TAC for topical anesthesia of extremity wounds in children. *Ann Emerg Med* 30:163–166, 1997.

Zenz M, Zenner D: Tramadol or ketamine for caudal analgesia? *Br J Anaesth* 85:805–807, 2000.

14 Pediatric Regional Anesthesia

Allison Kinder Ross

The practice of pediatric regional anesthesia has evolved over the past century from the study of spinal anesthetics in infants and children to an integral part of a sophisticated multispecialty practice involving continuous local anesthetic infusions with patient-controlled analgesia based on age-appropriate pharmacokinetics. Performing regional anesthetics in children may be perceived as difficult because of the age-related variations in anatomy and depth of structures. In addition, other issues, such as increased risk of toxicity of local anesthetics and lack of appropriate equipment, may present challenges to many practitioners when it comes to performing regional anesthesia in a child. To safely practice regional anesthesia in children, it is important to understand the safety issues regarding the pharmacokinetics of local anesthetics and their additives, to have knowledge of the anatomy in children of different ages, and to be aware of the indications and complications of the specific regional blocks.

SAFETY ISSUES

There are five major safety concerns regarding administering regional anesthesia to children:

1. Need for children to be anesthetized for placement of the regional block
2. Age-related changes regarding neurotoxicity
3. Risks of infection
4. Ability of regional anesthesia to mask an underlying compartment syndrome
5. Proper use of local anesthetics and risk of local anesthetic toxicity

REGIONAL ANESTHESIA IN THE ANESTHETIZED CHILD

Perhaps the biggest difference between adult and pediatric regional anesthesia other than the obvious size discrepancies is that children typically receive their regional anesthetic while they are under general anesthesia. This practice remains controversial outside of the pediatric arena (Bromage, 1996; Bromage and Benumof, 1998; Rosenquist and Birnback, 2003). Part of this criticism was based on a closed-claim case report of a woman who developed paraplegia following the placement of an epidural while she was under general anesthesia. As was pointed out in editorials by Fischer (1998) and by Krane and others (1998), this particular case, however, does not support the argument that the general anesthetic was the basis for the bad outcome. The actual cause of the paraplegia remains unknown, and there were many factors that could have led to such an outcome, such as previous lumbar laminectomy, unsuccessful initial attempts for epidural placement, placement of a thoracic epidural catheter, multiple episodes of intraoperative hypotension, and the presence of air in the thoracic region at the spinal cord on magnetic resonance imaging (MRI). Bromage and Benumof made the assumption that the patient could have warned the practitioners of a problem had she not been under general anesthesia. This also assumes that the patient's sedation would have been at a level that would have allowed her to provide warning signs. Although these assumptions may have some basis of defense, difficult block placement by inexperienced practitioners, use of air for loss of resistance, and intraoperative hypotension are all major risk factors for adverse outcome whether general anesthesia is present or not. Further, because of differences in patient cooperation, the practice of performing a regional anesthetic in children differs greatly from placing a block in an adult. The practice of performing regional anesthetic blocks during general anesthesia in children, including thoracic epidural blocks, is an accepted practice as long as the individual has the proper training and expertise. Over 50 international pediatric anesthesiologists signed the editorial by Krane and others to support the placement of blocks in anesthetized children. In fact, "it would be considered malpractice to perform such techniques in patients who were *not* fully anesthetized" (Dalens, 1999) and "any performance of a block in an agitated and moving child is not only unethical, but could be dangerous when the needle approaches the delicate nervous structures" (De Negri et al., 2002).

Rosenquist and Birnback wrote an editorial in response to a large retrospective study of 4298 adult thoracic surgical patients who underwent lumbar epidural catheter placement while under general anesthesia (Horlocker et al., 2003). In this large series, there were no neurologic complications including radicular symptoms or persistent paresthesias. Rosenquist and Birnback, however, echoed the sentiments of Bromage and Benumof that the risk-benefit ratio does not support the use of epidural blocks in anesthetized patients; they also stated that epidural blocks have been used in anesthetized children for over a decade and that "extrapolation of pediatric data to adult practice is not warranted and offers no reassurance" (2003).

In children who are under general anesthesia or who are heavily sedated, it may be difficult to recognize intravascular injection of a local anesthetic. For this reason, the practice of test dosing with a local anesthetic with the addition of epinephrine has been readdressed and should be a common practice (Tobias, 2001). It is also argued that an anesthetized child cannot warn the practitioner of a significant paresthesia and that there is the potential risk of neurologic injury from intraneural placement of a needle or anesthetic. This is a hypothetical risk that has not been supported by reports of large series of pediatric regional anesthetics (Pietropaoli et al., 1993; Goldman, 1995; Giaufre et al., 1996).

AGE-RELATED CHANGES IN NEUROTOXICITY

The use of local anesthetics and neurotoxicity on the developing nerve is an area that continues to be addressed. Animal data have demonstrated that all local anesthetics are potentially neurotoxic, and this neurotoxicity parallels their anesthetic potency (Selander, 1993). The factors that contribute to the mechanism of the neurotoxicity include the concentration of the local anesthetic and the time of exposure of the nerve to the local anesthetic. This is important in children, particularly in neonates, who may be at the greatest risk of direct neurotoxicity during nerve development and should not receive the higher concentrations of local anesthetics. Studies on rabbit nerve fibers have demonstrated an increased sensitivity to the blocking effects of local anesthetics in young nerves (Benzon et al., 1988). Additional in vitro biologic investigation has demonstrated that lidocaine, bupivacaine, mepivacaine, and ropivacaine all are capable of producing growth cone collapse and neurite degeneration (Radwan, 2002). However, the incidence of growth cone collapse with bupivacaine and ropivacaine is insignificant compared with lidocaine and mepivacaine. Additional investigation in this area is imperative to better understand the mechanisms behind neural injury and how it may affect nerves in children of different ages.

RISK OF INFECTION

Another safety consideration is the practice of preparing the skin before a regional block to reduce the risk of infection. Before placing any block, sterile preparation of the skin should be performed, but this is particularly important for central blocks to reduce the risk of meningitis or epidural abscess. The use of povidone-iodine, although useful for cleansing the skin before a regional block, may be harmful to the very sensitive skin of an infant. The povidone-iodine should also be allowed to dry and not be carried centrally with the needle into the epidural or subdural spaces. After the block has been placed, the iodine should be washed from the skin to avoid iodine burns. Chlorhexidine is recommended over the use of povidone-iodine as it has been shown to decrease colonization when used in young children for epidural catheter placement (Kinirons et al., 2001; Wagner and Prielipp, 2003). The actual risk of infection from regional techniques, however, is extremely low. For indwelling caudal catheters, the incidence of catheter tip colonization is 20% versus 4% for indwelling epidural catheters (McNeely et al., 1997). No patients with bacterial colonization of the catheters exhibited systemic signs of infection. Strafford and others (1995) studied 1620 children who received epidural catheters. There were no infections in the children who had the catheters placed for postoperative analgesia and only one significant infection in an immunosuppressed child who received a catheter on a long-term basis for pain secondary to her malignancy (Strafford et al., 1995). Giaufre and others (1996), in a prospective study of over 24,000 regional techniques performed in children by members of the French-Language Society of Pediatric Anesthesiologists, reported no infections.

COMPARTMENT SYNDROME

A concern often cited for failure to perform a regional anesthetic in pediatric patients for orthopedic procedures is the risk of an unrecognized compartment syndrome. The theory behind this concern is that the local anesthetic in the regional block may mask the initial symptoms of the sensation of pressure in the limb, which may lead to unrecognized compartment syndrome (Dunwoody et al., 1997). Case reports in children have demonstrated that a successful epidural block with a low concentration of local anesthetic does not mask the symptoms of compartment syndrome. They recommended that one should perform serial examinations on children to assess the operated extremity in the presence of good analgesia. Another option in a high-risk child is to measure compartmental pressures postoperatively in children who would clearly benefit from infusions of local anesthetic, such as those who have undergone microvascular surgery or amputation.

LOCAL ANESTHETICS IN CHILDREN

There are age-related changes in local anesthetic pharmacokinetics and pharmacodynamics. There are two classes of local anesthetics: the amides and the esters. Amides undergo enzymatic degradation in the liver. Local amide anesthetics should be used carefully in children, particularly in neonates and infants, as they may lack the ability to distribute and metabolize these agents effectively. Ester anesthetic agents are metabolized by plasma cholinesterase and have less age-related changes in metabolism.

Amide-class local anesthetics include lidocaine, etidocaine, prilocaine, mepivacaine, bupivacaine, levobupivacaine, and ropivacaine. Although all of these agents have been used for regional anesthesia in adults, etidocaine, mepivacaine, and prilocaine are rarely used in children. The choice of local anesthetic depends not only on the desired onset time and duration of action of the regional block but also on the safety of the agent.

Amide anesthetics are primarily protein bound in the plasma. Bupivacaine, levobupivacaine, and ropivacaine are more than 90% bound to the plasma proteins α_1-acid glycoprotein (high affinity for local anesthetics) and albumin (high volume and relatively

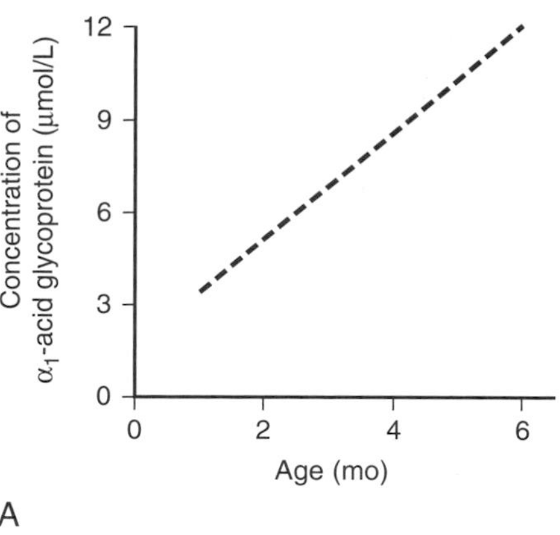

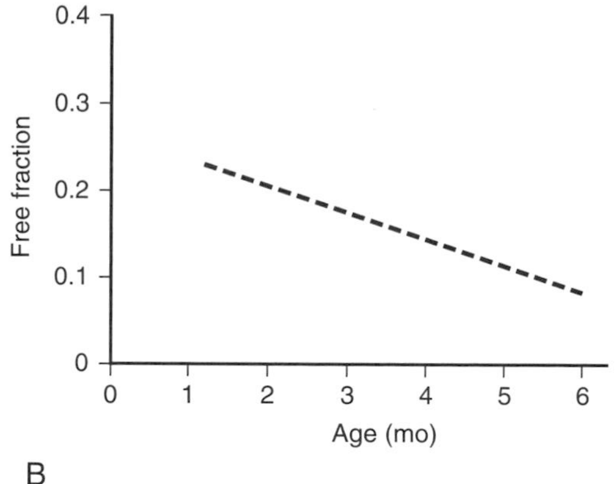

■ **FIGURE 14–1.** *A*, Age-related changes in the plasma concentration of α_1-acid glycoprotein. *B*, Age-related changes in the plasma free fraction of bupivacaine. (From Mazoit JX, Denson DD, Samii K: Pharmacokinetics of bupivacaine following caudal anesthesia in infants. *Anesthesiology* 68:387, 1988.)

low affinity for local anesthetics). It is the free or unbound fraction of the local anesthetic that is physiologically active and is responsible for its effect on the cardiovascular and central nervous systems. Infants less than 6 months of age have decreased levels of plasma proteins, which results in a larger free fraction of local anesthetic and consequently places this age group at a greater risk of toxicity from these agents (Lerman et al., 1989; Berde, 1992). As an infant matures, the plasma proteins increase and the plasma free fraction of the drug decreases. Adult levels of protein binding are reached at about 1 year of age (Fig. 14–1). Of interest is that α_1-acid glycoprotein levels increase in response to surgical stress, and the increased α_1-acid glycoprotein ultimately decreases the free fraction of local anesthetic agent. This occurs even when total plasma concentration appears to be near toxic levels (Tucker, 1994, 1996; Booker, 1996). Metabolism of amide local anesthetics occurs via the liver's cytochrome P450 system. These enzymes reach adult activity by the first year of life. The immaturity of liver enzymes in neonates and infants contributes to the decreased clearance of amide local anesthetics seen in this time period.

Ester anesthetics (e.g., chloroprocaine and tetracaine) depend on plasma esterases for their elimination. Similar to the decreased levels of plasma proteins in neonates and infants, there are decreased levels of plasma esterases as well (Zsigmond and Downs, 1971). This, however, has not been shown to be of clinical significance, and tetracaine is commonly used for spinal anesthetics in premature infants for inguinal hernia repairs. Chloroprocaine, although not a commonly used pediatric local anesthetic, has been used for caudal anesthesia. It is thought to afford a greater level of safety than amide anesthetics because of its rapid metabolism (Henderson et al., 1993; Tobias et al., 1996).

LOCAL ANESTHETICS AND RISKS OF TOXICITY

Children may be at increased risk of toxicity of local anesthetics because of their relatively increased cardiac output and increased systemic uptake of the agent. This increased systemic uptake may result in direct central nervous system (CNS) toxicity by increasing the amount of local anesthetic available to cross the blood-brain barrier. In addition, increased systemic uptake can cause direct cardiac toxicity. Lidocaine at plasma levels of 2 to 4 mcg/mL acts as an anticonvulsant, but at 10 mcg/mL, it produces convulsions (Dalens, 1995). Neonates, for example, manifest symptoms of neurotoxicity such as depressed Apgar scores from lidocaine at umbilical venous blood concentrations of 2.5 mcg/mL, significantly lower than the 5 mcg/mL that is associated with neurotoxicity in adults (Foldes et al., 1960; Shnider and Way, 1968; Ralston and Shnider, 1978; Tucker, 1986).

In unmedicated patients, initial symptoms of neurotoxicity include headache, somnolence, vertigo, and perioral or lingual paresthesia. These symptoms and any objective signs of neurotoxicity such as tremors, twitching, shivering, or actual convulsions may not be detected in infants and children under general anesthesia. Diagnosis of local anesthetic toxicity under general anesthesia can be made with indirect signs such as muscular rigidity, hypoxemia without other causes, unexplained tachycardia, dysrhythmias, or cardiovascular collapse. General anesthetics are protective from the CNS effects, but general anesthetics are not protective against cardiac toxicity and may even further contribute to the toxicity (Badgwell et al., 1990).

Cardiac toxicity occurs as the local anesthetic prevents the fast inward sodium channels in the myocardium from opening. Manifestations of toxicity from bupivacaine consist of dysrhythmias with evidence of high degree of conduction block, widening of the QRS, torsades de pointes, ventricular tachycardia related to reentry phenomena, or major cardiovascular collapse with decreased myocardial contractility (de La Coussaye et al., 1992). Bupivacaine may produce cardiac and CNS toxicity at serum concentrations of 2 mcg/mL in children (Tucker, 1986; Dalens and Mazoit, 1998). Although 2 mcg/mL is considered the toxic threshold for bupivacaine in children, and 4 mcg/mL in adults, the true toxic concentration of unbound bupivacaine is unknown in humans (Knudsen et al., 1997; Luz et al., 1998; Meunier et al., 2001; Berde, 1993).

Bupivacaine

Bupivacaine is a racemic mixture of equimolar amounts of *R*(+)-bupivacaine and *S*(−)-bupivacaine. Racemic bupivacaine had been the only amide local anesthetic with long duration and therefore the most commonly used amide local anesthetic in children. Pharmacokinetic studies of a single dose of racemic bupivacaine (2.5 mg/kg) injected in the caudal space have demonstrated differences between infants and children (Ecoffey et al., 1985; Desparmet et al., 1987; Mazoit et al., 1988). Infants have a greater volume of distribution (3.9 L/kg versus 2.7 L/kg), an increased elimination half-life (7.7 versus 4.6 hours), and decreased clearance (7.1 versus 10.0 mL/kg per min) compared with older children (Table 14–1). Although side effects from

■ **TABLE 14–1.** Summary of pharmacokinetics of local anesthetics in children

Agent	Block/Dose	Age of Child	C_{max} (mg/L)	T_{max} (min)	V_d (L/kg)	Cl (mL/kg per min)	$t_{1/2}$ (hr)	Reference
Bupivacaine	Caudal 2.5 mg/kg	1 to 6 mo	(0.55 to 1.93)	(10 to 60)	3.9 ± 2.0	7.1 ± 3.2	7.7 ± 2.4	Mazoit and others, 1988
	Epidural infusion 0.2 mg/kg per hr	11 mo to 15 yr	NM	NM	NM	6.49 (3.96 to 11.11)	3.36 ± 0.93	Desparmet and others, 1987
	Caudal 2.5 mg/kg	0 to 5 mo	1.109 (0.6 to 2.195)	60 (30 to 240)	NM	NM	2.75 (1.7 to 4.4)	Hansen and others, 2001
	Caudal 2.5 mg/kg plus epinephrine 2.5 mcg/mL		1.102 (0.449 to 1.909)	60 (60 to 360)			6.05 (3.97 to 8.95)	
	Ilioinguinal/ iliohypogastric 2 mg/kg (0.5%)	2 to 16 yr	2.2 ± 1.0	24 ± 11.9	NM	NM	3.6 ± 1.8	Ala-Kokko and others, 2002
Ropivacaine	Caudal 2 mg/kg	1 to 8 yr	0.47 ± 0.16	60 (12 to 249)	2.4 ± 0.7	7.4 ± 1.9	3.2 ± 0.8	Lonnqvist and others, 2000
	Caudal 2 mg/kg	<1 yr	0.73 ± 0.27	60 (15 to 90)	NM	NM	NM	Wulf and others, 2000
		1 to 5 yr	0.49 ± 0.21	52.5 (30 to 120)				
	Caudal 2 mg/kg	0 to 3 mo	0.748 (0.425-1.579)	NM	2.12 ± 0.75 (all infants)	3.1 ± 1.6 (all infants)	5.1 (all infants)	Hansen and others, 2001
		3 to 12 mo	0.604 (0.41-1.278)					
	Epidural 1.7 mg/kg	3 to 11 mo	0.61 (0.55 to 0.725)	60 (60 to 120)	2.37 (9%)	4.26 (9%)	NM	McCann and others, 2001
		1 to 4 yr	0.64 (0.54 to 0.75)	60 (30 to 90)	2.37 (9%)	6.15 (11%)	NM	
	Epidural infusion 0.4 mg/kg per hr	0.3 to 7.3 yr	NM	NM	3.1 (2.1 to 4.2)	8.5 (5.8 to 11.1)	4.9 (3 to 6.7)	Hansen and others, 2000
	Ilioinguinal/ iliohypogastric 2 mg/kg (0.75%)	2 to 16 yr	1.5 ± 0.8	35 ± 15.4	NM	NM	6.5 ± 4.4	Ala-Kokko and others, 2002
	Ilioinguinal/ iliohypogastric 3 mg/kg (0.5%)	1 to 12 yr	1.5 ± 0.93	45 (15 to 64)	NM	NM	2.0 ± 0.7	Dalens and others, 2001

Values are stated either with ±SD value, or with ranges or partition coefficients in parentheses.

C_{max}, peak plasma concentration; T_{max}, time to peak plasma concentration; V_d, volume of distribution; Cl, plasma clearance; $t_{1/2}$, terminal half-life; NM, not measured.

bupivacaine are rare, they can be serious, ranging from CNS excitation to cardiovascular collapse from direct cardiotoxicity. Case reports of possible toxicity of racemic bupivacaine secondary to continuous infusions of bupivacaine were reported in the early 1990s (Agarwal et al., 1992; McCloskey et al., 1992). In the report of McCloskey and others, children had continuous caudal infusions of 0.25% bupivacaine at doses between 1.67 and 2.5 mg/kg per hr. One neonate sustained bradycardia and hypotension, and two older children developed seizures. Bupivacaine serum concentrations at the time of the event ranged between 5.6 and 20.3 mcg/mL. In the cases reported by Agarwal and others (1992), one child who developed a seizure had an intrapleural catheter with a bupivacaine infusion rate of 0.5 mg/kg per hr. The seizure occurred with a plasma bupivacaine level of 5.6 mcg/mL. The other child in this report had a continuous bupivacaine epidural infusion at 1.25 mg/kg per hr, and seizures occurred with a plasma bupivacaine level of 5.4 mcg/mL. All children in the reports from McCloskey and Agarwal had plasma bupivacaine levels that exceeded the toxic threshold of bupivacaine (2-4 mcg/mL).

An editorial by Berde (1992) addresses the false generalization that children are more resistant to local anesthetic toxicity than are adults. Although earlier studies involving children noted no evidence of toxicity in patients with plasma concentrations of bupivacaine from 1 to 7 mcg/mL, the use of benzodiazepines in those children may have been protective (McIlvaine et al., 1988). Badgwell and others (1990) reported greater resistance to toxicity in 2-day-old piglets compared with older piglets. However, the direct application of this study to neonates is difficult because neonates have lower plasma protein concentrations and lower bupivacaine clearance. Berde recommended (1) that maximal allowable doses of local anesthetics should not be exceeded (Table 14–2), (2) infusion rates should be reduced in children with risk factors for seizures, and (3) the maximal allowable doses should be reduced by at least 30% for infants less than 6 months of age (Berde, 1992).

Levobupivacaine

Levobupivacaine is the *S*(–)-enantiomer of bupivacaine and is less toxic to the CNS or heart than is racemic bupivacaine (Mazoit et al., 1993; Graf et al., 1997; Huang et al., 1998). The decreased risk of cardiotoxicity from levobupivacaine has been shown in healthy adult volunteers after intravenous administration of either levobupivacaine or racemic bupivacaine (Bardsley et al., 1998). Although similar intravenous studies have not been done in children, animal and human studies suggest less toxicity and equipotency of levobupivacaine compared with bupivacaine (Mather and Chang, 2001; McLeod and Burke, 2001; Gristwood, 2002). Pharmacokinetic studies of levobupivacaine have not been completed in children.

Ropivacaine

Ropivacaine has shown promise in pediatric patients with the onset times similar to bupivacaine and durations of actions that are similar or perhaps slightly longer than bupivacaine (DaConceicao et al., 1998, 1999; Ivani et al., 1998, 2002; Lonnqvist et al., 2000; Hansen et al., 2001; Locatelli et al., 2005). There remains controversy as to the potency of ropivacaine compared with bupivacaine and adult studies do not correlate with pediatric studies (Ivani, 2002). Although not confirmed, ropivacaine at 0.2% exhibits the same analgesic effect as 0.25% in children, perhaps because of the intrinsic vasoconstrictive activity that is evident at the lower concentrations used in children (Ivani, 2002). Ropivacaine has less risk of CNS and cardiac toxicity than bupivacaine. In fact, inadvertent intravenous ropivacaine in a 1-year-old child failed to produce neurotoxic or cardiotoxic signs or symptoms (Thong et al., 2000). In a pharmacokinetic study of ropivacaine in children aged 1 to 8 who were administered 1 mL/kg 0.2% ropivacaine for caudal block, the free plasma concentrations were well below toxic levels (Lonnqvist et al., 2000). Clearance of the drug was 7.4 mL/kg per min and the terminal half-life was 3.2 hours. Hansen and others (2001) studied the pharmacokinetics of caudal ropivacaine in infants less than 1 year of age (see Table 14–1). In this study, infants less than 3 months of age were compared with the infants aged 3 months to 1 year (Hansen et al., 2001). Although the maximum free concentration of ropivacaine was significantly higher in the younger age group (99 mcg/L versus 38 mcg/L), the total and free plasma concentrations in all of the children less than 1 year old were within the range of concentrations previously reported in adults and older children (Lonnqvist et al., 2000; Wulf et al., 2000).

Reducing Risks of Toxicity

There are several safety measures that can reduce the risks of toxicity from local anesthetics in children. One primary safety measure is to avoid overdosing by adhering to recommendations for maximal allowable doses. For a bolus injection, the maximal recommended dose of lidocaine is 5 mg/kg. Because epinephrine decreases the uptake and absorption of local anesthetic, the dose of lidocaine can be increased to 7 mg/kg when epinephrine (5 mcg/mL) is added to the local anesthetic. Because levobupivacaine and ropivacaine have intrinsic vasoconstriction properties, the addition of epinephrine does not increase the maximal

TABLE 14–2. Maximal allowable dosing guidelines of local anesthetics

Local Anesthetic	Single Dose (mg/kg)	Continuous Infusion Rate (mg/kg per hr)	Continuous Infusion Rate in Infants <6 Months of Age‡ (mg/kg per hr)
Bupivacaine	3	0.4 to 0.5	0.2 to 0.25
Levobupivacaine	3*	0.4 to 0.5	0.2 to 0.25
Ropivacaine	3*	0.4 to 0.5	0.2 to 0.25
Lidocaine	5	1.6	0.8
Lidocaine with epinephrine†	7	NA	NA

Modified from Berde, 1992.
NA, not applicable.
*Maximal allowable dose may be up to 4 mg/kg (under investigation).
†Epinephrine added to local anesthetic at 5 mcg/mL or 1:200,000.
‡Rate should be reduced by additional 30% after 48 hours in infants.

recommended dose. The maximal allowable bolus dose for bupivacaine, ropivacaine, and levobupivacaine is 3 mg/kg (Agarwal et al., 1992; McCloskey et al., 1992). Recommendations for maximal dosing of continuous infusions are presented in Table 14–2 and are the same for bupivacaine, levobupivacaine, and ropivacaine (Berde, 1992). For epidural infusions, the infusion rates should not exceed 0.4 to 0.5 mg/kg per hr for patients greater than 6 months of age, and the recommendation for neonates is not to exceed 0.2 to 0.25 mg/kg per hr. Based on the clearance of bupivacaine and using the guidelines in Table 14–2, the plasma concentrations should remain below 2.5 mcg/mL and therefore below the toxic level of 4 mcg/mL in adults and recommended level of less than 2 mcg/mL in children. (Tucker, 1986; Desparmet et al., 1987; Mazoit et al., 1988; Berde, 1993). These infusions assume a loading dose of 2 to 2.5 mg/kg of bupivacaine and should be reduced by 25% in patients with risk factors for seizures (e.g., past history of febrile seizures, hypomagnesemia, and hyponatremia) (Agarwal et al., 1992; Berde, 1992).

In addition to dosing guidelines, the risk of toxicity is also affected by hypothermia, hypoxia, hypercarbia, acidosis, or hyperkalemia (Broadman, 1996). These factors enhance the toxicity of local anesthetics via different mechanisms. Another factor that leads to increased toxicity is the speed of injection of the local anesthetic agent. Rapid injections can cause toxicity by resulting in a high peak that may not allow for the adaptation of sodium channels against the local anesthetic action.

When combined, the toxicities of two local anesthetics are additive. If the maximal allowable dose of one local anesthetic has been reached, another local anesthetic agent should *not* be delivered (Giaufre et al., 1996). Although combinations of local anesthetics may be a common practice at some centers, maximal allowable dosing should be calculated for each of the anesthetics used and decreased based on the relative percentages of each.

The choice of local anesthetic is a clinical decision. In general, lower concentrations of local anesthetics such as 0.25% bupivacaine or levobupivacaine and 0.2% ropivacaine may be used in infants and small children, and higher concentrations such as 0.5% bupivacaine, levobupivacaine, or ropivacaine should be reserved for older children. Higher concentrations result in longer duration of action and increased motor block. In young children, there is a risk of direct local anesthetic toxicity on developing nerves (Selander, 1993; Lambert et al., 1994; Radwan et al., 2002). The age at which this is no longer a concern is unknown.

Test Dosing

Before injecting local anesthetics, it is essential to determine that the agent not be injected into the intravascular space. The absence of blood aspiration when administering a pediatric block is not a reliable indicator that the needle is not in a vessel. Infants, in particular, may be at greatest risk of intravascular injection (Freid et al., 1993; Ved et al., 1993; Flandin-Blety and Barrier, 1995). Although clinical practice has relied on a "test dose" to elicit a tachycardia when the test drug is inadvertently injected systemically, the test dose was often considered unreliable in the anesthetized patient (Desparmet et al., 1990). In the study of Desparmet and others of children anesthetized with halothane, only 16 of 21 children who received a test dose of 0.1% lidocaine with epinephrine 1:200,000 had an increase in heart rate that was greater than 10 beats per minute (bpm). When using halothane anesthesia, an increase of 20 bpm with prior administration of atropine improves the efficacy of the test dose. Isoproterenol has also been used as a test drug, and although it is a more reliable indicator of an intravascular injection in patients anesthetized with halothane (Perillo et al., 1993; Kozek-Langenecker et al., 1996), the safety of isoproterenol with neuraxial administration has not been determined. The validity of test dosing has been studied and reviewed (Tanaka and Nishikawa, 1998, 1999; Tobias, 2001). Using sevoflurane anesthesia, Tanaka and Nishikawa (1998, 1999) were able to demonstrate that an increase in heart rate of 10 bpm, an increase change in T-wave amplitude of 25%, or blood pressure increase of greater than 15 mm Hg defines a positive test dose. Prior administration of atropine did not affect these criteria.

A test dose can be a useful tool for identifying intravascular injection when the appropriate criteria are used. The test dose should not, however, be a replacement for slow incremental dosing of the total volume of the local anesthetic, attention to vital signs, and electrocardiographic monitoring throughout the drug administration. A recommended test dose under sevoflurane anesthesia is 0.1 mL/kg of the chosen local anesthetic with epinephrine 5 mcg/mL added but not to exceed 3 mL. A heart rate increase of 10 bpm, a systolic blood pressure increase of 15 mm Hg, a T-wave amplitude increase of greater than 25% from baseline, or bradycardia should alert the practitioner to possible intravascular injection (Tanaka and Nishikawa, 1998; 1999; Freid et al., 1993; Fisher et al., 1997; Tobias, 2001).

Another advantage of epinephrine administration in regional anesthesia is that, in addition to being a reliable marker for intravascular injection, the use of epinephrine decreases systemic absorption of the local anesthetic (Eyres et al., 1983, 1986). Children may be at increased risk of local anesthetic toxicity from increased systemic absorption because of their relatively higher cardiac output and regional blood flow. In a study comparing bupivacaine with epinephrine 5 mcg/mL to bupivacaine alone in children for fascia iliaca block, Doyle and others (1997) demonstrated that the peak plasma concentration was lower in the bupivacaine with epinephrine group (0.35 mcg/mL versus 1.1 mcg/mL) and that the time to peak concentration was more gradual (20 minutes versus 40 minutes from injection).

REVIEWS OF SAFETY OF REGIONAL ANESTHESIA IN CHILDREN

Despite the issues of the safety of regional anesthesia in children, as previously mentioned, studies have shown that the risks and complications in regional anesthesia in children are quite low and often preventable (Dalens and Hasnouai, 1989; Pietropaoli et al., 1993; Giaufre et al., 1996; Dalens and Mazoit, 1998). The largest of these studies was published by the French-Language Society of Pediatric Anesthesiologists (ADARPEF) (Giaufre et al., 1996). This prospective report covered 1 year and included 24,409 regional blocks in children. Central blocks accounted for greater than 60% of the blocks, whereas peripheral nerve blocks and local anesthetic techniques made up the remaining 38%. There were only 25 complications that occurred in the study, and all of the complications occurred in children who received central blocks. The overall complication rate of regional anesthesia was 0.9 per 1000.

The most common complications from regional blockade were inadvertent dural puncture (n=8), inadvertent intravascular injection of local anesthetic (n=6), technical problem (n=3), and overdosage of local anesthesia leading to dysrhythmias (n=2).

In addition, two children had transient paresthesias, one child had apnea after central morphine, and one child had a skin lesion after a caudal anesthetic administration. In this study, there were no deaths secondary to any of the complications. The conclusion from this study of regional anesthesia in children was that complications were rare and minor and that they occurred most often in the operating room where they were readily managed. In addition, when appropriate, a peripheral nerve block may be preferable to a central block.

The use of appropriately sized equipment for pediatric regional blocks cannot be overemphasized. The ease of performing a block in a small child is enhanced with the use of shorter, smaller-gauge needles that allow for exact placement. Eleven of the reviewed 23 complications in the large ADARPEF safety study could be contributed to the use of inappropriate equipment.

In a retrospective review of 24,005 regional anesthetics administered over a 10-year period, Flandin-Blety and Barrier (1995) reported 108 events without sequelae (0.45%). In this review, there were five events that resulted in severe neurologic injury, including tetraplegia in three children, paraplegia in one child, and one child with cerebral lesions. All five of the children were healthy and less than 3 months of age. Four of the five children had loss of resistance to air used for their technique to identify the epidural space. The true pathophysiologic causes for the neurologic injuries in these children are unknown, but the authors recommended that air not be used to identify the epidural space and that a lower concentration of epinephrine, such as 2.5 mcg/mL, be used to avoid possible ischemic injury. In addition, the authors recommended that the indications for regional anesthesia be reconsidered in children less than 18 months of age due to their incomplete myelination of neuronal fibers.

ADVANTAGES OF REGIONAL ANESTHESIA IN CHILDREN

There are advantages to the use of regional anesthesia that are evident and continue to increase the popularity of its practice. The use of regional anesthesia in combination with general anesthesia results in reduced concentrations of potent inhaled agents and reduced or absent use of opioids resulting in quick recovery times and less nausea and vomiting (Dalens and Hasnaoui, 1989; Yaster and Maxwell, 1989). In addition, regional anesthesia suppresses the neuroendocrine responses to surgery compared with general anesthesia alone (Murat et al., 1988; Wolf et al., 1993). Regional anesthesia as the sole technique for inguinal hernia repair has been shown to decrease the incidence of postoperative apnea in former preterm infants (Welborn et al., 1990, 1991; Cote et al., 1995; Krane et al., 1995). Although large numbers of outcome studies are lacking, regional anesthetic techniques have been shown to decrease the incidence of postoperative complications and reduce hospital stay (McNeely et al., 1997; Miller et al., 2002).

In addition to the advantages that regional anesthesia may offer, regional techniques have also been used for therapeutic purposes. Patients have received regional blocks for vascular insufficiency related to meningococcemia, Kawasaki's disease, erythromelalgia, and sickle cell disease (Edwards et al., 1988; Anderson et al., 1989; Tobias et al., 1989; D'Angelo et al., 1992; Yaster et al., 1994; Tobias, 2002). Lumbar sympathetic block has been used for infants and children with ischemic limbs secondary to arterial or intravenous infiltration (Sanchez et al., 1988), and stellate ganglion block has been effective for upper extremity ischemia (Lagade and Poppers, 1984; Parris et al., 1991). Regional anesthesia has also been a therapeutic tool in the treatment of postdural puncture headache. Epidural blood patches have been used successfully in a variety of children for this indication (Ylonen and Kokki, 2002).

CENTRAL NEURAXIAL BLOCKADE

Central blockade is performed in children for many of the same reasons that it is performed in adults, such as bilateral lower extremity, abdominal, and thoracic procedures. There are risks and benefits to performing central blocks that are inherent to the type of block chosen. Central blocks that are commonly performed in children include spinal blocks and epidural blocks. Epidural blocks may be placed at the caudal, lumbar, and thoracic levels. Contraindication to central blockade includes a child on anticoagulation therapy, a patient with a preexisting coagulopathy, or a patient or parent who refuses to consent to the procedure. Guidelines regarding regional anesthesia and anticoagulation therapy in adults may be useful for guiding the management of the child with similar concerns (Horlocker et al., 2003) (Table 14–3).

SPINAL ANESTHESIA

Spinal anesthesia was probably the earliest form of regional anesthesia that was considered a useful practice for children (Bainbridge, 1901; Tyrell-Gray, 1909). Since that time, spinal anesthetics have become an important anesthetic technique for reducing the incidence of postoperative apnea in premature and ex-premature infants (Harnik et al., 1986; Welborn et al., 1990; Krane et al., 1995; Somri et al., 1998). Infants who have continuing apnea at home or hematocrit less than 30% are at particular risk for postoperative apnea (Cote et al., 1995). Spinal anesthesia may also reduce the need for postoperative mechanical ventilation in those infants who are less than 60 weeks' postconceptual age after hernia repair (Huang and Hirshberg, 2001). The ability of a spinal anesthetic to densely block the dermatomes involved in inguinal hernia repair has kept this regional technique a popular choice in pediatric anesthesia for inguinal surgery. Often a spinal anesthetic combined with liberal clear liquids until 2 hours before the procedure and a pacifier intraoperatively are sufficient to keep an ex-premature infant comfortable while undergoing inguinal hernia repair. However, any ex-premature infant up to 44 weeks' postconceptual age, and up to 60 weeks' postconceptual age if the infant has risk factors such as anemia or ongoing apnea, should be a candidate for overnight monitoring after their surgery regardless of whether a pure regional technique was used.

Although spinal anesthesia may be used in any age group, there are relatively few true indications for a spinal anesthetic in older children. Older children may be at increased risk of postdural puncture headaches (Wee, 1996).

Anatomy

The anatomic differences between an infant and a young child or adult are clinically significant and must be taken into consideration when performing a spinal technique. The dural sac in a newborn ends at S3, and the conus medullaris may be located at L3 (Plate 14–1; color image is available on the DVD). To avoid the risk of spinal cord puncture in a neonate, a spinal

■ **TABLE 14–3.** American Society of Regional Anesthesia and Pain Medicine Guidelines for neuraxial anesthesia in patients receiving thromboprophylaxis

Antiplatelet Medication	Subcutaneous Heparin	Intravenous Heparin	Low-Molecular-Weight Heparin	Warfarin	Thrombolytics	Herbal Therapy
No contraindication with NSAIDs; discontinue ticlopidine 14 days, clopidogrel 7 days, GP IIb/IIIa inhibitors 8 to 48 hr in advance	No contraindication, consider delaying heparin until after block if technical difficulty anticipated	Heparinize 1 hr after neuraxial technique, remove catheter 2 to 4 hr after first heparin dose; no mandatory delay if traumatic	Twice-daily dosing: LMWH 24 hr after surgery, regardless of technique; remove neuraxial catheter 2 hr before first LMWH dose. Single daily dosing: Needle placement 12 hr after LMWH; first postoperative dose 4 to 12 hr; catheters removed 10 to 12 hr after LMWH and 4 hr prior to next dose; postpone LMWH 24 hr if traumatic	Document normal INR after discontinuation (prior to neuraxial technique): remove catheter when INR ≤1.5 (Initiation of therapy)	No data on safety interval for performance of neuraxial technique or catheter removal; follow fibrinogen level	No evidence for mandatory discontinuation prior to neuraxial technique; be aware of potential drug interactions

NSAIDs, nonsteroidal anti-inflammatory drugs; GP IIb/IIIa, platelet glycoprotein receptor IIb/IIIa; INR, international normalized ratio; LMWH, low-molecular-weight heparin.

Reprinted from Horlocker TT, Wadel DJ, Benson H, et al.: Regional anesthesia in the anticoagulated patient: defining the risks. *Reg Anesth Pain Med* 28:172, 2003. With permission from the American Society of Regional Anesthesia and Pain Management.

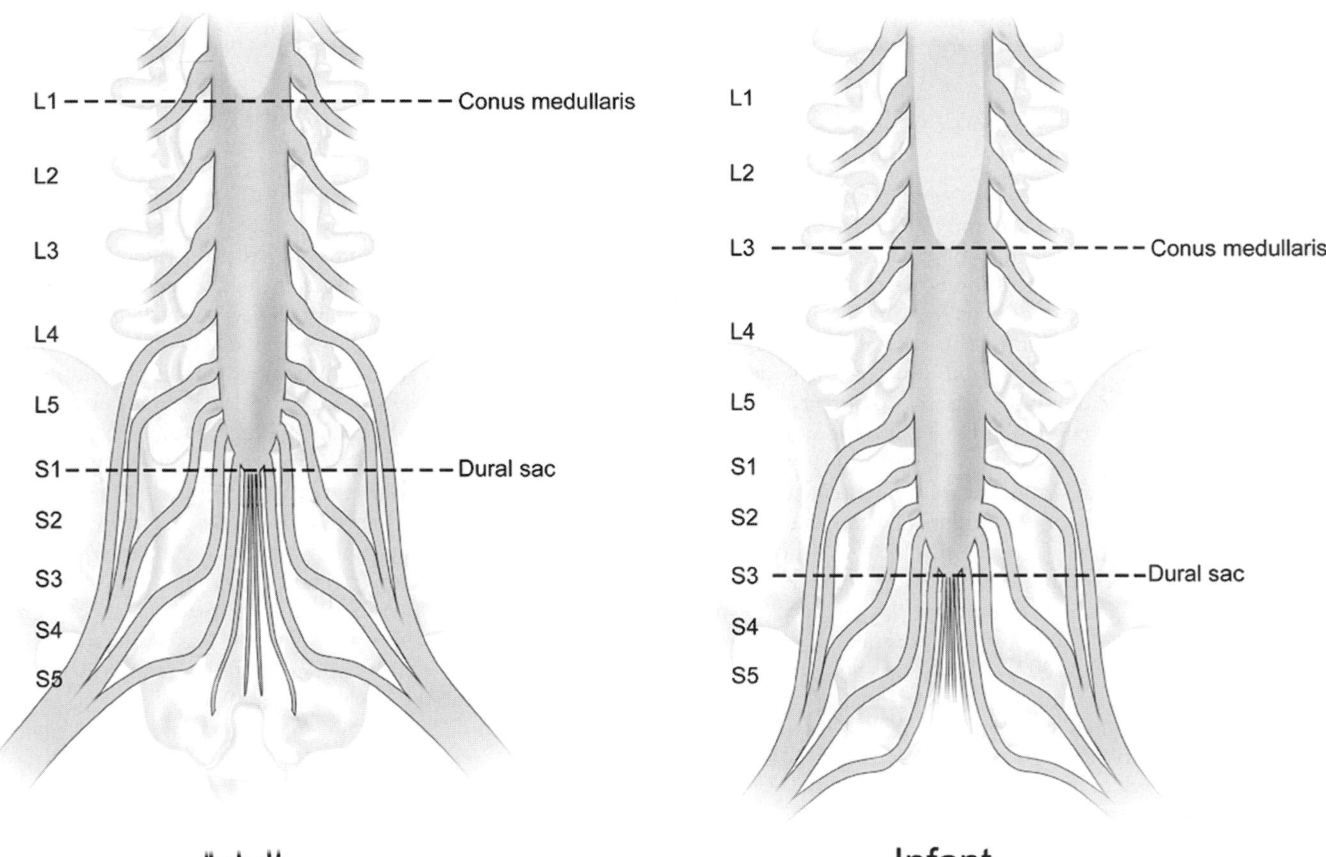

■ **PLATE 14–1.** Comparisons between levels of the conus medullaris and the dural sac in the infant versus the older child or adult. (Color image is available on the DVD.)

should be performed at the L4-5 interspace. After the first year of life, the spinal cord is in its adult position with the dural sac at S1 and conus medullaris at L1.

Technique

To perform a spinal anesthetic, one may position the infant on the side with the back flexed but with the head extended to avoid airway compromise. Some practitioners prefer to have the awake neonate or infant in the sitting position to improve success of the block by increasing the chance of good cerebrospinal fluid (CSF) flow through the needle by increasing the hydrostatic pressure. In either position, it is important that an assistant keep a firm grasp of the awake infant during the placement of the spinal block. An assistant with a firm hold increases the likelihood of a successful block and decreases the chance of complications.

A sterile prep and a clear plastic drape are used so that the anatomy may be seen. For neonates and infants, a $1^1/_2$-inch 22-gauge spinal needle is inserted at the L4-5 interspace (Plate 14–2; color image is available on the DVD). The stylet of the needle should be in place when inserted during the pass through the skin. This avoids the remote risk of an epidermoid tumor (Shaywitz, 1972; Barnitzky et al., 1977). Using this size needle in this age group, one should be able to feel the resistance as the needle enters the ligamentum flavum; then a "pop" should be felt as the needle enters the dura. The stylet is removed to check for the flow of CSF. In an infant positioned in the lateral position, if no CSF is evident after what seemed to be appropriate needle placement, the infant can be placed in the sitting position. This change in position may improve CSF flow once the subdural space is entered.

In children over 2 years of age, a longer needle with a smaller gauge may be used. The smaller gauge needle may decrease the incidence of PDPH but may also make it more difficult for the practitioner to feel the distinctive pop of the needle through the ligamentum flavum. In addition, the smaller size needle may inhibit the flow of CSF.

After confirmation of position into the subarachnoid space as evident by free flow of CSF through the needle, the local anesthetic solution is slowly injected. After the injection, the needle is removed and the child is placed in the supine position.

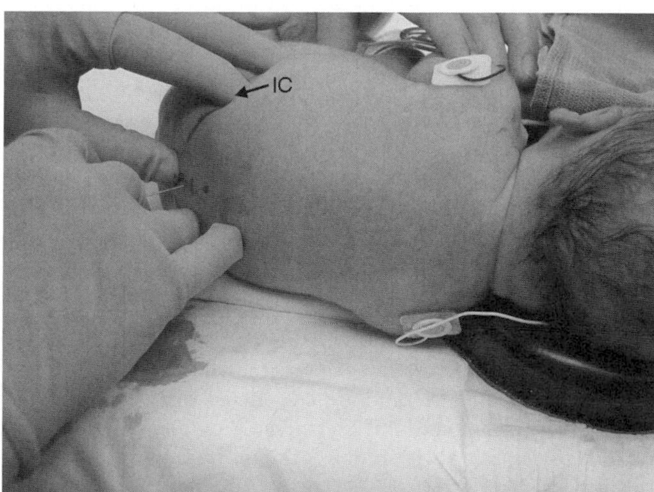

■ **PLATE 14–2.** Performance of spinal anesthetic in the neonate. Note how the back is flexed, but the neck remains extended for airway patency. IC, iliac crest. (Color image is available on the DVD.)

It is extremely important that the child remain supine and that the legs not be raised for any reason, including placement of an electrocautery pad. Lifting the child causes the local anesthetic to migrate and results in a high spinal level (Wright et al., 1990).

Dosing

The total volume of CSF in a neonate is 4 mL/kg compared with 2 mL/kg in an adult, and the hydrostatic pressure is 30 to 40 mm H_2O, lower than that of an adult. In addition, almost half of the total CSF volume is in the spinal subarachnoid space, whereas only one fourth of the total volume in adults is found in the spinal region. These factors play an important part of dosing spinal blocks as the local anesthetics are quickly diluted by the CSF in a neonate upon injection. Infants require higher volumes based on weight, but the duration of action of spinal blocks is shorter than that in adults (Rice et al., 1994).

Although there have been many different dosing regimens used over the years, tetracaine, either with or without epinephrine, is a commonly used local anesthetic for spinal anesthesia. Rice and others (1994) studied 100 infants to determine the duration of spinal block, and the authors compared three groups: lidocaine (3 mg/kg with epinephrine), tetracaine (0.4 mg/kg plain), and tetracaine (0.4 mg/kg with epinephrine). The duration in the lidocaine with epinephrine group was 56 ± 2.5 minutes; in the tetracaine plain group, 86 ± 4 minutes; and in the tetracaine with epinephrine group, 128 ± 3 minutes.

The following guidelines may be used for dosing spinal blocks in infants. If using 1% tetracaine, a dose of 0.5 mg/kg mixed in an equivalent amount of 10% dextrose to make the solution hyperbaric should provide at least 90 minutes of surgical analgesia. Yaster and Maxwell (1989) suggested that regardless of the infant's weight, 1.5 to 2 mg of tetracaine is the minimal effective dose (Yaster and Maxwell, 1989). To achieve 5 mg/mL tetracaine, mix 1 mL of 1% tetracaine with 1 mL of $D_{10}W$. The delivered volume is then 0.3 to 0.4 mL for infants less than 10 kg in weight. If 0.01 mL/kg of epinephrine is added to 0.75 to 1 mg/kg of hyperbaric tetracaine, surgical analgesia can be extended to 90 to 120 minutes. Bupivacaine can also be used for spinal blockade. A dose of bupivacaine, 0.5 to 0.6 mg/kg of either isobaric or hyperbaric bupivacaine, provides an average of 80 minutes of surgical analgesia (Dalens, 2000). Dosing of bupivacaine should be reduced for infants and young children who are greater than 5 kg in weight due to changes in CSF volume. For infants 5 to 15 kg, the dose of hyperbaric bupivacaine or tetracaine is 0.4 mg/kg or 0.08 mL/kg, and for children greater than 15 kg, the dose of bupivacaine or tetracaine is 0.3 mg/kg or 0.06 mL/kg (Dalens, 1995).

Complications

Complications during spinal anesthesia in children are uncommon. In the ADARPEF study, an intravascular injection during spinal anesthesia was the only reported complication in 506 cases (Giaufre et al., 1996). One complication that is associated with spinals, as well as with inadvertent subarachnoid entry during the administration of an epidural block, is post-dural puncture headache (PDPH). Although considered to be a rare occurrence in children, this event may actually be more common than originally thought. In fact, the incidence of PDPH following lumbar puncture has varied from 10% to 50% in children aged 10 to 18 years (Wee, 1995; Oliver, 2002). The onset of symptoms from a PDPH typically occurs within 48 hours with the hallmark symptom being a frontal or an occipital headache that is postural in nature. The cause of PDPH is most likely a persistent leakage of spinal fluid that causes a net decrease in CSF volume and intracranial pressure. The supine position helps to alleviate the symptoms of PDPH by decreasing the effect of gravity on the CSF leak. To reduce the risk of PDPH, smaller-gauge needles are used and the needle is inserted with the bevel parallel to the longitudinal fibers of the dura (Kokki and Hendolin, 1996). If a diagnosis of PDPH is made, simple measures such as bed rest and hydration can decrease the volume of CSF loss. In addition, analgesics to reduce the headache and intravenous caffeine may be administered. Caffeine is effective because of its ability to cause cerebrovascular vasoconstriction resulting in decreased cerebral blood flow. In one study, when caffeine was used prophylactically in adults, visual analog pain scores and analgesic demand following PDPH were lower (Yucel, 1999).

If conservative measures are ineffective in treating PDPH after 48 hours, an epidural blood patch should be considered. An epidural blood patch requires that blood be drawn in a sterile fashion from a peripheral vein. The blood is then injected into the epidural space under aseptic technique. An epidural blood patch is most effective 48 to 72 hours after the dural puncture and may be ineffective if performed immediately after dural tap due to high leakage of CSF that may interfere with blood clotting (Oliver, 2002). In a child who is awake during the placement of an epidural blood patch, the practitioner should stop the injection either once the child feels discomfort or pressure in the back. If a child is anesthetized during the performance of an epidural blood patch, no more than 0.3 mL/kg of blood should be injected into the epidural space (Ylonen, 2002).

Total spinal block with respiratory arrest and bradycardia is another complication of spinal anesthesia (Desparmet, 1990). The preganglionic sympathetic blockade that is commonly seen in adults secondary to a high spinal is not typically seen in children, particularly in infants (Oberlander et al., 1995; Finkel, 2003; Somri, 2003). Dohi and others (1979) were the first to describe the lack of hemodynamic changes following spinal block–induced sympathetic blockade in children. They found that children less than 5 years of age had little to no hemodynamic response to a T3 level tetracaine spinal anesthetic, whereas children greater than 8 years had cardiovascular responses that were more similar to those of adults. The mechanism for this lack of hemodynamic sympathectomy was postulated to be the immaturity of the sympathetic nervous system as well as differences in CSF volume and spinal cord surface area. In addition, it is also possible that the smaller blood volume that is present in the lower extremities of a young child compared with that of an adolescent or adult may account for less venous pooling and therefore less hemodynamic change (Dohi et al., 1979; Dohi and Seino, 1986). Despite the typical lack of cardiovascular compromise, neonates may occasionally require ventilatory support or pharmacologic intervention due to a high spinal with a resulting blockade of the cardiac accelerator fibers and/or decrease in stimulation of the right atrial stretch receptors (Wright et al., 1990). Investigation has shown that even former premature infants in the absence of fluid loading tolerate high spinal anesthesia with minimal autonomic changes (Oberlander et al., 1995).

CAUDAL ANESTHESIA

By far the most commonly used regional block in pediatric practice is the caudal epidural block. The reasons for the success of this regional technique are the ease of performing the block and the extensive safety record of its use in children. The caudal block is the easiest block to perform and to teach. Schuepfer and others (2000) evaluated the technical skills of residents in anesthesiology to determine the learning curve for performing a caudal block in a child. They found that there was a high success rate of performing a caudal anesthetic in a child after performing only a limited number of cases. Caudal blocks have great utility in ambulatory surgical patients and for inpatients. They can be administered as a single injection or as a continuous infusion. A caudal block can be used for any surgery that is performed on the lower abdomen or lower extremities, such as procedures involving innervation from the sacral, lumbar, and lower thoracic dermatomes. Commonly performed pediatric surgery such as inguinal hernia repair and orchiopexy with dermatomal distribution below T-10 makes the caudal block a useful adjunct to the anesthetic. Caudal blocks result in improved patient pain scores compared with scores of patients with general anesthesia alone (Londergan et al., 1994). Single-shot caudal anesthesia, when combined with postoperative ketorolac administration, allows children who have undergone intravesical ureteroneocystostomy to be discharged on postoperative day 1 (Miller et al., 2002). For outpatient urologic procedures, caudal block with light general anesthesia was superior to local nerve block or general anesthesia alone. Patients with caudal blocks had lower pain scores and lower postoperative pain medication requirements (Londergan et al., 1994). Single-shot caudal anesthesia has also been used in ex-premature infants as the sole anesthetic to decrease the incidence of postoperative apnea and to avoid the use of general anesthesia and narcotics (Bouchut et al., 2001).

The practice of placing a caudal block before incision would seem likely to improve postoperative care by providing preemptive analgesia. The benefits of providing preemptive analgesia through regional block have not been confirmed in pediatric caudal studies. Holthusen and others (1994) noted that there were no significant differences in cumulative postoperative analgesic requirements or cumulative pain scores between children having caudal blocks placed either before or after their circumcision. In a separate study comparing two groups of children who received caudal blocks for clubfoot repair, Goodarzi (1996) noted that there were no significant differences in the time to first postoperative analgesic administration or in cumulative analgesic requirements for the first 48 hours between the group that received the block before incision and the group that received the block after the incision. However, it should be realized that placing the caudal at the end of the procedure does not allow the benefit of lower inhaled anesthetic agent concentrations to be used intraoperatively.

There are relative contraindications to performing caudal anesthetics in children. These include the presence of a pilonidal cyst, or abnormal superficial landmarks at the sacral level. The presence of any of these may suggest that the dural sac and cord may not be in their normal anatomic positions. Absolute contraindications include true meningomyelocele of the sacrum or meningitis. Hydrocephalus and intracranial tumors decrease intracranial compliance and are considered relative contraindications to caudal or epidural anesthesia. Progressive degenerative neuropathy is not an absolute contraindication, but it carries medicolegal implications.

Anatomy

The caudal space is the result of a defect due to the nonfusion of the fifth sacral vertebral arch. This area of the nonfusion

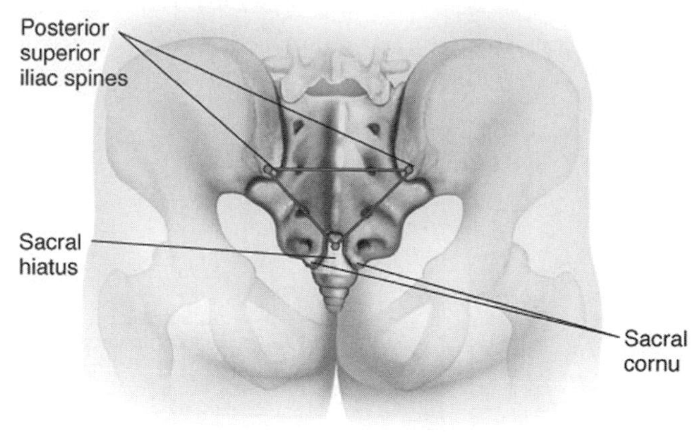

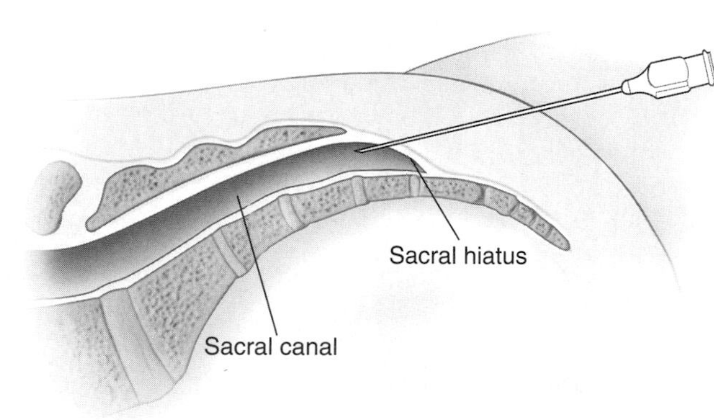

■ **PLATE 14–3.** *A,* Posterior anatomy of the caudal space. *B,* Lateral view of the caudal space and needle insertion. (Color image is available on the DVD.)

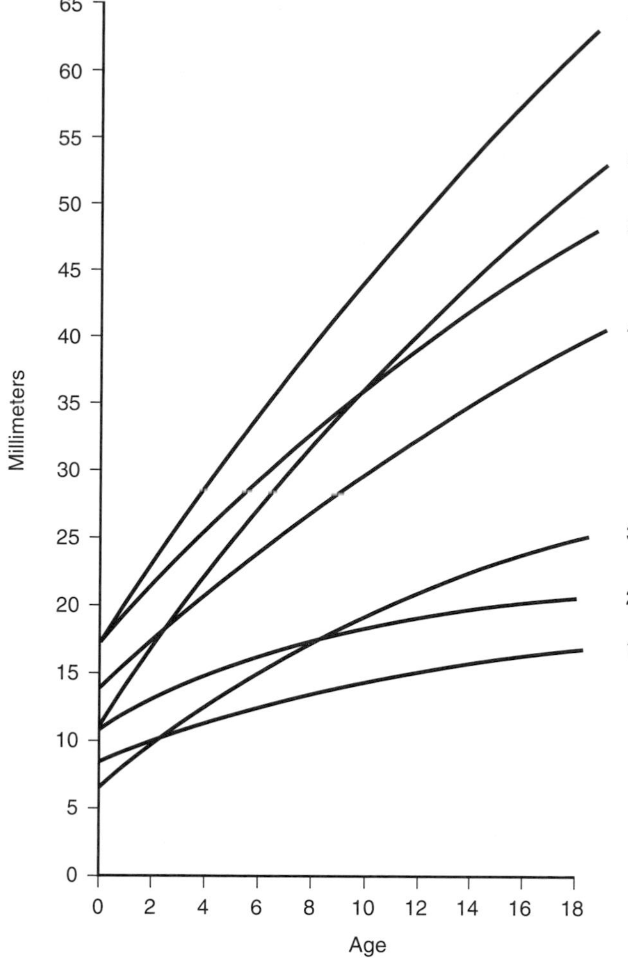

■ **FIGURE 14–2.** Depths to perineural, epidural and subarachnoid spaces according to age. (From Dalens B [ed]: *Regional Anesthesia in Infants, Children and Adolescents.* Philadelphia, Williams & Wilkins, 1995, p. 32.)

forms the sacral hiatus, the entry into the caudal epidural space. The landmarks around the sacral hiatus are the sacral cornua, the posterior superior iliac spines, and the coccyx (Plate 14–3*A, B*; color image is available on the DVD). To find the sacral hiatus, one palpates the sacral cornua and the indentation that is immediately caudal and in the midline. If the cornua are difficult to palpate, the general area of the sacral hiatus may be found by palpating the two posterior superior iliac spines, and assuming that a line between these would be the base of an equilateral triangle, the apex should be at the location of the sacral hiatus.

The caudal space itself lies underneath the sacrococcygeal ligament that runs through the sacral hiatus under the skin. Around 7 years of age, the child's caudal space begins to become more angulated and may be difficult to enter. Although it is possible to perform a caudal block in adolescents and adults, the formation of a presacral fat pad in puberty adds to the difficulty of placing the block. It should be remembered that the distance from the skin to the caudal space in neonates is minimal (Fig. 14–2) and that because the dural sac may extend to S3 in neonates, the possibility of entering the dural sac in this age group is increased.

Technique

The choice of needle to be used depends on whether the caudal anesthetic is to be a single-shot or whether additional dosing will be required. For a single-shot caudal, it is advantageous to use a short-beveled needle with a stylet. One may also use needles such as blunt 22-gauge or intravenous catheters that do not have stylets; however, there is a remote risk of developing an epidermal inclusion cyst or tumor if the epidermis is carried through the shaft of the needle into the neuraxial space (Shaywitz, 1972). A Crawford needle is similar to an epidural Touhy needle as it has a stylet and is blunt, but a Crawford needle's bevel is in alignment with the shaft of the needle so that a catheter exits the needle in a straight line rather than at an angle, such as with a Touhy. The Crawford needle is ideal for either single-shot local anesthetic injection or for placement of a caudal epidural catheter.

With the child in the lateral position, flex the hips with the dependent leg less flexed than the top leg for the Simm's position. Near the cephalad margin of the gluteal crease, feel for the

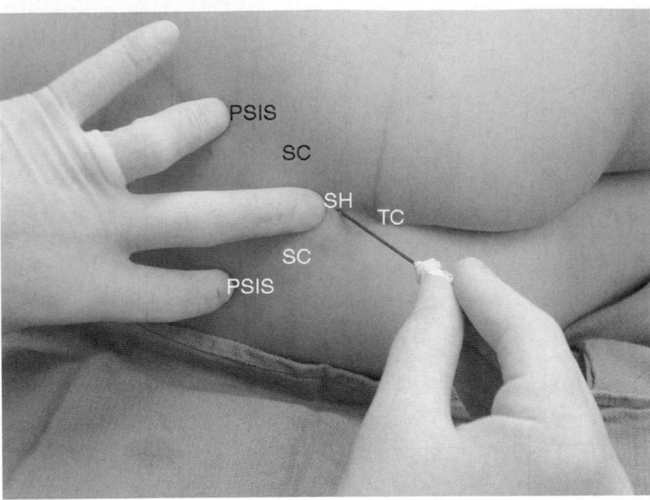

■ **PLATE 14–4.** Performance of caudal block. SC, sacral cornua; PSIS, posterior superior iliac spine; SH, sacral hiatus; TC, tip of coccyx. Note that an equilateral triangle is formed with the fingertips from PSIS to PSIS to needle insertion at SH. (Color image is available on the DVD.)

sacral cornua and the sacral hiatus, a depression immediately inferior to the cornua and in the midline. This is the sacral hiatus (Plate 14–4; color image is available on the DVD). After sterile preparation and drape, identify the sacral hiatus again with the nondominant gloved hand and place the needle into the skin in the midline at a 45° angle to the skin aiming cephalad. Resistance might be felt as the sacrococcygeal ligament is penetrated with a "pop" once the needle has passed into the epidural space. If using a single-injection technique, local anesthetic may be delivered once the sacrococcygeal ligament has been pierced. Frequent aspiration for blood and/or CSF should occur as small movements may result in misplacement of the tip of the needle. If using an intravenous catheter for entry into the caudal space, the angle of the needle must be dropped once the sacrococcygeal ligament has been pierced to align the needle and intravenous catheter with the epidural space. The needle should then be advanced approximately 2 to 3 more mm so that the catheter can be directly threaded into the epidural space. After a negative aspiration for blood and CSF, the local anesthetic should inject easily without resistance. A finger should palpate the skin cephalad to injection to ensure that the agent is not being injected subcutaneously. Although air has been used to check for crepitus after injection, this practice is not recommended due to the risk of air embolism (Guinard and Borboen, 1993; Schwartz and Eisenkraft, 1993).

Dosing

For a single-shot caudal anesthetic that does not have repeat dosing, the goal is to provide the appropriate intraoperative level and a prolonged postoperative analgesia (Plate 14–5; color image is available on the DVD). Although there have been formulas developed for determining levels for injection of a single-shot caudal, delivery of 1 mL/kg of local anesthetic with epinephrine 1:200,000 provides a thoracic level with a duration of 4 to 6 hours depending on the local anesthetic chosen (Armitage, 1979). Although one would never inject 1 mL/kg of local anesthetic in the epidural space of an adult, the anatomy of the caudal epidural space in a child is such that a high volume is needed in order to fill the loosely packed space and to spread

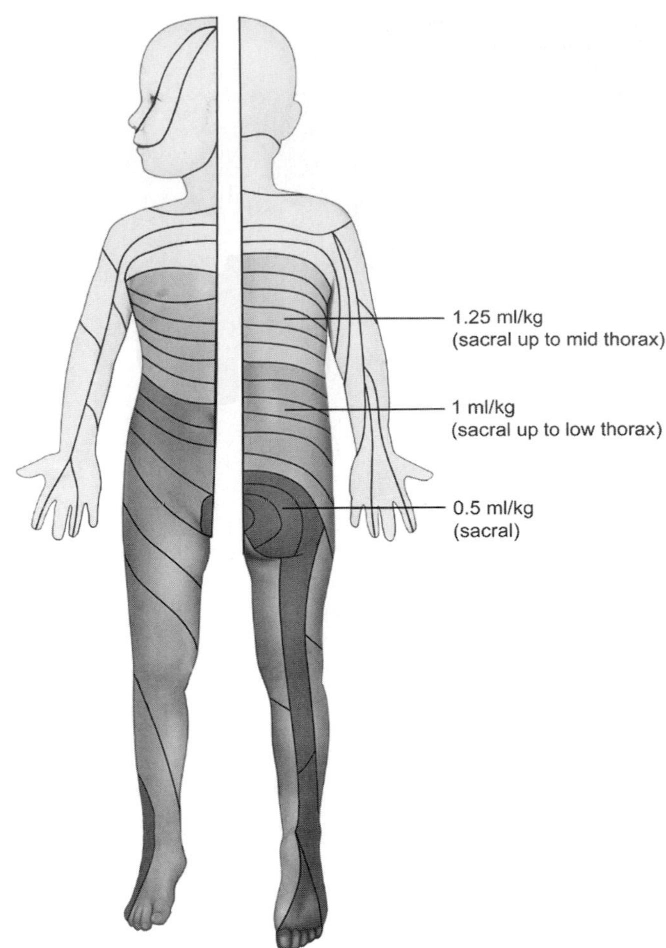

■ **PLATE 14–5.** Dermatomal distribution of different volumes of local anesthetic for single-shot caudal block. (Color image is available on the DVD.)

to reach the appropriate dermatomes. The caudal space communicates freely with the perineural spaces of the spinal nerves, which allows a lower concentration of local anesthetic to be effective. Dosing guidelines may be found in Table 14–4. Although convention suggests that an increased volume of local anesthetic should be required for adequate block and duration of action, a study found that there was no advantage to increasing the volume of local anesthetic over 0.7 mL/kg (Schrock et al., 2003). In children 1 to 6 years of age undergoing inguinal hernia repair, Schrock and others (2003) compared three groups, all of whom received 0.175% bupivacaine administered at different volumes (0.7 mL/kg, 1 mL/kg, and 1.3 mL/kg). The durations of action as determined by first postoperative analgesic were similar for all three groups: 4.2, 3.6, and 4.8 hours, respectively. In addition, there were no differences among the groups with regard to first time to void, ambulate, or discharge. However, in another study, Verghese and others (2002) noted that 1 mL/kg of 0.2% bupivacaine was more effective than a smaller volume of 0.8 mL/kg of 0.25% bupivacaine in blocking the peritoneal response of spermatic cord traction during orchidopexy. The quality of postoperative analgesia, however, was similar in the two groups.

The recommended concentration of bupivacaine for a single-shot caudal is 0.125% to 0.25%. However, Gunter and others (1991), in a dose-range study, concluded that 0.175% offered the

TABLE 14–4. Recommendations for dosing caudal and epidural blocks.

	Concentration	Dose	Possible Additives
Single-dose caudal	0.175% to 0.5%	0.75 to 1.25 mL/kg not to exceed 3 mg/kg	Epinephrine 2.5 to 5 mcg/mL
			Clonidine 1 to 2 mcg/kg Morphine 30 to 70 mcg/kg
Continuous caudal or lumbar epidural catheters	0.1% to 0.25%	0.4 mL/kg per hr or 0.2 to 0.4 mg/kg per hr	Fentanyl 2 to 5 mcg/mL Hydromorphone 5 to 10 mcg/mL
Continuous thoracic epidural	0.1% to 0.25%	0.3 mL/kg per hr or 0.1 to 0.2 mg/kg per hr	Fentanyl 2 to 5 mcg/mL Hydromorphone 5 to 10 mcg/mL

Bupivacaine, levobupivacaine, or ropivacaine may be used. Greater concentrations and larger doses should be reserved for levobupivacaine or ropivacaine. Doses and concentrations should be reduced in infants. Children less than 2 years of age who receive morphine centrally require 24-hour monitoring after its delivery.

best combination of analgesia and rapid recovery with the least number of side effects. When performing single shot caudal anesthesia in ex-premature infants for hernia repair, a combination of agents has been shown to be successful (Bouchut et al., 2001). A mixture of 0.5 mL/kg of 1% lidocaine, along with 0.5 mL/kg of 0.5% bupivacaine, was used in 25 infants. This combination provided surgical analgesia for 60 minutes. However, 1 of the 25 infants developed a total spinal block and 2 children developed postoperative apnea.

Some information is available on the use of the newer local anesthetics for caudal anesthesia in infants and children. Ropivacaine has been evaluated in children for caudal anesthesia and has been found to provide a similar onset and analgesic duration to bupivacaine (Ivani et al., 1998). In some studies, compared with bupivacaine, ropivacaine produced less of a motor block at 0.25% and 0.375% concentrations (DaConceicao and Coelho, 1998; DaConceicao et al., 1999). When 0.2% ropivacaine, 0.25% levobupivacaine, and 0.25% bupivacaine were compared in children for caudal anesthesia, postoperative analgesia was not significantly different among the groups, nor was the time for the first postoperative analgesic (Ivani et al., 2002). The only difference was a slight reduction in the incidence of motor block in the ropivacaine group.

When using 1 mL/kg of 0.2% ropivacaine, free plasma concentrations were well below toxic levels (Lonnqvist et al., 2000). To determine the effective concentration of ropivacaine for single-shot caudal analgesia, Bosenberg and others (2002) compared 1 mL/kg of 0.1%, 0.2%, and 0.3% ropivacaine in 110 children aged 4 to 12 years. The median time to first analgesic was 3.3, 4.5, and 4.2 hours in the groups, respectively. Pain scores were significantly higher in the 0.1% group compared with the 0.3% group. Motor block was 0%, 13%, and 28% in the 0.1%, 0.2%, and 0.3% groups, respectively. Bosenberg and others concluded that although 1 mL/kg of ropivacaine is effective for postoperative pain in children after inguinal surgery, the lower concentration of 0.1% is not effective, and the higher concentrations result in a higher rate of motor block.

In other dosing studies with ropivacaine, Koinig and others (1999) compared 0.75 mL/kg of 0.5% ropivacaine, 0.25% ropivacaine, and 0.25% bupivacaine in children aged 1.5 to 7 years undergoing inguinal hernia repair. The remarkable finding in this study was the duration of analgesia afforded by 0.5% ropivacaine. The duration in the ropivacaine 0.5% group was 1440 minutes, whereas the 0.25% ropivacaine and 0.25% bupivacaine groups were 208 minutes and 220 minutes, respectively.

Levobupivacaine, the *S*(–)-enantiomer of bupivacaine, has also been put into clinical practice as an alternative to bupivacaine. Ivani and others (2002) compared 1 mL/kg of caudal 0.25% levobupivacaine with 0.2% ropivacaine and 0.25% racemic bupivacaine in children and noted no significant difference in intraoperative or postoperative analgesia among the three groups (Ivani et al., 2002). In children less than 2 years of age, a dose of 2 mg/kg of 0.25% levobupivacaine had similar efficacy to racemic bupivacaine and levobupivacaine had a duration of action of 7.3 hours (Taylor et al., 2003). Ivani and others (2003) noted the optimum concentration of levobupivacaine at 1 mL/kg for single-shot caudal anesthesia without any additive was 0.2%. This dose provides 118 minutes of postoperative analgesia compared with 60 minutes with 0.125% and 158 minutes with 0.25%. The advantage of using 0.2% over 0.25% was the decreased incidence of motor blockade. Dosing guidelines for levobupivacaine are similar to those for bupivacaine (see Table 14–4).

Caudal Additives

One of the disadvantages of caudal anesthesia is the relatively short duration of postoperative analgesia in children, even when using long-acting local anesthetics. Many agents have been studied in an attempt to find an additive that would prolong the duration of analgesia for single-shot caudal anesthesia.

Epinephrine

The use of epinephrine for regional anesthetic techniques in children was discussed earlier in this chapter. It is recommended that epinephrine be added to single-dose local anesthetics at a dose of 5 mcg/mL or a concentration of 1:200,000. The hypothetical disadvantage of the use of epinephrine is vasoconstriction and possible cord ischemia from impaired flow to the artery of Adamkiewicz (Cook and Doyle, 1996). An epinephrine dose of 2.5 mcg/mL or a concentration of 1:400,000 may be used as an additive for central blocks (Flandin-Blety and Barrier, 1995).

Epinephrine serves as a marker for intravascular injection and decreased systemic absorption of local anesthetic. In addition, epinephrine may prolong the duration of a regional block. Warner and others (1987) compared children aged 3 months to 17 years receiving single-shot caudal block with 0.5 mL/kg bupivacaine 0.25%. One group received the bupivacaine plain and the other group had epinephrine 5 mcg/mL added to the local anesthetic. Epinephrine prolonged the duration of analgesia of the caudal block compared with the blocks that did not include epinephrine. The duration of analgesia decreased with increasing age with the greatest effect on children less than 5 years of age. Children aged 5 or less had a mean duration of analgesia 10 to 13 hours longer if epinephrine was in the solution. In children aged 6 to

10 years, epinephrine increased the duration of effect by 2 to 3 hours, whereas in children older than 11 years, epinephrine increased the block by 1 to 2 hours. However, in other studies, epinephrine has not been shown to prolong a caudal block with bupivacaine (Fisher et al., 1993; Cook et al., 1995).

Ketamine

Preservative-free ketamine has been described for caudal use in children to prolong a bupivacaine block following hernia surgery. Naguib and others (1991) compared three groups of children receiving either plain bupivacaine 0.25%, ketamine 0.5 mg/kg, or bupivacaine 0.25% plus ketamine 0.5 mg/kg. The group that received only ketamine 0.5 mg/kg had superior analgesia and longer duration of action than the group that had received plain 0.25% bupivacaine. The ketamine group also had similar analgesia and duration of action to the group that received the combination of ketamine and bupivacaine. No postoperative behavior changes were noted in the ketamine groups. These findings have been confirmed in subsequent studies using ketamine 0.5 mg/kg as an additive to either bupivacaine 0.25% or ropivacaine 0.2% in the caudal space (De Negri et al., 2001; Weber and Wulf, 2003). Cook and others (1995) studied children aged 1 to 10 years who received caudal anesthesia using 0.25% bupivacaine 1 mL/kg with the addition of either ketamine 0.5 mg/kg, clonidine 2 mcg/kg, or epinephrine 5 mcg/mL. The ketamine group had a mean duration of analgesia of 12.5 hours compared with 5.8 hours for the clonidine group and 3.2 hours for the epinephrine group. When used alone in the caudal space, ketamine at this dose of 0.5 mg/kg had a shorter duration of action than bupivacaine 0.25% with 1:200,000 epinephrine, but ketamine 1 mg/kg provided surgical and postoperative analgesia that was equivalent to bupivacaine (Marhofer et al., 2000).

Hager and others (2002) reported on the use of ketamine for caudal analgesia without local anesthetic and compared a group that received ketamine 1 mg/kg with two other groups who received, in addition to ketamine, clonidine 1 or 2 mcg/kg. The ketamine group had a mean duration of postoperative analgesia of 13.3 hours. When clonidine 1 mcg/kg or 2 mcg/kg was added to the ketamine, the mean duration was 22.7 hours and 21.8 hours, respectively. This particular study prompted a letter to the editor by Eisenach and Yaksh (2003) that stressed concern over the performance and publications of studies that subjected healthy children to agents that have not had adequate preclinical toxicity studies. Eisenach and Yaksh further discussed the potential risks of neurotoxicity using *S*(+)-ketamine in the epidural space without significant benefits to the otherwise healthy child. The response to this letter from the authors of the study defended their position with a number of reports on ketamine in the epidural space (Marhofer and Semsroth, 2003). The issue remains controversial as pointed out in a systematic review of nonopioid additives by Ansermino and others (2003). This review summarized the findings of randomized control trials performed on children using nonopioid additives in the caudal space and concluded that although clonidine, ketamine, and midazolam increase the duration of analgesia, the potential for neurotoxicity remains a concern with ketamine and midazolam. They also concluded that the routine use of nonopioid adjuvants for elective outpatient surgery had not been shown to improve patient outcome.

Clonidine

Clonidine, an α_2-adrenergic agonist, at 1 to 2 mcg/kg has been used with success and may result in an additional 4 to 6 hours of analgesia when combined with bupivacaine (Lee and Rubin, 1994; Constant et al., 1998). Ivani and others (2000) also demonstrated a beneficial effect of clonidine when added to ropivacaine. In this study, 0.1% ropivacaine plus clonidine 2 mcg/kg provided superior analgesic quality to a caudal block compared with 0.2% ropivacaine without clonidine. The true mechanism of analgesic action of clonidine remains unknown, but there is evidence that it has both central and peripheral sites of action (Ivani et al., 2002). Although clonidine may cause some sedation, particularly at the higher doses, and although the sedation has not been considered clinically significant in studies, caudal clonidine has been implicated in case reports as a cause of apnea in neonates (Breschan et al., 1999; Bouchut et al., 2001).

De Negri and others (2001) compared ketamine with clonidine to determine which agent would most effectively prolong a ropivacaine caudal anesthetic. Children 1 to 5 years of age received 0.2% ropivacaine 2 mg/kg, ropivacaine plus clonidine 2 mcg/kg, or ropivacaine plus ketamine 0.5 mg/kg for caudal anesthesia. Postoperative analgesia was significantly longer in the ropivacaine with ketamine group (701 minutes) compared with the ropivacaine with clonidine group (492 minutes) and the ropivacaine plain group (291 minutes). There were no clinically significant side effects in any of the groups. These findings were similar to the study by Cook and others (1995) that compared clonidine 2 mcg/kg with ketamine 0.5 mg/kg as additives to 0.25% bupivacaine caudal anesthesia.

Tramadol

Tramadol is an analgesic that acts centrally at opioid receptors and has been compared with bupivacaine alone and a tramadol-bupivacaine combination for caudal analgesia (Prosser et al., 1997; Batra et al., 1999; Gunduz et al., 2001). At a dose of 1 mg/kg of tramadol added to bupivacaine, patients had lower pain scores and longer durations of analgesia compared with bupivacaine alone (Batra et al., 1999). At a tramadol dose of 2 mg/kg added to bupivacaine, some children had sedative effects; however, this was not considered to be clinically significant (Gunduz et al., 2001). Caudal tramadol 2 mg/kg provides reliable postoperative analgesia similar to caudal morphine 30 mcg/kg for children undergoing herniorrhaphy (Ozcengiz et al., 2001).

Neostigmine

The use of neostigmine in the epidural space is a relatively new concept in children. Its action may be attributed to either direct action on the spinal cord via inhibition of the breakdown of acetylcholine in the dorsal horn or by peripheral antinociceptive effect (Shafer et al., 1998; Yang et al., 1998). A study in children compared three groups to determine the effectiveness of neostigmine 2 mcg/kg as a caudal analgesic for hypospadias repair, either alone or in combination with bupivacaine (Abdulatif and El-Sanabary, 2002). The groups received 1 mL/kg of either 0.25% bupivacaine plain, bupivacaine with neostigmine 2 mcg/kg, or neostigmine 2 mcg/kg plain. The combination of bupivacaine and neostigmine provided superior analgesia to either of the other two groups and a mean duration of 22.8 hours compared with 8.1 hours in the bupivacaine plain group and 5.2 hours in the neostigmine plain group.

Opioids

Opioids have been commonly used in caudal blocks with or without local anesthetic agents. There are two distinct classes of opioids: hydrophilic and lipophilic. In general, hydrophilic opioids such as morphine are capable of rostral spread, whereas lipophilic opioids such as fentanyl remain more localized to their area of injection. This difference accounts for the greater incidence of sedation and respiratory depression that occurs with hydrophilic agents.

Opioids may be used to improve the quality and duration of a block, but there are advantages and disadvantages to spinal axis opioids (Lonnqvist et al., 2002). The major disadvantage of opioid additives is the risk of respiratory depression. In children less than 1 year of age, the risk of respiratory depression from caudal morphine is significantly higher than that in children greater than 1 year of age (Valley and Bailey, 1991). In this study of 138 children who had received 70 mcg/kg of caudal morphine, the incidence of clinically significant respiratory depression was 8%. Ten of the 11 children with respiratory depression were less than 1 year of age and weighed less than 9 kg. Seven of the 11 patients also received intravenous opioids. All episodes of respiratory depression occurred within 12 hours of the caudal morphine injection. Therefore, spinal axis opioids are contraindicated in ambulatory surgical patients. Additionally, patients under 1 year of age and patients receiving supplemental intravenous opioids should be carefully monitored postoperatively.

Another disadvantage of neuraxial opioids is the increased incidence of postoperative pruritus, nausea, and vomiting. Although fentanyl 1 mcg/kg may prolong a caudal block, the incidence of pruritus and vomiting also increases (Constant et al., 1998). In one study, the investigation was actually halted due to the unacceptable incidence of postoperative vomiting in a group of children who had received caudal buprenorphine (Khan et al., 2002). Urinary retention is a side effect of caudal morphine and required urinary catheterization in 30% of children in one study using 70 mcg/kg morphine (Irving et al., 1993). Another reason for the avoidance of neuraxial opioids is the availability of alternative additives. As previously discussed, additives such as clonidine and ketamine have been used as adjuncts for central blockade with success and result in fewer side effects compared with opioids.

Despite the pitfalls of using opioids as a component of central blockade, the practice continues because of the relative advantages these agents offer. Preservative-free morphine more than doubles the duration of a single-shot bupivacaine caudal (Krane et al., 1987). In a study of children aged 1 to 16 years, there was a slightly greater incidence of urinary retention, pruritus, and nausea in the group that received caudal morphine, but there was no evidence of delayed respiratory depression even at doses of 100 mcg/kg in this age group. A caudal morphine dose of 30 mcg/kg has been recommended for children to provide the advantage of increased analgesic duration with decreased incidence of side effects, particularly respiratory depression (Krane et al., 1989). In children who were undergoing open-heart procedures, a dose of 75 mcg/kg morphine provided lower pain scores and decreased incidence of atelectatic changes on radiography compared with a control group that had not received caudal morphine (Rosen and Rosen, 1989). Plasma levels of morphine given via the caudal route peak at 21 ± 4.8 ng/mL approximately 10 minutes after injection (Wolf et al., 1991). These levels are lower than that associated with systemic administration of morphine.

Lipophilic opioids do not offer the same risk of respiratory depression as hydrophilic agents. The disadvantage of the lipophilic agents is the shorter duration of postoperative analgesia than what is provided by morphine, and there may actually be no benefit to the addition of fentanyl to local anesthetic for a single-shot caudal. In most reports, caudal fentanyl 1 mcg/kg has not been shown to increase the duration of analgesia produced by 0.125% bupivacaine, 0.25% bupivacaine, or 2% lidocaine (Jones et al., 1990; Campbell et al., 1992; Joshi et al., 1999; Baris et al., 2003). In contrast, Constant and others (1998) demonstrated the prolongation of analgesia in a study in which fentanyl 1 mcg/kg was added to a mixture of bupivacaine and lidocaine in children aged 6 to 108 months. The mean duration of analgesia in the fentanyl group was 253 ± 105 minutes compared with 174 ± 29 minutes in the control group without fentanyl. Vomiting occurred in 4 of 15 of the children who had extradural fentanyl and 0 of 14 in the children who had not received fentanyl.

Fentanyl and morphine were compared for efficacy and side effects in children aged 1 to 16 years (Lejus et al., 1994). The children all received a preincision epidural dose of 0.5% bupivacaine 0.75 mL/kg and then were divided into two groups. The morphine group received a preoperative bolus of epidural morphine 75 mcg/kg and the same morphine bolus dose 24 hours later. The fentanyl group received 2 mcg/kg before incision, followed by a continuous infusion of 5 mcg/kg per day. The group that received the fentanyl infusion had comparable analgesia to the morphine group with less pruritus (20% versus 53%) and less nausea and vomiting (0% versus 33%).

Complications

Complications from caudal anesthesia include risks during the performance of the block, risks from injection of local anesthetic, and side effects from the agents used. During the performance of a caudal block, the needle could be accidentally placed into the intravascular space, subarachnoid space, or sacral marrow. The incidence of intravascular injection should be decreased with the use of a short-beveled needle, and a test dose should provide information as to whether the needle is intravascular or in the vascular marrow (Dalens and Hasnaoui, 1989). The detection of a subarachnoid injection may be difficult if CSF is not clearly seen upon aspiration before local anesthetic injection. In the safety study of Giaufre and others (1996), inadvertent dural puncture was the most frequent complication. In the event the subarachnoid space has been entered, it is possible to reintroduce a needle for a caudal anesthetic; however, the agent should be injected very slowly to avoid the possible migration of local anesthetic solution into the subdural space through any previous puncture sites.

Children differ from adults in that hypotension secondary to centrally delivered local anesthetics is not generally a significant side effect from caudal or neuraxial regional anesthesia. Even without intravascular volume loading before the administration of a central blockade, hypotension is typically not observed in children less than 5 years of age (Dohi et al., 1979; Dohi and Seino, 1986). This may be due to either the immature sympathetic nervous system or the fact that the lower extremities, in proportion to overall body size, do not provide a significant volume for venous pooling.

Studies have been performed in children to investigate the hemodynamic response to caudal analgesia. Doppler studies to investigate hemodynamic changes have demonstrated that cardiac output does not change during caudal anesthesia in infants (Payen et al., 1987). However, a study to investigate pulmonary Doppler flow revealed that the pulmonary flow velocity changes during caudal anesthesia, presumably secondary to an increase in pulmonary artery resistance (Ozasa et al., 2002). Because the change may have reflected local anesthetic–induced vasoconstriction, the authors concluded that caudal epidural anesthesia is not recommended in children with pulmonary hypertension.

Urinary retention, although a concern, is not considered a frequent side effect in single-shot caudal anesthetics. Fisher and others (1993) reviewed the postoperative voiding interval in children who received either bupivacaine caudal blocks with and without epinephrine or ilioinguinal hypogastric nerve blocks. In this study, they noted no significant difference in the time to micturition among these groups. Although the range of times to first micturition varied widely from 25 to 630 minutes, no children required any intervention for urinary retention.

Complications from intravascular injection and accumulation of local anesthetics have previously been discussed.

CONTINUOUS CAUDAL CATHETERS

Intraoperatively, an indwelling catheter may be placed in the caudal epidural space. These catheters allow for additional dosing of the local anesthetic agents at the end of the procedure or in the recovery area before catheter removal. A repeat dose or a second dose of local anesthetic can safely be administered 90 to 120 minutes after the initial dose as long as maximal allowable dosing is not exceeded in that time period. In addition, continuous caudal block may be used as an alternative to spinal anesthesia in the ex-premature infant who is at risk for postoperative apnea while undergoing inguinal hernia repair. This technique has been used with success with and without a concomitant general anesthetic (Henderson et al., 1993; Peutrell and Hughes, 1993; Tobias et al., 1996).

The presence of a caudal catheter allows for continued postoperative pain management in children. Continuous infusions, although commonly used because of their ability to provide complete postoperative analgesia, have come under scrutiny because of a lack of prospective outcome studies that demonstrate benefit (Chalkiadis, 2003). Audits of postoperative infusions have demonstrated that 17% to 22% of patients require premature termination of the infusions. In 67% of these patients, the termination was due to an unacceptable rate of side effects or complications (Wilson and Lloyd-Thomas, 1993; Wood et al., 1994). This high rate leads one to question the benefit of neuraxial analgesia over intravenous analgesia (Chalkiadis, 2003). Side effects may be greater for lipophilic infused epidural opioids (e.g., fentanyl), because the catheter tip must be positioned at the interspace corresponding to the dermatomes of the surgical procedure. Another issue that argues against placing and maintaining a continuous epidural catheter includes the dissatisfaction in children of having a motor block. There may also be an increased incidence of postoperative urinary retention and pruritus in children who receive infusions of neuraxial opioids (Lloyd-Thomas and Howard, 1994).

Although these side effects are not necessarily dangerous, they do result in increased workload for medical staff, additional medications, and child/parent distress. More serious issues with continuous caudal infusions include the rare risks of epidural hematomas, epidural infection and abscesses, or respiratory depression from central opioids. In addition, there is the cost factor of the epidural catheter kits, the operative time to insert the caudal catheters, urinary catheters, and postoperative costs for pharmacy, nursing, on-call staff, and a pain service. For these reasons, it has been suggested that continuous infusions be reserved for those children who would truly receive a direct benefit.

Technique

The anatomy, a continuous catheter via the caudal route and entry into the caudal space have been described previously. In threading a caudal catheter, the space should first be dilated with a push of preservative-free normal saline. The catheter is then threaded through the needle until the tip of the catheter reaches the estimated desired level. The caudal approach to placing a lumbar or thoracic catheter in infants was described by Bosenberg and others (1988). Because of the loosely packed fat in the epidural space, a catheter should advance easily. If resistance is felt, it is most likely due to the catheter coiling or doubling back in the epidural space. In older children who may have more densely packed epidural fat, the use of a catheter with a stylet may increase the success rate (Gunter and Eng, 1992). In addition to using a catheter with a stylet, other means of improving success of this technique are to dilate the space with preservative-free normal saline before catheter placement, flexing the hips to straighten the spine, and utilizing fluoroscopy to ensure proper catheter tip position.

If an angiocath has been used for insertion of the catheter, the catheter may be withdrawn, twisted, and advanced through the plastic introducer until the desired position as determined by radiography is obtained. Catheters should not be withdrawn through metal needles due to the risk of shearing the catheter into the epidural space. Success in placing a thoracic catheter via the caudal route is variable. In a study of 86 infants who had caudal placement of a thoracic catheter that was confirmed by radiographs, the positions of 28 of these catheters were considered to be inadequate (Valairucha et al., 2002). Of the 28, 10 were determined to be in the high thoracic or cervical regions and were able to be pulled back, 17 were coiled in the lumbosacral area, and 1 was outside the epidural space in the presacral area. Radiographic confirmation of catheter tip position for thoracic catheters that are threaded from the caudal route is essential.

Dosing

Continuous caudal catheters that have their tip in the sacral or lower lumbar areas are dosed differently from those that have been threaded to the low to mid-thoracic levels. Suggestions for dosing may be found in Table 14–4. Continuous caudal catheters require large volumes of local anesthetic to fill the loose caudal epidural space and to spread the anesthetic cephalad to the desired dermatomal level. It is important to refer to the maximal allowable dosing recommendations so that these rates are not exceeded in an attempt to "drive up" the epidural block from the caudal space (see Table 14–2). Bupivacaine, ropivacaine, and levobupivacaine may be used for continuous caudal anesthesia, with or without additives. It is possible to improve the analgesia of a continuous caudal catheter by including a hydrophilic opioid such as preservative-free morphine or hydromorphone to the infusion.

In addition to a continuous infusion, there is the ability for children to benefit from patient-controlled epidural analgesia. Patient-controlled analgesia allows the patient to receive analgesia literally at the press of a button. Its popularity in children initially began in the late 1980s with intravenous opioids and has expanded to local anesthetic infusions for a variety of blocks. For patient-controlled analgesia to be effective, a patient or provider must be able to identify pain and push a button that signals a pump to deliver a preset amount of the local anesthetic solution. This pump is programmed in advance to deliver a bolus amount based on weight criteria and is set to adhere to specific time and dosage limits. In addition to the bolus that is delivered in response to the push of the button, the pump is capable of infusing a continuous background rate of local anesthetic solution. In a study of children who had undergone a total of 132 procedures in whom patient-controlled epidural analgesia was used postoperatively, more than 90% had satisfactory analgesia with no significant adverse effects (Birmingham et al., 2003). This study confirmed that children as young as age 5 have the cognitive ability to understand the use of patient-controlled analgesia.

Complications

Complications of continuous caudal infusions are typically secondary to the agent that is being delivered. The risk of local anesthetic toxicity has been discussed, and there is ample evidence that the use of bupivacaine at doses over 0.2 mg/kg per hr in infants and 0.4 mg/kg per hr in children greater than 6 months of age may lead to neurotoxicity or cardiovascular collapse (Agarwal et al., 1992; Berde, 1992, 1993; McCloskey et al., 1992).

In addition to the risk of serious complications, minor complications such as urinary retention, muscle weakness, itching, or nausea and vomiting can occur. Lowering the concentrations of local anesthetics and avoiding opioids in the central infusion can reduce the risk of these side effects. This regimen, however, puts the patient at greater risk of experiencing postoperative pain.

Continuous indwelling caudal catheters would seem to be an obvious setup for fecal contamination and infection. When caudal catheters have been compared with epidural catheters, caudal catheters were found to have a greater incidence of colonization of bacteria (20% versus 4%), with *Staphylococcus epidermidis* being responsible for the vast majority of colonization (McNeely et al., 1997). In addition, four of the nine caudal catheter tips that were colonized also involved gram-negative bacteria. Of interest, caudal catheter tip colonization was not predicted by duration of catheterization, skin inflammation, or dressing contamination. None of the children developed signs of epidural infection either in the hospital or during 3-month follow-up. Another study demonstrated the absence of epidural abscess or clinically significant infection from indwelling catheters for postoperative pain (Strafford et al., 1995). An option for children who are to have prolonged analgesia provided by a continuous caudal or epidural catheter is to tunnel the catheter under the skin (Aram et al., 2001). Catheters that have been tunneled under the skin should provide for a more long-term infusion of agents by providing decreased chance of catheter dislodgment and protection against colonization and infection.

EPIDURAL ANESTHESIA

Epidural anesthesia is commonly used for those procedures that involve surgery of the mid to upper abdomen and thorax that are less amenable to a continuous caudal anesthetic. Children who have procedures that have higher morbidity rates such as Nissen fundoplication may benefit from perioperative epidural analgesia (McNeely et al., 1997; Wilson et al., 2001). Postoperative complications and hospital stay may be reduced with the use of an epidural for this procedure compared with opioid analgesia alone. In addition, the use of epidural anesthesia is associated with a significantly reduced stress response to surgery in children, as determined by lower cortisol levels and plasma epinephrine levels (Murat et al., 1988; Wolf et al., 1993).

Although lumbar epidural blocks are commonly used, thoracic epidural blocks should be performed only by practitioners who are experienced in their use and should be reserved for children with pulmonary disease or those who are to undergo a surgical procedure in the thoracic area or upper abdominal area that is associated with significant postoperative pain. As discussed, under continuous caudal anesthesia, a catheter may be threaded from the caudal space cephalad to the thoracic region to provide more site-specific analgesia without the risks associated with placing a needle in the thoracic spine. However, threaded catheters from the caudal space are frequently malpositioned. In older children, a thoracic epidural inserted between T4 and T8 should attenuate the stress response associated with thoracic surgery and provide optimal postoperative analgesia (Hammer, 2001). Thoracic epidural catheters that are placed intraoperatively by the surgeon before wound closure for anterior spinal fusion and instrumentation for scoliosis have been shown to be safe and effective (Jason Lowry et al., 2001).

Anatomy

The epidural space in children is divided into sacral, lumbar, thoracic, and cervical levels. The caudal block enters at the sacral level. A lumbar epidural needle/catheter is typically placed at the L3-4 interspace, which in older children is found in the midline of a line that may be drawn between the two iliac crests. Although these landmarks are accurate in older children, the intercrestal line may actually cross the L5-S1 interspace in neonates and the L4-5 interspace in infants up to a year of age because of the lag of the growth of the spinal cord (see Plate 14–1). Because of the developmental changes that occur with the spinal cord and dural sac positions, placing an epidural catheter below the level of the intercrestal line (e.g., caudal area) may decrease the risk of a wet tap in a neonate or young infant.

Epidural pressures differ depending on the age of the patient. Infants have narrow epidural spaces and are more likely to exhibit leak around an epidural catheter from a backflow of solution if injected too quickly (Vas et al., 2001). Even at slow injection rates, epidural pressures in infants are higher than in adults.

The anatomy of the thoracic spine is similar to that of the lumbar spine with some exceptions. The spinous processes in the thoracic area are longer and the interspinous spaces narrower (Plate 14–6; color image is available on the DVD). These differences necessitate that the epidural needle be placed at a sharper angle in a cephalad direction. The ligaments in the thoracic area are more lax and may be more difficult to discern during needle placement compared with performing a lumbar needle insertion. Most important, the spinal cord occupies most of the spinal canal in the thoracic area, leaving little margin for error once the needle reaches the epidural space.

The depth to the epidural space at the L2-3 level is approximately 10 mm at birth, and this depth increases with age in a linear fashion. The approximate expected distance from the skin to the epidural space in children aged 6 months to 10 years is approximately 1 mm/kg body weight (Bosenberg, 1995). Approximate depths from the skin to the lumbar and thoracic epidural spaces for the different ages are referenced in Figure 14–2.

Technique

With the child in the lateral position and knees and hips flexed, the line that joins the two iliac crests crosses the body of S1 in

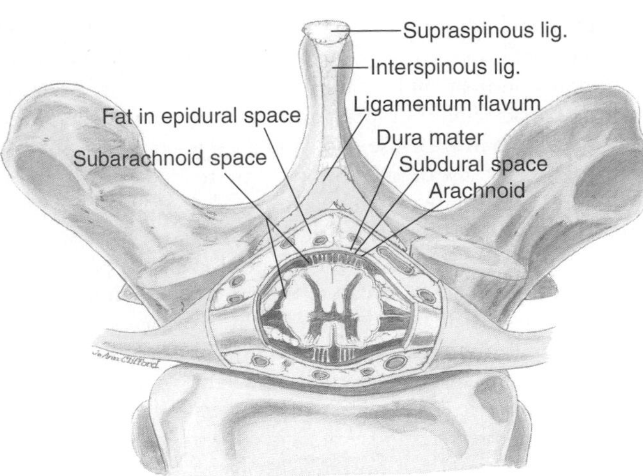

■ **PLATE 14–6.** Anatomy of the epidural space. (From Brown DL: *Atlas of Regional Anesthesia.* WB Saunders, Philadelphia, 1992, p. 286.) (Color image is available on the DVD.)

neonates, L5 in infants, L4-5 in young children, and L4 in older children and adolescents (Busoni and Messeri, 1989) (Plate 14–7; color image is available on the DVD). After sterile prep and drape, the needle should be placed in the midline between the spinous processes that are closest to the line that crosses the iliac crests. If performing a lumbar epidural puncture, the spinous processes require the needle to be directed slightly cephalad but mostly perpendicular to the skin. The needle is advanced slowly with one hand firmly against the child's back and holding the portion of the needle that is entering the child's skin. This is to avoid any inadvertent and rapid advancement of the needle. The needle passes through skin, subcutaneous tissue, supraspinous ligament, interspinous ligament, and then ligamentum flavum before entering the epidural space as illustrated in Plate 14–6. Because of the risk of air embolus, a continuous loss of resistance technique using saline rather than air to confirm the epidural space is the recommended approach (Sethna and Berde, 1993).

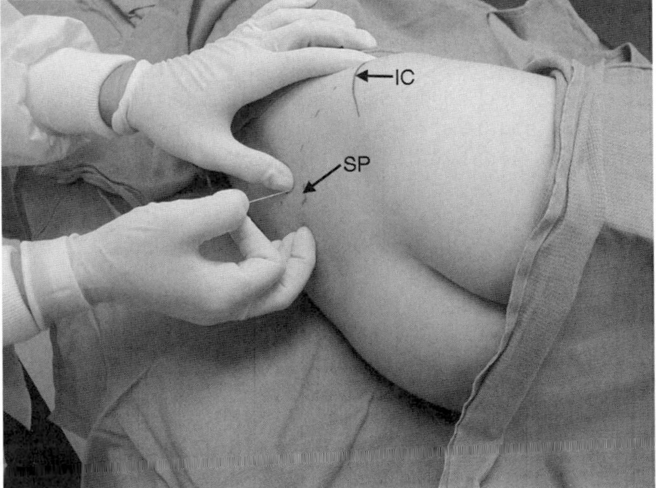

■ **PLATE 14–7.** Performance of the epidural block. IC, iliac crest; SP, spinous process. (Color image is available on the DVD.)

The ability to feel entry into the ligamentum flavum and the loss of resistance as the epidural space is entered are more subtle in infants than in adults. Once the epidural space is entered and there is negative aspiration for CSF or blood, the local anesthetic with epinephrine should be injected as an initial test dose before delivering the planned dose of local anesthetic. Compared with adults, epidural pressures differ in children, particularly in infants (Vas et al., 2001). Based on the relationship between the volume and rate of injection of local anesthetics in infants and the epidural pressure, a slow rate of injection is used, perhaps 0.5 mL/min.

To place a thoracic epidural, the child is placed in the lateral decubitus position. After sterile prep and drape, the point of needle insertion is the midpoint of the spinous processes at the chosen level. The needle should be at a 45- to 60-degree angle aiming cephalad until resistance is felt as the spinous ligaments are encountered. A syringe to detect loss of resistance to saline is attached and the needle is continuously advanced slowly with light pressure on the plunger of the syringe. A sudden loss of resistance indicates needle placement in the epidural space. One of the hallmarks of a successful thoracic epidural needle placement is the ease at which a catheter is threaded in this area. It should pass easily and without resistance.

Equipment

Appropriate-sized equipment is readily available for epidural placement in children. Short Touhy needles and small-gauge catheters, with and without metal helixes, are available. The main disadvantage of a small-gauge catheter is that they increase resistance to continuous infusions of local anesthetics. Postoperatively this can result in frequent alarm of the infusion pump.

Dosing

Epidural catheters are typically placed with the plan to continue their use in the postoperative period. Because the tip of the epidural catheter should be in close proximity to the level of surgery and because the lumbar/thoracic epidural space is more compact than the caudal space, the initial bolus of local anesthetic that is required for lumbar and thoracic epidural blocks is smaller (0.3 to 0.5 mL/kg) than the volumes required for a caudal injection. Approximately 90 minutes after the initial bolus, a continuous infusion may be initiated with care to stay within dosing guidelines (see Table 14–2). Commonly used local anesthetics for epidural analgesia are bupivacaine, levobupivacaine, and ropivacaine. Recommendations for epidural dosing may be found in Table 14–4.

When using 0.25% bupivacaine at a rate of 0.08 mL/kg per hr in the lumbar epidural space in children aged 11 months to 15 years, Desparmet and others (1987) demonstrated that the terminal half-life ranges from 164 to 270 minutes and that total body clearance is similar to that after single caudal injection. Larsson and others (1994) studied bupivacaine infusions in 12 infants. In infants, bupivacaine infusions at rates of 0.5 to 0.83 mg/kg per hr for 12 hours resulted in marked increases in plasma bupivacaine concentrations. Larsson also noted possible toxic reactions in 3 of the 12 infants and suggested these infusion rates were excessive for this age group.

The pharmacokinetics of epidural ropivacaine were assessed after a single injection of 1.7 mg/kg via a lumbar epidural catheter (McCann et al., 2001). The median peak plasma concentrations of ropivacaine were 610 mcg/L in infants aged 3 to 11 months and 640 mcg/L in children aged 12 to 48 months. In both groups of children the median peak plasma concentration was reached in 60 minutes. The calculated clearance of ropivacaine was 4.26 mL/kg per min in infants and 6.15 mL/kg/min in older children. There was no ropivacaine toxicity observed in either group. When ropivacaine 0.2% at 0.4 mg/kg per hr was delivered as a continuous lumbar or epidural infusion for 36 to 96 hours, Hansen and others (2000) noted no clinically significant side effects in 18 pediatric patients aged 4 months to 7 years. In this study, the volume of distribution of epidural ropivacaine was 3.1 L/kg, total clearance was 8.5 mL/kg per min, and the elimination half-life was 4.9 hours (see Table 14–1).

Epidural Additives

The advantage of adding clonidine to single-shot caudal blocks has been demonstrated, but only recently has there been investigation of its use for continuous epidural analgesia. In a study of 60 children who received a low lumbar epidural catheter for hypospadias repair, a postoperative infusion of ropivacaine alone versus ropivacaine with varying doses of clonidine was compared. In this study, plain ropivacaine 0.1% at 0.2 mg/kg per hr or ropivacaine 0.08% at 0.16 mg/kg per hr plus either clonidine 0.04, 0.08, or 0.12 mcg/kg/hr was evaluated (De Negri et al., 2001). The children who received the ropivacaine with the higher clonidine doses in the 0.08 to 0.12 mcg/kg per hr range had improved pain scores, longer time to first analgesic, and reduced total supplemental analgesics. In addition, these patients had no evidence of sedation or other side effects.

The use of neuraxial opioids was discussed in detail in the section on caudal analgesia. In a study designed to assess the efficacy of preoperative epidural morphine, 21 children were randomized to either receive 30 mcg/kg epidural morphine after induction of general anesthesia but before surgical incision or to not receive an epidural injection. Both groups were given intraoperative infusions of sufentanil and postoperative Patient Controlled Analgesia (PCA) with morphine. The group that had received preoperative epidural morphine, in comparison with the control group without epidural morphine, had lower pain scores and decreased total analgesic requirements postoperatively without increased side effects (Kiffer et al., 2001).

Epinephrine is a commonly used additive for single-shot epidural blocks because of its ability to decrease systemic absorption and perhaps prolong the block while adding an additional level of safety. For continuous infusions, these benefits must be weighed against the theoretical risks of vasoconstriction of spinal vessels. A study by Kokki and others (2002) compared a combination of ropivacaine and sufentanil with and without epinephrine 2 mcg/mL in a population of children. The group of children who had epinephrine in their postoperative epidural infusions had significantly lower infusion requirements and fewer side effects.

Complications

As discussed for caudal catheters, the risk of infection is very low. Although there have been case reports of epidural abscess, short-term epidural catheterization for postoperative courses do not appear to have the same risk of infection as those that may be placed for chronic pain (Strafford et al., 1995). In 1620 children studied over a 6-year period who received epidural catheters, there were no infections or epidural abscesses in catheters that had been placed for postoperative pain management. There was only one epidural abscess found in this study, and that was in an immunosuppressed child with terminal malignancy who had *Candida* colonization of the epidural space that had been invaded by tumor and who had an indwelling catheter for control of pain from her malignancy. When catheters have been removed and cultured, the incidence of catheter-tip colonization in epidural catheters is 4%, lower than that found in caudal catheters at 20% (McNeeley et al., 1997).

■ PERIPHERAL NERVE BLOCKS

The goal of placing peripheral nerve blocks (PNBs) is to specifically target analgesia to the location of the surgery so that side effects may be kept to a minimum (Ross et al., 2000). The safety of performing such blocks has been established, and it has been recommended by ADARPEF that peripheral blocks be used in place of central blocks when appropriate (Giaufre et al., 1996). In their safety study of regional anesthetics in children, there were no complications in the 9396 children who received PNBs or local anesthesia. Despite these findings, PNBs are underused in children, probably related to inexperience and the perception that they may be difficult to perform or may be hazardous.

Success of placing PNBs is often a function of knowledge of the anatomy and use of the appropriate equipment (Sethna and Berde, 1992). Insulated needles with a nerve stimulator are typically used for peripheral nerve blockade because they allow precise location of the nerve independent of the nerve's depth. With insulated needles, the field of current is localized to the needle's tip. Unsheathed needles may be less expensive and result in successful blocks, but the current is distributed not only to the needle's tip but also along the shaft of the needle. The required stimulatory current is greater (up to 2 mA) (Bosenberg, 1995). For upper extremity nerve blocks, a 1- or 2-inch insulated needle will suffice. Lower extremity blocks may require the use of longer needles, particularly for sciatic blocks in adolescents. Another practical consideration in performing a PNB with a nerve stimulator is that the use of neuromuscular blockers abolishes the ability to elicit muscle stimulation with a peripheral nerve stimulator. The peripheral nerve stimulator should be capable of delivering 0.1 to greater than 1.5 mA and be set to 2 Hz. The positive electrode of the nerve stimulator should be placed at least 10 cm from the nerve to be blocked and preferentially on the opposite limb.

To locate a nerve or plexus, one should begin with the nerve stimulator set at 1 to 1.2 mA and advance the needle until the desired motor response is achieved. The voltage may then be decreased. When the voltage is decreased to less than 0.5 mA, the motor response should be diminished but still present. One may need to make further fine adjustments in the needle's position in order to continue muscle stimulation of the appropriate muscle group at the lower voltage. However, an increase in voltage may be required to relocate the nerve if muscle stimulation is completely lost. Once the nerve stimulator's voltage is less than 0.5 mA and slight muscle stimulation results, then local anesthetic is injected. If the needle is in the correct position, the muscle stimulation should cease immediately. If there is intense muscle stimulation with 0.2 mA, the possibility of intraneural needle placement must be considered. Consequently, the needle should be withdrawn and readvanced carefully. In anesthetized children, the placement of a needle into a nerve would not be detected, so this warning sign of intense muscle stimulation at lower voltage is significant. In addition, one should look for other warning signs of intraneural injection such as difficulty with injection and increased heart rate with injection.

Surface nerve mapping has been used in children to improve the ability to locate a peripheral nerve or plexus and may be a useful practice, particularly in patients with abnormal anatomy and in infants who may be at higher risks of complications from regional anesthesia (Bosenberg, 2002). Nerve surface mapping is performed by setting the nerve stimulator at a frequency of 1 to 2 Hz and the current between 3 to 4 mA. The positive electrode should be at least 10 cm from the nerve to be mapped, and the negative electrode or alligator clamp that would normally be attached to the block needle is instead pressed against the skin at right angles across the suspected path of the nerve. Once a point of maximal motor response is found, a mark may be placed to indicate where the insulated needle may be inserted for regional blockade.

In children who are anesthetized, it is not possible to reliably test the success of a PNB; however, one may increase the voltage of the nerve stimulator after local anesthetic injection to determine that there is loss of stimulation. Although subtle, it is also possible to determine success of motor block by comparing the flaccidity of the blocked limb with the muscle tone of the contralateral extremity. Vasodilation and/or increased skin temperature, when present in the blocked limb, may be a more reliable indicator of a successful block, but its absence does not mean that the block is unsuccessful. The absolute determinant of a successful block is the absence of response to the surgical incision. Most PNBs, independent of the agent used, should provide total analgesia to the desired nerve or plexus within 20 minutes of the local anesthetic injection.

Dosing of PNBs is discussed with regard to the individual block. Independent of the local anesthetic delivered, the addition of epinephrine to the solution should provide additional safety when performing the block. As previously discussed, not only does the addition of epinephrine to the local anesthetic solution have the potential to serve as a marker for intravascular injection; it may also decrease overall absorption of the local anesthetic. In a study of 20 children who were to undergo unilateral surgery of the thigh, patients were administered a fascia iliaca block using 2 mg/kg bupivacaine either with or without epinephrine 5 mcg/mL (Doyle et al., 1997). The median maximum plasma bupivacaine concentration in the group without epinephrine was 1.1 mcg/mL compared with 0.3 mcg/mL in the group of patients in whom epinephrine was added to the bupivacaine. Not only did the epinephrine group have a significantly lower peak plasma level, but the onset time to peak plasma concentration was more gradual for the group with epinephrine.

The majority of PNB techniques are similar to those of adults. The differences from adult practice are presented here, along with blocks that are more directed to children.

■ UPPER EXTREMITY NERVE BLOCKS

Upper extremity blocks may be used for surgery of the shoulder, arm, and hand. Specifically, brachial plexus blocks below the clavicle, including the axillary approach, are suitable for surgery on the hand and those blocks above the clavicle are useful for surgery on the shoulder and upper arm (Plate 14–8; color image is available on the DVD). Depending on the approach to the plexus, it is also possible to provide total analgesia to the hand with blocks above the clavicle.

Anatomy

The brachial plexus contains the anterior branches of spinal roots C5 through T1 (Plate 14–9; color image is available on the DVD).

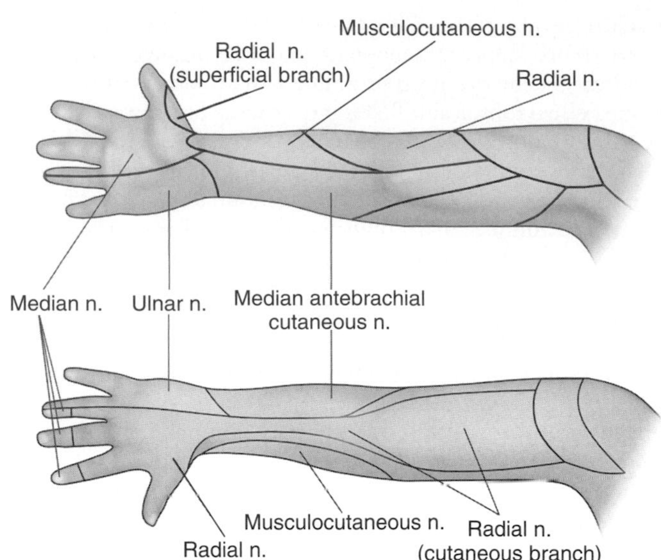

■ **PLATE 14–8.** Dermatomal distribution of brachial plexus. (Color image is available on the DVD.)

In the neck, these branches run between the anterior and middle scalene muscles and are enclosed in a fascial sheath. They then form three trunks (superior, middle, inferior) that exit the interscalene groove and run behind the subclavian artery. As they exit the interscalene groove, these cords form an anterior and a

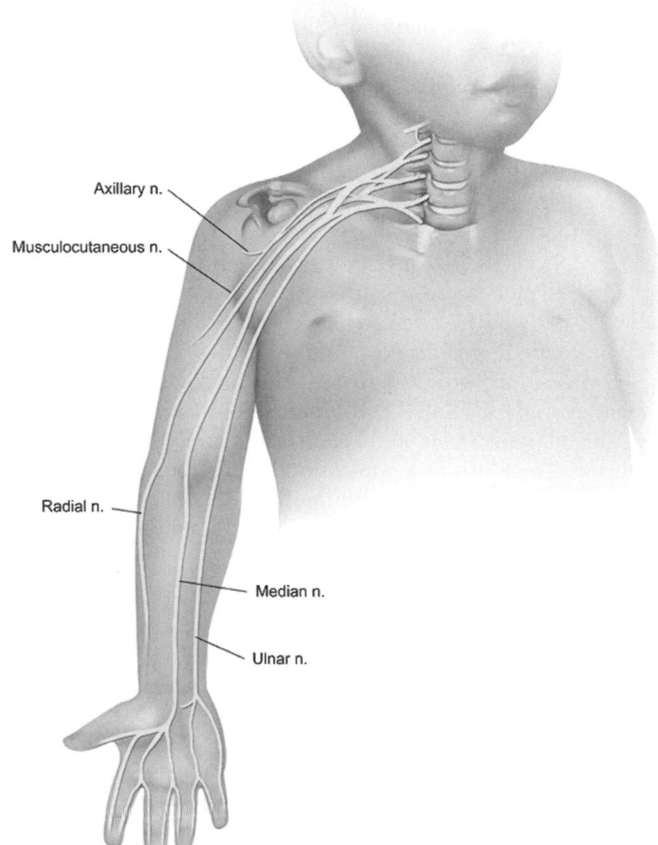

■ **PLATE 14–9.** Brachial plexus anatomy. (Color image is available on the DVD.)

posterior division. The divisions then unite to form lateral, posterior, and medial cords, depending on their relation to the axillary artery. There is a natural separation between the supraclavicular and infraclavicular plexus at the coracoid process that ultimately affects spread of local anesthetic (Vester-Andersen et al., 1986). At the level of the axilla exist the peripheral nerves that innervate the arm. The radial nerve supplies the dorsal aspect of the upper extremity below the shoulder including the thumb and dorsal aspects of the index, middle, and fourth fingers. The musculocutaneous nerve provides innervation to the biceps of the upper arm and cutaneous innervation to the lateral forearm. The median nerve innervates the majority of the forearm, as well as the ventral aspects of the second, third, and lateral portion of the fourth fingers, and the medial portion of the thumb. The ulnar nerve is more limited to the hand and innervates the lateral aspect of the fourth finger and all of the fifth finger.

Axillary Block

Axillary block is the most common approach to the brachial plexus in children and is suitable for procedures on the hand such as syndactyly repair and finger reimplantation (Plate 14–10; color image is available on the DVD). Advantages of performing an axillary block include the simplicity of the anatomy, ease of placement, and low risk of complications (Tobias 2001). Disadvantages include the need for a patient to be able to abduct the arm for access to the axilla and the inability to block the musculocutaneous nerve 40% to 50% of the time because it branches higher in the axilla than the ulnar, median, and radial nerves. Because the musculocutaneous nerve innervates the lateral side of the forearm, it may need to be blocked separately for surgical procedures that involve that nerve's distribution. Many approaches for an axillary block have been described and used in children. In a study to compare a single-injection versus a multiple-injection technique in children, unlike in adults, there was no difference in block quality found between the two techniques (Carre et al., 2000). This study also confirmed that using either technique, separate block of the musculocutaneous nerve is still required if necessary for the surgical site.

In a study to assess the efficacy of the timing of an axillary block, 55 children received 2 mg/kg of 0.25% bupivacaine either before surgical incision or immediately after surgery but before emergence (Altintas et al., 2000). Thirty-two percent of children in the presurgical group required no additional analgesics within the first 24 hours compared with 83% in the postsurgical group that required no additional analgesics. Although cumulative pain scores were higher in the presurgical group, both groups had effective analgesia.

Technique

A one-injection technique for axillary nerve block is accomplished by first palpating the axillary artery (Plate 14–11; color image is available on the DVD). The needle is then inserted immediately adjacent and superior to the artery high in the axilla, at a 30- to 45-degree angle aimed toward the midpoint of the clavicle (Plate 14–12; color image is available on the DVD). One may feel a "pop" as the plexus sheath is entered. Using a nerve stimulator, and after evidence of muscle stimulation in the hand is observed, local anesthetic is injected. A longitudinal swelling immediately beneath the skin as the local anesthetic fills the sheath may appear. This may occur especially in infants and young children. This swelling disappears quickly as the anesthetic spreads proximally into the sheath, and this swelling should not be confused with a subcutaneous injection. Subcutaneous injection does not have a longitudinal distribution and does not disappear quickly.

After the local anesthetic has been delivered and the needle removed, the arm should be adducted, thus releasing the pressure of the head of the humerus from the fossa. This motion along with holding distal pressure at the site of injection promotes proximal spread of the local anesthetic into the sheath. With a single-injection technique, all of the local anesthetic is delivered in one location. With a multiple-injection technique, the nerves are individually anesthetized by locating at least two

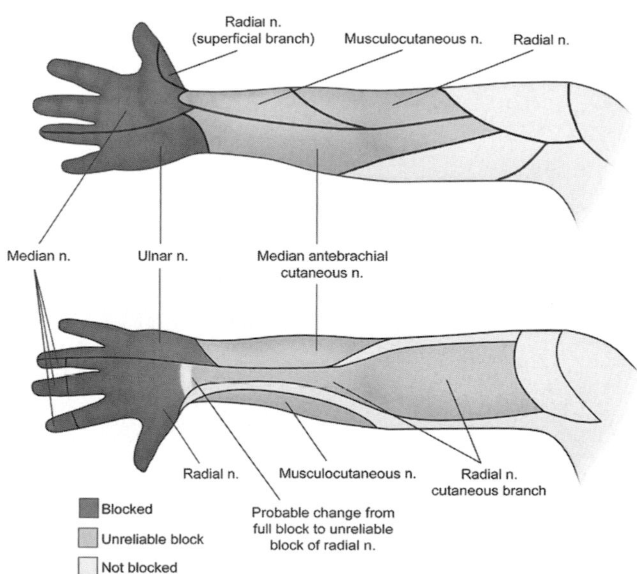

■ **PLATE 14–10.** Dermatomal distribution of axillary block. (Color image is available on the DVD.)

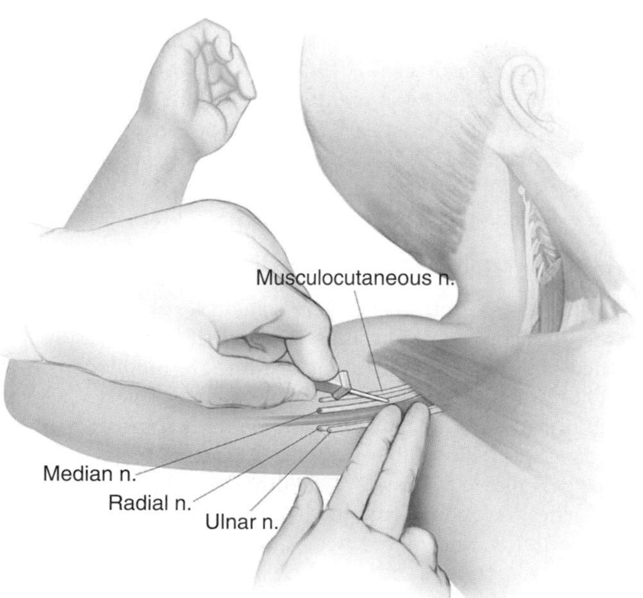

■ **PLATE 14–11.** Anatomy for axillary block. (Color image is available on the DVD.)

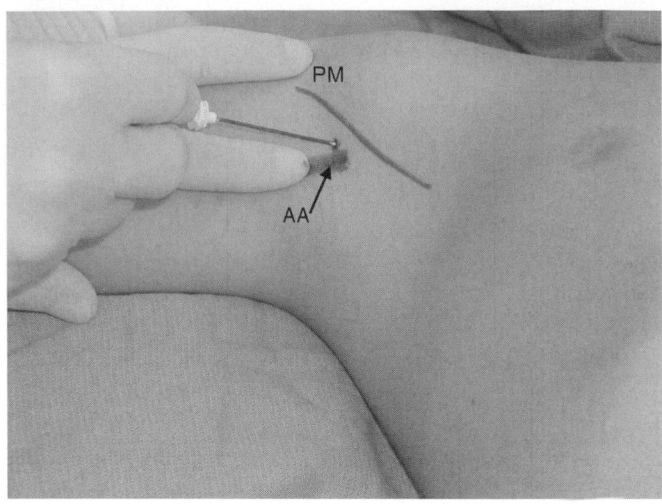

■ **PLATE 14–12.** Performance of the axillary block. AA, axillary artery; PM, pectoralis muscle. (Color image is available on the DVD.)

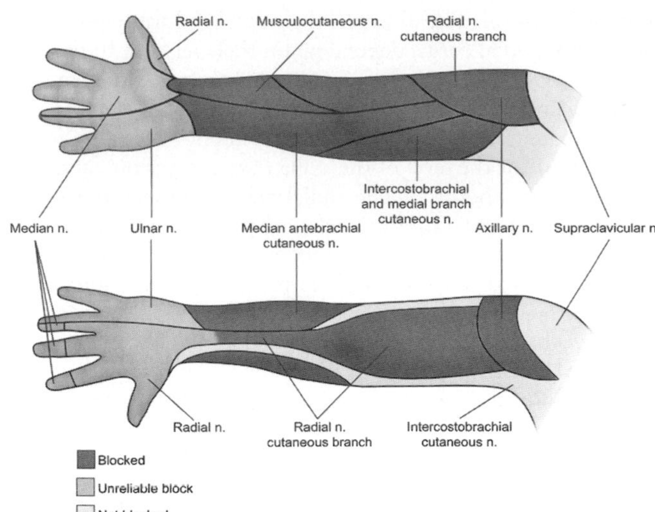

■ **PLATE 14–13.** Dermatomal distribution of lateral vertical infraclavicular brachial plexus block. (Color image is available on the DVD.)

of them individually using the nerve stimulator. Either technique may miss the musculocutaneous nerve because it exits the sheath proximal to the other three distal nerves. For this reason, a separate block of the musculocutaneous nerve is generally required. The musculocutaneous nerve is blocked by directly inserting the needle into the belly of the coracobrachialis muscle while looking for stimulation of biceps. In addition, if a surgical tourniquet is to be used and the patient is not having a general anesthetic, then the intercostobrachial nerve should be blocked. This is accomplished by placing a subcutaneous ring of local anesthetic high around the inner aspect of the arm.

Complications

There should be few complications when performing an axillary block. There is the rare risk of hematoma and nerve compression, and for this reason a transarterial approach may not be recommended in children. If inadvertent axillary artery puncture occurs, firm pressure should be applied for at least 5 minutes to avoid formation of hematoma and subsequent vascular insufficiency (Merril et al., 1981). Other complications may include relative distortion of anatomy after the first injection of local anesthetic in the axillary region or inadvertent overdosage of local anesthetic when multiple-injection techniques are used (Dalens, 1995). However, these complications were not reported in the pediatric study by Carre and others (2000).

Lateral Vertical Infraclavicular Block

A lateral vertical infraclavicular brachial plexus (LVIBP) block was introduced for pediatric use because the block can be performed without arm abduction. In addition, the block is more reliable in anesthetizing the musculocutaneous nerve, and the block provides better analgesia of upper arm compared with an axillary block (Fleischmann et al., 2003) (Plate 14–13; color image is available on the DVD). Although other infraclavicular approaches were considered too hazardous because of the risk of pneumothorax, the more lateral and vertical approach developed by Kapral and others (1999) provides a safe distance between puncture site and pleura. This technique has been used in adults and children and has been shown to provide a greater spectrum of block than the axillary approach (Kapral et al., 1999; Fleischmann et al., 2003). The indications for a lateral infraclavicular block are the same as those for axillary block.

Technique

With the child in the supine position, the upper arm should remain next to the trunk and the elbow flexed 90 degrees so that the forearm is on the abdomen. One palpates the coracoid process and, using a nerve stimulator, inserts a 1-inch 24-gauge insulated needle 0.5 cm distal to the coracoid process in a perpendicular or vertical direction while continuously aspirating for blood and/or air (Plates 14–14 and 14–15; color images are available on the DVD). Once appropriate stimulation has been determined and continuous aspiration for blood and/or air has been negative, local anesthetic solution is then injected. There is no need to block the musculocutaneous nerve separately when this approach is used.

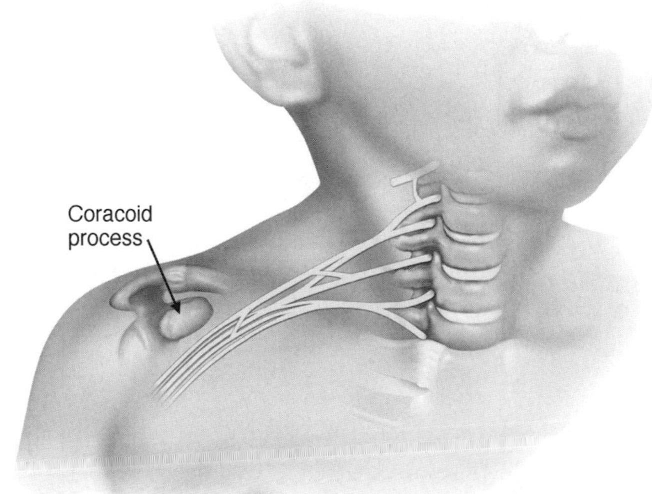

■ **PLATE 14–14.** Anatomy for lateral vertical infraclavicular brachial plexus block. (Color image is available on the DVD.)

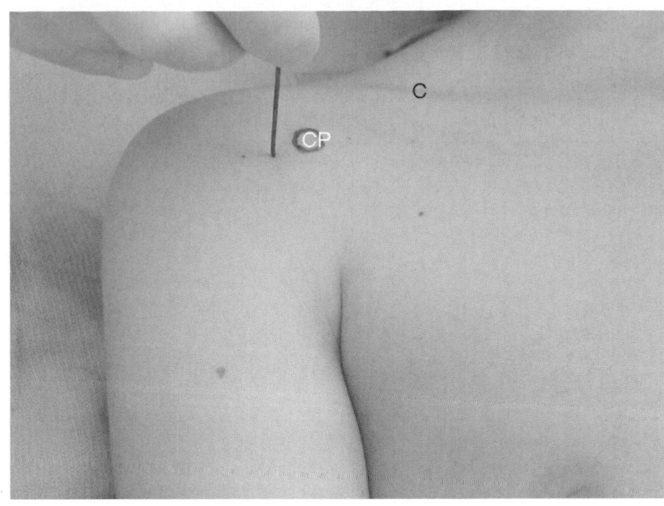

■ **PLATE 14–15.** Performance of lateral vertical infraclavicular brachial plexus block. CP, coracoid process; C, clavicle. (Color image is available on the DVD.)

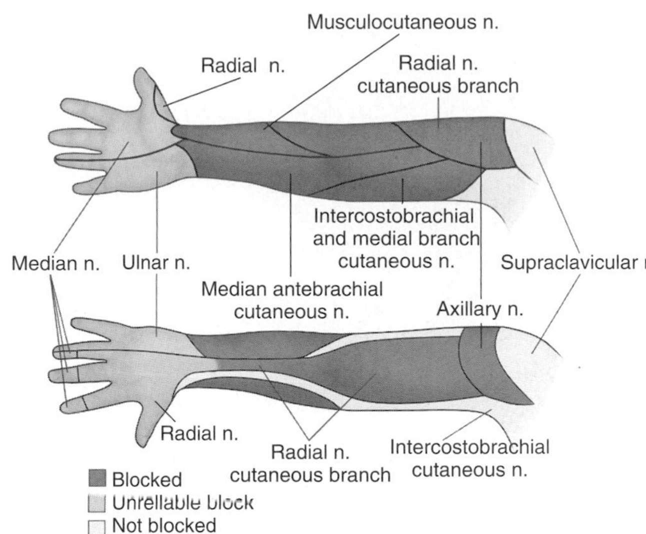

■ **PLATE 14–16.** Dermatomal distribution of parascalene block. (Color image is available on the DVD.)

Complications

Complications using this approach are rare. There may still be risk of inadvertent pleural or vascular puncture, but these risks should be less than with other approaches to the brachial plexus.

Interscalene Block

An interscalene block may be used for surgery of the shoulder and upper arm with success in children. An interscalene block also anesthetizes the musculocutaneous nerve reliably, but there is less reliability of blocking the ulnar nerve than with the other nerve blocks. This is because the ulnar nerve's origin is in the lower portion of the plexus. Interscalene blocks are used infrequently in children because of the perceived higher risk of complications and side effects.

Technique

With the patient supine and the head turned in the opposite direction, the posterior border to the sternocleidomastoid muscle may be palpated. Immediately inferior to this and at the level of the cricoid cartilage, the interscalene groove should be identified by rolling the fingers behind the sternocleidomastoid muscle. The needle is inserted at a 90-degree angle to the skin with a slight caudal angle to elicit distal contractions. If the phrenic nerve is stimulated, the diaphragm contracts, which indicates that the needle is too anterior. Once appropriate muscle stimulation is observed at the proper voltage, local anesthetic is injected.

Complications

Complications of interscalene block include pneumothorax, epidural injection, or intrathecal injection. Vertebral artery puncture may also occur with the risk of local anesthetic delivery directly to the CNS, resulting in CNS toxicity. In addition, there is a high risk of phrenic nerve block with paralysis of the hemidiaphragm. Phrenic nerve block is not well tolerated, especially in infants or patients with underlying respiratory compromise (Kempen et al., 2000). Unilateral vocal cord paralysis may also occur and result in airway compromise. Sympathetic blockade with Horner's syndrome is a common side effect of interscalene blocks.

Parascalene Block

The parascalene approach to the brachial plexus was developed by Dalens (1995) to provide effective analgesia to the shoulder and upper arm while minimizing the risks of vertebral artery puncture, dural puncture, and/or pneumothorax, that is, risks associated with an interscalene block. The parascalene block is similar to the interscalene approach, but by changing the insertion and direction of the needle, major structures in the neck are avoided (Plate 14–16; color image is available on the DVD). This block has been found to be easy to perform, with a 97% success rate in children on the first or second attempt (Dalens et al., 1987).

Technique

With the child supine and a roll under the shoulders, the arm should be adducted next to the trunk and the head turned to the opposite side. The primary landmarks are Chassaignac's tubercle (transverse process of C6) and the midpoint of the clavicle. Draw a line between these two structures and insert a needle at the junction of the upper two thirds and lower third of this line (Plates 14–17 and 14–18; color images are available on the DVD). This insertion spot should be at the level of the cricoid process near the external jugular vein. The approximate depth to the parascalene brachial plexus from the skin is different for different ages of children (see Fig. 14–2). Using low voltage, and once appropriate stimulation has been achieved, the local anesthetic solution is then injected.

Complications

Complications using the parascalene approach are rare but may include venous puncture, Horner's syndrome, and hemidiaphragmatic paralysis secondary to phrenic nerve paralysis.

Dosing of Upper Extremity Blocks

Various local anesthetics either alone or in combination have been used for upper extremity blocks. For prolonged analgesia, bupivacaine, levobupivacaine, or ropivacaine should be used. Because the brachial plexus is not highly vascular, the uptake

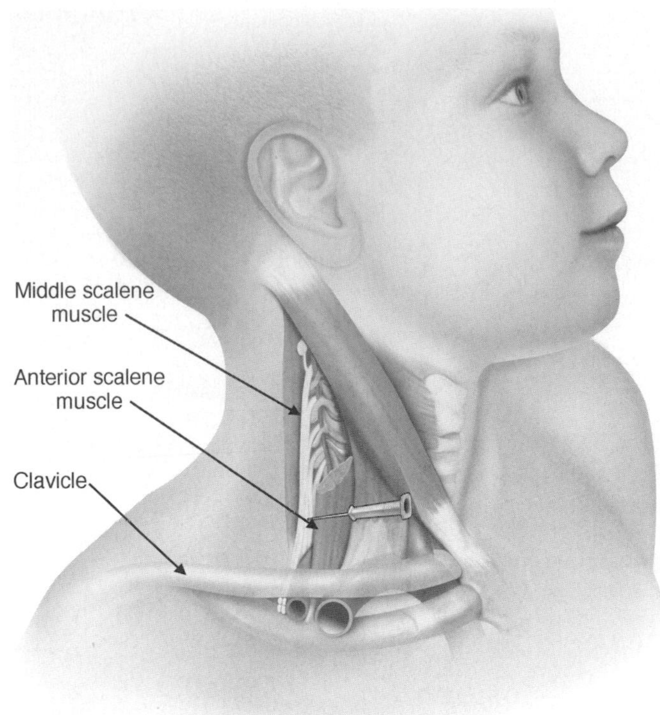

■ **PLATE 14–17.** Anatomy for parascalene block. (Color image is available on the DVD.)

of local anesthetic is less than that of pleural or central blocks; however, the maximal allowable doses of local anesthetic must be determined and the block dosed accordingly. When concentrations were compared, bupivacaine 2 mg/kg versus 3 mg/kg delivered for axillary block in children resulted in plasma levels of 1.35 mcg/mL and 1.84 mcg/mL, respectively (Campbell et al., 1986). These values are well below the toxic range. To compare 0.2% ropivacaine with 0.25% bupivacaine, Thornton and others (2003) administered 0.5 mL/kg to children for axillary block. There was no significant difference between the two groups in pain scores, time to first analgesic, or total analgesic in 24 hours. The median time to first dose of analgesic was 7.25 hours in the ropivacaine group and 9.3 hours in the bupivacaine group. In general, if using 0.25% to 0.5% bupivacaine or levobupivacaine or 0.2% to 0.5% ropivacaine, the lower concentrations should be used in children 5 years of age or less at a volume of 0.5 mL/kg. Epinephrine 5 mcg/mL should be added to the solution to assist in identifying intravascular injection and to decrease the absorption of the local anesthetic. Using these dosing guidelines, approximately 4 to 12 hours of analgesia should be achieved (Table 14–5).

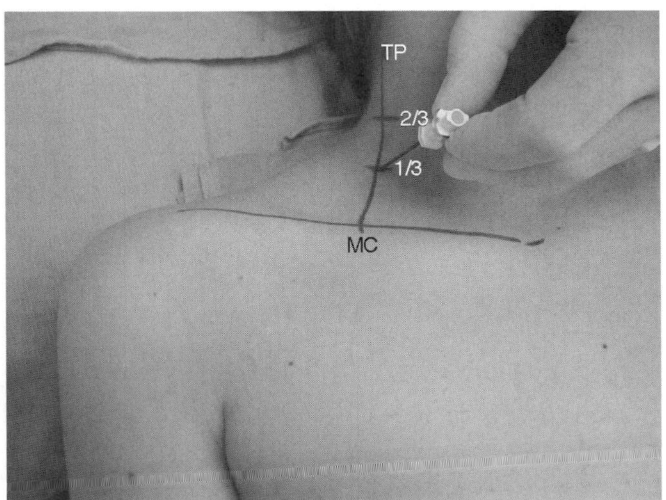

■ **PLATE 14–18.** Performance of parascalene block. TP, transverse process of C6; MC, midpoint of clavicle. (Color image is available on the DVD.)

■ **TABLE 14–5.** Recommendations for dosing of peripheral nerve blocks

Regional Technique	Bolus Dose (mL/kg)*	Continuous Infusion (mL/kg per hr)
Axillary	0.2 to 0.5	0.1 to 0.2
Parascalene	0.2 to 0.4	0.1 to 0.2
Femoral or lateral femoral cutaneous	0.3 to 1	0.15 to 0.3
Fascia iliaca	0.5 to 1	0.15 to 0.3
Lumbar plexus	0.5 to 1	0.15 to 0.3
Sciatic	0.3 to 1	0.15 to 0.3
Ilioinguinal/ iliohypogastric	0.25	NA
Penile block	0.1	NA
Paravertebral	0.5	0.2 to 0.25

NA, not applicable.

Bupivacaine, levobupivacaine, or ropivacaine may be used. For bolus dosing, lower concentrations such as 0.2% to 0.25% should be used in infants and young children, whereas concentrations of 0.375% to 0.5% should be used in children >5 to 8 years of age. For continuous infusions, lower concentrations such as 0.1% to 0.2% of all agents are acceptable.

*Epinephrine 1:200,000 should be added to single-shot peripheral nerve blocks except for penile block.

■ LOWER EXTREMITY NERVE BLOCKS

Although caudal block is the most commonly performed pediatric regional anesthetic technique, lower extremity nerve blocks often provide analgesia to the lower limbs with a more direct effect (McNicol, 1986; Dalens, 1995; Ross et al., 2000; Tobias, 2003). Lower extremity blocks are performed by anesthetizing the lumbar and/or sacral plexus.

The lumbar plexus is located in the psoas compartment that lies in the paravertebral space (Plate 14–19; color image is available on the DVD). The union of the anterior rami of lumbar nerves L1-4 constitutes the primary input of the lumbar plexus with a small portion of the twelfth thoracic nerve. As the plexus emerges from the paravertebral space, it divides into three nerves: the femoral, the lateral femoral cutaneous, and the obturator. Although the iliac vessels run anterior to the iliac fascia, these three nerves remain posterior to the fascia. The femoral nerve is a mixed nerve with motor innervation to the quadriceps muscles and sensory innervation to the anterior and medial thigh. A branch of the femoral nerve, the saphenous nerve, provides innervation below the knee to the medial aspect of the lower leg and foot near the saphenous vein. The lateral femoral cutaneous nerve is a sensory nerve with innervation to the lateral thigh, and the obturator nerve is primarily motor to the leg adductors with some sensory to the lower medial thigh and knee.

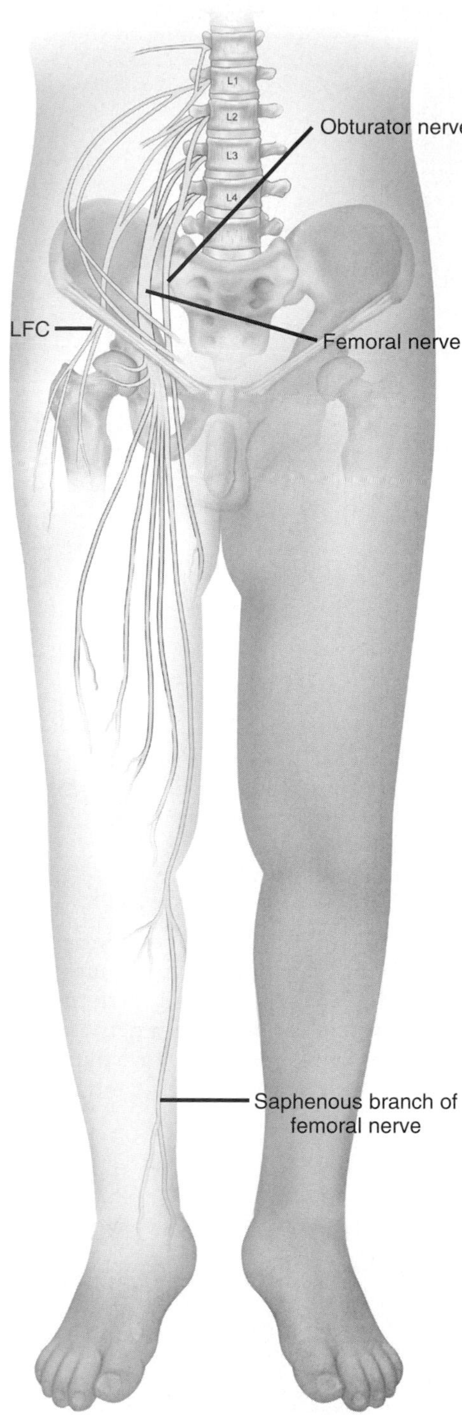

■ **PLATE 14–19.** Anatomy and distribution of lumbar plexus. LFC, lateral femoral cutaneous nerve. (Color image is available on the DVD.)

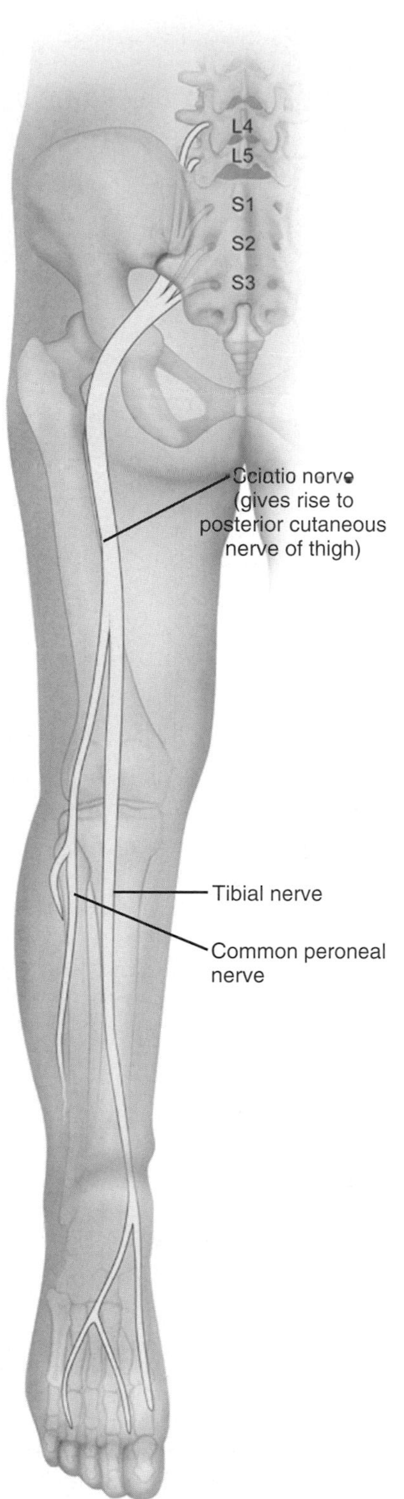

■ **PLATE 14–20.** Anatomy and distribution of sacral plexus. (Color image is available on the DVD.)

The sacral plexus is derived from the anterior rami of L4, L5, and S1-3 and gives rise to the sciatic nerve and the posterior cutaneous nerve of the thigh (Plate 14–20; color image is available on the DVD). The sciatic nerve is a mixed nerve that provides motor and sensory innervation to the posterior aspect of the thigh and the majority of the lower leg. As the sciatic nerve travels down the posterior thigh, it branches into the common peroneal and posterior tibial nerves.

Specific blocks of the lower extremity are described.

Lateral Femoral Cutaneous Nerve Block

Although an isolated block of the lateral femoral cutaneous nerve (LFC) is rarely needed, it may be blocked to provide analgesia for muscle biopsy of the vastus lateralis muscle during malignant hyperthermia testing (Wedel, 1989). An LFC block

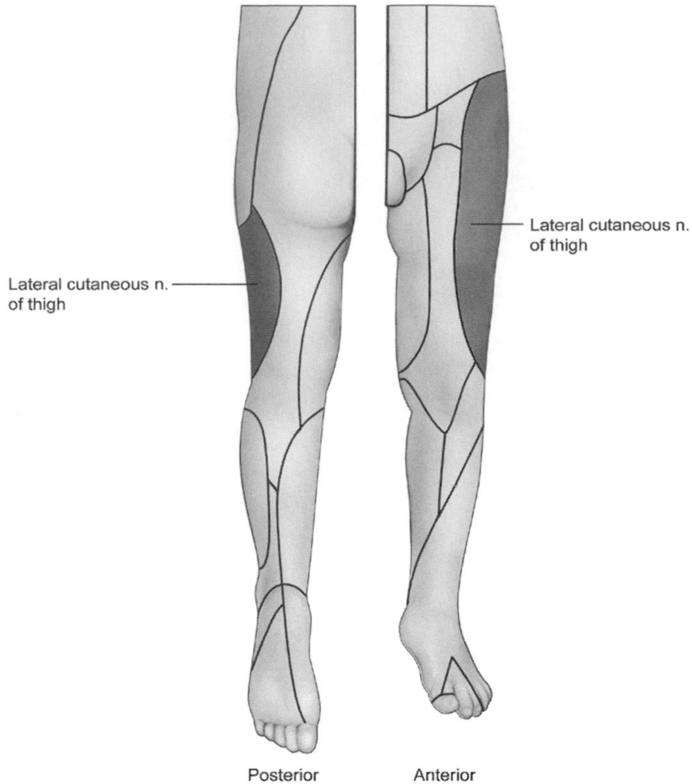

■ **PLATE 14–21.** Dermatomal distribution of lateral femoral cutaneous block. (Color image is available on the DVD.)

may also be used in combination with a femoral nerve block in high-risk children in place of a general anesthetic for complete analgesia for muscle biopsies of the thigh (Rosen and Broadman, 1986; Maccani et al., 1995).

Anatomy

The LFC arises from second and third lumbar nerves and travels deep to the iliacus fascia toward the anterior superior iliac spine until it emerges under the fascia lata in the upper thigh. It is a pure sensory nerve that innervates the lateral thigh to the knee, including some terminal branches at the patellar plexus. (Plate 14–21; color image is available on the DVD.)

Technique

No nerve stimulator is required to block the LFC as the LFC is purely a sensory nerve. In the infrainguinal approach, a blunt 22-gauge needle is inserted perpendicular to the skin aiming in the direction of the nerve inferolaterally 0.5 to 1 cm below the inguinal ligament and medial to the anterior superior iliac spine (Plate 14–22; color image is available on the DVD). A pop is felt as the needle pierces the fascia lata. Local anesthetic is then injected in a fanlike manner (McNicol, 1986).

Complications

There are no known serious complications from an isolated LFC except direct nerve trauma.

Femoral Nerve Block

A femoral nerve block may be used for any above-the-knee surgery of the lower extremity that requires analgesia of the majority of the thigh (Plate 14–23; color image is available on the DVD). This includes analgesia for femur fracture (Ronchi et al., 1989). The block is simple to perform either with or without a nerve stimulator; however, a nerve stimulator should not be used in an awake child with a femur fracture due to the pain that may occur with muscle contraction from nerve stimulation.

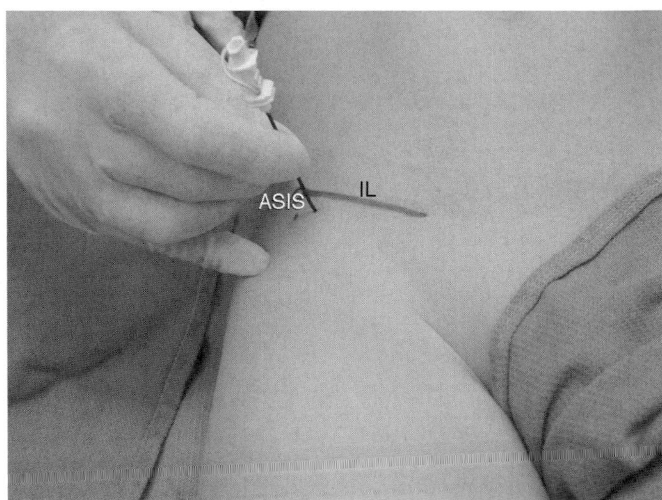

■ **PLATE 14–22.** Performance of lateral femoral cutaneous block. ASIS, anterior superior iliac spine; IL, inguinal ligament. (Color image is available on the DVD.)

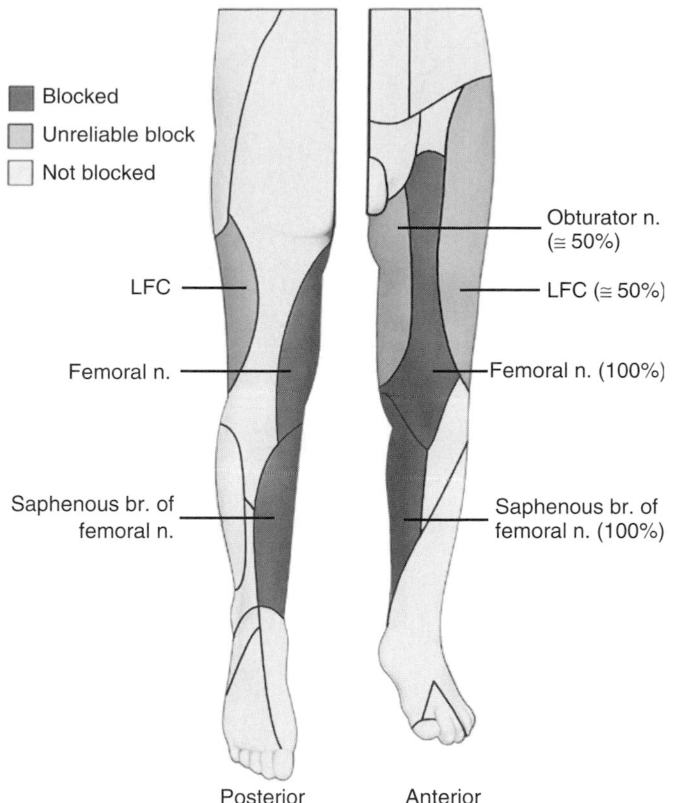

■ **PLATE 14–23.** Dermatomal distribution of femoral nerve block, "3 in 1," with percentages of complete block of individual nerves. LFC, lateral femoral cutaneous nerve. (Color image is available on the DVD.)

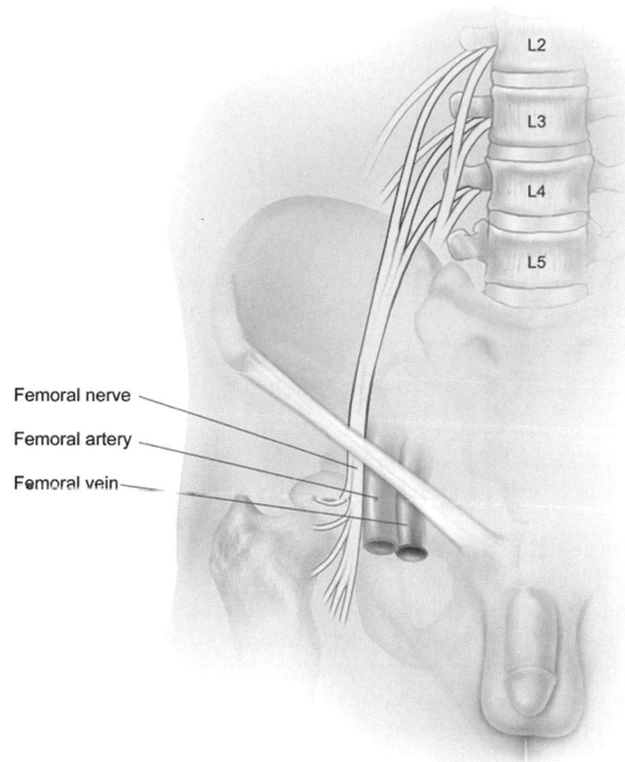

■ **PLATE 14–24.** Anatomy of femoral nerve block. (Color image is available on the DVD.)

Anatomy

The femoral nerve is derived from lumbar nerves 1 to 3 and enters the thigh within the femoral triangle below the inguinal ligament. The approximate depth to the femoral nerve from the skin should be reviewed (see Fig. 14–2). The nerve is immediately lateral to the femoral artery and is covered by the fascia lata and fascia iliaca (Plate 14–24; color image is available on the DVD).

Technique

With the child supine and the feet rotated outward, the femoral artery is palpated immediately below the inguinal ligament. The needle is inserted with a slight cephalad angle to the skin at 0.5 to 1 cm below the inguinal ligament and 0.5 to 1 cm lateral to the artery (Plate 14–25; color image is available on the DVD). As the needle pierces the fascia lata, a distinct pop is felt. If a nerve stimulator is used, the desired muscle response should be contraction of the mid quadriceps with a "patellar kick." If there is muscle stimulation medial to the mid patella at the thigh adductors, the needle is slightly adjusted laterally. If there is lateral muscle stimulation, the needle is adjusted slightly medially. Because of the close proximity of the femoral vessels, continuous aspiration for blood should be performed in order to detect intravascular entry. Once the desired location of the needle is achieved, local anesthetic is then injected.

A "3-in-1" block is a modification of a femoral nerve block. This technique anesthetizes the LFC and obturator nerve, which lie more proximal in the sheath. The 3-in-1 technique is accomplished by performing a femoral nerve block and promoting proximal spread. The landmarks and needle insertion are exactly the same as for a simple femoral block with the exception that the volume of local anesthetic is increased and distal pressure is used to promote cephalad spread to the lumbar plexus by means of using the femoral sheath as a conduit. When compared with a fascia iliaca compartment block (see later), a 3-in-1 approach can result in a higher failure rate (Dalens et al., 1989). In a study by Dalens and others, the 3-in-1 block was successful in anesthetizing the femoral nerve 100% of the time. However, completely

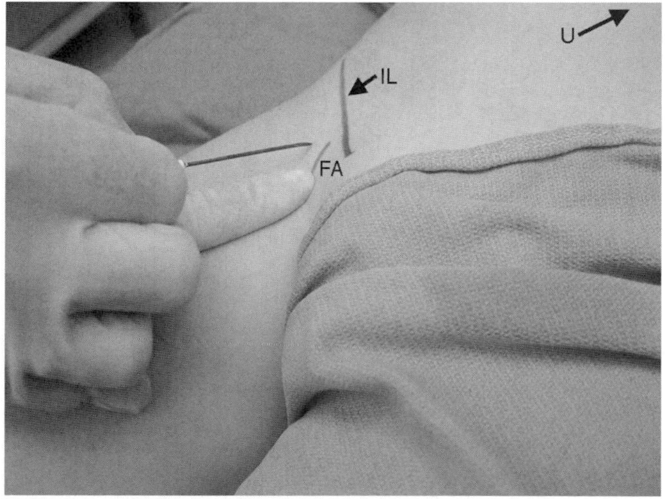

■ **PLATE 14–25.** Performance of femoral block. IL, inguinal ligament; FA, femoral artery; U, umbilicus. Needle insertion is 0.5 to 1 cm lateral to artery. (Color image is available on the DVD.)

blocking the LFC and obturator was successful in only 20% of the children. In this study, Dalens and others noted that the successful blocks of the LFC and obturator nerves in the 3-in-1 group were not due to proximal spread of the local anesthetic but instead may have been due to a fascia iliaca–like spread of the local anesthetic.

Complications

Complications from femoral or 3-in-1 blocks are uncommon but may include puncture of the femoral artery. In that event, pressure should be applied for at least 5 minutes to avoid the formation of a large hematoma.

Fascia Iliaca Compartment Block

The fascia iliaca block provides analgesia of the femoral, lateral femoral cutaneous, and obturator nerves (Plate 14–26; color image is available on the DVD). Compared with the 20% effectiveness of the 3-in-1 block, a fascia iliaca block may be effective in more than 90% of children (Dalens et al., 1989). Fascia iliaca blocks are useful for all above-the-knee lower extremity surgeries because of their ability to anesthetize this region in its entirety. In addition, the fascia iliaca block reliably anesthetizes the femoral branch of the genitofemoral nerve, the sensory nerve supply to Scarpa's triangle. Because of its ability to block the upper leg, the fascia iliaca compartment block can be used in combination with intravenous sedation or nitrous oxide for children who are undergoing muscle biopsy of the thigh.

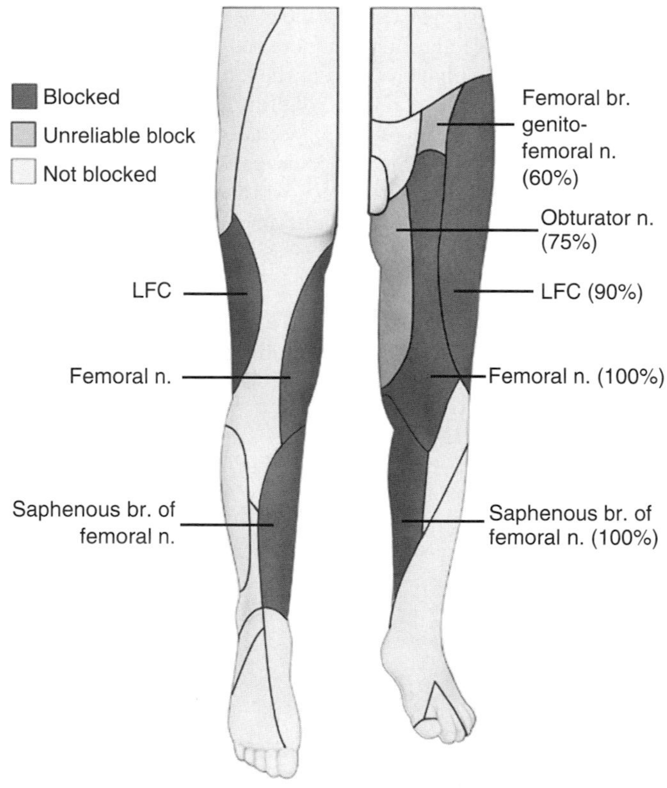

■ **PLATE 14–26.** Dermatomal distribution of fascia iliaca block, with relative percentages of successful block of individual nerves by this approach. LFC, lateral femoral cutaneous nerve. (Color image is available on the DVD.)

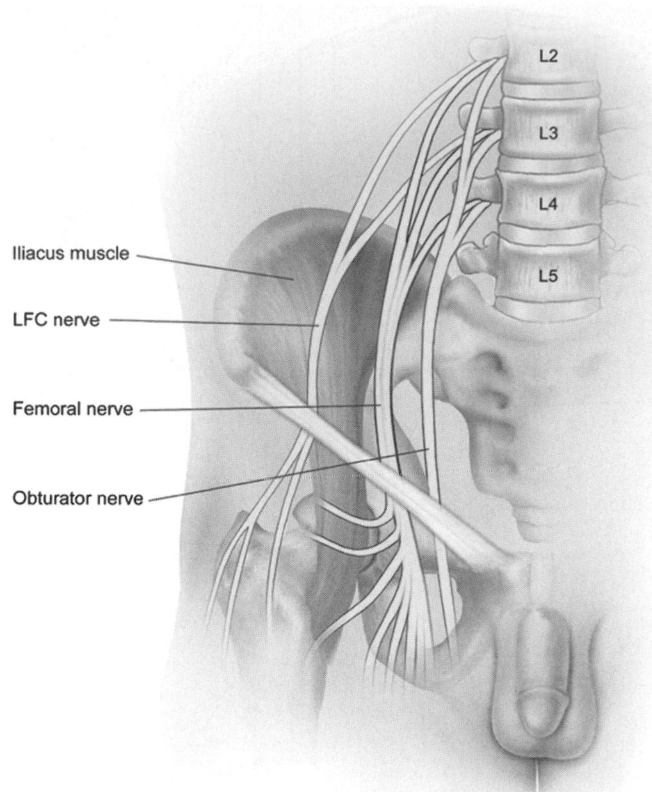

■ **PLATE 14–27.** Anatomy of fascia iliaca block. LFC, lateral femoral cutaneous nerve. (Color image is available on the DVD.)

Anatomy

The three distal nerves of the lumbar plexus—the femoral, lateral femoral cutaneous, and obturator nerves—all emerge from the psoas muscle and run along the inner surface of the fascia iliaca (Plate 14–27; color image is available on the DVD). A fascia iliaca compartment block delivers local anesthetic between the fascia iliaca and iliacus muscle, where it spreads to bathe the three nerves.

Technique

With the child in the supine position, the inguinal ligament is located by drawing a line from pubic tubercle to anterior superior iliac spine. Divide the inguinal ligament into thirds. At the junction of the lateral third and medial two thirds of the inguinal ligament, drop a line inferiorly 0.5 to 2 cm and perpendicular to the ligament. This is the point of needle insertion (Plate 14–28; color image is available on the DVD). A blunt needle is used and is inserted perpendicular to the skin. There is no need for a nerve stimulator because the goal is to find the area behind the iliacus fascia for anesthetic injection, not to locate a specific nerve. Two pops are felt as the needle first pierces the fascia lata and then the fascia iliaca. If light pressure is placed upon the plunger of the syringe, a loss of resistance is felt as the fascia iliaca is pierced. With the needle in the correct position, local anesthetic solution is injected.

Complications

Complications during a fascia iliaca block might include isolated femoral block if the injection is too medial; otherwise, there are

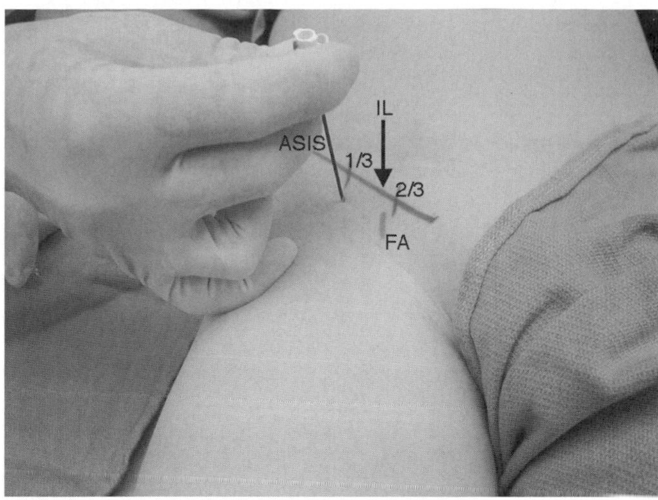

■ **PLATE 14–28.** Performance of fascia iliaca block. ASIS, anterior superior iliac spine; IL, inguinal ligament; FA, femoral artery. Needle insertion is 0.5 to 2 cm below inguinal ligament. (Color image is available on the DVD.)

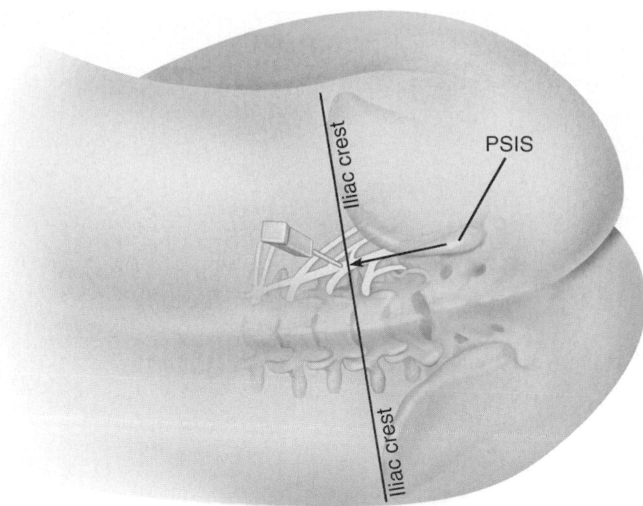

■ **PLATE 14–30.** Anatomy of lumbar plexus block. PSIS, posterior superior iliac spine. (Color image is available on the DVD.)

no known major complications from performing a fascia iliaca block.

Lumbar Plexus Block

Similar to the fascia iliaca compartment block, a lumbar plexus block provides analgesia to the three major nerves of the lumbar plexus (Plate 14–29; color image is available on the DVD). This block is useful for any surgery that may occur on the upper leg due to its complete ability to anesthetize that region. This block also anesthetizes the distal branches of the lumbar plexus, including the iliohypogastric, ilioinguinal, and genitofemoral nerves that innervate the groin area, applicable to many pediatric surgical procedures.

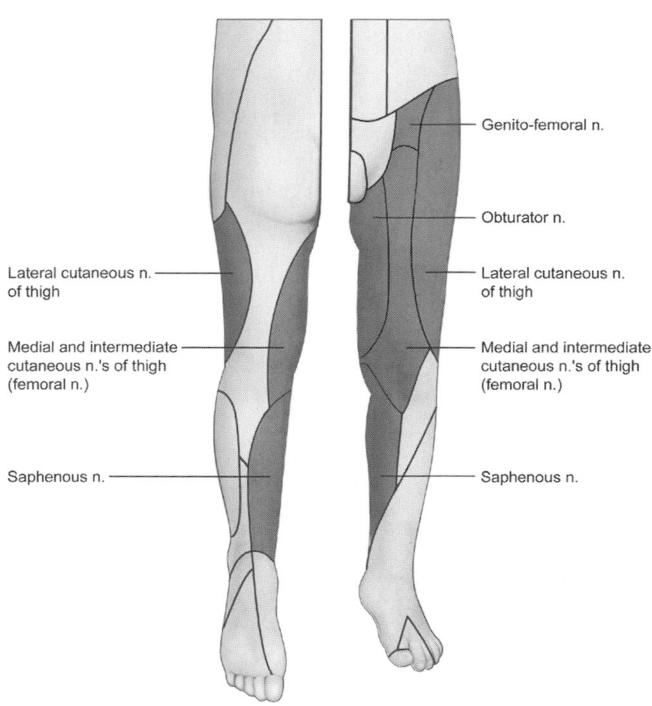

■ **PLATE 14–29.** Dermatomal distribution of lumbar plexus block. (Color image is available on the DVD.)

Anatomy

The lumbar plexus lies in the psoas compartment between the two masses of the psoas muscle that attach to the vertebrae and is surrounded by fascia that is derived from fascia iliaca (Plate 14–30; color image is available on the DVD). The approximate depth from the skin to the lumbar plexus in the different ages is noted (see Fig. 14–2).

Technique

In a study of 50 children aged 6 months to 16 years undergoing hip and upper lower extremity procedures, Dalens and others (1988) compared two techniques of lumbar plexus block. In group 1, a modification by Chayen of a psoas compartment block was used. In this technique a needle was inserted at the midpoint of a line connecting the spinous process of the fifth lumbar vertebra and the posterior superior iliac spine. There were difficulties with needle insertion in 7 of 25 children, and 23 of the 25 children had epidural spread of local anesthesia. In the second group, a modification of Winnie's approach was used. In this technique, a needle was inserted at the intersection of the line drawn to connect the iliac crests and a line drawn through the posterior superior iliac spine parallel to the spinous processes (Plate 14–31; color image is available on the DVD). There were no problems with needle insertion, and all 25 patients exhibited a unilateral lumbar plexus block distribution. Sacral distribution occurred in 23 of the 25 children as these two plexuses are found in the same anatomical plane.

Although both techniques provided effective analgesia to the lumbar plexus, the Chayen approach resulted in epidural spread rather than isolated lumbar plexus. Because of the greater ease of performance of the modified Winnie technique, this technique is further described for use in children.

Modified Winnie Approach to the Lumbar Plexus

With the child in the lateral position, block side up, the knees and thighs are flexed. Two lines are drawn (1) to connect the two iliac crests and (2) ipsilateral posterior superior iliac spine

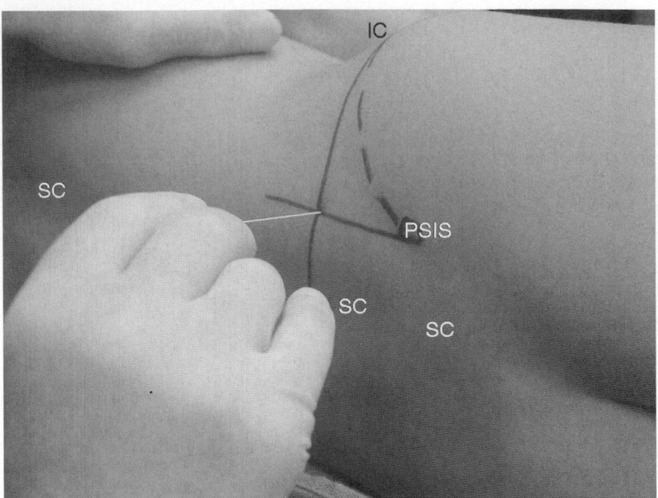

■ **PLATE 14–31.** Performance of lumbar plexus block. PSIS, posterior superior iliac spine; IC, iliac crest; SC, spinal column. Note that the needle is considerably lateral to spinal column. (Color image is available on the DVD.)

running cephalad and parallel to the spinous processes. The needle is inserted perpendicular to the skin at the intersection of the two lines (see Plate 14–31). The needle is advanced through the quadratus lumborum. If contact is made with a transverse process, the needle is then directed slightly more cephalad until a strong contraction of the mid (not lateral or medial) quadriceps with a "patellar kick" is apparent. If hamstring contractions are observed, the needle is then directed slightly more laterally. If there is isolated hip movement, the psoas has been directly stimulated. If the quadriceps and hamstrings are contracting simultaneously, the needle should be directed more cephalad to stimulate the lumbar rather than sacral plexus.

Complications

Although complications are rare, they may be serious if the needle is advanced too deeply into the retroperitoneum. Retroperitoneal hematoma is a significant risk, and continuous aspiration for blood should be done during performance of the block. The highest incidence of major bleeding after peripheral regional anesthetic techniques has been found to occur after a psoas compartment block (Horlocker et al., 2003).

Sciatic Nerve Block

A sciatic nerve block is indicated for surgical procedures that involve the lower extremity below the knee. When used in combination with blocks of the lumbar plexus, the lower extremity may be blocked in its entirety.

Anatomy

The sciatic nerve is derived from the anterior rami of L4-S3 and is the largest nerve in the body (see Plate 14–20). It emerges through the greater sciatic foramen to run between the greater trochanter of the femur and the ischial tuberosity before taking its position in the thigh posterior to the quadriceps femoris. If the sciatic nerve is blocked in its proximal position, this also anesthetizes the posterior femoral cutaneous nerve (a branch of ventral rami of S1-3). This nerve innervates the posterior thigh above the knee and the hamstring muscles. The sciatic nerve primarily consists of two nerves—the tibial and common peroneal nerves—which travel in a common sheath in the posterior upper portion of the leg. These nerves divide near the popliteal fossa and innervate the leg below the knee.

Approaches to the Sciatic Nerve

Several approaches to the sciatic nerve have been described in children. The posterior, anterior, and lateral approaches have been compared with respect to ease of performance, efficacy of block, and rate of complications (Dalens et al., 1990). The overall success rate of all three approaches exceeded 90%. However, there were fewer difficulties reported with the posterior approach. The posterior approach resulted in an 88% success rate on first attempt compared with 78% for lateral approach and only a 62% success rate on first attempt for anterior approach. In addition, vascular punctures occurred only in children who underwent an anterior approach. Because of the higher success rate of the posterior approach and the completeness of analgesia of sciatic and posterior branches (Plate 14–32; color image is available on the DVD), the posterior approach is described here. However, the reader is prompted to review the lateral approach especially for use in children who are unable to be positioned for the other approaches to the sciatic nerve (Dalens, 1995).

To block the sciatic nerve using the *posterior approach*, a modification of Labat's technique was developed by Dalens and others (1990). The child is placed in the lateral position with the side to be blocked uppermost and the upper leg flexed at both the hip and knee. Using a nerve stimulator and insulated needle, the point of needle insertion is at the midpoint of the line that extends from the tip of the coccyx to the greater trochanter of the femur. The needle should be perpendicular to the skin with slight angulation toward the lateral ischial tuberosity (Plates 14–33 and 14–34; color images are available on the DVD). The approximate depth to the sciatic nerve using the

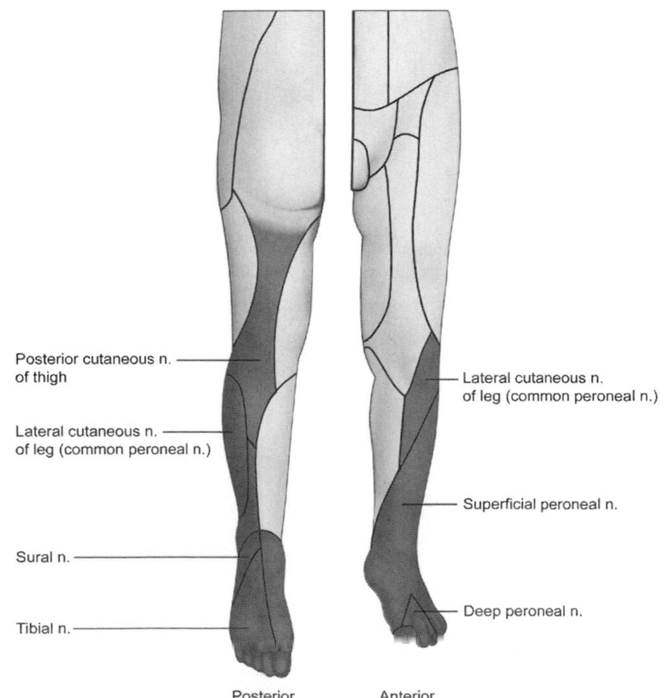

■ **PLATE 14–32.** Dermatomal distribution of posterior sciatic block. (Color image is available on the DVD.)

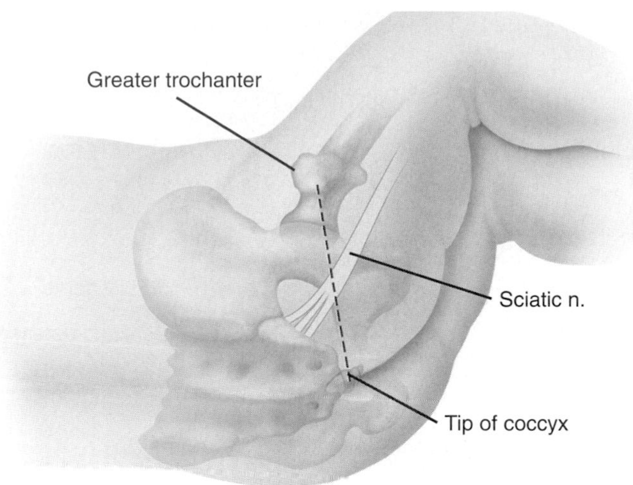

■ **PLATE 14–33.** Anatomy for posterior sciatic block. (Color image is available on the DVD.)

posterior approach changes with age (see Fig. 14–2). Using a nerve stimulator, the motor response is a movement in the patient's foot. Plantar flexion indicates stimulation of the tibial nerve. Dorsiflexion or eversion at the ankle indicates stimulation of the peroneal nerve. Once the appropriate muscle is elicited, local anesthetic is injected.

Complications of the posterior approach to the sciatic nerve include vascular puncture of gluteal vessels. Constant aspiration for blood should be maintained during performance of the block to avoid this complication.

The *Raj block* was developed in 1975 and is similar to the posterior approach (Raj et al., 1975). This approach anesthetizes the sciatic nerve slightly more distal than with the classic posterior approach (Plate 14–35; color image is available on the DVD). This block is performed in the supine child with the leg to be blocked lifted and flexed at the hip and knee (Plate 14–36; color image is available on the DVD). The needle is inserted at the midpoint between the ischial tuberosity and greater trochanter in the sciatic groove (Plate 14–37; color image is available on the DVD). Once appropriate muscle stimulation with less than 0.5 mA is seen at the foot, local anesthetic is injected. The advantage to this block is the reliability of the landmarks and simplicity of the block itself. By flexing the hip, the Raj technique brings the sciatic nerve closer to the skin. This improves the likelihood of a successful block, especially in obese children and adolescents.

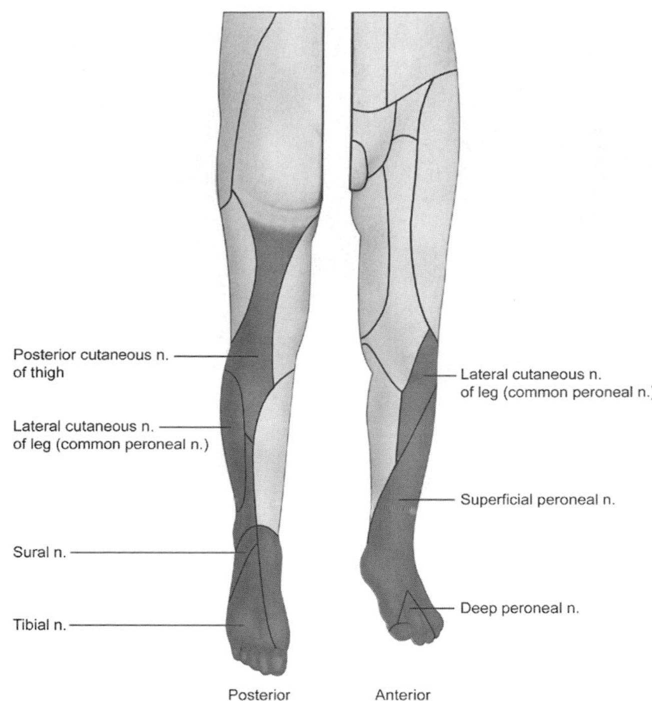

■ **PLATE 14–35.** Dermatomal distribution of Raj approach to sciatic nerve block. (Color image is available on the DVD.)

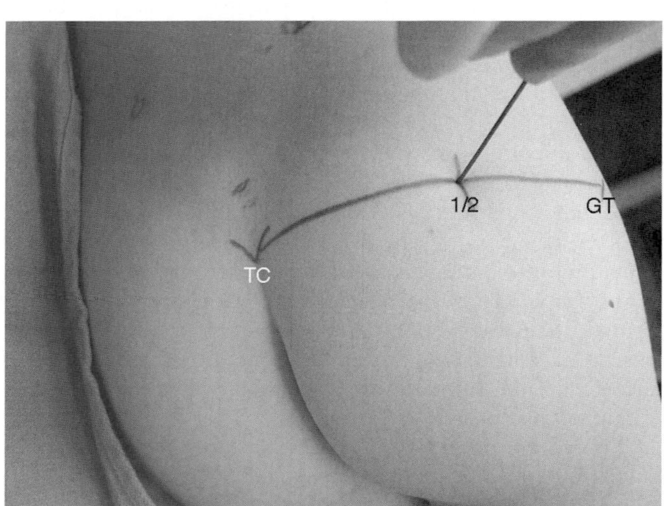

■ **PLATE 14–34.** Performance of posterior sciatic block. TC, tip of coccyx; GT, greater trochanter. (Color image is available on the DVD.)

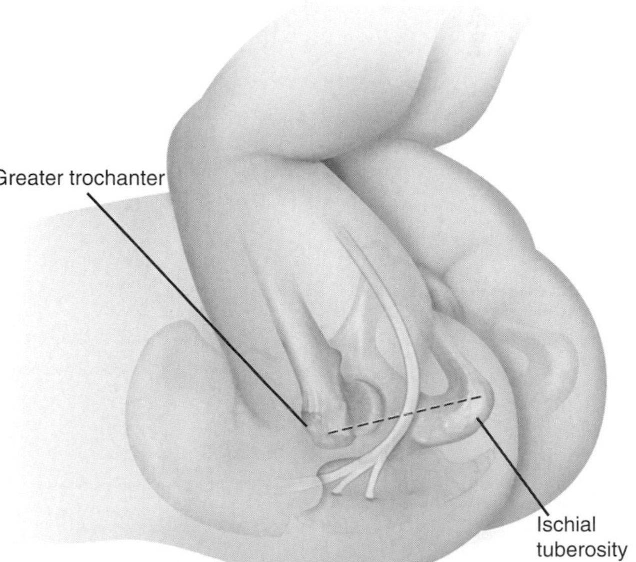

■ **PLATE 14–36.** Anatomy for Raj approach to sciatic nerve. (Color image is available on the DVD.)

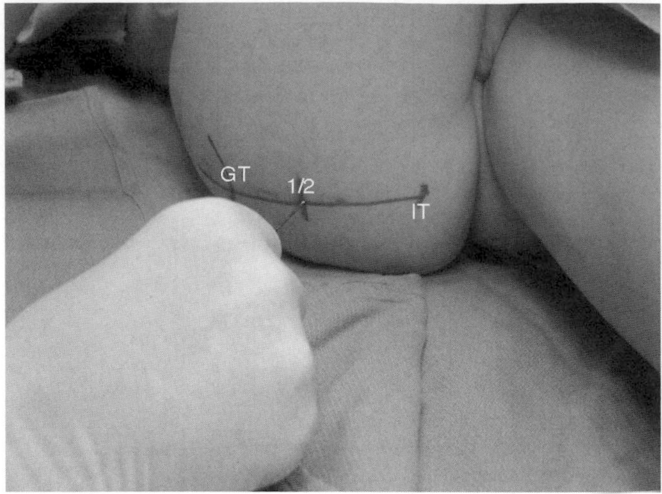

■ **PLATE 14–37.** Performance of Raj sciatic block. IT, ischial tuberosity; GT, greater trochanter. (Color image is available on the DVD.)

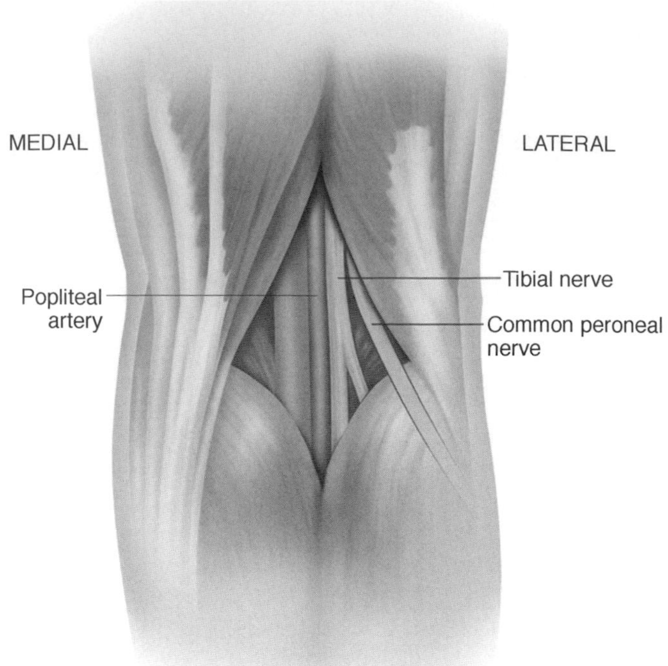

■ **PLATE 14–39.** Anatomy of popliteal fossa block. (Color image is available on the DVD.)

A *popliteal fossa block* may be used for procedures of the distal lower extremity and anesthetizes the sciatic nerve more distally in the leg and just proximal to the knee (Kempthorne and Brown, 1984) (Plate 14–38; color image is available on the DVD). Near the popliteal fossa, the sciatic nerve divides into the common peroneal nerve and posterior tibial nerve. The common peroneal nerve runs anteriorly to wrap around the head of the fibula, while the posterior tibial nerve travels down the posterior lower leg (Plate 14–39; color image is available on the DVD). In approximately 10% of the population, the branching of the sciatic nerve occurs more proximal to the popliteal fossa and high in the posterior thigh. For this reason, there may be a variable success rate in blocking the sciatic at this level, but both nerves are usually blocked by this approach due to a common epineural sheath that envelops the two nerves (Vloka et al., 1997). Advantages to the popliteal approach include the relative superficial location of the sciatic nerve to the skin and the decreased risk of intraneural injection, as the sciatic nerve is not fixed against any bony structures in this location. To easily access the popliteal fossa, the patient may remain in the supine position and the leg to be blocked is lifted with the knee and thigh flexed. The child may also be turned to the lateral position and the leg to be blocked positioned uppermost. The superior triangle of the popliteal fossa has as its boundaries the semimembranosus and semitendinosus tendons medially, the biceps femoris tendon laterally, and the popliteal crease inferiorly. The needle is inserted 45 degrees to the skin aiming cephalad and just lateral to the midline of the popliteal triangle (Plate 14–40; color image is available on the DVD).

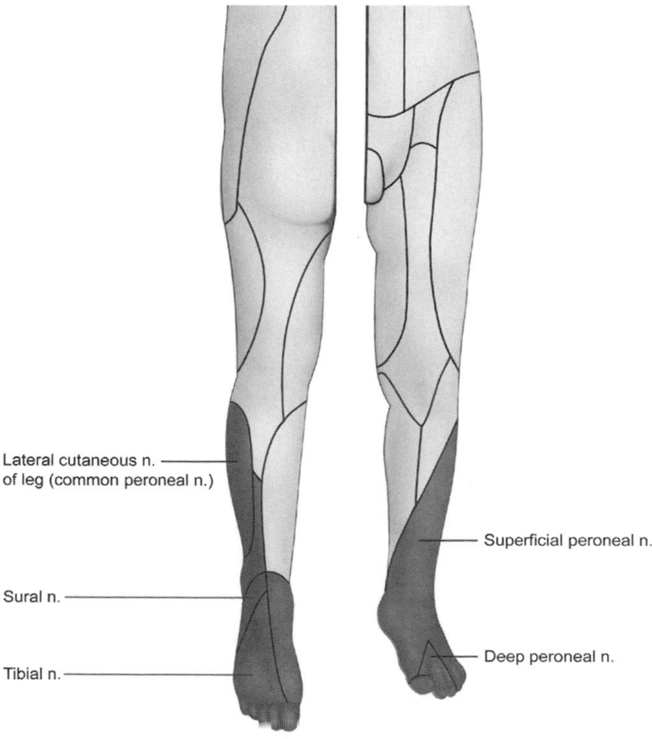

■ **PLATE 14–38.** Dermatomal distribution of popliteal fossa block. (Color image is available on the DVD.)

The distance from the popliteal fold to needle insertion is estimated based on weight. If the weight is less than 10 kg, the distance is 1 cm; if the weight is 10 to 20 kg, the distance is 2 cm (Konrad and Johr, 1998). Each 10 kg of body weight should move the needle cephalad in the triangle approximately 1 cm. Muscle stimulation of the foot in either the common peroneal or posterior tibial distribution is acceptable; however, posterior tibial stimulation may be a more reliable indicator of successful placement. Local anesthetic is injected once appropriate stimulation is apparent at less than 0.5 mA.

Konrad and Johr (1998) sought to determine a system for standardization of popliteal fossa block. They performed the block in 50 children between the ages of 2 months and 18 years. They determined that the minimal distance to the sciatic nerve in the popliteal fossa was 13 mm, and the depth did not vary

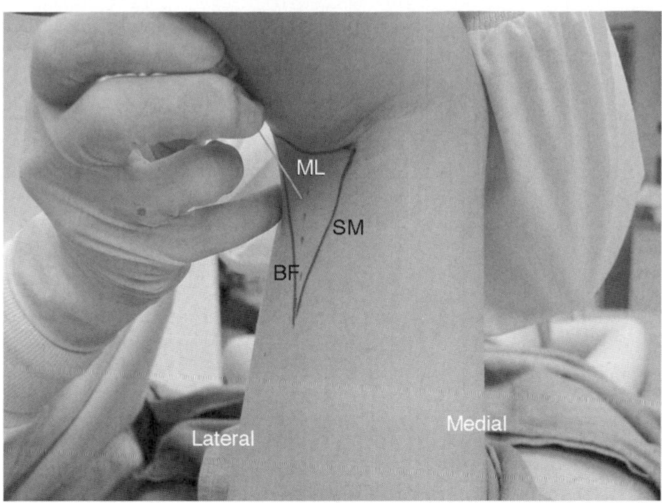

■ **PLATE 14–40.** Performance of popliteal block. SM, semimembranosus/semitendinosus tendons; BF, biceps femoris; ML, midline. (Color image is available on the DVD.)

significantly in patients weighing less than 35 kg but did increase for children weighing more than 35 kg. All of the blocks in the study were successful, and there were no complications. Vascular puncture was avoided due to the lateral position of the needle in relation to the popliteal vessels.

Tobias and Mencio (1999) provided analgesia in 20 children for foot and ankle surgery by performing popliteal fossa blocks at the completion of the surgical procedure. When using 0.75 mL/kg of 0.2% ropivacaine, the duration of analgesia was between 8 and 12 hours.

Ankle Block

An ankle block is a simple block that provides analgesia to the foot for procedures such as toe removal or simple reconstructive surgery.

Anatomy

There are five nerves that innervate the foot that must be blocked for analgesia of the foot in its entirety (Plate 14–41; color image is available on the DVD). The *saphenous nerve* is found near the saphenous vein on the medial side of the dorsum of the foot and is somewhat superficial in its location. It innervates the skin surrounding the medial malleolus. Following the dorsum of the foot, and near the anterior tibial artery, runs the *deep peroneal nerve*, which is responsible for the innervation of the web space between the first and second toes. As the name implies, this nerve runs deep and is found near the tibia and between the extensor hallucis longus and anterior tibial artery. Immediately lateral to the deep peroneal nerve, but found superficially, is the *superficial peroneal nerve*. This nerve innervates the medial and lateral aspects of the dorsum of the foot. The plantar innervation of the foot is supplied by the *tibial and sural nerves*. The tibial nerve is found immediately posterior to the posterior tibial artery and medial malleolus, and the *sural nerve* is located posterior to the lateral malleolus.

Technique

To perform an ankle block, each of the five nerves is blocked using a 25-gauge needle. With the child supine, the saphenous nerve is blocked by injecting 1 to 5 mL local anesthetic solution subcutaneously near the saphenous vein anterior to the medial malleolus. The deep peroneal nerve is blocked by inserting the needle lateral to the extensor hallucis longus tendon near the tibial artery and advancing the needle until it contacts the tibia. The needle should then be withdrawn slightly and 1 to 5 mL local anesthetic injected. The superficial peroneal nerve is blocked with a subcutaneous ring of local anesthetic across the lateral dorsum of the foot. The patient's foot then should be positioned so that the two posterior nerves may be blocked for complete analgesia of the foot. The tibial nerve is blocked midway between the medial malleolus and the calcaneus posterior to the tibial artery. The sural nerve is blocked midway between the lateral malleolus and the calcaneus. Each of the posterior nerves should receive 1 to 5 mL local anesthetic solution.

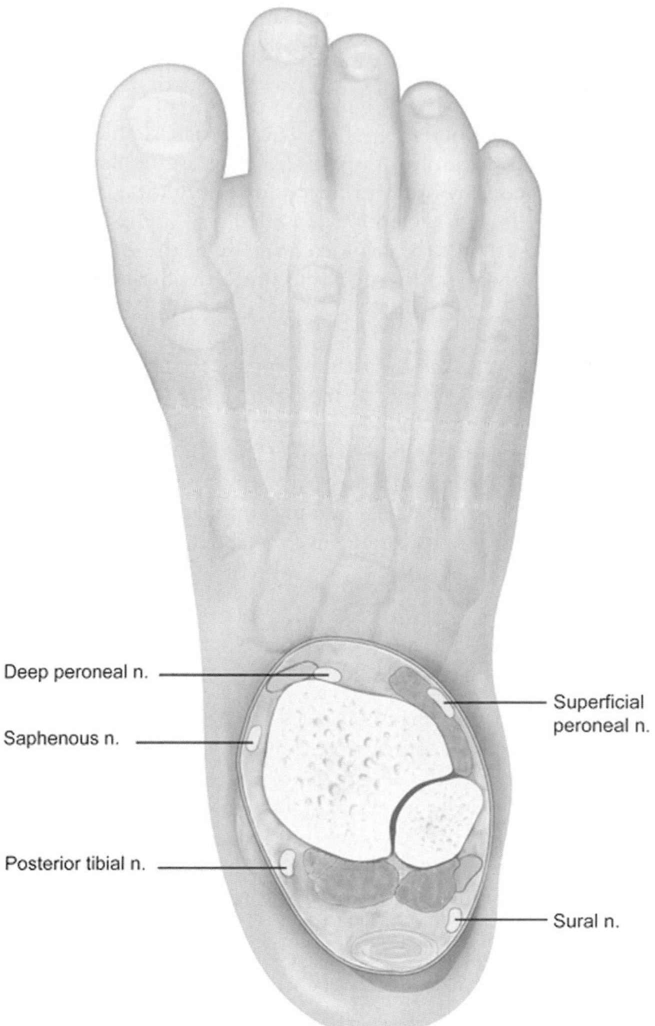

■ **PLATE 14–41.** Anatomy for ankle block. (Color image is available on the DVD.)

Dosing

To ensure complete analgesia to the foot with a duration of action greater than 4 hours, bupivacaine, ropivacaine, or levobupivacaine 0.5% should be used. The volumes delivered at each nerve depend on the age and size of the patient. The larger volumes are reserved for adolescents, but maximal dosing guidelines should not be exceeded. Epinephrine should not be added to the solution due to the risk of peripheral vasoconstriction.

Complications

Risks during performance of an ankle block should be rare. Because of the proximity of vessels, frequent aspiration for blood should be performed during injection. In addition, the use of epinephrine for an ankle block, particularly in an infant or a young child, should be avoided to reduce the possibility of ischemia secondary to loss of perfusion to the distal foot.

Dosing of Lower Extremity Blocks

The volumes of local anesthesia depend on the nerves to be blocked. For femoral nerve blocks, 0.3 to 0.75 mL/kg are administered, whereas for plexus blocks, volumes of 1 mL/kg are frequently needed (see Table 14–5). The duration of action of local anesthesia is dependent on the anesthetic concentration and age of the patient. When used in combination, local anesthetics are additive. It is important not to exceed maximal allowable dosing (see Table 14–2).

CONTINUOUS PERIPHERAL NERVE CATHETERS

Indwelling catheters may be placed for peripheral nerve analgesia for those procedures that result in significant and prolonged postoperative pain or when vascular insufficiency is a risk. Although there is no extensive literature on placing continuous catheters for peripheral nerves or plexus anesthesia in children, there is equipment available that is suitable for these younger patients. Options of catheter placement include a modification of a Seldinger technique with placement of a wire over a needle and then a catheter over the wire such as a 3 or 4 Fr Cook central line catheter. There are also commercially available continuous catheter kits that allow for catheter insertion after the plexus has been localized with a nerve stimulator. Examples of these kits that allow for continuous catheter placement in children include a system using a short 18-gauge insulated Touhy needle through which a 20-gauge catheter may be threaded (B. Braun, Bethlehem, PA). There are also systems available that use a catheter-over-needle approach where a 20-gauge introducing catheter similar to an intravenous cannula fits over a 22-gauge insulated needle. Once the stimulation is achieved, the cannula is inserted into the sheath, the needle removed, and then a styletted 24-gauge catheter is threaded into the sheath for continuous infusion.

There is little information on the continuous infusions of local anesthetics in upper extremity catheters in children, but dosing of an indwelling catheter for brachial plexus anesthesia should adhere to maximal allowable dosing guidelines as set forth in Table 14–2. Typical doses should start at 0.1 to 0.2 mL/kg per hr of either bupivacaine or levobupivacaine 0.125% to 0.25% or ropivacaine 0.1% to 0.2% (see Table 14–5). Increases in the infusion rate may be made as needed as long as the maximal infusion rate does not exceed 0.2 mg/kg per hr in infants less than 6 months or 0.4 mg/kg per hr in children older than 6 months. It would be unusual, however, for peripheral nerve catheter infusions to reach maximum limits. There has been a case report that describes the use of an axillary catheter for a child with epidermolysis bullosa simplex who required placement of an external fixator (Diwan et al., 2001). The practitioners managed this catheter for 2 days with bolus injections of 0.125% bupivacaine 0.5 mL/kg every 8 hours with success.

Continuous catheters have been used for the lower extremity in children, most commonly for femur fractures of patients in the intensive care unit setting (Johnson, 1994; Tobias, 1994). Johnson used an epidural catheter in the femoral sheath and delivered 0.125% bupivacaine at 0.3 mg/kg per hr. In these patients, plasma bupivacaine concentrations were well below toxic levels. Using a Seldinger technique and a 3 Fr 8-cm single-lumen central line catheter (Cook Critical Care, Bloomington, IN), Tobias administered continuous infusions of 0.15 mL/kg/hr of 0.2% bupivacaine to four children with femur fractures and closed head trauma. The catheters provided adequate analgesia in the intensive care unit setting for 4 to 6 days and there were no complications.

To provide more complete analgesia of the upper portion of the leg, catheters may also be placed in the lumbar plexus or fascia iliaca compartments. Sciard and others (2001), using nerve stimulation, placed 20-gauge plexus catheters (Pajunk, Albany, NY) in the lumbar plexus of children and administered continuous infusions of 0.2% ropivacaine at 0.33 to 0.4 mg/kg per hr. Paut and others (2001) inserted 20-gauge catheters (Contiplex; B. Braun, Melsungen, Germany) through 55-mm cannulas into the fascia iliaca compartment and administered continuous infusions of 0.1% bupivacaine at a rate of 0.135 ± 0.03 mg/kg per hour. The plasma bupivacaine levels at 24 and 48 hours were not significantly different at 0.71 mcg/mL and 0.84 mcg/mL, respectively. The authors concluded that the bupivacaine plasma concentrations at the rates used in their study for a continuous fascia iliaca block are within safety margins. Ivani and others (2003) reported a case of a 21-day continuous infusion via a continuous sciatic catheter in a 3-year-old boy with subtotal foot amputation. Using an infusion of 0.4 mg/kg per hr of 0.2% ropivacaine with clonidine 0.12 mcg/kg per hr, there was total pain relief and no complications.

The use of disposable pumps for continuous delivery via a peripheral catheter of local anesthetic solutions has become popular in the adult population for outpatient orthopedic surgery. Dadure and others (2003) described the use of the disposable elastomeric pumps in 25 children aged 1 to 15 years receiving continuous infusion via catheters in the popliteal, femoral, or axillary sheaths. A continuous infusion of 0.2% ropivacaine was used at a rate of 0.1 mL/kg per hr. The median pain score for all children was 0 up to 48 hours, and there were no adverse events.

ILIOINGUINAL/ILIOHYPOGASTRIC NERVE BLOCK

Ilioinguinal/iliohypogastric (ILIH) nerve block provides analgesia to the inguinal area and provides good perioperative pain relief for patients undergoing such procedures as inguinal hernia repair, orchiopexy, and hydrocelectomy (Hannallah et al., 1987; Casey et al., 1990; Fisher et al., 1993). Early studies compared the use of an ILIH block for children aged 1 to 7 years for inguinal hernia repair. The block was performed after induction of anesthesia but before surgical incision. When compared with general anesthesia without the block, the group of patients who received an ILIH nerve block ambulated earlier and required less analgesia in the immediate postoperative period. The ILIH block group also required less analgesia for the following 48 hours after surgery (Langer et al., 1987). Hannallah and others (1987) studied the efficacy of an ILIH block for orchiopexy surgery. They found no advantage to performing a caudal block over ILIH block for orchiopexy surgery as there were no significant differences between the groups in postoperative pain scores, postoperative vomiting, or time to meet discharge criteria. These results have been duplicated in other studies with no differences found between the ILIH groups and caudal groups with respect to postoperative pain scores, analgesic requirements, or times to micturition (Fisher et al., 1993; Splinter et al., 1995). However, in a similarly designed study, Somri and others (2002) noted that caudal anesthesia was significantly more effective than ILIH in decreasing plasma catecholamine levels for postorchidopexy.

Casey and others (1990) investigated the effectiveness of an ILIH nerve block for inguinal hernia repair and compared this with simple installation of bupivacaine into the surgical wound. There was no difference between the ILIH nerve block group and the wound installation group with regard to pain scores, analgesic requirements, or recovery or discharge times. In a study to assess the effectiveness of 0.5% bupivacaine (2 mg/kg) in patients receiving either an ILIH nerve block, wound infiltration, or a combination of wound infiltration and nerve block, Anatol and others (1997) noted that all three patient groups had effective analgesia and that there were no differences in pain scores or analgesic requirements among the three groups.

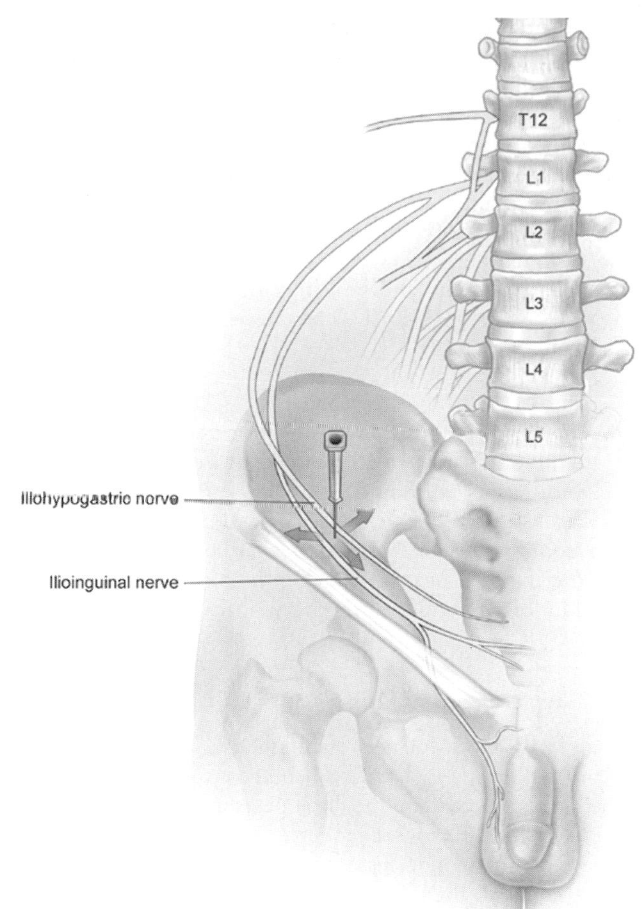

■ **PLATE 14–42.** Anatomy for ilioinguinal/iliohypogastric nerve block. (Color image is available on the DVD.)

Anatomy

The ilioinguinal and iliohypogastric nerves originate from the lumbar plexus and pierce the transversus abdominis muscle. The iliohypogastric nerve then takes its course between the transversus and internal oblique muscles and the ilioinguinal runs between internal oblique and external oblique. They pass superficial to transversus abdominus near the anterior superior iliac spine where they can be blocked before running their separate courses to innervate the inguinal region and upper scrotum (Plate 14–42; color image is available on the DVD). The spermatic cord also receives innervation from the genital branch of the genitofemoral nerve that originates from lumbar plexus, usually at L1 or L2.

Technique

The ilioinguinal and iliohypogastric nerves may be blocked in their location near the anterior superior iliac spine. If performed before incision, a sterile preparation of the skin is done and a blunt 22- or 25-gauge needle is inserted 1 cm superior and 1 cm medial to the anterior superior iliac spine (Plate 14–43; color image is available on the DVD). The needle is initially directed posterolaterally to contact the inner superficial lip of the ileum and then withdrawn while injecting local anesthetic during needle movement. Once the skin is reached, the needle is redirected toward the inguinal ligament (ensuring that the needle does not enter the ligament) and local anesthetic is injected after a "pop" is felt as the needle penetrates the oblique muscles. The needle should also be directed towards the ambilicus to deliver local anesthetic in the same plane. If the block is to be performed at the end of surgery, the surgeon may anesthetize the nerves under direct vision. The nerves lie at the lateral border of the incision. Lim and others (2002) determined that there is no added advantage to a single-shot versus double-shot ILIH nerve block.

Dosing

Bupivacaine 0.25% in a volume of 4 to 6 mL was used in a study by Hannallah and others (1987) that included males between the ages of 18 months and 12 years, while Casey and others (1990) used 0.25 mL/kg of bupivacaine 0.25% for children aged 2 to 10 years for hernia repair. Both of these studies cited good postoperative pain relief for these children. Although the maximum duration of analgesia is unknown from these studies, in the study by Casey and others (1990) effective analgesia was still present 180 minutes postoperatively. Levobupivacaine has been compared with placebo for patients aged 6 months to

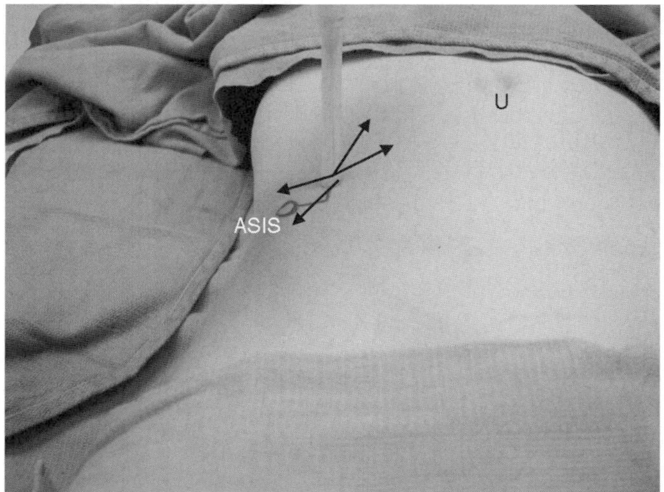

■ **PLATE 14–43.** Performance of ilioinguinal/iliohypogastric nerve block. ASIS, anterior superior iliac spine; U, umbilicus. A field block is performed in the direction of the arrows and inferiorly toward the inguinal ligament. (Color image is available on the DVD.)

12 years undergoing inguinal herniorrhaphy. In this study, Gunter and others (1999) noted that 0.25 mL/kg of 0.5% levobupivacaine was effective for ILIH block and was associated with a longer time to rescue analgesic administration and lower pain scores compared with children who had received no block. Dalens and others (2001) evaluated the effectiveness and pharmacokinetic profile of 0.5% ropivacaine 3 mg/kg for ILIH nerve block in children aged 1 to 12 years of age undergoing inguinal surgery. They noted that this dose provided satisfactory pain relief and peak ropivacaine plasma concentrations were 1.5 ± 0.93 mg/L. These levels were well below the toxic level.

Complications

Although complications from an ILIH nerve block are generally rare and minor, there have been case reports of colonic and small bowel perforation (Johr and Sossai, 1999; Amory et al., 2003). Inadvertent femoral nerve blockade and motor block of the quadriceps may occur if the local anesthetic solution spreads below the inguinal ligament during the block placement. This can yield a block similar to the fascia iliaca block (Roy-Shapiri et al., 1985).

PENILE NERVE BLOCK

A penile nerve block includes techniques such as subpubic nerve block, dorsal nerve block, and subcutaneous ring block and may be used for procedures on the distal penis including circumcision and uncomplicated hypospadias repair. Investigations have shown that newborns have a decreased stress response when undergoing circumcision with the benefit of a penile block. A ring block may be more effective than either a dorsal nerve block or local anesthetic cream (Maxwell et al., 1987; Stang et al., 1988; Lander et al., 1997; Butler-O'Hara et al., 1998; Hardwick-Smith et al., 1998). In addition, a subcutaneous ring block may result in a lower incidence of complications compared with a dorsal nerve block (Broadman et al., 1987). The subpubic nerve block blocks the nerves before they enter the base of the penis. This block is less likely to disrupt the vascular or penile structures. Holder and others (1997) compared the subcutaneous ring block in boys undergoing circumcision with a group of boys who had a subpubic block. The group anesthetized with the subpubic block had significantly lower pain scores. In addition, three boys in the subcutaneous ring block group had tissue distortion from the block that affected surgical conditions.

When using a penile block for boys undergoing hypospadias repair, Chhibber and others (1997) have shown that placing the block before incision and repeating the block at the end of surgery provided better postoperative pain control than did placing the block only once (i.e., either before or after the surgical procedure).

Anatomy

The distal two thirds of the penis is supplied by the dorsal nerves, which are branches of the pudendal nerve (Plate 14–44; color image is available on the DVD). The pudendal nerve arises from the sacral plexus. The dorsal nerves are located near the dorsal vessels and are surrounded by Buck's fascia.

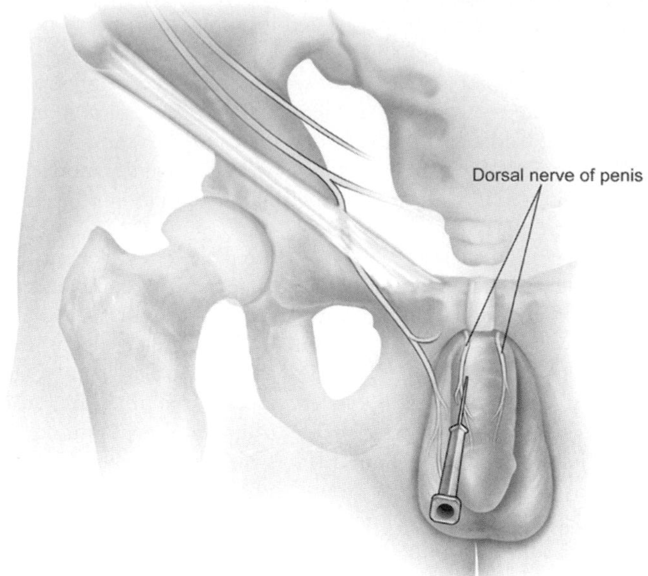

PLATE 14–44. Anatomy for dorsal nerve penile block. (Color image is available on the DVD.)

Technique

Subcutaneous Ring Block

A simple approach for blocking the dorsal nerves to the penis is the subcutaneous ring block. A skin wheel of local anesthetic (without epinephrine) is injected circumferentially around the base of the penis but superficial to Buck's fascia.

Dorsal Penile Block

A dorsal penile nerve block may be performed by injecting local anesthetic directly at the nerves as they run on each side of the penis at the level of the symphysis pubis (Plate 14–45; color image is available on the DVD). Using a 25-gauge needle, Buck's fascia is pierced and local anesthetic (without epinephrine) is injected at the 10:30 and 1:30 o'clock positions at the base of the penis. Due to the close proximity of the dorsal vessels, frequent aspiration for blood during the local anesthetic injection is necessary.

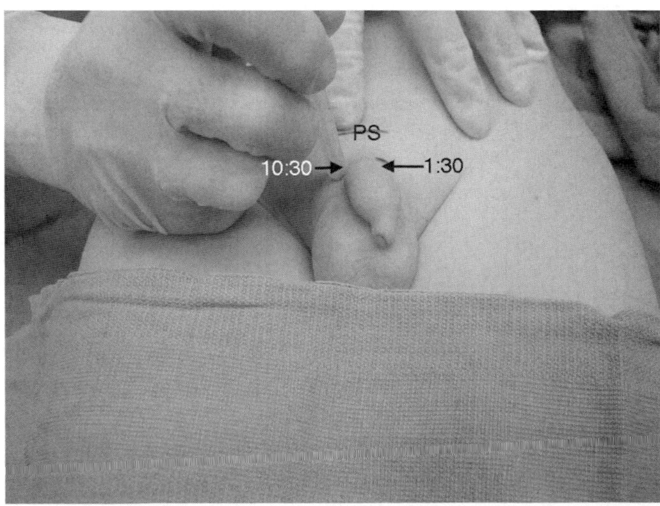

PLATE 14–45. Performance of dorsal nerve block. PS, pubic symphysis. Points of needle insertion are at 10:30 and 1:30 o'clock at the base of the penis. (Color image is available on the DVD.)

Subpubic Block

To perform a subpubic block, the penis is gently pulled downward and the needle is inserted perpendicular to the skin 0.5 to 1 cm lateral to the midline and caudal to the symphysis pubis. As the needle is advanced, it is directed slightly medially and caudally until Scarpa's fascia is crossed. Once that "give" is felt and assuming a negative aspiration for blood, local anesthetic is delivered.

Dosing

The most important point to remember about dosing a penile block is to NEVER USE EPINEPHRINE. The penis is an end organ and the use of epinephrine may lead to necrosis. For all techniques of providing penile nerve block, bupivacaine 0.25%, levobupivacaine 0.25%, or ropivacaine 0.2% may be used to provide analgesia with a duration of 4 to 6 hours. A subcutaneous ring block should be dosed so that there is subcutaneous evidence of local anesthetic injection around the base of the penis, but the dose must not exceed the maximal allowable recommendations for single injection (see Table 14–2). For a dorsal nerve block or subpubic block, approximately 0.1 mL/kg of local anesthetic is injected at each site. Sfez and others (1990) have shown that for a penile block, with 0.1 mL/kg at each injection site of either 0.25% bupivacaine or a 1:1 mixture of 0.25% bupivacaine with 1% lidocaine, serum local anesthetic concentrations were well below the toxic range.

Complications

As previously mentioned, epinephrine should never be used when performing a penile block as this may lead to significant vasoconstriction and ischemia (Berens and Pontus, 1990). Hematoma formation may occur from puncture of the dorsal vessels during dorsal nerve block. This can result in necrosis of the tip of the penis (Sara and Lowry, 1984). When performed properly, a subcutaneous ring block should be void of complications with the exception of tissue edema at the base of the penis. Tissue edema may affect the surgical conditions if the block is performed before the surgical procedure.

INTERCOSTAL BLOCK

Intercostal nerve block provides limited analgesia after thoracotomy, upper abdominal procedures, rib fractures, and insertion of chest tubes. An intercostal block may be useful for these indications in the perioperative arena or in an emergency department or intensive care unit setting.

Anatomy

The intercostal nerves arise paravertebrally from the first 11 thoracic spinal nerves and are located in a groove that is found underneath the corresponding rib and shared with the intercostal vessels (Plate 14–46; color image is available on the DVD). Gray and white rami communicantes branch off from the spinal

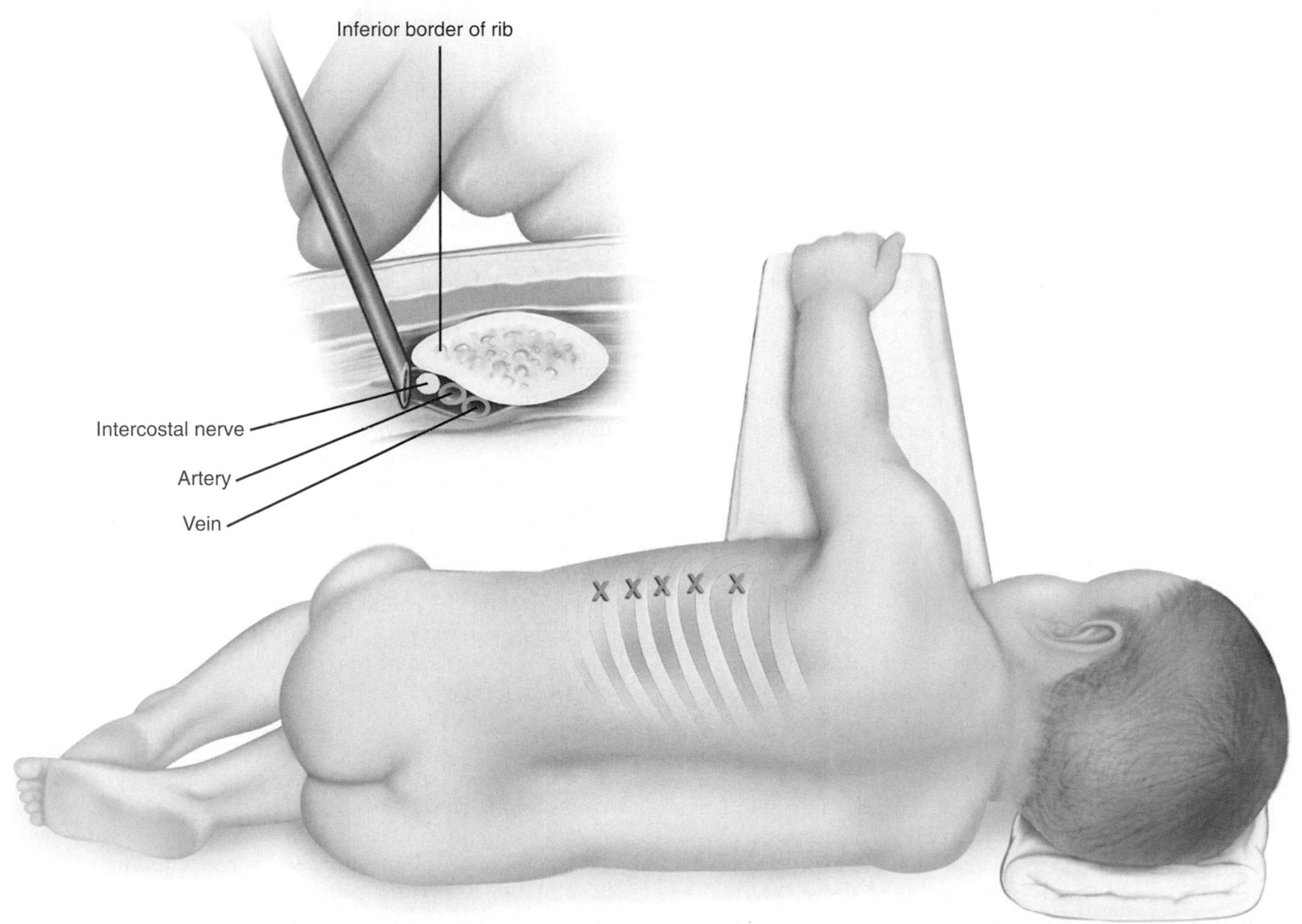

■ **PLATE 14–46.** Anatomy of intercostal nerves. (Color image is available on the DVD.)

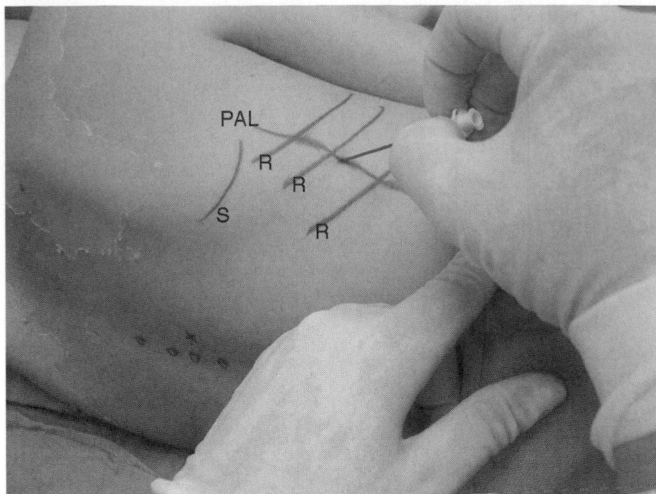

■ **PLATE 14–47.** Performance of intercostal block. PAL, posterior axillary line; S, scapula; R, inferior border of rib. Needle is directed to contact inferior border of each rib to be blocked and then "walked off" posteriorly. (Color image is available on the DVD.)

nerves and adjoin the sympathetic ganglia before entering the intercostal space. The intercostal space contains the intercostal nerve, artery, and vein and is bordered by the intercostal muscles.

Technique

To adequately anesthetize the intercostal nerves near their origin, the block is performed lateral to the paraspinous muscles toward the posterior axillary line. The child should be in the lateral decubitus position with the arm elevated so that the posterior axillary line is easily accessed (Plate 14–47; color image is available on the DVD). After sterile prep, insert a 25-gauge needle (length depends on age of child) through the skin, less than 1 cm below that of the lower border of the rib aiming cephalad to make contact with the rib itself. The needle is then withdrawn and advanced to "walk under" the inferior border of the rib until there is a feel of a slight loss of resistance as the muscles are penetrated (Fig. 14–3). The nerve is located immediately inferior to the vessels but in close proximity that requires frequent aspiration during injection of local anesthetic. To improve success of analgesia, the intercostal nerves two segments above and two segments below should be blocked in addition to the segment corresponding to incision. Although a single injection of an increased volume of 10 mL per segment has been shown to spread to multiple intercostal spaces in adults, this is not a common practice in children (Moorthy et al., 1992).

Dosing

A dose of 0.1 to 0.15 mL/kg per interspace (maximum of 3 mL per interspace) of local anesthetic agent is injected after negative aspiration. Bupivacaine 0.25%, levobupivacaine 0.25%, or ropivacaine 0.2% should provide 8 to 12 hours of analgesia.

Complications

Complications of intercostal block include pneumothorax, vascular puncture, and epidural or spinal local anesthetic spread. Spread of local anesthetic to the epidural or spinal spaces may occur if the injection travels through a dural sleeve covering the spinal root and may be more common in the posterior approach compared with more anterior approaches. In addition, there may

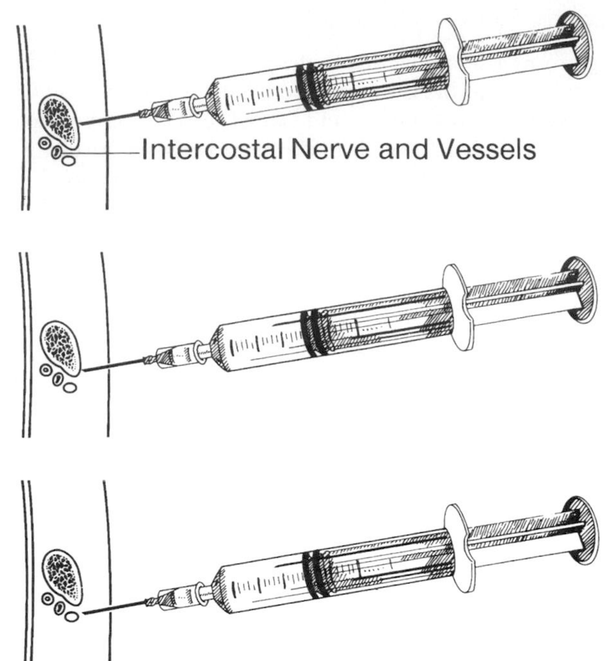

■ **FIGURE 14–3.** Needle advancement for performance of an intercostal nerve block.

be increased risk of local anesthetic toxicity from systemic uptake or inadvertent vascular puncture compared with other PNBs due to the close proximity of the intercostal vessels to the nerve.

■ PARAVERTEBRAL NERVE BLOCK

Paravertebral nerve block provides analgesia at specific dermatomes, and it is generally used for children who undergo unilateral procedures. Its use has been established in children and the main advantages include (1) localized pain control and (2) avoidance of large volumes of local anesthetic (Lonnqvist and Olsson, 1994; Lonnqvist et al., 1995; Richardson and Lonnqvist, 1998). Continuous paravertebral block has been shown to be effective for pain management for patients following thoracotomies, renal surgery, and cholecystectomy. Paravertebral blocks may be superior to epidural anesthesia in patients undergoing unilateral renal surgery, resulting in fewer morphine requirements in the postoperative period (Eng and Sabanathan, 1992; Lonnqvist, 1992; Lonnqvist and Olsson, 1994). Bolus injection of local anesthetic in the paravertebral space has been used successfully in children for inguinal surgery (Eck et al., 2002). Paravertebral blocks may be used in any patient where intercostal nerve blocks would be appropriate. Other advantages to performing paravertebral block include the spread of analgesia beyond one dermatome and the ease of catheter insertion for postoperative pain.

Anatomy

The paravertebral space is a wedge-shaped area along the vertebral column that contains the intercostal nerve, its dorsal ramus, the rami communicantes, and the sympathetic chain. The anterior boundary of the paravertebral space is the parietal pleura, and posterior to it is the superior costotransverse ligament and laterally, the posterior intercostal membrane (Fig. 14–4). There are equations to determine the depth of the paravertebral space

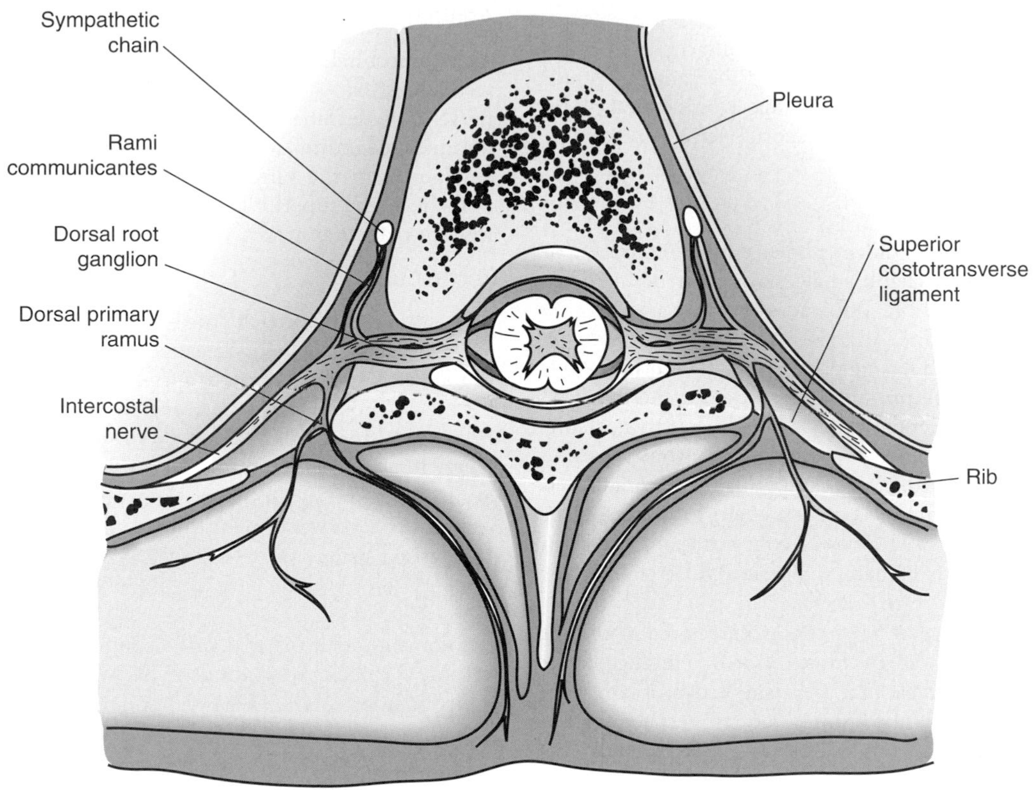

FIGURE 14–4. Anatomy of paravertebral space. (From Eason MJ, Wyatt R: Paravertebral thoracic block: A reappraisal. *Anaesthesia* 34:638–642, 1979.)

based on body weight (Lonnqvist and Hesser, 1993). The distance (in mm) from the spinous process to the paravertebral space = 0.12 × body weight (kg) + 10.2. The depth in mm from the skin to the paravertebral space = 0.48 × body weight (kg) + 18.7.

When injecting local anesthetic into the paravertebral space, the local anesthetic may spread several dermatomes due to the potential for free communication between adjacent spaces. The exception to this, however, may be at the T12 level where the psoas major muscle inserts into the vertebral column. In human cadavers, the psoas muscle may be a limiting factor in spread of local anesthesia from the thoracic region to segments below T12 (Lonnqvist and Hildingsson, 1992). For this reason, in the study of children undergoing paravertebral blocks for inguinal surgery, Eck and others (2002) administered two injections, one above T12 and the other injection below T12.

Technique

After sterile preparation and drape, with the child in the lateral position and the block side up, the spinous process of the level to be blocked is identified. The distance from the midline to the point of lateral puncture is approximately the same distance as the tip from one spinous process to another (Plate 14–48; color image is available on the DVD). If using a single-injection technique, a blunt spinal needle is used. If a catheter is to be threaded, a Touhy needle is necessary. Using a loss of resistance technique to saline, the needle is placed the proposed distance from the midline at the level of the spinous process. As the needle is inserted perpendicular to the skin, it makes contact with the corresponding transverse process. The needle is then "walked" over the cephalad margin of the transverse process. With gentle pressure on the syringe plunger, loss of resistance occurs once the needle crosses the costotransverse ligament and entry is gained into the paravertebral space. The loss of resistance is similar to, but less distinct than, that of going through the ligamentum flavum during epidural placement. Once the paravertebral space is identified, local anesthetic is injected into the space, and a catheter can be threaded if a continuous technique is desired.

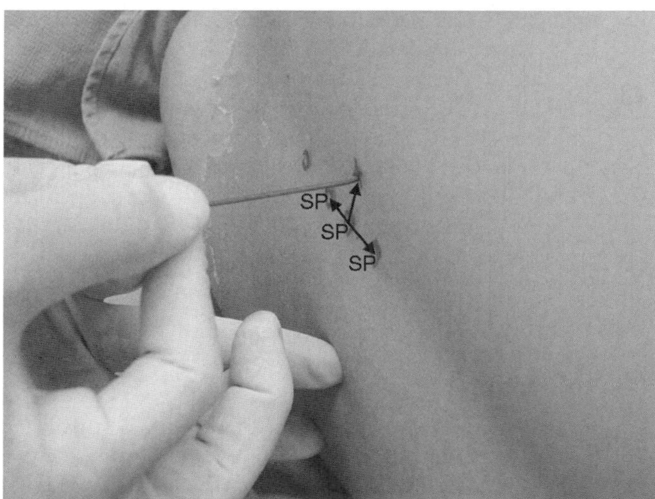

PLATE 14–48. Performance of paravertebral block. SP, spinous process. Lateral distance to point of needle insertion from midline should be equal to distance between spinous processes (*arrows*). (Color image is available on the DVD.)

Threading a catheter through a Touhy needle into the paravertebral space may require some manipulation and cephalad angulation of the bevel of the needle. In a child the catheter should not be threaded more than 2 to 3 cm. This avoids lateral placement of the catheter into an intercostal space and single dermatome analgesia.

Dosing

For a unilateral paravertebral block, a bolus dose of 0.5 mL/kg of local anesthetic provides reliable analgesia of four dermatomes (Lonnqvist and Hesser, 1993). Bupivacaine 0.25%, ropivacaine 0.2%, or levobupivacaine 0.25%, all with epinephrine 5 mcg/mL, may be used for single injection. If multiple levels are to be blocked, it is important not to exceed the maximal allowable dosing recommendations (see Table 14–2). For continuous infusions, bupivacaine, ropivacaine, or levobupivacaine can be infused at a rate of 0.25 mL/kg per hr for most children or 0.2 mL/kg per hr for infants (Cheung et al., 1997; Karmaker et al., 1996; Lonnqvist, 1992). Lower concentrations of 0.1 to 0.125% should provide adequate analgesia. Older children or adolescents may require 0.2 to 0.25%.

Infants with a mean age of 5.3 weeks who received a bolus of bupivacaine 0.25% followed by infusion at 0.5 mg/kg per hr had bupivacaine serum levels that were suggestive of considerable bupivacaine accumulation. Some patients reached potentially toxic levels (Karmaker et al., 1996). In a similar study in younger infants (median age of 1.5 weeks), Cheung and others (1997) used a lower concentration, lower infusion rate and added epinephrine 1:400,000 in an attempt to decrease the uptake of local anesthetic. With an initial 1.25 mg/kg bolus of 0.25% bupivacaine, and an infusion of 0.125% at 0.25 mg/kg per hr, the mean serum concentration was 1.60 mcg/mL. Three patients had plasma bupivacaine measurements of > 3 mcg/mL between 30 and 48 hours. None of these patients had any sequelae.

Complications

In one series of 367 patients for paravertebral block, the failure rate was 10.7% in adults and 6.2% in children (Lonnqvist et al., 1995). Complications of the block included hypotension (4.6%), vascular puncture (3.8%), pleural puncture (1.1%), and pneumothorax (0.5%). Of these complications, all the patients who had hypotension were adults, none of the patients who had a vascular puncture demonstrated local anesthetic toxicity, and only one of the patients who had a pleural puncture had a pneumothorax. This study suggested that the failure rate was comparable to that of epidural blocks but with a much lower incidence of hypotension and little risk of dural puncture. The overall safety of paravertebral blocks has been established, although this technique should be limited to those who are experienced in its use.

BLOCKS OF THE FACE AND SCALP

Infraorbital Nerve Block

The infraorbital nerve consists of four branches. These branches innervate the upper lip and mucosa along the upper lip, the vermilion, the lateral inferior portion of the nose, and the lower lid of the eye. Blocking the infraorbital nerve provides effective analgesia for cleft lip repair (Bosenberg and Kimble, 1995; Prabhu et al., 1999). This block is also useful for nasal procedures such as endoscopic sinus surgery, nasal septal reconstruction, and rhinoplasty.

Anatomy

The infraorbital nerve is a purely sensory nerve derived from the second maxillary division of the trigeminal nerve. The infraorbital nerve is a terminal branch that exits the skull through the foramen rotundum to enter the pterygopalatine fossa. Here it emerges from the infraorbital foramen to divide into its four branches—the superior labial, internal nasal, external nasal, and inferior palpebral nerves.

Technique

The intraoral approach to block the infraorbital nerve is achieved by advancing a 27-gauge needle along the inner surface of the lip and cephalad to the infraorbital foramen parallel to the maxillary premolar. To perform this block, first palpate the infraorbital foramen and pull the upper lip superiorly to allow room for the needle and syringe (Plate 14–49; color image is available on the DVD). Keep a finger on the infraorbital foramen during needle advancement to provide accurate measurement to the desired space.

Dosing

A total volume of 0.5 to 1 mL of bupivacaine 0.25%, levobupivacaine 0.25%, or ropivacaine 0.2% with 1:200,000 epinephrine added is injected after negative aspiration for blood.

Complications

The most common side effect from performance of an infraorbital nerve block is swelling around the eyelid. To avoid this, pressure should be applied at the site of injection for 5 minutes. Other complications are rare.

Great Auricular Nerve Block

The mastoid and external ear are innervated by the great auricular nerve. Analgesia for otoplasty and tympanomastoidectomy is

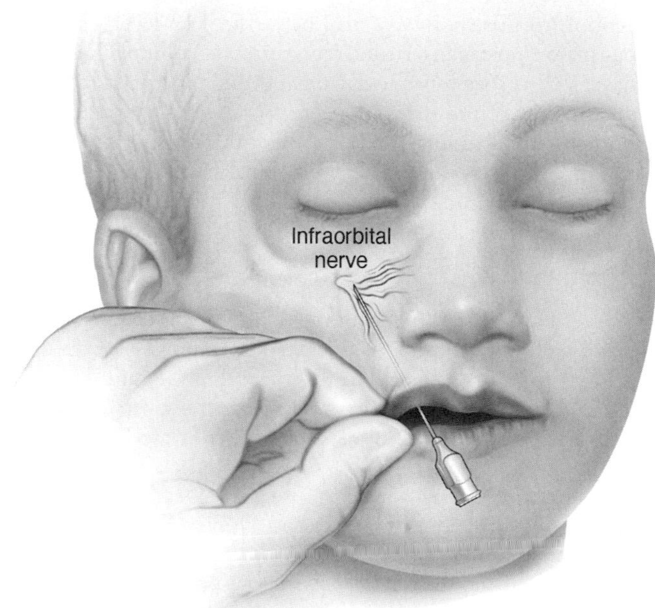

■ **PLATE 14–49.** Anatomy for infraorbital nerve block. (Color image is available on the DVD.)

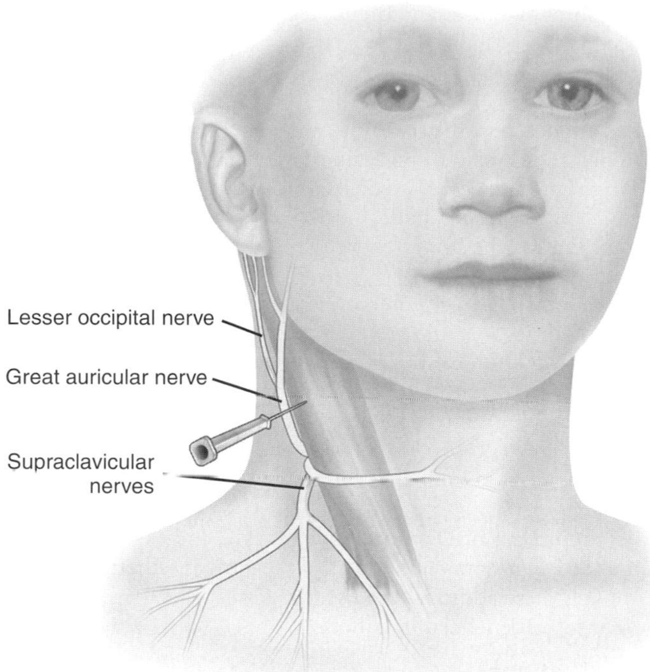

■ **PLATE 14–50.** Anatomy for great auricular nerve block. (Color image is available on the DVD.)

provided by blocking this nerve and leads to reduction in the perioperative use of opioids for these procedures (Cregg et al., 1996; Suresh and Wheeler, 2002).

Anatomy

The great auricular nerve is a sensory nerve branch of the superficial cervical plexus (C3). Its course at the level of the cricoid cartilage follows the posterior border of the belly of the clavicular head of the sternocleidomastoid muscle.

Technique

The great auricular nerve is blocked at the level of the cricoid cartilage (C6). The clavicular head of the sternocleidomastoid muscle is identified and local anesthetic is injected superficially along the belly of the muscle approximately 5 to 6 cm below the ear (Plate 14–50; color image is available on the DVD).

Complications

Complications from a great auricular nerve block may be significant and include intravascular injection due to the close proximity of the carotid artery and jugular veins. In addition, deep placement of the needle can result in phrenic nerve block, cervical plexus block, and Horner's syndrome.

Supraorbital and Supratrochlear Nerve Blocks

Anesthetizing the supraorbital and supratrochlear nerves can provide pain relief for procedures of the anterior scalp and forehead, including excision of skin lesions, neurosurgical procedures with incisions of the scalp or forehead, and laser therapy for hemangiomas (Suresh and Wheeler, 2002).

Anatomy

The supraorbital and supratrochlear nerves are terminal branches of the ophthalmic division of the trigeminal nerve (V_1).

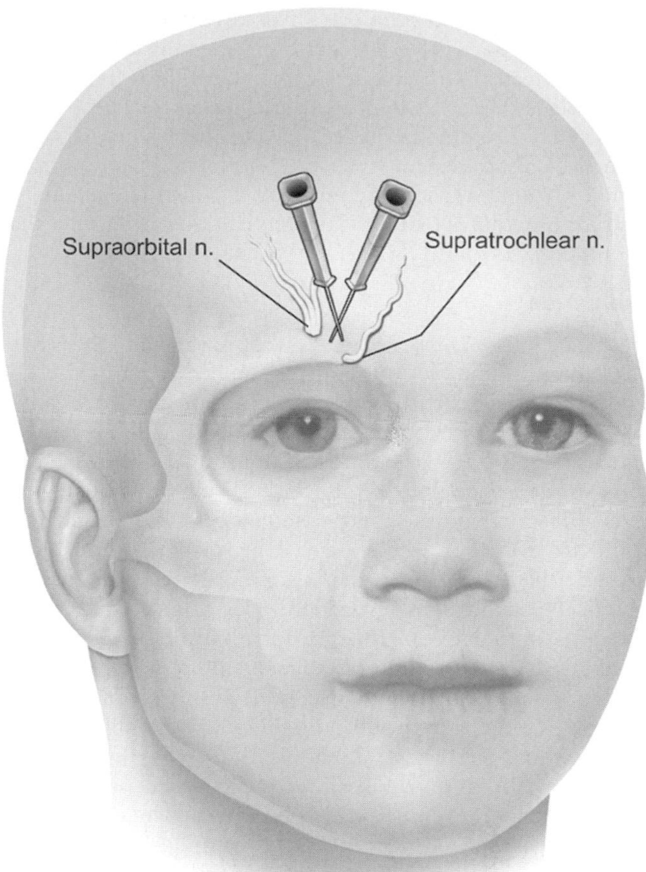

■ **PLATE 14–51.** Anatomy for supraorbital and supratrochlear nerve blocks. (Color image is available on the DVD.)

These nerves supply the forehead and the scalp anterior to the coronal suture. They are found immediately above the eyelid area, where the supraorbital nerve exits through the supraorbital foramen and the supratrochlear nerve exits the orbit between the trochlea and the supraorbital foramen (Plate 14–51; color image is available on the DVD).

Technique

These nerves are blocked using a 27-gauge needle. After identifying the supraorbital notch, the needle is inserted perpendicular to the skin at the notch until it contacts bone; it is then withdrawn slightly and local anesthetic is injected after negative aspiration. The supratrochlear nerve is blocked by withdrawing the needle back to the skin and aiming slightly medially.

Complications

Periorbital edema and ecchymosis are common side effects when performing blocks around the eye. To avoid this side effect, pressure can be applied to the supraorbital area for 5 minutes after the block has been placed.

■ INTRAVENOUS REGIONAL ANESTHESIA

Intravenous regional anesthesia (IVRA), or Bier block, describes a technique whereby an extremity is anesthetized by injecting local anesthetic intravenously and containing it within the extremity by using a tourniquet. This technique is useful only for intraoperative analgesia because the effect of the local anesthetic dissipates with release of the tourniquet. Intravenous regional anesthesia has been used in children for forearm fracture reduction and is considered safe and effective for most procedures of distal extremities that require pain relief for a short period of time (Davidson et al., 2002). IVRA should not be used for procedures that have a potential of lasting greater than 90 minutes.

Technique

A separate intravenous catheter is placed in the limb that is to be blocked and a double tourniquet is applied to this extremity. The limb should then be elevated and exsanguinated by wrapping the extremity with an elastic bandage beginning with the digits and proceeding toward the tourniquets (Plate 14–52; color image is available on the DVD). If the limb is fractured, exsanguination with the bandage should be deleted in an awake child to avoid excessive pain. The proximal tourniquet is then inflated to greater than 50 mm Hg above the baseline systolic blood pressure (Fitzgerald, 1976). If the operation is occurring on the lower extremity, inflation pressures should be closer to 100 mm Hg above systolic blood pressure. After proximal tourniquet inflation, local anesthetic is slowly injected into the venous cannula in the operative limb. Onset of block should occur within 5 minutes of injection. After testing for successful block, the procedure may begin. Once it is evident during the procedure that tourniquet pain is being experienced, the distal tourniquet is inflated. The proximal tourniquet may then be released. Tourniquet pain is typically not an immediate issue upon inflation of the distal tourniquet because that area remains anesthetized. Most children require sedation in addition to the IVRA.

At the end of the procedure, the distal tourniquet may be released for 15 seconds and then reinflated. The tourniquet may be released and reinflated two additional times. This allows some of the local anesthetic into the systemic circulation at short intervals to avoid local anesthetic toxicity from a large amount of local anesthetic being released all at once. There should remain at least one cuff inflated for at least 20 minutes after injection of the local anesthetic, regardless of the length of the procedure.

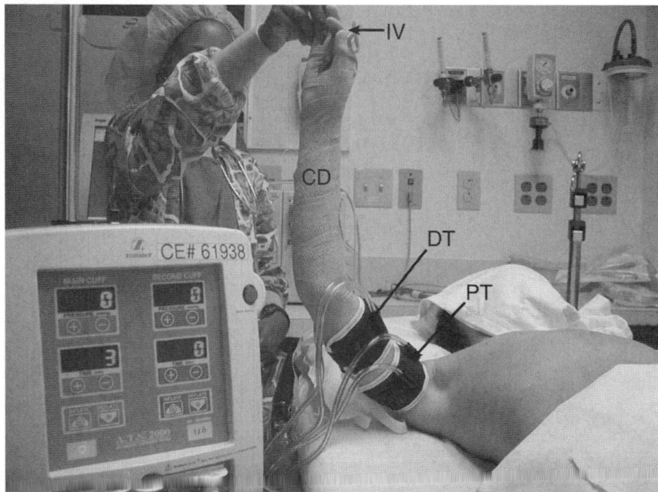

■ **PLATE 14–52.** Intravenous regional anesthetic. IV, intravenous catheter; CD, compression dressing; DT, distal tourniquet; PT, proximal tourniquet. (Color image is available on the DVD.)

Dosing

Either lidocaine or prilocaine may be used for intravenous regional anesthesia. Bupivacaine is contraindicated due to its ability to produce cardiotoxicity if it reaches the systemic circulation. When dosing lidocaine 0.5% or prilocaine 0.5%, use 0.6 mL/kg for the upper extremity and 1 mL/kg for the lower extremity.

In a study of 249 children over 3 years of age, either lidocaine 0.5% or prilocaine 0.5% was used for reduction of forearm fracture (Davidson et al., 2002). The dose used in this study was 0.6 mL/kg (or 3 mg/kg of local anesthetic). The group that had received the lidocaine had better analgesia than the prilocaine group with fewer cases of what was considered to be unacceptable pain during reduction of the fracture. There were no adverse events.

To improve block conditions, fentanyl 1 mcg/kg or pancuronium 0.01 mg/kg may be added to the local anesthetic solution. Although these additives are used in adults, they have not been proved to be beneficial in children.

Complications

Prilocaine can produce methemoglobinemia if injected systemically. Neurotoxicity and seizures may occur from lidocaine if the tourniquets fail or are released prematurely. For this reason, IVRA is not indicated for children with underlying seizure disorders. Children with sickle cell disease or vascular insufficiency should not receive IVRA because of the risk of prolonged tourniquet time.

■ TOPICAL ANESTHESIA

Topical anesthesia may be applied to a child either by using a cream or local infiltration to anesthetize the skin or by using topical application of local anesthetics directly to mucous membranes.

Topical local anesthetic cream was developed in the 1990s and has found popularity in the pediatric population due to its ability to anesthetize the skin before minor procedures. EMLA (Eutectic Mixture of Local Anesthetic) cream, a mixture of prilocaine and lidocaine, was the first commercially available agent that would anesthetize intact skin to a depth of 5 mm (Ehrenström et al., 1983). This mixture of prilocaine and lidocaine results in an oil-in-water emulsion that has a total local anesthetic concentration of 5%. EMLA cream has been found to be effective for superficial procedures such as venipuncture, laser treatment of port wine stains, and neonatal circumcision (Mannuksela and Korpela, 1986; Ashinoff and Geronemus, 1990; Taddio et al., 1997). EMLA cream has been found to reduce the neonatal physiologic response to circumcision compared with placebo, but it is not considered as effective as dorsal nerve block or penile ring block (Lander et al., 1997; Taddio et al., 1997; Howard et al., 1999).

EMLA cream is applied to intact skin at least 1 hour before the time of the procedure and covered with an occlusive dressing (Morgan-Hughes and Kirton, 2001). Heating the EMLA cream with an external heat pack after application has been shown to reduce the time to efficacy to 20 minutes, although a 60-minute waiting period is superior (Liu et al., 2003). EMLA cream should not be applied to traumatized or inflamed skin or on mucous membranes because of its potential for rapid absorption and systemic toxicity.

ELA-Max has become commercially available for use as a topical anesthetic for minor procedures and has been marketed as having the advantage of requiring only 30 minutes to be effective. ELA-Max is a cream consisting of 4% liposomal lidocaine. In a study of 120 children to compare ELA-Max with EMLA during venipuncture, the local anesthetic creams were applied at either 30 or 60 minutes before the procedure (Eichenfield et al., 2002). Both local anesthetic creams were effective, and the study demonstrated that a 30-minute application of ELA-Max without an occlusive dressing was as effective as a 60-minute application of EMLA with an occlusive dressing.

Local infiltration before minor procedures is effective as a method to provide pain relief during needle puncture or superficial incision. Although any local anesthetic can be used for injection, there is no benefit to using higher concentrations for most indications. Lidocaine 0.5% provides immediate analgesia to the site and is effective for 90 minutes. If a longer duration is desired for pain relief after the procedure, bupivacaine 0.25% may be used, which provides 2 to 3 hours of postprocedure analgesia. When using bupivacaine for local infiltration, one must be extremely careful to avoid injecting the local anesthetic into vascular structures. To decrease bleeding at the site during the procedure, epinephrine 2.5 to 5 mcg/mL is added to the local anesthetic solution. Plastic surgeons often increase the amount of epinephrine to 10 mcg/mL or 1:100,000 to keep the field clear of blood.

Maximal allowable dosing guidelines are the same for local infiltration as they are for other regional blocks. A total of 5 mg/kg of lidocaine, or 7 mg/kg lidocaine when epinephrine is added, can be used safely (Berde, 1993). When using bupivacaine either with or without epinephrine, 3 mg/kg is the maximal allowable dose. A simple rule of thumb when using bupivacaine 0.25% (2.5 mg/mL) is to not exceed 1 mL/kg of local anesthetic solution; therefore, the child never receives more than 2.5 mg/kg.

To use local infiltration in a child who is awake, measures to decrease the pain on injection must be taken for greater success. The child should be secured to decrease movement upon injection and during the procedure. A small-gauge needle such as a 27 gauge should be used and the injection performed slowly to minimize the pain that occurs with dissection of the superficial layers of the skin during injection. To further minimize pain, sodium bicarbonate is added to the solution at 1 mL/10 mL of lidocaine to increase the pH of the solution to physiologic values (Momsen et al., 2000). This buffered solution decreases the discomfort from the injection of the more acidic lidocaine without buffer (Christoph et al., 1988; Orlinsky et al., 1992).

Topical anesthesia may be applied to the *mucous membranes* of the nose and nasopharynx to decrease the discomfort associated with bronchoscopies, nasotracheal intubation, nasogastric tubes, or nasal airways. Topical anesthesia to the mucous membranes may be delivered by several methods. Lidocaine is available as a 5% ointment or 2% jelly. For mucous membranes, the 2% jelly is easy to apply and can be used for a greater surface area due to its lower concentration. The jelly may be simply applied to the nares and the tube for passage into the nose, and pledgets with the lidocaine jelly applied to the tip can be gently placed posteriorly in the nasopharynx to anesthetize that region. Although there are methods of delivering lidocaine as a nebulizer or spray, it is difficult to control the amount delivered, and at concentrations of 4%, it is easy to overdose a small child with this method. Peak plasma concentrations that are above the toxic levels are reached within 1 minute following the application of the 4% lidocaine spray due to fast absorption (Eyres et al., 1978). If this remains the preferred route for some practitioners, every attempt should be made to provide only the maximal allowable dose and to be alert for the potential of local anesthetic toxicity that can occur due to the high uptake from this vascular area.

MISCELLANEOUS PEDIATRIC REGIONAL ANESTHETIC BLOCKS

In addition to the described regional anesthetic techniques, there are certainly many more that have not been included in their entirety because of either low use or high complications. Some of these blocks, however, do have specific applications and may have been reported for this reason. An example of this is the cervical plexus block. It is not commonly used in children, but Tobias described its use in two adolescents who had known difficult airways and were scheduled to undergo neck surgery (1999).

For tonsillectomy patients, local anesthetic has been used to provide posttonsillectomy pain relief in children. Local bupivacaine infiltration of 5 mL per tonsillar pillar of 0.25% bupivacaine has been shown to lower pain scores in children (Jebeles et al., 1993). Smaller volumes, however, have not been shown to be as efficacious when 1.8 mL per tonsillar pillar has been used (Schoem et al., 1993). A glossopharyngeal nerve block for post-tonsillectomy pain was studied to determine its effectiveness and safety (Bean-Lijewski, 1997). The block consists of an injection of bupivacaine 0.25% to 0.5% into each lateral pharyngeal space using a 22-gauge spinal needle. This trial was terminated after two of the four children who had received the block developed severe upper airway obstruction after tracheal extubation. The conclusion was that the volume and concentration of bupivacaine resulted in blockade of the recurrent laryngeal nerves and/or the hypoglossal nerves. This technique, therefore, is not recommended.

SUMMARY

Regional anesthesia in children has progressed due to the development of improved local anesthetics, pediatric-sized equipment, and, most important, the knowledge that has been gained regarding patient safety and efficacy. As the field of regional anesthesia continues to develop, it may become the primary method of providing both intraoperative and postoperative analgesia, if strategies continue to diminish the risks and studies are carried out to promote the benefits (Goldman, 1995; Dalens and Mazoit, 1998).

Experienced practitioners in pediatric regional techniques provide an important service to children. Additional research must be directed at outcome studies to determine the true risks and benefits of these techniques in large populations of children. With the appropriate training and the use of appropriate agents and equipment, the practice of pediatric regional anesthesia as a means of providing superior analgesia should continue to be an essential part of the overall care of children in the perioperative period.

REFERENCES

Abdulatif M, El-Sanabary M: Caudal neostigmine, bupivacaine, and their combination for postoperative pain management after hypospadias surgery in children. *Anesth Analg* 95:1215, 2002.

Agarwal R, Gutlove DP, Lockhart CH: Seizures occurring in pediatric patients receiving continuous infusion of bupivacaine. *Anesth Analg* 75:284, 1992.

Ala-Kokko TI, Karinen J, Raiha E, et al.: Pharmacokinetics of 0.75% ropivacaine and 0.5% bupivacaine after ilioinguinal-iliohypogastric nerve block in children. *Br J Anaesth* 89:438, 2002.

Altintas F, Bozkurt P, Ipek N, et al.: The efficacy of pre versus postsurgical axillary block on postoperative pain in paediatric patients. *Paediatr Anaesth* 10:23, 2000.

Amory C, Mariscal A, Guyot E, et al.: Is ilioinguinal/iliohypogastric nerve block always totally safe in children? *Paediatr Anaesth* 13:164, 2003.

Anatol TI, Pitt-Miller P, Holder Y: Trial of three methods of intraoperative bupivacaine analgesia for pain after paediatric groin surgery. *Can J Anaesth* 44:1053, 1997.

Anderson CMT, Berde CB, Sethna NF, et al.: Meningococcal purpura fulminans: Treatment of vascular insufficiency in a 2 year old child with lumbar epidural sympathetic blockade. *Anesthesiology* 71:463, 1989.

Ansermino M, Basu R, Vanderbeek C, Montgomery C: Nonopioid additives to local anaesthetics for caudal blockade in children: A systematic review. *Paediatr Anaesth* 13:561, 2003.

Aram L, Krane EJ, Kozloski LJ, et al.: Tunneled epidural catheters for prolonged analgesia in pediatric patients. *Anesth Analg* 92:1432, 2001.

Armitage EN: Caudal block in children. *Anaesthesia* 34:396, 1979.

Ashinoff R, Geonemus RG: Effect of the topical anesthetic EMLA on the efficacy of pulsed dye laser treatment of port-wine stains. *J Dermatol Surg Oncol* 16:1008, 1990.

Badgwell JM, Heavner JE, Kytta J: Bupivacaine toxicity in young pigs is age-dependent and is affected by volatile anesthetics. *Anesthesiology* 73:297, 1990.

Bainbridge WS: Report on 712 operations on infants and young children under spinal anesthesia. *Arch Pediatr* 18:510, 1901.

Bardsley H, Gristwood R, Baker H, et al.: A comparison of the cardiovascular effects of levobupivacaine and rac-bupivacaine following intravenous administration to healthy volunteers. *Br J Clin Pharmacol* 46:245, 1998.

Baris S, Karakaya D, Kelsaka E, et al.: Comparison of fentanyl-bupivacaine or midazolam-bupivacaine mixtures with plain bupivacaine for caudal anaesthesia in children. *Paediatr Anaesth* 13:126, 2003.

Barnitzky S, Keucher TR, Mealey J Jr, et al.: Iatrogenic intraspinal epidermoid tumors. *JAMA* 237:148, 1977.

Batra YK, Prosad MK, Arya VK, et al.: Comparison of caudal tramadol versus bupivacaine for postoperative analgesia in children undergoing hypospadias surgery. *Int J Clin Pharmacol* 37:238, 1999.

Bean-Lijewski JD: Glossopharyngeal nerve block for pain relief after pediatric tonsillectomy: Retrospective analysis and two cases of life-threatening upper airway obstruction from an interrupted trial. *Anesth Analg* 84:1232, 1997.

Benzon HT, Strichartz GR, Gissen AJ, et al.: Developmental neurophysiology of mammalian peripheral nerves and age-related differential sensitivity to local anaesthetic. *Br J Anaesth* 61:754, 1988.

Berde CB: Bupivacaine toxicity secondary to continuous caudal epidural infusion in children. *Anesth Analg* 77:1305, 1993.

Berde CB: Convulsions associated with pediatric regional anesthesia. *Anesth Analg* 75:164-166, 1992.

Berens R, Pontus SP: A complication associated with dorsal penile nerve block. *Reg Anesth* 15:309, 1990.

Birmingham PK, Wheeler M, Suresh S, et al.: Patient-controlled epidural analgesia in children: can they do it? *Anesth Analg* 96:686, 2003.

Booker PD, Taylor C, Saba G: Perioperative changes in alpha$_1$-acid glycoprotein concentrations in infants undergoing major surgery. *Br J Anaesth* 76:365, 1996.

Bosenberg A, Thomas J, Lopez T, et al.: The efficacy of caudal ropivacaine 1, 2, and 3 mg/mL for postoperative analgesia in children. *Paediatr Anaesth* 12:53, 2002.

Bosenberg AT, Bland BAR, Schulte-Steinberg O, et al.: Thoracic epidural anesthesia via caudal route in infants. *Anesthesiology* 69:265, 1988.

Bosenberg AT, Gouws E: Skin epidural distance in children. *Anaesthesia* 50:894, 1995.

Bosenberg AT, Kimble FW: Infraorbital nerve block in neonates for cleft lip repair: Anatomical study and clinical application. *Br J Anaesth* 74:506, 1995.

Bosenberg AT, Raw R, Boezaart AP: Surface mapping of peripheral nerves in children with a nerve stimulator. *Paediatr Anaesth* 12:398, 2002.

Bosenberg AT: Lower limb nerve blocks in children using unsheathed needles and a nerve stimulator. *Anaesthesia* 50:206, 1995.

Bouchut JC, Dubois R, Foussat C, et al.: Evaluation of caudal anaesthesia performed in conscious ex-premature infants for inguinal herniotomies. *Paediatr Anaesth* 11:55, 2001.

Bouchut JC, Dubois R, Godard J: Clonidine in preterm-infant caudal anesthesia may be responsible for postoperative apnea. *Reg Anesth Pain Med* 26:83, 2001.

Breschan C, Krumpholz R, Likar R, et al.: Can a dose of 2 mcg/kg caudal clonidine cause respiratory depression in neonates? *Paediatr Anaesth* 9:81, 1999.

Broadman L, Hannallah RS, Belman AB, et al.: Post-circumcision analgesia: A prospective evaluation of subcutaneous ring block of the penis. *Anesthesiology* 67:399, 1987.

Broadman LM: Complications of pediatric regional anesthesia. *Reg Anesth* 21:64, 1996.

Bromage PR, Benumof JL: Paraplegia following intracord injection during attempted epidural anesthesia under general anesthesia. *Reg Anesth Pain Med* 23:104, 1998.

Bromage PR: Masked mischief. *Reg Anesth* 21:62, 1996.

Busoni P, Messeri A: Spinal anesthesia in children: Surface anatomy. *Anesth Analg* 68:418–419, 1989.

Butler-O'Hara M, Lemoine C, Guillet R: Analgesia for neonatal circumcision: A randomized controlled trial of EMLA versus dorsal penile block. *Pediatrics* 101:E5, 1998.

Campbell FA, Yentis AM, Fear DW, et al.: Analgesic efficacy and safety of a caudal bupivacaine-fentanyl mixture in children. *Can J Anaesth* 39:661, 1992.

Campbell RJ, Ilett KF, Dusci L: Plasma bupivacaine concentrations after axillary block in children. *Anaesth Intens Care* 14:343, 1986.

Carre P, Joly A, Field BC, et al.: Axillary block in children: Single or multiple injection? *Paediatr Anaesth* 10:35, 2000.

Casey WF, Rice LJ, Hannallah RS, et al.: A comparison between bupivacaine installation versus ilioinguinal/iliohypogastric nerve block for postoperative analgesia following inguinal herniorrhaphy in children. *Anesthesiology* 72:637, 1990.

Chalkiadis G: The rise and fall of continuous epidural infusions in children. *Paediatr Anaesth* 13: 91,2003.

Cheung SLW, Booker PD, Franks R, et al.: Serum concentrations of bupivacaine during prolonged paravertebral infusion in young infants. *Br J Anaesth* 79:9, 1997.

Chhibber AK, Perkins FM, Rabinowitz R, et al.: Penile block timing for postoperative analgesia of hypospadias repair in children. *J Urol* 158:1156, 1997.

Christoph RA, Buchanan L, Begalla K, Schwartz S: Pain reduction in local anesthetic administration through pH buffering. *Ann Emerg Med* 17:117, 1988.

Constant I, Gall O, Gouyet L, et al.: Addition of clonidine or fentanyl to local anaesthetics prolongs the duration of surgical analgesia after single-shot caudal block in children. *Br J Anaesth* 80:294, 1998.

Cook B, Doyle E: The use of additives to local anaesthetic solutions for caudal epidural blockade. *Paediatr Anaesth* 6:353, 1996.

Cook B, Grubb DJ, Aldridge LA, Doyle E: Comparison of the effects of adrenaline, clonidine, and ketamine on the duration of caudal analgesia produced by bupivacaine in children. *Br J Anaesth* 75:698, 1995.

Cote CJ, Zaslavsky A, Downes JJ, et al.: Postoperative apnea in former preterm infants after inguinal herniorrhaphy. *Anesthesiology* 82:809, 1995.

Cregg N, Conway F, Casey W: Analgesia after otoplasty: Regional nerve blockade versus local anaesthetic infiltration of the ear. *Can J Anaesth* 43:141, 1996.

DaConceicao JMJ, Coelho L: Caudal anaesthesia with 0.375% ropivacaine or 0.375% bupivacaine in paediatric patients. *Br J Anaesth* 80:507, 1998.

DaConceicao MJ, Coelho L, Khalil M: Ropivacaine 0.25% compared with bupivacaine 0.25% by the caudal route. *Paediatr Anaesth* 9:229, 1999.

Dadure C, Pirat P, Raux O, et al.: Perioperative continuous peripheral nerve blocks with disposable infusion pumps in children: A prospective descriptive study. *Anesth Analg* 97:687, 2003.

Dalens B (ed): *Regional Anesthesia in Infants, Children and Adolescents.* Baltimore, 1995, Williams and Wilkins.

Dalens B, Ecoffey C, Joly A, et al.: Pharmacokinetics and analgesic effect of ropivacaine following ilioinguinal/iliohypogastric nerve block in children. *Paediatr Anaesth* 11:415, 2001.

Dalens B, Hasnouai A: Caudal anesthesia in pediatric surgery: Success rates and adverse effects in 750 consecutive patients. *Anesth Analg* 68:83, 1989.

Dalens B, Tanguy A, Vanneuville G: Lumbar plexus block in children: A comparison of two procedures in 50 patients. *Anesth Analg* 67:750, 1988.

Dalens B, Tanguy A, Vanneuville G: Sciatic nerve blocks in children: comparison of the posterior, anterior, and lateral approaches in 180 pediatric patients. *Anesth Analg* 70:131, 1990.

Dalens B, Vanneuville G, Tanguy A: A new parascalene approach to the brachial plexus in children: Comparison with the supraclavicular approach. *Anesth Analg* 66:1264, 1987.

Dalens B, Vanneuville G, Tanguy A: Comparison of the fascia iliaca compartment block with the 3-in-1 block in children. *Anesth Analg* 69:705, 1989.

Dalens B: The expansion of paediatric anaesthesia. *Curr Opin Anaesth* 12:299, 1999.

Dalens BJ, Mazoit JX: Adverse effects of regional anaesthesia in children. *Drug Safety* 19:251, 1998.

Dalens BJ: Regional anesthesia in children. In Miller RD (ed): *Anesthesia.* Philadelphia, 2000, Churchill Livingstone.
D'Angelo R, Cohen IT, Brandom BW: Continuous epidural infusion of bupivacaine and fentanyl for erythromelalgia in an adolescent. *Anesth Analg* 74:142, 1992.
Davidson AJ, Eyres RL, Cole WG: A comparison of prilocaine and lidocaine for intravenous regional anaesthesia for forearm fracture reduction in children. *Paediatr Anaesth* 12:146, 2002.
De La Coussaye J, Brugada J, Allessie MA: Electrophysiologic and arrhythmogenic effects of bupivacaine. *Anesthesiology* 77:32, 1992.
De Negri P, Ivani G, Tirri T, et al.: New drugs, new techniques, new indications in pediatric regional anesthesia. *Minerva Anestesiologica* 68:420, 2002.
De Negri P, Ivani G, Visconti C, et al.: How to prolong postoperative analgesia after caudal anaesthesia with ropivacaine in children: S-Ketamine versus clonidine. *Paediatr Anaesth* 11:679, 2001.
De Negri P, Ivani G, Visconti C, et al.: The dose-response relationship for clonidine added to a postoperative continuous epidural infusion of ropivacaine in children. *Paediatr Anaesth* 93:71, 2001.
Desparmet J, Mateo J, Ecoffey C, et al.: Efficacy of an epidural test dose in children anesthetized with halothane. *Anesthesiology* 72:249, 1990.
Desparmet J, Meistelman C, Barre J, et al.: Continuous epidural infusion of bupivacaine for postoperative pain relief in children. *Anesthesiology* 67:108, 1987.
Desparmet JF: Total spinal anesthesia after caudal anesthesia in an infant. *Anesth Analg* 70:665, 1990.
Diwan R, Lakshmi V, Shah T, et al.: Continuous axillary block for upper limb surgery in a patient with epidermolysis bullosa simplex. *Paediatr Anaesth* 11:603, 2001.
Dohi S, Naito H, Takahashi T: Age-related changes in blood pressure and duration of motor block in spinal anesthesia. *Anesthesiology* 50:319, 1979.
Dohi S, Seino H: Spinal anesthesia in premature infants: Dosage and effects of sympathectomy. *Anesthesiology* 65:559, 1986.
Doyle E, Morton NS, McNicol LR: Plasma bupivacaine levels after fascia iliaca compartment block with and without adrenaline. *Paediatr Anaesth* 7:121, 1997.
Dunwoody JM, Reichert CC, Brown KLB: Compartment syndrome associated with bupivacaine and fentanyl epidural analgesia in pediatric orthopaedics. *J Pediatr Orthop* 17:285, 1997.
Eck JB, Cantos-Gustafsson A, Ross AK, et al.: What's new in pediatric paravertebral analgesia. *Tech Reg Anesth Pain Manage* 6:131, 2002.
Ecoffey C, Desparmet J, et al.: Bupivacaine in children: Pharmacokinetics following caudal anesthesia. *Anesthesiology* 63:447, 1985.
Edwards WT, Burney RG: Use of repeated nerve blocks in management of an infant with Kawasaki's disease. *Anesth Analg* 67:1008, 1988.
Ehrenström-Reiz G, Reiz S, Stockman O: Topical anaesthesia with EMLA, a new lidocaine-prilocaine cream and the Cusum technique for detection of minimal application time. *Acta Anaesth Scand* 27:510, 1983.
Eichenfield LF, Funk A, Fallon-Friedlander S, Cunningham BB: A clinical study to evaluate the efficacy of ELA-Max (4% liposomal lidocaine) as compared with eutectic mixture of local anesthetics cream for pain reduction of venipuncture in children. *Pediatrics* 109:1093, 2002.
Eisenach JC, Yaksh TL: Epidural ketamine in healthy children—What's the point? *Anesth Analg* 96:626, 2003.
Eng J, Sabanathan S: Continuous paravertebral block for postthoracotomy analgesia in children. *J Pediatr Surg* 27:556, 1992.
Eyres RL, Bishop W, Oppenheim RC, et al.: Plasma bupivacaine concentrations in children during caudal epidural analgesia. *Anaesth Intens Care* 11:20, 1983.
Eyres RL, Hastings C, Brown TCK, et al.: Plasma bupivacaine concentrations following lumbar epidural anaesthesia in children. *Anaesth Intens Care* 14:131, 1986.
Eyres RL, Kild J, Oppenheim R, et al.: Local anaesthetic plasma levels in children. *Anaesth Intens Care* 6:43, 1978.
Finkel JC, Boltz MG, Conran AM: Haemodynamic changes during high spinal anaesthesia in children having open heart surgery. *Paediatr Anaesth* 13:48, 2003.
Fischer HBJ: Regional anesthesia—Before or after general anesthesia. *Anaesthesia* 53:727, 1998.
Fisher QA, McComiskey CM, Hill JL, et al.: Postoperative voiding interval and duration of analgesia following peripheral or caudal nerve blocks in children. *Anesth Analg* 76:173, 1993.
Fisher QA, Shaffner DH, Yaster M: Detection of intravascular injection of regional anaesthetics in children. *Can J Anaesth* 44:582, 1997.
Fitzgerald B: Intravenous regional anaesthesia in children. *Br J Anaesth* 48:485, 1976.
Flandin-Blety C, Barrier G: Accidents following extradural analgesia in children. The results of a retrospective study. *Paediatr Anaesth* 5:41, 1995.
Fleischmann E, Marhofer P, Greher M, et al.: Brachial plexus anaesthesia in children: Lateral infraclavicular versus axillary approach. *Paediatr Anaesth* 13:103, 2003.
Foldes FF, Molloy R, McNall PG, et al.: Comparison of toxicity of intravenously given local anesthetic agents in man. *JAMA* 172:1493, 1960.
Freid EB, Bailey AG, Valley RD: Electrocardiographic and hemodynamic changes associated with unintentional intravascular injection of bupivacaine with epinephrine in infants. *Anesthesiology* 79:394, 1993.
Giaufre E, Dalens B, Gombert A: Epidemiology and morbidity of regional anesthesia in children: A one-year prospective survey of the French-language society of pediatric anesthesiologists. *Anesth Analg* 83:904, 1996.
Goldman L: Complications in regional anesthesia. *Paediatr Anaesth* 5:3, 1995.
Goodarzi M: The effect of perioperative and postoperative caudal block on pain control in children. *Paediatr Anaesth* 6:475, 1996.
Graf BM, Martin E, Bosnjak ZJ, et al.: Stereospecific effect of bupivacaine isomers on atrioventricular conduction in the isolated perfused guinea pig heart. *Anesthesiology* 86:410, 1997.
Gristwood RW: Cardiac and CNS toxicity of levobupivacaine: Strengths of evidence for advantage over bupivacaine. *Drug Safety* 25:153, 2002.
Guinard JP, Borboen M: Probable venous air embolism during caudal anesthesia in a child. *Anesth Analg* 76:1134, 1993.
Gunduz M, Ozcengiz D, Ozbek H, et al.: A comparison of single dose caudal tramadol, tramadol plus bupivacaine and bupivacaine administration for postoperative analgesia in children. *Paediatr Anaesth* 11:323, 2001.
Gunter JB, Dunn CM, Bennie JB, et al.: Optimum concentration of bupivacaine for combined caudal-general anesthesia in children. *Anesthesiology* 75:57, 1991.
Gunter JB, Eng C: Thoracic epidural anesthesia via the caudal approach in children. *Anesthesiology* 76:935, 1992.
Gunter JB, Gregg T, Varughese AM, et al.: Levobupivacaine for ilioinguinal/iliohypogastric nerve block in children. *Anesth Analg* 89:647, 1999.
Hager H, Marhofer P, Sitzwohl, et al.: Caudal clonidine prolongs analgesia from caudal S(+)-ketamine in children. *Anesth Analg* 94:1169, 2002.
Hammer GB: Pediatric thoracic anesthesia. *Anesth Analg* 92:1449, 2001.
Hannallah RS, Broadman LM, Belman AB, et al.: Comparison of caudal and ilioinguinal/iliohypogastric nerve blocks for control of post-orchiopexy pain in pediatric ambulatory surgery. *Anesthesiology* 66:832, 1987.
Hansen TG, Ilett KF, Lim SI, et al.: Pharmacokinetics and clinical efficacy of long-term epidural ropivacaine infusion in children. *Br J Anaesth* 85:347, 2000.
Hansen TG, Ilett KF, Reid C, et al.: Caudal ropivacaine in infants: Population pharmacokinetics and plasma concentrations. *Anesthesiology* 94:579, 2001.
Hansen TG, Morton NS, Cullen PM, Watson DG: Plasma concentrations and pharmacokinetics of bupivacaine with and without adrenaline following caudal anesthesia in infants. *Acta Anaesthesiol Scand* 45:42, 2001.
Hardwick-Smith S, Mastrobattista JM, Wallace PA, et al.: Ring block for neonatal circumcision. *Obstet Gynecol* 91:930, 1998.
Harnik EV, Hoy GR, Potolicchio S, et al.: Spinal anesthesia in premature infants recovering from respiratory distress syndrome. *Anesthesiology* 64:95, 1986.
Henderson K, Sethna NF, Berde CB: Continuous caudal anesthesia for inguinal hernia repair in former preterm infants. *J Clin Anesth* 5:120, 1993.
Holder KJ, Peutrell JM, Weir PM: Regional anesthesia for circumcision. Subcutaneous ring block of the penis and subpubic penile block compared. *Eur J Anaesthesiol* 14:495, 1997.
Holthusen H, Eichwede F, Stevens M, et al.: Pre-emptive analgesia: comparison of preoperative with postoperative caudal block on postoperative pain in children. *Br J Anaesth* 73:440, 1994.
Horlocker TT, Abel MD, Messick JM, et al.: Small risk of serious neurologic complications related to lumbar epidural catheter placement in anesthetized patients. *Anesth Analg* 96:1547, 2003.
Horlocker TT, Wedel DJ, Benzon H, et al.: Regional anesthesia in the anticoagulated patient: Defining the risks (The Second ASRA Consensus Conference on Neuraxial Anesthesia and Anticoagulation). *Reg Anesth Pain Med* 28:172, 2003.
Howard CR, Howard FM, Fortune K, et al.: A randomized, controlled trial of a eutectic mixture of local anesthetic cream (lidocaine and prilocaine) versus penile nerve block for pain relief during circumcision. *Am J Obstet Gynecol* 181:1506, 1999.
Huang JJ, Hirshberg G: Regional anaesthesia decreases the need for postoperative mechanical ventilation in very low birth weight infants undergoing herniorrhaphy. *Paediatr Anaesth* 11:705, 2001.
Huang YF, Pryor ME, Mather LE, et al.: Cardiovascular and central nervous system effects of intravenous levobupivacaine and bupivacaine in sheep. *Anesth Analg* 86:797, 1998.
Irving GA, Butt AD, Van der Veen B: A comparison of caudal morphine given pre- or post-surgery for postoperative analgesia in children. *Paediatr Anaesth* 3:217, 1993.

Ivani G, Codipietro L, Gagliardi F, et al.: A long-term continuous infusion via a sciatic catheter in a 3-year-old boy. *Paediatr Anaesth* 13:718, 2003.

Ivani G, Conio A, De Negri P, et al.: Spinal versus peripheral effects of adjunct clonidine: Comparison of the analgesic effect of a ropivacaine-clonidine mixture when administered as a caudal or ilioinguinal-iliohypogastric nerve blockade for inguinal surgery in children. *Paediatr Anaesth* 12:680, 2002.

Ivani G, De Negri P, Conio A, et al.: Comparison of racemic bupivacaine, ropivacaine and levobupivacaine for pediatric caudal anesthesia: Effects on postoperative analgesia and motor block. *Reg Anesth Pain Med* 27:157, 2002.

Ivani G, De Negri P, Conio A, et al.: Ropivacaine-clonidine combination for caudal blockade in children. *Acta Anaesthesiol Scand* 44:446, 2000.

Ivani G, De Negri P, Lonnqvist PA, et al.: A comparison of three different concentrations of levobupivacaine for caudal block in children. *Anesth Analg* 97: 368, 2003.

Ivani G, Mereto N, Lampugnani E, et al.: Ropivacaine in paediatric surgery: Preliminary results. *Paediatr Anaesth* 8:127, 1998.

Ivani G: Ropivacaine: Is it time for children? *Paediatr Anaesth* 12:383, 2002.

Jason Lowry K, Tobias J, Kittle D, et al.: Postoperative pain control using epidural catheters after anterior spinal fusion for adolescent scoliosis. *Spine* 26:1290, 2001.

Jebeles JH, Reilly JS, Gutierrez JF, et al.: Tonsillectomy and adenoidectomy pain reduction by local bupivacaine infiltration in children. *Int J Pediatr Otorhinolaryngol* 25:149, 1993.

Johnson CM: Continuous femoral nerve blockade for analgesia in children with femoral fractures. *Anaesth Intens Care* 22:281, 1994.

Johr M, Sossai R: Colonic puncture during ilioinguinal nerve block in a child. *Anesth Analg* 88:1051, 1999.

Jones RDM, Gunawardene WMS, Yeung CK: A comparison of lignocaine 2% with adrenaline 1:200,000 and lignocaine 2% with adrenaline 1:200,000 plus fentanyl as agents for caudal anaesthesia in children undergoing circumcision. *Anaesth Intens Care* 18:194, 1990.

Joshi W, Connelly NR, Dwyer M, et al.: A comparison of two concentrations of bupivacaine and adrenaline with and without fentanyl in paediatric inguinal herniorrhaphy. *Paediatr Anaesth* 9:317, 1999.

Kapral S, Jandrasits O, Schabernig C, et al.: Lateral infraclavicular plexus block vs axillary block for hand and forearm surgery. *Acta Anaesthesiol Scand* 43:1047, 1999.

Karmaker MK, Booker PD, Franks R, et al.: Continuous extrapleural paravertebral infusion of bupivacaine for post-thoracotomy analgesia in young infants. *Br J Anaesth* 76:811, 1996.

Kempen PM, O'Donnell J, Lawler R, et al.: Acute respiratory insufficiency during interscalene plexus block. *Anesth Analg* 90:1415, 2000.

Kempthorne PM, Brown TCK: Nerve blocks around the knee in children. *Anaesth Intens Care* 12:14, 1984.

Khan FA, Memon GA, Kamal RS: Effect of route of buprenorphine on recovery and postoperative analgesic requirements in paediatric patients. *Paediatr Anaesth* 12:786, 2002.

Kiffer F, Joly A, Wodey E, et al.: The effect of preoperative epidural morphine on postoperative analgesia in children. *Anesth Analg* 93:598, 2001.

Kinirons B, Mimoz O, Lafendi L, et al.: Chlorhexidine versus povidone iodine in preventing colonization of continuous epidural catheters in children: A randomized, controlled trial. *Anesthesiology* 94:239, 2001.

Knudsen K, Beckman Suurkula M, Blomberg S, et al.: Central nervous and cardiovascular effects of IV infusions of ropivacaine, bupivacaine and placebo in volunteers. *Br J Anaesth* 78:507, 1997.

Koinig H, Krenn CG, Glaser C, et al.: The dose-response of caudal ropivacaine in children. *Anesthesiology* 90:1339, 1999.

Kokki H, Hendolin H: Comparison of 25G and 29G Quincke spinal needles in paediatric day cases. *Paediatr Anaesth* 6:115, 1996.

Kokki H, Ruuskanen A, Karvinen M: Comparison of epidural pain treatment with sufentanil-ropivacaine infusion with and without epinephrine in children. *Acta Anaesthesiol Scand* 46:647, 2002.

Konrad C, Johr M: Blockade of the sciatic nerve in the popliteal fossa: A system for standardization in children. *Anesth Analg* 87:1256, 1998.

Kozek-Langenecker S, Chiari A, Semsroth M: Simulation of an epidural test dose with intravenous isoproterenol in awake and halothane-anesthetized children. *Anesthesiology* 85:277, 1996.

Krane EJ, Dalens BJ, Murat I, et al.: The safety of epidurals placed during general anesthesia. *Reg Anesth Pain Med* 23:433, 1998.

Krane EJ, Haberkern CM, Jacobson LE: Postoperative apnea, bradycardia and oxygen desaturation in formerly premature infants: Prospective comparison of spinal and general anesthesia. *Anesth Analg* 80:7, 1995.

Krane EJ, Jacobson LE, Lynn AM, et al.: Caudal morphine for postoperative analgesia in children: Comparison with caudal bupivacaine and intravenous morphine. *Anesth Analg* 66:647, 1987.

Krane EJ, Tyler DC, Jacobson LE: The dose response of caudal morphine in children. *Anesthesiology* 71:48, 1989.

Lagade MRG, Poppers PJ: Stellate ganglion block: A therapeutic modality for arterial insufficiency of the arm in premature infants. *Anesthesiology* 61:203, 1984.

Lambert LA, Lambert DH, Strichartz GR: Irreversible conduction block in isolated nerve by high concentrations of local anesthetics. *Anesthesiology* 80:1082, 1994.

Lander J, Brady-Fryer B, Metcalfe JB, et al.: Comparison of ring block, dorsal penile nerve block, and topical anesthesia for neonatal circumcision. *JAMA* 278:2157, 1997.

Langer JC, Shandling B, Rosenberg M: Intraoperative bupivacaine during outpatient hernia repair in children: A randomized double blind trial. *J Pediatr Surg* 22:267, 1987.

Larsson BA, Olsson GL, Lonnqvist PA: Plasma concentrations of bupivacaine in young infants after continuous epidural infusion. *Paediatr Anaesth* 4:159, 1994.

Lee JJ, Rubin AP: Comparison of a bupivacaine-clonidine mixture with plain bupivacaine for caudal analgesia in children. *Br J Anaesth* 72:258, 1994.

Lejus C, Roussiere G, Testa S, et al.: Postoperative extradural analgesia in children: Comparison of morphine with fentanyl. *Br J Anaesth* 72:156, 1994.

Lerman J, Stron A, LeDez KM, et al.: Effects of age on serum concentration of alpha-1 acid glycoprotein and the binding of lidocaine in pediatric patients. *Clin Pharmacol Ther* 46:219, 1989.

Lim S-L, SB AN, Tan G-M: Ilioinguinal and iliohypogastric nerve block revisited: Single shot versus double shot technique for hernia repair in children. *Paediatr Anaesth* 12:255, 2002.

Liu DR, Kirchner HL, Petrack EM: Does using heat with eutectic mixture of local anesthetic cream shorten analgesic time? *Ann Emerg Med* 42:27, 2003.

Lloyd-Thomas AR, Howard RF: A pain service for children. *Paediatr Anaesth* 4:3, 1994.

Locatelli B, Ingelmo P, Sonzogni V, et al.: Randomized, double-blind, phase III, controlled trial comparing levobupivacaine 0.25%, ropivacaine 0.25%, and bupivacaine 0.25% by the caudal route in children. *Br J Anaesth* 94:366, 2005.

Londergan TA, Hochman HI, Goldberger N: Postoperative pain following outpatient pediatric urologic surgery: A comparison of anesthetic techniques. *Urology* 44:572, 1994.

Lonnqvist PA, Hesser U: Location of the paravertebral space in children and adolescents in relation to surface anatomy assessed by computed tomography. *Paediatr Anaesth* 2:285, 1992.

Lonnqvist PA, Hesser U: Radiological and clinical distribution of thoracic paravertebral blockade in infants and children. *Paediatr Anaesth* 3:83, 1993.

Lonnqvist PA, Hildingsson U: The caudal boundary of the thoracic paravertebral space. *Anaesthesia* 47:1051, 1992.

Lonnqvist PA, Ivani G, Moriarty T: Use of caudal-epidural opioids in children: Still state of the art or beginning of the end? *Paediatr Anaesth* 12:747, 2002.

Lonnqvist PA, MacKenzie J, Soni AK, et al.: Paravertebral blockade. Failure rate and complications. *Anaesthesia* 50:813, 1995.

Lonnqvist PA, Olsson GL: Paravertebral vs. epidural block in children: Effects on postoperative morphine requirements after renal surgery. *Acta Anesthesiol Scand* 38:346, 1994.

Lonnqvist PA, Westrin P, Larsson BA, et al.: Ropivacaine pharmacokinetics after caudal block in 1-8 year old children. *Br J Anaesth* 85:506, 2000.

Lonnqvist PA: Continuous paravertebral block in children: Initial experience. *Anaesthesia* 47:607, 1992.

Luz G, Wieser C, Innerhofer P, et al.: Free and total bupivacaine plasma concentrations after continuous epidural anaesthesia in infants and children. *Paediatr Anaesth* 8:473, 1998.

Maccani RM, Wedel DJ, Melton A, et al.: Femoral and lateral femoral cutaneous nerve block for muscle biopsies in children. *Paediatr Anaesth* 5:223, 1995.

Mannuksela E-L, Korpela R: Double-blind evaluation of a lignocaine-prilocaine cream (EMLA) in children. *Br J Anaesth* 58:1242, 1986.

Marhofer P, Krenn CG, Plochl W, et al.: S(+)-Ketamine for caudal block in paediatric anaesthesia. *Br J Anaesth* 84:341, 2000.

Marhofer P, Semsroth M: Epidural ketamine in children—What's the point? (In Response) *Anesth Analg* 96:626, 2003.

Mather LE, Chang DH: Cardiotoxicity with modern local anaesthetics: Is there a safer choice? *Rev Drugs* 61:333, 2001.

Maxwell LG, Yaster M, Wetzel RC, et al.: Penile nerve block for newborn circumcision. *Obstet Gynecol* 70:415, 1987.

Mazoit JX, Boico O, Samii K: Myocardial uptake of bupivacaine. II. Pharmacokinetics and pharmacodynamics of bupivacaine enantiomers in the isolated perfused rabbit heart. *Anesth Analg* 77:477, 1993.

Mazoit JX, Denson DD, Samii K: Pharmacokinetics of bupivacaine following caudal anesthesia in infants. *Anesthesiology* 68:387, 1988.
McCann ME, Sethna NF, Mazoit JX, et al.: The pharmacokinetics of epidural ropivacaine in infants and young children. *Paediatr Anaesth* 93:893, 2001.
McCloskey JJ, Haun SE, Deshpande JK: Bupivacaine toxicity secondary to continuous caudal epidural infusion in children. *Anesth Analg* 75:287, 1992.
McIlvaine W, Knox RF, Fennessey PV, et al.: Continuous infusion of bupivacaine via intrapleural catheter for analgesia after thoracotomy in children. *Anesthesiology* 69:261, 1988.
McLeod GA, Burke D: Review: Levobupivacaine. *Anaesthesia* 56:331, 2001.
McNeely JK, Farber NE, Rusy LM, et al.: Epidural analgesia improves outcome following pediatric fundoplication. *Reg Anesth* 22:16, 1997.
McNeely JK, Trentadue NC, Rusy LM, et al.: Culture of bacteria from lumbar and caudal epidural catheters used for postoperative analgesia in children. *Reg Anesth* 22:428, 1997.
McNicol LR: Lower limb blocks for children. *Anaesthesia* 41:27, 1986.
Merril DG, Brodsky JB, Hentz RV: Vascular insufficiency following axillary block of the brachial plexus *Anesth Analg* 60:162, 1981.
Meunier J-F, Goujard E, Dubousset A-M, et al.: Pharmacokinetics of bupivacaine after continuous epidural infusion in infants with and without biliary atresia. *Anesthesiology* 95:87, 2001.
Miller OF, Bloom TL, Smith LJ, et al.: Early hospital discharge for intravesical ureteroneocystostomy. *J Urol* 167:2556, 2002.
Momson OH, Roman CM, Mohammed BA, Andersen G: Neutralization of lidocaine-adrenaline. A simple method for less painful application of local anesthesia. *Ugeskrift Laeger* 162:4391, 2000.
Moorthy SS, Dierdorf S, Yaw PB: Influence of volume on the spread of local anesthetic—Methylene blue solution after injection for intercostal block. *Anesth Analg* 75:389, 1992.
Morgan-Hughes NJ, Kirton CB: EMLA—Is one hour long enough? *Anaesthesia* 56:495, 2001.
Murat I, Walker J, Esteve C, et al.: Effect of lumbar anaesthesia on plasma cortisol levels in children. *Can J Anaesth* 66:729, 1988.
Naguib M, Sharif AMY, Seraj M, et al.: Ketamine for caudal analgesia in children: Comparison with caudal bupivacaine. *Br J Anaesth* 67:559, 1991.
Oberlander TF, Berde CB, Lam KH, et al.: Infants tolerate spinal anesthesia with minimal overall autonomic changes: Analysis of heart rate variability in former premature infants undergoing hernia repair. *Anesth Analg* 80:20, 1995.
Oliver A: Dural punctures in children: What should we do? *Paediatr Anaesth* 12:473, 2002.
Orlinsky M, Hudson C, Chan L, Deslauriers R: Pain comparison of unbuffered versus buffered lidocaine in local wound infiltration. *J Emerg Med* 10:411, 1992.
Ozasa H, Hashimoto K, Saito Y: Pulmonary Doppler flow velocity pattern during caudal epidural anaesthesia in children. *Paediatr Anaesth* 12:317, 2002.
Ozcengiz D, Gunduz M, Ozbek H, Isik G: Comparison of caudal morphine and tramadol for postoperative pain control in children undergoing inguinal herniorrhaphy. *Paediatr Anaesth* 11:459, 2001.
Parris WCV, Reddy BC, White HW, et al.: Stellate ganglion blocks in pediatric patients. *Anesth Analg* 72:552, 1991.
Paut O, Sallabery M, Schreiber-Deturmeny E, et al.: Continuous fascia iliaca compartment block in children: A prospective evaluation of plasma bupivacaine concentrations, pain scores, and side effects. *Anesth Analg* 92:1159, 2001.
Payen D, Ecoffey C, Carli P, et al.: Pulsed Doppler ascending aortic, carotid, brachial and femoral artery blood flows during caudal anesthesia in infants. *Anesthesiology* 67:681, 1987.
Perillo M, Sethna NF, Berde CB: Intravenous isoproterenol as a marker for epidural test-dosing in children. *Anesth Analg* 76:168, 1993.
Peutrell JM, Hughes DG: Epidural anaesthesia through caudal catheters for inguinal herniotomies in awake ex-premature babies. *Anaesthesia* 47:128, 1993.
Pietropaoli JA, Keller MS, Smail DF, et al.: Regional anesthesia in pediatric surgery. Complications and postoperative comfort level in 174 children. *J Pediatr Surg* 28:560, 1993.
Prabhu KP, Wig J, Grewal S: Bilateral infraorbital nerve block is superior to preincisional infiltration for analgesia after repair of cleft lip. *Scand J Plast Reconstr Surg Hand Surg* 33:83, 1999.
Prosser DP, Davis A, Booker PD, et al.: Caudal tramadol for postoperative analgesia in paediatric hypospadias surgery. *Br J Anaesth* 79:293, 1997.
Radwan IAM, Saito S, Goto F: The neurotoxicity of local anesthetics on growing neurons: A comparative study of lidocaine, bupivacaine, mepivacaine, and ropivacaine. *Anesth Analg* 94:319, 2002.
Raj PP, Parks RI, Watson TD, et al.: A new single-position supine approach to sciatic-femoral nerve block. *Anesth Analg* 54:489, 1975.
Ralston DH, Shnider SM: The fetal and neonatal effects of regional anesthesia in obstetrics. *Anesthesiology* 48:34, 1978.
Rice LJ, DeMars, PD, Whalen TV, et al.: Duration of spinal anesthesia in infants less than one year of age. *Reg Anesth* 19:325, 1994.
Richardson J, Lonnqvist PA: Thoracic paravertebral block. *Br J Anaesth* 81:230, 1998.
Ronchi L, Rosenbaum D, Athouel A, et al.: Femoral nerve blockade in children using bupivacaine. *Anesthesiology* 70:622, 1989.
Rosen KR, Broadman LM: Anaesthesia for diagnostic muscle biopsy in an infant with Pompe's disease. *Can Anaesth Soc J* 33:790, 1986.
Rosen KR, Rosen DA: Caudal epidural morphine for control of pain following open heart surgery in children. *Anesthesiology* 70:418, 1989.
Rosenquist RW, Birnback DJ: Epidural insertion in anesthetized adults: Will your patients thank you? *Anesth Analg* 96:1545, 2003.
Ross AK, Eck JB, Tobias JD: Pediatric regional anesthesia: beyond the caudal. *Anesth Analg* 91:16, 2000.
Roy-Shapiri A, Amoury RA, Ashcraft KW, et al.: Transient quadriceps paresis following local inguinal block for postoperative pain control. *J Pediatr Surg* 20:554, 1985.
Sanchez V, Segedin ER, Moser M, et al.: Role of lumbar sympathectomy in the pediatric intensive care unit. *Anesth Analg* 67:794, 1988.
Sara CA, Lowry CJ: A complication of circumcision and dorsal nerve block of the penis. *Anaesth Intens Care* 13:70, 1984.
Schoem SR, Watkins GL, Kuhn JJ, et al.: Control of early postoperative pain with bupivacaine in pediatric tonsillectomy. *Ear Nose Throat J* 72:560, 1993.
Schrock CR, Jones MB: The dose of caudal epidural analgesia and duration of postoperative analgesia. *Paediatr Anaesth* 13:403, 2003.
Schuepfer G, Konrad C, Schmeck J, et al.: Generating a learning curve for pediatric caudal epidural blocks: an empirical evaluation of technical skills in novice and experienced anesthetists. *Reg Anesth Pain Med* 25:385, 2000.
Schwartz N, Eisenkraft JB: Probable venous air embolism during epidural placement in an infant. *Anesth Analg* 76:1136, 1993.
Sciard D, Matuszczak M, Gebhard R, et al.: Continuous posterior lumbar plexus block for acute postoperative pain control in young children. *Anesthesiology* 95:1521, 2001.
Selander D: Neurotoxicity of local anesthetics: animal data. *Reg Anesth* 18:461, 1993.
Sethna NF, Berde CB: Pediatric regional anesthesia equipment. *Int Anesthesiol Clin* 30:163, 1992.
Sethna NF, Berde CB: Venous air embolism during identification of epidural space in children. *Anesth Analg* 76:925, 1993.
Sfez M, Mapihan YL, Mazoit X, et al.: Local anesthetic serum concentrations after penile block in children. *Anesth Analg* 71:423, 1990.
Shafer SL, Eisenach JC, Hood DD, Tong C: Cerebrospinal fluid pharmacokinetics and pharmacodynamics of intrathecal neostigmine methylsulfate in humans. *Anesthesiology* 89:1074, 1998.
Shaywitz BA: Epidermoid spinal cord tumors and previous lumbar punctures. *J Pediatr* 80:638, 1972.
Shnider SM, Way EL: The kinetics of transfer of lidocaine (Xylocaine) across the human placenta. *Anesthesiology* 29:944, 1968.
Somri M, Gaitini LA, Vaida SJ, et al.: Effect of ilioinguinal nerve block on the catecholamine plasma levels in orchidopexy: Comparison with caudal epidural block. *Paediatr Anaesth* 12:791, 2002.
Somri M, Gaitini LA, Vaida SJ, et al.: The effectiveness and safety of spinal anaesthesia in the pyloromyotomy procedure. *Paediatr Anaesth* 13:32, 2003.
Somri M, Vaida GS, Collins G, et al.: Postoperative outcome in high-risk infants undergoing herniorrhaphy: Comparison between spinal and general anaesthesia. *Anaesthesia* 53:762, 1998.
Splinter WM, Bass J, Komocar L: Regional anaesthesia for hernia repair in children: Local versus caudal anaesthesia. *Can J Anaesth* 42:197, 1995.
Stang HJ, Gunnar MR, Snellman L, et al.: Local anesthesia for neonatal circumcision. Effects on distress and cortisol response. *JAMA* 259:1507, 1988.
Strafford MA, Wilder RT, Berde CB: The risk of infection from epidural analgesia in children: A review of 1620 cases. *Anesth Analg* 80:234, 1995.
Suresh S, Wheeler M: Practical pediatric regional anesthesia. *Anesthesiol Clin North Am* 20:83, 2002.
Taddio A, Stevens B, Craig K, et al.: Efficacy and safety of lidocaine-prilocaine cream for pain during circumcision. *N Engl J Med* 336:1197, 1997.
Tanaka M, Nishikawa T: Evaluating T-wave amplitude as a guide for detecting intravascular injection of a test dose in anesthetized children. *Anesth Analg* 88:754, 1999.
Tanaka M, Nishikawa T: Simulation of an epidural test dose with intravenous epinephrine in sevoflurane-anesthetized children. *Anesth Analg* 86:952, 1998.

Taylor R, Eyres R, Chalkiadis GA, et al.: Efficacy and safety of caudal injection of levobupivacaine, 0.25%, in children under 2 years of age undergoing inguinal hernia repair, circumcision or orchidopexy. *Paediatr Anaesth* 13:114, 2003.

Thong WY, Pajel V, Khalil SN: Inadvertent administration of ropivacaine in a child. *Paediatr Anaesth* 10:563, 2000.

Thornton KL, Sacks MD, Hall R, et al.: Comparison of 0.2% ropivacaine and 0.25% bupivacaine for axillary brachial plexus blocks in paediatric hand surgery. *Paediatr Anaesth* 13:409, 2003.

Tobias JD, Haun SE, Helfaer M, et al.: Use of continuous caudal block to relieve lower-extremity ischemia caused by vasculitis in a child with meningococcemia. *J Pediatr* 115:1019, 1989.

Tobias JD, Mencio GA: Popliteal fossa block for postoperative analgesia after foot surgery in infants and children. *J Pediatr Orthop* 19:511, 1999.

Tobias JD, Rasmussen GE, Holcomb GW, et al.: Continuous caudal anaesthesia with chloroprocaine as an adjunct to general anaesthesia in neonates. *Can J Clin Anaesth* 43:69, 1996.

Tobias JD: Brachial plexus anaesthesia in children. *Paediatr Anaesth* 11:265, 2001.

Tobias JD: Caudal epidural block: A review of test dosing and recognition of systemic injection in children. *Anesth Analg* 93:1156, 2001.

Tobias JD: Cervical plexus block in adolescents. *JCA* 11:606, 1999.

Tobias JD: Continuous femoral nerve block to provide analgesia following femur fracture in a paediatric ICU population. *Anaesth Intens Care* 22:616, 1994.

Tobias JD: Regional anaesthesia of the lower extremity in infants and children. *Paediatr Anaesth* 13:152, 2003.

Tobias JD: Therapeutic applications of regional anaesthesia in paediatric-aged patients. *Paediatr Anaesth* 12:272, 2002.

Tucker GT: Perioperative changes in alpha1-acid glycoprotein concentrations. *Br J Anaesth* 77:130, 1996.

Tucker GT: Pharmacokinetics of local anesthetics. *Br J Anaesth* 58:717, 1986.

Tucker GT: Safety in numbers. The role of pharmacokinetics in local anesthetic toxicity: The 1993 ASRA lecture. *Reg Anesth* 19:155, 1994.

Tyrell-Gray HT: A study of spinal anaesthesia in children and infants. *Lancet* 2:913, 1909.

Valairucha S, Seefelder C, Houck CS: Thoracic epidural catheters placed by the caudal route in infants: The importance of radiographic confirmation. *Paediatr Anaesth* 12:424, 2002.

Valley RD, Bailey AG: Caudal morphine for postoperative analgesia in infants and children: A report of 138 cases. *Anesth Analg* 72:120, 1991.

Vas L, Raghavendran S, Hosalkar H, et al.: A study of epidural pressures in infants. *Paediatr Anaesth* 11:575, 2001.

Ved SA, Pinosky M, Nicodemis H: Ventricular tachycardia and brief cardiovascular collapse in two infants after caudal anesthesia using bupivacaine-epinephrine solution. *Anesthesiology* 79:1121, 1993.

Verghese ST, Hannallah RS, Rice LJ, et al.: Caudal anesthesia in children: Effect of volume versus concentration of bupivacaine on blocking spermatic core traction response during orchidopexy. *Anesth Analg* 95:1219, 2002.

Vester-Andersen T, Broby-Hohansen U, Bro-Rasmussen F: Perivascular axillary block. VI: The distribution of gelatine solution injected into the axillary neurovascular sheath of cadavers. *Acta Anaesthesiol Scand* 30:18, 1986.

Vloka JD, Hadzik A, Lesser JB, et al.: A common epineural sheath for the nerves in the popliteal fossa and its possible implications for sciatic nerve block. *Anesth Analg* 84:387, 1997.

Wagner CE, Prielipp RC: Chlorhexidine prep decreases catheter-related infections. *APSF Newsletter* 18:2, Spring 2003.

Warner MA, Kunkel SE, Offord KO, et al.: The effects of age, epinephrine, and operative site on duration of caudal analgesia in pediatric patients. *Anesth Analg* 66:995, 1987.

Weber F, Wulf H: Caudal bupivacaine and S(+)-ketamine for postoperative analgesia in children. *Paediatr Anaesth* 13:244, 2003.

Wedel DJ: Femoral and lateral femoral cutaneous nerve block for muscle biopsy in children. *Reg Anesth* 14:63, 1989.

Wee LH, Lam F, Cranston AJ: The incidence of PDPH in children. *Anaesthesia* 51:1164, 1996.

Welborn LG, Hannallah RS, Luban NL, et al.: Anemia and postoperative apnea in former preterm infants. *Anesthesiology* 74:1003, 1991.

Welborn LG, Rice LJ, Hannallah RS, et al.: Postoperative apnea in former preterm infants: Prospective comparison of spinal and general anesthesia. *Anesthesiology* 72:838, 1990.

Wilson GAM, Brown JL, Crabbe DG, et al.: Is epidural analgesia associated with an improved outcome following open Nissen fundoplication? *Paediatr Anaesth* 11:65, 2001.

Wilson PTJ, Lloyd-Thomas AR: An audit of extradural infusion analgesia in children using bupivacaine and diamorphine. *Anaesthesia* 48:718, 1993.

Wolf AR, Eyres RL, Laussen PC, et al.: Effect of extradural analgesia on stress responses to abdominal surgery in infants. *Br J Anaesth* 70:654, 1993.

Wolf AR, Hughes AD, Hobbs AJ, et al.: Combined morphine-bupivacaine caudals for reconstructive penile surgery in children: Systemic absorption of morphine and postoperative analgesia. *Anaesth Intens Care* 19:19, 1991.

Wood CE, Goresky GV, Klassen KA, et al.: Complications of continuous epidural infusions for postoperative analgesia in children. *Can J Anaesth* 41: 613, 1994.

Wright TE, Orr RJ, Haberkern CM, et al.: Complications during spinal anesthesia in infants: High spinal blockade. *Anesthesiology* 73:1290, 1990.

Wulf H, Peters C, Behnke H: The pharmacokinetics of caudal ropivacaine 0.2% in children. A study of infants aged less than 1 year and toddlers aged 1–5 years undergoing inguinal hernia repair. *Anaesthesia* 55:757, 2000.

Yang LC, Chen LM, Wang CJ, Buerkle H: Postoperative analgesia by intra-articular neostigmine in patients undergoing knee arthroscopy. *Anesthesiology* 88:334, 1998.

Yaster M, Maxwell LG: Pediatric regional anesthesia. *Anesthesiology* 70:324, 1989.

Yaster M, Tobin JR, Billett C, et al.: Epidural analgesia in the management of severe vaso-occlusive sickle cell crisis. *Pediatrics* 93:310, 1994.

Ylonen P, Kokki H: Management of postdural puncture headache with epidural blood patch in children. *Paediatr Anaesth* 12:525, 2002.

Yucel A, Ozyalcin S, Talu GK, et al.: Intravenous administration of caffeine benzoate for PDPH. *Reg Anesth Pain Med* 24:51, 1999.

Zsigmond EK, Downs JR: Plasma cholinesterase activity in newborns and infants. *Can Anaesth Soc J* 18:278, 1971.

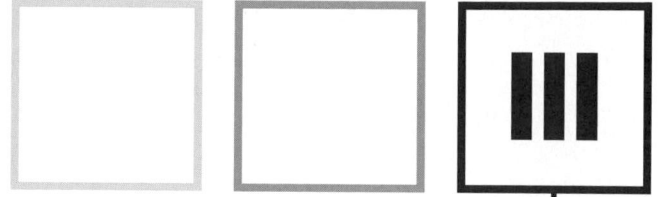

Clinical Management of Special Surgical Problems

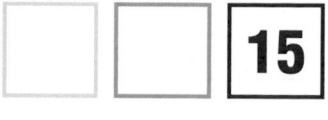

15 Anesthesia for Fetal Surgery

Jeffrey L. Galinkin • Uwe Schwarz • Etsuro K. Motoyama

Fetal surgery is an area of rapid and exciting growth. Ex-utero intrapartum therapy (EXIT), fetoscopic procedures, and open, midgestation procedures such as repair of myelomeningocele (MMC), congenital cystic adenomatoid malformations (CCAMs) of the lung, and sacrococcygeal teratoma (SCT) are now performed at multiple institutions around the world.

Fetal surgical techniques are based on years of animal and clinical research. In contrast, anesthesia for fetal surgery is based on clinical experience, case reports (Gaiser et al., 1997, 1999; O'Hara and Kurth, 1999; Rosen, 1999; Galinkin et al., 2000), and translation of responses to anesthetics in pregnant sheep (Motoyama et al., 1966, 1967; Palahniuk and Shnider, 1974; Biehl et al., 1983a, 1983b; Gregory et al., 1983; Bachman et al., 1986; Sabik et al., 1993). This chapter provides a review of the maternal and fetal anesthetic considerations for each type of fetal surgical procedure.

SURGICAL CONSIDERATIONS

Surgical intervention is considered when a fetus presents with a congenital lesion/condition that can compromise or disturb cardiovascular function or cause severe postnatal morbidity. Surgery is only performed when the risk to the mother is low and the risk of death or severe disability to the fetus outweighs no intervention. Contraindications for these procedures are medical conditions in the mother precluding surgery or lethal/disabling genetic defects in the fetus.

Fetal surgery can be divided into three distinct procedure groups (Table 15–1). Midgestation hysterotomy is performed on fetuses with well-defined congenital lesions. Surgery on the fetus is performed between 18 and 26 weeks through a hysterotomy. For these procedures, the fetus is exteriorized for surgical intervention and then placed back in the uterus to mature. Correction of these lesions is expected to either improve fetal survivability or enhance postgestation quality of life. If left untreated, these lesions result in severe disability or death.

Ex-utero intrapartum therapy (EXIT) procedures are hysterotomy-based procedures performed at or near term on fetuses with expected immediate postgestation airway or oxygenation compromise. Surgery on the fetus is done after hysterotomy but before cord clamping. Surgeons then assess the infant's airway through bronchoscopy and secure the airway via an endotracheal tube or tracheotomy before complete airway obstruction or ventilation failure. During this time, the fetus is maintained by placental transfer of oxygen and carbon dioxide.

Fetoscopic surgery is a minimally invasive technique that uses small-diameter trocars and laparoscopes placed percutaneously to access the uterus. This technique is most commonly used for the evaluation and treatment of twin reverse arterial perfusion sequence, twin-twin transfusion syndromes, amniotic band syndrome, and bladder outlet obstruction. Surgical devices such as electrocautery and lasers are used to ablate or cauterize vessels or tissue during these procedures. This technique is considered when fetal death or severe fetal morbidity is imminent or traditional therapeutic measures (e.g., amnioreduction) have failed.

OPEN FETAL SURGERY

Open fetal surgeries are usually performed on the midgestation fetus with MMC, CCAM, or SCT. To qualify as a surgical candidate, a mother must undergo extensive medical and psychosocial screening, have a fetus with disease that merits intervention, and be at low maternal risk for anesthesia and surgery.

Fetal surgery is performed through a low transverse abdominal incision. The uterus is exteriorized through this incision. Placental location is determined by ultrasonography, and a wide uterine incision is created with a specially designed absorbable stapler (Bond et al., 1989). This stapler allows performance of a "bloodless hysterotomy." After hysterotomy, the fetus or fetal part is exteriorized for fetal surgery. Once the defect has been repaired and returned to the uterus, a watertight two-layer uterine closure is made (Bianchi et al., 2000). Warm saline with

TABLE 15–1. Surgical approaches to fetal lesions: Timing and cause for treatment

Surgical Approach	Fetal Lesion/Anomaly	Reason for Treatment	Gestational Age
Open/hysterotomy	Congenital cystic adenomatoid malformation	Hydrops fetalis, lung hypoplasia	18 to 25 wk
	Myelomeningocele	Amniotic fluid neurotoxicity	22 to 26 wk
	Sacrococcygeal teratoma	Hydrops fetalis	18 to 25 wk
Ex-utero intrapartum therapy	Congenital or iatrogenic high airway obstruction	Secure airway	Near term
	Giant fetal neck mass	Secure airway, resect mass	Near term
Fetoscopic surgery	Twin–twin transfusion	Impending fetal death, hydrops fetalis	Midgestation
	Twin reversed arterial perfusion sequence	Impending fetal death, hydrops fetalis	Midgestation
	Bladder outlet obstruction	Hydronephrosis and renal hypoplasia	Midgestation

oxacillin is infused into the uterus to maintain uterine volume and decrease postoperative contractions. The skin is then closed and the maternal operation is completed.

ANESTHETIC CONSIDERATIONS

MATERNAL ANESTHETIC CONSIDERATIONS

Regional anesthesia is usually the technique of choice for obstetric anesthetic practice, but because the uterine relaxation required for fetal surgery is best provided by a high concentration of potent volatile agents, general anesthesia is the technique of choice for fetal surgery.

The maternal physiologic changes that occur during pregnancy contribute to increased anesthetic risk for both the mother and fetus. Pregnant patients undergoing general anesthesia are at increased risk for aspiration pneumonitis. Pregnancy decreases lower esophageal sphincter tone due in part to altered anatomic relationship of the esophagus to the diaphragm and stomach. In addition, pyloric displacement and increased gastric acid production result in an increased intragastric pressure. Rapid sequence induction is always performed for endotracheal intubation.

Pregnancy affects maternal pulmonary function. The cephalad encroachment of the gravid uterus reduces functional residual capacity, particularly the volumes of the lower lobes, and oxygen consumption increases to meet the increased demands of both the mother and the fetus. These factors increase the risk of hypoxia during rapid sequence induction. Decreases in capillary oncotic pressure and increases in capillary permeability increase the risk of pulmonary edema, especially postoperatively when magnesium sulfate is used for tocolysis.

The cardiovascular system is affected by pregnancy. A decrease in preload during supine positioning (supine hypotension syndrome), due to compression of the inferior vena cava, can cause maternal hypotension and fetal hypoxia. It is important to position the mother with left uterine displacement to displace the uterus from the inferior vena cava.

The parturient's central nervous system is also affected by pregnancy. During pregnancy, sensitivity to inhaled anesthetics is increased; minimum alveolar concentration (MAC) is significantly decreased; and sensitivity to muscle relaxants is also increased (Palahniuk et al., 1974; Strout and Nahrwold, 1981; Gin and Chan, 1994; Chan and Gin, 1995; Chan et al., 1996). Lower doses of volatile anesthetics and muscle relaxants are needed for surgery.

FETAL ANESTHETIC CONSIDERATIONS

The primary concern of anesthetic management is the maintenance of placental circulation and fetal cardiovascular stability. The combination of immature organ function and cardiovascular compromise predisposes the fetus to anesthetic difficulty. The fetal cardiovascular system is less able to compensate for hypoxia and hypovolemia than is that of a full-term infant. Lacking a functional pulmonary system to increase oxygen tension, the fetus relies on increased umbilical blood flow and cardiac output and blood flow redistribution to improve oxygen delivery to the vital organs. The Starling curve is shifted down in a fetus compared with a neonate, resulting in less cardiac output for a given stroke volume (Fig. 15–1). Cardiac output is more dependent on heart rate. Because of high vagal tone and low baroreceptor sensitivity, the fetus responds to stress with a decrease in heart rate.

Fetal circulating blood volume is relatively low; the midgestation fetus has an estimated fetoplacental blood volume of 50 to 70 mL (110 mL/kg) (Nicolaides et al., 1987; MacGregor et al., 1988). A small amount of surgical blood loss can precipitate hypovolemia. Inhaled anesthetics also destabilize the fetal cardiovascular system by causing direct fetal myocardial depression, vasodilation, and changes in arteriovenous shunting (Palahniuk and Shnider, 1974; Biehl et al., 1983; Bachman et al., 1986; Sabik et al., 1993).

Because of incomplete myelination and less synaptic activation, the fetus is more sensitive to inhaled agents. This increased sensitivity results in a decreased MAC compared with pregnant adults (Gregory et al., 1983; Bachman et al., 1986). Sensitivity to analgesics and muscle relaxants is also greater in the fetus compared with the neonate.

Fetal cutaneous heat and evaporative losses require warm ambient temperatures during fetal exposure. Limiting fetal surgical time and the use of warm irrigation fluids can prevent hypothermia.

Altered coagulation factors predispose to bleeding and cause difficulty in surgical hemostasis during fetal surgical manipulation.

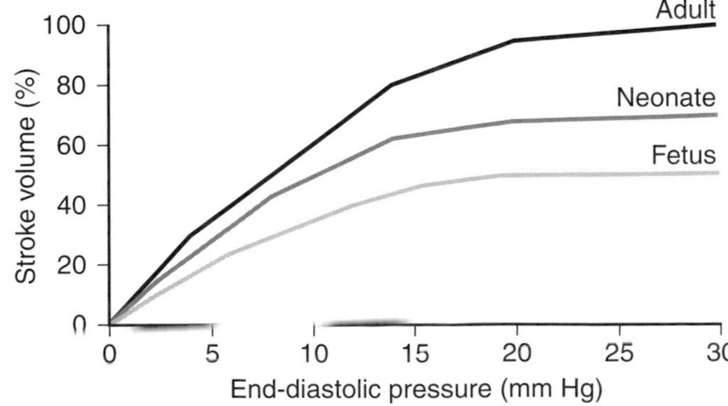

FIGURE 15–1. Stroke volume versus end-diastolic volume in the adult, neonate, and fetus.

The small blood volume of the fetus compounds this problem. Fetal hemoglobin can be assessed intraoperatively with central or percutaneous blood samples.

UTEROPLACENTAL ANESTHETIC CONSIDERATIONS

Uterine and umbilical blood flow and placental barriers to diffusion influence fetal oxygen delivery. Maternal systemic blood pressure and myometrial tone directly correlate with uterine artery blood flow. Volatile anesthetics decrease myometrial tone and tend to decrease maternal blood pressure and maternal placental blood flow. This can result in a decrease in fetal oxygenation (Heymann and Rudolph, 1967; Luks et al., 1996; Parry et al., 2001). Umbilical artery blood flow is influenced by fetal cardiac output and vascular resistance, both intrinsic and extrinsic (e.g., compression by a "nuchal cord"). Maintenance of a patent umbilical artery and a near-baseline maternal arterial pressure are critical (maternal systemic pressure within 10% of baseline).

Studies in fetal lambs have shown that fetal-placental blood flow is significantly affected by maternal arterial PCO_2 and pH. Maternal hypocapnea markedly reduces umbilical venous blood flow and results in fetal hypoxia and metabolic acidosis (Motoyama et al., 1966). In contrast, maternal hypercapnea ($PaCO_2 > 60$ mm Hg) and acidosis ($pH < 7.3$) increase umbilical venous blood flow and increase umbilical venous and fetal carotid PO_2 above the physiologic ranges (Motoyama et al., 1967). The results of this study also show that with the same maternal PCO_2, maternal hyperoxia was associated with an increase in fetal carotid PO_2 (Rivard et al., 1967). These findings in animal studies were corroborated in a clinical study in 38 parturient women during cesarean section under general inhalation anesthesia (Peng et al., 1972). In this study, the group of parturients, whose arterial PCO_2 ($PaCO_2$) was kept between 30 and 50 mm Hg with the addition of 2% CO_2, had significantly higher umbilical (postductal) arterial PO_2 and lower fetal base deficit than those who were ventilated with the equivalent ventilator setting but without added CO_2 and with lower $PaCO_2$ (20 to 30 mm Hg). There was a significant correlation between the maternal $PaCO_2$ and umbilical arterial PO_2 as well as fetal base deficit (Peng et al., 1972). Maternal hypocapnia should be avoided during maternal-fetal procedures. Possible efficacy of hypercapnea to enhance fetoplacental circulation should be explored in the future.

Control of myometrial tone by general inhalation anesthesia is necessary for open fetal surgery to provide optimal operative exposure. Epidural anesthesia alone does not provide uterine relaxation. Epidural anesthesia may help prevent premature labor in the postoperative period (Tame et al., 1999). Magnesium sulfate, terbutaline, nifedipine, and indomethacin are also used alone or in combination to maintain uterine quiescence in the postoperative period.

PREOPERATIVE EVALUATION AND PREPARATION

In the preanesthetic evaluation, maternal and family history of anesthetic problems, airway examination, maternal size/weight, placental location, and fetal cardiovascular function are all examined. The fetus is evaluated by ultrasonography, echocardiography, magnetic resonance imaging (MRI), and karyotype analysis. The mother must be able to comply with the intensive demands postoperatively including bed rest and compliance with medications. When the decision for surgery is made, a multidisciplinary team consisting of surgery, anesthesia, obstetrics, genetics, social work, and nursing personnel meet to discuss the plan and obtain consent.

Patients are admitted to the hospital on the day of surgery. In preparation for surgery, the operating room is warmed to 80°F (26.7°C), and type-specific packed red blood cells (for the mother) and O-negative packed red blood cells (for the fetus) are made available. Monitors include two pulse oximeters (maternal and fetal) and an arterial pressure transducer. Epinephrine 10 mcg/kg, atropine 20 mcg/kg, vecuronium 0.2 mg/kg, and fentanyl 20 mcg/kg are prepared in a sterile manner in 1-mL syringes for possible fetal intramuscular administration. After ensuring the nothing-by-mouth (NPO) status of the mother, a single large-bore intravenous catheter is inserted. Sodium bicitrate 30 mL PO and metoclopramide 10 mg IV are administered to the mother to decrease the risk of aspiration pneumonitis. An indomethacin suppository is administered for postoperative tocolysis. A lumbar epidural catheter is inserted and tested with lidocaine 1.5% with epinephrine 1:200,000. The parturient is then positioned on her left side or the operating room table is tilted to the left side to minimize supine hypotension syndrome.

INTRAOPERATIVE MANAGEMENT

Rapid sequence induction using intravenous sodium thiopental or propofol and succinylcholine is performed followed by tracheal intubation. General anesthesia is maintained with 0.5 MAC volatile anesthetic (isoflurane or desflurane) and 50% nitrous oxide. A radial arterial catheter, second intravenous catheter, nasogastric tube, and Foley catheter are inserted. Fetal status is monitored with sterile intraoperative echocardiography. Intravenous fluid is restricted to 500 mL total to reduce the risk of postoperative pulmonary edema.

Open hysterotomy procedures require low uterine tone to maintain fetal perfusion and optimize fetal exposure. Before the maternal skin incision, nitrous oxide is turned off to improve fetal oxygenation (Parpaglioni et al., 2002), and the inhalation agent is increased to 2.0 MAC to provide uterine relaxation and fetal anesthesia by the time of uterine and fetal incision. Ephedrine 5 to 10 mg IV or phenylephrine 1 to 2 mcg/kg IV is administered as necessary to maintain maternal systolic blood pressure within 10% of baseline.

Fetal anesthesia and analgesia are provided by a combination of placental passage of volatile anesthetics and intramuscularly administered opioids. Equilibration between mother and fetus with isoflurane (Biehl et al., 1983) (Fig. 15–2) and desflurane (Schwarz et al., 2003) (Fig. 15–3) reaches approximately 70% and 50% of maternal levels, respectively, in 1 hour. Before fetal incision, the fetus receives fentanyl 20 mcg/kg IM to supplement the anesthesia and provide postoperative analgesia.

Fetal well-being is assessed via both direct and indirect methods. For procedures in which a fetal extremity is accessed (CCAM and SCT resections), fetal arterial saturation is monitored by pulse oximetry. The pulse-oximetry probe is placed on the fetal hand and wrapped with foil to decrease ambient light exposure (Fig. 15–4). Normal fetal arterial saturation is 60% to 70% (Johnson et al., 1991); during fetal surgery, values greater than 40% represent adequate fetal oxygenation. Echocardiography is also used to monitor fetal heart rate and stroke volume.

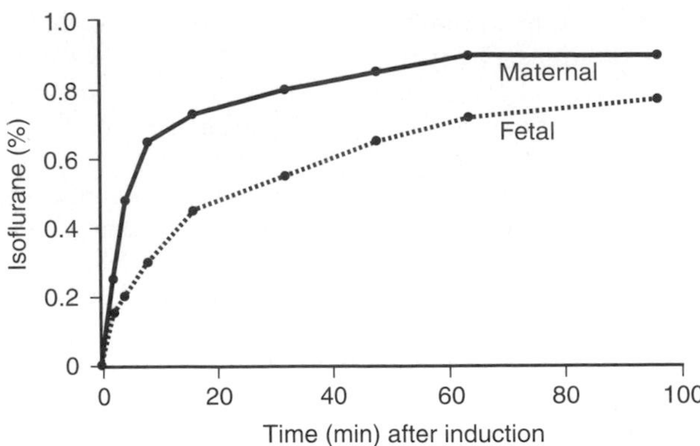

■ **FIGURE 15–2.** Isoflurane versus time for mother and fetus during maternal anesthesia.

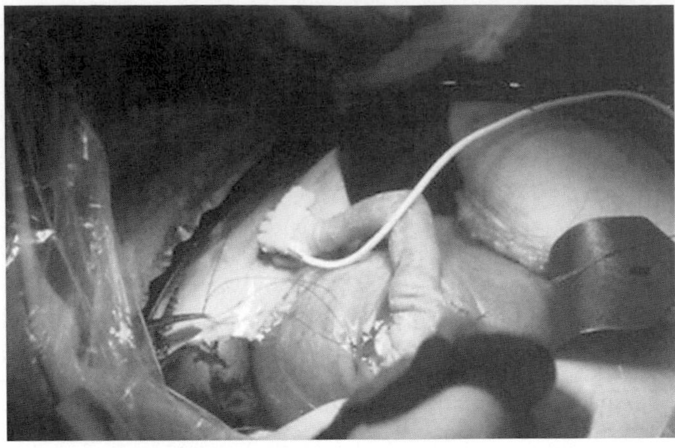

■ **FIGURE 15–4.** Fetal hand with pulse-oximetry probe.

Fetal distress, manifested by bradycardia, decreased saturations, or decreased stroke volume, is often a result of partial umbilical cord occlusion. Fetal arterial or venous blood gas samples may be obtained by the surgeons percutaneously or through umbilical or central vessel puncture to help guide therapy during periods of fetal distress. Warm, fresh O-negative blood can be administered to the fetus to correct anemia through a percutaneous peripheral venous line placed intraoperatively.

After closure of the uterus, the anesthetic is converted to a regional technique. As the final stitches are placed in the uterus, the volatile anesthetic is decreased to 0.5 MAC and the epidural catheter is dosed with local anesthetic and opioid (15 to 20 mL bupivacaine 0.25% and morphine 0.05 mg/kg). Tocolysis is instituted via a loading dose of magnesium sulfate 6 g IV followed by a magnesium sulfate IV infusion at 2 to 3 g/hr. The patient's trachea is extubated after skin closure, and she is then transferred to the obstetric floor for postoperative care.

POSTOPERATIVE MANAGEMENT

Key goals for postoperative management include prevention of premature labor and maintenance of maternal comfort. Magnesium sulfate is the drug of choice in the early postoperative period (18 to 24 hours) for tocolysis while a patient-controlled epidural infusion is used for analgesia. A well-functioning epidural analgesia may assist in the prevention of preterm labor (Tame et al., 1999). Indomethacin is continued for 48 hours postoperatively; fetal ductus arteriosus diameter is monitored daily. After discontinuation of the epidural block and magnesium sulfate, the first line of tocolysis is oral nifedipine. If this fails, terbutaline is administered via a subcutaneous route through an external pump. Bed rest is recommended for the remainder of the pregnancy. The patient is an obligate cesarean section for both this delivery and all subsequent deliveries due to the high uterine incision needed for these surgeries (Bianchi et al., 2000).

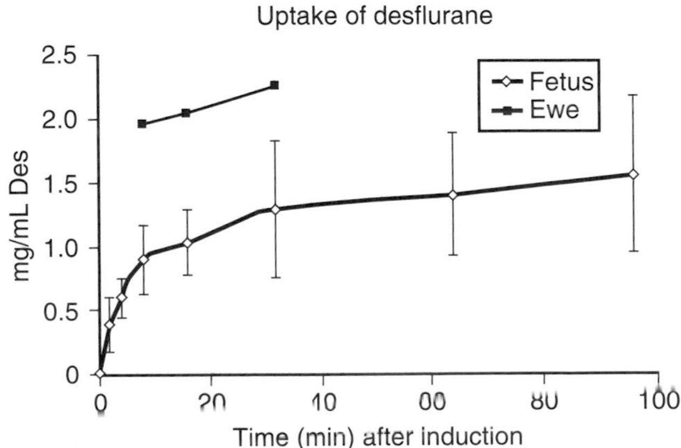

■ **FIGURE 15–3.** Desflurane versus time for mother and fetus during maternal anesthesia.

SURGICAL LESIONS ELIGIBLE FOR OPEN FETAL SURGERY

Myelomeningocele

A myelomeningocele (MMC) is a lumbosacral vertebral lesion that occurs when the dorsal portion of the spinal cord is not covered with skin (Fig. 15–5). The cord is exposed to the caustic amniotic fluid, causing a chronic chemical exposure. The open spinal cord is also exposed to traumatic injury via mechanical compression. The combination of these two exposures is thought

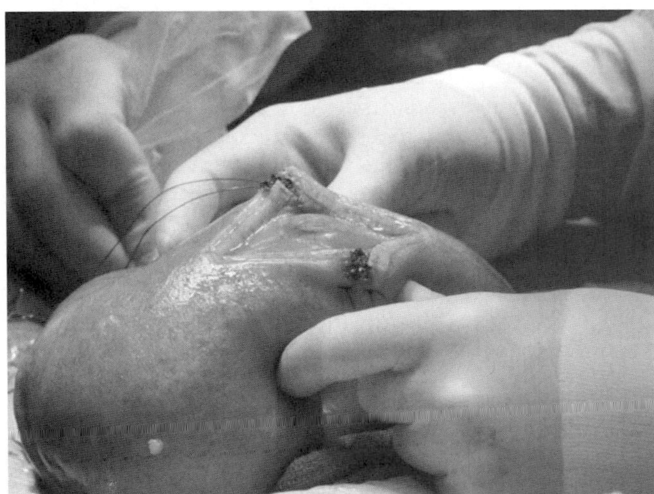

■ **FIGURE 15–5.** Surgical exposure of a fetal myelomeningocele in a 22-week-old fetus.

to be the underlying mechanism for progressive and irreversible damage to the spinal cord seen in these patients (Meuli et al., 1997). The long-term consequences of this lesion include paraplegia, hydrocephalus, incontinence, sexual dysfunction, skeletal deformities, and impaired mental development.

Maternal serum α-fetoprotein screening identifies more than 80% of fetuses with MMC by midgestation (Brock and Sutcliffe, 1972). Direct visualization of the fetal spine on ultrasonography can also aid in prenatal screening for fetuses greater than 16 weeks gestation. Other sonographic findings associated with MMC include frontal bone scalloping (lemon sign), abnormality of the cerebellum (banana sign), Chiari II malformation, hydrocephalus, microcephalus, and encephalocele.

The rationale for intrapartum midgestation MMC repair is based on the observation that lower extremity function during early pregnancy is progressively lost later in gestation (>20 weeks). In animals, intrauterine repair of MMC preserves peripheral neurologic function (Michejda, 1984; Heffez et al., 1990, 1993; Meuli et al., 1995a, 1995b; Hutchins et al., 1996) and decreases the incidence of hindbrain herniation (Chiari type II malformation) (Paek et al., 2000). A retrospective review of clinical experience confirmed these findings in humans (Adzick et al., 1998; Tulipan et al., 1998; Bruner et al., 1999a, 1999b; Sutton et al., 1999). Furthermore, intrauterine repair of MMC (fetal lesions below L-3) appeared to substantially reduce the incidence of shunt-dependent hydrocephalus compared with conventional treatment, even when lesion level was taken into account (Tulipan et al., 2003).

The surgical experience of fetal MMC repair is promising, but the varying natural history, lack of accurate prenatal indicators of neurologic function, and absence of matched controls and long-term follow-up hamper the risk/benefit assessment of prenatal intervention (Sutton et al., 1999). A multicenter long-term prospective randomized placebo-controlled trial began in 2003 to assess the overall usefulness of these procedures.

Congenital Cystic Adenomatoid Malformation

Congenital cystic adenomatoid malformation (CCAM) is a rare lesion characterized by a multicystic mass of pulmonary tissue with a proliferation of bronchial structures (Stocker et al., 1977; Miller et al., 1980). A CCAM results either from a failure of maturation of bronchiolar structures in early gestation (Stocker et al., 1977; Miller et al., 1980; Shanji et al., 1988) or as a focal pulmonary dysplasia (Leninger and Haight, 1973). Associated malformations include genitourinary anomalies, such as renal agenesis or dysgenesis; cardiac anomalies, including truncus arteriosus and tetralogy of Fallot; jejunal atresia; diaphragmatic hernia; hydrocephalus; and skeletal anomalies.

CCAMs can be detected on ultrasonography at as early as 16 weeks gestation and are the most common type of fetal thoracic masses detected in this manner. The majority of CCAMs are diagnosed before 22 weeks' gestation (Adzick et al., 1985) and represent a broad spectrum of clinical severity. They may enlarge significantly, may remain the same size, or may disappear in the prenatal period (Adzick et al., 1985, 2003; Rice et al., 1994).When sufficient cardiac and great vessel compression lead to cardiac failure, these lesions cause fetal death. Cardiac failure often manifests as hydrops fetalis, a condition consisting of polyhydramnios, ascites, skin edema, and effusions of the pericardial or pleural space.

A CCAM typically presents as a lobular lung lesion (Fig. 15–6). Rare cases have been reported of multilobar involvement of one lung or of bilateral lesions. Intrapartum fetal surgery for

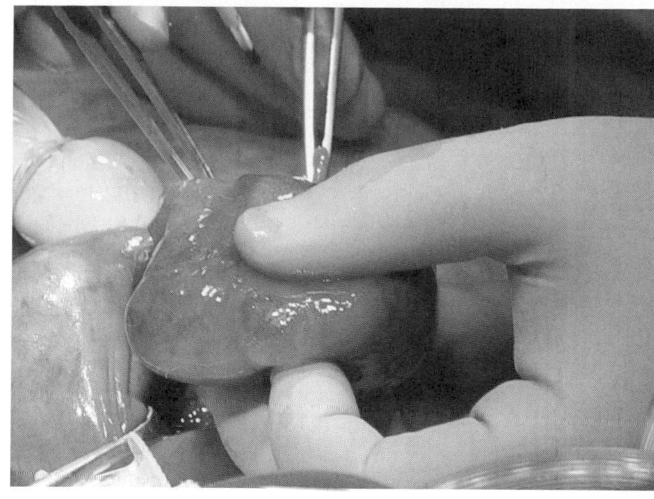

■ **FIGURE 15–6.** Surgical exposure of a fetal cystic adenomatous malformation.

thoracoamniotic shunting (in cases with a large predominant cyst) or lung lobectomy, with complete resection of the CCAM, is the treatment of choice for this disease process when fetal hydrops is present or if conservative treatment fails. The mortality rate for fetal lobectomy is about 50% (Adzick et al., 2003). In cases where there is extensive involvement of the entire lung, resection of multiple lobes or pneumonectomy may be necessary. Term or near-term fetuses with CCAMs that may not survive delivery secondary to mass size or expected fetal compromise at birth may qualify for an EXIT procedure with resection of the mass during EXIT with or without postoperative transfer to extracorporeal membrane oxygenation.

Sacrococcygeal Teratoma

A sacrococcygeal teratoma (SCT) is a neoplasm that can be composed of tissues of all three germ layers or multiple foreign tissues lacking organ specificity (Fig. 15–7). It occurs in

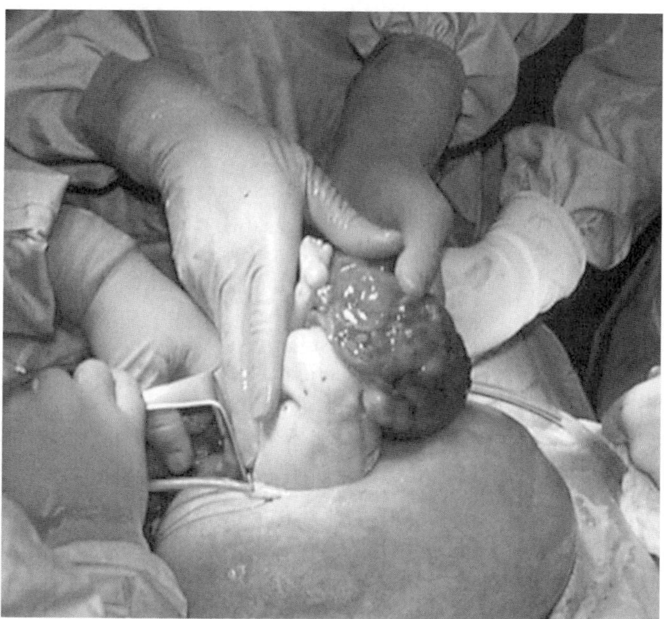

■ **FIGURE 15–7.** A sacrococcygeal teratoma at midgestation during fetal surgery.

approximately 1:35,000 live-births (Schiffer and Greenberg, 1956; Bale, 1984). Females are four times more likely to be affected as males, but development of malignancy is more often observed in males (Abbott et al., 1966; Conklin and Abell, 1967; Carney et al., 1972; Altman et al., 1974). Included in the differential diagnosis of SCT are lumbosacral myelomeningocele, neuroblastoma, glioma, hemangioma, neurofibroma, cordoma, leiomyoma, lipoma, melanoma, and other tumors and malformations of the sacrococcygeal region.

Prenatally diagnosed SCT is different from neonatal SCT. The mortality rate for SCT diagnosed in the antenatal period is 5%, whereas the mortality rate for SCT diagnosed in the perinatal period is close to 50% (Bond et al., 1990; Flake, 1993). Malignant invasion is the primary cause of death in neonatal SCT, but this occurs rarely in utero (Graf et al., 1998). High-output cardiac failure is the primary cause of death from fetal SCT secondary to a "vascular steal" phenomenon by the tumor (Bond et al., 1990). Hydrops fetalis occurs in 10% of fetal SCTs and results in fetal death if left untreated (Langer et al., 1989).

SCTs can also lead to a potentially devastating maternal complication—the maternal mirror syndrome (Ballantine syndrome) (Kuhlmann et al., 1987). In this syndrome, the mother experiences progressive symptoms suggestive of preeclampsia, including vomiting, hypertension, peripheral edema, proteinuria, and pulmonary edema, due to the release of placental vasoactive factors or endothelial cell toxins from the edematous placenta. This syndrome can be reversed only by delivering the child and the placenta but not by removing the SCT.

Prenatal diagnosis is made by ultrasonography or MRI and has been reported as early as 14 weeks' gestation (Holzgreve et al., 1985). Color flow Doppler ultrasonography of large vascular tumors can demonstrate markedly increased distal aortic blood flow and shunting of blood away from the placenta and toward the tumor.

The rationale behind the prenatal resection of SCT in utero is the devastating outcomes for these fetuses when the tumor is complicated by placentamegaly and hydrops fetalis. Currently, efforts are aimed at developing a minimally invasive approach to reverse the "vascular steal" physiology via coagulation of the tumor's major blood supply (Westerburg et al., 1998; Paek et al., 2001).

EX-UTERO INTRAPARTUM THERAPY

The EXIT procedure is used to achieve a patent fetal airway, to resect pulmonary masses, or to ensure adequate fetal oxygenation for diseases in which the fetus has a congenital or an acquired obstructive airway lesion. These procedures require general anesthesia to relax the uterus and anesthetize the fetus. EXIT procedures culminate with the delivery of the fetus. The newborn who underwent this surgery may require additional surgery and have special anesthetic needs.

PREOPERATIVE MANAGEMENT

Maternal preparation for EXIT is similar to that for open fetal surgery. Most of these patients are followed for an extended period of time because the fetal lesions were discovered on prenatal ultrasounds. Early prenatal diagnosis allows time for counseling and maternal and fetal testing that these patients require.

Anesthetic preparation is the same for the EXIT as for the open procedure with two notable exceptions: tocolytics are not used, and one additional operating room is available for direct postdelivery care and possible surgery of the newborn. Tocolytics are unnecessary because the procedure ends in delivery. Resuscitation equipment, neonatologists, and a second operating room are all made available for postdelivery care of the neonate.

INTRAOPERATIVE MANAGEMENT

The risks of aspiration and supine hypotensive syndrome are high in the term gestation mother with a large gravid uterus. After epidural placement, rapid sequence induction is performed, followed by orotracheal intubation. A second intravenous catheter, a nasogastric tube, and a Foley catheter are placed. The second intravenous catheter is placed in case the patient requires volume resuscitation for acute blood loss after delivery of the fetus. A maternal arterial cannula is placed when a fetus has end-stage disease manifesting as fetal hydrops due to lability of maternal blood pressure during these cases (unpublished observation).

Anesthesia for the EXIT is delivered via an inhalation-based technique. Sub-MAC concentrations (0.5 MAC) of volatile agents are used before maternal skin incision, and a high-level inhaled agent is used thereafter. Ephedrine and phenylephrine are used for maternal blood pressure maintenance. For rapid maternal and neonatal emergence after delivery, the preferred inhaled agent is desflurane because of its low blood-gas solubility.

During hysterotomy, it is important for the surgeons to only partially expose the fetus and to maintain the uterine volume at an appropriate level so that placental perfusion is maintained. Maternal hyperventilation should be avoided because maternal hypocapnia causes fetal placental vasoconstriction and fetal hypoxia (Motoyama et al., 1967; Peng et al., 1972). Fentanyl 20 mcg/kg IM is administered to the fetus to supplement fetal analgesia and provide postoperative analgesia. Fetal status is closely monitored via a pulse oximeter, sterile echocardiography, and visual inspection. Fetal blood gases are obtained as needed, and fresh O-negative blood is administered if necessary. Direct laryngoscopy and intubation of the fetus are performed by either the surgeons or the anesthesiologist. If the fetus cannot be intubated, partial resection of an obstructive lesion, tracheotomy, or both are performed by the surgeons. After the airway is secured and adequate fetal oxygenation with manual ventilation is ensured, the umbilical cord is clamped and the fetus is delivered.

After the delivery, it is important to quickly reverse uterine relaxation. Volatile agents are decreased after cord clamping, and the epidural catheter is dosed with local anesthetic and an opioid analgesic. Due to the anesthetic-induced uterine relaxation, uterine atony and significant blood loss are risks. The timing of cord clamping with respect to administration of oxytocin, methergine, and prostaglandin $F_{2\alpha}$ must be coordinated between anesthesiologist and surgeon. Blood loss is monitored, and cross-matched blood is administered if needed. Epidural analgesia is used for postoperative analgesia, and the trachea is extubated after surgical closure.

POSTDELIVERY/POSTOPERATIVE MANAGEMENT

After surgery/delivery, there are two patients for which to care. The mother is brought to a postpartum ward. The immediate disposition of the newborn infant is based on surgical need—a second operating room should be available in case further surgery is needed, such as for excision of a cervical teratoma. If surgery is not required immediately, a neonatology team resuscitates and transports the neonate to intensive care.

When further surgery is necessary, there are several considerations unique to the immediate newborn. First, it is essential to dry and clean the newborn to minimize evaporative heat loss and because of the inherent difficulty of monitors sticking to the newborn. Second, the immediate newborn has a lower MAC requirement. Third, these infants have a transitional cardiac circulation, which can be compromised by surgical manipulation of adjacent structures (see Chapter 3, Cardiovascular Physiology). Finally, the neonatal lungs are fluid filled, have low compliance, and are extremely susceptible to lung injury from hyperdistention (volutrauma). Vigorous resuscitation with high inflation pressure and volume can cause damage to the neonatal lung and adversely affect gas exchange (Jobe and Ikegami, 2001).

■ SURGICAL LESIONS ELIGIBLE FOR EX-UTERO INTRAPARTUM THERAPY

Lymphangioma (Cystic Hygroma)

A lymphangioma is a benign malformation composed of dilated cystic lymphatic tissue that most commonly occurs in the soft tissue of the neck, axilla, thorax, and lower extremities (Isaacs, 1997). The lesions vary in size from tiny subepidermal skin bubbles to large cystic masses filled with fluid, commonly referred to as cystic hygromas when presenting in the neck (Fig. 15–8).

Lymphangiomas are divided into two groups. The first group is identified by prenatal ultrasound examination in the second trimester; 60% of these fetuses have chromosomal abnormalities often associated with other structural anomalies and a high mortality rate (Cohen et al., 1989; Welborn and Timm, 1994). These cystic hygromas are usually situated at the posterior cervical triangle; associated structural anomalies include cardiac defects, hydronephrosis, neural tube defect, cleft lip and palate, multiple pterygium syndrome, skeletal anomalies, imperforate anus, and ambiguous genitalia.

The second group is diagnosed either at birth, as an isolated finding in an otherwise healthy infant, or as a new ultrasonographic finding in the third trimester. These lesions are a different entity than those seen in the first group. Lymphangiomas in these fetuses are located in the anterior cervical triangle, are not associated with other birth anomalies, and generally do not require emergent surgical resection.

The only fetal procedure that is indicated for large cystic hygromas is an EXIT procedure. The EXIT procedure allows the airway to be secured and a surgical resection of the cystic hygroma to be performed if immediately necessary. Although cyst aspiration can help to secure a fetal airway at birth of an unrecognized cystic hygroma, there are little data to support the use of in utero decompression of the fetal lesion (Kaufman et al., 1996). Intrauterine chemotherapy using OK-432 has also been attempted (Watari et al., 1996). The rationale for these fetal approaches was to prevent polyhydramnios, irreversible facial deformity, and hydrops fetalis.

Cervical Teratoma

Cervical teratomas (Fig. 15–9) are composed of tissues foreign to their normal anatomic sites. All three germ layers are represented within the tumor, whereas neural tissue is the most common histologic component. These tumors are extremely rare; fewer than 200 congenital cases have been described. Prenatal diagnosis of these lesions is usually made on ultrasonography (Bianchi et al., 2000).

Although cervical teratomas are most often malignant in adults, the vast majority of cervical teratomas in fetuses and infants are benign. The tumor leads to a high incidence of preterm labor and delivery, thought to be secondary to polyhydramnios (a complication in 20% to 40% of prenatally diagnosed cases) or tumor, or both, causing an increase in uterine size. Cesarean section often is recommended because of the abnormal fetal position. Airway obstruction and respiratory compromise can be life threatening after birth. Securing the airway via an EXIT procedure has become a standard procedure for fetal cases with cervical teratoma (Bianchi et al., 2000).

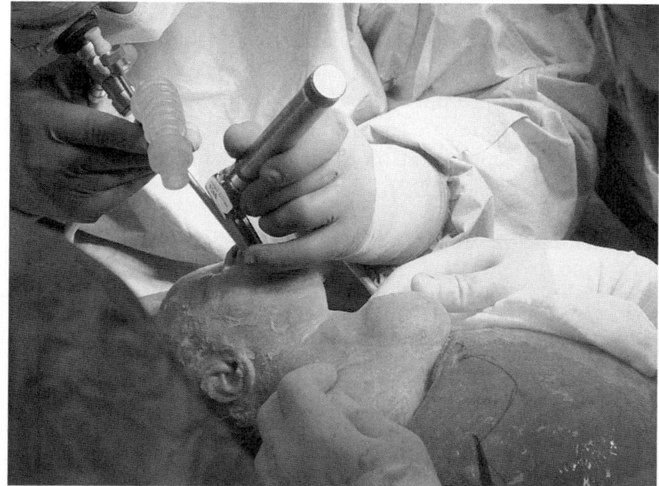

■ **FIGURE 15–8.** A fetus undergoing ex-utero intrapartum therapy (EXIT) procedure for cystic hygroma.

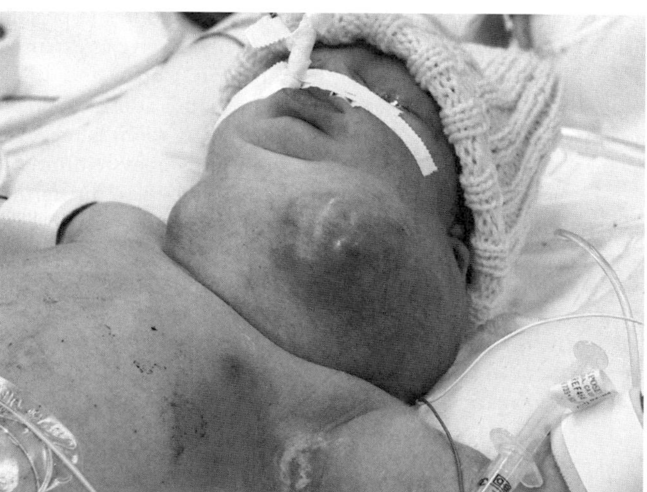

■ **FIGURE 15–9.** A fetus undergoing ex-utero intrapartum therapy (EXIT) procedure for cervical teratoma.

Congenital High Airway Obstruction Syndrome

Congenital high airway obstruction syndrome (CHAOS) is usually caused by laryngeal or tracheal atresia. CHAOS can also be caused by isolated tracheal stenosis or mucosal web or extrinsically by compression from a large cervical mass (e.g., teratoma, lymphangioma). CHAOS can be associated with hydrocephalus, vertebral anomalies, absent radius, bronchotracheal fistula, esophageal atresia, tracheoesophageal fistula, syndactyly, genitourinary anomalies, uterine anomalies, imperforate anus, cardiac anomalies, and anophthalmia. The main differential diagnosis for CHAOS is a bilateral CCAM.

Fetal upper airway obstruction prevents the clearance of lung fluid out of the airway and into the amniotic space. This fluid is normally produced under a pressure that favors its movement out of the fetal mouth. Ultrasonographic findings in CHAOS include large overdistended lungs that compress the mediastinum, bilaterally flattened or everted diaphragms, dilated large airways distal to the obstruction, and fetal ascites and/or hydrops fetalis due to heart and great vessel compression (Hedrick et al., 1994). Fetuses affected with CHAOS are delivered via an EXIT procedure. For fetuses that develop hydrops, early delivery or prenatal tracheostomy is an option, depending on gestational age.

■ FETOSCOPIC SURGERY

Fetoscopic surgical procedures are the most common fetal interventions and have the greatest potential to expand in scope of indications. These procedures involve the percutaneous placement of small trocars and fetoscopes into the uterus. Umbilical cord ligation and selective ablation of fetal connecting vessels are done for twin pregnancies complicated by twin reversed arterial perfusion sequence (TRAP) or twin-twin transfusion syndrome (TTTS), where the death of one or both twins is imminent and conventional therapy has failed. Bladder outlet obstruction can be treated using a fetoscope-guided laser to ablate posterior urethral valves, and amniotic bands can be ligated by fetoscopic technique. Also under investigation are fetoscopic techniques to assist in the management of fetuses with congenital diaphragmatic hernias (CDHs).

PREOPERATIVE MANAGEMENT

Because of the emergent nature of these procedures (especially for TTTS and TRAP), parturients may not receive as extensive preoperative evaluation as those undergoing open and EXIT procedures. Patients for fetoscopic surgery are admitted to the hospital on the day of surgery. The operating room is prepared as for an open procedure in the rare event a hysterotomy is required for surgical access. In the preoperative area, the mother receives sodium bicitrate PO, metoclopramide IV, and, if at high risk for preterm labor, indomethacin per rectum. Following placement of American Society of Anesthesiologists standard monitors, a lumbar epidural catheter is inserted and tested. The parturient is then positioned with left uterine displacement to prevent supine hypotension syndrome by compression of the inferior vena cava between the gravid uterus and the spine.

INTRAOPERATIVE MANAGEMENT

Anesthetic management of these cases depends on the location of the placenta, umbilical cord, and amniotic membranes (Galinkin et al., 2000). The location of these structures influences the difficulty of surgical exposure. In the patient with an anterior placenta, epidural anesthesia is often sufficient due to the ease of surgical access to the fetus and essential vessels. A complicating factor is severe polyhydramnios, which can make surgical exposure difficult, requiring general anesthesia to enable uterine manipulation to access the umbilical cord or other fetal structures. In a parturient with a posterior placenta, the uterus is easily accessible but the umbilical cord is often difficult to expose. The presence of a posterior placenta may necessitate a general anesthetic to allow for this additional uterine manipulation. Care should be taken to avoid maternal hyperventilation and hypocapnia, which may result in placental vasoconstriction and fetal hypoxia (Motoyama et al., 1966, 1967; Peng et al., 1972).

The risk for preterm labor increases with hysterotomy for a fetoscopic procedure or a maternal history of preterm labor. Preoperative uterine activity and intraoperative uterine manipulation guide the choice between a balanced general anesthetic, a deep general anesthetic (2 MAC isoflurane or desflurane), and the use of postoperative epidural analgesia. Deep inhalation anesthesia relaxes the uterus, whereas epidural analgesia postoperatively may decrease the risk of preterm labor (Tame et al., 1999). Prophylaxis of preterm labor also includes intraoperative administration of magnesium sulfate. Indomethacin is occasionally used for patients at high risk of preterm labor when cardiac failure is not present in the remaining fetus.

Anesthetic choice is guided by potential advantages and disadvantages for the mother and the fetus (Table 15–2). Epidural anesthesia is used for the majority of these cases and has the advantage of minimal effects on fetal hemodynamics (Hoffman et al., 1997), on uteroplacental blood flow (Alahuhta et al., 1991), and on postoperative uterine activity (Tame et al., 1999). The disadvantages include lack of uterine relaxation, lack of fetal anesthesia, and difficulty manipulating the uterus and cord while the fetus may be moving. A balanced inhalation–opioid anesthetic has the advantage of allowing uterine manipulation with an immobile and anesthetized fetus, yet should provide less fetal cardiovascular depression than deep inhalation anesthesia. General anesthesia also eliminates concerns associated with an awake patient, such as anxiety, combativeness, nausea, and emesis. The potential disadvantage of this technique is an inability to fully relax the uterus to access difficult cord positions. Deep inhalation anesthesia has the advantage of profound uterine relaxation, allowing externalization of the uterus and hysterotomy-based procedures. The disadvantages of this technique are fetal cardiovascular depression and decreased uteroplacental blood flow (Palahniuk and Shnider, 1974; Gaiser et al., 1999).

■ TABLE 15–2. Implications of anesthetic technique for fetoscopic surgery

	Fetal Depression	Uteroplacental Blood Flow	Uterine Relaxation
Regional anesthesia	–	–	–
Balanced general anesthetic, with/ without epidural	+	+/–	+/–
Deep general anesthetic with epidural	++	++	++

POSTOPERATIVE MANAGEMENT

As with the open hysterotomy cases, the most important aspect of postoperative management is tocolysis. Epidural catheters are removed after the surgery for these patients, unless they undergo hysterotomy-based procedures. Magnesium sulfate followed by either nifedipine or terbutaline is the mainstay of tocolytic management. Discharge from the hospital on postoperative day 1 to 2 is expected after these procedures.

SURGICAL LESIONS ELIGIBLE FOR FETOSCOPIC SURGERY

Twin Reverse Arterial Perfusion

Twin reverse arterial perfusion (TRAP) occurs only in the setting of a monochorionic pregnancy. This disease process complicates 1% of monochorionic pregnancies and 1:35,000 live births overall (James, 1977). The TRAP sequence is characterized by placental vascular arterioarterial anastomosis between twin fetuses, one being an acardiac/acephalic twin that receives its blood flow from the normal "pumping twin," thereby endangering the normal twin with high output cardiac failure. Reversal of normal umbilical cord blood flow occurs in the acardiac/acephalic twin, in that blood flows retrograde from the umbilical artery of the normal twin to the acardiac/acephalic twin and returns through the acardiac/acephalic twin's umbilical vein. The "pump" twin supplies the cardiac output for both twins. The acardiac twin is nonviable, and the perinatal mortality rate of the "normal" twin exceeds 50% due to high-output cardiac failure, fetal hydrops, and premature birth (Moore et al., 1990).

Management options for the TRAP sequence include observation, termination of the pregnancy, medical treatment of fetal hydrops and preterm labor, or surgical intervention (Hanafy and Peterson, 1997). Surgical cord coagulation by microlaparoscopic technique (fetoscopy) can be performed to interrupt (by laser or bipolar electrocautery) the umbilical artery perfusion to the abnormal twin (Yang and Adzick, 1998). The success for this treatment based on multiple case reports in the literature is 67% (Bianchi et al., 2000).

Twin-Twin Transfusion Sequence

Twin-twin transfusion sequence (TTTS) also occurs only in monochorionic twins. This syndrome has an incidence of 1 to 9:10,000 births (Bianchi et al., 2000). This disease results from an imbalance of blood flow across vascular anastomoses between the two fetal circulations. These twins are discordant in size, with oligohydramnios in the donor twin and polyhydramnios in the recipient twin (Fesslova et al., 1998). If fetal death occurs in the recipient, the co-twin is at very high risk of death (as high as 50%) or neurologic injury (van Heteren et al., 1998; Ries et al., 1999).

The severity of TTTS dictates the choice of surgical management technique. Selective fetoscopic laser photocoagulation (SFLP) of the twin-twin vascular anastomoses is performed when both twins can be saved. SFLP is used to selectively ablate vessels lying on the surface of the placenta that abnormally connect the vasculature of the twins. Umbilical cord coagulation is performed for twin gestations with end-stage TTTS, where one fetus is nonviable and threatens the life or neurologic state of the viable twin. This process separates the fetal circulations and protects the donor twin when the recipient twin is premorbid and not a candidate for SFLP.

Amniotic Bands

The amniotic band syndrome (ABS) consists of a group of congenital anomalies caused by constrictive bands that develop in the amniotic fluid. Deformities occur in the limbs, craniofacial regions, and trunk and appear as pseudosyndactyly, amputation, and/or craniofacial, visceral, or body wall defects. The incidence of these lesions is 1:1,200 to 1:15,000 live births (Chemke et al., 1973; Ho and Liu, 1987; Ray et al., 1988). It is believed that amniotic bands are caused by early rupture of the amnion, resulting in mesodermic bands that originate from the chorionic side of the amnion and insert on the fetal body. These bands have been replicated in an experimental model (Crombleholme et al., 1995) and can lead to amputations, constrictions, and postural deformities secondary to immobilization.

Fetoscopic surgery for the release of amniotic bands is a limb- and life-saving technique. The earlier the band occurs, the more severe is the resulting lesion. Amniotic rupture in the first weeks of pregnancy may result in craniofacial and visceral defects, whereas during the second trimester, the fetal morbidity ranges from formation of syndactyly to limb amputation. Threatened limb amputation may have devastating morphologic and functional effects on a limb, but it is not lethal. These patients are closely followed by repeated ultrasonographic evaluation. When limb compromise becomes an issue, fetoscopic surgery is performed to release these constricting bands. Umbilical cord constriction by amniotic bands can also occur with lethal consequences (Graf et al., 1997; Strauss et al., 2000) and is an emergent indication for fetal surgery. For this disease process, fetoscopic intervention can dramatically improve fetal outcome.

Congenital Diaphragmatic Hernia

Congenital diaphragmatic hernia (CDH) is a simple defect in the diaphragm in which abdominal viscera herniate into the chest, most often through a posterolateral defect in the diaphragm. It is thought to be due to failure of the pleuroperitoneal canal to close between 9 to 10 weeks of gestation. This lesion can result in pulmonary hypoplasia and pulmonary hypertension from compression of the developing lungs by the herniated viscera (Harrison et al., 1993). Despite advances in prenatal care, maternal transport, neonatal resuscitation, and the availability of extracorporeal membrane oxygenation, the physiologic consequences of the disease are associated with a high neonatal mortality rate and substantial long-term morbidity (Harrison et al., 1978).

The prenatal diagnosis of CDH is made on ultrasonographic demonstration of abdominal content such as bowel, stomach, or liver in the thorax. Because fetal pulmonary function cannot be assessed in utero, several sonographically detectable predictors of the severity of a CDH have been proposed. The two most important parameters are the lung-to-head ratio (LHR) (Lipshutz et al., 1997) and the position of the left lobe of the liver (Albanese et al., 1998). The LHR is the calculated volume of the contralateral lung (the ipsilateral lung cannot be identified with a CDH) indexed to head circumference to adjust for gestational age. Fetuses with an LHR of more than 1.4 have a relatively good prognosis with postnatal care and are not candidates for fetal intervention. Fetuses with a major portion of the left lobe of the liver herniated into the hemithorax have an approximately 50% survival rate, whereas those with the liver in normal abdominal position have a greater than 90% survival rate (Albanese et al., 1998).

The prenatal treatment strategy for CDH has undergone continuous development since the first attempted CDH repair in 1986 (Harrison et al., 1990, 1993). Open fetal surgery was associated with many technical problems. Data from a National Institutes of Health–funded prospective study demonstrated that repair of the diaphragm for those without liver herniation was no better than standard postnatal care (Harrison et al., 1997). Repair in cases with liver herniation was not technically feasible.

Knowledge from study of fetuses with CHAOS that resulted in hyperplastic lungs due to overdistention by lung fluid led to a new concept of CDH treatment (Hedrick et al., 1994). Midgestation tracheal occlusion was evaluated in human fetuses with severe CDH in an attempt to promote lung expansion. For this procedure, fetoscopically placed titanium clips were applied to temporarily occlude the fetal trachea (Bealer et al., 1995; Harrison et al., 1996, 1998; Skarsgard et al., 1996; VanderWall et al., 1996). The tracheal clips were removed in an EXIT procedure (Mychaliska et al., 1997). This technique was successful in increasing lung size but was abandoned due to poor fetal outcomes. A technique using a fetoscopically placed detachable tracheal balloon, which is removed at birth, was then developed, replacing the technique of tracheal clips through the anterior tracheal dissection of the fetus (Harrison et al., 2001).

A National Institutes of Health–sponsored randomized controlled trial of the detachable balloon technique was conducted between April 1999 and July 2001. The trial involved 24 pregnant women with a single fetus between 22 and 27 weeks of gestation and with left-sided CDH, liver herniation into the left hemithorax, and an LHR of less than 1.4 (Harrison et al., 2003). Under deep halothane anesthesia with nitroglycerin as needed, a 4-mm hysteroscope was passed through a 5-mm trocar and guided through the fetal vocal cords. The balloon was placed in the fetal trachea and inflated with isotonic contrast material. All 11 fetuses in the tracheal occlusion group were delivered by the EXIT procedure. Eight of 11 fetuses (73%) in the intervention group and 10 of 13 (77%) in the control group (neonatal surgery) survived more than 90 days. The rate of neonatal morbidity did not differ between the two groups, but premature rupture of the membrane and preterm delivery were significantly more common in the tracheal occlusion group (31 versus 37 weeks) (Harrison et al., 2003). Based on these results, fetal surgery for CDH was suspended in the United States in April 2001 with an indefinite moratorium.

Hydronephrosis—Bladder Outlet Obstruction

Obstructive uropathy occurs in 1:1,000 live births (Estes and Harrison, 1993). Unlike obstruction of the urinary tract at other levels, bladder outlet obstruction has the potential to affect the development of the whole urinary tract and the pulmonary system. Bladder outlet obstruction can lead to oligohydramnios and result in renal failure from renal dysplasia. Secondary pulmonary hypoplasia may also develop, leading to severe respiratory insufficiency at birth. Fetuses with obstructive uropathy can also have other associated nongenitourinary anomalies, chromosomal anomalies, and deformations related to oligohydramnios.

Prenatal intervention is possible for select fetuses with urinary tract obstruction. In cases of isolated bladder outlet obstruction due to posterior urethral valves, fetal vesicoamniotic shunting may be life saving. Fetuses are selected for this intervention based on three variables: fetal karyotype, detailed sonographic evaluation, and serial urine evaluation to determine the extent of underlying renal damage (Evans et al., 1991; Walsh and Johnson, 1999). The aim of prenatal intervention is to bypass or directly treat the obstruction, restoring amniotic fluid to normal levels.

Initially, open fetal surgery to place a vesicoamniotic shunt was performed for fetuses with severe bladder outlet obstruction. Unfortunately, this technique was abandoned due to the high complication rate for both mother and fetus (Crombleholme et al., 1988). Vesicoamniotic shunts have also been placed percutaneously under sonographic guidance, but catheter placement is not always successful and catheter displacement and obstruction occur in 25% of the cases. Fetoscopic ablation of posterior urethral valves is a technique developed in a fetal-lamb model that is now being used in humans (Quintero et al., 1995). This technique holds a great deal of promise for improving the treatment of urinary tract obstruction in utero (Estes et al., 1992). The technique involves in utero percutaneous cystoscopy followed by ablation of the posterior urethral valves by laser (Quintero et al., 1995). The use of this minimally invasive technique may greatly reduce the morbidity of in utero treatment of serious bladder outlet obstruction compared with standard therapy.

■ CONTROVERSIES

Fetal surgery is a new frontier of medicine. As with other emerging fields, such as stem cell research and gene therapy, controversy surrounds many aspects of these procedures. Anesthetic aspects are no exception. An editorial from *Anesthesiology* (Anand and Maze, 2001) questioned whether fetuses are appropriately anesthetized during fetal interventions. Based on animal and human literature, the fetus receives at least half the MAC concentration of anesthetic agent received by the mother (Palahniuk et al., 1974; Schwarz et al., 2003), and fentanyl administered intramuscularly to the fetus sufficiently blocks the fetal stress response (Fisk et al., 2001). Similarly, the lack of movement noted in the fetus during these procedures indicates adequate anesthesia. It is not known whether eliciting a stress response in a fetus causes any long-term effects or if the lack of long-term analgesia after fetal surgery is detrimental to outcome.

The use of volatile anesthetics as sole anesthetics for fetal surgery is a technique that has evolved over time and remains controversial. The traditional anesthetic technique for fetal surgery was a nitrous oxide–opioid technique that used intravenous nitroglycerin to provide uterine relaxation. This technique causes a labile maternal blood pressure and inconsistent uterine relaxation. The technique of deep general anesthesia evolved in response to these problems. Deep general anesthesia provides the benefit of profound uterine relaxation and predictable maternal decreases in blood pressure that are readily responsive to intravenous ephedrine. Traditionally, isoflurane and halothane were the inhalation agents of choice for this technique. Now, with the advent of more insoluble inhalation agents, desflurane is the primary agent used at many institutions for these cases due to ease of titratability. Unfortunately, there are little clinical or animal data showing superiority of maternal/fetal safety for any of these techniques.

Future research in fetal anesthesia is fraught with difficulty. Standardized assessment tools and blood "microsampling" techniques for the fetus need to be developed to allow further development of clinical protocols. Questions regarding fetal stress and optimal drug dosing in the fetus remain open to speculation until these techniques evolve to answer our questions.

■ SUMMARY

Anesthesia for fetal surgery continues to evolve. The anesthetic techniques that have emerged are safe for mother and fetus. Because of the myriad anesthetic and surgical issues that these cases generate, it is essential to have good communication and cooperation between surgeons, anesthesiologists, and perinatal physicians. This communication must exist from the preoperative period to the postoperative period to allow development of a cohesive anesthetic and surgical plan that can be used for the safe perioperative management of the fetal surgery patient.

REFERENCES

Abbott PD, et al.: Dystocia caused by sacrococcygeal teratoma. *Obstet Gynecol* 27:571–574, 1966.

Adzick NS, et al.: Fetal cystic adenomatoid malformation: Prenatal diagnosis and natural history. *J Pediatr Surg* 20:483–488, 1985.

Adzick NS, et al.: Successful fetal surgery for spina bifida. [comment]. *Lancet* 352(9141):1675–1676, 1998.

Adzick NS, et al.: Management of congenital lung lesions. *Semin Pediatr Surg* 12:10–16, 2003.

Alahuhta S, et al.: Effects of extradural bupivacaine with adrenaline for caesarean section on uteroplacental and fetal circulation [comments]. *Br J Anaesth* 67:678–682, 1991.

Albanese CT, et al.: Fetal liver position and perinatal outcome for congenital diaphragmatic hernia. *Prenat Diagn* 18:1138–1142, 1998.

Altman RP, et al.: Sacrococcygeal teratoma: American Academy of Pediatrics Surgical Section Survey–1973. *J Pediatr Surg* 9:389–398, 1974.

Anand KJ, Maze M: Fetuses, fentanyl, and the stress response: Signals from the beginnings of pain? [editorial] *Anesthesiology* 95:823–825, 2001.

Bachman CR, et al.: Isoflurane potency and cardiovascular effects during short exposures in the foetal lamb. *Can Anaesthet Soc J* 33:41–47, 1986.

Bale PM: Sacrococcygeal developmental abnormalities and tumors in children. *Perspect Pediatr Pathol* 8:9–56, 1984.

Bealer JF, et al.: The "PLUG" odyssey: Adventures in experimental fetal tracheal occlusion. *J Pediatr Surg* 30:361–364, 1995; discussion 364–365, 1995.

Bianchi DW, et al.: *Fetology: Diagnosis and management of the fetal patient.* New York, 2000, McGraw–Hill Companies Inc.

Biehl DR, et al.: Effect of halothane on cardiac output and regional flow in the fetal lamb in utero. *Anesth Analg* 62:489–492, 1983a.

Biehl DR, et al.: The uptake of isoflurane by the foetal lamb in utero: Effect on regional blood flow. *Can Anaesthet Soc J* 30:581–586, 1983b.

Bond SJ, et al.: Cesarean delivery and hysterotomy using an absorbable stapling device. *Obstet Gynecol* 74:25–28, 1989.

Bond SJ, et al.: Death due to high-output cardiac failure in fetal sacrococcygeal teratoma. *J Pediatr Surg* 25:1287–1291, 1990.

Brock DJ, Sutcliffe RG: Alpha-fetoprotein in the antenatal diagnosis of anencephaly and spina bifida. *Lancet* 2(7770):197–199, 1972.

Bruner JP, et al.: Endoscopic coverage of fetal myelomeningocele in utero. *Am J Obstet Gynecol* 180:153–158, 1999a.

Bruner JP, et al.: Fetal surgery for myelomeningocele and the incidence of shunt-dependent hydrocephalus [comment]. *JAMA* 282:1819–1825, 1999b.

Carney JA, et al.: Teratomas in children: Clinical and pathologic aspects. *J Pediatr Surg* 7:271–282, 1972.

Chan MT, Gin T: Postpartum changes in the minimum alveolar concentration of isoflurane. *Anesthesiology* 82:1360–1363, 1995.

Chan MT, et al.: Minimum alveolar concentrations of halothane and enflurane are decreased in early pregnancy. *Anesthesiology* 85:782–786, 1996.

Chemke J, et al.: The amniotic band syndrome. *Obstet Gynecol* 41:332–336, 1973.

Cohen MM, et al.: Antenatal detection of cystic hygroma. *Obstet Gynecol Surv* 44:481–490, 1989.

Conklin J, Abell MR: Germ cell neoplasms of sacrococcygeal region. *Cancer* 20:2105–2117, 1967.

Crombleholme TM, et al.: Amniotic band syndrome in fetal lambs. I: Fetoscopic release and morphometric outcome. *J Pediatr Surg* 30:974–978, 1995.

Crombleholme TM, et al.: Early experience with open fetal surgery for congenital hydronephrosis. *J Pediatr Surg* 23:1114–1121, 1988.

Estes JM, Harrison MR: Fetal obstructive uropathy. *Semin Pediatr Surg* 2: 129–135, 1993.

Estes JM, et al.: Fetoscopic surgery for the treatment of congenital anomalies. *J Pediatr Surg* 27:950–954, 1992.

Evans MI, et al.: Sequential invasive assessment of fetal renal function and the intrauterine treatment of fetal obstructive uropathies. *Obstet Gynecol* 77:545–550, 1991.

Fesslova V, et al.: Fetal and neonatal echocardiographic findings in twin-twin transfusion syndrome. *Am J Obstet Gynecol* 179:1056–1062, 1998.

Fisk NM, et al.: Effect of direct fetal opioid analgesia on fetal hormonal and hemodynamic stress response to intrauterine needling [comments]. *Anesthesiology* 95:828–835, 2001.

Flake AW: Fetal sacrococcygeal teratoma. *Semin Pediatr Surg* 2:113–120, 1993.

Gaiser RR, et al.: Anesthetic management of cesarean delivery complicated by ex utero intrapartum treatment of the fetus. *Anesth Analg* 84:1150–1153, 1997.

Gaiser RR, et al.: The cesarean delivery of a twin gestation under 2 minimum alveolar anesthetic concentration isoflurane: One normal and one with a large neck mass. *Anesth Analg* 88:584–586, 1999.

Galinkin JL, et al.: Anesthesia for fetoscopic fetal surgery: Twin reverse arterial perfusion sequence and twin-twin transfusions syndrome. *Anesth Analg* 91:1394–1397, 2000.

Gin T, Chan MT: Decreased minimum alveolar concentration of isoflurane in pregnant humans. *Anesthesiology* 81:829–832, 1994.

Graf JL, et al.: Chorioamniotic membrane separation: A potentially lethal finding. *Fetal Diagn Ther* 12:81–84, 1997.

Graf JL, et al.: A surprising histological evolution of preterm sacrococcygeal teratoma. *J Pediatr Surg* 33:177–179, 1998.

Gregory GA, et al.: Fetal anesthetic requirement (MAC) for halothane. *Anesth Analg* 62:9–14, 1983.

Hanafy A, Peterson CM: Twin-reversed arterial perfusion (TRAP) sequence: Case reports and review of literature [review]. *Aust N Z J Obstet Gynaecol* 37:187–191, 1997.

Harrison MR, et al.: Congenital diaphragmatic hernia: The hidden mortality. *J Pediatr Surg* 13:227–230, 1978.

Harrison MR, et al.: Correction of congenital diaphragmatic hernia in utero. V. Initial clinical experience. *J Pediatr Surg* 25:47–55, 1900; discussion 56–57, 1990.

Harrison MR, et al.: Correction of congenital diaphragmatic hernia in utero. VI. Hard-earned lessons. *J Pediatr Surg* 28:1411–1417, 1993; discussion 1417–1418, 1993.

Harrison MR, et al.: Correction of congenital diaphragmatic hernia in utero. VII: A prospective trial. *J Pediatr Surg* 32:1637–1642, 1997.

Harrison MR, et al.: Correction of congenital diaphragmatic hernia in utero. VIII. Response of the hypoplastic lung to tracheal occlusion. *J Pediatr Surg* 31:1339–1348, 1996.

Harrison MR, et al.: Correction of congenital diaphragmatic hernia in utero. IX. Fetuses with poor prognosis (liver herniation and low lung-to-head ratio) can be saved by fetoscopic temporary tracheal occlusion. *J Pediatr Surg* 33:1017–1022, 1998; discussion 1022–1023, 1998.

Harrison MR, et al.: Fetoscopic temporary tracheal occlusion by means of detachable balloon for congenital diaphragmatic hernia. *Am J Obstet Gynecol* 185:730–733, 2001.

Harrison MR, et al.: A randomized trial of fetal endoscopic tracheal occlusion for severe fetal congenital diaphragmatic hernia. *N Engl J Med* 349:1916–1924, 2003.

Hedrick MH, et al.: Plug the lung until it grows (PLUG): A new method to treat congenital diaphragmatic hernia in utero. *J Pediatr Surg* 29:612–617, 1994.

Hedrick MH, et al.: Congenital high airway obstruction syndrome (CHAOS): A potential for perinatal intervention. *J Pediatr Surg* 29:271–274, 1994.

Heffez DS, et al.: The paralysis associated with myelomeningocele: Clinical and experimental data implicating a preventable spinal cord injury. *Neurosurgery* 26:987–992, 1990.

Heffez DS, et al.: Intrauterine repair of experimental surgically created dysraphism. *Neurosurgery* 32:1005–1010, 1993.

Heymann MA, Rudolph AM: Effect of exteriorization of the sheep fetus on its cardiovascular function. *Circ Res* 21:741–745, 1967.

Ho DM, Liu HC: The amniotic band syndrome. Report of two autopsy cases and review of literature. *Chung Hua i Hsueh Tsa Chih [Chin Med J]* 39:429–436, 1987.

Hoffman CT, et al.: Effects of narcotic and non-narcotic continuous epidural anesthesia on intrapartum fetal heart rate tracings as measured by computer analysis. *J Matern-Fetal Med* 6:200–205, 1997.

Holzgreve W, et al.: Sonographic demonstration of fetal sacrococcygeal teratoma. *Prenat Diagn* 5:245–257, 1985.

Hutchins GM, et al.: Acquired spinal cord injury in human fetuses with myelomeningocele. *Pediatr Pathol Lab Med* 16:701–712, 1996.

Isaacs HJ: *Tumors of the fetus and newborn.* Philadelphia, 1997, WB Saunders.

James WH: A note on the epidemiology of acardiac monsters. *Teratology* 16:211–216, 1977.

Jobe AH, Ikegami M: Prevention of bronchopulmonary dysplasia. *Curr Opin Pediatr* 13:124–129, 2001.

Johnson N, et al.: Fetal monitoring with pulse oximetry. *Br J Obstet Gynaecol* 98:36–41, 1991.

Kaufman GE, et al.: Decompression of fetal axillary lymphangioma to prevent dystocia. *Fetal Diagn Ther* 11:218–220, 1996.

Kuhlmann RS, et al.: Fetal sacrococcygeal teratoma. *Fetal Ther* 2:95–100, 1987.

Langer JC, et al.: Fetal hydrops and death from sacrococcygeal teratoma: Rationale for fetal surgery [comment]. *Am J Obstet Gynecol* 160:1145–1150, 1989.

Leninger B, Haight C: Congenital cystic adenomatoid malformation of the left lower lobe with compression of remaining lung. *Clin Pediatr* 12:182–186, 1973.

Lipshutz GS, et al.: Prospective analysis of lung-to-head ratio predicts survival for patients with prenatally diagnosed congenital diaphragmatic hernia. *J Pediatr Surg* 32:1634–1636, 1997.

Luks FI, et al.: The effect of open and endoscopic fetal surgery on uteroplacental oxygen delivery in the sheep. *J Pediatr Surg* 31:310–314, 1996.

MacGregor SN, et al.: Prediction of fetoplacental blood volume in isoimmunized pregnancy. *Am J Obstet Gynecol* 159:1493–1497, 1988.

Meuli M, et al.: The spinal cord lesion in human fetuses with myelomeningocele: Implications for fetal surgery. *J Pediatr Surg* 32:448–452, 1997.

Meuli M, et al.: In utero surgery rescues neurological function at birth in sheep with spina bifida. *Nat Med* 1:342–347, 1995a.

Meuli M, et al.: Creation of myelomeningocele in utero: A model of functional damage from spinal cord exposure in fetal sheep [comment]. *J Pediatr Surg* 30:1028–1032, 1995b; discussion 1032–1033, 1995b.

Michejda M: Intrauterine treatment of spina bifida: Primate model. *Zeitschrift Kinderchir* 39:259–261, 1984.

Miller R, et al.: Congenital cystic adenomatoid malformation of the lung: A report of 17 cases and review of the literature. *Pathol Annu* 387–407, 1980.

Moore TR, et al.: Perinatal outcome of forty-nine pregnancies complicated by acardiac twinning. *Ann J Obstet Gynecol* 163:907–912, 1990.

Motoyama EK, et al.: Adverse effect of maternal hyperventilation on the foetus. *Lancet* 1(7432):286–288, 1966.

Motoyama EK, et al.: The effect of changes in maternal pH and P-CO2 on the P-O2 of fetal lambs. *Anesthesiology* 28:891–903, 1967.

Mychaliska GB, et al.: Operating on placental support: The ex utero intrapartum treatment procedure. *J Pediatr Surg* 32:227–230, 1997; discussion 230–231, 1997.

Nicolaides KH, et al.: Measurement of human fetoplacental blood volume in erythroblastosis fetalis. *Am J Obstet Gynecol* 157:50–53, 1987.

O'Hara I, Kurth CD: Anesthesia for fetal surgery. In Greeley WD, editor: *Pediatric anesthesia.* Philadelphia, 1999, Churchill Livingstone, pp 15.1–15.11.

Paek BW, et al.: Hindbrain herniation develops in surgically created myelomeningocele but is absent after repair in fetal lambs. *Am J Obstet Gynecol* 183:1119–1123, 2000.

Paek BW, et al.: Radiofrequency ablation of human fetal sacrococcygeal teratoma. *Am J Obstet Gynecol* 184:503–507, 2001.

Palahniuk RJ, Shnider SM: Maternal and fetal cardiovascular and acid-base changes during halothane and isoflurane anesthesia in the pregnant ewe. *Anesthesiology* 41:462–472, 1974.

Palahniuk RJ, et al.: Pregnancy decreases the requirement for inhaled anesthetic agents. *Anesthesiology* 41:82–83, 1974.

Parpaglioni R, et al.: Intraoperative fetal oxygen saturation during caesarean section: General anaesthesia using sevoflurane with either 100% oxygen or 50% nitrous oxide in oxygen. *Eur J Anaesthesiol* 19:115–118, 2002.

Parry AJ, et al.: *The impact of fetal exposure on hemodynamics, white cell activation, and stress response.* Pediatric Academic Societies Annual Meeting, Baltimore Convention Center, Baltimore, MD, 2001.

Peng AT, et al.: Effect of maternal hypocapnia v. eucapnia on the foetus during caesarean section. *Br J Anaesth* 44:1173–1178, 1972.

Quintero RA, et al.: Percutaneous fetal cystoscopy and endoscopic fulguration of posterior urethral valves. *Am J Obstet Gynecol* 172:206–209, 1995.

Quintero RA, et al.: Percutaneous fetal cystoscopy and endoscopic fulguration of posterior urethral valves [comment]. *Am J Obstet Gynecol* 172:206–209, 1995.

Quintero RA, et al.: In-utero percutaneous cystoscopy in the management of fetal lower obstructive uropathy. *Lancet* 346(8974):537–540, 1995.

Ray M, et al.: Amniotic band syndrome. *Int J Dermatol* 27:312–314, 1988.

Rice HE, et al.: Congenital cystic adenomatoid malformation: A sheep model of fetal hydrops. *J Pediatr Surg* 29:692–696, 1994.

Ries M, et al.: Rapid development of hydrops fetalis in the donor twin following death of the recipient twin in twin-twin transfusion syndrome. *J Perinatal Med* 27:68–73, 1999.

Rivard G, et al.: The relation between maternal and fetal oxygen tensions in sheep. *Am J Obstet Gynecol* 97:925–930, 1967.

Rosen MA: Anesthesia for fetal surgery. In *Obstetric anesthesia: Principles and practice.* St Louis, 1999, Mosby, pp 110–121.

Sabik JF, et al.: Halothane as an anesthetic for fetal surgery. *J Pediatr Surg* 28:542–546, 1993; discussion 546–547, 1993.

Schiffer M, Greenberg E: Sacrococcygeal teratoma in labor and the newborn. *Am J Obstet Gynecol* 72:1054–1062, 1956.

Schwarz U, et al.: The uptake of desflurane in fetal sheep: Preliminary results. Presented at the annual meeting of the Society of Pediatric Anesthesiology, 2003.

Shanji F, et al.: Cystic diseases of the lungs. *Surg Clin North Am* 68:581–618, 1988.

Skarsgard ED, et al.: Fetal endoscopic tracheal occlusion ('Fetendo-PLUG') for congenital diaphragmatic hernia. *J Pediatr Surg* 31:1335–1338, 1996.

Stocker JT, et al.: Congenital cystic adenomatoid malformation of the lung. Classification and morphologic spectrum. *Hum Pathol* 8:155–171, 1977.

Strauss A, et al.: Intra-uterine fetal demise caused by amniotic band syndrome after standard amniocentesis. *Fetal Diagn Ther* 15:4–7, 2000.

Strout CD, Nahrwold ML: Halothane requirement during pregnancy and lactation in rats. *Anesthesiology* 55:322–323, 1981.

Sutton LN, et al.: Improvement in hindbrain herniation demonstrated by serial fetal magnetic resonance imaging following fetal surgery for myelomeningocele [comment]. *JAMA* 282:1826–1831, 1999.

Tame JD, et al.: Level of postoperative analgesia is a critical factor in regulation of myometrial contractility after laparotomy in the pregnant baboon: Implications for human fetal surgery. *Am J Obstet Gynecol* 180:1196–1201, 1999.

Tulipan N, et al.: Reduced hindbrain herniation after intrauterine myelomeningocele repair: A report of four cases. *Pediatr Neurosurg* 29:274–278, 1998.

Tulipan N, et al.: The effect of intrauterine myelomeningocele repair on the incidence of shunt-dependent hydrocephalus. *Pediatr Neurosurg* 38:27–33, 2003.

van Heteren CF, et al.: Risk for surviving twin after fetal death of co-twin in twin-twin transfusion syndrome. *Obstet Gynecol* 92:215–219, 1998.

VanderWall KJ, et al.: Fetal endoscopic ('Fetendo') tracheal clip. *J Pediatr Surg* 31:1101–1103, 1996; discussion 1103–1104, 1996.

Walsh DS, Johnson MP: Fetal interventions for obstructive uropathy. *Semin Perinatal* 23:484–495, 1999.

Watari H, et al.: A case of intrauterine medical treatment for cystic hygroma. *Eur J Obstet Gynecol Reprod Biol* 70:201–203, 1996.

Welborn JL, Timm NS: Trisomy 21 and cystic hygromas in early gestational age fetuses. *Am J Perinatal* 11:19–20, 1994.

Westerburg B, et al.: Radiofrequency ablation of liver in the fetal sheep: A model for treatment of sacrococcygeal teratoma in the fetus. *Surg Forum* 49:461–463, 1998.

Yang EY, Adzick NS: Fetoscopy [review]. *Semin Laparosc Surg* 5:31–39, 1998.

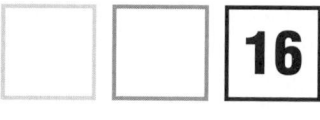

16 Anesthesia for Neonates and Premature Infants

Claire M. Brett • Peter J. Davis • George Bikhazi

The neonatal period, which encompasses the first month of extrauterine life, challenges the newborn infant in several respects. Once separated from the placenta, the newborn infant must function independently to adapt to the new environment. This adaptation involves anatomic, physiologic, and pharmacologic changes to maintain homeostasis and to ensure the infant's survival. Disease states, anesthesia, and surgery can interfere with these developmental changes and threaten survival. The anesthesiologist must understand the principles of neonatal anesthesia and surgery, the normal course of development, the pathophysiology of neonatal disease states, and the glossary of terms used to describe the neonates and their diseases (Box 16–1).

NEONATAL LESIONS REQUIRING SURGERY

Most neonatal lesions require emergency or urgent intervention. Infants born with congenital anomalies may have obvious malformations on physical examination or may show specific or nonspecific signs such as respiratory distress, gastrointestinal dysfunction, or temperature, hemodynamic, or metabolic instability. Of note, a neonate with one congenital anomaly may have coexisting anomalies that are not readily apparent. A detailed list of disease entities and coexisting anomalies has been described (Jones and Pelton, 1976; Lynn, 1985) (Box 16–2). An understanding of the congenital lesion(s) and its pathophysiology is essential to develop a logical and effective anesthetic plan. In addition, the general principles of care for all patients requiring surgery must be extrapolated to the newborn: positioning, blood loss, monitoring, fluid replacement, choice of anesthetic agents, and postoperative management.

PREANESTHETIC ASSESSMENT

Details of the newborn infant's perinatal course and delivery provide important information for the pediatric anesthesiologist. The preoperative assessment of the newborn should focus on the details of the labor and delivery and the infant's transition from fetal to newborn existence. Disease states, anesthetic agents, and surgical interventions can all influence the homeostatic mechanisms of adaptation.

MEDICAL HISTORY

The framework for developing an anesthetic plan for a newborn is centered on the specific medical history, current physical examination, and ongoing metabolic status. The medical history of a newborn requires a careful review of the mother's pregnancy (Box 16–3), analysis of the labor and delivery, and the events of the first hours/days of life. After the first few weeks of life, the details of the labor and delivery become less relevant, except to account for and understand why any residual medical sequelae exist.

Intrauterine Environment

The intrauterine environment has dramatic effects on the growth and the ability of the newborn to adapt to extrauterine life.

BOX 16–1 Glossary of Abbreviations

AGA: Appropriate for gestational age, >5th percentile, <90th percentile for gestational age
BPD: Bronchopulmonary dysplasia
CDH: Congenital diaphragmatic hernia
CLD: Chronic lung disease
ELBW: Extremely low birth weight, <1000 g
GFR: Glomerular filtration rate
LBW: Low birth weight, <2500 g
LGA: Large for gestational age, >90th percentile for gestational age
NEC: Necrotizing enterocolitis
NICU: Neonatal intensive care unit
PDA: Patent ductus arteriosus
Premature: <37 Weeks gestation
SGA: Small for gestational age, <5th percentile for gestational age
TEF: Tracheoesophageal fistula
Term: >37 Weeks gestation
VLBW: Very low birth weight, <1500 g

Although this impact is most obvious over the first few hours, days, and, in some cases, weeks of life, some intrauterine events may have lifelong consequences. For example, the effect of drugs on the development of the fetus can cause well-described multisystem influences producing specific syndromes (e.g., Dilantin [phenytoin], thalidomide, alcohol) or less dramatic but easily identifiable effects on total somatic growth (e.g., smoking, steroids) or produce syndromes of drug dependence/withdrawal (e.g., opioids, amphetamines). The effects of such exposure can have direct effects on morphogenesis, resulting in anomalies of the heart, pulmonary circulation, brain, and other organs (e.g., cleft lip and palate). In other cases, asphyxia from effects of drugs on placental blood flow or as a result of embolic infarction may result in poor growth of the fetus or premature labor producing indirect effects secondary to stress response, ischemia, and asphyxia. Such newborns may require vigorous resuscitation in the immediate neonatal period and have significant metabolic derangements (e.g., hypoglycemia, hypocalcemia).

Such a sequence is of vital significance to the anesthesiologist, because asphyxiated infants can manifest neurologic problems (e.g., seizures), transient cardiac dysfunction (e.g., cardiomyopathy, tricuspid insufficiency, pulmonary hypertension), renal insufficiency (e.g., acute tubular necrosis), and/or gastrointestinal/hepatic dysfunctions (e.g., necrotizing enterocolitis, clotting abnormalities). Thus, prenatal and perinatal events often provide important insight into the status of a neonate who is headed to the operating room.

Labor and Delivery and Perinatal Events

The infant who was born after a complicated labor and delivery may have metabolic, cardiovascular, and respiratory instability for variable lengths of time. These events are of particular importance to the anesthesiologist evaluating such an infant in the first 1 to 2 days of life but takes on lesser significance as the infant is stabilized. The preoperative assessment should include review of acid-base status, glucose and calcium requirements, temperature stability, urine output/renal function, and clotting function (platelet count, prothrombin time/partial thromboplastin time).

After an asphyxial event at birth, an infant may have significant glucose instability, especially if the infant is premature, large-for-gestational-age (LGA), or small-for-gestational-age (SGA). The rate of glucose infusion required to produce normal serum glucose (60 to 100 mg/dL) is important to note (see later).

Similarly, calcium hemostasis can be challenging to achieve in the asphyxiated, SGA, LGA, or preterm infant. The dose required over the previous 12 to 24 hours should be calculated

BOX 16–2 Commonly Encountered Lesions in the Neonate

Airway Lesions

Choanal atresia
Pierre Robin syndrome
Upper airway obstruction, for example:
- Cystic hygroma
- Upper airway cysts or webs
- Laryngeal stenosis
- Cleft lip and cleft palate

Thoracic Lesions

Tracheoesophageal fistula (TEF) and atresia
Congenital diaphragmatic hernia
Eventration of the diaphragm
Pneumomediastinum, pneumothorax, and pneumopericardium
Lobar emphysema
Congenital heart lesions
Mediastinal masses

Abdominal Lesions

Omphalocele
Gastroschisis
Intestinal atresia or stenosis
Pyloric stenosis
Malrotation and volvulus
Necrotizing enterocolitis (NEC)
Imperforate anus
Exstrophy of the cloaca or bladder
Incarcerated hernia
Megacolon
Biliary atresia
Hirschsprung's disease

Neurosurgical Lesions

Myelomeningocele
Encephalocele
Craniostenosis
Intracranial masses
Skull fractures
Hydrocephalus
Subdural hemorrhage
Spinal tumors

BOX 16–3 Maternal Factors Associated With Increased Perinatal Risk

- Hypertension
- Prolonged rupture of membranes
- Intravenous drug abuse
- Smoking
- Collagen vascular disease
- Diabetes
- Infection, inflammation

and the delivery method (intermittent bolus, constant infusion) noted. Infiltration of calcium into the subcutaneous space can produce skin sloughing and dehiscence. However, peripheral sites of infusion are difficult to observe when tiny infants are covered with surgical drapes. If an infusion of calcium is to be continued or delivery of a bolus is anticipated, the anesthesiologist must have reliable intravenous access in place.

For the first 2 to 3 hours of life, electrolyte levels of the newborn primarily reflect the mother's values as well as the perinatal events (e.g., asphyxia, placental or umbilical cord hemorrhage). If the newborn has required resuscitation, acidosis may persist for several hours, as perfusion to peripheral tissue is reestablished and gradually "washes out" lactate that had accumulated during the period of cardiovascular collapse. After the first few hours of life, lactate levels reflect a balance between oxygen delivery and normal metabolism (i.e., renal and hepatic function), ongoing metabolic derangements (e.g., sepsis, inherited metabolic diseases), or underlying congenital anomalies.

During the first 12 to 24 hours of life, sodium is generally not included in the intravenous fluid regimen. From day 2, the infusion of fluid is adjusted to reflect delivery of maintenance amounts of sodium (2 to 4 mEq/kg per day) as well as to replace any abnormal losses via the kidney or gastrointestinal tract, to compensate for abnormal water metabolism (e.g., syndrome of inappropriate antidiuretic hormone [ADH]), or to counter the effect of drugs (e.g., furosemide). In some cases where acidosis persists (e.g., inherited metabolic diseases, severe sepsis), an infusion of acetate (or even bicarbonate) is administered rather than chloride. Hyperkalemia and hyponatremia develop most commonly in the extremely low birth weight (ELBW) infant because of renal immaturity, asphyxia, and sepsis. In addition, premature infants tend to develop a mild metabolic acidosis and a renal tubular acidosis, because of their inability to absorb bicarbonate effectively in the proximal tubule.

Gestational Age

Perinatal problems can be related to an infant's gestational age and size. Full-term infants (37 to 42 weeks gestation) born weighing less than the 10th percentile for gestational age, possibly as a result of intrauterine malnutrition or infection, are considered SGA. SGA infants have different pathophysiologic problems from preterm infants (less than 37 weeks gestation) of the same weight (Lubchenco et al., 1963). Birth weight must be interpreted in the context of gestational age.

The well-accepted definition of "prematurity" is an infant less than 37 weeks gestation. Although infants less than 37 weeks gestation tend to share some common features, the physiologic variability between 24 and 36 weeks of gestation is enormous. In fact, a 36-week-gestation infant is more similar to a term infant than to a 24-, 26-, or 28-week-gestation infant. To more accurately analyze the preoperative evaluation and intraoperative management of "newborns," this age group is arbitrarily divided into more discrete subgroups based on gestational age.

Near-Term Infants (35 to 37 weeks gestation)

In the absence of congenital anomalies and without perinatal asphyxia, these infants usually have few of the major medical or surgical problems that are common in the more premature infant. A near-term infant may have some delay in establishing full feeds, whether breast or formula fed. Coincident with this, the incidence of nonhematologically based hyperbilirubinemia (e.g., not associated with positive Coombs or ABO/Rh incompatibility, etc.) is more common than in term infants. In the setting of the infant of a diabetic mother, pulmonary immaturity is common even at this late gestation. Otherwise, pulmonary function is similar to the term infant in most newborns born after 35 weeks gestation. Most surgical intervention in this developmental group is to treat congenital anomalies.

30 to 34 Weeks Gestation

For the sake of this general discussion, infants of 30 to 34 weeks gestation are considered to be similar. However, a 1200-g, 30-week-gestation infant has a greater incidence of the common problems of prematurity compared with a 2000-g, 34-week-gestation infant. Nonetheless, this range was chosen to simplify the specific discussion of preoperative evaluation.

Before exogenous pulmonary surfactant was introduced into clinical practice in 1990, this group of infants often developed respiratory distress syndrome (RDS), also known as hyaline membrane disease. Because of pulmonary immaturity, complications of respiratory supportive care developed, often in proportion to the severity of the RDS—pneumothorax, pulmonary interstitial emphysema, chronic lung disease, iatrogenic blood loss (sampling for blood analysis). With routine use of surfactant, the frequency and severity of classic RDS have decreased dramatically but have not been totally eliminated. The sequelae of pulmonary immaturity and its supportive care and the severity of subsequent chronic lung disease have changed from the presurfactant era. Nonetheless, the emergence of the "new bronchopulmonary dysplasia (BPD)" (see later) and the persistence of variations of chronic lung disease remain with an incidence as high as 20% to 25%.

Although uncommon in a 35-week-gestation infant, this age group of newborns may have marked temperature instability, especially if septic or asphyxiated. Feeding intolerance is common. Before enteral feeds are established, 30- to 34-week-gestation infants must be carefully monitored for metabolic problems, such as hypocalcemia and hypoglycemia. If total parenteral nutrition, either central or peripheral, is required for longer than 1 week, toxic effects (e.g., hepatic and renal) of intravenous alimentation may develop. The frequency of NEC is more common as gestational age decreases and when there is a coexisting patent ductus arteriosus (PDA).

The incidence of a PDA is high (20% to 30%) in these infants, but often the hemodynamic consequences are mild and spontaneous closure is common. In those infants with respiratory problems, the incidence of PDA is higher and more frequently requires either medical treatment (indomethacin) or surgical ligation. Similarly, the incidence of intracerebral bleeds increases with decreasing gestational age, and these intracranial hemorrhages are more common in the setting of other complications of prematurity—sepsis, asphyxia, or precipitous birth. Apnea is more frequent at this developmental stage and is most common in the presence of sepsis, temperature instability, metabolic abnormalities (hypoglycemia, hypocalcemia), and anemia.

27 to 29 Weeks Gestation

The complications of pulmonary, cardiovascular, gastrointestinal, and neurologic immaturity are magnified in this gestational age bracket in both incidence and severity. A key feature of these infants is the variability of diseases from one infant to another. Some infants are "growing preemies" after 1 to 2 weeks, whereas other infants develop multisystem dysfunction and poor growth.

In addition to the problems common in the greater-than-30-week-gestation infants, the impact of fragile skin and absence of subcutaneous tissue is increasingly important in infants of less than 30 weeks' gestation. Temperature instability, enormous caloric expenditure to maintain temperature, and significant transcutaneous fluid loss are of major significance when evaluating and planning for surgery at this developmental stage. Perioperative apnea is of major importance when planning for the postoperative monitoring and ventilatory support of such infants.

Less Than 26 Weeks Gestation

Infants of this gestational age are considered to be "on the edge of survivability." Pulmonary, neurologic, and gastrointestinal sequelae are frequent and occur more often than in the 27- to 29-week-gestation infant. Variability in the rate of clinical progress, in the incidence and severity of complications, and in the frequency/urgency of surgical procedures, is enormous in infants of less than 26 weeks gestation.

The immature central nervous system is fragile. Intracranial hemorrhage correlates with the infant's neurologic status and, eventually, defines the infant's general clinical outcome. Apnea and perioperative pulmonary insufficiency are of major significance in these infants for months after birth. Especially for the first few weeks and months of life, most infants at this developmental stage require postoperative ventilatory support, even when the infant has been without such intervention in the neonatal intensive care nursery before surgery and even when the procedure seems "trivial."

A history of perinatal resuscitation is not uncommon in both term and premature infants. Prolonged intubation is often necessary after meconium aspiration and hyaline membrane disease. In these infants, the airway should be evaluated for subglottic stenosis and lower airway obstruction.

PHYSICAL EXAMINATION

Newborns are classified according to gestational age and weight. The simplest classification is to group all infants less than 2.5 kg as "low birth weight." An infant of greater than 37 weeks gestational age is defined as "term." However, both of these labels are far too simplistic to provide any useful clinical information. Of more importance, the infant should be grouped according to weight as a function of gestational age. Birth weight in the 10th to 90th percentiles for gestational age is termed appropriate-for-gestational age (AGA), those less than the 10th percentile are SGA, and those greater than the 90th percentile are LGA. This, too, is a simplistic analysis, because differences in fetal growth can be marked when different populations are studied. For example, term infants born in Denver tend to be smaller than those born at sea level. Nonetheless, although the absolute value for birth weight at each gestational age is variable depending on geography, nutritional state, and other factors, the pattern of fetal growth is similar in all populations. That is, between 20 and 38 weeks, fetal growth is linear. Near term, fetal weight gain decelerates. Maternal nutrition, multiple gestation, maternal chronic disease, high altitude, genotype (chromosomal abnormalities), birth order, and male sex all have been clearly identified as affecting rate of fetal growth.

Although the topics of fetal growth and metabolism generally are not of major interest or significance to the anesthesiologist, "SGA" and "LGA" infants are at higher risk for a variety of metabolic and structural abnormalities (Box 16–4) that may be critical to analyze and understand before subjecting such a newborn to surgery and anesthesia. Monitoring such infants during surgery must be planned, because obtaining blood samples from infants under surgical drapes can be challenging. The assessment of the weight versus gestational age usually can be obtained from the patient's medical record or from the neonatologist. At other times, the pediatric anesthesiologist should be prepared to obtain this information via an abbreviated assessment such as that described by Ballard (1979) (Table 16–1). This method combines a neurologic and physical assessment to generate a score that estimates gestational age. The primary focus of the anesthesiologist for the physical examination of a newborn in the presurgical period is on the airway and the cardiopulmonary status.

REVIEW OF SYSTEMS AND DEVELOPMENTAL PHYSIOLOGY

Head and Neck

Abnormal anatomy of the head and neck should alert the anesthesiologist to possible difficulties in managing the airway. Those anesthetizing the newborn should appreciate the anatomy and embryology of the pediatric airway. A small jaw (micrognathia), a receding jaw, or both, as is seen in Pierre Robin and Treacher Collins syndromes may eliminate any

BOX 16–4 Common Metabolic and Structural Problems in Small- and Large-for-Gestational-Age (SGA and LGA) Infants

SGA
- Congenital anomalies
- Chromosomal abnormalities
- Chronic intrauterine infection
- Heat loss
- Asphyxia
- Metabolic abnormalities (hypoglycemia, hypocalcemia)
- Polycythemia/hyperbilirubinemia

LGA
- Birth injury (brachial, phrenic nerve, fractured clavicle)
- Asphyxia
- Meconium aspiration
- Metabolic abnormalities (hypoglycemia, hypocalcemia)
- Polycythemia/hyperbilirubinemia

■ **TABLE 16–1.** Physical examination to determine gestational age

	0	1	2	3	4	5
Skin	Gelatinous, red, transparent	Smooth, pink, visible veins	Superficial peeling &/or rash, few veins	Cracking, rare veins	Parchment, deep cracking, no vessels	Leathery, cracked, wrinkled
Lanugo	None	Abundant	Thinning	Bald areas	Mostly bald	
Plantar Creases	No crease	Faint red marks	Anterior transverse crease only	Anterior crease 2/3	Creases cover entire sole	
Breast	Barely present	Flat areola; no bud	Stippled areola, 1-2 mm bud	Raised areola, 3-4 mm bud	Full areola, 5-10 mm bud	
Ear	Pinna flat, stays folded	Slightly curved pinna with slow recoil	Well-curved pinna; soft but ready recoil	Formed & firm with instant recoil	Thick cartilage; ear stiff	
Genitals (male)	Scrotum empty; no rugae		Testes descending; few rugae	Testes down; good rugae	Testes pendulous; deep rugae	
Genitals (female)	Prominent clitoris & labia minora		Majora & minora equally prominent	Majora large; minora small	Clitoris & minora completely covered	

Score	**Gestational age (wks)**
5	26
10	28
15	30
20	32
25	34
30	36
35	38
40	40
45	42
50	44

For simplicity, the evaluation of neuromuscular maturity is not included. The maximum score for the physical maturity is 25, and the maximum for the neuromuscular maturity is also 25. Thus, 50 is correlated with the mature/postmature infant. In the setting of preoperative assessment, using only the physical maturity assessment, the correlation with gestational age will be estimated by multiplying by 2.

From Ballard JL, Novak KK, Driver M: A simplified score for assessment of fetal maturation of newly born infants. *J Pediatr* 95:769–774, 1979.

chance for a clear direct visualization of the upper airway. Intubation of the trachea often requires techniques beyond direct laryngoscopy.

1. Cleft lip with or without cleft palate occurs in 1:1000 live births. Associated congenital defects occur in up to 13% to 50% of patients with cleft palates and 7% to 13% of patients with cleft lips. Cleft palate may also complicate intubation.
2. Choanal atresia often is diagnosed in the delivery room when a catheter cannot be passed into the pharynx through the nostrils (see Chapter 23, Anesthesia for Otolaryngologic Surgery).

A subset of patients with choanal atresia has the CHARGE association. These associations include

C: Colobomatous malformation
H: Heart defect
A: Atresia choane
R: Retardation
G: Growth deficiency, Genital hypoplasia
E: Ear abnormalities

The neonate has been described as an obligate nasal breather, so that if both nostrils are obstructed, respiratory distress may develop. Hemangiomas, lymphangiomas, and hygromas of the neck can produce upper airway obstruction and must be evaluated carefully before induction of anesthesia.

Respiratory System

Differentiation of the lung can be divided into five phases: (1) the embryonic phase (weeks 4 to 6 of gestation) involves early airways formation; (2) the glandular stage (weeks 7 to 16) includes the formation of the lower conduction airways; (3) the canalicular phase (weeks 17 to 28) includes the appearance of the acinus; (4) the terminal sac period (weeks 28 to 36) is characterized by the appearance of the first respiratory units for gas exchange (terminal air sacs and surrounding capillaries); and (5) the alveolar phase (begins at about 36 weeks' gestation and continues until at least 18 months of age) (Burri, 1974; Langston et al., 1984). The timing of various malformations in utero can be estimated with knowledge of these phases of lung maturation. For example, all malformations of the conduction airways take place before 16 weeks gestation. Upper airway abnormalities take place between conception and 6 weeks of gestation. Bronchial malformations occur between 6 and 16 weeks of gestation, and lung hypoplasia becomes evident after 16 weeks gestation. In general, extrauterine viability is first likely after 26 weeks, when the respiratory saccules have developed and vascularization by capillaries has occurred. Before this time, vascular and pulmonary surface area is often inadequate for sufficient gas exchange.

Alveoli develop mainly after birth, increasing from 20 million terminal air sacs in the newborn to about 300 million at 18 months of age. In early gestation, the epithelial cells are simple and columnar in type. Specific cell types are not recognizable until the canalicular stage of development (17 to 28 weeks gestation). During the last 10% to 20% of gestation, type II pneumocytes can be identified. Although these cells have been identified in the human fetus between 22 and 26 weeks of gestation, these cells are more prominent after 34 to 36 weeks of gestation. The major change distinguishing these cells is the appearance of "osmophilic lamellar bodies." There is close correlation between the appearance of these lamellar bodies and the presence of surface-active material in lung extracts (i.e., surfactant).

By 16 weeks gestation, all subdivisions of the conducting airways have formed; that is, main stem bronchi as well as the conducting and terminal bronchioles are present. In the course of supportive care of a premature infant in an intensive care nursery, it is likely that oxygen, positive pressure ventilation, and infections each traumatizes and interferes with the normal but complex process of development of the immature airway. That the ex-premature infant has airway abnormalities consisting of increased resistance and reactivity is not surprising.

The first active inspiration after birth generates a negative intrapleural pressure as high as 70 to 80 cm H_2O. This is essential for lung expansion to overcome surface tension (Matoth et al., 1971). The volume of the first few breaths, ranging from 20 to 80 mL in full-term neonates, establishes the residual volume and the functional residual capacity (FRC) necessary for adequate gas exchange (Avery, 1974) (also see Chapter 2, Respiratory Physiology in Infants and Children).

The onset of breathing, marked by lung expansion and increased alveolar and arterial Po_2, dilates the pulmonary arterial circulation, decreases pulmonary vascular resistance (Strang, 1977), and increases pulmonary blood flow as well as arterial and mixed venous oxygen tensions. The perinatal increase in arterial oxygen tension (Pao_2 >50 mm Hg) is the initial stimulus for constriction of the ductus arteriosus and its functional closure within 10 to 15 hours after birth in the full-term infant. Mechanisms involving nitric oxide (NO) and prostaglandins lead to anatomic closure that usually occurs in 2 to 3 weeks (Born et al., 1956; Heymann and Rudolph, 1975; Seidner, 2001).

Gas exchange in the lungs is maintained fully after successful removal of the lung fluid from the airways and alveoli. Increased pulmonary lymphatic flow for several hours to days after birth (Humphreys et al., 1967) and the presence of surface-active phospholipids and surfactant specific proteins (surfactant) (King, 1982) contribute to the clearance of alveolar fluid (~30 mL/kg). Surfactant markedly reduces surface tension at the gas–liquid interface of the alveoli, maintaining the air spaces open even at end-expiration.

Immaturity of the respiratory control mechanisms can predispose the neonate, especially the premature infant, to life-threatening respiratory complications. The infant's response to hypoxia during the first 3 to 4 weeks of life is paradoxical (Cross and Oppe, 1952; Brady and Ceruti, 1966) in that a brief hyperpnea develops initially in response to hypoxia but is followed by respiratory depression; this initial hyperpnea can be prevented by hypothermia (Ceruti, 1966) (Fig. 16–1). Moreover, hypoxia, which normally increases the respiratory drive in response to hypercapnia, depresses the neonate's response to carbon dioxide (Rigatto et al., 1975). The sensitivity of an infant's ventilatory response to carbon dioxide increases with postnatal and gestational age (Rigatto et al., 1975) (see Chapter 2, Respiratory Physiology in Infants and Children).

The compliant rib cage of the newborn produces a mechanical disadvantage to effective ventilation. Negative intrapleural pressure of normal inspiratory effort tends to collapse the cartilaginous, compliant chest, which causes a paradoxical chest wall motion and limits air flow during inspiration (Knill et al., 1976). The circular configuration of the rib cage (versus ellipsoid in adults) and the horizontal angle of insertion of the diaphragm (versus oblique in adults) cause distortion of the rib cage and inefficient diaphragmatic contraction (Muller and Bryan, 1979).

Other factors also affect the infant's work and efficiency of breathing. Although the adult diaphragm contains 55% type I fibers (fatigue-resistant, slow-twitching, highly oxidative fibers), the diaphragm of the full-term infant has 25%, and that of the preterm infant, 10%. A lower proportion of type I fibers predisposes these primary respiratory muscles to fatigue (Keens et al., 1978). The intercostal muscles show a similar developmental pattern. Expression of various isoforms of the myosin heavy chains in muscle fibers of the diaphragm and the intercostals may contribute to easier fatigability in the newborn/young infant (Watchko and Sieck, 1993; Zhan et al., 1998). Less effective force–frequency (Richards et al., 1991), length–tension (Watchko and Sieck, 1993), and force–velocity relationships (Watchko et al., 1986) and mismatch of energy supply and demand characterize the immature muscle of the diaphragm and may predispose the newborn to fatigue, especially in the setting of decreased lung (e.g., RDS) or total chest wall compliance (e.g., total body edema).

Pulmonary surfactant effects dramatic changes in lung mechanics including distensibility and end expiratory volume stability. The development of RDS of the newborn correlates with insufficient (premature infants) or delayed (e.g., infants of diabetic mothers) synthesis of surfactant. A typical clinical feature of RDS is the early onset (within 6 hours) of symptoms that include tachypnea, retractions, grunting, and oxygen desaturation. The chest radiograph is also characteristic consisting of diffuse reticulogranular pattern with air bronchograms. A progressive worsening of symptoms with a peak severity by days 2 to 3 and recovery starting by 72 hours characterize the uncomplicated clinical course of RDS.

The discovery that surfactant deficiency is the primary pathophysiology of RDS eventually led to the development of commercially available surfactant. Delivery of surfactant either prophylactically or as a rescue technique has become the standard of care in the neonatal intensive care unit over the past two decades. In the neonatal intensive care unit, the usual practice is to deliver a dose of surfactant into the trachea of all newborns of

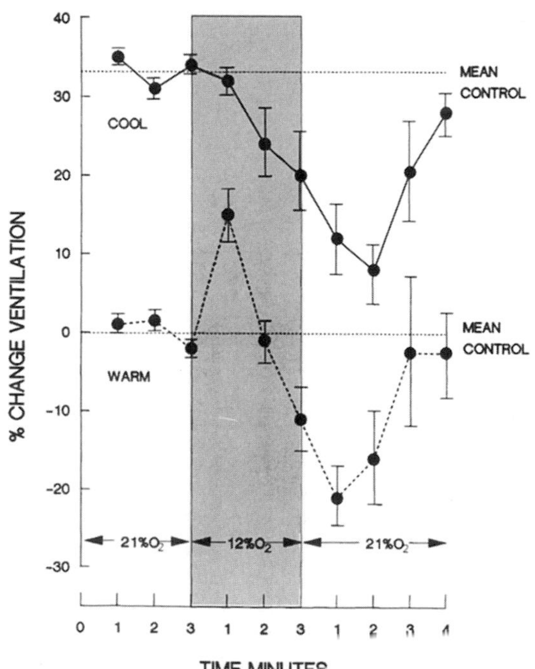

■ **FIGURE 16–1.** Percentage change in ventilation with normoxia and hypoxia in warm and cool environments plotted against time. (From Ceruti F: *Pediatrics* 37:556, 1966. Reproduced by permission of *Pediatrics,* copyright 1966 by AAP.)

less than 28 weeks gestational age. Another dose is given 12 hours later. If the infant remains mechanically ventilated, a third dose is administered about 12 hours after the second. If the trachea of a greater-than-28-week-gestation infant is intubated within the first several hours after birth, surfactant is given. Repeat doses are delivered if mechanical ventilation continues.

The sickest infants in the neonatal period are not always the ones who develop the most severe chronic lung disease. Due to the complexity of lung growth and development, chronic lung disease persists as a problem in about 20% of premature infants. This occurs even though artificial surfactant decreases the need for aggressive ventilatory support. Nonetheless, the most significant decrease in infant mortality observed in 20 years in the United States occurred in 1990, the year surfactant was released commercially. Surfactant therapy has been compared with vaccines from the standpoint of health economics (Long et al., 1995).

Oxygen toxicity, barotrauma (volume trauma) of positive pressure ventilation on immature lungs, and endotracheal intubation have been implicated as etiologic factors in the development of BPD (Philip, 1975). Infants who develop BPD continue to need supplemental oxygen and often have severe lower airway obstruction and air trapping, carbon dioxide retention, atelectasis, recurrent bronchiolitis, and bronchopneumonia. Maintaining normal gas exchange during anesthesia in these infants requires careful monitoring and increased respiratory support. A knowledge of the infant's acid-base status (that is, PCO_2, pH, PO_2) before surgery is essential for managing the infant's ventilation during anesthesia. Increased peak inspiratory pressure (PIP) and positive end-expiratory pressure (PEEP) may be needed to maintain adequate oxygenation. Reactive airway disease involving small airways is also a common feature of infants with BPD. A pneumothorax, mediastinal air leak, or interstitial emphysema may occur during mechanical or manual ventilation and must be considered in the differential diagnosis of sudden cardiorespiratory deterioration during anesthesia.

Infants with a history of RDS and endotracheal intubation who manifest stridor or a weak cry may have developed subglottic stenosis or subglottic granulomas (Hengerer, 1975). These lesions can cause significant narrowing of the trachea. Induction of anesthesia in the setting of critical impingement of the cross-sectional area of the upper airway may precipitate acute airway obstruction. The intraoperative and postoperative courses may be drastically affected by upper airway obstruction. For example, if the trachea is narrowed, the appropriate-sized endotracheal tube usually is smaller than that predicted for the infant's age and size. Secretions may be more difficult to suction, and mechanical ventilatory support may require unusual settings. In addition, special endotracheal tubes may be required (e.g., a 3.0-mm endotracheal tube that is longer than the routine 3.0 tube).

If this diagnosis is suspected preoperatively, the infant should be evaluated by experts such as a pediatric pulmonologist, surgeon, or otolaryngologist to formulate an organized evaluation. To some degree, the level of evaluation depends on the surgery planned and the severity of the infant's symptoms and signs. For example, computed tomography (CT) scanning, magnetic resonance imaging (MRI), or both might be performed to have a clear definition of the airway anatomy. The role of a diagnostic bronchoscopy also needs to be considered. In some cases, the decision might be to perform a bronchoscopy without a prior imaging study or in other cases, in addition to the radiologic studies. Finally, the possibility of a tracheostomy should be considered during the preoperative evaluation. Such an intervention has drastic effects on long-term care and therefore must be discussed in detail with the infant's family before proceeding with any surgical treatment.

Circulatory System

Transitional Circulation

The fetal circulation is characterized by increased pulmonary vascular resistance, decreased pulmonary blood flow, decreased systemic vascular resistance, and right-to-left blood flow through the PDA and the foramen ovale (Donovan, 1985). At birth, the onset of ventilation and the elimination of the placental circulation have dramatic effects on the relationship of systemic and pulmonary vascular resistances; that is, pulmonary vascular resistance decreases and pulmonary blood flow increases. Simultaneously, systemic vascular resistance increases, left atrial pressure increases, the foramen ovale closes functionally, and the right-to-left shunting ceases. However, bidirectional shunting through the ductus arteriosus may continue in the normal infant during the first 24 hours of life. If the ductus arteriosus remains patent, shunting eventually is predominantly left to right as pulmonary vascular resistance declines in the postnatal period. If anatomic closure is achieved and cardiac anatomy is normal, shunting through the ductus is eliminated.

On the other hand, arterial hypoxemia or acidosis in the newborn can precipitate return to a fetal pattern of circulation (i.e., pulmonary arterial vasoconstriction, pulmonary hypertension, reduced pulmonary blood flow). This combination leads to right atrial pressure increasing above left atrial pressure, resulting in right-to-left shunting through the foramen ovale and ductus arteriosus (Rudolph and Yuan, 1966). This return to a fetal circulatory pattern, termed persistent fetal circulation (PFC) or persistent pulmonary hypertension of the newborn (PPHN), further exacerbates the hypoxemia and acidosis. The control of the pulmonary circulation, especially during the transition from fetal to postnatal life, is complex and dependent on the interaction of a variety of mediators and factors, receptors, and neurologic, endocrine, and vascular control mechanisms (Kinsella and Abman, 1995) (Table 16–2). Although numerous treatments (hyperventilation, vasoactive agents) have been proposed over the past two to three decades, a selective and effective vasodilator of the pulmonary circulation has not been identified. In addition, PPHN may be an isolated phenomenon or may be associated with a variety of clinical scenarios including meconium aspiration, sepsis, polycythemia, diaphragmatic hernia, hypoxemia, acidosis, and severe hypotension. An echocardiogram is routinely performed in infants manifesting signs and symptoms of PPHN to definitively exclude structural cyanotic heart disease (Peckham and Fox, 1978; Murphy et al., 1981) (see Chapter 3, Cardiovascular Physiology in Infants and Children).

Myocardial Ultrastructure

The ability of the fetal and adult myocardium to contract and relax depends on the same basic process; namely, with activation, the cytosolic calcium concentration increases, inducing force generation and, as the calcium concentration decreases, relaxation occurs (Anderson, 1998). The membranes in the adult myocardium that control calcium flux and the contractile system that responds to calcium are present in the fetal heart; however, components of each system undergo qualitative and quantitative age-related changes. That is, progression toward adult myocardial function involves developmental changes in

■ **TABLE 16–2.** Factors that modulate pulmonary vascular resistance (PVR) in infants

Lowers PVR	Increases PVR
Endogenous Mediators and Mechanisms	
Oxygen	Hypoxia
Nitric oxide	Acidosis
PGI_7, E_2, D_2	Endothelin-I
Adenosine, ATP, magnesium	Leukotrienes
Bradykinin	Thromboxanes
Atrial natriuretic factor	Platelet-activating factor
Alkalosis	Ca^{2+} channel activation
K^+ channel activation	α-Adrenergic stimulation
Histamine	PGF_{2a}
Vagal nerve stimulation	
Acetylcholine	
β-Adrenergic stimulation	
Mechanical Factors	
Lung inflation	Overinflation or underinflation
Vascular cell structural changes	Excessive muscularization, vascular remodeling
Interstitial fluid and pressure changes	Altered mechanical properties of smooth muscle
Shear stress	Pulmonary hypoplasia
	Alveolar capillary dysplasia
	Pulmonary thromboemboli
	Main pulmonary artery distention
	Ventricular dysfunction, venous hypertension

PVR, pulmonary vascular resistance; PGI_2, E_2, D_2, prostaglandins I_2, E_2, and D_2; ATP, adenosine triphosphate; PGF_{2a}, prostaglandin F_{2a}.
From Kinsella JP, Abman SH: *J Pediatr* 126:853, 1995, with permission.

the sarcomere, myofibril, sarcoplasmic reticulum, extracellular matrix, membrane receptors, and sympathetic innervation.

Sarcomere

The immature myocardium develops less force against a load compared with the adult myocardium (Anderson et al., 1984). The premature and neonatal heart cannot maintain output against an arterial pressure that is "low" in the adult. In part, this reflects a smaller myocardial mass and a thinner-walled left ventricle. In addition, in the isolated immature myocyte, the velocity and quantity of sarcomere shortening are less than in the adult myocyte (Nassar et al., 1987).

Postnatally, the number and size of ventricular cells increase. The myocyte changes from a spheroidal shape to one where the cell has tapered ends, which makes contraction more efficient. The neonatal period is characterized by a major development of the left ventricle as the heart shifts from right to left predominance, with marked increase in left ventricular work secondary to higher stroke volume, systolic arterial pressure, and wall tension. Simultaneously, right ventricular work decreases secondary to the decrease in right ventricular systolic pressure. Left ventricular weight in relation to body weight increases; right ventricular weight decreases in relation to body weight. The increase in myocytes is more pronounced in the left than in the right ventricle. By the second month of life, increase in cell size rather than cell number becomes the predominant developmental phenomenon. This has major implications in the setting of congenital heart disease, especially lesions that obstruct outflow from either ventricle (Rudolph, 2000). Control of this postnatal development is not completely understood, but a role for α-agonist stimulation (Simpson, 1985), cortisol (Rudolph, 2000), thyroid hormone, and a variety of growth factors seems to be integral.

Isoforms of the sarcomeric proteins are expressed in developmental patterns, which, in part, determine myocardial function. For example, the activity of myosin ATPase has been correlated with the rate of cross-bridging, and a higher activity results in more efficient shortening velocity, a characteristic of the mature heart (Pagani and Julian, 1984). The expression of actin isoforms also varies during development. Cardiac, not skeletal, α-actin is expressed during human fetal life but the reverse is seen postnatally. The increase in skeletal α-actin has been linked to an increase in cardiac contractility after birth (Boheler et al., 1991). Another example of developmental importance of isoforms is the pattern of expression of tropomyosin, which has effects on diastolic relaxation; α-tropomyosin is the predominant isoform expressed in rapidly beating hearts (Muthuchamy et al., 1995).

The myocardial expression of isoforms of troponin I is of particular importance in the immature myocardium because this has been correlated with the relative resistance of the immature heart to acidosis (Solaro et al., 1988). The expression of slow skeletal muscle troponin I in fetal heart is linked to the newborn's ability to tolerate a greater degree of acidosis without myocardial depression. The response of the immature myocardium to sympathetic stimulation is similarly correlated with the expression of slow skeletal troponin I. Cardiac troponin is phosphorylated in response to β-stimulation. This phosphorylation decreases the sensitivity to calcium, facilitating diastolic relaxation. In the immature heart, the slow skeletal muscle isoform is not phosphorylated by β-adrenoceptor stimulation, which may have a negative effect on diastolic function (Noland et al., 1995). Finally, troponin T is expressed in many isoforms, and this too has been correlated with the responsiveness of myofilaments to calcium. If the newborn and adult myocardium have different abilities to respond to calcium and calcium channel–mediated pharmacologic agents, this may have major implications concerning pharmacologic therapy in the presence of disease (Anderson et al., 1995).

Myofibrils

The myofilament content of the myocyte increases, and their arrangement becomes more highly organized during postnatal maturation. In the fetus, the pattern of the myofilaments is chaotic, compared with the long parallel rows of cells seen in the adult myocardium (Nassar et al., 1987). The myofibrils are arranged in thin layers, which surround a collection of nuclei and mitochondria. This arrangement allows the trans-sarcolemmal movement of calcium, which is characteristic of the immature contractile process instead of an intracellular calcium release characteristic of contraction of the adult myocardium. The irregular arrangement of mitochondria in immature myocardium is likely to inhibit organized contractile activity, compared with the adult heart where the mitochondria alternate regularly within the sarcomere. In addition, the A and I bands of the sarcomere are irregular and the M band may be absent. The size of the Z band varies.

Sarcoplasmic Reticulum

The sarcoplasmic reticulum is the major intracellular organelle for controlling the cytosolic calcium during contraction. In the adult, only a small amount of extracellular calcium enters the myocyte and elicits the release of a larger amount of calcium from the sarcoplasmic reticulum. The immature heart has an underdeveloped sarcoplasmic reticulum. That is, the volume of sarcoplasmic reticulum within the cell and the ability to pump calcium increase with age. An increase in Ca^{2+}-ATPase activity has been linked to the increased function of the sarcoplasmic reticulum (Mahony and Jones, 1986; Mahony, 1988). A significant finding is that the newborn heart requires a higher extracellular calcium concentration to achieve maximal contractility (Jarmakani et al., 1982). Caffeine, which increases the release of calcium from the sarcoplasmic reticulum, has little effect on neonatal contractility, also suggesting that extracellular calcium, rather than intracellular calcium, has a primary role in control of contractility in the neonatal myocardium. With maturation, the quantity of sarcoplasmic reticulum, the number of specialized connections of the sarcoplasmic reticulum with other membranes, and the activity of Ca^{2+}-ATPase increases, as does the efficiency of pumping calcium.

Extracellular Matrix/Cytoskeleton

The immature myocardium is less compliant than that of the adult (Romero et al., 1972). This age-related increase in compliance is secondary to changes in the extracellular matrix and the cytoskeleton. Because of the low compliance, the systolic pressure and diastolic pressure of the right ventricle can significantly alter left ventricular function in the newborn heart. That is, the higher the right ventricular end-diastolic pressure, the less the left ventricle fills in response to the same filling pressure. A similar pattern occurs in the right ventricle when the left ventricular end-diastolic pressure is increased (Pinson et al., 1987).

The various proteins in the extracellular space important in attaching cell surfaces may contribute to suboptimal shortening of contractile elements. The distribution of various proteins important in this process changes with maturation. For example, desmin, a protein important in linking Z bands of myofibrils, is distributed throughout the subsarcolemma area. As the myocardium develops, the organization of this protein improves the connection of myofibrils with mitochondria facilitating the mechanics of contraction. The distribution of various proteins in the cytoskeleton and extracellular matrix probably explains the irregular pattern of the A and I bands as well as the indistinct or absent M band. Integrins, which are important in linking cell surfaces to extracellular matrix proteins, are distributed differently in the immature heart. The amount and types of collagen also follow a developmental pattern that is based on changes in the expression of various isoforms that improve resting load and passive state of the myocardium. Many of the changes in the cytoskeleton and extracellular matrix occur rapidly after birth (Robinson et al., 1983).

Membrane Receptors

Na^+,K^+-ATPase, the digitalis receptor, is a critical component of membrane function, regulating the cellular content of both sodium and calcium. The activity and quantity of this enzyme increase with maturation (Khatter and Hoeschen, 1982). The α-subunits undergo developmental changes that correlate with its activity. Of clinical importance, the decreased inotropic effects of glycosides on the newborn myocardium have been explained by this maturational change. Although less well defined, a maturational difference in the role of the Na^+–Ca^{2+} exchanger has been described, especially in species that are immature at birth (e.g., human, rat) (Nakanishi et al., 1987). This exchanger may contribute to the sensitivity of the newborn myocardium to changes in extracellular calcium concentration. For example, in the clinical setting of surgery and rapid delivery of blood, serum calcium concentration may decrease, affecting myocardial dysfunction (Sham et al., 1995).

Sympathetic Innervation

The sympathetic nervous system provides critical modulation of the developing myocardium at several levels: growth and differentiation of cells, regulation of calcium concentration, and response of contractile elements to calcium (Anderson et al., 1998). This system also undergoes extensive postnatal development. Both innervation of the heart and availability of catecholamines increase during maturation (Padbury et al., 1981; Nakanishi et al., 1987). On the subcellular level, the number and types of adrenoceptors and other membrane systems that are important in transmission of sympathetic stimuli are affected by maturational state but also vary from species to species. This emphasizes that caution is essential when extrapolating data from animals to clinical care of infants. For example, the fetal and neonatal myocardium of sheep has been shown to be more sensitive to norepinephrine (Friedman, 1972) than the myocardium of older animals. The reported increased sensitivity of the neonatal myocardium to norepinephrine has been compared with denervation sensitivity. In contrast, developmental responses to isoproterenol are not evident in sheep.

The differences in uptake systems for adrenergic agents as the innervation of the myocardium develops may in part explain these findings. Differences in the relative number of α- and β-adrenoreceptors have been described, but, as with other developmental systems, the characteristics vary from species to species. For example, both dogs and sheep have a developmental decrease in the number of α-adrenoreceptors (Wei and Sulakhe, 1979) and increase in β-receptors. In addition to changes in the population of receptors, the increase in adrenergic innervation of the myocardium and changes in the expression of isoforms of various G proteins (important in calcium current conduction) with development alters the response pattern to adrenergic stimuli.

Adrenergic stimuli are critical in normal growth and differentiation of the myocytes. The early high level of α-adrenoceptors may be critical in stimulating the left ventricular growth that develops in the early postnatal life. In fact, α_1-blockade interrupts the increase in protein synthesis seen in cultured myocytes exposed to α-stimulation (Robinson, 1996). Adenylate cyclase is an important enzyme that is involved in the intracellular transmission of β-stimulation. The activity of this system increases in concert with the increase in catecholamine levels. Similarly, developmental differences in the expression of isoforms of the regulatory subunit of G proteins have also been identified. The interaction of adrenergic innervation, catecholamine levels, and functional changes in multiple proteins that regulate responses to various agonists is complex and difficult to accurately extrapolate to clinical scenarios.

The newborn has the highest cardiac output per weight than any other age group (~200 mL/kg per min). Teitel and others (1985) hypothesized that the greater increase in performance with adrenergic stimulation observed in the older lamb is due to a "lesser resting β-adrenergic tone"; that is, the baseline state of the newborn myocardium is at a higher level of "β-adrenergic tone."

The fetus (i.e., preterm baby) may have impaired ventricular function secondary to decreased sympathetic innervation, decreased β-adrenoceptor concentration, immaturity of the sarcoplasmic reticulum structurally and functionally, and decreased number of myofibrils. This anatomy and physiology persist into the neonatal period, but cardiac output rapidly increases and cardiac performance is at a high level shortly after birth.

Myocardial Function

The major differences in myocardial function between the neonate and adult heart translate into important clinical applications (summarized in Box 16–5). The high content of collagen and high ratio of type I to type III collagen may account for the relative noncompliance of the neonatal heart and, consequently, its limited capacity to handle a volume load. Similarly, this nondistensible heart has limited capacity to increase stroke volume to augment cardiac output in response to increasing preload. The Frank-Starling response is considered to play a limited role and the heart rate a critical function in maintaining the cardiac output in the newborn. Over the first months of life, myocardial contractility gradually increases, which allows cardiac output to be maintained over a wider range of preload and afterload.

The initial step in evaluating the cardiovascular system of the newborn is a careful physical examination. Evaluating skin color, capillary filling time, trends in the blood pressure, heart rate, intensity of the peripheral pulses, presence of a murmur or S3 or S4, and decreased urine output or metabolic acidosis may provide the initial hint of abnormal cardiovascular function and lead to early detection of a congenital heart lesion. Murmurs, abnormal heart sounds, dysrhythmias, and cardiomegaly are rarely innocuous findings in the newborn. For example, the femoral pulses are decreased with coarctation of the aorta, whereas they are bounding in patients with a large shunt or PDA. Cardiomegaly is associated with left heart outflow obstruction and with a variety of metabolic abnormalities, including hypoglycemia, hypocalcemia, and birth asphyxia. Infants with these conditions should have a thorough cardiac evaluation, including a chest radiograph, an electrocardiogram, and an echocardiogram, especially if a surgical intervention is urgent. The interpretation of these studies allows rational planning for intraoperative monitoring, selection of anesthetic agents, delivery of fluids, postoperative recovery, and the extent of the surgical procedure (e.g., total correction or staged procedure).

Hematology

At birth, a full-term newborn normally has a hemoglobin concentration of 18 to 20 g/dL; a preterm infant usually has a lower hemoglobin concentration, ranging between 13 and 15 g/dL. Approximately 70% to 80% of the hemoglobin at birth is fetal hemoglobin (HgF), but the concentration of HgF decreases to physiologically insignificant levels by 3 to 6 months of age. The high affinity of HgF to oxygen shifts the hemoglobin-oxygen dissociation curve to the left, so that P_{50} (18 to 20 mm Hg) is less than in the adult value (27 mm Hg) (Smith and Nelson, 1976). Although high oxygen affinity improves the fetus' ability for oxygen uptake from the mother at the placental interface (Stern, 1973; Downes, 1974), after birth this same high affinity decreases the amount of oxygen released at tissue levels (Pang and Mellins, 1975). In the normal newborn, higher hemoglobin levels, greater blood volume, and increased cardiac output (per unit weight) compensate adequately for HgF. Such normal-term infants tolerate the gradual decrease in hematocrit over the first few months of life with the nadir as low as 9 to 10 g/dL. By comparison, the concentration of hemoglobin in the very-low-birth-weight (VLBW)/ELBW infant at birth normally ranges between 13 to 15 g/dL. Of note, the nadir of a premature (<30 weeks gestation) infant's hemoglobin may be as low as 6 to 7 g/dL by 3 to 4 months of age. However, erythropoietin is routinely administered to infants in the neonatal intensive care unit, thereby avoiding such a profound anemia (Soubasi et al., 1995; Al-Kharfy et al., 1996).

If a newborn is unstable secondary to congenital heart disease (especially cyanotic), sepsis, metabolic derangement, or other anomalies, the ability to compensate for HgF may be marginal. Such newborns with cardiovascular or respiratory instability often benefit from maintaining the hematocrit at greater than 40% to 45% to facilitate adequate oxygen delivery. Of note, after several transfusions with adult packed red blood cells (RBCs), the negative impact of HgF becomes less relevant. Blood loss exceeding 10% to 15% of the blood volume (or even less in some patients) may not be tolerated by newborns, especially the VLBW infants. Cross-matched blood should be available for any surgery, especially when blood loss is anticipated (see Chapter 2, Respiratory Physiology in Infants and Children).

Assessing clotting function should be considered before major surgery in the newborn for several reasons. First, the synthesis of prothrombin and factors II, VII, and X in the liver is immature. Second, perinatal asphyxia and septicemia affect function and concentration of both clotting factors and platelet count, resulting in coagulopathies. Before surgical intervention, the availability of the requirements for fresh frozen plasma, fibrinogen, and/or platelets must be assessed (see Chapter 32, Systemic Disorders in Infants and Children).

Renal Function

The fetal kidney is a passive organ, which at birth undergoes a transition to an active organ. Each day 200 to 1000 mL of urine is produced, depending on gestational age. Urine production increases from about 5 mL/hr at 20 weeks gestation, to 18 mL/hr at 30 weeks, and to 50 mL/hr at 40 weeks (Rabinowitz et al., 1989). The fetal kidney handles a large volume load and produces large amounts of hypotonic urine. However, the kidney is not essential for maintaining the normal fluid and electrolyte balance of the fetus in utero. Production of urine is important to maintain normal amnionic fluid volume, and, in that way, urine volume contributes to normal pulmonary and urinary tract development. The term newborn kidney usually has fetal lobulations but the full number of nephrons (i.e., 1×10^6/kidney) found in the adult kidney (McDonald and Emery, 1959) (see Chapter 4, Regulation of Body Fluids and Electrolytes in Infants and Children).

The renal function of the newborn compared with the adult is characterized by a decreased glomerular filtration rate

BOX 16–5 Comparison of Neonatal and Adult Myocardial Functions

	Neonate	Adult
Cardiac output	Rate dependent	Stroke volume and rate
Contractility	Reduced	Normal
Starling response	Limited	Normal
Catecholamine response	Reduced	Normal
Compliance	Reduced	Normal

(GFR), decreased solid excretion, and decreased concentrating power. In the first 24 hours of life, GFR may be as low as 4 mL/min per 1.73 m^2 in infants of less than 25 weeks gestational age. The GFR increases with gestational age, and by 34 to 36 weeks of gestation, values of 25 mL/min per 1.73 m^2 are achieved, similar to those reported for full-term infants (Svenningsen and Aronson, 1974). Over the first 3 months of life, GFR increases twofold to threefold. Thereafter, a slower rise is noted until adult values are reached by 12 to 24 months of life.

Renal function does respond to "demand" (solute exposure), and the newborn kidney improves its filtration and concentrating capacities if challenged. The high anabolic rate associated with growth does counteract the limited ability to excrete solute, because growth requires incorporation of calcium, nitrogen, sodium, phosphorus, and water into the new tissues. At 34 weeks gestational age, GFR increases markedly, whether the kidney is in utero or extrauterine. The GFR and tubular function of a 2-week-old 34-week-postconceptual age infant may be greater than a 1-day-old born at 34 weeks gestation. That is, the maturation of renal function in preterm infants after birth may be accelerated.

Maximum urinary osmolality after a DDAVP stimulation test was about 520 mOsm/kg in 30- to 35-week-gestation infants and 570 mOsm/kg in term infants at 4 to 6 weeks of age. In comparison, 1- to 2-year-old children responded to DDAVP by concentrating to 1300 to 1400 mOsm/kg (Svenningson and Aronson, 1974). The majority of infants are still not able to concentrate as well as adults by 6 to 12 months of life. The therapeutic index for fluid and electrolytes is narrow in the newborn, especially the VLBW infant in the first days after birth when insensible water loss may be enormous. In healthy children and adolescents, evaporation accounts for approximately 40% of total baseline water losses. However, in premature neonates, insensible water evaporation is several magnitudes greater because of marked transepidermal permeability as well as relatively large body surface area. Exposed premature infants have a 15 times more evaporative losses than do naked term infants during the first few days after birth (Hammarlund et al., 1983). An exposed VLBW infant can lose 10% of body weight during the first day of life by this route. Increased respiratory exchange in premature neonates can also contribute to water loss.

In addition to limited GFR, the tubular function of the neonatal kidney is immature. The discrepancy between the inner and the outer cortical nephrons is striking both anatomically and functionally. The inner nephrons (juxtamedullary) are more functional, as manifested by the length of the tubules when outer and inner cortical nephrons are compared. Because the site of filtering, the glomerulus, is uniform in its function, this leads to what is termed a "tubular/glomerular" imbalance. This imbalance in part explains why the urine of the newborn characteristically has a higher percentage of the filtered load (i.e., reabsorption at the proximal tubule has not occurred).

The limited tubular reabsorptive function of the kidney is the basis for the loss of bicarbonate and the "normal" acidosis that occurs in the newborn, particularly the premature (Vanpee et al., 1988) (sometimes called renal tubular acidosis, type 4). The pH of the urine may be greater than 5 despite a serum total carbon dioxide of 15 to 18. At some point, the threshold for bicarbonate loss is reached, the urine pH is 5.0 and a mild-moderate metabolic acidosis persists.

Similarly, proximal tubular reabsorption of sodium increases with gestational age; the percentage of filtered sodium excreted in the urine is at least 5% in the less-than-30-week-gestation infant and about 0.2% in the term infant (Vanpee et al., 1988). Of note, hypoxia, respiratory distress, and hyperbilirubinemia can increase fractional sodium excretion.

The distal tubular function also limits the ability of the kidney to excrete a sodium load. Until 34 weeks gestation, the level of aldosterone, the response to aldosterone, or both are low (Aperia et al., 1979). The premature proximal tubule fails to reabsorb sodium effectively and delivers a high load of sodium to the distal tubule, which is also unable to salvage this electrolyte. Furthermore, the preterm infant has high levels of circulating atrial natriuretic peptide, prostaglandins, and progesterone, all of which contribute to a negative sodium balance (Tulassay et al., 1986). High levels of ADH have been measured in the urine of both term and preterm infants in response to hypoxia, atelectasis, intraventricular hemorrhage, and BPD (Wiriyathian et al., 1986). In part, this nonosmotic secretion of ADH accounts for the dilutional hyponatremia of the newborn, especially the premature. The limited urinary concentrating ability in the fetus and newborn can be correlated with the immature medullary concentration gradient, decreased response to ADH, and an immature aldosterone system.

Finally, plasma rennin activity (PRA) is inversely related to gestational age, increasing slightly at 3 to 6 days of postnatal life and then decreasing over the next 3 to 6 weeks. Thereafter, a gradual decline is noted. The physiologic significance of the high PRA levels in the neonatal period may be related to the renal salt wasting and negative salt balance that occur in the first few weeks of extrauterine life.

Serum potassium levels of greater than 5.0 mmol/L are not uncommon in newborns, particularly premature infants with a mild metabolic acidosis. In addition to a relative hyperkalemia secondary to metabolic acidosis, nonoliguric hyperkalemia has been described in the ELBW infant (Mildenberger, 2002). The disorder is characterized by a rapid rise of serum potassium, usually in the first day of life and not later than 72 hours after birth. The proposed mechanism is a rapid shift of potassium from intracellular to extracellular compartments, but the etiology of the phenomenon is unclear. Treatment has included the well-accepted regimen (insulin/glucose and calcium/bicarbonate, as well as diuretics and binding resins).

Central Nervous System

Common derangements of early brain development correlate with abnormalities in one of the two major structures of embryogenesis: neural tube and prosencephalon (Volpe, 2001a). Primary neural tube (3 to 4 weeks) and prosencephalon (2 to 3 months) development are complete early in gestation. Neural tube anomalies that are associated with these early events are dramatic and often fatal: anencephaly, craniorachischisis totalis, myeloshisis, and encephalocele. Less severe defects include myelomeningocele, a restricted version of abnormal neural tube closure. This defect is the most clinically important, because the affected infants frequently survive. Hydrocephalus frequently accompanies myelomeningocele—60% in occipital, cervical, thoracic, or sacral lesions and about 90% in thoracolumbar, lumbar, or lumbosacral lesions. The Arnold-Chiari malformation is common in this second group of patients and frequently contributes to the development of the hydrocephalus via obstruction of fourth ventricular outflow or aqueductal stenosis. Similar to neural tube defects, severe prosencephalic anomalies (holoprosencephalies) are often fatal, especially those associated with chromosomal abnormalities (e.g., trisomy 13-15, trisomy/ring/deletion 18).

Less severe disorders such as agenesis of the corpus callosum and of the septum pellucidum are less often fatal but are frequently associated with abnormal neuronal migration and, in those cases, are accompanied by significant clinical abnormalities. Isolated agenesis of the corpus callosum can be asymptomatic. Partial agenesis syndromes are likely to have occurred later in development and are associated with a range of clinical syndromes correlated with coexistent migrational and structural disorders.

After the primary structure of the neural tube and the prosencephalon are established during the first 2 to 3 months of gestation, development of the central nervous system entails proliferation and migration. These developmental processes are likely to have the greatest effect on prognosis for the preterm infant.

Proliferation of neurons proceeds from the ventricular and subventricular regions at every level of the developing nervous system. From the second to the fourth month of gestation, some glia is forming but the primary process is neuronal proliferation. From the fifth month of gestation forward into adult life, glial multiplication is the primary process. This developmental process of moving from ventricle to subventricular site is of particular relevance when considering the pathophysiology of the preterm infant. Glial development does occur to a limited degree during early gestation, as these cells are vital for normal migration. Arterial and venous supply is established during neuronal proliferation. The two neuropathologic diagnoses that define the pattern of injury in the preterm infant are periventricular hemorrhagic infarction and periventricular leukomalacia.

Intracranial Hemorrhage-Germinal Matrix/Intraventricular Hemorrhage

The pathophysiology of this lesion is related to the structure of the immature brain (Volpe, 2001b and 1997; Lou et al., 2001). The proliferating region of the ventricular and subventricular areas of the developing nervous system is richly cellular and vascularized, and between 10 to 20 weeks of gestation is the site of origin of the neuroblasts. In the third trimester, this area is the source of glioblasts. The region is gelatinous in mid-gestation, but during the final 12 to 16 weeks of gestation, it gradually degenerates and is barely present in the term infant. The dense and well-developed vascular network at mid-gestation drains into a venous system that receives blood from the entire brain and terminates at the level of the head of the caudate nucleus, where the veins join the vein of Galen. The junction of capillaries with veins (rather than at arteries or arterioles) appears to be the site of bleeding in the premature brain. From 28 to 32 weeks gestation, the germinal matrix is most prominent at the level of the head of the caudate nucleus. This is the usual site of the germinal matrix hemorrhage.

Periventricular Leukomalacia

This bilaterally symmetrical, nonhemorrhagic lesion represents necrosis of white matter dorsal and lateral to the external angles of the lateral ventricles. More diffuse cerebral white matter injury has also been described. Periventricular leukomalacia is sometimes inappropriately described as a consequence of intraventricular hemorrhage, because both are frequently identified at the same time on the same scan. However, periventricular leukomalacia is a postischemic lesion, not a venous infarction (Takashima, 1986). Focal necrosis is seen pathologically. Tissue destruction may lead to formation of cavities and cysts. Eventually, with the loss of oligodendrocytes and abnormal myelination, the volume of white matter decreases and ventriculomegaly may develop. The most consistent clinical correlate of periventricular leukomalacia is spastic diplegia.

Autoregulation of Cerebral Blood Flow

Critically ill newborns often require mechanical ventilatory support, airway suctioning, and intravenous fluid boluses, all which may dramatically affect blood pressure, cardiac output, and heart rate. Episodes of metabolic instability (e.g., hypoglycemia, hypercarbia, hypocarbia, hypoxia, hyponatremia/hypernatremia, hypocalcemia) also can have dramatic effects on the hemodynamic status. Such fluctuation in blood pressure and cardiac output can have major impact on the central nervous system of the newborn, because the autoregulation of the cerebral blood flow is incomplete at this developmental stage compared with that seen in the adult. Autoregulation of cerebral blood flow seems to be intact over a wide range of arterial blood pressure of both preterm and term newborns (Fig. 16–2), but the range is narrower for the preterm infant. Of particular significance, the normal blood pressure of the preterm is at the lower range of the autoregulatory limit. With decreasing gestational age, this lower limit is closer and closer to normal blood pressure. Similarly, the upper range of autoregulation may be approached during later gestational development when arterial pressure increases (Papile et al., 1985). Furthermore, this normal range of autoregulation is disturbed or disrupted during hypoxia, acidosis, seizures, and with the low diastolic blood pressure of a PDA (Lou et al., 1979). A rapid increase in blood pressure may produce bleeding of the fragile vessels of the immature brain, whereas hypotension and low perfusion may produce ischemia (see Chapter 18, Anesthesia for Pediatric Neurosurgery).

Metabolic Requirements

Metabolic demands for growth are enormous in the newborn, especially the LBW infant. Adequate nutrition for growth and development must be analyzed from the viewpoint of both total calories and the appropriate ratio of fat, carbohydrate, and protein. These requirements vary enormously depending on gestational and postnatal age, cardiovascular status and perfusion, organ function (i.e., liver and kidney), infection, environmental temperature, metabolic rate, and other factors.

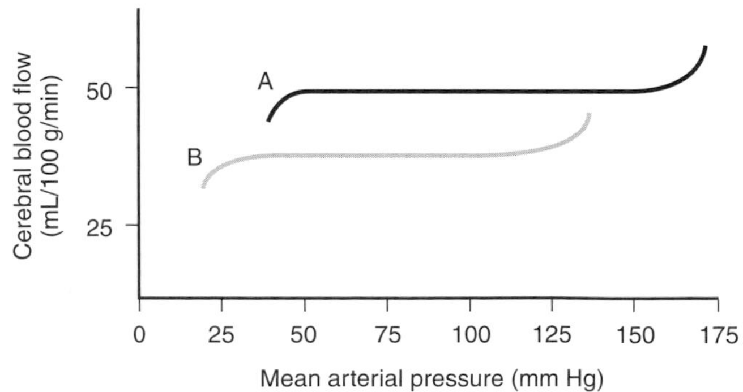

■ **FIGURE 16–2.** Autoregulation of cerebral circulation in neonates (curve B) and adults (curve A). (Redrawn from Harris MM: Pediatric neuroanesthesia. In Berry FA, editor: *Anesthetic management of difficult and routine pediatric patients,* 2nd ed. New York, 1990, Churchill Livingstone, pp 341–362. After data of Hernandez MJ, Brennan RW, Vannucci RC, Bowman GS: *Am J Physiol* 234:R209–R215, 1978.)

In addition, the major substrate to provide an adequate "energy source" varies from organ to organ. For example, brain and heart derive their energy from glucose metabolism. However, hepatic glycogen stores, the main source of glucose, are limited in the neonate, particularly those who are LGA or SGA. Thus, hypoglycemia in the neonatal period can be a major source of morbidity, causing apnea, hypotension, bradycardia, convulsions, and brain injury (Senior, 1973).

Neonates are NPO for hours to days prior to and after undergoing surgery for a variety of reasons, such as nonspecific ileus, a primary gastrointestinal anomaly, and/or cardiovascular instability secondary to sepsis (e.g., necrotizing enterocolitis). These infants must receive their nutrition (120 kcal/kg per day) via intravenous alimentation. Delivery of total parenteral nutrition (TPN) requires meticulous monitoring of body weight, urine output, electrolytes (sodium, potassium, chloride, magnesium, calcium, total carbon dioxide, etc.), total protein, albumin, blood urea nitrogen, and creatinine. The daily calculation of TPN is often uncomplicated, if the basic "rules" for increasing glucose, maintaining the appropriate nonprotein-to-protein ratio, and maintaining the relative percentage of total calories from fat and carbohydrate, are followed.

Calcium

Hypocalcemia is common in term infants who have not started oral feeds during the first day of life, have been asphyxiated, or have an underlying metabolic disorder (e.g., DiGeorge syndrome).

Slightly less than half of the total serum calcium is free or ionized, and most of the nonfree calcium is bound to protein (mostly albumin). The free calcium correlates with adequate cell function, so the ionized calcium concentration (1.0 to 1.3 mmol/L) is more physiologically relevant than the total calcium concentration. In older children and adults, the total calcium adequately estimates physiologic calcium. The serum calcium level in healthy full-term neonates averages 9 mg/dL during the first 40 hours of life (Root and Harrison, 1976), which is within the range of normal adult levels (8.7 to 10.1 mg/dL). Each 1 g/dL of albumin in the serum binds about 0.8 mg/dL of calcium, so that a low total calcium concentration may not be abnormal in the setting of significant hypoalbuminemia. Because total protein and albumin values are normally lower in the newborn and even lower in the VLBW infant, total calcium is an unreliable estimate of calcium status in the newborn.

Neonatal hypocalcemia is linked to the sudden cessation of active transplacental delivery of calcium (Tsang et al., 1973) (fetal levels are higher than those of the mother). Newborns may have a transient hypoparathyroidism secondary to the high fetal levels of calcium as well as refractoriness of the target cells to parathyroid hormone. Asphyxia elicits secretion of calcitonin, which also contributes to hypocalcemia of "sick" term or premature infants. The effect of these hormonal factors is further exacerbated by limited enteral intake by a "sick" and/or preterm infant. The incidence of hypocalcemia is inversely proportional to gestational age and birth weight and is common if adequate intake of calcium is not promptly established after birth. Infants of diabetic mothers have the additional factor of hypomagnesemia contributing to abnormal hypoparathyroid function (secondary hypoparathyroidism) and hypocalcemia. However, extrapolating these data to nonhealthy infants with abnormal blood volumes and multiorgan dysfunction is impossible. Other factors that contribute to neonatal hypocalcemia are abnormal intrauterine growth patterns (SGA, LGA), the administration of sodium bicarbonate, exchange transfusion with citrated blood, and alkalosis associated with hyperventilation (Bergman et al., 1974). In general, signs and symptoms of hypocalcemia are nonspecific and include hypotension, irritability, jitteriness, twitching, seizures, and, rarely, cyanosis and vomiting.

Glucose

SGA and LGA infants, especially those who are also preterm or have diabetic mothers, are at high risk for developing hypoglycemia. When enteral feeding is promptly established in the term infant, normal serum glucose levels range between 60 and 80 mg/dL. If the glucose level falls to less than 40 mg/dL, treatment should be initiated. Similar to hypocalcemia, hypoglycemia has nonspecific signs and symptoms—jitteriness, cyanosis, apnea, lethargy, hypotonia, and seizures. Hypoglycemic babies must be treated rapidly to prevent neurologic damage (Koivisto et al., 1972). In some cases (e.g., stable term infants), this may simply involve increasing oral intake and remeasuring the glucose every 30 to 60 minutes until the value is greater than 60 mg/dL for several hours and oral feedings are well established. In high-risk infants (e.g., infant of a diabetic mother) or those who are not likely to establish full enteral feedings (e.g., cleft palate, asphyxiated infants), intravenous treatment is preferred. In some cases, nasogastric feeds might be initiated.

The etiology of hypoglycemia is often clear—perinatal hypoxemia, sepsis, high circulating levels of insulin (Milner, 1972) in the infant of a diabetic mother, LGA or SGA, etc. In the preterm infant, inadequate glycogen stores and deficient gluconeogenesis are also important factors. In such high-risk infants, routine monitoring for hypoglycemia is critical because hypoglycemia is often asymptomatic or can be similar to symptoms and signs of other metabolic or systemic disorders. Treatment of hypoglycemia in LBW and critically ill infants consists of slow intravenous administration of a 250- to 500-mg/kg bolus of glucose as a D_5 or D_{10} solution, followed by an infusion of 10% to 15% dextrose solution to deliver 4 to 6 mg/kg per min and titrated to maintain the serum glucose at greater than 40 mg/dL, preferably 80 to 120 mg/dL (Box 16–6). Monitoring the glucose level is also critical to avoid hyperglycemia. A hyperosmolar state in a newborn, especially a VLBW infant, can result in intraventricular hemorrhage, osmotic diuresis, dehydration, and further release of insulin, leading to subsequent hypoglycemia.

Hyperinsulinism occurs infrequently in infants and is associated with erythroblastosis fetalis (Barrett and Oliver, 1968), Beckwith-Wiedemann syndrome, insulin-secreting pancreatic tumors, and polycythemia (Bedard and Kotagal, 1981).

Acid-Base Balance

Neonatal acid-base abnormalities can evolve from intrauterine problems (e.g., bleeding, infection, placental pathology) intrapartum events (e.g., umbilical cord prolapse, bleeding, prolonged or complicated labor), or intrinsic fetal anomalies (e.g., congenital heart disease, diaphragmatic hernia, upper airway or lung anomalies). A variety of etiologies may set the stage for cardiorespiratory depression in the newborn. Some neonatologists measure the pH, P_{O_2}, and P_{CO_2} from the umbilical vein (from the placenta) immediately after birth to assess the severity of the birth asphyxia. The acid-base status of the depressed newborn must be monitored serially to guide treatment (Table 16–3). Treatment and correction of acidosis (pH < 7.20) with intravenous sodium bicarbonate and glucose and mechanical ventilation can improve perfusion and oxygen delivery. Often acidosis clears as

BOX 16–6 Common Intravenous Fluid and Electrolyte Requirements in the Newborn

Glucose

Most newborns require 2 to 4 mg/kg per min.
Small-/large-for-gestational-age (SGA/LGA) infants may require >15 mg/kg per min on days 1 to 3 of life.
Glucose tolerance may fluctuate significantly in very low and extremely low birth weight (VLBW and ELBW) infants.

Sodium

Most newborns require no sodium for the first 24 hours of life.
On day 2 and beyond, most newborns receive 2 to 4 mEq/kg per day.
Sodium requirement may change dramatically in response to gastrointestinal, genitourinary, or transcutaneous losses, drug or metabolic effects.
The ELBW infant may have huge transcutaneous fluid losses, requiring meticulous monitoring and replacement.

Potassium

Requirements for potassium are minimal for the first 24 to 48 hours of life.
Subsequently, maintenance delivery is about 1 to 3 mEq/kg per day, always in the presence of a normal urine output.
Serum levels in the newborn, especially VLBW and ELBW, are higher than in older infants.
Replace gastrointestinal, genitourinary, or iatrogenic losses cautiously.

Calcium

Requirements for calcium range between 200 and 400 mg/kg per day (calcium gluconate).
Requirements for calcium vary with gestational age, history of asphyxia, growth disturbances (SGA, LGA).
Serum levels can be obtained for total Ca^{2+} and/or ionized Ca^{2+}.

perfusion is established with neonatal resuscitation. Establishing effective ventilation of the lungs with or without intubation of the trachea is the critical maneuver, but crystalloid or colloid infusion may also be necessary. Rarely are chest compressions or vasoactive medications (e.g., epinephrine) necessary. Sodium bicarbonate should only be given after ventilation is established and the PCO_2 is less than 35 mm Hg and the pH remains less than 7.20. Sodium bicarbonate is hyperosmolar and should be delivered slowly at a dose of 0.5 to 1 mEq/kg. Subsequent treatment with bicarbonate is based on frequent measurement of blood gases, serum electrolytes, and osmolality.

Electrolytes

The anesthesiologist must analyze the cardiorespiratory status, urine output, and laboratory values in the preoperative period to manage the neonate's fluid and electrolyte therapy. This is the framework for developing a rational plan for administering "maintenance fluid" during surgery.

Similar to the acid-base status, electrolyte abnormalities in the newborn are often secondary to intrauterine or intrapartum events or congenital anomalies that lead to asphyxia. That is, asphyxia is associated with hypocalcemia and hypoglycemia, renal failure (acute tubular necrosis), and myocardial depression. In addition, primary gastrointestinal malformations can lead to poor feeding and vomiting and dependence on intravenous fluids or TPN, predisposing to overhydration and other iatrogenic electrolyte problems.

Hypernatremia may occur in dehydrated infants if water loss is greater than sodium depletion, whereas hyponatremia occurs frequently in infants receiving salt-free solutions or water in excess of sodium. Inadequate or abnormal renal tubular function predisposes to serum sodium abnormalities. Hypokalemia can result from aggressive diuresis, respiratory alkalosis, and vomiting. Hyperkalemia may be caused by hypoperfusion states, massive blood transfusion, renal failure, or the administration of large amounts of potassium-containing solutions. Abnormalities in electrolyte balance may increase morbidity during anesthesia secondary to arrhythmias and, rarely, cardiac arrest.

Temperature Regulation

At birth, the newborn arrives abruptly into a cooler environment and loses thermal protection, and temperature regulation suddenly becomes an important and calorically expensive physiologic function. Once delivered, the infant loses heat via evaporation, convection, conduction, and radiation (see Chapter 5, Thermoregulation: Physiology and Perioperative Disturbances).

Neonates are homeotherms whose compensatory mechanisms to maintain core body temperature operate within a narrow

TABLE 16–3. Normal pH and blood gas values in umbilical arterial blood of the full-term neonate

	AGE OF NEWBORN			
	5 minutes	*1 hour*	*1 day*	*7 days*
pH	7.21 ± 0.05	7.33 ± 0.03	7.37 ± 0.03	7.37 ± 0.05
$PaCO_2$ (mm Hg)	46 ± 7	36 ± 4	33 ± 3	36 ± 3
Base excess (mmol/L)	–8 ± 2	–6 ± 1	–5 ± 1	–3 ± 1
PaO_2 (mm Hg)	50 ± 10	63 ± 11	73 ± 10	73 ± 10
Hematocrit (%)	53 ± 6	54 ± 5	55 ± 7	51 ± 8

Value are given as mean ± SD.
From Koch G, Wendel H: *Biol Neonate* 12:136, 1968, with permission from S. Karger AG, Basel.

environmental temperature range. In addition, many factors increase the neonate's tendency to lose heat: large surface area–to–body weight ratio, reduced subcutaneous fat, and an underdeveloped ability to shiver in response to cold. The major compensatory mechanism in response to cold stress is to produce heat by nonshivering thermogenesis. Nonshivering thermogenesis involves the release of norepinephrine, which initiates triglyceride and fatty acid metabolism in the energy-rich brown fat deposits of the newborn (Stern et al., 1965). Heat produced by this mechanism is extremely costly in the ill neonate because the energy available in brown fat is needed for growth and development.

Hypothermia increases oxygen consumption dramatically. The environmental temperature for the newborn in which oxygen consumption is minimal has been defined as the "neutral thermal environment." Oxygen consumption is minimal when the newborn's skin temperature is 36°C, and the environment temperature is between 32° and 34°C (Adamsons and Towell, 1965) (see Fig. 5–2, Chapter 5, Thermoregulation: Physiology and Perioperative Disturbances). Prematurity, hypoglycemia, and general anesthesia can exaggerate the neonate's metabolic responses to hypothermia (Swyer, 1975). Prolonged exposure to a hypothermic environment can place increased demands that may exceed the neonatal cardiopulmonary capacity for compensation. This can result in hypoventilation, inadequate oxygen delivery, tissue acidosis, and cardiovascular collapse (Gandy et al., 1965).

ANESTHETIC PHARMACOLOGY IN THE NEONATE

Increasing evidence indicates that the physiologic response of neonates to painful stimuli is similar to that of adults (see Chapter 13, Pain Management in Infants and Children). The response of the sympathetic nervous system to noxious stimulation includes tachycardia and hypertension, which in the setting of abnormal cerebral autoregulation predisposes the LBW infant to intraventricular hemorrhage and possibly pulmonary hypertension. The goal during anesthesia is to avoid pain and its cardiovascular and neurologic consequences. The response of newborns to narcotics and potent inhalation agents is variable, and meticulous titration is critical for neonates undergoing surgery to avoid cardiovascular collapse and to maintain acid-base balance but to eliminate awareness and pain.

Drug pharmacokinetics and pharmacodynamics are affected by anatomic factors relating to body composition and distribution of water as well as physiologic factors (metabolism [i.e., hepatic biotransformation], protein binding, and pathologic factors [disease, anesthesia, and surgery]). Maturational changes in distribution of total body water, in tissue composition, and in organ function contribute to the unique response of the newborn and young infant to various drugs. In early fetal development, water constitutes approximately 94% of body weight. As gestation continues, the total body water decreases so that at 32 weeks, 80% to 90% of body weight is water, and at term, total body water is approximately 70% to 75% of body weight. Adult proportions of fluid to body weight (55%) are reached between the age of 9 months and 2 years. The distribution of water between the extracellular and intracellular compartments also changes during fetal growth. Extracellular water (interstitial fluid plus plasma volume) decreases from 60% of body weight at the fifth month of fetal life to approximately 45% at term. Intracellular water increases from 25% in the fifth month of fetal life to 33% at birth. So, the extracellular fluid compartment of the newborn is equal to or greater than the intracellular fluid space. In adults, the intracellular and extracellular fluid compartments are approximately 40% and 20% of body weight, respectively. Because the plasma component of the extracellular fluid compartment remains at approximately 5% of body weight throughout life, it is the interstitial water that is greater in infancy (40%) and declines to 10% to 15% in the adult (Friis-Hansen, 1971).

Age-dependent changes in body composition also occur. At term, fat constitutes 11% of body weight. Fat content doubles by 6 months of age and is approximately 30% at 1 year. Teenage girls remain at approximately 20% to 30% fat, whereas teenage boys decrease to 10% to 15%. Moreover, the composition of fat tissue changes with age. Fat of the newborn may contain as much as 57% water and 35% lipids; adults have 26% water and 71% lipids (Friis-Hansen, 1971). Skeletal muscle comprises 25% of total body mass in a term newborn compared with 43% in an adult.

The binding of drugs to serum proteins depends on several factors, such as the concentration of protein, the number of binding sites on these proteins, and the affinity of the binding sites. The concentration of total serum protein, albumin, and α_1-acid glycoprotein is lower in early infancy and reaches adult levels by approximately 1 year (Pacifica and others, 1986). Albumin primarily binds acidic drugs; α_1-acid glycoprotein binds basic drugs. The concentration of these two proteins and their binding affinities are deficient in the newborn (Piafsky and Woolner, 1982).

The primary organ for drug biotransformation is the liver, but the kidney, intestine, lung, and skin also have minor roles. Hepatic oxidation, reduction, and hydrolysis (nonsynthetic, phase I reactions) mature rapidly, achieving adult rates by 6 months (Niems et al., 1976). Drugs metabolized via this cytochrome P450–dependent mono-oxygenase system include phenobarbital and phenytoin. Conjugation reactions (synthetic, phase II reactions) convert drugs into more polar compounds to facilitate renal excretion. These systems also mature postnatally.

The renal excretion of drugs is a function of glomerular filtration rate (GFR), active secretion, and passive reabsorption. GFR and secretion increase in an age-dependent manner. Renal blood flow (Hook and Bailie, 1979) and GFR (Arant, 1978) increase dramatically during the first postnatal week and more gradually during the next several months, and adult performance is achieved at approximately 6 to 12 months of age. Tubular secretory and reabsorptive capacity also mature postnatally (Fetterman et al., 1965).

Cardiac output and its distribution to various organs contribute to drug elimination. The perinatal adaptation to extrauterine life demands rapid changes in the circulation. This process may be inhibited as a result of congenital heart disease or acid-base problems. Drug metabolism and elimination may be drastically affected when cardiovascular function is abnormal.

INHALED ANESTHETIC AGENTS

Infants have a higher incidence of cardiovascular instability and cardiac arrest during induction of inhalation anesthesia than do older persons (Rackow et al., 1961; Friesen and Lichtor, 1982, 1983; Morray, 2000, 2002; Murat et al., 2004). This untoward effect of potent inhalation agents can be attributed to several factors, including faster equilibration, rapid myocardial uptake in infants, increased anesthetic requirement, and sensitivity of the neonatal myocardium. Infants attain a higher concentration of inhaled anesthetic agents in the heart and brain than do adults at the same inspired concentration. Moreover, the neonatal myocardium has decreased contractile mass, and the magnitude and velocity of fiber shortening are less than in the adult myocardium. These factors and the increased anesthetic requirement, which is inversely related to age, all produce a higher incidence of adverse cardiovascular effects in infants.

The rate of rise of the alveolar concentration of an inhaled anesthetic depends on several factors: the inspired concentration, alveolar ventilation, and uptake. The greater the alveolar ventilation, the faster is the rate of rise of the alveolar concentration. This effect of alveolar ventilation is affected by the size of the functional residual capacity (FRC). Infants and children have an FRC similar to that of the adult: 30 mL/kg per min. In contrast, alveolar ventilation is much higher in the infant (100 to 150 mL/kg per min) compared with the adult (60 mL/kg per min). This difference parallels the greater oxygen consumption of the infant. So, in the normal term newborn who weighs 3.0 kg, the ratio of alveolar ventilation to FRC is approximately 5:1, compared with the adult, in whom the same ratio is 1.5:1. As a result of this difference, the time constant of the inhaled anesthetic equilibrium for infants is much shorter than for the adult. Consequently, changes in concentrations of inspired gas are reflected rapidly in alveolar levels. In fact, it has been demonstrated that alveolar levels of inhalational anesthetic agents reach equilibrium faster in infants that in adults (see Chapter 6, Pharmacology of Pediatric Anesthesia).

The rise of the alveolar concentration of an inhaled anesthetic is opposed by uptake of the agent into lung tissue and, more important, blood. Three factors determine inhaled anesthetic uptake: cardiac output, the alveolar-to-mixed venous anesthetic partial pressure difference, and solubility. Each of these factors has unique aspects in the infant, compared with in the adult, and consequently affects the pharmacology of the uptake of inhaled agents.

The greater the cardiac output, the greater is the anesthetic uptake. The cardiac output of the newborn is 250 to 300 mL/kg per min; by 8 weeks, the cardiac output has decreased to 150 mL/kg per min. The cardiac output of young infants is approximately 3 to 6 times that of the normal adult (70 mL/kg per min). By itself, this high cardiac output should significantly decrease the rate of rise of the alveolar concentration of the soluble anesthetic agents. However, the newborn distributes a greater proportion of this cardiac output to the vessel-rich group of organs and less to the muscle and fat group. The equilibrium between the inspired and alveolar concentration of inhaled agent occurs more rapidly because uptake decreases faster.

Because the cardiac output is predominantly distributed to the vessel-rich group and because the muscle group is small, the arterial-venous partial pressure difference narrows quickly in the young and thereby decreases uptake.

Both left-to-right and right-to-left shunting occurs in infants. A left-to-right shunt results in an increase in total cardiac output. However, the shunted blood does not lose anesthetic to tissue; instead it returns to the lung with the same anesthetic partial pressure. This recycled blood cannot accept more anesthetic agent unless the alveolar partial pressure has risen. Thus, a left-to-right shunt has no effect on anesthetic uptake. A right-to-left shunt slows the rate of rise of the alveolar concentration of an inhaled anesthetic. The anesthetic-deficient–shunted blood dilutes the concentration of the anesthetic in the blood, decreasing the partial pressure of anesthetic in the arterial circulation. This slows the rate of rise of the anesthetic by slowing tissue uptake and equilibration.

Lerman and others (Lerman et al., 1984; Malviya and Lerman, 1990) reported that the blood-gas partition coefficient in newborns was consistently lower than that in adults by 18%. They also found that two or more serum constituents (albumin, globulin, triglyceride, cholesterol) are required to predict the blood-gas partition coefficient of isoflurane, enflurane, halothane, and methoxyflurane in all age groups. However, in a later study, blood-gas partition coefficients of isoflurane, halothane, and sevoflurane did not differ in preterm compared with term infants but were lower than in adults. Only serum cholesterol correlated with the blood-gas partition coefficients (Malviya and Lerman, 1990). The blood-gas partition coefficient is an important determinant of solubility and, therefore, the rate of rise of the alveolar concentration of an inhaled agent.

The effect of age on the solubility of the inhaled agents in tissue is also important in determining the rate of rise of the alveolar concentration of the agent—the rate of anesthetic induction. Data by Lerman and others (1986) are consistent with earlier work documenting that anesthetic solubility in brain, heart, liver, and muscle increases with age. An increase in solubility may prolong uptake, delay equilibration of the tissue partial pressure of anesthetic, and prolong the time of induction. Lerman and others found that the rate of increase in tissue anesthetic partial pressure, and, therefore alveolar anesthetic partial pressure, is approximately 30% more rapid in newborns than in adults.

Minimal alveolar concentration (MAC) is an estimate of anesthetic requirement. In the original study, Gregory and others (1969) reported that infants in the first 6 months of life had the highest MAC. In a later study, newborns were noted to require approximately 25% less halothane at MAC compared with infants who are between 1 and 6 months of age (Lerman et al., 1983) (see Chapter 6, Pharmacology of Pediatric Anesthesia).

INTRAVENOUS ANESTHETICS AND ANALGESICS

Several studies have shown an increased sensitivity to and more prolonged effects of barbiturates and morphine in the neonate and young infant (Kupferberg and Way, 1963; Way et al., 1965). These features have been attributed in part to the immaturity of the blood-brain barrier, allowing faster and greater penetration and therefore higher concentration of these drugs in the brain.

In 1981, Robinson and Gregory reported that, following a 10-mL/kg bolus of lactated Ringer's solution, 30 to 50 mcg/kg of fentanyl was a safe anesthetic for premature infants undergoing ligation of a PDA. Several years later, evidence was presented that infants who received fentanyl in combination with *d*-tubocurarine and nitrous oxide in oxygen had an improved perioperative course (Anand et al., 1987).

Plasma levels of fentanyl are lower in infants versus children versus adults (newborns were not studied) after similar intravenous doses (Singleton et al., 1987). Gauntlett and others (1988) noted in newborns that clearance of fentanyl increased during the first few weeks of life. Elimination half-life and volume of distribution did not change. In a study of newborns administered continuous fentanyl infusions, Saarenmaa and others (2000) noted that plasma clearance correlated with maturity (gestational age), whereas Santeiro and others (1997) noted a correlation of clearance with postnatal age. Koehntop and others (1986) have shown a highly variable disposition and elimination of fentanyl in neonates.

In addition, infants with increased intra-abdominal pressure (omphalocele, gastroschisis, septic ileus) appeared to have a further increase in the elimination half-life compared with infants undergoing repair of a PDA or myelomeningocele. Davis and others (1989) noted that the clearance of alfentanil in newborn premature infants was markedly reduced compared with older children (Fig. 16–3).

Koren and others (1985) have shown that the elimination half-life for morphine (13.9 hours) in human neonates is prolonged compared with that in older children and adults (2 hours). They also showed reduced clearance and higher serum concentration in neonates compared with those seen in older children after morphine infusion. Because of the large variability in clearance among neonates of different ages, the dose of opioids needs to be carefully titrated for each patient and each clinical setting.

Animal studies have shown a decreased ED_{50} for thiopental in the early weeks of life. Also, arousal in newborn rats occurred at lower brain levels of thiopental than in adult rats (Mirkin, 1975). Although this may suggest that lower doses of thiopental are needed in young neonates, studies by Jonmarker and others (1987) suggest the contrary. Similarly, ketamine requirements are greater (milligrams per kilogram of body weight) in infants than in older children (Lockhart and Nelson, 1974). Ketamine has been shown to produce apnea in infants with increased intracranial pressure (Lockhart and Jenkins, 1972). Ketamine produces hypertension and tachycardia, which some anesthesiologist have taken advantage of in caring for infants and children with congenital heart disease, cardiovascular instability, or both.

MUSCLE RELAXANTS

Developmental pharmacologic changes influence the requirements for muscle relaxants in infants and older children. Synaptic transmission is slow at birth, the rate at which acetylcholine is released during repetitive stimulation is limited, and neuromuscular reserve is reduced (Fig. 16–4). In addition, the reported sensitivity of infants to the effects of neuromuscular blocking agents has differed depending on whether drug administration was indexed to body weight or to body surface area. Because most neuromuscular blocking agents are distributed in the extracellular space and the extracellular space is related to the body surface area, dosage requirements for neuromuscular blocking agents frequently correlate with surface area rather than with body weight.

Fisher and others (1982) studied the infant's sensitivity to nondepolarizing muscle relaxants using the pharmacodynamic and pharmacokinetic properties of *d*-tubocurarine. These investigators determined the steady-state plasma concentration associated with 50% neuromuscular blockade (CP_{ss50}) and noted that infants had a lower CP_{ss50} than older children. Because the volume of distribution of *d*-tubocurarine in infants is significantly larger than that in older children, the dose (milligrams per kilogram of body weight) required to achieve the same degree of neuromuscular blockade appeared the same for infants and older children. Although the pharmacokinetic data reveal similar clearance values for infants and older children, the infant's larger volume of distribution and consequently longer elimination half-life suggest that infants need less frequent and smaller supplemental doses for continued neuromuscular relaxation. Although these data are specific for *d*-tubocurarine, the general principles can be extrapolated to other hydrophilic compounds that are primarily distributed to the "central compartment" (i.e., small volume of distribution).

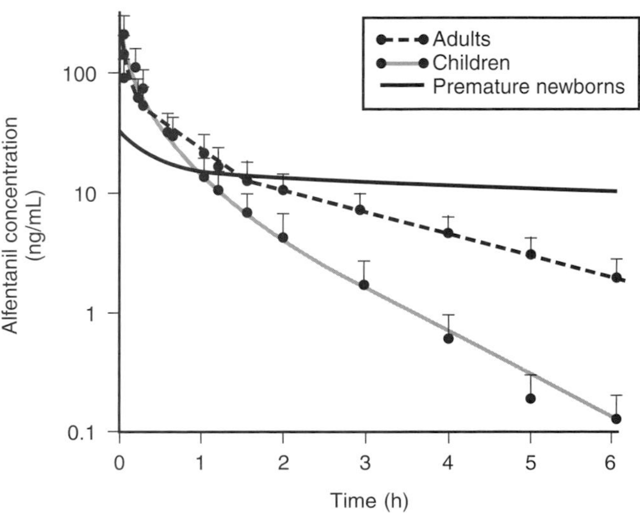

FIGURE 16–3. Age-related changes in alfentanil pharmacokinetics for premature infants, children, and adults. (From Davis CM, Brando M: Pediatric pharmacology. In Greely W, volume editor: *Atlas of anesthesiology*, vol. 7. Philadelphia, 1999, Churchill Livingstone.)

GENERAL PREANESTHETIC CONSIDERATIONS

FLUIDS

To devise a rational plan for administering fluid to the newborn during surgery requires the anesthesiologist to consider the same four components that are always relevant when analyzing what intravenous fluids are required: (1) estimating deficit, (2) calculating maintenance, (3) replacing ongoing losses, and (4) considering special losses/deficits/needs.

During the preoperative assessment, deficits should be recognized, and by the time surgery begins, dehydration or electrolyte imbalance should be reversed; that is, acidosis, low hemoglobin, poor urine output, poor perfusion, or other cardiovascular instability will have been treated appropriately. In some cases, acidosis and cardiorespiratory instability are the indications for surgery (e.g., necrotizing enterocolitis [NEC]), so that at some point,

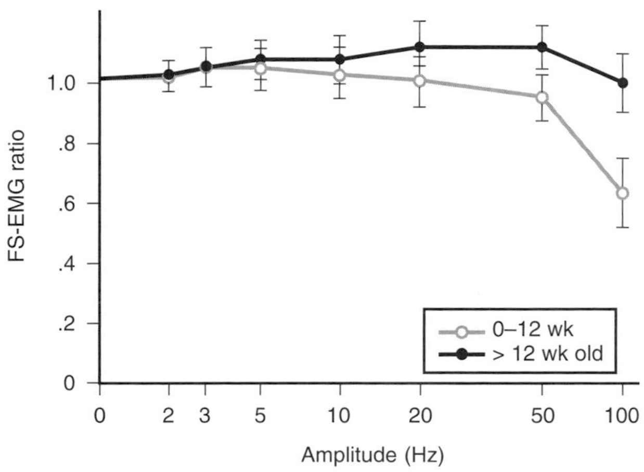

FIGURE 16–4. Tracings of the frequency sweep electromyogram (FS-EMG). (From Crumrine RS, Yodlowski EH: Assessment of neuromuscular function in infants. *Anestesiology* 54:29–32, 1981.)

proceeding with the surgery even with continuing acidosis or instability is the logical decision.

Neonates undergoing elective surgery can be fed until 4 hours before anesthesia and then given clear fluids until 2 hours before surgery. Formula is in the same category as solid food. Breast milk has been considered a "solid" by some and somewhere between a clear liquid and a solid by others. Many anesthesiologists chose an NPO range based on the frequency of routine feeding. That is, an infant feeding every 2 hours only needs to be NPO for 2 hours but another who is fed every 4 hours should be NPO for 4 hours. Few would emphasize replacing this amount of fluid before surgery.

Maintenance fluids for some infants include TPN. The anesthesiologist must note the amount of glucose/kg per minute as well as the amount of sodium, calcium, and potassium currently required by the infant (see Box 16–6) and ensure a reliable system to continue this regimen during surgery. If the TPN must be discontinued, a system for monitoring serum glucose must be incorporated into the anesthetic plan.

Third-space deficits should be replaced with infusions of an iso-osmotic solution, such as normal saline, lactated Ringer's, or Plasma-Lyte solution. That is, to avoid hyperglycemia, neither TPN nor any solution containing dextrose should be used to replace the ongoing fluid losses during surgery.

The point at which colloid should replace crystalloid varies with the patient, the surgical procedure, the anesthesiologist, and the surgeon. Most would infuse packed red blood cells after 10% to 20% of blood volume loss (10% to 20% of 100 mL/kg) or when hematocrit is less than 30% to 35% in a stable newborn. In the setting of continued instability, ongoing blood loss, and/or cyanotic heart disease, most would start blood replacement earlier. Other colloid (fresh frozen plasma, albumin, platelets) should be considered when laboratory or clinical evidence indicates that such therapy is required.

Defining what is "stable/normal" for each infant is essential before surgery. The anesthesiologist must know what the trends have been in blood pressure, heart rate, urine output, electrolytes, and ventilatory support and what interventions have been required to achieve stability. What is "stable/normal" may vary from patient to patient and from one point in time to another.

PREMEDICATION

Most newborns do not receive premedication before surgery. Some anesthesiologists might elect to premedicate certain infants—those with increased morbidity associated with transient bradycardia (e.g., cyanotic heart disease) or infants with marked airway secretions—with intravenous atropine (10 to 30 mcg/kg). The vagolytic effect of atropine has been reported to counteract the bradycardia and hypotensive effects of potent inhalation agents (Friesen and Lichtor, 1982). However, a relative overdose of inhaled agent is the most likely cause of bradycardia and hypotension during halothane anesthesia, and eliminating halothane, not delivering atropine, is the appropriate response. Careful titration of inhalational agents and relying on narcotic-based anesthesia, especially in the infant who will be mechanically ventilated postoperatively, have made this indication for atropine less relevant. The antisialagogue action of atropine also may be advantageous if copious secretions are noticed, because secretions can obstruct small endotracheal tubes and airways.

GENERAL APPROACH TO INTRAOPERATIVE MANAGEMENT

Safe and effective intraoperative management of the newborn depends on understanding basic principles of physiology and pharmacology, as well as understanding technical aspects of monitoring and the anesthesia equipment.

THERMAL PROTECTION

As already described, the newborn infant loses thermal protection after birth so that measures must be taken to protect against heat loss during surgery:

- Transport the baby in a heated "isolette."
- Warm the operating room to greater than 27°C (80°F).
- Use a warming mattress (water temperature of 40°C).
- Heat and humidify gases to 36°C (at the trachea).
- Use a radiant heat warmer with a servocontrol mechanism.
- Wrap noninvolved areas with plastic.
- Warm intravenous fluids and blood.
- Warm scrubbing and irrigation solutions.

MONITORING IN THE OPERATING ROOM

Attention must be paid to fine, seemingly insignificant details in the care of a sick neonate because the margin of safety is narrow. Although advanced electronic monitoring has contributed significantly to the safety of these babies, the anesthesiologist's clinical skills, judgment, and evaluation remain indispensable.

General Observation

Color (cyanosis, pallor), chest mobility (bilateral expansion, respiratory pattern, chest compliance), and palpation (warmth, pulses, peripheral perfusion) are often difficult to assess because of the patient's position and draping on the operating room bed. The use of specific monitors depends on the planned surgical intervention and the underlying disease state.

Circulatory Monitoring

A precordial stethoscope is a simple and effective means to assess the quality of heart sounds, rate, and rhythm. A change in the intensity of heart sounds indicates a decrease in blood pressure and possibly cardiac output. Depending on the surgical procedure and the airway management (mask versus LMA versus endotracheal tube), an esophageal stethoscope is an alternative monitor for noninvasive beat-to-beat cardiovascular monitoring. Although the sensitivity of the "stethoscope" has been discussed (Hubmayr, 2004), the simplicity and accuracy of the precordial and esophageal device to monitor heart tones and breath sounds during surgery involving pediatric patients cannot be denied.

The primary role for continuous electrocardiography during anesthesia for the newborn is to detect arrhythmias, especially in the setting of electrolyte disturbance or as evidence of adverse effects of various drugs. Simple monitoring of heart rate is available via the pulse oximeter, now a routine monitor for all patients in the operating room.

In most cases, the blood pressure can be accurately monitored with an automated device based on oscillometry (e.g., Dinamap) or ultrasonic flow (e.g., Arteriosonde) if the appropriate-sized cuff is available. Cuff inflation of the automatic devices should cycle no more frequently than every 3 to 4 minutes to avoid ischemia to the arm (Waugh and Johnson, 1984). Systolic blood pressure measurements correlate with the circulating blood volume and therefore are essential to monitor and guide fluid and blood replacement. Another alternative system is a Doppler ultrasonic transducer, which has a characteristic sound that decreases in intensity with a decrease in blood pressure.

An indwelling arterial cannula allows frequent blood sampling for cardiopulmonary and biochemical evaluation. A 22- or 24-gauge cannula can be inserted percutaneously or by cutdown into a variety of sites including the radial, dorsalis pedis, or posterior tibial artery. The adequacy of circulation to the hand should be assessed before the insertion of the catheter by applying a modified Allen's test (Brodsky, 1975). Rarely, the axillary artery is cannulated. In general, the umbilical artery can be cannulated in the first 4 to 7 days of life, but this is generally avoided after the first 2 days of life because of the risks of infection and vascular emboli. The umbilical catheter tip must be above the bifurcation of the aorta and below the level of the renal arteries. The placement of the catheter must be confirmed by a radiograph demonstrating the catheter tip to be between L4 and L5.

The risk for retinopathy of prematurity necessitates meticulous monitoring of oxygen saturation in the neonate, especially the VLBW infant. Most neonatologists would recommend adjusting the inspired oxygen to maintain oxygen saturation between 90% and 95%, depending on the underlying medical status, gestational age, hemoglobin, and postnatal age (i.e., quantity of HgF). Of importance, if blood is shunting right-to-left through a PDA, the oxygen saturation measured in the lower extremities or umbilical artery (postductal site) does not reflect the oxygen saturation in the retinal vessels (preductal site). To enable simultaneous monitoring of both preductal and postductal oxygen saturation, two pulse oximeters are placed, one on the right hand (preductal) and one on a lower extremity (postductal). During right-to-left shunting through the PDA, the preductal oxygen saturation is higher than the postductal value, and the difference depends on the amount of shunting. If blood is shunting right-to-left only via the foramen ovale or other intracardiac sites (e.g., ventriculoseptal defect), the preductal and postductal oxygen saturation are equal (see Chapters 2, 3, and 19, Respiratory Physiology in Infants and Children, Cardiovascular Physiology in Infants and Children, and Anesthesia for General Abdominal, Thoracic, Urologic, and Bariatric Surgery).

An arterial cannula must be connected to a pressure transducer and slowly and continuously infused with a small volume of dilute heparin solution (0.1 to 1 U/mL) at the rate of 0.5 to 1 mL/hr. In the ELBW infant, the flush volume should be measured and included in calculating the total daily fluid intake. In addition, extreme caution is critical while flushing an arterial cannula because retrograde embolization into the cerebral circulation is possible in the small infant, especially with a patent foramen ovale or ductus arteriosus.

A central venous catheter may be indicated to administer blood, fluid, TPN, and medications and to monitor central venous pressure (CVP). Using the Seldinger technique, a catheter can be inserted percutaneously into the subclavian, internal jugular, external jugular, or femoral vein. An indwelling umbilical vein catheter is not recommended because of its association with portal vein thrombosis. All central venous catheters are associated with significant morbidity including thrombosis, emboli, and infection. Central venous catheters in the LBW infant have additional risks, from malpositioning and from the disruption of venous flow (ratio of the size of vessel to the size of the catheter is low).

Ventilatory Monitoring

The combination of immature and fragile central nervous and cardiorespiratory systems coupled with unstable chest wall mechanics and variable responses to anesthetic agents frequently leads to mechanical ventilatory support both during and after surgery for the newborn. For each patient and for each procedure, the anesthesiologist must evaluate the needs and the requirements for mechanical ventilation. For some infants, the ventilatory status might be so precarious that using the ventilator from the neonatal intensive care unit intraoperatively might offer additional options for responding to intraoperative events affecting ventilatory status. Of note, if an infant is requiring a specific mode of ventilatory support such as high frequency or oscillation, the operating room strategy should be coordinated with the critical care team.

Manual ventilation has been proposed as a technique to allow the anesthesiologist to continuously sense changes in compliance of the chest and airways. However, Spears and others (1991) noted that manual ventilation can be extremely unreliable in sensing airway compliance changes. In addition to monitoring heart sounds, the precordial or esophageal stethoscope is a simple system to monitor ventilation and quality of breath sounds. Peak airway and end-expiratory pressure should also be measured. End-tidal carbon dioxide (mass spectrometers or infrared analyzers) devices are now the "standard of care" to continuously monitor the adequacy of respiratory exchange. These devices provide a breath-to-breath level of carbon dioxide tension, and the waveform of this measurement can provide information about rebreathing, ventilator disconnection, suspected air embolism, and hypermetabolic states (see Chapter 9, Anesthesia Equipment and Monitoring).

The pulse oximeter provides a precise, continuous readout of the hemoglobin oxygen saturation. During the first 1 to 2 weeks of life and without transfusion of autologous blood, the oxygen dissociation curve of HgF is shifted to the left of the adult curve so that hemoglobin saturation of 95% to 97% corresponds to PaO_2 of 52 to 77 mm Hg, assuming a P_{50} of 19. The hemoglobin saturation should be correlated with an arterial PO_2 measurement to ensure valid interpretation of oxygen saturation data in the operating room (see Chapter 2, Respiratory Physiology in Infants and Children).

Monitoring of the Neuromuscular Junction

Neuromuscular blockade can be monitored with a battery-operated nerve stimulator. The simple twitch and train-of-four are elicited by stimulating the ulnar nerve at the wrist or the posterior tibial nerve at the ankle. The neonate's neuromuscular response to nerve stimulation allows the anesthesiologist to titrate further doses of a muscle relaxant and avoid excessive neuromuscular blockade. However, neuromuscular monitoring is technically challenging for VLBW infants because of the small size of their muscles. Accurate data from the transcutaneous devices are often impossible to obtain. Inserting needles into a tiny infant's extremity should be justified because such trauma may cause bleeding or infection. Furthermore, even with needles in place, obtaining a reliable response using the standard battery-operated devices is unpredictable. Of significance, most of these infants require mechanical ventilation postoperatively, so that documenting full recovery to neuromuscular blockade is often unnecessary immediately after surgery.

Monitoring Urine Output

Devices that collect urine during surgery (specifically, Foley catheters or modifications) are helpful because, in the absence of glycosuria, urine output is a good indicator of hydration, circulating volume, and renal function. The desirable range of urine output in the neonate under anesthesia is 0.5 to 2.0 mL/kg per hr. Note that for a 1-kg infant, 0.5 to 2 mL of urine per hour is difficult to reliably collect in the setting of surgical drapes, lack of direct access to the patient, and easy kinking of drainage tubing secondary to pressure and positioning. Thus, in actual practice, accurately assessing urine output is difficult.

INDUCTION OF ANESTHESIA

The techniques for induction of anesthesia in the newborn vary with the infant's size, gestational age, medical status, surgical lesion, and the skill and experience of the anesthesiologist. For example, neonates with a full stomach should have tracheal intubation either "awake" or via a rapid sequence technique. Awake intubation has been associated with significant morbidity, including increased intracranial pressure, bradycardia, desaturation, breath holding (Raju et al., 1980; Hinkle, 1983; Marshall et al., 1984), apnea, and mechanical trauma to the airway. The use of an oxyscope (see Fig. 9–18), a laryngoscope designed to administer oxygen during laryngoscopy, can help to prevent hypoxemia during awake intubation (Hinkle, 1983). Titrating tiny intravenous doses of fentanyl (0.1 to 0.2 mcg/kg) or morphine sulfate (0.02 to 0.03 mg/kg) may diminish the trauma of awake intubation.

A rapid sequence induction in the premature infant is challenging. First, the small size of the face/mandible/upper airway and easily compressible trachea predispose to mechanical upper airway obstruction. Second, the inspired concentration of oxygen cannot be increased to 1.0 without introducing a risk for retinopathy of prematurity. This risk is constantly being weighed against the risk of hypoxemia. Even a short period of apnea can result in immediate oxygen desaturation. Of note, the "rapid sequence" technique is particularly risky in neonates with abdominal distention (i.e., low FRC) because any period of apnea promptly induces hypoxemia and positive pressure ventilation with a mask may be ineffective and may induce regurgitation. That is, abdominal distention may displace the diaphragm cephalad, decreasing lung volume (FRC) and compliance. This combination of factors prevents effective manual ventilation of the lungs via a mask and, at the same time, dilates the stomach (further compressing the diaphragm and lungs) and increases the risk for regurgitation, creating a cycle of events that can be disastrous as the anesthesiologist attempts to intubate the trachea.

Neonates with a high risk for a difficult visualization of the airway (micrognathia, macroglossia, protruding maxilla, cleft palate, or cysts obstructing the airway) must not be paralyzed until the ability to ventilate the infant's lungs with a mask is ensured. In such infants, an initial attempt at direct laryngoscopy with minimal sedation and the infant breathing spontaneously should be made before anesthetic agents or muscle relaxants are administered. In infants in whom direct laryngoscopy does not allow the larynx to be visualized, other techniques, such as bronchoscopy, must be considered (see Chapter 9, Anesthesia Equipment and Monitoring).

Direct laryngoscopy and endotracheal intubation of the neonate's trachea require head and neck positioning different from that recommended for the adult. The prominent occiput of the newborn results in an "automatic sniffing position" without the additional support of towels or blankets under the head/neck. The larynx of the newborn is one or two vertebral bodies cephalad to that of the adult, so that extension of the neck may impede visualizing the vocal cords. Gentle pressure (with the pinky finger, for example) can assist in moving the larynx into view during direct laryngoscopy. The Miller-0 straight laryngoscope blade is probably the most commonly recommended device for visualizing the airway of a tiny neonate (preterm or of low birth weight), and the Miller-1 is used in the full-term neonate. The Wis-Hipple 1.5 blade may be preferred in infants greater than 4 kg. Uncuffed 3.0- or 3.5-mm (inner diameter [ID]) Magill disposable endotracheal tubes with a Murphy eye are commonly the appropriate size to intubate the trachea in neonates. A 2.5-mm (ID) tube is usually used in infants less than 1200 g. To ensure that the endotracheal tube is not too large, inspired gas should leak around the endotracheal tube while delivering a manual positive breath (20 to 25 cm H_2O pressure). A tightly fitting tube can damage the subglottic mucosa, causing edema and postoperative stridor or possibly subglottic stenosis. The low perfusion pressure of the newborn may contribute to the higher risk for development of subglottic pressure necrosis in response to an endotracheal tube "pressing" on the tracheal mucosa in the infant.

Ensuring that the endotracheal tube is at the appropriate depth in the trachea of the LBW infant also requires attention. The distance from the vocal cords to the carina in the term infant is about 4 cm. One algorithm recommends that the 1-, 2-, 3-, and 4-kg infant should have an endotracheal tube taped with the 7-, 8-, 9-, and 10-cm mark, respectively, at the alveolar ridge. In VLBW infants, a chest radiograph may be needed to confirm the position of the endotracheal tube at the midtracheal level (see Chapters 8 and 9, Preoperative Preparation, and Anesthesia Equipment and Monitoring).

ANESTHETIC SYSTEMS

Several anesthetic delivery systems are safe and readily available for the care of neonates during surgery. Disposable, humidified pediatric circle systems have low compliance and thereby eliminate the problems previously described with the older, nondisposable, highly compliant circuits. Lightweight plastic valves have replaced the metal structures and eliminated the high resistance and "stickiness" associated with the older anesthesia machines. Because neonates are mechanically ventilated during surgery, the work of breathing associated with spontaneous ventilation is eliminated. The valveless, humidified, lightweight Mapleson D or E (Jackson Rees) systems are modifications of the Ayre T-piece or the Bain circuit (Bain and Spoerel, 1973).

All anesthetic delivery systems should incorporate a mechanism to heat and humidify the inspired gas mixture. The heating system must be regulated by a thermistor at the endotracheal tube connection to avoid hyperthermia and airway burns. The gas temperature at the monitoring site at the endotracheal tube must range from 36° to 37°C (Bain and Spoerel, 1973). Warm gases minimize damage to the tracheal mucosal cells associated with cold, dry gases. Heated inspired gases also decrease heat loss from the respiratory system. Alternatively, heat and moisture exchangers, known also as artificial noses, can be placed at the endotracheal tube connection to provide partial humidification and warming of the inspired gases. However, these artificial noses may be less efficient than devices incorporated in the anesthetic circuit.

During neonatal anesthesia, the anesthesia machine must be equipped to deliver air when nitrous oxide is contraindicated.

In addition, the anesthesia machine should have a mechanism to prevent the delivery of hypoxic gas mixtures and a monitor to measure inspired oxygen concentrations.

INTRAOPERATIVE FLUID MANAGEMENT

Calculating fluid requirements for newborns is an inexact science. Historically, caloric expenditure at rest has been the basis for calculating "maintenance" fluid requirements (Shires et al., 1961; Winters, 1973; Furman, 1987). Fluid requirements are based on the metabolic rate expressed in terms of caloric requirements (Holliday and Segar, 1957); that is, the energy requirements of a neonate are usually estimated to be 100 kcal/kg per 24 hours and 100 mL of fluid are consumed for every 100 calories metabolized per day. However, in some cases, during the first 2 to 3 days of life, the fluid requirements are considerably less. First, approximately 30 mL/kg of fluid is mobilized from the lungs into the extracellular fluid space. Second, urine output is often low in the first 24 hours after birth (see Chapter 4, Regulation of Body Fluids and Electrolytes in Infants and Children). On the other hand, these factors are countered by increased insensible loss through the highly permeable skin of the VLBW infant. The estimate for "maintenance" fluid in the newborn cannot be viewed as a simple calculation. Great variability among individual neonates related to gestational age, ambient temperature, exposure to radiant warmth, humidity, sepsis, physical activity, feeding pattern, disease, physiologic immaturity, and positive-pressure ventilation can dramatically alter fluid requirements.

These data for metabolic rate (100 kcal/kg per day and 100 mL/kg per day) are valid for infants weighing less than 10 kg. The metabolic rate decreases gradually with age such that an average adult consumes about 35 cal/kg per day. The important extension of the interaction of metabolic rate with fluid requirements gradually evolved to our current practice of estimating "maintenance" fluid as 4 mL/kg per hr for the first 10 kg, 2 mL/kg per hr for the next 10 kg, and 1 mL/kg for each kg over 20.

Maintenance electrolyte requirements are based on data from studies of basal metabolic rates. The requirements for sodium and potassium (chloride salts) have been reported to range between 2.5 to 3.0 mmol/100 kcal per 24 hr (Winters, 1973). Since chloride is included with both sodium and potassium, neonates may have an "extra" load of chloride. In addition, the tubular immaturity of the newborn allows renal loss of bicarbonate, exacerbating the metabolic acidosis associated with hyperchloremia. In some clinical settings, the hyperchloremia and associated metabolic acidosis are treated by infusing sodium acetate instead of sodium chloride.

Intraoperative fluid therapy has the same four components described for any clinical setting where intravenous treatment is considered: (1) maintenance fluid, (2) replacement of fluid deficit, (3) replacement of third-space loss, and (4) replacement of other losses.

Maintenance Fluids

Normal fluid losses consist primarily of insensible water loss from the respiratory system and evaporation from the skin. The average fluid loss from both lungs and skin can vary from 45 to 70 mL/100 cal. Changes in the respiratory rate and duration of crying can increase this value significantly (Zweymuller and Preining, 1970). Insensible water loss may be increased during phototherapy or when a radiant heater is used (Wu and Hodgman, 1974). Premature infants, especially those weighing less than 1500 g, have insensible water loss (Fanaroff et al., 1972) that can be as much as 3 times the loss in full-term infants secondary to a highly permeable epidermis and reduced subcutaneous fat. On the other hand, the mobilizing of fluid from the lungs over the first day of life decreases free water requirements over the first 24 hours of life.

Urinary losses are variable in the newborn but generally range between 45 to 65 mL/100 cal, depending on the solute load and fluid intake, as well as renal and cardiovascular function. Fecal loss of water and water expended for growth contributes a very small percentage (5 to 10 mL/100 kcal) to the total daily fluid loss. In summary, the variability for maintenance fluid over the first few days of life is enormous, but a total fluid loss of 95 to 145 mL/100 cal is a reasonable estimate.

Fluid Deficits

Fluid deficits are caused primarily by preoperative fasting or excessive gastrointestinal losses without parenteral replacement. Infants receiving adequate preoperative maintenance (and who have no additional fluid requirements) have no deficit. The volume of deficit is calculated by multiplying the hourly maintenance requirement by the number of hours since the last fluid intake. One algorithm recommends that intraoperative replacement of the fluid deficit be delivered over a period of 3 hours: 50% of the deficit volume is given in the first hour, 25% in the second hour, and 25% in the third hour (Furman et al., 1975). In some clinical settings (e.g., central nervous system injury), none or a fraction of the deficit is replaced. Deficit replacement may be carried into the postoperative period and is added to the regular hourly maintenance fluid.

Third-Space Fluid Loss

Surgical trauma can result in translocation of extracellular fluid from the intravascular space into the interstitial space (Shires et al., 1961) producing edema in the bowel wall and mesentery during intra-abdominal surgery (or pathology) or in the subcutaneous tissues and muscle following administration of large amounts of intravenous fluid. The magnitude of third-space loss depends on the site and extent of the surgical manipulation, is increased by inflammatory processes such as peritonitis, and occurs mostly during the first few hours of surgery. Guidelines for replacement of third-space losses include the following:

- During peripheral or superficial surgery: 1 to 3 mL/kg per hr
- During abdominal, chest, or hip surgery: 3 to 4 mL/kg per hr
- During extensive intra-abdominal surgery: 6 to 10 mL/kg per hr (or more)

Third-space loss must be replaced with an isotonic or iso-osmotic solution such as normal saline solution, lactated Ringer's solution, or other balanced salt solution such as Plasma-Lyte without dextrose. Neonates with severe peritonitis or a congenital lesion such as gastroschisis may need 25 to 100 mL/kg per hr for replacement of third-space losses. The state of hydration and degree of third-space loss should be reassessed continually by observing the status of fontanels, dryness of mucosa, and periorbital edema, as well as hemodynamic stability, CVP, and urine output.

Other Fluid Losses

Other fluid losses include those from suction or removal of gastric, intestinal, or pancreatic fluids, drainage of an ileostomy, diarrhea, or excessive sweat losses. In these cases, the electrolyte content of the fluid losses should be measured to determine replacement fluids.

Monitoring of Intraoperative Fluid Therapy

Although clinically assessing the volume status of the newborn during surgery is critical, supplemental data are often essential. Although neonates have limited renal concentrating and diluting capacities, they can excrete "concentrated" urine when dehydrated or dilute urine when overhydrated. Thus, in addition to measuring the total volume of urine (~0.5 to 2 mL/kg per hr is normal), urine osmolality and specific gravity add reliable data to assess the state of hydration and the needs for solute therapy. Urine osmolality in the neonate varies from 50 to 800 mOsm/L, with an average of 270 mOsm/L. Osmolality should be maintained between 200 to 400 mOsm/L, and specific gravity between 1.006 to 1.012.

Serum osmolality is also a useful monitor of electrolyte and fluid therapy. Increased osmolality reflects either reduced intake of water or increased intake of solute, chiefly sodium. A decrease in serum osmolality suggests an infusion of water in excess of sodium or insufficient delivery of, or excess loss of, sodium. Normal serum osmolality in the neonate ranges between 270 and 280 mOsm/kg (Rowe et al., 1974). Hyperosmolar states are particularly dangerous to the neonate because of the high risk for cerebral hemorrhage, kidney damage, or both. Hyperosmolarity can occur with rapid infusion of large quantities of sodium bicarbonate, tris(hydroxymethyl)aminomethane, hypertonic glucose, or hypertonic saline solution. Serum electrolytes must be measured concurrently with serum osmolality to guide electrolyte replacement.

Standard hemodynamic intraoperative monitoring contributes to assessing the adequacy of fluid therapy. Hypotension, diminished heart sounds, or tachycardia suggests compromised circulation and possibly inadequate fluid administration. If invasive monitors (i.e., indwelling arterial catheter or a CVP catheter) have been inserted, careful observation of their traces, in addition to the specific numerical readout, can provide valuable information about intravascular volume status. For example, if a patient is euvolemic, the arterial pressure tracing has a dicrotic notch in the middle third of the downstroke. If a patient is hypovolemic, the area under the arterial pressure curve decreases (i.e., waveform is narrow) and the dicrotic notch changes position. Similarly, when properly placed in the superior vena cava, the CVP catheter provides valuable data about volume status by monitoring right ventricular filling pressure, which is useful in guiding crystalloid and colloid infusions. Large variation in the CVP trace during positive pressure ventilation is common with hypovolemia. The balloon-tipped, flow-directed (Swan-Ganz) catheter, although not often used in the neonate, measures pulmonary arterial and left atrial pressures, which are reliable guides to adjusting fluid and pharmacologic therapy in critically ill infants.

Blood Replacement

Similar to older infants and children, the decision to deliver blood during surgery depends on the underlying and current cardiorespiratory status, ongoing blood loss, anticipated further blood loss, and baseline hemoglobin. In general, the hematocrit of a critically ill newborn undergoing surgery should be maintained at greater than 40% by delivering packed RBCs. Transfusion of other components of blood—platelets, fibrinogen, fresh frozen plasma—should be guided by a combination of laboratory studies and the clinical status.

MANAGEMENT OF COMMONLY ENCOUNTERED SURGICAL LESIONS

ABDOMINAL WALL DEFECTS: GASTROSCHISIS/OMPHALOCELE

Abdominal wall defects are rare, with an incidence of 0.3 to 2:10,000 births (Baird and MacDonald, 1981). Omphaloceles are more common (1:5000 to 1:7000). The diagnosis of an abdominal wall defect may first be suspected if the maternal serum α-fetoprotein is elevated. This laboratory value prompts an evaluation that includes a fetal ultrasound, which often confirms the presence of a lesion. With the frequency of fetal ultrasonography, an in utero definition of the anatomic defect can be made in about 95% of cases. The in utero diagnosis allows planned delivery at a medical center with resources for high-risk obstetric, surgical/anesthetic, and neonatal care.

Although omphalocele and gastroschisis appear to be similar on gross physical appearance, these lesions are distinct from each other. An omphalocele is a central defect of the umbilical ring, and the abdominal contents are within a sac, unless the sac ruptures in utero (Fig. 16–5). The umbilical cord is inserted into the sac, which is peritoneal membrane internally and amniotic membrane externally. The lesion has a fascial defect greater than 4 cm (<4 cm is often considered an umbilical hernia) and often as large as 10 to 12 cm. The sac often contains the stomach, loops of small and large intestine, and, in about 30% to 50%, the liver. A gastroschisis is an abdominal wall defect usually to the right of the umbilical cord (Fig. 16–6). This lesion is usually 2 to 5 cm in diameter and, in most cases, with only small and large bowel present. In rare cases, the liver may exit through the abdominal wall defect. The bowel is exposed to the intrauterine environment with no sac, so that the loops are matted, thickened, and often covered with an inflammatory coating or peel. Whether this exudative peel is secondary to a specific inflammatory pathway or just an effect of amniotic fluid is unclear. The umbilical cord is normal and separate from the defect. Cryptorchidism occurs with gastroschisis when the testes exit with the bowel through the abdominal wall (Weber et al., 2002).

Embryology

Although experimental models have been described (Correia-Pinto et al., 2001), the embryologic etiology of these lesions is not completely understood. Omphalocele has been described as a failure of the cephalic, lateral, and caudal folds to fuse (closure of the exocelomic space) and abnormal fusion and differentiation of myotomes to form abdominal wall musculature (7 to 12 weeks of gestation); the abdominal cavity is primarily underdeveloped. During weeks 7 to 12 of development, the midgut elongates and herniates into the umbilical cord. By week 12, the abdominal cavity is large enough for the developing gut to exit the cord and reenter the abdomen. Some believe that the simple failure of this return to the abdomen is a developmental arrest that results in an omphalocele and a small abdominal cavity. The abdominal cavity is small only because the gut remains in the umbilical sac.

Gastroschisis is considered to be an earlier embryologic event, resulting from an abnormality of the right omphalomesenteric artery or right umbilical vein development that results in ischemia to the right paraumbilical area. Abdominal wall defects have been ascribed to an abnormal relationship between cell proliferation and planned cell death (apoptosis) at the critical embryonic folding period. Inadequate mesoderm development may contribute to dysplastic abdominal wall growth. This underdeveloped

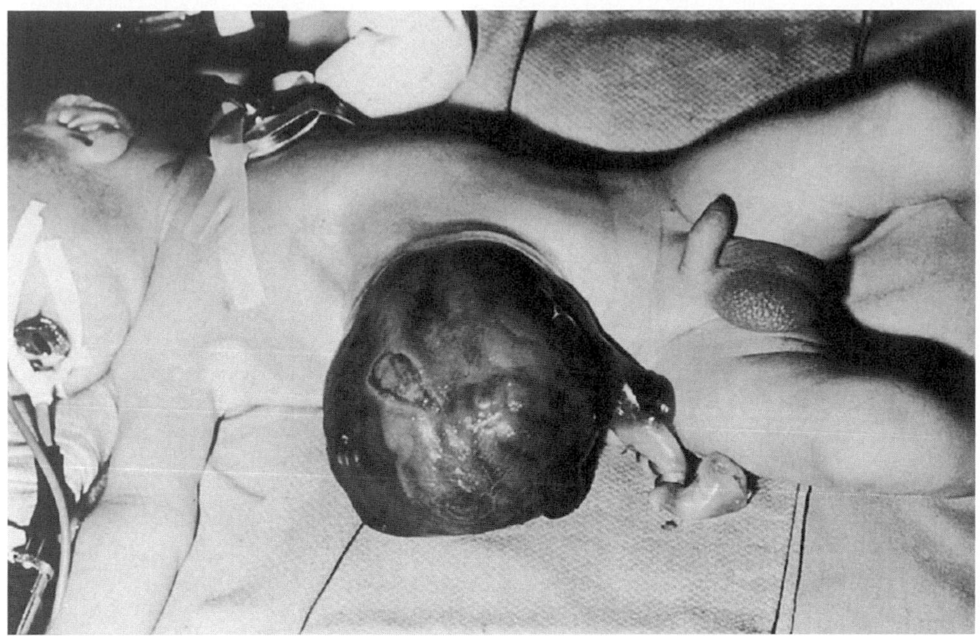

■ **FIGURE 16–5.** Newborn with large omphalocele, sac intact. Umbilical cord is seen emerging from mass. The major problem will be replacing the viscera in the small abdominal cavity.

site is commonly just to the right of the umbilicus and, with increased pressure of the growing intra-abdominal organs, ruptures. Similar defects in other areas may produce other lesions, such as exstrophy of the bladder.

Gastroschisis is usually an isolated lesion. The association of in utero exposure to acetaminophen, aspirin, and pseudoephedrine and the increased incidence of gastroschisis have been described (Werler et al., 2002; Baerg et al., 2003). In the case of either an omphalocele or gastroschisis, rotation of the gut is incomplete in utero. This results in various "malrotation" phenotypes. Intestinal atresias are common, especially in patients with gastroschisis.

Although neither gastroschisis nor omphaloceles are considered to be "familial," reports raise the possibility of familial occurrence (Yang et al., 1992; Torfs et al., 1994), and 50% to 75% of infants with an omphalocele have other anomalies and 20% to 30% have chromosomal abnormalities (Robinson and Abuhamad, 2000; Weber et al., 2002). For example, Beckwith-Wiedemann, Reiger, and prune belly syndromes are associated with omphaloceles, as are trisomy 13, 15, 18, and 21. If the omphalocele contains only bowel and if oligo- or polyhydramnios is present, the likelihood of an associated chromosomal abnormality increases. Syndromes of midline defects often include an omphalocele. One syndrome, pentalogy of Cantrell, includes an omphalocele, diaphragmatic hernia, sternal abnormalities, an ectopic and anomalous heart, and gene abnormalities at Xq25 to q26.1. Another syndrome involving the lower abdomen includes omphalocele, bladder or cloacal exstrophy,

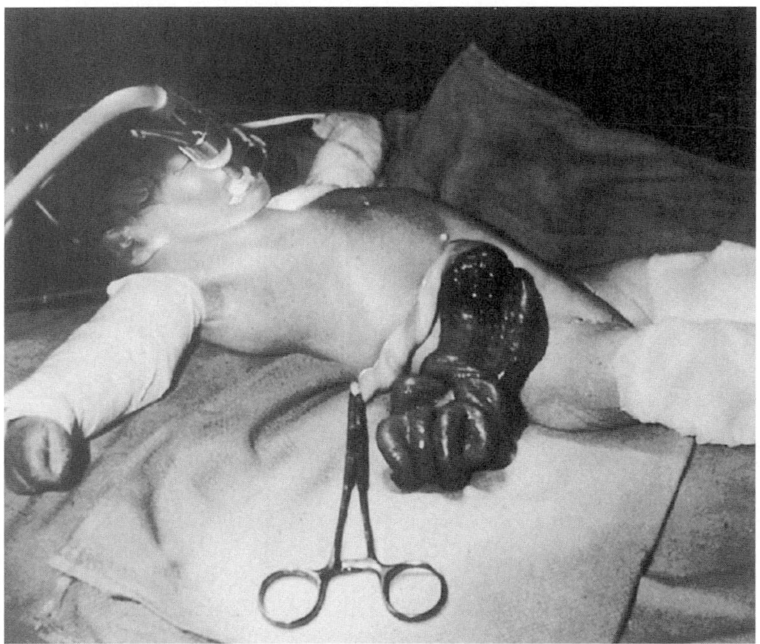

■ **FIGURE 16–6.** Gastroschisis, sometimes called ruptured omphalocele, but umbilical cord is intact. Heat loss, rapid dehydration, and infection are added to problems of omphalocele.

imperforate anus, colonic atresia, sacrovertebral anomalies, and meningomyelocele. No environmental or teratogenic associations have been proposed as etiologic causes.

Preoperative Management

The preoperative management of abdominal wall defects is concerned primarily with fluid resuscitation, minimizing heat loss, treating sepsis, and avoiding direct trauma to the herniated organs. Normothermia should be maintained or achieved by preventing heat loss from the exposed viscera. A bowel bag may be used for this purpose (Towne et al., 1980). Decompression of the stomach with an orogastric or nasogastric tube is important to prevent regurgitation, aspiration pneumonia, and further bowel distention. Broad-spectrum antibiotics are started, and intravenous fluid therapy, 2 to 4 times "maintenance," is infused to ensure adequate hydration and to compensate for a combination of peritonitis, edema, ischemia, protein loss, and significant third-space loss. Without such vigorous fluid resuscitation, hypovolemic shock, hemoconcentration, and metabolic acidosis may develop. A balanced salt solution (lactated Ringer's solution or 5% albumin) is used, and urine output is monitored. A urine output of 1 to 2 mL/kg per hr indicates adequate hydration. Because of the large fluid requirements, acid-base status and electrolyte levels should be monitored carefully by serial arterial or venous blood gas measurements. If severe metabolic acidosis develops despite fluid delivery, sodium bicarbonate, colloids, ventilatory support, and vasopressors may be administered in order to maintain the pH greater than 7.20.

Intraoperative Management

Surgical management is aimed at repairing the abdominal wall defect and reducing the protruded viscera. If primary closure is not possible, a staged repair is planned, including the use of the silo chimney or Silastic silo prosthesis (Schuster, 1967). The "silo" consists of a Silastic or Teflon mesh that is sutured to the fascia of the defect. The synthetic material used to cover the lesion and the specific mechanism for placing the organs into the abdomen (e.g., umbilical tapes, umbilical cord clamps) vary from center to center. After the silo is in place, the extra-abdominal organs are then gradually returned to the peritoneal cavity over 3 to 10 days (Fig. 16–7). Improved outcome has been claimed using the delayed repair approach after the nonoperative placement of a spring-loaded silo (Schlatter et al., 2003). These authors state that this procedure is accomplished in the neonatal intensive care nursery or delivery room and requires "no anesthesia." These authors claim that the time to both first and full feeds was shorter in the infants who underwent delayed closure. The prosthesis is then removed or reduced under general anesthesia, and eventually the defect is closed.

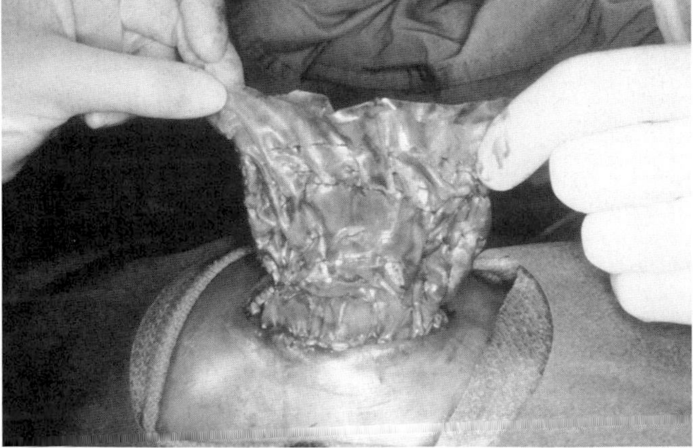

■ **FIGURE 16–7.** A silo is used to aid in the reduction of the abdominal contents when the abdominal cavity is too small. Over time the intestinal contents are gradually reduced back into the abdominal cavity.

Forcing the viscera into an underdeveloped abdominal cavity that cannot accommodate the herniated bowel and tight closure of the skin can restrict diaphragmatic excursion and possibly compress the lungs. The result is impaired ventilation and reduced return of vena caval blood. During abdominal closure, the anesthesiologist must monitor airway pressures and watch for decreased pulmonary compliance. The surgeon and the anesthesiologist should cooperate to assess the feasibility of a primary closure. Yaster and others (1988) noted that increases in intragastric pressure greater than 20 mm Hg and increases in CVP of greater than 4 mm Hg above baseline were frequently associated with reductions in venous return and cardiac index, requiring surgical decompression of the abdomen.

An arterial catheter facilitates blood sampling and continuous monitoring of blood pressure. A CVP catheter is probably more important than the arterial catheter, however, for evaluation of changes in blood volume and the degree of visceral compression during abdominal closure (Yaster et al., 1988). Metabolic monitoring is also important. Serial intraoperative glucose monitoring, especially in infants with Beckwith-Wiedemann syndrome, may be indicated. Fluid therapy consists of 5% to 10% dextrose in 0.2% saline at the maintenance rates stated earlier and lactated Ringer's solution (8 to 15 mL/kg, or more, per hour) for third-space loss. A warm environment must be maintained, as well as vigilant efforts at preventing heat loss (see Chapter 5, Thermoregulation: Physiology and Perioperative Disturbances).

After decompression of the stomach, anesthesia may be induced with inhalation or intravenous agents. Because it distends the bowel, nitrous oxide is avoided. The infant is paralyzed and ventilated with an air (or nitrogen) and oxygen mixture with low concentrations of an inhalation anesthetic. The inspired oxygen concentration must be adjusted to maintain oxygen saturation between 95% and 97% (the physiologic range of PaO_2 in the newborn, 50 to 70 mm Hg). Vane and others (1994) demonstrated that spinal anesthesia can be an effective anesthetic for the repair of gastroschisis in selected patients.

Postoperative Care

Postoperatively, except in infants with a small defect, mechanical ventilation should be maintained for 24 to 48 hours, or longer; thereafter, respiratory compliance usually improves dramatically (Nakayama et al., 1989, 1991). Infants with a small defect sometimes can be extubated at the conclusion of surgery. All of these patients must be carefully monitored for respiratory complications in an intensive care unit. Inferior vena caval compression, evident as "blue" lower limbs, or bowel ischemia (necrotizing enterocolitis) can occur as a result of increased abdominal pressure and may require surgical treatment. These infants are also at high risk for developing sepsis in the postoperative period.

The onset of peristalsis after repair of omphalocele or gastroschisis is usually delayed, and the resulting ileus may be prolonged (O'Neil and Grosfeld, 1974) so that TPN is generally required for days to weeks in the postoperative period.

Anticipating this, most infants with large lesions, especially gastroschisis, should have appropriate intravenous access established in the operating room to facilitate early postoperative nutritional support, which is essential for healing and recovery.

Outcome

Survival of infants born with anterior abdominal wall defects has improved dramatically secondary to prenatal diagnosis, improved surgical, anesthetic, and perioperative intensive care, and nutritional support. The advent of accurate prenatal imaging has allowed termination of a pregnancy when a fetus with multiple anomalies, chromosomal lesions, or a huge defect is identified. When the defect is isolated, 95% to 97% survival is expected. Mortality and long-term outcome are related to associated anomalies (e.g., cardiac, intestinal atresia, etc.), complications of treatment (bowel perforation, NEC, sepsis, short bowel syndrome), and the side effects of intravenous alimentation (liver failure, sepsis). Although specific data have been collected to stratify and predict outcome of patients with abdominal wall defects, the general pattern is that infants with a "simple" defect (no atresias, no extraintestinal anomalies, <5 to 6 cm) and no postoperative complications (obstruction, NEC, short gut syndrome) have a better prognosis than those with a "complex" lesion or postoperative course (Molik et al., 2001).

In a follow-up study of 23 infants (>16 years old) born with gastroschisis between 1972 and 1984 and who survived longer than 1 year, Davies and Stringer (1997) reported that 22 of these 23 infants were in good health and overall growth was normal. About one third of patients with gastroschisis had undergone surgery for adhesions, bowel obstruction, or scar complications related to their defect. Of note was that in 25% to 60% (Tunell, 1995; Davies and Stringer, 1997) of patients with anterior wall defects, the absence of an umbilicus was a distressing physical sign, especially during adolescence.

Other studies involving shorter follow-up periods have noted patients with chronic abdominal pain and gastroesophageal reflux (Fasching et al., 1996). An economic analysis of care of infants with gastroschisis emphasized that the cost of care is high and that on average 47 days of hospitalization were needed in to establish full feeds (Sydorak et al., 2002).

CONGENITAL DIAPHRAGMATIC HERNIA

Congenital diaphragmatic hernia (CDH) is a defect in the diaphragm that develops early in gestation and is associated with extrusion of intra-abdominal organs into the thoracic cavity (Fig. 16–8). The incidence of CDH ranges between 1:2500 and 1:3000 live births. The most common defect is posterolateral (Bochdalek) (90%), of which 75% are left-sided. Morgagni (anteromedial) and paraesophageal hernia and eventrations make up the remainder (Fig. 16–9). The anomaly is much more than a hole in the diaphragm. CDH is associated with

- Varying degrees of bilateral lung hypoplasia
- Pulmonary hypertension and arteriolar reactivity
- Congenital anomalies (e.g., cardiac, chromosomal anomalies)
- High mortality (30% to 50%)
- Significant morbidity, both short and long term

In addition to the marked abnormalities in both airway and vascular pulmonary development, striking dysfunction of the left ventricle has been noted. Karamanoukian and others (1995) noted that left ventricular mass and ventricular compliance may have a predictive value for outcome.

Prenatal diagnosis of CDH has increased from about 10% in 1985 to more than 50% at present. The most frequent findings include displacement of the heart and a fluid-filled stomach in the thorax. Of note, prenatal ultrasound evaluation can have a high incidence of false-negative results (Lewis et al., 1997).

Embryology

The diaphragm, lungs, and gastrointestinal tract develop synchronously. The lungs begin as a ventral bud of the foregut. Airway development and branching begin between the fourth and fifth weeks of gestation and progress until the terminal bronchioles are formed by the 17th week. The ventral (membranous) component of the diaphragm is formed between the third and fourth weeks of gestation. At about the eighth week of gestation, this portion envelops the esophagus, inferior vena cava, and aorta and fuses with the foregut mesentery to form the posterior and medial (membranous) portions of the diaphragm. The lateral margins of the diaphragm are derived from the muscular components of the body wall. The pleuroperitoneal canals close when all the membranous portions of the diaphragm fuse together, and by the ninth week of gestation, diaphragmatic closure is usually complete (Wells, 1954). If the closure (obliteration) of the pleuroperitoneal canals is delayed beyond the 9th to 10th

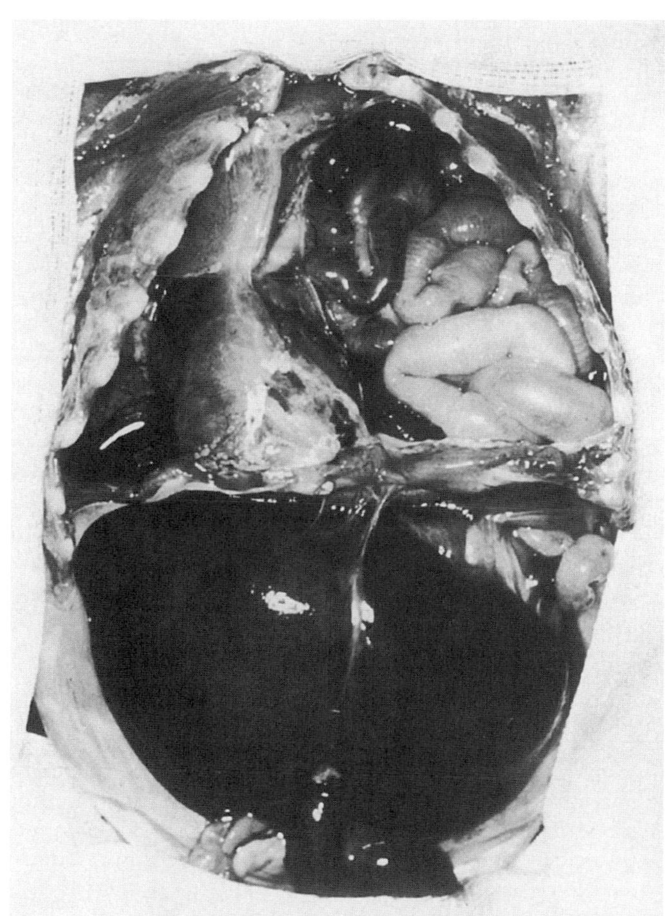

FIGURE 16–8. Diaphragmatic hernia at postmortem examination showing obliteration of left pleural cavity and severe compression of heart and right lung. (Courtesy Dr. Arnold Colodny, Boston, MA.)

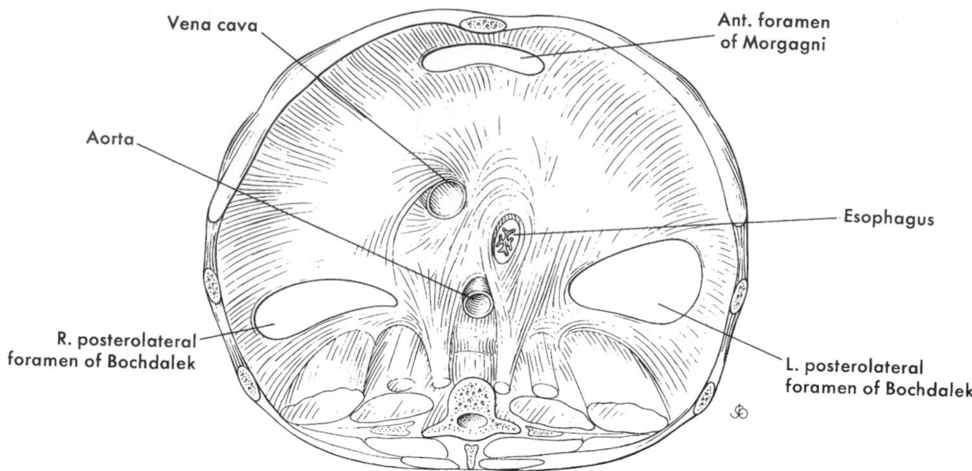

■ **FIGURE 16–9.** Diagram (from below) showing sites of congenital diaphragmatic hernia.

weeks of development or if the normal rotation and settling of the midgut occur before the 10th week or before the obliteration of the pleuroperitoneal canals, the midgut (abdominal viscera) herniates into the thoracic (pleural) cavity.

In the past, the defect has been attributed to an abnormal closure of the pleuroperitoneal canal, but investigation using the nitrofen-induced CDH model in the rat has allowed an innovative approach to reexamining the etiology of this lesion. CDH seems to be linked to a disordered formation of the pleuroperitoneal fold, a much earlier event (fourth week of gestation). The findings of an abnormal formation of the framework of mesenchyme, inhibiting muscular development of the diaphragm, has been linked to abnormalities in retinoid signaling pathway, suggesting that vitamin A may play a role in the pathophysiology of CDH (Greer et al., 2003).

Stillborn babies with CDH have a 95% incidence of other anomalies. Live-born infants have a 20% incidence of associated cardiovascular defects, most commonly PDA (Johnson et al., 1967). Others (Fauza and Wilson, 1994) have reported that hypoplastic left heart syndrome was the most frequently associated cardiac defect. Rarely, CDH is a part of a complex set of anomalies, Cantrell's pentalogy (Wesselhoeft and DeLuca, 1984), consisting of omphalocele, sternal cleft, ectopia cordis, and an intracardiac defect (ventricular septal defect or diverticulum of left ventricle). Although uncommon, CDH has been identified in the context of several syndromes including Fryns (Fryns et al., 1979), Goldenhar (Rollnick and Kaye, 1983), Brachmann-deLange (Jelsema et al., 1993), and Beckwith-Weidemann (Thornburn et al., 1970). From 5% to 18% of infants with CDH have associated chromosomal abnormalities (Cunniff et al., 1990; Bollman et al., 1995).

Preoperative Assessment

Pathophysiology

In the most common presentation, the herniated abdominal viscera, which include the midgut but may also include the stomach, parts of the descending colon, the left kidney, and the left lobe of the liver, occupy the left thoracic cavity and interfere with the development of the lung. In most cases, this produces some degree of pulmonary hypoplasia, the severity of which is related to how early in fetal development the herniation and compression occurred. The herniation of abdominal contents shifts the mediastinum to the right, which can cause compression and hypoplasia of the contralateral lung.

Several structural abnormalities of the pulmonary vasculature correlate with the pathophysiology of CDH. The low number of airways, the simple arterial branching pattern, the increase in smooth muscle mass at the level of the resistance vessels, and left ventricular abnormalities add to the cardiorespiratory dysfunction (Schwartz et al., 1994) produced by the hernia itself. Lung growth (alveolar) does occur postnatally, but growth at the preacinar level is limited in that the number of airway generations remains constant after mid-gestation (Geggel and Reid, 1984). Vascular remodeling provides larger and less muscular arteries, so that the pathology present at birth has been documented to reverse to some degree (Beals et al., 1992). The degree of pulmonary hypoplasia is predictive not only of survival but also of the development of chronic lung disease in the survivor.

Although the anatomic abnormalities of CDH are consistent with the phenomenon of persistent pulmonary hypertension, other factors are critical in determining the physiology of the pulmonary circulation of the newborn. For example, the fall in pulmonary vascular resistance and rise in pulmonary blood flow that are essential for the transition from the placental circulation to the postnatal pattern is dependent on adequate function of the endothelial cell. Imbalance in the production, release, and/or circulating levels of vasoconstrictors (leukotrienes C_4 and D_4, thromboxane A_2, platelet-activating factor) and vasodilators seems to be central to the right-to-left shunting observed with pulmonary hypertension associated with CDH (Furchgott and Zawadzki, 1980). Similarly, endothelins have taken a central role in defining and treating the newborn with pulmonary hypertension. These peptides are vasoconstrictors that are produced in response to inflammation, ischemia, and other stimuli. Multiple receptors have been localized both in the vascular smooth muscle and in the vascular endothelial cell. Of note, elevated levels of endothelin 1 have been described in infants with CDH (Rosenberg et al., 1993; Kobayashi and Puri, 1994). The release of these vasoactive agents appears to be the result of an inflammatory cascade produced in part by ventilator-induced epithelial and endothelial damage from hyperinflation of the hypoplastic lungs.

Clinical Presentation

Infants born with bilateral lung hypoplasia or severe unilateral hypoplasia exhibit symptoms in the first minutes to hours of life. Babies with less severe hypoplasia of the lung whose herniation occurred late in gestation generally present symptoms within

24 hours after birth. The classic triad of CDH consists of cyanosis, dyspnea, and apparent dextrocardia. Physical examination reveals a scaphoid abdomen, bulging chest, decreased breath sounds, distant or right-displaced heart sounds, and bowel sounds in the chest. Radiographic examination of the chest shows a bowel gas pattern in the chest, mediastinal shift and little lung tissue at the right costophrenic sulcus (Fig. 16–10).

Clinical presentation is related to survival. Infants with symptoms severe enough to require endotracheal intubation immediately after birth have a very poor prognosis. Infants weighing less than 1000 g, who are born at less than 33 weeks' gestation, or who have an PAO_2–PaO_2 gradient greater than 500 seldom survive (Raphaely and Downes, 1973). Antenatal diagnosis, neonatal stabilization and delayed surgery, and, most important, the avoidance of ventilator-induced lung injury have resulted in significant improvement in morbidity and mortality of infants with severe CDH.

Ultrasonography has made antenatal diagnosis of CDH possible. Sonographic determination of lung-to-head ratio and the presence or absence of liver herniation into the chest have been reported to correlate with postnatal outcome. Fetuses with liver herniation and a low lung-to-head ratio have high mortality and morbidity despite maximum care (NO, extracorporeal membrane oxygenation [ECMO], high-frequency ventilation [HFV], and delayed operative repair) (Albanese et al., 1998; Desfrere et al., 2000; Cacciari et al., 2001; Muratore et al., 2001a and b; Boloker et al., 2002; Stege et al., 2003). The reported survival rates for this lesion range from 40% to 90%, but these rates may be falsely elevated. Harrison (1978, 1994) noted that mortality may be "hidden" when in utero deaths and early postnatal deaths from extreme prematurity are not included in calculating mortality. The survival rate for all cases of isolated CDH approaches 70% in those without fetal surgery and 80% in those who do not require ECMO (Reickert et al., 1998).

In Utero Treatment

Because the fundamental pathophysiology of CDH is pulmonary hypoplasia, various fetal surgical techniques to improve the growth of hypoplastic lungs in utero have been reported (Harrison et al., 1990, 1993, 1997). Starting with animal models in the 1980s, Harrison and others gradually perfected the fetal surgical procedures, improved the treatment of preterm labor with tocolytics, and fine-tuned the anesthetic management to the point of establishing selection criteria for intervention in the human. Initially, a hysterotomy was performed and the fetus was partially exteriorized. The fetal circulation and, therefore, oxygenation were maintained via the placental circulation (ex utero intrapartum treatment [EXIT procedure]). The herniated viscera in the chest were reduced into the abdominal cavity by push-and-pull technique. The procedure was eventually drastically modified to a minimally invasive operation using fetoscopy to surgically occlude the trachea. Tracheal occlusion served to manipulate the physiology of fetal lung development. That is, the fetal lung development is physiologically accelerated by the airway expansion that results from accumulation of the lung fluid while the glottis is occluded. This tracheal occlusion technique has marginally improved the survival of the affected fetus but is associated with significant complications, including premature labor and delivery (Harrison et al., 2003). Meanwhile, the survival of the infants with CDH with conventional postnatal management (see later) had improved in the latter half of the 1990s. The National Institutes of Health–sponsored, controlled, comparative study did not show any increased survival after surgical treatment of fetuses with CDH (Harrison et al., 2003). Consequently, fetal surgery for the repair of CDH was suspended in 2001.

Timing of Surgery

CDH was considered a neonatal emergency and the infant with CDH was operated on as soon as possible after birth. The infant's lungs were hyperventilated with 100% oxygen circulation in an attempt to produce pulmonary vasodilation from hyperoxia and respiratory alkalosis. Although this combination of hyperoxia and respiratory alkalosis may produce transient pulmonary vasodilation, repetitious overdistention of the lung tissues results in damage to the alveolar and capillary membranes (barotrauma or, more accurately, volutrauma) and induces an inflammatory

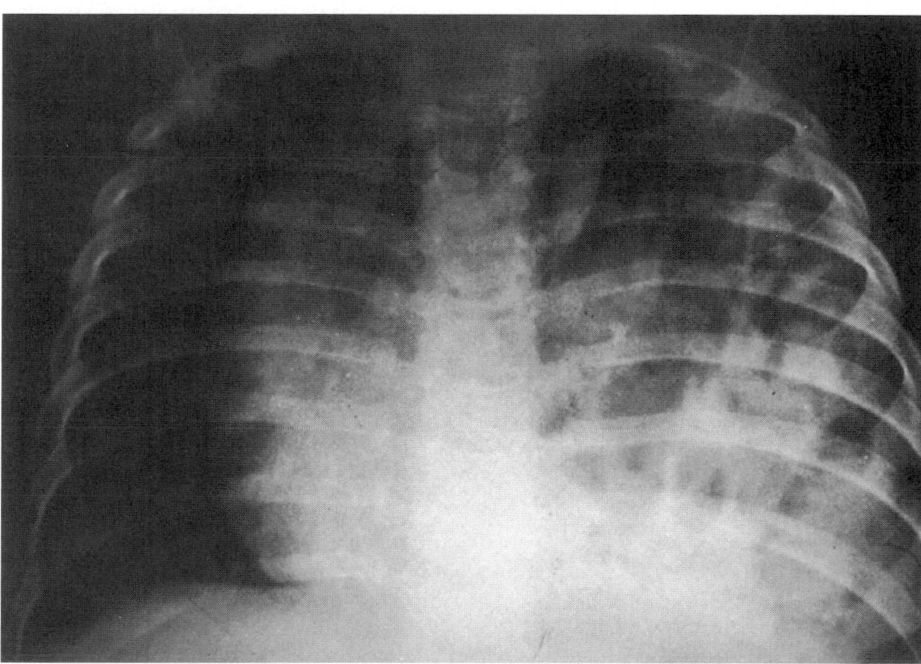

■ **FIGURE 16–10.** Diaphragmatic hernia. Radiograph shows loops of intestine in the left side of the chest, displacement of the heart to the right, and compression of the right lung.

reaction and the associated release of vasoactive mediators, eventually producing pulmonary vasoconstriction and pulmonary hypertension.

The goal of the initial management of CDH is to avoid a surgical intervention when the infant is hypoxic and acidotic (Levin, 1987). Instead, medical management is directed to stabilizing the cardiorespiratory status by improving oxygenation, correcting metabolic acidosis, reducing the right-to-left shunting, and increasing pulmonary perfusion (Miyasaka et al., 1984; Hazebroek et al., 1988). Sakai and others (1987) reported that the postoperative compliance of the respiratory system (C_{rs}), as measured with a noninvasive, passive mechanics technique (Lesouef et al., 1984), immediately decreased 10% to 77% from the preoperative value. The four infants with more than 50% decrease in compliance died after increased hypoxemia and acidosis. Respiratory mechanics in CHD, rather than improving, frequently deteriorate after repair of the hernia. Studies such as these prompted a revaluation of the practice of urgent surgery in this malformation.

Nakayama and others (1991) evaluated pulmonary function and outcome of 22 infants with severe CDH treated either with emergency repair or with preoperative stabilization for 2 to 11 days. Nine of 13 infants who underwent immediate repair of CDH received ECMO support postoperatively, and 6 of 13 infants (2 after ECMO) survived (46% survival). Six of nine infants whose surgery was delayed for preoperative stabilization immediately received ECMO support for 4 to 10 days; one died before surgery after an intraventricular hemorrhage. All other eight infants survived after surgery (89% survival). Seven days after surgery, respiratory system compliance (C_{rs}) for those infants operated on in the immediate repair group did not improve from the preoperative (immediate neonatal) values. In contrast, C_{rs} increased more than 60% from their baseline values in these infants who underwent preoperative stabilization. Although the duration of mechanical ventilation was similar in the survivors of the two groups, the preoperative stabilization group had higher postductal PaO_2, lower respiratory rates, lower peak and mean airway pressures, and lower FIO_2. Based on the physiologic and clinical evidence, these researchers concluded that preoperative stabilization is beneficial before the repair of CDH (Nakayama et al., 1991).

Preoperative Supportive Care

Preoperative care of an infant with severe CDH should start in the delivery room. Establishing effective ventilation in newborn infants often requires peak airway pressure greater than 30 cm H_2O. Bjorklund and others (1997) found that six manual inflations with a tidal volume of 35 to 40 mL/kg in preterm lambs resulted in persistent respiratory failure and pneumothorax despite surfactant treatment. Wada and others (1997) also found that ventilation of premature lambs at birth with a tidal volume of 20 mL/kg for only 30 minutes resulted in marked decreases in C_{rs} along with the development of poor gas exchange. In comparison, premature lambs ventilated with a tidal volume of 5 or 10 mL/kg maintained high C_{rs} and normal gas exchange. Although most infants with CDH are born at term or near term, these data from preterm lambs and the high incidence of chronic lung disease in survivors of CDH suggest that minimizing the barotrauma from positive pressure ventilation may be an important tactic from the first ventilatory intervention. In fact, some neonatologists advocate not only preoperative stabilization but also endotracheal intubation and high-frequency oscillatory ventilation (HFOV) immediately at birth. Preoperative stabilization is followed at least for several days. With this "lung protective" approach, Uezono (2003) reported a 90% survival rate after the repair of severe CDH.

Positive pressure ventilation by mask and bag is particularly risky for infants with CDH, because attempting to expand the noncompliant lungs may distend the stomach and intestines, which are in the left hemithorax, further decreasing chest compliance. Early intubation of the trachea and decompression of the stomach are important initial steps to prevent further distention of, and pulmonary compression by, the displaced abdominal viscera.

In the perioperative period, some infants exhibit a "honeymoon period," which is then followed by a sudden, often unexplained return to a state of persistent pulmonary hypertension and clinical deterioration (acidosis, hypoxemia, hypercapnia, pulmonary hypertension, and right-to-left shunting through the foramen ovale and the ductus arteriosus). Numerous efforts at manipulating the pulmonary vascular resistance have been used with varying degrees of success (or no success). In the 1970s/early 1980s, such measures included hyperventilation (often maintaining the pH > 7.50 and the PCO_2 < 25 mm Hg), ligation of the PDA, and pharmacologic therapy (e.g., isoproterenol, tolazoline). During the 1980s, other pharmacologic therapies were introduced, including prostacyclin, prostaglandins, NO, and ECMO (Goetzman et al., 1976; Clyman et al., 1977; Collins et al., 1977; Levy et al., 1977; Moodie et al., 1978; Soifer et al., 1982; Bohn et al., 1987; Langham et al., 1987; Pappert et al., 1995; Zwissler et al., 1995; Clark et al., 1998). More recently, therapeutic aims have been directed toward NO and ECMO.

Nitric Oxide (NO)

The role of NO in the treatment of CDH is a logical extension from the use of NO for infants with pulmonary hypertension, sepsis, and congenital heart disease (Kinsella et al., 1992; Roberts et al., 1992). NO diffuses across the alveolar capillary membranes and stimulates cyclic guanylate cyclase, which increases cyclic GMP, thereby causing vascular smooth muscle to relax (see Chapter 2, Respiratory Physiology in Infants and Children). At the present, a limited number of patients with CDH treated with NO have been reported. In a case report of premature infants with CDH, Lévêque and others (1994) noted that NO was a significant factor in the infants' survival. In a small series, Shah and others (1994) noted that patients with CHD may be more resistant to the effects of inhaled NO, whereas Karamanoukian and others (1994) reported that NO was effective in patients with hypoplastic lungs only after extracorporeal membrane oxygenation.

Extracorporeal Membrane Oxygenation

Frequently, infants with CDH for whom conservative medical management fails receive cardiorespiratory support with ECMO, which is similar to cardiopulmonary bypass (German et al., 1977; Hardesty et al., 1981; Bohn et al., 1987; Langham et al., 1987; Redmond et al., 1987). Several types of ECMO have been developed based on site of cannulation and the design of the ECMO circuit. The most common setup is a venoarterial circuit where the patient's internal jugular vein and common carotid artery are cannulated. In this system, blood is drained via gravity from the right atrium, oxygenated through the membrane oxygenator, and returned to the patient through the arterial cannulas. In patients who have undergone venovenous bypass, the patient's blood returns to the membrane oxygenator by gravity, is oxygenated in the membrane oxygenator, and then is returned to the venous system. In venovenous ECMO, adequate systemic oxygen delivery depends on the effective cardiac output, whereas in infants undergoing venoarterial ECMO, the bypass system can compensate for both pulmonary and myocardial dysfunction. Significant risks are associated with ECMO, including bleeding at surgical or chest tube insertion sites, intracranial hemorrhage, sepsis, hypertension, and brain death. Outcome data for neonates who have been supported with ECMO have been far more promising than the data from adults. Clearly, the underlying disease process influences the success rates of ECMO (Dalton, 1992) (Table 16–4). In general, because the mortality is higher and the likelihood of intracranial hemorrhage is higher in LBW infants, ECMO is limited to infants weighing more than 2.0 kg and of greater than 35 weeks' gestation.

In centers where ECMO support is available and entry criteria are followed, it is not surprising that survival in infants who do not require ECMO is higher than in those who do. For example, in one series of 30 infants with CDH who were surgically treated within the first day of life, the survival rate of the 18 who did not require ECMO was 83%. Of the 12 infants who underwent ECMO therapy for severe respiratory failure, 7 (58%) were weaned from ECMO and mechanical ventilation, and 6 (50%) were long-term survivors (Redmond et al., 1987). In a multicenter (n = 19) study including 93 infants with severe CDH who were treated with ECMO between 1983 and 1987, overall long-term survival was 58% (Langham et al., 1987).

The criteria for instituting ECMO vary and often are vague (failure of medical therapy, failure to respond to "maximal treatment," acute clinical deterioration making death appear likely). However, in most centers, stricter, specific guidelines are followed, including PAO_2–PaO_2 greater than 600 mm Hg for 8 hours, oxygen index ($[FIO_2 \times$ mean airway pressure$]/PaO_2$) of 51 for 5 hours, and cardiac arrest (Langham et al., 1987; Heiss et al., 1989; Norden et al., 1994; Steimle et al., 1994). Nonetheless, no selection criteria appear accurate in predicting which infants, if any, have sufficient pulmonary parenchyma to survive (Newman et al., 1990; Van Meurs, 1990; Charlton, 1993; Steimle et al., 1994). Steimle and others (1994) have shown that the application of ECMO to all patients resulted in overall decreased patient survival and only a modest (27%) survival rate for patients with severe cardiorespiratory compromise. In contrast, a multicenter study enrolled 632 of 730 neonates from the CDH Registry from January 1995 to November 1997. These infants had a complete data set and were eligible for ECMO by the weight criterion of greater than 2.0 kg. Of importance, the mortality risk of these infants was stratified according to previously validated independent predictors of survival: birth weight and 5-minute Apgar score. Five groups were defined based on increasing predictive mortality risk. ECMO significantly improved survival rates for those CDH neonates with a predictive mortality risk greater than or equal to 80%. Generally, the more critically ill the infant with CDH, the more likely that ECMO improves survival. Thus, before an intervention such as ECMO is considered, strict entry criteria must be followed. These criteria are not static, and as various modes of therapy are refined, the basis for initiating various therapies is likely to evolve (The Congenital Diaphragmatic Hernia Study Group, 1999).

Intraoperative and Postoperative Management

Usually, surgical repair is approached through an abdominal incision, but a transthoracic or thoracoabdominal approach is also possible. Infants with large defects may not tolerate primary closure of the abdomen after the hernia is reduced. In such a case, a chimney prosthesis or Silastic pouch is placed. In these infants, venous access in the lower extremities should be avoided because the inferior vena cava may be compressed after reduction of the hernia, limiting venous return. An internal jugular cannula provides more reliable access. This access allows CVP monitoring both intraoperatively and postoperatively and may be essential to deliver TPN postoperatively.

With rare exceptions, infants with a moderate or large CHD require ventilatory support preoperatively and most receive neuromuscular blockade. The goals of ventilation in the operating room are the same as preoperatively—to optimize pH and pulmonary blood flow with minimal barotrauma. Hyperventilation is reserved to initially treat an acute episode of pulmonary hypertension. If a sudden deterioration occurs in ventilation, hemodynamic status, or both, pulmonary hypertension must be quickly differentiated from a contralateral pneumothorax, because the treatment for a pneumothorax is needle thoracostomy and chest tube placement rather than hyperventilation.

All newborns deserve meticulous attention to temperature in the operating room, but infants with a CDH have dramatic risks associated with hypothermia (Nielson and Jorgensen, 1978), including an increase in pulmonary vascular resistance, which may increase right-to-left shunting through a PDA or the foramen ovale. Hypothermia increases oxygen consumption, and in the setting of marginal cardiorespiratory function, may result in inadequate oxygen delivery and acidosis, which then further increases pulmonary vasoconstriction and worsens arterial desaturation.

TABLE 16–4. International neonatal ECMO patient population (1973–1990)

	Survived	Died	Total
Patients Entered	3662 (83%)	769 (17%)	4431
Diagnosis			
Meconium aspiration syndrome	1575 (93%)	123 (7%)	1698 (38%)
RDS	551 (84%)	107 (16%)	658 (15%)
CDH	478 (61%)	306 (39%)	784 (18%)
Sepsis/pneumonia	433 (77%)	133 (23%)	566 (13%)
Air leak syndrome	12 (63%)	7 (23%)	19 (0.4%)
Pulmonary hypertension of the newborn	502 (88%)	71(12%)	573 (13%)
Other	111 (83%)	22 (17%)	133 (3%)

From Dalton HI, Thompson AE: Extracorporeal membrane oxygenation. In Fuhrman BP, Zimmerman J, editors: *Pediatric critical care.* St Louis, 1992, Mosby–Year Book. Reprinted with permission from *Neonatal ELSO (Extracorporeal Lift Support Organization) Registry Report,* Ann Arbor, MI, January 1991.

The selection of specific anesthetic agents must be based on cardiorespiratory status, the site for surgical repair (e.g., neonatal intensive care nursery or operating room), and the plans for intraoperative ventilatory support. Nitrous oxide is avoided in infants with CDH because most require high, inspired oxygen concentrations and because nitrous oxide can diffuse inside the viscera and exaggerate lung compression. If an anesthesia machine is available, low concentrations of inhalation anesthetics (sevoflurane or isoflurane) can be administered and increased if the patient is hemodynamically stable. In most cases, high-dose narcotics (usually, fentanyl) are administered and the narcotic infusion is continued into the postoperative period (Vacanti et al., 1984).

Outcome

Early reports of outcome in survivors of CDH noted a decreased total lung capacity and an increased residual volume (Reid and Hutcherson, 1976), as well as hyperinflation and reduced pulmonary perfusion on the affected side (Wohl et al., 1977). Imai and others (1994) noted a high incidence (>75%) of lower airway obstruction, air trapping, and reactive airway disease in those infants with severe CDH who required prolonged mechanical ventilation in the neonatal period. In addition, successful repair of CDH may be associated with gastroesophageal reflux (Nagaya et al., 1994; Sigalet et al., 1994). In a study by Lund and others (1994) on high-risk CDH survivors, 45% had developmental delay, 39% were below the fifth percentile for weight, 18% required a fundoplication, and 21% had a significant hearing loss.

TRACHEOESOPHAGEAL FISTULA AND ESOPHAGEAL ATRESIA

The incidence of this lesion is 1:4000 live births. Approximately 20% to 25% of these infants also have a congenital heart disease (ventricular septal defect, atrial septal defect, tetralogy of Fallot, atrioventricular canal, or coarctation of the aorta). Another 20% to 30% of infants with tracheoesophageal fistula (TEF) are premature, weighing less than 2000 g. Mortality associated with TEF generally depends on the severity of the underlying lung disease and associated anomalies. Improvements in anesthetic and surgical techniques allow greater than 90% survival in otherwise healthy full-term infants (Choudhury et al., 1999). In high-risk infants (<1800 g or with pneumonia) with TEF, mortality ranges from 15% to 60%.

In addition to cardiac anomalies, anorectal, genitourinary, vertebral, skeletal, and craniofacial abnormalities can occur with TEF. The VATER syndrome, described in 1973, is an association of the following anomalies: *V,* vertebral defects; *A,* anal defects; *T,* TEF; *E,* esophageal atresia; and *R,* radial or renal anomalies (Quan and Smith, 1973). Another acronym includes a "C" and "L" because cardiac and limb anomalies are also common. As many as 20% to 25% of infants with esophageal atresia have at least three of the lesions included in VACTERL (Rittler et al., 1996). Between 50% and 65% of infants with esophageal atresia with or without a TEF have at least one additional anomaly. Anomalies are more common in the isolated esophageal atresia type and least common in the H-type fistula.

Some infants may also have other anomalies as part of a generalized chromosomal syndrome. Clearly, the spectrum of presentation from an isolated TEF to a multisystem or chromosomal disorder has major implications for treatment options and surgical and anesthetic management.

Embryology

The embryogenesis of this set of lesions is not completely defined, but several aspects of the recent investigations are relevant to clinicians. The trachea and esophagus develop from a common site, the foregut, in the first 4 to 5 weeks of gestation. The high incidence of associated lesions within the trachea and the gastrointestinal tract is well known. For example, anomalies of the tracheobronchial tree occur in almost 50% of patients with TEF. The most common lesion is an ectopic right upper bronchus, but other lesions include congenital bronchial stenosis, congenital tracheal stenosis, tracheal web, and the absence of the right upper bronchus. Duodenal or ileal atresia, malrotation, and imperforate anus are common associated anomalies of the gastrointestinal system (Dave et al., 1999).

Both the esophagus and the trachea originate from the median ventral diverticulum of the primitive foregut. The TEF lesion results from failure of the two structures to separate during division of the endoderm. Esophageal atresia results when the tracheal structures assume most of the endoderm, and TEF results when the esophageal and tracheal ridges fail to develop, leaving a communication between the two structures.

An Adriamycin (doxorubicin)-induced TEF model in rats has allowed a careful examination of the distal esophageal development. This model results in the most common anatomic TEF: blind esophageal pouch and fistula between the trachea and the distal esophagus. The distal esophagus has been identified as being of tracheal origin by examining the expression of thyroid-transcription factor-1 (TTF-1), known to be specific to the respiratory tract. TTF-1 expression localizes to the lung bud but not to the esophagus early in gestation. TTF-1 was expressed in the fistula tract all through gestation. The distal "esophagus" appears to be of embryonic lung origin. This discovery is of major clinical relevance, explaining the pathophysiology and clinical findings of this disorder: poor esophageal motility, gastroesophageal reflux, esophageal stenosis, and pseudostratified columnar (respiratory epithelium) rather than squamous epithelium (esophageal epithelium) (Crisera et al., 1999a, 1999b). These same investigators have reported abnormal signaling of a glycoprotein (Sonic hedgehog) involved in embryologic processes including foregut development in human TEF tissue (Spilde et al., 2003).

Anatomy of Tracheoesophageal Fistula

The anatomic variations of TEF have been well described (Fig. 16–11, classification of Gross) and, in most cases (types B, C, and E), TEF and esophageal atresia occur together. The most common lesion (>90%) is type C, in which a fistula exists between the trachea and the lower esophageal segment at a point slightly above the carina, whereas the upper esophageal segment ends blindly in the mediastinum at the level of the second or third thoracic vertebra.

Clinical Presentation

TEF should be suspected in cases of maternal polyhydramnios and premature labor. Both conditions may result from esophageal obstruction that prevents the swallowing of amniotic fluid. The newborn infant exhibits excessive salivation, drooling, cyanotic spells, and coughing relieved by suctioning. The diagnosis of esophageal atresia can be confirmed in the delivery room by the inability to pass a catheter down the esophagus into the stomach. When a radiopaque catheter is used, a radiograph reveals the catheter in the blind upper pouch. If a TEF is

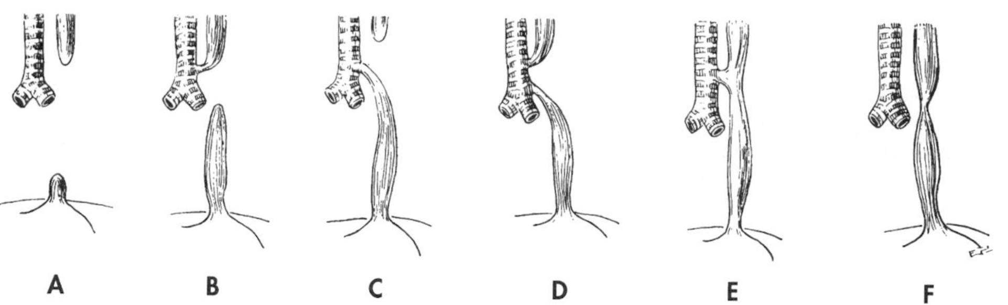

■ **FIGURE 16–11.** Types of congenital abnormalities of the esophagus. *A,* Esophageal atresia, no esophageal communication with the trachea. *B,* Esophageal atresia, upper segment communicating with the trachea. *C,* Esophageal atresia, lower segment communicating with the back of the trachea. More than 90% of all esophageal malformations fall into this group. *D,* Esophageal atresia, both segments communicating with the trachea. *E,* Esophagus has no disruption of its continuity but has a tracheoesophageal fistula. *F,* Esophageal stenosis. (From Gross RE: *The surgery of infancy and childhood.* Philadelphia, 1953, WB Saunders.)

present, a plain radiograph of the chest and abdomen reveals air or gas bubbles in the stomach and intestines that have entered through the fistula (Fig. 16–12). Ultrasonography is important to evaluate for any associated cardiac, renal, or genitourinary abnormalities.

Preoperative Management

The ligation of a TEF is urgent. Preoperatively, several interventions are undertaken promptly to protect the lungs from aspiration pneumonia, including

- Avoidance of feedings (NPO)
- Upright positioning of the infant to prevent gastroesophageal reflux
- Intermittent suctioning of the upper pouch
- Antibiotic therapy and physiotherapy in babies with contaminated lungs

Intraoperative Management

Optimally, a total repair can be accomplished as a one-stage procedure, in which the fistula is ligated and the esophagus is primarily anastomosed. In infants with significant associated anomalies or sepsis, a thoracotomy may be considered too risky and, instead, a palliative procedure, a gastrostomy, is performed under local or general anesthesia. Despite the lower morbidity associated with a gastrostomy, many anesthesiologists prefer to intubate the trachea to minimize the risks from aspiration during surgical manipulation. The definitive repair is performed within 24 to 72 hours, when the extent of other anomalies is defined, cardiovascular stability is established, and a clear surgical plan has been defined. The gastrostomy tube is kept patent to decompress the stomach and to minimize regurgitation into the lungs.

Unless the aortic arch is right-sided, the surgical approach for definitive repair is through a right thoracotomy using a posterolateral extrapleural approach. On occasion, the distal portion of the esophagus is either absent or too short to reach the proximal segment. In such cases, some surgeons may ligate the fistula and exteriorize the upper pouch through an esophagostomy. The infant is then fed via the gastrostomy until a weight of about 9 to 10 kg (20 lb) or 1 year of age has been reached. At that time, the two esophageal segments are surgically bridged with an interposed bowel segment or gastric tube graft.

A technique of "awake intubation" is generally considered as the safest approach to secure the airway in infants with TEF. This allows the appropriate positioning of the endotracheal tube without positive-pressure ventilation, as well as minimizing the

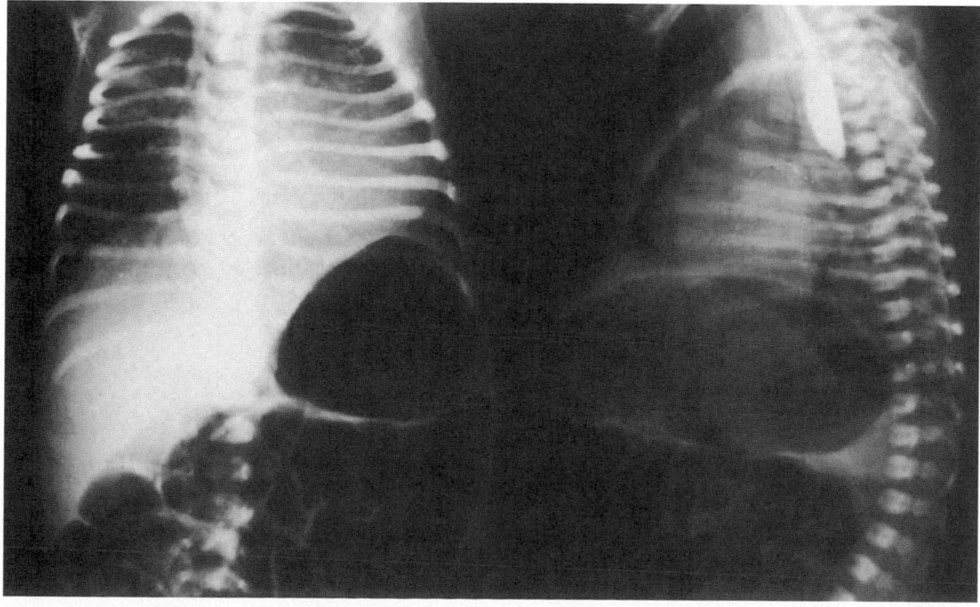

■ **FIGURE 16–12.** Gastric distention, in type C lesion, may require prompt relief. Note blindly ending esophagus on lateral view. (Courtesy Dr. Arnold Colodny, Boston, MA.)

risk of gastric distention from inspired gases passing through the fistula. Titrating small doses of fentanyl (0.2 to 0.5 mcg/kg) or morphine (0.02 to 0.05 mg/kg) before intubation is ideal, but this must be considered from the perspective of the infant's clinical status at the time of the procedure. An alternative induction technique includes an inhalation anesthetic with or without muscle relaxation with cautious, gentle positive-pressure ventilation.

After the endotracheal tube is in place, end-tidal carbon dioxide and oxygen saturation must be monitored, and the stomach and chest should be ausculated to ensure that the lungs are adequately ventilated and the stomach is not distended with inspired gases. If the endotracheal tube is positioned so that ventilation is entering the stomach via the fistula, or if the fistula itself has been intubated, the stomach may become distended and impair ventilation. Salem and others (1973) suggest distal positioning of the endotracheal tube, with the bevel facing anteriorly and the posterior wall of the endotracheal tube occluding the fistula, but this maneuver is challenging to achieve and maintain.

In patients with a gastrostomy, proper positioning of the endotracheal tube can be monitored by submerging the gastrostomy tube in a container of water so that gas bubbles are evident during ventilation of the fistula. If gas bubbling occurs, the endotracheal tube must be repositioned. Alternatively, the gastrostomy tube can be connected to a capnograph. When the endotracheal tube is proximal to the fistula, carbon dioxide is detected. When the endotracheal tube is distal to the fistula, no expiratory gases are detected.

Even with adequate positioning of the endotracheal tube, in some patients ventilation through the fistula still occurs. In patients without a gastrostomy, gastric distention may impair ventilation. Filston and others (1982) have suggested occluding the fistula with a Fogarty catheter placed through a bronchoscope. However, bronchoscopy, even without the challenge of precise positioning of a Fogarty, can be a difficult procedure in the newborn, especially if pulmonary compliance is abnormal.

In patients with a gastrostomy, gastric decompression may serve as a low resistance vent through which most of the tidal volume escapes. If this occurs, the gastrostomy tube should be clamped or, as Karl (1985) has reported, a retrograde Fogarty catheter can be inserted. Although theoretically possible, this technique is often impractical in the setting of small infants. Precisely positioning a Fogarty catheter so that the balloon is occluding only the fistula is difficult to achieve, and even if the positioning is perfect on initial attempt, maintaining this exact position of the catheter for any length of time is almost impossible. Furthermore, displacement of the balloon can be disastrous (e.g., occluding the trachea). The balloon is a high-pressure device that may impinge on small pulmonary vessels and/or airways compromising pulmonary blood flow or ventilation.

Once satisfactory ventilation is ensured, the chest is opened and the lungs are retracted. Lung retraction impairs ventilation, especially in infants with respiratory dysfunction from immature lungs, pneumonia, or congenital heart disease. Intermittent release of pressure by the surgeon to allow inflation of the right lung often improves oxygenation and ventilation. Blood clots or secretions may block the endotracheal tube, and frequent endotracheal suctioning may be required. Because the trachea is a soft structure in the newborn, surgical manipulation may kink the airway and further obstruct ventilation. Thus, interference with adequate oxygenation can occur as a result of the patient's anatomy, operative positioning, and surgical manipulations. Inspired concentration of oxygen must be closely monitored and adjusted, balancing the risks of oxygen toxicity with those of hypoxia. Close communication between the surgeon and anesthesiologist is essential.

After the TEF is ligated, the anesthesiologist is asked to pass a catheter through the nose or mouth into the blind upper pouch to identify the upper esophageal structure. The surgeon passes a catheter into the lower part of the esophagus, and the anastomosis is made over the catheter. When the anastomosis is complete, the catheter is withdrawn just above the suture line, and the proximal end of the catheter is marked at the mouth. The distance from the mouth to the distal tip is noted. Only catheters of this length should be used for suction in the postoperative period.

Intraoperative monitoring must be carefully planned. The precordial stethoscope is repositioned after induction of anesthesia into the left axilla. In infants with an unstable cardiorespiratory status or congenital heart disease, an arterial catheter (umbilical or right radial) should be placed. If an arterial catheter is not available, a noninvasive device is used. Other monitoring consists of an electrocardiogram, pulse oximetry, and end-tidal gas monitoring. In some infants, both preductal and postductal pulse oximeters are placed. The patient's temperature must also be monitored, and efforts must be made to prevent hypothermia.

Postoperative Management

Some term infants can be extubated after simple ligation of a TEF, but this is rare. Tracheomalacia or a defective tracheal wall at the site of the fistula can cause collapse of the airway and require reinsertion of the endotracheal tube. These specific problems with TEF, as well as the host of other cardiorespiratory problems of the newborn, generally require a period of postoperative ventilation for these infants, often for at least 24 to 48 hours. In addition, most surgeons request that ventilation with a mask and bag be avoided for at least several days postoperatively. Infants who have had repair of a "long-gap" atresia require postoperative ventilatory support for a longer (5 to 7 days) postoperative period. Neuromuscular blocking agents are administered during this time to eliminate any spontaneous ventilation. Postoperative ventilation is also planned for an infant whose lungs were contaminated, whose intraoperative course was complicated (e.g., tracheal perforation), or who has underlying lung disease associated with prematurity.

Outcome

TEF cannot be considered a simple anatomic problem cured by a surgical intervention. Many patients have anatomic narrowing of the esophagus either at the site of anastomosis or the fistula ligation, and this narrowing may progress to a severe stricture. Esophageal dysmotility and reflux are common, and may also lead to esophageal stricture. Recurrent upper and lower respiratory infections occur in 35% to 75% of patients (Dudley and Phelan, 1976). Pulmonary function studies 7 to 18 years after repair show a high incidence of obstructive and restrictive forms of lung disease (Milligan and Levison, 1979).

NECROTIZING ENTEROCOLITIS

Necrotizing enterocolitis (NEC) is a gastrointestinal emergency primarily affecting premature infants of gestational age less than 32 weeks; 80% of affected patients are preterm. The severity of the symptoms, complications, and mortality are inversely related to gestational age. Although centered in the gastrointestinal

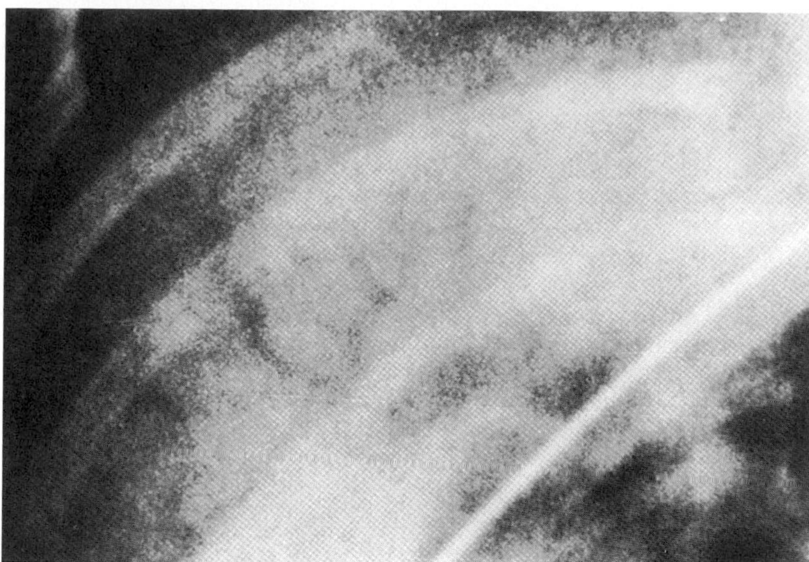

■ **FIGURE 16–13.** Air pattern in the portal venous system of the liver in an infant with necrotizing enterocolitis. (From Rowe MI: Necrotizing enterocolitis. In Welch KJ, Randolph JG, Ravitch MM, et al., editors: *Pediatric surgery*, 4th ed. Chicago, 1986, Year Book Medical Publishers.)

tract, NEC is a systemic process primarily related to the sepsis that accompanies the intestinal necrosis and increased mucosal permeability.

The etiology of NEC is considered to be multifactorial. The incidence of NEC (10% to 20%, in infants <1500 g) has not decreased and overall mortality has not improved over the past two to three decades. As the survival of the premature, especially the ELBW, infant has improved, the incidence of NEC has increased in some populations. The increased number of susceptible infants may explain the lack of improved overall survival in infants with NEC.

Bell and others (1978) described three stages of NEC. Stage 1 refers to mild disease with the infant having only nonspecific symptoms (vomiting, gastric residuals, apnea, bradycardia, guaiac-positive stools). There is no definitive radiologic evidence for NEC, and the state of the bowel is completely unknown. Stage 2 includes infants with definitive NEC. They have clinical symptoms similar to the infants in stage I, but on radiographs these infants have pneumatosis intestinalis or portal venous air (Figs. 16–13 and 16–14). These infants are suitable for medical management. Stage 3 includes infants with advanced disease. These infants have evidence of intestinal necrosis and/or perforation along with clinical signs of hemodynamic, respiratory, and/or hematologic instability. Although these three stages are not distinct and are actually a continuum of clinical disease, the three-stage concept helps define management strategies.

Pathophysiology

NEC is a paradoxical disease. Classically, it occurs in premature infants and in infants with LBW. Most infants with NEC weigh less than 2500 g and are less than 37 weeks gestational age at birth. However, NEC can also occur in full-term infants on the first day of life or months after birth. It can occur in fed or unfed infants, in a single patient, or as a nursery epidemic. Of note, term infants develop symptoms by day 2 to 3 of life, whereas the ELBW infants are more likely to develop NEC in the second week of life.

NEC is frequently linked to intestinal mucosal injury from ischemia caused by reduced mesenteric blood flow. Mesenteric blood flow may be compromised by a decreased cardiac output in the presence of fetal asphyxia, a PDA, postnatal apnea, heart failure, arrhythmia, or severe bradycardia and hypoxemia. Other factors that may contribute to the pathogenesis of NEC include enteral feeding of small preterm infants, use of a hyperosmolar formula, bacterial infection, intestinal dysfunction, gram-negative endotoxemia, polycythemia, congenital heart disease, and a history of umbilical arterial catheterization or exchange transfusion.

The most common anatomic site for NEC is the ileocolic region. However, NEC is frequently discontinuous, with patchy occurrence in both the small and large intestine in as many as 50% of cases. Large bowel involvement is most common in the term infant. Perforations often are multiple and commonly identified at the junction of a site of necrosis with more normal bowel but are also found within the affected areas.

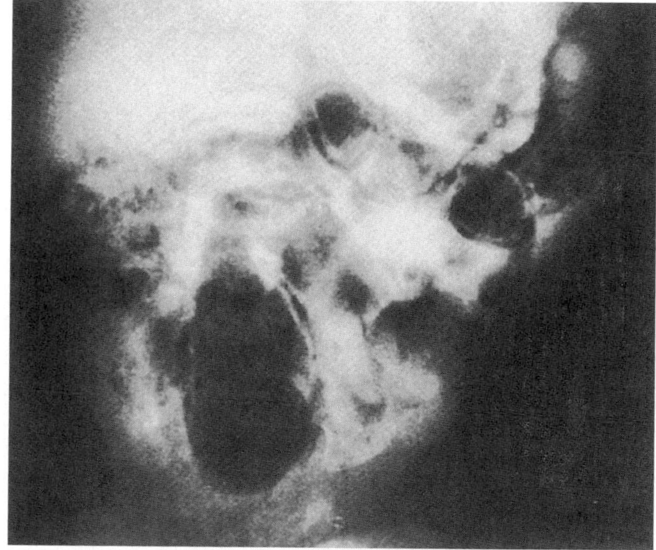

■ **FIGURE 16–14.** Pneumatosis intestinalis in an infant with necrotizing enterocolitis. (From Rowe MI: Necrotizing enterocolitis. In Welch KJ, Randolph JG, Ravitch MM, et al., editors: *Pediatric surgery*, 4th ed. Chicago, 1986, Year Book Medical Publishers. Reproduced with permission.)

The primary pathologic finding in NEC is coagulative or ischemic necrosis, but inflammation is prominent. The inflammatory response seems to be unique in that abscesses do not form, as seen in inflammatory bowel disease or infectious colitis or as a result of acute arterial occlusion. The combination of ischemia and bacteria seems to be essential. For example, NEC does not evolve after an episode of vascular injury in utero, when the bowel is sterile (Musemeche et al., 1986). Instead, an intestinal atresia or stenosis may develop. The formation of the gas bubbles (pneumatosis intestinalis) reflects fermentation of intraluminal substrate by bacteria. However, NEC is not associated with a specific organism or with particularly virulent bacteria. A wide range of organisms have been identified in the stool of infants with NEC, some who also have a bacteremia with the same organism—*Escherichia coli*, various strains of *Enterobacter, Klebsiella*, and *Pseudomonas*, and coagulase-negative staphylococci, and others.

Several "models" of NEC, emphasizing the role of inflammatory/vasoactive mediators, platelet-activating factor (PAF), and tumor necrosis factor (TNF) α have been developed (Fong et al., 1990; Sun and Hsueh, 1991; Sun et al., 1996; Wand et al., 1997; Tan et al., 2000). PAF is released by inflammatory cells as well as by bacteria and in high concentrations can induce hypotension and shock as well as increase gut permeability (Tan et al., 2000).

Elevated levels of PAF have been measured in infants with NEC (Rabinowitz et al., 2001). In addition, premature infants have low levels of PAF-degrading enzyme, acetylhydrolase (Caplan et al., 1990). Other mechanisms included in the pathogenesis of NEC include immature immunologic mechanisms, abnormal patterns of bacterial overgrowth, and deficient mesenteric blood flow regulation. Differences in the content of sialic acid and *N*-acetylglucosamine residues of the mucosa may affect anatomy and function of the microvilli, leading to certain types of bacterial colonization, bacterial adhesion, and, eventually, permeation of the gastrointestinal tract (Claud and Walker, 2001) (Fig. 16–15).

Preoperative Management

A typical infant with NEC is a preterm baby weighing less than 2500 g. These infants commonly have had perinatal asphyxia or other respiratory complications in the early postnatal period. Prenatal complications associated with NEC include premature rupture of the membranes, placenta previa, maternal sepsis, and toxemia of pregnancy (Touloukian, 1976; Uauy et al., 1991). A history of breech delivery or cesarean section are associated with 15% to 20% of NEC cases (Santulli et al., 1975). Infants with NEC may be acidotic, hypoxic, hypothermic, and in shock. The gastrointestinal signs appear between the 1st and 10th days of life in more than 90% of these babies (Touloukian, 1976). They include abdominal distention, retained gastric secretions (may be bile-tinged), vomiting, bloody or mucoid diarrhea, and occult blood loss in the stools. Bowel necrosis and perforation follow, and sepsis occurs, with thermal instability, lethargy, metabolic acidosis, jaundice, disseminated intravascular coagulation, and generalized bleeding. Most infants with NEC have a decreased platelet count (50,000 to 75,000/mm^3) and prolonged prothrombin and partial thromboplastin times. Abdominal radiographs may reveal dilated, fixed (adynamic ileus) loops of bowel, pneumatosis (intramural air in the intestine), gas in the portal venous system, and pneumoperitoneum. These are pathognomonic signs of NEC.

Unless there is evidence of intestinal necrosis or perforation, the initial treatment for NEC is nonoperative. Decompression of the stomach; cessation of feeding; broad-spectrum antibiotics; fluid and electrolyte therapy, including parenteral nutrition; and correction of hematologic abnormalities are the main components of medical therapy. Supportive therapy, including inotropic agents and steroids, may be used to treat endotoxic shock. Bowel perforation is the most important indication for surgery. Other relative indications include peritonitis, air in the portal system, bowel wall edema, ascites, and a progressively deteriorating cardiorespiratory status (Box 16–7).

The role for primary peritoneal drainage is not well defined. The effectiveness of peritoneal lavage in "buying time" for an infant to achieve hemodynamic, acid-base, and hematologic stability is actively debated. This procedure seems to be "palliative" because most infants eventually require surgery. The ELBW infant may benefit from such a temporizing procedure that would allow resuscitation and stabilization. If surgery is performed after the hemodynamic status improves, adequate gut perfusion to marginal segments of bowel might be established and, consequently, less bowel is resected. This might avoid excessive bowel resection and short gut syndrome (Ahmed et al., 1998).

The preoperative assessment of infants with NEC should focus on evaluating and correcting the respiratory, circulatory, metabolic, and hematologic disorders. Laboratory testing includes analysis of blood gases, glucose, electrolytes, and coagulation

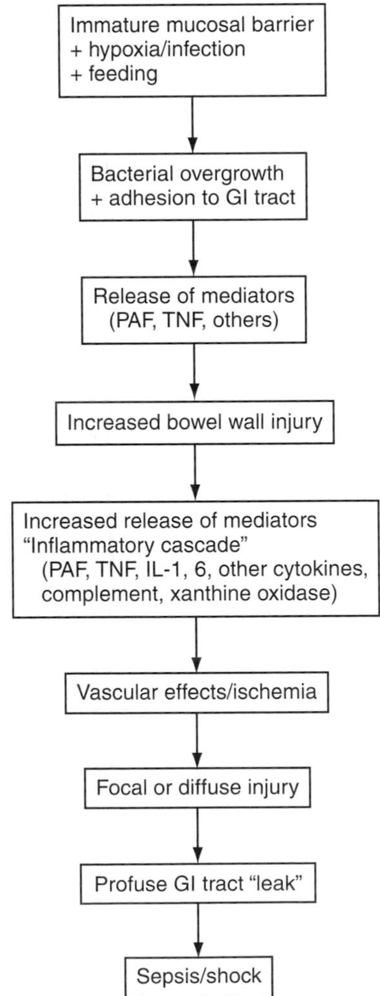

■ **FIGURE 16–15.** Schematic representation of the pathophysiology of necrotizing enterocolitis.

BOX 16–7 Indications for Operation

Absolute Indications

Pneumoperitoneum
Intestinal gangrene (positive results of paracentesis)

Relative Indications

Clinical deterioration
- Metabolic acidosis
- Ventilatory failure
- Oliguria; hypovolemia
- Thrombocytopenia
- Leukopenia; leukocytosis

Portal vein gas
Erythema of abdominal wall
Fixed abdominal mass
Persistently dilated loop

Nonindications

Severe gastrointestinal hemorrhage
Abdominal tenderness
Intestinal obstruction
Gasless abdomen with ascites

status, including platelet count. Increased fluid and crystalloid therapy may be needed in hypovolemic infants with massive third-space fluid losses. During fluid resuscitation, these infants must be monitored carefully for signs of PDA or congestive heart failure.

Intraoperative Management

Intraoperative monitoring should include arterial and central venous cannulas for continuous pressure monitoring, blood gas analysis, and other metabolic tests. Fresh frozen plasma, platelets, and red blood cells may be administered early in surgery in response to clinical and laboratory evidence of coagulopathy. Inspired oxygen concentration should be adjusted to produce an arterial oxygen tension of 50 to 70 mm Hg (Sp_{O_2}, 90% to 95%). Nitrous oxide must be avoided, especially in the presence of free air in the gastrointestinal and portal venous systems.

Potent inhalation agents are often poorly tolerated and often are only introduced in low concentrations to supplement narcotics or ketamine. Fentanyl or remifentanil combined with low-dose, inhaled anesthetic agents can provide infants with analgesia and amnesia as well as cardiovascular stability. Neuromuscular blocking agents facilitate surgical exposure. Inotropic agents occasionally are needed to support the cardiovascular system when fluid therapy alone fails to maintain adequate perfusion.

Because of the large fluid requirements, hypothermia is a frequent intraoperative complication. Usually the operating room and infused fluids are warmed to assist in maintaining adequate body temperature. In the surgical treatment of NEC, necrotic bowel is resected, and, usually, the marginally viable ends are exteriorized. The cardinal principles of surgery for NEC are to excise all necrotic bowel but preserve as much bowel length as possible by leaving "marginal" appearing bowel in place, decompressing the bowel, and removing pus, stool, and necrotic debris from the peritoneal cavity. Preserving bowel may require multiple segmental resections and second-look operations to reassess bowel viability. Selected patients may tolerate resection and primary reanastomosis. Bowel strictures often develop within days to months after the initial surgery, frequently necessitating further surgical intervention. In patients with enterostomies, closure can be attempted 4 weeks to 4 months later.

Postoperative Management

Postoperatively, mechanical ventilation and cardiovascular support are usually continued in the neonatal intensive care unit. Central venous parenteral nutrition is essential after sepsis is controlled and metabolic stability is established.

Outcome

Mortality from NEC is high, ranging between 10% and 30% (or higher in severely affected ELBW infants), depending on the gestational age, coexisting morbidity, and severity of the process. Infants who initially respond to medical management may eventually require surgery to treat bowel obstruction secondary to strictures or another episode of NEC. Similarly, those who initially respond to placement of an intraperitoneal drain for lavage may eventually require surgery. Infants who develop a spontaneous localized intestinal perforation are probably distinct from those with NEC and usually have a more benign course. The hospital course for preterm infants with NEC can be prolonged and characterized by repeated episodes of sepsis and long-term requirements for intravenous alimentation as enteral feedings are introduced slowly. A devastating complication in survivors of NEC is short bowel syndrome. In these cases, the extent of bowel resection is so extensive that the infant is unable to establish enteral feedings and inevitably develops hepatic failure secondary to intravenous alimentation.

Breast milk has been used in the preterm infant to prevent or at least decrease the incidence of NEC and its complications. The role for treatment with probiotics (Millar et al., 2003), nonspecific (steroids, indomethacin, magnesium, copper) and specific anti-inflammatory agents (e.g., PAF receptor blockers), growth factors (erythropoietin), or antibiotics remains speculative.

SACROCOCCYGEAL TERATOMA

Sacrococcygeal teratomas are the most common congenital neoplasm, occurring in 1:40,000 infants. Approximately 95% of infants are female.

Embryology/Diagnosis

The tumor is derived from pleuripotential cell lines and contains components consisting of all three germ layers. Perinatal mortality is high when the tumor is diagnosed antenatally. Postulated mechanisms of death include high output cardiac failure, preterm delivery secondary to polyhydramnios, anemia from hemorrhage into the tumor, dystocia, and tumor rupture.

Sacrococcygeal teratomas receive their blood supply from the middle sacral artery and branches of the internal iliac artery. A steal syndrome can shunt blood from the placenta and lead to high output cardiac failure and hydrops. Approximately 2% to 10% of sacrococcygeal tumors are malignant before the infant reaches 2 months of age, and 50% are malignant by 1 year of age. Serum α-fetoprotein levels are elevated in 70% of children with malignant tumors.

Sacrococcygeal tumors generally arise from the tip of the coccyx and vary with the amount of internal and/or external extension. These tumors are classified into four types according to their location (Box 16–8; Figs. 16–16 and 16–17).

BOX 16–8 Sacral Coccygeal Tumor Types

Type I	External with minimal pressure component
Type II	External considerable intrapelvic extension
Type III	External with pelvic and intra-abdominal extension
Type IV	Presacral; no external presentation

Intraoperative Management

Surgical treatment involves complete resection of both the tumor and coccyx. Failure to remove the coccyx completely can result in local recurrence. Treatment options in utero include open fetal surgery (Bullard and Harrison, 1995), endoscopic laser ablation (Hecher and Hackeloer, 1996), and radiofrequency ablation (Paek et al., 2001).

Anesthetic management for removal of tumors in the neonatal period requires an understanding of neonatal physiology and an appreciation for the possibility of cardiovascular instability, massive blood transfusion requirements, hypothermia, and coagulation dysfunction. Death during resection is often related to hemorrhage, hypothermia, coagulopathy, and the inability to provide adequate cardiopulmonary support during the intraoperative manipulation of the tumor. For large tumors, adequate venous access, central venous access, and invasive arterial pressure monitoring are essential.

Outcome

Predictors of poor outcome have been associated with (1) diagnosis before 20 weeks' gestation, (2) delivery before 30 weeks, (3) development of hydrops, (4) low birth weight, and (5) 5-minute Apgar score less than 7 (Chisholm et al., 1999).

IMPERFORATE ANUS (ANAL ATRESIA)

The incidence of anorectal malformations is 1:5000 live births. "Imperforate" anus can range from a mild stenosis to a complex syndrome with other associated congenital anomalies. The higher the anatomic relation of the terminal bowel to the puborectalis sling of the levator musculature, the greater is the incidence of associated anomalies. The frequency of additional genitourinary abnormalities is 48% but ranges from 14% in infants with perineal fistulas to 90% in infants with bladder fistulas. Twenty-four percent of infants have a tethered spinal cord (Levitt et al., 1997). Male infants with imperforate anus may require an operation soon after birth for relief of obstruction. In female infants, a rectovaginal fistula usually prevents total bowel obstruction so that surgical treatment is not an emergency.

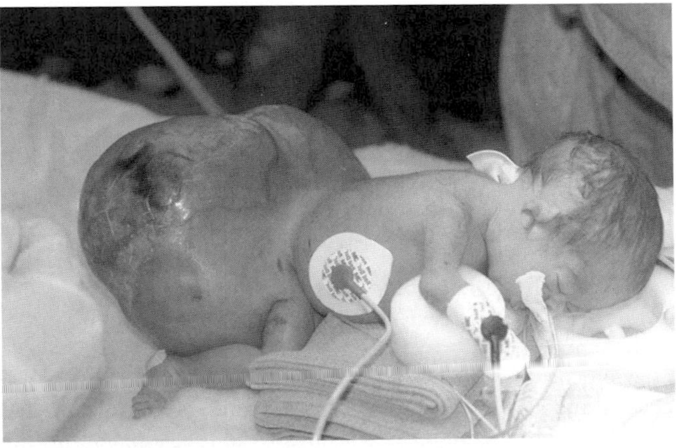

FIGURE 16–16. Sacrococcygeal teratoma type.

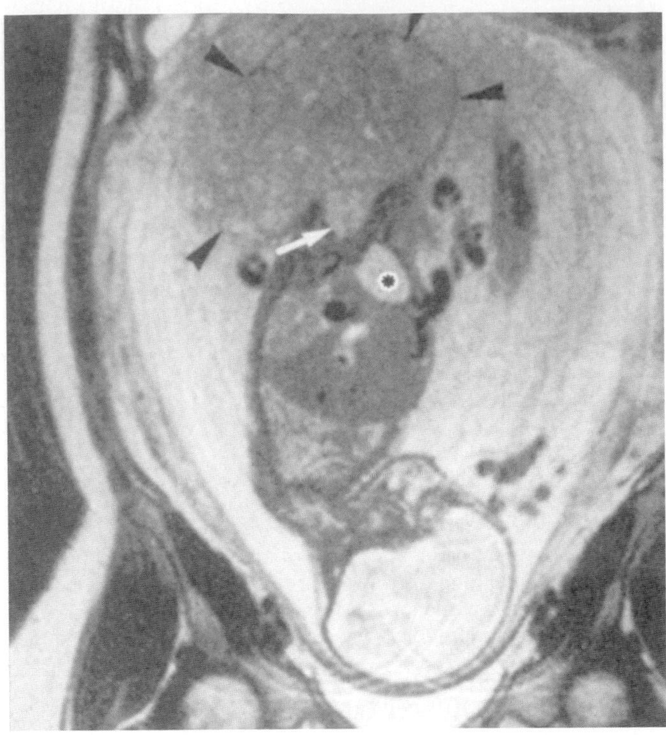

FIGURE 16–17. In utero diagnosis by magnetic resonance imaging. (From Auni et al.: *Am J Radiol* 178:179, 2002.)

Intraoperative Management

Anesthetic requirements vary depending on the severity of the abdominal distention and complexity of the surgery—a simple perineal anoplasty, a temporary colostomy, or an extensive abdominoperineal repair. Anorectal malformation can be classified by the presence or absence of a fistula and by the fistula's location (Pena and Hong, 2000) (Box 16–9). Perineal fistulas in both male and female infants represent the simplest defect, and treatment generally consists of an anoplasty performed in the neonatal period. Imperforate anus with no fistula is the least common presentation, whereas rectourethral fistulas are the most common with the exception of the perineal fistula. The standard surgical approach has generally involved three steps: (1) a diverting colostomy performed in the neonatal period, (2) the main repair done during infancy, and (3) a take-down colostomy performed later in infancy. Surgical trends, however, have been aimed at performing the primary repair without a colostomy. The primary repair involves a posterior surgical approach. Laparoscopic techniques have been used to assist in the pull-through technique (Georgeson, 2000).

Anesthetic considerations for neonates with intestinal obstruction from any etiology include airway management of a "full stomach," assessment of fluid status, correction of electrolyte disturbances, treatment of sepsis, and cardiorespiratory evaluation. Marked abdominal distention secondary to intestinal obstruction can impede diaphragmatic excursion and impair ventilation.

BOX 16–9 Therapeutic Classification of Anorectal Malformations

Males

Cutaneous fistula	No colostomy required
Anal stenosis	
Anal membrane	
Rectourethral fistula	Colostomy required
Bulbar	
Prostatic	
Rectovesical fistula	
Anorectal agenesis without fistula	
Rectal atresia	

Females

Cutaneous (perineal) fistula	No colostomy required
Vestibular fistula	Colostomy required
Vaginal fistula	
Anorectal agenesis without fistula	
Rectal atresia	
Persistent cloaca	

Gastric (or lower intestinal) contents often are incompletely emptied with nasogastric suction, so that the risk of aspiration is significant, especially in the setting of induction of general anesthesia.

Intubation of the trachea of infants with an apparently normal upper airway can be accomplished with an "awake" or rapid sequence technique. If the anesthesiologist suspects that the upper airway will be difficult to visualize, the usual airway precautions should be followed. That is, neuromuscular blocking agents, deep sedation, and general anesthesia are avoided and an "awake" technique is attempted. Supplemental support systems for the difficult airway (e.g., neonatal bronchoscopes, light wand, LMA) should be available (see Chapter 9, Anesthesia Equipment and Monitoring).

Anesthesia during the surgery can include potent inhalation anesthetics, narcotics, or both. In general, nitrous oxide is avoided because of the risk for increasing bowel distention. Intermediate- or long-acting nondepolarizing muscle relaxants often improve surgical conditions at lower inhaled anesthetic concentrations. If early postoperative extubation is planned, narcotics should be judiciously administered, but in many cases postoperative mechanical ventilation is required.

Imperforate anus is usually recognized early in the postnatal period, and in the group of infants without total bowel obstruction, massive distention may not develop and, therefore, the complications associated with intestinal obstruction are minimized, as are the complications from bowel ischemia, third-space fluid loss, electrolyte disturbances, and sepsis. Imperforate anus without a fistula can be associated with the development of total intestinal obstruction in utero, leading to severe abdominal distention, bowel perforation, sepsis, or a combination. In addition, other congenital anomalies often have a dramatic effect on the management of these infants. For example, imperforate anus is associated with tracheoesophageal fistula, renal anomalies, and heart disease.

During surgery, the management of fluids, blood replacement, and electrolyte delivery are similar to the principles discussed for NEC and for intestinal obstruction. As with any intra-abdominal surgery in the newborn, a major challenge is maintaining an adequate intravascular volume. The presence of radiopaque contrast agents, bowel manipulation, and peritonitis increases third-space fluid requirements. In such cases, 10 mL/kg per hr (or more) of isotonic saline solution or colloid is frequently needed intraoperatively. Monitoring urine output, quality of heart tones, heart rate, and blood pressure is a basic requirement to assess continuing fluid needs. Invasive monitors such as an arterial catheter and a CVP catheter generally are reserved for those with marked cardiorespiratory instability.

Postoperative Management

The preoperative and intraoperative courses and the effects of associated congenital anomalies set the stage for the postoperative course. Many infants require postoperative ventilatory support, total parenteral alimentation, cardiovascular support, and treatment of sepsis. The function and recovery of the gastrointestinal system vary enormously among infants with imperforate anus and seem to be related to whether the lesion is isolated and whether the complications of total bowel obstruction have developed.

Outcome

Intestinal obstruction has been one of the major causes of death after neonatal surgery. With more skilled pediatric management and the development of parenteral alimentation, mortality is now limited primarily to infants whose condition is diagnosed late and who require extensive excision of the small and large bowel. Long-term complications from anorectal malformations, especially a high imperforate anus, can be lifelong and involve sequelae related to fecal soiling, constipation, and sexual inadequacy.

INTESTINAL OBSTRUCTION

Intestinal obstruction is a surgical emergency in the newborn, requiring swift intervention after diagnosis. Bowel obstruction presents with symptoms and signs similar to those seen at other ages—vomiting, abdominal distention, decreased bowel sounds, and radiologic evidence of gas-filled loops of bowel. However, in the newborn the list of etiologies includes a unique set of congenital anomalies.

Delay in the diagnosis and treatment of such lesions may lead to various complications that can increase morbidity and mortality. As described for the infant with imperforate anus, delay in diagnosis leads to disturbance of fluid and electrolyte balance and increased abdominal distention, with subsequent respiratory embarrassment and high risk for aspiration pneumonitis. Intestinal perforation, necrosis of the bowel, and septicemia are other secondary consequences if intestinal obstruction is not managed promptly.

Distended bowel forces the diaphragm into a high, fixed position, limiting excursion, causing severe ventilatory compromise, and increasing the risk of aspiration. Although prompt surgical repair is imperative, optimizing the patient's metabolic status is critical before surgery. Initiation of corrective fluid and electrolyte therapy should precede the induction of anesthesia. Nasogastric suction may decrease gastric distention and the risk for aspiration, but, if the site of obstruction is below the duodenum, the abdominal distention is not drastically affected.

Although the underlying etiologies of intestinal obstruction are variable (annular pancreas, intestinal atresia or stenosis, duplication of intestine, meconium ileus, tumors, enterocolitis), the problems of anesthetic management for surgical correction of these lesions are similar.

Duodenal Obstruction

The incidence of duodenal obstruction in the neonate is 1:10,000 to 1:40,000 births and is frequently associated with other congenital anomalies such as Down syndrome, cystic fibrosis, renal anomalies, intestinal malrotation, and, especially, midline defects such as esophageal atresia and imperforate anus. An intraluminal diaphragm, a membranous web, or an annular pancreas can also be associated with obstruction of the duodenum. The degree of obstruction varies from severe or complete atresia to incomplete obstruction or stenosis. Air contrast films reveal a dilated stomach and a dilated proximal duodenum, resulting in the "double-bubble" appearance.

Infants with complete obstruction exhibit copious vomiting of bile or bile-stained gastric contents and minimal abdominal distention. The infant may or may not pass meconium in the first day of life. Infants who have incomplete obstruction have intermittent bile-stained vomiting and usually pass meconium. A delay in the treatment of this condition can result in dehydration, weight loss, and hypochloremic alkalosis.

Jejunoileal Atresia

Jejunoileal atresia causes complete obstruction in 1:5000 live births. In contrast to duodenal atresias, jejunoileal atresias are associated with few other anomalies. Prematurity is associated with 50% of cases, polyhydramnios with 25%, and cystic fibrosis with 20%.

The etiology of jejunoileal atresia is uncertain but is thought to involve intrauterine vascular accidents. Four types of atresia have been identified (Fig. 16–18). Type I is not a true atresia but actually is a membranous obstruction of the lumen in an intestine of otherwise normal length and diameter. Type II, a true atresia, consists of two blind ends frequently connected by a fibrous strand with slightly shortened intestinal length. Type IIIa lesions have blind ends separated by a mesenteric defect. The type IIIb lesion is also called "apple peel" or "Christmas tree" deformity, consisting of a long jejunal atresia with a very short remaining ileum. The superior mesenteric artery is missing, and the blood supply to the ileum is by retrograde flow via a branch of the ileocolic artery. Type 3b lesions are rare but have a very high mortality. Type IV lesions involve multiple intestinal atresias.

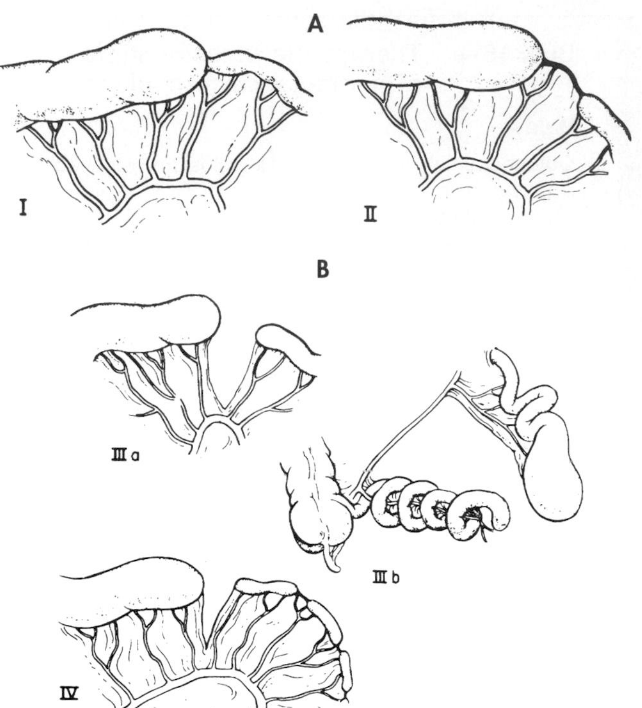

■ **FIGURE 16–18.** The various types of jejunal atresia. (With permission from Grosfeld JL: Jejunoileal atresia and stenosis. In Welch KJ, Randolph JG, Ravitch MM, et al., editors: *Pediatric surgery*, 4th ed. Chicago, 1986, Year Book Medical Publishers.)

Meconium Ileus

Meconium ileus is a luminal obstruction of the distal small bowel by abnormal meconium. Meconium ileus is found almost exclusively in patients with cystic fibrosis, but only 20% of patients with cystic fibrosis have meconium ileus. Because meconium ileus presents in the neonatal period, respiratory symptoms of cystic fibrosis generally are not present. Both surgical and nonsurgical therapies are used to relieve the obstruction. The nonsurgical approach involves diatrizoate meglumine (Gastrografin) enemas, which can be both diagnostic and therapeutic. Diatrizoate meglumine, a water-soluble contrast agent, loosens and softens the meconium, thereby facilitating its evacuation. When medical management does not succeed, surgery is performed. After the peritoneal cavity is entered and the obstruction is located, diatrizoate meglumine or acetylcysteine is injected into the bowel lumen and allowed to mix with the meconium. When the meconium has loosened, it is massaged into the colon. If this is unsuccessful, an enterostomy is performed, and the sterile meconium is evacuated from the small bowel.

Malrotation and Volvulus

Malrotations are rare and generally result from abnormalities in the rotation of the bowel, which usually occur during the 10th to 12th weeks of gestation. Consequently, areas of ischemia and atresia develop, along with volvulus, resulting in strangulation of bowel, bloody stools, abdominal distention, peritonitis, and hypovolemic shock. Nonrotation or malrotation is twice as common in boys as in girls and frequently produces symptoms of intestinal obstruction in the first 1 to 2 months after birth. In other cases, symptoms do not appear until later, even adulthood. Malrotations are often associated with duodenal stenosis or atresia or small intestinal atresia, as well as with cardiac, esophageal, urinary, and anal anomalies. Major anatomic defects of the abdominal wall (gastroschisis, omphalocele) and CDH universally have intestinal malrotation or nonrotation.

The operative procedure for a nonrotation complicated by volvulus consists of untwisting of the intestine and then a short intraoperative period of observation to evaluate recovery of vascular perfusion to the involved intestine. Areas of frank necrosis are excised, and a primary anastomosis is performed. If the patient has peritonitis or poor perfusion of the remaining bowel, proximal and distal enteral stomas are formed.

Children with less than 30 to 40 cm of small bowel generally develop short-gut syndrome and ultimately require total parenteral nutrition. If marginal areas of intestinal viability are present at operation, they may be left unresected in the hope that postoperative resuscitation improves their perfusion. Under these circumstances, a "second-look" operation usually is performed 24 to 48 hours later.

ANESTHESIA FOR THE PREMATURE AND EX-PREMATURE INFANT

Since the 1980s, vast improvement in prenatal care and better understanding of neonatal medicine have increased the survival of premature babies. Consequently, more premature infants or neonatal intensive care nursery graduates require surgical procedures.

Comparing mortality and short-term outcome among three time periods of 1987–1988, 1993–1994, and 1999–2000 provides a perspective on the impact of advances in obstetric and neonatal care since the 1980s (Fanaroff et al., 2003). Infants between 500 and 1500 g were studied, with separate emphasis on the 501- to 800-g infants. Although mortality decreased progressively from 1987 through 2000 for each gestational age bracket, survival without major morbidity (chronic lung disease, NEC, grade III/IV intraventricular hemorrhage) did not. Of note, these findings exist even with the administration of prenatal steroids increasing from 16% to 79%. Surfactant was given to 57% of all the infants in the 1999–2000 births and in 87% of those weighing 501 to 800 g. Inhaled nitric oxide did not affect mortality or BPD incidence, but it may improve developmental outcome in premature infants (Meurs et al., 2005; Van Mestan et al., 2005).

RESPIRATORY PROBLEMS OF THE PREMATURE INFANT AND EX-PREMATURE INFANT

The degree of pulmonary immaturity at birth depends on many factors but is primarily dependent on the gestational age. Anatomic and biochemical development are both essential for successful extrauterine adaptation of the respiratory system. In human fetuses, the alveoli develop from the primitive terminal air sacs after 36 weeks gestation; pulmonary surfactant in sufficient quantities normally is not produced in the type 2 pneumocytes and secreted onto the surface of the airspace until 32 to 34 weeks gestation, and this process depends on many factors (e.g., stress, cortisol, thyroid). Insufficient levels of surfactant result in alveolar wall instability and alveolar collapse at end-expiration.

Preterm infants are unable to maintain adequate rhythmic breathing after birth, and apneic episodes may be frequent. Moreover, preterm infants have increased work of breathing compared with full-term infants because a greater force is required to expand their alveoli and prevent collapse. The highly compliant thoracic cage prevents chest wall fixation during inspirations, so that negative intrathoracic pressure causes inward motion of the thorax and less effective expansion of the lung.

Full-term neonates respond to hypercapnia by increasing ventilation similar to adults. Although preterm babies initially hyperventilate, this response is transitory and overall they have a depressed carbon dioxide response curve (Frantz et al., 1976). The sensitivity to carbon dioxide increases with gestational age and postnatal age. A brief exposure to hypoxia is similar, and can result in transient hyperventilation but is followed by hypoventilation, periodic breathing, or apnea (Rigatto et al., 1975; Gerhardt and Bancalari, 1984).

The Hering-Breuer reflex (inflation of the lung resulting in apnea) is more prominent in preterm than in full-term infants. Transient apnea, lasting 5 to 10 seconds, is common, and prolonged apnea, exceeding 20 seconds, also occurs. Periodic breathing occurs in most preterm babies but becomes less frequent after 36 weeks gestation (Kelly and Shannon, 1981) (see Chapter 2, Respiratory Physiology in Infants and Children). Premature infants spend much of their time in rapid eye movement (REM) sleep, during which respiratory muscles relax and paradoxical movements of the rib cage and diaphragm develop. However, periodic breathing or apneic spells are more frequent during non-REM sleep. Even when they are awake, preterm infants have a large dead space–to–tidal volume (V_D/V_T) ratio because of uneven distribution of ventilation and capillary perfusion.

A high incidence of RDS (i.e., hyaline membrane disease) occurs among preterm infants because of an inadequate amount of pulmonary surfactant in immature lungs. Infants with RDS have increased Pa_{CO_2}, resulting in respiratory acidosis, and ventilation-perfusion imbalance, causing hypoxemia. Shunting through a PDA or foramen ovale may exaggerate hypoxemia. If congestive heart failure develops metabolic acidosis may follow. These infants often need respiratory support, including oxygen, and continuous positive airway pressure (CPAP) or intermittent positive-pressure ventilation (IPPV) with PEEP. The complications that occur during treatment of these infants include pneumothorax, pneumomediastinum, pulmonary interstitial emphysema, subglottic stenosis, and chronic lung disease. Although chronic lung disease is uncommon among term infants, disorders that require supplemental oxygen and mechanical ventilation, such as meconium aspiration and tracheoesophageal fistula, can produce a clinical picture similar to that seen in the ex-premature infant.

For the most part, chronic lung disease of infancy is a disorder that results from injury, repair, and abnormal development of premature lungs. Most infants who develop sequelae secondary to RDS are less than 30 weeks' gestation and require mechanical ventilatory support during the first week of life. The infant born at less than 26 weeks' gestation is at very high risk for the development of chronic lung disease.

Chronic Lung Disease Versus the "New Bronchopulmonary Dysplasia"

In 1967, Northway and others (1967) first described BPD, a chronic lung disease that developed in some preterm infants exposed to oxygen and positive pressure ventilation. In the original group of infants described by Northway and others, none were less than 31 weeks' gestation and only one weighed less than 1500 g.

Traditionally, the definition of BPD is based on the clinical and radiographic criteria proposed by Bancalari and others (1979), as follows:

1. Mechanical ventilation during more than 3 days in the first week of life
2. Persistence of oxygen dependence after 28 days
3. Radiographic abnormalities characterized by patchy density with areas of hyperlucency

The term "chronic lung disease" continues to evolve as the mortality of the less-than-28-week-gestation infant improves, as the physiology and pathology of the "new BPD" are defined, and as the use of oxygen is standardized for the ex-premature (Shennan et al., 1988).

The simplest strategy is to consider chronic lung disease of infancy as abnormal lung function with an abnormal chest radiograph identified in the first 3 to 4 months after birth.

This definition includes BPD. Classically, BPD was considered to be caused by RDS and to evolve as a consequence of the repair process. This repair process resulted in parenchymal fibrosis, chronic inflammation, airway epithelial metaplasia, and smooth muscle hypertrophy. The chest radiographs typically had areas of overinflation as well as areas of volume loss consistent with fibrosis (Fig. 16–19).

Current evidence confirms that a variety of factors interact synergistically to disrupt normal lung growth and development—genetics, hypoxia, hyperoxia, mechanical ventilation, steroids, and, unequivocally, inflammatory mediators. Chronic lung disease is the cumulative outcome of these multiple exposures (Jobe and Bancalari, 2001). As survival of ELBW infants has increased, and as the respiratory support of these infants has evolved in the era of surfactant therapy, a "new BPD" has been recognized both clinically and pathologically. First, these infants born after 1990 often are much less mature at birth than were the infants born in the 1970s and 1980s. That is, lung development at 24 to 27 weeks gestation is in the canalicular stage, and that at 31 to 34 weeks, the saccular stage. Second, because of artificial surfactant and prenatal glucocorticoids (betamethasone administered to the mother), the acute respiratory disease of the premature newborn is less severe. In fact, some infants who have never had classic RDS develop chronic lung disease. These infants develop oxygen dependency later and, in some cases, progress to require ventilatory support. Third, the characteristic fibroproliferative pattern of BPD is not seen in those surfactant-treated infants who have less severe acute pulmonary disease. Instead, the pathology in these infants is one of abnormal growth of both alveoli and vasculature (Hussain et al., 1998; Jobe and Bancalari, 2001). Alveoli are large and fewer in number, and the elastic tissue is abundant. Airways are free of epithelial metaplasia, and lung inflation is more uniform. This pattern has been documented in animal models and human infants (Chambers and Van Velzen, 1989; Coalson et al., 1999). The chest radiograph characteristically shows a uniform pattern, unlike that of "classic BPD" where there are areas of patchy density with areas of hyperlucency.

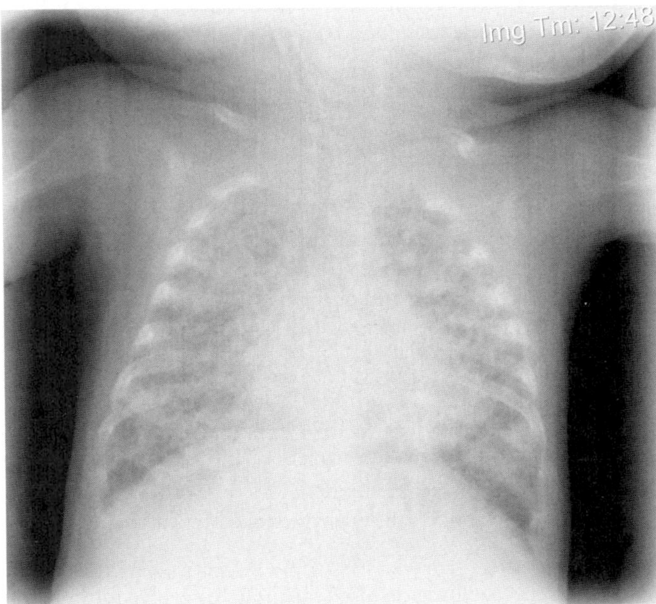

■ **FIGURE 16–19.** The pathologic description of classic chronic disease or "old BPD" is a fibroproliferative process with epithelial metaplasia, interstitial fibrosis, and air space obliteration from the fibrosis. This correlates with the radiologic findings of nonhomogeneity of the lung parenchyma with densities secondary to volume loss from fibrosis extending to the periphery coexisting with cystic emphysema (note cysts in both lung bases, right > left) and hyperinflation (note the flattened diaphragms). This is a pattern of repair of and response to injury.

The striking effects on alveolar growth in the "new BPD" imply a fundamental interference with a signaling pathway that is essential for normal lung development (Fig. 16–20). These signaling pathways can be affected by genetics, inflammation, infection, mechanical ventilation, and oxygen toxicity. The role of genetics has not been clearly defined, but fibroblast growth factor 10, transforming growth factor β, surfactant proteins, TNF-α converting enzyme, *hoxa5* gene, ENaC, cytochrome P450 1A2, and glucocorticoid receptors have all been associated with the disease (Nogee et al., 1994; Ramet et al., 2000; Copland and Post, 2002; Hallman and Haataja, 2003).

Infection and inflammation seem to play a critical role in the etiology of preterm delivery as well as subsequent chronic lung disease. Chorioamnionitis has been associated with preterm delivery, but its role in the subsequent development of chronic lung disease in this high-risk population has only been recently hypothesized (Gomez et al., 1998; Yoon et al., 1999; Schmidt et al., 2001). In addition to the high levels of interleukin (IL)-1 and IL-6 in fetal cord blood and a significant presence of inflammatory cells, IL-8 mRNA has been detected in the fetal lung of infants who later develop chronic lung disease (Schmidt et al., 2001).

Yoon and others (1999) noted that chorioamnionitis was easily detected in 92% of the placentas from preterm infants who developed BPD and 62% of those who did not. IL-1β, IL-6, and IL-8 were in the amniotic fluid within 5 days of preterm delivery and were predictive of subsequent development of BPD. Similar findings have been reported with TNF-α (Hitti et al., 1997). Chorioamnionitis may play a role in fetal lung injury as a result of systemic effects as well as direct effects on the lungs, as supported by the detection of such mediators in cord blood. Thus, chorioamnionitis may induce lung maturation in the fetus but simultaneously sets the stage for chronic lung disease (Shimoya et al., 2000).

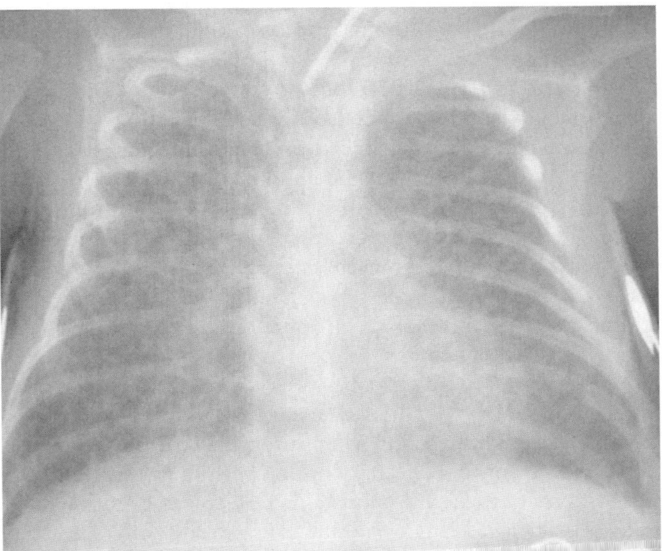

■ **FIGURE 16–20.** The abnormal pathology in the "new BPD" is abnormal growth of alveoli and vasculature, dilation of distal sites of gas exchange (alveolar ducts) but without prominent fibrosis. This correlates with a fine, hazy uniform parenchymal pattern with modest hyperinflation but no cysts. This is a pattern of arrested development.

In addition to the data relating chorioamnionitis to chronic lung disease, reports have proposed that proinflammatory cytokines are critical in the initial postnatal response to lung injury in the preterm infant (Groneck et al., 1994; Tullus et al., 1996; Jonsson et al., 1997). For example, in one report, TNF-α and several interleukins (IL-1β, IL-6, and IL-8) were measured daily in tracheobronchial aspirate fluid of 28 infants born at less than 34 weeks' gestation (Jonsson et al., 1997). Infants meeting appropriate criteria were treated with surfactant. In the 17 infants who developed chronic lung disease, significant increases in concentrations of TNF-α, IL-6, and IL-8 were obtained on days 2 and 3. TNF-α, IL-6, and IL-8 concentrations were significantly related to gestational age and duration of supplemental oxygen as well as to time receiving ventilatory support. IL-8 concentration decreased in infants with resolving RDS, whereas the infants who developed chronic lung disease had a sustained secretion of IL-8 (Groneck et al., 1994; Tullus et al., 1996; Jonsson et al., 1997). Other cytokine actors identified in high concentrations in the airways of infants with BPD include anaphylatoxin C5a, leukotriene C_4, platelet-activating factor, intercellular adhesion molecule-1 (ICAM-1), fibronectin, elastin degradation products, 5-hydroxyeicosatetranoic acid, IL-16, monocyte chemotactic protein, and macrophage inflammatory protein-1α.

Mechanical ventilation itself influences the development of chronic lung disease. Even after surfactant administration, mechanical ventilation initiates and sustains an inflammatory reaction. For example, the normal preterm lung is populated with few white cells (either macrophages or granulocytes). The influx of granulocytes into the alveoli of preterm infants after mechanical ventilation has been measured as soon as 1 hour of age; these infants have a higher incidence of BPD (Ferreira et al., 2000). Neutrophils release cytokines and initiate an inflammatory cascade that is associated with a higher incidence of BPD.

Hyperoxia produces lung injury at any stage of development but may be particularly insulting to the immature lung because of insufficiency of several systems that are important in protecting tissues from oxygen toxicity. This inadequate antioxidant state, coupled with exposure to higher oxygen concentrations than in the intrauterine environment, presents the premature infant with an excessive physiologic oxygen load. The resultant excess free radicals induce inflammation and damage to cellular lipids, proteins, and carbohydrates. Clearly, the preterm infant is predisposed to an oxidant/antioxidant imbalance. Of particular importance, antioxidant enzymes (superoxide dismutase, catalase, glutathione peroxidase, glutathione reductase) develop on a time scale similar to surfactant, so that the level of these antioxidants normally rises rapidly just before birth (Frank and Sosenko, 1987). In addition to its effects on antioxidant systems, hyperoxia inhibits surfactant synthesis, normal protein synthesis (Jornot et al., 1987), and DNA synthesis (Clement et al., 1985), as well as producing pulmonary vascular reactivity (Newman et al., 1983).

PULMONARY FUNCTION IN PREMATURE AND EX-PREMATURE INFANTS

Prematurity with or without RDS and with or without chronic lung disease is associated with long-term pulmonary sequelae. In addition to spirometric pulmonary assessments, exercise tolerance and diffusion of gases during exercise have helped define the functional impact of residual respiratory abnormalities in the ex-premature (Jacob, 1997). Seven- to 8-year-old children who had BPD after preterm birth had lower gas transfer compared with children who had been born at term or had been born prematurely but had no chronic lung disease (Mitchell et al., 1998). During exercise, only survivors of BPD had wheezing or oxygen desaturation. In a study by Jacob and others (1997), ex-premature infants with a history of *severe* BPD, ex-premature infants who had had RDS but no BPD, and healthy term infants were studied at ages 9 to 12 years. The BPD group used a greater percentage of their "ventilatory reserve" (VEmax/40 forced expiratory volume in 1 second [FEV_1]) during exercise, especially those children with the lowest FEV_1 (Jacob et al., 1997). Other studies (Bader et al., 1987; Parat et al., 1995; Santuz et al., 1995) have documented that children with a history of *mild* BPD do not have decreased exercise capacity compared with other survivors of neonatal mechanical respiratory support but that the BPD groups did have a greater incidence of oxygen desaturation during exercise.

Postmortem assessment of morphometric lung development has confirmed the drastic restriction in the number of alveoli in survivors of BPD compared with that in normal infants. The total number of alveoli in a 22-month-old (31.1 million) and a 28-month-old (40.4 million) was less than that in a normal 1-week-old (67.2 million) (Margraf et al., 1991). Of course, infants who die from chronic lung disease may have more dramatic morphometric abnormalities than the less severely affected survivors.

These postmortem studies of infants with chronic lung disease also documented an abnormal architecture of elastic fibers, the framework on which new alveoli develop. Elastic fiber damage is primarily linked to oxygen damage and an increased activity of elastase (Bruce et al., 1985). With damage to the cellular matrix, further deposition of collagen and elastin is erratic. Although the effects of prematurity on the molecular mechanisms of lung growth are not clearly defined, the consequences of decreased alveolar surface area and airway hyperreactivity have significant clinical implications.

Pulmonary Function During the First 2 Years After Preterm Birth

Chronic lung injury secondary to prematurity characteristically includes decreased vital capacity, obstruction of small airways, chest hyperinflation, and reactive airway disease. Over the first 1 to 2 years of life, the ex-premature infant often has respiratory compromise. Reactive airway disease is common and is exacerbated by frequent infections (Greenough et al., 1990; Parat et al., 1995; Smyth et al., 1995; Tarpy and Celi, 1995; Walther et al., 1995; Tait et al., 2001). Oxygen therapy may be necessary for months to years in order to maintain oxygen saturation between 90% and 95%. Bronchodilators and diuretics are often mainstays of therapy for these infants. Significant hypoxemia often accompanies respiratory infections, and hospital admission and readjustment of medications are frequently needed. Finally, aspiration associated with gastroesophageal reflux can lead to acute/recurrent pulmonary deterioration (Greenough et al., 1990; Radford et al., 1996).

Function in School-Aged and Older Ex-Premature Infants

In 1990, Northway and others (1990) presented follow-up of 26 patients from their original cohort (Northway et al., 1967). These patients were (Northway et al., 1990) between the ages of 14 and 23 years. None of these patients had been less than 1500 g or less than 30 weeks' gestation. Seventy-six percent had pulmonary dysfunction (i.e., abnormalities on pulmonary function tests or reactive airway disease, or both). Airway obstruction was noted in 68%, with 24% having fixed airway obstruction. Although all were "leading normal lives" and usually asymptomatic, the patients who had had BPD had more episodes of wheezing and pneumonia, limitation of exercise, and long-term medication use.

Now, 10 years after the introduction of surfactant and with improved modes of ventilation, studies have examined the pulmonary function of school-aged ex-premature infants. These infants can be divided into two groups: surfactant-treated ex-premature infants and non–surfactant-treated ex-premature infants. The pulmonary function tests in school-aged ex-premature infants with chronic lung disease who did not receive surfactant at birth were measured serially between 6 and 10 years of age and at 11 and 18 years of age. At the final testing period, pulmonary function tests revealed normal total lung capacity (TLC) and vital capacity (VC), but these values had improved over the time course of the repeated pulmonary function studies. Residual volume (RV) and RV/TLC decreased over time, suggesting gradual improvement in air trapping (Koumbourlis et al., 1996). The peak expiratory flow rate (PEFR), FEV_1, and the ratio FEV_1/FVC remained at or above the normal range in all patients. FEF_{25-75} (forced expiratory flow), FEF_{50}, and FEF_{75} were decreased in 50% of these patients. The lower values are suggestive of relatively small airways obstruction. Regardless, most children in both groups responded to inhaled bronchodilator treatment.

Lung volume abnormalities gradually normalized in this group of ex-premature infants with chronic lung disease, and this process continued well into adolescence. Chronic airflow obstruction is common but not present in all ex-premature infants with the diagnosis of chronic lung disease. That school-aged ex-premature infants who had the diagnosis of BPD as neonates have severe functional abnormalities is well established (Bertrand et al., 1985; MacLusky et al., 1986). What is of particular note is that prematurely born infants who had no significant lung disease in the newborn period may develop obstructive airway disease that persists into early childhood (MacLusky, 1986).

The pulmonary function tests in school-aged ex-premature infants who received surfactant at birth reveal that FVC, FEV_1, and FRC are within normal limits (similar to values obtained in a group who had not received surfactant). Airway resistance (Raw) was slightly elevated, and MEF_{25} (maximum expiratory flow, 25% lung volume) was slightly decreased, suggestive of mild lower airway obstruction. In addition, similar to studies in non–surfactant-treated VLBW infants, exercise challenge elicited bronchial reactivity. These data reveal little effect of surfactant on VLBW infants (25 to 30 weeks gestation) from the viewpoint of long-term pulmonary function at 6 to 7 years of age (Gappa et al., 1999).

In summary, (1) greater than 90% of children who had been diagnosed with chronic lung disease at 36 weeks postconceptual age had documented airway obstruction at follow-up; (2) the incidence of β-agonist responsive airway obstruction in ex-preterm infants is striking: 45% in surfactant-treated and 67% in the placebo group, compared with 0% in children who had been born at term; (3) the incidence of chronic lung disease was not different after surfactant treatment; and (4) the duration of intubation and oxygen therapy, with or without surfactant therapy, correlated with pulmonary outcome (Pelkonen et al., 1998).

Postanesthetic Apnea

Preterm and ex-premature infants ("ex-premies") undergoing elective surgery are more likely to encounter perioperative apnea (Gregory, 1981; Steward, 1982) than are term infants. Many such infants have a history of idiopathic apnea in the neonatal intensive care nursery, and this has been correlated with a higher susceptibility to life-threatening apnea in the postoperative period (Liu et al., 1983). Apnea (cessation of breathing for 20 seconds or longer) resulting in cyanosis and bradycardia occurs in 20% to 30% of preterm infants during the first month of life (American Academy of Pediatrics, 1978). Steward (1982) reported an 18% incidence of apnea in preterm infants (gestational age <38 weeks; postnatal age 3 to 28 weeks) during the first 12 hours after surgery.

A prospective study by Liu and others (1983) demonstrated that a history of apnea and a postconceptual age of less than 44 weeks were associated with prolonged postanesthetic apnea. Kurth and others (1987) found a 37% incidence of postanesthetic apnea (defined as cessation of breathing for longer than 15, rather than 20, seconds) in ex-premature infants whose postconceptual age varied from 32 to 55 weeks. The initial episode of apnea was found to occur as late as 12 hours after anesthesia. Kurth and others recommended that monitoring be continued in infants who develop apnea until they are apnea free for at least 12 hours if their postconceptual age is less than 60 weeks.

Welborn and others (1986) failed to demonstrate apnea in a group of healthy premature infants of less than 44 weeks postconceptual age undergoing general anesthesia for herniorrhaphy. They did find a 63.6% incidence of periodic breathing. Malviya and others (1993) noted that ex-premature infants younger than 44 weeks postconceptual age were at significantly greater risk for apnea than were infants older than 44 weeks. In the latter, Malviya and others determined the risk to be 3%. Coté and others (1995), in a combined analysis of 255 patients taken from previously published studies, noted that with logistic regression the incidence of apnea decreased to 1% at 55 to 56 weeks postconceptual age. In addition, in this meta-analysis of neonates with postoperative apnea, Coté and others (1995) noted that the incidence of apnea was inversely related to both gestational age and postconceptual age. Infants who are 55 weeks postconceptual age and younger are at greatest risk, and anemia further increases the risk (Fig. 16–21).

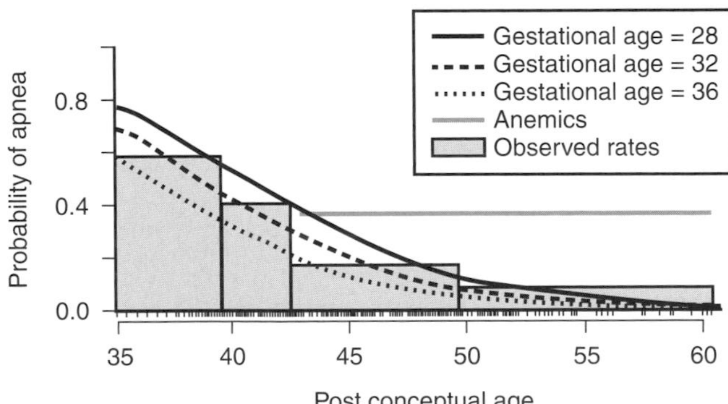

■ **FIGURE 16–21.** Predicted probability of apnea for all patients, by gestational age and weeks of postconceptual age. Patients with anemia are shown as the horizontal hatched line. Bottom marks indicate the number of data points by postconceptual age. The shaded boxes represent the overall rates of apnea for infants within that gestational age range. The probability of apnea was the same regardless of postconceptual age or gestational age for infants with anemia (horizontal hatched line). (Redrawn from Coté CJ, Zaslavsky A, Downes JJ, et al.: Postoperative apnea in former preterm infants after inguinal herniorrhaphy: A combined analysis. *Anesthesiology* 82:807, 1995.)

Other factors predisposing an infant, especially a premature, to apnea include hypoglycemia, hypoxia, hyperoxia, sepsis, anemia, hypocalcemia, and environmental temperature changes (Schute, 1977). Postoperative apnea occurring in preterm infants may also be related to the pharmacologic effects of general anesthesia and the immaturity of the central nervous system, including the respiratory center. In low concentrations, halothane can depress the chemoreceptor response to hypoxia (Knill and Gelb, 1978) and depress intercostal muscle preferentially, thus reducing the functional residual capacity and increasing the risk of hypoxemia (Tusiewicz et al., 1977; Motoyama et al., 1982). This, coupled with an immature response to hypoxia and hypercarbia, predisposes the premature infant to erratic respiratory responses in the perioperative period (Rigatto, 1982).

Residual anesthesia may be an important contributing factor to the occurrence of apnea in preterm infants in the postoperative period. Moreover, the cartilaginous upper airway of the preterm infants predisposes these infants to upper airway obstruction (Dransfield et al., 1983), which can be aggravated by the impact of residual anesthesia on the pharyngeal muscles. Elective surgery should be delayed, if possible, until the former preterm infant is older than 44 weeks postconceptual age (Gregory and Steward, 1983). Infants younger than 44 weeks postconceptual age who need surgery must be individually evaluated. The type of surgery and the patient's gestational age and postconceptual age, hematocrit, and current cardiorespiratory function (oxygen and/or diuretic dependent, chronic lung disease, neurologic status) are all factors that must be considered when developing a perioperative plan for the ex-premature infant—in particular, admission for 24 to 36 hours for postoperative monitoring.

NEUROLOGIC OUTCOME OF THE EX-PREMATURE INFANT

As an initial overview, neurologic morbidity associated with preterm birth can be divided into major and minor dysfunctions. The major impairments include "cerebral palsy," mental retardation, sensorineural hearing loss, and visual abnormalities. Hydrocephalus or seizures often accompany serious neurologic dysfunction. These major disorders are apparent before the age of 2 years and often earlier if the deficit is profound and occur 2 to 5 times more frequently in VLBW infants. Data document that approximately 50,000 infants who weigh less than 1500 g are born in the United States annually (Hack et al., 1996). At least 5% to 15% of these have spastic motor dysfunction, and intellectual abnormalities frequently accompany the motor problems. An additional 25% to 50% of VLBW infants have less significant ("minor") developmental abnormalities, such as isolated intellectual or cognition problems, speech and language disorders, learning disabilities, difficulties with balance and coordination, perceptual problems, emotional instability, social competence, and selective attention deficits (Volpe, 1997). In fact, these minor dysfunctions become more prevalent beyond infancy and with long-term follow-up are increasingly obvious.

From another viewpoint, 40% of all children with spastic motor deficits were born prematurely. In particular, spastic diplegia (with the legs more affected than the arms) is the most common syndrome of cerebral palsy seen in the ex-premature infant. About 70% of infants with spastic diplegia were born prematurely.

Discussing neurodevelopmental and functional outcome of the preterm infant without dividing this population into subgroups based on gestational age at birth provides limited insight into this important topic. Although follow-up data are limited and are available primarily for infants who are only 18 to 24 months past birth, these studies suggest that the group of infants born at the edge of survival (<500 to 600 g and 23 to 24 weeks gestational age) is at marked risk for neurologic and developmental problems.

The National Institute of Child Health and Human Development (NICHD) reported outcome studies at 18 to 22 months corrected age of 1480 ELBW infants according to 100-g weight categories (401 to 500, 501 to 600, 601 to 700, 701 to 800, 801 to 900, and 901 to 1000). For the entire cohort, 25% had an abnormal neurologic examination, 37% had a Bayley II Mental Developmental Index (MDI) of less than 70, and 29% had a Psychomotor Developmental Index (PDI) of less than 70 (Vohr, 2000).

In the many outcome studies across multiple developmental and behavioral domains, a consistent finding is that groups of premature children are less competent and score less well than do groups of full-term children (Piecuch, 1998; Vohr, 2000). On the other hand, individual premature children are not invariably less capable than individual full-term children; that is, individual developmental outcome remains difficult to accurately predict based on a type of neonatal course. Although the concept of "neurologic and developmental outcome" of the premature infant is extremely difficult to pinpoint during infancy, these developmental abnormalities are much more common when the birth weight of the AGA survivor moves further and further below 1000 g.

GASTROINTESTINAL FUNCTION IN THE EX-PREMATURE INFANT

Gastroesophageal reflux is a common event in infants but usually resolves by 4 months to 1 year of age. Since the 1980s, gastroesophageal reflux has been recognized more frequently because of an increased awareness and because of improved diagnostic techniques. Normal gastroesophageal function is complex and depends on effective esophageal motility, coordinated relaxation and contractility of the lower esophageal sphincter, intraluminal pressure of the stomach, and effective contractility, allowing emptying of the stomach. Patients with neurologic disorders appear to have a high incidence of autonomic neuropathy, which delays esophagogastric transit and gastric emptying. In fact, esophageal dysmotility has been recognized in approximately one third of children with severe gastroesophageal reflux. Another high-risk group of infants is those with congenital anomalies of the esophagus. Symptomatic gastroesophageal reflux is estimated to occur in 30% to 80% of infants who have required surgical repair of esophageal atresia.

The symptoms of gastroesophageal reflux often are related to esophagitis (emesis, irritability), but a wide spectrum of manifestations have been described. For example, if the refluxed material contacts the upper or lower airway, laryngospasm, stridor, laryngitis, recurrent laryngotracheitis, apnea, chronic cough, otitis media, asthma, recurrent bronchitis, pneumonia, or a combination may occur. Infants often present with "failure to thrive." Severe dental caries is an unusual, but not uncommon, presentation. Reflux occurs most commonly in the supine position, and thus is most common during sleep.

Neurologically impaired children are at high risk for having symptomatic gastroesophageal reflux, especially when the patient is fed via nasogastric tube or gastrostomy. In addition, delayed gastric emptying has been documented in infants and children with neurologic disorders and symptoms of gastroesophageal reflux. Although patients with upper airway obstruction and proximal gastroesophageal reflux can usually be managed successfully with medical therapy, some infants require fundoplication (Conley et al., 1995). Most who require surgery were either premature or developmentally delayed, or both. In another study, 75% of children with symptomatic gastroesophageal reflux and delayed gastric emptying were neurologically impaired (Papaila, 1989). Because of neurologic immaturity of the premature infant and higher incidence of neurologic abnormalities in the ex-premature infant, the incidence of gastroesophageal reflux is high in these groups and should be treated aggressively to minimize upper and lower respiratory complications in these populations who are already predisposed to pulmonary dysfunction.

PAIN IN THE NEONATE

The neonate's ability to experience pain has become a topic frequently discussed by anesthesiologists, pediatricians, and other scientists. Those involved with neonatal anesthesia have witnessed clinical evidence of increased sympathetic discharge (tachycardia and elevation of blood pressure) after surgical stimulation in an inadequately anesthetized infant. Moreover, facial grimacing and motor movements have been observed in the absence of paralysis.

Available evidence suggests that the cortical and peripheral centers necessary for pain perception, as well as the pain pathways, are well developed late in gestation (Anand and Hickey, 1987). Moreover, a neonate has an intact neuroendocrine response to stressful stimulation that is reflected in hormonal and metabolic changes. In a randomized, controlled trial of nitrous oxide-fentanyl (10 mcg/kg) anesthesia versus nitrous oxide alone in preterm neonates undergoing PDA ligation, the infants with nitrous oxide alone had a greater change in hormonal and fuel substrate levels in response to stress than did those treated with fentanyl (Anand et al., 1987). Moreover, the group without fentanyl was more likely to have postoperative circulatory or metabolic complications, such as bradycardia, hypotension, glycosuria, metabolic acidosis, the need for ventilatory support, and intraventricular hemorrhage. Alterations in sleep-wake patterns and behavior (e.g., irritability) have also been documented by different investigators during circumcision (Emde et al., 1971) or heel lancing (Field and Goldson, 1984) performed without anesthesia. These behavioral changes may have prolonged effects on the neurologic and psychological development of neonates. In VLBW preterm infants at risk for BPD, developmental outcomes were improved when the intensity of stressful stimulation and sensory input were reduced in the intensive care unit (Als et al., 1986).

Because of increased medical and public awareness regarding the adequacy of anesthetic techniques for premature infants and the physiologic alterations (increased right-to-left shunting, hypoxemia, acidosis, intraventricular hemorrhage) associated with stress and light anesthesia, anesthetic practices for neonates have been better defined. Consequently, several committees and sections of the American Academy of Pediatrics have proposed that anesthesia and analgesia be provided for neonates undergoing surgery. In moribund infants hemodynamically unable to tolerate anesthesia, the decision to withhold anesthetics should be based on the same medical criteria used for critically ill older patients (Poland et al., 1987).

DELIVERING ANESTHESIA TO PREMATURE INFANTS

Potent inhalation anesthetics can rarely be delivered to neonates, especially preterm infants, at a dose equivalent to or greater than MAC without producing unacceptable hemodynamic depression (Yaster, 1987), even when decreasing the dose to compensate for the lower MAC values in preterm infants (LeDez and Lerman, 1987; Lerman, 1988). In preterm infants who require postoperative ventilatory support, fentanyl, from 10 (Yaster, 1987) to 50 mcg/kg (Robinson and Gregory, 1981), has been a safe and effective anesthetic.

In the early days of intensive care of newborns (1970s), infants sometimes received only nitrous oxide with or without low doses of other inhaled anesthetics during surgical procedure. Furthermore, the trachea of an awake infant often was intubated without sedation or after the infant received only a neuromuscular blocker. These techniques do not provide adequate anesthesia to ablate the stress response to surgery (Booker, 1987; Hatch, 1987) or to other painful procedures. Premature and ex-premature infants may have dramatic responses to narcotics and potent inhaled anesthetics. Clearly, the benefit of providing adequate anesthesia and analgesia must be carefully balanced against the significant risk of cardiorespiratory depression in this fragile population. Titration of anesthetics to a desired effect, while carefully monitoring the cardiorespiratory status, is the goal. Developing and publishing simple protocols defining and recommending specific doses of drugs for this high-risk group of patients are impossible. These infants have wide variability in their responses to anesthetics and sedatives, and frequently experience exaggerated and unpredictable effects not observed in older infants and children.

REGIONAL ANESTHETIC TECHNIQUES

Since the 1990s, caudal epidural block with bupivacaine has been accepted as an effective and safe option to provide intraoperative and postoperative analgesia after lower abdominal surgery, particularly in preterm and ex-premature infants who had been treated for chronic respiratory failure in the neonatal intensive care unit (Booker, 1988; Rice et al., 1988; see also Chapter 13, Pain Management). Typically, such an infant undergoes an inhalational induction consisting of nitrous oxide and sevoflurane (low inhaled concentrations, titrated as tolerated) delivered by mask. After intravenous access is established, some anesthesiologists administer an intermediate-acting, nondepolarizing muscle relaxant in order to facilitate intubation of the trachea and to avoid high doses of a potent inhaled agent. For a noninvasive surgical procedure such as a hydrocele repair or an inguinal herniorrhaphy, routine monitors are adequate. After the trachea is intubated and the endotracheal tube is properly positioned and secured, anesthesia is maintained with nitrous oxide (60% to 70%) and a potent inhaled anesthetic in a concentration that preserves hemodynamic stability. The infant can then be placed in the lateral position and a caudal block placed using a 22-gauge "block" needle or an angiocath. In most cases, 1 mL/kg of 0.25% or 0.125% bupivacaine (1.25 to 2.5 mg/kg) is given as a bolus. An addition of epinephrine (5 mcg/mL) prolongs the analgesic effect to up to 3.5 hours.

The use of spinal anesthesia for herniorrhaphy in premature infants less than 36 weeks gestational age recovering from RDS is reportedly a safe and satisfactory alternative to general anesthesia. Respiratory problems occurred in 2 of 20 patients, however, and "intensive postoperative monitoring" was recommended (Harnik et al., 1986). The use of combined spinal and epidural anesthesia for major abdominal surgery in infants has also been reported by Williams and others (1997).

■ SUMMARY

For newborns to survive the transition from fetal to extrauterine life, critical multisystem developmental adaptation must occur. Congenital anomalies and acquired disease states requiring anesthetic and surgical intervention may deter this orderly physiologic transition. Those involved with anesthetic care of neonates must acquire and maintain an in-depth knowledge of developmental physiology as well as an understanding of the effects of immaturity on anesthetic and monitoring requirements. The pediatric anesthesiologist must assimilate this information and thoughtfully apply it to the practice of neonatal anesthesia.

REFERENCES

Adamsons K Jr, Towell ME: Thermal homeostasis in the fetus and newborn. *Anesthesiology* 26:531, 1965.

Ahmed T, Ein S, Moore A: The role of peritoneal drains in treatment of perforated necrotizing enterocolitis: recommendations from recent experience. *J Pediatr Surg* 33:1468–1470, 1998.

Albanese CT, Lopoo J, Goldstein RB, et al.: Fetal liver position and perinatal outcome for congenital diaphragmatic hernia. *Prenat Diagn* 18:1138–1142, 1998.

Al-Kharfy T, Smyth JA, Wadsworth L, et al.: Erythropoietin therapy in neonates at risk of having bronchopulmonary dysplasia and requiring multiple transfusions. *J Pediatr* 129:89–96, 1996.

Als H, Lawhon G, Brown E, et al.: Individualized behavioral and environmental care for the very low birth weight preterm infant at high risk for bronchopulmonary dysplasia: Neonatal intensive care unit and developmental outcome. *Pediatrics* 78:1123, 1986.

American Academy of Pediatrics Task Force on Prolonged Apnea: Prolonged apnea. *Pediatrics* 61:651, 1978.

Anand KJS, Hickey PR: Pain and its effects in the human neonate and fetus. *N Engl J Med* 317:1321, 1987.

Anand KJS, Sippel WG, Aynsley-Green A: Randomized trial of fentanyl anaesthesia in preterm babies undergoing surgery: Effects on the stress response. *Lancet* 1:243, 1987.

Anderson PAW: Physiology of the fetal, neonatal, and adult heart. In Polin RA, Fox WW, editors: *Fetal and neonatal physiology.* Philadelphia, 1998, WB Saunders, p 837.

Anderson PAW, Glick KL, Manring A, Crenshaw C Jr: Developmental changes in cardiac contractility in fetal and postnatal sheep: In vitro and in vivo. *Am J Physiol* 247:H371–H379, 1984.

Anderson PAW, Greig A, Mark TM, et al.: Molecular basis of human cardiac troponin T isoforms expressed in the developing, adult, and failing heart. *Circ Res* 76:681–686, 1995.

Anderson PAW, Kleinman CS, Lister G, Talner NS: Fetal and neonatal physiology. In Polin RI, Fox WW, editors: *Fetal and neonatal physiology.* Philadelphia, 1998, WB Saunders, p 856.

Aperia A, Broberger O, Herin P, Zetterstrom R: Sodium excretion in relation to sodium intake and aldosterone excretion in newborn pre-term and full-term infants. *Acta Paediatr Scand* 68:813–817, 1979.

Arant BS Jr: Developmental patterns of renal functional maturation compared in human neonates. *J Pediatr* 92:705–712, 1978.

Avery ME: *The lung and its disorders in the newborn infant,* ed 3. Philadelphia, 1974, WB Saunders.

Bader D, Ramos AD, Lew CD, et al.: Childhood sequelae of infant lung disease: Exercise and pulmonary function abnormalities after bronchopulmonary dysplasia. *J Pediatr* 110:693–699, 1987.

Baerg J, Kaban G, Tonita J, et al.: Gastroschisis: A sixteen-year review. *J Pediatr Surg* 38:771–774, 2003.

Bain JA, Spoerel WE: Flow requirements for a modified Mapleson D system during controlled ventilation. *Can Anaesth Soc J* 20:629, 1973.

Baird PA, MacDonald EC: An epidemiologic study of congenital malformations of the anterior abdominal wall in more than half a million consecutive live births. *Am J Hum Genet* 33:470–478, 1981.

Ballard JL, Novak KK, Driver M: A simplified score for assessment of fetal maturation of newly born infants. *J Pediatr* 95:769–774, 1979.

Bancalari E, Abdenour G, Feller R, Gannon J: Bronchopulmonary dysplasia: Clinical presentation. *J Pediatr* 95:819–823, 1979.

Barrett CT, Oliver TK Jr: Hypoglycemia and hyperinsulinism in infants with erythroblastosis fetalis. *N Engl J Med* 278:1260, 1968.

Beals DA, Schloo BL, Vacanti JP, et al.: Pulmonary growth and remodeling in infants with high-risk congenital diaphragmatic hernia. *J Pediatr Surg* 27:997–1002, 1992.

Bedard MP, Kotagal UR: Hypoglycemia in association with polycythemia. *Perinatol Neonatal* 5:83, 1981.

Bell MJ, Ternberg JL, Geigin RD, et al.: Neonatal necrotizing enterocolitis. Therapeutic decisions based upon clinical staging. *Ann Surg* 187:1–7, 1978.

Bergman L, Kjellmer I, Selstam U: Calcitonin and parathyroid hormone: Relation to early neonatal hypocalcemia in infants of diabetic mothers. *Biol Neonate* 24:151, 1974.

Bertrand JM, Riley SP, Popkin J, Coates AL: The long-term pulmonary sequelae of prematurity: The role of familial airway hyperreactivity and the respiratory distress syndrome. *N Engl J Med* 312:742–745, 1985.

Bjorklund LJ, Ingimarsson J, Curstedt T, et al.: Manual ventilation with a few large breaths at birth compromises the therapeutic effect of subsequent surfactant replacement in immature lambs. *Pediatr Res* 42:348–355, 1997.

Boheler KR, Carrier L, de la Bastie D, et al.: Skeletal actin mRNA increases in the human heart during ontogenic development and is the major isoform of control and failing adult hearts. *J Clin Invest* 88:323–330, 1991.

Bohn D, Tamura M, Perrin D, et al.: Ventilatory predictors of pulmonary hypoplasia in congenital diaphragmatic hernia, confirmed by morphologic assessment. *J Pediatr* 111:423, 1987.

Bollman R, Kalache K, Mau H, et al.: Associated malformations and chromosomal defects in congenital diaphragmatic hernia. *Fetal Diagn Ther* 10:52–59,1995.

Boloker J, Bateman DA, Wung JT, Stolar CJ: Congenital diaphragmatic hernia in 120 infants treated consecutively with permissive hypercapnia/spontaneous respiration/elective repair. *J Pediatr Surg* 37:357–366, 2002.

Booker PD: Management of postoperative pain in infants and children. *Curr Opin Anaesth* 1:1–7, 1988.

Booker PD: Postoperative analgesia for neonates. *Anaesthesia* 42:343, 1987.

Born GVR, Dawes GS, Mott JC, et al.: The constriction of the ductus arteriosus caused by oxygen and by asphyxia in newborn lambs. *J Physiol (Lond)* 132:304, 1956.

Brady JP, Ceruti E: Chemoreceptor reflexes in the newborn infant: Effects of varying degrees of hypoxia on heart rate and ventilation in warmer environment. *J Physiol* 184:631, 1966.

Brodsky JB: A simple method to determine patency of the ulnar artery intraoperatively prior to radial-artery cannulation. *Anesthesiology* 42:626, 1975.

Bruce MC, Wedig KE, Jentoft N, et al.: Altered urinary excretion of elastin cross-links in premature infants who develop bronchopulmonary dysplasia. *Am Rev Respir Dis* 131:568–572, 1985.

Bullard KM, Harrison MR: Before the horse is out of the barn: Fetal surgery for hydrops. *Semin Perinatol* 19:462–473, 1995.

Burri PH: The postnatal growth of the rat lung. III. Morphology. *Anat Rec* 178:711, 1974.

Cacciari A, Ruggeri G, Mordenti M, et al.: High-frequency oscillatory ventilation versus conventional mechanical ventilation in congenital diaphragmatic hernia. *Eur J Pediatr Surg* 11:3–7, 2001.

Caplan M, Hsueh W, Kelly A, Donovan M: Serum PAF acetylhydrolase increases during neonatal maturation. *Prostaglandins* 39:705–714, 1990.

Ceruti E: Chemoreceptor reflexes in the newborn infant: Effect of cooling on the response to hypoxia. *Pediatrics* 37:556, 1966.

Chambers H, Van Velzen D: Ventilator-associated pathology in the extremely immature lung. *Pathology* 21:79–83, 1989.

Charlton AJ: The management of congenital diaphragmatic hernia without ECMO (review). *Paediatr Anaesth* 3:201, 1993.

Chisholm CA, Heider AL, Kuller JA, et al.: Prenatal diagnosis and perinatal management of fetal sacrococcygeal teratoma. *Am J Perinatol* 16:89–92, 1999.

Choudhury SR, Ashcraft KW, Sharp RJ, et al.: Survival of patients with esophageal atresia: Influence of birth weight, cardiac anomaly and late respiratory complications. *J Pediatr Surg* 34:70–74, 1999.

Clark RH, Hardin WD Jr, Hirschl RB, et al.: Current surgical management of congenital diaphragmatic hernia: A report from the Congenital Diaphragmatic Hernia Study Group. *J Pediatr Surg* 33:1004–1009, 1998.

Claud EC, Walker WA: Hypothesis: Inappropriate colonization of the premature intestine can cause neonatal necrotizing enterocolitis. *FASEB J* 15:1398–1403, 2001.

Clement A, Hubscher U, Junod AF: Effects of hyperoxia on DNA synthesis in cultured porcine aortic endothelial cells. *J Appl Physiol* 59:1110–1116, 1985.

Clyman RI, Heymann MA, Rudolph AM: Ductus arteriosus responses to prostaglandin E_1 at high and low oxygen concentrations. *Prostaglandins* 13:219, 1977.

Coalson JJ, Winter VT, Siler-Khodr T, Yoder BA: Neonatal chronic lung disease in extremely immature baboon. *Am J Respir Crit Care Med* 160:1333–1346, 1999.

Collins DL, Pomerance JJ, Travis KW, et al.: A new approach to congenital posterolateral diaphragmatic hernia. *J Pediatr Surg* 12:149, 1977.

Conley SF, Werlin SL, Beste DJ: Proximal pH-metry for diagnosis of upper airway complications of gastroesophageal reflux. *J Otolaryngol* 24:295–298, 1995.

Copland IB, Post M: Understanding the mechanisms of infant respiratory distress and chronic lung disease. *Am J Respir Cell Mol Biol* 26:261–265, 2002.

Correia-Pinto J, Tavares ML, Baptista MJ, et al.: A new fetal rat model of gastroschisis: Development and early characterization. *J Pediatr Surg* 36:213–216, 2001.

Coté CJ, Zaslavsky A, Downes JJ, et al.: Postoperative apnea in former preterm infants after inguinal herniorrhaphy: A combined analysis. *Anesthesiology* 82:807, 1995.

Crisera CA, Connelly PR, Marmureanu AR, et al.: Esophageal atresia with tracheoesophageal fistula: Suggested mechanism in faulty organogenesis. *J Pediatr Surg* 34:204–208, 1999.

Crisera CA, Connelly PR, Marmureanu AR, et al.: TTF-1 and HNF-3β in the developing tracheoesophageal fistula: Further evidence for the respiratory origin of the 'distal esophagus'. *J Pediatr Surg* 34:1322–1326, 1999.

Cross KW, Oppe TE: The effect of inhalation of high and low concentrations of oxygen on the respiration of premature infants. *J Physiol* 117:38, 1952.

Cunniff C, Jones KL, Jones MC: Patterns of malformation in children with congenital diaphragmatic defects. *J Pediatr* 116:258–261, 1990.

Dalton HJ, Thompson AE: Extracorporeal membrane oxygenation. In Fuhrman BP, Zimmerman JJ: *Pediatric critical care.* St Louis, 1992, Mosby–Year Book.

Dave S, Bajpai M, Gupta DK, et al.: Esophageal atresia and tracheo-esophageal fistula: A review. *Indian J Pediatr* 66:759–772, 1999.

Davies BW, Stringer MD: The survivors of gastroschisis. *Arch Dis Child* 77:158–160, 1997.

Desfrere L, Jarreau PH, Dommergues M, et al.: Impact of delayed repair and elective high-frequency oscillatory ventilation on survival of antenatally diagnosed congenital diaphragmatic hernia: First application of these strategies in the more "severe" subgroup of antenatally diagnosed newborns. *Intensive Care Med* 26:934–941, 2000.

Donovan EF: Perioperative care of the surgical neonate. *Surg Clin North Am* 65:1061, 1985.

Downes JJ: Respiratory care of the newborn: ASA refresher course. *Anesthesiology* 2:65, 1974.

Dransfield DA, Spitzer AR, Fox WW: Episodic airway obstruction in premature infants. *Am J Dis Child* 137:441, 1983.

Dudley NE, Phelan PD: Respiratory complications in long term survivors of esophageal atresia. *Arch Dis Child* 51:279, 1976.

Emde RN, Harmon RJ, Metcalf D, et al.: Stress and neonatal sleep. *Psychosom Med* 33:491, 1971.

Fanaroff AA, Hack M, Walsh MC: The NICHD Neonatal Research Network: Changes in practice and outcomes during the first 15 years. *Semin Perinatol* 27:281–287, 2003.

Fanaroff AA, Wald M, Gruber HS, Klaus MH: Insensible water loss in low birth weight infants. *Pediatrics* 50:236, 1972.

Fasching G, Huber A, Uray E, et al.: Late follow-up in patients with gastroschisis. *Pediatr Surg Int* 11:103–106, 1996.

Fauza DO, Wilson JM: Congenital diaphragmatic hernia and associated anomalies: Their incidence, identification, and impact on prognosis. *J Pediatr Surg* 29:1113, 1994.

Ferreira PJ, Bunch TH, Albertine KH, Carlton DP: Circulating neutrophil concentration and respiratory distress in premature infants. *J Pediatr* 136:466–472, 2000.

Fetterman GH, Shuplock NA, Philip FJ, Gregg HS: The growth and maturation of human glomeruli and proximal convolutions from term to childhood. *Pediatrics* 35:601–619, 1965.

Field T, Goldson F: Pacifying effects of nonnutritive sucking on term and preterm neonates during heelstick procedures. *Pediatrics* 74:1012, 1984.

Filston HC, Chitwood WR Jr, Schkolne B, Blackmon LR: The Fogarty balloon catheter as an aid to management of the infant with esophageal atresia and tracheoesophageal fistula complicated by severe RDS or pneumonia. *J Pediatr Surg* 17:149, 1982.

Fisher DM, O'Keefe C, Stanski DR, et al.: Pharmacokinetics and pharmacodynamics of d-tubocurarine in infants, children, and adults. *Anesthesiology* 57:203, 1982.

Fong YM, Marano MA, Moldawer LL, et al.: The acute splanchnic and peripheral tissue metabolic response to endotoxin in humans. *J Clin Invest* 85: 1896–1904, 1990.

Frank L, Sosenko IR: Prenatal development of lung antioxidant enzymes in four species. *J Pediatr* 110:106–110, 1987.

Frantz ID III, Adler SM, Thach BT, et al.: Maturational effects on respiratory responses to carbon dioxide in premature infants. *J Appl Physiol* 41:41, 1976.

Friedman WF: Neuropharmacologic studies of perinatal myocardium. *Cardiovasc Clin* 4:43–57, 1972.

Friesen RH, Lichtor JL: Cardiovascular effects of inhalation induction with isoflurane in infants. *Anesth Analg* 62:411, 1983.

Friesen RH, Lichtor LJ: Cardiovascular depression during halothane anesthesia in infants: A study of three induction techniques. *Anesth Analg* 61:42, 1982.

Friis-Hansen B: Body composition during growth: In vivo measurements and biochemical data correlated to differential anatomical growth. *Pediatrics* 47(suppl):264–274, 1971.

Fryns JP, Moerman F, Goddeeris P, et al.: A new lethal syndrome with cloudy cornea, diaphragmatic defects and distal limb deformities. *Hum Genet* 50:65–70, 1979.

Furchgott RF, Zawadzki JV: The obligatory role of endothelial cells in relaxation of arterial smooth muscle by acetylcholine. *Nature* 288:373–376, 1980.

Furman EB: *Pediatric fluid management during anesthesia.* ASA Refresher Course Lectures, p 226, 1987.

Furman EB, Roman DG, Lemmer LAS, et al.: Specific therapy in water, electrolyte, and blood-volume replacement during pediatric surgery. *Anesthesiology* 42:187, 1975.

Gandy GM, Adamsons K, Cunningham N, et al.: Thermal environment and acid-base homeostasis in human infants during the first few hours of life. *Arch Dis Child* 40:465, 1965.

Gappa M, Berner MM, Hohenschild S, et al.: Pulmonary function at school-age in surfactant-treated preterm infants. *Pediatr Pulmonol* 27:191–198, 1999.

Gauntlett IS, Fisher DM, Hertzka RE, et al.: Pharmacokinetics of fentanyl in neonatal humans and lambs: effects of age. *Anesthesiology* 69:683–687, 1988.

Geggel Rl, Reid LM: The structural basis of PPHN. *Clin Perinatol* 2:525–549, 1984.

Georgeson KE, Inge TH, Albanese CT: Laparoscopically assisted anorectal pull-through for high imperforate anus—A new technique. *J Pediatr Surg* 35:927–930, 2000.

Gerhardt T, Bancalari E: Apnea of prematurity. I. Lung function and regulation of breathing. *Pediatrics* 74:58, 1984.

German JC, Gazzaniga AB, Amlie R, et al.: Management of pulmonary insufficiency in diaphragmatic hernia using extracorporeal circulation with a membrane oxygenator (ECMO). *J Pediatr Surg* 12:905, 1977.

Goetzman BW, Sunshine B, Johnson JD, et al.: Neonatal hypoxia and pulmonary vasospasm: Response to tolazoline. *J Pediatr* 89:617, 1976.

Gomez R, Romero R, Ghezzi F, et al.: The fetal inflammatory response syndrome. *Am J Obstet Gynecol* 179:194–202, 1998.

Greenough A, Maconochie E, Yuksel B: Recurrent respiratory symptoms in the first year of life following preterm delivery. *J Perinat Med* 18:489–494, 1990.

Greer JJ, Babiuk RP, Thebaud B: Etiology of congenital diaphragmatic hernia: the retinoid hypothesis. *Pediatr Res* 53:726–730, 2003.

Gregory GA: Outpatient anesthesia. In Miller RD, editor: *Anesthesia.* New York, 1981, Churchill Livingstone.

Gregory GA, Eger EI, Munson ES: The relationship between age and halothane requirements in man. *Anesthesiology* 30:488–491, 1969.

Gregory GA, Steward DJ: Life-threatening perioperative apnea in the ex-"premie." *Anesthesiology* 59:495, 1983.

Groneck P, Gotze-Speer B, Oppermann M, et al.: Association of pulmonary inflammation and increased microvascular permeability during the development of bronchopulmonary dysplasia: A sequential analysis of inflammatory mediators in respiratory fluids of high-risk preterm neonates. *Pediatrics* 93:712–718, 1994.

Hack M, Friedman H, Avroy A, Fanaroff MB: Outcomes of extremely low birth weight infants. *Pediatrics* 98:931–937, 1996.

Hallman M, Haataja R: Genetic influences and neonatal lung disease. *Semin Neonatol* 8:19–27, 2003.

Hammarlund K, Sedin G, Stromberg B: Transepidermal water loss in newborn infants. VIII. Relation to gestational age and postnatal age in appropriate and small for gestational age infants. *Acta Paediatr Scand* 72:721–728, 1983.

Hardesty RL, Griffith BP, Debski RF, et al.: Extracorporeal membrane oxygenation. Successful treatment of persistent fetal circulation following repair of congenital diaphragmatic hernia. *J Thorac Cardiovasc Surg* 81:556, 1981.

Harnik EV, Hoy GR, Potolicchio S, et al.: Spinal anesthesia in premature infants recovering from respiratory distress syndrome. *Anesthesiology* 64:95, 1986.

Harrison MR, Adzick NS, Bullard KM, et al.: Correction of congenital diaphragmatic hernia in utero. VII. A prospective trial. *J Pediatr Surg* 32:1637–1642, 1997.

Harrison MR, Adzick NS, Estes JM, Howell LJ: A prospective study of the outcome for fetuses with diaphragmatic hernia. *JAMA* 271:382–384, 1994.

Harrison MR, Adzick NS, Longaker MT, et al.: Successful repair in utero of a fetal diaphragmatic hernia after removal of herniated viscera from the left thorax. *N Engl J Med* 322:1582–1584, 1990.

Harrison MR, Bjordal RI, Langmork F, Knutrud O: Congenital diaphragmatic hernia: The hidden mortality. *J Pediatr Surg* 13:227–230, 1978.

Harrison MR, Keller RL, Hawgood SB, et al.: A randomized trial of fetal endoscopic tracheal occlusion for severe fetal congenital diaphragmatic hernia. *N Engl J Med* 349:1916–1224, 2003.

Harrison MR, Langer JC, Adzick NS: Correction of congenital diaphragmatic hernia in utero. VI. Hard-earned lessons. *J Pediatr Surg* 28:1411–1417, 1993.

Hatch DJ: Analgesia in the neonate. *Br Med J* 294:920, 1987.

Hazebroek FWJ, Tibboel D, Bos AP, et al.: Congenital diaphragmatic hernia: Impact of preoperative stabilization. A prospective pilot study in 13 patients. *J Pediatr Surg* 23:1139, 1988.

Hecher K, Hackeloer BJ: Intrauterine endoscopic laser surgery for fetal sacrococcygeal teratoma. *Lancet* 347:470, 1996.

Heiss K, Manning P, Oldham KT, et al.: Reversal of mortality for congenital diaphragmatic hernia with ECMO. *Ann Surg* 209:225, 1989.

Hengerer AS, Strome M, Jaffe BF: Injuries to the neonatal larynx from long-term endotracheal tube intubation and suggested tube modification for prevention. *Ann Otol Rhinol Laryngol* 84:764, 1975.

Heymann MA, Rudolph AM: Control of the ductus arteriosus. *Physiol Rev* 55:62, 1975.

Hinkle AJ: Awake neonatal laryngoscopy: Pre-oxygenation alone versus continuous oxygenation. *Anesthesiology* 59:A437, 1983.

Hitti J, Krohn MA, Patton DL, et al.: Amniotic fluid tumor necrosis factor-alpha and the risk of respiratory distress syndrome among preterm infants. *Am J Obstet Gynecol* 177:50–56, 1997.

Holliday MA, Segar WE: The maintenance need for water in parenteral fluid therapy. *Pediatrics* 19:823, 1957.

Hook JB, Bailie MD: Perinatal renal pharmacology. *Annu Rev Pharmacol Toxicol* 19:491–509, 1979.

Hubmayr RD: The times are a-changin'. *Anesthesiology* 100:1–2, 2004.

Humphreys PW, Normand ICS, Reynolds EOR, et al.: Pulmonary lymph flow and the uptake of liquid from the lungs of the lamb at the start of breathing. *J Physiol* 193:1, 1967.

Hussain AN, Siddiqui NH, Stocker JT: Pathology of arrested acinar development in postsurfactant BPD. *Hum Pathol* 29:710–717, 1998.

Imai T, Kurland G, Wiener E, et al.: Lung function in children after repair of severe neonatal congenital diaphragmatic hernia (CDH) and mechanical ventilation. *Am Rev Respir Dis* 149:A547, 1994.

Jacob SV, Lands LC, Coates AL, et al.: Exercise ability in survivors of severe bronchopulmonary dysplasia. *Am J Respir Crit Care Med* 155:1925–1929, 1997.

Jarmakani JM, Nakanishi T, Gerorge BL, Bers D: Effect of extracellular calcium ion myocardial mechanical function in the neonatal rabbit. *Dev Pharmacol Ther* 5:1–13, 1982.

Jelsema RD, Isada NB, Kazzi NJ, et al.: Prenatal diagnosis of congenital diaphragmatic hernia not amenable to prenatal or neonatal repair: Brachmann-de-Lange syndrome. *Am J Med Genet* 47:1022–1023, 1993.

Jobe AH, Bancalari E: Bronchopulmonary dysplasia. *Am J Respir Crit Care Med* 163:1723–1729, 2001.

Johnson DG, Deamer RM, Koop CE: Diaphragmatic hernia in infancy: Factors affecting the mortality rate. *Surgery* 62:1082, 1967.

Jones EP, Pelton DA: An index of syndromes and their anaesthetic implications. *Can Anaesth Soc J* 23:207–225, 1976.

Jonmarker C, Westrin P, Larsson S, Werner O: Thiopental requirements for induction of anesthesia in children. *Anesthesiology* 67:104, 1987.

Jonsson B, Tullus K, Brauner A, et al.: Early increase of TNF and IL-6 in tracheobronchial aspirate fluid indicator of subsequent chronic lung disease in preterm infants. *Arch Dis Child* 77:F198–F201, 1997.

Jornot L, Mirault ME, Junod AF: Protein synthesis in hyperoxic endothelial cells: Evidence for translational defect. *J Appl Physiol* 63:457–464, 1987.

Karamanoukian HL, Click PL, Zayek M, et al.: Inhaled nitric oxide in congenital hypoplasia of the lungs due to diaphragmatic hernia or oligohydramnios. *Pediatrics* 94:715, 1994.

Karamanoukian HL, Glick PL, Wilcox DT, et al.: Pathophysiology of congenital diaphragmatic hernia: XI. Anatomic and biochemical characterization of the heart in the fetal lamb CEH model. *J Pediatr Surg* 30:925–928, 1995.

Karl HW: Control of life-threatening air leak after gastrostomy in an infant with respiratory distress syndrome and tracheoesophageal fistula. *Anesthesiology* 62:670, 1985.

Keens TG, Bryan AC, Levison H, et al.: Developmental pattern of muscle fiber types in human ventilatory muscles. *J Appl Physiol Respir Environ Exerc Physiol* 44:909, 1978.

Kelly DH, Shannon DC: Treatment of apnea and excessive periodic breathing in the full-term infant. *Pediatrics* 68:183, 1981.

Khatter JC, Hoeschen RJ: Developmental increase of digitalis receptors in guinea pig heart. *Cardiovasc Res* 16:80–85, 1982.

King RJ: Pulmonary surfactant. *J Appl Physiol* 53:1, 1982.

Kinsella JP, Abman SH: Recent developments in the pathophysiology and treatment of persistent pulmonary hypertension of the newborn. *J Pediatr* 126:853, 1995.

Kinsella JP, Neish SR, Shaffer F, et al.: Low-dose inhaled nitric oxide in persistent pulmonary hypertension of the newborn. *Lancet* 340:819, 1992.

Knill R, Andrews W, Bryan AC, et al.: Respiratory load compensation in infants. *J Appl Physiol* 40:357, 1976.

Knill RL, Gelb AW: Ventilatory responses to hypoxia and hypercapnia during halothane sedation and anesthesia in man. *Anesthesiology* 49:244, 1978.

Kobayashi H, Puri P: Plasma endothelin levels in congenital diaphragmatic hernia. *J Pediatr Surg* 29:1258–1261, 1994.

Koch G, Wendel H: Adjustment of arterial blood gases and acid base balance in the normal newborn infant during the first week of life. *Biol Neonate* 12:136, 1968.

Koehntop DE, Rodman JH, Brundage DM, et al.: Pharmacokinetics of fentanyl in neonates. *Anesth Analg* 65:227, 1986.

Koivisto M, Blanco-Sequeiros M, Krause H: Neonatal symptomatic and asymptomatic hypoglycemia: A follow-up study of 151 children. *Dev Med Child Neurol* 14:603, 1972.

Koren G, Butt W, Chinyanga H, et al.: Post-operative morphine infusion in newborn infants: Assessment of disposition characteristics and safety. *J Pediatr* 107:963, 1985.

Koumbourlis AC, Motoyama EK, Mutich RL, et al.: Longitudinal follow-up of lung function from childhood to adolescence in prematurely born patients with neonatal chronic lung disease. *Pediatr Pulmonol* 21:28–34, 1996.

Kupferberg HJ, Way EL: Pharmacologic basis for the increased sensitivity of the newborn rat to morphine. *J Pharmacol Exp Ther* 141:105, 1963.

Kurth CD, Spitzer AR, Broennle AM, Downes JJ: Postoperative apnea in preterm infants. *Anesthesiology* 66:483, 1987.

Langham MR, Krummel TM, Bartlett RH, et al.: Mortality with extracorporeal membrane oxygenation following repair of congenital diaphragmatic hernia in 93 infants. *J Pediatr Surg* 22:1150, 1987.

Langston C, Kida K, Reed M, Thurlbeck WM: Human lung growth in later gestation and in the neonate. *Am Rev Respir Dis* 129:607, 1984.

LeDez KM, Lerman J: The minimum alveolar concentration (MAC) of isoflurane in preterm neonates. *Anesthesiology* 67:301, 1987.

Lerman J: Anaesthesia in preterm and ex-preterm infants. *Curr Opin Anaesth* 1:11, 1988.

Lerman J, Gregory GA, Willis MM, Eger EI II: Age and solubility of volatile anesthetics in blood. *Anesthesiology* 61:139–142, 1984.

Lerman J, Robinson S, Willis MM, Gregory GA: Anesthetic requirements for halothane in young children 0-1 months and 1-6 months of age. *Anesthesiology* 59:421–424, 1983.

Lerman J, Schmitt-Bantel BI, Gregory GA, et al.: Effect of age on solubility of volatile anesthetics in human tissues. *Anesthesiology* 65:307–311, 1986.

Lesouef PN, England SJ, Bryan AC: Passive respiratory mechanics in newborns and children. *Am Rev Respir Dis* 129:552–556, 1984.

Lévêque C, Hamza J, Berg AE, et al.: Successful repair of a severe left congenital diaphragmatic hernia during continuous inhalation of nitric oxide. *Anesthesiology* 80:1171, 1994.

Levin DL: Congenital diaphragmatic hernia: A persistent problem. *J Pediatr* 111:390–392, 1987.

Levitt MA, Patel M, Rodriguez G, et al.: The tethered spinal cord in patients with anorectal malformations. *J Pediatr Surg* 32:462, 1997.

Levy RJ, Rosenthal A, Freed MD, et al.: Persistent pulmonary hypertension in a newborn with congenital diaphragmatic hernia: Successful management with tolazoline. *Pediatrics* 60:740, 1977.

Lewis DA, Reickert C, Bowerman R, Hirschl RB: Prenatal ultrasonography frequently fails to diagnose congenital diaphragmatic hernia. *J Pediatr Surg* 32:352–356, 1997.

Liu LMP, Coté CJ, Goudsouzian NG, et al.: Life-threatening apnea in infants recovering from anesthesia. *Anesthesiology* 59:506, 1983.

Lockhart CH, Jenkins JJ: Ketamine-induced apnea in patients with increased intracranial pressure. *Anesthesiology* 37:92, 1972.

Lockhart CH, Nelson WL: The relationship of ketamine requirement to age in pediatric patients. *Anesthesiology* 40:507, 1974.

Long W, Zucker J, Kraybill E: Symposium on synthetic surfactant. II: Perspective and commentary. *J Pediatr* 126:S1–S4, 1995.

Lou HC, Lassen NA, Friis-Hansen B: Impaired autoregulation of cerebral blood flow in the distressed newborn infant. *J Pediatr* 94:118–121, 1979A.

Lou HC, Lassen NA, Tweed WA: Pressure passive cerebral blood flow changes and breakdown of the blood-brain barrier in experimental fetal asphyxia. *Acta Paediatr Scand* 68:57–63, 1979B.

Lou HC, Lassen NA, Tweed WA, Volpe JJ: Intracranial hemorrhage: Germinal matrix-intraventricular hemorrhage of the premature infant. In *Neurology of the newborn*, 4th ed. Philadelphia, 2001, WB Saunders, chap 11.

Lubchenco L, Hansman C, Dressler M: Intrauterine growth as estimated from liveborn birth-weight data at 24 to 42 weeks of gestation. *Pediatrics* 32:793, 1963.

Lund DP, Mitchell J, Kharasch V, et al.: Congenital diaphragmatic hernia: The hidden morbidity. *J Pediatr Surg* 29:258, 1994.

Lynn A: Unusual conditions in paediatric anaesthesia. *Clin Anesthesiol* 3:741, 1985.

MacLusky IB, Stringer D, Zarfen J, et al.: Cardiorespiratory status in long-term survivors of prematurity with and without hyaline membrane disease. *Pediatr Pulmonol* 2:94–102, 1986.

Mahony L: Maturation of calcium transport in cardiac sarcoplasmic reticulum. *Pediatr Res* 24:639–643, 1988.

Mahony L, Jones LR: Developmental changes in cardiac sarcoplasmic reticulum in sheep. *J Biol Chem* 261:15257–15265, 1986.

Malviya S, Lerman J: The blood/gas solubilities of sevoflurane, isoflurane, halothane, and serum constituent concentrations in neonates and adults. *Anesthesiology* 72:793–796, 1990.

Malviya S, Swartz J, Lerman J: Are all preterm infants younger than 60 weeks postconceptual age at risk for postanesthetic apnea? *Anesthesiology* 78:1076, 1993.

Margraf LR, Tomashefski JF, Bruce MC, Dahms BB: Morphometric analysis of the lung in bronchopulmonary dysplasia. *Am Rev Respir Dis* 143:391–400, 1991.

Marshall TA, Deeder R, Pai S, et al.: Physiologic changes associated with endotracheal intubation in preterm infants. *Crit Care Med* 12:501, 1984.

Matoth Y, Zaizov R, Varsano I: Postnatal chances in some red cell parameters. *Acta Paediatr Scand* 60:317, 1971.

McDonald MS, Emery JL: The later intrauterine and postnatal development of human glomeruli. *J Anat* 93:331–340, 1959.

Metkus AP, Esserman L, Sola A, et al.: Cost per anomaly: What does a diaphragmatic hernia cost? *J Pediatr Surg* 30:226, 1995.

Mestan KK, Marks JD, Hecox K, et al.: Neurodevelopmental outcomes of premature infants treated with inhaled nitric oxide. *N Engl J Med* 353:23–32, 2005.

Mildenberger E, Versmold HT: Pathogenesis and therapy of non-oliguric hyperkalaemia of the premature infant. *Eur J Pediatr* 161:415–422, 2002.

Millar M, Wilks M, Costeloe K: Probiotics for preterm infants? *Arch Dis Child Fetal Neonatal Ed* 88:F354–F358, 2003.

Milligan DWA, Levison H: Lung function in children following repair of tracheoesophageal fistula. *J Pediatr* 95:24, 1979.

Milner RDG: Neonatal hypoglycemia: A critical reappraisal. *Arch Dis Child* 47:679, 1972.

Mirkin BL: Perinatal pharmacology. *Anesthesiology* 43:156, 1975.

Mitchell SH, Teague WG, Robinson A: Reduced gas transfer at rest and during exercise in school-age survivors of bronchopulmonary dysplasia. *Am J Respir Crit Care Med* 157:1406–1412, 1998.

Miyasaka K, Sankawa H, Nakajo T, Akiyama H: Congenital diaphragmatic hernia: Is emergency radical surgery really necessary? *Jpn J Pediatr Surg* 16:1417, 1984.

Molik KA, Gingalewski CA, West KW, et al.: Gastroschisis: A plea for risk categorization. *J Pediatr Surg* 36:51–55, 2001.

Moodie DS, Telander RL, Kleinberg F, Feldt RH: Use of tolazoline in newborn infants with diaphragmatic hernia and severe cardiopulmonary disease. *J Thorac Cardiovasc Surg* 75:725, 1978.

Morray JP: Anesthesia-related cardiac arrest in children. An update. *Anesthesiol Clin North Am* 20:1–28, 2002.

Morray JP, Geiduschek JM, Ramamoorthy C, et al.: Anesthesia-related cardiac arrest in children: initial findings of the Pediatric Perioperative Cardiac Arrest (POCA) Registry. *Anesthesiology* 93:6–14, 2000.

Motoyama EK, Brinkmeyer SD, Mutich RL, et al.: Reduced FRC in anesthetized infants: Effect of low PEEP. *Anesthesiology* 57:A418, 1982.

Muller NL, Bryan AC: Chest wall mechanics and respiratory muscles in infants. *Pediatr Clin North Am* 26:503, 1979.

Murat I, Constant I, Maud'huy H: Perioperative anaesthetic morbidity in children: a database of 24,165 anaesthetics over a 30-month period. *Paediatr Anaesth* 14:158–166, 2004.

Muratore CS, Kharasch V, Lund DP, et al.: Pulmonary morbidity in 100 survivors of congenital diaphragmatic hernia monitored in a multidisciplinary clinic. *J Pediatr Surg* 36:133–140, 2001.

Muratore CS, Utter S, Jaksic T, et al.: Nutritional morbidity in survivors of congenital diaphragmatic hernia. *J Pediatr Surg* 36:1171 1176, 2001a.

Muratore CS, Utter S, Jaksic T, et al.: Pulmonary morbidity in 100 survivors of congenital diaphragmatic hernia monitored in a multidisciplinary clinic. *J Pediatr Surg* 36:133–140, 2001b.

Murphy ID, Rabinovitch M, Goldstein ID, Reid LM: The structural basis of persistent pulmonary hypertension of the new-horn infant. *J Pediatr* 98:962, 1981.

Musemeche CA, Kosloske AM, Bartow SA, Umland ET: Comparative effects of ischemia, bacteria and substrate on the pathogenesis of intestinal necrosis. *J Pediatr Surg* 21:536–538, 1986.

Muthuchamy M, Grupp II, Grupp G, et al.: Molecular and physiological effects of overexpressing striated muscle β-tropomyosin in the adult murine heart. *J Biol Chem* 270:30593–30603, 1995.

Nagaya M, Akatsuka H, Kato J: Gastroesophageal reflux occurring after repair of congenital diaphragmatic hernia. *J Pediatr Surg* 29:1447, 1994.

Nakanishi T, Okuda H, Kamata K, et al.: Development of myocardial contractile system in the fetal rabbit. *Pediatr Res* 22:201–207, 1987.

Nakayama DK, Motoyama EK, Tagge EM: Effect of preoperative stabilization on respiratory system compliance and outcome in newborn infants with congenital diaphragmatic hernia. *J Pediatr* 118:793, 1991.

Nakayama DK, Mutich R, Rowe MI, Motoyama EK: Pulmonary function following primary closure of abdominal wall defects in the newborn and its improvement with bronchodilators. *Surg Forum* 40:571, 1989.

Nassar R, Reedy MC, Anderson PA: Developmental changes in the ultrastructure and sarcomere shortening of the isolated rabbit ventricular myocyte. *Circ Res* 61:465–483, 1987.

Newman JH, Loyd JE, English DK, et al.: Effects of 100% oxygen on lung vascular function in awake sheep. *J Appl Physiol* 54:1379–1386, 1983.

Newman KD, Anderson KD, Van Meurs K, et al.: Extracorporeal membrane oxygenation and congenital diaphragmatic hernia: Should any infant be excluded? *J Pediatr Surg* 25:1048, 1990.

Nielson OH, Jorgensen AF: Congenital posterolateral diaphragmatic hernia: Factors affecting survival. *Z Kinderchir* 24:201, 1978.

Niems AH, Warner M, Loughnan PM, Aranda JV: Developmental aspects of the hepatic cytochrome P450 mono-oxygenase system. *Annu Rev Pharmacol Toxicol* 16:427–445, 1976.

Nogee LM, Garnier H, Dietz HC, et al.: A mutation in the surfactant protein B gene responsible for fatal neonatal respiratory disease in multiple kindreds. *J Clin Invest* 93:1860–1863, 1994.

Noland TA Jr, Guo X, Raynor RL, et al.: Cardiac troponin I mutants: Phosphorylation by protein kinases C and A and regulation of Ca^{2+}-stimulated MgATPase of reconstituted actomysin S-1. *J Biol Chem* 270:25445–25454, 1995.

Norden MA, Butt W, McDougall P: Predictors of survival for infants with congenital diaphragmatic hernia. *J Pediatr Surg* 29:1442, 1994.

Northway WH Jr, Moss RB, Carlisle KB, et al.: Late pulmonary sequelae of bronchopulmonary dysplasia. *N Engl J Med* 323:1793–1799, 1990.

Northway WH, Rosan RC, Porter DY: Pulmonary disease following respirator therapy of hyaline membrane disease. *N Engl J Med* 276:357–368, 1967.

O'Neil JA, Grosfeld JL: Intestinal malfunction after antenatal exposure of viscera. *Am J Surg* 127:129, 1974.

Pacifica GM, Biani A, Teddeucci-Brunelli G, et al.: Effects of development, aging, and renal and hepatic insufficiency as well as hemodialysis on the plasma concentrations of albumin and alpha 1 acid glycoprotein: Implications for binding of drugs. *Ther Drug Monit* 8:259–263, 1986.

Padbury JF, Diakomanolis ES, Lam RW, et al.: Ontogenesis of tissue catecholamines in fetal and neonatal rabbits. *J Dev Physiol* 3:297–303, 1981.

Paek BW, Jennings RW, Harrison MR, et al.: Radiofrequency ablation of fetal sacrococcygeal teratoma. *Am J Obstet Gynecol* 184:503–507, 2001.

Pagani ED, Julian FJ: Rabbit papillary muscle myosin isozymes and the velocity of muscle shortening. *Circ Res* 54:586–594, 1984.

Pang LM, Mellins RB: Neonatal cardiorespiratory physiology. *Anesthesiology* 43:171, 1975.

Papaila JG: Increased incidence of delayed gastric emptying in children with gastroesophageal reflux. A prospective evaluation. *Arch Surg* 124:933–936, 1989.

Papile L, Burnstein J, Burnstein R, et al.: Incidence and evolution of subependymal and intraventricular hemorrhage: A study of infants with birth weights less than 1500 grams. *J Pediatr* 92:529, 1978.

Papile LA, Rudolph AM, Heymann MA: Autoregulation of cerebral blood flow in the preterm fetal lamb. *Pediatr Res* 19:159–161, 1985.

Pappert D, Busch T, Gerlach H, et al.: Aerosolized prostacyclin versus inhaled nitric oxide in children with severe acute respiratory distress syndrome. *Anesthesiology* 82:1507, 1995.

Parat S, Moriette G, Delaperche M-F, et al.: Long-term pulmonary functional outcome of bronchopulmonary dysplasia and premature birth. *Pediatr Pulmonol* 20:289–296, 1995.

Peckham CJ, Fox WW: Physiologic factors affecting pulmonary artery pressure in infants with persistent pulmonary hypertension. *J Pediatr* 93:1005, 1978.

Pelkonen AS, Hakulinen AL, Turpeinen M, Hallman M: Effect of neonatal surfactant therapy on lung function at school age in children born very preterm. *Pediatr Pulmonol* 25:182–190, 1998.

Pena A, Hong A: Advances in the management of anorectal malformations. *Am J Surg* 180:370–376, 2000.
Philip AGS: Oxygen plus pressure plus time: The etiology of bronchopulmonary dysplasia. *Pediatrics* 55:44, 1975.
Piafsky KM, Woolner M: The binding of basic drugs to α_1-acid glycoprotein in cord serum. *J Pediatr* 100:820–823, 1982.
Piecuch RE, Leonard CH: Outcome of very preterm infants *Contemp Rev Obstet Gynecol* June:115–120, 1998.
Pinson CW, Morton MJ, Thornburg KL: An anatomic basis for fetal right ventricular dominance and arterial pressure sensitivity. *J Dev Physiol* 9: 253–269, 1987.
Poland RL, Roberts RJ, Gutierrez-Mazorra JF, Fonkalsrud EW: Neonatal anesthesia. *Pediatrics* 80:446, 1987.
Quan L, Smith DW: The VATER association: Vertebral defects, anal atresia, tracheoesophageal fistula with esophageal atresia, radial dysplasia. *Birth Defects* 8:75, 1973.
Quinn GE, Betts EK, Diamond GR, Schaeffer DB: Neonatal age (human) at retinal maturation. *Anesthesiology* 55:A326, 1981.
Rabinowitz R, Peters MT, Vyas S, et al.: Measurement of fetal urine production in normal pregnancy by real-time ultrasonography. *Am J Obstet Gynecol* 161:1264–1268, 1989.
Rabinowitz SS, Dzakpasu P, Piecuch S, et al.: Platelet-activating factor in infants at risk for necrotizing enterocolitis. *J Pediatr* 138:81–86, 2001.
Rackow H, Salanitre E, Green LT: Frequency of cardiac arrest associated with anesthesia in infants and children. *Pediatrics* 28:697, 1961.
Radford PJ, Stillwell PC, Blue B, Hertel G: Aspiration complications in bronchopulmonary dysplasia. *Chest* 107:185–188, 1996.
Raju TNK, Vidyasagar D, Torres C, et al.: Intracranial pressure during intubation and anesthesia in infants. *J Pediatr* 96:860, 1980.
Ramet M, Haataja R, Marttila R, et al.: Association between the surfactant protein A (SP-A) gene locus and respiratory-distress syndrome in the Finnish population. *Am J Hum Genet* 66:1569–1579, 2000.
Raphaely RC, Downes JJ Jr: Congenital diaphragmatic hernia: Prediction of survival. *J Pediatr Surg* 8:815, 1973.
Redmond C, Heaton J, Calix J, et al.: A correlation of pulmonary hypoplasia, mean airway pressure, and survival in congenital diaphragmatic hernia treated with extracorporeal membrane oxygenation. *J Pediatr Surg* 22:1143, 1987.
Reickert CA, Hirschl RB, Atkinson JB, et al.: Congenital diaphragmatic hernia survival and use of extracorporeal life support at selected level III nurseries with multimodality support. *Surgery* 123:305–310, 1998.
Reid IS, Hutcherson RJ: Long-term follow-up of patients with congenital diaphragmatic hernia. *J Pediatr Surg* 11:939, 1976.
Rice LJ, Pudimat MA, Hannallah RS: Timing of caudal block placement does not affect duration of postoperative analgesia in pediatric ambulatory surgical patients. *Anesthesiology* 69:A771, 1988.
Richards IS, Kulkarni A, Brooks SM: Human fetal tracheal smooth muscle produces spontaneous electromechanical oscillations that are Ca^{2+} dependent and cholinergically potentiated. *Dev Pharmacol Ther* 16:22–28, 1991.
Rigatto H: Apnea. *Pediatr Clin North Am* 29:1105–1116, 1982.
Rigatto H, Brady JP, Verduzco R: Chemoreceptor reflexes in preterm infants. II. The effect of gestational and postnatal age on the ventilatory response to inhaled carbon dioxide. *Pediatrics* 55:614, 1975.
Rigatto H, Verduzco RT, Cates DB: Effects of O_2 on the ventilatory response to CO_2 in preterm infants. *J Appl Physiol* 39:896, 1975.
Rittler M, Paz JE, Castilla EE: VACTERL association, epidemiologic definition and delineation. *Am J Med Gen* 63:529–536, 1996.
Roberts JD, Polaner DM, Lang P, et al.: Inhaled nitric oxide in persistent pulmonary hypertension of the newborn. *Lancet* 340:818, 1992.
Robinson JN, Abuhamad AZ: Abdominal wall and umbilical cord anomalies. *Clin Perinatol* 27:947–978, 2000.
Robinson RB: Review: Autonomic receptor-effector coupling during post-natal development. *Cardiovasc Res* 31:E68–E76, 1996.
Robinson S, Gregory GA: Fentanyl-air-oxygen anesthesia for ligation of patent ductus arteriosus in preterm infants. *Anesth Analg* 60:331–334, 1981.
Robinson TF, Cohen-Gould L, Factor SM: Skeletal framework of mammalian heart muscle: arrangement of inter- and pericellular connective tissue structures. *Lab Invest* 49:482–498, 1983.
Rollnick BR, Kaye CI: Hemifacial microsomia and variants: Pedigree data. *Am J Med Genet* 15:233–253, 1983.
Romero T, Covell J, Friedman WF: A comparison of pressure-volume relations of the fetal, newborn, and adult heart. *Am J Physiol* 222:1285–1290, 1972.
Root AW, Harrison HE: Recent advances in calcium metabolism. I. Mechanism of calcium homeostasis. *J Pediatr* 88:177–199, 1976.
Rosenberg AA, Kennaugh J, Koppenhafer SL, et al.: Elevated immunoreactive endothelin-1 levels in newborn infants with persistent pulmonary hypertension. *J Pediatr* 123:109–114, 1993.
Rowe MI, Lankau C, Newmark S: Clinical evaluation of methods to monitor colloid oncotic pressure in the surgical treatment of children. *Surg Gynecol Obstet* 139:889, 1974.
Rudolph AM: Myocardial growth before and after birth: Clinical implications. *Acta Paediatr* 89:129–133, 2000.
Rudolph AM, Yuan S: Response of the pulmonary vasculature to hypoxia and H^+ ion concentration changes. *J Clin Invest* 45:399, 1966.
Saarenmaa E, Neuvonen PJ, Fellman V: Gestational age and birth weight effects on plasma clearance of fentanyl in newborn infants. *J Pediatr* 136:767, 2000.
Sakai H, Tamura M, Hosokawa Y, et al.: Effect of surgical repair on respiratory mechanics in congenital diaphragmatic hernia. *J Pediatr* 111:432–438, 1987.
Salem MR, Wong AY, Lin YH, et al.: Prevention of gastric distention during anesthesia for newborns with tracheoesophageal fistulas. *Anesthesiology* 38:82–83, 1973.
Santeiro ML, Christie J, Stromquist C, et al.: Pharmacokinetics of continuous infusion fentanyl in newborns. *J Perinatol* 17:135–139, 1997.
Santulli TV, Schullinger JN, Heird WC, et al.: Acute necrotizing enterocolitis in infancy: A review of 64 cases. *Pediatrics* 55:376, 1975.
Santuz P, Baraldi E, Zaramella P, et al.: Factors limiting exercise performance in long-term survivors of bronchopulmonary dysplasia. *Am J Respir Crit Care Med* 152:1284–1289, 1995.
Schlatter M, Norris K, Uitvlugt N, et al.: Improved outcomes in the treatment of gastroschisis using a preformed silo and delayed repair approach. *J Pediatr Surg* 38:459–464, 2003.
Schmidt B, Cao L, Mackensen-Haen S, et al.: Chorioamnionitis and inflammation of the fetal lung. *Am J Obset Gynecol* 194:173–177, 2001.
Schuster SR: A new method for staged repair of large omphaloceles. *Surg Gynecol Obstet* 125:837, 1967.
Schute FJ: Apnea. *Clin Perinatol* 4:65, 1977.
Schwartz SM, Vermillion RP, Hirschl RB: Evaluation of left ventricular mass in children with left-sided congenital diaphragmatic hernia. *J Pediatr* 125:447–451, 1994.
Seidner SR, Chen YQ, Oprysko PR, et al.: Combined prostaglandin and nitric oxide inhibition produces anatomic remodeling and closure of the ductus arteriosus in the premature newborn baboon. *Pediatr Res* 50:365–373, 2001.
Senior B: Neonatal hypoglycemia. *N Engl J Med* 289:790, 1973.
Shah N, Jacob T, Exler R, et al.: Inhaled nitric oxide in congenital diaphragmatic hernia. *J Pediatr Surg* 29:1010, 1994.
Sham JS, Hatem SN, Morad M: Species differences in the activity of the Na(+)-Ca2+ exchanger in mammalian cardiac myocytes. *J Physiol* 488:623–631, 1995.
Shennan AT, Dunn MS, Ohlsson A, et al.: Abnormal pulmonary outcomes in premature infants: Prediction from oxygen requirement in the neonatal period. *Pediatrics* 82:527–532, 1988.
Shimoya K, Taniguchi T, Matsuzaki N, et al.: Chorioamnionitis decreased incidence of respiratory distress syndrome by elevating fetal interleukin-6 serum concentration. *Hum Reprod* 15:2234–2240, 2000.
Shires T, Williams J, Brown F: Acute change in extracellular fluids associated with major surgical procedures. *Ann Surg* 154:803, 1961.
Sigalet DL, Nguyen LT, Laberge JM, et al.: Gastroesophageal reflux associated with large diaphragmatic hernias. *J Pediatr Surg* 29:1262, 1994.
Simpson P: Stimulation of hypertrophy of cultured neonatal rat heart cells through an α1-adrenergic receptor and induction of beating through an α1-β1-adrenergic receptor interaction: evidence for independent regulation of growth and beating. *Circ Res* 56:884–894, 1985.
Singleton MA, Rosen JI, Fisher DM: Plasma concentrations of fentanyl in infants, children, and adults. *Can J Anaesth* 34:152–155, 1987.
Smith CA, Nelson NM: *The physiology of the newborn infant,* 4th ed. Springfield, IL, 1976, Charles C Thomas, Publisher.
Smyth J, Allen A, MacMurray B, et al.: Double-blind, randomized, placebo-controlled Canadian multicenter trial of two doses of synthetic surfactant or air placebo in 224 infants weighing 500-749 gm with respiratory distress syndrome. *J Pediatr* 126:S81–S89, 1995.
Soifer SJ, Morin FC III, Heymann MA: Prostaglandin D_2 reverses induced pulmonary hypertension in the newborn lamb. *J Pediatr* 100:458, 1982.
Solaro RJ, Lee JA, Kentish JC, Allen DG: Effects of acidosis on ventricular muscle from adult and neonatal rats. *Circ Res* 63:779–786, 1988.
Soubasi V, Kremenopoulos G, Diamanti E, et al.: Follow-up of very low birth weight infants after erythropoietin treatment to prevent anemia prematurity. *J Pediatr* 127:291–297, 1995.
Spears RS Jr, Yeh A, Fisher DM, Zwoss MS: The "educated hand." Can anesthesiologists assess changes in neonatal pulmonary compliance manually? *Anesthesiology* 75:693, 1991.
Spilde T, Bhatia A, Ostlie D, et al.: A role for sonic hedgehog signaling in the pathogenesis of human tracheoesophageal fistula. *J Pediatr Surg* 38:465–468, 2003.

Stege G, Fenton A, Jaffrey B: Nihilism in the 1990s: The true mortality of congenital diaphragmatic hernia. *Pediatrics* 112:532–535, 2003.

Steimle CN, Meric F, Hirschl RB, et al.: Effect of extracorporeal life support on survival when applied to all patients with congenital diaphragmatic hernia. *J Pediatr Surg* 29:997, 1994.

Stern L, Lees MH, Leduc J: Environmental temperature, oxygen consumption, and catecholamine excretion in newborn infants. *Pediatrics* 36:367, 1965.

Stern L: The use and misuse of oxygen in the newborn infant. *Pediatr Clin North Am* 20:447, 1973.

Steward DJ: Preterm infants are more prone to complications following minor surgery than are term infants. *Anesthesiology* 56:304, 1982.

Strang LB: *Neonatal respiration: Physiological and clinical studies.* Oxford, 1977, Blackwell Scientific Publications.

Sun X, Hsueh W: Platelet-activating factor produces shock, in vivo complement activation, and tissue injury in mice. *J Immunol* 147:509–514, 1991.

Sun XM, Qu XW, Huang W, et al.: Role of leukocyte beta 2-integrin in PAF-induced shock and intestinal injury. *Am J Physiol* 270:G184–G190, 1996.

Svenningsen NW, Aronson AS: Postnatal development of renal concentration capacity as estimated by DDAVP-test in normal and asphyxiated neonates. *Biol Neonate* 25:230–241, 1974.

Swyer PR: The intensive care of the newly born. *Physiological principles and practice. Monographs in Pediatrics,* vol 6. Basel, 1975, S Karger.

Sydorak RM, Nijagal A, Sbragia L, et al.: Gastroschisis: Small hole, big cost *J Pediatr Surg* 37:1669–1672, 2002.

Tait AR, Malviya S, Voepel-Lewis T, et al.: Risk factors for perioperative adverse respiratory events in children with upper respiratory tract infections. *Anesthesiology* 95:299–306, 2001.

Takashima S, Mito T, Ando Y: Pathogenesis of periventricular white matter hemorrhages in preterm infants. *Brain Dev* 8:25–30, 1986.

Tan XD, Chang H, Qu XW, et al.: PAF increases mucosal permeability in rat intestine via tyrosine phosphorylation of E-cadherin. *Br J Pharmacol* 129: 1522–1529, 2000.

Tarpy SP, Celi BR: Long-term oxygen therapy. *N Engl J Med* 333:710–714, 1995.

Teitel DF, Sidi D, Chin T, et al.: Developmental changes in myocardial contractile reserve in the lamb. *Pediatr Res* 19:948–955, 1985.

The Congenital Diaphragmatic Hernia Study Group: Does extracorporeal membrane oxygenation improve survival in neonates with congenital diaphragmatic hernia? *J Pediatr Surg* 34:720–724, 1999.

Thornburn MJ, Wright ES, Miller CG, Smith-Read E: Exomphalos-macroglossia-gigantism syndrome in Jamaican infants. *Am J Dis Child* 119:316–321, 1970.

Torfs CP, Velie EM, Oechsli FW, et al.: A population based study of gastroschisis: Demographic, pregnancy and lifestyle risk factors. *Teratology* 50:44–53, 1994.

Touloukian RJ: Neonatal necrotizing enterocolitis: An update on etiology, diagnosis, and treatment. *Surg Clin North Am* 56:281, 1976.

Towne BH, Peters G, Chang JHT: The problem of "giant" omphalocele. *J Pediatr Surg* 15:543, 1980.

Tsang RC, Light IJ, Sutherland JM, Kleinman LI: Possible pathogenetic factors in neonatal hypocalcemia of prematurity. The role of gestation, hyperphosphatemia, hypomagnesemia, urinary calcium loss, and parathormone responsiveness. *J Pediatr* 82:423–426, 1973.

Tulassay T, Rascher W, Seyberth HW, et al.: Role of atrial natriuretic peptide in sodium homeostasis in premature infants. *J Pediatr* 109:1023–1027, 1986.

Tullus K, Noack G, Burman L, et al.: Elevated cytokine levels in tracheobronchial aspirate fluids from ventilator treated neonates with bronchopulmonary dysplasia. *Eur J Pediatr* 155:112–116, 1996.

Tunell WP, Puffinbarger NK, Tuggle DW, et al.: Abdominal wall defects in infants: Survival and implications for adult life. *Ann Surg* 221:525–530, 1995.

Tusiewicz K, Bryan AC, Froese AB: Contributions of changing rib cage-diaphragm interactions to the ventilatory depression of halothane anesthesia. *Anesthesiology* 47:327, 1977.

Uauy RD, Fanaroff AA, Korones SB, et al.: Necrotizing enterocolitis in very low birth weight infants: Biodemographic and clinical correlates. *J Pediatr* 119:630, 1991.

Uezono S: Presented at the Joint Meeting of the Society of Pediatric Anesthesia and the Japanese Society of Pediatric Anesthesiologists. San Francisco, October 10, 2003.

Vacanti JP, Crone RK, Murphy JD, et al.: The pulmonary hemodynamic response to perioperative anesthesia in the treatment of high-risk infants with congenital diaphragmatic hernia. *J Pediatr Surg* 19:672, 1984.

Van Meurs KP, Newman KD, Anderson KD, Short BL: Effect of extracorporeal membrane oxygenation on survival of infants with congenital diaphragmatic hernia. *J Pediatr* 117:954, 1990.

Van Meurs KP, Wright LL, Ehrenkranz RA, et al.: Inhaled nitric oxide for premature infants with severe respiratory failure. *N Engl J Med* 353:13–22, 2005.

Vane DW, Abajian JC, Hong AR: Spinal anesthesia for primary repair of gastroschisis: A new and safe technique for selected patients. *J Pediatr Surg* 29:1234, 1994.

Vanpee M, Herin P, Zetterstrom R, Aperia A: Postnatal development of renal function in very low-birth-weight infants. *Acta Paediatr Scand* 77:191–197, 1988.

Vohr BR, Wright LL, Dusick AM, et al.: Neurodevelopmental and functional outcomes of extremely low birth weight infants in the National Institute of Child Health and Human Development Neonatal Research Network, 1993–1994. *Pediatrics* 105:1216–1226, 2000.

Volpe JJ: Brain injury in the premature infant: From pathogenesis to prevention. *Brain Dev* 19:519–534, 1997.

Volpe JJ: Intracranial hemorrhage: Germinal matrix-intraventricular hemorrhage of the premature infant. In *Neurology of the newborn*, 4th ed. Philadelphia, 2001b, WB Saunders, chap 11.

Volpe JJ: Neural tube formation and prosencephalic development. In *Neurology of the newborn*, 4th ed. Philadelphia, 2001a, WB Saunders, chap 1.

Wada K, Jobe Ah, Ikegami M: Tidal volume effects on surfactant treatment responses with the initiation of ventilation in preterm lambs. *J Appl Physiol* 83:1054–1061, 1997.

Walther FJ, Mullett M, Schumacher R, et al.: The American Exosurf Neonatal Study Group I: One-year follow-up of 66 premature infants weighing 500 to 699 grams treated with a single dose of synthetic surfactant or air placebo at birth: Results of a double-blind trial. *J Pediatr* 126:S13–S19, 1995.

Wand H, Tan X, Chang H, et al.: Regulation of platelet-activating factor receptor gene expression in vivo by endotoxin, platelet-activating factor, and endogenous tumour necrosis factor. *Biochem J* 322:603–608, 1997.

Watchko JF, Mayock DE, Standaert TA, Woodrum DE: Postnatal changes in transdiaphragmatic pressure in piglets. *Pediatr Res* 20:658–661, 1986.

Watchko JF, Sieck GC: Respiratory muscle fatigue resistance relates to myosin phenotype and SDH activity during development. *J Appl Physiol* 75: 1341–1347, 1993.

Waugh R, Johnson GG: Current considerations in neonatal anaesthesia. *Can Anaesth Soc J* 31:700, 1984.

Way WL, Costley EC, Way EL: Respiratory sensitivity of the newborn infant to meperidine and morphine. *Clin Pharmacol Ther* 6:454, 1965.

Weber TR, Au-Fliegner M, Downard CD, Fishman SJ: Abdominal wall defects. *Curr Opin Pediatr* 14:491–497, 2002.

Wei JW, Sulakhe PV: Regional and subcellular distribution of beta- and alpha-adrenergic receptors in the myocardium of different species. *Gen Pharm* 10:263–267, 1979.

Welborn LG, Ramirez N, Oh TH, et al.: Postanesthetic apnea and periodic breathing in infants. *Anesthesiology* 65:658, 1986.

Wells LJ: Development of the human diaphragm and pleural sacs. *Contrib Embryol* 35:109, 1954.

Werler MM, Sheehan JE, Mitchell AA: Maternal medication use and risks of gastroschisis and small intestinal atresia. *Am J Epidemiol* 155:26–31, 2002.

Wesselhoeft CW, DeLuca FG: Neonatal septum transversum diaphragmatic defects. *Am J Surg* 147:481, 1984.

Williams RK, McBride WJ, Abajian JC: Combined spinal and epidural anaesthesia for major abdominal surgery in infants. *Can J Anaesth* 44:511–514, 1997.

Winters RW: Maintenance fluid therapy. In Winters RW, editor: *The body fluids in pediatrics.* Boston, 1973, Little, Brown & Co.

Wiriyathian S, Rosenfeld CR, Arant BS Jr, et al.: Urinary arginine vasopressin: Pattern of excretion in the neonatal period. *Pediatr Res* 20:103–108, 1986.

Wohl MEB, Griscom NT, Strieder DJ, et al.: The lung following repair of congenital diaphragmatic hernia. *J Pediatr* 90:405, 1977.

Wu PYK, Hodgman JE: Insensible water loss in preterm infants: Changes with postnatal development and non-ionizing radiant energy. *Pediatrics* 54:704, 1974.

Yang P, Bealy TH, Khoury MJ, et al.: Genetic-epidemiologic study of omphalocele and gastroschisis: Evidence for heterogeneity. *Am J Med Genet* 44:668–675, 1992.

Yaster M: Analgesia and anesthesia in neonates. *J Pediatr* 111:394, 1987.

Yaster M, Buck JR, Dudgeon DL, et al.: Hemodynamic effects of primary closure of omphalocele/gastroschisis in human newborns. *Anesthesiology* 69:84, 1988.

Yoon BH, Romero R, Kim KS, et al.: A systemic fetal inflammatory response and the development of bronchopulmonary dysplasia. *Am J Obstet Gynecol* 181:773–779, 1999.

Zhan W-Z, Watchko JF, Prakash YS, Sieck GC: Isotonic contractile and fatigue properties of developing rat diaphragm muscle. *J Appl Physiol* 84:1260–1268, 1998.

Zweymuller E, Preining O: The insensible water loss of the newborn infant. *Acta Paediatr Scand* suppl:205, 1970.

Zwissler B, Rank N, Jaenicke U, et al.: Selective pulmonary vasodilation by inhaled prostacyclin in a newborn with congenital heart disease and cardiopulmonary bypass. *Anesthesiology* 82:1512, 1995.

17 Anesthesia for Cardiovascular Surgery

Frank H. Kern • Richard J. Ing • William J. Greeley

Creativity, innovation, hard work, and a bit of luck hallmark many of the scientific breakthroughs that have had a major impact on patient care. Nowhere is this more evident than the development of the heart-lung machine and the application of hypothermia for cardiac surgery. In the early 1950s in Minnesota, Bigelow's insights regarding hypothermia, Gibbon's first heart-lung pump, Lillihei's cross-circulation techniques, and Kirklin's refinements of the heart-lung machine and successful application formed the cornerstones for decades of success in cardiac surgery. This period of innovation marked dramatic breakthroughs for pediatric cardiology and surgery.

Stimulated by the earlier development of the Blalock-Taussig (BT) shunt for palliation of cyanotic heart disease and the development of extracorporeal circulation, a whole new era began in the management of congenital heart defects. Today, cardiac surgery has become an effective treatment for children with congenital heart defects. Through a cooperative effort between those in pediatric cardiology and cardiac surgery, significant progress in medical diagnosis and surgical treatment has been achieved. These advances encouraged the development of anesthesiologists with pediatric cardiovascular interests who understood the pathophysiology of congenital heart defects, the surgical procedures, and the required technology. This area of anesthetic expertise is distinguished by broad knowledge requirements in anesthesiology, pediatric medicine, and cardiology, along with an in-depth knowledge of cardiac and pediatric anesthesiology, intensive care medicine, congenital heart disease (CHD), and its surgical treatment. In addition, working with a multidisciplinary team with special interests and skills in managing patients with CHD and their families is fundamental to anesthetic practice. Once viewed primarily as a technical challenge, pediatric cardiac anesthesia has evolved into an exciting and demanding area based on sound physiologic principles and specialized skills.

■ UNIQUE ASPECTS OF PEDIATRIC CARDIAC ANESTHESIA

The process of repairing CHD pushes human physiology to its limits. Nowhere else in medicine are patients exposed to such biologic extremes as during congenital heart surgery.

Patients may be cooled to 15° to 18°C, be acutely hemodiluted to upward of 50% of their extracellular fluid volume, and undergo periods of total circulatory arrest. Managing patients with abnormal blood flow patterns exposed to these physiologic extremes is the challenge facing the anesthesiologist. Knowledge generated from operating rooms, intensive care units, catheterization and echocardiography laboratories, and animal experiments has been invaluable in improving care of these patients.

Clearly, the successful perioperative management of these patients cannot occur without a skilled group of multispecialty physicians, perfusionists, nurses, and respiratory therapists dedicated to the congenital cardiac patient. This team-oriented approach has evolved from an idealized construct to clear guidelines set forth by the American Academy of Pediatrics (AAP) (2002) to establish pediatric cardiovascular centers. Paramount to the AAP guidelines are dedicated facilities, personnel, and patient volume. The basis for these guidelines is provided by studies that have demonstrated a reduced mortality rate with increased hospital and surgical volume. Impact studies have demonstrated that regionalization reduces pediatric cardiac surgical deaths, with evidence-based studies outlining the benefits of referral to larger institutions and studies demonstrating a strong relationship between operator volume and outcomes with adult interventional catheterization procedures (Hannan et al., 1998; Malenka et al., 1999; Smith et al., 2002; Allen et al., 2003). Perhaps the most often quoted study of this group is the New York State review demonstrating that mortality for both high- and low-complexity pediatric cardiovascular procedures is significantly affected by case volume. Sixteen New York hospitals were evaluated. In hospitals performing fewer than 100 congenital cardiac surgeries a year, the mortality rate was 8.3% compared with a mortality rate of 6.0% for hospitals performing more than 100 cases per year. Mortality also correlated with the individual surgeon's annual case volume. Surgeons performing 75 or fewer operations a year had an in-hospital mortality rate of 8.8% versus 6.0% for surgeons with annual volumes of more than 75 operations per year (Hannan et al., 1998).

The increased expectation for better outcomes has been a driving force for the dedication of pediatric cardiac centers and the increasing interest in pediatric cardiac anesthesia support. This has had a dramatic impact on the volume of cases undergoing anesthesia in the operating room, catheterization laboratory, and echocardiography suite. It has become imperative for the anesthesia team to understand the principles underlying the management of patients with CHD and to apply them to the field of clinical anesthesia. This chapter provides an overview of some of the unique features of the pediatric patient, of CHD, and of the surgical procedures; addresses perioperative anesthetic management for procedures requiring cardiopulmonary bypass (CPB); and discusses closed heart procedures and anesthesia for interventional procedures.

DEVELOPMENTAL PHYSIOLOGY

Although many of the principles that govern modern pediatric cardiovascular anesthesia are similar to the principles applied to any pediatric patient, several important differences do exist (Box 17–1). Broadly speaking, certain characteristics of the cardiac system, CHD, and the surgical procedures account for the differences and are reviewed here. These differences result from the maturational effects of the developing heart, differing pathophysiologic conditions in CHD, the diversity of surgical repairs, and the use of specialized CPB techniques, such as deep hypothermia with or without total circulatory arrest.

BOX 17–1 Unique Characteristics of Pediatric Cardiac Anesthesia

Patient

- Normal organ system development and maturational changes of infancy
  - Cardiovascular: blood flow patterns of circulation at birth, myocardial compliance, systemic and pulmonary vasculature, β-adrenergic receptors
  - Pulmonary: respiratory quotient, closing capacity, chest compliance
  - Central nervous system: brain growth, cerebral blood flow, autonomic regulation
  - Renal: glomerular filtration rate, creatinine clearance
  - Hepatic: liver blood flow, microsomal enzyme activity
- Disease–growth interrelationship
  - Effects of systemic disease alter somatic and organ growth
  - Compensatory ability of developing organs for recovery from injury
- Immunologic immaturity of the infant
- Obligatory miniaturization, that is, small patient size and body surface area

Congenital heart disease

- Diverse anatomic defects and physiologic changes
- Altered ventricular remodeling owing to myocardial hypertrophy and ischemia
- Chronic sequelae of congenital cardiac disease

Surgical procedures

- Diversity of operations
- Frequent intracardiac and right ventricular procedures
- Use of deep hypothermia and circulatory arrest during repair
- Trend toward repair in early infancy
- Evolution of surgical techniques to avoid residua and sequelae
- Trend toward wider application of certain operations

Fetal Development

Organogenesis of the cardiovascular system is essentially complete by the sixth to eighth week of fetal life. All subsequent in utero cardiovascular growth and development are determined by flow patterns and intravascular/intracavitary pressures (Rudolph, 1985, 2001). When organogenesis is normal, early fetal flow patterns result in a pressure load on right ventricular ejection. The myocardium responds by developing a predominant right ventricular mass. In late fetal life, pressure differences between the right ventricle (RV) and the left ventricle (LV) are small, and at term the right and left ventricular chambers are of a similar mass. In utero, as well as postnatally, the ventricles undergo a modeling process that depends on pressure and flow characteristics of blood circulating through the heart (Perloff et al., 1982; Rudolph, 1985, 2001) (Fig. 17–1).

When cardiac morphogenesis is abnormal, loading conditions differ and the normal ventricular modeling process is altered (Perloff, 1982). Marked changes occur in ventricular size and function. The fetus is generally protected from the consequences

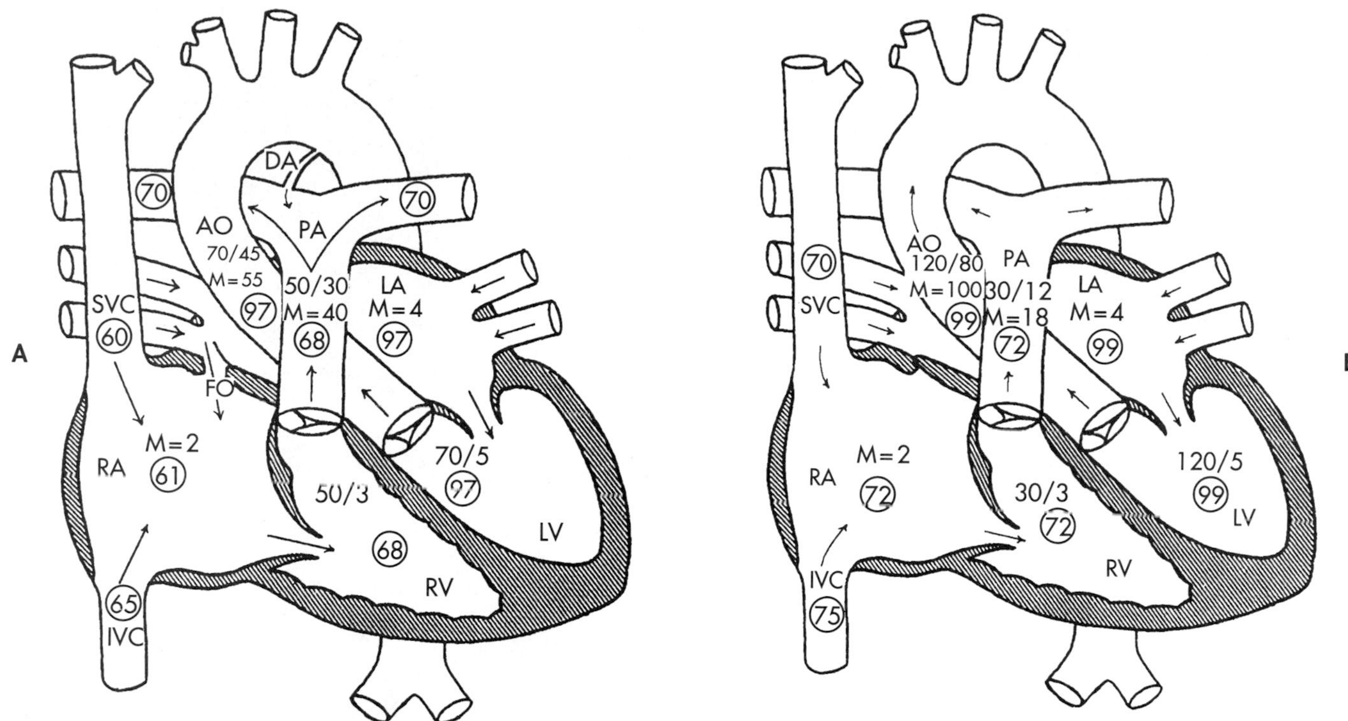

■ **FIGURE 17–1.** Comparison of the pressure and saturation data (circled values) for a normal neonatal *(A)* and adult *(B)* heart. Diagram of a postnatal heart is during transition to normal, mature type of circulation. Note the retrograde cardiac output through the ductus arteriosus and the pressure difference between the right atrium (RA) and left atrium (LA) and the right ventricle (RV) and left ventricle (LV). (Adapted from Rudolph AM: *Congenital diseases of the heart.* 1974, Year Book Medical Publishers, Chicago.)

of these changes because the lungs are not used for gas exchange, and in the parallel fetal circulation, both ventricles are recruited to pump blood to the systemic circulation. Also, the fetus is more adaptive in that ventricular muscle can increase cell number through cellular hyperplasia and cell mass through hypertrophy. Postnatally, separation of the circulations requires the ventricles to act independently or, if single-ventricle physiology exists, to suddenly increase pressure and volume workload by at least twofold, meeting the circulatory requirements of both pulmonary and systemic circulations (Rudolph, 1985, 2001).

Another factor complicating adaptation of the neonatal circulation at birth is the limited ability of the neonatal myocyte to augment its intrinsic contractility (Teital et al., 1991). The reduction in myocardial reserve is a function of the ultrastructure of the neonatal myocardium, β-adrenergic receptor density, and reactive pulmonary vascular physiology.

Immature Myocardium

The ultrastructure of the neonatal myocyte is dominated by organelles necessary for cellular synthetic function, resulting in a 50% reduction in the number of myofibrils and a nonlinear or chaotic arrangement to contractile elements (Legato, 1975). The neonatal myocytes lack a transverse tubular system, possess an immature sarcoplasmic reticulum (SR), and are rounder and more globular than mature myocytes. Intracellular calcium stores are maintained in the SR, a closed intracellular membranous network surrounding the myofibrils. Calcium is released from the SR and initiates cross-bridging between actin and myosin that occurs in a process known as *excitation–contraction coupling*. In the neonatal myocyte, intracellular calcium stores are reduced and the transport process is impaired. The ability of calcium release from the SR to affect actin–myosin binding is further weakened by the greater distance between the SR and the contractile unit of the myocyte (the sarcomere [actin, myosin], and the regulatory proteins [troponin and tropomyosin]) (Becker and Caruso, 1981; Humpherys and Cummings, 1984; Vetter et al., 1986; Nasser et al., 1987). The myocytic intracellular calcium stores are quantitatively less and calcium release is less effective than in a mature myocyte. The neonatal myocyte is more dependent on extracellular calcium and less dependent on intracellular calcium for contraction, making ionized calcium levels an important consideration in the neonate with myocardial dysfunction or complex congenital cardiac disease.

These ultrastructural changes reduce myocardial contractility and contribute to reduced ventricular compliance. In vitro experiments confirm that neonatal myocardium is both less compliant and less capable of stretch, a function of both the relative increase in noncontractile elements and the globular shape of neonatal myocytes (Becker and Caruso, 1981). Furthermore, the reduced myocardial compliance, together with an LV and an RV of equal mass and wall thickness, creates a greater ventricular interdependence so that failure of one ventricle results in shifting of the septum into the other ventricular chamber. The other low-compliance ventricle cannot readily compensate for the geometric changes, and in the neonate, univentricular heart failure rapidly becomes biventricular.

It has widely been accepted that immature myocardial contractile function is relatively poor in the fetus. Many texts and articles have stated over decades that fetal myocardium is unable to increase ventricular stroke volume when an increased myocardial preload is administered (Rudolph, 2001). However, work in fetal lambs demonstrated that at any level of mean arterial pressure, an increase in left atrial pressure *does* increase left ventricular stroke volume (Rudolph, 2001). The Starling curve for neonates is not flat and does not differ significantly from adults. This is more consistent with observed clinical practice and is an important correction of previously accepted dogma on neonatal cardiac physiology. What remains unresolved is whether the performances of the fetal and adult myocardium are comparable (Hawkins et al., 1989).

The neonatal heart appears to be more resistant to ischemia–reperfusion injury than is the normal adult heart. Much of this protection is due to a resistance to calcium influx during and after an ischemic event and to the larger energy stores in immature myocytes. Calcium influx, as discussed earlier, is reduced by the immature SR, thereby reducing calcium entry and subsequent cell injury (Chizzonite and Zak, 1981). In addition, the immature myocardium, by virtue of its growth requirements, has increased glycogen and amino acid stores, which increase cellular anaerobic capacity when nutrient delivery is reduced by ischemia (Hoerter, 1976; Julia et al., 1990, 1991). These factors appear to protect the normal immature myocardium from ischemic injury.

The cyanotic neonate or the neonate who presents in congestive heart failure appears to be less tolerant of ischemia than is the normal neonate (Jarmakani et al., 1978). Experimental evidence suggests that this is most likely due to impaired substrate delivery and marginal myocardial energy reserves (Jarmakani et al., 1978; Julia et al., 1991).

Normal Blood Flow Patterns

The cardiovascular system changes markedly at birth due to dramatic alteration in blood flow patterns (Rudolph, 1985, 2001) (Fig. 17–2). During fetal life, blood flow returning to the heart bypasses the nonventilated, fluid-filled lungs. Blood is then preferentially shunted across the patent foramen ovale (PFO) into the left atrium (LA) or passes from the RV across the patent ductus arteriosus (PDA) to the systemic circulation. At the time of birth, physiologic closure of the PDA and the foramen ovale brings about the normal adult circulatory pattern. The presence of certain congenital heart defects or pulmonary disease can disrupt this normal adaptive process, creating a transitional circulation where right-to-left shunting across the foramen ovale or the PDA persists (Rudolph, 1985, 2001). Under such circumstances, the continued presence of a transitional circulation leads to severe hypoxemia, acidosis, and hemodynamic instability, which are poorly tolerated in the neonate. On the other hand, when initially treating some forms of cyanotic CHD, the prolongation of this transitional circulation is actually beneficial, permitting pulmonary blood flow (PBF) and postnatal viability. An example of the latter is pulmonary atresia, where PBF is supplied via the PDA. Closure of the PDA results in a cessation of PBF with severe hypoxemia and death if ductal flow is not rapidly restored. Ductal patency can be maintained with the administration of prostaglandin E_1. Importantly, the transitional circulation can be manipulated by pharmacologic or mechanical ventilatory techniques to promote hemodynamic stability in the young patient.

Altered Blood Flow Patterns

The combination of low compliance, poor response to exogenously administered catecholamines, and a reduced response to β-adrenergic drugs places the neonate at a distinct disadvantage.

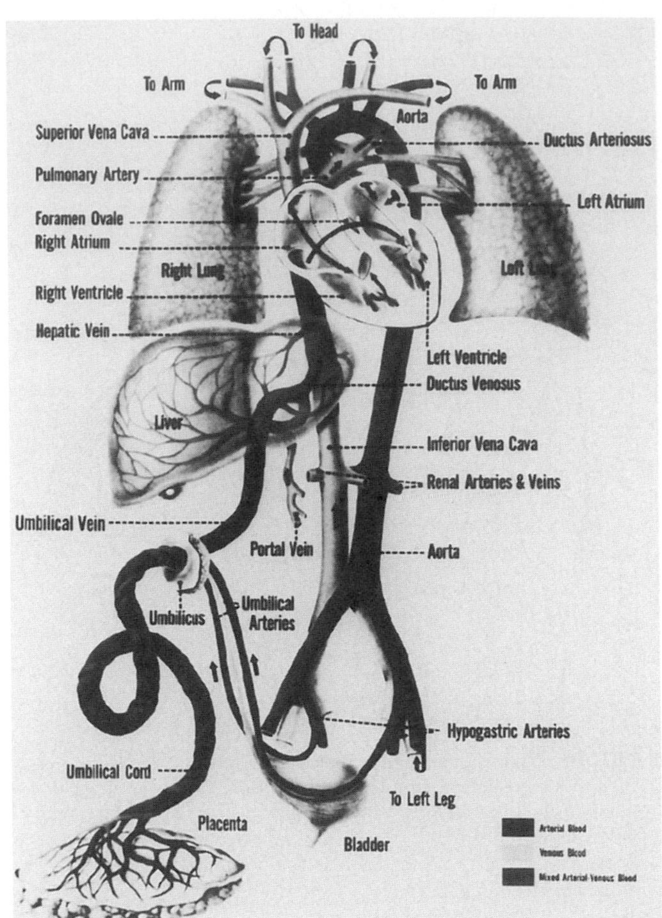

■ **FIGURE 17–2.** Course of the fetal circulation in late gestation. Note the selective blood flow patterns across the patent foramen ovale and the ductus arteriosus.

When combined with the altered circulatory patterns common in CHD, neonates face an increased likelihood of acute and severe heart failure.

Altered blood flow patterns become apparent at birth when the neonate must suddenly alter its loading conditions. Flow patterns change from a parallel circuit to a series circuit where each ventricle must supply flow independently in series to the systemic and pulmonic circulations (Baylen et al., 1977). Early ventricular failure may ensue, or, if the circulatory system can compensate for abnormal flow patterns, a persistent stimulus for further pathologic ventricular modeling occurs in the neonate or infant. An RV or LV with increased muscle mass and increased end-diastolic pressures causing abnormal systolic and diastolic functions is the net result (Jarmakani et al., 1971, 1972). Tetralogy of Fallot is a classic example of how persistent abnormal flow patterns affect cardiac function. Children in whom repair is delayed until 1 year of age demonstrate a propensity toward increased ventricular dysrhythmias in later life and have an increased incidence of late sudden death. This is presumed to be due to chronic cyanosis and hypoxemia in the hypertrophied right ventricular myocardium, resulting in multiple small ischemic areas (Franciosi and Blanc, 1968). When repair is delayed until the age of 3 years, a significant reduction in subsequent ventricular function can also be demonstrated (Borow et al., 1981; Graham, 1982). The sooner that normal flow patterns can be restored, the less stimuli there are for abnormal ventricular remodeling, and normal cardiac function can be preserved. Children with tetralogy of Fallot repaired earlier than 3 months of age have very good long-term outcomes but may have a transient, early postoperative period of greater inotropic support and fluid requirements (van Dongen et al., 2003).

The anesthesiologist needs to understand the impact of blood flow patterns on the neonatal circulatory system, because altered blood flow patterns at the time of surgery may have a negative effect on ventricular function. The extreme example is an arterial switch operation for transposition of the great arteries (TGA) in a child with an "unprepared" LV. Such a child cannot be weaned from CPB due to acute failure of the LV. This LV has insufficient muscle mass to handle systemic afterload because of a prolonged period of pumping against low pulmonary artery (PA) pressures before repair. The presence of an altered myocardial matrix and dysfunctional contractility should be given strong consideration in the perioperative management of the neonate and young child with CHD.

DEVELOPMENTAL PHARMACOLOGY

For many years, intravenous β-adrenergic receptor (βAR) agonist agents have been the mainstay of treatment for the pediatric patient with low cardiac output syndrome. However βAR agonists are less effective during the newborn period compared with their use in older children or adults (Teitel et al., 1985, 1991; Hausdorf et al., 1992). Dobutamine in doses of 6 to 20 mcg/kg per minute results in only a modest increase in load-independent measures of contractility. When propranolol, a β-adrenergic blocker, is administered, a severe reduction in load-independent measures of contractility ensues. In addition, a reduced βAR number and high circulating catecholamines are present in the normal neonate. At rest, neonatal animals have maximal binding of βARs, resulting in a reduced sensitivity to exogenous catecholamine administration.

Advances in molecular biology techniques have lead to improved understanding of the molecular mechanisms by which drugs and hormones work. With knowledge about the signal transmission pathways that influence myocardial contractility, it is clear that the neonatal heart differs significantly from myocardial responses at an older age. These findings have not only explained the less effective inotropic response to βAR agonist agents seen in neonates but also revealed new lines of investigation and the use of novel agents with improved therapeutic efficacy (Teitel et al., 1985; Anderson, 1989).

Although the basic mechanisms that control myocardial contractility appear to be the same in the fetal, neonatal, and adult heart, the maturational process of most myocardial signal transmission pathways is far from complete at birth. Variation in receptor systems with age have been measured at the level of function, quantity of signal transmission proteins within cells, and even differing relative expression of isoforms of the same signaling protein (protein isoforms often possess subtle functional differences) (Table 17–1).

Descriptions of the developmental pharmacology of the heart require knowledge of the signal transmission pathways mediating myocardial contractility. Of the many types of excitable transmembrane proteins found in the sarcolemma of myocytes, the majority belong to the G protein–coupled receptor family (Schwinn et al., 1991, 1994; Brodde et al., 1992). This group of receptors mediates several important signal pathways involved with cardiovascular homeostasis (e.g., adrenergic and muscarinic cholinergic receptor systems). Activated G protein–coupled receptors are linked via guanine nucleotide regulatory proteins (G proteins) to specific membrane effectors, which are responsible for the generation of cytoplasmic second messenger molecules. For example, stimulation of βARs in the myocardium causes activation of a stimulatory G protein (Gs) that in turn activates adenyl cyclase to increase generation of the second messenger cyclic adenosine monophosphate (cAMP). cAMP activates protein kinases in the sarcoplasm, which then phosphorylate target structures (e.g., myosin, ATPase, calcium channels) to cause increased myocardial contractility (Fig. 17–3). A second regulatory feedback process known as *desensitization* is simultaneously initiated with receptor activation in some receptor systems, which with continued receptor stimulation leads to blunted

TABLE 17–1. Comparison of molecular biology of neonatal and adult myocardial signal transmission pathways

Characteristics	Neonate	Adult
Hormone		
Myocardial NE levels	Decreased	Normal
NE release with stress (for example, CPB)	Increased	Normal
Receptor number		
βAR	Decreased	Normal
Angiotensin II	Increased	Normal
Second messenger		
cAMP (βAR stimulation)	Normal	Normal
Desensitization to catecholamines	No	Yes
Contractile elements		
Troponin I	80% Troponin Is isoform (TnIs) 20% Troponin Ic isoform (TnIc)	100% Troponin Ic isoform (TnIc)

NE, Norepinephrine; *CPB,* cardiopulmonary bypass; *βAR,* β-adrenergic receptor; *TnIs,* troponin Is slow skeletal muscle fiber isoform; *TnIc,* troponin I cardiac muscle fiber isoform.

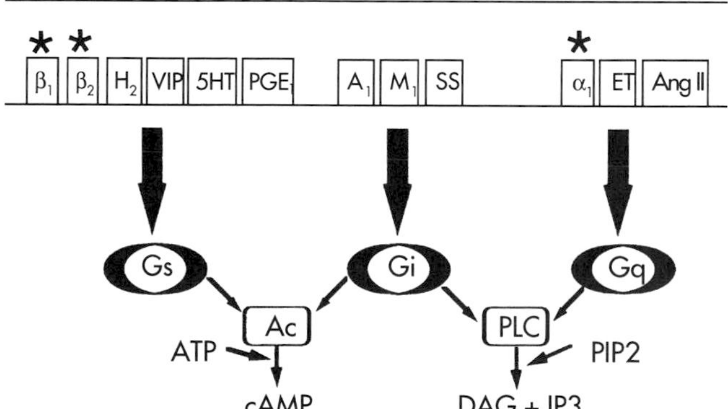

FIGURE 17–3. Schematic diagram of the 12-surface G protein–coupled receptors, β_1 and β_2, histamine 2 (H_2), vasoactive intestinal peptide (VIP), 5-hydroxytryptophan (5HT), and prostaglandin E_1 (PGE_1). All activate the Gs (or G stimulatory) protein and increase cAMP through stimulation of adenylyl cyclase, A1, M_1, and somatostatin (SS). All activate the Gi (or G inhibitory) protein, which inhibits adenylyl cyclase, reducing cytosolic levels of cAMP. The A_1, endothelin (ET), and angiotensin II (Ang II) receptors activate the Gq protein, which activates the second messenger phospholipase C and hydrolyses membrane lipids to produce diacylglycerol (DAG) and inositol triphosphate (IP3). IP3 and DAG activate protein kinases and mobilize calcium in a similar fashion as cAMP.

responsiveness and a decrease in receptor number (Schwinn et al., 1991; Schwinn, 1994). Prolonged βAR activation results in diminished cAMP generation for a given stimulus (uncoupling) and ultimately disappearance of receptors from the cell surface (sequestration and downregulation).

α_1ARs are present in human myocardium, where their stimulation has a more modest inotropic effect compared with βARs. α_1ARs are linked via Gq proteins and result in the hydrolysis of membrane phospholipids, resulting in diacylglycerol (DAG) and inositol triphosphate (IP3). IP3 and DAG activate protein kinases and mobilize calcium in a similar fashion as cAMP, resulting in a positive inotropic effect. The sarcolemma then becomes an important site of signal convergence for myocardial contractility, because several different receptor systems influence the generation of each "inotropic" second messenger at this site (Fig. 17–4).

Although βAR agonist agents mediate the most potent inotropic effect in adults (Brodde et al., 1992), they have not been as thoroughly investigated in the neonate. Because myocardial receptor systems that mediate contractility mature at different rates, it is possible that a more potent combination of receptor system and cardiotonic agents may be necessary for the treatment of low cardiac output in the neonate. For example, there are 12 known membrane receptors located on myocytes that possess inotropic properties. Current therapeutic approaches use only the βAR membrane receptor pharmacologically to augment inotropy.

In addition to membrane receptors, phosphodiesterase III inhibitors such as milrinone, enoximone, and amrinone appear to have impressive effects in some neonates who are refractory to high doses of βAR agonist agents (Hausdorf et al., 1992). These drugs improve myocardial inotropy via a mechanism that differs from β-adrenergic agonists. Phosphodiesterase III inhibitors decrease the rate of cAMP breakdown by inhibiting the action of the enzyme phosphodiesterase in the cytoplasm of the myocyte. By augmenting the length of action of cAMP, contractility is enhanced. Phosphodiesterase inhibitors have inotropic potential by augmenting the efficacy of endogenous catecholamines, and when used in conjunction with β-adrenergic agents, improved contractility should be anticipated (Hausdorf et al., 1992). Milrinone lactate (1,6-dihydro-2-methyl-6-oxo-[3,4′-bipyridine]-5-carbonitrile lactate) is a bipyridine inotrope/vasodilator.

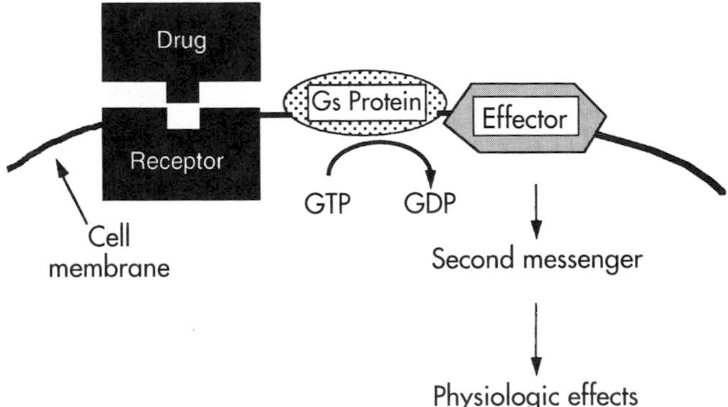

FIGURE 17–4. Schematic of G protein–coupled receptor. Drug binding to membrane receptors activates guanine nucleotide regulatory proteins, which activate a cytoplasmic second messenger through a specific membrane effector. An example is the Gs (G stimulatory protein), which in the presence of GTP activates adenylyl cyclase, a membrane effector molecule that generates cAMP. cAMP activates protein kinases and increases the intracellular calcium concentration necessary for excitation–contraction coupling.

TABLE 17–2. Inotropic potency of myocardial membrane G protein–coupled receptors

Receptor	Percent Inotropic Effect	Tissue Sample
$\beta_1 + \beta_2$	100	LV, RV
H_2	30–40	LV, RV
5-HT	50–60	RA
VIP	40	RV
α_1	10–15	LV
Angiotensin II	30–50	RA
ET	34	RA

5-HT, 5-Hydroxytryptamine; VIP, vasoactive intestinal peptide; ET, endothelin.

Milrinone selectively inhibits peak III cAMP phosphodiesterase and increases circulating cGMP, which facilitates vasodilation in the systemic and pulmonary bed. Peak III cAMP phosphodiesterase is the predominant isoform in cardiac and vascular smooth muscle. Inhibition of this enzyme results in increased cAMP, producing an increase in intracellular ionized calcium in cardiac muscle cells and relaxation of vascular smooth muscle. The effects of milrinone include increased myocardial lusitropy (energy-dependent relaxation), cAMP-mediated sarcolemmal calcium influx, inotropy, and cGMP-mediated smooth muscle vasodilation. Milrinone enhances cardiac contractility and cardiac relaxation and provides systemic and pulmonary afterload reduction.

In addition to conventional inotropic agents, clinical trials have demonstrated the inotropic potential of agents such as thyroxin, which works via several noncatecholamine mechanisms to augment contractility (Portman et al., 2000). The role of adrenal steroid depletion, particularly in stressed neonates, can be a factor in myocardial and vascular insensitivity to exogenously administered catecholamines. Although steroid depletion is uncommon, a brief trial of steroids pending the results of a cortisol level should be considered in neonates refractory to inotropes (Ng et al., 2001).

Still more theoretical is the potential of other receptor systems as angiotensin II receptors, which have only 30% to 50% of the inotropic potency of βARs in adult myocardium (Brodde et al., 1992) but are expressed at a 10-fold higher level than in the adult myocardium (Urata et al., 1989) (Table 17–2). Alternative approaches to inotropic support have been limited by drugs that are nonselective and therefore have additional untoward systemic effects. However, the recent interest in drugs such as vasopressin for cardiovascular support continues to raise interest as alternative options for patients with CHD (Mann et al., 2002).

CONGENITAL HEART DISEASE

The marked spectrum of intracardiac shunts, valve stenosis, disrupted great artery connections and the absence of cardiac chambers complicates a uniform anesthetic approach to patients with CHD. Moreover, there are myocardial changes resulting from the hemodynamic stress and increased cardiac work incurred by these defects. Functionally, these myocardial changes place the ventricles at great risk for the development of intraoperative ischemia and failure. An understanding of the isolated defect, associated myocardial changes, and hemodynamic consequences is fundamental to planning an appropriate anesthetic (Becker and Caruso, 1981). Too often, because of the complexity and diversity of the defects, the attentions of the anesthesiologist,

■ **TABLE 17–3.** Frequency of major cardiac lesions in first year of life among 2251 infants with heart disease

Diagnosis	Frequency (%)
Ventricular septal defect	16.6
D-Transposition of great arteries	10.5
Tetralogy of Fallot	9.4
Coarctation of aorta	8.0
Hypoplastic left ventricle	7.9
Patent ductus arteriosus	6.5
Endocardial cushion defect	5.3
Heterotaxias (dextro, meso-, levo-, asplenia)	4.2
Pulmonary stenosis	3.5
Pulmonary atresia	3.3
Atrial septal defect	3.1
Total anomalous pulmonary venous return	2.8
Tricuspid atresia	2.7
Single ventricle	2.6
Aortic stenosis	2.0
Double-outlet right ventricle	1.6
Truncus arteriosus	1.5

Modified from Flyer DC: *Pediatrics* 65(Suppl):377, 1980. Reproduced by permission of *Pediatrics* © 1980. Copyright © 1980 by AAP.

cardiologist, and surgeon are on the specific anatomic defect and the physiologic changes are ignored. It is imperative for the anesthesiologist not only to understand the anatomy but also to understand its hemodynamic and functional consequences on the cardiovascular system. Although an isolated heart defect may be identified, the entire cardiopulmonary system is usually affected.

Data compiled in the report of the New England Regional Infant Cardiac Program (Fyler, 1980) concerning the frequency of major cardiac lesions seen in the first year of life are given (Table 17–3). The first four lesions comprise almost 50% of all defects, whereas the first eight comprise almost 70%. Extracardiac anomalies are found in one fourth of patients with CHD. The frequency of extracardiac anomalies in infants with symptomatic cardiac disease is presented (Table 17–4).

PHYSIOLOGIC APPROACH TO CONGENITAL HEART DISEASE

The structural alterations seen in CHD comprise an encyclopedic list of malformations and prevent the development of a single,

■ **TABLE 17–4.** Frequency of extracardiac anomalies in symptomatic cardiac disease according to afflicted system

System	No.	%*
Musculoskeletal	137	8.8
Specific syndromes	132	8.5
Central nervous	107	6.9
Renal-urinary	83	5.3
Gastrointestinal	65	4.2
Respiratory	58	3.8
Endocrine	21	1.3
Immune-hematologic	10	<1
Reproductive	2	<1
Other	45	2.9

*Percent of total number of 1566 infants with cardiac abnormalities.
From Greenwood RD, Rosenthal A, Parisi L, et al. *Pediatrics* 55:485, 1975. Reproduced by permission of *Pediatrics* © 1975. Copyright © 1975 by the AAP.

■ **TABLE 17–5.** Classification of congenital heart defects

Physiologic Classification	Pulmonary Blood Flow	Comments
Shunts		
Left to right		
VSD	↑	Volume-overloaded ventricle
ASD		Develop CHF
PDA		
AV canal		
Right to left		
Tetralogy of Fallot	↓	Pressure-overloaded ventricle
Pulmonary atresia/VSD		Cyanotic
Eisenmenger's complex		Hypoxemia
Mixing Lesions		
Transposition/VSD	Generally ↓ but variable $\dot{Q}p/\dot{Q}s$	Variable pressure versus volume loaded
Tricuspid atresia		Usually cyanotic
Anomalous venous return		
Univentricular heart		
Obstructive Lesions		
Interrupted aortic arch		Ventricular dysfunction
Critical aortic stenosis		Pressure-overloaded ventricle
Critical pulmonic stenosis		Ductal dependence
Hypoplastic left heart syndrome		
Coarctation of the aorta		
Mitral stenosis		
Regurgitant Lesions		
Ebstein's anomaly		Volume overloaded
Other secondary causes		Develop CHF

ASD, atrial septal defect; AV, atrioventricular; CHF, congestive heart failure; PDA, patent ductus arteriosus; $\dot{Q}p$, pulmonary blood flow; $\dot{Q}s$, systemic blood flow; VSD, ventricular septal defect.

uniform anesthetic plan. A general physiologic classification is listed (Table 17–5). Fortunately, although structurally complex, these defects can be understood in a physiologic framework. Identification and classification on the basis of physiology provide an organized framework for the intraoperative anesthetic management and postoperative care of children with complex congenital cardiac defects. In general, congenital heart lesions fit into one of four categories: shunts, mixing lesions, outflow obstruction, and regurgitant lesions (see Table 17–5). Each lesion has a specific effect on PBF, systemic blood flow and ventricular function, which manifests as cyanosis, congestive heart failure, or problems with PA hypertension.

Shunt Lesions

Shunts are intracardiac connections between chambers or extracardiac connections between the aorta and PA, such as an atrial septal defect (ASD) or PDA. The direction of blood flow through the shunt is dependent on the relative pressures on either side of the shunt and the size of the shunt orifice (Berman, 1985). If the shunt is nonrestrictive and does not impede blood flowing freely in each direction, then the main determinant of blood flow is the resistance of the pulmonary and systemic vascular beds. The effect that a shunt lesion has on the cardiovascular system depends on its size and its direction, either right-to-left or left-to-right. Left-to-right shunts occur when the pulmonary vascular resistance (PVR) is less than the systemic vascular resistance (SVR) and blood flow is preferentially directed toward the lungs, resulting in increased PBF. In patients with large left-to-right shunts and low PVR, PBF can be significantly increased. This results in three pathophysiologic problems: (1) volume overload of the pulmonary circulation, (2) increased cardiac work for the LV that is required to increase stroke volume and heart rate to ensure adequate systemic perfusion, and (3) excessive PBF resulting in progressive elevation in PVR. The demand on the LV for increased cardiac output is limited in the infant, so that a large left-to-right shunt may outstrip the capacity of the left heart to maintain adequate systemic perfusion, and congestive heart failure results. Surgical closure of a hemodynamically significant defect such as a ventricular septal defect (VSD) with a large left-to-right shunt can produce worsening ventricular failure in the early postoperative period due to lack of a "pop off" because the VSD is now closed, requiring the LV and RV to pump blood solely against SVR and PVR, respectively. If the left-to-right shunt is left unrepaired, prolonged exposure to increased PBF results in progressive elevation in PVR. Fixed changes in pulmonary arterioles may develop, leading to pulmonary vascular obstructive disease. Common left-to-right shunt lesions are listed (see Table 17–5).

Right-to-left shunts occur when pulmonary vascular or outflow tract resistance exceeds SVR, thereby reducing PBF. The systemic circulation receives an admixture of deoxygenated blood via the shunt and results in cyanosis and hypoxemia. Pure right-to-left shunting due to raised PVR is seen in both Eisenmenger's complex and persistent pulmonary hypertension of the newborn. More commonly, PVR is low and a more complex lesion with obstruction to pulmonary outflow, proximal to the pulmonary vasculature, produces right-to-left shunting. Defects such as tetralogy of Fallot or pulmonary atresia with a VSD are classic right-to-left shunts. The shunting occurs through the VSD because of pulmonary outflow obstruction. Cardiac output is generally normal with right-to-left shunting lesions unless hypoxemia is severe and oxygen delivery to tissue is inadequate. There are two pathophysiologic problems: (1) reduced PBF resulting in systemic hypoxemia and cyanosis, and (2) an increased impedance to right ventricular ejection resulting in a pressure-overloaded RV and right ventricular dysfunction.

Mixing Lesions

Mixing lesions comprise the largest group of cyanotic congenital heart defects (see Table 17–5). In these defects, the mixing between the pulmonary and systemic circulation is so complete that the receiving chambers are considered a common chamber. The pulmonary-to-systemic blood flow ratio ($\dot{Q}p/\dot{Q}s$) is independent of shunt size and totally dependent on vascular resistance or outflow obstruction. The pulmonary and systemic circulations tend to be in parallel with one another rather than in series. In patients with no outflow obstruction, flow to the systemic or pulmonary circulation is dependent on the relative vascular resistances of both circuits, as in a univentricular heart or double-outlet RV. If SVR exceeds PVR in these defects, the tendency is toward excessive PBF and left-to-right shunting predominates. These patients have increased PBF, increased cardiac output, and a gradual elevation of PVR over time. If PVR exceeds SVR, as may occur episodically, in ductal-dependent lesions such as hypoplastic left heart syndrome (HLHS), systemic blood flow predominates, and PBF dramatically decreases, worsening hypoxemia (Table 17–6). In patients with a mixing lesion and left ventricular outflow obstruction, PBF may be so excessive that systemic perfusion is impaired.

TABLE 17–6. Ductal dependent lesions

PDA Provides Systemic Flow	PDA Provides Pulmonary Flow
Coarctation of the aorta	Pulmonary atresia
Interrupted aortic arch	Critical pulmonary stenosis
Hypoplastic left heart syndrome	Severe subpulmonic stenosis with VSD
Critical aortic stenosis	Tricuspid atresia with pulmonic stenosis

PDA, patent ductus arteriosus; VSD, ventricular septal defect.

Patients with mixing lesions and right ventricular outflow obstruction such as single ventricle with subpulmonic stenosis, systemic-to-pulmonary flow can vary from balanced flow to significantly decreased PBF and hypoxemia depending on the degree of obstruction. Typical mixing lesions include truncus arteriosus, univentricular heart, total anomalous pulmonary venous return, pulmonary atresia with large VSD, and single atrium.

Obstructive Lesions

Obstructive lesions usually occur across the ventricular outflow tracts and range from mild to severe. Severe lesions present in the newborn period with a pressure-overloaded, diminutive, and profoundly dysfunctional ventricle proximal to the obstruction. These lesions include critical aortic stenosis (AS), critical pulmonary stenosis (PS), coarctation of the aorta, interrupted aortic arch, and HLHS. In the left-sided obstructive defects, systemic perfusion is dependent on blood flow (desaturated) from the RV via the PDA and coronary perfusion is supplied by retrograde flow from the descending aorta. In right-sided obstructive lesions, PBF is supplied from the aorta via the PDA and right ventricular function is impaired. Pathophysiologic problems in left heart obstructive lesions include (1) profound left ventricular failure, (2) impaired coronary perfusion and ventricular ectopy, (3) hypotension, (4) PDA-dependent systemic circulation, and (5) systemic hypoxemia. The pathophysiologic problems of right heart obstructive lesions include (1) right ventricular dysfunction, (2) decreased PBF, (3) systemic hypoxemia, and (4) PDA-dependent PBF. Milder forms of outflow obstruction remain clinically asymptomatic for many years, such as with mild to moderate AS or PS, or asymptomatic coarctation of the aorta.

Regurgitant Lesions

Regurgitant lesions are uncommon as primary congenital defects. Ebstein's malformation of the tricuspid valve is the only pure regurgitant defect presenting in the newborn period. However, regurgitant lesions are frequently associated with an abnormality of valve structure, such as incomplete or partial atrioventricular canal defect, truncus arteriosus, or tetralogy of Fallot with an absent pulmonary valve. The pathophysiology of regurgitant lesions are (1) volume-overloaded circulation and (2) progression toward ventricular dilation and failure.

When considering the incidence of all of the congenital heart defects, three uncomplicated left-to-right shunts (VSD, ASD, and PDA) and two obstructive lesions (PS and coarctation) comprise 60% of all congenital cardiac defects. Mixing lesions, complicated obstructive defects, and right-to-left shunting lesions account for the vast majority of the remaining 40%. Interestingly, it is the latter group of defects that are more difficult to manage, are more labor intensive, and have a significantly higher morbidity and mortality rate. This observation is directly attributed to the complexity of the cardiovascular abnormalities seen in this group of patients where there is usually an absence of a chamber or a major ventricle–artery connection.

PHYSIOLOGIC CONSEQUENCES OF CONGENITAL HEART DISEASE

The chronic effects of CHD are a consequence of the imposed hemodynamic stress of the defect or the residua and sequelae after cardiac repair or palliation. These effects continue to alter normal growth and development of the cardiovascular system as well as of other organ systems throughout life (Graham, 1982).

Because complete surgical cures are rarely achieved and some repairs are palliative rather than corrective, abnormalities before and after repair produce long-term effects that affect the care of patients with CHD (Stark, 1989). Although the overall outlook for these patients is good in most instances, every defect has associated myocardial changes and every repair leaves certain obligatory abnormalities. The effects of altered myocardial loading conditions after cardiac surgery early in life require close follow-up. For example, after cardiac surgery for critical AS in infancy, subsequent operative or catheterization procedures often become necessary due to residual AS or insufficiency. Intervention limits volume and pressure overload and subsequent myocardial damage later in life (Brown et al., 2003).

Although many of the abnormalities are trivial and have no major import, others affect major organ system processes such as ventricular function, central nervous system growth, the conduction system of the heart, and PBF. Under these circumstances, the long-term quality of life is affected. Whether anesthetizing these patients for their primary cardiac repair or for noncardiac surgery, these chronic changes should be ascertained and be reflected in the anesthetic plan.

The myocardium is continually remodeled by specific hemodynamic stresses throughout life. Right ventricular growth and development are influenced by the low-resistance afterload of the pulmonary circulation. The LV is coupled to the high-resistance systemic circulation, which accelerates its rate of growth and development. This situation gives rise to the adult heart where left ventricular dominance of myocardial muscle mass occurs. This entire developmental process is referred to as *dynamic ventricular modeling* (Becker and Caruso, 1981). Abnormal hemodynamic loading conditions associated with CHD interrupt the normal ventricular modeling process (Perloff, 1982).

Abnormalities of ventricular performance at rest and with exercise can be detected in patients with chronic hemodynamic overload and complex cyanotic lesions. These abnormalities in ventricular function are the consequences of chronic ventricular pressure and/or volume overload, repeated episodes of myocardial ischemia, and residua or sequelae of surgical treatment (e.g., ventriculotomy, altered coronary artery supply, inadequate myocardial protection) (Graham, 1982). The modified Fontan procedure, for example, has a 40% increase in hydraulic power cost to move blood through the heart compared with the normal two-ventricle circulation. Power is the rate at which work is done. So although Fontan physiology is a significant improvement over shunt physiology, it still requires a 40% increase in myocardial work attributable to the lack of a pulmonary ventricle (Senzaki et al., 2002). The physiologic adaptive responses to chronic hypoxemia and ventricular pressure or volume overload are the primary stimuli producing the long-term ventricular dysfunction. For example, chronic volume overload of the LV as seen with left-to-right shunts or a chronic pressure-loaded LV due to left-sided obstructive lesions results in congestive heart failure. Chronic right ventricular volume overload as seen in pulmonic insufficiency after tetralogy of Fallot repair or a pressure-loaded RV such as with residual PS is also associated with chronic ventricular dysfunction and failure (Engle and Perloff, 1983). The mechanism for the dysfunction and failure in pressure-loaded ventricles is probably related to the development of myocardial hypertrophy as an adaptive response to chronic hemodynamic overload. The resultant myocardial hypertrophy outgrows vascular supply and results in ischemia and fibroblast proliferation. Permanent changes in myocardial structure and function are the end result. In patients with volume-overloaded ventricles, the heart contraction is inefficient due to extended sarcomere length and impaired actin–myosin cross-bridging.

In patients with cyanotic conditions, the long-term compensation for chronic cyanosis shows a major redistribution of organ perfusion with selected blood flow to the heart, brain, lung, and kidney and decreased flow to the splanchnic circulation, skin, muscle, and bone. Chronic cyanosis is associated with increased work of breathing in an attempt to increase oxygen uptake and delivery. The most dramatic complications are the decreased rate of somatic growth, increased metabolic rate, and increased hemoglobin concentration seen in cyanotic children with unrepaired defects.

Airway concerns are a major issue for children with congenital heart lesions. Airway pathology related to heart disorders fall into two broad categories: (1) disorders related to anomalous relationships between vascular structures and the tracheobronchial tree (e.g., vascular rings); this is discussed further in Anesthesia for Closed Heart Operations; and (2) disorders related to enlarged cardiac structures (e.g., dilated PAs, enlarged LA, ventricular dilation, and hypertrophy) (Kussman et al., 2004). Enlarged cardiac structures can result from increased left-to-right shunting, left atrial enlargement, right and left ventricular hypertrophy or dilation, and dilated PAs. The proximity of the PAs to the bronchi and the relationship of the LA to the distal trachea are shown (Fig. 17–5). Increases in left-to-right shunting can dilate PAs and result in airway compression at a number of sites: (1) PA enlargement can cause the aorta to compress the left lateral trachea. (2) PA dilation can cause compression of the left main bronchus at the origin of the upper lobe bronchus and at the junction of the right intermediate and right middle lobe bronchi. (3) Left atrial enlargement can affect the distal trachea and main stem bronchus. (4) Ventriculomegaly can compress the left main bronchus.

Symptoms of airway involvement include wheezing, stridor (expiratory or both inspiratory and expiratory), respiratory distress, and apnea. Incomplete obstruction can result in air trapping, atelectasis, pneumonia, and aspiration. Prolonged airway compression can cause tracheomalacia and/or bronchomalacia.

PREOPERATIVE EVALUATION

The anesthesiologist who cares for children with CHD is presented with a broad spectrum of anatomic and physiologic abnormalities. Patients range from young, healthy, asymptomatic children undergoing closure of a small ASD to the newborn infant with HLHS requiring aggressive perioperative hemodynamic and ventilatory support. Intertwined with the medical

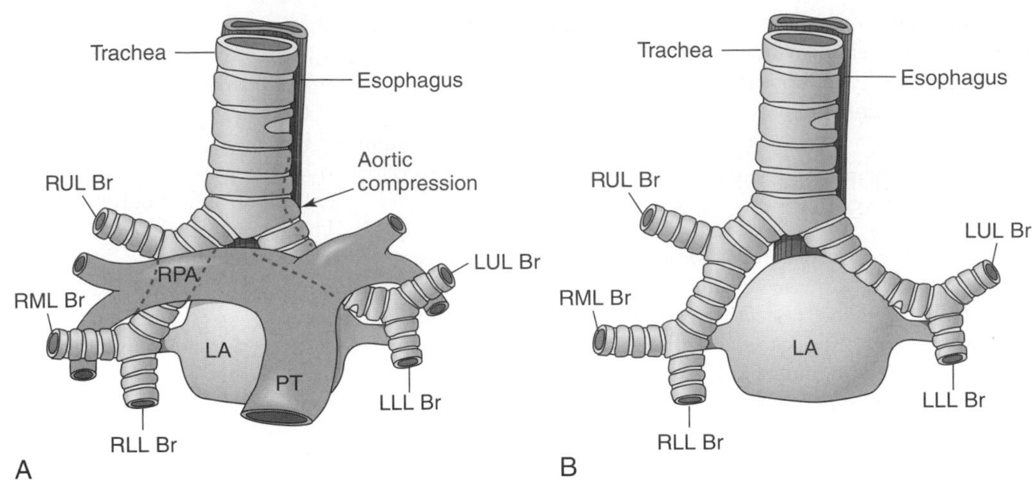

■ **FIGURE 17–5.** Relationship of the pulmonary arteries to the tracheobronchial tree. (Reproduced with permission from Berlinger et al.: Tracheobronchial compression in acyanotic congenital heart disease. *Ann Otol Rhinol Laryngol* 92:387–390, 1983.) (RUL, right upper lobe; LUL, left upper lobe; LLL, left lower lobe; PT, pulmonary trunk; LA, left atrium; RLL, right lower lobe; RML, right middle lobe; RPA, right pulmonary artery.)

diversity of these patients are the psychological issues of both the patient and the parents. Preparation of the patient and the family is time consuming, but omitting or compromising this aspect of patient care is a major deterrent to a successful outcome and patient/parental satisfaction. Cardiac surgeons, cardiologists, anesthesiologists, intensivists, and nurses must work as a team in preparing the patient and the family for surgery and postoperative recovery. This team-oriented approach also serves as a checkpoint to prevent errors and omissions in preoperative, intraoperative, and postoperative care necessitated by the complexity of cardiac surgery for CHD. The preoperative visit offers the family the opportunity to meet the surgeon and anesthesiologist and to begin preparing the patient and family for surgery.

The preoperative evaluation should always start with a careful history and physical examination. The history should concentrate on the cardiopulmonary system. Parents should be questioned about the general health and activity of their child. Fundamentally, a child's general health and activity reflect his or her cardiorespiratory reserve. Abnormalities may point toward cardiovascular or other organ system dysfunction that may pose anesthetic or surgical risk. Does the child have normal or impaired exercise tolerance? Is he or she gaining weight appropriately or exhibiting signs of failure to thrive on the basis of cardiac cachexia? Does the child exhibit signs of congestive heart failure (diaphoresis, tachypnea, poor feeding, or recurrent respiratory infections)? Is there progressive cyanosis or new onset of cyanotic spells? Any intercurrent illness such as a recent upper respiratory infection (URI) or pneumonia must also be ascertained. This may require delaying surgery, because of the negative impact airway reactivity and elevation of PVR may have on surgical outcome. It is becoming clear that a URI is not an innocuous problem when elective cardiac surgery is planned. A retrospective study of 713 children scheduled for elective cardiac surgery found that 96 had symptoms of a URI preoperatively. It was found that if symptomatic, they had a higher incidence of respiratory and multiple postoperative complications compared with children without a URI (29.2% versus 17.3% and 25% versus 10.3%, respectively; $P < .01$) and a higher incidence of postoperative bacterial infections (5.2% versus 1.0%; $P = .01$). These children with a URI also stay an average of 25 hours longer in the intensive care unit, although total hospital stay may not be prolonged. Parental confirmation of a URI is an important diagnostic indicator (Malviya et al., 2003).

Recurrent pneumonia, as mentioned previously, is a frequent finding in patients with congestive heart failure. In particular, patients with shunt physiology or mixing lesions with excessive PBF and altered lung compliance are at risk for viral and bacterial lung infections. Respiratory syncytial virus (RSV) is a particularly common and poorly tolerated lung infection in these patients.

A good history must delineate previous surgical interventions. The presence of shunts, patches, and conduits has an impact on the selected surgical and anesthetic approach. The presence of a left BT shunt is simply ligated intraoperatively, but accessing a left radial artery for invasive monitoring may be difficult and may not provide accurate or useful information. Current medications, previous anesthetic problems, and family history of anesthetic difficulties are equally important.

In the modern era of echocardiography and cardiac catheterization, physical examination rarely contributes additional information about the underlying cardiac lesion. However, the absence of a previous shunt murmur or the presence of a new murmur suggesting mitral regurgitation could suggest partial occlusion of a shunt or endocarditis, respectively.

It is extremely useful to assess the child's overall clinical condition. For example, an ill-appearing, cachectic child in respiratory distress has limited cardiorespiratory reserve, so the use of excessive premedication or a prolonged inhalational induction could result in significant hemodynamic instability and even cardiac arrest.

Laboratory evaluation should include hemoglobin, hematocrit, and serum electrolyte measurements if the patient is taking diuretics. An elevated hematocrit indicates the chronicity of a relative hypoxemia. Levels above 60% may predispose to capillary sludging and secondary end-organ damage, including stroke (Richardson and Clark, 1976). Harvesting patient blood just before the beginning of the procedure may reduce the need for transfusion after the procedure and provide "fresh whole blood" to treat postoperative coagulopathy in patients with a high preoperative hematocrit.

Echocardiography with Doppler color flow imaging (echo-Doppler) is invaluable, providing a noninvasive means of assessing intracardiac anatomy, blood flow patterns, and estimates of physiologic status (Sahn, 1985). For many cardiac defects, more invasive studies are generally not required if a good echocardiographic assessment is made. Echo-Doppler is especially helpful for defining intracardiac abnormalities. Extracardiac abnormalities, such as PA or vein stenosis, are sometimes more difficult to definitively define by echo-Doppler and may require cardiac catheterization or cardiac computed tomography or magnetic resonance imaging. The ability to accurately interpret anatomy and physiology requires a skilled echocardiographer and again points out the need for a well-integrated and interactive team. As intraoperative transesophageal echocardiography (TEE) is becoming an increasingly relied-on operative technique, the anesthesiologist must understand the anatomy and views offered by TEE and assist in the decisions based on the information available. In adult cardiovascular surgery, trained anesthesiologists have accurately assessed the intraoperative images in at least 95% of intraoperative echo studies after the surgical correction (Bettex et al., 2003). Although the complexity and variety of clinical defects are greater in children, the anesthesiologist needs to be involved in the interpretation, medical management, and additional operative interventions based on intraoperative echocardiogram.

Cardiac catheterization remains the gold standard for assessing anatomy and physiologic function in CHD (Rudolph, 1985, 2001). Important catheterization data for the anesthesiologist include the following:

1. Location, size, and direction of intracardiac shunting ($\dot{Q}p/\dot{Q}s$)
2. Pulmonary and systemic arterial pressures
3. Ventricular and atrial pressures with specific attention to left and right ventricular end-diastolic pressure
4. Oxygen saturation data
5. Intracardiac chamber size
6. Pulmonary vascular resistance
7. Valvular anatomy and function
8. Anatomy, location, and function of previously created shunts
9. Anatomic distortion of systemic or pulmonary arterial vessels, especially as it relates to previously placed shunts
10. Coronary artery anatomy

A careful review of the cardiac catheterization data and an understanding of how this information affects the operative and anesthetic plans are essential. Not all of the medical problems can be evaluated and corrected preoperatively; the surgeon and anesthesiologist must discuss potential management problems and any needs for further evaluation or intervention before operative intervention is considered. Appropriate communication and cooperation between the two physicians maximize patient care and facilitate perioperative clinical management. Typically, most institutions have a regularly scheduled, combined cardiology/cardiac surgery/anesthesiology/intensive care unit meeting to discuss candidates for surgery, during which all of the essential information regarding the previous list is displayed and discussed. Such a meeting is invaluable for learning about particular patients for surgery as well as providing a continuing educational opportunity to understand CHD and its medical, surgical, and interventional treatment options.

Premedication

The goal of premedication is to achieve adequate sedation in a nontraumatic fashion and to maintain respiratory and hemodynamic stability. In children with complex CHD, premedication is advocated. This improves oxygen saturation, diminishes myocardial oxygen consumption, and promotes a more satisfactory induction. Many premedication combinations have been used, including intramuscular opioids and sedatives, rectal barbiturates, a combination of a rectal barbiturate and an intramuscular opioid, or a combination of oral medications, including an opioid, a barbiturate, and/or a benzodiazepine. Rectal barbiturates are effective, but reports of apnea, bradycardia, and respiratory depression in 1% to 2% of patients mandate close observation by skilled personnel (Laishley et al., 1986). Bradycardia and apnea in particular are poorly tolerated in the child with CHD and may result in significant morbidity and mortality. Intramuscular medications cause pain and agitation, which generally result in increased myocardial oxygen consumption and arterial desaturation at the time of injection. Because this usually occurs before arrival into the operating suite and in the presence of the parents, most institutions have abandoned intramuscular injections for children entirely. Oral administration of premedication is effective and is the most widely accepted premedication for children with heart disease. In general, children younger than 6 months do not require a premedication agent. In children between the age of 6 and 9 months, midazolam (0.3 to 0.7 mg/kg) may be administered orally. In older children, 0.5 to 1.0 mg/kg (maximum dose, 20 mg) is effective. A calm, cooperative, sedated child is the usual result. In patients with known paradoxical responses to benzodiazepines, alternative agents such as pentobarbital (2 to 4 mg/kg) may be considered. Barbiturates have greater myocardial depressant effects, and dosages may need to be reduced in selective patients.

INTRAOPERATIVE MANAGEMENT

Operating Room Preparation

Advanced, careful preparation of the operating room is essential. The anesthesia machine must have the capacity to provide air as well as oxygen and nitrous oxide to help balance pulmonary and systemic blood flow. Intravenous tubing must be free from air bubbles to prevent air embolism to the left side of the circulation in patients with open communication, such as an ASD. Resuscitative drugs, labeled and ready for administration, should include calcium gluconate or calcium chloride, sodium bicarbonate, atropine, phenylephrine, lidocaine, and epinephrine. An inotropic infusion, usually dopamine, should be premixed and ready for administration for most cases, and additional infusions are made available if there is a strong suspicion for their need (epinephrine and milrinone). For all pediatric cases, certain anesthetic drugs are made available for use on an emergency basis (succinylcholine and atropine). These drugs are selected because of the potential for airway reactivity, hypotension, and bradycardia during anesthetic induction. In pediatric cardiac anesthesia, many of the patients have high endogenous catecholamines as an adaptive response to their underlying cardiac disease and have limited cardiovascular reserve. Thus, resuscitative drugs should be drawn up prior to anesthetic induction.

For congenital heart surgery, the ability to rapidly alter body temperature for cooling and rewarming is essential. During deep hypothermic CPB patients are cooled to 15° to 18°C. Surface cooling with a heating/cooling water mattress, warm air convection device, and an efficient room cooling/heating system are important in the operative management of these patients. The use of ice packs to the head is generally applied if circulatory arrest is part of the operative plan.

Physiologic Monitoring

The monitoring used for any particular patient should be dependent on the condition of the patient and the type and extent of the surgical procedure. The perioperative monitoring techniques available are listed (Box 17–2). Noninvasive monitoring devices are placed before the induction of anesthesia. In the crying pediatric patient, monitoring devices can be applied immediately after the induction of anesthesia, except for precordial stethoscope and pulse oximetry. Standard monitoring includes a precordial stethoscope five-lead electrocardiographic system, pulse oximetry, an appropriate-sized noninvasive blood pressure cuff, end-tidal CO_2 monitoring, and end-tidal gas monitoring. Additional monitoring includes an indwelling arterial catheter, central venous catheter, temperature probes, and TEE. Foley catheters are used in neonates and infants undergoing hypothermic circulatory arrest or reoperations and may be electively withheld in older children for less complex procedures unless dictated by renal insufficiency, prolonged procedures, significant fluid intake, or surgeon preference.

Continuous monitoring of arterial pressure is possible only through the use of an indwelling intra-arterial catheter. In young children, cannulation of the radial artery with a 22-gauge catheter is preferred. In older children and adolescents, a 20-gauge catheter may be substituted. Care must be taken to ensure that previous or currently planned operative procedures such as a radial artery cutdown, subclavian flap for coarctation repair, or a classic BT shunt do not interfere with the selected site of arterial pressure monitoring. Other sites available for cannulation include the ulnar, femoral, or axillary artery. Cannulation of the posterior tibial or dorsalis pedis artery is not usually performed for complex operative procedures. Peripheral arterial catheters of the distal lower extremities function poorly after CPB and do not reflect central aortic pressure when distal extremity temperature remains low (Stern et al., 1985). Alternatively, in patients with poor arterial access, a radial or an ulnar cutdown should be considered.

Myocardial and cerebral preservation is principally maintained through hypothermia, so the accurate and continuous monitoring of body temperature is crucial. Rectal or urinary and nasopharyngeal temperatures are monitored because they reflect core and brain temperatures, respectively. Monitoring of esophageal temperature is a good reflection of cardiac and thoracic temperatures. Tympanic probes are used successfully in some centers and are a useful reflection of cerebral temperature (Kern et al., 1992). They rarely cause tympanic membrane injury.

Pulse oximetry and capnography provide instantaneous feedback concerning adequacy of ventilation and oxygenation. They are useful in balancing shunt flow and providing data about surgically created shunts and PA bands, especially after the surgical procedure is completed. Peripheral vasoconstriction in patients undergoing deep hypothermia circulatory arrest (DHCA) sometimes renders digital oxygen saturation probes less reliable. Alternative sites such as the ear lobe or the tongue sensor have been used successfully in the newborn to provide a more central measure of oxygen saturation, with less temperature-related variability (Jobes and Nicolson, 1988).

The use of transthoracic (right atrium [RA], LA, or PA) or transvenous PA catheters is determined on an individual basis based on the disease process, surgical procedure, and needs of postoperative monitoring. For example, in neonates with PA hypertension or in children undergoing a Fontan procedure for tricuspid atresia or univentricular heart, these measurements can be especially useful. In the Fontan operation, no ventricle pumps blood to the lungs; adequacy of flow through the pulmonary bed is dependent on maintaining a gradient from the superior vena cava to the common atrium. Failure to maintain this gradient results in no forward flow, low cardiac output, and death. Monitoring of intracardiac common atrial pressure is useful in the intraoperative and postoperative management of these patients. In newborns, infants, and young children, transvenous PA catheters are more difficult to place.

As a general guideline, a transvenous PA catheter may be placed using the internal jugular approach in children weighing more than 7 kg. A 5.0 F PA catheter is used for patients with a body weight of 7 to 25 kg, and a 7.0 F PA catheter for children weighing more than 25 kg. For infants weighing less than 7.0 kg, percutaneous placement of a PA catheter can be performed from the femoral vein. The smaller transvenous catheters are difficult to float to the PA because of the extreme flexibility of the catheter, especially when they warm to body temperature. They therefore may require fluoroscopic guidance to place successfully. The use of intraoperative echo-Doppler has markedly reduced the need for placement of indwelling intracardiac catheters or transvenous PA catheters.

BOX 17–2 **Intraoperative Monitoring**

Cardiopulmonary System

Electrocardiogram
Standard seven-lead system, ST-T wave analysis
Pulse oximetry
Noninvasive blood pressure cuff
Capnograph, inhalational gas monitoring
Respiratory mechanics monitoring (peak inspiratory pressure, mean arterial pressure, peak end-expiratory pressure, tidal volume)
Indwelling arterial catheter
Central venous pressure catheter
Transthoracic pressure monitor
Left or right atrium, pulmonary artery
Transesophageal echocardiography with Doppler color flow imaging
Activated coagulation time monitor, blood gas monitoring, including lactate, pH, hematocrit

Central Nervous System

Peripheral nerve stimulator
Jugular venous bulb saturation
Transcranial Doppler
Processed electroencephalography, bispectral analysis
Near infrared spectroscopy, cerebral oxygenation index

Temperature

Nasopharyngeal, rectal, esophageal, tympanic

Renal Function

Foley catheter

Cardiac Monitoring

Echocardiography. In the late 1980s, echocardiography was introduced. The most promising was echocardiography with Doppler color flow imaging. Several reports from the late 1980s and early 1990s described the usefulness of intraoperative echo-Doppler during congenital heart surgery (Hagler et al., 1988; Ungerleider et al., 1989b; Muhiudeen et al., 1990, 1991). Two-dimensional echocardiography combined with pulsed-wave Doppler ultrasonography and color flow mapping demonstrates detailed morphologic as well as physiologic information in most cases.

The availability of biplane and omniplane TEE probes in smaller sizes has enabled TEE to become the standard modality for intraoperative echocardiography. The increased viewing angles available with these multiplane imaging probes have significantly improved the ability to evaluate the entire heart both before and after the repair. Epicardial echocardiography, which requires direct placement of the probe on the heart by the operative surgeon or cardiologist, is now infrequently used. Issues such as probe-induced arrhythmias, hemodynamic changes, and the risk of infection have always been considerations with this technique (Smallhorn, 2002). Further, the ability to obtain a variety of useful imaging views is limited by the amount of heart exposed and the probe angles available from an epicardial technique. In small neonates or when the surgeon attempts to provide smaller, more cosmetically appealing incisions, the exposed surface area of the heart is quite limited. Epicardial imaging is generally reserved for neonates weighing 2 to 2.5 kg or less or for a child with esophageal anomalies (tracheoesophageal fistula repair). Although monoplane probes are capable of being placed in infants weighing less than 2 kg, the available views remain limited, particularly in the more complex repairs performed in neonates.

With the use of TEE in the operating room, anatomic and physiologic data can be obtained before CPB. Occasionally, the preoperative evaluation may result in a revision of the initial diagnosis or identify an additional defect not previously recognized. This evaluation may refine the anesthetic and operative plans (Ungerleider et al., 1989a; Muhiudeen et al., 1991; Smallhorne, 2002; Bettex et al., 2003). Because of the unrestricted TEE approaches in anesthetized patients, new anatomic findings may be discovered and management plans changed accordingly. Postbypass echo-Doppler evaluation is able to immediately assess the quality of the surgical repair and to assess cardiac function by examining ventricular wall motion and systolic thickening (Ungerleider et al., 1989; Muhiudeen et al., 1992; Smallhorne, 2002; Bettex et al., 2003). This technique can show residual structural defects after bypass, which can be immediately repaired in the same operative setting and prevent the patient from leaving the operating room with significant residual structural defects that later require reoperation (Fig. 17–6). The ability to identify patients with new right and left ventricular contraction abnormalities after bypass, as determined by a change in wall motion or systolic thickening, allows for immediate and more thoughtful pharmacologic interventions when guided by TEE evaluation. Importantly, postbypass ventricular dysfunction and residual structural defects are identified by echo-Doppler assessment; left uncorrected, these are associated with an increased incidence of reoperation and greater morbidity and mortality (Ungerleider et al., 1992). This monitoring tool helps assess surgical outcome and identify operative risk factors.

Surgeons can demonstrate an operative learning curve with a reduced incidence of residual defects with experience. However, even when experienced surgeons perform the procedures, the use of an intraoperative echocardiogram can detect a 3% to 4% incidence of clinically significant residual disease that requires further surgical repair (Ungerleider et al., 1995). Patients leaving the operating room with residual disease have a considerable increase in hospital cost, length of stay, and need for further operative or interventional procedures. Cost and outcome benefits exist if residual anatomic disease is minimized by ensuring the most complete repair possible through the use of intraoperative TEE (Ungerleider et al., 1995).

The TEE probe is usually placed in the esophagus after the induction of anesthesia and intubation, so it is then available for monitoring. In a few centers, a prebypass image is not obtained and probe placement commences after weaning from CPB. The advantages of placing the probe at the beginning of the case are availability of a continuous monitor of cardiac structure and function and ability to monitor function at the time of weaning from CPB (Cyran et al., 1991; Muhiudeen et al., 1992). In addition, pharyngeal or esophageal bleeding is less likely when the probe is placed before heparin administration. Because of its ideal imaging location, biplane and multiplane TEE has been especially helpful in evaluating pulmonary venous return and the integrity of the left atrioventricular valve (AVV) after mitral valvuloplasty, complete AVV repair, and correction of complex CHD (Smallhorne, 2002). With the advent of smaller biplane and omniplane probes, enhanced viewing profiles have been achieved for most newborn infants (2 to 2.5 kg) requiring cardiac surgery (Decoodt et al., 1992). Potential complications of TEE in neonates include failure to insert the TEE probe, descending aorta and airway compression due to relatively large probe size or during probe flexion, accidental extubations particularly in orally intubated patients, and there has been one case of gastric incision described (Stevenson, 1995). In this case, the surgeon mistook the TEE probe for the end of the sternum. Many of the complications described are considered avoidable; with increased experience and more careful monitoring, these events should become increasingly rare (Stevenson, 1995).

The technique for intraoperative echocardiographic analysis in children using an epicardial approach is less commonly applied (Ungerleider et al., 1989a, 1992; Shah et al., 1992; Bengur et al., 1998). This approach requires that a clean, short-focused 5.0- or 7.0-MHz transducer be passed over the anesthesia screen, into a sterile sheath, where it then can be placed on the epicardial surface of the heart. This technique allows probe manipulations to optimally evaluate the major structures and dynamic function of the heart. The disadvantages of this approach include that sufficient operator skill and experience are required for probe manipulations (Ungerleider et al., 1992), views may be limited by the ability to place the probe on only selective regions of the heart, and the plane of the probe may provide off-angle and infrequently viewed cuts through the heart (Mochizuki et al., 1999).

Since the initial reports in the late 1980s, TEE has become a standard intraoperative approach in most major centers. Stevenson (2003) surveyed 70 congenital heart centers in the United States and Canada about their intraoperative use of echocardiography. Sixty-five centers responded, with 100% of them using intraoperative echocardiography (98% via TEE). Seventy-two percent of the centers used echocardiography (TEE) for all cases. The average duration of TEE experience for these centers was 6.1 years, and the majority of the centers relied on pediatric cardiologists trained in TEE to perform and interpret the studies.

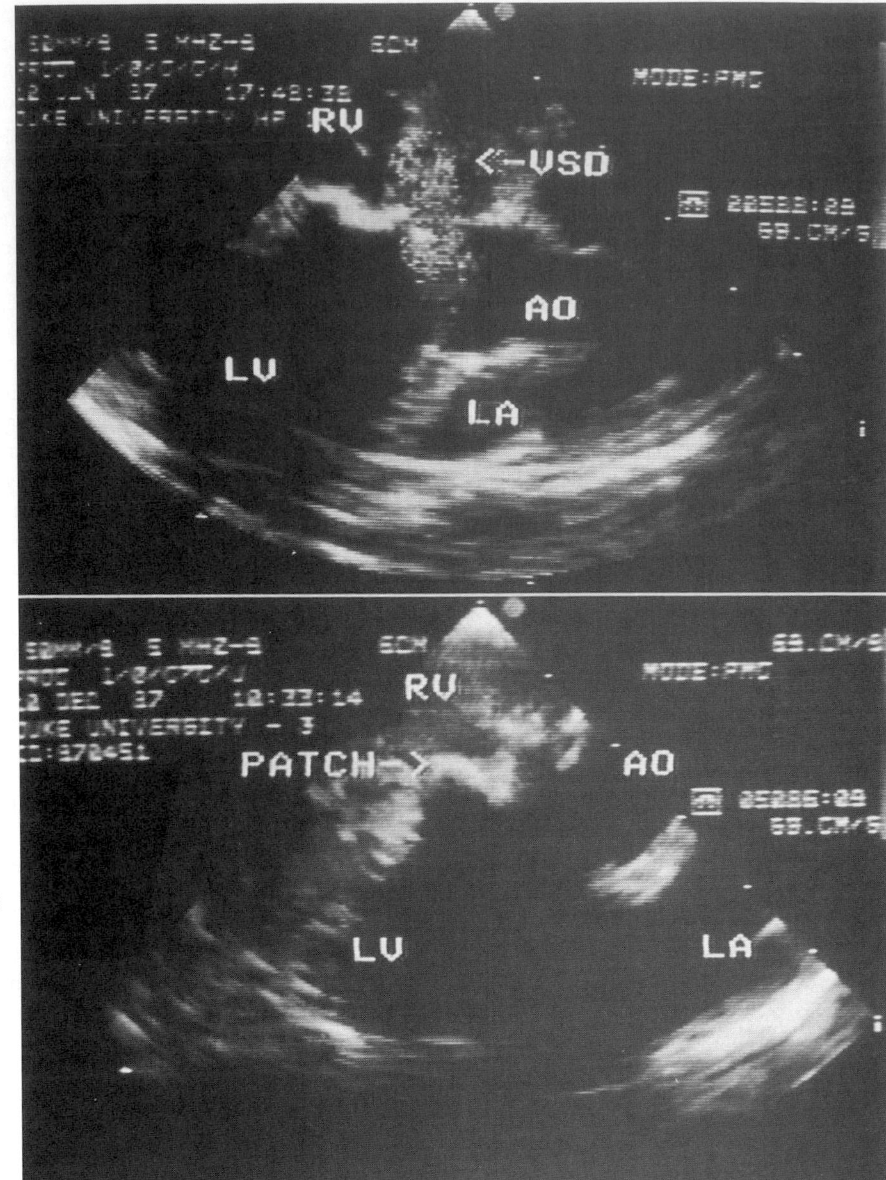

■ **FIGURE 17–6.** *(A)* Echocardiogram with a Doppler flow map in the long-axis view illustrating a residual ventricular septal defect (VSD) resulting from patch dehiscence after initial repair. Turbulent flow through the VSD appears as a mosaic of white particles *(arrow)*. This finding necessitated immediate reinstitution of CPB and rerepair. *(B)* Repeat Doppler flow map in the long-axis view illustrates patch closure *(arrow)* of the VSD after rerepair. Note the absence of turbulent flow with the loss of the mosaic of white. AO, aorta; LA, left atrium; LV, left ventricle; RV, right ventricle.

Central Nervous System Monitoring

The goals of brain monitoring are twofold. The first goal is to improve understanding of the cerebral function and dysfunction during cardiac surgery so that effective brain protection strategies can be developed. The second goal is to provide "online" cerebral monitoring to elucidate correctable cerebral perfusion abnormalities during CPB. Because many of the determinants of normal brain perfusion become externally controlled by the cardiac team during CPB (e.g., flow rate [cardiac output], perfusion pressure, temperature, hematocrit, arterial and venous cannula positions, and $PaCO_2$), knowledge of the effect of these factors on the brain in neonates, infants, and children is essential. Furthermore, examination of the brain under unusual biological circumstances, such as after total circulatory arrest or during continuous-flow CPB at deep hypothermia (15° to 18°C), permits a unique opportunity to describe cerebrovascular physiology and pathophysiology. Processed electroencephalography, transcranial Doppler (TCD), cerebral blood flow (CBF), jugular venous oxygen saturation, near infrared spectroscopy (NIRS), and cerebral metabolism measurements have provided important information during pediatric cardiovascular surgery (Austin et al., 1997).

Electroencephalography. This is helpful in monitoring physiologic function of the central nervous system during deep hypothermic bypass and total circulatory arrest. For example, during deep hypothermia and before total circulatory arrest, the electroencephalogram can identify residual cerebral electrical activity (Hickey and Wessel, 1987). Isoelectric silence can then be induced by further cooling. Because any residual electrical activity during arrest is associated with cerebral metabolism above basal activity, an isoelectric state may minimize ischemic injury to the brain during circulatory arrest. The use of drug-induced electrical silence does not have the same protective effect as hypothermia and may contribute to hemodynamic compromise in patients with postoperative myocardial dysfunction. In addition, the absence of electrical activity, particularly in newborns, does not necessarily correlate with optimal brain cooling. Case reports exist in which premature and near-term asphyxiated newborns have prolonged electrical silence with the eventual return of cortical electrical activity although with minimal neurologic recovery (Ashwal, 1997). Nonetheless, these observations suggest that electroencephalographic monitoring may not be as useful in newborns as has been suggested in adults to ensure optimal cerebral protection from hypothermia.

The electroencephalogram may also be useful in detecting the level and depth of anesthesia. In particular, the bispectral index (BIS), a processed electroencephalogram, has proved to be an effective monitor in older children and adults (Glass et al., 1997; Todd, 1998; Laussen et al., 2001). In newborns and infants, its reliability has been questioned, as processed electroencephalographic monitoring and its associated numerical correlation with anesthesia depth are based on adult electroencephalographic wave forms (Davidson et al., 2001). Evidence from studies in newborns suggests a much poorer correlation with the BIS number and the depth of anesthesia. Stimulus-induced elevations to the BIS occurred at much lower BIS levels in infants than in children during emergence from anesthesia (Davidson et al., 2001). Similarly, children with cerebral palsy and mental retardation demonstrate lower BIS values than matched normal children when awake and at similar levels of inhalational anesthetic (Choudhry et al., 2002).

After CPB, the presence of electroencephalogram-based seizures has been an indicator of significant neurologic injury (Rappaport et al., 1998; Bellinger et al., 1999). A strong correlation between post-CPB seizures and measured reductions in intelligence quotient later in life was demonstrated by the Boston Circulatory Arrest Study Group (Newburger et al., 1993; Rappaport et al., 1998). Possible seizure activity in the postoperative period should be suspected when physiologic parameters such as tachycardia or hypertension are seen. A low threshold for electroencephalographic evaluation or the use of antiepileptic agents as part of postoperative sedation (midazolam) should be strongly considered in the neonatal population. The etiology for post-CPB electroencephalographic seizures remains unclear. However, there is an increased risk with the presence of a VSD, suggesting that left-sided air and air embolism may be factors (Newburger et al., 1993).

Transcranial Doppler. TCD is one of a number of methods used to monitor CBF during pediatric cardiac surgery (Lundar et al., 1987; Hillier et al., 1991). TCD technology uses the Doppler principle to detect shifts in the frequency of reflected signals from blood in the middle cerebral artery to calculate blood flow velocity (Bishop et al., 1986). Because the diameter of this large cerebral artery is relatively constant, flow velocity should approximate CBF. The principal advantages of TCD include that it is noninvasive, it does not require radiation exposure, and it is a continuous monitor. An additional advantage of this technique is the capability of assessing rapid alterations in blood flow velocity due to temperature or perfusion changes, as commonly occur during cardiac surgery. The limitations of TCD monitoring include reproducibility, especially at low flows, where minute movement of the patient's head can dramatically alter signal intensity and alter baseline measurements; and the lack of validating studies of TCD during hypothermic CPB, where temperature, reduced flow rates, and the laminar flow characteristics of nonpulsatile perfusion may limit the accuracy of CBF velocity measurements. Although CBF velocity measurements by TCD have reasonable correlation with more standard measures of CBF during normothermia, there have been few studies examining its validity during hypothermic CPB.

TCD has been used to investigate the effect of CPB and deep hypothermic circulatory arrest (DHCA) on cerebral hemodynamics in children as well as to assess the incidence of cerebral emboli and the presence of flow reductions associated with cannula malplacement or perfusion abnormalities during bypass. Studies using TCD have enabled several investigative groups to provide important information regarding questions of normal and abnormal brain perfusion during cardiac surgery in children. Questions regarding cerebral perfusion pressure, autoregulation, and effect of $Pa{CO_2}$ and temperature have been addressed using TCD in children and are discussed later in Cardiopulmonary Bypass (Lundar et al., 1987; Hillier et al., 1991; Austin et al., 1997).

TCD has also provided qualitative and quantitative information regarding the presence of gaseous emboli in the middle cerebral artery during cardiac surgery (Padayachee et al., 1987; van der Linden et al., 1991). Quantification of this important mechanism of cerebral injury during cardiac surgery would be instructive, because it has been suggested to be a contributor to neurologic injury.

It also has been instructive as a method for determining optimal perfusion techniques. An example is a study in dogs (Cook et al., 2001) that suggested low-flow bypass actually results in a higher degree of gaseous emboli to the brain compared with high-flow bypass. The authors suggest that with higher SVR during low-flow CPB, an increased proportion of emboli is sent to the cerebral circulation. If supported by other studies, low-flow CPB may not be viewed as favorably as a preferred method of CPB management (Cook et al., 2001). Future investigations using TCD should address this mechanism of injury.

CBF studies in which xenon clearance technology was used have improved understanding of cerebrovascular dynamics in young children during CPB, especially during deep hypothermia and after periods of circulatory arrest (Greeley et al., 1988, 1989; Greeley and Ungerleider, 1991; Kern et al., 1991a, 1992b). In general, this investigational tool has been used to describe the effects of CPB, temperature, and various perfusion techniques on CBF and, indirectly, on brain metabolism. Studies in which this methodology was used have shown that some of the mechanisms of CBF autoregulation, such as pressure–flow regulation, are lost with deep hypothermia and that cerebral reperfusion is impaired after a period of total circulatory arrest (Fig. 17–7).

The capability of measuring cerebral metabolic activity during cardiac surgery has been applied both in immature animals and in neonates, infants, and children. Methods for monitoring cerebral metabolic activity include determining the cerebral metabolic rate for oxygen ($CMRO_2$) from CBF measurements, measuring jugular venous bulb saturation, and the use of NIRS. With $CMRO_2$ used as a metabolic index, the effects of temperature and DHCA on brain metabolism have been described (Greeley et al., 1991b). The primary effect of cooling during cardiac surgery is to reduce energy metabolism so that low-flow states and DHCA can be used. Monitoring the efficacy of brain cooling can be performed by measuring $CMRO_2$ or, more simply, by examining the venous oxygen saturation of the brain. The higher the saturation level during cooling, the greater are

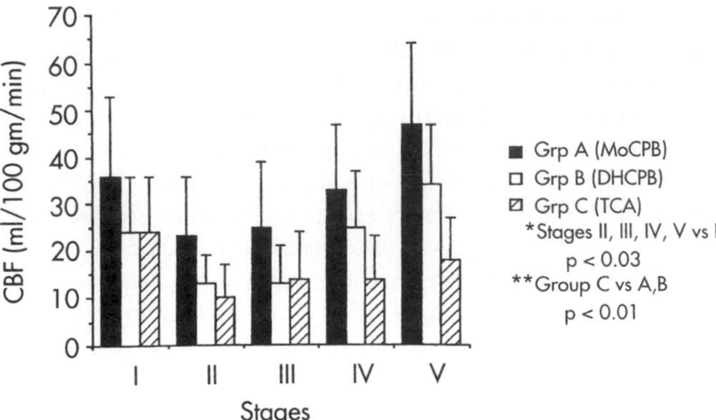

FIGURE 17–7. Bar chart of the changes in cerebral blood flow (CBF) before, during, and after cardiopulmonary bypass (CPB) in 67 infants and children (values are mean ± SD). Group (Frp) A underwent repair with moderate hypothermic CPB (MoCPB) at 28° to 32°C. Group B underwent deep hypothermic bypass (DHCPB) at 18° to 22°C. Group C underwent total circulatory arrest (TCA) at 18°C. Stage I, prebypass; stages II and III, during hypothermic bypass; stage IV, warming on bypass; stage V, after bypass. Note the impaired cerebral reperfusion after TCA (group C). (From Greeley WJ, Ungerleider RM, Smith L, et al.: The effects of deep hypothermic cardiopulmonary bypass and total circulatory arrest on cerebral blood flow in infants and children. *J Thorac Cardiovasc Surg* 97:737–745, 1989a, with permission.)

oxygen metabolic suppression and the protective cooling effects. A catheter can be placed in the right internal jugular vein, advanced retrograde to the venous bulb, and positioned to assess the cerebral venous effluent (Kern et al., 1992a). Using this technique, potential mechanisms for brain injury have been identified and effective protection strategies suggested, ensuring more complete brain cooling.

Near Infrared Spectroscopy. NIRS has the capability of measuring regional brain tissue oxyhemoglobin and cytochrome aa_3, the terminal mitochondrial enzyme in the respiratory chain. With the use of NIRS, intracellular brain tissue oxygen delivery and utilization during CPB have been preliminarily observed (Greeley et al., 1991). After promising animal studies indicating that mixed venous oxygen levels measured from the jugular bulb correlated linearly with cerebral mixed venous saturations measured with the NIRS monitor, commercial devices measuring oxyhemoglobin saturation and desaturation were approved by the U.S. Food and Drug Administration and are clinically available (Abdul-Khaliq et al., 2002). This device has two flexible pediatric disposable probes, which are easily applied to a patient's forehead. An oxyhemoglobin saturation index is measured in both hemispheres of the brain. Marked differences between perfusion to the right or the left side have suggested problems with adequate surgical arterial or venous cannulation placement. In addition, low cerebral oxygen delivery can be inferred by reductions in the measured oxyhemoglobin saturation index levels. Low oxyhemoglobin saturations are identified in patients undergoing hypoplastic left heart surgery during rewarming and after separation from CPB even when hemodynamics and arterial blood gases appear to be adequate. Efforts to increase cardiac output and oxygen-carrying capacity by raising the hematocrit and lowering the SVR generally improve cerebral oxygen saturation.

In addition to operative monitoring, there has been an increased interest in postoperative cerebral monitoring. The advantage of NIRS monitors is that the monitoring probes have longevity; the disposable flexible probes may be left in situ for up to 72 hours. Postoperatively in the intensive care unit, the data displayed may help determine adequate cerebral oxygenation trends. Clinically, NIRS may be used as an adjunctive continuous monitor of cerebral oxygen delivery, which at normothermia has a strong correlation with systemic oxygen delivery as measured by mixed venous saturations. Some congenital cardiac centers have begun to use a noninvasive cerebral oxygen saturation monitor as an adjunct for trends in effective cardiac output and oxygen delivery. The NIRS monitor is particularly useful in managing infants with single-ventricle anatomy after the Norwood procedure with or without the Sano modification in the intensive care unit when optimization of systemic cardiac output is crucial. However, the one disadvantage of the NIRS monitor is that it cannot be calibrated.

Induction and Mainteinance of Anesthesia

The principles of intraoperative management of cardiothoracic surgical procedures are based on an understanding of the pathophysiology of each disease process and a working knowledge of the effects of the various anesthetic and other pharmacologic interventions on the particular patient's condition. Selection of an induction technique is dependent on the degree of cardiac dysfunction, the cardiac defect, and the degree of sedation provided by the premedication. In children with good cardiac reserve, induction techniques can be quite varied as long as induction is careful and well monitored. The execution of induction is more important than the specific anesthetic technique in patients with reasonable cardiac reserve. A wide spectrum of anesthetic induction techniques with a variety of agents has been used safely and successfully; such as sevoflurane, sevoflurane and nitrous oxide, halothane, halothane and nitrous oxide, intravenous or intramuscular ketamine, or intravenous fentanyl, midazolam, propofol, or thiopental (Laishley et al., 1986; Williams et al., 1999; Russell et al., 2001). In patients with more limited cardiac reserve, the choice of induction agent becomes more important. In a prospective double-blind randomized study of inhalational agents in children undergoing congenital heart surgery, the use of halothane was compared with the use of sevoflurane for both induction and maintenance of anesthesia (Russell et al., 2001). Sevoflurane demonstrated a significant hemodynamic benefit compared with halothane. Primary outcome variables included bradycardia, severe hypotension (defined as a 30% decrease in the resting mean), and oxygen desaturation (>20% decrease) for at least 30 seconds. Patients receiving halothane experienced twice as many episodes of hypotension as did those receiving sevoflurane (P = .03) and more common use of therapeutic vasopressors to treat hypotension, particularly in patients with significantly altered cardiac physiology.

The most widely practiced intravenous induction techniques today include intravenous induction with a benzodiazepine such as midazolam and an opioid such as fentanyl or sufentanil. Alternative induction agents include etomidate, ketamine, and propofol. Etomidate provides hemodynamic stability and has been advocated for pediatric patients with limited cardiac reserve (Tobias, 2000). Ketamine is also an effective induction agent in children and has been advocated for patients with tetralogy of Fallot and other cyanotic lesions because it increases SVR, maintains cardiac output, and promotes left-to-right shunting across a VSD or intracardiac shunt. Ketamine can be administered intravenously or intramuscularly. An intramuscular injection, however, may result in pain, agitation, and subsequent arterial desaturation.

Propofol is also an effective induction agent in congenital cardiac patients. It does need to be titrated in patients with limited cardiac reserve because it causes a decrease in mean arterial pressure and SVR. In patients with single-ventricle shunt-dependent physiology, propofol induction and maintenance have been found to cause an increased right-to-left shunt with significantly decreased PBF (Williams et al., 1999). Another concern with propofol has been the association with severe metabolic acidosis after prolonged infusions described in children in the intensive care unit. This is rarely a problem if administered for less than 12 hours, but propofol kinetics are altered in infants recovering from cardiac surgery. An increased volume of distribution and reduced metabolic clearance after surgery cause prolonged elimination (Rigby-Jones et al., 2002).

The application of EMLA cream at the site of intravenous cannula insertion facilitates cannulation and minimizes patient pain and stress. EMLA is commonly applied 60 minutes before intravenous catheter placement when an intravenous induction is believed to be most suitable.

An inhalation induction is generally well tolerated and is the preferred approach in children without intravenous access. It should also be noted that parental presence in the operating room at the induction of anesthesia is an increasingly common practice. The use of inhalation inductions with parents present is easily orchestrated and well tolerated by the patient and observing parent.

Differential anesthetic uptake among patients with cyanotic versus acyanotic defects is common. Patients with reduced PBF have a delay in anesthetic uptake (see Chapter 6, Pharmacology of Pediatric Anesthesia). In extreme cyanosis, sevoflurane, because of its reduced solubility, may not achieve an adequate alveolar concentration to fully induce anesthesia. Halothane, because of its greater solubility, would be more efficacious in extreme cyanosis. In more conventional congenital cardiac patients, inhalation induction with halothane or sevoflurane can easily and safely be performed and the effect of right-to-left shunting on uptake and distribution is not clinically significant.

In patients who are at risk for right-to-left shunting and systemic desaturation, oxygenation is well maintained with a good airway and ventilation, even with halothane-induced hypotension (Greeley et al., 1986). Skilled airway management and effective ventilation are essential and take precedent over drug selection during anesthetic induction. It is essential to understand the complexities of shunts and vascular resistance changes, but airway, ventilation (CO_2), and oxygen effects on the cardiovascular system are of primary importance during the induction of anesthesia.

After anesthetic induction, intravenous access is established or a larger, more appropriate-sized indwelling intravenous catheter is placed. A nondepolarizing muscle relaxant is usually administered, and an intravenous opioid and/or inhalation agent is chosen for maintenance anesthesia. The child is preoxygenated with 100% oxygen, and an endotracheal tube is carefully positioned. Preoxygenation is done even in the ductal-dependent patient with increased PBF; this avoids desaturation during intubation. If the child arrives in the operating room with an endotracheal tube in place, replacement should be considered because inspissated secretions in a tube with a small internal diameter can cause significant obstruction to gas flow. During CPB, when humidified ventilation is discontinued, airway secretions increase and endotracheal tube obstruction can occur. This effect can be minimized by starting with a new endotracheal tube.

Due to the diverse array of congenital heart defects and surgical procedures, an individualized anesthetic management plan is essential. The maintenance of anesthesia in these patients depends on the age and condition of the patient, the nature of the surgical procedure, the anticipated duration of CPB, and the need for postoperative ventilatory support. Choice of a particular anesthetic agent is less important when the appropriate monitors are used and adherence to the physiologic guidelines mentioned earlier are met. More important than the specific anesthetic techniques and drugs is the skilled execution of the anesthetic plan, taking into account patient response to drugs, changes associated with surgical manipulation, and early recognition of intraoperative complications. In patients with complex defects requiring preoperative inotropic and ventilatory support, a carefully controlled induction and maintenance anesthetic with a potent opioid is usually chosen. In patients with a simple ASD or small perimembranous VSD, a potent inhalation agent alone or in combination with moderate opioid dosages is preferred as the principal anesthetic agent. This allows for extubation in the operating room or shortly after arrival in the intensive care unit and a less prolonged period of intensive care monitoring (Kloth and Baum, 2002). The reported changes in blood pressure and heart rate for the inhalation agents in normal children are observed in pediatric cardiac surgical patients as well.

Although sevoflurane, desflurane, halothane, and isoflurane decrease blood pressure in neonates, infants, and children, the vasodilatory properties of isoflurane and sevoflurane may improve overall cardiac output compared with those of halothane (Murray et al., 1986; Russell et al., 2001). Despite improved cardiac reserve with isoflurane and desflurane, the incidence of laryngospasm, coughing, and desaturation during induction of anesthesia limits their use as an induction agent in children with congenital heart defects (Friesen and Lichtor, 1983). Children with complex CHD and limited cardiac reserve require an anesthetic technique that provides hemodynamic stability. Inhalation agents are less well tolerated as a primary anesthetic in patients who have limited cardiac reserve, especially after CPB. Fentanyl and sufentanil are excellent induction and maintenance anesthetics for this group of patients.

Low to moderate doses of these opioids can be supplemented with incremental doses of inhalation anesthetics. The advantage of adding low concentrations of inhalation agents is a shortened period of postoperative mechanical ventilation while maintaining the advantage of intraoperative hemodynamic stability. Clearly, postoperative mechanical ventilation is required when a high-dose opioid technique is used. The hemodynamic effect of fentanyl at a dose of 25 mcg/kg with pancuronium given to infants in the postoperative period after operative repair of a congenital heart defect shows no change in left atrial pressure, PA pressure, PVR, and cardiac index and a small decrease in SVR and mean arterial pressure (Hickey et al., 1985a). Higher doses of fentanyl at 50 at 75 mcg/kg with pancuronium results in a slightly greater fall in arterial pressure and heart rate in infants undergoing repair for complex congenital heart defects (Hickey and Hansen, 1984). Fentanyl has also been shown to block stimulus-induced pulmonary vasoconstriction and contributes to the stability of the pulmonary circulation in neonates after congenital diaphragmatic hernia repair (Hickey et al., 1985a). The use of fentanyl appears to stabilize the pulmonary vascular responsiveness in newborns and young infants with reactive pulmonary vascular beds and to be helpful in weaning from CPB and stabilizing shunt flow.

TABLE 17–7. Sufentanil pharmacokinetics in pediatric cardiovascular patients*

Age Group	$t_{1/2}a$ (min)	$t_{1/2}b$ (min)	Clearance (mL/kg per min)	Vd_{ss} (L/kg)
1–30 days	23 ± 17	737 ± 346	6.7 ± 6.1	4.2 ± 1.0
1–24 mo	16 ± 5	214 ± 41	18.1 ± 2.7	3.1 ± 1.0
2–12 yr	20 ± 6	140 ± 30	16.9 ± 2.2	2.7 ± 0.5
12–18 yr	20 ± 6	209 ± 23	13.1 ± 0.4	2.7 ± 0.5

*All values are mean ± SD.
$t_{1/2}a$, Slow distribution half-life; $t_{1/2}b$, elimination half-life; Vd_{ss}, volume of distribution at steady state.

Sufentanil and pancuronium provide the same cardiovascular stability as fentanyl and pancuronium in pediatric cardiovascular patients. Children receiving a sufentanil induction as a single dose of 5 to 20 mcg have a stable preintubation period (Moore et al., 1985; Greeley et al., 1987a). Intubation and other stimuli such as sternotomy do not produce clinically significant alterations in hemodynamics, although changes are greater than with equipotent doses of fentanyl. Its use as an infusion produces fewer alterations in heart rate and blood pressure, which are particularly important in infants where marked hemodynamic changes are poorly tolerated. For neonates with critical CHD, a sufentanil anesthetic and continued postoperative infusion have been shown to reduce morbidity after cardiac surgery and to be superior to a halothane anesthetic and routine morphine postoperatively (Anand and Hickey, 1992). The blunting of the stress response observed in this study was believed to account for the differences in morbidity. Although high-dose intraoperative opioids followed by postoperative infusion had been the preferred approach in the 1980s and 1990s, evidence suggests no real advantage to high-dose opioids in reducing the stress response compared with moderate-dose opioids. Lower doses facilitate early extubation and limit the need for inotropes in the postoperative period (Gruber et al., 2001).

Alfentanil and remifentanil are short-acting potent opioids that have been used for cardiac surgery in children and show some promise in pediatric anesthesia cases because of their short elimination half-life and hemodynamic stability. A significantly slower heart rate has been observed in children anesthetized with remifentanil compared with fentanyl (Friesen et al., 2003).

As a primary anesthetic in children undergoing CPB, remifentanil and alfentanil must be administered via continuous infusion due to their short half-lives. When the infusion is discontinued, the patient's plasma concentration falls rapidly, particularly with remifentanil, and patients require supplements of longer-acting opioids such as fentanyl or morphine. The use of remifentanil and alfentanil is generally limited to repairs where early extubation in the operating room is planned. Remifentanil is an ultrarapid-acting opioid. Its unique metabolism by plasma and tissue esterases elimination makes it a more predictable drug. CPB can dramatically alter the pharmacokinetic profile of a drug. In adults, Hug and others (1994) have shown that CPB prolonged the elimination half-life of alfentanil and increased its central volume of distribution and volume of distribution at steady state. In a study of children undergoing CPB, Davis and others (1999) noted that for remifentanil, its volume of distribution and elimination half-life were unaffected by CPB.

Because of the widespread use of opioids in pediatric cardiac surgery and the availability of invasive monitoring, the pharmacokinetics and pharmacodynamics of these drugs have been well studied (Davis et al., 1987; Greeley et al., 1987a). In general, the clinical pharmacology of fentanyl and that of sufentanil share the same age-related pharmacokinetic and pharmacodynamic features (Table 17–7). Furthermore, sequential sufentanil anesthetics in neonates with CHD show marked increases in clearance and elimination between the first week and the third or fourth week of life (Greeley et al., 1988). The latter observation is most likely due to maturational changes in hepatic microsomal activity and improved hepatic blood flow from closure of the ductus venosus. The variability in clearance and elimination, coupled with limited cardiovascular reserve in the neonate during the first month of life, makes opioid dosing difficult in this age group. Careful titration of 5 to 10 mcg of fentanyl or 1 to 2 mcg of sufentanil or a continuous infusion technique provides the most reliable method of achieving hemodynamic stability and an accurate dose-response. CPB, different institutional anesthetic practices, and individual patient differences all influence pharmacokinetic and pharmacodynamic disposition of the opioids in ways that are not predictable. Even certain disease states, such as tetralogy of Fallot, alter pharmacokinetic processes (Koren et al., 1986).

An additional consideration is the success with circuit miniaturization and heparin-coated oxygenators and circuits (Darling et al., 1998; Olsson et al., 2000; Ozawa et al., 2000). As the circuit prime volume is reduced, the dilutional effects of bypass become less dramatic, and plasma concentrations of anesthetic drugs should be maintained at a higher level compared with earlier reports. Heparin and biological coatings designed to minimize activation of proinflammatory mediators and endothelial cell damage are applied to oxygenators and tubing. Reducing endothelial cell leakage should stabilize the patient's plasma volume and, by reducing renal and hepatic injury, improve drug clearance (Jensen et al., 2003).

CARDIOPULMONARY BYPASS

PHYSIOLOGIC DIFFERENCES BETWEEN PEDIATRIC AND ADULT PATIENTS

The management of CPB in neonates, infants, and children differs substantially from the adult patient. Pediatric patients are exposed to more severe biological extremes, including deep hypothermia (15° to 20°C), hemodilution (two- to fourfold dilution of circulating blood volume), low perfusion pressures (20 to 30 mm Hg), wide variation in pump flow rates (ranging from highs of 200 mL/kg per minute to total circulatory arrest), and wide ranging blood pH management (e.g., controlled [alpha stat, pH stat] and uncontrolled [post-TCA or post–low-flow CPB, when pH can be extremely and unpredictably low]). These physiologic stresses alter autoregulatory function. In addition to these prominent changes, subtle variations in glucose supplementation, cannula placement, presence of aortopulmonary collaterals, age, and size may impair effective perfusion during CPB.

■ **TABLE 17–8.** Differences between adult and pediatric cardiopulmonary bypass

Parameter	Adult	Pediatric
Hypothermic temperature	Rarely below 25° to 32°C	Commonly 15° to 20°C
Total circulatory arrest	Rarely used	Used but less common
Pump priming dose		
Blood volume dilution	25% to 33%	100% to 200%
Additives		Blood, albumin, FFP
Perfusion pressures	50 to 80 mm Hg	20 to 50 mm Hg
Influence of alpha stat versus pH stat management strategy	Minimal at moderate hypothermia	Marked at deep hypothermia
Measured $PaCO_2$ differences	30 to 45 mm Hg	20 to 80 mm Hg
Glucose regulation		
Hypoglycemia	Rare: requires significant hepatic injury	Common: reduced hepatic glycogen stores
Hyperglycemia	Frequent: generally easily controlled with insulin	Less common: rebound hypoglycemia may occur
Ultrafiltration	Conventional	Modified after CPB separation

Adult patients are rarely, if ever, exposed to these biological extremes. Temperature is rarely lowered below 25°C, hemodilution is more moderate, perfusion pressure is generally maintained at 30 to 80 mm Hg, flow rates are maintained at 50 to 65 mL/kg per minute, and pH management strategy is less influential because moderate hypothermic temperatures are commonly used, whereas deep hypothermia with or without circulatory arrest is rarely used (Table 17–8). Variables, such as glucose requirements and patient size, are more consistent in adults. Venous and arterial cannulas are larger and less deforming of the atria and aorta, and their placement is more predictable. Although superficially similar, the conduct of CPB in children is considerably different from that of adults. One would expect marked physiologic differences in the response to CPB in the child in general and in neonates and young infants in particular.

Clinical Application of Cardiopulmonary Bypass in Children

The CPB circuit must replace the function of both the heart and the lungs during cardiac surgery. Because of the use of nonpulsatile flow and the need for reduced perfusion flow rates to minimize blood return to the heart, hypothermia is required. Specifically, hypothermic CPB is used to preserve organ function during cardiac surgery and to prevent end-organ ischemia through a reduction in cellular metabolism and preservation of high-energy phosphate stores. As temperature is lowered, both basal and functional cellular metabolism is reduced and the rate of adenosine triphosphate (ATP) and phosphocreatine consumption is substantially reduced (Michenfelder and Theye, 1968; Swain et al., 1991). At deep hypothermia, cellular metabolism is so low and membrane fluidity reduced to such an extent that cellular basal metabolic needs and cellular membrane integrity can be maintained for a relatively prolonged period of time with minimal or no flow. Additional benefits include decreased production of putative mediators, a reduction in the rate of calcium influx into the cell due to the decreased fluidity of cellular membranes, and reduced rate of gene activation. These form the basis of the protective effects of deep hypothermia that allow for the implementation of low-flow deep hypothermic CPB and DHCA.

The degree of hypothermia selected is dependent on the need for reduced flow to enhance surgical repair. In general, three distinct methods of CPB are used: moderate hypothermia (25° to 32°C), deep hypothermia (15° to 20°C), or DHCA. The technique selected is based on the required surgical conditions, the patient size, the type of operation, and the potential physiologic impact on the patient.

Moderate hypothermic CPB (MHCPB) is the principal method of bypass used for older children and adolescents. In these patients, venous cannulas are less obtrusive and the heart can easily accommodate superior and inferior venae cavae (SVC and IVC, respectively) cannulation. Bicaval cannulation reduces right atrial blood return and improves the surgeon's ability to visualize intracardiac anatomy. The large cannulas used in older children are rigid and less likely to kink. Most surgeons are willing to cannulate the IVC and SVC in neonates and infants. However, in neonates and infants, this is technically more difficult and likely to induce brief periods of hemodynamic instability. In addition, the pliability of the cava and the rigidity of the cannulas may result in caval obstruction, reduced venous drainage, and elevated venous pressure in the mesenteric and cerebral circulations. When moderate hypothermia is used, perfusion flow rates must be high to meet metabolic demands of the patient. Recommendations for optimal pump flow rates for children are based on the patient's body mass and maintaining efficient organ perfusion as determined by arterial blood gases, acid-base balance, and whole body oxygen consumption during CPB (Fox et al., 1982; Hickey and Andersen, 1987). Table 17–9 lists recommended, albeit arbitrary, normothermic flow rates for children based on body weight. At hypothermic temperatures, metabolism is reduced and therefore pump flow rates may be reduced. A physiologic basis for low-flow CPB based on measurements of cerebral metabolism is presented later in this chapter.

Deep hypothermic CPB is generally reserved for neonates and infants requiring complex cardiac repairs. However, certain older children with complex cardiac disease or severe aortic or mitral valve regurgitation may require deep hypothermic temperatures. For the most part, deep hypothermia is selected to allow the

■ **TABLE 17–9.** Recommended pump flow rates for cardiopulmonary bypass in children

Patient Weight (kg)	Pump Flow Rate (mL/kg per min)
<3	150–200
3–10	125–175
10–15	120–150
15–30	100–120
30–50	75–100
>50	50–75

surgeon to operate under conditions of low-flow CPB or total circulatory arrest. Low-pump flows improve the operating conditions for the surgeon by providing a near bloodless field and generally allow the use of a single atrial cannula, facilitating better visualization of atrial anatomy and operative repairs performed through a right atriotomy.

Deep hypothermic CPB with total circulatory arrest allows the surgeon to remove the atrial and aortic cannula. With this technique, surgical repair is more precise because of the bloodless and cannula-free operative field. Arresting the circulation, even at deep hypothermic temperatures, introduces the question of how well deep hypothermia preserves organ function, with the brain being of greatest concern. Extensive clinical experience using DHCA has suggested the duration of a safe circulatory arrest period to be approximately 30 to 45 minutes, or longer (Kirklin and Barratt-Boyes, 1986; Wypij et al., 2003).

Formal experimental data evaluating the effect of DHCA on organ function are limited; however, organ preservation during the arrest period is primarily a function of hypothermia. Hypothermia preserves organ function by maintaining cellular ATP stores despite reduced delivery, reducing excitatory neurotransmitter release and preventing calcium entry into the cell even though energy-dependent calcium pumps are depleted of ATP stores. Normothermic ischemic injury and hypothermic protection are discussed in more detail in Deep Hypothermic Circulatory Arrest: Protection from Ischemic Injury.

PATHOPHYSIOLOGY OF HYPOTHERMIC CARDIOPULMONARY BYPASS IN CHILDREN

Pathophysiologic changes that occur during and after pediatric CPB relate to the nonendothelialized bypass circuit and oxygenator, hypothermia, the degree of hemodilution, nonpulsatile perfusion, the age of the patient, the preoperative myocardial substrate, the length of the ischemic period on the myocardium (cross-clamp time) or the entire body (low-flow CPB or total circulatory arrest), the type of anesthesia used, and the exaggerated inflammatory response present in the young child. The effects on the patient are both global and organ specific. Global hormonal and metabolic responses have been characterized as the *stress response* to hypothermic CPB.

General Effects of Cardiopulmonary Bypass

The release of a large number of metabolic and hormonal substances, including catecholamines, cortisol, growth hormone, cytokines, prostaglandins, leukotriene complements, glucose, insulin, beta endorphins, and other substances, characterize the stress response during hypothermic CPB (Hindmarsh et al., 1984; Greeley et al., 1986b, 1988). The likely causes for the elaboration of these substances include contact of blood with the nonendothelialized surface of the pump tubing and oxygenator (Bui et al., 1991), nonpulsatile flow, low perfusion pressure, hemodilution, and hypothermia. Other factors that may contribute to elevations of stress hormones include delayed renal and hepatic clearance during hypothermic CPB, myocardial injury, and exclusion of the pulmonary circulation from bypass. The lung is responsible for metabolizing and clearing many of these stress hormones. The stress response generally peaks during rewarming from CPB. There is evidence that the hormonal component of the stress response can be blunted, but not eliminated, by increasing the depth of anesthesia (Anand et al., 1987, 1990). Recent evidence suggests that the stress response in neonates and infants has less of an effect on outcome than was described in the early 1990s (Gruber et al., 2001).

It is unclear at what level elevated circulating stress hormones, normally an adaptive response, become detrimental. There is little question that these substances do mediate undesirable effects such as myocardial damage (catecholamines), systemic and pulmonary hypertension (catecholamines), pulmonary endothelial damage (cytokines, complement, eicosanoids, prostanoids), and pulmonary vascular reactivity (cytokines, prostanoids). The benefits of blunting the release of stress hormones and catecholamines with fentanyl in premature infants undergoing PDA ligation have been observed (Anand et al., 1987). Further, neonates with complex CHD who died in the postoperative period demonstrate much higher hormonal and metabolic responses during the intraoperative and postoperative periods than did survivors with similar cardiac defects (Anand et al., 1987, 1990).

The measured levels of stress hormones and catecholamines in neonates are generally an order of magnitude greater than those measured during CPB in the adult. Although blunting the extremes of the stress hormone response seems warranted, there is additional evidence suggesting that the newborn stress response, especially the endogenous release of catecholamines, may be an adaptive metabolic response necessary for survival at birth (Langercrantz and Slotkin, 1986). This suggests that complete elimination of an adaptive stress response may not be desirable, but modification of its extremes probably is desirable. To what extent acutely ill neonates with CHD are dependent on their stress response for maintaining hemodynamic stability during and after CPB is unknown.

The importance of adaptive versus maladaptive responses is even more relevant today. Earlier data from the late 1980s and early 1990s supported the concept that high-dose opioids blunt the stress hormone release and improve patient outcome (Anand et al., 1987, 1990). This was viewed as a significant advance to CPB management and necessary to preserve end-organ function in neonates and infants exposed to CPB. Reappraisals of the benefits of high-dose opioids to blunt the stress response to bypass for neonates have occurred. Data from Duncan and others (2000) suggest that moderate dosing of opioids (25 to 50 mcg/kg of fentanyl) is equally effective as the formerly recommended high-dose regimen (100 mcg/kg of fentanyl) with regard to blunting the stress response to CPB (Duncan et al., 2000). In another study by Gruber and others (2001), three different anesthetic regimens were evaluated: bolus fentanyl, fentanyl infusions, and a combination of fentanyl plus midazolam. All three regimens demonstrated high levels of stress hormone release. In fact, the magnitude of epinephrine release was 8 to 15 times higher than that reported in the study of Anand and others from a decade earlier. These findings suggest that catecholamines and stress hormones may not be as important as inflammatory mediators such as cytokines and leukotrienes. Despite this marked elevation in stress hormone release, there was no evidence of increased morbidity and mortality, The fact that lower doses of opioids have similar benefits as high-dose opioids in neonates and infants undergoing CPB suggests that the evolution of the heart-lung machine with reduced prime volume and heparin- or biocompatible material–coated oxygenators and circuits, the use of modified ultrafiltration to remove mediators, and improved prebypass and postbypass management strategies are having a positive impact on the outcome of neonates and infants undergoing CPB. The role of stress hormone modification appears less important today as a promotor for the activation of proinflammatory mediators.

Distinguishing maladaptive stress hormone release from adaptive release is the presence of mediators of systemic inflammation and endothelial injury. Complement activation, neutrophil activation, and release and activation of tumor necrosis factor and interleukins 1 and 6 have been well described during hypothermic CPB (Downing and Edmonds, 1992; Butler et al., 1993). These mediators of systemic inflammation, in conjunction with ischemia–reperfusion injury and the direct effects of hypothermia, account for organ injury during and after CPB. The main target of many of these mediators is the vascular endothelium. Endothelial injury results in altered microcirculatory function, which is responsible for elevations in PVR, cerebrovascular resistance (CVR), and SVR, commonly seen after hypothermic CPB. Endothelial injury impairs release of important vasodilators such as nitric oxide (NO) and prostacyclin and enhances the effect of vasoconstrictors such as endothelin (Aaronson et al., 2002). Direct endothelin antagonists such as BQ123 have been shown to reduce PVR after congenital heart surgery. Vascular endothelial damage associated with CPB is a prominent factor in post-CPB lung injury (Schulze-Neick et al., 2002).

In addition to these properties, the endothelial surface, pulmonary endothelium in particular, is responsible for metabolizing vasoconstrictors such as angiotensin, catecholamines, and eicosanoids (Aaronson et al., 2002). Injured endothelium, by virtue of reduced production of NO and impaired metabolism of mediators of vasoconstriction, promotes vasoconstriction. Endothelial cells also play an important regulatory role in water and solute transport. Abnormalities in endothelial function promote increased capillary permeability and increased interstitial edema (Greeley et al., 1988).

Evidence for microcirculatory dysfunction with nonpulsatile perfusion can be found in several studies. Ogata et al. (1960) directly observed that capillary flow in the omentum slowed and virtually ceased during nonpulsatile CPB at normothermia. At flow rates of 60 and 75 mL/kg per minute, nonpulsatile flow resulted in lower total body oxygen consumption, lower pH, and an increased base deficit than with pulsatile perfusion. Matsumato and others (1971) showed that at 37°C, nonpulsatile perfusion produced capillary sludging, dilation of the postcapillary venules, and increased edema formation in the conjunctival and cerebral microcirculation. In contrast, pulsatile CPB maintained capillary blood flow in the omentum, eliminated sludging in the conjunctival and cerebral microcirculation, and reduced jugular venous lactate levels (Matsumato et al., 1971; Geha et al., 1973). Studies of hypothermic low-flow CPB in a canine model demonstrated that converting low-flow nonpulsatile CPB at 25 mL/kg per minute to pulsatile perfusion improved brain pH, P_{CO_2}, and P_{O_2} (Watanabe et al., 1989). Measurements of $CMRO_2$ in neonates, infants, and children demonstrate that nonpulsatile perfusion accounts for a 9% reduction in brain metabolism (Greeley et al., 1991). Pulsatile perfusion may therefore improve cerebral perfusion at both normothermic and hypothermic temperatures. When low-flow CPB is used, the addition of pulsatile flow may provide improved microcirculatory perfusion and allow for better oxygen delivery to tissue at lower flow rates. Mechanistically, a lack of pulsatility alters the biomechanical forces exerted on the endothelium. This results in rather rapid changes in ion conductance, adenylate cyclase activity, and intracellular free calcium levels. These changes are similar to receptor-mediated changes in vascular tone seen with α- and β-receptor activity. If more prolonged exposure to nonpulsatile flow exists, changes in vascular tone may be augmented by release of local regulatory mediators such as endothelin.

Although improvements in microvascular flow and organ metabolism have been suggested with the addition of pulsatile flow, clinical studies have been inconclusive. Murkin and others (1987) observed a 13% improvement in CBF and cerebral oxygen consumption with pulsatile CPB in adults. In children, a small clinical trial of pulsatile CPB demonstrated no improvement in glucose, insulin, and cortisol responses during CPB (Mori et al., 1987). Although trials have been limited, it appears that the benefits of pulsatile perfusion would occur in patients with limited organ reserve or those exposed to more extreme perfusion variables such as low-flow CPB or DHCA. To date, clinical assessment of pulsatile perfusion during low-flow CPB or DHCA, which are more common to the pediatric patient, has not been elucidated fully. Also, the method in which pulsatility is mechanically produced is important. To be effective, the pulse wave must duplicate the mechanics of a normal cardiac cycle. Several pulsatile systems generate wave forms that are significantly different from a physiologic heartbeat.

During high-flow hypothermic CPB, peripheral vascular resistance increases in all vascular beds throughout the body. Flows to the kidneys, gastrointestinal tract, and brain are decreased and flow is preferentially shunted toward skeletal muscle (Lazenby et al., 1981). This is quite different from the intact patient who is not exposed to CPB but instead is surface cooled. These patients demonstrate an increase in peripheral vascular resistance and preferential flow to the brain, heart, and kidneys in response to a decrease in cardiac output. This difference between the hypothermic patient exposed to CPB and the surface-cooled hypothermic patient is dependent on the effects of hypothermia on cardiac output. During hypothermic CPB, when flow rates are maintained by the pump at high perfusion rates (flow rates of 3.0 L/min), blood is shunted away from the vital organs to the skeletal muscle. The vasculature of skeletal muscle serves as a large capacitance bed for excessive flow during high-flow hypothermic CPB. During low-flow hypothermic CPB, skeletal muscle vasculature constricts and total body blood flow is redistributed toward vital organs. Vital organ blood flow is maintained and provides effective oxygen delivery to maintain identical oxygen consumption at both full flow and after a 50% reduction in perfusion flow rates (Lazenby et al., 1981). In patients with aortopulmonary shunts (a common finding in patients with cyanotic heart disease who are undergoing CPB), there is a greater redistribution of blood flow away from the gastrointestinal tract and kidneys (Mavroudis et al., 1984). This excessive shunting may contribute to the higher incidence of end-organ injury observed in infants with large aortopulmonary shunts or aortopulmonary collaterals when exposed to prolonged periods of CPB.

pH Stat and Alpha Stat

The role of CO_2 management in CPB has been studied both experimentally and clinically. Based on the effect of CO_2 on arterial and intracellular pH at hypothermic temperatures, two divergent blood gas management strategies have been championed: alpha stat (temperature uncorrected) and pH stat (temperature corrected) (Norwood et al., 1979; Fox et al., 1984; Govier et al., 1984; Miyamoto et al., 1986; Swain et al., 1991). The concept of alpha stat and pH stat blood gas strategies is based on the effect temperature has on the balance between intracellular OH^- and H^+ ion concentrations. The intracellular balance between OH^- and H^+ concentration, electrochemical neutrality, is essential to maximize enzyme efficiency. At normothermia (37°C), intracellular electrochemical neutrality occurs at pH 7.40. As the temperature of the cell is decreased, however, maintaining electrochemical neutrality requires an increase in the OH^- ion concentration relative to the H^+ ion concentration (alkalosis). When an alkalotic milieu is not maintained during hypothermia, many investigators believed that enzymatic function is altered and intermediary metabolites become uncharged, more lipid-soluble, and freely diffusible across cellular membranes. The net effect would be altered intracellular metabolism. Maintaining an alkaline intracellular pH was believed to enhance cellular function. Swain and colleagues (1990, 1991) performed NMR studies in a piglet model and used sophisticated probes to assess intracellular pH differences between alpha stat and pH stat models. They found that the intracellular pH was in fact not dramatically different between the two blood gas management strategies. This finding put the alpha stat/pH stat issue of optimal management strategy into question. The blood gas management strategy that maintains an alkaline pH is the alpha stat strategy. The alpha stat strategy is implemented by maintaining pH 7.40 measured at 37°C without correction for the effects of temperature. This strategy allows the pH of the blood and the intracellular pH to become increasingly alkalotic during cooling through a reduction in intracellular H^+ ion concentration. In doing so, electrochemical neutrality is preserved. The reason uncorrected blood gas measurement is called *alpha stat* is because as body temperature cools, the normal blood buffers (NH_3, HCO_3^-, etc.) become ineffective. At hypothermic temperatures, intracellular and blood proteins become the only functional buffers. Buffering is necessary to decrease the concentration of H^+ ions during cooling. The alpha imidazole ring of the amino acid histidine accounts for the majority of buffering capacity at hypothermic temperature and is the reason why uncorrected blood gas management strategy is referred to as *alpha stat.*

Blood pH becomes increasingly alkalotic as it is cooled. To correct for this alkalotic "pH," CO_2 can be added to maintain a temperature-corrected pH of 7.40. The addition of CO_2 was believed to lower *intracellular* pH (pHi), resulting in an imbalance between H^+ and OH^- ions, that is, the loss of electrochemical neutrality. This approach of adding CO_2 to correct for the effect of cooling on blood pH is termed *pH stat.* Although pH stat was believed to alter cellular enzymatic function by lowering pHi, and altering electrochemical neutrality, it appears that cellular enzyme function is not impaired with pH stat. However, both pH and alpha stat markedly affect microcirculatory pH and CBF.

The current controversy over blood gas management strategy in congenital heart surgery remains unresolved. Two key areas have been critically evaluated using these techniques: (1) the neurologic effects of the two strategies and (2) myocardial function. Neurologic considerations relate to the effects of CO_2 on CBF, brain cooling, cerebral emboli, and the effect of pH on microcirculatory function. The pH stat strategy, by virtue of adding CO_2 during cooling, increases CBF. During cooling to deep hypothermia when low-flow bypass or circulatory arrest is being used, optimal brain cooling remains pivotal for cerebral protection. With this reasoning, pH stat may seem a more effective strategy. In contrast, we have already alluded to the concern of microembolic phenomenon and the fact that air emboli may be a significant contributor to neurologic morbidity, particularly in the congenital cardiac population, where left-sided air is a common concern. Increasing brain blood flow may also increase air emboli to the brain (Sungurtekin et al., 1999). In addition, if circulatory arrest is contemplated, starting the arrest period with a lower blood pH undoubtedly results in an even lower blood pH after the arrest period. The effect of a lower post–circulatory arrest pH on cerebral injury also must be considered.

In the mid 1990s, two key investigations in animals were performed evaluating alpha stat and pH stat using the percentage of cerebral metabolic recovery after circulatory arrest compared with the prearrest value as a marker for cerebral injury. In the first study by Skaryak and others (1995), piglets were cooled using alpha stat, pH stat, or pH stat followed by conversion to alpha stat strategy before undergoing a 90-minute period of circulatory arrest. The animals cooled with pH stat had a lower cerebral metabolic recovery than the alpha stat group, suggesting a greater injury. The crossover group cooled initially with pH stat and then converted to alpha stat before circulatory arrest had the greatest recovery of $CMRO_2$ of the three groups. These data imply that the pH stat does have a cooling benefit compared with the alpha stat, but the lower pH nullifies the benefit in animals with normal circulation. Switching over to alpha stat for a period of time before arrest optimizes pH before circulatory arrest and therefore maximizes the benefits of both strategies. The negative impact of low pH on the brain at deep hypothermia was also demonstrated by Ekroth and others (1989), when it was demonstrated that an increase in creatine kinase-BB bands occurred as the arterial pH fell below 7.1 (an uncorrected measurement using a pH stat strategy).

In a second series of experiments using a piglet model similar to that of Skaryak, Kirshbom and others (1995) surgically placed a 4-mm left subclavian–to–PA shunt on the animals before bypass and then ligated the shunt in half of the animals. The shunt was placed to simulate the effects of aortopulmonary collaterals. Collateral blood vessels are commonly present in cyanotic patients. The animals were then cooled with either a pH or an alpha stat strategy. The animals with a ligated shunt behaved similarly to those in the previous study. In contrast, the shunted animals cooled with alpha stat had significantly lower CBF, less effective brain cooling, and a significantly lower rate of metabolic recovery compared with the pH stat–cooled animals. The implication of this study was to demonstrate that pH stat strategy may have its greatest benefit in patients with cyanotic heart lesions. Cyanotic congenital cardiac defects have a tendency to develop aortopulmonary collateral blood vessels. The blood gas management strategy selected may not be equally applicable to all patients. Cyanotic patients may benefit from pH stat, whereas acyanotic lesions experimentally benefit from alpha stat. Other factors that were not evaluated by these studies include the role of intracardiac defects such as VSDs. VSDs may contribute to a greater opportunity for air to reach the left side of the circulation. With pH stat, cerebral air emboli may increase.

Hiramatsu and others (1995) evaluated the rate of pH recovery in an animal model using deep hypothermic circulatory arrest. In their study, the authors demonstrated a more rapid rate of recovery of blood pH with pH stat than with alpha stat. Although pH recovered more rapidly, the pH achieved immediately after circulatory arrest was substantially lower with pH stat. The question raised is, What is worse for the brain—the lowest pH or the rate of pH recovery?

In a clinical series designed to demonstrate a benefit for pH stat over alpha stat, Bellinger and others (2001) could not show a significant difference in neurologic outcome between alpha stat and pH stat blood gas strategies. Interestingly, a small subgroup of 16 patients with VSD had a significantly lower developmental outcome with pH stat compared with alpha stat. It was the only subgroup demonstrating a significant neurologic difference between the cooling strategies, and it favored alpha stat. The only clinical study to demonstrate a neurologic benefit to the pH stat strategy was a retrospective study of patients undergoing the Senning procedure for TGA (Jonas et al., 1993). These patients were operated on in the late 1970s and early 1980s. All of the patients were repaired using DHCA, and the average cooling time before initiation of circulatory was 14.5 minutes. Based on current knowledge, cooling times of less than 20 minutes have an increased risk of incomplete cerebral cooling using an alpha stat strategy (Kern et al., 1992). The brief cooling periods used in this study, even using a pH stat strategy, would never constitute optimal cooling and optimal cerebral protection based on current knowledge. Conclusions supporting pH stat strategy based on this analysis fail to account for the suboptimal approach to cerebral cooling.

These studies reinforce the benefits of a blood gas management strategy and one must take into account multiple factors, including bypass cooling strategy, the cardiac lesion, the presence of aortopulmonary collaterals, the presence of VSDs, the use of circulatory arrest, etc. In general, a consensus on the appropriate management strategy remains elusive. Most centers believe that cyanotic patients benefit from a pH stat strategy. Based on the data outlined earlier, alpha stat or a crossover strategy may be better for noncyanotic patients.

PATHOPHYSIOLOGY OF DEEP HYPOTHERMIC CIRCULATORY ARREST

All organs are at risk for hypoxic–ischemic injury, but the brain is the most sensitive and therefore the limiting factor when using DHCA. In contrast to the heart, where cardioplegic arrest has improved myocardial performance, a combination of hypothermia and nonpulsatile perfusion is the only modality of cerebral protection available. To understand the protective effects of hypothermic protection, a discussion of the pathophysiology of normothermic ischemia is warranted.

At normothermic temperatures, the energy-rich compounds (ATP and phosphocreatine) are maintained through oxidative metabolism. A majority of the ATP and phosphocreatine that are produced are utilized for maintaining ion homeostasis. In fact, it is estimated that 50% to 75% of high-energy phosphate expenditure is for the maintenance of transmembrane ionic gradients (Astrup, 1982; Hansen, 1985; Ericinska and Silver, 1989). Arresting the circulation at normothermia results in a rapid depletion of high-energy phosphate stores (Norwood et al., 1979a). After 2 minutes of complete ischemia, ATP levels fall to 10% of prearrest values (Norstrom and Siesko, 1978). In association with ATP depletion, there is a release of excitatory neurotransmitters such as glutamate and aspartate (Benveniste et al., 1984; Hagberg et al., 1987a, 1987b). Neurotransmitter release is not specific to ischemia; it can occur with other cerebral insults, such as hypoglycemia (Benveniste et al., 1984; Hagberg et al., 1987a, 1987b). Neurotransmitter release is thought, however, to represent a stereotypic response to ischemic injury.

Neurotransmitter release adversely affects membrane ionic permeability (Mutch and Hansen, 1984). ATP depletion in concert with excitatory neurotransmitter release signals a dramatic alteration in the maintenance of transmembrane ionic gradients. Electrochemical gradients for potassium, calcium, and sodium are lost, presumably due to unrestricted ion permeability across cell membranes (Hansen and Zeuthen, 1981). The loss of ionic gradients does not indicate a breakdown of cell membrane integrity, and although ATP levels are reduced, there is evidence to suggest that dysfunction of the energy-dependent ionic pumps does not occur within the first few minutes of normothermic ischemia (Mies and Paschen, 1984; Wieloch et al., 1984). However, low ATP levels may prevent the reestablishment of transmembrane ion gradients after the initial ion flux.

Calcium influx is the harbinger of permanent cellular damage. Approximately 95% of the calcium present in the extracellular space moves into the cell during the period of increased membrane permeability (Hansen and Zeuthen, 1981). Calcium influx results in accelerated cellular damage through the activation of calcium-dependent enzymes (phospholipases, nucleases, and xanthine oxidase). Phospholipases C and A_2 release free fatty acids (FFAs), such as arachidonic acid, from cell membrane phospholipids (Tang and Sun, 1985). FFAs uncouple oxidative phosphorylation and inhibit the exchange of adenosine diphosphate (ADP) for ATP across mitochondrial membranes. Arachidonic acid is metabolized to prostaglandins through the cyclooxygenase pathway and to leukotrienes through the 5-lipoxygenase pathway during post–ischemia–reperfusion. Ischemia alters the composition of prostaglandin production (Gaudet et al., 1980; Adesuyi et al., 1985). The potent vasoconstrictors prostaglandin GF_{2a} (PGF_{2a}) and thromboxane A_2 are produced in favor of vasodilators, such as prostacyclin (PGI_2). Thromboxane A_2 also promotes platelet aggregation, resulting in small vessel thrombosis.

Leukotrienes are undetectable in the nonischemic brain (Gaudet et al., 1980; Adesuyi et al., 1985). However, with ischemia and reperfusion, leukotriene levels and cytokines (tumor necrosis $factor_2$, interleukins, etc.) increase dramatically (Moskowitz et al., 1984). Like prostaglandins, leukotrienes are potent cerebral vasoconstrictors. In addition, leukotrienes are mediators of "secondary ischemic damage" through increased capillary permeability and promote leukocyte entry into the ischemic tissue. The probable result is an amplification of FFA-mediated cell injury, cerebral edema, activation of coagulation cascade, platelet plugging, and accelerated vascular thrombosis.

Nucleases become active after ischemia and have been implicated in creating single-stranded breaks in DNA. A majority of nucleases are calcium dependent, and thus calcium entry is an important cofactor for nuclease activity (Tullis and Rubin, 1982). In general, single-stranded DNA breaks are easily repaired (Ward et al., 1985). However, extensive single-stranded regions are prone to secondary breaks in the presence of oxygen free radicals. The conversion of single-strand breaks to double-strand breaks is considered lethal to the cell (Bryant, 1985; Radford, 1985).

The enzymatic breakdown of ADP and AMP not only wastes energy but also contributes to hypoxic cell damage (Guitierrez, 1991). AMP is either dephosphorylated to adenosine or deaminated to inosine monophosphate. Adenosine crosses the cell membrane through facilitated diffusion and acts as a potent local vasodilator. It is through adenosine release that the cell attempts to improve local oxygen delivery. During severe hypoxia, however, both inosine monophosphate and intracellular adenosine can be metabolized to hypoxanthine. Hypoxanthine in the presence of the enzyme xanthine oxidase is converted to the free radicals O_2^- and $H_2O_2^-$, important mediators of ischemic cerebral injury. Free radicals are catalyzed to potent oxidizing species that target proteins, unsaturated membrane lipids, and DNA. The result is extensive damage to cell membranes, nucleic acids, and enzyme systems (Aisen, 1980; Freeman and Crapo, 1982). A flow chart describing this cascade is shown (Fig. 17–8).

Hypothermia protects the brain from ischemic injury through preservation of high-energy phosphate stores, prevention of excitatory neurotransmitter release, restriction of membrane permeability, and prevention of calcium entry into the cell. By retarding ischemic injury, reperfusion can proceed uneventfully.

Several investigators examined the protective effect of deep hypothermia by measuring high-energy phosphate compounds with ^{31}P nuclear magnetic resonance (^{31}P-NMR) spectroscopy (Norwood et al., 1979a; Stocker et al., 1986; Chopp et al., 1989; Sutton et al., 1991; Jonas, 1993). These investigators reported that although ATP was rapidly depleted at normothermic temperatures, ATP levels were maintained at deep hypothermic temperatures (15° to 20°C) for a more prolonged period of time. At hypothermic temperatures, the rate of energy-dependent cellular enzyme systems such as Na^+,K^+-ATPase and Ca^{2+}-ATPase are drastically slowed. ATP and phosphocreatine utilization is reduced, excitatory neurotransmitter release is blunted, and ion homeostasis is maintained through both energy-dependent and -independent mechanisms. At hypothermic temperatures, ischemic events do not proceed concurrently.

Norwood and others (1979a) demonstrated that 25 minutes of DHCA significantly lowers creatine phosphate levels, but ATP stores are well maintained, in isolated perfused rat brains. In contrast, larger animal studies suggest that ATP levels reach their nadir after 21 to 33 minutes of hypothermic circulatory arrest (Norwood et al., 1979; Sutton et al., 1991; Swain et al., 1991; Jonas, 1993). After 1 hour of circulatory arrest, ^{31}P-NMR measurements suggested a delay in ATP recovery. In sheep, after 60 minutes of arrest at 15°C, ATP levels were reduced to 36% of control. Thirty minutes of normothermic reperfusion, however, restored ATP levels to 83% of control values (Swain et al., 1991). In a similar CPB model using piglets, intracellular pH did not recover from a 60-minute arrest period until after 40 minutes of normothermic reperfusion (Jonas, 1993). ATP and phosphocreatine levels recovered to 90% and 98% of baseline but required 3 hours of normothermic reperfusion. These studies of whole brain cerebral metabolism in both animals and children demonstrate a significant reduction in metabolism after DHCA, which is not found after low-flow CPB. Both cellular levels of ATP and global measures of cerebral metabolism are reduced after DHCA, suggesting organ dysfunction.

Studies of ischemic brain injury in the rat by Busto and others (1987, 1989), using a four-vessel occlusion model, demonstrated that ischemic injury results in an increased release in both glutamate and dopamine. When temperature was lowered from

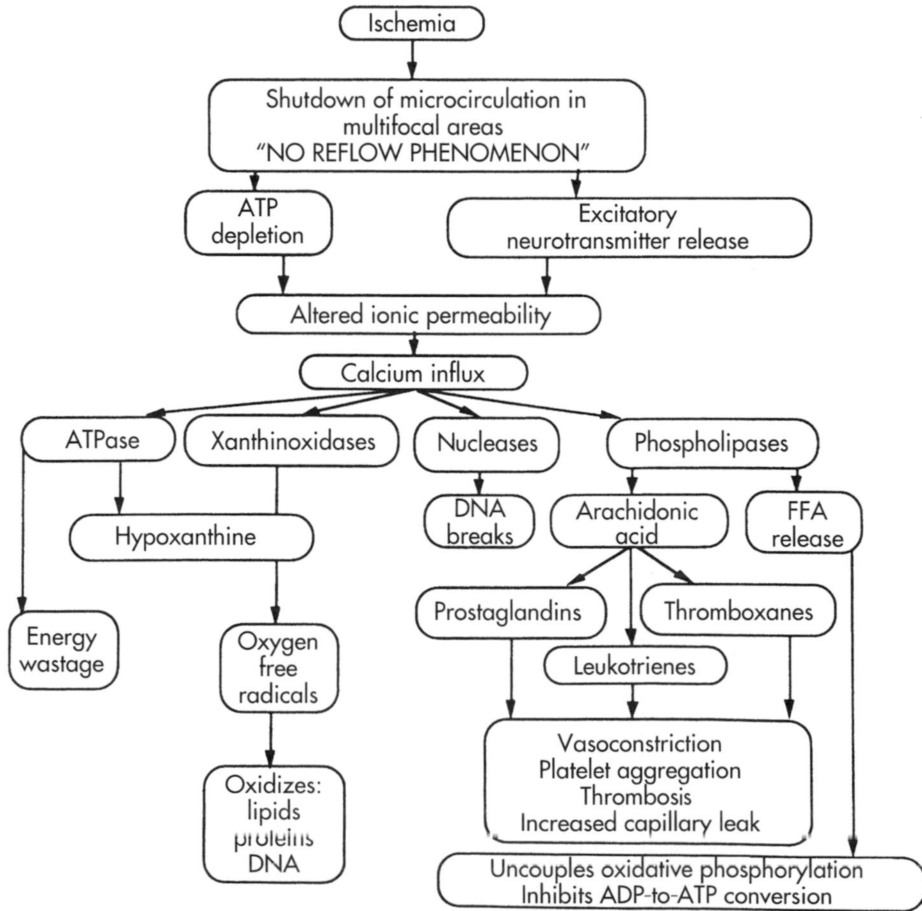

■ FIGURE 17–8. Flow chart describing the cellular events occurring during normothermic arrest.

36° to 33°C, the expected rise in glutamate release did not occur and dopamine levels decreased. Interestingly, minimal levels of hypothermia (34°C) have been shown to prevent the ischemic neuronal injury on the CA-1 layer of the hippocampus compared with normothermic controls. Moderate hypothermia of 27°C was no more protective than this slight level of hypothermia (Busto et al., 1987, 1989). This suggests that excitatory neurotransmitter release may act as an accelerator of neurologic injury by promoting the loss of transmembrane ionic gradients and enhancing calcium entry. More moderate levels of hypothermia may be sufficient to prevent the triggered release of excitatory neurotransmitters but do not reduce brain metabolism or alter transmembrane permeability to the same degree as more extreme hypothermic temperatures.

Deeper levels of hypothermia may provide additional protection from calcium entry through altering membrane fluidity. At deep hypothermic temperatures, cell membranes alter their permeability through changes in physical state of membrane lipids—in other words, less liquid and more semisolid (Rich and Langer, 1982). This may directly affect free ion movement across cellular membranes and provide additional protection once ATP-dependent mechanisms for ion homeostasis are lost.

As discussed later in this chapter, more efficient and rigorous cooling strategies, substitution of low-flow CPB for DHCA, reperfusion periods during the arrest period, higher hematocrits, pH stat cooling in select patients, and improved rewarming strategies may minimize the risk of low-flow CPB and DHCA and reduce neuropsychological injury. It should also be noted that to date, there has been no drug study that has demonstrated improved neurologic outcome in patients or animals undergoing CPB.

SPECIFIC ORGAN EFFECTS: MYOCARDIUM

CPB desensitizes cardiac βARs. Schwinn and others (1991) examined the effects of β-agonists on adenyl cyclase activity in canine left ventricular tissue and found that maximal isoproterenol stimulation resulted in a marked increase in β-receptor–mediated adenyl cyclase activity in the pre-CPB period. After 155 minutes of CPB, reexposure to the same isoproterenol infusion resulted in a significant decrease in βAR-stimulated adenyl cyclase activity. Thirty minutes after bypass, adenyl cyclase activity was greater than on prebypass measurements. Similar responses were obtained with submaximal infusions of isoproterenol and the β_2-selective drug zinterol. When β-receptor density was examined, it was found to be unchanged during CPB, suggesting that the reduction in function is related to the uncoupling of the β-receptor and adenylyl cyclase, which is the function of the Gs protein complex. It is interesting to note that 30 minutes after weaning from CPB, β-receptor number did begin to decrease, suggesting that β-receptor downregulation may play a role in the postoperative response to β-specific inotropic agents and, at least in older patients, downregulation occurs fairly quickly.

Schranz and others (1993) studied the effects of CPB on acyanotic pediatric patients and confirmed the experimental data obtained by Schwinn (1991, 1994). They demonstrated that after CPB, β-agonist–induced increases in cAMP were attenuated. However, when several non–β-receptor–dependent stimulators of adenylyl cyclase were examined, adenylyl cyclase activity increased in a normal fashion despite CPB. In addition, β_1- and β_2-receptor density was found to be unaltered by CPB. These studies suggest a primary role for the Gs protein complex in the desensitization of β-agonist action when weaning from CPB. Neonatal myocardium does not desensitize in response to high levels of circulating catecholamines. Several animal studies have demonstrated receptor signaling is different in early neonatal life. Instead of β-agonist administration producing desensitization of responses, it promotes receptor signaling by enhancing expression and/or catalytic efficiency of adenyl cyclase (Giannuzzi et al., 1995). Neonatal myocytes normally have a reduced number of β-receptors. Catecholamine responsiveness is reduced in the neonate. The lack of desensitization in the neonatal population means prolonged preoperative or postoperative catecholamine administration does not reduce myocardial responsiveness to these important inotropic agents.

Myocardial Protection

Although normal neonatal hearts may be more resilient to periods of ischemia, the effects of cyanosis and CPB offset these advantages. For this reason, most pediatric cardiac surgeons believe that the basic principles of myocardial preservation practiced during adult cardiac surgery should be followed in neonatal cardiac surgery.

Research in the field of myocardial preservation demonstrated that oxygenated blood is a better cardioplegic solution than crystalloid (Buckberg, 1979, 1990). Red blood cells contain large quantities of free radical scavengers and blood proteins contain histidine, an amino acid buffer that reduces intracellular acidosis during ischemia (Jennings and Reimer, 1983). Histidine is particularly important because it continues to function even at profound hypothermic temperatures (Bretschneider, 1980). In addition, the presence of red blood cells may increase oxygen delivery to myocardial tissue. Cold cardioplegia is generally preferred to warm cardioplegia. The rationale is similar to cerebral protection—preserving high-energy phosphate stores, preventing excitatory neurotransmitter release, restricting membrane permeability, and preventing calcium entry into the cell. Potassium is an important component of the cardioplegia solution because it maintains electrochemical quiescence. The nonbeating heart has decreased substrate utilization and allows for repletion of ATP and more homogeneous delivery of nutrients throughout the coronary system (Danforth et al., 1960; Domalik-Wawrzynski et al., 1987). This results in better global myocardial protection.

Other factors that have been shown to be beneficial in cardioplegia solutions include leukocyte depletion, reduced calcium content, the addition of the amino acids glutamate and aspartate, and oxygen radical scavengers (Lazar et al., 1980; Rozencrantz et al., 1982; Julia et al., 1988; Breda et al., 1989; Bolling et al., 1990; Chiba et al., 1993). Leukocytes and calcium play an important role in reperfusion injury. Glutamate and aspartate are amino acids that are intermediary metabolites of glycolysis and thereby provide substrate during reperfusion. Oxygen radical scavengers prevent membrane damage from ischemia-induced hydroxyl radicals. Blood cardioplegia has sufficient naturally occurring free radical scavengers to obviate the need for the addition of free radical scavengers to cardioplegia solution (Julia et al., 1988) (Table 17–10). Clermont and others (2002) indicated that systemic free radical activation may be a major contributor to myocardial oxidative stress related to CPB.

Some centers are adding low-concentration lidocaine to blood cardioplegia solutions. The rationale for this practice is to lengthen the time between cardioplegia doses, and there is some theoretical evidence of early sodium channel closure and less myocardial intracellular calcium damage during bypass. This lengthening of the

TABLE 17–10. Generic components of cardioplegia

Component	Effects
Normosol	Crystalloid vehicle
KCl	Electromechanical quiescence
Tham	Buffering capacity
CPD	Anticoagulant
$D_{5,25}W$	Substrate
Aspartate/glutamate	Provides substrate during reperfusion
Blood (hematocrit 15% to 20%)	Provides increased oxygen delivery, free radical scavenging, and pH buffering
Magnesium/lidocaine and mannitol	Decreased reperfusion injury
Low ionized calcium	Decreased reperfusion injury
Leukocyte depletion	Decreased reperfusion injury

inter–cardioplegia administration time points may allow a distinct surgical timing advantage in some small infants undergoing extensive aortic arch reconstructions. The rationale for this practice is shown largely in animal experimental data. Sunamori and others (1982) showed in dogs that a cardioplegia solution of lidocaine and magnesium had better myocardial preservation than cardioplegia without lidocaine. Clinical trials are needed, because a recent randomized trial in adult patients undergoing coronary revascularization has found no statistically significant improvement in myocardial preservation after the addition of lidocaine to a standard cardioplegia solution (Rinne et al., 1998).

Although blood cardioplegia appears beneficial, many surgical groups continue to use crystalloid cardioplegia in neonates with good success. This is particularly true when DHCA or continuous low-flow CPB at deep hypothermic temperatures is being used as part of the CPB management scheme. Deep hypothermic temperatures of 15° to 18°C are below typical cardioplegia temperatures of 22°C and provide myocardial protection.

The one exception to the use of cardioplegia is during the stage 1 repair of HLHS. Because of the risk of needle damage to the small ascending aorta, antegrade cardioplegia is avoided and cardioplegia is either not given or administered retrograde rather than prograde after aortic cross-clamping. In cases where cardioplegia is not used, the heart is protected by DHCA alone. Virtually all other patients receive cardioplegia.

One other factor in myocardial preservation comes from a study of myocardial troponin T levels in neonates and children undergoing CPB with either alpha stat or pH stat. In this study (Nagy et al., 2003), there is a suggestion that a pH stat cooling regimen may provide improved myocardial protection compared with alpha stat cooling regimens.

SPECIFIC ORGAN EFFECTS: BRAIN

During CPB, hypothermia is the most important factor that alters cerebral hemodynamic and metabolic parameters. Hypothermia produces a marked reduction in both CBF and brain metabolism ($CMRO_2$) at constant pump flow rates (Fig. 17–9). The coupling of flow to metabolism is an important concept in ensuring adequate oxygen delivery and limiting luxuriant perfusion to the brain. Variations in flow, metabolism, and their coupling are dramatically altered by hypothermic CPB (Julia et al., 1988; Greeley et al., 1988, 1989, 1991a, 1991b).

Cerebral Blood Flow

CBF falls in a direct linear relationship with temperature (see Fig. 17–9). In studies where CO_2, perfusion pressure, pump flow rate, and temperature were altered by the extracorporeal circulation, temperature is the most important factor influencing CBF during CPB in children (Greeley et al., 1988, 1989; Julia et al., 1988). Moderate hypothermia and deep hypothermia have different effects on CBF and its autoregulation.

Pressure–flow autoregulation, or the ability to maintain a constant CBF despite wide ranges in mean arterial pressures, has been shown to be intact during MHCPB (26° to 30°C) in adults and children when measured using alpha stat blood gas regulation (Govier et al., 1984; Murkin et al., 1987). In children, pressure–flow autoregulation remains intact over a range of mean arterial pressures of 15 to 80 mm Hg during MHCPB (Greeley et al., 1988). During moderate hypothermia, the cerebral vasculature maintains a normal physiologic response of dilation during low perfusion pressure and constriction when perfusion pressure is high. In contrast, at deep hypothermic temperatures of 15° to 20°C, pressure–flow autoregulation is lost (Greeley et al., 1989a). At deep hypothermic temperatures, CVR increases with temperature reduction. CVR remains high even when pump flow rates

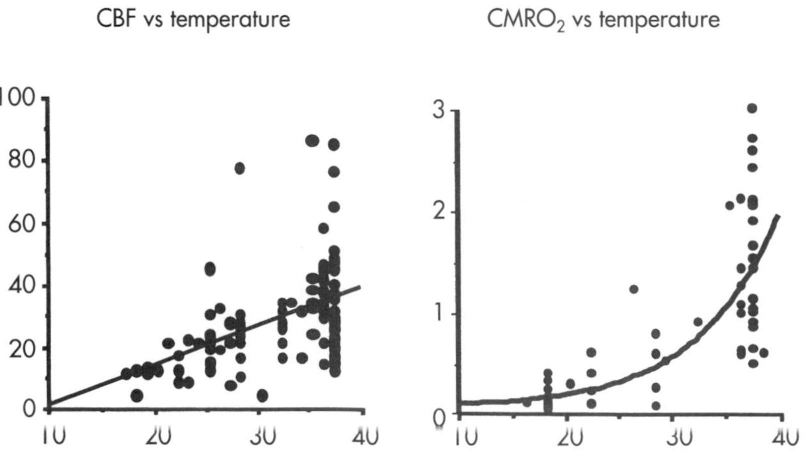

FIGURE 17–9. Effects of hypothermia on cerebral blood flow (CBF) and cerebral metabolism. There is a positive linear relationship between hypothermia and cerebral blood flow during pediatric cardiopulmonary bypass. In contrast, there is an exponential reduction in cerebral metabolism with temperature reduction during hypothermic cardiopulmonary bypass. $CMRO_2$, cerebral metabolic rate for oxygen.

and perfusion pressure are substantially reduced. Reduction in pump flow rates from 100 mL/kg per minute to as low as 30 mL/kg per minute does not significantly change CVR during deep hypothermic CPB. This loss of pressure-flow autoregulation is most likely due to the influence of deep hypothermic temperatures on vascular reactivity. Severe temperature reductions impair vascular relaxation (Civalero et al., 1962; Tanaka et al., 1988; Greeley et al., 1989a; Kern et al., 1991b). This has been described as a cold-induced "cerebrovasoparesis" (Greeley et al., 1989a, 1989b).

Cerebral Metabolism

CBF decreases in a linear fashion with reduction in brain temperature, but brain metabolism ($CMRO_2$) decreases exponentially (Greeley et al., 1991b; Milde, 1992) (see Fig. 17–9). A convenient expression of the effect of temperature on $CMRO_2$ is to calculate the ratio of metabolism at a temperature gradient of 10°C, called the *temperature coefficient*, or Q10 (Michenfelder and Theye, 1968). Cerebral oxygen consumption has been measured in a number of models during CPB (dog, monkey, and human) and has been shown to vary greatly between species and at differing ages within species (Bering, 1961; Michenfelder and Theye, 1968; Greeley et al., 1991b; Croughwell et al., 1993). In children and adults, Q10s of 3.65 and 2.8 have been reported, respectively (Greeley et al., 1991; Croughwell et al., 1993).

The increased metabolic suppression for younger patients may be due to more efficient cooling of the immature neurons and glial elements to hypothermia or may reflect greater brain mass as a percentage of body weight and more efficient brain cooling. Interspecies and intraspecies variability for Q10 may explain why variables other than temperature have been implicated as major contributors to cerebral protection during CPB. If adult-derived Q10 data are used, temperature-induced metabolic suppression would appear insufficient to explain clinically acceptable "safe" circulatory arrest periods.

Hypothermic protection alone may account for the majority of the protection seen during DHCA (Greeley et al., 1991b). Other variables, such as anesthetic agents, provide much smaller contributions to cerebral protection, once deep hypothermic temperatures (15° to 20°C) are reached (Michenfelder and Theye, 1968; Michenfelder, 1988). At more moderate temperatures, anesthetic agents and other cerebroprotective agents, such as calcium channel blockers, barbiturates, and *N*-methyl-D-aspartate antagonists, may be beneficial. If deep hypothermia is the only cerebroprotective agent used, factors that enhance cerebral cooling by modifying CBF, such as the addition of CO_2, may be important adjuncts to achieving uniform brain cooling and thereby improving global cerebral protection (Michenfelder and Theye, 1968; Michenfelder, 1988; Kern et al., 1991a, 1992a). These considerations are discussed later in this chapter.

Cerebral Blood Flow and Metabolism Coupling

CBF decreases linearly with reduction in temperature. In contrast, cerebral metabolism decreases exponentially with reduction in temperature. The flow–metabolism ratio must increase with decreasing temperature during CPB in children. In the awake healthy child, CBF and metabolism ($CMRO_2$) are regulated by the metabolic needs of regional areas of the brain. This has been termed *cerebral flow–metabolism coupling* and is an important regulatory feature of cerebral homeostasis (Kety, 1945; Scheinberg and Stead, 1949; Stullken et al., 1977). In humans, a mean CBF of 45 to 80 mL/100 g per minute is coupled to a $CMRO_2$ of 3.0 to 4.0 mL/100 g per minute, for a CBF/$CMRO_2$ ratio of 13 to 20:1 (Michenfelder, 1988; Greeley et al., 1991a). In neonates, $CMRO_2$, CBF, and the CBF/$CMRO_2$ ratios are generally higher than those for older children and adults. This is believed to be due to increased metabolic demand for neuronal growth, myelinization, etc. (Rosenberg et al., 1982). If CPB is managed using alpha stat blood gas regulation at a pump flow rate of 100 mL/kg per minute, the ratio of CBF to $CMRO_2$ increases with decreasing temperature, so that during MHCPB, the CBF/$CMRO_2$ ratio increases to 30:1. At deep hypothermic temperatures the ratio of the CBF to $CMRO_2$ extends to 75:1 (Greeley et al., 1991a). In contrast, pH stat blood gas regulation (the addition of CO_2 to the gas flow mixture) results in the CBF/$CMRO_2$ ratios of 60:1 at moderate hypothermia (Murkin et al., 1987), whereas at deep hypothermic temperatures, flow–metabolism ratios using pH stat strategy are unknown. Although alpha stat regulation has been believed to maintain flow-metabolism coupling at moderate hypothermia, CBF becomes increasingly luxuriant at lower temperatures in children, even using alpha stat blood gas regulation. Luxuriant flow becomes important when low pump flows are used in conjunction with deep hypothermic CPB.

LOW-FLOW CARDIOPULMONARY BYPASS

Guidelines for the safe implementation of low-flow CPB are not firmly established. Estimates for minimal acceptable pump flow rates (PFR) for children during CPB have been suggested based on metabolic measurements. Using Q10 data, one can predict $CMRO_2$ at different temperatures. For children at 37°C, the mean $CMRO_2 = 1.48$; at 28°C, the mean $CMRO_2 = 0.51$ (66% reduction); at 18°C, the mean $CMRO_2 = 0.16$ (89% reduction); and at 15°C, the mean $CMRO_2 = 0.11$ (93% reduction) (Greeley et al., 1991a). By comparing the reduction in $CMRO_2$ with proportional reductions in pump flow rates, an estimate of minimal acceptable flow rates can be predicted (Kern et al., 1993). The equation describing this relationship for infants is as follows:

$$MPFR(T) = e \cdot 1171(T - 37°C) \cdot (100\ mL/kg\ per\ minute)$$

where

MPFR(T) = minimal pump flow rate at temperature T
100 mL/kg per minute = Normothermic pump flow rate
$e \cdot 1171(T - 37°C) = CMRO_2$ at temperature T and at 37°C

Table 17–11 shows the calculated values derived from the MPFR(T) equation.

TABLE 17–11. Predicted minimal pump flow rates (MPFR)

Temperature (°C)	$CMRO_2$ (mL/100 g per min)	Predicted MPFR (mL/kg per min)
37	1.48	100
32	0.823	56
30	0.654	44
28	0.513	34
25	0.362	24
20	0.201	14
18	0.159	11
15	0.112	08

$CMRO_2$, cerebral metabolic rate for oxygen.

Both human and animal studies suggest that these data represent a reasonable approximation of acceptable minimal pump flow rates during hypothermic CPB. Swain and others (1991) using ^{31}P-NMR have demonstrated that flow rates of 10 mL/kg per minute at 15°C for periods of up to 2 hours in 8-week-old lambs maintain normal levels of ATP and phosphocreatine and normal brain pH. When flow is reduced to 5 mL/kg per minute at 15°C, organic phosphates become depleted and brain pH begins to fall. The effect of 5 mL/kg per minute flow rates on cerebral metabolism in these animals was indistinguishable from findings in a similar group of sheep undergoing 2 hours of circulatory arrest at 15°C. A calculated MPFR(T) of 7 mL/kg per minute is necessary to meet cerebral metabolic demands at this temperature.

In a neonatal piglet model, flow rates of between 5 and 10 mL/kg per minute at 18°C for 60 minutes resulted in only a modest reduction in metabolism (10%) after weaning from CPB compared with measurements obtained in thc prebypass period (Mault et al., 1993; Kern et al., 1993). These flow rates are just below the predicted flow rates of 11 mL/kg per minute, suggesting that these animals had borderline cerebral oxygen delivery for 18°C. Similar data in canines, monkeys, and humans have been derived and show surprisingly similar relationship between pump flow rate and metabolism at a variety of hypothermic temperatures (Fox et al., 1982; Miyamoto et al., 1986; Watanabe et al., 1989; Kern et al., 1993).

DEEP HYPOTHERMIC CIRCULATORY ARREST

Wernovsky and others (1992) demonstrated a higher incidence of transient postoperative seizures after 45 to 60 minutes of circulatory arrest compared with low-flow continuous perfusion. Their study results suggest that DHCA imparts a greater neurologic risk to neonates and infants compared with continuous-flow bypass. Bellinger and others (2003) reported on an 8-year neurologic assessment of 155 patients who had undergone the arterial switch procedure for TGA using either a low-flow bypass technique or a predominant DHCA strategy. In this study, full-scale IQ scores, academic achievement, memory, problem solving, visual-motor integration, and neurologic examination did not differ between the two groups. Children assigned to the circulatory arrest group performed statistically worse on motor function tests, including manual dexterity with the nondominant hand, speech apraxia, visual motor tracking, and phonologic awareness. Children who were assigned to the low-flow bypass group were associated with a more impulsive response style on continuous performance tests of vigilance and worse behavior as rated by teachers. The circulatory arrest group evaluated at 8 years out continued to demonstrate a greater motor impairment compared with the low-flow group. The low-flow group demonstrated greater behavioral problems and impulsive behavior. These findings suggest that methods to improve CPB management and the approach to DHCA could be improved based on the physiologic consequences outlined earlier. Furthermore, the approach used to implement and manage circulatory arrest in this study does not conform to, or adequately address, current techniques of brain protection and monitoring. Newer monitoring and protective strategies may significantly affect postarrest neurologic injury.

Deep Hypothermic Circulatory Arrest With Intermittent Perfusion Periods

Intermittent systemic perfusion between periods of DHCA has been suggested as an alternative to prolonged periods of DHCA.

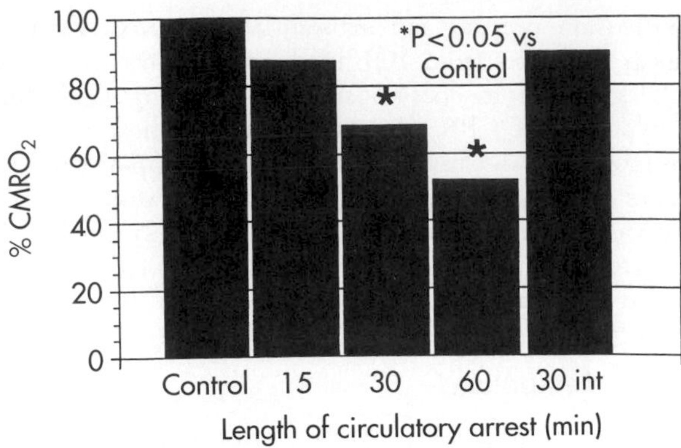

FIGURE 17–10. Percent cerebral metabolic rate for oxygen ($CMRO_2$) recovery after varying lengths of circulatory arrest in a piglet model. The longer the arrest period, the less recovery there is of $CMRO_2$. When a 60-minute period of circulatory arrest is interrupted for 1 minute and the animal is reperfused at 100 mL/kg per minute of flow, $CMRO_2$ returns to near-normal levels.

These periods of reperfusion may replete cerebral high-energy phosphate stores and preserve neurologic tissue. Data investigating this concept are limited. Reperfusion periods of 1 minute at deep hypothermic temperatures between two 30-minute circulatory arrest periods significantly improved metabolic recovery compared with a 60-minute period of circulatory arrest in neonatal piglet studies (Mault et al., 1992) (Fig. 17–10). This is consistent with NMR data, which suggest that high-energy phosphate compounds reach their nadir after approximately 30 minutes (Swain et al., 1991). In the study by Swain and others, sheep were exposed to a 30-minute period of reperfusion following a 60-minute period of circulatory arrest. There was partial restoration of intracellular pH, ATP, and phosphocreatine levels. A second 60-minute period of circulatory arrest, however, resulted in rapid depletion of ATP and phosphocreatine levels. After a second 60-minute period of circulatory arrest, ATP, phosphocreatine, and intracellular pH values were no different than after a continuous 2-hour arrest period. These studies support the conclusion that 30 minutes of arrest at deep hypothermic temperatures does not result in full depletion of cellular ATP and phosphocreatine. Replenishing cellular metabolic stores may occur more rapidly at hypothermic temperatures, especially if cellular levels of ATP are not fully depleted before reinstituting perfusion. In contrast, after 60 minutes of total circulatory arrest, a 30-minute reperfusion period at normothermia only partially restores the brain's metabolic reserve. Reperfusion after arrest periods of 20 to 30 minutes seems to have a greater benefit than reperfusion after 60 minutes of circulatory arrest. Several additional animal studies have demonstrated a benefit to intermittent perfusion (Langley et al., 1999; Strauc et al., 2003). Clinical data, however, remain elusive. Several clinical reports have described methods for both antegrade and retrograde cerebral perfusion principally in adults undergoing surgery for aortic arch aneurysm or dissection (Mass et al., 1997; Yoshii et al., 2003). Several studies comparing selective antegrade or retrograde cerebral perfusion in adults with ascending aortic arch disease were unable to demonstrate neurologic outcome improvement compared with circulatory arrest (Svensson et al., 2001). In one study of 289 adults undergoing ascending aortic arch surgery, DHCA was compared with selective antegrade cerebral perfusion. There was no statistical difference in neurologic outcome, but the selective perfusion group did have less renal dysfunction and were extubated earlier in the postoperative period (DiEusanio et al., 2003).

Cerebral Cooling Strategies

Accelerated rates of cooling (>1°C/min) during CPB using alpha stat regulation are associated with a lower developmental quotient in neonates undergoing DHCA (Bellinger et al., 1988). High cerebral oxygen extraction, low jugular venous bulb saturation, and a cerebral metabolic rate greater than that expected for 18°C suggest that inadequate cerebral perfusion from inefficient brain cooling is associated postoperatively with neurologic disability (Greeley et al., 1991b). Marked variability in cerebral cooling has been established in several clinical studies. When low jugular venous saturations were used as a marker for incomplete cerebral cooling, one third of patients demonstrated significantly slower brain cooling. When cooling techniques were varied, colder blood resulting in a larger temperature gradient between the blood and tissue contributed to more rapid and complete cerebral cooling (Kern et al., 1991a).

Temperature gradients occur between superficial temperature measurement and deep brain structures. Studies in the rat demonstrate temperature gradients of 2° to 6°C between deep brain structures and temporalis muscle in a study using a four-vessel occlusion model of cerebral ischemia (Busto et al., 1987; 1989). Significant differences in neuronal function, histopathology, free fatty acids, and excitatory neurotransmitter release were demonstrated based on regional differences in brain temperature (Busto et al., 1987, 1989; Okada et al., 1988). Animal studies also suggest that there are regional differences in the distribution of brain blood flow during hypercarbia. Deep brain structures (thalamus, brainstem, and cerebellum) receive a significantly greater percentage of CBF than do cortical structures (Hansen et al., 1984).

The ideal blood gas management strategy for children is not categorical. Just as the surgeon must decide the appropriate temperature for hypothermic bypass and whether to use moderate-flow, low-flow, or circulatory arrest, the appropriateness of a blood gas strategy depends on many modifiers. These modifiers include the degree of hypothermia, pump flow rate, use of DHCA, and cooling dynamics of the brain. Appropriate strategies can be hypothesized. During moderate hypothermia, selection of one blood gas management strategy over the other appears less critical because blood pH differences are small (Swan, 1984; Bashein et al., 1990). During deep hypothermia with or without circulatory arrest, the addition of CO_2 during active brain cooling could potentially improve the distribution of the cold perfusate to deep brain structures. Work by several investigators (Watanabe et al., 1989; Jonas, 1993; Skaryak et al., 1995) suggests that pH stat management enhances the distribution of extracorporeal perfusate to the brain and may help cool the brain more thoroughly and rapidly. Although improved cooling was demonstrated in these studies, metabolic recovery after circulatory arrest was shown to be impaired, suggesting that the acid load induced by pH stat had a negative effect on enzymatic or microcirculatory function after cerebral rewarming. To retain the benefits of pH stat on cooling and to eliminate its negative effects on enzymatic function suggest the use of a combined blood gas management strategy with pH and alpha stat in succession. In another study, a group of animals underwent initial cooling with pH stat followed by alpha stat to eliminate residual acid load before the initiation of DHCA (Skaryak et al., 1995). This group demonstrated improved metabolic suppression over alpha stat alone and a significant enhancement in metabolic recovery after rewarming. This suggests that initial cooling with pH stat, followed by alpha stat, may be preferable. A controlled clinical study evaluating this approach (combined pH/alpha stat cooling), however, is necessary before clinical benefits can be supported.

Other factors that may result in maldistribution of pump flow away from the cerebral circulation and contribute to inefficient cerebral cooling include anatomic variants (large aortic to pulmonary collaterals) and technical problems (aortic and venous cannula placement) (Spach et al., 1980; Kern et al., 1991a). Cyanotic patients, with known aortopulmonary collaterals, may benefit from the cerebrovasodilation of CO_2 during early cooling. Once cooled, however, if DHCA or deep hypothermia with low flow is planned, conversion to an alpha stat strategy before arrest may reduce postarrest cerebral acidosis.

At some centers, a period of hyperoxia is being used before initiation of DHCA. The rationale for this is based on studies of better neurologic histology after CPB in a group of animals exposed to hyperoxia and on the fact that dissolved oxygen is used by the brain to a greater extent than is oxygen bound to hemoglobin (Nollert et al., 1999).

Hematocrit and Neurologic Outcome

In a recent study, Jonas and others (2003) undertook a single-center randomized trial to assess the effects of hemodilution during CPB on neurologic and outcomes data. The patients were maintained at a hematocrit of 21.5% versus 27.8% during hypothermic CPB. The lower-hematocrit group had higher serum lactates at 1 hour after bypass and a significantly greater increase in total body water on the first postoperative day. At 1 year of age, the lower-hematocrit group had significantly worse scores on the Psychomotor Development Index. This suggests that higher hematocrits may be beneficial during hypothermic CPB (Jonas et al., 2003).

Corticosteroids

The use of stress-dose preoperative corticosteroids for infant CPB has increased during the past several years. Historically, methylprednisolone was added only to the pump prime. The addition of corticosteroids to the pump prime dates back to the 1950s. Administration of corticosteroids at the time CPB is initiated theoretically reduces efficacy, because it takes 6 to 8 hours to have a significant effect on modulation of the inflammatory response. In a neonatal piglet study, Lodge and others (1999) compared three groups of animals: those that received methylprednisolone 30 mg/kg administered intravenously 8 hours and 1.5 hours before bypass, those that received methylprednisolone administered in the pump prime, and a control group that did not receive steroids. The preoperative administration of steroids resulted in a significant improvement in lung compliance, alveolar-arterial P_{O_2} gradient, and PVR. There was a small improvement when steroids were administered to the pump prime–only group (Lodge et al., 1999). Other studies have involved the role of steroids on myocardial apoptosis. Although preoperative steroid administration was no different than administration to the prime alone (Pearl et al., 2002), steroids reduced the incidence of postcirculatory arrest, apoptosis, and cell death. In addition, preoperative steroids have also been shown to reduce total body edema, cerebral edema, and troponin I levels and improves $CMRO_2$ recovery after DHCA (Langley et al., 2000; Schwartz et al., 2003). Clinical studies have demonstrated a lower ratio of proinflammatory to anti-inflammatory cytokines and extravascular fluid after the administration of dexamethasone in adults (El Azab et al., 2002; Fillinger et al., 2002). The role of corticosteroids in pediatric cardiac surgery is still being investigated.

CARDIOPULMONARY BYPASS MANAGEMENT

INITIATION OF CARDIOPULMONARY BYPASS

Once the aortic and venous cannulas are positioned and connected to the arterial and venous limb of the extracorporeal circuit, bypass is initiated. The technique for initiating bypass varies depending on the size of the patient and the temperature of the perfusate.

In older children and adolescents, bypass is initiated slowly. The venous cannula is unclamped and blood is siphoned from the RA into the oxygenator via gravity drainage or occasionally by vacuum assist. When the more commonly used gravity drainage is instituted, the rate at which venous blood is drained from the patient is determined by the height difference between the patient and the oxygenator inlet, and the diameter of the venous cannula and line tubing. Venous drainage can be enhanced by increasing the height difference between the oxygenator and the patient. Venous drainage can be reduced by either decreasing the height difference between the oxygenator and the patient or by partially clamping the venous line. Vacuum-assist venous drainage (VAVD) is being used more frequently in pediatric CPB. It provides a gravity-independent means for maintaining venous return and can significantly increase venous blood return during CPB procedures. If perfusion vigilance for detecting air entrainment is adequately accounted for and arterial line filters are used, then VAVD is especially useful. With the current clinical trend toward smaller venous cannulas and lower prime and circuit volumes for neonatal CPB machines, VAVD is safe and increasingly becoming a standard for neonatal and infant CPB (Lau et al., 1999; Jegger et al., 2003).

Once venous blood begins to accumulate in the oxygenator, the arterial pump is slowly started. Its speed is gradually increased until full flow is reached. If return is diminished, line pressure is high, or mean arterial pressure excessive pump flow rates must be reduced. High line pressure and inadequate venous return are usually due to malposition or kinking of the arterial and venous cannulas, respectively.

In neonates and infants, when deep hypothermia is used, the pump prime is cold (18° to 22°C). When the cold perfusate contacts the myocardium, heart rate immediately slows and contraction is severely impaired. The contribution to total blood flow pumped by the heart rapidly diminishes. To sustain adequate systemic perfusion at or near normothermic temperatures, the arterial pump must reach full flows quickly. A major difference in the initiation of bypass in neonates and infants versus older children is the speed in which full support must be achieved. One method for initiating CPB in infants is to begin the arterial pump first; once the aortic flow is ensured, the venous cannula is unclamped and blood is siphoned out of the RA into the inlet of the oxygenator. Flowing before unclamping the venous cannula prevents the potential problem of patient exsanguination if aortic dissection or malplacement of the aortic cannula has occurred. Pump flow rates are then rapidly increased to sustain systemic perfusion. Because coronary artery disease is usually not a consideration, the myocardium should cool evenly. Exceptions to even myocardial cooling occur with coronary anomalies such as anomalous left coronary artery from the PA or pulmonary atresia with the presence of sinusoids. When a cold prime is used, caution must be exercised in using the pump to infuse volume before initiating CPB. Infusion of cold perfusate may result in bradycardia and impaired cardiac contractility before the surgeon is prepared to initiate CPB.

Once CPB begins, it is essential to observe the heart. Ineffective venous drainage can rapidly result in ventricular distention. This is especially true in infants and neonates where ventricular compliance is low and the heart may be intolerant of excessive preload augmentation. If distention occurs, pump flow must be reduced and the venous cannula repositioned. Alternatively, the heart may be vented or a pump sucker placed into the RA.

DISCONTINUATION OF CARDIOPULMONARY BYPASS

When a patient is weaned from CPB, the heart is allowed to fill by partially clamping the venous return tubing and reducing the arterial inflow until adequate blood volume is achieved. Blood volume is assessed by direct visualization of the heart and measuring cerebrovascular pressure and right atrial or left atrial filling pressures. When filling pressures are adequate, the venous cannula is clamped and the arterial inflow is stopped. The arterial cannula is left in place so that a slow infusion of residual pump blood can be used to optimize filling pressures. Myocardial function is assessed through direct cardiac visualization, central venous pressure or intracardiac monitoring, and intraoperative echocardiography. In corrected physiology, the pulse oximeter can also be used as a crude measure of cardiac output (Oshita et al., 1989). Low saturations or the inability of the oximeter probe to register a pulse may be a sign of very low output and high systemic resistance (Severinghaus and Spellman, 1990).

After the repair of some complex congenital heart defects, the anesthesiologist and surgeon may have difficulty separating a patient from CPB. Under these circumstances, a distinction must be made between residual anatomic disease, altered loading conditions on the heart induced by the repair or the effects of CPB on systemic and PVR, myocardial function, and pulmonary compliance. Anatomic problems should be evaluated by TEE. Having the patient leave the operating room with a clinically residual defect has been associated with a high mortality rate (Ungerleider, 1998). Simultaneously, the anesthesiologist should begin optimizing hemodynamics and interpreting monitored data to appropriately treat physiologic abnormalities. Echocardiography is helpful in assessing right ventricular and left ventricular function and evaluating PA pressure. A supplemental assessment of cardiac function performed in the operating room is an intraoperative "cardiac catheterization." This is done to assess isolated pressure measurements from the various chambers of the heart; catheter pull-back measurements are used to evaluate residual pressure gradients across valves, repaired sites of stenosis and conduits; and oxygen saturation data to look for residual shunts and assess cardiac output (SvO_2) (Gold et al., 1986). In combination with TEE, a complete intraoperative "picture" of a structural and functional evaluation of the postoperative cardiac repair can be obtained (Gold et al., 1986; Ungerleider et al., 1989a, 1989b; Muhiudeen et al., 1991, 1992; Stevenson et al., 1993). If structural abnormalities are found, the patient can be

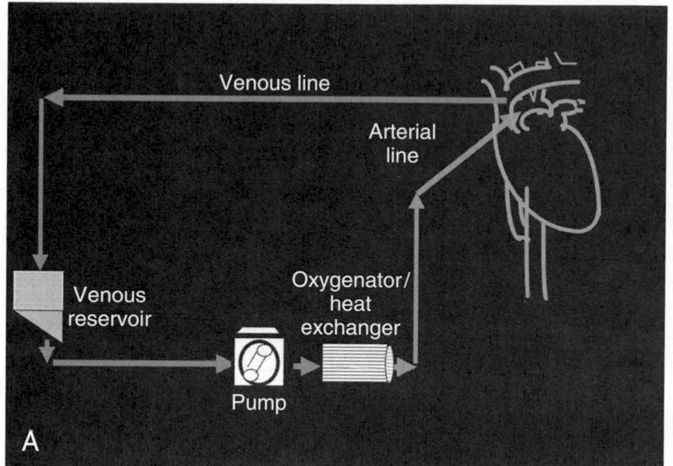

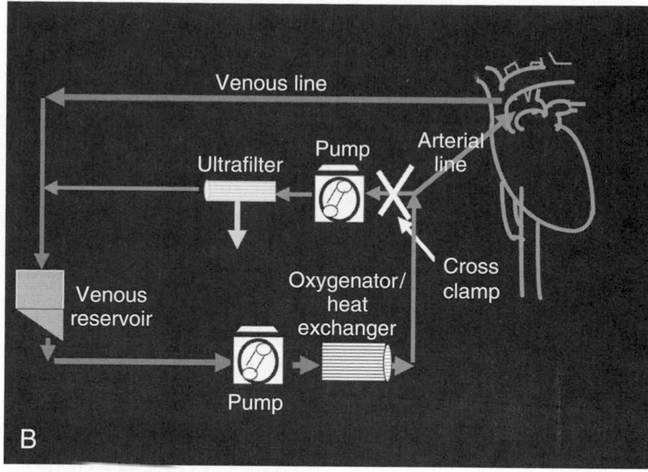

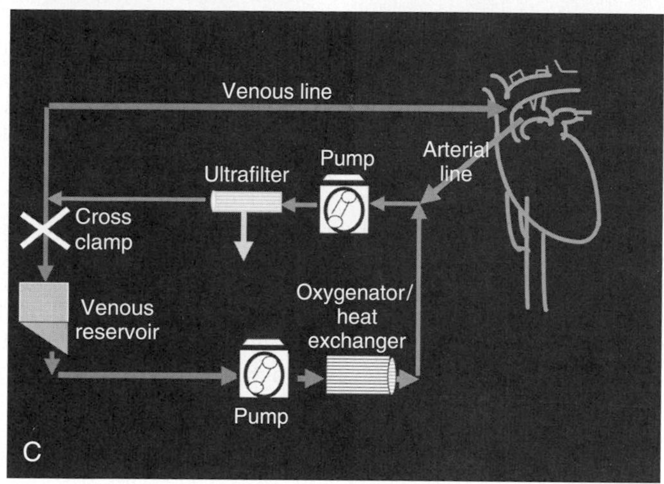

■ **FIGURE 17–11.** *(A)* Schematic of cardiopulmonary bypass (CPB). *(B)* Schematic of CPB with modified ultrafiltration (MUF) in line but clamped out of circuit. *(C)* Schematic of CPB with MUF in progress. After weaning from CPB, the MUF circuit is opened by removing the clamp from the ultrafiltration portion of the circuit and placing a clamp above the venous reservoir. The roller pump of the MUF circuit is turned on, and pulls approximately 5% to 10% of total cardiac output from the arterial cannula. The blood is pumped through the ultrafilter, fluid and mediators are removed in the ultrafiltrate, and blood is returned to the patient's circulation through the venous cannula. A cross-clamp is placed above the venous reservoir to prevent additional blood from entering the reservoir. If intravascular volume falls, blood can be added to the circuit at the venous reservoir and returned to the patient through the traditional portion of the bypass circuit.

placed back on CPB and residual defects can be repaired before leaving the operating room. Leaving the operating room with a significant residual structural defect adversely increases patient morbidity and affects survival (Goldet al., 1986; Ungerleider et al., 1989a, 1989b; Muhiudeen et al., 1990, 1991, 1992). Functional problems such as ventricular dysfunction may also be identified with echocardiography. Once diagnosed, therapy can be directed to the specific problem.

Modified Ultrafiltration

The use of modified ultrafiltration (MUF) after weaning from CPB has been advocated by a number of centers as a mechanism for removing inflammatory mediators, pulmonary vasoconstrictors, and excessive fluid at the end of CPB (Naik et al., 1991; Ungerleider, 1998; Hiramatsu et al., 2002). Animal and human studies using MUF have shown a consistent improvement in lung compliance, cerebral metabolic recovery, dilutional coagulopathy, hematocrit, and myocardial function (Skaryak et al., 1995; Keenan et al., 2000; Ootaki et al., 2002). Although long-term hemodynamic benefits have not been demonstrated, the acute improvement may reduce the need for more extraordinary support such as leaving the chest open or the institution of extracorporeal membrane oxygenation or ventricular assist device support in more marginal postbypass patients (Fig. 17–11).

■ MANAGEMENT STRATEGIES AFTER WEANING FROM CARDIOPULMONARY BYPASS

In this section on management strategies after weaning from CPB, we first discuss functional abnormalities common to all neonates, infants, and children after reparative or palliative operations for CHD. These include PA hypertension, right ventricular dysfunction, and left ventricular dysfunction. With this as background, approaches to specific congenital cardiac defects are noted. Because recognizing residual anatomic defects is an important part of the management of congenital heart patients who are difficult to wean from CPB, anesthesiologists must understand the repair and be cognizant of potential structural defects that may persist or become apparent after reconstructive heart surgery. The type, extent, and tolerance of residual cardiac defects are dependent on the method of repair and on whether the operation results in a complete anatomic and physiologic correction using the patient's native tissue, an anatomic and physiologic repair requiring artificial material to provide normal blood flow patterns (for children who are missing cardiac structures and require artificial material such as a conduit or a baffle), or a palliative operation necessitated by missing or diminutive ventricular chambers.

In patients receiving an anatomic and physiologic correction, residual defects are less common and occur at obvious locations. Because blood flow patterns are normal, mild to moderate anatomic defects are better tolerated in the postoperative period.

Patients who receive an anatomic and physiologic reconstruction but require prosthetic material to restore normal blood flow patterns are more likely to have anatomic problems because of the interposition of artificial material within the heart or great vessels. Residual anatomic defects are somewhat less well tolerated in this group due to the abnormal loading conditions that existed in the prerepair period and because extracardiac conduits may be positioned in a location that differs from the natural location of the great vessel it replaces. This reduces the efficiency of ventricular ejection.

In patients who have only a single ventricle and require palliative surgery, reconstruction is based first on having the single ventricle provide balanced blood flow to both the pulmonary and systemic circulation. A second procedure (or series of procedures) uses the single ventricle as a systemic ventricle. PBF is provided by channeling all of the systemic venous return directly to the PAs. PBF is maintained by a passive gradient from the systemic veins through the lungs and into the LA. This procedure known as the modified Fontan procedure is now widely applied to a variety of anatomic variants of single ventricle (Fontan et al., 1983). These patients are intolerant of residual anatomic gradients, regurgitant valves, and arrhythmias. They are also less responsive to physiologic problems after weaning from CPB.

PULMONARY ARTERY HYPERTENSION

Patients with elevated PVR are also quite sensitive to blood volume changes. A patient with PA hypertension has an increased right ventricular afterload. This may result in worsening right ventricular function. Under this circumstance, right ventricular end-systolic and diastolic volumes and pressures increase, resulting in a volume- and pressure-loaded RV. Increases in right ventricular pressure decrease coronary perfusion pressure to the RV, resulting in right ventricular ischemia. In addition, the volume-underloaded LV has decreased filling due to septal shift, resulting in decreased left ventricular stroke volume. Systemic perfusion is therefore quite dependent on left atrial preload, which requires a reduction in PVR to allow effective filling. Systemic hypotension may further affect right ventricular function by reducing coronary perfusion pressure.

Ventilation Strategies

Therapy for elevated PA pressures is aimed at lowering PVR and unloading the RV. Reductions in PVR are accomplished by altering ventilation, increasing inspired oxygen concentration, optimizing lung volumes, and using alkalinization, adequate sedation, nitric oxide, milrinone, occasionally α-blockers, and catecholamines.

Drummond and others (1981) showed that reducing $PaCO_2$ and increasing pH produces a consistent and reproducible reduction in PVR in infants with PA hypertension. Manipulating serum bicarbonate levels to achieve a pH between 7.5 and 7.6, while maintaining a $PaCO_2$ of 40 mm Hg, has equal salutary effects on PVR (Malik and Kidd, 1973; Lyrene et al., 1985). The increases in both arteriolar PO_2 and alveolar PO_2 decrease PVR. With intracardiac shunts, changes in FIO_2 have little effect on the PaO_2. Thus, by inference, a reduction in PVR induced by increasing the inspired oxygen concentration probably is a direct pulmonary vasodilatory effect of P_AO_2 rather than PaO_2. Experimental work by Custer and Hales (1985) showed that increased FIO_2 is a more potent vasodilator in neonatal than in adult animals. Similarly, an increase in FIO_2 has a vasodilatory effect on the pulmonary vascular bed of children with VSDs in the cardiac catheterization laboratory (Lock et al., 1982). Ventilatory mechanics also play a major role in reducing PVR (Nelson, 1966; Zapletal et al., 1976; Fagan, 1977). Newborns and infants have a high closing volume that is near functional residual capacity; therefore, at the end of a normal breath, some airway closure occurs (Mansell and Bryan, 1972). This process results in areas of lung that are perfused and unventilated. As these lung segments become increasingly hypoxemic, a secondary hypoxic vasoconstriction occurs (Rudolph and Yuan, 1966). The net effect is an increase in PVR. Careful inflation of the lungs to maintain functional residual capacity is beneficial to reduce PVR. In practice, because of increased anesthesia ventilator tubing compliance and endotracheal tube leaks, this may require a relatively large set tidal volume and the addition of 5 cm H_2O positive end-expiratory pressure (PEEP). After bypass, there is generally a reduction in lung compliance of approximately 20% in neonates; a higher pressure is necessary to achieve the same delivered tidal volume in most neonates.

In neonates with rapid heart rates, right ventricular output can be impaired by extending the inspiratory time beyond two cardiac cycles. With a more prolonged inspiratory time, a third consecutive heartbeat during inspiration has a marked reduction in the right ventricular stroke volume. Because PBF occurs predominantly during the expiratory phase of the respiratory cycle, the ventilatory pattern should be adjusted to allow an adequate distribution of gas throughout the lung during inspiration and a more prolonged expiratory phase to promote blood flow through the lungs.

End-expiratory pressure must be applied cautiously in patients with CHD. Low levels of PEEP (3 to 5 mm Hg) prevent narrowing of the capillary and precapillary blood vessels and reduce PVR (Kirklin et al., 1983; Taeed et al., 2001). Higher levels of PEEP or excessive mean airway pressure results in alveolar overdistention and compression of the capillary network in the alveolar wall and interstitium. This latter circumstance causes elevated PVR and reduced PBF (Jenkins et al., 1985).

The final and perhaps the least well recognized use of mechanical ventilation is to assist in unloading of the RV. During inspiration, intrathoracic pressure increases. Inspiration may therefore assist right ventricular systole by creating an increased pressure gradient from the lung to the LA. This ventilatory assist is commonly seen in patients with PA hypertension or right ventricular dysfunction. Typically, an augmentation of the arterial pressure trace during inspiration is seen. This concept is very similar to the thoracic pump mechanism of CPR (Weisfeldt and Halperin, 1986). The inspiratory assist must be balanced by the potential negative effects of increased mean airway pressure on PVR, that is, RV afterload. To maximize these cardiopulmonary interactions, inspiratory time should be limited to a time of two or fewer heartbeats, and mean airway pressure should be maintained at the lowest level possible to maintain effective lung volumes and functional residual capacity (FRC).

High-frequency jet ventilation (HFJV) is an uncommonly applied alternative mode of ventilation that has been successfully used in infants with pulmonary hypertension. HFJV eliminates CO_2 very efficiently and does so at a lower mean airway pressure. In patients with elevated PA pressure, HFJV reduces PVR and right ventricular afterload. The benefit of a reduced RV afterload occurs at a reduced airway pressure. For example, in postoperative Fontan patients whose cardiac output is directly linked to PVR and mean airway pressure, HFJV significantly decreases mean airway pressure, reduces PVR, and increases cardiac index (Andrew et al., 1987; Dietrich et al., 1993).

Another mode of ventilation, high-frequency oscillatory ventilation has been advocated for newborns with persistent pulmonary hypertension. It is an effective alternative mode of ventilation, but it may be poorly tolerated in the face of secondary right ventricular dysfunction as the high mean airway pressures required with this mode contribute to a right ventricular afterload and reduced right ventricular preload. If used, preload augmentation is required.

Pharmacology Strategies

Attempts to selectively manipulate PVR through pharmacologic interventions have been less than satisfying. Drugs that have shown the greatest promise both clinically and experimentally have been the phosphodiesterase inhibitors and NO.

Phosphodiesterase inhibitors, which have been used clinically and experimentally in treating elevations in PVR, include milrinone, enoximone, and amrinone. Some investigations have shown a reduction in PVR and SVR and an increase in right ventricular contractility (Henriksson et al., 1979; Colon-Otero et al., 1987; Vieira et al., 1991). Phosphodiesterase inhibitors have varying effects on cAMP and cyclic guanosine monophosphate (cGMP). cGMP is a more important mediator of pulmonary vascular smooth muscle. Amrinone, which is less commonly used today, has a more prominent effect on increasing cAMP than cGMP. It has a profound effect on SVR. Significant systemic hypotension may be seen with an amrinone loading dose. For this reason, milrinone has become the drug of choice for PA hypertension; it has a more prominent effect on cGMP, which results in pulmonary vascular relaxation. These variations in effect suggest adrenergic receptor subtypes may exist for phosphodiesterase type III inhibitors. In children, milrinone has been found to decrease SVR by 37% and PVR by 27% (Chang et al., 1995). Compared with catecholamines, milrinone has not been found to increase myocardial oxygen consumption (Chang et al., 1995). Milrinone also appears to have inotropic and lusitropic properties.

Nitric oxide (NO) is an endothelium-derived vasodilator of smooth muscle. The enzyme, nitric oxide synthase, converts L-arginine into NO and citrulline. NO diffuses across the endothelial cell to the adjacent smooth muscle, where it activates guanylate cyclase. The enzyme guanylate cyclase increases the production of cGMP. cGMP causes smooth muscle relaxation by preventing the release of calcium from the SR, thereby inhibiting muscle contraction. When NO diffuses into the intravascular space, it immediately binds with hemoglobin to form nitrosylhemoglobin, which is oxidized to methemoglobin. Methemoglobin is subsequently reduced to nitrates and nitrites and is excreted in the urine. The clinical importance of NO lies in the fact that it can be administered as an inhaled gas and delivered directly to the pulmonary vascular bed in contact with ventilating alveoli. The close proximity of the alveolus and the pulmonary vascular smooth muscle allows a direct effect of NO on pulmonary vascular smooth muscle. Because of the rapid binding and inactivation of NO by hemoglobin, minimal or no systemic effects occur. NO has been shown to bind 280 times faster to hemoglobin than carbon monoxide, which may explain why the systemic circulation is protected from its vasodilating properties. Clinically, reduction in PVR has been demonstrated in adult patients with mitral valve stenosis, in neonates with persistent pulmonary hypertension, and in children with reactive pulmonary hypertension after congenital heart surgery (Jobes and Nicolson, 1988; Girard et al., 1991; Horkay et al., 1992; Kern et al., 1992b; Roberts et al., 1993b; Wessel et al., 1997). Experience with NO in the operating room has shown it to be beneficial, although the degree of reduction in PVR is usually not as dramatic as initially hoped. NO is in general part of a group of therapies aimed at reducing PVR (Bender et al., 1997; Lillehei et al., 1999).

Sildenafil causes smooth muscle relaxation through the release of NO. Intravenous sildenafil has been shown to augment the pulmonary vasodilator effects of NO in infants early after cardiac surgery. However, sildenafil produced systemic hypotension and impaired oxygenation (Stocker et al., 2003). Oral sildenafil is undergoing safety and efficacy trials for primary pulmonary hypertension and chronic pulmonary hypertension. It has been shown to be as efficacious as NO in patients with a reactive component to chronic pulmonary hypertension (Michelakis et al., 2002). Sildenafil along with dyperidimole (which works through a cGMP mechanism) has been used to wean patients off NO.

Isoproterenol, a β_1- and β_2-adrenergic agonist, has mild PA vasodilating properties in the normal pulmonary circulation (Jobes et al., 1992). It causes mild PVR reduction in adult patients after cardiac transplant surgery, but there are minimal data supporting the efficacy of isoproterenol in treating PA hypertension in infants and young children after weaning from CPB. The minimal responsiveness of isoproterenol in treating PA hypertension is further complicated by the undesirable side effects of isoproterenol. Isoproterenol causes tachycardia, systemic vasodilation, and an increase in myocardial oxygen consumption (Harker, 1986). These effects may reduce coronary perfusion and result in myocardial ischemia. This may be especially problematic for the RV, which has to eject against a high PVR, with decreased coronary perfusion pressure and filling time.

PGE_1 and PGI_2 have a pulmonary vasodilating effect, but neither drug has effects that are limited to the pulmonary circulation (Woodman and Harker, 1990). Although PGE_1 has been used to treat pulmonary hypertensive crisis with varying degrees of success in newborns with persistent pulmonary hypertension, its beneficial effect following CPB is inconsistent. In addition, systemic vasodilation remains a common side effect, often requiring an inotropic infusion to maintain blood pressure. PGI_2 infusions have been used with some success in Europe (Saltzman et al., 1986). A report by Bush and others (1987) describes the successful use of PGI_2 in preventing pulmonary hypertensive crisis in five patients with congenital heart defects. Prostacyclin is currently investigational in the United States. Using a piglet model, Wauthy and others (2003) found NO to be a greater pulmonary vasodilator than prostacyclin.

Similar to NO are ultrashort-acting intravenous vasodilators. Ultrashort-acting intravenous vasodilators are nonspecific potent vasodilators with a half-life measured in seconds. Infusion of these drugs into the right side of the circulation produces a potent short-lived relaxation of PA smooth muscle. Once the drug reaches the systemic circulation, it is no longer functional. Adenosine and ATP-like compounds have these properties and may have clinical applicability in the treatment of PA hypertension (Horrow et al., 1990). Ng and others (2004) showed the vasodilatory properties of 50 mcg/kg per minute adenosine infusion together with 20 ppm of inhaled NO in newborns with persistent pulmonary hypertension.

Anesthesia Strategies

Reactive pulmonary vascular responses can be attenuated by increasing the depth of anesthesia (Hickey and Hansen, 1984, 1985a; Anand et al., 1990; Horrow et al., 1990). Opioid-based anesthetic regimens prevent sympathetic-mediated increases in PVR (Hickey and Hansen, 1984, 1985a). A continuous infusion of fentanyl, sufentanil, or combination of fentanyl/sufentanil plus midazolam may be particularly useful in patients who are prone to develop labile PA hypertension.

A study in newborn infants demonstrated that reactive pulmonary responses to endotracheal suction in the postoperative period can be minimized by the prior administration of fentanyl (Hickey et al., 1985). Because fentanyl does not block the effects of hypoxic pulmonary vasoconstriction, its effect is most likely due to the attenuated release of sympathomimetic mediators, which produce a direct vasoconstrictive effect on pulmonary arterial smooth muscle through cAMP and calcium release (Greeley et al., 1988; Anand et al., 1990).

RIGHT VENTRICULAR DYSFUNCTION

Primary right ventricular dysfunction is a common finding in neonates, infants, and children undergoing cardiac surgery. Hypertrophied RV in tetralogy of Fallot, surgically induced right ventricular dysfunction due to closure of a VSD through a right ventriculotomy, and the placement of a transannular patch across the right ventricular outflow tract (RVOT), causing acute pulmonary regurgitation and right ventricular volume overload, may present with right ventricular dysfunction after weaning from CPB in CHD patients (Friedman, 1972; Perloff, 1982; Berner et al., 1983; Hines and Barash, 1987).

The treatment of right ventricular dysfunction consists of increasing coronary perfusion pressure, preload augmentation (while avoiding marked increases in right ventricular end-diastolic pressure) (Friedman, 1972), and inotropic support with dopamine, epinephrine, and milrinone (Berner et al., 1983; Hines and Barash, 1987; McGovern et al., 2000; Hoffman et al., 2003). Mechanical ventilation should be adjusted to assist right ventricular function and minimize elevation in PVR.

In contrast to the LV, the low-pressure RV receives coronary blood flow during ventricular systole (Berne and Levy, 1981). In patients with right ventricular dysfunction, maintaining a normal to slightly elevated systolic pressure enhances coronary perfusion to the RV and augments contractility. Infusion of drugs such as dopamine and epinephrine, as well as intermittent doses of calcium and Neo-Synephrine (phenylephrine HCl), may be helpful in augmenting right ventricular perfusion pressure. If an increase in inotropic support persists, and frequent supplemental doses of calcium or Neo-Synephrine are required after weaning from CPB, a critical evaluation for other structural and/or functional abnormalities should be aggressively pursued. McGovern (2000)

TABLE 17–12. Effects of exogenous catecholamines on right ventricular injury

	Qp	PAP	PVR/Rin	TVE	PRSW
Dopamine	↑	No Δ	No Δ/no Δ	↓	↑
Dobutamine	↑	No Δ	↓/↓	No Δ	↑
Epinephrine	↑	↓	↓/↓	↑	↑

↑, Increase; ↓, decrease; No Δ, no change; PVR, pulmonary vascular resistance; TVE; transpulmonary vascular efficiency defined as measure of the ease of blood flow through the lungs; PRSW, load-independent measure of ventricular contraction; PAP, pulmonary artery pressure; Rin, intrinsic resistance.
(The key to this table is that only epinephrine improved the efficiency of moving blood through the lungs.)
(From McGovern JJ, Cheifertz IM, et al.: Right ventricular injury in young swine: Effects of catecholamines on right ventricular function and pulmonary vascular mechanics. *Pediatr Res* 48:763–769, 2000.)

reported the effects of dopamine, dobutamine, and epinephrine in a sophisticated piglet model of right ventricular dysfunction. In this model, epinephrine was the only inotropic agent to increase right ventricular contractility and reduce right ventricular afterload, suggesting that epinephrine may be the preferred inotropic agent in patients with right ventricular dysfunction (Table 17–12).

Preload should be maintained at a normal to slightly elevated level. Because right ventricular contractility is reduced, it is important to increase preload to optimize stroke volume as seen in Starling curve (Friedman, 1972). Excessive volume loading, however, is not well tolerated due to ventricular noncompliance. Excessive volume loading may result in elevated end-diastolic pressure, significant tricuspid regurgitation, and impaired forward flow. In general, a central venous pressure above 10 to 14 mm Hg is poorly tolerated in neonates and infants with right ventricular dysfunction unless the RV has marked hypertrophy and poor compliance (Rudolph, 1985).

If right ventricular dysfunction persists or worsens due to elevations in PA pressure or a low cardiac output state persists despite aggressive ventilatory and inotropic support, the surgical creation of a right-to-left shunt at the atrial level may significantly improve oxygen delivery. Typical patients who would benefit from this strategy include those undergoing neonatal repairs for tetralogy of Fallot and truncus arteriosus. In these patients, allowing an atrial communication to remain open with blood shunting in a right-to-left direction preserves cardiac output and oxygen delivery to the systemic circulation. Although these patients may remain cyanotic, their effective cardiac output is enhanced, systemic perfusion pressure is improved, and coronary perfusion to the RV is maintained. Over time, right ventricular pressure decreases, right-to-left shunting decreases, and systemic oxygen saturation improves. This same strategy of leaving an atrial communication to improve cardiac output has been extended to children with single-ventricle physiology through the fenestrated Fontan.

An additional strategy in neonates, infants, and children with significant postoperative right ventricular dysfunction is to leave the sternum open but covered with a Silastic membrane (Pearl et al., 1991). If mild ventricular distention has occurred and lung compliance is poor, eliminating the impedance imposed by the chest wall allows the lung to inflate at a lower mean airway pressure, decreasing right ventricular afterload. In addition, by reducing intrathoracic pressure, the right ventricular end-diastolic volume can increase at a lower end-diastolic pressure.

If right ventricular dysfunction persists despite these maneuvers, consideration should be given to extracorporeal life support (extracorporeal membrane oxygenation [ECMO]). When ECMO is used for circulatory support, venoarterial cannulation is chosen. Venovenous bypass provides gas exchange but does not provide cardiac output support. Venous and arterial access may be achieved through a large central artery and vein (usually the carotid and internal jugular) or by direct chest cannulation, a more common approach used in the operating room. Recovery from severe ventricular dysfunction is predicated on the concept that the myocardium sustained a transient injury and is capable of recovery with time, that is, *stunned myocardium* (Dietrich et al., 1989, 1990, 1991; Darling et al., 2001). ECMO is used to decrease ventricular wall tension, increase coronary perfusion pressure, and maintain systemic perfusion with oxygenated blood; the role of ECMO in patients with myocardial injury or pulmonary hypertension is to provide adequate systemic oxygen transport and systemic perfusion, while allowing the ventricle to "rest."

In patients without lung disease, reports of successfully using ECMO without the oxygenator has also been suggested as a way to use the ECMO system as a ventricular assist device and reduce the need for heparin in the immediate postbypass system (Darling et al., 2001). Theoretically, ECMO provides adequate systemic and coronary oxygen transport while reducing myocardial oxygen demand. This favorable shift in the oxygen supply/demand ratio may allow the heart to recover from reversible myocardial failure. In a review from the ECMO registry of all patients placed on ECMO for circulatory support, patients with tetralogy of Fallot, tetralogy-like physiology, or PA hypertension had the greatest likelihood of weaning from ECMO (Dietrich et al., 1993). Sixty-one percent of patients in this category were successfully weaned from mechanical support. This suggests that myocardial injury due to severe hypertrophy or PA hypertension may result in an ischemic ventricle that with extended rest, coronary reperfusion, and reduced right ventricular afterload will significantly recover function (Dietrich et al., 1993). For those patients placed on ECMO for left ventricular dysfunction, successful outcome is less common. Box 17–3 outlines a management strategy for patients with PA hypertension with right ventricular dysfunction. With use of technology derived from the operating room, ECMO circuits that used heparin-coated oxygenators and tubing have allowed the initiation and maintenance of ECMO without the administration of systemic heparin for periods of 8 to 24 hours. This is particularly beneficial in patients with significant postoperative coagulopathy or in the presence of central nervous system hemorrhage after placing the patient on ECMO. Nishinaka and others (2002) demonstrated that these heparin-coated circuits allowed for 34 days of ECMO without the need for systemic anticoagulants.

BOX 17–3 Management Strategy for Pulmonary Artery Hypertension With Right Ventricular Dysfunction

Diagnosis: Decreased oxygen delivery caused by pulmonary hypertension and decreased right ventricular cardiac output

First: Rule out residual anatomic defects or anaphylaxis.

Treatment: Decrease right ventricular afterload and improve right ventricular function.

Ventilatory Strategy

1. Increase alveolar and arterial oxygen.
2. Perform alkalinization (pH > 7.5).
3. Decrease $Paco_2$ (35 to 40 mm Hg).
4. Decrease mean airway pressure.

Pharmacologic Therapy

Optimize Coronary Perfusion.

1. Calcium
2. Phenylephrine or ?vasopressin
3. Dopamine
4. Epinephrine

Reduce Pulmonary Vascular Resistance/Right Ventricular Afterload.

1. Adequate anesthesia
2. Milrinone, amrinone
3. Nitric oxide
4. Sildenafil, prostacyclin, or adenosine possibly helpful

Surgical Interventions

1. Create atrial septal defect
2. Open chest

Additional Therapy

1. High-frequency jet or high-frequency oscillatory ventilation
2. Extracorporeal membrane oxygenation/right ventricular assist device

LEFT VENTRICULAR DYSFUNCTION

Pharmacologic Support

The contractile state of the LV may be impaired after pediatric cardiac surgery. When left ventricular ischemia is present, the causes include surgery-induced ischemia during the repair, the preoperative condition of the myocardium (myocardial hypertrophy, elevated end-diastolic pressures), and the effects of cardiopulmonary bypass with deep hypothermia and/or circulatory arrest on myocardial compliance (Mullins, 1989; Hellenbrand et al., 1990; Dietrich et al., 1992). Factors further complicating left ventricular function after cardiac surgery are reduced myocardial reserve, limited recruitable stroke work, and reduced compliance characteristic of the immature neonatal heart.

Left ventricular dysfunction can be treated by optimizing preload, increasing heart rate, increasing coronary perfusion pressure, correcting ionized calcium levels, and adding inotropic support. In the neonate, a greater dependence on heart rate, a reduction in myocardial compliance, and a diminished response to calcium and catecholamines must be considered. Inotropic support usually begins with dopamine (5 to 15 mcg/kg/minute) (Box 17–4).

Dopamine

Dopamine has the unique property of binding to dopaminergic receptors in the renal and mesenteric beds and improving perfusion to the gut and the kidneys. Dopamine augments cardiac contractility through two mechanisms: a direct stimulation of β_1-receptors in the heart and, more important, inducing norepinephrine release from sympathetic nerve endings (Lock et al., 1989). Several studies suggest that the effect of dopamine in children is age dependent. In young children after cardiac surgery,

BOX 17–4 Management Strategy for Left Ventricular Dysfunction

Diagnosis: Decreased oxygen delivery due to left ventricular dysfunction
First: Rule out residual anatomic defect.
Treatment: Optimize cardiac output (preload, contractility, and heart rate) and reduce afterload.

Optimize preload.

1. Measure right and left atrial pressures.
2. Maintain left atrial pressure at 8 to 12 mm Hg.
3. Shorten inspiratory times to augment left ventricular filling.

Augment cardiac output.

1. Optimize heart rate (A, AV sequential, or V pacing).
2. Inotropic support (dopamine, epinephrine, milrinone, dobutamine)
3. Calcium supplementation

Reduce afterload.

1. Milrinone, amrinone
2. Nitroprusside
3. Nicardipine

Reevaluate anatomic problems.

1. Transesophageal echocardiography
2. Intraoperative catheterization

Provide left ventricular mechanical support.

1. Extracorporeal membrane oxygenation/left ventricular assist device

dopamine increases cardiac output, and this effect correlates more with an elevation in heart rate than augmentation of stroke volume (Malviya et al., 1989; Hickey et al., 1992). In young adult patients, dopamine clearly increases stroke volume (Rothman et al., 1990). Nonetheless, infants and neonates respond favorably to dopamine infusion with an increase in systemic blood pressure and improved peripheral and renal perfusion. At higher doses, dopamine is converted to norepinephrine and acts as a combined β/α agonist.

Calcium

Calcium supplementation is also important in augmenting cardiac contractility. Although calcium has fallen into some disfavor due to concerns over reperfusion injury, calcium supplementation remains an important therapy after pediatric cardiac surgery. In particular, the underdeveloped SR in neonatal myocardium makes the neonatal heart more dependent on extracellular calcium concentrations than the adult myocardium (Okada et al., 1988). Because intracellular calcium concentration plays a central role in myocardial contractility, normal or even an elevated plasma level of ionized calcium may be necessary to augment stroke volume (Nakanishi et al., 1987). In addition, fluctuations in ionized calcium levels occur commonly after weaning from CPB. This effect is most often due to the relatively large transfusions of citrate and albumin-rich blood products such as whole blood, fresh frozen plasma (FFP), platelets, and cryoprecipitate necessary to promote postoperative hemostasis (Rebeyka et al., 1990). Routine monitoring of ionized calcium levels and regular calcium supplementation is helpful after weaning from CPB. This is especially true in patients with diminished left ventricular function. In patients with a slow sinus or junctional rate, calcium must be administered cautiously, as marked slowing of atrioventricular conduction may occur.

Epinephrine

Epinephrine is a potent α-, β_1-, and β_2-adrenergic agonist. In lower dosages of 0.03 to 0.1 mcg/kg per minute, β-mediated responses predominate. Dosages of 0.1 to 0.2 mcg/kg per minute have a mixed α/β effect; above 0.2 mcg/kg per minute, α-mediated responses predominate. Epinephrine is useful in patients with significant left ventricular dysfunction after cardiac repair who remain hypotensive or hypoperfused based on poor systemic perfusion or rising serum lactates (Bohn et al., 1980). It is effective in patients who do not respond to equivalent doses of dopamine or dobutamine, and it is particularly useful in patients with mild to moderate degrees of hypotension and echocardiographic or electrocardiographic evidence of ischemia.

Milrinone

Milrinone, enoximone, and amrinone are nonglycoside, noncatecholamine inotropic drugs. Their mechanism of action is mediated through the inhibition of phosphodiesterase type III (Henriksson et al., 1979; Colon-Otero et al., 1987; Vieira et al., 1991). Clinical studies addressing the use of phosphodiesterase III inhibitors in pediatric patients are limited. However, reports in neonates and young infants have shown a considerable benefit from the phosphodiesterase inhibitors, especially in patients whose myocardium is afterload sensitive, such as the postoperative arterial switch patient and the patient unresponsive to catecholamines (Vieira et al., 1991; Chang, 1995).

The optimal therapeutic plasma concentration of milrinone is 100 to 300 ng/mL (Levy et al., 2002). The Prophylactic Intravenous Use of Milrinone After Cardiac Operation in Pediatrics (PRIMACORP) study reported that a 50 mcg/kg intravenous loading dose followed by high-dose milrinone 0.75 to 1.0 mcg/kg per minute was safe and significantly decreased the risk of low cardiac output syndrome in this surgical population group (Hoffman et al., 2003). Milrinone has become an important agent to optimize left ventricular cardiac output in pediatric cardiac patients weaning from CPB. Bypass tends to increase SVR, and the combined inotropic, lusitropic, and afterload reduction of milrinone has been efficacious in treating left ventricular dysfunction after CPB. The loading dose is often administered in the operating room while the patient is on CPB.

Pharmacokinetic studies suggest that the loading dose for amrinone in children is twice the recommended adult dose (2 to 4.5 mg/kg) (Lawless et al., 1988). In clinical practice, however, amrinone in loading doses of 2 mg/kg and infusion rates of 10 to 15 mcg/kg per minute are very useful in the management of low cardiac output states in neonates, infants, and children. A higher dose (3 to 4 mg/kg) has been associated with profound systemic vasodilation in the postoperative cardiac patient. Because the onset of peripheral vasodilation precedes the increase in inotropy during the loading phase, a significant reduction in afterload and hypotension may occur if the dose is administered too quickly. This effect, coupled with its prolonged elimination half-life (approximately 3 to 15 hours), necessitates extreme caution when administering a loading dose of amrinone to children with borderline low blood pressure. In the postoperative period, loading doses of amrinone and milrinone are administered over a 20- to 30-minute period. Milrinone produces less systemic hypotension and is generally better tolerated than amrinone.

Dobutamine

Dobutamine is an effective, albeit weaker, inotropic agent in children. It has much less peripheral α-adrenergic effect than dopamine, and its β_1-adrenergic effect predominates, yielding a mild peripheral vasodilation. Although reported to have less chronotropic effects than dopamine, in neonates significant tachyarrhythmias may occur. This may relate to structural similarities between dobutamine and isoproterenol (Bohn et al., 1980). In children after cardiac surgery, dobutamine increases cardiac output primarily through increases in heart rate. The efficacy of dobutamine seems to be reduced in immature animals (Rothman et al., 1990). This is consistent with the previous discussion of reduced β receptors and a higher level of circulating catecholamines in newborns (Bohn et al., 1980; Berner et al., 1983).

Vasopressin

Synthetic 8-L-arginine vasopressin (AVP), acting at V_1 receptors, is administered as a continuous infusion for refractory hypotension following CPB in adults and has been used in children, particularly those in sepsis. In one study, the dosage of AVP was adjusted for patient size and ranged from 0.0003 to 0.002 U/kg per minute. During the first hour of treatment with AVP, systolic blood pressure rose from 65 ± 14 to 87 ± 17 mm Hg ($P < .0001$; n = 11). Infants with refractory low blood pressure and adequate cardiac function may benefit from AVP administration after cardiac surgery (Rosenzweig et al., 1999). No prospective data on the use of vasopressin are available to dictate its use in congenital heart surgery, but it is being used as an alternative agent when catecholamine-induced dysrhythmias, such as junctional ectopic tachycardia and hypotension, are present. AVP is also being recommended for the treatment of cardiac arrest. Preliminary data from out-of-hospital prospective resuscitation trials suggest that AVP is superior to epinephrine. Vasopressin may prove superior to epinephrine as a pressor agent during prolonged cardiopulmonary resuscitation in children as well (Mann et al., 2002).

Assist Devices for Left Ventricle

Compared with traditional ECMO, ventricular assist devices (VADs) may be a preferred means of circulatory support for children who are unable to be weaned from CPB due to primary left ventricular dysfunction and for patients with acute cardiomyopathy or myocarditis. Reinhartz and others (2003) showed a 72% survival rate for children of less than 1.3 kg/m^2 (mean, 1.09 kg/m^2; range, 0.73 to 1.29 kg/m^2) body surface area (BSA) placed on Thoratec LVAD (Thoratec Corp, Pleasanton, CA) for 0 to 120 days (mean, 42 days) because of cardiomyopathy or myocarditis. In this study, only one of seven patients with CHD survived.

VADs allow direct control of left atrial filling pressure and therefore left ventricular end-diastolic pressure can be minimized, allowing for a greater likelihood of left ventricular recovery. The most widely used device is the centrifugal pump, in which blood is moved by its entrainment against spinning blades and cones; an example is the Biomedicus pump. Centrifugal pumps require direct heart cannulation. A left ventricular assist device (LVAD) requires a left atrial venous cannula and an aortic cannula. Wire-reinforced cannulas are preferred, because kinking can result in marked reduction in cardiac output and/or ventricular distention. The cannulas are secured in place and connected via polypropylene tubing to the ports on the pump head. Long-term outcomes seem to be related to the underlying cardiac condition. The need for aortic cross-clamping before the patient is put on an LVAD has a negative impact on outcome (Schindler et al., 2003).

When the LVAD is activated, the flow rates are increased until the patient is completely weaned from CPB and the LVAD is providing full circulatory support. Left and right atrial monitoring catheters are strongly recommended during LVAD use. Because there is no venous reservoir in the centrifugal pump system, pressure monitoring is essential to ensure adequate intravascular volume to sustain pump flow rates and prevent pumping air. Low left atrial pressures may result from hypovolemia or right ventricular failure. A right atrial pressure monitor helps differentiate volume problems from right ventricular dysfunction. If right atrial pressures are high and left ventricular filling pressures are low, significant right ventricular failure is present and conversion to a biventricular assist device system or ECMO may be indicated. Box 17–4 outlines management strategies for left ventricular dysfunction.

■ SURGICAL PROCEDURES AND SPECIAL TECHNIQUES

The goals for congenital repair are the (1) physiologic separation of the pulmonary and systemic circulation, (2) relief of outflow obstruction, (3) preservation or restoration of ventricular mass and function, and (4) maintenance of the patient's quality of life and normalization of life expectancy. The available surgical procedures to accomplish these objectives are diverse and complex (Table 17–13). Compared with cardiac operations in adult patients, congenital heart repair involves more intracardiac surgery with a greater preponderance performed through the RA, RVOT, and left ventricular outflow tract (LVOT).

In general, operations performed for congenital heart defects can be divided into palliative and corrective procedures (Arciniegas, 1985). The type and timing of repair depend on the age of the patient, the specific anatomic defect, and the experience of the surgeon (see Table 17–13). Palliation in infancy is usually performed where there are missing anatomic parts such as in pulmonary atresia (absent RV and PA), tricuspid atresia (absent RV and tricuspid valve), HLHS (atretic or severely stenosed mitral and aortic valve and hypoplastic LV), univentricular heart (absent RV or LV), or mitral atresia (absent LV). These palliative procedures can be further subdivided into those that increase PBF, those that decrease PBF, and those that increase mixing. Palliative procedures that increase PBF include shunts (modified BT), outflow patch, or enlargement of the VSD. Those that decrease PBF include PA banding and ligation of a PDA. Those that improve intracardiac mixing include atrial septostomy or septectomy (balloon, blade, or Blalock-Hanlon).

With the improvements in surgical technique coupled with the advancements in anesthetic and technological support, repair in early infancy is more effective and has been the procedure of choice for many congenital cardiac defects (Castaneda et al., 1989). Neonatal repair is offered for a number of congenital heart defects (see Table 17–13), including total anomalous pulmonary venous return, interrupted aortic arch, and coarctation of the aorta, AS, PS, truncus arteriosus, and TGA. Atrioventricular septal defects (AVSDs) and tetralogy of Fallot are usually repaired in early infancy. In cases where pulmonary outflow obstruction

TABLE 17–13. Common congenital heart defects and surgical approaches

Anatomic Defect	Palliation	Complete Repair
Tetralogy of Fallot		VSD closure and RVOT patch
With PA atresia	Shunt	
With anomalous right coronary artery	Rastelli procedure	Patch above and below coronary artery
Hypoplastic left heart syndrome	Norwood followed by Fontan procedure	Transplantation
Transposition of the great arteries		Arterial switch
Unfavorable coronary anatomy	Atrial switch (Senning)	
Tricuspid atresia	Shunt followed by Fontan procedure	
Pulmonary atresia with VSD	Shunt followed by Fontan procedure	
With intact septum	Shunt followed by Fontan procedure	
Critical aortic or pulmonary stenosis		Valvotomy or catheterization laboratory balloon valvuloplasty
Interrupted aortic arch		End-to-end anastomosis
Total anomalous pulmonary venous return		Anastomosis pulmonary veins to left atrium and ASD closure
Single ventricle/normal PA	PA band followed by Fontan procedure	
With small PA	Shunt followed by Fontan procedure	
Truncus arteriosus		RV-PA conduit and VSD closure
Atrioventricular canal		Repair valve clefts/patch closure of ASD/attach valves to patch

ASD, atrial septal defect; PA, pulmonary artery; RV, right ventricle; RVOT, right ventricular outflow tract; VSD, ventricular septal defect.

is severe, tetralogy of Fallot requires neonatal repair. Repair in the neonatal period almost always requires a transannular patch, resulting in postoperative pulmonary insufficiency and a volume load on the previously pressure-loaded RV. Ventricular septal defects (VSDs) are not routinely closed in the newborn period, because many of these defects close on their own. Indications for early closure are usually related to unrelenting congestive heart failure despite medical management and impaired somatic growth. AVSDs are generally not repaired in infancy; patch closure and chordal reattachment are more readily performed in a larger heart. Occasionally, palliation is performed for some of these lesions in the newborn period with total correction later in life. Palliation is usually considered when closing the defect results in suboptimal chamber size, such as a patient with an unbalanced AVSD or with other severe congenital anomalies or when the patient is a poor candidate for CPB (birth asphyxia, intraventricular hemorrhage, etc.).

For well over a decade, the preferred approach to pediatric cardiovascular surgery has been to repair defects in infancy rather than to palliate (Castaneda et al., 1989). This trend is due to the increased morbidity and mortality associated with long-term medical management and the sequelae of multiple palliative operations. Early corrective surgery, if performed well, decreases the incidence of the chronic complications of CHD such as the problems associated with ventricular pressure or volume overload, cyanosis, and pulmonary vascular obstructive disease (Castaneda et al., 1989; Mahle et al., 2002). Complete repair, even in very low birth weight newborns weighing less than 1.5 kg, has been advocated by some (Reddy et al., 2000). In a series of 20 symptomatic low birth weight infants, early cardiac surgery with CPB resulted in an early infant mortality rate of 10%. At a median follow-up of 40 months, late mortality occurred in 5% and catheterization laboratory intervention was necessary in 25%. There was no evidence of intracranial hemorrhage after CPB. Although a higher surgical mortality rate was reported for low birth weight infants, prolonged medical management of these same patients generally purport a high morbidity and mortality (Reddy et al., 2000).

There may be a selective advantage of enhanced organ system protection during infant repair due to poorly understood factors promoting resistance to injury and enhanced recovery (i.e., enhanced organ plasticity and reserve) (Reddy et al., 1999). With the continued improvement in surgical techniques, bypass technology, interventional cardiology procedures, and the early treatment of CHD, specific organ systems such as the brain, heart, and lungs sustain less damage and may be spared the detrimental effects of chronic CHD and the effects of CPB.

Another trend observed in surgery for CHD is the continued evolution of new techniques to decrease long-term morbidity and enhance survival. For example, in the 1980s, the long-term problems with right ventricular dysfunction and failure associated with the Mustard and Senning procedures for repair of TGA encouraged many surgical groups to perform the arterial switch in the neonatal period as the procedure of choice (Castaneda et al., 1988). With the latter procedure, it was believed that a normal anatomic correction had better long-term results. A second example of the continuing evolution of technique is surgery for tetralogy of Fallot. Long-standing pulmonary insufficiency after right ventricular outflow repair for tetralogy of Fallot is associated with right ventricular dysfunction and failure. Preservation of the pulmonary valve at initial repair using a combined transatrial and transpulmonary approach during correction or the early insertion of a pulmonary homograft in the setting of pulmonary insufficiency is a technique that is used in the attempt to avoid the long-term problems of right ventricular dysfunction and failure (Pacifico et al., 1987).

Surgery for HLHS, once considered a fatal disease, has achieved significant long-term survival after a series of creative staging procedures initially described in the mid 1980s, and it achieved worldwide application by the early to mid 1990s (Norwood et al., 1991, 1992). Newer techniques evolved to minimize the morbidity of the Norwood procedure (Mahle et al., 2000), including the Sano modification (Sano et al., 2003). In this technique, first described by Imoto and others (2001), a conduit is sutured from the single RV to the PA instead of creating a shunt from the innominate artery to the PA. This modification preserves systemic diastolic blood pressure, and therefore coronary blood flow, in the postoperative period. Myocardial function improves, and both hemodynamics and end-organ perfusion appear better preserved in the early postoperative period (Mair et al., 2003; Pearl, 2003). Early pre-Glenn catheterization data have demonstrated a statistically significant finding of higher dP/dT (a measure of contractility) in the systemic ventricle after the Sano modification compared with the standard shunt approach (Mair et al., 2003). Studies of survivors of the Sano modification at 1 year after repair have found excellent outcomes that are comparable to those of the traditional modified BT shunt (Maher et al., 2003; Mahle et al., 2003; Mair et al., 2003; Pizarro et al., 2003, 2004; Sano et al., 2003). Also, the acute postoperative course may require less intensive management and patients may have improved mixed venous saturations. Long-term randomized outcome trials have been recommended to determine the risk of developing arrhythmias, the risk of thrombosis and infective endocarditis, and the long-term function of the single RV after a ventriculotomy incision in the systemic RV (Pearl, 2003).

Another interesting therapeutic option for the neonatal HLHS has been the use of a combined interventional cardiology and cardiac surgical approach. In the catheterization laboratory, an atrial septostomy is performed and a device is placed in the PA to restrict PBF. The patient is then taken to the operating room to have an innominate-to-PA shunt placed. Alternatively, a stent is placed in the ductus arteriosus in the catheterization laboratory. The combined interventional and operative approach to hypoplastic left heart surgery allows neonatal palliation to occur without the need of DHCA or bypass in many cases (Muller et al., 2003). The overall benefit is a reduced need for intensive care management and a reduced exposure to CPB. Innovations such as those outlined earlier continue to optimize the management of neonates with critical cardiac disease and reduce the long-term morbidity associated with palliative procedures and complex postoperative critical care management.

Other trends in surgical management include the broader application of surgical procedures initially designed for a specific defect. For example, the Fontan operation, which was originally devised for tricuspid atresia, has been used to repair complex univentricular hearts and HLHS (Gildein et al., 1990; Kopf et al., 1992). Attendant with this wider application of the Fontan operation for more complex defects once considered inoperable has been the rise in morbidity and mortality. Even this trend has been reversed in patients with higher-risk defects (Mayer et al., 1992).

In the early 1990s, the creation of a fenestration (or "hole") between the RA and LA at the time of the Fontan operation allowed right-to-left shunting, maintenance of cardiac output, and avoidance of ventricular failure in the early postoperative period. At a later time, once the patient has convalesced from the acute operative events, the fenestration was closed in the catheterization laboratory with an ASD closure device or, in some centers, at the bedside with a snare placed at the time of the operation. With the advent of a three-stage approach to the repair of single-ventricle patients, including a middle-stage procedure such as a bidirectional Glenn or hemi-Fontan, which allows the patient to maintain cardiac output by leaving the inferior vena cava (IVC) blood flow to return to the single ventricle and support cardiac output, the need for fenestration at the time of the Fontan procedure has been less. With the need for fenestration reduced, extracardiac conduits rather than intracardiac baffles with a fenestration (Kuroczynski et al., 2003) are used to complete the Fontan procedure. The long-term benefit of an extracardiac conduit reduces the exposure of the RA to high pressure and suture lines, of which both have been associated with an increased incidence of atrial arrhythmias (Fishberger et al., 1997; Kumar et al., 2003). The mortality and morbidity of atrial arrhythmias are significantly higher in the single-ventricle patient (Kumar et al., 2003).

Ingenuity, innovation, and continued refinement have permitted continued improvements in survival and quality of life for all patients with CHD. As the incisions in the myocardium become smaller, sutures are more precisely placed, and surgical techniques evolve, the complications of ventricular dysfunction, arrhythmias, and residual obstruction have declined and both life expectancy and life quality continue to improve.

One final difference unique to congenital heart surgery that has a major impact on anesthetic management relates to the type of cardiopulmonary support. Because of the complexity of repair in small patients, pediatric cardiac surgery involves operating at extreme biological conditions of temperature, hemodilution, and perfusion (Barratt-Boyes et al., 1971, 1980). Despite a long history of use, these techniques have pronounced physiologic effects on major organ system function and are far from understood with regard to long-term outcome.

COMPLETE ANATOMIC AND PHYSIOLOGIC REPAIRS

The postoperative management of the patient with a complete anatomic and physiologic correction is simplified because blood flow patterns after surgical correction are normal and, if an anatomic abnormality exists, the physiologic effect is more predictable and the location for the problem more obvious. Examples of complete anatomic repair include closure of an ASD or a VSD, repair of tetralogy of Fallot, and the arterial switch operation for TGA (see Table 17–13).

Atrial Septal Defects

Functional communications between the two atria are common congenital cardiac defects. ASDs are true defects, unlike a probe-patent PFO (which may be found in >20% of adults). ASDs comprise about 10% of all congenital anomalies in the pediatric population and are more common in females than in males (by 2:1). There are two main types: ostium secundum defects and ostium primum defects (Fig. 17–12). Secundum defects are the more common lesions and can be subdivided further into fossa ovalis defects, sinus venosus defects, and low ASDs. Fossa ovalis defects are located posteroinferiorly (midseptally) in the atrium, at the site of the fossa ovalis. Sinus venosus defects are located superiorly in the atrial septum at the opening of the SVC into the RA. This type is often associated with one or more pulmonary veins draining into the RA (partial anomalous pulmonary venous return). A low secundum ASD may, on occasion, have no inferior border. The defect is sitting over the entrance of the inferior vena cava into the RA (see Fig. 17–12). Some patients with ostium secundum defects have mitral valve prolapse (10%) or, very rarely, mitral stenosis (Lutembacher's syndrome).

Small septum secundum defects with PBF less than twice the systemic blood flow ($\dot{Q}p/\dot{Q}s < 1.5$ to 2) are well tolerated. Life expectancy is presumed to be normal, and symptoms are usually mild in childhood. In patients with a large septum secundum ($\dot{Q}p/\dot{Q}s > 2$), the PA pressure is normal or slightly increased, and the PVR remains normal. Systemic blood flow is usually slightly decreased because of impaired delivery of blood to the LV resulting from atrial shunting. If the ASDs are untreated, structural changes in the pulmonary vascular bed may occur over several decades and may result in pulmonary hypertension and congestive heart failure.

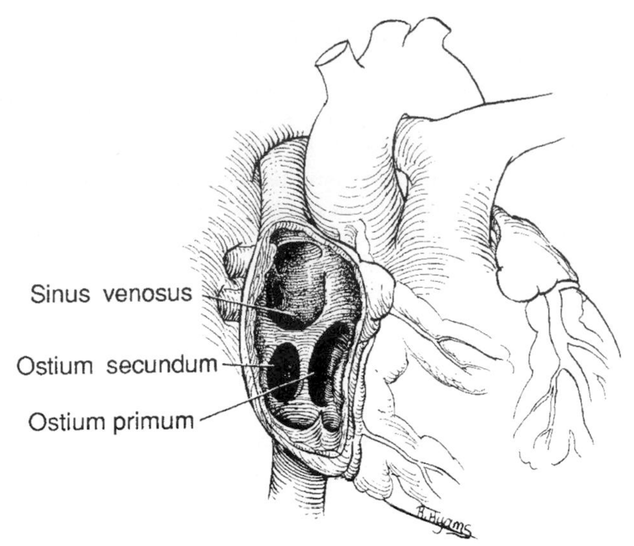

■ **FIGURE 17–12.** Drawing of interior of right atrium showing interatrial septum and position of three types of interatrial septal defects. (From Reed CC, Stafford TB, editors: *Cardiopulmonary bypass,* 2nd ed. Houston, 1985, Texas Medical Press, p 78.)

Because of the longstanding risks of pulmonary vascular disease, arrhythmias, and paradoxical emboli (especially in pregnant women), surgical repair is usually recommended. Surgery is usually performed in children between 2 and 5 years of age but may be done earlier in infants with ostium primum defects associated with mitral regurgitation and CHF.

ASDs are surgically repaired using CPB and patch closure if the defects are large. In addition, repair of the mitral or tricuspid valve or both may be required in patients with ostium primum defects. Primum defects usually have an associated cleft in the mitral valve, which requires suture closure. Surgical mortality is less than 1% in most centers, but the risk is increased in the presence of elevated PVR or congestive heart failure. Complications include complete heart block (<1%) and supraventricular arrhythmias. Residual mitral insufficiency may remain or even worsen in patients with ostium primum defects.

Total and Partial Anomalous Pulmonary Venous Connections

Anomalous pulmonary venous connection is a rare congenital heart defect that has a vast array of abnormalities. This condition occurs if one or more of the pulmonary veins connect to the RA. The physiologic result of the abnormal connections is abnormal return of the oxygenated pulmonary venous blood to the right side of the heart.

The anomalies of pulmonary venous connection are classified based on their anatomy and physiology (Hansen, 1985). If all of the pulmonary veins return to the RA, this condition is known as *total anomalous pulmonary venous connection* (TAPVC). If one or more, but not all, of the pulmonary veins connect to the RA, this condition is known as *partial anomalous pulmonary venous connection* (PAPVC). Approximately one third of patients with TAPVC have associated cardiac defects; prominent among associated defects are the heterotaxy syndromes.

The classification of TAPVC is based on the anatomic sight of the abnormal connection. TAPVC is usually classified according to the scheme proposed by Darling and others (1994), which is based on the anatomic site of an anomalous connection: type 1 is a supracardiac defect, type 2 is a cardiac defect, type 3 is an infracardiac defect, and type 4 is a mixed defect (Fig. 17–13).

The supracardiac type is the most common type, occurring in 41% to 49% of cases. In this type, the confluence of the

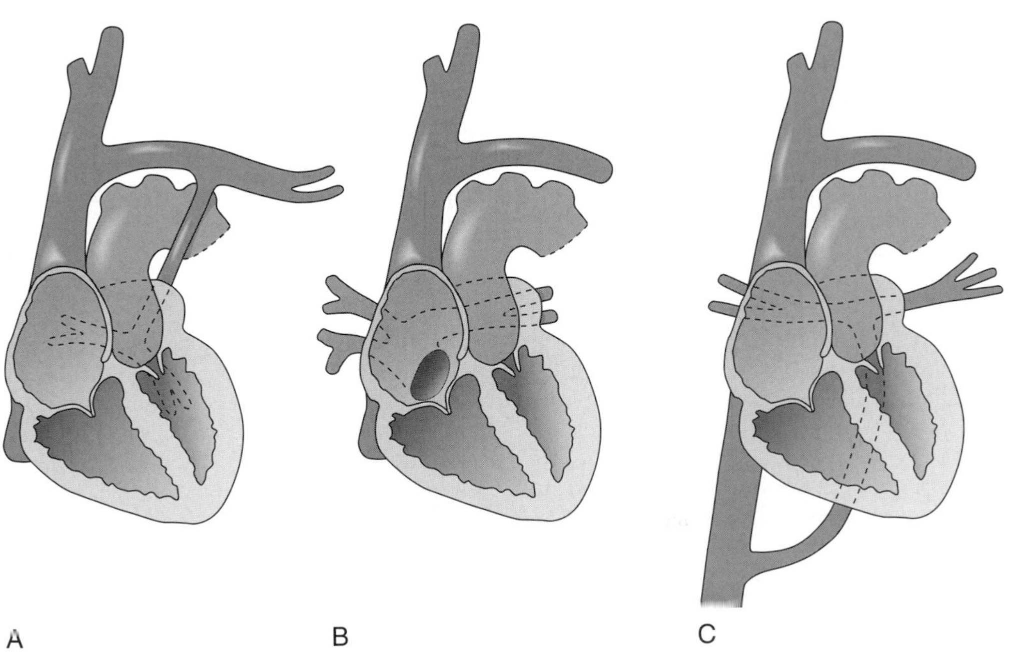

■ **FIGURE 17–13.** Type of total anomalous pulmonary venous connection. *(A)* Supracardiac type in which the pulmonary veins connect to the superior vena cava via a left vertical vein (persistent left superior vena cava). *(B)* Cardiac type in which the pulmonary veins drain into the coronary sinus. *(C)* Infracardiac type in which the pulmonary veins drain into a common pulmonary vein that passes through the diaphragm to enter the inferior vena cava.

pulmonary veins drains superiorly through a left superior vena cava (SVC) and, most often, enters the left innominate vein. Less frequently, there is connection of the ascending vein directly to the right SVC.

In the cardiac type of anomalous connection, the venous connection is to the coronary sinus or directly to the posterior wall of the RA. This type of TAPVC accounts for 18% to 31% of cases. Obstruction may occur at the point of entrance to the coronary sinus. A restrictive atrial communication may also occur with this type of defect.

With the infracardiac TAPVC, the distal site of connection is usually below the diaphragm, connecting with a vessel of the portal system. This type accounts for 13% to 24% of cases. In this defect, the pulmonary veins form a confluence behind the LA, and this confluence is drained through a connection that descends inferiorly, penetrates the diaphragm, and connects most frequently to the portal venous system, although connections to the ductus venosus, hepatic veins, or SVC have been reported. This type of abnormal pulmonary venous connection is usually associated with obstruction.

The mixed type of TAPVC occurs when there are two or more sites of anomalous venous connections. This type is rare, occurring in 5% to 10% of cases. Obstruction of one or more of the connections may occur.

With TAPVC, all pulmonary venous blood eventually returns to the RA. Because of the lower resistance of the pulmonary circulation, the majority of blood entering the RA is ejected out the RV into the pulmonary circulation. This situation results in right ventricular overload and may lead to symptoms and signs of congestive failure. An atrial level right-to-left shunt is obligatory to maintain cardiac output and systemic circulation. The amount of blood shunted to the LA is limited by the size of the interatrial connection and left atrial size. If there is no restriction of interatrial flow and left atrial compliance is normal, then the size of the right-to-left shunting is primarily determined by the relative compliance of the RV and LV. Dilation of the RV does occur, and PA pressure may range from being mildly elevated to systemic levels.

The presence of TAPVC with pulmonary venous obstruction results in raised pulmonary venous pressure and PA hypertension. PA hypertension is usually severe and results in decreased PBF and significant right-to-left shunting at both the atrial and ductal level. The right-to-left shunting produces severe hypoxemia in the neonatal period. The systemic hypoxemia is often serious enough to cause hemodynamic instability, resulting in hypotension, acidosis, and cardiac arrhythmias. Usually emergent surgical therapy to relieve obstruction or placement on ECMO to provide hemodynamic stability and multiorgan system resuscitation via reperfusion is necessary before operative intervention. The use of ECMO before the repair is associated with a higher mortality rate.

All patients with TAPVC require surgery. The urgency with which this surgery is performed is dictated by the anatomy, physiology, and clinical presentation, as discussed earlier. Patients with TAPVC who have pulmonary venous obstruction may be severely ill with noncompliant lungs and low cardiac output and require urgent surgical intervention. A cardiologic intervention in which the anomalous vein was opened with a stent allowed time for a patient to improve before surgical correction (Ramakrishnan and Kothari, 2004). Patients who lack pulmonary venous obstruction and who have an adequate-size ASD (to allow some flow to the LA and LV) may present with pulmonary congestion and tachypnea but without severe systemic acidosis and cyanosis and can be dealt with in a less emergent, but still urgent, fashion.

The goal of surgery is to connect the pulmonary venous return to the LA and obliterate the pathway connecting the pulmonary veins to the systemic venous system. In patients with the supracardiac and infracardiac types of anomalous drainage, there is ordinarily a confluence behind the LA to which all of the pulmonary veins converge (Delise et al., 1976; Eumel and Sreeram, 2004). This confluence drains into the systemic venous system by means of a connection that ascends toward the innominate vein (typical form of supracardiac TAPVC) or descends (through the diaphragm) toward the portal venous system (typical form of infracardiac TAPVC). For these anatomic types, surgical correction involves connection of the pulmonary venous confluence to the posterior aspect of the LA and ligation of the ascending or descending anomalous connection. The LA is almost always small in TAPVC. Embryologically, a significant portion of the LA is composed of the pulmonary venous connection derived from outgrowth from the fetal lungs. After surgical repair of TAPVC with obstruction, monitoring of both the PA and left atrial pressures is important, because these infants have a propensity to develop postoperative PA hypertension.

Ventricular Septal Defect

VSDs comprise 20% to 30% of all congenital heart defects. The interventricular septum is composed of three anatomic components: the membranous septum, the muscular septum, and the inlet septum. Anatomically, VSDs are classified according to their location. The term *crista supraventricularis* designates a muscular portion of the septum that separates the tricuspid and pulmonary valves and the pulmonary and aortic valves (Fig. 17–14). Supracristal VSDs (type I) lie just beneath the pulmonary valve and communicate with the RVOT above the supraventricular crest. Supracristal VSDs account for 5% to 8% of all VSDs and are associated with a significant incidence of aortic valve regurgitation. Membranous or infracristal VSDs (type II) constitute the most common type of VSD (75% to 80%) and are located in the membranous portion of the septum, immediately below the septal leaflet of the tricuspid valve. An inlet VSD (type III) is usually seen in atrioventricular defects where the defect is located in the posterior region of the septum, immediately below the inlet portion of the tricuspid valve. The incidence of this defect accounts for 4% of all VSDs. Defects located in the muscular portion of the septum (type IV) are frequently multiple and are found in 10% to 15% of VSDs.

A VSD is a condition of chronic volume overload in which a large increase in diastolic volume is tolerated with only minimal change in end-diastolic pressure (Graham, 1991). The left ventricular end-diastolic volume is usually twice normal, whereas left ventricular end-diastolic pressure and ejection fraction are unchanged. Right ventricular dilation also occurs with VSDs, but it is usually less severe (Graham, 1982). The effects of a persistent VSD on left and right ventricular function depend on the length of time the ventricle has been exposed to the chronic volume-overload state. Large VSDs left unrepaired for 2 to 3 years or longer have a greater incidence of permanent ventricular dysfunction. Patients with these disorders, along with neonates and infants with poorly compensated heart failure due to a large VSD, form a subset of patients at increased risk for postoperative ventricular dysfunction.

For the most part, the overwhelming majority of children undergoing closure of a VSD do well. Problems, however, can be

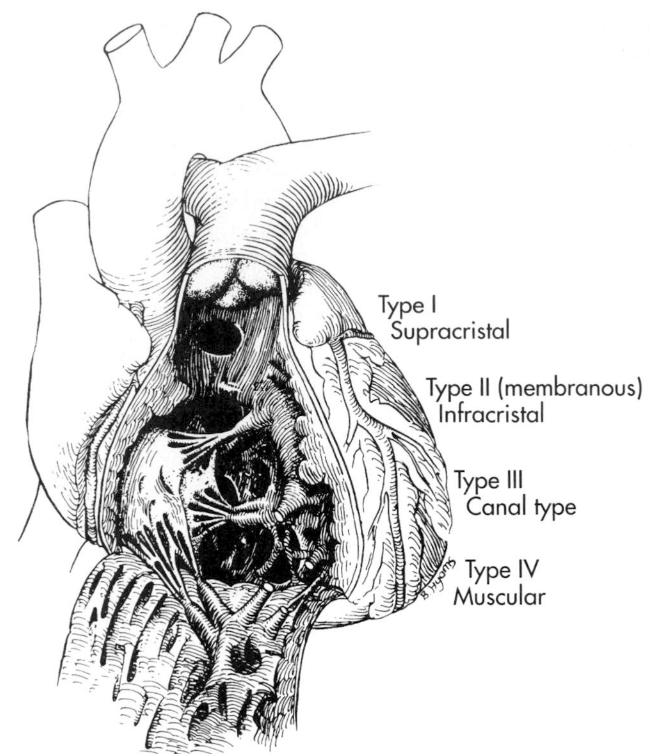

■ **FIGURE 17–14.** Classification of ventricular septal defects. (From Cooley DA, Norman JC: *Techniques in cardiac surgery.* Houston, 1975, Texas Medical Press, p 119.)

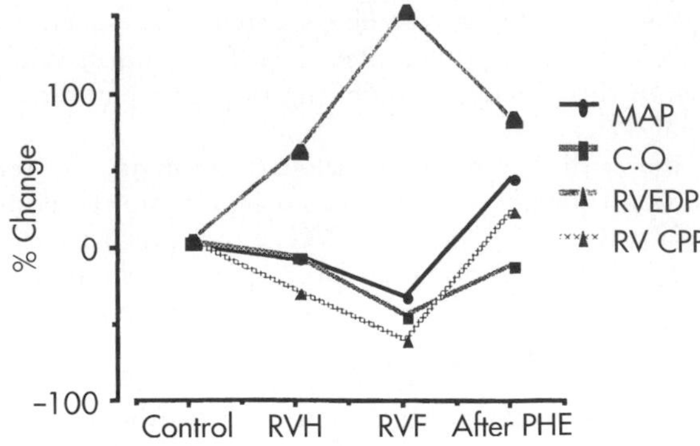

■ **FIGURE 17–15.** Sequential analysis of increasing pulmonary artery pressures in an experimental model. As pulmonary artery pressures are increased, the right ventricular (RV) end-diastolic pressure (EDP) increases RV hypertension (RVH), RV coronary perfusion pressure (RV CPP) decreases, and both cardiac output (CO) and mean arterial pressure (MAP) fall. As pulmonary artery hypertension increases, RV function worsens (increasing RVEDP), RV CPP narrows, and CO and MAP plummet. A bolus dose of phenylephrine (PHE) rapidly reverses RV dysfunction by improving coronary perfusion pressure to the RV. After PHE, RVEDP decreases and a statistically significant increase in CO and MAP is observed. (With permission from Vlahakes GJ, Turley K, Hoffman JI: The physiology of failure in acute right ventricular hypertension. *Circulation* 63:87–95, 1980.)

expected if a residual VSD remains, if significant preoperative congestive heart failure exists in infants, or if repair is associated with other cardiac anomalies such as coarctation of the aorta, interrupted aortic arch, or mitral or aortic valve anomalies (Pacifico et al., 1990).

Residual septal defects are diagnosed with intraoperative TEE. Previously undiagnosed defects are usually in the muscular septum. Residual defects around the patch are usually isolated to an area poorly visualized by the surgeon or near the conduction tissue (avoided to prevent heart block). Small residual defects less than 3 to 4 mm have a high likelihood of closing on their own, especially if the child is hemodynamically stable and on minimal support (Rychik et al., 1991).

Infants with a large VSD (Fig. 17–15) are susceptible to PA hypertensive crisis due to preexisting high PBF (Dietrich et al., 1992). After closure of the VSD, the RV must pump against increased PVR. The RV can no longer recruit the LV to assist in pumping against increased PVR. It must suddenly change from pumping against a volume load to supporting a pressure load. The change in loading conditions incurred by the cardiac surgery is an example of anticipated physiologic changes in cardiac loading. Similarly, the LV must pump a smaller-volume load against SVR without the luxury of pumping any extra volume through the VSD and into the lower-pressure right-sided circulation. The LV may be at a further disadvantage if PA pressures are high, the right ventricular dilates, and the septum shifts into the LV. This significantly alters left ventricular geometry and impairs left ventricular ejection (Meyer et al., 1972) (Fig. 17–16). Operative management is directed at reducing PVR and improving right ventricular contractility. These maneuvers improve blood return to the LV, restore left ventricular geometry, and improve cardiac output.

Patients undergoing repair at a late age or those with poor myocardial protection during repair are similarly subject to right and left ventricular dysfunction. Elevation in PA pressure may also be a component of their disease, but reactive PVR does not commonly occur with VSD after the early infancy period. PA pressures should decrease to one-half systemic in the operating room and generally decrease to one-third systemic within 24 hours of surgery. High PA pressure is very suggestive of a residual shunt, mitral regurgitation, or, less commonly, fixed changes associated with medial hypertrophy of the pulmonary arterioles. Echocardiographic evaluation is extremely helpful in these patients in the postoperative period.

Complete heart block is an uncommon finding today due to the precise anatomic knowledge concerning the location of the conduction tissue in different types of VSDs (Dickinson et al., 1982). Transient heart block, however, can occur. Stretching of the conduction tissue at the time of surgery to better visualize the defect, ion fluxes associated with cardioplegia solutions, and low calcium–containing primes are other contributing factors. Temporary ventricular pacing or, preferably, atrioventricular sequential pacing should be used in these patients. In many institutions, atrial and ventricular wires are routinely placed after all operations involving closure of a VSD.

Associated cardiac anomalies such as left-sided obstructive lesions (interrupted aortic arch and coarctation) result in a pressure-loaded, dysfunctional LV. These patients frequently require inotropic infusion to improve left ventricular contractility when being weaned from CPB.

Tetralogy of Fallot

Although the surgical approach to primary repair of tetralogy of Fallot has not changed significantly, the timing of repair has. Evidence has accumulated that a considerable portion of the myocardial, pulmonary, and central nervous system damage attributable to tetralogy of Fallot is more specifically due to

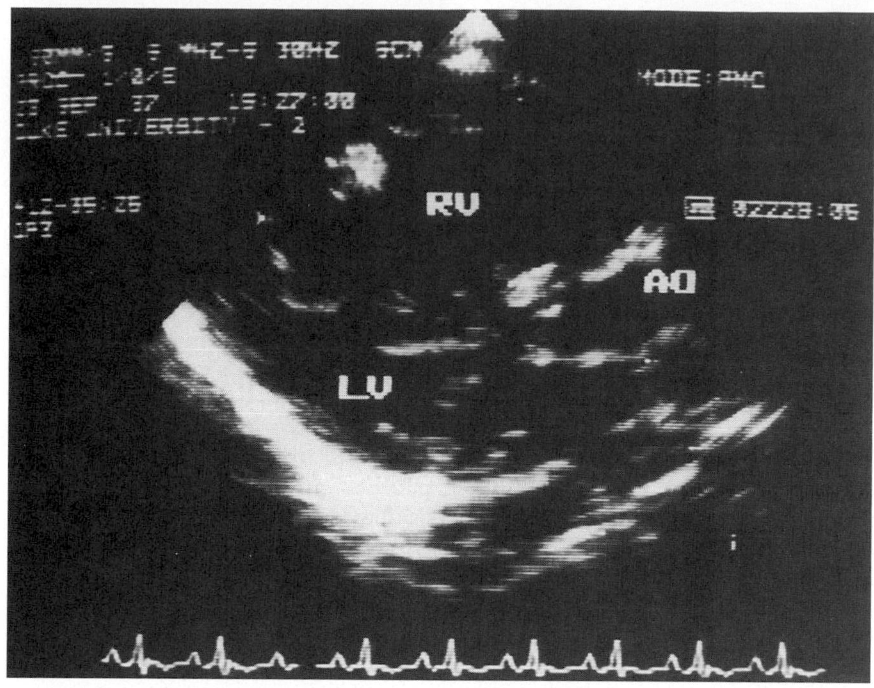

■ **FIGURE 17–16.** Echocardiogram demonstrating right ventricular (RV) dilation impinging on the left ventricle (LV). This alters left ventricular filling and geometry, secondarily reducing cardiac output. AO, aorta.

prolonged exposure to abnormal blood flow patterns, hypoxemia, and cyanosis (Borow et al., 1981; Castaneda et al., 1989; Newburger et al., 1993). Surgery involving multiple palliation procedures and long-term medical management does not alleviate these problems, and a marked increase in long-term morbidity and mortality has been demonstrated. For the past 15 years, there has been a greater impetus to repair rather than palliate these children in infancy (Castaneda et al., 1989). Most centers prefer to operate at 4 to 8 months of age, with a few opting for repair at earlier ages. A group from The Hospital for Sick Children in Toronto (van Dongen et al., 2003) reviewed their experience from 1997 through 1999. Seventy-eight consecutive patients were enrolled, and the mean age at operation was 8 months (range, 36 days to 18.5 months). The overall mortality was 1.3%, and intensive care unit stay was 2 days. Operative intervention at age younger than 3 months was associated with an increased need for inotropic support, higher postoperative fluid requirement, and higher incidence of secondary organ dysfunction.

The repair of tetralogy of Fallot includes a right ventriculotomy, patch closure of the VSD, resection of infundibular stenosis, and patch augmentation of the RVOT. The surgeon evaluates the size of the pulmonary valve and, if it is too small, the right ventricular incision is extended across the pulmonary valve annulus and onto the PA. A transannular patch creates pulmonary insufficiency, which may contribute a volume load to an already pressure-loaded RV (Ilbawi et al., 1987). The right ventriculotomy may also contribute to right ventricular dysfunction during weaning from CPB and may contribute to late right ventricular dysfunction or dysrhythmias (Atallah-Yunes et al., 1996). These concerns are more pronounced when surgery is performed in early infancy. An alternative surgical technique is to limit or eliminate the right ventricular incision by using a transatrial or combined transatrial/transpulmonary approach to resect muscle from the RVOT and to close the VSD (Pozzi et al., 2000). This approach has shown no increase in morbidity and mortality and has potential for lower long-term cardiac rhythm problems and sudden death, which is a concern in older patients who underwent repair decades earlier (Pozzi et al., 2000).

Repair in the first few months of life is usually necessary when severe RVOT obstruction, a small pulmonary valve orifice, and preoperative hypercyanotic spells are present. These patients commonly have a hypertrophied, noncompliant RV and frequently require a transannular patch across the RVOT. After repair, right ventricular systolic and diastolic dysfunction is common, as well as higher right-sided filling pressures and lower PBF. Consequently, the left ventricle receives less filling, and there is reduced stroke volume and decreased cardiac output. A reflex tachycardia occurs in an attempt to augment systemic perfusion.

Leaving the foramen ovale open or creating a small ASD at the time of surgery provides a right-to-left shunt at the atrial level. This shunt bypasses the noncompliant RV, preserving left ventricular filling and systemic perfusion. The patient is somewhat hypoxemic, but this is well tolerated in the face of improved systemic oxygen delivery. An alternate approach in patients with tetralogy of Fallot and diminutive PAs has been the placement of a fenestrated VSD patch. This approach has not been associated with increased mortality and has a low incidence of excessive right-to-left shunting (Marshal et al., 2003).

Persistently low cardiac output despite an atrial level shunt suggests either a residual anatomic problem or severe ventricular dysfunction. Intraoperative echocardiography and assessment of the adequacy of the right ventricular outflow patch by pressure measurements should be used to evaluate the repair for a residual VSD or inadequate relief of RVOT obstruction. If anatomic considerations persist, reoperation should be considered. If primary ventricular dysfunction exists, therapy should be directed toward right ventricular or left ventricular dysfunction as previously discussed and, rarely, the use of ECMO and VADs.

Anatomic variants in coronary artery anatomy alter the surgical approach and may affect anesthetic management in patients with tetralogy of Fallot. If the right coronary artery gives rise to the left anterior descending artery, the coronary courses directly across the RVOT. A standard transannular enlargement is not feasible because the right coronary would have to be transected. Under these circumstances, the surgeon must decide to either place a conduit over the outflow tract or resect as much infundibular tissue as possible and place a patch above and below the coronary artery (Hurwitz et al., 1980; Humes et al., 1987). In the latter case, the narrowest part of the RVOT is beneath the right coronary artery. Excessive preload may distend the RV, stretch the right coronary artery, and cause right ventricular ischemia. Although ischemic changes are uncommon in pediatric cardiac surgery, this anatomic arrangement of the coronary arteries substantially increases the likelihood of ventricular ischemia. Careful electrocardiographic observation for ischemic changes is essential when augmenting preload. Volume supplementation should be given in small increments, and right-sided filling pressures should be maintained within a narrow range to avoid right coronary stretch.

In the preoperative or the prebypass periods, tetralogy or hypercyanotic spells may occur. These episodes of acute cyanosis are due to an increase in subpulmonary infundibular spasm, a reduction in PBF, and an increase in right-to-left shunting across the VSD. Because the direction of intracardiac shunting is dependent on downstream resistance, hypercyanotic spells are due to increased resistance to blood flow across the RVOT.

Severe forms of tetralogy of Fallot present in early infancy with PS, annular stenosis, and diffuse hypoplasia of the RVOT (Lev and Eckner, 1964; Rabinovitch et al., 1981). This subset of tetralogy patients presents with severe cyanosis at birth that is poorly responsive to medical therapy. Classic hypercyanotic spells do not occur in this group because of fixed obstruction to the RVOT. Early operative intervention is required, and complete repair in infancy generally requires a transannular patch. More typically, tetralogy patients are electively repaired during the first 4 to 8 months of life. Early repair prevents significant cardiac hypertrophy and is best if performed before the onset of significant hypercyanotic spells.

Medical management for tetralogy spells is directed at reducing right-to-left shunting across the VSD by increasing SVR through the administration of phenylephrine and by decreasing the effective narrowing of the RVOT through volume loading, sedation, and, rarely, β-blockade to decrease contractility (this is not commonly applied in the operating room setting but has been used to stabilize patients preoperatively). Increasing SVR is a critical component of treating patients with tetralogy spells (Lang et al., 1980; Berner et al., 1989). Therapy is directed at reducing the infundibular obstruction through increasing preload and suppressing endogenous catecholamine release through increasing anesthetic depth or β-blockade. Increasing SVR rapidly reduces the right-to-left shunting across the VSD and restores oxygen saturation and oxygen delivery to acceptable levels.

The degree of ventricular shunting is dependent on the resistance to flow imposed at the level of the RVOT and the SVR. When the outflow tract resistance exceeds SVR, right-to-left shunting occurs. By increasing SVR, blood flow is preferentially in a left-to-right direction at the VSD and the hypercyanotic spell aborted. During surgery, opening the pericardium, manipulation of the RVOT, or atrial cannulation can alter preload and/or induce spasm of the infundibulum. In general, volume loading and administration of 25 to 100 mcg of phenylephrine are effective in restoring PBF and reducing right-to-left shunting at the VSD. However, occasionally severe cyanotic spells occur that are poorly responsive to medical therapy. Anesthetic management for these uncommon, yet life-threatening, events include correcting acidosis (sodium bicarbonate), increasing oxygen delivery to the tissue by increasing oxygen saturation through manipulations in SVR (phenylephrine), and increasing cardiac output through the administration of potent inotropic agents such as epinephrine via infusion or bolus to maintain cardiac output while the surgeon attempts to rapidly institute CPB. Once CPB is instituted, high flow rates should be established and maintained until the patient is fully resuscitated as judged by arterial and mixed venous blood gases and visual inspection of the heart.

Alternatively, a brief trial of placing a partial cross-clamp across the proximal aorta to reverse right-to-left shunting may be tried. This technique may increase PBF, reverse right-to-left shunting, and provide improved oxygen delivery before establishment of CPB. In patients with severe cyanotic spells, the administration of β-blocking agents may be counterproductive in that oxygen delivery may become compromised and myocardial ischemia or cardiac arrest may ensue. Hand ventilation with rapid ventilatory rates or high mean airway pressures should be discouraged during a hypercyanotic spell, because this increases intrathoracic pressure, reduces cardiac filling, and exacerbates dynamic obstruction at the RVOT.

Tetralogy of Fallot with an absent pulmonary valve is an unusual variant that occurs in 3% to 6% of tetralogy patients. The pulmonary valve is minuscule, dysplastic, and nonfunctional. Because of the absence of functional valve tissue, the RVOT remains widely patent despite moderate narrowing of the infundibulum. The associated VSD is large and malaligned. In the severe form of this disease, severe pulmonary regurgitation during gestation results in massive aneurysmal dilation of the main and branch PAs. The large conducting airways are compressed by these vessels, resulting in tracheobronchial malacia. In addition, the distal vessels do not branch in a typical segmental fashion but instead end in vascular tufts that entrap and compress the distal conducting airways. These patients present with excessive PBF, heart failure, and respiratory disease, characterized by obstruction of gas flow and increased airways resistance in the small, medium, and large airways (Fig. 17–17). Tetralogy of Fallot with absent pulmonary valve is associated with high morbidity and mortality.

Occasionally, palliation with a BT shunt is considered a preferred operation in tetralogy. In newborns with unrelenting hypercyanotic episodes and poor systemic perfusion who are either unresponsive or poorly responsive to medical management, a BT (or systemic-to-pulmonary) shunt can be placed. This is generally done off bypass. For newborns with tetralogy of Fallot who have hypoxic–ischemic encephalopathy or intraventricular hemorrhage, a BT shunt avoids the risks of heparinization and CPB. In general, however, exchanging tetralogy physiology for shunt physiology is not optimal. Prolonged exposure to shunt physiology risks the development of a dilated cardiomyopathy and/or pulmonary hypertension.

Atrioventricular Septal Defects

AVSDs are physiologically similar to large VSDs. AVSDs consist of an ostium primum ASD, an inlet VSD, and a cleft in the septal leaflets of the tricuspid and mitral valves (Figs. 17–18 and 17–19). The management of these patients is quite similar except they are more prone to PA hypertension. This is due to the large left-to-right shunt imposed by the septal defect. AVSDs are

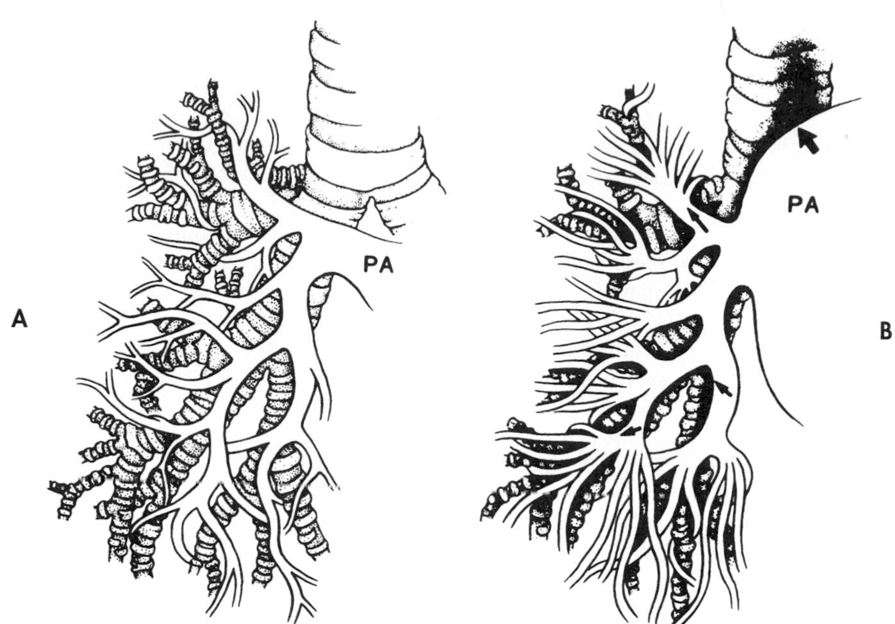

■ **FIGURE 17–17.** Diagrammatic representation of normal relationship between pulmonary artery and left bronchus *(A)* and compression of left main bronchus by the aneurysmal pulmonary artery *(B)* in the absent pulmonary valve syndrome. Note also compression of smaller bronchi that are entwined by tufts of abnormal vessels. (From Rabinovitch M, Grady S, David I, et al.: Compression of intrapulmonary bronchi by abnormally branching pulmonary arteries associated with absent pulmonary valves. *Am J Cardiol* 50:804, 1982. With permission from Excerpta Medica, Inc.)

commonly found in patients with trisomy 21. This genetic defect is associated with small peripheral airways in the lung and architecturally small PAs. Elevation in PVR may be due to an underdeveloped pulmonary vascular tree as well. Fixed PA hypertension has been described in trisomy 21 patients with AVSDs who are younger than 6 months (Frescura et al., 1987).

Valvular regurgitation is not an uncommon finding after AVSD repair (McGrath and Gonzales-Lavin, 1987). Mild to moderate regurgitation is generally well tolerated and is managed by decreasing systemic afterload. If concomitant ventricular dysfunction exists with AVV regurgitation, low-dose dopamine, dobutamine, or milrinone may be added. Milrinone is an extremely effective drug in this patient population. If severe AVV regurgitation exists, valve replacement may be necessary. Because the defect involves both annular and valve tissue, the artificial valve is difficult to position and there is a greater risk of perivalvular leaks. Complete heart block carries an increased risk after valve replacement in AVSDs, although it is generally uncommon (Kirklin and Barratt-Boyes, 1986a). This is due to a lack of normally developed annular tissue necessary to suture the mechanical valve in place and an increased likelihood of disrupting normal conduction tissue. Patients with AVSDs who do not have Down syndrome usually have greater dysplasia of valve tissue.

Transposition of the Great Arteries and Arterial Switch Operation

In TGA, the aorta arises from the RV and the PA arises from the LV. The arterial switch operation for TGA is the preferred surgical approach (Fig. 17–20); it allows the LV to be the systemic ventricle. Maintaining the LV as the systemic chamber

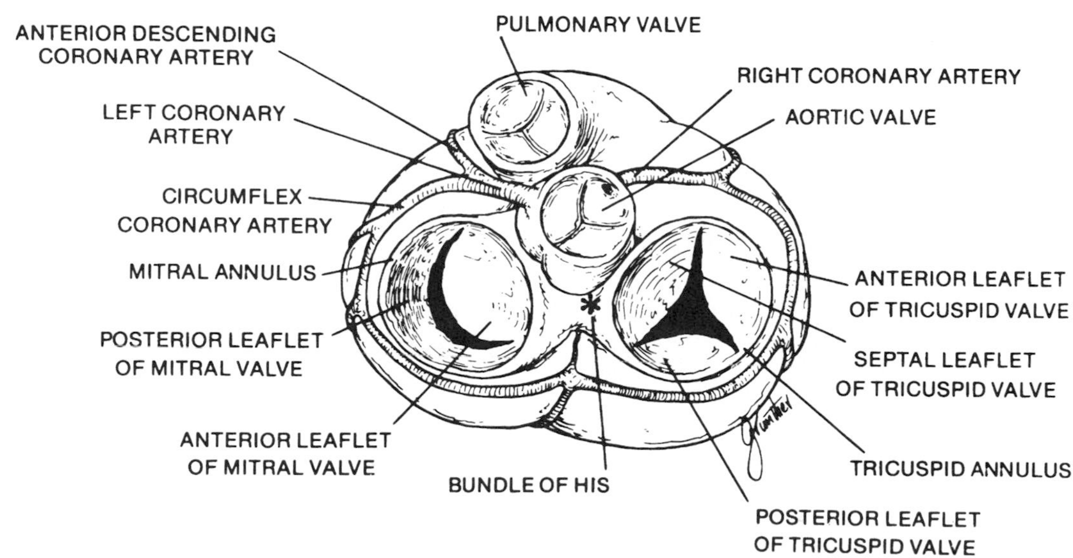

■ **FIGURE 17–18.** Normal atrioventricular valves consisting of leaflets that originate from an annulus and attach distally to papillary muscles by chordae tendinea. (From Lowe DA: Abnormalities of the atrioventricular valves. In Lake CL, editor: *Pediatric cardiac anesthesia.* Norwalk, CT, 1988, Appleton & Lange, p 300.)

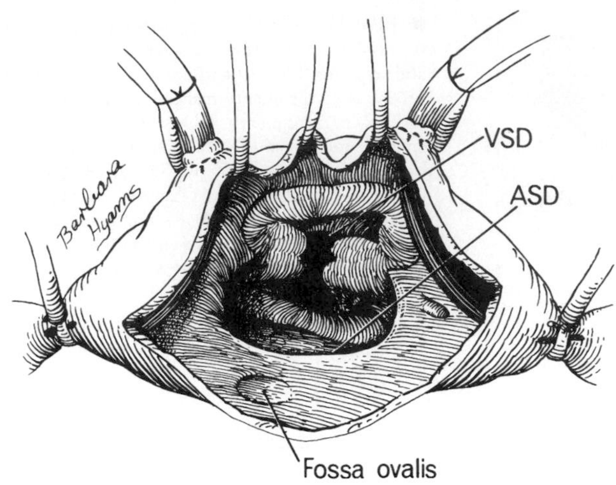

■ **FIGURE 17–19.** Complete atrioventricular canal in view from right atrium. ASD, atrial septal defect; VSD, ventricular septal defect. (From Cooley DA, Norman JC: *Techniques in cardiac surgery.* Houston, 1975, Texas Medical Press, p 128.)

improves ventricular longevity and reduces the incidence of systemic ventricular dysfunction. The cylindrical shape, the concentric contraction, and the location of the ventricular inlet and outlet at the base of the heart of the LV allow it to function better as a pressure pump and to account for improved long-term patient survival and reduced long-term morbidity compared with alternative surgical repairs.

Improvements in coronary transfer technique, myocardial preservation, and postoperative management have reduced perioperative mortality rates for this operation to less than 3% in simple transposition without other associated cardiac anomalies (Blume et al., 1999). In a report of 223 consecutive transposition patients, coronary artery anatomy was not found to be associated with increased mortality, although the presence of coronary abnormalities, including single right coronary, was associated with a longer duration of mechanical ventilation and need for delayed sternal closure (Blume et al., 1999). These low mortality rates rival those of the atrial switch procedure and are more impressive in view of the high incidence of late complications associated with atrial switch procedures (atrial dysrhythmias [50%], baffle stenosis [8% to 10%], pulmonary venous obstruction, [8% to 10%] and right [systemic] ventricular dysfunction [10% to 20%]) (Castaneda et al., 1989). The Congenital Heart Surgeons Society reviewed outcomes of 829 neonates from

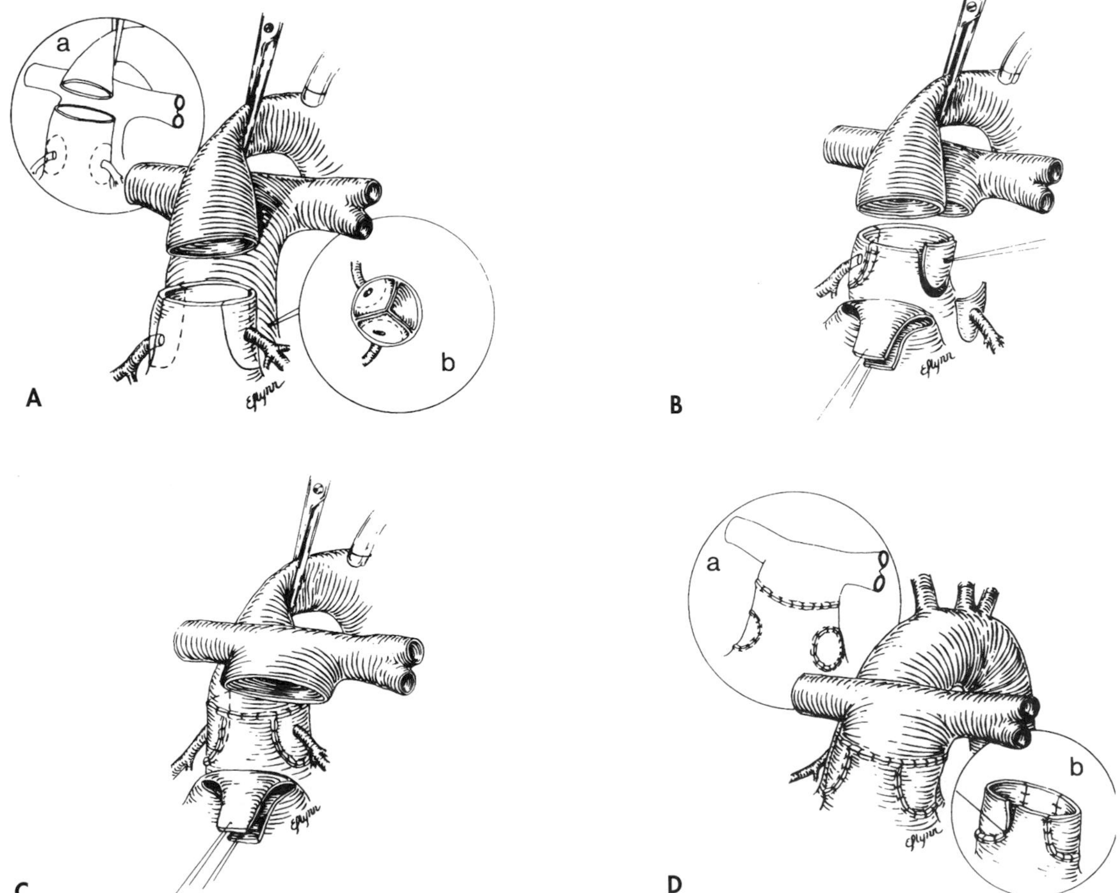

■ **FIGURE 17–20.** Arterial switch procedure. *(A)* Aorta is transected, and left and right coronary arteries and their bases are excised. *(B)* An equivalent segment of pulmonary arterial wall is excised, and coronary arteries are sutured to the pulmonary artery. *(C)* Distal pulmonary artery is brought anterior to ascending aorta, and the proximal pulmonary artery is anastomosed to the distal aorta. *(D)* Sites of coronary artery extraction are repaired with use of either (a) a patch of prosthetic material or (b) a segment of pericardium. Finally, proximal aorta is sutured to distal pulmonary artery. (Modified from Castaneda AR, Norwood WI, Jonas RA, et al.: Transposition of the great arteries and intact ventricular septum: anatomical repair in the neonate. *Ann Thorac Surg* 38:438, 1984, with permission from the Society of Thoracic Surgeons.)

24 institutions with complete TGA repaired during the years 1985 to 1989. This was the era when congenital heart centers began transitioning from the atrial switch procedure to the arterial switch procedure. In this review, the survival rate of the 516 children managed by an arterial switch operation was compared with the 285 atrial switch operation rate and found to be virtually identical (81% and 82%, respectively). In that era, the early mortality rate for the arterial switch procedure was 19%. The late mortality rate remained higher in the atrial switch group, accounting for the 15-year similarity in mortality (Williams et al., 2003).

The arterial switch operation involves mobilization of the PA and dissection onto the right and left PAs (see Fig. 17–20). The aorta and main PA are then transected. The aorta is divided above the coronary arteries and aortic valve. The LeCompte maneuver (the passage of the PA anterior to the aorta) is then performed. The coronary arteries are mobilized with 3 to 4 mm of surrounding aortic tissue and reimplanted onto the "neoaorta." Previously harvested patches of pericardium are used to close the defects resulting from removal of the coronary arteries.

Two factors dictate the survivability of a patient after an arterial switch operation: (1) global function of the LV and (2) focal ischemia (Wernovsky et al., 1988). Global ventricular function reflects how well the LV is prepared to pump against a systemic pressure load after the arterial switch procedure. In a patient who does not have VSD, the left ventricle pumps against the low resistance of the pulmonary circulation. In 2 to 4 weeks, the LV will lose its ability to pump against the systemic afterload after the arterial switch procedure (Danforth et al., 1960). In these patients, the LV must be either "prepared" by producing a pressure and volume load on the LV or by anticipating the need for a VAD or ECMO after weaning from CPB. The two-stage approach to preparing the LV is accomplished intraoperatively with PA banding, which creates a left ventricular pressure of 60% of systemic or greater, and the placement of a 4-mm aorta-to-pulmonary shunt in order to pressure and volume load the LV, respectively. These patients are frequently quite ill, but left ventricular function recovers to the point of being able to pump against systemic afterload. After the LV is "conditioned" over a period of 5 to 7 days, a second operation, an arterial switch operation, is immediately performed (Lacour-Gayet et al., 2001).

Inotropic support and afterload reduction are very effective in maximizing cardiac output after weaning patients from CPB after the arterial switch procedure. If inotropic support is excessive and cardiac output and systemic perfusion remain marginal, early introduction of a VAD or ECMO should be considered because myocardial function predictably worsens in the first 6 to 12 postoperative hours (Lacour-Gayet et al., 2001). Focal ischemia may also occur. Kinking, twisting, or excessive tension placed on the coronary arteries and compression of the coronary arteries because the main PA crosses tightly over the aorta (due to inadequate dissection of the branch PAs in combination with the LeCompte maneuver) are causes of focal ischemic changes in these patients. ST segment changes or regional wall motion abnormalities on intraoperative echocardiography should alert the anesthesiologist and surgeon to evaluate the coronary arteries and overlying structures.

Transposition of the Great Arteries: Senning or Mustard

Atrial repair of TGA is an example of a physiologic rather than a true anatomic correction (Fig. 17–21). Although indications

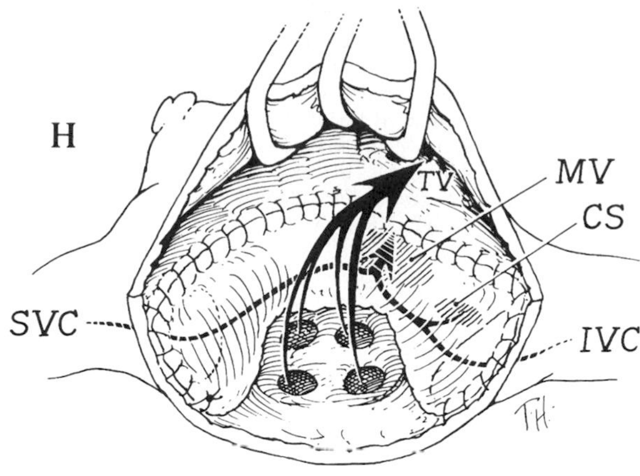

■ **FIGURE 17–21.** Diagram of interior of right atrium showing the baffle that rearranges and redirects atrial blood flow following Mustard procedure. Pulmonary vein openings are visualized. CS, coronary sinus; MV, mitral valve, IVC, inferior vena cava; TV, tricuspid valve. (From Reed CC, Stafford TB, editors: *Cardiopulmonary bypass,* 2nd ed. Houston, 1985, Texas Medical Press, p 78.)

for atrial-level repairs for transposition are becoming less and less common, unusual coronary anatomy, such as coronary arteries with an intramural course, have a higher risk for coronary transfer in the arterial switch operation. Under these circumstances, atrial level repair may be considered.

The Senning operation uses tissue from the right atrial wall and interatrial septum to fashion a conduit for the flow of deoxygenated (systemic venous) blood through the mitral valve and into the left (pulmonary) ventricle. The LV ejects this deoxygenated blood into the PA. The Mustard operation accomplishes the same physiologic correction as the Senning procedure, but it uses a pericardial or prosthetic baffle to redirect the flow of systemic venous blood (see Fig. 17–21).

Patients who underwent either the Mustard or the Senning procedure generally do well. Because the operative site is in the atrium, ventricular function is usually well preserved. In patients with low cardiac output after weaning from CPB, baffle obstruction versus primary myocardial dysfunction should be considered. Poor cardiac output and/or symptoms of SVC obstruction are highly suggestive of a baffle obstruction. The most common location for baffle obstruction is where the SVC channel crosses the atrial septum. Superior vena cava obstruction occurs in approximately 8% to 10% of patients (Pacifico et al., 1990). If there is good collateral venous drainage and the obstruction is not severe, it is usually well tolerated. However, an occasional patient requires revision of the baffle.

Dysrhythmias are the most common complication after atrial correction of transposition. The incidence of dysrhythmias ranges from 20% to 60%, with the higher number being more common with the Mustard repair (Gillette et al., 1980). Although bradycardia is most common, supraventricular tachyarrhythmias are also observed. In the Mustard repair, the wide excision of atrial tissue and long atrial suture line may damage the sinoatrial node or its blood supply. Temporary atrial and ventricular pacing wires should be routinely placed in these patients.

Rastelli Procedure

The Rastelli procedure (an operation for TGA with a VSD and an LVOT obstruction) combines an intracardiac baffle or tunnel from the VSD to the aorta and an extracardiac conduit to the

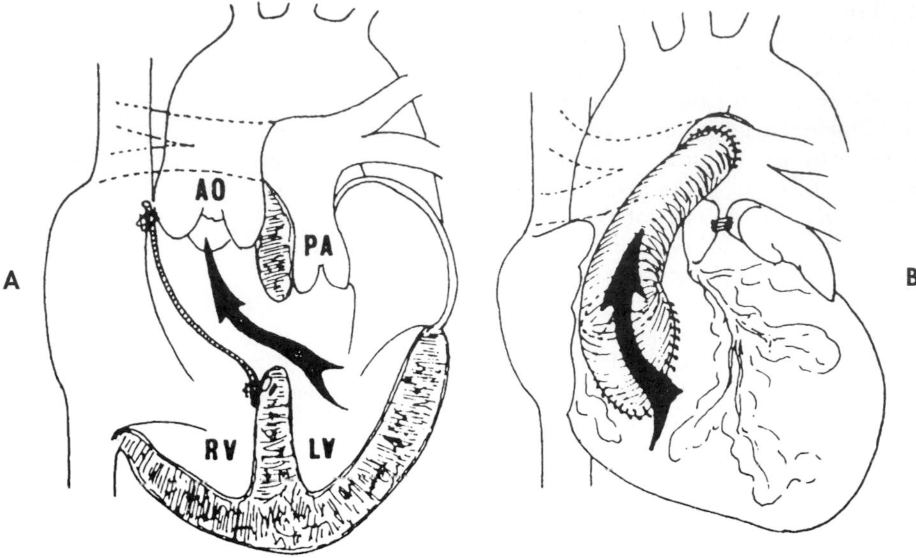

■ **FIGURE 17–22.** *(A)* In the Rastelli procedure, closure of ventricular septal defect results in the left ventricle (LV) ejecting blood into the aorta (AO). *(B)* An external right ventricle (RV)–to–pulmonary artery (PA) conduit is placed to provide pulmonary circulation. (From Strafford M: Transposition of the great vessels. In Lake CL, editor: *Pediatric cardiac anesthesia.* Norwalk, CT, 1988, Appleton & Lange, p 237.)

pulmonary artery (Fig. 17–22). The intracardiac baffle establishes continuity between the LV and the aorta. A large nonrestrictive VSD is required to allow uninterrupted flow between the LV and aorta. The VSD may have to be surgically enlarged during the operative procedure to prevent flow restriction. The extracardiac conduit establishes continuity between the RV and the PA.

Postoperatively, LVOT obstruction can occur due to inadequate enlargement of the VSD or obstruction of the intracardiac tunnel, resulting in an acute pressure load on the LV. High left-sided filling pressures, low cardiac output, high inotropic requirement, and a dilated poorly contractile LV are typical findings. Intraoperative echocardiography and pressure monitoring across the baffle and VSD are helpful to localize the area of left ventricular obstruction (VSD, baffle, etc.). During post-CPB assessment in patients with low cardiac output, the anesthesiologist must maintain preload, coronary perfusion pressures, systemic afterload, and contractility. Patients with baffle obstruction have customary signs of severe left-sided obstructive physiology (Kreselis et al., 1985).

The extracardiac RV-to-PA conduit can also be obstructed. Although this is more commonly seen in late follow-up, early postrepair obstruction may become apparent after chest closure. This results more commonly from extrinsic compression of the conduit by the sternum. The conduit can also drape across a coronary artery and, once the chest is closed, impinge on right coronary artery flow. Furthermore, the conduit can cause compression of the trachea or the right bronchus. Sudden changes in lung compliance, airways resistance, hypercarbia, or hypoxia suggest airway compression as a possible cause (Dekeon et al., 1992). Respiratory mechanics monitoring has been helpful in diagnosing this problem intraoperatively.

Heart block is an uncommon finding after Rastelli repair; however, if the VSD must be surgically enlarged, the risk of transient or permanent heart block increases. All patients undergoing VSD enlargement should have temporary atrial and ventricular pacing wires placed. It is important to ensure low pacing thresholds in the operating room, because postoperative myocardial edema usually results in increasing pacing thresholds. In neonates and infants with heart rate–dependent cardiac output, pacing wire failures resulting in a slow idioventricular rhythm are poorly tolerated and may become life threatening in the infant with marginal cardiac output in the early postoperative period.

Interrupted Aortic Arch

Interrupted aortic arch (IAA) is a congenital anomaly in which there is complete discontinuity between the ascending and descending aortas (Fig. 17–23). IAA almost always occurs in

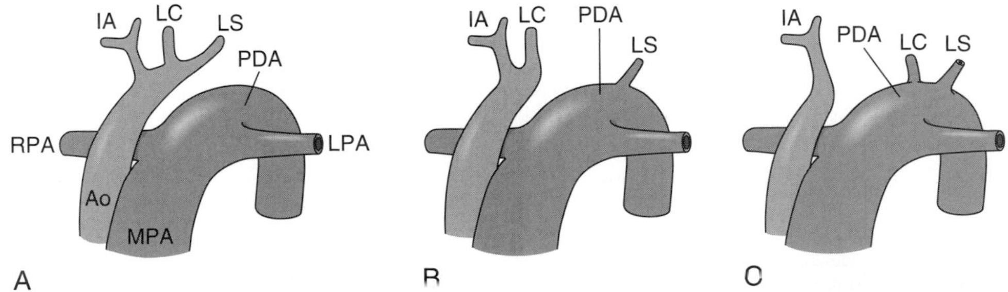

■ **FIGURE 17–23.** Types of aortic arch interruption. *(A)* In type A, the defect is distal to the left subclavian artery. *(B)* Type B has the interruption between the left subclavian (LS) and left carotid (LC) arteries. *(C)* Type C has the discontinuity between the innominate (IA) and left carotid arteries. Ao, aorta; LPA, left pulmonary artery; MPA, main pulmonary artery; PDA, patent ductus arteriosus; RPA, right pulmonary artery. (From Arciniegas E, editor: *Pediatric cardiac surgery.* Chicago, 1985, Year Book Medical, p 109, with permission.)

association with a VSD and a patent PDA. The PDA connects the PA to the descending aorta, supplying blood flow to the lower body. Occasionally, IAA may be associated with truncus arteriosus, and it is rarely associated with other cardiac defects such as double-outlet RV. There is often a stretched PFO or ASD. The stretched PFO probably develops as a result of the in utero left-to-right shunt from the downstream aortic obstruction. IAA is classified based on the location of the interruption. Type A interruption occurs at the isthmus, which is distal to the left subclavian; type B interruption occurs between the left common carotid artery and the left subclavian and is the most common type, with an incidence between 50% and 70% in most reported series. Type C interruption is between the innominate and the left common carotid artery (Celoria et al., 1959). If there is no associated VSD, then there may be an aortopulmonary window (a direct connection between the ascending aorta and the main PA). Interrupted aortic arch is rare and occurs in 1% of patients with CHD (Sandhu et al., 2002). Type B patients may have a higher incidence of chromosomal anomalies, including DiGeorge syndrome, with thymic hypoplasia and hypoparathyroidism (Schreiber et al., 2000).

Unless symptoms are detected prenatally with fetal echocardiography, they begin acutely with ductal closure, when infants acutely develop severe metabolic acidosis and poor peripheral perfusion. Descending aorta blood flow decreases dramatically as the lower body is dependent on a minimal amount of collateral blood flow. There is ischemia to the liver, kidney, and intestine, and lower extremity pulses are usually absent.

Resuscitation is dependent on reestablishing ductal patency through the administration of PGE_1 and correction of acidosis. Occasionally, the ductus may not close, in which case the child presents with congestive cardiac failure from a left-to-right shunt through the ductus.

After stabilization and optimization of organ function, the patient is usually maintained on a low FIO_2 to diminish left-to-right flow across the ductus and occasionally requires an elevated CO_2 through hypoventilation or exogenous CO_2 administration in order to optimize systemic blood flow. If instituted in the ICU, these management strategies should be continued through the pre-CPB period. After induction of anesthesia, placement of a lower limb and upper limb arterial catheters aids in CPB perfusion management and in the postbypass period helps to determine if a residual arch obstruction exists.

In most surgical centers a single stage repair with end-to-end anastomosis of the mobilized aorta and repair of all associated cardiac anomalies is preferred (Sell et al., 1988; Schreiber et al., 2000). Several studies have demonstrated a significantly higher mortality rate for staged repairs (Tlaskal et al., 1999; Schreiber et al., 2000). With adequate mobilization of the descending aorta, an interposition graft is rarely indicated.

Postsurgical complications include bleeding from dissection and mobilization of the aorta. If the aorta was stretched to complete the repair, the aorta may be under tension and obstruction of the left main bronchus can occur with evidence of air trapping on chest radiograph (Casteneda et al., 1994). Left ventricular dysfunction is common after repair. Residual LVOT obstruction occurs commonly, and may contribute to high postoperative afterload. Afterload reduction with vasodilators (nitroprusside or nicardipine) or milrinone is helpful when separating from CPB but is not helpful when a fixed obstruction exists at the site of the repair. Reoperative interventions or catheterization lab procedures are commonly required to treat arch obstruction (Sell et al., 1988; Castenada et al., 1994; Schreiber et al., 2000).

Ebstein's Anomaly

This is an uncommon cardiac defect of the tricuspid valve and RV. Posterior and septal leaflets of the tricuspid valve are displaced and dysplastic and the attachments to the tricuspid valve annulus are abnormal. The anterior leaflet is enlarged and often described as "sail like" in appearance. The effective tricuspid valve orifice is displaced apically into the RV. The RA is usually massively dilated and the junction between the RA and RV is enlarged. Because of the displacement of the tricuspid valve into the RV, the RV now consists of 2 parts. The inlet portion is described as "atrialized," its wall is thin and aneurysmal. The outlet portion is referred to as the "functional" portion of the RV (Fig. 17–24).

Ebstein's anomaly is a relatively rare defect accounting for less than 1% of all congenital cardiac defects. The pathophysiology depends on the extent of the tricuspid valve defect. In general, these patients have significant tricuspid valve regurgitation which reduces the volume of the blood entering the functional RV and creating a large regurgitant volume contributing to a dilated RA. If there is an associated ASD or a PFO, there is a right-to-left shunt at the atrial level. The small functional portion of the RV may have a limited stroke volume based on small size contributing to further tricuspid regurgitation. In infants with diastolic dysfunction in this small outlet portion of the RV, filling may be further impaired lessening forward flow of blood into the pulmonary circulation. An additional physiologic problem with this lesion relates to ventricular interactions. Because of the large RA and displacement of the tricuspid valve, the intraventricular septum tends to bow into the left ventricular cavity during diastole. This reduces left ventricular filling and decreases systemic cardiac output. Newborns with Ebstein's anomaly usually present with severe cyanosis. In less severe forms, they may present with supraventricular tachycardia or a murmur of tricuspid regurgitation.

Severe forms of Ebstein's anomaly presenting in neonates are usually fatal (Lerner et al., 2003). Several operative interventions are described for Ebstein's anomaly. The two-ventricle repair requires a tricuspid valve annuloplasty, radical reduction atrioplasty, and closure of ASD (most groups fenestrate the patch). In addition, the atrialized portion of the RV is plicated, obliterating the aneurysmal cavity, and the large anterior leaflet is allowed to function as a monocusp valve. Further, an RVOT patch is placed to create a normal-size (7- to 8-mm) outflow tract (Knott-Craig et al., 2002). Less commonly, right ventricular exclusion procedures may be performed. The RV size is reduced, the tricuspid valve is oversewn, and the coronary sinus is rerouted to the LA through an ASD (Sano et al., 2002).

Anesthetic management is directed at maintaining right ventricular contractility with inotropic support and right ventricular afterload reduction. Induction of anesthesia should be cautious. In general, an intravenous induction with midazolam and fentanyl is recommended. In the sick neonate, inhalation induction may be poorly tolerated, particularly with halothane because of the high risk of atrial and ventricular dysrhythmias. Supraventricular tachycardia occurs in approximately 30% of patients and those with ventricular tachyarrhythmias, including ventricular fibrillation, may occur commonly after separation from CPB. If ventricular ectopy is present, a lidocaine infusion starting at 40mcg/kg per minute should be administered.

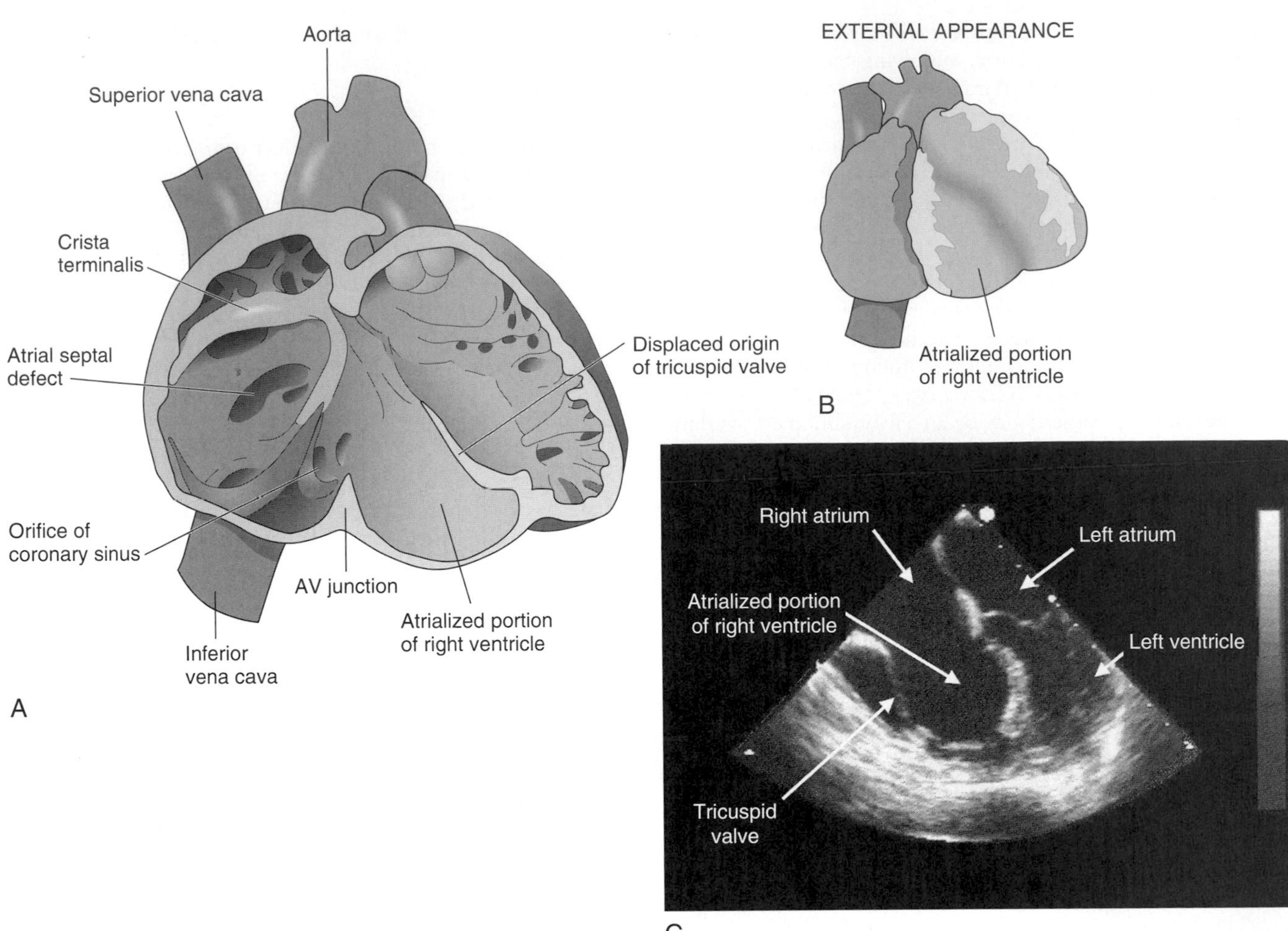

■ **FIGURE 17–24.** Anatomic features of Ebstein's anomaly. *(A)* Displacement of the posterior and septal leaflets into the right ventricle results in a large atrialized chamber and tricuspid valve incompetence. AV, atrioventricular. *(B)* External appearance. *(C)* Ebstein's anomaly, showing the atrialized portion of the right ventricle, with the tricuspid valve extending deep into the right ventricle and the intraventricular septum bowing into the left ventricle.

Alternative therapy includes procainamide or amiodarone. TEE should be used to evaluate the repair and the function of both the RV and LV. Particular attention should be given to the tricuspid valve, RVOT, and intraventricular septum.

PALLIATION SURGERY

Palliative surgery is reserved for cardiac lesions in which anatomic parts are missing, such as pulmonary atresia with intact septum (absent RV and PA), tricuspid atresia (absent RV and tricuspid valve), HLHS (absent mitral valve and small LV), mitral atresia (absent LV), or univentricular heart (absent RV or LV) (Castaneda et al., 1989). Underdeveloped or absent chambers and great vessels preclude complete reconstruction of a normal four-chambered heart. The intraoperative management of patients receiving palliative operations is not intuitive. These patients remain the most difficult group of patients to care for because blood flow patterns are abnormal, and the impact of preload augmentation, inotropic support, and afterload manipulations may redirect blood flow patterns as well as simply improve cardiac output and tissue oxygen delivery (Table 17–14). In addition, minor changes in PA pressure, PVR, AVV function, and ventricular performance may significantly increase postoperative morbidity (Pigott et al., 1988; Bridges et al., 1990).

The ultimate goal of palliative surgery is to separate the pulmonary and systemic circulation and in the case of a univentricular heart, to use the single ventricle as a systemic pumping chamber. The Fontan operation, initially described in 1971, and its modifications have been adapted to all forms of univentricular heart, including HLHS (Fontan et al., 1983; Mayer et al., 1986). The modified Fontan operation provides PBF by anastomosing all of the systemic venous return (SVC and IVC) to the PAs without an interposed pumping chamber. PBF is therefore dependent on maintaining a passive gradient from the systemic veins through the pulmonary vasculature and into the LA. This arrangement requires a low PVR and low left ventricular filling pressures. Since newborns have high PVR, they are not suitable candidates for a Fontan-type procedure. The goal in the newborn period is to achieve balanced blood flow between the pulmonary and systemic circulation until the PVR falls, rendering the child suitable for a modified Fontan procedure or more commonly a cavopulmonary anastomosis.

Hypoplastic Left Heart Syndrome

A palliative procedure is performed in the newborn period to limit excessive blood flow to the pulmonary circulation and provide balanced blood flow between the systemic and pulmonary circulation. In patients with two normal-sized great arteries this may be accomplished by placing a restrictive band around the main PA. If the main PA is very small or atretic and PBF is primarily from the ductus arteriosus, PBF is maintained by placing a restrictive PA-to-aorta shunt and ligating the ductus arteriosus, thereby limiting PBF and reducing the volume load on the single ventricle. In more complex anatomy, such as HLHS, the entire aorta must be reconstructed as well (Table 17–14).

In the HLHS, there is only a functional RV. The LV is severely hypoplastic, and the mitral valve is severely stenotic or atretic. In addition, the aortic valve is either atretic or severely stenotic, so much so that the PDA provides retrograde flow to the coronary circulation via the transverse and hypoplastic ascending arch and antegrade flow to the descending aorta. The single RV has to pump blood to both the pulmonary circulation (through the PA) and the systemic circulation (through the ductus arteriosus). The direction of predominant blood flow is dependent on downstream resistance, that is, the flow is determined by the PVR and the SVR. Ideally, balanced flow results in an equal portion of cardiac output going to both the systemic and pulmonary vascular beds, resulting in a 1:1 shunt (Fig. 17–25).

Operative repair for patients with HLHS requires a series of staged procedures culminating in the modified Fontan procedure. In infancy, the operative objective is to establish an outflow from the single RV to the systemic circulation. This is accomplished by performing an atrial septectomy to allow pulmonary venous blood to mix with systemic venous blood, transecting the main PA, creating a neoaorta using pulmonary homograft, and connecting it from the proximal pulmonary aorta to the hypoplastic ascending aorta (Norwood et al., 1983; Norwood and Murphy, 1990) (Fig. 17–26). This single great vessel provides systemic and coronary blood flow. PBF is provided by a Gore-Tex shunt from the innominate artery, subclavian artery, or, rarely, the neoaorta to the main PA. The Sano modification of the stage 1 Norwood palliative procedure uses a Gore-Tex shunt from the systemic ventricle to the PA (Sano et al., 2003). The first stage is a palliative procedure that eliminates the need for ductal patency. If not previously present, a large ASD is created intraoperatively, forming the RA and LA into a common chamber.

Perioperative management of patients with HLHS is based on maintaining effective systemic cardiac output and then balancing flow between the systemic and pulmonary circulations and minimizing the volume load on the heart—maintaining a pulmonary-to-systemic ratio of 1. This can be achieved by maintaining SaO_2 in the range of 70 to 80. In the preoperative period, excessive PBF is the most common problem; anesthetic management strategies are therefore directed at reducing PBF. Regardless of the anatomic lesion and the surgical technique required to achieve shunt-dependent blood flow, the physiologic goals are the same—to maintain effective systemic cardiac output, minimize volume load on the single ventricle, restrict excessive PBF, and maintain balanced flow between the pulmonary and systemic circulation (Hansen and Hickey, 1986; Norwood and Murphy, 1990; Norwood et al., 1991). If pulmonary resistance is low, then a greater proportion of the cardiac output is directed to the lungs and the single ventricle is required to increase its cardiac output by increasing stroke volume and heart rate (Pigott et al., 1988). The newborn heart has a reduced capacity to increase stroke volume, especially when volume loaded. When flow becomes unbalanced and a large left-to-right shunt provides a disproportionate amount of blood flow to the lungs, systemic hypoperfusion and metabolic acidosis result. Once low systemic perfusion is evident, therapy must be implemented to improve cardiac output, correct metabolic acidosis, and redistribute blood flow to the systemic circulation.

Postbypass and postoperative management are based primarily on increasing total cardiac output through the use of inotropes and phosphodiesterase type III inhibitors and, secondarily, on balancing blood flow between the systemic and pulmonary circuits if PBF is excessive (Table 17–15). A systemic arterial saturation of 75% to 80% with a mixed venous saturation of 50% to 60% gives a 1:1 shunt or balanced pulmonary/systemic flow. Lower mixed venous saturations are associated with poor cardiac output, and the inotrope support should be initiated or increased (Tweddell et al., 2000). Mixed venous oxygen saturation monitoring measured from the internal jugular venous catheter placed in the high SVC is an important monitor for assessing cardiac output and balancing pulmonary/systemic flow.

A balanced shunt can be calculated from the pulmonary/systemic flow equation:

$$\dot{Q}p/\dot{Q}s = (SaO_2 - SvO_2)\ (PvO_2 - PaO_2)$$

In this physiology, PA and aortic saturations are equal. Estimating balanced shunt flow just by the aortic saturations is not accurate because low mixed venous saturations and excessive shunt flow can result in systemic saturations of 75%. A reliable way of assessing shunt physiology intraoperatively is through continuous monitoring of arterial saturation with pulse oximetry and intermittent or continuous measures of mixed venous saturations. As a surrogate measure of continuous venous oximetry, a cerebral oximetry probe can be used in these patients. The absolute number may not be 100% accurate, but as a trend monitor, it may be useful. If mixed venous saturations are not monitored, low arterial saturations may reflect low total cardiac output rather than reduced PBF, as already noted.

TABLE 17–14. Single-ventricle anatomy and surgical palliation

Diagnosis	Surgical Therapy
Tricuspid atresia	Balloon atrial septostomy→cavopulmonary anastomosis→Fontan
Malaligned AV canal with hypoplastic right ventricle	Pulmonary artery band→cavopulmonary anastomosis→Fontan
Malaligned AV canal with hypoplastic left ventricle	DKS→cavopulmonary anastomosis→Fontan
Pulmonary atresia with intact ventricular septum	Modified BT shunt→cavopulmonary anastomosis→Fontan
Pulmonary atresia with discontinuous pulmonary arteries	Unifocalization with shunt→cavopulmonary anastomosis→Fontan
Double-outlet right ventricle with mitral atresia	DKS/Norwood/Sano→cavopulmonary anastomosis→Fontan
Double-inlet left ventricle	DKS→cavopulmonary anastomosis→Fontan
Hypoplastic left heart syndrome	Norwood/Sano→cavopulmonary anastomosis→Fontan
Critical aortic stenosis with hypoplastic left ventricle	Norwood/Sano→cavopulmonary anastomosis→Fontan
Subset of heterotaxy syndromes	Possible DKS→cavopulmonary anastomosis→Fontan

AV, Atrioventricular; BT, Blalock-Taussig; DKS, Damus-Kaye-Stanzel; Fontan procedure.

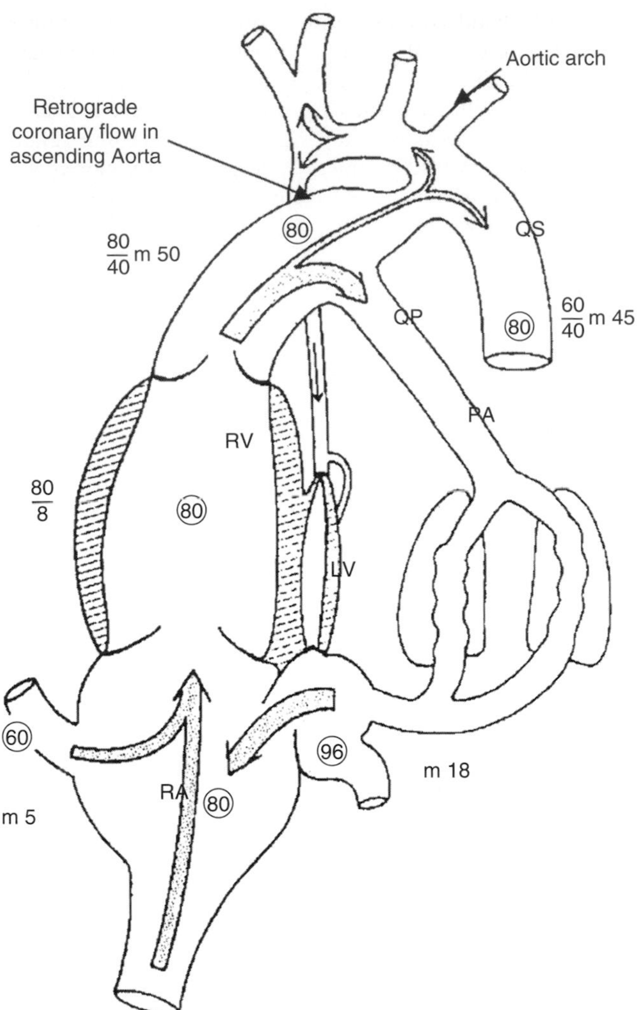

■ **FIGURE 17–25.** Hypoplastic left heart syndrome before surgery, showing the importance of maintaining a patent ductus arteriosus to maintain systemic cardiac output and balancing $\dot{Q}p/\dot{Q}s$. LV, left ventricle; PA, pulmonary artery; RA, right atrium; RV, right ventricle. (With permission from Rudolph A: *Congenital diseases of the heart*. Year Book Medical Publishers, Chicago. 1985, 2001.)

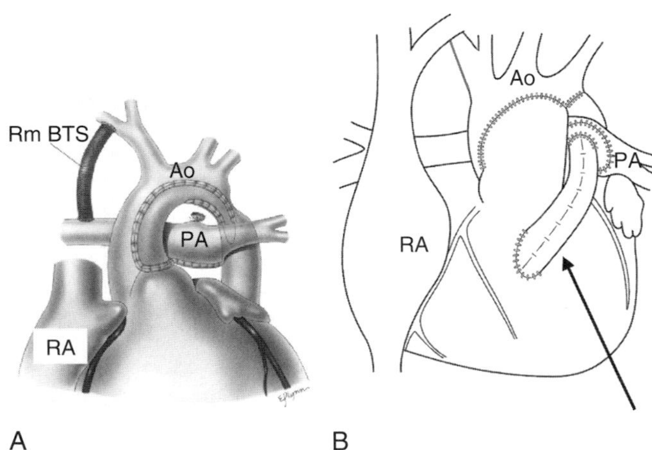

■ **FIGURE 17–26.** *(A)* Classic Norwood Stage 1 operation with a modified Blalock-Taussig shunt (BTS) from the innominate artery to the main pulmonary artery (PA). Also shown is reconstruction of the neoaorta and atrial septectomy. *(B)* Sano-modified Norwood operation, showing the right ventricle–to–PA conduit rather than a modified BT shunt. Ao, aorta; RA, right atrium.

Inotropic agents are important in improving systemic cardiac output in these patients. When comparing epinephrine, dopamine, and dobutamine, only epinephrine significantly improved systemic cardiac output and systemic oxygen delivery in a piglet model of HLHS; this is because epinephrine increased total cardiac output without increasing $\dot{Q}p/\dot{Q}s$. In contrast, dobutamine increased total cardiac output but increased $\dot{Q}p/\dot{Q}s$ to greater than 2:1 and therefore systemic oxygen delivery worsened. In this model dopamine had only a modest increase in total cardiac output and did not appear to affect $\dot{Q}p/\dot{Q}s$, so systemic oxygen delivery was statistically unchanged (Riordan et al., 1996). It has become increasingly apparent that increasing systemic cardiac output is critical in managing these patients and that inotropic support in conjunction with systemic afterload reduction is the preferred medical management strategy.

Another approach to the management of elevated SVR in the postbypass period is with the use of systemic vasodilators. Milrinone (0.5 mcg/kg per minute) in the postbypass and postoperative period and potent systemic vasodilators such as phenoxybenzamine (0.25 mg/kg) added to the bypass circuit represent two such strategies. The more commonly applied strategy initiates milrinone or other unloading agents shortly before separation from CPB and uses inotropic agents to

■ **TABLE 17–15.** Effects of aortic and mixed venous saturation on pulmonary and systemic flows in patients with single ventricles

Aortic Saturation (%)	Svo_2	Q_p/Q_s	Clinical Considerations
80	65	1:1	Balanced shunt
85	65	2:1	Mild reduction in systemic flow
90	65	5:1	Severe reduction in systemic flow
95	65	∞	Infinite shunt
75	65	1:2	Mild reduction in pulmonary flow
70	65	1:5	Severe reduction in pulmonary flow
80	50	2:1	Decreased cardiac ouput, increased $\dot{Q}_p$
80	30	>2:1	Decreased cardiac output, increased $\dot{Q}_p$

$\dot{Q}_p$, pulmonary blood flow; $\dot{Q}_s$, systemic blood flow.

optimize systemic cardiac output. The main advantage of this strategy is the ability to titrate increases in cardiac contractility and afterload reduction. The use of phenoxybenzamine on pump has the disadvantages that it is a potent noncompetitive antagonist of αARs that may take upward of 24 hours to regenerate, it is not titratable, and it may require low-dose norepinephrine (0.1 mcg/kg per minute) to increase mean blood pressure (Tweddell et al., 2000).

Ventricular dysfunction in the stage I Norwood patient with a systemic-to-pulmonary shunt is due to shunt-dependent volume overload and reduced coronary blood flow from diversion of blood through the systemic-to-pulmonary shunt. For this reason, there has been an increasing interest in alternative strategies to the initial surgical management of HLHS. The Sano modification, which replaced the systemic-to-pulmonary shunt with a shunt from the RV to the PA, preserves coronary perfusion by preventing diastolic runoff. Several small series have demonstrated significant improvement in diastolic blood pressure, myocardial function, and inotrope use (Maher et al., 2003; Mahle et al., 2003; Mair et al., 2003; Pizarro et al., 2003; Sano et al., 2003) (see Fig. 17–26*B*). Bicarbonate administration is also an important adjunct to low cardiac output in shunt-dependent patients. Sodium bicarbonate corrects metabolic acidosis and provides an optimal pH for inotropic effect.

Vasodilators such as nitroprusside reduce SVR and promote systemic cardiac output. In combination with ventilatory manipulations and bicarbonate administration, vasodilators should augment systemic perfusion. Vasodilators should be used cautiously, however, if systemic pressure is low. Volume support inotropic agents should be readily available when nitroprusside is administered. Milrinone is generally a preferred first-line drug, but if blood pressure is adequately supplemented with inotropic support, sodium nitroprusside can significantly augment systemic perfusion.

Studies have demonstrated the beneficial use of inhaled CO_2 as a pulmonary vasoconstrictor in patients with low PVR (Norwood et al., 1992; Bradley et al., 2001; Keidan et al., 2003). This technique has proved to be most useful in the prebypass period as opposed to the post-CPB period (Keidan et al., 2003). Patients almost always need to be paralyzed with a neuromuscular blocking agent when exogenous inhaled CO_2 is added. Sedation alone is usually ineffective. Intraoperative control of excessive PBF in the prerepair period is essential. Surface cooling and opening of the sternum reduce CO_2 production and decrease PVR, respectively. The administration of 1% to 2% CO_2 into the fresh gas flow may be beneficial in controlling PBF. The benefits of exogenous administration of CO_2 as opposed to controlled hypoventilation are that lung volumes can be maintained while PBF is restricted.

Hypoxic gas mixtures ($FIO_2 = 17\%$) have also been advocated to control PBF. The benefits of hypoxic gas mixtures are that they can be administered without the need for heavy sedation or the use of muscle relaxants. In centers where heart transplantation has been the preferred procedure for HLHS, newborns are extubated into hypoxic environments while waiting weeks to months for a donor heart. The disadvantage of a hypoxic gas mixture is decreased oxygen delivery. Impaired oxygen delivery becomes increasingly problematic if significant pulmonary edema, lung disease, or worsening ventricular function develops. In a randomized crossover controlled study, Tabbut and others (2001) noted that in 10 paralyzed and ventilated preoperative HLHS patients, 2.7% inspired CO_2 was found to improve delivery of oxygen compared with 17% FIO_2. A hypoxic gas mixture is rarely used after the first-stage repair for HLHS for reasons outlined earlier.

If PVR is significantly elevated, a more common occurrence during weaning from CPB, then inadequate PBF is the result and the patient becomes moderately to severely hypoxemic. Inspired FIO_2 of 1.0%, alkalinization, nitric oxide administration, and ensured adequate levels of anesthesia can reduce PVR and improve PBF. Persistent hypoxemia or significant hypercarbia unresponsive to ventilatory manipulations may be due to shunt dysfunction (clotting or kinking) and should be investigated by intraoperative echocardiography and visual inspection of the shunt. Urgent resumption of CPB is indicated if shunt flow remains inadequate despite these maneuvers.

Postbypass low cardiac output could be due to AVV regurgitation, neoaortic valve insufficiency, inadequate atrial septectomy, and coronary insufficiency due to kinking or poor flow through the native diminutive ascending aorta.

The end result of this first-stage procedure is the creation of a univentricular heart in which the single RV is directly connected to the systemic circulation. The newly created shunt connects either a branch of the aorta (innominate) to the PA or, in the Sano modification, a direct connection of the single ventricle to the PA. These procedures do not eliminate the need for balancing blood flow between pulmonary and systemic circulations but generally restrict PBF to a greater extent than the PDA. The palliative stage 1 procedure sets the stage for later correction with a cavopulmonary anastomosis with a bidirectional Glenn or hemi-Fontan procedure or, rarely, directly to a modified Fontan, as discussed later.

Another novel approach to the first-stage management of HLHS has been a combined cardiac catheterization and operating room approach to limit PBF and either place a stent to open the ductus or surgically place a modified BT shunt. This approach was first described by Gibbs and others (1993). A small series of eight patients with HLHS were reported by Muller and colleagues (2003) in which a catheterization laboratory–based approach to stage I palliation was used. In this series, the initial management included ductal stenting and balloon atrial enlargement if indicated. One to 3 days later, a surgically placed PA band was used to restrict PBF. There were no deaths in the initial palliation. The second-stage procedure requires a combined stage 1 and stage 2 operative intervention; this includes construction of a neoaorta and placement of a bidirectional Glenn. In this small series, there was one death after the combined stage 1 and 2 procedure (12.5% mortality).

The overall survival of the first-stage repair for HLHS (Norwood stage I) has been reported as 68% to 77% (Norwood and Murphy, 1990; Norwood et al., 1991, 1992; Bove et al., 1996; Kern et al., 1997). A comparison of survival rates from Children's Hospital of Philadelphia demonstrates the effects on survival of newer technical advances in the management of HLHS (Mahle et al., 2000) (Fig. 17–27). In particular, early survival (first 120 days) in the era of 1984 to 1988 was 56%; from 1995 to 1998 (pre-Sano), survival increased to 71%. Late survival statistics (after 120 days) has a strong correlation with the introduction of bilateral cavopulmonary anastomosis procedures (Glenn or hemi-Fontan). The impact on late survival was demonstrated with an increase in hospital survival from 96.3% for the bilateral cavopulmonary anastomosis in 1984 to 1988 to 100% in 1995 to 1998. For the Fontan procedure, the survival rates increased from 76% to 100% during this same timeframe.

With this evolution, the hospital discharge rate after the initial palliative procedure has continued to improve, with survival rates of 90% or higher reported in some series (Ghanayem et al., 2003). Home surveillance programs with strict attention to oxygen saturations with pulse oximetry and weight gain in infants following the HLHS first-stage repair are improving outcomes. Infants should achieve a minimum weight gain of 20 g during the course of 3 days, and home pulse oximetry monitoring to ensure saturations remain greater than 70% is advocated. This surveillance program has improved the survival of the interstage

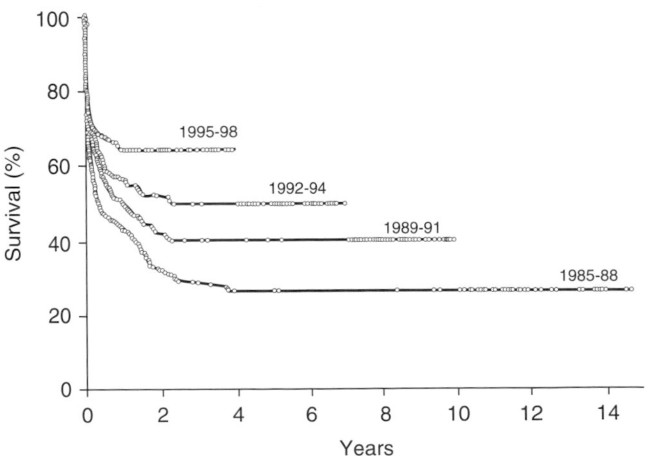

■ **FIGURE 17–27.** Graph depicting improved survival for the Norwood procedure from 1985 through 1998. The improved survival reflects the evolution of the operation. In particular, a cavopulmonary anastomosis is introduced as an interim operative procedure.

mortality between the Norwood operation and the subsequent cavopulmonary anastomosis (Ghanayem et al., 2003).

Truncus Arteriosus

Truncus arteriosus is a congenital cardiac defect that is characterized by a single great artery arising from the base of the heart with a single semilunar valve (van Praagh and van Praagh, 1965). This single artery gives rise to the systemic, pulmonary, and coronary circulations. The defect is classified by the location of the branch PAs, the presence or absence of a VSD, and the developmental characteristics of the ascending aorta and ductus arteriosus (Fig. 17–28). Type I truncus has a single, short main PA arising from the truncus that divides into left and right PAs, which follow a normal course into the hilum. In type II truncus arteriosus, the branch PAs arise from separate orifices off of the truncal artery. Type III truncus arteriosus is characterized by the right and left PAs arising from opposite lateral walls of the truncal artery. Type IV truncus arteriosus or hemitruncus is characterized by a single branch PA arising from the truncal artery and a second nonconfluent branch PA arising from aortopulmonary collateral vessels or the ductus arteriosus. Type IV truncus is commonly grouped with tetralogy of Fallot or pulmonary atresia. Truncus is also classified as type A (presence of a VSD) and type B (intact ventricular septum).

Patients with truncus arteriosus present with cyanosis, excessive PBF, heart failure, and truncal valve regurgitation. In the preoperative and prebypass period, management is directed at reducing PBF by increasing $PaCO_2$, maintaining FIO_2 at 0.21% and, if indicated, the use of exogenous CO_2 to reduce PBF. In addition, inotropic support may be necessary to augment systemic oxygen delivery by increasing systemic cardiac output (Qs) if PBF is excessive. Measures to reduce PBF may become increasingly important after opening the chest because this further reduces PVR by removing impedance of the chest wall.

Operative repair for truncus arteriosus is usually performed in the neonatal period. The operative procedure includes removing the PAs from the truncal artery, closing the VSD, and placing a valved homograft from the RV to the main PA. Regurgitation of the truncal valve is usually reduced by reducing the flow across the valve. Occasionally, however, severe truncal valve incompetence is present, necessitating truncal valve replacement. Severe regurgitation in the postbypass and postoperative periods is poorly tolerated, especially if moderate to severe myocardial dysfunction is present. Under these circumstances, truncal valve replacement is indicated. Postbypass management usually is directed at controlling PA hypertension and providing inotropic support for right and left ventricular dysfunction. Reactive PA hypertension is common in neonates with preoperative increased PBF, as is found in truncus arteriosus.

■ SINGLE VENTRICLE PROCEDURES

If total systemic venous return (SVC and IVC) is directed to the PAs, the arrangement is termed a *modified Fontan procedure*. In this operation, the IVC blood is directed to the SVC by the use of an intra-atrial tube graft or baffle (Jonas and Castaneda, 1988; Mayer et al., 1992) or an extracardiac conduit with or without fenestration (Stamm et al., 2002) (Fig. 17–29*A*, *B*). This surgical arrangement allows all systemic venous return to enter the pulmonary circulation. The cavopulmonary anastomosis is a "partial Fontan procedure"; that is, the SVC alone is anastomosed to the PAs and IVC flow is allowed to mix with pulmonary

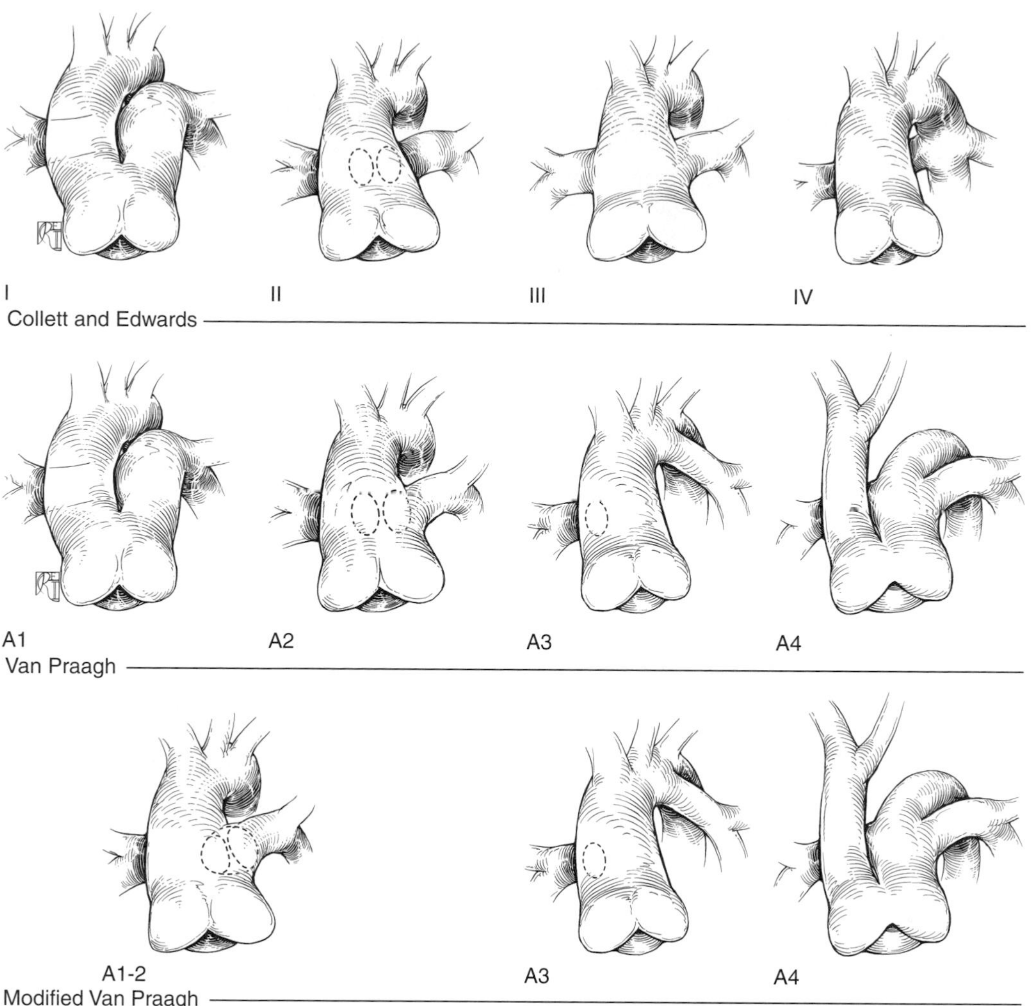

■ **FIGURE 17–28.** Truncus. There are similarities between the Collett and Edwards and the Van Praagh classifications of truncus arteriosus. Type I is the same as A1. Types II and III are grouped as a single type A2 because they are not significantly distinct embryologically or therapeutically. Type A3 denotes unilateral pulmonary artery with collateral supply to the contralateral lung. Type A4 is truncus associated with interrupted aortic arch (13% of all cases of truncus arteriosus). (From Mavroudis C, Backer CL, editors: *Pediatric cardiac surgery,* 3rd ed. Stamford, CT, 1999, Appleton & Lange, p 340, Chapter 19, Truncus Arteriosus.)

venous return. A classic Glenn shunt is a cavopulmonary anastomosis that connects the SVC directly to the right PA and oversews the SVC-RA junction. The left PA is left separated from the right PA and SVC, and therefore systemic venous blood flow from the SVC is directed only to the right lung. The classic Glenn is not used as a staging procedure for single-ventricle patients. The preferred forms of cavopulmonary anastomosis are the bidirectional Glenn shunt and hemi-Fontan. The bidirectional Glenn leaves the right PA and left PA in continuity (Fig. 17–30), and the SVC blood flow is distributed to both the right and left PAs. The SVC is disconnected from the RA. SVC flow enters into the common atrium (physiologic LA), mixes with pulmonary venous blood, and enters the single ventricle. An alternative intermediate-stage procedure is the hemi-Fontan, which anastomoses both PAs to the SVC. The SVC is left in continuity with the RA, and a partial tube graft is sewn in place below the SVC with a dam at the base of the tube graft. This arrangement facilitates the completion of the Fontan because the surgeon needs to open the RA, remove the dam, and complete the anastomosis between the partial tube graft and the IVC.

The advantage of the cavopulmonary anastomosis operation is maintaining cardiac output even if PBF is reduced. Poor functioning of a bidirectional Glenn in the operating room is characterized by desaturation. Cardiac output is well maintained unless PBF is severely reduced, resulting in inadequate myocardial oxygen delivery. Desaturation must be carefully assessed in the operating room to ensure adequate flow across the SVC and PA anastomosis, and avoiding an elevated PVR restrictive atrial septum, or obstructed pulmonary veins (Box 17–5).

Modified Fontan Procedure

The modified Fontan procedure can be completed by either a lateral tunnel procedure or an extracardiac conduit. The lateral tunnel procedure creates an intra-atrial tube graft between the SVC and IVC and is sewn so that the back wall of the atrium forms the posterior portion of the tube. Alternatively, an extracardiac conduit can be created. It connects the SVC to the IVC outside of the heart. The advantage of the lateral tunnel approach is that the posterior wall is native atrial tissue and allows the conduit to grow with the child. Also, the lateral tunnel conduit can be easily fenestrated. The extracardiac conduit is a solid tube and therefore does not grow with the patient; it also is difficult to fenestrate (see Fig. 17–29*B*). Fenestration requires a direct connection to the atrium. As atrial contraction occurs, it creates

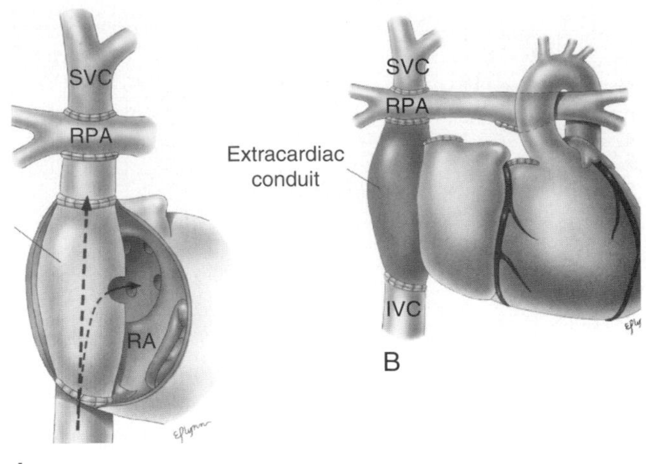

■ **FIGURE 17–29.** *(A)* The modified Fontan operation using a lateral tunnel approach. The lateral tunnel is created by placing an intra-atrial Gore-Tex tube graft extending from the inferior vena cava to the superior vena cava and sewn to the posterior atrial wall. Here, the lateral tunnel is fenestrated by placing a 4-mm punch hole in the Gore-Tex portion of the graft. This allows approximately 20% of cardiac output to enter the single (systemic) ventricle without having to pass through the lungs, thereby enhancing systemic oxygen delivery. *(B)* Modified Fontan operation using an extracardiac conduit rather than an intra-atrial lateral tunnel. This approach minimizes exposure of the atrial tissue to high pressure. The extracardiac conduit can be fenestrated but has a lower success rate of maintaining patency due to low flow and interruption of flow caused by atrial contraction. (With permission from O'Brien P, Boisurt JT: Current management of infants and children with single ventricle anatomy. *J Pediatr Nursing* 16:338–350, 2001.)

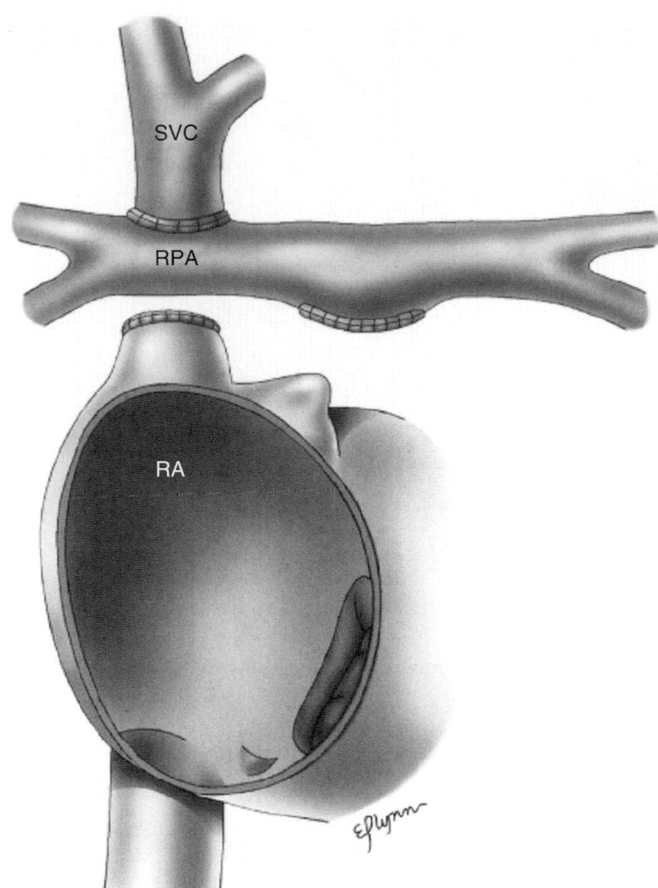

■ **FIGURE 17–30.** Bidirectional cavopulmonary anastomosis (bidirectional Glenn) demonstrating the connection of the superior vena cava (SVC) to the right pulmonary artery while maintaining continuity to both the right and left pulmonary arteries. The lower portion of the SVC is disarticulated from the right atrium, and the inferior vena cava blood flow enters the right atrium and mixes with left atrial blood through a widely patent atrial septectomy. RA, right atrium; RPA, right pulmonary artery. (With permission from O'Brien P, Boisurt JT: Current management of infants and children with single ventricle anatomy. *J Pediatr Nursing* 16:338–350, 2001.)

periods of low flow, and the fenestration commonly occludes early in the postoperative period. The main advantage of the extracardiac conduit is that atrial tissue is not exposed to high pressure and there are no suture lines in the atrium; atrial arrhythmias are less likely to occur in the long term. Acutely, there is also a higher incidence of effusions after the extracardiac Fontan procedure. Finally, the lack of a fenestration is generally well tolerated if a bidirectional Glenn or hemi-Fontan procedure preceded the modified Fontan procedure.

In the modified Fontan procedures, cardiac output is preload limited. Blood return to the single ventricle is dependent on maintaining a pressure gradient between the systemic veins, the pulmonary vasculature, and the single ventricle. Increased PVR, elevated PA pressures (>18 mm Hg), distortion of the PAs, obstruction of the SVC-to-PA anastomosis or intraatrial baffle, pulmonary venous obstruction, AVV regurgitation, or stenosis limits venous return to the single ventricle and decreases cardiac output (Bridges et al., 1990). Clinically, these abnormalities and systolic or diastolic single-ventricle dysfunction are manifest as low cardiac output in the Fontan patient. In the operating room, pressure monitoring, including systemic venous pressure, which reflects PA pressure, and left atrial or, more accurately, common atrial pressure are helpful in distinguishing causes for poor cardiac output and assists in optimally managing these patients (see Box 17–5). In addition, TEE may demonstrate residual anatomic problems such as flow obstruction through the conduit or baffle, valvular regurgitation, and pulmonary venous obstruction as well as ventricular functional abnormalities. The use of TEE can help target both medical and, if indicated, additional surgical treatment.

Fontan patients with good intraoperative hemodynamics have age-appropriate blood pressure when systemic venous pressure (measured in the SVC proximal to the SVC-PA anastomosis), which reflects PA pressure, ranges from 12 to 15 mm Hg and left atrial or common atrial pressure ranges from 5 to 8 mm Hg. Acutely, physiologic systemic venous pressures may be as high as 20 to 25 mm Hg in patients with persistent elevations in PA pressures. This elevated pressure (which is reflective of the PA pressure) may be tolerated for a short period of time in the postoperative period. However, these elevated pressures should decrease with medical management. When the systemic venous pressure exceeds 15 mm Hg, the common atrial pressure is high (10 to 15 mm Hg) and the transpulmonary gradient (systemic venous pressure-common atrial pressure) is less than 10 mm Hg, then ventricular dysfunction, AVV regurgitation, or ventricular outflow obstruction (aortic valve stenosis or supravalvar stenosis) must be ruled out. When the systemic venous pressure is high, the common atrial pressure is low, and the transpulmonary gradient is also low, then elevated PVR, PA hypertension, baffle obstruction, or previously unrecognized obstruction of the branch

BOX 17–5 Causes of Low Cardiac Output After Fontan Completion

	Systemic Venous Pressure	Common Atrial Pressure	Transpulmonary Gradient
Anatomic			
Pulmonary artery stenosis or obstruction	↑	↓	↑
Restrictive intra-atrial septum	↑	↑	↓
Systemic outflow tract obstruction	↑	↑	N to low
Superior vena cava clot or obstruction*	↑	↓	↑
Atrioventricular valve regurgitation or stenosis	↑	↑	N
Systemic aortic valve stenosis or regurgitation	↑	↑	N
Coarctation of the aorta	↑	↑	N
Pulmonary venous obstruction	↑	↓	↑
Physiologic			
Systemic ventricle dysfunction	↑	↑	N
Pulmonary hypertension	↑	↓	↑

*Superior vena cava–pulmonary artery pressure gradient >2 mm Hg.
Note: After the cavopulmonary anastomosis, because inferior vena cava blood flow enters the systemic ventricle without first having to pass through the lungs, any anatomic obstruction through the lungs will present with low oxygen saturation but a preserved cardiac output. (↑, increases; ↓, decreases; N, normal.)

PAs or pulmonary veins may be present. As previously mentioned, all of these problems are clinically manifest as low cardiac output.

High systemic venous and low common atrial pressures or a large gradient measured from the physiologic systemic venous catheter proximal to the anastomosis of the SVC and PAs in the Fontan patient may be a physiologic or an anatomic problem. Anatomic problems include baffle obstruction, obstructed pulmonary veins, and PA distortion. Baffle obstruction is easily remedied but must be diagnosed early before significant and irreversible consequences of abnormal hemodynamics occur. Baffle obstruction is best diagnosed by either TEE or measuring pressures in the IVC and SVC. Intraoperative echocardiography may not be able to visualize a narrowing or to appreciate minor pressure gradients within the atrial baffle or the SVC-to-PA anastomosis; this is particularly true if an extracardiac conduit is used. Mean pressure gradients as low as 3 to 4 mm Hg across the extracardiac conduit or intraatrial baffle are significant and suggest a clinically significant stenosis in the systemic venous-to-PA pathway.

Pulmonary venous obstruction can occur after Fontan operation, especially in patients with complex venous anatomy (e.g., heterotaxy syndromes) or in patients with a small LA (HLHS) (Mayer et al., 1986). This is more common in heterotaxy syndromes where the pulmonary veins enter the atrium at an unusual location and an intra-atrial baffle is used to complete the Fontan procedure. In these cases, most surgeons are performing an extracardiac connection between the SVC and IVC (Kumar et al., 2003). The use of a simple intra-atrial tube graft (lateral tunnel procedure) from the IVC to the SVC in patients with normal pulmonary veins and a single SVC minimizes the risk of pulmonary venous obstruction. If a left-sided SVC is also present, this may be directly anastomosed to the left PA and the left SVC-atrium junction oversewn. Obstructed, abnormal pulmonary veins are poorly tolerated physiologically in the Fontan procedure. In general, attempts are made to treat pulmonary venous obstruction by balloon dilation and/or placement of small stents in the cardiac catheterization laboratory. The results of this approach to treat pulmonary venous obstruction are poor in most cases but worth trying preoperatively.

PA distortion is usually due to a previous shunt procedure. This can be treated by balloon dilation or stenting in the catheterization laboratory before surgery, or the PA may need to be reconstructed in the operating room at the time of the Fontan procedure.

Physiologic problems resulting in high systemic venous and low common atrial pressures are generally due to an elevation in PVR or PA pressure. Fontan patients have a very limited ability to compensate for these changes and have diminished systemic perfusion and low cardiac output. Common treatable causes for increased PVR in the Fontan patient include hypoxia, hypercarbia, acidosis, excessive mean airway pressure or PEEP, and extrapleural compression of the lung due to pleural effusion, hemothorax, or pneumothorax. In the absence of a clearly reversible cause for increased PVR, therapy is directed toward controlling pH, $Paco_2$, Pao_2, and alkalinization. Reduced lung volumes should be treated with improving mechanical ventilation. High tidal volume ventilation with relatively short inspiratory times to achieve an arterial CO_2 of 33 to 38 mm Hg, along with systemic alkalinization with sodium bicarbonate, is effective in lowering PVR. Positive pressure ventilation, which results in high mean airway pressure or use of high end-expiratory pressure, has a negative impact on PBF. In general, it is important to provide a short inspiratory phase and a prolonged expiratory phase with low mean airway pressure. PBF predominates during exhalation, so an inspiratory-to-expiratory ratio of 1:3 or longer is preferred. PEEP may be used judiciously in Fontan patients to maintain functional residual capacity, as previously discussed. Excessive PEEP, however, is poorly tolerated in Fontan physiology. Jet ventilation is an effective alternative mode of ventilation that achieves alkalization at lower mean airway pressures and significantly improves cardiac output (Dietrich et al., 1993). Milrinone, epinephrine, and inhaled NO are useful therapeutic interventions. In addition, transfusion to hematocrits of 40% to 45% is useful in improving oxygen delivery.

There are three major causes for high systemic venous and high common atrial pressures in the Fontan patient: ventricular dysfunction (primarily diastolic dysfunction), AVV regurgitation, and ventricular outflow tract obstruction. The most troublesome consequence is diastolic dysfunction of the systemic ventricle. Because some preoperative Fontan candidates have a volume-loaded, hypertrophied ventricle, elevated ventricular end-diastolic pressures should be looked for after the Fontan operation (Nishioka et al., 1981; Sanders et al., 1982). The institution of the Glenn procedure at between 4 and 8 months and improved management of stage 1 Norwood procedure have significantly reduced the volume load on the single ventricle and contributed to preservation of myocardial function and better tolerance of Fontan physiology. Inotropic agents that improve systolic function such as epinephrine also have lusitropic properties and acutely benefit diastolic function. In the long term, inotropic agents impair ventricular relaxation. Vasodilators and phosphodiesterase type III inhibitors reduce ventricular volume and are beneficial in patients with diastolic dysfunction; however, in the postoperative Fontan patient, cardiac output is dependent on adequate preload and these patients are sensitive to a reduction in filling pressure. Drugs that promote ventricular relaxation or only minimally increase contractility and unload the heart such as nitroprusside, calcium channel blockers (e.g., nicardipine), and phosphodiesterase inhibitors (e.g., milrinone) may be helpful.

AVV regurgitation may be due to either a preexisting abnormal valve or the chronic volume load on the single ventricle in the pre-Fontan period (Nishioka et al., 1981; Sanders et al., 1982). In either case, AVV regurgitation is poorly tolerated in the postoperative Fontan patient because of the critical dependence of this physiology on ventricular filling. When valve replacement is combined with a Fontan operation, a higher-than-anticipated postoperative mortality has been observed (Kirklin and Barratt-Boyes, 1986). This may be related to the gradient that is present in an artificial valve and the consequent increase in left atrial pressure incurred. Most commonly, AVVs can be repaired successfully even with a circular annuloplasty to help control regurgitation, although there are some patients in whom the AVV regurgitation improves after the cavopulmonary anastomosis and a valvuloplasty is not justified. Patients with moderate or mild preoperative AVV regurgitation usually experience improvement and do not require a valvuloplasty (Mahle et al., 2001). Afterload reduction, coupled with preload augmentation and a mild increase in inotropy with a phosphodiesterase inhibitor, low-dose dopamine, or dobutamine, may be helpful in these patients.

Ventricular outflow tract obstruction results in a pressure load on a previously volume-loaded heart. This worsens ventricular systolic and diastolic function, increasing the risk of a poor outcome after Fontan. Interventional cardiac catheterization and balloon dilation of supravalvar AS are important components of preparing these patients for Fontan operation. In HLHS, aortic arch obstruction is not an uncommon finding after repair and is known to be an important factor that increases mortality after the Norwood operation. It may require close follow-up and ongoing reinterventions in the catheterization laboratory (Soongswang et al., 2001).

High common atrial pressure with low systemic venous pressure is not possible in Fontan physiology. Because blood flow through the lungs is passive (i.e., without the benefit of a pulmonary ventricle), reversing the pressure gradient would prevent filling of the single systemic ventricle and no systemic cardiac output would ensue. If readings are obtained in which the common atrial pressure is greater than the systemic venous pressure, this must be a technical monitoring problem. In Glenn physiology, because cardiac output is maintained through the IVC, it is possible to have SVC pressure below that of the common atrium and still maintain cardiac output. These patients are extremely cyanotic. The usual etiology for this rare condition is large aorta-to-pulmonary collaterals that result in reversal of flow from the collaterals through the proximal PAs and into the SVC. Treatments for this rare condition include coiling of the collaterals in the catheter laboratory or takedown of the Glenn and replacement with an aorta-to-pulmonary shunt.

Postoperatively, all patients undergoing Fontan procedures have elevated SVC pressures. Elevated pressures contribute to several complications, including pleural effusions, hepatic and renal dysfunction, ascites, and protein-losing enteropathy (Kirklin and Barratt-Boyes, 1986). High systemic venous and right atrial pressures result in diminished drainage through the thoracic duct and the release of atrial natriuretic factor, which may contribute to effusions. SVC flow may also be impaired and, when coupled with low cardiac output, systemic organ perfusion is significantly reduced. The net result is diminished perfusion pressure to the abdominal viscera, hepatic and renal dysfunction, a significant accumulation of ascites, and, less commonly, a protein-losing enteropathy. A poorly functioning Fontan with high systemic venous pressure may result in severe, acute, and fatal hepatic failure due to high hepatic venous pressure and a diminution in effective hepatic blood flow (see Box 17–5).

Staging Operations in Single Ventricle

The Fontan procedure has been applied to an increasing number of patients, many of whom have risk factors that historically have made them poor candidates for Fontan physiology. PA distortion, increased PVR, pulmonary hypertension, AVV regurgitation, diminished ventricular performance, ventricular hypertrophy, complex cardiac anatomy (other than tricuspid atresia), and complex systemic or pulmonary venous connections increase the mortality associated with a Fontan operation from 5% to 10% to rates of 20% to 30% in some series (Mayer et al., 1986; Bridges et al., 1990). Although the optimal management of these patients is in evolution, it is clear that continued palliation with an aorta-to-pulmonary shunt is a poor alternative, because ventricular function worsens with prolonged shunt physiology. Patients with tricuspid atresia have less ventricular dilation and hypertrophy after Fontan repair than do those who undergo a second aortopulmonary shunt procedure. Fontan candidates, due to greater distortion of the PA, experience deterioration of ventricular function and elevation of PVR (Mietus-Snyder et al., 1987; Mayer et al., 1992).

Staging operations such as the cavopulmonary anastomosis are being advocated as an interim procedure in patients with increased risk after a Fontan procedure (DeLeon et al., 1983; Mazzera et al., 1989). Cavopulmonary anastomosis or fenestrations are modifications that allow an atrial-level communication; that is, blood enters the systemic ventricle from the RA without passing through the lungs. The advantage of these procedures over the completed Fontan is that effective PBF is maintained while ventricular volume load is minimized and systemic oxygenation is improved over traditional shunting procedures (Mietus-Snyder et al., 1987). In addition, cardiac output is not limited by high pressure or flow resistance across the pulmonary vascular bed. In the cavopulmonary anastomosis (bidirectional Glenn or hemi-Fontan), the entire IVC flow enters into the physiologic LA, mixes with pulmonary venous blood, and enters the single ventricle (see Fig. 17–30). Cardiac output can be augmented because all of the IVC return goes directly to the systemic ventricle and is pumped to the systemic circulation. The bidirectional Glenn and hemi-Fontan have the added advantage of allowing for a technically simple conversion to a completed Fontan (Bridges et al., 1990; Mott et al., 2001).

The cavopulmonary anastomosis has had a major role in allowing the application of Fontan physiology to a broader array of patients who were considered poor Fontan candidates in the 1990s. This approach has a low operative mortality and facilitates adaptation to the completed Fontan physiology by limiting the damaging effects of prolonged exposure to shunt physiology (Mott et al., 2001). Although the bidirectional Glenn procedure is a marked improvement over forcing young infants into Fontan physiology, it is not an optimal long-term intervention. The main reason is as children grow, the contribution of venous return through the SVC becomes appreciably less and therefore PBF decreases. Also, prolonged exposure to the physiology of the cavopulmonary anastomosis results in the development of pulmonary arteriovenous malformations (AVMs) in approximately 25% of patients. AVMs result in a progressive increase in cyanosis. The mechanism for the development of AVMs is believed to be that the liver produces inhibitors of angiogenesis that are excluded from the pulmonary circulation, so proangiogenesis factors are left unchecked (Duncan et al., 2003).

A fenestrated Fontan is physiologically similar to the bidirectional Glenn procedure. In this arrangement, the Fontan operation is completed using an intra-atrial lateral tunnel, and a 4-mm punch hole is placed in the tube graft connecting the IVC to the SVC. The punch hole produces a right-to-left shunt that allows approximately 20% of venous return to cross directly from the RA to the LA, thereby increasing cardiac output with minimal reductions in systemic saturation (Bridges et al., 1990). This technique provides the added advantage of not requiring a second surgical procedure, because these small punch holes can be closed in the cardiac catheterization laboratory using catheter-positioned ASD closure devices, or, in many cases, the fenestration closes on its own (Lloyd et al., 1998).

The main physiologic advantage of a bidirectional Glenn procedure over a fenestrated Fontan is lower IVC pressure and a larger augmentation in cardiac output. In the fenestrated Fontan, higher IVC pressure results in reduced hepatic, renal, and mesenteric perfusion, and the approximate 20% increase in cardiac output afforded by the fenestration may not be adequate.

The postoperative management of these patients is similar to that of the completed Fontan patient. Systemic venous and common atrial pressures are monitored and similarly maintained. Systemic saturation is lower because of the right-to-left atrial shunt and is generally between 80% and 90%. A lower systemic saturation is generally well tolerated because of the increase in oxygen delivery and cardiac output (right-to-left shunt). Systemic saturations in the mid to high 90 percent values generally represent closure of the fenestration.

The bidirectional Glenn is also a useful "bailout" operation. If the child does not tolerate Fontan physiology in the early postbypass period and there is no anatomically correctable problem, the patient can be converted to a bidirectional Glenn if other support options are not demeaned valuable.

Complications immediately after the Glenn procedure or fenestrated Fontan are lower than after the completed Fontan. The incidence of pleural effusions, ascites, atrial dysrhythmias, and renal, hepatic, and mesenteric perfusion problems is diminished. Very low saturation values (50% to 60%) may be seen in some of these patients. If oxygen saturations remain very low, early cardiac catheterization is recommended, because extensive venous collaterals can be coil occluded in the cardiac catheterization laboratory (Bridges et al., 1990). If collaterals are not present, and there is no obstruction across the anastomosis or distortion of the pulmonary artery, then surgical options include conversion from a fenestrated Fontan to a bidirectional Glenn or placement of an aorta-to-pulmonary shunt to improve PBF.

Rhythm disturbances after the Fontan operation are common. The absence of sinus rhythm is a risk factor for Fontan operation, but evidence suggests that sinus rhythm is not an absolute requirement for successful outcome after the Fontan procedure (Balaji et al., 1991). Atrial pacing can improve cardiac output and systemic blood pressure, especially when junctional rhythm is present in the early postrepair period. Atrial pacing lowers left atrial pressure and provides an atrial kick that supplements systemic stroke volume (Alboliras et al., 1985). More significant rhythm disturbances such as atrial flutter and junctional ectopic tachycardia increase the risk of mortality in the early postrepair period. In a study by Balaji and others (1991), the presence of atrial tachyarrhythmias (atrial flutter, supraventricular atrial ectopic tachycardia, and junctional ectopic tachycardia) carried a very high mortality rate in the early postoperative period. By using a total cavopulmonary connection rather than an atriopulmonary connection, atrial tachyarrhythmias were less common and were more easily controlled with antiarrhythmic therapy, overdrive pacing, or DC cardioversion (Balaji et al., 1991). This finding suggests that a major contributor to postoperative arrhythmias in the Fontan patient is exposure of native atrial tissue to high pressure.

In a comparison of the hemi-Fontan with the Glenn procedure, the early postoperative incidence of sinus node dysfunction was higher in the hemi-Fontan patients. This is not surprising because the Glenn procedure is an extracardiac anastomosis (Cohen et al., 2000). High pressure explains the greater likelihood of atrial arrhythmias and why medical control is so difficult. With the bidirectional Glenn procedure and extracardiac Fontan connection, native atrial tissue is not exposed to elevated pressures. Atrial tissue is primarily exposed to common atrial pressure, which is substantially lower (generally 5 to 8 mm Hg) (Balaji et al., 1991; Kumar et al., 2003). The benefits from the extracardiac Fontan in terms of reducing cardiac dysrhythmias have led to the concept of converting lateral tunnel Fontan to an extracardiac Fontan and cryoablation surgery as an alternative to transplantation in those patients with a failing Fontan due to dysrhythmias. (Weinstein et al., 2003). Results have been encouraging. The presence of AVV regurgitation may also contribute as a risk factor for increased postoperative arrhythmias, again invoking high atrial pressures as a causative factor.

■ ANTICOAGULATION, HEMOSTASIS, AND BLOOD CONSERVATION

Modern pediatric cardiac anesthesia must include the principles and practice of effective anticoagulation, hemostasis, and blood conservation. Bleeding after CPB remains a significant problem in pediatric cardiac surgery (Manno et al., 1991).

Continuing blood loss after bypass, requiring blood component replacement, is associated with hemodynamic compromise as well as morbidity from multiple donor exposure. In pediatric patients, restoration of hemostasis has proved to be difficult, and diagnosis of the problem and treatment are marginally effective.

Neonates, infants, and children undergoing cardiac surgery with CPB have a higher rate of postoperative bleeding than do older patients (Manno et al., 1991). There are a number of causative factors. There is disproportionate exposure of blood to the area of nonendothelialized extracorporeal circuit. This exposure to the nonendothelialized circuit produces a heightened inflammation-like response and activates platelets. In addition, the CPB circuit and prime volume produce a dilutional coagulopathy (Kirklin et al., 1983). The inflammatory response is inversely related to patient age; the younger the patient, the more pronounced is the response (Greeley et al., 1988). Inflammation is known to be intimately related to activation of the coagulation system.

Complement and platelet activation is linked to the activation of other protein systems in the blood, such as the fibrinolytic system. This generalized protein system activation plays a major role during surgery and results in impaired hemostasis and an increased bleeding tendency. The most widely used monitor of anticoagulation during CPB is the activated coagulation time (ACT). The ACT does not correlate with circulating heparin levels (Culliford et al., 1981; Codispoti et al., 2001), particularly during hemodilution and deep hypothermia (Martindale et al., 1996). Also, the type of operations performed in neonates and infants usually involves more extensive reconstruction and suture lines, creating more opportunities for surgical bleeding (Dietrich et al., 1993; Martindale et al., 1996).

The immature coagulation system in neonates and young infants may also contribute to impaired hemostasis (Andrew et al., 1987). Although procoagulant and factor levels may be reduced in the young patient with cyanotic CHD due to immature or impaired hepatosynthesis (Colon-Otero et al., 1987), functional bleeding tendencies are not usually present before surgery. However, patients with cyanotic heart disease demonstrate an increased bleeding tendency after CPB for reasons that are not totally clear (Henriksson et al., 1979).

CPB is a significant thrombogenic stimulus that requires anticoagulation with heparin before initiation. Heparin is usually administered empirically based on patient weight, and its effect is followed by ACT monitoring. Because heparin effect is primarily due to coupling with anti–thrombin III (AT III) and because there are age-related differences in the level of circulating procoagulants and this inhibitor, variability of heparin dosing and effect has been a concern. High heparin sensitivity is observed in the first week of life and then decreases progressively until about 3 years of age, when values approach those observed in adults (Vieira et al., 1991). These findings are consistent with the variable quantities of circulating levels of procoagulants and inhibitors, especially prothrombin and AT III (Kern et al., 1992b). Heparin administration must also include a consideration of the quantity and composition of the priming volume for CPB, especially if FFP is added and the current trend continues of using smaller CPB circuits and prime volumes for neonates and infants. Recommendations for heparin are a dose of 300 to 400 U/kg plus an additional dose of 1 to 3 U/mL of prime and then maintaining the ACT at greater than 400 seconds. Deep hypothermia contributes to prolongation of the ACT, provides a false sense of adequate anticoagulation, and has led to an increased interest in using higher heparin doses, closer to 400 U/kg rather than the recommended 300 to 400 U/kg (Despotis et al., 1995).

Heparin is neutralized with protamine, and the dose of is calculated based on the dose of heparin given or on body weight. General requirements for protamine are 1 mg/100 U heparin administered or 5 to 7 mg/kg, and then the ACT is checked. It is unusual for a dose greater than 10 mg/kg to be required. However, the dose may have to be individualized based on the degree of observed surgical bleeding. This increased protamine requirement in young patients is indicative of the higher circulating heparin levels after CPB (Horkay et al., 1992). Delayed hepatic clearance of heparin due to organ immaturity and the predominant use of deep hypothermic CPB in this age group decrease metabolism and excretion of heparin. Interpatient variability mandates some form of individual assessment to guide drug dose, to prevent excess protamine administration (Jobes and Nicolson, 1988; Jobes et al., 1992).

As discussed, neonates and young infants with CHD have low circulating levels of procoagulants and inhibitors before surgery (Kern et al., 1992b). The thrombogenic and dilutional effects of CPB further contribute to hemostatic abnormalities after CPB. Formed blood elements such as leukocytes and platelets may be activated, and procoagulants diluted by CPB. DHCA causes greater fibrinolytic activity. The lower the temperature, the higher the degree of activation of the inflammatory and coagulation cascade. The causes of bleeding after CPB tend to be multifactorial. Injudicious use of blood products to separately correct individual coagulation abnormalities can further exacerbate the dilution of existing procoagulants. Severe reductions in hematocrit impair oxygen delivery and may contribute to neurologic pathology, especially after deep hypothermia.

Bleeding after CPB is not an unusual occurrence. The surgeon should first attempt to identify any obvious source of surgical bleeding at the sites of repair dissection and cannulation. Next, adequate protamine reversal of heparin is assessed by measuring the ACT. In general, standard coagulation tests show a prolongation of the bleeding time, partial thromboplastin time and prothrombin time, hypofibrinogenemia, and dilution of other procoagulants (Table 17–16). The most common reason for persistent bleeding is platelet dysfunction (Harker, 1986; Woodman and Harker, 1990; Tempe and Virmani, 2002).

Blood transfusion practices in the context of pediatric cardiac surgery vary widely, and no one approach has received broad acceptance (Kwiatkowski and Manno, 1999). In a CPB coagulation study in 494 pediatric patients undergoing cardiac surgery, the most reliable indicator of excessive bleeding and requirement for blood product transfusion after bypass was a platelet count of 108,000/μL or less (Williams et al., 1999). Low platelet counts in conjunction with active bleeding should be treated, first, with the administration of platelets. After platelets have been administered, if bleeding is still present, reassessment and repeat platelet infusion or the administration of cryoprecipitate in infants weighing less than 8 kg or of FFP in older children are considered. In a study of 75 pediatric patients undergoing CPB and cardiac surgery, children who weighed less than 8 kg had fewer postoperative requirements for transfusion products, if platelets were given followed by the administration of cryoprecipitate after separation from CPB. In those children administered FFP after a platelet transfusion, greater postoperative bleeding was observed (Miller et al., 1997). The excess bleeding after FFP transfusion was believed to be due to dilution

■ **TABLE 17–16.** Summary of coagulation tests during cardiopulmonary bypass (CPB) in infants

Assay	Pre-CPB	1 min on CPB	Cold CPB	Warm CPB	Postprotamine	Intensive Care Unit
Fibrinogen%	200 ± 59*	92 ± 18	94 ± 21	107 ± 24*	142 ± 28*	183 ± 33
Factor 2%	56 ± 13	30 ± 7	32 ± 8	33 ± 7§	48 ± 10	60 ± 33
Factor 5%	68 ± 20*	15 ± 4	17 ± 5	22 ± 7*	39 ± 11*	46 ± 10
Factor 7%	54 ± 11†	26 ± 5	27 ± 6	28 ± 5†	41 ± 8†	53 ± 16
Factor 8%	48 ± 20‡	0	0	0	32 ± 15‡	72 ± 45
Factor 9%	31 ± 13	20 ± 8	23 ± 5	31 ± 4	31 ± 9	40 ± 12
Factor 10%	52 ± 10	31 ± 7	31 ± 7	34 ± 8§	46 ± 10	47 ± 16
Platelets (k/mm^3)	225 ± 54*	65 ± 17	45 ± 8	93 ± 28*	120 ± 29*	
Antithrombin	49 ± 22	30 ± 12	29 ± 15	32 ± 13§	57 ± 28	68 ± 23
Heparin (units)	0.02 ± 0.03	0.41 ± 0.08	0.42 ± 0.08	0.42 ± 0.08	0.04 ± 0.04	0.07 ± 0.06
ACT (sec)	168 ± 20	>700	>700	>700	151 ± 31	

*$P < .0001$.
†$P < .002$.
‡$P < .005$.
§$P < .05$.

of platelets and red blood cells from the higher volume of FFP compared with cryoprecipitate. Under most circumstances, meticulous surgical technique, appropriate administration of protamine, adequate patient temperature, and platelet infusion correct excessive bleeding. In neonates, excessive bleeding, as well as the escalating dilutional effects of selective component therapy on the remaining procoagulants in small patients, makes the treatment of bleeding a difficult one. The use of fresh whole blood may be warranted under these circumstances. The administration of fresh whole blood (<48 hours old) after CPB can meet all of the hematologic requirements with minimum donor exposure. The efficacy of whole blood in restoring hemostasis and reducing blood loss after CPB has been demonstrated in patients younger than 2 years who are undergoing complex surgical repairs (Manno et al., 1991; Kwiatkowski and Manno, 1999). Most centers cannot obtain fresh whole blood due to screening requirements for blood-borne pathogens.

Many attempts have been made to reduce bleeding after CPB through pharmacologic interventions. Antifibrinolytics, ε-aminocaproic acid (EACA), and tranexamic acid (Horrow et al., 1990) have been used with fair success. One double-blind study in 41 repeat-surgery pediatric patients reported 24% less blood loss after cardiac surgery when tranexamic acid 100 mg/kg loading dose, followed by 10 mg/kg per hour, was administered intravenously (Reid et al., 1997). The most impressive results have been demonstrated with the use of aprotinin, a protease inhibitor (Royston et al., 1987). Aprotinin has antifibrinolytic properties in low concentrations and acts as a kallikrein inhibitor at higher levels. CPB causes increased kallikrein through contact activation, promoting thrombus and fibrin generation, which promotes fibrinolysis. The inhibition of kallikrein results in an inhibition of the contact phase of coagulation, and the inhibition of fibrinolysis reduces bleeding. Reduced thrombin generation leads to diminished platelet stimulation. Better preserved platelet function has been described for patients with aprotinin (Royston et al., 1987). Not surprisingly, then, aprotinin significantly reduces intraoperative and postoperative blood loss (Dietrich et al., 1989, 1990, 1991, 1992). Aprotinin use during pediatric cardiac surgery attenuates fibrinolytic activation in a dose-dependent fashion, attenuating the hemostatic activation during CPB with less plasmin formation and, because of inhibition of contact activation, less thrombin generation, thereby reducing fibrin split product formation (Dietrich et al., 1993). Higher doses of aprotinin reduce thrombin–AT III complex and F1/F2 fragments, supporting the hypothesis of suppression of clotting activation with higher aprotinin doses and plasma concentrations (Dietrich et al., 1993; Mossinger et al., 2003). Aprotinin use is recommended for reoperations and first operations in neonates where bleeding via extensive suture lines is anticipated. After a test dose, the recommended loading dose is 30,000 to 50,000 U/kg before sternotomy and then a CPB prime dose of 30,000 U/kg and continuous infusion of 7,000 to 10,000 U/kg per hour during surgery, aiming for a therapeutic plasma target range of 200 KIU/mL (Mossinger et al., 2003). Higher doses are generally used in neonates and infants due to the marked hemodilution of CPB in younger infants. Aprotinin is currently not approved by the Food and Drug Administration for use in children. However, aprotinin is being administered in many centers that care for pediatric cardiac surgical patients, including its use in DHCA (Tweddell et al., 2002). Anaphylaxis on reexposure of the drug is a risk (2.7% risk; 5% risk if reexposed within 6 months; 0.95% risk if reexposed after 6 months) (Laxenaire et al., 2000). Hypersensitivity reactions with aprotinin do occur; the drug should not be used in patients at risk for thromboembolism or in those with renal insufficiency.

The treatment of postbypass coagulopathy should be dictated more by clinical bleeding than by laboratory values alone. Isolated coagulation abnormalities are often present in the uncomplicated postoperative cardiac patient (see Table 17–15). Usually, these coagulation abnormalities self-correct themselves during the first postoperative day and are not associated with excessive bleeding. Routine correction of these abnormalities with infusion of blood products is *not* warranted. Blood products should not be administered unless there is clinical evidence of bleeding or a specific defect has been identified and specific component therapy used. Routine use of blood products for volume replacement is also to be avoided; Plasmanate, lactated Ringer's, or saline solution can be satisfactorily administered at a reduced cost without the hazards associated with transfusion. Another method of minimizing homologous blood transfusions is the adoption of a preoperative autologous blood donation program. Although autologous blood donation is not commonly done in children, it has been found to avoid the need for homologous blood transfusion in 94% of situations in a group of 80 older pediatric patients undergoing corrective cardiac surgery with CPB (Masuda et al., 1995).

ANESTHESIA FOR CLOSED HEART OPERATIONS

Early corrective repair in infancy with less palliation has significantly reduced the number of noncorrective closed heart operations. Noncorrective closed heart operations include PA banding, extracardiac shunts such as the modified BT shunt, and atrial septectomy. Corrective closed heart procedures include PDA ligation and repair of coarctation of the aorta. All of these procedures are performed without CPB. Venous access and intra-arterial monitoring are important in evaluating and supporting these patients, and the pulse oximeter remains an invaluable monitor during intraoperative management.

PATENT DUCTUS ARTERIOSUS

PDA ligation is performed through a left thoracotomy. The physiologic management is that of a simple shunt. Patients with a large PDA and low PVR generally present with excessive PBF and congestive heart failure. Neonates and premature infants also run the risk of having a large diastolic runoff to the PA, potentially impairing coronary perfusion. Patients range from an asymptomatic, healthy young child to the sick, ventilator-dependent premature infant on inotropic support. The former patient allows for a wide variety of anesthetic techniques and extubation in the operating room. The latter patient requires a carefully controlled anesthetic and fluid management plan. In general, a trial of medical management with indomethacin and fluid restriction is attempted in the premature infant before surgical correction. In the premature infant, transport to the operating room can be especially difficult and tedious, requiring great vigilance to avoid extubation, excessive patient cooling, and venous access disruption. For these reasons, many centers perform PDA ligation safely and cost-effectively in the neonatal intensive care unit (Mortier et al., 1996).

Intraoperatively, retractors may interfere with cardiac filling and ventilatory management so that hypotension, hypoxemia, and hypercarbia may occur. Complications include inadvertent ligation of the left PA or descending aorta, recurrent laryngeal nerve damage, and excessive bleeding due to inadvertent PDA disruption. After ductal ligation in premature infants, worsening pulmonary compliance and increased ventilatory support may occur, and an increase in left ventricular afterload should be anticipated. This is problematic if left ventricular dysfunction existed preoperatively.

COARCTATION OF THE AORTA

Coarctation accounts for about 8% of all CHD and ranks fourth or fifth among congenital cardiac anomalies. The incidence of coarctation has been reported to be 1:10,000, higher in males than in females (1.7:1). Extracardiac malformations are seen in about 7% of patients, the most frequent being Turner's syndrome (gonadal dysgenesis, webbed neck, and cubitus valgus), hypospadias, clubfoot, and ocular defects. Coarctation of the aorta is a narrowing of the descending aorta, almost always at the junction of the ductus arteriosus into the aortic arch. The posterior lateral shelf forming the localized narrowing is almost always directly across from the ductus. The term *juxtaductal* is used to describe the position of the coarctation.

Obstruction to left ventricular outflow results from coarctation, and this may range from severe obstruction with compromised systemic perfusion to mild upper extremity hypertension as the only manifestation. In neonates with a large posterior lateral shelf and a quickly developing obstruction, there is a sudden increase in left ventricular afterload that results in left ventricular failure. These patients usually become symptomatic in the first week of life. Left-to-right shunting occurs at the atrial level because of an enlarged and stretched foramen ovale. In the young infant with severe coarctation, systemic perfusion is dependent on right-to-left shunting across the PDA. In these circumstances, left ventricular dysfunction is very common and PGE_1 is often necessary to maintain systemic perfusion. When the ductus closes gradually and aortic obstruction develops over several months, left ventricular failure is less likely to occur. In older children, the presenting symptom of coarctation may be hypertension, intermittent claudication, cerebrovascular accident, or bacterial endocarditis involving the bicuspid aortic valve (a common associated finding).

In general, a larger peripheral intravenous catheter and an indwelling arterial catheter in the right upper extremity are recommended for intraoperative and postoperative management. In patients with left ventricular dysfunction, a central venous catheter may be placed intraoperatively for pressure monitoring and inotropic support. The surgical approach is through a left thoracotomy, where the aorta is cross-clamped and the coarctation is repaired with one of three techniques: an on-lay prosthetic patch, a subclavian artery flap or resection of the coarctation and an end-to-end anastomosis. The latter is the favored approach. Intravascular volume loading with 10 to 20 mL/kg of crystalloid is administered just before removal of the clamp. The anesthetic concentration is decreased, and additional volume support is given until the blood pressure rises. Additional anesthetic concerns include spinal cord damage, rebound hypertension, and pain control. Spinal cord injury occurs in less than 0.5% of patients. Associated lesions such as VSD and aberrant left subclavian artery, as well as intraoperative fever, have been associated with an increased risk of paralysis. Other associated factors include intraoperative hypertension and reoperation for coarctation, bicuspid aortic valve, subvalvar AS, and other cardiovascular disease (Attenhofer et al., 2002). The use of mild hypothermia has been advocated to lower oxygen consumption during aortic cross-clamping and to reduce the incidence of paralysis. In some centers, ice application in the surgical field is used. In older children, SSEP monitoring is frequently performed (see Chapter 9, Pediatric Anesthesia Equipment and Monitoring).

The other significant anesthetic concern is postrepair rebound hypertension. Hypertension after surgery is probably related to heightened baroreceptor reactivity and increased activation of the renin-angiotensin pathway. Perioperative hypertension is best treated with β-blockade (esmolol) or α/β-blockade (labetalol) or calcium channel blockade (nicardipine). Propranolol is useful in older patients, but it may cause severe bradycardia in infants and young children. Sodium nitroprusside does not appear to be useful except in very high doses; captopril or another angiotensin inhibitor is effective in controlling the hypertension. Most patients with coarctation are treated with β-blockers or captopril in the preoperative period.

EXTRACARDIAC SHUNTS

The placement of extracardiac shunts without CPB is managed by balancing pulmonary and systemic blood flows. Consideration should be given that the newly established shunt, depending on size, should offer greater resistance to PBF rather than the PDA.

In fact, the reason for placing a shunt in many cases is to replace a nonrestrictive ductus. Under these circumstances, attempts at manipulating PVR are less helpful. Central shunts are usually performed through a median sternotomy, and BT (subclavian artery–to–PA) shunts may be performed through a left or right thoracotomy. In patients in whom PBF is critically low, partial cross-clamping of the PA required for the distal anastomosis causes further reduction of PBF and desaturation. Pulse oximetry, as well as careful application of the cross-clamp to avoid PA distortion, is helpful in maintaining PBF. Rarely, severe desaturation and bradycardia occur with cross-clamping and necessitate the use of CPB to complete the procedure. Intraoperative complications include bleeding and severe systemic oxygen desaturation. During chest closure, shunt kinking or clotting can occur. In an attempt to avoid clotting of the shunt before cross-clamping, 50 to 100 U/kg heparin is administered. Pulmonary edema may result in the early postoperative period because of increased PBF from the surgically created shunt. Administering low FIO_2, increasing the $PaCO_2$, and manipulating PEEP may be helpful maneuvers to decrease PBF until the pulmonary circulation can adjust. Under such circumstances, early extubation is inadvisable.

PULMONARY ARTERY BANDING

PA banding is used to restrict PBF in infants who are deemed anatomically or physiologically uncorrectable at this time and have excessive PBF from a native PA. Most patients who require PA banding have complex anatomy and include heterotaxy syndromes and lesions that are RV dominant with normal-sized PAs and LV hypoplasia. Examples of a patient who may require PA banding include those with double-outlet RV with hypoplastic LV and patients with unbalanced AVSD and hypoplastic LV. These patients are generally in heart failure with reduced systemic perfusion and excessive PBF. The surgeon places a restrictive band across the main PA to reduce flow. Band placement is very imprecise and requires careful assistance from the anesthesia team to accomplish successfully. Many approaches have been suggested; one approach is to administer the patient a 21% inspired oxygen concentration and maintain the $PaCO_2$ at 40 mm Hg to simulate the postoperative state. Direct observation of an elevation of systemic blood pressure by 10 mm Hg and a reduction in PA pressure to one-half to two-thirds systemic suggest an appropriate band size. Following the end-tidal PCO_2 is helpful in ensuring that the band has had some impact on reducing PBF.

ATRIAL SEPTECTOMY

A Blalock-Hanlon atrial septectomy is an uncommon procedure for enlarging an intra-atrial connection. This procedure is done by occluding caval flow and creating an intra-atrial communication through the atrial septum. Balloon atrial septostomies (Rashkind procedure) and blade septectomies performed in the cardiac catheterization laboratory have replaced surgical intervention, except when LA size is very small or the atrial septum is thickened.

VASCULAR RINGS AND SLINGS

Vascular rings are anomalies of the great vessels and their branches that result in compression or obstruction of the esophagus and trachea (Kussman et al., 2004). Vascular rings may be complete or partial and are due to persistence of the normally obliterated component of the embryonic aortic arches (Fig. 17–31). The most common form of a complete vascular ring is a double aortic arch. In double aortic arch, the ascending aorta arises normally, but as it leaves the pericardium, it divides into a right and left arch, which join posteriorly to form the descending aorta. This complete vascular ring entraps both the esophagus and the trachea, creating proximal airway compression and dysphagia. These patients frequently present with inspiratory and expiratory stridor, occasional wheezing, swallowing difficulties, and, in severe forms, apnea and cyanosis. Although not commonly associated with other cardiac malformations, tetralogy of Fallot and TGA may be associated malformations.

Various types of right aortic arches may present with a complete vascular ring due to anomalous origin of the right subclavian artery from the right arch or persistence of the ligamentum arteriosus (closed fibrous portion of the ductus arteriosus). The ring formed by the anomalous vascular origin may compress the esophagus or the trachea. Similarly, a left aortic arch with an aberrant right subclavian artery passing posterior to the esophagus and right-sided ligamentum arteriosum may cause a partial vascular ring and result in dysphagia, although symptoms are uncommon.

Another form of vascular entrapment is caused by anomalous origin of the left PA, known as a *vascular sling*. In this malformation, the left PA arises from the right PA and courses behind the trachea at the carina but in front of the esophagus, causing obstruction of the distal intrathoracic portion of the trachea. Anomalous innominate artery, although technically not a vascular ring, can present clinically as similar to vascular rings. An anomalous innominate artery arises more distally and leftward from the aortic arch and as a result compresses the trachea anteriorly. Localized tracheomalacia can occur, and patients frequently present with stridor and apnea. Vascular slings present with obstruction of the intrathoracic large airways and result in symptoms on exhalation that include wheezing and expiratory stridor. Anesthetic management is predicated on managing patients with a narrowed tracheal bronchial airway. These patients benefit from PEEP during mechanical or mask-bag ventilation in order to distend the tracheobronchial airway. In addition, ventilatory benefits may be attained by applying mild cricoid pressure to prevent excessive gas flow into the esophagus and stomach. This maneuver prevents gastric distension, and promotes gas flow into the narrowed airway. Intubation is usually not difficult, because the problem is extrinsic compression of the airway by a vascular structure and, once positioned, the endotracheal tube effectively stents open the airway. In patients with severe airway obstruction, bag-mask ventilation may be difficult and may worsen with administration of neuromuscular blockade. An inhalation induction with spontaneous ventilation is the preferred induction in this subgroup of patients.

CARDIAC PACING

After repair of congenital cardiac defects, temporary pacing wires are generally placed to increase heart rate or provide atrioventricular synchrony in the early postbypass and postoperative periods. Temporary pacing augments cardiac output without the complications associated with pharmacologic therapy. β-Adrenergic agonists such as isoproterenol can increase heart rate; however, myocardial oxygen consumption is also increased. If the augmentation in heart rate does not effectively support

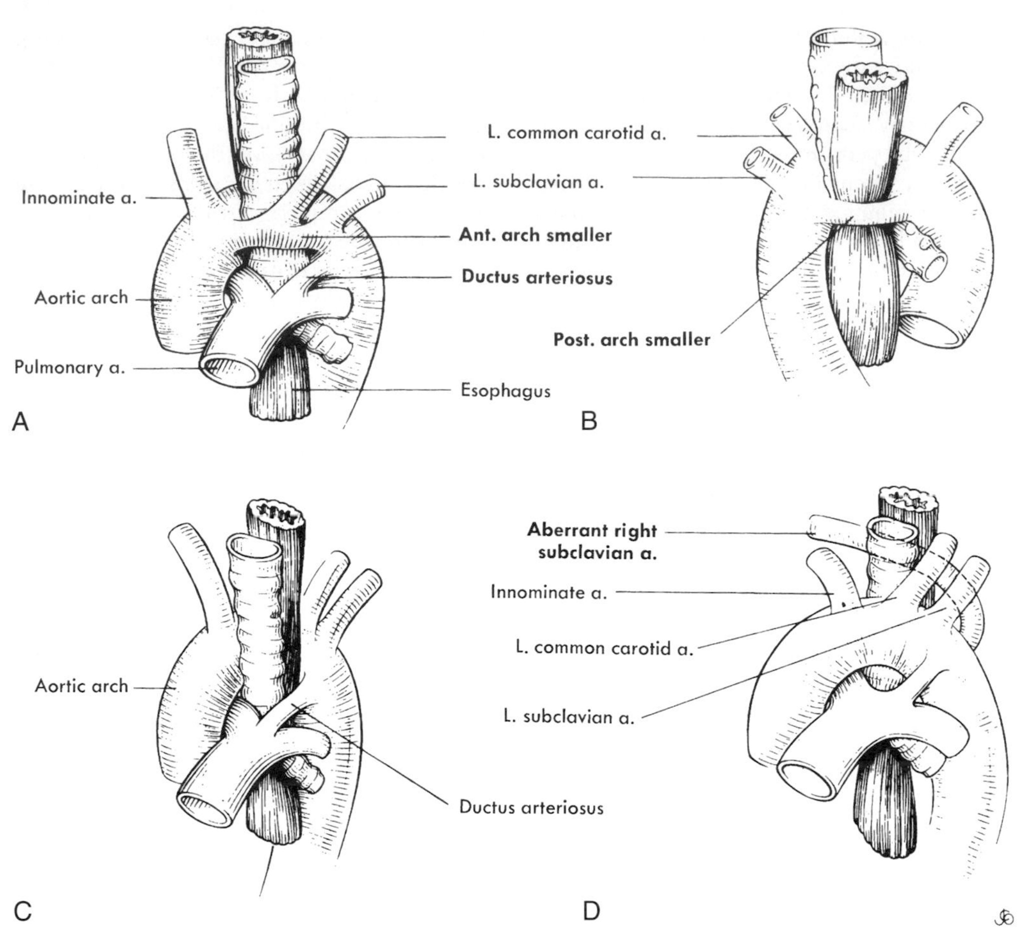

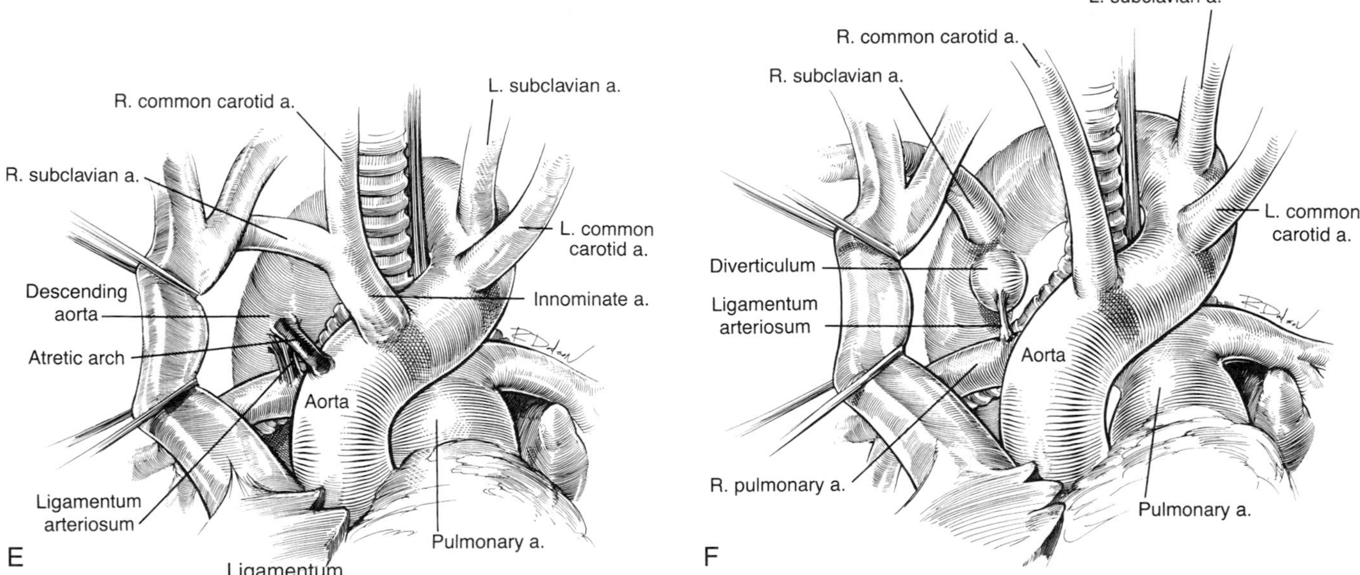

■ **FIGURE 17–31.** Anomalies of the aortic arch. *(A)* Double aortic arch, anterior view; note that posterior arch is larger. *(B)* Double aortic arch, posterior view; note that posterior arch is smaller. *(C)* Right aortic arch (going behind trachea and esophagus) with left ligamentum arteriosum or ductus arteriosus. *(D)* Aberrant right subclavian artery. *(E)* Schematic representation of a rare form of vascular ring comprised of a double aortic arch with an atretic right arch and a right ligamentum arteriosum. *(F)* Schematic representation of a vascular ring comprised of a left aortic arch, aberrant right subclavian artery, and right ligamentum arteriosum. (Reproduced with permission from Castaneda AR, Jonas RA, Mayer JE Jr, et al.: *Cardiac surgery of the neonate and infant.* Philadelphia, 1994, WB Saunders.)

oxygen delivery, myocardial ischemia may ensue. In children, increasing the heart rate to achieve age-appropriate levels or higher, or promoting atrioventricular synchrony through atrial or atrioventricular sequential pacing, may significantly improve cardiac output and oxygen delivery to tissues and is commonly used intraoperatively.

Temporary pacing may be either atrial, atrioventricular sequential, or ventricular pacing. Atrial pacing is preferred because it maintains a variable timing interval between atrial and ventricular contractions. Atrial pacing maximizes atrioventricular synchrony and augments the atrial contraction component of ventricular filling. If atrioventricular conduction is abnormal, atrioventricular sequential pacing may be used in either a synchronous (demand) mode or an asynchronous mode. In both modes, there is a fixed preset atrioventricular time interval that may or may not allow for maximal atrial contribution to cardiac output. A typical time interval used in infants is 150 milliseconds. Asynchronous pacing carries the potential for inducing ventricular tachyarrhythmias. However, this type of pacing may be the preferred method if the patient's intrinsic rhythm does not provide adequate cardiac output in a synchronized mode or competes with synchronized atrioventricular sequential pacing.

Distinguishing atrial from junctional dysrhythmias in the postoperative period is complicated by the intrinsically rapid heart rates of infants and further complicated by the use of rate-enhancing inotropic agents. In neonates with rapid heart rates (≥200 beats per minute), the P wave is typically buried in the T wave. Accurate diagnosis from a bedside monitor or 12-lead electrocardiogram is difficult. One of the most effective means of bedside electrocardiographic analysis is to use an atrial electrogram (Waldo, 1980). This is obtained by attaching two atrial pacing wires to the right and left arm leads of a standard electrocardiograph machine, while maintaining normal leg lead recordings. This configuration provides maximal accentuation of the P wave.

The most benign method of treating atrial tachycardias in the postbypass period is overdrive pacing, which avoids the negative inotropic effects of antiarrhythmic drugs. Several pacing techniques have been used to interrupt atrial tachycardias, including brief bursts of pacing above the atrial rate (usually 200 to 250 beats per minute), referred to as *burst suppression*; pacing 10 to 15 beats per minute above the supraventricular tachycardia rate and, once a rapid atrial rate is captured, gradual reduction in the pacing rate toward normal; and introducing a premature beat, which allows a sinus beat to occur during the refractory period of the reentry loop (this approach is generally the least efficacious). If pacing is unsuccessful and the patient is hemodynamically stable, drug therapy with digoxin, procainamide, adenosine, amiodarone, or verapamil may be useful. In patients with unstable hemodynamics, synchronized cardioversion is the procedure of choice.

The placement of permanent pacemakers in children requires general anesthesia. The preferred method of placement is through a transvenous approach. Patients with slow ventricular escape rates or poorly functioning permanent or temporary wires should have an external pacing system applied before induction. With the broader availability of external pacing systems within defibrillators, this should be available for all pacemaker cases. Isoproterenol infusions have historically been made available as a method to increase the ventricular rate by 10 to 20 beats per minute using low to moderate doses.

Permanent pacing systems have become increasingly sophisticated, including rate-adaptive pacemakers, which adjust their rate to the needs of the patient. A five-position pacemaker nomenclature has been developed to provide a precise understanding of pacemaker function. The first position describes the chamber or chambers being paced (A = atrial, V = ventricular, or D = dual [atrial and ventricular]) (Table 17–17). The second position defines the chamber being sensed by the pacemaker and is designated A, V, D, or 0 (none). The V designation means the R waves generated by the ventricle are sensed, and the A designation implies that the P waves generated by the atrium are sensed. The third position describes the response of the pacemaker after sensing the R or P wave and the designations are I (inhibit), T (trigger), D (dual), or 0 (none). An I designation implies the pacing circuit is inhibited. The fourth position describes the programmability of the pacemaker; designations are P (rate adaptive and output are programmable), M (multiprogrammable), R (rate adaptive), and 0 (none). Because almost all pacemakers are multiprogrammable, this designation is usually omitted. The fifth position designates arrhythmia control. The nomenclature includes P (pacing), S (shock), D (dual pacing and shocking), and 0 (none). This designation is for automatic implantable cardiac defibrillators (AICDs), which are not commonly used in pediatric patients. AICDs are implanted in children with prolonged QT interval or a history of ventricular tachycardia.

■ ANESTHESIA FOR INTERVENTIONAL CARDIAC PROCEDURES

Advances in interventional cardiac catheterization techniques are significantly changing the operative and nonoperative approaches to the patient with CHD. Intracardiac echocardiography, technological advancement in interventional devices (stents, closure devices, valves), and three-dimensional cardiac magnetic resonance imaging are greatly increasing the scope and complexity of nonoperative interventional cardiac catheterization and diagnostic procedures (Fogel, 2005; Thanopoulos et al., 2003; Zanchetta et al., 2003). As a result, less cardiac surgery and CPB are required for the safe closure of small secundum

■ **TABLE 17–17.** Pacemaker nomenclature

Pacers: Five-Letter Code	
First letter: chamber paced	A = atrium, V = ventricle, D = dual (A + V)
Second letter: chamber sensed	A = atrium, V = ventricle, D = dual (A + V), O = none
Third letter: response after sensing	I = pacing inhibited, T = pacing triggered, D = dual (I + T), O = none
Fourth letter: programmability	P = rate and output , M = multiprogrammable, C = communicating R = rate adaptive, O = none
Fifth letter: arrhythmia control	P = pacing, S = shock, D = dual (P + S), O = none
Examples	
AVI = atrial paced, ventricle sensed; pacing inhibited if beat sensed.	
VVIR = demand ventricular pacing with physiologic response to exercise.	
DDD = both atrium and ventricle paced, both sensed; pacing triggered in each chamber if beat not sensed.	

ASDs, VSDs, and PDAs. Stenotic aortic and pulmonic valves and recurrent aortic coarctations can be dilated in the catheterization laboratory, avoiding surgical intervention as well (Lock et al., 1989; Mullins, 1989; Hellenbrand et al., 1990; Hickey et al., 1992). These techniques shorten hospital stays and are particularly beneficial to patients with recurrent coarctation and muscular or apical VSDs, who are at a higher risk for surgical intervention. Many other patients with complex cardiac defects are poor operative risks. Innovative interventional procedures improve vascular anatomy, reduce pressure loads on ventricles, and decrease the repetitive operative risk for these patients. For example, in tetralogy of Fallot with hypoplastic PAs, balloon angioplasty and vascular stenting procedures create favorable PA anatomy and reduce proximal PA pressure and right ventricular end-diastolic pressure.

The anesthetic management of interventional procedures in the catheterization laboratory must include the same level of preparation that would apply in caring for these patients in the operating room. The patients have the same complex cardiac physiology and, in some cases, greater physiologic complexity and less cardiovascular reserve because of their poorer operative risks. Interventional catheterization procedures can impose acute pressure load on the heart during balloon inflation. Large catheters placed across mitral or tricuspid valves create acute valvular regurgitation or, in the case of a small valve orifice, transient valvular stenosis. When catheters are placed across shunts, severe reductions in PBF and marked cyanosis may occur (Malviya et al., 1989; Hickey et al., 1992). The anesthetic plan must consider the specific cardiology objectives of the procedure and the impact of anesthetic management in facilitating or hindering the interventional procedure. In general, there are three distinct periods involved in an interventional catheterization: the data acquisition period, the interventional period, and the postprocedural evaluation period.

During the data acquisition period, the cardiologist performs a hemodynamic catheterization to evaluate the need for and extent of the planned intervention. Catheterization data are obtained under baseline or normal physiologic conditions (i.e., room air, a physiologic $PaCO_2$, and either controlled or spontaneous ventilation). Because of the complexity of the interventional procedures and the need to maintain normal $PaCO_2$ and immobility, general anesthesia with controlled ventilation is increasingly required for children in the catheterization laboratory. Increased FIO_2 or changes in $PaCO_2$ may affect physiologic data. A secured airway allows the anesthesiologist to concentrate on hemodynamic issues. Positive pressure ventilation also reduces the risk of air embolism. During spontaneous ventilation, a large reduction in intrathoracic pressure may entrain air into vascular sheaths and result in moderate to large pulmonary or systemic air emboli. Precise device placement is also facilitated with controlled ventilation by reducing the respiratory shifting of cardiac structures.

Substantial blood loss and changes in ventricular function occur commonly during the intervention. Blood volume replacement and inotropic support may be necessary during or immediately after the interventional procedure. In the postprocedural period, the success and the physiologic impact of the intervention are evaluated. Blood pressure, mixed venous oxygen saturation, ventricular end-diastolic pressure, and cardiac output, when available, are used to assess the impact of the intervention. Postintervention recovery is generally done in an intensive care unit environment for monitoring and/or respiratory or cardiovascular support.

Because of the hemodynamic variability of many of these patients and the changing anesthetic requirements, continuous intravenous infusion with ketamine/midazolam, or propofol with fentanyl, alfentanil, or remifentanil is used. Many children with congenital cardiac disease may safely undergo induction of anesthesia with sevoflurane and then, after an intravenous cannula is secured, a maintenance infusion of propofol (50 to 125 mcg/kg per minute) along with remifentanil can be started. Potent inhaled anesthetics are generally not used as the primary anesthetic because of their negative inotropic effects; they are reserved for adjunctive anesthesia.

A brief description of some of the interventional procedures and the associated anesthetic implications are presented. The success and safety of these procedures, together with the miniaturization of intracardiac stents and closure devices, expand the therapeutic options for pediatric interventional cardiologists.

A fenestrated Fontan may have a closure device deployed if needed or a prematurely closed fenestration reopened and stented if necessary (Chatrath et al., 2003). Many of these procedures require TEE or intracardiac echocardiography (Zanchetta et al., 2003) to guide accurate stent or occluder deployment. The provision of anesthesia in the cardiac catheterization laboratory is challenging: the room is dark, the cardiac catheterization laboratory is generally poorly designed for anesthesia equipment, and communication can sometimes be less than ideal.

TRANSCATHETER CLOSURE FOR ATRIAL SEPTAL DEFECT

During the past 10 years, several different closure devices have reached the market, and most have been removed. Only the Amplatzer (AGA Medical Corporation, Golden Valley, MN) expanding heat-treated nickel-titanium double-wire disc is available in the United States (Fig. 17–32). The double disc flattens out once deployed with each side of the disc on opposite sides of the atrial septum. The original device used in the late 1980s and early 1990s was a collapsed, double-umbrella or clamshell device. This device had six arms within a meshed patch. The clamshell device was taken off the market because follow-up evaluation demonstrated cracks or breaks in some of the arms.

The ASD closure device is deployed by the cardiologist through a large introducer sheath that is placed in the femoral

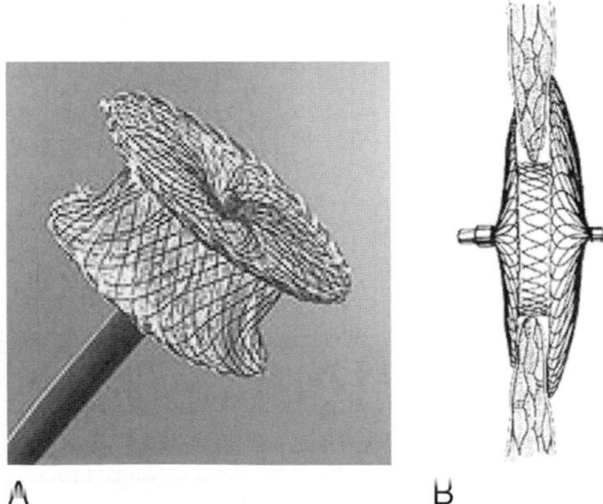

FIGURE 17–32. Amplatzer (AGA Medical Corporation, Golden Valley, MN) heat-treated nickel-titanium wires. *(A)* Open Amplatzer device. *(B)* Deployed Amplatzer device with the two flattened titanium-nickel discs that lie on each side of the atrial or ventricular wall after deployment for repair of an atrial or ventricular septal defect.

vein. A catheter containing the device is advanced from the femoral vein to the RA and placed across the ASD into the left atrial chamber. With the use of biplane fluoroscopy and TEE, the catheter is positioned in the LA away from the mitral valve (Lock et al., 1989). The sheath is pulled back to open the distal side of the device into the LA. The sheath and device are then pulled back so the distal side makes contact with the left atrial side of the septum. Fluoroscopy and TEE are used to confirm that the device is appropriately positioned and does not interfere with mitral valve motion. Once adequately seated, the sheath is pulled farther back to expose the proximal side of the device, which is then opened to engage on the right side of the atrial septum. When proper positioning is certain, the device is released (Lock et al., 1989). In a report of 122 children undergoing transcatheter ASD closures using the clamshell device, there was a 9% incidence of procedural complications resulting in hemodynamic complications requiring treatment (Hickey et al., 1992). Device embolization to either the right or left side of the circulation does occur and requires further interventions to retrieve them. One series reported an embolization incidence as high as 7% (Thanopoulos et al., 2003). There is an institutional learning curve with these newer devices, and most centers with experience can lower the incidence of device embolization to about 2% to 3% (Godart et al., 2003) (Table 17–18).

■ TABLE 17–18. Atrial septal defect (ASD) closure device

Complications	No. (%)	Therapy
Device embolization	6 (5)	Two retrieved in operating room
Air embolization	4 (3.3)	Pressors, atropine, volume, cardiopulmonary resuscitation seizure
Acute mitral regurgitation (MR), tricuspid regurgitation (TR)	2 (1.7)	Pressors reposition device
Chronic TR	1 (0.8)	Device removed in operating room; ASD closed
Brachial plexus injury	3 (2.5)	Transient
Dye reaction	(0.8)	Pressors and ventilation
Anesthetic	2 (1.7)	Apnea/airway obstruction

TRANSCATHETER CLOSURE FOR VENTRICULAR SEPTAL DEFECT

Most VSDs that are electively closed in the catheterization laboratory are midmuscular or apical VSDs, which are either difficult to close in the operating room or would require a left ventriculotomy. Left ventriculotomies are associated with a high incidence of late left ventricular dysfunction and have fallen into disfavor as a surgical option. The transcatheter approach requires a blade atrial septostomy and a retrograde catheter placed through the femoral artery and advanced to the LA. This catheter is pulled across the atrial septum into the RA and is used to guide an SVC catheter (placed through the internal jugular vein) across the created ASD into the LA, across the mitral valve, and into the LV. The VSD is approached from the left ventricular side. The left side of the intraventricular septum is smooth, whereas the right side is trabeculated. By placing the device on the left side, the VSD opening can be identified. The large sheath containing the closure device interferes with closure of the mitral valve, resulting in acute mitral regurgitation or, in cases where the VSD is large or the mitral annulus small, acute severe mitral valve obstruction. In this latter case, systemic outflow is decreased and a period of severe hypotension may be experienced. Judicious use of vasoconstrictors to maintain coronary perfusion during the catheter placement, followed by volume and inotropic resuscitation after the VSD device is secured, may be required.

BALLOON ANGIOPLASTY AND VALVOTOMY

One of the most important areas of interventional catheterization has been the dilation and stenting of hypoplastic or stenotic branch PAs. In patients with tetralogy of Fallot with hypoplastic PAs, pulmonary atresia, or single ventricle with surgically induced peripheral stenosis at the site of a previous shunt, the use of balloon angioplasty and stenting procedures creates favorable PA anatomy and reduces the risk of subsequent surgical repairs (Fig. 17–33). Balloon angioplasty is accomplished by tearing the vascular intima and media, allowing the vessel to remodel and heal with a larger diameter. The balloon is placed across the stenotic lesion so the middle of the balloon is at the stenosis. The balloon is inflated until the waist of the balloon is eliminated. Ideally, the most stenotic lesions are dilated first to

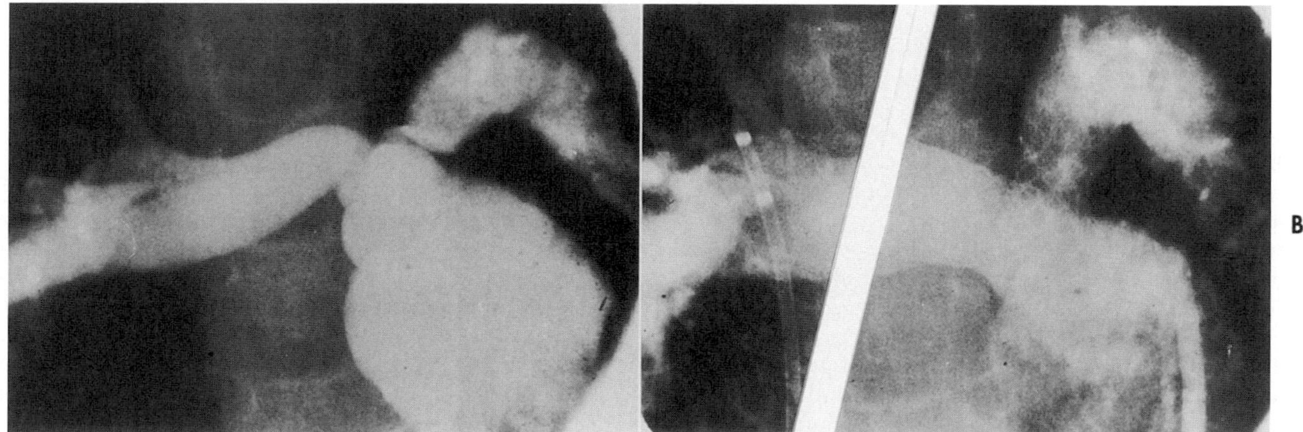

■ FIGURE 17–33. *(A)* Severe bilateral branch pulmonary artery stenosis at the distal end of a conduit in a patient with pulmonary atresia and ventricular septal defect. Stents were placed in the right and left pulmonary arteries. *(B)* Follow-up angiogram in the same projection and magnification showed marked improvement of both right and left pulmonary artery stenosis.

minimize the impact on PBF and cardiac output. When the balloon is inflated, PBF is reduced, right ventricular afterload is increased, and cardiac output falls. In patients with an associated VSD, right-to-left shunting and desaturation occur with balloon inflation. Occasionally, balloon catheters must be placed across aortopulmonary shunts, significantly reducing PBF. The procedure is successful in approximately 60% of patients. Complications include hypotension (40%), PA rupture (3%), unilateral reperfusion pulmonary edema (4%), aneurysmal dilation of the dilated pulmonary vessel (8%), death (1.5%), and transient postprocedural right ventricular dysfunction. Anesthetic support minimizes hemodynamic compromise by anticipating changes in blood flow patterns, treating transient hypotension, and providing airway support to minimize the risks of PA disruption and acute unilateral pulmonary edema (Rothman et al., 1990).

Balloon valvotomies are common interventional procedures. Acute inflation of the balloon results in a transient absence of forward flow and marked elevation in pressure in the chamber proximal to the valve. For aortic and pulmonary valvotomy, there may be acute ischemic injury to the ventricle with a drop in cardiac output. Measurement of the gradient across the valve may be artificially lower because of a reduction in flow across the valvular orifice. Successful balloon dilation of a stenotic valve also requires tearing of fused valve leaflets. Occasionally, the valve leaflets tear at nonfused regions, or the valves are damaged during the procedure, causing regurgitation. A mild degree of valvular regurgitation is well tolerated. Severe valvular regurgitation is generally poorly tolerated, because there is a rapid change in loading conditions from stenosis to severe valvular insufficiency. Patients with significant ventricular dysfunction before the intervention are particularly at risk for postprocedural hemodynamic instability.

RADIOFREQUENCY ABLATION OF ACCESSORY PATHWAYS

Radiofrequency ablation is a nonsurgical approach to eliminating atrial or ventricular reentrant tachyarrhythmias. The technique requires arrhythmia pathway mapping and precision ablation of the aberrant pathway using a radiofrequency ablation catheter. During the ablation, unexpected patient movement may result in catheter dislodgment and damage to normal conducting tissue, so general anesthesia is usually required in younger children. Anesthetic agents and techniques should be chosen to increase circulating catecholamines and avoid suppression of arrhythmogenesis so as to promote identification of the aberrant pathway. Several authors (Sharpe et al., 1994; Erb et al., 2002b) described the electrophysiologic effects of volatile anesthetics (enflurane, isoflurane, and halothane), propofol, and opioid-benzodiazepine–based anesthetics in patients undergoing radiofrequency ablation procedures. Volatile anesthetics prolonged the refractory periods of both normal atrioventricular conduction and the accessory pathway. Volatile anesthetic gases interfered with data interpretation and rendered postablative studies less reliable in judging the success of the procedure. The use of volatile anesthetics should be discouraged during electrophysiologic procedures. Conversely, patients with reentry tachycardias requiring anesthesia for noncardiac surgery may benefit from volatile anesthetic agents as they may reduce the incidence of supraventricular tachycardia during the operative procedure. Opioid-benzodiazepine anesthesia had no demonstrable effect on electrophysiologic measurements and therefore provided electrophysiologic data unencumbered by anesthetic effect.

A combination of propofol and opioids as a continuous intravenous anesthetic, along with nitrous oxide and neuromuscular blockade, does not affect the electrophysiology data. In addition, this anesthetic combination has been shown to decrease the incidence of postoperative nausea and vomiting compared with an inhalational anesthetic technique (Erb et al., 2002a, 2002b).

Rapid atrial pacing and, occasionally, an isoproterenol infusion are required during the mapping procedure. Severe postprocedural cardiomyopathy has been described, but it is very unusual. An underlying cardiomyopathy from frequent episodes of supraventricular tachycardia and myocardial oxygen imbalance caused by prolonged periods of rapid atrial pacing and isoproterenol infusions are the presumed causative factors.

Strict attention to arm support and padding of all pressure points are essential. Tension on the brachial plexus must be avoided, especially if arms are secured next to head at less than 90 degrees flexion/extension. Also, pressure on the radial nerve at the elbow can occur, especially for the longer radiofrequency arrhythmia ablation procedures. A peripheral arterial catheter is helpful during these lengthy procedures for continuous monitoring of arterial blood pressure and blood gases.

ANESTHESIA FOR NONCARDIAC SURGERY IN PATIENTS WITH CONGENITAL HEART DISEASE

Refinements in diagnostic and operative techniques, as well as advances in medical and anesthetic care, have resulted in marked improvement in survival of patients with CHD. Consequently, some of these patients may be subjected to elective or emergency noncardiac surgery either before or after correction of the cardiac anomaly. The anesthetic management of patients with uncorrected heart defects allows for little margin of error. It is essential that the anesthesiologist be knowledgeable not only of the basics of pediatric anesthesia but also of the pathophysiology of the cardiac lesions (Salem and Griffin, 1981).

The preoperative evaluation and preparation of patients with CHD for noncardiac surgery are not any different from the evaluation and preparation of those children undergoing repair of CHD (as described earlier). Because of the high incidence of associated congenital anomalies in patients with CHD, these anomalies must be ascertained, and the anesthetic plan must be altered appropriately (Moore, 1981; Salem and Griffin, 1981; Schwartz, 1985).

If the child has undergone one or more cardiac procedures in the past, it is essential to know whether the surgery was palliative or corrective, as well as if any complications or residual cardiac disease exists. For example, after repair of coarctation, some patients develop aortic stenosis or aortic insufficiency from the gradual thickening or everting of the bicuspid aortic valve. In some patients with repaired ASDs, 8% to 37% have angiographic evidence of mitral valve prolapse (Betrin et al., 1975). In patients who underwent a repair of tetralogy of Fallot, unifocal, multifocal, and repetitive premature ventricular contractions at rest or after exercise have been associated with ventricular tachycardia, ventricular fibrillation, and sudden death (Quattlebaum et al., 1976; Gillette et al., 1977). These patients with arrhythmias usually have residual hemodynamic abnormalities such as infundibular stenosis that are arrhythmogenic. Sinoatrial node dysfunction has been seen in patients after the Mustard procedure and ASD repair.

In children with uncomplicated CHD who undergo noncardiac procedures, surgery may be scheduled as an outpatient procedure. For patients with complex CHD, hospital admission

■ TABLE 17–19. Cardiac grid for common congenital heart lesions (desired hemodynamic changes)

	Preload	PVR	SVR	Heart Rate	Contractility
ASD	↑	↑	↓	N	N
VSD (left-to-right)	↑	↑	↓	N	N
VSD (right-to-left)	N	↓	↑	N	N
IHSS	↑	N	N↑	↓	↓
PDA	↑	↑	↓	N	N
Coarctation of the aorta	↑	N	↓	N	N
PS	↑	↓	N	↓	↑
AS	↑	N	↑	↓	N↑
MS	↑	N	N	↓	N↑
AR	↑	N	↓	N↑	N↑
MR	↑	N	↓	N↑	N↑

AR, aortic regurgitation; AS, aortic stenosis; ASD, atrial septal defect; IHSS, idiopathic hypertrophic subaortic stenosis; MR, mitral regurgitation; MS, mitral stenosis; PDA, patent ductus arteriosus; PS, pulmonary stenosis; PVR, pulmonary vascular resistance; SVR, systemic vascular resistance; VSD, ventricular septal defect.

should be considered the day before surgery, so that appropriate consultation and preparation can be made. In all patients, consultation with a pediatric cardiologist and access to recent echocardiography and catheterization data should be an integral part of the preoperative management. The anesthetic management decisions regarding induction technique, airway management, and maintenance of anesthesia are based on the patient's functional status, the pathophysiology of the underlying defect, the proposed operative procedure, and the anticipated hemodynamic response to the anesthetic agent. The cardiac grid (Table 17–19) may be used to construct an anesthetic plan.

Full resuscitative capabilities, including a defibrillator, must be available in the anesthetizing locations (Schwartz and Jobes, 1982). Resuscitation drugs must be readily accessible before anesthetic induction. These drugs should include epinephrine, sodium bicarbonate, atropine, lidocaine, and phenylephrine. The drugs may be drawn up and diluted to appropriate concentrations if the patient's clinical condition warrants it.

The only patients in whom antibiotic prophylaxis is not recommended are those with an isolated unrepaired secundum ASD, with a secundum ASD repaired with a patch, and with a previously ligated PDA.

Except in superficial and peripheral surgical procedures of short duration, controlled ventilation is desirable in these patients. Hypoventilation is poorly tolerated in CHD patients with limited cardiac reserve. In patients with tetralogy of Fallot, excessive mean airway pressure reduces cardiac filling and leads to increased right-to-left shunting across a VSD and cyanosis.

Preinduction monitoring of the child with cardiac disease for noncardiac surgery includes precordial stethoscope, electrocardiography, noninvasive blood pressure measurements, pulse oximetry, and temperature probe. Additional monitoring depends on the child's underlying cardiac status, disease state, and extent and duration of the anticipated surgery (Moore, 1981; Schwartz, 1985).

Postoperative respiratory support is dependent on the type and duration of surgery and/or the presence of significant cardiac or pulmonary dysfunction. Weaning from mechanical ventilatory support can gradually take place in the intensive care unit. For children in whom tracheal extubation is planned for at the end of the operative procedure, the criteria for extubation are similar to those for any child. The cardiovascular responses to reversal of neuromuscular blockade have been studied in healthy children and in children with cyanotic and acyanotic CHD (Salem et al., 1970; Wong et al., 1974). Despite slight changes in heart rate during reversal, cardiac output remains essentially unchanged during reversal (Sale et al., 1977). Antagonism of neuromuscular blockade need not be withheld for fear of arrhythmias. When the procedure is complete, the patient is transferred to the recovery room (or an intensive care environment if indicated) while oxygen is being administered. Close observation and monitoring of these children in the early postoperative period are essential.

■ ANESTHESIA FOR NONSURGICAL CARDIAC DISEASE

■ CARDIOMYOPATHY

Cardiomyopathies are defined as "diseases of the myocardium associated with cardiac dysfunction" (Richardson et al., 1996). They are classified based on newer pathophysiologic criteria. The five classes include dilated, hypertrophic, restrictive, arrhythmogenic RV, and unclassified. This classification is helpful to the anesthesiologist in optimizing an anesthetic plan for patients with cardiomyopathy. Cardiac surgery per se is not often performed in these children; however, they do present at end stage when cardiac transplantation or bridging to transplant is often the only alternative. Other patient encounters include placement of AICDs, central venous catheter placement, cardiac catheterization laboratory, muscle biopsies, dental rehabilitation, endoscopic diagnostic procedures, or childbirth.

Cardiomyopathies may be caused by ischemic heart disease (uncommon in children), toxin exposure, valvular heart disease, hypertension, inflammatory diseases (e.g., lupus), viral infections, metabolic diseases, and inherited disorders (e.g., glycogen storage disease type II, Pompe's disease). These etiologies usually fall into one of the pathophysiologic groups.

Dilated Cardiomyopathy

Systolic function is depressed usually with large ventricular volumes, elevated left ventricular end-diastolic pressures, high pulmonary venous pressures, and the presence of mitral or tricuspid valve regurgitation. The electrocardiogram may show bundle branch block, there may be ST-T wave abnormalities, and it is prudent to measure electrolytes before anesthesia, because these patients are on diuretics and possibly digoxin. Anesthetic management should focus on maintaining adequate preload, but overhydration causes pulmonary edema. Heart rate should be maintained at preinduction levels, because stroke volume is limited. The response to inotropes may be blunted, because stroke volume may increase minimally while heart rate increases excessively, resulting in impaired myocardial oxygen balance and ischemia. Mild afterload reduction is generally a preferred approach to enhance forward flow. Milrinone is a good inotrope and vasodilator for augmenting cardiac output in this type of cardiomyopathy. Afterload should be maintained at a normal-to-low SVR. A high afterload is not tolerated by a hypocontractile dilated cardiomyopathy. Etomidate 0.3 mg/kg is a hemodynamically stable induction agent; very low-dose maintenance inhalational agent may be used, together with fentanyl 2 to 5 mcg/kg and low-dose midazolam to prevent excessive SVR elevation. Monitoring may require a central venous catheter and an intra-arterial catheter to measure beat-to-beat blood pressure (Schechter et al., 1995).

Hypertrophic Cardiomyopathy

The pathophysiology associated with this diagnosis is noted for preservation of systolic function but poor diastolic function. Ventricular concentric or asymmetric hypertrophy usually develops, and over time, this decreases the ventricular cavity size. Frequently, the hypertrophied myocardium compresses endocardial blood vessels (Mohiddin et al., 2002). LVOT obstruction may be present. A reduction in preload increases dynamic obstruction and worsens cardiac output. An excessive decrease in SVR reduces coronary perfusion pressure and could result in ischemia. This sets up a downward spiral of diminished coronary blood flow, increased myocardial ischemia, and the risk of intraoperative ventricular fibrillation and sudden cardiac arrest. The anesthetic management of patients with this pathophysiology should be aimed at maintaining normal to slightly elevated SVR and preload at normal to moderately elevated levels. Heart rate is usually kept at a low to normal level to optimize diastolic filling time and enhance stroke volume. Inotropes are seldom needed and may decrease cardiac output in very severe hypertrophic cardiomyopathy, because systolic cavity obliteration may occur and diastolic filling time is reduced due to increased heart rate. Spontaneous ventilation is optimal for these patients because it preserves cardiorespiratory interactions. In the infantile form of glycogen storage disease type II or Pompe's disease, in which patients develop a severe form of hypertrophic cardiomyopathy, an anesthetic technique using spontaneous ventilation under ketamine and fentanyl titration with local or regional anesthesia has been found to be an alternative to inhalational general anesthesia (Ing et al., 2004). Propofol as the sole anesthetic agent in glycogen storage disease type II may not offer the safest anesthetic hemodynamic profile in the severe form of this cardiomyopathy (Ing et al., 2004), because it significantly decreases preload and SVR (Williams et al., 1999).

Restrictive Cardiomyopathy

This is a rare form of cardiomyopathy. It usually results in endomyocardial fibrosis with a severe decrease in ventricular compliance and poor ventricular filling. In the early stage of the disease, ejection fraction is maintained; as restriction progresses with time, left ventricular end-diastolic pressure increases, stroke volume significantly decreases, and cardiac output decreases. One of the distinguishing features of restrictive cardiomyopathy is the relentless progression of an elevated left ventricular end-diastolic pressure and resultant increase in PVR. By the time many children with a restrictive cardiomyopathy present with exercise intolerance, PVR is already greater than 10 to 15 Woods units; this prohibits them from being a recipient of a heart transplant (Weller et al., 2002).

The most common etiologies for restrictive cardiomyopathy in children are endomyocardial fibrosis and Loffler's endocarditis. Some believe them to be part of the same spectrum, but in Loffler's disease, intraventricular cavity thrombus formation is common, and eosinophilic infiltration into other organs causes small vessel arteritis. Endomyocardial fibrosis is characterized by fibrosis of the ventricular apex and mitral valve. LVOT obstruction is rare (Davies, 1960). The diagnosis is often made by echocardiography, showing small ventricles, massively dilated atria, and, rarely, pericardial effusion (Weller et al., 2002). The jugular venous pressure is often raised and can show a paradoxical increase in height during spontaneous inspiration. This is due to increased venous return into a noncompliant ventricle.

PERICARDITIS, PERICARDIAL EFFUSIONS, AND CARDIAC TAMPONADE

Acute Pericarditis

Acute pericarditis rarely causes restriction. It can occur in children at any age, and quite commonly the etiology is purulent pericarditis. *Staphylococcus* causes about 40% of cases; collagen vascular disease, 30%; virus, 20%; and radiation therapy and, rarely, neoplastic disease, 10% (Roodpeyma and Sadeghian, 2000; Kohli et al., 2001). A pericardiectomy is almost never required with acute pericarditis, but the pericardial cavity may need to be drained by a subxiphoid catheter that is usually inserted with transthoracic echocardiographic guidance in a sterile fashion under sedation. Propofol infusion with local anesthetic infiltration or occasionally ketamine is commonly used. Cardiac tamponade may be seen with associated acute carditis, but this is rare (Roodpeyama and Sadeghian, 2000).

Constrictive Pericarditis

Constrictive pericarditis is a chronic condition more commonly seen in the developing world. Tuberculosis is the number 1 offending pathogen. In more-developed nations, neoplastic disease, inflammatory conditions, and radiation therapy–induced constrictive pericarditis are more commonly seen (Kohli et al., 2001). Constrictive pericarditis is clinically suspected when there is a raised jugular venous pressure, hepatomegaly, pedal edema, pleural effusions, and massive ascites. Surgical therapy necessitates a pericardiectomy through a midline sternotomy, and although the heart may be cannulated for emergent CPB, all surgical attempts are made to complete the procedure without CPB because dissection of the adherent pericardium may cause myocardial stunning. Postoperatively, low cardiac output syndrome is commonly observed. Theoretically, the pericardium over the LV is removed first. It is argued that if the right side were released first, an increased ventricular volume may increase PBF and increase volume return to a small noncompliant LV, and this may cause pulmonary edema. This is rarely seen clinically, because as a practical matter, both ventricles are often released simultaneously as the surgical dissection steadily progresses.

Pericardial Effusion and Cardiac Tamponade

Postoperative tamponade may be caused by a rapidly increasing collection of fluid into the pericardial space if intact or directly into either the mediastinum or the pleural space if the pericardium is left open after cardiac surgery. A combination of fresh blood and formed clot is present and often requires urgent/emergent surgical reexploration for evacuation. The signs and symptoms are clinical and should be acted on before significant hemodynamic compromise occurs. If time permits, TEE should be obtained to confirm the diagnosis. The clinical presentation includes tachycardia, hypotension, central venous pressure elevation, worsening pulmonary compliance, and oxygen desaturation with poor peripheral perfusion. Early diagnosis and prompt therapy can ensure good outcome even in very small infants (Wirrell et al., 1993). In older children, pulsus paradoxus and distended neck veins are seen.

Anesthetic management of pericardial effusion depends on whether there is tamponade. In the presence of tamponade, a pericardial catheter should be placed using local anesthesia. If tamponade is not present based on echocardiographic evaluation, the use of a slow titration of anesthetic agents such as propofol is well tolerated. Patients should be volume loaded to optimize stroke volume before the administration of anesthetic drugs, and resuscitative agents should be available for use at the bedside.

A common source of unexpected cardiac tamponade in neonates, infants, and children is related to vascular or heart perforation from central lines. Line location has been looked at as a cause for cardiac perforation, with a higher risk identified for neonates. In neonates, general recommendations for the optimal placement of the distal tip of peripherally inserted central catheters, as well as percutaneously placed internal jugular or subclavian venous catheters, should lie at the SVC-RA junction (Nadroo et al., 2001). This corresponds to a level above T-2 as documented by chest radiography (Bargy et al., 1986).

In the operating room, central venous catheters are placed without radiologic confirmation. On arrival in the intensive care unit, a chest radiograph is obtained and the catheter placement is adjusted if indicated. Despite these recommendations, numerous reports exist of iatrogenic cardiac tamponade, often suspected as delayed migration or excessive movement of the catheter tip due to abduction of the arm or head flexion/extension changes. Catheter mobility of 3 to 5 cm has been described (Brandt et al., 1970) for subclavian and internal jugular central catheters, respectively. For peripherally placed central catheters, especially when crossing a joint area, greater degrees of movement have been documented, and it is recommended to limit limb movement (Henzel et al., 1971). This may explain the continued occurrence of cardiac tamponade despite appropriate catheter positioning. Although the recommendation for optimal placement of the catheter tip is at the SVC-RA juncture, it may actually be 1 cm within the RA. The rationale for this location is that the pericardium extends 1 to 2 cm proximal from the SVC RA juncture. The narrow SVC can be perforated by the tip of the catheter, leading to infusion of fluid into the pericardial space. By placing the tip within the wider opening of the RA, the tip swings freely and does not engage the wall of the RA, similar to a clapper in a bell.

Infants with catheter migration and gradual pericardial infusion of fluid usually present with sudden cardiac arrest; very few are successfully resuscitated with pericardiocentesis (Aiken et al., 1992; Nadroo, 2001). Retrospectively, it is sometimes noted that the patient may have been gradually deteriorating hemodynamically, with signs of dyspnea, tachycardia, or nausea misinterpreted for 12 to 24 hours before the cardiac arrest (Arbitman and Kart, 1979). For any patient with a central venous catheter in situ and a diagnosis of pericardial effusion, cardiac echocardiography with a small injection of agitated saline should be performed to confirm that the catheter tip is not the source of the pericardial infusion. If the catheter tip is seen in the pericardial space and that central catheter is used, any further injection of fluid worsens the effusion and contributes to worsening of the cardiac tamponade.

■ SUMMARY

The anesthetic management of children undergoing cardiac surgery requires a sound understanding of the basic principles of cardiovascular anesthesia, pediatric anesthesia, and intensive care and a working knowledge of the pathophysiology of congenital cardiac disease. Anesthesiologists must also know how to treat right ventricular dysfunction, left ventricular dysfunction, and PA hypertension and be aware of the potential residual anatomic problems associated with cardiac surgical interventions. This requisite knowledge, coupled with an open mind toward the ever-expanding strategies and techniques being developed worldwide for optimizing care of complex CHD patients, is essential. Through constant evolution and hard work, the overall life expectancy and life quality of the child with CHD continue to improve and we hope approach those of children born with a normal cardiovascular system.

REFERENCES

Aaronson PI, Robertson TP, Ward JP: Endothelium-derived mediators and hypoxic pulmonary vasoconstriction. *Respir Physiol Neurobiol* 132:107–120, 2002.

Abdul-Khaliq H, Troitzsch D, Schubert S, et al.: Cerebral oxygen monitoring during neonatal cardiopulmonary bypass and deep hypothermic circulatory arrest. *Thorac Cardiovasc Surg* 50:77–81, 2002.

Adesuyi S, Cockrell C, Gamache D, et al.: Lipoxygenase metabolism of arachidonic acid in brain. *J Neurochem* 45:770, 1985.

Aiken G, Porteous L, Tracy M, Richardson V: Cardiac tamponade from a fine Silastic central venous catheter in a premature infant. *J Paediatr Child Health* 28:325, 1992.

Aisen P: *The transferrins. Iron in biochemistry and medicine, II.* New York, 1980, Academic Press.

Alboliras E, Porter C, Danielson G, et al.: Results of the modified Fontan operation for congenital heart lesions in patients without preoperative sinus rhythm. *J Am Coll Cardiol* 6:228–235, 1985.

Allen SW, Gauvreau K, Bloom BT, et al.: Evidence-based referral results in significantly reduced mortality after congenital heart surgery. *Pediatrics* 112:24–28, 2003.

Alvis JM, Reves JG, et al.: Computer-assisted continuous infusions of fentanyl during cardiac surgery: Comparison with a manual method. *Anesthesiology* 63:41–50, 1985.

American Academy of Pediatrics, Section on Cardiology and Cardiac Surgery: Guidelines for pediatric cardiovascular centers. *Pediatrics* 109:544–549, 2002.

Anand KJS, Hansen DD, Hickey PR: Hormonal–metabolic stress response in neonates undergoing cardiac surgery. *Anesthesiology* 73:661, 1990.

Anand KJS, Hickey PR: Halothane-morphine compared with high-dose sufentanil for anesthesia and postoperative analgesia in neonatal cardiac surgery. *N Engl J Med* 326:1–9, 1992.

Anand KJS, Sippell WG, Aynsley-Green A: Randomized trial of fentanyl anesthesia in preterm neonates undergoing surgery: Effects on the stress response. *Lancet* 1:243, 1987.

Anderson PAW: Maturation and cardiac contractility. *Cardiol Clin* 7:209–225, 1989.

Andrew MB, Paes B, Milner R, et al.: Development of the human coagulation system in the full-term infant. *Blood* 70:165–172, 1987.

Arbitman M, Kart H: Hydromediastinum after aberrant central venous catheter placement. *Crit Care Med* 7:27–29, 1979.

Arciniegas E: *Pediatric cardiac surgery.* Chicago, 1985, Year Book Medical Publishers, Inc.

Ashwal S: Brain death in the newborn. *Curr Perspect Clin Perinatol* 24:859–882, 1997.

Astrup J: Energy-requiring cell functions in the ischemic brain. *J Neurosurg* 56:482, 1982.

Atallah-Yunes NH, Kavey RE, et al.: Postoperative assessment of a modified surgical approach to repair of tetralogy of Fallot: Long term follow up. *Circulation* 94(Suppl II):II-22–II-26, 1996.

Attenhofer Jost CH, Schaff HV, Connolly HM, et al.: Spectrum of reoperations after repair of aortic coarctation: Importance of individualized approach because of coexistent cardiovascular disease. *Mayo Clin Proc* 77:646–653, 2002.

Ausems ME, Hug CC, Stanski DR, et al.: Plasma concentrations of alfentanil required to supplement nitrous oxide anesthesia for general surgery. *Anesthesiology* 75:362–370, 1986.

Austin EH 3rd, Edmonds HL Jr, Auden SM, et al.: Benefit of neurophysiologic monitoring for pediatric cardiac surgery. *J Thorac Cardiovasc Surg* 114:707–715, 1997.

Balaji S, Gewillig M, Bull C, et al.: Arrythmias after the Fontan procedure: Comparison of total cavopulmonary connection and atriopulmonary connection. *Circulation* 84(Suppl III):III-162–III-167, 1991.

Bargy F, Barbet P, Houette G: The pericardium of the newborn infant. Anatomic and radioanatomic study with the view toward better positioning central catheters in the superior vena cava. *Bull Assoc Anat* 70:47, 1986.

Barratt-Boyes BG, Simpson M, Neutze JM: Intracardiac surgery in neonates and infants using deep hypothermia with surface cooling and limited cardiopulmonary bypass. *Circulation* 53:25–30, 1971.

Barratt-Boyes BG, Simpson MM, Neutze JM: Intracardiac surgery in neonates and infants using deep hypothermia. *Circulation* 62(Suppl III):III-73–III-80, 1980.

Barton P, Kalil AC, Nadel S, et al.: Safety, pharmacokinetics and pharmacodynamics of drotrecogin alfa (activated) in children with severe sepsis. *Pediatrics* 113(1 Pt (1)):7–17, 2004.

Bashein GBD, Townes BD, Nessly BS, et al.: A randomized study of carbon dioxide management during hypothermic cardiopulmonary bypass. *Anesthesiology* 72:7–15, 1990.

Baylen B, Meyer RA, Korfhagen J, et al.: Left ventricular performance in the critically ill premature infant with patent ductus arteriosus and pulmonary disease. *Circulation* 55:182–188, 1977.

Becker AE, Caruso G: *Congenital heart disease—a morphologist's view on myocardial dysfunction.* Edinburgh, 1981, Churchill Livingstone.

Bellinger DC, Wernovsky G, Rappaport L, et al.: Rapid cooling of infants on cardiopulmonary bypass adversely affects later cognitive function. *Circulation* 78:A358, 1988.

Bellinger DC, Wypij D, Kuban KC, et al.: Developmental and neurological status of children at 4 years of age after heart surgery with hypothermic circulatory arrest or low-flow cardiopulmonary bypass. *Circulation* 100:526–532, 1999.

Bellinger DC, Wypij D, du Plessis AJ, et al.: Developmental and neurologic effects of alpha-stat versus pH-stat strategies for deep hypothermic cardiopulmonary bypass in infants. *J Thorac Cardiovasc Surg* 121:374, 2001.

Bellinger DC, Bernstein JH, Kirkwood MW, et al.: Visual-spatial skills in children after open-heart surgery. *J Dev Behav Pediatr* 24:169–179, 2003.

Bellinger DC, Wypij D, duPlessis AJ, et al.: Neurodevelopmental status at eight years in children with dextro-transposition of the great arteries: The Boston circulatory arrest trial. *J Thorac Cardiovasc Surg* 26:1385–1396, 2003.

Bender KA, Alexander JA, Enos JM, et al.: Effects of inhaled nitric oxide in patients with hypoxemia and pulmonary hypertension after cardiac surgery. *Am J Crit Care* 6:127–131, 1997.

Bengur AR, Li JS, Herlong JR, et al.: Intraoperative transesophageal echocardiography in congenital heart disease. *Semin Thorac Cardiovasc Surg* 10:255–264, 1998.

Benveniste H, Drejer J, Schousboe A, et al.: Elevations of the extracellular concentrations of glutamate and aspartate in rat hippocampus during transient cerebral ischemia monitored by intracerebral microdialysis. *J Neurochem* 43:1369–1374, 1984.

Bering EAJ: Effect of body temperature change on cerebral oxygen consumption during hypothermia. *Am J Physiol* 200:417, 1961.

Berman W: *The hemodynamics of shunts in congenital heart disease.* New York, 1985 Raven Press.

Berne RM, Levy MN: Coronary circulation and cardiac metabolism. In Berne RM, Levy MN, editors: *Cardiovascular physiology.* St. Louis, 1981, The CV Mosby Co.

Berner M, Oberhansli I, Rouge J, et al.: Chronotropic and inotropic supports are both required to increase cardiac output early after corrective operations for tetralogy of Fallot. *J Thorac Cardiovasc Surg* 97:297–302, 1989.

Berner MJC, Rouge JC, Friedli B: The hemodynamic effect of phentolamine and dobutamine after open-heart operations in children: Influence of underlying heart defect. *Ann Thorac Surg* 35:643–650, 1983.

Bers D: *Excitation-contraction coupling and cardiac contractile force,* 2nd ed. Dordrecht, the Netherlands, 2001, Kluwer, pp 125–130.

Betrin A, Wyle E, Felderhof C, et al.: Prolapse of the posterior leaflet of the mitral valve associated with secundum atrial septal defect. *Am J Cardiol* 35:363, 1975.

Bettex DA, Schmidlin D, Bernath MA, et al.: Intraoperative transesophageal echocardiography in pediatric congenital cardiac surgery: A two-center observational study. *Anesth Analg* 97:1275–1282, 2003.

Bishop CCR, Powell S, Rutt D, et al.: Transcranial Doppler measurement of middle cerebral artery blood flow velocity: A validation study. *Stroke* 17:913–915, 1986.

Blume ED, Altmann K, Mayer JE, et al.: Evolution of risk factors influencing early mortality of the arterial switch operation. *J Am Coll Cardiol* 33:1702–1709, 1999.

Bohn DJ, Poirer CS, Edmonds JF: Efficacy of dopamine, dobutamine, and epinephrine during emergence from cardiopulmonary bypass in children. *Crit Care Med* 8:367–372, 1980.

Bolling SF, Bies LE, Bove E, et al.: Augmenting intracellular adenosine improves myocardial recovery. *J Thorac Cardiovasc Surg* 99:469–474, 1990.

Borow KM, Keane JF, Castaneda A, et al.: Systemic ventricular function in patients with tetralogy of Fallot, ventricular septal defect and transposition of the great arteries repaired during infancy. *Circulation* 64:878, 1981.

Bove EL, Lloyd TR: Staged reconstruction for hypoplastic left heart syndrome. *Ann Surg* 224:387, 1996.

Bradley SM, Simsic JM, Atz AM: Hemodynamic effects of inspired carbon dioxide after the Norwood procedure. *Ann Thorac Surg* 72:2088–2093, 2001.

Brandt RL, Foley WJ, Fink GH, et al.: Mechanism of perforation of the heart with production of hydropericardium by a venous catheter and its prevention. *Am J Surg* 119:311–316, 1970.

Breda MA, Drinkwater DC, Laks H, et al.: Prevention of reperfusion injury in the neonatal heart with leukocyte-depleted blood. *J Thorac Cardiovasc Surg* 97:654–658, 1989.

Bretschneider HJ: Myocardial protection. *Thorac Cardiovasc Surg* 28:295–299, 1980.

Bridges ND, Jonas RA, Mayer J, et al.: Bidirectional cavopulmonary anastomosis as interim palliation for high risk Fontan candidates: Early results. *Circulation* 82(Suppl IV):IV-170–IV-176, 1990.

Brodde O, Broede A, Daul A, et al.: Receptor systems in the non-failing human heart. *Basic Res Cardiol* 87(Suppl):1–14, 1992.

Brown JW, Ruzmetov M, Vijay P, et al.: Surgery for aortic stenosis in children: A 40-year experience. *Ann Thorac Surg* 76:1398–1411, 2003.

Bryant PE: Enzymatic restriction of mammalian cell DNA: Evidence for double-strand breaks as potentially lethal lesions. *Int J Radic Res* 48:55, 1985.

Buckberg GD: A proposed solution to the cardioplegia controversy. *J Thorac Cardiovasc* Surg 77:803–806, 1979.

Buckberg GD: Oxygenated cardioplegia: Blood is a many splendored thing. *Ann Thorac Surg* 50:175–177, 1990.

Bui KC, Hammerman C, Hirshl RB, et al.: Plasma prostanoids in neonates with pulmonary hypertension treated with conventional therapy and with extracorporeal membrane oxygenation. *J Thorac Cardiovasc Surg* 101:973–983, 1991.

Bush A, Busset C, Knight W, et al.: Modification of pulmonary hypertension secondary to congenital heart disease. *Am Rev Respir Dis* 136:767, 1987.

Busto R, Dietrich WD, Globus MY, et al.: Small differences in the intra-ischemic brain temperature critically determine the extent of ischemic neuronal injury. *J Cereb Blood Flow Metab* 7:729–736, 1987.

Busto R, Mordecai Y-T, Dietrich D, et al.: Effects of mild hypothermia on brain ischemia. *Stroke* 20:904–910, 1989.

Butler J, Rocker GM, Westaby S: Inflammatory responses to cardiopulmonary bypass. *Ann Thorac Surg* 55:552–559, 1993.

Castaneda AR, Mayer JEJ, Jonas RA, et al.: The neonate with critical congenital heart disease: Repair—a surgical challenge. *J Thorac Cardiovasc Surg* 98:869–875, 1989.

Castaneda AR, Trusler GA, Paul MA, et al.: The early results of treatment of simple transposition in the current era. *J Thorac Cardiovasc Surg* 95:4–22, 1988.

Casteneda AR, Jonas RA, Mayer JE, et al.: *Cardiac surgery of the neonate and infant.* Philadelphia, PA, WB Saunders, 1994, Chapter 22, pp 353–362.

Celoria GC, Patton RB: Congenital absence of the aortic arch. *Am Heart J* 58:407, 1959.

Chang AC, Atz AM, Wernovsky G, et al.: Milrinone: Systemic and pulmonary hemodynamic effects in neonates after cardiac surgery. *Crit Care Med* 23:1907, 1995.

Chiba Y, Muraoka R, Ihaya A, et al.: The effects of leukocyte depletion on the prevention of reperfusion injury during cardiopulmonary bypass. *J Thorac Cardiovasc Surg* 1:350–356, 1993.

Chizzonite R, Zak R: Calcium-induced cell death: Susceptibility of cardiac myocytes is age-dependent. *Science* 213:508–511, 1981.

Chopp M, Knight R, Tidwell CD, et al.: The metabolic effects of moderate hypothermia on global cerebral ischemia and recirculation in the cat: Comparison to monothermia and hypothermia. *J Cereb Blood Flow Metab* 9:141–148, 1989.

Choudry DK, Brenn BR: Bispectral index monitoring: A comparison between normal and children with quadriplegic cerebral palsy. *Anesth Analg* 95:1582–1585, 2002.

Civalero L, Moreno J, Senning A: Temperature conditions and oxygen consumption during deep hypothermia. *Acta Chir Scand* 123:179–188, 1962.

Clermont G, Vergely C, Jazayeri S, et al.: Systemic free radical activation is a major event involved in myocardial oxidative stress related to cardiopulmonary bypass. *Anesthesiology* 96:80–87, 2002.

Codispoti M, Ludlam CA, Simpson D, Mankad PS: Individualized heparin and protamine management in infants and children undergoing cardiac operations. *Ann Thorac Surg* 71:922, 2001.

Cohen MI, Bridges ND, Gaynor JW, et al.: Modifications to the cavopulmonary anastomosis do not eliminate early sinus node dysfunction. *J Thorac Cardiovasc Surg* 120:891–900, 2000.

Colon-Otero G, Gilchrist GS, Holcomb GR, et al.: Preoperative evaluation of hemostasis in patients with heart disease. *Mayo Clin Proc* 62:379–385, 1987.

Cook DJ: Con: Low-flow cardiopulmonary bypass is not the preferred technique for patients undergoing cardiac surgical procedures. *J Cardiothorac Vasc Anesth* 15:652–654, 2001.

Croughwell N, Smith L, Quill T, et al.: The effect of temperature on cerebral metabolism and blood flow in adults during cardiopulmonary bypass. *J Thorac Cardiovasc Surg* 103:549–554, 1993a.

Croughwell N, Newman MF, Blumenthal JA, et al.: Jugular venous saturation and cerebral arterial venous oxygen difference predict cognitive dysfunction after cardiac surgery. *Circulation* 88(Suppl II):II-289,1993b.

Culliford AT, Gitel SN, Starr N, et al.: Lack of correlation between activated clotting time and plasma heparin during cardiopulmonary bypass. *Ann Surg* 193:105, 1981.

Custer JR, Hales CA: Influence of alveolar oxygen on pulmonary vasoconstriction in newborn lambs vs sheep. *Am Rev Respir Dis* 132:326, 1985.

Cyran, SE, Myers JL, Gleason MM, et al.: Application of intraoperative transesophageal echocardiography in infants and small children. *J Cardiovasc Surg (Torino)* 32:318–321, 1991.

Danforth WH, Naegle S, Bing R: Effect of ischemia and reoxygenation on glycolytic reactions and adenosine triphosphate in heart muscle. *Circ Res* 8:965–969, 1960.

Darling EM, Shearer IR, Nanry K, et al.: Modified ultrafiltration in pediatric cardiopulmonary bypass. *J Extra Corpor Technol* 26:205–209, 1994.

Darling EM, Kaemmer D, Lawson S, et al.: Experimental use of an ultra-low prime neonatal cardiopulmonary bypass circuit utilizing vacuum-assisted venous drainage. *J Extra Corpor Technol* 30:184–189, 1998.

Darling EM, Kaemmer D, Lawson DS, et al.: Use of ECMO without the oxygenator to provide ventricular support after Norwood stage I procedures. *Ann Thorac Surg* 71:735–736, 2001.

Davidson AJ, McCann M, Devavaram P, et al.: The difference in the bispectral index between infants and children during emergence from anesthesia after circumcision surgery. *Anesth Analg* 93:326–330, 2001.

Davis PJ, Cook DR, Stiller RL, et al.: Pharmacodynamics and pharmacokinetics of high-dose sufentanil in infants and children undergoing cardiac surgery. *Anesth Analg* 66:203–210, 1987.

Davis PJ, Wilson AS, Siewers RD, et al.: The effects of cardiopulmonary bypass on remifentanil kinetics in children undergoing atrial septal defect repair. *Anesth Analg* 89:904, 1999.

Deal CW, Warden JC, Monk I: Effect of hypothermia on lung compliance. *Thorax* 25:105–109, 1970.

Decoodt P, Kacenelenbogen R, Bar JP, et al.: Clinical usefulness of biplane transesophageal echocardiography. *Echocardiogr J Cardiovasc Ultrasound Allied Techn* 9:257–264, 1992.

Dekeon M, Meldrum M, Meliones J, et al.: Pulmonary function testing demonstrates airway obstruction secondary to cardiovascular abnormalities. *Pediatr Crit Care Colloquium* Jan 30, 1992.

DeLeon S, Idriss F, Ilbawi M, et al.: The role of the Glenn shunt in patients undergoing the Fontan operation. *J Thorac Cardiovasc Surg* 85:669–677, 1983.

Delise G, Ando M, Calder AL, et al.: Total anomalous pulmonary veins connection: Report of 93 autopsied cases with emphasis on diagnostic and surgical considerations. *Am Heart J* 91:99–122, 1976.

DiEusanio M, Wesselink RM, Morshuis WJ, et al.: Hypothermic circulatory arrest and antegrade selective cerebral perfusion during ascending aorta hemiarch replacement: A retrospective comparison. *J Thorac Cardiovasc Surg* 125:849–854, 2003.

Dickinson D, Wilkinson J, Smith A, et al.: Variations in the morphology of the ventricular septal defect and disposition of the atrioventricular conduction tissues in tetralogy of Fallot. *Thorac Cardiovasc Surg* 30:243–247, 1982.

Dietrich W, Barankay A, Hahnel C, et al.: High-dose aprotinin in cardiac surgery: Three years' experience in 1,784 patients. *J Cardiothorac Vasc Anesth* 6:324–327, 1992.

Dietrich W, Henze R, Barankay A, et al.: High-dose aprotinin application reduces homologous blood requirement in cardiac surgery. *J Cardiothorac Anesth* 3:79–84, 1989.

Dietrich W, Mossinger H, Spannagl M, et al.: Hemostatic activation during cardiopulmonary bypass with different aprotinin dosages in pediatric patients having cardiac operations. *J Thorac Cardiovasc Surg* 105:712–720, 1993.

Dietrich W, Spannagl M, Jochum M, et al.: Influence of high-dose aprotinin treatment on blood loss and coagulation patterns in patients undergoing myocardial revascularization. *Anesthesiology* 73:1119–1126, 1990.

Dietrich W, Spannagl M, Schramm W, et al.: The influence of preoperative anticoagulation on heparin response during cardiopulmonary bypass. *J Thorac Cardiovasc Surg* 102:505–514, 1991.

Domalik-Wawrzynski LJ, Powell WR Jr, Guerrero L, et al.: Effect of changes in ventricular relaxation on early diastolic coronary blood flow in canine hearts. *Circ Res* 65:1751–1756, 1987.

Downing SW, Edmonds LH: Release of vasoactive substances during cardiopulmonary bypass. *Ann Thorac Surg* 54:1236–1243, 1992.

Drummond WH, Gregory GA, Heyman M, et al.: The independent effects of hyperventilation, tolazoline, and dopamine in infants with persistent pulmonary hypertension. *J Pediatr* 98:603–608, 1981.

Drummond WH, Lock JE: Neonatal pulmonary vasodilator drugs. *Dev Pharmacol Ther* 7:1, 1984.

Dubost C, Deloche A, Carpentier A, et al.: Endomyocardial fibrosis. *Chirurgie* 115:689–703, 1989.

Duncan BW, Desai S: Pulmonary arteriovenous malformations after cavopulmonary anastomosis. *Ann Thorac Surg* 76:1759–1766, 2003.

Duncan HP, Cloote A, Weir PM, et al.: Reducing stress response in the prebypass phase of open heart surgery in infants and young children: A comparison of different fentanyl doses. *Br J Anesth* 84:556–564, 2000.

El Azab SR, Rosseel PM, deLange JJ, et al.: Dexamethasone decreases the pro- to anti-inflammatory cytokine ratio during cardiac surgery. *Br J Anaesth* 88:496–501, 2002.

Emmel M, Sreeram N: Total anomalous pulmonary vein connection: Diagnosis, management and outcome. *Curr Treat Options Cardiovasc Med* 5:423–439, 2004.

Engle MA, Perloff JK: *Congenital heart disease after surgery: Benefits, residua, and sequelae.* New York, 1983, Yorke Medical Books.

Erb TO, Hall JM, Ing RJ, et al.: Postoperative nausea and vomiting in children and adolescents undergoing radiofrequency catheter ablation: a randomized comparison of propofol and isoflurane-based anesthetics. *Anesth Analg* 95:1577, 2002.

Erb TO, Kanter RJ, Hall JM, et al.: Comparison of electrophysiologic effects of propofol and isoflurane-based anesthetics in children undergoing radiofrequency catheter ablation for supraventricular tachycardia. *Anesthesiology* 96:1386, 2002.

Ericinska M, Silver IA: ATP and brain function. *J Cereb Blood Flow Metab* 9:2, 1989.

Fagan DG: Shape changes in V-P loops for children's lungs related to growth. *Thorax* 32:198, 1977.

Fillinger MP, Rassias AJ, Guyre PM, et al.: Glucocorticoid effects on the inflammatory and clinical responses to cardiac surgery. *J Cardiothorac Vasc Anesth* 16:163–169, 2002.

Fishberger SB, Wernovsky G, Gentles TL, et al.: Factors that influence the development of atrial flutter after the Fontan operation. *J Thorac Cardiovasc Surg* 113:80–86, 1997.

Fishberger SB, Wernovsky G, Gentles TL, et al.: Factors that influence the development of atrial flutter after the Fontan operation. *J Thorac Cardiovasc Surg* 11:70–74, 2003.

Fogel MA: Is routine cardiac catheterization necessary in the management of patients with single ventricles across staged Fontan reconstruction? No! *Pediatr Cardiol* May 5, 2005.

Fontan F, Deville C, Quagebeur J, et al.: Repair of tricuspid atresia in 100 patients. *J Thorac Cardiovasc Surg* 85:647, 1983.

Fox LS, Blackstone EH, Kirklin JW, et al.: Relationship of whole body oxygen consumption to perfusion flow rate during hypothermic cardiopulmonary bypass. *J Thorac Cardiovasc Surg* 83:239, 1982.

Fox L, Blackstone E, Kirklin J, et al.: Relationship of brain blood flow and oxygen consumption to perfusion flow rate during profound hypothermic cardiopulmonary bypass an experimental study. *J Thorac Cardiovasc Surg* 87:658–664, 1984a.

Fox L, Blackstone E, Kirklin J, et al.: Cerebral monitoring of somatosensory evoked potentials during profoundly hypothermic circulatory arrest. *Circulation* 1984b.

Fox L, Blackstone E, Kirklin J, et al.: Relationship of whole body oxygen consumption to perfusion flow rate during hypothermic cardiopulmonary bypass. *J Thorac Cardiovasc Surg* 83:239–248, 1984c.

Franciosi RA, Blanc WA: Myocardial infarction in infants and children. I. A necropsy study in congenital heart disease. *J Pediatr* 73:309, 1968.

Freeman BA, Crapo JD: Free radicals and tissue injury. *Lab Invest* 47:412, 1982.

Frescura C, Thiene G, Franceschini E, et al.: Pulmonary vascular disease in infants with complete atrioventricular septal defect. *Int J Cardiol* 15:91, 1987.

Friedman W: The intrinsic properties of the developing heart. *Prog Cardiovasc* Dis 15:87–111, 1972.

Friesen RH, Lichtor JL: Cardiovascular effects of inhalational induction with isoflurane in infants. *Anesth Analg* 62:411–417, 1983.

Friesen RH, Veit AS, Archibald DJ, et al.: A comparison of remifentanil and fentanyl for fast track paediatric cardiac anesthesia. *Paediatr Anaesth* 13:122–125, 2003.

Fyler D: Report of the New England Regional Infant Cardiac Program. *Pediatrics* 65(Suppl):376, 1980.

Gaudet RJ, Alam I, Levine L: Accumulation of cyclooxygenase products of arachidonic acid metabolism in gerbil brain during reperfusion after bilateral common carotid artery occlusion. *J Neurochem* 35:653–658, 1980.

Gaynor JW, Gerdes M, Zackai EH, et al.: Apolipoprotein E genotype and neurodevelopment sequelae of infant cardiac surgery. *J Thorac Cardiovasc Surg* 26:1736–1745, 2003.

Geha AS, Salaymeh MT, Abe T, et al.: Pressure-dependent cerebral ischemia during cardiopulmonary bypass. *Neurology* 23:521–529, 1973.

Ghanayem NS, Hoffman GM, Mussatto KA, et al.: Home surveillance program prevents interstage mortality after the Norwood procedure. *J Thorac Cardiovasc Surg* 126:1257, 2003.

Giannuzzi CE, Seidler FJ, Slotkin TA: Beta-adrenoceptor control of cardiac adenylyl cyclase during development: agonist pretreatment in the neonate uniquely causes heterologous sensitization, not desensitization. *Brain Res* 694:271, 1995.

Gibbs JL, Wren C, Watterson KG, et al.: Stenting of the arterial ductus combined with banding of the pulmonary arteries and atrial septostomy: A new approach to palliation for the hypoplastic left heart syndrome. *Br Heart J* 69:551–555, 1993.

Gildein HP, Ahmadi A, Fontan F, et al.: Special problems in Fontan-type operations for complex cardiac lesions. *Int J Cardiol* 29:21–28, 1990.

Gillette PC, Kugler JD, Garson AJ: Mechanisms of cardiac arrhythmias after the Mustard operation for transposition of the great arteries. *Am J Cardiol* 45:1225–1229, 1980.

Gillette PC, Yeoman M, Mullins C, et al.: Sudden death after repair of tetralogy of Fallot. Electrocardiographic and electrophysiologic abnormalities. *Circulation* 56:566, 1977.

Girard C, Lehot J, Clerc J, et al.: Inhaled nitric oxide (NO) in pulmonary hypertension following mitral valve replacement. *Anesthesiology* 75:A984, 1991.

Glass PS, Bloom M, Kearse L, et al.: Bispectral analysis measures sedation and memory effects of propofol, midazolam, isoflurane, and alfentanil in healthy volunteers. *Anesthesiology* 86:836–847, 1997.

Godart F, Rey C, Devos P, et al.: Transcatheter occlusion of moderate to large patent arterial ducts, having a diameter above 2.5 mm, with the Amplatzer duct occluder. Comparisons Rashkind buttoned devices and coils in 116 consecutive patients. *Cardiol Young* 13:413, 2003.

Gold JP, Jonas RA, Lang P, et al.: Transthoracic intracardiac monitoring lines in pediatric surgical patients: A ten year experience. *Ann Thorac Surg* 42:185, 1986.

Goldberg CS, Schwartz EM, Brunberg JA, et al.: Neurodevelopment outcome of patients after the Fontan operation: A comparison between children with hypoplastic left heart syndrome and other functional single ventricle lesions. *J Pediatr* 137:646–652, 2000.

Govier AV, Reves JG, McKay RD, et al.: Factors and their influence on regional cerebral blood flow during nonpulsatile cardiopulmonary bypass. *Ann Thorac Surg* 38:592–600, 1984.

Graham T: Ventricular performance in adults after operation for congenital heart disease. *Am J Cardiol* 50:612–620, 1982.

Graham TP: Ventricular performance in congenital heart disease. *Circulation* 84:2259–2274, 1991.

Greeley WJ, Bracey VA, Ungerleider RM, et al.: Recovery of cerebral metabolism and mitochondrial oxidation state is delayed after hypothermic circulatory arrest. *Circulation* 84(Suppl III):III-400–III-415, 1991a.

Greeley WJ, Bushman GA, Davis DP, et al.: Comparative effects of halothane and ketamine on systemic arterial oxygen saturation in children with cyanotic heart disease. *Anesthesiology* 65:666–668, 1986a.

Greeley WJ, Bushman G, Kong D, et al.: Effects of cardiopulmonary bypass on eicosanoid metabolism during pediatric cardiovascular surgery. *J Thorac Cardiovasc Surg* 95:842–849, 1988.

Greeley WJ, de Bruijn NP: Changes in sufentanil pharmacokinetics within the neonatal period. *Anesth Analg* 67:86–90, 1988.

Greeley WJ, de Bruijn NP, Davis DP: Sufentanil pharmacokinetics in pediatric cardiovascular patients. *Anesth Analg* 66:1067–1072, 1987a.

Greeley WJ, Kern FH, Meliones J, et al.: Monitoring the brain during cardiac surgery in children [editorial; comment]. *Can J Anaesth* 40:291–297, 1993.

Greeley WJ, Kern FH, Ungerleider RM, et al.: The effect of hypothermic cardiopulmonary bypass and total circulatory arrest on cerebral metabolism in neonates, infants, and children. *J Thorac Cardiovasc Surg* 101:783–794, 1991b.

Greeley WJ, Leslie JB, Reves JG: Prostaglandins and the cardiovascular system: A review and update. *J Cardiothorac Anesth* 1:331–349, 1987b.

Greeley WJ, Leslie JB, Reves JG, et al.: Eicosanoids (prostaglandins) and the cardiovascular system. *J Cardiol Surg* 1:357–378, 1986b.

Greeley WJ, Ungerleider RM: Assessing the effect of cardiopulmonary bypass on the brain [editorial; comment]. *Ann Thorac Surg* 52:417–419, 1991.

Greeley WJ, Ungerleider RM, Kern FH, et al.: Effects of cardiopulmonary bypass on cerebral blood flow in neonates, infants, and children. *Circulation* 80:1209–1215, 1989b.

Greeley WJ, Ungerleider RM, Smith L, et al.: The effects of deep hypothermic cardiopulmonary bypass and total circulatory arrest on cerebral blood flow in infants and children. *J Thorac Cardiovasc Surg* 97:737–745, 1989a.

Gruber EM, Laussen PC, Casta A, et al.: Stress response in infants undergoing cardiac surgery: A randomized study of fentanyl bolus, fentanyl infusion, and fentanyl-midazolam infusion. *Anesth Analg* 92:882–890, 2001.

Guitierrez G: Cellular energy metabolism during hypoxia. *Crit Care Med* 19:619–626, 1991.

Hagberg J, Andersson P, Kjellmer I, et al.: Extracellular overflow of glutamate, aspartate, GABA, and taurine in the cortex and basal ganglia of fetal lambs during hypoxia-ischemia. *Neurosci Lett* 78:311–317, 1987a.

Hagberg J, Andersson P, Lacarewicz J, et al.: Extracellular adenosine, inosine, hypoxanthine, and xanthine in relation to tissue nucleotides and purines in rat striatum during transient ischemia. *J Neurochem* 49:227, 1987b.

Hagler DJ, Tajik AJ, Seward JB, et al.: Intraoperative two-dimensional Doppler echocardiography. A preliminary study for congenital heart disease. *J Thorac Cardiovasc Surg* 95:516–522, 1988.

Hannan EL, Racz M, Kavey RE, et al.: Pediatric cardiac surgery: The effect of hospital and surgeon volume on in-hospital mortality. *Pediatrics* 101:963–969, 1998.

Hansen AJ: Effect of anoxia on ion distribution in the brain. *Physiol Rev* 65:101, 1985.

Hansen AJ, Zeuthen T: Extracellular ion concentrations during spreading depression and ischemia in the rat brain cortex. *Acta Physiol Scand* 113:437, 1981.

Hansen D, Hickey P: Anesthesia for hypoplastic left heart syndrome: Use of high-dose fentanyl in 30 neonates. *Anesth Analg* 65:127–132, 1986.

Hansen N, Brubakk A, Bratlid D, et al.: The effects of variations in PaCO2 on brain blood flow and cardiac output in the newborn piglet. *Pediatr Res* 18:1132–1136, 1984.

Harker LA: Bleeding after cardiopulmonary bypass. *N Engl J Med* 314:446–448, 1986.

Hausdorf G, Friedel N, Berjis F, et al.: Enoximone in newborns with refractory postoperative low output status. *Eur J Cardiothorac Surg* 6:311–317, 1992.

Hawkins J, Van Hare GF, Schmidt KG: Effects of increasing afterload on left ventricular output in fetal lambs. *Circ Res* 65:127–134, 1989.

Hellenbrand WE, Fahey JT, McGowan F, et al.: Transesophageal echocardiographic guidance for transcatheter closure of atrial septal defects. *Am J Cardiol* 66:207–213, 1990.

Henriksson P, Varendh G, Lundstrom NR: Haemostatic defects in cyanotic congenital heart disease. *Br Heart J* 41:23–27, 1979.

Henzel JH, DeWeese MS: Morbid and mortal complications associated with prolonged central venous cannulation. Awareness, recognition, and prevention. *Am J Surg* 121:600–605, 1971.

Hickey P, Andersen N: Deep hypothermic circulatory arrest: A review of pathophysiology and clinical experience as a basis for anesthetic management. *J Cardiothorac Anesth* 1:137–155, 1987.

Hickey P, Hansen D: Fentanyl and sufentanil-oxygen-pancuronium anesthesia for cardiac surgery in infants. *Anesth Analg* 63:117–124, 1984.

Hickey PR, Hansen DD, Wessel DL, et al.: Pulmonary and systemic hemodynamic responses to fentanyl in infants. *Anesth Analg* 64:483–490, 1985a.

Hickey PR, Hansen DD, Wessel DL, et al.: Blunting of stress responses in the pulmonary circulation of infants by fentanyl. *Anesth Analg* 64:1137–1143, 1985b.

Hickey PR, Wessel DL: *Anesthesia for treatment of congenital heart disease.* Miami, 1987, Grune & Stratton.

Hickey PR, Wessel DL, Streitz SL, et al.: Transcatheter closure of atrial septal defects: Hemodynamic complications and anesthetic management. *Anesth Analg* 74:44–50, 1992.

Hillier SC, Burrows FA, Bissonnette B, et al.: Cerebral hemodynamics in neonates and infants undergoing cardiopulmonary bypass and profound hypothermic circulatory arrest: Assessment by transcranial Doppler sonography. *Anesth Analg* 72:723–728, 1991.

Hindmarsh KW, Sankaran K, Watson V: Plasma beta-endorphin concentrations in neonates associated with acute stress. *Dev Pharmacol Ther* 7:198, 1984.

Hines R, Barash PG: *Right ventricular failure.* New York, 1987, Grune & Stratton.

Hiramatsu T, Miura T, Forbess JM, et al.: pH strategies and cerebral energetics before and after circulatory arrest. *J Thorac Cardiovasc Surg* 109:948–957, 1995.

Hiramatsu T, Imai Y, Kurosawa H, et al.: Effects of dilutional and modified ultrafiltration in plasma endothelin-1 and pulmonary vascular resistance after the Fontan procedure. *Ann Thorac Surg* 73:861–865, 2002.

Hoerter J: Changes in the sensitivity to hypoxia and glucose deprivation in the isolated perfused rabbit heart during perinatal development. *Pflugers Arch* 303:1–6, 1976.

Hardman J, Limbird L, editors: *Goodman and Gilman's pharmacological basis of therapeutics.* New York, 2001, McGraw-Hill, pp 136–146.

Hoffman TM, Wernovsky G, Atz AM, et al.: Efficacy and safety of milrinone in preventing low cardiac output syndrome in infants and children after corrective surgery for congenital heart disease. *Circulation* 107:996–1002, 2003.

Horkay F, Martin P, Rajah SM, et al.: Response to heparinization in adults and children undergoing cardiac operations. *Ann Thorac Surg* 53:822–826, 1992.

Horrow JC, Hlavacek J, Strong MD, et al.: Prophylactic tranexamic acid decreases bleeding after cardiac operations. *J Thorac Cardiovasc Surg* 99:70–74, 1990.

Hug CC Jr., Burm AG, de Lange S: Alfentanil pharmacokinetics in cardiac surgical patients. *Anesth Analg* 78:231, 1994.

Humes RA, Driscoll DJ, Danielson G, et al.: Tetralogy of Fallot with anomalous origin of the left anterior descending coronary artery. *J Thorac Cardiovasc Surg* 94:784–789, 1987.

Humpherys JE, Cummings P: Atrial and ventricular tropomyosin and troponin-I in the developing bovine and human heart. *J Mol Cell Cardiol* 16:643, 1984.

Hurwitz RA, Smith W, King H, et al.: Tetralogy of Fallot with abnormal coronary artery: 1967 to 1977. *J Thorac Cardiovasc Surg* 80:129–134, 1980.

Ilbawi MN, Idriss FS, DeLeon SY, et al.: Factors that exaggerate the deleterious effects of pulmonary insufficiency on the right ventricle after tetralogy repair: Surgical implications. *J Thorac Cardiovasc Surg* 93:36–41, 1987.

Ilke L, Hale K, Fashaw L, et al.: Developmental outcome of patients with hypoplastic left heart syndrome treated with heart transplant. *J Pediatr* 142:20–25, 2003.

Imoto Y, Kado H, Shiokawa Y, et al.: Experience with the Norwood procedure without circulatory arrest. *J Thorac Cardiovasc Surg* 122:879–882, 2001.

Jarmakani JM, Graham TP, Canent R: The effect of corrective surgery on heart volume and mass in children with ventricular septal defect. *Am J Cardiol* 27:254–258, 1971.

Jarmakani JM, Graham TP, Canent R: Left ventricular contractile state in children with successfully corrected ventricular septal defect. *Circulation* (Suppl I): I-102–I-110, 1972.

Jarmakani JM, Nagatomo T, Nakazawa M, et al.: Effect of hypoxia on myocardial high-energy phosphates in the neonatal mammalian heart. *Am J Physiol* 235:H475–H481, 1978.

Jegger D, Tevaearai HT, Mueller XM, et al.: Limitations using the vacuum-assist venous drainage technique during cardiopulmonary bypass procedures. *J Extra Corpor Technol* 35:207–211, 2003.

Jenkins J, Lynn A, Edmonds J, et al.: Effects of mechanical ventilation on cardiopulmonary function in children after open-heart surgery. *Crit Care Med* 13:77–80, 1985.

Jennings R, Reimer K: Factors involved in salvaging ischemic myocardium: Effect of reperfusion of arterial blood. *Circulation* 68(Suppl I):I-25–I-29, 1983.

Jensen E, Andreasson S, Bengtsson A, et al.: Influence of two different perfusion systems on inflammatory response in pediatric heart surgery. *Ann Thorac Surg* 75:919–925, 2003.

Jobes DR, Shaffer GW, Aitken GL: Heparin/protamine dosing guided by in vitro testing reduces blood loss and transfusion in cardiac surgery. *Anesthesiology* 77:A137, 1992.

Jobes JR, Nicolson SC: Monitoring of arterial hemoglobin oxygen saturation using a tongue sensor. *Anesth Analg* 67:186–193, 1988.

Jonas RA: Experimental studies of hypothermic circulatory arrest and low flow bypass. *Cardiol Young* 3:299–307, 1993.

Jonas RA, Castaneda AR: Modified Fontan procedure: Atrial baffle and systemic venous to pulmonary artery anastomotic techniques. *J Cardiol Surg* 3:91–96, 1988.

Jonas RA, Wypij D, Roth SJ, et al.: The influence of hemodilution on outcome after hypothermic cardiopulmonary bypass: Results of a randomized trial in infants. *J Thorac Cardiovasc Surg* 26:1765–1774, 2003.

Julia P, Kofsky E, Buckberg G, et al.: Studies of myocardial protection in the immature heart. I. Enhanced tolerance of immature vs adult myocardium to global ischemia with reference to metabolic differences. *J Thorac Cardiovasc Surg* 100:879–888, 1990.

Julia P, Kofsky E, Buckberg G, et al.: Studies of myocardial protection in the immature heart. III. Models of ischemic and hypoxic/ischemic injury in the immature puppy heart. *J Thorac Cardiovasc Surg* 101:14–19,1991.

Julia P, Partington M, Buckberg G, et al.: Superiority of blood cardioplegia in limiting reperfusion damage: Importance of endogenous oxygen free-radical scavengers in red blood cells. *Surg Forum* 39:221, 1988.

Keenan HT, Thiagarajan R, Stephens KE, et al.: Pulmonary function after modified venovenous ultrafiltration in infants: A prospective, randomized trial. *J Thorac Cardiovasc Surg* 119:501–505, 2000.

Keidan I, Mishaly D, Berkenstadt H, et al.: Combining low inspired oxygen and carbon dioxide during mechanical ventilation for the Norwood procedure. *Paediatr Anaesth* 13:58–62, 2003.

Kern F, Jonas R, Mayer J, et al.: Conventional temperature monitoring is a poor correlate of efficient brain cooling. *Anesthesiology* 75(Suppl):A57, 1991a.

Kern F, Morana N, Sears J, et al.: Coagulation defects in neonates during CPB. *Ann Thorac Surg* 54:541–546, 1992a.

Kern F, Ungerleider R, Quill T, et al.: Cerebral blood flow response to changes in PaCO2 during hypothermic cardiopulmonary bypass in children. *J Thorac Cardiovasc Surg* 101:618–622, 1991b.

Kern F, Ungerleider R, Reves J, et al.: The effect of altering pump flow rate on cerebral blood flow and cerebral metabolism in neonates, infants and children. *Ann Thorac Surg* 56:1366–1372, 1993.

Kern F, Jonas R, Mayer J, et al.: Temperature monitoring during infant CPB: Does it predict efficient brain cooling? *Ann Thorac Surg* 54:749–754, 1992b.

Kern F, Ungerleider R, Jacobs J, et al.: Computerized continuous infusion of intravenous anesthetic drugs during pediatric cardiac surgery. *Anesth Analg* 72:487–492, 1991c.

Kety SS: The determination of cerebral blood flow in man by the use of nitrous oxide in low concentrations. *Am J Physiol* 143:53, 1945.

Kirklin J, Westaby S, Blackstone EH, et al.: Complement and the damaging effects of cardiopulmonary bypass. *J Thorac Cardiovasc Surg* 86:845–852, 1983.

Kirklin JW, Barratt-Boyes BG: *Hypothermia, circulatory arrest, and cardiopulmonary bypass*. New York, 1986b, John Wiley & Sons.

Kirklin J, Barratt-Boyes B: *Cardiac surgery*. New York, 1986a, Churchill Livingstone.

Kirshbom PM, Skaryak LA, DiBernardo LR, et al.: Effects of aortopulmonary collaterals on cerebral cooling and cerebral metabolic recovery after circulatory arrest. *Circulation* 92(Suppl II):II-490–II-494, 1995.

Kloth RL, Baum VC: Very early extubation in children after cardiac surgery. *Crit Care Med* 30:787–791, 2002.

Knott-Craig CJ, Overholt ED, Ward KE, et al.: Repair of Ebstein's anomaly in the symptomatic neonate: An evolution of technique with 7-year follow-up. *Ann Thorac Surg* 73:1789–1792, 2002.

Kohli A, Rao KS, Nachiappan M, et al.: Pericardiectomy for constrictive pericarditis: Is prolonged inotropic support a bad omen? *J Indian Med Assoc* 99:499–501, 2001.

Kopf GS, Kleinman CS, Hijazi ZM, et al.: Fenestrated Fontan operation with delayed transcatheter closure of atrial septal defect—improved results in high-risk patients. *J Thorac Cardiovasc Surg* 103:1039–1048, 1992.

Koren G, Goresky G, Crean P, et al.: Unexpected alterations in fentanyl pharmacokinetics in children undergoing cardiac surgery: Age related or disease related? *Dec Pharmacol Ther* 9:183,1986.

Kreselis D, Rocchini A, Rosenthal A, et al.: Hemodynamic determinants of exercise induced ST segment depression in children with valvular aortic stenosis. *Am J Cardiol* 55:1133–1136, 1985.

Kumar SP, Rubinstein CS, Simsic JM, et al.: Lateral tunnel versus extracardiac conduit Fontan procedure: A concurrent comparison. *Ann Thorac Surg* 76:1389–1396, 2003.

Kuroczynski W, Kampmann C, Choi Y, et al.: The Fontan-operation: From intra- to extracardiac procedure. *J Thorac Cardiovasc Surg* 11:70–74, 2003.

Kussman BD, Geva T, McGowan FX: Cardiovascular causes of airway compression. *Paediatr Anaesth* 14:60, 2004.

Kwiatkowski JL, Manno CS: Blood transfusion support in pediatric cardiovascular surgery. *Transfus Sci* 21:63, 1999.

Lacour-Gayet F, Piot D, Zoghbi J, et al.: Surgical management and indication of left ventricular retraining in arterial switch for transposition of the great arteries with intact ventricular septum. *Eur J Cardiothorac Surg* 20:824–829, 2001.

Laishley RS, Burrows FA, Lerman J, et al.: Effects of anesthetic induction on oxygen saturation in cyanotic congenital heart disease. *Anesthesiology* 65:673–679, 1986.

Lakier J, Stanger P, Heymann M, et al.: Tetralogy of Fallot with absent pulmonary valve. Natural history and hemodynamic considerations. *Circulation* 50:167–173, 1974.

Lang P, Williams R, Norwood W: The hemodynamic effects of dopamine in infants after corrective cardiac surgery. *J Pediatr* 96:630, 1980.

Langercrantz H, Slotkin TA: The "stress" of being born. *Sci Am* 1:100–108, 1986.

Langley SM, Chai PJ, Jaggers JJ, et al.: Preoperative high dose methylprednisolone attenuates the cerebral response to deep hypothermic circulatory arrest. *Eur J Cardiothorac Surg* 17:279–286, 2000.

Langley SM, Chai PJ, Miller SE, et al.: Intermittent perfusion protects the brain during deep hypothermic circulatory arrest. *Ann Thorac Surg* 68:4–12, 1999.

Lau CL, Posther KE, Stephenson GR, et al.: Mini-circuit cardiopulmonary bypass with vacuum assisted venous drainage: Feasibility of an asanguineous prime in the neonate. *Perfusion* 14:389–396, 1999.

Laussen PC, Murphy JA, Zubrakowski D, et al.: Bispectral index monitoring in children undergoing mild hypothermic cardiopulmonary bypass. *Paediatr Anaesth* 11:567–573, 2001.

Lawless S, Burckart G, Diven W: Amrinone pharmacokinetics in neonates and infants. *J Clin Pharmacol* 28:283, 1988.

Lazar H, Buckberg G, Managanaro A, et al.: Reversal of ischemic damage with amino acid substrate enhancement during reperfusion. *J Thorac Surg* 80:350–354, 1980.

Lazenby W, Ko W, Zelano J, et al.: Effects of temperature and flow rate on regional blood flow and metabolism during cardiopulmonary bypass. *Ann Thorac Surg* 54:449–459, 1981.

Lefkowitz RJ: G protein-coupled receptor kinases. *Cell* 74:409–412, 1993.

Legato M: *Ultrastructural changes during normal growth in the dog and rat ventricular myofiber. Developmental and physiological correlates of cardiac muscle.* New York, 1975, Raven Press, p 249.

Lerner A, Dinardo JA, Comunale ME: Anesthetic management for repair of Ebstein's anomaly. *J Cardiothorac Vasc Anesth* 17:232–235, 2003.

Lev M, Eckner F: The pathologic anatomy of tetralogy of Fallot and its variants. *Dis Chest* 45:251–261, 1964.

Levy JH, Bailey JM, Deeb GM: Intravenous milrinone in cardiac surgery. *Ann Thorac Surg* 73:325–330, 2002.

Lillehei CW, Mayer JE Jr, Shamberger RC, et al.: Pediatric lung transplantation and "lessons from Green Surgery." *Ann Thorac Surg* 68(3 Suppl):S25–S27, 1999.

Lloyd TR, Rydberg A, Ludomirsky A, et al.: Late fenestration closure in the hypoplastic left heart syndrome: Comparison of hemodynamic changes. *Am Heart J* 136:302–306, 1998.

Lock J, Einjig S, Bass J, et al.: Pulmonary vascular response to oxygen and its influence on operative results in children with ventricular septal defects. *Pediatr Cardiol* 3:41, 1982.

Lock J, Rome J, Davis R, et al.: Transatrial closure of atrial septal defects: Experimental studies. *Circulation* 79:1091–1099, 1989.

Lodge AJ, Chai PJ, Daggett CW, et al.: Methylprednisolone reduces the inflammatory response to cardiopulmonary bypass in neonatal piglets: Timing of dose is important. *J Thorac Cardiovasc Surg* 117:515–522, 1999.

Lundar T, Lindberg H, Lindegaard KF, et al.: Cerebral perfusion during major cardiac surgery in children. *Pediatr Cardiol* 8:161–165, 1987.

Lyrene R, Welch K, Godoy G, et al.: Alkalosis attenuates hypoxic pulmonary vasoconstriction in neonatal lambs. *Pediatr Res* 19:126, 1985.

Maher KO, Pizarro C, Gidding SS, et al.: Hemodynamic profile after the Norwood procedure with right ventricle to pulmonary artery conduit. *Circulation* 108:782–784, 2003.

Mahle WT, Cohen MS, Spray TL, et al.: Atrioventricular valve regurgitation in patients with single ventricle: Impact of the bidirectional cavopulmonary anastomosis. *Ann Thorac Surg* 72:831–835, 2001.

Mahle WT, Cuadrado AR, Tam VK: Early experience with a modified Norwood procedure using right ventricle to pulmonary artery conduit. *Ann Thorac Surg* 76:1084–1088, 2003.

Mahle WT, Tavani F, Zimmerman RA, et al.: An MRI study of neurologic injury before and after congenital heart surgery. *Circulation* 106(Suppl):1109–1114, 2002.

Mahle WT, McBride MG, Paridon SM: Exercise performance in tetralogy of Fallot: The impact of primary complete repair in infancy. *Pediatr Cardiol* 23:224–229, 2002.

Mahle WT, Spray TL, Wernovsky G, et al.: Survival after reconstructive surgery for hypoplastic left heart syndrome: a 15-year experience from a single institution. *Circulation* 102:III136, 2000.

Mair R, Tulzer G, Sames E, et al.: Right ventricular to pulmonary artery conduit instead of modified Blalock-Taussig shunt improves postoperative hemodynamics in newborns after the Norwood operation. *J Thorac Cardiovasc Surg* 126:1378–1384, 2003.

Malhotra SP, Thelitz S, Riemer RK, et al.: Fetal myocardial protection is markedly improved by reduced cardioplegic calcium content. *Ann Thorac Surg* 75:1937–1941, 2003.

Malenka DJ, McGirth PD, Wennberg DE, et al.: The relationship between operator volume and outcomes after percutaneous coronary interventions in high volume hospitals in 1994-1996: The northern New England experience. Northern New England Cardiovascular Diseases Study Group. *J Am Coll Cardiol* 34:1471–1480, 1999.

Malik A, Kidd S: Independent effects of changes in H+ and CO2 concentrations on hypoxic pulmonary vasoconstriction. *J Appl Physiol* 34:318–323, 1973.

Malviya S, Voepel-Lewis T, Siewer M, et al.: Risk factors for adverse postoperative outcomes in children presenting for cardiac surgery with upper respiratory tract infections. *Anesthesiology* 98:628–632, 2003.

Malviya S, Burrows FA, Johnston A, et al.: Anaesthetic experience with paediatric interventional cardiology. *Can J Anaesth* 36:320–324, 1989.

Mann K, Berg RA, Nadkarni V: Beneficial effects of vasopressin in prolonged pediatric cardiac arrest: a case series. *Resuscitation* 52:149, 2002.

Manno CS, Hedberg KW, Kim HC, et al.: Comparison of the hemostatic effects of fresh whole blood, stored whole blood, and components after open heart surgery in children. *Blood* 77:930–936, 1991.

Mansell A, Bryan A: Airway closure in children. *J Appl Physiol* 33:711, 1972.

Marshall AC, Love BA, Lang P, et al.: Staged repair of tetralogy of Fallot and diminutive pulmonary arteries with a fenestrated ventricular septal patch. *J Thorac Cardiovasc Surg* 126:1427–1433, 2003.

Martindale SJ, Shayevitz JR, E'Errico D: The activated coagulation time: suitability for monitoring heparin effect and neutralization during pediatric cardiac surgery. *J Cardiothorac Vasc Anesth* 10:458, 1996.

Mass C, Kok R, Segers P, et al.: Intermittent antegrade/selective cerebral perfusion during circulatory arrest for repair of the aortic arch. *Perfusion* 12:127–132, 1997.

Masuda H, Moriyama Y, Yamaoka A, et al.: Preoperative autologous donation of blood in cardiac surgery—age related factors. *Jpn J Thorac Cardiovasc Surg* 46:267, 1998.

Matsota P, Livanios S, Marinopoulou E: Intercostal nerve block with bupivacaine for post-thoracotomy pain relief in children. *Eur J Pediatr Surg* 11:219–222, 2001.

Matsumato T, Wolferth CJ, Perlman M: Effects of pulsatile and non-pulsatile perfusion upon cerebral and conjunctival microcirculation in the dog. *Am Surg* 37:61–64, 1971.

Mault J, Ohtake S, Klingensmith M, et al.: Cerebral metabolism and circulatory arrest: Effects of duration and strategies for protection. *Ann Thorac Surg* 55:57–63, 1993.

Mault J, Whitaker E, Heinle J, et al.: *Intermittent perfusion during hypothermic circulatory arrest: A new and effective technique for cerebral protection.* New York, 1992, American College of Surgeons Clinical Congress, Surgical Forum.

Mavroudis C, Brown G, Katzmark S, et al.: Blood flow distribution in infant pigs subjected to surface cooling, deep hypothermia, and circulatory arrest. *J Thorac Cardiovasc Surg* 87:665–672, 1984.

Mayer J, Helgason H, Jonas R, et al.: Extending the limits of modified Fontan procedures. *J Thorac Cardiovasc Surg* 92:1021–1028, 1986.

Mayer JEJ, Bridges ND, Lock JE, et al.: Factors associated with marked reduction in mortality for Fontan operations in patients with single ventricle. *J Thorac Cardiovasc Surg* 103:444–451, 1992.

Mazzera E, Corno A, Picardo S, et al.: Bidirectional cavopulmonary shunts: Clinical applications as a staged or definitive palliation. *Ann Thorac Surg* 47:415–420, 1989.

McGoon DC, Mair DD: On the unmuddling of shunting, mixing and streaming. *J Thorac Cardiovasc Surg* 100:77, 1990.

McGovern JJ, Cheifetz IM, Craig DM, et al.: Right ventricular injury in young swine: Effects of catecholamines on right ventricular function and pulmonary vascular mechanics. *Pediatr Res* 48:763–769, 2000.

McGrath L, Gonzales-Lavin L: Actuarial survival, freedom from reoperation and other events after repair of atrioventricular septal defects. *Thorac Cardiovasc Surg* 94:582–586, 1987.

Mehta PA, Cunningham CK, Colella CB, et al.: Risk factors for sternal wound and other infections in pediatric cardiac surgery patients. *Pediatr Infect Dis J* 19:1000–1004, 2000.

Meliones J, Bove E, Dekeon M, et al.: High-frequency jet ventilation improves cardiac function after the Fontan procedure. *Circulation* 84(Suppl III): III-364–III-368, 1991.

Meyer R, Schwartz D, Benzing G, et al.: Ventricular septum in right ventricular volume overload. *Am J Cardiol* 30:349–354, 1972.

Michelakis E, Tymchak W, Lien D, et al.: Oral sildenafil is an effective and specific pulmonary vasodilator in patients with pulmonary arterial hypertension: Comparison with inhaled nitric oxide. *Circulation* 105:2398–2403, 2002.

Michenfelder J: *The hypothermic brain. Anesthesia and the brain.* New York, 1988, Churchill Livingstone, pp 23–34.

Michenfelder J, Theye R: Hypothermia: Effect of canine brain and whole-body metabolism. *Anesthesiology* 29:1107, 1968.

Mies G, Paschen W: Regional changes of blood flow, glucose, and ATP content determined on brain sections during a single passage of spreading depression in rat brain cortex. *Exp Neurol* 84:249, 1984.

Mietus-Snyder M, Lang P, Mayer J, et al.: Childhood systemic-pulmonary shunts: Subsequent suitability of Fontan operation. *Circulation* 76(Suppl III): III-39–III-46, 1987.

Milde LN: Clinical use of mild hypothermia for brain protection—A dream revisited. *J Neurosurg Anesthesiol* 4:211–215, 1992.

Miller BE, Mochizuki T, Levy JH, et al.: Predicting and treating coagulopathies after cardiopulmonary bypass in children. *Anesth Analg* 85:1196, 1997.

Mohiddin SA, Fananapazir L: Systolic compression of epicardial coronary and intramural arteries in children with hypertrophic cardiomyopathy. *Tex Heart Inst J* 29:290, 2002.

Miyamoto K, Kawashima Y, Matsuda H, et al.: Optimal perfusion flow rate for the brain during deep hypothermic cardiopulmonary bypass at 20°C. *J Thorac Cardiovasc Surg* 92:1065–1070, 1986.

Moore R: Anesthesia for the pediatric congenital heart patient for noncardiac surgery. *Anesthesiol Rev* 8:23, 1981.

Moore RA, Yang SS, McNicholas KW, et al.: Hemodynamic and anesthetic effects of sufentanil as the sole anesthetic for pediatric cardiovascular surgery. *Anesthesiology* 63:725–732, 1985.

Mori A, Tabata R, Nakamura Y, et al.: Effects of pulsatile cardiopulmonary bypass on carbohydrate and lipid metabolism. *J Cardiovasc Surg* 28:621–626, 1987.

Mortier E, Ongenae M, Vermassen F, et al.: Operative closure of patent ductus arteriosus in the neonatal intensive care unit. *Acta Chir Belg* 96:266, 1996.

Moskowitz M, Kiwak K, Hekimian K: Synthesis of compounds with properties of leukotrienes C4 and D4 in gerbil brains after ischemia and reperfusion. *Science* 224:886, 1984.

Mochizuki Y, Patel AK, Banerjee A, et al.: Intraoperative transesophageal echocardiography: Correlation of echocardiographic findings and surgical pathology. *Cardiol Rev* 7:270–276, 1999.

Mossinger H, Kietrich W, Braun SL, et al.: High-dose aprotinin reduces activation of hemostasis, allogeneic blood requirement, and duration of postoperative ventilation in pediatric cardiac surgery. *Ann Thorac Surg* 75:430, 2003.

Mott AR, Spray TL, Gaynor JW, et al.: Improved early results with cavopulmonary connections. *Cardiol Young* 11:3–11, 2001.

Muhiudeen IA, Kuecherer HF, Lee E, et al.: Intraoperative estimation of cardiac output by transesophageal pulsed Doppler echocardiography. *Anesthesiology* 74:9–14, 1991.

Muhiudeen IA, Roberson DA, Silverman NH, et al.: Intraoperative echocardiography in infants and children with congenital cardiac shunt lesions: Transesophageal versus epicardial echocardiography. *J Am Coll Cardiol* 16:1687–1695, 1990.

Muhiudeen IA, Roberson DA, Silverman NH, et al.: Intraoperative echocardiography for evaluation of congenital heart defects in infants and children. *Anesthesiology* 76:165–172, 1992.

Muller M, Akinturk H, Schindler E, et al.: Combined state 1 and 2 repair for hypoplastic left heart syndrome: Anaesthetic considerations. *Paediatr Anaesth* 13:360–365, 2003.

Mullins C: Pediatric and congenital therapeutic cardiac catheterization. *Circulation* 79:1153–1159, 1989.

Murkin JM, Farrar JK, Tweed WA, et al.: Cerebral autoregulation and flow/metabolism coupling during cardiopulmonary bypass: The influence of PaCO2. *Anesth Analg* 66:825–832, 1987.

Murray A, Glaria AP, Pearson DT, et al.: The protective effect of profound hypothermia on the canine central nervous system during one hour of circulatory arrest. *Ann Thorac Surg* 41:255–259, 1986.

Mutch W, Hansen AJ: Extracellular pH changes during spreading depression and cerebral ischemia: Mechanisms of brain pH regulation. *J Cereb Blood Flow Metab* 4:17, 1984.

Nadroo AM, Glass RB, Lin J, et al.: Changes in upper extremity position cause migration of peripherally inserted central catheters in neonates. *Pediatrics* 110:131, 2002.

Naik SK, Knight A, Elliott M: A prospective randomized study of a modified technique of ultrafiltration during pediatric open-heart surgery. *Circulation* 84(Suppl III):III-422–III-431, 1991.

Nagy ZL, Collins M, Sharpe T, et al.: Effect of two different bypass techniques on the serum troponin-T levels in newborns and children: Does pH-stat provide better protection? *Circulation* 108:577–582, 2003.

Nakanishi T, Seguchi M, Takao A: Intracellular calcium concentrations in the newborn myocardium. *Circulation* 76(Suppl IV):IV-455–IV-461, 1987.

Nasser R, Reedy MC, Anderson P: Developmental changes in the ultrastructure and sarcomere shortening of the isolated rabbit myocardium. *Circ Res* 61:465, 1987.

Nelson N: Neonatal pulmonary function. *Pediatr Clin North Am* 13:769, 1966.

Newburger JW, Jonas RA, Wernovsky G, et al.: A comparison of the perioperative neurologic effects of hypothermic circulatory arrest versus low-flow cardiopulmonary bypass in infant heart surgery. *N Engl J Med* 329:329–336, 1993.

Newburger JW, Wypij D, Bellinger DC, et al.: Length of stay after heart surgery is related to cognitive outcome at age 8 years. *J Pediatr* 143:67–73, 2003.

Ng C, Franklin O, Vaidya M, et al.: Adenosine infusion for the management of persistent pulmonary hypertension of the newborn. *Pediatr Crit Care Med* 5:10–13, 2004.

Ng PC, Lam CW, Fok T, et al.: Refractory hypotension in preterm infants with adrenocortical insufficiency. *Arch Dis Child Fetal Neonatal Educ* 84:F122–F124, 2001.

Nishioka K, Kamiya T, Ueda T, et al.: Left ventricular volume characteristics in children with tricuspid atresia before and after surgery. *Am J Cardiol* 47:1105–1107, 1981.

Nishinaka T, Tatsumi E, Taenaka Y, et al.: At least thirty-four days of animal continuous perfusion by a newly developed extracorporeal membrane oxygenation system without systemic anticoagulants. *Artif Organs* 26:548–551, 2002.

Nollert G, Nagashima M, Bucerius J, et al.: Oxygenation strategy and neurologic damage after deep hypothermic circulatory arrest. II. Hypoxic versus free radical injury. *J Thorac Cardiovasc Surg* 117:1172–1179, 1999.

Normal MG: Perinatal brain damage. *Perspect Pediatric Pathol* 4:41–92, 1978.

Norstrom C, Siesko B: Influence of phenobarbital on changes in the metabolites of the energy reserve of the cerebral cortex following complete ischemia. *Acta Physiol Scand* 104:271, 1978.

Norwood W: Hypoplastic left heart syndrome. *Ann Thorac Surg* 52:688–695, 1991.

Norwood W, Lang P, Hansen D: Physiologic repair of aortic atresia-hypoplastic left syndrome. *N Engl J Med* 308:23, 1983.

Norwood W, Norwood C, Castaneda A: Cerebral anoxia: Effect of deep hypothermia and pH. *Surgery* 86:203–209, 1979a.

Norwood W, Norwood C, Ingwall J, et al.: Hypothermic circulatory arrest: 31-Phosphorus nuclear magnetic resonance of isolated perfused neonatal rat brain. *J Thorac Cardiovasc Surg* 78:823–830, 1979b.

Norwood W, Murphy J: Hypoplastic left heart syndrome. In Sabiston DC, Spencer FC, editors: *Surgery of the chest*, 5th ed. Philadelphia, PA, 1990, WB Saunders, pp 1493–1502.

Norwood WIJ, Jacobs MI, Murphy JD: Fontan procedure for hypoplastic left heart syndrome. *Ann Thorac Surg* 54:1025–1029, 1992.

Ogata T, Ida Y, Nonoyama A, et al.: A comparative study of the effectiveness of pulsatile and nonpulsatile flow in extracorporeal circulation. *Arch Jpn Clin* 29:59, 1960.

Okada Y, Tanimoto M, Yoneda K: The protective effect of hypothermia on reversibility in the neuronal function of the hippocampal slice during long lasting anoxia. *Neurosci Lett* 84:277–282, 1988.

Ootaki Y, Yamaguchi M, Oshima Y, et al.: Effects of modified ultrafiltration on coagulation factors in pediatric cardiac surgery. *Surg Today* 32:203–206, 2002.

Olsson C, Siegbahn A, Henze A, et al.: Heparin-coated cardiopulmonary bypass circuits reduce circulating complement factors and interleukin-6 in paediatric heart surgery. *Scand Cardiovasc J* 34:33–40, 2000.

Oshita S, Uchimoto R, Oka H, et al.: Correlation between arterial blood pressure and oxygenation in tetralogy of Fallot. *J Cardiovasc Anesth* 3:597–600, 1989.

Ozawa T, Yoshihara K, Koyama N, et al.: Clinical efficacy of heparin-bonded bypass circuits related to cytokine responses in children. *Ann Thorac Surg* 69:584–590, 2000

Pacifico A, Kirklin J, Kirklin J: Surgical treatment of ventricular septal defect. In *Surgery of the chest,* 5th ed. Philadelphia, PA, 1990, WB Saunders, pp 1314–1331.

Pacifico AD, Sand ME, Bargeron LM, et al.: Transatrial-transpulmonary repair of tetralogy of Fallot. *J Thorac Cardiovasc Surg* 93:919–926, 1987.

Padayachee TS, Parsons S, Theobold R, et al.: The detection of microemboli in the middle cerebral artery during cardiopulmonary bypass: A transcranial Doppler ultrasound investigation using membrane and bubble oxygenators. *Ann Thorac Surg* 44:298–302, 1987.

Pearl J, Laks H, Drinkwater D, et al.: Repair of truncus arteriosus in infancy. *Ann Thorac Surg* 52:780–786, 1991.

Pearl JM: Right ventricular-pulmonary artery connection in Stage 1 palliation of hypoplastic left heart syndrome. *J Thorac Cardiovasc Surg* 126:1268–1270, 2003.

Pearl JM, Nelson DP, Schwartz SM, et al.: Glucocorticoids reduce ischemic-reperfusion induced myocardial apoptosis in immature hearts. *Ann Thorac Surg* 74:830–836, 2002.

Perloff J: Development and regression of increased ventricular mass. *Am J Cardiol* 50:605, 1982.

Picardo S, Testa G, La Vigna G, et al.: Post-thoracotomy analgesia in pediatric heart surgery: Comparison of 2 different techniques. *Minerva Anesthesiol* 61:277–282, 1995.

Pigott J, Murphy J, Barber G, et al.: Palliative reconstructive surgery for hypoplastic left heart syndrome. *Ann Thorac Surg* 45:122–128, 1988.

Pizarro C, Malec E, Maher KO, et al.: Right ventricle to pulmonary artery conduit improves outcome after stage 1 Norwood for hypoplastic left heart syndrome. *Circulation* 108(Suppl III):III-55–III-60, 2003.

Pizarro C, Mroczek T, Malec E, Norwood WI: Right ventricle to pulmonary artery conduit reduces interim mortality after Stage 1 Norwood for hypoplastic left heart syndrome. *Ann Thorac Surg* 78:1959, 2004.

Pizarro C, Norwood WI: Right ventricle to pulmonary artery conduit has a favorable impact on postoperative physiology after Stage I Norwood: preliminary results. *Eur J Cardiothorac Surg* 23:991, 2003.

Portman MA, Fearneyhough C, Ning XH, et al.: Triiodothyronine repletion in infants during cardiopulmonary bypass for congenital heart disease. *J Thorac Cardiovasc Surg* 120:604–608, 2000.

Pozzi M, Trivedi DB, Kitchner D, et al.: Tetralogy of Fallot: What operation, at which age? *Eur J Cardiothorac Surg* 17:631–636, 2000.

Quattlebaum T, Varghese J, Barber G, et al.: Sudden death among postoperative patients with tetralogy of Fallot. *Circulation* 54:671, 1976

Rabinovitch M, Herrera-DeLeon V, Castaneda A, et al.: Growth and development of the pulmonary vascular bed in patients with tetralogy of Fallot with and without pulmonary atresia. *Circulation* 64:1234, 1981.

Radford I: The level of induced DNA double strand breakage correlates with cell killing after x-radiation. *Int J Radiat Biol* 48:45, 1985.

Ramakrishnan S, Kothari SS: Preoperative balloon dilation of obstructed total anomalous pulmonary venous connection in a neonate. *Cathet Cardiovasc Interv* 61:128–130, 2004.

Rappaport LA, Wypij D, Bellinger DC, et al.: Relation of seizures after cardiac surgery in early infancy to neurodevelopmental outcome. Boston Circulatory Arrest Study Group. *Circulation* 97:773–779, 1998.

Rebeyka I, Yeh TJ, Hanan S, et al.: Altered contractile response in neonatal myocardium to citrate-phosphate-dextrose infusion. *Circulation* 82(Suppl IV): IV-367–IV-370, 1990.

Reddy VM, McElhinney DB, Sagrado T, et al.: Results of 102 cases of complete repair of congenital heart defects in patients weighing 700 to 2500 grams. *J Thorac Cardiovasc Surg* 117:324–331, 1999.

Reddy VM, Hanley FI: Cardiac surgery in infants with very low birth weight. *Semin Pediatr Surg* 9:91–95, 2000.

Reid RW, Zimmerman A, Laussen PC, et al.: The efficacy of tranexamic acid versus placebo in decreasing blood loss in pediatric patients undergoing repeat cardiac surgery. *Anesth Analg* 84:990, 1997.

Reinhartz O, Copeland JG, Farrar DJ: Thoratec ventricular assist devices in children with less than 1.3 m2 of body surface area. *ASAIO J* 49:727–730, 2003.

Rich T, Langer G: Calcium depletion in rabbit myocardium: Calcium paradox protection by hypothermia and cation substitution. *Circ Res* 51:131–141, 1982.

Richardson P: Task Force on the Definition and Classification of the Cardiomyopathies. *Circulation* 93:41, 1996.

Richardson JP, Clark CP: Tetralogy of Fallot: Risk factors associated with complete repair. *Br Heart J* 38:926–932, 1976.

Rigby-Jones AE, Nolan JA, Priston MJ, et al.: Pharmacokinetics of propofol infusions in critically ill neonates, infants, and children in an intensive care unit. *Anesthesiology* 97:1393–1400, 2002.

Rinne T, Kaukinen S: Does lidocaine protect the heart during coronary revascularization? *Acta Anaesthesiol Scand* 42:936–940, 1998.

Riordan CJ, Randsbaek F, Storey JH, et al.: Inotropes in the hypoplastic left heart syndrome: Effects in an animal model. *Ann Thorac Surg* 62:83–90, 1996.

Roberts J, Chen T, Kawai N, et al.: Inhaled nitric oxide reverses pulmonary vasoconstriction in the hypoxic and acidotic newborn lamb. *Circ Res* 72:246–254, 1993a.

Roberts J, Lang P, Bigatello L, et al.: Inhaled nitric oxide in congenital heart disease. *Circulation* 87:447–453, 1993b.

Roodpeyma S, Sadeghian N: Acute pericarditis in children: A 10-year experience. *Pediatr Cardiol* 21:363–367, 2000.

Rosenberg A, Jones M, Traystman R, et al.: Response of cerebral blood flow to changes in PCO2 in fetal, newborn and adult sheep. *Am J Physiol* 242:H862–H866, 1982.

Rosenzweig EB, Starc TJ, Chen JM, et al.: Intravenous arginine-vasopressin children with vasodilatory shock after cardiac surgery. *Circulation* 100(Suppl II): II-182–II-186, 1999.

Rothman A, Perry S, Keane J, et al.: Early results and follow-up of balloon angioplasty for branch pulmonary artery stenoses. *J Am Coll Cardiol* 15:1109–1117, 1990.

Royston D, Taylor KM, Bidstrup BP, et al.: Effect of aprotinin on need for blood transfusion after repeat open-heart surgery. *Lancet* 2:1289–1291, 1987.

Rozencrantz E, Okamoto F, Buckberg G, et al.: Advantages of glutamate-enriched cold blood cardioplegia in energy-depleted hearts. *Circulation* 66(Suppl II):II-151–II-156, 1982.

Rudolph AM (editor): *Congenital diseases of the heart: clinical-physiological considerations,* 2nd ed. New York, 2001, Armonk, Futura.

Rudolph A: Distribution and regulation of blood flow in the fetal and newborn lamb. *Circ Res* 57:811, 1985.

Rudolph A, Yuan S: Response of the pulmonary vasculature to hypoxia and H+ ion concentration changes. *J Clin Invest* 45:399, 1966.

Russell IA, Miller Hance WC, Gregory G, et al.: The safety and efficacy of sevoflurane anesthesia in infants and children with congenital heart disease. *Anesth Analg* 92:1152–1158, 2001.

Rychik J, Norwood W, Chil A: Doppler color flow mapping assessment of residual shunt after closure of large ventricular septal defects. *Circulation* 84(Suppl III):III-153–III-161, 1991.

Sabiston DJ, Theilen E, Gregg D: The relationship of coronary blood flow and cardiac output and other parameters in hypothermia. *Surgery* 38:498–505, 1955.

Sahn DJ: Real-time two-dimensional Doppler echocardiographic flow mapping. *Circulation* 71:849–853, 1985.

Salem M, Griffin A: Anesthetic considerations in patients with congenital heart disease for noncardiac surgery. In *Pediatric anesthesia: Current practice.* New York, 1981, Academic Press.

Salem M, Toyama T, Wong A, et al.: Hemodynamic response to antagonism of tubocurarine block with atrophine-neostigmine mixture in pediatric patients. *Br J Anaesth* 49:901, 1977.

Salem M, Ylagan L, Angel J, et al.: Reversal of curarization with atrophine-neostigmine mixture in patients with congenital heart disease. *Br J Anaesth* 42:991, 1970.

Saltzman E, Weinstein M, Weintraub R, et al.: Treatment with desmopressin acetate to reduce blood loss after cardiac surgery: A double-blind randomized trial. *N Engl J Med* 314:1402–1406, 1986.

Sanders S, Wright G, Keane J, et al.: Clinical and hemodynamic results of the Fontan operation for tricuspid atresia. *Am J Cardiol* 49:1733–1740, 1982.

Sandhu SK, Pettitt TW: Interrupted aortic arch. *Curr Treat Options Cardiovasc Med* 337–340, 2002.

Sano S, Ishino K, Kawanda M, et al.: Total right ventricular exclusion procedure: An operation for isolated congestive right ventricular failure. *J Thorac Cardiovasc Surg* 123:640–647, 2002.

Sano S, Ishino K, Kawada M, et al.: Right ventricle-pulmonary artery shunt in first-stage palliation of hypoplastic left heart syndrome. *J Thorac Cardiovasc Surg* 126:504–509, 2003.

Schechter WS, Kim C, Martinez M, et al.: Anesthetic induction in a child with end-stage cardiomyopathy. *Can J Anesth* 42:404–408, 1995.

Scheinberg P, Stead EA: The cerebral blood flow in male subjects as measured by the nitrous technique: Normal values for blood flow, oxygen utilization, glucose utilization, and peripheral resistance with observations on the effect of lilting and anxiety. *J Clin Invest* 28:1163–1168, 1949.

Schindler E, Muller M, Kwapisz M, et al.: Ventricular cardiac-assist devices in infants and children: Anesthetic considerations. *J Cardiothorac Vasc Anesth* 17:617–621, 2003.

Schmid ER, Burki C, Engel MH, et al.: Inhaled nitric oxide versus intravenous vasodilators in severe pulmonary hypertension after cardiac surgery. *Anesth Analg* 89:1108–1115, 1999.

Schrantz D, Droege A, et al.: Uncoupling of human cardiac beta-adrenoceptors during cardiopulmonary bypass with cardioplegic cardiac arrest. *Circulation* 87:422–426, 1993.

Schrantz D, Oelert H, Iverson S, et al.: Congenital mitral regurgitation caused by a perforation in the anterior leaflet. *Pediatr Cardiol* 11:93–95, 1990.

Schreiber C, Eicken A, Vogt M, et al.: Repair of interrupted aortic arch: Results after more than 20 years. *Ann Thorac Surg* 70:1896–1900, 2000.

Schulze-Neick I, Li J, Reader JA, et al.: The endothelin antagonist BQ123 reduces pulmonary vascular resistance after surgical intervention for congenital heart disease. *J Thorac Cardiovasc Surg* 124:435–441, 2002.

Schwartz A: *Anesthesia for non-cardiac surgery in the pediatric patient with congenital heart disease.* ASA Refresher Course Lectures, Park Ridge, IL, 1985.

Schwartz SM, Duffy JY, Pearl JM, et al.: Glucocorticoids preserve calpastatin and troponin I during cardiopulmonary bypass in immature pigs. *Pediatr Res* 54:91–97, 2003.

Schwartz A, Jobes D: Congenital heart disease-specific anesthetic considerations. In Kaplan JA: *Cardiac anesthesia.* Menlo Park, CA, 1982, Addison-Wesley.

Schwinn DA: Cardiac pharmacology. In *Cardiac anesthesia.* Philadelphia, PA, 1994, JB Lippincott, pp 21–60.

Schwinn D, Leone B, Spahn D, et al.: Desensitization of myocardial beta-adrenergic receptors during cardiopulmonary bypass. *Circulation* 84:2559–2567, 1991.

Sell JE, Jonas RA, Mayer JE, et al.: The results of a surgical program for interrupted aortic arch. *J Thorac Cardiovasc Surg* 96:864–877, 1988.

Senzaki H, Masutani S, Kobayashi J, et al.: Ventricular afterload and ventricular work in Fontan circulation: Comparison with normal two-ventricle circulation and single-ventricle circulation with Blalock-Taussig shunts. *Circulation* 105:2885–2892, 2002.

Severinghaus J, Spellman B: Pulse oximeter failure thresholds in hypotension and vasoconstriction. *Anesthesiology* 73:532–537, 1990.

Shah P, Stewart S, Calalang CC, et al.: Transesophageal echocardiography and the intraoperative management of pediatric congenital heart disease: Initial experience with a pediatric esophageal 2D color flow echocardiographic probe. *J Cardiothorac Vasc Anesth* 6:8–14, 1992.

Sharpe M, Dobkowski D, Murkin J, et al.: The electrophysiologic effects of volatile anesthetics and sufentanil on the normal atrioventricular conduction system and accessory pathways in Wolff-Parkinson-White syndrome. *Anesthesiology* 80:63–70, 1994.

Shigeaki O, Mault JR, et al.: Effect of a systemic-pulmonary artery shunt on myocardial function and perfusion in a piglet model. *Surg Forum* 42:200–203, 1991.

Skaryak L, Chai P, Kern F, et al.: Blood gas management and degree of cooling: Effects on cerebral metabolism before and after circulatory arrest. *J Thorac Cardiovasc Surg* 110:1649–1657, 1995.

Skaryak L, Chai P, Kern F, et al.: Combining alpha and pH stat blood gas strategy prior to circulatory arrest provides optimal recovery of cerebral metabolism. *Circulation* (Suppl I), 1993.

Skaryak LA, Kirshbom PM, DiBernardo LR, et al.: Modified ultrafiltration improves cerebral metabolic recovery after circulatory arrest. *J Thorac Cardiovasc Surg* 109:744–751, 1995.

Smallhorn JF: Intraoperative transesophageal echocardiography in congenital heart disease. *Echocardiography* 19:709–723, 2002.

Smith PC, Powell KR, Chang RKR, et al.: Can regionalization decrease the number of deaths for children who undergo cardiac surgery? A theoretical analysis. *Pediatrics* 110:849–850, 2002.

Somero G, White F: *Enzymatic consequences under alpha stat regulation.* Boston, 1985, Nijhoff.

Soongswang J, McCrindle BW, Jones TK, et al.: Outcomes of transcatheter balloon angioplasty of obstruction in the neo-aortic arch after the Norwood operation. *Cardiol Young* 11:54–61, 2001.

Spach M, Serwer G, Anderson P, et al.: Pulsatile aortopulmonary pressure-flow dynamics of patent ductus arteriosus in patients with various hemodynamic states. *Circulation* 61:110–122, 1980.

Stamm C, Friehs I, Duebener LF, et al.: Improving results of the modified Fontan operation in patients with heterotaxy syndrome. *Ann Thorac Surg* 74:1967–1977, 2002.

Stark, J: Do we really correct congenital heart defects? *J Thorac Cardiovasc Surg* 97:1–9, 1989.

Stern DH, Gerson J, Allen FB: Can we trust the direct radial artery pressure immediately following cardiopulmonary bypass? *Anesthesiology* 62:557–563, 1985.

Stevenson JG: Role of intraoperative transesophageal echocardiography during repair of congenital cardiac defects. *Acta Paediatr Suppl* 410:23–33, 1995.

Stevenson JG: Utilization of intraoperative transesophageal echocardiography during repair of congenital cardiac defects: A survey of North American centers. *Clin Cardiol* 26:132–134, 2003.

Stocker F, Herschkowitz N, Bossi E, et al.: Cerebral blood flow during cardiopulmonary bypass in man: Effect of arterial filtration. *Thorax* 41:386–395, 1986.

Stocker C, Penny DJ, Brizard CP, et al.: Intravenous sildenafil and inhaled nitric oxide: A randomized trial in infants after cardiac surgery. *Intensive Care Med* 29:1996–2003, 2003.

Strauc A, Spielvogel JT, Haldenwang PL, et al.: Cerebral physiology and outcome after hypothermic circulatory arrest followed by selective cerebral perfusion. *Ann Thorac Surg* 76:1972–1981, 2003.

Stullken EH Jr, Michenfenlder JD, et al.: The non-linear responses of cerebral metabolism to low concentrations of halothane, enflurane, isoflurane and thiopental. *Anesthesiology* 46:28, 1977.

Sunamori M, Amano J, Okamura T, et al.: Superior action of magnesium-lidocaine-1-aspartate cardioplegia in experimental myocardial protection. *Jpn J Surg* 12:372–380, 1982.

Sungurtekin H, Plochl W, Cook DJ: Relationship between cardiopulmonary bypass flow rate and cerebral embolization in dogs. *Anesthesiology* 91:1387–1393, 1999.

Sutton L, Clark B, Norwood C: Global cerebral ischemia in piglets under conditions of mild and deep hypothermia. *Stroke* 22:1567–1573, 1991.

Svensson LG, Nadolny EM, Penney DL, et al.: Prospective randomized neurocognitive and S-100 study of hypothermic circulatory arrest, retrograde brain perfusion and antegrade brain perfusion for aortic arch operations. *Ann Thorac Surg* 71:1905–1912, 2001.

Swain JA, McDonald TJJ, Balaban RS, et al.: Metabolism of the heart and brain during hypothermic cardiopulmonary bypass. *Ann Thorac Surg* 51:105–109, 1991.

Swain JA, McDonald TJ Jr., Robbins RC, Balaban RS: Relationship of cerebral and myocardial intercellular pH to blood pH during hypothermia. *Am J Physiol* 260:H1640, 1991.

Swain JA, Robbins RC, Balaban RS, et al.: The effect of cardiopulmonary bypass on brain and heart metabolism: a 31P NMR study. *Magn Reson Med* 15:446, 1990.

Swan H: The importance of acid-base management for cardiac and cerebral preservation during open heart operations. *Surg Gynecol Obstet* 158:391–414, 1984.

Syzmonowitcz W, Walker AM, Yu YH, et al.: Regional cerebral blood flow after hemorrhagic hypotension in the preterm, near term and term lamb. *Pediatr Res* 162:977–982, 1990.

Tabbutt S, Ramanoorthy C, Montenegro L, et al.: Impact of inspired gas mixtures on preoperative infants with hypoplastic left heart syndrome during controlled ventilation. *Circulation* (Suppl I):I-159–I-164, 2001.

Taeed R, Schwartz SM, Pearl JM, et al.: Unrecognized pulmonary venous desaturation early after Norwood palliation confounds Gp:Gs assessment and compromises oxygen delivery. *Circulation* 103:2699–2709, 2001.

Tanaka J, Shiki K, Asou T, et al.: Carbon dioxide, brain damage, and cardiac surgery [letter]. *Lancet* 1:353, 1988.

Tang W, Sun GY: Effects of ischemia on free fatty acids and diacylglycerols in developing rat brain. *J Dev Neurosci* 3:51–56, 1985.

Tavani F, Zimmerman RA, Clancy RR, et al.: Incidental intracranial hemorrhage after uncomplicated birth: MRI before and after neonatal heart surgery. *Neuroradiology* 45:253–258, 2003.

Teitel DF, Sidi D, Chin T, et al.: Developmental changes in myocardial contractile reserve in the lamb. *Pediatr Res* 19:948–955, 1985.

Teitel DF, Klautz R, Steendijk P, et al.: The end-systolic pressure-volume relationship in the newborn lamb: Effects of loading and inotropic interventions. *Pediatr Res* 29:473–482, 1991.

Tempe DK, Kirmani S: Coagulation abnormalities in patients with cyanotic congenital heart disease. *J Cardiothorac Vasc Anesth* 16:752, 2002.

Thanopoulos BD, Karanassios E, Tsaousis G, et al.: Catheter closure of congenital/acquired muscular VSDs and perimembranous VSDs using the Amplatzer devices. *J Interv Cardiol* 16:399, 2003.

Tlaskal T, Hucin B, Hruda J, et al.: Results of primary and two-stage repair of interrupted aortic arch. *Eur J Thorac Surg* 15:227–228, 1999.

Tobias JD: Etomidate: Applications in pediatric care and pediatric anesthesiology. *Pediatr Crit Care Med* 1:100–106, 2000.

Todd MM: EEGs, EEG processing, and the bispectral index. *Anesthesiology* 89:815–817, 1998.

Tullis R, Rubin H: Calcium protects DNase I from proteinase K: A new method for the removal of spin-trapped radicals in aqueous solution of pyrimidine nucleosides and nucleotides. Reaction of the hydroxyl radical. *Int J Radiat Biol* 41:241, 1982.

Tweddell JS, Hoffman GM, Fedderly RT, et al.: Patients at risk for low systemic oxygen delivery after the Norwood procedure. *Ann Thorac Surg* 69:1893–1899, 2000.

Ungerleider R, Greeley W, Sheikh K, et al.: The use of intraoperative echo with Doppler color flow imaging to predict outcome after repair of congenital cardiac defects. *Ann Surg* 210:526, 1989a.

Ungerleider R, Greeley W, Kanter R, et al.: The learning curve for intraoperative echocardiography during congenital heart surgery. *Ann Thorac Surg* 54:691–696, 1992.

Ungerleider R, Greeley W, Kisslo J: Intraoperative echocardiography in congenital heart disease surgery: Preliminary report on a current study. *Am J Cardiol* 63:3F–8F, 1989b.

Ungerleider R, Kisslo J, Greeley W, et al.: Intraoperative prebypass and postbypass epicardial color flow imaging in the repair of atrioventricular septal defects. *J Thorac Cardiovasc Surg* 98:90–99, 1989c.

Ungerleider R, Kisslo J, Greeley W, et al.: Intraoperative echocardiography during congenital heart operation: Experience from 1,000 cases. *Ann Thorac Surg* 60:539–542, 1995.

Ungerleider R: Effects of cardiopulmonary bypass and use of modified ultrafiltration. *Ann Thorac Surg* 65(6 Suppl):S35–S38, 1998.

Urata H, Healy B, Stewart R, et al.: Angiotensin II receptors in normal and failing human hearts. *J Clin Endocrinol Metab* 69:54–61, 1989.

van der Linden J, Casimir AH: When do cerebral emboli appear during open heart operations? A transcranial Doppler study. *Ann Thorac Surg* 51:237–241, 1991.

van Dongen EI, Glansdorp AG, Mildner RJ, et al.: The influence of perioperative factors on outcomes in children aged less than 18 months after repair of tetralogy of Fallot. *J Thorac Cardiovasc Surg* 126:703–710, 2003.

Van Praagh R, Van Praagh S: The anatomy of common aortopulmonary trunk (truncus arteriosus communis) and its embryologic implications. A study of 57 necropsy cases. *Am J Cardiol* 16:406–425, 1965.

Vetter R, Will H, Kuttner I, et al.: Developmental changes of Ca++ transport systems in chick heart. *Biomed Biochem Acta* 45:219, 1986.

Vieira A, Berry L, Ofoso F, et al.: Heparin sensitivity and resistance in the neonate: An explanation. *Thrombosis Res* 63:85–98, 1991.

Vlahakes GJ, Turley K, Hoffman JI: The physiology of failure in acute right ventricular hypertension. *Circulation* 63:87–95, 1980.

Waldo A: *Modes and methods of recording electrograms. Diagnosis and treatment of cardiac arrhythmias following open heart surgery.* Mt Kisco, NY, 1980, Futura Publishing, p 21.

Ward J, Blakeky W, Joner E: Mammalian cells are not killed by DNA single-strand breaks caused by hydroxyl radicals from hydrogen peroxide. *Radic Res* 103:383, 1985.

Watanabe T, Hrita H, Kobayashi M, et al.: Brain tissue pH, oxygen tension, and carbon dioxide tension in profoundly hypothermic cardiopulmonary bypass. *J Thorac Cardiovasc Surg* 97:396–401, 1989.

Wauthy P, Abdel Kafi S, et al.: Inhaled nitric oxide versus prostacyclin in chronic shunt-induced pulmonary hypertension. *J Thorac Cardiovasc Surg* 126: 1434–1441, 2003.

Weinstein S, Cua C, Chan D, et al.: Outcome of symptomatic patients undergoing extracardiac Fontan conversion and cryoablation. *J Thorac Surg* 126:529–536, 2003.

Weisfeldt ML, Halperin HR: Cardiopulmonary resuscitation: Beyond cardiac massage. *Circulation* 74:443–448, 1986.

Weller RJ, Weintraub R, Addonizio L, et al.: Outcome of idiopathic restrictive cardiomyopathy in children. *Am J Cardiol* 90:501–506, 2002.

Wernovsky G, Jonas R, Newburger J: The Boston Circulatory Arrest Study: Hemodynamics and hospital course after the arterial switch operation. *Circulation* 86(Suppl I):237A, 1992.

Wernovsky G, Hougen T, Walsh E, et al.: Mid-term results following the arterial switch operation for transposition of the great arteries with intact ventricular septum: Clinical, hemodynamic, echocardiographic, and electrophysiologic data. *Circulation* 77:1333, 1988.

Wernovsky G, Newburger JW: Neurologic and developmental morbidity in children with complex congenital heart disease. *J Pediatr* 142:6–8, 2003.

Wessel DL, Adatia I, Van Marter LJ, et al.: Improved oxygenation in a randomized trial of inhaled nitric oxide for persistent pulmonary hypertension of the newborn. *Pediatrics* 100:E7, 1997.

Wessel D, Triedman J, Wernovsky G, et al.: Pulmonary and systemic hemodynamics of amrinone in neonates following cardiopulmonary bypass. *Circulation* (Suppl II):II-488, 1989.

Wieloch T, Harris R, Symon L, et al.: Influence of severe hypoglycemia on brain extracellular calcium and potassium activities, energy, and phospholipid metabolism. *J Neurochem* 43:160, 1984.

Williams GD, Jones TK, Hanson KA, et al.: The hemodynamic effects of propofol in children with congenital heart disease. *Anesth Analg* 89:1411–1416, 1999.

Williams WG, McBride BW, Ashburn DA, et al.: Outcomes of 829 neonates with complete transposition of the great arteries 12-17 years after repair. *Eur J Cardio Surg* 24:1–10, 2003.

Wirrel EC, Pelausa EO, Allen AC, et al.: Massive pericardial effusion as a cause for sudden deterioration in a very low birth weight infant. *Am J Perinat* 10:419–423, 1993.

Wong A, Salem M, Mani M, et al.: Glycopyrrolate as a substitute for atropine in reversal of curarization in pediatric cardiac patients. *Anesth Analg* 53:412, 1974.

Woodman RC, Harker LA: Bleeding complications associated with cardiopulmonary bypass. *Blood* 76:1680–1697, 1990.

Wypij D, Newburger JW, Rappaport LA, et al.: The effect of duration of deep hypothermic circulatory arrest in infant heart surgery on late neurodevelopment: The Boston Circulatory Arrest Trial. *J Thorac Cardiovasc Surg* 126:1397–1403, 2003.

Yoshii S, Akashi O, Kobayashi M, et al.: Preliminary results of intermittent retrograde cerebral perfusion during proximal aortic arch surgery. *Jpn J Thorac Cardiovasc Surg* 51:588–593, 2003.

Zanchetta M, Onorato E, Rigatelli G, et al.: Intracardiac echocardiography-guided transcatheter closure of secundum atrial septal defect: a new efficient device selection method. *J Am Coll Cardiol* 42:1677, 2003.

Zapletal A, Paul T, Samenek M: Pulmonary elasticity in children and adolescents. *J Appl Physiol* 40:953, 1976.

18 Anesthesia for Pediatric Neurosurgery

Elliot J. Krane • Bridget M. Philip • Kelly K. Yeh • Karen B. Domino

The practice of anesthesia for pediatric neurosurgery encompasses the skills and knowledge of pediatric anesthesiology as well as the knowledge of cerebral pathophysiology. To provide optimal neuroanesthetic management and neurologic intensive care, the anesthesiologist must understand the physiology of the central nervous system, the effects of drugs on cerebral hemodynamics, and the physiology of the developing child.

NEUROPHYSIOLOGY

CEREBRAL BLOOD FLOW

Specific data on cerebral blood flow (CBF) in human infants and children are sparse, and many anesthetic principles must be inferred from the data in animals and adult humans. Total CBF in the adult is about 50 mL/100 g of brain tissue per min (Lassen and Christensen, 1976). The amount of flow varies in different anatomic areas. CBF is higher in gray matter (80 mL/100 g brain per min) than in white matter (20 mL/100 g brain per min). Lower CBF probably occurs in the developing brain of premature and newborn infants (30 to 40 mL/100 g per min), but in infants and older children, global CBF is higher than in adults (65 to 85 mL/100 g per min) (Settergren et al., 1980; Kreisman et al., 1989; Chiron et al., 1992).

Regional cerebral metabolic rate for oxygen ($CMRO_2$) is an important determinant of regional CBF because supply is closely linked to demand in both adults and children. CBF therefore increases with increased $CMRO_2$, such as that associated with seizures or fever. CBF also decreases with reduced $CMRO_2$, such as that caused by hypothermia or barbiturates. $CMRO_2$ is higher in children (5 mL/100 g per min) than in adults (3 to 4 mL/100 g per min) (Kennedy and Sokoloff, 1967).

Besides metabolic demand, CBF depends on cerebral perfusion pressure (CPP) and on arterial oxygen (PaO_2) and carbon dioxide ($PaCO_2$) tensions. CPP is equal to the mean arterial pressure (MAP) minus the cerebral venous pressure, which is well approximated by intracranial pressure (ICP) when the cranium is intact. The CBF is autoregulated to changes in MAP; that is, it remains constant when MAP is between 60 and 150 mm Hg in adults (Lassen and Christensen, 1976). Within this range, the cerebral blood vessels dilate at lower blood pressures and constrict at higher blood pressures to maintain a constant CBF. However, the autoregulatory response may take up to 2 minutes to occur. Because the MAP in infants is less than 60 mm Hg in the first year of life, the autoregulatory limits are probably lower. In neonatal lambs and dogs, the lower limit of autoregulation is 40 mm Hg (Purves and James, 1969; Hernandez et al., 1980; Rogers et al., 1980). One author extrapolated from animal data to describe the autoregulatory range as between 20 and 60 mm Hg in high-risk neonates (Pryds, 1991). In a study of 17 extremely low-birth-weight infants, Munro and others (2004) noted that cerebral autoregulation appears to be functional in normotensive but not hypotensive infants and that the lower limit of autoregulation appears to be a mean blood pressure of 30 mm Hg.

The true autoregulatory range in human premature infants, full-term newborns, infants, and children is undefined at the present, and the practitioner must do his or her best to extrapolate from newborn animal studies to humans and to interpolate between these and what is known to be the autoregulatory range in adults. Above and below the limits of autoregulation, CBF is passively dependent on CPP; inadequate CBF produces cerebral ischemia, and excessive CBF leads to edema formation and possibly intracranial hemorrhage.

The lower limit of autoregulation is lower with drug-induced hypotension than during hypovolemic hypotension (Fitch et al., 1973). Signs of cerebral ischemia generally do not occur when MAP is reduced to less than 60 mm Hg in adults during deliberate hypotension and general anesthesia. When blood pressure is increased above the autoregulatory range, large increases in CBF, disruption of the blood-brain barrier, and edema formation occur (Hatashita et al., 1986). Chronic hypertension raises the upper limit of autoregulation, although long-term antihypertensive therapy may restore the limit to normal (Hoffman et al., 1983). Autoregulation is attenuated by hypercapnia, hypoxia, high concentrations of volatile anesthetics, nitroprusside, and trauma. In local areas around brain tumors and in areas of focal cerebral ischemia, autoregulation is lost and perfusion is pressure dependent (Dong et al., 1996; Schmieder et al., 2000). Autoregulation is also impaired in premature infants with respiratory distress (Lou et al., 1979; Milligan, 1980; Daven et al., 1983; Ong et al., 1986).

In the adult, normal cerebral vessels dilate in response to increases in $PaCO_2$ and constrict in response to decreases in $PaCO_2$ (Lassen and Christensen, 1976). CBF varies linearly with $PaCO_2$ between 20 and 80 mm Hg, so that a 4% change in CBF occurs for each 1–mm Hg change in $PaCO_2$ within this range. At $PaCO_2$ greater than 80 mm Hg the cerebral vasculature is maximally dilated, and sensitivity to further increases in $PaCO_2$ decreases. As $PaCO_2$ decreases below 20 mm Hg, CBF does not decrease further, presumably because ischemia-induced metabolic changes override the response to CO_2. The mechanism of the response of the cerebral circulation to CO_2 involves changes in cerebrospinal fluid (CSF) and in periarteriolar pH. CO_2 crosses the blood-brain barrier more freely than do bicarbonate ions. Decreases in $PaCO_2$ acutely increase periarteriolar pH, which gradually normalizes owing to the subsequent movement of bicarbonate out of the CSF over the next 8 to 24 hours (Lassen and Christensen, 1976). CBF also returns to normal within 24 hours. With chronic hyperventilation, as occurs in patients in the intensive care unit, CSF pH is near normal despite low $PaCO_2$. If the $PaCO_2$ acutely rises to normal levels, the periarteriolar pH decreases, and CBF and ICP increase.

The cerebrovascular response to changes in $PaCO_2$ is not completely developed at birth (Rogers et al., 1980; Shapiro et al., 1980; Hansen et al., 1984). Hypercapnia increases CBF in newborn animals. The newborn brain is relatively insensitive to moderate degrees of hypocapnia. Brain blood flow does not decrease significantly from normocapnia until extreme degrees of hypocapnia ($PaCO_2$ <15 mm Hg) occur (Hansen et al., 1984).

The cerebral vasculature is less sensitive to changes in PaO_2. In adults, CBF does not increase until PaO_2 falls below 50 mm Hg (Lassen and Christensen, 1976). CBF then increases exponentially, with a fivefold increase occurring when PaO_2 is 25 mm Hg. Hyperoxia reduces adult CBF by approximately 10%. The fetal and neonatal circulation responds to small changes in PaO_2 (Rogers et al., 1980), perhaps because of the greater oxygen affinity of fetal hemoglobin. The age at which this heightened responsiveness decreases is unknown.

Other factors that affect CBF include hematocrit, body temperature, and autonomic tone. In the adult, increasing the hematocrit to greater than 50% reduces CBF by increasing blood viscosity and reducing the hematocrit to less than 30% increases CBF by decreasing viscosity (Wood et al., 1983). $CMRO_2$ and CBF are reduced by decreasing body temperature. Immaturity of the sympathetic nervous system in neonates may contribute to unusual CBF responses to the release of catecholamines (Rogers et al., 1980).

In summary, little is known about the physiology of the cerebral circulation in the newborn and infant human, although some studies have shown that in healthy full-term neonates, dynamic regulation of the cerebral circulation may occur on the first day of life (Mochalova et al., 1983). Data must be extrapolated from current knowledge of the physiology of human adults and animals. While normal newborn infants probably autoregulate CBF in response to changes in MAP, the autoregulatory limits are undefined; their cerebral circulation is less responsive to hypocapnia than is that of adults. In addition, vasomotor paralysis, in which the cerebral vessels normally do not autoregulate or respond to changes in $PaCO_2$, may occur in newborns with respiratory distress syndrome and in children with brain tumors, trauma, or brain ischemia.

INTRACRANIAL PRESSURE

In the adult the cranium is rigid. Brain tissue is noncompressible, and its volume is relatively constant. Increases in the volume of brain, CSF, or blood compartments must be compensated for by decreases in another compartment; this movement of blood or CSF from the cranial compartment occurs at the expense of an increase in ICP, creating a pressure gradient favoring such movement. Subsequently, further compensatory translocation of blood or fluid requires still greater gradients—that is, compliance diminishes. The compensatory mechanisms may fail when acute increases in intracranial volume (caused by hematoma or trauma, for example) occur rapidly. As a space-occupying lesion expands and the compensatory mechanisms fail, small increases in intracranial volume cause large increases in ICP. This phenomenon generates a typical pressure–volume, or compliance, curve (Fig. 18–1*A*).

In the infant, cranial decompression can also occur through expansion of the skull size. The anterior fontanel remains open until around 1 year of age, and the cranial sutures of a child's skull do not fuse until as late as the tenth year. Slow increases in intracranial volume can be offset by a slow increase in skull size before ICP increases. In contrast, skull diameter cannot increase with rapid changes in intracranial volume, such as after head injury. In these cases, ICP changes occur as in the adult.

The absence of intracranial hypertension says nothing about intracranial compliance, which may be severely impaired even if ICP is normal (Bruce et al., 1977; Wilkinson, 1981). Figure 18–1*A* illustrates this concept. During periods of diminished compliance but normal ICP (shaded area), small perturbations in intracranial volume are poorly tolerated and produce marked elevation of ICP and clinical deterioration. When intracranial compliance is known to be limited, patients should be treated with the appropriate techniques and safeguards as if intracranial hypertension were indeed present. Measures that reduce cerebral volume by dehydrating cerebral tissue (administration of mannitol or furosemide) or by reducing cerebral edema (as does dexamethasone) should also improve cerebral compliance (Fig. 18–1*B*).

Because a patient's intracranial compliance is seldom known, any patient with a space-occupying intracranial mass is assumed to have reduced intracranial compliance (meaning that small changes in intracranial volume result in large changes in pressure). The goal of neuroanesthetic management is to control CBF and cerebral blood volume (CBV) and, therefore, ICP.

EFFECTS OF DRUGS ON NEUROPHYSIOLOGY

The effects of the commonly used anesthetic agents on CBF, $CMRO_2$, and CSF dynamics are discussed in this section and are summarized in Table 18–1. There are no data on these effects

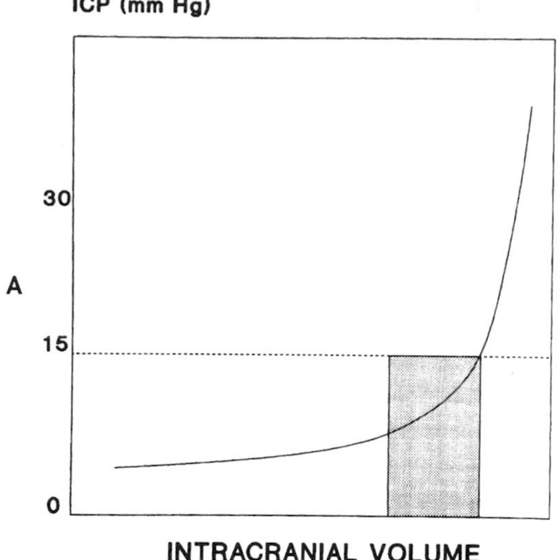

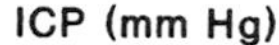

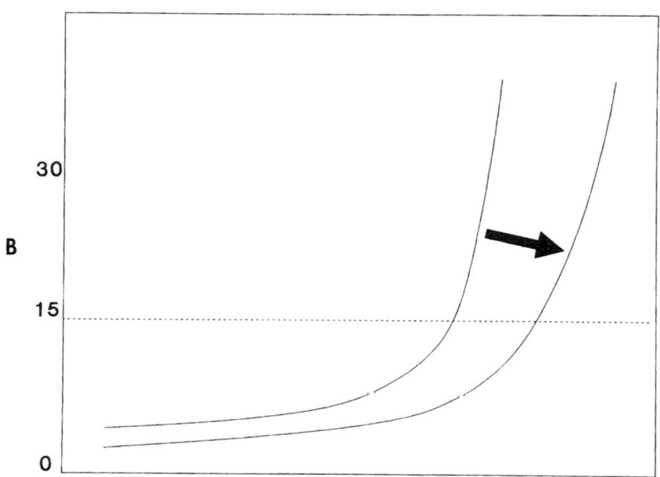

■ **FIGURE 18–1.** *A,* Ideal intracranial compliance curve. Note that if intracranial pressure (ICP) lies within the shaded area, ICP is normal, but intracranial compliance is limited. Relatively small changes in intracranial volume lead to relatively large increases in ICP. *B,* The intracranial compliance curve changes after a reduction in cerebral tissue volume, such as might occur after a dose of mannitol or after treatment of cerebral edema around a tumor with dexamethasone. Intracranial compliance increases in these circumstances.

in infants and children. The responses in children are assumed to be the same as those in adults.

■ INTRAVENOUS ANESTHETICS

Intravenous anesthetics generally reduce or do not alter CBF and ICP, with the exception of ketamine, which increases both CBF and ICP.

Propofol

Propofol is an intravenous induction agent with cerebrovascular properties similar to thiopental: both may depress systemic blood pressure but both potently decrease $CMRO_2$, CBF, and ICP (Van Hemelrijck et al., 1990; Warner et al., 1990; Fischer et al., 1992).

■ **TABLE 18–1.** Effects of anesthetic agents on cerebral metabolic rate for oxygen ($CMRO_2$), intracranial pressure (ICP), and cerebrospinal fluid (CSF) dynamics

Anesthetic Agent	CBF	$CMRO_2$	Autoregulation	ICP
Propofol	↓↓	↓↓	Preserved	↓↓
Thiopental	↓↓	↓↓	Preserved	↓↓
Opioids	—	—	Preserved	—
Etomidate	↓	↓	Preserved	↓
Lidocaine (nontoxic)	↓	↓↓	Preserved	↓
Benzodiazepines	↓	↓↓	Preserved	↓
Ketamine	↑↑	—	Unknown	↑↑*
Nitrous oxide	↑	↑	Preserved	↑
Isoflurane	↑	↓↓	Preserved	↑*
Halothane	↑↑	↓	Abolished	↑*
Sevoflurane	↑	↓↓	Preserved	↑*
Desflurane	↑	↓↓	Preserved	↑*

*Increase in ICP dose is related and blunted by hyperventilation.

Cerebral autoregulation and cerebral responsiveness to changes in arterial CO_2 tension (Fox et al., 1992; Petersen et al., 2003; Karsli et al., 2004) are well preserved during propofol anesthesia. Propofol is a good alternative to thiopental for induction of anesthesia for neurosurgery. In the presence of nitrous oxide and hypocapnia, propofol results in lower ICP and higher cerebral perfusion pressure (CPP) and in reduced cerebral cortical edema than isoflurane or sevoflurane. In patients with or at risk for intracranial hypertension and decreased cerebral perfusion, maintenance of anesthesia with propofol is superior to inhaled halogenated anesthetics, at least until the dura has been opened.

Barbiturates

The barbiturates decrease CBF, CBV, and $CMRO_2$ in a dose-dependent manner (Pierce et al., 1962; Michenfelder, 1974; Albrecht et al., 1977) and therefore reduce ICP. Neither CBF nor cerebral metabolism is significantly altered by subanesthetic doses of barbiturates. When the electroencephalogram (EEG) becomes isoelectric, CBF and $CMRO_2$ decrease to about 50% of normal, and additional doses of barbiturates have little further effect. Barbiturates may also be used to prevent increases in ICP that can occur with laryngoscopy and endotracheal intubation.

Autoregulation and the cerebrovascular response to changes in $PaCO_2$ remain intact during barbiturate anesthesia. The rate of CSF formation and the resistance to reabsorption of CSF are not altered by barbiturates (Mann et al., 1979). In doses that suppress the EEG, barbiturates reduce cerebral damage in animal and human models of focal cerebral ischemia (Smith et al., 1974; Nussmeir et al., 1986; Nehls et al., 1987). In animals, barbiturates also reduce the extent of cerebral edema after a cortical freeze injury. This decrease in edema is in contrast to the response observed with the volatile anesthetics (Smith and Macque, 1976).

Opioids

Opioids have little effect on CBF, CBV, or ICP unless respiration is depressed and $PaCO_2$ is increased (Miller et al., 1975; Misfeldt et al., 1976; Jobes et al., 1977; Moss et al., 1978a).

Fentanyl

When combined with nitrous oxide, fentanyl decreases CBF by 47% and $CMRO_2$ by 18% (Michenfelder, 1974).

Autoregulation and CO_2 responsiveness of the cerebral circulation are not altered. Fentanyl does not alter the rate of CSF formation, but it reduces the resistance to CSF reabsorption by 50% (Artru, 1983a, 1984b), the effect of which is to decrease CSF volume to a degree of unknown clinical significance. The neonatal cerebral circulation is also unaffected by fentanyl (Yaster et al., 1987).

Sufentanil and Alfentanil

Alfentanil in high doses (10 to 20 mcg/kg) reduces both CBF and $CMRO_2$ by 25% to 30% (Stephan et al., 1991; Warner et al., 1991), whereas at exceedingly high doses (10 to 200 mcg/kg), sufentanil may transiently increase CBF while reducing $CMRO_2$ (Milde et al., 1990). However, at conventional doses, sufentanil (Herrick et al., 1991; Weinstabl et al., 1991) and alfentanil (Mayberg et al., 1993) do not appear to have adverse effects on the cerebral vasculature or upon ICP in most patients. In a subset of patients with severe head injuries and very poor intracranial compliance, sufentanil may cause a small (e.g., <10 mm Hg) and transient increase in ICP that may be clinically significant in some settings (Sperry et al., 1992; Weinstabl et al., 1992; Albanese et al., 1993).

Remifentanil

Remifentanil is an ultra–short-acting opioid that is rapidly metabolized by plasma cholinesterases. The very short clinical duration of effect of remifentanil and its context-sensitive half-life that is independent of the duration of infusion (Minto et al., 1997, 2003) make it an appealing opioid for lengthy neurosurgical procedures after which rapid return of consciousness is desirable. As is the case with other opioids that have been studied, remifentanil does not increase CBF or ICP (Hoffman et al., 1993; Warner et al., 1996; Baker et al., 1997; Guy et al., 1997; Ostapkovich et al., 1998; Paris et al., 1998; Rizzi, 1998; Wagner et al., 2001; Lorenz et al., 2002; Gerlach et al., 2003; Klimscha et al., 2003; Lorenz et al., 2003; Engelhard et al., 2004; Lagace et al., 2004). Remifentanil, like other opioids, preserves cerebral autoregulation and CO_2 reactivity (Baker et al., 1997; Ostapkovich et al., 1998; Klimscha et al., 2003; Engelhard et al., 2004).

Return of consciousness is very rapid after remifentanil is discontinued, and the frequency of administration of naloxone to permit neurologic assessment is decreased (Guy et al., 1997). However, because remifentanil analgesia is very brief after its discontinuation, a long-acting opioid analgesic must be administered to prevent severe pain and rebound hypertension before or soon after remifentanil is discontinued (Domaingue, 2001; Gelb et al., 2003; Gerlach et al., 2003; Cafiero et al., 2004).

Other Intravenous Anesthetics

Etomidate reduces ICP by decreasing CBF and $CMRO_2$ by 34% and 45%, respectively. It, too, preserves the CO_2 responsiveness of the cerebral circulation (Renou et al., 1978; Moss et al., 1979). A side effect of etomidate administration is myoclonus. Myoclonus has been reported after prolonged continuous infusion of etomidate (Laughlin and Newberg, 1985). *Lidocaine* in clinical doses decreases CBF and reduces the increase in ICP associated with endotracheal intubation (Sakabe et al., 1974; Donegan and Bedford, 1980) and suctioning.

The *benzodiazepines* (diazepam, lorazepam, and midazolam) decrease CBF and $CMRO_2$ approximately 25% (Cotev and Shalit, 1975; Rockoff et al., 1980; Forster et al., 1982; Nugent et al., 1982; Nakahashi et al., 1991). Clinical doses of midazolam and diazepam do not alter ICP (Tateishi et al., 1981; Giffin et al., 1984).

Ketamine

In contrast to the other intravenous anesthetic agents, ketamine is a potent cerebrovasodilator. Ketamine increases CBF by 60% with little change in $CMRO_2$ (Dawson et al., 1971; Takeshita et al., 1972; Schwedler et al., 1982). The cerebrovascular response to administration of ketamine is thought to be the result of regional cerebral activation induced by the drug (Hougaard et al., 1974). Ketamine produces a marked increase in ICP, which can be reduced, but not prevented, by hyperventilation (Gardner et al., 1972; Sari et al., 1972; Shapiro et al., 1972). The increase in CBF, and presumably in ICP, can be blocked by previous administration of thiopental (Dawson et al., 1971). Ketamine has been associated with sudden elevation of ICP and clinical deterioration when used in patients with hydrocephalus and other intracranial pathology (Lockhart and Jenkins, 1972; Shapiro et al., 1972; Crumrine et al., 1975). Ketamine is not used in patients with reduced intracranial compliance.

INHALED ANESTHETICS

All currently used inhaled anesthetics, including nitrous oxide, are cerebrovasodilators to various degrees. The vasodilation can be minimized by the use of low concentrations and concomitant hyperventilation.

Nitrous Oxide

Nitrous oxide is a weak cerebrovasodilator whose effects on CBF are offset by hyperventilation and barbiturate anesthesia (Algotsson et al., 1992). The variability of effects that nitrous oxide has on CBF and ICP in different reports results from differences in experimental species and background anesthesia. In many animals, nitrous oxide in subanesthetic doses (60% to 70%) causes excitement and cerebral metabolic stimulation, with an accompanying increase in CBF (Theye and Michenfelder, 1968; Sakabe et al., 1978; Pelligrino et al., 1984; Todd, 1987).

Because nitrous oxide is not an adequate anesthetic in the absence of other inhalation or intravenous anesthetics, the modification of the cerebral effects of nitrous oxide by additional anesthetic drugs is particularly important. Seventy percent nitrous oxide does not, for example, cause a change in CBF, but it does reduce $CMRO_2$ by 15% to 20% during barbiturate and narcotic anesthesia (Sakabe et al., 1978). However, when nitrous oxide is added to a volatile anesthetic such as isoflurane (Cucchiara et al., 1974; Manohar and Parks, 1984) or halothane (Sakabe et al., 1976), both CBF and $CMRO_2$ increase. When nitrous oxide is added to sevoflurane, cerebral hyperemia increases and autoregulation is impaired (Iacopino et al., 2003). The cerebrovascular responses to changes in $PaCO_2$ and MAP are preserved during nitrous oxide anesthesia.

ICP may increase in response to nitrous oxide in patients with intracranial mass lesions and reduced intracranial compliance (Henriksen and Jorgensen, 1973; Moss and McDowall, 1979; Iacopino et al., 2003). The increase in ICP with nitrous oxide, however, is readily reversible by diazepam and barbiturate anesthesia and simultaneously initiated hyperventilation (Phirman and Shapiro, 1977).

The use of nitrous oxide for pediatric neuroanesthesia remains controversial. Some anesthesiologists prefer to avoid nitrous oxide because of its ability to increase $CMRO_2$ and reduce the cerebral protective effects of barbiturates. Others are concerned because nitrous oxide readily diffuses into collections of intracranial air and may increase ICP in the presence of pneumocephalus (Saidman and Eger, 1965; Artru, 1982; Skahen et al., 1986). Asymptomatic accumulation of intracranial air occurs commonly during craniotomies, especially those associated with posterior fossa surgery and drainage of CSF (Toung et al., 1986).

Some anesthesiologists discontinue nitrous oxide before closure of the dura to reduce the incidence of tension pneumocephalus. Others administer nitrous oxide throughout the procedure without any obvious detrimental effects, and indeed one randomized control trial comparing anesthetic techniques with and without nitrous oxide in patients undergoing sitting craniotomies showed no difference in the incidence of size of pneumocephalus between the three groups (Hernandez-Palazon et al., 2003). It may be that nitrous oxide equilibrates with intracranial air before the dura is closed. If so, ICP would not increase during craniodural closure because air pockets would already contain nitrous oxide. In addition, the discontinuance of nitrous oxide would decrease ICP, as nitrous oxide diffused back into the bloodstream (Skahen et al., 1986). Maintenance with nitrous oxide until the end of the surgery may be advantageous because it permits rapid awakening and may reduce the intracranial gas volume and the likelihood of delayed tension pneumocephalus.

Nitrous oxide is generally not contraindicated during sitting craniotomies despite the fact that the volume of a venous air embolus (VAE) expands in the presence of nitrous oxide. In fact, this phenomenon actually increases the sensitivity of monitoring for VAE by capnography (Losasso et al., 1992a), while at the same time nitrous oxide neither increases the risk of VAE (Losasso et al., 1992b) nor increases the hemodynamic consequences of VAE provided that nitrous oxide is discontinued when VAE is first detected (Losasso et al., 1992b).

Isoflurane

Isoflurane is the most popular of the volatile anesthetics for neuroanesthesia. Its popularity is based on the fact that it affects CBF less than does halothane at equivalent minimum alveolar concentration (MAC) doses (Todd and Drummond, 1984; Drummond and Todd, 1985; Algottson et al., 1988), the fact that 1 MAC isoflurane preserves cerebral autoregulation (McPherson and Traystman, 1988) and CO_2 responsiveness (McPherson et al., 1989), and the belief that it may provide cerebral protection (Newberg and Michenfelder, 1983; Newberg et al., 1983; Verhaegen et al., 1992). Cerebral autoregulation is less affected by isoflurane than by halothane (Todd and Drummond, 1984). In addition, isoflurane does not change CSF production, and it reduces the resistance to reabsorption of CSF (Artru, 1984a, 1984c). During hypocapnia, CBF is lower with 1.0 MAC isoflurane (with 75% nitrous oxide) than with nitrous oxide alone (Cucchiara et al., 1974; Drummond and Todd, 1985; Scheller et al., 1986). In contrast, 1.0 MAC halothane (with 75% nitrous oxide) increases CBF.

Despite their dissimilar effects on CBF, isoflurane and halothane increase ICP equally in an animal model of brain injury (Scheller et al., 1987). This is probably because isoflurane and halothane increase CBV to a similar degree (Artru, 1984d; Archer et al., 1987). In patients with reduced intracranial compliance, isoflurane increases ICP. The increase in ICP in these patients can be attenuated by simultaneous initiation of hyperventilation (Adams et al., 1981). Isoflurane may be safely used in patients with small supratentorial brain tumors (Madsen et al., 1987) but may cause dangerous increases in ICP in patients with large intracranial mass lesions that are associated with a midline shift evident on the computed tomography (CT) scan (Grosslight et al., 1985). As with halothane, isoflurane should be avoided in patients with reduced intracranial compliance until the dura is open, if ICP is not being monitored.

Isoflurane decreases $CMRO_2$ by 30%, and it causes an isoelectric EEG at concentrations above 2.0 MAC (Newberg et al., 1983). It is unique among the volatile agents in that it preserves normal cerebral energy states and aerobic metabolism at very low blood pressure (40 mm Hg), in contrast to the findings observed with hypotension induced by halothane, trimethaphan, or sodium nitroprusside (Newberg et al., 1984). In studies of mice exposed to 5% oxygen, isoflurane increased survival time and thus may have provided some degree of cerebral protection. In studies of incomplete global ischemia in isoflurane-anesthetized dogs, cerebral energy stores were increased, presumably through depression of cortical electrical activity and cerebral metabolism (Newberg and Michenfelder, 1983). Protective effects of isoflurane, however, were not observed in a primate model of regional cerebral ischemia (Nehls et al., 1987).

Sevoflurane

Sevoflurane is a fluorinated ether with a low blood-gas solubility. Studies in rabbits suggest that sevoflurane does not increase CBF at 0.5 to 1.0 MAC. Sevoflurane does cause increases in cerebral blood flow and ICP and a decrease in cerebral oxygen consumption (Scheller et al., 1988) and CPP similar to isoflurane (Petersen et al., 2003). Compared with isoflurane, sevoflurane allows more rapid emergence after lengthy neurosurgery, allowing more rapid neurologic assessment (Gauthier et al., 2002).

The increase in CBF with sevoflurane in normocapnic children is less than that with halothane (Monkhoff et al., 2001). Taken together, the available evidence suggests that sevoflurane is a more appropriate inhaled anesthetic than halothane during craniotomy and is equivalent in its cerebrovascular effects to isoflurane while allowing more rapid recovery after long anesthesia. As is the case with other halogenated agents, if ICP or intracranial compliance is compromised, sevoflurane should be withheld until the dura has been opened (Petersen et al., 2003).

Halothane

Halothane is a cerebral vasodilator that decreases cerebrovascular resistance (CVR) and increases CBF in a dose-dependent fashion (Wollman et al., 1964; Albrecht et al., 1977; Todd and Drummond, 1984; Brussel et al., 1991). The increase in CBF is transient; CBF decreases to baseline levels after 150 minutes of halothane anesthesia (Albrecht et al., 1983). CBV, however, remains elevated by 11% to 12% over a 3-hour period of halothane administration (Artru, 1983b). Halothane reduces $CMRO_2$ by 17% to 33% (Albrecht et al., 1977). The cerebral vasculature remains responsive to changes in arterial $PaCO_2$ (Alexander et al., 1964; Wollman et al., 1964; Drummond and Todd, 1985). Halothane in high concentrations (2.0 MAC) abolishes autoregulation of the cerebral circulation in response to changes in MAP in both adults (Miletich et al., 1976; Todd and Drummond, 1984) and infants (Messer et al., 1989). Halothane alters blood-brain barrier permeability, promoting the extravasation of plasma proteins into normal brain during periods of acute hypertension (Forster et al., 1978). Halothane reduces CSF formation by 30% in dogs and increases the resistance of reabsorption of CSF (Artru, 1983a, 1984b).

Because ICP is determined by CBV, CSF volume, and brain tissue volume, it is not surprising that ICP increases with halothane (Jennet et al., 1969; DiGiovanni et al., 1974). Peak increases are observed in 3 to 13 minutes, although the increase persists over 3 hours of halothane exposure (Artru, 1983b). The increase in ICP in patients with intracranial mass lesions can be attenuated, but not totally prevented, by establishing hyperventilation for 10 minutes before the introduction of halothane (Adams et al., 1972). If ICP is not being monitored, halothane should not be used in patients with reduced intracranial compliance until the dura is open and its effects on the brain can be seen.

Desflurane

Desflurane is an inhalation agent that is chemically similar to isoflurane. Its physicochemical properties are remarkable for a blood-gas partition coefficient even lower than that of nitrous oxide, permitting rapid uptake and washout of the gas. Desflurane effects on cerebral metabolism and hemodynamics are not as well studied as the effects of the other inhalation agents, but the existing animal studies suggest that its effects are not unique in any way. Desflurane at clinical concentrations is a potent cerebral vasodilator, increasing ICP (Artru, 1994; Artru et al., 1994), increasing CBF by 50% at 1.5 MAC, and reducing autoregulation of CBF (Lutz et al., 1990). However, cerebrovascular responsiveness to hypocapnia is preserved during desflurane anesthesia in laboratory animals, protecting the animal from increases in ICP if hyperventilation occurs during desflurane anesthesia (Lutz et al., 1991; Young, 1992). In patients with mass lesions, equivalent MAC doses of desflurane and isoflurane are similar in terms of absolute CBF, the response to increasing doses, and the preservation of CO_2 reactivity (Ornstein et al., 1993; Fraga et al., 2003). Desflurane effects on the EEG are also similar to those of isoflurane. At increasing concentrations, the electroencephalographic frequency decreases and the amplitude increases. Burst suppression appears at about 1.24 MAC (Rampil et al., 1991).

MUSCLE RELAXANTS

Succinylcholine

Succinylcholine is now very infrequently used in pediatric anesthesia, because of its association with life-threatening hyperkalemia and cardiac arrest in children with undiagnosed myopathies. This has led to a "black box warning" by the U.S. Food and Drug Administration, reserving its use in children for emergency intubation where securing the airway is necessary. Most often, the use of high-dose nondepolarizing neuromuscular blockers is appropriate even for emergently securing the airway in most children, but there are cases in which the most rapid and immediate pharmacologic paralysis is required, and succinylcholine remains the drug of choice in these circumstances.

Life-threatening hyperkalemia has also been associated with the administration of succinylcholine after many types of central nervous system disorders, including closed-head injury, even without motor deficits (Mazze et al., 1969; Thomas, 1969; Smith and Grenvik, 1970; Stone et al., 1970; Stevenson and Birch, 1979; Frankville and Drummond, 1987), cerebral hypoxia caused by near-drowning (Tong, 1987), subarachnoid hemorrhage (Iwatsuki et al., 1980), encephalitis (Cowgill et al., 1974), cerebrovascular accidents (Cooperman, 1970), and paraplegia (Cooperman et al., 1970; Tobey, 1970). The onset of the period of vulnerability is not well defined. It may begin as early as 24 to 48 hours after injury and may last up to 1 to 2 years after injury (Cooperman, 1970). Because the period of risk for succinylcholine-induced hyperkalemia after cerebral injury is undefined, succinylcholine should be avoided in these patients, except in the period immediately after injury.

Succinylcholine can increase CBF and ICP in patients with reduced intracranial compliance (Cottrell et al., 1983; Thiagarajah et al., 1985; Minton et al., 1986; Stirt et al., 1987a), probably because of cerebral stimulation from succinylcholine-induced increases in afferent muscle spindle activity (Lanier et al., 1986). The increases in CBF and ICP can be blunted by deep general anesthesia or by previous paralyzing or "defasciculating" doses of nondepolarizing muscle relaxants (Minton et al., 1986; Stirt et al., 1987a). In contrast, most nondepolarizing relaxants have little effect on CBV and ICP (Lanier et al., 1985; Minton et al., 1985; Rosa et al., 1986; Stirt et al., 1987b), unless associated with histamine release (*d*-tubocurarine, atracurium), which causes transient cerebrovasodilation and increased ICP (Tarkkanen et al., 1974; Vesely et al., 1987). Atracurium, in doses that do not release histamine, does not increase ICP, despite the accumulation of laudanosine, a major metabolic product of atracurium and a potential central nervous system arousal agent.

Nondepolarizing Muscle Relaxants

The presence of motor deficits or the administration of anticonvulsants may affect the dose of nondepolarizing muscle relaxant necessary in neurosurgical patients. Hemiplegia from an upper motor neuron lesion (such as a stroke or a brain tumor) is associated with resistance to nondepolarizing relaxants on the paretic side (Graham, 1980; Moorthy and Hilgenberg, 1980; Azar, 1984; Shayevitz and Matteo, 1985). Excessive doses of muscle relaxants may be given if dosage is guided by a nerve stimulator monitoring a hemiplegic extremity. In contrast, an increased response to nondepolarizing muscle relaxants is observed in paretic muscle lower motor neuron lesions (e.g., paraplegia and quadriplegia) (Brown and Charlton, 1975; Azar, 1984).

Acute administration of several anticonvulsants, including phenytoin, phenobarbital, trimethadione, and ethosuximide, enhances nondepolarizing neuromuscular blockade or delays its reversal (Ghandi et al., 1976; Spacek et al., 1999). Patients receiving chronic phenytoin or carbamazepine therapy are resistant to the effects of nondepolarizing relaxants, including pancuronium (Chen et al., 1983; Roth and Ebrahim, 1987), metocurine (Ornstein et al., 1985), vecuronium (Ong et al., 1986; Ornstein et al., 1987; Alloul et al., 1996), and rocuronium (Spacek et al., 1999; Hernandez-Palazon et al., 2001) but interestingly, not mivacurium or atracurium (Ornstein et al., 1987; Spacek et al., 1996, 1997). The cause of phenytoin-induced resistance to nondepolarizing muscle relaxants and the lack of the same effect with mivacurium or atracurium are unclear. Finally, no data have yet been published describing the interactions of the anticonvulsant felbamate, gabapentin, levetiracetam, tiagabine, topiramate, sodium valproate, or valproic acid with nondepolarizing neuromuscular blocking drugs.

VASODILATORS

The direct-acting vasodilators, including sodium nitroprusside, adenosine triphosphate (ATP), adenosine, nitroglycerin, diazoxide, and hydralazine, are cerebrovasodilators and may increase CBF and ICP (Stoyka and Schultz, 1975; Turner et al., 1977; Cottrell et al., 1978, 1980; Marsh et al., 1979; Ghani et al., 1989; McDowall, 1985). The calcium channel blockers also raise CBF and ICP (Cottrell et al., 1984; Mazzoni et al., 1985). These drugs should therefore be avoided in patients with reduced intracranial compliance, unless the dura is open or ICP is monitored. Indirect-acting antihypertensives, including trimethaphan (a ganglionic blocker), propranolol and esmolol (β-adrenergic blockers), and labetalol (a combined α/β-blocker), do not increase CBF or ICP (Magness et al., 1973; Turner et al., 1977; VonAken et al., 1982; McDowall, 1985). These agents are useful for the control of blood pressure in patients with elevated ICP. Trimethaphan may interfere with the neurologic examination by causing mydriasis, cycloplegia, or anisocoria.

Sodium nitroprusside lowers the range of cerebral autoregulation. Brain-surface oxygen tension is greater (Maekawa et al., 1979) and metabolic disturbances in brain biochemistry (e.g., lactate, pyruvate, and phosphocreatine levels) are less during nitroprusside-induced hypotension than with trimethaphan-induced or hemorrhage-induced hypotension (Michenfelder and Theye, 1977). In addition, cortical blood flow and electrical activity are better preserved at lower MAP with sodium nitroprusside (Ishikawa and McDowall, 1980). Nitroprusside, however, induces more pronounced blood-brain barrier dysfunction than does trimethaphan (Ishikawa et al., 1983). Because CBF, brain oxygen tension, neuronal function, and brain metabolism are better maintained with sodium nitroprusside than with trimethaphan at a MAP of 50 mm Hg, sodium nitroprusside is the preferred agent for deliberate hypotension.

PRINCIPLES OF PEDIATRIC NEUROANESTHESIA

PREOPERATIVE EVALUATION

The preoperative evaluation of the pediatric patient is discussed in Chapter 8, Preoperative Preparation. The general principles of preoperative assessment of children should be applied to the child with neurosurgical disease. In addition to these basic issues, the assessment and documentation of neurologic impairment and risk of intraoperative complications must be addressed. Of central importance in the preoperative assessment is for the anesthesiologist to determine whether elevated ICP is present, to assess whether a risk exists for regurgitation and aspiration, and to anticipate what surgical positioning will be required and to know its impact on anesthetic management.

The medical history may provide evidence of reduced intracranial compliance or elevated ICP. A history of headaches, especially postural headaches that are worse in a recumbent position or in the morning, is highly suggestive of intracranial hypertension. Although the child who is less than 3 years of age is not able to communicate the existence of headache, the parents frequently describe irritability, which suggests that headache may exist. Feeding intolerance or vomiting, especially in the morning and without attendant nausea, is also evidence of intracranial hypertension and should lead the anesthesiologist to check the serum electrolyte and blood urea nitrogen levels preoperatively. A history of protracted vomiting may also suggest that a significant risk of aspiration exists during the anesthetic induction and should prompt an appropriate modification of the induction technique (discussed later in this chapter). Table 18–2 outlines

TABLE 18–2. Signs of intracranial hypertension in infants and children

Infants	Children	Infants and Children
Irritability	Headache	Decreased consciousness
Full fontanel	Diplopia	Cranial nerve (III and VI) palsies
Widely separated cranial sutures	Papilledema	Loss of upward gaze (setting sun sign)
Cranial enlargement	Vomiting	Signs of herniation, Cushing's triad, pupillary changes

the clinical signs associated with intracranial hypertension in infants and children.

The preoperative history should also include medications, which frequently include anticonvulsant agents and steroids. In patients taking steroids, intraoperative and postoperative steroid administration is necessary both to treat cerebral edema and as replacement therapy for adrenal axis suppression.

The physical examination includes an assessment of the patient's airway, cardiovascular status, state of hydration, and neurologic status including an age-specific Glasgow Coma Scale (GCS) score (Table 18–3) (Reilly et al., 1988; Tatman et al., 1997), if consciousness is obtunded. If a cardiac murmur is detected during auscultation of the heart in a patient for whom a suboccipital craniotomy in the sitting position is planned, a formal cardiologic evaluation is indicated to rule out the existence of intracardiac shunting, which might lead to paradoxical air embolism (discussed later in this chapter), therefore relatively contraindicating use of the sitting position. Indeed, because approximately 20% to 25% of children without heart murmurs have a patent foramen ovale that would permit paradoxical air embolism in the event of a VAE (Schwarz et al., 1994; Fuchs et al., 1998), a cogent argument could be made for routine echocardiographic evaluation of all children in whom sitting craniotomies are planned to identify those individuals who should not be operated on in the sitting position (Fuchs et al., 1998).

The presence of intracranial hypertension may be deduced from the history, but when the medical history is brief, as in the case of head trauma, the existence of intracranial hypertension is sometimes more difficult to assess. The GCS (see Table 18–3) is very useful in the acute setting; a coma score of less than 6 in adults suggests the presence of acute intracranial hypertension (Bruce et al., 1977), and the GCS on presentation is well correlated with clinical outcome (Reilly et al., 1988; Grewal and Sutcliffe, 1991; Ong et al., 1996; Servadei et al., 1998; Coughlan et al., 2003) and the intraoperative development of a coagulopathy in children (Keller et al., 2001). In general, a patient who is comatose and has an abnormal response (decorticate posturing, decerebrate posturing, or flaccidity) to a painful stimulus (such as squeezing a digit) probably has elevated ICP, whereas the child who withdraws appropriately from a painful stimulus or who has a higher response to pain, such as eye opening, probably does not have elevated ICP at that time.

The elements of Cushing's triad—hyperventilation, bradycardia, and hypertension—are late sequelae of intracranial hypertension and portend impending cerebral herniation. Other late signs of intracranial hypertension associated with herniation syndromes include pupillary asymmetry; pupillary dilation or eccentricity; cranial nerve palsies, particularly third and sixth nerve paralysis; irregular respirations, particularly Cheyne-Stokes respirations; and hypotension (Bell and McCormick, 1978). These findings indicate a premortal condition and require immediate

■ TABLE 18–3. The Glasgow Coma Scale and Pediatric Glasgow Coma Scale

Glasgow Coma Scale (3 to 15 possible points)		
Best Motor Response		
6	Obeys commands	
5	Localizes pain	
4	Withdraws from pain	
3	Abnormal flexion	
2	Abnormal extension	
1	Flaccid	
Best Verbal Response		
5	Oriented	
4	Confused	
3	Inappropriate	
2	Incomprehensible	
1	None	
Eye Opening		
4	Spontaneous eye opening	
3	Opens eyes to voices	
2	Opens eyes to pain	
1	None	
Pediatric Glasgow Coma Scale (3 to 15 possible points) (Tatman et al., 1997)		
Best Motor Response	**>5 years**	**<5 years**
6	Obeys commands	Normal spontaneous movements
5	Localizes supraorbital pain	Withdraws to touch
4	Withdraws from nail bed pain	
3	Flexion to supraorbital pain	
2	Extension to supraorbital pain	
1	None	
Best Verbal Response	**>5 years**	**<5 years**
5	Oriented	Alert, babbles, coos, words to usual ability
4	Confused	Less than usual ability, irritable cry
3	Inappropriate words	Cries to pain
2	Incomprehensible sounds	Moans to pain
1	No response to pain	
T	Intubated	
Eye Opening		
4	Spontaneous	
3	To voices	
2	To pain	
1	None	
C	Closed (swelling, dressing)	

Pain should be made by pressing hard on the supraorbital notch (beneath medial end of eyebrow) with your thumb, except for M4, which is tested by pressing hard on the flat nail surface with the barrel of a pencil.

and decisive therapy, including endotracheal intubation and hyperventilation and the intravenous infusion of mannitol.

The remainder of the neurologic examination includes the assessment of cranial nerve function, peripheral tone and strength, deep tendon reflexes, plantar reflexes, and coordination. If a hemiparesis is present, it should be noted. The anesthesiologist need not perform a highly detailed neurologic examination, a task left for the attending neurosurgeon and the neurologist, but should focus on the neurologic functions important in planning the anesthetic management and postoperative care.

The laboratory studies of the neurosurgical patient include determination of the hematocrit and serum electrolyte levels, the latter to identify abnormalities of serum sodium and potassium associated with vomiting and dehydration, mannitol, or diuretic therapy or to detect the syndrome of inappropriate secretion of antidiuretic hormone, which may complicate intracranial pathology (see Chapter 4, Regulation of Body Fluids and Electrolytes). A blood sample should be sent to the blood bank for typing and cross-matching. Additional studies, such as an electrocardiogram, an echocardiogram, a coagulation profile, renal or hepatic function studies, blood gas analysis, or radiographic studies, may be indicated as well. Patients with suprasellar tumors such as craniopharyngiomas frequently have pituitary dysfunction and therefore should have a complete endocrine evaluation, including thyroid and adrenal function studies. Adrenal or thyroid replacement therapy can then be prescribed as indicated from the results of the studies.

■ PREMEDICATION

Premedication is often withheld from children undergoing neurosurgery. Sedatives and opioids should never be administered to an unobserved and unmonitored patient with elevated ICP, hypotonia, or central nervous system depression. Premedication in such patients may produce airway obstruction or respiratory depression and hypercapnia, with subsequent elevation of ICP. On the other hand, premedication, with a benzodiazepine such as midazolam, of children with diminished intracranial compliance is not associated with respiratory depression and eliminates anxiety and crying with their attendant cardiovascular changes, which themselves elevate ICP.

Children with intracranial aneurysms or arteriovenous malformations, who do not have increased ICP and who are at risk for intracranial bleeding if arterial hypertension occurs, should be sedated before transport to the operating room. Various premedications that may be used are discussed in Chapter 8, Preoperative Preparation. In older children with vascular malformations, preoperative β-adrenergic blockade with oral propranolol the night before and the morning of surgery helps to prevent tachycardia and hypertension during induction of anesthesia and laryngoscopy and is a useful adjunct when controlled hypotension is used. A total oral propranolol dose of 1 mg/kg divided into three or four doses at 6-hour intervals is usually effective. Alternatively, rapid intravenous β-blockade can be achieved before the induction of anesthesia with an intravenous infusion of esmolol (500-mcg/kg bolus followed by 50 to 200 mcg/kg per min). Although it is a drug to be avoided in patients with reduced intracranial compliance, intramuscularly delivered ketamine can be considered in patients who have no intravenous access, who will not tolerate an oral premedication, and who will benefit from premedication.

■ INDUCTION OF ANESTHESIA

Induction of general anesthesia should be planned to minimize the risk of inducing sustained, life-threatening intracranial hypertension. As a rule, acute neurosurgical patients have increased ICP and are at risk for gastric aspiration; they should have an intravenous cannula inserted preoperatively. Anesthesia in these children should be induced with an intravenous agent to minimize the risk of aspiration. Induction with a short-acting barbiturate or propofol and a muscle relaxant diminishes ICP and allows the anesthesiologist to induce hyperventilation early in the beginning of anesthesia. It usually is not feasible preoperatively to insert devices to monitor ICP using local anesthesia in children. Thus, ICP usually cannot be monitored before anesthetic induction.

If ICP is believed to be severely elevated, adjunctive measures should be instituted before induction. These include treatment with mannitol (0.25 to 0.5 g/kg) (Marshall et al., 1978) or with potent loop diuretics (furosemide, 0.25 to 1.0 mg/kg), steroid therapy in children with cerebral neoplasms (dexamethasone, 0.5 mg/kg), and drainage of CSF when possible in children with an indwelling ventriculoperitoneal or ventriculoatrial shunt (discussed later in this chapter).

Propofol (2 to 4 mg/kg) is also for induction of anesthesia. Sodium thiopental (4 to 7 mg/kg), sodium thiamylal (4 to 7 mg/kg), and methohexital (2 to 3 mg/kg) are short-acting barbiturates that are also appropriate for intravenous induction, and each markedly lowers ICP. Ketamine has no rational use as an induction agent in neurosurgical anesthesia (see earlier discussion).

It is not rare in the practice of pediatric anesthesia to have difficulty in establishing preoperative venous access. Occasionally, vascular access is extraordinarily difficult, and attempts to place an intravenous catheter result only in further crying and struggling, thereby exacerbating ICP. If no clinical deterioration ensues (that is, the child is still conscious), the intracranial compliance is probably adequate to allow modification of the anesthetic technique.

In the situation described, two alternatives exist. The first is to induce sleep with barbiturates administered by rectum. Thiopental (20 to 25 mg/kg as a 10% solution) may be used (see Chapter 10, Induction of Anesthesia). After about 5 to 10 minutes, when the child is well sedated, a vein is cannulated with the use of a subcutaneous infiltration of lidocaine or the preapplication of local anesthetic cream (EMLA [lidocaine/prilocaine] or Lidoderm [lidocaine]). Induction of general anesthesia then may proceed, with the rectal barbiturate augmented with an intravenous induction dose of propofol or barbiturate before relaxation and laryngoscopy.

The second alternative is to perform an inhalation induction. While there are some theoretical reasons why isoflurane may be preferable to sevoflurane or halothane as a neuroanesthetic (see earlier discussion), there is little question that inhalation inductions usually proceed more smoothly with sevoflurane or halothane, and the advantages of isoflurane are meager against the deleterious effects on ICP of coughing, breath holding, laryngospasm, and subsequent hypercapnia. These effects are more likely to occur during isoflurane inhalation inductions than during sevoflurane or halothane inductions. When consciousness is lost, ventilation should be controlled by the anesthesiologist, with hyperventilation initiated. The end-tidal concentration of the halogenated agent should not exceed 1 MAC, to minimize the risk of inducing intracranial hypertension. After intravenous access is secured, the anesthetic technique may be changed to a more conventional propofol/barbiturate–nitrous oxide–opioid–relaxant neuroanesthetic.

Neuromuscular blocking agents usually are administered to facilitate laryngoscopy and endotracheal intubation. If the planned procedure is a lengthy one and there is no concern of gastric aspiration, a nondepolarizing relaxant may be administered. Because histamine release transiently dilates the cerebral vasculature and elevates ICP, while simultaneously depressing systemic arterial pressure and CPP, drugs that do not release histamine are preferable. Vecuronium or pancuronium (0.08 to 0.15 mg/kg) and rocuronium (0.8 to 1.5 mg/kg) are nondepolarizing muscle relaxants that cause no histamine release.

When a significant risk of gastric aspiration exists, the most rapid intubation of the trachea possible is desirable. Succinylcholine may be used in this circumstance. Although succinylcholine may elevate ICP in patients with diminished intracranial compliance (Minton et al., 1985), the elevation of ICP is usually small, transient, and overshadowed by the clear adverse effects on ICP of retching, coughing, aspiration, and hypoventilation, which may occur with a more prolonged induction (Marsh et al., 1980). An alternative to the use of succinylcholine is high-dose rocuronium. At doses of 0.8 mg/kg, intubating conditions can be achieved in less than 1 minute (see Chapter 6, Pharmacology of Pediatric Anesthesia) and results in satisfactory conditions for intubation in about 1 minute. The duration of neuromuscular blockade after this dose is about 1 hour (Lennon et al., 1986).

Laryngoscopy is a potent stimulant and nearly always results in systemic and intracranial hypertension if anesthetic depth is inadequate (Moss et al., 1978b). Adjuvant drugs useful to blunt this response after induction of anesthesia are the rapid-acting opioid fentanyl (1 to 5 mcg/kg), sufentanil (0.2 to 1 mcg/kg), alfentanil (10 to 50 mcg/kg), and remifentanil (1 mcg/kg), or lidocaine (1.5 mg/kg), given intravenously 1 or 2 minutes before laryngoscopy (Bedford et al., 1980; Namill et al., 1981).

When a risk of aspiration exists, a modification of the rapid sequence induction technique is indicated. This modification calls for intravenous induction with propofol or thiopental, and a neuromuscular blocking drug, which may be either succinylcholine (preceded by a defasciculating drug), rocuronium, or high-dose vecuronium. Immediately after consciousness is lost, the patient is gently hyperventilated with oxygen while cricoid pressure is applied by the assistant. In so doing, ICP may be controlled while complete neuromuscular blockade and good conditions for intubation are awaited.

POSITIONING OF THE PATIENT

Certain considerations are common to all positions of the patient used during neurosurgery. If neurosurgery is known for one characteristic, it is its lengthy duration. This feature requires the anesthesiologist to carefully pad bony prominences such as the condyles of the elbows, the sacrum, and the ankles; to ensure that the limbs are in neutral positions; and to avoid stretching or compressing peripheral nerves. Eyes should be lubricated with a wetting agent or an antibiotic ointment to prevent corneal injury and should be carefully taped shut or padded. Urinary catheters are advisable for long surgical procedures to prevent bladder distention and to aid in fluid management.

As for most other pediatric surgical procedures, positioning a child for neurosurgery presents certain challenges. Although patients frequently disappear under surgical drapes and equipment, the anesthesiologist must make efforts to guarantee an unobstructed view of part of the patient, to have access to an extremity in case additional vascular catheters are needed, and, most important, to have access to the patient's airway and the anesthesia circuit in order to permit visual inspection of the airway and intermittent suctioning of the trachea. These goals may be achieved by suspending the drapes on bars or by tunneling the drapes.

Supratentorial procedures (such as parietal craniotomy or placement of a ventriculoperitoneal shunt) are generally performed with the patient lying supine and the head turned to one side. The anesthesiologist should secure the endotracheal tube to the nondependent side of the mouth to prevent oral secretions from loosening the adhesive tape used to fasten the endotracheal tube.

The prone position is used in pediatric neurosurgery for spine surgery and encephalocele repair and by some neurosurgeons for suboccipital craniotomy. In establishing the prone position, it is important to ensure that the patient's weight does not rest on the abdomen but rather is supported by bolsters under the pelvis and chest. Excessive abdominal pressure impedes ventilation of the lungs and leads to compression of the inferior vena cava and distention of the epidural venous plexus, either of which may increase surgical blood loss during spinal surgery. Flexion of the neck in the prone position can change the position of the endotracheal tube and cause intubation of a main stem bronchus.

In children older than about 4 years, explorations of the posterior fossa frequently are performed with the child in the sitting or semisitting position, to minimize intraoperative bleeding and tissue swelling and to facilitate surgical exposure. In younger children, these procedures are done with the child lying prone. Positioning in either the prone or the sitting position requires extreme flexion of the neck to expose the suboccipital skull, which frequently leads to intraoral kinking of the endotracheal tube. The use of armored endotracheal tubes minimizes this problem. Extreme neck flexion may also compromise venous or lymphatic drainage from the tongue and result in postoperative macroglossia. For this reason, oropharyngeal airways should not be in place while the patient is positioned (Albin et al., 1976).

The sitting position for suboccipital craniotomy is still preferred by some neurosurgeons for several reasons. This position facilitates exposure and use of the operating microscope; places the head above the heart, which favors venous drainage away from the surgical field; and reduces blood loss and edema formation. Although the seated position is advantageous to the neurosurgeon, it presents the anesthesiologist with two problems. The first is that cardiovascular stability is impaired during general anesthesia, and movement of the patient from the supine to the sitting position frequently results in postural hypotension. This can be prevented by wrapping the lower extremities with elastic bandages to minimize venous pooling, using a nitrous oxide–propofol–opioid technique, or limiting halogenated inhalation agents to less than 1 MAC before positioning (Marshall et al., 1984). Then the patient can be positioned slowly, in stages, while the anesthesiologist carefully monitors the patient's hemodynamics. The second problem for the anesthesiologist is more difficult to solve—that is, the occurrence of VAE (Bedford, 1983).

INTRAOPERATIVE MONITORING

Routine monitors for all pediatric anesthesia include precordial or esophageal stethoscope, pulse oximeter, continuous electrocardiogram, temperature thermistor, and noninvasive and/or intra-arterial measurement of blood pressure. Capnography for measurement of end-tidal CO_2 tension provides confirmation of endotracheal intubation, continuous monitoring of the patency of the breathing circuit, and a reliable trend monitor for guidance of hyperventilation of the neurosurgical patient.

Surgery within the cranial cavity, surgery expected to result in significant blood loss (loss of 20% of the estimated blood volume), or surgery with the potential for rapid blood loss (loss of 10% of the estimated blood volume in less than 15 minutes) requires the use of an arterial cannula to permit continuous monitoring of arterial blood pressure and episodic determination of arterial blood gases, electrolytes, hematocrit, etc.

Central venous cannulation via the internal jugular, external jugular, subclavian, or femoral vein is indicated for a craniotomy in the sitting position to permit aspiration of air from the right atrium and for other procedures in which major blood loss is anticipated. The use of the internal jugular vein is typically avoided in children with established, or at risk for, intracranial hypertension because of the potential to compromise cerebral venous drainage and further elevate ICP. Alternative sites are the external jugular, subclavian, and femoral veins.

Air can be successfully aspirated from central venous cannulas in 33% of episodes of VAE in children (Cucchiara and Bowers, 1982). Multiorifice central venous catheters specifically engineered for maximal aspiration of air, when properly positioned at the junction of the right atrium and superior vena cava, are used during sitting craniotomies in adults. These catheters are not commercially available in pediatric sizes or lengths, and their usefulness has not been demonstrated in pediatric neuroanesthesia.

Venous Air Embolism

Veins are thin-walled structures that collapse when incised if their pressure is subatmospheric. However, diploic veins, which bridge the scalp and the dura, are tethered open by bony connections in the skull and do not collapse when incised. The dural sinuses of the brain are also tethered open by dural and bony connections.

In the sitting position, there is a significant hydrostatic gradient between the head and the heart, and air may enter these open vessels. Venous air travels first to the heart and then to the lungs. Small amounts of air result in no physiologic change as long as there is no anatomic cardiac shunt (see later). Larger amounts of air become trapped in the lungs and result in pulmonary embolism: increased alveolar dead space and subsequent retention of CO_2, ventilation–perfusion mismatch and hypoxemia, and pulmonary hypertension (Adornato et al., 1978). Still larger amounts of venous air may become air-locked in the superior vena cava (Martin et al., 1984) or at the junction of the superior vena cava and the right atrium (Bunegin et al. 1981; Cucchiara et al., 1985), reduce cardiac output and blood pressure, and, in the extreme, produce pulseless electrical activity and cardiac arrest.

In the sitting position, the incidence of Doppler-detectable VAE in adults during craniotomies ranges from 20% to 40%, and roughly 40% of detectable air emboli are associated with hypotension (Michenfelder et al., 1972; Bithal et al., 2003). In children, the incidence of Doppler-detectable air emboli is about the same as in adults (Cucchiara and Bowers, 1982; Bithal et al., 2004), whereas VAE sufficient to decrease pulmonary blood flow and end-tidal CO_2 occurs in about 9% of cases, of which 21% are associated with hypotension (Harrison et al., 2002). In a pediatric patient, because a child's head makes up a greater surface area of the body, the incidence of VAEs during a craniotomy is at least the same (Cucchiara and Bowers, 1982; Bithal et al., 2004) or higher, approximately 66% to 80% (Soriano et al., 2002). In addition, in children, the frequency with which detectable air emboli are physiologically significant and produce hypotension may be much higher (Michenfelder et al., 1972).

The incidence of VAE during craniosynostosis repair in supine infants is as high as 67% to 83%, with hemodynamic changes occurring in one third of those in whom intravascular air is detected (Harris et al., 1987; Faberowski et al., 2000). The pediatric neuroanesthesiologist must monitor for venous air in children undergoing craniotomy in the sitting position, or craniosynostosis repair, and treat air entrainment promptly (see discussion of treatment of VAE later in this chapter).

If a cardiac shunt exists—that is, an atrial septal defect, a ventricular septal defect, a patent foramen ovale, or a patent ductus arteriosus, air may enter the left side of the heart and systemic circulation, embolizing vital organs (Perkins-Pearson et al., 1982; Albin et al., 1984; Mehta et al., 1984; Cucchiara et al., 1985; Soriano et al., 2002). This phenomenon is referred to as paradoxical air embolism (PAE) and, in the extreme, may result in cerebral or myocardial infarction. This may be likely if a significant bolus of venous air results in pulmonary arterial hypertension and elevation of right atrial pressure to levels exceeding left atrial pressure (Adornato et al., 1978; Perkins-Pearson et al., 1982). The sitting position is therefore relatively contraindicated when such an intracardiac septal defect is known to exist, unless the neurosurgeon has a compelling need to perform the surgery with the patient seated. Children with cardiac murmurs must be evaluated by echocardiography preoperatively to rule out septal defects. Routine preoperative contrast echocardiography before all sitting craniotomies in individuals with normal physical examinations is of unproved value in preventing PAE (Black et al., 1990).

A positive right-to-left atrial pressure gradient also may occur in the absence of a large air embolus; such a pressure gradient develops in many patients during prolonged anesthesia in the sitting position (Perkins-Pearson et al., 1982). This would allow even small volumes of air to move across a probe-patent foramen ovale into the systemic circulation. Because approximately 20% of the adult population have a probe-patent foramen ovale (Goss, 1973), the risk of PAE may be relatively great. This fact has prompted some to ask whether the sitting position for suboccipital craniotomy should not be abandoned altogether (Albin, 1984). Although this conclusion is not widely shared, certainly the risk of PAE mitigates against the sitting position if a septal defect is known to exist preoperatively.

VAE is not confined to neurosurgical procedures in the sitting position. It has been reported in children during craniosynostosis repair in either the supine (Harris et al., 1986, 1987; Phillips and Millikan, 1988) or the lateral (Joseph et al., 1985) position and in children undergoing posterior fossa explorations in the prone position (Meridy et al., 1974). It is, however, an unusual complication with these surgical positions and one that may be avoided by controlling ventilation, preventing negative intrathoracic pressure, maintaining adequate intravascular volume, and monitoring for venous air during craniosynostosis repair, particularly if a large osteotomy is anticipated (during craniofacial surgery, for example).

Air may enter the venous system slowly and insidiously, not altering physiology for a period of many minutes. On the contrary, although uncommon, air may enter rapidly in large volumes, producing immediate symptoms or even cardiac arrest if a large dural sinus has inadvertently been opened by the neurosurgeon. The goal of monitoring for VAE is to detect air entry well before physiologic changes occur, giving the anesthesiologist the time to inform the neurosurgeon early.

Several techniques and indicators may be used to detect VAE. In order of sensitivity and specificity (Fig. 18–2), they are transesophageal echocardiography (TEE), precordial Doppler ultrasonography, end-tidal capnography, end-tidal nitrogen detection, pulmonary artery pressure, central venous pressure, esophageal stethoscope, and measurement of systemic blood pressure (Gildenberg et al., 1981; Cucchiara et al., 1985; Black et al., 1990).

Of the various techniques for monitoring VAE, central venous pressure measurement, the esophageal stethoscope, and systemic blood pressure measurement cannot detect venous air until clinical deterioration is well established (Adornato et al., 1978). According to Bithal and others (2004), of 96 children scheduled to undergo a posterior craniotomy, capnometry detected 22% of air emboli (decrease in CO_2 tension of >0.7 kPa) and hypotension occurred in 33% of children (>20% change from baseline). Hence, more sensitive monitoring is required to detect smaller amounts of venous air before continuing embolization reaches physiologic significance.

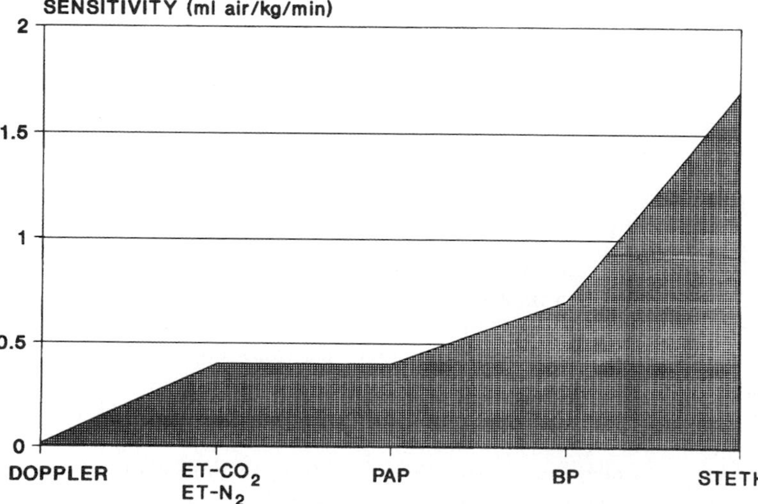

■ **FIGURE 18–2.** Relative sensitivities of different methods of monitoring for venous air embolism. The precordial Doppler is approximately 40 times more sensitive than the capnograph or pulmonary artery catheter in detecting vascular air. It will detect 1/100th of the amount of air associated with a change in blood pressure. (Data from Gildenberg PL, O'Brien RP, Britt WJ, et al.: *J Neurosurg* 54:75, 1981.)

Transesophageal echocardiography (TEE) has come into favor as the most sensitive, invasive, intraoperative instrument for detecting air emboli. In addition, it has the added benefit of identifying and localizing left atrial air.

In 1998, Mammoto and others (1998) described using TEE in 21 adult patients undergoing craniotomies in the sitting position to detect venous and paradoxical air emboli. VAEs were detected in every patient, whereas paradoxical air emboli appeared in only three patients with the most severe VAEs causing a reduction in end-tidal CO_2 and an increase in pulmonary artery pressures. Although TEE may be an excellent monitor for such intraoperative complications, especially in children, anesthesiologists must be aware of the potential for even bigger hazards with the use of this probe.

Particularly in children less than 10 kg, the placement of the TEE probe may be difficult and high resistance may be met with its passage into the esophagus. The anesthesiologist must take care to use a pediatric probe, lubricated well, and must never force the probe against resistance, as children are prone to esophageal perforation. In addition, the TEE probe may cause difficulty with ventilation and maintenance of adequate tidal volumes in smaller infants. Thus, although highly sensitive, the use of a TEE probe to detect air emboli in children during neurosurgical procedures may not be optimum and, to date, has not become the standard of practice.

Doppler ultrasound is the most sensitive noninvasive monitoring technique; it can detect minute quantities of venous air (Edmonds-Seal and Maroon, 1969; Maroon et al., 1969; Edmonds-Seal et al., 1970; Michenfelder et al., 1972; Maroon and Albin, 1974). In fact, the introduction of Doppler ultrasound into clinical practice transformed the once-held notion that VAE was a rare and catastrophic event to the present understanding that VAE is a common phenomenon. The Doppler detector should be placed in the second to fourth intercostal space to the right of the sternum; placement over the right atrium should be confirmed by rapid injection of saline solution into a peripheral intravenous catheter or into a central venous catheter. For those patients placed in the prone position and at risk for VAE, the posterior Doppler probe placement between the right scapula and spine can be effective for infants weighing less than 6 kg (Soriano et al., 1994). Because of the nearly continuous use of electrocautery, the Doppler apparatus is of limited use when air is most likely to embolize, that is, during the surgeon's entry into the cranial cavity. A second monitor is therefore necessary, one that is not affected by electrical interference in the operating room and one that is less sensitive than the Doppler apparatus, the capnograph. When a significant volume of air embolizes to the pulmonary vascular bed, alveolar dead space is created and the end-tidal CO_2 level decreases. A sudden decline in end-tidal CO_2 level is highly suggestive of VAE. If, however, the decreasing end-tidal CO_2 concentration is accompanied by a decrease in arterial blood pressure, the diagnosis may be obscured, because a reduction in cardiac output of any cause may diminish end-tidal CO_2 tension. If the anesthesiologist remains cognizant of this limitation, capnography is a valuable adjunctive technique for monitoring VAE.

When air embolizes to the pulmonary vascular bed, the nitrogen within the air embolism is exhaled by the lungs and may be detectable as end-tidal nitrogen by exhaled gas analysis (Drummond et al., 1985; Matjasko et al., 1985). The appearance of nitrogen in the end-tidal gases in association with decreasing end-tidal CO_2 tension is virtually pathognomonic of VAE (Losee et al., 1982).

Some authors have recommended placement of a pulmonary artery catheter both to detect and to treat VAE in adults. This practice is not used in children for three reasons. Pulmonary artery pressure monitoring is no more sensitive than capnography for detecting air embolism, pulmonary artery catheters are associated with significant risk, and the proximal lumen of a pulmonary artery catheter is too small for effective and rapid aspiration of cardiac air. Artru (1992) compared the volume of air embolism recovery using a multiorifice catheter and a 7F pulmonary artery catheter; he found a more than fivefold increase in gas recovery using the former. One can readily see how the volume of gas recovery would be further diminished through a pediatric 5F pulmonary artery catheter. If, however, a pulmonary artery catheter is inserted for other indications, the anesthesiologist should consider placing an additional central venous catheter specifically to treat air embolism or use a multiorifice introducer sheath for pulmonary artery catheters (Bowdle and Artru, 1988) that extends to the superior vena cava–right atrial junction and obviates the need for an additional central catheter.

In summary, all patients undergoing surgery that is associated with a risk of VAE should be monitored using a device to detect the entry of venous air, in addition to capnography and end-tidal gas analysis. The pulmonary artery catheter should not be used routinely for this purpose. Consideration should be given to placing an appropriately positioned central venous catheter to allow aspiration of venous air as well as to guide fluid therapy.

Confirming Placement of a Central Venous Cannula

The ability to aspirate air from the right atrium of a patient who has had a VAE was first recognized in 1965 (Michenfelder et al., 1966). After initial reports of successful air aspiration from a central venous catheter, the decision to place the central venous catheter in the mid portion of the right atrium was made intuitively (Michenfelder et al., 1969). Later, Bunegin and others (1981) showed that in an in vitro model of air aspiration, air was more likely to become trapped at the junction of the superior vena cava and the right atrium, which in adults is 3 cm above the sinoatrial node. This observation was confirmed in vivo several years later with the use of two-dimensional echocardiography during craniotomies performed in the sitting position (Cucchiara et al., 1985). The ideal position for the tip of the central venous catheter is, therefore, the junction of the superior vena cava and the right atrium. Catheter placement may be confirmed in one of three ways.

The first method of confirming correct catheter placement is fluoroscopy or a chest radiograph, both readily available in the operating room. The second method is to attach the catheter (via a metal hub or a stopcock) to the V lead of an electrocardiograph during placement (Martin, 1970). When the catheter tip is at the level of the sinoatrial node, large P waves have a characteristic biphasic conformation (Fig. 18–3). The catheter may then be withdrawn 1 to 3 cm (depending on the patient's age and size) to the level of the vena caval–right atrial junction. For the catheter to conduct electrocardiographic currents, it must be filled with an electrolyte solution. The solution may be either hypertonic saline solution or 8.4% sodium bicarbonate; the latter is more readily available in the operating room suite (Colley and Artru, 1984). The third method is to use pressure waveform monitoring while inserting the central venous catheter.

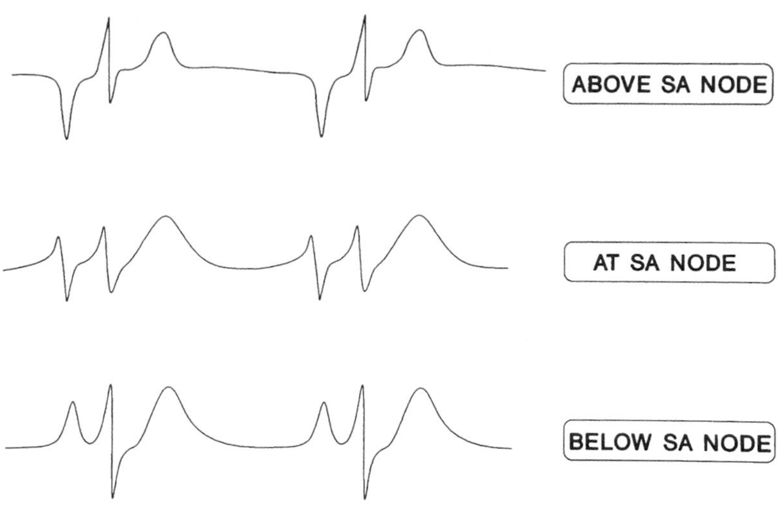

FIGURE 18–3. Continuous electrocardiographic monitoring of central venous catheter placement for craniotomy in the sitting position. The catheter is filled with hypertonic saline solution or 8.4% sodium bicarbonate and attached to a metal stopcock, which serves as the V lead of the electrocardiogram. When the catheter tip is above the sinoatrial (SA) node, the P wave has a negative deflection. When the catheter tip lies at the level of the SA node, the P wave is biphasic, with equal positive and negative voltages. When the catheter tip lies below the SA node, the P wave voltage is predominantly positive. In the adult, the correct position for the catheter tip is probably 1 to 3 cm above the SA node.

In this technique, the catheter is inserted until pressure monitoring demonstrates the tip to lie within the right ventricle. The catheter is withdrawn until the ventricular waveform disappears; then it is withdrawn an additional 4.3 cm in adult-sized patients. The catheter orifice then lies in the ideal position at the vena caval–right atrial junction (Mongan et al., 1992). Unfortunately, there are no data guiding this technique for pediatric patients.

Treatment of VAE

When a VAE is detected, treatment is initiated immediately; the treatment is tailored to the severity of the embolus. Figure 18–4 presents a treatment algorithm.

On detection of venous air, the surgeon is notified that air entrainment is occurring. The surgeon responds by identifying the points of air entry and sealing them or by flooding the surgical field with saline solution. Inspiratory hold after lung inflation (Valsalva maneuver) is useful both in preventing further air entry and in assisting the surgeon in identifying the source of air entry (Sharma and Tripathi, 1994). If the air embolus is physiologically significant, that is, it decreases end-tidal CO_2 or affects hemodynamics, nitrous oxide should be discontinued and the patient ventilated with 100% oxygen. Because nitrous oxide is less diffusible in blood than in gas, it diffuses into a pulmonary air embolus and enlarges its volume severalfold (Munson, 1971), causing further physiologic compromise (Mehta et al., 1984). Simultaneously, the anesthesiologist may compress the jugular veins under the surgical drapes to retard the rate of air entry into the central circulation until entry has been occluded. In cases of very severe VAE resulting in hypotension, the head of the operating table is lowered to increase venous return to the heart from the lower extremities, to decrease the rate of air entrainment, and to permit cardiopulmonary resuscitation in severe cases. When venous air is detected during a craniotomy performed in a sitting child, the success with which air may be aspirated varies from 38% to 60% (Cucchiara and Bowers, 1982).

Positive end-expiratory pressure (PEEP) is not indicated in the treatment of VAE. Theoretically, PEEP might decrease the rate of air entry by raising venous pressure but, in fact, Bedford and Perkins-Pearson (1982) found that PEEP (10 cm H_2O) did not elevate venous pressure sufficiently to stop air entry. It further impaired cardiac output and also raised right atrial pressures to levels exceeding left atrial pressures, thus potentially causing PAE in patients with patent foramen ovalae. The latter observation has been challenged by Pearl and Larson (1986), who demonstrated that PEEP (8 cm H_2O) did not increase right atrial pressures in excess of left atrial pressures in an animal model of VAE. Using a similar animal model, however, Toung and others (1988) found that PEEP (15 cm H_2O) did not raise cerebral venous pressure to above atmospheric pressure, whereas tourniquet compression of the veins of the neck did. The treatment of VAE, therefore, should include jugular compression but omit the use of PEEP. The possibility of PAE through an unsuspected patent foramen ovale mandates that aspiration of air be attempted during all episodes of air embolism. A central venous catheter should be placed in children undergoing a craniotomy in the sitting position.

After VAE has been treated, end-tidal CO_2 tension returns to baseline. At this point, nitrous oxide may be reintroduced if desired, whereas end-tidal CO_2 is carefully monitored for further changes. If the reintroduction of nitrous oxide causes end-tidal CO_2 to decrease, air persists in the pulmonary circulation, and

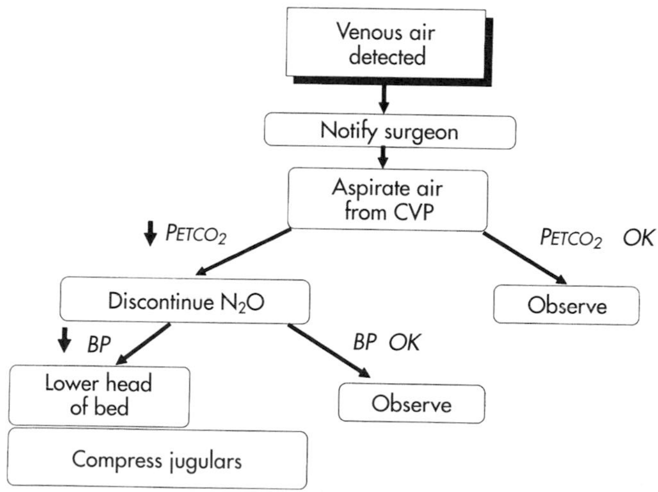

FIGURE 18–4. Decision algorithm for the management of venous air embolism during a craniotomy in the sitting position.

the nitrous oxide should be discontinued and an alternative anesthetic technique adopted (Shapiro et al., 1982).

NEUROPHYSIOLOGIC MONITORING

The purpose of neurophysiologic monitoring is to detect neurosurgical trauma or ischemia at a time at which neurologic injury is reversible, thus improving functional outcome. It is used in certain cases in which the risk of mechanical trauma to vital structures, or ischemia, is significant. When alterations in physiologic function occur, it alerts the neurosurgeon and anesthesiologist to alter the neurosurgical approach, or to restore hemodynamics (also see Chapter 9, Pediatric Anesthesia Equipment and Monitoring).

Although internationally accepted guidelines for intraoperative neurophysiologic monitoring (INM) are still far from being established, an article provides the following guidelines for such monitoring (Sala et al., 2002):

- INM is mandatory whenever neurologic complications are expected on a known pathophysiologic mechanism. INM should always be performed when any of the following are involved: supratentorial lesions in the central region and language-related cortex, brainstem tumors, intramedullary spinal cord tumors, conus-cauda equina tumors, rhizotomy for relief of spasticity, or spina bifida with tethered cord.
- Monitoring of motor evoked potentials (MEPs) is most appropriate to access functional integrity of descending motor pathways in the brainstem.
- Somatosensory evoked potential (SSEP) monitoring is of value in assessment of the functional integrity of sensory pathways leading to the sensory cortex.
- Monitoring of brainstem auditory evoked potentials remains a standard technique during surgery in the brainstem, cerebellopontine angle, and posterior fossa.
- Mapping of the motor nuclei of cranial nerves VII, IX, X, and XII on the floor of the fourth ventricle is valuable in identifying "safe entry zones" into the brainstem.

Electroencephalography

Electroencephalography is the most reliable intraoperative monitor for focal cerebral ischemia characterized by an attenuation of high-frequency activity and the appearance of slow delta waves (Soriano et al., 2002). In addition to monitoring the integrity of at-risk cerebral cortex, an intraoperative EEG is used to identify epileptiform foci for surgical excision. Cerebral hypoxia or ischemia causes the appearance of large-amplitude slow waves in the 1- to 4-Hz range in the regions affected. When electroencephalographic monitoring suggests the presence of ischemia, the cause must be identified and corrected, and differentiated from other benign sources of electroencephalographic changes such as increased anesthetic depth, hypocarbia, or hypothermia.

Somatosensory Evoked Potentials

SSEP monitoring is used most commonly during surgery on the spine, but it is also used during neurosurgery around the foramen magnum, or brainstem. During SSEP monitoring, electrical stimulation is made to the median or ulnar nerves at the wrists and the common peroneal or posterior tibial nerves at the ankles. Evoked electrical potentials can be measured overlying the spinal cord and the cerebral cortex. SSEPs are dependent on intact large myelinated peripheral sensory fibers, the posterior (dorsal) columns of the spinal cord, and the spinothalamic track. An absence, decreased amplitude, or increased latency of evoked potentials is highly suggestive of neurologic compromise (Sala et al., 2002).

SSEPs are extremely sensitive to volatile anesthetics and nitrous oxide. Total intravenous anesthesia is generally associated with better preservation of SSEPs than are low-dose volatile anesthetic techniques. Hypothermia also degrades the quality of SSEPs. The application of SSEP monitoring and the effects of anesthetics on SSEP monitoring are discussed in greater detail in Chapter 9, Pediatric Anesthesia Equipment and Monitoring.

Motor Evoked Potentials

MEPs are a top-down monitoring method of measuring brainstem and spinal cord integrity, whereas SSEPs are a bottom-up system. In other words, in MEP monitoring, the motor strips of the cerebral cortex or the motor fibers of the spinal cord are electrically or magnetically stimulated, whereas the resultant motor nerve action potentials or muscle action potentials that occur distally are recorded. MEPs demonstrate the integrity of the descending/anterior columns of the spinal cord, whereas SSEPs primarily monitor the integrity of the ascending/dorsal columns (Sala et al., 2004).

MEPs are even more sensitive to anesthetic agents than are SSEPs, and, of course, motor action potentials would disappear altogether if neuromuscular blocking agents were to be used. Even low-dose volatile anesthesia can obliterate MEPs (Kalkman et al., 1991). The role of MEP monitoring in pediatric neurosurgery is as yet undefined, as is the ideal anesthetic technique. In adults, an anesthetic technique using ketamine, alfentanil, and etomidate preserves MEPs better than volatile agents, nitrous oxide, or propofol (Kalkman et al., 1994; Ubags et al., 1997; Sihle-Wissel et al., 2000).

Transcranial Doppler

Transcranial Doppler measurement of middle cerebral artery blood velocity and, by extension, estimation of CBF is a technique that remains experimental in its clinical neurosurgical application. It has been clinically used by one investigator in adult patients during clipping of cerebral aneurysms, but it has no routine use in pediatric neurosurgery at the present time. It does have utility, however, as an experimental tool for the determination of the effects of anesthetic agents and physiologic changes on CBF and has emerged in the last decade as the best noninvasive method for the estimation of CBF in humans.

Transcranial Cerebral Oximetry

In the future, near infrared spectroscopy (NIRS), which measures cerebral oxygenation through an adhesive probe attached to the forehead, may become customary for neurosurgical procedures. It is a very sensitive monitor for cerebrovascular changes and assesses oxygen delivery and extraction, as well as CBV and CBF (Soriano et al., 2002). At the present time, this monitoring technique is experimental.

SELECTION OF ANESTHETIC AGENTS

Infiltration of the scalp with lidocaine or bupivacaine by the neurosurgeon is a simple and very useful technique for blunting the hemodynamic response to incision and craniotomy and for reducing the anesthetic requirement (Hillman et al., 1987).

Although nitrous oxide is a mild stimulant of cerebral metabolism and blood flow (Theye and Michenfelder, 1968; Dahlgren et al., 1981; Fitzpatrick and Gilboe, 1982), its effects on cerebral hemodynamics are overshadowed by previous administration of thiobarbiturates and concomitant hyperventilation (Phirman and Shapiro, 1977). Nitrous oxide may be used safely in patients with intracranial hypertension. Nitrous oxide has two disadvantages during neurosurgery: its effect on VAE and its effect on pneumocephalus—both are discussed in previous sections.

The effects of halogenated anesthetic agents on cerebral metabolism, blood flow, and ICP were discussed earlier. Halogenated inhalation anesthetics increase CBF, CBV, and ICP in a dose-dependent fashion, an effect that may be blunted or avoided by hyperventilation of the patient during their administration. In cases of preoperative intracranial hypertension or intracranial mass lesions, however, halogenated agents generally should be withheld until the dura is open unless ICP is monitored, so that the cerebral hemodynamic response may be observed.

In this circumstance, most neuroanesthesiologists would choose an anesthetic technique combining propofol or a barbiturate, nitrous oxide, opioids, and a nondepolarizing muscle relaxant. Such a "balanced" anesthesia technique is also associated with more rapid awakening after prolonged procedures than is typically seen with halogenated anesthetics, allowing earlier neurologic assessment of the neurosurgical patient.

Thiobarbiturates or propofol is usually administered intermittently during balanced anesthesia, a practice that reduces cerebral metabolism and blood flow and decreases ICP. Fentanyl is a commonly chosen opioid for neurosurgery because no histamine release is associated with this drug. Fentanyl analgesia requires 5 to 10 mcg/kg and is maintained with 1 to 3 mcg/kg per hr, either by intermittent bolus administration or by continuous infusion. For lengthy neurosurgical procedures, remifentanil, alfentanil, and sufentanil lead to more rapid awakening because of the more rapid metabolism and smaller volumes of distribution of the drugs (Shafer and Varvel, 1991; Youngs and Shafer, 1994). Of these short-acting opioids, remifentanil confers no residual analgesia whatever within a few minutes of the termination of its infusion; it is imperative that the anesthesiologist administer a long-acting opioid analgesic when, or soon after, discontinuing a remifentanil infusion to avoid the sudden onset of severe surgical pain, hypertension, etc.

Nondepolarizing muscle relaxants that do not release histamine (e.g., rocuronium, pancuronium, and vecuronium) are preferred for neurosurgery.

Adjunctive measures to control intracranial hypertension during neurosurgery include hyperventilation to a $PaCO_2$ of approximately 30 mm Hg, administration of mannitol or diuretics to reduce brain volume, and control of arterial blood pressure. Cerebral autoregulation is usually impaired in the presence of cerebral pathology and is blunted further by inhalation anesthetics. CBF, therefore, may fluctuate with alteration of arterial blood pressure. Maintenance of normotension is important in preserving CBF and preventing increases in ICP.

Antihypertensives that act by direct vasodilation (hydralazine, adenosine, sodium nitroprusside, nitroglycerin, and nitric oxide) are potent cerebral vasodilators and increase both CBF and ICP. Preferable are indirect-acting antihypertensives (fenoldopam, propranolol, esmolol, and labetalol), which can control hypertension in neurosurgical patients without increasing ICP.

Controlled, or deliberate, hypotension is used in procedures associated with the risk of significant intraoperative hemorrhage, such as craniofacial surgery, and cerebrovascular surgery of arterial aneurysms and arteriovenous malformations. Deliberate hypotension is contraindicated in the presence of intracranial hypertension or diminished intracranial compliance. Because the lower limit of cerebral autoregulation in children is not known, the lower limit of acceptable blood pressure in children during deliberate hypotension is also not known. In the absence of data to guide clinical decisions, the adopted practice is to decrease MAP by no more than 30% to 40% below the "awake" baseline but no less than 40 mm Hg for infants younger than 6 months and 50 mm Hg for older children. Deliberate hypotension and its complications are discussed in greater detail in Chapter 12, Blood Conservation in Infants and Children.

TEMPERATURE REGULATION

The maintenance of normal body temperature in children, once very challenging for pediatric anesthesiologists, has become second nature with the use of forced hot air warming mattresses and blankets, in concert with warming lights, heated humidification of inspired gases, and adjustment of ambient room temperature (indeed, gone are the days of working in rooms warmed to near-tropical degrees to maintain the temperatures of small infants undergoing lengthy procedures). The maintenance of normothermia and the avoidance of both hypothermia and hyperthermia are discussed elsewhere in this text (see Chapter 5, Thermoregulation: Physiology and Perioperative Disturbances).

In neurosurgical procedures, the induction of mild to moderate hypothermia (32° to 35°C) is used for cerebral protection during procedures in which there is a risk of intraoperative cerebral ischemia. For every 1°C below normal body temperature, the cerebral metabolic rate of oxygen consumption decreases 7% (Rosomoff and Holaday, 1954), which increases the ability of the cerebral tissue to tolerate periods of ischemia, and therefore is thought to improve surgical outcome. Whereas this has been experimentally demonstrated in animal models, it has not been so demonstrated in the human neurosurgical patient, although mild hypothermia has been shown to improve outcome in head-injured patients (Gal et al., 2002).

Deliberate Hypothermia

Biagas and Gaeta (1998) proposed that hypothermia can attenuate injury due to inflammation, excitotoxic amino acids (glutamate), nitric oxide, and free radicals. Marion (2002) showed a significant decrease in CSF glutamate and interleukin-1β levels in patients with a depressed GCS score maintained between 32° and 33°C for 12 hours compared with those maintained with a similar GCS score at a normothermic state. In addition, studies have shown that hypothermia is more effective than barbiturate therapy in lowering ICP in pediatric patients refractory to conventional therapy (Hayashi, 2000). Hypothermia may help to control elevated ICP in children, but it fails to arrest progression of infarction, such as that from an acute, subdural hematoma in a child (Inamasu et al., 2002).

Deliberate hypothermia may be induced in the child by not using the usual warming devices, leaving the child undraped in a cold operating room after induction of anesthesia and while inserting vascular catheters, positioning, and draping, and by using a cooling mattress, until the target temperature is achieved. Endovascular cooling of the brain has been described and offers superior cerebral cooling and rewarming compared with whole body cooling (Steinberg et al., 2004). Rewarming is achieved by using forced hot air warming mattresses and blankets and by raising the ambient room temperature. It is of great importance to achieve adequate rewarming to greater than 36°C before emergence and awakening to avoid the vasoconstriction, hypertension, and shivering that would occur in an emerging hypothermic child, followed by the hemodynamic instability that would be seen with the vasodilatation that accompanies rewarming later during the recovery period. Maintenance of general anesthesia is best continued until body temperature is sufficient for the child to tolerate emergence and awakening.

Complications of hypothermia and its reversal must be understood by the anesthesiologist; these include coagulopathy, immunodeficiency, and hyperglycemia. Children develop a coagulopathy during hypothermia, until normothermia is restored. Severe immunodeficiency and secondary infections can arise. For example, Lo and others (2002) cited a case of pancytopenia postoperatively in an 8-year-old child who had undergone resection of a craniopharyngioma under hypothermia. This condition resolved on further rewarming in the intensive care unit.

Moreover, it is critical to lower a high glucose value because glucose quickly penetrates the blood-brain barrier and increases pyruvate and lactate by inhibiting the tricarboxylic acid (TCA) cycle metabolism (Hayashi, 2000). In addition, children, like adults, are more difficult to awaken from general anesthesia if they are not normothermic and neuromuscular blockade is more difficult to reverse under hypothermic conditions. Finally, residual hypothermia on emergence causes shivering, and this increases basal, metabolic oxygen consumption dramatically. If this occurs, small doses of intravenous meperidine (0.1 to 0.2 mg/kg) may be effective in inhibiting shivering.

FLUID MANAGEMENT

The management of fluids in the neurosurgical patient is a clinical challenge because blood loss is difficult to measure. Inadequate fluid replacement leads to cardiovascular instability, and overhydration with hypo-osmotic solutions increases cerebral edema. Furthermore, diuretics used to reduce brain bulk cause intravascular volume shifts with electrolyte disturbances.

Blood-Brain Barrier Effects

Fluid and solute flux across the cerebral circulation is restricted by the blood-brain barrier. The blood-brain barrier is formed by cerebral capillary endothelial cells connected by a continuous, tight intercellular junction. Because of this tight junction, the cerebral capillary markedly restricts passage of most polar, hydrophilic molecules, except those with a specific carrier-mediated transport system (for example, glucose, essential amino acids). Small, polar molecules such as water move rapidly across the blood-brain barrier, with a 3-minute half-time for equilibration (Bering, 1952). In contrast, ions such as sodium move more slowly across the blood-brain barrier (half-time for equilibration is 2 to 4 hours) (Bakay, 1960); larger hydrophilic molecules such as albumin and mannitol are excluded from the brain by an intact blood-brain barrier.

Water movement across the blood-brain barrier depends on the osmotic gradient between plasma and brain. Water is removed from the brain's interstitial space when plasma osmotic pressure is increased, as with administration of mannitol or hypertonic saline solution. Water may move into the relatively hyperosmolar brain with rapid correction of hyperosmolar states (uremia, hyperglycemia) and with hyponatremia. Intravenous administration of free water causes a marked and prolonged increase in CSF pressure (Weed and McKibben, 1916). Administration of 5% dextrose solution is similar to giving free water because the uptake and metabolism of glucose are so rapid.

The blood-brain barrier becomes disrupted with many types of brain injury, including head trauma, subarachnoid hemorrhage, stroke, brain tumors, hypertension, hypercapnia, status epilepticus, and sodium nitroprusside administration (Pollay and Roberts, 1980). Movement of water across the blood-brain barrier then becomes a function more of hydrostatic pressure gradients than of osmotic gradients. The permeability of sodium, albumin, and mannitol is increased markedly. Fortunately, in most types of brain injury, large areas of intact blood-brain barrier remain.

Fluid Therapy Administration

The traditional approach to fluid management in neurosurgical patients is to restrict fluid intake in an attempt to prevent cerebral edema and subsequent increases in ICP (Shenkin et al., 1976). Like all postsurgical patients, neurosurgical patients transiently retain water and sodium postoperatively because of increased aldosterone and antidiuretic hormone (ADH) secretion, which may lead to hyponatremia and intravascular volume overload. Hypervolemia may cause hypertension, and a rebound increase in ICP may occur after administration of mannitol. Although hypervolemia should be avoided, there is little evidence to support the benefits of fluid restriction in neurosurgical patients. Even severe water restriction is only modestly effective in reducing brain water content in animals (Jelsma and McQueen, 1967). Fluid restriction has several detrimental effects, including hypovolemia and hypotension, especially in response to anesthetic agents and positive-pressure ventilation, inadequate renal perfusion, electrolyte and acid-base disturbances, lability while using vasodilators for deliberate hypotension, hypoxemia, and undesired reductions in CBF. Reductions in cardiac output increase pulmonary shunting and may cause hypoxemia in the presence of regional lung disease (e.g., atelectasis, pneumonia, pulmonary contusion) (Cheney and Colley, 1980). Decreases in PaO_2 have been observed in neurosurgical patients who are hypovolemic from osmotic diuresis and excessive fluid restriction. Clinical experience has shown that PaO_2 increases dramatically with volume administration in these patients.

Colloid-containing solutions often have been used during neurosurgery because albumin is excluded from the extracellular fluid of the brain in the presence of an intact blood-brain barrier. Many clinicians believe that the administration of large amounts of crystalloid itself can cause cerebral edema. This belief was supported by a study that noted an increase in brain water content and ICP when lactated Ringer's solution, but not hydroxyethyl starch, was used for fluid replacement during isovolemic hemodilution of normal rabbits (Todd et al., 1984). These results later were ascribed to differences in osmolality, rather than the colloid osmotic pressures, of the two solutions (Zornow et al., 1987). Brain water content in normal rabbits does not differ when volume is replaced with isotonic lactated Ringer's solution or hydroxyethyl starch of the same osmolality. Moreover, in a study involving patients 1 to 38 months, Paul and others showed a larger decrease in hemoglobin levels postoperatively after 20 mL/kg of 6% hydroxyethyl starch (a synthetic colloid) compared with 20 mL/kg of lactated Ringer's solution (a crystalloid) (Paul et al., 2003). Such studies demonstrate the superiority of colloids for plasma expansion in children but do not analyze the effects on the brain.

In contrast, brain water is increased when intravascular volume is replaced with a hypo-osmotic colloid solution. Osmolality, rather than colloid osmotic pressure, determines water movement across the intact blood-brain barrier. In the presence of a disrupted blood-brain barrier induced experimentally by a cortical freeze injury, however, albumin therapy is associated with less cerebral edema than is iso-osmotic crystalloid therapy (Albright et al., 1984).

In summary, it is unclear whether the best solution for use in patients with brain injury is isotonic colloid or crystalloid. Proponents of colloid emphasize that with most intracranial lesions, large areas of the brain still have an intact blood-brain barrier. In addition, the effect on brain water of the greater volume of crystalloid needed to restore intravascular volume is unknown. Proponents of crystalloid hypothesize that colloid might increase cerebral edema by holding additional fluid in the damaged area when it crosses the disrupted blood-brain barrier.

Because of the uncertainties just described, there is no clear advantage to using colloid or isotonic crystalloid for routine fluid therapy in neurosurgical patients. Hypertonic saline solutions may have some use in the resuscitation of head-injured patients; their use, however, is still experimental in the neuro-surgical setting. Hypotonic solutions are not used during neurosurgery because they increase brain edema: 5% dextrose, 5% dextrose in 0.2% saline solution, and 5% dextrose in 0.45% saline solution are all functionally hypotonic despite the tonicity out of the bottle, because the glucose is rapidly metabolized and is also transported into the brain, with the net effect of the hypotonic electrolyte solution remaining; administration of these solutions increases brain water content.

Furthermore, several studies in animals have demonstrated that dextrose administration, with or without hyperglycemia, augments brain damage in global (Lanier et al., 1987) and regional (Pulsinelli et al., 1982) cerebral ischemia. Increased blood glucose also appears to enhance postischemic neurologic damage in humans (Pulsinelli et al., 1983). Dextrose administration increases brain glucose and anaerobic metabolism of glucose in the presence of ischemia increases lactic acid, which causes neurologic damage. Because decreased cerebral perfusion and brain ischemia may occur with retraction in any intracranial procedure, routine glucose administration is not used in patients undergoing craniotomy who are not at risk for hypoglycemia.

Acceptable isotonic fluids are lactated Ringer's solution, normal saline, or any of the commercially available multiple-electrolyte balanced salt solutions that are designed to emulate the plasma water composition (e.g., Normosol, Abbott Pharmaceuticals). Normal saline is probably the most common crystalloid administered during pediatric craniotomies as it is slightly hyperosmolar (308 mOsm/kg) compared with serum osmolarity (285 to 290 mOsm/L) and therefore helps to prevent cerebral edema. However, anesthesiologists must use caution; large quantities of normal saline produce a hyperchloremic metabolic acidosis and hypernatremia in children (Constable, 2003). Lactated Ringer's (273 mOsm/L), on the other hand, is slightly hypo-osmolar and large quantities of intravenous infusion can increase cerebral edema formation.

Diuretics

Mannitol

Mannitol decreases brain water content by about 1% to 2% by increasing plasma osmolality, which creates an osmotic gradient across the intact blood-brain barrier. The amount of water that can be withdrawn from the brain depends on the magnitude of the osmotic gradient and the integrity of the blood-brain barrier. Mannitol is less effective with larger lesions. With a damaged blood-brain barrier, the concentration gradient moves mannitol into the brain, and this may account for the rebound increase in ICP occasionally seen after mannitol administration.

Mannitol causes a triphasic hemodynamic response. Transient (1 to 2 minutes) hypotension may occur after rapid administration of mannitol because of vasodilation (Coté et al., 1979). Subsequently, blood volume, cardiac index, and pulmonary capillary wedge pressure increase, reaching a maximum shortly after the termination of infusion (Rudehill et al., 1983). ICP may increase transiently because of increases in CBV and CBF. By 30 minutes after mannitol, blood volume returns to normal after diuresis, and pulmonary capillary wedge pressure and cardiac index decrease to less than normal levels.

Mannitol decreases blood viscosity and red blood cell rigidity, which may enhance perfusion of the brain's microcirculation. Mannitol transiently reduces hematocrit, increases serum osmolality, and causes hyponatremia, hypochloremia, acidosis resulting from bicarbonate ion dilution, and hyperkalemia after large (2 g/kg) doses. Prolonged and marked hyperosmolality with hyponatremia can occur in patients with acute and chronic renal failure.

Mannitol is the most efficient therapy for normalization of elevated cerebral extraction of oxygen representing oligemic ischemia in the presence of an elevated ICP. Mannitol is usually given in doses from 0.25 to 1.0 g/kg, which raises serum osmolality by 10 to 20 mOsm/kg (Soriano et al., 1996). Lower doses reduce ICP acutely and cause fewer electrolyte abnormalities but must be given more frequently (Marshall et al., 1978). The benefits and disadvantages of speed of administration and dose need to be weighed carefully in each patient.

Furosemide

Furosemide has been reported to lower ICP and brain water content when used alone in large (1 mg/kg) doses (Cottrell et al., 1977) or combined with mannitol in smaller doses (Pollay et al., 1983; Roberts et al., 1987). In contrast to mannitol, however, furosemide has been shown by some studies in normal and damaged brains to have little effect on ICP (Roberts et al., 1987). Furosemide may be preferred to mannitol in patients with cardiac or renal disease because it does not increase blood volume or ICP, nor does it cause electrolyte abnormalities as severe as those caused by mannitol. In large doses, furosemide reduces CSF formation and may reduce water and ion penetration across the blood-brain barrier (Pollay et al., 1983). Furosemide prolongs the effectiveness of mannitol by sustaining the induced increase in serum osmolality. Reductions in ICP and brain volume are consistently greater and last longer with mannitol plus furosemide than with either agent alone. However, hyponatremia, hypokalemia, hypochloremia, hyperosmolality, and a significantly greater rate of water and electrolyte excretion occur with the combination of diuretics.

ANESTHETIC MANAGEMENT FOR NEUROSURGICAL PROCEDURES

THE NEWBORN

Myelodysplasia

Myelodysplasia is a congenital failure of the neural tube to close, a process that normally occurs by 28 days' gestation. In its most common form, fusion fails in the middle or caudal neural groove, resulting in thoracic or lumbosacral meningomyelocele. When the site of failure is more cephalad, encephaloceles result. Anencephaly represents a defect in anterior closure of the neural groove. Figure 18–5 illustrates a newborn infant with a lumbosacral meningomyelocele with a partially epithelialized neural sac and exposed neuroplaque. With a meningomyelocele, the defective neural tissue is in open communication with the environment. Neurologic function very frequently is severely impaired distal to the defect. An encephalocele is a similar phenomenon usually involving the occipital skull and upper cervical spine (Fig. 18–6).

After closure of the neural tube, mesodermal and ectodermal structures complete the formation of the spinal column, skeletal muscles, and skin of the back. A defect in this process may result in herniation of dural elements posteriorly during morphogenesis, producing a meningocele (Fig. 18–7), which, unlike a meningomyelocele, contains no neural tissue. Although neurologic function is normal in children with meningoceles, the spinal cord is often tethered caudally by the sacral nerve roots. The tethered cord results in orthopedic or urologic symptoms in later childhood if it is not surgically corrected.

Congenital lesions of the central nervous system, unlike other types of congenital anomalies such as omphaloceles, are generally not associated with other anomalies or congenital heart disease; therefore, routine preoperative screening need not include a cardiologic evaluation. Most children with meningomyelocele also have an associated Arnold-Chiari malformation (see discussion later in this chapter), and hydrocephalus ultimately develops, necessitating a CSF shunt. The Chiari malformations involve the hindbrain and are classified into four types. Three of the four types involve hindbrain herniation, and the fourth type consists of cerebellar hypoplasia or aplasia (Box 18–1).

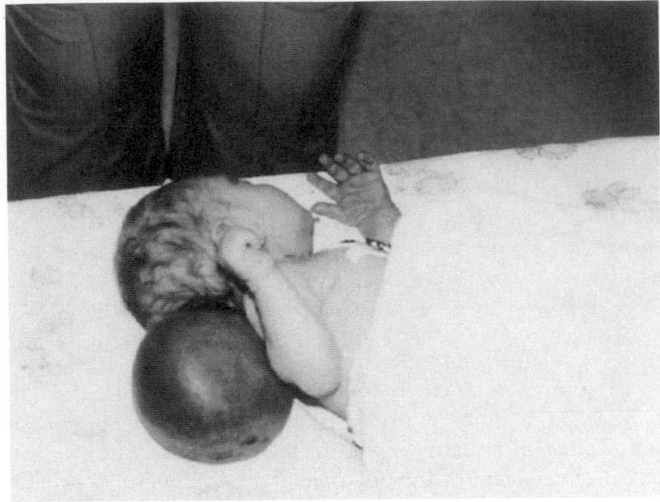

FIGURE 18–6. A newborn infant with an occipital encephalocele. Neurologic function was intact. The anesthesiologist's primary challenge is to control and intubate the airway in the lateral position to avoid traumatizing the lesion.

Anesthetic Considerations

Meningoceles and myelomeningoceles usually are repaired within the first day of life to minimize bacterial contamination of the exposed spinal cord and subsequent sepsis, which is the most common cause of death in this population. The anesthetic considerations relate to the concerns of anesthesia for newborns (described in Chapter 16, Anesthesia for Neonates and Premature Infants) and management of the airway.

As Figures 18–6 and 18–7 illustrate, intubation of the trachea may pose a challenge to the anesthesiologist. Endotracheal intubation may be performed with the infant in the left lateral

A

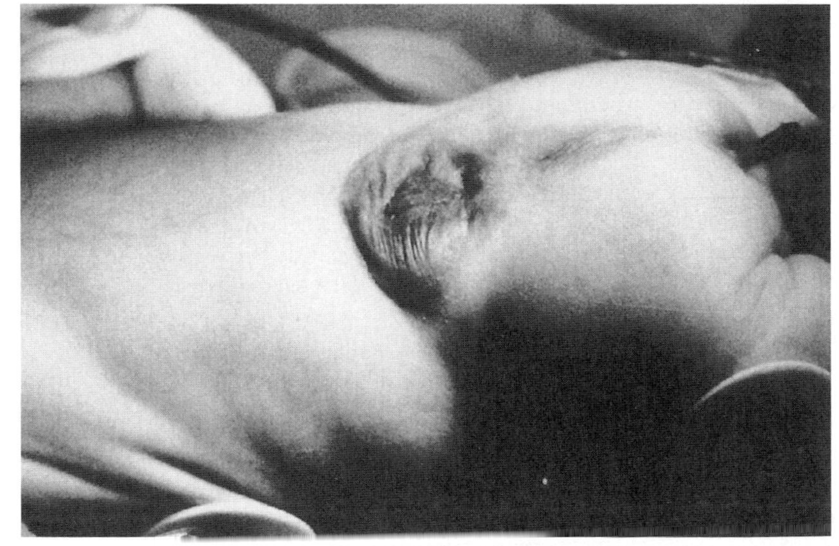

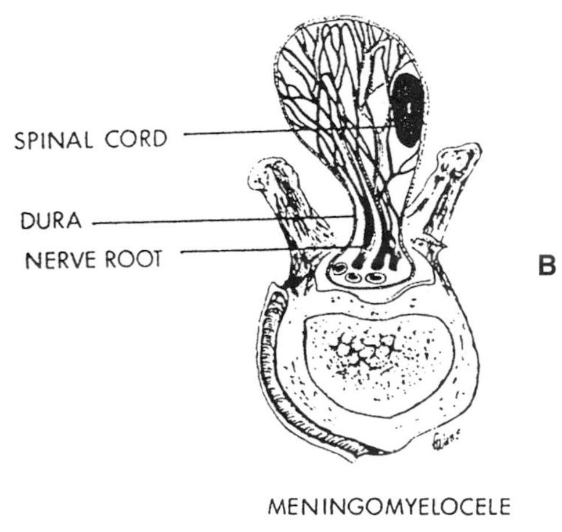

B

FIGURE 18–5. *A,* Newborn infant with a lumbosacral meningomyelocele. Note the partial epithelialization of the neural tissue, which is exposed to air centrally. Neurologic function was severely impaired distal to the defect. *B,* Schematic of meningomyelocele. (*B* from Carter S, Gold AP: Nervous system. In Rudolph AM, Barnett HL, Einhorn AH, editors: *Pediatrics,* 16th ed. Norwalk, CT, 1977, Appleton-Century-Crofts. Copyright © 1977 The McGraw-Hill Companies, Inc.)

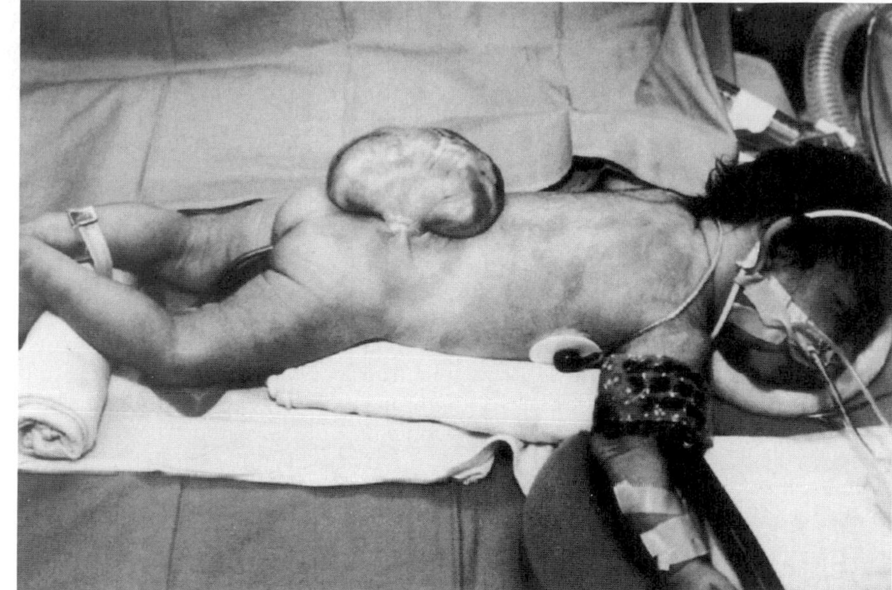

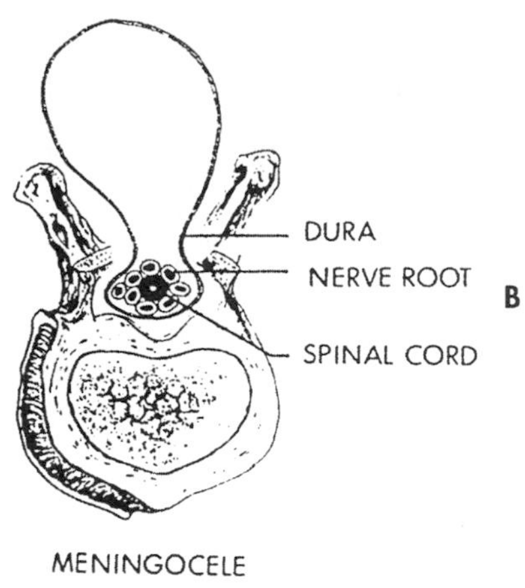

■ **FIGURE 18–7.** *A,* Newborn infant with a lumbar meningocele. No neural elements were within the sac, and neurologic function was normal distal to the lesion. *B,* Schematic of meningocele. (*B* from Carter S, Gold AP: Nervous system. In Rudolph AM, Barnett HL, Einhorn AH, editors: *Pediatrics,* 16th ed. Norwalk, CT, 1977, Appleton-Century-Crofts. Copyright © 1977 The McGraw-Hill Companies, Inc.)

decubitus position, with the head held in the midline by an assistant, or in the supine position, with the weight supported on the pelvis and portions of the spine not involved with the defect. An assistant must be available to ensure that no physical trauma to the neuroplaque occurs. In newborns in which a difficult airway is suspected, an awake intubation may be performed after atropine premedication (20 mcg/kg, minimum dose 0.1 mg) and preoxygenation. Otherwise, the induction may proceed by mask inhalation or by intravenous administration of propofol or thiopental and relaxant. If pancuronium is not the muscle relaxant of choice, atropine should precede intubation of the trachea. Future advancements in the management of myelomeningoceles lead to early correction through fetal neurosurgery, which involves a general anesthetic for a cesarean section for the mother (Sutton et al., 2001) (also see Chapter 15, Anesthesia for Fetal Surgery).

Blood loss during meningomyelocele repair usually is not excessive, averaging about 30 mL, or 10% of blood volume. If the lesion is extensive, however, the surgeon may find it necessary to undermine large areas of skin and fascia or to make fasciotomy incisions at the flanks to achieve primary closure of the defect. These practices will necessitate skin grafting over the fasciotomies and increase blood loss significantly.

Conservation of body heat is important for infants with a myelomeningocele, particularly because autonomic control below the level of the defect is abnormal. The operating room should be warmed to 27°C (80°F) before surgery and until the infant is draped. Radiant heat lamps are used during positioning and skin preparation until the infant is draped and again at the end of surgery, a forced hot air warmer is used to maintain body temperature, and humidification of inspired gases further prevents heat loss and minimizes pulmonary complications by humidification of the airway.

For poorly understood reasons, children with myelodysplasia have a significantly increased prevalence of allergy to latex in later childhood and adulthood (Kurup and Fink, 2001; Hepner and Castells, 2003). Thought at one time to be the consequence of frequent catheterization of neurogenic bladders by latex catheters or multiple previous surgical exposure to latex, it is now clear that latex allergy develops even in children without a history of multiple catheterizations or surgery (Hochleitner et al., 2001), although multiple previous surgeries have been identified as one risk factor, as well as a history of atopy, food allergies, and nonwhite race (Kelly et al., 1994). To prevent early sensitization to latex, newborns undergoing repair of myelomeningoceles and meningoceles should be treated as if they were latex allergic,

BOX 18–1 The Chiari Malformations

Chiari Type I

- Tonsillar herniation >5 mm below the plane of the foramen magnum
- No associated brainstem herniation or supratentorial anomalies
- Low frequency of hydrocephalus

Chiari Type II

- Caudal herniation of the vermis, brainstem, and fourth ventricle
- Associated with myelomeningocele and multiple brain anomalies
- High frequency of hydrocephalus and syringohydromyelia

Chiari Type III

- Occipital encephalocele containing dysmorphic cerebellar and brainstem tissue

Chiari Type IV

- Hypoplasia or aplasia of the cerebellum

using a latex-free surgical environment (Nieto et al., 2002) (see Chapter 32, Systemic Disorders).

Neonatal Hydrocephalus

Hydrocephalus itself is not a disease but rather is the consequence of many disease processes. In the newborn period, the two most common causes are anatomic anomalies associated with myelodysplasia and prematurity.

The Arnold-Chiari malformation is a collection of anatomic abnormalities that includes displacement of the cerebellar vermis through the foramen magnum, elongation of the brainstem and fourth ventricle, and noncommunicating hydrocephalus. Most children with meningomyelocele have an associated Arnold-Chiari malformation and ultimately develop hydrocephalus, usually in the first month of life.

Hydrocephalus frequently develops in premature infants who have had an intraventricular hemorrhage; this results in noncommunicating hydrocephalus from scarring or deposition of fibrinous deposits around the aqueduct of Sylvius. More often, hydrocephalus is the consequence of diminished CSF resorption from the arachnoid granulations from scar or fibrin deposition, and it is referred to as communicating hydrocephalus. Neonatal meningitis produces hydrocephalus by a similar mechanism.

Anesthetic management depends on whether ICP is elevated. Slow development of hydrocephalus in newborns is accompanied by increasing skull diameter to accommodate the increase in CSF volume, and, thus, normal ICP is maintained. Rapidly developing hydrocephalus outpaces gradual skull growth and results in rapid elevation of ICP and cerebral herniation unless it is treated. A tense anterior fontanel, irritability, vomiting, and ophthalmoplegia suggest intracranial hypertension.

Surgical management involves the shunting of CSF from a lateral ventricle to either the peritoneum (ventriculoperitoneal shunt) or sometimes into the right atrium (ventriculoatrial shunt). In the absence of abdominal pathology, the ventriculoperitoneal shunt is preferred. This allows the neurosurgeon to insert a redundant length of shunt tubing, which will accommodate the child's growth.

Anesthetic Considerations

Anesthetic management includes the usual considerations and depends on the presence or absence of intracranial hypertension. In the premature infant undergoing ventriculoperitoneal shunt placement, the inspired oxygen fraction should be limited to maintain PaO_2 and arterial oxygen tensions at 70 mm Hg and 95% to 97%, respectively. These levels minimize the risk of retinopathy of the premature infant. Ventilation should be controlled, with careful attention to inflation pressures to minimize the risk of pulmonary trauma, and measures should be taken to conserve body heat. In addition, serious dysrhythmias, especially bradycardias, may occur during ventriculostomies in children with obstructive hydrocephalus (El-Dawlatly et al., 1999). Besides using atropine to treat such bradyarrhythmias, simply alerting the surgeon of the bradycardia and pausing may resolve the problem without medications. The postoperative care of the premature or ex-premature infant who is less than 50 weeks' postconceptual age requires the use of a cardiorespiratory monitor or oximeter to detect postoperative apnea. Even if ICP is well controlled and a reservoir is placed, infants with a history of hydrocephalus may develop postoperative apneic spells, retractions, and/or vocal chord paralysis (Nishino et al., 1998).

Depressed Skull Fractures

Depressed skull fractures occur in the newborn when the infant's head descends through a narrow birth canal and is fractured by the mother's ischium; they usually are not the result of obstetric application of forceps (Bruce, 1980). A depressed skull fracture is a greenstick fracture, frequently resembling an indented table tennis or Ping-Pong ball, and is rarely associated with neurologic injury. Because of early concern regarding the administration of anesthetics to newborns, at one time such fractures were repaired using only local anesthesia, but modern anesthetic techniques make general anesthesia safe in newborns. Because the child is neurologically normal, no anesthetic considerations exist apart from those pertaining to all newborns. The surgeon introduces a periosteal elevator through a small incision in the coronal suture, advancing the instrument until it lies under the indentation in the skull. The elevator is then pushed up, and the scalp is sutured. More extensive or comminuted depressed skull fractures occasionally require a more extensive scalp flap and the use of titanium fixators to hold together the bone fragments.

INFANT AND CHILD

Craniosynostosis

Craniosynostosis, or craniostenosis, represents premature intrauterine fusion of one or more cranial sutures and causes an abnormal skull shape. Most often, it involves only the sagittal suture and results in a deformity that is primarily cosmetic. Development, intellect, and ICP are normal. However, if left uncorrected, many children experience cortex-associated retardation of intelligence. Occasionally, more than one suture is stenosed. Without treatment, this may result in intracranial hypertension as the brain grows and the skull does not. Multiple suture craniosynostosis is most commonly seen in association with craniofacial anomalies, particularly Apert's and Crouzon's syndromes, which are also associated with hypoplasia of the orbits and mid portion of the face.

Children with single-suture craniosynostosis are usually healthy. Surgery is most often performed between 2 and 6 months of life, a period that corresponds to the physiologic nadir of hemoglobin. The acceptable blood loss is very small, and blood transfusion is frequently needed. At least one intravenous catheter for volume infusion is necessary. Arterial cannulation for continuous monitoring is not routinely required for single-suture craniectomies but should be used for multiple-suture procedures.

Several reports have appeared describing VAE during craniosynostosis repair in infants (Harris et al., 1986, 1987). Most recently, using a precordial Doppler probe, Faberowski and coworkers demonstrated that of 23 patients undergoing craniectomies for craniosynostosis, 19 demonstrated 64 episodes of VAE without cardiovascular collapse (Faberowski et al., 2000). The incidence of clinically important air embolism during craniectomies is still undefined but is probably small. It may nevertheless be prudent to monitor patients with a precordial Doppler ultrasound device and to attempt central venous catheter placement to allow aspiration of venous air from the heart.

The surgery for sagittal synostosis is extradural and entails craniectomies on both sides of the sagittal suture. Blood loss begins with scalp incision early in surgery and is exceedingly difficult to quantify; thus, it is important for the anesthesiologist to begin transfusion early, before hypovolemia occurs. If an arterial or a central venous cannula has been placed, serial measurements of hematocrit guide transfusion and fluid therapy. A new surgical technique for sagittal suture craniosynostosis repair (spring-mediated cranial expansion) has been described that is associated with significantly less blood loss (Ririe et al., 2003). The place of this technique in the surgical armamentarium has yet to be defined. It is crucial for the anesthesiologist to anticipate which technique is used, as the former causes considerably more blood loss and, consequently, the patient is more likely to need a blood transfusion (Ririe et al., 2003).

Multiple-suture craniectomies are often performed in association with reconstruction of the midportion of the face and orbital advancement (see Chapter 20, Anesthesia for Pediatric Plastic Surgery). The associated blood loss is large, averaging 50% to 150% of total blood volume (Davies and Munro, 1975). This consideration necessitates the placement of two volume infusion catheters before the surgical incision, or one peripheral volume infusion catheter and one central venous catheter. An arterial cannula is necessary to monitor arterial pressure and for serial blood gas and hematocrit determinations. Central venous pressure monitoring aids fluid therapy and allows aspiration of venous air in the unusual event of air embolism.

The surgeon often ligates the endotracheal tube with silk suture or wire to the alveolar ridge to prevent its being dislodged under the drapes during surgery. If a nasotracheal tube is inserted in anticipation of prolonged postoperative ventilation in the intensive care unit, it should be sutured in place to the nares with silk suture. To prevent a corneal injury, the eyes should be lubricated with an antibiotic ointment or wetting agent and may be sutured closed with a tarsorrhaphy stitch or covered with a corneal shield.

Anesthetic Considerations

Either inhalation or balanced anesthesia is appropriate for craniofacial repairs. Intravenous anesthesia results in less cardiovascular depression and better postoperative analgesia. Moderate deliberate hypotension is usually used to reduce intraoperative bleeding (see Chapter 12, Blood Conservation).

Complicated craniofacial surgery involves intracranial surgery; a reduction of brain volume aids the surgical technique. This may be accomplished with hyperventilation, osmotic dehydration of the brain with mannitol, diuretic therapy with furosemide, or continuous CSF drainage with a lumbar, subarachnoid malleable needle or an epidural catheter placed through a Tuohy needle into the subarachnoid space.

The postoperative care depends on the extent of surgery and subsequent facial and airway edema. In surgery below the orbital ridge, extensive facial edema is common, and the endotracheal tube can be left in place for 48 hours after surgery until resolution of facial and airway edema. To ensure the security of the endotracheal tube, the child can be heavily sedated during this time to maintain neuromuscular blockade and ventilate the lungs mechanically until edema resolves and permits extubation of the trachea.

Vascular Malformations

Arteriovenous Malformations

Arteriovenous malformations (AVMs) are congenital nests of abnormal blood vessels. They may occur anywhere within the body, but when they occur in the brain, they present in four different manners: in the newborn as congestive heart failure (CHF), and in the older child as seizures, hydrocephalus, or, most commonly and tragically, intracranial hemorrhage (Millar et al., 1994; Newfield and Hamid, 2001).

AVMs, unless they are very large, are usually occult in newborns. According to Millar and others, only 18% of AVMs become symptomatic before the age of 15 and symptoms vary from hemorrhage (50%) to seizures and hydrocephalus (36%) in infants and children, whereas newborns may present with high-output, congestive heart failure (18%) (Millar et al., 1994). AVMs are associated with a mortality rate of greater than 90% when CHF is present, and the anesthesiologist should assess signs and symptoms of CHF preoperatively. Although newborn malformations often are not amenable to surgical intervention, the anesthesiologist will nonetheless be called on to anesthetize the child for cerebral diagnostic angiography, embolization, microsurgery, or stereotactic radiosurgery. In addition, the role of endovascular therapy for intracranial aneurysms is rapidly evolving and, in the near future, thrombolytic intra-arterial therapy in children will become more common.

Anesthetic Considerations

Anesthetic management should minimize cardiovascular depression and wide fluctuations in arterial blood pressure to decrease the risk of spontaneous intracranial hemorrhage. Intracranial hypertension usually is not present, but many lesions obstruct CSF pathways and cause hydrocephalus. Local anesthesia, with an infusion of propofol, usually suffices for angiography. More invasive procedures, such as attempts at embolization, require a deeper general anesthesia, endotracheal intubation, and neuromuscular blockade to ensure immobility. Invasive cardiovascular monitoring and controlled hypotension are requirements. Arteriovenous malformations may pose a risk of VAE if a venous structure is opened by the surgeon, and therefore devices to monitor for an embolism should be in place.

As discussed previously, it is often useful to establish preanesthetic β-adrenergic blockade before inducing anesthesia. Anesthetic induction often uses a technique of graded stimuli. An intravenous induction with thiopental and/or propofol and opioid is followed by the introduction of nitrous oxide with or without a potent inhaled anesthetic by mask. Then stimuli of increasing intensity are introduced, and the cardiovascular response to each is judged. If a stimulus produces an increase in blood pressure or heart rate, the anesthetic depth is increased. A potent and rapidly acting hypotensive agent, such as sodium nitroprusside, esmolol, or fenoldopam, should be at hand for the rapid treatment of resultant hypertension. After several milder stimuli, the trachea finally is intubated after anesthesia has been augmented with a further dose of propofol and intravenous lidocaine. A suitable sequence of graded stimuli might be vascular cannulas, oral airway, bladder catheter, laryngoscopy with lidocaine spray, intubation, Mayfield head tongs, and, finally, surgical incision. One technique combines opioid-based anesthetics with neuromuscular blockade and low-dose inhalation anesthesia to control blood pressure.

High inspired concentrations of halogenated anesthetic have an unpredictable effect on arterial blood pressure in the newborn, particularly in the presence of CHF. An alternative and very satisfactory technique is total intravenous anesthesia (TIVA) using an infusion of propofol and remifentanil, with a neuromuscular blocking agent to provide absolute immobility. This technique allows the most rapid emergence with the ability to perform an early postembolization neurologic examination.

Moyamoya Syndrome

During the past decade, major, tertiary centers are seeing an increase in the number of cases of moyamoya disease in adults and children alike, and the etiology is still unknown. Moyamoya is an idiopathic, chronic vaso-occlusive disorder of the distal, internal carotid arteries and circle of Willis that presents as transient ischemic attacks or recurrent strokes in children. *Moyamoya* means "hazy puff of smoke" in Japanese and refers to the angiographic appearance of the abnormal network of vessels that develop at the base of the brain and basal ganglia to supply a collateral route of blood flow (Suzuki and Takaku, 1969). An increase in elastin gene expression has been identified, suggesting the importance of overproduction of elastin in the pathophysiology (Yamamoto et al., 1997).

Moyamoya syndrome is not a distinct entity but rather the syndromic consequence of a number of individual disease processes, and hence may be seen with previous cranial radiation, Alagille syndrome and other causes of hypercholesterolemia, neurofibromatosis, and trisomy 21, to name some of the more common associations (Jacob and Kausalya, 1990; Horn et al., 2004; Kamath et al., 2004; Kim et al., 2004; Spetzler, 2004).

Interestingly, patients with Alagille syndrome develop vascular lesions such as moyamoya, and anesthesiologists need to be aware of the comorbidities associated with this syndrome before formulating an anesthetic plan for neurosurgical procedures. Alagille syndrome is classically composed of five characteristics: typical peculiar facies, chronic cholestasis, posterior embryotoxon, butterfly-like vertebral-arch defects, and cardiovascular malformations (most commonly peripheral or branch pulmonary artery stenosis) (Alagille, 1996). The 20-year mortality is 75%, and factors contributing to mortality are complex congenital heart disease (15%), intracranial bleeding (25%), and hepatic disease or hepatic transplantation (Emerick et al., 1999). Hyperlipidemia is common in patients with Alagille syndrome. However, hyperlipidemia alone is not adequate to explain the severe vascular abnormalities and unidentified genetic factors that predispose Alagille patients to develop vasculopathy (Woolfenden et al., 1999). It is important for anesthesiologists to keep in mind that patients with Alagille syndrome who present with focal cerebral ischemic symptoms in their preoperative history should be evaluated for moyamoya syndrome or more proximal carotid lesions with magnetic resonance imaging or angiography.

The anesthetic management for revascularization is not complicated by considerations of ICP, the effects of anesthetics on CBF, and so on, but requires careful maintenance of normal physiologic blood hemodynamics and of normocarbia, because both hypocarbia and hypercarbia can produce vascular steal phenomena and result in ischemia to marginally perfused cerebral tissue (Sumikawa and Nagai, 1983; Bingham and Wilkinson, 1985; Chadha et al., 1990; Martino and Werner, 1991; Kurehara et al., 1993; Petty, 1993; Soriano et al., 1993; Henderson and Irwin, 1995; Kansha et al., 1997; Sato et al., 1999). As for other cerebrovascular surgical procedures in which cerebral ischemia is a risk, the induction of mild to moderate hypothermia is frequently used.

Epilepsy Surgery

According to the Epilepsy Foundation, 300,000 American children under the age of 14 have epilepsy, and for those with seizures not controlled by medications there are now therapeutic options. When medication fails to adequately control seizures, neurologists may place children on ketogenic diets or implant vagus nerve stimulators. In refractory cases, one option is surgical resection of the epileptic cortex. 20% to 30% of patients with intractable epilepsy may benefit from a surgical procedure.

Epilepsy surgery is most beneficial in patients with partial epilepsy due to a structural lesion, which most frequently lies within the temporal lobe. The standard surgical procedures for patients with epilepsy include focal resection, corpuscallostomy, hemispherectomy, and vagal nerve stimulation. The most common operation for patients with intractable seizures is a partial temporal lobectomy. When the epileptic focus lies in the left hemisphere, a Wada test (an intracarotid injection of a barbiturate in the awake or sedated patient) may be performed to determine if the site of the surgery is indeed dominant and contains the speech center. If in fact the side of the lobectomy is within the speech center and the child is old enough to follow directions appropriately, the craniotomy may be performed under deep sedation with electrocorticographic monitoring (Tobias and Jimenez, 1997; Domaingue, 2001; Ard et al., 2003). With propofol and low-dose remifentanil, as well as appropriate local wound infiltration by the surgeon, the patient can be awakened intraoperatively to interact with the surgeon once the seizure focus is exposed. This minimizes the risk of surgical damage to the speech center. More often, however, children are not appropriate subjects for an awake craniotomy, and the epileptic focus is electrically mapped preoperatively and then subsequently resected.

In this instance, children undergo magnetic resonance imaging before a craniotomy for placement of an electrode grid followed at some time later by a craniotomy and surgical placement of surface and/or depth grids marking the epileptic foci. The earlier discussions regarding craniotomies may be used as a guideline for anesthetic management; there are generally no concerns regarding the management of ICP or CBF, the primary considerations being the effects of chronic administration of anticonvulsants on the pharmacodynamics and pharmacokinetics of neuromuscular blockers, and the relative resistance of the patient to these agents (Alloul et al., 1996; Hernandez-Palazon et al., 2001). In addition, patients may experience a seizure at any time before, during, or after the anesthesia, and provisions must be at hand for the rapid treatment of the seizure with a short-acting barbiturate, benzodiazepine, or propofol. After the surgical placement of electrical cortical grids and recovery from the anesthetic, patients are monitored for several days in the hospital, using continuous electroencephalography and other neurologic testing, to map the epileptic foci.

After cortical mapping and identification of the seizure focus, the patient returns to the operating room for the definitive cortical resection. The anesthetic management includes the principles involved with craniotomies. In addition, epilepsy surgery frequently requires manipulation and stimulation of structures that can cause acute and severe bradycardia, sinus arrest, and hypotension (Sato et al., 2001; Sinha et al., 2004). The structures most sensitive to stimulation, especially by temperature changes from irrigation, include the amygdala, insular cortex, and brainstem. Despite surgical cortical resection of the epileptic focus, patients remain at risk during emergence and recovery from anesthesia for seizures. Provisions must always be at hand for the rapid treatment of a seizure and for control of the patient's airway should a seizure compromise respiration.

Vagal nerve stimulation (VNS) is another surgical alternative to treatment of medically intractable seizures. Because seizures are highly synchronized patterns on the EEG, the thought is that appropriately timed stimulation of the vagus nerve can blunt the paroxysmal epileptiform activity. The device is programmed to provide baseline stimulation of the left vagus nerve. Implantation of the device involves creating an infraclavicular subcutaneous pocket to house the impulse generator, tunneling the electrodes subcutaneously to a left anterior cervical incision and connecting the electrodes to the left vagus nerve. The principles of the VNS are similar to those of cardiac pacemakers, and consequently, for patients returning to surgery for other reasons, the VNS unit needs to be turned off so there will be no interference with the electrocautery device. Side effects of VNS involve vocal cord paralysis, bronchoconstriction, bradycardia, and asystole (Patwardhan et al., 2000; Smyth et al., 2003, Bijwadia et al., 2005).

Finally, for those children who present for anesthesia who have been managed with a ketogenic diet, the anesthetic management requires the use of glucose-free intravenous solutions, and periodic measurement of serum pH and bicarbonate to detect and allow the early treatment of metabolic acidosis.

Spinal Cord Surgery

Spinal surgery in children is necessary to correct various congenital or acquired conditions such as tethered spinal cords, myelomeningoceles, primary or metastatic tumors, Chiari malformations, and herniated discs. Presenting symptoms usually include progressive gait abnormalities, paresis, neuropathic pain, and/or changes in bowel or bladder function. A laminectomy may be performed before the onset of the neurologic symptoms or to alleviate existing symptoms.

Preoperative anesthetic considerations for laminectomies include a detailed history and physical examination of the patient, including accurate documentation of any sensory or motor deficits and other neurologic symptoms prior to surgery. As discussed in the section on myelodysplasias, patients with myelomeningoceles have a high incidence of allergy to latex, so appropriate precautions should be taken (Kurup and Fink, 2001; Hepner and Castells, 2003).

The focus of intraoperative management is minimizing spinal cord ischemia and compression on the spinal cord. These are accomplished by maintenance of spinal cord perfusion pressure through control of blood pressure and minimizing venous congestion through careful positioning of the patient to prevent compression of the abdomen.

Blood loss during most neurosurgical laminectomies is minor; however, highly vascular tumors may cause substantial bleeding, which can be especially significant over several hours of surgical time. In addition to routine monitoring and vascular access, placement of an intra-arterial line should be strongly considered in surgical cases that are expected to last several hours, especially if for tumor resection, because the blood loss can be insidious, significant, and difficult to assess. Placement of a urinary catheter should also be used in these cases as an additional measure of fluid status and to avoid postoperative bladder distention.

New neurologic deficits occur as a complication of spinal cord surgery. Intraoperative neuromonitoring of spinal cord function is often used by surgeons for early detection of spinal cord compromise. The intraoperative wake-up test is the traditional method for assessing the integrity of the spinal cord, but this can be impossible in an infant or a young child who is not able to follow commands appropriately (Soriano et al., 2002). SSEPs and MEPs provide a moment-to-moment assessment of spinal cord function, but use of the two has implications for anesthetic management as both are sensitive to anesthetic agents (Sala et al., 2002, 2004; Soriano et al., 2002; Strahm et al., 2003). Abrupt changes in volatile anesthetic concentration can affect the signals for SSEPs and MEPs (Soriano et al., 2002). Mapping MEPs precludes the use of neuromuscular blocking drugs. The anesthetic management of patients undergoing surgery under SSEP or MEP monitoring is discussed in Chapters 7, 9, and 21.

Positioning of the child for spinal cord surgery carries risks discussed previously in the section on prone positioning. Of great importance is the prevention of abdominal compression, which has the effect of raising inferior caval pressure and causing the shunting of venous blood into the epidural venous plexus from the cava. The chest and pelvis must be placed on bolsters to elevate the abdomen from the operating room table. The head may be turned to one side or maintained on a headrest in the midline, with care being taken to avoid overflexion or overextension of the neck. After final positioning has been achieved, breath sounds must be auscultated to confirm repositioning has not changed the endotracheal tube position. Pressure points must all be padded, and assurance must be made that there is no compression of the male genitalia or the female breasts, the orbits, and the auricles of the ears. The eyes and ears should be rechecked routinely and periodically as part of the intraoperative monitoring.

Lesions Usually Associated with Elevated Intracranial Pressure

Hydrocephalus

Hydrocephalic children with ventriculoperitoneal or ventriculoatrial shunts frequently experience shunt malfunction or failure and come to medical attention when intracranial pressure becomes elevated. Early symptoms of shunt malfunction are headache and irritability, and later symptoms include lethargy, seizure, vomiting, and ophthalmoplegia (Fig. 18–8). Most commonly, the shunt malfunction occurs in the distal shunt tubing within the atrium or peritoneum, or in the valve in the scalp. If the malfunction is not in the proximal intraventricular portion of the shunt, the neurosurgeon, pediatrician, or anesthesiologist can place a needle in the shunt reservoir (which is easily palpable under the scalp) and withdraw an aliquot of CSF, thereby lowering ICP. This maneuver may be lifesaving. Placing a needle in the reservoir also provides the anesthesiologist the ability to monitor ICP (Fig. 18–9). In a select group of patients with noncommunicating hydrocephalus and preservation of the pathway between the subarachnoid space and the venous system, a third ventriculostomy can be performed and alleviate the need for a shunt. Complications of the third ventriculostomy include third cranial nerve paresis, hemiparesis, and bradycardia (El-Dawlatly et al., 2000). Because the fenestration of the third ventricular floor is in close proximity to the basilar artery, traumatic hemorrhage can also occur.

Anesthetic Considerations. The anesthetic technique depends on whether intracranial hypertension exists. If so, no opioid premeditation should be given, and an intravenous induction with propofol or a thiobarbiturate and nondepolarizing agent is appropriate, as discussed earlier. Hyperventilation and avoidance

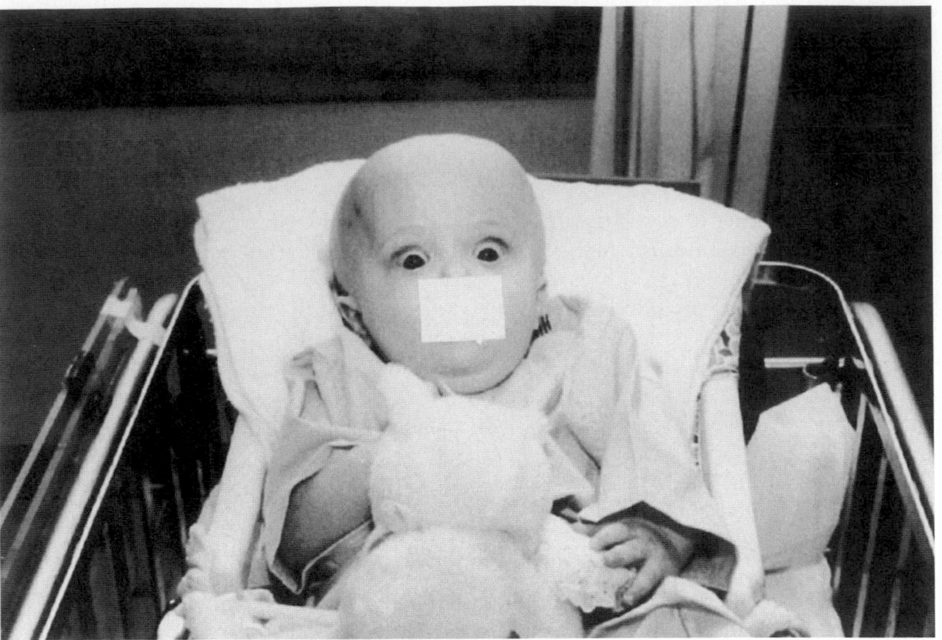

■ **FIGURE 18–8.** An infant with hydrocephalus. Note enlarged head and the downward gaze (the setting sun sign). The latter suggests the presence of intracranial hypertension.

of potent inhalation agents help to control ICP. Once the ventricles have been decompressed, a halogenated agent may be introduced and hyperventilation discontinued.

Brain Tumors

Cancer is the most common nontraumatic cause of death in children, and brain tumors are the most common solid tumor of childhood. In adults, two thirds of brain tumors are supratentorial; the opposite is true in children, in whom two thirds of brain tumors occur in the posterior fossa (Table 18–4). Astrocytomas (including glioblastomas) of various degrees of malignancy, and medulloblastomas together account for more than half of pediatric central nervous system tumors (Walker, 1976).

Some children with brain tumors have significant elevation of ICP because of the mass effect of the tumor, cerebral edema, or secondary hydrocephalus if the tumor obstructs CSF pathways. Others have minimal alteration in cerebral dynamics but have come to medical attention while the tumor is small and causing symptoms as a result of destruction or compression of neural structures.

Anesthetic Considerations. Planning the anesthetic care hinges on whether ICP is elevated. Supratentorial tumor resections require invasive monitoring and an anesthetic technique designed to control ICP (Fig. 18–10). Suboccipital craniotomies for explorations of the posterior fossa or brainstem present the anesthesiologist with several unique problems associated with

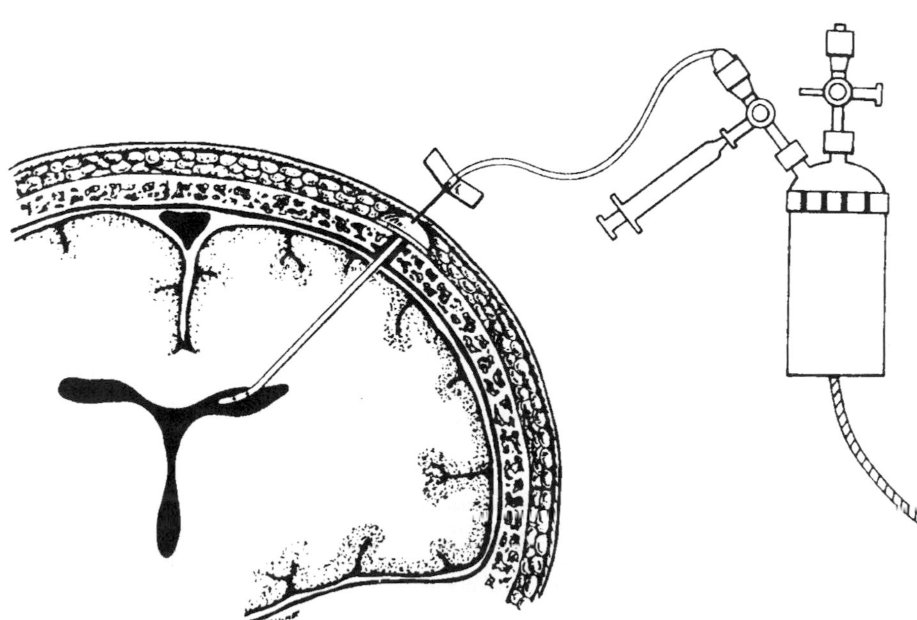

■ **FIGURE 18–9.** Technique for inserting a needle in the reservoir of a ventriculoatrial or ventriculoperitoneal shunt, to remove cerebrospinal fluid or to monitor intracranial pressure. (From Wilkinson HA: Intracranial pressure monitoring: Techniques and pitfalls. In Cooper PR, editor, *Head injury.* Baltimore, 1981, Williams & Wilkins.)

■ **TABLE 18–4.** Distribution of common brain tumors in children, according to location and histologic appearance

Location and Type of Tumor	Percentage of All Brain Tumors*
Infratentorial	**45 to 60**
Primitive neuroectodermal tumor (medulloblastoma)	20 to 25
Low-grade cerebellar astrocytoma	12 to 18
Ependymoma	4 to 8
Malignant brainstem glioma	3 to 9
Low-grade brainstem astrocytoma	3 to 6
Other	2 to 5
Supratentorial Hemispheric	**25 to 40**
Low-grade astrocytoma	8 to 20
Malignant glioma	6 to 12
Ependymoma	2 to 5
Mixed glioma	1 to 5
Ganglioglioma	1 to 5
Oligodendroglioma	1 to 2
Choroid-plexus tumor	1 to 2
Primitive neuroectodermal tumor	1 to 2
Meningioma	0.5 to 2
Other	1 to 3
Supratentorial Midline	**15 to 20**
Suprasellar	6 to 9
Craniopharyngioma	4 to 8
Low-grade chiasmatic-hypothalamic glioma	1 to 2
Germ-cell tumor	1 to 2
Pituitary adenoma	0.5 to 2.5
Pineal	**2 to 6**
Low-grade glioma	1 to 2
Germ-cell tumor	0.5 to 2
Pineal parenchymal tumor	0.5 to 2

*Percentages are derived from reviews of population-based and institutional tumor registries (and Pollack IF, et al., unpublished data). With permission from Pollack IF: *N Engl J Med* 331:1500, 1994.

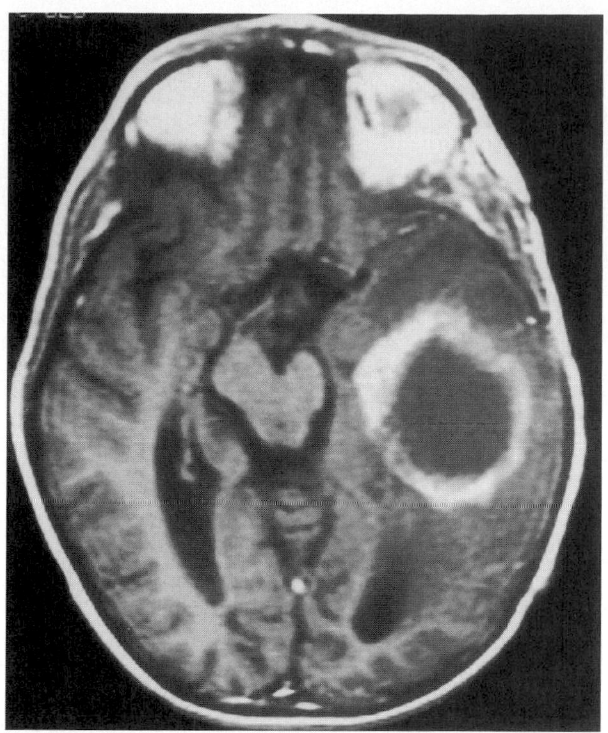

■ **FIGURE 18–10.** Magnetic resonance image of supratentorial tumor. High-grade gliomas are generally less well circumscribed with irregular enhancement.

positioning and maintenance of the airway (discussed earlier) and with changes in respiratory and cardiovascular function associated with brainstem compression (Allan et al., 1970) (Fig. 18–11). Neurosurgeons commonly place the child's head in a Mayfield head frame for tumor resection and, thus, the anesthesiologist must keep in mind the potential for skull fractures, dural tears, and intracranial hematomas from the pins in pediatric patients (Soriano et al., 2002).

A common intraoperative complication to posterior fossa exploration is associated with surgical trauma of the brainstem, especially when surgery is within the fourth ventricle. Brainstem compression or retraction may alter the respiratory pattern or

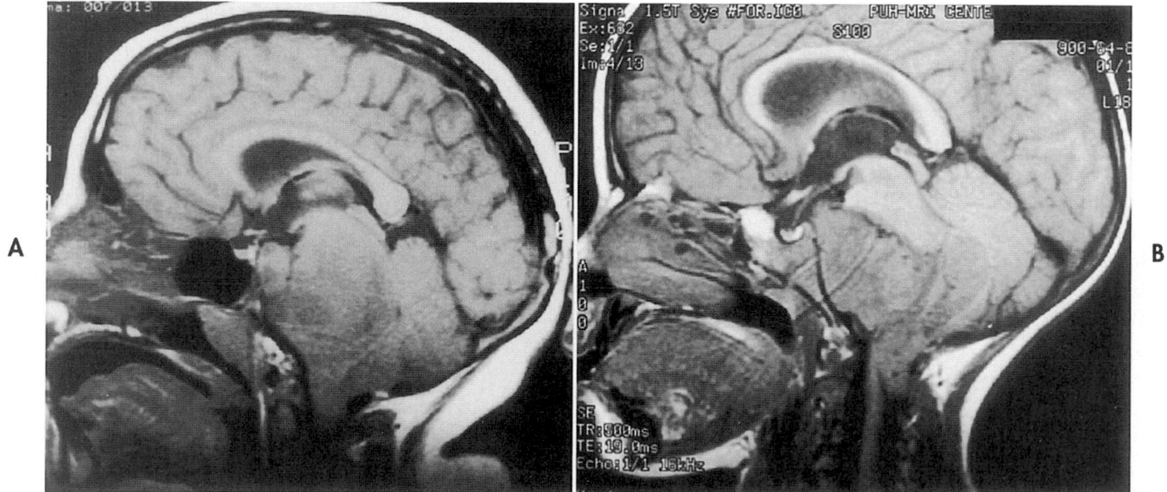

■ **FIGURE 18–11.** Magnetic resonance image of infratentorial tumors. *A,* Brainstem glioma. *B,* Ependymoma displacing the pons and medulla.

cause hiccoughs or apnea. To facilitate monitoring for these events, spontaneous breathing was once advocated. The risk of spontaneous ventilation and negative thoracic pressure in promoting VAE, however, outweighs its benefit (Michenfelder et al., 1969). Brainstem compression also may be detected by its effects on cardiovascular function. Arrhythmias occur simultaneously with alterations in ventilatory control, particularly sudden tachycardia, premature ventricular beats, nodal arrhythmias, and bradyarrhythmias (Michenfelder et al., 1969; Millar, 1972; Davies and Munro, 1975; Albin et al., 1976; Pollack, 1994) and occur in as many as 14% of pediatric patients (Meridy et al., 1974). There also may be a sudden alteration in vascular tone, resulting in sudden hypotension or hypertension. Notifying the neurosurgeon to discontinue the manipulation is generally the only intervention needed, although postoperative brainstem dysfunction may follow.

Occasionally, intraoperative surgical trauma to the brainstem during tumor resection results in postoperative dysfunctions. These include delayed awakening or prolonged unresponsiveness, impaired respiratory drive and central hypoventilation, loss of protective airway reflexes, and vocal cord paralysis. For these reasons, postoperative extubation of the trachea should follow spontaneous ventilation and return of consciousness, although some authors advocate extubation during spontaneous ventilation and deep anesthesia to minimize coughing (Allan et al., 1970). Shortly after extubation, the integrity of airway reflexes should be assessed. Immediate stridor after extubation suggests vocal cord paralysis, whereas delayed stridor is more consistent with postextubation croup. Fiberoptic transnasal laryngoscopy is useful for assessment of vocal cord function when the diagnosis is unclear.

Postoperative craniotomy patients are observed at least overnight in an intensive care setting. Latent complications, such as intracranial bleeding, must be detected early, evaluated, and treated expeditiously to minimize neurologic sequelae. Bleeding in the posterior fossa usually produces dramatic alterations in consciousness and rapid deterioration. Seizures and inappropriate secretion of antidiuretic hormone, with subsequent hyponatremia, also are occasional delayed complications of craniotomies.

Craniopharyngiomas

Craniopharyngiomas are histologically benign suprasellar tumors, the morbidity of which result from local destruction or compression of nearby important structures, notably the hypothalamus, the optic chiasm, and the pituitary gland. They are the third most common intracranial tumor in children and are treated by resection and decompression followed by radiation therapy (Gonc et al., 2004).

These patients often have endocrine abnormalities, and thyroid and adrenal function studies are obtained preoperatively. In a study review of 66 children with craniopharyngiomas, growth retardation or pubertal delay seems to be one of the first findings. Moreover, there is commonly a delayed diagnosis as evidenced by the presence of nausea and vomiting due to elevated ICP from tumor size (Gonc et al., 2004). If resection of the tumor is urgent, that is, if compression of the optic chiasm threatens vision, adrenal insufficiency is assumed to be present and is treated accordingly. Hydrocephalus and intracranial hypertension also may be present, necessitating ventriculostomy placement before resection of the tumor. In view of the hazards of surgical resection, predominantly cystic tumors can be treated with intracavity irradiation (phosphorus 32). Perioperative morbidity is low, and the cyst involutes in the majority of patients (Pollack, 1994) (Fig. 18–12).

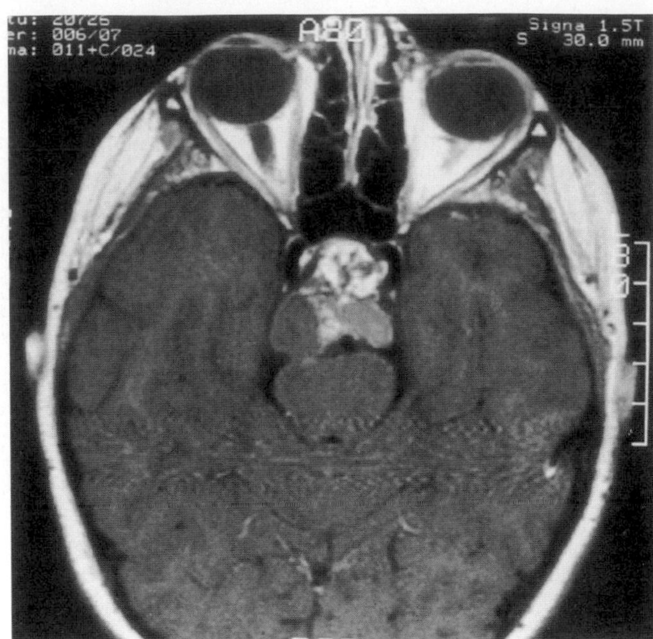

■ **FIGURE 18–12.** Magnetic resonance image of craniopharyngiomas demonstrating both cystic and solid components.

The usual surgical approach to craniopharyngiomas in children is a frontal craniotomy, with dissection under a frontal lobe through an olfactory nerve to reach the optic chiasm. Microscopic technique is usually used, and surgery is often long and laborious.

Postoperative problems are common. Diabetes insipidus occurs frequently, usually within hours of surgery. Occasionally, diabetes insipidus may become evident intraoperatively; its treatment in either event is the same. The diagnosis of diabetes insipidus may be made if there are large urinary losses with associated euvolemia or hypovolemia, increasing serum sodium and serum osmolality, and inappropriately dilute urine osmolality (urine osmolality is usually less than 200 mOsm/L during diabetes insipidus). The diuresis of diabetes insipidus must be replaced on an hourly basis with an appropriately dilute intravenous fluid; 2.5% dextrose in 0.2 normal saline solution is appropriate, but even this low concentration of glucose frequently produces hyperglycemia. If fluid replacement of urine loss alone is inadequate to maintain euvolemia or results in unacceptable elevation of the serum glucose level, as is usually the case, diabetes insipidus must be treated pharmacologically with an aqueous vasopressin infusion, intranasal desmopressin (1-desamino-8-D-arginine vasopressin [DDAVP]), or intravenous DDAVP. Aqueous vasopressin often produces hypertension and decreased splanchnic blood flow because of the vasopressor effect of vasopressin, whereas DDAVP is free of cardiovascular side effects but its duration of action is longer than that of vasopressin. Vasopressin is started at an infusion rate of 0.5 mU/kg per hr. The rate may be successively doubled until the desired antidiuresis is achieved. The pediatric intranasal dose of DDAVP is 0.05 to 0.3 mL/day divided into two doses (5 to 30 mcg/day). The intravenous dose is 0.5 to 3 mcg/day, also divided into two doses.

Neurosurgery around the hypothalamus is also associated with cerebral salt wasting, which also causes massive diuresis.

Easily confused with diabetes insipidus, cerebral salt wasting causes natriuresis, hyponatremia (unlike diabetes insipidus), and markedly elevated urine sodium concentration (50 to 150 mEq/L). The syndrome resolves spontaneously, but it may persist for weeks. Therapy is supportive, consisting of salt replacement to compensate for the natriuresis.

Anesthetic Considerations. In addition to the concerns regarding diabetes insipidus and cerebral salt wasting, an ongoing controversy among neurosurgeons and neuroanesthesiologists is whether the trachea should be extubated with the patient awake or deeply anesthetized after craniotomy. Extubation when the patient is awake ensures the presence of intact airway reflexes and allows rapid evaluation of neurologic function by the neurosurgeon. Deep extubation in the presence of halogenated agents is often associated with less coughing and bucking on emergence but leaves the patient at risk for airway obstruction, reflux and aspiration of gastric contents, and delays in awakening and neurologic assessment. The anesthesiologist must reach his or her own accord with the neurosurgeon. However, extubation when the patient is awake generally is preferred. It may be accomplished with little or no coughing and bucking if (1) an adequate level of narcosis exists at the end of surgery, (2) neuromuscular relaxation is maintained until just before awakening is desired, (3) intravenous lidocaine is given just before nitrous oxide inhalation is terminated, and (4) no halogenated inhalation agents (which delay emergence) are present during awakening. If these conditions are met, patients frequently respond to commands shortly after nitrous oxide is terminated and will not cough. If coughing does occur, it may be treated with intravenous lidocaine and a short-acting synthetic opioid.

Head Trauma

Accidents are the most common cause of death in childhood, and most children dying of traumatic injuries have head trauma. The outcome of childhood head trauma is superior to its outcome in adults (Bruce et al., 1978; Kraus et al., 1987). The Glasgow Coma Scale (see Table 18–3) is a useful predictor of outcome: mortality associated with a score of less than 8 is 59% (Bruce et al., 1981; Kraus et al., 1987). Global cerebral reactivity to CO_2 is preserved in many children with a Glasgow Coma Scale score of greater than 4 (Meyer et al., 1999).

Children with head trauma are different from adults with head trauma in three important ways. The first is the epidemiology of the lesions. The second is the phenomenon of "malignant brain edema" seen commonly in children but rarely in adults. The third is the hemodynamic response to cranial hemorrhage in children.

Only a minority of children with head trauma require surgical intervention to remove an intracranial hematoma (Kraus et al., 1987). Most head-injured children have cerebral concussions or contusions. Epidural hematoma accounts for fewer than 10% of pediatric head injuries, and subdural hematomas are equally uncommon. More common is diffuse axonal cerebral injury accompanied by cerebral swelling, or "malignant brain edema." This is a notable problem in children from birth to 16 years of age who seem to be prone to the development of acute, diffuse brain swelling, even in association with a seemingly minor closed head injury (Bruce, 1980; Bruce et al., 1981). At the cellular level, brain injury initiates an excitotoxic cascade, which increases CSF glutamate. This cascade also activates the *N*-methyl-D-aspartate (NMDA) receptors, which are involved in the modulation of intracellular secondary messengers. The end result is an increase in intracellular calcium and a cascade of intracellular destructive reactions that include proteolysis, lipid peroxidation, free radical formation, and degeneration of neurons.

Brain swelling in this setting is caused by dramatic increases in cerebral metabolism, CBF, and CBV rather than to primary edema formation, which follows secondarily (Kasoff et al., 1972; Bruce et al., 1981). One might intuitively conclude that therapy designed to minimize cerebral metabolism and control arterial blood pressure would be most effective, but experimental confirmation of the best treatment is lacking.

Arterial hypertension is a common sequel to head trauma. Hypertension may be caused by pain, agitation, or intracranial hypertension. Arterial hypertension may in turn contribute to cerebral edema formation, particularly in regions of the brain with vasomotor paralysis and increased CBF (Durward et al., 1983), in which blood flow is passively pressure dependent. Control of arterial blood pressure then becomes an important consideration. If arterial hypertension is secondary to acute elevation of ICP, therapy should first be directed toward lowering ICP. If acute intracranial hypertension has been ruled out as the cause, analgesics and sedatives may suffice. Arterial hypertension unresponsive to these initial measures may, however, be a nonspecific response to intracranial injury. As such it is frequently associated with increased cardiac stimulation and increased serum catecholamine levels. In this setting, propranolol and labetalol are useful agents for control of hypertension and tachycardia and do not elevate ICP (Feibel et al., 1981; Robertson et al., 1983).

When hypotension is associated with a head injury in a child, the first consideration is acute blood loss from associated lesions as small as scalp lacerations, as more than 50% of the severely head-injured children are multiple trauma patients (Orliaguet et al., 1998). In the absence of blood losses, "neurogenic hypotension" could be the cause of hypotension. Its precise mechanism has not been clearly elucidated, but exhaustion of endogenous catecholamines after a massive release following trauma has been suggested as an explanation (Chesnut et al., 1998). As is the case in adults, when hypotension is associated with a head injury in a child, one should search for an associated injury in the thorax and abdomen, but unlike the adult patient, a cranial hematoma may contain one third to one half of an infant's blood volume. Small children with skull fractures and associated epidural or subgaleal hematomas can have significant hemorrhage into the hematoma and subsequent hypovolemia and hypotension, which may be further aggravated by preoperative mannitol or diuretic therapy. Head injuries in adolescents and adults are not associated with blood loss of such a relative magnitude, and hypotension in this population is caused most often by a second injury.

Spinal cord injuries in children may exist concurrently with head injuries and must be ruled out. Plain radiographs of the spine in preschool-aged children are difficult to interpret because of incomplete ossification of the spine, and occult cervical fractures may be present. The best way to make this determination is during the cranial CT scan, by scanning the cervical spine as well. If a spine injury is suspected or known to be present, the trachea must be intubated only while an assistant, preferably a neurosurgeon, holds and stabilizes the head and neck, preventing excessive flexion or extension of the spine. If the head- and spinal cord–injured patient also has an airway compromised by facial trauma, a tracheostomy under local anesthesia is the safest way to avoid loss of the airway and further injury to the spinal cord.

Anesthetic Considerations. The anesthetic care of the child with a head injury often begins in the emergency department or the trauma ward. Evaluation of the airway and endotracheal intubation are of course the first priorities. The awake or arousable child may be watched closely. The unresponsive child should have an endotracheal tube inserted and be hyperventilated. ICP rarely is monitored at this point, but intracranial hypertension should be assumed to be present and the effects of laryngoscopy and intubation on ICP should be borne in mind. These potent stimuli should follow a sleep dose of a short-acting propofol (2 to 3 mg/kg) or thiobarbiturate (4 to 7 mg/kg) and succinylcholine (after defasciculation). Intravenous lidocaine (1 to 2 mg/kg) and a potent synthetic opioid (e.g., fentanyl, sufentanil, or remifentanil) are useful adjunctive drugs to blunt the cerebral hemodynamic response to laryngoscopy and intubation. If hypovolemia exists or is suspected, the dose of propofol or barbiturate should be reduced , or midazolam (0.1 to 0.6 mg/kg) may be substituted for hypnosis and amnesia. Midazolam should be avoided in the presence of overt hypovolemia. With facial or airway trauma, a difficult intubation is possible, and neuromuscular blockade usually is withheld. Intubation may be performed after topical anesthesia, a laryngeal nerve block, and sedation with lorazepam or midazolam. Nasotracheal intubation should not be performed when a basilar skull fracture is suspected. The management of the difficult airway is discussed in Chapter 10, Induction of Anesthesia.

The child with head trauma who requires neurosurgery should be fully monitored, with the use of invasive cardiovascular monitors (arterial cannula and a central venous catheter). Adequate quantities of banked blood must be available in the operating room, and an intravenous cannula of sufficient size for fluid resuscitation should be placed. The choice of anesthetic agents should take into account the likelihood of intracranial hypertension, and this is discussed in preceding sections. Sharples and others noted that almost 30% of the children dying within the first hours following head trauma could have been saved if adequate evaluation and prompt treatment of hypoventilation and hypotension had been initiated earlier (Cruz, 1996). Hypotension alone and hypotension with associated hypoxemia triple and quadruple the mortality of pediatric brain injuries (Pigula et al., 1993).

SUMMARY

Anesthesia for the pediatric neurosurgical patient requires a knowledge of cerebral pathophysiology and an understanding of the interaction between anesthetic agents and cerebral physiology. It is crucial for the anesthesiologist, neurosurgeon, and radiologist to work together to provide a team-structured approach toward diagnosis, resection, and treatment for pediatric patients, especially because children gain 80% of their brain weight between 6 and 12 months and this time is so critical for a good, positive outcome (Kang and Lee, 1999). For the anesthesiologist caring for neurosurgical patients, careful attention to detail is important in ensuring optimal outcome for each child.

REFERENCES

Adams RW, Cucchiara RF, Gronert GA, et al.: Isoflurane and cerebrospinal fluid pressures in neurosurgical patients. *Anesthesiology* 54:97, 1981.

Adams RW, Gronert GA, Sundt TM Jr, et al.: Halothane, hypocapnia, and cerebrospinal fluid pressure in neurosurgery. *Anesthesiology* 37:510, 1972.

Adornato DC, Gildenberg PL, Ferrario CM, et al.: Pathophysiology of intravenous air embolism in dogs. *Anesthesiology* 49:127, 1978.

Alagille D: Alagille syndrome today. *Clin Invest Med* 19:325, 1996.

Albanese J, Durbec O, Viviand X, et al.: Sufentanil increases intracranial pressure in patients with head trauma. *Anesthesiology* 79:493, 1993.

Albin M: The paradox of paradoxic air embolism. *Anesthesiology* 61:222, 1984.

Albin MS, Babinski M, Maroon JC, et al.: Anesthetic management of posterior fossa surgery in the sitting position. *Acta Anaesthesiol Scand* 20:117, 1976.

Albrecht RF, Miletich DJ, Madala JR: Normalization of cerebral blood flow during prolonged halothane anesthesia. *Anesthesiology* 58:26, 1983.

Albrecht RF, Miletich DJ, Rosenberg R, et al.: Cerebral blood flow and metabolic changes from induction to onset of anesthesia with halothane or pentobarbital. *Anesthesiology* 47:252, 1977.

Albright AL, Latchaw RE, Robinson AG: Intracranial and systemic effects of osmotic and oncotic therapy in experimental cerebral edema. *J Neurosurg* 60:481, 1984.

Alexander SC, Wollman H, Cohen PJ, et al.: Cerebrovascular response to Pa_{CO_2} during halothane anesthesia in man. *J Appl Physiol* 19:561, 1964.

Algotsson L, Messeter K, Nordstrom CH, et al.: Cerebral blood flow and oxygen consumption during isoflurane and halothane anesthesia in man. *Acta Anaesthesiol Scand* 32:15, 1988.

Algotsson L, Messeter K, Rosen I, et al.: Effects of nitrous oxide on cerebral haemodynamics and metabolism during isoflurane anaesthesia in man. *Acta Anaesthesiol Scand* 36:46, 1992.

Allan D, Kim H, Cox JM: The anaesthetic management of posterior fossa explorations in infants. *Can Anaesth Soc J* 17:227, 1970.

Alloul K, Whalley DG, Shutway F, et al.: Pharmacokinetic origin of carbamazepine-induced resistance to vecuronium neuromuscular blockade in anesthetized patients. *Anesthesiology* 84:330, 1996.

Archer DP, Labrecque P, Tyler JL, et al.: Cerebral blood volume is increased in dogs with administration of nitrous oxide or isoflurane. *Anesthesiology* 67:642, 1987.

Ard J, Doyle W, Bekker A: Awake craniotomy with dexmedetomidine in pediatric patients. *J Neurosurg Anesthesiol* 15:263, 2003.

Artru AA: Relationship between cerebral blood volume and CSF pressure during anesthesia with isoflurane or fentanyl in dogs. *Anesthesiology* 60:575, 1984d.

Artru AA, Powers K, Doepfner P: CSF, sagittal sinus, and jugular venous pressures during desflurane or isoflurane anesthesia in dogs. *J Neurosurg Anesthesiol* 6:239, 1994.

Artru AA: Effects of enflurane and isoflurane on resistance to reabsorption of cerebrospinal fluid in dogs. *Anesthesiology* 61:529, 1984a.

Artru AA: Effects of halothane and fentanyl anesthesia on resistance to reabsorption of CSF. *J Neurosurg* 60:252, 1984b.

Artru AA: Effects of halothane and fentanyl on the rate of CSF production in dogs. *Anesth Analg* 62:581, 1983a.

Artru AA: Intracranial volume/pressure relationship during desflurane anesthesia in dogs: Comparison with isoflurane and thiopental/halothane. *Anesth Analg* 79:751, 1994.

Artru AA: Isoflurane does not increase the rate of CSF production in the dog. *Anesthesiology* 60:193, 1984c.

Artru AA: Nitrous oxide plays a direct role in the development of tension pneumocephalus intraoperatively. *Anesthesiology* 57:59, 1982.

Artru AA: Relationship between cerebral blood volume and CSF pressure during anesthesia with halothane or enflurane in dogs. *Anesthesiology* 58:533, 1983b.

Artru AA: Venous air embolism in prone dogs positioned with the abdomen hanging freely: Percentage of gas retrieved and success rate of resuscitation. *Anesth Analg* 75:715, 1992.

Azar I: The response of patients with neuromuscular disorders to muscle relaxants: A review. *Anesthesiology* 61:173, 1984.

Bakay L: Studies in sodium exchange. *Neurology* 10:564, 1960.

Baker KZ, Ostapkovich N, Sisti MB, et al.: Intact cerebral blood flow reactivity during remifentanil/nitrous oxide anesthesia. *J Neurosurg Anesthesiol* 9:134, 1997.

Bedford RF, Parsing JA, Pobereskin L, et al.: Lidocaine or thiopental for rapid control of intracranial hypertension. *Anesth Analg* 59:435, 1980.

Bedford RF, Perkins-Pearson NAK: PEEP for treatment of venous air embolism. *Anesthesiology* 57:A379, 1982.

Bedford RF: Venous air embolism: A historical perspective. *Semin Anesth* 2:169, 1983.

Bell WE, McCormick WF: Transtentorial and cerebellar herniations. In Schaffer AJ, Markowitz M, editors: *Major problems in clinical pediatrics, vol 8, Increased intracranial pressure in children: Diagnosis and treatment.* Philadelphia, 1978, WB Saunders.

Bering EA Jr: Water exchange of central nervous system and cerebrospinal fluid. *J Neurosurg* 9:275, 1952.

Biagas KV, Gaeta ML: Treatment of traumatic brain injury with hypothermia. *Curr Opin Pediatr* 10:271, 1998.

Bijwadia JS, Hoch RC, Dexter DD: Identification and treatment of bronchoconstriction induced by a vagus nerve stimulator employed for management of seizure disorder. *Chest* 127:401, 2005.

Bingham RM, Wilkinson DJ: Anaesthetic management in moya-moya disease. *Anaesthesia* 40:1198, 1985.

Bithal P, Dash HH, Vishnoi N, et al.: Venous air embolism: Does the site of embolism influence the hemodynamic changes? *Neurol India* 51:370, 2003.

Bithal PK, Pandia MP, Dash HH, et al.: Comparative incidence of venous air embolism and associated hypotension in adults and children operated for neurosurgery in the sitting position. *Eur J Anaesthesiol* 21:517, 2004.

Black S, Muzzi DA, Nishimura RA, et al.: Preoperative and intraoperative echocardiography to detect right-to-left shunt in patients undergoing neurosurgical procedures in the sitting position. *Anesthesiology* 72:436, 1990.

Bowdle TA, Artru AA: Treatment of air embolism with a special pulmonary artery catheter introducer sheath in sitting dogs. *Anesthesiology* 68:107, 1988.

Brown JC, Charlton JE: Study of sensitivity to curare in certain neurological disorders using a regional technique. *J Neural Psychiatry* 38:34, 1975.

Bruce DA, Alavi A, Bilaniuk L, et al.: Diffuse cerebral swelling following head injuries in children: The syndrome of "malignant brain edema." *J Neurosurg* 54:170, 1981.

Bruce DA, Berman WA, Schut L: Cerebrospinal fluid pressure monitoring in children: Physiology, pathology and clinical usefulness. *Adv Pediatr* 24:233, 1977.

Bruce DA, Schut L, Bruno LA, et al.: Outcome following severe head injury in children. *J Neurosurg* 48:679, 1978.

Bruce DA: Special considerations in the pediatric age group. In Cooper PR, editor *Head injury.* Baltimore, 1980, Williams & Wilkins.

Brussel T, Fitch W, Brodner G, et al.: Effects of halothane in low concentrations on cerebral blood flow, cerebral metabolism, and cerebrovascular autoregulation in the baboon. *Anesth Analg* 73:758, 1991.

Bunegin L, Albin MS, Helsel PE, et al.: Positioning the right atrial catheter: A model for reappraisal *Anesthesiology* 55:343, 1981.

Cafiero T, Burrelli R, Latina P, et al.: Analgesic transition after remifentanil-based anesthesia in neurosurgery. A comparison of sufentanil and tramadol. *Minerva Anesthesiol* 70:45, 2004.

Chadha R, Singh S, Padmanabhan V: Anaesthetic management in moyamoya disease. *Anaesth Intensive Care* 18:120, 1990.

Chen J, Kim YD, Dubois M, et al.: The increased requirement of pancuronium in neurosurgical patients receiving Dilantin chronically. *Anesthesiology* 59:A288, 1983.

Cheney FW, Colley PS: The effect of cardiac output on arterial Wood oxygenation. *Anesthesiology* 52:496, 1980.

Chesnut RM, Gautille T, Blunt BA, et al.: Neurogenic hypotension in patients with severe head injuries. *J Trauma* 44:958, 1998.

Chiron C, Raynaud C, Maziere B, et al.: Changes in cerebral blood flow during brain maturation in children and adolescents. *J Nucl Med* 33:696, 1992.

Colley PS, Artru AA: ECG-guided placement of Sorenson CVP catheters via arm veins. *Anesth Analg* 63:953, 1984.

Constable PD: Hyperchloremic acidosis: The classic example of strong ion acidosis. *Anesth Analg* 96:919–922, 2003.

Cooperman LH, Strobel GE Jr, Kennell EM: Massive hyperkalemia after administration of succinylcholine. *Anesthesiology* 32:161, 1970.

Cooperman LH: Succinylcholine-induced hyperkalemia in neuromuscular disease. *JAMA* 213:1867, 1970.

Coté CJ, Greenhow E, Marshall BE: The hypotensive response to rapid intravenous administration of hypertonic solutions in man and rabbit. *Anesthesiology* 50:30, 1979.

Cotev S, Shalit MN: Effects of diazepam on cerebral blood flow and oxygen uptake after head injury. *Anesthesiology* 43:117, 1975.

Cottrell JE, Giffin JP, Hartung J, et al.: Intracranial pressure during nifedipine-induced hypotension. *Anesth Analg* 62:1078, 1984.

Cottrell JE, Gupta B, Rappaport H, et al.: Intracranial pressure during nitroglycerin-induced hypotension. *J Neurosurg* 53:309, 1980.

Cottrell JE, Hartung J, Giffin JP, et al.: Intracranial and hemodynamic changes after succinylcholine administration in cats. *Anesth Analg* 62:1006, 1983.

Cottrell JE, Patel K, Turndorf H, et al.: Intracranial pressure changes induced by sodium nitroprusside in patients with intracranial mass lesions. *J Neurosurg* 48:329, 1978.

Cottrell JE, Robustelli A, Post K, et al.: Furosemide- and mannitol induced changes in intracranial pressure and serum osmolality and electrolytes. *Anesthesiology* 47:28, 1977.

Coughlan MD, Fieggen AG, Semple PL, et al.: Craniocerebral gunshot injuries in children. *Childs Nerv Syst* 19:348, 2003.

Cowgill DB, Mostello LA, Shapiro HM: Encephalitis and a hyperkalemic response to succinylcholine. *Anesthesiology* 40:409, 1974.

Crumrine RS, Nulsen FE, Weiss MH: Alterations in ventricular fluid pressure during ketamine anesthesia in hydrocephalic children. *Anesthesiology* 42:758, 1975.

Cruz J: Adverse effects of pentobarbital on cerebral venous oxygenation of comatose patients with acute traumatic brain swelling: Relationship to outcome. *J Neurosurg* 85:758, 1996.

Cucchiara RF, Bowers B: Air embolism in children undergoing suboccipital craniotomy. *Anesthesiology* 57:338, 1982.

Cucchiara RF, Seward JB, Nishimura RA, et al.: Identification of patent foramen ovale during sitting position craniotomy by transesophageal echocardiography with positive airway pressure. *Anesthesiology* 63:107, 1985.

Cucchiara RF, Theye RA, Michenfelder JD: The effects of isoflurane on canine cerebral metabolism and blood flow. *Anesthesiology* 40:571, 1974.

Dahlgren N, Ingvar M, Yokoyama H, et al.: Influence of nitrous oxide on local cerebral blood flow in awake, minimally restrained rats. *J Cereb Blood Flow Metab* 1:211, 1981.

Daven JR, Milstein JM, Guthrie RD: Cerebral vascular resistance in premature infants. *Am J Dis Child* 137:328, 1983.

Davies DW, Munro IR: The anesthetic management and intraoperative care of patients undergoing major facial osteotomies. *Plast Reconstr Surg* 55:50, 1975.

Dawson B, Michenfelder JD, Theye A: Effects of ketamine on canine cerebral blood flow and metabolism: Modification by prior administration of thiopental. *Anesth Analg* 50:443, 1971.

DiGiovanni AJ, Goodnick J, Neign JL, et al.: The effect of halothane anesthesia on intracranial pressure in the presence of intracranial hypertension. *Anesth Analg* 53:823, 1974.

Domaingue CM: Propofol/remifentanil in neurosurgery. *Anaesth Intensive Care* 29:205, 2001.

Donegan MF, Bedford RF: Intravenously administered lidocaine prevents intracranial hypertension during endotracheal suctioning. *Anesthesiology* 52:516, 1980.

Dong ML, Kofke WA, Policare RS, et al.: Transcranial Doppler ultrasonography in neurosurgery: Effects of intracranial tumour on right middle cerebral artery flow velocity during induction of anaesthesia. *Ultrasound Med Biol* 22:1163, 1996.

Drummond JC, Prutow RJ, Scheller MS: A comparison of the sensitivity of pulmonary artery pressure, end-tidal carbon dioxide, and end-tidal nitrogen in the detection of venous air embolism in the dog. *Anesthesiology* 64:688, 1985.

Drummond JC, Todd MM: The response of the feline cerebral circulation to Pa_{CO_2} during anesthesia with isoflurane and halothane and during sedation with nitrous oxide. *Anesthesiology* 62:268, 1985.

Durward QJ, Del Maestro RF, Amacher AL, et al.: The influence of systemic arterial pressure and intracranial pressure on the development of cerebral vasogenic edema. *J Neurosurg* 59:803, 1983.

Edmonds-Seal J, Maroon JC: Air embolism diagnosed with ultrasound. *Anaesthesia* 24:438, 1969.

Edmonds-Seal J, Prys-Roberts C, Adams AP: Transcutaneous Doppler ultrasound flow detectors for diagnosis of air embolism. *Proc R Soc Med* 63:831, 1970.

El-Dawlatly AA, Murshid W, El-Khwsky F: Endoscopic third ventriculostomy: A study of intracranial pressure vs. haemodynamic changes. *Minim Invasive Neurosurg* 42:198, 1999.

El-Dawlatly AA, Murshid WR, Elshimy A, et al.: The incidence of bradycardia during endoscopic third ventriculostomy. *Anesth Analg* 91:1142–1144, 2000.

Emerick KM, Rand EB, Goldmuntz E, et al.: Features of Alagille syndrome in 92 patients: Frequency and relation to prognosis. *Hepatology* 29:822, 1999.

Engelhard K, Reeker W, Kochs E, et al.: Effect of remifentanil on intracranial pressure and cerebral blood flow velocity in patients with head trauma. *Acta Anaesthesiol Scand* 48:396, 2004.

Faberowski LW, Black S, Mickle JP: Incidence of venous air embolism during craniectomy for craniosynostosis repair. *Anesthesiology* 92:20, 2000.

Feibel JH, Baldwin CA, Joynt RJ: Catecholamine-associated refractory hypertension following acute intracranial hemorrhage: Control with propranolol. *Ann Neurol* 9:340, 1981.

Fischer M, Moskopp D, Nadstawek J, et al.: Totale intravenose Anaesthesia mit Propofol und Alfentanil verringert im Gegensatz zu einer kombinierten Inhalationsanaesthesie fie Fließgeschwindigkeit inder A. cerebri media. *Anaesthetist* 41:15, 1992.

Fitch W, Ferguson GG, Sengupta D, et al.: Autoregulation of cerebral blood flow during controlled hypotension. *Stroke* 4:324, 1973.

Fitzpatrick JH, Gilboe DD: Effects of nitrous oxide on the cerebrovascular tone, oxygen metabolism, and EEG of the isolated perfused canine brain. *Anesthesiology* 57:480, 1982.

Forster A, Judge O, Morel D: Effects of midazolam on cerebral blood flow in human volunteers. *Anesthesiology* 56:453, 1982.

Forster A, VanHorn K, Marshall LF, et al.: Anesthetic effects on blood-brain barrier function during acute arterial hypertension. *Anesthesiology* 49:26, 1978.

Fox J, Gelb AW, Enns J, et al.: The responsiveness of cerebral blood flow to changes in arterial carbon dioxide is maintained during propofol-nitrous oxide anesthesia in humans. *Anesthesiology* 77:453, 1992.

Fraga M, Rama-Maceiras P, Rodino S, et al.: The effects of isoflurane and desflurane on intracranial pressure, cerebral perfusion pressure, and cerebral arteriovenous oxygen content difference in normocapnic patients with supratentorial brain tumors. *Anesthesiology* 98:1085, 2003.

Frankville DD, Drummond JC: Hyperkalemia after succinylcholine administration in a patient with closed head injury without paresis. *Anesthesiology* 67:264, 1987.

Fuchs G, Schwarz G, Stein J, et al.: Doppler color-flow imaging: Screening of a patent foramen ovale in children scheduled for neurosurgery in the sitting position. *J Neurosurg Anesthesiol* 10:5, 1998.

Gal R, Cundrle I, Zimova I, et al.: Mild hypothermia therapy for patients with severe brain injury. *Clin Neurol Neurosurg* 104:318, 2002.

Gardner AE, Dannemiller FJ, Dean D: Intracranial cerebrospinal fluid pressure in man during ketamine anesthesia. *Anesth Analg* 51:741, 1972.

Gauthier A, Girard F, Boudreault D, et al.: Sevoflurane provides faster recovery and postoperative neurological assessment than isoflurane in long-duration neurosurgical cases. *Anesth Analg* 95:1384, 2002.

Gelb AW, Salevsky F, Chung F, et al.: Remifentanil with morphine transitional analgesia shortens neurological recovery compared to fentanyl for supratentorial craniotomy. *Can J Anaesth* 50:946, 2003.

Gerlach K, Uhlig T, Huppe M, et al.: Remifentanil-propofol versus sufentanil-propofol anaesthesia for supratentorial craniotomy: A randomized trial *Eur J Anaesthesiol* 20:813, 2003.

Ghandi IC, Jindal MN, Patel VK: Mechanism of neuromuscular blockade with some antiepileptic drugs. *Arzneimittelforschung* 26:258, 1976.

Ghani GA, Sung YF, Weinstein MS, et al.: Effects of intravenous nitroglycerin on the intracranial pressure and volume pressure response. *J Neurosurg* 58:562, 1989.

Giffin JP, Cottrell JE, Shwiry B, et al.: Intracranial pressure, mean arterial pressure, and heart rate following midazolam or thiopental in humans with brain tumors. *Anesthesiology* 60:491, 1984.

Gildenberg PL, O'Brien RP, Britt WJ, et al.: The efficacy of Doppler monitoring for the detection of venous air embolism. *J Neurosurg* 54:75, 1981.

Gonc EN, Yordam N, Ozon A, et al.: Endocrinological outcome of different treatment options in children with craniopharyngioma: A retrospective analysis of 66 cases. *Pediatr Neurosurg* 40:112, 2004.

Goss CM: *Gray's anatomy,* 29th ed. Philadelphia, 1973, Lea & Febiger.

Graham DH: Monitoring neuromuscular block may be unreliable in patients with upper-motor-neuron lesions. *Anesthesiology* 52:74, 1980.

Grewal M, Sutcliffe AJ: Early prediction of outcome following head injury in children: An assessment of the value of Glasgow Coma Scale score trend and abnormal plantar and pupillary light reflexes. *J Pediatr Surg* 26:1161, 1991.

Grosslight K, Foster R, Colohan AR, et al.: Isoflurane for neuro-anesthesia: Risk factors for increases in intracranial pressure. *Anesthesiology* 63:533, 1985.

Guy J, Hindman BJ, Baker KZ, et al.: Comparison of remifentanil and fentanyl in patients undergoing craniotomy for supratentorial space-occupying lesions. *Anesthesiology* 86:514, 1997.

Hansen NB, Brubakk AM, Brattid D, et al.: The effect of variations in $Pa{CO_2}$ on brain blood flow and cardiac output in the newborn piglet *Pediatr Res* 18:1132, 1984,

Harris MH, Strafford MA, Rowe RW, et al.: Venous air embolism and cardiac arrest during craniectomy in a supine infant. *Anesthesiology* 65:547, 1986.

Harris MH, Yemen TA, Strafford MA, et al.: Venous embolism during craniectomy in supine infants. *Anesthesiology* 67:816, 1987.

Harrison EA, Mackersie A, McEwan A, et al.: The sitting position for neurosurgery in children: A review of 16 years' experience. *Br J Anaesth* 88:12, 2002.

Hatashita S, Hoff JT, Isbii S: Focal brain edema associated with acute hypertension. *J Neurosurg* 64:643, 1986.

Hayashi N: [Brain hypothermia treatment for the management of severe pediatric brain injury]. *No To Hattatsu* 32:122, 2000.

Henderson MA, Irwin MG: Anaesthesia and moyamoya disease. *Anaesth Intensive Care* 23:503, 1995.

Henriksen HT, Jorgensen PB: The effect of nitrous oxide on intracranial pressure in patients with intracranial disorders. *Br J Anaesth* 45:486, 1973.

Hepner DL, Castells MC: Latex allergy: An update. *Anesth Analg* 96:1219, 2003.

Hernandez MJ, Brennan RW, Bowman GS: Autoregulation of cerebral blood flow in the newborn dog. *Brain Res* 184:199, 1980.

Hernandez-Palazon J, Tortosa JA, Martinez-Lage JF, et al.: Rocuronium-induced neuromuscular blockade is affected by chronic phenytoin therapy. *J Neurosurg Anesthesiol* 13:79, 2001.

Hernandez-Palazon J, Martinez-Lage JF, de la Rosa-Carrillo VN, et al.: Anesthetic technique and development of pneumocephalus after posterior fossa surgery in the sitting position. *Neurocirugia (Astur)* 14:216, 2003.

Herrick IA, Gelb AW, Manninen PH, et al.: Effects of fentanyl, sufentanil, and alfentanil on brain retractor pressure. *Anesth Analg* 72:359, 1991.

Hillman DR, Rung GW, Thompson WR, et al.: The effect of bupivacaine scalp infiltration on the hemodynamic response to craniotomy under general anesthesia. *Anesthesiology* 67:1001, 1987.

Hochleitner BW, Menardi G, Haussler B, et al.: Spina bifida as an independent risk factor for sensitization to latex. *J Urol* 166:2370, 2001.

Hoffman WE, Cunningham F, James MK, et al.: Effects of remifentanil, a new short-acting opioid, on cerebral blood flow, brain electrical activity, and intracranial pressure in dogs anesthetized with isoflurane and nitrous oxide. *Anesthesiology* 79:107, 1993.

Hoffman WE, Miletich DJ, Albrecht RF: Cerebrovascular response to hypotension in hypertensive rats: Effect of antihypertensive therapy. *Anesthesiology* 58:326, 1983.

Horn P, Pfister S, Bueltmann E, et al.: Moyamoya-like vasculopathy (moyamoya syndrome) in children. *Childs Nerv Syst* 20:382, 2004.

Hougaard K, Hansen A, Brodersen P: The effect of ketamine on regional cerebral blood flow in man. *Anesthesiology* 41:562, 1974.

Iacopino DG, Conti A, Battaglia C, et al.: Transcranial Doppler ultrasound study of the effects of nitrous oxide on cerebral autoregulation during neurosurgical anesthesia: A randomized controlled trial. *J Neurosurg* 99:58, 2003.

Inamasu J, Ichikizaki K, Matsumoto S, et al.: Mild hypothermia for hemispheric cerebral infarction after evacuation of an acute subdural hematoma in an infant. *Childs Nerv Syst* 18:175, 2002.

Ishikawa T, Funatsu N, Okamoto K, et al.: Blood-brain barrier dysfunction following drug-induced hypotension in the dog. *Anesthesiology* 59:526, 1983.

Ishikawa T, McDowall DG: Electrical activity of the cerebral cortex during induced hypotension with sodium nitroprusside and trimethaphan in the cat. *Br J Anaesth* 53:605, 1980.

Iwatsuki N, Kuroda N, Keisuke A, et al.: Succinylcholine-induced hyperkalemia in patients with ruptured cerebral aneurysms. *Anesthesiology* 53:64, 1980.

Jacob R, Kausalya R: Moyamoya disease. *Anaesth Intensive Care* 18:582, 1990.

Jelsma LF, McQueen JD: Effect of experimental water restriction on brain water. *J Neurosurg* 26:35, 1967.

Jennett WB, Barker J, Fitch W, et al.: Effect of anaesthesia on intracranial pressure in patients with space-occupying lesions. *Lancet* 1:61, 1969.

Jobes DR, Kennell EM, Bush GL, et al.: Cerebral blood flow and metabolism during morphine-nitrous oxide anesthesia in man. *Anesthesiology* 47:16, 1977.

Joseph MM, Leopold GA, Carillo JF: Venous air embolism during repair of craniosynostosis in the lateral position. *Anesth Rev* 12:46, 1985.

Kalkman CJ, Drummond JC, Patel PM, et al.: Effects of droperidol, pentobarbital, and ketamine on myogenic transcranial magnetic motor-evoked responses in humans. *Neurosurgery* 35:1066, 1994.

Kalkman CJ, Drummond JC, Ribberink AA: Low concentrations of isoflurane abolish motor evoked responses to transcranial electrical stimulation during nitrous oxide/opioid anesthesia in humans. *Anesth Analg* 73:410, 1991.

Kamath BM, Spinner NB, Emerick KM, et al.: Vascular anomalies in Alagille syndrome: A significant cause of morbidity and mortality. *Circulation* 109:1354, 2004.

Kang JK, Lee KS: Comparison between pediatric and adult neurosurgery: Management and future perspectives. Tethered cord syndrome, hydrocephalus, craniosynostosis. *Childs Nerv Syst* 15:795, 1999.

Kansha M, Irita K, Takahashi S, et al.: Anesthetic management of children with moyamoya disease. *Clin Neurol Neurosurg* 99(suppl 2):S110, 1997.

Karsli C, Luginbuehl I, Bissonnette B: The cerebrovascular response to hypocapnia in children receiving propofol. *Anesth Analg* 99:1049, 2004.

Kasoff SS, Zingesser LH, Shulman K: Compartmental abnormalities of regional cerebral blood flow in children with head trauma. *J Neurosurg* 36:463, 1972.

Keller MS, Fendya DG, Weber TR: Glasgow Coma Scale predicts coagulopathy in pediatric trauma patients. *Semin Pediatr Surg* 10:12, 2001.

Kelly KJ, Pearson ML, Kurup VP, et al.: A cluster of anaphylactic reactions in children with spina bifida during general anesthesia: Epidemiologic features, risk factors, and latex hypersensitivity. *J Allergy Clin Immunol* 94:53, 1994.

Kennedy C, Sokoloff L: An adaptation of the nitrous oxide method to the study of the circulation in children; normal values for cerebral blood flow and metabolic rate in childhood. *J Clin Invest* 36:1130, 1967.

Kim SK, Seol HJ, Cho BK, et al.: Moyamoya disease among young patients: Its aggressive clinical course and the role of active surgical treatment. *Neurosurgery* 54:840, 2004.

Klimscha W, Ullrich R, Nasel C, et al.: High-dose remifentanil does not impair cerebrovascular carbon dioxide reactivity in healthy male volunteers. *Anesthesiology* 99:834, 2003.

Kraus JF, Fife D, Conroy C: Pediatric brain injuries: The nature, clinical course, and early outcomes in a defined United States population. *Pediatrics* 79:501, 1987.

Kreisman NR, Olson JE, Home DS, et al.: Cerebral oxygenation and blood flow in infant and young adult rats. *Am J Physiol* 256:R78, 1989.

Kurehara K, Ohnishi H, Touho H, et al.: Cortical blood flow response to hypercapnia during anaesthesia in moyamoya disease. *Can J Anaesth* 40:709, 1993.

Kurup VP, Fink JN: The spectrum of immunologic sensitization in latex allergy. *Allergy* 56:2, 2001.

Lagace A, Karsli C, Luginbuehl I, et al.: The effect of remifentanil on cerebral blood flow velocity in children anesthetized with propofol. *Paediatr Anaesth* 14:861, 2004.

Lanier W, Stangland KJ, Scheithauer BW, et al.: The effects of dextrose infusion and head position on neurologic outcome after complete cerebral ischemia in primates: Examination of a model. *Anesthesiology* 66:39, 1987.

Lanier WL, Milde JH, Michenfelder JD: Cerebral stimulation following succinylcholine in dogs. *Anesthesiology* 64:551, 1986.

Lanier WL, Milde JH, Michenfelder JD: The cerebral effects of pancuronium and atracurium in halothane-anesthetized dogs. *Anesthesiology* 63:589, 1985.

Lassen NA, Christensen MS: Physiology of cerebral blood flow. *Br J Anaesth* 48:719, 1976.

Laughlin TP, Newberg LA: Prolonged myoclonus after etomidate anesthesia. *Anesth Analg* 64:80, 1985.

Lennon RL, Olson RA, Gronert GA: Atracurium or vecuronium for rapid sequence endotracheal intubation. *Anesthesiology* 64:510, 1986.

Lo L, Singer ST, Vichinsky E: Pancytopenia induced by hypothermia. *J Pediatr Hematol Oncol* 24:681, 2002.

Lockhart CH, Jenkins JJ: Ketamine-induced apnea in patients with increased intracranial pressure. *Anesthesiology* 376:92, 1972.

Lorenz IH, Kolbitsch C, Hinteregger M, et al.: Remifentanil and nitrous oxide reduce changes in cerebral blood flow velocity in the middle cerebral artery caused by pain. *Br J Anaesth* 90:296, 2003.

Lorenz IH, Kolbitsch C, Hormann C, et al.: The influence of nitrous oxide and remifentanil on cerebral hemodynamics in conscious human volunteers. *Neuroimage* 17:1056, 2002.

Losasso TJ, Black S, Muzzi DA, et al.: Detection and hemodynamic consequences of venous air embolism. Does nitrous oxide make a difference? *Anesthesiology* 77:148, 1992a.

Losasso TJ, Muzzi DA, Dietz NM, et al.: Fifty percent nitrous oxide does not increase the risk of venous air embolism in neurosurgical patients operated upon in the sitting position. *Anesthesiology* 77:21, 1992b.

Losee JM, Sherrill D, Virtue RW, et al.: Quantitative detection of venous air embolism in the dog by mass spectrometry measurement of end tidal nitrogen. *Anesthesiology* 57:A146, 1982.

Lou HC, Lassen NA, Friis-Hansen B: Impaired autoregulation of cerebral blood flow in the distressed newborn infant. *J Pediatr* 94:118, 1979.

Lutz LJ, Milde JH, Milde LN: The cerebral functional, metabolic, and hemodynamic effects of desflurane in dogs. *Anesthesiology* 73:125, 1990.

Lutz LJ, Milde JH, Milde LN: The response of the canine cerebral circulation to hyperventilation during anesthesia with desflurane. *Anesthesiology* 74:504, 1991.

Madsen JB, Cold GE, Hansen ES, et al.: The effect of isoflurane on cerebral blood flow and metabolism in humans during craniotomy for small supratentorial cerebral tumors. *Anesthesiology* 66:332, 1987.

Maekawa T, McDowall DG, Okuda Y: Brain-surface oxygen tension and cerebral cortical blood flow during hemorrhage and drug-induced hypotension in the cat. *Anesthesiology* 51:313, 1979.

Magness A, Yashon D, Locke G, et al.: Cerebral function during trimethaphan-induced hypotension. *Neurology* 23:506, 1973.

Mammoto T, Hayashi Y, Ohnishi Y, et al.: Incidence of venous and paradoxical air embolism in neurosurgical patients in the sitting position: Detection by transesophageal echocardiography. *Acta Anaesthesiol Scand* 42:643, 1998.

Mann JD, Mann ES, Cookson SL: Differential effects of pentobarbital, ketamine hydrochloride, and enflurane anesthesia on CSF formation rate and outflow resistance in the rat. *Neurosurgery* 4:482, 1979.

Manohar M, Parks C: Regional distribution of brain and myocardial perfusion in swine while awake and during 1.0 and 1.5 MAC isoflurane anesthesia produced without and with 50% nitrous oxide. *Cardiovasc Res* 18:344, 1984.

Marion DW: Moderate hypothermia in severe head injuries: The present and the future. *Curr Opin Crit Care* 8:111, 2002.

Maroon JC, Albin MS: Air embolism diagnosed by Doppler ultrasound. *Anesth Analg* 53:399, 1974.

Maroon JC, Edmonds-Seal J, Campbell RL: An ultrasonic method for detecting air embolism. *J Neurosurg* 31:196, 1969.

Marsh ML, Dunlop BJ, Shapiro HM, et al.: Succinylcholine intracranial pressure effects in neurosurgical patients. *Anesth Analg* 59:550, 1980.

Marsh ML, Shapiro HM, Smith RW, et al.: Changes in neurological status and intracranial pressure associated with sodium nitroprusside administration. *Anesthesiology* 51:336, 1979.

Marshall LF, Smith RW, Rauscher LA, et al.: Mannitol dose requirements in brain-injured patients. *J Neurosurg* 48:169, 1978.

Marshall WK, Bedford RF, Miller ED: Cardiovascular responses in the seated position-impact of four anesthetic techniques. *Anesth Analg* 62:648, 1984.

Martin JT: Neuroanesthetic adjuncts for patients in the sitting position. III. Intravascular electrocardiography. *Anesth Analg* 49:793, 1970.

Martin RW, Ashleman B, Colley PS: Effects of cardiac output on the clearance of air emboli from the superior vena cava. *Anesthesiology* 60:580, 1984.

Martino JD, Werner LO: Hypocarbia during anaesthesia in children with moyamoya disease. *Can J Anaesth* 38:942, 1991.

Matjasko J, Petrozza P, Mackenzie CF: Sensitivity of end-tidal nitrogen in venous air embolism detection in dogs. *Anesthesiology* 63:418, 1985.

Mayberg TS, Lam AM, Eng CC, et al.: The effect of alfentanil on cerebral blood flow velocity and intracranial pressure during isoflurane-nitrous oxide anesthesia in humans. *Anesthesiology* 78:288, 1993.

Mazze RI, Escue HM, Houston JB: Hyperkalemia and cardiovascular collapse following administration of succinylcholine to the traumatized patient. *Anesthesiology* 31:540, 1969.

Mazzoni P, Giffin JP, Cottrell JL, et al.: Intracranial pressure during diltiazem-induced hypotension in anesthetized dogs. *Anesth Analg* 64:1001, 1985.

McDowall DG: Induced hypotension and brain ischaemia. *Br J Anaesth* 57:110, 1985.

McPherson RW, Briar JE, Traystman RJ: Cerebrovascular responsiveness to carbon dioxide in dogs with 1.4% and 2.8% isoflurane. *Anesthesiology* 70:843, 1989.

McPherson RW, Traystman RJ: Effects of isoflurane on cerebral autoregulation in dogs. *Anesthesiology* 69:493, 1988.

Mehta MP, Sokoll MD, Gergis DS: Effects of venous air embolism on the cardiovascular system and acid base balance in the presence and absence of nitrous oxide. *Acta Anaesthesiol Scand* 28:226, 1984.

Meridy HW, Creighton RE, Humphreys RP: Complications during neurosurgery in the prone position in children. *Can Anaesth Soc J* 21:445, 1974.

Messer J, Haddad J, Bientz J, et al.: Influence of anesthetics on cerebral blood flow velocity in infancy. Effects of halothane versus thiopental-fentanyl. *Dev Pharmacol Ther* 13:145, 1989.

Meyer P, Legros C, Orliaguet G: Critical care management of neurotrauma in children: New trends and perspectives. *Childs Nerv Syst* 15:732, 1999.

Michenfelder JD, Martin JT, Altenburg BM, et al.: Air embolism during neurosurgery: An evaluation of right-atrial catheters for diagnosis and treatment. *JAMA* 208:1353, 1969.

Michenfelder JD, Miller RH, Gronert GA: Evaluation of an ultrasonic device (Doppler) for the diagnosis of venous air embolism. *Anesthesiology* 36:164, 1972.

Michenfelder JD, Terry HR, Daw EF, et al.: Air embolism during neurosurgery: A new method of treatment. *Anesth Analg* 45:390, 1966.

Michenfelder JD, Theye RA: Canine systemic and cerebral effects of hypotension induced by hemorrhage, trimethaphan, halothane, or nitroprusside. *Anesthesiology* 46:188, 1977.

Michenfelder JD, Theye RA: Effect of fentanyl, droperidol and Innovar on canine cerebral metabolism and blood flow. *Br J Anaesth* 43:630, 1971.

Michenfelder JD: The interdependency of cerebral function and metabolic effects following massive doses of thiopental in the dog. *Anesthesiology* 41:231, 1974.

Milde LN, Milde JH, Gallagher WJ: Effects of sufentanil on cerebral circulation and metabolism in dogs. *Anesth Analg* 70:138, 1990.

Miletich DJ, Ivankovich AD, Albrecht RF, et al.: Absence of auto-regulation of cerebral blood flow during halothane and enflurane anesthesia. *Anesth Analg* 55:100, 1976.

Millar C, Bissonnette B, Humphreys RP: Cerebral arteriovenous malformations in children. *Can J Anaesth* 41:321, 1994.

Millar RA: Neuroanaesthesia in the sitting position. *Br J Anaesth* 44:495, 1972.

Miller R, Tausk HC, Stark DCC: Effect of Innovar, fentanyl and droperidol on the cerebrospinal fluid pressure in neurosurgical patients. *Can Anaesth Soc J* 22:502, 1975.

Milligan DWA: Failure of autoregulation and intraventricular haemorrhage in preterm infants. *Lancet* 1:896, 1980.

Minto CF, Schnider TW, Gregg KM, et al.: Using the time of maximum effect site concentration to combine pharmacokinetics and pharmacodynamics. *Anesthesiology* 99:324, 2003.

Minto CF, Schnider TW, Shafer SL: Pharmacokinetics and pharmacodynamics of remifentanil. II. Model application. *Anesthesiology* 86:24, 1997.

Minton MD, Grosslight K, Stirt JA, et al.: Increases in intracranial pressure from succinylcholine: Prevention by prior nondepolarizing blockade. *Anesthesiology* 65:165, 1986.

Minton MD, Stirt JA, Bedford RF: Increased intracranial pressure from; succinylcholine: Modification by prior nondepolarizing blockade. *Anesthesiology* 63:A391, 1985.

Misfeldt BB, Jorgensen PB, Spotoff H, et al.: The effects of droperidol and fentanyl on intracranial pressure and cerebral perfusion pressure in neurosurgical patients. *Br J Anaesth* 48:963, 1976.

Mochalova, LD, Khodov DA, Zhukova TP: Cerebral circulation control in healthy full-term neonates. *Acta Paediatr Scand Suppl* 311:20, 1983.

Mongan P, Peterson RE, Culling RD: Pressure monitoring can accurately position catheters for air embolism aspiration. *J Clin Monit* 8:121, 1992.

Monkhoff M, Schwarz U, Gerber A, et al.: The effects of sevoflurane and halothane anesthesia on cerebral blood flow velocity in children. *Anesth Analg* 92:891, 2001.

Moorthy SS, Hilgenberg JC: Resistance to nondepolarizing muscle relaxants in paretic upper extremities of patient with residual hemiplegia. *Anesth Analg* 59:624, 1980.

Moss E, McDowall DG: ICP increases with 50% nitrous oxide in oxygen in severe head injuries during controlled ventilation. *Br J Anaesth* 51:757, 1979.

Moss E, Powell D, Gibson RM, et al.: Effect of etomidate on intracranial pressure and cerebral perfusion pressure. *Br J Anaesth* 51:347, 1979.

Moss E, Powell D, Gibson RM, et al.: Effects of fentanyl on intracranial pressure and cerebral perfusion pressure during hypocapnia. *Br J Anaesth* 50:779, 1978a.

Moss E, Powell D, Gibson RM, et al.: Effects of tracheal intubation on intracranial pressure following induction of anaesthesia with thiopentone or althesin in patients undergoing neurosurgery. *Br J Anaesth* 50:353, 1978b.

Munro MJ, Walker, AM, Parfield CP: Hypotensive extremely low birth weight infants have reduced cerebral blood flow. *Pediatrics* 114:1591–1596, 2004.

Munson ES: Effect of nitrous oxide on the pulmonary circulation during venous air embolism. *Anesth Analg* 50:785, 1971.

Nakahashi K, Yomosa H, Matsuzawa N, et al.: Effect on cerebral blood flow of midazolam during modified neurolept-anesthesia. *Masui* 40:1787, 1991.

Namill JF, Bedford RF, Weaver DC, et al.: Lidocaine before endotracheal intubation: Intravenous or laryngotracheal? *Anesthesiology* 55:578, 1981.

Nehls DG, Todd MM, Spetzler RF, et al.: A comparison of the cerebral protective effects of isoflurane and barbiturates during temporary focal ischemia in primates. *Anesthesiology* 66:453, 1987.

Newberg LA, Michenfelder JD: Cerebral protection by isoflurane during hypoxemia or ischemia. *Anesthesiology* 59:29, 1983.

Newberg LA, Milde JH, Michenfelder JD: Systemic and cerebral effects of isoflurane-induced hypotension in dogs. *Anesthesiology* 60:541, 1984.

Newberg LA, Milde JH, Michenfelder JD: The cerebral metabolic effects of isoflurane at and above concentrations that suppress cortical electrical activity. *Anesthesiology* 59:23, 1983.

Newfield P, Hamid RK: Pediatric neuro-anesthesia. Arteriovenous malformations. *Anesthesiol Clin North Am* 19:229, 2001.

Nieto, A, Mazon A, Pamies R, et al.: Efficacy of latex avoidance for primary prevention of latex sensitization in children with spina bifida. *J Pediatr* 140:370, 2002.

Nishino H, Kinouchi K, Fukumitsu K, et al.: [Anesthesia and perioperative management in infants with Chiari type ii malformation]. *Masui* 47:982, 1998.

Nugent M, Artru AA, Michenfelder JD: Cerebral metabolic, vascular and protective effects of midazolam maleate. *Anesthesiology* 56:172, 1982.

Nussmeier NA, Arlund C, Slogoff S: Neuropsychiatric complications after cardiopulmonary bypass. Cerebral protection by a barbiturate. *Anesthesiology* 64:165, 1986.

Ong BY, Bose D, Palahniuk RJ: Acidemia impairs autoregulation of cerebral blood flow in newborn lambs. *Can Anaesth Soc J* 33:5, 1986.

Ong L, Selladurai BM, Dhillon MK, et al.: The prognostic value of the Glasgow Coma Scale, hypoxia and computerised tomography in outcome prediction of pediatric head injury. *Pediatr Neurosurg* 24:285, 1996.

Orliaguet GA, Meyer PG, Blanot S, et al.: Predictive factors of outcome in severely traumatized children. *Anesth Analg* 87:537, 1998.

Ornstein E, Matteo RS, Schwartz AE, et al.: The effect of phenytoin on the magnitude and duration of neuromuscular block following atracurium or vecuronium. *Anesthesiology* 67:191, 1987.

Ornstein E, Matteo RS, Young WL, et al.: Resistance to metocurine-induced neuromuscular blockade in patients receiving phenytoin. *Anesthesiology* 63:294, 1985.

Ornstein E, Young WL, Fleischer LH, et al.: Desflurane and isoflurane have similar effects on cerebral blood flow in patients with intracranial mass lesions. *Anesthesiology* 79:498, 1993.

Ostapkovich ND, Baker KZ, Fogarty-Mack P, et al.: Cerebral blood flow and CO_2 reactivity is similar during remifentanil/N_2O and fentanyl/N_2O anesthesia. *Anesthesiology* 89:358, 1998.

Paris A, Scholz J, von Knobelsdorff G, et al.: The effect of remifentanil on cerebral blood flow velocity. *Anesth Analg* 87:569, 1998.

Patwardhan RV, Stong B, Begin EM, et al.: Efficacy of vagal nerve stimulation in children with medically refractory epilepsy. *Neurosurgery* 47:1353, 2000.

Paul M, Dueck M, Joachim Herrmann H, et al.: A randomized, controlled study of fluid management in infants and toddlers during surgery: Hydroxyethyl starch 6% (HES 70/0.5) vs lactated Ringer's solution. *Paediatr Anaesth* 13:603, 2003.

Pearl RG, Larson CP: Hemodynamic effects of positive end-expiratory pressure during continuous venous air embolism in the dog. *Anesthesiology* 64:724, 1986.

Pelligrino DA, Miletich DJ, Hoffman WE, et al.: Nitrous oxide markedly increases cerebral cortical metabolic rate and blood flow in the goat. *Anesthesiology* 60:405, 1984.

Perkins-Pearson NAK, Marshall WK, Bedford RF: Atrial pressures in the seated position: Implication for paradoxical air embolism. *Anesthesiology* 57:493, 1982.

Petersen KD, Landsfeldt U, Cold GE, et al.: Intracranial pressure and cerebral hemodynamic in patients with cerebral tumors: A randomized prospective study of patients subjected to craniotomy in propofol-fentanyl, isoflurane-fentanyl, or sevoflurane-fentanyl anesthesia. *Anesthesiology* 98:329, 2003.

Petty LA: Anesthetic management of a patient with moyamoya disease: A case report. *Aana J* 61:277, 1993.

Phillips RJ, Mulliken JB: Venous air embolism during a craniofacial procedure. *Plast Reconstr Surg* 82:155, 1988.

Phirman JR, Shapiro HM: Modification of nitrous oxide-induced intracranial hypertension by prior induction of anesthesia. *Anesthesiology* 46:150, 1977.

Pierce EC, Lambertsen CJ, Deutsch S, et al.: Cerebral circulation and metabolism during thiopental anesthesia and hyperventilation in man. *J Clin Invest* 41:1664, 1962.

Pigula FA, Wald SL, Shackford SR, et al.: The effect of hypotension and hypoxia on children with severe head injuries. *J Pediatr Surg* 28:310, 1993.

Pollack IF: Brain tumors in children (review). *N Engl J Med* 331:1500, 1994.

Pollay M, Fullenwider C, Roberts PA, et al.: Effect of mannitol and furosemide on blood-brain osmotic gradient and intracranial pressure. *J Neurosurg* 59:945, 1983.

Pollay M, Roberts PA: Blood-brain barrier: A definition of normal and altered function. *Neurosurgery* 6:675, 1980.

Pryds O: Control of cerebral circulation in the high-risk neonate. *Ann Neurol* 30:321, 1991.

Pulsinelli WA, Levy DE, Sigsbee B, et al.: Increased damage after ischemic stroke in patients with hyperglycemia with or without established diabetes mellitus. *Am J Med* 74:540, 1983.

Pulsinelli WA, Waldman S, Rawlinson D, et al.: Moderate hyperglycemia augments ischemia brain damage: A neuropathologic study in the rat. *Neurology* 32:1239, 1982.

Purves MJ, James IM: Observations on the control of cerebral blood flow in sheep fetus and newborn lamb. *Circ Res* 25:651, 1969.

Rampil IJ, Lockhart SH, Eger EI, et al.: The electroencephalographic effects of desflurane in humans. *Anesthesiology* 74:434, 1991.

Reilly PL, Simpson DA, Sprod R, et al.: Assessing the conscious level in infants and young children: A paediatric version of the Glasgow Coma Scale. *Childs Nerv Syst* 4:30, 1988.

Renou AM, Vernhiet J, Macrez P, et al.: Cerebral blood flow and metabolism during etomidate anaesthesia in man. *Br J Anaesth* 50:1047, 1978.

Ririe DG, David LR, Glazier SS, et al.: Surgical advancement influences perioperative care: A comparison of two surgical techniques for sagittal craniosynostosis repair. *Anesth Analg* 97:699, 2003.

Rizzi RR: No difference between remifentanil and fentanyl in patients undergoing craniotomy. *Anesthesiology* 88:271, 1998.

Roberts PA, Pollay M, Engles C, et al.: Effect on intracranial pressure of furosemide combined with varying doses and administration rates of mannitol. *J Neurosurg* 66:440, 1987.

Robertson CS, Cliftonn GL, Taylor AA, et al.: Treatment of hypertension associated with head injury. *J Neurosurg* 59:455, 1983.

Rockoff MA, Naughton KVH, Shapiro HM, et al.: Cerebral, circulatory, and metabolic responses to intravenously administered lorazepam. *Anesthesiology* 53:215, 1980.

Rogers MC, Nugent SK, Traystman RJ: Control of cerebral circulation in the neonate and infant. *Crit Care Med* 8:570, 1980.

Rosa G, Orfei P, Sanfilippo M, et al.: The effects of atracurium besylate (Tracrium) on intracranial pressure and cerebral perfusion pressure. *Anesth Analg* 65:381, 1986.

Rosomoff HL, Holaday DA: Cerebral blood flow and cerebral oxygen consumption during hypothermia. *Am J Physiol* 179:85, 1954.

Roth S, Ebrahim ZY: Resistance to pancuronium in patients receiving carbamazepine. *Anesthesiology* 66:691, 1987.

Rudehill A, Lagerkransen M, Lindquist C, et al.: Effects of mannitol on blood volume and central hemodynamics in patients undergoing cerebral aneurysm surgery. *Anesth Analg* 62:875, 1983.

Saidman LJ, Eger EI II: Changes in cerebrospinal fluid pressure during pneumoencephalography under nitrous oxide anesthesia. *Anesthesiology* 26:67, 1965.

Sakabe T, Kuramoto T, Inoue S, et al.: Cerebral effects of nitrous oxide in the dog. *Anesthesiology* 48:195, 1978.

Sakabe T, Kuramoto T, Kumagae S, et al.: Cerebral responses to the addition of nitrous oxide to halothane in man. *Br J Anaesth* 48:957, 1976.

Sakabe T, Maekawa T, Ishikawa T, et al.: The effects of lidocaine on canine cerebral metabolism and circulation related to the electroencephalogram. *Anesthesiology* 40:433, 1974.

Sala F, Krzan MJ, Deletis V: Intraoperative neurophysiological monitoring in pediatric neurosurgery: Why, when, how? *Childs Nerv Syst* 18:264, 2002.

Sala F, Lanteri P, Bricolo A: Motor evoked potential monitoring for spinal cord and brain stem surgery. *Adv Tech Stand Neurosurg* 29:133, 2004.

Sari A, Okuda Y, Takeshita H: The effects of thalamonal on cerebral circulation and oxygen consumption in man. *Br J Anaesth* 44:330, 1972.

Sato K, Shirane R, Kato M, et al.: Effect of inhalational anesthesia on cerebral circulation in moyamoya disease. *J Neurosurg Anesthesiol* 11:25, 1999.

Sato K, Shamoto H, Yoshimoto T: Severe bradycardia during epilepsy surgery. *J Neurosurg Anesthesiol* 13:329, 2001.

Scheller MS, Tateishi A, Drummond JC, Zornow MH: The effects of sevoflurane on cerebral blood flow, cerebral metabolic rate for oxygen, intracranial pressure, and the electroencephalogram are similar to those of isoflurane in the rabbit. *Anesthesiology* 68:548, 1988.

Scheller MS, Todd MM, Drummond JC, et al.: The intracranial pressure effects of isoflurane and halothane administered following cryogenic brain injury in rabbits. *Anesthesiology* 67:507, 1987.

Scheller MS, Todd MM, Drummond JC: Isoflurane, halothane and regional cerebral blood flow at various levels of $Pa{CO_2}$ in rabbits. *Anesthesiology* 64:598, 1986.

Schmieder K, Schregel W, Harders A, et al.: Dynamic cerebral autoregulation in patients undergoing surgery for intracranial tumors. *Eur J Ultrasound* 12:1, 2000.

Schwarz G, Fuchs G, Weihs W, et al.: Sitting position for neurosurgery: Experience with preoperative contrast echocardiography in 301 patients. *J Neurosurg Anesthesiol* 6:83, 1994.

Schwedler M, Miletich DJ, Albrecht RF: Cerebral blood flow and metabolism following ketamine administration. *Can Anaesth Soc J* 29:222, 1982.

Servadei F, Nasi MT, Cremonini AM, et al.: Importance of a reliable admission Glasgow Coma Scale score for determining the need for evacuation of posttraumatic subdural hematomas: A prospective study of 65 patients. *J Trauma* 44:868, 1998.

Settergren G, Lindblad BS, Persson B: Cerebral blood flow and exchange on oxygen, glucose, ketone bodies, lactate, pyruvate and amino acids in anesthetized children. *Acta Paediatr Scand* 69:457, 1980.

Shafer SL, Varvel JR: Pharmacokinetics, pharmacodynamics, and rational opioid selection. *Anesthesiology* 74:53, 1991.

Shapiro HM, Greenberg JH, Van Horn Naughton K, et al.: Heterogeneity of local cerebral blood flow-$Pa{CO_2}$ sensitivity in neonatal dogs. *J Appl Physiol* 49:113, 1980.

Shapiro HM, Wyte SR, Harris AB: Ketamine anaesthesia in patients with intracranial pathology. *Br J Anaesth* 44:1200, 1972.

Shapiro HM, Yoachim J, Marshall LF: Nitrous oxide challenge for detection of residual intravascular pulmonary gas following venous air embolism. *Anesth Analg* 61:304, 1982.

Sharma K, Tripathi M: Detection of site of air entry in venous air embolism: Role of Valsalva maneuver. *J Neurosurg Anesthesiol* 6:209, 1994.

Sharples PM, Eyre JA: Head injury—how community paediatricians can help. *Arch Dis Child* 66:908,1991.

Shayevitz JR, Matteo RS: Decreased sensitivity to metocurine in patients with upper motoneuron disease. *Anesth Analg* 64:767, 1985.

Shenkin HA, Bezier HS, Bouzarth WF: Restricted fluid intake: Rational management of the neurosurgical patient. *J Neurosurg* 45:432, 1976.

Sihle-Wissel M, Scholz M, Cunitz G: Transcranial magnetic-evoked potentials under total intravenous anaesthesia and nitrous oxide. *Br J Anaesth* 85:465, 2000.

Sinha PK, Neema PK, Manikandan S, et al.: Bradycardia and sinus arrest following saline irrigation of the brain during epilepsy surgery. *J Neurosurg Anesthesiol* 16:160, 2004.

Skahen S, Shapiro HM, Drummond JC, et al.: Nitrous oxide withdrawal reduces intracranial pressure in the presence of pneumocephalus. *Anesthesiology* 65:192, 1986.

Smith A, Hoff J, Nielsen S, et al.: Barbiturate protection in acute focal cerebral ischemia. *Stroke* 5:1, 1974.

Smith AL, Macque JJ: Anesthetics and cerebral edema. *Anesthesiology* 45:64, 1976.

Smith RB, Grenvik A: Cardiac arrest following succinylcholine in patients with central nervous system injuries. *Anesthesiology* 33:558, 1970.

Smyth MD, Tubbs RS, Bebin EM, et al.: Complications of chronic vagus nerve stimulation for epilepsy in children. *J Neurosurg* 99:500, 2003.

Soriano SG, Eldredge EA, Rockoff MA: Pediatric neuro-anesthesia. *Anesthesiol Clin North Am* 20:389, 2002.

Soriano SG, McCann ME, Laussen PC: Neuro-anesthesia. Innovative techniques and monitoring. *Anesthesiol Clin North Am* 20:137, 2002.

Soriano SG, McManus ML, Sullivan LJ, et al.: Cerebral blood flow velocity after mannitol infusion in children. *Can J Anaesth* 43:461, 1996.

Soriano SG, McManus ML, Sullivan LJ, et al.: Doppler sensor placement during neurosurgical procedures for children in the prone position. *J Neurosurg Anesthesiol* 6:153, 1994.

Soriano SG, Sethna NF, Scott RM: Anesthetic management of children with moyamoya syndrome. *Anesth Analg* 77:1066, 1993.

Spacek A, Neiger FX, Spiss CK, et al.: Atracurium-induced neuromuscular block is not affected by chronic anticonvulsant therapy with carbamazepine. *Acta Anaesthesiol Scand* 41:1308, 1997.

Spacek A, Neiger FX, Spiss CK, et al.: Chronic carbamazepine therapy does not influence mivacurium-induced neuromuscular block. *Br J Anaesth* 77:500, 1996.

Spacek A, Nickl S, Neiger FX, et al.: Augmentation of the rocuronium-induced neuromuscular block by the acutely administered phenytoin. *Anesthesiology* 90:1551, 1999.

Sperry RJ, Bailey PL, Reichman MV, et al.: Fentanyl and sufentanil increase intracranial pressure in head trauma patients. *Anesthesiology* 77:416, 1992.

Spetzler RF: Moyamoya. *J Neurosurg Spine* 100:541; author reply 541, 2004.

Steinberg GK, Ogilvy CS, Shuer LM, et al.: Comparison of endovascular and surface cooling during unruptured cerebral aneurysm repair. *Neurosurgery* 55:307, 2004.

Stephan H, Groger P, Weyland A, et al.: Einflu von Sufentanil aug Hirndurchblutung, Hirnstoffwechsel und die CO2-Reaktivitat der menschlichen Hirngefaße. *Anaesthesist* 40:153, 1991.

Stevenson PH, Birch AA: Succinylcholine-induced hyperkalemia in a patient with a closed head injury. *Anesthesiology* 51:89, 1979.

Stirt JA, Grosslight KR, Bedford RF, et al.: "Defasciculation" with metocurine prevents succinylcholine-induced increases in intracranial pressure. *Anesthesiology* 67:50, 1987a.

Stirt JA, Maggio W, Haworth C, et al.: Vecuronium: Effect on intracranial pressure and hemodynamics in neurosurgical patients. *Anesthesiology* 67:570, 1987b.

Stone WA, Beach TP, Hamelberg W: Succinylcholine: Danger in the spinal-cord-injured patient. *Anesthesiology* 32:168, 1970.

Stoyka WW, Schultz H: The cerebral response to sodium nitroprusside and trimethaphan controlled hypotension. *Can Anaesth Soc J* 22:275, 1975.

Strahm C, Min K, Boos N, et al.: Reliability of perioperative SSEP recordings in spine surgery. *Spinal Cord* 41:483, 2003.

Sumikawa K, Nagai H: Moyamoya disease and anesthesia. *Anesthesiology* 58:204, 1983.

Sutton LN, Sun P, Adzick NS: Fetal neurosurgery. *Neurosurgery* 48:124, 2001.

Suzuki J, Takaku A: Cerebrovascular "moyamoya" disease. Disease showing abnormal net-like vessels in base of brain. *Arch Neurol* 20:288, 1969.

Takeshita H, Okuda Y, Sari A: The effects of ketamine on cerebral circulation and metabolism in man. *Anesthesiology* 36:69, 1972.

Tarkkanen L, Laitinen L, Johanssen G: Effects of *d*-tubocurarine on intracranial pressure and thalamic electrical impedance. *Anesthesiology* 40:247, 1974.

Tateishi A, Maekawa T, Takeshita H, et al.: Diazepam and intracranial pressure. *Anesthesiology* 54:335, 1981.

Tatman A, Warren A, Williams A, et al.: Development of a modified paediatric coma scale in intensive care clinical practice. *Arch Dis Child* 77:519, 1997.

Theye RA, Michenfelder JD: The effect of nitrous oxide on canine cerebral metabolism. *Anesthesiology* 29:1113, 1968.

Thiagarajah S, Sophie S, Azar I, et al.: Effect of succinylcholine on the ICP of cats with and without thiopental pretreatment. *Anesthesiology* 63:A392, 1985.

Thomas ET: Circulatory collapse following succinylcholine: Report of a case. *Anesth Analg* 48:333, 1969.

Tobey RE: Paraplegia, succinylcholine, and cardiac arrest. *Anesthesiology* 32:359, 1970.

Tobias JD, Jimenez DF: Anaesthetic management during awake craniotomy in a 12-year-old boy. *Paediatr Anaesth* 7:341, 1997.

Todd MM, Drummond JC: A comparison of the cerebrovascular and metabolic effects of halothane and isoflurane in the cat. *Anesthesiology* 60:276, 1984.

Todd MM, Tommasino C, Moore S, et al.: The effects of acute isovolemic hemodilution on the brain: A comparison of crystalloid and colloid solutions. *Anesthesiology* 61:A122, 1984.

Todd MM: The effects of $Pa{CO_2}$ on the cerebrovascular response to nitrous oxide in the halothane-anesthetized rabbit. *Anesth Analg* 66:1090, 1987.

Tong TK: Succinylcholine-induced hyperkalemia in near-drowning. *Anesthesiology* 66:720, 1987.

Toung TJK, Miyabe M, McShane AJ, et al.: Effect of PEEP and jugular venous compression on canine cerebral blood flow and oxygen consumption in the head elevated position. *Anesthesiology* 68:53, 1988.

Toung TSK, McPherson RW, Donham RT, et al.: Pneumocephalus: Effects of patient position on the incidence and location of aerocele after posterior fossa and upper cervical cord surgery. *Anesth Analg* 65:65, 1986.

Turner JM, Powell D, Gibson RM, et al.: Intracranial pressure changes in neurosurgical patients during hypotension induced with sodium nitroprusside or trimethaphan. *Br J Anaesth* 49:419, 1977.

Ubags LH, Kalkman CJ, Been HD, et al.: The use of ketamine or etomidate to supplement sufentanil/N_2O anesthesia does not disrupt monitoring of myogenic transcranial motor evoked responses. *J Neurosurg Anesthesiol* 9:228, 1997.

Van Hemelrijck J, Fitch W, Mattheussen M, et al.: Effect of propofol on cerebral circulation and autoregulation in the baboon. *Anesth Analg* 71:49, 1990.

Verhaegen MJ, Todd MM, Warner DS: A comparison of cerebral ischemic flow thresholds during halothane/N2O and isoflurane/N2O anesthesia in rats. *Anesthesiology* 76:743, 1992.

Vesely R, Hoffman WE, Gil KSL, et al.: The cerebrovascular effects of curare and histamine in the rat. *Anesthesiology* 66:519, 1987.

VonAken H, Puchstein C, Schweppe ML, et al.: Effect of labetalol on intracranial pressure in dogs with and without intracranial hypertension. *Acta Anaesthesiol Scand* 26:615, 1982.

Wagner KJ, Willoch F, Kochs EF, et al.: Dose-dependent regional cerebral blood flow changes during remifentanil infusion in humans: A positron emission tomography study. *Anesthesiology* 94:732, 2001.

Walker MD: Diagnosis and treatment of brain tumors. *Pediatr Clin North Am* 23:131, 1976.

Warner C, Hoffman WE, Baughman VL, et al.: Effects of sufentanil on cerebral blood flow, cerebral blood flow velocity, and metabolism in dogs. *Anesth Analg* 72:177, 1991.

Warner C, Hoffman WE, Segil IJ, et al.: Propofol decreases cerebral and spinal cord blood flow and maintains autoregulation in rats. *J Neurosurg Anesthesiol* 2:220, 1990.

Warner DS, Hindman BJ, Todd MM, et al.: Intracranial pressure and hemodynamic effects of remifentanil versus alfentanil in patients undergoing supratentorial craniotomy. *Anesth Analg* 83:348, 1996.

Weed LH, McKibben PS: Pressure changes in the cerebrospinal fluid following intravenous injection of solutions of various concentrations. *Am J Physiol* 48:512, 1916.

Weinstabl C, Mayer N, Richling B, et al.: Effect of sufentanil on intracranial pressure in neurosurgical patients. *Anaesthesia* 46:837, 1991.

Weinstabl C, Mayer N, Spiss CK: Sufentanil decreases cerebral blood flow velocity in patients with elevated intracranial pressure. *Eur J Anaesthesiol* 9:481, 1992.

Wilkinson HA: Intracranial pressure monitoring: Techniques and pitfalls. In Cooper PR, editor: *Head injury.* Baltimore, 1981, Williams & Wilkins.

Wollman H, Alexander SC, Cohen PJ, et al.: Cerebral circulation of man during halothane anesthesia. *Anesthesiology* 25:180, 1964.

Wood JH, Simeone FA, Fink EA, et al.: Hypervolemic hemodilution in experimental focal cerebral ischemia. *J Neurosurg* 59:500, 1983.

Woolfenden AR, Albers GW, Steinberg GK, et al.: Moyamoya syndrome in children with Alagille syndrome: Additional evidence of a vasculopathy. *Pediatrics* 103:505, 1999.

Yamamoto M, Aoyagi M, Tajima S, et al.: Increase in elastin gene expression and protein synthesis in arterial smooth muscle cells derived from patients with moyamoya disease. *Stroke* 28:1733, 1997.

Yaster M, Koehler RC, Traystman RJ: Effects of fentanyl on peripheral and cerebral hemodynamics in neonatal lambs. *Anesthesiology* 66:524, 1987.

Young WL: Effects of desflurane on the central nervous system. *Anesth Analg* 75:S32, 1992.

Youngs EJ, Shafer SL: Pharmacokinetic parameters relevant to recovery from opioids. *Anesthesiology* 81:833, 1994.

Zornow MH, Todd MM, Moore SS: The acute cerebral effects of changes in plasma osmolality and oncotic pressure. *Anesthesiology* 67:936, 1987.

19 Anesthesia for General Abdominal, Thoracic, Urologic, and Bariatric Surgery

Greg Hammer • Steven Hall • Peter J. Davis

In this chapter, the anesthetic considerations of the most common general abdominal, thoracic, urologic, and bariatric procedures are summarized. Common surgical problems with practical suggestions and discussions of anesthetic technique and anesthetic concerns are offered.

For the most part, anesthetic considerations for pediatric general surgery are similar to those for adults. Inhalation anesthesia supplemented with muscle relaxants can provide adequate operating conditions. Nitrous oxide should be avoided in the presence of a bowel obstruction and in situations where one-lung anesthesia may render the patient hypoxemic. For those in whom aspiration of gastric contents is a major concern, either rapid-sequence induction or awake intubation should be performed. Because children about to undergo urgent emergency surgery frequently have fluid and electrolyte imbalances as well as underlying hemodynamic instability, a thorough preoperative assessment of the patient is essential. In addition to the selection of anesthetic agents to render the patient unconscious, the role of regional anesthesia in providing the child with perioperative pain relief has assumed dramatic opportunity in children. The details of these regional techniques of caudal, lumbar epidural anesthesia, ilioinguinal/iliohypogastric nerve block, penile nerve block, and intercostal nerve block are discussed in Chapter 14, Pediatric Regional Anesthesia. The last factor that influences anesthetic management is the planned operative approach. As the frontiers of minimally invasive surgery expand, these new techniques can markedly influence the patient's cardiorespiratory stability and consequently the choice of anesthetic agents.

■ VIDEO ENDOSCOPY

With the development of smaller instruments, progress in video technology, and growing experience among pediatric surgeons, video endoscopic surgery is being performed for an increasing number of pediatric surgical indications. Benefits of video laparoscopy and thoracoscopy include small incisions and scars, reduced surgical intervention and postoperative pain, earlier return of bowel function, and more rapid recovery (Box 19–1) (Reddick and Olsen, 1989; Soper et al., 1992; Soper et al., 1994; Steiner et al., 1994; Sawyers, 1996; Hunter, 1997; Danelli et al., 2002). Fiberoptic endoscopes that can be passed through a needle are now manufactured, and digital video signals can be electronically modified to yield sharp, detailed, color images with a minimum light intensity. Digital cameras are designed to maintain an image in an upright orientation regardless of how the telescope is rotated. They are also equipped with an optical or a digital zoom to magnify the image or give the illusion of moving the telescope closer to the object of interest. The smallest of telescopes use fiberoptics and are less than 2 mm in diameter. Two-millimeter disposable ports, mounted on a Veress needle, are used for introduction of these small instruments. Larger instruments and ports are used in larger patients and for more complex cases.

BOX 19–1 Advantages of Video Endoscopic Surgery in Infants and Children

- Improved visualization
- Decreased surgical stress
- Decreased postoperative pain
- Decreased ileus/earlier return to enteral feeding
- Shorter hospitalization
- Quicker return to normal activity (parents and patient)
- Fewer long-term complications
- Cosmetically superior

Another major advance in video endoscopic surgery is the development of the endoscopic suite in which all necessary wiring is in equipment booms, ceilings, and walls. The manipulation of digital images is controlled by voice or touch-screen command either from the operative field or at a conveniently located station nearby. High-quality digital images are displayed on flat panel monitors that can be positioned within a comfortable viewing range. Remote-controlled cameras can direct any view in the room to any of the monitors or to a remote site. Digital radiographs can be routed from the radiology department to the operating room, and consultants in remote locations can be viewed on monitors in the operating room so that the surgeon can see to whom they are speaking.

An additional feature of newer endoscopy suites is voice-controlled bed positioning. Robotic tools can be vocally directed to position telescopes in the surgical field for optimal viewing; these surgical "telemanipulators" facilitate microsurgery in confined spaces even in small infants. Other endoscopic robots are being developed for a wide range of surgical applications.

GENERAL ABDOMINAL SURGERY

Abdominal and thoracic pathologic conditions requiring surgical intervention may be caused by metabolic or endocrine disturbances, tumors, inflammatory processes, or embryologic disorders. Box 19–2 lists abdominal conditions commonly encountered in pediatric general surgery.

LAPAROSCOPY

Laparoscopic surgery involves the intraperitoneal or extraperitoneal insufflation of carbon dioxide through a Veress needle. A variable-flow insufflator terminates flow at a preset intra-abdominal pressure of up to 15 mm Hg. Once the abdomen is filled with carbon dioxide, the Veress needle is replaced by a cannula through which a video laparoscope is inserted. Additional ports are placed according to the surgical procedure undertaken.

The laparoscopic procedures that can be performed in infants and children are virtually unlimited. A list of operations currently being performed is shown in Box 19–3. As surgeons gain experience with laparoscopic surgery, the time required to complete these operations decreases (Fig. 19–1). The safety and efficacy of commonly performed laparoscopic procedures compared with alternative approaches (e.g., endoscopic, open surgical techniques) have been compared.

Laparoscopic gastrostomy involves placement of an umbilical port and a left subcostal cannula (the future site of the gastrostomy). The stomach is pulled to the abdominal wall and the gastrostomy is performed using the Seldinger technique (Fig. 19–2). Operative time is approximately 30 minutes (Tomicic et al., 2002). The risks may be less than those for percutaneous endoscopic gastrostomy (PEG) in small children because the procedure is done under direct vision. There is less trauma than with open surgery, and feedings are initiated within 24 hours. *Laparoscopic fundoplication* for the treatment of gastroesophageal reflux disease (GERD) is associated with a complication and recurrence rate comparable to or less than that for open surgery (Esposito et al., 2000).

The laparoscopic treatment of appendicitis in children has been controversial, particularly in complicated cases (e.g., gangrene, perforation). Experience indicates, however, that *laparoscopic appendectomy* is not associated with an increased risk compared with open surgery, even in the presence of perforation (Meguerditchian et al., 2002). The incidence of wound infections and intra-abdominal abscesses may be less in laparoscopic versus open appendectomy (Paya et al., 2000). Surgical times are comparable and postoperative pain and length of hospital stay are diminished (Canty et al., 2000; Lintula et al., 2001). Comparable results have been reported for *laparoscopic cholecystectomy* (Esposito et al., 2001) and *laparoscopic splenectomy* in pediatric patients (Danielson et al., 2000; Park et al., 2000). Diagnostic laparoscopy and *laparoscope-guided cholangiography* are being used in the evaluation of neonatal conjugated hyperbilirubinemia, avoiding the need for laparotomy and operative cholangiography (Hay et al., 2000).

The role of laparoscopy in the treatment of solid neoplasms is evolving. Indications include biopsy of suspected malignancies, staging or determination of resectability, "second-look" procedures to help determine response to chemotherapy, and diagnosis of

BOX 19–2 Abdominal Surgical Conditions Commonly Encountered in Pediatric Patients

- Abdominal-intestinal obstruction
- Atresia
- Stenosis
- Duplication
- Volvulus
- Meconium ileus
- Tumor
- Pyloric stenosis
- Appendicitis
- Meckel's diverticulum
- Regional enteritis
- Acute necrotizing enterocolitis
- Inguinal or umbilical hernia
- Biliary atresia
- Liver cysts or tumors
- Neuroblastoma
- Wilms tumor
- Hirschsprung's disease
- Portal hypertension
- Splenomegaly
- Ruptured viscus
- Exstrophy of bladder
- Tumors of bladder
- Adrenogenital syndrome
- Ovarian cyst or tumors

BOX 19–3 Laparoscopic Procedures in Infants and Children

- Abdominal exploration
  - Infection
  - Mass
  - Trauma
  - Abdominal pain
- Adrenalectomy
- Appendectomy
- Bariatric procedures
- Biopsy
  - Abscess
  - Mass
  - Liver, kidney
- Cholecystectomy
- Colectomy
- Drainage
  - Abscess
  - Cyst
  - Biliary tract
- Diaphragmatic hernia repair
- Fundoplication
- Gastrostomy
- Herniorrhaphy
- Intestinal atresia repair
- Intussusception repair
- Jejunostomy
- Kasai procedure
- Ladd's procedure
- Liver resection
- Nephrectomy
- Oophorectomy
- Orchidopexy
- Orchiectomy
- Ovarian cystectomy
- Pancreatectomy
- Posterior urethral valve repair
- Pull-through
  - Hirschsprung's
  - Imperforate anus
- Splenectomy
- Tenckhoff catheter placement
- Ventriculoperitoneal shunt placement
- Vesicoureteral reimplantation

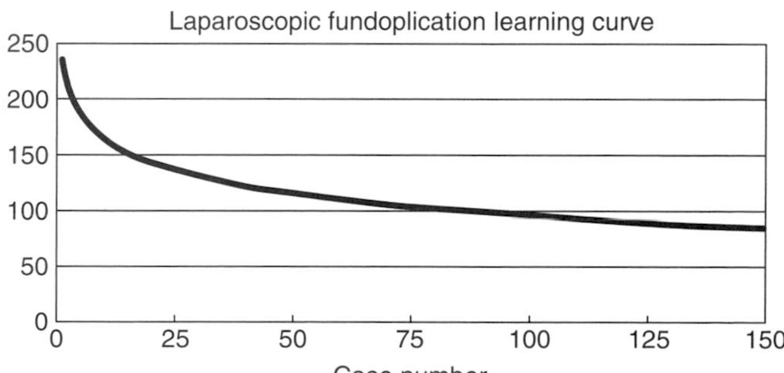

■ **FIGURE 19–1.** The "learning curve" for laparoscopic fundoplication. (Adapted from Georgeson KE, Inge TH, Albanese CT: Laparoscopically assisted anorectal pull-through for high imperforate anus: A new technique. *J Pediatr Surg* 35:927, 2000.)

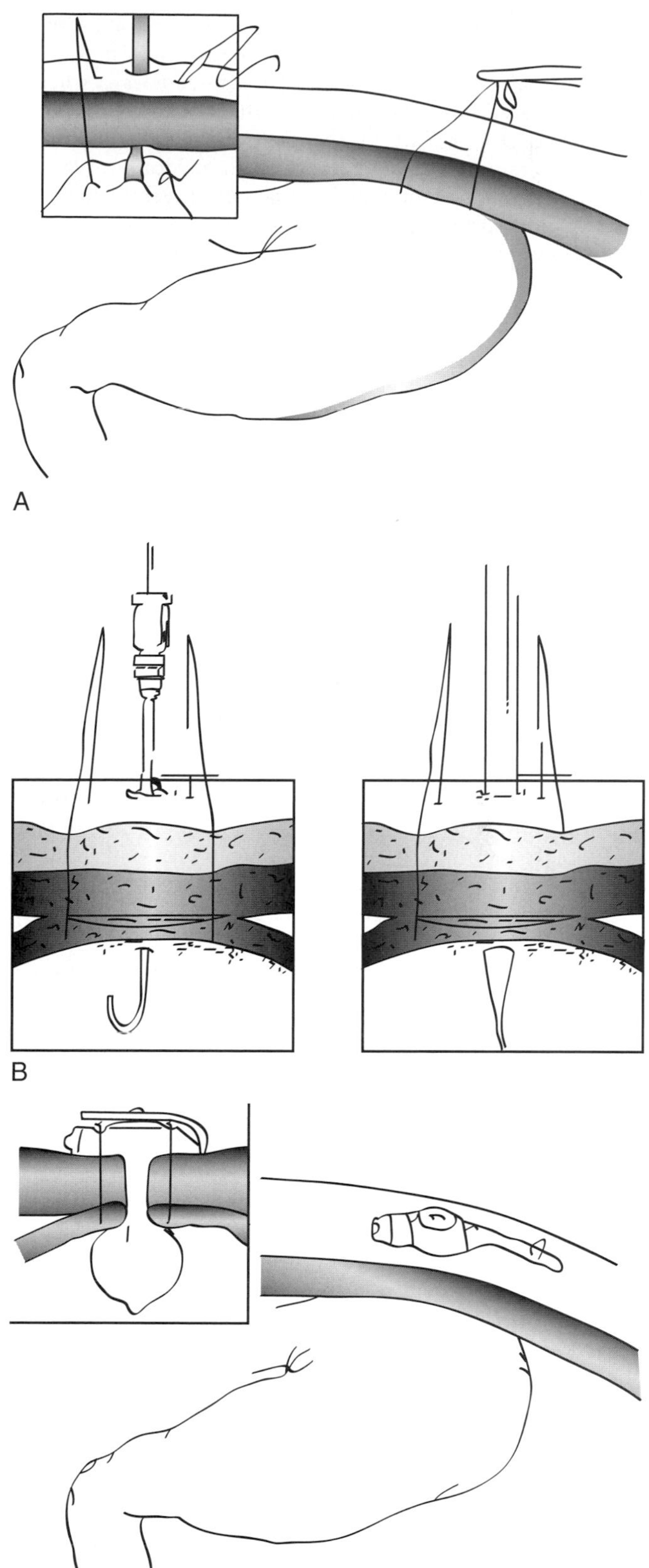

■ **FIGURE 19–2.** Laparoscopic gastrostomy. The stomach is entered and pulled up to the anterior abdominal wall (*A*) and is sutured in place (*B*). The gastrostomy tube is then placed (*C*).

recurrent or metastatic disease (Sailhamer et al., 2003). *Laparoscopic tumor ablation* or *curative resection* may have a role in selected cases. Open surgery may be required in cases wherein complete resection of the intact specimen with delineation of surgical margins is part of the protocol design in patients enrolled in multicenter studies. Although advocates of laparoscopic surgery maintain that laparoscopic surgery can reduce hospital costs, promote earlier patient discharge, produce less postoperative pain, improve cosmetic results, and allow patients a more rapid return to full activity, evidence for this is questionable so far (Rangel et al., 2003).

ANESTHETIC CONSIDERATIONS

Although regional anesthesia may be used alone in older children, general anesthesia is nearly always used for laparoscopic procedures. The use of the laryngeal mask airway (LMA) has been described in adults undergoing laparoscopy. The reliability of the standard LMA to provide adequate gas exchange during positive pressure ventilation is controversial (Maltby et al., 2000; Lu et al., 2002). More favorable ventilation and a reduction in inadvertent gastric insufflation have been reported with the LMA-ProSeal (The Laryngeal Mask Company Limited, Henley on Thames, UK; Maltby et al., 2002). In infants and children, however, endotracheal tube (ETT) placement remains the standard.

Following tracheal intubation, the stomach is suctioned with an orogastric tube to decrease the risk of visceral injury during trocar insertion. The surgeon may prefer to place the patient near the foot of the table, especially for procedures in infants. The table position itself may need to be changed repeatedly during the operation, and both the Trendelenburg and the reverse Trendelenburg positions are often used. Accordingly, care must be taken to secure the patient to the table (e.g., using rolls of gauze and tape) while ensuring that the extremities are well padded and are not subject to inadvertent movement and untoward pressure during the operation. Inadvertent endobronchial intubation may occur due to cephalad displacement of the diaphragm associated with the Trendelenburg position and/or abdominal insufflation with gas. As a part of routine monitors, a precordial stethoscope should be placed over the left chest to readily detect this complication.

A variety of general anesthetic techniques have been used for laparoscopic surgery. Regional anesthesia is not commonly used as an adjunct to general anesthesia in pediatric patients unless the laparoscopy is converted to an open procedure. The use of nitrous oxide is controversial. Concerns have been raised that nitrous oxide may cause bowel distention, compromising visibility and exposure during surgery (Eger and Saidman, 1965; Cunningham and Brull, 1993). In addition, nitrous oxide may exacerbate the already increased incidence of nausea and vomiting following laparoscopy (Divatia et al., 1996; Tramer et al., 1996), although the findings of several studies have failed to confirm these effects of nitrous oxide (Taylor et al., 1992; Jensen et al., 1993). However, nitrous oxide can also support combustion. Because of its antiemetic effect, propofol has been recommended for maintenance of anesthesia during laparoscopy (Song et al., 1998). The combination of propofol and remifentanil has been advocated due to rapid emergence without an increase in postoperative nausea and vomiting compared with the use of inhalation anesthesia (Grundmann et al., 2001). Because of the increased incidence of postoperative nausea and vomiting associated with laparoscopy, prophylactic treatment with antiemetics and histamine blockers (droperidol, metoclopromide) have been commonly used. Orogastric suctioning at the end of the operation may also help reduce the risk of postoperative nausea and vomiting.

Because of the reduced postoperative pain associated with laparoscopy compared with open surgery, postoperative analgesia can usually be achieved with intravenous and oral agents. Although diminished compared with open surgery, pain following laparoscopic surgery is associated with incision, visceral manipulation, irritation and traction of nerves, vascular traction and injury, presence of residual gas in the abdomen, and inflammatory mediators (Alexander, 1997). Pain is frequently localized to the back or shoulder.

A variety of approaches to prevent and treat pain after laparoscopy have been described. Bupivacaine infiltration at incision sites before skin incision has been shown to decrease postoperative pain (Kato et al., 2000; Moiniche et al., 2000). Bupivacaine infiltration has been found to be superior to intravenous fentanyl or tenoxicam in reducing postoperative pain (Salman et al., 2000). "Low-dose" intrathecal morphine and bupivacaine also decrease postoperative pain (Motamed et al., 2000). Intraperitoneal local anesthetic instillation and mesosalpinx block may diminish postoperative pain after laparoscopy and may be beneficial in reducing postoperative shoulder pain (Kiliç et al., 1996). Intraperitoneal instillation of both bupivacaine and meperidine has been shown to be more efficacious than the combination of intraperitoneal bupivacaine and intramuscular meperidine (Colbert et al., 2000).

Caution must be used to avoid toxic plasma concentrations of local anesthetics due to systemic absorption in infants and children, however. Perioperative acetaminophen, nonsteroidal anti-inflammatory agents, and other nonopioid analgesics should be used in combination with opioids as needed for postoperative analgesia. Clonidine has been shown to reduce the requirement for postoperative opioids and also has the advantage of decreasing the tachycardia associated with pneumoperitoneum (Yu et al., 2003).

Physiologic changes during laparoscopic surgery are related to positioning (Trendelenburg, reverse Trendelenburg), increased abdominal pressure due to gas insufflation, and increased arterial carbon dioxide tension associated with insufflation. The magnitude of physiologic changes associated with laparoscopic surgery is influenced by the patient's age, underlying myocardial function, and anesthetic agents. The reverse Trendelenburg position may cause hypotension, especially in the anesthetized patient with intravascular hypovolemia. The Trendelenburg position causes cephalad displacement of the diaphragm, restricting lung excursion and posing the risk of endobronchial intubation. In addition, central venous pressure and heart rate increase, and systemic arterial pressures and cardiac output decrease (Hirvonen et al., 1995). The pulmonary effects depend on the patient's age, weight, pulmonary function, degree of Trendelenburg position, anesthetic agents, and ventilation technique. Atelectasis and a decrease in functional residual capacity and pulmonary compliance may be observed. Ventilation/perfusion mismatch may result in decreased arterial oxygen tension. Neuromuscular blockade, endotracheal intubation, and positive pressure ventilation may help to reduce the pulmonary effects of Trendelenburg position. As long as intra-abdominal pressure is kept below 15 mm Hg, oxygen saturation can generally be maintained during position changes and pneumoperitoneum despite adverse changes in respiratory mechanics (Sprung et al., 2003). Significant hypercarbia may occur despite adjustments in mechanical ventilation, especially in infants.

Both pneumoperitoneum and the Trendelenburg position reduce femoral venous flow, increasing the risk of thrombotic complications (Rosen et al., 2000). Cardiovascular instability associated with laparoscopy has also been attributed to hypercarbia-induced arrhythmias, venous gas embolus, compression of the vena cava, pneumothorax, and pneumomediastinum. Insufflation to an intra-abdominal pressure of 12 mm Hg can cause septal hypokinesis, and left ventricular wall motion abnormalities (Huettmann et al., 2003; Hoymork et al., 2003). The increase in intra-abdominal pressure associated with gas insufflation results in increased intrathoracic pressure and increased pulmonary and systemic vascular resistances, and decreased cardiac output (Hirvonen et al., 1995; Hirvonen et al., 2000). Arterial blood pressure may be decreased, maintained, or even elevated by an increase in systemic vascular resistance. Reduction in splanchnic, hepatic, and renal blood flow and increases in the plasma concentrations of catecholamines, cortisol, prolactin, growth hormone, and glucose levels have been reported with carbon dioxide pneumoperitoneum (Hashikura et al., 1994; Mikami et al., 1998; Ishizuka et al., 2000).

Hypothermia is avoided by warming the insufflating gas and/or maintaining insufflating flows of less than 2 L/min.

A new technique known as gasless laparoscopy eliminates the risks of pneumoperitoneum by using mechanical retraction (Canestrelli et al., 1999). Reduced visualization is associated with this technique, however, and its application to pediatrics remains uncertain (Lukban et al., 2000).

INGUINAL HERNIORRHAPHY AND UMBILICAL HERNIORRHAPHY

During the seventh month of gestation, the testicle descends from the abdomen through the inguinal wall into the scrotum. The processus vaginalis, a peritoneal covering, encloses the testicles during their descent. In term infants, the processus vaginalis is usually closed at birth, but it remains patent in 15% to 37% of people. In premature infants, the incidence is much higher depending on the gestational age at the time of birth. The continued patency of the processus vaginalis is the principal factor in the development of congenital hernias and hydroceles.

Inguinal hernia repair is the most frequent general surgical procedure performed by pediatric surgeons. Males are more frequently affected than females, and the incidence of inguinal hernia is highest in the first year of life. Right-sided hernias (60%) occur more frequently than left-sided (30%) and bilateral (10%) hernias. Other risk factors associated with inguinal hernias are prematurity, chronic respiratory illness, and excessive intraperitoneal fluid (ventriculoperitoneal shunts, ascites, peritoneal dialysis).

The surgical technique for this procedure is well described (Rowe and Lloyd, 1986). Laparoscopic techniques have also been described (Lobe and Schropp, 1992; Lee and Liang, 2002; Schier et al., 2002), as well as needleoscopic techniques (Prasad et al., 2003). The overall complication rate after elective hernia repair is about 2% and increases to 14% after operations for incarcerated hernia. A major surgical issue in patients with a unilateral inguinal hernia is whether the contralateral side should be explored, thereby subjecting the patient to possible unnecessary damage to the contralateral vas deferens and spermatic cord. In a number of studies, a patent contralateral processus vaginalis occurs about 60% of the time. However, this patency appears age related, with the highest rate occurring in infants (63%) and incidence decreasing until 2 years of age, when it appears to plateau at 41% (Rowe and Lloyd, 1986). Despite the high incidence of patent processus vaginalis, the incidence of contralateral hernias is about 15%. The development of a contralateral hernia is also age dependent. If the initial hernia developed in the first year of life, there is a fourfold greater chance that a contralateral hernia will develop compared with children whose initial hernia presented after 1 year of age. In girls with unilateral inguinal hernias, the incidence of positive explorations for contralateral hernias is 60%. Consequently, girls almost always undergo contralateral exploration. Laparoscopy without a separate incision has been advocated to examine the contralateral side when the ipsilateral hernia sac is of sufficient width to allow passage of a laparoscope (Yerkes et al., 1998).

Herniorrhaphies are commonly performed as elective procedures; however, in children with incarceration and signs of bowel obstruction, a rapid-sequence induction with application of cricoid pressure is needed.

The following discussion pertains to elective, uncomplicated hernias. Anesthesia can be induced by mask inhalation of volatile agents or by rectal or intravenous techniques. Endotracheal intubation is usually unnecessary for herniorrhaphy except in infants under 1 year of age, in whom it may be difficult to maintain an adequate airway with bag and mask ventilation without distending the stomach. However, the use of the LMA in these patients may make tracheal intubation unnecessary. The patient must be well anesthetized when the spermatic cord is being manipulated. Inadequate depth of anesthesia at this stage can result in laryngospasm and/or bradycardia. Caudal epidural anesthesia or ilioinguinal/iliohypogastric nerve block can be quite effective both in providing postoperative pain relief and in diminishing the intraoperative anesthetic requirements (Markham et al., 1986). Premature infants have a particularly high incidence of inguinal hernias. In these infants, in whom an inhalation anesthetic may have increased risks, spinal anesthesia (Harnik et al., 1986) and caudal epidural (Spear et al., 1988) anesthesia have been used successfully to avoid general anesthesia and endotracheal intubation.

ORCHIOPEXY

Cryptorchidism affects approximately 0.8% of 1-year-old boys. The undescended testicle may lie within the abdomen, the inguinal canal, or the external ring just proximal to the scrotum. Although the undescended testicle is usually associated with a hernia, the most significant medical risk for the patient is the chance of developing a malignancy, which is 10-fold greater than in a normally descended one.

The objectives of repair for undescended testicles are to alter the course of the spermatic artery from the renal pedicle to the internal ring to the external ring and to create in its place a direct line from the renal pedicle to the scrotum. However, the surgical approach to patients with undescended testes is not uniform (Hinman, 1987; Heiss et al., 1992). The general approach to patients with a nonpalpable testis is inguinal exploration. If neither the testis nor proof of its absence is found, the lower posterolateral surface of the peritoneal cavity is explored. When the testis is found, it is either removed or surgically placed in the scrotum. This can be accomplished by a staged orchiopexy, autotransplantation of the testis, or Fowler-Stephens procedure. The Fowler-Stephens approach takes advantage of the vascular arcades between the deferential and spermatic arteries within the cord. Because of this collateral blood flow, high ligation of the testicular vessels can preserve the testicular blood supply and provide the surgeon with mobility in bringing the testicle down into the scrotum. The Fowler-Stephens approach has undergone modification and is now generally done in two stages. The first stage involves clipping of the spermatic vessel, whereas the second stage, performed months later, involves the formal orchiopexy. With the advent of laparoscopic surgery, both stages of the Fowler-Stephens approach can be done with the aid of a laparoscope (Atlas and Stone, 1992; Bogaert et al., 1993).

The anesthetic considerations are similar to those for inguinal hernia repair. Because of the traction and manipulation of the spermatic cord and testicle, the incidence of intraoperative bradycardia and laryngospasm is somewhat increased. Consequently, a deeper level of anesthesia is required. However, the need for a deeper plane of anesthesia and the risk of bradycardia and laryngospasm can be lessened by the use of intraoperative nerve blocks or regional anesthesia. If an intra-abdominal exploration or the use of laparoscopy is anticipated, or both, the trachea is generally intubated. Because the incidence of postoperative nausea and pain is significant, caudal nerve blocks and prophylactic antiemetics, such as ondansetron, 0.1 mg/kg, are recommended.

SURGERY FOR PYLORIC STENOSIS

Pyloric stenosis is one of the most common gastrointestinal abnormalities presenting in the first 6 months of life. This disorder has a polygenic mode of inheritance and occurs 4 times more commonly in males and more frequently in white infants. The frequency of this disorder ranges from 1.4 to 8.8:1000 live births (Zeidan et al., 1988; Dubé et al., 1990; Saunders and Williams, 1990; Bissonnette and Sullivan, 1991; Murtagh et al., 1992). There is some controversy regarding the associated risk of pyloric stenosis with the maternal postnatal exposure to macrolides (Louik et al., 2002; Sorensen et al., 2003). Pyloric stenosis has been associated with cleft palate and esophageal reflux.

The cardinal features of pyloric stenosis condition are projectile vomiting, visible peristalsis, and a hypochloremic, hypokalemic, metabolic alkalosis. Although hypokalemia is a frequent finding, Schwartz and others (2003) reported in a retrospective chart review that 36% of patients with pyloric stenosis were noted to have hyperkalemia. Nonbilious vomiting is the classic presenting symptom and generally occurs between 2 and 8 weeks of age. Jaundice occurs in less than 5% of patients and is thought to be associated with caloric deprivation and hepatic gluconyltransferase deficiency. The jaundice resolves after successful treatment. Diagnosis is made by palpation of an olive-sized mass in the upper abdomen and is frequently confirmed by radiographic studies. Although false-positive studies are rare, false-negative findings can occur in up to 19% of the ultrasound examinations and in 10% of the contrast studies.

The pathologic condition involves gross thickening of the circular muscles of the pylorus, resulting in a gradual obstruction of the gastric outlets. Vanderwinden and others (1992) noted a deficiency of nitric oxide synthetase in the muscle layers of infants with pyloric stenosis. The pathophysiology of pyloric stenosis frequently leads to hypovolemia and a hypochloremic metabolic alkalosis.

Winters (1973) outlines the pathophysiology that leads to hypochloremic, hypokalemic metabolic alkalosis. In pyloric stenosis, persistent vomiting results in a loss of gastric juices rich in hydrogen and chloride ions and, to a lesser extent, sodium and potassium ions. Because the obstruction is at the level of the pylorus, the vomitus does not contain the usual alkaline secretions of the small intestine; the patient develops a metabolic alkalosis.

As an increased bicarbonate load is presented to the kidney, the resorptive capacity of the proximal tubule is overwhelmed and an increased amount of $NaHCO_3$ and water is delivered to the distal tubule. Because $NaHCO_3$ cannot be reabsorbed in the distal tubule, aldosterone secretion occurs. Increased aldosterone increases sodium reabsorption and kaliuresis. Potassium loss is further exacerbated by potassium being exchanged in the tubule for hydrogen in an effort to maintain normal plasma pH.

With persistent vomiting and intravascular volume depletion, the renal response shifts to maintain the patient's intravascular volume and sodium conservation occurs. Increased secretion of aldosterone promotes sodium conservation and potassium excretion. In the distal tubule, sodium is also conserved in exchange for hydrogen ions. This may result in a paradoxical aciduria and worsening metabolic alkalosis.

Surgical pyloromyotomy, a relatively simple procedure in the hands of skilled pediatric surgeons, is curative (Fig. 19–3). The operative mortality of 10% has declined to less than 0.5%. The surgery can be performed either laparoscopically or as an open procedure. In a comparative study, Campbell and others (2002) noted that laparoscopic pyloromyotomy has become the dominant approach. However, laparoscopic pyloromyotomy is associated with an increased rate of complications, higher hospital charges, and a reduction in the general surgical resident's operating experience (Campbell et al., 2002). Pyloromyotomy for pyloric stenosis is not a medical emergency that requires immediate surgical intervention. The major anesthetic considerations are recognizing and treating dehydration and acid-base abnormalities before beginning anesthesia. In addition, the patient is at risk for aspirating gastric contents.

The initial therapeutic approach is aimed at repletion of intravascular volume and correction of electrolyte and acid-base abnormalities (e.g., 5% dextrose in 0.45% NaCl with 40 mmol/L of potassium infused at 3 L/m^2 per 24 hr). Most children respond to therapy within 12 to 48 hours, after which surgical correction can proceed in a nonemergency manner.

Once the child is satisfactorily hydrated and after the appropriate monitors (precordial stethoscope, electrocardiogram, pulse oximeter, and blood pressure cuff) are placed, the infant is ready for induction of anesthesia. The obstructed pylorus and associated vomiting increase the possibility of aspirating gastric contents during induction of anesthesia. A thorough evacuation of the stomach contents through a nasogastric or an orogastric tube, with proper preoxygenation and monitoring, greatly reduces the chance of regurgitation during induction, although it does not completely eliminate the possibility of aspiration (Cook-Sather et al., 1997). Infants with pyloric stenosis are thus considered by some anesthesiologists to be in an equivalent status to infants with a full stomach. Thus, a rapid sequence induction is preferred to secure the airway and minimize the risks of aspiration (Dierdorf and Krishna, 1981; Battersby et al., 1984). On the other hand, mask inhalation induction preceded by careful emptying of the stomach has been used safely in several pediatric centers (MacDonald et al., 1987). In a prospective nonrandomized observational study of 76 infants with pyloric stenosis, Cook-Sather and others (1998) compared three techniques: awake intubation, rapid sequence intubation, and modified rapid sequence intubation (ventilation through cricoid pressure). In this study, awake intubation was not superior to anesthetized, paralyzed intubations. Awake intubation prevented neither bradycardia nor oxygen desaturations.

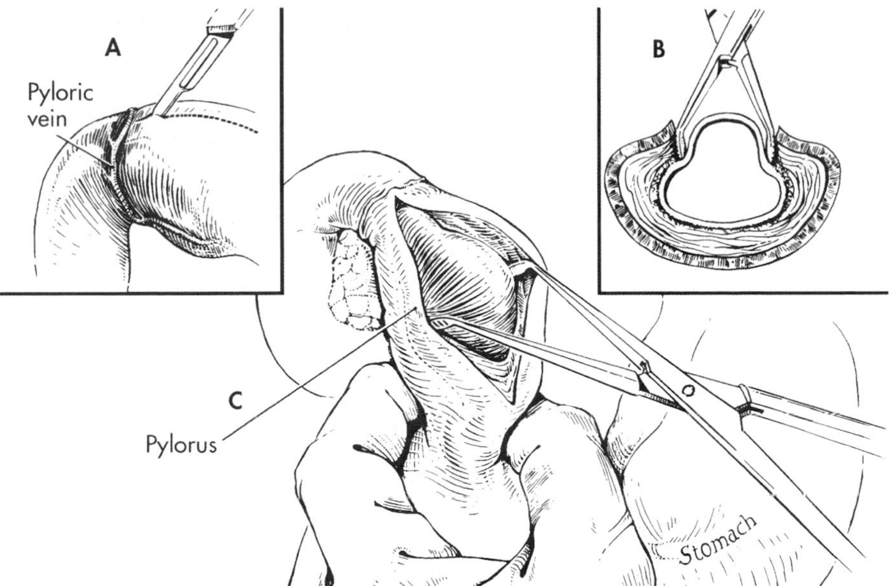

■ **FIGURE 19–3.** Pyloric stenosis. Operative technique of pyloromyotomy. *A*, Incision made on anterosuperior surface through avascular area. *B*, Cross section of hypertrophied pylorus after operation has been completed. *C*, Circular muscle is separated, allowing submucosa to bulge. (From Benson CO: Infantile hypertrophic pyloric stenosis. In Welch KJ, et al., editors: *Pediatric surgery,* 4th ed. Chicago, 1986, Year Book Medical Publishers.)

After induction and intubation of the trachea, a nasogastric or an orogastric tube is reinserted and left in place during the operative procedure. This allows the surgeon to test the integrity of the pyloric mucosa after pyloromyotomy. A small volume of air is injected down the nasogastric tube, and the surgeon manipulates the air bubble into the duodenum and occludes the bowel lumen both proximal and distal to the incision. Mucosal perforation is indicated if there is air leakage. After the operation, which usually requires less than 30 minutes, the effects of any nondepolarizing muscle relaxant are reversed. Then the infant can be safely extubated when fully awake and with intact protective airway reflexes. Some believe that opioid analgesia is seldom necessary (Battersby et al., 1984) and may predispose patients to a prolonged emergence from anesthesia (MacDonald et al., 1987). It is not unusual to encounter lethargy or drowsiness in these infants in the immediate postoperative period. Respiratory depression has been noted to occur postoperatively and is possibly related to cerebrospinal fluid pH and hyperventilation (Andropoulos et al., 1994). Rare occurrences of hypoglycemia, apnea, convulsions, and cardiac arrest in the early postoperative period have also been cited. These events have been ascribed to the cessation of intravenous glucose infusions and the depletion of liver glycogen in these infants (Shumake, 1975). Infants usually begin oral feedings 8 hours after the procedure. The choice of maintenance anesthetic agent for infants with pyloric stenosis has been studied (Wolf et al., 1996; Chipps et al., 1999; Davis et al., 2001; Galinkin et al., 2001).

In the study by Wolf and others, clinical postoperative apnea occurred in 3 of 11 infants anesthetized with isoflurane and in none of the 9 infants anesthetized with desflurane. In a multicenter study comparing halothane and remifentanil, where both drugs were administered to similar clinical end points, remifentanil was not associated with postoperative respiratory depression. In this study, all infants received both preoperative and postoperative pneumograms, and remifentanil (as opposed to halothane) was not associated with new pneumogram abnormalities in the postoperative period (Davis et al., 2001; Galinkin et al., 2001).

WILMS TUMOR PROCEDURES

Wilms tumor is the most common childhood abdominal malignancy, occurring in an incidence, consistent throughout the world, of 5.0 to 7.8 per 1 million children under 15 years of age. Wilms tumor accounts for about 6% of all malignancies in childhood. The incidence is equal in the two sexes. The peak age at diagnosis is between 1 and 3 years. Wilms tumor occurs bilaterally in 5% of patients. Patients with Wilms tumor frequently have associated anomalies (aniridia, 1%; hemihypertrophy, 2%; genitourinary abnormalities, 5%; ectopic and solitary kidneys [horseshoe kidneys, ureteral duplications, hypospadias]). Other associated conditions include Beckwith-Wiedemann syndrome and neurofibromatosis. The signs and symptoms associated with Wilms tumor are variable. The most frequent finding is an increasing abdominal girth with a palpable abdominal mass (85%). Hypertension occurs in 60% of patients, and hematuria is present in 10% to 25%.

Wilms tumor generally is located in the upper or lower renal pole. It may involve the renal vein and extend up the vena cava to the right atrium. Prognosis of the disease is related to its staging (Table 19–1). Patients with favorable staging have an 80% to 90% chance of cure, whereas patients with metastasis have a 50%

■ **TABLE 19–1.** Wilms tumor staging

Staging	Description
I	Tumor limited to the kidney and excised.
II	Tumor extending beyond the kidney, but completely excised. The tumor may have been biopsied or there may have been local spillage of tumor confined to the flank.
III	Residual nonhematogenous tumor confined to the abdomen. Lymph node involvement in the abdomen. Diffuse peritoneal contamination by spillage or tumor growth that has penetrated through the peritoneal surface.
IV	Hematogenous metastases. Lymph node involvement beyond the abdominal cavity.
V	Bilateral renal involvement at diagnosis.

chance of long-term survival. Risk factors for local recurrence of Wilms tumor include an advanced local stage (involvement of the para-aortic lymph nodes), unfavorable histology, and spillage of tumor at the time of resection (Shamberger et al., 1999). Therapy for Wilms tumor includes surgery, chemotherapy, and radiotherapy. Depending on the size of the tumor and the staging, chemotherapy may be started either before or after surgery. Chemotherapy generally involves vincristine, actinomycin, and anthracycline (doxorubicin).

Preoperative evaluation of the patient is related to the presence of metastases and the patient's cardiopulmonary function. If the patient has had prior chemotherapy with Adriamycin, cardiac function should be assessed by echocardiogram (see Chapters 3 and 32, Cardiovascular Physiology and Systemic Disorders). Serum electrolyte levels should be assessed if there is a history of vomiting. Renal dysfunction is unusual even in patients with bilateral Wilms tumor.

Anesthetic considerations revolve around the issue of abdominal distention with delayed gastric emptying and potentially large intraoperative blood losses. Abdominal distention may place the patient at risk for aspiration of gastric contents, so full-stomach precautions should be taken at the induction of anesthesia. Intraoperative blood loss can be a significant factor because of the tumor's location and possible involvement of the renal vein and vena cava. Two large-bore intravenous catheters are recommended. Because of the possibility that the vena cava may be cross-clamped (either to be explored for extension of tumor or to control hemorrhage), the large-bore catheters should be preferentially inserted above the diaphragm.

Pulmonary function may be compromised because of metastasis, tumor embolization, abdominal distention, or surgical traction. Monitoring of the patient should include pulse oximetry and capnography as well as the standard monitors of electrocardiograph, blood pressure, and esophageal stethoscope. Arterial catheters are generally reserved for patients with large tumors, patients with previous intra-abdominal surgery (increased number of adhesions), and patients with significant cardiorespiratory depression.

After induction, anesthesia is maintained with potent inhalation anesthetic agents. Nitrous oxide is avoided because of the bowel distention, and opioids are administered to reduce the anesthetic requirements. An alternative approach that provides both excellent operative conditions and postoperative pain control is the use of combined general anesthesia with a continuous epidural infusion.

NEUROBLASTOMA PROCEDURES

Neuroblastoma is the most common extracranial solid tumor of childhood and involves the postganglionic sympathetic nervous system. Fifty percent of tumors arise in the adrenal, 30% occur below the diaphragm, and 20% occur in cervical or thoracic sites. Neuroblastoma accounts for 8% to 10% of pediatric cancers. The median age of presentation is 22 months, with 37% of patients presenting under 1 year of age, and 51% of patients being less than 4 years of age. Clinical presentation may be related to the primary tumor, to its metastasis, or to the associated paraneoplastic syndromes (Table 19–2). Metastases from neuroblastoma occur in lymph nodes, liver, cortical bone, bone marrow, orbits, and skin. The paraneoplastic syndromes can present with hypertension secondary to catecholamine release and/or kidney displacement with renal artery stretching

TABLE 19–2. Presenting signs and symptoms of neuroblastoma

Primary tumor	Abdominal mass or pain; respiratory distress or dysphagia; vocal cord paralysis; bowel or bladder dysfunction; Horner's syndrome; heterochromia of iris on affected side; incidental finding on chest radiograph
Metastatic disease	Hepatomegaly; lymphadenopathy; bone pain; periorbital ecchymoses; subcutaneous nodules; marrow replacement with anemia, fever, or bruising from low blood counts; systemic illness; failure to thrive; fever of unknown origin
Paraneoplastic syndromes	1. Vasoactive intestinal peptide (VIP) syndrome: Chronic watery diarrhea and abdominal distention 2. Opsoclonus-myoclonus or cerebellar ataxia syndrome 3. Excessive catecholamine syndrome: hypertension, headaches, flushing, sweating, tachycardia, palpitations

and renin-angiotensin stimulus. The gastrointestinal symptoms (diarrhea, flushing, abdominal distention) are attributed to vasoactive intestinal peptides, whereas the etiology of opsoclonus and ataxia is unclear.

Tumor prognosis has been related to age of presentation, extent of disease (staging) (Fig. 19–4), degree of tumor differentiation, amount of catecholamine metabolites, serum ferritin level, lactate dehydrogenase level, neuron-specific enolase level, serum lymphocyte count, ganglioside presence, *N*-myc amplification, deletion of chromosome 1p, additional copies of chromosome 17q, and TRKA expression (Smith et al., 1989; Hiyama et al., 1991; Berthold et al., 1992; Eckschlager, 1992; Murakami et al., 1992; Qualman et al., 1992; Shuster et al., 1992; Haase et al., 1999). However, patient age and tumor stage are the two most important independent variables. The Evans staging system uses tumor location, lymph node involvement, and presence of metastases, whereas the Pediatric Oncology Group (POG) system emphasizes tumor resectability and identification of residual disease to predict survival and treatment.

Treatment involves surgical resection and chemotherapy. Although neuroblastoma is radiosensitive, 45% of patients present with metastasis so that its use is sometimes limited in primary therapy. In a series of adrenal neuroblastomas less than 6 cm not associated with adjacent vessel or organ involvement, DeLaagause and others (2003) reported successful tumor removal with laparoscopic techniques. The anesthetic considerations depend on the planned surgical procedure, the location and size of the tumor, and the metabolic effects of the tumor. Electrolyte imbalance may result from vomiting and diarrhea caused by excessive production of vasoactive intestinal peptide (VIP). Despite the production of catecholamines, significant hypertension has been reported in 9% to 30% of patients (Weinblatt et al., 1983; Haberkern et al., 1992).

Intraoperatively, blood loss and third-space fluid losses can accompany the resection of tumor. Haberkern and others (1992) noted in a retrospective review that 45% of patients had hypotension after the tumor excision, whereas fewer than 3% of the patients had cardiovascular signs of increased catecholamine release during tumor resection. Although in patients with mediastinal neuroblastoma airway complications are rare owing to the tumor's location in the posterior mediastinum, airway compromise can occur, and evidence of airway compression by the tumor should be evaluated before starting the anesthetic induction. Intravenous or inhalational inductions may be performed.

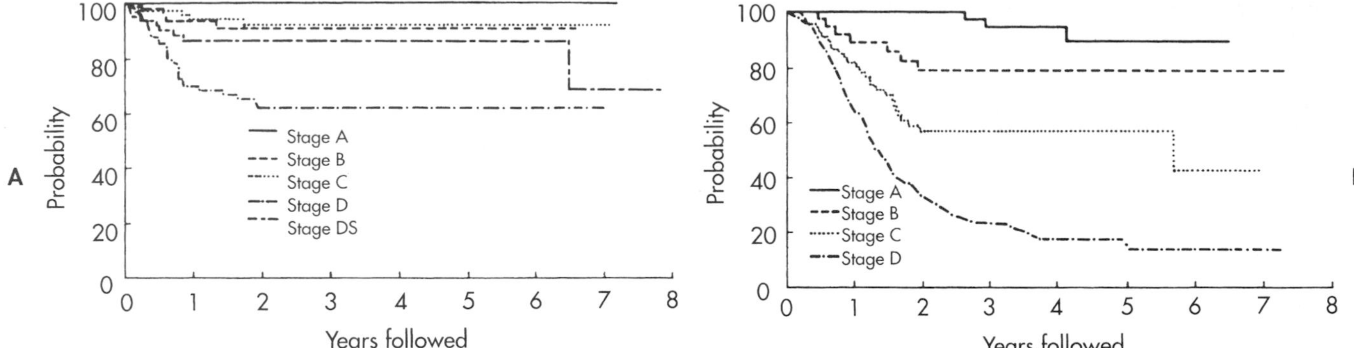

FIGURE 19–4. Prognosis of neuroblastoma related to age and staging. *A*, Children under 1 year of age. *B*, Children over 1 year of age. The staging is according to the Pediatric Oncology Group (POG) system. *Stage A:* Complete gross resection of primary tumor, with or without microscopic residual. Intracavitary lymph nodes, not adhered to and removed with primary (nodes adhered to or within tumor resection may be positive for tumor without upstaging patient to stage C), histologically free of tumor. If primary in abdomen or pelvis, liver histologically free of tumor. *Stage B:* Grossly unresected primary tumor. Nodes and liver are the same as for stage A. *Stage C:* Complete or incomplete resection of primary. Intracavitary nodes not adhered to primary histologically positive for tumor. Liver as in stage A. *Stage D:* Any dissemination of disease beyond intracavitary nodes: extracavitary nodes, liver, skin, bone marrow, bone. *Stage D(S):* Would be Evans stage I or II except for metastatic tumor in liver, bone marrow, or skin. *Evans stage I:* Tumor confined to the organ of structure of origin. *Evans stage II:* Tumor extending in continuity beyond the organ or structure of origin but not crossing the mid-line. Regional lymph nodes on the ipsilateral side may be involved. (Data courtesy of Dr. Jonathan J. Shuster and the Pediatric Oncology Group. From Brodeur GM: Neuroblastoma and other peripheral neuroectodermal tumors. In Fernbach DJ, Viett TJ, editors: *Clinical pediatric oncology,* St. Louis, 1991, Mosby.)

Both volatile agents and opioids have been safely used along with combined regional and general anesthetic techniques (Haberkern et al., 1992).

ANTIGASTROESOPHAGEAL REFLUX PROCEDURES

Gastroesophageal reflux (GER) involves a dysfunction of the esophageal sphincter mechanism that allows gastric contents to return into the esophagus and consequently may place an anesthetized patient at risk for aspiration. The clinical spectrum of GER can range from patients who are completely asymptomatic to patients with severe esophagitis, esophageal bleeding, esophageal stricture, malnutrition, and respiratory compromise. Although in the pediatric population GER can be physiologic secondary to an immature maturation of the lower esophageal sphincter mechanism, this aspect of GER generally resolves by 15 months of age. GER is also seen in children who are neurologically compromised as well as patients who have survived diaphragmatic hernias, tracheoesophageal fistula, and esophageal atresia repairs. GER has also been noted in about 10% of patients who have undergone successful treatment of pyloric stenosis.

In normal children, reflux of gastric contents is prevented by the gastroesophageal junction. This junction is composed of a lower esophageal sphincter (LES). The LES is a high-pressure zone in the distal esophagus that lies in both the mediastinum and abdomen and becomes functionally mature by 6 weeks of postnatal age. Factors that affect the valve mechanism of the LES include the cardioesophageal angle of His; the esophageal hiatus, a sling of muscle that is part of the diaphragm; and the phrenoesophageal ligament. The degree of reflux, the duration of acid exposure within the esophagus, the ability of the esophagus to clear its contents, and the extent of mucosal damage are the primary factors that determine the degree of esophagitis and consequently its clinical and pathologic significance.

In pediatric patients, the complications of GER include respiratory compromise (bronchospasm, chronic aspiration with pneumonitis, reactive airway disease and apnea) and esophagitis (esophageal metaplasia, Barrett's esophagus, stricture, dysphagia). Diagnostic evaluation includes an upper gastrointestinal series, nuclear scan, upper endoscopy, and esophageal pH probe.

Treatment of GER may involve both medical and surgical therapies. Medical therapy consists of both conservative and pharmacologic interventions (thickened feedings, avoidance of overfeeding, postcibal position therapy). The use of medication is aimed at blocking acid secretions using H_2-blocker agents (e.g., ranitidine) and improving gastroesophageal motility and gastric emptying (e.g., metoclopramide, bethanechol). Cisapride, a dopamine antagonist, is also used as a motility drug. Its mode of action is postulated to increase the release of acetylcholine from the myenteric plexus and to increase receptor sensitivity to acetylcholine.

The surgical procedures are aimed at establishing an intra-abdominal segment of esophagus and creating a physiologic angle of His (Fig. 19–5). The two common procedures are the 360-degree fundoplication of Nissen and the partial wrap of Thal-Nissen. To avoid the gas bloat syndrome (aerophagia, gastric distention, inability to belch or vomit) associated with Nissen fundoplications, the Thal-Nissen partial wrap is frequently used.

The surgical procedure can be performed as either an open or a laparoscopic procedure (Georgeson, 1993; Rothenberg, 1998; Bourne et al., 2003; Esposito et al., 2003; Steyaert et al., 2003). In the children undergoing laparoscopic antireflux procedures, the physiological perturbations of pneumoperitoneum, increased intra-abdominal pressure, and the associated absorption of carbon dioxide need to be considered.

Surgical success rates approach 95% in pediatric patients with normal neurologic development, but in children who are neurologically impaired, morbidity and mortality remain high. It is important in these patients to determine if their underlying symptoms result from GER as opposed to nasopharyngeal incoordination and/or esophageal or antral dysmotility (Flake et al., 1991; Martinez et al., 1992; Smith et al., 1992). The presence of GER places the patient at risk for aspiration during induction of anesthesia. Preoperative preparation with H_2-blockers and motility drugs should be continued. A rapid sequence

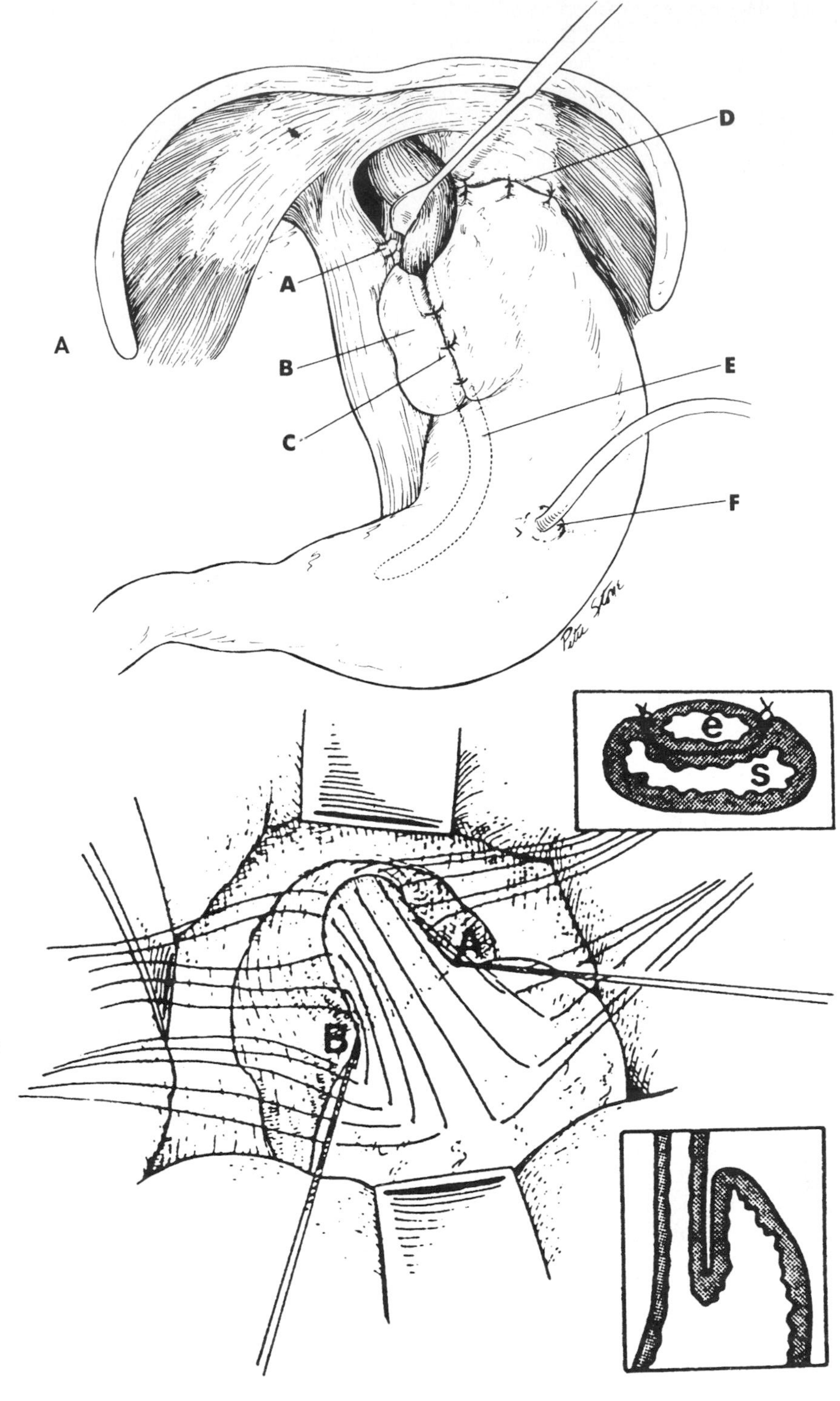

■ **FIGURE 19–5.** *A*, Salient features of Nissen fundoplication in infants. A, Crural sutures to reduce hiatus. B, Generous loose, adequate tissue in the wrap. C, Sutures placed through seromuscular depth of both gastric and esophageal walls. D, Sutures to fix the fundus to the diaphragm. E, Appropriately sized mercury-filled dilator to ensure adequate lumen. F, Gastrostomy in all infants and whenever there is any question of gastric outlet problems. *B*, The Thal fundoplication. A partial wrap of the fundus is performed anteriorly around the lower esophageal segment. (*A* from Randolph JG: *Ann Surg* 198:579, 1983. Illustrated by Peter Stone. *B* from Ashcraft KW: Thal fundoplication. In Ashcraft KW, Holder TM, editors: *Pediatric esophageal surgery.* Orlando, 1986, Grune & Stratton, Inc.)

induction should be used, providing a difficult airway is not anticipated. At least one large-bore intravenous catheter should be placed, although fluid and blood losses are minimal. However, pneumothorax, lacerated spleen, puncture or compression of the vena cava or aorta, and lacerated hepatic veins can occur.

Other anesthesia concerns in patients with GER focus on the degree of neurologic and respiratory compromise of the patient. Because these children frequently have seizure disorders, preoperative concern should be directed at proper anticonvulsant therapy. Oral anticonvulsants generally cannot be administered for 48 to 72 hours in the postoperative period. Consequently, patients requiring carbamazepine and valproic acid need alternate medicines so that breakthrough seizures do not occur.

For children with severe respiratory compromise or neuromuscular disease, postoperative ventilatory support may be necessary. In children without significant preoperative pulmonary compromise, extubation may be delayed after surgery and supplemental oxygen is given as needed.

SURGERY FOR BILIARY ATRESIA

Biliary atresia is characterized by a lack of gross patency of the extrahepatic bile duct. It occurs in 1:15,000 live births (Shim et al., 1974), and in 10% to 15% of the patients, other abnormalities are associated with embryologic development, including absent inferior vena cava, intestinal malrotation, polysplenia, and preduodenal portal vein (Lilly and Chandra, 1974). Although biliary atresia is often considered a congenital lesion, it has dynamic properties as well. In microscopic studies of the biliary anatomy obtained from patients at 2 and 4 months of age, the histologic results suggest that biliary structures gradually disappear and are replaced by fibrous tissue. In addition, the success rate for the palliative surgical procedure has been reported as 50% in infants operated on before 4 months of age and 80% in those undergoing surgery before 2 months of age (Ohi et al., 1985).

Kasai and others (1989), in a review of 245 patients undergoing corrective procedures over a 35-year period, noted that 10-year survival was 74% in infants operated on before 60 days of life. However, Tan and others (1994) have questioned whether earlier corrective surgery is associated with ductal patency. In a series of 205 patients, Tan and others noted that survival may be more closely related to the severity of intrahepatic biliary cholangiopathy.

In a 27-year review of 81 patients with biliary atresia, Wildhaber and others (2003) noted that direct bilirubin less than 2.0, the absence of bridging liver fibrosis, and the number of cholangitis episodes were predictive factors in the success of the Kasai portoenterostomy. Popovic and others (2003) noted that cholinesterase levels can be a useful index of liver function (protein synthesis) early after the Kasai procedure and is independent of albumin synthesis.

Clinically, biliary atresia presents in infants from 1 to 6 weeks of age. About 50% are anicteric until the second or third week of life. The diagnosis of biliary atresia is confirmed either by liver biopsy or by exploratory laparotomy. Surgical palliation for biliary atresia involves hepatic portoenterostomy (Kasai procedure) (Fig. 19–6).

Complications of the surgical repair and from the underlying disease state include cholangitis, portal hypertension, and fat-soluble vitamin deficiency (Kasai et al., 1975). For the anesthesiologist, these complications take on greater significance in patients who return to the operating room for further surgical revision of biliary drainage, treatment of intra-abdominal sepsis, or relief of an intestinal obstruction. Because these complications occur frequently and because end-stage liver disease can follow the Kasai procedure, the role of liver transplantation as a primary treatment of biliary atresia has been raised. Kasai and others (1989) suggested that liver transplantation as a primary form of treatment may be indicated for patients older than 3 months with an enlarged, hard liver. Laurent and others (1990) noted that although Kasai's operation does improve the prognosis of biliary atresia, it is not a definitive cure and 80% of these patients become candidates for liver transplantation.

Anesthetic management for a Kasai procedure (Kasai, 1974) in patients with biliary atresia follows the basic principles of pediatric anesthesia. In infants in whom venous access is already present, induction is achieved with a hypnotic agent, such as propofol (2 to 3 mg/kg), and a muscle relaxant (cisatracurium 0.2 mg/kg). In infants without an intravenous catheter in place, inhalation induction is performed with oxygen, nitrous oxide, and sevoflurane. Once the child is adequately anesthetized, an intravenous catheter is inserted and a muscle relaxant is administered to facilitate endotracheal intubation and to decrease the concentration of potent inhalation anesthetic. After induction, anesthesia is maintained with an oxygen-air-isoflurane mixture along with intravenous opioids. Because of bowel distention, nitrous oxide is avoided.

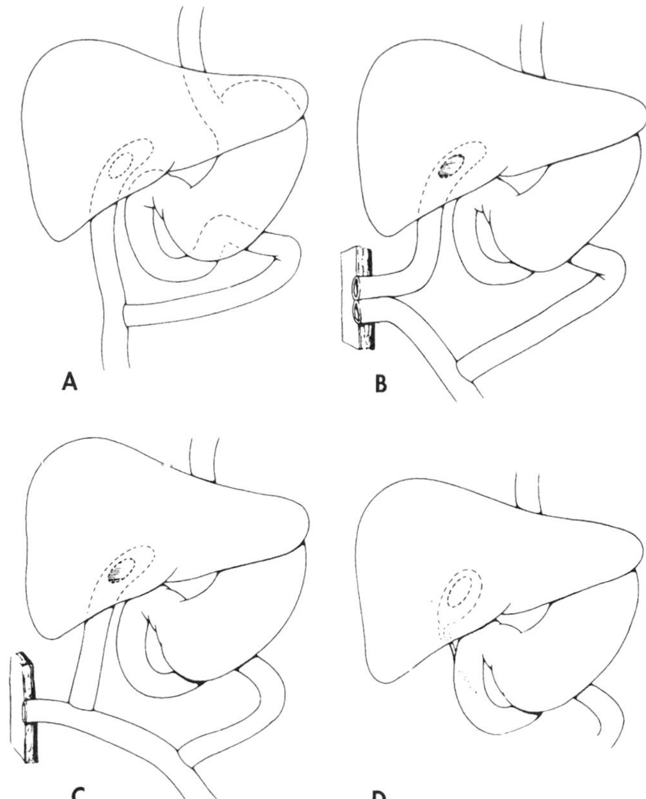

■ **FIGURE 19–6.** Illustrations of the Kasai procedure and its various modifications. *A*, Original Kasai. *B*, Kasai H-double-barreled vent. *C*, "Bishop-Koop" vent. *D*, Gallbladder "Kasai." (From Filston HC, Izant RJ Jr: *The surgical neonate, evaluation, and care.* Norwalk, CT, 1985, Appleton-Century-Crofts.)

Gelman and others (1984) have shown that hepatic blood flow and oxygen supply are better maintained during isoflurane than during halothane anesthesia. Consequently, isoflurane in an oxygen and air mixture is most commonly administered to patients undergoing surgery for biliary atresia.

Anesthesia monitoring for the patient undergoing a Kasai procedure is similar to that used for other pediatric surgical procedures. Arterial cannulation and central venous pressure monitors are rarely used and are generally reserved for patients with other coexisting problems, such as sepsis, pneumonia, cholangitis, and severe cirrhosis. In general, hemodynamic stability is well maintained and the need for intraoperative vasoactive agents is rare. Sometimes the surgical approach involves dividing the triangular and coronary ligaments and displacing the whole liver anteriorly. Although this technique may facilitate exposure, it may compress the inferior vena cava and thereby result in hypotension by decreasing venous return. Ventilation is controlled, and end-tidal gases are monitored for carbon dioxide, oxygen, and volatile anesthetic agents. Adequacy of oxygenation is monitored by the pulse oximeter.

The operative procedures generally last 3 to 4 hours, and major blood loss does not occur. Perioperative fluid therapy involves replacement of maintenance and deficit fluids as well as provision for the calculated third-space losses. Third-space losses may vary from 6 to 10 mL/kg per hr. Generally, lactated Ringer's solution is used to restore third-space losses.

Prevention of hypothermia is a major concern for the anesthesiologist. The large surface-to-volume ratio of infants, their relative lack of insulation tissue, coupled with the cold operating room, exposure of body cavities to low environmental temperatures, infusions of cold fluid, and ventilation with dry gases, all increase the potential for hypothermia during surgery. Consequently, great effort must be applied both before and during surgery to protect against heat loss. Methods of preventing heat loss are discussed in Chapter 5, Thermoregulation: Physiology and Perioperative Disturbances.

The pharmacology of anesthetic agents in infants and children with hepatic disease has not been fully evaluated. Although the liver is the major site of drug biotransformation, the effects of hepatic dysfunction on drug elimination and disposition are inconsistent. The degree of liver dysfunction and the drug's ability to bind to plasma proteins are important variables in determining drug kinetics in patients with liver disease.

In general, liver function is fairly well preserved in the first few months of life in children with biliary atresia. As the children get older and ductal fibrosis begins, liver dysfunction ensues. Consequently, in children who return for repeat surgical procedures, the pharmacology of intravenous anesthetic agents and adjuncts may be altered.

In infants with biliary atresia undergoing the Kasai procedure, if major fluid shifts have not occurred, blood loss has been minimal, and the patient is warm, all efforts are made to reverse the muscle relaxation and extubate the trachea at the end of the procedure. In children with other organ system failures (specifically sepsis, cholangitis, or pneumonia), those who are cold at the end of the procedure (<35°C), or those who have undergone transfusion of more than one blood volume, extubation is delayed until warmth and hemodynamic stability are restored. In these children, postoperative recovery and monitoring are carried out in an intensive care setting.

LIVER TUMOR PROCEDURES

Liver tumors in children are uncommon, but malignant tumors comprise 72% of pediatric primary hepatic tumors. Of these malignant tumors, hepatoblastoma and hepatocarcinoma are the predominant tissue types (Table 19–3). Hepatoblastoma commonly affects white boys under 2 years of age. An abdominal mass that has increased in size is usually the presenting symptom.

TABLE 19–3. Malignant hepatic tumors

Hepatomas	Hepatoblastoma	129
	Hepatocellular carcinoma	98
Other	Mixed mesenchymal tumor	9
	Rhabdomyosarcoma	6
	Angiosarcoma	4
	Undifferentiated sarcoma	3
	Teratocarcinoma	1
	Cholangiosarcoma	1
	Malignant histiocytoma	1

From Exelby PR, Filler RM, Grosfeld JL: Liver tumors in children in the particular reference to hepatoblastoma and hepatocellular carcinoma: American Academy of Pediatrics Surgical Section Survey—1974. *J Pediatr Surg* 10:329, 1975.

Anemia, jaundice, and ascites are infrequent findings. Liver function test results are frequently normal. From 2% to 3% of patients may have an associated hemihypertrophy (Geiser et al., 1970). Hepatoblastoma has also been associated with isosexual precocity as a result of the liver's ectopic gonadotropic production and the Beckwith-Wiedemann syndrome (Sotelo-Avita et al., 1976), polyposis coli, Wilms tumor, and fetal alcohol syndrome.

An increased incidence of hepatoblastomas has been associated with low birth weight (Ikeda et al. 1997; Feusner et al., 1998). Between 1973 and 1997, the rate of hepatoblastoma increased. This is in contrast to the decreased incidence observed for hepatocarcinoma (Darbari et al., 2003). Hepatoblastomas are derived from primitive epithelial parenchyma and are classified by the predominant epithelial component. Among the variants are fetal, embryonal, macrotrabecular, and anaplastic. Survival is related to the histology and completeness of the surgical resection. Fetal histology has a greater than 90% survival rate compared with a 50% survival rate for embryonal histology. A few survivors have anaplastic histology.

Hepatocellular carcinoma appears to have two age peaks: under 4 years of age and between 12 and 15 years of age (Leventhal, 1987). As in adults with hepatocellular carcinoma, the prognosis of survival in children with the disease is 5% to 10%. Typically, patients with hepatocellular carcinoma have the systemic symptoms of weight loss, jaundice, fever, and lethargy. As opposed to adults with this tumor, only about 5% of children have associated cirrhosis (Jones, 1960). Other associated diseases include von Gierke's disease, type I glycogenesis, cystinosis, extrahepatic biliary atresia, α_1-antitrypsin deficiency, hypoplasia of intrahepatic bile ducts, Wilson's disease, giant cell hepatitis, and Solo's syndrome (Zangeneh et al., 1969; Palmer and Wolfe, 1976; Weinberg et al., 1976; Dehner, 1978).

Anesthetic management for pediatric patients undergoing hepatic lobe resection or tumor resection involves the same principles as for patients with biliary atresia. Efforts at maintaining adequate alveolar ventilation, temperature homeostasis, cardiovascular stability, and fluid management have previously been described. Some patients receive adjunct chemotherapy before surgery. The chemotherapeutic protocol must be reviewed. Frequently, Adriamycin, an anthracycline, is a major component of hepatic cancer chemotherapy and has been associated with a dose-dependent irreversible cardiomyopathy. All patients receiving anthracycline chemotherapy should undergo history, physical examination, electrocardiogram, chest radiograph, and echocardiogram to further evaluate signs and symptoms of cardiac toxicity and cardiac reserve (see Chapters 3 and 32, Cardiovascular Physiology and Systemic Disorders).

Because the potential for massive blood loss exists in patients undergoing hepatic resection, adequate venous access and invasive monitoring are essential to patient management. Two or three large-bore peripheral intravenous catheters are inserted, and a central venous pressure catheter is placed to monitor cardiac filling pressures. Either the radial or the femoral artery is cannulated, not only to monitor blood pressure but also to determine blood gas levels, chemistry, and coagulation profile. Because of the potential for large fluid shifts, a Foley catheter is placed to measure urine output and assist in assessing the adequacy of fluid resuscitation.

Massive blood volume replacement is a frequent component of the anesthetic resuscitation in children undergoing hepatic resection. Massive blood volume replacement may create physiologic derangements that have anesthetic and surgical consequences.

These physiologic alterations include disorders of coagulation, acid-base imbalance, electrolyte imbalance, hypothermia, and decreased tissue oxygen delivery.

Many children undergoing tumor resection require postoperative ventilatory support. The anesthetic plan should permit early tracheal extubation in the operating room. However, in the event that intraoperative findings reveal unresectable tumor, postoperative care should include observation in the pediatric intensive care unit and attention to changes in intravascular volume and blood pressure. Continued bleeding may require transfusion of blood or fresh frozen plasma, or even return to the operating room for surgical control.

HIRSCHSPRUNG'S DISEASE PROCEDURES

The basic pathology underlying congenital megacolon, or Hirschsprung's disease, is a gangliosis, or total absence of ganglion cells, in the intrinsic nerve supply of the bowel. The aganglionic area extends proximally from the anal sphincter and involves varying lengths of colon. The normal nerve supply, consisting of Auerbach's plexuses and Meissner's plexuses, which together form the myenteric nerve complex of the bowel, usually becomes an increasingly diffuse network in the descending and terminal portions of the bowel. Absence of the ganglion cells, which occurs in approximately 1:10,000 infants, causes a condition resembling spasm in the area without ganglion cells, whereas the normal bowel proximal to the spastic portion undergoes tremendous distention, with retention of feces and intestinal obstruction or, in less serious cases, prolonged bouts of constipation. Although the cause of Hirschsprung's disease is unknown, defects in non-adrenergic, noncholinergic innervations may prevent relaxation of the aganglionic segment. Bealer and others (1994) have demonstrated that nitric oxide synthetase is deficient in the aganglionic colon of patients with Hirschsprung's disease and that this deficiency may prevent smooth muscle relaxation of the aganglionic segment. On a molecular level, mutations in the RET proto-oncogene have been found (Sancandi et al., 2000).

In 10% to 20% of patients with Hirschsprung's disease, it is clinically present at birth. Symptomatic infants have delayed passage of meconium, irritability, failure to thrive, and abdominal distention. Older children may present with constipation, fecal soiling, and diarrhea. The major complication from Hirschsprung's disease is acute enterocolitis, a potentially life-threatening event. Diagnosis of Hirschsprung's disease is made by radiographic examination and confirmed by suction biopsy specimens from the rectum. Surgery is usually a two-stage procedure, with the initial procedure being a colostomy. The definitive surgical procedure is generally performed when the child is older (>1 year of age). The surgical approaches are varied and over time have undergone modifications (Fig. 19–7). Attention has focused on the use of a one stage transoral endorectal pull-through approach (Elhalaby et al., 2004). Each surgical technique has its own associated intraoperative and perioperative complications, but enterocolitis, wound dehiscence, anastomotic leakage, intestinal obstruction, and fecal soiling are common to all. All of these surgical procedures aim either to excise or to bypass the aganglionic portion of the bowel and to free and advance the remaining normal portion of bowel toward the rectum. These procedures are often long (6 to 8 hours) and involve surgical explorations through the perineum and abdomen.

Laparoscopic surgery has also been used in the treatment of Hirschsprung's disease (Jona et al., 1998; Wulkan and Georgeson, 1998; Georgeson et al., 1999). The minimally invasive assisted pull-through technique is generally used for patients where the aganglianotic segment is confined to the rectum sigmoid or proximal left colon (Georgeson, 2002). Anesthetic concerns for patients with Hirschsprung's disease are similar to those for any child having surgery. Maintaining body temperature and providing appropriate fluid therapy (for replacement of large third-space losses) are the major challenges for the anesthesiologist.

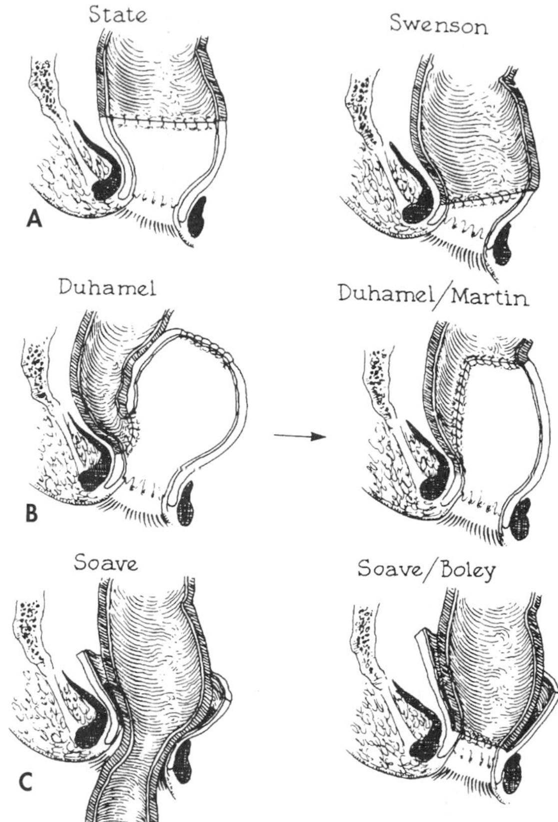

FIGURE 19–7. Graphic representation in lateral view of the three major operative procedures for Hirschsprung's disease. Evolution of each from left to right. Unshaded native rectum is aganglionic. Shaded, pulled-through bowel contains ganglion cells. *A*, State's procedure was a prototypic anterior resection of dilated rectosigmoid. Lengthy aganglionic segment remained. In Swenson's procedure an oblique anastomosis resulted in ganglion cells within 1 cm of the verge posteriorly. *B*, In the original Duhamel's operation, the oversewn native rectum enlarged as a blind loop, which resulted in a fecaloma that caused partial obstruction. In Martin's modification, the blind loop is obviated by complete division of the septum and anastomosis of the anterior walls of the native rectum and pulled-through colon. Bowel that contains ganglion cells reaches within 1 cm of the anal verge posteriorly. *C*, In the original Soave's procedure, full-thickness colon that contained ganglion cells was advanced through the demucosalized native rectal sleeve. Excess colon extended from the anus for several weeks before transection and delayed anastomosis. In the Boley modification, a primary anastomosis is done 1 cm above the verge. Ganglion cells are present circumferentially at that level. (From Philappart AI: Hirschsprung's disease. In Ashcraft KW, Holder TM: *Pediatric surgery*, 2nd ed. Philadelphia, 1993, WB Saunders.)

Anesthesia induction can be either by inhalation or intravenous means. Because of the surgical bowel manipulation and the relative obstructive nature of the underlying disease, nitrous oxide is discontinued after induction, and anesthesia is maintained with a mixture of air, oxygen, and potent inhalation agent. Long-term follow-up of patients with Hirschsprung's disease suggests that 25% of patients will require a reoperation and that between 19% and 25% of patients will develop enterocolitis (Fortuna et al., 1996).

SURGERY FOR APPENDICITIS

Acute appendicitis is a common condition in children. Although the mortality from acute appendicitis is rare (case-fatality ratio, 0.3%) (Addiss et al., 1990), morbidity (peritonitis, abscess formation, wound infection) is related to the state of the appendix at the time of the operation. The highest incidence of appendicitis is found in patients aged 10 to 19 years. The incidence of perforation of the appendix in children appears to be about 30% to 45%, but in preschool children and infants it can be as high as 80%. The incidence of appendicitis appears to be affected by race and sex. The incidences of appendicitis is 1.4 to 1.6 times greater in whites than nonwhites, whereas the perforation rate for nonwhites is 22% compared with 18% for whites (Addiss et al., 1990).

The signs and symptoms of appendicitis are variable. The incidence of negative appendectomy (surgery performed without positive appendicitis) is significant. In males, the negative appendectomy rate is about 9%, whereas in females, it is about 22%. In females, diagnostic accuracy decreases during childbearing years, whereas in males, diagnostic accuracy does not appear to be affected by age. Classically, the patient presents with periumbilical pain that eventually localizes to the right lower quadrant. Anorexia, nausea, and vomiting are frequent, as is a low-grade fever. Continued progression of the inflammatory course results in increased tenderness in the right lower quadrant as well as referred pain to the right lower quadrant on palpation of other areas of the abdomen. With advanced disease, gangrene and perforation of the appendix occur with ensuing peritonitis and possible abscess formation.

The pathophysiology of appendicitis is thought to be related to an obstruction of the lumen of the appendix with subsequent bacterial overgrowth and distention of the appendix. In untreated cases, distention and overgrowth lead to gangrene and rupture. Although there is some urgency in making the diagnosis and surgically removing the appendix, the operation is never so urgent that a proper review of the patient's medical history and physical assessment cannot be performed.

Preoperative anesthetic management of the child with diagnosed appendicitis includes concerns regarding fluid and electrolyte disorders. Because these children may have been vomiting and may be febrile, signs and symptoms of dehydration should be assessed and any fluid or electrolyte deficits corrected.

Once the child has been adequately volume resuscitated and a normal airway is anticipated, an intravenous rapid sequence induction with cricoid pressure is performed. Anesthetic technique (inhalation agents versus opioid-based techniques) may depend on the surgical technique used to remove the appendix. Although frequently the appendix is removed by laparotomy, the role of laparoscopy (especially in females) in both diagnosis and management is increasing (Gilchrist et al., 1992; Kuster and Gilrey, 1992; Olsen et al., 1993). In a study by McAnena and others (1992), the median postoperative hospitalization stay was one half and the rate of wound infection one third in patients undergoing laparoscopic appendectomy compared with patients undergoing open appendectomy. In a study involving 30 pediatric hospitals, Pansky and others (2003) noted significant variability in practice and resource utilization among the institutions. In addition, the length of stay did not differ between those patients who underwent an open or a laparoscopic appendectomy.

Regardless of surgical technique, monitoring of the patient includes electrocardiogram, pulse oximeter, temperature probe, blood pressure cuff, pre-cordial stethoscope, and end-tidal gas measurements. Depending on the patient's body temperature, active cooling techniques (cooling blanket, rectal acetaminophen suppositories, cool intravenous fluids, and cool intra-abdominal irrigations) may be needed to help lower the patient's temperature. The addition of inhalational anesthetic gases may also augment cooling by promoting cutaneous vasodilation with subsequent increased heat loss.

INTUSSUSCEPTION REPAIR

Intussusception is produced by the invagination or telescoping of one portion of the intestine into another (Fig. 19–8). It tends to occur more frequently in males than females. Over 50% of cases occur in children under 1 year of age, and less than 10% of cases occur in children older than 5 years. Ninety percent of cases have idiopathic causes, which are frequently seen in children less than 1 year of age. Older children are more likely to have Meckel's diverticulum, intestinal polyp, lymphoma, adhesions, trauma hemolytic uremic syndrome, or ectopic pancreatic nodule as an etiology. Intussusception has also been reported postoperatively and after blunt abdominal trauma (Linke et al., 1998; Komadina and Smrkolj, 1998). In addition, there has been a reported association of rotavirus vaccine and intussusception (Zanardia et al., 2001).

The clinical presentation of acute intussusception involves sudden paroxysms of abdominal pain, bloody stools and an abdominal mass, although in one series of patients, 18% of the children had painless intussusception (Hutchison et al., 1980). In a review of 14 published reports, Losek (1993) noted that

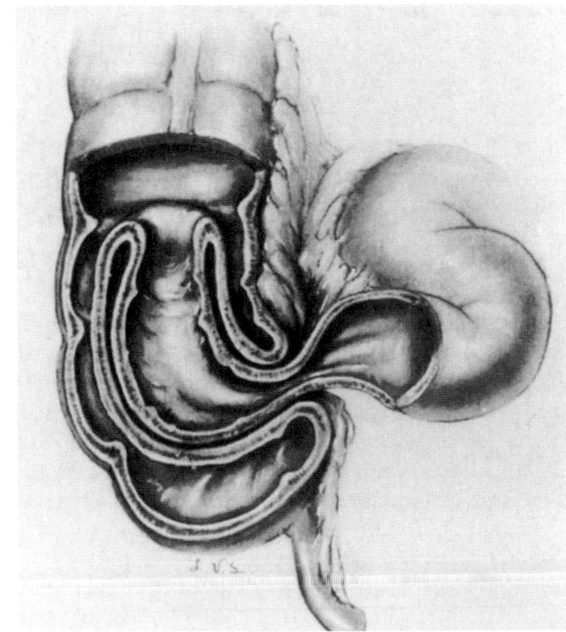

FIGURE 19–8. Intussusception. (From deLorimier AA, Harrison MR: Pediatric surgery. In Dunphy JE, Way LW: *Current surgical diagnosis and treatment.* Los Altos. CA, 1979, Lange Medical Publisher.)

bloody stools were present in 42% of patients. Occult blood was noted in 43% and abdominal masses were present in 62% of patients. Intussusception can also present with neurologic findings (lethargy, apnea, seizures, hypotonia, opisthotonus) similar to a picture of septic encephalopathy (Conway, 1993). Other symptoms and signs may include diarrhea, vomiting, fever, and dehydration. In other children, intussusception can present as a chronic entity that may mimic gastroenteritis (Shekhawat et al., 1992), whereas in neonates, intussusception may mimic necrotizing enterocolitis (Price et al., 1993).

About 90% of intussusceptions are ileocolic, with the remainder being ileoileal and colocolic. Treatment for intussusception involves the administration of appropriate fluids to combat dehydration and radiologic or surgical attempts to reduce the invaginated bowel. Hydrostatic enemas with barium or air have been reported to be successful in 80% of patients. However, enemas are contraindicated in patients with evidence of peritonitis, shock, and intestinal perforation. Surgical laparotomy with manual reduction and/or resection as well as laparoscopic approaches have been described for the surgical management in patients with unsuccessful radiologic reduction and in patients with signs of intestinal perforation, peritonitis, and shock.

Anesthetic considerations include restoring electrolyte and fluid deficits. Shock should be treated before commencing anesthesia. The intravascular deficits may be further exacerbated by the presence of barium in the gastrointestinal tract. The child with an intussusception should also be considered at risk for aspiration, and because of the intestinal obstruction, nitrous oxide should be avoided. Anesthesia should be induced with intravenous agents. If hemodynamic instability is a concern, ketamine or etomidate should be used as the hypnotic agent for induction.

■ GENERAL THORACIC SURGERY

Thoracic surgery in children is performed for a wide variety of congenital, neoplastic, infectious, and traumatic lesions; these lesions are listed in Box 19–4. The patient may be a few hours old with a congenital cystadenamatous malformation (CCAM) and life-threatening respiratory distress or an adolescent with an asymptomatic mediastinal tumor. Regardless of age or disease, four principles are common to all patients undergoing general anesthesia for thoracic surgery, as follows:

1. Preoperative evaluation and preparation can minimize intraoperative problems and improve the safety of the anesthetic.
2. The anesthesiologist must be aware of potential intraoperative problems.
3. Modern monitoring techniques have increased the safety with regard to anesthetic management.
4. Surgical approaches and techniques are constantly changing as efforts are made by surgeons to use minimally invasive procedures.

A thorough preoperative evaluation is essential in caring for the pediatric patient scheduled for thoracic surgery. Appropriate imaging and laboratory studies should be performed preoperatively according to the lesion involved. Guidelines for fasting, choice of premedication, and preparation of the operating room are used as for other infants and children scheduled for major surgery. Following induction of anesthesia, placement of an intravenous catheter, and tracheal intubation, arterial catheterization should be performed for most patients undergoing thoracotomy as well as those with severe lung disease having thoracoscopic surgery. This facilitates monitoring of arterial blood pressure during manipulation of the lungs and mediastinum as well as arterial blood gas tensions during single lung ventilation (SLV). For thoracoscopic procedures of relatively short duration in patients without severe lung disease, the insertion of an arterial catheter is not required. Placement of a central venous catheter is generally not indicated if peripheral intravenous access is adequate for projected fluid and blood administration.

Inhaled anesthetic agents are commonly administered in 100% O_2 during maintenance of anesthesia. Isoflurane may be preferred due to less attenuation of hypoxic pulmonary vasoconstriction (HPV) compared with other inhaled agents, although this has not been studied in children (Benumof et al., 1987). Nitrous oxide is avoided. Use of intravenous opioids may facilitate a decrease in the concentration of inhaled anesthetics used and thereby limit impairment of hypoxic pulmonary vasoconstriction. Alternatively, total intravenous anesthesia may be used with a variety of agents. The combination of general anesthesia with regional anesthesia and postoperative analgesia is particularly desirable for thoracotomy but may also be beneficial for thoracoscopic procedures, especially when thoracostomy tube drainage, a source of significant postoperative pain, is used following surgery. A variety of regional anesthetic techniques have been described for intraoperative anesthesia and postoperative analgesia, including intercostal and paravertebral blocks, intrapleural infusions, and epidural anesthesia (see Chapter 14, Regional Anesthesia).

In awake patients, except for young infants, ventilation is normally distributed preferentially to dependent regions of the lung, so that there is a gradient of increasing ventilation from the most nondependent to the most dependent lung segments. Because of gravitational effects, perfusion normally follows a similar distribution, with increased blood flow to dependent lung segments; therefore, ventilation and perfusion are normally well matched. However, controlled ventilation under general anesthesia with decreased functional residual capacity and absent diaphragmatic contractions result in a reverse distribution of ventilation (see Chapter 2, Respiratory Physiology). During thoracic surgery,

BOX 19–4 Common Thoracic Surgical Procedures in Children

Empyema
Chest wall deformities
Chest wall masses
Lung abscess
Bronchiectasis
Lobar emphysema
Tumor (primary or metastatic)
Pulmonary sequestration
Congenital adenomatoid malformation
Congenital cysts of the lung
Bronchogenic cysts
Esophageal lesions
Mediastinal masses
Scoliosis

these and other factors act to increase ventilation/perfusion ($\dot{V}/\dot{Q}$) mismatch. Compression of the dependent lung in the lateral decubitus position may cause atelectasis. Surgical retraction, SLV, or both result in collapse of the operative lung. Hypoxic pulmonary vasoconstriction (HPV), which acts to divert blood flow away from underventilated lung regions, thereby minimizing $\dot{V}/\dot{Q}$ mismatch, may be diminished by the use of inhaled anesthetic agents and other vasodilating drugs. These factors apply similarly to infants, children, and adults. The overall effect of the lateral decubitus position on $\dot{V}/\dot{Q}$ mismatch, however, is different in infants than in older children and adults.

In adults with unilateral lung disease, oxygenation is optimal when the patient is placed in the lateral decubitus position with the healthy lung dependent ("down") and the diseased lung nondependent ("up") (Remolina et al., 1981). Presumably, this is related to an increase in blood flow to the dependent, healthy lung and a decrease in blood flow to the nondependent, diseased lung due to the hydrostatic pressure (i.e., gravitational) gradient between the two lungs. This phenomenon promotes $\dot{V}/\dot{Q}$ matching in the adult patient undergoing thoracic surgery in the lateral decubitus position.

In infants with unilateral lung disease, however, oxygenation is improved with the healthy lung "up" (Heaf et al., 1983). Several factors account for this discrepancy between adults and infants. Infants have a soft, easily compressible rib cage that cannot fully support the underlying lung. Functional residual capacity is closer to residual volume, making airway closure likely to occur in the dependent lung even during tidal breathing (Mansell et al., 1972).

Finally, the infant's increased oxygen requirement, coupled with a small functional residual capacity, predisposes to hypoxemia. Infants normally consume 6 to 8 mL of O_2/kg per min compared with a normal O_2 consumption in adults of 2 to 3 mL/kg per min (Dawes, 1973). For these reasons, infants are at an increased risk of significant oxygen desaturation during surgery in the lateral decubitus position.

THORACOSCOPY

During the past decade, the use of video-assisted thoracoscopic surgery has dramatically increased in both adults and children (see discussion under "Video Endoscopy"). As with laparoscopy, reported advantages of thoracoscopy include smaller chest incisions, reduced postoperative pain, and more rapid postoperative recovery compared with thoracotomy (Weatherford et al., 1995; Angellilo et al., 1996; Mouroux et al., 1997).

Thoracoscopic surgery is being used extensively for pleural debridement in patients with empyema, lung biopsy and wedge resections for interstitial lung disease, mediastinal masses, and metastatic lesions. More extensive pulmonary resections, including segmentectomy and lobectomy, have been performed for lung abscess, bullous disease, sequestrations, lobar emphysema, CCAM, and neoplasms. Other thoracoscopic procedures are listed in Table 19–4.

Thoracoscopy can be performed while both lungs are being ventilated using CO_2 insufflation and placement of a retractor to displace lung tissue in the operative field. However, SLV is extremely desirable during thoracoscopy because lung deflation improves visualization of thoracic contents and may reduce lung injury caused by the use of retractors (Benumof, 1995).

TABLE 19–4. Thoracoscopic procedures in infants and children

Anterior spinal fusion
Aortopexy
Biopsy
Abscess
Interstitial lung disease
Mass
Cyst excision
Decortication/debridement of empyema
Diaphragmatic plication
Diaphragmatic hernia repair
Drainage
Abscess
Cyst
Esophageal atresia repair
Exploration
Infection
Mass
Trauma
Foregut duplication resection
Hiatal hernia repair
Lobectomy
Mediastinal mass excision
Patent ductus arteriosus (PDA) ligation
Segmentectomy
Sequestration resection
Sympathectomy
Tracheoesophageal (TE) fistula ligation
Thymectomy
Thoracic duct ligation

SURGERY FOR CHEST WALL DEFORMITIES

Pectus excavatum (funnel chest) (Fig. 19–9) and the less common pectus carinatum (pigeon breast) deformities are congenital abnormalities of the sternum, ribs, and costal cartilages. These deformities are usually minimal at birth but progress with age. A higher incidence of both deformities occurs in children with Marfan's syndrome or congenital heart disease and in families in which other children have the defect (Rubicsek, 2000).

These children often appear asymptomatic but occasionally have cardiac or pulmonary abnormalities related to the deformity. Patients with pectus excavatum generally present with normal or modestly reduced forced vital capacity and total lung capacity and, in severe cases, $\dot{V}/\dot{Q}$ mismatch. The heart is displaced to the left and compressed, lending to arrhythmias, right-axis deviation on electrocardiogram, a functional murmur, and reduced stroke volume most noticeable in the standing position and during exercise, explaining the mild exercise intolerance experienced by some patients. The cardiac and pulmonary abnormalities are in most instances benign and may worsen as the child ages but may be improved by surgical repair. There also is an increased incidence of mitral valve prolapse in patients with pectus deformities.

Preoperative assessment focuses on exercise tolerance and other signs of cardiopulmonary compromise, such as lung infections. Laboratory evaluation includes a chest radiograph with pulmonary function tests, arterial blood gases, or electrocardiogram added only if there is clinical evidence of significant underlying disease. Echocardiography is now commonly performed to detect the presence of mitral valve prolapse. If the child has mitral valve prolapse, prophylaxis for subacute bacterial endocarditis is administered. Patients are often emotionally distressed by the appearance of chest deformity and may benefit from preoperative counseling and, if needed, premedication.

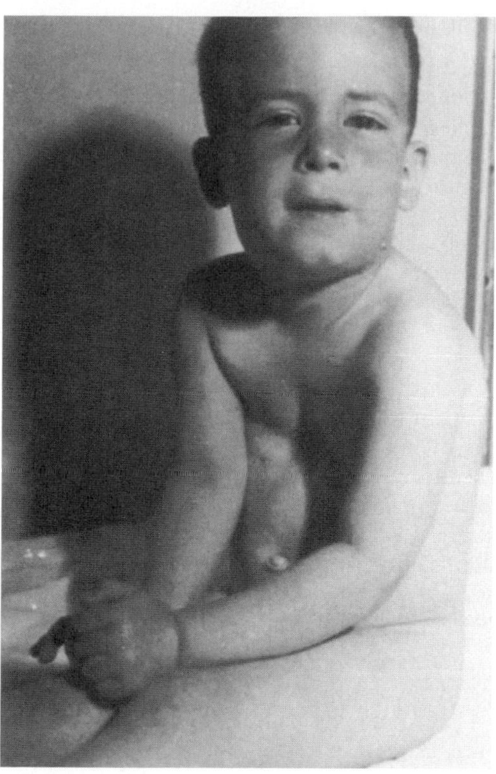

■ **FIGURE 19–9.** Pectus excavatum deformity becomes most obvious when the child is in the sitting position.

Classic operative repair involves extrapleural excision of the sternocostal cartilages and mobilization of the sternum and ribs. The most common complications of operative repair are pneumothorax, flail chest, and postoperative atelectasis; blood loss is usually minimal to moderate. Intraoperative monitors include temperature, blood pressure, pulse, heart and breath sounds, airway pressure, and oxygen saturation or tension. Capnography is also useful, while arterial catheterization is needed only if there is a specific indication. General anesthesia with controlled ventilation is the method of choice, with no agents specifically indicated or contraindicated because of the operation itself. Oxygen by facemask is administered in the recovery room, but it is usually not needed after the child fully awakens. Although patient-controlled analgesia is commonly used for postoperative analgesia, both intercostal nerve blocks and thoracic epidural analgesia have become increasingly popular for children undergoing pectus repair (Robicsek, 2000).

A thoracic epidural catheter provides more reliable analgesia to the operative area than a lumbar epidural that has been threaded up a great distance. However, thoracic epidural catheters are not as easy to insert as lumbar catheters, and many practitioners are not comfortable with their routine use. Although a technique using electrocardiographic guidance and insertion from the caudal space has been described, it is not widely used (Tsui, 2002). An additional issue with the thoracic catheters is the safety of their insertion under general anesthesia (Horlocker, 2003). Although some children allow insertion before induction (McBride, 1996), many younger children are not likely to remain cooperative for the procedure, mandating insertion after induction (Hammer, 2002; Birmingham, 2003). Moreover, several centers have actively and successfully used thoracic epidural techniques in anesthetized children for thoracic and cardiac procedures without complications related to insertion after induction (Cassady, 2000; Birmingham, 2003). Solutions of both bupivacaine with fentanyl and fentanyl alone have been used successfully, including in the patient-controlled mode for appropriately mature children (Birmingham, 2003; Caudle, 1993) (see Chapter 14, Pediatric Regional Anesthesia).

Another approach has used a minimally invasive technique in which the costal cartilages are preserved and the sternum is elevated with a bar. Under direct vision and through a thorascope, a transmediastinal tunnel is created and a prebent bar is passed behind the sternum with the convex side down. The bar is then rotated 180 degrees in order to elevate the sternum (Nuss et al., 1998; Nuss, 2002). Borowitz and others (2003) have shown that static pulmonary function and ventilatory response to exercise was normal both before and after surgery, thereby suggesting that placement of the bar does not result in an increased chest wall restriction. In addition, Lawson and others (2003) noted that the surgical repair of the pectus excavatum following the Nuss procedure had a positive impact on both the patient's physical and emotional well-being. Complications of this minimally invasive approach include atelectasis, subcutaneous emphysema, pericardial and pleural effusions, myocardial perforation, diaphragmatic perforation, and dislocation of the stabilizing bar (Willekes, 1999; Molik, 2001; Moss, 2001; Hosie et al., 2002; Uemura et al., 2003). Postoperative pain following the Nuss procedure is significant. Thoracic epidural analgesia for 2 to 3 days followed by oral opioid therapy is appropriate.

THORACOTOMY, LOBECTOMY, AND PNEUMONECTOMY

Thoracotomy in the infant or child can be indicated for congenital abnormalities (cysts), tumors (mediastinal teratomas), trauma (gunshot wounds), or infective lesions (bronchiectasis). Subsegmental resection is used for biopsy and removal of metastatic tumors, whereas lobectomy is most commonly used for removal of congenital anomalies and extensive tumor metastasis. Pneumonectomy in children is done for various tumors, congenital abnormalities, and inflammatory lesions, such as bronchiectasis. Perioperative management differs dramatically, depending on the indication for surgery.

Surgical Lesion

If a space-occupying lesion is present, the patient is examined for signs of decreased cardiac output, diminished lung volume and reserve, and airway compression (Keon, 1981). History focuses not only on general exercise tolerance but also on signs of intermittent airway obstruction (stridor, cyanosis, or wheezing). Physical examination includes checking for a shift in the trachea, asymmetric chest movement, wheezing, and any signs of respiratory distress. Laboratory assessment should include a chest radiograph, but additional studies, such as tomograms, angiography, or computed tomography (CT), often provide more exact data about vascular or airway compression and compromise. It is crucial to determine the extent of airway compression and physiologic compromise because impairment may worsen with induction of anesthesia as sympathetic and muscular tones are reduced.

If the intrathoracic lesion is a primary or metastatic tumor, the history concentrates on previous treatment (Baldeyrou et al., 1984). Previous treatment for the tumor, especially chemotherapy and radiation, is important. Special attention is given to anthracycline (cardiac toxicity), bleomycin (pulmonary toxicity), and steroid (adrenal suppression) therapy. If there is any question about functional disability caused by this treatment, consultation with the child's oncologist is useful. Anemia, thrombocytopenia, and malnutrition are common in these patients and should be improved before surgery (Beattie, 1984). A special consideration is the immunocompromised patient with an unknown pulmonary infiltrate. This is usually assumed to be an opportunistic infection, but because it may represent metastasis, a biopsy is occasionally requested. These patients are often in poor general condition, and they may require postoperative ventilatory support, especially if they had only marginal compensation before surgery (Imoke et al., 1983; Prober et al., 1984).

Assessment

General assessment of the child starts with vital signs and overall appearance. Because children tolerate the loss of large amounts of usable lung tissue without obvious distress, the appearance of dyspnea or diminished exercise tolerance is an ominous sign. The history in older children focuses on complaints of dyspnea, cyanosis, wheezing, coughing, and weight loss. Infants often show less specific signs, such as poor feeding, irritability, choking, or change in sleep habits. If the child has had previous surgery, the perioperative course should be examined. The chest is inspected for asymmetric expansion and use of accessory muscles and then is auscultated for wheezes, rales, rhonchi, and absent breath sounds in both the supine and sitting positions. Physical assessment of the cardiovascular system concentrates on the presence of a gallop, murmurs, arrhythmias, and adequate peripheral pulses.

Preparation

Preparation for surgery starts with a discussion of the proposed anesthetic with the parents and, if appropriate, the child. The anesthetic plan, including monitors, possible complications, and potential for postoperative ventilation, is discussed. It is best to delay surgery until any infection or bronchospasm has been brought under optimal medical control with antibiotics, chest physiotherapy, and bronchodilators, as needed (Sutton et al., 1983). It may be difficult or impossible to eradicate infections or bronchospasm completely in destructive lesions such as bronchiectasis. If this is the case, it is acceptable to proceed after reasonable medical therapy has optimized the patient's status so that no further improvement is anticipated.

Monitoring

At a minimum, thoracotomy requires monitoring of inspired oxygen, blood pressure, heart and breath sounds, airway pressure, and temperature, as well as an electrocardiogram. Oxygen saturation by pulse oximeter or, less commonly, by transcutaneous oxygen tension (PO_2) monitor (Harnick et al., 1983) is vital for detection of sudden changes in oxygenation from lung compression or kinking of the airway. Capnography is particularly useful for detecting sudden changes in effective ventilation. Arterial cannulation for pressure and arterial blood samples is useful and is needed if extensive blood loss or resection of lung tissue is expected or if the child is already critically ill. Percutaneous arterial cannulas (24 gauge in neonates, 22 gauge in children up to 8 to 10 years of age, and 20 gauge in preadolescents and older) can be inserted in children and should be used whenever indicated. Central venous monitoring is used less commonly but can be helpful for guiding extensive volume replacement. Urinary drainage is a consideration for particularly long procedures.

Positioning

Positioning of the patient has often been used to minimize spillage of lung contents because double-lumen tubes are impractical in smaller patients (Conlan et al., 1986). Suction through the ETT may not be adequate to control large quantities of pus freed during surgical manipulation. The prone and lateral positions are the most commonly used. Positioning can cause significant ventilatory changes in children. Functional residual capacity (FRC) decreases during general anesthesia (Motoyama et al., 1982) but actually increases when the child is turned to the lateral position. The increase in FRC and ventilation occurs mainly in the uppermost part of the lung. The FRC falls dramatically once the pleura is opened (Larsson et al., 1987). The practical problems of dislodgment of the ETT with movement and adequate padding in these positions are especially important in children. Open-celled foam with adhesive backing (Reston; 3M, St. Paul, MN) can be applied to the thorax, pelvic rim, and other pressure points to minimize the effects of positioning. Also, the tube position must be rechecked each time the patient is moved.

Anesthesia

General endotracheal anesthesia presents various challenges to the anesthesiologist. A quiet, smooth inhalation induction is often used in infants and smaller children, whereas an intravenous induction is used in the older child. If there is concern about spillage of lung contents, rapid securing of the airway with intravenous induction is preferred to minimize coughing. The choice of appropriate anesthetic agents depends on both the patient's status and the surgical lesion. Nitrous oxide can accumulate in cysts with air-fluid levels and should be avoided in these patients or in patients requiring a high fraction of inspired oxygen (FIO_2). Volatile agents are especially useful in patients with bronchospastic disorders. The rate of rise of inhalational anesthetics may be slowed in the presence of intrapulmonary shunting. Precipitous hypotension is another potential problem with volatile agents in patients with low cardiac reserve. Muscle relaxants are routinely used along with controlled ventilation employing humidified gases. Although mechanical ventilators are usually acceptable, manual ventilation provides useful information to the anesthesiologist about changes in compliance or airway resistance, especially in infants or in procedures where there is recurrent obstruction of the airway.

Single-Lung Ventilation Techniques

Single-Lung Ventilation Using a Single-Lumen Endotracheal Tube. The simplest means of providing SLV is to intentionally intubate the ipsilateral mainstem bronchus with a conventional single-lumen ETT (Rowe et al., 1994). When the left bronchus is to be intubated, the bevel of the ETT is rotated 180 degrees and the head is turned to the right (Kubota et al., 1987). The ETT is advanced into the bronchus until breath sounds on the operative side disappear. A fiberoptic bronchoscope may be passed through or alongside the ETT to confirm or guide placement. When a cuffed ETT is used, the distance from the tip of the tube to the distal cuff must be shorter than the length of the bronchus so that the ETT does not occlude the upper lobe bronchus (Lammers et al., 1997) (Fig. 19–10). This technique is simple and requires no special equipment other than a fiberoptic bronchoscope. This may be the preferred technique of SLV in emergency situations such as airway hemorrhage or contralateral tension pneumothorax.

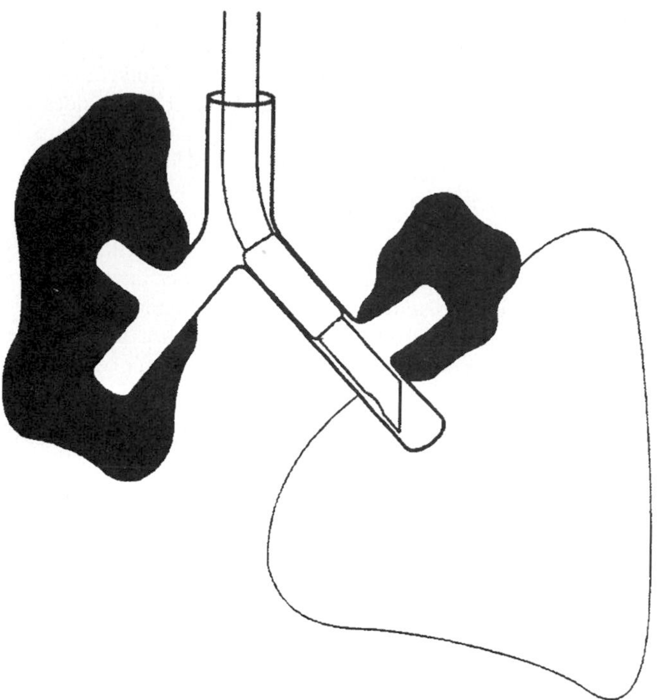

■ **FIGURE 19–10.** Obstruction of the left upper lobe bronchus with a cuffed endotracheal tube used for left-sided single-lung ventilation.

Problems can occur when using a single-lumen ETT for SLV. If a smaller, uncuffed ETT is used, it may be difficult to provide an adequate seal of the intended bronchus. This may prevent the operative lung from adequately collapsing or fail to protect the healthy, ventilated lung from contamination by purulent material from the contralateral lung. The operative lung cannot be suctioned using this technique. Hypoxemia may occur due to obstruction of the upper lobe bronchus, especially when the short right mainstem bronchus is intubated.

Single-Lung Ventilation Using a Balloon-Tipped Bronchial Blocker. A Fogarty embolectomy catheter or an end-hole, balloon wedge catheter may be used for bronchial blockade to provide SLV (Fig. 19–11) (Ginsberg, 1981; Lin and Hackel, 1994; Hammer et al., 1996; Turner et al., 1997). Placement of a Fogarty catheter is facilitated by bending the tip of its stylette toward the bronchus on the operative side. A fiberoptic bronchoscope is used to reposition the catheter and confirm appropriate placement. When an end-hole catheter is placed outside the ETT, the bronchus on the operative side is initially intubated with an ETT. A guidewire is then advanced into that bronchus through the ETT. The ETT is removed and the blocker is advanced over the guidewire into the bronchus. An ETT is then reinserted into the trachea alongside the blocker catheter. The catheter balloon is positioned in the proximal mainstem bronchus under fiberoptic visual guidance. With an inflated blocker balloon, the airway is completely sealed, providing more predictable lung collapse and better operating conditions than with an ETT in the contralateral bronchus.

A potential problem with this technique is dislodgment of the blocker balloon into the trachea. The inflated balloon then blocks ventilation to both lungs, prevents collapse of the operated lung, or both. The balloons of most catheters currently used for bronchial blockade have low-volume, high-pressure properties and overdistention can damage or even rupture the airway (Borchardt et al., 1998). A study, however, reported that bronchial blocker cuffs produced lower "cuff to tracheal" pressures than double-lumen tubes (Guyton et al., 1997). When closed tip bronchial blockers are used, the operative lung cannot be suctioned and continuous positive airway pressure (CPAP) cannot be provided to the operative lung if needed.

When a bronchial blocker is placed outside the ETT, care must be taken to avoid injury caused by compression and resultant ischemia of the tracheal mucosa. The sum of the catheter diameter and the outer diameter of the ETT should not exceed the tracheal diameter. Outer diameters for pediatric ETTs are shown in Table 19–5.

Adapters have been used that facilitate ventilation during placement of a bronchial blocker through an indwelling ETT (Takahashi et al., 2000; Arndt et al., 1999). Use of a 5F endobronchial blocker that is designed for use in children with a multiport adapter and fiberoptic bronchoscope (FOB) has been described (Cook Critical Care, Inc., Bloomington, IN) (Hammer et al., 2001). The balloon is elliptical in shape so that it conforms to the bronchial lumen when inflated. The blocker catheter has a maximum outer diameter of 2.5 mm (including the deflated balloon), a central lumen with a diameter of 0.7 mm, and a distal balloon with a capacity of 3 mL. The balloon has a length of 1.0 cm, corresponding to the length of the right mainstem bronchus in children approximately 2 years of age (Scammon, 1923). The blocker is placed coaxially through a dedicated port in the adapter, which also has a port for passage of an FOB and ports for connection to the anesthesia breathing circuit and ETT (Fig. 19–12). The FOB port has a plastic sealing cap, whereas the blocker port has a Tuohy-Borst connector, which locks the catheter in place and maintains an air-tight seal. Because oxygen can be administered during passage of the blocker and FOB, the

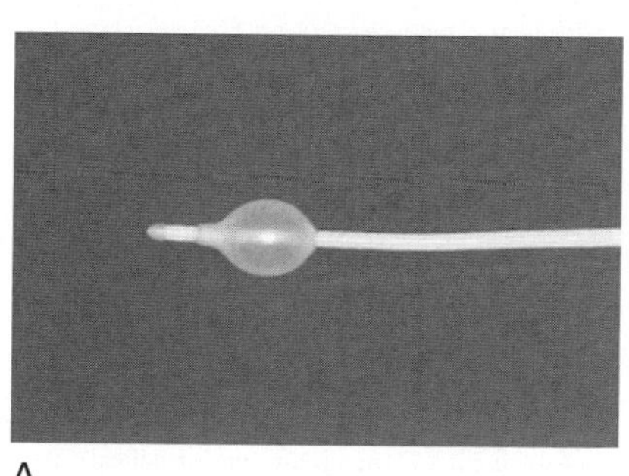

A

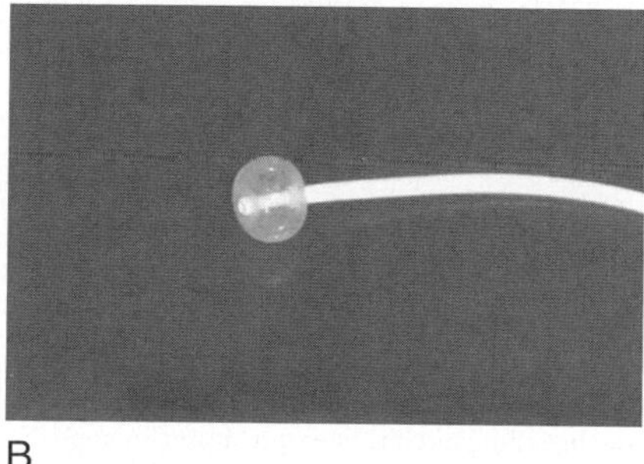

B

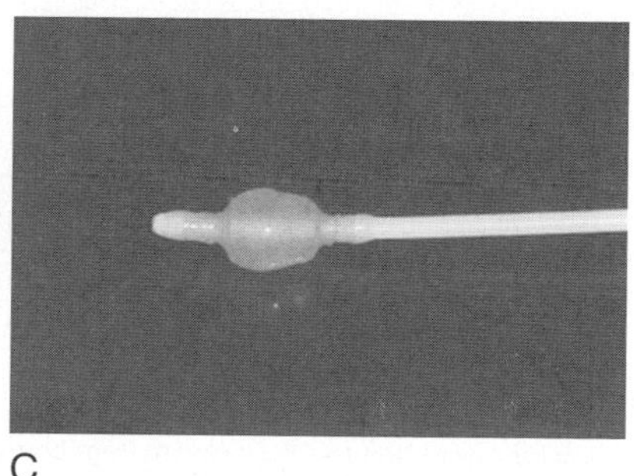

C

■ **FIGURE 19–11.** Balloon-tipped catheters used as bronchial blockers for single-lung ventilation. *A*, Fogarty catheter. *B*, Arrow balloon wedge catheter. *C*, Cook endobronchial blocker.

■ TABLE 19–5. Diameters of pediatric endotracheal tubes

ID (mm)	OD (mm)*
3.0	4.3
3.5	4.9
4.0	5.5
4.5	6.2
5.0	6.8
5.5	7.5
6.0	8.2
6.5	8.9
7.0	9.6

ID, internal diameter.
Cuffed tubes have approximately 0.5-mm additional outer diameter (OD).
*Sheridan Tracheal Tubes, Kendall Healthcare, Mansfield, MA.

risk of hypoxemia during blocker placement is diminished, and repositioning of the blocker may be performed with fiberoptic guidance during surgery.

When the placement of a bronchial blocker inside the ETT is guided by an FOB, both the blocker catheter and FOB must pass through the indwelling ETT. The inner diameter of the ETT through which the catheter and FOB are to be placed must be larger than the sum of the outer diameters of the catheter and the FOB. The 5F blocker catheter and an FOB with a 2.2-mm diameter, for example, may be inserted through an ETT as small as 5.0-mm internal diameter (ID). For children with an indwelling ETT smaller than 5.0 mm ID, a blocker catheter can be positioned under fluoroscopy (Fig. 19–13).

Single-Lung Ventilation Using a Univent Tube. The Univent tube (Fuji Systems Corporation, Tokyo, Japan) is a single-lumen ETT with a second lumen containing a small blocker catheter that can be advanced into a bronchus (Fig. 19–14) (Kamaya and Krishna, 1985; Kawande, 1987; Gayes, 1993). A balloon located at the distal end of this small tube serves as a blocker. Univent tubes require a fiberoptic bronchoscope for successful placement. Univent tubes are now available in sizes as small as 3.5- and 4.5-mm ID for use in children over 6 years of age (Table 19–6) (Hammer et al., 1998). Because the blocker tube is firmly attached to the main ETT, displacement of the Univent blocker balloon is less likely than when other blocker techniques are used. The blocker of the 4.5 Univent tube has a small lumen, which allows egress of gas and can be used to insufflate oxygen or suction the operated lung.

A disadvantage of the Univent tube is the large amount of cross sectional area occupied by the blocker channel, especially in the smaller-size tubes. Smaller Univent tubes have a disproportionately high resistance to gas flow (Slinger and Lesiuk, 1998). The Univent tube's blocker balloon has low-volume, high-pressure characteristics so mucosal injury can occur during normal inflation (Benumof et al., 1992; Kelley et al., 1992).

Single-Lung Ventilation Using a Double-Lumen Tube. All double-lumen tubes (DLTs) are essentially two tracheal tubes of unequal length molded longitudinally together. The shorter tube ends in the trachea, and the longer tube, in the bronchus. Marrarro (1994) described a bilumen tube for infants. DLTs for older children and adults have cuffs located on the tracheal and bronchial lumens. The tracheal cuff, when inflated, allows positive pressure ventilation. The inflated bronchial cuff allows ventilation to be diverted to either or both lungs and protects each lung from contamination from the contralateral side.

Conventional plastic DLTs, once only available in adult sizes (35F, 37F, 39F, and 41F), are now available in smaller sizes (Table 19–7). The smallest cuffed DLT is 26F (Rusch, Duluth, GA), which may be used in children as young as 8 years of age. DLTs are also available in sizes 28F and 32F (Mallinckrodt Medical, Inc., St. Louis, MO) suitable for children 10 years of age and older.

DLTs are inserted in children using the same technique as in adults (Brodsky and Mark, 1983). The tip of the tube is inserted just past the vocal cords and the stylette is withdrawn. The DLT is rotated 90 degrees to the appropriate side and then advanced into the bronchus. In the adult population, the depth of insertion is directly related to the height of the patient

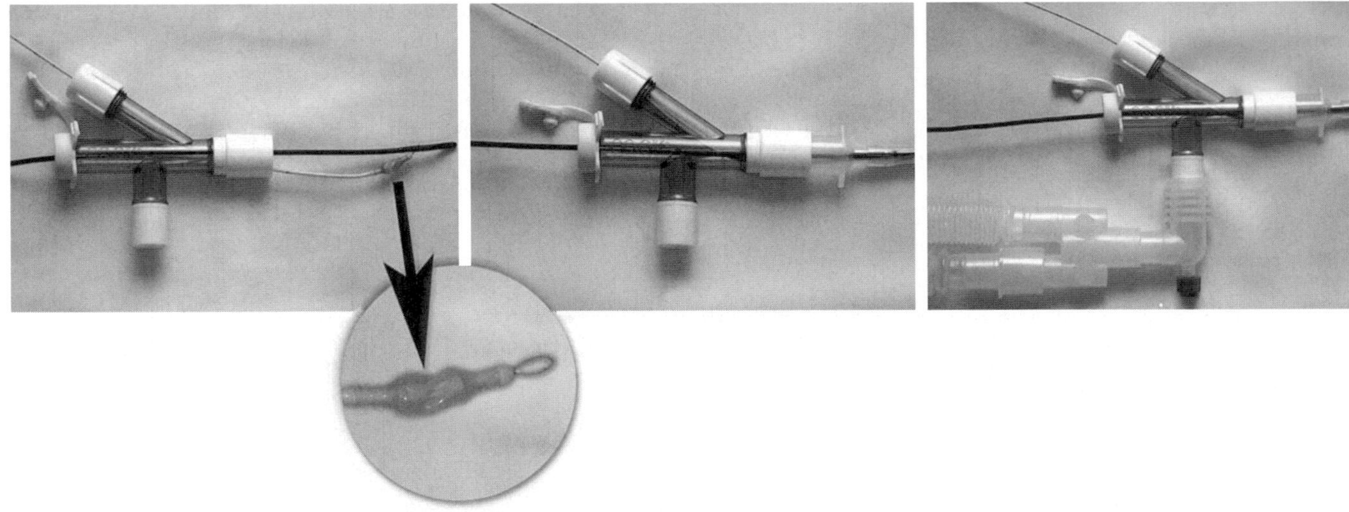

■ FIGURE 19–12. The Cook 5F endobronchial catheter is shown inserted in the multiport adapter (Cook Critical Care, Inc., Bloomington, IN). The adapter has four ports for connection to (*A*, clockwise from bottom) the breathing circuit, fiberoptic bronchoscope (FOB), endobronchial catheter, and endotracheal tube. After the FOB and endobronchial catheter have been inserted through the multiport adaptor, the FOB is placed through the monofilament loop at the distal end of the catheter (*arrow*). The multiport adaptor is then attached to the indwelling endotracheal tube (*B*) and the breathing circuit (*C*). The FOB is directed into the mainstem bronchus on the operative side. The catheter is then advanced until the monofilament loop slides off the end of the FOB into the bronchus.

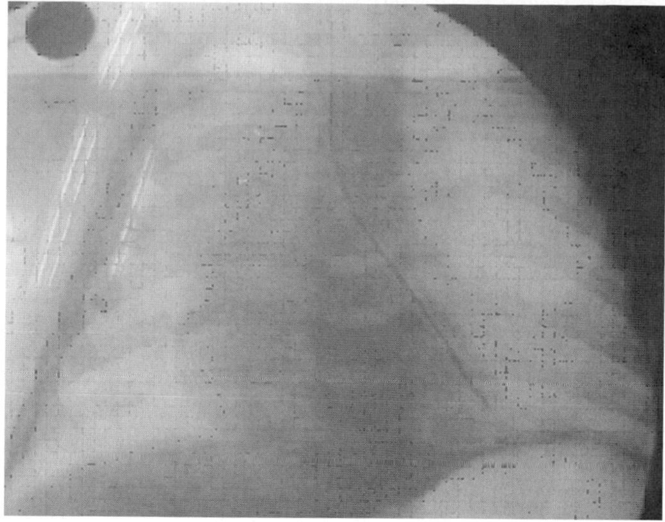

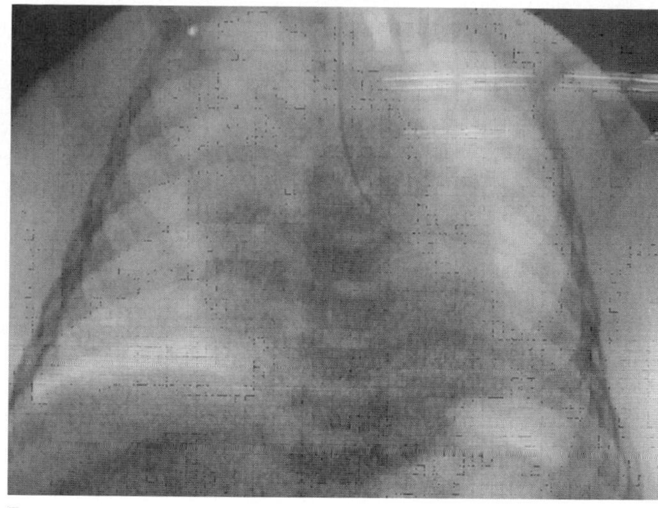

■ **FIGURE 19–13.** Positioning of a bronchial blocker under fluoroscopy. *A*, The catheter has been advanced into a segmental bronchus on the left. *B*, The catheter has been pulled back so that the balloon is in the left mainstem bronchus.

(Brodsky et al., 1996). No equivalent measurements are yet available in children. If fiberoptic bronchoscopy is to be used to confirm tube placement, an FOB with a small diameter and sufficient length must be available (Slinger, 1989).

A DLT offers the advantage of ease of insertion as well as the ability to suction and oxygenate the operative lung with CPAP. Left DLTs are preferred to right DLTs because of the shorter length of the right main bronchus (Benumof et al., 1987). Right DLTs are more difficult to accurately position because of the greater risk of right upper lobe obstruction. DLTs are safe and easy to use. There are very few reports of airway damage from DLTs in adults, and none in children. Their high-volume, low-pressure cuffs should not damage the airway if they are not overinflated with air or distended with nitrous oxide while in place. Guidelines for selecting appropriate tubes (or catheters) for SLV in children are shown in Table 19–7. There is significant variability in overall size and airway dimensions in children, particularly in teenagers. These recommendations are based on average values for airway dimensions. Larger DLTs may be safely used in adult-size teenagers.

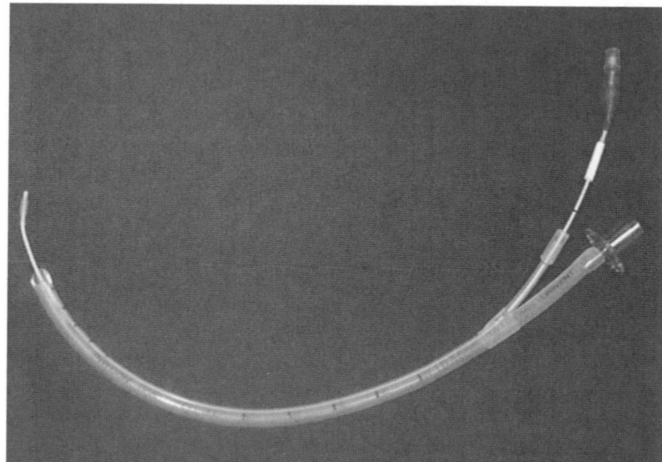

■ **FIGURE 19–14.** The Univent tube is a single-lumen endotracheal tube with a second lumen containing a small blocker catheter.

Postoperative Care

Tracheal extubation at the completion of surgery is often possible after simple subsegmental resection or lobectomy. However, the patient's underlying cardiopulmonary reserve, the course of the surgery, and the expected postoperative course may preclude extubation. Although postoperative pain can cause significant splinting, intercostal or epidural blocks, coupled with judicious parenteral opioids, can minimize the discomfort (see Chapters 13 and 14, Pain Management and Regional Anesthesia). Whether in the operating room or in the intensive care area, before extubation the patient must be awake, breathing well, able to cough and maintain an airway, and able to maintain acceptable oxygenation with no more than 40% inspired oxygen. A chest radiograph should be obtained as soon as possible after surgery to detect any significant pneumothorax or atelectasis. Atelectasis is common and usually responds to humidity, encouragement to cough, CPAP, and, if necessary, endotracheal suction.

■ **TABLE 19–6.** Univent tube diameters

ID (mm)	OD (mm)*
3.5	7.5/8.0
4.5	8.5/9.0
6.0	10.0/11.0
6.5	10.5/11.5
7.0	11.0/12.0
7.5	11.5/12.5
8.0	12.0/13.0
8.5	12.5/13.5
9.0	13.0/14.0

ID, internal diameter; OD, outer diameter.
*Sagittal/transverse.

■ **TABLE 19–7.** Tube selection for single-lung ventilation in children

Age (yr)	ETT (ID)*	BB (F)	Univent†	DLT (F)
0.5 to 1	3.5 to 4.0	2‡		
1 to 2	4.0 to 4.5	3‡		
2 to 4	4.5 to 5.0	5§		
4 to 6	5.0 to 5.5	5§		
6 to 8	5.5 to 6	5§	3.5	
8 to 10	6.0 Cuffed	5§	3.5	26‖
10 to 12	6.5 Cuffed	5§	4.5	26‖ to 28¶
12 to 14	6.5 to 7.0 Cuffed	5§	4.5	32¶
14 to 16	7.0 Cuffed	5§	6.0	35¶
16 to 18	7.0 to 8.0 Cuffed	9§	7.0	35¶

BB, bronchial blocker; ETT, endotracheal tube; ID, internal diameter; DLT, double-lumen tube; F, French.
*Sheridan Tracheal Tubes, Kendall Healthcare, Mansfield, MA.
‡Edwards Lifesciences LLC, Irvine, CA.
§Cook Critical Care, Inc., Bloomington, IN.
†Fuji Systems Corporation, Tokyo, Japan.
‖Rusch, Duluth, GA.
¶Mallinckrodt Medical, Inc., St. Louis, MO.

The expected postoperative course depends on both the surgical procedure and the underlying diseases. After simple lobectomy, most children develop normally and have normal exercise tolerance (McBride et al., 1980). Children who have undergone pneumonectomy may have more problems (Buhain and Brody, 1973). With time, overinflation of the remaining lung occurs, with a demonstrable decrease in vital capacity. These children may have significant exercise intolerance for a prolonged period after surgery.

SURGERY IN CONGENITAL LOBAR EMPHYSEMA, PULMONARY SEQUESTRATION, AND CYSTIC LESIONS

Congenital Lobar Emphysema

Congenital lobar emphysema is a rare cause of sudden respiratory distress in infants (Leape and Longino, 1964). Hyperinflation and progressive air trapping cause expansion of the affected lobe, along with compression of other lung tissue, mediastinal shifting, and impaired venous return. The most commonly affected is the left upper lobe, followed by the right middle and upper lobes. Occasionally more than one lobe is affected. The cause of the obstruction is unknown in most cases, although many show evidence of deficient and disordered bronchial cartilage. In some cases there are identifiable causes of bronchial compression, such as aberrant blood vessels, bronchial cysts, and bronchial stenosis. Finally, some patients have widespread lung disease with poor elastic recoil throughout (Ryckman and Rosenkrantz, 1985).

Congenital lobar emphysema usually appears clinically between the newborn period and the first 6 months of life (Murray, 1967) with tachycardia and retractions. The child may have rapid, progressive accumulation of gas in the affected lobe. Physical examination reveals asymmetric expansion of the thorax, wheezing, displacement of the cardiac impulse, hyperresonance to percussion, and diminished breath and heart sounds. Chest radiographs (Fig. 19–15) show overdistention of the affected lobe, mediastinal shift, and atelectasis in other lobes. The chest radiograph can help differentiate lobar emphysema from pneumothorax or congenital cysts by the presence of faint bronchovascular markings and herniation of the affected lobe across the midline.

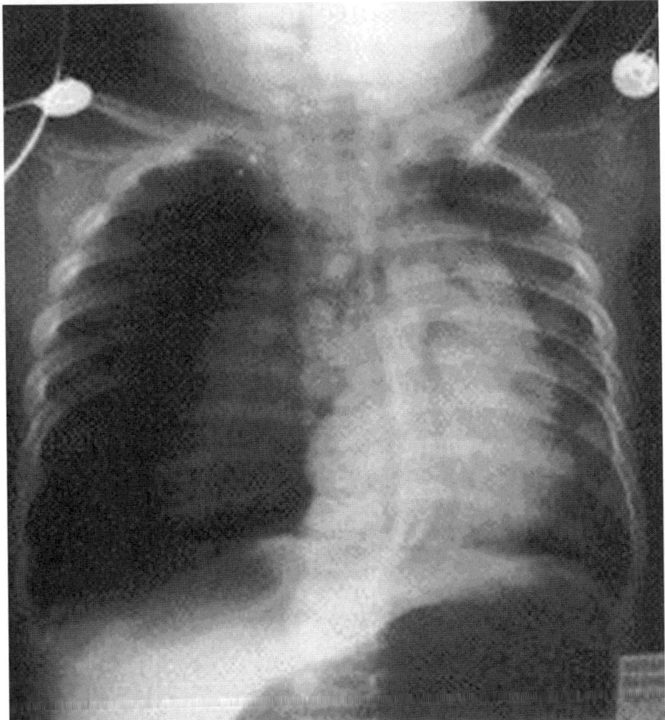

A

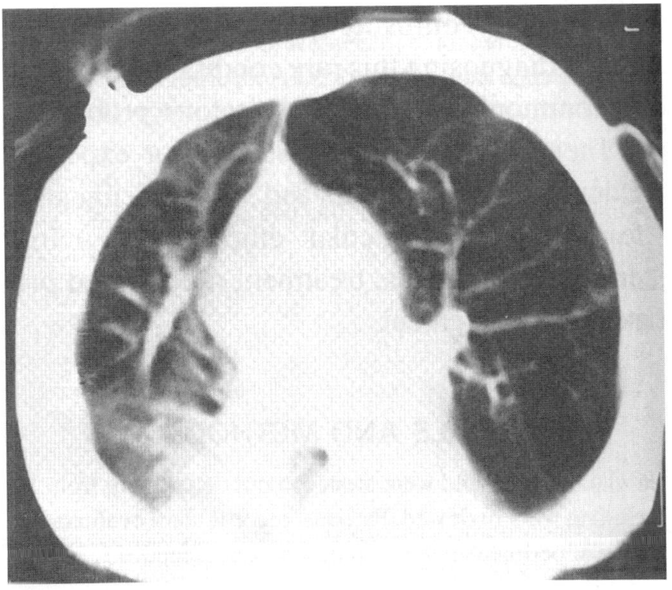

B

■ **FIGURE 19–15.** Right-sided congenital lobar emphysema. *A,* The right lung appears hyperinflated and lucent and may be mistaken for a pneumothorax. *B,* Computed tomography scan reveals markedly hyperexpanded right lung, mediastinal shift to the left, and compression of the left lung.

Infants who show rapid deterioration constitute a surgical emergency to relieve the expanding lobe with its ventilatory and cardiac impairment. Many patients do not have a clear clinical picture, however, but rather have a vague history of intermittent cyanosis or respiratory distress, failure to thrive, or unusual respiratory distress with feeding or a cold. Lobar emphysema is also seen in preterm infants with respiratory distress who are undergoing mechanical ventilation, which most frequently develops in the right upper lobe.

Preoperative evaluation depends on the degree of patient distress (Payne et al., 1984). If there is rapid deterioration, evaluation is limited. Chest tube placement, needle aspiration of the trapped air, and vigorous mechanical ventilation have been tried as palliative procedures but are associated with a much higher mortality than thoracotomy and lobectomy. If the patient is stable and there is any question about the diagnosis, procedures such as radioisotope perfusion scans, angiography, or CT imaging can be used before proceeding with definitive surgery. During preanesthetic evaluation, cardiopulmonary stability of the patient is the prime concern. The degree of distress, its progression, and the need for supplemental oxygen are key components of the examination. Cardiac evaluation is important because these patients have a higher incidence of congenital heart disease, especially ventricular septal defect.

Monitoring includes pulse oximetry to detect rapid changes in oxygenation, especially with induction. In deteriorating patients, there may be little time to establish intra-arterial monitoring before incision. Doppler-assisted or automated blood pressure cuffs increase the accuracy of measurements and are especially useful in infants. After intubation, capnography is helpful.

Induction of anesthesia in infants with congenital lobar emphysema is a critical phase in the anesthetic management. The crying, struggling infant can increase the amount of trapped gas, whereas positive-pressure ventilation or positive airway pressure by the anesthesiologist can also increase the emphysema. A smooth inhalation induction with sevoflurane and oxygen is often used, with positive-pressure ventilation minimized until the chest is open (Coté, 1978). Controlled or assisted ventilation is added if unacceptable hypoventilation develops, whereas intubation is performed with or without muscle relaxants, depending on the patient's tolerance of positive-pressure ventilation. High-frequency ventilation has been used successfully in infants with lobar emphysema (Goto et al., 1987) and should be considered if the practitioner is familiar with the technique. The low airway pressures are especially suitable for these patients. Nitrous oxide is avoided because it can expand the emphysematous areas (Payne et al., 1984). If the lobe expands suddenly, the surgeon should be ready to open the chest immediately and relieve the pressure. Raghavendran and others (2001) have also described a technique involving caudal epidural catheter threaded to the thoracic level in spontaneously breathing patients who were anesthetized with potent inhaled anesthetic agents.

An alternative induction approach, especially for unstable infants, is sedation with intravenous ketamine (1 to 2 mg/kg) and local anesthetic infiltration of the incision site (Coté, 1978). After the intrathoracic pressure has been relieved, general anesthesia can proceed with any technique appropriate to the patient's underlying status. Older children who are stable often undergo bronchoscopy before thoracotomy to rule out a foreign body or other correctable lesions. After induction with oxygen and a volatile agent, thorough topical anesthesia with 2% to 4% lidocaine (not more than 4 to 6 mg/kg) smoothes the course. As with the younger patient, rapid surgical decompression may be needed as the case proceeds.

In most patients, the trachea can be extubated at the end of the lobectomy. Humidity, coughing, and early increases in activity or ambulation minimize atelectasis in the immediate postoperative period. These children do well clinically after surgery but have reduced forced vital capacity and delayed forced expiration, not only in the immediate postoperative period but throughout childhood (Eigen et al., 1976; McBride et al., 1980).

Pulmonary Sequestrations

Pulmonary sequestrations result from disordered embryogenesis producing a nonfunctional mass of lung tissue supplied by anomalous systemic arteries. Presenting signs include cough, pneumonia, and failure to thrive and often present during the neonatal period, usually before the age of 2 years. Diagnostic studies include CT scans of the chest and abdomen and arteriography. Magnetic resonance imaging (MRI) may provide high-resolution images, including definition of vascular supply. This may obviate the need for angiography. Surgical resection is performed following diagnosis. Pulmonary sequestrations do not generally become hyperinflated during positive pressure ventilation. Nitrous oxide administration may result in expansion of these masses, however, and should be avoided.

Congenital Cystic Lesions

Congenital cystic lesions in the thorax may be classified into three categories (Kravitz, 1994). *Bronchogenic cysts* result from abnormal budding or branching of the tracheobronchial tree. They may cause respiratory distress, recurrent pneumonia, and/or atelectasis due to lung compression. *Dermoid cysts* are clinically similar to bronchogenic cysts but differ histologically, as they are lined with keratinized, squamous epithelium rather than respiratory (ciliated columnar) epithelium. They usually present later in childhood or adulthood. *Cystic adenomatoid malformations* (CCAM) are structurally similar to bronchioles but lack associated alveoli, bronchial glands, and cartilage (Ryckman and Rosenkrants, 1985). Because these lesions communicate with the airways, they may become overdistended due to gas trapping, leading to respiratory distress in the first few days of life. When they are multiple and air filled, CCAM may resemble congenital diaphragmatic hernia (CDH) radiographically. Treatment is surgical resection of the affected lobe. As with CDH, prognosis depends on the amount of remaining lung tissue, which may be hypoplastic due to compression in utero (Schwartz and Ramachandran, 1997).

■ SURGERY FOR DISEASES OF THE MEDIASTINUM

Surgical problems of the mediastinum fall into three major categories: masses, infections, and pneumomediastinum. The mediastinum is functionally divided into anterior, middle, and posterior segments. This classification is useful diagnostically in evaluating defects because of the propensity of lesions to develop primarily in only one of the divisions (Table 19–8).

Masses in the anterior portion of the mediastinum tend to be lymphomas, lymphangiomas (cystic hygroma), and teratomas. Thymomas and thymic cysts can appear here but are rare in childhood. Lymphomas are primarily of the Hodgkin's type, and biopsy of them is done only for diagnostic purposes. The survival of the child with mediastinal lymphoma depends on the

TABLE 19–8. Mediastinal masses

Location	Presentation
Anterior Division	
Lymphomas Lymphangiomas (cystic hygroma) Teratomas Thymomas and thymic cysts	Superior vena cava syndrome Cardiac tamponade Tracheal and lung compression
Middle Division	
Bronchogenic cysts Granulomas Lymphomas	Airway obstruction Stridor Obstructive emphysema
Posterior Division	
Enteric cysts, duplications Neuroblastoma Ganglioneuroma, neurofibroma	Airway obstruction Recurrent pneumonias Dysphagia

systemic spread of the tumor and not on the amount of lymphoma present in the mediastinum. Lymphangiomas are often extensions of cystic hygromas from the cervical region into the mediastinum. If not all of the lymphangioma is removed at initial resection, further extension may occur. Anterior mediastinal masses can present in various ways. Although they may be asymptomatic and detected incidentally on a chest radiograph, they may also present as compression of pulmonary or vascular structures. Superior vena cava syndrome, cardiac tamponade, and both tracheal and lung compression can be prominent characteristics (Levin et al., 1985; Northrip et al., 1986).

Bronchogenic cysts, granulomas, and lymphomas predominate in the middle division. Bronchogenic cysts comprise 7.5% of all mediastinal masses (Fig. 19–16). They may be asymptomatic or have symptoms of airway obstruction or recurrent pulmonary infection (Birmingham et al., 1993; Landsman et al., 1994). Bronchogenic cysts usually are next to the trachea or mainstem bronchi at the level of the carina, but they can also be intrapulmonary. They can produce sudden, life-threatening airway obstruction at any age. Lesser degrees of obstruction appear initially as wheezing, stridor, or unilateral obstructive emphysema.

In the posterior division, enteric cysts and tumors of neurogenic origin (neuroblastoma, ganglioneuroma, neurofibroma) predominate. Enteric cysts and duplications are lined with secretory epithelium and can enlarge rapidly and cause dysphagia, ulceration, or bleeding. In rare cases they can ulcerate directly into the tracheobronchial tree. Neurogenic tumors are usually asymptomatic and detected on a routine chest radiograph, although they can be responsible for tracheobronchial compression, recurrent pneumonias, and, rarely, stigmata of pheochromocytoma.

Mediastinal infections and inflammation are less common today than in the past (Campbell and Lilly, 1983). Modern antibiotic therapy dramatically reduced the incidence of suppurative mediastinitis caused by *Staphylococcus* and other organisms, whereas the incidence of tuberculosis and other similar infections in the general population has diminished. Although mediastinitis can result from extension of cervical node infections or hematogenous spread, the more likely cause is perforation of the trachea or esophagus. Foreign bodies can be responsible for perforation of the larynx, trachea, or esophagus; instrumentation of the trachea (endotracheal intubation or suction) or esophagus (esophageal dilation) can also be responsible.

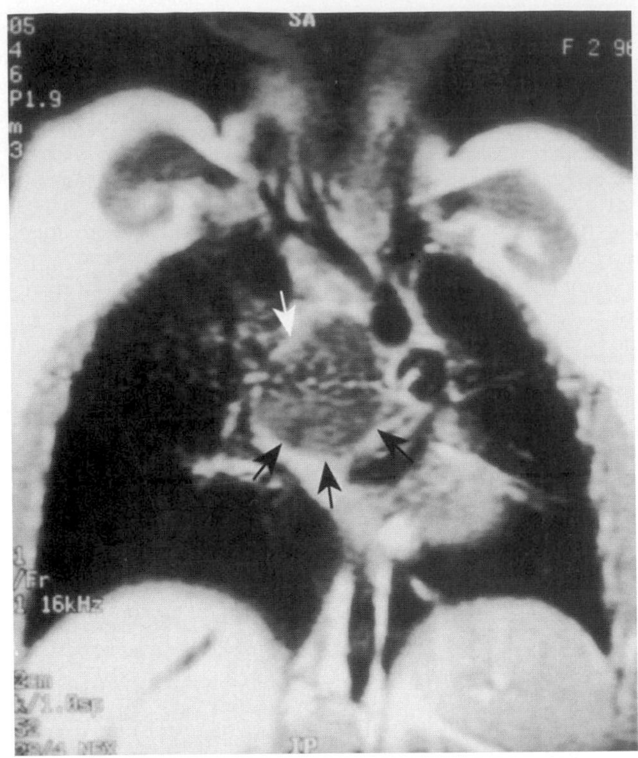

FIGURE 19–16. Magnetic resonance imaging of the chest; coronal section through the trachea and bronchogenic cyst (*black arrows*) located in the subcrinal area. The cyst is shown compressing the right mainstem bronchus (*white arrow*). (From Landsman IS, Bronert BJ, Wiener ES, Ford HR: *Anesth Analg* 79:803, 1994.)

Pneumomediastinum is an accumulation of air, usually in the superior anterior division. This occurs in trauma patients and as a result of mechanical ventilation, especially in newborns who undergo long-term ventilation and children with severe asthma. Pneumomediastinum is usually asymptomatic, but it may be responsible for tamponade and hypotension. These patients need urgent decompression by thoracostomy. Pneumomediastinum can be accompanied by pneumopericardium, which may need to be drained urgently as well. The intrathoracic pressure generated by pneumomediastinum can impede venous drainage of the head and result in increased intracranial pressure.

Anesthetic management of children with mediastinal diseases demands careful preoperative evaluation (Mackie and Watson, 1984). The location and nature of the disease are crucial to both preparation and management. The airway is considered first (Todres et al., 1976; Keon, 1981). If there is evidence of obstruction, the site and degree must be assessed. History and physical examination should focus not only on signs such as cyanosis and stridor but also on maneuvers or circumstances that change the signs. The practitioner should determine if sleep, excitement, position, movement of the head and neck, or coughing changes the degree of obstruction. Although chest radiographs and barium studies provide some information, CT scans are best at delineating the obstruction. These scans have the added advantage of demonstrating extension of infection or tumor into structures such as the pericardium. If a foreign body is responsible for the problem, the location and stability of the object are assessed.

Signs of lower airway disease can be caused by mediastinal tumors (Sibert et al., 1987). Compression of the lower airways and lung tissue can be responsible for wheezing, atelectasis,

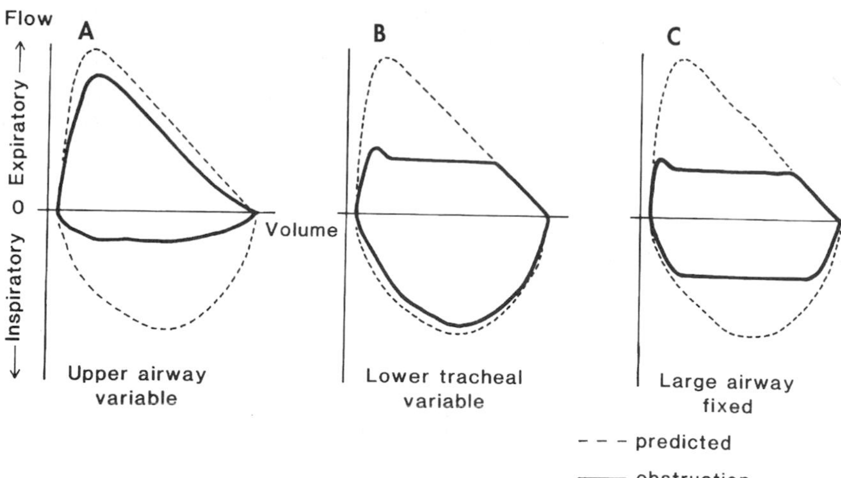

■ **FIGURE 19–17.** Schematic tracing of maximum expiratory–inspiratory flow–volume curves. *A*, Variable upper airway obstruction caused by papillomatosis of the larynx. *B*, Variable central (intrathoracic) airway obstruction caused by tracheomalacia. *C*, Fixed-type obstruction caused by tracheal stenosis. (From Motoyama EK: Physiologic: Alterations in tracheostomy. In Myers EN, Stool SE, Johnson JT, editors: *Tracheostomy*. New York, 1985, Churchill Livingstone.)

obstructive emphysema, and recurrent pneumonias. This is important because wheezing caused by compression of lower airways and lung tissue usually does not respond to bronchodilators, nor will atelectasis caused by compression respond to chest physical therapy. Repeat chest radiographs or pulmonary function tests can help delineate the degree of functional impairment. In older, more cooperative children, maximal inspiratory and expiratory flow-volume loops obtained with the patient upright and supine can quantitate the functional degree of impairment and help distinguish fixed from variable obstructions (Fig. 19–17).

Cardiovascular involvement may be related to direct compression of the heart or of the great vessels. Echocardiography or CT scanning can delineate impingement. The important determination is assessment of functional impairment. If the child has arrhythmias, pulsus paradoxus, hypotension, or superior vena cava syndrome, the risk of general anesthesia increases dramatically.

Induction of anesthesia may remove compensatory efforts by the patient (Neuman et al., 1984). The child's position, pattern of ventilation, or sympathetic tone while awake may have been responsible for barely maintaining adequate cardiopulmonary function (Bray and Fernandes, 1982; Prakash et al., 1988) (Fig. 19–18). In these situations, the anesthesiologist and surgeon must determine alternative approaches to the lesion (Mackie and Watson, 1984). If the child has a better airway, easier ventilation, or less hypotension in one position, efforts are made to keep him or her in this position. Biopsy of accessible lesions under local anesthesia should be considered if there is significant cardiopulmonary compromise. In extreme cases, radiation therapy quickly shrinks the tumor mass, allowing a biopsy to be done later with less risk to the patient (Piro et al., 1976). If general anesthesia is used, the surgeon should be present at induction and prepared for interventions such as passage of a rigid bronchoscope or immediate release of a pneumomediastinum via subxiphoid thoracostomy. Of utmost importance is that patients, family, pediatrician, and surgeon all understand the risk of cardiovascular and respiratory compromise that exists in performing tissue biopsies under general anesthesia (Fig. 19–19).

Mask induction with a volatile agent and 100% oxygen is appropriate if there is concern about airway obstruction. The negative intrathoracic pressure of spontaneous breathing and any beneficial effect this has on maintenance of airway patency are preserved (Sibert et al., 1987). In some cases, airway obstruction worsens with positive-pressure ventilation; it may be necessary to maintain spontaneous or assisted ventilation. Two important monitors during induction are breath sounds from the precordial stethoscope and continuous oxygen saturation monitoring from a pulse oximeter. Nitrous oxide is avoided in all cases of

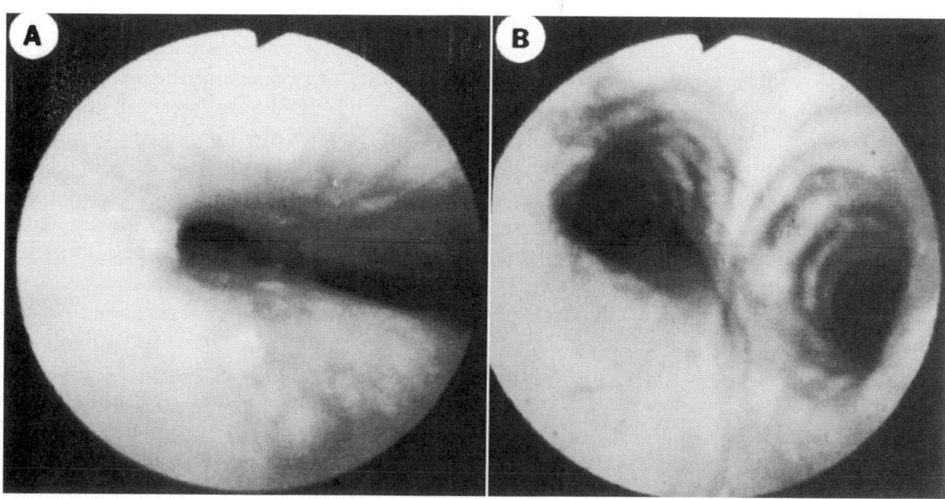

■ **FIGURE 19–18.** The effects of anesthesia on tracheal compression in a patient with a mediastinal mass. (From Prakash UBS, Abel MD, Hubmayr RD: Mediastinal mass and tracheal obstruction during general anesthesia. *Mayo Clin Proc* 63:1004, 1988.)

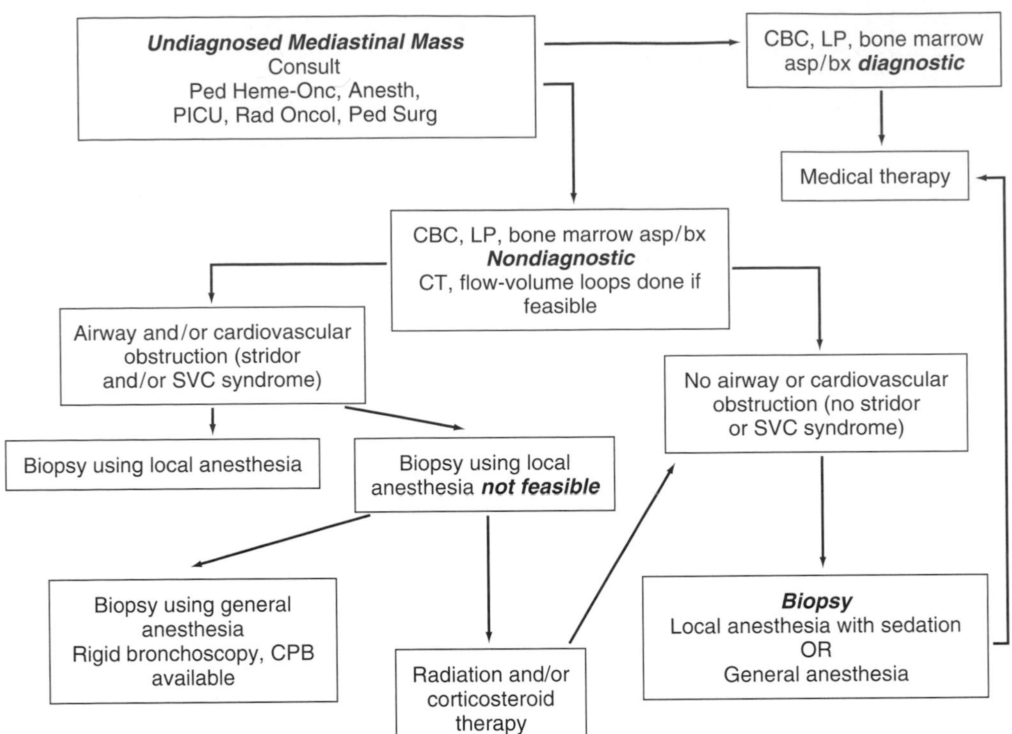

■ **FIGURE 19–19.** Algorithm for mediastinal mass.

pneumomediastinum or obstructive emphysema and in patients who have significant $\dot{V}/\dot{Q}$ abnormalities from lung compression (Mackie and Watson, 1984). The role of nitrous oxide in patients with asymptomatic bronchogenic cysts is unclear. Because these cysts are air filled, they may expand on exposure to nitrous oxide and cause airway compromise. In rare cases of severe airway impingement, intubation in the awake, sedated patient may be necessary to secure the airway safely for general anesthesia. If cardiac compression is of primary concern, narcotic-based anesthesia with or without ketamine for induction is a useful technique.

Thoracotomy or thoracostomy is usually the operative procedure performed in these patients. Major complications include massive blood loss, further obstruction or perforation of the airway, and lung compression (Barash et al., 1976; Neuman et al., 1984). There continue to be sporadic reports of death during the induction and maintenance of anesthesia in children with mediastinal masses, emphasizing the need for meticulous preoperative evaluation and intraoperative care. From review of the 44 pediatric patients with mediastinal masses, Ferrari and Bedford (1990) noted that significant anesthesia-related problems occurred in the patients who were symptomatic before surgery. They noted that general anesthesia could be administered with the following caveats: spontaneous ventilation must be performed, induction of anesthesia should be in the sitting position, intravenous access should be in the lower extremity, and a rigid bronchoscope and experienced bronchoscopist must be available. The anesthesiologist not only must be prepared for each complication but also must notify the surgeon immediately if there is loss of airway, difficulty in ventilation, or sudden hypotension.

■ UROLOGIC SURGERY

There is a wide range of surgical lesions that require the expertise of a pediatric urologist (Box 19–5). Although the anesthetic requirements for the different surgical lesions vary, the preoperative anesthetic assessment focuses on several important considerations. First, does the child have a known syndrome that has multiple anesthetic considerations? Second, does the child have other congenital anomalies, such as cardiac abnormalities, that require evaluation? Last, does the child have signs or symptoms of any underlying renal insufficiency? (See Table 19–9.) In general, renal failure is divided into acute and chronic components. Acute renal failure is the sudden loss of the kidney's ability to excrete water, electrolytes, and waste products in sufficient quantities to maintain the body's homeostasis. The causes of acute renal failure are numerous but are divided into four broad categories—prerenal, renal parenchymal, renal tubule, and obstructive. Regardless of its cause, management of acute renal failure is aimed at ensuring that the patient has an adequate circulating blood volume and avoiding fluid overload.

Congestive heart failure occurs when more than insensible fluid losses and urinary output are replaced. Although either a normal or reduced urinary output can occur with acute renal failure, with the onset of anuria or oliguria, hyperkalemia and hypocalcemia can occur. Hyperkalemia is the major life-threatening complication of acute renal failure and therefore must be treated immediately. Because of the kidney's inability to excrete cellular waste products, acidosis also develops in acute renal failure. Although most patients with acute renal failure have reversible conditions, some patients go on to develop chronic failure (see Chapter 4, Regulation of Body Fluids and Electrolytes).

Chronic renal failure or end-stage renal disease (ESRD) results in a 95% loss of creatinine clearance. A 50% loss of nephrons generally results in no biochemical abnormalities and a glomerular filtration rate of about 80%. The biochemical manifestations of ESRD result in inability of the kidney to regulate water and electrolytes and to excrete acid waste products. Because the kidney is also an exocrine organ, progressive renal failure is also

BOX 19–5 **Genitourinary Conditions Requiring Surgery During Infancy and Childhood**

- Congenital anomalies
  - Ureteral valves
  - Double renal pelvis and ureters
  - Ectopic ureter
  - Megaureter
  - Ureterocele
  - Neurogenic bladder
  - Exstrophy of bladder
  - Undescended testes
  - Hypospadias, epispadias
  - Phimosis
  - Vaginal anomalies
- Cysts and tumors
  - Wilms tumor
  - Cystic kidney
  - Neuroblastoma
  - Ganglioneuroma
  - Adrenogenital tumors
  - Pheochromocytoma
  - Retroperitoneal teratoma
  - Ovarian tumor
- Trauma
  - Ruptured kidney
  - Ruptured bladder
  - Urethral injuries
- Renal failure (operative procedures)
  - Renal biopsy
  - Nephrectomy
  - Shunt and fistula creation
  - Parathyroidectomy
  - Renal transplantation
- Infections
  - Cystitis
  - Urethritis
  - Paraphimosis
- Other
  - Renal and bladder calculi and stones

accompanied by abnormalities in the excretion of vitamin D, parathyroid hormone, and erythropoietin. ESRD, through its biochemical and hormonal mediators, affects all organ systems (see Chapter 4).

In addition to the pathophysiologic problems that accompany patients with renal and urologic abnormalities, the anesthesiologist must be cognizant of potential emotional difficulties that children have when faced with genitourinary surgery. Not infrequently, some of these patients have deep-seated emotional problems, and the anesthesiologist should be sensitive to their needs. Issues involving the psychologic preparation of the patient are explored in Chapter 7, Psychological Aspects.

In the child with normal renal function, anesthesia for urologic surgery is similar to anesthesia for most other types of surgery. In patients with renal insufficiency, nephrotoxic drugs should be avoided or their dosage reduced. The differences in distribution and excretion of drugs that are renally excreted should be remembered. This primarily applies to neuromuscular blockers, because there is little evidence that the volatile agents are materially different in patients with renal insufficiency. There is

TABLE 19–9. Signs and symptoms of patients with renal insufficiency

System	Signs and symptoms
Cardiovascular	Hypertension Increased cardiac output/high output failure Atherosclerosis/hyperlipidemia Pericarditis Variable increase in 2,3-diphosphoglycerate levels
Pulmonary	Hypoxemia Pulmonary edema Pleuritis
Hematologic	Anemia secondary to erythropoietin deficiency Anemia secondary to blood loss, decreased iron absorption, and folic acid deficiency Platelet dysfunction Decreased antithrombin III levels Increased factor VIII and fibrinogen
Neurologic	Irritability, confusion, anxiety, memory loss, encephalopathy, and psychosis Seizures, coma Peripheral neuropathy
Gastrointestinal	Anorexia, nausea, vomiting, gastroparesis
Metabolic/ endocrine	Renal osteodystrophy secondary to hyperparathyroidism, hyperkalemia, hypocalcemia, metabolic acidosis, hypernatremia, and hyponatremia
Infectious disease	Hepatitis B or non-A, non-B hepatitis Cytomegalovirus and human immunodeficiency virus

a well-known risk of prolongation of action with morphine and, especially, meperidine, but the synthetic opioids are used more commonly in this population. Among the muscle relaxants, a delayed onset and slight resistance to vecuronium have been reported in renal failure patients (Hunter, 1984), as well as delayed onset with rocuronium (Driessen, 2002). However, these differences are modest, even in children with complete renal failure.

Urologic procedures frequently require patients to be positioned in the lateral, prone, or lithotomy position. Each of these positions can be associated with compression-type injuries, as well as compromise of ventilation and venous return. Consequently, anesthetic management requires not only diligence to patient monitoring but also attention to appropriate patient positioning, padding, and rechecking of positioning.

CYSTOSCOPY

Cystoscopy is commonly performed in children under the general anesthesia to evaluate abnormalities of the urethra, bladder, and ureters. This is a relatively brief procedure; however, positioning the patient away from the anesthesia machine, extending the anesthetic tubings and monitor cables, maintaining a possibly difficult airway at the far end of the operating table, and exposing the patient to a cold room and irrigating solutions may complicate the delivery of anesthesia. Mask inhalation anesthesia is usually satisfactory, and endotracheal intubation or laryngeal mask airway is not necessary beyond infancy, as long as a satisfactory airway can be maintained. It is important, however, to maintain a relatively deep plane of anesthesia before insertion of the cystoscope because the urethral stimulation may precipitate laryngospasm (Breuer-Lockhart reflex) (Stehling and Furman, 1980). Regional anesthesia is infrequently used as the primary anesthetic for cystoscopy, but can be used for postoperative analgesia. However, most children experience little discomfort on awakening.

CIRCUMCISION

Circumcision is the most frequently performed surgical procedure in the world (Klauber and Sant, 1985). Most circumcisions are performed during the newborn period, and many are done without any anesthesia. However, there is increasing attention paid to providing analgesia for the procedure, including the use of the simple penile nerve block by obstetricians, family practitioners, and pediatricians (Maxwell, 1987; Howard et al., 1998). Simple techniques can significantly decrease cardiovascular and behavioral responses to pain in these neonates (Holliday, 1999). With increased education, especially at the resident level, there should be an increase in these techniques being used by primary care practitioners.

Beyond the newborn period, circumcision is usually performed under general anesthesia. Mask inhalation anesthesia with sevoflurane or isoflurane in nitrous oxide and oxygen is commonly used. A penile nerve block can be performed either immediately after anesthetic induction or at the end of the operation. It may be advantageous to place the block before the circumcision because the anesthetic requirement is decreased and emergence is more rapid. Caudal epidural anesthesia is also efficacious, although penile nerve block is preferred by some because less local anesthetic is given and less time is taken to perform the block. Others have suggested that the time, expense, and risk of caudal block are not justified for circumcision, because parenteral opioid administration is equally effective (Martin, 1982).

A comparison of different modalities for analgesia, with a focus on caudal analgesia, found that although the need for rescue analgesia is reduced in the early postoperative period when caudal block is compared with parenteral analgesia, there is a paucity of data in the literature to accurately compare both the short- and long-term effectiveness of caudal block versus other modalities such as parental analgesia, penile block, or topical anesthetic gel or cream (Allan, 2003). This analysis points out a problem in analyzing almost all the work on analgesia for urologic procedures—there are insufficient studies available that compare all available modalities in a consistent, uniform manner, thereby allowing direct comparison of risks and benefits.

HYPOSPADIAS REPAIR

Hypospadias occurs in approximately 8:1000 male births (Belman, 1985). Associated anomalies that cause difficulties for the anesthesiologist are rare. Hypospadias is repaired either as a single-stage or a multistage procedure, depending on the complexity of the anatomic abnormality. The surgical procedure usually requires several hours, so most anesthesiologists prefer endotracheal intubation rather than mask anesthesia for patient safety and for convenience. The laryngeal mask airway (LMA) may also be useful in these procedures. Blood loss is usually not significant, and transfusion is rarely required. Induction of anesthesia can be achieved by any of the techniques commonly used in children. Intraoperatively, anesthesia can be maintained using either an inhalation or a balanced technique. General anesthesia combined with a conduction block provides excellent intraoperative conditions and postoperative pain relief.

Caudal epidural block may be the optimal choice because it provides complete intraoperative and postoperative analgesia. Penile block is less effective than caudal epidural anesthesia for postoperative analgesia after hypospadias repair, especially in cases of proximally located hypospadias (Blaise and Roy, 1986). When only a distal penile hypospadias is present, penile nerve block may be as effective as caudal epidural anesthesia. In children under 1 year of age, a single caudal epidural injection of bupivacaine (0.25% with 5 mcg/mL epinephrine; 1.2 mL/kg) is administered after the induction of general anesthesia (Hannallah, 1987). Some practitioners prefer 0.2% or 0.125% bupivacaine to give greater volume with less risk of motor blockade. The caudal block is repeated at the end of the surgery if more than 1 hour has elapsed since the first caudal epidural injection. For children older than 1 year, it can be worthwhile to place a catheter for continuous caudal block using a commercially available epidural catheter kit. With the availability of smaller epidural catheters, a continuous infusion of local anesthetic may also be practical for younger patients (see Chapter 14, Pediatric Regional Anesthesia).

URETERAL REIMPLANTATION AND BLADDER NECK SURGERY

Reimplantation of one or both ureters is performed for treatment of vesicoureteral reflux whether it occurs congenitally or results from repeated urinary tract infections. The duration of the procedure may vary from 2 to 5 hours, so general anesthesia and endotracheal intubation are indicated. A caudal or lumbar epidural catheter can be used to provide supplemental regional anesthesia intraoperatively, minimizing the general anesthetic requirement as well as providing for postoperative analgesia and prevention of bladder spasm. The surgical procedure usually precludes the ability to measure urine output accurately. In those patients for whom the surgery is anticipated to take a long time, a central venous pressure catheter can be placed. For shorter surgical procedures, losses can be estimated by observation of the surgical field and vital signs. Serial hematocrit values should be measured whenever blood loss appears excessive. As with other urologic procedures, regional anesthesia via the caudal or epidural approach can be very useful for both intraoperative and postoperative pain relief.

PRUNE-BELLY SYNDROME PROCEDURES

The prune-belly syndrome (Eagle-Barrett syndrome) occurs in 1:40,000 births, mostly in boys, and results from distal urinary tract obstruction that leads to multiple secondary organ dysfunction (Jones, 1988). Figure 19–20 outlines the proposed sequence of events in the urethral obstruction malformation complex that leads to the classic manifestations, namely, abdominal muscular deficiency, renal dysplasia, excel abdominal skin, and cryptorchidism. Other variable features include colonic malrotation, persistent urachus, and lower limb abnormalities. Figure 19–21 shows the typical physical appearance of a child with prune-belly syndrome.

A classification system has been devised according to the severity of disease in prune-belly syndrome (Woodhouse, 1982). Group I children have severe renal disease, pulmonary hypoplasia, or both, which is incompatible with survival. Group II children are seen as neonatal emergencies with severe uropathy and urinary tract infection and require multiple corrective surgical procedures. Group III patients have minimal problems in the newborn period but are prone to infections in later childhood. The prognosis in group II and III children is good, with as many as half of the children in group II developing normally and exhibiting good renal function.

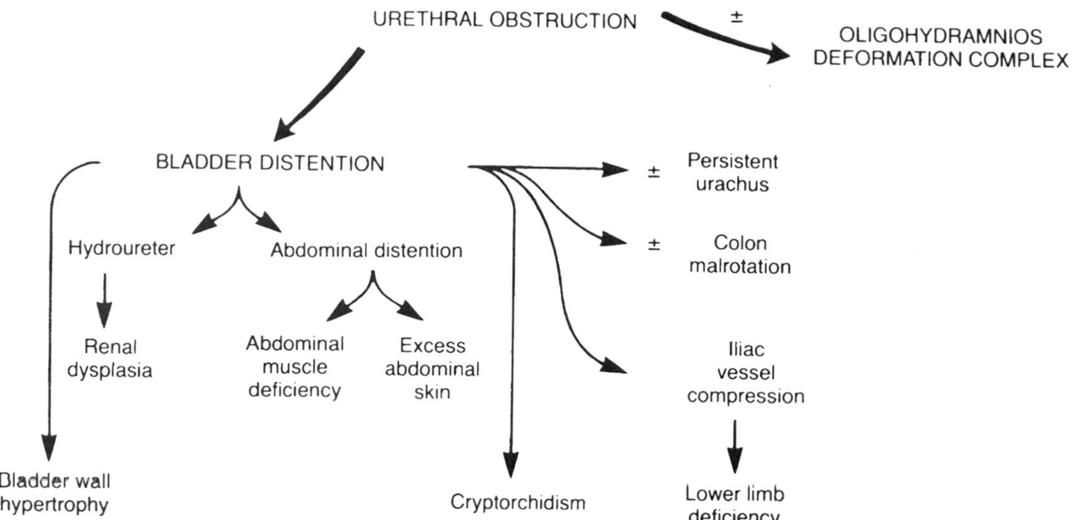

■ **FIGURE 19–20.** Developmental pathogenesis of early urethral obstruction sequence. (From Jones KL, editor: *Smith's recognizable patterns of human malformation.* Philadelphia, 1988, WB Saunders.)

These patients have a depressed cough mechanism resulting from deficient abdominal musculature, so preoperative sedation is best avoided. Because aspiration is a risk, administration of an H_2-antagonist (such as ranitidine) and sodium citrate may be indicated to raise gastric pH, and rapid sequence induction may be recommended. Controlled ventilation is necessary intraoperatively to prevent hypoventilation. Anesthesia can be maintained with inhalation agents or intravenous techniques, although muscle relaxation is usually unnecessary. Tracheal extubation should be performed only when the patient is awake and meets appropriate criteria. A review of 120 anesthetic cases suggested that intraoperative morbidity was rare, despite allowing spontaneous breathing in half of the cases (Henderson, 1987).

Postoperatively, respiratory infections occurred in approximately 7% of cases; one patient died from postoperative aspiration pneumonitis (Henderson, 1987). These patients require close observation and aggressive pulmonary toilet. Caudal, epidural, or spinal anesthesia in awake or mildly sedated patients may be useful for procedures such as cystoscopy or herniorrhaphy. After abdominal procedures, caudal or lumbar epidural administration of local anesthetic may be indicated to minimize postoperative pain. Postoperative mechanical ventilation may be required for patients who undergo extensive abdominal procedures or when significant pulmonary disease is present.

A wide variety of urologic abnormalities are found in prune-belly syndrome, including renal dysplasia, dilated and tortuous ureters, enlarged and dysfunctional bladder, urethral obstruction, and prostatic hypoplasia (Barrett and Mansoni, 1987). Despite severe urologic abnormalities, renal function may be well preserved. The surgical approach has become more conservative with the appreciation of the relatively good outcome in these patients. The standard surgical approach includes acceptance of the dilated upper urinary tract without extensive ureteral remodeling procedures and maintenance of adequate bladder drainage with urethral surgery (Barrett and Mansoni, 1987).

REPAIR OF EXSTROPHY OF THE BLADDER

Exstrophy of the bladder is a rare anomaly, occurring in 1:30,000 births, most commonly in boys. This anomaly can be subdivided into classic exstrophy, cloacal exstrophy, and epispadias. Classic exstrophy is most common, with an absence of the anterior wall of the bladder and overlying abdominal wall, epispadias, and separation of the symphysis pubis. Many urologists prefer to perform a staged repair, with the initial stage scheduled

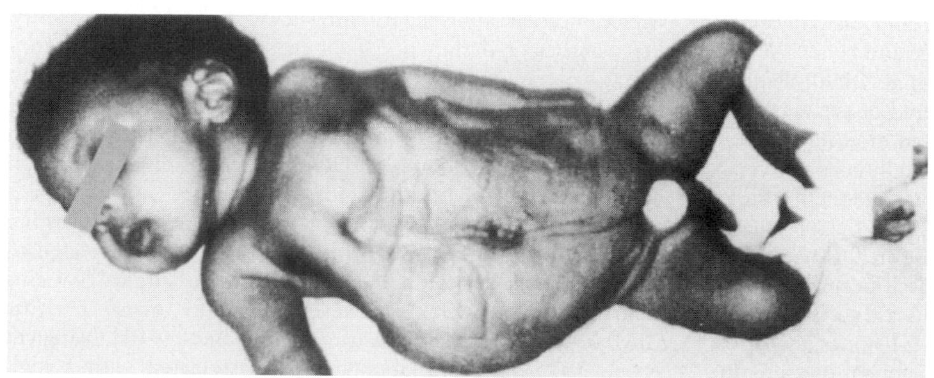

■ **FIGURE 19–21.** Infant with prune-belly syndrome. Note lax abdominal skin. (From Jones KL, editor: *Smith's recognizable patterns of human malformation.* Philadelphia, 1988, WB Saunders.)

during the newborn period. This allows approximation of the symphysis pubis without the need for iliac osteotomies. Multiple procedures are usually necessary in the first years of life to achieve complete repair. To formulate an appropriate anesthetic plan, including an accurate prediction of blood loss, the anesthesiologist must discuss the surgical plan preoperatively with the urologist.

During the newborn period, blood loss, evaporative losses, and third-space fluid losses can be excessive during bladder exstrophy repair. It is recommended that two intravenous catheters or a central venous catheter be placed before surgery. An arterial catheter may be useful for monitoring blood pressure and allowing the sampling of blood for measurement of glucose levels, hematocrit, and blood gas analysis. In addition, significant heat loss is common during these procedures, demanding close attention to temperature levels and active warming, usually through a forced-air heating system. A combined general anesthetic-epidural technique is increasingly popular for these cases, with the epidural catheter providing excellent analgesia into the postoperative period (Wee, 1999). Bupivacaine or ropivacaine is commonly used, but an opioid is not often added in the neonatal period because of the risk of respiratory depression, unless prolonged mechanical ventilation is anticipated. Postoperatively, careful attention must be focused on maintaining fluid and electrolyte homeostasis, as well as preventing anemia, hypotension, and hypoxia, as in any other case.

BARIATRIC SURGERY

OBESITY IN CHILDREN AND ADOLESCENTS

Obesity is the most common health problem facing U.S. children today. Data suggest that the prevalence of obesity continues to increase rapidly. Results from the National Health and Nutrition Examination Survey III reveal that approximately 14% of children in the United States are obese, as defined by body mass index (BMI) greater than the 95th percentile (Centers for Disease Control and Prevention Update, 1997). The prevalence is increasing approximately 47% to 73% faster among black and Hispanic children than among non-Hispanic white children. As of 1998, the prevalence of obesity in children had increased to 21.5% among African Americans, 21.8% among Hispanics, and 12.3% among non-Hispanic whites (Strauss and Pollack, 2001).

Childhood obesity has been defined variously by absolute weight, weight-for-height percentiles, percentiles of ideal body weight, triceps skinfolds, and BMI (weight in kilograms divided by height in meters squared). The most recent recommendations from the Centers for Disease Control and Prevention (CDC) suggest that BMI is the most appropriate and easily available method to screen for childhood obesity. Age and gender cutoffs for BMI have been published (Kuczmarski et al., 2000). Patients with a BMI of greater than 30 are considered obese, and those with a BMI of greater than 40 are considered morbidly obese.

Although many of the adverse effects of childhood obesity may not become apparent for decades, even young children may suffer severe morbidity. Psychological problems include low self-esteem, self-consciousness, helplessness, and depression. Hypertension, hypercholesterolemia, and hyperinsulinism all occur in young, obese children, leading to coronary artery disease and diabetes in adulthood. Obese children may develop gallstones, hepatitis, obstructive sleep apnea, and increased intracranial pressure due to pseudotumor cerebri (Strauss, 2002). The adverse effects of obesity in childhood are shown in Box 19–6. These complications may result in the need for surgery (e.g., gallstones, slipped epiphysis, bariatric surgery) and complicate the anesthetic management during surgery (airway obstruction or reactivity, hyperglycemia, systemic or intracranial hypertension).

BOX 19–6 Adverse Effects of Obesity in Childhood

- Hypertension
- Dyslipidemia
- Orthopedic
  - Slipped capital femoral epiphysis
  - Blount's disease (tibia vara)
- Endocrine
  - Diabetes
  - Insulin resistance
  - Polycystic ovary syndrome, irregular menses
- Gastroenterologic
  - Gallstones
  - Steatohepatitis
- Respiratory
  - Asthma
  - Sleep apnea
- Neurologic
  - Pseudotumor cerebri

PHYSIOLOGIC CONSIDERATIONS

Obesity is associated with many physiologic disturbances of concern to anesthesiologists. Work of breathing is increased, and fatty chest and abdominal walls decrease chest compliance. FRC and airway closing capacity are significantly reduced, causing hypoxemia due to intrapulmonary shunting. Exacerbations of hypoxemia due to sleep apnea may lead to pulmonary hypertension, cor pulmonale, and heart failure. A small number of morbidly obese patients have somnolence, cardiac enlargement, polycythemia, hypoxemia, and hypercapnia (Pickwickian syndrome). Morbidly obese patients with preoperative pulmonary dysfunction have higher morbidity following bariatric surgery but may subsequently have significant improvement in sleep apnea, gas exchange abnormalities, pulmonary hypertension, and cardiac function (Sugerman et al., 1992).

Cardiac reserve is decreased in obese patients. Even normotensive morbidly obese patients have increased preload and afterload, increased pulmonary artery pressures, and elevated right and left ventricular stroke work compared with nonobese patients. The degree of cardiac abnormality correlates with the degree of obesity. Left ventricular dysfunction is often present in young, asymptomatic obese patients. Right ventricular failure is common in older patients (Brodsky and Vierra, 2000). Weight loss, whether through diet or bariatric surgery, can reverse cardiac dysfunction and hypertension (Jones, 1996). Hypertension is common among morbidly obese adolescents and adults.

The gastric contents of unpremedicated, nondiabetic, fasting obese patients (BMI > 30) without GER are not increased in volume or acidity compared with nonobese surgical patients (Harter et al., 1998). However, morbidly obese patients (BMI > 40) do have large gastric volumes and low pH (Vaughan et al., 1975). Morbid obesity is also associated with a high incidence of GER, with 70% of patients complaining of heartburn (Hagen et al., 1987).

Other gastrointestinal abnormalities in morbidly obese patients include steatohepatitis, cirrhosis, and gallstones (Clain et al., 1987). Approximately 30% of patients who do not have gallstones at the time of bariatric surgery develop gallstones within 3 to 6 months after surgery, prompting many surgeons to perform a cholecystectomy at the time of the bariatric procedure.

Endocrine and genetic abnormalities are associated with obesity and short stature. Hirsutism, increased muscle mass, and acanthosis nigricans are associated with polycystic ovary syndrome. Obesity associated with mental retardation may signify a congenital syndrome such as Prader-Willi, Laurence-Moon-Biedl, or Cohen's syndromes. Females with short stature and obesity may be diagnosed with Turner's syndrome. Recurrent headaches, especially if associated with vomiting, may be caused by pseudotumor cerebri; papilledema may be seen on fundoscopic examination.

BARIATRIC SURGICAL PROCEDURES

Gastric bypass and other types of bariatric surgery have been considered appropriate for selected adults with a BMI of 40 or of 35 in the presence of comorbid conditions (Consensus Development Conference Panel, 1991; National Institutes of Health, 1998). Few data and no guidelines exist for bariatric surgery in adolescents. In 1975, Soper and others (1975) reported on 18 morbidly obese adolescents and young adults (age < 20 years) who underwent either gastric bypass or gastroplasty. The median weight loss was approximately 25% of body weight by 3 years following surgery. A similar report in 1980 described an average weight loss of 40 kg at 3 years and 26 kg at 5 years after surgery (Anderson et al., 1980). Major early postoperative complications occurred in more than one third of the patients, including one death from an anastomotic leak. Since these early reports, the gastric bypass procedure has undergone significant modifications. Surgical stapling devices allow compartmentalization of the stomach without complete transection (Kellum et al., 1998). "Long limb" gastric bypass has also been used in patients with BMI of greater than 50, with improved weight loss compared with conventional bypass procedures (Brolin et al., 1992).

Strauss and others (2001) reported their results in 10 adolescents, aged 15 to 17 years, who underwent gastric bypass surgery. All patients were highly motivated and had demonstrated serious attempts at weight loss in diet and behavior modification programs. All adolescents were behaviorly and genetically normal and were more than 100% and 100 pounds above their ideal body weight. Obesity-related morbidities included sleep apnea, hypertension, vertebral fracture, and severe school avoidance. No perioperative complications were reported. Satisfactory weight loss was achieved in 9 of 10 patients, with a mean weight loss of greater than 50 kg. Late complications included protein-calorie and micronutrient malnutrition in one patient, an abdominal wall hernia requiring surgical repair in one patient, cholecystectomy in two patients, and small bowel obstruction requiring surgery in one patient.

Abu-Abeid and others (2003) reported their experience with 11 adolescents, aged 11 to 17 years, who underwent laparoscopic adjustable gastric banding (LAGB). Unlike gastric bypass operations, LAGB involves no anastomoses and no bypass of functional bowel, and the operation is reversible. The authors cited no perioperative or late complications; the mean decrease in BMI was from 46.6 to 32.1 kg/m^2. One patient with heart failure and pulmonary hypertension had significant functional improvement during the 23-month follow-up period.

ANESTHETIC MANAGEMENT

Preoperative Considerations

In preparation for surgery, a thorough history and physical examination should be performed. Review of systems is focused on medical complications of obesity shown in Box 19–6. Medications taken for weight loss and other conditions are noted. Blood pressure and oxygen saturation should be recorded. Airway examination may reveal large tonsils and a small pharyngeal airway. Cardiac and lung auscultation may reveal signs of heart failure, pulmonary hypertension, wheezing, and low lung volumes. An electrocardiogram may show findings of cor pulmonale. An echocardiogram should be considered if cardiac dysfunction is suspected. In association with frequent urination, nocturia, and fatigue, blood glucose values may confirm the diagnosis of diabetes.

Administration of premedication should be followed by monitoring of oxygen saturation as ventilatory depression and airway obstruction may occur. An H_2-receptor antagonist and metoclopramide may be given 60 to 90 minutes prior to anesthetic induction to decrease gastric volume and acidity. A nonparticulate oral antacid may be given immediately prior to induction.

Intraoperative Management

Many obese patients become hypoxemic in the supine position due to upper airway obstruction and diminished FRC. Elevating the head of the operating room table may diminish these changes. Noninvasive blood pressure measurements may be inaccurate, prompting the need for intra-arterial monitoring. Measurement of arterial blood gases at baseline and during general anesthesia is recommended, especially for lengthy surgeries. Because venous access may be limited, placement of a central venous catheter, although technically challenging, may be required. Meticulous attention to positioning and padding of the head, neck, and extremities is essential in order to prevent injury during surgery. Patients must be well secured to the operating room table in anticipation of the use of the Trendelenburg and reverse Trendelenburg positions as well as lateral rotation of the operating room table.

Because the risk of aspiration is high in morbidly obese patients, tracheal intubation should be performed when general anesthesia is administered even for brief procedures. Rapid sequence induction or awake fiberoptic-guided intubation should be performed to minimize the risk of pulmonary aspiration of gastric contents. Although most patients can be intubated with appropriate body positioning and direct laryngoscopy, two anesthesiologists and a "difficult airway" cart should be present during induction and intubation. Preoxygenation should be performed until the oxygen saturation had been 100% for several minutes. Patients should be ventilated with 100% oxygen with 10 to 15 mL/kg tidal volumes based on ideal weight. Moderate levels of positive end-expiratory pressure (PEEP) should be added to minimize airway closure, atelectasis, and oxygen desaturations. High levels of PEEP may depress cardiac output. Hypoxemia may occur due to placement of abdominal packs or retractors, gas insufflation during laparoscopic procedures, and use of the lithotomy or Trendelenburg positions. In extreme cases, the panniculus may need to be mechanically displaced to improve compliance and reduce physiologic shunt during surgery (Wyner et al., 1981).

Drug and fluid administration should be based on ideal body weight. Doses of selected drugs may need to be increased compared with those administered to lean patients, however, due to increases in blood volume and cardiac output in the obese patient (Brodsky and Vierra, 2000). Thiopental and midazolam have increased volumes of distribution in obese patients. Dosing regimens based on ideal body weight for propofol have been recommended (Servin et al., 1993). A nerve stimulator should be used to guide the dosing of muscle relaxants and to monitor complete reversal of their effect. Excessive fat overlying the nerves may render surface electrodes ineffective, and needle electrodes may occasionally be required.

Although technically more difficult in obese patients, regional anesthetic techniques should be considered with or without general anesthesia. Local anesthetics may eliminate the need for muscle relaxants and their reversal. Even when general anesthesia is used in combination with regional anesthesia, decreased concentrations and doses of inhalation and intravenous agents allow for more rapid awakening and spontaneous airway control. Postoperative analgesia with epidural infusions facilitates improved pulmonary function.

Regional blocks can be difficult because important anatomic landmarks are often obscured. Long spinal or epidural needles are needed. The depth of insertion is difficult to predict; BMI alone is not an accurate predictor for depth of the epidural space (Watts, 1993). Accordingly, the incidence of inadvertent dural puncture is increased in obese patients. Morbidly obese patients, however, have a decreased incidence of postdural puncture headache. Because the spread of local anesthetics is directly related to BMI, local anesthetic doses should be reduced by 20% to 25% for both epidural and subarachnoid blocks in obese patients (Pitkanen, 1987; Taivainen et al., 1990). Insulated needles and a nerve stimulator may be helpful in identifying the appropriate nerves for peripheral nerve blocks.

Postoperative Care

Postoperative mechanical ventilation is infrequently needed except in the presence of significant cardiac disease, massive intraoperative fluid resuscitation, sepsis, or airway trauma during intubation. Tracheal extubation in hemodynamically stable, morbidly obese patients should be performed with the upper body elevated 30 to 45 degrees. The patient should be maintained in this position for transport in order to maximize FRC and oxygenation (Vaughan et al., 1976). Supplemental oxygen should be administered via nasal cannula or mask for at least 3 days after abdominal or thoracic procedures (Taylor et al., 1985). Nasal continuous positive airway pressure (N-CPAP) or bilevel positive airway pressure (Bi-PAP) via nasal mask is used for patients with sleep apnea; these modalities may normalize breathing during sleep and prevent nocturnal oxyhemoglobin desaturation (Series et al., 1992; Rennotte et al., 1995). Nasogastric tubes used during surgery must be removed before the application of N-CPAP or Bi-PAP. A potential complication of these therapies is gastric distention and disruption of bowel anastomoses, although this risk appears to be small.

Thromboembolism is a major cause of postoperative morbidity in obese surgical patients. Pulmonary emboli occur in as many as 5% of obese patients following laparotomy (Brodsky and Vierra, 2000). The risk of thromboembolism can be reduced with heparin, pneumatic compression devices, or both (Fasting et al., 1985). If an epidural catheter is to be used, it should be placed prior to initiation of heparin therapy and removed at least 12 hours after the last dose of heparin (Horlocker et al., 2003).

Deep breathing, coughing, and early ambulation must be encouraged, and effective postoperative analgesia is essential. Patient-controlled analgesia with an intravenous opioid or epidural opioid with or without local anesthetic may be used. Analgesic drugs should be dosed according to ideal body weight. Vigilant monitoring for signs of excessive sedation and respiratory depression is required.

■ SUMMARY

The pediatric patient presenting for abdominal, genitourinary, or thoracic surgery spans the pathophysiologic spectrum. Both acute and elective clinical presentations, coupled with age-related nuances of the disease, dictate the perioperative anesthetic care of the patient. Advances in intraoperative techniques and postoperative pain management have enabled the surgical frontiers in those specialties to advance.

REFERENCES

Abu-Abeid S, Gavert N, Klausner JM, Szoid A: Bariatric surgery in adolescence. *J Pediatr Surg* 38:1379, 2003.

Addiss DG, Shaffer N, Fowler BS, Tauxe RV: The epidemiology of appendicitis and appendectomy in the United States. *Am J Epidemiol* 132:910, 1990.

Adelman S, Benson CD: Bochdalek hernias in infants: Factors determining mortality. *J Pediatr Surg* 11:569–573, 1976.

Alexander JI: Pain after laparoscopy. *Br J Anaesth* 79:369–378, 1997.

Allan CY, Jacqueline PA, Shubhda JH: Caudal epidural block versus other methods of postoperative pain relief for circumcision in boys. *Cochrane Database Syst Rev* 2:CD003005, 2003.

Altman RP, Chandra R, Lilly JR: Ongoing cirrhosis after successful porticoenterostomy in infants with biliary atresia. *J Pediatr Surg* 10:685, 1975.

Anderson AE, Soper RT, Scott DH: Gastric bypass for morbid obesity in children and adolescents. *J Pediatr Surg* 15:876, 1980.

Andropoulos DB, Heard MB, Johnson KL, et al.: Postanesthetic apnea in full-term infants after pyloromyotomy. *Anesthesiology* 80:216, 1994.

Angelillo Mackinlay TA, Lyons GA, Chimondeguy DJ, et al.: VATS debridement versus thoracotomy in the treatment of loculated postpneumonia empyema. *Ann Thorac Surg* 61:1626–1630, 1996.

Arndt GA, De Lessio ST, Kranner PW, et al.: One-lung ventilation when intubation is difficult—Presentation of a new endobronchial blocker. *Acta Anaesthesiol Scand* 43:356–358, 1999.

Atlas I, Stone N: Laparoscopy for evaluation of cryptorchid testis. *Pediatr Urol* 40:256, 1992.

Azarow KS, Pearl RH, Zurcher R, et al.: Primary mediastinal masses: A comparison of adult and pediatric populations. *J Thorac Cardiovasc Surg* 106:67–72, 1993.

Azizkhan RG, Dudgeon DL, Colombani PM, et al.: Life-threatening airway obstruction as a complication to the management of mediastinal masses in children. *J Pediatr Surg* 20:816–822, 1985.

Bachland R, Audet J, Meloche R, et al.: Physiologic changes associated with unilateral pulmonary ventilation during operations on the lung. *Can Anaesth Soc J* 22:659, 1975.

Baldeyrou P, Lemoine G, Zucker GM, et al.: Pulmonary metastases in children: The place of surgery. *J Pediatr Surg* 19:121, 1984.

Baraka A, Dajani A, Maktabi M: Selective contralateral bronchial intubation in children with pneumothorax or bronchopleural fistula. *Br J Anaesth* 55:901, 1983.

Baraka A, Slim M, Dajani A, et al.: One-lung ventilation of children during surgical excision of hydatid cysts of the lungs. *Br J Anaesth* 54:23, 1982.

Baraka A: Selective bronchial intubation for one lung ventilation in children. *Middle East J Anesthesiol* 9:9, 1987.

Barash PG, Tsai B, Kitahata LM: Acute tracheal collapse following mediastinoscopy. *Anesthesiology* 44:67, 1976.

Barratt TM, Manzoni GA: The dilated urinary tract. In Holliday MA, Barratt TM, Vernier RL, editors: *Pediatric nephrology.* Baltimore, 1987, Williams & Wilkins.

Barry JE, Auldist AW: The VATER association: One end of a spectrum of anomalies. *Am J Dis Child* 128:769–771, 1974.

Battersby EF, Facer E, Glover WJ, et al.: Ketamine anaesthesia for pyloromyotomy (letter). *Anaesthesia* 39:381, 1984.

Bealer JF, Natuzzi ES, Buscher C, et al.: Nitric oxide synthetase is deficient in the aganglionic: colon of patients with Hirschsprung's disease. *Pediatrics* 93:647, 1994.

Beattie EJ: Surgical treatment of pulmonary metastases. *Cancer* 54:2729, 1984.

Beebe DS, Swica H, Carlson N, et al.: High levels of carbon monoxide arc produced by electro-cautery of tissue during laparoscopic cholecystectomy. *Anesth Analg* 77:338, 1993.

Belman AB: Anomalies of the urinary tract, urethra. In Kelalis PP, King LR, Belman AB, editors: *Clinical pediatric urology*, ed 2. Philadelphia, 1985, WB Saunders.

Benumof JF, Augustine SD, Gibbons JA: Halothane and isoflurane only slightly impair arterial oxygenation during one-lung ventilation in patients undergoing thoracotomy. *Anesthesiology* 67:910–914, 1987.

Benumof JL, Gaughan SD, Ozaki GT: The relationship among bronchial blocker cuff inflation volume, proximal airway pressure, and seal of the bronchial blocker cuff. *J Cardiothorac Vasc Anesth* 6:404–408, 1992.

Benumof JL: Lung separation: a final, final word. *J Cardiothorac Vasc Anesth* 9:618, 1995.

Berthold F, Trechow R, Utsch S, Zieschang J: Prognostic factors in metastatic neuroblastoma. A multivariate analysis of 182 cases. *Am J Pediatr Hematol Oncol* 14:207, 1992.

Birmingham PK, Uejima T, Luck SR: Anesthetic management of the patient with a bronchogenic cyst: A review of 24 cases. *Anesth Analg* 76:879, 1993.

Birmingham PK, Wheeler M, Suresh S, et al.: Patient-controlled epidural analgesia in children: Can they do it? *Anesth Analg* 96: 686–691, 2003.

Bissonnette B, Sullivan PJ: Pyloric stenosis. *Can J Anaesth* 38:668, 1991.

Blaise G, Roy WL: Postoperative pain relief after hypospadias repair in pediatric patients: Regional analgesia versus systemic analgesics. *Anesthesiology* 65:84, 1986.

Bloch EC, Filston HC: A thin fiberoptic bronchoscope as an aid to occlusion of the fistula in infants with tracheoesophageal fistula. *Anesth Analg* 67:791–793, 1988.

Bloch EC: Tracheo-bronchial angles in infants and children. *Anesthesiology* 65:236, 1986.

Bogaert GA, Kogan BA, Mevorach RA: Therapeutic laparoscopy for intra-abdominal testes, *Pediatr Urol* 42:182, 1993.

Borchardt RA, LaQuaglia MP, McDowall, Wilson RS: Bronchial injury during lung isolation in a pediatric patient. *Anesth Analg* 87:324–325, 1998.

Borowitz D, Cerny F, Zallen G, et al.: Pulmonary function and exercise response in patients with pectus excavatum after Nuss repair. *J Pediatr Surg* 38:544–547, 2003.

Bouchut JC, Dubois R, Moussa M, et al.: High frequency oscillatory ventilation during repair of neonatal congenital diaphragmatic hernia. *Paediatr Anaesth* 10:377–379, 2000.

Bourne MC, Wheeldon C, MacKinlay GA, et al.: Laparoscopic Nissen fundoplication in children: 2-5 year follow-up. *Pediatr Surg Int* 19:537–539, 2003.

Bray RJ, Fernandes FJ: Mediastinal tumour causing airway obstruction in anaesthetized children. *Anaesthesia* 37:571, 1982.

Brecher ME, Rosenfeld M: Mathematical and computer modeling of acute normovolemic hemodilution. *Transfusion* 34:176, 1994.

Brodsky JB, Macario A, Mark JBD: Tracheal diameter predicts double-lumen tube size: A method for selecting left double-lumen tubes. *Anesth Analg* 82:861–864, 1996.

Brodsky JB, Mark JBD: A simple technique for accurate placement of double-lumen endobronchial tubes. *Anesth Rev* 10:26–30, 1983.

Brodsky JB, Vierra MA: Anesthetic management of the obese patient. *Adv Anesth* 17:149–171, 2000.

Brolin RE, Kenler HA, Gorman JH, Cody RP: Long-limb gastric bypass in the superobese. *Ann Surg* 215:387, 1992.

Brooks JG, Bustamante SA, Koops BL, et al.: Selective bronchial intubation four the treatment of severe localized pulmonary interstitial emphysema in newborn infants. *J Pediatr* 91:648, 1977.

Buckland RW, Manners JM: Venous air embolism during neurosurgery: A comparison of various methods of detections in man. *Anaesthesia* 31:633, 1976.

Buhain WJ, Brody JS: Compensatory growth of the lung following pneumonectomy. *J Appl Physiol* 35:898, 1973.

Bunegin L, Albin MS, Hesel PE, et al.: Positioning the right atrial catheter: A model for reappraisal. *Anesthesiology* 55:343, 1981.

Campbell BT, McLean K, Barnhart DC, et al.: A comparison of laparoscopic and open pyloromyotomy at a teaching hospital. *J Pediatr Surg* 37:1068, 2002.

Campbell DN, Lilly JR: The changing spectrum of pulmonary operations in infants and children. *J Thorac Cardiovasc Surg* 83:680, 1983.

Canestrelli M, Canni M, Mori R, et al.: The new techniques of gynaecologic laparoscopy: Gasless, open Hanson, optic trocar. *Panminerva Med* 41: 371–377, 1999.

Caudle CL, Freid EB, Bailey AG: Epidural fentanyl infusion with patient-controlled epidural analgesia for postoperative analgesia in children. *J Pediatr Surg* 28:554–558, 1993.

Canty TG, Collins D, Losasso B, et al.: Laparoscopic appendectomy for simple and perforated appendicitis in children: The procedure of choice? *J Pediatr Surg* 35:1582–1585, 2000.

Cassady JF Jr, Lederhaas G, Cancel DD, et al.: A randomized comparison of the effects of continuous thoracic epidural analgesia and intravenous patient-controlled analgesia after posterior spinal fusion in adolescents. *Reg Anesth Pain Med* 25:246–253, 2000.

Caudle CL, Freid EB, Bailey AG, et al.: Epidural fentanyl infusion with patient-controlled epidural analgesia for postoperative analgesia in children. *J Pediatr Surg* 28:554, 1993.

Cay DL, Csenderits LE, Lines V, et al.: Selective bronchial blocking in children. *Anaesth Intensive Care* 3:117, 1975.

Centers for Disease Control and Prevention Update: Prevalence of obesity among children, adolescents, and adults—United States, 1988–1994. *MMWR Morb Mortal Wkly Rep* 46:199, 1997.

Chipps BE, Moynihan R, Schieble T, et al.: Infants undergoing pyloromyotomy are not at risk for postoperative apnea. Staff of Sutter Community Hospital Sleep Disorders Center. *Pediatr Pulmonol* 27:278–81, 1999.

Clain DJ, Lefkowitch JH: Fatty liver disease in morbid obesity. *Gastroenterol Clin North Am* 16:239, 1987.

Clark RH, Hardin WD Jr, Hirschl RB: Current surgical management of congenital diaphragmatic hernia: A report from the Congenital Diaphragmatic Hernia Study Group. *J Pediatr Surg* 33:1004–1009, 1998.

Colbert ST, Moran K, O Hanlon DM, et al.: An assessment of the value of intraperitoneal meperidine for analgesia postlaparoscopic tubal ligation. *Anesth Analg* 91:667–670, 2000.

Conlan AA, Moyes DG, Schutz J, et al.: Pulmonary resection in the prone position for suppurative lung disease in children. *J Thorac Cardiovasc Surg* 92:890, 1986.

Consensus Development Conference Panel: Gastrointestinal surgery for severe obesity. *Ann Intern Med* 115:956, 1991.

Conway EE Jr: Central nervous system findings and intussusception: How are they related? *Pediatr Emerg Care* 9:15, 1993.

Cook-Sather SD, Tulloch HV, Liacouras CA, Schreiner MS: Gastric fluid volume in infants for pyloromyotomy. *Can J Anaesth* 44:278, 1997.

Coté CJ: The anesthetic management of congenital lobar emphysema. *Anesthesiology* 49:296, 1997.

Cullum AR, English CW, Branthwaite MA: Endobronchial intubation in infancy. *Anaesthesia* 28:66–70, 1973.

Cumming WA: Esophageal atresia and tracheoesophageal fistula. *Radiol Clin North Am* 13:277–295, 1975.

Cunningham AJ, Brull SJ: Laparoscopic cholecystectomy: Anesthetic implications. *Anesth Analg* 76:1120, 1993.

Cushing H: Some experimental and clinical observations concerning states of increased intracranial tension. *Am J Med Sci* 124:375, 1902.

Danelli G, Berti M, Perotti V, et al.: Temperature control and recovery of bowel function after laparoscopic or laparotomic colorectal surgery in patients receiving combined epidural/general anesthesia and postoperative epidural anesthesia. *Anesth Analg* 95:467–471, 2002.

Danielson PD, Shaul DB, Phillips JD, et al.: Technical advances in pediatric laparoscopy have a beneficial impact on splenectomy. *J Pediatr Surg* 35: 1578–1581, 2000.

Darbari A, Sabin KM, Shapiro CN, et al.: Epidemiology of primary hepatic malignancies in U.S. children. *Hepatology* 38:560–565, 2003.

Davis PJ, Galinkin J, McGowan FX, et al.: A randomized multicenter study of remifentanil compared with halothane in neonates and infants undergoing pyloromyotomy. I. Emergence and recovery profiles. *Anesth Analg* 93: 1380–1386, 2001.

Dawes GS: *Fetal and neonatal physiology.* Chicago, 1973, Year Book Medical.

Dehner LP: Hepatic tumors in the pediatric age group: A distinctive clinicopathologic spectrum. *Perspect Pediatr Pathol* 4:217, 1978.

De Lagausie P, Berrebi D, Michon P, et al.: Laparoscopic adrenal surgery for neuroblastomas in children. *J Urol* 170:932–935, 2003.

Dierdorf ST, Krishna G: Anesthetic management of neonatal surgical emergencies. *Anesth Analg* 60:204, 1981.

Divatia JV, Vaidya JS, Badwe RA, Hawaldar RW: Omission of nitrous oxide during anesthesia reduces the incidence of postoperative nausea and vomiting. *Anesthesiology* 85:1055–1062, 1996.

Donnelly LF, Sakurai M, Klosterman LA: Correlation between findings on chest radiography and survival in neonates with congenital diaphragmatic hernia. *AJR Am J Roentgenol* 173:1589–1593, 1999.

Driessen JJ, Robertson EN, Egmond JV, Booij LHDJ: Time-course of action of rocuronium 0.3 mg/kg in children with and without endstage renal failure. *Paediatr Anaesth* 12:507–510, 2002.

Dubé S, Dubé P, Hardy JF, Rosenfeld RE: Pyloromyotomy of Ramstedt: Experience of a nonspecialized centre. *Can Assoc Clin Surg* 33:95, 1990.

Eckschlager T: Lymphocyte count as a prognostic factor in childhood cancer. *Pediatr Hematol Oncol* 9:99, 1992.

Eger EL 2nd, Saidman LJ: Hazards of nitrous oxide anesthesia in bowel obstruction and pneumothorax. *Anesthesiology* 26:61, 1965.

Eigen J, Lemon RJ, Waring WW: Congenital lobar emphysema: Long term evaluation of surgically and conservatively treated children. *Am Rev Respir Dis* 113:823, 1976.

Elhalaby EA, Hashish A, Elbarbary MM, et al.: Transanal one-stage endorectal pull-through for Hirschsprung's disease: a multicenter study. *J Pediatr Surg* 39:345–351, 2004.

Esposito C, Gonzalez Sabin MA, Corcione F, et al.: Results and complications of laparoscopic cholecystectomy in childhood. *Surg Endosc* 15:890–892, 2001.

Esposito C, Montupet P, Amici G, Desruelle P: Complications of laparoscopic antireflux surgery in childhood. *Surg Endosc* 14:622–624, 2000.

Esposito C, Van Der Zee DC, Settimi A, et al.: Risks and benefits of surgical management of gastroesophageal reflux in neurologically impaired children. *Surg Endosc* 17:708–710, 2003.

Fasting H, Andersen K, Kraemmer Nielsen H, et al.: Prevention of postoperative deep venous thrombosis: Low-dose heparin versus graded pressure stockings. *Acta Chir Scand* 151:245, 1985.

Feusner J, Buckley JD, Robinson L, et al.: Prematurity and hepatoblastoma: more than just an association? *J Pediatr* 133:585–586, 1998.

Ferrari LR, Bedford RF: General anesthesia prior to treatment of anterior mediastinal masses in pediatric cancer patients. *Anesthesiology* 72:991, 1990.

Filston HC, Chitwood WR Jr, Schkolne B, et al.: The Fogarty balloon catheter as an aid to management of the infant with esophageal atresia and tracheoesophageal fistula complicated by severe RDS or pneumonia. *J Pediatr Surg* 17:149–151, 1982.

Fisher DM: When is the ex-premature infant no longer at risk for apnea? (editorial) *Anesthesiology* 82:807, 1995.

Flake AW, Shopene C, Ziegler MM: Anti-reflux gastrointestinal surgery in the neurologically handicapped child. *J Pediatr Surg* 6:92, 1991.

Forbes AR, Cohen WH, Eger EI II: Pancuronium reduces halothane requirement in man. *Anesth Analg* 58:497, 1977.

Fortuna RS, Weber TR, Tracy TF Jr., et al.: Critical analysis of the operative treatment of Hirschsprung's disease. *Arch Surg* 131:520–524, 1996.

Franken EA Jr, Smith JA, Smith WL: Tumors of the chest wall in infants and children. *Pediatr Radiol* 6:13–18, 1977.

Frenckner B, Ehren H, Granholm T: Improved results in patients who have congenital diaphragmatic hernia using preoperative stabilization, extracorporeal membrane oxygenation, and delayed surgery. *J Pediatr Surg* 32:1185–1189, 1997.

Galinkin JL, Davis PJ, McGowan FX, et al.: A randomized multicenter study of remifentanil compared with halothane in neonates and infants undergoing pyloromyotomy. II. Perioperative breathing patterns in neonates and infants with pyloric stenosis. *Anesth Analg* 93:1387–1392, 2001.

Gayes JM: The Univent tube is the best technique for providing one-lung ventilation. Pro: One-lung ventilation is best accomplished with the Univent endotracheal tube. *J Cardiothorac Vasc Anesth* 7:103–105, 1993.

Geary MP, Chitty LS, Morrison JJ: Perinatal outcome and prognostic factors in prenatally diagnosed congenital diaphragmatic hernia. *Ultrasound Obstet Gynecol* 12:107–1011, 1998.

Geiser CF, Baez A, Schindler AM, Shik VE: Epithelial hepatoblastoma associated with congenital hemihypertrophy and cystathionuria. *Pediatrics* 46:66, 1970.

Gelman S, Fowler KC, Smith LR: Liver circulation and function during isoflurane and halothane anesthesia. *Anesthesiology* 61:726, 1984.

Georgeson KE: Laparoscopic gastrostomy and fundoplication. *Paediatr Ann* 92:675–677, 1993.

Georgeson KE, Cohen RD, Hebra A, et al.: Primary laparoscopic-assisted endorectal colon pull-through for Hirschsprung's disease: A new gold standard. *Ann Surg* 229:678, 1999.

Georgeson KE, Inge TH, Albanese CT: Laparoscopically assisted anorectal pull-through for high imperforate anus: A new technique. *J Pediatr Surg* 35:927, 2000.

Georgeson KE: Laparoscopic-assisted pull-through for Hirschsprung's disease *Semin Pediatr Surg* 11:205, 2002.

Gilchrist BF, Lobe TE, Schropp KP, et al.: Is there a role for laparoscopic appendectomy in pediatric surgery? *J Pediatr Surg* 27:209, 1992.

Ginsberg RJ: New technique for one-lung anesthesia using a bronchial blocker. *J Thorac Cardiovasc Surg* 82:542–546, 1981.

Goto H, Boozalis ST, Benson KT, et al.: High-frequency jet ventilation for resection of congenital lobar emphysema. *Anesth Analg* 66:684, 1987.

Grant DM, Thompson GE: Diagnosis of congenital tracheoesophageal fistula in the adolescent and adult. *Anesthesiology* 49:139–140, 1978.

Grundmann U, Silomon M, Bach F, et al.: Recovery profile and side effects of remifentanil-based anaesthesia with desflurane or propofol for laparoscopic cholecystectomy. *Acta Anaesthesiol Scand* 45:320–326, 2001.

Guyton AC: *Textbook of medical physiology,* 7th ed. Philadelphia, 1985, WB Saunders.

Guyton DC, Besselievre TR, Devidas M, et al.: A comparison of two different bronchial cuff designs and four different bronchial cuff inflation methods. *J Cardiothorac Vasc Anesth* 11:599–603, 1997.

Haase GM, Perez C, Atkinson JB: Current aspects of biology, risk assessment, and treatment of neuroblastoma. *Semin Surg Oncol.* 16:91–104, 1999.

Haberkern CM, Coles PG, Morray JP, et al.: Intraoperative hypertension during surgical excision of neuroblastoma. Case report and review of 20 years' experience. *Anesth Analg* 75:854, 1992.

Haberkern M, Dangel P: Normovolemic haemodilution and intraoperative autotransfusion in children: Experience with 30 cases of spinal fusion. *Eur J Pediatr Surg* 1:30, 1991.

Hagen J, Deitel M, Khanna RK, et al.: Gastroesophageal reflux in the massively obese. *Int Surg* 72:1, 1987.

Hammer GB, Brodsky JB, Redpath J, Cannon WB: The Univent tube for single lung ventilation in children. *Paediatr Anaesth* 8:55–57, 1998.

Hammer GB, Harrison TK, Vricella LA, et al.: Single lung ventilation using a new pediatric bronchial blocker. *Paediatr Anaesth* 12:69, 2002.

Hammer GB, Lammers CR: Pediatric otolaryngology. In Jaffe RA, Samuels SI, editors: *Anesthesiologist's manual of surgical procedures.* Philadelphia, 1999, Lippincott Williams & Wilkins, pp 872–875.

Hammer GB, Manos SJ, Smith BM, et al.: Single lung ventilation in pediatric patients. *Anesthesiology* 84:1503–1506, 1996.

Hammer GB: Pediatric thoracic anesthesia. *Anesthesiol Clin North Am* 20:153–180, 2002.

Hannallah RS, Broadman LM, Belman AB, et al.: Comparison of caudal and ilioinguinal/iliohypogastric nerve blocks for control of postorchiopexy pain in pediatric ambulatory surgery. *Anesthesiology* 66:832, 1987.

Harnick E, Kulezycki L, Gomes MN: Transcutaneous oxygen monitoring during bronchoscopy and washout for cystic fibrosis. *Anesth Analg* 62:357, 1983.

Harnik EV, Hoy GR, Potolicchio S, et al.: Spinal anesthesia in premature infants recovering from respiratory distress syndrome. *Anesthesiology* 64:95, 1986.

Harrison MR, Bjordal RI, Langmark F, et al.: Congenital diaphragmatic hernia: The hidden mortality. *J Pediatr Surg* 13:227–230, 1978.

Harter RL, Kelly WB, Kramer MG, et al.: A comparison of the volume and pH of gastric contents of lean and obese patients. *Anesth Analg* 86:147–152, 1998.

Hashikura Y, Kawasaki S, Munakata Y, et al.: Effects of peritoneal insufflation on hepatic and renal blood flow. *Surg Endosc* 8:759–761, 1994.

Hay SA, Kabesh AA, Soliman HA, Abdelrahman AH: Idiopathic intussusception: The role of laparoscopy. *J Pediatr Surg* 34:577, 1999.

Hay SA, Soliman HE, Sherif HM, et al.: Neonatal jaundice: The role of laparoscopy. *J Pediatr Surg* 35:1706–1709, 2000.

Heaf DP, Helms P, Gordon MB, Turner HM: Postural effects on gas exchange in infants. *N Engl J Med* 28:1505–1508, 1983.

Hebra A, Swoveland B, Egbert M, et al.: Outcome analysis of minimally invasive repair of pectus excavatum: Review of 251 cases. *J Pediatr Surg* 35:252–257, 2000.

Heiss KF, Shandling B: Laparoscopy for the impalpable testes: Experience with 53 testes. *J Pediatr Surg* 27:175, 1992.

Henderson AM, Vallis CJ, Summer E: Anaesthesia in the prune-belly syndrome, a review of 36 cases. *Anaesthesia* 42:54, 1987.

Hinman F Jr: Management of the intra-abdominal testis. *Eur J Pediatr* 146(suppl 2):549–550, 1987.

Hirvonen EA, Nuutinen LS, Kauko M: Hemodynamic changes due to Trendelenburg positioning and pneumoperitoneum during laparoscopic hysterectomy. *Acta Anaesthesiol Scand* 39:949–955, 1995.

Hirvonen EA, Poikolainen EO, Pääkkönen ME, Nuutinen LS: The adverse hemodynamic effects of anesthesia, head-up tilt, and carbon dioxide pneumoperitoneum during laparoscopic cholecystectomy. *Surg Endosc* 14:272–277, 2000.

Hiyama E, Hiyama K, Yokoyama T, Ishii T: Immunohistochemical analysis of N-myc protein expression in neuroblastoma. Correlation with prognosis of patients. *J Pediatr Surg* 26:838, 1991.

Hogg CE, Lorhan PH: Pediatric bronchial blocking. *Anesthesiology* 33:560, 1970.

Holder TM, Ashcraft KW, Sharp RJ, et al.: Care of infants with esophageal atresia, tracheoesophageal fistula, and associated anomalies. *J Thorac Cardiovasc Surg* 94:828–835, 1987.

Holliday MA, Pinckert TL, Kiernan SC, et al.: Dorsal penile nerve block vs topical placebo for circumcision in low-birth-weight neonates. *Arch Pediatr Adolesc Med* 153:476–480, 1999.

Horlocker TT, Abel MD, Messick JM Jr, et al.: Small risk of serious neurologic complications related to lumbar epidural catheter placement in anesthetized patients. *Anesth Analg* 96:1547–1552, 2003.

Horlocker TT, Wedel DJ, Benzon H, et al.: Regional anesthesia in the anticoagulated patient: Defining the risks (the second ASRA Consensus Conference on Neuraxial Anesthesia and Anticoagulation). *Reg Anesth Pain Med* 28:172, 2003.

Hosie S, Sitkiewicz T, Petersen C, et al.: Minimally invasive repair of pectus excavatum-the Nuss procedure. A European multicenter experience. *Eur J Pediatr Surg* 12:235, 2002.

Howard CR, Howard FM, Garfunkel LC, et al.: Neonatal circumcision and pain relief: current training practices. *Pediatrics* 101:423–428, 1998.

Hoymork SC, Raeder J, Brimsmo B, Steen PA: Bispectral index, serum drug concentrations and emergence associated with individually adjusted target-controlled infusions of remifentanil and propofol for laparoscopic surgery. *Br J Anaesth* 91:773, 2003.

Huettemann E, Sakka SG, Petrat G, et al.: Left ventricular regional wall motion abnormalities during pneumoperitoneum in children. *Br J Anaesth* 90:733–736, 2003.

Humphreys GH, Hogg BM, Ferrer J: Congenital atresia of the esophagus. *J Thorac Surg* 32:332–348, 1956.

Hunter JG: Advanced laparoscopic surgery. *Am J Surg* 173:14–18, 1997.

Hunter JM, Jones RS, Utting JE: Comparison of vecuronium, atracurium and tubocurarine in normal patients and in patients with no renal function. *Br J Anaesth* 56:941–950, 1984.

Hutchison IF, Olayiwola B, Young DG: Intussusception in infancy and childhood. *Br J Surg* 67:209, 1980.

Ikeda H, Matsuyama S, Tanimura M: Association between hepatoblastoma and very low birth weight: a trend or a chance? *J Pediatr* 130:557–560, 1997.

Imoke E, Dudgeon DL, Colombani P, et al.: Open lung biopsy in the immunocompromised pediatric patient. *J Pediatr Surg* 18:816, 1983.

Ishizuka B, Kudo Y, Amemiya A, et al.: Plasma catecholamine responses during laparoscopic gynecologic surgery with CO2 insufflation. *J Am Assoc Gynecol Laparosc* 7:37–43, 2000.

Ivy DD, Ziegler JW, Kinsella JP, et al.: Dipyridamole attenuates rebound pulmonary hypertension after inhaled nitric oxide withdrawal in postoperative congenital heart disease. *J Thorac Cardiovasc Surg* 115:875–882, 1998.

Jensen AG, Prevedoros H, Kullman E, et al.: Preoperative nitrous oxide does not influence recovery after laparoscopic cholecystectomy. *Acta Anaesthesiol Scand* 37:683–686, 1993.

Jona JZ, Cohen RD, Georgeson KE, Rothenberg SS: Laparoscopic pull-through procedure for Hirschsprung's disease. *Semin Pediatr Surg* 7:228, 1998.

Jones DR, Graeber GM, Tanguilig GG, et al.: Effects of insufflation on hemodynamics during thoracoscopy. *Ann Thorac Surg* 55:1379, 1993.

Jones DW: Body weight and blood pressure: Effects of weight reduction on hypertension. *Am J Hypertens* 9:50S, 1996.

Jones E: Primary carcinoma of the liver with associated cirrhosis in infants and children. Report of a case. *Arch Pathol* 75:5, 1960.

Jones KL: *Smith's recognizable patterns of malformation*, 4th ed. Philadelphia, 1988, WB Saunders.

Kaapa P, Koivisto M, Ylikorlaka O, Kouvalainen K: Prostacyclin in the treatment of neonatal pulmonary hypertension. *J Pediatr* 107:951–953, 1985.

Kamaya H, Krishna PR: New endotracheal tube (Univent tube) for selective blockade of one lung. *Anesthesiology* 63:342–323, 1985.

Kasai M, Mochizuki I, Ohkohchi N, et al.: Surgical limitation for biliary atresia: Indication for liver transplantation. *J Pediatr Surg* 24:851, 1989.

Kasai M, Watanabe I, Ohi R: Follow-up studies of long-term survivors after hepatic portoenterostomy for "noncorrectable" biliary atresia. *J Pediatr Surg* 10:173, 1975.

Kasai M: Treatment of biliary atresia with special reference to hepatic portoenterostomy and its modifications. *Prog Pediatr Surg* 6:519, 1974.

Kasai T, Yaegashi K, Hirose M, Tanaka Y: Spinal cord injury in a child caused by an accidental dural puncture with a single-shot thoracic epidural needle. *Anesth Analg* 96:65–67, 2003.

Kato J, Ogawa S, Katz J, et al.: Effects of presurgical local infiltration of bupivacaine in the surgical field on postsurgical wound pain in laparoscopic gynecologic examinations: A possible preemptive analgesic effect. *Clin J Pain* 16:12–17, 2000.

Kelley JG, Gaba DM, Brodsky JB: Bronchial cuff pressures of two tubes used in thoracic surgery. *J Cardiothorac Vasc Anesth* 6:190–194, 1992.

Kellum JM, DeMaria EJ, Sugarman HJ: The surgical treatment of morbid obesity. *Curr Probl Surg* 35:795, 1998.

Keon TP: Death on induction of anesthesia for cervical node biopsy. *Anesthesiology* 55:471, 1981.

Khoo ST: Anaesthesia for fiberoptic bronchoscopy in children. *Anaesthesia* 45:248–249, 1990.

Kiliç A, Basgül E, Özdemir A, Erdem MK: The efficacy of intraperitoneal bupivacaine application on early postoperative pain and blood gas values after laparoscopic cholecystectomy. *Agri Dergisi* 8:20–26, 1996.

Klauber GT, Sant GR: Disorders of the male external genitalia. In Kelalis PP, King LR, Belman AB, editors: *Clinical pediatric urology*, 2nd ed. Philadelphia, 1985, WB Saunders.

Komadina R, Smrkolj V: Intussusception after blunt abdominal trauma. *J Trauma* 45:615, 1998.

Kravitz RM: Congenital malformations of the lung. *Pediatr Clin North Am* 41:453–472, 1994.

Kubota H, Kubota Y, Toshiro T, et al: Selective blind endobronchial intubation in children and adults. *Anesthesiology* 67:587–589, 1987.

Kubota Y, Toyoda Y, Nagata N, et al.: Tracheo-bronchial angles in infants and children. *Anesthesiology* 64:374, 1986.

Kuczmarski RJ, Ogden CL, Grummer-Strawn LM, et al.: *CDC growth charts: United States. Advance data from vital and health statistics.* Washington, DC, 2000, National Center for Health Statistics, 2000. Publication No. 314.

Kuster G, Gilroy S: The role of laparoscopy in the diagnosis of acute appendicitis. *Am J Surg* 58:627, 1992.

Laborde F, Noirhomme P, Karam J, et al.: A new video-assisted thoracoscopic surgical technique for interruption of patent ductus arteriosus in infants and children. *J Thorac Cardiovasc Surg* 102:279, 1993.

Lamberty JM, Rubin BK: The management of anaesthesia for patients with cystic fibrosis. *Anaesthesia* 40:448, 1985.

Lammers CR, Hammer GB, Brodsky JB, Cannon WB: Failure to isolate the lungs with an endotracheal tube positioned in the bronchus. *Anesth Analg* 85:946, 1997.

Landsman IS, Gronert BJ, Wiener ES, Ford HR: Fluoroscopy as an aid to anesthetic management for bronchogenic cyst resection. *Anesth Analg* 79:803, 1994.

Larsson A, Jonmarker C, Jogi P, et al.: Ventilatory consequences of the lateral position and thoracotomy in children. *Can J Anaesth* 43:141, 1987.

Laurent J, Gauthier F, Bernard O, et al.: Long-term outcome after surgery for biliary atresia. Study of 40 patients surviving for more than 10 years. *Gastroenterology* 99:1793, 1990.

Lawson ML, Cash TF, Akers R, et al.: A pilot study of the impact of surgical repair on disease-specific quality of life among patients with pectus excavatum. *J Pediatr Surg* 38:916, 2003.

Leape LL, Longino LA: Infantile lobar emphysema. *Pediatrics* 34:246, 1964.

Lee Y, Liang J: Experience with 450 cases of micro-laparoscopic herniotomy in infants and children. *Pediatr Endosurg Innov Techn* 6:25–28, 2002.

Lee BY, Thoden WR, McCann WJ Jr, et al.: Intraoperative anticoagulation during arterial reconstructive procedures. *Surg Gynecol Obstet* 155:809, 1982.

Lester LA, Egge A, Hubbard VS, et al.: Aspiration and lung abscess in cystic fibrosis. *Am Rev Respir Dis* 127:786, 1983.

Leventhal BG: Neoplasms and neoplasm-like structures. In *Nelson's textbook of pediatrics*. Philadelphia, 1987, WB Saunders.

Leveque C, Hamza J, Berg AE, et al.: Successful repair of a severe left congenital diaphragmatic hernia during continuous inhalation of nitric oxide. *Anesthesiology* 1994; 80:1171–1175.

Levin H, Bursztein S, Heifetz M: Cardiac arrest in a child with an anterior mediastinal mass. *Anesth Analg* 64:1129, 1985.

Levy M, Gick B, Springer C, et al.: Bronchoscopy and bronchography in children. *Am J Dis Child* 137:14, 1983.

Lewiston NJ: Bronchiectasis in childhood. *Pediatr Clin North Am* 31:865, 1984.

Lilly JR, Chandra RS: Surgical hazards of co-existing anomalies in biliary atresia. *Surg Gynecol Obstet* 139:49, 1974.

Lin YC, Hackel A: Paediatric selective bronchial blocker. *Paediatr Anaesth* 4:391–392, 1994.

Lincoln JC, Stark J, Subramanian S, et al.: Congenital lobar emphysema. *Ann Surg* 173:55–62, 1971.

Linke F, Eble F, Berger S: Postoperative intussusception in children. *Pediatr Surg Int* 14:175, 1998.

Lintula H, Kokki H, Vanamo K: Single-blinded randomized clinical trial of laparoscopic versus open appendicectomy in children. *Br J Surg* 88:510–514, 2001.

Lobe TE, Schropp KP: Inguinal hernias in pediatrics: Initial experience with laparoscopic inguinal exploration of the asymptomatic contralateral side. *J Laparoendosc Surg* 2:135–140, 1992.

Lonie DS, Harper NJN: Nitrous oxide, anaesthesia and vomiting: The effect of nitrous oxide anaesthesia on the incidence of vomiting following gynaecological laparoscopy. *Anaesthesia* 41:703, 1986.

Losek JD: Intussusception: Don't miss the diagnosis! *Pediatr Emerg Care* 9:46, 1993.

Louik C, Werler MM, Mitchell AA: Erythromycin use during pregnancy in relation to pyloric stenosis. *Am J Obstet Gynecol* 186:288, 2002.

Lu PP, Brimacombe J, Yang C, et al.: ProSeal versus the Classic laryngeal mask airway for positive pressure ventilation during laparoscopic cholecystectomy. *Br J Anaesth* 88:824–827, 2002.

Lukban JC, Jaeger J, Hammond KC, et al.: Gasless versus conventional laparoscopy. *N J Med* 97:29–34, 2000.

MacDonald NJ, Fitzpatrick GJ, Moore KP, et al.: Anaesthesia for congenital hypertrophic pyloric stenosis. *Br J Anaesth* 59:672, 1987.

Mackie AM, Watson CB: Anesthetic management of mediastinal masses. *Anesth Analg* 63:698, 1984.

Malek MH, Fonkalsrud EW, Cooper CB: Ventilatory and cardiovascular responses to exercise in patients with pectus excavatum. *Chest* 124:870–882, 2003.

Maltby JR, Beriault MT, Watson NC, et al.: Gastric distension and ventilation during laparoscopic cholecystectomy: LMA-Classic vs. tracheal intubation. *Can J Anaesth* 47:622–626, 2000.

Maltby JR, Beriault MT, Watson NC, et al.: The LMA-ProSeal is an effective alternative to tracheal intubation for laparoscopic cholecystectomy. *Can J Anaesth* 49:857–862, 2002.

Mansell A, Bryan C, Levison H: Airway closure in children. *J Appl Physiol* 33:711–714, 1972.

Marco AP, Yeo CJ, Rock P: Anesthesia for a patient undergoing laparoscopic cholecystectomy. *Anesthesiology* 73:1268, 1990.

Mariani G, Barefield ES, Carlo WA: The role of nitric oxide in the treatment of neonatal pulmonary hypertension. *Curr Opin Pediatr* 8:118–125, 1996.

Markham SJ, Tomlinson J, Hain WR: Ilioinguinal nerve block in children, a comparison with caudal block for intra- and postoperative analgesia. *Anaesthesia* 41:1098, 1986.

Marraro G: Selective bronchial intubation in paediatrics: The Marraro paediatric bilumen tube. *Paediatr Anaesth* 4:255–258, 1994.

Martin LVH: Postoperative analgesia after circumcision in children. *Br J Anaesth* 54:1263, 1982.

Martin TM, Nicholson SC, Bargas MS: Propofol anesthesia reduces emesis and airway obstruction in pediatric outpatients. *Anesth Analg* 76:144, 1993.

Martinez DA, Ginn-Pease ME, Caniano DA: Sequelae of antireflux surgery in profoundly disabled children. *J Pediatr Surg* 27:267, 1992.

Maxwell LG, Yaster M, Wetzel RC, Niebyl JR: Penile nerve block for newborn circumcision. *Obstet Gynecol* 70:415, 1987.

McAnena OJ, Austin O, O'Connell PR, et al.: Laparoscope versus open appendectomy: A prospective evaluation. *Br J Surg* 79:818, 1992.

McBride J, Wohi ME, Strieder DJ, et al.: Lung growth and airway function after lobectomy for congenital lobar emphysema. *J Clin Invest* 66:962, 1980.

McBride WJ, Dicker R, Abajian JC, Vane DW: Continuous thoracic epidural infusions for postoperative analgesia after pectus deformity repair. *J Pediatr Surg* 31:105–107, 1996.

McLellan I. Endobronchial intubation in children. *Anaesthesia* 29:757–758, 1974.

Meguerditchian AN, Prasil P, Cloutier R, et al.: Laparoscopic appendectomy in children: A favorable alternative in simple and complicated appendicitis. *J Pediatr Surg* 37:695–698, 2002.

Michenfelder JD, Miller RH, Gronect GA: Evaluation of an ultrasonic device (Doppler) for the diagnosis of venous air embolism. *Anesthesiology* 36:164, 1972.

Miguet D, Claris O, Lapillonne A, et al.: Preoperative stabilization using high-frequency oscillatory ventilation in the management of congenital diaphragmatic hernia. *Crit Care Med* 22:S77–S82, 1994.

Mikami O, Fujise K, Matsumoto S, et al.: High intra-abdominal pressure increases plasma catecholamine concentrations during pneumoperitoneum for laparoscopic procedures. *Arch Surg* 133:39–43, 1998.

Miller KA, Woods RK, Sharp RJ, et al.: Minimally invasive repair of pectus excavatum: A single institution's experience. *Surgery* 130:652–657, 2001.

Miller RD, Brzica SM Jr: Blood, blood components, colloids, and autotransfusion therapy. In Miller RD, editor: *Anesthesia*, 2nd ed. New York, 1986, Churchill Livingstone.

Miller RD, Robbins TO, Tong MJ, et al.: Coagulation defects associated with massive blood transfusions. *Ann Surg* 174:794, 1971.

Moiniche S, Jorgensen H, Wetterslev J, Dahl JB: Local anesthetic infiltration for postoperative pain relief after laparoscopy: A qualitative and quantitative systematic review of intraperitoneal, port-site infiltration and mesosalpinx block. *Anesth Analg* 90:899–912, 2000.

Molik KA, Engum SA, Rescorla FJ, et al.: Pectus excavatum repair: Experience with standard and minimal invasive techniques. *J Pediatr Surg* 36:324–328, 2001.

Moss AJ: The cardiovascular system in cystic fibrosis. *Pediatrics* 70:728, 1982.

Moss RL, Albanese CT, Reynolds M: Major complications after minimally invasive repair of pectus excavatum: Case reports. *J Pediatr Surg* 36:155–158, 2001.

Motamed C, Bouaziz H, Franco D, Benhamou D: Analgesic effect of low-dose intrathecal morphine and bupivacaine in laparoscopic cholecystectomy. *Anaesthesia* 55:118–124, 2000.

Motoyama EK, Hen J, Tamas L, Dolan TF: Spirometry with positive airway pressure: A simple method to evaluate obstructive lung disease in children. *Am Rev Respir Dis* 126:766, 1982.

Mouroux J, Clary-Meinesz C, Padovani B, et al.: Efficacy and safety of video-thoracoscopic lung biopsy in the diagnosis of interstitial lung disease. *Eur J Cardiothorac Surg* 11:22–26, 1997.

Muir JJ, Warner MA, Offord KP, et al.: Role of nitrous oxide and other factors in postoperative nausea and vomiting: A randomized and blinded prospective study. *Anesthesiology* 66:513, 1987.

Mulder DS: Pain management principles and anesthesia techniques for thoracoscopy. *Ann Thorac Surg* 56:630, 1993.

Murakami T, Ohmori H, Katoh T, et al.: Differences of L-myc polymorphic patterns of neuroblastoma in patients under 1 year versus older ages: A preliminary report. *J Pediatr Surg* 27:1442, 1992.

Murray GF: Congenital lobar emphysema. *Surg Gynecol Obstet* 124:611, 1967.

Murtagh K, Perry P, Corlett M, Eraser I: Infantile hypertrophic pyloric stenosis. *Dig Dis* 10:190, 1992.

Mychaliska GB, Bullard KM, Harrison MR: In utero management of congenital diaphragmatic hernia. *Clin Perinatol* 23:823–841, 1996.

National Institutes of Health: Clinical guidelines on the identification, evaluation, and treatment of overweight and obesity in adults. *Obes Res* 6(suppl 2):51S, 1998.

Neuman GG, Sidebotham G, Negoianu E, et al.: Laparoscopy explosion hazards with nitrous oxide. *Anesthesiology* 78:875, 1993.

Neuman GG, Weingarten AE, Abramowitz RM, et al.: The anesthetic management of the patient with an anterior mediastinal mass. *Anesthesiology* 60:144, 1984.

Nichols DC, Yaster Y, Lynn AM, et al.: Disposition and respiratory effects of intrathecal morphine in children. *Anesthesiology* 79:733, 1993.

Nishibayashi SW, Andrassy RJ, Wooley MM: Congenital cystic adenomatoid malformation: A 30 year experience. *J Pediatr Surg* 16:704, 1981.

Nonoyama A, Tanaka K, Osako T, et al.: Surgical treatment of pulmonary abscess in children under 10 years of age. *Chest* 85:358, 1984.

Northrip DR, Bowman KB, Tsueda K: Total airway occlusion and superior vena cava syndrome in a child with an anterior mediastinal tumor. *Anesth Analg* 65:1079, 1986.

Nuss D, Croitoru DP, Kelly RE Jr, et al.: Review and discussion of the complications of minimally invasive pectus excavatum repair. *Eur J Pediatr Surg* 12:230–234, 2002.

Nuss D, Kelly RE, Croitoru DP, Katz ME: A 10-year review of a minimally invasive technique for the correction of pectus excavatum. *J Pediatr Surg* 33:545, 1998.

Ohi R, Hanamatsu M, Mochizuki I, et al.: Progress in the treatment of biliary atresia. *World J Surg* 9:285, 1985.

Olsen JB, Myren CV, Haahr PE: Randomized study of the value of laparoscopy before appendectomy. *Br J Surg* 80:922, 1993.

Palmer PE, Wolfe JH: α_1-Antitrypsin deposition in primary hepatic carcinomas. *Arch Pathol Lab Med* 100:232, 1976.

Park A, Heniford BT, Hebra A, Fitzgerald P: Pediatric laparoscopic splenectomy. *Surg Endosc* 14:527–531, 2000.

Paya K, Fakhari M, Rauhofer U, et al.: Open versus laparoscopic appendectomy in children: A comparison of complications. *JSLS* 4:121–124, 2000.

Payne K, Van Zyl W, Richardson M: Anaesthesia for congenital lobar emphysema resection. *South Afr Med J* 66:421, 1984.

Peña A, Hong A: Advances in the management of anorectal malformations. *Am J Surg* 180:370, 2000.

Piro AJ, Weiss DR, Hellman S: Mediastinal Hodgkin's disease: A possible danger for intubation anesthesia. *Int J Radial Oncol Biol Phys* 1:415, 1976.

Pitkanen MT: Body mass and spread of spinal anesthesia with bupivacaine. *Anesth Analg* 66:127, 1987.

Popovic L, Batinica S, Mestrovic T, et al.: The value of cholinesterase activity after Kasai operation. *Pediatr Surg Int* 19:605–607, 2003.

Prakash UBS, Abel MD, Hubmayr RD: Mediastinal mass and tracheal obstruction during general anesthesia. *Mayo Clin Proc* 63:1004, 1988.

Prasad R, Lovvorn HN, III, Wadie GM, et al.: Early experience with needle-scopic inguinal herniorrhaphy in children. *J Pediatr Surg* 38:1055–1058, 2003.

Price KJ, Roberton NRC, Pearse RG: Intussusception in preterm infants. *Arch Dis Child* 68:41, 1993.

Prober CG, Whyte H, Smith CR: Open lung biopsy in immunocompromised children with pulmonary infiltrates. *Am J Dis Child* 138:60, 1984.

Qualman SJ, O'Dorisio MS, Fleshman DJ, et al.: Neuroblastoma. Correlation of neuropeptide expression in tumor tissue with other prognostic factors. *Cancer* 70:2005, 1992.

Rabinovitch M: Pulmonary hypertension. In Adams FH, Emmanouilides GC, Riemenschneider TA, editors: *Moss' heart disease in infants, children, and adolescents*, 4th ed. Baltimore, 1989, Williams & Wilkins.

Raghavendran S, Kiwan R, Shah T, Vas L: Continuous caudal epidural analgesia for congenital lobar emphysema: A report of three cases. *Anesth Analg* 93:348, 2001.

Randolph JG: Experience with the Nissen fundoplication for correction of gastroesophageal reflux in infants. *Ann Surg* 198:579, 1983.

Rangel SJ, Henry MCW, Brindle M, Moss RL: Small evidence for small incisions: Pediatric laparoscopy and the need for more rigorous evaluation of novel surgical therapies. *J Pediatr* Surg 38:1429, 2003.

Rao CC, Krishna G, Grosfeld JL, et al.: One-lung pediatric anesthesia. *Anesth Analg* 60:450, 1981.

Raynor AC, Capp MP, Sealy WC: Lobar emphysema of infancy: Diagnosis, treatment, and etiologic aspects. *Ann Thorac Surg* 4:374–385, 1967.

Reddick EJ, Olsen DO: Laparoscopic laser cholecystectomy: A comparison with mini-lap cholecystectomy. *Surg Endosc* 3:131, 1989.

Remolina C, Khan AU, Santiago TV, Edelman NH: Positional hypoxemia in unilateral lung disease. *N Engl J Med* 304:523–525, 1981.

Rennotte MT, Baele P, Aubert G, et al.: Nasal continuous positive airway pressure in the perioperative management of patients with obstructive sleep apnea submitted to surgery. *Chest* 107:367, 1995.

Roberts JD, Polaner DM, Lang P, Zapol WM: Inhaled nitric oxide in persistent pulmonary hypertension of the newborn. *Lancet* 340:818–819, 1992.

Robicsek F. Surgical treatment of pectus excavatum. *Chest Surg Clin N Am*. 10:277–296, 2000.

Rodgers BM: Pediatric thoracoscopy: Where have we come and what have we learned? *Ann Thorac Surg* 56:704, 1993.

Rogers DA, Philippe PG, Lobe TE, et al.: Thoracoscopy in children: An initial experience with an evolving technique. *J Laparoendosc Surg* 2:7, 1992.

Rosen DM, Chou DC, North L, et al.: Femoral venous flow during laparoscopic gynecologic surgery. *Surg Laparosc Endosc Percutan Tech* 10:158–162, 2000.

Rothenberg S: Experience with 220 consecutive laparoscopic Nissen fundoplications in infants and children. *J Pediatr Surg* 33:274–278, 1993.

Rowe MI, Lloyd DA: Inguinal hernia. In Welch K, editor: *Pediatric surgery*, ed 4. Chicago, 1986, Yearbook Medical Publishers.

Rowe R, Andropoulos D, Heard M, et al.: Anesthetic management of pediatric patients undergoing thoracoscopy. *J Cardiothorac Vasc Anesth* 8:563, 1994.

Ryckman FC, Rosenkrantz JG: Thoracic surgical problems in infancy and childhood. *Surg Clin North Am* 65:1423, 1985.

Sailhamer E, Jackson CCA, Vogel AM, et al.: Minimally invasive surgery for pediatric solid neoplasms. *Am Surg* 69:566–568, 2003.

Salman MA, Yücebas ME, Coskun F, Aypar Ü: Day-case laparoscopy: A comparison of prophylactic opioid, NSAID or local anesthesia for postoperative analgesia. *Acta Anaesthesiol Scand* 44:536–542, 2000.

Sancandi M, Ceccherini I, Costa M, et al.: Incidence of RET mutations in patients with Hirschsprung's disease. *J Pediatr Surg* 35:139, 2000.

Saunders MP, Williams CR: Infantile hypertrophic pyloric stenosis: Experience in a district general hospital. *J Coll Surg Edinb* 35:36, 1990.

Sawyers JL: Current status of conventional (open) cholecystectomy versus laparoscopic cholecystectomy. *Ann Surg* 223:1–3, 1996.

Scammon RE: Dimensions of the respiratory tract at various ages in man. In Abt IA, editor: *Pediatrics*. Philadelphia, 1923, WB Saunders, p 257.

Scheinin B, Lindgren L, Scheinin TM: Preoperative nitrous oxide delays bowel function after colonic surgery. *Br J Anaesth* 64:154, 1990.

Schier F, Montupet P, Espositio C: Laparoscopic inguinal herniorrhaphy in children: A three-center experience with 933 repairs. *J Pediatr Surg* 37:395–397, 2002.

Schwartz D, Connelly NR, Manikantan P, Nichols JH: Hyperkalemia and pyloric stenosis. *Anesth Analg* 97:355, 2003.

Schwartz MZ, Ramachandran P: Congenital malformations of the lung and mediastinum: A quarter century of experience from a single institution. *J Pediatr Surg* 32:44–47, 1997.

Schwartz N, Eisencraft JB: Positioning of the endotracheal tube in an infant with tracheoesophageal fistula. *Anesthesiology* 69:289–290, 1988.

Series F, Cournier Y, La Forge J, et al.: Mechanisms of the effectiveness of continuous positive airway pressure in obstructive sleep apnea. *Sleep* 15:47S, 1992.

Servin F, Farinotti R, Haberer J-P, et al.: Propofol infusion for the maintenance of anesthesia in morbidly obese patients receiving nitrous oxide. *Anesthesiology* 57:48, 1993.

Shamberger RC, Guthrie KA, Ritchey ML, et al.: Surgery-related factors and local recurrence of Wilms tumor in National Wilms Tumor Study 4. *Ann Surg* 229:292–297, 1999.

Shamberger RC, Welch KJ, Sanders SP: Mitral valve prolapse associated with pectus excavatum. *J Pediatr* 111:404, 1987.

Shamberger RC, Welch KJ: Surgical correction of pectus carinatum. *J Pediatr Surg* 22:48, 1987.

Shekhawat NS, Prabhakar G, Sinha DD, et al.: Nonischemic intussusception in childhood. *J Pediatr Surg* 27:1433, 1992.

Shim WKT, Kasai M, Spence MA: Racial influence on the incidence of biliary atresia. *Progr Pediatr Surg* 6:53, 1974.

Shumake LB: Postoperative hypoglycemia in congenital hypertrophic pyloric stenosis. *South Med J* 68:223, 1975.

Shuster JJ, McWilliams NB, Castleberry R, et al.: Serum lactate dehydrogenase in childhood neuroblastoma. A pediatric oncology group recursive partitioning study. *Am J Clin Oncol* 15:295, 1992.

Sibert KS, Biondi JW, Hirsch NP: Spontaneous respiration during thoracotomy in a patient with a mediastinal mass. *Anesth Analg* 66:904, 1987.

Slinger PD, Lesiuk L: Flow resistances of disposable double-lumen, single-lumen, and Univent tubes. *J Cardiothorac Vasc Anesth* 12:142–144, 1998.

Slinger PD: Fiberoptic bronchoscopic positioning of double-lumen tubes. *J Cardiothorac Anesth* 3:486–496, 1989.

Smith CD, Othersen HB, Gogan NJ, Walker JD: Nissen fundoplication in children with profound neurologic disability. High risks and unmet goals. *Ann Surg* 215:654, 1992.

Smith EI, Haase GM, Seeger RC, Brodeur GM: A surgical perspective on the current staging in neuroblastoma: The International Neuroblastoma Staging System Proposal. *J Pediatr Surg* 24:386, 1989.

Song D, Whitten CW, White PF, et al.: Antiemetic activity of propofol after sevoflurane and desflurane anesthesia for outpatient laparoscopic cholecystectomy. *Anesthesiology* 89:838–843, 1998.

Soper NJ, Barteau JA, Clayman RV, et al.: Comparison of early postoperative results for laparoscopic versus standard open cholecystectomy. *Surg Gynecol Obstet* 174:114, 1992.

Soper NJ, Brunt LM, Kerbl K: Laparoscopic general surgery. *N Engl J Med* 330:409, 1994.

Soper RT, Mason EE, Printen KJ, Zellweger H: Gastric bypass for morbid obesity in children and adolescents. *J Pediatr Surg* 10:51, 1975.

Sorensen HT, Skriver MV, Pedersen L, et al.: Risk of infantile hypertrophic pyloric stenosis after maternal postnatal use of macrolides. *Scand J Infect Dis* 35:104, 2003.

Sotelo-Avila C, Gooch WM III: Neoplasms associated with the Beckwith-Wiedemann syndrome. *Perspect Pediatr Pathol* 3:255, 1976.

Spear RM, Deshpande JK, Maxwell LG: Caudal anesthesia in the awake, high-risk infant. *Anesthesiology* 69:407, 1988.

Sprung J, Whalley DG, Falcone T, et al.: The impact of morbid obesity, pneumoperitoneum, and posture on respiratory system mechanics and oxygenation during laparoscopy. *Anesth Analg* 94:1345–1350, 2002.

Stehling LC, Furman EB: Anesthesia for congenital anomalies of the genitourinary system. In Stehling LC, Zauder HL, editors: *Anesthetic implications of congenital anomalies in children*. New York, 1980, Appleton-Century-Crofts.

Steiner CA, Bass EB, Talamini MA, et al.: Surgical rates and operative mortality for open and laparoscopic cholecystectomy in Maryland. *N Engl J Med* 330:403, 1994.

Steyaert H, Al Mohaidly M, Lembo MA, et al.: Long-term outcome of laparoscopic Nissen and Toupet fundoplication in normal and neurologically impaired children. *Surg Endosc* 17:543–546, 2003.

Stocker JT, Madewell JE, Drake RM: Congenital cystic adenomatoid malformation of the lung. Classification and morphologic spectrum. *Hum Pathol* 8:155, 1977.

Stool SE, Randall P: Unexpected ear disease in infants with cleft palate. *Cleft Palate J* 4:99, 1967.

Strauss RS, Bradley LJ, Brolin RE: Gastric bypass surgery in adolescents with morbid obesity. *J Pediatr* 138:499, 2001.

Strauss RS, Pollack HA: Epidemic increase in childhood overweight, 1986–1998. *JAMA* 286:2845, 2001.

Strauss RS: Childhood obesity. *Pediatr Clin North Am* 49:175, 2002

Sugerman HJ, Fairman RG, Sood RK, et al.: Long-term effects of gastric surgery for treating respiratory insufficiency of obesity. *Am J Clin Nutr* 55:597S, 1992.

Sumner E, Frank JD: Tolazoline in the treatment of congenital diaphragmatic hernias. *Arch Dis Child* 56:350–353, 1981.

Sutton PP, Lopez-Vidriero M, Pavia D, et al.: Effect of chest physiotherapy on the removal of mucus in patients with cystic fibrosis. *Am Rev Respir Dis* 127:390, 1983.

Taivainen T, Tuominen M, Rosenberg PM: Influence of obesity on the spread of spinal anesthesia after injection of plain 0.5% bupivacaine at the L3-4 or L4-5 interspace. *Br J Anaesth* 64:542, 1990.

Takahashi M, Horinouchi T, Kato M, et al.: Double-access-port endotracheal tube for selective lung ventilation in pediatric patients. *Anesthesiology* 93:308–309, 2000.

Tan CEL, Davenport M, Driver M, Howard ER: Does the morphology of the extrahepatic biliary remnants in biliary atresia influence survival? A review of 205 cases. *J Pediatr Surg* 29:1459, 1994.

Taylor E, Feinstein R, White PF, Sopor N: Anesthesia for laparoscopic cholecystectomy: Is nitrous oxide contraindicated? *Anesthesiology* 76:541, 1992.

Taylor RR, Kelly TM, Elliot CG, et al.: Hypoxemia after gastric bypass surgery for morbid obesity. *Arch Surg* 120:1298, 1985.

Todres ID, Reppert G, Hall D, et al.: Management of critical airway obstruction in a child with mediastinal tumor. *Anesthesiology* 45:1000, 1976.

Tomicic JT, Luks FI, Shalon L, Tracy TF: Laparoscopic gastrostomy in infants and children. *Eur J Pediatr Surg* 12:107–110, 2002.

Tramer M, Moore A, McQuay H: Omitting nitrous oxide in general anaesthesia: Meta-analysis of intraoperative awareness and postoperative emesis in randomized controlled trials. *Br J Anaesth* 76:186, 1996.

Truog RD, Schena JA, Hershenson MB, et al.: Repair of congenital diaphragmatic hernia during extracorporeal membrane oxygenation. *Anesthesiology* 72: 750–753, 1990.

Tsui BC, Seal R, Koller J: Thoracic epidural catheter placement via the caudal approach in infants by using electrocardiographic guidance. *Anesth Analg* 95:326–330, 2002.

Turner MWH, Buchanon CCR, Brown SW: Paediatric one lung ventilation in the prone position. *Paediatr Anaesth* 7:427–429, 1997.

Uemura S, Nakagawa Y, Yoshida A, Choda Y: Experience in 100 cases with the Nuss procedure using a technique for stabilization of the pectus bar. *Pediatr Surg Int* 19:186, 2003.

Vanderwinden JM, Mailleux P, Schiffman SN, et al.: Nitric oxide synthase in infantile hypertrophic pyloric stenosis. *N Engl J Med* 327:511, 1992.

Vaughan RW, Bauer S, Wise L: Volume and pH of gastric juice in obese patients. *Anesthesiology* 43:686, 1975.

Vaughan RW, Bauer S, Wise L: Effect of position (semirecumbent versus supine) or postoperative oxygenation in markedly obese subjects. *Anesth Analg* 55:37–41, 1976.

Vinograd I, Klim B, Efrati Y: Airway obstruction in neonates and children: Surgical treatment. *J Cardiovasc Surg* 35:7–12, 1994.

Watson CB, Bowe EA, Burk W: One-lung anesthesia for pediatric thoracic surgery: A new use for the fiberoptic bronchoscope. *Anesthesiology* 56:314–315, 1982.

Watts RW: The influence of obesity on the relationship between body mass index and the distance to the epidural space from the skin. *Anaesth Intensive Care* 21:309, 1993.

Weatherford DA, Stephenson JE, Taylor SM, et al.: Thoracoscopy versus thoracotomy: Indications and advantages. *Ann Surg* 61:83–86, 1995.

Weber TR, Vane DW, Krishna G, et al.: Neonatal lung abscess. Resection using one-lung anesthesia. *Ann Thorac Surg* 36:464, 1983.

Wee l, Stokes MA: Bladder exstrophy in a neonate at risk of transient myasthenia gravis: A role for remifentanil and epidural analgesia. *Br J Anaesth* 82:774–776, 1999.

Weinberg AG, Mize CE, Worthen HG: The occurrence of hepatoma in the chronic form of hereditary tyrosinemia. *J Pediatr* 88:434, 1976.

Weinblatt ME, Heisel MA, Siegel SE: Hypertension in children with neurogenic tumors. *Pediatrics* 71:947, 1983.

Weir PM, Munro HM, Reynolds PI: Propofol infusion and the incidence of emesis in pediatric outpatient strabismus surgery. *Anesth Analg* 76:760, 1993.

Welch KJ, Randolph JG, Ravitch MM, et al., editors: *Pediatric surgery,* 4th ed. Chicago, 1986, Year Book Medical Publishers.

Wilcox S, Vandam LD: Alas, poor Trendelenburg and his position! A critique of its uses and effectiveness. *Anesth Analg* 67:574, 1988.

Wildhaber BE, Coran AG, Drongowski RA, et al.: The Kasai Portoenterostomy for biliary atresia: A review of a 27-year experience with 81 patients. *J Pediatr Surg* 38:1480–1485, 2003.

Willekes CL, Backer CL, Mavroudis C: A 26-year review of pectus deformity repairs, including simultaneous intracardiac repair. *Ann Thorac Surg* 67:511, 1999.

Winters RW: Metabolic alkalosis of pyloric stenosis. In Winters RW, editor: *The body fluids in pediatrics.* Boston, 1973, Little, Brown & Co.

Wolf AR, Lawson RA, Dryden CM, et al.: Recovery after desflurane anesthesia in the infant: comparison with isoflurane. *Br J Anaesth* 76:362–4, 1996.

Woodhouse CRJ, Ransley PG, Innes-Williams D: Prune-belly syndrome: Report of 47 cases. *Arch Dis Child* 57:856, 1982.

Wulkan ML, Georgeson KE: Primary laparoscopic endorectal pull-through for Hirschsprung's disease in infants and children. *Semin Laparosc Surg* 5:9, 1998.

Wyner J, Brodsky JB, Merrell RC: Massive obesity and arterial oxygenation. *Anesth Analg* 60:691, 1981.

Yeh TF, Pildes RS, Salem MR: Treatment of persistent tension pneumothorax in a neonate by selective bronchial intubation. *Anesthesiology* 49:37–38, 1978.

Yerkes EB, Brock JW 3rd, Holcomb GW III, et al.: Laparoscopic evaluation for a contralateral patent processus vaginalis: part III. *Urology* 51:480–483, 1998.

Yu HP, Hseu SS, Yien HW, et al.: Oral clonidine premedication preserves heart rate variability for patients undergoing laparoscopic cholecystectomy. *Acta Anaesthesiol Scand* 47:185–190, 2003.

Zanardi LR, Haber P, Mootrey GT, et al.: Intussusception among recipients of rotavirus vaccine: reports to the vaccine adverse event reporting system. *Pediatrics* 107:E97, 2001. Available at: http://www.pediatrics.org/cgi/content/full/107/6/e97.

Zangeneh F, Limbeck GA, Brown BI, et al.: Hepatorenal glycogenosis (type I glycogenosis) and carcinoma of the liver. *J Pediatr* 74:73, 1969.

Zeidan B, Wyatt J, Mackersie A, Brereton RJ: Recent results of treatment of infantile hypertrophic pyloric stenosis. *Arch Dis Child* 63:1060, 1988.

20 Anesthesia for Pediatric Plastic Surgery

Jayant K. Deshpande • Kevin Kelly • Matthew B. Baker

In this chapter, the anesthetic considerations of the most common plastic surgical procedures are summarized. Common surgical problems with practical suggestions and discussions of anesthetic technique and anesthetic concerns are offered.

Plastic surgical procedures range from minor cosmetic repairs to extensive major reconstructive surgery. Frequently, reconstructive surgery is a staged procedure. Consequently, these patients make numerous visits to the operating room. The anesthesiologist should visit the patient preoperatively to assess the child's fears and anxieties. In addition, the anesthesiologist should provide reassurance and, when necessary to assessing the child, provide adequate premedication (see Chapters 7 and 10, Psychological Aspects of Pediatric Anesthesia and Induction of Anesthesia and Maintenance of the Airway).

CRANIOFACIAL RECONSTRUCTION

Children who undergo craniofacial reconstruction may have disorders ranging from synostosis of a single cranial suture with resultant abnormal skull formation to congenital anomalies, such as Apert's, Crouzon's, and other syndromes, which may involve multiple skull sutures and other facial anatomic anomalies (Box 20–1). Despite the sometimes significant craniofacial deformations present in these children, their underlying neurodevelopmental status and general health are often quite normal (Figs. 20–1 to 20–4 (see Color plates, DVD, for Figure 20–4 C and D). The goal of surgical intervention is to improve the anatomy and geometry of the cranium and face and thereby permit normal brain growth and to minimize subsequent abnormal psychosocial development. Since the 1990s, surgical and anesthetic techniques have evolved sufficiently to allow repair to be performed during late infancy or early toddlerhood. Early repair has resulted in excellent surgical outcomes and possibly psychosocial development of the child.

The perioperative care of children undergoing craniofacial reconstruction requires an informed and collaborative team of health care providers. Pediatric plastic surgeons and neurosurgeons work in tandem to remove and rearrange the skull deformity while avoiding potential trauma to the underlying brain, venous sinuses, and blood vessels. Specialists in cranio-oromaxillofacial surgery and otolaryngology often comprise active members of the team, particularly if reconstruction of the midface or jaw is required. Experienced anesthesiologists are crucial members of the team, as perioperative management requires balancing possible conflicting issues, such as brain protection and reducing cerebral edema while maintaining an adequate circulating blood volume (Box 20–2). Timely postoperative care, including anticipating and preventing complications, requires that the pediatric intensivist and critical care nurses are familiar with the surgical and perioperative management plan. Children who have undergone plastic surgery of the head and neck often need speech therapy, physiotherapy, and possible psychological support after surgery. The child's primary care physician, along with the plastic surgeon, must know how to deal with these complex issues and how to act as the child's and family's advocate in order to coordinate the multiple care providers.

BOX 20–1 Partial List of Syndromes and Conditions Commonly Associated With Craniofacial Anomalies

Apert's syndrome
Cleidocranial dysostosis
Congenital craniosynostosis
Craniofacial hemangioma/other vascular malformations
Crouzon's syndrome
Goldenhar's syndrome
Hemifacial microsomia
Mandibular dysostosis
Maxillofacial deformities
Neurofibromatosis
Pfeiffer's syndrome
Plagiocephaly
Treacher Collins syndrome

PREOPERATIVE MANAGEMENT

During the preoperative visit, the anesthesiologist should become familiar with the child's underlying pathophysiology, as well as the parents' expectations and anxieties and the child's personality (see Chapter 7, Psychological Aspects of Pediatric Anesthesia). The history should provide information regarding current medications, allergies, asthma, recent upper respiratory tract infections, and previous anesthetic and surgical experiences. Difficult intubation is a major concern in these patients. The anesthesiologist should be aware that previous reconstructive surgery may have altered the airway anatomy dramatically (e.g., development of temporomandibular joint [TMJ] ankylosis). The presence of

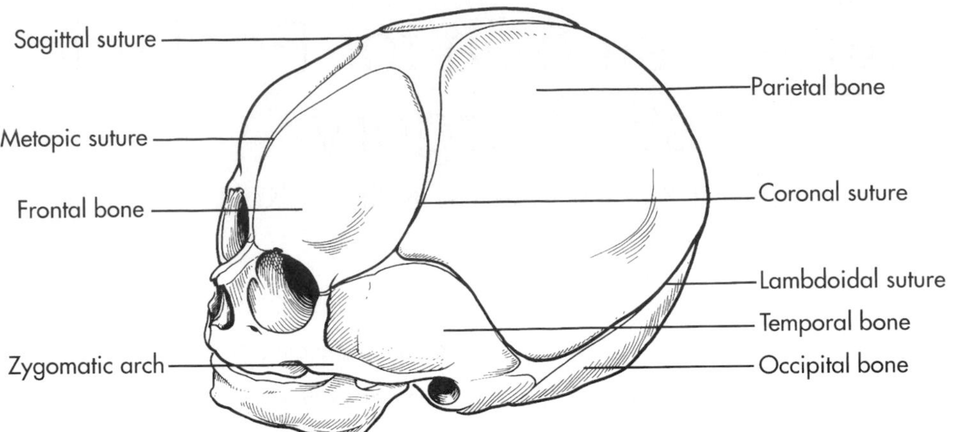

■ **FIGURE 20–1.** Cranium with normal sutures and skull bones.

somnolence, nausea, vomiting, episodes of apnea or bradycardia, or cranial nerve dysfunction (especially visual disturbances) suggests increased intracranial pressure.

Fortunately, young children with craniosynostosis rarely develop intracranial pressure problems because the skull can expand in another direction during the postnatal period in order to compensate for the decreased growth perpendicular to the suture that is fused (Heeckt et al., 1993; Siddiqi et al., 1995). This skull expansion does, however, add to the skull deformity. Hydrocephalus can be seen in children with cranial stenosis and should be treated prior to cranial reconstruction to avoid complications. If hydrocephalus is present and a history of seizures is documented, then blood levels of anticonvulsant should be determined proportionately. Some congenital syndromes may also be associated with anomalies of the heart or lungs; in these instances, details of any cardiopulmonary involvement must be elicited.

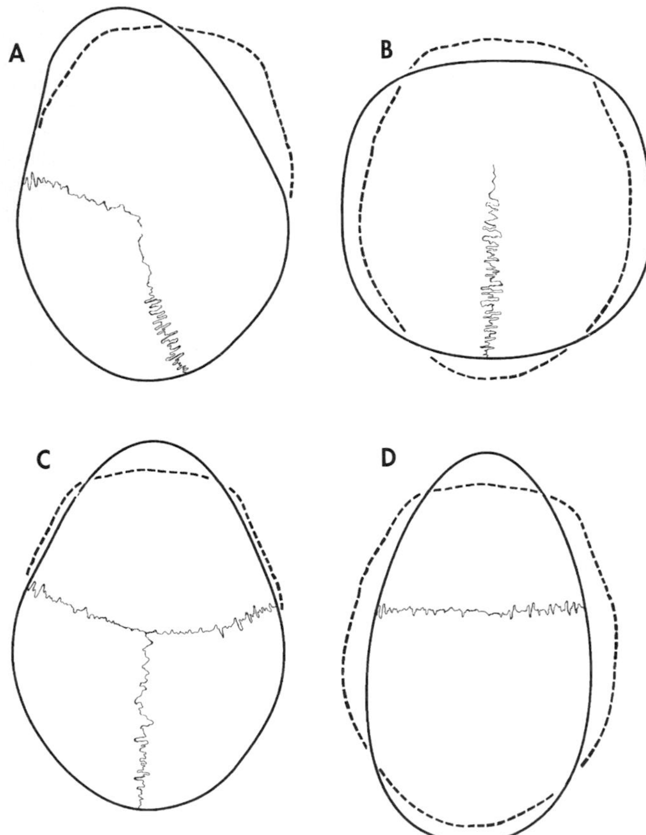

■ **FIGURE 20–2.** Craniosynostosis results in abnormal skull growth with the deformity determined by which suture is prematurely fused. Skull growth is inhibited perpendicular to the fused suture. The dotted line represents the normal skull configuration. *A*, Unilateral fusion of the coronal suture producing a flattening of the affected side and contralateral frontal bossing. *B*, Bilateral coronal synostosis causing a widened foreshortened skull. *C*, Metopic craniosynostosis produces a triangularly shaped forehead. *D*, Sagittal synostosis causes an elongation and narrowing of the cranium.

The physical examination includes evaluation of the patient's mental status and vital signs. Any signs and symptoms of increased intracranial pressure must be noted. Cushing's triad—apnea, bradycardia, and hypertension (Cushing, 1902)—is rarely present in these children, but "sundowning" (which means pressing on an open fontanel causes the gaze to fall) or wide sutures are not uncommon in children with elevated intracranial pressure (see Fig. 18–8 in Chapter 18, Anesthesia for Neurosurgery). Preoperative neurologic deficits should be documented. The examination of airway patency is also extremely important. The child may have limited ability to open the mouth, and the pharynx may be difficult to visualize. Micrognathia, retrognathia, or mandibular hypoplasia, commonly associated with syndromes such as Pierre Robin, Treacher Collins, Beckwith-Wiedemann, or Crouzon's, can make intubation difficult. Patients who have long-standing upper airway obstruction because of choanal atresia, mandibular hypoplasia, or other causes may have chronic hypoventilation and hypoxia. Patients with craniofacial anomalies and associated hydrocephalus may experience episodes of apnea and recurrent hypoxia (Handler, 1985). Such situations can produce pulmonary hypertension and subsequently lead to cor pulmonale (Rabinovitch, 1989; Rosen, 1996). The evaluation of these patients should include an electrocardiogram and, possibly, an echocardiogram.

Preoperative laboratory evaluation includes determination of hematocrit and hemoglobin concentrations and, if there has been significant vomiting, determination of electrolyte levels. A therapeutic drug level should be documented for any patient receiving anticonvulsants. The results of other studies, including chest radiographs, electrocardiograms, and electroencephalograms, must be reviewed. Finally, the anesthesiologist should

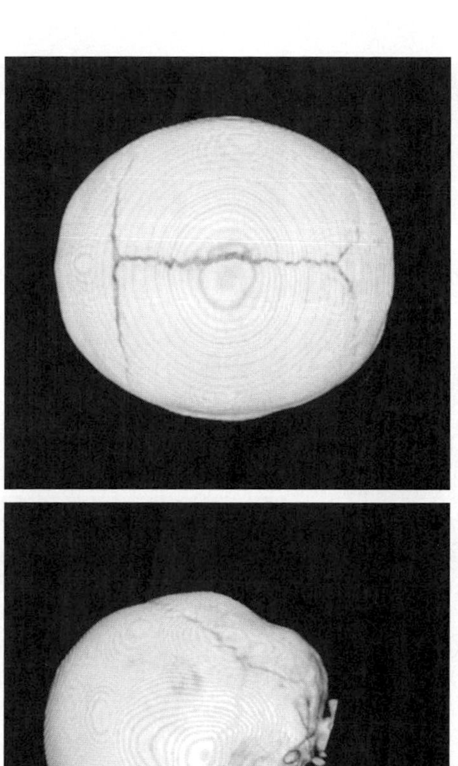

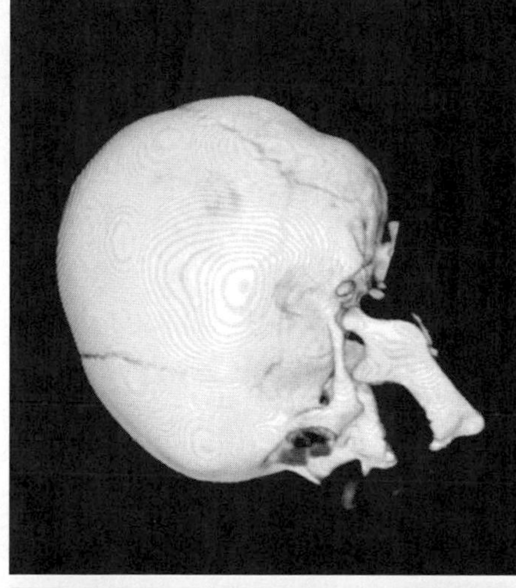

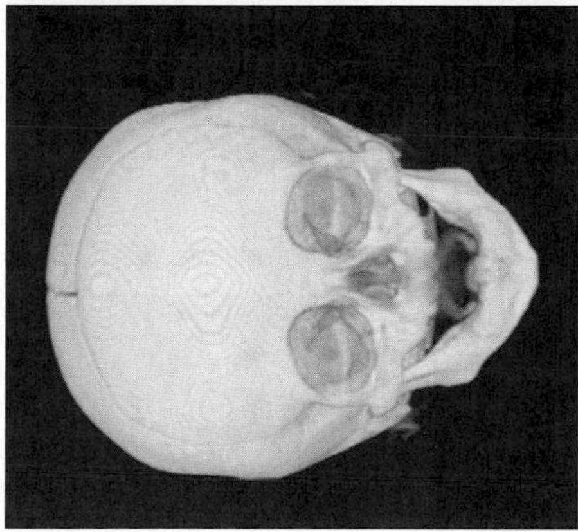

■ **Figure 20–3.** These 3-DCT scans of a child's skull show the location of normal sutures. Concentric circles are imaging artifacts.

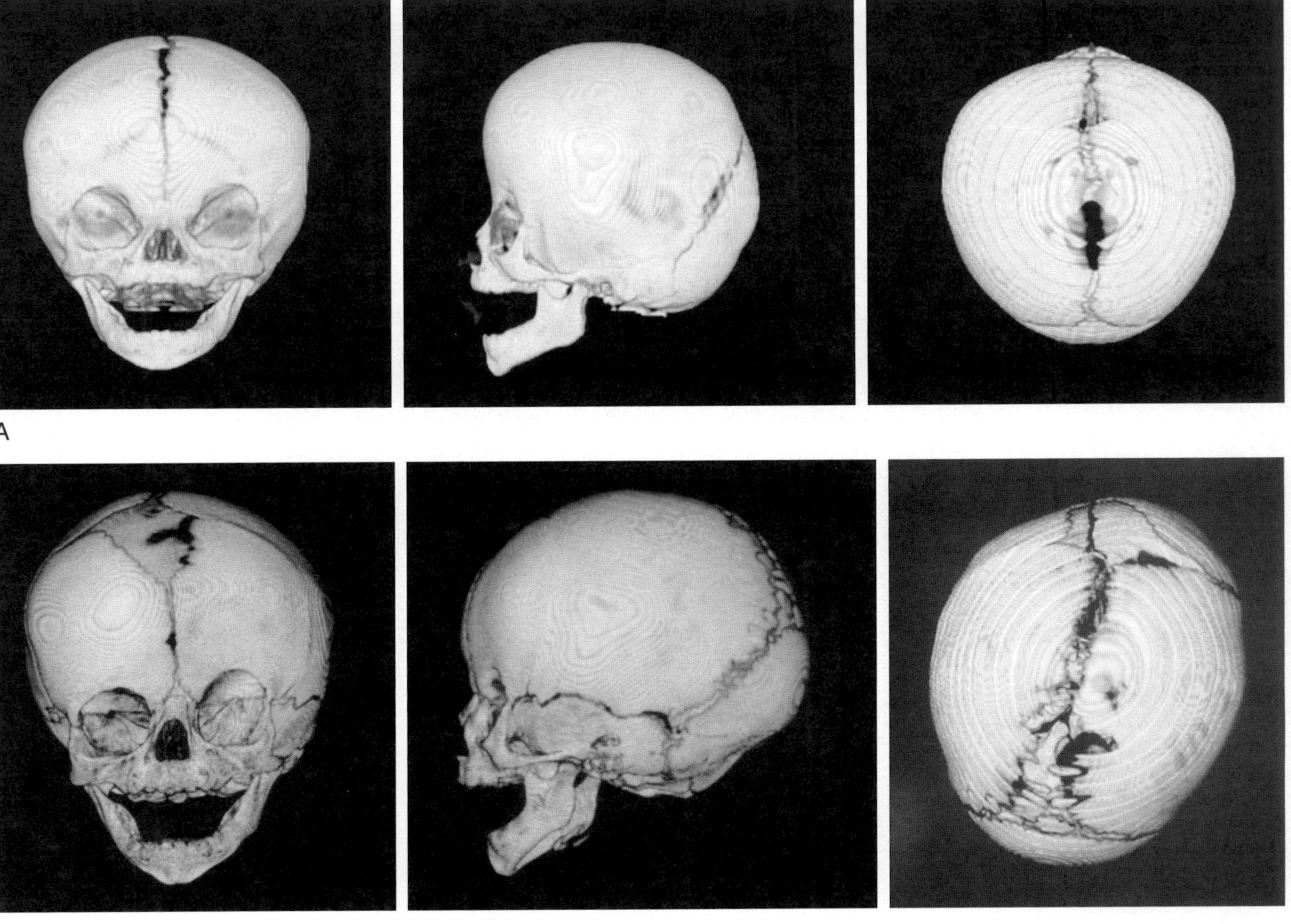

■ **Figure 20–4.** Six 3-DCT scans of the heads of children with cranial deformities. Concentric circles are imaging artifacts. *A*, Brachycephaly with bilateral coronal suture synostosis; *B*, plagiocephaly or unilateral coronal synostosis; *C*, scaphocephaly or sagittal suture synostosis; and *D*, trigonocephaly or metopic suture synostosis. (See Color Plates, DVD for Figures 20–4 C and D.)

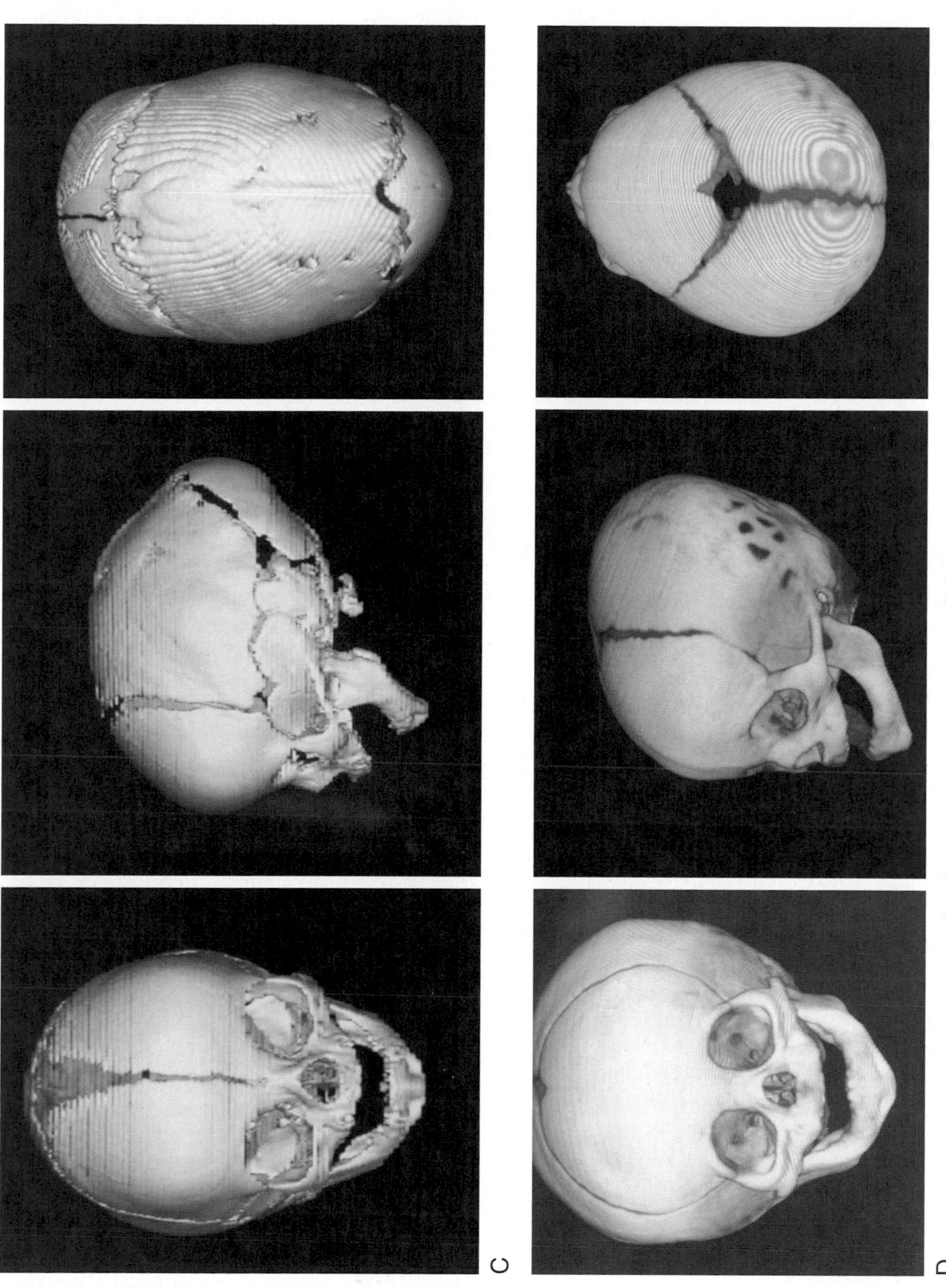

■ **Figure 20–4. cont'd**

BOX 20–2 Common Perianesthetic Challenges of Craniofacial Surgery

Difficult airway
- Difficult to maintain patent airway during surgery

Field avoidance
- Head position often 90 to 180 degrees away from anesthesiologist

Massive blood loss
- Can approach or exceed 1 blood volume

Massive fluid shifts and difficult fluid management
- As a result of considerable blood loss, and significant evaporative losses from exposed dura and brain during long procedure

Temperature control
- Hypothermia likely because of exposed dura and brain during long procedure

Potential positional trauma from prolonged procedure
- Precautions must be taken to prevent nerve and skin injury

Risk of air embolism from exposed skull and venous channels

Postoperative care issues
- Including ongoing coagulopathy
- Management of the difficult airway
- Potential need for mechanical ventilation
- Family support and care

confirm that at least one blood volume equivalent of packed red blood cells is available in the blood bank before surgery.

Oral medications can be continued (especially anticonvulsant medications) up to and including the morning of surgery. In patients not at risk for increased intracranial pressure or significant airway obstruction, an oral preoperative sedative, such as midazolam (0.25 to 0.5 mg/kg), may be useful to ease anxiety and increase the ease of inhalation induction.

Before formulating a plan for intraoperative care, the anesthesiologist should have a clear understanding of the surgical plan. The surgical team frequently includes both a neurosurgeon and a plastic and reconstructive (craniofacial) surgeon. The anesthesiologist must know the nature and extent of the surgical procedure planned and the position the patient will be in on the operating table. The anesthetic plan should incorporate the usual considerations for any anesthetic in a child and must allow for special concerns relevant to the condition (see later discussion). These patients usually do not have a concomitant disease, such as gastroesophageal reflux, and fast preoperatively for a sufficient duration (i.e., clear fluid up to 2 hours prior to anesthesia) so that induction of anesthesia can proceed routinely.

INDUCTION OF ANESTHESIA

Anesthesia usually can be induced by inhalation of volatile agents. Sevoflurane has evolved to be the preferred agent because of its rapid uptake and its association with relatively few airway complications during induction (see Chapter 10, Induction of Anesthesia). Two large-bore peripheral intravenous catheters and an arterial cannula are placed after anesthesia induction. Occasionally a central venous catheter may be needed if peripheral venous access is insufficient or if the child's hemodynamic status is tenuous. Muscle relaxants facilitate intubation. A preformed oral (RAE) tube or an armored (anode) tube of the appropriate size is inserted and secured with benzoin and tape. Alternatively, the surgeon may wire the endotracheal tube in place around the teeth or to the mandible or maxilla. Occasionally, nasotracheal tubes are required for the operative procedure. These tubes are often secured by placing a suture firmly around the wall of the endotracheal tube and into the nasal septum. After the position of the tube is verified, the child can be mechanically ventilated. The eyes must be lubricated and the eyelids taped shut or sutured closed by the surgeon. Alternatively, scleral shields may be placed in both eyes to provide protection without interfering in the surgical field of vision. In addition to arterial blood pressure, heart tones, breath sounds, pulse oximetry (SpO_2), end-tidal carbon dioxide tension ($PETCO_2$), urine output, and body temperature are continually monitored. In patients with preexisting increased intracranial pressure, anesthetic management is modified to preserve cerebral perfusion pressure (see Chapter 18, Anesthesia for Neurosurgery).

Induction of anesthesia in patients with airway abnormalities presents some distinct difficulties. The anatomic defects can restrict mouth opening, distort pharyngeal and laryngeal anatomy, and hinder the placement and securing of the endotracheal tube. For these children, intravenous access must be established before induction. In the presence of significant airway abnormality, the fiberoptic bronchoscope can be an effective tool used to place an endotracheal tube even in small infants (see Chapter 10, Induction of Anesthesia). In experienced hands, a Bullard laryngoscope (see Chapter 10 and Chapter 23, Anesthesia for Otorhinolaryngology Surgery) is an alternative adjunct for difficult intubation. Rarely, one may need to perform awake intubation or tracheostomy under sedation and local anesthesia. Tracheostomy in infants, and particularly those with an abnormal airway, and without an endotracheal tube in place, is an extremely difficult procedure at best and should be attempted only by a surgical team with experience in performing tracheostomies in infants and children.

Craniofacial reconstructive procedures can be time consuming, lasting many hours; patients should be positioned on the operating room table with great care. Most commonly, the child is supine during the procedure with the head slightly elevated. The neck may be flexed in an extreme position to provide better access to the occiput while keeping the child supine. Eye protection can be provided by placement of scleral shields. Additional protective padding should be used at pressure points and sensitive areas, including eyes, forehead, elbows, genitalia, and knees. In some cases, it may be necessary to place the child in a prone or lateral position. In these instances, the anesthesiologist should take additional caution to ensure that the airway is secure, the eyes are appropriately protected, and the pressure points are well padded. Rolls of bed sheets or other padding are used to distribute the pressure over the shoulders and hips to ensure good excursion of the chest and abdomen. In order to allow maximum surgical access to the head and face for the procedure, the head of the table (and thus the child) often is rotated 90 to 180 degrees away from the anesthesia field. The anesthesia care team has extremely limited access to the child and particularly the airway. A warm-water heating pad under the patient and a forced air warming device to cover the extremities and trunk help maintain body temperature (see Chapter 9, Anesthesia Equipment and Monitoring).

INTRAOPERATIVE MANAGEMENT

Craniofacial reconstruction often involves extensive craniotomies and exposure of large areas of brain encased in the dura (Figs. 20–5 and 20–6; see Color Plates, DVD, for Fig. 20–6). Direct pressure and trauma on these exposed surfaces during surgery can cause brain swelling and increased intradural pressure, which can further compromise regional cerebral blood flow. The signs of significant increases in intradural pressure include a taut dura and loss of dural pulsation. A lumbar cerebrospinal fluid drain occasionally may be necessary. The drain can be placed after the induction of anesthesia (usually in the L4-5 interspace) and is used to periodically withdraw cerebrospinal fluid during surgery. However, lumbar cerebrospinal fluid drains are contraindicated in patients with preexisting increased intracranial pressure. A commercially available kit for continuous epidural anesthesia can be used to perform a "wet" tap with an 18-gauge Crawford (or Huested) needle. All spinal catheters must be clearly labeled to avoid the accidental injection of drugs into the intrathecal space. Recent body of evidence supports the use of moderate hypothermia to reduce potential neuronal injury. Maintaining the body temperature between 35° to 37°C may be neuroprotective without increasing the risk of cardiovascular or hematologic abnormalities.

Anesthesia can be maintained using an inhalational anesthetic, intravenous anesthesia, or a combination of both. If a head-up or sitting position is used, nitrous oxide should not be used because of the concern of air embolism (see below). Infusions of remifentanil help provide sufficient anesthesia during prolonged surgery and yet are associated with a rapid emergence at the end of the procedure (Chiaretti et al., 2000). Most patients also require supplemental volatile anesthetic, such as isoflurane (commonly 0.25 to 0.5 MAC). Physiologic variables, including body temperature, arterial blood pressure, heart rate, arterial blood gas tensions, pH, P_{ETCO_2}, Sp_{O_2}, hematocrit, platelet count, blood glucose levels, and urine output, are monitored through the course of the procedure.

Craniofacial surgery requires attention to fluid homeostasis. The child has a larger body surface area-to-volume ratio compared with the adult. The child's head comprises nearly 18%

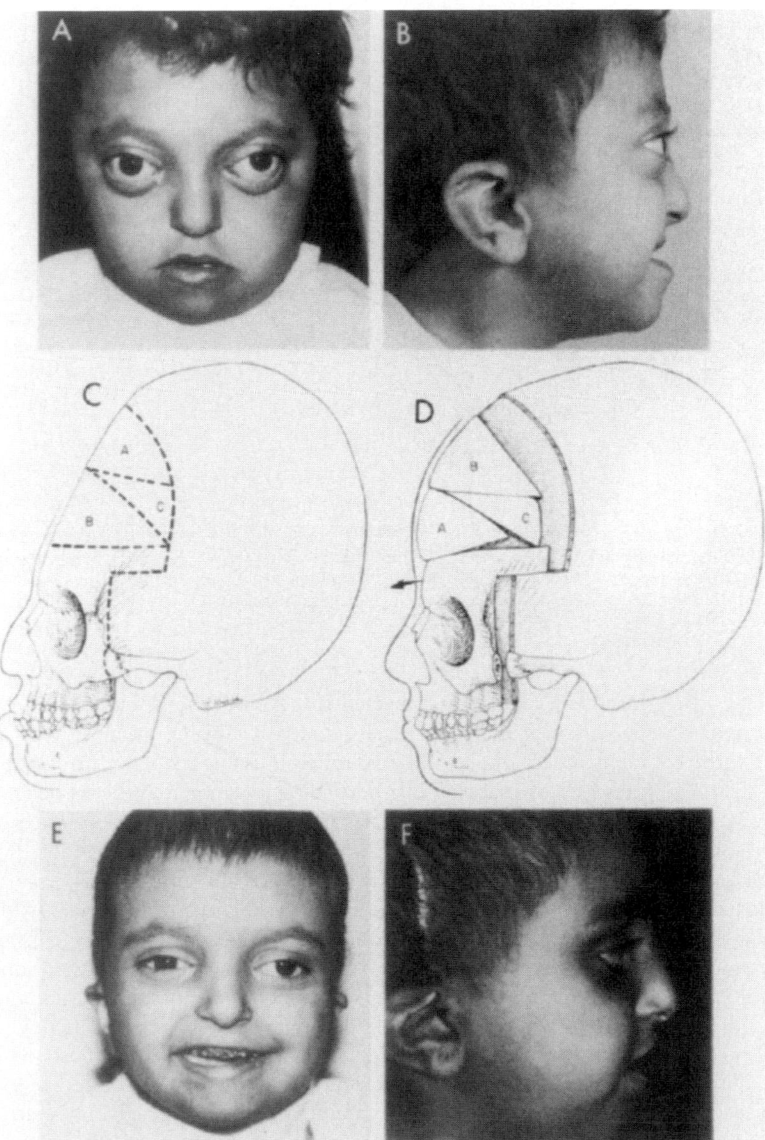

FIGURE 20–5. Presentation and correction of craniofacial abnormalities in a 4-year-old child with Crouzon's syndrome. (From Welch KJ, Randolph JG, Ravitch MM, et al., editors: *Pediatric surgery,* vol 1, 4th ed. Chicago, 1986, Year Book Medical Publishers, p 433.)

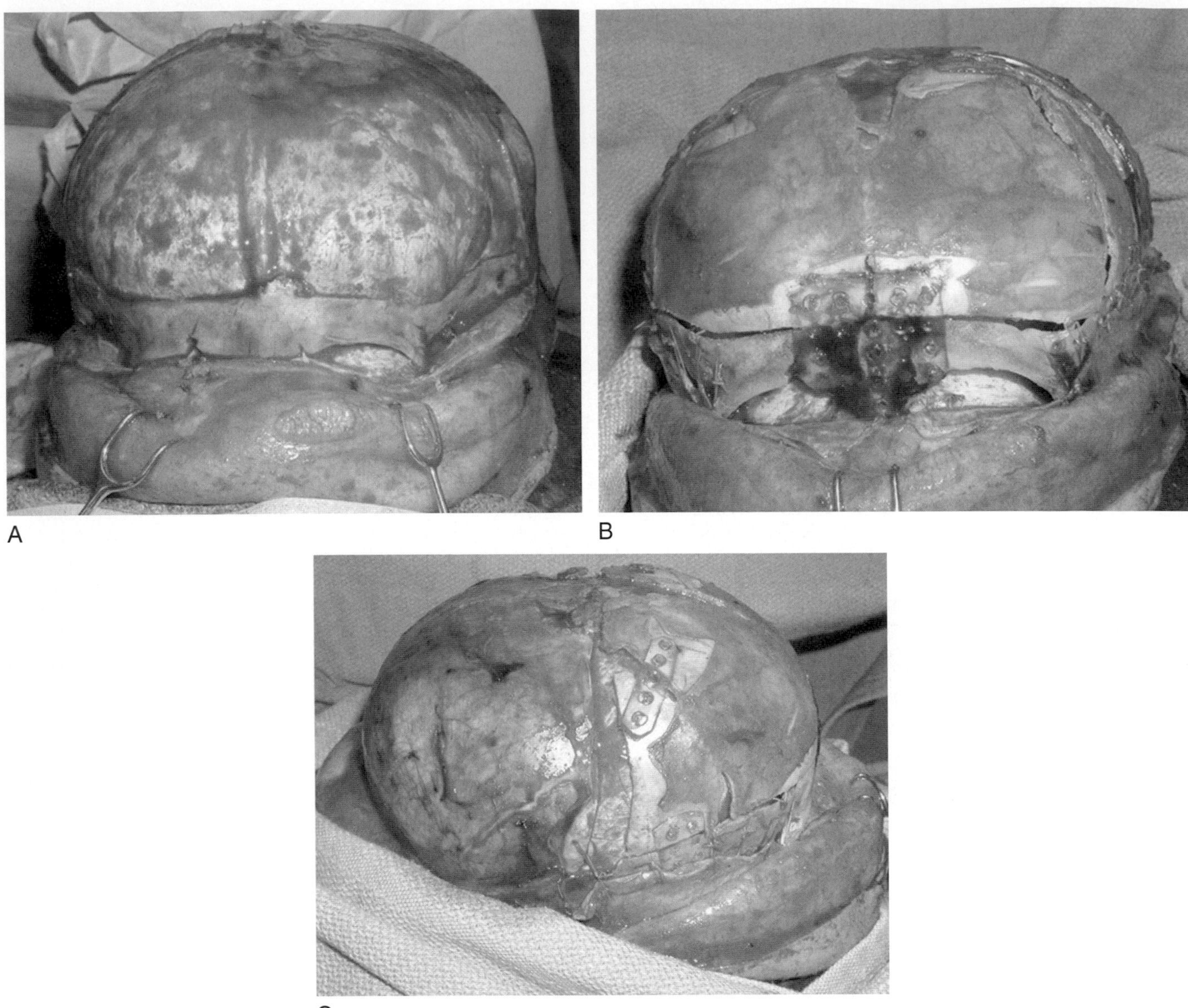

■ **FIGURE 20–6.** Intraoperative dissection for craniofacial reconstruction. Note the extensive dissection that can be associated with significant blood loss, heat loss, and potential risk to brain. *A*, Frontal view: anterior skull bones removed in preparation for reconstruction. The underlying dura over the frontal cortex is exposed. *B*, Frontal view: anterior skull reconstruction using previously removed cranial bones. Note the screw holes in the absorbable plates visible in the midline of skull. *C*, Lateral view (forehead on right): note the intricate joining of re-formed skull fragments using absorbable plates and screws to reconstruct the forehead. Skin hooks used to retract the covering soft tissues are visible. (See Color Plates, DVD.)

of the surface area, whereas the adult's comprises only 9%. This larger surface area results in fluid and heat losses that are proportionately greater in the child. If the procedure is extradural, third-space fluid losses may equal 6 to 8 mL/kg per hr or more. If the (fibrous) dura mater is opened, the fluid losses are greater, 10 to 12 mL/kg per hr or more. In addition, these procedures are commonly associated with large intraoperative blood losses (see later). Intravascular volume must be maintained to achieve adequate perfusion of tissue beds and prevent venous air embolism. Fluid restriction and dehydration, common in adult neurosurgical patients, can create a potentially hazardous situation.

Because of the factors confounding intraoperative fluid therapy, the anesthesiologist must rely on various indicators to monitor fluid requirements and therapy. The urine output, along with central venous pressure measurement when available, can help guide intraoperative fluid therapy. A child who has adequate intravascular fluid is expected to have urine output of 1 mL/kg per hr or greater. However, urine output alone may not accurately reflect intravascular volume status and renal perfusion. The presence of diabetes insipidus or glycosuria may be associated with continued "satisfactory" urine output in the presence of reduced intravascular volume. In addition, if mannitol or other diuretics have been administered to reduce intradural pressure, urine output may not reflect intravascular volume status.

Craniofacial reconstruction is often associated with large intraoperative blood losses. The blood loss usually is via venous or bony oozing and generally accumulates in the drapes; estimations of blood loss are often inaccurate. Serial hematocrits, combined with an appreciation of the child's intravascular volume status, should guide transfusion therapy. The decision to transfuse red blood cells is based on the need to maintain the oxygen-carrying capacity of the blood at levels that meet the patient's metabolic demands.

This decision is also influenced by the rate of ongoing surgical blood losses. Traditionally, hemoglobin levels less than 8 to 10 g/dL were thought to be insufficient to maintain adequate tissue oxygen delivery (Fontana et al., 1995); a patient was routinely transfused to maintain the hematocrit above 30%. However, with the use of normovolemic hemodilution, it may be possible to maintain adequate tissue substrate delivery with hematocrits as low as 20%. Haberkern and Dangel (1991) found that hemodilution below this value is associated with decreased mixed venous oxygenation, indicating a significant increase in oxygenation extraction, tissue dysoxia, or ischemia (Dishart et al., 1998). Because of the relatively small allowable blood loss in infants and small children, this technique usually does not reduce the exposure risk to a unit of autologous blood (Brecher and Rosenfeld, 1994). Advances in hemostasis have reduced intraoperative blood loss. The use of fibrin glue on the bone margins may substantially decrease ongoing intraoperative blood loss (Valbonesi et al., 2002; Panfilov, 2003).

Coagulopathies may occur for several reasons. Coagulation factors may be consumed rapidly because of ongoing blood loss (Williams et al., 2001). Tissue thromboplastin is released by surgical manipulation and inadvertent trauma to the brain and dura. Massive infusion of fluid aimed at keeping up with evaporative losses and transfusion of red cells to replace blood loss can result in dilutional coagulopathies. Any one or a combination of these etiologies can produce the bleeding disorder seen in patients undergoing craniofacial repair. Fresh frozen plasma is reserved for factor-deficient bleeding diatheses documented by a prolongation of the prothrombin time (PT) or activated partial thromboplastin time (aPTT). If coagulation studies can be performed at the point of care or are available in a timely manner, the transfusion of FFP can be based on appropriate laboratory studies. In the absence of such timely results, empiric transfusion of FFP may be necessary. One study in children undergoing craniofacial reconstruction found that the PT is prolonged in up to 19% of cases, lending support to the intraoperative use of FFP transfusion. When necessary, 10 to 20 mL/kg of FFP should correct the prolonged PT (Williams et al., 2001).

Thrombocytopenia, not factor deficiency, is more commonly the source of the bleeding disorder in the presence of significant blood loss, and serial platelet counts are used to guide transfusion therapy. Platelet transfusion in infants with platelet levels less than 75,000/mm^3 should minimize bleeding caused by thrombocytopenia. A new therapy for reducing blood loss during craniofacial surgery is the use of aprotinin, a serine protease inhibitor (D'Errico et al., 2003). Aprotinin was administered as a loading dose (240 mg/m^2) followed by an infusion (56 mg/m^2 per hr) for the duration of the procedure. The patients who received aprotinin experienced significantly less blood loss than did those who were administered a placebo infusion.

The use of deliberate hypotension and patient positioning also may minimize intraoperative blood loss (see Chapter 12, Blood Conservation). Positioning with the head above the heart (approximately 30 degrees) improves venous drainage, decreases the blood loss, and may optimize the surgical exposure. The addition of deliberate hypotension decreases cerebral perfusion pressure and increases the risk of venous air embolism.

Maintaining body temperature in the desired range can be a significant problem in children in any lengthy procedure involving exposure of a large surface area. Heat loss may be reduced by warming all intravenous fluids, wrapping the nonexposed body parts in plastic sheets, using a forced-air warmer, and placing the child on a heating pad. In addition, heated humidifiers or heat-moisture exchange (HME) devices are used in the airway circuit to minimize evaporative heat loss from the respiratory tree, as well as to prevent dehydration of central airway mucosa. A radiant warmer is often useful when the child first arrives in the operating room and is uncovered during anesthesia induction and monitor placement. The goal of intraoperative temperature maintenance is body temperature of 35° to 37°C, as mentioned earlier.

Craniofacial reconstruction may also present risks specific to the central nervous system, such as air embolism and cerebral trauma. Air embolism can occur when venous structures, which develop subatmospheric intravascular pressure, are exposed to the atmosphere and air is entrained intravascularly (Souder, 2000). Signs of small amounts of venous air embolism can be quite subtle. Mass spectroscopy of end-tidal gases offers the most sensitive indication, with an elevation of the end-tidal nitrogen concentration. More commonly available is PETCO_2. A sudden decrease in PETCO_2 is nearly as sensitive an indicator of air embolism as is the end-tidal nitrogen concentration. Monitoring for emboli with precordial Doppler stethoscopes has been recommended in adults (Bedford et al., 1981). When positioned properly on the patient's chest, these stethoscopes are extremely sensitive, detecting small venous air embolisms (VAEs) by a characteristic murmur. In infants and small children, however, this technique is extremely cumbersome to use because of the child's small chest and heart size and offers little benefit. Monitoring of blood pressure and oxygenation is relatively insensitive for the detection of VAEs, as is the monitoring of pulmonary artery pressure. If a VAE is suspected or diagnosed, 100% oxygen should be administered to the patient, and the surgical field must be flooded with fluid, so that fluid, and not air, is entrained. Efforts are made to elevate venous pressures by placing the patient in a head-down (Trendelenburg) position and administering intravenous fluids. The central venous catheter may serve a special purpose in the treatment of VAEs. Specifically, in the face of a large VAE, it may be possible to aspirate out air. This effort is most effective if the tip of the catheter is placed within the right atrium at its junction with the superior vena cava (Bunegin el al., 1981).

Although these procedures are usually extradural, the brain may be subject to surgical trauma or hypoperfusion. The anesthetic technique should be designed to reduce these risks. Steps include maintaining adequate intravascular volume and systemic perfusion pressure and mild hypothermia.

The pharmacologic maneuvers for brain protection are not clearly delineated because the basic mechanisms of neurologic injury are not completely understood. Central nervous system damage may result from direct cerebral trauma, cerebral edema, or regional hypoxia or hypoperfusion (ischemia). Central nervous system damage induces a common set of reactions, including release of toxic neurotransmitter substances (excitotoxins such as glutamate and aspartate), opening of calcium channels, and influx of calcium into neurons. In turn, these effect detrimental reactions in the neuronal cytosol, such as release of arachidonic acid and other free fatty acids and production of oxygen free radicals that can damage the cell and mitochondrial membranes (Clausen and Bullock, 2001). Despite improved understanding and effort, no current drug or therapeutic modality has been demonstrated to provide clear protection against, nor cure for, such neurologic injury (also see Chapter 18, Anesthesia for Neurosurgery).

POSTOPERATIVE MANAGEMENT

After surgery, these patients usually are allowed to emerge from anesthesia and resume spontaneous ventilation. Most patients meet extubation criteria soon after surgery is completed and the trachea is extubated. The child then can be transported to the pediatric intensive care unit (PICU) directly or alternatively taken to the postanesthetic care unit (PACU) for immediate postoperative care and then transported to the PICU. During transport, the child's respiratory and hemodynamic status should be continuously monitored. Occasionally, patients may need to remain intubated for ventilatory support in the immediate postoperative period because of the possibility of hypoventilation, resulting from prolonged anesthesia, hypothermia, or brain edema from trauma or fluid shifts. In addition, the surgical procedure may include manipulation of the mandible, maxilla, or another part of the airway, which can result in mucosal swelling or hematoma that can compromise the airway. All of these children require close observation in the PICU for at least 24 to 48 hours postoperatively. The patient's neurologic status should be assessed frequently for the development of somnolence, confusion, irritability, or other signs of altered mental status. Deterioration may be caused by hypoxia, hypercapnia, cerebral edema, acute or subacute shifts of intracranial contents, intracranial bleeding, hypoglycemia, or electrolyte imbalances, which must be appropriately and quickly treated to prevent further complications.

Postoperative bleeding or fluid losses because of ongoing fluid shifts (from intravascular to interstitial) may compromise systemic and brain perfusion. Transfusion of blood products or isotonic fluid therapy may be necessary to treat decreased peripheral perfusion and systemic hypotension. Additional doses of FFP or platelets may be needed to correct ongoing coagulopathy. The patient's skin perfusion, temperature, arterial blood pressure, blood gas levels, serial hematocrit, coagulation profiles, and urine output must be continually monitored.

Advances in technology have resulted in improved materials for surgical repair of the cranial defect. Absorbable plates and screws were first used in orthopedic surgery and now are commonly used in craniofacial repair. The materials are made from polyglycolic and polylactic acid. The screw and plates dissolve in 1 to 1.5 years, leaving no hardware remaining in the child's skull. The process may reduce the number of repeat operations the patient requires (Turvey et al., 2002).

EXTERNAL FIXATION AND OSSEOUS DISTRACTION DEVICES

Improvements in technology have permitted staged repairs of midfacial, maxillary, and mandibular defects. Osseous distraction is a technique that has been developed over the past 10 to 15 years. Ilizarov (1990) first reported the use of distraction osteogenesis induced by placement of an external fixator to permit proper growth and alignment in long bones. The technique applies tension to distract bone and stimulate new bone formation in a slow progressive nature. The goal is to stimulate soft tissue and bony changes in the craniofacial skeleton. This technique can be applied to the mandible, the maxilla, or the frontal region of the skull. The surgeon performs an osteotomy, usually through one cortex of a bony area that needs to be expanded. Pins are then set on both sides of the osteotomy and a distraction device is applied to the pins. Slow (1 mm/day) distraction tension is applied to stimulate bony formation in the region of the osteotomy. Because the slow tension is also applied to the soft tissues, this facilitates soft tissue mobilization as well. The method is particularly useful in children who have hypoplastic mandibles or hypoplastic midfaces.

After the desirable distraction has been obtained over weeks or months, the device is left in position for several months to allow the bone, which has been formed, to consolidate and create a solid union across the osteotomy site. Once consolidation is completed, the patient is brought back to the operating room (or, for older patients, the office) and the distraction device is removed under anesthesia or intravenous sedation. Devices can be placed externally, like an external fixator (Fig. 20–7; see Color Plates, DVD), or internally, buried under the skin. Some of these devices can be very cumbersome, consisting of a head frame with bars extending in front of the patient's face.

The larger head frame devices pose a real challenge for the anesthesiologist as airway management, including intubation, can be quite difficult. After the procedure, swelling around the osteotomy sites may be present but resolves over 24 to 48 hours.

Although helpful in improving surgical results and reducing the risk of repeat major operations, these devices pose potential and real postoperative risks to the patient, as well as nursing challenges. Admission to the intensive care unit (ICU) should be planned ahead of time and postoperative management discussed with the ICU staff. Often, the surgical repair involves wire fixation of the maxilla and mandible, producing a "locked jaw with clenched teeth" that cannot be opened easily. The patient's airway may or may not be patent via the nasal route. Children often mouth breath through teeth clenched in place. Emergent care and access to the airway may require cutting the wires to open the mouth. In these children, wire cutters should be readily available (taped to the bedside). However, this maneuver poses its own risks because of an unstable midface or mandible. Furthermore, if disturbed during routine or emergent care, the metal parts may cause bleeding from areas that are difficult to see and control. Initial postoperative care must be provided in the pediatric ICU. In addition, the anesthesiologist or intensivist should be available and be familiar with the use of equipment to secure a patent airway (e.g., transtracheal jet ventilation, cricothyrotomy, and management of the difficult airway).

Complications that can occur with the distraction devices include infections along pin sites and mobilization of the pins prior to the completion of the distraction, making it necessary to remove them prematurely. In addition, patients must live with these devices for weeks to months, creating possible psychological problems for them at home and school. Osseous distraction of the facial skeleton has been a very popular and successful technique. It is most often useful in children who have a hypoplastic mandible, midface, or both.

SPECIAL CONSIDERATIONS FOR PIERRE ROBIN SEQUENCE

The syndrome of micrognathia and glossoptosis and cleft palate is known as the Pierre Robin sequence (Robin, 1934). Because of the anatomic anomalies, infants often present with respiratory distress shortly after birth. Because of the small mouth cavity and relatively large tongue, the infant can experience partial or profound airway obstruction. In most infants, airway patency can be achieved through changes in the position of the head and neck in relation to the body. Often, placement in the

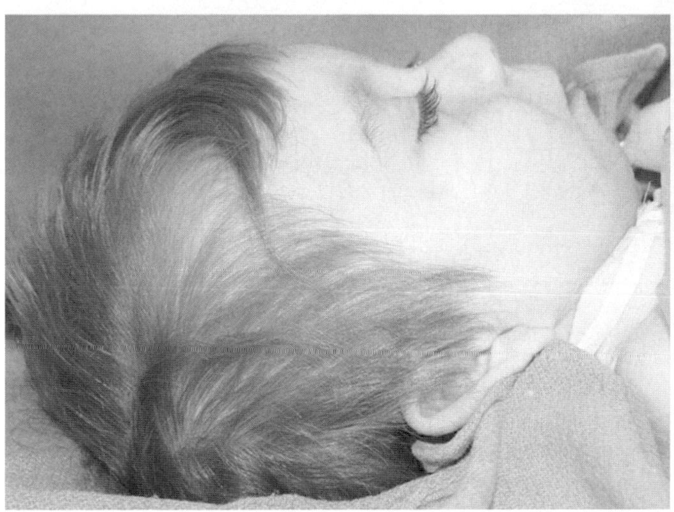

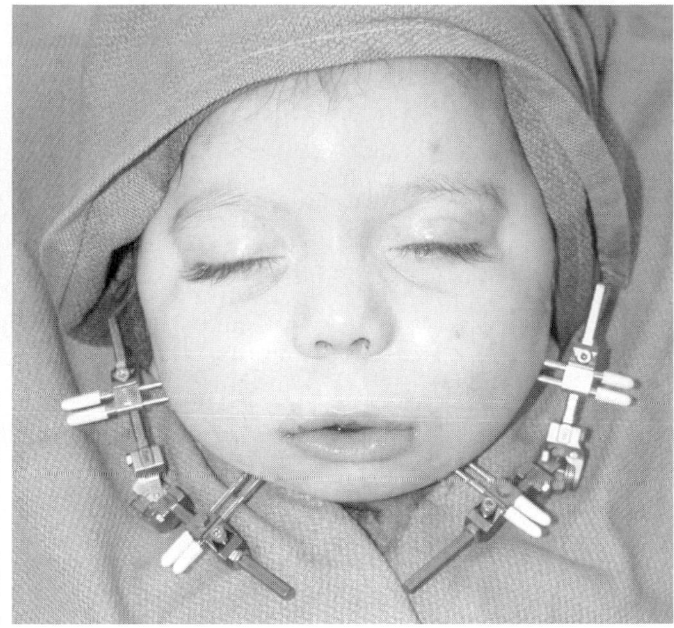

A B

■ **FIGURE 20–7.** *A*, Infant with Pierre Robin sequence. *B*, External fixation of the midface following surgery for repair in a patient with Pierre Robin sequence. (See Color Plates, DVD.)

prone position relieves the barrier to airflow. The placement of a nasopharyngeal airway may permit the child to breath relatively normally and provides a temporizing intervention. The airway problems are less likely to be life threatening with age and usually, after 6 months of age, are not a cause of significant concern (Benjamin and Walker, 1991). On occasion, the obstruction is severe enough to require urgent intubation and, possibly, surgical intervention. Airway management may be extremely difficult in these children because of the distorted anatomy related to the small jaw, the large tongue, and cleft palate.

Children with Pierre Robin sequence may present in the neonatal period for tracheostomy if the mandibular hypoplasia is severe. More commonly, these patients present later in infancy or toddlerhood for corrective surgery of the cleft palate and for mandibular reconstruction. Anesthetic considerations in these children are similar to those undergoing cleft palate repair (see later). Children with Pierre Robin sequence who undergo mandibular reconstruction with an osseous distraction device are susceptible to the same perioperative issues discussed earlier.

■ CLEFT LIP AND CLEFT PALATE REPAIR

Cleft lip and cleft palate may occur together or separately (Westmore and Willging, 1996). Cleft lip with or without cleft palate occurs in 1:1000 births; cleft palate alone occurs in approximately 1:2500 births. The syndrome of cleft lip (with or without cleft palate) is more common in males, whereas isolated cleft palate is more common in females. In addition to the lip and palate abnormalities, these patients have a higher incidence of other congenital malformations (Table 20–1). Middle ear disease is extremely common in patients with cleft palate (Stool and Randall, 1967). Siblings and offspring of persons who have cleft palate or cleft lip are also at greater risk of having one or the other.

The cleft lip deformity may be as mild as a small defect in the vermilion border or may manifest as much as a complete separation that involves the nasal floor. The clefts may be unilateral or bilateral and may involve the alveolar ridge (Fig. 20–8; see Color Plates, DVD). In addition, associated dental abnormalities may also be seen. Cleft palate may occur as an isolated deformity or in association with cleft lip. Isolated cleft palate is commonly a midline defect involving simply the uvula or may manifest more extensively as a defect of the soft and hard palates. If cleft lip is associated, the cleft palate defect may expose either one or both of the nasal cavities to the oral cavity. Such obvious defects of the upper airway predispose the child to difficulties in swallowing and repeated aspiration and pulmonary infection.

Before surgery, the clinical management is aimed at reducing the chance of aspiration and pulmonary compromise by feeding these infants in an upright position with either an infant or a "premie" nipple. The Haberman nipple is the most successful for feeding these children because the child does not have to generate suction to get the fluid from the nipple. In some situations, it may be appropriate to feed the child through a nasogastric tube. However, this is less than ideal. The anesthesiologist should know if there is or has been pulmonary compromise. In addition, any associated congenital anomalies should be noted.

Anesthesia may be induced via mask or intravenous techniques. In general, the more severe the cleft palate, the less chance there is for airway obstruction; in patients with hypoplastic mandibles or cleft palates wide enough that the tongue can

■ **TABLE 20–1.** Congenital anomalies associated with cleft lip with or without cleft palate

Frequent	Occasional
Fetal hydantoin syndrome	Cri du chat syndrome
Mohr syndrome	Larsen's syndrome
Fetal trimethadione syndrome	Facioauriculovertebral anomalad
Orofaciodigital syndrome	Meckel-Gruber syndrome
Roberts' syndrome	Oculodentodigital syndrome
Trisomy 18 syndrome	Trisomy 18 syndrome
4 p-syndrome	Waardenburg's syndrome

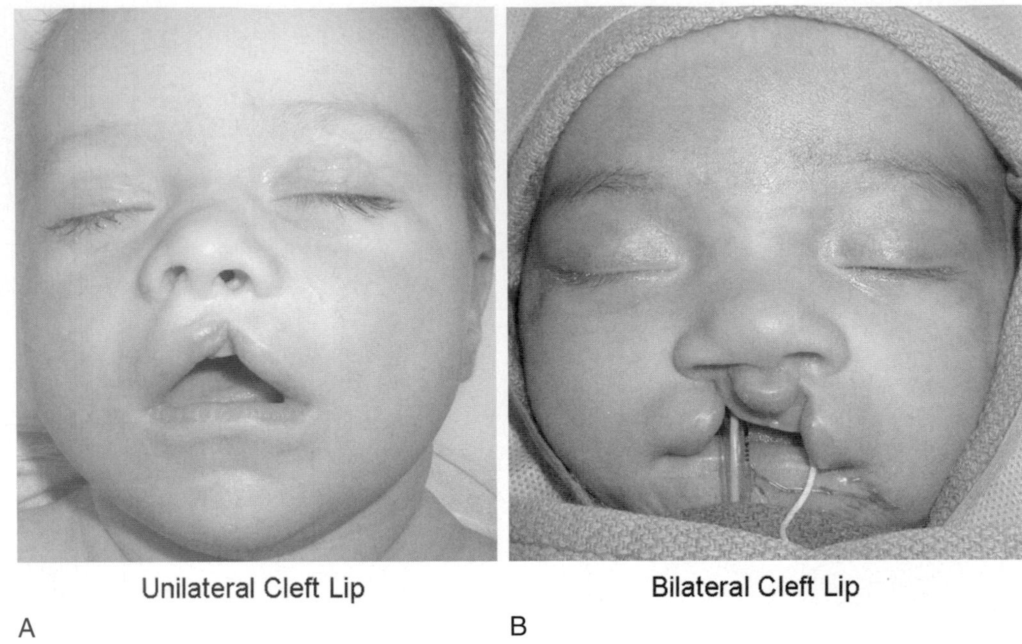

■ **FIGURE 20–8.** Infants with single or unilateral *(A)* and double bilateral cleft lip *(B)*. Presence of the clefts, especially with the free premaxilla and double cleft, makes intubation difficult. (See Color Plates, DVD.)

prolapse into the nasopharynx, airway obstruction can occur and pose a significant problem during the induction of anesthesia. With adequate preparation and experience in caring for these children, induction of anesthesia and endotracheal intubation can be performed quite safely. After induction, endotracheal intubation can proceed with the placement of an appropriately sized oral RAE endotracheal tube. After proper intratracheal positioning is confirmed, the tube may be secured with benzoin and taped to the middle chin. Ventilation during the procedure may be assisted or mechanically controlled. Before surgery begins, the eyes should be securely taped shut to prevent trauma or other damage.

Maintenance of anesthesia may be accomplished using inhalation agents alone or in combination with opioids. Nondepolarizing muscle relaxants may decrease the total amount of volatile anesthetics needed (Fogdall and Miller, 1975). The duration of the repair is usually 60 to 120 minutes.

Before beginning the repair, the surgeon places a throat pack in the posterior portion of the pharynx. In addition, a Dingman gag is used in cleft palate repair to hold the mouth open during surgery (Fig. 20–9; see Color Plates, DVD). This apparatus contains a groove in which the endotracheal tube should sit without being occluded. Malposition of the gag in relation to the endotracheal tube, however, can lead to partial or complete obstruction of the tube. The anesthesiologist must be particularly aware of the breath sounds and chest compliance during placement and manipulation of the gag. Cleft lip repair is associated with only modest amounts of blood loss. The repair of cleft palate, however, may be associated with moderate bleeding, but rarely is there a need for blood transfusion.

After the repair is complete, the inhalation anesthetics are discontinued and the child is allowed to emerge from anesthesia. If muscle relaxants have been used, appropriate reversal is accomplished with neostigmine (0.07 mg/kg) or edrophonium (1.0 mg/kg), and atropine (0.02 to 0.03 mg/kg) or glycopyrrolate (0.01 mg/kg). When the child exhibits good spontaneous ventilation, a negative inspiratory force of −30 cm H_2O or greater, and a good leg or head lift, he or she can be safely extubated. Any posterior pharynx throat pack must be removed and an oropharyngeal airway may be inserted before extubation. In addition, the oropharynx should be suctioned to remove pooled blood or secretions. The patient should be fully awake before extubation, because partial or complete upper airway obstruction with soft tissue is common after repair of cleft palate. After the child has been extubated, he or she is placed in the lateral position to optimize air movement and to minimize the chance of aspiration. Usually, nasal passages are blocked postoperatively, and

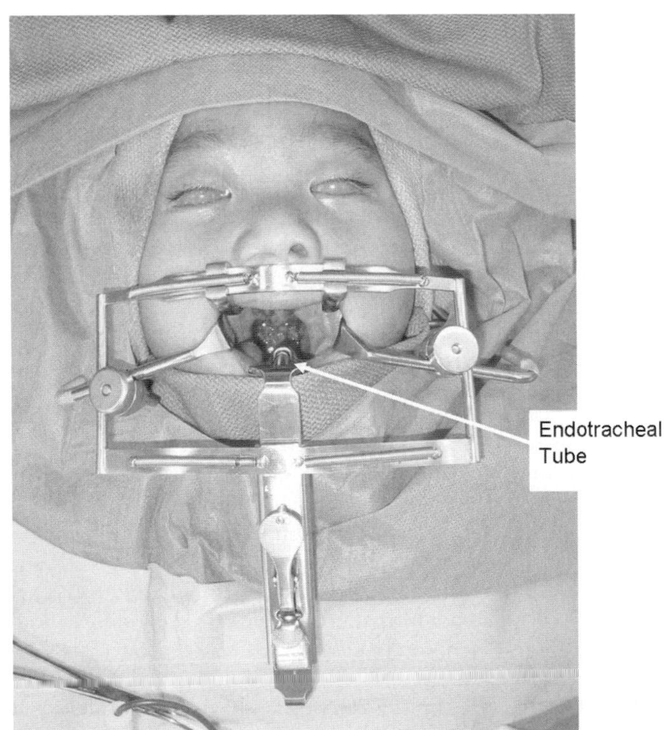

■ **FIGURE 20–9.** Management of cleft palate repair. Tongue blade of Dingman gag holds endotracheal tube in place and provides exposure for the surgeon. Eyes are covered with scleral shields for protection. (See Color Plates, DVD.)

the infant may experience difficulty breathing through the mouth before readjusting to oral breathing.

In the postoperative period, arm restraints, which prevent elbow flexion, are routinely used to keep the child's hands away from the child's face. Care should be taken to provide adequate fluid therapy to maintain hydration. In addition, the child may experience further bleeding from the operative site, particularly if a cleft palate has been repaired. More important, partial or complete airway obstruction may occur because of mucosal swelling in the hypopharynx. Use of a mouth gag is the most frequent cause of postoperative tongue swelling, and the degree and frequency of swelling appear to be associated with the duration of tongue compression by the mouth gag blade. Other causes of postoperative airway obstruction include subglottic edema, flap edema, increased oral secretion, posterior displacement of the tongue, and an overlooked throat pack. The child should be closely monitored for at least the first 24 hours.

Children who have undergone cleft palate repair may develop difficulty with speech during the toddler years. Although most children have satisfactory speech patterns, some may manifest velopharyngeal incompetence. These children should be evaluated aggressively with the use of speech recordings, airflow studies, video fluoroscopy, and endoscopy. If velopharyngeal incompetence is diagnosed, surgery may be indicated, as this condition does not resolve with nonsurgical treatment. Velopharyngeal incompetence can be treated by various surgical options, including complete revision or re-repair of the palate deformity, a pharyngeal flap, or a sphincter pharyngoplasty. The superiorly based pharyngeal flap is commonly performed when the lateral wall motion is good to excellent (Fig. 20–10). The flap is elevated down to prevertebral fascia and up to the base near the midpoint of the tonsillar fossa. The palate is split and the nasal mucosa dissected into two posterior flaps. Any operation on the palate can cause edema and potential airway obstruction.

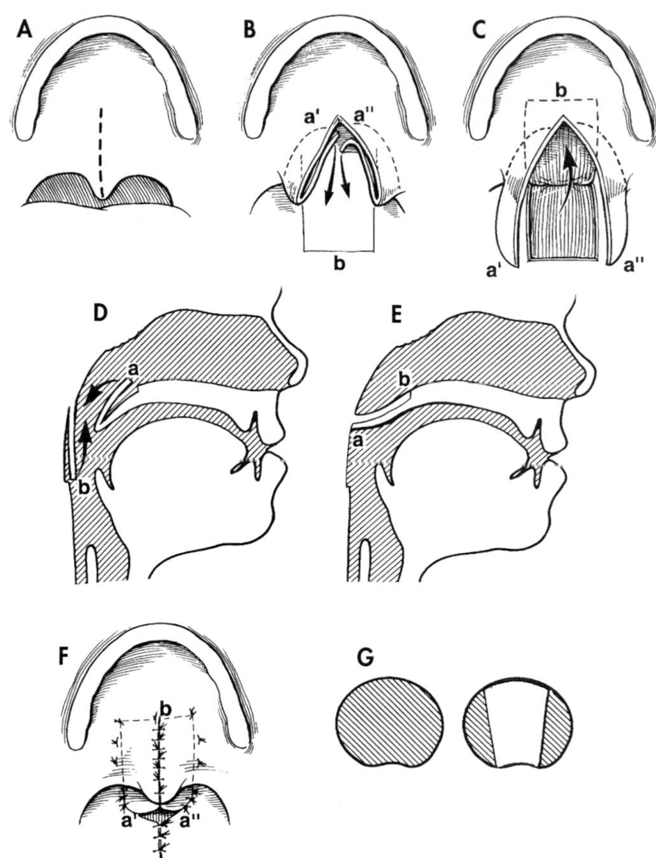

■ **FIGURE 20–10.** The superior velopharyngeal flap. The soft palate is divided *(A)* and the nasal layer flaps are dissected *(B)*. The flap is elevated and attached to the nasal aspect of the soft palate *(C)*. The nasal layer flaps *(a)* and the pharyngeal flap *(b)* are approximated *(D)* and the soft palate is closed *(E)*. *F* shows the relative positions of the pharyngeal and nasal flaps. The relative position of the pharyngeal flap in the pharynx is shown in *G*. (Adapted from Johnson P, Pirruccello FW: Surgical repair of cleft lip and palate. In Pirruccello, editor: *Cleft lip and palate plastic surgery: Genetics and the team approach.* FW Charles C Thomas, 1987. Courtesy of Charles C Thomas Publisher, Ltd., Springfield, IL.)

The sphincter pharyngoplasty may be performed in patients who have poor lateral pharyngeal wall movement but good motility of the palate (Hofer et al., 2002). The procedure involves elevating the posterior faucial pillars with the underlying muscles. In addition, a transverse incision is made. The medial walls of the faucial flaps are sutured to the superior aspect of the posterior wall incisions. Subsequently, the lateral edges of the flap are sutured closed to reduce the velopharyngeal defect. Stumps of the palatal pharyngeous muscles are sutured closed. Such a procedure again involves a posterior oral pharynx and involves extensive soft tissue dissection. The airway patency during the immediate postoperative period is of great concern to the anesthesiologist.

The anesthetic management and the approach to the airway during surgery for velopharyngeal incompetence are similar to those in the child with a primary cleft palate. Postoperative problems specific to the child with a pharyngeal flap and sphincter pharyngoplasty include possible airway obstruction because of swelling of the oropharynx, intraoral bleeding, and obstruction or aspiration of blood. Postoperative coughing on emergence may increase venous pressures and the chance of postoperative bleeding. Great caution should be used to minimize the chance of postoperative coughing and vomiting. The child must be closely monitored, usually overnight, as with primary closure.

■ SUMMARY

Plastic surgery in infants and children is primarily aimed at repairing anomalies of bony growth—primarily of the head and face. Surgical procedures are aimed at relieving airway obstruction and modeling the bones and soft tissues of the skull and face so that they grow and develop normally. Anesthetic management of these patients is challenging for many reasons, including the presence of airway abnormalities and perioperative airway compromise, massive intraoperative bleeding and coagulopathies, and potentially difficult postoperative course. Proper care of these infants requires a knowledgeable anesthesia care team as part of the whole craniofacial team.

REFERENCES

Bedford RF, Marshall WK, Butler A, Welsh JE: Cardiac catheters for diagnosis and treatment of venous air embolism: A prospective study in man. *J Neurosurg* 55:610–614, 1981.

Benjamin B, Walker P: Management of airway obstruction in the Pierre Robin sequence. *Int J Pediatr Otorhinolaryngol* 22:29–37, 1991.

Brecher ME, Rosenfeld M: Mathematical and computer modeling of acute normovolemic hemodilution. *Transfusion* 34:176–179, 1994.

Bunegin L, Albin MS, Hesel FE, et al.: Positioning the right atrial catheter: A model for reappraisal. *Anesthesiology* 55:343, 1981.

Chiaretti A, Pietrini D, Piastra M, et al.: Safety and efficacy of remifentanil in craniosynostosis repair in children less than 1 year old. *Pediatr Neurosurg* 33:83–88, 2000.

Clausen T, Bullock R: Medical treatment and neuroprotection in traumatic brain injury. *Curr Pharmaceut Design* 7:1517–1532, 2001.

Cushing H: Some experimental and clinical observations concerning states of increased intracranial tension. *Am J Med Sci* 124:375, 1902.

D'Errico CC, Munro HM, Buchman SR, et al: Efficacy of aprotinin in children undergoing craniofacial surgery. *J Neurosurg* 99:287–290, 2003.

Dishart MK, Schlichtig R, Tonnessen TI, et al.: Mitochondrial redox state as a potential detector of liver dysoxia in vivo. *J Appl Physiol* 84:791–797, 1998.

Fogdall RP, Miller RD: Neuromuscular effects of enflurane, alone and combined with d-Tubocurarine, pancuronium, and succinylcholine, in man. *Anesthesiology* 42:173–178, 1975.

Fontana JL, Welborn L, Mongan PD, et al.: Oxygen consumption and cardiovascular function in children during profound intraoperative normovolemic hemodilution. *Anesth Analg* 80:219–225, 1995.

Haberkern M, Dangel P: Normovolaemic haemodilution and intraoperative auto-transfusion in children: Experience with 30 cases of spinal fusion. *Eur J Plastic Surg* 1:30–35, 1991.

Handler SD: Upper airway obstruction in craniofacial anomalies: Diagnosis and management. *Birth Defects Orig Artif Ser* 21:15–31, 1985.

Heeckt P, Muhlbauer W, Anderl H, et al: Early radical treatment of pancraniofacial synostosis. *Ann Plastic Surg* 30:312–319, 1993.

Hofer SO, Dhar BK, et al.: A 10-year review of perioperative complications in pharyngeal flap surgery. *Plast Reconstr Surg* 110:1393–1397, 2002; discussion 1398–1400, 2002.

Ilizarov GA: Clinical application of the tension-stress effect for limb lengthening. *Clin Orthop* 250:8–26, 1990.

Panfilov DE: MIDI face-lift and tricuspidal SMAS-flap. *Aesthetic Plast Surg* 27:27–37, 2003.

Rabinovitch M: Pulmonary hypertension. In Adams FH, Emmanouilides CC, Riemenschneider TA, editors: *Moss' heart disease in infants, children, and adolescents,* 4th ed. Baltimore, 1989, Williams & Wilkins.

Robin P: Glossoptosis due to atresia and hypotrophy of the mandible. *Am J Dis Child* 48:541–547, 1934.

Rosen CL: Obstructive sleep apnea syndrome (OSAS) in children: Diagnostic challenges. *Sleep* 19:S274–S277, 1996.

Siddiqi SN, Posnick JC, Buncic R, et al.: The detection and management of intracranial hypertension after initial suture release and decompression for craniofacial dysostosis syndromes. *Neurosurgery* 36:703–708, 1995; discussion, 708–709, 1995.

Souder JE: Pulmonary air embolism. *J Clin Monit Comput* 16:375–383, 2000.

Stool SE, Randall P: Unexpected ear disease in infants with cleft palate. *Cleft Palate J* 4:99–103, 1967.

Turvey TA, Bell RB, Tejera TJ, Proffit WR: The use of self-reinforced biodegradable bone plates and screws in orthognathic surgery. *J Oral Maxillofac Surg* 60:59–65, 2002.

Valbonesi M, Giannini G, Migliori F, et al.: The role of autologous fibrin-platelet glue in plastic surgery: A preliminary report. *Int J Artif Organs* 25:334–338, 2002.

Westmore RF, Willging JP: The oral cavity and oropharynx. In Rudolph AM, Rudolph JIE, Rudolph CD, editors: *Rudolph's pediatrics,* 20th ed. Stanford, CT, 1996, Appleton & Lange, pp 962–964.

Williams GD, Ellenbogen RG, Gruss JS: Abnormal coagulation during pediatric craniofacial surgery. *Pediatr Neurosurg* 35:5–12, 2001.

21 Anesthesia for Pediatric Orthopedic Surgery

Aaron L. Zuckerberg • Myron Yaster

Anesthesia for pediatric orthopedic surgery encompasses the entire age and medical spectrum of pediatrics. It includes the newborn and the adolescent, the otherwise normal, the chronically ill, the patient with multiple complex congenital anomalies, the emergent trauma patient, and the elective inpatient and outpatient. Orthopedic surgeons operate on virtually every area of the body from the cervical spine to the pelvis to the toes. In many instances, the perioperative anesthetic plan for pediatric orthopedic patients depends more on the child's age and on the site and emergent nature of surgery than on the underlying disease or the specifics of the surgical procedure. In other cases, the underlying medical condition, associated anomalies, pathophysiology, and surgical procedure dictate the anesthetic plan. Frequently, the anesthesiologist must be aware of unusual associated syndromes that have obvious orthopedic implications and syndromes with underlying clinical significance unrelated to the orthopedic condition. Table 21–1 lists conditions that are commonly encountered in pediatric orthopedic surgery and describes their anesthetic implications.

A common feature of children with orthopedic diseases, particularly patients with congenital anomalies, generalized constitutional diseases of bone and cartilage, or connective tissue disorders, is the significant disability that affects their everyday lives. Some of these children must undergo repeated hospitalization and may require multiple anesthetics and surgical procedures. These children may have overwhelming fear and apprehension, and they may be completely terrorized by the hospital experience ("hospitalitis"). Simply approaching these children in hospital clothing may elicit screams of terror. Others, with diseases such as cerebral palsy, may be of normal intelligence but are often treated as if they were mentally incapacitated because of their inability to communicate clearly. The approach to the orthopedic patient must be individualized.

Orthopedic surgery is among the most common types of surgery performed in the United States. Technological advances permit more sophisticated orthopedic diagnoses, and they have vastly expanded the range of treatment options and operations available to the orthopedic surgeon. The technological, physiologic, and pharmacologic advances in anesthesiology have allowed the orthopedic surgeon to contemplate longer, more extensive, and more innovative operations on younger and sicker patients than was ever before possible. Regardless of the underlying condition, almost all orthopedic surgical procedures have recurring anesthetic concerns, including positioning, airway management, blood loss and fluid replacement, conservation of body temperature, and postoperative pain management. The anesthesiologist must have knowledge of the particular surgeon, the operation, the positioning of the patient, and the duration of the procedure.

■ SCOLIOSIS

Scoliosis, derived from the Greek root meaning "crooked," is a lateral and rotational deformity of the thoracolumbar spine. With progression of the lateral spinal curvature, the spinous processes rotate toward the concave side of the curve. The ribs on the convex side are pushed posteriorly by the rotating spine, forming the characteristic gibbous deformity. The ribs on the concave side become prominent anteriorly and are crowded together. Occasionally, scoliosis is associated with kyphosis (Fig. 21–1).

TABLE 21–1. Anesthetic implications of commonly encountered orthopedic disorders

Disease	Surgical Interventions	Anesthetic Implications
Congenital Malformations		
Amniotic band constriction	Soft tissue release	May have facial clefts
Clubfoot	Tendon lengthening, release	Dictated by associated malformations
Klippel-Feil syndrome	Release, scoliosis	Limited C-spine mobility, heart defects
Radial dysgenesis	Tendon lengthening, pollicization release	Dictated by associated malformations
Sprengel's deformity		Only associated Klippel-Feil syndrome
Acquired Conditions		
Charcot-Marie-Tooth disease	Tendon transfer	None known
Legg-Calvé-Perthes disease	Osteotomies, pinning	As per associated diseases (sickle cell)
Osteomyelitis	Culture, aspiration	Systemic bacterial infection
Septic arthritis	Culture, irrigation	Systemic bacterial infection
Slipped femoral capital epiphysis	Pinning	Obesity
Tumors		
Benign	Excision, curettage	Blood loss may be significant, pathologic fracture
Malignant	Radical excision, amputation	Blood loss; metastasis: CNS, lung; chemotherapy cardiotoxicity
Syndromes, Inherited Conditions		
Apert's syndrome	Syndactyly repair	Airway usually normal, occasional cardiac defect
Ellis-van Creveld syndrome	Polydactyly	Cardiac defects, bronchial collapse
Holt-Oram syndrome	As in radial dysgenesis	Cardiac defects (ASD, VSD)
Marfan syndrome	Kyphosis	Cardiac defects (AI, MR), aortic aneurysm
Moebius sequence	Syndactyly	Micrognathia, cleft palate, cranial nerve palsy
Osteogenesis imperfecta	Pathologic fractures, scoliosis	Fractures on positioning or intubation; hypermetabolic fever, platelet dysfunction
VATER association	As in radial dysgenesis	Cardiac defects, tracheoesophageal fistula
Dwarfism		
Achondroplasia	Spinal fusion, decompression	Poor cervical mobility, restrictive lung disease
Morquio-Ullrich disease	C-spine fusion	Unstable C-spine, restrictive lung disease
Systemic Disease		
Juvenile rheumatoid arthritis	Varies	TMJ ankylosis, C-spine immobility or instability, carditis, occasional pulmonary involvement
Neurofibromatosis	Scoliosis	CNS tumors, occasional pheochromocytoma
Sickle cell anemia	Osteomyelitis, Legg-Calvé-Perthes disease, pathologic fracture	Anemia, sickle crisis: hypothermia, hypoxia, hypovolemia, avoid tourniquet when possible
CNS Diseases		
Arthrogryposis multiplex	Releases, scoliosis	TMJ ankylosis, C-spine immobility, GE reflux, postoperative upper airway obstruction
Cerebral palsy	Releases	GE reflux, postoperative upper airway obstruction
Myelomeningocele	Lower extremity tendon releases	Hydrocephalus
Werdnig-Hoffmann disease	Scoliosis	Respiratory insufficiency, bulbar involvement—poor secretion handling, succinylcholine-induced hyperkalemia
Myopathies		
Duchenne's muscular dystrophy	Releases, scoliosis	Respiratory insufficiency, cardiomyopathy, succinylcholine-induced hyperkalemia, malignant hyperthermia
Myotonia dystrophica	Releases	Succinylcholine-induced myotonic spasm, cardiac conduction system involvement, avoid direct muscle stimulation

AI, aortic insufficiency; ASD, atrial septal defect; CNS, central nervous system; C-spine, cervical spine; GE, gastroesophageal; MR, mitral regurgitation; TMJ, temporomandibular joint; VSD, ventricular septal defect; VATER association (vertebral defects, imperforate anus, tracheoesophageal fistula, radial and renal dysplasia).

The progression of scoliosis and the severity of its systemic manifestations correlate with the angle of curvature measured by the Cobb method (Table 21–2). This is the angle between the upper surface of the "top-end" vertebra and the lower surface of the "bottom end" vertebra. The end vertebrae are those that are maximally tilted. Perpendicular lines are extended from these end vertebrae to the center of the curve. The angle formed by the intersecting perpendiculars determines the angle of curvature (Fig. 21–2). The curve is defined as facing to the right or to the left, depending on the convexity of the curve. A lateral curve of greater than 10 degrees is abnormal. Respiratory impairment rarely occurs with a curvature of less than 60 degrees.

EPIDEMIOLOGY AND ETIOLOGY

The overall prevalence of spinal deformities in the North American population is between 1% and 2% (Weinstein et al., 2003). In the past, polio or tuberculosis infection was the most common cause

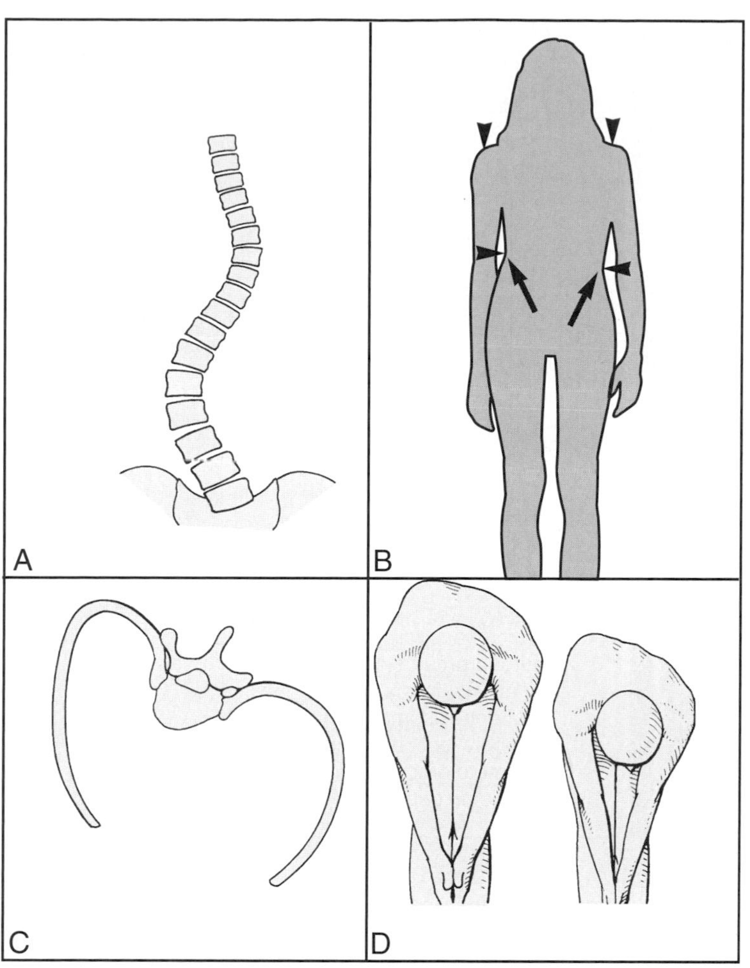

■ **FIGURE 21–1.** Structural changes in idiopathic scoliosis. *A*, As curvature increases, alterations in body configuration develop in the primary and compensatory curve regions. *B*, Asymmetry of shoulder height, waistline, and elbow-to-flank distance are common findings. *C*, Vertebral rotation and associated posterior displacement of the ribs on the convex side of the curve are responsible for the characteristic deformity of the chest wall in scoliosis patients. *D*, In the school screening examination for scoliosis, the patient bends forward at the waist. Rib asymmetry of even a small degree is obvious. (From Scoles PV: Spinal deformity in childhood and adolescence. In Behrman RE, Vaughn VC III, editors: *Nelson textbook of pediatrics*, Update 5. Philadelphia, 1989, WB Saunders.)

of this disease. Today, most cases of scoliosis are classified as idiopathic because the basic pathophysiology remains unknown. Pedigree analysis suggests that scoliosis is a sex-linked trait with variable expression and incomplete penetrance (Xiong and Sevastik, 1998; Lowe et al., 2000). The most common types of scoliosis are listed in Box 21–1.

Congenital scoliosis is a curvature of the spine that is the result of a rib or vertebral anomaly. Idiopathic scoliosis is the most common of the spinal deformities and has three periods of onset, all coincident with periods of rapid growth spurts: infantile (<3 years old), juvenile (3 to 10 years old), and adolescent (>10 years old). Progression of the deformity depends on the age of onset. Infantile idiopathic scoliosis has been associated with an increased incidence of mental retardation, inguinal hernias, congenital dislocation of the hip, and congenital heart disease.

■ **TABLE 21–2.** Correlation of angle of curve and symptoms in patients with scoliosis

Angle of Curvature	Significance
<10	Normal curvature
>25	Echocardiographic evidence of increased pulmonary artery pressures
>40	Surgical intervention
>65	Restrictive lung disease
>100	Symptomatic lung disease, dyspnea on exertion
>120	Alveolar hypoventilation

Juvenile idiopathic scoliosis can usually be managed conservatively (Lowe et al., 2000). Adolescent idiopathic scoliosis is the most common form of scoliosis and occurs most commonly in girls (Weinstein et al., 2003). The curve may resolve, remain stable, or progress in severity. The most significant prognosticators of curve progression in girls are age at onset, premenarchal status, and bone age (Table 21–3) (Ahn et al., 2002; Lowe et al., 2000).

NATURAL HISTORY

The natural history of scoliosis varies according to the cause and the pattern of vertebral involvement. If uncorrected, scoliosis is marked by curve progression, cosmetic deformity, back pain, and compromise of physiologic function (Weinstein et al., 2003). In most cases of idiopathic scoliosis, the spinal curvature remains small, and conservative nonoperative management is appropriate (Ascani et al., 1986). In 0.2% to 0.5% of cases, the curve is progressive and requires surgical intervention (Ahn et al., 2002). In patients with idiopathic scoliosis, only those with thoracic apices and curves of more than 100 degrees are at increased risk of death from cor pulmonale and right ventricular failure (Weinstein et al., 1981). In most patients with idiopathic scoliosis, the grim prognosis of early death and respiratory failure is untrue (Weinstein et al., 1981, 2003). When to perform this surgery is controversial. The worse the curve and the more compromised the cardiorespiratory function, the greater is the risk of perioperative morbidity and mortality.

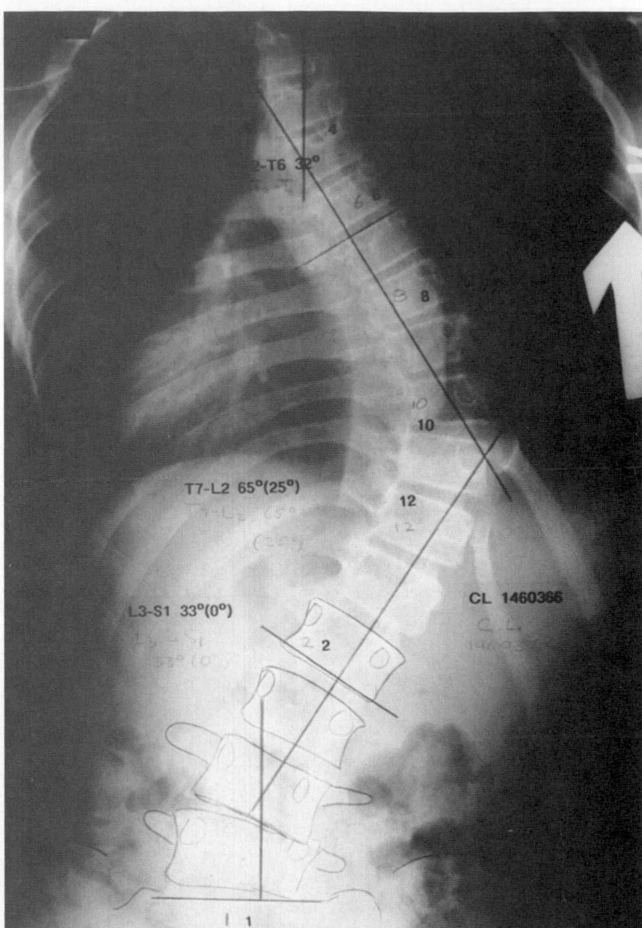

■ **FIGURE 21–2.** Standing posteroanterior radiograph of a 13-year-old girl with a severe right thoracic section. Notice the Cobb measurement technique. The Cobb angle is derived by drawing lines parallel to the superior surface of the proximal-end vertebra and the inferior surface of the distal-end vertebra. Perpendiculars to these lines are erected, and the angle of intersection of these lines is measured. The numbers in parentheses indicate the degree of correction of the deformity on side-bending radiographs. (From Thompson GH: The spine. In Behrman RE, editor: *Nelson textbook of pediatrics*, 16th ed. Philadelphia, 2004, Elsevier.)

BOX 21–1 **Classification of Scoliosis**

Congenital scoliosis
- Vertebral anomalies
- Rib anomalies
- Spinal dysraphism

Idiopathic scoliosis
- Infantile (<3 years of age)
- Juvenile (3 to 10 years of age)
- Adolescent (>10 years of age)

Scoliosis associated with neuromuscular disease
- Cerebral palsy
- Poliomyelitis
- Myopathies
- Muscular dystrophies
- Syringomyelia
- Friedreich's ataxia

Traumatic scoliosis
- Fractures
- Irradiation
- Burns
- Surgery

Syndromes associated with scoliosis
- Neurofibromatosis (von Recklinghausen's disease)
- Marfan syndrome
- Osteogenesis imperfecta
- Mucopolysaccharidosis
- Rheumatoid arthritis

Neoplastic disease

RESPIRATORY SEQUELAE OF SCOLIOSIS

As the degree of curvature progresses, vertebral rotation results in narrowing of the thoracic cage. Lung volumes and pulmonary compliance are inversely related to the degree of this curve. Nevertheless, even asymptomatic patients have demonstrable abnormalities in pulmonary function. When the scoliotic curve is greater than 65 degrees, respiratory function is compromised. Pulmonary function tests demonstrate the characteristic pattern of restrictive lung disease. The vital capacity (normal, 60 mL/kg) is severely reduced, often to less than 60% of predicted. Of the subdivisions of vital capacity, inspiratory capacity is affected to a greater extent than expiratory reserve volume. Functional residual capacity and residual volume are not as severely affected. These alterations in lung volumes are caused by changes in chest wall compliance and the resting position of the thoracic cage, rather than parenchymal changes.

The impairment in pulmonary function occurring in scoliosis from neuromuscular disease is exacerbated by coexisting abnormalities in central respiratory drive, coordination of swallowing, and innervation of the upper airway and respiratory musculature. Pulmonary dysfunction in these patients is exacerbated by the increased frequency of respiratory infections, predilection to aspiration, and impaired ability to clear pulmonary secretions. Patients with abnormal pulmonary function test results, particularly a forced vital capacity (FVC) of less than 50%, or who have hypercapnia preoperatively will probably require postoperative (or chronic) ventilation. Maximum inspiratory and expiratory mouth pressures (PImax, PEmax) that the patient can generate against airway occlusion are the important indices for his or her ability to reexpand the lungs (sighs, PImax < −40 cm H_2O) and to expel secretions (coughs, PEmax > +40 cm H_2O). Unless the patient can generate more than these threshold pressures preoperatively, postoperative admission to the intensive care unit for ventilatory support should be planned ahead of time.

CARDIOVASCULAR SEQUELAE OF SCOLIOSIS

Mitral valve prolapse is found in 25% of patients with scoliosis but in less than 10% of age-matched controls. Echocardiographic evidence for increased pulmonary artery pressures has been demonstrated in individuals with only modest degrees of scoliosis in the absence of abnormal pulmonary function (Primiano et al., 1983). Patients with angles of curvature greater than 70 degrees develop pulmonary hypertension on exercise;

■ **TABLE 21–3.** Incidence of scoliotic curve progression at the time of diagnosis of a 10-degree curve in girls

Age	Menarchal Status	Bone Maturity
<11 years (88%)	Premenarche (53%)	Immature (68%)
>15 years (29%)	Postmenarche (11%)	Mature (18%)

patients with curves greater than 110 degrees have mean pulmonary artery hypertension at rest. Kafer has proposed that this increase in pulmonary vascular resistance is not just the result of lung compression from thoracic cage abnormalities but also an increased incidence of hypoxic pulmonary vasoconstriction (Kafer, 1980; Schur et al., 1984). Rather, development of the pulmonary vascular bed may be impaired, resulting in a fundamental reduction in the number of functional vascular units per lung (Kafer, 1980; Schur et al., 1984).

Any child with a myopathy or borderline respiratory status should have an electrocardiogram and an echocardiogram performed to assess the presence of cor pulmonale, ventricular wall motion, ejection fraction, and ventricular wall thickness. Many myopathies, particularly Duchenne's muscular dystrophy, involve cardiac muscle and skeletal muscle (Milne and Rosales, 1982; Miller et al., 1998). Duchenne's muscular dystrophy is the most common muscular dystrophy occurring in children presenting for surgery. An X-linked recessive disorder, this progressive, debilitating disease affects skeletal, cardiac, and smooth muscle. Typically, afflicted boys become wheel chair dependent by the age of 10 years, and death from respiratory or cardiac failure occurs before the age of 20. Scoliosis is common, and surgery is often performed to improve the quality of life.

Numerous anesthetic challenges occur in patients with Duchenne's muscular dystrophy. Clinically significant cardiomyopathies and rhythm disturbances manifest by 10 years of age (see Chapter 32, Systemic Disorders). Many of these children are obese because of muscle weakness, fatty degeneration of muscle fibers, and lack of exercise. Succinylcholine can cause a fatal hyperkalemia in these patients, who may present for surgery before the diagnosis has been definitively made, and the routine use of this muscle relaxant is no longer recommended in all children (Solares et al., 1986; Sullivan et al., 1994).

PREOPERATIVE EVALUATION

The most important aspects of the preoperative evaluation include determination of the location and degree of the spinal curvature, the cause of the scoliosis, the patient's history of exercise tolerance, respiratory symptoms, and the presence of coexisting diseases. A directed physical examination of the cardiorespiratory system should evaluate the presence of tachypnea, crackles, wheezing, and signs of right heart failure, such as hepatomegaly, jugular venous distention, and peripheral edema. Any preoperative neurologic deficits should be recorded. Based on the severity of the curve and the degree of respiratory impairment, the preoperative laboratory studies listed in Box 21–2 should be requested.

Right heart involvement is reflected in the findings of right ventricular hypertrophy and right axis deviation on the electrocardiogram. Estimates of the degree of pulmonary hypertension may be made by evaluating the right systolic time interval and the velocity of tricuspid regurgitation on the echocardiogram. Pulmonary function tests are useful in establishing the risk of pulmonary complications in the immediate postoperative period. An FVC of less than 30 mL/kg (or less than 50% of predicted) or a forced expiratory volume at 1 second (FEV_1) less than 50% of predicted usually indicates postoperative respiratory insufficiency and the need for prolonged postoperative mechanical ventilation. Peak inspiratory and expiratory forces with the airway occluded of at least −30 cm H_2O and +40 cm H_2O, respectively, are needed for effective sighs and postoperative coughing and expulsion of secretions.

BOX 21–2 Preoperative Tests for Scoliosis Surgery

- Chest radiograph
- Electrocardiogram
- Echocardiogram
- Pulmonary function tests
  - Arterial blood gas
  - Spirometry
    - Forced vital capacity (FVC)
    - Forced expiratory volume at 1 second (FEV_1), FEV_1/FVC
    - Peak expiratory flow rate (PEFR)
    - Peak inspiratory pressure ($P_I max$)
    - Peak expiratory pressure ($P_E max$)
- Coagulation studies
  - Platelet count
  - Prothrombin time, partial thromboplastin time
- Electrolyte panel
- Liver function tests

Children with myelodysplastic syndromes are likely to develop an allergy to latex products (Kelly et al., 1994; Brock-Utne, 2003). All children with a myelodysplastic syndrome should be considered allergic to latex, and nonlatex products (e.g., tourniquets, sterile and nonsterile gloves) should be substituted for the latex equivalents. Corticosteroids and antihistamines are not administered prophylactically.

SURGICAL TECHNIQUES

The treatment of spinal curvature is dictated by the type of scoliosis and by the surgeon's expertise and preferences. Very few cases of congenital scoliosis can be managed conservatively. The mainstay of therapy for congenital scoliosis is posterior spinal fusion without instrumentation, followed by prolonged immobilization. Instrumentation in these patients has been associated with a prohibitively high rate of paraplegia, which is presumed to be the result of coexisting cord and vertebral anomalies. Although conservative therapy is the most frequently employed treatment for idiopathic scoliosis, when rapid curve progression is anticipated, surgical intervention is employed for severe truncal deformities and for pain unrelieved by medical therapy (Weinstein et al., 2003).

Posterior Spinal Fusion

The goal of scoliosis surgery is to achieve a spinal fusion and stabilization of the curve. After incision through the supraspinal ligament, the paraspinous musculature is reflected. The vertebral laminae are decorticated, the facet joints are destroyed, and the spinous processes are removed so that raw cancellous bone is exposed. Bone graft obtained from the iliac crest, ribs on the convex side, or the bone bank is cut into matchstick-sized strips and packed over the decorticated surfaces, mainly on the concave side. The fusion extends from one vertebra above the curve to the second vertebrae below. Instrumentation is usually inserted to hold the spine in the best possible position while fusion is accomplished. Without a properly performed fusion, the instrumentation will ultimately fatigue.

Several instrumentation techniques are available for treatment of the scoliotic spine. The Harrington rod is a stainless steel rod that is connected to the inferior facets and pedicles of the spine by multiple ratchet hooks that are placed at the terminal aspects of the curve. Distraction is adjusted using the ratchet principle (Harrington, 1988; Harrington and Dickson, 1976). The incidence of neurologic complications after this technique is 0.23%. The disadvantages of the Harrington rod include two-dimensional correction, curvature distraction by the end hooks, and the need for prolonged postoperative immobilization. Because of these problems, this technique is rarely used.

Segmental spinal instrumentation was introduced to improve three-dimensional correction and the ability to achieve differential distraction at multiple levels. The Luque instrumentation system consists of sublaminar wires on each side of the spinous process and a long, L-shaped rod that can be contoured three-dimensionally. The curve is corrected as the wires are tightened (Luque, 1986; Luque and Rapp, 1988). The internal fixation achieved is more rigid than that obtained with the Harrington system, and it can be extended to the pelvis. The most common deficit after Luque rod instrumentation is a sensory dysesthesia, which is usually observed late (2 to 6 days) in the postoperative period. The proposed mechanism for these findings is expansion of an epidural hematoma in the area of the sublaminar wires (Johnston, 1986).

The Cotrel-Dubousset segmental spinal instrumentation system uses multiple laminar and pedicular hooks attached to a double-rod frame (Richards and Johnston, 1987). This enables three-dimensional correction of complex curves and obviates the need for postoperative immobilization. It is more time consuming than the Harrington system, increases intraoperative blood loss, and has a lower incidence (0.6%) of neurologic complications than Luque rods. Double-curve patterns are more complex and require multiple hooks at multiple fixation sites, necessitating more extensive decortication and contributing to additional blood loss. The limitation of posterior spinal fusion with or without instrumentation is that the anterior growth plates, which play a major role in the development of the deformity, are not affected. Late torsional deformities can result.

Anterior Spinal Surgery

The anterior approach to spinal deformities has been advocated for several specific deformities, including severe kyphosis and lordotic paralytic curves in patients with cerebral palsy. Surgery consists of discectomies with or without instrumentation, performed alone or in combination with a posterior spinal fusion. Video-assisted thoracoscopic surgery can be used for this procedure if instrumentation is not being used (Newton et al., 1997; Sucato, 2003). The surgical approach used to expose the anterior portion of the spine depends on the exact spinal deformity. Thoracic curves are usually approached through a left thoracotomy, and the procedure is facilitated by insertion of a double-lumen endotracheal tube and one-lung ventilation. Alternatively, single-lung ventilation in young children is performed by advancing a tracheal tube into the main stem bronchus opposite the side of surgery or by positioning a bronchial blocker into the main stem bronchus on the operative side. Multiple techniques for placing a variety of bronchial blockers outside the tracheal tube have been described for use in children (Hammer et al., 1999, 2002) (see Chapter 19, Anesthesia for General, Thoracic, and Urologic Surgery). The combined curve of the thoracolumbar spine is exposed transdiaphragmatically by means of a high subcostal incision that necessitates taking the diaphragm down from its bony insertion. Lumbar curves can be approached extraperitoneally or transabdominally. In general, complications of the anterior approach include great vessel disruption, hemothorax, pneumothorax, paralytic interruption of spinal cord perfusion, and excessive angulation or compression of the spinal cord by rapid distraction of the curvature. Spinal cord injury can result from mechanical damage by a screw or disruption of segmental spinal arteries.

One-Stage versus Two-Stage Anterior-Posterior Spinal Fusion

The combined anterior and posterior spinal fusion maximizes curve correction and minimizes recurrence and pseudoarthrosis formation by obtaining a circumferential fusion. Whether to combine these procedures into a single operation or to perform them in a staged manner is controversial. The staged approach frequently requires prolonged hospitalization and allows recovery from extensive anterior procedures before proceeding with the posterior fusion (Brown et al., 1982). If complications preclude continuation of the staged procedure, premature anterior fusion may compromise the ultimate correction of the curve. A single operation provides recovery that is more rapid, shorter hospitalization, longer operative times, greater blood loss, and possibly more immediate postoperative respiratory complications. O'Brien and others (1992) compared the results of a one-stage versus two-stage anterior-posterior fusion in 26 patients with progressive neuromuscular scoliosis. The mean operative time for the one-stage procedure was 6.6 hours and 7.9 hours for the two-stage procedure. There were no differences in the percentage of curve correction, blood requirements, or postoperative complications between the two groups. However, patients undergoing the one-stage correction experienced a shorter anesthetic time, were extubated more quickly, and required fewer days of hyperalimentation than the two-stage group (Shufflebarger et al., 1991; O'Brien et al., 1992). Overall, the number of intensive care and hospital days was 60% of those for patients undergoing the two-stage repair.

Staged Segmental Scoliosis Surgery

Occasionally, the surgeon and anesthesiologist are confronted by a patient whose physical status precludes a general anesthetic. Dalens and others (1993) reported the successful performance of a staged segmental spinal correction under regional anesthesia. Based on the findings of Rao and others (1990), who demonstrated that the spinal canal can be safely exposed under local anesthesia, epidural or subarachnoid anesthesia was provided over a 3-month period for segmental correction of three to five vertebrae at a time in six patients with American Society of Anesthesiologists (ASA) physical status 4 and with angles of curvature of 75 to 130 degrees. The duration of each procedure was 90 minutes. Neurologic function was evaluated by performing neurologic examination in awake patients and assessing painful sensations and limb mobility. Of 44 regional anesthetics, 13 were epidural, and 31 were subarachnoid. In 14 instances, subarachnoid blockade was achieved after surgical exposure under local anesthesia. The average duration of the procedure was 140 minutes. Bupivacaine and morphine were used in most instances. The administration of 0.125% bupivacaine intrathecally resulted in complete pain relief at the surgical site without any evidence of motor blockade. There were no episodes of respiratory depression in the perioperative period, and patients were discharged from the hospital within 4 days (Dalens et al., 1993; Tobias, 2004).

ANESTHETIC MANAGEMENT OF SCOLIOSIS SURGERY

Monitoring

Dramatic hemodynamic instability and substantial blood and heat loss are the hallmarks of scoliosis surgery. In addition to the monitors routinely used in conducting a pediatric general anesthetic, an indwelling arterial catheter and central venous cannula are recommended. These invasive catheters allow monitoring of beat-beat changes in blood pressure, adequacy of oxygenation, ventilation, and intravascular volume, and they provide a direct route for administering cardiotonic medications. A pulmonary artery catheter may be substituted for a central venous catheter if significant myocardial dysfunction is found during the preoperative cardiac evaluation. Body temperature may decrease during the course of a spinal procedure, and continuous monitoring and meticulous thermoprotective strategies are required to prevent intraoperative hypothermia.

Monitoring Intraoperative Complications

Scoliosis surgery is high-risk surgery. Complications are related to the surgery and prone position and include cardiovascular collapse resulting from extensive blood loss, inadequate venous return, air embolism, or latex anaphylaxis (Weinstein et al., 2003); coagulopathies, acid-base imbalance, and electrolyte disturbances (e.g., hyperkalemia, hypocalcemia) from massive blood transfusions (Lowe et al., 2000); inability to ventilate or oxygenate because of endotracheal tube malposition or obstruction (Xiong and Sevastik, 1998), chest or tracheal compression in the prone position, and pneumothorax or hemothorax resulting from surgery (Ahn et al., 2002); myoglobinuria and renal insufficiency caused by rhabdomyolysis; and visual loss and pressure-point injuries from the prone position (Ascani et al., 1986). Common intraoperative problems and the monitoring used for these problems are described in Table 21–4.

Hypotension and cardiovascular collapse are common during this surgery, making it among the highest-risk procedures performed in pediatric surgery and anesthesia. *Physicians always should presume that hypotension is caused by hypovolemia until proved otherwise.* Other causes are far less common and include latex (or rarely drug) anaphylaxis, anesthetic overdose, pneumothorax or hemothorax (particularly in a single-staged anterior posterior procedure), impaired venous return resulting from the prone position, surgical manipulation, and venous air embolism. Air embolism can occur because the epidural veins are exposed during surgery and are above the level of the heart. The outcome from a massive air embolus is almost uniformly fatal.

Because cardiopulmonary resuscitation is virtually impossible to perform in the prone position, a battle plan to turn the patient supine must be well established and rehearsed. As in any emergency, it is the anesthesiologist's responsibility to declare the emergency and to call for help. Because the surgeon needs time to pack and cover the open wound with sterile towels and adhesive plastic, it is always better to begin the process early, rather than waiting until the last possible moment.

Neurologic Monitoring

Postoperative paralysis or sensory loss is the most devastating and often unpredictable complication of scoliosis surgery (Owen, 1999). Neurologic injury may result from direct injury to the spinal cord or nerves during instrumentation, from excessive traction during distraction, or from compromised perfusion of the spinal cord. Because the ramifications associated with motor deficit are significantly greater than those of sensory deficit, surgically induced paraplegia has always been the major concern of scoliosis surgery.

TABLE 21–4. Potential intraoperative complications during scoliosis repair and precautionary monitoring regimen

Problem	Solution
I. Endotracheal tube malposition in the prone position	A. Securely tape the tube before turning 1. Benzoin 2. Waterproof tape B. After turning prone, 1. Listen to both lung fields; do not allow the stretcher to leave the operating room until satisfied that the tube has not migrated. C. Arterial blood gas determination every hour D. Esophageal stethoscope
II. Alteration in pulmonary compliance in the prone position	A. Arterial blood gas determination every hour B. Proper position on frame, to ensure that the chest can expand unimpeded
III. Alteration in cardiac function in the prone position	A. Proper position on frame, to ensure that venous return is not compromised B. Indwelling arterial catheter C. Central venous catheter
IV. Acute hypovolemia	A. Indwelling arterial catheter B. Central venous catheter C. Bladder catheter D. Two large-bore peripheral intravenous catheters in addition to the central venous catheter
V. Extensive blood loss, often occult	A. Beat-to-beat blood pressure monitoring B. Hemoglobin measurement every hour C. Weigh sponges
VI. Development of coagulopathy	A. Platelet count every 1 to 2 hours B. Prothrombin time, aPTT, and fibrin split products every 2 hours
VII. Electrolyte abnormalities from transfusions	A. Frequent measurement of Na^+, K^+, and ionized Ca^{2+} B. Avoid using "old" packed red blood cells
VIII. Excessive heat loss	A. Core temperature measurements B. Heat conservation (plastic bags; heated, humidified gas) C. Active heating (warm air)
IX. Neurologic injuries	A. Proper positioning, particularly the eyes and elbows (brachial plexus injury) B. Intraoperative neurologic assessment of cord function

Spinal Cord Blood Flow

The organization of the spinal cord blood supply is segmental in a cross-sectional and rostral-caudal fashion (Fig. 21–3). The intrinsic spinal cord vasculature consists of the anterior median and the paired posterior spinal arteries. The vasculature supplying these vessels arises from the segmental arteries of the aorta and branches of the subclavian—the vertebral arteries—and the internal iliac arteries. The solitary anterior median spinal artery runs along the entire length of the cord in the anterior sulcus, giving off penetrating branches that supply the ventral two thirds of the spinal cord. Blood flow in the anterior spinal artery is not continuous throughout its span; instead, the anterior spinal artery functions as an anastomotic channel between the terminal branches of successive radicular arteries. Blood leaving the terminal aspects of these radicular arteries courses upward and downward in the anterior spinal artery. Between adjacent radicular arteries, there are points where blood flows in either direction. The paired posterior spinal arteries, which supply the dorsal third of the cord, also have discontinuous segments and appear more like a plexus of pial vessels than paired arteries.

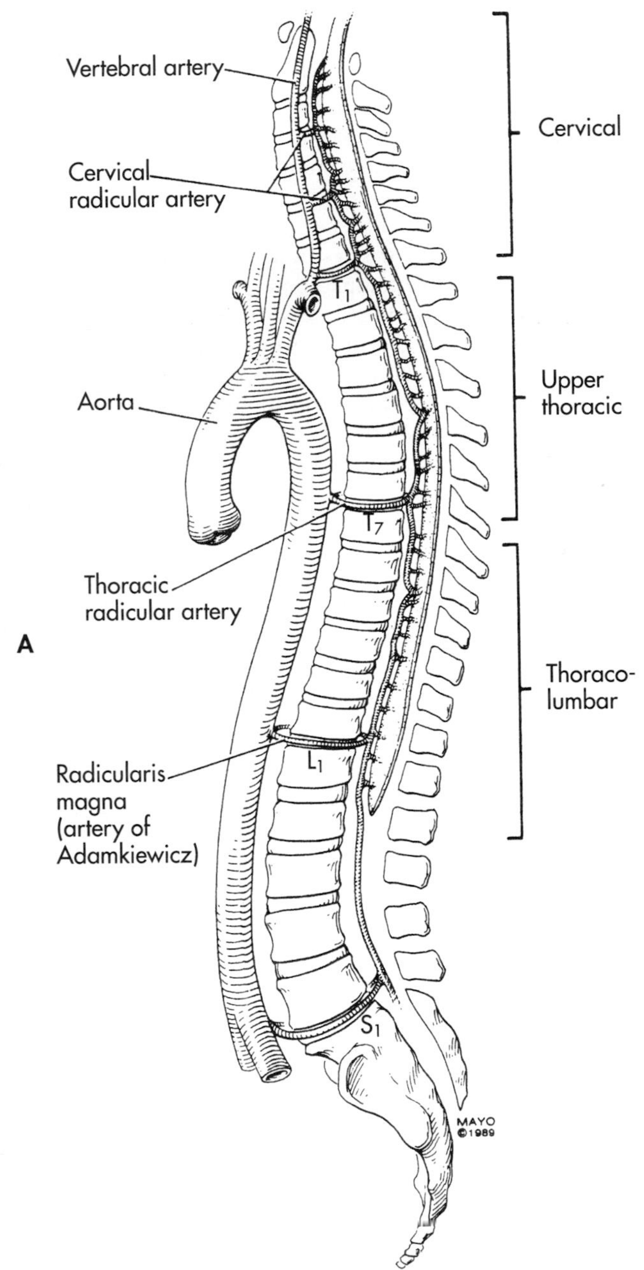

■ **FIGURE 21–3.** The anatomy of blood flow to the spinal cord is distinctive in the vertical and horizontal distributions. *A*, Segmental blood flow along the cord axis.

These three perimedullary vessels give rise to the intramedullary arterial system: the central arteries that supply the gray matter and the deep portions of the white matter and the radial arteries that supply most of the white matter. Nonfunctional anastomotic links exist between the central arterial supply and the radial arterial supply at a given spinal segment. This border zone and the radial circulation appear at highest risk for ischemic insult.

The regional circulation of the spinal cord is divided into four segments. The cervical and lumbosacral regions each receive double the blood flow of the thoracic region (see Fig. 21–3). Although each vertebral level has paired segmental arteries, only six to eight important medullary arteries are formed. These medullary arteries join the spinal arteries. The segmental arteries at all other levels are functionally nonsuppliers of blood to the spinal cord itself. The vertebral arteries form the rostral origins of the anterior and posterior spinal arteries and represent the principal supply to the cervical cord. Branches of the thyrocervical and costovertebral arteries supply the lower cervical and upper thoracic cord. A radicular artery arising from T7 provides perfusion for the middle thoracic cord. The most consistent and important of the anterior medullary arteries is the artery of Adamkiewicz, the arteria radicularis magna, which usually joins the anterior spinal artery between T8 and L3. This artery is the predominate source of blood supply to the lower two thirds of the spinal cord. The implications of this design dictate the clinical manifestations of impaired cord perfusion. Watershed areas, subject to ischemia during low-flow states, exist between the anterior and posterior circulations and between the four different spinal segments. The segments of T4-7 appear to be highly susceptible to injury during periods of hypoperfusion. The dependence of the lower two thirds of the cord on the artery of Adamkiewicz puts this region at particular risk during surgical manipulation of the thoracolumbar aorta and spinal column, the lumbar artery enlargement syndrome. Although the clinical picture of this syndrome is not constant, it is marked by the development of flaccid paraplegia or quadriplegia (depending on the level of the lesion) and dissociated sensory impairment in which heat and pain sensations are affected, while deep sensation is spared.

The same principles that regulate the cerebral blood flow are operative in the control of spinal cord blood flow. As such, cord blood flow depends on the perfusion pressure (i.e., mean arterial pressure or cerebrospinal fluid pressure), integrity of the circulation, microcirculatory autoregulation, and intrinsic regulation. If the perfusion pressure falls below 50 mm Hg, spinal cord blood flow is reduced. Spinal cord blood flow autoregulates within the range of a mean arterial pressure of 60 to 150 mm Hg. Spinal cord blood flow is also regulated on an intrinsic basis in response to arterial oxygen and carbon dioxide tensions, pH, and cord temperature in a fashion identical to that of the cerebral circulation. Hypercapnia increases flow, whereas a PaO_2 below 60 mm Hg results in a vasodilatation that overrides the effects of hypocarbia and autoregulation (see Chapter 18, Anesthesia for Neurosurgery).

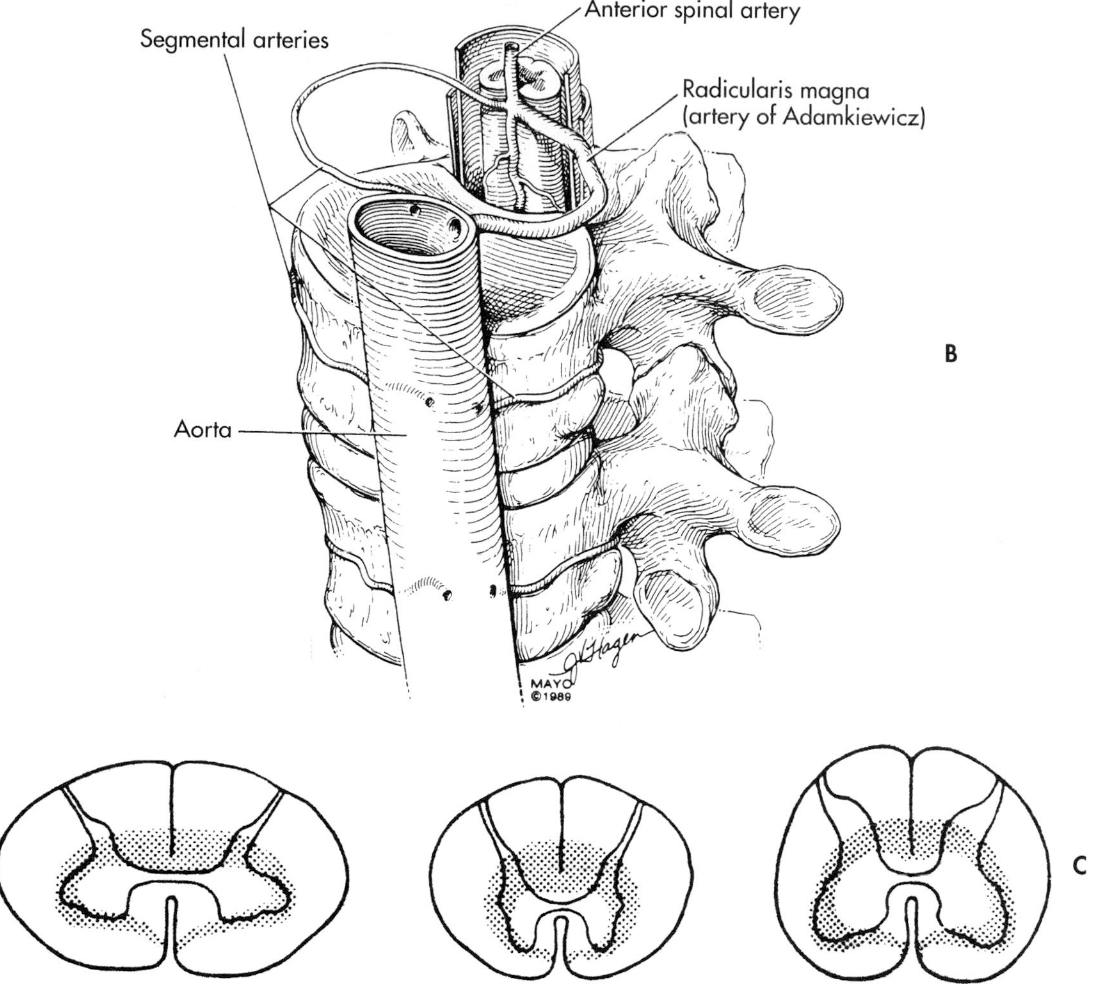

■ **FIGURE 21–3, Cont'd.** *B,* The thoracic cord depends on flow from a number of thoracic radicular arteries, principally the artery of Adamkiewicz. *C,* The cross-sectional distribution of blood flow is distinctive. The outer zone of the cord (white matter) is supplied by the radial arteries; the inner zone (gray and white matter) is supplied by the central arteries. Tissue in the *shaded region* is supplied by both sources. (*A* and *B,* from Cucchiara RF, Michenfelder JD, editors: *Clinical neuroanesthesia.* New York, 1990, Churchill Livingstone; *C,* from Vinken PJ, Bruyn GW, editors: *The handbook of clinical neurology,* vol 12. New York, 1972, North Holland.)

Minimizing Postoperative Neurologic Complications

The estimated risk of postoperative neurologic injury in patients undergoing spinal instrumentation is 0.72% to 1.6% (MacEwen et al., 1975; Dawson et al., 1991; Nuwer et al., 1995; Cervellati et al., 1996). In a study of 7885 patients who underwent instrumentation or fusion without instrumentation, 87 patients developed acute neurologic changes, and 36% of these patients recovered without sequelae. Individuals with nonidiopathic scoliosis are at higher risk for neurologic injury. Children with congenital scoliosis suffer neurologic complications disproportionately (MacEwen et al., 1975; Cervellati et al., 1996).

To minimize the risk of these devastating neurologic injuries, a variety of methods of intraoperative neurologic monitoring have been used. The goal of this monitoring is to identify and herald the onset of neurologic impairment and to provide the surgeon and anesthesiologist with the opportunity to implement appropriate interventions that may minimize permanent damage. These approaches include wake-up tests and the use of neurophysiologic monitoring.

Wake-up Test

Vauzelle and others (1973) first described the use of the wake-up test to assess the integrity of the spinal cord. In this technique, patients are awakened intraoperatively to assess spinal cord motor function. The wake-up test requires an anesthetic that allows rapid recovery of consciousness and motor function. Ideally, the wake-up test should be rehearsed preoperatively. During rehearsal, the patient is informed that he or she will be momentarily awakened at the time of rod insertion to test the function of the spinal cord. Patients must be reassured that they will neither remember the event nor experience pain while they are "awake." Preoperative preparation increases the speed and success of the test.

When a wake-up test is performed, the operating room must be quiet, the surgeon must stop operating, and an observer is positioned (usually under the drapes) to look for foot movement. After discontinuation of the anesthetic, the patient is first asked to move his or her hands ("squeeze my fingers") to evaluate the level of consciousness and then asked to move his or her feet ("wiggle your toes"). If the patient is unable to move his or her feet but can move his or her hands, spinal cord compromise is presumed, and the spinal rod instrumentation is removed immediately. Spinal cord perfusion is maximized by raising the mean arterial blood pressure, increasing the hemoglobin concentration, and normalizing arterial carbon dioxide and oxygen tensions (Vauzelle et al., 1973). In one series of 166 patients in whom the wake-up test was used, 3 patients had demonstrable neurologic deficits when awakened. These deficits disappeared immediately on release of the distracting force (i.e., rods) (Hall et al., 1978; Nuwer et al., 1995).

Hazards associated with the wake-up test include accidental extubation, air embolization produced by deep inspirations, falling off the operating room table, and dislodgment of spinal instrumentation rods and vascular catheters (Ben David, 1988). There are many other limitations to this test. It tests only the anterior spinal cord (motor function) and not the dorsal column (sensory). It requires patient cooperation and has limited use in patients with baseline cognitive dysfunction. The wake-up test provides a snapshot of a single moment of spinal cord function and can realistically be performed only once or twice during a procedure. A spinal injury may be missed because it occurred after the wake-up test was performed. Depending on the anesthesiologist's skill and the anesthetic technique employed, it may take 5 to 45 minutes after a wake-up test is requested by the surgeon before wake-up status can be achieved.

Neurometric Monitoring

Sensory Evoked Potentials. Electrophysiologic (neurometric) monitoring provides a real-time, continuous assessment of spinal cord function and does not require patient movement, arousal, or cooperation (see Chapter 9, Equipment and Monitoring). The most common technique uses somatosensory evoked potentials (SEPs), in which the cortical and subcortical responses to peripheral nerve stimulation are monitored (Nash and Brown, 1989). Typically, a peripheral mixed nerve (i.e., posterior tibial nerve, peroneal nerve, and median nerve) is stimulated at fixed intervals during a procedure. SEPs are recorded repeatedly during surgery, and their amplitude (height) and latency (time of occurrence) are compared with baseline values. Based on changes in these characteristics, it is possible to determine the functional status of the spinal cord sensory tracts. SEP monitoring requires specialized technology and expertise. To resolve the very-low-amplitude evoked potentials from background random or spontaneous cortical activity, computer signal averaging of repetitive sensory responses is required. The processed evoked potential waveform is plotted as voltage against time and is characterized by the post-stimulus latency and amplitude. The post-stimulus latency reflects the time required for impulse transmission from the site of sensory stimulation. A reduction in amplitude of more than 50% or an increase in latency of less than 10% relative to baseline values is generally considered significant.

SEPs monitor only the dorsal columns of the spinal cord and provide no direct evidence of loss of motor function or anterior spinal cord injury. Motor deficits may occur in the absence of alterations in SEPs, and numerous case reports have recorded the postoperative finding of paralysis despite unchanged intraoperative SEPs (i.e., false-negative results) (Lesser et al., 1986). The most comprehensive information regarding the false-negative rate of SEPs comes from a survey of spine surgeons by the Scoliosis Research Society and the European Spinal Deformity Society, in which 342 postoperative neurologic deficits were reviewed from a collection of 33,000 cases. Of these, 28% were not detected by SEP monitoring (Dawson et al., 1991). When SEP monitoring

TABLE 21–5. Effects of anesthetic agents on somatosensory evoked potentials

Agent	Amplitude	Latency
Halothane	↓	↑
Desflurane	↓	↑
Isoflurane	↓	↑
Sevoflurane	↓	↑
Nitric oxide (N_2O)	↓	↔
Barbiturates	↓	↑
Etomidate	↑	↔
Ketamine	↑	↔
Midazolam	↓	↔
Opioids	↔	↔
Propofol	↔	↔

↓, Decreases; ↑, increases; ↔, remains the same.

is equivocal, many recommend an intraoperative wake-up test to assess motor function (Grundy, 1983).

Many pharmacologic and physiologic variables affect the latency and amplitude of SEPS and have been estimated to account for up to 44% of intraoperative SEP changes. The most important of these are the anesthetic agents, blood pressure, and body temperature, and these variables are summarized in Table 21–5 (Grundy et al., 1981; Grundy, 1983). Nitrous oxide has no effect on SEP latency but does decrease its amplitude by 50% (Sloan and Koht, 1985; Lam et al., 1994). All of the potent inhaled anesthetic agents produce dose-dependent increases in latency and decreases in amplitude (Sloan, 1998). Substantial recovery of latency and amplitude are achievable with discontinuance of nitrous oxide and the inhaled vapors (Peterson et al., 1986; Lam et al., 1994; Schindler et al., 1998; da Costa et al., 2001). In a similar fashion, the intravenous anesthetic agents increase SEP latency and decrease amplitude, with the exceptions of midazolam, ketamine, etomidate, propofol, and opioids. Midazolam has no effect on latency (Sloan et al., 1990); ketamine (Schubert et al., 1990; Langeron et al., 1997) and etomidate (Thakor et al., 1991) augment SEP amplitude. Propofol has no effect on amplitude or latency, and it is highly recommended as a component of total intravenous anesthesia for scoliosis surgery (Maurette et al., 1988; Scheepstra et al., 1989; Sloan, 1996, 1998; Rundshagen et al., 2000).

Fentanyl appears to have minimal effect on SEP waveform (Pathak et al., 1983; Kimovec et al., 1990). The amplitude and latency of the waveform are also affected by age, preexisting neurologic deficits, body temperature, $PaCO_2$, hypoxia, and blood pressure (Fig. 21–4) (Grundy, 1983; Lubicky et al., 1989; Sloan, 1996, 1998). The reliability of spinal cord monitoring may be dramatically affected by the variability of the evoked responses. Spontaneous variability in the amplitude and latency of SEP is increased and the amplitude of the waveform diminished during anterior fusions compared with posterior fusions (Grundy, 1983; Lubicky et al., 1989). Muscle relaxants have no direct deleterious effects on the SEP but may produce a more reliable recording by providing "quieter" conditions.

An anesthetic milieu that is compatible with adequate neurometric monitoring and that allows rapid awakening can be created using a variety of approaches. McPherson and others (1985) demonstrated that fentanyl-isoflurane (0.25% to 1.0%) plus oxygen and fentanyl-enflurane (0.25% to 1.0%) plus oxygen preserves SEPs better than fentanyl-nitrous oxide (50%) plus oxygen. Eliminating nitrous oxide appears to be the key

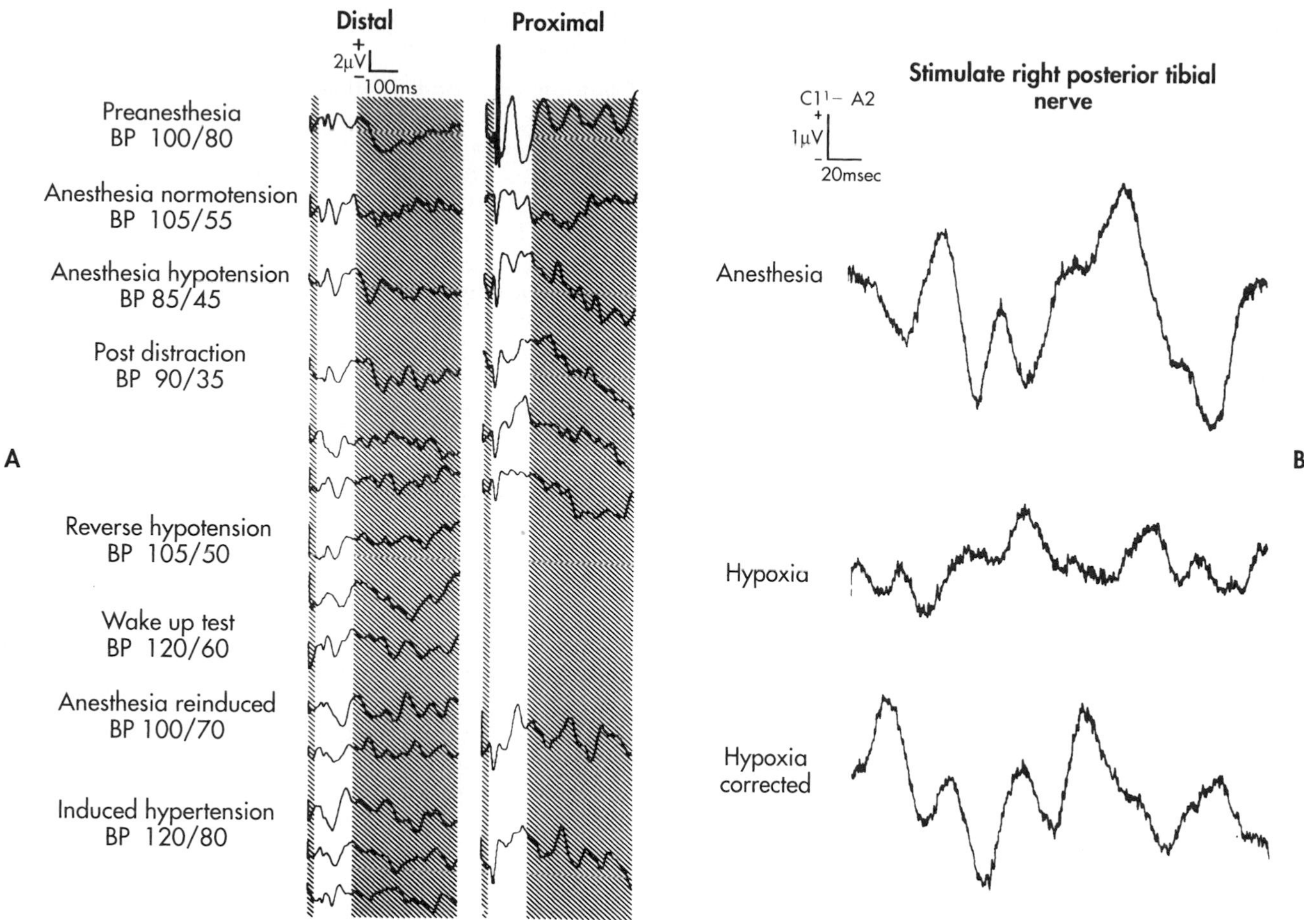

■ **FIGURE 21–4.** Somatosensory evoked potentials (SEPs) change with hypotension and hypoxia. *A,* During the combination of distraction and hypotension, distal SEPs were unchanged. Resumption of normotension restored the SEP to baseline. *B,* SEP responses are exquisitely sensitive to hypoxia (PO_2 = 41 mm Hg). Resumption of normoxia restored the SEP to baseline.

(Kalkman et al., 1991a, 1991b). Substituting desflurane or sevoflurane for isoflurane (or enflurane) and a remifentanil infusion produces ideal SEPs and still allows for rapid wake-up if a wake-up test is required. Alternatively, the physician can substitute a continuous propofol infusion for nitrous oxide or the potent inhaled anesthetics (e.g., desflurane, isoflurane) in combination with an opioid (Kalkman et al., 1991a, 1991b). When using a continuous propofol infusion, some method of titration (i.e., BIS monitor or target-controlled infusion pump) is invaluable to prevent excessive dosing and accumulation of propofol (Gale et al., 2001; Varveris and Morton, 2002). Because etomidate augments SEP amplitude, it is particularly useful in patients with abnormal preoperative SEPs. These individuals are at greatest risk for the development of postoperative neurologic catastrophes (Sloan et al., 1988; Samra and Sorkin, 1991). Pentobarbital at doses sufficient to result in electroencephalographic burst suppression or isoelectricity preserves SEP (Drummond et al., 1987).

Baseline SEP recordings are made after turning the patient to the prone position. After the patient is prone, the anesthetic depth, end-tidal carbon dioxide (CO_2) levels (35 to 45 mm Hg), temperature, and blood pressure (mean arterial pressure > 60 mm Hg) should be maintained to minimize these effects on the SEPs during surgery. Throughout the surgical procedure, a physiologic and pharmacologic steady state must be maintained to effectively use SEPs as monitors of spinal cord function. Deepening the anesthetic depth during critical operative moments when the risk of neurologic compromise is highest must be avoided to minimize the potential for pharmacologically induced false-positive changes. The intraoperative changes of increased latency, decreased amplitude, or complete loss of waveform must be attributed to spinal cord injury rather than an anesthetic-induced effect.

When the baseline is being established, knowledge of the various effects of anesthetic drugs on SEPs can be advantageously used to produce optimal signal acquisition. In the setting of less than optimal baseline SEP acquisition, a strategic change in the anesthetic regimen may result in improvement of the quality of the SEP signal. For example, discontinuing nitrous oxide or desflurane, or both, and substituting an etomidate or propofol infusion can significantly improve SEP acquisition.

Using the criterion of more than 40% amplitude decrease as a significant change, excellent specificity and sensitivity are achievable. In patients with idiopathic scoliosis (i.e., neurologically intact), SEPs are reliable and can be obtained in more than 98% of patients (Dawson et al., 1991; Padberg et al., 1998). However, in patients with preexisting diseases such as neuromuscular scoliosis, the reliability of the SEP is less than 75% but can be improved with the addition of motor evoked potential (MEP) monitoring (Ashkenaze et al., 1993). Precise communication and coordination of efforts among the surgeon, the anesthesiologist, and the neurometric specialist are imperative when a change in SEP is observed. Normalization of the SEPs may occur spontaneously, with relaxation of the distraction instrumentation, or by improving spinal cord perfusion (e.g., increasing blood pressure, arterial carbon dioxide blood levels).

Motor Evoked Potentials. SEPs are not the method of choice for monitoring motor tract function or for detecting the presence of a surgically induced motor deficit. To avoid any type of postoperative neurologic deficit, SEPs should be monitored in conjunction with some other measurement of motor tract function. The most obvious is the use of MEPs. In this technique, direct monitoring of motor function uses myogenic or neurogenic responses (Owen et al., 1988, 1989, 1991; Edmonds et al., 1989; Aglio et al., 2002). The myogenic motor evoked potential (MMEP) relies on direct stimulation of the spinal cord, resulting in an electromyographic response ("twitch") (Owen et al., 1988, 1989, 1991; Owen, 1999). Because a twitch must be elicited, MMEPs necessitate an anesthetic involving no or incomplete neuromuscular blockade (<30% return of twitch height in a train of four). Incomplete paralysis is potentially hazardous during delicate surgical procedures performed on prone patients suspended on positioning frames, particularly if patients are lightly anesthetized.

Alternatively, neurogenic motor evoked potentials (NMEPs) can be used to assess the integrity of the spinal cord motor pathways (Edmonds et al., 1989; Aglio et al., 2002). In this technique, stimulating electrodes are placed percutaneously above the site of operation at the base of adjacent spinous processes, or a magnetic coil is placed over the scalp, stimulating the motor cortex with a magnetic impulse. This results in electrical transmission down the motor nerve tracts. This neural conduction can be recorded from the lateral column of the spinal cord, from the spinal epidural space using percutaneous needles, from the peripheral spinal nerves (e.g., sciatic nerve), and from muscle. The recording of MEPs from muscle has the serious disadvantage of being highly sensitive to all volatile and other anesthetics, muscle relaxants, and several other drugs commonly used in the operating room (Schmid et al., 1992). Anesthetic agents have less of an effect when NMEPs are recorded from the spinal epidural space or peripheral nerves (Owen et al., 1991). Monitoring of NMEPs is difficult because of the efficiency of the central nervous system (CNS) in conducting impulses through the spinal cord and peripheral nerves to muscle groups. These extremely small electrical impulses are difficult to record over the spinal cord or peripheral nerves. Improvement in computer amplification of these signals has overcome many of these technical shortcomings. The motor response elicited from MEPs may be so significant that it may hinder the surgical procedure or move the patient's position on the frame. MEP monitoring is usually used intermittently or at specific points during the surgical procedure when pathways amenable to MEP monitoring are at risk.

Both forms of motor evoked potentials are sensitive to the effects of anesthetics (Herdmann et al., 1996; Sihle-Wissel et al., 2000). Compared with SEPs, the use of MMEPs and NMEPs in the operating room remains in its infancy, and the effects of anesthetic agents on these monitors is unclear and based on studies involving small numbers of patients. All of the potent inhaled vapors produce dose-dependent increases in latency and decreases in amplitude (Yamada et al., 1994). Like the SEPs, amplitudes and latencies of MEPs are significantly affected by nitrous oxide (Sihle-Wissel et al., 2000). Of the four most commonly used intravenous anesthetic agents, continuous infusions of etomidate and methohexital preserve MEP amplitude to a greater extent than thiopental and propofol (Taniguchi et al., 1993).

Choosing the Best Method. The ability to monitor the descending motor pathways is intuitively appealing. Animal studies suggest that MEPs are more sensitive than SEPs in identifying spinal cord compromise. Using an experimental model of overdistraction in hogs, Owen and others (1988, 1991) demonstrated that abolition of NMEP waveforms occurred 4 to 5 minutes earlier than SEP changes and that the wake-up test was positive only 5 to 6 minutes after NMEP changes. In other words, the spinal cord injury can be identified earlier with NMEP than with SEP monitoring, and this early warning occurs before gross evidence for neural dysfunction (i.e., wake-up test result). In the series of hog studies, the SEP false-negative rate was 13.6%, and the NMEP false-negative rate was 0% when the animals were evaluated by the wake-up test 5 minutes later (Owen et al., 1991; Owen, 1999).

Glassman described a patient with a severe spinal deformity undergoing spinal instrumentation in whom the MEPs were abolished at the moment of maximal distraction, but the SEPs remained unaltered. A wake-up test confirmed the absence of motor function (Glassman et al., 1993). However, there is no consensus about which stimulatory modality (electrical or magnetic) and which evoked potential (neurogenic or electromyographic) is superior in detecting early changes in spinal cord function. Clinical comparisons of the various MEP methods with SEP and wake-up tests during spinal distraction are needed.

Blood Loss

The vast area of decorticated, raw cancellous bone that is exposed during spinal surgery results in extensive blood loss that can exceed 25 mL/kg even in uncomplicated surgery. Children with neuromuscular scoliosis often require more extensive procedures, including pelvic stabilization, than children with idiopathic scoliosis and can easily have blood losses that exceed a blood volume (Meert et al., 2002). However, even if the extent of surgery is controlled, patients with neuromuscular diseases have an almost seven times higher risk of losing more than 50% of their estimated total blood volume during scoliosis surgery than normal controls (Edler et al., 2003).

An estimation of circulating blood volume should be made before the induction of anesthesia. The estimated blood volume (EBV) is calculated by multiplying the patient's weight by the approximate blood volume based on age (Table 21–6). From the EBV, the initial hematocrit (Hct), and the minimum acceptable hematocrit, an estimation can be made of the maximum allowable blood loss (MABL) before packed red blood cell transfusions are indicated (Kallos and Smith, 1974):

$$\mathrm{MABL} = \frac{(\mathrm{EBV})\left(\mathrm{Hct}_{\mathrm{initial}} - \mathrm{Hct}_{\mathrm{accepted}}\right)}{\dfrac{\left(\mathrm{Hct}_{\mathrm{initial}} + \mathrm{Hct}_{\mathrm{accepted}}\right)}{2}}$$

TABLE 21–6. Approximate blood volume

Age	Total Blood Volume (mL/kg)
Premature infant	90 to 105
Term newborn	80 to 85
1 to 12 months	70 to 80
Older child	70 to 80
Adult	60 to 70

The decision to transfuse red blood cells should be based on the balance between oxygen supply and demand, which depends on the oxygen content of the blood, cardiac output, regional distribution, and metabolic needs. The trigger to transfuse is then based on the patient's risk for developing inadequate oxygenation.

Because blood loss may be difficult or impossible to accurately assess, we estimate blood loss by measuring the hemoglobin concentration hourly and by assuming that changes in central venous pressure reflect ongoing blood loss. As blood loss progresses and exceeds a blood volume, medical causes of bleeding, such as dilutional thrombocytopenia or loss of clotting factors V and VIII, become increasingly important in accounting for the inability of the surgeon to achieve hemostasis. Platelet counts and coagulation profiles (i.e., prothrombin time, partial thromboplastin time, fibrinogen, and fibrin split products) should be obtained at regular intervals when extensive blood loss occurs.

Multiple strategies have been described to minimize blood loss and the need for blood transfusions in the perioperative period. These approaches include attempts at reduction of intraoperative blood loss and reduction of transfusion of homologous blood products. Techniques that may decrease intraoperative blood loss include induced hypotension, alteration of the operative position, changes in surgical technique, and administration of desmopressin (1-desamino-8-D-arginine vasopressin [DDAVP]) and aprotinin. Techniques aimed at decreasing the use of homologous blood products include intraoperative blood salvage, preoperative autologous blood donation, and perioperative hemodilution and apheresis (Laupacis and Fergusson, 1997; Bryson et al., 1998; Huet et al., 1999). Each of these techniques has demonstrated efficacy in some clinical situations.

Predonation of autologous blood is increasingly accepted by surgeons and families and has been used extensively in children (Helfaer et al., 1998). The primary limitation of this method is the number of units that a child or adolescent can donate (Goodnough et al., 1989). Recombinant erythropoietin, which increases red cell mass, has been used in the weeks immediately preceding surgery to maximize a patient's ability to donate autologous blood and halves the risks of needing a homologous blood transfusion (Vitale et al., 1998, 2002; Goodnough, 2001).

Alternatively, perioperative hemodilution and apheresis, sometimes referred to as *isovolumic hemodilution*, can substitute for or augment autologous blood donation (Hur et al., 1992; Bryson et al., 1998; Copley et al., 1999). Before incision, the patient's blood is withdrawn from a large-bore peripheral intravenous canula or from a central venous catheter and replaced with an isotonic balanced salt solution or colloid in a ratio of 3:1. When using this technique, oxygen extraction increases, and oxygen delivery decreases; careful attention to acid-base balance (i.e., lactate levels) is essential when using this technique (Copley et al., 1999). The removed blood is stored in anticoagulated bags, and it is administered as needed to maintain the hematocrit at a predetermined level, usually above 20%. Complications of this technique include postoperative pulmonary edema, anasarca, and prolonged postoperative mechanical ventilation. Perioperative salvage of blood (i.e., use of Cell Saver system) allows blood lost in the operative field to be returned to the patient in the perioperative period (Huet et al., 1999). How efficient this technique is, how long the salvaged red blood cells survive, and its place in limiting blood transfusion are unclear (Ray et al., 1986; Blais et al., 1996; Abildgaard et al., 2001; Vitale et al., 2002). When using salvaged blood, it is imperative that the blood be processed and washed adequately to avoid life-threatening bleeding and pulmonary complications caused by transfusion of cellular and tissue debris. Salvaged blood can also result in profound hypotension (e.g., citrate, air embolism) and hemolytic and bleeding complications from centrifugation, cellular debris, or anticoagulant overdosage.

DDAVP increases plasma factor VIII and von Willebrand factor concentration when given intravenously, thereby decreasing the activated partial thromboplastin time and enhancing fibrinolysis by increasing levels of plasminogen activator. DDAVP has been used successfully to prevent bleeding during surgical procedures in patients with mild to moderate hemophilia or von Willebrand disease. Infusions of DDAVP have shortened or normalized bleeding times in patients with chronic renal failure. This apparent improvement in qualitative platelet function lasts between 4 and 8 hours. Despite early reports by Kobrinsky and others (1987) that demonstrated a 25% reduction in operative blood loss when DDAVP was administered preoperatively to patients undergoing scoliosis repair, others have not been able to reproduce these findings. There is no evidence that DDAVP reduces the blood loss incurred by patients undergoing scoliosis repair (Guay et al., 1992; Theroux et al., 1997; Alanay et al., 1999; Henry et al., 2001).

Deliberate Hypotension

The most common blood-preservation technique is deliberate hypotension (Yaster et al., 1986; Petrozza, 1990; Tobias, 2002) (see Chapter 12, Blood Conservation). Numerous techniques to reduce blood pressure have been used, typically with drugs that are direct venous and arterial vasodilators, such as nitroprusside and nitroglycerin. Ganglionic-blocking drugs (e.g., trimethaphan), α_2-adrenergic agonists (e.g., clonidine), β- and α_1-antagonists (e.g., propranolol, esmolol, prazosin, hydralazine), dopamine agonists (e.g., fenoldopam), inhaled anesthetics (e.g., halothane, isoflurane, sevoflurane, desflurane), major conduction blockade (i.e., epidural), and calcium channel blockers (e.g., nicardipine) are used alone or in combination with the direct-acting venous and arterial vasodilators to lower blood pressure (Yaster et al., 1986; Hersey et al., 1997; Post and Frishman, 1998; Tobias, 1998, 2000, 2002; Degoute et al., 2003; Hackmann et al., 2003).

Deliberate hypotension can be used in any patient who is otherwise healthy. It is contraindicated if there is any evidence of end-organ injury or ischemia. Blood pressure is usually lowered to mean arterial pressures of 50 to 60 mm Hg. In the past, the most commonly used technique was a continuous infusion of nitroprusside (1 to 8 mcg/kg per minute) combined with β-blockade, using propranolol (1 to 2 mg), labetalol, or an esmolol infusion (Tinker and Michenfelder, 1976). β-Blockade is necessary when hypotension is induced with nitroprusside because nitroprusside produces a reflex tachycardia and increases cardiac index. These combine to limit the ability of nitroprusside to lower blood pressure (Yaster et al., 1986). Nitroglycerin, which is often used for deliberate hypotension in adults, fails to reduce mean arterial blood pressures below 60 mm Hg in children when administered in doses as high as 40 mcg/kg per minute (Yaster et al., 1986). Potent inhalation agents, such as halothane or sevoflurane, also can be used to induce hypotension in children and adolescents but may interfere with evoked potential monitoring (Tobias, 1998) and delay the ability to rapidly perform a wake-up test. When combined with low-dose sevoflurane or desflurane, remifentanil is extremely effective. Regardless of the technique used to induce deliberate hypotension, the appropriate use of adjuvants in the anesthetic technique can aid achieving the desired effect of hypotension. Children can be premedicated with oral clonidine (4 to 8 mcg/kg) 2 hours before surgery to reduce anxiety and to facilitate the induction and maintenance of hypotension during surgery (Hackmann et al., 2003).

Although deliberate hypotension clearly reduces blood loss, provides a relatively bloodless surgical field, and facilitates surgical dissection, its use in scoliosis surgery is controversial. Animal studies have suggested an additive effect of hypotension and surgical pressure on the spinal cord in producing neurologic injury (Brodkey et al., 1972). In dogs, Griffiths and others (1979) have shown that cord compression can alter dorsal column conduction at perfusion pressures that did not affect blood flow. Use of deliberate hypotension mandates normocarbia and adequate oxygen carrying capacity.

Vigilant monitoring is essential when deliberate hypotension is used. An arterial catheter for beat-beat monitoring of blood pressure and for frequent arterial blood gas sampling and hematocrit determinations is essential. Because patients must remain normovolemic at all times, a central venous pressure catheter is a useful monitor. Nitroprusside has been shown to decrease arterial oxygen tension in children and to increase the $PAO_2 - PaO_2$ (Yaster et al., 1986). We can assume that the lowered oxygen carrying capacity of low-hematocrit blood, when coupled with hypoxemia and hypocapnia from overzealous ventilation, can only exacerbate cord ischemia caused by surgical traction or hypotension. Other end organs that must be protected from hypotension include the heart and kidney. The heart is easily monitored by following the ST segment of the V_5 lead of the electrocardiogram. The kidney is monitored by bladder catheterization and measuring urine output hourly. Renal perfusion pressure can be assumed to be inadequate if urine output falls to less than 1 ml/kg per hour.

Aprotinin

A number of investigators have examined the role of aprotinin and other antifibrinolytics as hemostatic agents in limiting perioperative blood loss and transfusion requirements (Kannan et al., 2002; Cole et al., 2003). Aprotinin is a serine protease inhibitor that acts on the clotting cascade as an antifibrinolytic, an antiinflammatory, and a platelet membrane stabilizer. The hemostatic effect of aprotinin is ascribed to its antifibrinolytic properties and its ability to preserve platelet function. In particular, in high doses it inhibits the kallikrein-kinin system, decreasing its activation in the presence of tissue trauma. It also may involve, conserve, and restore platelet function with a protective effect on specific platelet receptors (Royston, 1992, 1995). Aprotinin may play a protective role against disseminated intravascular coagulopathy through its anti-VIIa activity. Aprotinin dosages are variably expressed: 1 mL = 1.4 mg = 10,000 kallikrein inhibitor units (KIU).

In a randomized, double-blind, controlled trial, Cole and others (2003) found a 40% reduction in blood loss in children at high risk for blood loss, such as those with neuromuscular scoliosis or those undergoing reoperation. In that study, after a test dose of 1 mL (10,000 KIU) given 10 minutes before the loading dose, aprotinin was administered as a 240-mg/m^2 load over 30 minutes before incision. The loading dose was followed by a continuous infusion of 56 mg/m^2 per hour throughout the case and was maintained for 4 hours after surgery (Cole et al., 2003). If a patient had more than 1 m^2 of body surface area, the maximum dose, 280 mg (200-mL vial), was given as the loading dose, and maintenance was 70 mg (50 mL)/hour (see Chapter 32, Systemic Disorders).

Positioning

An anesthetized patient is extremely vulnerable during positioning for scoliosis surgery. The patient is unable to feel the extreme discomfort of certain positions that alter the normal mechanics of the body. Vulnerable parts, such as peripheral (ulna) nerves, male genitalia, the nipples, and the anterior superior iliac spine (to protect the lateral femoral cutaneous nerve of the thigh), must be especially protected to avoid injury by pressure or stretching. Of the peripheral nerves, the brachial plexus is most vulnerable to stretch in the prone position (Martin, 1997). Stretching of the lower trunks of the brachial plexus is most likely to occur when the head is turned to the contralateral side, the ipsilateral shoulder is abducted, and ipsilateral elbow is bent. Although efforts to prevent neuropathies are frequently debated, there is little hard evidence to support specific management recommendations.

The patient's eyes are vulnerable to corneal abrasion and to optic vein engorgement and retinal ischemia. Postoperative visual loss is a devastating and poorly understood injury. Over the past decade, there has been much speculation that the frequency of perioperative blindness has been increasing among patients undergoing major spine surgery. Roth and others (1996) found a much higher incidence of blindness (1 in 600) among patients undergoing complex spinal surgery. A report from the Mayo Clinic did not support this finding (Nuttall et al., 2001). To help analyze the risk factors involved, the American Society of Anesthesiologists has established an anonymous, postoperative visual loss registry (www.asaclosedclaims.org).

Ischemic optic neuropathy, which affects the anterior or posterior portions of the optic nerve, is the most common cause of postoperative visual loss. Visual loss may also be caused by retinal arterial occlusion and cortical blindness. Awakening with visual impairment may be one of the most frightening and catastrophic postanesthetic complications that a patient could sustain. It is also an enormous medicolegal liability problem. Commonly cited risk factors in patients undergoing scoliosis surgery in the prone position include hypotension, anemia, and external compression of the eye. Unfortunately, blindness has occurred even when these risk factors did not occur (Lee and Lam, 2001; Roth and Barach, 2001).

Decreased perfusion pressure in the retina or optic nerve may be caused by decreased mean arterial pressure or increased pressure in the venous drainage of the retina or optic nerve. Prolonged decreases in blood pressure, especially in patients with disturbed autoregulation, may be deleterious. Increased venous pressure (i.e., with internal jugular vein compression or ligation, prolonged head-down position, or large quantities of fluid infusion) also decreases perfusion. With prone positioning, increases in intraocular pressure might be potentiated by these factors. The combination of decreased blood pressure and increased venous pressure seems to pose the greatest risk.

The prone position increases intraabdominal pressure, which impairs ventilation by decreasing chest compliance and by limiting chest expansion. It also engorges epidural veins, which increases intraoperative bleeding and potentially increases the risk of postoperative epidural hematoma formation. Increased intraabdominal pressure leads to compression of the inferior vena cava, which impedes venous return to the heart. This decreases cardiac output and engorges epidural veins. To facilitate venous return and avoid increased intraabdominal pressure, specially designed frames have been developed that allow the abdomen to hang free and facilitate respiratory movement (Relton and Hall, 1967; Nuttall et al., 2000).

Turning the anesthetized patient from the supine to the prone position requires careful orchestration by the entire surgical and anesthesia team. Cervical spine injury, dislodgement of intravascular and urinary catheters, accidental endotracheal tube extubation or dislodgement, inability to ventilate once prone, and dramatic changes in cardiac output can easily occur. During the turn, monitoring, with the exception of an esophageal stethoscope, is difficult. Once turned, auscultation of both lung fields is imperative. The adequacy of pressure-point padding (e.g., elbows, breasts, scrotum, feet) must be ensured to avoid peripheral nerve compression (i.e., ulnar nerve) and soft tissue damage.

The surgical plan and preference determine the patient's position and the device used to stabilize the patient's head. A pin-type or horseshoe-shaped holder may be employed and requires careful application and padding to avoid catastrophic oculofacial injuries. Alternatively, the head may be rested on a securely arranged stack of pillows to avoid exaggerated neck flexion, rotation, or ear trauma.

Anesthetic Techniques

Given the potential complications of neurologic injury and profound hemorrhage associated with spinal surgery, the anesthetic technique employed should have minimal effects on neurophysiologic monitoring, allow for a wake-up test, and provide for hemodynamic stability to minimize complications. The combination of remifentanil with desflurane or propofol allows for SEP and NMP monitoring and for a rapid wake-up response if necessary.

Patients with preexisting neurologic deficits, such as cerebral palsy, paralytic scoliosis, and congenital scoliosis, have variable SEP waveforms of weak amplitude. The use of an etomidate infusion in these patients can augment the amplitude of the evoked responses and increase the reliability of SEP monitoring (Lubicky, 1989). Etomidate suppresses the adrenal cortical stress response for 8 to 24 hours after its use (Wagner et al., 1984; Kenyon et al., 1985). Whether patients administered etomidate should be prophylactically treated with corticosteroid replacement continues to be debated (Wagner et al., 1984). Vitamin C supplementation may be an attractive therapeutic alternative because it increases cortisol concentrations during etomidate infusions (Boidin et al., 1986).

■ POSTOPERATIVE MANAGEMENT

Although pulmonary failure and the need for postoperative ventilation are the primary problems of scoliosis surgery, other common postoperative concerns include ongoing blood loss, disseminated intravascular coagulation, hypovolemia, and development of syndrome of inappropriate secretion of antidiuretic hormone (SIADH), paralytic ileus, and pain. The most important initial decision at the conclusion of surgery is whether to extubate the trachea. This decision is based in large part on the patient's preoperative pulmonary function and on the intraoperative course. Scoliosis surgery produces an immediate and transient decrease in vital capacity of 40% or more in all patients (Schur et al., 1984). These changes in vital capacity have been demonstrated in patients more than 24 months after repair (Upadhyay et al., 1993). Patients with preoperative FVC levels of less than 50% of predicted and patients with nonidiopathic scoliosis should be extubated in the pediatric intensive care unit after cognitive faculties and respiratory muscle strength have returned to baseline. Other common pulmonary complications in the postoperative period include atelectasis, pneumothorax, and pleural effusions.

Syndrome of inappropriate antidiuretic hormone (SIADH) is common and manifests as hyponatremia, hypo-osmolality, decreased urine output, and increased urine osmolality. The increased plasma volume reduces the hemoglobin concentration and can be identified by following the red blood cell's mean corpuscular volume (MCV). As the level of ADH increases, plasma water increases, resulting in free water entry into red blood cells. The MCV increases, and the hemoglobin and mean corpuscular hemoglobin content (MCHC) decrease. In contrast, the MCV should not change in the face of postoperative blood loss (Mason et al., 1989).

Because the surgery is so extensive, pain is an expected complication in all scoliosis patients. Postoperative pain can be treated with intravenous opioid therapy (i.e., patient-controlled analgesia [PCA]) or regional anesthetic techniques, or both (Tobias, 2004). For PCA use, patients are started on a basal infusion of morphine (0.02 mg/kg per hour) or hydromorphone (0.004 mg/kg per hour), combined with a low-dose (0.25 mcg/kg per hour) naloxone infusion (Gan et al., 1997; Maxwell and Yaster, 2003). The patient or nurse can trigger the PCA machine's bolus button, which provides an additional dose of morphine (0.02 mg/kg) or hydromorphone (0.004 mg/kg) (Yaster et al., 1997; Monitto et al., 2000). Many centers are using neuraxial techniques for postoperative analgesia (Tobias, 2004). Typically, a single epidural catheter is inserted by the surgeon at the T8-9 level before wound closure. Alternatively, two catheters are placed at the top and bottom of the wounds by the surgeon. These catheters are intermittently or continuously infused with opioids (i.e., morphine, hydromorphone, or fentanyl) or local anesthetics (i.e., 0.625% to 1.25% bupivacaine solutions), or both.

Nonsteroidal antiinflammatory drugs (NSAIDs), such as ketorolac, have a morphine-sparing effect and result in fewer opioid-induced side effects such as somnolence, constipation, and pruritus (Reuben et al., 1997, 1998). The use of ketorolac does not increase bleeding, the need for transfusions, or reoperation (Reuben et al., 1998; Vitale, 2003). Nevertheless, for reasons that are discussed later, the use of ketorolac in scoliosis patients should be avoided, because in human and laboratory studies, NSAIDs significantly inhibit spinal fusion (Glassman et al., 1998; Martin et al., 1999).

NSAIDs such as ketorolac are thought to have deleterious effects on bone healing and fracture repair, although the actual clinical effects appear to be controversial at this point (Huo et al., 1991; Dimar et al., 1996; Glassman et al., 1998). In some studies, chronic NSAID use for more than 3 months was associated with lower fusion and success rates (Deguchi et al., 1998; Glassman et al., 1998; Harder and An, 2003).

The effects of NSAIDs are thought to principally affect the bone morphogenetic proteins (BMPs) (Harder and An, 2003). The BMPs are a class of osteoinductive proteins that play an important role in bone growth and are essential for the growth and development of skeletal tissue and for bone regeneration during fracture repair (Bostrom and Camacho, 1998; Khan et al, 2000).

Martin and others (1999), using a rabbit model of spinal fusion, investigated the effects of ketorolac on graft healing. Compared with a saline control group, less than one half of the rabbits receiving ketorolac had a stable bone graft. However, the coadministration of a recombinant BMP with ketorolac to a third group of rabbits resulted in 100% successful fusion rate. The investigators concluded that the effects of the NSAID could be completely reversed by the administration of a BMP (Martin et al., 1999). Clinical trials using recombinant BMPs to improve graft healing are only in the preliminary stage (Khan et al., 2002; Sandhu and Khan, 2003). Initial studies evaluating the effects of cyclooxygenase-2 (COX-2)–specific inhibitors on bone healing have produced similar results (Gilron et al., 2003). The healing of stabilized tibial fractures in COX-2–deficient mice was significantly delayed, as was intramembranous calvarial bone formation. These bone-healing deficiencies were reversed by the administration of prostaglandin E_2 and by BMP-2 (Zhang et al., 2002). In some studies, COX-2 inhibition seemed to have less severe effects on bone healing compared with nonspecific COX-1 and COX-2 NSAIDs (Gerstenfeld, 2003). In a retrospective analysis of more than 300 patients undergoing spinal fusion who received a COX-2 inhibitor, ketorolac, or no NSAIDs for the first 5 postoperative days, patients who received ketorolac had a threefold increase in nonunion rate compared with COX-2 recipients or controls (Maxy and Glassman, 2001; Gajraj, 2003a, 2003b).

JOINT DISORDERS

ARTHROGRYPOSIS MULTIPLEX CONGENITA

Arthrogryposis multiplex congenita (AMC) consists of a heterogeneous group of nonprogressive conditions which have in common fetal akinesia. This results in the birth of a baby with multiple, congenitally curved, rigid joints. The incidence is 1 in 3000 live births. Because of their extensive contractures, tense skin, and minimal muscle mass and subcutaneous tissue, these children have been described as looking like "thin, wooden dolls."

Arthrogryposis is a physical sign resulting from many different medical conditions. In the past, an in utero, self-limited anterior horn cell disease was proposed (O'Flaherty, 2001; Bonilla-Musoles et al., 2002). Efforts are being made to distinguish between myogenic and neurogenic causes of AMC. AMC has been associated with maternal myasthenia gravis, in which there is transplacental transfer of maternal anti–acetylcholine receptor antibody to the fetus early in gestation, limiting fetal movements (Riemersma et al., 1996; Jacobson et al., 1999; Polizzi et al., 2000). AMC has also been associated with a mutation in rapsyn, a receptor-associated protein at the synapse that is responsible for the maintenance of specific structures at the synapse of the neuromuscular junction (Burke et al., 2003). Neurogenic AMC can result from focal cerebral deficits and produce asymmetrical limb involvement (Takano et al., 2001).

Most children with AMC have quadrimelic limb involvement. Joint involvement is symmetrical, increases distally, and results in severe contractures and joint rigidity. The most common orthopedic deformities include talipes equinovarus, dislocated hip, dislocated patella, and scoliosis. Surgical management is directed at correcting all lower extremity deformities that delay ambulation. These are ideally performed before the patient is 2 years old. Upper extremity surgery is designed to improve hand function.

The anesthetic management of children with arthrogryposis multiplex congenita (AMC) is complicated by associated congenital abnormalities, an abnormal upper airway, and positioning difficulties. Arthrogryposis is associated with congenital heart disease, pulmonary hypertension–cor pulmonale, and urogenital anomalies (Oberoi et al., 1987). Case reports highlight associated renal tubular acidosis, cholestasis, gastroschisis, and Hirschsprung's disease (Eastham et al., 2001; Sooriyabandara and Aluwihare, 2001). Decreased pulmonary reserve resulting from pulmonary hypoplasia and scoliotic restrictive lung disease may potentiate hypoxemia and may necessitate postoperative ventilatory support. Despite these associated anomalies, it must be emphasized that these children have normal intelligence and can expect to live a nearly normal life span.

Patients with arthrogryposis have micrognathia, a high arched palate, and a short and rigid neck making tracheal intubation difficult and at times impossible (Oberoi et al., 1987; Szmuk et al., 2001). Direct laryngoscopy and intubation become more difficult as the patient ages because craniofacial involvement often progresses with growth. Alternatives to direct laryngoscopy and tracheal intubation, such as the use of the laryngeal mask airway, with or without the use of a tube exchanger, or fiberoptics, have been used successfully in this disorder (Nguyen et al., 2000; Szmuk et al., 2001; Thomas and Parry, 2001). The extensive contractures, tense skin, and minimal muscle mass and subcutaneous tissue pose challenges for intraoperative positioning and intravenous access.

Children with arthrogryposis may have altered responses to neuromuscular relaxants and are akin to other patients with anterior horn cell diseases. Although hyperkalemic responses to succinylcholine have not been reported, prudence mandates avoiding the routine use of depolarizing muscle relaxants. Although the response to nondepolarizing relaxants has been reported to be extremely variable, the use of short-acting nondepolarizing agents in association with careful monitoring of neuromuscular function has been successful in these patients.

The association of intraoperative hyperthermic crises with AMC has been sporadically reported in the literature. Hopkins and others (1991), in reporting three cases of hyperpyrexia, reviewed the literature of nine additional cases. In nine cases, hyperthermia, tachycardia, and hypercarbia were observed intraoperatively. Six episodes were assumed to be malignant hyperthermia, and dantrolene therapy was immediately instituted. Two cases responded rapidly to aggressive cooling. One patient received a nontriggering anesthetic. The halothane contracture test was not performed in any of these reported cases. Conversely, Baines and others (1986) reported no case of malignant hyperthermia among 67 patients with AMC anesthetized with triggering agents. In light of the absence of laboratory confirmation, the occurrence of a hyperthermic crisis without exposure to triggering agents, and a large number of affected patients without a hyperthermic response, Hopkins and others (1991) concluded that these hypermetabolic responses are distinct from malignant hyperthermia. The association between AMC and malignant hyperthermia may be unfounded.

JUVENILE RHEUMATOID ARTHRITIS

Juvenile rheumatoid arthritis (JRA) is the most common rheumatic disease of childhood (Jarvis, 2002; Schneider and Passo, 2002). It is defined as the presence of peripheral arthritis beginning before the patient is 16 years old and having a duration of at least 6 weeks. The estimated incidence is 14 cases per 100,000 children per year.

JRA is divided into three subsets based on the symptoms at onset. Oligoarthritis, representing approximately 50% of all JRA, is common in girls, with the peak age of onset at 2 years. During the first 6 months of the disease, fewer than five joints are affected, typically the knees and less commonly the ankles and wrists. Seventy-five percent of these patients have a positive antinuclear antibody (ANA) titer. Oligoarthritis is rarely destructive. Polyarticular JRA, representing 20% to 40% of JRA cases, is also more common in girls, with a peak age of onset of 3 years. In this variant, five or more joints are affected, commonly the small joints of the hand. Only 40% of these patients have a positive ANA result, and 10% have positive test results for rheumatoid factor. Polyarticular JRA has associated subcutaneous nodules and erosions. The arthritis is destructive in 15% of patients. Moderate systemic manifestations of anemia and growth retardation are seen. Systemic JRA, also known as Still's disease, manifests with fever, macular rash, leukocytosis, lymphadenopathy, and hepatomegaly. Symmetrical polyarthritis is seen in these children. Boys and girls are affected equally, and they can present for treatment at any age. The cervical spine, jaw, hands, hips, and shoulders can be involved. Only 10% of these children have positive ANA results. The arthritis can be destructive in 25% of cases. Patients with systemic JRA can have pericarditis, pleuritis, uveitis, splenomegaly, and abdominal pain. Common surgical procedures include various joint arthroplasties and synovectomies, correction of uveitis, scoliosis surgery, limb length–discrepancy surgery, and limb and mandibular osteotomies.

Anesthetic considerations in the child with JRA are principally focused on airway management. The mandibular head and the temporomandibular joint (TMJ) can be destroyed in JRA, limiting mouth opening. TMJ disease can also affect mandibular growth, resulting in micrognathia. Cervical spine disease is commonly seen in the systemic and the polyarticular forms of JRA, sometimes resulting in spinal fusion, reducing cervical mobility. Cervical stiffness is reported in 46% to 60% of patients. Radiographic changes are usually seen in the late stages of the disease and only in children with severe involvement. As a component of atlantoaxial rotatory subluxation or as a solitary manifestation, torticollis can develop, further increasing the degree of difficulty of these patients' airway management (Subach et al., 1998; Uziel et al., 1998). Cricoarytenoiditis, an unusual manifestation of systemic JRA, can result in airway obstruction and in severe distortion of the glottic anatomy (Jacobs and Hui, 1977; Vetter, 1994). Children with JRA should undergo a complete preoperative evaluation of the TMJ and the cervical spine, looking for evidence of limited range of motion. The assessment should include dynamic radiographs.

MARFAN SYNDROME

Marfan syndrome is an autosomal dominant connective tissue disorder caused by mutations of genes on chromosome 15 that encode fibrillin, a complex glycoprotein that helps maintain the elastic properties of the soft connective tissues. These tissues are all lax, resulting in joint subluxation (Dietz et al., 1991a, 1991b; Dietz and Pyeritz, 1995). Marfan syndrome patients have abnormalities of their cardiovascular, skeletal, and ocular systems. The cardiovascular complications of Marfan syndrome, including aortic root dilatation and dissection, are thought to be consequences of the alterations in the fibrillin-rich aortic tunica media. Aortic disease is the major cause of morbidity and premature death of these patients (Gott et al., 2002).

Aortic size appears to correlate with central pulse pressure, and children with Marfan syndrome maintained on β-blockade and calcium antagonist therapy have slower aortic root growth than do those who are unmedicated (Jondeau et al., 1999; Rossi-Foulkes et al., 1999). Long-term medical therapy in combination with prophylactic cardiac surgery when the ascending aorta exceeds 50 mm has increased the long-term survival of patients with Marfan syndrome (Finkbohner et al., 1995; Gott et al., 1999). The incidence of mitral valve prolapse is increased among persons with Marfan syndrome.

In addition to the cardiovascular anomalies, patients with Marfan syndrome have a high incidence of pectus excavatum and spontaneous pneumothoraces. The inward depression of the sternum that results from excessive growth of costochondral cartilages, in combination with severe scoliosis, produces a precarious physiologic state in which respiratory compromise can result from lung compression, or cardiovascular collapse can occur from impeded venous return or distortion of the great vessels or diminished coronary perfusion. Pizov and others (1997) observed that after inexplicable cardiovascular collapse during posterior spinal instrumentation, mild sternal compression was sufficient to disrupt coronary artery blood flow as visualized by echocardiography in his patient with severe, concurrent scoliosis and pectus excavatum.

Marfan syndrome affects the spine in several ways. Scoliosis has been reported in 40% to 70% of patients with the syndrome. These patients are at risk for atlantoaxial translation with neck flexion and extension (Hobbs et al., 1997). Patients undergoing seemingly routine uneventful direct laryngoscopy and endotracheal intubation can develop atlantoaxial rotatory subluxation manifested as unresolved torticollis and neck pain in the postoperative period. These events are thought to result from abnormal bone morphology, from the abnormal shape of the atlantoaxial facet, or from the laxity of ligaments (Herzka et al., 2000). In a series of 100 patients with Marfan syndrome, more than 50% had evidence of increased atlantoaxial translation. The preadolescent population had a greater range of motion than did the adolescent or adult groups (Hobbs et al., 1997). Atlantoaxial subluxation has been reported as a cause of sudden death of patients with Marfan syndrome (MacKenzie and Rankin, 2003).

Anesthetic management of patients with Marfan syndrome starts with a preoperative cardiovascular and cervical spine evaluation. Patients who are destined to undergo prone procedures should have the effects of sternal compression evaluated by echocardiography preoperatively. The anesthesiologist should consult with the patient's cardiologist to determine whether the doses of β-blockade and calcium channel antagonism are appropriate. The anesthetic technique should aim to decrease myocardial contractility and avoid sudden increases in blood pressure, to minimize the risk for aortic dissection or rupture. In the setting of mitral valve prolapse, hypovolemia and tachycardia should be avoided. Nasotracheal fiberoptic intubation may be useful in patients with underlying disease and those with atlantoaxial instability.

SYNDROMES OF DISPROPORTIONATE SHORT STATURE: DWARFISM

Children with dwarfism are unified solely by their phenotype of disproportionate short stature and associated limb deformities.

More than 35,000 dwarfs are estimated to live in the United States, and the individual osteochondrodysplasias and mucopolysaccharidoses that produce this phenotype number well over 100 (Berkowitz et al., 1990). Achondroplasia, the most common form of dwarfism, has an incidence of 150 per 1 million live births (Orioli et al., 1986). Many other forms are rare. The mucopolysaccharidoses (MPS) (i.e., Hurler's syndrome [MPS I-H], Hunter's syndrome [MPS II], Morquio's syndrome [MPS IV], and Scheie's syndrome [MPS V]) are few in number but pose significant anesthetic challenges. At one time, dwarfs were considered social curiosities who possessed an aura of mystery and played a prominent role in folklore and mythology. Improved societal support for this disability has resulted in an enormous number of orthopedic procedures that are performed on these patients. Limb-lengthening techniques (Yasui et al., 1997; Aldegheri and Dall'Oca, 2001), cervical decompression, joint replacement, limb realignment, and bone marrow transplantation for patients with mucopolysaccharidoses are but a few of the procedures that are increasingly being performed on these patients. The number of diseases that constitute the dwarfing syndrome is enormous, and the limited anecdotal anesthetic experience for many of these precludes an encyclopedic review of all of the syndromes. Nevertheless, the common pathologic conditions to a large number of the dwarfing syndromes listed in Box 21–3 should be evaluated in the preoperative preparation of an affected patient.

AIRWAY ABNORMALITIES

Characteristics

The anesthetic management of dwarfs is frequently complicated by anatomic abnormalities of the upper airway and by difficulty in visualization of the larynx during direct laryngoscopy. Inability to intubate is the major cause of morbidity and mortality when anesthetizing dwarfs (Berkowitz et al., 1990). Upper airway obstruction is frequently a result of thickened pharyngeal and laryngeal structures, narrowed nasal passages, micrognathia, copious secretions, pharyngeal hypoplasia, and tracheal narrowing. This is seen most frequently in patients with mucopolysaccharidoses, diastrophic dysplasia, camptomelic dysplasia, severe diastrophic dysplasia, and dwarfs with Russell-Silver syndrome. Some patients demonstrate upper airway obstruction even in the awake state. Airway patency can be severely affected by positional changes alone. Some patients with achondroplasia, Morquio's syndrome, and metatropic dysplasia maintain a patent airway with the neck extended but completely obstruct when the neck is flexed. Sedation and general anesthesia often result in complete upper airway obstruction. Direct laryngoscopy and tracheal intubation are extremely difficult to perform in many dwarfs. Endotracheal intubation is often hampered by inadequate laryngeal exposure, infiltration of the glottic structures with abnormal mucopolysaccharide, and tracheal and subglottic narrowing. In contrast, the patient with achondroplasia may have narrow nasal passages and pharyngeal hypoplasia because of dysplasia and angulation of the cranial base and hypoplasia of the maxilla, but the airway is rarely obstructed, and it can be easily managed with a facemask (Monedero et al., 1997).

Anesthetic Management

Preoperative sedative drugs should be avoided in patients prone to upper airway obstruction. Before induction, intravenous access

---

BOX 21–3 Systemic Manifestations of the Dwarfing Syndromes

Upper Airway Abnormalities—Mucopolysaccharidoses, Achondroplasia

Macroglossia
Micrognathia (mesomelic dysplasia, diastrophic dysplasia, dwarf with Russell-Silver syndrome)
Small oral opening
Temporomandibular joint immobility
Tonsillar and adenoidal hypertrophy
Narrow nasopharynx
Laryngomalacia

Difficult Laryngoscopy—Mucopolysaccharidoses

Abnormal glottic structures
Short neck, cervical scoliosis (Morquio syndrome, metatropic dysplasia, diastrophic dysplasia, spondyloepiphyseal dysplasia)
Copious secretions

Upper Airway Obstruction—Mucopolysaccharidoses

Abnormal neck position
Abnormal upper airway
Laryngomalacia
Copious secretions

Pulmonary Dysfunction—Mucopolysaccharidoses, Achondroplasia, Asphyxiating Thoracic Dystrophy

Restrictive lung disease
Thoracic dystrophy
Scoliosis
Pulmonary hypertension
Obstructive sleep apnea

Cardiovascular Dysfunction—Osteogenesis Imperfecta, Mucopolysaccharidoses, Asphyxiating Thoracic Dystrophy, Achondroplasia

Congenital heart disease
Acquired valvular disease
Cor pulmonale
Restrictive lung disease
Obstructive sleep apnea

Neurologic Complications—Achondroplasia, Osteogenesis Imperfecta

Atlanto-occipital instability, odontoid hypoplasia
Cervicomedullary compression
Intracranial hypertension
Deafness

Hematologic Dysfunction—Osteogenesis Imperfecta

Disorder platelet aggregation

Other Manifestations—Osteogenesis Imperfecta

Propensity for bony fractures
Hypermetabolism

is obtained, and an antisialagogue is administered. If the potential for severe upper airway obstruction and difficult intubation is anticipated, the equipment and personnel required for establishment of an emergency airway should be present before the induction of anesthesia (see Chapter 10, Induction of Anesthesia). Spontaneous ventilation is mandatory. Often, the only way to identify the glottis is by observation of the air bubbles during spontaneous ventilation. An inhalational induction with high concentrations of oxygen and sevoflurane or a continuous intravenous infusion of propofol or ketamine is an equally effective approach in this situation. After an adequate anesthetic plane is achieved, endotracheal intubation can be accomplished by direct laryngoscopy or by fiberoptic-guided bronchoscopy. Alternatives include the lightwand and fiberoptic intubation by means of a laryngeal mask airway. Neuromuscular relaxants are avoided until the airway is secured. Rarely, a tracheostomy performed while the patient is awake may be the safest approach. The examiner must avoid neck manipulation, particularly neck flexion during laryngoscopy, in patients with atlantoaxial instability or foramen magnum stenosis.

PULMONARY DYSFUNCTION

Characteristics

The pulmonary dysfunction common to children with the dwarfing syndromes is multifactorial in origin. Restrictive lung disease is a consequence of thoracic cage dystrophy (e.g., Jeune's syndrome) or scoliosis, and it results in reduced lung volumes, ventilation-perfusion mismatching, progressive hypoxemia, and hypercarbia. Obstructive or central sleep apnea causes pulmonary hypertension, substantial morbidity, and sudden death (Sisk et al., 1999). Structural abnormalities, particularly in MPS, may cause intrathoracic obstruction. The preoperative assessment of these patients must include an evaluation of pulmonary function and a sleep study. The finding of central apnea necessitates a neuroradiologic evaluation of the cervical spine and foramen magnum. The presence and severity of pulmonary hypertension can be determined by an electrocardiogram and echocardiography.

Anesthetic Management

The degree of pulmonary dysfunction discovered during preoperative evaluation has profound implications on intraoperative and postoperative management. Severe obstructive sleep apnea may preclude an inhalational induction of anesthesia or the use of premedicants. Significant restrictive lung diseases with attendant ventilation-perfusion mismatch, proclivity to atelectasis, and development of increased $PAO_2 - PaO_2$ may necessitate placement of an indwelling arterial catheter to ensure adequate gas exchange throughout the perioperative period. The severity of restrictive lung disease dictates the necessity for continued intubation and ventilation postoperatively.

CARDIAC DYSFUNCTION

Characteristics

Children with dwarfing syndromes have a variety of causes for cardiac dysfunction. There is a high incidence of coexisting structural heart disease, such as atrial septal defects, in a number of the dysplasias. Acquired valvular heart disease is a common complicating feature of children with MPS and is occasionally found in osteogenesis imperfecta. Ischemic heart disease may result from infiltrative mucopolysaccharides or from the consequences of cor pulmonale and long-standing pulmonary hypertension. Physical examination, chest radiography, electrocardiography, and echocardiography are useful in diagnosing pulmonary hypertension. The most reliable indicators of pulmonary hypertension are the presence of tricuspid regurgitation and prolongation of the right systolic time interval. The electrocardiogram should be reviewed for evidence of myocardial ischemia, particularly in patients with Hurler's syndrome or Hunter's syndrome.

Anesthetic Management

The anesthetic management of a patient with dwarfism, impaired myocardial dysfunction, and pulmonary hypertension must be meticulously planned and executed. Invasive monitoring of arterial, central venous, and in severe cases, pulmonary artery pressures is frequently necessary. The use of intraoperative transesophageal echocardiography may be warranted in patients with severe valvular dysfunction or those who have evidence of ischemic heart disease. Modest hypoxemia and hypovolemia can exacerbate preexisting pulmonary hypertension and borderline right ventricular function, and they must be avoided. The need to maintain an adequate anesthetic depth, crucial in avoiding intraoperative pulmonary hypertensive crises, must be balanced by the limitations imposed by compromised ventricular function. Attention must also be directed to the effects of changes in heart rate, blood pressure, filling pressures, and systemic vascular resistance on myocardial function. In light of these challenges, an opioid-based anesthetic in combination with adrenergic-modulating agents may provide the most stable intraoperative milieu for this subset of patients. The use of opioids in patients at risk for postoperative airway obstruction may result in postoperative intubation and mechanical ventilation.

NEUROLOGIC DYSFUNCTION

Characteristics

Cervicomedullary compression and hydrocephalus are the main neurologic concerns in patients with dwarfism. The causes of cervical cord compression include atlanto-occipital instability, foramen magnum stenosis, and, infrequently, cervical scoliosis. Foramen magnum stenosis is a frequent complication of achondroplasia. Physical findings or a history consistent with upper motor neuron weakness (e.g., progressive weakness, hyperreflexia, abnormal plantar response), sleep apnea, cyanosis, or respiratory distress is suggestive of cervicomedullary compression. Flexion and extension neck films should be obtained to determine the degree of cervical spine instability in affected patients.

Anesthetic Management

Improper positioning of the head, neck, and shoulders during the induction of anesthesia, laryngoscopy, and surgery may lead to catastrophic intraoperative cord ischemia. Patients with Morquio's syndrome, diastrophic dysplasia, and achondroplasia are at greatest risk. The maintenance of in-line traction during intubation or fiberoptic intubation may be advisable. Cervical stabilizing devices such as a halo cast or a Milwaukee brace may be applied before anesthesia to avoid cervical subluxation and dislocation. Unfortunately, these devices may make direct laryngoscopy impossible. Succinylcholine should be avoided if there is any evidence of pyramidal tract signs, muscle wasting, or paresis. Autonomic hyperreflexia may be a potential problem in patients with cervical cord compression or myelopathy.

The coexistence of intracranial hypertension and a difficult airway is particularly challenging to the anesthesiologist. The conventional approaches of inhalational or intravascular induction may have salutary effects on one element of management but catastrophic consequences on the other. Balancing these conflicting requirements must be done on a case-by-case approach. One approach is to use an intravenous infusion of propofol to place a laryngeal mask airway, through which a fiberoptic bronchoscope is passed. Once identification of the glottic structures is assured, an intubating dose of propofol is administered to blunt the intracranial pressure response to endotracheal intubation.

OSTEOGENESIS IMPERFECTA

Osteogenesis imperfecta represents a subpopulation of dwarfs with unique problems. Osteogenesis imperfecta is a disease resulting from a defect in type I collagen, and this group of disorders manifests with abnormalities in bone, teeth, sclera, and ligaments (Chevrel and Meunier, 2001; Cohen, 2002; Zeitlin et al., 2003). The four clinical subtypes are listed in Table 21–7.

The hallmarks of this disease are bony fragility and multiple fractures after even innocuous trauma. Scoliosis and kyphosis are common. Medical management includes the use of bisphosphonate drugs (Chevrel and Meunier, 2001; Glorieux, 2001; Zeitlin et al., 2003). These are anti–bone-resorptive drugs that may reduce fracture frequency, increase bone density, promote remodeling of previously crush-fractured vertebrae, reduce chronic pain, and improve mobility in children and infants with osteogenesis imperfecta.

The hallmark of anesthetic management is to handle these patients very gently. Fractures may occur from simple procedures such as applying a tourniquet or taking a blood pressure or while positioning the patient on the operating room table. Airway management may cause fractures, and the physician must pay particular attention to the teeth, mandible, and cervical spine. Occasionally, visualization of the airway is difficult, and the use of a laryngeal mask airway may be very helpful (Kostopanagiotou et al., 2000). Osteogenesis imperfecta patients have a hypermetabolic state and become hyperthermic during anesthesia (Porsborg et al., 1996). This is not malignant hyperthermia, even though a few case reports of true malignant hyperthermia have been reported in these patients (Cole et al., 1982). The routine pediatric anesthetic practice of preventing intraoperative hypothermia, such as using warming blankets and heated, humidified gasses, should be tempered, and antimuscarinics such as atropine and glycopyrrolate should be used judiciously.

Some patients with osteogenesis imperfecta bruise easily as a result of a presumed platelet abnormality. Bleeding and hemorrhage are rare, but approximately 30% of these patients have abnormal bleeding times, capillary fragility, and reduced levels of factor VIII.

OSTEOPETROSIS

Osteopetrosis (i.e., marble bone disease) is an inherited disease in which bone cannot be resorbed or remodeled, and it is associated with significant physiologic derangements. The severity of osteopetrosis can be predicted by its inheritance pattern; the autosomal recessive form is very severe and predominately affects infants and children. Benign autosomal recessive osteopetrosis is associated with cerebral calcifications and renal tubular acidosis (Gerritsen et al., 1994). Children with the malignant form of recessive osteopetrosis frequently suffer from airway compromise, intracranial hypertension, and pancytopenia with a compensatory hepatosplenomegaly (Geyser et al., 1982; Fasth and Porras, 1999). Persons with all forms of osteopetrosis are at risk for pathologic fractures. Patients with osteopetrosis frequently require anesthetics for bone biopsies to assess the efficacy of interferon therapy and for treatment of their pathologic fractures (Key et al., 1995).

Burt and others (1999), in a series of 65 anesthetics for children with osteopetrosis, reported that the rate of airway management difficulties was much higher in this group of children compared with the other children anesthetized at their institution. Mandibular abnormalities and temporomandibular joint immobility contributed to the difficulty of orotracheal intubation, and abnormalities of the nasal turbinates made nasotracheal intubation difficult. Cervicomedullary stenosis limited optimal head positioning, and concurrent thrombocytopenia exacerbated airway instrumentation and limited the options of a regional anesthetic. No particular anesthetic technique was deemed superior, except for an emphasis on meticulous preoperative airway preparation with the ready availability of the resources for emergency airway management.

CEREBRAL PALSY

Cerebral palsy is a static encephalopathy that may be defined as a nonprogressive disorder of posture and movement. It is often associated with epilepsy and abnormalities of speech, vision, and

TABLE 21–7. Subtypes of osteogenesis imperfecta

Type	Features
I	Mildest form of osteogenesis imperfecta (OI); mild bone fragility; bimodal fracture curve (first peak between 1 year and puberty; second, smaller peak postmenopausally in women and after 70 years in men); normal stature; blue sclerae; deafness in some cases, most commonly occurring in second decade; dominant inheritance
II	Most severe form of OI; perinatal lethal form; one half do not survive day 1, and 90% are dead by 1 week; extreme short stature; short, bowed long bones, particularly lower limbs; ribs have beaded appearance from recurrent fractures; respiratory insufficiency; absence of calvarial mineralization; dominant mutation
III	Progressively deforming type; many fractures; thin ribs with discrete fractures; curvature of spine that may be severe enough to reduce pulmonary reserve; severe short stature; deafness; dentinogenesis imperfecta; dominant mutation; rare recessives unlinked to type I collagen genes
IV	Mild to moderate bone fragility; short stature; deafness in some cases; dentinogenesis imperfecta; dominant inheritance

Adapted from Cohen MM Jr: Some chondrodysplasias with short limbs: Molecular perspectives. *Am J Med Genet* 112:304–313, 2002.

TABLE 21–8. Four classification systems for cerebral palsy

Physiologic	Topographic	Etiologic	Functional
Spastic	Monoplegia	Prenatal (e.g., infection, metabolic, anoxia, toxic, genetic)	Class I: no limitation of activity
Athetoid	Paraplegia	Perinatal (e.g., anoxia)	Class II: slight to moderate limitation
Rigid	Hemiplegia	Postnatal (e.g., toxins, trauma, infection)	Class III: moderate to great limitation
Ataxic	Triplegia		Class IV: no useful physical activity
Tremor	Quadriplegia		
Atonic	Diplegia		
Mixed	Double hemiplegia		
Unclassified			

intellect resulting from a defect or lesion of the developing brain (Kuban and Leviton, 1994). It is the most common childhood motor disability, occurring in 2 of 1000 live births (Grether et al., 1996; Nelson and Grether, 1999). Multiple causes of CNS damage result in the phenotype of cerebral palsy. In premature infants, periventricular leukomalacia is commonly associated with the development of cerebral palsy. In term infants, early antenatal insults are attributed to be the cause of the CNS injury and can manifest as events at the time of delivery. The most common etiologic factors are prematurity and birth weight above or below ideal weight for gestational age (Jarvis et al., 2003).

Cerebral palsy may be classified by a description of the motor handicap in terms of physiologic (major motor abnormality), topographic (extremity involved), etiologic, and functional capacity (Table 21–8). Although the CNS lesion is static, the degree of impairment can change with time. Cerebral palsy is commonly associated with a spectrum of developmental disabilities, including mental retardation, epilepsy, and visual, hearing, speech, cognitive, and behavioral abnormalities. The motor handicap may be the least of the child's problems. The need to treat each patient's individual problems uniquely and to avoid generalization cannot be overemphasized. Some children with cerebral palsy may be of normal intelligence but limited in their ability to communicate. Others with marked developmental delay may be difficult to separate from their parents because of natural fear and an inability to reason in a way expected of children with normal intelligence.

Patients with cerebral palsy often require multiple surgical procedures. Orthopedic operations to improve function of the extremities are common, and some patients require surgical correction of progressive spinal deformities. Common procedures include surgical soft tissue procedures that reduce muscle spasm around the hip girdle, including an adductor tenotomy or psoas transfer and release.

Several drugs are commonly used in treating spasticity, athetosis, dystonia, and seizures in cerebral palsy patients, and many of these drugs have significant anesthetic implications. Drugs used to treat spasticity include dantrolene, benzodiazepines, and baclofen. Incapacitating athetosis is treated with levodopa and dystonia with carbamazepine and trihexyphenidyl. Seizures are commonly treated with phenobarbital, phenytoin, clonazepam, carbamazepine, and sodium valproate.

The muscle spasticity of cerebral palsy is thought to be caused by inadequate release of the inhibitor γ-aminobenzoic acid (GABA) in the dorsal horn of the spinal cord, resulting in a relative excess of excitatory glutamate on the alpha motor neurons that produces simultaneous contraction of agonist and antagonist muscle groups (Albright et al., 1991; Albright, 1996; Albright and Shultz, 1999). The symptoms of spastic diplegia can be treated surgically with rhizotomy, a procedure in which the roots of the spinal nerves are divided. Spasticity can also be treated medically by the administration of a continuous intrathecal infusion of baclofen or by local intramuscular injection of botulinum toxin. Baclofen is a GABA agonist on the receptors located in the dorsal horn of the spinal cord, and it can reduce the pain and muscle spasms. Continuous intrathecal baclofen infusions have been successfully used to treat ambulating children with inadequate leg strength and patients with upper and lower extremity spasticity, improving their function and comfort levels (Albright et al., 1991; Albright, 1996; Albright and Shultz, 1999). Botulinum toxin is taken up in the presynaptic terminal, and it inhibits acetylcholine release into the neuromuscular junction, functionally denervating muscle fibers within 2 to 3 cm of the injection for up to 2 to 6 months (Denislic and Meh, 1995; Forssberg and Tedroff, 1997). Tight heel cords may be treated surgically by tenotomy of the Achilles tendon.

Preoperative concerns for children with cerebral palsy focus on their pulmonary, gastrointestinal, and neurologic problems. Children with cerebral palsy are prone to aspiration pneumonia from gastroesophageal reflux and nasopharyngeal aspiration. Many have chronic lung disease with a reactive component, and they suffer from frequent respiratory infections (Toder, 2000). Obstructive sleep apnea is seen in 20% to 50% of this patient population (Kotagal et al., 1994). Obstructive sleep apnea has many causes, including bulbar dysfunction, neurogenic laryngomalacia, and laryngeal dystonia (Worley et al., 2003).

Airway management can be complicated by restricted TMJ range of motion and by poor and malpositioned dentition. Cerebral palsy patients commonly have gastroesophageal reflux disease, dysfunctional swallowing, and severe food refusal, all contributing to suboptimal nutritional status that portends increased perioperative complications. Children with cerebral palsy have a higher incidence of latex allergy than the general population (Nakamura et al., 2000). Thirty percent of children with cerebral palsy require antiepileptic medications (Singhi et al., 2003).

Perioperative seizure management in the patient with cerebral palsy is the same as for any patient with a seizure disorder. Most anesthetic agents are anticonvulsants, and they can be used safely in patients with underlying seizure disorders. A few anesthetic agents, such as enflurane, etomidate, ketamine, methohexital, EMLA (i.e., eutectic mixture of local anesthetics, 2.5% lidocaine and 2.5% prilocaine), and normeperidine (i.e., active metabolite of meperidine), are proconvulsants and should be avoided if alternatives are available. Most of these proconvulsant anesthetic agents actually raise the seizure threshold in normal patients and are proconvulsant only in patients with underlying seizure disorders. Patients should take their chronic anticonvulsants on the day of surgery. Virtually all anticonvulsants have long half-lives of elimination (24 to 36 hours), and if blood anticonvulsant levels are within the therapeutic range, a 24-hour period can elapse without taking the anticonvulsant and without increasing the risk of a seizure.

In most orthopedic surgical procedures performed in cerebral palsy patients, almost any anesthetic technique and combination of drugs can be used. Potent inhaled anesthetics, muscle relaxants (including succinylcholine), hypnotics, sedatives, opioids, and local anesthetics have been used safely. Children with cerebral palsy appear to have a lower minimum alveolar concentration (MAC) than unaffected children (Frei et al., 1997). Succinylcholine does not cause hyperkalemia, and it can be safely administered to cerebral palsy patients. These patients have a slightly increased sensitivity to succinylcholine compared with normal children (Dierdorf et al., 1985; Theroux et al., 1994). Resistance to nondepolarizing muscle relaxants and rapid recovery from neuromuscular blockade have been reported in cerebral palsy patients, which may be explained by the increase in extrajunctional acetylcholine receptors (Theroux et al., 2002).

Postoperative pain management is important in the care of cerebral palsy patients. The surgical procedures, particularly those for relieving spasticity, are extremely painful. The severely affected child with cerebral palsy may be unable to communicate his or her pain, and health care providers are often unable to accurately assess the severity of postoperative pain. Parents and other routine caretakers are invaluable in assessing the pain of these patients. The Non-communicating Children's Pain Checklist—Postoperative Version has been validated for children with intellectual disabilities (Breau et al., 2002, 2003). Postoperative pain is treated with continuous epidural (caudal or lumbar) infusions. Lidocaine (1.5 to 2.0 mg/kg per hour) plus fentanyl (0.5 mcg/kg per hour), chloroprocaine (3 mg/kg per hour) plus fentanyl (0.5 mcg/kg per hour), and bupivacaine (0.625 to 1 mg/mL, 0.2 to 0.4 mg/kg per hour) with or without fentanyl (0.5 mcg/kg per hour) or hydromorphone (2 to 4 mcg/kg per hour) have all been used. Muscle spasms are virtually universal and are treated prophylactically with intravenous diazepam. The addition of clonidine to the postoperative epidural infusion at a dose of 0.08 to 0.12 mcg/kg per hour is also effective at relieving muscle spasms (Nolan et al., 2000). The management of posterior rhizotomy requires special attention. Often used in severe spasticity, this surgical procedure requires stimulation of the dorsal roots intraoperatively and observation of muscle response (Peacock and Staudt, 1990; Abbott et al., 1993) (see Chapter 18, Anesthesia for Neurosurgery).

ILIZAROV METHOD

HISTORY

Professor G.A. Ilizarov introduced the concept of distraction osteogenesis in the 1950s. Working as a general practitioner in Siberia, he found himself treating many patients with chronic osteomyelitis associated with bone loss and many World War II veterans who had developed fracture nonunions. Using materials from the metal factories at which many of his patients were employed, he fashioned external fixators and transosseous wires to induce the formation of new bone between freshly cut osseous surfaces that are gradually pulled apart. Using this technique, he was able to salvage limbs that otherwise would have been amputated. For many years, he worked in isolation, with his techniques remaining unknown in most of the world (Fig. 21–5).

Over the past 20 years, this method has undergone significant refinements, and it is now employed in the treatment of congenital limb and other skeletal deformities, acquired short limbs, and angular deformities and the reconstruction of large bony defects resulting from trauma, tumor excision, infection, and fracture nonunions (Herbert et al., 1995). Distraction osteogenesis has also been used to treat the numerous syndromes associated with micrognathia and retrognathia, such as the Pierre Robin sequence, Treacher Collins syndrome, Nager's syndrome, velocardiofacial syndrome, and Pfeiffer's syndrome, that can result in airway obstruction (McCarthy et al., 2001; Sidman et al., 2001).

The success of the Ilizarov technique of distraction osteogenesis depends on adherence to the principles of tension-stress phenomena. These include a low-energy osteotomy to preserve periosteal blood supply; a slow, incremental distraction rate to preserve soft tissue blood supply; and maintenance of full function of the extremity. Bone healing is promoted by the biologic stress of walking on or flexing a broken limb, causing a trampoline-like effect of pulling and contracting that stimulates bone growth and healing. Using a corticotomy that preserves blood flow to the periosteum and the medullary canal, a gap between healthy, vascular-sufficient bone is created. Wires are inserted into the bone above and below the osteotomy and are attached under tension to an external fixator at 90-degree angles to the plane of the deformity. After an initial latency period, the osteotomy is gradually distracted at a rate of 1 mm per day in four incremental steps. The external fixator serves as the distracting device and provides optimal mechanical stability so that weight bearing and range of motion on the operative limb are possible on the second hospital day. The early functional use of the affected limb stimulates callus formation and osteoblastic activity (Aronson, 1997).

ANESTHETIC CONSIDERATIONS

Because the Ilizarov procedure is applied to children with a wide spectrum of diseases, including those with complex congenital musculoskeletal anomalies, the anesthetic implications of their coexisting diseases often take precedence over those of the operative procedure. These operative procedures are often long and complex, but they are plagued with few hemodynamic perturbations and only modest blood loss. The perioperative complications of the Ilizarov procedure that are affected by anesthetic management include nerve injury and the need for intact motor function and optimal analgesia in the postoperative period. Nerve injury can occur during pin placement and during the distraction process. To recognize inadvertent surgical trauma to nerves in the operative field, neuromuscular relaxation is avoided so that muscle contractions can be recognized. Postoperative surgical pain can be intense in the first 48 hours, and these patients are encouraged to begin physical therapy on the first postoperative day with an emphasis on passive range of motion and weight bearing (Paley, 1990).

Children undergoing an Ilizarov procedure are often anesthetized with a general anesthetic supplemented with an epidural catheter. In most cases, endotracheal intubation is accomplished with short-acting neuromuscular blockade or with deep inhalational or intravenous anesthesia. Children with concurrent airway or cervical spine anomalies are intubated with a fiberoptic bronchoscope or with a laryngeal mask airway–guided approach during spontaneous breathing. After the induction of general anesthesia, an epidural catheter is placed, and a continuous epidural infusion of 0.8 to 1 mg/mL of bupivacaine with 1 mcg/mL of fentanyl is begun in the operating room at an infusion rate of 1 mL/kg per hour. Anesthesia is maintained with

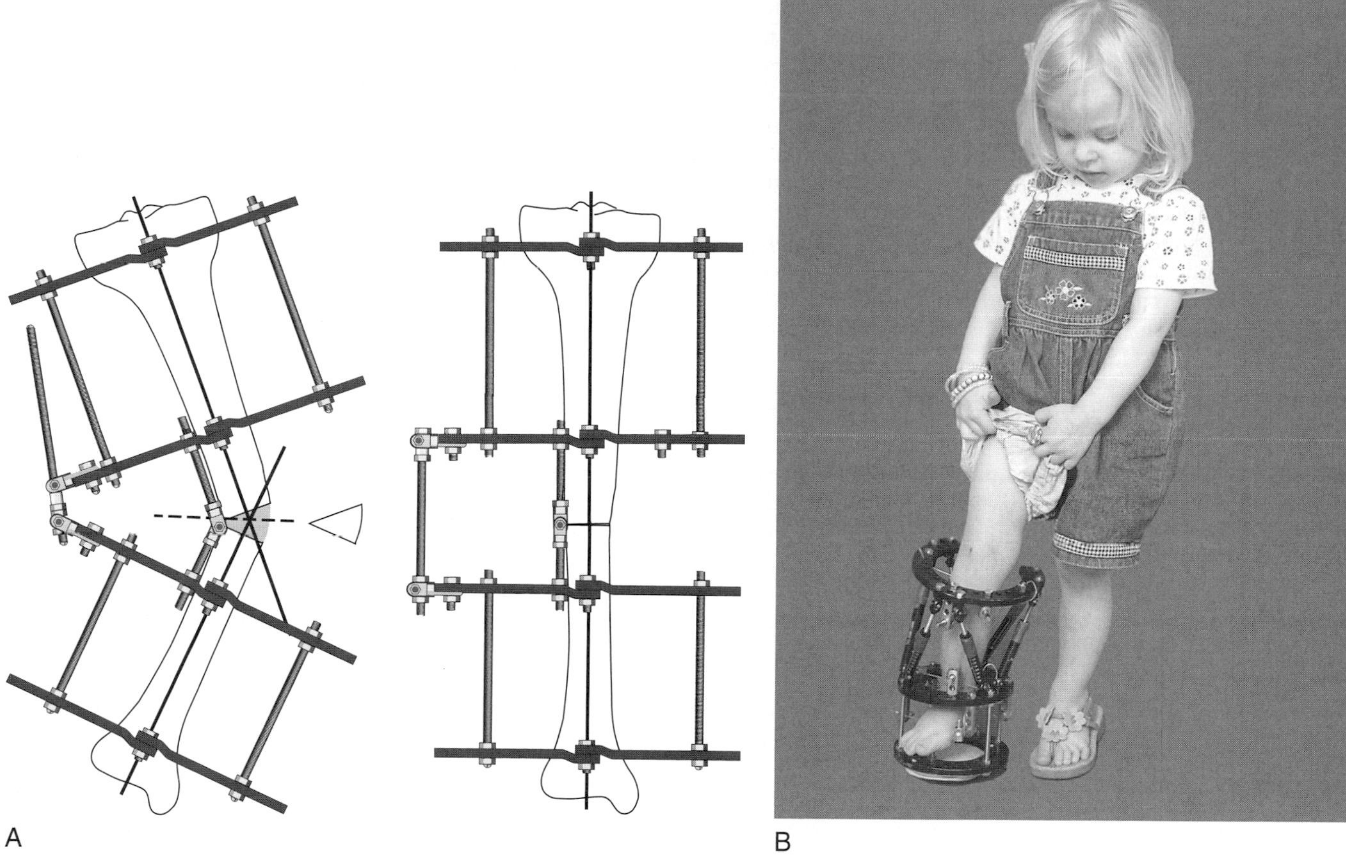

■ **FIGURE 21–5.** *A,* Wedge osteotomy *(right)* after application of an Ilizarov apparatus to correct a rotational deformity. With the external fixator in place *(left)*, the rotational deformity has been corrected, and the bone is ready for lengthening by slow adjustment of the diaphyseal rings. *B,* Children with external fixators are encouraged to resume as much normal function as possible.

small amounts of opioids and a low concentration of inhaled anesthetic agents. The epidural infusion of bupivacaine and fentanyl is continued for the first 24 to 36 hours postoperatively and augmented with acetaminophen. Postoperative analgesia is maintained with the epidural catheter. In patients without an epidural catheter in place, intravenous PCA is used.

■ TOURNIQUETS

Pneumatic tourniquets are commonly used to provide a dry operative field and limit intraoperative blood loss during extremity surgery (Kam et al., 2001). Modern pneumatic tourniquets consist of three basic components: a cuff, similar to a blood pressure cuff, which is wrapped around a patient's limb and then inflated; a compressed gas source; and a mechanism with a pressure gauge, designed to maintain pressure in the cuff at a set value. After elevation and application of an Esmarch bandage to exsanguinate the limb, the tourniquet is applied over smooth padding and inflated to a pressure of 100 mm Hg above systolic pressure for the lower extremity and 50 mm Hg above systolic pressure for the upper extremity (Patterson and Klenerman, 1979). To prevent accidental injury, the cuff should have a width that is greater than one half of the limb's diameter and an accurate pressure gauge. The duration of inflation should be carefully monitored.

How long the tourniquet can remain safely inflated is controversial. The most common recommendation, 2 hours, is based on the finding that cellular ischemic changes, such as mitochondrial swelling, myelin degeneration, glycogen storage depletion, and Z-line lysis, are reversible if the tourniquet is inflated for no more than 1 to 2 hours (Patterson and Klenerman, 1979). The deleterious effects of tourniquet inflation include pain while the tourniquet is inflated ("tourniquet pain"), metabolic and hemodynamic changes that occur during tourniquet inflation and deflation, and nerve injury and damage to blood vessels and muscle if the tourniquet is inflated for excessive periods.

In awake patients undergoing extremity surgery under regional anesthetic blockade, tourniquet pain is described as a dull, ill-defined ache that occurs approximately 45 to 60 minutes after a tourniquet is inflated. Over time, this pain becomes unbearable, but it subsides immediately after tourniquet deflation. This pain occurs despite adequate regional anesthesia for the surgical procedure itself. The cause of tourniquet pain remains uncertain. Early intervention in the treatment of tourniquet pain is imperative. Intravenous opioids have limited efficacy, and induction of general anesthesia or deflation of the cuff is the only effective solution to this problem. Prophylaxis may be possible. The addition of opioids to local anesthetic solutions at the time of neural blockade appears to decrease the incidence of tourniquet pain in patients undergoing a regional anesthetic.

The hemodynamic consequences of tourniquet application include increases in blood and central venous pressures. Kaufman and Walts (1982) reported an overall 30% increase in blood pressure during tourniquet inflation. The blood pressure response is more exaggerated in patients under general anesthesia than in those undergoing regional blockade (Valli et al., 1987). Tourniquet-induced hypertension can be prevented by the preoperative administration of 0.25 mg/kg of ketamine (Satsumae et al., 2001). Limb exsanguination and tourniquet inflation can redistribute 15% of the total blood volume to the general circulation rapidly. Central venous pressure increases of up to 14 mm Hg have been reported in adults with the application of bilateral tourniquets. The clinical significance of central venous pressure reduction that accompanies tourniquet deflation primarily depends on the presence of preexisting cardiac dysfunction.

The metabolic changes that accompany tourniquet use include an increase in core temperature during tourniquet inflation and the development of transient metabolic acidemia and hypercarbia after tourniquet release (Dickson et al., 1990; Kam et al., 2001). The increased output of carbon dioxide and lactic acid from the ischemic limb causes a transient decrease in arterial pH, with a maximum decrease within 4 minutes, returning to baseline values within 10 to 30 minutes. The sudden release of carbon dioxide into the circulation when lower limb tourniquets are released can markedly increase intracranial pressure in head trauma patients (Eldridge and Williams, 1989; Kam et al., 2001). Normocapnia maintained by hyperventilation after tourniquet deflation can prevent increased cerebral blood flow velocity and intracranial pressure.

Tourniquet-induced hyperthermia, usually 1°C to 2°C, occurs within 90 minutes of tourniquet inflation and appears to be the result of decreased cutaneous heat loss from skin distal to the tourniquet (Bloch et al., 1992). The metabolic acidosis and hypercarbia that occurs after tourniquet release is the result of reperfusion and the washing out and reentry into the central circulation of lactic acid, potassium, and other toxic substances that accumulated in tissues during tourniquet-induced limb ischemia. Accompanying hemodynamic effects include hypertension and hypotension, tachycardia, bradycardia, and rarely, ventricular arrhythmias. These effects are self-limiting and usually resolve over a few minutes. Other than increasing minute ventilation in patients who are being mechanically ventilated, most pediatric patients rarely or never require specific therapy for tourniquet deflation.

CLUBFOOT

Clubfoot (i.e., talipes equinovarus) is a relatively common congenital deformity that occurs in 1 of 1000 live births. Most clubfoot deformities are bilateral and can occur in otherwise normal children who have no syndrome, cytogenetic abnormality, or extrinsic cause for the deformity (Drvaric et al., 1989; Cummings et al., 2002). Clubfoot is commonly seen in patients with neuropathies and myopathies such as myelodysplasia, cerebral palsy, arthrogryposis, spinal muscular atrophy, and muscular dystrophy (Drvaric et al., 1989; Cummings et al., 2002). There are degrees of severity of clubfoot and the treatment is individualized in each patient. In some patients, manipulation and casting can restore the bony architecture. In others, surgery is required. When to perform surgery is controversial. Some surgeons prefer to operate on neonates; others operate when the child is 3 months, 6 months, or older than 1 year.

The patient is positioned prone (Cincinnati and two-incision technique) or supine (Turco incision), and the procedure is performed with a tourniquet. The surgery involves soft tissue release, including posterior, medial, plantar, and lateral releases; tendon transfer and lengthening; and pin fixation (Drvaric et al., 1989; Cummings et al., 2002). At the completion of surgery, the foot and the calf to the middle thigh are well padded and casted. Postoperatively, patients experience intense pain. Virtually any general anesthetic technique can and has been used for this surgery. Because postoperative pain is such an important aspect of the care of these patients, a combined regional (epidural or sciatic nerve block) and general anesthetic technique is commonly used. The epidural catheter is used intraoperatively and postoperatively.

The percutaneous Ponseti approach to the clubfoot involves weekly stretching of the deformity, followed by application of a long leg cast. By 4 to 5 weeks, all components of the deformity are corrected, with the exception of the equinus. The equinus is addressed with a percutaneous Achilles tenotomy, followed by a final long leg cast (Herzenberg et al., 2002; Ponseti, 2002; Ippolito, 2003; Lehman et al., 2003).

DEVELOPMENTAL DYSPLASIA OF THE HIP

Developmental dysplasia of the hip (i.e., congenital hip dislocation) is a spectrum of abnormalities of the developing hip joint that ranges from shallowness of the acetabulum to capsular laxity and instability to frank dislocation (Bauchner, 2000; Eastwood, 2003; Scherl, 2004). Developmental dysplasia of the hip is relatively common, occurring in 1 of 1000 live births. Previously known as congenital hip dislocation, it is now understood to be a condition that is not purely congenital but develops over time. It is common in children born by breech delivery. Screening in the newborn period consists of looking for asymmetries in skin folds, range of abduction, and height of the knees, as well as using provocative testing. The latter, known as the Ortolani test, elicits a click or clunk as the femoral head is moved in and out of the acetabulum. In the absence of other developmental disabilities, developmental dysplasia of the hip does not cause significant functional disability even if the diagnosis is missed or delayed, but untreated, it can lead to degenerative hip arthritis.

Treatment is designed to relocate and stabilize the femoral head in the acetabulum. Bracing (with the Pavlik harness) (Mubarak and Bialik, 2003) and body casting are used for the first 6 months to 1 year of life, after which most patients require surgery to reseat the hip. Virtually any general anesthetic technique can and has been used for casting and surgery.

SLIPPED CAPITAL FEMORAL EPIPHYSIS

Slipped capital femoral epiphysis (SCFE) is a displacement of the femoral head in relation to the femoral neck through the growth plate during a period of rapid growth in adolescence (Loder et al., 2001; Scherl, 2004). SCFE is common in obese teenagers and manifests with pain localized to the groin or to the knee or distal thigh (Kocher et al., 2004). On physical examination, these children limp, and the diagnosis made by obtaining anteroposterior and frog leg lateral radiographs of the pelvis. In 20% of patients, SCFE is bilateral on presentation, although only one side may be symptomatic.

Surgical management consists of placing one or two screws across the growth plate of the affected hip to prevent further slip. The pinning is made in situ, meaning that no attempt is made to reduce the epiphysis back to its original position; such maneuvers damage the blood supply to the femoral head and lead to avascular necrosis (Boero et al., 2003). Virtually any general anesthetic technique can and has been used for this surgery. Many of these patients have full stomachs when they present emergently and are therefore at risk for pulmonary aspiration of gastric contents.

FRACTURES

Children with fractures are among the most common patients seen by orthopedic surgeons. Most fractures are simple and treated without an anesthesiologist present. However, major blunt trauma often involves fractures of the long bones in children. These patients should be carefully examined for evidence of trauma involving other organ systems, particularly the cervical spine. In very young infants, fractures are rare. When present, child abuse must be considered in the differential diagnosis.

How to anesthetize a patient with a fracture depends on the urgency of the procedure, the risk of vomiting and aspiration, the child's maturity, and the wishes of the parents and surgeon. Regional or general anesthesia is possible. Regional anesthesia may make it impossible to evaluate motor function even if dilute concentrations of local anesthetics are used. When using general anesthesia, "full stomach" precautions should be used to minimize the risks of vomiting and pulmonary aspiration of gastric contents. This necessitates the use of rapid-sequence induction and airway protection with an endotracheal tube.

UPPER EXTREMITY BLOCKS

The upper extremity is innervated by the brachial plexus. The nerves are enclosed in a perineurovascular sheath that is divided into a supraclavicular (interscalene) and an infraclavicular (axillary) compartment. This fascial compartmentalization limits the spread of local anesthetics. An interscalene block provides more extensive blockade than an axillary approach, even if the amounts of local anesthetics used are identical (Dalens et al., 1987; Ross et al., 2000; Suresh and Wheeler, 2002). This occurs because more nerve fibers are blocked with a supraclavicular approach than with an axillary approach. If the upper arm is fractured, the axillary approach to the brachial plexus may not provide sufficient analgesia.

The axillary approach is a preferred technique because it is virtually free of all complications, does not require paresthesias to provide superior blockade, and is simple to perform (Yaster and Maxwell, 1989). In contrast to the effects in adults, this technique blocks the radial and musculocutaneous branches of the brachial plexus in children. Several techniques have been described. Because the axillary artery lies within the fascial sheath of the brachial plexus and the spread of local anesthetic within the fascia results in neural blockade, local anesthetic solutions deposited anywhere near the axillary artery produce a nerve block.

One technique is shown in Figure 21–6 (Yaster and Maxwell, 1989). The patient's arm is abducted at a right angle, with the forearm and hand supinated. The elbow is flexed and the hand held in a "saluting" position. The axillary artery is used as the landmark. After aseptic preparation of the skin, the anesthesiologist's nondominant hand is positioned such that the middle finger lies directly over the artery and compresses it and the brachial plexus against the humerus. A wheal of local anesthetic is deposited directly over the pulsating artery. Using a 25-gauge needle, local anesthetic is deposited on each side of the artery, staying as close as possible to the border of the artery. On the initial pass on each side of the artery, the needle is inserted slowly, aspirating constantly for arterial blood. If no blood is aspirated, 1 mL of local anesthetic is injected as the needle is withdrawn. In a fanlike manner, 1 mL of local anesthetic is injected on each sweep away from the artery. Usually, 5 mL of local anesthetic is deposited on each side of the artery (see Chapter 14, Regional Anesthesia).

LOWER EXTREMITY BLOCKS

The femoral nerve block is the quickest, easiest, and most effective technique of relieving the pain of a femoral shaft fracture (Yaster and Maxwell, 1989). When bupivacaine without epinephrine is used in a femoral nerve block, patients with fractures are provided with adequate anesthesia for the application of traction and for the necessary (and usually painful) manipulations that occur during radiologic examinations. The duration of analgesia is approximately 3 hours, and peak plasma levels of bupivacaine average less than 1 mcg/mL.

The femoral nerve, composed of nerve roots from L2, L3, and L4, is a mixed sensory and motor nerve located just under the inguinal ligament, lateral to the femoral artery in the femoral sheath (Fig. 21–7). After aseptic preparation of the skin, a 25- or 22-gauge, short-bevel needle is inserted perpendicular to the surface approximately 3 to 5 mm lateral to the artery and 1 to 2 cm inferior to the inguinal ligament. The needle is advanced until a pop is felt, indicating penetration of the fascia of the femoral sheath. This occurs at a depth that is clearly deeper than the artery. After a negative aspiration for blood, the needle is immobilized, and 1 to 5 mL of local anesthetic is deposited slowly. The needle is withdrawn to the skin and then redirected laterally and deep to the arterial pulsation. After aspirating for blood on each pass, more local anesthetic is injected in a fanlike manner away from the artery. This ensures adequate local anesthetic deposition in the fascia surrounding the nerve and thereby provides effective sensory blockade. The maximum dosage of 0.25% bupivacaine is 1 mL/kg. Higher concentrations of local anesthetic are rarely used because they produce motor blockade. The resulting anesthesia usually lasts 3 to 6 hours. This block can be repeated as often as is needed.

Alternatively, a fascia iliaca block can be performed (Dalens et al., 1989). This 3-in-1 block provides outstanding analgesia and provides coverage of the areas innervated by the femoral nerve, the lateral femoral cutaneous nerve, and the obturator nerve. A line is drawn outlining the skin projection of the inguinal ligament from the anterior superior iliac spine to the spine of the pubic bone. This line is then measured and divided into thirds. A short-bevel needle is inserted perpendicularly to the skin, 0.5 to 1 cm below at the outer third skin mark. A first give (with loss of resistance if gentle pressure is exerted on the barrel of the syringe) is felt as the tip of the needle crosses the fascia lata, and a second one occurs as the fascia iliaca is pierced. After aspirating for blood, the anesthetic solution is injected. A catheter can also be inserted and thereby provide continuous analgesia (see Chapter 14, Regional Anesthesia).

FAT EMBOLISM SYNDROME

FES is a collection of respiratory, hematologic, neurologic, and cutaneous symptoms and signs associated with trauma and other disparate surgical and medical conditions such as sickle cell acute chest syndrome and acute pancreatitis (Vichinsky et al., 1994, 2000). The incidence of the clinical syndrome is low (<1% in retrospective reviews), and embolization of marrow fat appears to be an almost inevitable consequence of long bone fractures (Mellor and Soni, 2001; Parisi et al., 2002). It is characterized by pulmonary insufficiency (i.e., hypoxemia), petechiae, and

■ **FIGURE 21–6.** The axillary block. The anesthesiologist's nondominant hand is positioned such that the middle finger lies directly over the brachial artery *(A)*, compressing the brachial plexus against the humerus. After placement of a skin wheal directly over the artery, fanlike injections of local anesthesia are made on each side of the artery as close as possible to the lateral border of the artery. Approximately five sweeps are made on each side of the artery, and 1 mL of local anesthetic is deposited on each sweep.

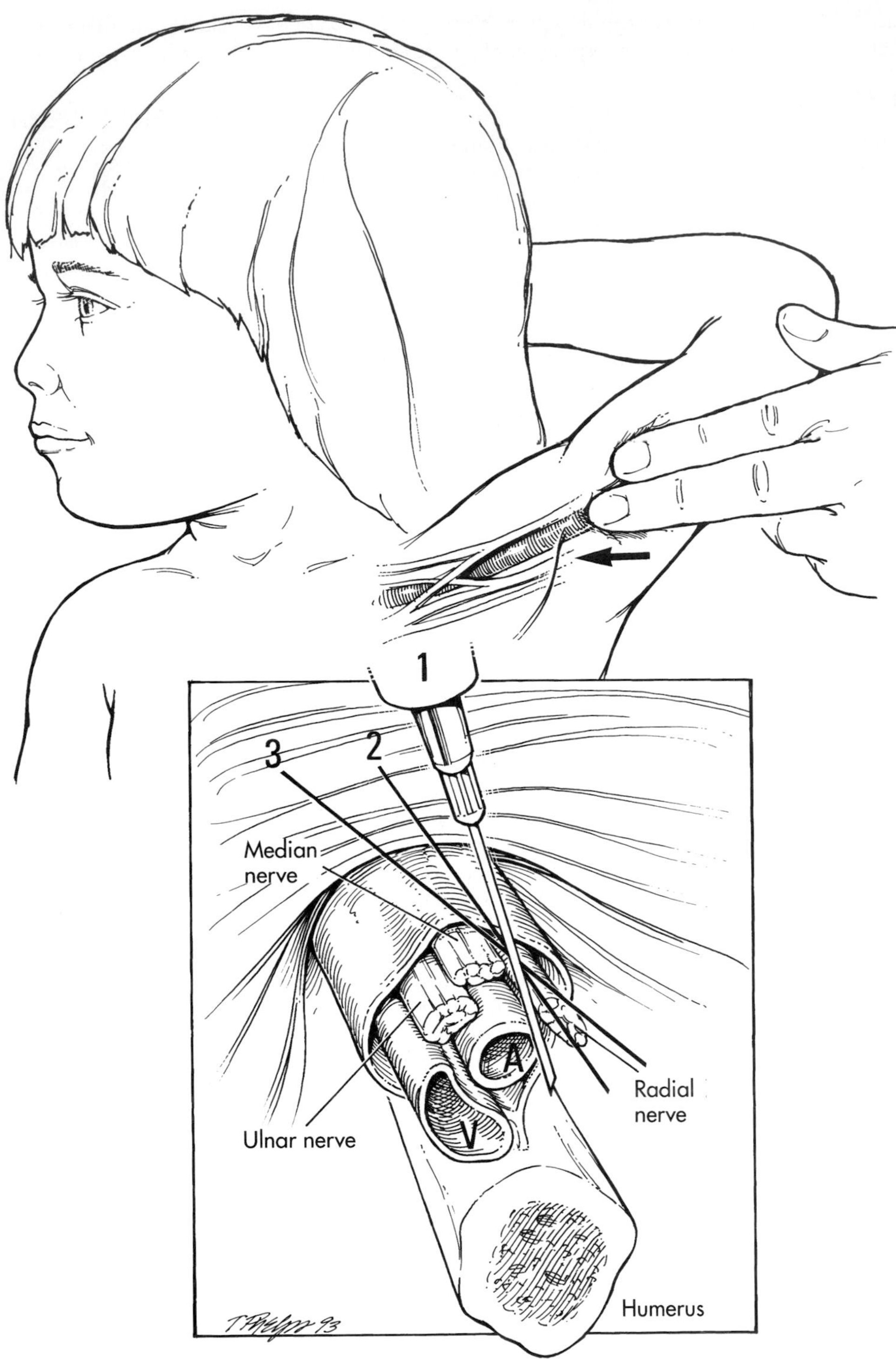

neurologic dysfunction (Box 21–4). The challenge to the pediatric anesthesiologist is to recognize the intraoperative manifestations of FES in a multiple-trauma patient or in a patient with an isolated long bone fracture.

■ PATHOPHYSIOLOGY

The physiopathologic mechanisms that produce the FES remain controversial. In the most accepted mechanical hypothesis, bone injury results in adipose tissue and blood vessel disruption and in hematoma formation. Increasing tissue pressure from hematoma expansion drives fat globules into the peripheral circulation. Chylomicrons are destabilized by the effects of fat intravasation and form very large, circulating fat globules. Fat can be detected in pulmonary arterial samples in up to 70% of patients with long bone or pelvic fractures, especially if the pulmonary artery catheter is wedged (Byrick et al., 1989). In the pulmonary vascular bed, these fat particles are hydrolyzed to free fatty acids, which produce pulmonary vasculitis and hemorrhagic pneumonitis. Surfactant activity is compromised, functional residual capacity is decreased, and endothelial integrity is violated. As a result, a large $PAO_2 - PaO_2$ value is generated, pulmonary

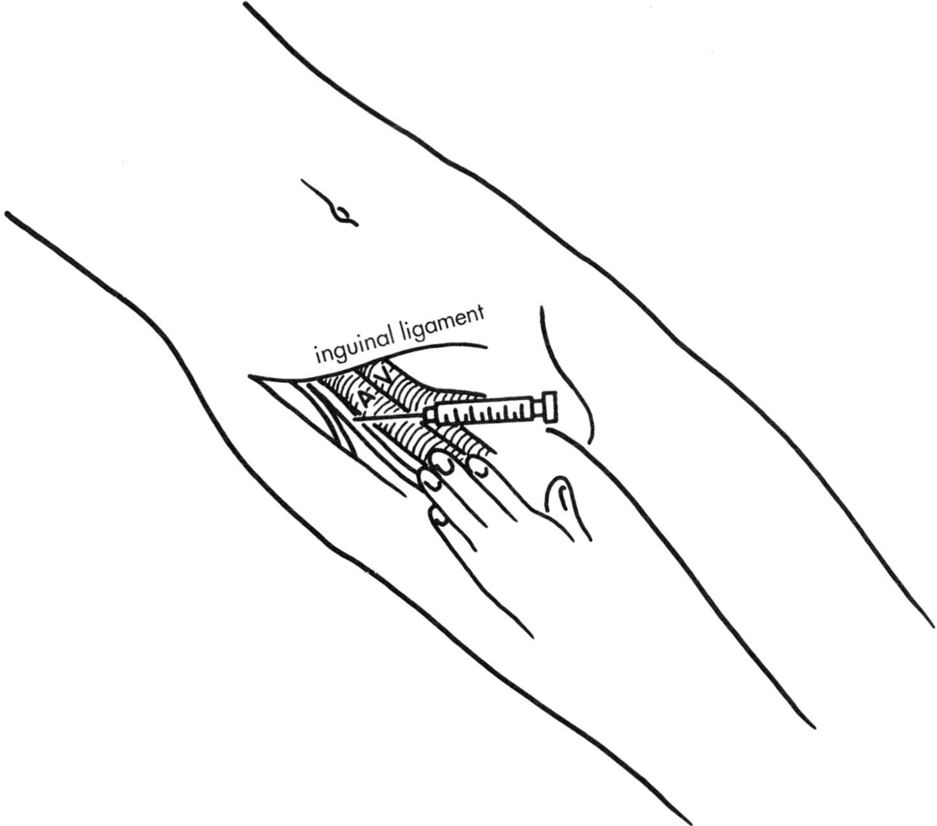

■ FIGURE 21–7. The femoral nerve block. After placing a skin wheal, the anesthesiologist's nondominant hand compresses the femoral artery and nerve against the underlying tissue and bone immediately below the inguinal ligament. A 22- to 25-gauge needle is then inserted perpendicularly, approximately 0.05 to 1 cm lateral to the pulsation of the femoral artery (A), into the femoral nerve's fascial sheath.

vascular resistance is increased, and pulmonary compliance is decreased. Fat particles and free fatty acids can enter the systemic circulation through pulmonary arteriovenous shunts to generate the central, renal, and cutaneous manifestations of this syndrome.

BOX 21–4 Diagnostic Criteria for Fat Embolism Syndrome

Major Criteria

- Pulmonary insufficiency
  - $Pa_{O_2} < 60$ mm Hg
- Neurologic dysfunction
  - Confusion
  - Disorientation
  - Lethargy
  - Focal deficits
  - Seizures
  - Coma
- Petechiae

Minor Criteria

- Fever
- Thrombocytopenia
- Anemia
- Tachycardia
- Elevated erythrocyte sedimentation rate
- Retinal changes

PRESENTATION

FES can be demonstrated in 90% of patients with long bone fractures, but symptomatic FES occurs in only 10% to 22% of patients with long bone or pelvic fractures. Classically, it develops 24 to 72 hours after an injury and is characterized by acute respiratory insufficiency with diffuse pulmonary infiltrates, global neurologic dysfunction, and petechiae. The pulmonary compromise is usually followed by the neurologic changes. If a petechial rash develops, it occurs 48 to 72 hours after the onset of FES. This complete presentation is seen in less than 10% of cases. Respiratory insufficiency may be the only manifestation of this syndrome, and it may occur in only one third of patients. This unexplained hypoxia is how FES manifests during general anesthesia (van Besouw and Hinds, 1989). Few patients with FES have a fulminant course in which severe pulmonary hypertension and progressive right heart failure develop within hours of the injury. Vasopressor infusions are frequently required when this occurs.

The diagnosis of FES is a clinical one, and it may be difficult to establish (Georgopoulos and Bouros, 2003). Supportive laboratory tests include an inexplicable drop in Pa_{O_2}, hematocrit, platelet counts, and fibrinogen levels. The characteristic radiograph of bilateral fluffy pulmonary infiltrates may not be apparent for 24 to 48 hours after the onset of FES. Fat is seen in the urine in 50% of patients within 3 days. The utility of serum and urinary measurements of fat and lipase activity are limited by their poor sensitivity and specificity and by a lack of availability. Identification of fat droplet cells in bronchoalveolar lavage is the only rapid and specific method of identifying the development of this syndrome (Chastre et al., 1990; Mimoz et al., 1995). The retinal changes of bilateral cotton-wool spots and intraretinal hemorrhages are seen in 60% of patients with FES.

In the operating room, the time of highest risk for the development of FES occurs during the transfer of the fracture patient from the stretcher to the operating room table. Fulminant FES can manifest within 30 minutes of this transfer, and it is recognized by inexplicable, progressive oxygen desaturation and increasing peak inspiratory pressures. A high index of suspicion is necessary to make the diagnosis. Other manifestations of FES during anesthesia include sudden hypotension, tachycardia, bradycardia, dysrhythmia, decreased lung compliance, pulmonary edema, and severe, unexplained surgical bleeding or oozing from multiple sites resulting from disseminated intravascular coagulation.

End-tidal CO_2 monitoring does not seem to be as sensitive to fat emboli as it is in other embolic states. Although end-tidal CO_2 does change with a massive fat embolism, end-tidal CO_2 monitoring has not been as effective as echocardiography in detecting smaller emboli. Transesophageal echocardiography can detect fat emboli during surgical manipulation of the operative bone, and it can demonstrate the regional wall motion abnormalities and right ventricular dilatation that are harbingers of the FES physiologic perturbations (Capan and Miller, 2001).

After FES develops, the treatment is nonspecific and supportive. It consists of early resuscitation and stabilization, administration of 100% oxygen, application of positive end-expiratory pressure, and the use of inverse-ratio ventilation. Bronchoscopy and bronchoalveolar lavage are useful in establishing a diagnosis and in removing the intraluminal debris and hemorrhagic exudate that accompany a fulminant presentation. An adequate intravascular volume must be maintained, and inotropic infusions and red blood cell transfusions are often required. Historically, advocated therapies have included intravenous alcohol, heparin, low-molecular-weight dextrans, and steroids. Limited data support the efficacy of any of these therapies once FES has begun. Early administration of methylprednisolone may decrease the incidence of FES (Lindeque et al., 1987). A 10% mortality rate has been reported for all patients; among children, the mortality rate is 33%.

SUMMARY

The orthopedic patient presents multiple challenges to the anesthesiologist. In many instances, the perioperative anesthetic plan for pediatric orthopedic patients depends more on the child's age and on the site and emergent nature of surgery than on the underlying disease or the specifics of the surgical procedure. In other cases, the underlying medical condition, associated anomalies, pathophysiology, and surgical procedure dictate the anesthetic plan. The anesthetic plan must address these issues and the recurring themes of positioning, airway management, blood loss and fluid replacement, conservation of body temperature, and postoperative pain management. In the future, the continued technologic, physiologic, and pharmacologic advances in our specialty will allow for longer, more extensive, and more innovative operations on younger and sicker patients than was possible in the past.

REFERENCES

Abbott R, Johann-Murphy M, Shiminski-Maher T, et al.: Selective dorsal rhizotomy: Outcome and complications in treating spastic cerebral palsy. *Neurosurgery* 33:851–857, 1993.

Abildgaard L, Aaro S, Lisander B: Limited effectiveness of intraoperative autotransfusion in major back surgery. *Eur J Anaesthesiol* 18:823–828, 2001.

Aglio LS, Romero R, Desai S, et al.: The use of transcranial magnetic stimulation for monitoring descending spinal cord motor function. *Clin Electroencephalogr* 33:30–41, 2002.

Ahn UM, Ahn NU, Nallamshetty L, et al.: The etiology of adolescent idiopathic scoliosis. *Am J Orthop* 31:387–395, 2002.

Alanay A, Acaroglu E, Ozdemir O, et al.: Effects of deamino-8-D-arginin vasopressin on blood loss and coagulation factors in scoliosis surgery: A double-blind randomized clinical trial. *Spine* 24:877–882, 1999.

Albright AL: Intrathecal baclofen in cerebral palsy movement disorders. *J Child Neurol* 11(Suppl 1):S29–S35, 1996.

Albright AL, Cervi A, Singletary J: Intrathecal baclofen for spasticity in cerebral palsy. *JAMA* 265:1418–1422, 1991.

Albright AL, Shultz BL: Plasma baclofen levels in children receiving continuous intrathecal baclofen infusion. *J Child Neurol* 14:408–409, 1999.

Aldegheri R, Dall'Oca C: Limb lengthening in short stature patients. *J Pediatr Orthop B* 10:238–247, 2001.

Aronson J: Limb-lengthening, skeletal reconstruction, and bone transport with the Ilizarov method. *J Bone Joint Surg Am* 79:1243–1258, 1997.

Ascani E, Bartolozzi P, Logroscino CA, et al.: Natural history of untreated idiopathic scoliosis after skeletal maturity. *Spine* 11:784–789, 1986.

Ashkenaze D, Mudiyam R, Boachie-Adjei O, et al.: Efficacy of spinal cord monitoring in neuromuscular scoliosis. *Spine* 18:1627–1633, 1993.

Baines DB, Douglas ID, Overton JH: Anaesthesia for patients with arthrogryposis multiplex congenita: What is the risk of malignant hyperthermia? *Anaesth Intensive Care* 14:370–372, 1986.

Bauchner H: Developmental dysplasia of the hip (DDH): An evolving science. *Arch Dis Child* 83:202, 2000.

Ben David B: Spinal cord monitoring. *Orthop Clin North Am* 19:427–448, 1988.

Berkowitz ID, Raja SN, Bender KS, et al.: Dwarfs: Pathophysiology and anesthetic implications. *Anesthesiology* 73:739–759, 1990.

Blais RE, Hadjipavlou AG, Shulman G: Efficacy of autotransfusion in spine surgery: Comparison of autotransfusion alone and with hemodilution and apheresis. *Spine* 21:2795–2800, 1996.

Bloch EC, Ginsberg B, Binner RA Jr, et al.: Limb tourniquets and central temperature in anesthetized children. *Anesth Analg* 74:486–489, 1992.

Boero S, Brunenghi GM, Carbone M, et al.: Pinning in slipped capital femoral epiphysis: Long-term follow-up study. *J Pediatr Orthop B* 12:372–379, 2003.

Boidin MP, Erdmann WE, Faithfull NS: The role of ascorbic acid in etomidate toxicity. *Eur J Anaesthesiol* 3:417–422, 1986.

Bonilla-Musoles F, Machado LE, Osborne NG: Multiple congenital contractures (congenital multiple arthrogryposis). *J Perinat Med* 30:99–104, 2002.

Bostrom MP, Camacho NP: Potential role of bone morphogenetic proteins in fracture healing. *Clin Orthop* S274–S282, 1998.

Breau LM, Camfield CS, McGrath PJ, et al.: The incidence of pain in children with severe cognitive impairments. *Arch Pediatr Adolesc Med* 157:1219–1226, 2003.

Breau LM, Finley GA, McGrath PJ, et al.: Validation of the Non-communicating Children's Pain Checklist—postoperative version. *Anesthesiology* 96:528–535, 2002.

Brock-Utne JG: Clinical manifestations of latex anaphylaxis during anesthesia differ from those not anesthesia/surgery-related. *Anesth Analg* 97:1204–1205, 2003.

Brodkey JS, Richards DE, Blasingame JP, et al.: Reversible spinal cord trauma in cats. Additive effects of direct pressure and ischemia. *J Neurosurg* 37:591–593, 1972.

Brown JC, Swank S, Specht L: Combined anterior and posterior spine fusion in cerebral palsy. *Spine* 7:570–573, 1982.

Brown RH, Schauble JF, Hamilton RG: Prevalence of latex allergy among anesthesiologists: Identification of sensitized but asymptomatic individuals. *Anesthesiology* 89:292–299, 1998.

Bryson GL, Laupacis A, Wells GA: Does acute normovolemic hemodilution reduce perioperative allogeneic transfusion? A meta-analysis. The International Study of Perioperative Transfusion. *Anesth Analg* 86:9–15, 1998.

Bulger EM, Smith DG, Maier RV, Jurkovich GJ: Fat embolism syndrome. A 10-year review. *Arch Surg* 132:435–439, 1997.

Burke G, Cossins J, Maxwell S, et al.: Rapsyn mutations in hereditary myasthenia: Distinct early- and late-onset phenotypes. *Neurology* 61:826–828, 2003.

Burt N, Haynes GR, Bailey MK: Patients with malignant osteopetrosis are at high risk of anesthetic morbidity and mortality. *Anesth Analg* 88:1292–1297, 1999.

Byrick RJ, Kay JC, Mullen JB: Capnography is not as sensitive as pulmonary artery pressure monitoring in detecting marrow microembolism. Studies in a canine model. *Anesth Analg* 68:94–100, 1989.

Capan LM, Miller SM: Monitoring for suspected pulmonary embolism. *Anesthesiol Clin North Am* 19:673–703, 2001.

Cervellati S, Bettini N, Bianco T, et al.: Neurological complications in segmental spinal instrumentation: Analysis of 750 patients. *Eur Spine J* 5:161–166, 1996.

Chastre J, Fagon JY, Soler P, et al.: Bronchoalveolar lavage for rapid diagnosis of the fat embolism syndrome in trauma patients. *Ann Intern Med* 113:583–588, 1990.

Chevrel G, Meunier PJ: Osteogenesis imperfecta: Lifelong management is imperative and feasible. *Joint Bone Spine* 68:125–129, 2001.

Cohen MM Jr: Some chondrodysplasias with short limbs: Molecular perspectives. *Am J Med Genet* 112:304–313, 2002.

Cole JW, Murray DJ, Snider RJ, et al.: Aprotinin reduces blood loss during spinal surgery in children. *Spine* 28:2482–2485, 2003.

Cole NL, Goldberg MH, Loftus M, et al.: Surgical management of patients with osteogenesis imperfecta. *J Oral Maxillofac Surg* 40:578–584, 1982.

Copley LA, Richards BS, Safavi FZ, et al.: Hemodilution as a method to reduce transfusion requirements in adolescent spine fusion surgery. *Spine* 24:219–222, 1999.

Croteau S, Rauch F, Silvestri A, et al.: Bone morphogenetic proteins in orthopedics: From basic science to clinical practice. *Orthopedics* 22:686–695, 1999.

Cucchiara RF, Michenfelder JD, editors: *Clinical neuroanesthesia*. New York, 1990, Churchill Livingstone.

Cummings RJ, Davidson RS, Armstrong PF, et al.: Congenital clubfoot. *Instr Course Lect* 51:385–400, 2002.

da Costa VV, Saraiva RA, de Almeida AC, et al.: The effect of nitrous oxide on the inhibition of somatosensory evoked potentials by sevoflurane in children. *Anaesthesia* 56:202–207, 2001.

Dalens B, Vanneuville G, Tanguy A: A new parascalene approach to the brachial plexus in children: Comparison with the supraclavicular approach. *Anesth Analg* 66:1264–1271, 1987.

Dalens B, Vanneuville G, Tanguy A: Comparison of the fascia iliaca compartment block with the 3-in-1 block in children. *Anesth Analg* 69:705–713, 1989.

Dalens BJ, Khandwala RS, Tanguy A: Staged segmental scoliosis surgery during regional anesthesia in high risk patients: A report of six cases. *Anesth Analg* 76:434–439, 1993.

Dawson EG, Sherman JE, Kanim LE, et al.: Spinal cord monitoring. Results of the Scoliosis Research Society and the European Spinal Deformity Society survey. *Spine* 16:S361–S364, 1991.

Degoute CS, Ray MJ, Gueugniaud PY, et al.: Remifentanil induces consistent and sustained controlled hypotension in children during middle ear surgery. *Can J Anaesth* 50:270–276, 2003.

Deguchi M, Rapoff AJ, Zdeblick TA: Posterolateral fusion for isthmic spondylolisthesis in adults: Analysis of fusion rate and clinical results. *J Spinal Disord* 11:459–464, 1998.

Denislic M, Meh D: Botulinum toxin in the treatment of cerebral palsy. *Neuropediatrics* 26:249–252, 1995.

Dickson M, White H, Kinney W, et al.: Extremity tourniquet deflation increases end-tidal P_{CO_2}. *Anesth Analg* 70:457–458, 1990.

Dierdorf SF, McNiece WL, Rao CC, et al.: Effect of succinylcholine on plasma potassium in children with cerebral palsy. *Anesthesiology* 62:88–90, 1985.

Dietz HC, Cutting GR, Pyeritz RE, et al.: Marfan syndrome caused by a recurrent de novo missense mutation in the fibrillin gene. *Nature* 352:337–339, 1991a.

Dietz HC, Pyeritz RE, Hall BD, et al.: The Marfan syndrome locus: Confirmation of assignment to chromosome 15 and identification of tightly linked markers at 15q15-q21.3. *Genomics* 9:355–361, 1991b.

Dietz HC, Pyeritz RE: Mutations in the human gene for fibrillin-1 (FBN1) in the Marfan syndrome and related disorders. *Hum Mol Genet* 4:1799–1809, 1995.

Dimar JR, Ante WA, Zhang YP, et al.: The effects of nonsteroidal anti-inflammatory drugs on posterior spinal fusions in the rat. *Spine* 21:1870–1876, 1996.

Drummond JC, Todd MM, Schubert A, et al.: Effect of the acute administration of high dose pentobarbital on human brain stem auditory and median nerve somatosensory evoked responses. *Neurosurgery* 20:830–835, 1987.

Drvaric DM, Kuivila TE, Roberts JM: Congenital clubfoot. Etiology, pathoanatomy, pathogenesis, and the changing spectrum of early management. *Orthop Clin North Am* 20:641–647, 1989.

Eastham KM, McKiernan PJ, Milford DV, et al.: ARC syndrome: An expanding range of phenotypes. *Arch Dis Child* 85:415–420, 2001.

Eastwood DM: Neonatal hip screening. *Lancet* 361:595–597, 2003.

Edler A, Murray DJ, Forbes RB: Blood loss during posterior spinal fusion surgery in patients with neuromuscular disease: Is there an increased risk? *Paediatr Anaesth* 13:818–822, 2003.

Edmonds HL Jr, Paloheimo MP, Backman MH, et al.: Transcranial magnetic motor evoked potentials (tcMMEP) for functional monitoring of motor pathways during scoliosis surgery. *Spine* 14:683–686, 1989.

Eldridge PR, Williams S: Effect of limb tourniquet on cerebral perfusion pressure in a head-injured patient. *Anaesthesia* 44:973–974, 1989.

Fasth A, Porras O: Human malignant osteopetrosis: Pathophysiology, management and the role of bone marrow transplantation. *Pediatr Transplant* 3(Suppl 1): 102–107, 1999.

Finkbohner R, Johnston D, Crawford ES, et al.: Marfan syndrome: Long-term survival and complications after aortic aneurysm repair. *Circulation* 91:728–733, 1995.

Forssberg H, Tedroff KB: Botulinum toxin treatment in cerebral palsy: Intervention with poor evaluation? *Dev Med Child Neurol* 39:635–640, 1997.

Frei FJ, Haemmerle MH, Brunner R, et al.: Minimum alveolar concentration for halothane in children with cerebral palsy and severe mental retardation. *Anaesthesia* 52:1056–1060, 1997.

Gajraj NM: Cyclooxygenase-2 inhibitors. *Anesth Analg* 96:1720–1738, 2003a.

Gajraj NM: The effect of cyclooxygenase-2 inhibitors on bone healing. *Reg Anesth Pain Med* 28:456–465, 2003b.

Gale T, Leslie K, Kluger M: Propofol anaesthesia via target controlled infusion or manually controlled infusion: Effects on the bispectral index as a measure of anaesthetic depth. *Anaesth Intensive Care* 29:579–584, 2001.

Gan TJ, Ginsberg B, Glass PS, et al.: Opioid-sparing effects of a low-dose infusion of naloxone in patient-administered morphine sulfate. *Anesthesiology* 87:1075–1081, 1997.

Georgopoulos D, Bouros D: Fat embolism syndrome: Clinical examination is still the preferable diagnostic method. *Chest* 123:982–983, 2003.

Gerritsen EJ, Vossen JM, van Loo IH, et al.: Autosomal recessive osteopetrosis: Variability of findings at diagnosis and during the natural course. *Pediatrics* 93:247–253, 1994.

Gerstenfeld LC, Thiede M, Seibert K, et al.: Differential inhibition of fracture healing by non-selective and cyclooxygenase-2 selective non-steroidal anti-inflammatory drugs. *J Orthop Res* 21:670–675, 2003.

Geyser PG, Hugo JM, Ingram H: Anaesthetic management in sclerosteosis. A case report. *S Afr Med J* 61:488, 1982.

Gilron I, Milne B, Hong M: Cyclooxygenase-2 inhibitors in postoperative pain management: Current evidence and future directions. *Anesthesiology* 99:1198–1208, 2003.

Glassman SD, Johnson JR, Shields CB, et al.: Correlation of motor-evoked potentials, somatosensory-evoked potentials, and the wake-up test in a case of kyphoscoliosis. *J Spinal Disord* 6:194–198, 1993.

Glassman SD, Rose SM, Dimar JR, et al.: The effect of postoperative nonsteroidal anti-inflammatory drug administration on spinal fusion. *Spine* 23:834–838, 1998.

Glorieux FH: The use of bisphosphonates in children with osteogenesis imperfecta. *J Pediatr Endocrinol Metab* 14(Suppl 6):1491–1495, 2001.

Goodnough LT, Rudnick S, Price TH, et al.: Increased preoperative collection of autologous blood with recombinant human erythropoietin therapy. *N Engl J Med* 321:1163–1168, 1989.

Goodnough LT: Erythropoietin therapy versus red cell transfusion. *Curr Opin Hematol* 8:405–410, 2001.

Gott VL, Cameron DE, Alejo DE, et al.: Aortic root replacement in 271 Marfan patients: A 24-year experience. *Ann Thorac Surg* 73:438–443, 2002.

Gott VL, Greene PS, Alejo DE, et al.: Replacement of the aortic root in patients with Marfan's syndrome. *N Engl J Med* 340:1307–1313, 1999.

Grether JK, Nelson KB, Emery ES III, et al.: Prenatal and perinatal factors and cerebral palsy in very low birth weight infants. *J Pediatr* 128:407–414, 1996.

Griffiths IR, Trench JG, Crawford RA: Spinal cord blood flow and conduction during experimental cord compression in normotensive and hypotensive dogs. *J Neurosurg* 50:353–360, 1979.

Grundy BL: Intraoperative monitoring of sensory-evoked potentials. *Anesthesiology* 58:72–87, 1983.

Grundy BL, Nash CL Jr, Brown RH: Arterial pressure manipulation alters spinal cord function during correction of scoliosis. *Anesthesiology* 54:249–253, 1981.

Guay J, Reinberg C, Poitras B, et al.: A trial of desmopressin to reduce blood loss in patients undergoing spinal fusion for idiopathic scoliosis. *Anesth Analg* 75:405–410, 1992.

Hackmann T, Friesen M, Allen S, et al.: Clonidine facilitates controlled hypotension in adolescent children. *Anesth Analg* 96:976–981, 2003.

Hall JE, Levine CR, Sudhir KG: Intraoperative awakening to monitor spinal cord function during Harrington instrumentation and spine fusion. Description of procedure and report of three cases. *J Bone Joint Surg Am* 60:533–536, 1978.

Hammer GB, Fitzmaurice BG, Brodsky JB: Methods for single-lung ventilation in pediatric patients. *Anesth Analg* 89:1426–1429, 1999.

Hammer GB, Harrison TK, Vricella LA, et al.: Single lung ventilation in children using a new paediatric bronchial blocker. *Paediatr Anaesth* 12:69–72, 2002.

Harder AT, An YH: The mechanisms of the inhibitory effects of nonsteroidal anti-inflammatory drugs on bone healing: A concise review. *J Clin Pharmacol* 43:807–815, 2003.

Harrington PR: The history and development of Harrington instrumentation. *Clin Orthop* 227:3–5, 1988.

Harrington PR, Dickson JH: Spinal instrumentation in the treatment of severe progressive spondylolisthesis. *Clin Orthop* 117:157–163, 1976.

Helfaer MA, Carson BS, James CS, et al.: Increased hematocrit and decreased transfusion requirements in children given erythropoietin before undergoing craniofacial surgery. *J Neurosurg* 88:704–708, 1998.

Henry DA, Moxey AJ, Carless PA, et al.: Desmopressin for minimising perioperative allogeneic blood transfusion. *Cochrane Database Syst Rev* 2:CD001884, 2001.

Herbert AJ, Herzenberg JE, Paley D: A review for pediatricians on limb lengthening and the Ilizarov method. *Curr Opin Pediatr* 7:98–105, 1995.

Herdmann J, Deletis V, Edmonds HL Jr, et al.: Spinal cord and nerve root monitoring in spine surgery and related procedures. *Spine* 21:879–885, 1996.

Hersey SL, O'Dell NE, Lowe S, et al.: Nicardipine versus nitroprusside for controlled hypotension during spinal surgery in adolescents. *Anesth Analg* 84:1239–1244, 1997.

Herzenberg JE, Radler C, Bor N: Ponseti versus traditional methods of casting for idiopathic clubfoot. *J Pediatr Orthop* 22:517–521, 2002.

Herzka A, Sponseller PD, Pyeritz RE: Atlantoaxial rotatory subluxation in patients with Marfan syndrome. A report of three cases. *Spine* 25:524–526, 2000.

Hobbs WR, Sponseller PD, Weiss AP, et al.: The cervical spine in Marfan syndrome. *Spine* 22:983–989, 1997.

Hopkins PM, Ellis FR, Halsall PJ: Hypermetabolism in arthrogryposis multiplex congenita. *Anaesthesia* 46:374–375, 1991.

Huet C, Salmi LR, Fergusson D, et al.: A meta-analysis of the effectiveness of cell salvage to minimize perioperative allogeneic blood transfusion in cardiac and orthopedic surgery. International Study of Perioperative Transfusion (ISPOT) investigators. *Anesth Analg* 89:861–869, 1999.

Huo MH, Troiano NW, Pelker RR, et al.: The influence of ibuprofen on fracture repair: Biomechanical, biochemical, histologic, and histomorphometric parameters in rats. *J Orthop Res* 9:383–390, 1991.

Hur SR, Huizenga BA, Major M: Acute normovolemic hemodilution combined with hypotensive anesthesia and other techniques to avoid homologous transfusion in spinal fusion surgery. *Spine* 17:867–873, 1992.

Ippolito E, Farsetti P, Caterini R, et al.: Long-term comparative results in patients with congenital clubfoot treated with two different protocols. *J Bone Joint Surg Am* 85:1286–1294, 2003.

Jacobs JC, Hui RM: Cricoarytenoid arthritis and airway obstruction in juvenile rheumatoid arthritis. *Pediatrics* 59:292–294, 1977.

Jacobson L, Polizzi A, Morriss-Kay G, et al.: Plasma from human mothers of fetuses with severe arthrogryposis multiplex congenita causes deformities in mice. *J Clin Invest* 103:1031–1038, 1999.

Jarvis JN: Juvenile rheumatoid arthritis: A guide for pediatricians. *Pediatr Ann* 31:437–446, 2002.

Jarvis S, Glinianaia SV, Torrioli MG, et al.: Cerebral palsy and intrauterine growth in single births: European collaborative study. *Lancet* 362:1106–1111, 2003.

Johnston CE, Happel LT Jr, Norris R, et al.: Delayed paraplegia complicating sublaminar segmental spinal instrumentation. *J Bone Joint Surg Am* 68:556–563, 1986.

Jondeau G, Boutouyrie P, Lacolley P, et al.: Central pulse pressure is a major determinant of ascending aorta dilation in Marfan syndrome. *Circulation* 99:2677–2681, 1999.

Kafer ER: Respiratory and cardiovascular functions in scoliosis and the principles of anesthetic management. *Anesthesiology* 52:339–351, 1980.

Kalkman CJ, ten Brink SA, Been HD, et al.: Variability of somatosensory cortical evoked potentials during spinal surgery. Effects of anesthetic technique and high-pass digital filtering. *Spine* 16:924–929, 1991a.

Kalkman CJ, Traast H, Zuurmond WW, et al.: Differential effects of propofol and nitrous oxide on posterior tibial nerve somatosensory cortical evoked potentials during alfentanil anaesthesia. *Br J Anaesth* 66:483–489, 1991b.

Kallos T, Smith TC: Replacement for intraoperative blood loss. *Anesthesiology* 41:293–295, 1974.

Kam PC, Kavanagh R, Yoong FF, et al.: The arterial tourniquet: Pathophysiological consequences and anaesthetic implications. *Anaesthesia* 56:534–545, 2001.

Kannan S, Meert KL, Mooney JF, et al.: Bleeding and coagulation changes during spinal fusion surgery: A comparison of neuromuscular and idiopathic scoliosis patients. *Pediatr Crit Care Med* 3:364–369, 2002.

Kaufman RD, Walts LF: Tourniquet-induced hypertension. *Br J Anaesth* 54: 333–336, 1982.

Kawaguchi M, Sakamoto T, Inoue S, et al.: Low dose propofol as a supplement to ketamine-based anesthesia during intraoperative monitoring of motor-evoked potentials. *Spine* 25:974–979, 2000.

Kelly KJ, Pearson ML, Kurup VP, et al.: A cluster of anaphylactic reactions in children with spina bifida during general anesthesia: Epidemiologic features, risk factors, and latex hypersensitivity. *J Allergy Clin Immunol* 94:53–61, 1994.

Kenyon CJ, McNeil LM, Fraser R: Comparison of the effects of etomidate, thiopentone and propofol on cortisol synthesis. *Br J Anaesth* 57:509–511, 1985.

Key LL Jr, Rodriguiz RM, Willi SM, et al.: Long-term treatment of osteopetrosis with recombinant human interferon gamma. *N Engl J Med* 332:1594–1599, 1995.

Khan SN, Bostrom MP, Lane JM: Bone growth factors. *Orthop Clin North Am* 31:375–388, 2000.

Khan SN, Sandhu HS, Lane JM, et al.: Bone morphogenetic proteins: Relevance in spine surgery. *Orthop Clin North Am* 33:447–463, ix, 2002.

Kimovec MA, Koht A, Sloan TB: Effects of sufentanil on median nerve somatosensory evoked potentials. *Br J Anaesth* 65:169–172, 1990.

Kobrinsky NL, Letts RM, Patel LR, et al.: 1-Desamino-8-D-arginine vasopressin (desmopressin) decreases operative blood loss in patients having Harrington rod spinal fusion surgery. A randomized, double-blinded, controlled trial. *Ann Intern Med* 107:446–450, 1987.

Kocher MS, Bishop JA, Weed B, et al.: Delay in diagnosis of slipped capital femoral epiphysis. *Pediatrics* 113:e322–e325, 2004.

Kostopanagiotou G, Coussi T, Tsaroucha N, et al.: Anaesthesia using a laryngeal mask airway in a patient with osteogenesis imperfecta. *Anaesthesia* 55:506, 2000.

Kotagal S, Gibbons VP, Stith JA: Sleep abnormalities in patients with severe cerebral palsy. *Dev Med Child Neurol* 36:304–311, 1994.

Kuban KC, Leviton A: Cerebral palsy. *N Engl J Med* 330:188–195, 1994.

Lam AM, Sharar SR, Mayberg TS, et al.: Isoflurane compared with nitrous oxide anaesthesia for intraoperative monitoring of somatosensory-evoked potentials. *Can J Anaesth* 41:295–300, 1994.

Langeron O, Lille F, Zerhouni O, et al.: Comparison of the effects of ketamine-midazolam with those of fentanyl-midazolam on cortical somatosensory evoked potentials during major spine surgery. *Br J Anaesth* 78:701–706, 1997.

Laupacis A, Fergusson D: Drugs to minimize perioperative blood loss in cardiac surgery: Meta-analyses using perioperative blood transfusion as the outcome. The International Study of Peri-operative Transfusion (ISPOT) Investigators. *Anesth Analg* 85:1258–1267, 1997.

Lee LA, Lam AM: Unilateral blindness after prone lumbar spine surgery. *Anesthesiology* 95:793–795, 2001.

Lehman WB, Mohaideen A, Madan S, et al.: A method for the early evaluation of the Ponseti (Iowa) technique for the treatment of idiopathic clubfoot. *J Pediatr Orthop B* 12:133–140, 2003.

Lesser RP, Raudzens P, Luders H, et al.: Postoperative neurological deficits may occur despite unchanged intraoperative somatosensory evoked potentials. *Ann Neurol* 19:22–25, 1986.

Lindeque BG, Schoeman HS, Dommisse GF, et al.: Fat embolism and the fat embolism syndrome. A double-blind therapeutic study. *J Bone Joint Surg Br* 69:128–131, 1987.

Loder RT, Aronsson DD, Dobbs MB, et al.: Slipped capital femoral epiphysis. *Instr Course Lect* 50:555–570, 2001.

Lowe TG, Edgar M, Margulies JY, et al.: Etiology of idiopathic scoliosis: Current trends in research. *J Bone Joint Surg Am* 82:1157–1168, 2000.

Lubicky JP, Spadaro JA, Yuan HA, et al.: Variability of somatosensory cortical evoked potential monitoring during spinal surgery. *Spine* 14:790–798, 1989.

Luque ER: Segmental spinal instrumentation of the lumbar spine. *Clin Orthop* 126–134, 1986.

Luque ER, Rapp GF: A new semirigid method for interpedicular fixation of the spine. *Orthopedics* 11:1445–1450, 1988.

MacEwen GD, Bunnell WP, Sriram K: Acute neurological complications in the treatment of scoliosis. A report of the Scoliosis Research Society. *J Bone Joint Surg Am* 57:404–408, 1975.

MacKenzie JM, Rankin R: Sudden death due to atlantoaxial subluxation in Marfan syndrome. *Am J Forensic Med Pathol* 24:369–370, 2003.

Manolagas SC: Birth and death of bone cells: Basic regulatory mechanisms and implications for the pathogenesis and treatment of osteoporosis. *Endocr Rev* 21:115–137, 2000.

Martin GJ Jr, Boden SD, Titus L: Recombinant human bone morphogenetic protein-2 overcomes the inhibitory effect of ketorolac, a nonsteroidal anti-inflammatory drug (NSAID), on posterolateral lumbar intertransverse process spine fusion. *Spine* 24:2188–2193, 1999.

Martin JT: The ventral decubitus (prone) position. In Martin JT, Warner MA, editors. *Positioning in anesthesia and surgery*. Philadelphia, 1997, WB Saunders, pp155–195.

Mason RJ, Betz RR, Orlowski JP, et al.: The syndrome of inappropriate antidiuretic hormone secretion and its effect on blood indices following spinal fusion. *Spine* 14:722–726, 1989.

Maurette P, Simeon F, Castagnera L, et al.: Propofol anaesthesia alters somatosensory evoked cortical potentials. *Anaesthesia* 43(Suppl):44–45, 1988.

Maxwell LG, Yaster M: Effects of a low-dose naloxone infusion on opioid-induced side effects and analgesia in children and adolescents treated with intravenous patient-controlled analgesia: A prospective, randomized, controlled, double-blind study. *Anesthesiology* 99:A1453, 2003.

Maxwell LG, Kaufmann SC, Bitzer S, et al.: The effects of a small-dose naloxone infusion on opioid-induced side effects and analgesia in children and adolescents treated with intravenous patient-controlled analgesia: a double-blind, prospective, randomized, controlled study. *Anesth Analg* 100: 953–958, 2005.

Maxy RJ, Glassman SD: The effect of nonsteroidal anti-inflammatory drugs on osteogenesis and spinal fusion. *Reg Anesth Pain Med* 26:156–158, 2001.

McCarthy JG, Stelnicki EJ, Mehrara BJ, et al.: Distraction osteogenesis of the craniofacial skeleton. *Plast Reconstr Surg* 107:1812–1827, 2001.

McPherson RW, Mahla M, Johnson R, et al.: Effects of enflurane, isoflurane, and nitrous oxide on somatosensory evoked potentials during fentanyl anesthesia. *Anesthesiology* 62:626–633, 1985.

Meert KL, Kannan S, Mooney JF: Predictors of red cell transfusion in children and adolescents undergoing spinal fusion surgery. *Spine* 27:2137–2142, 2002.

Mellor A, Soni N: Fat embolism. *Anaesthesia* 56:145–154, 2001.

Miller F, Moseley CF, Koreska J, et al.: Pulmonary function and scoliosis in Duchenne dystrophy. *J Pediatr Orthop* 8:133–137, 1998.

Milne B, Rosales JK: Anaesthetic considerations in patients with muscular dystrophy undergoing spinal fusion and Harrington rod insertion. *Can Anaesth Soc J* 29:250–254, 1982.

Mimoz O, Edouard A, Beydon L, et al.: Contribution of bronchoalveolar lavage to the diagnosis of posttraumatic pulmonary fat embolism. *Intensive Care Med* 21:973–980, 1995.

Monedero P, Garcia-Pedrajas F, Coca I, et al.: Is management of anesthesia in achondroplastic dwarfs really a challenge? *J Clin Anesth* 9:208–212, 1997.

Monitto CL, Greenberg RS, Kost-Byerly S, et al.: The safety and efficacy of parent-/nurse-controlled analgesia in patients less than six years of age. *Anesth Analg* 91:573–579, 2000.

Mubarak SJ, Bialik V: Pavlik: The man and his method. *J Pediatr Orthop* 23:342–346, 2003.

Nakamura CT, Ferdman RM, Keens TG, et al.: Latex allergy in children on home mechanical ventilation. *Chest* 118:1000–1003, 2000.

Nash CL Jr, Brown RH: Spinal cord monitoring. *J Bone Joint Surg Am* 71:627–630, 1989.

Nelson KB, Grether JK: Causes of cerebral palsy. *Curr Opin Pediatr* 11:487–491, 1999.

Newton PO, Wenger DR, Mubarak SJ, et al.: Anterior release and fusion in pediatric spinal deformity. A comparison of early outcome and cost of thoracoscopic and open thoracotomy approaches. *Spine* 22:1398–1406, 1997.

Nguyen NH, Morvant EM, Mayhew JF: Anesthetic management for patients with arthrogryposis multiplex congenita and severe micrognathia: Case reports. *J Clin Anesth* 12:227–230, 2000.

Nolan J, Chalkiadis GA, Low J, et al.: Anaesthesia and pain management in cerebral palsy. *Anaesthesia* 55:32–41, 2000.

Nuttall GA, Garrity JA, Dearani JA, et al.: Risk factors for ischemic optic neuropathy after cardiopulmonary bypass: A matched case/control study. *Anesth Analg* 93:1410–1416, 2001.

Nuttall GA, Horlocker TT, Santrach PJ, et al.: Predictors of blood transfusions in spinal instrumentation and fusion surgery. *Spine* 25:596–601, 2000.

Nuttall GA, Stehling LC, Beighley CM, et al.: Current transfusion practices of members of the American Society of Anesthesiologists: A survey. *Anesthesiology* 99:1433–1443, 2003.

Nuwer MR, Dawson EG, Carlson LG, et al.: Somatosensory evoked potential spinal cord monitoring reduces neurologic deficits after scoliosis surgery: Results of a large multicenter survey. *Electroencephalogr Clin Neurophysiol* 96:6–11, 1995.

Oberoi GS, Kaul HL, Gill IS, et al.: Anaesthesia in arthrogryposis multiplex congenita: Case report. *Can J Anaesth* 34:288–290, 1987.

O'Brien CA, Jia D, Plotkin LI, et al.: Glucocorticoids act directly on osteoblasts and osteocytes to induce their apoptosis and reduce bone formation and strength. *Endocrinology* 145:1835–1841, 2003.

O'Brien T, Akmakjian J, Ogin G, et al.: Comparison of one-stage versus two-stage anterior/posterior spinal fusion for neuromuscular scoliosis. *J Pediatr Orthop* 12:610–615, 1992.

O'Flaherty P: Arthrogryposis multiplex congenita. *Neonatal Netw* 20:13–20, 2001.

Orioli IM, Castilla EE, Barbosa-Neto JG: The birth prevalence rates for the skeletal dysplasias. *J Med Genet* 23:328–332, 1986.

Owen JH: The application of intraoperative monitoring during surgery for spinal deformity. *Spine* 24:2649–2662, 1999.

Owen JH, Bridwell KH, Grubb R, et al.: The clinical application of neurogenic motor evoked potentials to monitor spinal cord function during surgery. *Spine* 16:S385–S390, 1991.

Owen JH, Jenny AB, Naito M, et al.: Effects of spinal cord lesioning on somatosensory and neurogenic-motor evoked potentials. *Spine* 14:673–682, 1989.

Owen JH, Laschinger J, Bridwell K, et al.: Sensitivity and specificity of somatosensory and neurogenic-motor evoked potentials in animals and humans. *Spine* 13:1111–1118, 1988.

Padberg AM, Wilson-Holden TJ, Lenke LG, et al.: Somatosensory- and motor-evoked potential monitoring without a wake-up test during idiopathic scoliosis surgery: An accepted standard of care. *Spine* 23:1392–1400, 1998.

Paley D: Problems, obstacles, and complications of limb lengthening by the Ilizarov technique. *Clin Orthop* 250:81–104, 1990.

Parisi DM, Koval K, Egol K: Fat embolism syndrome. *Am J Orthop* 31:507–512, 2002.

Pathak KS, Brown RH, Nash CL Jr, et al.: Continuous opioid infusion for scoliosis fusion surgery. *Anesth Analg* 62:841–845, 1983.

Patterson S, Klenerman L: The effect of pneumatic tourniquets on the ultrastructure of skeletal muscle. *J Bone Joint Surg Br* 61:178–183, 1979.

Peacock WJ, Staudt LA: Spasticity in cerebral palsy and the selective posterior rhizotomy procedure. *J Child Neurol* 5:179–185, 1990.

Peterson DO, Drummond JC, Todd MM: Effects of halothane, enflurane, isoflurane, and nitrous oxide on somatosensory evoked potentials in humans. *Anesthesiology* 65:35–40, 1986.

Petrozza PH: Induced hypotension. *Int Anesthesiol Clin* 28:223–229, 1990.

Pizov R, Kaplan L, Floman Y, et al.: Temporary right coronary artery flow disruption during instrumented correction of the spine. *Anesthesiology* 86:1210–1211, 1997.

Polizzi A, Huson SM, Vincent A: Teratogen update: Maternal myasthenia gravis as a cause of congenital arthrogryposis. *Teratology* 62:332–341, 2000.

Ponseti IV: The Ponseti technique for correction of congenital clubfoot. *J Bone Joint Surg Am* 84:1889–1890, 2002.

Porsborg P, Astrup G, Bendixen D, et al.: Osteogenesis imperfecta and malignant hyperthermia. Is there a relationship? *Anaesthesia* 51:863–865, 1996.

Post JB, Frishman WH: Fenoldopam: A new dopamine agonist for the treatment of hypertensive urgencies and emergencies. *J Clin Pharmacol* 38:2–13, 1998.

Practice Guidelines for blood component therapy: A report by the American Society of Anesthesiologists Task Force on Blood Component Therapy. *Anesthesiology* 84:732–747, 1996.

Primiano FP Jr, Nussbaum E, Hirschfeld SS, et al.: Early echocardiographic and pulmonary function findings in idiopathic scoliosis. *J Pediatr Orthop* 3:475–481, 1983.

Rao S, Yadav A, Galvan R: Posterior cervical spine stabilization under local anesthesia. *J Spinal Disord* 3:250–254, 1990.

Ray JM, Flynn JC, Bierman AH: Erythrocyte survival following intraoperative autotransfusion in spinal surgery: An in vivo comparative study and 5-year update. *Spine* 11:879–882, 1986.

Relton JE, Hall JE: An operation frame for spinal fusion. A new apparatus designed to reduce haemorrhage during operation. *J Bone Joint Surg Br* 49:327–332, 1967.

Reuben SS, Connelly NR, Lurie S, et al.: Dose-response of ketorolac as an adjunct to patient-controlled analgesia morphine in patients after spinal fusion surgery. *Anesth Analg* 87:98–102, 1998.

Reuben SS, Connelly NR, Steinberg R: Ketorolac as an adjunct to patient-controlled morphine in postoperative spine surgery patients. Reg Anesth 22:343–346, 1997.

Richards BS, Johnston CE: Cotrel-Dubousset instrumentation for adolescent idiopathic scoliosis. *Orthopedics* 10:649–654, 1987.

Riemersma S, Vincent A, Beeson D, et al.: Association of arthrogryposis multiplex congenita with maternal antibodies inhibiting fetal acetylcholine receptor function. *J Clin Invest* 98:2358–2363, 1996.

Ross AK, Eck JB, Tobias JD: Pediatric regional anesthesia: Beyond the caudal. *Anesth Analg* 91:16–26, 2000.

Rossi-Foulkes R, Roman MJ, Rosen SE, et al.: Phenotypic features and impact of beta blocker or calcium antagonist therapy on aortic lumen size in the Marfan syndrome. *Am J Cardiol* 83:1364–1368, 1999.

Roth S, Barach P: Postoperative visual loss: Still no answers—yet. *Anesthesiology* 95:575–577, 2001.

Roth S, Thisted RA, Erickson JP, et al.: Eye injuries after nonocular surgery. A study of 60,965 anesthetics from 1988 to 1992. *Anesthesiology* 85:1020–1027, 1996.

Royston D: Blood-sparing drugs: Aprotinin, tranexamic acid, and epsilon-aminocaproic acid. *Int Anesthesiol Clin* 33:155–179, 1995.

Royston D: High-dose aprotinin therapy: A review of the first five years' experience. *J Cardiothorac Vasc Anesth* 6:76–100, 1992.

Rundshagen I, Schnabel K, Schulteam EJ: Midlatency median nerve evoked responses during recovery from propofol/sufentanil total intravenous anaesthesia. *Acta Anaesthesiol Scand* 44:313–320, 2000.

Samra SK, Sorkin LS: Enhancement of somatosensory evoked potentials by etomidate in cats: An investigation of its site of action. *Anesthesiology* 74:499–503, 1991.

Sandhu HS, Khan SN: Recombinant human bone morphogenetic protein-2: Use in spinal fusion applications. *J Bone Joint Surg Am* 85(Suppl 3):89–95, 2003.

Satsumae T, Yamaguchi H, Sakaguchi M, et al.: Preoperative small-dose ketamine prevented tourniquet-induced arterial pressure increase in orthopedic patients under general anesthesia. *Anesth Analg* 92:1286–1289, 2001.

Scheepstra GL, de Lange JJ, Booij LH, et al.: Median nerve evoked potentials during propofol anaesthesia. *Br J Anaesth* 62:92–94, 1989.

Scherl SA: Common lower extremity problems in children. *Pediatr Rev* 25:52–62, 2004.

Scheufler KM, Zentner J: Motor-evoked potential facilitation during progressive cortical suppression by propofol. *Anesth Analg* 94:907–912, 2002.

Schindler E, Muller M, Zickmann B, et al.: Modulation of somatosensory evoked potentials under various concentrations of desflurane with and without nitrous oxide. *J Neurosurg Anesthesiol* 10:218–223, 1998.

Schmid UD, Boll J, Liechti S, et al.: Influence of some anesthetic agents on muscle responses to transcranial magnetic cortex stimulation: A pilot study in humans. *Neurosurgery* 30:85–92, 1992.

Schneider R, Passo MH: Juvenile rheumatoid arthritis. *Rheum Dis Clin North Am* 28:503–530, 2002.

Schubert A, Licina MG, Lineberry PJ: The effect of ketamine on human somatosensory evoked potentials and its modification by nitrous oxide. *Anesthesiology* 72:33–39, 1990.

Schur MS, Brown JT, Kafer ER, et al.: Postoperative pulmonary function in children. Comparison of scoliosis with peripheral surgery. *Am Rev Respir Dis* 130:46–51, 1984.

Scoles PV: Spinal deformity in childhood and adolescence. In Behrman RE, Vaughn VC III, editors: *Nelson textbook of pediatrics*, Update 5. Philadelphia, 1989, WB Saunders.

Shufflebarger HL, Grimm JO, Bui V, et al.: Anterior and posterior spinal fusion: Staged versus same-day surgery. *Spine* 16:930–933, 1991.

Sidman JD, Sampson D, Templeton B: Distraction osteogenesis of the mandible for airway obstruction in children. *Laryngoscope* 111:1137–1146, 2001.

Sihle-Wissel M, Scholz M, Cunitz G: Transcranial magnetic-evoked potentials under total intravenous anaesthesia and nitrous oxide. *Br J Anaesth* 85:465–467, 2000.

Singhi P, Jagirdar S, Khandelwal N, et al.: Epilepsy in children with cerebral palsy. *J Child Neurol* 18:174–179, 2003.

Sisk EA, Heatley DG, Borowski BJ, et al.: Obstructive sleep apnea in children with achondroplasia: Surgical and anesthetic considerations. *Otolaryngol Head Neck Surg* 120:248–254, 1999.

Sloan TB: Anesthetic effects on electrophysiologic recordings. *J Clin Neurophysiol* 15:217–226, 1998.

Sloan TB: Evoked potential monitoring. *Int Anesthesiol Clin* 34:109–136, 1996.

Sloan TB, Fugina ML, Toleikis JR: Effects of midazolam on median nerve somatosensory evoked potentials. *Br J Anaesth* 64:590–593, 1990.

Sloan TB, Koht A: Depression of cortical somatosensory evoked potentials by nitrous oxide. *Br J Anaesth* 57:849–852, 1985.

Sloan TB, Ronai AK, Toleikis JR, et al.: Improvement of intraoperative somatosensory evoked potentials by etomidate. *Anesth Analg* 67:582–585, 1998.

Solares G, Herranz JL, Sanz MD: Suxamethonium-induced cardiac arrest as an initial manifestation of Duchenne muscular dystrophy. *Br J Anaesth* 58:576, 1986.

Sooriyabandara S, Aluwihare AP: Arthrogryposis multiplex congenita distal type II associated with facial abnormality, renal abnormality, polydactyly and Hirschsprung's disease. *Ceylon Med J* 46:156–157, 2001.

Subach BR, McLaughlin MR, Albright AL, et al.: Current management of pediatric atlantoaxial rotatory subluxation. *Spine* 23:2174–2179, 1998.

Sucato DJ: Thoracoscopic anterior instrumentation and fusion for idiopathic scoliosis. *J Am Acad Orthop Surg* 11:221–227, 2003.

Sullivan M, Thompson WK, Hill GD: Succinylcholine-induced cardiac arrest in children with undiagnosed myopathy. *Can J Anaesth* 41:497–501, 1994.

Suresh S, Wheeler M: Practical pediatric regional anesthesia. *Anesthesiol Clin North Am* 20:83–2113, 2002.

Szmuk P, Ezri T, Warters DR, et al.: Anesthetic management of a patient with arthrogryposis multiplex congenita and limited mouth opening. *J Clin Anesth* 13:59–60, 2001.

Takano T, Aotani H, Takeuchi Y: Asymmetric arthrogryposis multiplex congenita with focal pachygyria. *Pediatr Neurol* 25:247–249, 2001.

Taniguchi M, Nadstawek J, Langenbach U, et al.: Effects of four intravenous anesthetic agents on motor evoked potentials elicited by magnetic transcranial stimulation. *Neurosurgery* 33:407–415, 1993.

Tenbrock K, Kruppa S, Mokov E, et al.: Analysis of muscle strength and bone structure in children with renal disease. *Pediatr Nephrol* 14:669–672, 2000.

Thakor NV, Vaz CA, McPherson RW, et al.: Adaptive Fourier series modeling of time-varying evoked potentials: Study of human somatosensory evoked response to etomidate anesthetic. *Electroencephalogr Clin Neurophysiol* 80:108–118, 1991.

Theroux MC, Akins RE, Barone C, et al.: Neuromuscular junctions in cerebral palsy: Presence of extrajunctional acetylcholine receptors. *Anesthesiology* 96:330–335, 2002.

Theroux MC, Brandom BW, Zagnoev M, et al.: Dose response of succinylcholine at the adductor pollicis of children with cerebral palsy during propofol and nitrous oxide anesthesia. *Anesth Analg* 79:761–765, 1994.

Theroux MC, Corddry DH, Tietz AE, et al.: A study of desmopressin and blood loss during spinal fusion for neuromuscular scoliosis: A randomized, controlled, double-blinded study. *Anesthesiology* 87:260–267, 1997.

Thomas PB, Parry MG: The difficult paediatric airway: A new method of intubation using the laryngeal mask airway, Cook airway exchange catheter and tracheal intubation fibrescope. *Paediatr Anaesth* 11:618–621, 2001.

Thompson GH: The spine. In Behrman RE, editor: *Nelson textbook of pediatrics*, 16th ed. Philadelphia, 2004, Elsevier.

Tinker JH, Michenfelder JD: Sodium nitroprusside: Pharmacology, toxicology and therapeutics. *Anesthesiology* 45:340–354, 1976.

Tobias JD: A review of intrathecal and epidural analgesia after spinal surgery in children. *Anesth Analg* 98:956–965, 2004.

Tobias JD: Controlled hypotension in children: A critical review of available agents. *Paediatr Drugs* 4:439–453, 2002.

Tobias JD: Fenoldopam for controlled hypotension during spinal fusion in children and adolescents. *Paediatr Anaesth* 10:261–266, 2000.

Tobias JD: Sevoflurane for controlled hypotension during spinal surgery: Preliminary experience in five adolescents. *Paediatr Anaesth* 8:167–170, 1998.

Toder DS: Respiratory problems in the adolescent with developmental delay. *Adolesc Med* 11:617–631, 2000.

Upadhyay SS, Ho EK, Gunawardene WM, et al.: Changes in residual volume relative to vital capacity and total lung capacity after arthrodesis of the spine in patients who have adolescent idiopathic scoliosis. *J Bone Joint Surg Am* 75:46–52, 1993.

Uziel Y, Rathaus V, Pomeranz A, et al.: Torticollis as the sole initial presenting sign of systemic onset juvenile rheumatoid arthritis. *J Rheumatol* 25:166–168, 1998.

Valli H, Rosenberg PH, Kytta J, et al.: Arterial hypertension associated with the use of a tourniquet with either general or regional anaesthesia. *Acta Anaesthesiol Scand* 31:279–283, 1987.

van Besouw JP, Hinds CJ: Fat embolism syndrome. *Br J Hosp Med* 42:304–301, 1989.

van't Hof RJ, Ralston SH: Nitric oxide and bone. *Immunology* 103:255–261, 2001.

Varveris DA, Morton NS: Target controlled infusion of propofol for induction and maintenance of anaesthesia using the Paedfusor: An open pilot study. *Paediatr Anaesth* 12:589–593, 2002.

Vauzelle C, Stagnara P, Jouvinroux P: Functional monitoring of spinal cord activity during spinal surgery. *Clin Orthop* 93:173–178, 1973.

Vetter TR: Acute airway obstruction due to arytenoiditis in a child with juvenile rheumatoid arthritis. *Anesth Analg* 79:1198–1200, 1994.

Vichinsky E, Williams R, Das M, et al.: Pulmonary fat embolism: A distinct cause of severe acute chest syndrome in sickle cell anemia. Blood 83:3107–3112, 1994.

Vichinsky EP, Neumayr LD, Earles AN, et al.: Causes and outcomes of the acute chest syndrome in sickle cell disease. National Acute Chest Syndrome Study Group. *N Engl J Med* 342:1855–1865, 2000.

Vinken PJ, Bruyn GW, editors: *The handbook of clinical neurology,* vol 12. New York, 1972, North Holland.

Vitale MG, Choe JC, Hwang MW, et al.: Use of ketorolac tromethamine in children undergoing scoliosis surgery. an analysis of complications. *Spine J* 3:55–62, 2003.

Vitale MG, Levy DE, Park MC, et al.: Quantifying risk of transfusion in children undergoing spine surgery. *Spine J* 2:166–172, 2002.

Vitale MG, Stazzone EJ, Gelijns AC, et al.: The effectiveness of preoperative erythropoietin in averting allogenic blood transfusion among children undergoing scoliosis surgery. *J Pediatr Orthop B* 7:203–209, 1998.

Wagner RL, White PF, Kan PB, et al.: Inhibition of adrenal steroidogenesis by the anesthetic etomidate. *N Engl J Med* 310:1415–1421, 1984.

Weinstein SL, Dolan LA, Spratt KF, et al.: Health and function of patients with untreated idiopathic scoliosis: A 50-year natural history study. *JAMA* 289:559–567, 2003.

Weinstein SL, Zavala DC, Ponseti IV: Idiopathic scoliosis: Long-term follow-up and prognosis in untreated patients. *J Bone Joint Surg Am* 63:702–712, 1981.

Worley G, Witsell DL, Hulka GF: Laryngeal dystonia causing inspiratory stridor in children with cerebral palsy. *Laryngoscope* 113:2192–2195, 2003.
Xiong B, Sevastik JA: A physiological approach to surgical treatment of progressive early idiopathic scoliosis. *Eur Spine J* 7:505–508, 1998.
Yamada H, Transfeldt EE, Tamaki T, et al.: The effects of volatile anesthetics on the relative amplitudes and latencies of spinal and muscle potentials evoked by transcranial magnetic stimulation. *Spine* 19:1512–1517, 1994.
Yaster M, Billett C, Monitto C: Intravenous patient controlled analgesia. In Yaster M, Krane EJ, Kaplan RF, et al., editors: *Pediatric pain management and sedation handbook*. St. Louis, 1997, Mosby Year Book, pp 89–112.
Yaster M, Maxwell LG: Pediatric regional anesthesia. *Anesthesiology* 70:324–338, 1989.
Yaster M, Simmons RS, Tolo VT, et al.: A comparison of nitroglycerin and nitroprusside for inducing hypotension in children: A double-blind study. *Anesthesiology* 65:175–179, 1986.
Yasui N, Kawabata H, Kojimoto H, et al.: Lengthening of the lower limbs in patients with achondroplasia and hypochondroplasia. *Clin Orthop* 298–306, 1997.
Zeitlin L, Fassier F, Glorieux FH: Modern approach to children with osteogenesis imperfecta. *J Pediatr Orthop B* 12:77–87, 2003.
Zhang X, Schwarz EM, Young DA, et al.: Cyclooxygenase-2 regulates mesenchymal cell differentiation into the osteoblast lineage and is critically involved in bone repair. *J Clin Invest* 109:1405–1415, 2002.

22 Anesthesia for Pediatric Ophthalmic Surgery

Michael Winn Hauser • Robert D. Valley • Ann G. Bailey

Anesthesia for ophthalmologic procedures in children requires an understanding of several physiologic and pharmacologic concepts that are unique to this population. The majority of ophthalmic procedures are brief and noninvasive, but the spectrum extends to more invasive procedures in patients with significant comorbid disease. Caring for otherwise healthy children undergoing nasolacrimal duct probing or strabismus surgery may be relatively straightforward, but the pediatric anesthesiologist is also required to care for vulnerable infants born prematurely or with congenital disorders and associated pathology of the eye. Each year in the United States, approximately 4%, or 160,000, of the 4.3 million pediatric procedures performed are for ophthalmic disease (Hall and Lawrence, 1998; Hall and Owings, 2002).

Anesthesiologists with a particular interest in ophthalmologic anesthesia can find valuable resources through the Ophthalmic Anesthesia Society (http://www.eyeanesthesia.org/) and the British Ophthalmic Anaesthesia Society (http://www.boas.org/home.html).

A glossary of terms is given in Box 22–1.

■ ANATOMY AND PHYSIOLOGY

Knowledge of the anatomy and physiology of the eye is paramount to understanding the array of ophthalmic procedures performed, the influence that anesthesia may have on normal and abnormal ocular physiology, and the systemic effects that surgical manipulation of the eye may have on the patient.

■ ANATOMY OVERVIEW

The eye is an extension of the central nervous system (the diencephalon) that rests in the orbit, is cushioned by fat, and is suspended by ligaments and fascial structure.

The orbit is formed by a complex arrangement of seven cranial bones: frontal, zygomatic, sphenoid, maxilla, palatine, lacrimal, and ethmoid (Fig. 22–1). The optic foramen transmits the optic nerve, the ophthalmic artery and vein, and the sympathetic contributions from the carotid plexus. The superior orbital fissure transmits branches from four other cranial nerves (oculomotor, trigeminal, trochlear, and abducens) and the superior and inferior ophthalmic veins. The infraorbital fissure (representing the weakest aspect of the orbit) transmits the infraorbital and zygomatic nerves. The infraorbital foramen (located below the orbital rim) transmits the infraorbital nerve, artery, and vein.

The globe is composed of three contiguous layers: sclera, uveal tract, and retina. The sclera is the dense outer covering that provides the fibrous structure necessary for maintaining the shape of the globe. The anterior portion of the sclera (the cornea) is transparent and avascular, permitting transmission of light to the retina. The highly vascular uveal tract is composed of the iris, ciliary body, and choroid, enveloping the posterior aspect of the globe. The iris divides the anterior segment of the eye into the anterior and posterior chambers. The ciliary body is the site of aqueous humor production and contains the ciliary muscles, which are responsible for accommodation of the lens. The choroid is the highly vascular layer of the globe that provides blood supply to the retina. The retina is a delicate membrane composed of 10 distinct layers that are involved in the conversion of light to neural impulses. The axons of the retinal ganglion nerves converge at the optic disc and pierce the sclera to form the optic nerve.

The aqueous humor occupies the anterior and posterior chambers of the eye (Fig. 22–2) and is responsible for providing nutrients to the avascular lens and the endothelial aspect of the cornea. The volume of aqueous humor (0.3 mL in the adult) is primarily responsible for intraocular pressure (IOP) regulation.

BOX 22–1 Glossary of Ophthalmologic Terms

Blepharospasm: Tonic spasm of the orbicularis oculi muscle, producing more or less complete closure of the eyelids

Buphthalmos: Enlargement and distention of the fibrous coats of the eye

Cyclocryotherapy: Freezing of the ciliary body; done in the treatment of glaucoma

Epiphora: Abnormal overflow of tears; also known as *illacrimation*

Episcleritis: Inflammation of tissues overlying the sclera; also inflammation of the outermost layers of the sclera

Gonioscopy: Examination of the angle of the anterior chamber of the eye

Goniotomy: Operation for glaucoma characterized by an open angle and normal depth of the anterior chamber; consists of the opening of Schlemm's canal under direct vision secured by a contact glass

Tonometry: Measurement of tension or pressure frequently assessed by the *applanation*

Tonometer: Instrument that measures intraocular pressure by determination of the force necessary to flatten a corneal surface of constant size

Trabeculectomy: Creation of a fistula between the anterior chamber of the eye and the subconjunctival space by surgical removal of a portion of the trabecular meshwork

From *Dorland's Illustrated Medical Dictionary*, 2000.

The vitreous humor, created embryologically between months 1 and 4, is a hydrophilic gel that accounts for 80% of the volume of the globe. The vitrous humor is 99% water, although in the presence of hyaluronic acid (a mucopolysaccharide), its viscosity is twice that of water. The volume of the vitreous humor is more constant than that of the aqueous humor, although it may be slightly influenced by hydration status and osmotically active medications.

The optic nerve (cranial nerve II) is the nerve of vision and may be thought of as a diverticulum of the forebrain. The oculomotor nerve (cranial nerve III) provides motor innervation to four of the six extraocular muscles and the levator palpebrae superioris as well as parasympathetic innervation to the pupillary sphincter (miosis) and ciliary muscles (accommodation). The two other extraocular muscles are innervated by the trochlear and abducens nerves. The ophthalmic division of the trigeminal nerve (cranial nerve V) transmits all of the nonvisual sensory innervation from the eye and orbit and provides sympathetic innervation to the pupillary dilators (mydriasis). The temporal and zygomatic branches of the facial nerve (cranial nerve VII) innervate the orbicularis oculi (Ellis and Feldman, 1997).

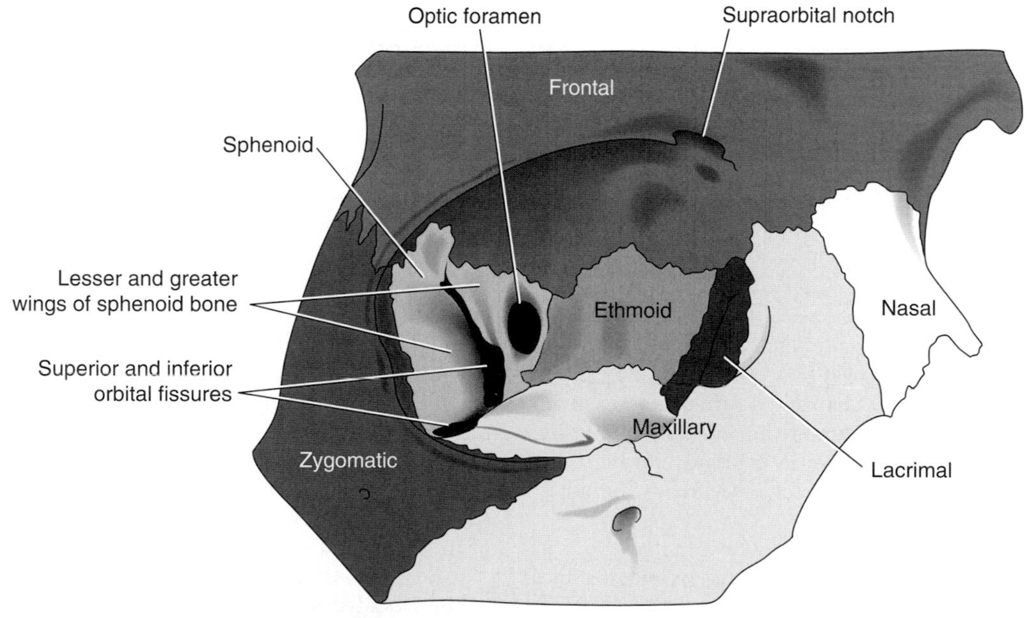

FIGURE 22–1. Skeletal anatomy of the orbit.

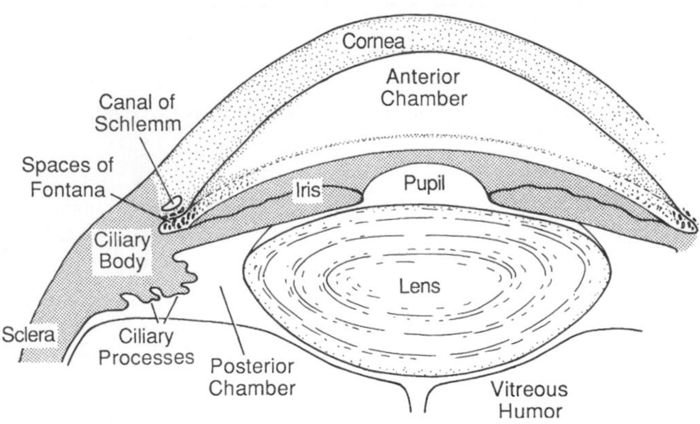

FIGURE 22–2. Anatomy of the anterior eye. (From McGoldrick KE: Anesthesia for ophthalmic surgery. In Motoyama ES, Davis PJ, editors: *Smith's anesthesia for infants and children*, 6th ed. Philadelphia, 1996, Mosby, p 633, with permission.)

Blood is supplied to the eye and orbit through branches of the internal and external carotid arteries. The first branch of the intracranial carotid artery, the ophthalmic artery, divides into the central retinal artery as well as the long and short posterior ciliary arteries to nourish the retina. The long and short posterior ciliary arteries converge to supply the choriocapillaris, the capillary layer within the choroid that supplies 60% to 80% of the oxygen to the retina. The anterior portion of the optic nerve is perfused by the posterior ciliary arteries. It is this network of arteries that is subject to significant individual variation, predisposing some patients to anterior ischemic optic neuropathy after periods of hypotension. The posterior optic nerve is perfused by pial vessels branching from the ophthalmic artery. Superior and inferior ophthalmic veins drain the orbit, and the central retinal vein provides ocular drainage. All venous drainage is subsequently transmitted to the cavernous sinus (Williams, 2002).

PHYSIOLOGY OVERVIEW

The physiology of the eye is quite complex, but an understanding of the physiologic and pharmacologic control of IOP is of primary importance to the anesthesiologist. The ability to avoid deviations in IOP is key to providing satisfactory anesthesia for all intraocular procedures and in caring for the patient with glaucoma and traumatic injury to the globe.

Normal IOP varies between 10 and 20 mm Hg and may differ by as much as 5 mm Hg between the two eyes. Normal pressures are somewhat lower in the newborn (average, 9.5 mm Hg) but approximate adult pressures by 5 years of age (Pensiero et al., 1992). A pressure above 25 mm Hg at any age is considered abnormal (Johnson and Forrest, 1994). Transient changes in IOP are well tolerated in the intact eye, although chronic elevations may be detrimental to normal retinal perfusion and vision.

Three primary determinants of IOP are (1) external pressure, (2) venous congestion, and (3) changes in intraocular volume. The volume and exertional pressure of the aqueous humor are carefully regulated in the normal eye to maintain normal IOP. As mentioned previously, the volume of the vitreous humor is usually constant.

The aqueous humor is formed primarily by the ciliary bodies, where secretion is facilitated by the carbonic anhydrase and cytochrome oxidase systems. The feedback control of aqueous humor formation is poorly understood, although production of aqueous humor is known to be augmented by sympathetic stimulation and suppressed by parasympathetic control. Variations in the osmotic pressure of the aqueous humor and plasma influence aqueous humor formation, as illustrated by the following equation:

$$IOP = \kappa[(OP_{aq} - OP_{pl}) + Pc]$$

where κ is the coefficient of outflow, OP_{aq} and OP_{pl} are the osmotic pressures of the aqueous humor and plasma, respectively, and Pc is the capillary prefusion pressure. The benefit of hypertonic solutions in lowering IOP is realized through an understanding of this equation.

Most of the aqueous humor produced in the posterior chamber flows through the pupil into the anterior chamber, exiting the eye through Schlemm's canal (a thin vein that extends circumferentially around the eye) and into the orbital venous system.

Fluctuations in aqueous humor outflow also dramatically alter IOP. The prime factor determining outflow of aqueous humor is the diameter of Fontana's spaces as illustrated by the following equation based on the Hagen-Poiseuille Law:

$$A = \frac{r^4(P_{iop} - P_v)}{8\eta l}$$

where A is the volume of aqueous humor outflow per unit of time, r is the radius of Fontana's spaces, P_{iop} is IOP, P_v is venous pressure, η is viscosity, and l is length of Fontana's spaces.

With mydriasis, Fontana's spaces narrow, resistance to outflow is increased, and IOP rises. Mydriasis is a threat in both closed-angle and open-angle glaucoma. Hence, a miotic such as pilocarpine hydrochloride is often efficacious when applied conjunctivally before surgery in patients with glaucoma.

The α_1-stimulation or sympathetic stimulation leads to mydriasis, a decrease in aqueous outflow and an increase in IOP. Most of the agents used to produce mydriasis also modestly increase IOP. β-stimulation has no effect on pupillary diameter, but paradoxically both β-agonists and β-antagonists may decrease IOP. Cholinergic stimulation or parasympathetic stimulation produces miosis and a decrease in IOP such that glaucoma patients are frequently treated with miotic agents.

The arterial circulation of the eye is autoregulated. Only marked deviations in systemic arterial pressures affect IOP. Elevated venous pressures, on the other hand, can dramatically increase IOP, primarily by augmenting the choroidal blood volume and tension of the orbit. Coughing, vomiting, and Valsalva maneuvers may increase IOP to 40 mm Hg or more. Respiratory acidosis increases IOP, whereas metabolic acidosis has the opposite effect. Conversely, respiratory alkalosis decreases IOP, whereas metabolic alkalosis increases IOP (Calobrisi and Lebowitz, 1990). Hypoxia is capable of increasing IOP by dilating intraocular vessels while hyperoxia appears to decrease IOP (Johnson and Forrest, 1994).

Three ophthalmic reflexes that should be recognized by the anesthesiologist caring for the ophthalmic patient include (1) the oculocardiac reflex (OCR), (2) the oculorespiratory reflex (ORR), and (3) the oculoemetic reflex (OER). All three reflexes are elicited by pressure or torsion on the extraocular muscles transmitting afferent impulses through the ophthalmic division of the trigeminal nerve.

The OCR, through its vagal efferent pathway, may manifest as sinus bradycardia, ectopy, and sinus arrest. Death secondary to the OCR in otherwise healthy children has been described

(Lang and Van der Wal, 1994; Smith, 1994). A more thorough description of this reflex, prophylaxis, and therapy are provided later in the discussion of intraoperative complications.

The ORR has also been recognized for nearly 100 years but is less often appreciated with the use of controlled ventilation. Through a postulated connection between the trigeminal nerve, the pneumotaxic center of the pons, and the medullary respiratory centers, pressure on the extraocular muscles may result in tachypnea or respiratory arrest (Johnson and Forrest, 1994). This reflex is not inhibited by the use of atropine or glycopyrrolate. A review of the ORR and its potential for causing hypercapnia and hypoxia (potentially aggravating the OCR) has heightened awareness of the reflex and led some investigators to recommend controlled ventilation during strabismus surgery (Blanc et al., 1988).

The OER is admittedly more theoretical than the other two reflexes but would explain the high incidence of nausea and emesis after strabismus surgery. An association between the OCR and the OER has been demonstrated such that patients who exhibit the OCR intraoperatively are 2.6 times more likely to experience postoperative vomiting than those without OCR manifestations (Allen et al., 1998). Anticholinergic therapy does not decrease the incidence of postoperative nausea and vomiting (PONV). Appropriate prophylaxis and treatment of PONV have been studied extensively and are thoroughly reviewed later in this chapter.

GENERAL CONSIDERATIONS IN CARING FOR THE OPHTHALMOLOGIC PATIENT

The anesthesiologist caring for the ophthalmologic patient should be familiar with the disorders and syndromes frequently associated with ocular pathology, the effects of ophthalmic medications used preoperatively and intraoperatively, and the ocular effects of the anesthetic agents to be used during the perioperative period.

ASSOCIATED CONGENITAL AND METABOLIC CONDITIONS

Ophthalmologic disorders may be inherited as isolated defects in autosomal recessive, autosomal dominant, and X-linked recessive fashion. An additional large number of metabolic defects, congenital syndromes, and chromosomal abnormalities are also associated with ocular pathology. The anesthesiologist caring for the ophthalmologic patient must be aware of these associations. An overview of the commonly encountered syndromes and disorders along with their ocular manifestations and potential anesthetic implications is given (McGoldrick, 1992; Baum and O'Flaherty, 1999; Butera et al., 2000) (Table 22–1).

OPHTHALMOLOGIC MEDICATIONS AND THEIR SYSTEMIC EFFECTS

There are a variety of medications used by pediatric ophthalmologists in the outpatient and perioperative settings that may have important anesthetic ramifications. As with all medications, the ophthalmic agents have both desirable and undesirable effects that may be more pronounced and ominous in the pediatric patient by virtue of greater systemic absorption and/or higher dosing relative to body weight and pharmacologic compartment. The anesthesiologist must be familiar with every medication used in the perioperative period while paying particular attention to the total dose administered and potential for deleterious effects. An overview of the ophthalmic medications is provided (Table 22–2).

The topical ophthalmologic agents have greater use than systemic agents in the pediatric and adult populations, primarily by diminishing most of the side effects that would be consequential to systemic administration. Nevertheless, the excess from ocular application invariably enters the lacrimal system, reaching the nasopharyngeal mucosa where systemic absorption is greatly enhanced compared with that at the conjunctival sac. While a single drop from a commercial eye dropper may have a volume ranging between 50 and 75 μL, maximal ocular bioavailability is reached by instillation of only 20 μL (McGoldrick, 1992). It has been recommended that digital pressure over the lacrimal duct for 5 minutes after instillation may reduce systemic absorption by 67% (Zimmerman et al., 1984). Keeping the eye gently closed for 5 minutes may afford similar benefit, yet both techniques are understandably difficult in the conscious and fretful child.

CYCLOPLEGIC AND MYDRIATIC AGENTS

Those agents used most commonly in the perioperative setting include cycloplegic and mydriatic agents. The agents are necessary for performing certain procedures, cycloplegic refraction, and funduscopy. The cycloplegic agents act via parasympatholytic action to block the muscarinic receptors of the ciliary body, paralyze the ciliary muscles, and inhibit accommodation. Outside of the perioperative period, the cycloplegic agents are also used to decrease the discomfort of ciliary body spasm common to a variety of inflammatory conditions.

Cyclopentolate, a commonly used cycloplegic agent, has a peak effect within 20 to 45 minutes and residual effects that persist for as long as 36 hours (Cooper et al., 2000). Mild gastrointestinal discomfort and feeding intolerance are the most frequently encountered side effects, although more severe atropine-like toxicity with symptoms ranging from vomiting, ileus (Bauer et al., 1973), hyperthermia, delirium, and grand mal seizures (Kennerdell and Wucher, 1972) has also been reported.

Tropicamide is a belladonna alkaloid that is also used as a topical cycloplegic agent. Maximal cycloplegic effect takes place within 20 to 40 minutes, and residual effects may persist for 6 hours. Because tropicamide is less reliable than cyclopentolate, it is most often used in combination with cyclopentolate and/or phenylephrine.

Atropine and homatropine are extremely potent antiaccommodative agents that are rarely used for pediatric patients in the perioperative setting. The agents are more commonly used for intraocular inflammation and amblyopia therapy; they may also be used for prolonged mydriasis after cataract extraction to prevent the formation of synechiae. Common side effects include thirst, tachycardia, and hyperthermia (McGoldrick, 1992), although more severe symptoms may result with overzealous administration.

Mydriasis is usually produced as a secondary effect of the cycloplegic agents (by paralyzing the constrictors of the iris), yet additional mydriatic agents are often used to maximize peripheral and anterior retinal visualization. The mydriatic agents are sympathomimetic agents that mimic the effects of endogenous epinephrine and norepinephrine.

Ophthalmic phenylephrine (available in 2.5% and 10% concentrations) is commonly used for mydriasis and vasoconstriction during various procedures. Maximal effects are generally

TABLE 22–1. Congenital syndromes and chromosomal abnormalities with associated ocular manifestations

Disorder or Syndrome	Ocular Manifestations	Anesthetic Implications
Acute intermittent porphyria	Cataracts, retinal degeneration, optic atrophy	Various medications, including barbiturates and etomidate, may trigger attacks.
Apert's syndrome	Glaucoma, cataracts, strabismus, hypertelorism, proptosis	Possibly difficult intubation, possible choanal stenosis, cervical spine fusion, CHD (10% incidence)
Cri du chat syndrome	Strabismus	Micrognathia and possibly difficult intubation, hypotonia, prone to hypothermia, CHD (33% incidence)
Crouzon's disease	Glaucoma, cataracts, strabismus, hypertelorism, proptosis	Possibly difficult intubation, possible elevated intracranial pressure
Cystinosis	Corneal clouding, retinal degeneration	Chronic renal failure, possible diabetes mellitus, esophageal varices, recurrent epistaxis, hyperthermia
Down syndrome	Cataracts, strabismus	Trisomy 21, airway obstruction, atlantoaxial instability, CHD (50% incidence), may be more sensitive to atropine
Ehlers-Danlos syndrome	Retinal detachment, blue sclera, ectopia lentis, keratoconus	Laryngeal trauma possible with intubation, careful positioning, avoid arterial and central venous lines
Goldenhar's syndrome	Glaucoma, cataracts, strabismus, lacrimal drainage defects	Hemifacial microsomia and possible cervical spine abnormalities, possible difficult mask and intubation, rare CHD and hydrocephalus
Hallerman-Streiff syndrome	Congenital cataracts, coloboma, microphthalmia, glaucoma	Major craniofacial abnormalities with likely difficult intubation, upper airway obstruction, chronic lung disease
Homocystinuria	Ectopia lentis, pupillary block glaucoma, retinal detachment, optic atrophy, central retinal artery occlusion, strabismus	Marfanoid habitus with kyphoscoliosis and sternal deformity, prone to thromboembolic complications and hypoglycemia
Hunter's syndrome	Retinal degeneration, optic atrophy	Frequent difficult intubation, copious secretions, macroglossia, stiff temporomandibular joint, limited neck mobility, possible ischemic or valvular heart disease
Hurler's syndrome	Corneal clouding, retinal degeneration, optic atrophy	Frequent difficult intubation and difficult mask, possible cervical spine instability, possible ischemic or valvular heart disease
Jeune syndrome	Retinal degeneration	Limited thoracic excursion, pulmonary hypoplasia, possible renal and hepatic insufficiency
Lowe's syndrome	Cataracts, glaucoma (hydrophthalmia)	Renal failure, renal tubular acidosis
Marfan syndrome	Ectopia lentis, glaucoma, retinal detachment, cataracts, strabismus	Aortic or pulmonary artery dilation, aortic and mitral valve disease, pectus excavatum, risk for pneumothorax
Moebius sequence	Strabismus, ptosis, congenital nerve VI and VII palsy	Possibly difficult intubation, micrognathia, copious secretions, possible cervical spine anomalies
Myotonia congenita	Cataracts, blepharospasm	Prone to myotonic contractions, sustained contraction with succinylcholine
Myotonic dystrophy	Cataracts, ptosis, strabismus	Prone to myotonic contractions, succinylcholine-associated contractions and hyperkalemia, frequent cardiac conduction abnormalities, sensitive to central nervous system depressants
Rubella syndrome	Cataracts, microphthalmos, glaucoma, optic atrophy	Neonatal pneumonia, anemia, and thrombocytopenia; CHD, hypopituitarism, diabetes mellitus
Sickle cell disease	Retinal detachment, vitreous hemorrhage, retinitis proliferans	Tendency for sickling occurs with high hemoglobin S concentrations, hypoxemia, cold, stasis, dehydration and infection
Smith-Lemli-Opitz syndrome	Congenital cataracts	Possibly difficult intubation, micrognathia, pulmonary hypoplasia, CHD, gastroesophageal reflux, seizure disorders
Stickler syndrome	Vitreous degeneration, retinal detachments, cataracts, strabismus	Possibly difficult intubation, micrognathia, mitral valve prolapse, marfanoid habitus, scoliosis, kyphosis
Sturge-Weber syndrome	Choroidal hemangioma, glaucoma, ectopia lentis	Angiomas of the airway, CHD and high output failure, seizure disorders, hyperkalemic response to succinylcholine in those with hemiplegia
Treacher Collins syndrome	Lid defects, microphthalmia	Frequently difficult intubation, mandibular hypoplasia, CHD
Turner syndrome	Ptosis, strabismus, cataracts, corneal scars, blue sclera	Possibly difficult intubation and intravenous access, CHD
von Hippel–Lindau syndrome	Retinal hemangioma	Possible increased intracranial pressure, possible pheochromocytoma, cerebellar tumors may also produce episodic hypertension
von Recklinghausen's disease	Ptosis, proptosis, optic glioma and meningioma, optic atrophy, glaucoma, Lisch nodules	Possibly difficult mask ventilation and intubation, possible airway tumors, restrictive lung disease, renovascular hypertension, possible pheochromocytoma, sensitive to neuromuscular blockers
Zellweger syndrome	Glaucoma, cataracts, optic atrophy, optic nerve hypoplasia	Micrognathia, possible CHD, renal and adrenal insufficiency

CHD, congenital heart disease.

TABLE 22–2. Commonly used ophthalmic medications

Type	Medication	Concentration	Pertinent Systemic and Ocular Effects
Cycloplegic			
	Cyclopentolate	0.5%, 1%, 2%	Muscarinic antagonist—side effects include gastrointestinal disturbance, atropine-like toxicity, and inhibition of plasma cholinesterase (in vitro).
	Tropicamide	0.5%, 1%	Muscarinic antagonist—side effects are minimal.
	Atropine	1%	Muscarinic antagonist with the most potent ocular effects and a duration of action of longer than 1 week—side effects are numerous.
	Homatropine	2%, 5%	Muscarinic antagonist with a shorter onset and duration of action than atropine—side effects are numerous.
	Scopolamine	0.25%	Muscarinic antagonist that is not frequently used for diagnostic cycloplegia and mydriasis and for the treatment of iridocyclitis—side effects include an increase in intraocular pressure such that intravenous or intramuscular scopolamine as a premedication should not be used in the glaucomatous patient.
Mydriatic			
	Phenylephrine	2.5%, 10%	α-agonist used for maximal mydriasis and vasoconstriction without cycloplegia—potential side effects include hypertension, tachycardia or reflex bradycardia, pulmonary edema, cardiac arrhythmia, cardiac arrest, and subarachnoid hemorrhage.
	Hydroxyamphetamine	1%	Sympathomimetic used in combination with tropicamide primarily for differentiating preganglionic and postganglionic lesions producing Horner's syndrome.
Miotic			
	Acetylcholine	1%	Cholinergic agonist used intraocularly to produce complete miosis after cataract surgery, keratoplasty, other anterior segment surgery—side effects include bradycardia, hypotension, and bronchospasm.
Glaucoma Agent			
	Pilocarpine	1% to 8%	Cholinomimetic or parasympathomimetic used to produce miosis and a decrease in intraocular pressure for chronic and acute angle-closure glaucoma—side effects include gastrointestinal disturbance, diaphoresis, and brow pain.
	Echothiophate iodide	0.125%	Long-acting anticholinesterase agent used to produce miosis for open-angle glaucoma—side effects include bradycardia, hypotension, nausea, vomiting, diarrhea, weakness, and inhibition of plasma cholinesterase for up to 6 weeks after discontinuation.
	Timolol, levobunolol	0.25%, 0.5%	Nonselective β-antagonists that reduce intraocular pressure by decreasing aqueous humor production and possibly outflow—side effects include bronchospasm, bradycardia, hypotension, and apnea in neonates.
	Betaxolol	0.5%	Selective β_1-antagonist—side effects are possible but less commonly observed in contrast to the nonselective β-antagonists.
	Apraclonidine	0.5%, 1%	Selective alpha-2 agonist incapable of crossing the blood-brain barrier and used to reduce aqueous secretion—side effects are minimal.
	Brimonidine	0.15%, 0.2%	Selective α_2-agonist capable of crossing the blood-brain barrier—side effects include apnea, bradycardia, hypotension, hypothermia, and somnolence with an incidence as high as 83%.
	Latanoprost, bimatoprost, travoprost	Varies	Prostaglandin F_2 analogues that increase aqueous humor outflow and decrease intraocular pressure in open-angle glaucoma—side effects are minimal and usually limited to ocular side effects.
	Acetazolamide	Varies	Systemic competitive inhibitor of carbonic anhydrase that reduces formation of aqueous humor—side effects include acidosis, hypokalemia, hyponatremia, and allergic reactions.
	Dorzolamide, brinzolamide	Varies	Topical carbonic anhydrase inhibitors that reduce the production of aqueous humor—side effects are uncommon.
	Mannitol	25%	Inert sugar that increases plasma osmotic pressure and decreases the volume of aqueous humor—side effects include transient hypervolemia followed by hypovolemia and potential for hypotension.
Miscellaneous			
	Proparacaine, tetracaine	0.5%	Ester local anesthetics frequently used intraoperatively and during examination—side effects are minimal and usually limited to burning and possible epithelial damage.
	Cocaine	4%, 10%	Ester local anesthetic with vasoconstrictive properties—side effects include tachycardia, hypertension, dysrhythmias, hyperthermia, and seizures.
	Naphazoline	0.01%, 0.1%	α-agonist used primarily for intraoperative vasoconstriction.
	Fluorescein	NA	Intravascular dye used to evaluate the integrity of retinal vasculature—side effects include hypertension, nausea, and vomiting.
	Sulfur hexafluoride	NA	Intraocular gas known to persist for up to 4 weeks after injection.
	Perfluoropropane, carbon octofluorine	NA	Intraocular gases known to persist for up to 6 weeks after injection.
	Botulinum toxin	NA	Neurotoxin produced by *Clostridium botulinum,* which inhibits release of acetylcholine used for treatment of strabismus and blepharospasm.

observed within 15 minutes, and residual effects may persist for 4 hours after administration. The generally accepted dosing limit for pediatric patients is one drop of the 2.5% solution in each eye per hour (Borromeo-McGrail et al., 1973). One drop (50 μL) of the 2.5% solution contains approximately 1.25 mg of phenylephrine. The potential for severe hypertension, pulmonary edema, cardiac arrhythmia, cardiac arrest, and subarachnoid hemorrhage with topical phenylephrine is well appreciated by surgeons and anesthesiologists alike. With careful application of the 2.5% solution, systemic effects are typically mild, well tolerated, and generally observed within 1 to 20 minutes after application (Fraunfelder et al., 2002). Although one study demonstrated no significant difference in the mydriatic effects of cyclopentolate versus phenylephrine (both administered in combination with tropicamide) (Rosales et al., 1981), many ophthalmologists still rely on the medication either primarily or when additional dilation is needed after the administration of other preparations.

GLAUCOMA PHARMACOLOGIC THERAPY

Unlike the management of adult glaucoma, the primary treatment for pediatric glaucoma is surgical. Medical therapy may occasionally be instituted perioperatively in an effort to minimize IOP. There are an expansive number of medications and combination products available, but none are formally approved for pediatric use. Convenient classifications for the glaucoma medications include the direct- and indirect-acting parasympathomimetics, sympathomimetics, β-antagonists, selective α_2-agonists, carbonic anhydrase inhibitors, prostaglandin analogues, and hypertonic solutions.

Pilocarpine is a parasympathomimetic agent that produces miosis and a fall in IOP that is thought to result from an increase in aqueous humor outflow. It is rarely used for temporary treatment before surgery in children but should be discontinued on the evening before surgery for adequate assessment of pressure (Khaw et al., 2000). At recommended dosages, side effects are thought to be rare but may include gastrointestinal disturbances and diaphoresis. More severe cardiovascular effects (hypotension, bradycardia, and atrioventricular block) are occasionally observed in the geriatric patient (Everitt and Avorn, 1990).

The long-acting anticholinesterase drugs (echothiophate iodide and demecarium bromide) are infrequently used in the pediatric patient. They are occasionally used in the adult refractory to other glaucoma therapy. These agents are of particular interest to the anesthesiologist because of their ability to profoundly inhibit the metabolism of succinylcholine, mivacurium, and the ester anesthetics for up to 6 weeks after discontinuation of therapy.

Topical epinephrine and its prodrug, dipivefrin, are sympathomimetic agents historically used in the treatment of glaucoma. Topical epinephrine is occasionally used by ophthalmologists in the intraoperative setting and is known to potentiate dysrhythmias in the myocardium sensitized by the volatile agents. Halothane clearly has the greatest dysrhythmogenic potential, although one study has demonstrated that the pediatric heart may be more resistant to the interactions between halothane and exogenous epinephrine (Karl et al., 1983; Ueda et al., 1983). At equipotent concentrations, isoflurane has three times less the dysrhythmogenic potential of halothane (Marshall and Longnecker, 2001). Desflurane and sevoflurane are thought to be similar to isoflurane in this regard (Moore et al., 1993; Navarro et al., 1994).

The β-blocking agents timolol, levobunolol, and betaxolol act by decreasing the production of aqueous humor and are occasionally used postoperatively in children. The agents should not be used in the neonatal and infant populations in light of several reports of apnea with the use of timolol (Olson et al., 1979; Bailey, 1984). In older children and adults, the use of betaxolol, which is selective for the β_1-receptors, is associated with fewer complications involving the pulmonary system, although dyspnea and bronchospasm have been reported (Everitt and Avorn, 1990). Lethargy, bradycardia, and heart block are possible with all of the topical β-blocking agents (Gross and Pineyro, 1997).

Apraclonidine and brimonidine are topical α_2-agonists that decrease sympathetic tone and subsequently reduce aqueous humor production. Brimonidine, unlike apraclonidine, is capable of crossing the blood-brain barrier and should be used with great caution in young children. Bradycardia, hypotension, hypothermia, hypotonia, and apnea have all been reported with the use of brimonidine (Enyedi and Freedman, 2001).

Newer topical agents, including the prostaglandin analogues (latanoprost, bimatoprost, and travoprost) and the topical carbonic anhydrase inhibitors (dorzolamide and brinzolamide), are generally very safe in the pediatric population but are believed to be less effective than they are in adults (Beck, 2001). The topical carbonic anhydrase inhibitors, like systemic acetazolamide, are sulfonamide derivatives that should be avoided in the patient with sulfa sensitivity.

MISCELLANEOUS OPHTHALMOLOGIC AGENTS

Topical anesthetics, including cocaine, tetracaine, and proparacaine, are occasionally used by ophthalmologists in the perioperative setting. Cocaine is rarely used, but it is unique among the local anesthetics because of its vasoconstrictive properties. The potential for serious cardiovascular and central nervous system effects should be recognized by both the surgeon and anesthesiologist. The accepted maximum dose is 3 mg/kg, with 1.5 mg/kg being preferable in the presence of volatile anesthetics. One drop of the 4% formulation contains approximately 1.5 mg of cocaine (McGoldrick, 1992). The drug should not be used in patients with cardiovascular disease or in the presence of additional adrenergic-modifying medications such as monoamine oxidase inhibitors and tricyclic antidepressants.

Intraocular gases, including sulfur hexafluoride, perfluoropropane, and carbon octofluorine, are poorly diffusible inert gases that may be injected during certain vitreoretinal procedures. When nitrous oxide is present during injection, the nitrous oxide equilibrates with these new gas spaces to increase the volume and pressure of the intraocular injection, potentially compromising retinal perfusion. Animal studies, case reports, and mathematical models have demonstrated the necessity of (1) discontinuing nitrous oxide not less than 15 minutes before intraocular gas injection and (2) avoiding subsequent use of nitrous oxide for at least 4 weeks after the use of sulfur hexafluoride and 6 weeks after the use of perfluoropropane or carbon octofluorine (Wolf et al., 1983; McGoldrick, 1992; Seaberg et al., 2002).

EFFECTS OF VARIOUS ANESTHETIC AGENTS ON INTRAOCULAR PRESSURE

It is important to understand the ocular effects of the various anesthetic agents. An anesthetic plan should be chosen that provides optimal surgical conditions for intraocular procedures and minimizes risk of morbidity in those patients with preexisting intraocular hypertension and traumatic injury to the globe.

The central nervous system depressants (benzodiazepines, barbiturates, and opioids) frequently used by the anesthesiologist decrease IOP in both normal and glaucomatous eyes. The agents commonly used for preoperative anxiolysis in the pediatric population are associated with minor decreases in IOP that should not affect diagnostic measurements and likewise should not be relied on to attenuate the increase in IOP attributable to the use of succinylcholine and laryngoscopy. Effects specific to the use of oral or rectal midazolam in the pediatric population have not been delineated, although two studies of the use of intravenous midazolam in adults demonstrate minimal effects on IOP (Virkkila et al., 1992; Carter et al., 1999).

With the possible exception of ketamine, all of the intravenous induction agents are associated with a significant decrease in IOP. Thiopental and propofol reduced IOP by 40% and 53%, respectively, in one study (Mirakhur and Shepherd, 1985), although both agents are unable to completely attenuate increases that are secondary to succinylcholine and laryngoscopy (Mirakhur et al., 1987). Etomidate diminished IOP more profoundly than thiopental in one adult study (Calla et al., 1987), but it is difficult to eliminate the possibility of myoclonus with etomidate. This could be hazardous to the patient with traumatic injury and bothersome to the ophthalmologist. Early studies of the effects of ketamine uniformly demonstrated an increase in IOP, but subsequent studies in adults and children (Peuler et al., 1975; Ausinsch et al., 1976) have demonstrated either insignificant changes or minor decreases in IOP. There is no clear consensus regarding the effects of ketamine on IOP, although its association with blepharospasm and nystagmus makes other induction agents more useful for the ophthalmologic patient.

All of the volatile anesthetics are associated with a dose-dependent decrease in IOP. Various postulated mechanisms include a reduction in aqueous humor production with a concomitant increase in outflow, relaxation of the supporting musculature, and depression of the central nervous system control center for IOP (McGoldrick, 1992). As was previously demonstrated with halothane (Watcha et al., 1990), reliable measurements of IOP may be made for approximately 10 minutes after mask induction with sevoflurane (Yoshitake et al., 1993).

The deleterious effects of succinylcholine on IOP and the various methods of attenuating these effects have been evaluated by numerous investigators for several decades. The augmentation of IOP is thought to be mediated not only by tonic contractions of the extraocular muscles but also by dilation of the choroidal vasculature and relaxation of the orbital smooth muscle (Calobrisi and Lebowitz, 1990). In a study of patients undergoing elective enucleation, Kelly and others (1993) noted that after succinylcholine administration, the IOP did not change in the eye where the extraocular muscles were detached. It does not appear that extraocular muscle contraction significantly contributes to the increase in IOP after succinylcholine administration. In adult patients with normal IOP, succinylcholine at doses between 1.5 and 2 mg/kg increased pressures by no more than 9 mm Hg, with peak effects demonstrated within 3 minutes after administration (Pandey et al., 1972). In patients who were not intubated, IOP was restored to baseline within 6 minutes, although other studies have demonstrated mild elevations that may persist for 30 minutes after succinylcholine administration. While these effects of succinylcholine are significant in comparison to the effects of the nondepolarizing agents, they are clearly insignificant in comparison to the increase in IOP that is possible with laryngoscopy, coughing, and retching.

Numerous methods of blunting the rise in IOP secondary to succinylcholine and laryngoscopy have been evaluated, although none have demonstrated consistent or reliable efficacy. The results of early studies of pretreating patients with small doses of the nondepolarizing agents were promising (Miller et al., 1968) but later refuted (Meyers et al., 1978). In two adult studies, the use of alfentanil was demonstrated to significantly attenuate the response to succinylcholine and intubation (Polarz et al., 1992; Eti et al., 2000). Another study comparing the effects of fentanyl and alfentanil demonstrated that although both agents were effective in attenuating the response to succinylcholine, fentanyl did not significantly attenuate the increase in IOP secondary to laryngoscopy (Sweeney et al., 1989). Early studies concerning the benefit of lidocaine before succinylcholine were discouraging (Smith et al., 1979), but lidocaine had favorable effects on IOP during laryngoscopy and intubation in subsequent investigations (Mahajan et al., 1987; Warner et al., 1989). The opioids and lidocaine may also facilitate gentle extubations after intraocular procedures and in patients with elevated IOP.

More contemporary methods of controlling IOP with the use of succinylcholine and laryngoscopy have been promising. Premedication with sublingual nifedipine (Indu et al., 1989) and oral clonidine (Ghignone et al., 1988; Polarz et al., 1993) has demonstrated efficacy in the elderly population. Intramuscular dexmedetomidine also effectively reduced IOP during regional anesthetic procedures in adults (Virkkila et al., 1994). None of these methods have been evaluated in the pediatric population.

More information regarding airway management and the effects on IOP are discussed in "Traumatic Injury and the Ruptured Globe." In addition, Vachon and others (2003) review the use of succinylcholine and the open globe.

GENERAL ANESTHETIC CONSIDERATIONS

PREMEDICATION

The value of premedication is well appreciated by all physicians providing anesthetic care to children. Premedication is useful to ease separation from parents and to provide for a smooth induction. Children between the ages of 1 and 6 years frequently benefit from premedication. Older children, especially those subject to repeated procedures, may also benefit from premedication. Oral midazolam (0.25 to 0.5 mg/kg) is commonly used and is generally effective within 10 to 20 minutes after administration (Coté et al., 2002). Nasal midazolam (0.2 mg/kg) may be useful in the patient refusing oral administration, but the acidity of the formulation is associated with a 71% incidence of burning and crying on administration (Karl et al., 1993). Oral clonidine (2 to 4 mcg/kg) also provides adequate anxiolysis within 30 minutes and has been demonstrated to decrease the incidence of PONV after strabismus surgery in two investigations (Mikawa et al., 1995; Handa and Fujii, 2001). Neither midazolam nor clonidine consistently decreases the incidence of emergence delirium (Fazi et al., 2001; Valley et al., 2003). At recommended doses, neither of the agents should prolong the time required for discharge from the postoperative recovery unit.

GENERAL ANESTHESIA

General anesthesia for ophthalmologic procedures in children is similar to that provided for other brief surgical procedures.

Many ophthalmologic procedures may be performed on an outpatient basis when the age of the patient does not mandate postoperative monitoring. Mask induction with nitrous oxide and sevoflurane or halothane is common for young patients who do not require rapid sequence induction. Clear communication with the ophthalmologist can delineate which procedure may be performed with mask anesthesia or requires the use of a laryngeal mask airway or endotracheal tube. Consideration should be given to the proposed duration of the procedure and the possibility that access to the airway may be difficult.

Anesthesia can be maintained with any of the volatile agents, but the incidence of emergence delirium may be higher with the newer, less-soluble agents (Welborn et al., 1996; Lapin et al., 1999). Nitrous oxide is avoided if inert gas is to be injected into the eye. Nitrous oxide has been associated with an increased incidence of PONV in some adult studies (Hartung, 1996; Tramer et al., 1996, 1997), although similar effects cannot be demonstrated in the pediatric population. One study demonstrated no correlation between the use of nitrous oxide and the incidence of PONV in pediatric strabismus patients (Kuhn et al., 1999). Maintenance with propofol may also be used, but three studies have demonstrated a higher incidence of dysrhythmias attributable to the OCR with propofol anesthesia (Watcha et al., 1991; Larsson et al., 1992; Tramer et al., 1998). Neuromuscular blockade is often indicated for intraocular procedures to ensure that the field remains motionless and that coughing or bucking does not result in damage to the eye and untoward increases in IOP.

A smooth emergence from anesthesia is desired after ophthalmologic procedures. This may be facilitated by deep extubation in the lateral position. Any of the inhaled agents may be safely used for deep extubation, although slightly more airway complications may occur with the use of desflurane (Valley et al., 2003). Small doses of intravenous lidocaine (0.5 to 1 mg/kg) may be administered before extubation if the depth of anesthesia is unclear.

LOCAL AND REGIONAL ANESTHESIA

The primary methods of administering local anesthetics for ocular procedures include topical application, infiltration, and regional blockade. Conjunctival injection is often used to provide anesthesia for the treatment of retinopathy of prematurity. Topical application or infiltration may be useful in the cooperative older child to perform otherwise uncomfortable examinations and simple procedures such as foreign body removal and laceration repair. Solitary regional techniques, including retrobulbar, peribulbar, and sub-Tenon's blocks, are effectively used in adults for a variety of ophthalmologic procedures, but they generally are avoided in children younger than 18 years (Johnson and Forrest, 1994). The benefits of regional techniques as adjuncts to general anesthesia in children are controversial.

The retrobulbar or intraconal block was first described in 1884. The block involves injection of local anesthetic into the posterior cone of the extraocular muscles and is effective in producing anesthesia and akinesia by blocking the ciliary ganglion and the oculomotor and abducens nerves. Hyaluronidase is a commonly used adjuvant that decreases the time for onset. The retrobulbar technique is not frequently used in the pediatric population. Complications of the retrobulbar block include stimulation of the OCR, retrobulbar hemorrhage, penetration of the optic nerve, intravascular injection, and brainstem anesthesia (McGoldrick, 1992). One study evaluating the efficacy of retrobulbar blocks in combination with general anesthesia for pediatric strabismus surgery demonstrated no significant benefit, although the sample size was relatively small (Ates et al., 1998).

The peribulbar or periconal block has been increasingly used since it was first described in 1986. Because the cone of the extraocular muscles is not entered, the potential for intraocular and intradural injection is minimized and the risk of retrobulbar hemorrhage and direct nerve injury is virtually eliminated (McGoldrick, 1992). Disadvantages of the peribulbar block include a slightly higher failure rate (10% incidence) and an increased forward pressure on the globe secondary to the larger volumes of local anesthetic required (Zahl, 1992). Two pediatric studies (Deb et al., 2001; Subramaniam et al., 2003) that compared peribulbar blocks with intravenous meperidine for vitreoretinal and strabismus surgery demonstrated superior analgesia and significantly less PONV for up to 24 hours after surgery. Parental satisfaction was also greater for those patients receiving adjunctive regional blocks.

Regional techniques are not suitable for most pediatric patients, but regional ophthalmologic anesthesia may be appropriate for some children. Although it is unlikely that the pediatric anesthesiologists will ever be expected to perform such procedures, a general understanding of the techniques and potential complications is important.

INTRAOPERATIVE AND POSTOPERATIVE COMPLICATIONS

OCULOCARDIAC REFLEX

The OCR was first described by two independent observers in 1908. The OCR is reported to occur at an incidence as high as 70% to 79% during pediatric ophthalmologic surgery (particularly strabismus surgery) without the use of prophylaxis (Ruta et al., 1996; Allen et al., 1998). The reflex is most often elicited by traction on the extraocular muscles but is also elicited by pressure on the eye and after intraorbital or retrobulbar injections. The reflex has been observed in the congenitally anophthalmic child (Ward and Bass, 2001) and in the patient with an empty orbit after enucleation (Kerr and Vance, 1983). The anesthesiologist should be aware of the OCR and its potential consequences.

The OCR is mediated by the afferent ophthalmic division of the trigeminal and the efferent vagal nerves (Fig. 22–3). The most common manifestation of the reflex is sinus bradycardia, but more ominous manifestations, including atrioventricular block, ventricular bigeminy, ventricular tachycardia, and asystole, have been described. Most studies define significant OCR-related bradycardia as a 10% to 20% decrease in the resting heart rate that is sustained for 5 seconds or longer. With sustained traction on one of the extraocular muscles, a counterregulatory adrenergic phase and restoration of heart rate occur, which may be followed by a further increase in heart rate once traction is released (Braun et al., 1993). Most often, the initial bradycardia is associated with a variable degree of hypotension, although bradycardic hypertensive responses are also possible (Hahnenkamp et al., 2000).

When the reflex occurs intraoperatively, release of the stimulus is usually effective in ablating dysrhythmias within 10 to 20 seconds. If bradycardia persists or is worrisome, the patient may be given atropine (10 to 20 mcg/kg IV) or glycopyrrolate (10 mcg/kg IV). The initial effects of atropine should be evident within 20 seconds, and the maximal response is observed after 80 seconds (Braun et al., 1993). In the event that intravenous

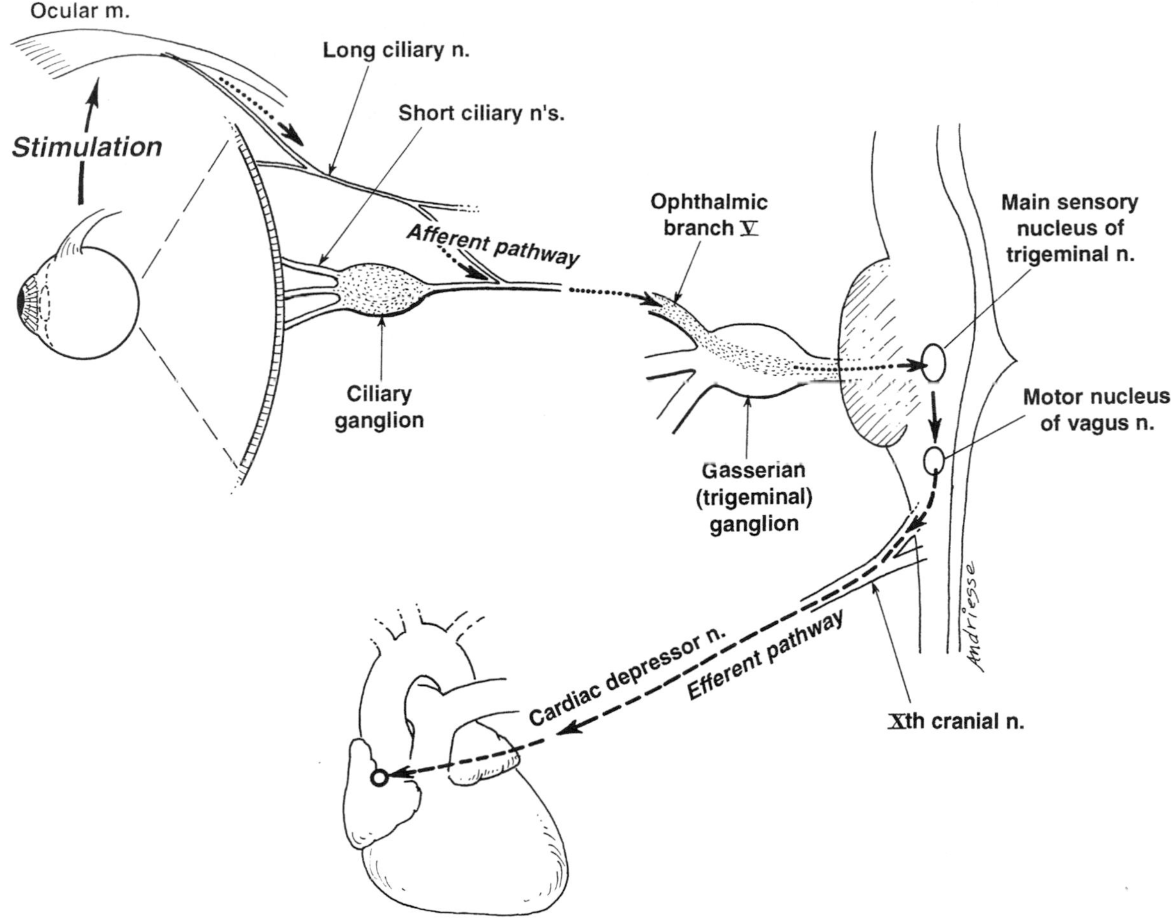

■ **FIGURE 22–3.** Anatomy and physiology of the oculocardiac reflex. (From Vassallo SA, Ferrari LR: Anesthesia for ophthalmology. In Coté CJ, Ryan JF, Todres ID, et al., editors: *A practice of anesthesia for infants and children,* 2nd ed. Philadelphia, 1993, WB Saunders, p 325, with permission.)

access is not available or is unreliable, one study has determined that intraglossal administration is superior to the intramuscular route and in fact may be superior to intravenous administration (Arnold et al., 2002). It is generally safe to proceed with surgery once normal sinus rhythm at a rate within 10% of baseline is restored.

The value of prophylaxis has been debated for many years; there clearly is no method of completely eliminating the occurrence of OCR. The current consensus is that most pediatric patients (but not adults) undergoing strabismus surgery should be treated with intravenous atropine at a dose of 20 mcg/kg before manipulation (Steward, 1983). Intravenous glycopyrrolate at a dose of 10 mcg/kg also has demonstrated efficacy with slightly less pronounced tachycardia. One randomized study of 120 children demonstrated a reduction in the incidence of OCR to 5% with glycopyrrolate and 2% with atropine given immediately after induction (Chisakuta and Mirakhur, 1995). Preoperative treatment by oral or intramuscular routes is generally not warranted and is probably less effective (Mirakhur et al., 1982; Mirakhur, 1991). Opponents to prophylaxis with atropine maintain that possible dysrhythmias secondary to atropine itself (ventricular tachycardia, ventricular fibrillation, and left bundle branch block) may be more ominous and difficult to treat than the dysrhythmias associated with the OCR (Massumi et al., 1972; McGoldrick, 1992). These effects are much more common in the adult patient. In otherwise healthy children, the tachycardic effects of atropine or glycopyrrolate should be safe and well tolerated.

Retrobulbar blocks are effective in preventing the OCR (Taylor et al., 1963; Braun et al., 1993; Deb et al., 2001); regional blocks are not frequently used during pediatric procedures and have triggered the reflex during placement. Topical lidocaine, applied directly to the medial rectus at 1 mg/kg, decreased the incidence of the OCR to 19% (versus 79% in the control population); this technique has not been investigated since the initial study of 36 pediatric patients (Ruta et al., 1996).

The reflex may occur during regional and general anesthesia, and the depth of anesthesia is thought to be irrelevant. Hypercarbia and hypoxemia, which may be more likely in the spontaneously breathing patient, are associated with a greater incidence of the bradycardic response. At least four studies have demonstrated that the choice of maintenance agents may influence the incidence or severity of the OCR. In one study of 39 pediatric patients mechanically ventilated through laryngeal mask airways, propofol anesthesia was associated with the greatest decrease in heart rate during a standardized traction of an extraocular muscle. Ketamine was associated with the least decrease in heart rate, whereas halothane and sevoflurane were associated with intermediate effects (Hahnenkamp et al., 2000). In another study of spontaneously breathing normocarbic patients who were not pretreated with atropine, sevoflurane was associated with a 38% incidence of OCR, whereas halothane was associated with an incidence of 79% (Allison et al., 2000).

POSTOPERATIVE PAIN

Many of the common ophthalmologic procedures have minimal postoperative analgesic requirements. Examinations under anesthesia, nasolacrimal duct probing, and cataract extraction are associated with negligible postoperative discomfort. The various procedures performed for glaucoma and strabismus are associated with moderate postoperative pain. The requirements for analgesia should be reviewed with the surgeon, the patient, and the family during the formulation and general discussion of the anesthetic plan.

For patients requiring minimal analgesia, rectal acetaminophen (30 to 40 mg/kg) may be administered after induction and followed with subsequent doses (20 mg/kg) at 6-hour intervals (Birmingham et al., 2001). Up to 120 minutes may be required to achieve peak serum levels. Intravenous ketorolac (0.5 mg/kg) yields consistent analgesia for those procedures resulting in moderate postoperative pain (Dsida et al., 2002). Two studies of ketorolac administered for strabismus surgery have demonstrated analgesia equivalent to that provided by fentanyl (1 mcg/kg) or morphine (0.1 mg/kg) with a substantial reduction in PONV (Munro et al., 1994; Mendel et al., 1995).

Opioid analgesics should not be withheld from patients requiring more intensive analgesia. More painful procedures include cryotherapy (for various disorders), ablation, and enucleation for patients with retinoblastoma. Nausea, vomiting, and respiratory depression can complicate postoperative recovery, but the opioid agents provide greater facility for titration, may minimize coughing and bucking at extubation, and attenuate the incidence of emergence delirium.

POSTOPERATIVE NAUSEA AND VOMITING

Nausea and vomiting after ophthalmologic procedures is so common that it often serves as a model for the evaluation of various prophylactic techniques. Several large-scale studies report that PONV occurs in children at an incidence of 13% to 42% after general anesthesia for all procedures (Rose and Watcha, 1999). The incidence of PONV in untreated children after strabismus surgery ranges from 40% to 88% (Lerman, 1995). Older children and those receiving opioid analgesics are at greater risk. Prophylaxis versus symptomatic treatment is debated for low-risk procedures in children, but it is generally accepted that prophylaxis should be provided for children undergoing strabismus surgery and all intraocular procedures regardless of demographics and the anesthetic technique used. Retching and vomiting may be particularly detrimental after surgical or traumatic trespass of the globe. A summary of prophylactic measures is provided (Box 22–2).

The efficacy of droperidol, a butyrophenone, has been demonstrated in numerous studies since the 1980s. Low doses (20 mcg/kg) given after induction are as effective as higher doses (75 mcg/kg) and are less likely to prolong recovery time (Brown et al., 1991). Lower doses (15 mcg/kg) in combination with ondansetron (100 mcg/kg IV) are more effective than either drug given individually (Shende et al., 2001). The Food and Drug Administration issued a black box warning in 2001 regarding the potential for fatal dysrhythmias associated with prolonged QTc intervals in rare patients administered droperidol. No significant complications have been reported in children with the use of low-dose droperidol. However, the pediatric anesthesiologist may find it easier to use alternative drugs as PONV prophylaxis than to comply with the rigorous monitoring recommendations made by the Food and Drug Administration.

BOX 22–2 Prophylaxis for Postoperative Nausea and Vomiting

Demonstrated Benefit

Clonidine premedication 4 mcg/kg PO

Avoiding opioid analgesics

Avoiding nitrous oxide (controversial)

Dexamethasone 0.15 to 1 mg/kg IV

Ondansetron 50 to 200 mcg/kg IV

Metaclopramide 100 to 250 mcg/kg IV

Withholding oral intake postoperatively

No Demonstrated Benefit

Anticholinergic therapy

Gastric content evacuation before emergence

Ondansetron is a serotonin (5-hydroxytryptamine [5-HT])$_3$ receptor antagonist commonly used for prophylaxis and rescue therapy at doses ranging from 50 to 200 mcg/kg IV. The half-life in children is slightly shorter than it is in adults (2.5 versus 3.8 hours), and side effects are unusual in all populations (Culy et al., 2001). Administration either before or after surgical manipulation is acceptable with equivalent benefit (Madan et al., 2000). It has been demonstrated that doses of 75 mcg/kg are as effective as higher doses in the immediate postoperative period (Sadhasivam et al., 2000). Two studies have demonstrated that higher doses (150 to 200 mcg/kg) are required for significant benefit carried through the initial 24-hour postoperative period (Rose et al., 1994; Bowhay et al., 2001).

Other 5-HT$_3$ receptor antagonists have been developed since 1991, primarily in an effort to increase the duration of action of ondansetron (Rose and Watcha, 1999). Both granisetron (20 to 40 mcg/kg IV or PO) and ramosetron (6 mcg/kg IV) have demonstrated efficacy in the pediatric strabismus population, although the costs of both drugs are slightly prohibitive (Munro et al., 1999; Fujii et al., 2001).

Evaluations of dexamethasone have been favorable primarily in light of the agent's low risk, low cost, long duration of action (up to 48 hours), and potential for augmenting postoperative analgesia (Splinter and Rhine, 1998). A study by Subramaniam and others (2001) compared high-dose dexamethasone at 1 mg/kg (maximum, 25 mg) with ondansetron at 100 mcg/kg (maximum, 4 mg) and demonstrated a similar incidence of PONV during the initial 6 hours but significantly less during the subsequent 18 postoperative hours in those treated with dexamethasone. The severity of PONV and the number of patients requiring rescue medication were also significantly less in the dexamethasone group. The greatest reduction in PONV after surgery for strabismus was reported in a study using a lower dose of dexamethasone (150 mcg/kg; maximum, 8 mg) in combination with ondansetron (50 mcg/kg) after induction (Splinter, 2001). Facial flushing is possible after dexamethasone, but there is no evidence in the literature for more detrimental side effects (hyperglycemia, delayed wound healing, adrenal suppression) after single-dose therapy (Subramaniam et al., 2001).

Metoclopramide is a dopaminergic antagonist that provides central antiemetic action as well as increased gastric emptying and increased tone at the lower esophageal sphincter. There is inconsistent support in the literature for the use of metoclopramide for PONV prophylaxis. Two randomized studies have demonstrated moderate benefit with metoclopramide at a dose of 250 mcg/kg given after induction (Broadman et al., 1990; Lin et al., 1992), although two later studies failed to demonstrate any significant benefit (Shende and Haldar, 1998; Kathirvel et al., 1999).

Four early studies that compared propofol anesthesia with halothane demonstrated a significant attenuation of PONV after strabismus surgery when propofol was used (Watcha et al., 1991; Larsson et al., 1992; Reimer et al., 1993; Weir et al., 1993). Benefit was demonstrated primarily during the immediate postoperative period, and two of these studies found a much higher incidence of OCR-related bradycardia with propofol. One later study compared propofol with isoflurane anesthesia and failed to demonstrate any significant benefit with propofol (Hamunen et al., 1997).

Other modalities of prophylaxis for PONV continue to emerge in response to an appropriate focus on cost effectiveness and patient and parental satisfaction. It is left to each clinician to determine what risk is tolerable and which patient population may derive the greatest benefit from therapy.

SPECIFIC PATHOLOGY AND SURGICAL AND ANESTHETIC MANAGEMENT

EXAMINATION UNDER ANESTHESIA

Although some centers perform simple examinations and minor procedures for young children under procedural sedation, many ophthalmologists prefer general anesthesia to perform more thorough and accurate examinations. Common evaluations include tonometry, funduscopy, and the assessment of visual evoked potentials. Most examinations take no more than 5 to 10 minutes, but a sufficient depth of anesthesia must be provided. Premedication and anxiolysis are most beneficial to children who require a series of examinations over time.

For healthy children, mask induction and maintenance of spontaneous ventilation provide adequate conditions for the ophthalmologist while also affording accurate control of anesthetic depth and a smooth emergence from anesthesia. Accurate measurements of IOP can be made for the initial 10 minutes after induction and maintenance with both sevoflurane and halothane (Watcha et al., 1990; Yoshitake et al., 1993). More lengthy examinations, including photographic retinal mapping and assessment of visual evoked potentials, may be performed with either propofol sedation or spontaneous ventilation with inhaled anesthetic agents and laryngeal mask airway.

RETINOPATHY OF PREMATURITY

Retinopathy of prematurity (ROP) is a multifactorial disease defined as the failure of retinal vascular development. The infant with ROP may require anesthetic care for procedures both related and unrelated to ocular pathology. ROP is of particular interest to the pediatric anesthesiologist because the routine management of the infant at risk may alter the development or progression of the disease itself.

Associations with ROP include low birth weight, prematurity, neonatal oxygen exposure, recurrent apnea, exchange transfusion, and vitamin E deficiency. ROP occurs in approximately 70% of infants who weigh less than 1,000 g at birth. Fortunately, 80% to 90% of these infants have spontaneous regression of their retinal changes (Simons and Flynn, 1999; Moore, 2000). It is clear that supplemental oxygen and relative hyperoxia are not the only factors responsible for development of the disease. Nevertheless, the immature retina is indisputably more susceptible to damage from the higher ex utero concentrations of oxygen and subsequent free radical liberation.

The immature retina responds to elevated oxygen tension (or another insult) by arrest of normal vasculogenesis and later by neovascularization and fibrous tissue formation in the retina and vitreous humor. Retinal tears and detachment may occur secondary to contraction of the vitreous humor. Vasculogenesis takes place between 16 and 44 weeks after conception. In the normal developing retina, there is no clear border dividing the vascular and avascular tissue. This border becomes more prominent in those patients with ROP and forms the basis for staging the disease. The International Classification of Retinopathy of Prematurity (ICROP) was established in 1984 to uniformly describe the anatomic zone involved and the severity or stage of disease (Committee for the Classification of Retinopathy of Prematurity, 1984). Definitions for the various stages are provided (Box 22–3). Threshold ROP, defined by specific ICROP criteria, is the stage of progression that is amenable to treatment.

Investigations have demonstrated the benefit of extremely limited oxygen supplementation in premature infants without ROP and the potential benefit of more liberal oxygen therapy in older infants with established prethreshold disease (Sinha and Tin, 2003). At one institution, rigorous guidelines restricting the use of oxygen greatly diminished the occurrence of advanced ROP and abolished the need for laser therapy over a 5-year

BOX 22–3 International Classification of Retinopathy of Prematurity Stages

Stage 1:	Fine demarcation line is visible between vascular and avascular regions
Stage 2:	Broad ridge divides the vascular and avascular regions
Stage 3:	Neovascularization is noted at the ridge, on the posterior surface and anteriorly toward the vitreous cavity
Stage 4:	Subtotal retinal detachment
Stage 5:	Total retinal detachment in an open or closed funnel configuration

From Committee for the Classification of Retinopathy of Prematurity: An international classification of retinopathy of prematurity. *Pediatrics* 74:127, 1984.

period (Chow et al., 2003). The STOP-ROP multicenter controlled trial revealed that patients with established prethreshold disease are not harmed by oxygen supplementation and that a subset of these patients may benefit from higher arterial saturations (STOP-ROP Multicenter Study Group, 2000).

It is prudent to the anesthesiologist to limit oxygen supplementation in those infants without a diagnosis of ROP during the period of retinal vascularization. Older infants (>44 weeks postconceptional age) and those with established prethreshold disease are probably less vulnerable to higher oxygen tensions commonly provided during transports and general anesthesia. Anesthesia provided for nonophthalmologic procedures was once believed to increase the risk of ROP, but controlling for other risk factors has revealed that such a population is at no greater risk (Flynn, 1984).

Infants with threshold ROP are treated by cryotherapy or laser photocoagulation depending on specific clinical findings. Cryotherapy involves placement of a probe chilled with nitrous oxide on the outer surface of the globe. Cryonecrosis of the underlying retinal tissues results in a decrease in the incidence of retinal detachment. Laser procedures (diode and argon lasers) are the preferred modality of therapy but require greater visualization than the cryotherapy technique. Both procedures may be performed with atropine, opioids, and local anesthetic injection, although many ophthalmologists prefer the benefits of general anesthesia and a protected airway. Elective intubations are performed in those infants not currently requiring ventilatory support. Cryotherapy may require adequate analgesia during and after the procedure. Sullivan and others (1995) have advocated intubation for all patients undergoing cryotherapy to better meet the needs of these patients and the surgeon. Careful monitoring is mandatory, and neonatologists or anesthesiologists must be available, if not directly involved, in the event of cardiorespiratory disturbances, which occur in 5% to 9% of all cases (Brown et al., 1990; Haigh et al., 1997).

STRABISMUS

Strabismus has a prevalence of 3% to 5% in the pediatric population (Vivian, 2000). The disorder is most often idiopathic but may be associated with poor vision, cataracts, trauma, neuromuscular disorders, or one of several congenital syndromes (see Table 22–1). Surgical correction involves isolation of one or more of the extraocular muscles with subsequent recession (transection and reinsertion) or resection (shortening) of the muscle. Contemporary techniques involving botulinum toxin injection and postoperative adjustable sutures are not frequently used in the pediatric population. Amblyopia develops in approximately 50% of all patients with congenital esotropia and should be treated with occlusion therapy before surgical correction for strabismus (Guthrie and Wright, 2001).

General anesthesia may be provided by a flexible laryngeal mask airway, although endotracheal intubation with controlled ventilation may lessen the risk of hypercarbia and hypoxemia, which are known to increase the incidence and severity of the OCR (Blanc et al., 1988). Many ophthalmologists request the use of paralytic agents for performance of the forced duction test to more clearly differentiate paretic and restrictive disorders before surgical correction. This possibility should be discussed with the surgeon before formulating the anesthetic plan. Prolonged contractions of the extraocular muscles associated with the use of succinylcholine interfere with interpretation of the forced duction test for at least 15 minutes after administration (France et al., 1980). Its use is relatively contraindicated.

Masseter muscle rigidity after succinylcholine administration is four times more common in children anesthetized for strabismus surgery than in the general pediatric surgical population (Carroll, 1987). Because of the association of masseter muscle rigidity with malignant hyperthermia and an increased incidence of malignant hyperthermia in patients undergoing strabismus surgery, these patients are thought to be at a greater risk for the development of malignant hyperthermia (Strazis and Fox, 1993) (see Chapter 31, Malignant Hyperthermia).

Prophylaxis for both the OCR and PONV are critical for the patient undergoing strabismus repair. Postoperative pain is generally mild and of conjunctival origin. Rectal acetaminophen, intravenous ketorolac, or both are usually effective. Topical analgesics (ketorolac, diclofenac, and oxybuprocaine) have been evaluated in the strabismus population, and clear advantages over systemic agents and uniform efficacy have not been demonstrated (Morton et al., 1997; Bridge et al., 2000).

LACRIMAL APPARATUS DYSFUNCTION

Congenital nasolacrimal duct obstruction is present in 60% to 70% of all infants at birth; spontaneous resolution is observed in 96% of these children by 1 year of age (Freitag and Woog, 2000). Congenital obstructions are most often isolated findings but may be associated with a variety of syndromes and craniofacial defects (see Table 22–1). Acquired nasolacrimal duct obstruction is infrequently encountered in the pediatric population but may be secondary to trauma, granulomatous disease, and systemic neoplasms (leukemia and lymphoma). The anatomy of the nasolacrimal duct system is illustrated (Fig. 22–4).

The initial surgical management of congenital obstruction usually requires only simple probing to establish patency. A small Bowman probe is inserted through one or both of the puncti, through the lacrimal sac, and subsequently into the nasolacrimal duct to pierce the valve of Hasner beneath the inferior turbinate (Freitag and Woog, 2000). The procedure is frequently atraumatic, requires no more than 5 to 10 minutes, and has been performed successfully in the office setting in children younger than 6 months. Usually, the procedure is performed with general mask anesthesia. As with similar noninvasive procedures, intravenous access is not absolutely required for patients who are easily mask ventilated. Patients with significant comorbidities may be more safely cared for with intravenous access, and it has been demonstrated that those at risk for endocarditis should receive appropriate antibiotic prophylaxis (Eippert et al., 1998).

The lacrimal system may be irrigated with saline or fluorescein after the procedure to demonstrate patency. Preventing excessive pooling, possible laryngospasm, and aspiration may require only head-down positioning and careful suctioning through the ipsilateral naris or oropharynx. Some anesthesiologists believe that these patients are better managed with intubation to provide optimal protection of the airway (Johnson and Forrest, 1994). Analgesic requirements after nasolacrimal probing and irrigation are negligible.

Secondary surgical management of nasolacrimal obstruction may include infracture of the inferior turbinate, placement of silicone tubing that remains in place for 3 to 12 months, and dacryocystorhinostomy (Freitag and Woog, 2000). Dacryocystorhinostomy is a procedure used to bypass the nasolacrimal duct by creating an anastomosis between the lacrimal

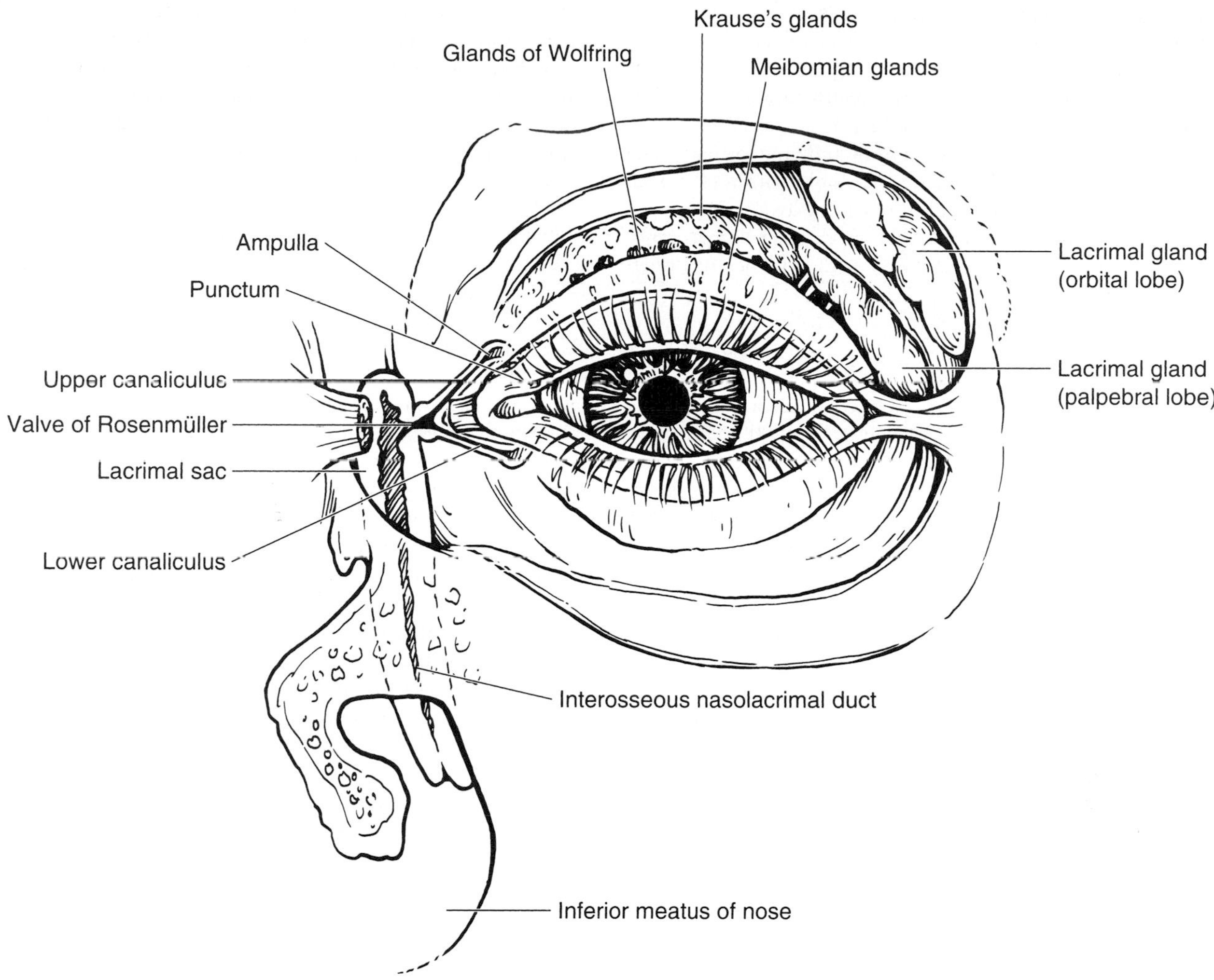

■ **FIGURE 22–4.** Anatomy of the lacrimal duct apparatus. (From Nowinski TS: Anatomy and physiology of the lacrimal system. In Bosniak S, editor: *Principles and practice of ophthalmic plastic and reconstructive surgery*, vol 2. Philadelphia, 1996, WB Saunders, p 732, with permission.)

sac and the nasal mucosa beneath the middle turbinate. A small incision is made just medial to the medial canthus and overlying the lacrimal sac. These more complex procedures may require up to 2 hours to perform and may be complicated by appreciable blood loss. They require general anesthesia with endotracheal intubation. Topical vasoconstrictors may be used to minimize bleeding at the highly vascular nasal mucosa, and pharyngeal packing is usually beneficial. Acetaminophen, ketorolac, or small doses of opioids should provide adequate postoperative analgesia.

■ CATARACTS

The prevalence of pediatric cataracts is between 1.2 and 6 per 10,000 live births. Bilateral cataracts are most commonly associated with systemic disease (see Table 22–1), whereas unilateral cataracts are more often idiopathic (Russell-Eggitt, 2000; Fallaha and Lambert, 2001). Surgery for bilateral congenital cataracts must be performed within the first several weeks of life to allow for normal retinal development. Unilateral congenital disease requires surgical attention within the first 4 months of life to prohibit the development of irreversible amblyopia.

Lens extraction is performed after maximal mydriasis with one or more of the topical agents. Ultrasonic phacoemulsification (commonly used in adults) is infrequently used in the pediatric population because of the pliable nature of the immature lens. Vitrectomy instrumentation is the preferred method of extraction in young children; the entire procedure is typically performed with only one intraocular instrument. Capsular opacification occurs frequently in children such that a capsulectomy is usually performed at the time of primary surgery. Intraocular lens implants are commonly provided to children older than 6 months with unilateral disease and children older than 1 year with bilateral disease (Fallaha and Lambert, 2001).

Anesthesia for lens extraction should provide complete akinesia and meticulous control of IOP. Because most of these patients are infants, controlled ventilation with muscle relaxants provides optimal operating conditions. The anesthesiologist should be aware of associated systemic disease and the potential systemic effects of the topical preparations used by the ophthalmologist. Rarely, maximal pupillary dilation requires an infusion of epinephrine (1:200,000) delivered and then continuously aspirated from the anterior chamber. Attention to the electrocardiogram tracing permits detection of systemic absorption, which fortunately is uncommon (McGoldrick, 1992). Analgesic requirements are usually minimal and under normal circumstances may be met with rectal acetaminophen.

Postoperative apnea has been reported in the otherwise healthy full-term infant after cataract surgery (Tetzlaff et al., 1988). Speculation has associated ocular pathology or procedures with postoperative apnea in the otherwise healthy infant, but this association has yet to be clearly described.

Surgical postoperative complications include the formation of secondary membranes, glaucoma, and endophthalmitis (Fallaha and Lambert, 2001). Endophthalmitis may be avoided by treating nasolacrimal duct obstruction before cataract surgery and postponing cataract surgery in children with evidence of upper respiratory tract infection.

GLAUCOMA

Pediatric glaucomas are a diverse group of disorders with a prevalence of 1:10,000 live births (Khaw et al., 2000). Pediatric glaucoma is most often a congenital abnormality inherited in an autosomal recessive pattern that is slightly more prevalent in males (McGoldrick, 1992). Only 10% of pediatric glaucoma diagnoses are associated with systemic disease, congenital disorders, or other ocular abnormalities. The diagnosis may be suspected in the patient presenting with buphthalmos, epiphora, photophobia, or corneal clouding (Khaw et al., 2000). The definitive diagnosis is made only by tonometry, corneal examination, funduscopy, and gonioscopy (examination of the iridocorneal angle).

Open-angle glaucoma is diagnosed when a normal trabecular meshwork is visible on gonioscopy. Closed-angle glaucoma is diagnosed when the iridocorneal angle is obstructed by the iris. Infantile glaucoma develops before the age of 3 and is a primary disorder in approximately 50% of all cases. Juvenile glaucoma refers to disease that develops after the age of 3 and is most often secondary to or associated with other ocular or systemic disorders.

Surgical management varies between patients and is dependent on the measurements and observations made under general anesthesia. Corrective procedures include goniotomy, trabeculotomy, trabeculectomy, and cyclocryotherapy (Beck, 2001). Goniotomy is a relatively brief procedure; the other surgical techniques may require longer periods of general anesthesia. Patients often require frequent evaluations, because surgical correction is typically incremental and performed in carefully monitored stages.

The anesthetic management is quite similar for all procedures. A careful review of the past medical history, comorbid conditions, and concurrent pharmacologic therapy is crucial (see Tables 22–1 and 22–2). Premedication with atropine or glycopyrrolate is acceptable, but the use of scopolamine is generally contraindicated in the glaucomatous patient. Mask inductions are acceptable and followed by gentle laryngoscopy and placement of an oral RAE endotracheal tube. Stable IOP and complete akinesia must be maintained throughout the surgical procedure. Neostigmine with glycopyrrolate or atropine may be safely administered for reversal of neuromuscular blockade; both agents have only minimal ocular effects at the routinely recommended doses. Unlike many other ocular procedures, surgery for glaucoma (particularly cyclocryotherapy) may be associated with moderate to severe postoperative pain. Opioids, in conjunction with prophylaxis for PONV, should be incorporated into the anesthetic plan.

RETINOBLASTOMA

Retinoblastoma is the most common intraocular malignancy in the pediatric population with a prevalence of 1:20,000 live births. Fifty percent of all cases are secondary to mutations of the retinoblastoma gene, although only 25% of patients with the heritable form of the disease have a positive family history (Moore, 2000). The diagnosis is generally made by 3 years of age. Children with a positive family history have a 5% risk for developing retinoblastoma; these patients require frequent examinations until the age of 5.

Therapy for retinoblastoma varies depending on the severity of disease and has evolved dramatically since the 1970s. Treatment modalities may include combinations of enucleation, external beam radiation, localized radiotherapy, laser ablation, thermotherapy, cryotherapy, and chemotherapy (Uusitalo and Wheeler, 1999). Through early diagnosis, chemoreduction, and focal ablation methods, many children with retinoblastoma are spared enucleation and serial external beam radiotherapy (Shields and Shields, 1999). Candidates for external beam radiotherapy include patients with bilateral disease requiring enucleation of the more involved eye and patients with diffuse vitreous and subretinal seeding.

Anesthetic requirements for enucleation are similar to those for other moderately complex ophthalmic procedures. The incidence of OCR-mediated dysrhythmias is high, and appropriate prophylaxis with atropine or glycopyrrolate is warranted. Intraoperative blood loss can be significant, and controlled hypotension has been provided at many centers (Johnson and Forrest, 1994). Contemporary surgical techniques effectively minimize blood loss such that the need for transfusion is uncommon. Postoperative pain is frequently significant.

External beam radiotherapy may require as many as 24 radiation sessions and anesthetics over the course of 4 to 6 weeks. Each session is of a few minutes' duration, but the session requires the patient to remain motionless. Various anesthetic methods have been used, including rectal or intramuscular methohexital, intravenous or intramuscular ketamine, and brief inhalation anesthetics by insufflation methods, laryngeal mask airways, and endotracheal intubation (McGoldrick, 1992). When a central venous catheter has been placed for adjuvant chemotherapy, a single bolus of propofol is probably the most effective method of providing the required 2 to 3 minutes of anesthesia with minimal recovery requirements.

VITREORETINAL DISORDERS

Retinal tears and detachment in the pediatric population are most often secondary to ROP but may also result from trauma and vitreous degeneration common to certain syndromes (see Table 22–1). Small tears may be amenable to laser therapy or cryopexy; more significant tears and detachment often require complex surgical management and up to 3 hours of general anesthesia. Surgical options include scleral buckling (in combination with cryopexy), closed vitrectomy, and open-sky vitrectomy (Hunter et al., 2000).

The scleral buckle procedure involves the attachment of a tiny sponge or silicone band that constricts the sclera and holds the retina in position (Fig. 22–5). The scleral buckle remains permanently attached to the eye and may restrict normal growth of the child's eye if tension is not released with subsequent surgery. Vitrectomy may be considered in the presence of a failed scleral buckle, for high retinal detachment, and for media opacification. The closed vitrectomy is slightly more difficult in the pediatric population and involves lensectomy for segmentation and removal of the vitreous by microvitreoretinal blades

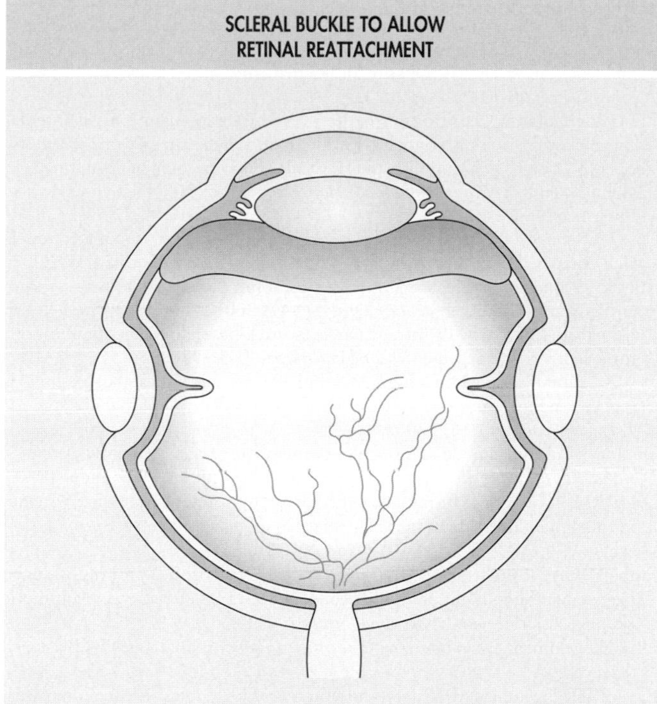

■ **FIGURE 22–5.** Scleral buckle. Open-angle glaucoma, also known as chronic simple glaucoma, is a condition of elevated IOP in an eye with an anatomically open anterior chamber angle. The trabecular meshwork is thought to be sclerosed, resulting in inefficient aqueous filtration and drainage. Closed-angle glaucoma is a mechanical closing of the pathway for aqueous egress for the eye. The iris may move into direct contact with the posterior surface of the cornea, impeding the aqueous outflow path, or the crystalline lens may swell, resulting in papillary blocking. In the latter case, the lens blocks the route for aqueous humor to travel from the posterior to the anterior chamber. (From Sears J, Capone A: Retinopathy of prematurity. In Yanoff M, Duker JS, editors: *Ophthalmology.* Philadelphia, 1999, Mosby, p 19.1, with permission.)

and vitrectomy instruments. The open-sky technique involves complete removal of the cornea, lensectomy, and en bloc removal of the fibrous mass filling the funnel of the detached retina (Hunter et al., 2000).

Anesthetic considerations for such procedures include prophylaxis for the OCR (the extraocular muscles are often bridled to permit optimal positioning), complete neuromuscular blockade, and the potential need to lower IOP with agents such as mannitol and acetazolamide. Silicone oil or one of the long-acting inert gases (see Table 22–2) may be injected into the vitreous chamber at the conclusion of the procedure in an effort to improve surgical success.

■ TRAUMATIC INJURY AND RUPTURED GLOBE

The optimal management for the patient presenting with ocular injury has been widely debated for many years, although many contemporary pundits consider the controversy mundane. Ophthalmic injuries are most often superficial, but a disproportionate number of serious penetrating injuries occur in children (Johnson and Forrest, 1994). It is often difficult to differentiate the emergent case (penetrating injury) from the nonemergent (nonpenetrating injury) case in children without examination under general anesthesia.

The pressure in the ruptured globe becomes atmospheric, and any external pressure or increase in internal pressure may lead to prolapse of the intraocular contents and a diminished possibility for recovery of vision. The possibility of salvaging the eye after penetrating injury requires surgical intervention within several hours of the injury. Traditional periods of fasting are not acceptable.

The importance of maintaining a quiet environment in the preoperative period cannot be overemphasized. Crying and thrashing can have devastating effects on IOP. Forceful eyelid closure may increase IOP by as much as 70 mm Hg (McGoldrick, 1993). Venous cannulation can be facilitated by pentobarbital, oral or rectal midazolam, and transdermal anesthetics. Access subsequently permits the administration of additional anxiolytics, analgesics, and prophylaxis for aspiration. Once sedation is adequate, the injured eye should be patched to provide comfort and minimize ocular movement.

When intravenous access is available, the anesthesiologists must consider the risks and benefits of succinylcholine (Vachon et al., 2003). Current consensus remains in favor of succinylcholine for rapid provision of optimal intubating conditions and reliable attenuation of coughing and bucking immediately after the endotracheal tube is secured. It is widely accepted that succinylcholine increases IOP despite various methods of blunting the response, but it is also clear that the succinylcholine-induced rise in IOP is inconsequential in relation to the possible rise with laryngoscopy and intubation (Cunningham and Barry, 1986). Support for the use of succinylcholine is derived from feline models of both anterior and posterior segment trauma (Moreno et al., 1991) and retrospective chart reviews and testimonials from the Wills Eye Hospital and the Massachusetts Eye and Ear Infirmary (Libonati et al., 1985; Donlon, 1986).

Some anesthesiologists use nondepolarizing neuromuscular blockers for modified rapid sequence inductions in patients with penetrating ocular injuries. The nondepolarizing agents provide either no effect on or a slight decrease in IOP. Three described methods for accelerating the onset of the older nondepolarizing agents include (1) divided doses of pancuronium (Mehta et al., 1985), (2) high-dose vecuronium (Abbott and Samuel, 1987), and (3) synergism with *d*-tubocurarine and pancuronium (Abdulla, 1993). Most anesthesiologists concede that none of these techniques provide the speed and reliability of succinylcholine. Rocuronium (1.2 mg/kg) has been demonstrated to have no effect on IOP (Mitra et al., 2001) and may provide intubating conditions comparable to succinylcholine within 60 seconds (Mazurek et al., 1998; Perry et al., 2003). Rocuronium is probably the most effective alternative to succinylcholine, especially for patients with comorbid conditions that mandate avoidance of the agent.

Although isolated ocular injuries are more common in children, the anesthesiologist should be aware of other injuries that may compromise the patient's condition. Liberal doses of either propofol or thiopental, adjuvant agents, and neuromuscular monitoring are paramount before attempted laryngoscopy and placement of the endotracheal tube. A gastric tube should be placed to evacuate the contents of the stomach only after the airway is protected and paralysis is complete. Complex surgical repairs may not be performed during the initial presentation, and surgical time may vary from 1 hour to several hours. Complete paralysis and attention to IOP are mandatory throughout the procedure. Deep extubation is an option for patients not considered at risk for aspiration.

■ SUMMARY

The pediatric population provides the anesthesiologist with a wide variety of ophthalmologic pathology. The anesthetic challenges are considerable. An understanding of the pertinent physiologic and pharmacologic principles, as well as an appreciation of the continued advancement in surgical therapy, affords optimal patient management and favorable outcomes.

REFERENCES

Abbott MA, Samuel JR: The control of intra-ocular pressure during the induction of anaesthesia for emergency eye surgery. A high-dose vecuronium technique. *Anaesthesia* 42:1008, 1987.

Abdulla WY: The synergistic effect of two different nondepolarizing muscle relaxants on intraocular pressure. *J Clin Anesth* 5:5, 1993.

Allen LE, Sudesh S, Sandramouli S, et al.: The association between the oculocardiac reflex and post-operative vomiting in children undergoing strabismus surgery. *Eye* 12(Pt 2):193, 1998.

Allison CE, De Lange JJ, Koole FD, et al.: A comparison of the incidence of the oculocardiac and oculorespiratory reflexes during sevoflurane or halothane anesthesia for strabismus surgery in children. *Anesth Analg* 90:306, 2000.

Arnold RW, Farah RF, Monroe G: The attenuating effect of intraglossal atropine on the oculocardiac reflex. *Binocul Vis Strabismus Q* 17:313, 2002.

Ates Y, Unal N, Cuhruk H, et al.: Postoperative analgesia in children using preemptive retrobulbar block and local anesthetic infiltration in strabismus surgery. *Reg Anesth Pain Med* 23:569, 1998.

Ausinsch B, Rayburn RL, Munson ES, et al.: Ketamine and intraocular pressure in children. *Anesth Analg* 55:773, 1976.

Bailey PL: Timolol and postoperative apnea in neonates and young infants. *Anesthesiology* 61:622, 1984.

Bauer CR, Trottier MC, Stern L: Systemic cyclopentolate (Cyclogyl) toxicity in the newborn infant. *J Pediatr* 82:501, 1973.

Baum V, O'Flaherty J: *Anesthesia for genetic, metabolic and dysmorphic syndromes of childhood.* Philadelphia, 1999, Lippincott Williams and Wilkins.

Beck A: Diagnosis and management of pediatric glaucoma. *Ophthalmol Clin North Am* 14:2001.

Birmingham PK, Tobin MJ, Fisher DM, et al.: Initial and subsequent dosing of rectal acetaminophen in children: A 24-hour pharmacokinetic study of new dose recommendations. *Anesthesiology* 94:385, 2001.

Blanc VF, Jacob JL, Milot J, et al.: The oculorespiratory reflex revisited. *Can J Anaesth* 35:468, 1988.

Borromeo-McGrail V, Bordiuk JM, Keitel H: Systemic hypertension following ocular administration of 10 per cent phenylephrine in the neonate. *Pediatrics* 51:1032, 1973.

Bowhay AR, May HA, Rudnicka AR, et al.: A randomized controlled trial of the antiemetic effect of three doses of ondansetron after strabismus surgery in children. *Paediatr Anaesth* 11:215, 2001.

Braun U, Feise J, Muhlendyck H: Is there a cholinergic and an adrenergic phase of the oculocardiac reflex during strabismus surgery? *Acta Anaesthesiol Scand* 37:390, 1993.

Bridge HS, Montgomery CJ, Kennedy RA, et al.: Analgesic efficacy of ketorolac 0.5% ophthalmic solution (Acular) in paediatric strabismus surgery. *Paediatr Anaesth* 10:521, 2000.

Broadman LM, Ceruzzi W, Patane PS, et al.: Metoclopramide reduces the incidence of vomiting following strabismus surgery in children. *Anesthesiology* 72:245, 1990.

Brown G, Tasman W, Naidoff M, et al.: Systemic complications associated with retinal cryoablation for retinopathy of prematurity. *Ophthalmology* 97:855, 1990.

Brown R Jr, James D, Weaver R, et al.: Low-dose droperidol versus standard-dose droperidol for prevention of postoperative vomiting after pediatric strabismus surgery. *J Clin Anesth* 3:306, 1991.

Butera C, Plotnik J, Bateman J: Ocular genetics. In Gallin P, editor: *Pediatric ophthalmology*. New York, 2000, Thieme Medical Publishing, Inc, p 78.

Calla S, Gupta A, Sen N, et al.: Comparison of the effects of etomidate and thiopentone on intraocular pressure. *Br J Anaesth* 59:437, 1987.

Calobrisi BL, Lebowitz P: Muscle relaxants and the open globe. *Int Anesthesiol Clin* 28:83, 1990.

Carroll JB: Increased incidence of masseter spasm in children with strabismus anesthetized with halothane and succinylcholine. *Anesthesiology* 67:559, 1987.

Carter K, Faberowski LK, Sherwood MB, et al.: A randomized trial of the effect of midazolam on intraocular pressure. *J Glaucoma* 8:204, 1999.

Chisakuta AM, Mirakhur RK: Anticholinergic prophylaxis does not prevent emesis following strabismus surgery in children. *Paediatr Anaesth* 5:97, 1995.

Chow LC, Wright KW, Sola A: Can changes in clinical practice decrease the incidence of severe retinopathy of prematurity in very low birth weight infants? *Pediatrics* 111:339, 2003.

Committee for the Classification of Retinopathy of Prematurity: An international classification of retinopathy of prematurity. *Pediatrics* 74:127, 1984.

Cooper K, Singh K, Zimmerman T: Ocular pharmacology in children. In Gallin P, editor: *Pediatric ophthalmology.* New York, 2000, Thieme Medical Publishers, Inc, p 92.

Coté CJ, Cohen IT, Suresh S, et al.: A comparison of three doses of a commercially prepared oral midazolam syrup in children. *Anesth Analg* 94:37, 2002.

Culy CR, Bhana N, Plosker GL: Ondansetron: A review of its use as an antiemetic in children. *Paediatr Drugs* 3:441, 2001.

Cunningham AJ, Barry P: Intraocular pressure—physiology and implications for anaesthetic management. *Can Anaesth Soc J* 33:195, 1986.

Deb K, Subramaniam R, Dehran M, et al.: Safety and efficacy of peribulbar block as adjunct to general anaesthesia for paediatric ophthalmic surgery. *Paediatr Anaesth* 11:161, 2001.

Donlon J: Succinylcholine and open eye injury. *Anesthesiology* 64:524, 1986.

Dorland's illustrated medical dictionary. Philadelphia, 2000, WB Saunders.

Dsida RM, Wheeler M, Birmingham PK, et al.: Age-stratified pharmacokinetics of ketorolac tromethamine in pediatric surgical patients. *Anesth Analg* 94:266, 2002.

Eippert GA, Burnstine RA, Bates JH: Lacrimal-duct-probing-induced bacteremia: Should children with congenital heart defects receive antibiotic prophylaxis? *J Pediatr Ophthalmol Strabismus* 35:38, 1998.

Ellis H, Feldman S: *Anatomy for anaesthetists.* Oxford, UK, 1997, Blackwell Science.

Enyedi LB, Freedman SF: Safety and efficacy of brimonidine in children with glaucoma. *J AAPOS* 5:281, 2001.

Eti Z, Yayci A, Umuroglu T, et al.: The effect of propofol and alfentanil on the increase in intraocular pressure due to succinylcholine and intubation. *Eur J Ophthalmol* 10:105, 2000.

Everitt DE, Avorn J: Systemic effects of medications used to treat glaucoma. *Ann Intern Med* 112:120, 1990.

Fallaha N, Lambert S: Pediatric cataracts. *Ophthalmol Clin North Am* 14:2001.

Fazi L, Jantzen EC, Rose JB, et al.: A comparison of oral clonidine and oral midazolam as preanesthetic medications in the pediatric tonsillectomy patient. *Anesth Analg* 92:56, 2001.

Flynn JT: Oxygen and retrolental fibroplasia: Update and challenge. *Anesthesiology* 60:397, 1984.

France NK, France TD, Woodburn JD Jr, et al.: Succinylcholine alteration of the forced duction test. *Ophthalmology* 87:1282, 1980.

Fraunfelder FW, Fraunfelder FT, Jensvold B: Adverse systemic effects from pledgets of topical ocular phenylephrine 10%. *Am J Ophthalmol* 134:624, 2002.

Freitag S, Woog J: Congenital nasolacrimal obstruction. *Ophthalmol Clin North Am* 13:2000.

Fujii Y, Tanaka H, Ito M: Ramosetron compared with granisetron for the prevention of vomiting following strabismus surgery in children. *Br J Ophthalmol* 85:670, 2001.

Ghignone M, Noe C, Calvillo O, et al.: Anesthesia for ophthalmic surgery in the elderly: The effects of clonidine on intraocular pressure, perioperative hemodynamics, and anesthetic requirement. *Anesthesiology* 68:707, 1988.

Gross R, Pineyro A: Current use of ophthalmic beta blockers. *J Glaucoma* 6:188, 1997.

Guthrie ME, Wright K: Congenital esotropia. *Ophthalmol Clin North Am* 14, 2001.

Hahnenkamp K, Honemann CW, Fischer LG, et al.: Effect of different anaesthetic regimens on the oculocardiac reflex during paediatric strabismus surgery. *Paediatr Anaesth* 10:601, 2000.

Haigh PM, Chiswick ML, O'Donoghue EP: Retinopathy of prematurity: Systemic complications associated with different anaesthetic techniques at treatment. *Br J Ophthalmol* 81:283, 1997.

Hall M, Lawrence L: *Ambulatory surgery in the United States, 1996.* Advance data from Vital and Health Statistics; No. 300. Hyattsville, MD, 1998, National Center for Health Statistics.

Hall M, Owings M: *National hospital discharge survey.* Advance data from Vital and Health Statistics; No. 329. Hyattsville, MD, 2002, National Center for Health Statistics.

Hamunen K, Vaalamo MO, Maunuksela EL: Does propofol reduce vomiting after strabismus surgery in children? *Acta Anaesthesiol Scand* 41:973, 1997.

Handa F, Fujii Y: The efficacy of oral clonidine premedication in the prevention of postoperative vomiting in children following strabismus surgery. *Paediatr Anaesth* 11:71, 2001.

Hartung J: Twenty-four of twenty-seven studies show a greater incidence of emesis associated with nitrous oxide than with alternative anesthetics. *Anesth Analg* 83:114, 1996.

Hunter DG, Mukai S, Hirose T: Advanced retinopathy of prematurity. In Albert DM, Jakobiec FA, editors: *Principles and practice of ophthalmology.* Philadelphia, 2000, WB Saunders, p 1936.

Indu B, Batra YK, Puri GD, et al.: Nifedipine attenuates the intraocular pressure response to intubation following succinylcholine. *Can J Anaesth* 36:269, 1989.

Johnson R, Forrest F: *Local and general anaesthesia for ophthalmic surgery.* Oxford, UK, 1994, Butterworth-Heinemann Medical.

Karl HW, Rosenberger JL, Larach MG, et al.: Transmucosal administration of midazolam for premedication of pediatric patients. Comparison of the nasal and sublingual routes. *Anesthesiology* 78:885, 1993.

Karl HW, Swedlow DB, Lee KW, et al.: Epinephrine-halothane interactions in children. *Anesthesiology* 58:142, 1983.

Kathirvel S, Shende D, Madan R: Comparison of anti-emetic effects of ondansetron, metoclopramide or a combination of both in children undergoing surgery for strabismus. *Eur J Anaesthesiol* 16:761, 1999.

Kelly RE, Dinner M, Turner LS, et al.: Succinylcholine increases intraocular pressure in the human eye with the extraocular muscles detached. *Anesthesiology* 79:948, 1993.

Kennerdell JS, Wucher FP: Cyclopentolate associated with two cases of grand mal seizure. *Arch Ophthalmol* 87:634, 1972.

Kerr WJ, Vance JP: Oculocardiac reflex from the empty orbit. *Anaesthesia* 38:883, 1983.

Khaw P, Narita A, Armas R, et al.: The paediatric glaucomas. In Moore A, editor: *Fundamentals of clinical ophthalmology: Paediatric ophthalmology.* London, 2000, BMJ Books, p 92.

Kuhn I, Scheifler G, Wissing H: Incidence of nausea and vomiting in children after strabismus surgery following desflurane anaesthesia. *Paediatr Anaesth* 9:521, 1999.

Lang SA, Van der Wal M: Death from the oculocardiac reflex. *Can J Anaesth* 41:161, 1994.

Lapin SL, Auden SM, Goldsmith LJ, et al.: Effects of sevoflurane anaesthesia on recovery in children: A comparison with halothane. *Paediatr Anaesth* 9:299, 1999.

Larsson S, Asgeirsson B, Magnusson J: Propofol-fentanyl anesthesia compared to thiopental-halothane with special reference to recovery and vomiting after pediatric strabismus surgery. *Acta Anaesthesiol Scand* 36:182, 1992.

Lerman J: Are antiemetics cost-effective for children? *Can J Anaesth* 42:263, 1995.

Libonati MM, Leahy JJ, Ellison N: The use of succinylcholine in open eye surgery. *Anesthesiology* 62:637, 1985.

Lin DM, Furst SR, Rodarte A: A double-blinded comparison of metoclopramide and droperidol for prevention of emesis following strabismus surgery. *Anesthesiology* 76:357, 1992.

Madan R, Perumal T, Subramaniam K, et al.: Effect of timing of ondansetron administration on incidence of postoperative vomiting in paediatric strabismus surgery. *Anaesth Intensive Care* 28:27, 2000.

Mahajan RP, Grover VK, Munjal VP, et al.: Double-blind comparison of lidocaine, tubocurarine and diazepam pretreatment in modifying intraocular pressure increases. *Can J Anaesth* 34:41, 1987.

Marshall B, Longnecker D: General anesthetics. In Hardman J, Limbird L, editors: *Goodman and Gilman's the pharmacologic basis of therapeutics.* New York, 2001, McGraw-Hill Medical Publishing, p 295.

Massumi RA, Mason DT, Amsterdam EA, et al.: Ventricular fibrillation and tachycardia after intravenous atropine for treatment of bradycardias. *N Engl J Med* 287:336, 1972.

Mazurek AJ, Rae B, Hann S, et al.: Rocuronium versus succinylcholine: Are they equally effective during rapid-sequence induction of anesthesia? *Anesth Analg* 87:1259, 1998.

McGoldrick K: Anatomy and physiology of the eye. In McGoldrick K, editor: *Anesthesia for ophthalmic and otolaryngologic procedures.* Philadelphia, 1992a, WB Saunders, p 176.

McGoldrick K: Anesthetic ramifications of ophthalmic drugs. In McGoldrick K, editor: *Anesthesia for ophthalmic and otolaryngologic surgery.* Philadelphia, 1992b, WB Saunders, p 227.

McGoldrick K: Anesthetics and intraocular pressure: Management of penetrating eye injuries. In McGoldrick K, editor: *Anesthesia for ophthalmic and otolaryngologic surgery.* Philadelphia, 1992c, WB Saunders, p 183.

McGoldrick K: Ocular pathology and systemic diseases: Anesthetic implications. In McGoldrick K, editor: *Anesthesia for ophthalmic and otolaryngologic surgery.* Philadelphia, 1992d, WB Saunders, p 210.

McGoldrick K: Ophthalmologic and systemic complications of surgery and anesthesia. In McGoldrick K, editor: *Anesthesia for ophthalmic and otolaryngologic surgery.* Philadelphia, 1992e, WB Saunders, p 272.

McGoldrick K: Pediatric ophthalmic surgery: Anesthetic considerations. In McGoldrick K, editor: *Anesthesia for ophthalmic and otolaryngologic surgery.* Philadelphia, 1992f, WB Saunders, p 190.

McGoldrick K: The open globe: Is an alternative to succinylcholine necessary? *J Clin Anesth* 5:1, 1993.

Mehta MP, Choi WW, Gergis SD, et al.: Facilitation of rapid endotracheal intubations with divided doses of nondepolarizing neuromuscular blocking drugs. *Anesthesiology* 62:392, 1985.

Mendel HG, Guarnieri KM, Sundt LM, et al.: The effects of ketorolac and fentanyl on postoperative vomiting and analgesic requirements in children undergoing strabismus surgery. *Anesth Analg* 80:1129, 1995.

Meyers EF, Krupin T, Johnson M, et al.: Failure of nondepolarizing neuromuscular blockers to inhibit succinylcholine-induced increased intraocular pressure, a controlled study. *Anesthesiology* 149:48, 1978.

Mikawa K, Nishina K, Maekawa N, et al.: Oral clonidine premedication reduces vomiting in children after strabismus surgery. *Can J Anaesth* 42:977, 1995.

Miller RD, Way WL, Hickey RF: Inhibition of succinylcholine-induced increased intraocular pressure by non-depolarizing muscle relaxants. *Anesthesiology* 29:123, 1968.

Mirakhur RK: Anticholinergic drugs in anaesthesia. *Br J Hosp Med* 46:409, 1991.

Mirakhur RK, Jones CJ, Dundee JW, et al.: IM or IV atropine or glycopyrrolate for the prevention of oculocardiac reflex in children undergoing squint surgery. *Br J Anaesth* 54:1059, 1982.

Mirakhur RK, Shepherd WF: Intraocular pressure changes with propofol (Diprivan): Comparison with thiopentone. *Postgrad Med J* 61(suppl 3):41, 1985.

Mirakhur RK, Shepherd WF, Darrah WC: Propofol or thiopentone: Effects on intraocular pressure associated with induction of anaesthesia and tracheal intubation (facilitated with suxamethonium). *Br J Anaesth* 59:431, 1987.

Mitra S, Gombar KK, Gombar S: The effect of rocuronium on intraocular pressure: A comparison with succinylcholine. *Eur J Anaesthesiol* 18:836, 2001.

Moore A: Disorders of the vitreous and retina. In Moore A, editor: *Fundamentals of clinical ophthalmology: Paediatric Ophthalmology.* London, 2000, BMJ Books, p 121.

Moore A: Intraocular tumors. In Moore A, editor: *Fundamentals of clinical ophthalmology: Pediatric ophthalmology.* London, 2000, BMJ Books, p 143.

Moore M, Weiskopf R, Eger E, 2nd, et al.: Arrhythmogenic doses of epinephrine are similar during desflurane or isoflurane anesthesia in humans. *Anesthesiology* 79:943, 1993.

Moreno RJ, Kloess P, Carlson DW: Effect of succinylcholine on the intraocular contents of open globes. *Ophthalmology* 98:636, 1991.

Morton NS, Benham SW, Lawson RA, et al.: Diclofenac vs oxybuprocaine eye drops for analgesia in paediatric strabismus surgery. *Paediatr Anaesth* 7:221, 1997.

Munro HM, Riegger LQ, Reynolds PI, et al.: Comparison of the analgesic and emetic properties of ketorolac and morphine for paediatric outpatient strabismus surgery. *Br J Anaesth* 72:624, 1994.

Munro HM, D'Errico CC, Lauder GR, et al.: Oral granisetron for strabismus surgery in children. *Can J Anaesth* 46:45, 1999.

Navarro R, Weiskopf RB, Moore MA, et al.: Humans anesthetized with sevoflurane or isoflurane have similar arrhythmic response to epinephrine. *Anesthesiology* 80:545, 1994.

Olson RJ, Bromberg BB, Zimmerman TJ: Apneic spells associated with timolol therapy in a neonate. *Am J Ophthalmol* 88:120, 1979.

Pandey K, Badola RP, Kumar S: Time course of intraocular hypertension produced by suxamethonium. *Br J Anaesth* 44:191, 1972.

Pensiero S, Da Pozzo S, Perissutti P, et al.: Normal intraocular pressure in children. *J Pediatr Ophthalmol Strabismus* 29:79, 1992.

Perry J, Lee J, Wells G: Rocuronium versus succinylcholine for rapid sequence induction intubation (Cochrane Review). *Cochrane Database Syst Rev* CD002788, 2003.

Peuler M, Glass DD, Arens JF: Ketamine and intraocular pressure. *Anesthesiology* 43:575, 1975.

Polarz H, Bohrer H, Fleischer F, et al.: Effects of thiopentone/suxamethonium on intraocular pressure after pretreatment with alfentanil. *Eur J Clin Pharmacol* 43:311, 1992.

Polarz H, Bohrer H, Martin E, et al.: Oral clonidine premedication prevents the rise in intraocular pressure following succinylcholine administration. *Ger J Ophthalmol* 2:97, 1993.

Reimer EJ, Montgomery CJ, Bevan JC, et al.: Propofol anaesthesia reduces early postoperative emesis after paediatric strabismus surgery. *Can J Anaesth* 40:927, 1993.

Rosales T, Isenberg S, Leake R, et al.: Systemic effects of mydriatics in low weight infants. *J Pediatr Ophthalmol Strabismus* 18:42, 1981.

Rose JB, Martin TM, Corddry DH, et al.: Ondansetron reduces the incidence and severity of poststrabismus repair vomiting in children. *Anesth Analg* 79:486, 1994.

Rose JB, Watcha MF: Postoperative nausea and vomiting in paediatric patients. *Br J Anaesth* 83:104, 1999.

Russell-Eggitt I: Disorders of the lens. In Moore A, editor: *Fundamentals of clinical ophthalmology: Paediatric ophthalmology.* London, 2000, BMJ Books, p 111.

Ruta U, Mollhoff T, Markodimitrakis H, et al.: Attenuation of the oculocardiac reflex after topically applied lignocaine during surgery for strabismus in children. *Eur J Anaesthesiol* 13:11, 1996.

Sadhasivam S, Shende D, Madan R: Prophylactic ondansetron in prevention of postoperative nausea and vomiting following pediatric strabismus surgery: A dose-response study. *Anesthesiology* 92:1035, 2000.

Seaberg RR, Freeman WR, Goldbaum MH, et al.: Permanent postoperative vision loss associated with expansion of intraocular gas in the presence of a nitrous oxide-containing anesthetic. *Anesthesiology* 97:1309, 2002.

Shende D, Bharti N, Kathirvel S, et al.: Combination of droperidol and ondansetron reduces PONV after pediatric strabismus surgery more than single drug therapy. *Acta Anaesthesiol Scand* 45:756, 2001.

Shende D, Haldar M: Prophylactic metoclopramide administered immediately after the induction of anesthesia has no effect on the incidence of postoperative emesis after strabismus surgery. *Ind Pediatr* 35:237, 1998.

Shields CL, Shields JA: Recent developments in the management of retinoblastoma. *J Pediatr Ophthalmol Strabismus* 36:8, 1999.

Simons BD, Flynn JT: Retinopathy of prematurity and associated factors. *Int Ophthalmol Clin* 39:29, 1999.

Sinha SK, Tin W: The controversies surrounding oxygen therapy in neonatal intensive care units. *Curr Opin Pediatr* 15:161, 2003.

Smith RB: Death and the oculocardiac reflex. *Can J Anaesth* 41:760, 1994.

Smith RB, Babinski M, Leano N: The effect of lidocaine on succinylcholine-induced rise in intraocular pressure. *Can Anaesth Soc J* 26:482, 1979.

Splinter WM: Prevention of vomiting after strabismus surgery in children: Dexamethasone alone versus dexamethasone plus low-dose ondansetron. *Paediatr Anaesth* 11:591, 2001.

Splinter WM, Rhine EJ: Low-dose ondansetron with dexamethasone more effectively decreases vomiting after strabismus surgery in children than does high-dose ondansetron. *Anesthesiology* 88:72, 1998.

Steward DJ: Anticholinergic premedication for infants and children. *Can Anaesth Soc J* 30:325, 1983.

STOP-ROP Multicenter Study Group: Supplemental therapeutic oxygen for prethreshold retinopathy of prematurity (STOP-ROP), a randomized, controlled trial. I: Primary outcomes. *Pediatrics* 105:295, 2000.

Strazis KP, Fox AW: Malignant hyperthermia: A review of published cases. *Anesth Analg* 77:297, 1993.

Subramaniam B, Madan R, Sadhasivam S, et al.: Dexamethasone is a cost-effective alternative to ondansetron in preventing PONV after paediatric strabismus repair. *Br J Anaesth* 86:84, 2001.

Subramaniam R, Subbarayudu S, Rewari V, et al.: Usefulness of pre-emptive peribulbar block in pediatric vitreoretinal surgery: A prospective study. *Reg Anesth Pain Med* 28:43, 2003.

Sullivan TJ, Clarke MP, Tuli R, et al.: General anesthesia with endotracheal intubation for cryotherapy for retinopathy of prematurity. *Eur J Ophthalmol* 5:187, 1995.

Sweeney J, Underhill S, Dowd T, et al.: Modification by fentanyl and alfentanil of the intraocular pressure response to suxamethonium and tracheal intubation. *Br J Anaesth* 63:688, 1989.

Taylor C, Wilson F, Roesch R: Prevention of the oculo-cardiac reflex in children. *Anesthesiology* 24:646, 1963.

Tetzlaff JE, Annand DW, Pudimat MA, et al.: Postoperative apnea in a full-term infant. *Anesthesiology* 69:426, 1988.

Tramer M, Moore A, McQuay H: Omitting nitrous oxide in general anaesthesia: Meta-analysis of intraoperative awareness and postoperative emesis in randomized controlled trials. *Br J Anaesth* 76:186, 1996.

Tramer M, Moore A, McQuay H: Meta-analytic comparison of prophylactic antiemetic efficacy for postoperative nausea and vomiting: Propofol anaesthesia vs omitting nitrous oxide vs total i.v. anaesthesia with propofol. *Br J Anaesth* 78:256, 1997.

Tramer MR, Sansonetti A, Fuchs-Buder T, et al.: Oculocardiac reflex and postoperative vomiting in paediatric strabismus surgery. A randomised controlled trial comparing four anaesthetic techniques. *Acta Anaesthesiol Scand* 42:117, 1998.

Ueda W, Hirakawa M, Mae O: Appraisal of epinephrine administration to patients under halothane anesthesia for closure of cleft palate. *Anesthesiology* 58:574, 1983.

Uusitalo M, Wheeler S: New approaches in the clinical management of retinoblastoma. *Ophthalmol Clin North Am* 12:1999.

Vachon CA, Warner DO, Bacon DR: Succinylcholine and the open globe. Tracing the teaching. *Anesthesiology* 99:220, 2003.

Valley RD, Freid EB, Bailey AG, et al.: Tracheal extubation of deeply anesthetized pediatric patients: A comparison of desflurane and sevoflurane. *Anesth Analg* 96:1320, 2003.

Virkkila M, Ali-Melkkila T, Kanto J: Premedication for outpatient cataract surgery: A comparative study of intramuscular alfentanil, midazolam and placebo. *Acta Anaesthesiol Scand* 36:559, 1992.

Virkkila M, Ali-Melkkila T, Kanto J, et al.: Dexmedetomidine as intramuscular premedication for day-case cataract surgery. A comparative study of dexmedetomidine, midazolam and placebo. *Anaesthesia* 49:853, 1994.

Vivian A: The management of childhood strabismus. In Moore A, editor: *Fundamentals of clinical ophthalmology: Paediatric ophthalmology.* London, 2000, BMJ Books, p 177.

Ward B, Bass S: The oculocardiac reflex in a congenitally anophthalmic child. *Paediatr Anaesth* 11:372, 2001.

Warner LO, Bremer DL, Davidson PJ, et al.: Effects of lidocaine, succinylcholine, and tracheal intubation on intraocular pressure in children anesthetized with halothane-nitrous oxide. *Anesth Analg* 69:687, 1989.

Watcha MF, Chu FC, Stevens JL, et al.: Effects of halothane on intraocular pressure in anesthetized children. *Anesth Analg* 71:181, 1990.

Watcha MF, Simeon RM, White PF, et al.: Effect of propofol on the incidence of postoperative vomiting after strabismus surgery in pediatric outpatients. *Anesthesiology* 75:204, 1991.

Weir PM, Munro HM, Reynolds PI, et al.: Propofol infusion and the incidence of emesis in pediatric outpatient strabismus surgery. *Anesth Analg* 76:760, 1993.

Welborn LG, Hannallah RS, Norden JM, et al.: Comparison of emergence and recovery characteristics of sevoflurane, desflurane, and halothane in pediatric ambulatory patients. *Anesth Analg* 83:917, 1996.

Williams EL: Postoperative blindness. *Anesthesiol Clin North Am* 20:367, 2002.

Wolf GL, Capuano C, Hartung J: Nitrous oxide increases intraocular pressure after intravitreal sulfur hexafluoride injection. *Anesthesiology* 59:547, 1983.

Yoshitake S, Sendaya K, Mizutani A, et al.: The changes of intraocular pressure during sevoflurane anesthesia in children. *Masui* 42:52, 1993.

Zahl K: Selection of techniques for regional blockade of the eye and adnexa. In McGoldrick K, editor: *Anesthesia for ophthalmic and otolaryngologic surgery.* Philadelphia, 1992, WB Saunders, p 235.

Zimmerman TJ, Kooner KS, Kandarakis AS, et al.: Improving the therapeutic index of topically applied ocular drugs. *Arch Ophthalmol* 102:551, 1984.

23 Anesthesia for Pediatric Otorhinolaryngologic Surgery

Ira S. Landsman • Jay A. Werkhaven • Etsuro K. Motoyama

The care of children requiring anesthesia for otorhinolaryngology or ear, nose, and throat (ENT) surgery is described in this chapter. Most pediatric otorhinolaryngologic surgical procedures are of short to intermediate duration, and most of the children in whom they are performed are in reasonably good health. However, the anesthesiologist often encounters children with potentially life-threatening upper airway obstruction (e.g., acute epiglottitis) or with severe pulmonary insufficiency requiring diagnostic or therapeutic ENT procedures. New surgical techniques, such as laryngeal laser surgery, have challenged pediatric anesthesiologists to develop innovative approaches for the protection and maintenance of the patent upper airway.

The art and science of anesthesia must be well integrated in caring for the child undergoing ENT anesthesia. Many procedures, including adenoidectomy, rigid bronchoscopy, and laser removal of papillomas, require short intervals of deep planes of anesthesia and limited movement of the patient. To effectively manage operating room services, the patient must awake in a timely manner without airway irritability. Some of the major changes in pediatric anesthesia over the past decade include the abandonment of halothane in favor of sevoflurane. Although sevoflurane appears to be a safer anesthetic agent than halothane, sevoflurane-induced postoperative delirium continues to challenge the pediatric anesthesiologist.

Propofol has many properties that make it a useful anesthetic agent for ENT surgery. Propofol causes less airway irritability than thiopental. Propofol may be protective against and therapeutic for laryngospasm (Brown et al., 1991; Scanlon et al., 1993; Allsop et al., 1995; Afshan et al., 2002). Propofol also has useful antiemetic properties and a low incidence of emergence delirium (Uezono et al., 2000; Moore et al., 2003; Voepel-Lewis et al., 2003), making this anesthetic a good choice for ENT anesthesia.

■ ANESTHESIA FOR OTOLOGIC PROCEDURES

Otitis media is the most frequently diagnosed childhood malady, with the highest incidence occurring among children between the ages of 6 and 18 months. The frequency of otitis media decreases after the first year of life. By age 7 years, otitis media becomes a less frequent pediatric diagnosis. Otitis media is inflammation of the middle ear, without reference to pathogenesis or cause. The other areas of the temporal bone that are contiguous with the middle ear, including the mastoid, petrous apex, and perilabyrinthine air cells, also may be involved. Statistically, in those who have had a single episode of acute otitis media, residual middle ear fluid remains in up to 40% of patients at 1 month, 20% at 2 months, and 10% at 3 months (Pelton et al., 1977; Teele et al., 1980; Gluckman, 1990).

Many children with persistent middle ear effusion continue to be clinically symptomatic with recurrent acute otitis media, pain, fever, vertigo, disturbed sleep, or significant hearing loss. These symptoms are the most common indications for middle ear effusion drainage by myringotomy and tympanostomy tubes. Myringotomy and insertion of tympanostomy tubes may also be helpful in patients with recurrent acute otitis or atelectasis of the tympanic membrane. Tympanostomy tubes may prevent permanent structural damage and/or cholesteatoma. Myringotomy with aspiration of the middle ear effusion but without tube placement may be appropriate in children with severe otalgia or when culture of the middle ear fluid is required in the evaluation of a child with fever of unknown origin. If the patient will require multiple myringotomy procedures, placement of a tympanostomy tube may be considered.

Many patients with congenital anomalies are candidates for myringotomy tubes. Patients with cleft palate, craniofacial malformations, Down syndrome, Turner's syndrome, and human immunodeficiency virus (HIV) infection have a higher incidence of otitis media and therefore have a greater need for myringotomy and insertion of tympanostomy tubes than the general population (Bluestone and Klein, 2001). These children have other airway and medical issues that complicate the usual approach to the healthy child requiring myringotomy tubes. Critically ill patients with a history of prolonged nasotracheal intubation have a high incidence of persistent middle ear effusions requiring middle ear ventilation.

Adenoidectomy for chronic otitis media with effusion may benefit some children. The effectiveness of adenoidectomy for chronic otitis media with effusion is not directly related to adenoid size. For children who have recurrent or chronic otitis media with effusion and who had one or more myringotomy and tympanostomy tube insertion procedures in the past, adenoidectomy may be a reasonable option (Paradise et al., 2003). Upper airway obstruction, recurrent acute or chronic adenoiditis, and sinusitis are additional indications for adenoidectomy in children who have chronic otitis media with effusion.

MYRINGOTOMY AND INSERTION OF TYMPANOSTOMY TUBES

Candidates for myringotomy and tube insertion can present with subacute or chronic upper respiratory tract infection with or without fever. In these children, surgical intervention appears to improve the symptoms of upper respiratory infection postoperatively (Tait and Knight, 1987). However, the finding by these investigators is applicable only to myringotomy for children with middle ear effusion; it should not be generalized or applied to children with upper respiratory infection (especially in its acute phase with fever) who are scheduled for other surgical procedures (Hinkle, 1989).

In expert hands, the performance of uncomplicated bilateral myringotomies and tube insertions requires only 5 to 10 minutes of operating time; the procedure, however, may take considerably more time when performed by inexperienced trainees or in patients with narrow ear canals. Myringotomy is almost exclusively performed on an outpatient basis.

Preoperative sedation should be administered based on the child's anxiety level. Mask induction of anesthesia with nitrous oxide, oxygen, and sevoflurane (or halothane) provides effective and smooth induction and maintenance anesthesia with prompt emergence. Preoperative or intraoperative analgesia is advocated for early postoperative pain relief. Because these children are usually anesthetized without intravascular access, preoperative administration of oral acetaminophen or nonsteroidal anti-inflammatory drugs (NSAIDs) (Watcha et al., 1992) and intraoperative intranasal fentanyl or butorphanol (Bennie et al., 1998; Galinkin et al., 2000; Finkel et al., 2001) or intramuscular ketorolac (Pappas et al., 2003) has been studied and recommended. It appears intraoperative ketorolac (1 mg/kg, up to 30 mg) administered by the intramuscular route provides superior analgesia than oral or rectal acetaminophen. Ketorolac is associated with less vomiting and minimal sedation compared with intranasal butorphanol and perhaps with fentanyl. However, ketorolac, along with other NSAIDs, should be used with caution because ketorolac affects platelet function, and increased postoperative bleeding during adenoidectomy has been reported (Dahl and Kehlet, 1994; Nikanne et al., 1997).

Because children undergoing myringotomy commonly have adenoidal hypertrophy, they may exhibit signs of nasal and upper airway obstruction (Bluestone and Klein, 2001). These children may require continuous positive airway pressure (CPAP) during inhalational induction and an oropharyngeal airway after reaching a surgical plane of anesthesia to maintain a patent airway (see Chapter 2, Respiratory Physiology, and Chapter 10, Induction of Anesthesia). Although myringotomy and tube insertion may last less than 10 minutes, it should be performed with standard monitoring (i.e., using a precordial stethoscope, pulse oximeter, electrocardiogram, thermometer, and automated blood pressure cuff). Myringotomy is one of few exceptions in modern pediatric anesthesia practice in the United States for which intravenous infusion is not routinely administered.

Postoperative hypoxemia occurs frequently in infants and children during transport (Patel et al., 1988) and in the recovery room, even after minor surgical procedures such as myringotomy (Motoyama and Glazener, 1986). After myringotomy, patients are prone to upper airway obstruction, and these children should be transferred to the recovery room in the lateral position while receiving supplemental oxygen (see Chapter 11, Intraoperative and Postoperative Management).

MASTOIDECTOMY AND TYMPANOPLASTY

The clinical importance of the mastoid process is related to its contiguous structures, which include the posterior and middle cranial fossa, the sigmoid and lateral sinuses, the facial nerve, the semicircular canals, and the petrous tip of the temporal bone. The distal part of the middle ear and mastoid are connected by the aditus ad antrum, making the mastoid susceptible to infection by infectious processes from the middle ear. With improved medical and surgical management of otitis media, mastoidectomy for mastoiditis has declined considerably over the past several decades. However, mastoidectomies may also be performed in association with cholesteatoma removal and tympanoplasty. Tympanoplasty is performed in patients with chronic perforation or atelectasis of the tympanic membrane (Bluestone and Klein, 2003). Deep retraction pockets may lead to squamous epithelium within the middle ear and mastoid cavities, causing a cholesteatoma that may grow by the enzymatic activity of the skin tissues and accumulation of squamous debris.

Tympanoplasty is an operation to reconstruct the tympanic membrane with or without grafting. The primary indications for tympanoplasty are repair of tympanic perforation; stabilization or improvement of hearing; removal or prevention of congenital, iatrogenic, or primary or secondary acquired cholesteatoma; and removal of atelectatic or diseased areas of the tympanic membrane (Haynes and Harley, 2002). Grafting materials include fat, fascia, perichondrium, periosteum, cartilage, vein, and paper patch.

Mastoidectomy involves the surgical exposure and removal of mastoid air cells. There are several types of mastoidectomy (Bluestone and Klein, 2003). In a complete simple "cortical" mastoidectomy, the mastoid air-cell system is removed, but the canal wall is left intact. The operation is performed for acute or chronic mastoid osteitis, and it is frequently part of the surgical procedure advocated by some surgeons for cholesteatoma.

Posterior tympanotomy or facial recess tympanotomy involves removal of mastoid air cells, followed by formation of an opening between the mastoid and middle ear created in the posterior wall of the middle ear lateral to the facial nerve and medial to the chorda tympani. This procedure allows better visualization of the facial recess without removing the canal wall, and it is primarily advocated for ears in which a cholesteatoma has formed.

With a modified radical mastoidectomy, a portion of the posterior ear canal wall is removed, and a permanent mastoidectomy cavity is created, but the tympanic membrane and some or all of the ossicles are left intact. The procedure is usually performed when a cholesteatoma cannot be removed without removing the canal wall; some function may be preserved.

Radical mastoidectomy involves removal of all mastoid air cells, the posterior ear canal wall, the tympanic membrane, and the ossicles except part or all the stapes. No attempt is made to preserve function. Removal of the posterior ear canal wall allows communication among the exenterated mastoid cellular area, middle ear, and external auditory canal, forming a common single cavity. The procedure is indicated when there is extensive cholesteatoma in the middle ear and mastoid that cannot be removed by a less radical procedure. The operation may be indicated for a suppurative complication of otitis media.

Tympanomastoidectomy with tympanoplasty is the term used when a tympanoplasty is performed in conjunction with a mastoidectomy. Mastoidectomies that leave the posterior ear canal wall intact are closed cavity, canal wall up, or intact canal wall procedures, whereas those in which the posterior canal is partially removed are open cavity or canal wall down procedures.

Anesthetic Management

All children should be monitored with the standard monitoring that includes a pulse oximeter, end-tidal carbon dioxide (CO_2) monitor, precordial stethoscope, electrocardiogram, thermometer, and automated blood pressure cuff. Often, electromyography is used to avoid injury to the facial nerve. In these circumstances, neuromuscular blockade is avoided. Standard no oral intake (NPO) guidelines should be followed in nonemergent situations.

For mastoidectomy and tympanoplasty, the patient is positioned supine, with the head laterally rotated away from the affected side. It is important to carefully rotate the neck of a patient under general anesthesia because of the risk of atlantoaxial rotational subluxation (Brisson et al., 2000). Induction of anesthesia may proceed by inhalational or intravenous induction. The anesthesiologist should consider endotracheal intubation without muscle relaxation or with short-acting muscle relaxation so the facial nerve can be monitored during surgery. The use of nitrous oxide may be contraindicated during and after placement of the tympanic graft, because nitrous oxide accumulates in a closed gas space and increases the ambient pressure; some surgeons believe this tends to lift the graft away from its new site (Koivunen et al., 1996; Doyle and Banks, 2003).

The most common postoperative complication requiring unscheduled admission to the hospital for children undergoing tympanomastoidectomy is postoperative nausea and vomiting (PONV) (Megerian et al., 2000). PONV has been attributed to surgical stimulation of the vestibular labyrinth, anesthetic techniques, or a combination of the two (Jellish et al., 1995; Dornhoffer and Manning, 2000). Propofol has antiemetic properties (Ved et al., 1996; Erb et al., 2002b). It appears that propofol used for induction and maintenance of anesthesia is superior to isoflurane or sevoflurane in reducing PONV after middle ear surgery (Jellish et al., 1995, 1999; Moore et al., 2003). The use of intravenous dexamethasone during surgery appears to decrease PONV in patients after undergoing tympanomastoid surgery (Liu et al., 2001).

COCHLEAR IMPLANTS

Cochlear implantation has become a feasible choice for profoundly hearing-impaired children (Figs. 23–1 and 23–2). Profoundly deaf children's auditory nerve fibers remain intact, but the sensory neuroepithelium in the cochlea is absent. This damage occurs because of a genetic defect, infection, cochlear ossification, or aging (Fischetti, 2003). Cochlear implants bypass the damage by receiving and converting sound into signals sent along electrodes to cells adjacent to the auditory nerve. Hearing aids are ineffective because sound cannot be converted into an electrical impulse. Cochlear implants have 8 to 22 electrodes that are placed through a cochleostomy. Sounds received from an external microphone are converted to an electric signal that is received and transmitted by the cochlear nerve (Balkany et al., 2001; Miyamoto and Kirk, 2003). Because the cochlea is full size at birth, there is no anatomic difficulty with electrode insertion in very young children.

Surgery requires 2 to 3 hours, and it is performed through an extended postauricular incision along with a mastoidectomy. Anesthetic considerations are the same as for mastoidectomy, including the avoidance of the muscle relaxants so the facial nerve can be monitored. The anesthesiologist should establish the patient's level of hearing dysfunction so that a method of communication can be established. It is helpful to have a parent or sign language specialist accompany the child to the operating room. If the child reads lips, masks should be kept down from the anesthesiologist's lips until after induction of anesthesia.

OTOPLASTY

Otoplasty is a cosmetic procedure to reconstruct or restructure the auricle. Anesthetic considerations are similar to those in other head and neck cosmetic procedures, with one minor modification. Otoplasty is frequently bilateral, requiring both sides to be simultaneously prepared and draped. To ensure symmetry, simultaneous visualization requires frequent head motion and the endotracheal tube must be well secured.

ANESTHESIA FOR RHINOLOGIC PROCEDURES

REDUCTION OF NASAL FRACTURE

A nasal fracture may cause considerable bleeding, and the blood may be swallowed into the stomach. These patients therefore are assumed to have a full stomach, regardless of the time of last food intake. Reduction of a nasal fracture may take only a few moments, but in the acute situation, an oral endotracheal tube is mandatory to protect the airway from pulmonary aspiration. More commonly, surgery is delayed for several days after an isolated nasal fracture to allow swelling to subside. In these cases, a flexible laryngeal mask airway (LMA) can be substituted for an endotracheal tube. The LMA cannot prevent aspiration of stomach contents into the lungs, but it can prevent blood from the nose passing through the vocal cords (John et al., 1991; Williams and Bailey, 1993). The LMA may be removed either when the patient is deeply anesthetized or when awake.

NASAL POLYPECTOMY

This procedure is performed under general anesthesia, often using a preformed RAE endotracheal tube, which was originally

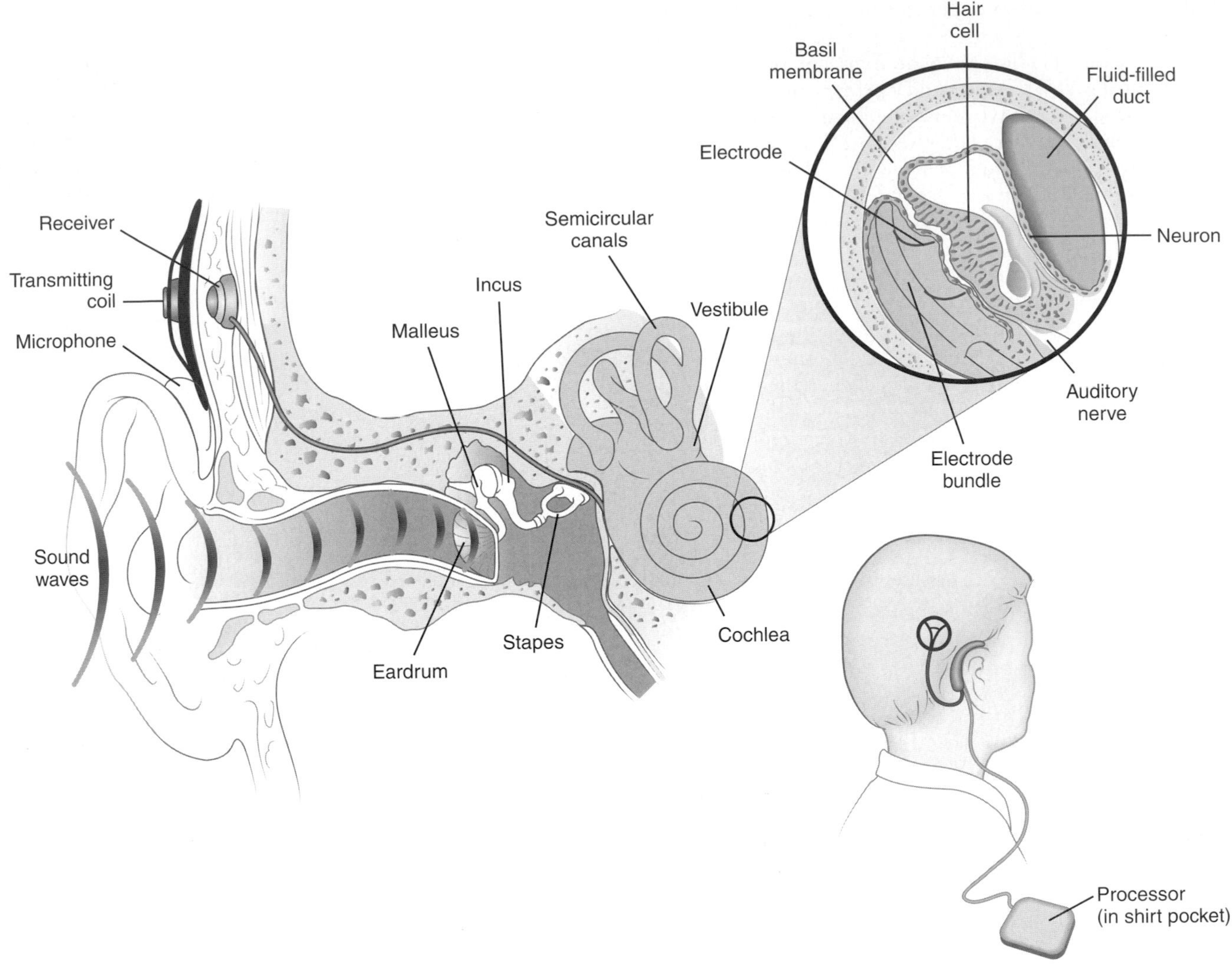

■ **FIGURE 23–1.** The outer ear collects the pressure waves of a sound, which the eardrum converts into mechanical vibrations in tiny bones in the middle ear. The oscillating stapes sets off pressure waves within the fluid in the cochlea, which stimulates nerve cells on the auditory nerve that leads to the brain. The cochlea transmits pressure waves through its duct fluid, displacing the basilar membrane, which bends hair cells to various degrees. The cells release neurotransmitters that cause attached neurons to fire, telling the brain where along the duct the bending has occurred, which corresponds to the frequency of the original sound, and communicating the amplitude of the bending, which indicates the loudness. The cochlear implant uses a microphone worn behind the ear to pick up sound and send it to a processor, where integrated circuits and algorithms amplify, digitize, and filter the sound into a coded signal sent to the transmitter coil. The coil sends the signal by radio waves through the skin to an implanted receiver. The receiver converts the waves into electrical impulses that travel along electrodes that end at cells at certain points along the cochlea. A magnet in the transmitter holds it against the implanted receiver. (From Fischetti M: Cochlear implants. To hear again. *Sci Am* 288:82–83, 2003.)

developed by Ring and colleagues (1975) (see Chapter 9, Anesthetic Equipment and Monitoring). Packing of the pharynx is indicated in most intranasal procedures. One end of the oropharyngeal gauze packing should be tagged with a hemostat and left hanging externally at one corner of the mouth. A note should be prominently placed in the room for all to see, or a labeled tape should be placed across the exit door, reminding all operating room personnel that a throat pack is in place and needs to be removed. Historically, as much as 10 mcg/kg of epinephrine, usually in a 1:200,000 solution (5 mcg/mL), can be used in children for homeostasis under halothane anesthesia without apparent myocardial irritability (Karl et al., 1983; Ueda et al., 1983). However, most clinicians have changed their choice of maintenance anesthetic to isoflurane, sevoflurane, desflurane, propofol, or remifentanil, regardless of the epinephrine dose (see Chapter 11, Intraoperative and Postoperative Management).

Special consideration should be given to the management of children with cystic fibrosis, in whom nasal polyps often occur (Hulka, 2000) (see Chapter 32, Systemic Disorders). The polyps are multiple and recur after removal. These children often have severe obstructive lung disease with recurrent pulmonary infection and thick, tenacious secretions. They are frequently hypoxemic in room air. During general anesthesia, the cystic fibrosis patient may require frequent endotracheal lavage with saline and deep suctioning. Secretions can hamper oxygenation and ventilation; a rise in the peak inspiratory pressure intraoperatively may indicate that the endotracheal tube requires suctioning. An inhaled bronchodilator should be immediately available to treat bronchospasm. Inhaled anesthetics and nitrous oxide or opioids and a relaxant may be used for patients with mild to moderate airway obstruction. Nitrous oxide should be avoided in those with severe lower airway obstruction with air trapping

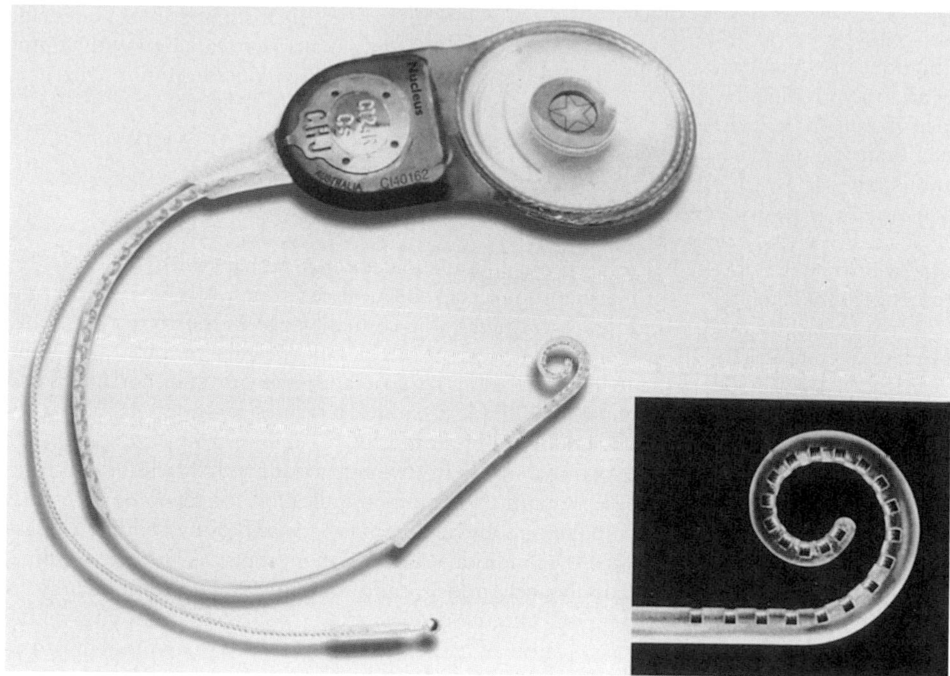

■ **FIGURE 23–2.** In the Nucleus 24 Counter implant, the active intracochlear electrode array is precurved to wrap around the modiolus. A stylus is used to straighten the electrode during insertion. (From Miyamoto RT, Kirk KI: Cochlear implants in children. In Bluestone CD, Stool SE, Alper CM, et al., editors: *Pediatric otolaryngology*, 4th ed. Philadelphia, 2003, WB Saunders, p 809.)

because of possible hyperinflation of trapped air spaces and alveolar rupture.

In addition to pulmonary pathology, upper airway obstruction frequently occurs in these patients. During induction, the mouth must be kept open because nasal air passages may be completely blocked by the polyp. Nasal packing, usually placed at the completion of the surgical procedure, may lead to further problems in ventilation and oxygenation in the postoperative period. This situation is partially relieved if the surgeon first introduces a nasopharyngeal airway and then packs around it. If preoperative pulmonary function is poor, the physician should consider transferring the patient to the intensive care unit, with the endotracheal tube in place, for immediate postoperative respiratory care.

■ SINUS SURGERY

Sinus surgery is indicated for children who have failed maximum medical therapy. Children with allergy or gastroesophageal reflux disease should receive maximal medical therapy and should rarely require surgery (Goldsmith and Rosenfeld, 2003). Children with immune deficiency, immotile cilia syndrome (i.e., Kartagener's syndrome), or cystic fibrosis (Gysin et al., 2000) are at high risk for chronic sinusitis. Unfortunately, because of their underlying disease, these children have a significant surgical failure rate (Herbert and Bent, 1998).

In children with recurrent sinusitis without chronic disease, adenoidectomy should be the initial procedure if the quantity of adenoid tissue visualized on endoscopy is considered sufficient to serve as a reservoir of bacterial pathogens. Adenoidectomy or adenotonsillectomy is usually the first-line surgical intervention for preschoolers, and it is often appropriate in older children. The expected rate of improvement is 70% to 80% (Goldsmith and Rosenfeld, 2003).

Endoscopic sinus surgery (ESS) should be performed only when children have failed previous therapies. In contrast to older traditional techniques of sinus surgery, ESS focuses on enlarging the natural ostia of the maxillary and ethmoid sinuses, while preserving most or all of the sinus mucosa (Goldsmith and Rosenfeld, 2003). In addition to children with chronic sinusitis who fail medical management, Lusk (2003) lists the accepted indications for ESS as complete nasal obstruction in patients with cystic fibrosis, antrochoanal polyp, intracranial complications, mucoceles and mucopyoceles, orbital abscess, traumatic injury in the optic canal, dacrocystorhinitis due to sinusitis, fungal sinusitis, certain neoplasms, and meningoencephalocele. In properly selected children, the results are good, with an expected improvement of 80% (Lusk, 2003). Preoperative computed tomography (CT) is essential in defining the specific diseased sinuses and in looking for anatomic abnormalities that need to be addressed, including septal deviation, concha bullosa cells, obstructing Haller air cells, and abnormal middle turbinates (Goldsmith and Rosenfeld, 2003).

ESS is performed under general anesthesia using an oral preformed (RAE) or standard endotracheal tube. Many of these children have chronic disease or upper airway obstruction. The anesthetic approach is similar to that described for nasal polypectomy and adenotonsillectomy. The surgeon may elect to use topical oxymetazoline (0.25% to 0.50%) for initial vasoconstriction and then infiltrate the tissue with lidocaine (0.5%) and epinephrine (1:100,000 solution) for hemostasis. The surgeon and the anesthesiologist should be aware that the duration of vasoconstriction usually does not last longer than 1.5 hours, and when surgical procedures are not completed within this period, mild bleeding may make visualization of the surgical site difficult and present a potential problem postoperatively. Some surgeons routinely pack the nose with gauze after the procedure for hemostasis, and the patient becomes an obligate mouth breather. Other surgeons may elect to use Surgicel or FloSeal to obtain hemostasis, and each of these may have the potential for migration into the lower airway.

CHOANAL ATRESIA

Choanal atresia is a congenital malformation in which no connection exists between the nasal cavity and the aerodigestive tract (Prasad et al., 2002); it has an incidence of 1 in 7000 births. The atresia is bony (30%) or mixed membranous and bony (70%). The existence of purely membranous atresia has come into question (Brown et al., 1996). Choanal atresia is unilateral in 50% to 60% of patients. Syndromes associated with choanal atresia include Apert's syndrome, DiGeorge syndrome, trisomy 18, Treacher Collins syndrome, camptomelic dysplasia, and CHARGE association (i.e., coloboma, heart defects, atresia choanae, retardation of growth and development, genitourinary problems, and ear anomalies) (Telfick et al., 1997).

The symptoms caused by choanal atresia depend on whether the obstruction is unilateral or bilateral. Because neonates are obligatory nasal breathers, those with bilateral disease present with acute respiratory distress. Respiratory distress can be attenuated if the mouth is kept open with an oral airway strapped in place or by a large rubber nipple with a large hole cut in it and kept in place with an umbilical tape around the neck (McGovern, 1961; Hengerer and Wein, 2003). For the neonate with bilateral choanal atresia, surgical nasal correction or tracheostomy must be performed within the first few days of life. Other infants may have only unilateral atresia, with minimal symptoms that can go undiagnosed for months or even years. The most common complaint is intractable unilateral anterior nasal discharge.

A number of surgical procedures have been described for the correction of choanal atresia, including endoscopic, transnasal, transseptal, and transpalatal procedures (Holland and McGuirt, 2001). Timing of surgery for bilateral choanal atresia varies, and it depends on the infant's ability to adapt to oral breathing and acquire adequate nutrition. Hengerer and Wein (2003) state that some surgeons advocate "a rule of tens" to guide the timing of surgical intervention. The child must reach 10 weeks of age, weigh 10 pounds, and have a hemoglobin level of 10 g. Other surgeons have demonstrated routine success in newborns 48 to 72 hours old and weighing as little as 1900 g (Werkhaven J, personal communication, 2003).

The anesthetic approach depends on the child's condition. In general, intravenous induction with a muscle relaxant of intermediate duration, endotracheal intubation with an oral RAE tube, and maintenance with an inhaled agent and opioid or propofol and remifentanil infusion suffice. Rarely, algorithms for difficult neonatal intubation must be used for securing the airway in infants with bilateral choanal atresia. After the atresia is surgically corrected, the surgeon is often faced with the problem of restenosis (Pirsig, 1986). Two innovations have created optimism that the restenosis rate can be reduced. Newer endoscopic techniques with powered instrumentation have enhanced safety and efficacy for choanal atresia repair (Prasad et al., 2002). Mitomycin-C, an aminoglycoside and alkylating agent used as an intravenous antineoplastic agent, can be used topically after choanal atresia repair. Topical application inhibits fibroblast growth and migration and granulation tissue formation responsible for restenosis (Holland and Mcguirt, 2001). Topical mitomycin has not caused systemic effects and has not contributed to anesthetic complications.

Postoperatively, patients with unilateral obstruction usually do well and require no special monitoring. However, infants undergoing bilateral repair can exhibit partial or intermittent upper airway obstruction that persists for some time. The infant should be observed closely in the intensive care unit with appropriate monitoring until breathing dynamics have normalized.

ANESTHESIA FOR PHARYNGEAL AND LARYNGEAL PROCEDURES

TONSILLECTOMY AND ADENOIDECTOMY

Tonsillectomy and adenoidectomy (perhaps with the exception of myringotomies) are the most common pediatric surgical procedures performed in the United States. Although tonsillectomy and adenoidectomy are frequently performed procedures, the benefits in relation to cost and risk are still hotly debated (Paradise, 2003). Just about every indication has its advocates and detractors (Bluestone, 2001; Paradise, 2003).

Nocturnal upper airway obstruction, with or without obstructive sleep apnea, is a common indication for adenotonsillectomy. A mild, partial obstruction in otherwise healthy children is exacerbated by conditions such as achondroplasia, Down syndrome, mucopolysaccharidosis, and obesity. Adenotonsillectomy is considered curative when adenotonsillar hypertrophy is the primary cause of childhood sleep-related breathing disorders (Schechter, 2002). Indications for tonsillectomy include recurrent pharyngotonsillitis, chronic tonsillitis, hemorrhagic tonsillitis, peritonsillar abscess, streptococcal carriage, dysphagia, abnormal dentofacial growth, halitosis, and suspicion of malignant disease (i.e., tonsil asymmetry) (Darrow and Siemans, 2002). Additional indications for adenoidectomy include recurrent or chronic rhinosinusitis or adenoiditis, and recurrent otitis media (Darrow and Siemans, 2002). Adenotonsillar hypertrophy with resultant upper airway obstruction is the most frequent cause of obstructive sleep apnea in children (Fig. 23–3).

Obstructive Sleep Apnea Syndrome

Obstructive sleep apnea syndrome (OSAS) is a disorder of breathing during sleep characterized by prolonged partial upper airway obstruction or intermittent complete obstruction (i.e., obstructive apnea) that disrupts normal sleep-time breathing and normal sleep patterns (American Thoracic Society, 1996). OSAS also occurs in children with upper airway narrowing due to craniofacial anomalies and in those with neuromuscular diseases, including cerebral palsy and muscular dystrophy (Marcus, 2001).

Adenotonsillar hypertrophy is the most common cause of OSAS in children. Many published papers, primarily case reports and case series, support the idea that tonsillectomy with or without adenoidectomy is often the cure for OSAS (Schechter et al., 2002).

The peak prevalence of OSAS occurs at 2 to 8 years, which is the age the tonsils and adenoids are proportionately large in relation to the child's upper airways. The site of collapse is most commonly at the level of the adenoids or velopharynx (Isono et al., 1998). Although OSAS is associated with adenotonsillar hypertrophy, there must be other neuromuscular factors involved. These patients usually do not obstruct while awake, implying sleep induces another dimension to OSAS. Some otherwise normal children with OSAS with smaller tonsils and adenoids are cured by adenotonsillectomy, whereas others with larger tonsils and adenoids are not (Marcus, 2001). The patency of pharyngeal airway is maintained by tonic and phasic contractions of the upper airway dilator muscles, such as the genioglossus, geniohyoid, and velopalatine muscles. Compared with other inspiratory muscles (i.e., diaphragm and intercostal muscles),

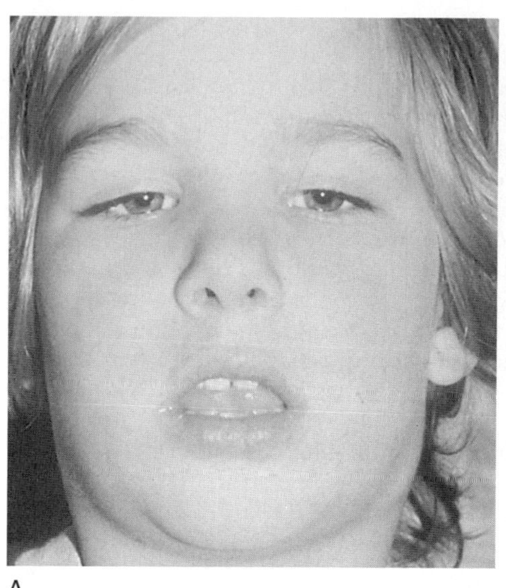

A

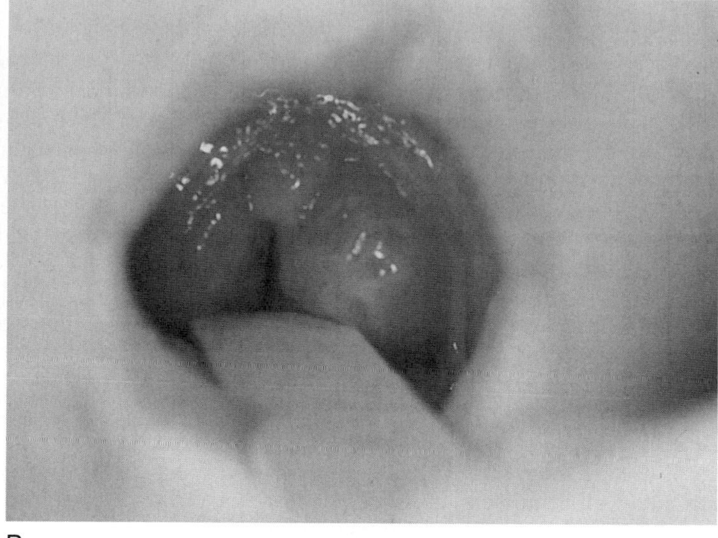

B

■ **FIGURE 23–3.** Adenoidal and tonsillar hypertrophy. *A,* Dull expression of a child with marked adenotonsillar hypertrophy and nasal obstruction (i.e., adenoid facies). He must keep his mouth open to breathe and shows signs of fatigue as a result of obstructive sleep apnea caused by upper airway obstruction. *B,* On examination of the pharynx, his enlarged tonsils are seen meeting in the midline. (From Yellon RB, McBride TP, Davis HW: Otolaryngology. In Zitelli BJ, Davis HW, editors: *Atlas of pediatric physical diagnosis,* 4th ed. St. Louis, 2002, Mosby, p 836.)

these upper airway muscles are preferentially depressed with sleep, sedatives, and general anesthetics (Ochiai, Guthrie, Motoyama, 1989, 1992) (see Chapter 2, Respiratory Physiology). It is hypothesized that children with OAS may have abnormal centrally mediated activation of their airway muscles, leading to a more collapsible upper airway (Marcus et al., 1994).

Symptoms of OSAS include nocturnal snoring, breathing pauses, gasping, use of accessory muscles of respiration, enuresis, and excessive sweating (Messner, 2003). The diagnosis of OSAS is based on a thorough history and physical examination along with appropriate sleep studies, including polysomnography. Snoring, increased respiratory efforts, periodic obstructive apnea, and oxygen desaturation while sleeping are the universal features of OSAS, which must be differentiated from the benign condition referred to as *primary snoring*. Although definitive diagnosis of OSAS is made by a positive polysomnogram, many children are not tested because the polysomnography laboratories specializing in children are few in number, and the tests are expensive and require an overnight stay (Sterni and Tunkel, 2003). Most children are diagnosed by recommendations set forth by the section of Pediatric Pulmonology Subcommittee on Obstructive Sleep Apnea, sans Polysomnography. This committee's recommendations for otherwise healthy children older than 1 year are as follows (Schechter, 2002):

1. All children should be screened for snoring. As part of routine health care maintenance for all children, pediatricians should ask whether the patient snores. An affirmative answer should be followed by a more detailed evaluation.
2. Complex, high-risk patients should be referred to a specialist.
3. Patients with cardiorespiratory failure cannot await elective evaluation. It is expected that these patients will be in an intensive care setting and will be treated by a specialist; these patients are not covered in this practice guideline.
4. Thorough diagnostic evaluation should be performed. History and physical examination have been shown to be poor in discriminating between primary snoring and OSAS. Polysomnography is the only method that quantifies ventilatory and sleep abnormalities, and it is recommended as the diagnostic test of choice. Other diagnostic techniques, such as videotaping, nocturnal pulse oximetry, and daytime nap studies, may be useful in discriminating between primary snoring and OSAS. However, they do not assess the severity of OSAS, which is useful for determining treatment and follow-up.
5. Adenotonsillectomy is the first line of treatment for most children. CPAP is an option for those who are not candidates for surgery or do not respond to surgery.

Children with OSAS have a host of sequelae, which are usually reversible after adenotonsillectomy but can lead to perioperative complications during and after surgery. Children with OSAS may present with failure to thrive, although the cause of this growth failure is unclear (Sterni and Tunkel, 2003). Many of these children experience a growth spurt after surgery. Children with OSAS may have neurocognitive deficits such as poor learning, behavioral problems, and lower grades in school than non-OSAS children. Adenotonsillectomy improves functioning in these children (Marcus, 2001).

Severe, untreated OSAS may lead to pulmonary hypertension and cor pulmonale caused by nocturnal hypoxia and hypercarbia resulting in compensatory changes in the pulmonary vasculature. Pulmonary vascular resistance increases, causing increased right ventricular strain. Severe cases may progress to pulmonary hypertension, arrhythmias, and cor pulmonale, which are reversible by performing early adenotonsillectomy (Miman and Kirazli, 2000). Children with OSAS also tend to have higher diastolic blood pressures. The cardiovascular changes appear to be the result of an increase in sympathetic tone that results from obstructive respiratory events (Marcus et al., 1998). Fortunately, few children develop clinically significant heart failure. It is prudent to pursue an aggressive cardiac evaluation if the child has a loud second heart sound, has exercise intolerance, or has diastolic hypertension. Because children are diagnosed earlier today, significant heart disease is rarely an issue (Marcus, 2001). Tonsillectomies, adenoidectomies, and adenotonsillectomies are performed on an outpatient basis, except for patients with a history of OSAS.

Preoperative Preparations

A careful review of the history, laboratory data, and physical examination results are essential for the optimal outcome of adenotonsillectomy. Careful evaluation of coagulation status is important before performing this procedure. If there is a history of easy bruisability, frequent epistaxis, or positive family history, the prothrombin time (PT), partial thromboplastin time (PTT), and platelet count should be obtained to rule out coagulopathies. In many pediatric institutions, a coagulation profile is obtained routinely for patients scheduled for adenotonsillectomy. However, in a prospective study of hemostatic assessment of patients before tonsillectomy, routine measurements of a coagulation profile were not useful predictors of postoperative bleeding (Close et al., 1994).

Although relatively mild, von Willebrand's disease (i.e., reduced factor VIII, decreased platelet adhesiveness because of deficient von Willebrand factor) is the most common coagulopathy seen among patients scheduled for adenotonsillectomy. Children with von Willebrand's disease or mild hemophilia A are treated preoperatively with desmopressin (1-desamino-8-D-arginine vasopressin [DDAVP]) (Prinsley et al., 1993). DDAVP is a synthetic analogue of vasopressin, which, in addition to its antidiuretic effect, stimulates endothelial cells and releases stored factor VIII and von Willebrand factor (Manucci, 1988). The intravenous dose of DDAVP is 0.3 mcg/kg, given over 20 minutes before anesthetic induction.

The examiner should elicit a history of drug ingestion, especially acetylsalicylic acid (ASA). If the patient was given ASA-containing drugs recently, surgery should be postponed, because these drugs cause platelet dysfunction for as long as 10 days and may cause excessive bleeding intraoperatively and postoperatively (Davies and Steward, 1977; Paradise, 2003).

During the preoperative visit, the patency of oral and nasal air passages is carefully examined. The patient's mouth should be inspected for the degree of tonsillar hypertrophy or inflammation. The examiner should also have the child breathe with the mouth closed to evaluate the degree of nasal airway obstruction and estimate adenoidal hypertrophy. It is important to inspect the teeth routinely, because tonsillectomy is often performed on children who are losing their primary dentition. Any teeth missing preoperatively should be noted carefully. A tooth that is loose should be pointed out to the parent and child, with the explanation that it may be necessary to remove it while the child is anesthetized (it must then be saved). It is also possible for the surgeon to dislodge or chip teeth in the application of a mouth gag or during other intraoperative manipulations.

Anesthetic Management

All children should be monitored with a pulse oximeter, end-tidal CO_2 precordial stethoscope, electrocardiogram, thermometer, and automated blood pressure. Oxygen saturation is determined in room air before the induction of anesthesia to establish the baseline value. If neuromuscular blockade is required, a nerve stimulator should be used to track the depth of paralysis. Standard NPO guidelines should be followed in nonemergent situations.

Children who are anxious preoperatively may receive sedation with oral midazolam. In older children scheduled for intravenous induction, EMLA cream (i.e., eutectic mixture of local anesthetics, 2.5% lidocaine and 2.5% prilocaine) is applied to the dorsum of both hands and sealed with plastic adhesives at least 1 hour before intravenous catheter insertion (see Chapter 8, Preoperative Preparation, and Chapter 10, Induction of Anesthesia).

The anesthetic approach to tonsillectomy or adenoidectomy is similar to the methods described for myringotomies. Adenoidectomy is a relatively short procedure (15 to 45 minutes), and many centers perform anesthesia without neuromuscular blockade and with less opioid than suggested in the following descriptions. Anesthesia is induced most commonly with oxygen and nitrous oxide followed by sevoflurane. As with those undergoing myringotomies, children with adenotonsillar hypertrophy often have partial or complete nasal airway obstruction. The mouth must be kept open during the induction of anesthesia until the gag reflex is abolished and the oral airway is inserted. Moderate CPAP (10 to 15 cm H_2O) during induction before the oral airway insertion helps to prevent pharyngeal airway collapse as a result of the relaxation of upper airway muscle tone (Reber et al., 2001; Bruppacher et al., 2003) (see Chapter 2, Respiratory Physiology, and Chapter 10, Induction of Anesthesia).

After the intravenous route is established, atropine or glycopyrrolate may be given for its anticholinergic effects. The patient's trachea is intubated with a preformed oral (RAE) tube under deep inhalational anesthesia, inhalational anesthesia supplemented with propofol, or with the aid of an intermediate-acting, nondepolarizing muscle relaxant (e.g., cisatracurium, vecuronium). In older children, anesthesia may be induced intravenously with propofol (2 to 3 mg/kg) mixed with lidocaine (1 to 2 mg/mL of propofol) to reduce pain at injection site, with or without anticholinergic agent or a muscle relaxant. If thiopental is used for induction then it must be supplemented with an inhaled anesthetic or muscle relaxant before intubating the trachea. Inhalation anesthetic or propofol infusion is continued thereafter with spontaneous or controlled ventilation. A cuffed endotracheal tube is preferred to reduce the chance of aspiration of blood and secretions and to reduce gas leaks around the tube. A cuffed endotracheal tube, 0.5 to 1.0 mm ID smaller than the age-appropriate size, should be chosen to accommodate the passage of the cuff through the subglottis (Khine et al., 1997; James, 2001; Fine and Borland, 2004). The endotracheal tube is immobilized with adhesive tape over the middle of the lower lip (Fig. 23–4). The breath sounds on both sides of the chest should be auscultated carefully to avoid endobronchial intubation. The endotracheal tube is then held in place by the groove-bladed tongue depressor that is a part of the Ring adaptation of the Brown-Davis mouth gag (Fig. 23–5).

Anesthesia is maintained with supplemental opioids to reduce the requirement of the anesthetic maintenance agent and to provide postoperative analgesia. The physician may start with a loading dose of 1 to 2 mcg/kg of fentanyl, 50 to 100 mcg/kg of morphine, or 10 to 20 mcg/kg of hydromorphone given intravenously, with additional doses administered as needed. There is evidence that high doses of dexamethasone (up to 1 mg/kg, 25 mg maximum) reduce postoperative swelling and pain and decrease the incidence of PONV without apparent adverse effects attributable to dexamethasone (Pappas et al., 1998). Children receiving dexamethasone are more likely to advance to a soft-solid diet on the first postoperative day (Steward et al., 2003).

Bleeding during tonsil and adenoid surgery seldom is excessive, but massive hemorrhage has occurred with tearing of the

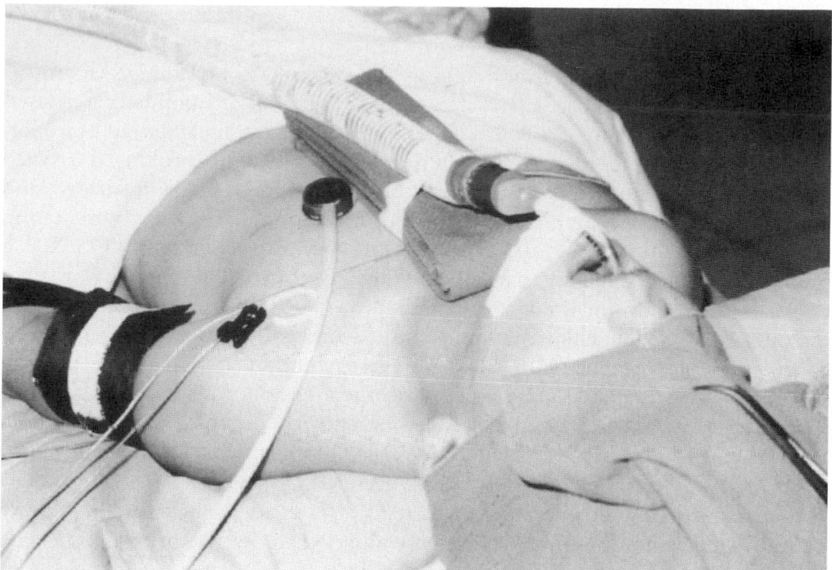

■ **FIGURE 23–4.** For tonsillectomy or adenoidectomy, an oral RAE endotracheal tube is fixed over the middle of the lower lip.

carotid vessels (Smith, 1972, 1980). Homeostasis is usually obtained using electrocautery. There have been several reports of fires due to electrocautery-induced ignition of the endotracheal tube or packing during tonsillectomy. Fires are caused by combustible material in an oxygen-rich environment (Mattucci and Militana, 2003); management of airway fires is discussed in a later section.

At the conclusion of surgery, the surgeon usually suctions the pharynx and larynx under direct vision to prevent bleeding caused by agitation of raw mucosal surfaces by a suction catheter. Some surgeons elect to superficially infiltrate 0.25% bupivacaine into the tonsillar fossa to aid in postoperative pain relief. This practice, however, has been associated with airway obstruction after extubation. The anesthesiologist should always use a plastic tonsil suction tip and should never blindly suction the nasopharynx or oropharynx after adenoidectomy or tonsillectomy. Before a child regains active reflexes toward the completion of surgery, the anesthesiologist should auscultate both sides of the chest to rule out the presence of aspirated blood or secretions and, under direct laryngoscopic visualization, examine the mouth and pharynx for blood and other debris that could cause irritation after extubation.

Laryngospasm may occur when the patient is extubated after tonsillectomy. Methods for avoiding this problem include extubating the trachea while the child is deeply anesthetized (not recommended for children with OSAS) or almost completely awake (see Chapter 11, Intraoperative and Postoperative Management). Although intravenous lidocaine has not consistently proved helpful in preventing laryngospasm, application of local anesthetic before intubation or manipulation of the airway can reduce the incidence of laryngospasm during intubation and after extubation (Leicht et al., 1985; McCulloch et al., 1992; Landsman, 1997). It appears that lidocaine deposited locally in the laryngeal area suppresses laryngeal mucosa neuroreceptor transmission.

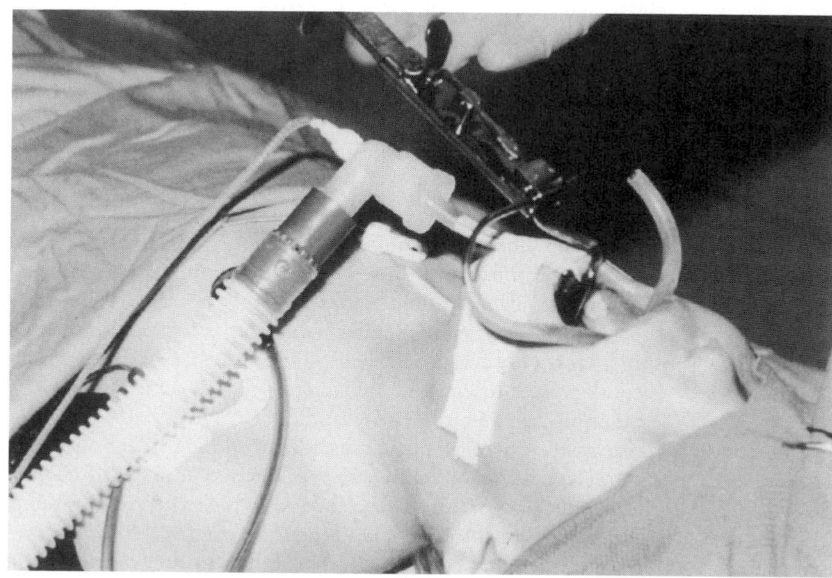

■ **FIGURE 23–5.** Patient in position for tonsillectomy. A Brown-Davis mouth gag holds the mouth open. An oral RAE endotracheal tube is fixed to the middle of the lower lip and is held in the groove of the tongue blade.

However, lidocaine's duration of action at laryngeal receptor sites is only 30 minutes, and its administration before intubation may not protect against laryngospasm at the time of extubation (Warner, 1996).

Conventional "preoxygenation" with 100% oxygen before extubation, which has been practiced for decades, may cause more atelectasis than breathing oxygen mixed with air. An air mix (FIO_2 of 0.5 to 0.7) together with slow deep sighs (or vital capacity maneuvers) before extubation can minimize the development of atelectasis after general anesthesia (Benoit et al., 2002; Tusman et al., 2003). These authors suggest that the patient should breathe a 1:1 to 1:2 air-oxygen mixture (60% to 73% oxygen) instead of 100% oxygen. The lungs are then slowly inflated to a peak pressure of 30 to 35 cm H_2O several times (i.e., vital capacity maneuvers) to eliminate atelectasis that has developed during the course of general anesthesia. This can be achieved by closing and reopening the exhaust valve of the anesthesia circuit while the patient breathes spontaneously against CPAP. The endotracheal tube is left in place until the child reestablishes adequate rhythmic breathing on air-oxygen mixture. The child is then extubated as the anesthesiologist squeezes the bag by hand with the exhaust valve nearly closed, so that a moderate positive pressure (15 to 20 cm H_2O) is maintained to the endotracheal tube and the lungs. Positive extending pressure on the airway walls also attenuates the excitation of the superior laryngeal nerve and may diminish the risk of laryngospasm (Suzuki and Sasaki, 1977; Sasaki, 1979) (see Chapter 2, Respiratory Physiology). Positive airway pressure at the moment of extubation causes a coughing motion, which helps expel secretions around the vocal cords; lungs filled with a high concentration of oxygen maintain oxygenation of the child for several minutes in the event of laryngospasm. The mouth is suctioned again to remove blood and secretions brought up by the endotracheal tube during its removal. For the management of laryngospasm, see Chapter 10 (Induction of Anesthesia) and Chapter 11 (Intraoperative and Postoperative Management).

Postoperative Management

Children with hypertrophic tonsils and adenoids tend to have increased airway obstruction immediate postoperatively. The presence of blood and secretions in the pharynx and larynx may provoke upper airway reflexes. These patients tend to become hypoxemic more often and perhaps more severely during the first several hours after surgery than patients undergoing procedures not involving the upper airways (Motoyama and Glazener, 1986). However, they seem to maintain their preoperative levels of oxygen saturation in room air thereafter, as determined with pulse oximetry (Motoyama and Borland, unpublished observations). Fortunately, serious complications after adenotonsillectomy are infrequent. Postoperative hemorrhage, however, does occur and can become a life-threatening catastrophe (discussed later). Postoperative emesis is relatively common because of pharyngeal mucosal irritation from surgery and bloody secretions that are swallowed. It is therefore prudent for the anesthesiologist to administer antiemetics (i.e., ondansetron or metoclopramide) prophylactically in addition to dexamethasone before the end of surgery (Pappas et al., 1998). Pain after tonsillectomy is mild to moderate and may be controlled by opioids given intraoperatively as part of anesthetic management or by supplementation (morphine, 50 mcg/kg; fentanyl, 0.5 to 1.0 mcg/kg; hydromorphone, 10 mcg/kg) in the postanesthetic care unit. Postoperative pain after adenoidectomy is relatively mild. Acetaminophen is a good adjunct to pain control in these patients.

Children undergoing adenotonsillectomy for OSAS require close observation after surgery and are not candidates for same-day surgery. These children have a higher incidence of postoperative respiratory complications, including prolonged oxygen requirements, airway obstruction requiring nasal airway, and major respiratory compromise requiring airway instrumentation (Biavati et al., 1997; Wilson et al., 2002). Because OSAS is a disorder of anatomic and dynamic factors of upper airway function, it is not surprising a procedure that is curative in many of these children would cause significant postoperative respiratory complications. Because these children are presumed to have impaired neuromuscular control of upper airway patency, residual anesthetic effects combined with blood, edema and residual lymphoid tissue obstructing the postsurgical airway can lead to postoperative respiratory events (Wilson et al., 2002). McColley and others (1992) reported a 58% incidence of severe respiratory compromise in children younger than 3 years that was associated with severe oxygen desaturation ($SpO_2 < 70\%$) or hypoventilation from upper airway obstruction. Among children with obstructive sleep apnea undergoing adenotonsillectomy (mean age, 5 years), intraoperative and postoperative complications are particularly high among those who were born prematurely (85% versus 25% to 34% in full-term infants). Children with OSAS tend to emerge from anesthesia slower than children without OSAS. This may be explained by their deficit in sleep arousal mechanisms. They seem to have elevated sleep arousal mechanisms in response to hypercarbia and increased upper airway obstruction (Marcus et al., 1998, 1999). Other subtle disturbances of sleep architecture may be present (Bandla et al., 1999).

A rare complication of adenotonsillectomy in children with severe OSAS is pulmonary edema resulting from relief of upper airway obstruction. The exact cause is unknown. Galvis and others (1980) hypothesized that during obstructed breathing, extreme negative pressures occur in the intrapleural and intrathoracic compartments. Intubation results in sudden equalization of pressure. The pulmonary venous pressure is suddenly much higher than intrathoracic pressure, resulting in pulmonary hyperemia and edema. Furuhashi-Yanaha and colleagues (2000) hypothesized that the abrupt switch from nasal to oral breathing during emergence from anesthesia might create acute obstruction, which creates an increase in negative intrapleural pressure leading to pulmonary edema. Regardless of the cause, these children require oxygen, diuretic therapy, and possible reintubation to provide CPAP or positive end-expiratory pressure (PEEP). This condition usually resolves in 24 to 48 hours (Carcillo, 2003).

Posttonsillectomy Bleeding

Occasionally, bleeding continues or recurs after tonsillectomy, and the child must be anesthetized to suture or pack the bleeding area. Posttonsillar bleeding is classified as primary or secondary bleeding. Primary bleeding occurs within the first 24 hours after surgery; primary bleeding is usually more brisk and profuse than secondary bleeding. Most fatal hemorrhages occur within the first 24 hours after surgery (Randall and Hoffer, 1998). Most posttonsillectomy bleeding occurred within the first 6 hours after surgery (Crysdale and Russel, 1986; Carithers et al., 1987; Guida and Mattucci, 1990). It is therefore desirable to keep the patients undergoing tonsillectomy and adenoidectomy in the same-day surgery setting for up to 6 to 8 hours to minimize the risk of hemorrhage after discharge from the hospital (Carithers et al., 1987; McGoldrick, 1993).

Secondary bleeding usually occurs 24 hours to 5 to 10 days after surgery, when the eschar covering the tonsillar bed sloughs (Verghese and Hannallah, 2001). Allen and others (1973) reported a 0.1% incidence of posttonsillectomy bleeding necessitating repeat exploration in the operating room. Crysdale and Russel (1986) reported a 2.15% incidence of bleeding during the overnight stay in the hospital for 9400 children undergoing tonsillectomy with or without adenoidectomy. Of these, 3% (0.06% of all patients) required reexploration under general anesthesia.

The child with tonsillar bleeding may be brought back to the anesthesia service several hours postoperatively or even days or weeks after the surgery. Because primary bleeding tends to be more rigorous, bleeding may obstruct the view of the larynx and emergent tracheostomy may be needed. The otolaryngologist should be present before anesthetic induction. Whether the bleeding is primary or secondary, the following issues must be addressed before induction of anesthesia. The child usually is hypovolemic, anemic, agitated, or in shock, with a stomach full of blood clots and often without an intravenous catheter. This is one of the most dangerous and challenging situations in pediatric anesthesia practice, and the failure to initiate prompt action has been one of the main causes of death associated with tonsillectomy (Alexander et al., 1965).

Under these circumstances, intravenous access must be reestablished, unless it is still in place to rehydrate or transfuse without delay. It is frequently difficult to find a suitable vein for insertion of a large enough catheter (at least 22 gauge for infants, 20 gauge for children) for rapid hydration and transfusion in an agitated and hypovolemic child with extreme cutaneous vasoconstriction. An intraosseous infusion or surgical cutdown may be indicated in some patients.

It may be difficult to estimate the extent of blood loss and dehydration. The patient may be tachycardic and have an elevated blood pressure caused by the release of endogenous catecholamines from hemorrhage, hypovolemia, or fear and excitement. If the child is sitting up and talking without feeling dizzy, hypovolemia is only mild to moderate; there is enough time to evaluate his or her volume status with the determination of hemoglobin, hematocrit, and urine specific gravity and to obtain additional information on his or her overall physical status. If the child is lying down and has pale conjunctivae, hypotension, and diminished consciousness, he or she may be on the verge of hypovolemic shock and volume resuscitation must begin without delay. In most cases, tonsillar bleeding is not massive, and the child should be rehydrated and transfused as needed before the induction of anesthesia. Hematocrit values should be rechecked after rehydration to have a more accurate estimate of blood loss.

The anesthesiologist must be aware that the child and parents are extremely frightened. If the patient's condition permits, he or she may be sedated with intravenous midazolam to relieve anxiety. Before the induction of anesthesia, all the precautions and preparations for the patient with a full stomach should be made. These include at least one, but preferably two, well-functioning suction apparatuses with large-bore suction tubes, extra laryngoscope handles and blades, and several cuffed endotracheal tubes with lubricated stylets in place. An experienced assistant should always be available to help the anesthesiologist and to apply cricoid pressure during the rapid-sequence induction (see Chapter 10, Induction of Anesthesia).

After preoxygenation, atropine (0.02 mg/kg) and a defasciculating dose of nondepolarizing muscle relaxant in older children, the child is intubated most commonly with a rapid sequence technique using sodium thiopental (3 to 6 mg/kg), propofol (2 mg/kg), etomidate (0.3 to 0.4 mg/kg), or ketamine (2mg/kg), with doses guided by the patient's hemodynamic status, and succinylcholine (2 mg/kg), with cricoid pressure. Alternatively, rocuronium (1.2 mg/kg) may be used. When using thiopental and rocuronium for induction, significant precipitation will occur if they are given together without flushing the intravenous tubing between the two drugs. If the child is still anemic or dehydrated before induction, ketamine (2 mg/kg) may be used instead of propofol or thiopental, because the latter two drugs may cause profound myocardial depression and hypotension. A cuffed endotracheal tube is used in these cases to prevent blood from entering the trachea around the uncuffed tube (Berry, 1982).

Management of anesthesia during maintenance and emergence in these patients focuses on hypovolemia and a full stomach. A large-bore gastric tube is introduced through the mouth to decompress the stomach, although it is not possible to evacuate all blood clots and solid food. Both sides of the chest are carefully auscultated, and the endotracheal tube is suctioned to rule out aspiration of blood or gastric contents. When there is doubt, fiberoptic bronchoscopy may be performed before extubation, and a portable chest radiograph is taken in the operating room or in the postanesthetic care unit. The endotracheal tube is left in place until the child is fully awake and normal gag and cough reflexes have returned.

The death of a child as a consequence of tonsil and adenoid surgery is particularly tragic because the operation in most cases is elective in nature and the child is in relatively good health. Mortality rates reported in the literature range from 1 in 1000 to 1 in 27,000 (Bluestone et al., 1975; Avery and Harris, 1976). The anesthesia-related mortality unadjusted for age is reported to be 1 in 14,000 (Avery and Harris, 1976).

Peritonsillar Abscess

Peritonsillar cellulitis and abscess occur more frequently in older children and adults than in young children. Most infections appear to originate in the tonsil and spread to the peritonsillar space between the tonsillar capsule and the superior constrictor muscle. The infection may spread upward into the palate but usually does not invade the posterior tonsillar pillar or the posterior pharyngeal wall (Teele, 1983). The patient presents with complaints of severe sore throat, difficulty in swallowing, and high fever. Progressive difficulty in opening the mouth may develop because of spasm of the pterygoid muscles. It is therefore imperative to determine the extent of limitation of mouth opening preoperatively. The affected tonsillar area is markedly inflamed and swollen, and the uvula is displaced to the opposite side (Cook, 1982). In older children and adolescents, it is possible to perform incision and drainage of a peritonsillar abscess with intravenous sedation using an opioid and topical or local anesthesia, with the patient in a head-down position and his or her head turned to the side of the abscess. If this is not possible, general endotracheal anesthesia is necessary.

The child should be well sedated. Anesthesia is induced with oxygen, nitrous oxide, and sevoflurane by mask or with intravenous sodium thiopental or propofol. Anesthesia is deepened in oxygen without nitrous oxide while spontaneous breathing is maintained and assisted in a head-down tilt with the head turned toward the affected side. Under deep inhalational anesthesia, the larynx is exposed carefully with the laryngoscope blade for intubation with a cuffed endotracheal tube. It is advantageous to let the patient breathe spontaneously and maintain the upper airway muscle tone and airway patency. Muscle relaxants should not be given until the anesthesiologist is certain that the airway can be maintained by mask and bag. Two large-bore suction catheters and tonsil suction tips should be on hand in case the abscess ruptures during the process of laryngoscopy and intubation.

Use of the Laryngeal Mask Airway During Adenotonsillectomy

Since the early 1990s, there have been several reports (but no scientific studies) describing the use of the armored LMA rather than an endotracheal tube for airway support during tonsil or adenoid surgery. The armored LMA can be held within the Boyle-Davis gag and remain patent (Alexander, 1990) (Fig. 23–6). The reported benefits of using the LMA are avoiding tracheal intubation with its associated complications of trauma, cardiovascular stimulation, endobronchial intubation, coughing, laryngospasm, and subglottic edema (Hatcher and Stack, 1999). The disadvantages of the armored LMA include the risk of aspiration of stomach contents and the risk of inadequate positioning (Hatcher and Stack, 1999).

Hern and others (1999) reported the surgeon's perspective on the use of LMA for tonsillectomy. In their study, 44 children were anesthetized using an LMA, and 47 patients were anesthetized using an endotracheal tube before tonsillectomy. There was an 11.4% failure rate for the LMA, requiring change to an endotracheal tube before the end of the procedure. The LMA was reported to hamper the surgeon's visualization of the field and might have led to removal of less tonsillar tissue in the LMA group. It is difficult to suggest that the LMA is a superior choice for airway management during tonsillectomy. Additional objective data must be accumulated before recommending this technique.

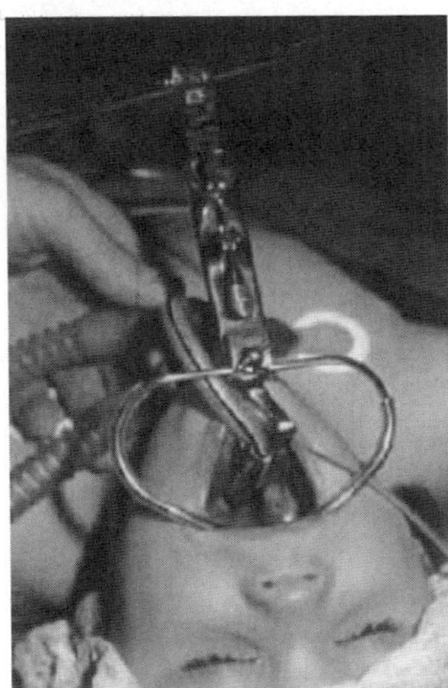

FIGURE 23–6. Armored laryngeal mask airway is used for adenotonsillectomy in a child. (From Kretz FJ, Reimann B, Stelzner J, et al.: The laryngeal mask in pediatric adenotonsillectomy. A meta-analysis of medical studies [in German]. *Anaesthesist* 49:706, 2000. With permission of Springer Science and Business Media.)

LASER SURGERY OF THE LARYNX

The laser (*l*ight *a*mplification by the *s*timulated *e*mission of *r*adiation) has been used increasingly in otolaryngology since the introduction of the CO_2 laser for laryngeal surgery (Strong et al., 1973). The laser is a beam of coherent electromagnetic radiation that can be focused to a very small spot with precision, resulting in controlled coagulation, incision, or vaporization of the target tissue without it affecting the neighboring tissues (Geffin et al., 1986; Keon, 1988). Clinical uses of the laser for upper and lower airways and its anesthetic implications have been reviewed elsewhere (Beamis et al., 1991; Rampil, 1992; Pashayan, 1994).

The principal components of a laser system include a lasing medium (gaseous or solid) that holds the molecules whose electrons create the laser light, resonating mirrors to boost lasing efficiency, and an energy source that pumps the lasing molecules into producing laser light (Fig. 23–7) (Rampil, 1992). Some lasers use a gaseous lasing media, such as CO_2, argon, or helium-neon, whereas other lasers use solid rods of laser-passive material that contain small quantities of ionic impurities, such as chromium (for ruby laser) and neodymium (Nd). A synthetic gem crystal, yttrium-aluminum-garnet (YAG), is commonly used as a passive host matrix (Rampil, 1992). Fiberoptic bundles are used for beam delivery of lasers of visible and near-infrared wavelength. For the CO_2 laser with invisible far-infrared wavelength, an articulated arm containing front-surface mirrors at each junction is used together with a low-powered visible helium-neon gas laser beam through the same optical path as a guide (Rampil, 1992; Pashayan, 1994). Physical characteristics of commonly used lasers are described in Table 23–1.

The most commonly used laser for laryngeal surgery is the CO_2 laser. The CO_2 laser, which has a long, far-infrared wavelength, is completely absorbed by the bending frequency of the water molecules; it is absorbed completely in the first few layers of cells and produces very little scatter of energy. The powerful, focused CO_2 laser beam therefore produces explosive vaporization of the target tissue surface with minimal damage to the underlying tissues (Beamis et al., 1991; Rampil, 1992). The thermal effect (i.e., coagulation lateral to the zone of vaporization) can be varied between 80 and 400 μm. The thermal effect is diminished with increasing water content or vascularity of the tissue or by the use of less power. Thermal coagulation also decreases with shorter pulse duration. The CO_2 laser beam is delivered to the target tissue by means of an articulated arm and a micromanipulator attached to the microscope or a bronchoscope coupler for tracheobronchial applications (Werkhaven, 1995). The micromanipulator allows surgical precision on the order of 250 μm.

The potassium (kalium) titanyl phosphate (KTP) laser and argon laser operate in the green and blue-green wavelength range of the spectrum. The KTP and argon laser beams are transmitted through clear substances and are well absorbed by pigments in the tissues, especially melanin and hemoglobin. They therefore have widespread applications for certain lesions, such as hemangiomas and granulation tissue (Werkhaven, 1995). The energy scatter is intermediate between the CO_2 and Nd:YAG laser beams. Because the depth of thermal damage produced by a laser beam beyond the immediate vaporization site partially depends on scatter, it produces vaporization (but less than that of the CO_2 laser) in addition to coagulation and cutting (Beamis et al., 1991). The depth of tissue penetration is 0.5 to 2 mm (Pashayan, 1994). KTP and argon laser beams,

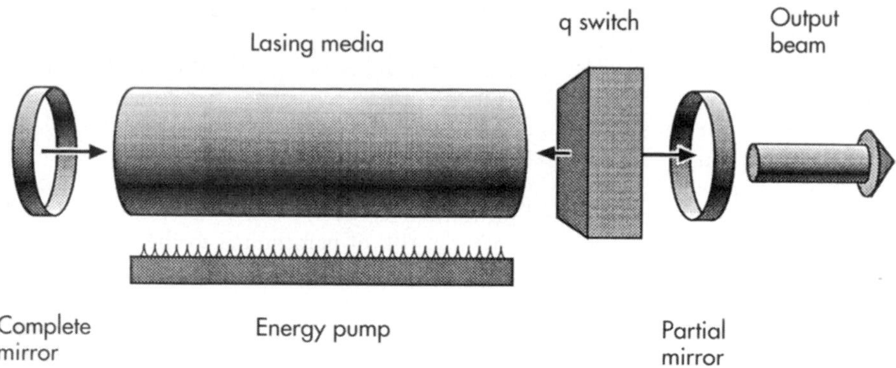

■ **FIGURE 23–7.** The central component is the lasing medium itself. This may, for example, be a solid crystal of yttrium-aluminum-garnet (YAG) with a small concentration of neodymium (Nd) or a tube containing carbon dioxide. The energy pump provides the means of obtaining a population inversion of orbital electrons. It may consist of a xenon flash lamp or an electric spark generator. A pair of axial mirrors allows separated passes of collimated photons through the media, enabling maximum amplification by stimulated emission. The mirror on the right is not 100% reflective, allowing the beam to escape eventually. The optional Q-switch increases efficiency of pulsed lasers by allowing a small delay to increase the pumping. (Adapted from Rampil IJ: Anesthetic considerations for laser surgery. *Anesth Analg* 74:424, 1992.)

as well as the Nd:YAG beam, can be transmitted by means of fiberoptic bundles through the rigid or flexible bronchoscope to vaporize or coagulate lesions in the tracheobronchial lumen (Geffin et al., 1986; Ward, 1992).

The Nd:YAG laser has a near-infrared wavelength, is transmitted through clear fluids, and is readily absorbed by proteins. It is absorbed much less by water, and the beam is transmitted and scattered through much larger volumes of tissue. The energy of the Nd:YAG laser beam is therefore widely disseminated and produces less vaporization and more thermal coagulation. The depth of tissue penetration may range from 2 to 6 mm (Pashayan, 1994). The Nd:YAG laser is transmitted by means of flexible optic fibers that can be directed through the side suction port of ventilating bronchoscope. The ablation of granulation tissue, mixed capillary-cavernous hemangioma, or obstructive vascular tumor in the tracheobronchial wall may be accomplished successfully with the Nd:YAG laser (Werkhaven, 1995).

Risks Associated with Laser Surgery

Because of potential danger with the use of laser beams in the operating room, the users and other operating room personnel should follow the safety guidelines established by the American National Standard for the Safe Use of Laser in Health Care Facilities and published by the American National Standard Institute (ANSI, 1430 Broadway, New York, NY 10018; ANSI Z136). Doors to operating rooms where laser surgery is in progress should be clearly marked to prevent unprotected personnel from accidentally straying into the path of laser beams. Warning signs should specify the class and type of the laser being used as well as appropriate protective measures specific for the wavelength (Rampil, 1992; Pashayan, 1994).

All laser beams for medical use are transmitted through air and are well reflected by smooth metal surfaces. Patients and health care personnel involved in laser surgery are at risk for laser injury, particularly of the eyes. The nature and extent of eye injury depend on the wavelength of the laser beam and its energy. Because the laser beam of far-infrared wavelength is absorbed by the surface it first encounters, errant CO_2 laser beams can cause serious cornea ulcerations and scar formation (Liebowitz and Peacock, 1980). Visible and near-infrared lasers (e.g., KTP, argon, Nd:YAG) penetrate through the transparent cornea and anterior chamber of the eye, are absorbed by the retina, and cause serious damage. The anesthetized patient's eyes should be taped closed and covered with saline-soaked eye pads or metal shields, or both (Keon, 1988). Operating room personnel must wear safety goggles that are specific for the laser wavelength in use. Safety goggles should provide wrap-around protection from reflected beams (Rampil, 1992). For CO_2 lasers, any plastic or regular eyeglasses (not contact lenses nor thin plastic splash protection shields) will suffice as protection (provided that lateral aspects of the eye are also covered), because far-infrared beams are completely absorbed. Visible and near-infrared lasers require specific filters for particular laser wavelengths.

Incandescent debris resulting from the explosive vaporization of the tissue in contact with the laser beam produces a plume of smoke with fine particulates (0.1 to 0.8 μm), which may contain infectious or mutagenic viral particles (Nezhat et al., 1987; Kokosa and Eugene, 1989). Fragments of DNA have been found in the smoke plume, but only one study has found viral transmission from the laser plume (Garden, 2002). The same risk actually exists for the smoke plume from electrocautery. Ordinary surgical masks do not effectively filter particles smaller than 3.0 μm; special high-efficiency masks are therefore needed to filter laser plume particles (Rampil, 1992).

A laser beam can ignite inflammable materials used for general anesthesia, such as endotracheal tubes, anesthesia circuits, oil-based lubricants, ointments, sponges, and drapes (Snow et al., 1976; Cozine et al., 1981; Hermens et al., 1983). All materials used for endotracheal tubes, with the exception of special metallic tubes, are quite vulnerable to laser impact (Geffin et al., 1986; Sosis, 1989a, 1989b). Polyvinyl chloride (PVC) tubes appear to be more easily punctured and ignited by CO_2 laser than red-rubber tubes, and to produce more toxic combustion fumes (Ossoff et al., 1983), although black smoke from burning rubber is probably just as damaging to the airway mucosa. Wolf and Simpson (1987) found that once PVC is ignited, it is less flammable than silicone or red rubber, with a flammability

■ **TABLE 23–1.** Lasers commonly used for airway surgery

Laser Medium	Color	Wavelength (nm)	Tissue Penetration (mm)
CO_2	Far infrared	10,600	<0.25
Nd:YAG	Near infrared	1064	2 to 6
KTP	Green	532	0.5 to 2
Argon	Blue/green	488/515	0.5 to 2

Adapted from Rampil IJ: *Anesth Analg* 74:424, 1992; and Pashayan AG: *Anesthesia for laser surgery, Annual Refresher Courses,* No. 221, 1994, ASA.

index (i.e., FIO_2 at which the material ignites) of 0.26, compared with silicone (0.19) and red rubber (0.18); this means silicone and rubber tubes continue to burn in room air, whereas PVC tubes do not. Red-rubber tubes, however, are more resistant to puncture than PVC tubes (41 versus 0.8 seconds with PVC at the same power density) and intramural fires are less likely to occur (Ossoff, 1989). For these reasons, metal tubes are preferred overall.

During laser surgery, when a nonmetallic endotracheal tube is used, the inspired concentration of oxygen should be reduced to 30% or less, as long as the patient is adequately oxygenated, to reduce combustibility of endotracheal tubes (Hermens et al., 1983). Oxygen may be diluted by nitrogen or helium to reduce inflammability of endotracheal tubes (Pashayan and Gravenstein, 1985; Simpson et al., 1990). Oxygen concentrations up to 60% may be used if helium is the diluent gas. Nitrous oxide supports combustion above 450°C and should therefore be avoided (Wolf and Simpson, 1987; Keon, 1988). It is imperative that the patient be immobilized during laser surgery. The choice of anesthetics depends largely on the technique of ventilation during the laser surgery.

Airway Fire

An airway fire is potentially the worst complication to occur with the use of the laser. Although uncommon, the risk should be appreciated by the anesthesiologist and surgeon, and appropriate responses should be planned before the procedure. Airway fires also have been reported with the use of electrocautery for tonsillectomy and tracheotomy.

Although fires can occur in the operating room environment if the laser accidentally contacts flammable material, airway fires may occur only if flammable materials are present within the airway. Materials such as endotracheal tubes or cottonoid pledgets within the airway are the most common sources of combustion. In the absence of flammable materials, an airway fire cannot be sustained. Although the use of the laser on tissue may generate combustible breakdown products such as methane, the amounts are too small to produce enough heat to self-generate other combustible products. As noted, the concentration of oxygen should be kept as low as possible in the presence of combustible materials.

In the unfortunate event of an airway fire, a mnemonic of the four Es— *extract, eliminate, extinguish*, and *evaluate*—may help guide management. In the event of an airway fire, immediately *extract* all combustible materials from the airway such as pledgets or endotracheal tubes, even if they are still burning. Second, *eliminate* the source of oxygen being delivered to the endotracheal tube. The continued delivery of oxygen to a combustible source produces a blowtorch effect that can further ignite material in the vicinity. Third, *extinguish* any other fires in the vicinity. If a combustible material such as a pledget is still in the airway and cannot be removed, saline flush should be used to extinguish the fire. Fourth, *evaluate* any damage that may have been caused by the fire or the combustion byproducts. The operative field needs to be examined along with the lower tracheobronchial tree. Standards and guidelines for the management of surgical fires, including airway fires, have been published (A clinician's guide to surgical fires, 2003).

Ventilatory Management During Laser Surgery

Numerous anesthetic approaches have been reported for airway management during laryngeal laser surgery. Transtracheally, general anesthesia through a preexisting tracheostomy is the easiest and probably the safest method. It is performed by replacing the preexisting tracheostomy cannula with a metal tracheostomy tube. Manually operated intermittent jet ventilation (Rontal et al., 1980; Scamman and McCabe, 1986; Ravussin et al., 1987) or high-frequency jet ventilation (Smith et al., 1975) by means of a needle or a catheter through the cricothyroid membrane has been used. These techniques, however, have a potential risk of barotrauma to the upper airways and overdistension of lungs (e.g., pneumothorax, pneumomediastinum), particularly when the laryngeal airway is obstructed. Subcutaneous emphysema and pneumomediastinum also may occur because of needle misplacement or a direct leak at the tracheal puncture site (Borland and Reilly, 1987). Without tracheostomy or transtracheal puncture, the maintenance of airways and pulmonary ventilation during laser surgery can be accomplished by means of manual jet ventilation (i.e., Saunder's jet) without an endotracheal tube. A combination of intravenous propofol, topical lidocaine, and small doses of opioids (i.e., fentanyl or remifentanil infusion) has been used successfully with the patient breathing spontaneously (Borland LM, unpublished data).

Nonflammable Endotracheal Tubes

Red-rubber tubes wrapped with reflective aluminum or copper adhesive-backed tape, originally described by Snow and others (1974), have been used effectively (Norton et al., 1976), but the use of these homemade, laser-resistive tubes has decreased considerably over the past decade with the advent of commercially available nonflammable endotracheal tubes. Before wrapping a red-rubber tube with a metal tape, the tube should be wiped with alcohol to remove greasy or oily residues that interfere with adhesion. It should also be wiped with tincture of benzoin or an equivalent before spiral wrapping with a metal tape (Rampil, 1992). There should be no windows of exposed tube; care should be taken to prevent wrinkles, which may cause abrasion of the laryngotracheal mucosa.

Certain metallic tapes do not sufficiently prevent the CO_2, Nd:YAG, or KTP laser beams from penetrating the endotracheal tube and igniting a blowtorch fire. The CO_2 laser can ignite the adhesive backing of all these tapes and perforate the aluminum tapes within 0.1 second (Sosis, 1989a). Other aluminum tapes (3M No. 425 and 433, 3M Corp., St. Paul, MN) and a copper foil tape (Venture Tape Corp, Rockland, MA; 3M Corp.) are effective in shielding at least 60 seconds of direct exposure (ECRI, 1990; Sosis and Dillon, 1990). A metallic foil wrap for endotracheal tubes, specifically manufactured for the laser, is also available (Laser Guard, Merocel Corp., Mystic, CT) and is approved by the U.S. Food and Drug Administration (FDA). This metal-based surgical sponge provides protection against CO_2, argon, and KTP lasers but not against Nd:YAG lasers, according to the study by the Emergency Care Research Institute (ECRI, 1990). It also provides a smoother surface than metal tapes on the endotracheal tube for better airway mucosal protection but is bulky, adding about 2 mm to the diameter of the endotracheal tube.

A number of laser-resistant endotracheal tubes with metal exteriors have become available for clinical use. The Laser Flex tube (Mallinckrodt, St. Louis, MO; Bivona, Gary, IN) is a stainless steel spiral with a PVC tip, with or without two distal saline-inflatable cuffs (Fig. 23–8). This tube is resistant to CO_2 and the Nd:YAG laser (ECRI, 1990, 1992). The Fome Cuff tube

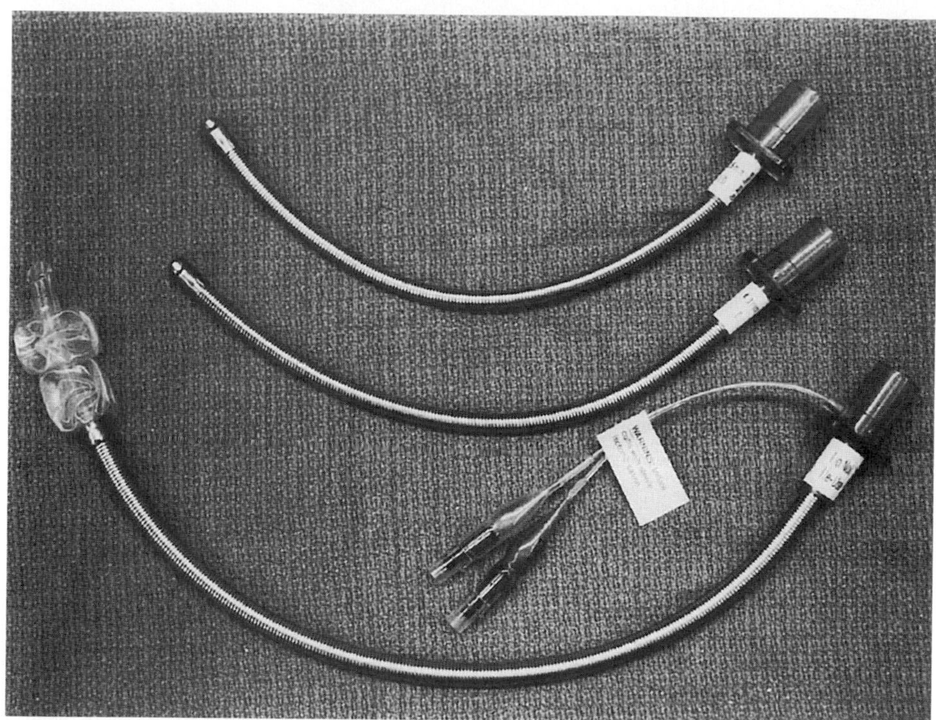

■ **FIGURE 23–8.** Flexible stainless steel (Laser Flex) tubes. *Top to bottom*, A 3.5-mm-ID, uncuffed tube; a 4.0-mm-ID, uncuffed tube; and a 5.0-mm, double-cuffed tube. (Courtesy of Mallinckrodt Medical Inc., St. Louis, MO.)

(Bivona, Gary, IN) is an aluminum spiral tube with an outer coating of silicone that is approved by the manufacturer for the CO_2 laser only. This tube has a self-inflating foam sponge-filled cuff. The foam in the cuff prevents deflation of the cuff after puncture, but damage to the filling tube may cause difficulty in deflating the cuff (Rampil, 1992). The Laser Shield II (Medtronic/Xomed, Jacksonville, FL) is silicon-based endotracheal tube wrapped with metal foil and then wrapped in polytetrafluoroethylene tape to smooth the tube. These tubes are available only in two sizes, and the smallest size (5.0) has an outside diameter with cuff roughly equivalent to a size 5.5 endotracheal tube.

Anesthesia with Nonflammable Endotracheal Tubes

For laser resections of laryngeal papillomas in a child, anesthesia may be induced by mask with nitrous oxide and sevoflurane with the standard monitors, including a precordial stethoscope, pulse oximeter, a capnograph, electrocardiogram, blood pressure cuff, and nerve stimulator. After intravenous access is secured and an intermediate-acting muscle relaxant is given, the child is intubated with a laser-resistant endotracheal tube. Nitrous oxide is then replaced with air or a helium-oxygen mixture (i.e., heliox). Anesthesia is maintained with a volatile anesthetic or propofol infusion with nitrogen and oxygen, and inspired oxygen concentration is kept at 30% or less as long as oxygen saturation can be maintained at or above 98%. The patient's eyes are taped closed and then covered with saline-soaked gauze pads; the portion of the endotracheal tube not metal coated is also covered with saline-soaked towels to avoid the fire hazard of the laser beam while a Jako-type suspension laryngoscope is being positioned. The child is paralyzed, and ventilation is controlled manually or mechanically with a ventilator. Supplemental opioids may be added intravenously to reduce the need for the inhaled anesthetic. Dexamethasone (0.4 mg to 1 mg/kg) may be used prophylactically to minimize postoperative mucosal swelling.

Anesthesia with Manual Jet Ventilation

A more commonly accepted and practiced method for ventilation during laryngeal laser surgery is the use of a Venturi apparatus (i.e., Sanders' jet injector), originally described by Sanders (1967) and Spoerel and others (1971) and applied in pediatric patients by Miyasaka and others (1980) as well as others (Johans and Reichert, 1984; Scamman and McCabe, 1986; Borland and Reilly, 1987). The apparatus consists of an injector and tubing, a toggle switch, a reducing valve or regulator, and a tubing and connector to a high-pressure wall oxygen supply (50 psi) (Figs. 23–9 and 23–10). After a precordial stethoscope, a pulse oximeter sensor, electrocardiogram leads, and a blood pressure cuff are positioned on the child, anesthesia is induced usually by mask with nitrous oxide, sevoflurane, and oxygen. An intravenous catheter is inserted, an axillary or rectal temperature probe is placed, and a nerve stimulator is positioned. Cisatracurium (or other intermediate-acting muscle relaxant), fentanyl (2 to 3 mcg/kg), and lidocaine (1 mg/kg) are injected intravenously. Midazolam may be given to ensure amnesia during the laser surgery. Alternatively, anesthesia may be switched to intravenous propofol with or without a small dose of fentanyl. Nitrous oxide is discontinued, and the patient is ventilated with 100% oxygen for several minutes before the mask is removed. The surgeon positions the child's head and inserts a Jako suspension laryngoscope to secure a patent laryngeal airway.

In children, supraglottic jet ventilation is used. Subglottic jet ventilation is rarely used in children, because it requires extremely delicate skills to assess adequate egress of air between pulses, or pneumothorax or pneumomediastinum results (Fumsaker, 1944).

For supraglottic ventilation, a 10-French metal injector is inserted into the side channel of the suspension laryngoscope and is secured with the distal end 1 to 2 cm above the glottic opening; the metal injector is readjusted as needed to obtain the optimal distance and direction. Oxygen concentration of the jet injector is adjusted with an oxygen blender to reduce the inspired

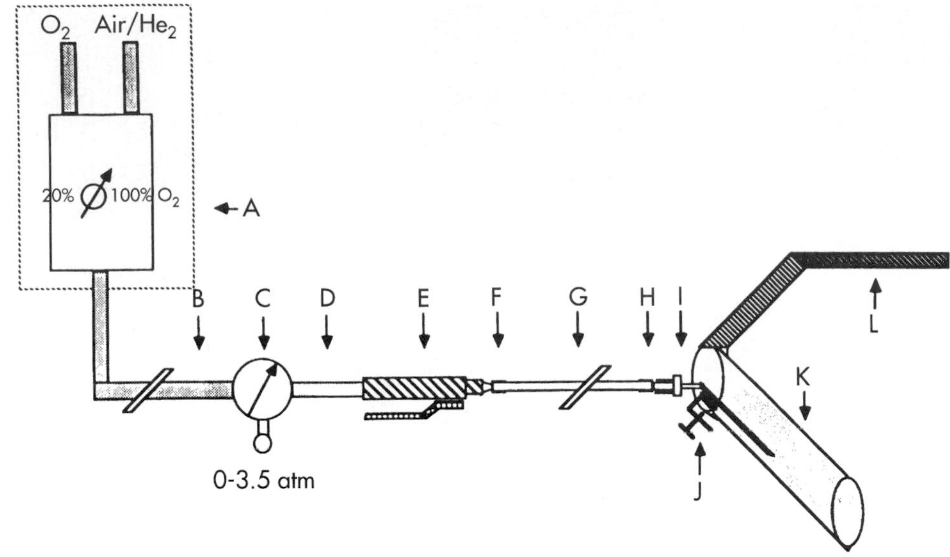

FIGURE 23–9. The Venturi ventilation apparatus with injector needle-on-clamp. *A*, High-pressure gas source with optional oxygen–nitrous oxide or helium blender. *B*, High-pressure tubing. *C*, Reducing valve and pressure gauge. *D*, Short piece of high-pressure tubing. *E*, Manual, all-or-none trigger valve. *F*, Tapered metal connector of the pop-off type. *G*, Low-pressure plastic tubing. *H*, Optional Luer-Loc fitting on tapered metal connector of the pop-off type. *I*, An adapted, curved stainless steel needle, 12 to 18 gauge. *J*, Screw clamp to fit on the edge of the operating laryngoscope. *K*, Schematic outline of the operating laryngoscope. *L*, Laryngoscope handle that fits the suspension apparatus. It should be possible for fittings *F* and *H* to pop off when high-pressure is inadvertently transmitted through the low-pressure tubing (i.e., when *C* or *E*, or both, are failing) or when an obstruction occurs distally. (Adapted from Van Der Spek AF, Spargo PM, Norton ML: The physics of lasers and implications for their use during airway surgery. *Br J Anaesth* 60:709, 1988.)

oxygen concentration with room air entrainment to 30% or less, provided that oxygen saturation on the pulse oximeter is 98% or higher. The anesthesiologist begins jet ventilation by intermittently squeezing the toggle switch. Short bursts of inspiration with air entrainment (1 to 2 seconds) with the driving pressure of 15 psi or less (the pressure may vary with different setups), followed by enough expiration time (2 to 4 seconds) to complete exhalation, provides adequate pulmonary ventilation. Close observation of the child's chest motion during each breath is crucial to prevent air trapping, hyperinflation, and volutrauma to the lungs (Borland and Reilly, 1987). Inspired oxygen concentration is decreased as low as possible by adjusting the oxygen-blender to maintain S_pO_2 between 98% and 100% throughout the procedure. If passive exhalation is unusually prolonged, measures to improve airway patency must be taken immediately. This can usually be accomplished by readjusting or redirecting the injector. Occasionally, when papillomatous growth about the glottis is extensive, the child may require intubation with a small tube and manual ventilation while the surgeon improves the glottic aperture by debulking papillomas on and around the vocal cords.

After the laryngeal surgery is completed, ventilation is maintained with 100% oxygen by mask and bag, or the airway is secured by intubation with a small cuffed or uncuffed orotracheal tube. Neuromuscular blockade is reversed in the usual manner. The endotracheal tube is removed after neuromuscular blockade is completely reversed and the child is breathing satisfactorily.

The manual jet ventilation technique offers several advantages in laryngeal laser surgery, including adequate ventilation, excellent surgical access to the larynx (especially to the anterior and posterior commissures where an endotracheal tube obliterates the exposure),

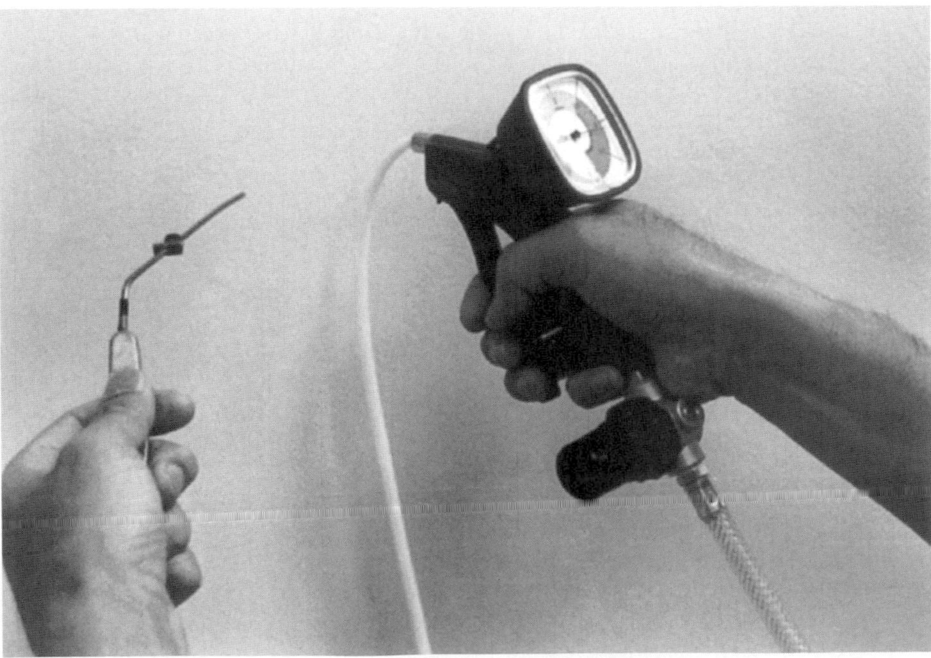

FIGURE 23–10. A Saunders-type, hand-held jet ventilation apparatus. (Courtesy of Manujet III, VBM Medizintechnik, Sulz am Neckar, Germany.)

and the absence of ignitable material in the surgical field (Norton et al., 1976; Goforth et al., 1983). Potential risks of this technique include pneumothorax, pneumomediastinum, distension of the stomach and regurgitation, aspiration of resected material, and dehydration of mucosal surface (Lines, 1973; Norton et al., 1976; Rontal et al., 1980; Ruder et al., 1981; Keon, 1988).

Anesthesia with Spontaneous Breathing

Anesthesia for airway laser surgery can be managed by experts with a combination of carefully administered intravenous anesthesia and topical lidocaine. Anesthesia may be induced with inhalation of sevoflurane with a nitrous oxide-oxygen mixture while the patient is allowed to breathe spontaneously. After an intravenous catheter is inserted and the patient positioned with a suspension laryngoscope, topical lidocaine is sprayed under the direct vision. Inhaled anesthetics are turned off and an infusion of propofol is started. During laser surgery, high-dose propofol (300 to 400 mcg/kg per minute) is supplemented with intermittent doses of morphine (up to 0.1 mg/kg) or an infusion of fentanyl (2 to 3 mcg/kg per hour) to prevent tachypnea. The concentration of oxygen insufflations should be limited to less than 30% for safety while the patient's breathing is continuously monitored with a precordial stethoscope and oxygen saturation is monitored with a pulse oximeter. A manual jet ventilator (Sanders) should be readily available for supraglottic jet ventilation as needed if the patient's breathing is too depressed or he or she becomes apneic. Alternatively, total intravenous anesthesia (TIVA) may be administered with a combination of remifentanil and propofol infusions. This combination appears to make spontaneous breathing more difficult to maintain.

Laser Bronchoscopy

The laser may be used coupled to a ventilating bronchoscope. If the CO_2 laser is used, higher oxygen concentrations may be employed, because there is no flammable material within the airway. The fibers used for KTP and Nd:YAG laser delivery may support combustion, and when used through a bronchoscope, the inspired oxygen concentration should be less than 40%.

TRACHEOSTOMY

Tracheostomy is indicated in numerous situations before development of respiratory distress (Stool and Eavey, 1990). The three primary indications for the creation of an artificial airway are airway obstruction, chronic assisted ventilation, and pulmonary toilet (Wetmore et al., 1999; Carron et al., 2000). Table 23–2 lists conditions for which tracheotomy has been advocated in pediatric patients (Wetmore, 2003).

The ideal tracheotomy tube conforms to the trachea and neck without causing undo pressure or injury to the skin or

TABLE 23–2. Conditions for which tracheotomy has been advocated

	Allergy	**Metabolic**	**Prophylactic**	**Degenerative; Idiopathic**	**Sleep Disorders**
Upper airway obstruction	Angioneurotic edema Anaphylaxis		Head and neck surgery Neurosurgery Cardiac surgery Prolonged endotracheal tube placement	Vocal cord paralysis	Pharyngeal musculature collapse Tonsilloadenoid hypertrophy
Pulmonary toilet assisted ventilation	Asthma	Cystic fibrosis Coma due to diabetes, Reye syndrome, uremia, etc. Respiratory distress syndrome		Central nervous system or neuromuscular failure as in Guillain-Barré syndrome, polymyositis, myasthenia gravis, botulism, cardiac arrest, respiratory arrest	
	Congenital	**Trauma**	**Toxic**	**Infection**	**Neoplastic**
Upper airway obstruction	Choanal atresia Macroglossia Cleft palate Pierre Robin anomaly Laryngomalacia Laryngeal stenosis Vocal cord paralysis Laryngeal webs, cysts Subglottic stenosis Vascular ring Tracheal hypoplasia	Facial injury Oral injury Foreign body Burns (steam, smoke, thermal) Laryngeal edema Recurrent laryngeal nerve injury Laryngeal fracture	Corrosives	Epiglottitis Laryngotracheitis (croup) Gingivostomatitis Diphtheria Retropharyngeal abscess Ludwig angina Neek cellulitis Tetanus Rabies Plague	Laryngeal tumors Tracheal tumors Tumors of pharynx and tongue: papilloma, hemangioma, lymphangioma, sarcoma
Pulmonary toilet, assisted ventilation	Congenital heart disease Congenital heart failure Esophageal atresia due to tracheoesophageal fistula Hypoplastic lung due to diaphragmatic hernia Adjunct to craniofacial surgery	Head trauma Crushed chest Shock lung Intrapulmonary hemorrhage Pneumothorax After lung bypass	Coma due to toxins (e.g., phenobarbital) Hydrocarbon lung Aspiration syndromes such as from meconium	Meningitis Encephalitis Brain abscess Pneumonia Bronchiolitis Poliomyelitis Pulmonary aspiration necessitating laryngeal closure	Brain tumors Spinal cord tumors

From Werkhaven J: Laser surgery. In Bluestone CD, Stool SE, Alper CM, et al., editors. *Pediatric otolaryngology*, 4th edition. WB Saunders, 2003, Philadelphia, pp 1573–1598, Table 93–1.

tracheal mucosa. Plastic tracheotomy tubes are commonly used because they cause minimal tissue reaction. Tracheotomy tubes should be manufactured in metric sizes that correspond to endotracheal tube sizes. However, metal tracheotomy tubes are still measured in French sizes (Wetmore, 2003). Table 23–3 compares the sizes of the endotracheal tubes and commonly used tracheotomy tubes in infants and children (Wetmore, 2003).

Anesthetic Approach for Tracheostomy

The need for tracheotomy may occur emergently, urgently, or electively. It is essential for the surgeon and anesthesiologist to establish a plan before surgery. Some situations, including laryngeal trauma, massive facial injuries, upper airway obstruction, and oropharyngeal distortion, require emergency tracheostomy for airway management. This procedure is usually performed outside the operating room and fortunately rarely in the pediatric population.

Urgent tracheotomy may be required in neonates for congenital airway defects and for older children because of upper airway trauma, corrosive ingestion, infections, and tumors (see Table 23–2). Although these children may initially maintain oxygenation and ventilation, they are at risk for acute respiratory failure. They may have airway anomalies that contribute to difficult or impossible tracheal intubation. The location of the obstruction will dictate the surgical and anesthetic approach. The anesthesiologist must establish whether the child can maintain a patent airway under anesthesia and whether they can be intubated by standard laryngoscopy or fiberoptic bronchoscopy. Sedation with ketamine may also be an option. Otherwise, anesthesia is induced with an inhaled anesthetic agent (i.e., propofol or ketamine) after preoxygenation in the position in which the child is most comfortable, often the sitting position. If there is no intravenous catheter in place an intravenous catheter is inserted, and atropine (0.01 to 0.02 mg/kg) or glycopyrrolate (0.01 mg/kg) is injected intravenously after induction of anesthesia. Unless a normal, unobstructed airway can be maintained, muscle relaxants should not be used because total upper airway obstruction may result. After the child is anesthetized but spontaneously breathing, topical lidocaine (up to 5 mg/kg) may be sprayed on the larynx to ablate laryngeal reflexes before laryngoscopy. If intubation is impossible, an LMA may be used to maintain an airway until the tracheotomy is performed. Tracheotomy is best performed in infants with an endotracheal tube or a rigid bronchoscope in place to ensure adequate pulmonary gas exchange. The endotracheal tube also helps the surgeon to identify the trachea. Many surgeons prefer to use a rigid bronchoscope held in place rather than an endotracheal tube. The rigid bronchoscope allows for a firmer anatomic reference for the trachea, but it cannot be taped in place and must be held by hand. Elective tracheotomy is usually performed in children already intubated for chronic ventilation or pulmonary toilet or performed in combination with tumor removal or repair of tracheal abnormalities.

For tracheotomy, the patient is positioned with the shoulders elevated by placing a roll underneath the neck so that the neck is hyperextended. Some surgeons request that the anesthesiologist hold the chin with the left hand to keep the neck stretched so that soft tissue over the trachea is stabilized (Fig. 23–11) (Stool and Eavey, 1990). The surgeon palpates the neck to identify the thyroid and cricoid cartilages, sometimes with difficulty. The trachea is palpated down to the sternal notch, guided by the presence of an endotracheal tube. A skin incision is made about 1 fingerbreadth above the sternal notch, either horizontally or vertically. When the fascial layer is incised under the subcutaneous fat and the trachea is identified, a pair of stay sutures, one on each side of the tracheal incision, is placed for traction during the cannulation of the tracheotomy tube. The stay sutures also serve to prevent asphyxiation in the event that the tracheotomy tube becomes displaced in the immediate postoperative period

■ TABLE 23–3. Size comparison of endotracheal and plastic tracheostomy tubes

Cannula	Approx. French	Inner Diameter (mm)	Outer Diameter (mm)	Overall Length
Endotracheal Tube*				
2.5		2.5	3.6	12 cm
3.0		3.0	4.3	14 cm
3.5		3.5	4.9	16 cm
4.0		4.0	5.6	18 cm
4.5		4.5	6.2	20 cm
5.0		5.0	6.9	22 cm
5.5		5.5	7.5	25 cm
6.0		6.0	8.2	26 cm
Bivona†				
2.5	12	2.5	4.0	30 mm
2.5	12	2.5	4.0	38 mm
3.0	14	3.0	4.7	32 mm
3.0	14	3.0	4.7	39 mm
3.5	16	3.5	5.3	34 mm
3.5	16	3.5	5.3	40 mm
4.0	18	4.0	6.0	36 mm
4.0	18	4.0	6.0	41 mm
4.5	20	4.5	6.7	42 mm
5.0	22	5.0	7.3	44 mm
5.5	24	5.5	8.0	46 mm
Franklin‡				
3.5		3.5	5.0	44 mm
4.0		4.0	6.0	44 mm
4.5		4.5	6.7	48 mm
5.0		5.0	8.0	51 mm
5.5		5.5	8.5	54 mm
6.0		6.0	9.3	57 mm
Portex				
3.0		3.0	5.0	36 mm
3.5		3.5	5.8	40 mm
4.0		4.0	6.5	44 mm
4.5		4.5	7.1	48 mm
5.0		5.0	7.7	50 mm
5.5		5.5	8.3	52 mm
Shiley‖				
00 Neonatal		3.1	4.5	30 mm
00 Pediatric		3.1	4.5	39 mm
0 Neonatal		3.4	5.0	32 mm
0 Pediatric		3.4	5.0	40 mm
1 Neonatal		3.7	5.5	34 mm
1 Pediatric		3.7	5.5	41 mm
2 Pediatric		4.1	6.0	42 mm
3 Pediatric		4.8	7.0	44 mm
4 Pediatric		5.5	8.0	46 mm

*The endotracheal tubes are marked with the inner diameter, usually with the outer diameter, and with the length.

†The Bivona tube is manufactured by the Bivona Corporation of Gray, IN. Both the inner and outer diameters are marked on the tubes.

‡The Franklin tube is of the Great Ormond Street design, manufactured in England and distributed by Inmed Corporation, Norcross, GA. The tubes are stamped with just the inner diameter.

‖The Shiley tube is manufactured by Shiley Laboratories, Irvine, CA. The tubes are stamped with the size and inner and outer diameters.

From Werkhaven J: Laser surgery. In Bluestone CD, Stool SE, Alper CM, et al., editors. *Pediatric otolaryngology*, 4th edition. WB Saunders, 2003, Philadelphia, pp 1573–1598, Table 93–3.

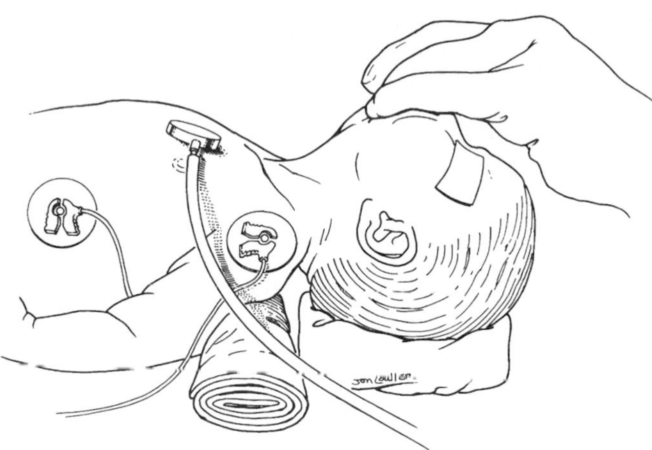

■ **FIGURE 23–11.** Schematic of a child positioned for tracheostomy with the shoulders elevated, the neck hyperextended, and the chin pulled up by hand.

before the tract has formed (Myers et al., 1985). Before the tracheotomy cannula is inserted in the tracheal incision, the endotracheal tube or bronchoscope is slowly pulled back to accommodate the insertion. The endotracheal tube or bronchoscope should not be removed completely until successful ventilation is demonstrated through the tracheotomy. The anesthesia delivery tube is then disconnected from the endotracheal tube under the drapes and reconnected to the proximal universal adapter end of the tracheotomy tube over the operative field.

An esophageal stethoscope or a nasogastric tube has occasionally been misidentified as an endotracheal tube in the trachea by the surgeon, and inadvertent esophageal incision has been made (Schwartz and Downes, 1977); esophageal stethoscopes therefore should be avoided during tracheotomy. The child is monitored with a precordial stethoscope, pulse oximeter, capnograph, electrocardiogram, automated blood pressure cuff, and rectal or skin thermometer.

Major intraoperative and postoperative complications of tracheotomy include hemorrhage, subcutaneous emphysema, pneumothorax, and pneumomediastinum. The neck and shoulders of the child should be palpated for the typical crepitus to rule out subcutaneous emphysema. Then both sides of the chest are auscultated. In most hospitals, the patient is transferred to the intensive care unit for observation and a chest radiograph to ensure proper tracheotomy tube positioning and the absence of pneumothorax.

■ LARYNGEAL STENOSIS

Laryngeal stenosis may occur in the supraglottis, glottis, or subglottis. Clinically, subglottic stenosis is most common. Supraglottic stenosis is rare in children. It usually is a consequence of thermal or chemical injury or iatrogenic injury after previous reconstructive airway surgery.

Subglottic Stenosis

Neonatal subglottic stenosis can be categorized as congenital or acquired. The incidence of congenital subglottic stenosis is 5%; the remaining cases are acquired. Subglottic stenosis in the full-term infant is defined as a subglottic airway diameter of less than 4 mm at the level of the cricoid cartilage and less than 3 mm in the premature infant (Walner et al., 2001). This narrowing can be compared with the reference point of a neonatal endotracheal tube. The outer diameter of a 2.5 endotracheal tube is 3.6 mm, and the outer diameter of a 3.0 endotracheal tube is 4.2 mm (Rutter et al., 2003). The diagnosis of subglottic stenosis is made by rigid endoscopy while the patient is anesthetized. The extent of the subglottic stenosis is determined by placement of an endotracheal tube that allows an airway leak between 10 and 25 cm H_2O (Table 23–4). This leak allows accurate measure of the airway size. The airway stenosis is then graded as follows: grade I, less than 50% obstruction; grade II, 51% to 70% obstruction; grade III, 71% to 91% obstruction; and grade IV, no detectable lumen (Gerber and Holinger, 2003).

In the absence of trauma, an abnormality of the cartilage or subglottic tissues is usually considered congenital. The cause of congenital subglottic stenosis is thought to be a failure of the laryngeal lumen to recanalize after completion of normal epithelial fusion at the end of the third month of gestation (Walander, 1955). Congenital subglottic stenosis lies on a continuum of embryologic failure that includes laryngeal atresia, stenosis, and webs. In its mildest form, congenital subglottic stenosis merely represents a normal appearing cricoid with a smaller-than-average diameter, usually with an elliptical shape. Infants and children with mild subglottic stenosis may present with a history of recurrent upper respiratory infections, often diagnosed as croup, in which minimal glottic swelling precipitates airway obstruction. The location of the stenosis is usually 2 to 3 mm below the true vocal cords (Rutter et al., 2003).

Severe congenital subglottic stenosis can be a life-threatening airway emergency manifesting immediately after the infant is delivered. If endotracheal intubation is successful, the patient may require intervention before extubation. In more severe cases,

■ **TABLE 23–4.** Obstruction of laryngotracheal stenosis estimated by endotracheal tube sizing

Age of Patient	ID 2.0	ID 2.5	ID 3.0	ID 3.5	ID 4.0	ID 4.5	ID 5.0	ID 5.5
Premature	40*	—	—	—	—	—	—	—
	58	30	—	—	—	—	—	—
0-3 mo	68	48	26	—	—	—	—	—
3-9 mo	75	59	41	22	—	—	—	—
9 mo to 2 yr	80	67	53	38	20	—	—	—
2 yr	84	74	62	50	35	19	—	—
4 yr	86	78	68	57	45	32	17	—
6 yr	89	81	73	64	54	43	30	16

*Endotracheal tube sizing is used for characterizing firm, mature subglottic stenosis. The size is determined by placement of an endotracheal tube that leaks 10 to 25 cm H_2O. The numbers in the columns indicate the percent of obstruction.

ID, internal diameter of the endotracheal tube.

Adapted from Gerber ME, Holinger LD: Congenital laryngeal anomalies. In Bluestone CD, Stool SE, editors: *Pediatric otolaryngology.* New York, 2003, WB Saunders, pp 1460–1472.

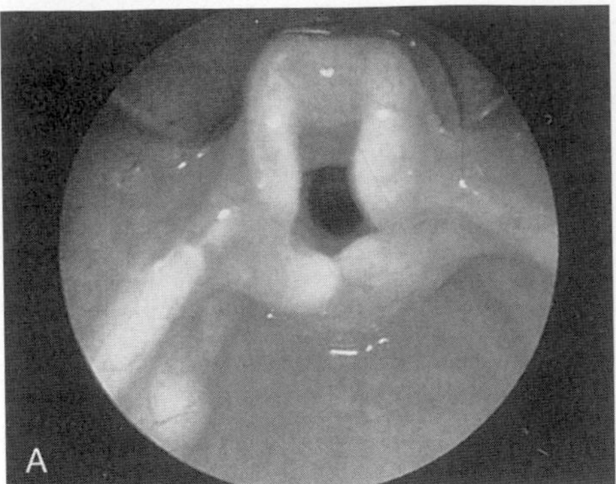

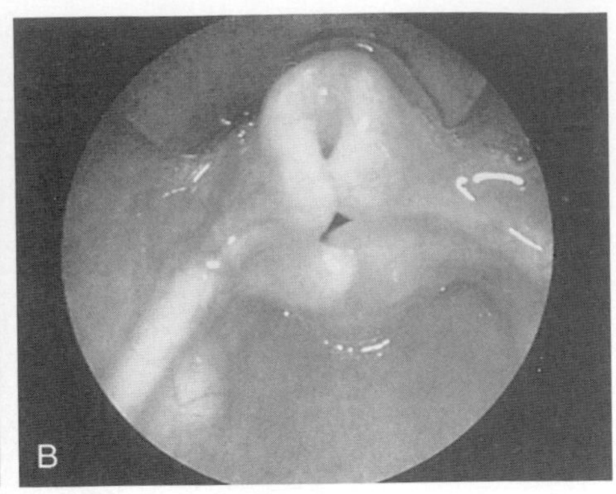

FIGURE 23–12. Laryngomalacia. *A,* The larynx during expiration; the omega-shaped epiglottis and the arytenoid cartilages appear normal. *B,* The larynx during inspiration; the force of the inspiratory airflow leads to collapse of the laryngeal inlet. Infolding of the epiglottic surface and the arytenoids causes severe upper airway obstruction. (From Yellon RF, McBride TP, et al.: Otolaryngology. In Zitelli BJ, Davis HW, editors: *Atlas of pediatric physical diagnosis,* 4th ed. St. Louis, 2002, Mosby, p 863.) (See also Color illustrations, DVD.)

tracheotomy can be life saving at the time of delivery. Infants with congenital subglottic stenosis may have surprisingly few symptoms and may not present for treatment for weeks or months after birth (Rutter et al., 2003). After the initial management of congenital subglottic stenosis, the larynx will grow with the patient and may not require further surgical intervention.

Laryngomalacia is a congenital condition of excessive flaccidity of the laryngeal structures, especially the epiglottis and arytenoids, most likely caused by the lack of neural control of laryngeal muscles. Laryngomalacia accounts for more than 70% of persistent stridor in neonates and young infants (Fig. 23–12); the remaining 10% of neonatal stridor is caused by vocal cord paralysis (Fig. 23–13) (Yellon et al., 2002).

In the mid-1960s, long-term intubation was introduced as the preferred artificial airway in neonates (McDonald and Stocks, 1965). With increasing neonatal survival rates, subglottic stenosis occurred as a frequent morbidity caused by long-term tracheal intubation. Acquired subglottic stenosis results from intubation trauma and accompanying inflammatory responses. Factors suspected in contributing to this problem include prematurity, the size and amount of movement of the endotracheal tube, duration of intubation, laryngeal or tracheal injury during intubation, and presence of infection during the course of tracheal intubation. The incidence of acquired subglottic stenosis has decreased over the past decade by minimizing the issues known to exacerbate subglottic injury (Walner et al., 2001). Patients presenting to the otolaryngologist for diagnosis or treatment for subglottic stenosis are intubated in the neonatal intensive care unit, have a tracheotomy in place with an established diagnosis, or are examined on an outpatient basis for symptoms suggesting subglottic stenosis (Cotton, 2000).

Surgical Management of Acquired Subglottic Stenosis in the Neonate

Neonatal subglottic stenosis unresponsive to nonoperative therapy may require tracheotomy or an anterior cricoid split procedure. Tracheotomy is performed if in addition to severe subglottic injury there is substantial glottic and/or tracheal involvement. After tracheotomy and without the endotracheal tube to act as a stent, the stenosis becomes more severe. Over the next 2 years, the airway may heal, allowing for decannulation, but more often, surgical reconstruction of the trachea will be necessary (Rutter et al., 2003).

The anterior cricothyroidotomy or cricoid split is an effective treatment for some cases of acquired neonatal subglottic stenosis in the absence of substantial glottic or tracheal or pulmonary pathology (Rutter et al., 2003). The neonate must meet the following criteria (Cotton, 2000):

1. Failure of extubation on at least two occasions
2. Body weight greater than 1500 g
3. Absence of assisted ventilation for 10 days
4. Supplemental oxygen requirement less than 30%
5. Absence of heart failure for at least 1 month
6. No evidence of an upper or lower respiratory infection
7. No antihypertensive medication required

The procedure is performed under general anesthesia with muscle relaxation. The shoulders are elevated, and the neck is extended as in the tracheotomy position (see Fig. 23–11). A horizontal incision is made in the skin over the cricoid cartilage. The cricoid cartilage, upper trachea, and lower edge of the thyroid cartilage are exposed. An incision is made through the

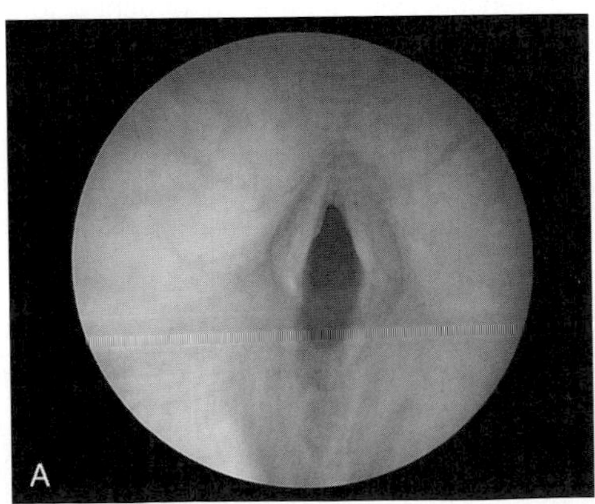

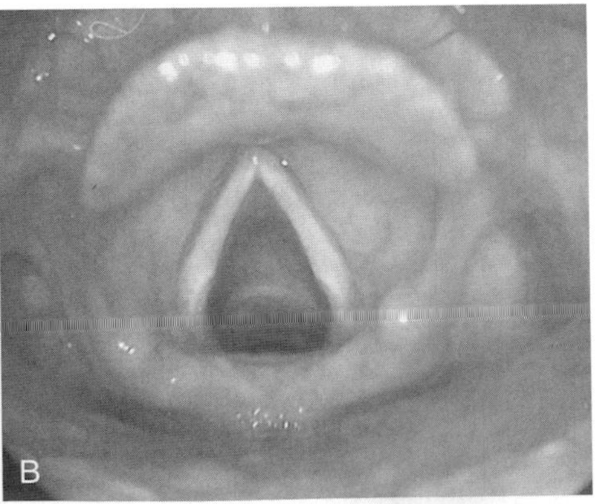

FIGURE 23–13. *A,* Congenital bilateral vocal cord paralysis. The marked narrowing of the aperture between the vocal cords stems from the loss of ability to abduct on inspiration. *B,* Normal neonatal vocal cords with a wide opening during inspiration. (From Yellon RF, McBride TP, Davis HW: Otolaryngology. In Zitelli BJ, Davis HW, editors: *Atlas of pediatric physical diagnosis,* 4th ed. St. Louis, 2002, Mosby, p 863.) (See also Color illustrations, DVD.)

cricoid ring and underlying mucosa through the first two tracheal rings and the lower one third of the thyroid cartilage. Stay sutures are placed on both severed edges of the cricoid cartilage, as in a tracheotomy (Healy, 1995b). The endotracheal tube, which has been used for anesthesia and airway management is then removed. It is replaced while the larynx is still split with a nasotracheal tube, which is one size (0.5 mm) larger than that predicted for the patient's age and body size. The surgeon helps guide the nasotracheal tube into position through the open incision. The wound is closed loosely with a drain. The nasotracheal tube is left in place for 7 days to stent the subglottic aperture. The patient is kept well sedated with or without mechanical ventilation in the pediatric intensive care unit. A modification of the anterior cricoid split is to place a cartilage graft over the split in an effort to allow the airway to seal more rapidly, leading to earlier extubation. Thyroid alar cartilage and occasionally auricular cartilage are used (Rutter et al., 2003).

Laryngotracheal Reconstruction in Children

Chronically ventilated infants who have undergone tracheotomy because of prolonged intubation and subglottic stenosis most likely will require laryngeal reconstructive surgery. Children with greater than 70% obstruction of their laryngeal lumen usually require this surgery to allow for decannulation (Rutter et al., 2003).

Laryngotracheal reconstruction has become the standard of care for symptomatic subglottic stenosis in the pediatric age group. The five stages involved with laryngotracheal reconstruction are characterization of the stenosis, expansion of the tracheal lumen, stabilization of the framework, healing of the airway, and decannulation (Rothschild et al., 1995). The procedure has evolved to include a variety of techniques for expanding the laryngotracheal complex to provide a stable airway of sufficient size. These include, but are not limited to, anterior cartilage graft with the tracheotomy left in place without stent; long-term (several months) stenting with or without cartilage grafts; and short-term (4 to 6 weeks) stenting with anterior or posterior cartilage grafts (Cotton, 2000).

Anterior cartilage graft with a tracheotomy left in place without a stent is indicated primarily for isolated anterior subglottic stenosis with no or relatively mild posterior subglottic components. A variation of this procedure is to remove the tracheotomy at the time of surgery and perform a single stage laryngotracheoplasty. Posterior division of the cricoid plate and the introduction of a cartilage graft in between the cut ends are indicated particularly for children with persistent posterior glottic pathology or primarily posterior subglottic pathology (Cotton, 2000).

Single-stage laryngotracheal reconstruction (LTR) uses cartilage grafts to obtain stability of the reconstructed airway. Single-stage LTR may include an anterior cartilage graft, a posterior cartilage graft, or both, and reconstruction often includes a cartilage graft at the former stoma site. The grafts are supported temporarily by a full-length endotracheal tube fixed in position through the nasal route (Cotton et al., 2000). The optimal time for extubation has not been established definitively. In general, children remain intubated for 7 to 10 days for anterior cartilage grafts alone, and 12 to 14 days if a posterior and anterior graft is required (Cotton, 2000).

The patient may be anesthetized by the intravenous route or through a tracheotomy cannula. Standard monitoring includes pulse oximetry, precordial stethoscope, capnography, anesthetic gas monitoring, electrocardiogram, blood pressure apparatus, peripheral nerve stimulator, and axillary or rectal temperature monitor. The patient is placed in the tracheotomy position with the shoulders elevated and the neck hyperextended. A tracheotomy tube is replaced with a sterile cuffed armored (anode) endotracheal tube through the tracheostomy stoma and is covered under an adhesive drape to minimize contamination of the surgical field.

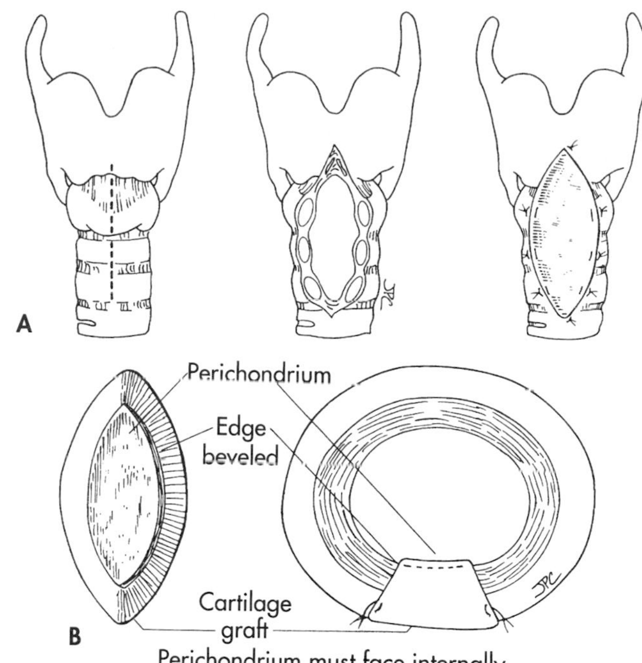

■ **FIGURE 23–14.** Schematic of laryngotracheoplasty for subglottic stenosis. *A,* Laryngotracheal incision with upper and lower extension, depending on the extent of stenosis, and a cartilage graft. *B,* Cartilage graft is shown with the perichondrium internalized. A graft is sutured in position. (From Healy GB: Surgery of the larynx and trachea. In Bluestone CD, Stool SE, editors: *Atlas of pediatric otolaryngology.* Philadelphia, 1995b, WB Saunders.)

Through a horizontal skin incision over the cricoid cartilage, laryngeal structures are exposed. A vertical incision is made through the lower thyroid cartilage, the cricoid cartilage, and the upper tracheal rings (Fig. 23–14*A*). The rib cartilage graft, which had been taken from the anterior chest wall with the external perichondrium intact, is used for the anterior or posterior grafts (see Fig 23–14*B*). Auricular cartilage and septal cartilage have also been used as graft materials. Toward the conclusion of surgery, the armored tube is removed from the tracheotomy stoma and replaced with a cuffed nasotracheal tube, one size larger than is appropriate for the patient's age and size, to stent the larynx. This intraoperative transition needs to be carefully coordinated between the anesthesiologist and the surgeon.

One requirement of single-stage LTR is meticulous postoperative management of the patient's condition in the intensive care unit. The nasotracheal airway must be maintained securely during the time of extended stenting without accidental extubation. The postoperative management of single-stage LTR patients is not standardized (Cotton, 2000). Some centers use sedation to prevent agitation and accidental self-extubation and to avoid pharmacologic paralysis (Rothschild et al., 1995). However, many children do not tolerate nasotracheal intubation and require prolonged sedation and neuromuscular blockade to ensure maintenance of an airway with minimal trauma during healing (Brandom, 1997; Yellon et al., 1997). If neuromuscular blockade is used, daily recovery of neuromuscular function and the avoidance of prolonged use of corticosteroids will be associated with less muscle weakness after extubation (Yellon et al., 1997). Prolonged sedation with benzodiazepines or opioids can lead to withdrawal syndrome, and close observation after weaning these agents is paramount.

Acute Supraglottitis or Epiglottitis

Acute infectious epiglottitis or supraglottitis is a relatively uncommon but truly life-threatening disease of childhood. Acute epiglottitis is an acute bacterial infection principally involving supraglottic structures, including the lingular surface of the epiglottis, the aryepiglottic folds, and the arytenoids, with little or no involvement of subglottic structures, including the laryngeal surface of the epiglottis. It is therefore more appropriate to call it *supraglottitis*. Until the late 1980s, before the vaccination became available, *Haemophilus influenzae* type b (Hib) was the causative organism in more than 75% of cases. Group A β-hemolytic streptococci account for most of the rare cases of epiglottitis (Gorelick and Baker, 1994). With the advent of effective Hib conjugate vaccines in 1988, the incidence of Hib disease has declined dramatically in the United States (Adams et al., 1993; Hoekelman, 1994). The age-specific incidence of Hib disease among children younger than 5 years old decreased by 71% and that of Hib meningitis by 82% between 1985 and 1991 (Adams et al., 1993). Similarly, the incidence of acute epiglottitis, one of the most dreaded childhood emergencies, has declined by 84% (Gorelick and Baker, 1994).

Until the late 1980s, before the era of Hib conjugate vaccination, preschool children between the ages of 2 and 6 years had the highest incidence of supraglottitis, although it occurred in infants, in older children, and occasionally in adults (Schloss et al., 1979; Blackstock et al., 1987; Crysdale and Sendi, 1988). The highest number of cases is reported in the spring and fall, but sporadic cases are reported in other seasons. The condition usually begins with complaints of severe sore throat associated with dysphagia and a thick, muffled voice without a preceding history of runny nose. Rarely is there a croupy or barking cough, except in atypical cases in infants (Blackstock et al., 1987). The symptoms rapidly progress, and typical pathognomonic signs of *d*ysphagia, *d*ysphonia, *d*yspnea, and *d*rooling (i.e., the four Ds) appear (Diaz, 1985).

In most children presenting with stridor in the emergency room, the most common symptoms found in those with acute epiglottitis are drooling, agitation, and absence of spontaneous cough (Mauro et al., 1988). The child looks toxic and usually has a high fever and tachycardia. The disease progresses very rapidly and may be fatal, with severe airway obstruction within 6 to 12 hours, unless immediate steps are taken to restore the patient's upper airway patency. Classically, the child is sitting up, is dyspneic with the mouth open and drooling, and resists attempts to get him or her to lie down. There is forward chin thrust, slight cervical flexion, and forward flexion at the waist, together with tripod placement of the arms to support this posture. The inspiratory phase is slow, with stridor and retraction, whereas the expiratory phase is unobstructed. The inspiratory sound has been compared with that of a quacking duck.

As soon as acute supraglottitis is diagnosed in the emergency room, a pediatric anesthesiologist or intensive care staff and otolaryngologist should be called. The child should never be left unattended by one of these physicians, because the disease can progress so rapidly that complete upper airway obstruction may ensue within minutes. The patient is kept in a sitting or tripod position with an oxygen mask in place and with a pulse oximeter monitoring. The child is transferred to the operating room without delay and is accompanied by an anesthesiologist or an intensivist and an otolaryngologist.

A laryngoscope with several blades, endotracheal tubes with stylets, a bronchoscope, and a self-inflating bag with facemask and oxygen must accompany the patient for emergency intubation (Oh and Motoyama, 1977). Throat examination should not be attempted in the emergency room, because the risk of complete airway obstruction is great. If the child's condition permits or when the diagnosis is questionable, the patient may be transferred to the pediatric intensive care unit, where a radiograph of the lateral neck is taken with a portable x-ray machine (Butt et al., 1988). In the intensive care unit, all the help and expertise needed for an emergency should be readily available. In most patients, a swollen epiglottis obstructing the air (shadow) is seen on the lateral neck radiograph (Fig. 23–15*A*). Negative radiographs, however, do not necessarily rule out supraglottitis.

Compared with acute supraglottitis, the onset of laryngotracheobronchitis (subglottic croup) is insidious. The child starts with the symptoms of upper respiratory infection, with rhinorrhea, cough, sore throat, and low-grade fever for several days before developing the symptoms of upper airway obstruction characterized by inspiratory stridor and barky or seal-like coughs (i.e., croup). The symptoms may last from a few days to more than a week, with various degrees of severity that is worse at night in the supine position. In severe cases, endotracheal intubation under general anesthesia is required.

A lateral neck radiograph typically shows a narrowing of the airway shadow below the vocal cords (see Fig. 23–15*B*). An anteroposterior radiograph of the neck may show a long area of airway narrowing resembling a steeple of a church ("steeple sign") (Fig. 23–16).

Anesthetic Management of Acute Supraglottitis

In the operating room, anesthesia is induced with halothane (historically) or sevoflurane and oxygen in a sitting position while the child is monitored with a precordial stethoscope, pulse oximeter, and electrocardiogram. The child in respiratory distress usually breathes continually, uninterrupted by breath holding. A moderate continuous positive pressure (10 to 15 cm H_2O) must be maintained to minimize the inspiratory collapse of laryngeal airways by the Venturi effect, and ventilation must be assisted with moderate continuous positive airway pressure while avoiding inflating the stomach with excessive pressure. An intravenous access is established as soon as the child is sufficiently obtunded, and atropine (0.02 mg/kg) is given to block vagally mediated slowing of the heart; bradycardia in an atropinized child is a sign of severe hypoxia.

The induction may take much longer, even with a higher concentration of an anesthetic, to reach the state where relaxation and centrally fixed pupils indicate that the child is ready for intubation. The use of muscle relaxants is contraindicated, even when the maintenance of the airway with mask and bag seems reasonable, because their use often results in the relaxation of pharyngeal muscles and complete obstruction of the laryngeal airway; frantic attempts to ventilate the child with high pressure cause gastric distension, regurgitation, and further asphyxia.

Endotracheal intubation is performed orally with a styletted tube one or two sizes smaller than usual. Visualization of the classic cherry-red epiglottis under direct laryngoscopy confirms

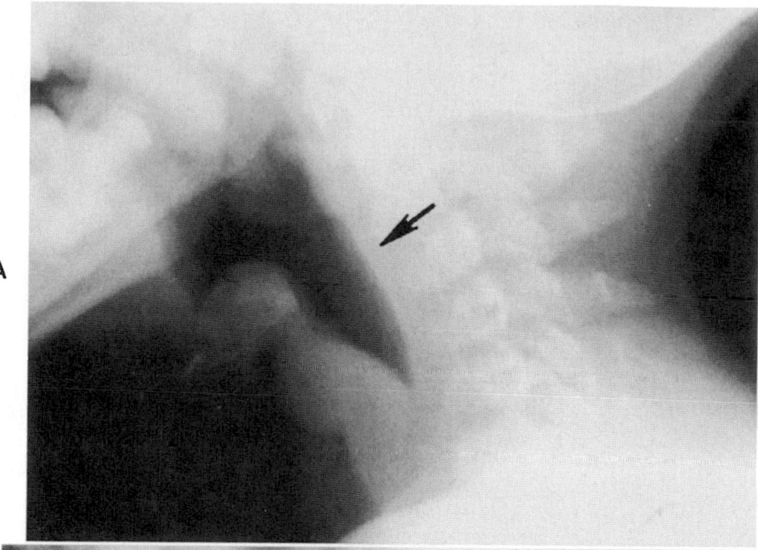

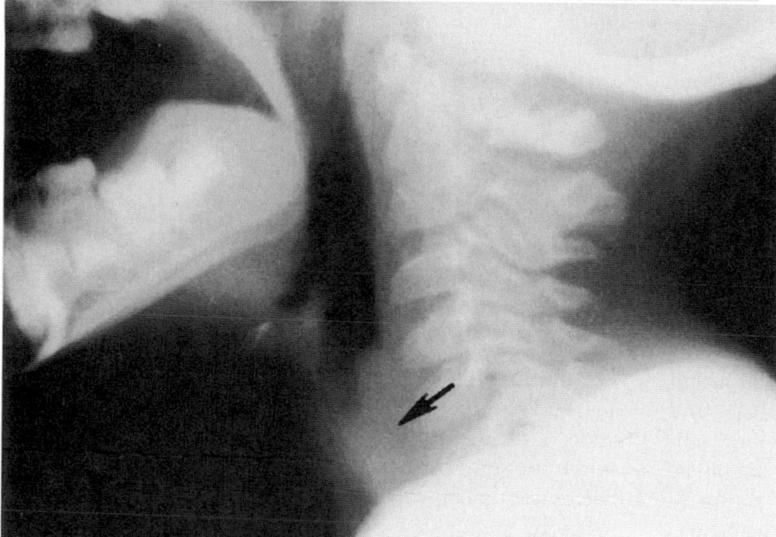

■ **FIGURE 23–15.** Radiographs of the lateral area of the neck. *A*, Supraglottitis. The upper airway is obstructed by marked swelling of the epiglottis and other supraglottic structures. Notice the loss of normal curvature of the cervical spine. *B*, Laryngotracheitis. Arrows point to airway constriction below the vocal cords. (Courtesy of Dr. K.S. Oh, Department of Radiology, The Children's Hospital of Pittsburgh, PA.)

the diagnosis (Fig. 23–17). However, the picture may be atypical or only part of the epiglottis may be inflamed or swollen. Inflammatory swelling of other supraglottic structures, including the uvula, arytenoids, aryepiglottic folds, and false vocal cords, also causes severe obstruction. To visualize the vocal cords for intubation, the epiglottis is lifted by the curved tip of a straight laryngoscope blade (e.g., Phillips 1). In children with severe obstruction and mucosal swelling, identification of supraglottic structures and glottic opening with a laryngoscope blade may be extremely difficult. Under these circumstances, forcible manual chest compression by the assistant may open up the expiratory passages momentarily (or produce a few bubbles of expired air). By aiming the tip of the endotracheal tube at that spot and advancing the tube with a gentle twisting motion, the physician may be successful in inserting the tube in the glottis (Smith, 1980). In case intubation proves to be impossible, a surgeon who can perform an emergency tracheotomy in the operating room with the surgical instruments and various tracheotomy tubes should be immediately available.

After the endotracheal tube is in place, breath sounds are checked on both sides of the chest, and the tube is fixed with adhesive tapes. The breath sounds are monitored carefully with the precordial stethoscope while continuous positive pressure (10 to 15 cm H_2O) is maintained, because pulmonary edema may occur after the relief of severe upper airway obstruction (Travis et al., 1977; Galvis et al., 1980), with an incidence of about 7% (Davis et al., 1981). Throat and blood cultures are taken during this period of stabilization but not before the intubation and restoration of adequate pulmonary gas exchange.

After the child's condition is stabilized after the restoration of adequate alveolar ventilation, some anesthesiologists replace the orotracheal tube by a nasotracheal tube that has a leak at or below 30 cm H_2O (Oh and Motoyama, 1977). This is not a necessary step, and the physician should be confident that the switch could be made without losing the airway. Because acute epiglottitis has become an uncommon phenomenon, many anesthesiologists are happy with the oral intubation and leave the tube in place. The child can be deeply sedated for 24 hours to avoid premature extubation.

Since the mid-1970s, the management of epiglottitis with tracheotomy has been replaced by the less invasive long-term nasotracheal or orotracheal intubation as the standard treatment

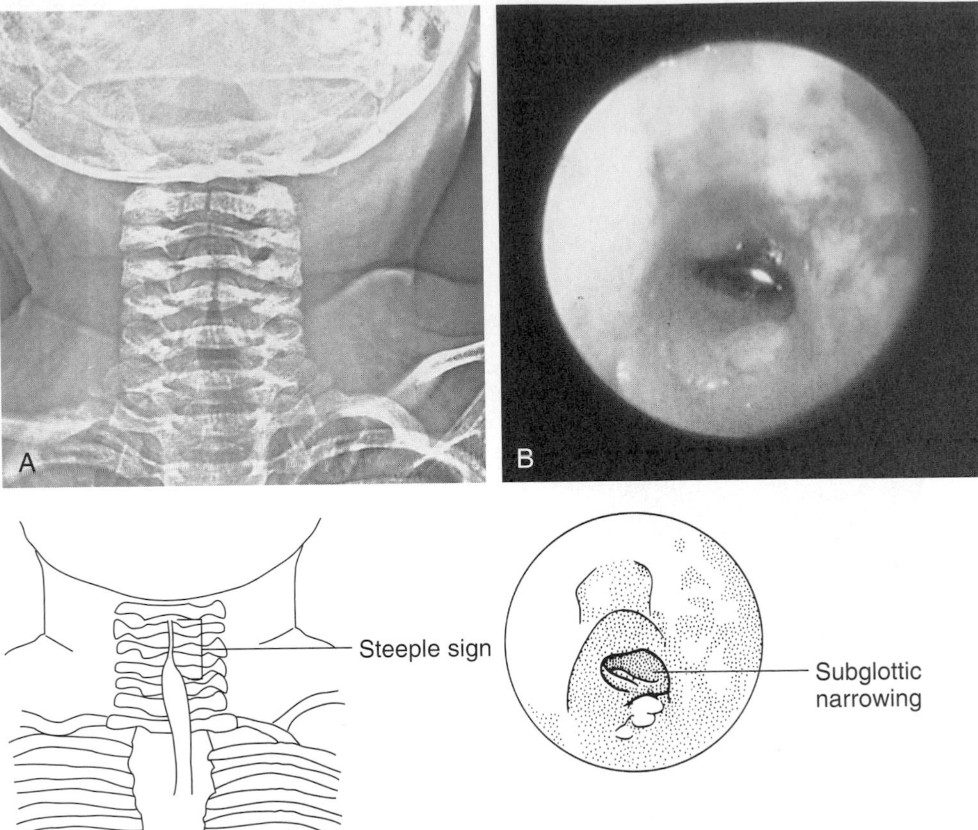

■ **FIGURE 23–16.** Subglottic croup (i.e., laryngotracheobronchitis). *A,* Anteroposterior radiograph of the neck reveals a long area of the airway *(shadow)* narrowing and extending well below the normally narrowed area at the level of the vocal cords. This finding often is called the *steeple sign. B,* In this child, direct visualization using a bronchoscope revealed subglottic narrowing that was so severe that it would require endotracheal intubation or tracheostomy to establish an adequate airway. (Courtesy of Sylvan Stool, M.D., Children's Hospital of Pittsburgh, PA.) (From Yellon RF, McBride TP, Davis HW: Otolaryngology. In Zitelli BJ, Davis HW, editors: *Atlas of pediatric physical diagnosis,* 4th ed. St. Louis, 2002, Mosby, p 860.) (See also Color illustrations, DVD.)

of choice. This has significantly reduced the duration of hospital stay for children with acute supraglottitis (Oh and Motoyama, 1977; Schloss et al., 1983). Accidental or self-extubation is a potentially disastrous complication. Careful taping of the tube and proper restraint of elbows and hands can prevent untimely extubation. Because most children are bacteremic, antimicrobial therapy, consisting of ampicillin with sulbactam, cefotaxime, or ceftriaxone, is started after blood and throat cultures are obtained. Any fluid deficits should be corrected parenterally. After the emergence from anesthesia, the child often falls back to sleep for some time because of sleep deprivation and exhaustion. After this period, most patients require minimal or no sedation (Oh and Motoyama, 1977), although deep sedation has been used in some centers. Usually, it is possible to extubate these patients in 24 to 48 hours. A return of normal body temperature and increased leaks around the nasotracheal tube are major signs of recovery. The epiglottis may be examined under direct vision, with intravenous propofol or thiopental to determine the time for extubation. Alternatively, a flexible fiberoptic bronchoscope may be used transnasally with intravenous sedation.

■ ANESTHESIA FOR ENDOSCOPY

Anesthesia for rigid and flexible bronchoscopy in infants and children requires meaningful cooperation and communication between the endoscopist and anesthesiologist (Donlon, 1996). The surgeon and the anesthesiologist are both working in the same anatomic field. The anesthesiologist is concerned about maintaining a patent airway, oxygenation, adequate ventilation, preventing

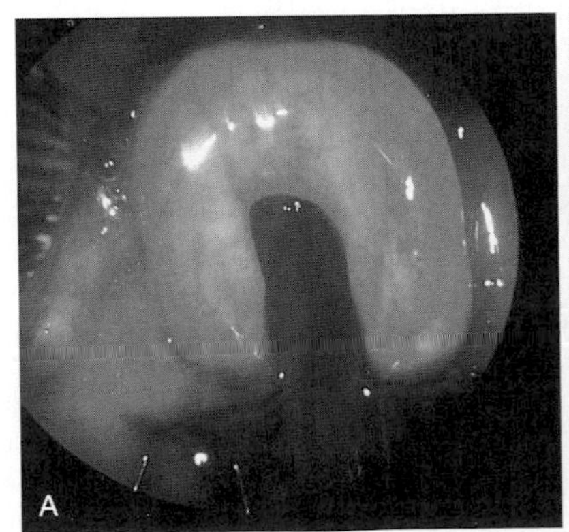

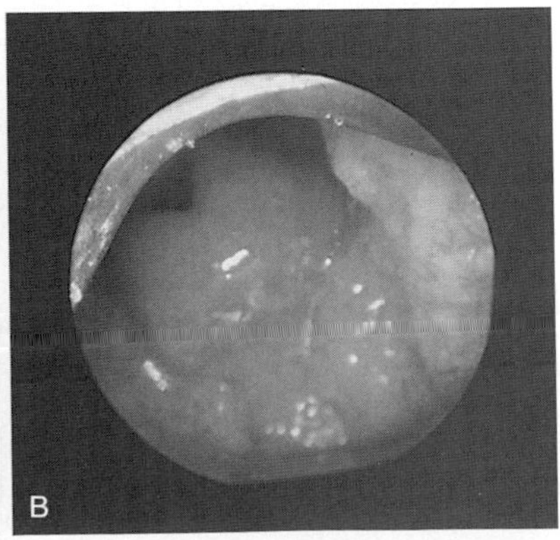

■ **FIGURE 23–17.** A bright red and swollen epiglottis in a patient with acute supraglottitis. It may retain its omega shape *(A)* or resemble a cherry *(B)*. (From Yellon RF, McBride TP, Davis HW: Otolaryngology. In Zitelli BJ, Davis HW, editors: *Atlas of pediatric physical diagnosis,* 4th ed. St. Louis, 2002, Mosby, p 858.) (See also Color illustrations, DVD.)

aspiration, minimizing laryngeal motion, and preventing cardiac dysrhythmias, and the surgeon needs a clear view of a motionless field for a reasonable time. Sometimes, these goals may conflict. Donlon (1996) has eloquently described the anesthetic goals during bronchoscopy:

- Control of the airway
- Decreased airway reflexes
- Topical anesthesia
- Amnesia
- Unobstructed view of immobile surgical field
- No time restriction on surgeon inherent in the anesthetic technique
- Prevention of aspiration
- Smooth emergence
- Safe extubation
- Minimization of secretions
- Prevention of adrenergic reflexes

To achieve these goals, anesthetic management must be individualized based on the patient's age, concurrent illnesses, goals of endoscopy, skill of the anesthesiologist, and the proven track record of the anesthetic technique.

Rigid bronchoscopy has broad applications in the diagnostic and therapeutic arenas. Common indications for pediatric patients include investigation of stridor, upper and central airway obstruction, gastroesophageal reflux disease, and removal of airway foreign bodies (Hoeve and Rombout, 1992; Cohen et al., 2001). Flexible bronchoscopy is frequently used for examination of the nasal cavity, nasopharynx, larynx, trachea, and bronchi in motion. Technological advances, such as smaller instruments and improved forceps, will continue to expand the diagnostic and therapeutic role of the flexible bronchoscopy (Cohen et al., 2001). Flexible and rigid bronchoscopies are used complementarily, and these procedures are often performed during the same examination. Table 23–5 lists the common indications for fiberoptic and rigid bronchoscopy. Many scenarios exist when either instrument can be used for the same indication.

The Storz-Hopkins rigid bronchoscope, with a ventilating sidearm, provides excellent visibility for pediatric bronchoscopy (Szekely and Farkas, 1978; Johnson et al., 1986). This bronchoscope consists of several components: Storz bronchoscope (sizes 3.0 to 6.0); Hopkins glass rod telescope (2.8 and 4.0 mm ED); antifog sheath for the telescope; adapter for anesthesia circuit connecting to the sidearm, which shares the same narrow channel for aspiration and instrumentation; glass obturator cap; and the light source attached to the telescope and prism (Fig. 23–18). The pediatric Storz rigid bronchoscopes are available in three lengths and various diameters (Fig. 23–19). A variety of forceps is available for biopsy and foreign body removal.

It is important to use the smallest optical telescope through the rigid bronchoscope to not completely occlude or unduly increase airflow resistance. For example, use of the standard optical telescope (4 mm OD), as recommended in the literature (Szekely and Farkas, 1978), almost completely occludes the lumen of small bronchoscopes (size 3.5 and smaller). The total airway resistance increases six to sevenfold (Widlund, et al., 1982) unless a smaller telescope (2.8 mm OD) is used (Table 23–6). When airway resistance is too high, neither spontaneous nor controlled ventilation is sufficient for adequate gas exchange during rigid bronchoscopy. High airway resistance would be expected to cause hyperinflation of the lungs and respiratory acidosis (Rah et al., 1979). Spontaneous breathing during rigid bronchoscopy, especially in neonates and infants, should be limited primarily to evaluations of the larynx and documentation of tracheobronchomalacia in the patient with stridor. The high resistance caused by the telescope within the bronchoscope, together with central respiratory depression caused by general anesthesia, makes spontaneous breathing nearly impossible in these young children (Motoyama, 1992).

With the advances in fiberoptic technology, diagnostic bronchoscopy can be performed with a flexible fiberoptic bronchoscope during spontaneous breathing with topical anesthesia and minimal sedation even in the sick premature infant. Bronchoscopy also may be performed under general anesthesia through an endotracheal tube or LMA by means of a right-angle

TABLE 23–5. Indications for flexible or rigid bronchoscopy

Indications for Fiberoptic Laryngoscopy	Indications for Fiberoptic Bronchoscopy
Evaluation of stridor	*Diagnostic*
Hoarseness or weak cry	Stridor
Difficult preextubation of epiglottitis	Tracheotomy surveillance
Indications for Rigid Microlaryngoscopy and Bronchoscopy	Persistent wheezing
Stridor	Persistent atelectasis
Tracheotomy surveillance	Persistent pneumonia/diffuse infiltrates
Foreign body evaluation/management	Chronic cough
Interval evaluation following laryngotracheal reconstruction	Infiltrates in the immunocompromised host bronchoalveolar lavage
Chronic cough	Mild hemoptysis
Severe hemoptysis	Lung lesion of unknown cause
Management of severe laryngotracheal infections	Selective bronchography
Airway trauma	Assessment of toxic inhalation/aspiration
Assessment of toxic inhalation/aspiration	Monitor after lung transplantation
Evaluation of laryngeal pathology	*Therapeutic*
Management of mass lesions of the airway, including recurrent respiratory papillomatosis	Confirmation of endotracheal tube position
	Acute lobar aelectasis
	Cystic fibrosis management
	Removal of mucous plugs

From Hartnick CJ, Cotton RT: Stridor and airway obstruction. In Bluestone CD, Stool SE, Alper CM, et al., editors. *Pediatric otolaryngology*, 4th edition. WB Saunders, 2003, Philadelphia, pp 1437–1447, Table 81–4.

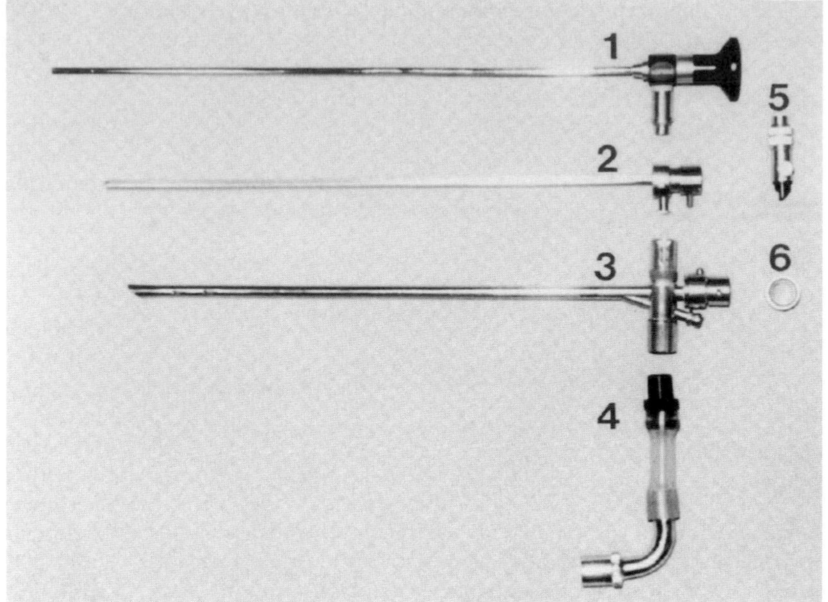

■ **FIGURE 23–18.** Storz-Hopkins pediatric bronchoscopy assembly. 1, Hopkins glass rod telescope. 2, Antifog sheath for the telescope shown in 1. 3, Storz ventilation bronchoscope, which accommodates the telescope and antifog sheath. 4, Adapter for the anesthesia circuit. 5, Prism. 6, Glass obturator cap.

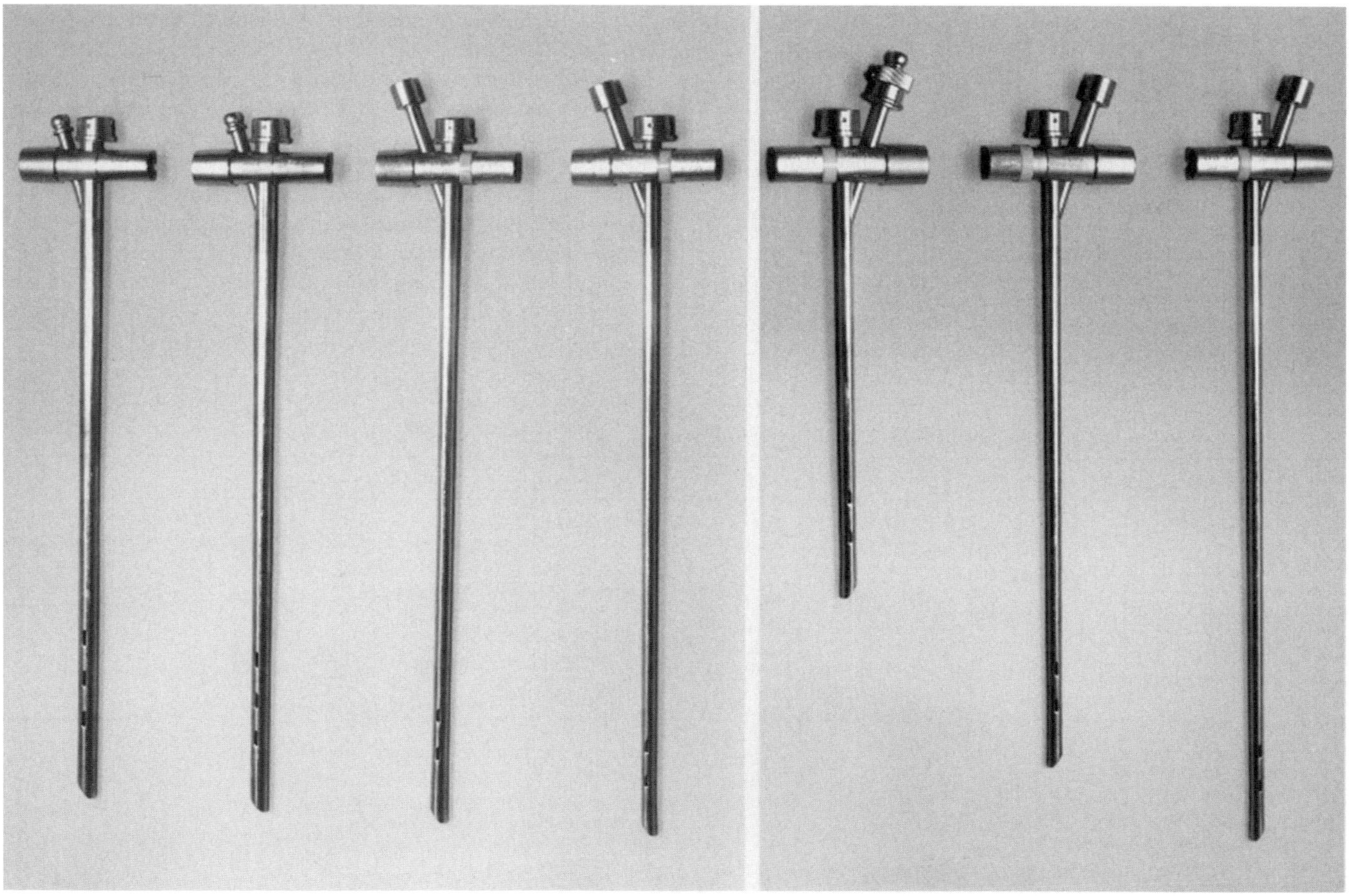

■ **FIGURE 23–19.** Different bronchoscope sizes (3.5 to 6.0) *(left)* and lengths (20, 26, and 30 cm) *(right)* are shown. (From Casselbrant ML, Alper CM: Methods of examination. In Bluestone CD, Stool SE, editors: *Pediatric otolaryngology*, 4th ed. New York, 2003, WB Saunders, pp 1379–1394.)

TABLE 23–6. Flow resistance of Storz bronchoscope in relation to estimated airway resistance (cm H_2O/L/sec) in infants and children

Age	Airway Resistance (R_{aw})	Bronchoscope Size	BRONCHOSCOPE RESISTANCE		Ratio R_{sa-2}/R_{aw}
			R_{sa-1}*	R_{sa-2}†	
1 wk	29	3.0	17	31	4.1
6 mo	19	3.5	12	134	7.0
3 yr	10	4.0	14	37	5.7
5 yr	8	5.0	10	17	3.1
10 yr	5	6.0	16	19	4.3

*Flow resistance through breathing sidearm (R_{sa}) at 0.4 L/sec without telescope.
†R_{sa} at 0.4 L/sec with telescope (4.0 mm OD) engaged in bronchoscope.
Based on data from Widlund B, Walczak S, Motoyama EK: Flow-pressure characteristics of pediatric Storz-Hopkins bronchoscopes. *Anesthesiology* 57:A417, 1982.

adapter with a diaphragm (Maekawa et al., 1981; Wood and Postma, 1988). The use of the flexible fiberoptic bronchoscope for difficult intubation is described in Chapter 10 (Induction of Anesthesia).

LARYNGOSCOPY AND BRONCHOSCOPY FOR STRIDOR

Stridor in pediatric patients may have a congenital or acquired cause. Most cases are of extrathoracic origin, but some originate in the large intrathoracic airways (i.e., trachea and major bronchi) (Box 23–1) (Maze and Bloch, 1979). Stridor may be caused by fixed obstruction (i.e., airway cross section does not change with transmural pressure) or various degrees of obstruction (i.e., airway caliber responds to changes in transmural pressure). These children must be examined while they are actively breathing to document underlying pathophysiology.

The anesthetic approach should be individualized, with good communication between the endoscopist and anesthesiologist. All children should be monitored with a pulse oximeter, end-tidal CO_2 monitor, precordial stethoscope, electrocardiogram, and automated blood pressure and thermometer. Oxygen saturation is determined in room air before the induction of anesthesia to establish the baseline value. If neuromuscular blockade is required, a nerve stimulator should be used to track the depth of paralysis. Standard NPO guidelines should be followed.

In the newborn infant, flexible and rigid forms of bronchoscopy are used to determine the cause of stridor. Flexible bronchoscopic examination of the infant's larynx by the nasal approach is possible when the child is awake. The infant should be swaddled for restraint. Information about cord mobility and laryngeal dynamics can be made without much stress to the infant. Atropine or glycopyrrolate can be used as an antisialogue and to prevent vagally mediated bradycardia. The nasal mucosa can be anesthetized with topical lidocaine to prevent discomfort during the transnasal approach, but the vocal cords should not be sprayed, because topical anesthesia affects their motion. Midazolam or low-dose propofol may be helpful to reduce the infant's excessive movement while still maintaining breathing dynamics. Because the upper airway muscles, including the vocal cords (i.e., cricoarytenoid muscles), are extremely sensitive to the depressant effect of sedatives and anesthetics (Ochiai et al., 1989, 1992), anesthesia should be maintained at a minimal level. Otherwise, the vocal cord motions will cease.

Alternatively, anesthesia is induced with an inhaled agent (i.e., sevoflurane or halothane) without assisting ventilation and intravenous access is established. After atropine or glycopyrrolate is infused and a nasal topical decongestant (i.e., oxymetazoline) and lidocaine is sprayed, the anesthetic is discontinued while flexible nasopharyngoscopy is performed as the infant starts to wake up and the motion of the vocal cords return before the diagnosis of vocal cord paralysis is made. This approach is superior, especially for the diagnosis of laryngomalacia. The infant breathes actively and may move, but he or she is still unconscious during the flexible laryngoscopy. The patient is then reanesthetized with an inhaled anesthetic or with propofol for rigid tracheobronchoscopy.

Only by rigid bronchoscopy under the controlled conditions of general anesthesia can a magnified clear view of the larynx and lower airways be achieved (Hartnick and Cotton, 2003). The use of the rigid bronchoscope allows for lower airway inspection while maintaining complete and secure control over oxygenation and ventilation. After airway dynamics are inspected by fiberoptic or rigid bronchoscopy, the child can be paralyzed with an intermediate muscle relaxant. Anesthesia can be maintained with an inhaled anesthetic agent or total intravenous anesthesia. Communication must continue with the bronchoscopist to maintain adequate oxygenation and ventilation. When the lower airways are explored, the endoscopist may need to be reminded to intermittently to return above the carina for the anesthesiologist to ventilate and oxygenate both lungs.

In older infants and children, spontaneous breathing may be maintained during the entire procedure. This technique for laryngoscopy and bronchoscopy with spontaneous breathing is useful for the evaluation of stridor, laryngomalacia, and tracheobronchomalacia. It is also a technique some anesthesiologists advocate for foreign body removal from the airway. Maintenance of spontaneous breathing can be achieved with an inhalational or an intravenous anesthetic technique. For example, after inhalational induction, the concentration of sevoflurane in oxygen is maintained at 2 or 3 minimum alveolar concentration (MAC) for about 5 minutes to establish a sufficient tissue level of anesthesia to allow endotracheal instrumentation (Smith, 1980). An alternative is to discontinue the inhaled anesthetic, slowly provide a bolus (2 to 3 mg/kg) of propofol, and begin a propofol infusion between 200 and 400 mcg/kg per minute while maintaining spontaneous breathing. Supplementation with fentanyl or morphine can further ablate laryngeal responses. Before endoscopy, the glottis and trachea are topically anesthetized with 2% to 4% lidocaine (up to 5 mg/kg) under the direct vision.

The otolaryngologist then proceeds, using a ventilating bronchoscope and a telescope in situ. Initially, the endoscopist

BOX 23–1 Causes of Stridor in the Pediatric Patient

Congenital Stridor

Craniofacial dysmorphology (with micrognathia and glossoptosis)
- Pierre Robin syndrome
- Treacher Collins syndrome (mandibulofacial dysostosis)
- Hallermann-Streiff (oculomandibular) syndrome
- Moebius syndrome
- De Lange's syndrome
- Freeman-Sheldon syndrome (whistling face)

Macroglossia
- Beckwith's syndrome
- Congenital hypothyroidism
- Glycogen storage diseases
- Down syndrome
- Diffuse muscular hypertrophy of the tongue
- Localized lingual tumors
- Laryngomalacia

Congenital subglottic stenosis
Congenital laryngeal webs
Laryngotracheoesophageal cleft
Congenital vocal cord paralysis
Vascular rings and slings
Congenital tracheal anomalies
Congenital tumors and cysts
- Congenital subglottic hemangroma
- Laryngeal lymphangioma and cystic hygroma
- Cysts and laryngoceles
- Miscellaneous congenital tumors

Birth trauma: edema
Metabolic stridor: laryngismus stridulus
Immunologic stridor: hereditary angioneurotic edema
Neurogenic stridor: reflex laryngospasm

Acquired Stridor

Infectious stridor
- Supraglottitis
- Subglottic group
- Acute spasmodic laryngitis
- Diphtheria
- Retropharyngeal abscess

Immunologic stridor—juvenile rheumatoid arthritis
Foreign bodies
Postintubation stridor
Laryngeal trauma: mechanical, thermal, chemical
Neoplasia
- Laryngeal papillomatosis
- Miscellaneous tumors and nodes

Modified from Maze A, Bloch E: Stridor in pediatric patients. *Anesthesiology* 50:132, 1979.

inspects the appearance and motion (widening) of vocal cords with inspiration and the motion of the soft tissues surrounding the inlet to the larynx. The tip of the bronchoscope is held above the inlet to the larynx without touching the pharyngeal or laryngeal soft tissues. After the bronchoscope is introduced past the vocal cords, the anesthesia circuit is connected to the side arm of the bronchoscope allowing for continued spontaneous ventilation or supplemental controlled ventilation. At the end of bronchoscopy, the bronchoscope is removed, and the anesthetic agents are discontinued. If the patient has been spontaneously breathing throughout the anesthesia, the patient can be maintained with oxygen by means of a mask and CPAP. If the patient is apneic or neuromuscular blockade was required, the child may be intubated and ventilated until clinically ready for extubation.

BRONCHOSCOPY FOR FOREIGN BODY ASPIRATION

Foreign body aspiration occurs most frequently in children between 1 and 3 years of age. Common aspirated objects include peanuts, seeds, and other food particles and less frequently plastic and metal particles (Baraka, 1974; Blazer et al., 1980). Foreign bodies are embedded more commonly in the right main bronchus than in the left and less frequently in the larynx and trachea (Blazer et al., 1980; Cohen et al., 2001). Symptoms and signs associated with bronchial aspiration include coughing, wheezing, dyspnea, and decreased air entry in the affected side, whereas dyspnea, stridor, coughing, and cyanosis are more common with laryngeal or tracheal foreign bodies (Blazer et al., 1980).

In addition to the usual preoperative assessment, physical examination should focus on the location, degree of airway obstruction, and gas exchange. A review of the latest chest radiographs is helpful in determining the location of the foreign body and for evidence of secondary pathologic changes such as atelectasis, air trapping, or pneumonia (Fig. 23–20). If significant hyperinflation of one lung or lobe exists, nitrous oxide should be withheld because of the potential danger of further increase in gas volume and possible rupture of the affected lung. Although it is desirable to keep the child NPO 6 or more hours for solids and 2 hours for clear liquids, the patient's condition determines the timing of the bronchoscopic examination. If foreign body aspiration causes life-threatening respiratory distress, its removal takes precedence over NPO guidelines.

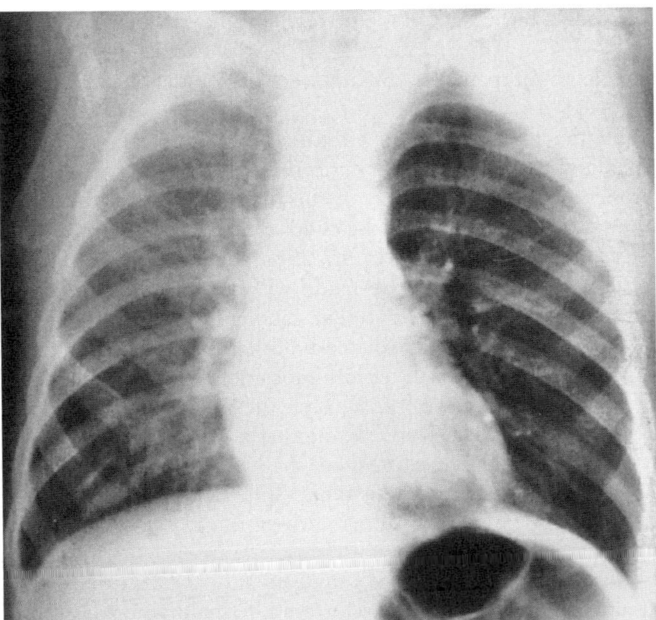

FIGURE 23–20. Foreign body in the left bronchus with hyperinflation of the ipsilateral portion of the lung. (Courtesy of Dr. K.S. Oh, Department of Radiology, The Children's Hospital of Pittsburgh, PA.)

A major controversy in the anesthetic management of patients undergoing bronchoscopy for foreign body removal is whether to control ventilation or to maintain spontaneous ventilation (Verghese and Hannallah, 2001). There are few data to justify one technique over the other. Woods (1990) prefers spontaneous ventilation, and Kosloske (1982) advocates neuromuscular blockade and controlled ventilation. The risk of controlled ventilation is to force the foreign body deeper into the small airways, and the risk for the spontaneously breathing patient is unexpected movement or cough (Donlon, 1996). In a report of four patients in whom the bronchoscopist had the foreign body slip from the forceps back into the airway, neither controlled ventilation with muscle paralysis nor spontaneous breathing under a deep plane of anesthesia played a role in the mishaps. It was thought that the experience of the endoscopist and the availability of proper equipment were more important factors than the method of ventilation (Pawar, 2000).

Muscle relaxation is particularly useful for bronchoscopy involving the removal of a foreign body distal to the carina especially because the duration of these procedures can extend to more than an hour. If the spontaneous ventilation technique is employed, meticulous topical anesthesia of the vocal cords with lidocaine can decrease the risk of coughing and laryngospasm. Propofol-based total intravenous anesthesia would be a superior choice over inhalational anesthesia because propofol provides a steady level of anesthesia regardless of ventilation and perfusion mismatches (Verghese and Hannallah, 2001).

The anesthetic approach to the child who has aspirated a foreign body must be individualized. All children should be monitored with a pulse oximeter, end-tidal CO_2 precordial stethoscope, electrocardiogram, thermometer, and automated blood pressure. Oxygen saturation is determined in room air before the induction of anesthesia to establish the baseline value. If neuromuscular blockade is required, a nerve stimulator should be used to track the depth of paralysis.

Foreign bodies in the larynx are more likely to cause total airway obstruction than are foreign bodies below the glottis. Foreign bodies located in the bronchi may dislodge from cough or change in position and cause total obstruction (Woods, 1990). In case of acute respiratory distress and hypoxemia with a laryngeal foreign body, anesthesia is induced with the patient in a sitting position with an inhaled anesthetic and oxygen while the patient is monitored with a precordial stethoscope, pulse oximeter, and electrocardiogram. Spontaneous breathing is preferable; positive pressure ventilation may cause the foreign body to be displaced and further obstruct the airway (Darrow and Holinger, 2003). After inhalational induction, intravenous access is established (if not already available), and a vagolytic dose of atropine (0.02 to 0.03 mg/kg) is administered. After intravascular access is established, inhalational anesthesia may be switched to total intravenous anesthesia with propofol with or without opioids (e.g., fentanyl, remifentanil). For children in stable condition with foreign body aspiration presumed to be in the bronchus, an intravenous catheter is inserted before the induction, and the child is monitored in the usual manner. If a full stomach is suspected, the physician must weigh the risk of aspiration against loss of a patent airway before rapid sequence with succinylcholine and cricoid pressure is considered.

As soon as the child is anesthetized, the endoscopist must ensure that no foreign body is present above the vocal cords. If the laryngeal outlet is clear, the larynx is sprayed with 2% to 4% lidocaine, and a bronchoscope is inserted through the laryngeal inlet. Fortunately, it is rare for an anesthesiologist to encounter a foreign body in the larynx and upper trachea that causes dyspnea and life-threatening hypoxia.

Immediately after the bronchoscope passes the glottis, the anesthesia circuit is connected to the breathing sidearm of the bronchoscope, and manual ventilation or spontaneous breathing with manual assist is resumed. It is important to remember that, with extremely high flow resistance through the side arm of the bronchoscope, spontaneous breathing is all but ineffective and the respiratory rate (especially the expiratory phase) must be kept very slow to allow sufficient time for passive exhalation. Inspiratory gas flow is adjusted to accommodate for the leak around the bronchoscope.

During the procedure, the anesthesiologist's attention should be focused on the breath sounds detected by the precordial stethoscope, the symmetry of respiratory excursion, and oxygen saturation measured by a pulse oximeter. Close communication and cooperation between the bronchoscopist and the anesthesiologist are essential throughout bronchoscopy. It is important to remember that the lumen of the bronchoscope is narrowed by the telescope and the use of instruments, especially when a suction catheter is inserted through the side port, the same narrow channel through which the patient must be ventilated (Cotton and Reilly, 1990). The rate of rise in end-tidal PCO_2 in apneic infants and young children is extremely high, at the rate of approximately 9 mm Hg/min (Motoyama et al., 2001). The period of apnea or severe hypoventilation therefore should be closely observed and communicated with the endoscopist. The physician must make sure that after each period of hypoventilation or apnea the telescope, forceps, or endobronchial suction catheter through the bronchoscope's side arm is removed. The distal end of the bronchoscope should be pulled above the carina, and the proximal open end of the bronchoscope is occluded with the endoscopist's thumb or a glass obturator cap (see Fig. 23–18), so that the child can be hyperventilated before instrumentation is resumed. Keep in mind that during the crucial moment of foreign body retrieval, ventilation sometimes must be held until the oxygen saturation begins to fall.

When the foreign body or its fragment is successfully grasped with the forceps, the forceps and the bronchoscope are carefully pulled out of the trachea and the larynx together as a single unit. It is imperative that the upper airway and glottis are totally relaxed allowing the foreign body to pass through without being dislodged prematurely. The patient is mask ventilated until the bronchoscope is reintroduced into the trachea. This maneuver may be repeated when the foreign body is fragmented. If a large, obstructive foreign body is removed from the bronchus but is dislodged in the trachea or larynx during the process of retrieval, it can cause serious obstruction of the entire respiratory system unless it is removed immediately. If prompt removal is not possible, the foreign body should be pushed back into one of the main bronchi so that ventilation can be resumed with at least one lung.

Intraoperative complications include laryngospasm, bronchospasm, hypoxia, arrhythmias, and pneumothorax. They are preventable by maintaining adequate anesthesia, oxygenation, ventilation, and muscle relaxation. Premature ventricular contraction, although rare, can usually be treated with hyperventilation, intravenous lidocaine (1 mg/kg), and by avoiding halothane. Pneumothorax, although infrequent, must be kept in mind if acute deterioration of ventilation and gas exchange occurs. A portable chest radiograph is diagnostic, and a chest tube is inserted to reexpand the lung.

After the completion of bronchoscopy for foreign body retrieval, the child is usually intubated with an endotracheal tube. Tracheal intubation allows for tracheobronchial suction, lung expansion, and for oxygenation and ventilation until adequate reversal of muscle relaxation and return to spontaneous breathing. Dexamethasone (0.4 to 1.0 mg/kg, up to 20 mg/kg) is given prophylactically to prevent laryngeal edema (Tunnessen and Feinstein, 1980; Postma et al., 1987). Postoperative croup is treated with inhalation of racemic epinephrine (0.5 mL of 2.25% solution diluted in 3 mL of saline solution) (Adair et al., 1971).

ENDOSCOPY FOR FOREIGN BODY INGESTION

According to the National Safety Council, suffocation from foreign body ingestion and aspiration is the third leading cause of accidental death in children younger than 1 year and the fourth leading cause in children between 1 and 6 years old. Ingestions are often asymptomatic, unrecognized, and self-resolving. Because retained esophageal foreign bodies are so much more common than aspirations, procedures for removal outnumber those for aspirated foreign bodies (Manning and Stool, 2003). The most commonly ingested foreign body is a coin followed by food or bones. Other foreign bodies include buttons, batteries, pins, safety pins, thumbtacks, and small toys (McGahren, 1999). Once in the stomach or bowel, coins usually pass through the remainder of the gastrointestinal tract. Many coins, however, become lodged in the esophagus. The most frequent symptoms of upper esophageal foreign body include dysphagia, drooling, gagging, retching, and vomiting. The child may also experience coughing, choking, and significant airway compromise. Serious complications, such as esophageal erosion, caused by retained esophageal coins are rare and occur only after a coin has been lodged more than 24 hours. Soprano and others (1999) recommend that children with a single coin in any part of the esophagus who have no history of esophageal disease, or respiratory compromise on presentation to the emergency department, be observed for 12 to 24 hours. These authors found that within 24 hours there is a 28% chance of spontaneous passage of the coin into the stomach, regardless of esophageal location (Soprano et al., 1999).

A chest radiograph should be obtained in all cases of suspected foreign body ingestion. Ingested foreign bodies are predisposed to lodge in three areas of anatomic constriction in the esophagus: the proximal esophagus at the level of the cricopharyngeal muscle and thoracic inlet (the foreign body is seen at the level of the clavicles on chest radiograph), the middle esophagus at the level of the carina and the aortic arch, and the distal esophagus just proximal to the esophageal gastric junction (the foreign body is seen two to four vertebral bodies above the stomach bubble on chest radiography). The most common site for foreign bodies to lodge is at the upper esophagus at the level of the thoracic inlet. If the foreign body is a coin, it will be oriented in a transverse position because the opening of the esophagus is widest in a transverse position (McGahren, 1999).

Removal of a foreign body from the esophagus is not usually a complicated procedure. As long as the child is not dyspneic, the physician should wait 4 to 6 hours after the last meal, depending on the child's age, until the stomach is empty. The child should be well sedated, and anesthesia is induced with inhaled or intravenous anesthetics. During esophagoscopy, the mucosa over the cricoid cartilage may be traumatized by compression between the endotracheal tube anteriorly and the rigid esophagoscope posteriorly. A prospective review involving more than 50,000 general pediatric anesthetic cases revealed that the incidence of postintubation croup after esophagoscopy was 20 times higher than that of the general pediatric surgical population during the same time period (Moro, Borland, and Motoyama, unpublished observations). A reduced-size endotracheal tube may be helpful to minimize subglottic swelling (Smith, 1980). Dexamethasone (0.4 to 1 mg/kg up to 20 mg) may also reduce the incidence of postoperative stridor.

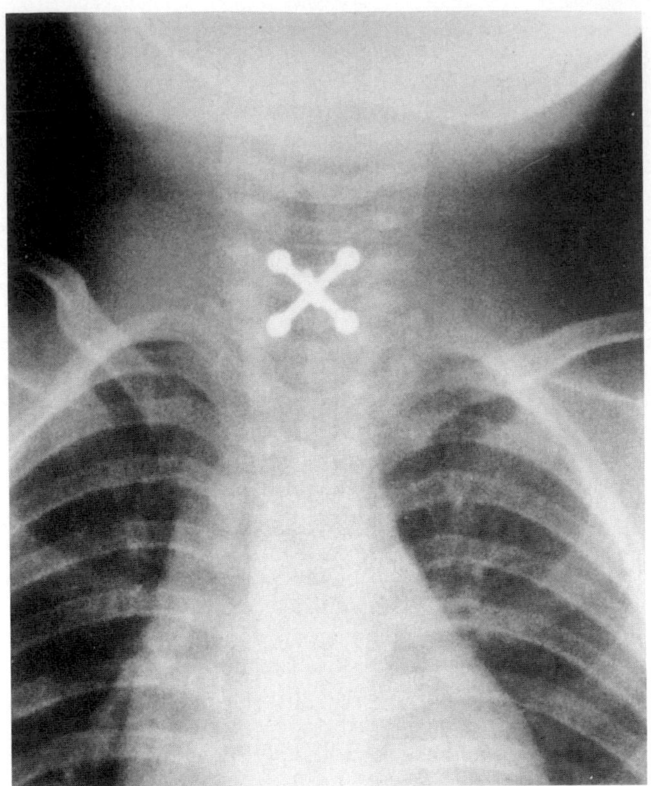

FIGURE 23–21. A jack is lodged high in the esophagus of a 4-year-old boy. (Courtesy of Dr. J. Medina, Department of Radiology, The Children's Hospital of Pittsburgh, PA.)

The only potential and major hazard with foreign body ingestion is the situation in which the foreign body, usually a coin, is held in the hypopharynx, and on gagging and coughing, it dislodges and slips into the larynx, completely occluding the airway. When a radiograph of the neck demonstrates a foreign body high in the esophagus (Fig. 23–21), the child is sedated heavily with an opioid and a sedative to avoid excitement, gagging, and coughing. After intravenous access is established and atropine is given, the trachea is intubated under deep inhalational anesthesia or propofol with or without muscle relaxation. The use of neuromuscular blockade is determined by the ability to ventilate the child with positive pressure. Cricoid pressure is avoided under these circumstances because it may irritate the upper airway or dislodge the foreign body.

SUMMARY

Surgical procedures involving the ear, nose, and throat are the most frequently performed procedures requiring general anesthesia in infants and children. Most procedures are of short duration and involve relatively healthy patients. However, there is a subset of patients with congenital abnormalities and OSAS that presents with difficult airways and significant upper airway obstruction. Improved monitoring technology, newer anesthetic agents (e.g., sevoflurane, propofol), and shorter-acting muscle relaxants have made care of these patients safer and more efficient.

Over the past 2 decades, a drastic decline of acute supraglottitis, the most dreaded of childhood emergencies for pediatric anesthesiologists, has been witnessed with the development of the Hib vaccine. Technological advances in laser surgery and laryngoplasty have continued to challenge pediatric anesthesiologists to develop approaches to meet the needs of advancing otolaryngologic technology.

REFERENCES

A clinician's guide to surgical fires: How they occur, how to prevent them, how to put them out. *Health Devices* 32:5, 2003.

Aberdeen E, Downes JJ: Artificial airways in children. *Surg Clin North Am* 54:1155, 1974.

Adair JC, Ring WH, Jordan WS, et al.: Ten-year experience with IPPB in the treatment of acute laryngotracheobronchitis. *Anesth Analg* 50:649, 1971.

Adams WG, Deaver KA, Cochi SL, et al.: Decline of childhood *Haemophilus influenzae* type b (Hib) disease in the Hib vaccine era. *JAMA* 269:221, 1993.

Afshan G, Chohan U, Qamar-UL, et al.: Is there a role of a small dose of propofol in the treatment of laryngeal spasm? *Paediatr Anaesth* 12:625, 2002.

Airway fires: Reducing the risk during laser surgery. *Health Devices* 19:109, 1990.

Alexander CA: A modified Intravent laryngeal mask for ENT and dental anaesthesia. *Anaesthesia* 45:892, 1990.

Alexander DW, Graff TW, Kelley E: Factors in tonsillectomy mortality. *Arch Otolaryngol* 82:409, 1965.

Allen TH, Steven IM, Sweeney DB: The bleeding tonsil: Anesthesia for control of haemorrhage after tonsillectomy. *Anaesth Intensive Care* 1:517, 1973.

Allsop E, Innes P, Jackson M, et al.: Dose of propofol required to insert the laryngeal mask airway in children. *Paediatr Anaesth* 5:47, 1995.

American Thoracic Society: Standards and indications for cardiopulmonary sleep studies in children. *Am J Respir Crit Care Med* 153:866, 1996.

Avery AD, Harris LJ: Tonsillectomy, adenoidectomy, and tonsillectomy with adenoidectomy: Assessing the quality of care using short-term outcome measures. Quality of medical care assessment using outcome measures: Eight disease-specific applications. Santa Monica, CA, 1976, Rand Corp.

Balkany TJ, Hodges A, Miyamoto RT, et al.: Cochlear implants in children. *Otolaryngol Clin North Am* 34:455, 2001.

Bandla HP, Hopkins RL, Beckerman RC, et al.: Pulmonary risk factors compromising postoperative recovery after surgical repair for congenital heart disease. *Chest* 116:740, 1999.

Baraka A: Bronchoscopic removal of inhaled foreign bodies in children. *Br J Anaesth* 46:124, 1974.

Beamis JE Vergos K, Rebeiz EE, et al.: Endoscopic laser therapy for obstructive tracheobronchial lesions. *Ann Otol Rhinol Laryngol* 100:413, 1991.

Benoit Z, Wicky S, Fischer J-F, et al.: The effect of increased FIO_2 before tracheal extubation on postoperative atelectasis. *Anesth Analg* 95:1477, 2002.

Bennie RE, Boehringer LA, Dierdorf SF, et al.: Transnasal butorphanol is effective for postoperative pain relief in children undergoing myringotomy. *Anesthesiology* 89:385, 1998.

Berry FA: Post-tonsillectomy bleeding. In *Common problems in pediatric anesthesia.* Chicago, 1982, Year Book Medical Publishers.

Biavati MJ, Manning SC, Phillips DL: Predictive factors for respiratory complications after tonsillectomy and adenoidectomy in children. *Arch Otolaryngol Head Neck Surg* 123:517, 1997.

Blackstock D, Adderley RJ, Steward DJ: Epiglottitis in young infants. *Anesthesiology* 67:97, 1987.

Bland JW Jr, Edwards FK: Pulmonary hypertension and congestive heart failure in children with chronic upper airway obstruction. New concepts of etiologic factors. *Am J Cardiol* 23:830, 1969.

Blazer S, Naveh Y, Friedman A: Foreign body in the airway. A review of 200 cases. *Am J Dis Child* 134:68, 1980.

Bluestone CD: Controversies in tonsillectomy, adenoidectomy and tympanostomy tubes. In Bailey B, editor: *Head and neck surgery—otolaryngology.* Philadelphia, 2001, Lippincott Williams & Wilkins, pp 993–1006.

Bluestone CD, Klein JO: Intracranial Complications of otitis media. In Bluestone CD, Stool SE, editors: *Pediatric otolaryngology.* Philadelphia, 2003, WB Saunders, pp 765–778.

Bluestone CD, Klein JO: *Pediatric otolaryngology.* Philadelphia, 2001, WB Saunders.

Bluestone CD, Klein JO: *Pediatric otolaryngology.* Philadelphia, 2003, WB Saunders.

Bluestone CD, Paradise JL, Kass EH, et al.: The workshop on tonsillectomy and adenoidectomy. *Ann Orol Rhinol Laryngol* suppl.19:84, 1975.

Borland LM, Reilly IS: Jet ventilation for laser laryngeal surgery in children. Modification of the Saunders jet ventilation technique. *Int J Pediatr Otorhinolaryngol* 14:65, 1987.

Brandom BW: Postoperative management of laryngotracheal reconstruction. *Int Anesthesiol Clin* 35:127, 1997.

Brisson P, Patel H, Scorpio R, et al.: Rotary atlanto-axial subluxation with torticollis following central-venous catheter insertion. *Pediatr Surg Int* 16:421, 2000.

Brown GW, Patel N, Ellis FR: Comparison of propofol and thiopentone for laryngeal mask insertion. *Anaesthesia* 46:771, 1991.

Brown OE, Pownell P, Manning SC: Choanal atresia: A new anatomic classification and clinical management applications. *Laryngoscope* 106:97, 1996.

Bruppacher H, Reber A, Keller JP, et al.: The effects of common airway maneuvers on airway pressure and flow in children undergoing adenotonsillectomies. *Anesth Analg* 97:29, 2003.

Butt W, Shann F, Walker C, et al.: Acute epiglottitis: A different approach to management. *Critical Care Medicine* 16:43, 1988

Carcillo J: Intensive care management of infection-related acute upper airway obstruction in children. In Bluestone CD, Stool SE, editors: *Pediatric otolaryngology.* Philadelphia, 2003, WB Saunders, pp 1599–1604.

Carithers JS, Gebhart DE, Williams JA: Postoperative risks of pediatric tonsilloadenoidectomy. *Laryngoscope* 97:422, 1987.

Carron JD, Derkay CS, Strope GL, et al.: Pediatric tracheotomies: Changing indications and outcomes. *Laryngoscope* 110:1099, 2000.

Casselbrant ML, Alper CM: Methods of examination. In Bluestone CD, Stool SE, Alper CM, et al., editors: *Pediatric otolaryngology*, 4th ed. Philadelphia, 2003, WB Saunders, pp 1379–1394.

Cayler GG, Johnson EE, Lewis BE, et al.: Heart failure due to enlarged tonsils and adenoids. The cardiorespiratory syndrome of increased airway resistance. *Am J Dis Child* 118:708, 1969.

Close HL, Kryzer TC, Nowlin JR, et al.: Hemostatic assessment of patients before tonsillectomy: A prospective study. *Otolaryngol Head Neck Surg* 111:733, 1994.

Cohen S, Pine H, Drake A: Use of rigid and flexible bronchoscopy among pediatric otolaryngologists. *Arch Otolaryngol Head Neck Surg* 127:505, 2001.

Cook DR: Peritonsillar abscess and hyperthyroidism. In Sterling LC, editor: *Common problems in pediatric anesthesia.* Chicago, 1982, Year Book Medical Publishers.

Coté CJ, Goldstein EA, Coté MA, et al.: A single-blind study of pulse oximetry in children. *Anesthesiology* 68:184, 1988.

Coté CJ, Roll N, Liu LMP, Gousouzian NG: A single-blind study of pulse oximetry and capnography in children. *Anesthesiology* 74:984, 1991.

Cotton RT: Advancing the quality of care for children. *Arch Otolaryngol Head Neck Surg* 116:33, 1990.

Cotton RT: Management of subglottic stenosis. *Otolaryngol Clin North Am* 33:111, 2000.

Cotton RT, Reilly JS: Congenital malformations of the larynx. In Bluestone CD, Stool SE, editors: *Pediatric otolaryngology*, 2nd ed. Philadelphia, 1990, WB Saunders, pp 1121–1128.

Cozine K, Rosenbaum LM, Askanazi J, et al.: Laser-induced endotracheal tube fire. *Anesthesiology* 55:583, 1981.

Crysdale WS, Russel D: Complications of tonsillectomy and adenoidectomy in 9,409 children observed overnight. *Can Med Assoc J* 135:1139, 1986.

Crysdale WS, Sendi K: Evolution in the management of acute epiglottitis: a 10-years experience with 242 children. *Int Anesthesiol Clin* 26:32–38, 1988.

Crysdale WS, Sendi KS, Yoo J: Esophageal foreign bodies in children: 15-year review of 484 cases. *Ann Otol Rhinol Laryngol* 100:320, 1991.

Dahl JB, Kehlet H: Non-steroidal anti-inflammatory drugs: Rationale for use in severe postoperative pain. *Br J Anaesth* 72:375, 1994.

Darrow DH, Holinger LD: Foreign bodies of the larynx, trachea, and bronchi. In Bluestone CD, Stool SE, editors: *Pediatric otolaryngology.* Philadelphia, 2003, WB Saunders, pp 1543–1557.

Darrow DH, Siemens C: Indications for tonsillectomy and adenoidectomy. *Laryngoscope* 112:6, 2002.

Davies DW, Steward DJ: Unexpected excessive bleeding during operation: Role of acetylsalicylic acid. *Can Anaesth Soc J* 24:452, 1977.

Davis HW, Gartner JC, Galvis AG, et al.: Acute upper airway obstruction: Croup and epiglottitis. *Rev Pediatr Clin North Am* 28:859, 1981.

Diaz JH: Croup and epiglottitis in children: The anesthesiologist as diagnostician. *Anesth Analg* 64:621, 1985.

Donlon JV, Benumof JL: *Anesthetic and airway management of laryngoscopy and broncoscopy.* St Louis, 1996, Mosby.

Dornhoffer J, Manning L: Unplanned admissions following outpatient otologic surgery: The University of Arkansas experience. *Ear Nose Throat J* 79:710, 2000.

Doyle WJ, Banks JM: Middle ear pressure change during controlled breathing with gas mixtures containing nitrous oxide. *J Appl Physiol* 94:199, 2003.

Emhardt JD, Weisberger ED, Dierdorf SF, et al.: The rise of arterial carbon dioxide during apnea in children. *Anesthesiology* 69:779, 1988.

Erb TO, Hall JM, Ing RJ, et al.: Postoperative nausea and vomiting in children and adolescents undergoing radiofrequency catheter ablation: A randomized comparison of propofol- and isoflurane-based anesthetics. *Anesth Analg* 95:1577, 2002b.

Erb TO, Schulman SR, Sugarman J: Permission and assent for clinical research in pediatric anesthesia. *Anesth Analg* 94:1155, 2002a.

Fine GF, Borland LM: The future of the cuffed endotracheal tube. *Paediatr Anaesth* 14:38–42, 2004.

Finkel JC, Cohen IT, Hannallah RS, et al.: The effect of intranasal fentanyl on the emergence characteristics after sevoflurane anesthesia in children undergoing surgery for bilateral myringotomy tube placement. *Anesth Analg* 92:1164, 2001.

Fischetti M: Cochlear implants. To hear again. *Sci Am* 288:82, 2003.

Funsaker DH: Anesthesia for microlaryngeal surgery: The case for subglottic jet ventilation. *Laryngoscope* 104:1–30, 1944.

Furuhashi-Yanaha A, Dohi S, Oshima T, et al.: Acute pulmonary edema caused by impaired switching from nasal to oral breathing in the emergence from anesthesia. *Anesthesiology* 92:1209, 2000.

Galinkin JL, Fazi LM, Cuy RM, et al.: Use of intranasal fentanyl in children undergoing myringotomy and tube placement during halothane and sevoflurane anesthesia. *Anesthesiology* 93:1378, 2000.

Galvis AG, Stool SE, Bluestone CD: Pulmonary edema following relief of acute upper airway obstruction. *Ann Otol Rhinol Laryngol* 89:124, 1980.

Garden JM, O'Banion MK, Bakus AD, et al.: Viral disease transmitted by laser-generated plume (aerosol). *Arch Dermatol* 138:1303, 2002.

Geffin B, Shapshay SM, Bellack GS, et al.: Flammability of endotracheal tubes during Nd-YAG laser application in the airway. *Anesthesiology* 65:5 11, 1986.

Gerber ME, Holinger LD: Congenital laryngeal anomalies. In Bluestone CD, Stool SE, editors: *Pediatric otolaryngology*. Philadelphia, 2003, WB Saunders, pp 1460–1472.

Gluckman IL: Inflammatory diseases of the mouth and pharynx. In Bluestone CD, Stool SE, editors: *Pediatric otolaryngology*, 2nd ed. Philadelphia, 1990, WB Saunders.

Goforth AJ, Cooke JE, Putney FJ: An anesthesia technique for laser surgery of the larynx. *Laryngoscope* 93:822, 1983.

Goldsmith AJ, Rosenfeld RM: Treatment of pediatric sinusitis. *Pediatr Clin North Am* 50:2, 2003.

Gorelick MH, Baker MD: Epiglottitis in children, 1979 through 1992. Effects of *Haemophilus influenzae* type b immunization. *Arch Pediatr Adolesc Med* 148:47, 1994.

Guida RA, Mattucci KF: Tonsillectomy and adenoidectomy: An inpatient or outpatient? *Laryngoscope* 100:491, 1990.

Gysin C, Alothman GA, Papsin BC: Sinonasal disease in cystic fibrosis: Clinical characteristics, diagnosis, and management. *Pediatr Pulmonol* 30:481, 2000.

Hartnick CJ, Cotton RT: Stridor and airway obstruction. In Bluestone CD, Stool SE, editors: *Pediatric otolaryngology*. Philadelphia, 2003, WB Saunders, pp 1437–1447.

Hatcher IS, Stack CG: Postal survey of the anaesthetic techniques used for paediatric tonsillectomy surgery. *Paediatr Anaesth* 9:311, 1999.

Haynes DS, Harley DH: Surgical management of chronic otitis media: Beyond tympanotomy tubes. *Otolaryngol Clin North Am* 35:827, 2002.

Healy GB: The appropriateness of tympanostomy tubes for children. *JAMA* 273:700, 1995a.

Healy GB: Surgery of the larynx and trachea. In Bluestone CD, Stool SE, editors: *Atlas of pediatric otolaryngology*. Philadelphia, 1995b, WB Saunders.

Hengerer AS, Wein RO: Congenital malformations of the nose and paranasal sinuses. In Bluestone CD, Stool SE, editors: *Pediatric otolaryngology*. Philadelphia, 2003, WB Saunders, pp 979–994.

Herbert RL, Bent JP: Meta-Analysis of outcomes of pediatric functional endoscopic sinus surgery. *Laryngoscope* 108:796, 1998.

Hermens JM, Bennett MJ, Hirshman CA: Anesthesia for laser surgery. *Anesth Analg* (Paris) 62:218, 1983.

Hern JD, Jayaraj SM, Sidhu VS, et al.: The laryngeal mask airway in tonsillectomy: The surgeon's perspective. *Clin Otolaryngol Allied Sci* 24:122, 1999.

Hinkle AJ: What wisdom is there in administering elective general anesthesia to children with active upper respiratory tract infection? *Anesth Analg* 68:413, 1989.

Hoekelman RA: Epiglottitis: Another dying disease? *Pediatr Ann* 23:229, 1994.

Hoeve LJ, Rombout J: Pediatric laryngobronchoscopy: 1332 procedures stored in a database. *Int J Pediatr Otorhinolaryngol* 24:73, 1992.

Holland BW, McGuirt WF Jr: Surgical management of choanal atresia: Improved outcome using mitomycin. *Arch Otolaryngol Head Neck Surg* 127:1375, 2001.

Hulka GF: Head and neck manifestations of cystic fibrosis and ciliary dyskinesia. *Otolaryngol Clin North Am* 33:1333, 2000.

Hwang J, St John WM, Bartlett D: Respiratory related hypoglossal nerve activity: Influence of anesthetics. *J Appl Physiol* 55:785, 1983.

Isono S, Shimada A, Utsugi M, et al.: Comparison of static mechanical properties of the passive pharynx between normal children and children with sleep-disordered breathing. *Am J Respir Critical Care Med* 157:1204, 1998.

James I: Cuffed tubes in children. *Paediatr Anaesth* 11:259, 2001.

Jellish WS, Jensen RL, Anderson DE, et al.: Intraoperative electromyographic assessment of recurrent laryngeal nerve stress and pharyngeal injury during anterior cervical spine surgery with Caspar instrumentation. *J Neurosurg* 91:170, 1999.

Jellish WS, Leonetti JP, Murdoch JR, et al.: Propofol-based anesthesia as compared with standard anesthetic techniques for middle ear surgery. *J Clin Anesth* 7:292, 1995.

Johans TG, Reichert TI: An insufflation device for anesthesia during subglottic carbon dioxide laser microsurgery in children. *Anesth Analg* 63:368, 1984.

John RE, Hill S, Hughes TJ: Airway protection by the laryngeal mask: A barrier to dye placed in the pharynx. *Anaesthesia* 46:366, 1991.

Johnson JT, Schuller DE, Silver F, et al.: Antibiotic prophylaxis in high-risk head and neck surgery: One-day vs. five-day therapy. *Otolaryngol Head Neck Surg* 95:554, 1986.

Karl HW, Swedlow DB, Lee KW, Downes JJ: Epinephrine interactions in children. *Anesthesiology* 58:142, 1983.

Keon TP: Anesthetic considerations for laser surgery. *Int Anesthesiol Clin* 26:50, 1988.

Khine HH, Corddry DH, Kettrick RG, et al.: Comparison of cuffed and uncuffed endotracheal tubes in young children during general anesthesia. *Anesthesiology* 86:627, 1997.

Koivunen P, Alho OP, Uhari M, et al.: General anesthesia with and without nitrous oxide (N_2O) and the weight of middle ear effusion in children undergoing adenoidectomy and tympanostomy. *Laryngoscope* 106:724, 1996.

Kokosa I, Eugene I: Chemical composition of laser-tissue interaction smoke plume. *J Laser Appl* 2:59, 1989.

Kosloske AM: Bronchoscopic extraction of aspirated foreign bodies in children. *Am J Dis Child* 136:924, 1982.

Kretz FJ, Reimann B, Stelzner J, et al.: The laryngeal mask in pediatric adenotonsillectomy. A meta-analysis of medical studies [in German]. *Anaesthesist* 49:706, 2000.

Krishna P: Post-tonsillectomy bleeding: A meta-analysis. *Laryngoscope* 111:1358, 2001.

Landsman IS: Mechanisms and treatment of laryngospasm. *Int Anesthesiol Clin* 35:67, 1997.

Laser-resistant tracheal tubes. *Health Devices* 21:4, 1992.

Leicht P, Wisborg T, Chraeinrner-Jorgensen B: Does intravenous lidocaine prevent laryngospasm after extubation in children? *Anesth Analg* 64:1193, 1985.

Liebowitz HM, Peacock GR: Cortical injury produced by carbon dioxide laser radiation. *Arch Ophthalmol* 52:993, 1980.

Lines V: Anaesthesia for laryngoscopy and microlaryngeal surgery in children. *Anaesth Intensive Care* 1:507, 1973.

Liu YH, Li MJ, Wang PC, et al.: Use of dexamethasone on the prophylaxis of nausea and vomiting after tympanomastoid surgery. *Laryngoscope* 111:1271, 2001.

Lusk R: Surgical management of chronic rhinosinusitis. In Bluestone CD, Stool SE, editors: *Pediatric otolaryngology*. Philadelphia, 2003, WB Saunders, pp 1013–1020.

Maekawa S, Fukuda K, Yamauchi T, et al.: Follow-up study of pharyngeal carriers of beta-hemolytic streptococci among school children in Sapporo City during a period of 2 years and 5 months. *J Clin Microbiol* 13:1017, 1981.

Manning SC, Stool SE: Foreign bodies of the pharynx and esophagus. In Bluestone CD, Stool SE, editors: *Pediatric otolaryngology*. Philadelphia, 2003, WB Saunders, pp 1324–1337.

Mannucci PM: Desmopressin: A non-transfusional form of treatment for congenital and acquired bleeding disorders. *Blood* 72:1449, 1988.

Marcus CL: Sleep-disordered breathing in children. *Am J Respir Crit Care Med* 164:16, 2001.

Marcus CL, Greene MG, Carroll JL: Blood pressure in children with obstructive sleep apnea. *Am J Respir Crit Care Med* 157:1098, 1998.

Marcus CL, Lutz J, Hamer A, et al.: Developmental changes in response to sub atmospheric pressure loading of the upper airway. *J Appl Physiol* 87:626, 1999.

Marcus CL, McColley SA, Carroll JL, et al.: Upper airway collapsibility in children with obstructive sleep apnea syndrome. *J Appl Physiol* 77:918, 1994.

Mattucci KF, Militana CJ: The prevention of fire during oropharyngeal electrosurgery. *Ear Nose Throat J* 82:107–109, 2003.

Mauro RD, Poole SR, Lockhart CH: Differentiation of epiglottitis from laryngotracheitis in the child with stridor. *Am J Dis Child* 142:679, 1988.

Maze A, Bloch E: Stridor in pediatric patients. *Anesthesiology* 50:132, 1979.

McColley SA, April MM, Carroll JL, et al.: Respiratory compromise after adenotonsillectomy in children with obstructive sleep apnea. *Arch Otolaryngol Head Neck Surg* 118:940, 1992.

McCulloch TM, Richardson MA, Flint PW, et al.: Lidocaine effects on the laryngeal chemoreflex, mechanoreflex, and afferent electrical stimulation reflex. *Ann Otol Rhinol Laryngol* 101:583, 1992.

McDonald IH, Stocks JG: Prolonged nasotracheal intubation: A review of its development in a pediatric hospital. *Br J Anaesth* 37:161, 1965.

McGahren ED: Esophageal foreign bodies. *Pediatr Rev* 20:129, 1999.

McGoldrick KE: Tonsillectomy and adenoidectomy: Avoiding complications. *Day Surg Patient* 2:1, 1993.

McGovern PH: Bilateral choanal atresia in newborns: A new method of medical management. *Laryngoscope* 71:480, 1961.

McGowan FX, Kenna MA, Fleming JA, et al.: Adenotonsillectomy of upper airway obstruction carries increased risk in children with a history of prematurity. *Pediatr Pulmonol* 13:222, 1992.

Megerian CA, Reily J, O'Connell FM, et al.: Outpatient tympanomastoidectomy: Factors affecting hospital admission. *Arch Otolaryngol Head Neck Surg* 126:1345, 2000.

Messner AH: Treating pediatric patients with obstructive sleep disorders: An update. *Otolaryngol Clin North Am* 36:519, 2003.

Miman MC, Kirazli T, Ozyurek R: Doppler echocardiography in adenotonsillar hypertrophy. *Int J Pediatr Otorhinolaryngol* 54:21, 2000.

Miyamoto RT, Kirk KI: Cochlear implants in children. In Bluestone CD, Stool SE, editors: *Pediatric otolaryngology*. Philadelphia, 2003, WB Saunders, pp 808–816.

Miyasaka K, Sloan IA, Froese AB: An evaluation of the jet injector (Sanders) technique for bronchoscopy in paediatric patients. *Can Anaesth Soc J* 27:117, 1980.

Moore JK, Moore EW, Elliott RA, et al.: Propofol and halothane versus sevoflurane in paediatric day-case surgery: Induction and recovery characteristics. *Br J Anaesth* 90:461, 2003.

Motoyama EK: Anesthesia and the upper airway in infants and children. *Int Anesthesiol Clin* 30:17, 1992.

Motoyama EK, Fine GF, Jacobson KH, et al.: Accelerated increases in end-tidal CO_2 ($P_{ET}CO_2$) in anesthetized infants and children during rebreathing. *Anesthesiology* 94:A1276, 2001.

Motoyama EK, Glazener CI: Hypoxemia after general anesthesia in children. *Anesth Analg* 65:267, 1986.

Myers EN, Stool SE, Johnson JT: Technique of tracheotomy. In Myers EN, Stool SE, Johnson JT, editors: *Tracheotomy*. New York, 1985, Churchill Livingstone.

Nezhat C, Winen WK, Nezhat C, et al.: Smoke from laser surgery: Is there a health hazard? *Laser Surg Med* 7:376, 1987.

Nikanne E, Kokki H, Tuovinen K: Perioperative ketoprofen in small children during adenoidectomy. *Br J Anaesth* 78:24, 1997.

Noonan JA: Reversible cor pulmonale due to hypertrophied tonsils and adenoids; studies in two cases. *Circulation* 32:164, 1965.

Norton ML: Anesthesia for laser surgery in laryngobronchoesophagology. *Otolaryngol Clin North Am* 16:785, 1983.

Norton ML, deVos P: New endotracheal tube for laser surgery of the larynx. *Ann Otol Rhinol Laryngol* 87:554, 1978.

Norton MI, Strong MS, Baughan CW, et al.: Endotracheal intubation and Venturi (jet) ventilation for laser microsurgery of the larynx. *Ann Otol Rhinol Laryngol* 85:656, 1976.

Nowill WK, Ridall EG: Blood loss during adenotonsillectomy. *Surgery* 66:856, 1969.

Ochiai R, Guthrie RD, Motoyama EK: Differential sensitivity to halothane anesthesia of the genioglossus, intercostals and diaphragm in kittens. *Anesth Analg* 74:338, 1992.

Ochiai R, Guthrie RD, Motoyama EK: Effects of varying concentrations of halothane on the activity of the genioglossus, intercostals, and the diaphragm in cats: An electromyographic study. *Anesthesiology* 70:812, 1989.

Oh TH, Motoyama EK: Comparison of nasotracheal intubation and tracheostomy in management of acute epiglottitis. *Anesthesiology* 46:214, 1977.

Ossof RH: Laser safety in otolaryngology—head and neck surgery: Anesthetic and educational considerations for laryngeal surgery. *Laryngoscope* 99:1, 1989.

Ossof RH, Duncavage IA, Eisenman TS, et al.: Comparison of tracheal damage from laser-ignited endotracheal tube fires. *Ann Otol Rhinol Laryngol* 92:333, 1983.

Palel R, Norden J, Hannallah RS: Oxygen administration prevents hypoxemia during postanesthetic transport in children. *Anesthesiology* 69:616–618, 1988.

Pappas AL, Fluder EM, Creech S, et al.: Postoperative analgesia in children undergoing myringotomy and placement equalization tubes in ambulatory surgery. *Anesth Analg* 96:1621, 2003.

Pappas AL, Sukhani R, Hotaling AJ, et al.: The effect of preoperative dexamethasone on the immediate and delayed postoperative morbidity in children undergoing adenotonsillectomy. *Anesth Analg* 87:57, 1998.

Paradise JL: Tonsillectomy and adenoidectomy. In Bluestone CD, Stool SE, editors: *Pediatric otolaryngology*. Philadelphia, 2003, WB Saunders, pp 1210–1222.

Paradise JL, Bluestone CD, Rogers KD, et al.: Efficacy of adenoidectomy for recurrent otitis media in children previously treated with tympanostomy-tube placement results of parallel randomized and nonrandomized trials. *JAMA* 263:2066, 1990.

Paradise JL, Feldman HM, Campbell TF, et al.: Early versus delayed insertion of tympanostomy tubes for persistent otitis media: Developmental outcomes at the age of three years in relation to prerandomization illness patterns and hearing levels. *Pediatr Infect Dis J* 22:309, 2003.

Pashayan AG: *Anesthesia for laser surgery. ASA Refresher Course,* No. 221. Park Ridge, IL, 1994, American Society of Anesthesiologists.

Pashayan AG, Gravenstein JS: Helium retards endotracheal tube fires from carbon dioxide lasers. *Anesthesiology* 62:274, 1985.

Pawar DK: Dislodgement of bronchial foreign body during retrieval in children. *Paediatr Anaesth* 10:333, 2000.

Pelton SI, Shurin PA, Klein JO: Persistence of middle ear effusion after otitis media. *Pediatr Res* 11:504, 1977.

Pirsig W: Surgery of choanal atresia in infants and children: Historical notes and updated review. *Int J Pediatr Otorhinolaryngol* 11:153, 1986.

Postma DS, Prazma J, Woods CI, et al.: Use of steroids and a long-acting vasoconstrictor in the treatment of postintubation croup. A ferret model. *Arch Otolaryngol Head Neck Surg* 113:844, 1987.

Prasad M, Ward RF, April MM, et al.: Topical mitomycin as an adjunct to choanal atresia repair. *Arch Otolaryngol Head Neck Surg* 128:398, 2002.

Prinsley P, Wood M, Lee CA: Adenotonsillectomy in patients with inherited bleeding disorders. *Clin Otolaryngol* 18:206, 1993.

Rah KH, Salzberg AM, Boyan CP, et al.: Respiratory acidosis with the small Storz-Hopkins bronchoscopes: Occurrence and management. *Ann Thorac Surg* 27:197, 1979.

Rampil IJ: Anesthetic considerations for laser surgery. *Anesth Analg* 74:424, 1992.

Randall DA, Hoffer ME: Complications of tonsillectomy and adenoidectomy. *Otolarygol Head Neck Surg* 118:61, 1998.

Ravussin P, Bayer-Berger M, Monnier P, et al.: Percutaneous transtracheal ventilation for laser endoscopic procedures in infants and small children with laryngeal obstruction: Report of two cases. *Can J Anaesth* 34:83, 1987.

Reber A, Pagonini R, Frei FJ: Effect of common airway manoeuvres on upper airway dimensions and clinical signs in anaesthetized, spontaneously breathing children. *Br J Anaesth* 86:217, 2001.

Ring WH, Adair JC, Elwyn RA: The new pediatric endotracheal tube. *Anesth Analg* 54:237, 1975.

Rontal M, Rontal E, Wenokur M: Jet insufflation anesthesia for endolaryngeal surgery. *Laryngoscope* 90:1162, 1980.

Rothschild MA, Cotcamp D, Cotton RT: Postoperative medical management in single-stage laryngotracheoplasty. *Arch Otolaryngol Head Neck Surg* 121:1175, 1995.

Ruder CB, Raphael NL, Abramson AL, et al.: Anesthesia for carbon dioxide laser microsurgery of the larynx. *Otolaryngol Head Neck Surg* 89:732, 1981.

Rutter MJ, Yellon RF, Cotton RT: Management and prevention of subglottic stenosis in infants and children. In Bluestone CD, Stool SE, editors: *Pediatric otolaryngology*. Philadelphia, 2003, WB Saunders, pp 1519–1542.

Sanders RD: Two ventilating attachments for bronchoscopes. *Del Med J* 39:170, 1967.

Sasaki CT: Development of laryngeal function: Etiologic significance in the sudden infant death syndrome. *Laryngoscope* 89:1964, 1979.

Scamman FL, McCabe BF: Supraglottic jet ventilation for laser surgery of the larynx in children. *Ann Otol Rhinol Laryngol* 95:142, 1986.

Scanlon P, Carey M, Power M, et al.: Patient response to laryngeal mask insertion after induction of anaesthesia with propofol or thiopentone. *Can J Anaesth* 40:816, 1993.

Schechter MS: Section on pediatric pulmonology, Subcommittee on Obstructive Sleep Apnea Syndrome. Technical report: Diagnosis and management of childhood obstructive sleep apnea syndrome. *Pediatrics* 109:69, 2002.

Schloss MD, Hannallah R, Baxter JD: Acute epiglottitis: 26 years' experience at the Montreal Children's Hospital. *J Otolaryngology* 8:259, 1979.

Schloss MD, Pham-Dang H, Rosales JK: Foreign bodies in the tracheobronchial tree—a retrospective study of 217 cases. *J Otolaryngol* 12:212, 1983.

Schwartz AJ, Downes JJ: Hazards of a simple monitoring device, the esophageal stethoscope. *Anesthesiology* 47:64, 1977.

Seliman OL, Patel RI, Hannallah RS: Change in arterial oxygen saturation in the pediatric patient during postoperative transport. *Anesthesiology* 65:447, 1986.

Shprintzen RJ: Pierre Robin, micrognathia, and airway obstruction: The dependency of treatment on accurate diagnosis. *Int Anesthesiol Clin* 26:64, 1988.

Simpson JI, Schiff GA, Wolf GL: The effect of helium on endotracheal to be flammability. *Anesthesiology* 73:538, 1990.

Smith RB, Schaer WB, Pfaeffle H: Percutaneous transtracheal ventilation for anesthesia and resuscitation: a review and report of complications. *Can Anesth Soc J* 22:607–612, 1975.

Smith RM: Anesthesia for pediatric otolaryngology. In Ferguson CE, Kendig EL Jr, editors: *Pediatric otolaryngology*. Philadelphia, 1972, WB Saunders.

Smith RM: *Anesthesia for infants and children*, 4th ed. St Louis, 1980, CV Mosby.

Snow JC, Kripke BJ, Strong MS, et al.: Anesthesia for carbon dioxide laser microsurgery on the larynx and trachea. *Anesth Analg (Cleve)* 53:507, 1974.

Snow JC, Norton ML, Suluja IS, et al.: Fire hazard during CO_2, laser microsurgery on the larynx and trachea. *Anesth Analg* 55:146T, 1976.

Soprano JV, Fleisher GR, Mandl KD: The spontaneous passage of esophageal coins in children. *Arch Pediatr Adolesc Med* 153:1073, 1999.

Sosis MB: Evaluation of five metallic tapes for protection of endotracheal tubes during CO laser surgery. *Anesth Analg* 68:392, 1989a.

Sosis MB: What is the safest endotracheal tube for Nd-YAG laser surgery? A comparative study. *Anesth Analg* 69:802, 1989b.

Sosis M, Dillon F: What is the safest foil tape for endotracheal tube protection during Nd-YAG laser surgery? A comparative study. *Anesthesiology* 72:553, 1990.

Spoerel WE, Narayanan PS, Singh NP: Transtracheal ventilation. *Br J Anaesth* 43:932, 1971.

Sterni LM, Tunkel DE: Obstructive sleep apnea in children: An update. *Pediatr Clin North Am* 50:427, 2003.

Steward DL, Welge JA, Myer CM: Steroid for improving recovery following tonsillectomy in children. *Cochrane Database Syst Rev* 1: CD003997, 2003.

Stool SE, Eavey R: Tracheostomy. In Bluestone CD, Stool SE, editors: *Pediatric otolaryngology*, 2nd ed. Philadelphia, 1990, WB Saunders.

Stool SE, Eavey RD: Tracheotomy. In Bluestone CD, Stool SE, editors: *Pediatric otolaryngology*. Philadelphia, 2003, WB Saunders, pp 1226–1243.

Strong MS, Jako EJ, Polyani T, et al.: Laser surgery in the aerodigestive tract. *Am J Surg* 126:529, 1973.

Suzuki M, Sasaki CT: Laryngeal spasm: A neurophysiologic redefinition. *Ann Otol Rhinol Laryngol* 86:150, 1977.

Szekely E, Farkas E, Matyas G, et al.: Comparative studies of the IgA content of bronchial secretion, nasal secretion and serum in children with chronic respiratory tract diseases. *Kinderarztl Prax* 46:67, 1978.

Tagaito Y, Isono S, Nishino T: Upper airway reflexes during a combination of propofol and fentanyl anesthesia. *Anesthesiology* 88:1459, 1998.

Tait AR, Knight PR: The effects of general anesthesia on upper respiratory tract infections in children. *Anesthesiology* 67:930, 1987.

Teele DW: Inflammatory diseases of the mouth and pharynx. In Bluestone CD, Stool SE, editors: *Pediatric otolaryngology*. Philadelphia, 1983, WB Saunders.

Teele DW, Healy GB, Tally FP: Persistent effusions of the middle ear: Cultures for anaerobic bacteria. *Ann Otol Rhinol Laryngol* 89:102, 1980.

Telfik TL, Kaloustian VM: *Congenital anomalies of the ear, nose and throat*. New York, 1997, Oxford Press, pp 218–219.

Travis KW, Todres ID, Shannon DC: Pulmonary edema associated with croup and epiglottitis. *Pediatrics* 59:695, 1977.

Tunnessen WW Jr, Feinstein AR: The steroid-croup controversy: An analytic review of methodologic problems. *J Pediatr* 96:751, 1980.

Tusman G, Bohn SH, Tempra A, et al.: Effect of recruitment maneuver on atelectasis in anesthetized children. *Anesthesiology* 98:14, 2003.

Ueda W, Hirakawa M, Mae O: Appraisal of epinephrine administration to patients under halothane anesthesia for closure of cleft palate. *Anesthesiology* 58:574, 1983.

Uezono S, Goto T, Terui K, et al.: Emergence agitation after sevoflurane versus propofol in pediatric patients. *Anesth Analg* 91:563, 2000.

Van Der Spek AF, Spargo PM, Norton ML: The physics of lasers and implications for their use during airway surgery. *Br J Anaesth* 60:709, 1988.

Ved SA, Walden TL, Montana J, et al.: Vomiting and recovery after outpatient tonsillectomy and adenoidectomy in children. Comparison of four anesthetic techniques using nitrous oxide with halothane or propofol. *Anesthesiology* 85:4, 1996.

Verghese ST, Hannallah RS: Pediatric otolaryngologic emergencies. *Anesthesiol Clin North Am* 19:237, 2001.

Voepel-Lewis T, Malviya S, Tait AR: A prospective cohort study of emergence agitation in the pediatric postanesthesia care unit. *Anesth Analg* 96:1625, 2003.

Walander A: The mechanism of origin of congenital malformation of the larynx. *Acta Otolaryngol* 45:426, 1955.

Walner DL, Loewen MS, Kimura RE: Neonatal subglottic stenosis–incidence and trends. *Laryngoscope* 111:48, 2001.

Ward RF: Treatment of tracheal and endobronchial lesions with the potassium titanyl phosphate laser. *Ann Otol Rhinol Laryngol* 10:205, 1992.

Warner DO: Airway pharmacology. In Benumof JL, editor: *Airway management*. Boston, 1996, Mosby, p 74.

Watcha MF, Ramirez-Ruiz M, White PF, et al.: Perioperative effects of oral ketorolac and acetaminophen in children undergoing bilateral myringotomy. *Can J Anaesth* 39:649, 1992.

Werkhaven JA: Laryngotracheal laser surgery. In Bluestone CD, Stool SE, editors: *Atlas of pediatric otolaryngology*. Philadelphia, 1995, WB Saunders.

Wetmore RF: Tracheotomy. In Bluestone CD, Stool SE, editors: *Pediatric otolaryngology*. Philadelphia, 2003, WB Saunders, pp 1583–1598.

Wetmore RF, Marsh RR, Thompson ME, et al.: Pediatric tracheostomy: A changing procedure? *Ann Otol Rhinol Laryngol* 108:695, 1999.

Widlund B, Vlaczak S, Motoyama E: Flow pressure characteristics of pediatric Storz-Hopkins bronchoscope. *Anesthesiology* 54:341, 1983.

Widlund B, Walczak S, Motoyama E: Flow-pressure characteristics of pediatric Storz-Hopkins bronchoscopes. *Anesthesiology* 57:A417, 1982.

Williams PJ, Bailey PM: Comparison of the reinforced laryngeal mask airway and tracheal intubation for adenotonsillectomy. *Br J Anaesth* 70:30, 1993.

Wilson JW, Robertson CF: Angiogenesis in paediatric airway disease. *Paediatr Respir Rev* 3:219, 2002.

Wolf GL, Simpson II: Flammability of endotracheal tubes in oxygen and nitrous oxide-enriched atmosphere. *Anesthesiology* 67:236, 1987.

Wood RE, Postma D: Endoscopy of the airway in infants and children. *J Pediatr* 112:1, 1988.

Woods AM: Pediatric endoscopy. In Berry FA, editor: *Anesthetic management of difficult and routine pediatric patients*, 2nd ed. New York, 1990, Churchill Livingstone, pp 199–242.

Yellon RF, McBride TP, Davis HW: Otolaryngology. In Zitelli BJ, Davis HW, editors: *Atlas of pediatric physical diagnosis*, 4th ed. St Louis, 2002, Mosby, pp 818–865.

Yellon RF, Parameswaran M, Brandom BW: Decreasing morbidity following laryngotracheal reconstruction in children. *In Anesthesiol Clin* 35:145, 1997.

24 Anesthesia for Pediatric Dentistry

Andrew Herlich

In view of the advances in health care, dental disease is still among the most prevalent of diseases, according to the Centers for Disease Control and Prevention. For instance, the incidence of dental caries in children is 7 times more common than hay fever and 5 times more common than asthma in children. Maternal nutritional and behavioral influences are so strong that the mother will likely pass caries to her infant (American Academy of Pediatrics, 2003). The impact of caries is pervasive; poor nutrition may cause them or be the result of them. However, fluoridation of community water supplies, use of children's vitamins containing fluoride, and increased awareness of dental hygiene have produced a significant reduction in dental caries in the general population.

Despite the advances in preventive dentistry, there are still conditions that require more than local anesthesia to facilitate dental treatment. General anesthesia may be required to treat children with severe systemic disease or disabling congenital anomalies and infants or toddlers with milk-bottle caries who require partial or complete oral rehabilitation. General anesthesia may also be required for those children and adolescents with severe developmental delay who require a safe and effective environment to render the necessary dental treatment. In addition, the fearful or combative child may require procedural sedation when behavior modification techniques have not succeeded. A glossary of commonly used dental terminology is shown in Box 24–1.

HUMAN DENTITION

DENTAL DEVELOPMENT

Initial calcification of the primary tooth buds may be seen in the fourth month of prenatal life. In general, by the end of the sixth prenatal month, all of the primary teeth have begun to develop. The newborn infant is edentulous, with the rare exception of a mandibular central incisor. This natal or neonatal tooth tends to be quite mobile and, in the past, was thought to require immediate extraction. Recent data suggest that by the end of the neonatal period, this mobile tooth becomes quite stable and capable of normal masticatory function. It is indeed fortunate for the infant, because these neonatal teeth are frequently the only primary teeth that develop in that position (King and Lee, 1989; Cunha et al., 2001).

The sequence of eruption of human teeth may critically affect infant feeding, behavioral, and masticatory skills. Major changes in the appearance of the dentition in the oral cavity probably alter important aspects of neurobehavioral development (Wright, 2000). As an example of eruption sequence alterations, premature infants and neonates requiring prolonged orotracheal intubation have significant defects in both oral and dental structures that may persist up to age 5 years, despite the absence of the orotracheal tube (Fadavi et al., 1992).

The order of appearance of the teeth in the oral cavity tends to follow generalized patterns. Usually the teeth erupt in pairs. A mandibular right central incisor erupts approximately at the same time as the mandibular left central incisor, at approximately 6 to 7 months of age. The mandibular teeth usually precede their maxillary counterparts; the maxillary incisors erupt approximately 1 month later than the mandibular incisors. The eruption sequence continues and is usually complete by age 2 to 2 $^1/_2$ years. The last tooth to erupt is the deciduous second molar, or "2-year molar," so named because of its appearance at age 2 years. The order of appearance of the primary or deciduous teeth is shown in Table 24–1.

When completed, the primary dentition totals 20 teeth (Wright, 2000). As the toddler's growth continues, the mandible and maxilla enlarge, causing separations, also known as diastemata, between the primary teeth (Zwemer, 1993). The diastemata increase as the primary teeth are beginning to exfoliate and the permanent or succedaneous teeth begin to erupt. The separations also permit sufficient room for the proper alignment of the permanent dentition.

The maintenance of the health and hygiene of the primary teeth is essential to avoid premature tooth loss. When primary teeth are prematurely lost as a result of decay or trauma, the space needed for the permanent tooth eruption is also lost because the natural tendency of the tooth is to tip mesially (toward the midline) in the oral cavity. Subsequently, dental malocclusions tend to occur. Finally, the primary teeth may also function as the permanent teeth if the permanent analogous tooth fails to develop (Wright, 2000).

The transition period between exfoliation of the primary teeth and eruption of the permanent teeth is called the mixed-dentition phase. This phase continues until the last primary

BOX 24–1 Glossary of Common Dental Terminology

Proper Name	Common name/defination
Abutment	Tooth/teeth on either side of an edentulous area supporting a bridge
Amalgam	Silver-coated restoration
Bicuspid	Premolar tooth (older term)
Bitewing	Dental radiograph that views several adjacent maxillary and mandibular teeth simultaneously; especially useful in evaluating dental caries
Bruxism	Involuntary tooth grinding
Bur	Drill bit used to prepare a tooth for caries restoration
Caries	Dental cavity
Composite	Tooth-colored restoration
Crown	Portion of the tooth seen in the mouth above the gum line; also, term used for the dental restoration of the same anatomic region; popularly known as a cap
Cuspid	Canine tooth (older term)
Diastemata	Separations between the teeth; commonly seen between the maxillary central incisors
Dry socket	Nonhealing extraction site
Endodontic therapy	Root canal therapy
Exfoliation	Spontaneous loss of a tooth
Exodontia	Dental extraction
Eye tooth	Canine tooth (familiar term)
Gingivitis	Inflammation of superficial aspects of the peridontium
Handpiece	Dental drill
Ludwig's angina	Dental infection of the floor of the mouth involving the submandibular, submaxillary, and submental spaces bilaterally
Milk tooth	Primary or baby tooth
Occlusion	Patient's "bite"
Oral prophylaxis	Dental cleaning
Overbite	Degree of vertical overlap of the maxillary teeth over the mandibular teeth
Overjet	Degree of horizontal projection of the maxillary teeth beyond the mandibular teeth
Periapical	Structures surrounding the apex of the root; a periapical dental radiograph also includes the clinical crown of the tooth
Periodontium	Soft and hard tissues surrounding and supporting teeth
Pulpotomy	Therapeutic removal of the coronal portion of the dental pulp
Pyorrhea	Common name for periodontal or gum disease; except for gingivitis, periodontal disease is rare in children
Rubber dam	Square latex or vinyl sheet used to isolate the teeth from the oral cavity during dental treatment

tooth is normally exfoliated or extracted. Unlike the primary teeth, the permanent teeth normally erupt so that there is tooth-to-tooth contact.

The first molars, or 6-year molars, are the first permanent teeth to erupt. Similar to their primary counterparts, the mandibular teeth usually precede the maxillary teeth. The permanent incisors, beginning at approximately age 6 to 7 years. Unlike the primary dentition, where there is usually a variability of several months in the timing of eruption, the permanent teeth may vary as much as 1 to 2 years in eruption sequence. The general eruption sequence of permanent teeth is noted (see Table 24–1). At the completion of the eruption sequence, the permanent dentition consists of 32 teeth (Wright, 2000) (see Table 24–1).

The third molars, also commonly known as "wisdom teeth," have the least predictable eruption sequence of any of the human dentition. They may erupt as early as age 15 to 16 years, as late as age 25 years, or not at all. Quite commonly, the third molars fail to erupt because of dental germinal pattern alterations or impactions within the soft or hard tissues. Impactions usually occur because of insufficient bony growth of the maxilla or mandible in proportion to the individual's full dental complement.

In addition to the frequently absent third molars, two other permanent tooth forms are sometimes congenitally absent. The mandibular premolars and the maxillary lateral incisors may be congenitally absent, either singly or in symmetric pairs (Neville et al., 2002). Occasionally, a tooth that is thought to be congenitally absent is actually impacted within the soft tissues or alveolar bone.

Just as there are congenitally absent teeth, there are supernumerary or accessory teeth. The most common supernumerary tooth is the mesiodens, a conically shaped tooth consistently located in the midline between the maxillary central incisors. Other supernumerary teeth are the third premolars and fourth maxillary molars (Neville et al., 2002).

DENTAL IDENTIFICATION

There are two principal universal dental identification systems. In both systems, the primary teeth are designated by letters and the permanent teeth are designated by numbers. These systems differ in the way that the dental arches (mandible and maxilla) are divided. The first system uses a sequential means for identification, with the primary maxillary right second molar designated as tooth A and followed sequentially around the contralateral side of the maxilla to the left second molar, which is tooth J. The primary mandibular left second molar is tooth K, and the system is completed upon reaching the mandibular right second molar, tooth T. Similarly, the numbering system for the permanent dentition starts with the maxillary right third molar as tooth 1 and continues to the maxillary left third molar, tooth 16.

TABLE 24–1. Eruption sequence of the human dentition

Tooth	Eruption	Age When Root Completed (yr)
Primary Dentition		
Maxillary		
Central incisor	7 ½ mo	1 ½
Lateral incisor	9 mo	2
Cuspid	18 mo	3 ¼
First molar	14 mo	2 ½
Second molar	24 mo	3
Mandibular		
Central incisor	6 mo	1 ½
Lateral incisor	7 mo	1 ½
Cuspid	16 mo	3 ¼
First molar	12 mo	2 ¼
Second molar	20 mo	3
Permanent Dentition		
Maxillary		
Central incisor	7 to 8 yr	10
Lateral incisor	8 to 9 yr	11
Cuspid	11 to 12 yr	13 to 15
First bicuspid	10 to 11 yr	12 to 13
Second bicuspid	10 to 12 yr	12 to 14
First molar	6 to 7 yr	9 to 10
Second molar	12 to 13 yr	14 to 16
Mandibular		
Central incisor	6 to 7 yr	9
Lateral incisor	7 to 8 yr	10
Cuspid	9 to 10 yr	12 to 14
First bicuspid	10 to 12 yr	12 to 13
Second bicuspid	11 to 12 yr	13 to 14
First molar	6 to 7 yr	9 to 10
Second molar	11 to 13 yr	14 to 15

From Schour I, Massler M: The development of the human dentition. *JADA* 28:1153, 1941. Reprinted by permission of ADA Publishing Co.

The system continues with the mandibular left third molar, tooth 17, and is completed with the mandibular right third molar, tooth 32 (Herlich, 1990). Both pediatric and general dentists commonly use this system of tooth identification.

The second designation system divides the dental arch into quadrants. All primary central incisors are tooth A and follow distally or posteriorly, so that all primary second molars are tooth E. To make the designation more specific, the quadrant is also named. For example, the primary maxillary right lateral incisor would be designated maxillary right B. Similarly, the permanent dentition is divided into quadrants. All central incisors are tooth 1 and continue posteriorly, so that all third molars are tooth 8. This system is most commonly used by orthodontists (Fig. 24–1, *A* and *B*).

DENTAL ANATOMY AND PHYSIOLOGY

The tooth is composed of a crown, which is usually visible for clinical examination, and a root, which is not seen during routine clinical examination. They are separated by the cementoenamel junction or cervical region of the tooth (Fig. 24–2). The cementoenamel junctions are seen more commonly in adult dentition if gingival ("gum") recession occurs. The crown is responsible for the slicing, ripping, and grinding of foodstuffs (incisors, canines, and molars, respectively). The root structure imparts stability to the tooth in its surrounding tissues. The anterior teeth, the incisors and the canines, are single-rooted with a conical shape. The posterior teeth, the premolars and molars, are multirooted and impart most of their stability by both the number of roots and the subtle divergent directions in which the roots may grow.

Surrounding the root structure of the tooth is the periodontium. The periodontium is composed of three structures as follows:

1. The most external portion is a combination of the gingival and alveolar mucosa, which constitute the soft tissue covering for the remainder of the periodontal structures.
2. The periodontal ligament attaches the external surface of the root to the alveolar bone, acting as a shock absorber and anchor during masticatory function.
3. The bony component is called the alveolar bone or tooth socket. It should be noted that beneath the alveolar bone rests the supporting basal or skeletal bone. Basal bone is the part seen in edentulous patients and forms the skeletal support for full or partial dentures. When the tooth structure is lost, alveolar bone is also lost and is not naturally regenerated.

The individual teeth are composed of enamel, dentin, dental pulp, and cementum (Wright, 2000) (see Fig. 24–2). The enamel covers the external surface of the dental crown. It is the hardest substance in the human body and, unlike bone, has no living cells. When intact, enamel functions as a thermal insulator and an impervious barrier to chemicals and microorganisms.

On the internal surface of the enamel lies the dentin. It is composed of microtubules and has living cells within the dentinal structure. When tooth decay is advanced, noxious stimuli are readily transmitted via the dentinal tubules to the underlying dental pulp. The neurovascular supply of the individual teeth is contained within the dental pulp. Pain is easily elicited by many different stimuli—thermal, tactile, or liquid. The pain is transmitted from the dental pulp through the root apices to the alveolar bone and subsequently to the body's pain receptors.

The final portion of the tooth structure is the dental cementum, which covers the external surface of the roots. Because it is not nearly as hard and impervious to the surroundings as is enamel, noxious stimuli are perceived when the cementum is exposed. The cementum is similar to the dentin of the tooth. Patients who enjoy good dental health usually do not have exposed cementum. However, with gingival and alveolar recession, root structure and its investing cementum may be exposed to the external environment.

Some morphologic differences exist between deciduous and succedaneous teeth. The most obvious difference exists in the absolute size of the teeth in general. The deciduous teeth are significantly smaller than their permanent counterparts. With respect to the molars, the buccal-lingual dimensions are proportionately more narrow. In contrast, the mesial-distal dimensions are proportionately larger.

Another difference between the sets of dentition rests in the color of the enamel. The primary teeth are "milky white" or opalescent; hence, the name "milk teeth" may be used. The permanent teeth, on the other hand, are significantly less "milky" because of the pigment absorption that has occurred during their development or has been acquired during the intraoral lifetime of the tooth (Wright, 2000). Two examples are tetracycline staining (developmental) and caffeine staining (acquired).

The pulp chambers of the primary teeth are proportionately larger than the permanent teeth because of the relative thinness of the deciduous enamel and dentin (Wright, 2000). Less than

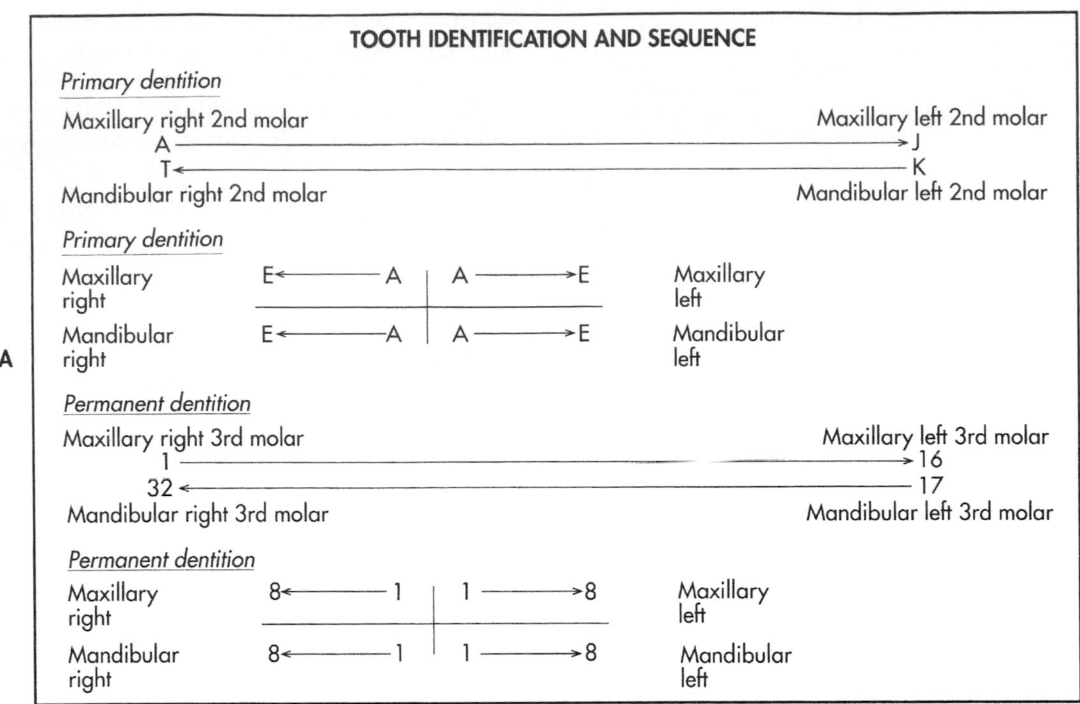

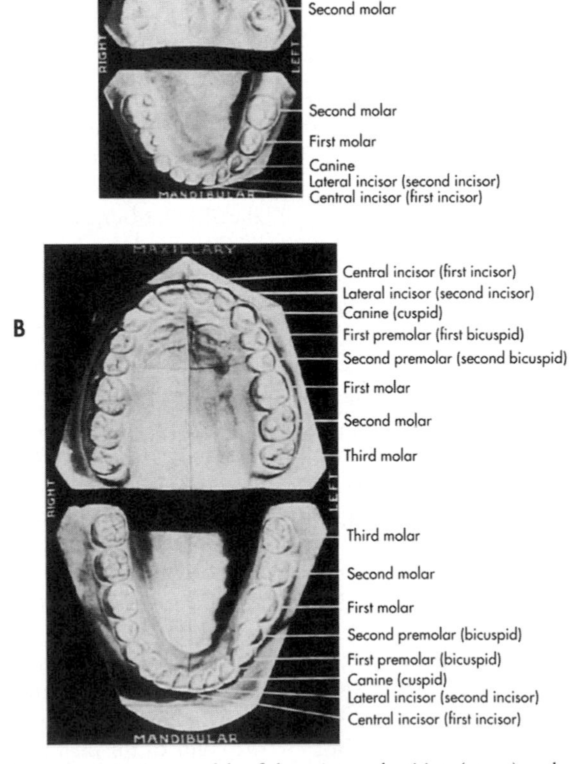

■ **FIGURE 24–1.** *A*, Tooth identification and sequence. *B*, Cast models of the primary dentition (upper) and permanent dentition (lower). (*A* from Herlich A: Dental complications of anesthesia. *Prog Anesthesiol* 11:250, 1990. *B* from Ash MM Jr [ed]: *Wheeler's dental anatomy, physiology, and occlusion,* 7th ed. Philadelphia, 1993, WB Saunders, p 2.)

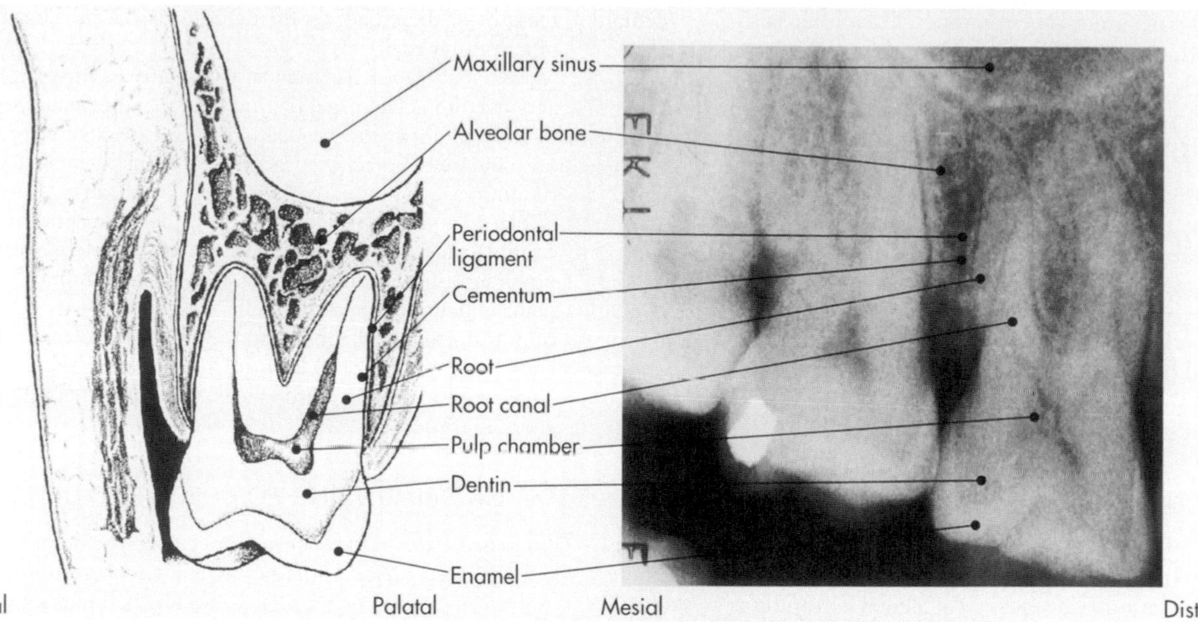

■ **FIGURE 24–2.** A schematic (*left*) and radiographic (*right*) view of a right maxillary molar. (Modified with permission from Ash MM Jr [editor]: *Wheeler's dental anatomy, physiology, and occlusion,* 7th ed. Philadelphia, 1993, WB Saunders, p 6.)

meticulous dental restorations or large carious lesions may predispose the primary teeth to pulpal or endodontic therapy earlier than their permanent counterparts.

The root structures of the primary molars are more saber shaped and extend laterally beyond the crown width. This unique root structure allows adequate room for the permanent tooth bud to develop and mature until the exfoliative process is completed for the primary tooth (Wright, 2000).

■ PATIENT SPECTRUM

The population base of the pediatric dentist or pedodontist is generally comprised of healthy children who are able to comprehend and follow simple directions by the pedodontist and their staff. However, during their training of 2 years or longer, pediatric dentists are trained to treat the following patient groups:

- Physically handicapped adolescents and adults
- Neonates, young infants, and toddlers too young to cooperate with routine dental care
- Fearful, unmanageable, or psychologically challenged children
- The entire spectrum of medically compromised children
- Children with dental problems in a hospital critical care unit
- Children with orofacial trauma
- Children requiring interceptive or minor orthodontic care

The physically handicapped patient most likely to appear for treatment by the pedodontist has athetoid cerebral palsy, postencephalitis syndrome, profound mental retardation, or autistic behavior (Dougherty et al., 2001; Shenkin et al., 2001; Waldman and Perlman, 2001). For instance, patients with cerebral palsy may be wheelchair bound and have significant difficulty in controlling the athetoid motion. The use of nitrous oxide, which depresses involuntary movement in cerebral palsy, may ensure a higher success rate in dental treatments for the patients (Kauffman et al., 1991). The pedodontist is specially trained to deal with these problems in the kindest and most expedient methods available regardless of the clinical setting (Rosenstein, 1978; Pope and Curzon, 1991).

The pedodontist may be called on to fabricate a presurgical appliance for cleft lip and palate infants in the newborn period. These presurgical appliances facilitate surgical closure of the palate. They also improve sucking and feeding in the cleft lip and palate patient. Some toddlers may have developed circumoral burns from child abuse or domestic accidents. As a result, they may need an acrylic prosthesis to protect the child from shrinkage of circumoral tissues.

Emotionally impaired children or those who are too fearful to undergo routine treatment by a general dentist frequently are referred to the pediatric dentist who is both familiar with and comfortable in the treatment of such patients.

On a routine basis, the pediatric dentist is called on to treat the medically compromised child or adolescent with whom the general practitioner is reluctant to get involved in treatment. For instance, the pediatric dentist primarily treats the child with congenital heart disease, the insulin-dependent diabetic, the patient with craniofacial anomalies, or the child with oncologic diseases in conjunction with the pediatrician or primary care physician. Both fear and lack of training may cause the general dentist to feel quite uncomfortable in treating the compromised child or adolescent. In addition, the general dental practitioner frequently lacks the physical resources, such as specialized equipment, to care for these patients. The pediatric dentist is usually quite comfortable in recommending and prescribing antibiotic prophylaxis for subacute bacterial endocarditis, for example, and keeps current with appropriate timing in dosage, effectiveness, and relative risks (Wahl, 1994; Hayes and Fasules, 2001; American Academy of Pediatric Dentistry, 2000, 2002).

A few unfortunate children may develop such severe illnesses or injuries that they require prolonged admissions in critical care units. These severely ill children also need dental care, which takes place at the bedside. As an example, the child who has sustained significant head injuries may develop neuropathic chewing, which damages dental tissues, specifically by wearing down teeth via grinding action, or damages soft tissues such as tongue or cheek maceration. The pedodontist can fabricate an intraoral acrylic appliance to prevent further damage to oral tissues.

Finally, the pediatric dentist may be called to the emergency department of a hospital to treat orofacial trauma. This situation is more common in pediatric hospitals, where pediatric dental house officers are on 24-hour call with attending supervision. In general hospitals without specified pediatric dental services, the oral and maxillofacial surgeon usually handles pediatric dental trauma.

DENTIST'S NEEDS AND TECHNIQUES

The pediatric dental patient requiring anesthesiology services usually needs many dental procedures during a single anesthetic administration. The quality of dental restorations is probably improved under general anesthesia (Tate et al., 2002; Al-Eheideb and Herman, 2003). In addition, the parents of children who have had general anesthesia for pediatric dental care have greater satisfaction than those parents of children who did not have general anesthesia (Acs et al., 2001). After induction of general anesthesia and protection of the airway, the anesthesiologist, the anesthesia machine, and the anesthesia equipment cart are positioned at either the patient's head or side.

The dentist's first step is to obtain necessary intraoral radiographs of the teeth (periapical, bitewing, and occlusal radiographs). Subsequently, the dentist performs a clinical examination. After placement of a pharyngeal pack (which should be noted on the anesthesia record), dental impressions may be taken if future orthodontic treatment is anticipated. Also, the dentist usually places a rubber dam around the dental arch to be treated. The rubber dam is more commonly nonlatex despite its name. Nevertheless, in the latex-sensitive patient, care must be taken to ensure that nonlatex products are being used. The rubber dam is held in place by a metal clamp that grasps the dental crown. A substantial length of dental floss or umbilical tape is tied around the clamp before its placement to prevent inadvertent loss in the aerodigestive tract. Except for extractions and oral prophylaxis, the remainder of the treatment is performed with the rubber dam in place. Caries removal and tooth restoration take place with silver amalgam, tooth colored composite, or preformed crowns. The rubber dam affords the dentist a dry environment in which the dental materials optimally cure and achieve their greatest compressive and tensile strength. The rubber dam also is a barrier to protect the patient from iatrogenic dental trauma, including the accidental loss of dental materials or broken instruments and their possible entrance into the aerodigestive tract. The application of topical fluorides takes place after all of the restorative dentistry is completed with the rubber dam still in place (Mathewson and Primosch, 1995).

When severe malocclusion, facial skeleton dysmorphism, or tooth loss prevents rubber dam placement, the dentist still needs to maintain a dry intraoral environment. Injection of glycopyrrolate (0.007 to 0.01 mg/kg) or atropine (0.01 to 0.02 mg/kg) immediately after the placement of the intravenous cannula affords satisfactory intraoral conditions. The pedodontist places cotton rolls along the buccal and lingual or facial and palatal margins of the adjacent soft tissues to assist in the achievement of a dry oral cavity.

Pediatric dentistry may also encompass the need for oral and maxillofacial surgery. Oral and maxillofacial surgeons frequently perform the procedures with extensive training. Many oral and maxillofacial surgeons have dual dental and medical training, as well as fellowship training in head and neck surgery or plastic and reconstructive surgery. Because children may have craniofacial anomalies, including orofacial clefts, orthognathic problems, tumors, and blunt or penetrating trauma, such surgical management requires the ability to combine cosmesis, restoration of normal occlusion, and the promotion of normal growth and development of the entire facial skeleton (Kaban, 1993; Vig and Fields, 2000; Ord et al., 2002; Oza et al., 2002; Zeltser et al., 2003).

CLINICAL SETTING FOR PEDIATRIC DENTISTS

Most pediatric dental treatment occurs in the dental office without the need for psychologic or pharmacologic intervention to address the child's fear and anxiety. The hallmark of dental pain management is a kind practitioner and staff and the responsible use of adequate local/topical anesthesia. For one group of patients, simple behavior modification techniques improve the level of cooperation in the dental chair. These techniques include the tell-show-do method and voice control for the fearful, hostile, or disruptive child. The tell-show-do technique involves explaining before the procedure, demonstrating the procedure outside of the child's mouth, and then actually performing the procedure on the patient. This technique removes the fear of the unknown from the procedure (Lenchner and Wright, 1975). Voice control involves modulation of both the volume and tone of the dentist's voice to achieve positive behavioral results (Wilson, 1994). A preschool child, for whom behavior modification is deemed necessary, should rationally be scheduled during the morning because the child's longest attention span and optimal level of cooperation are early in the day. Additional "behavior modification techniques" have been used by the dentist to physically restrain frightened children. Included in these techniques are hand-over-mouth exercise, passive physical restraint with a rigid board (Papoose Board), and active physical restraint by dental personnel. These techniques are controversial because of their potential psychologic trauma and legal implications (Nathan, 1989; Wilson, 1994; Wright, 1994). Despite its controversy, the "hand-over-mouth" technique is an acceptable technique by the American Academy of Pediatric Dentistry provided written consent is obtained from the legal guardian before its use (American Academy of Pediatric Dentistry, 2002).

Local anesthetic blocks are the greatest proportion of analgesia for pediatric dental procedures. Most blocks are local infiltration in the maxillary region or mandibular nerve blocks in the mandible. Adverse reactions seldom occur to local anesthesia when administered alone. Most commonly they are related to a relative overdose or lapse in technique. However, it may take a small dose inappropriately injected to cause palpitations, diaphoresis, or even dizziness (Kaufman et al., 2000). Rarely does vasomotor collapse occur. True allergic reactions are probably the smallest proportion of untoward reactions, including allergy to metabisulfite or other preservatives of local anesthesia, including *para*-aminobenzoic acid (Campbell et al., 2001).

Behavior modification may include such novel approaches as hypnosis or music therapy. Highly motivated, intelligent, attentive, or anxious children may have a good emotional and analgesic response to hypnosis when other forms of behavior modification, including pharmacologic forms, are precluded (Kleinhauz and Eli, 1993). Children as young as 3 to 4 years of age may be successfully hypnotized in the dental office (Lampshire, 1975). Music did not diminish pain, anxiety, or disruptive behavior in a recent study (Aitken et al., 2002) despite anecdotal beliefs of pediatric dentists and parents. Nevertheless, in this study, the patients enjoyed listening to the music and chose to listen to music in subsequent visits.

Electroanesthesia (transcutaneous electronic nerve stimulation [TENS]) has been successfully used in children in the dental office setting. TENS is reported to be effective based on several interrelated theories. These pain control theories include gate control, endorphin release, and serotonin release. For dental procedures, disposable electrode pads are placed bilaterally in the treated dental arch after drying the buccal mucosa. Using a dentally specific TENS device, a pulse rate of 110 Hz, and a pulse width of 225 microseconds in the normal mode, amplitude is slowly increased until the desired response is obtained. Twitching of the lower lip is the amplitude end point in the mandibular arch, and twitching of the orbicularis oculi is the amplitude end point in the maxillary arch. Children are instructed to raise a hand if the amplitude is too uncomfortable, and it is subsequently diminished (te Duits et al., 1993). This technique works best in the area of restorative dentistry in the teeth that have relatively shallow lesions with respect to the dentoenamel junction (Quarnstrom, 1992; te Duits et al., 1993).

There are no published data that have accurately quantified the numbers of pediatric patients requiring either oral or parental sedation or general anesthesia. The spectrum of use of sedation is illustrated by the fact that medication including nitrous oxide is being used less than in previous years and studies. The most recent study by Houpt (2002) suggests that although more sedation is being used, it is being used by fewer practitioners on more patients in the United States. A retrospective review of pediatric sedation management suggests that at one U.S. dental school pediatric dental clinic, nonpharmacologic behavioral management is favored more frequently because of greater success (Eid, 2002). One British study has estimated that more than 300,000 general anesthetics are still being administered for dentistry in the Great Britain, mostly for children. This same study suggests that the number of general anesthetics available for dentistry is much less than it was in the 1970's (Blayney et al., 1999). It is implied that most general anesthetics in Great Britain, however, are provided in a hospital setting, as opposed to the United States.

Most pediatric dentists and those treating handicapped patients are experienced in the use of nitrous oxide and oral premedication when necessary in the dental office. The reported advantages of nitrous oxide delivered via a Goldman nasal mask include analgesia and sedation (Nathan et al., 1988). The incidence of diffusion hypoxia is minimal after the use of nitrous oxide and oxygen alone as opposed to nitrous oxide supplementation to parenteral or oral sedatives (Quarnstrom et al., 1991; Dunn-Russell et al., 1993). Hypoxemia in general may occur when 30% to 50% nitrous oxide is added to chloral hydrate sedation (Litman et al., 1998). In children with enlarged tonsils, oral midazolam 0.5 mg/kg and 50% nitrous oxide resulted in significant upper airway obstruction and implied hypoxia (Litman et al., 1998).

The American Society of Anesthesiologists Physical Status I and II patients are appropriate candidates for treatment with pharmacologic adjuncts within the dental office setting. If a child's Physical Status is III or beyond, the hospital setting is probably a wiser choice. Again, it must be emphasized that the pediatric dentist should use local anesthesia to optimize analgesia and anesthesia for the patient. Local anesthesia may add to the potential complications of polypharmacy if attention is not paid to doses that are age and weight appropriate. This is especially true in the pediatric age group. The pediatric dentist rarely uses intramuscular or intravenous sedation while serving as both the operator and the practitioner administering the sedation.

There are reports of severe adverse outcomes, including hypoxic brain damage and occasional deaths, with the use of nitrous oxide, local anesthesia, and other premedicants. Invariably, these adverse outcomes result from relative or absolute overdosage of one or a combination of nitrous oxide, local anesthetic, or parenteral medication (Goodson and Moore, 1983; Doyle and Goepferd, 1989; Coté et al., 2000a). Because of the widely publicized adverse outcomes of dental office sedation and general anesthetics, the trend in this type of care has been to move away from the dental office unless guidelines by the American Academy of Pediatric Dentistry are followed. These guidelines were promulgated in 1985 and restated in 2001 to promote and ensure that the public is aware and the pediatric patient is protected. The guidelines describe which practitioner is able to administer general anesthesia/deep sedation and where it can be provided.

In the United Kingdom, a group of investigators has performed several retrospective analyses during the 1970s and 1980s. Retrospective data obtained from a national data bank indicated that dental office deaths are infrequent and that the number has decreased substantially in the second survey. The decreases in deaths probably result from two factors. First, fewer general anesthetics are being administered in the dental office. Second, the concept of the single dental practitioner/anesthetist is becoming less frequent because of warnings and suggestions from the General Dental Council of Great Britain. The anesthetist and dental practitioner are more commonly two individuals, each of whose attention is directed toward a single task. Also, the British survey indicated that the person providing anesthesia is more commonly a physician (Coplans and Curson, 1982, 1993). In the United States, closed claims morbidity and mortality involving oral surgeons suggest that during the period of 1988 to 1999, there were 22 deaths in the office and 136 anesthesia-related claims in total. It was calculated that the death rate was 1 in every 747,732 (0.013:10,000) administrations of anesthesia in the dental office (Deegan, 2001).

In the United States, opposing forces create difficulties for the pediatric dental patient. Economic issues tend to restrict hospital-based procedures, including payment for only the dental service without payment for the anesthesia service, payment for the anesthesia service without payment for the dental service, and frequently no or only partial payment for the hospital service. Frequently, the patient's family is faced with a significant out-of-pocket expense, which many can ill afford to pay. On the other hand, the litigious nature of our society has prevented the rational expansion of anesthesia services in the office environment beyond sedation. Mandated equipment and monitors and the cost of liability insurance may be prohibitive for the office practitioner.

Another issue that has significant economic concerns is the cost of multiple treatments in the dental office with procedural sedation as opposed to a single session in the operating room of the hospital under general anesthesia. In healthy patients aged 24 to 60 months, the investigators found that a patient who required more than three treatment visits with procedural sedation had more cost-effective treatment when all of the treatments were provided in a single visit under general anesthesia (Lee et al., 2001).

A reasonable compromise may be a well-equipped hospital-based or surgicenter dental clinic with standard monitoring devices and resuscitation equipment. Pediatric patients with American Society of Anesthesiologists status I through IV may be suitable candidates. With the use of proper equipment and appropriately trained personnel, a large diversity of patients may be safely and satisfactorily treated on an outpatient basis. If the clinic is rationally designed, including recovery areas equipped with oxygen, suction apparatus, and essential monitoring devices, the anesthesiologist may safely administer the anesthetic outside of the traditional operating room setting. It allows for more efficient use of time and space as well as reduced cost. From the perspective of the parent and child, outpatient treatment permits more rapid return to familiar surroundings and activities of daily living (Zuckerberg, 1994). Only the patients with disease or physical conditions that preclude off-site clinical practice need to be treated in the operating room in today's environment. Some examples of the patients who may need the traditional operating room setting include those with difficult airways, patients with coagulopathies, and those with complex anomalies or cardiovascular disease for whom more than standard monitoring is necessary.

SEDATION AND ANESTHESIA FOR DENTAL PROCEDURES

The key to success in anesthetic management is a good history and physical examination of the patient. The parent or caregiver of the child should be able to relate relevant data such as previous anesthetic successes and failures. These anesthetic experiences should also be related for any family members. Birth history, growth, and development, including psychological issues and the child's emotional status, may be helpful in conducting a safe and pleasant dental experience. If the child has significant fears or behavioral problems that warrant premedication, the historical background permits the anesthesiologist to select an appropriate premedication agent.

The physical examination of the child must include the airway. Despite plans for nasotracheal intubation, the oral cavity must also be examined, because nasotracheal intubation may not be successful. Loose teeth, enlarged tonsils and adenoids, or herpes labialis all affect the anesthesiologist's management of the airway. Issues of nasal obstruction or sinus disease also have a great impact on the decision-making process for airway management. Cardiac murmurs should be investigated as to their relative seriousness. Most cardiac murmurs are in fact innocent flow murmurs; however, reasonable percentages are pathologic conditions and warrant prophylaxis for endocarditis. Other factors, such as coagulation status, neurologic history, and recent viral syndromes, may also affect the anesthesiologist's decision-making process.

PROCEDURAL SEDATION

In 1985, The American Academy of Pediatric Dentistry established goals for sedation of the pediatric dental patient. These goals are as follows:

- To permit the practitioner to provide quality care
- To manage behavior that is disruptive to the surrounding environment
- To promote and provide a beneficial psychologic response to treatment
- To promote the overall welfare of the patient
- To produce a postoperative patient who safely meets discharge criteria in a positive psychologic state

With these goals in mind, procedural sedation of the pediatric dental patient may be considered. The foundations of pharmacologic sedation for the pediatric dental patient are monitoring standards to which all practitioners should adhere (Wilson, 2000). Minimum or moderate procedural sedation intended in the sensitive patient may become deep sedation or general anesthesia if vigilance is not applied. These standards have been promulgated by several organizations, including the American Society of Anesthesiologists (2002), the American Academy of Pediatrics (1985), the American Society of Dental Anesthesiologists, and the American Academy of Pediatric Dentistry (2002) (Consensus Conference, National Institutes of Health, 1985; Rosenberg and Campbell, 1991; Council on Scientific Affairs, American Medical Association, 1993). The American Academy of Pediatric Dentistry guidelines suggest that children who are status ASA III or IV should have treatment that necessitates sedation performed in a hospital environment.

Even with 50% nitrous oxide/oxygen, pulse oximetry and a precordial stethoscope are strongly encouraged by the American Academy of Pediatric Dentistry. Additionally, a full E cylinder of oxygen and a self-inflating bag and mask capable of delivering 15 L/min of oxygen must be available in the care facility. An important monitor is a trained individual whose sole duty is to pay attention to the electronic and mechanical monitors in place and who is prepared to act upon untoward events. As previously mentioned, the treating dentist should not be the person administering the anesthetic.

Before any sedation is administered, which includes nitrous oxide/oxygen, appropriate fasting guidelines must be given to the parents or guardians of the patient. Data suggest that prolonged fasts meant to reduce the likelihood of vomiting and aspiration are somewhat deleterious to patient outcome. Guidelines for fasting from solid foods, milk, and milk products remain at a minimum of 8 hours. However, clear liquids, including *pulpless* juices, plain gelatin, and ice Popsicles, are encouraged and acceptable until 2 hours before the anticipated arrival in the care facility. The pediatric patient is more cooperative and the parents are more satisfied as a result of these suggested guidelines (Schreiner, 1994). All of these guidelines are predicated upon normal gastrointestinal function. If the patient has abnormal gastrointestinal function, more conservative NPO orders must be considered.

Oral, intranasal/transoral, parenteral, and rectal routes for administration of sedative medications are used during procedural sedation. Pediatric dentists have traditionally and preferentially used the oral route to administer premedication (Primosch and Bender, 2001). The old practice of having the parents administer a prescribed oral medication at home has been fraught with danger in the toddler and young child. Airway obstruction and emesis with aspiration were real complications of that practice. For reasons of safety, practice has changed. Children are now brought to the treatment facility or dental office 1 hour ahead of the scheduled procedure time, and the oral premedication is administered under the guidance of the pediatric dentist. Two of the most popular agents have been hydroxyzine (1 to 2 mg/kg) and chloral hydrate (50 to 75 mg/kg; maximum dose, 2 g). These agents have had a good success rate and a reasonable margin of safety. In addition, nitrous oxide may be given in conjunction with the usual administration of local anesthetic blocks (Moore et al., 1984; Shapira et al., 1992). More potent oral agents, such as ketamine, meperidine, promethazine, diazepam, and midazolam, are also given in the treatment facility or dental office. The practitioner must allow for a reasonable time for onset of action before dental treatment (Sullivan et al., 2001). Oral midazolam has gained widespread popularity because of its reasonable margin of safety in addition to its rapid onset for either premedication before general anesthesia or as the main agent for procedural sedation (Kupietzky and Houpt, 1993; Levine et al., 1993). These agents may be given alone or with another agent—frequently, it is promethazine (Dallman et al., 2001; Bui et al., 2002; Nathan and Vargas, 2002).

Transmucosal fentanyl has been used successfully by one group of investigators in an oralet form. The fentanyl oralet permitted satisfactory separation from parents and mask induction of general anesthesia (Moore et al., 2000). The very high rate of emesis has limited the use of fentanyl oralets.

In many cases, mild oxygen desaturation was noted and easily treated with supplemental oxygen and repositioning of the patient's airway. In some cases, when nitrous oxide was added to the oral premedication, the degree of hypoxemia increased (Litman et al., 1998). The use of traditional monitors such as clinical observation, blood pressure, and pulse was clearly insufficient to assess the degree of hypoxemia. Pulse oximetry, capnography, and precordial stethoscopes have become necessary to adequately assess and prevent poor outcomes despite limitations in the pediatric dental environment (Anderson and Vann, 1988; Poiset et al., 1990; Wilson, 1990; Dunn-Russell et al., 1993). The use of supplemental oxygen also helps to reduce hypoxemia. Novel means of improving oxygenation include the delivery of supplemental oxygen via the saliva injector and the use of external nasal dilators (Milnes, 2002; Moses and Lieberman, 2003).

Intranasal or transoral administration of water-soluble agents such as ketamine, midazolam, or sufentanil produces effective sedation and premedication for procedural sedation. However, sufentanil produces a significantly high incidence of respiratory depression, even in relatively small doses (1.0 mcg/kg) and is not recommended (Abrams et al., 1993). Midazolam (0.5 mg/kg orally, or 0.3 mg/kg intranasally) is ideal for creating a milieu in which the child is easily separated from the parent. It also transforms a disruptive child into a quiescent child in the dental chair with minimal desaturation (Abrams et al., 1993; Levine et al., 1993). However, once the handpiece (dental drill) was activated, the noise distracted the child sufficiently that the pediatric dentist could not efficiently treat the child (Theroux et al., 1994). Despite the popularity of oral sedation, one group of investigators found that there was no relationship between oral sedation and behavior of the children in the dental office on subsequent visits (McComb et al., 2002).

The rectal route of administration for procedural sedation and premedication has enjoyed popularity with only a small number of practitioners. Midazolam (1.0 mg/kg or even higher doses) has been used for procedural sedation and for premedication. Onset of action usually occurs within 15 to 30 minutes (Roelofse and Van Der Bijl, 1991). The main drawback to rectal administration of these agents is the risk of expulsion of the sedative and the unreliable uptake for the distal colonic mucosa.

Many drugs have been used as parenteral agents for procedural sedation in pediatric dentistry. Opioids, benzodiazepines, antihistamines, ultra short-acting barbiturates, and dissociatives have been used successfully. All have had some negative features as well. Short-acting agents with acceptable margins of safety in dental sedation include methohexital, meperidine, ketamine, diazepam, and midazolam. Respiratory depression and concomitant hypoxia have been the recurrent theme in parenteral sedation by pediatric dentists (Allen, 1992; Coté et al., 2000a, 2000b). As previously mentioned, clinical observation was insufficient and the airway was subsequently lost. Because of the fine line between moderate procedural sedation, deep sedation, and general anesthesia, the dentist and assistant who administer procedural sedation must be experienced in recognizing and handling cardiorespiratory depression. Electrocardiography, pulse oximetry, blood pressure, capnography, and precordial stethoscope are essential monitors (Herlich, 1996).

Other drawbacks to intravenous sedation in pediatric dentistry have been the potential for inflicted pain to achieve intravenous access and the lack of familiarity with drug combinations on the part of the practitioner. The child's fear of pain from a needle puncture has been successfully addressed by inhalation of nitrous oxide in oxygen or the transmucosal administration of midazolam. Use of EMLA cream or transdermal lidocaine before venipuncture has been successful in reducing or eliminating needle puncture pain (Nilsson et al., 1994). Also, EMLA- and lidocaine-impregnated patches have been used intraorally with varying success before local anesthetic blocks and local procedures before the insertion of rubber dam clamps (Stecker et al., 2002). The main disadvantage of the use of transdermal local anesthetics is that it requires that EMLA be placed at least 45 minutes to 1 hour before a painful procedure.

In general, children undergoing sedation as opposed to general anesthesia underwent the same behavioral changes postoperatively. Their levels of stress and anxiety were essentially the same (Camm et al., 1987).

GENERAL ANESTHESIA

Induction and Maintenance

For children in whom procedural sedation is unsuccessful because of psychologic or medical factors, general anesthesia is required for dental procedures. Examples include patients with developmental delays, coagulopathies, or compromised cardiovascular systems in whom sophisticated monitoring techniques are necessary. In addition, general anesthesia is indicated in children for extensive or prolonged procedures such as complete oral rehabilitation for those with milk-bottle caries syndrome. Common conditions and procedures that require general anesthesia are listed (Box 24–2).

The traditional induction technique for general anesthesia in the pediatric age group in the United States has been inhalational anesthesia. The anesthesia mask is coated with a pleasant scent such as a fruit-scented lip balm. Sevoflurane, nitrous oxide and oxygen, or, less commonly, halothane nitrous oxide and oxygen is administered using high flows and concentrations

BOX 24–2 Conditions That May Require General Anesthesia in Pediatric Dentistry

- A child of less than 2 or 3 years of age with extensive dental caries such as milk bottle caries syndrome
- A neonate with a cleft palate who needs dental impressions for a presurgical appliance (before cleft lip and palate surgery). It may require only the presence of an anesthesiologist.
- Uncorrected or partially corrected congenital heart disease or other similarly advanced cardiopulmonary compromise
- Neurologic disorders such as poorly controlled seizures, athetoid cerebral palsy, or postencephalitic syndromes where patient movement is involuntary and uncontrollable
- Blood dyscrasias and coagulopathies
- Craniofacial anomalies in the toddler and young primary school–aged child such as Treacher Collins, Apert's, or Crouzon's syndrome or other severe orofacial clefting
- Any patient with receptive and/or expressive communication disorders such as moderate to severe mental retardation and autism
- Profound fear, anxiety, disruptive behavior, or other personal maladaptive behavior in the dental office where other pain or behavior control modalities have failed
- Severe orofacial trauma or infection requiring dental care such as incision and drainage, control of hemorrhage, or reduction of dental or bony fractures and dislocations
- Socioeconomic situations that preclude multiple return visits to the dentist wherein extensive dental treatment is needed
- Extensive dental care in a patient who is a candidate for major organ transplantation

while the anesthesiologist tells a story or provides another diversion. Intravenous induction techniques may include the use of a transdermal local anesthetic followed by the insertion of an intravenous cannula and subsequent administration of an appropriate intravenous agent, most commonly propofol or thiopental (Zuckerberg, 1994). Propofol may be mixed with lidocaine (1 mL of 1% lidocaine added to 9 mL of 1% propofol) to minimize local irritation and pain (see Chapter 10, Induction of Anesthesia). Other techniques for the induction of general anesthesia include rectal administration of methohexital, thiopental, ketamine, or midazolam (Martone et al., 1991; Roelofse and Van Der Brijl, 1991; Zuckerberg, 1994). The nasal or oral transmucosal administration of water-soluble agents such as ketamine or midazolam has also been used (Levine et al., 1993).

In children with intellectual or emotional handicaps in whom all other attempts have been futile, an intramuscular injection of ketamine/glycopyrrolate with or without midazolam is used. These techniques should only be attempted with appropriate monitoring and with the availability of oxygen, self-inflating resuscitation bag, and suction.

Once general anesthesia is induced, intravenous access and the airway are secured. All monitors may be placed before or after induction of anesthesia, depending on the cooperation of the patient. When possible, the first monitors that are placed, regardless of the timing of their placement, should be pulse oximetry and a precordial stethoscope. Careful positioning, padding, and application of thermal conservation devices must be accomplished before the beginning of dental treatment (see Chapter 10, Induction of Anesthesia).

The maintenance of general anesthesia may be accomplished with a volatile agent with nitrous oxide and oxygen, all intravenous agents, or a combination of intravenous and inhalational agents. If an intravenous agent is chosen for maintenance, an ideal agent may be propofol. It has the advantage of a short duration of action along with its antiemetic benefits (Coté, 1994). Remifentanil is also an appropriate choice.

Concerns have been raised over the appropriateness of the use of halothane versus sevoflurane for dental anesthesia with respect to cardiac arrhythmias. A study in the United Kingdom suggested that there were far more arrhythmias from the use of halothane than there were from the use of sevoflurane. An accompanying commentary in the same publication suggested that technique in terms of spontaneous versus controlled ventilation as well as the use of an endotracheal tube versus nasal mask would reduce or prevent such problems. Also, the use of anticholinergics may reduce these arrhythmias regardless of the use of halothane or sevoflurane (Blayney et al., 1999; Brandom and Herlich, 1999) (see Chapter 6, Pharmacology, and Chapter 10, Induction of Anesthesia).

Analgesia may be provided by morphine (0.10 mg/kg), meperidine (0.5 to 1.0 mg/kg), or fentanyl (1 to 4 mcg/kg). The nonsteroidal anti-inflammatory agent ketorolac (0.5 to 1.0 mg/kg) given intravenously as a single dose may be quite helpful. The untoward side effects of ketorolac, especially postoperative bleeding—are rare for dental procedures, especially with a single dose. Ketorolac should be avoided after extensive dental extractions (see Chapter 11, Intraoperative and Postoperative Management).

AIRWAY MANAGEMENT

Management of the airway during general anesthesia for dentistry is most commonly achieved via nasotracheal intubation. This route permits the dentist the greatest degree of freedom to treat the patient without the immediate presence of an orotracheal tube within the treatment area. The use of a preformed nasotracheal tube, such as the nasal RAE tube, maintains a low profile across the patient's nose and forehead. Care must be taken to prevent retraction pressure around the external nares when securing the tube. In addition, the eyes must be protected and the forehead padded. Caveats to nasotracheal intubation are the same for dental treatment as for any other nasotracheal intubation. Due to the higher incidence of bacteremia after nasal intubation in relation to oral intubation, as well as the high incidence of bacteremia following dental extraction and rehabilitation, it is imperative that children with congenital heart disease be given prophylactic antibiotics to prevent subacute bacterial endocarditis (Herlich, 1996) (see Chapter 10, Induction of Anesthesia).

Unusual intranasal foreign bodies, such as a piece of a toy, are occasionally seen in the pediatric age group. Careful inspection of the nares before nasotracheal intubation may reveal these foreign bodies. In addition, active upper respiratory tract or sinus infections, acutely inflamed turbinates, previous nasal surgery, cleft palate repair with pharyngeal flap, and hemorrhagic diathesis all present the anesthesiologist with the need to assess the relative risks to nasotracheal intubation. Previous craniofacial trauma with ongoing basilar skull disruption is a relative contraindication to nasotracheal intubation. Fiberoptic guidance of nasotracheal intubation helps reduce some of the attendant comorbidities that the anesthesiologist may face (Herlich, 1991). Complications of nasotracheal intubation include bacteremia, dislodgment of adenoidal tissue, and laceration of aerodigestive mucosa with subsequent false passage. Turbinate ulceration may also occur. Awake fiberoptic nasotracheal intubation may become the technique of choice when the child presents for urgent repair of maxillofacial trauma (Kaban, 1993). After adequate preparation of the patient, careful awake fiberoptic intubation may safely secure the airway with minimal alteration of the surrounding craniofacial structures (Gendelman and Herlich, 1993).

Fiberoptic intubation may become the rule rather than the exception in patients with mandibulofacial dysostosis (Treacher Collins syndrome), Pierre Robin sequence, Goldenhar's syndrome, and other congenital craniofacial anomalies. These patients frequently have palatal clefts and severe dental problems that require dental therapy as well as the possibility of orthognathic surgery (Gendelman and Herlich, 1993). If a fiberoptic laryngoscope is not readily available, a suction catheter may be placed inside of the nasotracheal tube to guide it through the nasal passages and act as an obturator (Herlich, 1996). Both techniques help reduce the risk or severity of epistaxis when topical vasoconstrictors are ineffective or contraindicated.

High-frequency jet ventilation has been used successfully in pediatric dentistry under general anesthesia under limited circumstances. After induction of general anesthesia, a No. 10 French suction catheter is passed into one of the nares; then high-frequency jet ventilation is initiated (Nazif and Sarner, 1991). The reported advantages of the technique include its rapidity and minimal trauma to the nasal passages with reduced risk of epistaxis. It also has the advantage of ease in patients with craniofacial syndromes such as Treacher Collins syndrome or patients with hemorrhagic diathesis. From the dentist's point of view, the small catheter used for high-frequency jet ventilation has the advantage of a very low profile and minimal interference with intraoral and extraoral radiographs. There are disadvantages to the technique that should not be overlooked. The airway is poorly protected with a small suction catheter used for ventilation. Also, because of the size of the catheter, inadvertent extubation occurred in several patients. Finally, the greatest disadvantage for the operating dentist is the difficulty in treating posterior teeth with advanced caries because of the posterior displacement of the tongue (Nazif and Sarner, 1991). Posterior dental extractions also presented with similar problems.

If nasotracheal intubation is precluded, an orotracheal tube is acceptable, provided the dentist and the anesthesiologist are aware of the need to frequently change the position of the endotracheal tube within the oropharynx and resecure the tube each time it is repositioned. A preformed orotracheal tube, such as the oral RAE tube, may be disadvantageous because it is designed to be a midline tube. Moving the preformed tube to either side of the mouth may cause an eccentric position within the trachea. An endobronchial intubation may also be possible creating difficulties in ventilation. If orotracheal intubation is needed, a conventional endotracheal tube easily moves to either side of the mouth and oropharynx with the compensatory eccentric tracheal position of the tube. The advantages of the orotracheal route of intubation in pediatric dentistry are the usual lack of associated trauma and the speed with which it may be accomplished. The disadvantages of orotracheal intubation for dental procedures include the necessity of moving the tube from one side of the mouth to the other and the decreased ability for the dental operator to place a rubber dam and complete dental treatment efficiently. Suboptimal position and placement of dental instruments may also occur when an orotracheal tube is in place. A pharyngeal pack reduces the likelihood that blood and debris are introduced into the aerodigestive tract. Notation of the time of insertion and pack removal from the pharynx on the anesthesia record saves needless airway embarrassment postoperatively.

The armored version of the laryngeal mask airway (LMA), or flexible LMA, may be indicated in some pediatric dental patients who need dental care under general anesthesia. The advantages of the LMA are its ease of placement and tolerance in the spontaneously ventilating patient. Similar to an orotracheal tube, its disadvantages include its presence in the oral cavity, the interference with rubber dam placement, and its larger size in comparison with a standard orotracheal tube. With a skilled pediatric dentist performing restorative dentistry or surgical procedures, minimal hemorrhage may be seen on the LMA at the end of the procedure (Alexander, 1990; Webster et al., 1993).

Despite meticulous technique on the part of the pediatric dentist and the placement of a rubber dam, dental materials may lodge in the oropharynx and subsequently enter the laryngotracheobronchial tree. Hence, a gentle but thorough cleaning and suctioning of the oropharynx before extubation are mandatory.

■ POSTOPERATIVE PROBLEMS

Most postoperative problems related to pediatric dentistry are common to many other surgical procedures. Postoperative pain, prolonged emergence difficulties with voiding and ambulation, and nausea and vomiting are all seen in pediatric dental patients. However, even after brief general anesthetics for dental procedures, significant hypoxemia may be encountered that is not relieved by administering supplemental oxygen alone. A British study demonstrated that experienced postanesthesia care nursing for dental procedures was the most effective means of preventing and treating hypoxemia after dental procedures (Lanigan, 1992).

Postoperative pain may be obviated by the early use of intraoperative administration of analgesics such as morphine (0.1 mg/kg), fentanyl (1 to 2 mcg/kg), or meperidine (1 to 2 mg/kg). In addition, an acetaminophen suppository (30 to 40 mg/kg), given shortly before the end of the procedure, confers additional analgesia with minimal side effects. Oral acetaminophen (10 to 15 mg/kg) may be even more effective if given preoperatively (Yaster et al., 1994).

Postoperative nausea and vomiting has numerous etiologies in the pediatric dental population. A common cause is swallowed blood. Once intraoral bleeding has ceased, the nausea and vomiting from this cause usually abate. Opioid use and abdominal distention caused by bag-mask ventilation with upper airway obstruction or with excessive pressure may also produce postoperative nausea and vomiting. Nitrous oxide is a controversial cause of postoperative nausea and vomiting. A cause of emesis or nausea unique to dentistry is the inadvertent ingestion of intraoperatively administered topical fluorides to reduce dental caries (Mathewson and Primosch, 1995).

With prolonged postoperative nausea and vomiting, increased hydration and antiemetics may be administered with their attendant caveats, including bladder distention, extrapyramidal effects, and prolonged sedation (Herlich, 1996). Ondansetron 100 to 150 mcg/kg is effective in lessening the severity of postoperative nausea and vomiting. Metoclopramide (50 to 100 mcg/kg) is also used but is less effective than ondansetron (Johnson, 1993). At the time of this writing, droperidol has been under the cloud of a "black box" warning from the Food and Drug Administration, and its use has essentially been curtailed. Nevertheless, it is still an effective and cost-effective antiemetic. Dexamethasone (0.1 to 0.2 mg/kg, up to a maximum of 10 mg) is another highly effective medication for the prevention and treatment of postoperative nausea and vomiting, especially in conjunction with ondansetron (see Chapter 11, Intraoperative and Postoperative Management). If the emesis is severe enough to warrant admission to the hospital for control and rehydration, the pediatric dentist requires the services of a primary care physician (presumably a pediatrician) to assume the overall management of the pediatric dental patient. Fluid and electrolyte management, as well as general patient welfare issues, may be beyond the scope and comfort level of the pediatric dentist. Also, hospital privileges may mandate co-management by the pediatric dentist and primary care physician.

Some postoperative problems appear more frequent among patients who have had dental rehabilitation, surgical removal of impacted teeth, or other surgical lesions. Postoperative hyperpyrexia seems to occur with greater frequency in patients in whom intraoral dental procedures have been performed. One group investigated preschool-aged children to ascertain the etiology of such febrile states. In a randomized fashion, some children were given oral antibiotics 1 hour before their procedure. All children received general anesthesia with nasotracheal intubation and subsequent packing of the oropharynx to reduce the incidence of aspiration of gastric contents and blood. Ventilation was controlled to reduce the likelihood of atelectasis as a cause of postoperative temperature elevation. Intravenous fluid therapy was administered to both groups to reduce the contribution of dehydration as a cause of postoperative temperature elevation. Both groups were found to have an equal rate of significant postoperative temperature elevation. The authors had suggested that other perioperative etiologies should be investigated, including anesthetic effects on temperature regulation during dental procedures (Holan et al., 1993). There may be certain dentally induced pyrogens, or a broader spectrum of antibiotic may be needed to cover an organism causing the hyperpyrexic bacteremia.

Nasotracheal intubation, as previously described, is the preferred method of airway protection. However, transient postoperative epistaxis is not uncommon in patients with boggy turbinates, traumatic intubation or extubation, or relatively stenotic nares (Herlich, 1996). Usually, direct pressure adequately treats the problem. Rarely, vasoconstrictors and intranasal packing are needed to treat the epistaxis.

Other sequelae of traumatic intubations or extubations, such as croup or generalized laryngeal edema, may need to be treated with intravenous dexamethasone (0.4 mg/kg) immediately after a traumatic or oversized intubation, and possible vasoconstrictors such as racemic epinephrine may be used after extubation.

Postobstruction or negative pressure pulmonary edema may be seen in children with large muscle mass or obesity. The patients are usually of the adolescent age group, but it can occur in children as young as 5 years (Van Kooy and Gargiulo, 2000; Ciavarro et al., 2002).

Postoperative oral bleeding should be treated with direct intraoral pressure if a site can be located. Generalized oozing of blood may be treated with gauze dental packs that have large extraoral tails for the purpose of retrieval. The oral packs act as compression dressings, which should be left in place for 2 hours and not be replaced unless there is significant ongoing hemorrhage. Premature removal or replacement dislodges clots that have not sufficiently matured and retracted into the dental socket. Persistent, minor oral hemorrhage after extraction may also be created.

Dislodgment of recently cemented crowns or appliances, inadvertent movement of dental packs, or avulsion of loose teeth not previously extracted may require the presence of the dentist in the postanesthesia care unit to treat the problem.

■ DENTAL COMPLICATIONS OF ANESTHESIA

The dental complications of anesthetic care are varied, usually minor, but a frequent source of malpractice claims. Most minor injuries are settled without going through malpractice litigation. In one study of a large tertiary medical center, the frequency of perianesthetic dental trauma requiring repair, stabilization, or removal of the tooth was approximately 1 in 4500 cases (Warner et al., 1999). Nevertheless, the anesthesiologist must be aware of the potential pitfalls and take appropriate safeguards. If a dental complication of anesthesia does occur, a dental consultation should be obtained as soon as possible. Also, the chief of the anesthesia department, the hospital's risk manager, and the patient's family should be notified. Patients old enough to understand what has transpired should also be informed.

The neonate is not immune from the dental complications of anesthesia. Laryngoscopy of the neonatal oral cavity may result in excoriation or laceration of the gum pads. Unilateral right- or left-sided hypoplastic enamel defects may be seen in the primary maxillary incisors as a result of laryngoscopy during the neonatal period (Angelos et al., 1989). Oropharyngeal airways, as well as suction devices, may also cause lacerations or excoriation of the intraoral soft tissues. Prophylactic use of water-soluble lubricants or saline solution applied to any of these devices before their placement reduces the likelihood of intraoral trauma.

Many of the children and their parents are aware of loose primary teeth during the preoperative visit. However, a careful examination, including a mobility check of each primary tooth before induction of general anesthesia, is appropriate (Maxwell et al., 1994).

If an excessively loose primary tooth is noted during the exfoliative phase, the parents should be informed, and it may be safely removed by the anesthesiologist once general anesthesia has been induced. In this increasingly litigious society, a separate, written consent may be necessary for removal of the loose primary tooth by the anesthesiologist. A gauze barrier is placed lingually to prevent inadvertent introduction of the tooth into more distal locations within the respiratory or gastrointestinal tract. Subsequently, the second gauze is wrapped around the loose tooth to be extracted. With a twisting and snapping action, the tooth is easily removed. The tooth is usually missing most or all of its root structure. The reason for the root structure loss is the natural resorptive processes that occur from the underlying permanent tooth that is beginning to erupt. If some of the root structure remains in the extraction site, no attempt should be made to retrieve it. The retrieval process may cause damage to the erupting permanent tooth bud. Also, the remaining root fragment naturally and harmlessly sequesters into the oral cavity (Herlich et al., 1996).

Conditions that may predispose the pediatric patient to dental avulsions under general anesthetic conditions include the scissors-like action of the anesthesiologist's fingers in the mouth opening before laryngoscopy. If this maneuver is accomplished using the incisors, the likelihood of inadvertent avulsion is increased. The mouth-opening maneuvers should be accomplished by using the molars whenever possible to take advantage of their inherent dental stability as well as to effect the largest opening possible. The use of oropharyngeal airways in the pediatric or adult patient as a bite block should be avoided for similar reasons. The anterior teeth are single rooted. If the patient closes the mouth with excessive force, the force transmission by the tooth is essentially perpendicular to the airway and leads to increased risk of avulsion or fracture. The ideal technique uses gauze bite blocks with a long retrieval tag placed along the molar teeth. The forces are now directed toward softer material and the multirooted molar teeth, which are more likely to sustain and evenly disperse the vertical, shear forces (Herlich, 1990; Herlich et al., 1996).

The inadvertent avulsion of loose primary teeth may nevertheless be unavoidable during airway manipulations. If a primary tooth is avulsed, it is imperative that it be retrieved. The tooth is usually found elsewhere in the mouth or outside of the oral cavity. It may also be found on the patient's gown or bed sheets or on the floor. If it cannot be located in these likely places, anteroposterior and lateral thoracoabdominal radiographs are necessary to locate the tooth. If the tooth is found in the digestive tract, it should pass without incident within several days. If the tooth is found in the tracheobronchial tree, however, it must be retrieved by whatever means necessary, including thoracotomy. The sequelae of leaving a foreign body in the tracheobronchial tree are extremely dangerous (Herlich, 1990; Herlich et al., 1996).

If a primary tooth was lost and then retrieved, it should not be reimplanted. Such attempts are usually futile because of its advanced root resorption before exfoliation. Reimplantation of a primary tooth may also cause significant damage to the underlying permanent tooth bud. However, if the avulsed tooth is a permanent tooth and morphologically intact, attempts should be made to reimplant it as soon as possible. The success of dental reimplantation depends on early reimplantation. Because the periodontal ligament has remnants attached to the tooth that are crucial to the success of reimplantation, the avulsed tooth should not be scrubbed with any material. Ideal preparation consists of *gentle rinsing* of the tooth in cool physiologic saline solution to remove crude debris and gross clots. Subsequently, the tooth should be placed in a cool saline-soaked gauze pad until a dentist can reimplant it either in the operating room or as early as possible during the postoperative period.

Reimplantation also includes splinting of the tooth to one or two adjacent teeth on each side of the reimplanted tooth to confer stability. Despite early reimplantation, failures exist and may necessitate root canal therapy or extraction at an unspecified later date. The time course of reimplantation failure is unpredictable (Herlich, 1990).

Pediatric dentistry has made many advances to conserve tooth structure and space if deciduous teeth are lost prematurely. Various polymer and metal crown structures may be bonded or cemented in place. Normal intraoral forces or untoward unnatural forces may cause these prosthetic devices to be loosened or avulsed during airway manipulations. For the most part, they may be easily recemented or bonded postoperatively. Most hospital dental consultants are able to rebond or recement these prostheses in place without difficulty.

Interceptive orthodontic appliances, such as mandibular lingual arch wires, maxillary segmental orthodontic wires, or both, are bonded by brackets to the teeth. These appliances may become loosened or avulsed during airway maneuvers. Similar to other prosthetic devices, they may also be recemented or bonded postoperatively with little harm to the patient or dentition (Herlich, 1990).

In general, a thorough preoperative history and examination and prudent warnings to the parent reduce dissatisfaction when inadvertent dental complications do occur. Congenital craniofacial anomalies, such as palatal clefts, mandibulofacial dysostosis (Treacher-Collins syndrome), Pierre Robin sequence, and hemifacial microsomia, may indeed increase the likelihood of dental complications because of intubation difficulties. Congenital dental anomalies, such as amelogenesis imperfecta or dentinogenesis imperfecta, may subject the patient to dental fracture with even the most trivial airway manipulations.

Acquired dental problems, such as milk-bottle caries syndrome, occur on the lingual surfaces of teeth in children who are regularly put to bed with a bottle of milk, formula, or glucose water. These carious lesions tend to require extensive pediatric dental rehabilitation in very young patients for whom prolonged dental visits are not feasible. As previously mentioned, those lesions may also be subject to the dental complications of anesthesia.

Pharmacologic agents such as oncologic chemotherapy, chronic inhaled or systemic steroids, diphenylhydantoin, and nifedipine may also cause intraoral or dental damage. A child with a blood dyscrasia or one who has had head and neck radiotherapy may also be subject to dental complications of anesthesia. Blood dyscrasias predispose the child to increased intraoral hemorrhage even during daily oral hygiene activities such as tooth brushing.

Head and neck radiation result in significant xerostomia (dry mouth) because of the destruction of the salivary glands. Because normal salivary flow has been eliminated, these children are at a very high risk for cervical (gumline) caries and possible dental complications during anesthesia. Regardless of the severity or nature of the injury, any head, neck, and oral trauma may predispose a patient to dental complications of anesthesia. With proper planning and care, the patient will have fewer and less severe dental complications (Herlich et al., 1996).

SUMMARY

A diverse and potentially challenging pediatric population requires dental care. For the most part, the dental needs of children are largely unknown by the physician population at large, short of their personal experience in the dental chair. This chapter addresses dental issues from the viewpoint of anatomy, physiology, and dental growth and development. The dentist's needs and technical confinements are elaborated to prepare for collaboration with the anesthesiologist in dealing with the spectrum of dental procedures. Particular attention is paid to the behavioral and physiologic needs of the pediatric dental population. Nonpharmacologic, pharmacologic, and practical technical strategies are suggested for both the dental operatory and operating room setting. The pitfalls and complications of each anesthetic technique are given to reduce the learning curve and the anesthesiologist's anxiety when problems do arise. Gentility and understanding of the pediatric dental patient are required to meet the challenges facing the anesthesiologist and ultimately improve patient care, as well as provide a background for future clinical research.

REFERENCES

Abrams R, Morrison JE, Villasenor A, et al.: Safety and effectiveness of intranasal administration of sedative medications (ketamine, midazolam, or sufentanil) for urgent brief pediatric dental procedures. *Anesth Prog* 40: 63, 1993.

Acs G, Pretzer S, Foley M, et al.: Perceived outcomes and parental satisfaction following rehabilitation under general anesthesia. *Pediatr Dent* 23:419, 2001.

Aitken JC, Wilson S, Coury D, et al.: The effect of music distraction on pain, anxiety, and behavior in pediatric dental patients. *Pediatr Dent* 24:114, 2002.

Al-Eheideb AA, Herman NG: Outcomes of dental procedures performed on children under general anesthesia. *J Clin Dent* 27:181, 2003.

Alexander CA: A modified Intavent laryngeal mask for ENT and dental anaesthesia [letter]. *Anaesthesia* 45: 892, 1990.

Alfonzo-Echeverria EC, Berg JH, Wild TW, et al.: Oral ketamine for pediatric outpatient dental surgery and sedation. *Pediatr Dent* 15: 182; 1993.

Allen GD: Diagnosis and treatment of respiratory problems in sedation and anesthesia in dentistry. *Anesth Prog* 39: 150, 1992.

American Academy of Pediatric Dentistry: Guideline on antibiotic prophylaxis for patients at risk. Revised 2002. *Pediatr Dent* 24:107, 2002.

American Academy of Pediatric Dentistry: Guideline on behavior management. *Pediatr Dent* 24:68, 2002.

American Academy of Pediatric Dentistry: Guideline on prevention of bacterial endocarditis. *Pediatr Dent* 24:109, 2002.

American Academy of Pediatric Dentistry: Guidelines for the elective use of conscious sedation, deep sedation and general anesthesia in pediatric dental patients. *Pediatr Dent* 24:74, 2002.

American Academy of Pediatrics: Oral health risk assessment timing and establishment of the dental home. *Pediatrics* 111:1113, 2003.

American Society of Anesthesiologists: Practice guidelines for sedation and analgesia by non-anesthesiologists: An updated report by the American Society of Anesthesiologists task force on sedation and analgesia by non-anesthesiologists. *Anesthesiology* 96:1004, 2002.

Anderson JA, Vann WF Jr: Respiratory monitoring during pediatric sedation: Pulse oximetry and capnography. *Pediatr Dent* 10:94, 1988.

Angelos G, Smith DR, Jorgenson R, et al.: Oral complications associated with oral tracheal intubation. *Pediatr Dent* 11:133, 1989.

Blayney MR, Malins AF, Cooper GM: Cardiac arrhythmias in children during outpatient general anaesthesia for dentistry: A prospective randomized trial. *Lancet* 354:1864, 1999.

Brandom BW, Herlich A: Safety of outpatient dental anaesthesia for children [commentary]. *Lancet* 354:1836, 1999.

Bui T, Redden RJ, Murphy S: A comparison study between ketamine and ketamine-promethazine in pediatric dental patients. *Anesth Prog* 49:14, 2002.

Camm JH, Mourino AP, Cobb EJ, et al.: Behavioral changes of children undergoing dental treatment using sedation versus general anesthesia. *Pediatr Dent* 9:229 1987.

Campbell JR, Maestrello CL, Campbell RL: Allergic response to metabisulfite in lidocaine anesthetic solution. *Anesth Prog* 48:21, 2001.

Canfield DW, Reiber K, Bennett CR: Oversedation in a pediatric patient: Case report. *Pediatr Dent* 9:111, 1987.

Cauldwell CB, Fisher DM: Sedating pediatric patients: Is propofol a panacea? *Radiology* 186:9, 1993.

Ciavarro C, Kelly JPW: Postobstructive pulmonary edema in an obese child after an oral surgery procedure under general anesthesia: A case report. *J Oral Maxillofac Surg* 60:1503, 2002.

Clokie C, Metcalf I, Holland A: Dental trauma in anaesthesia. *Can J Anæsth* 36:675, 1989.

Committee on Drugs, American Academy of Pediatrics: Consensus Conference; Guidelines for the elective use of conscious sedation, deep sedation and general anesthesia in pediatric patients. *Pediatrics* 76:317, 1985.

Consensus Conference, National Institutes of Health: Anesthesia and sedation in the dental office. *JAMA* 254:1073, 1985.

Coplans MP, Curson I: Deaths associated with dentistry and dental disease 1980-1989. *Anaesthesia* 48:435, 1993.

Coplans MP, Curson I: Deaths associated with dentistry. *Br Dent J* 153:357, 1982.

Coté CJ, Karl HW, Notterman DA, et al.: Adverse sedation events in pediatrics: Analysis of medications used for sedation. *Pediatrics* 106:633, 2000a.

Coté CJ, Notterman DA, Karl HW, et al.: Adverse sedation events in pediatrics: A critical incident analysis of contributing factors. *Pediatrics* 105:805, 2000b.

Coté CJ: Sedation for the pediatric patient. *Pediatr Clin North Am* 41:31, 1994.

Council on Scientific Affairs, American Medical Association: The use of pulse oximetry during conscious sedation. *JAMA* 270:1463, 1993.

Cunha RF, Carrilho-Boer FA, Dias-Torriani D, et al.: Natal and neonatal teeth: review of the literature. *Pediatr Dent* 23:158, 2001.

Dallman JA, Ingelzi MA Jr, Briskie DM: Comparing the safety, efficacy and recovery of intranasal midazolam vs. oral chloral hydrate and promethazine. *Pediatr Dent* 23:424, 2001.

Davis M: Conscious sedation practices in pediatric dentistry: A survey of members of the American Board of Pediatric Dentistry College of Diplomates. *Pediatr Dent* 10:328, 1988.

Deegan AE: Anesthesia morbidity and mortality, 1988-1999: Claims statistics from AAOMS National Insurance Company. *Anesth Prog* 48:89, 2001.

Dougherty N, Romer M, Lee RS: Trends in special care training in pediatric dental residencies. *J Dent Child* 68:384, 2001.

Doyle KA, Goepferd SJ: An allergy to local anesthetics? The consequences of misdiagnosis. *J Dent Child* 56:103, 1989.

Dunn-Russell T, Adair SM, Sams D, et al.: Oxygen saturation and diffusion hypoxia in children following nitrous oxide sedation. *Pediatr Dent* 15:88, 1993.

Eid H: Conscious sedation in the 21st century. *J Clin Pediatr Dent* 26:179, 2002.

Fadavi S, Adeni S, Dziedzic K, et al.: The oral effects of orotracheal intubation in prematurely born preschoolers. *J Dent Child* 59:420, 1992.

Finley GA, Mac Manus B, Sampson SE, et al.: Delayed seizures following sedation with propofol. *Can J Anæsth* 40:863, 1993.

Gendelman MS, Herlich A: Anesthesia for oral and maxillofacial surgery. *Prog Anesthesiol* 7:18, 1993.

Goldbeck LO: General anesthesia in dental offices. *JAMA* 255:1567, 1986.

Goodson JM, Moore PA: Life-threatening reactions after pedodontic sedation: An assessment of narcotic, local anesthetic, and antiemetic drug interaction. *J Am Dent Assoc* 107:239–245, 1983.

Goupil MT: Occupational health and environmental emergencies. In Bennett JD, Rosenberg MB, editors: *Medical emergencies in dentistry.* Philadelphia, 2002, WB Saunders, pp 513–524.

Hayes PA, Fasules J: Dental screening of pediatric cardiac surgical patients. *J Dent Child* 68:255, 2001.

Hennes HM, Wagner V, Bonadio WA, et al.: The effect of oral midazolam on anxiety of preschool children during laceration repair. *Ann Emerg Med* 19:1006, 1991.

Herlich A, Garber JG, Orkin FK: Dental and salivary complications. In Gravenstein N, Kirby RR editors: *Complications in anesthesiology*, 2nd ed. Philadelphia, 1996, Lippincott-Raven, pp 163–174.

Herlich A: Anesthesia for dentistry. In Motoyama EK, Davis PJ editors: *Smith's anesthesia for infants and children,* 6th ed. St Louis, 1996, Mosby–Year Book, pp 677–691.

Herlich A: Dental complications of anesthesia. *Prog Anesthesiol* 11:250, 1990.

Herlich A: Fiberoptic for head and neck patients. *Anesthesiol Clin North Am* 9:111, 1991.

Hersh EV, Helpin ML, Evans OB: Local anesthetic mortality: Report of a case. *J Dent Child* 58:489, 1991.

Holan G, Kadari A, Engelhard D, et al.: Temperature elevation in children following dental treatment under general anesthesia with or without prophylactic antibiotics. *Pediatr Dent* 15:99, 1993.

Holzman R: Morbidity and mortality in pediatric anesthesia. *Pediatr Clin North Am* 41:239, 1994.

Houpt M: Project USAP 2000–Use of sedative agents by pediatric dentists: A 15-year follow-up survey. *Pediatr Dent* 24:4, 2002.

Iwasaki J, Vann WF Jr, Dilley DCH, et al.: An investigation of capnography and pulse oximetry as monitors of pediatric patients sedated for dental treatment. *Pediatr Dent* 11:111, 1989.

Johnson R: Hospital treatment of the handicapped dental patient. In Wessels KE, Gardner AE, editors: *Dentistry and the handicapped patient.* Postgraduate dental handbook series, No. 5, Littleton, MA, 1979, PSG Publishing.

Kaban LB: Diagnosis and treatment of fractures of the facial bones in children 1943-1993. *J Oral Maxillofac Surg* 51:722, 1993.

Kaufman E, Goharian S, Katz Y: Adverse reactions triggered by dental local anesthetics: A clinical survey. *Anesth Prog* 47:134, 2000.

Kaufman E, Meyer S, Wolnerman JS, et al.: Transient suppression of involuntary movements in cerebral palsy patients during dental treatment. *Anesth Prog* 38:200, 1991.

Kleinhauz M, Eli I: When pharmacologic anesthesia is precluded: The value of hypnosis as a sole anesthetic agent in dentistry. *Spec Care Dent* 13:15, 1993.

Kupietzky A, Houpt MI: Midazolam: A review of its use for conscious sedation of children. *Pediatr Dent* 15:237, 1993.

Lampshire EL: Hypnosis in dentistry for children. In Wright GZ, editor: *Behavior management in dentistry for children.* Philadelphia, 1975, WB Saunders, pp 115–128.

Lanigan CJ: Oxygen desaturation after dental anesthesia. *Br J Anaesth* 68:142, 1992.

Lee JY, Vann WF Jr, Roberts MW: A cost analysis of treating pediatric dental patients using general anesthesia versus conscious sedation. *Anesth Prog* 48:82, 2001.

Lenchner V, Wright GZ: Nonpharmaco-therapeutic approaches to behavior management. In Wright GZ, editor: *Behavior management in dentistry for children.* Philadelphia, 1975, WB Saunders, pp 91–114.

Levine MF, Spahr-Schopfer IA, Hartley E, et al.: Oral midazolam premedication in children: The minimum time for separation from parents. *Can J Anæsth* 40:726, 1993.

Litman RS, Kottra JA, Berkowitz RJ, et al.: Upper airway obstruction during midazolam/nitrous oxide sedation in children with enlarged tonsils. *Pediatr Dent* 20:318, 1998.

Litman RS, Kottra JA, Verga KA, et al.: Chloral hydrate sedation: The additive sedative and respiratory depressant effects of nitrous oxide. *Anesth Analg* 86:724, 1998.

Loeffler PM: Oral benzodiazepines and conscious sedation: A review. *J Oral Maxillofac Surg* 50:989, 1992.

Martone CH, Nagelhout J, Wolf SM: Methohexital: A practical review for outpatient dental anesthesia. *Anesth Prog* 38:195, 1991.

Mathewson RJ, Primosch RE: *Fundamentals of pediatric dentistry,* 3rd ed. Chicago, 1995, Quintessence Publishing Co, Inc.

Maxwell LG, Deshpande JK, Wetzel RC: Preoperative evaluation of children. *Pediatr Clin North Am* 41:93, 1994.

McComb M, Koenigsberg SR, Broder HL, et al.: The effects of oral conscious sedation on future behavior and anxiety in pediatric dental patients. *Pediatr Dent* 24:3, 2002.

Milnes AR: Delivering supplemental oxygen during sedation via a saliva injector. *Pediatr Dent* 24:340, 2002.

Moore PA, Cuddy MA, Magera JA et al.: Oral transmucosal fentanyl pretreatment for outpatient general anesthesia. *Anesth Prog* 47:29, 2000.

Moore PA, Mickey EA, Hargreaves JA, et al.: Sedation in pediatric dentistry: A practical assessment procedure. *J Am Dent Assoc* 109:564, 1984.

Moses AJ, Lieberman M: The effect of external nasal dilators on blood oxygen levels in dental patients. *J Am Dent Assoc* 134:97, 2003.

Nathan JE, Vargas KG: Oral midazolam with and without meperidine for management of the difficult young pediatric dental patient: A retrospective study. *Pediatr Dent* 24:129, 2002.

Nathan JE, Venham LL, West MS, et al.: The effects of nitrous oxide on anxious young pediatric patients across sequential visits: A double-blind study. *J Dent Child* 55:220, 1988.

Nathan JE: Management of the difficult child: A survey of pediatric dentists' use of restraints, sedation, and general anesthesia. *J Dent Child* 56:293, 1989.

Nazif MM, Sarner JB: High frequency jet ventilation in complete oral rehabilitation. *J Dent Child* 58:248, 1991.

Neville BW, Damm DD, Allen CM, et al.: *Oral and maxillofacial pathology,* 2nd ed. Philadelphia, 2002, WB Saunders, pp 69–106.

Nilsson A, Boman I, Wallin B, et al.: The EMLA patch: A new type of local anaesthetic application for dermal analgesia for children. *Anaesthesia* 49:70, 1994.

Ord RA, Blanchaert RH Jr, Nikitakis NG, et al.: Ameloblastoma in children. *J Oral Maxillofac Surg* 60:762, 2002.

Oza N, Agarwal K, Panda KN: An unusual mode of injury: Implantation of a broken toothbrush medial to ramus: Report of a case. *J Dent Child* 68:193, 2002.

Phero JC: Pharmacologic management of pain, anxiety, and behavior: Conscious sedation, deep sedation, and general anesthesia. *Pediatr Dent* 15:429, 1993.

Poiset M, Johnson R, Nakamura R: Pulse rate and oxygen saturation in children during routine dental procedures. *J Dent Child* 57:279, 1990.

Pope JEC, Curzon ME: The dental status of cerebral palsied children. *Pediatr Dent* 13:156, 1991.

Primosch RE, Bender F: Factors associated with administration route when using midazolam for pediatric conscious sedation. *J Dent Child* 68:233, 2001.

Quarnstrom F: Electronic dental anesthesia. *Anesth Prog* 39:162, 1992.

Quarnstrom FC, Milgrom P, Bishop MJ, et al.: Clinical study of diffusion hypoxia after nitrous oxide analgesia. *Anesth Prog* 38:21, 1991.

Roelofse JA, Van Der Bijl P: Adverse reactions to midazolam and ketamine premedication in children [letter]. *Anesth Prog* 38:73, 1991.

Rosenberg M: Oral ketamine for deep sedation of difficult-to-manage children who are mentally handicapped: A case report. *Pediatr Dent* 13:221, 1991.

Rosenberg MB, Campbell RL: Guidelines for intraoperative monitoring of dental patients undergoing conscious sedation, deep sedation, and general anesthesia. *Oral Surg Oral Med Oral Pathol* 71:2, 1991.

Rosenstein S: *Dentistry in cerebral palsy and related handicapping conditions.* Springfield, IL, 1978, Charles C Thomas.

Sams DR, Thornton JB, Wright JT: The assessment of two oral sedation drug regimens in pediatric dental patients. *J Dent Child* 59:306, 1992.

Schreiner MS: Preoperative and postoperative fasting in children. *Pediatr Clin North Am* 41:111, 1994.

Seiler CL, Shellhart WC, Casamassimo PS: Efficacy and safety of intravenous ketamine for the severely handicapped. *J Dent Child* 57:263, 1990.

Shapira J, Holan G, Guelmann M, et al.: Evaluation of the effect of nitrous oxide and hydroxyzine in controlling the behavior of the pediatric dental patient. *Pediatr Dent* 14:167, 1992.

Shenkin JD, Davis MJ, Corbin SB: The oral health of special needs children: Dentistry's challenge to provide care. *J Dent Child* 68:201, 2001.

Stecker SS, Swift JQ, Hodges JS, et al.: Should a mucoadhesive patch (Dentipatch) be used for gingival anesthesia in children? *Anesth Prog* 49:3, 2002.

Sullivan DC, Wilson CFG, Webb MD: A comparison of two oral ketamine-diazepam regimens for the sedation of anxious pediatric dental patients. *Pediatr Dent* 23:223, 2001.

Sykes P: Accidents do not happen—They are caused. *Anesth Prog* 39:111, 1991.

Tate AR, Ng MW, Needleman HL, et al.: Failure rates of restorative procedures following dental rehabilitation under general anesthesia. *Pediatr Dent* 24:69, 2002.

te Duits E, Goepfor S, Donly K, et al.: The effectiveness of electronic dental anesthesia in children. *Pediatr Dent* 15:191, 1993.

Theroux MC, West DW, Corddry DH, et al.: Efficacy of intranasal midazolam in facilitating dental procedures in preschool children. *SAMBA Mtg Abstract* 9:2, 1994.

Trapp LD: Techniques for induction of general anesthesia in the pediatric dental patient. *Anesth Prog* 39:138, 1992.

Tyler DC: Pharmacology of pain management. *Pediatr Clin North Am* 41:59, 1994.

Van Kooy MA, Gargiulo RF: Postobstructive pulmonary edema. *Am Fam Phys* 62:401–404, 2000.

Veerkamp JS, Gruythuysen RJ, van Amerongen WE, et al.: Dental treatment of fearful children using nitrous oxide. Part II: The parent's point of view. *J Dent Child* 59:115, 1992.

Vermeulen M, Vinckier F, Vandenbroucke J: Dental general anesthesia: Clinical characteristics of 933 patients. *J Dent Child* 58:27, 1991.

Vig KWL, Fields HW: Facial growth and management of orthodontic problems. *Pediatr Clin North Am* 47:1085, 2000.

Wahl MJ: Myths of dental-induced endocarditis. *Arch Intern Med* 154:137, 1994.

Waldman HB, Perlman SP: Children with both mental retardation and mental illnesses live in our communities and need dental care. *J Dent Child* 68:360, 2001.

Warner ME, Benefeld SM, Warner MA, et al.: Perianesthetic dental injuries: Frequency, outcomes, and risk factors. *Anesthesiology* 90:1302, 1999.

Webster AC, Morley-Forster PK, Dain S, et al.: Anaesthesia for adenotonsillectomy: A comparison between tracheal intubation and the armoured laryngeal mask airway. *Can J Anaesth* 40:1171, 1993.

Wei SHY: *Pediatric dentistry: Total patient care.* Philadelphia, 1988, Mosby–Year Book, pp 306–391.

Whitehead BG, Durr DP, Adair SM, et al.: Monitoring of sedated pediatric dental patients. *J Dent Child* 55:329, 1988.

Wilson S: Conscious sedation and pulse oximetry: False alarms? *Pediatr Dent* 12:228, 1990.

Wilson S: Nonpharmacologic issues in pain perception and control. In Pinkham JR, editor: *Pediatric dentistry: Infancy through adolescence,* 2nd ed. Philadelphia, 1994, WB Saunders, pp 88–97.

Wilson S: Pharmacologic behavior management for pediatric dental treatment. *Pediatr Clin North Am* 47:1159, 2000.

Wright GZ, Chiasson RC: The use of sedation agents by Canadian pediatric dentists. *Pediatr Dent* 9:308, 1987.

Wright GZ: Psychologic management of children's behaviors. In McDonald RE, Avery DR, editors: *Dentistry for the child and adolescent,* 6th ed. St Louis, 1994, Mosby–Year Book, pp 32–52.

Wright JT: Normal formation and development of defects of the human dentition. *Pediatr Clin North Am* 47:975, 2000.

Yaster M, Kost-Byerly S, Maxwell LG: Opioid agonists and antagonists. In Schechter NL, Berde CB, Yaster M, editors: *Pain in infants, children, and adolescents,* ed 2. Philadelphia, 2002, Lippincott Williams & Wilkins, pp 181–224.

Yaster M, Sola JE, Pegrolli W Jr, et al.: The night after surgery. Postoperative management of the pediatric outpatient-surgical and anesthetic aspects. *Pediatr Clin North Am* 41:199, 1994.

Zeltser R, Kalter A, Casap N, et al.: Oropharyngeal impalement injuries in children: Report of 2 cases. *J Oral Maxillofac Surg* 61:510, 2003.

Zuckerberg AL: Perioperative approach to children. *Pediatr Clin North Am* 41:15, 1994.

Zwemer TJ: *Boucher's clinical dental terminology,* 4th ed. St Louis, 1993, Mosby–Year Book.

25 Anesthesia and Sedation for Procedures Outside the Operating Room

Keira P. Mason • Steven E. Zgleszewski • Robert S. Holzman

Advances in diagnostic technology, increasing populations of patients surviving critical medical or surgical illness, requests from medical colleagues for support during prolonged or high-risk procedures, and concern about liability exposure have lead to an increased demand for the professional services of anesthesiologists outside the operating room (Fig. 25–1). The limited space and supply of operating rooms in some institutions have further contributed to anesthetic delivery out of the operating room. Nonanesthesiologists have expressed increased interest and willingness in providing sedation and analgesia services outside of the operating room, often using anesthesia codes to bill for their services. Most anesthesiologists do not condone this practice, although no legal action to date has been taken to discourage it. Pediatric radiologists, oncologists, dentists, gastroenterologists, pulmonologists, and others provide the majority of sedation for their procedures. Monitoring techniques, available personnel, and oral intake (NPO) guidelines vary among institutions, and many sedation protocols do not conform to the sedation guidelines of the American Academy of Pediatrics (AAP) (Committee on Drugs, 1992).

Providing and delivering anesthesia outside of the operating room can be challenging and hazardous. The department of anesthesia may not want to commit limited financial resources to providing state-of-the-art anesthesia equipment and monitors in an extramural location with a limited caseload. Consequently, the anesthesia machine and monitors may consist of operating room leftovers and undesirables. Support personnel working in nonsurgical areas may have little experience with anesthesia care, delivery, and needs, particularly in the case of an emergency. Acquiring insurance approval may be difficult because third party insurers do not always understand the justification for an anesthesiologist's services. Likewise, few anesthesiologists are familiar with the specific procedures, nuances, and risks associated with all interventional radiologic, gastroendoscopic, or radiation treatment procedures. Conflicts may arise among physicians, administrative personnel, and third party insurers.

ADMINISTRATIVE REQUIREMENTS FOR EXTRAMURAL LOCATIONS

ORGANIZATION AND ADMINISTRATION

A good relationship between the extramural department and the department of anesthesiology is critical to providing safe anesthetic coverage. Each department has its own needs, goals, and guidelines. It is ideal to designate a team of anesthesiologists

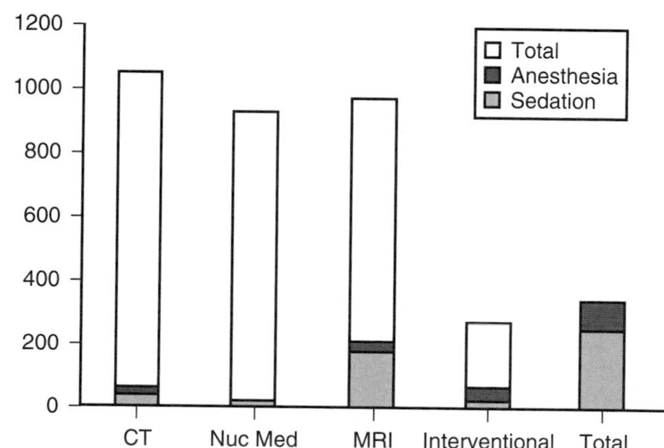

FIGURE 25–1. Average monthly caseload: anesthesia support for radiology at Children's Hospital Boston (November 1999 through April 2003). The overwhelming majority of radiology studies are accomplished without anesthesia or sedation, but a significant minority (>3,000 per year) involve anesthesiologists directly or by consultation. CT, computed tomography; Nuc Med, nuclear medicine; MRI, magnetic resonance imaging.

committed to providing extramural anesthesia care and troubleshooting the logistical challenges of providing anesthesia in the various locations. Each member should rotate through the different extramural sites to maintain familiarity with the procedures, to foster a relationship with the physicians and ancillary personnel, and to understand the anesthesia demands unique to each site.

Few extramural locations are configured to deliver anesthetics. Ideally, anesthesiologists should be involved in the early stages of site design to ensure that minimum standards for anesthesia delivery are met and to troubleshoot engineering issues and advocate for adequate space for anesthetic induction and emergence (Committee on Drugs, 1992; American Academy of Pediatrics, 1999). Physical plant considerations for magnetic resonance imaging (MRI) site planning have been previously described (Koskinen, 1985). When anesthesia services are requested, these sites may not meet minimum standards (House of Delegates et al., 1994) and require reengineering to include the minimum requirements stated by the American Society of Anesthesiologists (ASA). The anesthesia machine should be equipped with back-up supplies of E cylinders filled with oxygen and nitrous oxide. If pipeline oxygen is not available, oxygen should be supplied from H cylinders (6,600 L) rather than from the smaller E tanks (659 L).

Scavenging systems should be carefully evaluated in the extramural location. Unlike the operating room, passive scavenging systems may not always be possible. A safe means of active scavenging may be provided by the vacuum at the wall or wall suction canisters. A scavenging system should be dedicated solely to waste gases. Most MRI scanners do not have wall suction because MRI-compatible wall suction is not widely available. If the suction is located outside the MRI suite, a mouse-sized hole may be created in the suite's wall to allow suction tubing to be passed inside (Koskinen, 1985).

Electrical circuitry and lighting in extramural locations may not be up to operating room standards; even if the outlets are grounded and up to hospital grade, there may still be plug incompatibility. Adaptors and conversion plugs should always be available. Although some extramural locations carry a minimal risk of electrical shock or electrocution, these sites do not have line-isolation monitors (LIMs) and do not warn of excess leakage of current. Supplemental lighting for record-keeping, label verification, establishment of intravenous access, and visualization of the patient is critical. Even under the best circumstances, for example, lighting is dim in the MRI scanner and monitoring by simple clinical observation can be limited. Anesthesia personnel may not always remain in the imaging suite, particularly during MRI, computed tomography (CT) scanning, and radiation therapy. Remote television monitoring or hardwiring through reinforced walls can allow remote video display of the patient and monitors within.

A storage area large enough to stock anesthesia equipment and supplies must be easily and quickly accessible. This area should be routinely checked and restocked and kept locked when anesthesia services are not required. The need for redundancy of nondisposable supplies is a matter of philosophy. Are two laryngoscopes sufficient, or should there be a third? Is one electrocardiographic monitor sufficient, or should there be a battery-operated monitor for backup and transport? Drugs should be checked per the usual operating room routine, and expired medications replaced. Gas cylinder supplies must be reliable, especially in areas without piped oxygen. A code cart should be conveniently located in an area known to all physicians and ancillary personnel. This cart should be routinely checked and restocked.

Finally, extramural anesthetizing locations are often distant from the operating room. Patients may need to remain anesthetized during transport to or from the extramural location. For these circumstances, ensured elevator access with key-controlled emergency overrides is a must. All anesthesiologists who deliver extramural services should be familiar with their surroundings. Checklists are invaluable to guarantee consistent patient care, anesthesia monitoring, equipment, documentation, and backup assistance.

PERSONNEL, SUPPORT, AND LOGISTICS

Support and medical personnel in nonsurgical areas may not be familiar with the requirements of an anesthesiologist, thereby providing an important educational and training opportunity. Proper training facilitates teamwork and minimizes chaos in critical situations. A standard anesthesia cart at each anesthetizing location should be fully stocked with essential medications, necessary adjuvant equipment, spare self-inflating Ambu bag (Ambu Inc., Linthicum, MD), endotracheal tubes, laryngeal mask airways (LMAs), suction catheters, intravenous supplies, laryngoscope handles and blades, and a variety of oral and nasopharyngeal airways.

A director of anesthesia services at an extramural location can orchestrate, facilitate, and coordinate anesthesia services. This director can also serve as a consultant for the nonanesthesia medical and nursing staff. By being available to answer questions, provide on-site consults, examine patients, and provide backup support or emergency airway expertise, the anesthesiologist can also support a nurse-administered sedation program. Nurses who provide sedation under the supervision of the ordering extramural physician (gastrointestinal, radiology, dental) should be regularly certified in pediatric advanced life support (PALS) and basic life support (BLS). The Joint Commission on Accreditation of Healthcare Organizations (JCAHO) *Anesthesia and Sedation Manual* sets guidelines for credentialing all personnel (physicians and nurses) who administer sedation. All children scheduled for nursing sedation should receive a prescreen telephone call from a radiology nurse the day before the scheduled scan. Often, these telephone calls are made after business hours to ensure that a parent is home. The nurse reviews the medical history, relays NPO instructions, and reminds the parents to administer the child's routine medications with a sip of clear fluid. The supervising physician must give final approval for sedation, after reviewing the child's medical history and current medical status, before ordering the medications. To minimize the chance of drug delivery error or miscalculation, it is helpful to have preprinted order sheets.

It is crucial to know who to call for assistance if a problem arises. A speed-dial system should be available from all extramural anesthetizing location sites to immediately request emergency backup.

PERIPROCEDURAL PATIENT CARE

STANDARDS OF PRACTICE AND QUALITY ASSURANCE

The practice standards adopted by the ASA in 1986 for basic intraoperative monitoring apply as well to extramural locations.

Practice standards and guidelines promulgated by the AAP (Committee on Drugs, 1992; American Academy of Pediatrics, 1999) are exceeded by established practice standards in anesthesiology (AAP, Section on Anesthesiology, 1999). Significant variances may exist when nonanesthesiologists provide sedation (Keeter et al., 1990). Practice Standards for Non-Anesthetizing Locations were adopted by the ASA in 1994 (House of Delegates et al., 1994).

As recommended by the JCAHO, the department of anesthesia should oversee all sedation protocols and meet on a regular basis to review adverse events, policies, and procedures and to make recommendations for improvements. Ideally, adverse events such as failed or prolonged sedations, paradoxical reactions, hypoxia, emesis, unscheduled admission, and cardiac or respiratory events are identified and entered into a computerized database. In addition, the extramural nurse should call all patients and families within 24 hours to follow up on patient outcome and identify any delayed adverse events.

SCHEDULING AND PREPARATION OF PATIENTS

Appropriate planning for providing anesthesia begins with a familiarity with the procedure. The requesting service orders the procedure and then leaves the logistics of scheduling to the extramural service. The referring physician should not schedule the procedure because he or she may not realize the subtle logistics of the procedure or its duration. Radiologists, in particular, recognize that involvement with anesthesia lengthens their total time commitment to a patient and potentially limits the number of procedures accomplished in a day (Winter, 1978; Cremin, 1990). A well-coordinated system to screen patients on the day of procedure is important. Experienced personnel, usually a certified nurse practitioner (CRNP), should be designated to take initial vital signs, review recent medical history, insert intravenous catheter, if necessary, and familiarize the family with the upcoming anesthesia procedure.

Screening patients for extramural procedures may be time consuming and challenging. Many children are chronically ill, nutritionally impaired, and medically complicated. These issues must be carefully addressed through attention to the patient's history, physical examination, previous medical records, outside consultations, and close communication with other medical colleagues. Several consultants may need to confer to fully understand the patient's current state of health. Not every procedure is elective. For example, urgent procedures may be required *despite* an upper respiratory tract infection (URI), ongoing pneumonia, deteriorating physical status, untreated gastroesophageal reflux, sepsis, or hemodynamic instability. In these situations, consultation among the anesthesiologist, the requesting physician, and the radiologist should confirm urgency. Anesthesia plans should be modified to accommodate the requirements of the procedure (breath-holding for chest CT scan) and the patient's medical condition.

It is not always possible for an anesthesiologist to provide sedation and anesthesia for all children when there is a large volume of cases. A structured nursing sedation program can provide safe and effective sedation. As recommended by the JCAHO, the department of anesthesia at each facility should work with the department of radiology and nursing to develop and oversee a sedation program. In actuality, the sedation program begins with the triaging of patients before scheduling the procedure.

TABLE 25–1. "Red flags" for sedation

Red Flag	Indications
Apnea	Documented by sleep study, strong clinical history, or apnea monitor
Unstable cardiac disease	Cyanotic, depressed myocardial function, significant stenotic or regurgitation lesions
Respiratory compromise	Recent (<8 weeks) pneumonia, bronchitis, asthma, respiratory infection
Craniofacial defect History of a difficult airway	Potential for difficult airway
Active gastroesophageal reflux or vomiting	In poor control, with or without medical or surgical treatment
Hypotonia and lack of head control	Patient may not be able to maintain his or her airway without assistance
Allergies to barbiturates	Usually the mainstay of a sedation protocol; also allergy to other sedatives to be administered
Prior failed sedation	Unable to be sedated or unsuccessful imaging study because of excessive movement
Tremors	Unlikely to be ablated with sedation

A radiology nurse screens the patient by reviewing the past and current medical history and gathering any relevant laboratory or clinical studies. She or he then contacts the family or referring physician for clarification if needed. After this review, the nurse, in the majority of cases, is able to make an appropriate referral for either general anesthesia or procedural sedation. Because MRI is a unique environment, it is more efficient to have the MRI nurses screen the patient before and on the day of the procedure. To ensure consistent decision making, the departments of anesthesia and radiology should develop a set of guidelines and "red flags" (Table 25–1) to help in this triaging process. If there are any questions or additional medical history or studies that need clarification, the nurse and anesthesiologist confer before making the final decision regarding general anesthesia or procedural sedation.

In addition to the usual preanesthetic evaluation issues, chronically ill children often have electrolyte disturbances, coagulation and hematologic abnormalities, and hemodynamic instability. A consent for the administration of general anesthesia or procedural sedation must be obtained.

Is gastroesophageal reflux a contraindication to procedural sedation? Because gastroesophageal regurgitation is common in infants, a detailed clinical history should be taken with regard to the incidence and timing of the regurgitation. If the reflux is predictable (i.e., only associated with mealtimes or soon thereafter), children are usually approved for procedural sedation. NPO guidelines are adjusted to minimize the risk of reflux. For example, if the infant refluxes within 2 hours of solid feeds but never after 3 hours, then the NPO guidelines for this infant may be extended to 6 hours for solids.

SELECTION OF AGENTS AND TECHNIQUES

The selection of an anesthetic technique in an extramural location depends on the patient's underlying medical condition, age, drug tolerance, and anticipated procedure. The airway management may be influenced by the procedure itself, anticipated postprocedural course (intensive care unit, postprocedural intubation), and past anesthetic course (difficult intubation). The assistance of the department of anesthesia is often sought when sedation administered by the radiologist has failed (Hubbard et al., 1992). Beware that parents and radiologists may have the unrealistic expectation that anesthesia provides ideal conditions and ensures successful completion of the procedure.

Premedication has many purposes—the relief of anxiety, easy separation from parents, sedation, analgesia, amnesia, reduction of salivary and gastric secretions, elevation of gastric pH, and decreased cardiac vagal activity. Medications should be adjusted to the psychological and physiologic conditions of both the patient and family. Parent-present inductions may be offered when the presence of a parent has a calming effect on the child. In the event of potentially detrimental parent anxiety, premedication may be preferable to a parent-present induction (Kain et al., 2001). (See Chapter 7, Psychological Aspects, and Chapter 8, Preoperative Preparation.)

Barbiturates may be useful as a sole method of providing sedation. Pentobarbital (Nembutal), for example, has the advantage of providing sedation, minimal respiratory and circulatory depression, and rare adverse events (Karian et al., 2002). Barbiturates have no analgesic properties. They can produce paradoxical reactions, especially in children. No antagonist to barbiturates is available; dosing should be carefully titrated. Intravenous pentobarbital via titration has been used successfully by radiologists while monitoring oral and nasal airflow, oxygen saturation (with a pulse oximeter [SpO_2]), end-tidal carbon dioxide, and cardiac rate and rhythm, with transient decreases in SpO_2 in up to 7.5% of patients; interventions have included stimulation and head repositioning (Strain et al., 1988; Connor et al., 2003). Other studies have described the use of pentobarbital in both the oral and intravenous forms (Chung et al., 2000; Mason et al., 2001). For infants younger than 1 year, oral pentobarbital is more successful and carries a lower rate of adverse events compared with chloral hydrate (Rooks et al., 2003). The long half-life of pentobarbital (≈24 hours) mandates careful and conservative recovery and discharge guidelines. The dosage of pentobarbital is 2 to 6 mg/kg PO, up to 9 mg/kg in patients who are receiving barbiturate therapy.

Sodium thiopental in a mean induction dose of 6 mg/kg and a mean total dose of 8.5 ± 3 mg/kg has been used successfully as the sole anesthetic for CT/MRI in 200 children from 1 month to 12 years of age (Spear et al., 1993). Methohexital has a shorter recovery time than thiopental and is more effective than oral chloral hydrate (Manuli and Davies, 1993). Methohexital-induced seizures in patients with temporal lobe epilepsy have been reported; thiopental or pentobarbital is an alternative for these patients (Rockoff and Goudsouzian, 1981). For patients taking barbiturate-containing anticonvulsant medications, a higher dose limit is generally more successful. Methohexital has also been used intramuscularly for radiotherapy at doses of 8 to 10 mg/kg. The onset time via this route is often twofold to threefold longer than that for rectally administered methohexital (Jeffries, 1988).

Opiates reduce anesthetic and preprocedural and postprocedural analgesic requirements. They are reversible with naloxone. Narcotics may be unnecessary for purely nonpainful diagnostic procedures, but they may be very useful for therapeutic interventions, especially for those patients with postprocedural pain. They are also useful following anthracycline chemotherapy, with documented impaired myocardial function (Burrows et al., 1985). Because narcotics depress the ventilatory response to CO_2, this respiratory depression may be of particular concern for children with increased intracranial pressure (ICP). Narcotics may also worsen preexisting nausea and vomiting.

Benzodiazepines have the advantage of anxiolysis with minimal vomiting and cardiorespiratory depression. Intravenous injection of diazepam (Valium) is painful and may lead to thrombophlebitis; midazolam (Versed) is water soluble and therefore may be more suitable for intravenous or intramuscular injection. The elimination half-life of midazolam averages 2.5 hours compared with 20 to 70 hours for diazepam (Greenblatt et al., 1981; Reves et al., 1985). Young patients or patients with significant liver disease may have prolonged duration and exaggerated effect of the benzodiazepines.

Preparation of the stomach and aspiration prophylaxis are of particular concern for urgently scheduled cases (outside of NPO guidelines) or when the medical history suggests aspiration risk. If H_2-receptor antagonists are used, bronchospasm may occur in asthmatic patients because of the relative increased availability of H_1-receptors. H_2-blockers may also inhibit metabolism of other concurrently administered medications. Metoclopramide accelerates gastric emptying and increases tone in the lower esophageal sphincter but is associated with a significant incidence of extrapyramidal side effects in children. Ondansetron works synergistically with other agents through its vagal blocking actions in the gastrointestinal tract as well as through its inhibition of the chemoreceptor trigger zone via serotonin receptor antagonism, particularly for patients undergoing radiation therapy with pulses of chemotherapy (Burnette and Perkins, 1992; Figg et al., 1993).

Ketamine has been very popular since the 1970s for sedation, analgesia, or anesthesia outside the operating room due to its support of the cardiovascular and respiratory systems. Ketamine-induced nightmares, hallucinations, delusions, and agitation are rare in children (Sussman, 1974; Hostetler and Davis, 2002). Mason and others (2002) reported on a ketamine sedation program for use in interventional radiology. In this program, intravenous or intramuscular ketamine was administered in the intervention radiology suite by credentialed radiology nurses and radiologists to patients undergoing selected procedures. This protocol has allowed painful procedures to be tolerated by patients who previously would have required general anesthesia (Mason et al., 2002).

Although propofol does not have a labeled indication for children younger than 3 years, propofol has been used in this age group as a means of providing sedation or anesthesia. Propofol sedation via bolus and continuous infusion for brain MRI (total dosage, 5 mg/kg per hour) has provided successful imaging conditions and allowed patients to meet discharge criteria within 20 minutes (Vangerven et al., 1992). Fatal metabolic acidosis and myocardial failure associated with lipemic serum have been reported in five children admitted to the intensive care unit for respiratory support for URIs while being sedated with continuous-infusion propofol (Parke et al., 1992). For radiation therapy patients, propofol has been successfully used when administered through a catheter by a syringe pump calibrated to deliver milliliters per hour. Bloomfield and others (1993) suggested that the syringe pump begin at the maximum infusion rate of 99 mL/hr until the patients fell asleep (usually over 1 to 3 minutes); then the infusion rate was gradually decreased during treatment until it was shut off at the end (Fig. 25–2). Patients were typically awake, alert, and taking clear liquids 20 minutes later (Bloomfield et al., 1993).

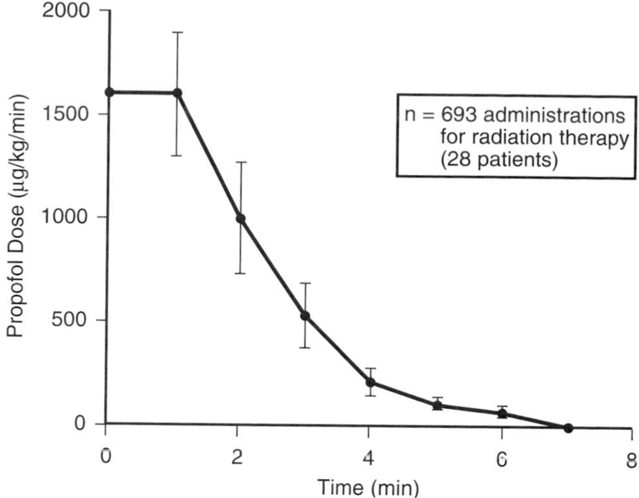

FIGURE 25–2. Propofol dosing via continuous infusion.

Some patients require general anesthesia because of previous sedation failures, the need for a secure airway, or procedural logistics. Newer, less-soluble anesthetic agents such as sevoflurane and desflurane have pharmacokinetic profiles that compare favorably with propofol in adults (Van Hemelrijck et al., 1991); there is little reason to believe that would not be the case with children, although pediatric anesthesiologists usually avoid using desflurane because of its pungency and ability to cause airway irritability. Repeat halothane anesthetics have been associated with veno-occlusive disease in children undergoing total body irradiation, alkylating agent chemotherapy, and preparation for bone marrow transplantation (Gentet et al., 1988; Griswold et al., 1988). The ideal volatile agent for repeat anesthetics is unclear; halothane has its potential disadvantages based on reports of hepatitis (Kenna et al., 1987) and bromism (Goudsouzian et al., 1988; Morrison and Friesen, 1990). Isoflurane produces no measurable change in liver function tests during daily anesthesia for several weeks for radiotherapy (Jones et al., 1991), but its ability to cause airway irritability limits its usefulness during induction of anesthesia. Since its introduction to clinical practice in the mid 1990s, sevoflurane has become the volatile anesthetic of choice in children. Its lack of airway irritability and its ability to provide children with stable hemodynamic function coupled with its rapid onset and offset make sevoflurane a useful agent for children.

Volatile agent vaporizer performance in the MRI suite has been studied. The output of a Fortec II vaporizer (Fraser Harlake, Orchard Park, NY) varied according to vaporizer location and orientation of the bimetallic strip within the magnetic field (Kross and Drummond, 1991). The movements of the bimetallic ferromagnetic temperature compensator within the MRI magnetic field altered vaporizer output by as much as 91% of the dialed output concentration. Several other vaporizers (Ohio Forane, Ohio Medical Products, Madison; WI; Ohmeda Isotec IV vaporizer, Ohmeda, Steeton, England; and Forane Vapor 19.1, Dragerwerk AG, Lubeck, Germany) were incompatible with the MRI environment because of stronger ferromagnetic internal component content or the location of a ferromagnetic spring within the temperature compensator. Measuring inspired and end-tidal levels of volatile agents when delivering a general anesthetic in the MRI environment may provide reassurance.

Regional anesthesia, although still relatively rare in pediatric operating room practice and even rarer outside the operating room, remains a valid choice in some circumstances. Intercostal nerve blocks may be very useful for lung or rib biopsies, placement of chest tubes, biliary or subphrenic drainage procedures, and insertion of biliary stents. Nerve block of the brachial plexus via the axillary, interscalene, or supraclavicular route has been reported for the brachial approach to catheterization (Eggers et al., 1967; Ross and Williams, 1970), and neuraxial block of the lower extremities, for femoral catheterizations and percutaneous approaches to the kidney (Lind and Mushlin, 1987). Spinal anesthesia has been successfully used for repeat painful radiotherapy on lower extremities, in conjunction with regional hyperthermia and limb exsanguination (Spencer and Barnes, 1980).

Indwelling central catheters are implanted in the majority of radiotherapy patients and can be utilized for induction and maintenance of anesthesia, blood draws, intravenous fluid administration, and chemotherapy. Dressing changes are oftenaccomplished in conjunction with the sedation or anesthesia. Antiseptic preparation of all injection sites with povidone-iodine (Betadine) and alcohol is critical. At the end of the session, the catheter should be carefully flushed with heparinized saline. An alternative to central lines is the use of a heparin lock peripheral intravenous line, changed weekly, with careful parental instruction. Smoothness of emergence is particularly important after angiographic procedures because of the risk of dislodging a clot or bleeding at the puncture site. Some of these patients have been heparinized without protamine reversal. Unlike in adults, sandbags and weights are not routinely applied to angiographic cannulation sites of children.

A final word—the best choice may be no medication. Occasionally, the loss of self-control with sedation produces dysphoria and some patients fare better when completely awake. Minimal medication may be preferable in patients with complicated and unstable medical conditions who may not tolerate the anesthesia or sedation. Some procedures (unilateral carotid barbiturate injection or Wada test) may require conversation, interaction, and responsiveness of the patient. In these situations, no sedation may be the best alternative.

POSTANESTHESIA CARE

Recovery criteria and the recovery room environment after procedural sedation or general anesthesia administered in an extramural location must be no different than the postanesthesia care delivered to children after an operative procedure. JCAHO guidelines must be followed at extramural anesthesia recovery sites. Each site must have sources of supplemental oxygen, ability to deliver positive pressure ventilation, available perioperative suction and monitoring equipment, and a nursing staff trained in postanesthesia care. Discharge criteria should be established by an anesthesiologist in conjunction with the extramural service and its nursing staff.

Analgesic requirements after the procedure are extremely variable. Groin puncture may be only mildly annoying for adults, but the inability to move about and the ache of blood dissecting subcutaneously cause considerable discomfort in children. After angiography, all children require a minimum pediatric acute care unit stay of 4 hours to ensure that the puncture site does not bleed or a hematoma does not develop. Ideally, the patient should be pain free and resting supine and motionless to minimize the risk of a groin-puncture bleed or hematoma. Experienced nursing staff can recognize, manage, and call for extra help when they encounter unexpected agitation, delirium, or obtundation.

The anesthesiologist may be asked to participate in the perioperative care of patients for embolization procedures. These patients frequently experience pain or swelling after the procedure. The degree of pain depends on the extent of embolization, agent used for embolization, postembolic swelling, and amount of tissue necrosis. A variety of analgesic techniques are available, and the use of steroids perioperatively, while not directly decreasing pain, may be of benefit in reducing edema and postembolic neuritis. Postembolic swelling influences perioperative airway management for procedures in the head and neck. Pediatric patients in particular may need to remain intubated after such procedures, particularly when visible edema in the floor of the mouth, tongue, hypopharynx or oropharynx, or anterior neck could compromise a patent airway.

Nausea or vomiting may, because of the Valsalva maneuver, increase venous blood pressure, which can aggravate bleeding and swelling in puncture sites or after head and neck procedures. Hypothermia is a risk at some extramural locations because the MRI, CT, and interventional radiology equipment requires a cool environment. Heating lamps and forced-air heaters may be used when safe and appropriate. Finally, with the use of iodine-containing radiocontrast media (RCM) and sclerosing and embolizing agents, consideration must be given to adequate volume resuscitation, the risk of a contrast media reaction, and bladder catheterization for detection of oliguria, polyuria, or hematuria.

RESUSCITATION

Each extramural anesthetizing location is unique with regard to conducting resuscitation. Redundancy of monitoring devices and equipment is important; one should not be limited to a single item that could malfunction at the time of resuscitation. Patients with multiple allergies, shellfish allergies, or atopic disease are at increased risk of exhibiting anaphylaxis to iodine-containing contrast media. These patients may benefit from pretreatment with steroids and antihistamines. Areas with restricted access, MRI suites in particular, should have designated adjacent locations to perform full resuscitation. These areas should be equipped with wall oxygen, suction, and full monitoring and resuscitation capability. A Laerdal (Laerdal Medical Corp., Wappingers Falls, NY) self-inflating silicone bag (with no ferromagnetic working parts) or nonferrous Jackson-Rees circuit (Meridian Medical Technologies, Columbia, MD) should always be kept inside the MRI suite.

The physicians, nurses, anesthesiologists, technologists, and support personnel must know the location of a readily accessible code cart. In addition, a hard board to be placed under the patient during resuscitation should be available. Mock codes should be performed regularly to ensure adequate flow, teamwork, and delineation of responsibilities in the event of an emergency. The MRI scanner poses a special problem; codes should never be conducted in the scanner because as support personnel rush inside to assist, nonremoved ferrous materials become projectiles and impose an even more hazardous situation. Quenching a magnet should not be an alternative. Quenching requires a minimum of 3 minutes to eliminate the magnetic field. In addition, inadequate exhaust during a quench has been known to produce hypoxic conditions in the scanner and has resulted in a patient's death. A "black quench" could melt the MRI coils and require replacement of the scanner, a costly and time-consuming undertaking. Defibrillators are not MRI compatible and may not function properly when exposed to the magnetic field (Snowdon, 1989). In an emergency, the patient should be removed from the scanner to an area outside of the magnetic field. This designated area is a safe place for resuscitation and should have not only a wall oxygen source for a self-inflating (Ambu) bag but also access to appropriate monitors.

SPECIFIC EXTRAMURAL SITES

RADIOLOGY

Computerized Tomography Scanning

CT differentiates between high-density (calcium, iron, bone, and contrast-enhanced vascular and cerebrospinal fluid [CSF] spaces) and low-density (oxygen, nitrogen, carbon in air, fat, CSF, muscle, white matter, gray matter, and water-containing lesions) structures. Because the scan time is quick, CT may be preferable for patients who are medically unstable and in need of rapid diagnosis, such as a child being evaluated for abuse, an intracranial hemorrhage, or an abdominal or a thoracic mass. Other indications for emergency CT scans include encephalopathy and a change in neurologic status. In these situations, the issues of a full stomach and increased ICP usually necessitate a rapid sequence induction with tracheal intubation. Head CT scan is often the preferred study in emergency situations where head trauma is involved (Blankenberg et al., 2000).

The actual scanning sequences are short and can range from 10 to 40 seconds. These short scan times enable many children to complete a CT scan without any sedation, especially with parental presence and distraction techniques. When an anesthesiologist is involved, it is often for airway or failed sedation issues or for a medically complicated patient. An important aspect of some CT scans is to visualize the sinuses, ears, inner auditory canal, and temporomandibular bones and to evaluate for choanal atresia or craniofacial abnormalities. These scans may require direct coronal imaging with extreme head extension (off the end of the table between a 40- to 70-degree angle) or absolute immobility for three-dimensional reconstruction.

Any patient who is at risk for cervical instability should be properly screened before neck extension. Children with Down syndrome are at risk for atlantoaxial instability; the incidence of instability varies from 12% to 32% (Blankenberg et al., 2000). Many children with Down syndrome require cervical spine radiographs before entering grade school or participation in the Special Olympics. Usually, the parents are well aware of the radiologic findings. The cervical spine films, however, do not indicate whether the child is at risk for dislocation (Davidson, 1988). Rather, children who exhibit neurologic signs or symptoms such as abnormal gait, increased clumsiness, fatigue with ambulation, or a new preference for sitting games are at risk. In infants, developmental milestones (crawling, sitting up, reaching for objects, etc.) should be examined. Physical signs may include clonus, hyperreflexia, quadriparesis, neurogenic bladder, hemiparesis, ataxia, and sensory loss. The asymptomatic Down syndrome child with radiologic evidence of instability may be approved for procedural sedation, but unnecessary neck movement should be avoided. It is important to recognize that any child who displays neurologic signs or symptoms should not be sedated by either a nurse or an anesthesiologist until neurosurgical or orthopedic consultation is obtained.

Radiologists use Gastrografin (diatrizoate meglumine/diatrizoate sodium [48.29% total iodine]) when evaluating abdominal masses. Gastrografin diluted to a concentration of 1.5% is usually considered a clear liquid. The volume that is administered orally is significant: infants younger than 1 month receive 60 to 90 mL, infants between 1 month and 1 year of age may receive up to 240 mL, and children between the ages of 1 and 5 years receive between 240 and 360 mL. Because sedation or anesthesia should usually be accomplished within a window of 1 to 2 hours after ingestion of the contrast media, most "elective" NPO guidelines would be violated, yet radiologists insist that the scan must be completed while the Gastrografin is still in the gastrointestinal tract. There are no published data on optimal induction or sedation techniques as they relate to aspiration risk in these circumstances. Full-strength (3%) Gastrografin is hyperosmolar and hypertonic. All Gastrografin should be diluted to an isomolar and isotonic 1.5% concentration of neutral pH. There is one case report of 1.5% Gastrografin aspiration in a child (Friedman et al., 1986) with no adverse sequelae; the risk of using a 1.5% concentration of Gastrografin seems low (Wells et al., 1991).

Embolization Procedures

Interventional techniques include nonvascular and vascular intervention (Towbin and Ball, 1988). In vascular interventions, embolization and sclerotherapy have become important techniques for treating vascular malformations, aneurysms, fistulas, and hemorrhage and accomplishing renal ablation. Percutaneous transluminal angioplasty and fibrinolytic therapy are gaining popularity in pediatric institutions. Even in the smallest babies, great success is being reported, and the important contribution that adequate sedation and analgesia can make to ultimate outcome has been recognized (Diament et al., 1985). The basic indications for embolization are occlusion of vascular malformations, management of uncontrollable hemorrhage, medical renal ablation, and presurgical embolization of hypervascular masses.

Vascular malformations are congenital aberrant connections between blood vessels. Vascular malformations may be composed of lymphatic, arterial, and venous connections. These lesions, although present at birth, are often discrete and not clearly visible. As the child grows, the vascular malformation may expand rapidly, growing with the child. This rapid proliferative phase may occur in response to hormonal changes (pregnancy, puberty), trauma, or other stimuli (Jackson et al., 1993). Vascular malformations may be high-flow or low-flow lesions, depending on which vessels are involved. High-flow lesions include arteriovenous fistulas, some large hemangiomas, and arteriovenous malformations (AVMs). Particularly with large lesions, high-output cardiac failure and congestive heart failure with the potential for pulmonary edema should be anticipated and sought in the medical history and physical examination. Low-flow lesions consist of venous, intramuscular venous, and lymphatic malformations. Surgical resection of symptomatic vascular malformations may be hazardous as well as unsuccessful: any vascular element that is not resected may enlarge and cause further problems. For this reason, the combination of invasive angiography and embolization is becoming an alternative to surgical resection.

Because vascular malformations enlarge over time, even those lesions that are asymptomatic may require intervention. Patients with symptoms may experience pain, tissue ulceration, disfigurement, airway or cardiovascular compromise, impairment of limb function, coagulopathy, claudication, hemorrhage, and progressive nerve degeneration or palsy. Because large vascular lesions require multiple embolization procedures, parents and patients are often comforted by seeing familiar anesthesiologists. Especially with these complicated patients, familiarity with the patient is another benefit of having a core group of anesthesiologists in the radiology suites. Vascular embolization is also used as a bridge to surgical resection. Successful embolization and sclerotherapy decrease the size of the malformation and reduce blood flow to the lesion, thereby decreasing surgical risks.

During embolization of vascular malformations, radiologists often strive to cut off not only the feeding vessels but also the central confluence (nidus). It is at the nidus that much of the arterial shunting occurs. Embolic agents include stainless steel minicoils, absorbable gelatin pledgets and powder, detachable silicone balloons, polyvinyl alcohol foam, cyanoacrylate glue, and ethanol. The choice of agent depends on the clinical situation and the size of the blood vessel. When permanent occlusion is the goal, polyvinyl alcohol foam and ethanol are often used. Both occlude at the level of the arterioles and capillaries. Medium-sized to small arteries may be occluded with coils, which are the equivalent of surgical ligation. Particularly in trauma situations, when only temporary (days) occlusion is the goal, absorbable gelatin pledgets or powder is used (Coldwell et al., 1994).

Large hemangiomas may be associated with the coagulopathy of Kasabach-Merritt syndrome. In this condition, the hemangioma traps and destroys platelets and other coagulation factors, resulting in thrombocytopenia and an increased risk of bleeding. As the hemangioma involutes, the coagulation status improves (Mulliken and Young, 1988). A condition described as systemic intravascular coagulation (SIC) can occur after the embolization of extensive vascular malformations. This condition is marked by an elevated prothrombin time (PT) with a decrease in coagulation factors and platelets.

Absolute ethanol is injected in vascular malformations to promote sclerosis. Ethanol may produce a coagulum of blood and cause endothelial necrosis (Becker et al., 1984). Sclerotherapy or embolization with absolute (99.9%) ethanol increases the risk of a postprocedural coagulopathy (Mason et al., 2001) marked by positive D-dimers, elevated PT, and decreased platelets. Ethanol causes thrombosis because it injures the vascular endothelium. Ethanol also denatures blood proteins. Extensive ethanol injections can cause hematuria, and urinary catheters should be inserted to monitor urine output, diuresis, and hematuria. Especially with children scheduled for day surgery, liberal fluid replacement ensures that the hematuria clears before discharge. Ethanol can cause neuropathy and tissue necrosis if not injected selectively. Using selective catheterization and direct percutaneous puncture, care is taken not to expose normal blood vessels to the ethanol. In addition to the risk of hematuria, ethanol can cause significant serum alcohol levels. Mason and others (2000) note that up to 1 mL/kg of ethanol can be administered and that serum ethanol levels have been greater than the intoxication level of 0.008 mg/dL. Patients with high serum ethanol levels are either sedated or extremely agitated, depending on their particular response to intoxication.

Embolization or balloon occlusion of AVMs, vascular tumors, intracranial aneurysms, and fistulas carries considerable risk of catastrophic results. Such risks include a sudden intracranial hemorrhage, acute cerebral ischemia, and catheter or balloon migration. If the patient is sedated, he or she may require urgent airway management. Procedures that take very long require a urinary catheter, especially if contrast media is used.

Cerebral angiography requires the patient to be motionless and requires exquisite control of ventilation. Anesthetic technique, both in choice of agent and in control of arterial CO_2 tension, may affect cerebral blood flow and hence the quality of the scan. Cerebral angiography in children may be performed for the diagnosis or follow-up of Moyamoya disease, and these children should have anesthetic techniques that minimize the risk of transient ischemic attacks and stroke during the procedure (Soriano et al., 1993). (See Chapter 18, Neurosurgery.) Other considerations include controlled hypercarbia to promote vasodilation and to facilitate access and visualization of the vasculature for the radiologist. In the event of vasospasm or difficult access of small, tortuous vessels, locally administered (through the catheter) nitroglycerin in small doses (25 to 50 mcg) may facilitate visualization and access. Occlusion of the venous portion of the AVMs without complete occlusion of the arterial inflow vessels could result in acute swelling and bleeding. Vascularity reduction through occlusion of major feeder vessels is the goal of embolization of large AVMs before planned surgical excision. This may be accomplished as a staged procedure over several days, involving repeat anesthesia or sedation sessions.

Angiographic imaging may be enhanced through the use of glucagon. Glucagon is efficacious for digital subtraction angiography, visceral angiography, and selective arterial injection in the viscera. Glucagon, when needed, is administered in divided doses of 0.25 mg to a maximum of 1.0 mg intravenously. Risks include glucagon-induced hyperglycemia, vomiting (particularly when administered rapidly), gastric hypotonia, and provocation signs of pheochromocytoma (McLoughlin et al., 1981; Chernish and Maglinte, 1990; Jehenson, 1991). Children who receive glucagon should be routinely administered prophylactic antiemetics.

The ability to intermittently assess neurologic function and mental status is invaluable during embolization procedures but may not be practical in children because of fear, pain, and movement. General anesthesia permits easier control of blood pressure and ventilation and eliminates concern about patient movement. For children, general anesthesia is often preferred during high-risk procedures that require immobility and periods of breath-holding. Preprocedural assessment should include any history of seizures, bleeding, treatment with anticonvulsants or anticoagulants, neurologic symptoms, and evaluation of ICP status. It is important to determine whether the patient has had any transient ischemic attacks or evidence of cerebrovascular occlusion. Vasodilator agents (calcium channel blockers) and/or nitrate derivatives may have to be administered after embolization. Because many patients are anticoagulated during the procedure, a preoperative coagulation profile should be obtained. A variety of anticoagulants may have to be on hand as well to provide prophylaxis for thrombosis (Bidabe et al., 1990)

The potential morbidity associated with embolization is not negligible. AVMs involving the head and neck frequently require cannulation of the external carotid artery branches and the thyrocervical trunk. All patients scheduled for embolization should be typed and cross-matched for blood. Patients who undergo embolizations of AVMs of the head and neck are at risk for stroke, cranial nerve palsies, skin necrosis, blindness, infection, and pulmonary embolism (Riles et al., 1993). It is important to document full return of neurologic status after the patient is extubated.

Ultrasound-Directed Procedures

Needle biopsies and drainage procedures are directed with ultrasound guidance for diagnostic examination (kidney, liver, lung, muscle, unknown mass, unknown fluid). Percutaneous drainage of abscesses, cysts, pancreatic pseudocysts, and other fluid-containing structures can often be accomplished with ultrasound guidance. Ultrasound is useful for placement of difficult central venous catheters (CVLs) and peripherally inserted central catheters. The requirement for general anesthesia versus procedural sedation for ultrasound-guided procedures depends in part on the duration of the procedure, the location involved, the risks associated with the procedure, and any procedural requirements. The need for controlled ventilation with breath-holding may mandate an endotracheal tube and general anesthesia. Associated secondary effects of the end-organ disease must be kept in mind in the overall anesthesia care plan.

Magnetic Resonance Imaging

Atoms with an odd number of protons and/or neutrons are capable of acting as magnets. When they are aligned in a static magnetic field, they can be subjected to radiofrequency (RF) energy that alters their original orientation. With removal of the RF pulse, the nuclei rotate back to their original alignment (relaxation), and the energy released can be detected and transformed into an image. Hydrogen is the atom most often used for imaging, because it is present in most tissues as water and long-chain triglycerides.

MRI is used for the evaluation of central nervous system neoplasms, nonhemorrhagic trauma, and vascular and hemorrhagic lesions (Barnes, 1992). Brain MRI is frequently performed to evaluate developmental delay, behavioral disorders, seizures, failure to thrive, apnea/cyanosis, hypotonia, and mitochondrial/metabolic disorders. Magnetic resonance angiography (MRA) is especially helpful in evaluating vascular flow and can often replace invasive angiography in follow-up evaluations of vascular malformations, interventional therapy, or radiotherapy (Edelman and Warach, 1993a, 1993b). MRA does not involve the injection of intravascular contrast media and thereby avoids any risk of contrast reaction.

The most common cause of image degradation when performing MRI in children is patient movement. Techniques for monitoring anesthetized or critically ill patients during MRI have been described in several excellent reports (Karlik et al., 1988; Peden et al., 1992; Tobin et al., 1992). It is important to decide at the outset whether the anesthesia support should be within the magnetic field or outside of it; this will determine the configuration and composition of the equipment. Equipment located outside the magnetic field (e.g., outside of the 30- to 50-Gauss (G) line) can consist of standard equipment with long monitoring leads, and ventilation and gas aspiration tubing. The risks are related to disconnection and impaired direct contact monitoring. When placed close to the magnet, the anesthesia machine and its components must be nonferrous, with power supplied by filtered sources. All battery-operated equipment must be securely fixed in position and not moved during the examination because the homogeneity of the magnetic field is affected and the diagnostic images degraded. Most intravenous needles and catheters with metallic hubs are composed of high-grade stainless steel, which is not ferromagnetic. Infusion pumps can be placed outside of the magnetic field; the pump itself may malfunction under the influence of the strong magnetic field.

When placed outside the magnetic field, extra-long small-bore tubing is required for infusion. Intravenous or inhalation general anesthesia may be used effectively; there is some suggestion that the MRI signal may be altered under the influence of general inhalation anesthetics. Sedation can be problematic in the MR environment when so little of the patient is directly visible. MRI-compatible stethoscopes and flashlights are also helpful. Intubation in the MRI scanner can be accomplished without investing in MRI-compatible laryngoscopes; the only component of the laryngoscope that is not MRI compatible is the battery in the handle, but lithium-containing batteries are MRI compatible. Be aware that some batteries labeled as "lithium" may be tainted with a ferrous-containing substance. To identify this situation, the anesthesiologist should carefully bring the battery into the MRI scanner to confirm compatibility. Nonferrous laryngoscopes should be clearly identified to minimize the risk of a projectile injury in the scanner.

Anesthetic management of children in the MRI suite is highly dependent on the availability of MRI, compatible monitors, and anesthesia gas machines and proximity of the anesthetic provider to the patient and MRI unit. Anesthetic management also depends on the availability of support personnel, the personal style and comfort level of the anesthesiologist, and, of course, the patient's particular medical history. Requiring a general anesthetic to complete a noninvasive procedure is often a frightening concept for parents. Parents do not realize that although there is no pain or discomfort involved in the procedure, the child may still need a general anesthetic to remain motionless for the scan. It is the rare child who is able to remain motionless after oral midazolam or intramuscular ketamine. One technique for general anesthesia is to perform an inhalation induction followed by placement of an LMA. During the scan, the patient maintains spontaneous ventilation. Lidocaine gel (2%) on the LMA cuff is a useful adjunct, in that the lidocaine gel can decrease the incidence of sore throat (Keller et al., 1997) and retching (Chan and Tham, 1995). A retrospective study of 200 patients demonstrated the usefulness of this approach (Brimacombe et al., 1995). In children with upper respiratory infections, there was a lower incidence of mild bronchospasm, laryngospasm, breath-holding, and major oxygen desaturation (<90%) in the group with LMAs compared with the group with endotracheal anesthesia (Tait et al., 1998). In the MRI suite, temperature monitoring can be accomplished by liquid crystal display (skin temperature).

Anesthesiologists must be aware of many personal items taken for granted—clipboards, pens, watches, scissors, clamps, credit cards, eyeglasses, paperclips, etc. Laryngoscopes and blades are not ferromagnetic, but the batteries contained within the handle are ferromagnetic. As an alternative, a plastic laryngoscope can be powered by a single, paper-covered nonmagnetic 3-V lithium battery or a DC light source (Karlik et al., 1988; Peden et al., 1992; Tobin et al., 1992). Conventional electrocardiographic monitoring is not possible because as the lead wires traverse the magnetic fields, image degradation occurs; electrocardiography by telemetry is often chosen. Nonferrous pulse oximeters are available, and in some circumstances, fiberoptically cabled pulse oximeters may be shielded by aluminum foil to minimize magnetic field degradation. Burns have resulted from pulse oximetry monitoring in MRI (Shellock and Slimp, 1989; Brow et al., 1993).

Any wire in the magnet bore that is a sizable portion of a wavelength may absorb a considerable amount of energy from the transmitting coil, and large voltages may build up on the surface of the wire with no discharge path other than free space. If the wire is poorly insulated or partly exposed, the voltage may discharge through space into the skin, causing significant local burns. Precordial stethoscopes made of nonferrous materials are acceptable, but the amount of noise generated during RF pulsing and the length of tubing required render auscultation ineffective. The use of infrared transmission of breath and heart sounds with a special microphone has been described (Henneberg et al., 1992). Average noise levels of 95 dB have been measured in a 1.5-T MRI machine, comparable to noise levels of very heavy traffic (92 dB) or light road work (90 to 110 dB). Exposure to this level of noise has not been considered hazardous if limited to less than 2 hours per day (Gangarosa et al., 1987). There are case reports, however, of both temporary (Brummett et al., 1988) and permanent (Kanal et al., 1990) hearing loss after an MRI scan. Earplugs or MRI-compatible headphones should be offered to all pediatric patients.

Although studies in mice (Sperber et al., 1984) and dogs (Shuman et al., 1988) suggest that exposure to magnetic fields may increase body temperature, it is unlikely that static magnetic fields up to 1.5 T have any effect on core body temperature in adult humans (Shellock et al., 1986). To date, there have been no definitive studies to determine whether magnetic fields increase body temperature in the anesthetized or sedated pediatric patient. RF heating is a potential risk. The specific absorption rate (SAR) is measured in Watts per kilogram and is used to follow the effects of RF heating. The Food and Drug Administration allows an SAR of 0.4 W/kg averaged over the whole body. Ex vivo exposure of large metal prostheses to fields over six times that experienced in MRI have not revealed any appreciable heating (Davis et al., 1981). There are no appreciable problems with RF in magnets less than 2 T (Anonymous, 1988).

There are focal heating concerns with respect to monitoring equipment in the MRI scanner. For example, electrocardiographic leads must not have frayed or exposed wires. Any coils or loops in a conductor can cause tissue burns. There are case reports of first-, second-, and third-degree burns after MRI (Shellock and Slimp, 1989). To prevent patient injury, care must be used to avoid creating a conductive loop between the patient and a conductor (electrocardiographic monitoring/gating leads, plethysmographic gating wire, and fingertip attachment). During the scan, exposed wires or conductors cannot touch the patient's skin and no imaging coil can be left unconnected to the magnet.

The biologic effect of MRI should be considered when offering parent-present induction. To date there are no reports implicating MRI for any defects in chromosomal aberration, spermatogenesis, cell growth, or behavior and memory. Studies in amphibians demonstrate that exposure to a 4-T magnetic field does not cause any defects in embryologic development (Prasad et al., 1990). Most hospital MRI machines are 1.5 T. Despite these studies, pregnant mothers are usually not allowed in the scanner, regardless of their desire to be present for induction.

The characteristics of internal compression volume and respiratory minute volume in a 9-m breathing circuit in children and infants have been studied, and nomograms have been established to provide "long distance" mechanical ventilatory support for patients undergoing MRI (Neumark et al., 1989). Breathing circuits should be extra-long to ensure continuity of the circuit during movement of the gantry in and out of the scanner bore. A ventilator (225/SIMV; Monaghan Medical Corp., Plattsburg, NY) specifically designed for MRI has become available, which may be particularly important for use in patients who would be adversely affected by the length of circuit needed in this circumstance (Smith et al., 1986).

The American College of Radiology has established guidelines to avoid mishaps in the MRI environment (Kanal et al., 2002). Special care should be taken to distinguish ferrous from nonferrous oxygen tanks. Complications and deaths have occurred due to the accidental introduction of a ferrous cylinder into the MRI environment (Chaljub et al., 2001).

Additional MRI safety issues include implanted objects (i.e., cardiac pacemakers), ferromagnetic attraction creating "missiles," noise, biologic effects of the magnetic field, thermal effects, equipment issues, and claustrophobia. Some stainless steel may contain ferritic, austenitic, and martensitic components (Steels, 1961; Dujovny et al., 1985; Persson and Stahlberg, 1985). Martensitic alloys contain fractions of a crystal phase known as martensite, which has a body-centered cubic structure, is prone to stress corrosion failure, and is ferromagnetic. Austenite is formed in the hardening process of low carbon and alloyed steels and has ferromagnetic properties. Iron, nickel, and cobalt are also ferromagnetic. For this reason, the components of any implanted device should be carefully researched before entering the magnet. Stainless steel or surgical stainless objects interacting with an external magnetic field may produce translational (attractive) and rotational (torque) forces. Intracranial aneurysm clips, cochlear and stapedial implants, shrapnel, intraorbital metallic bodies, and prosthetic limbs may move and dislodge. Some eye makeup and tattoos may contain metallic dyes and therefore cause ocular, periorbital, and skin irritation (Scherzinger and Hendee, 1985; Prasad et al., 1990). Some tissue expanders that are used in reconstructive surgery have a magnetic port to help identify the location for intermittent injections of saline (Liang et al., 1989). Personal experience has also demonstrated that Bivona (Bivona Medical Technologies, Division of UroQuest Medical Corporation, Gary, IN) tracheostomy tubes may pose a risk in the MRI environment. Although not listed on the package insert, there is ferrous material within the Bivona tracheostomy tube itself. This may not only produce rotational and translational motion but may also prove to be a thermal hazard.

The magnetic field may affect the electrocardiogram. The changes in the T wave are not due to biologic effects of the magnetic field but rather to superimposed induced voltages. This effect of the magnetic field on the T wave is not related to cardiac depolarization, because no changes to the P, Q, R, or S wave have ever been observed in patients exposed to fields up to 2 T. There are no reports of MRI affecting heart rate (Beischer, 1969), electrocardiographic recording (McRobbie and Foster, 1985), cardiac contractility (Gulch and Lutz, 1986), or blood pressure (Tenforde et al., 1983). One study, however, found that humans exposed to a 2-T magnet for 10 minutes developed a 17% increase in the cardiac cycle length (CCL). The CCL reverted to preexposure length within 10 minutes of removing the patient from the magnetic field (Jehenson et al., 1988). The implications of this finding are unclear. This change in CCL in patients with normal hearts may be of no consequence. The implications of this finding for patients with fragile dysrhythmias or sick sinus syndrome, however, have yet to be determined.

Cardiac pacemakers present a special hazard in and around the MRI scanner, especially in patients who are pacemaker dependent. Most pacemakers have a reed relay switch that can be activated when exposed to a magnet of sufficient strength (Pavlicek et al., 1983). This activation could convert the pacemaker to the asynchronous mode. There are at least two known cases of patients with pacemakers who died from cardiac arrest while in the MRI scanner. The autopsy of one patient determined that the death was the result of an interruption of the pacemaker in the magnetic environment (Health, 1989). In addition to the risk of pacemaker malfunction, there is the chance that torque on the pacer or pacing leads may create a disconnect or microshock (Erlebacher et al., 1986). Caution should be taken so that the patient with the pacemaker avoids both the MRI suite and the immediate surroundings, to a fringe area of less than 5 G. Heart valves, unlike cardiac pacemakers, are not ferromagnetic and are not a contraindication to MRI. It is critical that everyone entering the vicinity of the MRI scanner fills out a screening form that specifically lists every possible implantable device, alerting the MRI staff to any potential hazards.

Projectiles are a hazard in the MRI suite. In the presence of an external magnetic field, a ferromagnetic object can develop its own magnetic field. The attractive forces that are created between the intrinsic and extrinsic magnetic fields can propel the ferromagnetic object toward the MRI scanner. Placing a magnet outside the MRI scanner is a helpful way to test any objects as to their attraction to a magnet and avoid disasters in the MRI scanner. Some objects that have been attracted to the MRI magnet are a metal fan, pulse oximeter, shrapnel, wheelchair, cigarette lighter, stethoscope, pager, hearing aid, vacuum cleaner, calculator, hair pin, oxygen tank, prosthetic limb, pencil, insulin infusion pump, keys, watches, and steel-tipped/heeled shoes (Kanal, 1992). Large objects may have so much attractive force with the MRI scanner that quenching the magnet may be the only way to release the object once it is attached to the scanner. Quenching the magnet is not without risk; this action fills the scanner with noxious helium gas, mandates extensive follow-up technical support to restart the magnet, and requires a minimum of 48 hours to regenerate the magnetic field.

Some patients experience claustrophobia and have difficulty cooperating during the study. Anxiety reactions (Granet and Gelber, 1990) have been estimated to occur in 4% to 30% of patients (Melendez and McCrank, 1993). Patients with extreme skeletal abnormalities such as advanced scoliosis or flexion contractures may be unable to lie motionless or supine for the duration of the scan; these patients may require general anesthesia for positioning and comfort.

NUCLEAR MEDICINE

Nuclear medicine is one of the oldest functional imaging disciplines. These scans are useful for identification of epileptic foci in refractory epilepsy, evaluation of cerebrovascular (Moyamoya) disease, and evaluation of cognitive and behavior disorders (O'Tuama and Treves, 1993). Anesthesiologists become involved when the child's medical history suggests that procedural sedation would not be appropriate; to complete these scans, the child must remain motionless for at least 1 hour.

The two most common nuclear medicine studies that require the administration of an anesthetic are single-photon emission computed tomography (SPECT) and positron emission tomography (PET). SPECT scans use single-photon γ-emitting radioisotopes and rotating gamma cameras to produce three-dimensional brain images. SPECT scans involve the use of radiolabeled technetium-99m (^{99m}Tc; half-life, 6 hours), which has a high rate of first-pass extraction as well as intracellular trapping in proportion to regional cerebral blood flow (Chiron et al., 1989). This scan is ideal when seeking seizure foci, which are associated with alterations in regional cerebral blood flow and metabolism. This scan often precedes surgical resection of the identified focus. The technetium radionuclide is ideal because it remains intracellular and can be visualized on scan hours after a seizure has occurred. Ideally, the child should be scanned within 1 to 6 hours of the seizure. The radionuclides are physiologically harmless and nonallergenic. Caretakers, however, should wear gloves to minimize contact with radiation-containing secretions.

PET scans use PET and radionuclide tracers of metabolic activity, such as oxygen or glucose metabolism (Chugani, 1993; Griffeth et al., 1993). Unlike SPECT scans, PET scans should be performed during the seizure itself. Because of the short half-life of the glucose tracer (110 minutes), the scan is best completed during the seizure or within 1 hour thereafter.

RADIATION ONCOLOGY

Radiation therapy for children uses ionizing photons to destroy lymphomas, acute leukemias, Wilms' tumor, retinoblastomas, and tumors of the central nervous system. Repeat sessions are typical, requiring reliable motionlessness to precisely aim the beam at malignant cells while sparing healthy cells and remote monitoring with a child in isolation. A planning session in a simulator is often scheduled before the initiation of radiation therapy so that fields to be irradiated can be plotted and marked.

Radiation therapy is usually very brief and nonpainful and may be approached with a variety of plans for rendering the patient temporarily motionless. The key issue is the anesthesiologist's limited access to the patient. Remote video monitoring and electrocardiography and pulse oximetry are crucial. Two or three video cameras are used to look at the monitors, the chest, and the face of the patient. A CVL in young children undergoing a long course of radiation therapy helps immensely. It is important to remember that infants undergoing radiation therapy after a prolonged fast are at risk for hypoglycemia; delayed awakening or tremulousness should prompt a Dextrostix determination.

Fractionated radiation therapy is the principle of dividing the total radiation therapy course into discrete daily sessions, allowing normal tissue repair between sessions while the tumor burden is lessened or destroyed. Hyperfractionated, or multiple-session daily, radiation therapy is a modality reported primarily in adults for head and neck cancer. The rationale for twice-daily fractionation in children is that fractionation to growing bone in rats reduces the growth deficit by 25% to 30%. The hope is that other normal tissues may be similarly spared during growth (Eifel, 1988; Eifel et al., 1990). One successful approach has been to give children an initial formula feeding 6 hours before their first treatment and keep them NPO until recovery from their second anesthetic 6 hours after the first (Menache et al., 1990). However, with the current liberalization of NPO guidelines, another approach is to give children clear liquids during their recovery from the first anesthetic until 3 hours before the second anesthetic.

Stereotactic radiosurgery (gamma knife) is a major advance in the treatment of selected intracranial AVMs and tumors in children (Loeffler et al., 1990). Stereotactic radiosurgery differs from external beam radiotherapy in several important ways. A focused single large fraction of radiation is used instead of smaller, daily fractions. Stereotactic radiosurgery uses relatively weak intensity γ-rays produced by 201 cobalt-60 sources, which intersect at a single point; all 201 beams converge to destroy tumors, vascular malformations, or abnormal tissue sites within the brain. Normal brain tissue surrounding the abnormality is relatively protected from radiation effects. In children and adults, most radiosurgery had originally concentrated on the treatment of small, histologically benign lesions such as vascular malformations, acoustic neuromas, and pituitary adenomas. This focus has been expanded to include malignant tumors such as solitary metastases, ependymomas, glioblastomas, and several other tissue types. For optimal results, the tumor volume is small (≤ 14 cm^3) (Coffey et al., 1992; Lunsford and Linskey, 1992).

Stereotactic radiosurgery requires coordination among members of the departments of radiology, radiation therapy, neurosurgery, and anesthesia. The stereotactic procedure begins in either the CT or MRI suite. The child is placed in a stereotactic head frame that is screwed into the cranium. Most adults are able to tolerate this entire procedure with local anesthesia or sedation. The neurosurgeon infiltrates the skin with a local anesthetic before applying the head frame. Adults and older children who tolerate this procedure with sedation alone may vomit as a result of the anxiety, the headache, or the location of the tumor itself. Because the head frame is heavy and cumbersome, it is difficult for the vomiting patient to turn his or her head to protect the airway. Pediatric patients (including most teenagers) typically require a general anesthetic. General anesthetic with tracheal intubation is induced and a nasogastric tube is placed before placement of the head frame. The key for removal of the head frame is taped to the frame itself.

Calculations for dose and the three-dimensional coordinates for the beam may take several hours to compute following the initial radiologic study and head frame placement. A variety of anesthetic techniques are used, including continuous infusion, volatile anesthetics, or combinations of both. Some patients do well with sedation and spontaneous breathing, but younger patients are usually mechanically ventilated. An initial CT scan is followed by computer calculations. Once the calculations are complete, the patient is transferred to the radiosurgery suite for irradiation. After irradiation, the patient is allowed to emerge from the anesthetic (Loeffler et al., 1990). The most common perioperative problem is nausea and vomiting, probably due to sensitivity of the chemoreceptor trigger zone centers to radiation.

Stereotactic radiation therapy is more precise localization of the fractionated radiation dose over the same duration of time as conventional radiation therapy, with the adjunctive use of a head frame. Considerations for the head frame include ease of application, reliability, ability to deliver supplemental oxygen and support the airway with a facemask if needed, and rapid removal of the facial restraint should it become necessary.

Total body irradiation (TBI) is associated with vomiting. Factors involved with postprocedural emesis include patient movement, single-dose (compared with fractionated) radiation, and patient age of greater than 10 years. Sedation has been found to decrease the incidence of vomiting with TBI, as has general endotracheal anesthesia (Whitwam et al., 1978; Westbrook et al., 1987). Propofol sedation might be ideal, given its sedative, recovery, and antiemetic properties.

Anesthesia may alter the radiosensitivity of tumors. A biphasic response to tumor radiosensitivity has been found in mice under ketamine and diazepam anesthesia (Nias and Perry, 1989). Although cellular oxygen metabolism is reduced by the anesthetic as well as by hypothermia, the blood supply to the mouse tumors remained intact and therefore enhanced radiosensitivity after 25 minutes, with less radiosensitivity at 10 minutes.

Oxygen enrichment tended to enhance sensitivity with time as well. A radioprotective effect and shorter tumor growth delay have been found in phenobarbital-anesthetized mice compared with ketamine-anesthetized mice undergoing radiotherapy based on decreased tumor blood volume. Hypoxic cell sensitizers have been found to decrease the protective influence of anesthetics on normal lung tissue of previously anesthetized mice, whereas they do not alter the sensitivity of normal lung tissue in unanesthetized mice (Down et al., 1983).

CLINIC AND OFFICE PROCEDURES

Endoscopic Procedures

Gastrointestinal endoscopy has become a routine part of patient care, and as such it constitutes the bulk of procedures performed by a pediatric gastroenterologist (Fox, 1998). Depending on the patient and the type of procedure contemplated (therapeutic versus diagnostic), children may require no or minimal to moderately deep sedation or general anesthesia. Minimal sedation may impair cognitive function and coordination while ventilatory and cardiovascular functions are relatively unaffected. However, pediatric patients often are uncooperative and do not tolerate endoscopic procedures with minimal or moderate sedation, necessitating deeper sedation or general anesthesia to successfully accomplish the procedure (ASA, 2002).

The inability to independently maintain ventilatory function and to respond purposefully increases the risk involved with deep sedation. It has been recommended that deep sedation and general anesthesia be performed by an anesthesiologist (Saint-Maurice, 1992; Wolfe and Rao, 1992; Hassall, 1993, 1994; Dillon et al., 1998; Bouchut et al., 2001; Koh et al., 2001). Furthermore, if the majority of these cases could be done in the endoscopy suite rather than the operating room, then multiple advantages can be realized—increased operating room use for surgical procedures and improved efficiency and turnover in scheduling in the smaller and more manageable endoscopy suite. Children with more complex medical problems, anticipated airway difficulties, morbid obesity, or behavioral problems can undergo their procedure in the operating room. Regardless of the site of the procedure, all patients scheduled for endoscopy should be evaluated before the procedure to confirm that they are appropriate candidates. In addition, the anesthetic technique depends on the procedure, the patient, and the skill of the endoscopist as well as the limitations and capabilities of the endoscopy suite (e.g., total intravenous anesthesia techniques in the absence of appropriate scavenging).

Procedural sedation is readily achieved with an intravenous anesthetic combining a sedative (e.g., midazolam), an opioid (e.g., fentanyl, alfentanil, remifentanil), and a hypnotic (e.g., propofol). Spontaneous ventilation without the patient's airway being intubated has been shown to be a safe and effective technique (Bouchut et al., 2001; Koh et al., 2001). The majority of complications are respiratory and usually occur during an esophagogastroduodenoscopy (EGD); these complications include apnea, laryngospasm, bronchospasm, and airway obstruction. Most problems resolve after withdrawal of the endoscope and positive pressure ventilation with a tightly fitting mask, but some patients require endotracheal intubation to secure an airway and have the procedure safely completed.

Esophagogastroduodenoscopy

Access to the airway is obviously limited once a transoral endoscope is in place. It is important to maintain spontaneous ventilation during deep sedation because any airway intervention needed typically requires the removal of the endoscope. The two most stimulating portions of the EGD are transoral and transpyloric passage of the endoscope. A smooth endoscope insertion can be aided by topical spray of local anesthesia to the oropharynx to help eliminate coughing and gagging.

A majority of the respiratory complications noted previously occur during EGD, especially in infants and younger children, compared with colonoscopy. It has been suggested that this results from a combination of factors that include the large size of the endoscope and partial airway obstruction resulting in hypoxemia. Abdominal distention secondary to air introduced into the stomach may impair diaphragmatic excursion and lead to hypoventilation. This has led several groups to select 6 months as the age before which general anesthesia with endotracheal intubation is required for the procedure, due to a higher respiratory complication rate in this age group (Wolfe et al., 1992; Koh et al., 2001).

Colonoscopy

Access to the airway is unimpeded during a colonoscopy. Deep sedation can be achieved more readily, and if respiratory problems occur, airway interventions are straightforward to manage. Patients undergoing colonoscopy also experience increased stimulation during certain parts of the procedure, such as traversing the colon to the cecum. At times, abdominal pressure is applied to help guide the colonoscope. The depth of the anesthetic should be adjusted accordingly.

Endoscopic Retrograde Cannulation of the Pancreas

Although many institutions report success of procedural sedation in pediatric patients undergoing ERCP (Teng et al., 2000; Prasil et al., 2001), general anesthesia with endotracheal intubation may make the procedure easier to perform, especially if the procedure is long, the patient has significant comorbid diseases, or the procedure is performed with the patient in the prone position.

Psychiatric Interviews

Intravenous sodium amobarbital has a long history as an adjunct to psychotherapy, having found its peak use during World War II and immediately thereafter in aiding soldiers to deal with the stresses and trauma of combat (Zonana, 1979). This technique has had a resurgence for diagnostic and therapeutic interventions in adults, but pediatric reports are rare. Weller and others (1985) reported success in the diagnosis and treatment of prepubertal children and emphasized the "backup" of an anesthesiologist. The induction of a tranquil state until signs of sedation occur, such as slurred speech, a sense of fatigue, difficulty counting backwards, and "basal" vital signs, are not unlike our daily efforts at anxiolysis during monitored anesthesia care. The use of a bispectral index (BIS) monitor may prove to be a useful adjunct as well (Palmer et al., 2001). The psychiatric interview process under these conditions is fascinating to participate in, if only as an observer. Memory retrieval, such as the uncovering of relationships between current psychopathology and earlier traumatic life events, and symptom removal via therapeutic suggestions are examples of interventions facilitated by the pharmacologically induced relaxed state made possible by the anesthesiologist during the interview.

SAFETY ISSUES FOR PATIENTS AND THEIR ANESTHESIOLOGISTS

As anesthesiologists find themselves participating in the care of patients requiring increasingly sophisticated imaging technology, it is appropriate to examine the risks for patients and staff exposed to the types of high energies and contrast agents used.

USE OF CONTRAST MEDIA

In a comprehensive review, Goldberg (1984) noted approximately 5% of radiologic examinations with RCM are complicated by adverse reactions, with one third of these being severe and requiring immediate treatment. Reactions occur most commonly in patients between 20 and 50 years of age and are relatively rare in children. The male/female ratio is about 2.5:1, not dissimilar to the gender distribution of other allergies such as latex, aspirin, and neuromuscular blocking agents. With a history of atopy or allergy, the risk of a reaction is increased 1.5- to 10-fold. Reactions vary from mild, subjective sensations of restlessness, nausea, and vomiting to a rapidly evolving, angioedema-like picture accompanied by bronchospasm, arrhythmias, and cardiac arrest. Because of the high osmolar concentration of these agents (often >1,000 mOsm and sometimes >2,000 mOsm), caution should be exercised with patients who have a limited cardiovascular reserve such as patients in congestive heart failure or those with cardiomyopathy. In addition, volume-depleted young children who have been kept NPO for prolonged intervals or who have had bowel preps should be hydrated before RCM administration.

Patients dependent on a full intravascular volume status (patients with sickle cell disease, restricted pulmonary circuit volume with cyanotic congenital heart disease, with arteriovenous shunts, etc.) should be monitored carefully for an initial rise in filling pressures and intravascular volume and subsequent diuresis following an osmolar load. Patients with impaired excretory mechanisms, such as those in renal failure, must be monitored closely following high osmolar loads. Low osmolar RCM are relatively safe with regard to life-threatening reactions, but moderate non–life-threatening reactions that require some treatment occur 0.2% to 0.4% of the time and a severe life-threatening reaction can occur in 0.04% of patients (Thomsen and Bush, 1998).

RCM contain iodine because its high density and low toxicity make it an ideal agent for visualization and differentiation. The iodine is filtered through the glomeruli and is not reabsorbed by either the glomeruli or the tubules. Because the contrast agent is hypertonic relative to plasma, an initial hypertensive response is usually followed by a hyperosmotic diuresis with the potential for hypotension. Equilibration with the extracellular fluid compartment occurs within 10 minutes, heralded by the onset of diuresis. Special attention should be paid when administering iodine RCM to any child with a history of congestive heart failure. The initial increase in blood volume may precipitate cardiovascular compromise. Patients with hepatic or renal dysfunction should be observed closely for signs of impaired excretion of the RCM. Sickle cell disease presents its own inherent risks associated with RCM.

After administration, the increase in blood osmolarity may precipitate shrinkage, clumping, and, ultimately, sickling of erythrocytes. One theoretical concern in patients with sickle cell disease is sickle crisis and vascular occlusion. Sickled cells are known to align with external magnetic fields to which they are exposed; it is unknown how this theoretical concern compares, for example, with the normal forces of deformation imposed on red cells of patients with sickle cell disease in their normal course through the vascular tree (Kanal et al., 1990).

Gadolinium dithylenetriaminepentaacetic acid (DTPA) is a low osmolar ionic contrast medium used for MRI, with a slower clearance in neonates and young infants than in adults, yielding longer windows for imaging (Elster, 1990). Free gadolinium has a biologic half-life of several weeks, with uptake and excretion taking place in the kidneys and liver. Unfortunately, free gadolinium is quite toxic and is chelated to another structure that restricts the ion and decreases its toxicity. The clinical safety profiles for the three available MRI contrast agents are quite comparable, with the most common reactions being nausea, vomiting, hives, and headache. Local injection site symptoms include irritation, focal burning, or a cool sensation. Transient elevations in serum bilirubin (3% to 4% of patients) have been reported, and a transient elevation in iron for Magnevist and Omniscan (15% to 30% of patients) occurs, which tends to reverse spontaneously within 24 to 48 hours (Van Wagoner and Worah, 1993). Anaphylactoid reactions occur in 1:100,000 to 1:500,000 of doses and are rarer in children.

The earlier literature states that patients who have had anaphylactic reactions to shellfish are at increased risk of anaphylactoid reaction to RCM. The irony of the statement is that it may be correct, but for nonobvious reasons. The original rationale was that shellfish contain high quantities of iodine and therefore it was assumed that there would be a risk of cross-reactivity. However, neither shellfish allergy nor RCM reactions are due to iodine. Atopy per se is a risk factor; the association between atopy, anaphylactic reactions to shellfish, and a possible predisposition to an RCM reaction may indeed be valid.

The treatment of severe allergic reactions, whether anaphylactoid or anaphylactic, is no different than that for any other allergic reaction. Epinephrine, aminophylline, atropine, diphenhydramine, and steroids have all been used to control varying degrees of adverse reactions. A patient who requires RCM administration and who has had a previous reaction to RCM has an increased (35% to 60%) risk for a reaction on reexposure. Pretreatment of these high-risk patients with prednisone and diphenhydramine 1 hour before RCM administration reduces the risk of reactions to 9%; the addition of ephedrine 1 hour before RCM administration further reduces the rate to 3.1% (Kelly et al., 1978; Greenberger, 1984).

Allergic reactions rarely occur with oral agents. The incidence of severe anaphylactoid reactions to gastrointestinally administered agents is approximately 1:2,500,000 and the causes remain unknown. There are no pretreatment protocols established for these types of reactions and no well-defined risk factors. Gastrointestinal complications include nausea, vomiting, and diarrhea. One of the factors that may protect against having an allergic reaction is the poor absorption of oral iodinated contrast agents. Indeed, disruption of the gastrointestinal mucosa is recognized as causing an increase in absorption of oral contrast and the urinary excretion of contrast in a gastrointestinal study is a well-recognized sign. Yet rarely, they are associated with bronchospasm, flushing, periorbital edema, pruritis, rash, rhinitis, and urticaria.

IONIZING RADIATION

Radiation exposure is directly proportional to the duration of the procedure and inversely proportional to the square of the distance from the source. Henderson and others (1991) monitored the radiation exposure of 16 pediatric anesthesia fellows during a 2-month period. Fellows assigned to the cardiac catheterization laboratory had fluoroscopy exposure times of 14 to 85 minutes per case, typically for two or three cases per day. For these anesthesiologists, badge readings ranged from 20 to 180 mrem/month. All noncardiac anesthesia fellows had undetectable (<10 mrem/month) levels. All fellows wore lead aprons, 50% wore a thyroid shield, and one stepped at least 10 feet away from the source during every exposure; this latter fellow had a reading of 30 mrem, despite having spent 26 hours in the catheterization laboratory. The annual maximum permissible dose (MPD) for nonradiation workers (including anesthesiologists) is 100 mrem or 1 milli-Sievert (mSv, Systeme Internationale Units). For comparison, the MPD for radiation workers is 50 mSv annually and 10 mSv times age cumulatively. MPD during pregnancy for radiation workers (per gestation) is 5 mSv.

HIGH-INTENSITY MAGNETIC FIELDS

MRI exposes the patient (and the health care workers surrounding the patient) to a static magnetic field, a rapid switched spatial gradient magnetic field, and RF magnetic fields. The static magnetic field, which causes alignment of unpaired tissue protons, may cause movement of ferromagnetic devices such as vascular clips, ventricular shunt connectors, casings for pacemakers, and control devices for pacemakers. Metallic devices in other areas, particularly when invested with fibrous tissue, are less problematic (Shellock and Crues, 1988; Shellock, 1989). As mentioned previously, tissue expanders may have magnetic ports to facilitate identification of the injection site. Despite their low mass, such ports have a potential for torque and movement in the presence of a strong magnetic field; the specific type of tissue expander should be identified before patient entry into the MRI suite (Liang et al., 1989). Assessment of risk in patients with implants or other possibly ferromagnetic devices or objects consists of a careful history that includes penetrating wounds, physical examination to look for scars, and possibly a plain radiograph of the region in question (Pohost et al., 1992). Other concerns have been increased blood pressure, cardiac arrhythmias, and impaired mental function. While these issues have been described or theorized on an experimental basis, little clinical documentation is available.

The magnetic field generates an electrical current that is 2 to 3 orders of magnitude less than that of a defibrillator (10 mA/M^2 compared with 1,000 to 10,000 mA/M^2). This current strength may nevertheless reprogram a programmable pacemaker and interfere with its function (Erlebacher et al., 1986). Exposure to a strong external magnetic or electromagnetic field can lead to conversion of a demand pulse generator from synchronous to asynchronous mode, damage to the reed switch (which activates the fixed-rate pulse generator), reprogramming of pacemaker parameters, induction of currents in the electrode wires, or displacement of the generator itself. Indeed, it is the sensitivity of some reed switches that has determined the "safety boundary" of magnetic resonance devices as being 5 G (5×10^{-4} T). Patients with implantable defibrillators-cardioverters, implantable infusion (e.g., insulin) pumps, cochlear implants, and neurostimulators are all at risk for having the implant device reprogrammed on exposure to the magnetic field. Defibrillator failure has been reported in the MRI environment (Snowdon, 1989).

As stated previously, RF pulses cause heat production in metallic implants and coiled wires such as electrocardiographic cables or pulse oximeter cables if they are looped and laying on the patient's skin. Patients with compromised thermoregulatory abilities, such as those with cardiac problems or fever or taking certain drugs, may be at particular risk. Included in this group are infants, whose SAR is greater than that of adults because of the greater ratio of body surface area to body mass. SAR refers to the energy absorption (e.g., increasing body temperature) with an increase in the total amount of RF energy absorbed (Fitzsimmons, 1992).

Increased reports of vertigo, nausea, and a metallic taste have been found in a study on human exposure to a 4-T magnetic field (whole body scanner) (Schenck et al., 1992). Fertilized frog embryos exposed to a 4-T magnetic field did not demonstrate any adverse effects on early development (Prasad et al., 1990). An increase in cardiac cycle length of 17% was found in healthy volunteers in a 2-T environment after 10 minutes of exposure, causing speculation about the effect of the 2-T environment on the sinus node (Jehenson et al., 1988). This may be of particular concern in patients with a preexisting arrhythmia history. Of more significant concern in pediatric patients is the potential for hypothermia because of the airflow directed through the scanner cavity and the inability to control room temperature or use radiant warmers. The use of warm intravenous fluid bags, thermal packs, and blankets can decrease heat loss. Excellent reviews of monitoring considerations and equipment choices in the MRI environment as well as patient safety principles are available (Kanal et al., 1990; International Non-Ionizing Radiation Committee of the International Radiation Protection Association, 1991; Fitzsimmons, 1992; Menon et al., 1992; New York Academy of Sciences, 1992; Patteson and Chesney, 1992; Pohost et al., 1992), and the American College of Radiology published a white paper on magnetic resonance safety (Kanal et al., 2002).

MRI and spectroscopy do not use ionizing radiation. Secondary harmful effects, such as magnetic objects becoming projectiles within the magnetic field as they approach the bore of the magnet and potentially causing injury, are a consideration (Chu and Sangster, 1986; Chaljub et al., 2001). Patients (and anesthesiologists!) with metallic implants such as vascular clamps, hemostatic clips, dental devices, heart valve prostheses, intravascular coils, filters and stents, ocular implants, orthopedic implants, otologic implants, shrapnel, penile implants, and vascular access ports must be individually evaluated for their risk in the MRI environment (Cahalan et al., 1987; Shellock and Curtis, 1991).

As with individual precautions, equipment precautions should be taken for all ferromagnetic objects such as intravenous stands, oxygen and nitrous oxide cylinders, and monitoring equipment. The anesthesia machine, if used in the scanning room, should be outfitted with aluminum gas cylinders and kept in the corner of the room. Anesthesia machines especially designed to be MRI compatible are readily available.

DIFFICULT AIRWAY MANAGEMENT IN THE RADIOLOGY SUITE

If a child with a known difficult airway requires intubation to complete the scheduled procedure, it is wise to perform the anesthetic induction in the operating room, an area where access to emergency airway equipment is readily available. Regardless of an anesthesiologist's comfort level and familiarity with extramural environments, the same depth of backup coverage is simply not available.

The unrecognized difficult airway is problematic in a remote location; it is important to have LMAs stocked in all extramural anesthesia carts. If a child cannot be intubated or mask ventilated, LMAs can provide a successful alternative. Case reports describe the successful use of LMAs in children with difficult craniofacial anomalies, such as Goldenhar's syndrome (Fan et al., 1995; Haxby and Liban, 1995) and even Pierre Robin association (Hansen et al., 1995). Similarly, a lightwand may facilitate endotracheal intubation in the child with a difficult airway (Holzman et al., 1988).

It is important to recognize that the airway that had not been difficult on induction may become difficult on emergence following sclerotherapy with alcohol and subsequent tissue edema, particularly at the base of the tongue, the neck, or the mediastinum (Furst et al., 1996; Ohlms et al., 1996; Fishman, 1999). These patients often require several days of airway support and ongoing evaluation in the intensive care unit until airway swelling is no longer a concern.

BLOOD LOSS MANAGEMENT OUT OF THE OPERATING ROOM

Transfusion requirements are rare in extramural locations, yet preprocedural anemia, accidental perforation of vascular structures, or medical transfusion requirements such as sickle cell disease or prematurity may require transfusion therapy. Equipment familiar to the anesthesiologist and identical to that available in the operating room is a welcome sight in a life-threatening emergency. Calling for additional help, establishing additional vascular access, and coordinating with the blood bank are crucial. Having a runner available may be critical when there is no designated "circulating nurse." It may become necessary to involve a surgeon urgently and transport the patient to the operating room, in which case it would be optimal to have another anesthesia team set up the operating room while the patient is being prepared for transport.

SUMMARY

We reviewed some general issues as well as some specific situations for anesthetizing children outside the operating room. There is no "correct technique" for delivering anesthesia to patients in these areas. Versatility must be maintained to adapt to many different clinical situations and remote locations. Because of the evolution of specialized equipment and procedures for radiology in particular, it is likely that the involvement of anesthesiologists in caring for children outside of the operating room will increase in years to come.

REFERENCES

American Academy of Pediatrics, Section on Anesthesiology: Guidelines for the pediatric perioperative anesthesia environment. *Pediatrics* 103:512, 1999.

American Society for Metals Committee for Wrought Stainless Steels: *Wrought stainless steels.* Metals Park, OH, 1961, American Society for Metals.

American Society of Anesthesiologists, ASA Task Force on Sedation and Analgesia by Non-anesthesiologists: Practical guidelines for sedation and analgesia by non-anesthesiologists. *Anesthesiology* 96:1004, 2002.

Anonymous: Consensus conference. Magnetic resonance imaging. *JAMA* 259:2132, 1988.

Barnes P: Imaging of the central nervous system in pediatrics and adolescence. *Pediatr Clin North Am* 39:743, 1992.

Becker GJ, Holden RW, Clatte EC: Therapeutic embolization with absolute ethanol. *Semin Intervent Radiol* 1:118, 1984.

Beischer DE: Vectorcardiogram and aortic blood flow of squirrel monkeys in a strong superconductive electromagnet. In Barnothy M, editor: *Biological effects of magnetic fields*, vol 2. New York, 1969, Plenum, p 241.

Bidabe AM, Greselle JF, Gin AM, et al.: Protocole de preparation, d'anesthesie et de surveillance en angiographie therapeutique. *Agressologie* 31:280, 1990.

Blankenberg F, Loh N, Bracci P, et al.: Sonography, CT, and MR imaging: A prospective comparison of neonates with suspected intracranial ischemia and hemorrhage. *AJNR Am J Neuroradiol* 21:213, 2000.

Bloomfield EL, Masaryk TJ, Caplin A, et al.: Intravenous sedation for MR imaging of the brain and spine in children: Pentobarbital versus propofol. *Radiology* 186:93, 1993.

Bouchut J, Godard J, Lachaux A: Deep sedation for upper gastrointestinal endoscopy in children. *J Pediatr Gastroenterol Nutr* 32:108, 2001.

Brimacombe J, Tucker P, Simons S: The laryngeal mask airway for awake diagnostic bronchoscopy. A retrospective study of 200 consecutive patients. *Eur J Anaesthesiol* 12:357, 1995.

Brose WG, Samuels SI, Steinberg GK: Cardiorespiratory arrest following initiation of cranial irradiation for treatment of a brain stem tumor. *Anesthesiology* 71:450, 1989.

Brow TR, Goldstein B, Little J: Severe burns resulting from magnetic resonance imaging with cardiopulmonary monitoring. Risks and relevant safety precautions. *Am J Phys Med Rehabil* 72:166, 1993.

Brummett R, Talbot J, Charuhas P: Potential hearing loss resulting from MR imaging. *Radiology* 169:539, 1988.

Burnette PK, Perkins J: Parenteral ondansetron for the treatment of chemotherapy and radiation-induced nausea and vomiting. *Pharmacotherapy* 12:120, 1992.

Burrows FA, Hickey PR, Colan S: Perioperative complications in patients with anthracycline chemotherapeutic agents. *Can Anaesth Soc* J 32:149, 1985.

Cahalan MK, Litt L, Botvinick EH, et al.: Advances in noninvasive cardiovascular imaging: implications for the anesthesiologist. *Anesthesiology* 66:356, 1987.

Chaljub G, Kramer L, Johnson RR, et al.: Projectile cylinder accidents resulting from the presence of ferromagnetic nitrous oxide or oxygen tanks in the MR suite. *AJR Am J Roentgenol* 177:27, 2001.

Chan S, Tham C: The effects of 2% lignocaine gel on incidence of retching with the use of the laryngeal mask airway. *Anaesthesia* 50:257, 1995.

Chernish SM, Maglinte DD: Glucagon: Common untoward reactions—review and recommendations. *Radiology* 177:145, 1990.

Chiron C, Raynaud C, Dulac O, et al.: Study of the cerebral blood flow in partial epilepsy of childhood using the SPECT method. *J Neuroradiol* 16:317, 1989.

Chu WK, Sangster W: Potential impacts of MRI accidents. *Radiol Technol* 58:139, 1986.

Chugani H: PET in preoperative evaluation of intractable epilepsy. *Pediatr Neurol* 9:411, 1993.

Chung T, Hoffer F, Connor L, et al.: The use of oral pentobarbital sodium (Nembutal) versus oral chloral hydrate in infants undergoing CT and MR imaging—a pilot study. *Pediatr Radiol* 30:332, 2000.

Coffey RJ, Lunsford LD, Flickinger JC: The role of radiosurgery in the treatment of malignant brain tumors. *Neurosurg Clin North Am* 3:231, 1992.

Coldwell D, Stokes K, Yakes W: Embolotherapy: Agents, clinical applications, and techniques. *Radiographics* 14:623, 1994.

Committee on Drugs, American Academy of Pediatrics: Guidelines for monitoring and management of pediatric patients during and after sedation for diagnostic and therapeutic procedures. *Pediatrics* 89:1110, 1992.

Connor L, Burrows P, Zurakowski D, et al.: Effects of intravenous pentobarbital with or without fentanyl on end-tidal carbon dioxide levels during deep sedation of pediatric patients undergoing MRI scans. *AJR Am J Roentgenol* 181:1691, 2003.

Cremin BJ: Sedation for CT examinations in children. *Br J Radiol* 63:316, 1990.

Davidson R: Atlanto-axial instability in Down syndrome: A fresh look at the evidence. *Pediatrics* 81:857, 1988.

Davis P, Crooks L, Arakawa M, et al.: Potential hazards in NMR imaging: Heating effects of changing magnetic fields and RF fields on small metallic implants. *AJR Am J Roentgenol* 137:857, 1981.

Department of Health and Human Services, Food and Drug Administration: *Guidelines for evaluating electro-magnetic exposure risk for trials of clinical NMR systems.* Washington, DC, 1982, Food and Drug Administration.

Diament MJ, Boechat MI, Kangarloo H: Interventional radiology in infants and children: Clinical and technical aspects. *Radiology* 154:359, 1985.

Dillon M, Brown S, Casey W: Colonoscopy under general anesthesia in children. *Pediatrics* 102:381, 1998.

Down JD, Collis CH, Jeffery PK, et al.: The effects of anesthetics and misonidazole on the development of radiation-induced lung damage in mice. *Int J Radiat Oncol Biol Phys* 9:221, 1983.

Dujovny M, Kossovsky N, Kossowsky R, et al.: Aneurysm clip motion during magnetic resonance imaging: In vivo experimental study with metallurgical factor analysis. *Neurosurgery* 17:543, 1985.

Edelman RR, Warach S: Magnetic resonance imaging (Part I). *N Engl J Med* 328:708, 1993a.

Edelman RR, Warach S: Magnetic resonance imaging (Part II). *N Engl J Med* 328:785, 1993b.

Eggers GW, Metzgar MT, Plumlee JE: Axillary block and sedation for cardiac catheterization. *Anesthesiology* 28:936, 1967.

Eifel PJ: Decreased bone growth arrest with hyperfractionated irradiation in weanling rats. *Int J Radiat Oncol Biol Phys* 15:141, 1988.

Eifel PJ, Sampson CM, Tucker SL: Radiation fractionation sensitivity of epiphyseal cartilage in a weanling rat model. *Int J Radiat Oncol Biol Phys* 19:661, 1990.

Elster AD: Cranial MR imaging with Gd-DTPA in neonates and young infants: Preliminary experience. *Radiology* 176:225, 1990.

Erlebacher J, Cahill P, Pannizzo F, et al.: Effect of magnetic resonance imaging on DDD pacemakers. *Am J Cardiol* 57:437, 1986.

Fan S, Lee T, Chen L: Long-term propofol infusion and airway management in a patient with Goldenhar's syndrome. *Acta Anaesthesiol* 5:33, 1995.

Figg WD, Graham CL, Hak LJ, et al.: Ondansetron: A novel antiemetic agent. *South Med J* 86:497, 1993.

Fishman S: Vascular anomalies of the mediastinum. *Semin Pediatr Surg* 8:92, 1999.

Fitzsimmons JR: The design of RF systems for patient safety. *Ann N Y Acad Sci* 649:313, 1992.

Fox V: Clinical competency in pediatric endoscopy. *J Pediatr Gastroenterol Nutr* 26:200, 1998.

Friedman B, Hartenberg M, Mulroy J, et al.: Gastrografin aspiration in a 3 3/4-year-old girl. *Pediatr Radiol* 16:506, 1986.

Furst S, Burrows P, Holzman R: General anesthesia in a child with a dynamic, vascular anterior mediastinal mass. *Anesthesiology* 84:976, 1996.

Gangarosa R, Minnis J, Nobbe J, et al.: Operational safety issues in MRI. *Magn Reson Imaging* 5:287, 1987.

Gentet JC, Bernard JL, Aimard L, et al.: Veno-occlusive disease in children after intensive chemo- and radiotherapy and repeated halothane anesthesias. *Acta Oncol* 27:579, 1988.

Goldberg M: Systemic reactions to intravascular contrast media. A guide for the anesthesiologist. *Anesthesiology* 60:46, 1984.

Goudsouzian NG, Alifimoff JK, Cote CJ: Isoflurane for radiotherapy in children? *Anesthesiology* 68:648, 1988.

Granet RB, Gelber LJ: Claustrophobia during MR imaging. *N J Med* 87:479, 1990.

Greenberger P: Contrast media reactions. *J Allerg Clin Immunol* 74:600, 1984.

Greenblatt DJ, Locniskar A, Ochs HR, et al.: Automated gas chromatography for studies of midazolam pharmacokinetics. *Anesthesiology* 55:176, 1981.

Griffeth L, Rich K, Dehdashti F, et al.: Brain metastases from non-central nervous system tumors: Evaluation with PET. *Radiology* 186:37, 1993.

Griswold JD, Vacanti FX, Goudsouzian NG: Twenty-three sequential out-of-hospital halothane anesthetics in an infant. *Anesth Analg* 67:779, 1988.

Gulch R, Lutz O: Influence of strong static magnetic fields on heart muscle contraction. *Phys Med Biol* 31:763, 1986.

Hansen T, Joensen H, Henneberg S: Laryngeal mask airway guided tracheal intubation in a neonate with the Pierre Robin syndrome. *Acta Anaesthesiol Scand S* 39:129, 1995.

Hassall E: Should pediatric gastroenterologists be i.v. drug users? *J Pediatr Gastronterol Nutr* 16:370, 1993.

Hassall E: Who should perform pediatric endoscopic sedation? *J Pediatr Gastroenterol Nutr* 18:114, 1994.

Haxby E, Liban J: Fiberoptic intubation via a laryngeal mask in an infant with Goldenhar syndrome. *Anaesth Intensive Care* 23:753, 1995.

Health C: *MR product reporting program and medical device report program.* Washington, DC, 1989, U.S. Food and Drug Administration.

Henderson KH, Lu JK, Rockoff MA, et al.: Radiation exposure of anesthesiologists. *Anesthesiology* 75:A896, 1991.

Henneberg S, Hok B, Wiklund L, et al.: Remote auscultatory patient monitoring during magnetic resonance imaging. *J Clin Monit* 8:37, 1992.

Holzman R, Nargozian C, Florence F: Lightwand intubation in children with abnormal upper airways. *Anesthesiology* 69:784, 1988.

Hostetler M, Davis C: Prospective age-based comparison of behavioral reactions occurring after ketamine sedation in the ED. *Am J Emerg Med* 20:463, 2002.

House of Delegates: *Guidelines for nonoperating room anesthetizing locations.* Annual meeting of the American Society of Anesthesiologists, San Francisco, CA, 1994, American Society of Anesthesiologists.

Hubbard AM, Markowitz RI, Kimmel B, et al.: Sedation for pediatric patients undergoing CT and MRI. *J Comput Assist Tomogr* 16:3, 1992.

International Non-Ionizing Radiation Committee of the International Radiation Protection Association: Protection of the patient undergoing a magnetic resonance examination. *Health Phys* 61:923, 1991.

Jackson I, Carreno R, Potparic Z, et al.: Hemangiomas, vascular malformations, and lymphovenous malformations: Classification and methods of treatment. *Plast Reconstr Surg* 91:1216, 1993.

Jeffries G: Radiotherapy and children's anaesthesia. *Anaesthesia* 43:416, 1988.

Jehenson P, Duboc D, Lavergne T, et al.: Change in human cardiac rhythm induced by a 2-T static magnetic field. *Radiology* 166(1 Pt 1):227, 1988.

Jehenson PM: Reducing doses of glucagon used in radiologic examinations. *Radiology* 179:286, 1991.

Jones RM, Diamond JG, Power SJ, et al.: A prospective study of liver function in infants and children exposed to daily isoflurane for several weeks. *Anaesthesia* 46:1087, 1991.

Kain Z, Mayes L, Caramico L, et al.: Parental presence during induction of anesthesia. A randomized controlled trial. *Anesthesiology* 84:1060, 2001.

Kanal E: An overview of electromagnetic safety considerations associated with magnetic resonance imaging. *Ann N Y Acad Sci* 649:204, 1992.

Kanal E, Borgstede J, Barkovich A, et al.: American College of Radiology White Paper on MR Safety. *AJR Am J Roentgenol* 178:1335, 2002.

Kanal E, Shellock F, Talagala L: Safety considerations in MR imaging. *Radiology* 176:593, 1990.

Karian V, Burrows P, Zurakowski D, et al.: The development of a pediatric radiology sedation program. *Pediatr Radiol* 32:348, 2002.

Karlik SJ, Heatherley T, Pavan F, et al.: Patient anesthesia and monitoring at a 1.5 T MRI installation. *Magn Reson Med* 7:210, 1988.

Keeter S, Benator RM, Weinberg SM, et al.: Sedation in pediatric CT: National survey of current practice. *Radiology* 175:745, 1990.

Keller C, Sparr H, Brimacombe J: Laryngeal mask lubrication. A comparative study of saline versus 2% lignocaine gel with cuff pressure control. *Anaesthesia* 52:592, 1997.

Kelly J, Patterson R, Lieberman P: Radiographic contrast media studies in high risk patients. *J Allerg Clin Immunol* 62:181, 1978.

Kenna JG, Neuberger J, Mieli-Vergani G, et al.: Halothane hepatitis in children. *Br Med J* 294:1209, 1987.

Koh J, Black D, Leatherman I: Experience with an anesthesiologist interventional model for endoscopy in a pediatric hospital. *J Pediatr Gastroenterol Nutr* 33:314, 2001.

Koskinen MF: Magnetic resonance imaging (MRI) site planning and economics. *Med Instrum* 19:244, 1985.

Kross J, Drummond JC: Successful use of a Fortec II vaporizer in the MRI suite: A case report with observations regarding magnetic field-induced vaporizer aberrancy. *Can J Anaesth* 38:1065, 1991.

Liang M, Narayanan K, Kanal E: Magnetic ports in tissue expanders—a caution for MRI. *Magn Reson Imaging* 7:541, 1989.

Lind LJ, Mushlin PS: Sedation, analgesia and anesthesia for radiologic procedures. *Cardiovasc Intervent Radiol* 10:247, 1987.

Loeffler J, Rossitch EJ, Siddon R, et al.: Role of stereotactic radiosurgery with a linear accelerator in treatment of intracranial arteriovenous malformations and tumors in children. *Pediatrics* 85:774, 1990.

Lunsford LD, Linskey ME: Stereotactic radiosurgery in the treatment of patients with acoustic tumors. *Otolaryngol Clin North Am* 25:471, 1992.

Manuli MA, Davies L: Rectal methohexital for sedation of children during imaging procedures. *AJR Am J Roentgenol* 160:577, 1993.

Mason K, Michna E, DiNardo J, et al.: Evolution of a protocol for ketamine-induced sedation as an alternative to general anesthesia for interventional radiologic procedures in pediatric patients. *Radiology* 225:457, 2002.

Mason K, Michna E, Zurakowski D, et al.: Serum ethanol levels in children and adults after ethanol embolization or sclerotherapy for vascular anomalies. *Radiology* 217:127, 2000.

Mason K, Neufeld E, Karian V, et al.: Coagulation abnormalities in pediatric and adult patients after sclerotherapy or embolization of vascular anomalies. *AJR Am J Roentgenol* 177:1359, 2001.

Mason K, Zurakowski D, Karian V, et al.: Sedatives used in pediatric imaging: Comparison of IV pentobarbital with IV pentobarbital with midazolam added. *AJR Am J Roentgenol* 177:427, 2001.

McLoughlin MJ, Langer B, Wilson DR: Life-threatening reaction to glucagon in a patient with pheochromocytoma. *Radiology* 140:841, 1981.

McRobbie D, Foster M: Cardiac response to pulsed magnetic fields with regard to safety in NMR imaging. *Phys Med Biol* 30:695, 1985.

Melendez JC, McCrank E: Anxiety-related reactions associated with magnetic resonance imaging examination. *JAMA* 270:745, 1993.

Menache L, Eifel PJ, Kennamer DL, et al.: Twice-daily anesthesia in infants receiving hyperfractionated irradiation. *Int J Radiat Oncol Biol Phys* 18:625, 1990.

Menon DK, Peden CJ, Hall AS, et al.: Magnetic resonance for the anaesthetist. Part I: Physical principles, applications, safety aspects. *Anaesthesia* 47:240, 1992.

Morrison JE, Friesen RH: Elevated serum bromide concentrations following repeated halothane anaesthesia in a child. *Can J Anaesth* 37:801, 1990.

Mulliken J, Young A: *Vascular birthmarks, hemangiomas, and malformations.* Philadelphia, PA, 1988, WB Saunders.

Neumark J, Petricek W, Schramm W: Patientenferne beatung und Narkose bei der Kernspintomographie. *Anaesthetist* 38:273, 1989.

New York Academy of Sciences: Principles for the protection of patients and volunteers during clinical magnetic resonance diagnostic procedures. *Ann N Y Acad Sci* 31:372, 1992.

Nias AHW, Perry PM: Variation of tumour radiosensitivity with time after anaesthetic. *Br J Radiol* 62:932, 1989.

Ohlms L, Forsen J, Burrows P: Venous malformation of the pediatric airway. *Int J Pediatr Otorhinolaryngol* 37:99, 1996.

O'Tuama L, Treves S: Brain single-photon emission computed tomography for behavior disorders in children. *Semin Nucl Med* 23:255, 1993.

Palmer G, Davidson A, Sethna N, et al.: Use of the Bispectral Index monitor to aid titration of propofol during a drug-assisted interview. *Paediatr Anaesth* 11:245, 2001.

Parke TJ, Stevens JE, Rice ASC, et al.: Metabolic acidosis and fatal myocardial failure after propofol infusion in children: Five case reports. *Br Med J* 305:613, 1992.

Patteson S, Chesney JT: Anesthetic management for magnetic resonance imaging: Problems and solutions. *Anesth Analg* 74:121, 1992.

Pavlicek W, Geisinger M, Castle L, et al.: The effects of nuclear magnetic resonance on patients with cardiac pacemakers. *Radiology* 147:149, 1983.

Peden CJ, Menon DK, Hall AS, et al.: Magnetic resonance for the anaesthetist, Part II: Anaesthesia and monitoring in MR units. *Anaesthesia* 47:508, 1992.

Persson B, Stahlberg F: Safety aspects of magnetic resonance examinations. *Int J Technol Assess Health Care* 1:647, 1985.

Pohost GM, Blackwell GG, Shellock FG: Safety of patients with medical devices during application of magnetic resonance methods. *Ann N Y Acad Sci* 649:302, 1992.

Prasad N, Wright D, Ford J, et al.: Safety of 4-T MR imaging: Study of effects on developing frog embryos. *Radiology* 174:251, 1990.

Prasil P, Laberge J, Barkun A, et al.: Endoscopic retrograde cholangiopancreatography in children: A surgeon's perspective. *J Ped Surg* 36:733, 2001.

Reves JG, Fragen RJ, Vinik HR, et al.: Midazolam: Pharmacology and uses. *Anesthesiology* 62:310, 1985.

Riles T, Berenstein A, Fisher F, et al.: Reconstruction of the ligated external carotid artery for embolization of cervicofacial arteriovenous malformations. *J Vasc Surg* 17:491, 1993.

Rockoff MA, Goudsouzian NG: Seizures induced by methohexital. *Anesthesiology* 54:333, 1981.

Rooks V, Chung T, Connor L, et al.: Comparison of oral pentobarbital sodium (Nembutal) and oral chloral hydrate for infant sedation during radiologic imaging. *AJR Am J Roentgenol* 180:1125, 2003.

Ross DM, Williams DO: Combined axillary plexus block and basal sedation for cardiac catheterization in young children. *Br Heart J* 32:195, 1970.

Saint-Maurice C: Sedation techniques in pediatric anesthesia. *Curr Opin Anesthesiol* 5:1, 1992.

Schenck JF, Dumoulin CL, Redington RW, et al.: Human exposure to 4.0 Tesla magnetic fields in a whole-body scanner. *Med Physics* 19:1089, 1992.

Scherzinger A, Hendee W: Basic principles of magnetic resonance imaging—an update. [review]. *West J Med* 143:782, 1985.

Shellock FG: Biological effects and safety aspects of magnetic resonance imaging. *Magn Reson Q* 5:243, 1989.

Shellock FG, Crues JV: MRI: Safety considerations in magnetic resonance imaging. *Magn Reson Imaging Decis* 2:25, 1988.

Shellock FG, Curtis JS: MR imaging and biomedical implants, materials and devices: An updated review. *Radiology* 180:541, 1991.

Shellock FG, Schaefer DJ, Gordon CJ: Effect of a 1.5 T static magnetic field on body temperature of man. *Magn Reson Med* 3:644, 1986.

Shellock FG, Slimp GL: Severe burn of the finger caused by using a pulse oximeter during MR imaging. *AJR Am J Roentgenol* 153:1105, 1989.

Shuman W, Haynor D, Guy A, et al.: Superficial- and deep-tissue temperature increases in anesthetized dogs during exposure to high specific absorption rates in a 1.5-T MR imager. *Radiology* 167:551, 1988.

Smith DS, Askey P, Young ML, et al.: Anesthetic management of acutely ill patients during magnetic resonance imaging. *Anesthesiology* 65:6, 1986.

Snowdon S: Defibrillator failure in a magnetic resonance unit [letter]. *Anaesthesia* 44:359, 1989.

Soriano S, Sethna N, Scott R: Anesthetic management of children with Moyamoya syndrome. *Anesth Analg* 77:1066, 1993.

Spear RM, Waldman JY, Canada ED, et al.: Intravenous thiopentone for CT and MRI in children. *Paediatr Anaesth* 3:29, 1993.

Spencer HT, Barnes PJ: Spinal anaesthesia for paediatric radiotherapy. *Anaesth Intensive Care* 8:214, 1980.

Sperber D, Oldenbourg R, Dransfeld K: Magnetic field induced temperature change in mice. *Naturwissenschaften* 71:100, 1984.

Stokes M, Soriano S, Tarbell N, et al.: Anesthesia for stereotactic radiosurgery in children. *J Neurosurg Anesthesiol* 7:100, 1995.

Strain JD, Campbell JB, Harvey LA, et al.: IV Nembutal: Safe sedation for children undergoing CT. *AJR Am J Roentgenol* 151:975, 1988.

Sussman D: A comparative evaluation of ketamine anesthesia in children and adults. *Anesthesiology* 40:459, 1974.

Tait A, Pandit U, Voepel-Lewis T, et al.: Use of the laryngeal mask airway in children with upper respiratory tract infections: A comparison with endotracheal intubation. *Anesth Analg* 86:706, 1998.

Tenforde T, Gaffey C, Moyer B, et al.: Cardiovascular alterations in Macaca monkeys exposed to stationary magnetic fields: Experimental observations and theoretical analysis. *Bioelectromagnetics* 4:1, 1983.

Teng R, Yokohata K, Utsunomiya N: Endoscopic retrograde cholangiopancreatography in infants and children. *J Gastroenterol* 35:39, 2000.

Thomsen H, Bush WJ: Treatment of the adverse effects of contrast media. *Acta Radiol* 39:212, 1998.

Tobin JR, Spurrier EA, Wetzel RC: Anaesthesia for critically ill children during magnetic resonance imaging. *Br J Anaesth* 69:482, 1992.

Towbin RB, Ball WS: Pediatric interventional radiology. *Radiol Clin North Am* 26:419, 1988.

Van Hemelrijck J, Smith I, White PF: Use of desflurane for outpatient anesthesia. A comparison with propofol and nitrous oxide. *Anesthesiology* 75:197, 1991.

Van Wagoner M, Worah D: Gadodiamide injection. First human experience with the nonionic magnetic resonance imaging enhancement agent. *Invest Radiol* 28:S44, 1993.

Vangerven M, Van Hemelrijck J, Wouters P, et al.: Light anaesthesia with propofol for paediatric MRI. *Anaesthesia* 47:706, 1992.

Weller EB, Weller RA, Fristad MA: Use of sodium amytal interviews in prepubertal children: Indications, procedure, and clinical utility. *J Am Acad Child Psychol* 24:747, 1985.

Wells H, Hyrnchak M, Burbridge B: Direct effects of contrast media on rat lungs. *Can Assoc Radiol J* 42:261, 1991.

Westbrook C, Glaholm J, Barrett A: Vomiting associated with whole body irradiation. *Clin Radiol* 38:263, 1987.

Whitwam JG, Owen JR, Spiers ASD, et al.: General anaesthesia for high-dose total-body irradiation. *Lancet* 1(8056):128, 1978.

Winter J: Efficiency of utilization of a computed tomography scanner. *AJR Am J Roentgenol* 131:89, 1978.

Wolfe T, Rao C: Anesthesia for selected procedure. *Semin Pediatr Surg* 1:74, 1992.

Zonana HV: Hypnosis, sodium amytal, and confessions. *Bull Am Acad Psychiatry Law* 7:18, 1979.

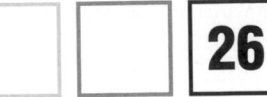

26 Office-Based Pediatric Anesthesia

Richard Berkowitz

"A pediatrician's dream of the ideal world would be to have individuals knowledgeable about the special needs of infants and children assembled wherever children are to be treated" (Avery, 1975). Little did Dr. Avery know back in 1975, as she wrote these words in the journal *Anesthesiology* as a guest editor introducing a symposium on pediatric anesthesia, to what extent and in what places children were to be anesthetized and by whom. The prophetic nature of her question, "Where will pediatric surgery be done in the future?" and her statement, "Surely the anesthetist should contribute to the definition of what can be done in what setting," is astounding when considering how rapidly the surgical and anesthetic care of children has progressed from the hospital to the ambulatory surgery center to the office-based setting over the past 15 to 20 years (Avery, 1975).

The concept of office-based anesthesia and surgery is not a novel one, as dentists, oral surgeons, and plastic surgeons have been office based for decades. In fact, dentists and oral surgeons have been at the forefront of office anesthesia and surgery dating back to one of the first office-based anesthetics, involving Colton and Wells in 1844, for an extraction of a wisdom tooth (Jacobsohn, 1995; Yagiela, 1999).

We have now come full circle, as prior to the early 1900s many surgical procedures were performed in offices. Subsequently, as surgical procedures became more complex, the hospital became the major site for surgery (Yagiela, 1999). Despite this shift, the development of ambulatory anesthesia continued throughout the 20th century with the development of the first free-standing surgical center in 1916, by Waters (White, 1997), and ultimately with the first ambulatory surgery center established by Reed and Ford in the late 1960s.

Over the past several years, the concept of office-based anesthesia and surgery is well publicized. In addition to the increasing number of clinical reports looking at the efficacy or regarding the subject of office-based anesthesia (Laurito, 1998; Tang et al., 1999; Arens, 2000; Joshi, 2003), there are, unfortunately, numerous reports of significant morbidity and mortality both in the medical literature (de Jong, 1999; Rao et al., 1999; Morrell, 2000; Stoelting, 2000) and the lay press (LaMendola, 1998; Schulte et al., 1998; Vogt, 2000; Neergaard, 1999; Hilton, 2001). This should be compelling evidence for the anesthesiologist to realize that office-based surgery and anesthesia has arrived and may be here to stay. In addition, for skeptics, a published closed claims analysis of office-based anesthesia and surgery, which lends itself to the fact that the process exists and can be an impetus to process improvement, is the convincing evidence (Domino, 2001).

Interest in office-based anesthesia is also, in part, manifested by the increasing number of societies—specifically, the Society for Ambulatory Anesthesia (SAMBA), and the Anesthesia Patient Safety Foundation (APSF)—that promulgate educational and safety literature in this relatively new arena for anesthesiologists. Also, the American Society of Anesthesiologists (ASA), as well as other groups, including, but not limited to, The American College of Surgeons and its various subspecialties, the American Dental Association, the American Academy of Pediatric Dentistry, and the American Association of Nurse Anesthetists, have published guidelines specifically addressing office-based anesthesia or surgery or both (Table 26–1). However, in some cases these guidelines address only the issue of sedation/analgesia with other organizations updating their sedation/analgesia policies to include general anesthesia (American Academy of Pediatric Dentistry, 2004). All of these societies have developed guidelines or policies in response to the overwhelming interest and growing participation by their memberships in this area, as well as an overall common concern for patient safety.

Also significant and perhaps legitimizing the presence of office-based anesthesia and surgery in present day medicine is the ever-increasing number of states developing legislation that specifically address this area. Consequent to this dynamic period of law making and law revision is that the ASA Office of Legal Affairs is continuing to compile information pertinent to the states that have developed and those that are developing legislation regulating office-based anesthesia and surgery.

Simply stated, office-based anesthesia is the practice of anesthesia in the free-standing physician's office and is defined as the provision of anesthesia service in an operating area or a procedure room that is not licensed as an ambulatory surgery center. It is the most "liberated" form of anesthesia practice and is at the farthest end of the spectrum of "out of the operating room" anesthesia. In a sense, it is anesthesia for the most remote location

TABLE 26–1. Specialty-specific guidelines for sedation/analgesia and office anesthesia and surgery*

Organization	Document	Adopted	Revised
American Society of Anesthesiologists (ASA)	Guidelines for Ambulatory Anesthesia and Surgery	1973	2003
	Guidelines for Nonoperating Room Anesthetizing Locations	1994	2003
	Practice Guidelines for Sedation and Analgesia by Non-Anesthesiologists	1995	2001
	Guidelines for Office-Based Anesthesia	1999	2004
	Continuum of Depth of Sedation	1999	2004
	Qualifications of Anesthesia Providers in an Office-Based Setting	1999	2004
American College of Surgeons (ACS)	Guidelines for Optimal Ambulatory Surgical Care and Office-Based Surgery†	1994	2000
American Academy of Pediatrics (AAP)	Guidelines for Monitoring and Management of Pediatric Patients During and After Sedation for Diagnostic and Therapeutic Procedures	1985	2002
	Guidelines for the pediatric perioperative environment	1999	NA
American Academy of Pediatric Dentistry (AAPD)	Guideline on the Elective Use of Minimal, Moderate, and Deep Sedation and General Anesthesia in Pediatric Dental Patients	1985	2004
	Guideline on the Use of Anesthesia Trained Personnel in the Provision of General Anesthesia/Deep Sedation to the Pediatric Dental Patient	2001	NA
American Dental Association (ADA)	ADA Policy Statement: The Use of Conscious Sedation, Deep Sedation and General Anesthesia in Dentistry	1999	2002
American Society of Dental Anesthesiologists (ASDA)	Policy Statement on Practice Parameters	1998	
American Society of Plastic Surgery (ASPS)	Patient Safety in Office-Based Surgery Facilities: I. Procedures in the Office-Based Setting, II. Patient Selection‡ Practice Advisory	2001	NA
	on Liposuction§	2003	NA
American Association of Nurse Anesthetists (AANA)	Standards for Office-Based Anesthesia	1997	2002

*Not a complete list, as other professional societies may also have related guidelines.
†These guidelines specify surgery by facility class (A, B, C) depending on the invasiveness of the surgery and type of anesthesia used.
‡Practice advisory only.
§In this practice advisory, the ASPS recommends that in the event that sedation/analgesia is used, the surgeon follow the ASA Guidelines for Sedation and Analgesia by Non-Anesthesiologists.

(except, perhaps, for those individuals delivering anesthesia care in isolated areas of Third World countries).

Traditionally, office-based anesthesia has been the realm of various specialists including, but not limited to, dentists, oral surgeons, plastic surgeons, podiatrists, certified registered nurse anesthetists (CRNAs), and, in some instances, gastroenterologists. Until recently, few anesthesiologists dared to venture out of their conventional roles as hospital-based or ambulatory surgery-based physicians.

To what extent has the office-based surgical volume increased that it is requiring or necessitating the rapid development of this new "subspecialty" of ambulatory anesthesia? According to one marketing study (SMG Marketing-Verispan, L.L.C., 2002), the total number of outpatient procedures exceeded 30 million in the year 2000 and was estimated to break the 35 million mark in 2003 (Fig. 26–1). Office-based surgical procedures representing approximately 10 million office-based procedures were performed in 2003, comprising almost 30% of the total number of outpatient procedures (see Fig. 26–1).

Exact numbers pertaining to pediatric procedures occurring in office-based settings are difficult to obtain, but in 1996 the National Center for Health Statistics (NCHS) estimated that approximately 8.5% of ambulatory surgical procedures were performed on children less than 15 years old (Hall et al., 1998). Although many different types of surgical procedures, including otolaryngologic (Siegel et al., 2000; Garin et al., 2001; Friedman et al., 2002), urologic (Cartwright et al., 1996; Smith et al., 2000), cosmetic (Grevelink et al., 1997), and ophthalmologic (Goldblum et al., 1996), are performed on children in the office-based setting, the majority of procedures requiring anesthesia or sedation in the office setting for children are dental procedures (Yagiela, 1999; Ross et al., 2002).

The most common reason for children to require dental procedures is related to dental caries, and furthermore, a majority of dental caries disease in the United States occurs in a small proportion of the pediatric population (Yagiela, 1999). It is estimated that close to 500,000 children per year require some level of anesthesia for their dental disease. Yagiela (1999) reports that a survey by the American Academy of Pediatric Dentistry estimated in 1995 that this number is probably closer to 200,000, with the discrepancy being due to a paucity of access to the appropriate care secondary to a lack of insurance coverage.

WHY OFFICE-BASED SURGERY AND ANESTHESIA?

As one can see from the marketing data previously presented (see Fig. 26–1), there is a compelling need to be able to provide quality surgical and anesthesia services in the office-based setting. The actual reasons as to why this boom has occurred and continues to evolve and why anesthesiologists are more aggressively entering this arena are severalfold.

Ostensibly, the most persuasive argument for a shift to the office-based setting is financial. Limitations in reimbursement due to health care reform and economic constraints have caused physicians to become more creative in facilitating cost-effective approaches to surgery. One may reduce costs by reducing or eliminating facility fees that ordinarily accompany the cost sharing charges at hospital-based and ambulatory surgery–based centers. Because much of office-based surgery, especially cosmetic surgery, is performed on a cash-payment, fee-for-service basis, cost containment by limiting facility fee overhead becomes crucial to patient affordability. This affordability is crucial in the case of pediatric dental procedures, where in many instances neither

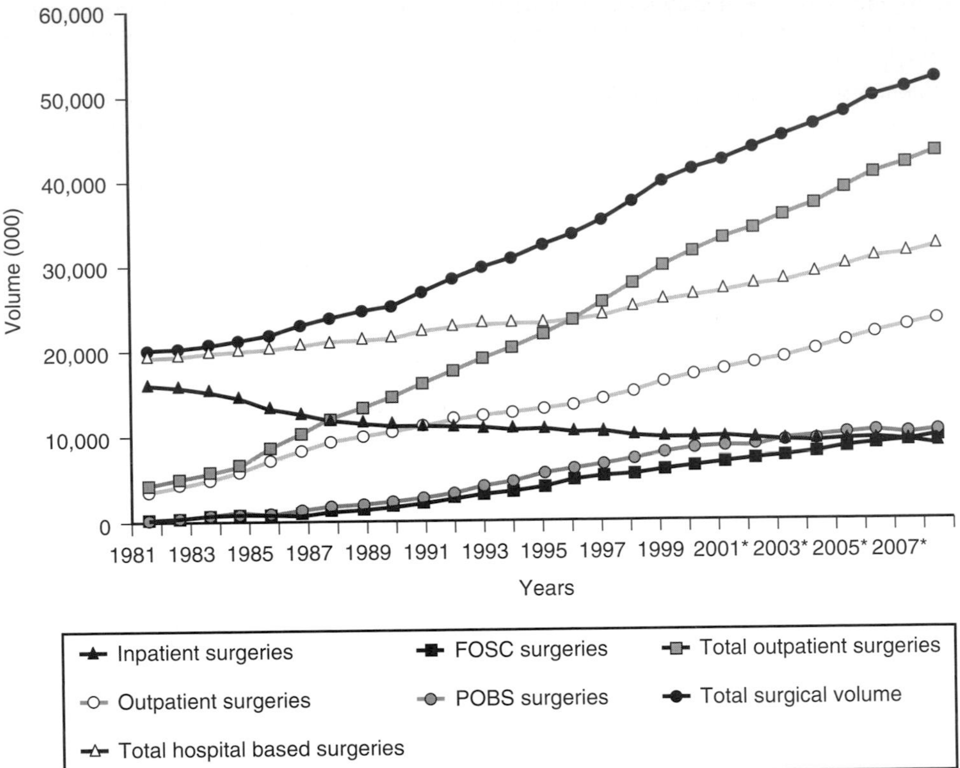

■ **FIGURE 26–1.** This graph represents past and future trends in surgical volumes in specific patient care sites. Notice increasing surgical volumes in the FOSC (freestanding outpatient surgery center) and POBS (physician office–based surgery center). (Courtesy of SMG Marketing–Verispan, L.L.C., 2002, Chicago, IL.)

dental nor medical insurance covers out-of-office dental procedures and anesthesia costs (Ross et al., 2002).

Although the lack of a facility fee is ideal and helps provide the surgeon with a cheaper alternative for the patient, the reality of the situation is that surgeons often include a facility fee in their global fee to the patient to offset the overhead (personnel, supplies, etc.) required to run an office-based practice. In some instances, insurance companies may reimburse physicians a facility fee, but the cost to the third party payers may still be less than if the procedure is performed in a hospital- or surgery center–based setting. Consequently, the procedure becomes financially advantageous for the surgeon, the anesthesiologist, the insurance company, and the patient.

One surgical study from the United States in the early 1990s compares the cost of performing an inguinal herniorrhaphy in the hospital with that of the cost in an office setting. This study finds the latter a more cost-effective alternative regardless of the technique used. The total cost for a laparoscopic approach to repair in the hospital outpatient setting and the office setting was $5,500 and $1,500, respectively. For a standard open repair, the total cost for the hospital setting was $2,200, and for the office setting, $895 (Schultz, 1994).

Operating in the office affords the surgeon not only financial but also logistical advantages. Office-based surgical practice virtually eliminates the lost time caused by turnover delays, bumping cases secondary to emergencies, overscheduled cases, and travel times between facilities. In the office-based setting, whatever turnover delays do occur can be quickly remedied by the surgeon, as he or she has total control over the personnel and the facility.

The ability of the surgeon to schedule on-site clinic visits between surgical cases allows for the efficient use of time. This eliminates the usual routine of having to rush back to the office between procedures or having office hours at the conclusion of a long and busy day at the hospital or surgery center.

Another advantage of office-based procedures is the more private, less stressful, and more familiar environment. For the anesthesiologist, office-based anesthesia may allow for an enhanced income, a better work environment (working with a limited number of surgeons or, in some instances, the same surgeon), and, in most practices, the lack of a night call schedule. Whether these potential advantages of establishing or taking part in an office-based practice prevail over the relative disadvantages of working in an extremely remote environment, routinely providing anesthesia care for cases of decreased complexity (compared with those cases in a hospital setting), providing anesthesia services under itinerant conditions, and perpetually competing with other anesthesiologists and anesthesia providers for business, becomes an individual decision.

■ SAFETY AND OUTCOME

With the medical community, third party payers, and the consumers (our patients) pushing for more expeditious and cost-effective (and hence potentially more profitable) ways in which to provide surgical and anesthesia services, the anesthesia services are moving farther from the hospital safety net. Dr. Ervin Moss, who is the impetus behind tighter regulation of office-based anesthesia and surgery in the state of New Jersey, stated that, "Some say the major difference between the office-based and hospital-based anesthesiologist is that the former must be more courageous or foolhardy" (Moss, 1998).

Whether or not Dr. Moss's characterization of the office-based anesthesiologist holds true, the fact remains that we must provide anesthesia care that is as safe, if not safer, than hospital-based or surgery center–based anesthesia. Others have questioned whether the convenience of office-based surgery and anesthesia is worth the risk (Arens, 2000).

Although the risk of death from anesthesia has decreased and is quoted to be anywhere from 1:20,000 to 1:250,000 (Arens, 2000; Biboulet et al., 2001; Newland et al., 2002) and the incidence of cardiac arrest in children is described to be 1.4:10,000 (Morray et al., 2000), an accurate assessment of the safety profile of office-based anesthesia and surgery relative to the pediatric population is difficult secondary to the paucity of information. Mandatory reporting for morbidity and mortality related to office procedures does not exist. To make an assessment of the relative safety of office-based anesthesia and surgery, it is imperative to look at data reviewing the safety of pediatric ambulatory surgery, pediatric dental office surgery, and pediatric sedation/analgesia, as well as the adult literature that reviews this topic.

Many of the cases brought to the attention of the medical, dental, and lay community involved children undergoing office dental procedures (Morell, 2000). This information not only is tied intimately with the present topic but also is the point of origin for much of the controversy over the safety and efficacy of office-based anesthesia for children.

In two reports from the United States, Coté and others (2000a, 2000b) retrospectively analyzed information obtained from the Food and Drug Administration, the U.S. Pharmacopoeia, and a survey of pediatric specialists to report on contributing factors to critical incidents and medications used in sedation as they relate to adverse sedation events in children undergoing diagnostic and therapeutic procedures.

Coté and others (2000a) reported on 95 incidents. Over half of these incidents resulted in death (n = 51) and permanent neurologic injury (n = 9). The remaining patients either had prolonged hospitalization without injury (n = 21) or sustained no harm as a result of the adverse event (n = 14). Of note was that those children who were cared for in non–hospital-based facilities (older and healthier) had a much higher rate of death and permanent neurologic injury (93%) than did those cared for in hospital-based facilities (37%). The authors also reported inadequate resuscitation was a major factor in the non–hospital-based facilities (57%) compared with the hospital-based setting (2.5%) and that patients cared for in the nonhospital setting were more likely to sustain a cardiac arrest as the second or third event compared with those in the hospital setting ($P < .001$).

In the second report, Coté and others (2000b) used the same 95 incidents to determine if there was a relationship between medications and adverse events. Although the authors noted no relationship between the class of drug used, the route of administration, and the incidence of death and permanent neurologic injury, they did note that adverse outcomes were associated with the administration of drug overdoses and administration of three or more sedating medications. Furthermore, 11 of 12 patients (all younger than 6 years) sustained adverse outcomes either at home or in a car. Two of the 12 patients, who had received sedative medication at home prior to their procedure, sustained an adverse event at home before the scheduled procedure.

Of note was that over one third of the reported events occurred during sedation for dental procedures (n = 32). Twenty-nine of these resulted in death or permanent neurologic injury. Most of the involved practitioners were either oral surgeons or dentists, three were pedodontists, and one was a nurse anesthetist under the supervision of a dentist. None of the practitioners were anesthesiologists (Coté et al., 2000b).

The dental practices were the only sites in these reports to have used nitrous oxide. In addition to the greater tendency toward the use of nitrous oxide, there was a greater tendency for these practitioners to use multiple drugs (more than three) compared with other practitioners: 39% and 13%, respectively. The authors conclude that many of these adverse events may have been prevented by consistency between monitoring guidelines and by practice and training requirements among health care professionals of differing specialties who administer sedation and anesthesia.

Although there are anecdotal reports (Denman et al., 1968; Johnson et al., 2001; Manoharan et al., 2001) and studies (Yee et al., 1985; Blayney et al., 1999; Girdler et al., 1999) of adverse outcomes, complications, and side effects related to sedation and anesthesia in the dental literature, others have reported on a safety record that is as good as, if not better than, that of the anesthesia community (Laskin, 1999; Saxen et al., 1999; Whitmire, 1999; Yagiela, 2001). The incidence of mortality rates in dental anesthesia is reported to be anywhere from 1:250,000 in the United Kingdom (Cartwright, 1999) to 1:300,000 (D'Eramo, 1999) to less than 1:1 million in the United States (Brandom and Herlich, 1999; Laskin, 1999).

As if there is not enough controversy within the anesthesia community, within the dental community there is also debate over who can best serve the patient requiring anesthesia for a dental procedure. Yagiela points out that members of the American Society of Dental Anesthesiologists, those who provide "approximately 25,000 pediatric general anesthetics per year," subscribe closely to the American Academy of Pediatrics and American Society of Anesthesiologists guidelines for sedation and anesthesia (Yagiela, 2001). He also states that "since the organization's inception 2 decades ago, there have been no known incidents of mortality or significant morbidity in children managed in the dental office by a dentist anesthesiologist" and intimates that safety may be improved in dental offices with a greater adherence to these guidelines by the dental community as a whole (Yagiela, 2001).

In contrast to the paucity of information about the safety and outcomes related to office-based anesthesia, the efficacy of anesthesia in pediatric ambulatory surgery in general is well known. As reported by Willetts (1997), outpatient surgery may date back to James H. Nicoll, a Glasgow surgeon who, in the early 1900s, successfully performed several thousand ambulatory procedures on young children at the West Graham Street Dispensary for Children. Contemporary authors also show that for many surgical procedures, the ambulatory setting for surgery and anesthesia is safe, cost effective, and therefore preferable to in-patient surgery (Moir et al., 1987; Postuma et al., 1987; Patel et al., 1988; Hannallah, 1991; Ghosh et al., 1994).

In one prospective study examining the efficacy of pediatric day surgery at the Children's Hospital of Eastern Ontario, the overall complication rate was very low. The investigators, over a 5-year period, prospectively studied children undergoing various outpatient procedures including myringotomy, tonsillectomy and adenoidectomy, dental procedures, and inguinal hernia repairs. Most of the children were between 2 and 7 years old, and the total number of cases approached 25,000. The reported complication rate was 1.6% per year. The most common complication was postoperative bleeding, primarily secondary to tonsillectomy and adenoidectomy. None of the complications resulted in permanent disability (Letts et al., 2001).

Much of the information relative to the outcomes for office-based anesthesia and surgery is anecdotal. In a retrospective report, specifically looking at outcomes for plastic surgical procedures,

Hoefflin and others (2001) reported no significant morbidity and no mortality in more than 23,000 procedures over an 18-year period in which general anesthesia was used. The anesthesia was physician administered, and the facility was certified by the American Association for Accreditation of Ambulatory Surgical Facilities (AAAASF) (Hoefflin et al., 2001). In this report, most of the patients underwent cosmetic surgery, with some patients having multiple procedures. The only incidents reported as significant by the authors were the rare occurrence of electrocardiograph and oxygen monitor failure. None of these events resulted in any patient complications, although three patients were hospitalized for custodial care. Minor anesthetic complications included nausea and vomiting (<5%), postextubation sore throat (<5%), shivering, one case of dental damage, one case of delayed (10 days) deep vein thrombosis, and one case of carpal tunnel syndrome following intravenous catheter infiltration.

In another report, Coldiron (2001, 2002) reviewed critical surgical incidents that occurred in physicians' offices in the state of Florida subsequent to a mandatory reporting in February 2000. This mandatory reporting resulted from several newspaper article accounts of poor patient outcomes and questions of whether office anesthesia and surgery were safe. Those incidents requiring reporting are listed in Box 26–1.

In the data obtained from Florida's Agency for Health Care Administration, there were 43 reported complications by 41 different physicians. These complications included eight deaths (Table 26–2). The most common complications were adverse drug reactions, several of which were anaphylactic in nature. Unfortunately, the total number of patients undergoing office-based procedures was not reported, so a true incidence could not be determined.

Coldiron (2001, 2002) noted that the reported deaths and complications were unrelated to whether the physician was board certified, whether the physician had similar surgical privileges in a hospital, and whether the facility was certified by one of the accrediting bodies—the AAAASF, the American Society of Plastic and Reconstructive Surgery (ASPRS), or the American Association for Ambulatory Health Care (AAAHC).

Bitar and others (2003) retrospectively reviewed close to 5000 office-based plastic surgery procedures that were performed under monitored anesthesia care with sedation. The procedures in this study were performed by board-certified plastic surgeons, and anesthesia was provided by a CRNA. Nearly all patients were reported to be American Society of Anesthesiologists (ASA) Class I or II (99.9%), and the majority of patients were adult females (92%). The most common complications reported in this study were dyspnea (0.05%, n = 2), protracted nausea and vomiting (0.2%, n = 6), and unplanned hospital admission (0.05%, n = 2). One patient required intubation without prolonged sequelae. The author reported no cardiac arrests, deaths, or any incidence of deep vein thrombosis or pulmonary embolus. The author concluded that office anesthesia and surgery were safe when using appropriate protocols and patient selection.

BOX 26–1 Incidents in Surgical Offices Requiring Reporting by the State of Florida

- Death
- Brain damage
- Wrong patient surgery
- Wrong site surgery
- Wrong procedure
- Surgery to remove an unplanned foreign object from a surgical procedure
- Transfer of a patient to a hospital
- Spinal damage
- Surgical repair of injuries or damage resulting from a planned surgical procedure

From Coldiron B: Office surgical incidents: 19 Months of Florida data. *Dermatol Surg* 28:710, 2002.

TABLE 26–2. Cause of death and specialist involved in Florida report

Surgery	Anesthesia Type/Provider	Etiology	No. of Patients*
Liposuction	General/M.D. or CRNA	Pulmonary embolus	3
Breast reduction	General/M.D.	Bronchospasm	1
Chin lift	Deep sedation/CRNA	Asystole	1
Peritoneal dialysis catheter	Local/radiologist	Unspecified	1
Radiology procedure	None	Contrast reaction	1

*The eighth death occurred due to exsanguination in an anesthesiologist's office 10 days postoperatively after a tonsillectomy in a hospital. The fact that the death occurred in an office mandated reporting.

From Coldiron B: Office surgical incidents: 19 Months of Florida data. *Dermatol Surg* 28:710, 2002.

In a review, Koch (2003) reported on several office-based anesthesia practices from various regions of the United States that were performed between 1981 and 2002. In this report, Koch noted no intraoperative deaths in over 64,000 anesthesia cases. Furthermore, in a subset of pediatric patients that comprised this report, one Chicago-based office anesthesia practice reported no intraoperative deaths, significant perioperative morbidity, or emergent hospital transfers in over 600 pediatric anesthesia cases. Children in this subset ranged in age from 18 months to 17 years. Most of the children were less than 6 years old and were classified as ASA Class I or II patients (D. Barinholtz, Mobile Anesthesiologists, L.L.C., personal communication, September 4, 2003).

In a review of the ASA's Closed Claims Project database, Domino (2001) compared claims made against anesthesiologists in the office setting (n = 14) with those made in other ambulatory surgery settings (n = 753). Claims for dental damage and for nonoperative pain management were excluded from this analysis.

Although patient demographics were similar in both groups (Table 26–3), most of the claims in the office-based setting were related to plastic surgery or dental procedures, whereas in the ambulatory setting, most claims were related to procedures other than plastic or dental.

The severity of injury appeared greater in the office-based setting compared with other ambulatory sites. Most of the claims made in other ambulatory sites (62%) were for "temporary or nondisabling injury," whereas most of the claims from the office-based setting were for death (64%). The author pointed out, however, that without a denominator, a true risk assessment for each site cannot be ascertained.

In both office-based settings and ambulatory settings, Domino noted respiratory events were most common (Table 26–4).

■ TABLE 26–3. Patient characteristics in analysis of claims made in office-based anesthesia incidents

	Ambulatory Anesthesia (n = 753)	Office Based (n = 14)
Age (mean yr)	41	45
Female (%)	58	64
ASA Class I/II (%)	82	89
Elective surgery (%)	97	100
Anesthesia type		
General (%)	66	71
‡MAC (%)	10	14
Surgical procedure		
Dental (%)	3	21
Plastic surgery (%)	32*	64*
Other (%)	64†	14†

*$P < 0.05$ Ambulatory versus office based.
†$P < 0.01$ Ambulatory versus office based.
‡MAC, monitored anesthesia care.
From Domino KB: *Office-based anesthesia: Lessons learned from the Closed Claims Project.* ASA Newsletter 2001 reprinted with permission from the American Society of Anesthesiologists, 520 N. Northwest Highway, Park Ridge, IL 60068-2573.

A summary of airway-related complications and drug-related complications in office-based claims is shown in Table 26–4. Although the timing for injury was similar for both sites, there tended to be fewer claims for events occurring after discharge in the other ambulatory claims (7%) than for the office-based claims (21%).

The Closed Claims Project analysis also revealed that a greater number of office-based claims were deemed to be potentially preventable by better monitoring. Also, a greater percentage of office-based claims involved substandard care compared with other ambulatory settings (not statistically significant), and payment was made in a higher percentage of claims (92% versus 59%) and for a higher median payment ($200,000 versus $85,000) for office-based claims than for other ambulatory settings, respectively.

■ LEGISLATION AND REGULATIONS

There are many entities presently imparting their influences on the practice of office-based anesthesia and surgery. These include, but are not limited to, state regulatory bodies; federal regulatory agencies such as the Centers for Medicare and Medicaid Services (CMS) and the Office of the Inspector General (OIG); national medical professional societies; national medical and safety organizations such as the Federation of State Medical Boards (FSMB), the National Committee for Quality Assurance (NCQA), and the National Patient Safety Foundation (NPSF); accrediting organizations such as the American Association for Accreditation of Ambulatory Surgery Facilities, Inc. (AAAASF), the Accreditation Association for Ambulatory Health Care, Inc. (AAAHC), and the Joint Commission on Accreditation of Healthcare Organizations (JCAHO); and the insurance industry.

The main problem with regulation and legislation concerning office-based surgery and anesthesia is the wide regulatory variability that exists among states. Some states are highly regulated, whereas other states have no regulations (Table 26–5). In the states that do have regulations, these regulations are frequently ambiguous. State regulations regarding facility structure, personnel, equipment, and credentialing of individual practitioners differ widely. A more complete compendium of state regulations is available through the ASA Office of Governmental and Legal Affairs. In addition to state agencies and legislation, professional societies can regulate practice by establishing practice guidelines, practice standards, and/or advisories. The disadvantage of professional societies is that they run the risk of being self-interest groups. Consistent regulatory control could also be achieved by recognizing established accrediting bodies as oversight organizations. The organizations most commonly involved in the accreditation of ambulatory surgery centers (ASCs) are AAAASF, AAAHC, and JCAHO.

Historically, AAAASF, formerly known until the early 1990s as the American Association for Accreditation of Ambulatory Plastic Surgery Facilities, Inc. (AAAAPSF), was initially created to accredit only outpatient plastic surgery facilities. However, as other medical specialties moved procedures to free-standing outpatient settings, this organization became active in accrediting these facilities as well (AAAASF, 2003).

In contrast to AAAHC and JCAHO, AAAASF accredits facilities over a much narrower spectrum of medical specialties. The surgical specialties include colon and rectal, obstetrics and gynecology, ophthalmology, orthopedic, otolaryngology, plastic surgery, general surgery, and urology. AAAASF is particularly restrictive in its practitioner credentialing. This organization requires all surgeons to be certified by the American Board of Medical Specialties (ABMS) and requires all of its surgeons practicing at an ambulatory or office-based facility to have hospital privileges for the same procedures being performed in the office facility (AAAASF, 2003).

JCAHO and AAAHC, in addition to the facilities mentioned for AAAASF, approve facilities where oral and maxillofacial, dental, dermatologic, podiatric, cosmetic, vascular, and pain procedures are performed. Although these two organizations are not as restrictive on the practitioner privilege issue as the AAAASF, their credentialing policies are very complete.

In addition to defining requirements for surgical personnel, all three organizations offer accreditation processes that outline expectations for the facilities as they relate to meeting standards for the facility physical plant (e.g., by ensuring that state, Occupational Safety and Health Administration [OSHA], and National Fire Protection Association regulations are followed), anesthesia administration, monitoring, equipment and personnel, ancillary staff, patient transfer policies, patient safety and emergency resuscitation issues, quality improvement, and patient satisfaction issues. A summary of some of the similarities and

■ TABLE 26–4. Damaging events in office-based anesthesia claims

	Ambulatory Anesthesia (n = 666)		Office Based (n = 12)	
Type of Event	*No.*	*%*	*No.*	*%*
Respiratory	150	22	6	50
Cardiovascular	67	10	1	8
Equipment	74	11	1	8
Drug related	58	9	3	25
Block-needle trauma	41	6	1	8

From Domino KB: *Office-based anesthesia: Lessons learned from the Closed Claims Project.* ASA Newsletter 2001 reprinted with permission from the American Society of Anesthesiologists, 520 N. Northwest Highway, Park Ridge, IL 60068-2573.

■ **TABLE 26–5.** Summary of state activities on office-based anesthesia/surgery regulation*

State	Regulations in Place	Regulations in Development†	Enforceable, Yes/No	Comments	Governor Opt-out‡
Alabama	No	Yes	No	Regulations/guidelines proposed	No
Arizona	Yes (limited)	No	Yes	Offices exempt from regulation/licensure unless using general anesthesia or where general anesthesia is covered under dentistry rules	No
California	Yes	NA	Yes	Accreditation required	No
Colorado	No (guidelines and policy statement only)	No	No	Voluntary	No§
Connecticut	Yes	NA	Yes	Accreditation required for all facilities using a minimum of moderate sedation/analgesia	No
District of Columbia	Yes (limited)	No	No	Medical board advisory to follow ASA guidelines; offices must be licensed as health facilities if complex surgery performed	—
Florida	Yes	NA	Yes	Accreditation or annual state inspection required	No
Georgia	No	Yes	No	Legislation introduced requiring accreditation	No
Illinois	Yes	No	Yes	Only address scope of anesthesia, not surgery	No
Iowa	No	Yes	No	Legislation proposed; annual licensure would be required	Yes
Kansas	No	Yes	No	Medical society adopted regulations/guidelines that encourage accreditation for offices	Yes
Louisiana	No	Yes	No	State medical board approved draft; no final rule	No
Massachusetts	No (guidelines only)	Yes	No	Guidelines endorsed by state board of registration in medicine; legislation introduced requiring licensure or accreditation of ambulatory surgical facilities	No
Mississippi	Yes	No	Yes	Not comprehensive, but does provide for alternate pathway for credentialing of surgeons for procedures outside specific specialty	No
New Jersey	Yes	NA	Yes	Regulations require accreditation by state	No
New York	No	Yes	No	Voluntary guidelines only, urge accreditation; recent legislation proposed specifically addressing office-based surgery	No
North Carolina	No	Yes	No	Guidelines outlined in medical board position statement; noncompliance could result in medical board sanctions	No
Ohio	Yes	NA	No	Medical board regulations effective January 2004	No
Oklahoma	No	No	No	State medical board guidelines only	No
Oregon	Yes	No	Yes	Regulations only	No§
Pennsylvania	Yes	NA	Yes	Accreditation required for Class A facilities; for Class B, C facilities state inspection and licensure required	No
Rhode Island	Yes	NA	Yes	Accreditation required	No
Tennessee	No	Yes	No	Regulations proposed by medical board	
South Carolina	No	Yes	No	Guidelines only, which require accreditation and urge legislation on enforceability	No
Texas	Yes	No	Yes	Regulations for anesthesia practitioners; accredited outpatient facilities exempt	No
Virginia	Yes	Yes	Yes	Outlines rules for anesthesia administration and educational requirements for nonanesthesiology physicians	No
Washington	No	Yes	No	State medical society guidelines only; regulations being developed	No§

*Adapted from Barinholtz D: American Society of Anesthesiologists, 2003.

†NA, not applicable and means that state regulations are extensive. With states that have guidelines or regulations, "No" means that these are not extensive and presently there are no plans to change them.

‡There are other states where the governor has opted out of the CMS rule on supervision of nurse anesthetists, but only those states presently addressing the office-based setting are mentioned here.

§Opt-out by state's governor is being considered.

differences between the three most visible accrediting organizations is given in Table 26–6.

Whether accreditation affects outcomes in office-based surgery and anesthesia is uncertain. In a survey study, the AAAASF sent a questionnaire to its accredited facilities that addressed patient safety in plastic surgical office facilities. Two hundred forty-one of 418 facilities responded to the questionnaire. Over a 5-year period that included over 400,000 surgical procedures, the authors reported the risk of significant complications to be 1 of 213 cases and the risk of death to be 1 of 57,000 cases. They concluded that overall risk in an accredited office is comparable to that of other ambulatory surgical sites (free-standing or hospital based) (Morello et al., 1997). In a retrospective review of an accredited office-based plastic surgery facility, Byrd and others (2003) reported no deaths in over 5000 cases. However, these authors noted that several patients required hospital admission for various medical problems.

■ **TABLE 26–6.** Similarities and differences between various accreditation organizations

Accreditation Body	AAAASF	AAAHC	JCAHO
Medicare deemed status	Yes	Yes	Yes
Requires board certification of surgeon	Yes	No	No
Requires physician supervision of anesthesia*	Yes	Yes	Yes
Additional educational requirements for nonanesthesiologists supervising	Yes	No	No
Accreditation cycle	3 Years	6 Months, 1 year, or 3 years	3 Years
Approximate base cost†	$675 to $1000	$2990	$3975
Corporate Web site	www.aaaasf.org/	www.aaahc.org/	www.jcaho.org/

AAAASF, American Association for Accreditation of Ambulatory Surgical Facilities; AAAHC, American Association for Ambulatory Health Care; JCAHO, Joint Commission on Accreditation of Healthcare Organizations.

*This requirement may not apply in the event a state's governor has opted out of the physician supervision of nonanesthesiologist anesthesia providers requirement.

†Cost for an accreditation survey may be influenced by the number of offices to be accredited, the number of surgeons and surgical specialties, and whether a facility is asking for Medicare "deemed" status.

■ CLINICAL ASPECTS

Particular attention must be paid to patient and case selection, preoperative preparation, special problems related to anesthetic administration, and postoperative care. Absence of a plan by the anesthesiologist caring for a child in the office, specifically related to these issues, can lead to a practice that is fraught with safety dilemmas and logistic and scheduling problems that negatively impact the success of an office-based anesthesia practice. Time constraints are the rule rather than the exception in office-based practice.

■ PATIENT AND PROCEDURE SELECTION

The decision process that occurs when deciding which patients are appropriate to care for in the office-based setting does not differ greatly from that of caring for patients in the "free-standing" ambulatory surgery center. The factors that most commonly determine whether a child is an appropriate candidate for office-based anesthesia and surgery are patient age, associated medical illnesses and ASA physical status, type of surgery, potential for blood loss, potential for significant postoperative complications, and duration of surgery.

Because most office-based procedures for pediatric patients involve dental procedures, a majority of the children undergoing these procedures are older than 1 year. However, as the realm of office-surgery for children expands and because there are no prospective studies as yet in the office-based anesthesia literature looking at outcomes and patient age for children undergoing office-based surgery, it seems that present guidelines for other ambulatory surgery venues should be used. When taking this latter point into consideration, the minimum age requirement (other parameters such as type of procedure not withstanding) for children undergoing office-based procedures can be determined by whether a child requires prolonged postoperative monitoring based on postconceptual age or the administration of opiate analgesics and other respiratory depressant agents (Welborn et al., 1994; Galinkin et al., 1998). Although postanesthesia care unit complications may be more common in neonates and infants resulting from respiratory complications (Westman, 1999), any other minimum age requirements are often arbitrary and may reflect the comfort level of office staff and anesthesia personnel caring for the child (Ross et al., 2002). Adherence to policies and guidelines set forth for minimum age requirements for outpatient anesthesia in ambulatory surgery centers and hospital-based ambulatory surgery departments is critical.

Most children cared for in the office-based setting are ASA Class I and II patients. In some situations, it may be acceptable to provide anesthesia care for those children with stable comorbidities who are ASA Class III patients despite the fact that these patients, in general, may be more susceptible to adverse outcomes from anesthesia (Morray, 2002). Some of the pediatric comorbidities considered high risk for the office-based surgical suite include obstructive sleep apnea, labile asthma and other significant pulmonary disease, complex congenital heart disease, labile diabetes mellitus, significant neurologic and neuromuscular disorders, sickle cell disease, and upper respiratory tract infection.

In one prospective study looking at prolonged recovery stay and unplanned hospital admission following ambulatory surgery in pediatric patients, the authors reported annual rates of approximately 4% and 2%, respectively. PONV and respiratory complications were the most common factors leading to prolonged recovery stay, whereas respiratory complications (32%) and surgical reasons (30%) were the factors most commonly responsible for unplanned hospital admission. These authors also found that higher ASA physical status had a direct relationship to unplanned hospital admission and adverse respiratory events (D'Errico et al., 1998).

Dornhoffer and others (2000), in a retrospective chart review, evaluated unplanned hospital admission following four types of otologic procedures (not including myringotomy tube placement) in adult and pediatric outpatients. The unplanned hospital admission rates for children and adults were 5.7% and 2.3%, respectively. The most common reasons for unplanned hospital admission were postoperative nausea and/or vomiting.

In addition, Dornhoffer and others (2000) noted that tympanomastoidectomy with ossicular reconstruction, procedures lasting longer than 2 hours, and asthma were increased risk factors. In contrast to this study, Mingus and others (1997) reported that surgical cases lasting as little as 1 hour may be associated with a higher rate of unplanned hospital admission.

In a study by Fortier and others (1998) involving over 15,000 patients, unplanned hospital admission following ambulatory surgery was related to longer duration of anesthesia and surgery, higher ASA physical status (Classes II and III), postoperative bleeding, excessive pain, and nausea and vomiting. Of note was that surgical reasons were identified to be more commonly responsible for hospital admission than were anesthesia-related issues (38% and 25%, respectively). The fact that the office-based setting is best suited for those children who are healthy without significant comorbidity and are undergoing minimally invasive procedures may inherently result in few postoperative complications.

PREOPERATIVE PREPARATION

Preanesthetic Interview

As is the case with ambulatory surgery in general, rarely is the preanesthetic interview for office-based surgery for pediatric patients conducted in person. For the anesthesiologist who works in a limited number of offices, preanesthetic interviews may be possible during the patient's presurgical office visit if the anesthesiologist should be attending that particular office on the same day. This is the exception rather than the rule when anesthesiologists provide itinerant care for a multitude of offices. Although some authors have advocated surgical evaluation in certain instances on the same day of surgery (Overdyk et al., 1999), most preanesthetic interviews will be initiated by telephone prior to the day of surgery.

The preanesthetic interview for office-based procedures does not differ much from that described for other ambulatory settings (Welborn, 1996). However, a few important points should be made relative to the preanesthetic interview for an office-based procedure.

First, the anesthesiologist should make some initial contact with a child's parents or guardian prior to the day of surgery. Unlike the ambulatory surgery center or hospital-based ambulatory surgery department, the parents often cannot associate their child's scheduled procedure with the community-acquired reputation of a particular private or academic institution. An anesthesiologist's reputation in the office-based environment is based on the advocacy of the child's private physician, surgeon, or dentist and unfortunately is only as good as the anesthesiologist's last case (or self-advocacy literature). The initial telephone interview must be used as a way to instill confidence in his or her abilities and to alleviate parental anxiety by relating one's level of experience or training background or by discussing a cogent and acceptable anesthetic plan. These few "public relations" minutes are invaluable.

Second, the interview process must elicit enough of a history to determine whether a child is a candidate for the scheduled office-based procedure or whether the procedure needs to be delayed. The same-day cancellation leaves an undesirable block of open time for the anesthesiologist and the surgeon. Finally, in many instances, the preanesthetic telephone interview is used not only as the mechanism by which parents receive final preoperative instructions (e.g., NPO guidelines, medication instructions) but also to make final financial arrangements.

Preoperative Laboratory Testing

Because most children receiving office-based anesthesia services are healthy and are undergoing minimally invasive procedures, the necessity for preoperative laboratory testing is rare. As is advocated by other authors, any laboratory testing should be determined on an individual patient basis by clinical need following the preanesthetic interview (Roizen et al., 1987; Welborn, 1996; Monaghini, 1990, Friedberg, 2003). Despite agreement on the lack of clinical utility and increased cost of routine preoperative laboratory screening among anesthesia professionals, an anesthesiologist providing office-based anesthesia services must be aware of any state and local government mandates for such testing. Additionally, each practitioner must establish his or her policy in determining the cost-to-benefit yield (especially in the office setting where cost savings are a key advantage) on more controversial laboratory testing such as pregnancy testing in adolescents and teenagers (Azzam et al., 1996; Hennrikus et al., 2001).

Preoperative Sedation

Despite the somewhat less intimidating environment of the office, the anxiety that pediatric patients undergoing office-based procedures experience is probably no less than that in other surgical environments. The need for preoperative sedation or some other useful mechanism by which the anesthesiologist can reduce preoperative anxiety is critical. In fact, the space-limited environment of many office practices and the close proximity to office waiting rooms and other patients may make preoperative sedation of children most at risk for preoperative anxiety even more important.

The group of children most likely to undergo a mask induction of anesthesia is also the age group of children most likely to experience preoperative anxiety (Kain et al., 1996; McCann et al., 2001; Kain et al., 2002; Watson et al., 2003). Most children receiving preoperative sedation receive midazolam (McCann et al., 2001). Although various routes of administration are advocated, including intranasal (Davis et al., 1995; Griffith et al., 1998) and rectal (Marhofer et al., 1999), oral administration of midazolam is the most common (Levine et al., 1993; McGraw et al., 1998). Ease of administration as determined by acceptance by the child in most instances dictates the route of administration. Most often in practice, a dose of 0.5 to 1.0 mg/kg (maximum dose, 20 mg) orally is effective.

Although some have found that certain routes of administration of midazolam have no impact on discharge times (Davis et al., 1995; Kain et al., 2000), others find that there are significant delays in recovery or discharge times with the use of orally administered midazolam in combination with various anesthetic techniques (Viitanen et al., 1999). Also, the use of combination preoperative sedation, such as intramuscular ketamine and midazolam, in uncooperative children may be inappropriate for the office-based setting due to prolonged discharge times (Verghese et al., 2003).

For children tolerating preoperative intravenous catheter placement (with or without application of local anesthetic cream), the use of midazolam may not be necessary. Small repeated doses (0.25 to 0.5 mg/kg) of intravenous propofol under constant monitoring provide excellent preoperative anxiolysis without respiratory depression and in many instances provide excellent amnesia to the immediate preoperative period. This technique is especially advantageous in short surgical procedures. However, propofol is associated with pain on injection and lidocaine may have to be added to the infusion.

Although the benefits of parental presence are questionable (to the child and parent), especially compared with pharmacologic approaches to preoperative anxiety reduction (McCann et al., 2001; Kain et al., 2003), the office-based environment may provide an excellent opportunity for parental presence during induction of anesthesia, especially in cases where sterility concerns are minimal such as for dental restoration procedures.

When the administration of a preoperative sedative is indicated, the anesthesiologist must take into consideration whether the benefit of sedation (to the patient, parents, waiting patients, and office staff) outweighs the chance that the sedative will delay discharge following anesthesia. This is particularly true in instances where a physician must be present until the patient is discharged home.

INTRAOPERATIVE CARE

The intraoperative care of the pediatric patient in the office-based setting relative to induction and maintenance of anesthesia does not differ much from that in other ambulatory settings. Despite the minimal standards set forth by most states relative to office-based anesthesia, from the anesthesiologist's perspective, monitoring, and equipment standards and guidelines must not be different for the office than for other surgical and anesthesia sites. One should adhere to the Standards for Basic Anesthetic Monitoring (ASA, 2004) and Guidelines for Office-Based Anesthesia (ASA, 2003) (see Chapter 9, Anesthesia Equipment and Monitoring). With this in mind, one's anesthetic technique is limited only by the equipment, supplies, and resources of the physical plant that he or she has available.

Most office-based surgical procedures using anesthesia require intravenous access and hydration. The child's fluid deficit is based on the NPO period and is replaced with lactated Ringer's solution.

Despite liberalizing the NPO period (clear liquids 2 to 3 hours prior to anesthesia), administration of intravenous fluids both during and after the surgical procedure is important. There is evidence in both adult and pediatric populations that aggressive intraoperative fluid management (Yogendran et al., 1995; Elhakim et al., 1998) and delaying oral intake after surgery (Schreiner et al., 1992), especially when perioperative opioids are administered (Kearney et al., 1998), decrease the incidence of postoperative nausea and vomiting (PONV).

ANESTHETIC TECHNIQUE

The concept of "rapid onset, rapid recovery, and minimal side effects," used often to describe the important characteristics of an appropriate anesthetic technique in an ambulatory setting, is equally important for the office setting. Although all types of anesthesia can be used in the office setting, including regional anesthesia (Rosenquist, 2001), general anesthesia and varying levels of sedation are most often used in children.

Even though anesthesiologists debate the clinical (safety and outcome) and cost efficacy of newer anesthetic agents (sevoflurane, desflurane, remifentanil, and propofol) compared with some of the older agents (halothane, isoflurane), these newer agents offer a distinct advantage as it relates to their predictability (Tang et al., 1999; Moore et al., 2002; Fishkin et al., 2003). All levels of the continuum of anesthesia (minimal sedation to general anesthesia) are used in the office setting. The type of anesthesia is determined by the age and cooperation level of the child, the type of procedure, the ease with which local anesthetic can be administered and its efficacy in a particular surgical procedure, and, as stated previously, the available equipment.

General anesthesia can be accomplished by using a pure volatile technique, a total intravenous technique, or a combination of the two (volatile induction with intravenous maintenance) techniques. The former and latter obviously depend on the availability of an anesthesia machine and on whether a specific office can comply with OSHA requirements relative to appropriate gas scavenging. Some surgical offices, depending on surgical volume and cost efficacy, may provide the anesthesiologist with a standard anesthesia machine; in other instances, the anesthesiologist may transport a single-vaporizer-equipped portable anesthesia machine to each office (D. Barinholtz, Mobile Anesthesiologists, L.L.C., personal communication, September 4, 2003).

All of the newer volatile agents have been shown to be efficacious in pediatric ambulatory surgery (Welborn et al., 1996; Moore et al., 2002). However, if one is transporting a machine with single-vaporizer capability, then sevoflurane may be the agent of choice due to its efficacy in both induction and maintenance of anesthesia, as well as its rapid onset and offset characteristics. Although some advocate the use of desflurane for maintenance of anesthesia for ambulatory surgery because of its predictability relative to emergence (Fishkin et al., 2003), it is impractical as a complete office-based anesthetic agent in children due to its lack of efficacy for inhalation induction (Zwass et al., 1992; Olssen, 1995; Smiley, 1996). Similarly, the intravenous agents propofol (Hannallah et al., 1994; Cohen et al., 2001) and remifentanil (Davis et al., 1997, 2000, 2001; Pinsker, 1999) are shown to be useful in the ambulatory setting.

Although remifentanil can be used successfully in an ambulatory setting when the airway is secured with an endotracheal tube, evidence suggests this narcotic should be used cautiously when the airway is not secured. Litman (1999) evaluated the use of remifentanil for moderate sedation in 17 patients (20 procedures) aged 2 to 12 years who were undergoing short, painful procedures. All patients received intravenous midazolam, 50 mcg/kg, in combination with remifentanil 1 mcg/kg followed by an initial infusion of remifentanil of 0.1 mcg/kg per min. The remifentanil infusion was then titrated every 5 minutes to provide adequate sedation and analgesia. The average appropriate dose of remifentanil utilized was 0.4 mcg/kg per min. Although the author reported successful use of this technique in 17 of 20 procedures, 1 child became unresponsive requiring assisted ventilation, and hypoxemia was avoided in 10 of 13 children by continuous stimulation during the procedure.

In adults, the combination of a propofol infusion, titrated to bispectral analysis (BIS) number, and intermittent ketamine boluses has been reported (Friedberg, 2003). In children (propofol 100 to 200 mcg/kg per min, titrated by BIS; ketamine 0.5- to 1.0-mg/kg boluses) undergoing dental restoration procedures, D. Barinholtz (Mobile Anesthesiologists, L.L.C., personal communication, September 4, 2003) noted that combining propofol (100 to 200 mcg/kg per min) with ketamine boluses completely avoided the need for opiate analgesics.

Although any agent can be safely used in the office-based setting, it is imperative that the office-based anesthesiologist develop an anesthetic routine that allows for an expeditious induction with appropriate maintenance levels of anesthesia while at the same time affording a rapid emergence. It is also essential that this anesthetic routine minimize the incidence of postoperative side effects, nausea and vomiting.

Another critical aspect of intraoperative anesthesia care in the office-based setting is airway management. Although multiple factors determine the type of airway, any type of airway from a mask to laryngeal mask airway to endotracheal tube may be appropriate. For some procedures, especially when using only sedation, airway intervention is usually minimal, but deciding on the appropriate airway intervention in some cases may be difficult. This is particularly true when providing anesthesia for dental or other intraoral procedures.

Despite the fact that many dental cases are performed with oral sedation and nitrous oxide (Saxen et al., 1999; Ross et al., 2002), longer dental restoration procedures may necessitate the use of an endotracheal tube (D. Barinholtz, Mobile Anesthesiologists, L.L.C., personal communication, September 4, 2003). This is most often true in offices where the anesthesiologist may have limited access to the patient's airway due to positioning or cramped quarters. Subsequently, ventilation is controlled by hand or mechanical means or the patient can breathe spontaneously. One must be judicious in the use of muscle relaxants to facilitate intubation. Prolonged effects of these agents may lead to delayed emergence and consequently delayed discharge and turnover for subsequent cases.

LEVEL OF CONSCIOUSNESS MONITORING

The central theme of office-based anesthesia is to accomplish excellent, safe, time-efficient, and cost-effective anesthesia. One must look favorably on any technology that can possibly aid in achieving these goals.

The BIS monitor (Aspect Medical, Newton, MA) is described to be able to determine the level of sedation, predict the loss of consciousness, and thus perhaps diminish intraoperative awareness when used with various anesthetic agents (Glass et al., 1997). Despite previous evidence that BIS is shown to decrease anesthetic use and hasten recovery in adult patients (Glass et al., 1997; Song et al., 1997), the use of the BIS monitor is only recently making its way into the realm of pediatric anesthesia (Denman et al., 2000; Bannister et al., 2001; McCann et al., 2002; Religa et al., 2002).

In one study, Denman and others (2000) found that in children aged 0 to 12 years who were anesthetized with sevoflurane, the BIS value correlated to the depth of anesthesia. Furthermore, this study also confirmed that for a particular level of anesthesia (BIS = 50), children younger than 2 years had a significantly higher end-tidal concentration of sevoflurane than did children aged 2 to 12 years (1.55% versus 1.25%, respectively).

Bannister and others (2001) studied the effect of BIS on anesthetic use and recovery in 240 children. They noted in patients aged 0 to 6 months that the BIS had no effect on anesthetic emergence. However, in older children, BIS was associated with less anesthetic administration and an earlier emergence time.

Religa and others (2002) evaluated the association between BIS and level of consciousness in pediatric patients (age range, 3 to 6 years) undergoing dental procedures using a sedation protocol. These authors found that there was a significant association between behavioral responses and levels of sedation. However, the authors noted that BIS offered no advantage over routine clinical monitoring and behavioral assessment in this setting.

POSTANESTHESIA CARE

As in any ambulatory setting, the patient undergoing office-based surgery must meet established criteria prior to discharge home, with the goal being to discharge the patient as quickly and as safely as possible (Patel et al., 2001). Actual discharge criteria include an adequate level of consciousness, good pain control, good hydration, minimal to no nausea, and a defined period of time since the last emesis (Ross et al., 2002; Fishkin et al., 2003). Furthermore, the appropriate personnel (at a minimum of that outlined by the ASA Guidelines for Office-Based Anesthesia, 2003) must remain with the child until discharge-ready status is reached.

The causes for delayed discharge can be either anesthesia or surgery related, but in the ambulatory setting two of the most common non-life-threatening reasons are inadequate pain control and PONV. Unlike the typical ambulatory setting, which often has the capability to care for patients with a prolonged recovery period, the office-based setting has little margin for error relative to these two problems.

POSTOPERATIVE PAIN CONTROL

The goals for postoperative pain control in the office setting are not dissimilar from the overall goals for office-based anesthesia and surgery. In situations where the use of local anesthesia is not possible or feasible, one must use analgesic agents that are efficacious, have minimal side effects, and will not delay patient discharge.

Despite the fact that various opiate analgesics are routinely used and can be administered via conventional (intravenous, intramuscular while asleep, oral) and less conventional (intranasal) routes (Galinkin et al., 2000; Finkel et al., 2001) in traditional ambulatory surgery settings, their use in the office setting is often minimized or eliminated to help avoid PONV that is drug (Weinstein et al., 1994) and dose (Anderson et al., 2000) related. Furthermore, because a preponderance of complications leading to unplanned hospital admission following ambulatory surgery in infants is related to the respiratory system (Westman, 1999), opiate use in this age group, leading to respiratory depression, could potentially exacerbate these numbers.

Standard use of nonopioid analgesics such as the nonsteroidal anti-inflammatory drugs (NSAIDs) and acetaminophen, when not contraindicated, is advocated. Ketorolac is found to be useful for postoperative analgesia in a variety of pediatric surgical procedures when postoperative bleeding is not a concern, and it can be administered intravenously in a dose of 0.5 to 0.8 mg/kg (maximum dose, 30 mg).

Purday and others (1996) compare three alternative doses of ketorolac, 0.75 mg/kg, 1.0 mg/kg, and 1.5 mg/kg, with morphine 0.1 mg/kg in pediatric patients aged 2 to 12 years who are undergoing dental restoration procedures. The authors found that ketorolac, in all three doses, was as efficacious as morphine sulfate in the management of postoperative pain and was associated with statistically less PONV. Similarly, Maunuksela and others (1992) noted ketorolac to be as efficacious as morphine following pediatric eye surgery.

Ibuprofen can also be used to treat postoperative pain, but reports on its effectiveness for some surgical procedures are mixed. Kokki and others (1994) showed that preoperative administration of rectal ibuprofen, 40 mg/kg, divided into 4 equal doses, was effective in the treatment of postoperative pain in children aged 1 to 4 years in that it reduced the need for supplemental morphine postoperatively. In contrast, Bennie and others (1997), in a double-blind, placebo-controlled study of children older than 6 months who were undergoing bilateral myringotomy and tube placement, found no benefit to the preoperative oral administration of ibuprofen (10 mg/kg) or acetaminophen (15 mg/kg) in the treatment of postoperative pain compared with a placebo group. Joshi and others (2003) reported success with preoperatively administered oral rofecoxib, a newer cyclooxygenase 2 NSAID, given in a dose of 1 mg/kg, in treating postoperative pain and reducing PONV in children (3 to 11 years old) undergoing tonsillectomy.

Acetaminophen administration was also effective for postoperative analgesia, especially in procedures resulting in mild or moderate pain (Tobias, 2000). Although high-dose acetaminophen (40 mg/kg), administered rectally, has been shown to be effective and has opiate-sparing effects (Korpela et al., 1999), the restrictive quarters of some offices may make this route of administration somewhat prohibitive. Similarly, preoperative high-dose acetaminophen (40 mg/kg), administered orally in a one-time dose is shown to be effective in the treatment of postoperative pain following myringotomy and tube placement in children ages 17 months to 6 years, without reaching toxic plasma levels (Bolton et al., 2002). This is contrary to the aforementioned studies (Bennie et al., 1997), where oral acetaminophen in standard doses (15 mg/kg) was shown to be ineffective.

Opiate analgesics are not totally precluded from office-based surgery and may in fact at times be necessary. When either NSAIDs or acetaminophen is inadequate in the treatment of postoperative pain, then traditional combination drugs such as acetaminophen with codeine (0.5 to 1.0 mg/kg of the codeine component) may be appropriate.

POSTOPERATIVE NAUSEA AND VOMITING

PONV remains a major cause of prolonged discharge time and unanticipated hospital admission following ambulatory surgery (Fortier et al., 1998) and plays a significant role in patient dissatisfaction with the perioperative experience (Myles et al., 2000). In one report, approximately 20% of patients surveyed expressed the potential for PONV as their primary concern (Shevde et al., 1991). The optimal treatment of this problem, whether prophylactic or rescue, is essential due to the negative influence it can have on an office-based practice (Tang et al., 1999).

Tang and others (2001) compared the use of propofol-N_2O anesthesia with the use of desflurane-N_2O anesthesia plus antiemetic prophylaxis on the incidence of PONV in patients undergoing brief, superficial surgical procedures in an office setting. Patients in the propofol group received no PONV prophylaxis, whereas those in the desflurane group received ondansetron (4 mg), droperidol (0.625 mg), and metoclopramide (10 mg) intravenously at the end of surgery. Neither group received opiate analgesics nor muscle relaxants, and all patients received local anesthetic at the surgical site and ketorolac for postoperative pain management. The overall incidence of nausea and vomiting was very low in both groups and did not differ statistically. Patient satisfaction in both groups was excellent.

In another office-based study, Tang and others (2003) compared the addition of 5-hydroxytryptamine$_3$ (5-HT_3) receptor antagonists to a control regimen in patients receiving desflurane-N_2O maintenance anesthesia following propofol induction. All patients received droperidol (0.625 mg) and dexamethasone (4 mg) as baseline antiemetic prophylaxis. Subsequently, patients were randomly assigned to receive placebo, dolasetron (12.5 mg), or ondansetron (4 mg) intravenously prior to emergence from anesthesia. The results of this study show that the incidence of nausea and vomiting was the same in all groups.

The best regimen for prophylaxis against PONV in children and adults is not known, although dexamethasone has been shown to be an excellent choice for various procedures in the pediatric and adult populations either by itself (Subramaniam, 2001) or in combination with 5-HT_3 receptor antagonists (Splinter et al., 1998; Rose et al., 1999; Henzi et al., 2000; Splinter, 2001; Negri et al., 2002; Sukhani, 2002). The dose range for dexamethasone in pediatric patients is reported to be from 0.1 mg/kg when used with ondansetron (Splinter et al., 1998) to 1.5 mg/kg when used alone (Henzi et al., 2000). In a quantitative systematic review, Henzi and others (2000) found the use of dexamethasone to be safe in otherwise healthy patients.

Those children at high risk are probably most benefited by prophylactic treatment of PONV. Those at high risk include patients with a previous history of PONV, a history of motion sickness, those undergoing certain surgical procedures (strabismus repair, inguinal herniorrhaphy, orchiopexy), and those receiving perioperative opiate analgesics.

Several authors advocate the use of multiple drug regimens in the treatment of PONV in pediatric and adult ambulatory surgical patients (Rose et al., 1999; Scuderi et al., 2000; Negri et al., 2002; Gan et al., 2003). However, whether prophylactic treatment of PONV, single drug or multiple drug, in all patients undergoing office-based surgery and anesthesia is clinically and economically efficacious as opposed to only treating patients who are at risk can only be determined by further study of patients in this more restrictive setting.

ESTABLISHING AN OFFICE-BASED PRACTICE

The individual or hospital-based surgery center group must decide whether committing resources to this type of practice is a worthwhile endeavor. The initial investment for this type of practice in the United States can be prohibitive, as the cost may run as high as $100,000 to $200,000 (D. Barinholtz, Mobile Anesthesiologists, L.L.C., personal communication, September 4, 2003). These costs include, but are not limited to, those for equipment and supplies, professional accreditation discussed earlier, legal services for incorporation of the group, malpractice coverage, professional staff (physician, nursing, biomedical, secretarial, and billing), policy and procedure development, and marketing.

One must also consider the type of office-based practice that should be initiated. The group or individual can be committed to one surgeon's office, depending on case volume, or can be committed to several surgeons, traveling to various office locations. From a logistic perspective, the former is easier because it allows for centralization of resources, the most important of which are equipment and medications.

A group practice considering an office-based venture must decide if it can designate a specific number of full-time equivalent staff to this site and still be able to provide sufficient clinical coverage to fulfill its contractual obligation to its home facility. If not, the group must then decide whether the cost of hiring new staff (physicians, recovery nurses, technical staff) will be offset by the potential revenue generated by the new practice. For the solo practitioner who may be caught up in the excitement of a new practice, overcommitment to too many surgeons may result in scheduling nightmares and a failure to meet obligations.

The individual or group must also meet the challenge of being able to market against other physicians or physician groups, as well as alternative and perhaps less expensive anesthesia providers in this competitive arena. Can the group provide a unique service, such as pediatric anesthesia coverage, that will make it more attractive to a particular surgeon or dentist?

Finally, and probably as important as any of the other issues related to establishing an office-based practice, the potential political fallout related to a new practice cannot be overemphasized. An anesthesia group with obligations to specific hospital or surgery center facilities must be ready to justify to administrators its practice of providing office-based anesthesia services to surgeons

BOX 26–2 General Categories of Required Supplies Transported by the Office-Based Anesthesiologist

Anesthesia supply box	Defibrillator (w/appropriate sized paddles)
Recovery supply box	Anesthesia drug box
Pediatric supply box	Recovery drug box
Airway box	Emergency airway equipment (LMAs, fiberoptic bronchoscope, cricothyrotomy kits, etc.)
Portable suction equipment	
Monitoring equipment with disposables	
Malignant hyperthermia tray	Portable anesthesia machine with vaporizer
Positive pressure ventilation system	Oxygen "E" cylinders
Miscellaneous (batteries, records, etc.)	

Courtesy of D. Barinholtz, Mobile Anesthesiologists, L.L.C., 2003.

who typically operate in these administrators' facilities. This diversion of income-generating surgical procedures may be construed as a violation of a group's service agreement and consequently prompt administrators to solicit the services of a new group.

EQUIPMENT AND SUPPLIES

Essentially all of the standard anesthesia equipment that is required in hospital ambulatory facilities (operating room and off-site) and surgery centers is required for office-based practice. All monitoring standards must be met in the office-surgical suite. Monitoring equipment must have battery backup capability as some offices may not have emergency generator capabilities in the event of power failure. Working in one facility where the equipment is capitalized by the surgeon or capitalized by the anesthesiologist and stored in the surgeon's office is much easier to deal with than the more common alternative of the anesthesiologist bringing the anesthesia workroom from place to place. Box 26–2 outlines general categories of supplies, standard and emergency, that must be transported to surgical sites by the office-based anesthesiologist.

For those practitioners who provide total intravenous anesthesia, an anesthesia machine is not necessary, but the presence of equipment capable of delivering positive pressure ventilation with oxygen is mandatory. For those anesthesiologists providing care to pediatric patients, a vaporizer-containing anesthesia machine is invaluable. Most anesthesia machines are moveable, but there are a few machines that are truly portable and available for care of pediatric and adult patients in the office setting. One such machine is the OBA-1 (OBAMED, Inc., Cardinal Medical Specialties, Inc., Louisville, KY), which weighs approximately 35 pounds, is vaporizer equipped, and is MRI compatible (Fig. 26–2). The OBA-1 allows only spontaneous or manually controlled ventilation, as it is not equipped with an internal ventilator. The Magellan-2200, Model 1/M (Oceanic Medical Products, Inc., Atchison, KS) and the Narkomed-Mobile (Draeger Medical, Inc., Telford, PA) are also marketed for office

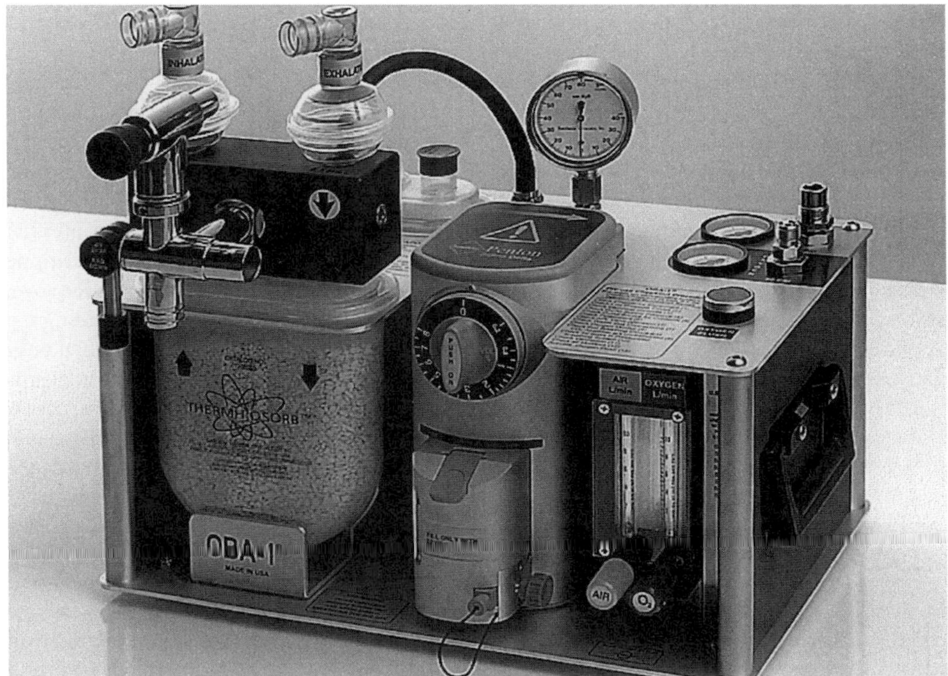

FIGURE 26–2. The OBA-1 portable, MRI-compatible anesthesia machine. (Courtesy of Charles A. Smith, Vice-President Operations, Research and Development, Cardinal Medical Specialties, Inc., Louisville, KY.)

anesthesia and both contain an internal ventilator. The latter machine, despite its ability to be rolled, is a much heavier unit and may not be practical for the anesthesiologist who is changing office venues on a daily basis.

Regardless of the type of machine one chooses to use, caution must be used during transport; maintaining the machine's vaporizer in an upright position is essential to avoid spillage and the administration of an inappropriately high concentration of volatile agent. Often, draining the vaporizer prior to transport minimizes this risk. Furthermore, familiarity with state and federal safety guidelines relative to the transportation of medical gases is critical.

Whenever a volatile agent or succinylcholine is to be used, one must be prepared to treat malignant hyperthermia (MH). A stock supply of dantrolene must be available, and it is the responsibility of the anesthesiologist or a representative of the practice to proactively educate the surgeon and the surgeon's office personnel on appropriate protocol in the event of an MH episode (see Chapter 31, Malignant Hyperthermia).

Finally, the office-based anesthesiologist must become aware of and be in compliance with the rules and regulations (federal and state specific) relative to the delivery, transport, clerical requirements (dispensing, wastage), and storage of opiates and other controlled substances that are used in the office setting.

STAFFING

In the United States, the providers of office-based anesthesia services presently fall into one of three major categories (exclusive of the operator-anesthetist scenario): physician anesthesiologists, dentist anesthesiologists (2 years of anesthesia training following completion of dental school), and CRNAs. The conditions under which each of these three groups can practice are determined by state regulations regarding the administration of anesthesia in dental and surgical offices. Consequently, the composition of office-based anesthesia groups may vary by geographic location and can be comprised of and owned by all physicians, all dentist anesthesiologists, CRNA groups with and without collaborating physician medical directors, or various combinations of these individuals.

Beyond the anesthesia providers, however, are the ancillary personnel who are necessary to make a busy office-based practice successful. The individuals who are often required include nursing staff, biomedical/technical staff, and billing and clerical staff. The number of anesthesia sites a practice covers simultaneously and the volume of cases usually determine the staffing for a particular organization.

In some practices, an anesthesiologist or a CRNA may travel solo to a site. In this instance, the anesthesia provider is responsible for preoperative, intraoperative, and postanesthesia care of the child and requires the assistance of the surgical nursing staff. When multiple cases are performed at a single site, then a surgical office nurse is responsible for monitoring a patient during recovery.

In anesthesiologist-only practices, the preferred scenario is to have a staff nurse, employed by the group, available to assist with induction of anesthesia and to be responsible for monitoring the postanesthesia care of the child. Nurses with critical care or postanesthesia care unit (PACU) experience, who are ACLS-PALS certified, are best suited for this type of position. Anesthesia practices are sometimes able to procure reimbursement for the professional services rendered by these nurses to the PACU care of patients.

Having such personnel relieves the surgical ancillary staff from any anesthesia-related patient care responsibility and facilitates timely turnover when multiple cases are being performed in a single office. Experienced nurses may also be used to initiate telephone screening to provide patients with their preoperative anesthesia and surgical instructions, coordinate anesthesia scheduling, assist in purchasing supplies and equipment, and educate surgical staff on the specifics of the anesthesia process.

REIMBURSEMENT

Mentioned earlier is the potential for cost savings by moving surgical cases from hospital outpatient or ambulatory surgical facilities to the office. Unfortunately, in some arenas, anesthesia-requiring office procedures are the rule due to the lack of insurance coverage for these procedures. This is especially true in pediatric dentistry, where dentists have had their proverbial "backs against the wall." With few exceptions in the United States, dental and medical insurance policies traditionally failed to cover the cost of anesthesia and/or hospitalization for children requiring dental procedures (Saxen et al., 1999; Yagiela, 1999). This has forced dentists to minimize costs, for these children and their families, by performing procedures in the office with or without the aid of an anesthesia provider.

However, the American Dental Association reports that there are at least 29 states, since the mid-1990s, that have passed laws requiring that medical insurance plans pay for hospital and connected medical expenses (e.g., general anesthesia services) when the dental treatment occurs in the hospital, ambulatory surgery center, or dental office (Box 26–3) (J. Hansen, American Dental Association, personal communication, August 25, 2003).

Some of the elements of these state laws are similar and often determine which children are eligible to receive coverage based on minimum and maximum age and medical/behavioral conditions. Many of these laws, despite mandating coverage, also outline that any provisions of the existing policy, such as meeting prior authorization requirements by showing medical necessity or payable deductibles, still hold true.

Some states also determine the acceptable facilities where the procedure can be performed by mandating insurance coverage only for procedures performed in the hospital or surgery center. Some laws also exempt dental-only insurance plans from their provisions. The number of states requiring coverage for the anesthesia portion of dental care may continue to increase, resulting in increased access to care for those children having the greatest need, regardless of qualified surgical site.

Reimbursement and collections for anesthesia and surgery in offices are somewhat complex and often work differently for the surgical provider and the anesthesia provider (Koch et al., 2003). Fee-for-service reimbursement can be lucrative for the anesthesiologist in a high-volume cosmetic surgeon's office. However, because patients undergoing cosmetic surgery are often charged a set global fee for a specific procedure, some surgeons may look toward a lower-cost anesthesia provider, so the surgeon may recover a greater amount of the preset fee. This may intensify competition among anesthesia providers for these types of procedures.

Reimbursement from third-party payers is at negotiated rates that usually vary by geographic location and payer. Despite the fact that some payers reimburse anesthesia practices for professional fees and supplies/equipment, there are those that invoke the CMS policy that a facility be licensed by the state in order to bill for the latter. Consequently, this may mean a greater cost

BOX 26–3 States Adopting Laws or Regulations Requiring Medical Plans to Pay for Hospitalization/General Anesthesia When Dental Treatment Must Be Performed in the Hospital or Medical Expenses Incurred When Treatment Is in the Dental Office (Some States)

California (1998)
Colorado (1998)
Connecticut (1998)
Florida (1998)
Georgia (1999)
Illinois (2002)
Indiana (1999)
Iowa (2000)
Kansas (1999)
Kentucky (2002)
Louisiana (1997)
Maine (2001)
Maryland (1998)
Michigan (2001)
Minnesota (1995)
Mississippi (1999)
Missouri (1998)
Nebraska (2000)
New Hampshire (1998, 2003)
New Jersey (1999)
North Carolina (1999)
North Dakota (1999)
Oklahoma (1998)
South Dakota (1999)
Tennessee (1997)
Texas (1997)
Virginia (2000)
Washington (2001)
Wisconsin (1997)

burden to the patient (D. Barinholtz, Mobile Anesthesiologists, L.L.C., personal communication, September 4, 2003). Koch and others (2003) point out that office-based anesthesia practices may become even more ubiquitous and successful by duplicating cost recovery strategies of surgeons—namely, better collection of facility fees and site of service differentials that provide for greater reimbursement for procedures performed in offices.

SUMMARY

Anesthesiologists have become increasingly involved in the practice of office-based anesthesia and surgery. Consequently, anesthesiologists must be proactive in ensuring that patient safety is the principal concern for all professionals providing anesthesia services in the office setting. It seems unlikely that the various professional societies, whose memberships are actively involved in office anesthesia and surgery, will agree on a specific set of anesthesia delivery guidelines. Consistency between states in the regulation of this practice is crucial and may be the only viable alternative in helping to ensure that "the standard of care is the standard of care." This standard should be applicable regardless of surgical setting or patient age. Only further study will aid in determining whether the safety and cost profiles for office-based anesthesia are comparable to those of other ambulatory settings and ultimately whether office-based anesthesia will continue to be a worthwhile venture.

REFERENCES

Accreditation Association for Ambulatory Health Care (AAAHC): Summary of state activities on office-based surgery. August 2003 update. Personal communication, September 29, 2003.

American Academy of Pediatric Dentistry: *Clinical guidelines on the elective use of minimal, moderate, and deep sedation and general anesthesia in pediatric dental patients,* 2004. Available at http:// www. aapd.org/media/Policies_Guidelines/G_Sedation.pdf

American Association for Accreditation of Ambulatory Surgery Facilities (AAAASF), 2003. Available at http://www.aaaasf.org/history.php

American Association of Nurse Anesthetists: Standards for office-based anesthesia practice, 2002. Available at http://www.aana.com/crna/prof/obstandards.asp

American College of Surgeons: *Guidelines for optimal ambulatory surgical care and office based surgery,* 3rd ed. Chicago, 2000, American College of Surgeons.

American Society of Anesthesiologists: Continuum of depth of sedation. Definition of general anesthesia and level of sedation—analgesia, 2004. Available at http://www.asahq.org/publicationsAndServices/Standards/20.pdf

American Society of Anesthesiologists: Guidelines for ambulatory anesthesia and surgery, 2003. Available at http://www.asahq.org/publicationsAndServices/standards/04.pdf

American Society of Anesthesiologists: Guidelines for nonoperating room anesthetizing locations, 2001. Available at http://www.asahq.org/publicationsAndServices-Standards/14.pdf

American Society of Anesthesiologists: Guidelines for office-based anesthesia, 2004. Available at http://www.asahq.org/publicationsAndServices/standards/12.pdf

American Society of Anesthesiologists Office of Governmental and Legal Affairs: *Office based surgery and anesthesia, statutes, regulations and guidelines* (rev. ed.). Washington, D.C., 2003, American Society of Anesthesiologists.

American Society of Anesthesiologists: Practice guidelines for sedation and analgesia by nonanesthesiologists, 2001. Available at http://www.asahq.org/publicationsAndServices/sedation1017.pdf

American Society of Anesthesiologists: Standards for basic anesthetic monitoring, 2004. Available at http://www.asahq.org/publicationsAndServices/standards/02.pdf

American Society of Anesthesiologists: Statement on qualifications of anesthesia providers in an office-based setting, 2004. Available at http://www.asahq.org/publicationsAndServices/Standards/29.pdf

American Society of Plastic Surgery (ASPS) Committee on Patient Safety: *Practice advisory on liposuction: Executive summary.* Arlington Heights, IL, 2003, ASPS.

Anderson BJ, Ralph CJ, Stewart AW, et al.: The dose-effect relationship for morphine and vomiting after day-stay tonsillectomy in children. *Anaesth Intensive Care* 28:155, 2000.

Arens JF: Anesthesia for office-based surgery: Are we paying too high a price for access and convenience? *Mayo Clinic Proc* 75:225, 2000.

Avery ME: Editorial views: A pediatrician's perspective. *Anesthesiology* 43:142, 1975.

Azzam FJ, Padda GS, DeBoard JW, et al.: Preoperative pregnancy testing in adolescents. *Anesth Analg* 82:4, 1996.

Bannister CF, Brosius KK, Sigl JC, et al.: The effect of bispectral index monitoring on anesthetic use and recovery in children anesthetized with sevoflurane in nitrous oxide. *Anesth Analg* 92:877, 2001.

Bennie RE, Boehringer LA, McMahon S, et al.: Postoperative analgesia with preoperative oral ibuprofen or acetaminophen in children undergoing myringotomy. *Paediatr Anaesth* 7:399, 1997.

Biboulet P, Aubas P, Dubourdieu J, et al.: Fatal and non fatal cardiac arrests related to anesthesia. *Can J Anaesth* 48:326, 2001.

Bitar G, Mullis W, Jacobs W, et al.: Safety and efficacy of office based surgery with monitored anesthesia care—sedation in 4778 consecutive plastic surgery procedures. *Plast Reconstr Surg* 111:150, 2003.

Blayney MR, Malins AF, Cooper GM: Cardiac arrhythmias in children during outpatient general anaesthesia for dentistry: A prospective randomised trial. *Lancet* 354:1864, 1999.

Bolton P, Bridge HS, Montgomery CJ, et al.: The analgesic efficacy of preoperative high dose (40 mg x kg^{-1}) oral acetaminophen after bilateral myringotomy and tube insertion in children. *Paediatr Anaesth* 12:29, 2002.

Brandom BW, Herlich A: Safety of outpatient dental anaesthesia for children (commentary). *Lancet* 354:1836, 1999.

Byrd HS, Barton FE, Orenstein HH, et al.: Safety and efficacy in an accredited outpatient plastic surgery facility: A review of 5316 consecutive cases. *Plast Reconstr Surg* 112:636, 2003.

Cartwright D: Death in the dental chair. *Anaesthesia* 54:105, 1999.

Cartwright PC, Snow BW, McNees DC: Urethral meatotomy in the office using topical EMLA cream for anesthesia. *J Urol* 156:857, 1996.

Coldiron B: Office surgical incidents: 19 Months of Florida data. *Dermatol Surg* 28:710, 2002.

Coldiron B: Patient injuries from surgical procedures performed in medical offices. *JAMA* 285:2582, 2001.

Cohen IT, Hannallah RS, Goodale DB: The clinical and biochemical effects of propofol infusion with and without EDTA for maintenance anesthesia in healthy children undergoing ambulatory surgery. *Anesth Analg* 93:106, 2001.

Coté CJ, Notterman DA, Karl HW, et al.: Adverse sedation events in pediatrics: A critical incident analysis of contributing factors. *Pediatrics* 105:805, 2000.

Coté CJ, Karl HW, Notterman DA, et al.: Adverse sedation events in pediatrics: Analysis of medications used for sedation. *Pediatrics* 106:633, 2000.

Coté CJ: Pediatric, dental communities concerned about safe sedation for kids. *AAP News* 21:204, 2002.

Croasdale M: Florida opens loophole in office surgery rule, 2002. Available at http://www.ama-assn.org/amednews/2002/08/12/prsd0812.htm. Accessed May 1, 2005.

Davis PJ, Finkel JC, Orr RJ, et al.: A randomized, double blinded study of remifentanil versus fentanyl for tonsillectomy and adenoidectomy surgery in pediatric ambulatory surgical patients. *Anesth Analg* 90:863, 2000.

Davis PJ, Lerman J, Suresh S, et al.: A randomized multicenter study of remifentanil compared with alfentanil, isoflurane, or propofol in anesthetized pediatric patients undergoing elective strabismus surgery. *Anesth Analg* 84:982, 1997.

Davis PJ, Tome JA, McGowan FX, et al.: Preanesthetic medication with intranasal midazolam for brief pediatric surgical procedures: Effect on recovery and hospital discharge times. *Anesthesiology* 82:2, 1995.

de Jong RH: Mega-dose lidocaine dangers seen in "tumescent" liposuction. *Anesth Patient Safety Found Newsletter* 14:25, 1999.

Denman JH, Hingson RA, Tomaro AJ: Cardiac resuscitation in the dental office: Report of case. *J Oral Surg* 26:470, 1968.

Denman WT, Swanson EL, Rosow D, et al.: Pediatric evaluation of the bispectral index (BIS) monitor and correlation of BIS with end tidal sevoflurane concentration in infants and children. *Anesth Analg* 90:872, 2000.

D'Eramo EM: Mortality and morbidity with outpatient anesthesia: The Massachusetts experience. *J Maxillofac Surg* 57:531, 1999.

D'Errico C, Voepel-Lewis TD, Siewert M, et al.: Prolonged recovery stay and unplanned admission of the pediatric surgical outpatient: An observational study. *J Clin Anesth* 10:482, 1998.

Domino KB: Office-based anesthesia: Lessons learned from the Closed Claims Project. *Am Soc Anesthesiol Newsletter* 65:9, 2001.

Dornhoffer J, Manning L: Unplanned hospital admissions following outpatient otologic surgery: The University of Arkansas experience. *Ear Nose Throat J* 79:712, 2000.

Elhakim M, el-Sebiae S, Kaschef N, et al.: Intravenous fluid and postoperative nausea and vomiting after day-case termination of pregnancy. *Acta Anaesthesiol Scand* 42:216, 1998.

Federation of State Medical Boards: Report of the Special Committee on Outpatient (Office-Based) Surgery: Executive summary, 2002. Available at http://www.fsmb.org/Policy%20Documents%20and%20White%20Papers/outpatient_surgery_cmt_rpt.htm

Finkel JC, Cohen IT, Hannallah RS, et al.: The effect of intranasal fentanyl on the emergence characteristics after sevoflurane anesthesia in children undergoing surgery for bilateral myringotomy tube placement. *Anesth Analg* 92:1164, 2001.

Fishkin S, Litman RS: Current issues in pediatric ambulatory anesthesia. *Anesthesiol Clin North Am* 21:305, 2003.

Fortier J, Chung F, Su J: Unanticipated admission after ambulatory surgery: A prospective study. *Can J Anaesth* 45:612, 1998.

Friedberg BL: Anesthesia for cosmetic facial surgery. *Int Anesthesiol Clin* 41:13, 2003.

Friedberg BL, Sigl JC: Clonidine premedication decreases propofol consumption during bispectral index (BIS)-monitored propofol ketamine technique for office based surgery. *Dermatol Surg* 26:848, 2000.

Friedman O, Deutsch ES, Reilly JS, et al.: The feasibility of office based laser assisted tympanic membrane fenestration with tympanostomy tube insertion: The duPont Hospital experience. *Int J Pediatr Otorhinolaryngol* 62:31, 2002.

Galinkin JL, Fazi LM, Cuy RM, et al.: Use of intranasal fentanyl in children undergoing myringotomy and tube placement during halothane and sevoflurane anesthesia. *Anesthesiology* 93:1378, 2000.

Galinkin JL, Kurth D: Neonatal and pediatric apnea syndromes. *Probl Anesth* 10:444, 1998.

Gan TJ, Meyer T, Apfel C, et al.: Consensus guidelines for managing postoperative nausea and vomiting. *Anesth Analg* 97:62–71, 2003.

Ganzberg SI, Weaver JM: Anesthesia for office-based oral and maxillofacial surgery. *Dent Clin North Am* 43:547, 1999.

Garin P, Ledeghen S, Van Prooyen-Keyser S, et al.: Office-based CO_2 laser assisted tympanic membrane fenestration addressing otitis media with effusion. *J Clin Laser Med Surg* 19:185, 2001.

Ghosh S, Sallam S: Patient satisfaction and postoperative demands on hospital and community services after day surgery. *Br J Surg* 81:1635, 1994.

Girdler NM, Smith DG: Prevalence of emergency events in British dental practice and emergency management skills of British dentists. *Resuscitation* 41:159, 1999.

Glass PS, Bloom M, Kearse L, et al.: Bispectral analysis measures sedation and memory effects of propofol, midazolam, isoflurane, and alfantanil in healthy volunteers. *Anesthesiology* 86:836–847, 1997.

Goldblum TA, Summers CG, Egbert JE, et al.: Office probing for congenital nasolacrimal duct obstruction: A study of parental satisfaction. *J Pediatr Ophthalmol Strabismus* 33:244, 1996.

Grazer F, de Jong RH: Fatal outcomes from liposuction. Census survey of cosmetic surgeons. *Plast Reconstr Surg* 105:436, 2000.

Grevelink JM, White VR, Bonoan R, et al.: Pulsed laser treatment in children and the use of anesthesia. *J Am Acad Dermatol* 37:75, 1997.

Griffith N, Howell S, Mason DG: Intranasal midazolam for premedication of children undergoing day-case anaesthesia: Comparison of two delivery systems with assessment of intraobserver variability. *Br J Anaesth* 81:865, 1998.

Hall MJ, Lawrence L: Ambulatory surgery in the United States, 1996-1998 advance data. The National Center for Health Statistics, 300, 1–16. Available at http://www.cdc.gov/nchs/data/ad/ad300.pdf. Accessed March 20, 2005.

Hannallah RS: Selection of patients for paediatric ambulatory surgery. *Can J Anaesth* 38:887, 1991.

Hannallah RS, Britton JT, Schafer PG, et al.: Propofol anesthesia in pediatric ambulatory surgery patients: A comparison with thiopentone and halothane. *Can J Anaesth* 41:12, 1994.

Hennrikus WL, Shaw BA, Gerardi JA: Prevalence of positive preoperative pregnancy testing in teenagers scheduled for orthopedic surgery. *J Pediatr Orthop* 21:677, 2001.

Henzi I, Walder B, Tramèr MR: Dexamethasone for the prevention of postoperative nausea and vomiting: A quantitative systematic review. *Anesth Analg* 90:186, 2000.

Hilton L: Office surgery moratorium has doctors debating issue, January 8, 2001. Available at http://bizjournals.com/jacksonville/stories/2001/01/08/story7.html

Hoefflin SM, Bornstein JB, Gordon M: General anesthesia in an office-based plastic surgical facility: A report on more than 23,000 consecutive office-based procedures under general anesthesia with no significant anesthetic complications. *Plast Reconstr Surg* 107:243, 2001.

Iverson RE, Apfelbaum JL, Brunner JG, et al.: Patient safety in office-based surgery facilities: I. Procedures in the office-based setting. *Plast Reconstr Surg* 110:1337, 2002.

Iverson RE, Lynch DJ, Apfelbaum J, et al.: Patient safety in office-based surgery facilities: II. Patient selection. *Plast Reconstr Surg* 110:1785, 2002.

Jacobsohn PH: Horace Wells, discoverer of anesthesia. *Anesth Prog* 42:73, 1995.

Johnson EL, Roberts MW, Prasad R: Complication associated with general anesthesia: Report of case. *ASDC J Dent Child* 68:332, 2001.

Joshi GP: The Society for Ambulatory Anesthesia:17th Annual meeting report. *Anesth Analg* 96:903, 2003.

Joshi W, Connelly NR, Reuben SS, et al.: An evaluation of the safety and efficacy of administering rofecoxib for postoperative pain management. *Anesth Analg* 97:35, 2003.

Kain ZN, Caldwell-Andrews A, Wang SM: Psychological preparation of the parent and pediatric surgical patient. *Anesthesiol Clin North Am* 20:29, 2002.

Kain ZN, Caldwell-Andrews AA, Mayes LC, et al.: Parental presence during induction of anesthesia. Physiological effects on parents. *Anesthesiology* 98:58, 2003.

Kain ZN, Mayes LC, O'Connor TZ, et al.: Preoperative anxiety in children: Predictors and outcomes. *Arch Pediatr Adolesc Med* 150:1238, 1996.

Kain ZN, Mayes L, Wang S et al.: Parental presence and a sedative premedicant for children undergoing surgery: A hierarchical study. *Anesthesiology* 92:939, 2000.

Kearney R, Mack C, Entwistle L: Withholding oral fluids from children undergoing day surgery reduces vomiting. *Paediatr Anaesth* 8:331, 1998.

Keenan R, Shapiro J, Dawson K: Frequency of anesthetic cardiac arrests in children. Effect of pediatric anesthesiologists. *J Clin Anesth* 3:433, 1991.

Keenan R, Shapiro J, Kane F, et al.: Bradycardia during anesthesia in infants: An epidemiologic study. *Anesthesiology* 80:976, 1994.

Koch ME, Dayan S, Barinholtz D: Office-based anesthesia: An overview. *Anesthesiol Clin North Am* 21:417, 2003.

Kokki H, Hendolin H, Maunuksela EL, et al.: Ibuprofen in the treatment of postoperative pain in small children. A randomized double-blind-placebo controlled parallel group study. *Acta Anaesthesiol Scand* 38:467, 1994.

Korpela R, Korvenoja P, Meretoja OA: Morphine-sparing effect of acetaminophen in pediatric day-case surgery. *Anesthesiology* 91:442, 1999.

LaMendola, B: No surgery ever routine, student's death from cosmetic surgery examined. Fort Lauderdale Sun Sentinel, 1998. Available at http://pqasb.pqarchiver.com/sun_sentinel/. Accessed July 7, 2003.

Laskin DM: The risks of itinerant anesthesia services (editorial). *J Oral Maxillofac Surg* 57:363, 1999.

Laurito CE: Report of educational meeting. The Society for Office-Based Anesthesia, Orlando, Florida, March 7, 1998. *J Clin Anesth* 10:445, 1998.

Letts M, Davidson D, Splinter W, et al.: Analysis of the efficacy of pediatric day surgery. *Can J Surg* 44:193, 2001.

Levine M, Spahr-Schopfer I, Hartley E, et al.: Oral midazolam premedication in children: The minimum time interval for separation from parents. *Can J Anaesth* 40:726, 1993.

Litman RS: Conscious sedation with remifentanil and midazolam during brief painful procedures in children. *Arch Pediatr Adolesc Med* 153:1085, 1999.

MacCallum PL, MacRae DL, Sukerman S, et al.: Ambulatory adenotonsillectomy in children less than 5 years of age. *J Otolaryngol* 30:75, 2001.

Manoharan G, Moohan V, Adgey J: Ventricular fibrillation in a 12-year-old boy recovering from dental anaesthesia. *Int J Cardiol* 81:271, 2001.

Marhofer P, Glaser C, Krenn CG, et al.: Incidence of therapy of midazolam induced hiccups in paediatric anaesthesia. *Paediatr Anaesth* 9:295, 1999.

Maunuksela EL, Kokki H, Bullingham RE: Comparison of intravenous ketorolac with morphine for postoperative pain in children. *Clin Pharmacol Ther* 52:436, 1992.

McCann ME, Brustowicz RM, Bacsik J, et al.: The bispectral index and explicit recall during the intraoperative wake-up test for scoliosis surgery. *Anesth Analg* 94:1474, 2002.

McCann ME, Kain ZN: The management of preoperative anxiety in children: An update. *Anesth Analg* 93:98, 2001.

McGraw T, Kendrick A: Oral midazolam premedication and postoperative behavior in children. *Paediatr Anaesth* 8:117, 1998.

Medical Society of the State of New York (January 7, 2002): Office based surgery guidelines. Supreme Court declares DOH office-based surgery guidelines null and void. Available at http://www.mssny.org/members_only/prac_man/OBSguidelines.htm. Accessed April 20, 2003.

Meneghini L, Zadra N, Zanette G, et al.: The usefulness of routine preoperative laboratory tests for one-day surgery in healthy children. *Paediatr Anaesth* 8:11, 1998.

Mingus ML, Bodian CA, Bradford CN, et al.: Prolonged surgery increases the likelihood of admission of scheduled ambulatory surgery patients. *J Clin Anesth* 9:446, 1997.

Moir CR, Blair GK, Fraser GC, Marshall RH: The emerging pattern of pediatric day-care surgery. *J Pediatr Surg* 22:743, 1987.

Moore EW, Pollard BJ, Elliott RE: Anaesthetic agents in pediatric day case surgery: Do they affect outcome? *Eur J Anaesthsiol* 19:9, 2002.

Morell RC: OBA questions, problems just now recognized, being defined. *Anesth Patient Safety Newsletter* 15:1, 2000.

Morello DC, Colon GA, Fredericks S, et al.: Patient safety in accredited office surgical facilities. *Plast Reconstr Surg* 99:1496, 1997.

Morray JP: Anesthesia-related cardiac arrest in children. An update. *Anesthesiol Clin North Am* 20:1, 2002.

Morray JP, Geiduschek JM, Ramamoorthy MB, et al.: Anesthesia-related cardiac arrest in children. Initial findings of the Pediatric Perioperative Cardiac Arrest (POCA) registry. *Anesthesiology* 93:6, 2000.

Moss E: Revelations: New Jersey office regulations adopted. *Am Soc Anesthesiol Newsletter* 62:17, 1998.

Myles PS, Williams DL, Hendrata M, et al.: Patient satisfaction after anaesthesia and surgery: Results of a prospective survey of 10,811 patients. *Br J Anaesth* 84:6, 2000.

Neergaard L: Sedation safety alert. Anesthesia in doctor's office riskier. *Chicago Sun-Times* Friday, March 19, 1999.

Negri PD, Ivani G: Management of postoperative nausea and vomiting in children. *Paediatr Drugs* 4:717, 2002.

Newland MC, Ellis SJ, Lydiatt CA, et al.: Anesthesia-related cardiac arrest and its mortality. A report covering 72,959 anesthetics over 10 years from a US teaching hospital. *Anesthesiology* 97:108, 2002.

Olsson GL. Inhalational anaesthesia at the extremes of age: Paediatric anaesthesia. *Anaesthesia* 50(suppl):34, 1995.

Overdyk FJ, Napoleon B, Tagge EP, et al.: "One-stop" surgery: implications for anesthesiologists of an expedited pediatric surgical process. *South Med J* 92:308, 1999.

Patel RI, Hannallah RS: Anesthetic complications following pediatric ambulatory surgery: A 3-yr study. *Anesthesiology* 69:1009, 1988.

Patel RI, Verghese ST, Hannallah RS, et al.: Fast-tracking children after ambulatory surgery. *Anesth Analg* 92:918, 2001.

Percy L: Personal communication, ASA Office of Governmental and Legal Affairs, May 9, 2003.

Pinsker MC, Caroll NV: Quality of emergence from anesthesia and incidence of vomiting with remifentanil in a pediatric population. *Anesth Analg* 89:71, 1999.

Postuma R, Ferguson CC, Stanwick RS, et al.: Pediatric day-care surgery: A 30 year hospital experience. *J Pediatr Surg* 22:304, 1987.

Purday JP, Reichert CC, Merrick PM: Comparative effects of three doses of intravenous ketorolac or morphine on emesis and analgesia for restorative dental surgery in children. *Can J Anaesth* 43:221, 1996.

Rao RB, Ely SF, Hoffman RS: Deaths related to liposuction. *N Engl J Med* 340:1471, 1999.

Religa ZC, Wilson S, Ganzberg SI, et al.: Association between bispectral analysis and level of conscious sedation of pediatric dental patients. *Pediatr Dent* 24:221, 2002.

Roizen MF, Kaplan EB, Schreider BD, et al.: The relative roles of the history and physical examination and laboratory testing in preoperative evaluation for outpatient surgery: The "Starling" curve of preoperative laboratory testing. *Anesthesiol Clin North Am* 5:15, 1987.

Rose JB, Watcha MF: Postoperative nausea and vomiting in paediatric patients. *Br J Anaesth* 83:104, 1999.

Rosenquist R: Regional anesthesia for office-based surgery. *ASA Newsletter* 65:12, 2001.

Ross AK, Eck JB: Office-based anesthesia for children. *Anesthesiol Clin North Am* 20:195, 2002.

Saxen MA, Wilson S, Paravecchio R: Anesthesia for pediatric dentistry. *Dent Clin North Am* 43:231, 1999.

Schreiner MS, Nicolson SC, Martin T, et al.: Should children drink before discharge from day surgery? *Anesthesiology* 76:528, 1992.

Schulte F, Bergal J: For these patients, the ultimate price. Cosmetic surgery: The hidden dangers, 1998. Available at http//pqasb.pqarchiver.com/sun_sentinel/. Accessed July 7, 2003.

Schultz LS: Cost analysis of office surgery clinic with comparison to hospital outpatient facilities for laparoscopic procedures. *Int Surg* 79:273, 1994.

Scuderi PE, James RL, Harris L, et al.: Multimodal antiemetic management prevents early postoperative vomiting after outpatient laparoscopy. *Anesth Analg* 91:1408, 2000.

Shevde K, Panagopoulos G: A survey of 800 patients' knowledge, attitudes, and concerns regarding anesthesia. *Anesth Analg* 73:190, 1991.

Siegel G, Brodsky L, Waner M, et al.: Office-based laser assisted tympanic membrane fenestration in adults and children: Pilot data to support an alternative to traditional approaches to otitis media. *Int J Pediatr Otorhinolaryngol* 53:111, 2000.

SMG Marketing-Verispan, L.L.C.: Freestanding outpatient surgery center market report, 2002 edition. Yardley, PA, 2002, Verispan.

Smiley RM: An overview of induction and emergence of characteristics of desflurane in pediatric, adult, and geriatric patients. *Anesth Analg* 75:S38, 1996.

Smith C, Smith DP: Office pediatric urologic procedures from a parental perspective. *Urology* 55:272, 2000.

Song D, Joshi GP, White PF: Titration of volatile anesthetics using bispectral index facilitates recovery after ambulatory anesthesia. *Anesthesiology* 87:842–848, 1997.

Splinter WM: Prevention of vomiting after strabismus surgery in children: Dexamethasone alone versus dexamethasone plus low-dose ondansetron. *Paediatr Anaesth* 11:591, 2001.

Splinter WM, Rhine EJ: Low-dose ondansetron with dexamethasone more effectively decreases vomiting after strabismus surgery in children than does high-dose ondansetron. *Anesthesiology* 88:72, 1998.

Stoelting RK: Special Issue: OBA safety. Office-based anesthesia provokes safety fears. *Anesth Patient Safety Found Newsletter* 15:1, 2000.

Subramaniam B, Madan R, Sadhasivam S, et al.: Dexamethasone is a cost-effective alternative to ondansetron in preventing PONV after paediatric strabismus repair. *Br J Anaesth* 86:84, 2001.

Sukhani R, Pappas AL, Lurie J, et al.: Ondansetron and dolasetron provide equivalent postoperative vomiting control after ambulatory tonsillectomy in dexamethasone-pretreated children. *Anesth Analg* 95:1230, 2002.

Tang J, Chen L, White PF, et al.: Recovery profiles, costs, and patient satisfaction with propofol and sevoflurane for fast-track office-based anesthesia. *Anesthesiology* 91:253, 1999.

Tang J, Chen X, White PF, et al.: Antiemetic prophylaxis for office-based surgery. Are the 5-HT_3 receptor antagonists beneficial? *Anesthesiology* 98:293, 2003.

Tang J, White PF, Wender RH, et al.: Fast-track office-based anesthesia: A comparison of propofol versus desflurane with antiemetic prophylaxis in spontaneously breathing patients. *Anesth Analg* 92:95, 2001.

Tobias JD: Weak analgesics and non-steroidal anti-inflammatory agents in the management of children with acute pain. *Pediatr Clin North Am* 47:527, 2000.

Twersky RS: Standards for office anesthesia vary widely or do not exist, 2000. Available at http://www.apsf.org/resource_center/newsletter/2000/spring-105-Twersky.htm

Verghese ST, Hannallah RS, Patel R, et al.: Ketamine and midazolam is an inappropriate preinduction combination in uncooperative children undergoing brief ambulatory procedures. *Paediatr Anaesth* 13:228, 2003.

Viitanen H, Annila P, Viitanen M, et al.: Midazolam premedication delays recovery from propofol-induced sevoflurane anesthesia in children 1-3 yr. *Can J Anaesth* 46:766, 1999.

Vogt A: $4.5 Million dollars in boy's death, 2000. Available at http://pqasb.pqarchiver.com/chicagotribune/.

Watson AT, Visram A: Children's preoperative anxiety and postoperative behaviour. *Pediatr Anaesth* 13:188, 2003.

Weinstein MS, Nicolson SC, Schreiner MS: A single dose of morphine sulfate increases the incidence of vomiting after outpatient inguinal herniorrhaphy. *Anesthesiology* 81:572, 1994.

Welborn LG: Pediatric outpatient anesthesia. In Motoyama EK, Davis PJ, editors: *Smith's anesthesia for infants and children.* St Louis, 1996, Mosby–Year Book, pp 709–725.

Welborn LG, Greenspun JC: Anesthesia and apnea. Perioperative considerations in the former premature infant. *Pediatr Clin North Am* 41:188, 1994.

Westman HR: Postoperative complications and unanticipated hospital admissions. *Semin Pediatr Surg* 8:23, 1999.

White PF: Ambulatory anesthesia and surgery: Past, present and future. In White PF, editor: *Ambulatory anesthesia and surgery.* London, 1997, WB Saunders, pp 3–34.

Whitmire HC Jr: Medicolegal considerations for office-based anesthesia in dentistry. *Dent Clin North Am* 43:361, 1999.

Willetts IE, James H, Nicoll, et al.: Pioneer pediatric surgeon. *Ann R Coll Surg Engl* 79(suppl):164, 1997.

Yagiela J: Adverse sedation events in pediatrics (letter). *Pediatrics* 107:1494, 2001.

Yagiela JA: Office-based anesthesia in dentistry. *Dent Clin North Am* 43:201, 1999.

Yee KF, Holland RB, Carrick A, et al.: Morbidity following day-stay dental anaesthesia. *Aust Dent J* 30:333, 1985.

Yogendran S, Asokumar B, Cheng DC, et al.: A prospective randomized double-blinded study of the effect of intravenous fluid therapy on adverse outcomes on outpatient surgery. *Anesth Analg* 80:682, 1995.

Zwass MS, Fisher DM, Welborn LG, et al.: Induction and maintenance characteristics of anesthesia with desflurane and nitrous oxide in infants and children. *Anesthesiology* 76:373, 1992.

Anesthesia for Pediatric Same-Day Procedures

David M. Polaner

Outpatient procedures continue to constitute the majority of anesthetic procedures performed in children in the United States. It is estimated that more than 60% of anesthetic procedures in children are performed on outpatients, and this number is considerably higher in some practice settings. Although the practice of outpatient anesthesia and surgery for children is not new—reports in the medical literature have documented the practice for nearly 100 years—advances in drugs and techniques are transforming how we care for our day surgery patients. Procedures that previously required overnight stays can often be performed on a same-day basis. We are able to reduce the incidence of troubling side effects of anesthetics that may have prevented the discharge of patients in the past, and better postoperative analgesic regimens may allow earlier discharge. Changes in facility designs have improved our ability to provide outpatient care in an efficient and cost-effective manner, while simultaneously enhancing and simplifying the perioperative experience for our patients and their families. Nevertheless, along with these advances have come new challenges. The envelope of what patient and procedure are appropriate for same-day surgery has continued to stretch, while resources may be shrinking under the managed care environment in North America. The pressure to increase performance and throughput places greater stresses on the perioperative system, and great care must be taken to avoid cutting corners for the illusionary benefits of efficiency and cost containment alone.

Historical reports of outpatient surgery date back to the early twentieth century, when Nicholl reported nearly 9000 operations on ambulatory children at Glasgow's Royal Hospital for Sick Children (Nicholl, 1909). Other early reports from the United States soon followed, but it was not until the 1970s that studies were published looking at same-day surgery from a systems perspective. In addition to examining the patient population, complication rates, and surgical procedures, these reports began to look at issues such as cost and delivery of care, as well as the optimization of the nursing and support staff, organization, and physical plant for outpatient surgery. Attention to these details continues to play a central role in the increased utilization and success of outpatient surgery. In the current economic climate of health care in the United States, there is and will continue to be a major emphasis on cost savings. In addition to the economic advantages of savings on hospital resources, a primary driving force in the popularity of pediatric outpatient surgery is satisfaction of the patients and their parents. There are obvious advantages for many parents and children to avoid even overnight hospitalization and to have the child back in his or her familiar home environment on the same day. The decisions that are made in planning the outpatient system will have a major impact on how parents perceive ease of use and quality of care of the entire system and, as a result, its success. Factors that are not medical (ease of parking, efficiency of check-in, waiting time, parental presence during induction of anesthesia, and early admission to the postanesthetic care unit [PACU]) may make impressions on the parent that are equal to the obvious medical issues, such as complication rates, postoperative analgesia, nausea and vomiting, and rapid return to the preoperative mental state.

■ PROCEDURES AND PATIENTS AMENABLE TO OUTPATIENT SURGERY AND ANESTHESIA

Many operative procedures are well suited to be performed on pediatric outpatients, and all share several common characteristics. They all are peripheral procedures that do not involve violation

BOX 27–1 Operations Commonly Performed as Outpatient Surgical Procedures by Specialty

Otolaryngology

Myringotomy and ventilating tubes, adenoidectomy (see text), tonsillectomy (see text), frenulectomy, branchial cleft cysts, endoscopic sinus surgery, examinations under anesthesia including some bronchoscopy

Ophthalmology

Examination under anesthesia, strabismus repair, nasolacrimal duct probe, intraocular lens implantation, trabeculectomy

General pediatric surgery and urology

Herniorrhaphy and hydrocelectomy, orchiopexy, uncomplicated hypospadias, cystoscopy and cystoscopic surgery, circumcision, esophagoscopy, lumps and bumps

Gastroenterology

Endoscopy

Plastic surgery

Cleft lip and some cleft palate repairs, placement of tissue expanders, scar revisions, minor reconstructive procedures (otoplasty, septorhinoplasty, etc.)

Orthopedics

Hardware removal, casting, percutaneous tenotomies, arthrograms

Radiology

Imaging studies, radiation therapy

Dentistry

of a body cavity. They all have a limited duration, generally less than 2 hours, and have minimal or moderate amounts of postoperative pain that can easily be managed with oral analgesics or the one-time administration of a regional block. They do not result in major physiologic perturbations or blood loss, nor do they disturb the ability to take oral fluids and nutrition in the immediate postoperative period. They do not require postoperative monitoring beyond the capability of the parents and home. Commonly performed outpatient procedures are listed and categorized in Box 27–1.

CONTRAINDICATIONS FOR OUTPATIENT ANESTHESIA

There are few firm contraindications to outpatient surgery for amenable procedures, but there are some patients who have medical issues that make it advisable to consider an overnight ("23-hour") admission rather than a discharge on the day of surgery. In the majority of these cases, monitoring is required because of anesthetic-related risks, or because of exceptional risks related to the operative procedure or postoperative care in susceptible individuals.

EX-PREMIES AND APNEA

The risk of postanesthetic apnea in former premature infants has been well described since the early 1980s, when Liu and others (1983) published the first prospective study of premature infants anesthetized between 41 and 46 weeks postconceptual age (postconceptual age = gestational age at birth + current age in weeks). In this report, a group of premature infants was compared with a control group of term infants of similar ages. The incidence of apnea, defined as pauses in breathing lasting longer than 15 seconds, was 20%. Subsequent studies have approximated this incidence, although some have placed the at-risk period as far out as 60 weeks postconceptual age (Welborn et al., 1986; Kurth et al., 1987; Warner et al., 1992). It is now established that infants born before 36 weeks of conception are at risk of apnea after general anesthesia. It appears that this is due to immaturity in control of breathing by the brainstem after exposure to general anesthetics, and there may be similar risks after exposure to sedative-hypnotic agents and neuroleptic agents such as ketamine. Numerous studies have tried to define the period of susceptibility in the at-risk population. Several investigators have stratified the risk depending on postconceptual age and gestational age at birth, and a meta-analysis of eight studies has reported that the postconceptual age required to reduce the risk to less than 1% with 95% confidence was 54 weeks in infants born at 35 weeks gestational age and 56 weeks in those born before 32 weeks (Malviya et al., 1993; Coté et al., 1995). In this meta-analysis, anemia was also associated with increased apnea risk, even in infants older than 42 weeks postconceptual age. The patients in the numerous studies that were included in this meta-analysis may not have all been comparable in terms of underlying state of health, so one must approach these data (as in all meta-analyses) with some caution. Several investigators have suggested that the use of regional anesthesia may eliminate the risk, and a few even advocate discharge of these patients on the day of surgery if no other agents have been administered (Veverka et al., 1991; Webster et al., 1991; Sartorelli et al., 1992; Krane et al., 1995). However, uncontrolled case reports of apnea after spinal anesthesia have been published (Watcha et al., 1989; Tobias et al., 1998). Because these are case reports and there were no control pneumograms, it is unknown if the apnea was related to the anesthetic, but these reports have still prompted most clinicians and consultants to continue to recommend admission and monitoring of these patients for 24 hours after any anesthetic. Caffeine, which has a long history of effective use in apnea of prematurity, has also been suggested to increase central respiratory drive after anesthesia in these patients, although this is still not commonly used (Welborn et al., 1988, 1989).

OBSTRUCTIVE SLEEP APNEA

One of the most common indications for tonsillectomy is upper airway obstruction during sleep. In many centers, obstructive sleep apnea (OSA) accounts for 50% or more of all children presenting for tonsillectomy and adenoidectomy (Messner, 2003). These children may have abnormal ventilatory responses to both hypoxia and hypercarbia due to the chronic exposure to hypoxic and hypercarbic conditions during sleep (Strauss et al., 1999; Kerbl et al., 2001). These responses can take up to several weeks to revert to normal after resolution of the obstruction. There are concerns, therefore, about the ability to maintain adequate breathing and oxygenation after the exposure to general anesthetics and to opioids given for postoperative analgesia. A study of 15 otherwise normal children, aged 1 to 18, with mild OSA used preoperative and postoperative pneumograms to assess respiratory status on the night after adenotonsillectomy. Nine of these children received a halothane-based anesthetic, and six received a fentanyl-based technique. The number of obstructive events decreased and the nadir of oxygen saturation improved from 78% to 92% with fentanyl-based technique. The authors concluded that in cases of mild OSA without other underlying disorders, intensive postoperative monitoring is not necessary (Helfaer et al., 1996). In a group of 134 children selected for outpatient tonsillectomy, of whom 83% carried the diagnosis and indication for surgery of OSA, 11 (8.2%) were admitted for overnight observation after experiencing respiratory problems in the postanesthetic care unit (Lalakea et al., 1999). These patients as a group were significantly younger than those discharged home (average age, 4 versus 6.3 years). Preoperative evaluation and assessment of OSA were not described. Most otolaryngologists consider significant (as opposed to mild) OSA to be a contraindication to outpatient management of adenotonsillectomy, especially in children younger than 3 years, although in one small study the postoperative complications in these younger children were not related to obstructive events (Slovik et al., 2003). Those investigators suggested that the severity of OSA, rather than patient age, may be a more predictive factor, but this is in conflict with other reports, which recommend that age of less than 3 years should be considered an independent discriminator (Shott et al., 1987; Biavati et al., 1997). The only criterion that appears to be accurate in the diagnosis and stratification of severity in OSA is polysomnography; the history or pulse oximetry alone is neither specific nor sensitive enough (American Thoracic Society, 1996; Schechter, 2002; Subcommittee on Obstructive Sleep Apnea American Academy of Pediatrics, 2002).

PREOPERATIVE EVALUATION AND PLANNING

The evaluation of outpatients for surgical procedures presents a significant organizational challenge to the anesthesiologist. Because one of the primary goals of outpatient surgery is both efficiency and rapid throughput, there is a great disincentive to require preoperative visits before the day of surgery. At the same time, an efficient system demands an absolute minimum of cancellations on the day of surgery. Such pressures put both the anesthesiologist and the system as a whole at increased risk of proceeding with cases in which the patient may not be optimally prepared for surgery and anesthesia. There is also a stress of "production pressure"—the urgency to move patients rapidly through the preoperative queue and into the operating room on schedule. This, too, is in competition with the need to provide the best and most complete evaluation and care of the patient. To avoid these situations, a system of preoperative screening must be instituted that provides the most accurate, up-to-date, and complete information to the anesthesiologist so that he or she may make well-informed decisions about patient management. Fortunately, both technological and nontechnological aids exist to streamline this process.

The implications of cancellation, particularly on the day of surgery, go far beyond the efficiency of the operating room. A survey by Tait and others (1997) found that nearly half of parents whose children's operations were cancelled on the day of scheduled surgery missed a day of work and that about half of these parents went unpaid as a result. Many drove long distances to get to the hospital, and nearly 25% were frustrated or angry as a result of the cancellation. A small number of dissatisfied or angry parents can have an adverse impact on the success of an outpatient surgery program well out of proportion to their numbers, and great attention must be paid to minimize these events by using systems that work effectively.

In many cases, a preoperative visit to the anesthesiologist is neither practical nor necessary. Because the majority of children presenting for same-day surgery are relatively healthy, screening tools such as telephone interviews and self-reporting can be implemented. Coordination with the surgeon's office may reduce both redundancy in paperwork and repeated questioning of the patient's family. The efficiency in combining surgical, anesthetic, and nursing evaluation can be greatly enhanced if a computerized record is used. With these systems, which are finally maturing after years of development, data from one evaluation can automatically populate another linked database. This can greatly streamline the evaluation process. Even in the majority of institutions where paper records remain the standard, systems using secure e-mail, facsimile, or even common forms can be designed to eliminate redundancy. The elimination of needless paperwork can be a great aid in increasing patient throughput, as well as in reducing the frustration of staff and parents alike.

The initial step in preoperative planning and evaluation begins when the surgeon books the case. This is the first opportunity for the system to alert the anesthesiologist of any unusual conditions or underlying illnesses that the patient may have. A short list of check boxes on the booking form suffices and need not involve great detail. This information can be reviewed by an anesthesiologist to detect any cases that might benefit from especially extensive consultation or planning before the day of surgery.

Because the surgeon's office is the initial contact point of the patient's family with the perioperative system, it also provides an excellent opportunity to present the parents with introductory information about the anesthetic. A pamphlet describing generalities such as the role of the pediatric anesthesiologist in caring for the child, NPO instructions, contact telephone numbers, and other information specific to the hospital or outpatient surgical center can be a useful reference for the family. Having a written reference for NPO guidelines is especially helpful, because lack of adherence to these instructions is a common cause of case delay or cancellation. Parents should be given a telephone number to call both for questions about the anesthetic agent that they feel cannot wait until the preoperative assessment and for consultation with an anesthesiologist should an intercurrent illness develop between the time of the visit to the surgeon and the day of surgery.

A preoperative visit to the surgeon alone, however, does not optimize the preoperative evaluation process for the anesthesiologist or for the same-day surgery process as a whole. A case-control study of pediatric outpatient cancellations found that 10% of same-day surgery patients at a children's hospital were cancelled on the day of surgery, and half of those were for preventable reasons. Cancelled patients who had inadequate preoperative preparation were more likely to have been seen only in the surgeon's office and not in the hospital's preoperative program (MacArthur et al., 1995). It is clear that further screening is necessary to address general medical and anesthetic concerns.

A short telephone interview with the patient's parent before scheduled surgery, whether conducted by the anesthesiologist or a nurse practitioner, not only can be a source of clinical information about the patient and about the parent's concerns but also can forestall unanticipated problems that can cause delays, cancellations, or complications on the day of surgery. Knowing in advance, for example, that an asthmatic child had a mild upper respiratory tract infection (URI) the week before allows the anesthesiologist to prescribe a short course of steroids with ample time for the drug to take effect. The child who has sickle cell disease with an active URI, on the other hand, might have his or her operation postponed, thus saving the parents a trip to the hospital and allowing the schedule to be rearranged before the day begins. A well-organized system for conducting these calls should be established so that patients are not missed and communication with the anesthesiologists scheduled to care for them can be easily accomplished. It is important to organize the system so that the calls are most effective. As could be expected, a study of over 5000 patients conducted at National Children's Hospital in 1992 found that calls made during the evening were far more likely to successfully reach the parents (Patel and Hannallah, 1992). In the United Kingdom and in some hospitals in the United States, preoperative clinics, rather than telephone screening, are used, but this may necessitate an additional visit by the family. The inconvenience may outweigh the advantages of a face-to-face visit for some families, and success may be predicated upon ease of use of the system. Preoperative screening and evaluation can also improve throughput on the day of surgery, particularly if there is a long list of very short-duration cases, such as myringotomy and tube placement. The duration of those cases is so short that the time it takes to do a preoperative evaluation may be longer than the operative time. Saving even 10 or 15 minutes per hour might allow the team to perform an additional operative procedure each hour.

Other methods of communication, including secure Web sites and e-mail, have been used for similar purposes. The ability of a family to access a secure server and enter preoperative interview information will likely become increasingly attractive in coming years. Although the personal interaction with a knowledgeable professional can never be replaced, certain standard data can be entered with great efficiency in this manner. Intranet-based kiosks at the hospital, where patients' families can use either keyboard or touch screen technology to enter information that is now entered on paper questionnaires at the time of admission, will become increasingly important modalities as hospitals move from paper-based records to digital ones.

It is particularly important that reports of previous operative procedures or consultations by specialists be available to the anesthesiologist during the preoperative assessment. A computerized repository of this information is the best solution, as it allows immediate access from any location, but many institutions have not yet migrated to completely digital medical records. A day surgery coordinator should have the responsibility of ensuring that necessary outside and internal records are readily available the day before surgery, to avoid delays. Such information also must be immediately accessible to the anesthesiologist on the day of surgery.

In some locations, it is common for a child's pediatrician to be responsible for "clearing" the child for surgery. This can be a considerable help, as the pediatrician often has the best knowledge of the child's underlying illnesses and conditions. The pediatrician, however, often has little understanding of the issues that are of greatest concern to the anesthesiologist and may actually miss or ignore problems that can affect anesthetic management, to the detriment of the preoperative evaluation process. The anesthetic implications and preoperative optimization of airway anatomy and function, gastroesophageal reflux, upper respiratory illness, and asthma, as well as of syndromes and chronic conditions such as trisomy 21 and the former premature infant, all may be underappreciated by pediatricians who do not work in the operating room or administer anesthesia and who usually have had little or no training in perioperative medicine (Fisher, 1991). Several reviews by pediatric anesthesiologists in the pediatric literature have discussed the preoperative screening process and what the pediatrician needs to know about preparing the child for anesthesia (Fisher, 1991; Fisher et al., 1994; Maxwell et al., 1994; Section on Anesthesiology, 1996). If a hospital or surgicenter relies on pediatricians as a major link in the preoperative assessment chain, the pediatricians must be familiar with this literature and should have ongoing communication with their anesthesiologist colleagues.

PREOPERATIVE TESTING

Policies on preoperative testing have been completely reassessed, and abandonment of the routine use of tests has become the norm. This is driven by both the growing number of studies that demonstrated little or no value in such testing and economic concerns that mandate the elimination of unnecessary expenditures.

Urinalysis

A 1990 study of nearly 500 children scheduled for elective surgery found abnormalities in 15%; however, more than 80% of those were historically known, clinically insignificant, or false-positive results. The authors concluded that preoperative urinalysis should not be routinely performed on healthy children for preoperative assessment (O'Conner and Drasner, 1990).

Pregnancy Testing

Sexual activity in adolescence is increasingly common, and, as a result, the risk of undiagnosed first trimester pregnancy may be increased in adolescents undergoing elective surgery. A survey of members of the Society for Pediatric Anesthesia found that nearly half of the respondents routinely test for pregnancy in postpubertal patients (Patel et al., 1997). Other investigators have found a low yield of positive results, especially in girls under 15 years of age, but their study had a relatively small number of subjects, and some investigators who care for patients in different geographical regions have reported far higher rates of pregnancy in very young adolescents (Kempen, 1997;

Kempen et al., 1997; Wheeler and Coté, 1999). All of these investigators determined that history is an unreliable indicator of pregnancy, so that despite the small number of positive pregnancy test results, there is no reasonable alternative to testing. Pregnancy testing, which in most institutions is performed using urinary β-human chorionic gonadotropin (β-hCG), is reliable, inexpensive, and quick. Elective procedures should be cancelled if the result of the test indicates pregnancy, and appropriate referral and consultation should be obtained. With these facts in mind, routine testing for pregnancy in postpubertal girls is likely warranted. The ethical, legal, and criminal implications of positive findings are beyond the scope of this chapter but are discussed in the cited references.

Hematocrit/Complete Blood Cell Count

Unless an operation is expected to result in significant blood loss (highly unlikely for outpatient surgery), the screening complete blood cell count (CBC) has little or no value (Roy et al., 1990; Hackmann et al., 1991; Roy et al., 1991). These studies have demonstrated that the presence of mild to moderate anemia has little to no effect on the conduct of anesthesia or outcome of children undergoing same-day surgical procedures. The presence of anemia in former premature infants under 54 weeks of postconceptual age has been found to correlate with an increased risk of postanesthetic apnea, and it is possible that screening for anemia in this population may detect those at increased risk (Welborn et al., 1991). It is not known, however, if the anemia is the cause of increased apnea or only an associated finding. The neonatal literature is in conflict regarding the effect of transfusion on apnea of prematurity, with several studies demonstrating decreased apnea after transfusion, and several reporting no change (Joshi et al., 1987; Hume, 1997). Of additional interest is the finding by Poets and others (1997) that there was a 3% increase in oxygen saturation after transfusion, although the frequency of apneic events did not diminish. Bifano and others (1992) found fewer apneic events both in the transfusion-treated group and in the control group who received volume expansion with 5% albumin, suggesting that improved cerebral circulation on the basis of hemodynamic effects, not increased oxygen carrying capacity, may be the benefit of this intervention. It must be recognized that these studies looked specifically at apnea of prematurity, not postanesthetic apnea in premature infants, and it may not be accurate to generalize their findings to the perioperative population. All at-risk former premature infants should be admitted for postoperative monitoring in any case; thus, screening may not alter clinical practice. Children with sickle cell disease (not trait) need to have a hemoglobin level measured, as both management and outcome of these patients are dependent on an adequate level of hemoglobin A or F (see later).

Sickle Cell Testing

In many states, newborns in at-risk populations are screened for sickle cell disease, so the sickle cell status of all infants and children in those locations is known. In locations where such newborn screening is not universal, it is prudent to obtain sickle cell testing in any infant of at-risk ethnicity whose status is unknown, at least under the age of 3 years. Children older than this are likely to have had symptoms if affected. In children who do have sickle cell disease, a preoperative hemoglobin level is mandated to determine the need for preoperative transfusion. A large multicenter trial found that simple transfusion, if the hemoglobin was less than 10 g/dL, is as effective as exchange transfusion in these patients (Vichinsky et al., 1995). Although one study has found that minor surgical procedures could be performed in sickle cell patients without preoperative transfusion, complication rates were significantly higher in those undergoing abdominal, thoracic, or airway procedures (Griffin and Buchanan, 1993). Sickle cell trait, which usually does not cause any symptoms or illness, has rarely been associated with complications of surgery and anesthesia (Konotey-Ahulu, 1969; McGarry and Duncan, 1973; Atlas, 1974; Gibson and Love, 1974), but hemoglobin determination in these patients is unnecessary (also see Chapter 32, Systemic Disorders in Infants and Children).

Heart Murmurs and Cardiology Consultation

At least 25% of healthy children have an audible heart murmur at some time during childhood, and the question of when to refer a child to a pediatric cardiologist for the evaluation of a new murmur is often raised during the preoperative evaluation. The vast majority of these are functional "innocent" murmurs, not associated with any structural heart disease. Innocent murmurs are soft (less than grade 3), blowing, and loudest along the left sternal border. They tend to decrease or disappear during inspiration. Most congenital heart lesions present before the first several months of life, so in the absence of symptoms a murmur in an older child is less likely (but not entirely unlikely) to be significant. Exceptions include atrial septal defects, small ventricular septal defects, some cases of coarctation of the aorta, some hemodynamically insignificant valvular lesions that are still endocarditis risks, and, in rare instances, other lesions. The ability of a pediatric cardiologist to distinguish between a functional murmur and one caused by a structural heart lesion by examination alone was evaluated and found to be high, so more extensive (and expensive) evaluation, such as echocardiography, is rarely necessary (Newburger et al., 1983). If the child is older than 6 months, without any symptoms referable to the cardiac system, most skilled clinicians should be able to evaluate these murmurs and rule out hemodynamically significant congenital heart disease. Cardiomyopathy can also present with a new murmur, so a previously undetected murmur accompanied by symptoms suggestive of impaired myocardial performance or irritability, such as dysrhythmias, especially if they follow a viral illness, should be evaluated by a cardiologist.

Many children with congenital heart lesions require antibiotic prophylaxis for the prevention of endocarditis when undergoing at-risk operations. The American Heart Association recommendations are available at http://www.americanheart.org/presenter.jhtml?identifier=1745. One should note that for optimal treatment, the intravenous antibiotic should be administered at least 30 minutes before the procedure's start, which can pose a considerable problem in day surgery when an intravenous catheter is not present before induction. For procedures on the respiratory tract, intraoral procedures, or moderate risk patients for genitourinary procedures, oral antibiotics can be given 1 hour before the procedure, thereby eliminating the problem of timing in these cases. For genitourinary procedures in high-risk patients, this timing is more problematic, because there are no good oral alternatives. A reasonable approach is to begin to administer the antibiotics as soon as intravenous access is obtained but to be mindful of the need to administer gentamicin over a minimum of 10 to 15 minutes (also see Chapter 32, Systemic Disorders in Infants and Children).

■ UNDERLYING ILLNESSES AND COMPLICATING FACTORS

There are numerous underlying conditions that exist commonly in relatively healthy children that do not preclude outpatient surgery but that have implications regarding the preoperative preparation and anesthetic management.

UPPER RESPIRATORY TRACT INFECTIONS

Probably the most common problem to confront the anesthesiologist caring for children in outpatient surgery is the child with a URI and has been reviewed by Tait and Malviya (2005). Viral respiratory tract illness is virtually ubiquitous in children, particularly during the winter months when close indoor contact in school and daycare with other children with colds is impossible to avoid. The average preschool child contracts between six and eight URIs per year. Both upper and lower respiratory tract viral infections can increase airway inflammation, irritability, and respiratory tract secretions via mechanisms as diverse as increased production and decreased degradation of tachykinins and other neuropeptides, virus-induced damage to M2 muscarinic receptors in the airways leading to vagal-mediated hyperreactivity, and increased volume and viscidity of airway secretions causing subsegmental atelectasis (Empey et al., 1976; Dusser et al., 1989; Barclay et al., 1992). Increased airway reactivity and hyperresponsiveness occur in the lower airways even in patients with respiratory viral illness clinically limited to the upper airway and even in those with no history of asthma (de Kluijver et al., 2002). After the apparent resolution of the URI, increased airway hyperresponsiveness and irritability may persist for as long as 6 to 8 weeks (Empey et al., 1976; Empey, 1983). In children with underlying respiratory disease, such as asthma, bronchopulmonary dysplasia, or other chronic lung diseases, these responses may be further exaggerated. Other risk factors that may be associated with more serious or frequent complications are age of less than 1 year and sickle cell disease (Cohen and Cameron, 1991). In what is perhaps one of the most comprehensive investigations of URI and anesthesia, 1078 infants and children were prospectively studied (Tait et al., 2001). Independent risk factors for respiratory complications were endotracheal intubation, history of prematurity, reactive airways disease, parental smoking, airway surgery, nasal congestion and the presence of copious secretions. Of interest is that the history of prematurity was a risk factor even in children who were several years old and no longer had ongoing problems referable to their premature birth.

Numerous studies have documented that children who either have URIs or have recently recovered from one have more minor airway complications during or after anesthesia compared with healthy children. Mild oxygen desaturation and coughing, as well as more potentially serious complications such as bronchospasm, laryngospasm, and respiratory failure, are particularly likely to occur if the airway is stimulated. Tait and Knight (1987) prospectively studied a large cohort of children undergoing myringotomy and ventilating tube placement for chronic or recurrent otitis media. There was no significant increase in respiratory problems in the children with intercurrent URIs, and the severity of respiratory illness, as well as the duration of URI symptoms, actually decreased in the group receiving halothane anesthesia by mask without instrumentation of the airway. These beneficial results may have been influenced by the effects of myringotomy and drainage on the course of the infection. Coté and colleagues (Coté et al., 1991; Rolf and Coté, 1992), in their investigation of the utility of capnometry and pulse oximetry in detecting adverse events during anesthesia and in a subsequent report further analyzing these data, found that children with URIs commonly had mild oxygen desaturation both during surgery and in recovery. Others have noted that postoperative oxygen requirements in these children are commonly but transiently increased (Levy et al., 1992). It is possible that the cause is related to subsegmental atelectasis from increased quantity and viscidity of secretions, and that with deep breathing and coughing after emergence, reexpansion of these segments occurs. In the prospective study cited earlier, patients with current or recent URI had a greater incidence of respiratory complications, including breath-holding and desaturation of less than 90%, although none of the complications were associated with long-term sequelae. Both the authors and an accompanying editorial concluded that most children with URIs who were not overtly ill and had no other complicating medical issues could, with judicious attention to anesthetic technique, be safely anesthetized with increased risk for only mild transient sequelae (Coté, 2001; Tait et al., 2001).

The potential for more serious complications in children with URI should not be overlooked. A prospective study of over 15,000 children found that children who developed laryngospasm were twice as likely to have a URI (Schreiner et al., 1996). The investigators found that the incidence of laryngospasm was most clearly related to the parent's subjective assessment of a URI, and that younger age and surgeries involving the airway were additive risk factors. A prospective case-control study of 1283 children with URI who underwent general anesthesia found a 2- to 7-fold increase in respiratory complications during the perioperative course compared with their counterparts without URI (Cohen and Cameron, 1991). The incidence was 11-fold higher if the patient was intubated. A very small minority of children with URI who do not appear to be very ill during the preoperative examination develop acute respiratory failure after the induction of anesthesia or sometime during the anesthetic course. Severe hypoxia, bronchospasm, ventilatory insufficiency, and diminution of compliance may occur, requiring postoperative ventilatory support and critical care management. Some of these children have underlying lower respiratory tract disease, such as pneumonia, and others may experience shunt and ventilation/perfusion mismatch from atelectasis and pulmonary collapse due to inspissation of secretions and mucus plugging (Campbell, 1990; Barclay et al., 1992). In rare instances, cardiomyopathy follows viral illness. There are several reports of cardiac dysrhythmias after induction of general anesthesia in patients thought to have postviral myocarditis. The onset of abnormal rhythms on the electrocardiograph tracing or sudden deterioration of blood pressure or perfusion should alert the anesthesiologist to this possibility (Brampton and Jago, 1990; Terasaki et al., 1990).

It should be borne in mind that all of the ill patients who are included in these studies had mild to moderate URIs—children who were more severely ill were cancelled by the clinicians responsible for their care and were never enrolled in the study. Thus, clinical judgment remains crucial in deciding whether to cancel a case. Firm criteria for when to proceed and when to cancel are hard to discern, but the following can be used as guidelines.

- Laboratory tests are usually not useful; clinical impression is more reliable, such as the presence of toxicity, fever, purulent nasal discharge, productive cough, or wheezing. If physical examination suggests pneumonia, a chest radiograph may be confirmatory.
- Ex-premature infants, infants with pulmonary disease (asthma, bronchopulmonary dysplasia, etc.), infants under 1 year of age, and children with sickle cell disease are more at risk.

- Patients undergoing airway surgery are more at risk.
- Endotracheal intubation increases the risk of complications. Data suggest that the risk of airway complications in children with URI is lowest with a conventional facemask, intermediate with a laryngeal mask airway (LMA), and greatest with an endotracheal tube (Tait et al., 1998, 2001).
- Airway hyperresponsiveness exists for 3 to 4 weeks after the resolution of the URI.
- Transient oxygen requirements or other mild respiratory symptoms frequently occur and PACU discharge time may be delayed.

ASTHMA

The prevalence and severity of asthma continue to increase in the United States and other industrialized countries. As of 1998, 6.4% of the U.S. population carried the diagnosis of asthma, and two thirds of those cases are children. Nearly one-half million patients are hospitalized yearly with exacerbations of asthma, and almost half of those are children. The prevalence has increased by about 60% since the 1980s. The death rate, although low, more than doubled from 1975 to 1995 (Molfino and Slutsky, 1994; Sears, 1995). Children with a history of asthma can be safely and effectively anesthetized for same-day surgery, but careful preoperative preparation and evaluation, and intraoperative management, are crucial to avoid exacerbations and complications. Although it is common to think of asthma in terms of bronchospasm, current definitions of the disease emphasize the role or airway inflammation in pathogenesis, progression, and management. A consensus conference of the National Institutes of Health National Heart, Lung, and Blood Institute (2002) defined *asthma* as a chronic inflammatory disorder of the airways that involved many cell types beyond those structural elements of the airways themselves, including mast cells, eosinophils, and T lymphocytes. The inflammatory processes that are involved in both the pathogenesis of the disorder and the progression of disease are now addressed much more effectively in therapy for all asthmatics, not only those with severe disease. The mainstay of therapy in the past was the chronic use of bronchodilator therapy, with anti-inflammatory drugs reserved for the more severe cases; current thinking is that first-line treatment should target inflammation (Spahn and Szefler, 2002; Kemp, 2003; Liu and Szefler, 2003).

Anesthetizing the child with a history of asthma for outpatient surgery involves the same general principles as for inpatient procedures (Pradal et al., 1995). It is critical for the asthmatic patient to closely adhere to his or her medication regimen before surgery. Inhaled steroids and agents such as leukotriene inhibitors and cromolyn all require chronic use for efficacy. The patient must use these medicines regularly and faithfully in the days and weeks before anesthesia. For those who have required systemic steroids in the past, a short course of steroids, beginning 24 hours before the induction of anesthesia, may be advisable, particularly if intubation of the trachea is required. Preoperative and intraoperative treatment with a short-acting β-agonist such as nebulized albuterol may be helpful as well, even if the patient is not symptomatic, because events may occur during surgery that are likely to provoke airway irritability, especially intubation (Maslow et al., 2000). Much like the child with a URI, avoidance of intubation and airway stimulation, if possible, reduces the potential for exacerbation of airway irritability.

Volatile anesthetics, which have bronchodilatory properties, have obvious advantages in the asthmatic child. Propofol, which has been shown to relax tracheal smooth muscle in vitro and to decrease airway resistance in both healthy and asthmatic subjects during induction of anesthesia, is an excellent choice when an intravenous induction is used (Pizov et al., 1995; Eames et al., 1996). This effect on airway smooth muscle has been shown to be even greater than that of ketamine (Pedersen et al., 1993) and was also demonstrated during maintenance when an infusion was continued during the anesthetic. A propofol-based anesthetic, combined with either regional anesthesia or a non–histamine-releasing opioid, is a good alternative to volatile anesthesia when a total intravenous technique is indicated or desired. Caution must be taken with the sulfite-containing preparation of propofol—one study in adults demonstrated a significant increase in airway resistance with this formulation compared with the non–sulfite-containing drug (Rieschke et al., 2003).

Emergence from anesthesia is perhaps the most vulnerable period. Although the stimulation of intubation at induction is unquestionably a time of increased risk, the ability to treat bronchospasm by deepening the anesthetic in response to airway hyperreactivity is not present at emergence. There is, therefore, an advantage to deep extubation when a volatile technique is used, because the patient can awaken without the endotracheal tube (a highly potent stimulus to the airway) in place. Judicious timing of extubation during emergence from total intravenous anesthesia can accomplish the same goal (also see Chapter 11, Intraoperative and Postoperative Management; and Chapter 32, Systemic Disorders).

The risk of anesthesia in a child with an active exacerbation of asthma is certainly increased, and careful attention must be given to postponing procedures in these patients until baseline control of the disease is regained. The child with severe asthma who is never fully "clear" can still be a suitable candidate for outpatient surgery if (1) his or her clinical management is optimized; (2) aggressive preoperative treatment, such as a short course of systemic steroids, increased bronchodilator therapy, and strict avoidance of airway irritants like tobacco smoke, is instituted; and (3) contingency plans for admission are made in the event of an exacerbation.

DIABETES

Type 1 diabetes in children is not uncommon, occurring in approximately 1 in 500 school-aged children, but data on the optimal intraoperative management of children with this disease are scant. Perianesthetic management of diabetes mellitus in children has been reviewed (Chadwick and Wilkinson, 2004; Ahmed et al., 2005). Although many of the problems involved in anesthetizing adults relate to the late complications of this condition (damage to many end-organ systems, autonomic dysfunction), these problems are less prevalent in children, and the most common issue is that of glucose control. Children with diabetes can be safely anesthetized as outpatients if great care is taken to maintain good glucose homeostasis. In the recent past, it was often recommended to administer half of the usual insulin dose on the morning of surgery and to begin a glucose-containing intravenous solution soon thereafter. Better options, however, are now the norm for management (McAnulty et al., 2000; McAnulty and Hall, 2003; Chadwick and Wilkinson, 2004; Ahmed et al., 2005). In most patients, it is easiest to schedule their surgery early in the day and to administer no insulin at all on the morning of surgery, with the exception of insulin glargine. It is a recombinant human insulin analogue for basal control with no true peak and a very long duration of action of about 24 hours, which can be administered in the usual dose.

The blood glucose level should be obtained under general anesthesia, once intravenous access has been established, and upon awakening and again 2 to 3 hours later. Intravenous infusions containing 5% glucose have often been recommended for intraoperative fluid management, but it is easier to use a non–glucose-containing intravenous fluid into which a glucose-containing intravenous catheter is "piggybacked." In this manner, the patient's fluid requirements and glucose requirements can be independently regulated. Because the most potentially catastrophic complication of diabetes during surgery is unrecognized hypoglycemia, blood glucose levels should be measured periodically during the procedure. Hypoglycemia should be treated promptly by reducing or stopping any insulin administration and increasing the intravenous glucose rate, and hyperglycemia treated with a continuous insulin infusion titrated to effect, usually beginning at a rate of 0.05 unit/kg per hour. The very short duration of action of intravenous regular insulin (about 5 minutes) makes glucose control much easier with this method (Barnett et al., 1980). The same management scheme is continued in the PACU until the patient is awake and taking oral fluids without difficulty. At that time, a dose of subcutaneous regular insulin can be administered, and an oral diet begun. Blood glucose levels should be measured frequently during the postoperative day, because the stress of surgery often alters insulin requirements, and adjust the dose accordingly. The usual insulin regimen can often be restarted on the day after surgery (see Chapter 32, Systemic Disorders).

MALIGNANT HYPERTHERMIA

The advent of improved and short-acting intravenous anesthetics has made the management of patients with malignant hyperthermia (MH) considerably simpler. Current recommendations for the care of MH patients no longer includes prophylactic therapy with dantrolene, and the use of nontriggering techniques coupled with proper preparation of the anesthesia machine can ensure that these patients are not exposed to triggering agents. A 10-year review of 303 patients with the diagnosis of MH who underwent trigger-free anesthesia found that none developed fever in the perioperative period that was attributable to an MH crisis, and none required treatment with dantrolene (Yentis et al., 1992). The authors concluded that MH-susceptible patients are suitable candidates for outpatient anesthesia (see Chapter 31, Malignant Hyperthermia).

SICKLE CELL ANEMIA

Children with sickle cell disease have increased risks in the perioperative period. Preoperative testing and management of transfusion were discussed earlier. The major risk factors for inducing a crisis in the perioperative period are dehydration, hypoxia, diminished perfusion, and acidosis. If close attention is paid to avoiding these, most sickle cell patients can be managed as outpatients for suitable operations. In particular, good hydration and analgesia are important for stable recovery. One must be more strict than usual in ensuring that the child can take oral fluids without difficulty before discharge home. The use of surgical tourniquets for orthopedic surgery in sickle cell patients is controversial (Adu-Gyamfi et al., 1993) but should probably be avoided in outpatient surgery where postoperative acid-base status, perfusion, and the development of late-onset complications cannot be closely followed. Tonsillectomy and adenoidectomy in sickle cell patients with obstructive sleep apnea appear to entail increased risks and should not be performed on an outpatient basis (Sidman and Fry, 1988; Derkay et al., 1991; Halvorson et al., 1997) (see Chapter 32, Systemic Disorders).

PREOPERATIVE PREPARATION OF THE CHILD AND FAMILY

FAMILY-CENTERED CARE

There is an increasing emphasis in pediatric care on the care of the child within the context of the family. This is in part behind the current vogue for including the parents of the patient in the experience of induction of anesthesia and early parental admission to the PACU. When one considers outpatient surgery, however, this concept is extended even further, because the family is more intimately involved in the postoperative care of the child than ever before. The parent or primary caregiver becomes the surrogate nurse once the child is discharged home and therefore must be involved to a greater degree in the postoperative experience even before discharge from the day surgery unit. It has become the norm in most pediatric institutions and general hospitals that have sizable pediatric surgical programs for parental involvement to include preoperative tours of the operating room and PACU, parental presence during induction of anesthesia, and admission of the parents to the PACU very soon after the child's arrival and emergence from anesthesia. In most cases, experience with these programs has found them to ease, not complicate, the care of the child, and disruptive parents are the rare exception (Schofield and White, 1989).

PREOPERATIVE TEACHING AND PARENTAL PRESENCE

Outpatient surgery is an intense experience for both parents and children. Many things happen in a very short time span, and the emphasis on efficiency and throughput can limit the time that staff can spend in preparing parent and child for all that will occur. Preoperative teaching programs have become common methods of education to help families understand what to expect on the day of surgery. These programs include preoperative tours of the outpatient surgery center, preoperative telephone calls, written brochures, and videotapes (Karl et al., 1990; Kleinfeldt, 1990; O'Byrne et al., 1997; Cassady et al., 1999; Bellew et al., 2002; Koinig, 2002). While the explicit goal of these programs is education and the efficient transmission of information, an implicit goal is the reduction in anxiety of patients as well as their parents and undesirable behavioral consequences of the stress of the perioperative experience (Margolis et al., 1998). The first objective of education and transmission of information can be met by many, if not all, of these programs, but teaching and tour programs may not be as effective in reducing anxiety and improving behavior as commonly thought. A study of 143 children aged 2 to 6 years who were randomized to receive either an interactive teaching book or no intervention found more, not less, preoperative anxiety in the children who had received the book but less aggression during induction and fewer behavioral changes 2 weeks after surgery (Margolis et al., 1998).

A well-controlled and designed study found that preoperative teaching programs of various modalities had an effect of anxiolysis only in the holding area on the day of surgery; that effect did not extend effectively to the induction period itself (Kain et al., 1998) (see Chapter 7, Psychological Aspects of Pediatric Anesthesia).

Although parental satisfaction was clearly increased by parental presence during induction and highly anxious children benefited from presence of a parent during induction, children's anxiety and behavior were more effectively modulated by the use of premedication (Kain et al., 1996, 1998). While these data might suggest that the expense and effort of elaborate teaching programs, when examined in a critical and rigorous manner, may not be as cost-effective as more modest programs combined with premedication, one must recognize that limited benefits have value as well. For the parent and child who are waiting for an hour in the preoperative area, a reduction in stress for that period alone is meaningful.

Part of the art of pediatric anesthesia, of course, is the ability to rapidly establish effective and reassuring communication with parent and child. The rapport and trust that the anesthesiologist create during the preoperative interview also provides an important and effective method of reassurance and anxiolysis that can enhance the transition to the operating room. In the outpatient setting, where time is more constrained, the value of a quick game, magic trick, kind word, or even brief induction of hypnotic suggestion should not be underestimated. The child may be additionally comforted by bringing a security item, such as a blanket or favorite toy, into the operating room. Having this item immediately available at the time of emergence may also be helpful (also see Chapter 7, Psychological Aspects of Pediatric Anesthesia, and Chapter 10, Induction of Anesthesia and Maintenance of the Airway).

PREOPERATIVE FASTING

In preparation of a child for anesthesia and surgery, it is extremely important to properly instruct the parents in regard to food and fluid intake. A number of studies in the 1990s demonstrated that clear fluids with or without sugar are rapidly cleared from the stomach and that the gastric fluid pH and volume are independent of the duration of fasting beyond 2 hours, provided that only clear fluids are consumed on the day of surgery (Schreiner et al., 1990; Splinter and Schaefer, 1990, Litman et al., 1994). The liberalization of guidelines for preoperative fluid administration offers the benefit of improved patient comfort. It also means that fewer infants and children demonstrate signs of hypoglycemia or dehydration at the time of anesthetic induction (Welborn et al., 1993). Over the last decade, most pediatric institutions have altered and shortened the fasting period for clear liquids to 2 to 3 hours prior to induction of anesthesia for all ages, although approaches to infants on breast-feeding tend to vary among different institutions (Ferrari et al., 1999).

Infants less than 6 months of age on breast milk require 4 hours of fasting. Breast milk or infant formula should be considered as solid food because the fat is the main determinant delaying gastric emptying (Litman et al., 1994). Older infants over 6 months of age on milk or infant formula should be fasted for 6 hours; children on solid food, including cereal, toast, and juice with pulp (e.g., orange juice), are usually fasted for 8 hours (or NPO after midnight) prior to induction of anesthesia.

PREMEDICATION

As was noted earlier, the use of sedative premedication has been shown to be the most effective means of reducing preoperative anxiety, postoperative recall, and maladaptive behavior in children undergoing outpatient surgery. Oral midazolam has become the most commonly used premedicant in the United States since the 1990s. Significant reduction in postoperative recall and establishment of anterograde amnesia has been demonstrated with 0.5 mg/kg of midazolam administered orally as soon as 10 minutes before induction (Kain et al., 2000). Oral doses as low as 0.25 mg/kg have been demonstrated to be as effective as larger doses with only a slightly slower time of onset (Coté et al., 2002). Of particular concern in the outpatient setting, however, is the problem of delayed emergence. Several studies using 0.5 mg/kg of oral midazolam have found that the drug delayed recovery (Bevan et al., 1997; Viitanen et al., 1999a, 1999b), but the actual time of discharge from the hospital was not prolonged. In institutions where the PACU is divided into phase I (initial recovery from the operating room until the child has reached an awake state, with stable vital signs and is ready to take oral fluids) and phase II (less intensive observation and readying for discharge home) areas, this translates to a longer stay in phase I recovery only. Such delays have the potential to affect throughput and cause bottlenecks for patients arriving from the operating room but do not affect total hospital time. The use of lower doses may reduce this problem, but data are not yet available.

The benefits of oral administration, fairly rapid onset, and reliability of effect give midazolam considerable advantage over other agents. It does have several disadvantages, however, that must be considered. Midazolam has an extremely bitter and unpleasant taste. Although both the commercially available oral product and products compounded by the hospital mask the flavor to some degree, acceptance by some children remains poor. Alternative nonparenteral routes of administration have been studied, including nasal (0.2 to 0.3 mg/kg), transmucosal (0.2 mg/kg), and rectal (0.3 mg/kg), but each of these also has disadvantages, so that the oral administration remains the most commonly used and best tolerated for the majority of children (Saint-Maurice et al., 1986; Karl et al., 1993; Pandit et al., 2001).

Other agents and routes of administration, although less commonly used, have a place in the armamentarium. Other medications have been used in conjunction with midazolam, notably ketamine (Funk et al., 2000). Its advantage over a single-drug regimen appears to be in the child who is exceptionally uncooperative and requires a deeper level of sedation resulting from a dissociative state. Oral and transmucosal fentanyl have been used with success as well. Both the oral administration of the intravenous preparation and the commercially available oral transmucosal fentanyl "lollypop" have been shown to be effective, but postoperative nausea may be increased compared with other agents, limiting its usefulness in the outpatient setting (Howell et al., 2002; Tamura et al., 2003). Similar results have been seen with nasally administered sufentanil, which also may cause nasal burning and chest wall rigidity. This agent appears to be less useful than others for these reasons and has largely fallen out of favor with most pediatric anesthesiologists. Intramuscular administration of premedication is uncommonly used in children for obvious reasons—children have an intense dislike of needles. In some cases, however, when a child is exceedingly uncooperative and unmanageable, there may be no better alternative, and it is safer and more humane to administer a quick intramuscular injection with a small needle than to force the anesthesia mask on the face of an awake, struggling child for what will surely appear to be a very long 60 seconds. Ketamine, often in combination with midazolam and glycopyrrolate, is the most commonly used agent. The usual doses range from 2 to 3 mg/kg; lower doses are administered in combination with 0.1 mg/kg of midazolam. A high concentration (100 mg/mL) of ketamine should be used to minimize the injected volume (see Chapter 8, Preoperative Preparation).

ANESTHETIC TECHNIQUES

The operative procedure and underlying condition of the patient remain the primary decisive factors when choosing an anesthetic plan, but the disposition of the patient, that is, discharge on the day of surgery, is an important consideration as well. An outpatient anesthetic has, in addition to all of the other usual goals, the priority of rapid return to baseline function with minimal untoward effects. It is only with these objectives in mind that patients can be effectively discharged home in a timely fashion.

INDUCTION

Although clinical indications may on occasion dictate the safest induction technique, in many instances the older child may be given a choice, usually between inhalation and intravenous induction. Most children prefer an inhalation induction, but there are some who find the mask intolerable and prefer to have an intravenous catheter started with EMLA cream or local anesthetic. In cooperative school-aged children, this can often be accomplished without difficulty and may be offered to appropriate children as an option (also see Chapter 10, Induction of Anesthesia and Maintenance of the Airway in Infants and Children).

The vast majority of children in the United States have an inhalation induction of anesthesia for outpatient procedures. The advantages are obvious—relatively rapid induction without any painful stimulus. Most children are needle-phobic and are quite relieved when informed that they need not have anything painful done to them while conscious. The technique of inhalation induction is described in detail in Chapter 10 (Induction of Anesthesia). If the child uses a pacifier, it may be kept in his or her mouth until consciousness is lost, and the facemask placed over it. Scented oils such as bubble gum or fruit flavors may be added to the facemask to disguise the odor of the volatile agent. The room should be otherwise quiet and free from conversation or other distractions; the anesthesiologist should maintain continuous verbal contact with the child, telling a story in a soft, soothing modulated voice until the child falls asleep.

Sevoflurane has largely supplanted halothane as the agent of choice for induction. It has several advantages over halothane as an induction agent. Primary among these is the far greater hemodynamic stability of this agent. Sevoflurane induces far fewer problems with hypotension and diminished cardiac output than halothane does, even in the child who has a relatively long fasting period. Although some of this is due to the properties of the drug, some is also due to the construction of the vaporizer, because fewer minimum alveolar concentration (MAC) multiples can be given, preventing the anesthesiologist from delivering as deep an anesthetic. Dysrhythmias are also less common, because the drug does not cause the same degree of sensitization of the myocardium to catecholamines. Induction is rapid, and because sevoflurane is nonpungent, it causes very little airway irritation and coughing. It is possible to quickly increase the inspired concentration of sevoflurane or even begin with the vaporizer set at 8% and still avoid coughing. Sevoflurane does have a mildly unpleasant odor, but it is still easier to breathe than halothane, the only other agent suitable for inhalation induction. Sevoflurane does have several disadvantages as an induction agent compared with halothane. It causes more interference with ventilatory drive and respiratory muscle function, reducing the effectiveness of spontaneous ventilation (Brown et al., 1998). Because the vaporizers are calibrated to give fewer MAC multiples than halothane vaporizers, overpressure to achieve rapid depth of anesthesia is more difficult. There is a considerable economic penalty as well—sevoflurane is more than 20 times as expensive as halothane. In many cases, even if a total intravenous anesthetic is planned, an inhalation induction with sevoflurane is performed until intravenous access can be established.

In the United States, intravenous induction is a less commonly used technique for children. Propofol (3.5 mg/kg) has many attributes that make it an ideal intravenous induction agent for outpatient anesthesia. Not only does it have a very rapid onset of action, but its termination of action is similarly fast, with a characteristic rapid return to baseline function. The drug has antiemetic properties, a highly desirable asset in outpatient anesthesia. Its only drawback is pain on injection. Although this may be moderated with lidocaine (1 to 2 mg/kg), injected before or mixed with the propofol, it can be quite painful, especially if injected into a small vein.

Rectal induction with a barbiturate such as methohexital, thiopental, or thiamylal has the advantage of being able to be performed in an induction area outside of the operating room. This allows the parents to be present without having to actually enter the operating room itself and can be administered easily to most toddlers. Rectal induction with barbiturates in general has a significant disadvantage in outpatient anesthesia—a very prolonged elimination half-life. Because of this, this technique is infrequently used in this setting.

AIRWAY MANAGEMENT

There are numerous options for management of the airway in outpatient anesthesia. In many cases, a conventional anesthesia mask is used, such as during myringotomy and tube placement. This minimizes the risk of airway irritation but requires that at least one of the anesthesiologist's hands be occupied. It is contraindicated in the event of a full stomach and may be problematic in cases of easy airway obstruction, such as adenotonsillar hypertrophy.

The endotracheal tube remains the gold standard for the secured airway, although other devices are also commonly used. Many pediatric anesthesiologists intubate their patients "deep"—without the use of neuromuscular relaxants. This eliminates the need for reversal or for concerns of residual neuromuscular blockade postoperatively but mandates skillful judgment of anesthetic depth to avoid cord injury or laryngospasm. Just as with any anesthetic, one must choose the endotracheal tube size carefully so as to avoid producing injury or irritation to the vocal cords and trachea. It is particularly important to avoid any degree of postextubation croup in a patient who is going to be

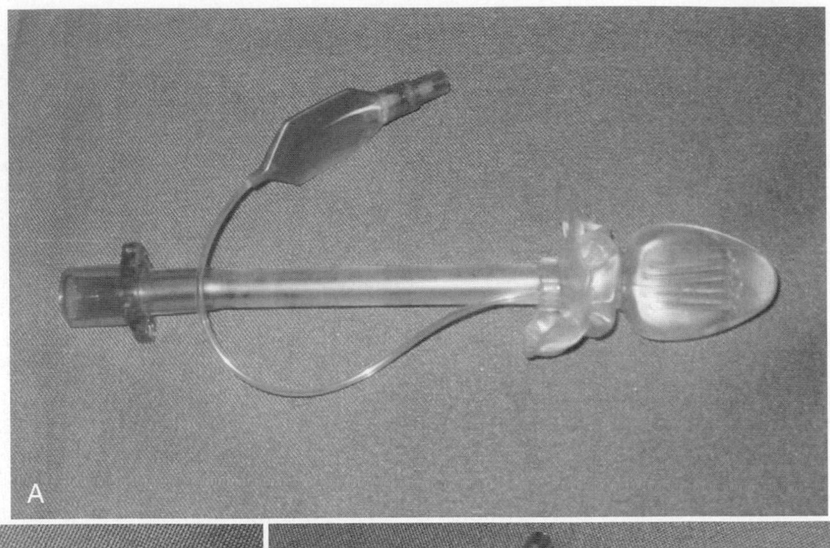

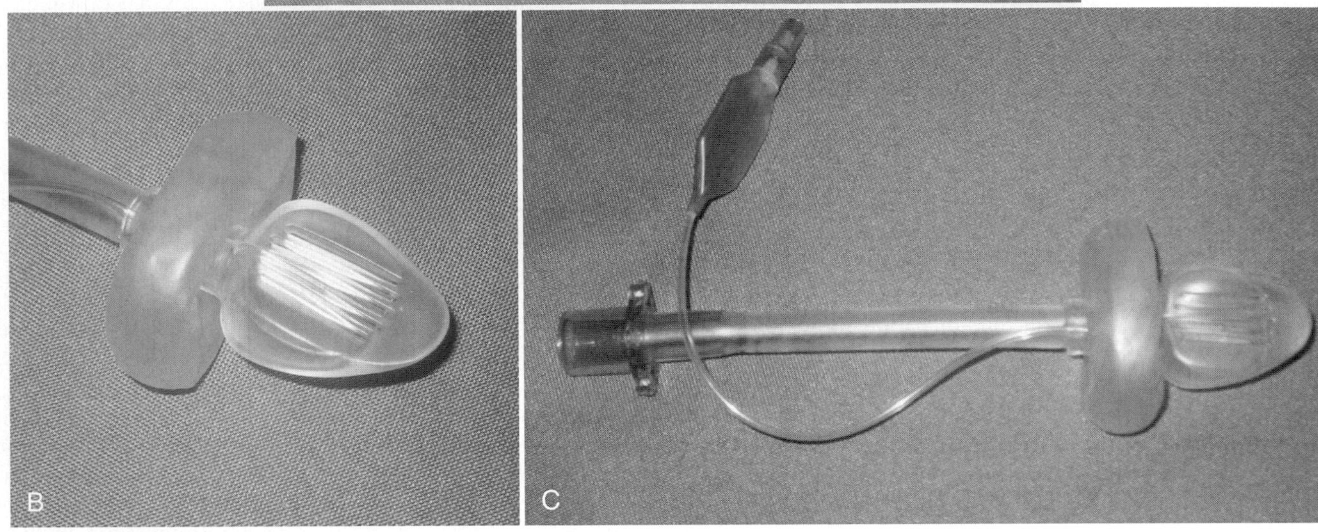

■ **FIGURE 27–1.** Cobra perilaryngeal airway (PLA). (*A*) The device with the cuff deflated ready for insertion. (*B*) A view of the laryngeal surface of the device. (*C*) The inflated cuff, which fills and conforms to the pharynx when in place.

discharged home the same day. Certain outpatient surgery cases may still benefit from the placement of an endotracheal tube, such as herniorrhaphy, when the contralateral side is examined laparoscopically.

Supraglottic airway devices cause less laryngeal irritation than an endotracheal tube, and can be placed without visualization of the airway (Brimacombe, 1995). The laryngeal mask airway (LMA), developed by Brain, is the first of these devices and is available in multiple pediatric sizes. Several competitors, including the Cobra perilaryngeal airway (PLA; Engineered Medical Systems, Tri-Anim Corp.) (Fig. 27-1*A* to *C*) and the cuffed oropharyngeal airway (COPA; Mallinckrodt, Inc.) (Fig. 27-2*A* and *B*), are now marketed (Robbins and Connelly, 2000; Bussolin and Busoni, 2002). All of these devices offer a less stimulating means of maintaining the airway while freeing the hands of the anesthesiologist for other tasks (see Chapter 9, Anesthetic Equipment and Monitoring). As was mentioned, a number of studies have demonstrated that the ability to maintain a stable airway without stimulating the larynx and trachea can decrease the incidence of adverse respiratory events in children with active or recent URIs (Tait et al., 1998). The same is likely to be true for patients with asthma. Although the LMA may diminish lower respiratory tract stimulation, it does not appear to decrease the incidence of postoperative sore throat (Splinter et al., 1994). There are no data that compare the different supraglottic devices. The findings by Tait and others (1998) that endotracheal tubes are more stimulating than LMAs, which are in turn more stimulating than a facemask, may serve to guide the decision of how to manage the airway if all other factors are equal (see Chapter 10, Induction of Anesthesia and Maintenance of the Airways in Infant and Children).

■ ANESTHETIC MAINTENANCE

The ideal maintenance regimen for outpatient anesthesia would have three defining characteristics: ease of titration, rapid offset, and minimal residual side effects. While it can be argued that several techniques or contemporary agents fit this definition, none are entirely free of all side effects or are ideal agents in every situation.

Inhalation anesthesia is still the most commonly used maintenance technique and has numerous advantages to commend it. No organ or enzymatic metabolism is necessary for its elimination; it is simply breathed away. Volatile agents are easily titrated to effect, and anesthetic depth can be adjusted with

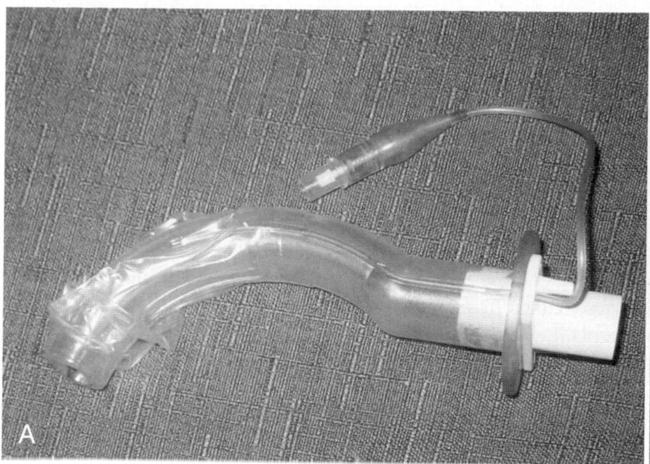

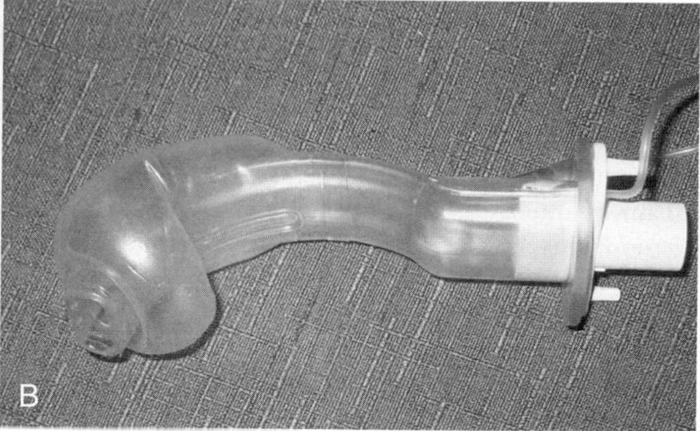

■ **FIGURE 27–2.** Cuffed oropharyngeal airway (COPA). The device is sized and inserted like a conventional oropharyngeal airway with the cuff deflated (*A*) and the cuff inflated (*B*). The end of the device has a standard 15-mm connector to attach to the breathing circuit.

relative rapidity. They are relatively economical, especially compared with newer intravenous agents, and they have beneficial effects on reactive airways, a common problem in children. There are several significant disadvantages that may diminish the claim for volatile agents as the ideal agents for outpatient anesthesia.

Halothane has in many places been replaced by sevoflurane as the primary volatile anesthetic in children. It has been claimed that the lower blood-gas solubility coefficient of sevoflurane gives it significant advantage over halothane for emergence, where a more rapid return to consciousness is desired in the outpatient setting. Data, however, do not confirm this contention and may actually give halothane several advantages over sevoflurane as a maintenance agent (Bacher et al., 1997). While return to wakefulness may indeed be quicker with sevoflurane when both agents are discontinued simultaneously, the speed to awakening can be adjusted by merely turning off the halothane sooner. Perhaps more important, time to awakening has no relationship to time to discharge from the hospital (Lerman et al., 1996; Sury et al., 1996; Welborn et al., 1996). The latter is the metric that reflects both day surgery unit efficiency and cost savings, and anesthesia with sevoflurane has not been shown to produce shorter discharge times, which is generally related to other factors, including premedication, complications of recovery such as postoperative nausea and vomiting (PONV), and analgesic needs (Bacher et al., 1997).

Sevoflurane has one additional characteristic that limits its effectiveness as a maintenance agent in outpatient anesthesia—the problem of emergence agitation. Several investigators have studied this problem, which can be exceedingly disruptive and disturbing for PACU caregivers and parents. With the increased use of sevoflurane, it became apparent that there was an increase in emergence agitation or delirium in the PACU (Rieger et al., 1996; Beskow and Westrin, 1999; Cravero et al., 2000). The child with emergence agitation appears wild and incoherent; he is inconsolable and does not appear to recognize familiar people. This phenomenon has clearly been distinguished from inadequate analgesia. Cravero and others (2000) compared emergence characteristics of sevoflurane anesthesia with those of halothane anesthesia in children undergoing magnetic resonance imaging. This prospective randomized study design effectively eliminated pain or dysphoria of neural blockade as potential confounding variables, leaving only the choice of volatile agent as a factor (Cravero et al., 2000). Using either low- or high-threshold criteria to define agitation and delirium, the investigators found much higher rates (33% versus 0% with high-threshold criteria and 88% versus 12% with low-threshold criteria) with sevoflurane than with halothane. Any time advantage due to more rapid emergence was eliminated by the difficulty in caring for the agitated child in the PACU, and hospital discharge times were not different.

Another study of sevoflurane in 100 children undergoing myringotomy and tube placement found that even with very short anesthetics, the incidence of emergence agitation was unacceptably high (Lapin et al., 1999). Although discharge times in this study were faster in the sevoflurane group, 67% demonstrated emergence agitation, leading them to conclude that sevoflurane was unsuitable for use as a sole agent for this procedure. They found that the addition of midazolam reduced this problem while lengthening recovery but not discharge times. The use of an opioid may have a similar or even more beneficial effect. It is possible that the cause is related to the different effects of these agents on brain function that has been noted on electroencephalography (Constant et al., 1999).

Desflurane is another new volatile agent with rapid onset and offset characteristics due to an exceptionally low blood-gas partition coefficient and solubility. It, too, appears to have a higher incidence of emergence agitation than older agents (Davis et al., 1994; Welborn et al., 1996; Valley et al., 2003). Emergence is significantly faster than with sevoflurane, however, due to its low solubility in tissues such as muscle and brain. Because sevoflurane is similar to halothane in its solubility in vessel-rich tissue groups, after discontinuance of the agent, significant blood concentrations are maintained as the agent returns from these depot storage sites to the bloodstream along its concentration gradient. This does not occur to a significant degree with desflurane because of its low tissue solubility, thereby speeding emergence time. Desflurane has also been found to decrease the ability to maintain spontaneous ventilation at concentrations greater than 1 MAC (Behforouz et al., 1998). Although desflurane is a potent airway irritant and is contraindicated for inhalation induction due to a very high incidence of severe laryngospasm, it does not appear to cause problems with deep extubation (Zwass et al., 1992; Sneyd et al., 1998; Valley et al., 2003) (see Chapter 11, Intraoperative and Postoperative Management).

Nitrous oxide continues to be used as an adjunctive agent for outpatient anesthesia in combination with both volatile and intravenous agents. It is useful as a sedative while placing intravenous cannulas in situations where a pure intravenous technique is used, and it can ease the introduction of more pungent volatile agents when performing inhalation induction. Its use as an agent for maintenance, however, is limited by its capacity to increase the incidence of PONV. For this reason, its use in the outpatient setting has been debated (Divatia et al., 1996).

The development of propofol heralded a new era in the maintenance of anesthesia in the same-day surgery setting. It is not hyperbole to suggest that it thrust total intravenous anesthesia (TIVA) into the mainstream of anesthetic techniques, allowing rapid titration of anesthetic depth and prompt emergence without the use of volatile agents. Propofol is a potent antiemetic, and it can reduce the incidence of nausea and vomiting when used in combination with both other anesthetic agents and other antiemetics (Sneyd et al., 1998; Barst et al., 1999). Despite the rapid emergence characteristics, the incidence of delirium and agitation is very low compared with sevoflurane or desflurane. The major limitation of propofol is its limited analgesic properties, and it must be used with an opioid or a regional technique to provide adequate depth of anesthesia for most painful procedures. It is an excellent and perhaps the ideal agent for use in imaging, radiation treatment, or invasive radiologic procedures where there is a minimum or absence of stimulation (Aldridge and Gordon, 1992; Martin et al., 1992; Vangerven et al., 1992; Frankville et al., 1993). It is particularly attractive for anesthesia for radiation therapy, where children require daily repeated general anesthetics for up to 6 consecutive weeks. In this situation, children are able to be ready for discharge home within 20 minutes of the end of the treatment session and, in contrast to the use of other agents such as barbiturates, have no evidence of either drug accumulation or development of tolerance and dose escalation (Glauber and Audenaert, 1987; Mills and Lord, 1992; Fassoulaki et al., 1994).

Remifentanil is a unique intravenous opioid with very rapid onset and elimination. In contrast to other opioids, its degradation is independent of organ metabolism, instead relying on hydrolysis by plasma esterases. The drug permits the anesthesiologist to provide intense intraoperative levels of opioid analgesia with no residual respiratory depression after emergence (Roulleau et al., 2003). Other postoperative side effects usually associated with opioids, such as nausea and vomiting, excessive sedation, and respiratory depression, are absent (Pinsker and Carroll, 1999). Intraoperative conditions are notable for hemodynamic stability, although both bradycardia and hypotension can occur at higher infusion rates. The most significant caveat to the use of remifentanil is that its rapid degradation provides no postoperative analgesia (Davis et al., 2000). It is essential, therefore, to use another agent or technique for this purpose, such as a long-acting opioid, regional block, or a nonsteroidal anti-inflammatory drug (NSAID) such as ketorolac, and to administer it with adequate time for action before dissipation of the effect of remifentanil (see Chapter 11, Intraoperative and Postoperative Management).

Perhaps the most effective manner in which to use remifentanil is to combine it with propofol. The combination of the two agents provides a balanced anesthetic that is easily titratable and results in significant reductions in the dose of both (Grundmann et al., 1998; Keidan et al., 2001). The two drugs can be mixed in the same syringe and administered via syringe pump. Because remifentanil degrades in propofol over time, aliquots small enough to be infused within 1 hour should be used (Stewart et al., 2000). For procedures of mild to moderate noxious stimulation, 10 mcg of remifentanil/mL in 1 mL (10 mg) of propofol is used, with infusion rates beginning at 100 mcg of propofol/kg per minute (0.1 mcg of remifentanil/kg per minute). This concentration permits the maintenance of spontaneous ventilation in most patients (Peacock et al., 1998; Reyle-Hahn et al., 2000). For more stimulating or painful procedures, the remifentanil concentration is doubled to 20 mcg per 1 mL of propofol, and the infusion begun at the same rate of 100 mcg of propofol per minute (0.2 mcg of remifentanil/kg per minute). Many patients breathe spontaneously with this concentration as well, although slow respiratory rates are common, and one must be vigilant to avoid hypoventilation. This technique provides a very stable intraoperative course, combined with an exceptionally smooth emergence and very rapid return to baseline function.

Regional anesthesia (usually in combination with a general anesthetic) can be used to great advantage in same-day surgery. The prime advantage and reason for its use is the provision of postoperative analgesia, but the modest reduction in the depth of general anesthesia can speed recovery and reduce the incidence of opioid-related untoward effects. Partial motor blockade is a not uncommon side effect of regional blocks, but, in most cases, it is not a contraindication to discharge home and can be reduced or eliminated by the use of low-concentration local anesthetics, and most children have their motor block resolved before discharge from the PACU (Burns et al., 1990). Other reported advantages of regional blockade include decreased intraoperative blood loss and improved operating conditions during hypospadias repair (Gunter et al., 1990). For operations less than 1 hour in duration, preoperative blockade did not affect the duration of postoperative analgesia compared with blockade administered at the end of the procedure (Rice et al., 1990).

Nearly all regional anesthetics in children are administered after the induction of general anesthesia. The reader is referred to Chapter 14 (Pediatric Regional Anesthesia) for details on performing the various regional blocks. In most cases, regional blockade for ambulatory surgery is performed with local anesthetics only, omitting opioids and adjuvant agents, such as clonidine and ketamine. This eliminates the risks of respiratory depression that can occur with those additives, an important safety consideration in the patient who will not be monitored after discharge from the PACU.

NEUROMUSCULAR BLOCKADE

In most outpatient procedures in infants and children, neuromuscular blockade is not necessary. The majority of surgical procedures that are performed in this setting can be performed without it, and intubation can most commonly be achieved with inhalation anesthesia with or without topical lidocaine, perhaps combined with a single dose of propofol in older children. When muscle relaxants are used, one should best avoid any of the longer-acting nondepolarizers and rely on intermediate-acting drugs such as mivacurium, cisatracurium, and vecuronium. These agents are discussed in detail in Chapter 6 (Pharmacology for Pediatric Anesthesia). When used, adequacy of reversal must be ensured. An investigation in adults found that incomplete reversal and mild degrees of residual neuromuscular blockade were common (Debaene et al., 2003). At least with some agents, children are less prone to inadequate spontaneous reversal. In children receiving mivacurium, residual weakness was not observed, whereas the finding was present in the adults (Bevan et al., 1996). Nevertheless, stringent criteria for adequacy of spontaneous reversal must be sought, and reversal agents administered if necessary (Baurain et al., 1998; Ali, 2003).

FLUIDS

As the allowable NPO times for clear liquid become shorter, the consequences of preoperative fasting are less problematic, but there remain occasional patients who come to surgery with varying degrees of dehydration (Coté, 1990; Cook-Sather et al., 2003). Additionally, the patient who is to be discharged home may not be interested in drinking large amounts of fluids in the hours immediately after surgery. It is useful, therefore, to provide adequate intravenous hydration not only to correct the fluid deficit but also to provide a cushion for the postoperative period. This is particularly the case for operations that may disrupt the ability to drink easily, such as tonsillectomy. Isotonic fluids should be administered, and the intravenous catheter may be kept in place until just before discharge. It is rarely necessary to provide glucose supplementation in the intravenous fluids (Sandstrom et al., 1993). One should try to replete the deficit plus current maintenance requirements within 2 to 3 hours. In some cases, children are discharged home before that, but those are generally the ones at least risk for inadequate intake.

EMERGENCE

The management of patients during emergence and the techniques of awake versus deep extubation and their comparison are detailed elsewhere (see Chapter 11, Intraoperative and Postoperative Management). The management of emergence from anesthesia in the outpatient setting is largely a question about the intubated child and whether the endotracheal tube should be removed when the patient is deep or awake. Certainly the contraindications to deep extubation (full stomach, difficult airway, blood in the pharynx) are no different in the outpatient or inpatient setting. Those who prefer awake extubation are primarily concerned about the loss of airway and of the development of laryngospasm. There are certain advantages of deep extubation in the same-day surgery settings provided that the PACU staff is adept and experienced at dealing with the patient who has been extubated deep. The patient awakens from anesthesia in the PACU without the noxious stimulus of an endotracheal tube in place and may have a smoother emergence. The child with reactive airways disease does not have the airway stimulation that may precipitate a potentially severe episode of bronchospasm. Operating room efficiency is enhanced, because the patient is able to leave the operating room within a minute of the end of the surgery, and room turnover can proceed at a more rapid pace. Several caveats, in addition to the contraindications mentioned, are crucial to increase the safety of this practice. The tube should not be withdrawn unless the patient is breathing spontaneously and has been demonstrated to have no alteration in breathing pattern with stimulation of the trachea (usually accomplished by gently moving the endotracheal tube). In most cases, this requires at least a 2 MAC value of inhaled anesthetic. The patient should be placed on his or her side after extubation to prevent oropharyngeal secretions from collecting in the hypopharynx either stimulating the larynx or causing aspiration. Supplemental oxygen and close attention to airway patency are necessary during transport to the PACU. It is best to leave the child undisturbed in the PACU until he awakens on his own.

POSTOPERATIVE ANALGESIA

No child can be discharged to home if the pain cannot be adequately managed by the parents using simple interventions. Inadequate analgesia has been identified in several studies as one of the most common causes for unanticipated admission to the hospital after surgery (Grenier et al., 1998). In another study, postoperative pain was identified by parents as the major problem they encountered after discharge home (Kokinsky et al., 1999). Only 28% of the patients in this study had received regional blocks.

REGIONAL AND LOCAL ANESTHESIA

Regional and local anesthesia has become one of the key modalities for postoperative analgesia for amenable procedures (see Chapter 14, Pediatric Regional Anesthesia). Among the commonly performed operations in pediatric outpatient surgery that are associated with significant postoperative pain, only adenotonsillectomy is not suitable for local or regional anesthesia. A prospective randomized study in children of glossopharyngeal nerve block, previously reported as an effective technique in adults, was stopped before its completion due to a 50% incidence of upper airway obstruction in the treatment group. The authors terminated the study and concluded that glossopharyngeal block is dangerous in children after tonsillectomy due to the common occurrence of inadvertent blockade of the vagus and recurrent laryngeal nerves (Bean-Lijewski, 1997).

Strict attention to the limits of local anesthetic dose must be observed with any regional block, and aspiration should precede any injection. When large volumes of local anesthetic are injected for any regional block, both a test dose and incremental injection technique should be used to minimize the risk of intravascular injection. A maximum of 2.5 mg/kg of bupivacaine can be administered to children over 6 months of age; younger infants should have the dose reduced by 30% (1.8 mg/kg) due to decreased levels of plasma binding proteins (Lerman et al., 1989; Luz et al., 1998). In addition, there appears to be an increased toxicity risk during general anesthesia with volatile agents (Badgwell et al., 1990). In these younger infants, an additional margin of safety may be gained by the use of levo-bupivacaine or ropivacaine, which appears to have less toxic potential (Bardsley et al., 1998; Kohane et al., 1998; Gunter et al., 1999; Morrison et al., 2000).

Although usually performed by the surgeon, the value of wound infiltration with local anesthetic should not be underestimated. There are numerous minor procedures for which a regional nerve block would be more intervention than necessary, such as simple hardware removals in orthopedics, excisional biopsies of small lesions, etc., where infiltration of the wound can be used to great advantage. Blood levels with this technique have been found to be low when dose limits are adhered to (Mobley et al., 1991). When a peripheral nerve or regional block can be performed, however, those techniques may offer superior analgesia. A study of caudal analgesia compared with wound infiltration for analgesia after inguinal herniorrhaphy found not only better analgesia but also quicker emergence times, fewer pain-related behaviors, and earlier hospital discharge times with the caudal block. Less supplementation with systemic analgesics was required with caudal block than with local infiltration (Conroy et al., 1993).

CAUDAL ANESTHESIA

Caudal anesthesia is probably the most commonly performed block in pediatric anesthesia practice. It is usually easy to administer, has an acceptably low incidence of complications, and is highly effective for surgical procedures below the level of the umbilicus (Dalens and Hasnaoui, 1989). The duration of effective analgesia is considerably longer than one would expect based on the usual length of action of the local anesthetic alone. A study that compared 0.25% bupivacaine with and without epinephrine found that the addition of epinephrine markedly prolonged the analgesia and that prolonged duration of analgesia was correlated with both younger age and lower surgical site (penoscrotal versus inguinal) (Warner et al., 1987). Duration of analgesia ranged from as short as 5 hours (inguinal surgery, older than 11 years) to as long as 23 hours (penoscrotal operation, 1 to 5 years old) as judged by the time to first requirement for supplemental analgesia. In a study of caudal blockade for analgesia after clubfoot repair, analgesia lasted at least 8 hours (Foulk et al., 1995).

Side effects of caudal block in children are unusual. Multiple studies have confirmed that urinary retention does not occur after caudal block using local anesthetic without central neuraxis opioids (Warner et al., 1987; Fisher et al., 1993). No differences in side effects were seen between caudal block and ilioinguinal-iliohypogastric nerve block; PACU stays were longer by less than 5 minutes and hospital stay by less than 10 minutes with the caudal blockade (Splinter et al., 1995). Motor function is not significantly impaired at the time of discharge and does not preclude or delay discharge (Burns et al., 1990).

Although one study found that placing the block at the end of the case resulted in better analgesia (Holthusen et al., 1994), other well-controlled studies have shown that there is no decrement in the duration of analgesia with caudal blocks administered at the beginning or end of surgery for procedures lasting less than 1 hour (Rice et al., 1990). A study of 0.5 mL/kg versus 1 mL/kg of 0.125% bupivacaine with epinephrine for penile and scrotal surgery found no difference in the duration of analgesia up to 8 hours postoperatively (Malviya et al., 1992).

Peripheral nerve blocks can be used with considerable efficacy for outpatient surgery in children and can be administered either by the anesthesiologist or by the surgeon on the operative field. Ilioinguinal-iliohypogastric nerve block combined with wound infiltration showed similar efficacy to a caudal block for analgesia after inguinal herniorrhaphy in two randomized studies (Schindler et al., 1991; Splinter et al., 1995). Paraumbilical block was shown to provide excellent analgesia for umbilical herniorrhaphy, although the duration of analgesia was less than 8 hours in 3 of 11 subjects (Courreges et al., 1997). Fascia iliaca block is a very effective and easy-to-place block for surgery of the leg above the level of the knee (Dalens et al., 1989). Ophthalmic surgery is often associated with considerable postoperative pain. Placement of a peribulbar block (Coppens et al., 2002; Subramaniam et al., 2003) or a subconjunctival injection (Ates et al., 1998) has been shown to provide long-lasting analgesia with a minimum of side effects in pediatric patients. Peripheral nerve blocks are often used in older patients undergoing distal hypospadias repairs or for circumcision. The dorsal nerve block has been shown to result in better postoperative analgesia than a penile ring block (Holder et al., 1997). Greater auricular nerve block has been shown to be efficacious after tympanomastoid surgery (Suresh et al., 2002).

INTRAVENOUS AGENTS

The development of parenterally administered NSAIDs, principally ketorolac, has allowed the anesthesiologist to administer nonopioid analgesics of equipotency to opioid analgesia. There is a sizable literature on the use of ketorolac in pediatric patients over the age of 1 year. The use of a cycloxygenase-2 (COX-2) inhibitor for analgesia in pediatric surgical patients has been reviewed (Farrar and Lerman, 2002; Kokki, 2003; Morris et al., 2003). However, clinical studies to date of COX-2 inhibitors in pediatric patients have been limited. Many of these studies have specifically examined the role of ketorolac in outpatient surgery. Ketorolac has been shown to have several advantages over opioid analgesics for postoperative analgesia in pediatric outpatients. There is a significant reduction in nausea and vomiting in patients receiving ketorolac compared with morphine, fentanyl, or other opioids (Mendel et al., 1995; Purday et al., 1996). The duration of a single dose of ketorolac is longer (6 hours) than that of most of the commonly used opioid analgesics (Dsida et al., 2002). Lack of respiratory depression is one of ketorolac's major advantages over opioids. A major problem with the use of ketorolac in outpatient analgesia is that it causes reversible dysfunction of platelet adhesion, and bleeding problems have been noted to be more common in children undergoing adenotonsillectomy (Gallagher et al., 1995; Judkins et al., 1996; Splinter et al., 1996; Splinter and Roberts, 1996). Bleeding problems have not been reported in other types of surgery, but one should use caution in administering ketorolac after other oral surgical procedures. Ketorolac appears to offer significant benefits to the pediatric outpatient after selected operations.

Opioids remain the gold standard for postoperative analgesia for moderate to severe pain, and they are still commonly prescribed for pediatric outpatients, both parenterally during anesthesia and via oral, transmucosal, and other routes for postoperative analgesia. Their principal disadvantages are the side effects of nausea, vomiting, and respiratory depression; at the doses prescribed for outpatients, ileus is rarely a problem. Even a single dose of morphine administered for postoperative analgesia after inguinal surgery has been reported to increase the incidence of postoperative nausea and vomiting (PONV) (Weinstein et al., 1994). For this reason, the author recommends that when opioids are used in outpatient surgery, multimodal prophylactic antiemetic therapy should be administered.

Intranasal fentanyl (2 mcg/kg, administered intraoperatively) has been used primarily for analgesia after myringotomy and tube surgery. Because these procedures are commonly performed without obtaining intravenous access, this provides an easy route for the administration of a potent analgesic. In a study comparing intranasal fentanyl with placebo, postoperative conditions were superior with fentanyl (Henderson et al., 1988). Children who received intranasal fentanyl not only were more comfortable and less agitated but also did not have an increase in PONV, a problem that has been noted with intranasal sufentanil (Henderson et al., 1988; Galinkin et al., 2000).

Numerous oral opioid analgesics are used for postoperative analgesia in children. In the majority of cases, these drugs are prescribed by the surgeon, not the anesthesiologist. Commonly used agents include oxycodone (0.1 to 0.2 mg/kg PO every 3 to 4 hours), hydrocodone (0.5 mg/kg PO every 3 to 4 hours), and codeine (1 mg/kg PO every 3 to 4 hours). All of these agents can be given in combination with acetaminophen and/or NSAIDs for added efficacy. These agents are generally administered for 1 to 3 days.

PEDIATRIC ACUTE CARE UNIT/ RECOVERY/DISCHARGE ISSUES

NAUSEA AND VOMITING

Postoperative nausea and vomiting (PONV) is perhaps the most common complication after anesthesia, although the reported incidence varies widely from approximately 8% to 50% (Heyland et al., 1997; Villeret et al., 2002). The variance is most likely due to study methodology and definitions. It is usually not an intractable problem but certainly is the cause of considerable distress and, if not well controlled, may be a cause of unanticipated overnight admission (Patel et al., 1997; Rose and Watcha, 1999). Numerous factors have been identified as increasing the risk of vomiting after anesthesia and surgery—some related to the surgical procedure, and some related to the anesthetic. The most common of these are listed in Table 27–1. Because discharge home is so dependent on the child returning to a baseline condition that allows the intake of fluids and nutrients, it is essential that nausea and vomiting be kept to a minimum for outpatient surgeries.

Anesthetic technique has been correlated with the incidence of PONV, with propofol-based techniques having the lowest incidence (Sneyd et al., 1998; Barst et al., 1999; Gurkan et al., 1999). The use of volatile agents, opioids, nitrous oxide, and cholinergic drugs for the reversal of neuromuscular blockade all increase the risk, although one study found that desflurane had less PONV than reported with other volatile anesthetics (Mendel et al., 1995; Divatia et al., 1996; Kuhn et al., 1999). Remifentanil, in contrast with other opioids, did not increase PONV (Pinsker and Carroll, 1999).

There have been studies of both treatment and prophylaxis of PONV in children undergoing outpatient surgery and anesthesia. One of the drugs commonly studied, droperidol, is no longer commonly used because of a rare association with cardiac dysrhythmias, so it is not discussed here. The most commonly used drugs for treatment and prophylaxis are the 5-HT3 antagonists (ondansetron, granisetron), dexamethasone, and metoclopramide. All have been shown to be effective for both prophylaxis and treatment in at least one study.

TABLE 27–1. Common causes of postoperative nausea and vomiting in outpatients

Surgical Factors	Anesthetic Factors	Patient Factors
Adenotonsillectomy Middle ear surgery Testicular surgery Laparoscopic surgery Insufflation of the bowel (endoscopy)	Use of volatile agents Use of nitrous oxide Use of opioids Insufflation of the stomach (difficult mask ventilation) Reversal of neuromuscular blockade (cholinergics) Unrelieved pain	Prior history of postoperative nausea and vomiting History of motion sickness Age >2 years Girls > boys

Dose-response studies of ondansetron suggest that for maximal efficacy, prophylactic doses of 0.1 to 0.15 mg/kg up to 4 mg should be administered (Rose et al., 1996; Patel et al., 1997; Sadhasivam et al., 2000). Lower doses were either not as effective or no more effective than placebo. Timing the dose before or after manipulation of the extraocular muscles in strabismus surgery (one of the most "emetogenic" operations) did not appear to make a difference (Madan et al., 2000). Another HT-3 antagonist, granisetron, was effective when 0.2 mg/kg was administered orally before the induction of anesthesia (Munro et al., 1999). When a single dose is not adequate, controversy exists as to whether a second dose is efficacious (Rose and Martin, 1996; Kovac et al., 1999). Dexamethasone is effective at preventing PONV and has the additional advantage of costing a very small fraction of the price of the HT-3 antagonists (Splinter and Roberts, 1996; Subramaniam et al., 2001). Dosing recommendations vary widely, but most studies recommend between 0.2 and 1.0 mg/kg, to not exceed 20 mg. Metoclopramide acts by increasing gastric emptying. Although it appears to be effective, some investigators have found it to be less so than ondansetron. It has a higher incidence of side effects, primarily sleepiness and occasional extrapyramidal effects, than either of the other agents (Broadman et al., 1990; Furst and Rodarte, 1994). Cisapride, which also is a prokinetic agent, was found to be ineffective in treating PONV (Cook-Sather et al., 2002).

The use of multiple agents in combination for those at greatest risk of PONV is recommended by several investigators. It appears that combining multiple drugs with different mechanisms of action yields the best results (Rose and Watcha, 1999). Similarly, the use of a low-risk anesthetic, especially propofol, which appears to have antiemetic properties of its own, in combination with prophylaxis, may result in the lowest incidence of all (Barst et al., 1999).

An additional factor that has been found to promote PONV is the insistence on oral intake in the PACU before discharge. While it appears sensible to want to demonstrate that a child is able to take and retain oral intake before discharge home, investigators found that insistence on oral intake before discharge increased the incidence of PONV and lengthened hospital stay (Schreiner et al., 1992; Schreiner and Nicolson, 1995). This common practice probably deserves a critical reexamination (see Chapter 11, Intraoperative and Postoperative Management).

INADEQUATE ANALGESIA

One of the common reasons for unanticipated admission, acceptable levels of analgesia are a necessity before discharge. No child can leave the hospital unless one is sure that the caregivers at home will be able to manage postoperative pain. More potent oral analgesics are often adequate to enable discharge, but in the event that it is not the case, admission and parenteral medications may be necessary. When the level of pain seems out of proportion to either the procedure performed or the experience of the clinicians, causes other than the obvious ones should be sought, although it must also be remembered that pain is a subjective experience and pain thresholds can vary widely.

EXCESSIVE SOMNOLENCE

This is rarely a cause for admission but may be a cause for a prolonged PACU stay. Common reasons include excessive narcosis, sedative or opioid drug errors (unintentional or patient sensitivity), unusual sensitivity to inhaled anesthetics, and drug interactions.

■ COMPLICATIONS AND UNANTICIPATED ADMISSION

Even when all care issues have been optimized, there inevitably are patients who develop complications that prevent discharge home and require hospitalization. Inadequate analgesia, inability to take adequate oral fluids, PONV, excessive somnolence, respiratory deterioration in children with URI or occult lower tract disease, or surgical complications all occur at some point. What is most important is that there is a system in place to streamline these admissions. In some institutions, this may be overnight admission to a short-stay unit, which may be on the ward, in the PACU, or in the emergency department. In others, it will mean a bed on the regular ward. In all cases, it is essential that adequate follow-up be maintained by both the surgical and anesthetic team so that the issues that mandated admission are properly and adequately addressed.

■ FACILITY DESIGN AND PATIENT THROUGHPUT

Because such a large percentage of children undergoing surgery are cared for as outpatients, it is very common that their surgery takes place not in a separate outpatient facility but in the main operating room. Even though these facilities are not usually designed with outpatients in mind, and using them in this manner may be awkward at times, there are still numerous changes in organization that can reap benefits both in parent and patient satisfaction and in efficiency and throughput.

Patient throughput can be improved through the design of separate intake and discharge areas—one for inpatient and same-day admissions and a second for day surgery patients. In this manner, the routing through the admissions process could be streamlined, with optimized procedures for each. The two facilities enable staff to work more efficiently, as they can each focus on only a single function. All patients who are operated on in the main operating room are still routed through the same PACU, but same-day surgery patients are sent to the phase II recovery area in the same-day surgery area as soon as they are ready. This enables "fast tracking" and more rapid discharge of these patients. The same concept can be used for anesthesia for outpatient imaging, with those patients discharged home directly from a recovery area in the radiology department. Focusing on these systems issues can enable more patients to be cared for in a smoother and more professional manner.

■ SUMMARY

The number of children in the United States undergoing outpatient anesthesia has surpassed the number of inpatient cases. Many of the considerations for the care of these patients are identical to that of inpatients, but there are unique issues that must be addressed to enable children to go home on the day of surgery and anesthesia. Careful case selection, both on the basis of the child's underlying condition and for the planned surgical procedure, is critical in ensuring the success of an outpatient program. Whether these procedures are performed in the day surgery unit of a hospital or in a freestanding surgical center, the same level of same-day perioperative services for children should be available. One must have a well-designed systematic approach to organization, throughput, and clinical care to achieve both efficiency and safety.

REFERENCES

Adu-Gyamfi Y, Sankarankutty M, Marwa S: Use of a tourniquet in patients with sickle-cell disease. *Can J Anaesth* 40:24–27, 1993.

Ahmed Z, Lockhart CH, Weiner M, and Klingensmith G: Advances in diabetes management: Implications for anesthesia. *Anes Analg* 100:666–669, 2005.

Aldridge LM, Gordon NH: Propofol infusions for radiotherapy. *Paediatr Anaesth* 2:133–137, 1992.

Ali HH: Criteria of adequate clinical recovery from neuromuscular block. *Anesthesiology* 98:1278–1280, 2003.

American Thoracic Society: Standards and indications for cardiopulmonary sleep studies in children. *Am J Respir Crit Care Med* 153:866–878, 1996.

Ates Y, Unal N, Cuhruk H, et al.: Postoperative analgesia in children using preemptive retrobulbar block and local anesthetic infiltration in strabismus surgery. *Reg Anesth Pain Med* 23:569–574, 1998.

Atlas SA: The sickle cell trait and surgical complications. A matched-pair patient analysis. *JAMA* 229:1078–1080, 1974.

Bacher A, Burton AW, Uchida T, et al.: Sevoflurane or halothane anesthesia: Can we tell the difference? *Anesth Analg* 85:1203sP6, 1997.

Badgwell J, Heavner J, Kytta J: Bupivacaine toxicity in young guinea pigs is age-dependent and is affected by volatile anesthetics. *Anesthesiology* 73:297–303, 1990.

Barclay K, Williams AJ, Major E: Propofol infusion in children [letter; comment]. *BMJ* 305:953; discussion 953–954, 1992.

Bardsley H, Gristwood R, Baker H, et al.: A comparison of the cardiovascular effects of levobupivacaine and rac-bupivacaine following intravenous administration to healthy volunteers. *Br J Clin Pharmacol* 46:245–249, 1998.

Barnett AH, Robinson MH, Harrison JH, et al.: Mini-pump: Method of diabetic control during minor surgery under general anaesthesia. *Br Med J* 280:78–79, 1980.

Barst SM, Leiderman JU, Markowitz A, et al.: Ondansetron with propofol reduces the incidence of emesis in children following tonsillectomy. *Can J Anaesth* 46:359–362, 1999.

Baurain MJ, Hennart DA, Godschalx A, et al.: Visual evaluation of residual curarization in anesthetized patients using one hundred-hertz, five-second tetanic stimulation at the adductor pollicis muscle. *Anesth Analg* 87:185–189, 1998.

Bean-Lijewski JD: Glossopharyngeal nerve block for pain relief after pediatric tonsillectomy: retrospective analysis and two cases of life-threatening upper airway obstruction from an interrupted trial. *Anesth Analg* 84:1232–1238, 1997.

Behforouz N, Dubousset AM, Jamali S, et al.: Respiratory effects of desflurane anesthesia on spontaneous ventilation in infants and children. *Anesth Analg* 87:1052–1055, 1998.

Bellew M, Atkinson KR, Dixon G, et al.: The introduction of a paediatric anaesthesia information leaflet: an audit of its impact on parental anxiety and satisfaction. *Paediatr Anaesth* 12:124–130, 2002.

Beskow A, Westrin P: Sevoflurane causes more postoperative agitation in children than does halothane. *Acta Anaesthesiol Scand* 43:536–541, 1999.

Bevan DR, Kahwaji R, Ansermino JM, et al.: Residual block after mivacurium with or without edrophonium reversal in adults and children. *Anesthesiology* 84:362–367, 1996.

Bevan JC, Veall GR, Macnab AJ, et al.: Midazolam premedication delays recovery after propofol without modifying involuntary movements. *Anesth Analg* 85:50–54, 1997.

Biavati MJ, Manning SC, Phillips DL: Predictive factors for respiratory complications after tonsillectomy and adenoidectomy in children. *Arch Otolaryngol Head Neck Surg* 123:517–521, 1997.

Bifano EM, Smith F, Borer J: Relationship between determinants of oxygen delivery and respiratory abnormalities in preterm infants with anemia. *J Pediatr* 120(2 Pt 1):292–296, 1992.

Brampton WJ, Jago RH: Acute viral myocarditis. A death associated with anaesthesia. *Anaesthesia* 45:215–217, 1990.

Brimacombe J: The advantages of the LMA over the tracheal tube or facemask: A meta-analysis. *Can J Anaesth* 42:1017–1023, 1995.

Broadman LM, Ceruzzi W, Patane PS, et al.: Metoclopramide reduces the incidence of vomiting following strabismus surgery in children. *Anesthesiology* 72:245–248, 1990.

Brown K, Aun C, Stocks J, et al.: A comparison of the respiratory effects of sevoflurane and halothane in infants and young children. *Anesthesiology* 89:86–92, 1998.

Burns AM, Shelly MP, Dewar AK: Caudal analgesia for pediatric day case surgery: Assessment of motor function prior to discharge. *J Clin Anesth* 2:27–30, 1990.

Bussolin L, Busoni P: The use of the cuffed oropharyngeal airway in paediatric patients. *Paediatr Anaesth* 12:43–47, 2002.

Campbell NN: Respiratory tract infection and anaesthesia. Haemophilus influenzae pneumonia that developed under anaesthesia. *Anaesthesia* 45:561–562, 1990.

Cassady JF Jr, Wysocki TT, Miller KM, et al.: Use of a preanesthetic video for facilitation of parental education and anxiolysis before pediatric ambulatory surgery. *Anesth Analg* 88:246–250, 1999.

Chadwick V, Wilkinson KA: Diabetes mellitus and the pediatric anesthetist. *Paediatr Anaesth* 14:716–723, 2004.

Cohen MM, Cameron CB: Should you cancel the operation when a child has an upper respiratory tract infection? *Anesth Analg* 72:282–288, 1991.

Conroy JM, Othersen HB Jr, Dorman BH, et al.: A comparison of wound instillation and caudal block for analgesia following pediatric inguinal herniorrhaphy. *J Pediatr Surg* 28:565–567, 1993.

Constant I, Dubois MC, Piat V, et al.: Changes in electroencephalogram and autonomic cardiovascular activity during induction of anesthesia with sevoflurane compared with halothane in children. *Anesthesiology* 91:1604–1615, 1999.

Cook-Sather SD, Harris KA, Chiavacci R, et al.: A liberalized fasting guideline for formula-fed infants does not increase average gastric fluid volume before elective surgery. *Anesth Analg* 96:965–969, table of contents, 2003.

Cook-Sather SD, Harris KA, Schreiner MS: Cisapride does not prevent postoperative vomiting in children. *Anesth Analg* 94:50–54, table of contents, 2002.

Coppens M, Versichelen L, Mortier E: Treatment of postoperative pain after ophthalmic surgery. *Bull Soc Belge Ophthalmol* 27–32, 2002.

Coté C: The upper respiratory tract infection (URI) dilemma: Fear of a complication or litigation? *Anesthesiology* 95:283–285, 2001.

Coté CJ: NPO after midnight for children—A reappraisal. *Anesthesiology* 72:589–592, 1990.

Coté CJ, Cohen IT, Suresh S, et al.: A comparison of three doses of a commercially prepared oral midazolam syrup in children. *Anesth Analg* 94:37–43, table of contents, 2002.

Coté CJ, Rolf N, Liu LM, et al.: A single-blind study of combined pulse oximetry and capnography in children. *Anesthesiology* 74:980–987, 1991.

Coté CJ, Zaslavsky A, Downes JJ, et al.: Postoperative apnea in former preterm infants after inguinal herniorrhaphy. A combined analysis. *Anesthesiology* 82:809–822, 1995.

Courreges P, Poddevin F, Lecoutre D: Para-umbilical block: A new concept for regional anaesthesia in children. *Paediatr Anaesth* 7:211–214, 1997.

Cravero J, Surgenor S, Whalen K: Emergence agitation in paediatric patients after sevoflurane anaesthesia and no surgery: A comparison with halothane. *Paediatr Anaesth* 10:419–424, 2000.

Dalens B, Hasnaoui A: Caudal anesthesia in pediatric surgery: Success rate and adverse effects in 750 consecutive patients. *Anesth Analg* 68:83–89, 1989.

Dalens B, Vanneuville G, Tanguy A: Comparison of the fascia iliaca compartment block with the 3-in-1 block in children [published erratum appears in *Anesth Analg* 70:474, 1990]. *Anesth Analg* 69:705–713, 1989.

Davis PJ, Cohen IT, McGowan FX Jr, et al.: Recovery characteristics of desflurane versus halothane for maintenance of anesthesia in pediatric ambulatory patients. *Anesthesiology* 80:298–302, 1994.

Davis PJ, Finkel JC, Orr RJ, et al.: A randomized, double-blinded study of remifentanil versus fentanyl for tonsillectomy and adenoidectomy surgery in pediatric ambulatory surgical patients. *Anesth Analg* 90:863–871, 2000.

de Kluijver J, Grunberg K, Sont JK, et al.: Rhinovirus infection in nonasthmatic subjects: Effects on intrapulmonary airways. *Eur Respir J* 20:274–279, 2002.

Debaene B, Plaud B, Dilly MP, et al.: Residual paralysis in the PACU after a single intubating dose of nondepolarizing muscle relaxant with an intermediate duration of action. *Anesthesiology* 98:1042–1048, 2003.

Derkay CS, Bray G, Milmoe GJ, et al.: Adenotonsillectomy in children with sickle cell disease. *South Med J* 84:205–208, 1991.

Divatia JV, Vaidya JS, Badwe RA, et al.: Omission of nitrous oxide during anesthesia reduces the incidence of postoperative nausea and vomiting. A meta-analysis. *Anesthesiology* 85:1055–1062, 1996.

Dsida RM, Wheeler M, Birmingham PK, et al.: Age-stratified pharmacokinetics of ketorolac tromethamine in pediatric surgical patients. *Anesth Analg* 94:266–270, table of contents, 2002.

Dusser D, Jacoby D, Djokic T, et al.: Virus induces airway hyperresponsiveness to tachykinins: Role of neutral endopeptidase. *J Appl Physiol* 67:1504–1511, 1989.

Eames WO, Rooke GA, Wu RS, et al.: Comparison of the effects of etomidate, propofol, and thiopental on respiratory resistance after tracheal intubation. *Anesthesiology* 84:1307–1311, 1996.

Empey DW: Effect of airway infections on bronchial reactivity. *Eur J Respir Dis Suppl* 128(Pt 1):366–368, 1983.

Empey DW, Laitinen LA, Jacobs L: Mechanisms of bronchial hyperreactivity in normal subjects after upper respiratory infections. *Am Rev Respir Dis* 113:131–139, 1976.

Farrar MW, Lerman J: Novel concepts for analgesia in pediatric surgical patients. Cyclooxygenase-2 inhibitors, alpha 2-agonists, and opioids. *Anesthesiol Clin North Am* 20:59–82, 2002.

Fassoulaki A, Farinotti R, Mantz J, et al.: Does tolerance develop to the anaesthetic effects of propofol in rats? *Br J Anaesth* 72:127–128, 1994.

Ferrari LR, Rooney FM, Rockoff MA: Preoperative fasting practices in pediatrics. *Anesthesiology* 90:978–980, 1999.

Fisher QA: Clear for surgery: Current attitudes and practices of pediatricians [published erratum appears in *Clin Pediatr (Phila)* 30:326, 1991]. *Clin Pediatr (Phila)* 30:35–41, 1991.

Fisher QA, Feldman MA, Wilson MD: Pediatric responsibilities for preoperative evaluation. *J Pediatr* 125(5 Pt 1):675 685, 1994.

Fisher QA, McComiskey CM, Hill JL, et al.: Postoperative voiding interval and duration of analgesia following peripheral or caudal nerve blocks in children. *Anesth Analg* 76:173–177, 1993.

Foulk DA, Boakes J, Rab GT, et al.: The use of caudal epidural anesthesia in clubfoot surgery. *J Pediatr Orthop* 15:604–607, 1995.

Frankville DD, Spear RM, Dyck JB: The dose of propofol required to prevent children from moving during magnetic resonance imaging. *Anesthesiology* 79:953–958, 1993.

Funk W, Jakob W, Riedl T, et al.: Oral preanaesthetic medication for children: Double-blind randomized study of a combination of midazolam and ketamine vs midazolam or ketamine alone. *Br J Anaesth* 84:335–340, 2000.

Furst SR, Rodarte A: Prophylactic antiemetic treatment with ondansetron in children undergoing tonsillectomy. *Anesthesiology* 81:799–803, 1994.

Galinkin JL, Fazi LM, Cuy RM, et al.: Use of intranasal fentanyl in children undergoing myringotomy and tube placement during halothane and sevoflurane anesthesia. *Anesthesiology* 93:1378–1383, 2000.

Gallagher JE, Blauth J, Fornadley JA: Perioperative ketorolac tromethamine and postoperative hemorrhage in cases of tonsillectomy and adenoidectomy. *Laryngoscope* 105:606–609, 1995.

Gibson IH, Love SH: Sickle cell trait: A rare cause of post-operative death in Northern Ireland. *Ulster Med J* 43:143–147, 1974.

Glauber DT, Audenaert SM: Anesthesia for children undergoing craniospinal radiotherapy. *Anesthesiology* 67:801–803, 1987.

Grenier B, Dubreuil M, Siao D, et al.: Paediatric day case anaesthesia: Estimate of its quality at home. *Paediatr Anaesth* 8:485–489, 1998.

Griffin TC, Buchanan GR: Elective surgery in children with sickle cell disease without preoperative blood transfusion. *J Pediatr Surg* 28:681–685, 1993.

Grundmann U, Uth M, Eichner A, et al.: Total intravenous anaesthesia with propofol and remifentanil in paediatric patients: A comparison with a desflurane-nitrous oxide inhalation anaesthesia. *Acta Anaesthesiol Scand* 42:845–850, 1998.

Gunter JB, Forestner JE, Manley CB: Caudal epidural anesthesia reduces blood loss during hypospadias repair. *J Urol* 144(2 Pt 2):517–519; discussion 530, 1990.

Gunter JB, Gregg T, Varughese AM, et al.: Levobupivacaine for ilioinguinal/iliohypogastric nerve block in children. *Anesth Analg* 89:647–649, 1999.

Gurkan Y, Kilickan L, Toker K: Propofol-nitrous oxide versus sevoflurane-nitrous oxide for strabismus surgery in children. *Paediatr Anaesth* 9:495–499, 1999.

Hackmann T, Steward DJ, Sheps S: Anemia in pediatric day-surgery patients: prevalence and detection. *Anesthesiology* 75, 1991.

Halvorson DJ, McKie V, McKie K, et al.: Sickle cell disease and tonsillectomy. Preoperative management and postoperative complications. *Arch Otolaryngol Head Neck Surg* 123:689–692, 1997.

Helfaer MA, McColley SA, Pyzik PL, et al.: Polysomnography after adenotonsillectomy in mild pediatric obstructive sleep apnea. *Crit Care Med* 24:1323–1327, 1996.

Henderson JM, Brodsky DA, Fisher DM, et al.: Pre-induction of anesthesia in pediatric patients with nasally administered sufentanil. *Anesthesiology* 68:671–675, 1988.

Heyland K, Dangel P, Gerber AC: Postoperative nausea and vomiting (PONV) in children. *Eur J Pediatr Surg* 7:230–233, 1997.

Holder KJ, Peutrell JM, Weir PM: Regional anaesthesia for circumcision. Subcutaneous ring block of the penis and subpubic penile block compared. *Eur J Anaesthesiol* 14:495–498, 1997.

Holthusen H, Eichwede F, Stevens M, et al.: Pre-emptive analgesia: Comparison of preoperative with postoperative caudal block on postoperative pain in children. *Br J Anaesth* 73:440–442, 1994.

Howell TK, Smith S, Rushman SC, et al.: A comparison of oral transmucosal fentanyl and oral midazolam for premedication in children. *Anaesthesia* 57:798–805, 2002.

Hume H: Red blood cell transfusions for preterm infants: The role of evidence-based medicine. *Semin Perinatol* 21:8–19, 1997.

Joshi A, Gerhardt T, Shandloff P, et al.: Blood transfusion effect on the respiratory pattern of preterm infants. *Pediatrics* 80:79–84, 1987.

Judkins JH, Dray TG, Hubbell RN: Intraoperative ketorolac and posttonsillectomy bleeding. *Arch Otolaryngol Head Neck Surg* 122:937–940, 1996.

Kain ZN, Caramico LA, Mayes LC, et al.: Preoperative preparation programs in children: A comparative examination. *Anesth Analg* 87:1249–1255, 1998.

Kain ZN, Hofstadter MB, Mayes LC, et al.: Midazolam: Effects on amnesia and anxiety in children. *Anesthesiology* 93:676–684, 2000.

Kain ZN, Mayes LC, Caramico LA, et al.: Parental presence during induction of anesthesia. A randomized controlled trial. *Anesthesiology* 84:1060–1067, 1996.

Kain ZN, Mayes LC, Wang SM, et al.: Parental presence during induction of anesthesia versus sedative premedication: Which intervention is more effective? *Anesthesiology* 89:1147–56; discussion 9A-10A, 1998.

Karl HW, Pauza KJ, Heyneman N, et al.: Preanesthetic preparation of pediatric outpatients: The role of a videotape for parents. *J Clin Anesth* 2:172–177, 1990.

Karl HW, Rosenberger JL, Larach MG, et al.: Transmucosal administration of midazolam for premedication of pediatric patients. Comparison of the nasal and sublingual routes. *Anesthesiology* 78:885–891, 1993.

Keidan I, Berkenstadt H, Sidi A, et al.: Propofol/remifentanil versus propofol alone for bone marrow aspiration in paediatric haemato-oncological patients. *Paediatr Anaesth* 11:297–301, 2001.

Kemp JP: Recent advances in the management of asthma using leukotriene modifiers. *Am J Respir Med* 2:139–156, 2003.

Kempen PM: Preoperative pregnancy testing: A survey of current practice. *J Clin Anesth* 9:546–550, 1997.

Kempen PM, Norton P, Vu H: A risk index for pregnancy during anesthesia. *J Clin Anesth* 9:194–199, 1997.

Kerbl R, Zotter H, Schenkeli R, et al.: Persistent hypercapnia in children after treatment of obstructive sleep apnea syndrome by adenotonsillectomy. *Wien Klin Wochenschr* 113(7-8):229–234, 2001.

Kleinfeldt AS: Preoperative phone calls. Reducing cancellations in pediatric day surgery. *AORN J* 51:1559–1564, 1990.

Kohane DS, Sankar WN, Shubina M, et al.: Sciatic nerve blockade in infant, adolescent, and adult rats: A comparison of ropivacaine with bupivacaine. *Anesthesiology* 89:1199-208; discussion 10A, 1998.

Koinig H: Preparing parents for their child's surgery: Preoperative parental information and education. *Paediatr Anaesth* 12:107–109, 2002.

Kokinsky E, Thornberg E, Ostlund AL, et al.: Postoperative comfort in paediatric outpatient surgery. *Paediatr Anaesth* 9:243–251, 1999.

Kokki H: Nonsteroidal anti-inflammatory drugs for postoperative pain: a focus on children. *Paediatr Drugs* 5:103–123, 2003.

Konotey-Ahulu FI: Anaesthetic deaths and the sickle-cell trait. *Lancet* 1:267–268, 1969.

Kovac AL, O'Connor TA, Pearman MH, et al.: Efficacy of repeat intravenous dosing of ondansetron in controlling postoperative nausea and vomiting: A randomized, double-blind, placebo-controlled multicenter trial. *J Clin Anesth* 11:453–459, 1999.

Krane EJ, Haberkern CM, Jacobson LE: Postoperative apnea, bradycardia, and oxygen desaturation in formerly premature infants: Prospective comparison of spinal and general anesthesia. *Anesth Analg* 80:7-13, 1995.

Kuhn I, Scheifler G, Wissing H: Incidence of nausea and vomiting in children after strabismus surgery following desflurane anaesthesia. *Paediatr Anaesth* 9:521–526, 1999.

Kurth CD, Spitzer AR, Broennle AM, et al.: Postoperative apnea in preterm infants. *Anesthesiology* 66:483–438, 1987.

Lalakea ML, Marquez-Biggs I, Messner AH: Safety of pediatric short-stay tonsillectomy. *Arch Otolaryngol Head Neck Surg* 125:749–752, 1999.

Lapin SL, Auden SM, Goldsmith LJ, et al.: Effects of sevoflurane anaesthesia on recovery in children: A comparison with halothane. *Paediatr Anaesth* 9:299–304, 1999.

Lerman J, Davis PJ, Welborn LG, et al.: Induction, recovery, and safety characteristics of sevoflurane in children undergoing ambulatory surgery. A comparison with halothane. *Anesthesiology* 84:1332–1340, 1996.

Lerman J, Strong HA, LeDez KM, et al.: Effects of age on the serum concentration of alpha 1-acid glycoprotein and the binding of lidocaine in pediatric patients. *Clin Pharmacol Ther* 46:219–225, 1989.

Levy L, Pandit UA, Randel GI, et al.: Upper respiratory tract infections and general anaesthesia in children. Peri-operative complications and oxygen saturation. *Anaesthesia* 47:678–682, 1992.

Litman RS, Wu CL, Quinlivan JK: Gastric volume and pH in infants fed clear liquids and breast milk prior to surgery. *Anesth Analg* 79:482–485, 1994.

Liu AH, Szefler SJ: Advances in childhood asthma: Hygiene hypothesis, natural history, and management. *J Allergy Clin Immunol* 111(3 Suppl):S785–S792, 2003.

Liu LMP, Coté CJ, Goudsouzian NG, et al.: Life-threatening apnea in infants recovering from anesthesia. *Anesthesiology* 59:506–510, 1983.

Luz G, Wieser C, Innerhofer P, et al.: Free and total bupivacaine plasma concentrations after continuous epidural anaesthesia in infants and children. *Paediatr Anaesth* 8:473–478, 1998.

MacArthur AJ, MacArthur C, Bevan JC: Determinants of pediatric day surgery cancellation. *J Clin Epidemiol* 48:485–489, 1995.

Madan R, Perumal T, Subramaniam K, et al.: Effect of timing of ondansetron administration on incidence of postoperative vomiting in paediatric strabismus surgery. *Anaesth Intensive Care* 28:27–30, 2000.

Malviya S, Fear DW, Roy WL, et al.: Adequacy of caudal analgesia in children after penoscrotal and inguinal surgery using 0.5 or 1.0 ml.kg-1 bupivacaine 0.125%. *Can J Anaesth* 39(5 Pt 1):449–453, 1992.

Malviya S, Swartz J, Lerman J: Are all preterm infants younger than 60 weeks postconceptual age at risk for postanesthetic apnea? *Anesthesiology* 78:1076–1081, 1993.

Margolis JO, Ginsberg B, Dear GL, et al.: Paediatric preoperative teaching: Effects at induction and postoperatively. *Paediatr Anaesth* 8:17–23, 1998.

Martin LD, Pasternak LR, Pudimat MA: Total intravenous anesthesia with propofol in pediatric patients outside the operating room. *Anes Analg* 74:609–612, 1992.

Maslow AD, Regan MM, Israel E, et al.: Inhaled albuterol, but not intravenous lidocaine, protects against intubation-induced bronchoconstriction in asthma. *Anesthesiology* 93:1198–1204, 2000.

Maxwell LG, Deshpande JK, Wetzel RC: Preoperative evaluation of children. *Pediatr Clin North Am* 41:93–110, 1994.

McAnulty GR, Hall GM: Anaesthesia for the diabetic patient. *Br J Anaesth* 90:428–429, 2003.

McAnulty GR, Robertshaw HJ, Hall GM: Anaesthetic management of patients with diabetes mellitus. *Br J Anaesth* 85:80–90, 2000.

McGarry P, Duncan C: Anesthetic risks in sickle cell trait. *Pediatrics* 51:507–512, 1973.

Mendel HG, Guarnieri KM, Sundt LM, et al.: The effects of ketorolac and fentanyl on postoperative vomiting and analgesic requirements in children undergoing strabismus surgery. *Anesth Analg* 80:1129–1133, 1995.

Messner AH: Treating pediatric patients with obstructive sleep disorders: An update. *Otolaryngol Clin North Am* 36:519–530, 2003.

Mills DC, Lord WD: Propofol for repeated burns dressings in a child: A case report. *Burns* 18:58–59, 1992.

Mobley KA, Wandless JG, Fell D: Serum bupivacaine concentrations following wound infiltration in children undergoing inguinal herniotomy. *Anaesthesia* 46:500–501, 1991.

Molfino NA, Slutsky AS: Near-fatal asthma. *Eur Respir J* 7:981–990, 1994.

Morris JL, Rosen DA, Rosen KR: Nonsteroidal anti-inflammatory agents in neonates. *Paediatr Drugs* 5:385–405, 2003.

Morrison SG, Dominguez JJ, Frascarolo P, et al.: A comparison of the electrocardiographic cardiotoxic effects of racemic bupivacaine, levobupivacaine, and ropivacaine in anesthetized swine. *Anesth Analg* 90:1308–1314, 2000.

Munro HM, D'Errico CC, Lauder GR, et al.: Oral granisetron for strabismus surgery in children. *Can J Anaesth* 46:45–48, 1999.

Newburger JW, Rosenthal A, Williams RG, et al.: Noninvasive tests in the initial evaluation of heart murmurs in children. *N Engl J Med* 308:61–64, 1983.

National Heart, Lung, and Blood Institute: *National Asthma Education and Prevention Program Expert panel report: guidelines for the diagnosis and management of asthma*, 2002.

Nicholl J: The surgery of infancy. *Br Med J* 2:753, 1909.

O'Byrne KK, Peterson L, Saldana L: Survey of pediatric hospitals' preparation programs: Evidence of the impact of health psychology research. *Health Psychol* 16:147–154, 1997.

O'Conner ME, Drasner K: Preoperative laboratory testing of children undergoing elective surgery. *Anes Analg* 70:176–180, 1990.

Pandit UA, Collier PJ, Malviya S, et al.: Oral transmucosal midazolam premedication for preschool children. *Can J Anaesth* 48:191–195, 2001.

Patel RI, DeWitt L, Hannallah RS: Preoperative laboratory testing in children undergoing elective surgery: Analysis of current practice. *J Clin Anesth* 9:569–575, 1997.

Patel RI, Hannallah RS: Preoperative screening for pediatric ambulatory surgery: Evaluation of a telephone questionnaire method. *Anesth Analg* 75:258–261, 1992.

Peacock JE, Luntley JB, O'Connor B, et al.: Remifentanil in combination with propofol for spontaneous ventilation anaesthesia. *Br J Anaesth* 80:509–511, 1998.

Pedersen CM, Thirstrup S, Nielsen-Kudsk JE: Smooth muscle relaxant effects of propofol and ketamine in isolated guinea-pig trachea. *Eur J Pharmacol* 238:75–80, 1993.

Pinsker MC, Carroll NV: Quality of emergence from anesthesia and incidence of vomiting with remifentanil in a pediatric population. *Anesth Analg* 89:71–74, 1999.

Pizov R, Brown RH, Weiss YS, et al.: Wheezing during induction of general anesthesia in patients with and without asthma. A randomized, blinded trial. *Anesthesiology* 82:1111–1116, 1995.

Poets CF, Pauls U, Bohnhorst B: Effect of blood transfusion on apnoea, bradycardia and hypoxaemia in preterm infants. *Eur J Pediatr* 156:311–316, 1997.

Pradal M, Vialet R, Soula F, et al.: The risk of anesthesia in the asthmatic child. *Pediatr Pulmonol Suppl* 11:51–52, 1995.

Purday JP, Reichert CC, Merrick PM: Comparative effects of three doses of intravenous ketorolac or morphine on emesis and analgesia for restorative dental surgery in children. *Can J Anaesth* 43:221–225, 1996.

Reyle-Hahn M, Niggemann B, Max M, et al.: Remifentanil and propofol for sedation in children and young adolescents undergoing diagnostic flexible bronchoscopy. *Paediatr Anaesth* 10:59–63, 2000.

Rice LJ, Pudimat MA, Hannallah RS: Timing of caudal block placement in relation to surgery does not affect duration of postoperative analgesia in paediatric ambulatory patients. *Can J Anaesth* 37(4 Pt 1):429–431, 1990.

Rieger A, Schroter G, Philippi W, et al.: A comparison of sevoflurane with halothane in outpatient adenotomy in children with mild upper respiratory tract infections. *J Clin Anesth* 8:188–197, 1996.

Rieschke P, LaFleur BJ, Janicki PK: Effects of EDTA- and sulfite-containing formulations of propofol on respiratory system resistance after tracheal intubation in smokers. *Anesthesiology* 98:323–328, 2003.

Robbins L, Connelly NR: An evaluation of the cuffed oropharyngeal airway for elective pediatric anesthesia. *J Clin Anesth* 12:555–557, 2000.

Rolf N, Coté CJ: Frequency and severity of desaturation events during general anesthesia in children with and without upper respiratory infections. *J Clin Anesth* 4:200–203, 1992.

Rose JB, Brenn BR, Corddry DH, et al.: Preoperative oral ondansetron for pediatric tonsillectomy. *Anesth Analg* 82:558–562, 1996.

Rose JB, Martin TM: Posttonsillectomy vomiting. Ondansetron or metoclopramide during paediatric tonsillectomy: Are two doses better than one? *Paediatr Anaesth* 6:39–44, 1996.

Rose JB, Watcha MF: Postoperative nausea and vomiting in paediatric patients. *Br J Anaesth* 83:104–117, 1999.

Roulleau P, Gall O, Desjeux L, et al.: Remifentanil infusion for cleft palate surgery in young infants. *Paediatr Anaesth* 13:701–707, 2003.

Roy WL, Lerman J, McIntyre BG: Preoperative hemoglobin values in minor paediatric surgery. *Can J Anaesth* 37(4 Pt 2):S7, 1990.

Roy WL, Lerman J, McIntyre BG: Is preoperative haemoglobin testing justified in children undergoing minor elective surgery? [see comments]. *Can J Anaesth* 38:700–703, 1991.

Sadhasivam S, Shende D, Madan R: Prophylactic ondansetron in prevention of postoperative nausea and vomiting following pediatric strabismus surgery: A dose-response study. *Anesthesiology* 92:1035–1042, 2000.

Saint-Maurice C, Meistelman C, Rey E, et al.: The pharmacokinetics of rectal midazolam for premedication in children. *Anesthesiology* 65:536–538, 1986.

Sandstrom K, Nilsson K, Andreasson S, et al.: Metabolic consequences of different perioperative fluid therapies in the neonatal period. *Acta Anaesthesiol Scand* 37:170–175, 1993.

Sartorelli KH, Abajian JC, Kreutz JM, et al.: Improved outcome utilizing spinal anesthesia in high-risk infants. *J Pediatr Surg* 27:1022–1025, 1992.

Schechter MS: Technical report: Diagnosis and management of childhood obstructive sleep apnea syndrome. *Pediatrics* 109:e69, 2002.

Schindler M, Swann M, Crawford M: A comparison of postoperative analgesia provided by wound infiltration or caudal analgesia. *Anaesth Intensive Care* 19:46–49, 1991.

Schofield NM, White JB: Interrelations among children, parents, premedication, and anaesthetists in paediatric day stay surgery. *BMJ* 299:1371–1375, 1989.

Schreiner MS, Nicolson SC: Pediatric ambulatory anesthesia: NPO—before or after surgery? *J Clin Anesth* 7:589–596, 1995.

Schreiner MS, Nicolson SC, Martin T, et al.: Should children drink before discharge from day surgery? *Anesthesiology* 76:528–533, 1992.

Schreiner MS, O'Hara I, Markakis DA, et al.: Do children who experience laryngospasm have an increased risk of upper respiratory tract infection? *Anesthesiology* 85:475–480, 1996.

Schreiner MS, Triebwasser A, Keon TP: Ingestion of liquids compared with preoperative fasting in pediatric outpatients. *Anesthesiology* 72:593–597, 1990.

Sears MR: Changing patterns in asthma morbidity and mortality. *J Investig Allergol Clin Immunol* 5:66–72, 1995.

Section on Anesthesiology, American Academy of Pediatrics: Evaluation and preparation of pediatric patients undergoing anesthesia. *Pediatrics* 98:502–508, 1996.

Shott SR, Myer CM 3rd, Cotton RT: Efficacy of tonsillectomy and adenoidectomy as an outpatient procedure: A preliminary report. *Int J Pediatr Otorhinolaryngol* 13:157–163, 1987.

Sidman JD, Fry TL: Exacerbation of sickle cell disease by obstructive sleep apnea. *Arch Otolaryngol Head Neck Surg* 114:916–917, 1988.

Slovik Y, Tal A, Shapira Y, et al.: Complications of adenotonsillectomy in children with OSAS younger than 2 years of age. *Int J Pediatr Otorhinolaryngol* 67:847–851, 2003.

Sneyd JR, Carr A, Byrom WD, et al.: A meta-analysis of nausea and vomiting following maintenance of anaesthesia with propofol or inhalational agents. *Eur J Anaesthesiol* 15:433–445, 1998.

Spahn JD, Szefler SJ: Childhood asthma: New insights into management. *J Allergy Clin Immunol* 109:3–13, 2002.

Splinter WM, Bass J, Komocar L: Regional anaesthesia for hernia repair in children: local vs caudal anaesthesia. *Can J Anaesth* 42:197–200, 1995.

Splinter WM, Schaefer JD: Unlimited clear fluid ingestion two hours before surgery in children does not affect volume of pH of stomach contents. *Anesth Intensive Care* 18:522–526, 1990.

Splinter WM, Rhine EJ, Roberts DW, et al.: Preoperative ketorolac increases bleeding after tonsillectomy in children. *Can J Anaesth* 43:560–563, 1996.

Splinter WM, Roberts DJ: Dexamethasone decreases vomiting by children after tonsillectomy. *Anesth Analg* 83:913–916, 1996.

Splinter WM, Smallman B, Rhine EJ, et al.: Postoperative sore throat in children and the laryngeal mask airway. *Can J Anaesth* 41:1081–1083, 1994.

Stewart JT, Warren FW, Maddox F, et al.: The stability of remifentanil hydrochloride and propofol mixtures in polypropylene syringes and polyvinylchloride bags at 22 degrees to 24 degrees. *Anesth Analg* 90:1450, 2000.

Strauss SG, Lynn AM, Bratton SL, et al.: Ventilatory response to CO2 in children with obstructive sleep apnea from adenotonsillar hypertrophy. *Anesth Analg* 89:328–332, 1999.

Subcommittee on Obstructive Sleep Apnea, American Academy of Pediatrics: Clinical practice guideline: diagnosis and management of childhood obstructive sleep apnea syndrome. *Pediatrics* 109:704–712, 2002.

Subramaniam B, Madan R, Sadhasivam S, et al.: Dexamethasone is a cost-effective alternative to ondansetron in preventing PONV after paediatric strabismus repair. *Br J Anaesth* 86:84–89, 2001.

Subramaniam R, Subbarayudu S, Rewari V, et al.: Usefulness of pre-emptive peribulbar block in pediatric vitreoretinal surgery: a prospective study. *Reg Anesth Pain Med* 28:43–47, 2003.

Suresh S, Barcelona SL, Young NM, et al.: Postoperative pain relief in children undergoing tympanomastoid surgery: is a regional block better than opioids? *Anesth Analg* 94:859–862, table of contents, 2002.

Sury MR, Black A, Hemington L, et al.: A comparison of the recovery characteristics of sevoflurane and halothane in children. *Anaesthesia* 51:543–546, 1996.

Tait AR, Knight PR: The effects of general anesthesia on upper respiratory tract infections in children. *Anesthesiology* 67:930–935, 1987.

Tait AR, Malviya S: Anesthesia for the child with an upper respiratory tract infection: still a dilemma? *Anesth Analg* 100:59–65, 2005.

Tait AR, Malviya S, Voepel-Lewis, et al.: Risk factors for perioperative adverse respiratory events in children with upper respiratory tract infections. *Anesthesiology* 95:299–306, 2001.

Tait AR, Pandit UA, Voepel-Lewis T, et al.: Use of the laryngeal mask airway in children with upper respiratory tract infections: a comparison with endotracheal intubation. *Anesth Analg* 86:706–711, 1998.

Tait AR, Voepel-Lewis T, Munro HM, et al.: Cancellation of pediatric outpatient surgery: economic and emotional implications for patients and their families. *J Clin Anesth* 9:213–219, 1997.

Tamura M, Nakamura K, Kitamura R, et al.: Oral premedication with fentanyl may be a safe and effective alternative to oral midazolam. *Eur J Anaesthesiol* 20:482–486, 2003.

Terasaki F, Kitaura Y, Hayashi T, et al.: Arrhythmias in Coxsackie B3 virus myocarditis. Continuous electrocardiography in conscious mice and histopathology of the heart with special reference to the conduction system. *Heart Vessels Suppl* 5:45–50, 1990.

Tobias JD, Burd RS, Helikson MA: Apnea following spinal anaesthesia in two former pre-term infants. *Can J Anaesth* 45:985–989, 1998.

Valley RD, Freid EB, Bailey AG, et al.: Tracheal extubation of deeply anesthetized pediatric patients: a comparison of desflurane and sevoflurane. *Anesth Analg* 96:1320–1324, table of contents, 2003.

Vangerven G, Van Hemelrijch J, Wouters P, et al.: Light anesthesia with propofol for paediatric MRI. *Anaesthesia* 47:706–707, 1992.

Veverka TJ, Henry DN, Milroy MJ, et al.: Spinal anesthesia reduces the hazard of apnea in high-risk infants. *Am Surg* 57:531–534; discussion 534–535, 1991.

Vichinsky EP, Haberkern CM, Neumayr L, et al.: A comparison of conservative and aggressive transfusion regimens in the perioperative management of sickle cell disease. The Preoperative Transfusion in Sickle Cell Disease Study Group [see comments]. *N Engl J Med* 333:206–213, 1995.

Viitanen H, Annila P, Viitanen M, et al.: Premedication with midazolam delays recovery after ambulatory sevoflurane anesthesia in children. *Anesth Analg* 89:75–79, 1999a.

Viitanen H, Annila P, Viitanen M, et al.: Midazolam premedication delays recovery from propofol-induced sevoflurane anesthesia in children 1-3 yr. *Can J Anaesth* 46:766–771, 1999b.

Villeret I, Laffon M, Duchalais A, et al.: Incidence of postoperative nausea and vomiting in paediatric ambulatory surgery. *Paediatr Anaesth* 12:712–717, 2002.

Warner LO, Teitelbaum DH, Caniano DA, et al.: Inguinal herniorrhaphy in young infants: perianesthetic complications and associated preanesthetic risk factors. *J Clin Anesth* 4:455–461, 1992.

Warner M, Kunkel S, Offord K, et al.: The effects of age, epinephrine, and operative site on duration of caudal analgesia in pediatric patients. *Anesth Analg* 66:995–998, 1987.

Watcha MF, Thach BT, Gunter JB: Postoperative apnea after caudal anesthesia in an ex-premature infant. *Anesthesiology* 71:613–615, 1989.

Webster AC, McKishnie JD, Kenyon CF, et al.: Spinal anaesthesia for inguinal hernia repair in high-risk neonates [see comments]. *Can J Anaesth* 38:281–286, 1991.

Weinstein MS, Nicolson SC, Schreiner MS: A single dose of morphine sulfate increases the incidence of vomiting after outpatient inguinal surgery in children. *Anesthesiology* 81:572–577, 1994.

Welborn LG, de Soto H, Hannallah RS, et al.: The use of caffeine in the control of post-anesthetic apnea in former premature infants. *Anesthesiology* 68:796–798, 1988.

Welborn LG, Hannallah RS, Fink R, et al.: High-dose caffeine suppresses postoperative apnea in former preterm infants. *Anesthesiology* 71:347–349, 1989.

Welborn LG, Hannallah RS, Luban NL, et al.: Anemia and postoperative apnea in former preterm infants. *Anesthesiology* 74:1003–1006, 1991.

Welborn LG, Hannallah RS, Norden JM, et al.: Comparison of emergence and recovery characteristics of sevoflurane, desflurane, and halothane in pediatric ambulatory patients. *Anesth Analg* 83:917–920, 1996.

Welborn LG, Norden JM, Seiden N, et al.: Effect of minimizing preoperative fasting on perioperative blood glucose homeostasis in children. *Paediatr Anaesth* 3:167, 1993.

Welborn LG, Ramirez N, Oh TH, et al.: Postanesthetic apnea and periodic breathing in infants. *Anesthesiology* 65:658–661, 1986.

Wheeler M, Coté CJ: Preoperative pregnancy testing in a tertiary care children's hospital: a medico-legal conundrum. *J Clin Anesth* 11:56–63, 1999.

Yentis SM, Levine MF, Hartley EJ: Should all children with suspected or confirmed malignant hyperthermia susceptibility be admitted after surgery? A 10-year review. *Anesth Analg* 75:345–350, 1992.

Zwass MS, Fisher DM, Welborn LG, et al.: Induction and maintenance characteristics of anesthesia with desflurane and nitrous oxide in infants and children. *Anesthesiology* 76:373–378, 1992.

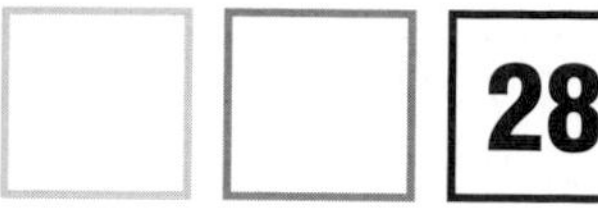

28 Anesthesia for Pediatric Organ Transplantation

Kerri M. Robertson • Avinash C. Shukla • Francis X. McGowan, Jr. • David S. Beebe • Kumar G. Belani • Victor L. Scott

With the exception of kidney transplantation, which became standard therapy by the mid 1970s, solid organ transplantation has only recently achieved status as an accepted treatment for a multitude of systemic organ dysfunctions. The introduction of cyclosporine in the early 1980s spurred rapid growth in transplantation. However, the number of cases worldwide has plateaued as donor-limited maximum levels have been reached (UNOS, 2005). Approximately 27,000 solid organ transplantations are performed in the United States each year. As of spring 2005, the number of patients on the waiting list by the United Network of Organ Sharing (UNOS) is 87,750, and this list only continues to increase in volume yearly (UNOS, 2005). Because the incidence of end-stage organ disease increases with age, children account for only a small, yet ever increasing, fraction (5% to 7%) of the total number of transplant recipients. Nevertheless, this means that approximately 2000 children undergo solid organ transplantation each year (Table 28–1).

In 1973, the U.S. Congress legally recognized organ donation as a voluntary gift by adopting the Uniform Anatomical Gift Act. In addition, the Omnibus Budget Reconciliation Act (implemented in October 1987) stipulates that hospitals will not receive reimbursement from Medicare or Medicaid unless written protocols for the identification of potential organ donors are established. Physicians now are routinely expected to approach families of terminally ill patients and request organ donation. Since 1987, the UNOS established uniform policies and standards, with a guarantee of equitable access of member institutions to available donor organs. Patients under this system are classified according to the severity of disease on a scale from UNOS 1 to 4.

- A UNOS 1 patient is the sickest and is confined to an intensive care unit (ICU).
- A UNOS 2 patient is one who is hospitalized but does not require ICU care.
- UNOS 3 and 4 patients do not require hospitalization; however, the status 3 patient is more debilitated than the status 4 patient, conceivably with secondary organ dysfunction by the particular disease process.

This system of stratification has been more refined for each organ system in the 2000s and is elaborated on in each section of this chapter as it pertains to the specific organ systems.

Organs procured in a local region must first be offered to patients within that particular geographic region, based on their UNOS status, before they can be sent elsewhere. Arizona is the only state that prevents its organs being sent out without being first offered to a patient specifically within that state. There are

TABLE 28–1. Number of solid organ transplants in the United States, 1990–2004

	All Ages	Pediatric	Percent of Transplants
1990-2004	336,359	26,607	7.9%
2004	27,022	1,816	6.8%
2003	25,462	1,794	6.7%
2002	24,897	1,749	6.6%
2001	24,208	1,719	6.5%
2000	23,236	1,604	6.0%
1999	22,012	1,654	6.2%
1998	21,511	1,653	6.2%
1997	20,300	1,647	6.2%
1996	19,748	1,595	6.0%
1995	19,389	1,608	6.0%
1994	18,296	1,553	5.8%
1993	17,631	1,533	5.8%
1992	16,133	1,378	5.2%
1991	15,754	1,456	5.5%
1990	15,001	1,397	5.3%

Data from UNOS.
Recipients with unknown ages were not included.

BOX 28–1 **Brain Death Guidelines in Children**

1. Diagnosis of irreversible coma
   Exclude all potentially reversible causes of coma: drug intoxication (barbiturates, sedatives, hypnotics, and alcohol)
2. Physical examination
   a. Coma
   b. Apnea (determined by standardized testing)
   c. Absence of brainstem function (no cough, gag, or sucking reflexes; no *oculocephalic* or *cold* caloric-induced eye movements)
   d. Normothermia
   e. Normotension
   f. Flaccid tone, absence of spontaneous movement
   g. Atropine resistance (failure to increase the heart rate by more than 5 beats per minute after atropine sulfate is given intravenously
3. Consistent physical examination during period of observation, as follows:
   a. Seven days to 2 months of age: two exams and isoelectric electroencephalograms (EEGs) 48 hours apart
   b. Two months to 1 year of age: two exams and isoelectric EEGs 24 hours apart, or one exam and isoelectric EEG, plus radionuclide angiogram showing absence of cerebral blood flow
   c. Over 1 year of age: two exams 12 to 24 hours apart, EEGs and isotope angiography optional, physiologic support measures established usually in the ICU. These measures include administration of inotropes, blood volume replacement and blood product transfusions

From Hosenpud and others, 1994.

236 kidney, 88 liver, 67 pancreas, 151 heart, 43 heart-lung, and 55 lung transplantation centers across the United States (UNOS, 2005). UNOS reports a total of 256 Solid Organ Transplantation Centers in the United States managed by 11 Organ Procurement and Transplantation Networks (OPTNs), which includes all states inclusive of Hawaii, Puerto Rico, and Alaska (UNOS, 2005).

Although collectively transplantation procedures are relatively uncommon, there are many published reports devoted to care of organ donors and recipients reflecting the broad experience accumulated with kidney, liver, heart, heart-lung, and isolated lung transplantation. Maintenance of physiologic homeostasis during the removal of a failed native organ and the subsequent allograft reperfusion period is among the most challenging of endeavors for anesthesiologists and surgeons alike. This chapter discusses the current body of knowledge for each type of major solid organ transplantation, with a specific focus on special considerations for clinical management of children. In addition, attention is focused on xenotransplantation, immunosuppression, graft-versus-host disease (GVHD), and posttransplant lymphoproliferative disease (PTLD), as well as artificial assist devices currently being used in the treatment of end-organ failure or as bridges to transplantation.

DETERMINATION OF BRAIN DEATH IN CHILDREN

Brain death is defined as the absence of cortical and cerebral function without preservation of brainstem function. Cerebral blood flow measured in this setting must also be absent. Publication of brain death criteria specifically addressing findings in infants and children has clarified most of the ambiguities created by age-related neurologic differences (Report of Special Task Force, Pediatrics, 1988). The currently accepted guidelines for determination of brain death in neonates, infants, and children are summarized (Box 28–1). Detailed reviews of this topic providing a thorough discussion of these guidelines and their application have been published (Ashwal and Schneider, 1991; Ashwal, 1993). Prospective donors must fully meet the age-appropriate criteria and be declared legally brain dead before personnel attempt to obtain consent for organ donation from the family. A physician must record the official time of death in the chart before transferring the donor to the operating room for the organ procurement procedure. Although the donor is officially dead, the care of an anesthesiologist is required to continue all needed procedures to maintain cardiac output and organ perfusion, at least until the viscera have been flushed with the cold preservative solution. At this point, ventilation can be discontinued and the responsibility of the anesthesiologist is concluded.

One area that remains particularly controversial is the appropriateness of organ donation from anencephalic newborns. This tragic developmental anomaly results in the absence of the cerebral cortex and upper brainstem, so that these infants possess no potential for normal neurologic development. Despite the uniformly fatal outcome in these cases, such infants can never meet the usual criteria for brain death (Baird, 1984). The use of prenatal ultrasonography has made the intrauterine diagnosis of anencephaly commonplace, thus providing the significant advantage of "planned donation." Because neonatal-sized organs are in extremely short supply, many professionals look to anencephalic neonates as a potential source to alleviate this shortage (Peabody, 1989). In addition, the positive aspects of organ donation for the parents of an anencephalic infant, which can be realized, is another benefit. However, there is no legal framework in the United States allowing the use of anencephalic infants as organ donors, and the ethical questions surrounding this practice are far from being resolved. Although at least one country has established legal parameters allowing organ procurement from these infants (Girvin, 1993), a significant change in societal attitudes must occur before such a practice becomes legal.

DONOR MANAGEMENT

Successful donor-directed strategies for the 2000s focus on increasing the size of the donor pool through expansion of acceptable donor criteria, adoption of a comprehensive donor management strategy, and innovative surgical techniques that allow organ sharing. Few cadaveric pediatric donors exist, so organ availability for transplantation is increasingly dependent on living donors (kidney, liver, lung, small bowel, and pancreas), split-liver transplantation, and asystolic, non-heart-beating donors.

Recovery of organs from the cadaveric/deceased donors requires continuing care of the patient's preexisting condition, with a shift in primary emphasis from minimizing neurologic injury and preserving life to protection of specific organs. Principles of pediatric donor care are comparable to those of adults, but meticulous adjustments are necessary due to special physiologic needs of children. The leading causes of death in children are asphyxia and trauma, and as such, a history of cardiac resuscitation, hypotension, and hypoxemia is frequent in this donor population (Fischer-Froehlich et al., 2002).

The primary responsibility of the intensivist and anesthesiologist is to direct therapy toward maintaining the normal physiologic sequelae of brain death and normalizing gross alterations in physiologic and biochemical parameters. Organs from cadaveric/deceased donors may be injured or damaged from preexisting comorbid factors, hemodynamic instability, endocrine, metabolic and electrolyte imbalances, hypoxemia, endotoxin release, and immune activation inherent in the brain death process (Jawan et al., 2002; Zaroff et al., 2002) (Table 28–2). By implementing an aggressive approach to donor care, it is possible to increase the donor retrieval rate by 30% without prejudicing outcome (Wheeldon, 1995). Use of the UNOS Critical Pathway for the Organ Donor has resulted in an 11.3% increase in the number of organs transplanted per 100 donors (Hommquist et al., 1999; Rosendale et al., 2002).

ORGAN RETRIEVAL

Organ procurement is usually completed in 6 hours or less, depending on the operating team's experience, the number of organs intended for retrieval, and the presence of variations in the vascular anatomy. In the face of worsening hypoxemia, coagulopathy, or refractory hypotension, the organ recovery surgery should be expedited to prevent ischemic injury to transplantable organs. The specific organ(s) to be retrieved determine type of fluid management and ideal central venous pressure (CVP), FIO_2, and the choice of allowable maximum doses for inotropic or vasoactive support. Management decisions are dictated by which organs are being considered, as, for example, hemodynamic goals preferred by surgeons transplanting abdominal organs are occasionally directly opposed to those of thoracic transplant surgeons.

Preoperative donor evaluation includes determining hemodynamic stability and vasopressor support, electrolytes and therapy for diabetes insipidus, pulmonary status, renal function and urine output, coagulopathy, and the degree of hypothermia. Routine anesthetic monitoring is supplemented with the placement of an intra-arterial catheter in an upper extremity to facilitate sampling and monitoring of the arterial blood pressure. The need for measuring CVP is especially important if the heart and lungs are being considered for donation. Arterial blood

TABLE 28–2. Normal physiologic sequelae of brain death

Sequela	Cause	Management
Hypotension	Neurogenic shock, hypovolemia, hypothermia, electrolyte disorders, endocrine abnormalities, myocardial dysfunction	Mean arterial pressure >60 mm Hg CVP 4 to 12 mm Hg PCWP 8 to 12 mm Hg SVR 800 to 1200 dyne/s per cm^5 Cardiac index >2.4 L/min per m^2 Inotropic support in order of preference (in mcg/kg per min): Dopamine <10 Dobutamine <10 Epinephrine <0.1 Norepinephrine and renal-dose dopamine Infrarenal aortic cross-clamp
Endocrine abnormalities	Disruption of the hypothalamic pituitary axis resulting in adrenal insufficiency; hypothyroidism, or diabetes insipidus	Volume replacement: correct electrolytes; inotropic support Steroids: methylprednisolone 15 mg/kg T3: 4-mcg bolus and 3 mcg/hr infusion Arginine vasopressin 1-U bolus, then continuous infusion at 0.5 to 4 U/h, titrated to a systemic vascular resistance of 800 to 1200 dyne/s per cm^5 Insulin: 1 U/hr minimum. Titrate to maintain blood sugar 120 to 180 mg/dL
Hypothermia	Loss of hypothalamic, neural, or endocrine regulation; resuscitation with cold fluids or blood products	Early aggressive warming to maintain the temperature above 36°C At <30°C may be unresponsive ACLS drug therapy, defibrillation, or pacing
Anemia coagulopathies	Hemorrhage, hemodilution DIC, fibrinolysis, dilutional hypothermia	Transfuse to keep hematocrit >30% Factor replacement, transfusion rewarming, early organ retrieval

Modified from Rosengard, 2002.

gases, hematocrit, electrolytes, blood glucose, and osmolality are assessed every hour, or more frequently as needed.

Strict asepsis is observed, prophylactic antibiotics are administered, and the donor is positioned and prepared surgically. The eyelids are taped shut and covered with cold saline compresses or ice packs for corneal protection. After 300 U/kg of heparin is administered and cardioplegia is achieved, the liver, intestines, and kidneys are flushed with cold preservation solution and sequential removal of organs can proceed. The spleen and omental lymph nodes are removed for tissue typing, and the aorta, inferior vena cava, and common carotid and iliac vessels are taken for vascular grafts. Anesthetic support of the organ donor is necessary until the proximal aorta is surgically occluded, and in situ flushing of organs has begun. Subsequently, the ventilator should be disconnected and monitoring discontinued as electrocardiographic (ECG) activity may persist for up to 70 minutes following cardiac arrest (Oakmne, 1975; Logigian and Ropper, 1985).

To avoid reflex muscular contractions and facilitate surgical exposure, a long-acting muscle relaxant is administered intravenously. The declaration of brain death requires the loss of cerebral and brainstem reflexes, but spinal reflexes may remain intact. Complex movements of the limbs and trunk can be confused with reflex movements of cerebral origin and may create tremendous anxiety for the operating room personnel.

In addition to spinal reflexes, a reflex pressor response to nociceptive stimuli is sometimes observed. This pressor response may lead to excessive operative blood loss and damage to the renal grafts. Management requires a reduction in preload, afterload, or both, while minimizing any possible adverse drug toxicity, especially to the liver and kidneys. Thus antihypertensive agents such as nitroglycerin or nitroprusside may be required if the volatile anesthetic, preferably isoflurane, is not successful in ablating this response.

Because brain death results in the loss of central mechanisms that control the endocrine and autonomic nervous systems, despite maximum physiologic support, cardiac death usually occurs within 48 to 72 hours. Up to 25% of potential brain-dead organ donors are lost each year in North America due to cardiovascular collapse (Jenkins et al., 1999). Hypotension and hemodynamic instability secondary to neurogenic shock and hypovolemia, due to the absence of brainstem function, should be anticipated in all donors and aggressively treated.

Intravascular Volume Management

Brainstem injury produces a sequence of hemodynamic events evolving from an initial increase in parasympathetic tone to a massive catecholamine surge with hypertension and tachycardia. Despite an increased perfusion pressure, the resulting vasoconstriction may cause tissue ischemia that disrupts the production of ATP, generates oxygen free radicals, increases cytosolic calcium concentration, and activates various enzymatic cascades, such as endonucleases or nitric oxide syntheses (Kunzendorf et al., 2002). A subsequent hypotensive phase caused by loss of autonomic regulation of the peripheral vasculature and unopposed vasodilatation may further reduce the oxygen supply to tissues. Hypovolemia is seen with inadequate replacement of blood and fluid losses, uncontrolled diabetes insipidus, and osmotic diuresis caused by hyperglycemia, mannitol, or systemic radiocontrast dyes administered during the evaluation process.

Aggressive fluid replacement therapy with colloid or crystalloid solutions and cytomegalovirus (CMV)-negative blood products directed at restoring and maintaining the intravascular volume is the first step in donor resuscitation. The hemodynamic status and adequacy of intravenous fluid resuscitation should be monitored continuously with arterial and central venous pressure catheters. In adults, hemodynamic targets include systolic blood pressure greater than 85 mm Hg, mean arterial pressure greater than 60 mm Hg, CVP of 6 to 10 mm Hg, and heart rate less than 100 beats per minute, with a urine output greater than 1 to 2 mL/kg/hr. The hematocrit should be maintained at 30%. The choice of crystalloid- or colloid-containing solutions usually depends on institutional preference and the sensitivity of the liver and lungs to low osmotic pressure-mediated tissue edema. When only the kidneys are to be harvested, the donor can be maximally fluid-loaded. For lung or heart-lung retrieval, relative hypovolemia is preferred. Infusion of colloids is recommended, with limited use of crystalloid and early initiation of inotropic support to maintain a systolic blood pressure above 90 mm Hg and CVP between 6 and 8 mm Hg. During the initial echocardiographic evaluation, if left ventricular ejection fraction is less than 45%, aggressive management with placement of a pulmonary arterial catheter, if possible, and hormonal (steroids, vasopressin, and T_3 or T_4) resuscitation is strongly recommended (Zaroff, 2002).

Hemodynamic Support

The goals of hemodynamic support are to achieve euvolemia, to adjust vasoconstrictors and vasodilators to maintain a normal afterload, and to optimize cardiac output without relying on high doses of β-agonists or other inotropes, which increase myocardial oxygen consumption and deplete the myocardium of high-energy phosphates (Zaroff, 2002). With persistent hypotension, despite volume replacement, vasopressor therapy should be initiated. Dopamine up to 10 mcg/kg per min is the preferred drug of choice because the glomerular filtration rate is increased as well as cardiac output while dilating the renal, mesenteric, and coronary vasculature.

When dopamine is used for inotropic support in infants, doses significantly higher than those needed in the adult may be required, presumably because of catecholamine receptor immaturity or deficiency (Kelly et al., 1984). At these higher doses (15 mcg/kg per min), no adverse effects on glomerular filtration rate or urine output are apparent (Outwater and Rockoff, 1984). An infusion of phenylephrine, epinephrine, and norepinephrine may be useful to increase peripheral vascular tone, but they have the inherent risk of causing marked peripheral vasoconstriction or an increase in pulmonary artery pressure (PAP). An infusion of vasopressin starting at 0.5 mU/kg per hr, then doubling every 30 minutes to effect or maximum infusion of 10 mU/kg per hr, may be efficacious in the setting of hypotension and low systemic vascular resistance (SVR), especially in combination with an inotropic infusion such as epinephrine. There is evidence that dopamine may reduce allograft rejection, not only through support of blood pressure but possibly also through more complex mechanisms that inhibit expression of adhesion molecules, which are required for leukocyte migration into the graft, to produce acute rejection (Carlos et al., 1997; Schnuelle et al., 1999). Dobutamine should be used where cardiac output is decreased because of reduced myocardial contractility and pulmonary hypertension.

It has been recognized that the state of brain death is a dynamic inflammatory process. The activation of inflammatory mediators leads to a nonspecific immune response, which may be associated with accelerated acute graft rejection and poorer long-term outcome (Kunzendorf, 2002). In addition, a significant part of organ injury after storage and cold ischemia is caused by reperfusion, initiated by leukocyte adhesion to endothelial cells and the production of oxygen-derived free radicals and peroxides.

ECG abnormalities are common during the brain death process, such as marked ST-T wave abnormalities or other ischemic changes, inverted T waves, widened QRS complexes, and prolonged QT interval. In addition, atrial and ventricular arrhythmias and various degrees of conduction abnormalities may occur. These arrhythmias usually result from autonomic instability (catecholamine storm and loss of the vagal motor nucleus) compounded by electrolyte abnormalities (e.g., low magnesium and potassium), acid-base disturbances (Newsome, 1979), or increased intracranial pressure (ICP) (Cushing's reflex). The difficulty lies in differentiating these transient findings from those of catecholamine-induced myocardial injury or irreversible ischemia, which can produce decreased biventricular systolic and diastolic function and contractility. Bradycardia is not a problem unless it contributes to hypotension. It may be treated with any inotropic agents or temporary transthoracic or venous pacing.

Eventually, the heart stops. Despite all therapeutic efforts, the arrhythmias encountered are usually resistant to therapy (Logigian and Popper, 1985). Bradyarrhythmias leading to asystole rather than ventricular fibrillation, as seen in adults, are the terminal cardiac rhythms in pediatric patients. The propensity for this particular dysrhythmia may be related to an immature autonomic nervous system and small muscle mass in the pediatric donor (Walsh and Krongrad, 1983). In the event of a sudden cardiac arrest during the procurement procedure, cardiopulmonary resuscitation should be started to facilitate organ perfusion, and liver, pancreas, intestines, and kidney procurement should proceed rapidly with cross-clamping of the aorta at the diaphragm and infusion of cold preservation solution into the distal aorta and portal vein.

Pulmonary Management

All potential organ donors require mechanical ventilation, usually for a period of several days. Subsequent deterioration of lung function may result from pulmonary contusions due to trauma, aspiration pneumonitis, fat emboli, and pulmonary edema (cardiogenic and neurogenic). Any of these may result in hypoxia, putting all organs at risk. In addition, infectious complications, oxygen toxicity, barotrauma, and atelectasis may contribute to an increase in the alveolar-arterial gradient $A-aDO_2$. Only approximately 25% of cadaveric/deceased donors of other organs are satisfactory lung donors. High-dose methylprednisolone administration has been shown to significantly improve oxygenation and increase donor lung recovery (Follette et al., 1998). The beneficial effects of steroids probably result from attenuation of the effects of proinflammatory cytokines released as a consequence of brain death (Glasser et al., 2001). As the total lung water increases from a combination of pulmonary capillary leakage and disruption of the Starling forces in the lung, pulmonary compliance decreases with resultant impedance of alveolar gas exchange. Neurogenic pulmonary edema is easily managed with positive end-expiratory pressure (PEEP). Lung protective strategies include maintenance of an arterial saturation of 95% or a PaO_2 greater than 100 mm Hg with the lowest possible FIO_2 setting, preferably no higher than 40%. Limiting high distention pressures in the lung during volume control modes of ventilation using small tidal volumes, low peak inspiratory pressure (PIP) and avoiding PEEP in excess of 7.5 cm H_2O is desirable. $PaCO_2$ (30 to 35 mm Hg) and pH (7.35 to 7.45) should be normalized. The maintenance of a mild to moderate alkalemia has been reported by some to reduce the likelihood of ventricular fibrillation (Becker et al., 1981).

Diabetes Insipidus

Diabetes insipidus (DI) occurs in the vast majority of brain-dead donors. It is a direct result of hypothalamic-pituitary dysfunction, with a resultant deficiency of antidiuretic hormone (ADH) from the posterior lobe of the pituitary. Typically DI is clinically manifested by a frequently massive urine output that bears no relationship to the intravascular fluid volume with urine hypo-osmolarity, serum hyperosmolarity, normal sodium excretion, and worsening hypernatremia. This massive hypotonic diuresis (>4 mL/kg per hr) then leads to dehydration, hypotension, and oliguria (Newsome, 1979).

Once the diagnosis is confirmed, treatment should begin with appropriate fluid and hormone replacement. Therapeutic intervention includes replacement of urinary losses with warmed isotonic or hypotonic crystalloid solutions on a volume-for-volume basis. In addition, vasopressin (controlled intravenous low-dose infusion of L-arginine vasopressin [AVP] at 2 to 10 mcg/kg per min) or desmopressin acetate (DDAVP) when the urine output exceeds 3 mL/kg per hr is administered (Levitt et al., 1984). DDAVP is an analog of AVP that is highly selective for the vasopressin V_2 receptor subtype found in the renal collecting duct and without the vasopressor activity in humans that is mediated by V_1 receptors on vascular smooth muscle. There are several mechanisms regulating the release of AVP. Hypovolemia, as occurs during hemorrhage, results in a decrease in atrial pressure. Specialized stretch receptors within the atrial walls and large veins (cardiopulmonary baroreceptors) entering the atria decrease their firing rate when there is a fall in atrial pressure. Afferent nerve fibers from these receptors synapse within the nucleus tractus solitarius of the medulla, which sends fibers to the hypothalamus, a region of the brain that controls AVP release by the pituitary gland. Atrial receptor firing normally inhibits the release of AVP by the posterior pituitary. With hypovolemia or decreased CVP, the decreased firing of atrial stretch receptors leads to an increase in AVP release. Hypothalamic osmoreceptors sense extracellular osmolarity and stimulate AVP release when osmolarity rises, as occurs with dehydration. Finally, angiotensin II receptors located in a region of the hypothalamus regulate AVP. Therapy should always be guided by serum electrolyte and osmolality measurements made every 2 to 4 hours. Several investigators have demonstrated prolonged hemodynamic stability in donors with the addition of an infusion of AVP to existing pressor support. Donors without clinically apparent DI can demonstrate a baroreflex-mediated defect of vasopressin secretion and pressor hypersensitivity to exogenous hormones. In these patients, low-dose vasopressin significantly increases blood pressure (Chen et al., 1999). Absence of AVP may be a predominant factor responsible for the eventual cardiac arrest in all brain-dead patients.

Vasopressin is a potent vasoconstrictor. Its hemodynamic effects are dose dependent and include generalized systemic vasoconstriction, increased blood pressure, decreased cardiac output, diminished coronary and renal blood flow, bradycardia, and arrhythmias. These effects potentially may cause irreversible ischemia to donor organs. Therefore, it is desirable to discontinue the infusion at least 1 hour before surgery. An infusion of nitroglycerin or nitroprusside is occasionally recommended to prevent myocardial ischemia and the potential untoward renal effects of diminished renal perfusion. Vasopressin supplementation (2 to 10 mcg/kg per min continuous infusion) in a porcine model of brain-dead potential organ donors resulted in physiologic levels of the hormone, with normal plasma osmolarity and serum sodium levels, and decreased urine output, potassium needs, and fluid requirements without effects on the peripheral vascular resistance or microscopic evidence of organ ischemia (Blaine et al., 1984). The benefits of early treatment for the polyuria of DI with a vasopressin infusion appear to outweigh the potential detrimental effects.

Endocrine and Metabolic Functions

Despite disruption of the hypothalamic-pituitary axis, hormone production from the anterior lobe of the pituitary gland persists in most brain-dead patients. Rapid depletion of vasopressin, cortisol, insulin, T_4, and free T_3 occurs in experimental animal models of brain death (Novitzky et al., 1984), but endocrine dysfunction in humans is usually solely manifested as DI (Wijdicks et al., 2001). Novitzky and others (1987) claim that true hypothyroidism exists as evidenced by a decrease in free T_3. They have shown that hormonal replacement therapy (T_3, cortisol, and insulin with glucose) improves cardiac output and reduces the need for pressor support. As such, many transplant groups administer thyroid hormones to hemodynamically "rescue" unstable donors who show evidence of anaerobic metabolism or profound hypotension refractory to volume resuscitation and therapy with multiple vasopressors. Three-drug hormonal resuscitation (steroids, vasopressin, and T_3 or T_4) has been shown to increase the number of organs transplanted per donor by 22.5% (Rosendale et al., 2003). Intravenous T_4 has the disadvantage of a slower and unpredictable onset of action. As a result of the inconsistent findings reported in the literature, the indication for T_3 or T_4 therapy is unclear. In fact, evaluation of a complete thyroid panel assay reveals a characteristic picture of euthyroid sick syndrome with T_3, T_4, free T_4 index, and free T_4 decreased or borderline, reverse T_3 increased, and a normal thyroid-stimulating hormone level (Robertson et al., 1988). One should keep in mind that while T_3 may rescue the donor heart, it may have detrimental effects, including tachycardia, arrhythmia, metabolic acidosis, and profound hypotension. Moreover, potentially many of the noted physiologic responses may in fact be a result of the absence of brain-blood flow in the brain-dead patient even with the partial circulation of the cavernous sinus system.

Electrolyte disturbances are routine, most being iatrogenic, as a result of treatment of the original injury or in response to physiologic perturbations during the brain death process. Hypernatremia is inevitable as a result of DI and a variety of strategies used to treat elevated ICP. The liver is exquisitely sensitive to hypernatremia (>155 mEq/L) with increased levels correlating with primary graft loss after transplantation (Figueras, 1996). Serum potassium, magnesium, calcium, and phosphate levels are often depleted and require prompt replacement therapy. Hyperglycemia may be due to peripheral insulin resistance or administration of large amounts of dextrose-containing solution for fluid resuscitation.

Hypothermia

Hypothermia is universal due to loss of thermal regulation by the central nervous system (CNS) (rendering the patient poikilothermic), exposure to a cold ambient temperature, and massive infusions of cold intravenous fluids. Although a mild degree of hypothermia may be beneficial to organ protection and preservation, the consequences of hypothermia, which are clinically significant, include diuresis, hyperglycemia, coagulopathy, arrhythmias, myocardial depression, pulmonary hypertension, hypotension, and eventually cardiac arrest (Reuler, 1978). Hypothermia further complicates the process of certification of brain death by causing the pupils to appear fixed and dilated. Active rewarming measures to maintain a core temperature above 36°C are mandatory and should be initiated early.

ORGAN PRESERVATION

Traditionally, optimal organ preservation has been achieved by the combination of maximizing donor hemodynamics, using improved surgical procurement techniques with minimal dissection of vascular structures, cannulation of the abdominal aorta for rapid in situ core cooling, en bloc removal of abdominal organs with separation of graft components on the back table. Cold storage techniques with a hyperkalemic hyperosmolar solution at a temperature of 4°C and treating the donor or recipient pharmacologically can preserve the kidneys for up to 72 hours but rarely do well in the recipient after 36 to 48 hours. The heart and lungs should be transplanted within 4 to 6 hours and the pancreas preferably within 6 to 12 hours. The preservation solution introduced from the University of Wisconsin (UW solution) in 1988 has allowed extension of the safe preservation time of the donor liver from 8 to 24 hours (Jamieson et al., 1988) (Box 28–2). Iced storage and core cooling result in a slowing of cellular metabolism and energy consumption; glucose or hydrogen ion buffers prevent cellular acidosis; and donor heparinization (30,000 U or 300 U/kg) prevents microvascular thrombosis, promoting even organ flushing and reperfusion. The use of hypertonic solutions or impermeates suppresses hypothermic-induced cell swelling. Addition of antioxidants and free radical scavengers protect against reperfusion injury. Pharmacologic manipulations available for pediatric donors include allopurinol (free radical scavenger), prostaglandin E_1 (vasodilation, membrane stabilization, antiplatelet effect), and methylprednisolone (Belzer and Southard, 1988).

BOX 28–2 University of Wisconsin (UW) Solution Composition

Potassium lactobionate: 100 mmol/L
KH_2PO_4: 25 mmol/L
$MgSO_4$: 5 mmol/L
Raffinose: 30 mmol/L
Adenosine: 5 mmol/L
Glutathione: 3 mmol/L
Allopurinol: 1 mmol/L
Hydroxyethyl starch: 50 g/L
Adjust pH to 7.4 with KOH
Add before use: dexamethasone (8 mg/L), insulin (40 units/L), penicillin (200,000 U/L)
Final values: $Na^+ = 25 \pm 5$ mmol/L; $K^+ = 120 \pm 5$ mmol/L; mOsm/L $= 320 \pm 10$

■ LIVING-RELATED ORGAN TRANSPLANTATION

Over the past several years, a consistently widening gap has become evident between the demand for and supply of transplantable organs. At the end of 2002, there were 2307 pediatric transplant candidates on the waiting lists for various organs, which was a small decline from 2382 candidates from the previous year. This was the first decline in 10 years and reflects a decrease in the size of the liver and lung waiting lists, with the majority of children wait-listed for liver and kidney organs. Unfortunately, the number of cadaveric pediatric donors has steadily decreased from a high of 1214 in 1995 to 805 in 2004 (OPTN/UNOS, January 1988 to October 2004). Pediatric cadaveric/deceased donors are more likely to donate each specific organ compared with adult cadaveric/deceased donors, as evident in data reported from 2002: kidneys (92%), livers (87%), lungs (16%), heart (50%), pancreas (40%), and intestine (9%) (UNOS/OPTN, 2005). With this serious shortage of donor organs of appropriate size and suitability for infants and small children, the waiting times for some organs has increased dramatically. For example, with only 20% of lungs from cadaveric/deceased donors meeting stringent donor criteria, the waiting period varies with 42% of pediatric patients waiting less than 1 year to 15% listed for 5 or more years. In 2004, 179 children registered on the waiting list died before a suitable organ was identified.

This chronic shortage has prompted the development of programs for living-related organ donation. The original concept was developed for renal transplantation in the early 1950s, and currently in the United States, 49% of pediatric transplants are from living donors (Seikaly et al., 2001). Justification was relatively easy, because a healthy relative could "safely" donate one of his or her two kidneys without jeopardizing renal function in the remaining solitary kidney and the results from living related pediatric renal transplantation had been superior to those of cadaveric transplantation, at all ages. Later, techniques were developed to use one or more left lateral segments of a parent's liver that would be suitable for a small child with chronic liver disease (Broelsch et al., 1991; Lang et al., 2004). Lessons learned from "split" or "reduced-size" cadaveric adult livers for implantation into children were used in the development of living-related liver transplantation programs, which can accommodate large children and small adults using the right lobe of the liver. From 1989 to 2004, 941 pediatric liver transplants from living donors were performed in the United States (see Table 28–1).

With similar methodology, living donor transplantation has been successfully developed for pancreas, lung (unilateral and bilateral lower lobes), and small bowel transplantation. In addition, there has been increasing interest in donation after cardiac death (DCD) with a National Consensus Conference in April 2005 and the hope of expanding this pool from 200 to 1000 donors per year in the United States. Although pediatric donors constitute close to 20% of the total DCD donor pool, very few of the kidneys (3 of 291) and livers (1 of 78) recovered are allocated to pediatric recipients (UNOS/OPTN, 2005). This practice may reflect concerns regarding long-term graft function, given the limited outcomes data available.

Living-related organ donation has, for the most part, been performed from parent to child. The use of children for living kidney donation remains highly controversial, and in general, most transplant programs will not use a donor younger than 18 years of age except in very limited circumstances, such as identical twins or an emancipated minor for his or her own child (Abecassis et al., 2000). Living-related donor procedures have several advantages, including the fact that they can be electively scheduled when the recipient is in optimal condition. However, with the exception of living-related renal transplantation, which has excellent outcomes with 1-year graft survival in children older than 1 year of age ranging from 94% to 96%, due to the relatively small number of transplants performed, the long-term functional outcome of living lung, pancreas, and small intestine transplants remains to be established. The incidence of mortality and graft loss is less for children younger than 2 years if they receive a liver allograft from a living donor compared with a decreased donor (Reding et al., 2003). In addition, many troubling ethical issues arise, such as the risk to the donor and recipient, validity of informed consent, and concerns about donor privacy and confidentiality.

Uncomplicated unilateral nephrectomy has an exceedingly low mortality (<0.1%), but the same is not true for right lobe liver donors (0.2% to 1%), left segment/lobe liver donors (0.06% to 0.2%), and right lobectomy of the lung (<5% mortality) (Middleton et al., 2005). Between 2000 and 2004, there were three mishaps in the United States in the field of living-related organ transplantation, and in one instance, the hospital's liver transplantation program was forced to close because an organ donor died due to seemingly avoidable causes. These cases have highlighted the significant risks associated with these procedures and why some have called for a moratorium in living-related organ transplantation (Stagg-Elliott V, *Am Med News.* April 2002; Grady D, *NY Times.* January 2002). Also, the true number of living related donor deaths remains in a quandary as worldwide there have been fewer than 20 deaths reported in donors for all organ transplants, hence, the skepticism of the known, unpublished data (Hayashi and Trotter, 2002; Trotter et al., 2002).

■ IMMUNOSUPPRESSION

Since the early 1980s, organ transplantation has emerged from an experimental therapy to a highly successful treatment for end-organ failure of multiple causes. The single most important factor in this progression has been the development of effective immunosuppressive regimens. This section focuses on the various immunosuppressive agents used, complications, and the emergence of newer agents.

History

The idea of organ transplantation dates from the early 1900s, and it has only been with the development of immunosuppressive agents that the viability of this field has reached its zenith today. Prior to 1981, patient survival was poor because of inadequate immunosuppressive regimens. Corticosteroids and azathioprine were the mainstays of therapy, with graft survival only in the 30% to 50% range. The introduction of the calcineurin inhibitors cyclosporine, in 1981, and, subsequently, tacrolimus revolutionized the field of solid organ transplantation with 1-year graft and patient survival rates as high as 90% and greater in some organ systems (UNOS, 2005). The main goal of any effective immunosuppression regimen is the prevention of organ rejection with minimal side effects and complications. This section reviews the various immunosuppressive agents commonly used for induction (primary) therapy, maintenance therapy, and treatment of rejection after organ transplantation; although varied for the different organ systems, the applied principles are almost identical. There is an emphasis on the calcineurin inhibitors cyclosporine and tacrolimus, the major agents used by most transplant centers worldwide.

DRUGS FOR IMMUNOSUPPRESSION

Corticosteroids

Corticosteroids were the initial mainstay of therapy for organ transplantation, although their use is on the decline. They are effective particularly in both prevention and treatment of acute rejection episodes. Their predominant mechanisms of action include the inhibition of interleukin (IL)-1 and IL-2 production, suppression of helper and suppressor T cells, suppression of cytotoxic T cells, and reduction in the migration and activity of neutrophils (Cohen, 2002). The use of long-term corticosteroids has been questioned because of their adverse side effects, particularly in the pediatric population. The trend since the 1900s is to use fewer steroids for maintenance therapy (Ascher, 1995; Margarit et al., 1989). Many centers do not currently use steroids as part of their long-term regimens. The first report of steroid withdrawal after transplantation was published in 1989 (Margarit et al., 1989). Everson and associates (Stegall et al., 1997; Everson et al., 1999) published a literature review that demonstrated that greater than 50% to 85% of patients can be withdrawn from steroids without changes in acute rejection episodes, patient survival, or graft survival rates. This percentile difference is noted depending on the antirejection agent used for maintenance therapy (i.e., tacrolimus versus cyclosporine). Steroid withdrawal is preferable as it is associated with significantly less incidence of hypertension, hypercholesterolemia, and diabetes mellitus; it is less likely to result in cushingoid features and delayed development and obesity in the pediatric patient. Despite controversy over their use in maintenance therapy, corticosteroids remain the first-line agents for the treatment of acute rejection. The response rates vary depending on organ system and depending on whether the patient is maintained on cyclosporine or tacrolimus (The U.S. Multicenter FK506 Liver Study Group, 1994).

Azathioprine

Azathioprine, the imidazole derivative of 6-mercaptopurine, was introduced in the late 1950s and early 1960s. Its mechanism of action is by the inhibition of differentiation and proliferation of T- and B-lymphocytes by blocking DNA and RNA synthesis. The net effect is a resultant reduction in the numbers of circulating white cells, both lymphocytes and granulocytes. One notable advantage of this agent is its steroid-sparing effect, allowing lower doses of steroids to be used with equal efficacy and fewer side effects. The use of this agent is limited, however, by noteworthy side effects, particularly hematologic and gastrointestinal. As many as 50% of patients present with bone marrow suppression and exhibit a profound leukopenia and/or thrombocytopenia while on treatment with this agent (Cattaral et al., 2000). Gastrointestinal side effects include pancreatitis, nausea, vomiting, and hepatotoxicity. Patients are at increased risk for opportunistic infections. An increased risk of malignancy, especially lymphomas and its reported incidence, however, remains controversial. The primary pathway of metabolism is by its inactivation of this molecule by xanthine oxidase, an enzyme blocked by allopurinol. The recommended dose of azathioprine is 1 to 2 mg/kg per day. Blood levels are not monitored for this agent.

Mycophenolate Mofetil

Mycophenolate mofetil (MMF; CellCept) is a morpholinoethyl ester of mycophenolate. It is well absorbed orally and hydrolyzed to its active form mycophenolic acid. Mycophenolic acid acts by competitively inhibiting inosine monophosphate dehydrogenase and hence blocks de novo synthesis of purines, primarily guanine. Lymphocytes, in contrast to other rapidly replicating cells, depend entirely on this pathway for purine synthesis. Hence, MMF's primary mechanism of action is the selective inhibition of lymphocyte proliferation. This drug is one of the newer agents introduced in the past 10 years and has been shown to be more efficacious than azathioprine in combination therapy (Fisher et al., 1998). There is also some experimental evidence to suggest that MMF may reduce the risk of chronic allograft rejection, which has been attributed to its antiproliferative activity against B-lymphocytes and arterial smooth-muscle cells (Azuma et al., 1995; Schmid et al., 1995). The most common side effects are gastrointestinal, including nausea, abdominal pain, anorexia, gastritis, and diarrhea. Diarrhea affects as many as 30% of patients but usually responds to a decrease in dose. MMF also causes leukopenia and thus should be avoided in combination with azathioprine. The usual dosage is 600 mg/m^2 per day orally in two divided doses. Like azathioprine, blood levels are not monitored with this agent. The antivirals acyclovir and ganciclovir increase MMF levels, and antacids decrease MMF absorption (Cohen, 2002).

Calcineurin Inhibitors

These agents are the primary immunosuppressive pharmaceuticals that have been developed to date, and they include tacrolimus and cyclosporine. Their effectiveness is via their interaction with calcineurin. The single most important cytokine in the immunology of transplantation rejection appears to be IL-2. It is produced through a sequence of events, which commence when a recipient antigen-processing cell comes into contact with the donor cell's major histocompatibility antigens (MHCs). The donor MHC fragment is processed and placed on the antigen-processing cell surface. When an appropriate recipient T cell is encountered, the T-cell receptor and the donor MHC bind. This initiates a cascade of enzymatic intracellular reactions via phosphorylation and calcium stores are released, which then combine with calmodulin. This calcium-calmodulin complex then activates calcineurin. Calcineurin appears to be directly involved in the pathway that induces the production of the IL-2 molecule. Cyclosporine and tacrolimus primarily act by binding calcineurin via the cyclosporine-cyclophilin complex or the tacrolimus-FK binding protein complex, respectively. Binding of calcineurin by either of these complexes inhibits its enzymatic action, preventing the dephosphorylation of nuclear factor of activated T cells. This nuclear factor of activated T cells must be dephosphorylated to enter the nucleus, where it is required for IL-2 gene transcription.

Cyclosporine

Cyclosporine is a neutral lipophilic cyclic endocapeptide extracted from the fungus *Tolypocladium inflatum* in the early 1970s. Cyclosporine is poorly absorbed from the gastrointestinal tract, and there is considerable variation in its bioavailability as biliary flow is essential for absorption of the drug. Neoral (Novartis Pharmaceuticals Corp., East Hanover, NJ), the microemulsion formula of cyclosporine, is much less dependent on bile production and flow than is Sandimmune (Novartis Pharmaceuticals Corp.), the standard preparation. Neoral gives a more consistent level of cyclosporine and is associated with less evidence of rejection (Graziadei et al., 1997; Pinson et al., 1998). Recommended oral dose is 10 to 15 mg/kg per day (3× IV dose). The IV dose is 3 to 5 mg/kg over a 20 hr continuous infusion. Neoral has replaced Sandimmune in most major transplant centers worldwide. Cyclosporine is metabolized by the cytochrome P-450-3A system (Cantarovich et al., 1998). Agents that induce these enzymes increase the metabolism of cyclosporine, resulting in lower blood levels. Conversely, agents that inhibit P-450 activity will result in higher circulating cyclosporine levels. In addition, cyclosporine can interfere with the metabolism of other medications.

Digoxin, lovastatin, and prednisolone can have significantly decreased clearance with resultant toxicity. The side effects associated with cyclosporine are numerous. Nephrotoxicity is one of the most significant side effects of cyclosporine, and it may present as acute and/or chronic renal pathologic alterations. The acute nephrotoxicity, which often resolves on reduction or discontinuation of the medication, probably results from afferent arteriolar vasoconstriction with resulting decreased glomerular filtration rate. The chronic nephrotoxicity, which does not appear to be reversible, is associated with arteriolar hyalinosis, tubular vacuolization, interstitial nephritis, and cortical atrophy. Neurotoxicity is another common side effect seen in as many as 50% of patients. This can range from headaches and tremors to seizures and coma. Due to variations in absorption and metabolism, cyclosporine levels tend to fluctuate. Dosing (10 to 15 mg/kg P.O. per day) should be adjusted based on the formulation used (i.e., Neoral versus Sandimmune) and serum or blood levels. Several techniques exist for the measurement of cyclosporine levels, including radioimmunoassay and high-pressure liquid chromatography. The levels can be measured in whole blood, serum, or plasma. Most centers use whole blood trough levels by the radioimmunoassay technique. A level of 100 to 200 ng/mL is generally desirable in the first 3 to 6 months after transplant depending on the organ transplanted. The level can usually be maintained at lower levels thereafter, again depending on the organ transplanted.

Tacrolimus

This calcineurin inhibitor, initially researched and brought to market under the name FK506, is a novel immunosuppressant isolated from *Streptomyces tsukubaensis* in 1985 (Kino et al., 1987; Starzl et al., 1989). Tacrolimus (FK506; Prograf) shares many similarities with cyclosporine, including their basic mechanism of action and metabolism by cytochrome P-450-3A, in addition to the side effect profiles. However, significant differences exist between these drugs, which have been elucidated in the past decade. Tacrolimus is 10 to 100 times more potent than cyclosporine, possesses hepatotrophic properties, and does not rely on bile for its absorption. Renal impairment, neurotoxicity, and hypertension occur with similar frequencies in both cyclosporine- and tacrolimus-based regimens. Tacrolimus is associated with more hyperglycemia. Reportedly, as many as 20% of tacrolimus recipients become insulin-dependent diabetics because of the agent's direct effect on pancreatic beta cells and peripheral insulin receptors. Tacrolimus appears to have a higher incidence of post-transplant lymphoproliferative disease (PTLD). Considering that accelerated atherosclerosis is an important issue after solid organ transplantation, it is important to note that tacrolimus produces less hyperlipidemia and thus results in a less adverse cardiovascular risk profile than cyclosporine. Statistically significant improvements have been seen in total cholesterol, low-density lipoprotein cholesterol, and triglyceride levels when patients were switched from cyclosporine to tacrolimus. A dose of 0.1 mg/kg b.i.d. is given orally (Manzarbeitia et al., 2001). Tacrolimus is given at an oral dose of 0.1 mg/kg b.i.d. Tacrolimus levels are usually measured in whole blood specimens by enzyme immunoassay techniques. As with cyclosporine, drug levels of 5 to 15 ng/mL are desirable in the first few months after transplantation depending on the organ system transplanted.

Efficacy of Cyclosporine and Tacrolimus

After its introduction, cyclosporine became the drug of choice for the prevention of allograft rejection. Tacrolimus, initially reserved for use as rescue therapy in refractory rejection, has now become a first-line immunosuppressive agent in many centers worldwide. Large multicenter U.S. and European randomized clinical trials have been performed to compare tacrolimus and cyclosporine (Sandimmune) for primary and maintenance immunosuppression (European FK506 Multicenter Liver Study Group, 1994; The U.S. Multicenter FK506 Liver Study Group, 1994; Wiesner, 1998). In the European trial, patient and graft survival rates were similar; however, significantly lower rates of acute rejection were seen in the tacrolimus group in some organ systems. More episodes of acute and steroid-resistant rejection were seen in the cyclosporine group. The tacrolimus group had a lower cumulative steroid exposure and fewer requirements for monoclonal antibody therapy (European FK506 Multicenter Liver Study Group, 1994). Patients on tacrolimus, however, had significantly more medication-related adverse effects.

At 5-year follow-up, tacrolimus recipients showed less rejection but there was no overall improvement in patient or graft survival for all solid organ transplants. Many of these large trials used Sandimmune as the cyclosporine preparation, hence confounding some of the data to date. Neoral has been shown to be superior to Sandimmune (Freeman et al., 1995; Mirza et al., 1997). Tacrolimus appears to be superior to cyclosporine for the treatment of rejection episodes. Episodes of acute rejection, even steroid-resistant episodes, may resolve when patients are switched from cyclosporine- to tacrolimus-based therapy (Jonas et al., 1996; Millis et al., 1996a,b; 1998). Also, chronic rejection has shown a response in more than half of patients converted from cyclosporine to tacrolimus for some solid organ transplants (Klintmalm et al., 1993; Wiesner, 1998). The choice of calcineurin inhibitor tends to be a matter of institutional preference. Many units are using tacrolimus-based therapy, citing less rejection, less steroid use, less OKT3 needed for immunosuppression, and less hyperlipidemia. However, many centers still advocate the use of cyclosporine (usually Neoral) based on equivalent patient/graft survival rates and a lower incidence of diabetes mellitus and PTLD.

Rapamycin

Rapamycin (sirolimus) is a macrolide antibiotic isolated from the fungus *Streptomyces hygroscopicus*. It effectively inhibits both B- and T-cell activity (Poon et al., 1996; Poston et al., 1999). Rapamycin is structurally similar to tacrolimus. It uses the same intracellular binding protein as tacrolimus but blocks B- and T-cell activation at a later stage than the calcineurin inhibitors. Rapamycin and cyclosporine appear to act synergistically to inhibit lymphocyte proliferation (Kimball et al., 1991). The oral bioavailability of rapamycin is variable. Like the calcineurin inhibitors, it is metabolized by the cytochrome P-450-3A system. The efficacy of rapamycin in solid organ transplantation was initially shown in the renal transplant population (Groth et al., 1999; Kahan et al., 1999; McAlister et al., 2000). Small studies in liver transplant patients have shown rapamycin to be an effective agent when combined with a calcineurin inhibitor (Watson et al., 1999; Trotter et al., 2001). Most of these patients could be maintained on steroid-free regimens. Acute rejection episodes were significantly decreased compared with historical controls (30% versus 70%) (Kahan et al., 1999, 2000).

The main role of rapamycin may be in allowing calcineurin inhibitor dose reduction in those patients with evidence of tacrolimus or cyclosporine toxicity (Brattstrom et al., 1998; Groth et al., 1999). The most frequent dose-related adverse effects include hyperlipidemia, leukopenia, thrombocytopenia, oral ulcerations, and joint pains. Both cholesterol and triglyceride levels can significantly increase and should be monitored while on therapy. An increased risk exists of lymphocele. A "black box' warning of its associated risk of thrombotic episodes in its first month of use is given. Calcineurin inhibitor levels, especially those of cyclosporine, have been shown to significantly increase while on rapamycin therapy and should also be closely monitored.

Antilymphocyte and Antithymocyte Globulins

Antilymphocyte globulin (ALG) and antithymocyte globulin (ATG) are produced by extracting immunoglobulins from animals (usually horse or rabbit) that have been immunized with human lymphocytes or thymocytes, respectively. The patient should be premedicated with acetaminophen (10 mg/kg, P.O.), diphenyl hydramine (1 mg/kg, P.O.), and methyl prednisone (2 mg/kg, I.V.) to prevent allergic or hypersensitivity reactions. The intravenous administration of these polyclonal antibodies (the dose of ATG, 5 mg/kg given over 6 hours) causes rapid and profound depletion of peripheral lymphocytes. A major limitation of all polyclonal antilymphocyte preparations is batch-to-batch heterogeneity, which results in unpredictable side effects and, importantly, variable efficacy. ALG and ATG are not typically used as first-line agents for immunosuppression. They appear to delay the onset of the first episodes of organ rejection, but the overall rates of rejection are similar to those seen with calcineurin inhibitors (Neuhaus et al., 2000). The focus of this form of therapy is as the primary immunosuppression in patients unable to tolerate calcineurin inhibitors (i.e., significant pretransplant renal insufficiency) and in the treatment of steroid-resistant (and possibly OKT3-resistant) rejection. Commonly observed side effects include allergic reactions, serum sickness, fever, and thrombocytopenia as with OKT3 and other systemically infused immunoglobulins. Cytokine release syndrome (cardiovascular collapse with a hemodynamic profile similar to septic shock, pulmonary edema, seizures, and renal failure) may be seen with the administration of these agents similar in kind to that sometimes seen with OKT3 or any other immunoglobulin. The incidence of lymphoproliferative disease is also increased among patients who have received ALG and ATG.

OKT3

OKT3 (Orthoclone-muromonab-CD3) is a monoclonal antibody specifically directed against the CD3 complex of the cell membrane of lymphocytes; it is an antibody specifically directed at the T3 antigen of human T cells—those cells that directly attack the transplanted organ—and is unlike the polyclonal antibody preparations. Intravenous infusion (0.1 mg/kg/day for 10 to 14 days) results in tremendous lymphocyte depletion. Induction with OKT3 has not shown any significant benefit over the calcineurin inhibitors (McDiarmid et al., 1991). Because of its toxicity and the availability of less toxic agents, OKT3 is generally reserved for patients with severe steroid resistant rejection (Portela et al., 1995; Wall and Adams, 1995). OKT3, ALG, and ATG provide 60% to 90% graft salvage rates for acute rejection in various organ system transplants. The side effect profile of OKT3 is similar to that of ALG and ATG, including the cytokine release syndrome, infectious complications, and malignancy potential. This protein, not unlike ALT and ATG, preferably is administered to a patient monitored for over 4 to 6 hours. Lymphocyte and platelet counts must be closely monitored.

Interleukin-2 Receptor Antagonists

As discussed earlier, IL-2 is the most noteworthy cytokine known to be involved in the rejection of transplanted solid organs. Although calcineurin inhibitors decrease the amount of IL-2 produced, IL-2 receptor antagonists prevent the protein itself from binding to the active lymphocytes by competitive inhibition. Unlike ALG, ATG, and OKT3, which target the entire lymphocyte population, IL-2 receptor antagonists specifically target the actively dividing cells by binding to the IL-2 receptor's CD25 moiety, which is only expressed in active cells (Langrehr et al., 1998). There are two available IL-2 receptor antagonists: basiliximab and daclizumab. Given its recent introduction into the armamentarium for immunosuppression, these agents have not been fully studied. However, early studies have indicated that these agents need to be combined with calcineurin inhibitors to be effective (Vincenti et al., 1998). No significant data exist at the time of this writing regarding the treatment of rejection episodes with these agents. While awaiting further studies, however, these agents should probably be used for induction of immunosuppression (Eckhoff et al., 2000) in those patients at high risk for calcineurin inhibitor-related toxicity. Also, they appear to be well tolerated without significant adverse effects. Dosing and timing for administration of these agents vary depending on the organ system to be transplanted. Moreover, it appears that IL-2 receptor antagonists are needed only immediately at the time of the transplantation (immediately before or after reperfusion of the transplanted organ), with a second dose at approximately 4 days in the immediate immunosuppressive induction period.

HEART, LUNG, AND HEART-LUNG TRANSPLANTATION

HEART TRANSPLANTATION

History

Christian Barnard conducted the first heart transplantation on December 3, 1967. The patient lived for 18 days before succumbing to a fatal bout of pneumonia (Barnard et al., 1967). The first pediatric cardiac heart transplantation was carried out within a week of this landmark achievement. The group was led by Adrian Kantrowitz, and the patient was a 3 week old child with Ebstein's anomaly and pulmonary atresia. The procedure involved immersion of both the donor and recipient in iced water to achieve topical cooling. As the recipient's chest was opened, the heart fibrillated and thus open cardiac massage was undertaken until such time as the patient's temperature was low enough to commence circulatory arrest (Kantrowitz et al., 1968). Over the next few years, about 100 more heart transplantations were conducted, with a mean survival of 1 month (Mendeloff et al., 2002). The poor outcomes were probably due to inadequate technological advancements in key areas such as surgical techniques, cardiopulmonary bypass, immunosuppression, and the clinical diagnosis and management of rejection.

The preliminary understanding of the immunobiology of organ rejection and its role in transplantation failure, the development of the bioptome and a grading system for rejection, and the isolation of a fungal extract with immunosuppressive properties that came to be developed as cyclosporine: all helped spur renewed interest in transplantation (Caves et al., 1973). Adult transplantation programs began to be established; pediatric transplantation during this early period was mostly in adolescents and was conducted under the aegis of adult programs. Infant and pediatric cardiac transplantation did not become established as a separate entity until the mid-1980s, when transplantation was recommended as a primary therapy for lethal congenital lesions, and successful heart transplantation in an 8-month-old was performed by Cooley and colleagues (Bailey et al., 1985a; Cooley et al., 1986).

There was a steady increase in the number of pediatric patients undergoing heart transplantation in the 1980s and early 1990s, with the rate peaking in the mid-1990s. According to the International Society for Heart and Lung Transplantation, 5002 pediatric heart transplants were performed in the period 1982 through 2002, representing just less than 8% of all heart transplants. Currently approximately 300 to 350 pediatric heart transplantations are carried out per year (compared with 3122 adult transplants in 2001). Mortality figures have improved significantly, with a 75% actuarial survival at 4 years for the period, in comparison with less than 55% for the early era of transplantation. As indications have continued to expand (see later), continued growth in pediatric heart transplantation has been limited primarily by the availability of donor hearts. In response, particularly for neonates, most programs have opted, whenever possible, for staged palliation of congenital heart defects, in order to avoid the uncertainty (and potential death) that placement on the transplant waiting list entails.

The issue of transplantation versus palliation in early infancy is far from settled. Proponents of transplantation believe that infant transplantation may be associated with enhanced engraftment and induction of tolerance, reducing the amount of immunosuppression required. Neonates in particular may experience a "window of immune tolerance," with a lower likelihood of rejection and the ability to use less aggressive immunosuppression (Boucek et al., 1990). Heart transplantation is technically more difficult and may be associated with higher mortality in those who have undergone prior palliative cardiac surgery. Transplantation as a primary therapy also may reduce the risk of progressive organ deterioration, particularly of the pulmonary parenchyma and vasculature, that can result from some palliative procedures or severe cardiac dysfunction arising after failed congenital procedures. On the other hand, the limited donor supply makes attempts at surgical correction the only option for many patients. Advocates of staged reconstruction argue that transplantation is a waste of resources in those for whom an alternative is available. Transplantation carries the attendant complications of rejection, immunosuppression, drug toxicity, infection, malignancy, and the need for retransplantation.

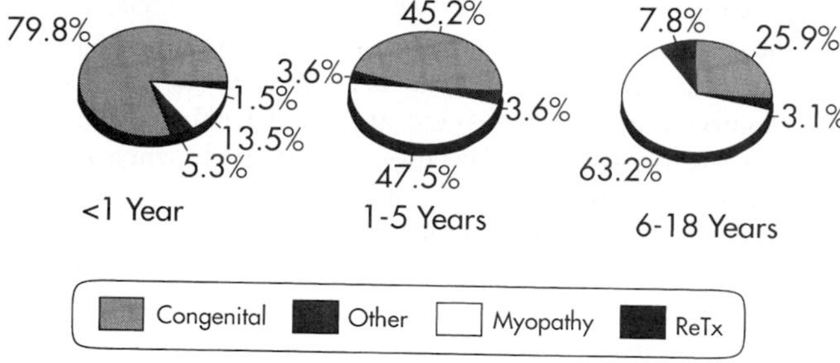

■ **FIGURE 28–1.** Indications for pediatric heart transplantation. (From Hosenpud JD, Novick RJ, Breen TJ, et al.: The registry of the International Society for Heart and Lung Transplantation: Eleventh official report. *J Heart Lung Transplant* 13:561, 1994. With permission from the International Society for Heart and Lung Transplantation.)

Hypoplastic left heart syndrome (HLHS) is an example that outlines the nature of this conflict. Five-year survival for this lesion following heart transplantation (including deaths while waiting for a donor) and the staged reconstruction procedures (Stage I Norwood palliation, bidirectional Glenn cavopulmonary shunt, and modified Fontan procedure) are essentially the same. The transplanted heart is structurally normal but is associated with all of the complications of antirejection therapy and, when done in neonates, may require one or more retransplantations due to chronic rejection and graft failure. Staged reconstruction for HLHS mandates life with Fontan physiology, and thus a significant likelihood of severe dysrhythmias and late ventricular dysfunction, potentially resulting in a need for transplantation.

Patient Demographics

Children younger than 1 year continue to make up the majority of the transplants performed (Fig. 28–1). There then appears to be a decreasing number of transplants for the 5- to 7-year-old age group followed by a second peak in the teenage years. This distribution is closely linked to etiology, with congenital heart disease as the major indication for transplantation in the first year of life and cardiomyopathy the primary indication in the older age groups. In 2001, 76% of pediatric transplants in children less than 1 year of age were for congenital heart disease, whereas in the 1- to 10-year-old and 11- to 17-year-old age groups, the percentages undergoing transplantation for cardiomyopathy were 51% and 63%, respectively. The majority of heart transplants in older patients with congenital heart disease are performed as these patients' palliative or reconstructive surgeries become inadequate to sustain a quality of life (ventricular failure, dysrhythmias, etc.). Valvular heart disease, coronary artery disease associated with hyperlipidemia, and myocardial tumors are less frequent (<2%) indications for heart transplantation in children. Drug-induced cardiomyopathy (especially anthracycline) is another infrequent indication, although there is some evidence that this may become a more frequent problem in pediatric patients as they age. Retransplantation accounted for 4% of all transplantations; this rate has not changed appreciably in the past several years.

Surgical Indications for Heart Transplantation

The development of cyclosporine and other immunosuppressive agents has enabled heart transplantation to become a viable therapy for end-stage heart failure regardless of etiology. Indeed, according to the International Society for Heart and Lung

Transplantation, survival at 4 years now exceeds 75%. It may thus be considered an alternative treatment to standard surgical procedures for certain congenital heart defects such as HLHS and pulmonary atresia with intact interventricular septum. The decision to perform transplantation is best made when patient survival is known to be unlikely or of short duration and other options have failed. As mentioned previously, the mortality rate of pediatric heart transplantation and concerns about long-term graft survival and immunosuppression must still be balanced against the natural history of the disease process and the results of alternative surgical repairs. For example, in the instance of dilated cardiomyopathy, particularly in children who are older than 2 years, heart transplantation may offer the only alternative to death. The case for transplantation for HLHS is somewhat different. For infants with HLHS treated with heart transplantation, data indicate 1-year and overall survival rates of 84% and 63%, respectively (Bailey and Gundry, 1990), which is similar to the survival figures for staged reconstructive procedures (Norwood and Jacobs, 1992; Norwood et al., 1992). In the current era, both of these techniques would have to be considered palliative.

Of note, data from the Pediatric Heart Transplant Study Group suggest that if one were to list all neonates with HLHS for transplantation, less than 10% would receive a heart. It has been argued that using a scarce resource for conditions that can be palliated diverts donor organs from those for whom transplantation is the only option (Morrow et al., 1997; Fricker et al., 1999).

Patient Selection

Congenital Heart Disease

Certain groups of infants have conditions that cannot be palliated. An example of this would be the child with HLHS that consists of aortic atresia and a perforated mitral valve. These children have abnormal coronary artery anatomy and coronary myointimal hyperplasia that can predispose to systemic (right) ventricular dysfunction after staged reconstruction. Infants with this anatomic variant might therefore be better candidates for transplantation, although this remains controversial (Freedom, 1983; Weinberg et al., 1985; Pigott et al., 1988). Other lesions in neonates and infants that may be considered relatively strong indications in favor of heart transplantation include pulmonary atresia with intact ventricular septum, univentricular heart, and unbalanced forms of atrioventricular septal defect or double-outlet right ventricle. Although these conditions can usually be palliated with staged reconstructive techniques, transplantation is often favored for these infants because of the high perioperative mortality rates (the result of problematic cardiac anatomy) and because outcome studies have shown poor long-term results of the palliative procedures.

Patients with poor outcome after palliative or staged reconstructive attempts are another group with congenital heart disease who may require subsequent transplantation. Examples include (1) patients with univentricular heart physiology in whom ventricular dysfunction has developed, thus precluding a Fontan procedure (some of these patients will also develop pulmonary hypertension necessitating a heart-lung transplantation); (2) patients who had undergone a Fontan procedure and now present with end-stage ventricular dysfunction; (3) patients with significant myocardial damage in association with anomalous left coronary artery; and (4) patients with ventricular failure following an atrial baffle procedure (such as a Mustard or Senning procedure) for transposition of the great arteries.

Dilated Cardiomyopathy

Dilated cardiomyopathy is the most frequent type of cardiomyopathy encountered in children. Although most cases are believed to result from a viral or an inflammatory etiology, definitive proof is often lacking. Dilated cardiomyopathy can result from other metabolic and genetic defects as well. Potentially treatable causes of heart failure such as carnitine deficiency and other metabolic abnormalities should be excluded. Children diagnosed with dilated cardiomyopathy at ages greater than 2 have a worse prognosis (Griffin et al., 1988; Chen et al., 1990); overall mortality exceeds 50% within 1 year of diagnosis. Factors other than age that are associated with poor outcome include severe cardiomegaly, decreased ejection fraction, and low cardiac output. These children usually present with systolic dysfunction (usually biventricular), congestive heart failure symptoms, and/or dysrhythmias. Occasionally, sudden death may be the first sign. Empirical treatment with diuretics, inotropes, and vasodilators is usually initiated. Although these therapies may provide some symptomatic improvement, it is unclear whether even maximal medical management can alter the natural course of the disease process. A subset of patients with dilated cardiomyopathy can present with acute fulminant myocarditis, which further exacerbates their condition. Some (approximately one third) patients with dilated cardiomyopathy may substantially improve after a period of intensive medical or mechanical (e.g., extracorporeal membrane oxygenation [ECMO] or ventricular assist device) cardiac support.

Dilated cardiomyopathy can also occur after the use of doxorubicin in patients who have undergone chemotherapy regimens for a variety of pediatric leukemias and solid tumors. Doxorubicin is particularly toxic to cardiac muscle, at least in part due to free radical-mediated mitochondrial injury. In addition to the total dose administered (especially in excess of 250 to 400 mg/m^2), other risk factors appear to be female sex and an age less than 4 years when treated (Lipschultz et al., 1991, 1995). It appears that early myocyte loss results in an inability of the heart to successfully adapt to the demands of growth and increasing afterload. These patients frequently present for heart transplantation a decade or more after cancer treatment (Wallace, 2003). One major unresolved concern regarding transplantation for this group is the risk of cancer recurrence in the setting of intensive immunosuppression. It is believed that a candidate who has no evidence of the primary malignancy 1 year after treatment has an acceptable risk for the introduction of immunosuppression. (Fricker et al., 1999).

Hypertrophic Cardiomyopathy

Hypertrophic cardiomyopathy is another major form of cardiomyopathy that occurs with some frequency in the pediatric population. A study found that hypertrophic cardiomyopathy made up 42% of all new presentations of cardiomyopathy during a 3-year period (Lipshultz et al., 2003). Left ventricular outflow obstruction and diastolic dysfunction as a result of increased ventricular mass secondary to left ventricular hypertrophy characterize this condition. Sudden death, most likely due to ventricular tachycardia, may also be the first presenting feature. Increased risk may be associated with young age at presentation, a family history of hypertrophic cardiomyopathy, and a history of syncope (McKenna et al., 1981; Maron et al., 1987). There does not appear to be a good correlation between the severity of ventricular outflow obstruction and the risk of fatal arrhythmia.

Furthermore, although symptomatic improvement may occur with the use of β-adrenergic blockers or calcium channel antagonists, these therapies (as well as others that may be used to improve symptoms arising from outflow obstruction such as asynchronous biventricular pacing and ventricular myomectomy) do not appear to have a significant effect on mortality (Wigle et al., 1985), thus making the identification of at-risk patients and the timing for transplantation extremely problematic.

Relative Contraindications to Pediatric Heart Transplantation

A number of variables must be assessed before referring any patient for heart transplantation. The presence of increased pulmonary vascular resistance (PVR), active infection, irreversible organ damage, pulmonary emboli or infarction, other severe systemic disease, active malignancy, and significant psychosocial limitations are the major factors to be considered.

Particular attention is given to the degree of pulmonary hypertension, as it is a key determinant of function of the donor right ventricle after transplantation and hence of overall outcome. The incidence of increased pulmonary vascular resistance in children who are admitted for heart transplantation is probably greater than that in adults because of the number of congenital pediatric lesions that can be associated with increased pulmonary blood flow or raised left atrial pressure. Increased left atrial pressure can also be a frequent contributor to elevated PVR in patients with cardiomyopathy. In adults, PVR of greater than 6 Wood units is usually considered to be a relative contraindication for heart transplantation. The upper limit of PVR that precludes successful heart transplantation in children has not been firmly established (Benson et al., 1991). It has been shown that right ventricular dysfunction or critical pulmonary hypertension after transplantation is unlikely in children whose preoperative PVR is less than 6 Wood units (Addonizio and Rose, 1987). This same group suggests that PVR index (PVRI) rather than PVR be used, in that the former allows some correction for body size. Others suggest that the transpulmonary gradient (TPG) is a more accurate predictor of early transplant mortality than PVR and that a TPG of greater than 15 mm Hg is associated with an increased risk, at least in adults (Murali et al., 1993). In the present era, most centers view increased PVR as only a relative contraindication, and successful heart transplantation has occurred in children with a PVRI between 7 and 15 Wood units. In such patients, one approach has been to attempt to distinguish a fixed, irreversible pulmonary vascular disease from pulmonary hypertension with a reactive component that resolves with insertion of a well-functioning heart. This distinction is frequently attempted on the basis of PVR response to vasodilators such as oxygen, nitroglycerin, prostaglandin (PG)E_1, or inhaled nitric oxide in the catheterization laboratory.

Previously, children in whom the PVR was reduced to less than 8 Woods units after 1 to 2 weeks of prostaglandin therapy were also considered for transplantation (Baum et al., 1991; Benson et al., 1991). Evidence suggests that long-term (months rather than weeks) continuous intravenous prostacyclin (PGI_2) can significantly reduce PVR, thus reducing right ventricular afterload and allowing for heart transplantation in a previously excluded group (Rosenzweig et al., 1999; Kao et al., 2001; Dandel et al., 2003). Another approach to transplantation in the presence of pulmonary hypertension in infants and children is to use an “oversize” donor heart (1.5 to 2 times the size of the recipient). The oversize gives the recipient a greater right ventricular mass to respond to the elevated PVR (Addonizio et al., 1989). However, the usefulness of this approach has not been statistically confirmed.

Patients with truly fixed and overly severe pulmonary hypertension are not candidates for orthotopic heart transplantation. Options include either heterotopic transplantation (the recipient's heart remains in place to assist with right ventricular work) or heart-lung transplantation. Both alternatives are less desirable. The operative and long-term mortality rates of heterotopic transplantation are increased (5-year survival, 54%) compared with orthotopic transplantation (5-year survival, ≈75%) (Kriett and Kaye, 1991). Survival after heterotopic transplantation is better compared with heart-lung transplantation.

Viral Infection

Cytomegalovirus (CMV) infection, in particular, is a significant cause of morbidity and mortality in transplant patients, as well as being a likely major contributor to the manifestations and severity of chronic heart transplant rejection (see later). However, the limited donor pool has made it impossible from a practical standpoint to exclude the transplantation of hearts from CMV-positive donors into CMV-negative recipients. Use of anti-CMV therapies such as ganciclovir has become a standard component of most transplantation regimens.

Whether hepatitis C viruses (HCVs) in the donor or recipient should be a contraindication remains undetermined. In a survey of 72 thoracic transplantation centers, 64% do list HCV-positive patients for heart transplantation and 74% use HCV-positive organs (albeit in either HCV-positive recipients or UNOS 1 recipients) (Lake et al., 1997). Those in favor suggest that HCV acquisition is better than the alternative (i.e., death without transplantation). The argument against is that a significant proportion of infected posttransplant patients begin to have progressive liver dysfunction within 5 to 10 years after transplantation. In addition, antiviral therapy appears to be less reliable; there also is an increased incidence of hepatocellular carcinoma in this subgroup (Fishman et al., 1996). A full evaluation of liver function should be conducted on a potential HCV-positive recipient before listing and the use of HCV-positive organs should follow the practice stated above (Fricker et al., 1999). There is a limited number of case studies of heart transplant patients with preexisting or acquired HIV infection, making definitive recommendations problematic. Despite the fact that these individuals may be immunocompromised and be more susceptible to opportunistic infections than other candidates, results in HIV-positive recipients seem to be encouraging (Calabrese et al., 2003; Morgan et al., 2003).

Psychosocial

Psychosocial problems and noncompliance are significant issues in the pediatric population, particularly in adolescents. Severe psychiatric disorders that cannot be controlled are a contraindication to the procedure. However, postoperative noncompliance can be difficult to predict and is an important risk factor for rejection and other complications. Reliable caretakers and a stable family structure are extremely important to the success of transplantation in infants and children because of the requirements for and stresses of frequent hospital visits, procedures, numerous medications, and chronic illness.

Donor Selection

Donors are matched largely according to blood type and body size. Typically, donor weight approximates that of the recipient.

As mentioned previously, if the PVR is increased, a donor up to 2.5 times the weight of the recipient may be sought. Human lymphocyte antibody (HLA) typing and donor lymphocyte cross-matching are usually done retrospectively.

Most infant and pediatric donors are trauma victims (motor vehicle accidents, child abuse); occasionally they result from sudden infant death syndrome or intracranial hemorrhage. Hypotension requiring pressor support (catecholamines, vasopressin) is common in victims with severe brain injury or brain death; it should not be inferred that it indicates myocardial dysfunction. Significant myocardial damage can result directly from trauma or secondarily from hypotension, hemorrhage, or ischemia. Routine donor screening includes a chest radiograph, electrocardiogram, and echocardiogram; mild contractile dysfunction is usually not an absolute contraindication to donation. There is some evidence that increased blood concentrations of cardiomyocyte proteins such as the cardiac-specific isoform of troponin I in donor blood is predictive of graft failure (Grant, 1994). Many centers administer T_3 (triiodothyronine) to the donor before harvest, based on evidence that it is associated with improved graft contractile function in the recipient (Novitzky et al., 1990).

In an effort to expand the potential donor pool, some centers have extended the conventional limits for ischemic times. One study compared ischemic times of greater than 8 hours with less than 90 minutes in pediatric heart transplants. They found no difference in early or late recipient outcome between the two groups (Scheule et al., 2002). Current practice recommendations suggest, limiting the ischemia time of the donor heart to less than 6 hours, and preferably to less than 4 hours, is likely to produce the least amount of myocardial preservation injury and acceptable graft function.

Infection, such as evidence of pneumonia, in the donor is relatively common. In general, rather than being a contraindication for the use of the organ, positive cultures in the donor are used to guide postoperative antibiotic management in the recipient.

Perioperative Management of the Pediatric Heart Transplant Recipients

Preoperative Considerations

In potential recipients, blood is typed to ensure ABO compatibility and a panel reactive antibody test (PRA [tests recipient reactivity to antigens in a panel of *random*, not donor, sera]) is conducted. In children with a negative PRA test, matching is done solely on the basis of blood typing. In children who react to more than 10% of random sera, a negative prospective lymphocyte crossmatch is ideal. However, this is not always possible, and strategies for the recipient with a highly reactive PRA include pretransplantation and posttransplantation plasmapheresis of the recipient, often in combination with intravenous pooled immunoglobulin (Leech et al., 2003). In general, preoperative blood transfusions should be avoided whenever possible so as not to stimulate antibody production; and obviously, transfused blood should be CMV negative for CMV-negative recipients.

The approach to the perioperative management of patients with congenital heart disease for heart transplantation should be based on a comprehensive understanding of the patient's cardiovascular pathophysiology. Outflow obstruction is characterized by increased pressure work, chamber hypertrophy, and a reduced ability to increase output. Optimal function is achieved by ensuring adequate preload and controlling the heart rate to allow adequate time for chamber filling and ejection. Left ventricular outflow obstruction requires the maintenance of SVR in the face of fixed cardiac output and coronary blood flow. Right ventricular obstruction may also benefit from reducing the afterload (PVR) where possible. In the instance of significant hypertrophy of either ventricle (or both ventricles), it is important to maintain coronary perfusion pressure (and hence aortic blood pressure) and oxygen-carrying capacity (i.e., hematocrit) to ensure adequate myocardial oxygen delivery to the hypertrophied muscle mass.

Valvular regurgitation may occur as a result of congenital lesions or severe dilated cardiomyopathy. Increased ventricular volume loading is the end result. Contractile function is preserved by keeping the heart rate normal to somewhat increased, in order to decrease ventricular filling time and volume and to optimize cardiac output. Other possible maneuvers include afterload reduction and inotropic support ("inodilators" such as milrinone or dobutamine), which tend to decrease chamber size and wall tension, as well as increase forward flow, and reduce the regurgitant fraction.

Large left-to-right shunts impose both volume and pressure loads on the right ventricle and pulmonary circulation as well as a volume load on the left ventricle. Systemic hypoperfusion, ventricular dysfunction, acidosis, oliguria, and eventual circulatory collapse can be induced by maneuvers that increase the magnitude of the left-to-right shunt, $\dot{Q}_p/\dot{Q}_s$ (i.e., decrease PVR and/or increase SVR). The increased pulmonary blood flow may also result in left atrial hypertension and pulmonary edema. Management involves the maintenance of PVR and preventing increased pulmonary flow with subsequent "steal" from the systemic circulation. Inotropic therapy may be required to maintain contractility and blood pressure.

Different principles apply to patients with cyanotic lesions associated with decreased pulmonary blood flow. Adequate oxygenation is dependent on the balance of PVR to SVR, as well as overall cardiac output. Increasing PVR or decreasing SVR can severely compromise pulmonary blood flow. A subset of children admitted for heart transplantation are dependent on surgical systemic-to-pulmonary shunts for pulmonary blood flow. The flow through these shunts may be marginal at the time of transplantation, either because of growth or due to partial occlusion or narrowing of the shunt. Under these circumstances, systemic oxygen saturation is increased by increased cardiac output and SVR; significant increases in PVR should be avoided. The approach to shunts that are large with substantial pulmonary blood flow (best indicated clinically by high systemic oxygen saturation for the lesion [typically >85% to 90%] and wide pulse pressure) follows that described above for large left-to-right shunt lesions.

Cardiac function in end-stage dilated cardiomyopathy occurs at the extremes of the LaPlace and Frank-Starling relation. This means that wall tension is maximal, subendocardial perfusion is easily compromised, and even minor changes in heart rate, contractility, preload, and afterload can lead to myocardial decompensation. The early addition of inotropic support may prevent bradycardia, augment contractility, augment myocardial blood flow, and minimize the negative inotropic effect of anesthetic agents. Positive-pressure ventilation can affect ventricular performance (Badke, 1982; Kaul, 1986). High intrathoracic pressure and large lung volumes can compress alveolar capillaries and thus increase PVR and right ventricular afterload. These effects can decrease right ventricular function. By the mechanism of ventricular interdependence, left ventricular filling and function can also be compromised. Hypoventilation may also increase

PVR by producing hypoxia, hypercarbia, and atelectasis (West, 1974). At appropriate lung volumes, positive-pressure ventilation often improves function of the failing systemic ventricle by reducing afterload (ventricular transmural pressure is decreased by the increase in intrathoracic pressure, thereby reducing afterload as per LaPlace's law).

The management of the child with HLHS awaiting transplantation merits specific discussion (see Chapter 17, Anesthesia for Cardiovascular Surgery). To maintain systemic perfusion via the ductus arteriosus, an infusion of PGE_1 (0.05 to 0.10 mcg/kg per min) is usually begun shortly after birth. Systemic perfusion may require further augmentation with inotropes and volume replacement. Any metabolic acidosis is monitored and also treated aggressively. A balloon atrial septostomy may be performed to ensure unimpeded left-to-right atrial flow.

The major goals of preoperative management of HLHS are to maintain systemic perfusion, promote optimal systemic oxygen delivery, and prevent excessive pulmonary blood flow; large increases in PVR are also to be avoided. Thus, a careful balance must be maintained between the ratio of pulmonary-to-systemic blood flow ($\dot{Q}_p/\dot{Q}_s$). Hyperventilation, alkalosis, and hyperoxia all decrease PVR and increase pulmonary blood flow ($\dot{Q}_p$), with a subsequent decrease in systemic blood flow ($\dot{Q}_s$). Therapeutic efforts are directed to maintaining normocarbia, normal pH, and the arterial oxygen saturation at approximately 75% to 80%. This range of SpO_2 is generally indicative of a "balanced circulation" (i.e., acceptable $\dot{Q}_p/\dot{Q}_s$ ratio) and generally favors appropriate systemic oxygen delivery, adequate myocardial contractility and blood pressure. If excessive pulmonary blood flow arises, nitrogen is added to the inspired gas mixture (delivered via either endotracheal tube or head box) in order to provide a hypoxic gas mixture (<21%). Intubation, paralysis, and induced hypercarbia (usually via carbon dioxide added to the breathing circuit in conjunction with normal minute ventilation) can also be used to decrease excessive pulmonary blood flow while improving systemic oxygen delivery and cerebral oxygenation (Tabbutt et al., 2001; Ramamoorthy et al., 2002).

Bridge to Heart Transplantation

A significant number of children die while awaiting heart transplantation. The number varies according to age, etiology, and degree of heart failure at the time of presentation but ranges from 23% to 70% (McGiffin et al., 1997; Morrow et al., 1997; Mital et al., 2003). Mechanical extracorporeal life support (ECLS) using either venoarterial extracorporeal membrane oxygenation (ECMO) or a paracorporeal ventricular assist device (VAD) has been proved to minimize myocardial oxygen consumption and permit myocardial recovery (Kirshbom et al., 2002). In children with end-stage heart failure awaiting transplantation, the major problem is duration of mechanical support. In the setting of transplantation, these techniques have increasingly been successful in supporting the failing circulation as a bridge to transplantation (Kanter et al., 1987; Delius et al., 1990; del Nido et al., 1992; Levi et al., 2002). Additional indications for ECLS include postoperative ventricular or pulmonary failure that prevents weaning from cardiopulmonary bypass, severe pulmonary arterial hypertension despite maximal medical support (alkalinization, inotropic agents, inhaled nitric oxide), and refractory postoperative ventricular or pulmonary dysfunction.

The selection of technique depends on patient size and site(s) of dysfunction (see later). When using mechanical support in the postoperative setting, care must be taken to exclude anatomic causes of graft dysfunction that require operative intervention. The ability of mechanical support to facilitate recovery also requires that organ dysfunction be reversible. These factors mandate both appropriate patient selection and the institution of mechanical support before irreversible organ injury occurs. The importance of the latter consideration was demonstrated in early studies of ECMO treatment of respiratory failure in adults, where prolonged mechanical ventilatory support before ECMO use was associated with pathologic evidence of irreversible lung injury, minimal improvement during ECMO, and poor outcome (Gille and Bagniewski, 1976; Zapol et al., 1979).

Extracorporeal Membrane Oxygenation

ECMO reduces ventricular work by reducing wall tension and maintains systemic perfusion and oxygenation. It is the preferred means of mechanical support in very small infants with myocardial failure and in patients who require supported gas exchange. Arteriovenous cannulation is usually used, although venovenous bypass may be used in a patient only requiring ventilatory support. The most frequent cannulation sites are mediastinal, using single right atrial and ascending aortic cannulas, and in the neck, with cannulas in the internal jugular vein and carotid artery. Left atrial decompression is required in any patient in whom left ventricular ejection is inadequate and/or whose left atrium is not decompressed (i.e., via a patent foramen ovale or atrial septal defect). This can be achieved via a separate left submammary approach to the apex of the heart or right anterior thoracotomy to the left atrium if the chest is closed. The femoral and iliac vessels in infants and young children (<10 to 15 kg) cannot usually accommodate cannulas of sufficient size to permit complete circulatory support. ECMO should be instituted early before significant nonthoracic end-organ damage has occurred, and complications such as pulmonary edema and infection should be treated aggressively.

The minimal circuit volume is usually 300 to 400 mL, and the whole system consists of tubing, a reservoir, a membrane oxygenator, and heat exchanger. Before cannulation, heparin (100 to 200 units/kg) is administered intravenously with confirmation that systemic administration has occurred by measurement of the activated clotting time (ACT). The ACT is usually maintained between 180 and 200 seconds with a heparin infusion. Larger than usual doses of heparin, as well as other drugs that are lipophilic (such as fentanyl or midazolam), may be required because of binding to the circuit and oxygenator (Rosen et al., 1990). Perfusion flow rates range from 100 to 125 mL/kg per min for full circulatory support. An increased flow rate is required in the presence of a patent shunt, which also may need to be narrowed or occluded if systemic perfusion remains inadequate. Appropriate blood products are used to maintain the hematocrit between 35% and 45% and the platelet count greater than 100,00/mm^3. Fresh-frozen plasma or cryoprecipitate may be needed to maintain adequate concentrations of clotting factors. If possible, the skin should be closed over the chest and cannulas, or a surgical membrane should be used instead. Echocardiography may be used frequently during ECMO to assess cardiac structure, global contractile function, and the need for left atrial venting or the evacuation of fluid and blood collections.

Once ECMO is established, levels of inotropic support are reduced. Ventilatory support and the FIO_2 are also decreased, although infrequent lung expansion (4 to 6 breaths/min) and low levels of PEEP are used to stabilize lung volumes, prevent alveolar collapse, and limit inactivation of alveolar surfactant.

Greater amounts of PEEP may be indicated in the presence of significant pulmonary disease (Keszler et al., 1989). Mechanical ventilation of surfactant-deficient lungs may exacerbate lung injury (Jobe et al., 1985). Exogenous surfactant administration may have a role in improving pulmonary function and facilitating weaning from ECMO in patients with lung injury (Lewis and Jobe, 1993; McGowan et al., 1993).

ECMO has been used successfully as a bridge to cardiac transplantation, as well as a mechanism to permit recovery in instances of severe postcardiotomy myocardial failure, including acute cardiac allograft failure (del Nido, 1994; Duncan, 1998). In one study (Delius et al., 1990), all (three of three) patients placed on ECMO while awaiting transplantation died. Del Nido (1996) reported on 14 children who were considered candidates for heart transplantation and were placed on ECMO as a bridge to transplantation. In this series, eight children had postcardiotomy myocardial dysfunction, three had dilated cardiomyopathy, and three had acute viral myocarditis. Five of the 14 patients were placed on ECMO during cardiopulmonary resuscitation. Nine patients underwent a heart transplant and seven patients had long-term survival. One patient with viral myocarditis recovered spontaneously. Four patients died of sepsis while on ECMO, and one late death occurred from PTLD.

Poor outcome associated with ECMO is usually due to the presence of significant coexisting disease or injury. Complications from ECMO include hemorrhage, renal dysfunction, neurologic injury, infection, dysrhythmias, and difficulties with maintaining adequate nutrition (Kanter et al., 1987; Weinhaus et al., 1989; Delius et al., 1990; Pennington and Swartz, 1993).

ECMO may also be used to support the failing heart after transplantation. Delius and others (1990) reported on the early survival of two of three patients placed on ECMO postoperatively for acute rejection or graft dysfunction. In patients with congenital heart disease requiring postoperative ECMO support, overall survival was between 40% and 70% (Kanter et al., 1987; Rogers et al., 1989; Weinhaus et al., 1989). Outcome appears to be substantially better in children who are placed on ECMO postoperatively after an initial period without circulatory support compared with those who require ECMO in the operating room to wean from CPB. This may reflect a more serious degree of irreversible cardiac injury in those patients requiring ECMO to wean from CPB. Major bleeding complications also appear to be less in this setting if the patient has some period off of CPB and before institution of ECMO. Sustained dysrhythmias are also likely to indicate severe myocardial injury and poor outcome. Left atrial decompression to reduce left ventricular end-diastolic pressure (LVEDP) and increase subendocardial perfusion may improve myocardial and pulmonary function in these patients.

ECMO is not designed for long-term use, and after a period of greater than 6 weeks, the risk of bleeding, sepsis, and end-organ dysfunction becomes prohibitive. VADs have been demonstrated in the adult population to be capable of supporting patients for many months without end-organ damage (Farrar et al., 1994). Both systems are not exclusive of one another and many children may be placed on ECMO in the emergent situation and converted to a VAD on an elective basis. Despite the successful use of small-size adult VADs in children (Helman et al., 2000; Reinhartz et al., 2001), until recently, the only choice for mechanical support in neonates was ECMO. However, the development of miniature pediatric-sized VADs has permitted the use of pulsatile mechanical support in neonates and children, and the number and types of these devices that are available for long-term ventricular support of infants and children is increasing (Hetzer et al., 1998; Schindler, 2003). In an outcome study following transplantation, Stiller and others (2003) noted no significant difference in short- or long-term mortality, neurologic outcome or acute rejection in those patients who had a VAD device placed compared with those who did not.

Partial Ventriculectomy

Another method that deserves mention as a bridge to transplantation is the use of partial ventriculectomy and mitral valve repair. This method has been used successfully to provide a biological rather than mechanical bridge in the period before transplantation in the child with dilated, end-stage cardiomyopathy (Hsu et al., 2002).

Anesthetic Management

The anesthetic management of the pediatric heart transplant recipient requires a thorough understanding of the pathophysiology of the particular condition. One begins with an analysis of the patient's anatomy and assessment of cardiopulmonary function. It is useful to then outline the events that will improve or destabilize contractile function, pulmonary blood flow, and systemic perfusion. One can then formulate an anesthetic plan based on these variables and the predicted responses to anesthetic agents, cardiovascular drugs, and ventilatory manipulations.

Premedication

Most children coming for heart transplantation, regardless of whether they have fasted, should probably be considered to have full stomachs because of their debilitated state and poor perfusion. Therefore, the administration of nonparticulate antacids or H_2 antagonists and metoclopramide may be advisable. Sedative premedication is avoided or administered cautiously in those patients with severe ventricular dysfunction. In addition to limiting anxiety, reoperative sedation can decrease PVR and myocardial oxygen demand and increase systemic saturations.

Monitoring

Standard noninvasive monitors, including a precordial stethoscope, pulse oximeter, three-lead ECG, and a noninvasive automated blood pressure monitor, are placed before induction. Arterial and central venous catheters and temperature monitors are generally placed after the induction of anesthesia and intubation of the patient's trachea. If the child has significant ventricular dysfunction, the arterial catheter may be placed using local anesthesia before induction. The avoidance of right internal jugular cannulation to preserve the vessel for subsequent endomyocardial biopsies is advocated by some. Routine pulmonary arterial catheterization before CPB has not been found to be beneficial (Martin et al., 1989). In those patients in whom such monitoring may be warranted (e.g., those with a potential for increased PVR), one practice is to insert the vascular sheath after induction. A thermodilution/oximetric catheter (4 Fr or greater) can then be passed into the pulmonary artery with surgical assistance before terminating CPB.

Induction and Maintenance of Anesthesia

Agents should be selected according to their effects on heart rate, contractility, and vascular resistance (see Chapter 3, Cardiovascular Physiology in Infants and Children, and Chapter 6, Pharmacology). Intravenous induction agents are generally preferred. Among intravenous agents, ketamine, etomidate, and high-dose synthetic opioids have all been used in pediatric patients. Ketamine or etomidate can be combined with succinylcholine or high-dose rocuronium/ vecuronium if a rapid sequence induction is required. Ketamine will effectively preserve myocardial contractility and SVR in patients with relatively normal myocardial function and adrenergic tone. In patients with severe cardiomyopathy, the ability to increase stroke volume is absent, adrenergic receptors are downregulated as a result of increased circulating catecholamines, and sympathetic tone is already maximal. Ketamine may then reduce cardiac output as a result of its direct negative inotropic effects; if ketamine administration is accompanied by increased SVR, stroke volume, particularly by the myopathic heart, may be reduced further (Gutzke et al., 1989). Etomidate probably produces minimal effects on contractility and vascular resistances at standard induction doses, although Pagel and others (1998) noted in experimental animals that etomidate-induced increases in aortic impedance could potentially reduce the contractility of the failing systemic ventricle. The opioids fentanyl and sufentanil are generally well tolerated in children. A delay in the time to peak effect of fentanyl and perhaps increased sensitivity to the drug are apparent in patients with severely reduced ventricular function (Benowitz and Meister, 1976; Wynands et al., 1983). These factors mandate slow administration and careful titration in children with congestive heart failure. Larger doses of fentanyl (25 to 75 mcg/kg) and sufentanil (5 to 10 mcg/kg) can effectively blunt increases in PVR and provide extended hemodynamic stability.

Pancuronium may be a useful muscle relaxant to offset the vagotonic and bradycardic effects of fentanyl and sufentanil. Vecuronium or rocuronium may be used in patients in whom minimal effects on heart rate and blood pressure are preferred. Severe bradycardia and even asystole have been reported from the use of vecuronium and sufentanil in combination (Starr et al., 1986).

Scopolamine may be useful for providing amnesia if a narcotic technique is used. Benzodiazepines can cause significant reductions in myocardial contractility and SVR when given in combination with potent opioids (Tomicheck et al., 1983). Barbiturates decrease SVR and myocardial contractility. They should be avoided unless ventricular function is known to be preserved.

Inhalation induction is used infrequently in this group of patients because of the hemodynamic side effects of myocardial depression and hypotension as well as the increased risk of aspiration (Borland, 1985; Demas et al., 1986). An inhalation induction with sevoflurane and careful airway management can be a satisfactory approach for the infant with congenital heart disease and preserved ventricular function. Nitrous oxide is usually avoided in older children with cardiomyopathy or increased PVR because of potentially significant reductions in myocardial contractility and uncertain effects on PVR (Lappas et al., 1975; Schulte-Sasse et al., 1982). However, in infants, Hickey and others (1986) showed that N_2O does not produce the elevations in PAP and pulmonary artery resistance seen in adults.

A right-to-left shunt will slow the rate of inhalation induction because less anesthetic is taken up from the lungs. The magnitude of slowing is less when using more soluble agents because rapid uptake of soluble agents makes alveolar delivery the rate-limiting step. For insoluble agents such as nitrous oxide and sevoflurane, right-to-left shunts slow induction appreciably (see Chapter 6, Pharmacology). Of note, anesthetic removal rates and the ability to change anesthetic depth are similarly slowed, and thus inhaled anesthetic excess will be difficult to reverse in patients with significant right-to-left shunts. Left-to-right shunts do not affect the rate of inhaled induction in an appreciable manner (Tanner et al., 1985).

In summary, the potential for circulatory collapse during induction of anesthesia and conversion to positive-pressure ventilation should be anticipated in the patient with severely compromised ventricular function or circulatory instability, regardless of the chosen anesthetic technique. In patients with relatively severe contractile dysfunction, it may be helpful to institute inotropic support before induction. Response to volume expansion, inotropic support, defibrillation, and other resuscitative measures is infrequent when it occurs in this setting in the severely compromised heart. The ability to proceed immediately to CPB should be available.

Operative Management

The surgical technique of pediatric heart transplantation is similar to that used in adults (Figs. 28–2 and 28–3). Increased technical difficulty and risk of hemorrhage before bypass should be expected in children who have had previous heart surgery. Hypothermic CPB is standard. A period of deep hypothermia with circulatory arrest is often required in young infants (e.g., HLHS) and those requiring extensive aortic or other vascular reconstruction (Mavroudis et al., 1988; Bailey et al., 1989). The usual duration of circulatory arrest is less than 1 hour; longer periods increase the risk for some degree of irreversible cerebral insult.

For infants with HLHS, the pulmonary artery is cannulated as the arterial inflow site for CPB (systemic blood flow occurs via the ductus arteriosus). Complicated repairs with extensive suture lines and anastomoses may be necessary in infants with HLHS (because of aortic hypoplasia), abnormalities of the pulmonary arteries (because of pulmonary atresia, truncus arteriosus, previous banding, or Fontan procedures), or abnormalities of the superior vena cava (after a Glenn anastomosis). Such reconstruction increases the overall risk of the procedure by prolonging the duration of bypass and circulatory arrest and also increasing the severity of postbypass bleeding.

Acute right ventricular dysfunction is one of the major problems in the transplanted heart immediately after CPB. The initial approach is to minimize PVR in order to reduce right ventricular afterload. Ventilatory manipulations are initially used to reduce PVR and optimize right ventricular (and consequently, left ventricular) performance. Before termination of CPB, the endotracheal tube is suctioned and several vital capacity inflations are performed to expand atelectatic lungs. Moderate hyperventilation with 100% oxygen is then used to maximize alveolar and arterial oxygen tension and achieve a $Pa{CO_2}$ in the range of 25 to 30 mm Hg. While no specific mode of ventilation can be universally recommended, in general the use of larger tidal volumes (e.g., >10 mL/kg) and slower respiratory rates frequently appears to provide the best balance between minute ventilation and deleterious effects on right ventricular filling and function. The use of PEEP to improve gas exchange usually does not adversely affect PVR. In addition to hyperoxia and alkalinization (via both ventilation and supplemental sodium bicarbonate), inhaled nitric oxide can be a valuable therapy in the transplant patient at risk for post-CPB pulmonary hypertension. Other maneuvers to support the failing right ventricle include ensuring adequate coronary perfusion pressure, preload, and use of

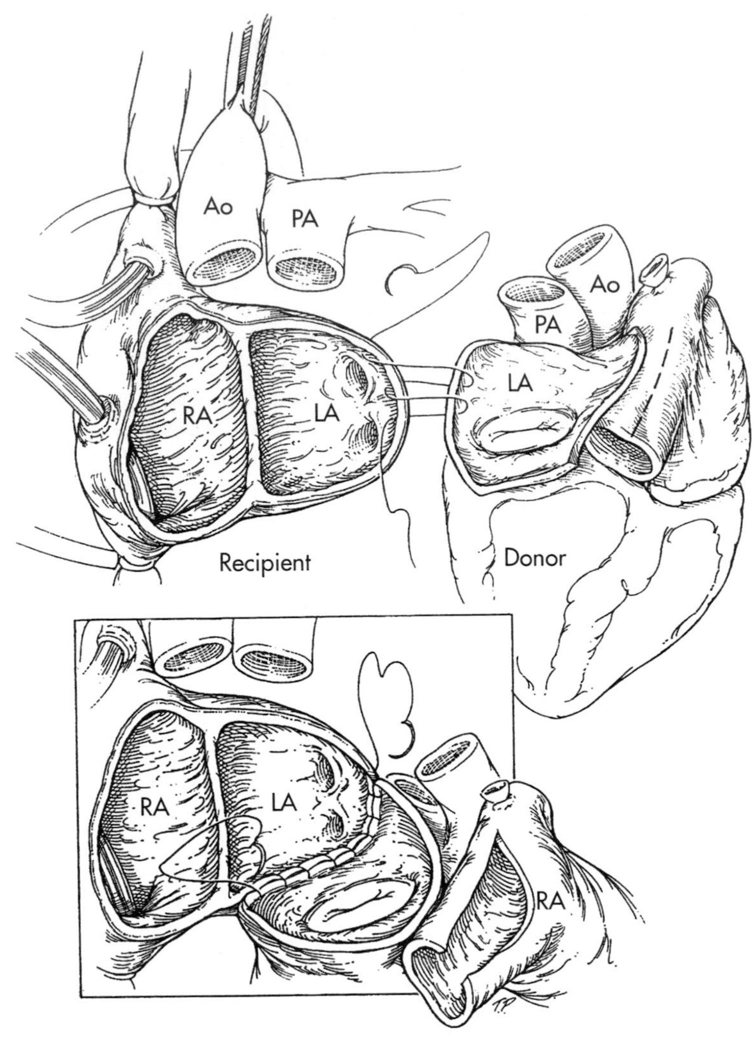

FIGURE 28–2. Cardiac implantation after recipient cardiectomy. The venous cannulas are shown entering the superior and inferior vena cavae with retained cuffs of the right and left atrial tissue. The pulmonary artery (PA) is transected and the aorta is cross-clamped with aortic (Ao) cannula out of the field of view. The *inset* details the first atrial anastomosis along the inferior margin of the left atrium (LA), showing the mitral valve of the donor heart. The aortic perfusion cannula is not shown. RA, right atrium. (From the Handbook of Cardiac Transplantation, 1995, with permission of the American College of Cardiology Foundation.)

inotropes and inodilators (see Chapter 17, Anesthesia for Cardiovascular Surgery).

Usually, a modest level of inotropic support (e.g., 5 to 10 mcg/kg per min of dopamine) is sufficient, unless there has been more extensive preservation and/or reperfusion injury, RV failure, or technical problems with the graft. Typically, right and left atrial filling pressures are similar; filling pressures in the range of 10-15 cm H_2O are necessary to support cardiac output. Higher values and/or significant discrepancies between right and left atrial pressures should arouse suspicions of pulmonary hypertension, right ventricular failure (increased right atrial pressure), or severe left ventricular dysfunction (increased left atrial pressure).

A situation peculiar to infant and pediatric transplantation is the occasional use of hearts from donors of relatively smaller body size than the recipient. Such "undersizing" of the donor may be associated with apparent graft insufficiency or failure, manifested as low cardiac output and systemic perfusion despite optimal or maximal filling pressures and inotropic support. Pulmonary hypertension and significant preservation injury exacerbate the hemodynamic instability. ECMO may be needed to permit a period of myocardial recovery in this setting of acute postoperative graft dysfunction.

In addition to having ischemia-reperfusion injury, the donor heart is also denervated. In the absence of sinus rhythm or if the chronotropic response to vasoactive drugs is insufficient, atrial or atrioventricular sequential pacing is often needed in the immediate postbypass period to facilitate adequate heart rate, cardiac output, and control of ventricular filling. It is unusual for pacing to be required for more than several days posttransplantation. The continued need for pacing suggests more significant damage to the organ.

Postoperative bleeding is another frequent problem. The potential causes are multiple. Extensive scarring and adhesions from previous palliative procedures are common. Pediatric patients may require some degree of aortic or pulmonary artery reconstruction at the time of transplantation, creating potentially extensive high-pressure suture lines that are not found in other heart transplantation settings. Chronic cyanosis may be associated with coagulation factor deficiencies, accelerated fibrinolysis, platelet function abnormalities, and an increased number and size of collateral vessels. Abnormalities in a variety of coagulation proteins also have been found in patients with single-ventricle physiology (Odegard, 2002, 2003). Many patients receive chronic anticoagulant therapy (aspirin, warfarin [Coumadin], etc.), which cannot be discontinued in sufficient time to allow recovery of the coagulation profile before transplantation. Significant hemodynamic shear stress (e.g., aortic stenosis) can result in an acquired form of von Willebrand disease by promoting degradation of active, high molecular weight von Willebrand multimers into inactive monomers. Cardiopulmonary bypass induces

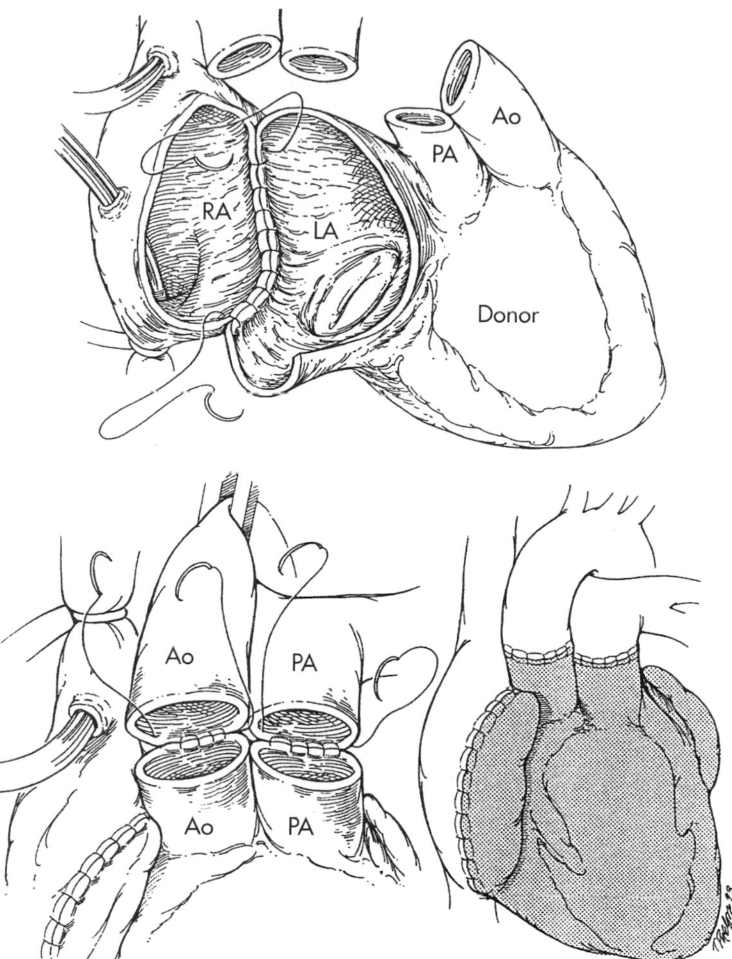

■ **FIGURE 28–3.** Anastomosis of the right atrial suture line. The *upper panel* shows the right atrial anastomosis following which, in the *lower panel*, the heart is swung over into position to complete the atrial free wall suture. The great artery anastomoses are made, after which the heart is de-aired and the cross clamp is removed. The aortic perfusion cannula is not shown. PA, pulmonary artery; Ao, aorta; RA, right atrium; LA, left atrium. (From the Handbook of Cardiac Transplantation, 1995, with permission of the American College of Cardiology Foundation.)

bleeding in infants and small children. The causes for bleeding are multifactorial and include hemodilution of coagulation factors, higher flow rates, higher shear stress (resulting in increased activation and consumption of platelets and coagulation and fibrinolytic proteins), greater blood trauma, use of colder temperatures, and an increased systemic inflammatory response.

In general, after protamine has been given to neutralize the heparin, platelets are given and are followed by cryoprecipitate (Miller, 1997). Specific patients, such as those receiving warfarin preoperatively or with clinically significant preoperative coagulopathy due to hepatic dysfunction or malabsorption/protein-losing enteropathy, may also benefit from the administration of fresh frozen plasma. Use of antifibrinolytic agents such as tranexamic acid or aprotinin may also be beneficial, particularly in small infants and patients with a history of one or more prior thoracic procedures. Aprotinin may also have some beneficial effects on inflammation and reperfusion injury.

Immunosuppression in Heart Transplantation

In brief, the rejection process begins when recipient CD4 T cells recognize foreign antigen in the donor heart. Recognition leads to activation of the larger T-cell pool, with subsequent IL-2 secretion, thereby triggering activation of monocytes/macrophages, B cells, and cytotoxic CD8 cells.

Induction of immunotherapy is targeted toward the prevention of T-cell activation. This can occur by depleting the T-cell pool with monoclonal or polyclonal antibodies or by using monoclonal antibodies to prevent IL-2 secretion. OKT3 is a murine monoclonal antibody used in clinical practice. This agent binds to the CD3 molecule on the T-cell surface. This complex is closely linked to the antigenic recognition site of the T-cell receptor. Within minutes of the commencement of OKT3, the T-cell population decreases dramatically (Delmonico and Cosimi, 1988). T-cells reappear within 3 to 5 days, but without the CD3 molecule. Although OKT3 was originally used in the context of acute rejection, its current use also includes induction of immunosuppression. When OKT3 is used in this fashion, the administration of cyclosporine or tacrolimus may be delayed by 5 to 7 days. This is particularly useful in the context of patients with borderline renal function where calcineurin inhibitors and their nephrotoxic properties can further compromise renal function. Other side effects of OKT3 include chills, fever, diarrhea, dyspnea, and wheezing. Pulmonary edema and cardiac arrest have also been reported (Thistlethwaite et al., 1988).

ATG and ALG are polyclonal antibodies prepared from thymocytes and lymphoblasts, respectively. They are both IgG antibodies, and while the precise mechanism of action has yet to be elucidated, their administration causes profound lymphocytolysis. Side effects include chills, febrile reactions, erythema, and pruritus. Thrombocytopenia occurs in over 50% of patients, and serum sickness and Steven Johnson syndrome have also occurred secondary to ATG or ALG therapy.

Basiliximab and daclizumab are both monoclonal antibodies to the alpha chain of the IL-2 receptor. The receptor has three noncovalently bound chains. The alpha chain is specific for IL-2 and once activated by IL-2, the T cell begins its rejection amplification cascade (Kovarik et al., 1999). The binding of these monoclonal antibodies effectively and rapidly prevents activation of the cascade. Furthermore, the alpha chain is not present in inactivated T cells, and thus only activated T cells are targeted (Denton et al., 1999). There is some concern that these agents may be associated with an increased incidence of superimposed infections such as CMV and possibly the development of PTLD.

Maintenance of Immunosuppression

Three classes of drugs are available for maintenance immunosuppression. Corticosteroids are nonspecific anti-inflammatory agents. Their effects are numerous and include inhibiting cytokine and cell surface molecule gene transcription in monocytes, inhibiting phospholipase A_2 enzyme activity and thus reducing the inflammatory cell activation, signaling, and inflammatory molecule production. Steroids also inhibit the nuclear transcription factor NF-κB, thus reducing IL-2 gene transcription and the production of several other proinflammatory cytokines and signaling and recognition molecules (Auphan et al., 1995).

Antiproliferative agents prevent the expansion of activated T-cell and B-cell clones. The original agent used for this purpose, azathioprine, is being replaced by newer agents such as mycophenolate mofetil (MMF) and sirolimus (rapamycin). The toxic effects of azathioprine include bone marrow depression leading to marked leukopenia, possible liver damage, and the development of pancreatitis.

MMF is a selective inhibitor of the de novo pathway of purine biosynthesis, thus inhibiting cell proliferation. It is administered as a morpholinoethylester prodrug of mycophenolic acid, which is metabolized to the active compound. Its mechanism of action is the result of reversible noncompetitive inhibition of inosine-monophosphate-dehydrogenase activity (IMDPH). It thereby targets proliferating lymphocytes, which are dependent on the availability of guanine nucleotides, which are no longer generated (Allison et al., 1993; Brazelton et al., 1996; Shaw et al., 1999). Side effects of MMF include nausea and vomiting; but it lacks significant bone marrow and renal toxicity. There is a concern, however, about the possible development of invasive CMV infection during the use of MMF.

Rapamycin (sirolimus) is a newer antiproliferative agent that, despite binding to FK506-binding protein 12, confers its action by inhibiting cellular proliferation without inhibiting calcineurin. Side effects appear to be dose-dependent elevation of triglyceride levels and dose-dependent bone marrow suppression.

Calcineurin Inhibitors. Calne's first published use of cyclosporine as an immunosuppressive agent was in 1979, and it continues to be one of the primary drugs used for the prevention of rejection in many transplant programs (Calne et al., 1979). The mechanism of action of cyclosporine involves binding to cyclophilin in the T-cell cytosol. This cyclosporine/cyclophilin complex then binds to calcineurin and prevents calcineurin from promoting transcription of the IL-2 gene, thus preventing further IL-2 production (Liu et al., 1991; Flanagan et al., 1991; Schreiber et al., 1992; Schreier et al., 1993). The most significant side effect of cyclosporine therapy is nephrotoxicity; other significant side effects include liver dysfunction, hypertension, hyperlipidemia, and PTLD.

Tacrolimus (FK506) is a macrolide that also acts as a calcineurin inhibitor. It forms a complex with an immunophilin, FK-binding protein, and this complex subsequently binds to calcineurin to prevent IL-2 gene transcription (Sigal et al., 1992; Liu et al., 1991). Side effects include nephrotoxicity, glucose intolerance, and an increased incidence of PTLD.

Calcineurin inhibitors, antimetabolites, and corticosteroids are the mainstays of antirejection therapies. While the use of cyclosporine still predominates, tacrolimus use is increasing. The nephrotoxicity of both drugs is significant. Use of azathioprine appears to be decreasing in favor of MMF or sirolimus. The use of sirolimus will increase further if suggestions of reduced transplant vasculopathy associated with its use are confirmed (Mancini et al., 2003). The use of steroids remains at fairly constant levels, but increased acceptance of the newer agents is likely to lead to more rapid weaning and lower dosing of corticosteroids and thereby limit the side effects of growth retardation, hypertension, and glucose intolerance.

Data from the International Society for Heart and Lung Transplantation suggest that fewer than 40% of children receive induction immunotherapy. The most common induction therapy includes either ATG or ALG followed by a specific IL-2 receptor antagonist. A small proportion of children also receive OKT3. There are as yet no randomized multicenter studies to determine the benefits of induction therapy, but one retrospective multicenter's study determined that children given polyclonal ATG had lower mortality than those given no induction agent or OKT3 (Boucek et al., 1999). In general, the use of induction therapy allows the initiation of calcineurin inhibitors to be delayed for a few days postoperatively, which may be most beneficial in those patients with some degree of renal dysfunction.

Complications

Complications following heart transplantation can be divided into those associated with rejection and those arising from other causes. Acute rejection generally occurs in the first year posttransplantation and is the most frequent cause of death during this time period. Late-onset acute rejection also occurs in a significant number of children beyond the first posttransplant year. Acute rejection remains a source of morbidity and correlates with the ongoing need for immunosuppression. Although risk factors for acute rejection have been sought, results have been conflicting (Kirklin et al., 1992; Chartrand et al., 2001; Webber, 2003). Overall, it would appear that an older age at the time of transplantation increases the risk of acute rejection and that an episode of acute rejection in the first year increases the risk of subsequent episodes (Webber et al., 2003).

Clinical detection of rejection remains difficult, as signs and symptoms are subtle and nonspecific; these include general malaise, fever, change in activity or appetite, tachycardia, and conduction or voltage changes on the surface ECG. More severe bouts may be accompanied by symptomatic reductions in graft function. Other relatively noninvasive tests, such as various myocardial or inflammatory markers in blood, echocardiography, and cardiac magnetic resonance imaging, continue to be investigated, but none of the tests have shown the necessary sensitivity and specificity. As a result, endomyocardial biopsy remains the gold standard for diagnosis of rejection (Boucek, 2000; Wagner et al., 2000). It is performed at scheduled intervals as a surveillance tool, to guide immunosuppression regimens and dosing, and to diagnose acute rejection episodes.

Chronic rejection and associated posttransplantation coronary artery disease are the leading causes of death among late survivors of heart transplantation. According to data from the International Society for Heart and Lung Transplantation, approximately 20% of all pediatric transplant patients have some degree of posttransplantation coronary artery disease at 5 years posttransplantation. This accelerated vasculopathy can affect infants, children, and adults alike. The mortality following diagnosis is substantial. The histologic appearance is that of concentric myointimal proliferation that ultimately results in luminal occlusion. In addition to repeated bouts of rejection, CMV infection is likely to be a contributing risk factor. Efforts have been made to more aggressively control other etiologic factors present in these patients that can contribute to the development of atherosclerosis, such as hypertension, hyperlipidemia, and glucose intolerance. At present, the effects of these efforts are uncertain.

As the transplanted heart is denervated, chest pain caused by myocardial ischemia is a rare presenting complaint; progressive deterioration in graft function, heart failure, or sudden death are the primary presentations for rejection. For this reason, transplant recipients are routinely screened (usually on a yearly basis) for this development. Although coronary angiography was long thought to be the most sensitive means of detecting the development of graft vasculopathy, it underestimates the presence of early or mild disease. As a result, many centers have begun to use dobutamine stress echocardiography as the primary means of screening for coronary artery disease in transplant recipients. Intracoronary ultrasound may also be useful (Dent et al., 2000; Pahl et al., 1999; Costello et al., 2003).

Treatment of posttransplant coronary artery disease is palliative coronary artery stenting (which is of limited benefit given the diffuse nature and involvement of distal vessels) or retransplantation. Rapamycin, which appears to slow the progression of transplant vasculopathy, has shown some benefit, either as an additional immunosuppressive treatment or in the form of rapamycin-coated coronary stents (Mancini et al., 2003; Morice et al., 2002). Retransplantation for graft vasculopathy and resulting graft failure is associated with greater risk and diminished success.

Infection following heart transplantation is usually caused by bacterial pathogens that do not cause disease in the immunocompetent host. Immunosuppression makes the severity of infection much worse, and even with early aggressive therapy, such infections are a significant cause of morbidity and mortality in the transplant patient. In addition to bacterial pathogens, other opportunistic pathogens such as fungi and viruses (CMV, Ebstein-Barr, and adenovirus), cause significant morbidity. Infection with Ebstein-Barr virus has been associated with the development of PTLD (Webber et al., 2003). This may be treated initially with reduction in immunosuppressive therapy and, failing this, with chemotherapeutic agents. Other complications in heart transplant patients are mostly secondary to immunosuppressive regimens and include diabetes, growth retardation, hypertension, and renal dysfunction.

Outcome After Pediatric Heart Transplantation

Data from the International Society for Heart and Lung Transplantation show the actuarial 10-year survival for all pediatric heart recipients exceeds 50% (Boucek et al., 2002). The mortality rate is higher in infants in the first year of life but is followed by a slightly lower mortality rate of less than 2% per year in the 4- to 10-year period. If one excludes first-year mortality, the conditional actuarial survival in infants exceeds 80%. Adolescents have a slightly higher average mortality of 4% per year. In comparing the actuarial survival in the first 4 years posttransplant by era, significant progress has occurred. During the period 1982 through 1987, the actuarial 4-year survival was just below 60%, whereas in the current era (1998 through 2001), the 4-year actuarial survival approaches 80%.

The greatest risk factor for first-year mortality was the diagnosis of congenital heart disease. Other risk factors for poor first-year outcome included ventilatory support before transplantation, hospitalization before transplantation, and the need for retransplantation. Recipient age was also found to be a risk factor. Those patients younger than 6 years and older than 12 years were at increased risk.

Recipient factors not associated with increased risk during the first year include the need for inotropic support, use of prostaglandin, use of ECMO, prior sternotomy, height, the need for dialysis, recent infection, or a history of malignancy. Although age did affect first-year mortality risk, weight as an independent factor posed no additional risk.

Overall, the leading cause of death in transplant recipients under the age of 3 is acute rejection, and over 3 years of age is coronary artery vasculopathy (Boucek et al., 2002). Among survivors, over 95% of patients report no limitation of activity at the 5-year follow-up. However, with formal exercise testing, as many as 50% may have mild to moderate limitations in exercise and aerobic capacity. In the absence of rejection, in general myocardial and somatic growth are normal in most pediatric transplant recipients (de Broux et al., 2001).

LUNG TRANSPLANTATION

Demographics and Indications

At present, more than 1200 pediatric lung transplantations have been performed (Boucek, 2002). As with pediatric heart transplantation, available data suggest that the annual number of pediatric lung transplants conducted since the late 1980s has decreased, since a peak in the late 1990s. Waiting times have increased overall; adolescents may wait as long as 1 or 2 years for cadaveric lungs (average waiting time, 20 months), while younger children aged 1 to 10 years wait an average of approximately 6 to 12 months. Organ donation and viability continue to be major limitations (Sweet, 2003; Burch and Aurora, 2004).

Early pediatric transplantation efforts emerged directly from adult experience, and the majority of the recipients were older children with cystic fibrosis (CF), primary pulmonary hypertension, secondary pulmonary hypertension (e.g., from congenital heart disease), and pulmonary fibrosis. With increasing experience and the development of pediatric lung transplant centers, transplantation in infants and younger children has grown, and children younger than 2 to 3 years may now comprise 10% to 20% of lung transplant recipients. In infants and young children, the most common diagnoses include interstitial lung disease, primary pulmonary hypertension, severe pulmonary vein obstruction, and alveolar proteinoses.

Contraindications

Absolute contraindications to pediatric lung transplantation include hepatitis B or C virus infection, HIV infection, active malignancy within the past 1 to 2 years, and irreversible neurologic or neuromuscular disorders. Significant liver, heart, or renal dysfunction (requiring dialysis) is also an absolute contraindication; lung-liver or heart-lung transplantation may be considered with the first two of these conditions. Some issues such as prior thoracotomies or pleurodeses, steroid dependence, or colonization with a variety of organisms (especially in patients with CF) are no longer absolute contraindications in many centers. Relative contraindications can include significant musculoskeletal disease, invasive ventilation (which has been linked to increased risk in older patients, potentially less so in infants and young children), colonization with various fungi or atypical mycobacteria, poor nutritional status (<70% or >130% of ideal body weight), and an inability to wean from or significantly reduce dependency on systemic corticosteroids. As with heart transplantation, significant psychological and behavioral disturbances in the potential recipient, or social and familial circumstances that could hinder access to care and/or compliance with complex medical regimens, may also preclude transplantation.

Organ Preservation

Achieving successful lung preservation continues to be a difficult problem. Lung ischemic time is a major factor in the development of posttransplant lung injury. The optimal duration of preservation is between 3 and 4 hours, although lungs with ischemic times as long as 9 hours have been implanted successfully (Kaiser et al., 1991). During organ harvest, the lungs and pericardium are exposed and a prostaglandin infusion is begun. Prostaglandin is believed to cause pulmonary dilation and thereby improves the distribution of preservation solution. The vena cavae are then transected, the left atrial appendage is incised, and then the aorta is cross-clamped. This harvesting sequence prevents any left atrial hypertension, and thus reduces the risk of pulmonary edema. A cold crystalloid preservation solution (Euro-Collins) with a high potassium concentration is infused into the pulmonary artery while cardioplegia is administered into the aortic root. Ventilation is discontinued and the lungs are allowed to deflate. For single- or sequential double-lung transplantation, the left atrium is divided such that a cuff of atrial tissue surrounds the right and left pulmonary veins. The pulmonary veins may be excised in a single atrial cuff for double-lung transplantation. If both the heart and lung(s) are to be used (but in different recipients), adequate segments of the left atrium and pulmonary artery must be allocated to each (Griffith and Zenati, 1990). During transportation, the lungs are generally kept deflated, although there is some experimental evidence that intermittent inflation prolongs the allowable ischemic time (Toledo-Pereyra, 1977). In addition, some centers believe that donor cooling with CPB also extends the permissible ischemic time (Heritier et al., 1992).

Single-Lung Transplantation

Single-lung transplantation is performed infrequently in pediatric patients. One general reason is that the ability of the transplanted lung to grow remains uncertain. Most practitioners believe it is wise to implant as much "normal" lung tissue as possible to meet the demands of future somatic growth in children. Second, the most frequent indication for pediatric lung transplantation is CF, and there is great concern about the transplanted lung being contaminated by the chronically infected native lung.

When a single-lung transplant is performed, the most important decision is the determination of laterality, usually determined by chest radiograph, chest computed tomography, and/or scans. The side that appears to have the less affected lung and/or that has better ventilation/perfusion scan is kept; the opposite side is transplanted. If possible, implantation is done on the side opposite to any previous thoracotomy. Typically, a more emphysematous lung is removed (or volume reduced) so as not to compress the allograft on the opposite side. A more fibrotic lung might remain, so as to favor ventilation and blood flow distribution to the transplanted lung.

Omentum may be fashioned to provide a "vascular cuff" around the bronchial anastomosis in order to improve bronchial blood supply. In such cases, a midline laparotomy is performed first, in order to mobilize omentum with an attached pedicle. This is tunneled through the diaphragm and the incision is closed (Fig. 28–4). Single-lung ventilation is then instituted (see later). A thoracotomy is performed, and the pulmonary artery, pulmonary veins, and mainstem bronchus are exposed. The pulmonary artery is then test-occluded while gas exchange, PAP, and hemodynamic status are observed. The lung is removed if the patient tolerates this procedure. Allograft implantation involves connecting the donor atrial flap containing the pulmonary vein orifices to an area of recipient left atrial tissue that is isolated within a clamp. The pulmonary artery anastomosis is completed. The technique of telescoping bronchial anastomosis is used more frequently (Calhoon et al., 1991). To perform this, the smaller of the two bronchial ends is placed inside the other one to a depth of one cartilaginous ring, and then the connection is oversewn. This method provides sufficient blood flow for high-quality bronchial healing and precludes the need for an omental cuff. The lung is then gently inflated. Air within the vascular spaces is removed either via the pulmonary artery (with the left atrium partially occluded, the proximal end of the pulmonary artery clamped, and its distal end vented) or via the left atrial cuff (with the pulmonary artery unclamped and the left atrial cuff vented). Pulmonary blood flow and ventilation are then established simultaneously.

Double-Lung Transplantation

Double-lung transplantation is the type of lung transplant operation performed most frequently in pediatric patients. The technique most often used involves sequentially implanting each lung. This method has several advantages compared with en bloc implantation, which was done previously by some (Pasque et al., 1990; Kaiser et al., 1991). The lungs are harvested individually, each with a separate pulmonary artery, mainstem bronchus, and two pulmonary veins encompassed within a cuff of the donor's left atrium. A bilateral anterior thoracosternotomy is performed extending across the midline by transverse sternotomy. This approach ("clamshell" incision) allows the anterior thoracic cage to be swiveled upward, providing full access to the bilateral hilar structures (Fig. 28–5). Each set of pulmonary arteries and mainstem bronchi are anastomosed end to end, and each left atrial cuff is anastomosed to the recipient's left atrium. CPB is almost always used in pediatric patients, although it is possible to perform bilateral sequential lung transplantation without CPB. Omental flaps may be mobilized for each bronchial connection, although most current techniques use telescoping bronchial anastomoses (de Hoyos and Mauer, 1992). Both methods appear to result in improved healing of the airway connections, compared with tracheal anastomoses (as are used with the en bloc method). This is presumably due to enhanced blood flow (Pinsker et al., 1979).

Living Donor Lung Transplantation

The shortage of donor organs has led to the development of living donor lobar lung transplantation, which requires that two separate donors each undergo lobectomies to provide right and left lower lobes. Outcomes of living donor lung transplants have been comparable to cadaveric lung transplants (Starnes, 1999).

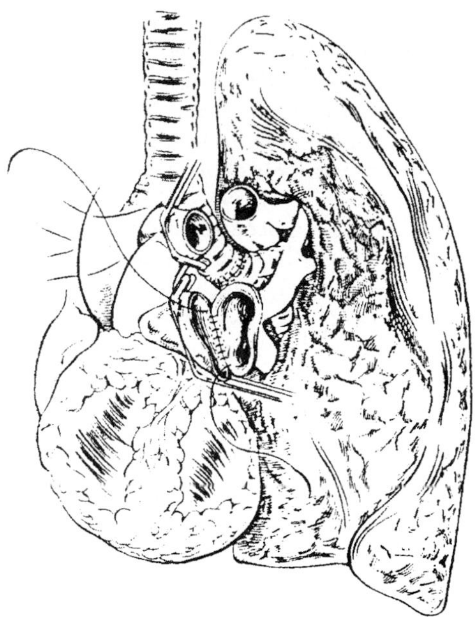

■ **FIGURE 28–4.** The bronchial anastomosis is first completed, followed by the vascular anastomoses. The vessel is reconstructed from posterior to anterior with the suture untied, allowing for de-airing through the anastomosis later. (From Kirby TJ, Birnbaum PL: Technique of single-lung transplantation. In Patterson GA and Couraud L (eds): *Current topics is general thoracic surgery*, Vol. 3, Lung Transplantation, Amsterdam, 1995, Elsevier Science B.V.)

The technique of living related lung transplants also overcomes some of the inherent difficulties of attempting to predict the clinical course of various types of lung disease and the appropriate timing for listing the patient for transplantation. Size limitations can be problematic: adult lobes are usually too large for children under 5 years, and, conversely, the amount of lung tissue may be insufficient for well-grown adolescents. The various anastomoses, particularly those of the pulmonary veins, can be technically difficult and prone to stenosis. The operation obviously poses more than minimal risk to the donors, and truly informed consent may be difficult to determine in such an emotionally difficult situation. The ethical issues are therefore complex, and this procedure is infrequently performed.

■ HEART-LUNG TRANSPLANTATION

Because of early problems with the integrity of bronchial anastomoses, many patients with terminal lung disease received heart-lung transplants, with the possibility of their (normal) heart going to a heart transplant recipient in a "domino" procedure. Since the development of techniques to promote healing of bronchial anastomoses, the frequency of heart-lung transplantation has decreased substantially. At present, in pediatric patients it is only considered for patients with pulmonary hypertension or other end-stage lung disease when there is also congenital heart disease that cannot be repaired and in patients with end-stage lung disease and severe left ventricular or right ventricular dysfunction. Pulmonary hypertension with right heart dysfunction is no longer considered an indication, unless the

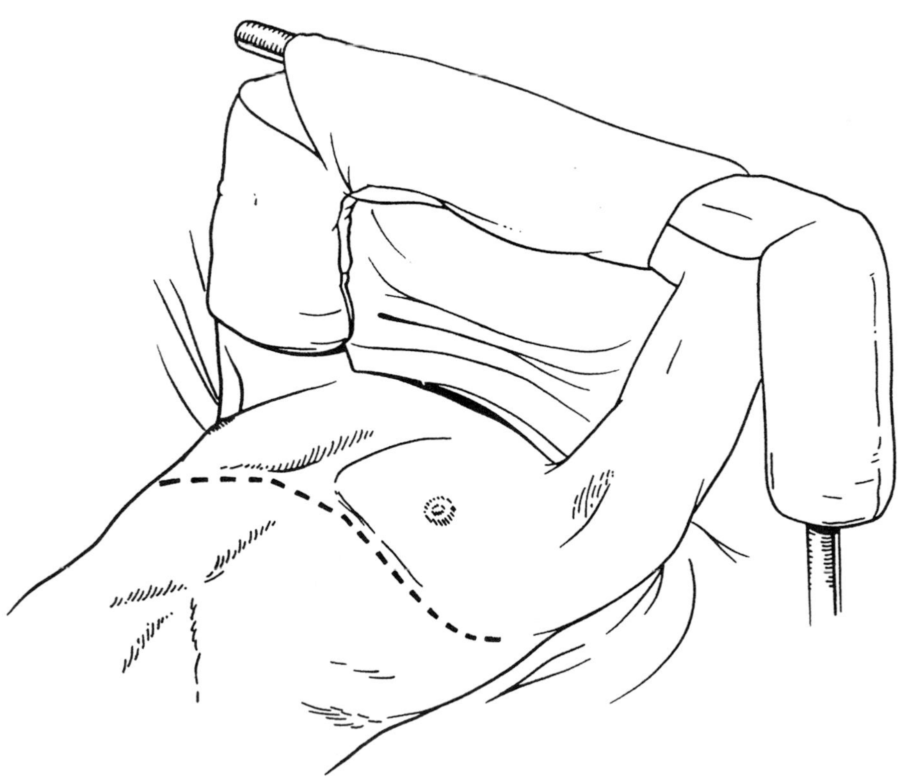

■ **FIGURE 28–5.** Clam shell position with the arms at 90 degrees.

right ventricular dysfunction is severe, as it often improves after successful lung transplantation.

Anesthetic Management

It should be noted that these patients are often critically ill by the time they come for lung transplantation. This is due to several factors, including the nature of the underlying disease, and reticence on the part of both physicians and patients/families to undergo such a procedure, as well as the long waiting time required for cadaveric organs. For example, the clinical course of CF is very unpredictable. Most centers initiate the transplantation process when a CF patient's FEV_1 falls below 30% to 40% of predicted value; however, most centers would not actually transplant patients at this point if the patient thinks that his or her quality of life is acceptable (Yankaskas, 2002). Thus, the CF patient is likely to be quite compromised (pulmonary, nutrition, etc.) by the time of actual transplantation. In children with pulmonary hypertension, survival has been inversely related to right atrial and pulmonary artery pressures, as well as to the product of right atrial pressure and PVR (Clabby, 1997). However, it is likely that prostacyclin therapy (and perhaps newer agents such as endothelin receptor antagonists) will improve survival and prevent or at least delay the need for lung transplantation in some children with pulmonary hypertension (McLaughlin, 2002).

Patients with end-stage COPD or restrictive lung disease are often hypoxic and hypercarbic and may be dependent on supplemental oxygen. Their ventilatory effort is at least partially sustained by increased circulating catecholamine concentrations. Sedation can reduce ventilatory drive and cause hypotension and is best avoided. If necessary, small increments of midazolam may be titrated until the desired effect is achieved. Although sedative medication may be useful as an adjunct to control pulmonary vascular responses during induction, this should only be given in the immediate preoperative period with full monitoring in situ. If undertaken, small increments of midazolam are administered until the desired effect is achieved.

The preoperative assessment of the patients is focused on the cardiopulmonary status as well as dysfunction in other organ systems. The CF patient undergoing lung transplantation is usually already on maximal medical therapy. This may include oral or inhaled bronchodilators, supplemental oxygen, nebulized antibiotics, *N*-acetylcysteine or DNase, and chest physiotherapy. These are continued through the time of surgery. It is important to have recent information about right ventricular function and PAP (both usually with echocardiography). Baseline liver and renal function, as well as coagulation status (potentially compromised by malabsorption), should also be determined.

Monitoring and Vascular Access

Noninvasive monitoring is instituted before induction. An arterial catheter may also be inserted under local anesthesia before induction. However, this is usually performed following induction in young children. Although cannulation of the central venous circulation may be difficult in the patient with severe obstruction or fibrosis, due to the large negative intrathoracic pressures generated during spontaneous ventilation, it is usually possible before induction. Pulmonary artery catheterization before pneumonectomy is essential if assessing the response to pulmonary arterial cross-clamping is required (i.e., single-lung transplantation or bilateral sequential transplantation without cardiopulmonary bypass). The catheter may either be floated into the appropriate artery using transesophageal echocardiography (TEE) guidance, or the surgeon may place the tip by palpation. It is essential to withdraw the catheter tip into the main pulmonary artery before pneumonectomy in patients undergoing bilateral lung transplantation. If present, TEE may be used to visualize the effects of pulmonary artery occlusion and mechanical ventilation on ventricular function (Triantafillou and Heerdt, 1991). TEE can also provide valuable information about ventricular function and volume status after transplantation.

Intraoperative and postoperative bleeding can be significant. This may be exacerbated by extensive adhesions, especially in patients with long-standing lung inflammation (e.g., CF) or those who have undergone prior thoracic surgery. Thus, it is important to have large-bore vascular access to facilitate rapid volume resuscitation. Often, the use of a rapid infusion device is quite helpful. Almost all pediatric lung transplantations are performed with the patient supine and the patient's arms raised over the head and flexed at the elbows (see Fig. 28–5). This position may occlude catheters placed in the antecubital fossae, and thus other sites are recommended. Epidural catheters can provide excellent postoperative analgesia and facilitate ventilatory effort and pulmonary toilet. Although the use of both lumbar or thoracic approaches are adequate, the decision to place the catheter while the child is awake or after induction remains unresolved. In addition, the placement of an epidural catheter for a child who is to undergo lung transplantation using CPB is also contentious. An alternative approach is to place the epidural catheter on the first or second postoperative day, before extubation, when the coagulation status has normalized.

Induction and Maintenance of Anesthesia

A child who is to undergo lung transplantation has precarious physiology and minimal reserve and is usually frightened and thus has elevated levels of circulating endogenous catecholamines. Thus it is important that the anesthetic induction have minimal effects on the pulmonary and cardiovascular systems. Myocardial depression and increased pulmonary vascular tone should be avoided, whereas bronchodilation and pulmonary vascular dilation are desirable. Etomidate, ketamine, propofol, and thiopental have all been used successfully for intravenous induction (Triantafillou and Heerdt, 1991). However, should a rapid sequence induction be required, etomidate may provide the best overall combination of hemodynamic stability and rapid airway control. Ketamine is useful in those patients prone to airway reactivity. The effect of ketamine on PVR is controversial; it probably does not increase PVR if hypoxia and hypercarbia are avoided (Hickey et al., 1985). Ketamine does, however, have some direct negative inotropic effects, and it should be avoided in patients with severe pulmonary hypertension or significant right ventricular dysfunction.

Potent synthetic opioids such as fentanyl are frequently used for both induction and maintenance of anesthesia. In addition to providing relative hemodynamic stability, opioids are effective in attenuating sympathetic stimulation in those patients prone to pulmonary hypertensive crises. In order to avoid the chest wall rigidity (and limitation to ventilation) that may occur with these agents, it is usually preferable to perform an intravenous induction with etomidate, establish neuromuscular blockade, and then titrate the opioids to achieve the desired effect. Although the vagolytic effects of pancuronium may be useful in conjunction with synthetic opioid administration, vecuronium or rocuronium also may be used.

There is some evidence that nitrous oxide may increase PVR and impair hypoxic pulmonary vasoconstriction (Sykes et al., 1977; Schulte-Sasse et al., 1982), and thus it is probably best avoided. Inhaled anesthetics are usually used in moderate concentrations as anesthetic adjuncts and to provide amnesia; bronchodilation and perhaps some degree of pulmonary vasodilation secondary to abolishment of pulmonary vascular vasoconstriction may be other benefits. All volatile anesthetics are likely to impair hypoxic pulmonary vasoconstriction to some degree, which may be a particular problem if single-lung ventilation is used and also in patients with significant lung disease, $\dot{V}/\dot{Q}$ mismatch, and/or intrapulmonary shunting (Benumof, 1985).

A standard single-lumen endotracheal tube of an appropriate size is used for lung transplantation with CPB. An appropriate double-lumen endotracheal tube is inserted after induction for single-lung transplantation or bilateral sequential transplantation without CPB. It is placed to provide differential lung isolation, and its position may be confirmed by flexible bronchoscopic examination (Benumof, 1985). At all times, the possibility of tube obstruction due to inspirated secretions and blood clots must be kept in mind. If a double-lumen endotracheal tube is used, it is exchanged for a standard endotracheal tube at the completion of the procedure.

Usually the initial inspiratory oxygen concentration is set at 100%. This can then be adjusted according to pulse oximetry and blood gases. Ventilatory parameters are set according to the pathophysiology of the disease involved. The patient with restrictive lung disease is best ventilated with higher rates and lower-than-normal tidal volumes to minimize peak airway pressures, whereas the patient with obstructive lung disease may benefit from longer expiratory times to allow complete expiration and to prevent "stacking" of breaths. In some situations it may be necessary to manually ventilate the patient in order to establish the optimal ventilatory pattern. The addition of PEEP may improve gas exchange. It should be remembered that excessive PEEP may compromise the patient's cardiovascular status. Volume resuscitation and inotropic support may be necessary to counter the negative hemodynamic effects of PEEP. In patients with CF, frequent suctioning of the endotracheal tube should be performed to keep it clear of copious and tenacious secretions.

Intraoperative Concerns

The group of patients undergoing lung transplantation have, by definition, severely compromised cardiorespiratory function. If the intention is to conduct either a single-lung or sequential bilateral lung transplantation without using CPB, there needs to be constant reassessment of the patient's underlying cardiorespiratory status, because single-lung ventilation frequently leads to unacceptable levels of CO_2 and cardiac instability (Triantafillou and Heerd, 1991). If at any point the situation becomes untenable, the patient is placed on CPB in order to complete the procedure.

There are two events that must be critically evaluated. First, with the onset of single-lung ventilation, an immediate increase in airways resistance occurs in all patients. In those patients with restrictive lung disease, these changes are more pronounced. High airway pressure will both inhibit venous return and reduce pulmonary blood flow. The initial respiratory management is an adjustment of the ventilatory setting and the possible addition of inotropic agents to augment support for right ventricular function. If gas exchange and hemodynamic status are not improved, then it is important to reinstitute two-lung ventilation while plans for CPB are instituted.

The second intervention that needs to be evaluated is when the pulmonary artery is occluded during single-lung ventilation. Occlusion of the pulmonary artery during one-lung ventilation leads to an improvement in gas exchange. This occurs because the shunt passing through the collapsed lung is removed and the $\dot{V}/\dot{Q}$ matching in the perfused lung is improved by minimizing physiologic dead space. However, PAP is increased, with a concomitant increase in afterload. This increased afterload is best treated with pulmonary vasodilation using agents such as prostaglandin, milrinone, or nitric oxide. Maintaining coronary perfusion of the hypertensive right ventricle is essential to preserving its function. Thus, adequate preload and inotropic support (alone or in combination with α-adrenergic agonists) may also be necessary. If right ventricular failure cannot be managed with preload and inotropic support, then the pulmonary artery should be unclamped and CPB instituted.

Double sequential lung transplantation performed on CPB does not have these physiologic difficulties. The lungs are reperfused individually as soon as the anastomoses are complete. Following the implantation of the first lung, there is often a "honeymoon" period of excellent gas exchange. However, this may be short-lived. Gas exchange may worsen due to factors that include reperfusion injury, pulmonary edema, and reduced compliance. Pulmonary hypertension may also occur due to hyperinflation in an open thoracic cavity. These two problems can usually be resolved with ventilatory adjustment and the use of moderate levels of PEEP. Inotropic support is frequently required. Blood products, including platelets and clotting factors, may be required (occasionally in quite substantial amounts) to correct for ongoing bleeding at surgical sites, adhesions as a result of CPB, and/or preexisting coagulation abnormalities. Use of antifibrinolytic agents, particularly aprotinin, may have beneficial effects with regard to the inflammatory response and the reperfusion injury.

Patients with "septic lungs" (e.g., CF patients) can occasionally develop sepsis or a syndrome resembling septic shock, probably from bacteremia and/or release of inflammatory mediators during removal of their native lungs, in the early postbypass period. The outcome is frequently poor, despite intensive therapy with inotropes, antibiotics, etc.

Early Postoperative Complications

Acute Graft Dysfunction

Acute dysfunction of the transplanted lung immediately after implantation or over the ensuing several hours continues to be a significant problem, occurring in up to 30% to 40% of recipients. The primary mechanism is believed to be related to ischemia-reperfusion injury, and in fact its appearance and severity are generally associated with a longer duration of ischemia. The contribution of other factors, such as duration of donor support and occult lung injury (e.g., trauma, infection, multiple transfusions), or recipient factors, such as chronic infection/colonization or use of CPB, is unclear. Acute graft dysfunction typically resembles an acute respiratory distress syndrome or noncardiogenic pulmonary edema, with key features that include markedly decreased lung compliance and impaired gas exchange (especially oxygenation).

The primary treatment is preventive, aiming to keep lung ischemic times less than 5 to 6 hours whenever possible. The other major focus is mechanical ventilation, with appropriate use of airway pressures and PEEP. In general, ventilatory parameters should be adjusted to maintain normocarbia or mild hypocarbia with adequate but not excessive lung expansion. Peak and mean airway pressures are kept at the minimum required to maintain gas exchange while protecting the bronchial anastomoses and limiting the possibility of volutrauma. Inspired oxygen concentration is kept as low as practical such that PaO_2 is below 120 mm Hg in order to limit oxygen toxicity and reperfusion injury. In the case of single-lung transplantation, the two differing cardiorespiratory requirements make hypoxia due to $\dot{V}/\dot{Q}$ mismatching more likely (Triantafillou and Heerd, 1991). It may, on occasion, be necessary to use differential lung ventilation in order to address the ventilatory requirements of the two lungs independently (Smiley et al., 1991; Todd, 1990). Fluid and blood product administrations are limited as much as possible. Inhaled nitric oxide may be beneficial in some circumstances to improve the matching of ventilation to perfusion and to reduce PVR. ECMO has been used successfully in some cases of acute graft failure (Meyers et al., 2000).

Infection

Infection is a significant problem in the immediate postoperative period. There are multiple risk factors. In addition to extensive surgical sites and invasive catheters, the patient is often nutritionally compromised and has begun receiving high-potency immunosuppressive agents. The transplanted lung is denervated. The cough reflex is therefore lost below the level of the anastomosis. Airway ciliary function is also likely to be severely impaired in the posttransplant period. It is essential that chest physiotherapy and tracheobronchial suction be performed routinely to prevent accumulation of blood and secretions, which can obstruct the endotracheal tube or airways and contribute to infection. Bronchoscopy may be necessary at times to clear the airway of the debris. An absence of lymphatic drainage from the donor lung(s) contributes to the tendency to accumulate lung water and develop infection and acute graft dysfunction (Montefusco and Veith, 1986; Todd, 1990).

Use of prophylactic antibiotics is routine and is guided by the donor's and recipient's colonization status and by subsequent surveillance cultures in the recipient. Ganciclovir (for CMV) and antifungal agents are given when these pathogens exist in either donor or recipient. Infection with parainfluenza, adenovirus, and herpesvirus can be life threatening in pediatric lung transplant recipients (Bridges, 1996).

Postoperative hemorrhage is one of the most frequent major complications, with the surgical anastomoses and adhesions within the chest being the most common sites. A high degree of suspicion must be maintained to quickly diagnose anastomotic obstruction or ischemia (bronchial anastomoses). Echocardiography and nuclear medicine perfusion scans can be effective in detecting obstruction of the pulmonary arterial or venous connections (the latter may be a particular problem in lobar transplantation, and in either setting can be heralded by copious amounts of pink, frothy secretions after reperfusion). The bronchial anastomoses are usually inspected toward the end of the procedure using flexible bronchoscopy. Airway necrosis and dehiscence are frequently fatal. Increasing scarring and stenosis can also occur. Therefore, regular fiberoptic bronchoscopy is also conducted after surgery to screen for these problems (Todd et al., 1990; de Hoyos et al., 1992).

Rarely, recurrent laryngeal or phrenic nerve damage can become apparent in the postoperative period, most likely as a consequence of the surgical procedure. These are often transient, although permanent vocal cord or hemidiaphragmatic paralysis can occur; the latter may require plication of the diaphragm.

Later Complications

Although the principal cause of death during the first 30 days after transplantation is graft failure, infection in the setting of sustained immunosuppression is a leading cause of death in the first year; it continues to be a significant cause of mortality after that period (Boucek, 2002). Symptoms of infection in the transplant patient are often difficult to distinguish from those of rejection. Both can present with fever, dyspnea, decreased oxygenation, and pulmonary infiltrates. Definitive diagnosis for most entities requires bronchial lavage and culture; some patients may need a lung biopsy to rule out infection or rejection. Prevention of infection is a primary goal in the management of lung transplant recipients.

Cytomegalovirus (CMV) is one of the most frequent causes of infection in the transplant patient, especially in the CMV-negative recipients who have received organs from CMV-positive recipients. CMV infection may be asymptomatic or symptomatic and may cause pneumonitis (where it is associated with fever, respiratory distress, decreased pulmonary function, hypoxemia, and patchy interstitial infiltrates), gastrointestinal disease (abdominal pain, fevers, and increased liver function enzymes), or viremia. It may also present a sepsis-like picture that can progress to multiple organ failure. CMV infection has been associated with acute cellular rejection and also an increased frequency and severity of chronic rejection (Duncan et al., 1992). Aggressive treatment with antiviral agents, with possible reduction in immunosuppressive therapy, is usually successful. Diagnosis is usually based on positive antibody staining in lung tissue specimens, although newer assays that detect antigenemia may allow for earlier and less invasive diagnosis (Kusne, 1999). The use of ganciclovir has decreased the incidence and severity of CMV-related disease in these patients. Prophylactic treatment is usually used in patients where either the donor or recipient is CMV positive.

Overall, patients are constantly at risk for bacterial lung infection. Patients with CF are more susceptible to bacterial infection with agents such as *Pseudomonas aeruginosa* or fungal organisms such as *Aspergillus*. These infectious agents should be actively sought (using bronchoalveolar lavage and transbronchial lung biopsy), especially in patients who do not respond to empiric therapy. Infection with Ebstein-Barr virus is of note because of its association with malignancy (see later).

Another significant and often insidious complication is the development of airway obstruction due to scarring and granuloma formation, usually at the bronchial anastomosis suture line. The lesion can progress over several months and typically presents as wheezing and shortness of breath. Flow-volume loops and large airway flow rates are usually reduced. The diagnosis is confirmed by bronchoscopy and is treated with dilation and/or stenting.

Delayed gastric emptying and gastroparesis may frequently follow lung transplantation, perhaps due to surgical injury to the vagus nerve. In addition to the obvious aspiration risk at the time of subsequent surgeries, gastroesophageal reflux has been linked to occult (or overt) aspiration, lung injury, graft failure, and bronchiolitis obliterans (Berkowitz et al., 1995; Huddleston, 1996).

Acute Rejection

Acute rejection is most frequent in the first year and particularly the first several months after transplantation, declining substantially thereafter (Sweet, 1997, 2003). It is often initially asymptomatic; symptoms include fever, dyspnea, and desaturation. Positive laboratory tests can include pleural effusions and/or perihilar infiltrates on chest radiography, and lower airway obstruction with decreased FVC and FEV_1 on spirometry. The diagnosis is made (and attempts to differentiate from infection) using bronchoalveolar lavage and transbronchial biopsy. The diagnosis of acute rejection requires the presence of lymphocytic bronchitis or bronchiolitis with associated perivascular mononuclear infiltrates. Acute rejection is most often treated with high-dose steroids, to which patients usually respond rapidly with improvements in symptoms and pulmonary function tests. More persistent or severe episodes are typically treated with OKT3 or ATG. Although most lung transplant patients will experience at least one episode of rejection in the first year, additional episodes should prompt reevaluation of the immunosuppressive regimen. Acute rejection episodes are believed to be a major risk factor for the later development of bronchiolitis obliterans.

Bronchiolitis Obliterans

The major manifestation of chronic rejection is obliterative bronchiolitis (bronchiolitis obliterans). Bronchiolitis obliterans syndrome affects greater than 50% of all pediatric recipients more than 5 years posttransplantation, and bronchiolitis obliterans is the most common cause of death after 1 year. As with patients following heart transplantation, all lung transplant patients are followed with transbronchial biopsies, initially every 3 months and with increasing intervals to evaluate the presence of rejection. Pulmonary function tests are also performed to rule out or follow the progression of bronchiolitis obliterans. Respiratory symptoms of bronchiolitis obliterans are not dissimilar to those of asthma involving small airways; it sometimes responds mildly to bronchodilators even though the transplanted lungs are denervated. However, as time progresses, the airway obstruction becomes irreversible. Histologic examination confirms the diagnosis, although progressive reductions in FEV_1 and maximum expiratory flow rates (FEF_{25-75}, FEF_{75}) are sufficient to make the diagnosis without histologic evidence. An association has been shown of bronchiolitis obliterans with increased episodes of acute rejection and/or infection (particularly CMV) and the onset of chronic rejection. The primary therapy is aimed at immunosuppressive prevention of acute rejection and prompt treatment of CMV (Sharples et al., 1996).

Although increased immunosuppressive therapy has been used to attempt to halt the progress of the disease, no solution except retransplantation has been shown to be beneficial. Unfortunately, the 1-year survival rate for a retransplanted lung recipient is only 26% (Sharples et al., 1996).

Immunosuppression for Lung Transplantation

There is substantial variability among pediatric lung transplant centers in terms of standard immunosuppressive regimens for preventing rejection. Induction immunosuppression is used in approximately 40% of patients, typically with an IL-2 receptor antagonist or ATG. All centers use combination therapy for chronic immunosuppression, typically a steroid, a calcineurin inhibitor (cyclosporine or tacrolimus), and an inhibitor of T-cell proliferation (mycophenolate mofetil or azathioprine). Complications arising from the use of these agents have been largely summarized earlier and, as with heart transplantation, significant morbidity is associated with the use of these drugs. Hypertension, hyperlipidemia, diabetes, and renal dysfunction are all present to varying extents. Diabetes is a particular problem in CF patients who have undergone a lung transplant, most likely due to pancreatic injury as a result of their underlying disease; as noted earlier, steroids (which cause insulin resistance) and tacrolimus (postulated to have a direct pancreatic effect) are additional risk factors. In addition, PTLD affects up to 15% of patients (Armitage et al., 1995). Those treated with tacrolimus may have an even higher incidence of PTLD.

Outcome

The overall actuarial survival for single-lung transplants approximates to 25% at 5 years compared with 40% at 5 years with a double-lung transport. This difference reflects the better pulmonary reserve and larger pulmonary vascular bed in double-lung transplants compared with single-lung transplants (UNOS/OPTN, 2005).

When survival is compared by age group, children less than 1 year of age have an actuarial survival at 7 years of greater than 40%, whereas those greater than 1 year have an actuarial 7-year survival of less than 35%. Unfortunately, the actuarial survival in the current era of transplantation shows no significant improvement compared with the past decade. Mortality in the first month posttransplantation is usually secondary to graft failure, whereas mortality in the first year beyond the first month is predominantly due to infection.

Chronic rejection in the form of bronchiolitis obliterans affects more than 50% of transplant recipients after the first year and becomes the main cause of death. On a slightly more optimistic note, of those patients who survive, more than 80% show no limitation of activity at 1, 3, and 5 years.

LIVER TRANSPLANTATION

The first successful pediatric liver transplant was performed in 1967 (Starzl et al., 1968). Between 1989 and 2004, almost 1000 pediatric patients have successfully undergone liver, pancreas, or intestinal transplantation in the United States. Before 1980, with the use of the immunosuppressive agents azathioprine and prednisone, the 5-year survival in the pediatric patient following liver transplantation was a dismal 20% (Gordon and Bismuth, 1991; Gordon et al., 1991). After the introduction of cyclosporine in 1980, long-term survival after liver transplantation became a reality. For the first time, 5-year patient survival began to exceed that of the life expectancy related to the specific disease process. Graft survival has progressively improved since 1992, with, for example, a 1-year graft survival of 81% in 2001 (6- to 10-year recipient age) compared with 68% a decade ago (UNOS/OPTN, 2005). Patient survival for this age group is estimated at 1 year at 90.5%; 3 years, 85.9%; and 5 years, 83.8%. Patient survival in the first year after transplant is similar for all age groups except children younger than 1 year, who have the highest annual death rate. For these infant recipients transplanted in 2001 and 2002, there was a marked decline in 1-year death rate, which is also seen as a trend for children aged 1 to 5 years and those aged 11 to 17 years. Improvements in patient and graft survival rates have been attributed to new immunosuppressive regimens consisting of tacrolimus (FK506, Prograf), MMF, and rapamycin with diminished use of cyclosporine, azathioprine, and corticosteroids and improved access to the donor pool using reduced grafts, living donors, and a new UNOS scoring system (Pediatric End-Stage Liver Disease [PELD] scale) for estimating medical urgency.

The age distribution in pediatric patients varies, with the majority of liver transplants performed in patients 5 years of age or younger. In the pediatric patient population to date, 28% of grafts have been given to patients less than 1 year old, 37% transplanted in patients 1 to 5 years old, and the remaining 35% in children 6 to 17 years old. From 1988 to 2004, a total of 8951 pediatric liver transplants have been performed in the United States (UNOS/OPTN, 2005).

Liver transplantation, as well as multivisceral and small bowel transplantation, has become a widely accepted therapy for organ failure of the abdominal viscera. Although small bowel transplantation is still in its infancy, it has gained recognition as an acceptable therapy for intestinal dysfunction of various etiologies. For all ages, 126 intestinal transplantations were performed in 2004, of which 77 patients were less than 18 years old.

General Indications and Contraindications

The recognition of orthotopic liver transplantation (OLT) as a viable alternative for pediatric patients with liver failure has increased the number of potential recipients. By the same token, the past decade has also revealed diseases now considered absolute contraindications to OLT, having failed to provide demonstrable improvement in patient survival.

The indications for OLT can be classified in general as follows:

1. End-stage liver disease (ESLD) expected to progress to death
2. Secondary disease not confined to the liver
3. Prevention of the complications of major metabolic disorders
4. Nonprogressive liver disease in which mortality is greater than the risk of OLT
5. Fulminant hepatic failure

Disease-specific indications for OLT are shown in Box 28–3.

With improvements in surgical and medical expertise the absolute and relative contraindications to pediatric OLT continue to evolve. There are very few absolute contraindications to OLT: the presence of any active, untreated bacterial, fungal, or viral infection at the time of transplantation; cancer outside the liver or those liver tumors not meeting cure criteria; actively replicating HBV infection; AIDS; or technically not feasible. The relative contraindications are more variable and tend to be transplant center specific. Examples include a child with ESLD and advanced cardiopulmonary disease, epilepsy, or multisystem organ failure and with HIV-positive serology.

BOX 28–3 Disease-Specific Indications for Orthotopic Liver Transplantation (Percent of UNOS Pediatric Recipients 1995–1999)

- Biliary atresia (46%)
  - Biliary hypoplasia
  - Alagille's syndrome
  - Extrahepatic
- Metabolic diseases (12%)
  - Tyrosinemia
  - Glycogen storage disease types I and II
  - α_1-Antitrypsin deficiency
  - Wilson's disease
  - Primary oxalosis/oxaluria
  - Hemochromatosis-hemosiderosis
  - Hyperlipidemia-II-homozygous
  - Cystic fibrosis
- Cholestatic and noncholestatic cirrhosis (14%)
- Malignant neoplasms and benign tumors
- Acute hepatic necrosis (14%)
- Miscellaneous
  - Budd-Chiari syndrome
  - TPN/hyperalimentation-induced liver disease
  - Neonatal hepatitis
  - Congenital hepatic fibrosis
  - Familial cholestasis
  - Trauma
  - Graft-versus-host disease secondary to nonliver transplant

PATHOPHYSIOLOGY OF END-STAGE LIVER DISEASE

ESLD is an irreversible process that results in diffuse fibrosis and cirrhosis with loss of functional hepatocytes. The clinical manifestations are independent of the etiology but are primarily related to the degree of liver dysfunction. This dysfunction is secondary to structural changes that the liver undergoes after it sustains any type of significant damage. Irrespective of the cause of the hepatic insult, there is cell necrosis followed by an attempt at regeneration by the liver. If the damage is of a chronic nature, this regeneration leads ultimately to fibrosis, further necrosis, and micronodular and/or macronodular cirrhosis. Interestingly, the liver is the only solid organ in the body that can fully regenerate after sustaining up to 80% destruction of its functional capacity or similarly a resection of up to 80% of the organ.

There are two main mechanisms through which structural changes lead to hepatic failure: cellular dysfunction and portal hypertension. In cellular dysfunction, liver cell mass decreases as hepatocytes become necrotic. As the liver attempts to regenerate, fibrosis develops, with the eventual disruption of the portal triads. The end result is formation of intrahepatic shunts, sinusoidal thickening, and an overall increase in the resistance to blood flow. This constellation of abnormalities results in the development of portal hypertension and varices. Similarly, biliary drainage becomes abnormal, leading to the intracellular accumulation of byproducts that are normally secreted (proteins, bile). Altogether these changes lead to abnormal hepatocyte energy metabolism, defects in protein and lipid synthesis, and alterations in substrate clearance.

Portal hypertension develops as a result of the increased resistance to blood flow through the disrupted sinusoids. In addition to this increase in resistance, there is an increase in splanchnic arterial blood flow caused by the development of arteriovenous shunts and vasodilatation as liver failure progresses. Worsening portal hypertension is manifested by ascites, splenomegaly, and portasystemic shunts (varices, hemorrhoids, telangiectasia). These portasystemic shunts lead to decreased clearance of previously metabolized substrates by the liver. Cellular function is further compromised as oxygen is shunted away, leading to a potentially dysoxic environment (Dishart et al., 1998). Irrespective of the cause of liver failure, the pathophysiologic derangements are manifested in a similar fashion in the cardiovascular, pulmonary, renal, neurologic, and hematologic systems.

Child-Pugh Classification

The Child-Pugh classification is a universal scoring system of the degree of liver failure in patients with cirrhosis. Traditionally assigning patients to Child-Pugh class A, B, or C has been used as a predictive index for operative mortality rate in adult patients undergoing portosystemic shunting procedures. The estimated

TABLE 28–3. Child-Pugh scoring system for cirrhosis

Score	Bilirubin (mg/dL)	Albumin (g/dL)	PT (sec > control)	Hepatic Encephalopathy	Ascites (grade)
1	<2	>3.5	<4	None	None
2	2 to 3	2.8 to 3.5	4 to 6	1 to 2	Mild
3	>3	<2.8	>6	3 to 4	Severe
Child class: A = 5 to 6; B = 7 to 9; C = 10 to 15 points.					

1- and 5-year survival rates are 95% and 75% for patients with Child-Pugh class B and 85% and 50% for patients with Child-Pugh class C, respectively. After the onset of the first major medical complication (ascites, variceal bleeding, jaundice, or encephalopathy), survival rates for these patients are significantly reduced. Variables measured by this system include ascites, encephalopathy, serum albumin, serum bilirubin, and prothrombin time. Points are subsequently assigned to different degrees of each variable, and the total points are used to assign a grade within the Child-Pugh scoring system (Table 28–3). Although a liver biopsy is often helpful in assessing histologic activity and the amount of fibrosis in patients with chronic hepatitis, it is not a criterion for the determination of the Child-Pugh class. Until February 2002, the Child-Pugh score was used by transplant centers to group patients into one of four medical urgency categories: blood type, patient size, medical urgency, and waiting time determined liver allocation.

Pediatric End-Stage Liver Disease (PELD) Scale

The PELD numerical scale is currently used by UNOS for liver allocation for ages less than 12 years. PELD replaced the previous status 2B and 3 for pediatric patients, while status 1 is not affected by PELD. PELD is based on bilirubin, INR, albumin, growth failure, and age when patients are listed for transplantation, and it is used to calculate a value on a numerical scale, which is an accurate predictor of 3-month mortality, independent of the complications of portal hypertension and the etiology of the liver disease. The MELD (Model for End-stage Liver Disease) is a similar numerical scale ranging from 6 (less ill) to 40 (gravely ill) that is used for ages 12 and older (UNOS/OPTN, 2005). The score indicates how urgently the patient needs a transplant in the next three months. The number is calculated from three routine laboratory test results: bilirubin, INR, and creatinine (Edwards and Harper, 2001, 2002; Kremers et al., 2004).

SYSTEMIC MANIFESTATIONS OF END-STAGE LIVER DISEASE

ESLD is associated with unique systemic physiologic alterations (Robertson, 1998) (Table 28–4).

Cardiovascular System

Progressive liver failure is characterized by a hyperdynamic circulation with a left ventricular ejection fraction greater than 65%, fixed low total peripheral resistance, and a compensatory increase in cardiac output, impaired circulatory reserve, and diminished response to catecholamines. High-risk patients are those with cardiomyopathy and dysrhythmias, congestive heart failure from fluid and reverse electrolyte imbalances, and moderate to severe pulmonary hypertension.

Systemic vascular resistance (SVR) is low because of peripheral vasodilatation and shunting (cutaneous, intrapulmonary, portopulmonary, and pleural). This profound vasodilatation may result from abnormal levels of vasodilator substances, possibly originating in the splanchnic circulation, that would otherwise be cleared by the liver. The most likely mediators include nitric oxide, tumor necrosis factor-α, and endothelium-derived relaxing factor. Activation of the renin-aldosterone-angiotensin system causes an increase in extracellular fluid volume through salt and water retention, and release of AVP results in a decrease in free water excretion, despite an overall central hypovolemia.

TABLE 28–4. Cardiovascular, pulmonary, and renal complications of advanced cirrhosis

Cardiovascular
"Hyperdynamic circulation"
Increased cardiac index and stroke volume
Decreased systemic vascular resistance
Low to normal mean arterial pressure (widened pulse pressure)
Increased heart rate
Central hypovolemia
Increased circulating blood volume
Decreased effective plasma volume
Increased sympathetic tone
Hyporesponsiveness of the vasculature to pressor therapy
Flow-dependent oxygen consumption
Hepatic and splanchnic vasculature
Portal hypertension
Portal-systemic collateral circulation
Decreased hepatic blood flow
Alcoholic cardiomyopathy (reduced LVEF)
Cirrhotic cardiomyopathy (impaired cardiac contractility, defective excitation contraction coupling, systolic and diastolic function, prolonged QTc interval, autonomic dysfunction, impaired β-adrenergic function and postreceptor defect, decreased responsiveness to catecholamines, conductance abnormalities)
Arrhythmias
Pulmonary
Arterial hypoxemia (PaO_2 <70 mm Hg)
Hepatopulmonary syndrome
Portopulmonary hypertension
Impaired hypoxic pulmonary vasoconstriction
Increased pulmonary blood flow
Parenchymal abnormalities
Restrictive ventilatory pattern due to ascites limiting diaphragmatic excursion, pleural effusions, or chest wall deformity due to osteoporosis
Obstructive airway disease, emphysema, bronchitis-bronchiectasis
Interstitial lung disease (infection, pneumonitis, pulmonary edema)
Renal
Renin-angiotensin-aldosterone activation: impaired sodium handling, water excretion, potassium metabolism, and concentrating ability
Impaired renal acidification
Prerenal insufficiency (ascites or diuretics)
Acute renal failure (acute liver failure, biliary obstruction, sepsis)
Hepatorenal syndrome
Glomerulopathies

Similarly, the sympathetic nervous system is activated in an attempt to cause peripheral vasoconstriction to maintain adequate circulating volume. Mixed venous oxygen saturation (SvO_2) is elevated in the pulmonary artery (blood blended in the right ventricle from the IVC and SVC and coronary circulation) and is dependent on SaO_2, cardiac output, hemoglobin, and oxygen consumption. The increase in SvO_2 results from poor oxygen extraction and correlates somewhat with cardiac index (Jugan et al., 1992; Steib et al., 1993).

Of the metabolic or inherited disorders, several have associated cardiovascular malformations. For example, Alagille's syndrome is an autosomal dominant disorder characterized by chronic cholestasis and cardiac anomalies, including, most commonly, peripheral pulmonary stenosis, tetralogy of Fallot, coarctation of the aorta, atrial or ventricular septal defect, patent ductus arteriosus, or pulmonary atresia.

Respiratory System

Cirrhotic patients are predisposed to arterial hypoxemia from intrapulmonary shunting due to capillary vasodilatation, restrictive lung disease caused by ascites or pleural effusions, impaired hypoxic pulmonary vasoconstriction, increased pulmonary blood flow and a rightward shift in the oxygen-dissociation curve due to decreased levels of 2,3-diphosphoglycerate (2,3-DPG). Respiratory compromise may also result from the hepatopulmonary syndrome, portopulmonary hypertension, defects in alveolar oxygen diffusion or pulmonary manifestations of systemic disease (e.g., CF, autoimmune disease, or α_1-antitrypsin deficiency). These defects are compensated for by an increase in mixed venous oxygen saturation and resting cardiac output (Schott et al., 1999; Teramoto et al., 2000). Arterial hypoxemia usually responds to supplemental oxygen and positive-pressure ventilation. Depressed airway reflexes, delayed gastric emptying, hiatus hernia, and massive ascites increase the risk of aspiration. Pulmonary edema, atelectasis, and pneumonia are not uncommon.

The frequency of hepatopulmonary syndrome (chronic liver disease, increased alveolar-arterial gradient $A\text{–}aDO_2$ while breathing room air, and intrapulmonary vasodilatation) is reported between 4% and 29% (Naeije, 2003; Mazzeo et al., 2004). Patients with liver disease may develop progressive and refractory hypoxemia due to abnormal intrapulmonary vascular dilatation causing anatomic shunting and diffusion-perfusion abnormalities (Hoeper et al., 2004). These patients are at risk for systemic arterioembolization causing stroke, intracranial hemorrhage, or brain abscess. The prognosis of the hepatopulmonary syndrome is poor, and a mortality rate of 41% within 2 to 5 years has been reported (Krowka et al., 1993). In contrast, up to 20% of cirrhotic patients are at risk of developing portopulmonary hypertension (portal hypertension and increased pulmonary vascular resistance). Severe pulmonary hypertension may cause acute right ventricular failure and sudden cardiac death. Preoperative therapy with epoprostenol, nitric oxide, and sildenafil may improve outcome in this group if right ventricular function is preserved and treatment results in a decrease in pulmonary pressures and vascular remodeling. (Ghofrani et al., 2002; Makisalo et al., 2004)

Renal System

Renal dysfunction is common in patients with ESLD, and the kidneys are very susceptible to insult and prone to failure. Fluid and electrolyte imbalances are secondary to diuretic therapy, hypoalbuminemia, and portal hypertension causing generalized ascites, progressive edema, hypovolemia, dilutional hyponatremia, and hypokalemic metabolic alkalosis. Three main mechanisms singularly or in combination contribute to renal insufficiency: prerenal causes, acute tubular necrosis (ATN), and hepatorenal syndrome. Renal insufficiency not only complicates the management of liver failure patients but, more importantly, may contribute to mortality. Thus it is important to aggressively evaluate and treat reversible causes of renal insufficiency (Table 28–5). Renal function is often difficult to assess in these patients because reduced muscle mass and hepatic synthesis of creatine reduces the serum creatinine. Creatinine clearance will overestimate the glomerular filtration rate.

TABLE 28–5. Strategic plan for optimizing renal function and prevention of hepatorenal syndrome

Initial Management
Homeostatic environment (electrolytes, acid-base status, hematocrit)
Cardiovascular stability (euvolemia, mean arterial pressure >60 mm Hg)
Identify intrinsic renal parenchymal disease
Treat bacterial infections and complications related to liver disease, i.e., ascites, dilutional hyponatremia, and variceal bleeding
Avoidance of nephrotoxic agents (e.g., NSAIDs or aminoglycosides)
Optimize Renal Perfusion
Intravascular volume expansion
Drug therapy (splanchnic vasoconstriction or renal vasodilators): vasopressin analogues, α-adrenergic agonists, endothelin antagonists, antioxidants
Strategies
Transjugular intrahepatic portosystemic shunt
Spontaneous bacterial peritonitis: albumin and antibiotic therapy

Modified from Gines P, Guevara M, Arroyo V, Rodes J: Hepatorenal syndrome. *Lancet* 362:1819–1827, 2003.

Prerenal azotemia is most commonly associated with aggressive use of diuretic therapy in the treatment of ascites. With a decreased effective blood volume, patients are more susceptible to the volume-depletion effects of diuretics and large volume paracentesis without adequate intravascular volume replacement. As with other types of prerenal azotemia, the urine sodium level will be low (<15 mEq/L) with a fractional excretion of sodium (FE_{Na}) of less than 1%. This type of renal failure is amenable to careful volume replacement.

The kidneys in patients with liver failure are also at increased risk for developing ATN as a result of decreased renal perfusion. This decreased perfusion is a consequence of a relative decrease in central blood volume due to splanchnic pooling, which activates secretion of vasopressin, in combination with other compensatory mechanisms attempting to restore mean arterial pressure such as increased sympathetic tone and renin-angiotensin activity. Renal perfusion is further compromised because prostaglandin synthesis is reduced in advanced liver disease. Prostaglandins are the most potent renal arteriolar vasodilators (Govindarajan et al., 1987; Claria and Arroyo, 2003). Hence, tubular function is much closer to an ischemic threshold in liver failure patients. This low ischemic threshold renders the kidneys more susceptible to nephrotoxic drugs such as intravenous contrast dye or aminoglycosides used to treat infectious complications. Additionally, in the patient with "tense" ascites, renal cortical perfusion may also be diminished due to an abdominal compartment syndrome. Urine sodium in this setting is usually greater than 20 mEq/L with an FE_{Na} of greater than 1% (Epstein, 1985). Treatment should be directed at minimizing additional renal injury, optimizing renal perfusion, and maintaining urine output, with some form of dialysis possibly introduced until the ATN resolves. This usually occurs within 10 to 14 days. It is not uncommon, however, for the hepatorenal syndrome to become superimposed once the patient develops ATN.

The most consequential form of renal dysfunction with a very poor prognosis is the hepatorenal syndrome. This syndrome is characterized by a rapid deterioration in renal function associated with profound sodium retention and low urinary sodium excretion. It is usually precipitated by a major physiologic event, such as gastrointestinal hemorrhage, sepsis, or surgery. It is differentiated from prerenal azotemia by the lack of responsiveness to volume expansion. The pathogenesis is severe renal vasoconstriction with absence of cortical blood flow. Interestingly, this vasoconstriction is reversible if the kidney is transplanted into a host with normal hepatic function (Koppel et al., 1969). This form of renal failure requires dialysis to sustain life but may be reversible with liver transplantation (Iwatsuki et al., 1973).

Hematologic Complications

Anemia, thrombocytopenia, and coagulopathy are the expected findings in the patient with liver failure. Anemia is usually a result of bone marrow suppression, vitamin deficiency, hemorrhage, and diminished erythropoietin production caused by renal insufficiency. Thrombocytopenia (platelet count $<100{,}000/mm^3$) is seen in 70% (Kang et al., 1985) of patients with liver disease and is primarily a result of portal hypertension with platelet sequestration in the spleen; however, bone marrow suppression, abnormalities in platelet metabolism, inadequate production of thrombopoietin, or autoimmune causes may also be contributing factors (Peck-Radosavljevic, 2000). Impaired platelet aggregation and clot retraction due to qualitative platelet defects are also seen in patients with liver disease and renal failure.

The tissue factor pathway of coagulation is classically assessed by measuring the partial thromboplastin time (PTT) and the prothrombin time (PT). The liver is the main site of synthesis of all coagulation factors except von Willebrand's factor, which is produced primarily in the vascular endothelium. Failure of bile salt secretion results in poor absorption of vitamin K, which is a cofactor necessary for the posttranscriptional γ-carboxylation and activation of factors II, VII, IX, and X. In cirrhotic patients the levels of fibrinogen and factor VIII are usually supranormal with the production of all other clotting factors diminished. Additionally, approximately 80% of patients with liver failure also produce an abnormal fibrinogen molecule (dysfibrinogenemia) (Martinez et al., 1978; Cunningham et al., 2002). Control of coagulation therefore depends on the balance of hepatic synthesis of clotting factors and its clearance of activated clotting factors, plasminogen activators, and fibrinolytic proteins.

Neurologic Complications

Hepatic encephalopathy is a frequent metabolic complication of acute or chronic liver disease. The neuropsychiatric abnormalities are often reversible with the clinical presentation ranging from subtle personality changes to frank coma. Neuromuscular symptoms include tremor, hyperreflexia, and decerebrate posturing. There are three theories regarding the pathogenesis of hepatic encephalopathy: (1) ammonia toxicity with accumulation of toxins in the brain, (2) alteration in plasma amino acid composition with accumulation of false neurotransmitters, and (3) increase in neuroinhibitory substances, manganese, monoamines, or endogenous opiates. Various studies have supported aspects of each hypothesis, yet none has been conclusively established. In patients who have died in hepatic coma, neuropathologic findings occur in the astrocytes, rather than neuronal changes. Positron emission tomography studies show decreased glucose utilization in the cerebral cortex, which may explain the neuropsychiatric abnormalities. (Butterworth, 1996).

Forty percent of ammonia is generated in the intestine from ingested nitrogenous substances and subsequently metabolized in the liver into urea, which is excreted through the kidneys and into the colon. With liver failure and portosystemic shunting, ammonia, which is a known neurotoxin, accumulates and readily diffuses into the brain, where it exerts its neurotoxicity. The lack of a strong correlation between blood ammonia levels and the degree of hepatic encephalopathy, the presence of this condition in the absence of elevated ammonia levels, and the neuroexcitatory effects of low ammonia concentration have been used as arguments against ammonia being the sole factor in the pathogenesis. Other metabolic byproducts, such as mercaptans and short-chain fatty acids, have also been implicated.

With progressive liver failure, the ratio of branched-chain amino acids to aromatic amino acids decreases. These aromatic amino acids cross the blood-brain barrier and may competitively inhibit "normal" neurotransmitters and favor the generation of false neurotransmitters (octopamine), which have an inhibitory effect on cerebral function.

GABA is a major inhibitory neurotransmitter in the central nervous system that regulates the chloride channel. It has been suggested that elevated ammonia levels enhance GABAergic neurotransmission and synergistically augment the action of benzodiazepine receptor agonists (Basile and Jones, 1997). This theory is supported by the fact that hepatic encephalopathy can at times be improved by the benzodiazepine receptor antagonist flumazenil.

Among the multiple precipitating factors in hepatic encephalopathy are azotemia, drugs (sedatives, tranquilizers, analgesics), gastrointestinal bleeding, excess dietary protein, metabolic alkalosis, infection, and constipation (Abou-Assi and Vlahcevic, 2001). Treatment consists of reducing dietary protein, avoiding sedatives, administering lactulose (converts ammonia to nonabsorbable ammonium and modifies the colonic flora), correction of hypokalemia, discontinuation of diuretics, treating infection, and volume expansion.

Endocrine dysfunction is common in ESLD. Oversecretion of growth hormone and glucagon leads to peripheral and hepatic insulin resistance and impaired glucose metabolism, with lipid utilization as a preferred energy substrate. Hypoglycemia is an ominous sign indicative of depletion of glycogen stores in the liver and survival limited to days without intravenous glucose supplementation and transplantation.

Fulminant Hepatic Failure

Fulminant hepatic failure (FHF) is the most severe, life-threatening complication of liver failure. The differentiation of acute fulminant liver failure versus an acute exacerbation of chronic liver disease is important with regard to therapeutic and prognostic implications, as not all acute liver failure patients are the same. Fulminant hepatic failure is usually defined as rapidly progressive liver failure with the onset of encephalopathy within 8 weeks of the onset of jaundice in patients without a previous history of liver disease. However, no uniform definition of FHF in children has been established. One definition that is widely accepted is the sudden onset of liver failure with altered mental status and coagulopathy in an otherwise healthy child (Nazer and Nazer, 2004). In the pediatric age group, the incidence of FHF is estimated to be 50 cases per year in the United States. FHF was the primary diagnosis in 15% of pediatric patients transplanted from 1995 to 2000.). Viral hepatitis and drug-induced hepatotoxity are the two most common causes, but in most cases, the exact etiology remains unidentified. For the majority of fulminant failure patients, survival ultimately depends on medical stabilization and urgent liver transplantation, as mortality rates may reach 80% to 90%.

The etiology of FHF is quite varied. In approximately 50% of patients FHF is caused by acute viral hepatitis (A, B, C, D, E, and non A-E). Of note, HCV infection is not a significant cause of FHF in children. Many other viruses are also recognized, including Epstein-Barr virus (EBV), CMV, paramyxovirus, varicella-zoster virus, herpesvirus types 1, 2, and 6, parvovirus, and adenovirus. Less common causes include hepatotoxic drugs (acetaminophen, salicylates, chlorinated hydrocarbons, halothane, isoniazid, intravenous tetracycline, sodium valproate, methanol, *Amanita* mushroom poisoning), ischemia, vascular obstruction (Budd-Chiari syndrome), massive steatosis (Reye's syndrome), and metabolic causes (Wilson's disease in older children; in neonates: inborn errors of metabolism and hemochromatosis).

Jaundice is the most common presenting symptom, with mental changes occurring over the next 2 weeks in most patients. The condition then progresses in as many as 80% of patients to coma, with development of ascites, cerebral edema, decorticate and decerebrate posturing, severe coagulopathy, gastrointestinal bleeding, and hemodynamic instability.

Cerebral edema appears to be the major cause of morbidity in patients with FHF and contributes to the high mortality rates. Early signs and symptoms include increased muscle tone, arterial hypertension, seizures, agitation, and sluggish papillary response to light. Infants may present with poor feeding, irritability, and altered sleep patterns. The mechanism of cerebral edema is unknown, although both vasogenic and cytotoxic etiologies have been proposed. Whatever the cause, cerebral edema ultimately leads to intracranial hypertension, impairment of cerebral perfusion, irreversible neurologic brain injury, uncal herniation, and death (Hanid et al., 1979). Encephalopathy may be classified according to the scheme in Table 28–6. This is useful to judge the effects of treatment and assess the progression of the disease process.

Medical treatment is generally supportive until either recovery with hepatocyte regeneration, liver transplantation (cadaveric, split, or living related donor), or death. Experimental approaches have been tried using liver-assist devices. Supportive measures are directed at minimizing morbidity and mortality from serious complications. This includes monitoring in a critical care unit; endotracheal intubation for airway protection; an infusion of 10% to 20% glucose to prevent hypoglycemia and replacement of calcium phosphorous and magnesium; antibiotic treatment of infections, peritonitis, and pneumonia; maintaining urine output and avoidance of nephrotoxic drugs with surveillance for renal insufficiency; H_2-blockers for stress ulcer prophylaxis; correction of coagulopathy with vitamin K, plasmapheresis, and platelets, with fresh frozen plasma reserved for patients with active bleeding, as normalization of PT is often used as a prognostic indicator for recovery of synthetic function; avoidance of volume overload; and, most important, management of intracranial hypertension. Protein intake is restricted, with lactulose enemas and oral neomycin given to decrease enteric bacteria that produce ammonia and evacuate the bowels. If a causative agent is identified, then specific treatment should be initiated early: *N*-acetylcysteine for acetaminophen overdose.

Initial management of cerebral edema should begin with a computed tomography (CT) scan of the brain to assess cerebral blood flow (Aggarwal et al., 1994). If there is evidence of cerebral edema and compromise of cerebral blood flow without carbon dioxide responsiveness, continuous monitoring of ICP is vital, especially in stage 3 or 4 encephalopathy. Therapeutic measures to reduce ICP include head-up positioning, ventilatory support with moderate hyperventilation and mannitol for a documented ICP greater than 30 mm Hg with progressive edema (Aggarwal et al., 2005). It may be efficacious to place a jugular bulb catheter so that adequate assessment of cerebral metabolism is possible (Lassen and Lane, 1961). The important parameters that aid in management are the arteriovenous oxygen content difference ($AVDO_2$), glucose, and lactate across the brain (Aggarwal et al., 1993, 1994, 2005). Mild hypothermia to 34°C and barbiturate coma remain controversial topics with respect to the management of the patient with hepatic coma. Barbiturate coma should be reserved until all therapeutic interventions have failed to reduce ICP. Continuous electroencephalographic (EEG) monitoring is advisable in this instance, since the goal is to achieve EEG silence. Proceeding to liver transplantation will be inherent on the likelihood of neurologic recovery.

Serial abdominal computed tomography scans may be useful in assessing the hepatic size and morphology. A transjugular liver biopsy is invaluable but may not provide a definitive diagnosis and results correlate poorly with prognosis. Histologic findings are of two types: extensive necrosis of the peripheral hepatocytes with little or no regeneration (drugs and viral hepatitis) and microvesicular steatosis and centrilobular necrosis (Reye's syndrome and metabolic disorders). Serum levels of liver enzymes do not correlate with the severity of the disease. Typically, conjugated hyperbilirubinemia is present, with hyponatremia, hyperkalemia, respiratory alkalosis, and metabolic acidosis.

Prognostic criteria include the patient's age, cause of liver disease, onset and degree of encephalopathy relative to the appearance of jaundice, serum bilirubin level, PT/INR, serum creatinine, factor V level, and arterial pH. A sensitive predictor of outcome

TABLE 28–6. Staging (grading) of hepatic encephalopathy

Stage	Mental Status	Tremor (Asterixis)	Electroencephalogram
I	Euphoria, altered sleep, slurred speech	Slight	Δ and α irregularities
II	Drowsiness, incontinence	Marked	Slow α and Δ
III	Arousable from sleep, confused	Diminished	τ wave prevalent
IV	Responsive to painful stimuli	Absent	Slow Δ to flat
V	Unresponsive to pain	Absent	Flat

is the INR value. With an INR of 4 or greater, the mortality rate reaches 86%; with an INR of less than 4, it may be as low as 27% (Nazer and Nazer, 2004).

PREOPERATIVE EVALUATION

Risk assessment of the patient scheduled for OLT is still in its evolutionary stage. The primary focus for the anesthesiologist is to evaluate the whole patient for systemic manifestations of ESLD as well as predictable disease-specific extrahepatic manifestations (such as pulmonary involvement with CF).

Cardiovascular Evaluation

Cardiac evaluations of pediatric candidates for OLT should be tailored according to the underlying cause of cirrhosis. Inherited metabolic liver disorders rank second behind biliary atresia as an indication of OLT in children; as such, possible myocardial involvement should be considered in patients with oxalosis, glycogen storage disease type III, Gaucher's disease, Niemann-Pick disease, Wilson's disease, neonatal iron storage disease, and amyloidosis. The physical examination and diagnostic work-up should focus on cardiac auscultation, the presence or absence of cyanosis (arterial oxygen saturation SpO_2 and PaO_2) or clubbing, and transthoracic echocardiography. Detection of a cardiac anomaly may then require cardiac catheterization.

Cardiac function in adults with cirrhosis has been extensively investigated, but there is little information available on children. A study of 22 children with cirrhosis compared with a control-group of healthy age- and sex-matched children (mean age, 4.1 ± 3.5 years) reported that pediatric OLT candidates have normal left ventricular systolic function unless their hearts were primarily involved in the underlying disease. In advanced liver failure, left ventricular systolic function may be impaired. These children also had increased systolic LVPWT (left ventricular posterior wall thickness), which may reflect left ventricular hypertrophy and impaired diastolic function. Left ventricular ejection fraction is usually normal or increased at rest in adults with cirrhosis unaccompanied by ascites (Grose et al., 1995; Laffi et al., 1997). The presence of ascites adversely affects cardiac function in adults (Valeriano et al., 2000). In contrast, most pediatric patients with ascites have normal left ventricular systolic function. Cyanosis is not a reliable sign of hypoxemia in children because of changes due to crying, anemia, and jaundice. Clubbing in patients with chronic liver disease is a common finding, with a prevalence ranging from 23% to 32% (Ozcay et al., 2002). Given the physiologic stresses inherent in liver transplant surgery, cardiac problems may emerge perioperatively that contribute to significant morbidity and mortality in patients with cirrhosis and mild or latent cardiomyopathy (Myers and Lee, 2000).

Pulmonary Evaluation

Patients have various degrees of pulmonary impairment, including normal PaO_2 and reduced DLCO, significant arterial hypoxemia, hepatopulmonary syndrome, portopulmonary hypertension, and preexisting lung disease. The question that has not been definitively answered is, "What values of FEV_1, DLCO, and PaO_2 identify the high-risk pediatric patient scheduled for liver transplant surgery?" Investigative studies include chest radiography, pulmonary function studies, high-resolution computed tomography studies of the lung, contrast transthoracic echocardiography with saline, and arterial blood gas measurements.

Cirrhosis affects the pulmonary circulation, lung parenchyma, and pleural spaces. Reduced alveolar-capillary diffusion may be seen in the absence of significant hypoxemia, especially in patients with HCV cirrhosis. This anatomic derangement of the alveolar-capillary membrane worsens with disease progression with DLCO abnormal at less than 80% predicted value. A reduced diffusion capacity may persist up to 15 months after transplantation (Ewert et al., 1999). Of interest, the Hepatitis C Association is supporting a no-smoking policy for teens and adults, as smoking has been determined to be an independent risk factor associated with elevated ALT levels among anti-HCV-seropositive patients (Wang et al., 2002; Hezode et al., 2003).

Mild arterial hypoxemia is common in patients with cirrhosis and, primarily caused by a decrease in FRC and total lung capacity (ascites, pleural effusions), impaired diffusion capacity, and pulmonary arteriovenous shunting (Liu and Lee, 1999). In advanced liver diseases, ventilation/perfusion ($\dot{V}/\dot{Q}$) defect is an important cause of hypoxemia. The arterial blood gas analysis while standing and breathing 100% FIO_2 is of particular importance because severe hypoxemia patients with at least a moderate response to breathing 100% oxygen on standing (PaO_2 >150 mm Hg) are thought to have an adequate pulmonary reserve and may be safely oxygenated intraoperatively (Krowka et al., 1997; Mohamed et al., 2002). Nonresponsive individuals should be suspected of having a fixed shunt, and transplantation should be delayed pending further evaluation.

Hepatopulmonary syndrome (HPS) was once considered a contraindication to transplantation, but now it is considered an indication for early liver transplantation, as there is no successful long-term medical treatment. Patients typically present with progressive exertional dyspnea and hypoxemia. HPS is characterized by the triad of chronic liver disease, hypoxemia, and intrapulmonary shunting in the absence of primary cardiac or pulmonary disease. The exact incidence in the pediatric patient population is unknown. The pathoanatomic defects causing arterial hypoxemia include intrapulmonary vascular dilatation due to dilated precapillaries, direct arteriovenous communications, and engorged pleural blood vessels. This results in decreased oxygen diffusion into the dilated vessels (diffusion-perfusion impairment) along with decreased intrapulmonary transit time and decreased hypoxic pulmonary vasoconstriction. This is actually not a true "anatomic" shunt, as the patient with the more common type I lesions will demonstrate a significant PaO_2 response to 100% oxygen.

Appropriate preoperative evaluation should include a chest radiograph, an arterial blood gas level measurement with the patient breathing room air and then 100% FIO_2, and one of several imaging techniques: perfusion lung scanning, contrast-enhanced (microbubble) transthoracic echocardiography, lung scintiscan, or pulmonary angiography (identifies type I O_2 reactive versus type II O_2 nonreactive lesions). With liver transplantation, HPS is reversible (Liang et al., 2001), but regression of vascular abnormalities in patients with true anatomic shunts and those with marked precapillary dilatation and evidence of poor response to supplemental oxygenation is not predictable (Lange and Stoller, 1995). Treatment of HPS type II presents a dilemma, although liver transplantation with concomitant lung transplantation is a possible choice (Yuan et al., 2003).

Pulmonary arterial hypertension as a consequence of liver dysfunction is termed portopulmonary hypertension (PPH). This is a pulmonary vasoproliferative and vasoconstrictive process leading to pulmonary hypertension (increased PVR and normal PCWP or LVEDP) and right heart failure frequently not reversible by liver transplantation. This disorder is uncommon (up to 20% of patients with cirrhosis of the liver), and its existence in the pediatric population is not well described. How rapidly PPH can develop varies, as reports indicate anywhere from 3 weeks to 5 years. Remarkably, a review of published PPH cases through 1999 documented that 65% of diagnoses were first recognized during the liver transplant procedure (Krowka et al., 2004). The clinical presentation is subtle and includes exertional dyspnea, fatigue, ankle edema, chest pain, and syncope. Arterial hypoxemia is reported in 80% of patients with moderate to severe disease, with an increased alveolar-arterial oxygen gradient $A\text{–}aDO_2$, reduced diffusion capacity, and accentuated respiratory alkalosis (Kuo et al., 1997; Cotton et al., 2002). Transthoracic contrast-enhanced echocardiography is the screening procedure of choice, with right heart catheterization the gold standard for making the diagnosis and assessing right ventricular function. The best prognosis is in patients with mild symptoms, preserved heart function, and pulmonary arteries responsive to vasodilator therapy.

Treatment options include inhaled nitric oxide, calcium channel blockers, anticoagulation, digoxin, diuretics, supplemental oxygen, and intravenous prostacyclin. The significance of this disease entity is its high perioperative morbidity and mortality in patients undergoing OLT. The data available to date indicate a perioperative mortality of greater than 70% with an mPAP of 45 mm Hg or higher and up to 100% if the mean pressure is greater than 50 mm Hg at the time of transplant. There is no increase in mortality risk if the mPAP is 35 mm Hg. The national liver transplant database reports an overall mortality perioperatively of 36%. The key to survival is good right ventricular function. Even after OLT, the pulmonary vascular abnormalities may progress unless long-term pulmonary vasodilator therapy is instituted.

Pulmonary involvement in the patient with α_1-antitrypsin deficiency or CF is not uncommon in the pediatric patient. α_1-antitrypsin has a reported incidence of liver involvement in 10% to 20% of patients, primarily those who are PIZZ homozygotic (Psacharopoulos et al., 1983). The incidence of this phenotype is 1:7000 in the United States and 1:2000 in Scandinavia (Schwarzenberg and Sharp, 1990). Males are affected more frequently than females. About 10% to 20% of PIZZ individuals develop neonatal cholestasis, and jaundice is often the first presentation of this disease. α_1-antitrypsin deficiency is also associated with cirrhosis and primary liver cancer and may be associated with coexisting obstructive lung disease. Appropriate assessment should be obtained in this particular group of patients with liver failure.

Renal Evaluation

Renal dysfunction in conjunction with worsening hepatic function is common. Acute renal failure requiring hemodialysis is a strong predictor of mortality in these patients. Bartosh and others (1997) reported abnormal renal function in one third of children following liver transplantation, with acute renal failure requiring dialysis (6.2%) a predictor of a high mortality rate (85%). The etiology of renal insufficiency in the patient with ESLD is usually multifactorial. Possible causes include hepatorenal syndrome, disturbances of salt and water clearance, ATN, renal pathology associated with the underlying liver diseases, and diminished intravascular volume causing prerenal azotemia. Exposure to nephrotoxic drugs such as intravenous contrast dyes, aminoglycosides, and nonsteroidal anti-inflammatory agents may also contribute to ATN.

Urine sodium handling is an important variable during evaluations. Both prerenal azotemia and hepatorenal syndrome are characterized by normal urinary sediment, very low urine sodium concentrations (<10 mEq/L), azotemia, and oliguria; it is important to exclude hypovolemia. Specifically, hepatorenal syndrome does not respond to a fluid change with diuresis, whereas the expected response in the patient with prerenal azotemia is diuresis and a subsequent decrease in the serum creatinine and urea nitrogen levels. ATN tends to be salt wasting at its initial presentation, with urine sodium concentrations characteristically greater than 30 mEq/L. An important diagnostic test is the FENa, which also aids in the distinction between these two disease processes. Obtaining an accurate GFR using creatinine clearance in patients with cirrhosis and ascites may give spurious results, as GFR measurements may range from high values to those diagnostic of end-stage renal disease despite the presence of a normal serum creatinine (Papadakis and Arieff, 1987).

Renal ultrasonography is a simple (noninvasive), useful adjunct in the evaluation of azotemia. Kidney size and structural abnormalities should be ascertained for evidence of obstructive uropathy. If a renal biopsy demonstrates irreversible renal disease, then a combined liver and kidney transplant should be considered. Prerenal azotemia due to hypovolemia usually resolves with judicious volume replacement. ATN is usually self-limited and runs a 7- to 14-day course with appropriate support. However, the hepatorenal syndrome is usually not reversible without liver transplantation (Gonwa et al., 1989).

Biliary atresia is the main indication for liver transplantation in infants and children. A palliative surgical hepatoportoenterostomy (Kasai procedure), as opposed to a primary curative OLT, may be performed preferably in the first 60 days of life to restore biliary flow. The natural progression of this disease to cirrhosis and death may then be markedly delayed, with survival reported up to 20 or 30 years. Portal hypertension occurs in at least two thirds of children after portoenterostomy even with complete restoration of biliary flow and return of the serum bilirubin to normal values. In addition, the subsequent development HPS or pulmonary hypertension has been reported.

SURGICAL TECHNIQUE

There are a few significant differences between the surgical techniques for liver transplantation between children and adults. Size discrepancies affect the choice of donor liver, biliary drainage procedure, primary or delayed abdominal closure, the feasibility of using venovenous bypass, and the incidence of hepatic artery thrombosis and other vascular thrombotic complications.

Previous surgery for biliary atresia (Kasai procedure) or open liver biopsy or the use of segmental grafts increases the risk of perioperative bleeding. Donor-recipient size mismatch, especially for children younger than 2 years, has necessitated the utilization of reduced-size and split-liver cadaveric/deceased donors grafts (in situ or ex vivo) and segmental grafts from living donors. Blood loss must be kept to a minimum, given the small total blood volume of the child. The arterial anastomosis is a major challenge because of its small diameter, so there must be creative use of vascular grafts (iliac, carotid, and aortic conduits), which requires partial cross-clamping of the abdominal aorta. Two basic liver transplant techniques are described.

Classic OLT requires placing clamps on the portal vein and suprahepatic and infrahepatic vena cava, and the diseased liver is

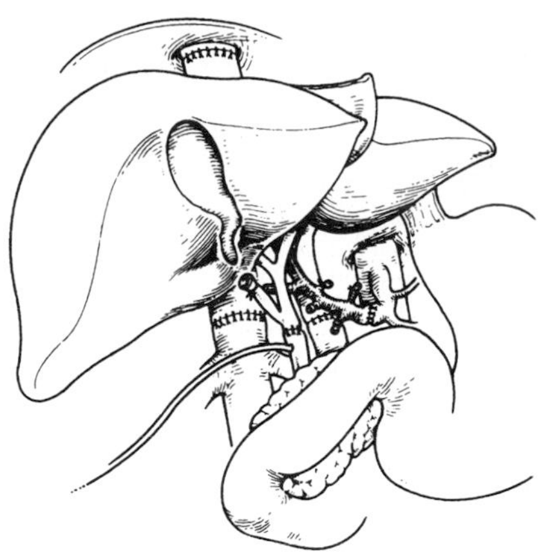

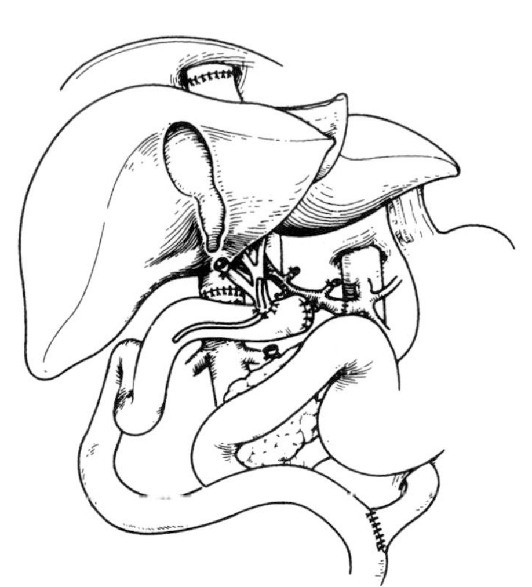

■ **FIGURE 28–6.** Biliary tract reconstruction with choledochojejunostomy, using a Roux limb. (From Starzl TE, Iwatsuki S, VanThiel DH, et al.: *Hepatology* 2:614, 1982; with permission of the American Association for the Study of Liver Diseases.)

then removed en bloc (Starzl et al., 1984; Starzl and Iwatsuki, 1987) (Fig. 28–6). In most cases, with sufficient collateral circulation and preload and pressor support, the patient tolerates 90 minutes of cross-clamping. Otherwise, hemodynamic stability is maintained in larger children and adults with venovenous bypass. The new liver is placed starting with the vascular outflow anastomosis first, which includes the suprahepatic vena cava and infrahepatic vena cava, followed by the vascular inflow of the portal vein and finally the hepatic artery. Biliary reconstruction depends on the underlying diagnosis and size discrepancy of the recipient and donor bile ducts. A Roux-en-Y (hepaticojejunostomy) with or without a stent is most common.

The second approach is referred to as the "piggyback hepatectomy technique." The liver is dissected away from the retrohepatic vena cava, which eliminates the need for total caval clamping and facilitates the use of different size-matched grafts. This has become the preferred technique in pediatric liver transplantation. The diseased liver is mobilized with sequential ligation of the portal vein, short hepatic veins from the IVC to the liver, and the left/right/middle hepatic veins. In this technique, there are only two vascular anastomoses that need to be completed before the reestablishment of blood flow to the donor liver: the suprahepatic cava of the donor liver to the native hepatic veins (end-to-side) or the donor IVC to the recipient IVC (end-to-side) with partial clamping of the IVC and the portal vein anastomosis (Tzakis et al., 1989) (Fig. 28–7). The piggyback technique requires a longer operative time but offers the advantages of greater hemodynamic stability and reduced red blood cell transfusion, intraoperative fluids, and requirement for vasoactive drugs (Moreno-Gonzalez et al., 2003).

The surgical procedure is divided into four distinct stages. Stage I, *the liver dissection phase,* occurs from induction of anesthesia to devascularization of the diseased liver. Stage II, the *anhepatic phase,* begins with removal of the native liver and ends when the IVC and portal vein anastomoses are complete. Stage III, the *reperfusion phase,* occurs with reperfusion of the donor liver by release of the clamps on the portal vein and IVC. Hepatic arterial reconstruction is performed after portal reperfusion, surgical hemostasis, and hemodynamic stability are established. Stage IV is biliary reconstruction with either a duct-to-duct anastomosis or choledochojejunostomy to a Roux-en-Y limb.

The routine use of venovenous bypass during the anhepatic phase of OLT with or without preservation of the cava remains controversial. In early experiments of OLT in a noncirrhotic dog model, it was discovered that clamping of the portal vein or IVC resulted in death of the animal within 30 minutes (Shaw et al., 1985). Although it was later found that most patients can tolerate caval and portal vein clamping remarkably well, Shaw and others (1984) reported in 1984 a 10% intraoperative mortality due to hemodynamic instability in adults during the anhepatic phase. Because of this, a bypass system was developed consisting of heparin-bonded tubing and a centripetal-force pump, allowing cannulation of the femoral and portal veins and diversion of mesenteric and IVC blood to the SVC through the subclavian or axillary veins (Griffith et al., 1985) (Fig. 28–8). Over the years the technique of veno-venous bypass (VVB) has undergone simplification, but unfortunately, there are no published randomized clinical trials of specific outcomes to evaluate its potential benefits. VVB is not without associated morbidity, and Kuo and others (1995) demonstrated that omission of VVB saved 3 hours of operative time, perfusion charges, and circuit costs.

Results from a survey conducted in 1998 of 50 major liver transplant centers indicated that the use of VVB in North America was decreasing, with 91% routinely using VVB in 1987 and 42% of the same programs in 1997 (Chari et al., 1998). Children have a high tolerance to caval cross-clamping. This is a great advantage because it is very inconvenient or impossible to use VVB in patients weighing less than 25 kg (Shaw et al., 1984, 1985). The prerequisite VVB blood flow is usually 20% to 40% of the cardiac output or greater than 1 L/min (Griffith et al., 1985). As these children are not heparinized, the extremely low-flow states that result in children less than 20 kg would predispose to almost certain formation of emboli.

■ ANESTHETIC MANAGEMENT

Most liver transplantation centers develop their own practice of intraoperative care and utilization of clinical resources.

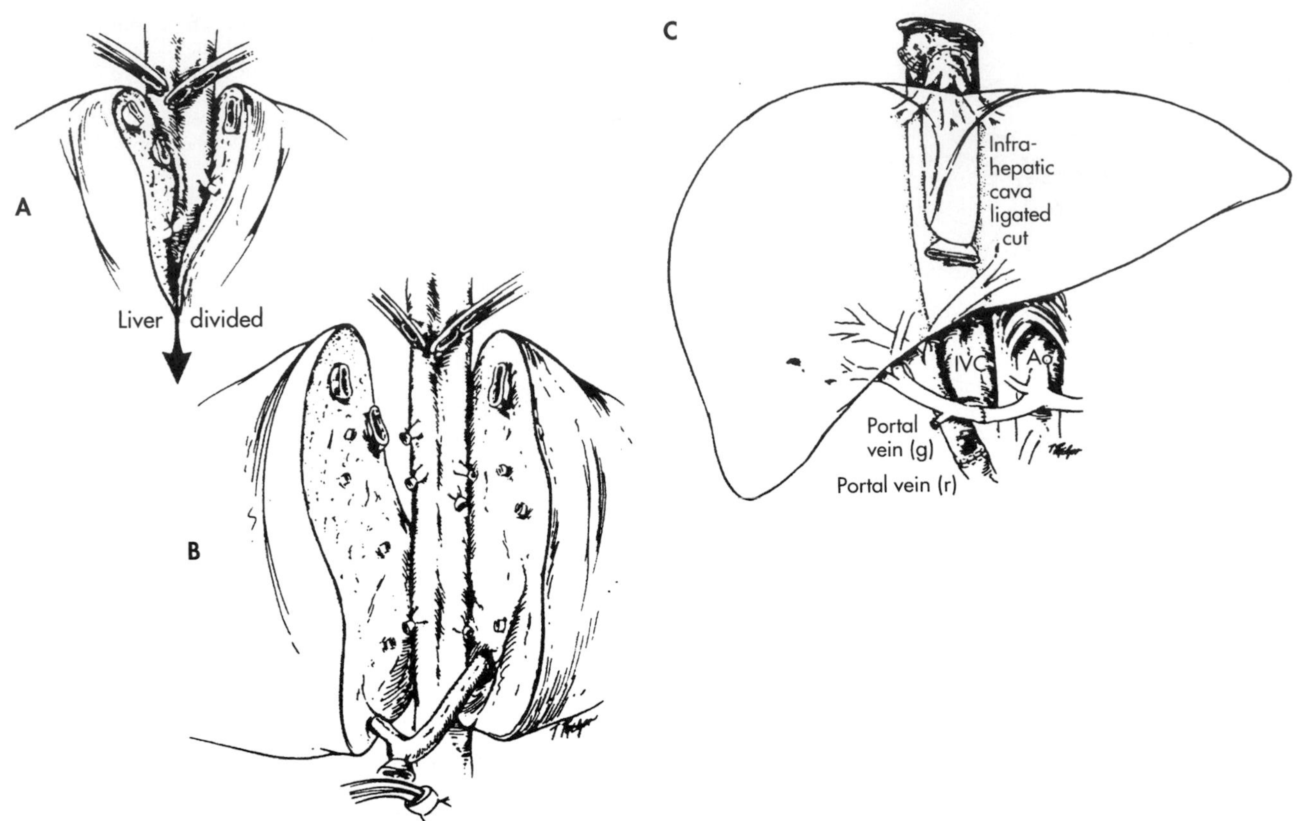

■ **FIGURE 28–7.** The native liver is dissected away from the IVC and the vascular pedicle of the hepatic veins is isolated. The native liver, after being devascularized, may then be transected to allow intraparenchymal exposure of the hepatic veins (**A** and **B**). The final appearance of the recipient liver is illustrated with the native IVC intact and the confluence of the recipient's hepatic veins at the suprahepatic cava, being anastomosed to the donor's intact IVC (**C**). (From Tzakis A, Todo S, Starzl TE: Orthotopic liver transplantation with preservation of the inferior vena cava. *Ann Surg* 210:649–652, 1989.)

A survey of intraoperative resource utilization in anesthesia for liver transplantation in the United States during 2002 indicated that pediatric only programs were distinctly different in personnel, equipment, monitoring, and VVB utilization when compared with adult or mixed-age programs (Schumann, 2003). Pediatric only programs always monitored platelets and traditional coagulation studies (PT, INR, PTT, fibrinogen, D-dimer), with less than 30% of these programs using ACT and TEG to monitor coagulation. Intraoperative metabolic monitoring included ionized calcium in all pediatric programs; magnesium, 46.2%; phosphate, 30.8%; and lactate, none. Measuring arterial blood gases, electrolytes (sodium, potassium), and blood glucose level took place in all programs primarily using operating room satellite laboratories with a turnaround time of less than 5 minutes. The majority of pediatric only programs deployed two anesthesia personnel per case. Anesthesia fellows were used significantly more often and ancillary personnel significantly less often than at mixed-age centers. This observation may be explained by a reduced need for VVB and rapid large-volume infusion: rapid infusion system in 15.4%, level 1 in 46.2%, and no rapid infusion device in 38.5%. This is a significant deviation that is practiced from adult-only or mixed-age centers. None of the 11.3% of centers using transesophageal echocardiography were pediatric only centers. Only a small number used continuous cardiac output monitoring (7.7%), bispectral index (BIS) (15.4%), VVB (7.7%), and more than one arterial catheter (15.4%).

Anesthetic management can be compartmentalized into four distinct stages corresponding to the four surgical stages previously described. An understanding of the pathophysiologic changes that occur in each stage of the surgery allows the anesthesiologist to anticipate and appropriately diagnose, manage, and treat the cardiovascular, hematologic, metabolic, and other derangements encountered throughout the surgery (Borland et al., 1985; Carlier et al., 1987; Kang and Gelman, 1987; Lindop and Farman, 1983; Carton et al., 1994a, 1994b). Liver transplantation in the pediatric patient is very similar to adults from a technical point of view, but there are distinct differences in transfusion requirements and strategies for minimizing blood loss, perioperative coagulation, hemodynamic consequences of caval clamping and reperfusion of the liver, monitoring, vascular access, incidence of thrombosis of the hepatic artery, retransplantation rate, and postoperative pain relief.

Induction and Maintenance of Anesthesia

Liver transplantation has essentially become a semiurgent or elective procedure. The recipient is premedicated with oral, intravenous, or intranasal midazolam. In the operating room, standard monitors are placed and the patient is preoxygenated. Patients without serious cardiac disease or multisystem organ failure will tolerate routine induction of anesthesia followed by endotracheal intubation. Rapid-sequence intravenous induction includes atropine (0.01 to 0.02 mg/kg); a sedative/hypnotic agent using thiopental (3 to 5 mg/kg), propofol (2 mg/kg), etomidate (0.2 to 0.3 mg/kg), or ketamine (1 to 2 mg/kg); fentanyl (2 to 3 mcg/kg); rocuronium (1.0 mg/kg); or succinylcholine (2 mg/kg). The airway is secured with an oral endotracheal

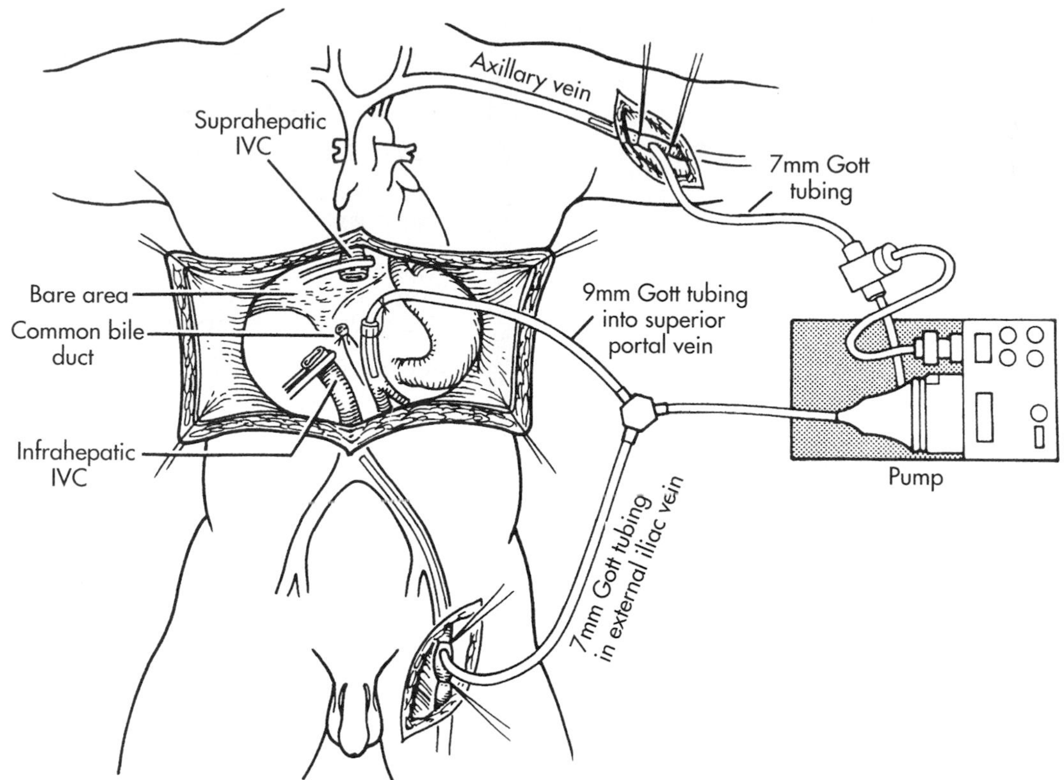

■ **FIGURE 28–8.** This technique was developed to augment cardiac output and diminish vascular congestion during the anhepatic stage of the surgery. Note the placement of the cannulas, joined by a connector, into the portal vein and the femoral veins. Blood drained from the splanchnic and systemic venous systems is then returned to the right heart through the axillary vein with the aid of a pump. (From Kang Y, Gelman S: Liver transplantation. In Gelman S, editor: *Anesthesia and organ transplantation,* Philadelphia, 1987, WB Saunders.)

tube (preferably cuffed), which is then anchored to the face with tincture of benzoin and adhesive tape. Choosing the appropriate size of endotracheal tube and proper positioning is especially important. Placement of an uncuffed tracheal tube of insufficient diameter may result in inadequate alveolar ventilation, especially as chest compliance is reduced during surgery by upper abdominal retraction, tissue edema of the lung parenchyma, surgeons leaning on the chest wall, and placement of a large liver graft. In anticipation of these factors, a tracheal tube with a leak at an inflating pressure greater than 15 to 20 cm H_2O should be placed with the tip approximately 2 cm proximal to the carina.

Succinylcholine has been used traditionally for intubation in pediatric patients at risk for aspiration. Today, this practice is a controversial issue. The "black box warning" indicates that there are rare reports of ventricular dysrhythmias and cardiac arrest secondary to acute rhabdomyolysis with hyperkalemia in apparently healthy children who received succinylcholine. Many of these children were subsequently found to have a skeletal muscle myopathy whose clinical signs were not obvious. Because it is difficult to identify which patients are at risk, it is recommended that the use of succinylcholine in children should be reserved for emergency intubation or where immediate securing of an airway is necessary as succinylcholine has the fastest onset (30 to 60 seconds) compared with other muscle relaxants (see Chapter 6, Pharmacology; Chapter 10, Induction of Anesthesia).

Alternatively, using a relatively large dose of a nondepolarizing muscle relaxant permits securing the airway rapidly without placing the patient at risk for hyperkalemia. The ideal drug in patients with end-stage liver or kidney disease is cis atracurium, as it undergoes spontaneous breakdown at physiologic temperature and pH (Hoffmann elimination), as well as ester hydrolysis. In patients with hepatorenal syndrome, nondepolarizing muscle relaxants should be administered cautiously and titrated to effect. Muscle relaxants requiring significant renal excretion include pancuronium (40%), metocurine (43%), tubocurarine (45%), doxacurium (30%), and pipecuronium (38%). Vecuronium and pancuronium also have 3-OH metabolites, which accumulate in renal failure. The 3-OH metabolite of vecuronium is 50% as potent as the parent compound, and that of pancuronium has two thirds the potency of the parent compound. Muscle relaxants that are metabolized in the liver include pancuronium, vecuronium, rocuronium, and pipecuronium. Vecuronium and rocuronium also have significant biliary excretion. Pancuronium has an increased volume of distribution, prolonged elimination half-life, and decreased plasma clearance in patients with cirrhosis. These patients may need more pancuronium initially to achieve muscle relaxation, and they have a prolonged recovery of blockade between doses (Duvaldestin et al., 1978). In patients with biliary obstruction, the initial dose of pancuronium required is unchanged, whereas the duration of action of each dose is similarly prolonged (Duvaldestin et al., 1978). This may be advantageous because the operative procedure is lengthy and ventilation is usually required for at least 24 hours postoperatively.

The patient is positioned on the operating table supine with the arms abducted and elbows flexed. It is essential to keep the patient covered, warm, and dry. Strategies include warming blanket, heated humidified gases, intravenous fluid warmers, wrapping extremities, Mylar foil wrapping, and using a thick cotton mattress pad below with a U-shaped surround Bair Hugger (Arizant Inc., Eden Prairie, MN) forced-air warming device. Care should be taken to avoid stretch injury of the brachial plexus or pressure necrosis of the occiput, ears, heels, sacrum, or elbows. After the induction of anesthesia, additional monitoring is established: end-tidal CO_2, rectal and esophageal temperature probes, an esophageal stethoscope, an indwelling urinary catheter, a peripheral nerve stimulator, and systemic arterial and central venous pressure cannulas. Access to arterial pressure monitoring above the diaphragm is essential because cross-clamping of the abdominal aorta may be necessary during the hepatic arterial anastomosis.

A radial and femoral (or brachial) arterial line is often used during surgery if there is concern about the accuracy of the radial arterial blood pressure compared with central blood pressure during hemodynamic instability (Kamath et al., 2001), as well as the need for frequent blood sampling necessitating interruption of the pressure tracing. One or two additional large intravenous cannulas (preferably 18-gauge or larger) are then inserted in the upper extremities, either percutaneously or by surgical cutdown. Routine use of VVB in larger children will preclude use of the left arm for venous access. If placement of vascular access in the arms is difficult, the lower extremities may be used, with the understanding that during the anhepatic stage venous return to the heart depends on collateral flow or VVB. A central venous catheter is placed in the external or internal jugular vein. In smaller children, the surgeon will often insert a Hickman catheter (large-bore double-lumen central venous line). The use of a sheath-type catheter in larger children will allow for the rapid infusion of large volumes of blood components and the insertion of a flow-directed balloon-tipped pulmonary artery catheter. Technical difficulties in placing a pulmonary artery catheter and subsequent displacement or migration by surgical maneuvers may preclude its routine use in pediatric patients.

The patient is ventilated with a tidal volume and respiratory rate adjusted to maintain a normal end-tidal CO_2 and arterial carbon dioxide level of 35 to 40 mm Hg. Tidal volume and minute ventilation may be improved using a pressure-limited mode. Air-oxygen is used with an inspiratory oxygen concentration sufficient to maintain adequate oxygenation. PEEP of 5 cm H_2O is routinely added because progressive atelectasis is common. Nitrous oxide is avoided because of its sympathomimetic effects; propensity to cause bowel distention, which may make surgical exposure and closure of the abdomen difficult; and limiting effect on increasing the inspiratory concentration of oxygen.

During anesthesia, all factors inducing arterial hypotension should be avoided. General anesthesia and surgery decrease hepatic blood flow and jeopardize oxygen supply to the liver. Intraoperative reductions in the arterial blood pressure and cardiac output decrease portal blood flow. Contributing factors include anesthetic drugs (inhalational anesthetics, vasodilators, β-blockers, α_1-agonists, H_2-blockers, and vasopressin), hypovolemia, ventilatory mode, hypoxemia, hypercarbia, and acidosis. Surgical manipulation in the right upper quadrant can reduce hepatic blood flow up to 60% from sympathetic activation or direct compression of the vena cava and splanchnic vessels. Compensatory vasodilatation of the hepatic artery in response to decreased portal inflow is diminished by volatile anesthetic agents in a dose-related manner (and absent in a denervated liver), and consequently blood flow becomes pressure dependent. Isoflurane has the least detrimental effect on liver blood flow. A simultaneous decrease in the liver's metabolic demand tends to balance the oxygen supply-uptake ratio. A study of hepatic circulation in pigs during surgical stress and anesthesia suggested that fentanyl and light isoflurane provided adequate hepatic oxygen supply, whereas anesthesia with higher concentrations of isoflurane (which decrease blood pressure >30%) or with halothane in any concentrations studied resulted in inadequate hepatic oxygen supply (Gelman et al., 1987).

BOX 28–4 Anesthetic Management Problems During the Four Stages of Surgery

Stage I: Recipient Hepatectomy

Blood loss, anemia, coagulation abnormalities
Hypotension
Hypoxemia
Hypothermia
Hyperkalemia, hypocalcemia, acidosis
Encephalopathy with raised intracranial pressure

Stage II: Anhepatic Stage

Hemodynamic changes with caval clamping and total hepatic vascular exclusion
Acidosis, hypocalcemia, hypothermia, hypoglycemia
VVB
Urine output and renal function
Backwashing of the liver

Stage III: Reperfusion

Reperfusion syndrome
Postreperfusion hyperkalemia
Fibrinolysis
Pulmonary thromboembolism
Pulmonary hypertension
Fluid overload, ventricular dysfunction, pulmonary edema
Systemic hypotension
Hypothermia

Stage IV: Biliary Reconstruction

Primary nonfunction or delayed primary function of the graft
Abdominal closure
Hypokalemia
Coagulation status, bleeding
Renal dysfunction
Hyperglycemia, metabolic alkalosis, hypomagnesemia

When administering drugs to patients with chronic liver disease, all drug dosages should be decreased and carefully titrated until the desired effect is achieved. Experts currently recommend that isoflurane alone or in combination with small doses of fentanyl be used as the method of choice provided adequate pulmonary ventilation, cardiac output, and arterial pressure are maintained. Anesthetic management problems during the four stages of surgery are listed in Box 28–4.

Cardiovascular Changes

During stage I, hypotension is secondary to major fluid shifts, bleeding, and ionized hypocalcemia (Jawan et al., 2003). Transient decreases in mean arterial pressure are not unusual in this stage from surgical manipulation of the liver and compression of the IVC transiently precluding venous return to the heart. Drainage of ascites may result in hypotension if the patient is not adequately hydrated before incision of the peritoneum.

Factors contributing to blood loss include adhesions from prior operations, coagulopathy (factor deficiency, low platelets, abnormal fibrinogen, or disseminated intravascular coagulopathy), portal hypertension and collateral venous circulation, and lack of surgical hemostasis (especially a hole in the IVC). Placement of the suprahepatic caval clamp may be associated with arrhythmia, and in one instance I have witnessed hypotension and hypoxemia due to acute right ventricular outflow tract obstruction, as the pericardium and a portion of the right ventricle were included in the clamp. Hypotension that is unresponsive to intravenous pressors should raise suspicions of absolute or relative hypovolemia (limited preload due to vascular clotting or torsion of the liver on its vascular pedicle), acidosis, sepsis, or vasoparesis.

During stage II, classic OLT requires a trial of portal vein and IVC clamping. The hemodynamic response is characterized by a decrease in cardiac output, CVP, and PAP and compensatory increase in heart rate and SVR (Eyraud et al., 2002). Hemodynamic instability may result from decreased venous return (modified by VVB or piggyback technique) and insufficient physiologic compensation by the patient for this acute change. Therapeutic strategies then polarize into the "flooders" and the "squeezers," each with associated morbidity for the patient. Colloid or crystalloid boluses are administered, followed by dopamine or norepinephrine (phenylephrine or epinephrine) for pressor support. The goal is to maintain the lowest filling pressures compatible with an acceptable mean arterial pressure in anticipation of an increase in PAP with removal of the caval and portal vein clamps. Pulmonary hypertension may result due to an increase in venous return from the gut and lower extremities and reactive changes in pulmonary vascular resistance with the release of vasoactive hormones which are recirculated systemically. The donor liver is flushed either with crystalloid or colloid or by backwashing the liver. The procedure for backwashing involves insertion of a red rubber cannula into the recipient/donor IVC, and the clamp is removed from the portal vein, allowing washing of the liver with autologous blood retrograde from the portal vein through the donor liver, exiting through the cannula into a stainless steel graduated cylinder.

Communication with the surgeon at this point is imperative as one does not hear the sound of the suction or observe blood filling the canisters, but the patient becomes immediately and dramatically hypotensive. Hypotension associated with this maneuver can be ameliorated with the prophylactic administration of phenylephrine or epinephrine boluses, gentle fluid administration, or transfusion of packed red blood cells if the hematocrit is low. The elimination of air bubbles, hyperkalemic preservation solution, hormones, or other "evil humors" has been credited for decreasing the incidence of subsequent reperfusion syndrome in adult patients that may occur with reperfusion of the liver (Fukuzawa et al., 1994). The goal for warm ischemia time (time from liver up into the surgical field until reperfusion in the recipient) is usually less than 60 minutes, so managing hypotension and preparing for reperfusion occur over a relatively short period. Reactivation of HCV has been shown to be less if the warm ischemia time can be kept under 35 minutes, which shortens the target time for completing this portion of the operation even further (Clavien et al., 2004).

During stage III, severe hemodynamic instability may occur immediately after reperfusion of the transplanted liver, including severe hypotension, bradycardia, supraventricular and ventricular arrhythmias, variable cardiac output, and occasionally cardiac arrest (0% to 5%). These changes are due to recirculation of the residual hyperkalemic preservation solution from the donor liver directly to the recipient's heart or the postreperfusion syndrome (defined as a decrease in mean arterial pressure >30% from baseline for at least 1 minute within 5 minutes of reperfusion). The incidence of this postreperfusion syndrome in adults may be as high as 30%, and epinephrine boluses are usually required to prevent cardiovascular collapse (Aggarwal et al., 1987). Immediately after reperfusion left ventricular function may be impaired and pulmonary capillary wedge pressure, CVP, and PAP usually increase with a major decrease in SVR, while TEE monitoring shows a stable or even decreased left ventricular end-diastolic volume. These contradictory findings may be due to a period of deteriorated left ventricular compliance or "cardioplegia" on reperfusion (Suriani et al., 1996; De Wolf, 1999).

The etiology of postreperfusion syndrome remains unclear, but it may be caused by the release of vasoactive mediators from the ischemic liver or decompressed portal circulation, changes in the rate of venous return (volume overload), and perhaps an increase in serum potassium. Possible mediators that are highly suspect include nitric oxide and TNF-α with demonstrable increased levels after graft reperfusion (Nishimura et al., 1993) and xanthine oxidase, a generator of cytotoxic oxygen radicals that may produce myocardial dysfunction and cellular damage. Vasoactive drugs for pressor support (norepinephrine, epinephrine, dopamine) may be required, and a balance is reached between a lowered mean arterial pressure and often very low SVR, permitting increased flow to perfusable organs at a lower perfusion pressure. Prophylactic use of aprotinin has been reported to ameliorate the postreperfusion syndrome in liver transplantation, as reflected by a significant reduction in vasopressor requirements (Milroy et al., 1995; Molenaar et al., 2001). High filling pressures should be avoided that may cause congestion of the donor liver, bleeding from surgical sites, and biventricular dysfunction with pulmonary edema. Therapies for reducing filling pressures include limiting intravenous infusions, furosemide-induced diuresis, vasodilatation (intravenous nitroglycerin or morphine), nitric oxide, or PGE_1.

Blood Loss, Coagulation, and Hemostasis

During liver transplant surgery, the effects of fibrinolysis, thrombocytopenia, coagulation factor, and fibrinogen deficiency on clinical bleeding are not always predictable and transfusion requirements are variable. Portal hypertension with fragile venous collaterals, adhesions from prior operations, and lack of surgical hemostasis contribute to the complexity of massive blood loss and hemostatic management. Independent predictors of increased transfusion requirements include the severity of liver disease or Child-Pugh classification (especially those hospitalized for inpatient support), preoperative PT, history of abdominal operations, preoperative hematocrit and factor V levels, portal vein hypoplasia, reduced-size liver graft, and operative time as a marker for more difficult surgery (Ozier et al, 1995; Maurer and Spence, 2004). Usually, the greatest operative blood loss occurs during vascular dissection and the hepatectomy phase. During this stage, there is a progressive degradation of the coagulation cascade. A dilutional coagulopathy results along with progressive thrombocytopenia. The range of blood loss may be from 0.5 to 25 times the blood volume (Borland et al., 1985).

Alterations of coagulation in the pediatric patient during OLT have been studied (Kang et al., 1989). Classic hourly monitoring of the prothrombin time, activated partial thromboplastin time (aPTT), and platelet counts demonstrates a progressive prolongation of the PT and PTT, as well as a significant decrease of all clotting factors. On graft reperfusion, there may be profound prolongation of the PTT, usually to greater than 100 seconds. Besides the standard coagulation tests (PT, aPTT, fibrinogen, platelets, and D-dimer), the TEG (thromboelastogram) and Sonoclot (coagulation and platelet function analyzer) are used in the evaluation of coagulation. The TEG is performed using whole blood; it assesses clot formation until an end point of clot lysis or retraction is determined. TEG findings have correlated with clinical bleeding and can assist in treating intraoperative hemorrhage by identifying the cause of the bleeding diathesis (factor deficiency, fibrinolysis, heparin effect, thrombocytopenia, or platelet dysfunction) (Kang, 1986; Zuckerman et al., 1981) (Fig. 28–9). Abnormalities of the reaction time (r), the alpha angle (a), or the maximum amplitude (MA) may indicate decreased clotting factors, diminished factor VIII and fibrinogen, or diminished platelet function or number, respectively (Kang et al., 1989). Conversely, a short reaction time is indicative of a hypercoagulable state. This has occasionally been observed in patients who have developed thrombosis after graft reperfusion (Kang, 1995; Gologorsky et al., 2001; Planinsic et al., 2004).

Increased fibrinolytic activity is observed in patients with ESLD as a result of increased tissue plasminogen activator (TPA) activity and reduced synthesis of fibrinolysis inhibitors. TPA further increases during the anhepatic stages and peaks immediately after graft reperfusion. Various antifibrinolytic agents have been used to counter this accelerated fibrinolysis evident immediately on graft reperfusion in up to 80% of patients, but their precise role remains undefined. These include aprotinin, ε-aminocaproic acid (EACA), and tranexamic acid. Aprotinin is a serine protease inhibitor that prevents the lysis of fibrinogen by inhibiting plasmin, kallikrein, and leukocyte elastase. Studies have reported a significant reduction in blood loss (60%) and packed red blood cell transfusion requirements compared with control subjects, with no increase in thrombotic complications (Porte et al., 2000; Dalmau et al., 2003; Porte, 2004). Other studies have not reported a benefit with aprotinin use. EACA (Kang et al., 1987) and tranexamic acid prevent fibrinolysis by inhibiting plasminogen and plasmin, thus preventing the eventual degradation of fibrin. In addition, a significant heparin effect may be seen immediately on graft reperfusion for up to 30 minutes. This effect is caused by the release of endogenous heparinoids from the liver, as well as residual heparin from the preservation solution. Calcium is an important coenzyme in the coagulation cascade. During the dissection and anhepatic phases of liver transplantation, hypocalcemia may develop, especially when large amounts of fresh frozen plasma have been given. In many transplant centers, continuous calcium infusions and magnesium supplements are routine therapy.

The approach to blood product replacement differs in children from adults because of two important concerns: thrombosis

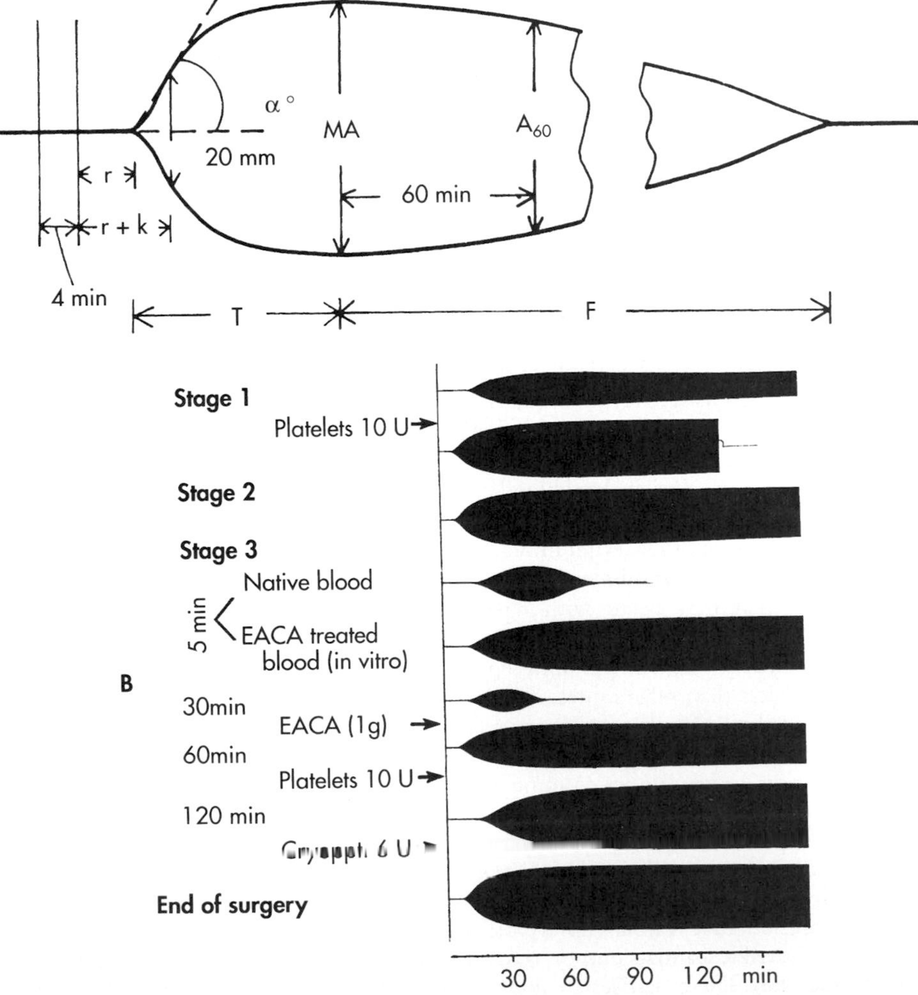

■ **FIGURE 28–9.** Thromboelastogram (TEG). A, This is a representation of the normal parameters that are measured and analyzed for interpretation of the TEG. B, This figure illustrates the coagulation alterations that are noted during OLT. Note the elements of low platelets that improve the MA after administration of platelets, the development of fibrinolysis, which is treated by EACA and detected early on the TEG at the time of graft reperfusion. In addition, the diminished alpha angle in stage 3 is treated with administration of cryoprecipitate, with noted improvement of coagulation. (From Kang Y, Gelman S: Liver transplantation. In Gelman S, editor: *Anesthesia and organ transplantation.* Philadelphia, 1987, WB Saunders.)

of the hepatic artery and postoperative hypercoagulability. Thrombosis of the hepatic artery is the most common serious complication after liver transplantation in children and as such, less fresh frozen plasma and platelets are routinely administered. Following reperfusion, ideally the hematocrit should be maintained at 20% to 30% to minimize the increase in blood viscosity and to limit the risk of thrombotic complications (Tisone et al., 1988). Children have been reported to be at greater risk for hepatic artery thrombosis compared with adults due to small arterial size, no use of intraoperative microscope, and postoperative hypercoagulable state (Heffron et al., 2003). The incidence of hepatic artery thrombosis has been reported in 15% of the mixed-ages pediatric series (Otte et al., 1990); however, it appears to be directly related to the size of the hepatic artery (smaller arteries and livers from neonates or infants having the highest incidence of this complication) (Mazzaferro et al., 1989; Jurim et al., 1995; Mas et al., 2003; Martin et al., 2004) and technical complications during the vascular reconstruction. When a split liver is used, thrombosis is relatively rare (5% to 8%) and similar to the adult rate (Gridelli et al., 2003). Thus, in some institutions, aggressive correction of coagulation is pursued only when there is diffuse bleeding after graft reperfusion or if monitoring reveals fibrinolysis that was not reversed by the new liver. Many transplant centers use the normalization of the PT and platelet count as indicators of recovery of donor liver graft function. Persistent hypothermia, coagulopathy with bleeding, hypocapnia, hyperkalemia, acidosis, absence of bile duct production, hyperglycemia, renal insufficiency, and hemodynamic instability may suggest suboptimal graft function.

Following liver transplantation in children, a decrease occurs in protein C and antithrombin III levels to below 50% of normal values and persists for 10 days. This prolonged decrease is not seen in adults. Immediately after surgery, a 10-fold increase in plasminogen activator inhibitor occurs, with a further increase 6 to 9 days later. Therefore, in the immediate postoperative period between days 4 and 10, children are at an increased risk of thrombosis (Harper et al., 1988). An attempt to minimize this occurrence has resulted in administration of anticoagulation therapy: intravenous heparin, dextran 40, aspirin, and antithrombin III (Abengochea et al., 1995). There are also differences in coagulation between the infant and adult. In the normal neonate, there is a deficiency of vitamin K-dependent clotting factors for several weeks. Protein C is significantly reduced for at least 6 months (Andrew et al., 1987), and protein S concentrations do not increase to within the normal adult range until 3 months of age (Donaldson et al., 1991). Protein C inhibits the function of factors VIII and V and enhances fibrinolysis, which is enhanced by protein S.

In the child whose body weight is greater than 20 kg, use of the rapid infusion system (RIS) facilitates the rapid replacement of blood products. In this instance, however, blood product replacement is similar to that for an adult. A unit each of red blood cells, fresh frozen plasma, and 250 mL of either normal saline solution or neutral pH-balanced salt solution (Plasmalyte) is mixed in the cardiotomy reservoir of the RIS. This mixture mimics whole blood with a hematocrit of 28% to 30%. Blood replacement may occur at a rate of up to 1500 mL/min if needed.

Hypothermia and hypocalcemia are known to contribute to coagulopathy (Kang, 1995). Altered platelet function and an increased incidence of fibrinolysis are recognized consequences. Thus temperatures below 35°C are best avoided. Finally, cell salvage may be beneficial in the patient undergoing OLT. Blood recovery of up to 30% is expected, but the need for rapid volume replacement limits its use. In addition, the use of the cell saver is contraindicated in patients with viral or bacterial infections, tumors, or FHF without an identifiable cause of the liver failure. Massive blood transfusion has an associated morbidity of more frequent bouts of sepsis, a prolonged stay in the intensive care unit, a higher rate of severe CMV infection, and higher rates of graft failure and patient mortality (Maurer and Spence, 2004).

Metabolic Function

Hepatic failure can result in impairment of numerous complex metabolic functions that may significantly impact anesthetic care. The liver plays a critical role in maintaining a normal blood glucose level; hypoglycemia frequently results from failure of gluconeogenesis, insufficient insulin degradation, and a depletion of glycogen stores. Most patients with chronic liver disease are undernourished and fat stores are diminished with impairment of lipid transport and the integrity of cellular membranes.

Altered Glucose Metabolism

Hypoglycemia is rarely seen unless the patient presents with acute FHF or has exhausted their liver glycogen stores. Patients may also be at risk during catecholamine infusions or those requiring insulin for the management of hyperkalemia. During the anhepatic phase, there are several sources of glucose available to the patient such as a significant amount of free glucose (84 mg/dL by day 35 of storage) contained in packed red blood cells (Miller, 2000), 5% dextrose in water (D_5W) solution used as a carrier for drug infusions, and the administration of intravenous methylprednisolone for induction of immunosuppression during the portal anastomosis. Hyperglycemia after graft reperfusion is common due to glucose release from ischemic hepatocytes, steroid-induced insulin resistance, and decreased glucose metabolism in hypothermic patients (DeWolf et al., 1987). As such, hourly monitoring of blood glucose levels is essential (Fig. 28–10).

Acute Ionized Hypocalcemia and Magnesium

Ionized hypocalcemia results from the rapid transfusion of large volumes of blood products containing citrate, especially during periods of hypothermia and acidosis. Citrate chelates both calcium and magnesium and other divalent cations. Hypotension is usually not significant until an ionized calcium level of 0.56 mmol/L (Marquez et al., 1986, Martin et al., 1990). The consequence of acute ionized hypomagnesemia (Scott et al., 1996) is not yet apparent, although it may result in a higher incidence of atrial arrhythmias and decreased myocardial contractility. Replacement of calcium with either calcium chloride or gluconate in equivalent calcium doses is equally effective. Administration of calcium chloride in the central line may result in transient arrhythmia, but deposition into tissues from an extravasated peripheral line will result in severe tissue necrosis. The recipient routinely receives sodium bicarbonate and calcium chloride about 1 minute before reperfusion to counteract anticipated hyperkalemia and hypotension.

Hypokalemia is the norm in chronic liver failure. It results from the use of diuretics, altered aldosterone metabolism, and metabolic alkalosis. If ventricular arrhythmias are noted during stages I and II, magnesium replacement is recommended. Potassium replacement is avoided because there is an expected transient twofold to threefold increase in potassium concentration

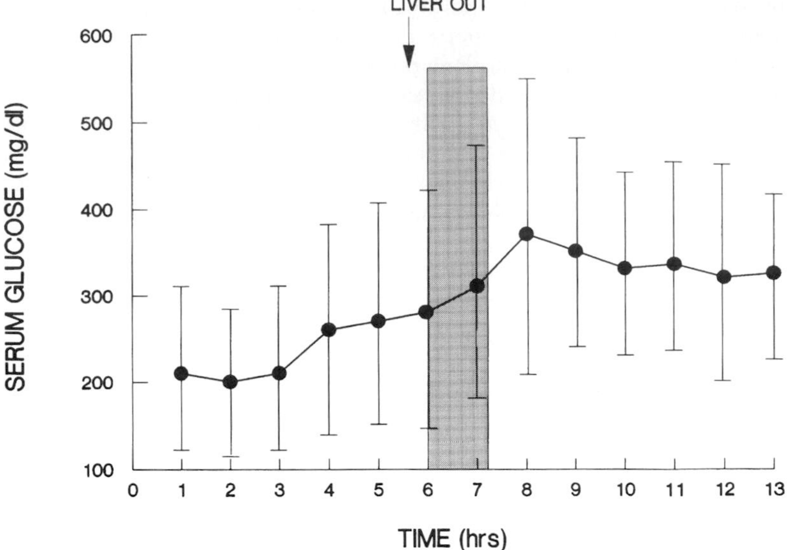

■ **FIGURE 28–10.** Glucose versus time. Mean and SD values are represented. *Shaded area* represents the anhepatic phase. (Reprinted with permission from International Anesthesia Research Society from Anesthesia for Pediatric Orthotopic Liver Transplantation by Borland LM, Roule M, Cook DR: *Anesth Analg* 64:117, 1985.)

immediately on graft reperfusion. Hypokalemia is common after graft reperfusion, usually as a result of diuresis, receptor stimulation with the use of epinephrine, and uptake of potassium by the new liver. Cautious replacement during the biliary reconstruction phase is appropriate if the patient has no preexisting renal insufficiency and evidence of adequate urine output.

Hyperkalemia should be treated aggressively at any point during the surgery. This electrolyte disturbance usually results from massive transfusion of red blood cells that have an estimated potassium content of 76 mEq/L by day 35 of cold storage or from renal failure (Miller, 2000). The judicious use of diuretics as well as an infusion of glucose and insulin may be of benefit in reducing the potassium load (De Wolf et al., 1993). This is most crucial before revascularization of the donor liver. Postreperfusion hyperkalemia (7 to 12 mEq/L) is transitory, with redistribution occurring in 1 to 2 minutes, which seldom needs pharmacologic intervention other than prophylactic sodium bicarbonate and calcium intravenously (Nakasuji and Bookallil, 2000). Washed red blood cells prevent the further development of this problem. When hyperkalemia is life threatening, the use of venovenous hemofiltration or removal of part of the patient's blood volume and washing by the cell saver may be beneficial.

Metabolic acidosis is progressive during OLT and peaks during graft reperfusion. It results from transfusion of blood products and becomes accentuated during the anhepatic stage when liver metabolism of citrate, lactate, and other acids is absent. Whether tissue hypoperfusion is a contributing factor remains unclear; however, this should be balanced by the fact that overall body oxygen consumption is reduced during the anhepatic stage. The threshold for bicarbonate administration is a base deficit of −5 mEq/L. Associated morbidity includes hypernatremia, hypercarbia, and hyperosmolality. Acidosis usually resolves after reperfusion of the graft. Sodium bicarbonate should be administered as indicated and any ongoing problem identified (poor perfusion with lactic acidosis or delayed primary/nonfunction of the graft). Metabolic alkalosis is common postoperatively due to potassium and diuretic therapy and metabolism of citrate or lactate. This may delay weaning of the patient from mechanical ventilation.

Hyponatremia and Hyperosmolarity

Dilutional hyponatremia is common and worrisome at serum sodium levels less than 125 mEq/L. Central pontine myelinolysis (CPM) is a frequently symmetric noninflammatory demyelinating disorder within the brainstem pons. In at least 10% of patients, demyelination also occurs in extrapontine areas. Clinical manifestations are characterized by postoperative confusion and/or weakness or a "locked-in" syndrome after transplantation (Estol et al., 1989; Wszolek et al., 1989). The most frequent findings are delirium, pseudobulbar palsy, and spastic quadriplegia, which may result in permanent neurologic deficits. CPM occurs inconsistently as a complication of severe and prolonged hyponatremia, particularly when the sodium is corrected too rapidly. A study by Singh and others (1994) demonstrated that CPM was present in 29% of postmortem examinations of adult liver transplant patients. Risk factors included serum sodium less than 120 mEq/L for more than 48 hours, aggressive intravenous fluid therapy with hypertonic saline solutions, and hypernatremia during treatment.

Empirical data show that CPM is likely to occur when the total perioperative increase in sodium concentration is above 15 to 20 mEq/L (Estol et al., 1989; Yu et al., 2004). In these patients, the choice of crystalloid should be Plasmalyte or 0.45% NaCl. Hyperosmolality has also been considered as a contributor to the development of CPM. In the presence of either of these metabolic derangements, the judicious use of THAM is recommended because the osmolality of THAM is 308 mOsm/L, whereas that of sodium bicarbonate is 2000 mOsm/L. In addition, the sodium content of bicarbonate buffer is 8.4% compared with 0.9% NaCl in intravenous solutions.

Temperature Regulation

The most effective means of cooling a man is to give him an anesthetic… .

—Pickering, 1958

Surgical procedures that place these patients at risk for unintentional hypothermia are those involving exposure of large skin, serosal, and mucosal surfaces during lengthy procedures under general anesthesia in a cold operating room, especially with no humidification of gases and infusion of cold intravenous fluids. Disruption of the hypothalamic thermoregulatory center causes the patient to become poikilothermic. The most significant contributors to hypothermia in the pediatric patient undergoing OLT are radiant and evaporative heat losses. In addition, the use of venovenous bypass may result in a 0.5° to 1.0°C temperature loss when a heat exchanger is not used. Preservation of the donor liver is inherent on rendering the organ metabolically inert by reducing the core temperature to 4°C through cold preservation techniques. To further extend this cooling period while performing the vascular anastomosis in the recipient, the liver may be wrapped in cold compresses or ice, which will further reduce the core temperature of the patient. With reperfusion, a hypothermia-induced cardiac arrhythmia and arrest may result if the perfusate of the liver is allowed to further cool the sinus node. Modest hypothermia to 35°C is well tolerated with minimal effects on coagulation, but platelet dysfunction, fibrinolysis, and bleeding begin to increase in a linear fashion as the core temperature decreases. Mild hypothermia may be beneficial as a reduction in metabolic oxygen requirements may limit warm ischemia and cerebral and myocardial injury. In pediatric patients, the detrimental physiologic effects of mild hypothermia (32° to 35°C) and the increased risk of infection clearly outweigh these minimal benefits.

Attention should be directed to aggressively maintaining a normal body temperature. This may be achieved by using forced air warming (Bair Hugger) or raising the ambient temperature of the operating theater. In addition, protective barriers should be strategically placed to prevent the operating room table from becoming wet, because this will result in conductive cooling of the patient. Heating of the humidified gases is also an important maneuver.

Pulmonary Function

Hypoxemia is common in pediatric patients with ESLD due to ascites and pleural effusions causing a decrease in FRC and total lung capacity, impaired diffusion capacity, and pulmonary arteriovenous shunting. After the induction of anesthesia, difficulties in ventilation and oxygenation may occur with diaphragmatic paralysis resulting in an acute restrictive lung effect. The increased A–aDO_2 usually improves after the abdominal cavity is opened. If relative hypoxemia persists, other causes of venous admixture should be sought.

Factors that may worsen oxygenation during the surgical procedure include clot or air emboli, progression of acute respiratory distress syndrome, transfusion-related acute lung injury, HPS, and pulmonary edema from excessive fluid administration. Finally, extubation of the patient at the end of the procedure is not recommended no matter how short the surgery because 50% to 55% (McAlister et al., 1993) of patients will develop right diaphragmatic paralysis postoperatively, and 25% will have pleural effusions, which compromise pulmonary function. The fast-track approach to anesthetic care may reduce the requirement for postoperative mechanical ventilation but does not reduce the intensive care unit stay after liver transplantation (Gurakar et al., 1995; Findlay et al., 2002).

Renal Function

Renal insufficiency is a common finding in patients undergoing OLT and contributes significantly to postoperative morbidity, as well as being an independent predictor of postoperative mortality (Gonwa, 2005). The patient who comes to the operating room with hepatorenal syndrome or ATN should not be expected to show improvement of renal function until after the graft functions (McCauley et al., 1990). Information collected by the National Institute of Diabetes and Digestive and Kidney Diseases (NIDDK) Liver Transplantation Database support the conclusion that renal insufficiency in fulminant hepatic failure and those patients requiring preoperative dialysis or liver-kidney transplantation in cirrhosis predicts lower posttransplant patient and graft survival rates (Brown et al., 1996).

A progressive decline in urine output is expected, with little or none during the anhepatic portion of the surgery without preservation of the IVC or use of VVB. This physiologic alteration has been thought to be secondary to congestion of the kidney from increased renal venous pressures with total cross-clamping of the infrahepatic IVC (Gunning et al., 1991). Whether the incidence of postoperative renal insufficiency is as frequent in the patient in whom the piggyback technique is used remains unclear. The judicious use of the diuretics (mannitol and furosemide) is recommended in the patient who develops oliguria (Polson et al., 1987). If furosemide is used, it should be noted that it may be ineffective in the patient with a low albumin level (average albumin in the patient with liver failure for OLT is 1.8 to 2.5 mg/dL). Although a renal dose of dopamine not exceeding 1.5 mcg/kg per min is often recommended, there is no clear benefit from its use as a renal protective agent (Polson et al., 1987; Gray et al., 1991; Swygert et al., 1991; Kellum and Decker, 2001). The incidence of renal complications postoperatively in all patients undergoing OLT remains the same with or without the use of venovenous bypass and/or diuretic therapy (Schwarz et al., 2001; Cabezuelo et al., 2003). Acute renal insufficiency is estimated to occur after liver transplantation in up to 67% of recipients (Rimola et al., 1987). Contributing factors include preexisting renal insufficiency, intraoperative complications (suboptimal renal perfusion associated with hypotension, massive transfusion, increased caval pressures), early graft dysfunction, sepsis, and administration of cyclosporine or tacrolimus in the immediate posttransplant period.

GRAFT REDUCTION AND SPLIT-LIVER TRANSPLANTATION

With the plateau in organ availability in the past 5 years and the increased indications for OLT, newer creative techniques have been developed to increase organ availability to pediatric patients. These three techniques—living-related, split livers, and graft reduction—account for up to 30% of all pediatric OLT in some centers. Living related organ transplantation has been discussed earlier.

Reduced-size liver transplantation (graft reduction) was first performed by Bismuth and Houssin (1984) and Broelsch and others (1991). This procedure involves the dissection of the graft at the back table with preparation of either the right lobe, left lobe, or left lateral segment graft, depending on the size of the recipient. The choice of lobe is related to the size of the recipient. With a recipient-to-donor size discrepancy of 1:2, a right lobe graft is chosen. Similarly, if the recipient-to-donor size discrepancy is 1:4 or 1:8 (Thistlethwaite et al., 1991), a left lobe graft or a left lateral segment graft is chosen, respectively. Because this technique, as with split livers, requires the preparation of the graft at the back table, it lends itself to an increased cold ischemic time of the liver. Vascular anastomoses for this procedure are usually end-to-end with the occasional need for a piggyback technique or the direct anastomosis of the hepatic veins to the vena cava.

In split-liver transplantation, the liver is divided into left and right lobes and transplanted into two recipients (Emond et al., 1990; Otte et al., 1990; Renz et al., 2004) (Fig. 28–11). The division results in the right lobe containing the portal vein, hepatic artery, IVC, and common bile duct, while the left lobe includes the left lobar branches of the vessels and the left hepatic duct. Transplantation of the left lobe may necessitate the use of interposition vascular grafts, whereas the right lobe is transplanted in a fashion similar to that used for the whole organ. Most frequently, biliary reconstruction is by the Roux-en-Y technique because of the size discrepancy of the donor and recipient bile ducts.

Living-related liver transplantation from parent to child was described in 1991 by Brolesch, Whitington and others (1991) and has the potential advantages of increasing the availability of organs, reducing the waiting times and deaths on the recipient waiting list, allowing medical optimization of the recipient while minimizing the risk of clinical deterioration, and limiting

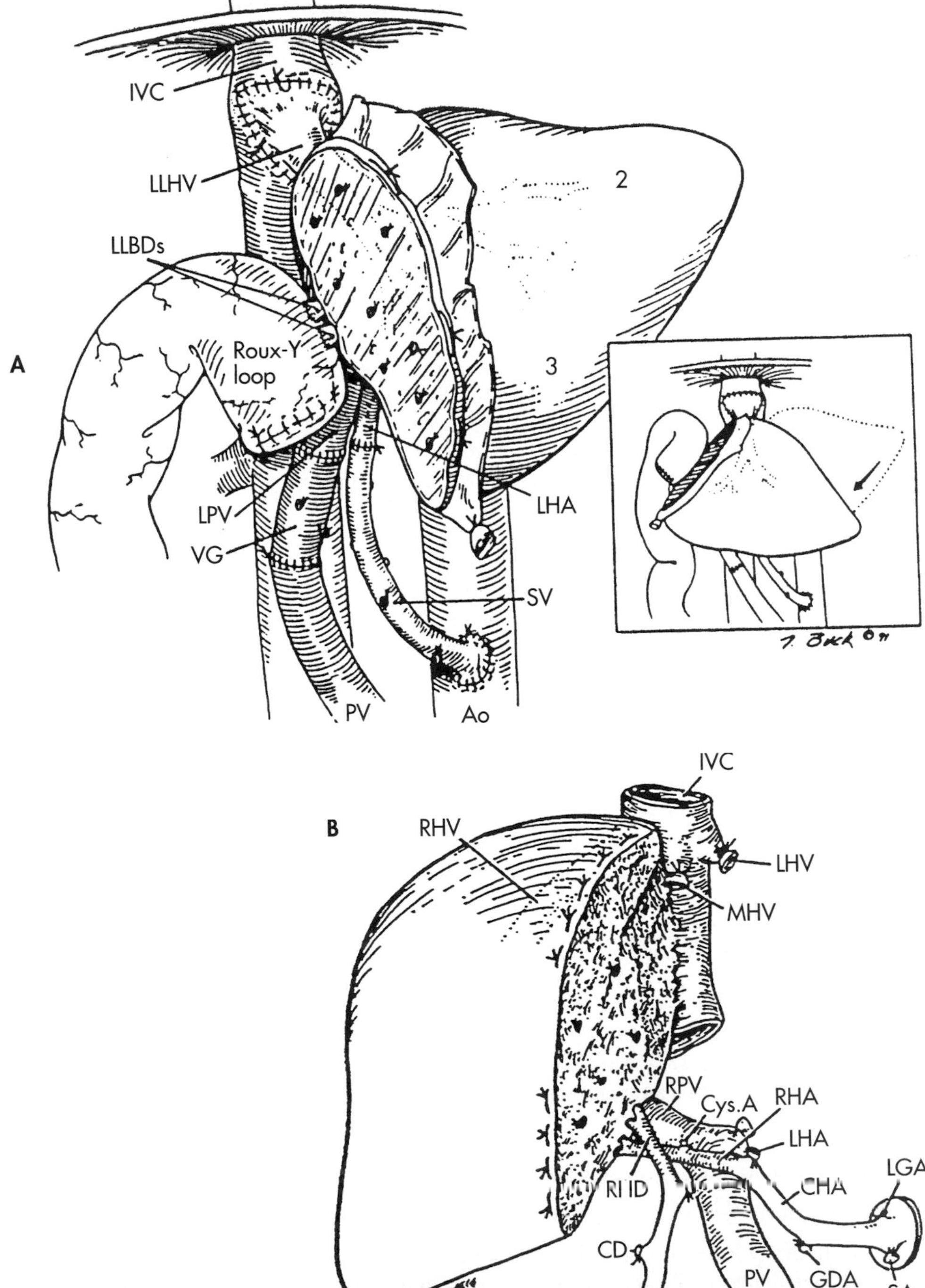

■ **FIGURE 28–11.** Split liver transplantation. Demonstrated here is the use of either a right or left hepatic lobe. Note that the right lobe retains the native donor IVC whereas the left lobe is connected to the recipient IVC by the use of the left hepatic vein. (**A** from Broelsch CE, et al.: Liver transplantation in children from living-related donors. *Ann Surg* 214:428, 1991; **B** from Broelsch CE, Emond JC, Thistlewaite JR, et al.: Liver transplantation, including the concept of reduced-size liver transplants in children. *Ann Surg* 208:410–420, 1988.)

immunosuppressive therapy by decreasing the immunogenicity of the transplanted organ. In addition, societies in which the criteria for death differ from those previously described (Tanaka et al., 1993) are now able to offer organ transplantation in a socially acceptable manner. Until 1998, the majority of all living donor grafts in the United States went to children under 1 year of age. Living donation is not without risk. Mortality among healthy donors is low, but complications in the donor are relatively common.

These findings then raise the issues of safety and ethics. Potential risks to the donor include transfusion, biliary complications, negative psychosocial aspects (out-of-pocket expenses, loss of income, stress on the donor and donor family, change in body image, inability to work for at least 4 to 8 weeks after donation, and poor recipient outcome), and death. Up to 20% of donors may experience complications related to major abdominal surgery, including pneumonia, atelectasis, wound infection, small-bowel obstruction, incisional hernia, pressure ulcers, phlebitis, neuropraxia or peroneal nerve palsy, and reoperation. Until 1994, all living-donor liver transplants were performed with a left-lateral segmentectomy of one or more lobes or left lobectomy (20% of liver) from parent-to-child or adult-to-small adult. Adult-to-adult transplantation of the right hepatic lobe (60% of liver) was first reported in Japan in 1994, and in the United States a total of 62 live donor liver transplants were completed in 1996, peaking at 506 in 2001, then 355 in 2002, 315 in 2003, and 244 in 2004, for a total of 2518 living liver donors from 1989 to present (UNOS/OPTN, 2005). An estimated 5% of patients on the transplant waiting list would be able to identify a suitable donor, resulting in approximately 750 living-donor liver cases in the United States each year. Adult-sized pediatric patients undergoing A2ALDLT may require a right hepatic lobe to provide sufficient liver mass for the recipient. In 1999, increasing numbers of older children (aged 11 to 17 years) began to receive living donor grafts, which by 2001 accounted for 18 of 107 pediatric living-donor recipients. This change paralleled the increasing number of adult living donor recipients. The donor is left with approximately half or less of their hepatic mass following hepatectomy, but due to the large functional reserve of the liver and its regenerative capacity, clinical evidence of hepatic insufficiency is rare.

Prolonged prothrombin time, elevated serum aminotransferase levels, and increased bilirubin level normalize after 1 week. The donor's native liver can regenerate to its original size within several weeks. The greatest concern for donor safety is the risk for donor death, which has been estimated at 0.28% to 2% to 3%, with 10 reported cases due to technical errors, sepsis, and pulmonary embolism (Hayashi and Trotter, 2002; Trotter et al., 2002). The actual mortality rates are probably higher than the number of reported cases. A survey indicated that the lay public would be willing to undergo right hepatectomy as a liver donor, even with a marginal outcome in the recipient. In addition, the respondents were willing to accept a mortality rate among donors that was nearly 100 times the current rate (Trotter et al., 2002). On October 7, 2002, the National Institutes of Health launched the A2ALL (adult-to-adult living liver donor) registry, which enables data collection from 10 U.S. centers over 7 years to allow adequately powered studies to examine outcomes and determine the risk-benefit ratio to the donor and recipient.

All three of these techniques have associated complications, with split-liver grafts having the highest rates of associated complications and mortality. Because the integrity of the transected surface of the liver cannot be fully assessed until after reperfusion of the graft, these procedures all have an associated increased (Moreno et al., 1991) blood loss in comparison to whole organ transplantation. In addition, bile duct leaks and seroma formations are not uncommon in the transected liver. Although this specific complication was initially associated with split-liver transplantations, alterations of the surgical techniques have resulted in bile leak complications similar to those seen with reduced-size liver transplantation. The incidence of hepatic artery and portal vein thrombosis is clearly reduced with the use of these techniques. Survival of grafts and of patients at 1 year is better after living-related liver transplantation (81%) (Epstein, 1985) than with split-livers (67%) (Broelsch et al., 1991); however, overall 5-year survival with all of these procedures is similar.

ARTIFICIAL LIVER ASSIST DEVICES

Acute liver failure (ALF) is a disease with a high mortality with standard therapy at present being OLT. Liver transplantation, however, is hindered by the increasing shortage of organ donors even in the setting of an increased volume of living related and unrelated liver transplantation. ALF has a high mortality on the order of 50% to 80%, depending on the inciting event that has resulted in hepatocellular destruction (Lee et al., 2001; Liu et al., 2001). For over five decades, liver assist therapies have been explored as alternative therapy for ALF. The bioartificial liver (BAL) therapy appears to be the most promising revelation as a solution to this problem to act as a bridge for ALF patients to obtain liver transplantation or to liver regeneration, as these systems showed significant survival improvement in experimental studies. The ultimate goal of these devices is to prevent the ultimate complication of ALF, which is hepatic encephalopathy, cerebral edema with uncal herniation, and ultimately death.

Nonbiologic Liver Support

The biology of ALF seems to be a result of a number of lower and middle molecular weight toxic substances that are no longer cleared by the dysfunctional hepatocytes or, conversely, the lack of production of hepatotrophic proteins and other molecules essential for cellular homeostasis. Many attempts have been made to develop nonbiologic liver support therapies based on detoxification of the patient's blood (Mito, 1986; Rahman and Hodgson, 1999; Stockmann et al., 2000; Davenport, 2001; Kjaergard et al., 2003). In the 1950s, hemodialysis was introduced in an attempt to remove toxins; however, no improved survival was appreciated (Jones et al., 1959; Kiley et al., 1958; Knell and Dukes, 1976; Opolon et al., 1976; Matsubara et al., 1990). Hemofiltration showed limited outcome (Bellomo and Ronco, 2000; Agarwal and Farber, 2002). With the introduction of hemoperfusion and plasma perfusion, a more aggressive approach was also undertaken for the removal of protein-bound substances (Schlechter et al., 1958; Mori et al., 2002). Various types of resins have also been used (Rozenbaum et al., 1971; Juggi, 1973) and were particularly effective in the removal of lipophilic substances. Additionally, activated charcoal as an adsorbent of possible toxin has been used. However, the varied combination of filters, methodologies with charcoal and cation exchange resins, did not improve ultimate survival, although there were invariable reports of clinical improvement as well as survival (Yarmush et al., 1992; Ash, 1994; Flendrig, 1998).

The most promising nonbiologic support therapies to date combine detoxification of water-soluble and protein-bound toxins in a dialysis system, such as the molecular adsorbents recirculating system (MARS) (Mitzner et al., 2000; Schmidt et al., 2001; Stange et al., 2002; Steiner and Mitzner, 2002).

Only MARS treatment to date has shown significantly improved survival in a controlled trial of a subgroup of patients with hepatorenal syndrome. MARS uses a system that integrates charcoal hemoperfusion in parallel with a system for removal of albumin-bound molecules perfused across an albumin exchange chamber. However, the imprecise removal of compounds by these systems and their lack of capacity to synthesize liver-specific proteins and other hepatotrophic factors probably account for their limited effect. Mortality rates in the control group were 100% at day 7 compared with 63% of the MARS-treated group in the aforementioned trial (Mitzner et al., 2000) in ALF patients treated with MARS to date. As with biological support devices, however, a significant number of patients have also been transplanted while being treated, hence limiting the understanding of the true efficacy of this system. The ability to proceed with a true randomized double-blind controlled prospective study in this population of patients raises a number of ethical questions. Clearly there is an approved therapy for ALF, which is OLT. To withhold this treatment with the likelihood that a patient may die as part of the randomized study would be less than ethical, given the mortality rate of 80% in this patient population when left untreated by liver transplantation.

Biologic Liver Support

Biologic approaches for the treatment of ALF rely on the functionality of livers or hepatocytes from xenogeneic or human origin that can be exploited to support the patient's liver. These functions consist of detoxification, numerous metabolic functions, synthesis of proteins (e.g., coagulation cascade proteins and albumin), and various other molecules. Additionally, approximately 70% of the body stores of potassium is maintained in the liver. In 1956, it was demonstrated that fresh bovine liver homogenate could be used to metabolize salicylic and barbituric acids and ketone bodies and produce urea from ammonium chloride (Sorrentino, 1956). The many different biologic approaches that followed thereafter engaged xenogenic cross-hemodialysis, in which the patient's blood was dialyzed against blood of a living animal (Kimoto, 1959) or animal liver tissue preparations (Mikami et al., 1959; Nose et al., 1963). Although these techniques could be beneficial to patients with liver failure, they were not considered to be suitable for clinical application because of the complexity of the procedure and the rapid loss of efficacy. Moreover, xenogeneic extracorporeal liver perfusion in humans temporarily had been shown to improve biochemical parameters and the patient's clinical neurologic condition (Abouna et al., 1999; Horslen et al., 2000).

A major concern with all nonhuman biological liver assist devices is the potential for xenozoonoses. Xenozoonoses are pathogens that may be transmitted to humans from animal species, in this instance, swine. With porcine cells being the preferential substrate of choice, the concern here is for the introduction of porcine endogenous retrovirus (PERVs), which could prove deadly to humans. Controlled clinical trials indicating survival improvement have as yet not been reported (Eiseman et al., 1965; Stockmann et al., 2000). Liver support, however, as mentioned earlier, can be provided by human cross-circulation (Burnell et al., 1967), although the potential toxicities and adverse reactions in the human donor severely limited this approach. Also, significant moral and ethical questions have again been raised, hence forcing researchers to look at other venues and possibilities. Exchange transfusion, another seemingly logical and brilliant maneuver, was associated with reversal of hepatic coma (Yamazaki et al., 1987; Kondrup et al., 1992; Clemmesen et al., 2001). This treatment in combination with hemodialysis improved survival from 18% to 50% (four of eight patients) in one uncontrolled, nonrandomized trial (Brunner and Losgen, 1987). A major problem with exchange transfusion is the need for a large amount of plasma. Furthermore, this technique might at the same time remove essential hepatotrophic factors. Moreover, the administration of plasma to the patients nullifies any possibility of determining if there is improvement of hepatocellular function by the measurement through the routine measurement of the coagulation system; plasma exchange transfusion will ultimately correct the coagulation defects of ALF (Brunner and Losgen, 1987).

Isolated liver cells have been used in a variety of configurations in the development of the BAL: suspended, substrate attached, and encapsulated in semipermeable membranes. Hepatocytes used for liver support can be divided into two categories: implantable systems and extracorporeal systems. Several case reports and case series concerning transplantation of human hepatocytes have shown beneficial effects in liver failure (Strom and Fisher, 2003). In 1987, Matsumura and others reported the first application of a BAL support system in a patient. The principle of this BAL support system was against a suspension of functioning cryopreserved rabbit hepatocytes. Two years later, Margulis and others (1989) reported a controlled trial that included 126 patients. The BAL device that was used contained porcine hepatocytes in a polychlorovinyl capsule. This BAL treatment was relatively simple and cheap. There was no mention of specified pathogen-free status of the animals from which the hepatocytes were harvested for the two aforementioned systems. What is astonishing is that there have been no further published reports in the literature concerning patient treatment with the Matsamura or Margulis systems.

Use of xenogeneic hepatocytes for hepatocyte replacement and transplantation in humans has not yet been reported. The BAL systems are extracorporeal systems, temporarily connected to the circulation of the patient. BAL systems consist of an artificial component (i.e., the bioreactor and its equipment) and a biocomponent (i.e., hepatocytes, most often xenogenic). Although an increasing number of BAL devices have been produced or are currently under development, only 11 different BAL devices have thus far been exploited clinically. Significant prolongation of survival has been shown in animal studies with BAL systems, and therefore clinical application of a BAL has high expectations (Flendrig et al., 1999; Suh et al., 1999; Berry and Phillips, 2000; Gerlach et al., 2001; Sosef et al., 2002).

Hybrid and Modular Assist Devices

Another possibility and consideration for a support device has been to bridge the artificial and bioartificial xenogenic devices given the varying degrees of reported success with the technologies independently. Hence, the Liver Support System (LSS) device (Gerlach, 1996; Sauer et al., 2001; Mundt et al., 2002) was first developed in Berlin, Germany. This device consists of a specially designed bioreactor endeavored at improving cellular oxygenation and mass exchange. The system is fabricated by a multitude of interwoven hollow fiber membranes, creating a three-dimensional framework over which hepatocyte aggregates are distributed. The LSS is the only system that has been used in clinical studies with primary porcine hepatocytes as well as primary human hepatocytes derived from discarded donor livers. Porcine endogenous retrovirus (PERV) transmission was tested and found to be negative in these clinical trials (Gerlach et al., 2002).

The modular extracorporeal liver support (MELS) system, seemingly the preeminent hybrid of MARS and BAL, combines different extracorporeal therapy units, tailored to suit the individual clinical needs of each individual patient (Sauer et al., 2002). The MELS consists of the LSS system combined with a Detox Module based on single-pass albumin dialysis for removing albumin-bound toxins. The human hepatocytes used were harvested from cadaveric/deceased donors livers that were being discarded because of steatosis, cirrhosis, fibrosis, or mechanical injury. This system has been used in a limited number of patients to date and has shown no profound improvement in morbidity or mortality in the patients treated. No adverse events were observed. Albeit, in all cases, neurologic status improved, and slight improvement of coagulation was observed during the treatment period.

Biochemical Improvement Following Bioartificial Liver Treatment

Hitherto, biochemical improvement as a result of BAL treatment, as judged by elimination of ammonia and bilirubin, was reported in most clinical studies by the varied devices used in the research protocols. According to Mundt and others (2002), the assessment of only biochemical variables before and after liver support treatment might fail to detect a beneficial effect, because of continuing deterioration of the patient. Ellis and others (1996), Hughes and Williams (1995), and Colletti and others (1994) emphasized that any additional function provided by the device is difficult to assess because changes in blood tests may not discriminate between synthetic and detoxification functions of the liver assist device and those of the native liver. Comparing plasma samples from the inlet and outlet of the device at the same time can also be used to assess efficacy of the BAL treatment. Except for the ELAD system, which was associated with an increase in ammonia and bilirubin levels, application of other systems, tested experimentally, was associated with more or less a biochemical improvement. Nonetheless, it is imperative to elucidate whether the noted clinical improvements are in fact due to the devices or simply a result of washout of molecules and substances being measured. The expectation should be, as with all systems that use large-volume plasma exchange for several hours, that the serum levels of molecules such as bilirubin and ammonia will be diminished as they diffuse down their concentration gradients.

Everything considered, the concept of BAL support has proved to be successful in experimental animal studies. In addition, clinical application of BAL devices has proved to be safe by the current methodology of practice. Clinical evaluation of BAL treatment is rather mired by the variation in the patient groups studied. Additionally, the fact that most patients undergo subsequent OLT prevents any clear understanding as to whether or not these systems significantly improve morbidity and mortality. However, neurologic and biochemical parameters appeared to improve after treatment with different BAL systems. To ultimately determine the effect of BAL treatment on survival, controlled, randomized trials in an appropriate animal model or controlled clinical trials in large patient groups will be required to yield statistically significant outcomes. A multicenter human clinical trial, however, raises several ethical and moral dilemmas as previously discussed, given that there is an approved effective treatment for the disease entity to be investigated, that is, liver transplantation. In parallel, BAL research should focus on the replacement of hepatocytes of animal origin by hepatocytes of human origin, either primary hepatocytes or immortalized cell lines, to overcome possible immunologic reactions and xenozoonosis

■ MULTIVISCERAL AND INTESTINAL TRANSPLANTATION

The technical feasibility of intestinal transplantation was first described in 1905 by Alexis Carrel. Given the early successes with kidney transplantation in identical twins during the early 1960s, Lillehei and others described experimental transplantation of the stomach, intestine, and pancreas (1967). Simultaneously, Starzl and Kaupp (1960) described transplantation of multiple abdominal viscera in dogs and, many years later, in humans (Starzl et al., 1989). Until the late 1980s, there were no long-term survivors of small bowel transplantation beyond 6 months. With the introduction of cyclosporine and tacrolimus, as well as an improved understanding of graft rejection in pigs, successful long-term survival was possible (Grant et al., 1990). This procedure has a high rate of morbidity and mortality. The major cause of graft failure is due to acute or chronic rejection (small bowel transplant [SBT] 79%; small bowel/liver transplant [SB/LT] 71%; multivisceral transplant [MVT] 56%). Infection, CMV enteritis, lymphoproliferative disease, and multisystem organ failure are major causes of death. The rate of GVHD after intestinal transplantation is 0% to 16% (Pirenne et al., 1997; Abu-Elmagd et al., 1998; Reyes et al., 1998; Sudan et al., 2000). Patient and graft survival rates are lower than for solid organ transplantation, with approximately one half of the patients receiving intestinal transplants surviving 5 years.

Multivisceral transplantation may include SBT in isolation, in combination with liver transplantation (SB/LT), or in combination with multiple organs (MVT) (Starzl et al., 1991a, 1991b). An isolated SBT is typically recommended for patients on home parenteral nutrition (HPN) who have exhausted their venous access. Combined SBT/LT is recommended for patients with irreversible HPN cirrhosis or intestinal failure associated with a hypercoagulable state that can be corrected by a simultaneous liver transplant. MVT is for patients with locally aggressive tumors that necessitate evisceration of the abdominal organs (duodenal fistulas, locally aggressive tumors, multiorgan failure with a nonreconstructable gastrointestinal tract) or in the patient with benign conditions involving the liver, pancreas, or stomach (Tzakis et al., 1989).

The Health Care Financing Administration's (HCFA) clinical indications for intestinal transplantation implemented in 2001 include impending liver failure due to HPN, thrombosis of major central venous channels, frequent line infection and sepsis, and frequent episodes of severe dehydration. Significant bone disease, metabolic disorders, failure to thrive, and significant limitations on social and personal activities are not considered indications. As most patients function well on HPN, the risks of intestinal transplantation are only warranted with failure of HPN therapy. The goal of intestinal transplantation is to eliminate the need for TPN and to reverse or prevent TPN-associated liver disease. The first year of waiting list candidates for intestinal transplantation with UNOS was 1993.

General Indications

In the pediatric population, chronic intestinal failure results from massive bowel resection (short bowel syndrome) or functional impairment of the bowel due to disturbances in motility or extensive parenchymal disorders (Okada et al., 1994).

Necrotizing enterocolitis, intestinal atresia (Todo et al., 1994a, 1994b), midgut volvulus, gastroschisis, microvillus inclusion disease, Hirschsprung disease, and intestine pseudoobstruction are the primary causes of isolated small intestinal failure. This is in marked contrast to the adult population, in which intestinal failure is caused primarily by Crohn's disease and thrombotic episodes involving the major splanchnic vessels. If the length of the small bowel is less than 60 to 70 cm, parenteral nutrition is required (normal length of a small bowel in the infant being 200 to 250 cm). For the patient to survive, HPN is essential. HPN has significant metabolic sequelae, the foremost being liver failure and bone disease (Bowyer et al., 1985; Colomb et al., 1994; Sondheimer et al., 1998; Chan et al., 1999; Wasa et al., 1999; Cavicchi et al., 2000).

The hepatic dysfunction in the patient on long-term TPN includes, most commonly, hepatic steatosis and cholestasis, phospholipidosis, or cirrhosis, which is observed in 15% to 40% of patients after 3 years. Up to 100% of patients have biliary sludge or gallstones after 6 weeks. In the pediatric population this is a reversible form of liver dysfunction (Grosfeld et al., 1986) if the bilirubin level is less than 30 mg/dL and the patient is returned to total enteral feeding. Patients are followed through the North American Home Parenteral and Enteral Nutrition Patient Registry supported by the Oley Foundation (formerly the OASIS registry, started in 1984) (Howard et al., 1991). This registry reports survival for patients on long-term HPN to be 87% to 96% at 1 year and 70% to 90% at 3 years. The majority of deaths are related to progression of the underlying disease.

In 2001, the majority of the 111 intestinal transplants were performed in only four transplant centers in the United States, with short gut syndrome accounting for more than 60% of these cases. Sixty-one intestinal transplants were performed in pediatric patients. Children younger than 6 years were the recipients of almost half of all intestine transplants, with 74% of registrants on the waiting list 17 years old or younger, and half of these between the ages of 1 and 5 years. Patient and graft survival were 62% and 34%, respectively, at 3 years posttransplant in the 1- to 5-year age group (UNOS/OPTN, 2005). There is no significant difference in outcomes between recipients of SB/LT versus those of isolated SB transplants. The International Transplant Registry and several large centers have shown that 77% to 93% of surviving recipients remain independent of parenteral nutrition beyond 6 to 12 months after transplantation (Abu-Elmagd et al., 1998; Grant, 1999; Sudan et al., 2000).

The majority of multivisceral transplantations have been performed in adults. The efficacy of these procedures is still undetermined, as only a few procedures have been done worldwide. At the University of Pittsburgh the combined survival of all procedures is approximately 65% at 4 years (Todo et al., 1995). Graft survival is 50% to 60%, with the best survival in patients receiving multivisceral or liver and intestinal grafts. Transplantation of the colon together with the rest of the viscera appears to diminish overall graft survival.

PREOPERATIVE ASSESSMENT

The patient should be evaluated specifically for progressive liver disease and evidence of portal hypertension. Extrahepatic manifestation of the primary disease causing the patient's intestinal failure should be identified. Complications of TPN should be elucidated (infection, catheter occlusion, and hepatic disease). Comorbid conditions such as infection, renal disease, electrolyte abnormalities, and gastroparesis predisposing to regurgitation and aspiration should be considered. Appropriate evaluation of patency of the large vessels of the neck (subclavian and internal jugular veins) is essential because repeated central vein cannulation or long-term indwelling catheter use for the administration of HPN may lead to loss of vascular access due to venous thrombosis (Grosfeld et al., 1986). Doppler ultrasonography is sometimes useful to access central venous access, although the gold standard is a venogram.

Knowledge of the patient's prior surgeries as well as the abdominal vascular anatomy is important, particularly in a patient scheduled for a multivisceral transplant, because these are the most technically complex surgical procedures. A discussion with the surgical team regarding the planned approach is essential, particularly because multiple blood vessels may be partially or fully cross-clamped during the operation. Because of the high rate of postoperative infectious complications, broad-spectrum antibiotics, antifungal drugs, and ganciclovir prophylaxis are routinely administered.

SURGICAL TECHNIQUE: RECIPIENT OPERATION

The final decision to proceed with either a multivisceral or an intestinal transplant is ultimately made after a laparotomy and a meticulous inspection of the native vessels and abdominal organs. Thus, continuous communication between the donor and recipient teams is essential. In addition, procurement of both the donor iliac artery and vein (Starzl et al., 1991a, 1991b) as well as the thoracic aorta is essential for vascular reconstruction of the graft. The graft is usually preserved with cold University of Wisconsin (UW) solution. The length of time the organ is kept in the preservation solution should be minimized because intestinal mucosal damage occurs in UW solution due to increased lipid peroxidation (Takeyoshi et al., 2001).

The operation begins with a midline incision, which is extended to either a unilateral or bilateral transverse subcostal incision. The choice of incision depends on the planned operation, with a bilateral incision used preferentially in the multivisceral transplant. The procedure continues as described by Todo and others (Fig. 28–12); in the patient receiving an isolated intestinal transplantation, the superior mesenteric artery is anastomosed exclusively to the infrarenal aorta. Venous blood from the isolated small bowel graft is drained into the mesenteric venous system at one of three sites: the donor superior mesenteric vein (SMV) to the distal end of the recipient SMV, SMV to the hilar portion of the main portal vein, or donor SMV to the confluence of the SMV and splenic vein (Todo et al., 1994a, 1994b).

In the recipient of liver-intestine or multivisceral graft, the use of venovenous bypass is usually impossible because of vascular thromboses of the major vessels seen with the long-term use of HPN. The liver is usually placed in a piggyback fashion, and occasionally a temporary portacaval shunt is used to decompress the abdominal viscera. Vascular anastomoses are performed as illustrated in Figure 28–13. The arterial and venous anastomoses are performed before reperfusion of the graft. Arterial anastomoses in this instance are usually with a Carrel patch (see Fig. 28–13), containing both the celiac and superior mesenteric artery for the combined intestinal and multivisceral graft to the infrarenal abdominal aorta. In some instances, an aortic conduit may be used to facilitate the anastomoses of the superior mesenteric artery (SMA) and celiac axis to the abdominal aorta. If a portacaval

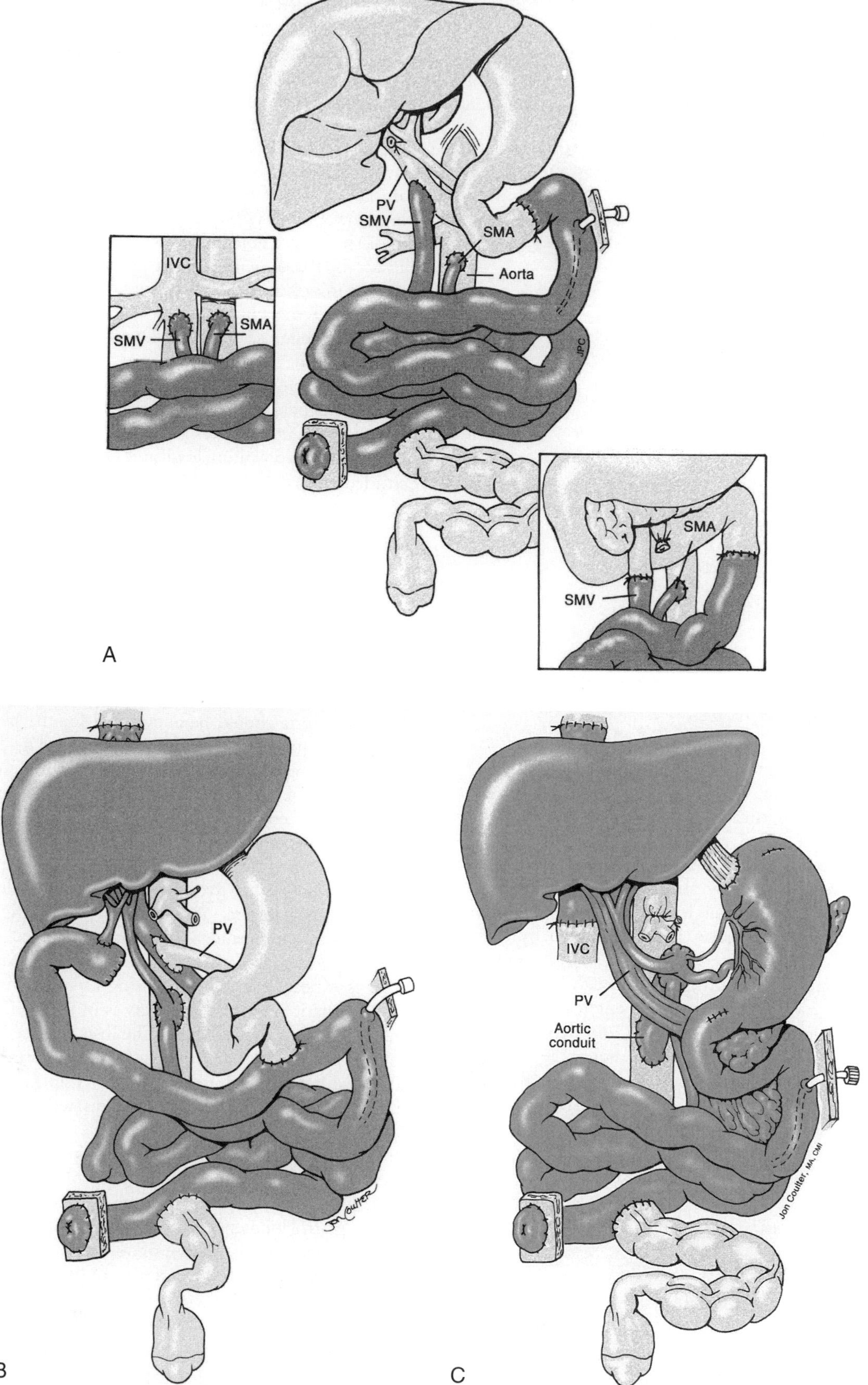

■ **FIGURE 28–12.** Varied forms of intestinal and multivisceral transplantations. **A,** Isolated intestinal transplantation. **B,** Combined liver-intestine. **C,** Full multivisceral with resection of the native retrohepatic vena cava with multivisceral transplantation. PV, portal vein; SMV, superior mesenteric vein; SMA, superior mesenteric artery; VC, vena cava; IVC, inferior vena cava. (From Todo S, Tzaki AG, Abu-Elmagd K, et al.: Intestinal transplantation in composite visceral graft or alone. *Ann Surg* 216:223–234, 1992, with permission.)

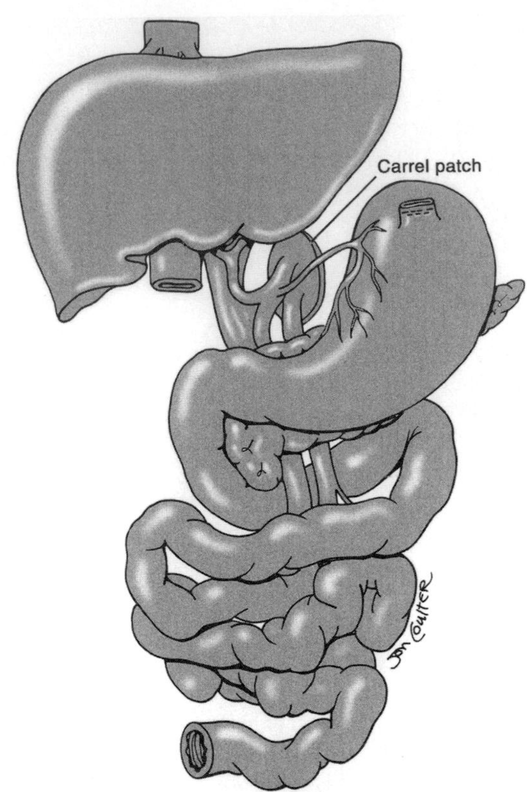

■ **FIGURE 28–13.** Multivisceral allograft with the utilization of the Carrel patch with the superior mesenteric artery and the celiac axis origins. (From Todo S, Tzakis A, Abu-Elmagd K, et al.: Current status of intestinal transplantation. *Adv Surg* 27:295–316, 1994.)

shunt is performed, it is subsequently converted to a portaportal anastomosis to facilitate perfusion of the liver with the splanchnic hepatotropic factors.

After completion of the vascular anastomoses, the gastrointestinal continuity is reestablished by anastomosing the appropriate donor intestine to recipient bowel. In the multivisceral recipient, proximal intestinal reconstruction is accomplished by anastomosing the distal esophagus to the anterior wall of the donor stomach. A pyloroplasty is routinely preformed, followed by a gastrostomy, the first of three essential enterotomies, which helps to prevent delayed gastric emptying and decompress the intestine. A jejunostomy is performed for enteral feeding. The final enterotomy is achieved by exteriorization of the distal end of the donor intestine in a chimney fashion. The recipient ileum or colon is then anastomosed to the side of the graft distal to the stoma. Finally, a cholecystectomy follows, as well as biliary reconstruction by a choledochojejunostomy or Roux-en-Y procedure.

■ ANESTHETIC MANAGEMENT

Small Bowel Transplantation

In the patient scheduled for isolated small bowel transplantation, the anesthetic management is similar to that for other major abdominal surgeries. The patient usually has a central venous catheter, although it is sometimes placed in an unconventional site if the subclavian and internal jugular veins are thrombosed (right atrial, transhepatic, or direct inferior vena caval catheters). These procedures are lengthy and lend themselves to significant third space losses and major fluid shifts. Two large-bore intravenous catheters above the diaphragm and a radial arterial catheter are recommended. CVP should also be monitored as a guide for fluid replacement. If central vein cannulation is impossible, it is best to proceed without its use; femoral vein cannulation may be used for volume replacement. All blood products should be CMV-negative and irradiated to minimize the risk of GVHD.

The choice of anesthetic agents depends on the patient's underlying disease and hemodynamic status. Nitrous oxide should be avoided because it may cause additional bowel distention. The choice of fluids remains controversial in patients undergoing bowel surgery. Not infrequently, significant bowel swelling and distention are noted after reperfusion of the graft. Frequently, diuresis is recommended as a means to treat this problem, although it is often ineffective. Moreover, the etiology of the intestinal edema is most likely related to the preservation of the organ. The use of colloids, preferentially albumin, is recommended in patients who have a low albumin level preoperatively.

Reperfusion of the isolated small bowel graft usually has minimal hemodynamic effects. The reperfusion syndrome seen with liver transplantation is absent in this instance as a result of the relatively low potassium load and the low volume of effluent extruded from the graft. Hemodynamic stability is the norm, and coagulopathy or metabolic derangements are unusual.

Multivisceral Transplantation

Anesthetic considerations for the patient scheduled for multivisceral transplantation are identical to those for the patient undergoing OLT. There are, however, unique and specific considerations with respect to planned vascular anastomoses (Todo et al., 1995; Starzl, 1993) (see Fig. 28–13). The liver is usually placed in a piggyback fashion in this instance. A partial cross-clamping of the abdominal aorta should be anticipated for the placement of the arterial anastomosis using a Carrel patch (see Fig. 28–13).

The surgical procedure is divided into three stages, similar to those with solitary liver transplantation. Completion of the abdominal viscera exenteration during the preanhepatic stage is the period of greatest blood loss (De Wolf, 1991). Hemodynamic alterations during this period are related to complications of massive transfusion and manipulation of the abdominal viscera. Ionized hypocalcemia, hypomagnesemia, lactic acidosis, and progressive hypothermia should be anticipated. In addition, a progressive coagulopathy, as seen in the patients undergoing OLT, is expected. Thus monitoring of coagulation is essential. The anhepatic stage of the surgery is usually performed without the use of venovenous bypass. The liver is placed in a piggyback fashion, and vascular anastomosis of the intestine follows. A significant difference with respect to reperfusion of the multivisceral graft from that of the liver is that the arterial anastomoses must be performed before graft reperfusion. The graft is flushed with 50 mL/kg of saline solution before reperfusion to reduce the potassium load from the preservation solution.

Reperfusion of the multivisceral graft is similar to that of the hepatic graft. Hypotension and bradycardia are the usual observations secondary to the release of a large volume of hypothermic, hyperkalemic acidotic preservation solution into the right heart. These changes are usually short lived, with normalization of the hemodynamics within minutes after reperfusion. The incidence of the postreperfusion syndrome in this group of patients is not well defined.

■ KIDNEY TRANSPLANTATION

The earliest kidney transplant in a child was performed by Michon and colleagues in Paris on Christmas Eve in 1952. A 16-year-old boy had just undergone nephrectomy for a right ruptured kidney after a fall. Unfortunately, it was discovered he had no left kidney. An ABO-compatible kidney from his mother was placed in the iliac region. Initially, the kidney excreted urine and had good renal function. However, on posttransplant day 21, abrupt anuria occurred, indicating rejection and the patient died. Two years later, Murray and colleagues performed the first successful kidney transplant between two identical twins. The first successful pediatric transplant was performed by Goodwin, Mims, and Kaufman at the University of Oregon in 1959 between pediatric identical twins, one of whom had glomerulonephritis. Eighteen years posttransplant, the kidney was still functioning with normal morphology by biopsy (Papalois and Najarian, 2001).

Routine kidney transplantation in pediatric patients, however, awaited the development of effective immunosuppressive agents. Potent corticosteroids, calcineurin inhibitors such as cyclosporine or tacrolimus, monoclonal antibodies, antimetabolites like azathioprine, and the purine synthetase inhibitor MMF have all been used successfully in pediatric patients to prevent rejection (Papalois and Najarian, 2001). Superior survival and improved long-term growth and development can be obtained with kidney transplantation compared with chronic hemo- or peritoneal dialysis. Newer immunosuppressive regimens relying less on high-dose corticosteroids have further improved the growth and development of children receiving a renal transplant. In addition, pediatric patients who receive a kidney transplant are much more likely to have a normal lifestyle compared with those requiring hemodialysis (So et al., 1987; Beebe et al., 1991; Turenne et al., 1997; Benfield et al., 1999; Elshihabi et al., 2000; Healy et al., 2000; McDonald et al., 2000; Qvist et al., 2000; Papalois and Najarian, 2001; Qvist et al., 2002; Smith et al., 2002).

Approximately 300 pediatric patients undergo living related kidney transplantation a year in the United States and 150 to 200 receive a cadaveric transplant. Infants and small children (<15 kg) constitute between 10% and 15% of both cadaveric and living related transplants in the pediatric age group (Elshihabi et al., 2000; McDonald et al., 2000).

Numerous studies have shown that the overall success rate for renal transplantation in children and teenagers is similar to that of adults (Elshihabi et al., 2000; McDonald et al., 2000; Smith et al., 2002). The most recent 1- and 5-year patient survival rates in patients receiving living related kidney transplants were 97% and 94%, respectively. The graft survival rates over the same time periods were 91% and 78% (McDonald et al., 2000). The patient survival rates for recipients of cadaveric organs are slightly lower: 96% at 1 year and 91% at 5 years. However, the graft survival rates at 1 (81%) and 5 years (64%) are much lower in recipients of cadaveric organs. Rejection is the main cause of graft loss (Elshihabi et al., 2000).

In contrast, most reports show that the 1-year patient survival following transplantation is lower if the recipient is less than 2 years of age compared with older children following living-related transplantation (89%); graft survival is also less (≈85%). Both the mortality and graft loss are greater in cadaveric transplantation as well (Elshihabi et al., 2000; McDonald et al., 2000). Vascular thrombosis is much more likely to be a cause of graft loss in infants than older children or adults. Although renal transplantation has been successful in very small children (<10 kg), clearly infants and small children constitute a high-risk group for kidney transplantation (Beebe et al., 1991; Singh et al., 1997; Benfield et al., 1999; Elshihabi et al., 2000; Healy et al., 2000; McDonald et al., 2000; Neipp et al., 2002).

Unique Characteristics of Pediatric Recipients

Recipients of renal transplants differ from their adult counterparts in several ways. Obstructive nephropathy or hypoplastic kidneys are common causes for transplantation in the pediatric age group. Glomerulonephritis is less common, and, in contrast to adults, diabetes as a cause of renal failure in this age group is rare (Benfield et al., 1999) (Table 28–7). Consequently, many of the diseases that cause renal failure in children do not recur and successful transplantation could, in theory, be a permanent solution. Also, although most adults have received dialysis before transplantation, up to 35% of children who receive a transplant have never had dialysis before. Of the children who are on dialysis, one half are receiving peritoneal and one half hemodialysis (Elshihabi et al., 2000; McDonald et al., 2000). Finally, kidney transplantation using infants or small children as donors has a lower success rate because of the small size of the donor vasculature. Therefore, children usually receive a transplant from someone who is an adult or large child, often much larger than the recipient. In recipients who are infants or small children, the kidney may be many times larger than they would normally have (Miller et al., 1983; Beebe et al., 1991; Healy et al., 2000).

Infants less than 2 years of age are an important subset of pediatric patients because they are at higher risk for graft loss. Unlike older children or adults, rejection in infants is not the primary cause of failure of the transplanted kidney. The main reason for graft loss in the younger recipient is vascular thrombosis (Beebe et al., 1991; Singh et al., 1997; Healy et al., 2000; Neipp et al., 2002).

Infants also have a higher incidence of delayed function of the renal allograft. This is important because infants and children with delayed graft function have an increased incidence of graft

■ TABLE 28–7. Causes of renal dysfunction in the 4898 children undergoing kidney transplantation from the 1997 North American Pediatric Renal Transplant Cooperative Study

Diagnosis	n (N = 4898)	%
Obstructive uropathy	804	16.4
Aplastic/hypoplastic/dysplastic kidneys	783	16
Focal segmental glomerulosclerosis	582	11.9
Reflux nephropathy	274	5.6
Systemic immunologic disease	232	4.7
Chronic glomerulonephritis	206	4.2
Syndrome of agenesis of abdominal musculature	138	2.8
Congenital nephrotic syndrome	132	2.7
Polycystic kidney disease	131	2.7
Medullary cystic disease/juvenile nephrosclerosis	131	2.7
Familial nephritis	116	2.4
Pyelo/interstitial nephritis	112	2.3
Cystinosis	111	2.3
Membranoproliferative glomerulonephritis type 1	111	2.3
Renal infarct	87	1.8
Idiopathic crescentic glomerulonephritis	84	1.7
Membranoproliferative glomerulonephritis type 2	47	1
Oxalosis	33	0.7
Wilms tumor	30	0.6
Membranous nephropathy	27	0.6
Drash syndrome	27	0.6
Sickle cell nephropathy	9	0.2
Diabetic glomerulonephritis	5	1
Other	326	6.7
Unknown	235	4.8

From Benfield MR, McDonald R, Sullivan EK, et al.: The 1997 Annual Renal Transplantation in Children Report of the North American Pediatric Renal Transplant Cooperative Study (NAPRTCS). *Pediatr Transplant* 3:152, 1999.

loss in the years following transplantation. Kidneys with delayed function are likely to have sustained permanent injury and are susceptible to failure following rejection or other insult. Providing adequate perfusion of a very large kidney relative to the recipient size to prevent vascular thrombosis and delayed graft function is one of the main challenges for the pediatric anesthesiologist caring for an infant or a small child undergoing renal transplantation (Tejani et al., 1999).

PATHOPHYSIOLOGY OF RENAL FAILURE

The effects of chronic renal failure on infants and children result from the kidney's role as a filter of metabolic waste products and fluid regulation and its active role in hormone production. As the glomerulofiltration rate becomes reduced, the kidney's ability to clear acids, urea, and potassium diminishes; overall poor nutrition is the result. Therefore, infants and children with renal failure have growth retardation and often have developmental delay. Chronic metabolic acidosis, hyperkalemia, and phosphatemia develop. The elevated phosphorus binds to the serum calcium and magnesium, resulting in hypocalcemia and magnesemia. Fractures in active children can occur as calcium is leached from the bones. Chronic uremia can result in central nervous system depression and congestive heart failure and can impair platelet function. Seizures and permanent neurologic damage may be a consequence of electrolyte imbalances and fluxes from renal insufficiency and dialysis therapy. Volume overload can result as the kidney's ability to clear sodium and free water diminishes (Belani and Palahniuk, 1991).

Hormone function of the kidney is affected by renal failure as well. Erythropoietin production may be severely reduced and cause anemia. Renin production becomes elevated as the kidney senses diminished perfusion, resulting in hypertension. Similarly parathyroid hormone levels become elevated as the parathyroid gland responds to a reduced serum calcium level. These changes are present in infants and small children to various degrees despite adequate dialysis and the administration of exogenous erythropoietin and vitamin supplementation. The net effect is a child who is small and frail, hypertensive, and chronically acidotic (Belani and Palahniuk, 1991; Beebe et al., 1991).

PREOPERATIVE ASSESSMENT

All systems are affected by end-stage renal disease. Attention must be paid to the extent of renal failure and its effects on organ function and to the child's growth and development. Smaller tracheal tube sizes and intravascular catheters may be needed if the child has not been growing adequately. The cause of renal failure, if a systemic disorder such as oxalosis exists, also affects other organ function. Agenesis or dysplasia of the kidneys may be associated with other congenital disorders such as ventricular septal defects. The presence of cardiac failure or congestive heart disease should be determined. Although most children with renal failure have a hyperdynamic circulation from chronic anemia, some do develop cardiac insufficiency from concurrent congenital heart disease, uremia, or chronic volume overload. The parents should be asked about frequent episodes of dyspnea or asthma attacks. In addition to usual reactive airway disease in children, asthma attacks in children with renal insufficiency may suggest volume overload. The presence of wheezing, rales, dyspnea, an enlarged liver, and hypertension on physical examination suggests fluid overload that may require dialysis before surgery. A history of frequent fractures suggests the child may have brittle bones from hypocalcemia and be at risk for dental injury during anesthesia. Finally, the parents and/or patient should be asked if the child has symptoms of acid reflux or delayed gastric emptying because those conditions are quite common with renal insufficiency (Belani and Palahniuk, 1991; Beebe et al., 1991).

When examining the airway, the anesthesiologist must pay particular attention to the teeth, which may be fragile from chronic hypocalcemia. Vascular access is also often difficult in these patients because of frequent hospitalizations and repeated blood drawing and catheterizations. The extremities should be examined to plan where to obtain vascular access and place an arterial catheter, if indicated (Belani and Palahniuk, 1991; Beebe et al., 1991).

Preoperative Dialysis

One of the things the anesthesiologist and surgeon need to ascertain before surgery is if the patient needs dialysis. The day of the last dialysis and type of dialysis, hemodialysis or peritoneal, should be determined. Some patients who have not previously dialyzed are chronically hyperkalemic. Potassium can be transfused from the donor kidney as it is reperfused, particularly if it has been filled with a high potassium preservative, such as the UW solution. It is therefore best to reduce the potassium to normal levels either via dialysis or ion exchange resins (Kayexalate) before transplantation in the chronically hyperkalemic patient (Belani and Palahniuk, 1991; Beebe et al., 1991).

If the patient is hyperkalemic (potassium >6.0 mmol/L), acidotic, or volume overloaded, the surgery should be delayed and dialysis performed. Although peritoneal dialysis may be adequate for the daily treatment of patients and is commonly used in children, it may be inadequate to prepare children for surgery. Therefore, children often are converted from peritoneal to hemodialysis several weeks before transplantation to ensure adequate dialysis. The large-bore (2 mm ID) Hickman catheters are usually used for hemodialysis in infants and young children; they also provide excellent vascular access for the renal transplant procedure (Beebe et al., 1991).

SURGICAL TECHNIQUE

The surgical technique has been described in detail elsewhere (Miller et al., 1983). In relatively larger children (>20 kg), the kidney is placed in the pelvis as in an adult renal transplant. A lower flank incision is used with a retroperitoneal approach. Systemic heparinization is usually not required because heparin can be applied directly by the surgeon through the arteriotomy and venotomy and the anastomoses are performed quickly. The renal artery is anastomosed to the common iliac or hypogastric artery. The renal vein is usually attached to the common iliac or external iliac vein. The ureter is then anastomosed to the bladder (Fig. 28–14A). In this approach, only one lower extremity is without circulation before reperfusion. Occasionally, hypotension results from revascularization of the kidney in the older child or teenager. In general, the hemodynamic changes are minimal.

In contrast when transplanting an adult kidney into an infant or small child (<20 kg), the kidney is sewn directly on to the aorta and vena cava (Fig. 28–14B). Usually the peritoneum is opened and both the aorta and inferior vena cava are cross-clamped. Because the major vessels are clamped, low-dose heparinization (50 to 100 mg/kg) is often used. The lower extremity is deprived of both arterial perfusion and venous drainage during the anastomoses. Because the kidney is much

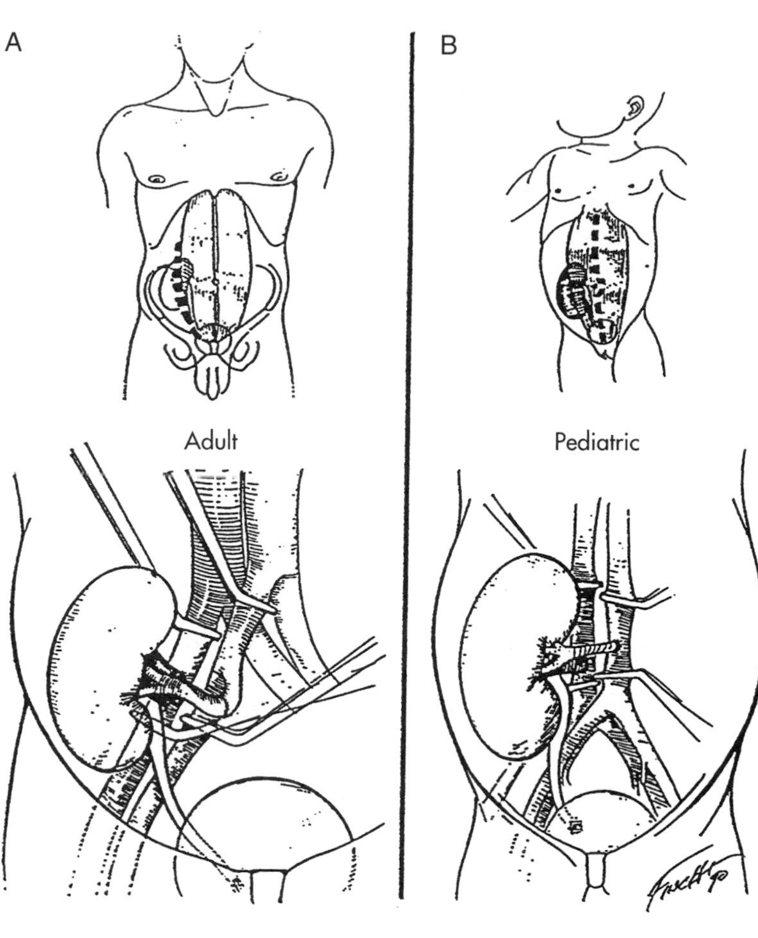

■ **FIGURE 28–14.** Surgical placement of renal allograft in adults and older children (**A**) versus infants. (**B**) The vascular anastomosis with the use of an adult-size organ in the pediatric patient is to the aorta and vena cava. (From Belani KG, Polahniuk RJ: Kidney transplantation. *Internat Anesth Clin* 29:17–29, 1991.)

larger relative to the recipient than in the older child or adult, the hemodynamic changes in an infant on reperfusion can be profound (Beebe et al., 1991).

Infants and small children usually require other concurrent operations in addition to the kidney transplant. For example, if the cause of renal failure is vesicoureteral reflux with recurrent urinary tract infections, bilateral nephrectomies are often performed simultaneously to prevent graft sepsis. Concurrent splenectomy, although no longer routine, are occasionally performed if the spleen is enlarged to allow room for the kidney. A large-bore Hickman dialysis catheter is also placed in infants before beginning the transplantation if not already present for intravenous access and CVP monitoring (Beebe et al., 1991).

■ ANESTHETIC MANAGEMENT

There are many anesthetic techniques that have been used successfully in the anesthetic management of renal transplantation in children. However, when planning the anesthetic, several items unique to renal transplantation must be kept in mind. (1) The patient suffers from chronic renal failure and may manifest many of its effects, including anemia, hyperkalemia, and hypervolemia. (2) The transplanted kidney may not function effectively initially. Therefore, muscle relaxants, such as pancuronium, and other drugs dependent primarily on the kidney for excretion should not be used. (3) Immunosuppressive drugs need to be administered. Allergic reactions and hypotension may occur with some of the agents. (4) The kidney has been ischemic before transplantation, which may increase its vulnerability to further injury. Potentially nephrotoxic agents such as enflurane should be avoided. (5) Adequacy of the intravascular volume status before and following reperfusion of the allograft must be ensured. (6) The anesthesiologist must be prepared to deal with hyperkalemia, hyperglycemia, hypocalcemia, and other electrolyte disorders that may arise over the course of the operation and perioperative period (Belani and Palahniuk, 1991; Beebe et al., 1991).

Induction and Maintenance of Anesthesia

In general, most children without an intravenous catheter in place receive preoperative sedation with either oral or rectal midazolam (0.5 mg/kg). Ketamine (3 mg/kg) and atropine (20 mcg/kg) may be added to rectal midazolam if a greater level of sedation is desired (Beebe et al., 1992). If an intravenous catheter is in place, midazolam 0.1 to 0.2 mg/kg intravenously may be administered for sedation.

An inhaled induction of anesthesia with sevoflurane with or without nitrous oxide may be used in stable patients with normal gastric function who have been NPO for an adequate length of time. Halothane also has been used for both induction and maintenance of anesthesia in children undergoing renal transplantation. However, hypotension and myocardial depression are more common with inhaled inductions using halothane, and it is the agent most often associated with hepatotoxicity. Therefore, halothane rarely is used since the advent of newer inhaled agents (Belani and Palahniuk, 1991; Beebe et al., 1991).

Often an intravenous induction of anesthesia is used in children undergoing renal transplantation, particularly if there is a concern that the patient may be unstable and require vasopressors or other drugs. Also, transplant surgeons often order oral immunosuppressive agents preoperatively. Sometimes the children will only take the drugs with milk or juice. If the medications are necessary and the surgery cannot be delayed, an intravenous induction and aspiration precautions are required (Belani and Palahniuk, 1991; Beebe et al., 1991).

Intravenous thiopental or propofol may be used in healthy children. Ketamine (1 to 3 mg/kg) has proved useful as an induction agent in infants and children suspected to be hypovolemic from recent dialysis. Ketamine maintains the autonomic tone and blood pressure while the volume status is corrected. Maintenance of the blood pressure and a strong pulse with ketamine is also useful when attempting to place an arterial catheter (Belani and Palahniuk, 1991; Beebe et al., 1991).

Tracheal intubation and skeletal muscle relaxation are always provided by an agent not dependent on the kidney for excretion, such as cisatricurium. Intermediate-acting steroidal muscle relaxants such as vecuronium or rocuronium may also be used, but their action may be prolonged because of partial renal excretion. Succinylcholine is usually not administered except in emergencies because it can raise the serum potassium concentration by 0.5 to 0.7 mmol/L. This could be dangerous in patients who are already hyperkalemic. Also, drugs dependent on renal excretion, such as pancuronium, should not be used because prolonged neuromuscular blockade can result if the kidney does not function properly in the perioperative period (Belani and Palahniuk, 1991; Beebe et al., 1991).

Following the induction of general anesthesia and tracheal intubation, anesthesia is maintained with isoflurane or desflurane. Even if sevoflurane has been used for an inhaled induction of general anesthesia, it usually is not used for maintenance because of concerns about nephrotoxicity with sevoflurane from fluoride ion and/or compound A production. Although nephrotoxicity in normal kidneys from sevoflurane in humans has never been demonstrated, its effects on transplanted kidneys are unknown (Artru, 1998). Either isoflurane or desflurane is therefore usually used for maintenance of anesthesia.

Nitrous oxide had been used frequently in the past and may still be used in older children. An air-oxygen mixture is usually used in infants to prevent bowel distention that may occur with nitrous oxide in an abdomen that will be quite full with an adult kidney. Opioids such as fentanyl are also administered in moderate doses to reduce the amount of inhaled agent required and to provide postoperative pain relief (Belani and Palahniuk, 1991; Beebe et al., 1991).

Monitoring

In addition to standard monitors (ECG, pulse oximetry, noninvasive blood pressure, end-tidal gas analysis, temperature), all children undergoing renal transplantation need their CVP monitored. This helps ensure that the children have had adequate volume administered before perfusion of the allograft as well as providing a means to administer immunosuppressive agents that can only be given centrally (thymoglobulin, OKT3, etc.). As noted earlier, in infants, the CVPs are often monitored through a large-bore Hickman catheter. This also serves as an excellent, high-flowing catheter to allow transfusion directly into the central circulation as well as a means to provide dialysis should the kidney initially fail (Belani and Palahniuk, 1991; Beebe et al., 1991).

Arterial catheters are also useful in infants and small children who require cross-clamping of the aorta. Reperfusion of the kidney in this situation can result in profound hypotension. The beat-to-beat data provided by an arterial catheter allow more rapid correction of hypotension and greater stability. Arterial blood gases obtainable from an arterial catheter are also often helpful. However, because the lower extremity is not perfused during anastomosis, the arterial catheter must be placed in an upper extremity (Belani and Palahniuk, 1991; Beebe et al., 1991).

Care During Perfusion of the Allograft

In older children who receive a kidney that is appropriately sized for their body weight, patient care during reperfusion is relatively straightforward. The hemoglobin level and electrolytes are checked following induction of general anesthesia. Older children usually do not require blood unless the hemoglobin level is less than 8 mg/dL. Similarly, children with renal failure often have a chronic metabolic acidosis; sodium bicarbonate is rarely required unless the pH is less than 7.25 despite mild hyperventilation. To ensure adequate hydration before reperfusion, normal saline or albumin is administered, provided the hematocrit is adequate until the CVP is 12 to 14 mm Hg. The systolic blood pressure is also allowed to rise to approximately 100 to 120 mm Hg before reperfusion to prevent hypotension when the clamps are released. Sodium mannitol (0.5 g/kg) and furosemide (1 mg/kg) are also administered to stimulate a diuresis. If the systolic blood pressure falls below 90 mm Hg, administration of a vasopressor such as ephedrine may be necessary. Rarely, dopamine may be administered by infusion for persistent hypotension (Belani and Palahniuk, 1991).

Management of perfusion of an adult kidney in an infant is more challenging. Unlike in older children or adults, both the aorta and inferior vena cavae are cross-clamped. Also unlike in adults, low-dose systemic heparinization (50 U/kg) is required before clamping the vessels. Since blood pools in the unperfused lower extremities while the kidney is sutured into place, release of the cross clamps causes ischemic byproducts in both the kidney and lower extremities to enter the central circulation. The adult kidney itself can initially absorb up to 300 mL of blood. Vasodilatation from ischemia can cause a large fraction of the infant's cardiac output to shunt through the new kidney. Occasionally potassium from the preservative solution from the new kidney is transfused rapidly into the central circulation of the infant, resulting in cardiac arrhythmias, hypotension, and sometimes arrest. Surgeons try to prevent this by perfusing the kidney with normal saline to wash out the hyperkalemic preservative solution (UW solution) but are not always successful. Also, in all cases, the kidney has been kept cold to preserve the organ while ischemic. Revascularization can result in significant hypothermia. Hypothermia may subsequently depress cardiac function and interfere with cardiac contractility that is needed to increase the cardiac output to perfuse the new kidney. Hypothermia also interferes with platelet and coagulation function, thereby predisposing the infant or child to increased perioperative bleeding (Belani and Palahniuk, 1991; Beebe et al., 1991).

In the past, infants receiving this operation had a high incidence of profound hypotension with perfusion of the allograft. This was often followed by vascular thrombosis or ATN. Subsequent experience in infants receiving an adult kidney has been much more successful (Beebe et al., 1991; Healy et al., 2000; Humar et al., 2001).

The main difference in the care of infants for reperfusion of the kidney received by an infant compared to an older child or adult is that the central venous pressure must be raised to a much higher level, at least 18 mm Hg, before reperfusion. Packed red blood cells and colloids (5% albumin and/or fresh frozen plasma if clotting parameters are diminished) all can be used to achieve this before reperfusion. The systemic blood pressure must also be at least 20% higher than the preoperative value for the infant to tolerate cross-clamp release. Often this is achieved with transfusion to elevate the CVP and lowering the anesthetic concentration to 0.5 MAC. However, some infants require an infusion of dopamine (3 to 5 mcg/kg per min). As in older children and adults, sodium mannitol 0.5 to 1.0 g/kg is administered before cross-clamp release, as well as Lasix (0.5 to 1 mg/kg) (Beebe et al., 1991).

The amount of volume required to raise the CVP to 18 mm Hg is often impressive. Many times greater than 100% of the infant's calculated blood volume is administered before reperfusion of the kidney. Additional volume is often required after reperfusion to replace ongoing blood loss and/or support the blood pressure if still inadequate (Beebe et al., 1991).

One must keep in mind that all blood products administered through the Hickman catheter during kidney transplantation in children require warming because transfusion of cold blood into the central circulation can result in myocardial depression as well as worsen hypothermia (Beebe et al., 1991).

Forced air surface warming with a device such as the Bair Hugger is also helpful to prevent hypothermia in kidney transplantation in children. However the lower extremities should not be warmed until unclamping of renal vessels has been accomplished. Warming of the lower extremists using forced-air surface warming during aortic cross-clamping in animals resulted in hypotension, pulmonary hypertension, and myocardial depression. This was thought to result from greater production of ischemic byproducts in lower extremities warmed during aortic cross-clamping (Beebe et al., 1993).

Immediately before cross-clamp release, atropine (20 mcg/kg) and calcium chloride (10 mg/kg) are administered. Atropine is administered because infants can occasionally develop vagally mediated profound bradycardia with the sudden loss of SVR. Calcium is important because potassium may immediately be transfused into the central circulation from the kidney if it has not been flushed of the high-potassium preservative solution (UW solution) before reperfusion. Often sodium bicarbonate is administered as well (1 mmol/kg) to neutralize the acid that develops in the ischemic lower extremities and new kidney. The dopamine infusion may need to be increased and other inotropes (e.g., epinephrine 1 mcg/kg as single aliquots) may be necessary immediately after reperfusion, but generally the pressure stabilizes at the initial, preoperative value (Beebe et al., 1991) (Fig. 28–15).

In both infants and older children, the urine output is replaced milliliter per milliliter with one-half normal saline solution as soon as it can be measured. This solution is chosen because this is the concentration of sodium excreted by a kidney with some degree of ATN and/or having received large doses of diuretics. Replacement of all the urine output with intravenous fluid ensures a brisk diuresis, and it is continued for up to 2 days following surgery. Dextrose is not added to the replacement solution because, if large volumes are administered due to a brisk urine output, hyperglycemia often results (Belani and Palahniuk, 1991; Beebe et al., 1991).

Postoperative Care

Following closure of the wounds, virtually all older children can have skeletal muscle relaxants reversed and be extubated as soon as they are awake and strong. Pain relief is achieved by means of patient-controlled analgesia with morphine, fentanyl, or hydromorphone. Most older children are cared for in the transplantation unit or ward. Rarely is intensive care unit admission

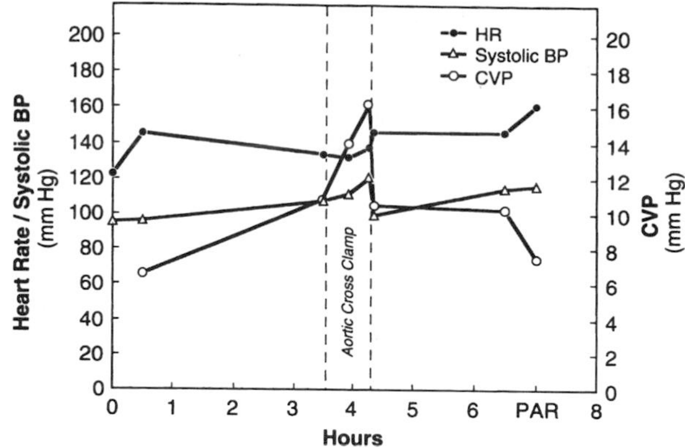

■ **FIGURE 28–15.** The systolic blood pressure (BP), heart rate (HR), and central venous pressure (CVP) during renal transplantation in infants. (From Beebe DS, Belani KG, Mergens P, et al.: Anesthetic management of infants receiving an adult kidney transplant. *Anesth Analg* 73:725–730, 1991, with permission.)

required, although most infants and small children require care in the pediatric intensive care unit overnight. Urine is replaced milliliter per milliliter with one-half normal saline for 2 days postoperatively. After this time, these children are allowed to begin oral intake and diuresis is no longer forced. Discharge to home varies with the patient's ability to tolerate oral feedings, but is usually within 1 week of surgery (Belani and Palahniuk, 1991; Beebe et al., 1991).

Infants usually can be extubated in the operating room or recovery room as well despite the presence of a large adult kidney, which causes obvious abdominal distention. Chest radiographic evidence of pulmonary edema due to the large amounts of fluid administered to infants is present in at least 25% of patients in the recovery room. Despite this, less than 10% of infants require mechanical ventilation in the intensive care unit postoperatively. Fluid management is similar to older children, but the amount of urine output from the adult kidney can be profound (i.e., 80 mL/kg per hr). Electrolytes therefore must be closely monitored. Eventually over several days the kidney adjusts to the smaller size of the recipient and produces the proper amount of urine (Beebe et al., 1991).

■ PANCREAS AND ISLET CELL TRANSPLANTATION

Diabetes mellitus (DM) has reached epidemic levels in the United States, given the increased incidence of obesity estimated at 62% in both the pediatric and adult populations. In 2004, there were a documented 13 million people living with DM and an estimated 5 million undiagnosed or untreated patients in the United States (Diabetes Control and Compilation Trial Research Group, 1993). Worldwide, the disease incidence of DM is astronomical and is noted to be in the top five causes of morbidity and mortality in the industrialized world. This multisystem disease process results in end organ dysfunction in not only the kidneys, but in the neurological, ophthalmologic, cardiovascular, and vascular systems predominantly; it spares no organ system, including the hematologic, from its negative deleterious effects. This all occurs as a result of hyperglycemia, a consequence of the inability of the beta-islet cells of Langerhans of the pancreas to secrete insulin, or inaction at the insulin receptor. Remarkably, the aggregate mass of the islet cells of the adult pancreas weighs only 1 to 1.5 grams. With this seemingly simple genetic or acquired defect of this ostensibly tiny, yet important, mass of cells, DM results in complications with the consequences of blindness in 15%, renal failure and myocardial infarctions in approximately 20%, and strokes and amputations in an estimated 10% and 12%, respectively, of patients afflicted. Given these complications, the costs estimates in 2002 alone were approximately $132 billion spent in for medical care and lost productivity owing to DM (Diabetes mellitus, 2004). With these estimates and noted disease complications, it is then simple to rationalize the need for alternative therapies, such as pancreas, islet cell, and kidney-pancreas transplantation, as potential treatments for patients with DM.

The first clinical pancreas transplantation was performed in 1966, with a simultaneous kidney transplant in a uremic, diabetic patient at the University of Minnesota by Kelly, Lillehei and others (Lillehei et al., 1970, Sutherland 1979). Since that initial event, simultaneous kidney pancreas (SPK), pancreas after kidney transplant (PAK), pancreas transplant alone (PTA), and islet cell transplantation have taken a quantum leap ahead in the field of solid organ transplantation. Over 100 institutions in the United States and nearly the same number worldwide have performed these procedures in the latter part of the 20th century (Gruessner and Sutherland, 1997, 2003). With the rapid growth of these procedures and their relative success since 1980, and with the introduction of newer immunosuppressive drugs as well as immunosuppressive regimens, the International Pancreas Transplant Registry was created in 1980. Simultaneously, there has been data tracking by UNOS, as mandated by this governmental agency since 1987. In the United States, the Center for Medical Services–Medicare deemed pancreas transplantation to be a reimbursable procedure. The longest survivor of a SPK transplant, in a procedure performed at the University Hospital in Zurich on April 10, 1981, is still alive and well as of 2005 with both organs functional. It has been more than 24 years since the procedure, performed when the patient was 30 years old. Initially, poor success and survival was noted in the 1980s; however, by the early 1990s, over 1000 pancreatic transplants were being performed annually, as the surgical procedure was refined and many of the inherent complications were resolved.

Pediatric patients, however, account for a very small percentage (less than 3%) of all pancreas transplant procedures, and are the smallest relative percentile group of any solid organ transplant. As of April 1, 2005, UNOS reported a total of 147 pancreas (PTA+PAK) and 23 simultaneous kidney pancreas transplants (SKP) performed since 1988 in the pediatric patient population; a total of 170 of the cumulative 27,682 pediatric solid organ transplants performed to date in the United States (UNOS, 2005). Data compiled by the International Pancreas Transplant Registry (IPTR) at the University of Minnesota (tracked to June, 2003) indicate more than 19,600 pancreas transplants reported. The majority (14,300) were performed in the United States.

The total number of pediatric candidates on the waiting list as of April 2005 was 22 for pancreas and 3 for kidney pancreas. These data are in significant contradistinction to those of the adult population: on the UNOS waiting list, at the same time period, there were 1694 and 2455 candidates awaiting pancreas (PTA+PAK) or SKP transplant procedures, respectively. The reason for these disparate numbers is intuitively evident, given the fact that organ transplantation, in most cases, is reserved for patients with end organ damage and complications, a process that may take some 10 to 20 years to develop in the diabetic patient.

In the United States, from 1988 through 2002, 79% of these transplant patients underwent SPK. Approximately 14% of these patients per year underwent PAK, whereas only 6% underwent PTA (data from the IPTR, University of Minnesota). The one-year graft survival for SPK is approximately 86% to 91%, PTA is 83.8%, and PAK is 78.4%. The one-year patient survival data are the following: 95.9% for SKP, 99.2% for PTA, and 96.6% for PAK. These data are the best of any solid organ, transplant patient population, except the living-related kidney transplant patient population. Long-term insulin independence is achieved in 70% to 80% of pancreas transplant recipients (Bland, 2003; Kahl, Bechstein and Redi, 2001).

Islet cell transplantation, first performed in 1974, is still in its infancy, yet a successful procedure was accomplished with the first case. This procedure, similar in kind to bone marrow transplantation, is dependent on the total mass or number of transplanted islet cells. Most notably, islet allotransplantation had not been consistently successful until the early 1990s (Gruessner and Sutherland, 2003), with the ability of patients to achieve sustained insulin independence. Moreover, success was achieved recently for a repetitive series of multiple consecutive recipients. The number of procedures performed worldwide to date has been reported to be over 450, with patient and graft survival at 75% and 65%, respectively. The majority of procedures have been performed in the United States; and in Europe, the majority of cases have been performed in Giessen, Germany, and Milan, Italy. Although it is possible that islet cell transplantation may become the dominant form of beta islet cell replacement in the near future, the need for SKP, PTA, and PAK will remain, since only 4% of patients with islet cell transplantation are currently insulin independent at one year. This unsettling result may indeed be related to the aforementioned low beta cell transplanted mass and has been demonstrated clinically at the University of Edmonton in Alberta and the University of Miami. At these institutions, strategies to improve beta cell mass have been undertaken by the use of more than one donor per patient. By these means, insulin independence has occurred after the second or third transplant. The acquisition of insulin independence is improved in islet allotransplantation after kidney transplantation (IAK), 45% at one year, and in simultaneous islet and kidney transplantation (SIK), 74% at one year with normalized glycosylated (glycated) hemoglobin. These data have been reported by the Giessen Group (Meyer et al., 1998; International Transplant Registry [ITR] News Letters #8, 1999; #9, 2001).

ISLET CELL TRANSPLANTATION

Islet cell transplantation has gained recognition as an acceptable potential cure for type 1 DM. The Diabetes Control and Complications Trial Group demonstrated the value of maintaining near normal blood glucose levels with intensive insulin therapy, for the prevention or delay of the devastating long-term complications related to diabetic neuropathy micro- and macroangiopathy (Diabetes Control and Complications Trial Research Group, 1993; Manske et al., 1999; Sollinger et al., 1998; Gruessner and Sutherland, 2003). Pancreas transplantation can achieve long-term glucose metabolic control, in a state of complete insulin independence, as noted previously (Diabetes mellitus, 2004). Unfortunately, pancreas transplantation is still associated with some morbidity and mortality (Powers, 2001), hence, the endeavors undertaken to achieve beta cell transplantation. Islet cell transplantation presents the great advantages of a fast and easy procedure with virtually absent or minimal perioperative morbidity, but its success has yet to match those of pancreas transplantation.

Although restricted to the few institutions where the technique is available, the indications for allogeneic islet cell transplantation are currently the same as those for whole organ pancreas transplantation. The procedure is primarily offered to type-1 diabetic patients with end-stage renal failure and is performed as either a simultaneous islet-kidney (SIK) or an islet-after-kidney (IAK) procedure. Another potential indication for islet transplantation is after pancreatic graft failure, as retransplantation is associated with an increased incidence of graft failure (Federlin et al., 1999). Patients with DM due to cystic fibrosis or hemochromatosis are also candidates for islet transplantation although exocrine pancreatic function is also required (Hering and Ricordi, 1999). Transplantation of islets alone in patients with functioning kidneys, in order to prevent the development of diabetic complications, is not yet considered a reasonable option, because of the burden of lifelong immunosuppression and the significant associated risk of developing severe infections and malignancies.

The field of islet cell transplantation made revolutionary progress in the late 1980s by automated islet cell isolation with the use of a computerized centrifugation system and continuous enzymatic digestion of the pancreas for islet purification in discontinuous gradients (Ricordi et al., 1988; Kahl et al., 2001). This increased the yield of the islet isolation procedure and allowed for the first time recovery of a critical mass of beta cells from a single donor sufficient for transplantation in a diabetic recipient (Linetsky et al., 1997; Ricordi et al., 1992).

Islet cell infusion into the liver is the most common technique and site for this procedure. Other sites of implantation include the peritoneal cavity, epiploic flaps, and the spleen, but without the significant success seen with hepatic implantation. Numerous advantages are associated with the use of the liver: it is easily and readily accessible via the portal route and considered to be immunologically protective. Moreover, functioning islets have been demonstrated to survive there for several years after transplantation, which is similar to dendritic cells (Ricordi et al., 1996).

Monitored anesthesia care (MAC) is all that is required, as with many invasive radiological procedures. Implantation of the islets is performed via a minimally invasive radiological procedure. The portal vein is cannulated by a transhepatic percutaneous approach with angiographic guidance. Alternatively, for SIK transplantation, an open procedure may be performed after completion of kidney transplantation via a midline incision. In this case, the portal system is usually accessed by catheterization of a mesenteric vein. The purified islet suspension is slowly infused with continuous monitoring of the intraportal hydrostatic pressure (Oberholzer et al., 1999).

The morbidity and mortality associated with intraportal islet infusion are minimal. Among 215 recipients of an islet allograft reported to the International Islet Transplant Registry (ITR) from 1990 through 1996, one patient died as a direct consequence of the procedure because of an inadvertent hepatic arterial injury, resulting in a fatal hemorrhage (ITR News Letter #9, 2001). Four nonlethal complications have been reported: perforation of the gallbladder requiring laparoscopic cholecystectomy; tear of the splenic capsule requiring splenectomy; bacteremia due to infusion of a contaminated islet preparation; and portal vein thrombosis in a simultaneous liver-islet transplant procedure (Hering et al., 1999).

Through December 2000, greater than 450 islet allografts have been performed worldwide, including 306 since 1990, as a result of the breakthrough due to the automated method of islet isolation (ITR News Letter #9, 2000; Oberholzer, 1999). Cumulative 1-year patient and graft survival of 96% and 35%, respectively, were obtained in 200 C-peptide negative, type-1 diabetic patients who underwent transplantation from 1990 through 1997. The persistence of graft function can be assessed by measurable levels of basal serum C-peptide, at a threshold of 0.5 ng/ml. The observation that 32% of recipients lose graft function within 1 month of transplantation (and 46% within 3 months) indicates that primary nonfunction might be a major cause of islet graft loss (ITR Newsletter #9, 2000; Meyer et al., 1998).

Although the evidence of measurable C-peptide in the serum indicates unequivocal survival of the islet graft, it does not necessarily imply that patients can achieve lasting survival without supplemental insulin. However, it must be emphasized that islet graft function in the absence of insulin independence is still associated with markedly improved metabolic control, glucose counter regulation, and hypoglycemia awareness (Meyer et al., 1998).

Analysis of parameters reported to the ITR has allowed identification of four determinants of persisting graft function at 1 year and insulin independence for more than 7 days. The four criteria derived from these findings that form the basis for state-of-the-art islet allotransplantation are (1) transplantation of an islet mass (6000 islet equivalents [IEQ]/kg body weight; IEQ is the calculated number of islets if all had an ideal diameter of 150 μm); (2) cold ischemia time of the pancreas (< 8 h); (3) immunosuppression induction with antilymphocyte or antithymocyte globulins, or anti-IL-2R monoclonal antibodies, as opposed to OKT3 or none; and (4) liver as the site of islet graft implantation. A significantly beneficial effect is obtained especially when all four criteria are fulfilled (ITR News Letter #8, 1999).

Remarkable results have been obtained by the Giessen group with the implementation of new strategies aimed at promoting islet engraftment and transplant survival (ITR News Letter #8, 1999). The Giessen protocol included, in addition to fulfillment of the four aforementioned criteria, strategies based on observations made in experimental animal models, namely the use of endotoxin-free reagents, the use of antioxidant agents (nicotinamide), and the administration of IV insulin starting 2 to 3 days prior to transplant in order to diminish metabolic demand on the graft. With this protocol, insulin independence has been achieved in approximately 30% of transplanted patients (Beebe et al., 1995).

As already highlighted, the majority of islets are lost early after transplantation. The early events leading to graft loss are collectively termed primary nonfunction and are not related to an immune phenomenon. Rather, they result from poor intrinsic quality of the islet preparation or from interaction of the islets with inflammatory elements of the hepatic microenvironment in which they are implanted. Direct islet damage provoked by cytokines and nitric oxide released by activated Kuppfer cells and sinusoidal endothelial cells, as a result of islet implantation, has been clearly demonstrated (Kaufman et al., 1990). Islets are an essentially avascular graft, which renders them particularly prone to hypoxia, at least during the few days it takes before neovascularization ensues for the islets (Bretzel et al., 1999).

A second set of problems arises from the high metabolic demand imposed on the islet graft, which results from several factors. A normal pancreas consists of approximately 1 million islets, a figure that is far from being matched with the threshold of 6000 IEQ/kg considered necessary for graft function. When one considers that a significant number of transplanted islets are lost to the noxious inflammatory environment, it is evident that the engrafted islet mass is by and large marginal for its insulin release workload. To make matters worse, islet transplantation currently necessitates conventional immunosuppression, based on the association of several drugs consisting of a calcineurin inhibitor (such as cyclosporin A or tacrolimus) and steroids. All three drugs have long been known to have a diabetogenic effect, which further increases the metabolic load on the islets (Shapiro et al., 1998).

Islet grafts are also prone to destruction by recurrence of autoimmunity in addition to allorejection. There has been no clear indication so far that islets are more susceptible to allorejection than are whole pancreas transplants. The inflammatory insult to islets in a microenvironment of activated macrophages leads to a situation of increased availability of islet allopeptides and antigen-presenting cells, which may enhance alloantigen presentation to host T-cells and, thus, promote ensuing immune graft loss (Halloran et al., 1997; Sutherland et al., 1989). Although immune rejection and recurrence of autoimmunity are exceedingly difficult to distinguish, there is strong evidence that the latter is a significant mechanism of islet graft loss despite adequate conventional immunosuppression (Jaeger et al., 1997).

Renewed enthusiasm has arisen from the improved results of clinical islet transplantation. Marvelously, the advent of newer immunosuppressive agents has resulted in a reduction of the need for the administration of diabetogenic calcineurin inhibitors. Notably, due to the synergistic actions of rapamycin and cyclosporin, the dosage of both drugs can be lowered significantly with optimal immunosuppressive properties but minimal toxicity (Hricik et al., 1998; Kahan et al., 1998). Protocols using mycophenolate mofetil also allow early tapering and withdrawal of steroids in the immunosuppressive regimen (Hricik et al., 1998). Induction protocols including anti-IL-2 receptor monoclonal antibodies (basiliximab, daclizumab) are under evaluation (Basadonna et al., 1998).

One major potential advantage of islet grafts over whole pancreas is the possibility of expanding the pool of transplant tissue. Several alternate sources are being explored, such as cell lines or in vitro expansion of cultured cells. However, porcine xenogeneic islets are likely to become an important alternate source of insulin-producing tissue. The rationale for choosing the pig as an islet donor for humans is manifold: (1) its supply is "unlimited" and it is easy to raise in a controlled fashion in a clean environment; (2) its size and weight match those of humans; and (3) the sequence of porcine insulin differs from the human sequence by only one amino acid and adequately substitutes for human insulin.

The difficulties observed in isolating and culturing adult porcine islets can be partially overcome by using fetal or neonatal piglets as islet donors. Mechanisms of islet xenorejection and immunosuppressive regimens are under investigation in several animal models; and ten type-1 diabetic patients have received fetal porcine islet xenografts infused in the portal bloodstream or under the kidney capsule in a Swedish pilot clinical trial (Groth et al., 1994; Berney et al., 1999; Soon-Shiong et al., 1994). Although no patient became insulin-independent, evidence of porcine islet function for 200 to 400 days was obtained by the detection of porcine C-peptide in the urine of four of the recipients. These results, published in 1994 and obtained under a classic cyclosporin/azathioprine-based regimen, are an encouraging baseline, considering the advances in transplantation immunology and immunosuppression made in the past 10 years (Ricordi et al., 1996, 1997). A major concern remains regarding the safety of xenotransplantation. The risk of xenozoonoses, notably porcine endogenous retroviruses (PERVs), is under acute scrutiny and is at the center of a debate that goes beyond purely scientific issues. In this regard, it is noteworthy that the ten Swedish recipients of porcine fetal islets screened negative for PERV in a study conducted by the Centers for Disease Control and Prevention in Atlanta 5 to 8 years after transplantation (Heneine et al., 1998; Groth et al., 1994).

PANCREAS AND KIDNEY-PANCREAS TRANSPLANTATIONS

Diabetes mellitus is a pathogenic process, which results in hyperglycemia. Typically, type 1 DM (insulin dependent diabetes mellitus [IDDM]) is usually the result of the synergistic effects of genetic, environmental, infectious, and immunologic factors leading to pancreatic beta cell destruction and the resultant absolute absence of insulin production or secretion (Powers, 2001). Its incidence appears to be on the order of approximately 30,000 new onset cases per year in the United States, and it has been the predominant cause of DM in the pediatric population until the end of the past decade.

Type 2 DM (non-insulin dependent diabetes mellitus [NIDDM]) is most often associated with obesity and seen in the elderly population, albeit not exclusively, as it has been noted to be occurring with increasing frequency in the pediatric population, linked to the increased incidence of obesity. Furthermore, genetic differences exist between both IDDM and NIDDM as evidenced by twin studies (Barnett et al., 1981). In this classic publication, the concordance rate (both twins affected) of IDDM was 50% as contrasted with a concordance rate of greater than 90% for twins having NIDDM, demonstrating the importance of genetic factors playing a much larger role in this variant of the disease.

Approximately 5% to 10% of diagnosed cases of diabetes are type 1 diabetes mellitus (Clinical Topic Tours, 2004; Powers, 2001). Acute complications include diabetic ketoacidosis, in addition to coronary artery disease, peripheral vascular disease, cerebrovascular disease, nephropathy, autonomic and peripheral neuropathy, and retinopathy (Diabetes Control and Complications Trial Research Group, 1993; The Diabetes Control and Complications Trial Research Group, 2000; Ladikta et al., 2001; Rabbat et al., 2003). The usual treatment of type 1 DM is the lifelong administration of exogenous insulin. Pancreas transplantation offers patients who have IDDM an endogenous source of insulin, hence its importance for this variant of DM particularly. Type 2 DM (NIDDM) is managed by exercise, weight loss, diet, oral hypoglycemic agents, or exogenous insulin administration (Powers, 2001). It is distinctive by its noted insulin resistance without an absolute insulin deficiency. Acute complications include hyperosmolar non-ketotic coma, but ketoacidosis may also be a mode of presentation.

The primary objective of pancreas or beta-islet cell transplantation is to restore endogenous insulin secretion to a diabetic individual, by the provision of the missing normal beta cell function, in order to achieve euglycemia as well as glucagon response to hypoglycemia, allowing patients to be insulin-free, eat a regular diet, and ultimately prevent the multisystem organ complications previously noted. Occasionally, exocrine pancreatic function is also desired to restore both types of hormonal functions of the pancreas as a result of possibly total pancreatectomy or cystic fibrosis (Powers, 2001; Kahl et al., 2001; Hakim, 2003; Kiberd and Larson, 2000; Paty et al., 2001; Coosemans and Pirenne, 2003). Carbohydrate, fat, and protein metabolism is expected to normalize after pancreas transplantation and may eventually stabilize and even prevent the development of microvascular disease (Coosemans and Pirenne, 2003). An additional goal of all pancreas transplants is to improve the patients' quality of life (Hakim, 2003; Kiberd and Larson, 2000; Kalathil et al., 2000). Although exogenous insulin administration with tight glucose control has been shown to delay and even prevent the progression and complications of DM (infections, diabetic retinopathy, nephropathy, and neuropathy), the mean serum glucose was only normalized to 155 + 30 mg/dL, and the primary adverse effect was a two- to threefold increase in the incidence of hypoglycemic episodes (Diabetes Control and Complications Trial Research Group, 1993). Patients who are "brittle diabetics" are best treated with the beta-islet cell replacement therapy.

Unfortunately, progression of macrovascular disease has occurred despite successful kidney and pancreas transplantation. This might be a result of the vascular drainage of insulin from the transplanted graft, directly into the systemic circulation, bypassing the normal portoenteric circulation with drainage of insulin into the liver, its principal site of action (Nankivell et al., 2000). The hyperinsulinemia has been postulated to be pathogenic in this regard.

For diabetic patients with imminent or established end-stage renal disease (ESRD) who have had, or plan to have, a renal transplant, the American Diabetes Association now recommends pancreas transplantation as an acceptable therapeutic alternative to exogenous insulin therapy (American Diabetic Association, 2003). Diabetic patients should be considered for pancreas transplantation (PTA) in the absence of indications for kidney transplantation in the setting of frequent, acute, and severe metabolic complications, incapacitating clinical and emotional problems with exogenous insulin therapy, and consistent failure of insulin-based management to prevent complications. In the majority of cases, pancreas transplantation is performed in the setting of type 1 DM with end stage renal disease. Patients for PTA or PAK procedures must have stable and adequate kidney function at the time of transplant, as both the operative procedure and the immunosuppressive agent may result in a further decline in the patient's renal function. As beta-islet cell transplantation is still in the developmental stage, and should be performed only in a controlled setting where facilities for this procedure are available, it should be reserved for patients who may not be appropriate surgical candidates for the previously mentioned procedures.

Absolute contraindications to transplantation of any type include active malignancy or infection; recently treated malignancy not meeting the minimum disease-free observation period as suggested by the Clinical Practice Guidelines of the American Society of Transplantation (Diabetes Control and Complications Trial Research Group, 2000); psychiatric disease so severe or unstable that the stress of this surgery would likely result in marked decompensation; and patients unable or unwilling to take immunosuppressant medications regularly such that graft failure would be certain.

As with kidney transplantation, patients with pancreatic failure for any of the group of procedures for beta-islet cell replacement will require a thorough evaluation, given the constellation of complications of hyperglycemia in diabetic patients. These include ischemic heart disease, cardiomyopathy, renal failure, autonomic neuropathy and gastroparesis, hypertension, cerebrovascular, ophthalmologic, and macrovascular diseases. A meticulous review of the current list of medications and allergies must be undertaken. The patient selected to receive a cadaveric/deceased donor organ requires urgent attention, evaluation, and preparation for the procedure, as the procured organ has a limited life in the preservation solution, usually not to exceed 24 hours. Hence, the anesthetic evaluation, if not previously completed as part of the pretransplant evaluation, will require a de novo thorough evaluation in a timely manner.

The degree of renal dysfunction, if any, is of particular importance, as it will in essence dictate the particular type of procedure that the patient should receive; that is, SPK versus PTA, given the fact that SPK transplants account for 79% of pancreas transplants, and PAK transplants account for 14% of transplants. Most often this decision has been made as part of the preoperative evaluation in order to have the patient placed on the waiting list. Moreover, a determination of the patient's acid-base status, daily serum glucose, electrolyte concentrations, and time of last hemodialysis is of great importance. Anemia associated with ESRD, due to diminished production of erythropoietin and chronic bone marrow suppression, is often associated with an increased morbidity and a diminished graft success (Koehntop, Beebe, and Belani, 2000).

The principal cause of perioperative mortality in adult pancreas recipients is coronary artery disease (Bland, 2003). Hence, screening tests that are mandatory for the preoperative cardiovascular evaluation include coronary angiography in addition to the usual noninvasive studies, which often may include a dobutamine stress echocardiogram (Rabbat et al., 2003; Boston et al., 2002). Moreover, depending on the findings, pretransplantation coronary revascularization reduces the risk of subsequent cardiac events (Rabbat et al., 2003).

The pediatric patient for pancreas transplant, however, is usually devoid of cardiovascular and significant renal complications, as his or her disease process is usually not of as long a duration as in the adult patient. Nonetheless, it is imperative that all end organ damage be fully assessed and excluded from the history.

A history of gastroparesis needs to be addressed appropriately in the pediatric patient as this may warrant an IV rapid sequence induction as opposed to an inhalation induction. Aspiration prophylaxis with H_2 receptor antagonists, metoclopramide, and possibly a nonparticulate antacid should be considered. Autonomic neuropathy, which results in gastroparesis, may predispose these patients to episodes of hypotension during the transplant or any anesthetic.

Airway evaluation is of special importance, but adult diabetics have an increased incidence of difficult intubations (Hogan, Rusy and Springman, 1988). This correlates with the longevity of the disease and may prove irrelevant in children.

Surgical Procedures

Several surgical techniques for pancreas transplantation have been described. However, the approach taken for a patient is dependent on the type of procedure chosen. Initially considered, is the recipient to receive an SKP or PTA? After the appropriate blood and tissue typing for human lymphocyte antigen (HLA) markers and ABO compatibility, the organ is prepared on the back table, and vascular grafts, if needed, are also anastomosed at this time, while the organ is maintained in cold preservation solution (a measure to minimize warm ischemic preservation injury).

Postinduction of general anesthesia and placement of the standard monitors including an arterial and a central venous catheter, a surgical midline incision is made in order to facilitate implantation of the pancreas graft as well as the kidney if necessary. The right colon is mobilized by incising the peritoneal reflection, allowing its positioning cephalad. The right iliac vessels are then dissected, and in patients undergoing bladder drainage (BD) technique, the right iliac vein is completely mobilized by ligating and dividing all posterior branches. Mobilizing the sigmoid colon and reflecting it medially then accomplishes exposure of the left iliac system. Ligating and dividing the posterior branches as on the right side then allows mobilization of the iliac vein. The graft is then implanted with the head of the pancreas and the duodenum directed toward the pelvis. In BD grafts, the site for the vascular anastomosis is usually the common iliac vein and the common iliac artery. The graft with duodenal "button" is then anastomosed to the bladder as noted in Figure 28-16.

Compared with BD pancreatic allografts, the vascular anastomoses of enteric drainage (ED) grafts are achieved using the more proximal iliac vasculature. Usually, the venous anastomosis is performed in the area of the distal inferior vena cava and the arterial anastomosis is to the proximal right common iliac artery. The organ is then anastomosed to a proximal portion of the jejunum as noted in Figure 28-17.

A crucial element at the time of graft reperfusion is the sequence of release of the vascular clamps slowly. Over the course of several minutes, the vascular clamps are removed in the following sequence: proximal venous clamp, distal arterial clamp, proximal arterial clamp, and distal venous clamp. After each clamp is removed, careful hemostasis of bleeding vessels on the surface of the pancreas and at each vascular anastomosis, if necessary, is accomplished before any further clamps are removed.

The surgical approach to pancreas engraftment is dependent on whether or not exocrine secretions will be managed by either enteric (ED) or bladder drainage (BD). From 1987 to 1995, over 90% of pancreas transplants were performed using bladder drainage, initially described by Salinger and others and later modified by Corry and others to include the aforementioned duodenal "button," which acts as a reinforcement of the anastomosis of the graft to the bladder. This approach allows for serial measurements of urinary amylase, one method for monitoring graft rejection (Bland, 2003; Cooseman and Pirenne, 2003; Bloom et al., 1997; Cattral et al., 2000). Pancreatic biopsies are relatively effortless and less risky as the organ is placed lower in the pelvis (see Fig. 28-16).

Chronic loss of pancreatic secretions into the bladder can result in associated complications of metabolic acidosis, a finding in the majority of patients with BD, and perhaps dehydration. Electrolyte abnormalities, which are the result of the loss of sodium bicarbonate-rich pancreatic secretions, are not infrequent. Moreover, local bladder irritation, hematuria, urethritis, bladder leak, neurogenic bladder, chemical cystitis, urethritis, allograft pancreatitis, duodenitis, bladder calculi, urethral erosions, prostatitis, urethral strictures, and infections are all inherent possible complications (Kahl et al., 2001; Bloom et al., 1997; Cattral et al., 2000). In fact, the frequency of urological complications is high, (50% to 77% with this approach), but it rarely affects either patient mortality or graft loss.

The kidney, if implanted as during a SKP, is positioned in the left iliac fossa and an ureteroneocystostomy is performed. Vascular anastomoses are to the dissected left iliac vessels in the child over 20 kg (see Fig 28-17). However, in the infant less than 20 kg, the graft is implanted with anastomoses of the vasculature to the aorta and vena cava.

The enteric drainage technique has become the surgical technique of choice given the reputed constellation of complications (Bland, 2003; Cooseman and Pirenne, 2003; Bloom et al., 1997; Cattral et al., 2000). Initially, enteric drainage was associated with a high morbidity rate because of peritoneal leakage and the need for frequent reoperations. In this procedure, the pancreatic duct is inserted into the small bowel using a "button" of duodenum or a roux-en-Y limb (see Fig. 28-17). Although Roux-en-Y was used predominantly for enteric drainage at most centers, its

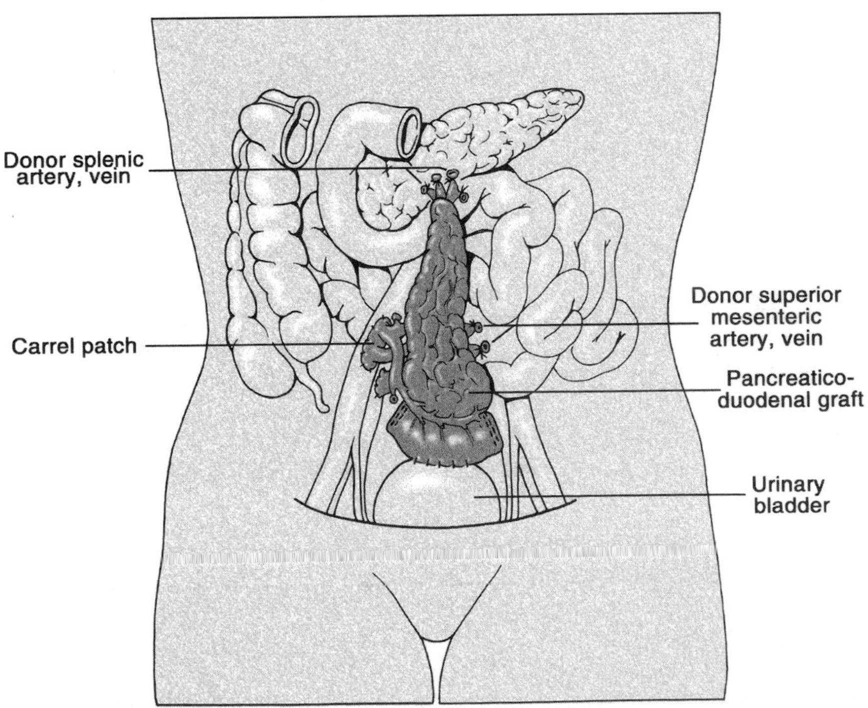

■ **FIGURE 28–16.** Solitary pancreas transplant (PTA) with the urinary bladder being utilized for exocrine drainage (bladder drainage [BD] technique). Note the native pancreas is in situ (see text).

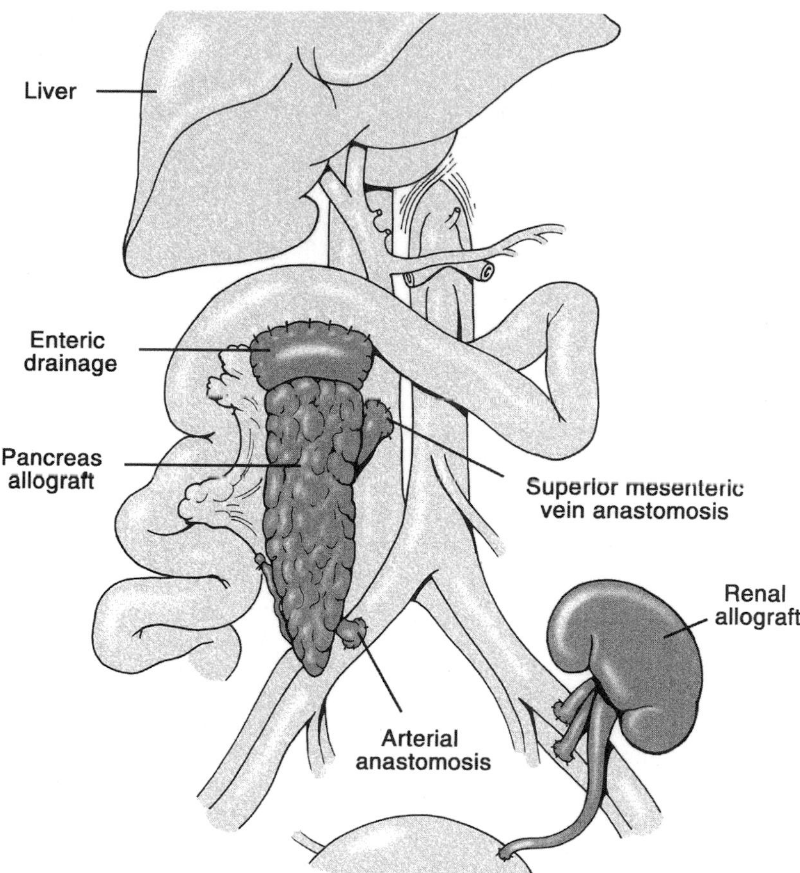

■ **FIGURE 28–17.** Pancreas and kidney transplants (PAK or SKP) with the donor pancreas vascularized to facilitate enteric exocrine drainage to a proximal portion of the jejunum (enteric drainage [ED] technique). The donor kidney is implanted in the left iliac fossa anastomosed to the femoral vessels and a uretero-neocystostomy is performed. (see text).

role has diminished. This is primarily a result of the reduced need for monitoring of graft rejection as immunosuppressive regimens have improved with a contemporaneous reduction in the frequency of rejection episodes. Currently over 55% to 77% of pancreas transplants are with enteric drainage as reported to UNOS for the period from 1999 to 2002.

Enteric drainage, by nature, avoids the complications associated with bladder drainage (Coosemans and Pirenne, 2003; Bloom et al., 1997; Cattral et al., 2000). Vascular management of the pancreatic graft has also evolved. Venous graft effluent can be drained into either the systemic or portal circulation. Portal venous drainage was used in approximately 25% of pancreas transplants from 1996 to 2002 (Bland, 2003). Both portal and systemic drainage are associated with excellent glycemic control; however, fasting serum insulin levels are significantly lower in portal drainage without effect on graft survival rates at 1 year for SPK or PAK (Bland, 2003; Cattral et al., 2000). PTA has a slightly higher graft survival rate with portal drainage (Bland, 2003). A postulated advantage of portal venous drainage is the avoidance of hyperinsulinemia, which has been associated with advanced atherosclerosis and vasculopathy. Pancreas grafts have been associated with the highest surgical complication rate of all routinely transplanted solid organs. Causes for technical failure of the cadaveric/deceased donor primary pancreas transplants include vascular thrombosis, pancreatitis, anastomotic leak, bleeding, rejection, and infections (Laftavi et al., 1998; Troppman et al., 1998; Humar et al., 2000; Sutherland et al., 2001; Michalek et al., 2002).

Vascular thrombosis is the most commonly cited cause of graft failure and previously was assumed to be associated with technical complications of the operation. After a thorough pathological evaluation of sequential cases of massive thrombosis, it is now evident that unrecognized hyperacute rejection is far more common than had been appreciated in this setting. Hence, organ rejection may in fact be the most common cause of graft loss and the culprit to blame. Significant risk factors for graft loss include older donor age, re-transplantation, re-laparotomy for infection, leakage, and bleeding (Troppman et al., 1998; Humar et al., 2000). The quality of a cadaveric/deceased donor graft can directly affect graft performance. As experience with pancreas transplant has increased, the incidence of re-laparotomy has decreased (Humar et al., 2000). Risk factors for recipient death include older recipients, re-transplantation, re-laparotomy for thrombosis, infection, leakage, and bleeding (Troppman et al., 1998).

Anesthetic Management

After appropriate positioning and placement of the standard monitors, anesthesia is induced, either with an intravenous technique or an inhalation technique with agents appropriate for the patient's baseline metabolic condition, followed by orotracheal intubation. In children, a central venous catheter and preferably a radial arterial catheter are inserted (as both iliac arteries may potentially be used for vascular anastomoses). Following the induction, the volatile anesthetic agent should be isoflurane or desflurane in patients with renal dysfunction, as they appear to be virtually devoid of nephrotoxicity and physiologically do not diminish renal arteriolar blood flow. Nitrous oxide is avoided as it increases the size of gas-containing spaces such as the bowel. A balanced anesthesia technique may also be used to maintain general anesthesia.

Morphine-6-glucuronide and normeperidine, the metabolites of morphine and meperidine, respectively, may accumulate in renal failure. The accumulation of normeperedine in this setting causes seizures. Hydromorphone may be used in preference to these agents, as it is less dependent on renal excretion. However, intraoperatively and immediately postoperatively, fentanyl is the opioid of choice; it has minimal associated hemodynamic alterations. The choice of muscle relaxant is dependent on the degree of renal impairment.

In patients with significant cardiovascular disease, direct arterial pressure monitoring and right heart monitoring with a pulmonary artery catheter should be considered as well as continuous transesophageal echocardiogram (TEE) as needed. These measures, however, are rarely necessary in the pediatric patient. Serum glucose levels must be carefully monitored at least hourly during general anesthesia, particularly after graft reperfusion, with maintenance of the serum glucose between 100 and 200 mg/dL (Koehntop, Beebe and Belani, 2000), as hyperglycemia will trigger early islet cell dysfunction (Clark et al., 1982; Imamura et al., 1988). Maintaining serum glucose levels in an acceptable range is accomplished by continuous infusion of regular insulin at a rate of 0.1 U/kg/h, with concurrent dextrose infusion when serum glucose levels are 150 mg/dL. The addition of dextrose ensures uninterrupted intracellular fuel to avoid perioperative ketosis. Pancreatic beta cells may function as early as 5 minutes after reperfusion with the release of insulin (Troppman and Gruessner, 2004). Delayed graft function may be treated postoperatively with an insulin infusion titrated to keep blood glucose levels 150 mg/dL (Sealey, 1988). Somatostatin may also be administered to decrease exocrine pancreatic secretion (Bloom et al., 1997).

Prior to allograft reperfusion with release of the vascular clamps, the hemodynamics are optimized to ensure adequate perfusion and prevent hypotension. Intravenous fluids, either crystalloid or colloid, are administered to achieve a central venous pressure in the range of 12 to 14 mm Hg and a systolic blood pressure of at least 140 mm Hg (Koehntop, Beebe, and Belani, 2000). Alternatively, in patients with a pulmonary artery catheter, careful titration of volume versus filling pressures and cardiac output can be used to optimize intravascular fluid status before vascular unclamping. The end tidal concentration of the inhaled agents may need to be reduced, as reperfusion of both grafts may result in short-lived hypotension as a result of vasodilation, cytokine release, transient myocardial dysfunction, and metabolic acidosis. This may require the administration of fluids, vasopressor (preferably dopamine), intravenous bicarbonate or thamasol, and blood products when appropriate.

It is imperative to maintain adequate and even supranormal perfusion pressure and blood flow to the new allograft. This may help to prevent graft vessel thrombosis, the most common cause of technical pancreatic graft failure (Bland, 2003). This complication more than likely is related to organ rejection. Most patients should preferably be extubated in the operating room at the end of surgery if the usual criteria are met. Serum glucose, hemoglobin, electrolytes, and troponin levels should be checked along with a baseline arterial blood gas for the determination of any residual acidosis immediately upon arrival in the intensive care unit or the recovery room. A patient with a bladder anastomosis often requires supplemental sodium bicarbonate to treat the metabolic acidosis caused by the loss of pancreatic secretions into the bladder (Sudan, Sudan, and Stratta, 2000; Kahl, Bechstein, and Redi, 2001; Coosemans and Pirenne, 2003; Troppman and Gruessner, 2004). Postoperatively, patients receive 5% dextrose in 0.45% saline as maintenance fluid. Nasogastric and urine output losses are replaced in equivalent amounts with half (0.45%) normal saline.

Pancreas transplant recipients have a higher incidence of acute rejection and immunologic graft loss than any other solid organ recipients. There were four main protocols of initial maintenance immunosuppression from 1996 to 2002 for cadaveric primary pancreas transplants in the United States: azathioprine, cyclosporine, mycophenolate mofetil, and tacrolimus; one other additional agent is sirolimus (Bland, 2003). There is great variation in immunosuppression induction therapy: namely, T-cell depleting polyclonal antibodies (Atgam, lymphocyte immune globulin) versus T-cell depleting monoclonal antibodies (OKT3) versus T-cell nondepleting antibodies (anti-CD25–directed daclizumab [Zenapax] and basiliximab [Simulect]) (Van der Pijl et al., 1996; Gruessner et al., 1997; Cattral et al., 2000; Kahl et al., 2001; Stegall et al., 2001; Knight et al., 2003). In the United States, the most common induction protocol uses an antibody induction in combination with tacrolimus, mycophenolate mofetil, and steroids (Bland, 2003). Pancreas transplant recipients are at risk of developing infection for numerous reasons, including immunosuppression, contamination from the duodenal segment of the graft, and serum glucose irregularity because of DM (Troppman et al., 2004). Infection prophylaxis with broad spectrum antibiotics targeting staphylococci, gram-negative bacteria, anaerobes, and cytomegalovirus is routine in many centers (Bloom et al., 1997; Humar et al., 2000; Coosemans and Pirenne, 2003). Prophylaxis against vascular thrombosis consists of either low-dose intravenous heparin (300–500 U/h) or subcutaneous administration of heparin followed by aspirin (Humar et al., 2000; Coosemans and Pirenne, 2003).

Pancreas transplantation is now an established procedure for the surgical treatment of diabetes mellitus. It is most commonly performed simultaneously during kidney transplantation. Islet cell transplantation will no doubt be the procedure of choice once it becomes a more routine procedure because of the minimal surgery involved and particularly so, as the scientific obstacles to transform this procedure into one which is customary seem to have been overcome. The perioperative care of patients for pancreas transplantation involves understanding of the pathophysiology of DM and renal failure and the goals of the procedure.

BONE MARROW TRANSPLANTATION

Bone marrow transplantation was first performed in an infant in 1968, when a 2-year-old boy received bone marrow from his sister to treat Wiskott-Aldrich syndrome. Since that time, bone marrow transplantation is increasingly used to treat a variety of hematologic, metabolic, genetic, and oncologic disorders in pediatric patients. Although the death rate from graft failure, infection, and GVHD is still high (approximately 40%), the success rate has improved over time with advances in immunosuppression, chemotherapy, antibiotics, and supportive care (Beebe et al., 1995). The number of children receiving bone marrow transplantation for various disorders is increasing approximately 10% per year (Goldman and Horowitz, 2002).

Patients can receive bone marrow from a relative or unrelated donor (allogenic transplants) or syngeneic donor (identical twins) or can receive their own marrow back following a course of chemotherapy (Stein et al., 1990; Beebe et al., 1995). The cord blood of newborn donors has become popular as a marrow source for both pediatric patients and adults. There is minimal risk of viral exposure with cord blood, and the donor is not placed at risk. The primary benefit to cord blood transplantation, however, is for reasons probably related to the immaturity of the newborn stem cell; the incidence of GVHD is markedly lower than standard bone marrow or peripheral stem cell transplants (Cohena and Nagler, 2003).

Prior to receiving a bone marrow transplant, children require bone marrow ablation with chemotherapy and occasionally total body irradiation. The processed donor marrow or stem cells from peripheral or cord blood are administered intravascularly, where they circulate and settle into the patient's bone marrow beds. Occasionally engraftment will fail to occur. Even if engraftment is successful, complications are frequent and include (1) infection, (2) GVHD, (3) toxicity from chemotherapy or radiation therapy, or (4) veno-occlusive disease of the liver (Gentet and Bernard, 1988; Stein et al., 1990; McDowall, 1993; Beebe et al., 1995; Schure and Holzman, 2000; Wah et al., 2003).

Infection is one of the main causes of morbidity and mortality in bone marrow transplant recipients. Ablation of the bone marrow renders a patient neutropenic for as long as several weeks before full engraftment occurs. T- and B-cell function may also be depressed for several months following bone marrow transplantation and cause recipients to be susceptible to viral and fungal infections (Stein et al., 1990; Beebe et al., 1995).

GVHD occurs when the T-lymphocytes derived from the donor's bone marrow react against the host. Acute GVHD occurs between 2 and 10 weeks posttransplantation and may manifest itself as skin rash, watery or bloody diarrhea, or hepatic involvement with hyperbilirubinemia. Chronic GVHD develops 3 to 15 months after bone marrow transplantation. It occurs most commonly in patients who have previously had acute GVHD. Chronic GVHD may present with scleroderma, oral mucositis, interstitial pneumonitis, and polymyositis (Stein et al., 1990; Beebe et al., 1995; Schure and Holzman, 2000; Wah et al., 2003).

Total body irradiation may cause pneumonitis, restrictive cardiomyopathy, pulmonary fibrosis, and oral mucositis. Chemotherapeutic agents such as doxorubicin can result in cardiomyopathy or other toxicities. In addition, veno-occlusive disease of the liver may develop following intensive chemotherapy and radiation therapy. This complication, which is most often fatal, occurs approximately 2 weeks posttransplantation when the small hepatic venules become fibrotic and develop pericentral hepatocyte necrosis and congestion (Gentet and Bernard, 1988).

Before receiving a bone marrow transplant, pediatric patients often require anesthesia for indwelling central venous catheterization, bone marrow biopsies, and total body irradiation. Following transplantation, children often require anesthesia for (1) biopsies to evaluate the status of the bone marrow transplant and determine if GVHD has developed and (2) treatment of the surgical complications that may follow this procedure. Most patients undergoing bone marrow transplantation tolerate anesthesia for these procedures without difficulty. However, complications can occur, particularly in those recipients less than 2 years of age, and anesthesiologists must keep in mind the unique medical problems associated with children undergoing bone marrow transplantation (Stein et al., 1990; Beebe et al., 1995).

PREOPERATIVE ASSESSMENT

Prior to administering anesthesia, bone marrow recipients must be examined both for potential difficulties from the patient's underlying disease as well the complications arising from the bone marrow transplant. For example, tracheal intubation and airway care are often difficult in patients with the metabolic disorder Hurler syndrome, which is treated with bone marrow transplantation (Belani et al., 1993).

The airway on all children receiving a bone marrow transplant must be examined for the presence of mucositis. Mucositis develops in bone marrow transplant recipients when they are neutropenic before the time the marrow becomes functional. Neutropenia leads to the development of oral infections and mucositis. Mucositis has been a cause of difficult intubation in pediatric bone marrow recipients. Mucositis also may increase the incidence of postextubation laryngeal edema in the postoperative period (Beebe et al., 1995).

Thrombocytopenia is also common in children before the time engraftment occurs and may require platelet transfusions during surgery. Other coagulopathies may also be present, particularly in the presence of hepatic dysfunction (Stein et al., 1990; Beebe et al., 1995).

Infection and/or GVHD may result in pneumonitis. Chronic GVHD can cause permanent restrictive pulmonary dysfunction. Preoperative examination of the pulmonary system is therefore important in these children and can help anesthesiologists plan for potential intraoperative complications and postoperative ventilation strategies (Stein et al., 1990; Beebe et al., 1995; Schure and Holzman, 2000; Wah et al., 2003). Although chemotherapy may result in cardiac dysfunction, practically, this rarely is a concern in the pediatric transplant recipients (Stein et al., 1990; Beebe et al., 1995).

Finally, radiation and/or chemotherapy and GVHD can result in nausea and vomiting. Tracheal intubation and airway protection may therefore be required (Stein et al., 1990; Beebe et al., 1995).

ANESTHETIC MANAGEMENT

There are a variety of anesthetic techniques that can safely be used to anesthetize a child undergoing bone marrow transplantation. No drug, agent, or technique is absolutely contraindicated (Stein et al., 1990; Beebe et al., 1995). Some anesthesiologists have raised concern about the use of nitrous oxide in bone marrow recipients because of its known suppression of the enzyme methionine synthetase, which is required for nucleotide synthesis. However, a randomized study of cellular function and bone marrow engraftment of bone marrow recipients exposed to nitrous oxide anesthesia failed to show any deleterious effects of the agent (Lederhaas et al., 1995).

The concern that is unique to bone marrow recipients is the high incidence and potential morbidity from mucositis that occurs when patients are neutropenic. Pediatric anesthesiologists must assume that patients are at risk for developing mucositis at some time during their treatment. Techniques should be chosen, when possible, that minimize potential for mucosal damage in the oropharynx. For example, intravenous propofol has proved useful for sedation for total body irradiation using spontaneous ventilation without airway instrumentation. Propofol also has a rapid recovery profile and antiemetic effects. Propofol may therefore allow earlier feeding and better nutrition in infants undergoing radiation therapy than other intravenous agents such as ketamine or thiopental (Beebe et al., 1995).

The laryngeal mask has also been recommended to provide a more secure airway in infants and small children undergoing total body irradiation. However, damage to the posterior pharyngeal wall has been reported in an infant undergoing total body irradiation (Marjot, 1991). It can prove useful for children with Hurler syndrome or other causes of a difficult airway undergoing total body irradiation or other procedures requiring anesthesia (Haynes and Morton, 1993).

Patients who have already developed mucositis and require anesthesia present a challenge to the pediatric anesthesiologist. Most of these children require tracheal intubation to prevent aspiration of infected mucus. The preoperative airway examination may be difficult due to pain. For the same reason, awake intubation may be impossible as well. Movement and struggling during the procedure may cause bleeding and edema and obscure the laryngeal inlet. A rapid sequence induction usually provides the best conditions for an atraumatic tracheal intubation as well as minimizing the time aspiration of infected secretions may occur. However, in patients with mucositis who develop stridor or other signs of airway obstruction, an inhaled induction of general anesthesia with sevoflurane and oxygen similar to that used with a child with acute supraglottitis may be required. In all cases, the pediatric anesthesiologist must be prepared with adequate suction and several tracheal tube sizes if the laryngeal inlet is narrowed due to edema (Beebe et al., 1995).

Care must be taken with extubation as well. Most patients with mucositis can be extubated when fully awake. Often these patients develop croup in the postoperative period, and may require treatment with dexamethasone (0.5 to 1 mg/kg) and one or more courses of racemic epinephrine treatment. However, patients with mucositis and severe edema of the laryngeal inlet may require prolonged intubation until the edema resolves (Beebe et al., 1995).

■ POSTTRANSPLANT LYMPHOPROLIFERATIVE DISEASE

PTLD is one of the most life-threatening complications of immunosuppressive therapy in this era of organ transplantation even with the use of newer immunosuppressive agents as well as regimens for induction and maintenance. It is seen after both solid organ and bone marrow transplantation. Patients receiving bone marrow, liver, or kidney transplants have an estimated incidence of 1% to 3%, whereas recipients of heart and heart-lung transplantation have an incidence of 5% to 13%. EBV is confirmed in over 50% of pediatric and 85% of adult patients. The time to presentation of this disease ranges from 1 to 150 months after transplantation.

The most common sites of involvement are the lymph nodes and gastrointestinal tract, with homograft involvement dependent on the organ transplanted. The heart is usually spared from involvement with heart transplantation. However, with heart-lung transplantation, the lungs are the most frequently involved sites (Sklarin, 1991). Similarly, the liver is a frequent site of involvement in recipients of bone marrow transplantation.

Because lymphoproliferative disease requires the active infection of the B cell with the virus, it seems that pediatric patients have a higher likelihood for the development of lymphoproliferative disease, the rationale being that pediatric patients have not been exposed to the virus and thus have no antibodies for the prevention of infection. Cyclosporin A–induced suppression of the suppressor T-lymphocyte is responsible for continued uncontrolled polyclonal proliferation of the transformed B-lymphocyte, infected with the episomal EBV DNA. Tumors generated in response to the virus are varied. Non-Hodgkin's lymphomas are the rule with lymphomas.

Treatment of PTLD is by several modalities with reduction of the immunosuppressive agent being the most efficacious. This allows for the improvement of immunosurveillance; however, the reestablishment of the host defense may exacerbate organ rejection. Approximately two thirds of patients will be responsive to this maneuver in EBV-related PTLD. Alternatively, cytokines and immune globulin have been used to enhance the immune response. Fischer-Froehlich and others (2002) reported the use of anti-B-cell antibodies in controlling B-cell lymphomas. α-Interferon in conjugation with gamma globulin has also proved to be efficacious. Surgical resection of tumors has also improved survival in selected cases, with survival reported at 74% relative to the 31% overall survival after the presentation of PTLD (Stieber, 1991). Acyclovir inhibits EBV replication. Prophylaxis with this agent may prove to be beneficial because the drug does not prevent proliferation of EBV-infected cells already transformed.

Immunosuppression under tacrolimus apparently does not appear to confer protection from the development of PTLD. The time to development of the disease with its use appears to be similar to CyA; however, enough experience has not yet been gained with the use of this agent.

PTLD holds no special consideration for the anesthesiologist in the immediate preoperative period of the graft transplantation. Because these patients often return to the hospital for additional procedures posttransplantation, several points are noteworthy. Tonsillar hypertrophy is a frequent presentation of this disease in the pediatric patient and often requires bilateral tonsillectomy for diagnosis of the disease as well as management of upper airway obstruction. Occasionally these patients may have been treated with chemotherapeutic agents, which possibly resulted in additional organ dysfunction.

■ INFECTIOUS DISEASES

The risk of infection in the transplant patient is directly influenced by two factors: the patient's environmental exposure and the patient's immunosuppressive regimen. The spectrum of causative agents varies with viral infections, with CMV being the most deleterious (Ho, 1991; Patel et al., 1996). Antirejection therapy is the most important contributor to the development of infection, with CyA at the top of the list of implicated agents. A clear example of this is the incidence of CMV infection, which has increased from 15% in the pre-CyA era to over 50% today (Rubin and Tolkoff-Rubin, 1991). Evolving evidence also demonstrates that immunosuppressive regimens with identical antirejection effects can have a different spectrum of infection.

The spectrum of presentation of CMV infection is bimodal and has two sources. The virus may be reactivated from a latent phase, or there may be active infection. Although prior infection confers acquired immunity, this may also be the source of latent infection in the immunosuppressed patient. The donor organ has been shown to act as a source of latent infection. The effects of CMV infection may be quite devastating, and damage to the grafted organ is frequently encountered. Obliterative bronchiolitis, chronic coronary atherosclerosis, and vanishing bile duct syndrome are often attributed to CMV infection of the lungs, heart, and liver, respectively.

Other viral infections with significant consequence to the host are hepatitis B and C virus and HIV infection. There is a significant reinfection rate of the hepatic graft in patients known to be ε-antigen positive before transplantation. This has raised the question as to whether this group of patients should have transplants. Hepatitis B is devastating to all graft recipients; a higher-than-normal rate of overwhelming hepatic failure is the rule. Hepatitis C is also a significant problem, with approximately 10% of solid organ recipients acquiring the virus. Data now suggest that up to 50% of organ recipients from donors who are antibody positive progress to develop active infection.

Fungal infections remain a major concern in organ transplantation (Castaldo et al., 1991a, 1991b). Divided into two categories, these infections may be either invasive and opportunistic or represent geographically restricted systemic mycosis. Amphotericin, the mainstay of therapy for systemic infections, has now been joined by fluconazole. Fluconazole is far less toxic than amphotericin and represents a significant advance in antifungal therapy.

Bacterial infections have a devastating consequence, cover a wide spectrum, and include atypical agents such as *Nocardia asteroides* and *Mycobacterium*. Prophylactic therapy for several infections has gained wide acceptance. For example, low-dose trimethoprim-sulfamethoxazole has been quite efficacious in the prevention of *Pneumocystis carinii* infection in all organ transplants, as well as in the prevention of urosepsis in the renal transplant patient.

GRAFT-VERSUS-HOST DISEASE AND CHIMERISM

GVHD is a major complication of bone marrow transplantation. It occurs in 30% to 40% of patients and is fatal in a third of the patients afflicted (Pienne, 1991). The disease is caused by an immunologic attack of the donor cytotoxic T-lymphocytes on the target organs and tissues of the recipient, frequently sites involving the skin, liver, and gastrointestinal tract. Therapy and prevention for this disease are immunosuppression of the response mediated by the cytotoxic T cells. Since CyA selectively suppresses this response, it has become the therapy of choice. Drug therapy is usually required for 6 to 12 months. T-lymphocyte depletion before transplantation is now being explored as an alternate therapy; however, potential problems include graft rejection and leukemic relapse. An additional approach to the prevention of GVHD is the use of monoclonal antibodies to paralyze the recipient immune system.

In the past decade, with the noted subgroup of patients who no longer required immunosuppression, along with clinical understanding of GVHD, genesis of the idea of chimerism began to take hold. It became evident that solid organ transplant recipients were transformed into chimeras, to varying degrees irrespective of the organ transplanted. A chimera is defined as the acquisition by the recipient of the donor leukocytes and lymphoid and dendritic cells, which spread through vascular routes to the host's lymphoid tissue from the transplanted organ. Conversely the engrafted organ will acquire the recipient's immune system and a population of the recipient's leukocytes. This is clearly demonstrated in liver transplantation in which the entire macrophage system, including the Kupffer cells of the graft, is replaced by that of the host (Starzl et al., 1992), which was the first actual biochemical realization of a chimera (Fig. 28–18).

The early thoughts and dismissal of leukocyte chimerism-associated mechanisms were diversionary, in view of the early recognition that implanted organ allografts promptly become mixtures of donor and recipient cells (i.e., organ chimerism). The evidence was first presented in 1968 by karyotyping studies of livers that had been transplanted to female recipients from male cadaveric/deceased donors (Kashiwagi et al., 1969). Whereas the rest of the allograft remained male, the bone marrow-derived passenger leukocytes including Kupffer cells were largely replaced with recipient female cells within 100 days of transplantation. These alterations were incorrectly assumed to be a unique feature of the transplanted liver until it was demonstrated in 1991 that most

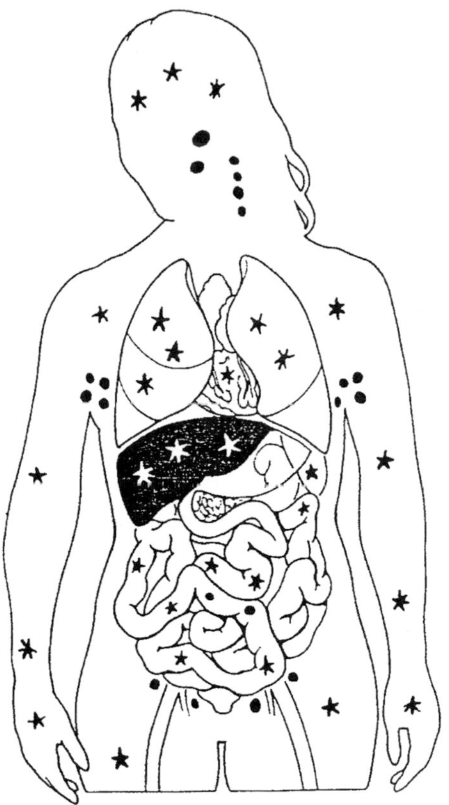

FIGURE 28–18. Result of traffic of the donor and recipient lymphoreticular cell traffic after successful liver transplantation (white, recipient cells; black, donor cells). (From Starzl TE, Demetris A, Murase N, et al.: Cell migration, chimerism, and graft acceptance. *Lancet* 339:1579–1582, 1992a.)

of the lymphoid tissues of the engrafted rat (Murase et al., 1991) and human intestine (Iwaki et al., 1991) were replaced by recipient cells of the same lineages. An epiphany occurred when comparable findings were confirmed in successfully transplanted human kidney, pancreatic (Starzl, Demetris, et al., 1993; Randhawa et al., 1993), and thoracic organ allografts (Randhawa et al., 1993), and thus it became unambiguously clear that all engrafted organs were chimeric structures.

In reality the first evidence, although circumstantial, of chimerism was first noted in the early era of organ transplantation (1962-1963 at the University of Colorado) when recipients who were noted to be PPD (purified protein derivative [tuberculin]) negative were transplanted with organs from donors who were PPD positive. In this series of patients, 77% of the recipients eventually converted to become PPD positive. Yet at the same time these recipients did not develop active tuberculosis. What accounted for this phenomenon? Some postulated that there must be adoptive transfer of donor cellular immunity by leukocytes in the renal graft vasculature and hilar lymphoid tissue (Kirkpatrick and Wilson, 1964). However, this postulate was almost unanimously discounted because neither the large quantity of passenger leukocytes nor the fact that these cells migrated was appreciated at the time.

Additional insight and understanding of chimerism were revealed within the past decade by a series of patients who had received solid organ transplantation but could be weaned successfully from the need for daily immunosuppression. In fact, a number of patients are now on chronically reduced levels and intervals for dosing of immunosuppressants or simply none at all as graft tolerance has occurred due to the evident microchimerism.

This two-way cell traffic seen in all forms of organ transplantation appears to be essential in the development of tolerance. In fact, the distinct differences in the amount of lymphoid cell transplanted from the donor along with the graft may confer the likelihood of that organ being rejected, as well as the likelihood for the development of GVHD, as seen with the small bowel transplant donor with its large reservoir of lymphoid tissue. The initial concerns for GVHD in multivisceral and intestinal transplantation, due to the large lymphoid tissue load in the mesenteric organs, have not been shown to be ones of significance. In fact, the increased incidence of GVHD seen in these particular types of solid organ transplantation may be related to the transplantation of lymphoid depleted organs. Indeed, the first two successful kidney (and the first successful transplantations of any species on the planet) was accomplished by sublethal total lymphoid irradiation of the recipients. The epochal events were performed in January and June 1959, first by Joseph Murray and colleagues in Boston (Merrill et al., 1960; Murray et al., 1964) and then by a Paris team led by Hamburger (1959). There had been no leukocyte infusions given to the recipients and the organs were donated by fraternal (not identical) twins and functioned for 20 and 26 years without maintenance immunosuppression. These results were and still remain astonishing and marked the cornerstone event yet unknowingly as the first insight into the mechanism of chimerism (Starzl, 1992). That the two-way cell traffic was essential in the prevention of GVHD in all solid organ transplantation was evident by the early 1990s (Murase, 1995).

Given these observations, it would seem evident that transplantation of the donor's bone marrow simultaneously with the graft may play a role in the induction of immunotolerance and the prevention of graft rejection. Infusion of donor-derived cells can improve organ allograft survival in animal models (Fontes et al., 1994, 1996). Under certain conditions, it can even induce tolerance (i.e., unlimited organ survival without any maintenance immunosuppressive therapy) (Starzl et al., 2004). Among the numerous experimental protocols leading to tolerance of solid organs in animal models, how can we find our bearings in human transplantation? Numerous problems have yet to be solved: the type and amount of donor-derived cells (including stromal cells) to be used, the timing for infusion of donor cells in keeping with organ transplantation, the route of infusion (should it be intravenous, into the portal vein?), and the conditioning regimen. The first clinical trials would appear to indicate that tolerance induction in humans using donor-derived cells is a relatively safe solution that is both promising and realistic. A number of clinical experiments have demonstrated that this simultaneous transplantation has in fact conferred variable immunotolerance on the engrafted organ in all types of solid organ transplantation (Shapiro et al., 1996).

The need became evident for minimal immunosuppression in transplantation, as overimmunosuppression clearly led to the prevention of the establishment of the chimera or microchimerism. Central to this clinical trial is the harvesting of the recipient's bone marrow for storage to be later used for bone marrow rescue in the event that there is the development of GVHD. Albeit the current data appear to be muddy, as the methodologies of induction of immunosuppression have changed as well as the agents being used for maintenance of therapy. The realization of the need to alter the prior practice has now lengthened the time frame of the clinical trials given this change.

XENOTRANSPLANTATION

As already outlined, the significant advances achieved in the field of organ transplantation, in the past three decades particularly, have led to an increased demand for organs, creating a wide gap between organ availability and supply. While the number of transplants performed worldwide is limited by this dramatic donor shortage, alternative sources need to be explored where a wider availability of organs would allow an expansion rather than a contraction of the indication for transplantation and at the same time a relaxation of the patient selection criteria. Hence, the renewed interest in xenotransplantation, which has been observed in the last decade (Evans et al., 1992; Cooper et al., 1997).

Before the concept of xenotransplantation advances to a clinical reality, at least three practical challenges must be overcome. The first consists of the immunologic barriers as will be noted. The second issue is related to the potential risk of the introduction of novel and earth-shattering infectious organisms into the human recipient (and possibly into the human population at large) via the xenotransplant, often referred to as xenozoonoses. Last, xenotransplantation raises issues and concerns in several different fields, most notably theological and anthropological, with psychological, ethical, and legal considerations (Caplan, 1985; Reemtsma, 1985). This commentary mainly focuses on the immunologic issues of xenotransplantation as well as on the risk of exposing the general public to novel infectious agents, xenozoonoses.

The pig, although considered to be the most suitable animal source of organs for humans, has significant obstacles associated with this endeavor as there are three main rejection mechanisms preventing the clinical application of a pig-to-human xenotransplantation procedure: hyperacute rejection (HAR), acute humoral xenograft rejection (AHXR), and cellular xenograft rejection (CXR). These immunologic barriers are significantly more difficult to overcome in a pig-to-human xenotransplant compared with a primate-to-human xenotransplant (e.g., baboon-to-human). In 1964, Reemtsma and others described six human recipients of chimpanzee kidneys, the longest survivor of whom died of causes unrelated to rejection 9 months after xenotransplantation (Reemtsma et al., 1964; Reemtsma, 1991).

The first cardiac xenotransplantation, performed by Hardy and others in 1964, also represented the first attempt at cardiac transplantation in humans, predating Barnard's report by nearly 4 years. Since 1964, when Hardy and others at the University of Mississippi performed the world's first heart xenotransplant using a chimpanzee as a donor, there have been eight documented attempts at clinical heart xenotransplantation. Five of these donors were nonhuman primates (two baboons, three chimpanzees), and three were domesticated farm animals (one sheep, two pigs) (Hardy et al., 1964; Cooley et al., 1968; Marion, 1969; Shapiro, 1969; Barnard et al., 1977). However, by the time the first human neonatal cardiac xenotransplantation was performed by Bailey in 1984 (the so-called "Baby Fae" case), there had been only limited experimental experience with prolonged graft survival in the newborn xenotransplant recipient. Baby Fae was a newborn infant with HLHS and became the longest survivor (Cooper et al., 2000) (Table 28–8). This recipient heart of an ABO-blood group mismatched baboon functioned for 20 days (Bailey et al., 1986). Studies presented by Bailey and others shortly before the Baby Fae case described a mean survival time of 72 days in newborn lamb-to-goat xenotransplants, with one survivor living to 165 days (Bailey et al., 1985a,b).

■ TABLE 28–8. World experience in clinical heart xenotransplantation

Case	Year	Surgeon	Institution	Donor	Type of Transplant	Outcome	Reference Source
1	1964	Hardy	University of Mississippi, Jackson, Mississippi, US	Chimpanzee	OHT	Functioned 2 hours (heart too small to support circulation)	Hardy JD et al., 1964
2	1968	Ross	National Heart Hospital, London, UK	Pig	HHT	Cessation of function within 4 minutes (vascular function)	Ross DN, 1969 Cooper DKC, 1995
3	1968	Ross	National Heart Hospital, London, UK	Pig	Perfused with human blood but not transplanted	Immediate cessation of function (vascular function)	Ross DN, 1969 Cooper DKC, 1997
4	1968	Cooley	Texas Heart Institute, Houston, Texas, US	Sheep	OHT	Immediate cessation of function (vascular rejection)	Cooley DA et al., 68 Cooley DA, 1969
5	1969	Marion	Lyon, France	Chimpanzee	OHT	Rapid failure (raised pulmonary vascular resistance)	Marion P, 1969
6	1977	Barnard	University of Cape Town, Cape Town, South Africa	Baboon	HHT	Functioned 5 hours (heart too small to support circulation)	Barnard CN et al., 1977
7	1977	Barnard	University of Cape Town, Cape Town, South Africa	Chimpanzee	HHT	Functioned 4 days (failed from probable vascular rejection)	Barnard CN et al., 1977
8	1984	Bailey	Loma Linda University, Loma Linda, California, USA	Baboon	OHT	Functioned 20 days (failed from vascular rejection)	Bailey LL et al., 1985
9	1991	Religa	Silesian Academy of Medicine, Sosnowiec, Poland	Pig	OHT	Functioned <24 hours	Czaplicki et al., 1992
10	1996	Baruah	India	Pig	OHT	Functioned <24 hours	Unpublished

OHT, orthotopic heart transplantation; HHT, heterotopic heart transplantation.

Modified from Tanigichi S, Cooper DKC: Clinical xenotransplantation—past, present and future. *Ann R Coll Surg Engl* 79:13–19, 1977. (Copyright © The Royal College of Surgeons in England. Reproduced with permission.)

Czaplicki and others in 1992 described a case in which they attempted the xenotransplantation of a pig heart into a human recipient with Marfan's syndrome.

In 1992, Makowka and colleagues (unpublished) in Los Angeles transplanted a pig liver into a 26-year-old woman dying of acute liver failure from autoimmune hepatitis and fulminant hepatic failure. Subsequently, also in the early 1990s, two baboon-to-human liver xenotransplantations were performed in Pittsburgh (Marino et al., 1994). These experiences demonstrated that a human might live with a baboon liver. However, while in the past nonhuman primates have been preferred as a source of organs for humans, the transplant community and regulatory agencies (U.S. Food and Drug Administration) in the countries dealing with this issue currently are more auspiciously looking to pigs. This is because nonhuman primates potentially carry an increased risk of infection transmission and also because of a variety of other ethical and practical concerns (e.g., organ size and species on the endangered lists). The reality is that in the two cases of baboon-to-human liver xenotransplantation mentioned, it was possible to demonstrate only a single case of a baboon pathogen (a CMV), which was apparently transferred to a patient, and for all other primate xenotransplantation, there have been no reports of other zoonoses. Notwithstanding, this event did not result in a disease process (Michaels and Simmons, 1994), and the death of both patients was unrelated to any sort of xenozoonoses. In both recipients, evidence was found of an adequately functioning liver mass, sufficient to sustain life. On the other hand, even though proved feasible, the use of baboons is complicated mainly by limited availability, inadequate size of organs for adult human beings, and high costs as well as the political and ethical issues raised.

Another nonhuman primate, the chimpanzee, is most likely the perfect donor for human transplantation, biologically speaking, primarily due to the very small genetic differences between this species and humans, or rather the enormous amount of genetic homology shared by the two; approximately 98% of the DNA of both species appears to be identical. Hence the patient, a woman as reported above in 1964, lived for 9 months (Reemtsma et al., 1964) without dialysis with a functioning chimpanzee kidney and died free of rejection, possibly due to this shared genetic homology. The endangered status of the chimpanzee, however, prevents their widespread use for clinical purposes. In the United States, only 25 to 50 chimpanzees may be used annually for biomedical research, and it is estimated that only 70 chimpanzees per year would be available worldwide as potential organ donors. Therefore, their use (as well as the use of other great apes such as the gorilla) would further jeopardize these species and would raise insurmountable ethical concerns without solving or greatly impacting the organ shortage problem.

In the past decade, the use of genetic engineering has resulted in a marked improvement of the survival time of a pig organ transplanted in a nonhuman primate model (Cozzi et al., 1995). Nevertheless, substantial immunologic barriers still exist, and strategies to prevent HAR and AHXR in a pig-to-primate need to be developed further. Although the use of genetic engineering has resulted in significant improvement in survival time for a pig organ in a nonhuman primate (close to 3 months), these survival times do not yet approach that of human organ allotransplantation. The ultimate goal here is obviously to obtain immunologic tolerance of the graft by the recipient organism and hence enhanced graft and patient survival.

The barrier to successful xenotransplantation of vascularized porcine organs into humans is antibody and complement-mediated HAR, mostly as a result of naturally occurring anti-Gal(1,3) Gal antibodies. This carbohydrate epitope, which is not found in humans or Old World monkeys, may be induced by gut bacteria, which possess a related Gal(1,3)Gal structure (Galili et al., 1988). The strategies to deal with these include transgenic approaches designed to reduce the antibody titer and to express either membrane-bound or soluble complement regulators, most notably, CD46, CD55, and CD-59. These approaches may be combined with attempts to modify the donor animals by the inactivation of their galactosyl transferase genes so as to diminish the synthesis of Gal(1,3)Gal, although this is still experimental in the pig. Such a strategy will probably also require nuclear transfer technology for the production of pigs with "knockout genes" or composite transgenic technology with multiple gene transfer (Lambrigits et al., 1998; Sandrin and Mckenzie, 1999). In this regard preliminary evidence of these approaches shows that it appears to attenuate experimental hyperacute rejection.

Successful xenotransplantation may also require the induction of T-cell tolerance with the use of deliberate mixed hemopoietic chimerism using donor and recipient bone marrow; an approach that has been used successfully in baboons to transiently suppress anti-Gal responses in marrow transplant (Ohdan et al., 1999). Human-to-baboon bone marrow transplantation has already been performed, after conditioning the donor marrow with nonlethal irradiation. It remains to be seen if incomplete or even full chimerism will change the image of animal organs sufficiently to make them immunologically be viewed as "allografts" by humans.

Newer approaches are of necessity complex if we are to entirely eliminate the offending epitope principally involved in xenografting. Cloning of pigs with inactivated Gal glycosyltransferase systems by a combination of available technology (notably cloning of animals from somatic cells) and modification of candidate genes in such clones by homologous recombination may provide an alternative to stem cell approaches (Wilmut et al., 1997; McGrath et al., 2000).

There are also a number of other concerns limiting the wide application of xenotransplantation in a clinical setting. The most important of these is the infectious disease risks posed by xenozoonoses as outlined previously. The critical question is whether in our attempts to save individual human life through a xenotransplantation, are we putting the population at large at an increased risk from novel infectious disease. On one side of this debate there are those who believe that any chance of introducing new infectious organisms into the human population is far too great a risk to pay for the introduction of this technology and that, as a consequence, xenotransplantation should not be performed at all (Butler, 1998, 1999). On the opposite side, however, others are convinced that there should not be any further delay in using this technology for life-saving procedures such as transplanting an animal liver or heart as a "bridge" solution in the treatment of a fulminant hepatitis or acute cardiomyopathy with HLHS, respectively, while awaiting a suitable human organ.

The true risk to humans of swine-related viral infection is unclear, but given views concerning the cross-species genesis of AIDS, variant Creutzfeldt-Jakob disease (commonly known as the prion implicated mad cow disease), chicken Hong Kong HSNI influenza virus, and the current Southeast Asian pandemic of Nipah virus (probably reservoired in fruit bats but transmitted to humans by swine contact and responsible for a number of recent fatal deaths in Malaysia and Singapore), a general social concern seems justified (Hahn et al., 2000). Moreover, xenotransplantation could change the dynamics of infection by the breaching of the physical barrier towards cross-species infection (through surgical implantation), by attendant immunosuppression, and by human proteins, which normally modulate HAR serving as viral receptors and protecting against complement-directed antiviral attack (Weiss, 1998).

The porcine endogenous retroviruses (PERVs) are viewed as carrying the most significant risk of xenozoonoses in clinical xenotransplantation, where it has been reported that PERVs are capable of infecting human cells in vitro (Patience et al., 1997). The importance of the PERV agent is its capacity for vertical transmission, where the genome is incorporated into the genome of the host. Such a replication-competent virus has a potential for infecting totally unrelated species. These PERVs were originally detected being released from porcine renal cell cultures and are retroviruses that share homology with murine leukemia viruses (Armstrong et al., 1971). Since the types of pigs used for xenotransplantation contain at least 50+ PERVs incorporated into their genome, until these are cloned and sequenced, it will be difficult to determine how replication competent they are and consequently what is their infectious potential (Rogel-Gilliard et al., 1999). It is so far evident that in a large cohort of patients either receiving xenografts or undergoing extracorporeal perfusion of their blood through pig organs that none have shown evidence of PERV infection, either by seroconversion of PERV antibodies (using serologic assays or polymerase chain reaction viral genomic primers) or by the presence of PERV DNA detectable in peripheral blood monocytes (Paradis et al., 1999). This, however, has been associated with the presence of porcine mitochondrial and centromeric DNA sequences in some patients often detectable for many years following extracorporeal therapies, which suggests that these viruses have little true contagious potential. These results need to be viewed with caution because it is possible that PERVs themselves may result in immune dysfunction (Tackle et al., 2000). The hope of breeding PERV-free animals seems to be a realistic prospect for the not-too-distant future (Stoye, 1997).

If, on the one hand, the obstacles discouraging the practice of xenotransplantation are well known to both clinicians and scientists (HAR, AHXR, and xenozoonoses), there are also undeniably strong arguments in support of xenotransplantation, which go beyond the mere problem of organ shortage. Xenotransplantation may offer many other clinical opportunities exceeding the simple idea of treating patients with end-stage organ diseases. In theory, a pig-to-human hepatic xenograft might be less susceptible to re-infection with HCV or of recurrence of an autoimmune disorder where xenotransplantation could be used to cure such diseases more effectively than allotransplantation.

It would be essentially unethical in fact to proceed with xenotransplantation research without putting in place strict principles, which limit these new risks as much as possible. In this context given all the clinical implications, the issue of xenotransplantation needs to be discussed in the social arena, in order to research the widest agreement on such a delicate matter involving philosophical, cultural, religious, and scientific themes (Daar, 1997;

Fishman et al., 1998). Such a debate will effectively parallel the recent debate, which has been carried out on the legislative and parliamentary floors in many countries concerning stem cell and human embryonic cloning research (Toledo-Pereyra, 2003). The outcomes of such legislation will affect not only the direction of approved research activity (a restriction hitherto little experienced by researchers) but also the make-up of high-quality personnel involved (Crawford, 2002). The wrong decisions here will simply drive researchers to other countries or to other fields of endeavor or underground, as has happened in the past. Individual and collective informed consent for xenotransplantation will require public dialogue (Barker and Polcrak, 2001), a process that has so far been somewhat waiting on the runaway train of legislation.

■ SUMMARY

Since the 1970s, solid organ transplantation has gained notoriety and acceptability as a viable form of medical therapy for many forms of end-stage organ disease in the pediatric patient as well as early therapy for congenital anomalies and varied inherited genetic diseases otherwise without a cure. Scientific advances in the development of better immunosuppression protocols have allowed enhanced survival of children from otherwise deadly diseases. The challenge for the future will be the development of more specific immunomodulation, better understanding of chimerism, and application of xenotransplantation where appropriate. Clearly, at this juncture, our understanding of the immunologic milieu has allowed us to offer cellular transplantation as a cure for genetic disease, as with bone marrow transplantation for the treatment of sickle cell disease (Vichinsky, 2002). In addition, the application of an artificial cardiac and liver assist device will become invaluable in reducing the mortality of patients with fulminant hepatic failure and in the treatment of congenital cardiovascular anomalies.

Challenges for the anesthesiologist will remain having a greater impact on the perioperative care in this group of patients given the long duration of the procedures as well as the need for the transfusion of blood products, all of which alter the immunology of the recipient; these procedures often lend themselves to significant blood loss. Will the anesthesiologist be able to affect this immunologic environ by better optimization of hemostasis? If so, will this eventually affect the episodes of early organ rejection and infectious complications? With all of the knowledge gained, we are now left with significant ethical dilemmas as we now begin to push the limits of living related and unrelated organ transplantation. The proposal by UNOS to allow living related and unrelated donors who are not perfectly matched to their particular cohort recipient to trade organs to appropriately matched unknown recipients has created a new conundrum within the area of transplantation. The prospect of xenografts has yet to be realized, but this along with the potential of stem cell research for the treatment of several diseases cannot be ignored.

REFERENCES

A blinded, randomized clinical trial of mycophenolate mofetil for the prevention of acute rejection in cadaveric renal transplantation. The Tricontinental Mycophenolate Mofetil Renal Transplantation Study Group. *Transplantation* 61:1029–1037, 1996.

Abecassis M, Adams M, Adams P, et al.: Consensus statement on the live organ donor. *JAMA* 284:2919–2926, 2000.

Abengochea A, Vila JJ, Jimenez J, et al.: Pediatric liver transplantation. *Anesth Analg* 80:851–852, 1995.

Abou–Assi S, Vlahcevic ZR: Hepatic encephalopathy: Metabolic consequence of cirrhosis often is reversible. *Postgrad Med* 109:52–54, 57–60, 63–55, 2001.

Abouna GM, Ganguly PK, Hamdy HM, et al.: Extracorporeal liver perfusion system for successful hepatic support pending liver regeneration or liver transplantation: A preclinical controlled trial. *Transplantation* 67:1576–1583, 1999.

Abu-Elmagd K, Reyes J, Todo S, et al.: Clinical intestinal transplantation: New perspectives and immunologic considerations. *J Am Coll Surg* 186:512–525; discussion 525–527, 1998.

Abu-Elmagd K, Todo S, Tzakis A, et al.: Three years clinical experience with intestinal transplantation. *J Am Coll Surg* 179:385–400, 1994.

Addonizio LJ, Hsu DT, Fuzesi L, et al.: Optimal timing of pediatric heart transplantation. *Circulation* 80:III84–89, 1989.

Addonizio LJ, Rose EA: Cardiac transplantation in children and adolescents. *J Pediatr* 111:1034–1038, 1987.

Advisory Group on the Ethics of Xenotransplantation: *Animal tissue into humans*. London, 1996: Stationary Office.

Agarwal R, Farber MO: Is continuous veno-venous hemofiltration for acetaminophen-induced acute liver and renal failure worthwhile? *Clin Nephrol* 57:167–170, 2002.

Aggarwal S, Kang Y, DeWolf A, et al.: Transcranial Doppler: Monitoring of cerebral blood flow velocity during liver transplantation. *Transplant Proc* 25:1799–1800, 1993.

Aggarwal S, Kang Y, Freeman JA, et al.: Postreperfusion syndrome: cardiovascular collapse following hepatic reperfusion during liver transplantation. *Transplant Proc* 19(4 Suppl 3):54–55, 1987.

Aggarwal S, Kramer D, Yonas H, et al.: Cerebral hemodynamic and metabolic changes in fulminant hepatic failure: A retrospective study. *Hepatology* 19:80–87, 1994.

Agarwal S, Obrist W, Yonas H, et al.: Cerebral hemodynamic and metabolic profiles in fulminant hepatitis failure. *Liver Transplant* In press.

Allan JS: Xenotransplantation at a crossroads: Prevention vs. progress. *Nature* 2:18–21, 1996.

Allison AC, Kowalski WJ, Muller CD, Eugui EM: Mechanisms of action of mycophenolic acid. *Ann N Y Acad Sci* 1993; 696:63–87, 1993.

American Diabetes Association: Pancreas transplantation for patients with type 1 diabetes. *Diabetes Care* 26(Suppl 1):S120, 2003.

Andrew M, Paes B, Milner R, et al.: Development of the human coagulation system in the full–term infant. *Blood* 70:165–172, 1987.

Armitage JM, Kurland G, Michaels M, et al.: Critical issues in pediatric lung transplantation. *J Thorac Cardiovasc Surg* 109:60–64; discussion 64–65, 1995.

Armstrong JA, Porterfield JS, De Madrid AT: C type virus particles in pig kidney cell lines. *J Gen Virol* 10:195–198, 1971.

Artru AA: Renal effects of sevoflurane during conditions of possible increased risk. *J Clin Anesth* 10:531, 1998.

Ascher N: Rejection of the transplanted liver. In Madrey WC, Sorrell MF, editors: *Transplantation of the liver*, 2nd ed. Norwalk, CT, 1995, Appleton and Lange, pp 225–245.

Ash SR: Hemodiabsorption in treatment of acute hepatic failure and chronic cirrhosis with ascites. *Artif Organs* 18:355–362, 1994.

Ashwal S, Schneider S: Pediatric brain death: Current perspectives. In Barness LA, editor: *Advances in pediatrics*. Chicago, 1991, Mosby–Year Book.

Ashwal S: Brain death in early infancy. *J Heart Lung Transplant* 12:S176–178, 1993.

Auphan N, DiDonato JA, Rosette C, et al.: Immunosuppression by glucocorticoids: Inhibition of NF-kappa B activity through induction of I kappa B synthesis. *Science* 270:286–290, 1995.

Azeka E, Marcial MB, Jatene M, et al.: Eight-year experience of pediatric heart transplantation: Clinical outcome using non-invasive methods for the evaluation of acute rejection. *Pediatr Transplant* 6:208–213, 2002.

Azuma H, Binder J, Heemann U, et al.: Effects of RS61443 on functional and morphological changes in chronically rejecting rat kidney allografts. *Transplantation* 59:460–466, 1995.

Badke FR: Left ventricular dimensions and function during right ventricular pressure overload. *Am J Physiol* 242:H611–618, 1982.

Bailey LL, Gundry SR: Hypoplastic left heart syndrome. *Pediatr Clin North Am* 37:137–150, 1990.

Bailey LL, Jan J, Johnson W, Jolley WB: Orthotopic cardiac xenografting in the newborn goat. *J Thorac Cardiovasc Surg* 89:242–247, 1985b.

Bailey L, Kahan B, et al.: Session V: The neonatal immune system: window of opportunity? *J Heart Lung Transplant* 10:828–840, 1991.

Bailey LL, Nehlsen-Cannarella SL, Doroshow RW, et al.: Cardiac allotransplantation in newborns as therapy for hypoplastic left heart syndrome. *N Eng J Med* 315: 949–951, 1986.

Bailey LL, Nehlsen Cannarella SL, Concepcion W, et al.: Cardiac xenotransplantation in a neonate. *JAMA* 254:3321–3329, 1985a.

Bailey LL, Wood M, Razzouk A, et al.: Heart transplantation during the first 12 years of life. Loma Linda University Pediatric Heart Transplant Group. *Arch Surg* 124:1221–1225, 1989.

Baird PA, Sadovnick AD: Survival in infants with anencephaly. *Clin Pediatr* 23:268–271, 1984.

Barker JH, Polcrak L: Respect for persons, informed consent and the assessment of infectious disease risks in xenotransplantation. *Med Health Care Philos* 4: 53–70, 2001.

Barnard CN, Wipowitz A, Losman JG: Heterotopic cardiac transplantation with a xenograft for assistance of the left heart in cardiogenic shock after cardiopulmonary bypass. *S Afr Med J* 52:1035, 1977.

Barnard CN: The operation. A human cardiac transplant: An interim report of a successful operation performed at Groote Schuur Hospital, Cape Town. *S Afr Med J* 41:1271–1274, 1967.

Barnett AH, et al.: Diabetes in identical twins: A study of 200 pairs. *Diabetologia* 20:57, 1981.

Bartosh SM, Alonso EM, Whitington PF: Renal outcomes in pediatric liver transplantation. *Clin Transplant* 11(5 pt 1):354–360, 1997.

Basile AS, Jones EA: Ammonia and GABA-ergic neurotransmission: Interrelated factors in the pathogenesis of hepatic encephalopathy. *Hepatology* 25:1303–1305, 1997.

Basadonna GP, Auersvald L, Khuong CQ, et al.: Antibody-mediated targeting of CD45 isoforms: a novel immunotherapeutic strategy. *Proc Natl Acad Sci U S A* 95:3821–3826, 1998.

Baum D, Bernstein D, Starnes VA, et al.: Pediatric heart transplantation at Stanford: results of a 15-year experience. *Pediatrics* 88:203–214, 1991.

Becker H, Vinten-Johansen J, Buckberg GD, et al.: Myocardial damage caused by keeping pH 7.40 during systemic deep hypothermia. *J Thorac Cardiovasc Surg* 82:810–821, 1981.

Beebe DS, Belani KG, Chang PN, et al.: Effectiveness of preoperative sedation with rectal midazolam, ketamine, or their combination in young children. *Anesth Analg* 75:880, 1992.

Beebe DS, Belani KG, Mergens P, et al.: Anesthetic management of infants receiving an adult kidney transplant. *Anesth Analg* 73:725, 1991.

Beebe DS, Gauthier RL, Demars JJ, et al.: Lower extremity hypothermia is beneficial during infra-renal cross clamping in pigs. *Anesth Analg* 77:241, 1993.

Beebe DS, Kim S, Belani KG, et al.: Endotoxemia during small bowel transplantation in pigs. *Transplant Proc* 27:593–594, 1995.

Beebe DS, Liao JC, Belani KG: Pathophysiology of diabetes mellitus. In: Klinck JR, Lindop MJ, editors: *Anesthesia and intensive care for organ transplantation.* New York, Chapman and Hall Medical, 1998.

Beebe DS, Urban M, Belani KG: Anaesthetic management of bone marrow transplant recipients less than two years of age. *Paediatr Anaesth* 5:107, 1995.

Belani KG, Krivitt W, Carpenter BLM, et al.: Children with mucopolysaccharidosis: Perioperative care, morbidity, mortality, and new findings. *J Pediatr Surg* 28:403, 1993.

Belani KG, Palahniuk RJ: Kidney transplantation. *Int Anesth Clin* 29:17, 1991.

Bellomo R, Ronco C: Continuous hemofiltration in the intensive care unit. *Crit Care* 4:339–345, 2000.

Belzer FO, Southard JH: Principles of solid-organ preservation by cold storage. *Transplantation* 45:673–676, 1988.

Benfield MR, McDonald R, Sullivan EK, et al.: The 1997 Annual Renal Transplantation in Children Report of the North American Pediatric Renal Transplant Cooperative Study (NAPRTCS). *Pediatr Transplant* 3:152, 1999.

Benowitz NL, Meister W: Pharmacokinetics in patients with cardiac failure. *Clin Pharmacokinet* 1:389–405, 1976.

Benson L, Freedom RM, Gersony W, et al.: Cardiac replacement in infants and children: indications and limitations. *J Heart Lung Transplant* 10:791–801, 1991.

Benumof JL: One-lung ventilation and hypoxic pulmonary vasoconstriction: implications for anesthetic management. *Anesth Analg* 64:821–833, 1985.

Berkowitz N, Schulman LL, McGregor C, et al.: Gastroparesis after lung transplantation. Potential role in postoperative respiratory complications. *Chest* 108:1602–1607, 1995.

Berney T, Ricordi C: Immunoisolation of cells and tissues for transplantation. *Cell Transplant* 8:577–579, 1999.

Bernuau J, Rueff B, Benhamou JP: Fulminant and subfulminant liver failure: Definitions and causes. *Semin Liver Dis* 6:97–106, 1986.

Berry MN, Phillips JW: The isolated hepatocyte preparation: 30 Years on. *Biochem Soc Trans* 28:131–135, 2000.

Bismuth H, Houssin D: Reduced-sized orthotopic liver graft in hepatic transplantation in children. *Surgery* 95:367–370, 1984.

Blaine EM, Tallman RD Jr, Frolicher D, et al.: Vasopressin supplementation in a porcine model of brain-dead potential organ donors. *Transplantation* 38:459–464, 1984.

Bland B: Pancreas transplant worldwide. International Pancreas Transplant Registry 2003. Available at http://www.iptr.umn.edu/ar_midyear2003/03_midyear_update_page2.htm.

Bloom R, Olivares M, Rehman L, et al.: Long-term pancreas allograft outcome in simultaneous pancreas-kidney transplantation: a comparison of enteric and bladder drainage. *Transplantation* 64:1689–1695, 1997.

Borland LM: Anesthesia for organ transplantation in children. *Int Anesthesiol Clin* 23:173–199, 1985.

Boucek MM, Kanakriyeh MS, Mathis CM, et al.: Cardiac transplantation in infancy: donors and recipients. Loma Linda University Pediatric Heart Transplant Group. *J Pediatr* 116:171–176, 1990.

Borland LM, Roule M, Cook DR: Anesthesia for pediatric orthotopic liver transplantation. *Anesth Analg* 64:117–124, 1985.

Boucek MM, Edwards LB, Keck BM, et al.: The Registry of the International Society for Heart and Lung Transplantation: Fifth Official Pediatric Report–2001 to 2002. *J Heart Lung Transplant* 21:827–840, 2002.

Boucek MM: Surveillance endomyocardial biopsy in pediatric heart transplantation: Fashion or foible? *Pediatr Transplant* 4:173–176, 2000.

Boucek RJ, Jr, Naftel D, Boucek MM, et al.: Induction immunotherapy in pediatric heart transplant recipients: a multicenter study. *J Heart Lung Transplant* 18:460–469, 1999.

Bowyer BA, Fleming CR, Ludwig J, et al.: Does long-term home parenteral nutrition in adult patients cause chronic liver disease? *JPEN J Parenter Enteral Nutr* 9:11–17, 1985.

Brattstrom C, Wilczek H, Tyden G, et al.: Hyperlipidemia in renal transplant recipients treated with sirolimus (rapamycin). *Transplantation* 65:1272–1274, 1998.

Brazelton TR, Morris RE: Molecular mechanisms of action of new xenobiotic immunosuppressive drugs: Tacrolimus (FK506), sirolimus (rapamycin), mycophenolate mofetil and leflunomide. *Curr Opin Immunol* 8:710–720, 1996.

Bretzel RG, Brandhorst D, Brandhorst H, et al.: Improved survival of intraportal pancreatic islet cell allografts in patients with type-1 diabetes mellitus by refined peritransplant management. *J Mol Med* 77:140–143, 1999.

Bridges ND, Mallory GB, Huddleston CB, et al.: Lung transplantation in infancy and early childhood. *J Heart Lung Transplant* 15:895–902, 1996.

Broelsch CE, Edmond JC, Whitington PF, et al.: Application of reduced size liver transplants as split grafts, axillary orthotopic grafts, and living-related segmental transplants. *Ann Surg* 212:368–375, 1990.

Broelsch CE, Whitington PF, Emond JC, et al.: Liver transplantation in children from living related donors: Surgical techniques and results. *Ann Surg* 214:428–437; discussion 429–437, 1991.

Brown RS Jr, Lombardero M, Lake JR: Outcome of patients with renal insufficiency undergoing liver or liver-kidney transplantation. *Transplantation* 62:1788–1793, 1996.

Brunner G, Losgen H: Benefits and dangers of plasma with fulminant hepatic failure. In Oda T, Shiokawa Y, Inoue N, editors. *Therapeutic plasmapheresis VI.* Cleveland, 1987, ISAO Press, pp 187–191.

Burch M, Aurora P: Current status of paediatric heart, lung, and heart-lung transplantation. *Arch Dis Child* 89:386–389, 2004.

Burnell JM, Dawborn JK, Epstein RB, et al.: Acute hepatic coma treated by cross-circulation or exchange perfusion. *N Engl J Med* 276: 935–943, 1967.

Butler D: FDA warns on primate xenotransplants. *Nature* 398:549, 1999.

Butler D: Last chance to stop and think on risks of xenotransplants. *Nature* 391:320–324, 1998.

Butterworth RF: The neurobiology of hepatic encephalopathy. *Semin Liver Dis* 16:235–244, 1996.

Cabezuelo JB, Ramirez P, Acosta F, et al.: Does the standard vs piggyback surgical technique affect the development of early acute renal failure after orthotopic liver transplantation? *Transplant Proc* 35:1913–1914, 2003.

Calabrese F, van der Wal AC, Levi M: Infection and inflammation in the cardiovascular system. *Cardiovasc Res* 60:1–4, 2003.

Calhoon JH, Grover FL, Gibbons WJ, et al.: Single lung transplantation. Alternative indications and technique. *J Thorac Cardiovasc Surg* 101:816–824, 1991.

Cantarovich M, Barkun JS, Tchervenkov JI, et al.: Comparison of neoral dose monitoring with cyclosporine through levels versus 2-hr postdose levels in stable liver transplant patients. *Transplantation* 66:1621–1627, 1998.

Calne RY: Immunosuppression for organ grafting. *Int J Immunopharmacol* 1:163–164, 1979.

Caplan AL: Ethical issues raised by research involving xenografts. *JAMA* 254:3339–3343, 1985.

Carlier M, Veyckemans F, Scholtes JL, et al.: Anesthesia for pediatric hepatic transplantation: Experience of 33 cases. *Transplant Proc* 19:3333–3337, 1987.

Carlos TM, Clark RS, Franicola–Higgins D, et al.: Expression of endothelial adhesion molecules and recruitment of neutrophils after traumatic brain injury in rats. *J Leukoc Biol* 61:279–285, 1997.

Carrel A: The transplantation of organs: A preliminary communication. *JAMA* 45:1654, 1905. (correct)

Carton EG, Plevak DJ, Kranner PW, et al.: Perioperative care of the liver transplant patient: Part 2. *Anesth Analg* 78:382–399, 1994a.

Carton EG, Rettke SR, Plevak DJ, et al.: Perioperative care of the liver transplant patient: Part 1. *Anesth Analg* 78:120–133, 1994b.

Castaldo P, Stratta RJ, Wood RP et al.: Clinical spectrum of fungal infections after orthotopic liver transplantation. *Arch Surg* 126:149–156, 1991a.

Castaldo P, Stratta RJ, Wood RP et al.: Fungal disease in liver transplant recipients: A multivariate analysis of risk factors. *Transplant Proc* 23(1 pt 2): 1517–1519, 1991b.

Cattral M, Bigam D, Hemming A, et al.: Portal venous and enteric exocrine drainage versus systemic venous and bladder exocrine drainage of pancreas grafts: clinical outcome of 40 consecutive transplant recipients. *Ann Surg* 232:688–695, 2000.

Cattaral MS, Lilly LB, Levy GA: Immunosuppression in liver transplantation. *Semin Liver Dis* 20:523–531, 2000.

Caves PK, Stinson EB, Griepp RB, et al.: Result of 54 cardiac transplants. *Surgeon* 74:307–314, 1973.

Cavicchi M, Beau P, Crenn P, et al.: Prevalence of liver disease and contributing factors in patients receiving home parenteral nutrition for permanent intestinal failure. *Ann Intern Med* 132:525–532, 2000.

Celli S, Valdivia LA, Fung JJ, et al.: Long-term survival of heart and liver xenografts with splenectomy and FK506. *Transplant Proc* 25:647–8, 1993.

Chan S, McCowen KC, Bistrian BR, et al.: Incidence, prognosis, and etiology of end-stage liver disease in patients receiving home total parenteral nutrition. *Surgery* 126:28–34, 1999.

Chari RS, Gan TJ, Robertson KM, et al.: Venovenous bypass in adult orthotopic liver transplantation: Routine or selective use? *J Am Coll Surg* 186:683–690, 1998.

Chen SC, Nouri S, Balfour I, et al.: Clinical profile of congestive cardiomyopathy in children. *J Am Coll Cardiol* 15:189–193, 1990.

Chartrand C, Servando ES, Chartrand S: Risk factors for acute rejection after pediatric heart transplantation. *Transplant Proc* 33(1–2):1732–1734, 2001.

Chen JM, Cullinane S, Spanier TB, et al.: Vasopressin deficiency and pressor hypersensitivity in hemodynamically unstable organ donors. *Circulation* 100(suppl II):244–246, 1999.

Clabby ML, Canter CE, Moller JH, Bridges ND: Hemodynamic data and survival in children with pulmonary hypertension. *J Am Coll Cardiol* 30: 554–560, 1997.

Claria J, Arroyo V: Prostaglandins and other cyclooxygenase-dependent arachidonic acid metabolites and the kidney in liver disease. *Prostaglandins Other Lipid Mediat* 72(1–2):19–33, 2003.

Clavien PA, Camargo CA Jr, Croxford R, et al.: Definition and classification of negative outcomes in solid organ transplantation: Application in liver transplantation. *Ann Surg* 220:109–120, 1994.

Clavien PA, Emond J, Vauthey JN, et al.: Protection of the liver during hepatic surgery. *J Gastrointest Surg* 8:313–327, 2004.

Clemmesen JO, Kondrup J, Nielsen LB, et al.: Effects of high-volume plasmapheresis on ammonia, urea, and amino acids in patients with acute liver failure. *Am J Gastroenterol* 96:1217–1223, 2001.

Cohen MG: Current immunosuppression in liver transplantation. *Am J Therapeutics* 9:119–125, 2002.

Cohena Y, Nagler A: Hematopoietic stem-cell transplantation using umbilical-cord blood. *Leuk Lymphoma* 44:1287, 2003.

Colletti LM, Johnson KJ, Kunkel RG, et al.: Mechanisms of hyperacute rejection in porcine liver transplantation: Antibody-mediated endothelial injury. *Transplantation* 57:1357–1363, 1994.

Colomb V, Goulet O, De Potter S, et al.: Liver disease associated with long-term parenteral nutrition in children. *Transplant Proc* 26:1467, 1994.

Cooley DA, Frazier OH, van Buren CT, et al.: Cardiac transplantation in an 8-month-old female infant with subendocardial fibroelastosis. *JAMA* 256: 1326–1329, 1986.

Cooley DA, Hallman GL, Bloodwell RD, et al.: Human heart transplantation: Experience with 12 cases. *Am J Cardiol* 22:804, 1968.

Cooper DKC, Kemp E, Platt JL, White DJG: *Xenotransplantation: The transplantation of organs and tissues between species,* 2nd ed. Berlin/Heidelberg, 1997, Springer-Verlag.

Cooper DKC, Keogh AM, Brink J, et al.: Report of the Xenotransplantation Advisory Committee of the International Society for Heart and Lung Transplantation: The present status of xenotransplantation and its potential role in the treatment of end-stage cardiac and pulmonary disease. *J Heart Lung Transplant* 19:1125–1165, 2000.

Coosemans W, Pirenne J: Pancreatic transplantation. *Acta Chir Belg* 103:73–80, 2003.

Costello JM, Pahl E: Prevention and treatment of severe hemodynamic compromise in pediatric heart transplant patients. *Paediatr Drugs* 4:705–715, 2002.

Costello JM, Wax DF, Binns HJ, et al.: A comparison of intravascular ultrasound with coronary angiography for evaluation of transplant coronary disease in pediatric heart transplant recipients. *J Heart Lung Transplant* 22:44–49, 2003.

Cotton CL, Gandhi S, Vaitkus PT, et al.: Role of echocardiography in detecting portopulmonary hypertension in liver transplant candidates. *Liver Transpl* 8:1051–1054, 2002.

Council of Europe recommendation on xenotransplantation, 1997.

Cozzi E, White DJ: The generation of transgenic pigs as potential organ donors for humans. *Nat Med* 1:964, 1995.

Crawford LM, Jr: Xenotransplantation Advisory. *JAMA* 288:688, 2002.

Cunningham MT, Brandt JT, Laposata M, et al.: Laboratory diagnosis of dysfibrinogenemia. *Arch Pathol Lab Med* 126:499–505, 2002.

Czaplicki J, Blonska B, Religa Z: The lack of hyperacute xenogeneic heart transplant rejection in a human. *J Heart Transplant* 11:393–396, 1992.

Daar AS: Ethics of xenotransplantation: Animal issues, consent and likely transformation of transplant ethics. *World J Surg* 21:975–982, 1997.

Dalmasso AP, Vercellotti GM, Platt JL, et al.: Inhibition of complement-mediated endothelial cell cytotoxicity by decay-accelerating factor: Potential for prevention of xenograft hyperacute rejection. *Transplantation* 52:530, 1991.

Dalmau A, Sabate A, Koo M, et al.: The prophylactic use of tranexamic acid and aprotinin in orthotopic liver transplantation: A comparative study. *Liver Transpl* 10:279–284, 2003.

Dandel M, Kemper D, Weng Y, et al.: Primary pulmonary hypertension: survival benefits of therapy with prostacyclin analogs and transplantation. *Transplant Proc* 35:2117–2120, 2003.

Davenport A: Artificial hepatic support: Where are we now? *Blood Purif* 19:1–3, 2001.

de Broux E, Huot CH, Chartrand S, et al.: Growth after pediatric heart transplantation. *Transplant Proc* 33(1–2):1735–1737, 2001.

De Hoyos A, Maurer JR: Complications following lung transplantation. *Semin Thorac Cardiovasc Surg* 4:132–146, 1992.

de Hoyos A, Maurer JR: Complications following lung transplantation. *Semin Thorac Cardiovasc Surg* (Review) 4:132–146, 1992.

del Nido PJ, Dalton HJ, Thompson AE, et al.: Extracorporeal membrane oxygenator rescue in children during cardiac arrest after cardiac surgery. *Circulation* 86:II300–304, 1992.

del Nido PJ, Armitage JM, Fricker FJ, et al.: Extracorporeal membrane oxygenation support as a bridge to pediatric heart transplantation. *Circulation* 90(5 Pt, 2):II66–69, 1994.

del Nido PJ: Extracorporeal membrane oxygenation for cardiac support in children. *Ann Thorac Surg* 61:336–339, 1996.

de Rave S, Tilanus HW, van Der LJ, et al.: The importance of orthotopic liver transplantation in acute hepatic failure. *Transpl Int* 15:29–33, 2002.

Delius RE, Zwischenberger JB, Cilley R, et al.: Prolonged extracorporeal life support of pediatric and adolescent cardiac transplant patients. *Ann Thorac Surg* 50:791–795, 1990.

Delmonico FL, Cosimi AB: Monoclonal antibody treatment of human allograft recipients. *Surg Gynecol Obstet* 166:89–98, 1988.

Demas K, Wyner J, Mihm FG, Samuels S: Anaesthesia for heart transplantation. A retrospective study and review. *Br J Anaesth* 58:1357–1364, 1986.

Dent CL, Canter CE, Hirsch R, et al.: Transplant coronary artery disease in pediatric heart transplant recipients. *J Heart Lung Transplant* 19:240–248, 2000.

Denton MD, Magee CC, Sayegh MH: Immunosuppressive strategies in transplantation. *Lancet* 353:1083–1091, 1999.

DeRoover A, Langnas A: Surgical methods of small bowel transplantation. *Curr Opin Organ Transplant* 4:335–342, 1999.

deWolf A, Frenette L, Kang Y, et al.: Insulin decreases the serum potassium concentration during the anhepatic stage of liver transplantation. *Anesthesiology* 78:677–682, 1993.

deWolf A: Transesophageal echocardiography and orthotopic liver transplantation: General concepts. *Liver Transpl Surg* 5:339–340, 1999.

DeWolf AM: Multiviscera and pancreas transplantation. *Int Anesthesiol Clin* 29:111–136, 1991.

DeWolf AM, Kang YG, Todo S, et al.: Glucose metabolism during liver transplantation in dogs. *Anesth Analg* 66:76–80, 1987.

Diabetes mellitus. Clinical Topic Tours, updated May 17, 2004, MD Consult. Available at http:// home.mdconsult.com/das/stat/view/40323679-2/ctt.

Dishart MK, Schlichtig R, Tonnessen TI, et al.: Mitochondrial redox state as a potential detector of liver dysoxia in vivo. *J Appl Physiol* 84:791–797, 1998.

Donaldson VH, et al.: Hemorrhagic disorders of neonates. In Ratnoff OD, Forbes CD, editors. *Disorder of hemostasis.* Philadelphia, 1991, WB Saunders, pp 423–458.

Duncan BW, Ibrahim AE, Hraska V, et al.: Use of rapid-deployment extracorporeal membrane oxygenation for the resuscitation of pediatric patients with heart disease after cardiac arrest. *J Thorac Cardiovasc Surg* 116:305–311, 1998.

Duncan SR, Paradis IL, Yousem SA, et al.: Sequelae of cytomegalovirus pulmonary infections in lung allograft recipients. *Am Rev Respir Dis* 146:1419–1425, 1992.

Duvaldestin P, Agoston S, Henzel D, et al.: Pancuronium pharmacokinetics in patients with liver cirrhosis. *Br J Anaesth* 50:1131–1136, 1978.

Eckhoff DE, McGuire B, Sellers M, et al.: The safety and efficacy of a two-dose daclizumab (Zenapax) induction therapy in liver transplant recipients. *Transplantation* 69:1867–1872, 2000.

Edwards EB, Harper AM: Application of a continuous disease severity score to the OPTN liver waiting list. *Clin Transpl* 19–24, 2001.

Edwards EB, Harper AM: The impact of MELD on OPTN liver allocation: preliminary results. *Clin Transpl* 21–28, 2002.

Eiseman B, Liem DS, Raffucci F: Heterologous liver perfusion in treatment of hepatic failure. *Ann Surg* 162:329–345, 1965.

Ellis AJ, Hughes RD, Wendon JA, et al.: Pilot-controlled trial of the extracorporeal liver assist device in acute liver failure. *Hepatology* 24:1446–1451, 1996.

Elshihabi I, Chavers B, Donaldson L, et al.: Continuing improvement in cadaver donor graft survival in North American children: The 1998 Annual Report of the North American Pediatric Renal Transplant Cooperative Study (NAPRTCS). *Pediatr Transplant* 4:235, 2000.

Emond JC, Whitington PF, Thistlethwaite JR, et al.: Transplantation of two patients with one liver: Analysis of a preliminary experience with 'split-liver' grafting. *Ann Surg* 212:14–22, 1990.

Epstein M: Renal complications of liver disease. *Clin Symp* 37:1–32, 1985.

Estol CJ, Faris AA, Martinez AJ, et al.: Central pontine myelinolysis after liver transplantation. *Neurology* 39:493–498, 1989.

Ethics Committee of the Transplantation Society: The Transplantation Society and xenotransplantation (draft guidelines). *Transplant Soc Bull* 6:11–14, 1997.

European FK506 Multicenter Liver Study Group: Randomized trial comparing tacrolimus (FK506) and cyclosporine in prevention of liver allograft rejection. *Lancet* 344:423–428, 1994.

Evans RW, Orians CE, Ascher NL: The potential supply of organ donors. An assessment of the efficacy of organ procurement efforts in the United States. *JAMA* 267:239–246, 1992.

Everson GT, Trouillot T, Wachs M, et al.: Early steroid withdrawal in liver transplantation is safe and beneficial. *Liver Transpl Surg* 5:S48–S57, 1999.

Ewert R, Mutze S, Schachschal G, et al.: High prevalence of pulmonary diffusion abnormalities without interstitial changes in long-term survivors of liver transplantation. *Transpl Int* 12:222–228, 1999.

Eyraud D, Richard O, Borie DC, et al.: Hemodynamic and hormonal responses to the sudden interruption of caval flow: Insights from a prospective study of hepatic vascular exclusion during major liver resections. *Anesth Analg* 95:1173–1178, 2002.

Farmer DG, Anselmo DM, Ghobrial RM, et al.: Liver transplantation for fulminant hepatic failure: Experience with more than 200 patients over a 17-year period. *Ann Surg* 237:666–676, 2003.

Farrar DJ, Hill JD, Gray LA, Jr., et al.: Heterotopic prosthetic ventricles as a bridge to cardiac transplantation. A multicenter study in 29 patients. *N Engl J Med* 318:333–340, 1988.

Farrar DJ, Hill JD: Recovery of major organ function in patients awaiting heart transplantation with Thoratec ventricular assist devices. Thoratec Ventricular Assist Device Principal Investigators. *J Heart Lung Transplant* 13:1125–1132, 1994.

Federlin K, Pozza G: Indications for clinical islet transplantation today and in the foreseeable future—the diabetologist's point of view. *J Mol Med* 77:148–152, 1999.

Figueras J, Busquets J, Grande L, et al.: The deleterious effect of donor high plasma sodium and extended preservation in liver transplantation: A multivariate analysis. *Transplantation* 61:410–413, 1996.

Findlay JY, Jankowski CJ, Vasdev GM, et al.: Fast track anesthesia for liver transplantation reduces postoperative ventilation time but not intensive care unit stay. *Liver Transpl* 8:670–675, 2002.

Fischer-Froehlich D, Eichmann E, Weber M, et al.: The paediatric organ donor: Coordination pitfalls. *Organs and Tissues* 3:153–158, 2002.

Fisher RA, Ham JM, Marcos A et al.: A prospective randomized trial of mycophenolate mofetil with Neoral or tacrolimus after orthotopic liver transplantation. *Transplantation* 66:1616–1621, 1998.

Fishman J, Sachs D, Shaikh R Editors: Xenotransplantation: Scientific frontiers and public policy. *Ann NY Acad Sci* 862:1–251, 1998.

Fishman JA, Rubin RH, Koziel MJ, et al.: Hepatitis C virus and organ transplantation. *Transplantation* 62:147–154, 1996.

Flanagan WM, Corthesy B, Bram RJ, et al.: Nuclear association of a T-cell transcription factor blocked by FK-506 and cyclosporin A. *Nature* 352:803–807, 1991.

Flendrig LM, Calise F, Di Florio E, et al.: Significantly improved survival time in pigs with complete liver ischemia treated with a novel bioartificial liver. *Int J Artif Organs* 22:701–709, 1999.

Flendrig LM: Development of a novel bioartificial liver assist device (thesis). Academic Medical Center, University of Amsterdam, Amsterdam, the Netherlands, 1998.

Follette DM, Rudich SM, Babcock WD: Improved oxygenation and increased lung donor recovery with high-dose steroid administration after brain death. *J Heart Lung Transplant* 17:423–429, 1998.

Fontes P, Rao AS, Demetris AJ, et al.: Bone marrow augmentation of donor-cell chimerism in kidney, liver, heart, and pancreas islet transplantation. *Lancet* 344:151–155, 1994.

Fontes P, Rao AS, Reyes J, et al.: Concomitant infusion of unmodified donor bone marrow into unconditioned recipients of intestinal allografts. *Transplant Proc* 28: 2757–2758, 1996.

Food and Drug Administration Center for Biologics Xenotransplantation Advisory Subcommittee to Examine Ongoing Clinical Trials, 1997.

Freedom RM, Pongiglione G, Williams WG, et al.: Palliative right ventricular outflow tract construction for patients with pulmonary atresia, ventricular septal defect and hypoplastic pulmonary arteries. *J Thorac Cardiovasc Surg* 86: 24–36, 1983.

Freeman D, Grant D, Levy G, et al.: Pharmacokinetics of a new oral formulation of cyclosporine in liver transplant recipients. *Ther Drug Monit* 17:213–216, 1995.

Fricker FJ, Addonizio L, Bernstein D, et al.: Heart transplantation in children: Indications. Report of the Ad Hoc Subcommittee of the Pediatric Committee of the American Society of Transplantation (AST). *Pediatr Transplant* 3:333–342, 1999.

Fukuzawa K, Schwartz ME, Acarli K, et al.: Flushing with autologous blood improves intraoperative hemodynamic stability and early graft function in clinical hepatic transplantation. *J Am Coll Surg* 178:541–547, 1994.

Galili U, Mandrell RE, Hamadeh RM, et al.: Interaction between human natural anti-alpha-galactosyl immunoglobulin G and the bacteria of the human flora. *Infect Immuno* 56:1730–1737, 1988.

Gelman S, Dillard E, Bradley EL Jr: Hepatic circulation during surgical stress and anesthesia with halothane, isoflurane, or fentanyl. *Anesth Analg* 66:936–943, 1987.

Gentet JC, Bernard JL, Aimard L, et al.: Veno-occlusive disease in children after intensive chemo and radiotherapy and repeated halothane anesthesias: A report of 2 cases. *Acta Oncol* 27:579, 1988.

Gerlach JC, Botsch M, Kardassis D, et al.: Experimental evaluation of a cell module for hybrid liver support. *Int J Artif Organs* 24:793–798, 2001.

Gerlach JC, Zeilinger K, Sauer IM, et al.: Extracorporeal liver support: Porcine or human cell based systems? *Int J Artif Organs* 25:1013–1018, 2002.

Gerlach JC: Development of a hybrid liver support system: A review. *Int J Artif Organs* 19:645–654, 1996.

Ghofrani HA, Wiedemann R, Rose F, et al.: Combination therapy with oral sildenafil and inhaled iloprost for severe pulmonary hypertension. *Ann Intern Med* 136:515–522, 2002.

Gille JP, Bagniewski AM: Ten years of use of extracorporeal membrane oxygenation (ECMO) in the treatment of acute respiratory insufficiency (ARI). *Trans Am Soc Artif Intern Organs* 22:102–109, 1976.

Gines P, Guevara M, Arroyo V, et al.: Hepatorenal syndrome. *Lancet* 362:1819–1827, 2003.

Girvin J: Brain death criteria must be revised so that society can readily benefit from families who offer their anencephalic infants as organ donors. *J Heart Lung Transplant* 12:S369, 1993.

Glasser M, Waaga AM, Laskowski IA, et al.: Organ transplantation. From brain-dead donors: its impact on short- and long-term outcome revisited. *Transplant Rev* 15:1–10, 2001.

Goldman JM, Horowitz MM: The International Bone Marrow Transplant Registry. *Int J Hematol* 76:393, 2002.

Gologorsky E, De Wolf AM, Scott V, et al.: Intracardiac thrombus formation and pulmonary thromboembolism immediately after graft reperfusion in 7 patients undergoing liver transplantation. *Liver Transpl* 7:783–789, 2001.

Gonwa TA, Poplawski S, Paulsen W, et al.: Hepatorenal syndrome and orthotopic liver transplantation. *Transplant Proc* 21(1 pt 2):2419–2420, 1989.

Gonwa TA: Management of nephrologic complications in the liver transplant patient. 2005. Available at: http://www.centerspan.org/pubs/liver/gonwa1.htm

Gordon RD, Bismuth H.: Liver Transplant Registry report. *Transplant Proc* 23 (1 pt 1):58–60, 1991.

Gordon RD, Todo S, Tzakis AG, et al.: Liver transplantation under cyclosporine: A decade of experience. *Transplant Proc* 23(1 pt 2):1393–1396, 1991.

Govindarajan S, Nast CC, Smith WL, et al.: Immunohistochemical distribution of renal prostaglandin endoperoxide synthase and prostacyclin synthase: Diminished endoperoxide synthase in the hepatorenal syndrome. *Hepatology* 7:654–659, 1987.

Grant D, Wall W, Mimeault R, et al.: Successful small-bowel/liver transplantation. *Lancet* 335:181–184, 1990.

Grant JW, Canter CE, Spray TL, et al.: Elevated donor cardiac troponin I. A marker of acute graft failure in infant heart recipients. *Circulation* 90:2618–2621, 1994 (erratum in *Circulation* 91:3027, 1995).

Grant D: Intestinal transplantation: 1997 Report of the International Registry. Intestinal Transplant Registry. *Transplantation* 67:1061–1064, 1999.

Gray PA, Bodenham AR, Park GR: A comparison of dopexamine and dopamine to prevent renal impairment in patients undergoing orthotopic liver transplantation. *Anaesthesia* 46:638–641, 1991.

Graziadei IW, Wiesner RH, Marotta PJ, et al.: Neoral compared with Sandimmune is associated with a decrease in histologic severity of rejection in patients undergoing primary liver transplantation. *Transplantation* 64:726–731, 1997.

Green TP, Isham-Schopf B, Irmiter RJ, et al.: Inactivation of heparin during extracorporeal circulation in infants. *Clin Pharmacol Ther* 48:148–154, 1990.

Gridelli B, Spada M, Petz W, et al.: Split-liver transplantation eliminates the need for living-donor liver transplantation in children with end-stage cholestatic liver disease. *Transplantation* 75:1197–1203, 2003.

Griffin ML, Hernandez A, Martin TC, et al.: Dilated cardiomyopathy in infants and children. *J Am Coll Cardiol* 11:139–144, 1988.

Griffith BP, Shaw BW Jr, Hardesty RL, et al.: Veno-venous bypass without systemic anticoagulation for transplantation of the human liver. *Surg Gynecol Obstet* 160:270–272, 1985.

Griffith BP, Zenati M: The pulmonary donor. *Clin Chest Med* 11:217–226, 1990.

Grose RD, Nolan J, Dillon JF, et al.: Exercise-induced left ventricular dysfunction in alcoholic and non-alcoholic cirrhosis. *J Hepatol* 22:326–332, 1995.

Grosfeld JL, Rescorla FJ, West KW: Short bowel syndrome in infancy and childhood: Analysis of survival in 60 patients. *Am J Surg* 151:41–46, 1986.

Groth CG, Backman L, Morales JM et al.: Sirolimus (rapamycin)-based therapy in human renal transplantation: similar efficacy and different toxicity compared with cyclosporine. Sirolimus European Renal Transplant Study Group. *Transplantation* 67:1036–1042, 1999.

Groth CG, Korsgren O, Tibell A, et al.: Transplantation of porcine fetal pancreas to diabetic patients. *Lancet* 344:1402–1404, 1994.

Gruessner AC, Sutherland DE: Pancreas transplant outcomes for the United States (US) and non-US cases reported to the United Network for Organ Sharing (UNOS) and the International Pancreas Transplant Registry (IPTR) as of October, 2002. In Cecka JM, Terasaki PI, editors: *Clinical transplants 2002*. Los Angeles, UCLA Immunogenetic Center; 2003, pp. 42–69.

Gruessner R, Sutherland D, Najarian J, et al.: Solitary pancreas transplantation for nonuremic patients with labile insulin-dependent diabetes mellitus. *Transplantation* 64:1572–1577, 1997.

Gunning TC, Brown MR, Swygert TH, et al.: Perioperative renal function in patients undergoing orthotopic liver transplantation: A randomized trial of the effects of verapamil. *Transplantation* 51:422–427, 1991.

Gurakar A, Hassanein T, van Thiel DH: Right diaphragmatic paralysis following orthotopic liver transplantation. *J Okla State Med Assoc* 88:149–153, 1995.

Gutzke GE, Shah KB, Glisson SN, et al.: Cardiac transplantation: a prospective comparison of ketamine and sufentanil for anesthetic induction. *J Cardiothorac Anesth* 3:389–395, 1989.

Hahn BH, Shaw DM, DeCock KM, et al.: AIDS as a zoonosis: Scientific and public health implications. *Science* 287:607, 2000.

Hakim NS: Pancreatic transplantation for patients with type 1 diabetes. Exp Clin Transplant Proc 35:2801–2802, 2003.

Halloran PF, Homik J, Goes N, et al.: The "injury response": a concept linking nonspecific injury, acute rejection, and long-term transplant outcomes. *Transplant Proc* 29:79–81, 1997.

Hamburger J, Vaysse J, Crosnier J, et al.: *Presse Med* 67:1771–1775, 1959.

Hanid MA, Mackenzie RL, Jenner RE, et al.: Intracranial pressure in pigs with surgically induced acute liver failure. *Gastroenterology* 76:123–131, 1979.

Hardy JD, Chavez CM, Kurrus FE, et al.: Heart transplantation in man: Developmental studies and report of a case. *JAMA* 188:114–122, 1964.

Harper PL, Edgar PF, Luddington RJ, et al.: Protein C deficiency and portal thrombosis in liver transplantation in children. *Lancet* 2:924–927, 1988.

Hastillo A, Hess ML: Heart xenografting: A route not yet to trod. *J Heart Lung Transplant* 12:3–4, 1993.

Hayashi PH, Trotter JF: Review article: Adult-to-adult right hepatic lobe living donor liver transplantation. *Aliment Pharmacol Ther* 16:1833–1841, 2002.

Haynes SR and Morton: The laryngeal mask airway: A review of its use in paediatric anaesthesia. *Paediatr Anaesth* 56:65, 1993.

Health Canada: Report of the National Forum. Xenotransplantation: Clinical, ethical, and regulatory issues. Health Canada, 1997.

Healy PJ, McDonald R, Waldhausen JHT, et al.: Transplantation of adult living donor kidneys into infants and small children. *Arch Surg* 135:1035, 2000.

Heffron TG, Pillen T, Welch D, et al.: Hepatic artery thrombosis in pediatric liver transplantation. *Transplant Proc* 35:1447–1448, 2003.

Helman DN, Addonizio LJ, Morales DL, et al.: Implantable left ventricular assist devices can successfully bridge adolescent patients to transplant. *J Heart Lung Transplant* 19:121–126, 2000.

Heneine W, Tibell A, Switzer WM, et al.: No evidence of infection with porcine endogenous retrovirus in recipients of porcine islet-cell xenografts. *Lancet* 352:695–699, 1998.

Hering B, Ricordi C: Islet transplantation for patients with type 1 diabetes: results, research priorities, and reasons for optimism. *Graft* 2:12–27, 1999.

Heritier F, Madden B, Hodson ME, Yacoub M: Lung allograft transplantation: indications, preoperative assessment and postoperative management. *Eur Respir J* 5:1262–1278, 1992.

Hetzer R, Loebe M, Potapov EV, et al.: Circulatory support with pneumatic paracorporeal ventricular assist device in infants and children. *Ann Thorac Surg* 66:1498–506, 1998.

Hezode C, Lonjon I, Roudot-Thoraval F, et al.: Impact of smoking on histological liver lesions in chronic hepatitis C. *Gut* 52:126–129, 2003.

Hickey PR, Hansen DD, Cramolini GM, et al.: Pulmonary and systemic hemodynamic responses to ketamine in infants with normal and elevated pulmonary vascular resistance. *Anesthesiology* 62, 287–293, 1985.

Hickey PR, Hansen DD, Strafford M, et al.: Pulmonary and systemic hemodynamic effects of nitrous oxide in infants with normal and elevated pulmonary vascular resistance. *Anesthesiology* 65:374–378, 1986.

Ho M: Cytomegalovirus infection and indirect sequelae in the immunocompromised transplant patient. *Transplant Proc* 23:2–7, 1991.

Hoeper MM, Krowka MJ, Strassburg CP: Portopulmonary hypertension and hepatopulmonary syndrome. *Lancet* 363:1461–1468, 2004.

Hommquist M, Chabalewski F, Blount T, et al.: A critical pathway: Guiding care for organ donors. *Crit Care Nurse* 19:84–100, 1999.

Horslen SP, Hammel JM, Fristoe LW, et al.: Extracorporeal liver perfusion using human and pig livers for acute liver failure. *Transplantation* 70:1472–1478, 2000.

Hosenpud JD, Novick RJ, Breen TJ, et al.: The Registry of the International Society for Heart and Lung Transplantation: Eleventh official report–1994. *J Heart Lung Transplant* 13:561–570, 1994.

Howard L, Heaphey L, Fleming CR, et al.: Four years of North American registry home parenteral nutrition outcome data and their implications for patient management. *JPEN J Parenter Enteral Nutr* 15:384–393, 1991. (http://www.nih–a2all.org/contact.asp)

Hricik DE: Withdrawal of immunosuppression: implications for composite tissue allograft transplantation. *Transplant Proc* 30:2721–2723, 1998.

Hsu RB, Chen RJ, Wu MH, et al.: Non–transplant cardiac surgery for end-stage dilated cardiomyopathy in small children. *J Heart Lung Transplant* 22:94–97, 2003.

Hsu RB, Chien CY, Wang SS, et al.: Nontransplant cardiac surgery as a bridge to heart transplantation in pediatric dilated cardiomyopathy. *Tex Heart Inst J* 29:213–215, 2002.

Huddleston CB: Surgical complications of lung transplantation in children. *Semin Thorac Cardiovasc Surg* 8:296–304, 1996.

Hughes RD, Williams R: Evaluation of extracorporeal bioartificial liver devices. *Liver Transpl Surg* 1:200–206, 1995.

Humar A, Arrazola L, Mauer M, et al.. Kidney transplantation in children: Should there be a minimum age? *Pediatr Nephrol* 16:941, 2001.

Institute of Medicine workshop (U.S.): Xenotransplantation–Science, ethics and public policy. Washington, DC, 1996, National Academy Press.

Iwaki Y, Starzl TE, Yagihashi A, et al.: Replacement of donor lymphoid tissue in small-bowel transplants. *Lancet* 337:818–819, 1991.

Iwatsuki S, Popovtzer MM, Corman JL, et al.: Recovery from "hepatorenal syndrome" after orthotopic liver transplantation. *N Engl J Med* 289:1155–1159, 1973.

Jaeger C, Brendel MD, Hering BJ, et al.: Progressive islet graft failure occurs significantly earlier in autoantibody-positive than in autoantibody-negative IDDM recipients of intrahepatic islet allografts. *Diabetes* 46:1907–1910, 1997.

Jamieson NV, Sundberg R, Lindell S, et al.: Successful 24- to 30-hour preservation of the canine liver: A preliminary report. *Transplant Proc* 20(suppl 1): 945, 1988.

Jawan B, de Villa V, Luk HN, et al.: Ionized calcium changes during living-donor liver transplantation in patients with and without administration of blood-bank products. *Transpl Int* 16:510–514, 2003.

Jawan B, Goto S, Lia C, et al.: The effect of hypernatremia on liver allografts in rats. *Anesth Analg* 95:1169–1172, 2002.

Jenkins DH, Reilly PM, Schwab CW: Improving the approach to organ donation: A review. *World J Surg* 23:644–649, 1999.

Jobe A, Jacobs H, Ikegami M, et al.: Lung protein leaks in ventilated lambs: effects of gestational age. *J Appl Physiol* 58:1246–1251, 1985.

Jonas S, Bechstein WO, Tullius SG, et al.: Indications for tacrolimus anti-rejection therapy in liver allograft recipients. *Transpl Int* 9:S164–S170, 1996.

Jones RC, Strader LD, Berry WC: Peritonela dialysis in liver coma. *US Armed Forces Med J* 10:977–982, 1959.

Jugan E, Albaladejo P, Jayais P, et al.: Continuous monitoring of mixed venous oxygen saturation during orthotopic liver transplantation. *J Cardiothorac Vasc Anesth* 6:283–286, 1992.

Juggi JS: Extracorporeal cation-exchange circuits in the treatment of hyperammonaemia of hepatic failure. *Med J Aust* 1:926–930, 1973.

Jurim O, Csete M, Gelabert HA, et al.: Reduced-size grafts—The solution for hepatic artery thrombosis after pediatric liver transplantation? *J Pediatr Surg* 30:53–55, 1995.

Kahan BD: Rapamycin: personal algorithms for use based on 250 treated renal allograft recipients. *Transplant Proc* 30:2185–2188, 1998.

Kahan BD for the Rapamune U.S. Study Group: Efficacy of sirolimus compared with azathioprine for reduction of acute renal allograft rejection. *Lancet* 356:194–202, 2000.

Kahan BD, Julian BA, Pescovitz MD, et al.: Sirolimus reduces the incidence of acute rejection episodes despite lower cyclosporine doses in Caucasian recipients of mismatched primary renal allografts: A phase II trial. Rapamune Study Group. *Transplantation* 68:1526–1532, 1999.

Kahl A, Bechstein WO, Frei U: Trends and perspectives in pancreas and simultaneous pancreas and kidney transplantation. *Curr Opin Urol* 11:165–174, 2001.

Kaiser LR, Pasque MK, Trulock EP, et al.: Bilateral sequential lung transplantation: the procedure of choice for double-lung replacement. *Ann Thorac Surg* 52:438–446, 1991.

Kalathil K, Sureshkumar TM, Nabil M, et al.: Assessment of quality of life after simultaneous pancreas-kidney transplantation. *Am J Kidney Dis* 39:1300–1306, 2000.

Kamath GS, et al.: Is brachial preferable to radial arterial pressure measurement in liver transplantation (abstract). *Liver Transplant* 7:C24, 2001.

Kang Y, Borland LM, Picone J, et al.: Intraoperative coagulation changes in children undergoing liver transplantation. *Anesthesiology* 71:44–47, 1989.

Kang Y, Gelman S: Liver transplantation. In Gelman S, editor: *Anesthesia and organ transplantation.* Philadelphia, 1987, WB Saunders, pp 139–185.

Kang Y, Lewis JH, Navalgund A, et al.: Epsilon-aminocaproic acid for treatment of fibrinolysis during liver transplantation. *Anesthesiology* 66:766–773, 1987.

Kang Y: Blood coagulation during liver, kidney, and pancreas transplantation. In Lake CL, Moore RA, editors: *Blood: Hemostasis, transfusion, and alternatives in the perioperative period.* New York, 1995, Raven Press, pp 529–537.

Kang Y: Thromboelastography in liver transplantation. *Semin Thromb Hemost* 21(Suppl 4):34–44, 1995.

Kang YG, Martin DJ, Marquez J, et al.: Intraoperative changes in blood coagulation and thromboelastographic monitoring in liver transplantation. *Anesth Analg* 64:888–896, 1985.

Kang YG: Monitoring and treatment of coagulation. In Winter PM, Kang YG, editors: *Hepatic transplantation: Anesthetic and perioperative management.* New York, 1986, Prueger, pp 151–173.

Kanter KR, Pennington G, Weber TR, et al.: Extracorporeal membrane oxygenation for postoperative cardiac support in children. *J Thorac Cardiovasc Surg* 93:27–35, 1987.

Kantrowitz A, Haller JD, Joos H, et al.: Transplantation of the heart in an infant and an adult. *Am J Cardiol* 22:782–90, 1968.

Kao B, Balzer DT, Huddleston CB, et al.: Long-term prostacyclin infusion to reduce pulmonary hypertension in a pediatric cardiac transplant candidate before transplantation. *J Heart Lung Transplant* 20:785–788, 2001.

Kashiwagi N, Porter KA, Penn I, et al.: Studies of homograft sex and of gamma globulin phenotypes after orthotopic homotransplantation of the human liver. *Surg Forum* 20:374–376, 1969.

Kaufman DB, Platt JL, Rabe FL, et al.: Differential roles of Mac-1+ cells, and CD4+ and CD8+ T lymphocytes in primary nonfunction and classic rejection of islet allografts. *J Exp Med* 172:291–302, 1990.

Kaul S: The interventricular septum in health and disease. *Am Heart J* 112:568–581, 1986.

Kawauchi M, Gundry SR, de Begona JA, et al.: Prolonged orthotopic xenoheart transplantation in infant baboons. *J Thorac Cardiovasc Surg* (in press).

Kellum J, Decke J: Use of dopamine in acute renal failure: meta-analysis. *J Crit Care Med* 29:1526–1531, 2001.

Kelly KJ, Outwater KM, Crone RK: Vasoactive amine in infants and children. *Clin Anaesthesiol* 2:427, 1984.

Keszler M, Subramanian KN, Smith YA, et al.: Pulmonary management during extracorporeal membrane oxygenation. *Crit Care Med* 17:495–500, 1989.

Khoury GF, Brill J, Walts L, et al.: Atypical serum cholinesterase eliminated by orthotopic liver transplantation. *Anesthesiology* 67:273–274, 1987.

Kiberd B, Larson T: Estimating the benefits of solitary pancreas transplantation in nonuremic patients with type 1 diabetes mellitus: a theoretical analysis. *Transplantation* 70:1121–1127, 2000.

Kiley JE, Gundermann KJ, Lie TS: Ammonia intoxication treated by hemodialysis. *N Engl J Med* 25:1156–1161, 1958.

Kimball PM, Kerman RH, Kahan BD: Production of synergistic but nonidentical mechanisms of immunosuppression by rapamycin and cyclosporine. *Transplantation* 51:486–490, 1991.

Kimoto S: The artificial liver: Experiments and clinical application. *Trans Am Soc Artif Intern Organs* 5:102–112, 1959.

Kino T, Hatanaka H, Hashimoto M, et al.: FK506, a novel immunosuppressant isolated from a Streptomyces. I: Fermentation, isolation, and physico-chemical and biological characteristics. *J Antibiot* 40:1249–1255, 1987.

Kirklin JK, Naftel DC, Bourge RC, et al.: Rejection after cardiac transplantation. A time-related risk factor analysis. *Circulation* 86:II236–241, 1992.

Kirkpatrick CH, Wilson WE, Talmage DW: Immunologic studies in human organ transplantation. I. Observation and characterization of suppressed cutaneous reactivity in uremia. *J Exp Med* 119:727–742, 1964.

Kirshbom PM, Bridges ND, Myung RJ, et al.: Use of extracorporeal membrane oxygenation in pediatric thoracic organ transplantation. *J Thorac Cardiovasc Surg* 123:130–136, 2002.

Kjaergard LL, Liu J, Als-Nielsen B, et al.: Artificial and bioartificial support systems for acute and acute-on-chronic liver failure: A systematic review. *JAMA* 289:217–222, 2003.

Klintmalm GB, Goldstein R, Gonwa T, et al.: Use of Prograf (FK506) as rescue therapy for refractory rejection after liver transplantation. U.S. Multicenter FK506 Liver Study Group. *Transplant Proc* 25:679–688, 1993.

Knell AJ, Dukes DC: Dialysis procedures in acute liver coma. *Lancet* 2:402–403, 1976.

Koehntop DE, Beebe DS, Belani K: Perioperative anesthetic management of the kidney-pancreas transplant recipient. *Current Opinions in Anaesthesiology* 13:341–347, 2000.

Kondrup J, Almdal T, Vilstrup H, et al.: High volume plasma exchange in fulminant hepatic failure. *Int J Artif Organs* 15:669–676, 1992.

Koppel MH, Coburn JW, Mims MM, et al.: Transplantation of cadaveric kidneys from patients with hepatorenal syndrome: Evidence for the functional nature of renal failure in advanced liver disease. *N Engl J Med* 280:1367–1371, 1969.

Kovalik JM, Kahan BD, Rajagopalan PR, et al.: Population pharmacokinetics and exposure-response relationships for basiliximab in kidney transplantation. The U.S. Simulect Renal Transplantation Study Group. *Transplantation* 68: 1288–1294, 1999.

Kremers WK, van IJperen M, Kim WR, et al.: MELD score as a predictor of pretransplant and posttransplant survival in OPTN/UNOS status 1 patients. *Hepatology* 39:764–769, 2004.

Kriett JM, Kaye MP: The Registry of the International Society for Heart and Lung Transplantation: Eighth Official Report—1991. *J Heart Lung Transplant* 10:491–498, 1991.

Krowka MJ, Dickson ER, Cortese DA: Hepatopulmonary syndrome: Clinical observations and lack of therapeutic response to somatostatin analogue. *Chest* 104:515–521, 1993.

Krowka MJ, Mandell MS, Ramsay MA, et al.: Hepatopulmonary syndrome and portopulmonary hypertension: A report of the multicenter liver transplant database. *Liver Transpl* 10:174–182, 2004.

Krowka MJ, Porayko MK, Plevak DJ, et al.: Hepatopulmonary syndrome with progressive hypoxemia as an indication for liver transplantation: Case reports and literature review. *Mayo Clin Proc* 72:44–53, 1997.

Kunzendorf U, Hohenstein B, Oberbarnscheid M, et al.: Duration of donor brain death and its influence on kidney graft function. *Am J Transplant* 2:292–294, 2002.

Kuo PC, Alfrey EJ, Garcia G, et al.: Orthotopic liver transplantation with selective use of venovenous bypass. *Am J Surg* 170:671–675, 1995.

Kuo PC, Plotkin JS, Johnson LB, et al.: Distinctive clinical features of portopulmonary hypertension. *Chest* 112:980–986, 1997.

Kusne S, Grossi P, Irish W, et al.: Cytomegalovirus PP65 antigenemia monitoring as a guide for preemptive therapy: a cost effective strategy for prevention of cytomegalovirus disease in adult liver transplant recipients. *Transplantation* 68:1125–1131, 1999.

Kusne S, Shapiro R, Fung J: Prevention and treatment of cytomegalovirus infection in organ transplant recipients. *Transpl Infect Dis* 1:187–203, 1999.

Laditka S, Mastanduno M, Laditka J: Health care use of individuals with diabetes in an employer-based insurance population. *Arch Intern Med* 161:1301–1308, 2001.

Laffi G, Barletta G, La Villa G, et al.: Altered cardiovascular responsiveness to active tilting in nonalcoholic cirrhosis. *Gastroenterology* 113:891–898, 1997.

Laftavi M, Gruessner A, Bland B, et al.: Diagnosis of pancreas rejection: cytoscopic transduodenal versus percutaneous computed tomography scan-guided biopsy. *Transplantation* 65:528–532, 1998.

Lake KD, Smith CI, LaForest SK, et al.: Policies regarding the transplantation of hepatitis C-positive candidates and donor organs. *J Heart Lung Transplant* 16:917–921, 1997.

Lambrigits D, Sachs DH, Cooper DKC: Discordant organ xenotransplantation primates; world experience and current status. *Transplantation* 66:547–561, 1998.

Lang H, Radtke A, Liu C, et al.: Extended left hepatectomy—Modified operation planning based on three-dimensional visualization of liver anatomy. *Langenbecks Arch Surg* 389:306–310, 2004.

Lange PA, Stoller JK: The hepatopulmonary syndrome. *Ann Intern Med* 122:521–529, 1995.

Langrehr JM, Glanemann M, Guckelberger O, et al.: A randomized, placebo-controlled trial with anti-interleukin-2 receptor antibody for immunosuppressive induction therapy after liver transplantation. *Clin Transplant* 12:303–312, 1998.

Lappas DG, Buckley MJ, Laver MB, et al.: Left ventricular performance and pulmonary circulation following addition of nitrous oxide to morphine during coronary-artery surgery. *Anesthesiology* 43:61–69, 1975.

Larson-Wadd K, Belani KG: Pancreas and islet cell transplantation. *Anesthesiology Clin N Am* 22:663–674, 2004.

Lassen NA, Lane MH: Validity of internal jugular blood for study of cerebral blood flow and metabolism. *J Appl Physiol* 16:313–320, 1961.

Lederhaas G, Brock-Utne JG, Negrin RS, et al.: Is nitrous oxide safe for bone marrow harvest? *Anesth Analg* 80:770, 1995.

Lee WS, McKiernan P, Beath SV, et al.: Fulminant hepatic failure in children in the United Kingdom: Etiology and outcome. *Hepatology* 34:291A, 2001.

Leech SH, Lopez-Cepero M, LeFor WM: Plasmapheresis and IVIG in the management of the sensitized cardiac recipient. *Hum Immunol* 64(10 Suppl):S27, 2003.

Levi D, Marelli D, Plunkett M, et al.: Use of assist devices and ECMO to bridge pediatric patients with cardiomyopathy to transplantation. *J Heart Lung Transplant* 21:760–770, 2002.

Levitt MA, Fleischner AS, Meislin HW: Acute post-traumatic diabetes insipidus: Treatment with continuous intravenous vasopressin. *J Trauma* 24:532, 1984.

Lewis JF, Jobe AH: Surfactant and the adult respiratory distress syndrome. *Am Rev Respir Dis* 147:218–233, 1993.

Liang CD, Chen CL, de Villa VH, et al.: Successful liver transplantation in a child with biliary atresia and hepatopulmonary syndrome. *J Formos Med Assoc* 100:403–406, 2001.

Lidofsky SD, Bass NM, Prager MC, et al.: Intracranial pressure monitoring and liver transplantation for fulminant hepatic failure. *Hepatology* 16:1–7, 1992.

Lillehei RC, Idezuki Y, Feemster JA, et al.: Transplantation of stomach, intestine, and pancreas: experimental and clinical observations. *Surgery* 62:721–741, 1967.

Lillehei RC, Simmons RL, Najarian JS, et al.: Pancreatico-duodenal allotransplantation: experimental and clinical experience. *Ann Surg* 172:405–436, 1970.

Linetsky E, Bottino R, Lehmann R, et al.: Improved human islet isolation using a new enzyme blend, liberase. *Diabetes* 46:1120–1123, 1997.

Lindop MJ, Farman JV: Anaesthesia: assessment and intraoperative management. In Calne R, editor: *Liver transplantation.* New York, 1983, Grune & Stratton, pp 121–145.

Lipshultz SE, Colan SD, Gelber RD, et al.: Late cardiac effects of doxorubicin therapy for acute lymphoblastic leukemia in childhood. *N Eng J Med* 324: 808–815, 1991.

Lipshultz SE, Lipsitz SR, Mone SM, et al.: Female sex and drug dose as risk factors for late cardiotoxic effects of doxorubicin therapy for childhood cancer. *N Engl J Med* 332:1738–1743, 1995.

Lipshultz SE, Sleeper LA, Towbin JA, et al.: The incidence of pediatric cardiomyopathy in two regions of the United States. *N Engl J Med* 348:1647–1655, 2003.

Liu E, Dobyns E, Narkewicz M, et al.: Acute hepatic failure in children: A seven year experience at a children's hospital. *Hepatology* 34:197A, 2001.

Liu J, Farmer JD, Jr, Lane WS, et al.: Calcineurin is a common target of cyclophilin-cyclosporin A and FKBP-FK506 complexes. *Cell* 66:807–815, 1991.

Liu H, Lee SS: Cardiopulmonary dysfunction in cirrhosis. *J Gastroenterol Hepatol* 14:600–608, 1999.

Logigian EL, Ropper AH: Terminal electrocardiographic changes in brain-dead patients. *Neurology* 35:915–918, 1985.

Makisalo H, Koivusalo A, Vakkuri A, Hockerstedt K: Sildenafil for portopulmonary hypertension in a patient undergoing liver transplantation. *Liver Transpl* 10:945–950, 2004.

Malago M, Rogiers X, Broelsch CE: Liver splitting and living donor techniques. *Br Med Bull* 53:860–867, 1997.

Mancini D, Pinney S, Burkhoff D, et al.: Use of rapamycin slows progression of cardiac transplantation vasculopathy. *Circulation* 108:48–53, 2003.

Manske CL: Risks and benefits of kidney and pancreas transplantation for diabetic patients. *Diabetes Care* 22(Suppl 2):B114–20, 1999.

Manzarbeitia C, Reich DJ, Rothstein KD, et al.: Tacrolimus conversion improves hyperlipidemic states in stable liver transplant recipients. *Liver Transplant* 7:93–99, 2001.

Margarit C, Martinez-Ibanez V, Tormo R, et al.: Maintenance immunosuppression without steroids in pediatric liver transplantation. *Transplant Proc* 21:2230–2231, 1989.

Margulis MS, Erukhimov EA, Andreiman LA, et al.: Temporary organ substitution by hemoperfusion through suspension of active donor hepatocytes in a total complex of intensive therapy in patients with acute hepatic insufficiency. *Resuscitation* 18:85–94, 1989.

Marino IR, Doyle HR, Nour B, et al.: Baboon liver Xenotransplantation in humans: Clinical experience and principles learned. *Transplantation* 57:1, 1994.

Marion P: Les transplantations cardiques et les transplantation hepatiques. *Lyon Med* 222:585, 1969.

Marjot R: Trauma to the posterior pharyngeal wall caused by a laryngeal mask airway. *Anaesthesia* 46:589, 1991.

Maron BJ, Bonow RO, Cannon RO, III, et al.: Hypertrophic cardiomyopathy. Interrelations of clinical manifestations, pathophysiology, and therapy. *N Engl J Med* 316:780–789, 1987.

Marquez J, Martin D, Virji MA, et al.: Cardiovascular depression secondary to ionic hypocalcemia during hepatic transplantation in humans. *Anesthesiology* 65:457–461, 1986.

Martin RD, Parisi F, Robinson TW, Bailey L: Anesthetic management of neonatal cardiac transplantation. *J Cardiothoracic Anesth* 3:465–469, 1989.

Martin SR, Atkison P, Anand R, et al.: Studies of Pediatric Liver Transplantation 2002: Patient and graft survival and rejection in pediatric recipients of a first liver transplant in the United States and Canada. *Pediatr Transplant* 8:273–283, 2004.

Martin TJ, Kang Y, Robertson KM, et al.: Ionization and hemodynamic effects of calcium chloride and calcium gluconate in the absence of hepatic function. *Anesthesiology* 73:62–65, 1990.

Martinez J, Palascak JE, Kwasniak D: Abnormal sialic acid content of the dysfibrinogenemia associated with liver disease. *J Clin Invest* 61:535–538, 1978.

Mas VR, Fisher RA, Maluf DG, et al.: Hepatic artery thrombosis after liver transplantation and genetic factors: Prothrombin G20210A polymorphism. *Transplantation* 76:247–249, 2003.

Matsubara S, Okabe K, Ouchi K et al.: Continuous removal of middle molecules by hemofiltration in patients with acute liver failure. *Crit Care Med* 18:1331–1338, 1990.

Matsumoto N, Rorie DK, Van Dyke RA: Hepatic oxygen supply and consumption in rats exposed to thiopental, halothane, enflurane, and isoflurane in the presence of hypoxia. *Anesthesiology* 66:337–343, 1987.

Matsumura KN, Guevara GR, Huston H, et al.: Hybrid bioartificial liver in hepatic failure: preliminary clinical report. *Surgery* 101:99–103, 1987.

Maurer J, Spence RK: Transfusion requirements in liver transplantation. September 3, 2004. Retrieved 2/12/2005, 2005, from http://www.emedicine.com/med/topic3508.htm.

Mavroudis C, Harrison H, Klein JB, et al.: Infant orthotopic cardiac transplantation. *J Thorac Cardiovasc Surg* 96:912–924, 1988.

Mazzaferro V, Esquivel CO, Makowka L, et al.: Hepatic artery thrombosis after pediatric liver transplantation—A medical or surgical event? *Transplantation* 47:971–977, 1989.

Mazzeo AT, Lucanto T, Santamaria LB: Hepatopulmonary syndrome: a concern for the anesthetist? Pre-operative evaluation of hypoxemic patients with liver disease. *Acta Anaesthesiol Scand* 48:178–186, 2004.

McAlister VC, Gao Z, Peltekian K, et al.: Sirolimus tacrolimus combination immunosuppression. Lancet 355:376–377, 2000.

McAlister VC, Gao Z, Peltekian K, et al.: Sirolimus tacrolimus combination immunosuppression. *Lancet* 355:376–377, 2000.

McAlister VC, Grant DR, Roy A, et al.: Right phrenic nerve injury in orthotopic liver transplantation. *Transplantation* 55:826–830, 1993.

McCauley J, Van Thiel DH, Starzl TE, et al.: Acute and chronic renal failure in liver transplantation. *Nephron* 55:121–128, 1990.

McDiarmid SV, Busuttil RW, Levy P, et al.: The long-term outcome of OKT3 compared with cyclosporine prophylaxis after liver transplantation. *Transplantation* 52:91–97, 1991.

McDonald R, Donaldson L, Emmett L, et al.: A decade of living donor transplantation in North American children: The 1998 annual report of the North American Pediatric Transplant Cooperative Study (NAPRTCS). *Pediatr Transplant* 4:221, 2000.

McDowall RH: Anesthesia considerations for pediatric cancer. *Semin Surg Oncol* 9:478, 1993.

McGiffin DC, Naftel DC, Kirklin JK, et al.: Predicting outcome after listing for heart transplantation in children: comparison of Kaplan-Meier and parametric competing risk analysis. Pediatric Heart Transplant Study Group. *J Heart Lung Transplant* 16:713–722, 1997.

McGowan FX, Jr, Ikegami M, del Nido PJ, et al.: Cardiopulmonary bypass significantly reduces surfactant activity in children. *J Thorac Cardiovasc Surg* 106:968–977, 1993.

McGrath KJ, Howcroft J, Campbell KHS, et al.: Production of gene targeted sheep by nuclear transfer from cultured somatic cells. *Nature* 405:1066–1069, 2000.

McKenna W, Deanfield J, Faruqui A, et al.: Prognosis in hypertrophic cardiomyopathy: role of age and clinical, electrocardiographic and hemodynamic features. *Am J Cardiol* 47:532–538, 1981.

McKenzie IPC, Koulmanda M, Mandrell TE, et al.: Pig Islet xenografts are susceptible to anti-pig, but not Gala alpha(1,3)Gal antibody plus complement in Gal o/o mice. *J Immunol* 161:5116–5119, 1998.

McLaughlin VV: Medical management of primary pulmonary hypertension. *Expert Opin Pharmacother* 3:159–165, 2002.

Medicare Announces Intention to Cover Intestinal and Multivisceral Transplantation. 2005. Available at: http://c4isr.com/oley/lifeline/trans.html

Mendeloff EN: The history of pediatric heart and lung transplantation. *Pediatr Transplant* 6:270–279, 2002.

Merrill JP, Murray JE, Harrison JH, et al.: *N Engl J Med* 262:1251–1260, 1960.

Meyer C, Hering BJ, Grossmann R, et al.: Improved glucose counterregulation and autonomic symptoms after intraportal islet transplants alone in patients with long-standing type I diabetes mellitus. *Transplantation* 66:233–240, 1998.

Meyers BF, Sundt TM III, Henry S, et al.: Selective use of extracorporeal membrane oxygenation is warranted after lung transplantation. *J Thorac Cardiovasc Surg* 120:20–26, 2000.

Micheals MG, Simmons RL: Xenotransplant associated zoonoses: Strategies for prevention. *Transplantation* 57:1, 1994.

Michler RE, McManus RP, Sadeghi AN, et al.: Prolonged primate cardiac xenograft survival with cyclosporine. *Surg Forum* 359–60, 1985.

Middleton P, Duffield M, Lynch S, et al.: Live donor liver transplantation adult outcomes: A systematic review. 2005. Available at: http://nhscrd.york.ac.uk/online/hta/20040902.htm

Mikami J, Moto M, Nishimuro A, et al.: Surgical treatment of acute liver failure. II: An experimental study of extracorporeal metabolism in the artificial liver using slices of canine liver. *Jpn J Gastroenterol* 56:1022, 1959.

Miller BE, Mochizuki T, Levy JH, et al.: Predicting and treating coagulopathies after cardiopulmonary bypass in children. *Anesth Analg* 85:1196–1202, 1997.

Miller CC, Luan CT, Bock GH, et al.: Transplantation of the adult kidney into the very small child: Technical considerations. *Am J Surg* 145:243, 1983.

Miller RD: Transfusion Therapy. In Miller RD, editor: *Anesthesia,* 5th ed. Philadelphia, 2000, Churchill Livingstone, pp 1613–1644.

Millis JM, Bruce DS, Newell KA, et al.: Treatment of steroid-resistant rejection with tacrolimus before OKT3 in liver transplant recipients. *Transplant Proc* 28:1014, 1996a.

Millis JM, Cronin DC, Newell KA, et al.: Successful use of tacrolimus for initial rejection episodes after liver transplantation. *Transplant Proc* 30:1407–1408, 1998.

Millis JM, Woodle ES, Piper JB, et al.: Tacrolimus for primary treatment of steroid–resistant hepatic allograft rejection. *Transplantation* 61:1365–1369, 1996b.

Milroy SJ, Cottam S, Tan KC, et al.: Improved haemodynamic stability with administration of aprotinin during orthotopic liver transplantation. *Br J Anaesth* 75:747–751, 1995.

Mirza DF, Gunson BK, Soonawalla Z, et al.: Reduced acute rejection after liver transplantation with Neoral based triple immunosuppression. *Lancet* 349:701–702, 1997.

Mital S, Addonizio LJ, Lamour JM, et al.: Outcome of children with end-stage congenital heart disease waiting for cardiac transplantation. *J Heart Lung Transplant* 22:147–153, 2003.

Mito M: Hepatic assist: Present and future. *Artif Organs* 10:214–218, 1986.

Mitzner SR, Stange J, Klammt S, et al.: Improvement of hepatorenal syndrome with extracorporeal albumin dialysis MARS: Results of a prospective, randomized, controlled clinical trial. *Liver Transpl* 6:277–286, 2000.

Mohamed R, Freeman JW, Guest PJ, et al.: Pulmonary gas exchange abnormalities in liver transplant candidates. *Liver Transpl* 8:802–808, 2002.

Molenaar IQ, Begliomini B, Martinelli G, et al.: Reduced need for vasopressors in patients receiving aprotinin during orthotopic liver transplantation. *Anesthesiology* 94:433–438, 2001.

Montefusco CM, Veith FJ.: Lung transplantation. *Surg Clin North Am* 66:503–515, 1986.

Moreno E, Garcia I, Loinaz C, et al.: Reduced-size liver transplantation in children and adults. *Transplant Proc* 23:1953, 1991.

Moreno-Gonzalez E, Meneu-Diaz JG, Fundora Y, et al.: Advantages of the piggy back technique on intraoperative transfusion, fluid consumption, and vasoactive drugs requirements in liver transplantation: A comparative study. *Transplant Proc* 35:1918–1919, 2003.

Morgan JA, Bisleri G, Mancini DM: Cardiac transplantation in an HIV-1-infected patient. *N Engl J Med* 349:1388–1389; author reply 1388–1389, 2003.

Mori T, Eguchi Y, Shimizu T, et al.: A case of acute hepatic insufficiency treated with novel plasmapheresis plasma diafiltration for bridge use until liver transplantation. *Ther Apher* 6:463–466, 2002.

Morice MC, Serruys PW, Sousa JE, et al.: A randomized comparison of a sirolimus-eluting stent with a standard stent for coronary revascularization. *N Engl J Med* 346:1773–1780, 2002.

Morrow WR, Naftel D, Chinnock R, et al.: Outcome of listing for heart transplantation in infants younger than six months: predictors of death and interval to transplantation. The Pediatric Heart Transplantation Study Group. *J Heart Lung Transplant* 16:1255–1266, 1997.

Mundt A, Puhl G, Muller A, et al.: A method to assess biochemical activity of liver cells during clinical application of extracorporeal hybrid liver support. *Int J Artif Organs* 25:542–548, 2002.

Murali S, Kormos RL, Uretsky BF, et al.: Preoperative pulmonary hemodynamics and early mortality after orthotopic cardiac transplantation: the Pittsburgh experience. *Am Heart J* 126:896–904, 1993.

Murase N, Demetris AJ, Woo J, et al.: Lymphocyte traffic and graft-versus-host disease after fully allogeneic small bowel transplantation. *Transplant Proc* 23:3246–3247, 1991.

Murase N, Starzl TE, Tanabe M, et al.: Variable chimerism, graft-versus-host disease, and tolerance after different kinds of cell and whole organ transplantation from Lewis to brown Norway rats. *Transplantation* 60:158–171, 1995.

Murray JE, Sheil AG, Moseley R, et al.: Analysis of mechanism of immunosuppressive drugs in renal homotransplantation. *Ann Surg* 160:449–473, 1964.

Myers RP, Lee SS: Cirrhotic cardiomyopathy and liver transplantation. *Liver Transpl* 6(4 Suppl 1):S44–S52, 2000.

Naeije R: Hepatopulmonary syndrome and portopulmonary hypertension. *Swiss Med Wkly* 133:163–169, 2003.

Nakasuji M, Bookallil MJ: Pathophysiological mechanisms of postrevascularization hyperkalemia in orthotopic liver transplantation. *Anesth Analg* 91:1351–1355, 2000.

Nankivell B, Lau S-G, Chapman J, et al.: Progression of macrovascular disease after transplantation. *Transplantation* 69:574–581, 2000.

Nazer H, Nazer D: Fulminant hepatic failure. 2004. Available at: http://www.emedicine.com/PED/topic808.htm

Neipp M, Offner G, Luck R, et al.: Kidney transplant in children weighing less than 15 kg: Donor selection and technical considerations. *Transplantation* 73:409, 2002.

Neuhaus P, Nashan B, Clavien P, et al.: Basiliximab reduces the rate and severity of acute rejection in adult liver transplant recipients (abstract). *Transplantation* 69S:118, 2000.

Newsome HH: Vasopressin: Deficiency, excess and the syndrome of inappropriate antibiotic hormone secretion. *Nephron* 23:125, 1979.

Nishimura Y, Takei Y, Kawano S, et al.: Long-term storage of liver grafts is associated with a postoperative elevation of tumor necrosis factor: A possible role in the pathogenesis of primary nonfunction of the graft and pulmonary complications. *Transplant Proc* 25(1 pt 1):130–131, 1993.

Norwood WI, Jr, Jacobs ML, Murphy DJ: Fontan procedure for hypoplastic left heart syndrome. *Ann Thorac Surg* 54:1025–1029, 1992.

Nose Y, Mikami J, Kasai N, et al.: An experimental artificial liver using extracorporeal metabolism with sliced or granulated canine liver. *ASAIO Trans* 9:358, 1963.

Novitzky D, Cooper DK, Chaffin JS, et al.: Improved cardiac allograft function following triiodothyronine therapy to both donor and recipient. *Transplantation* 49:311–316, 1990.

Novitzky D, Cooper DK, Reichart B: The value of hormonal therapy in improving organ viability in the transplant donor. *Transplant Proc* 19(1 pt 3): 2037–2038, 1987.

Novitzky D, Wicomb WN, Cooper DKC, et al.: Electrocardiographic, haemodynamic and endocrine changes occurring during experimental brain death in the chacma baboon. *Heart Transplant* 4:63, 1984.

Oaknine G: Bedside procedures in the diagnosis of brain death. *Resuscitation* 4:159–177, 1975.

Oberholzer J, Triponez F, Lou J, et al.: Clinical islet transplantation: a review. *Ann N Y Acad Sci* 875:189–199, 1999.

Odegard KC, McGowan FX, Jr, DiNardo JA, et al.: Coagulation abnormalities in patients with single-ventricle physiology precede the Fontan procedure. *J Thorac Cardiovasc Surg* 123:459–465, 2002.

Odegard KC, McGowan FX, Jr, Zurakowski D, et al.: Coagulation factor abnormalities in patients with single-ventricle physiology immediately prior to the Fontan procedure. *Ann Thorac Surg* 73:1770–1777, 2002.

Odegard KC, McGowan FX, Jr, Zurakowski D, et al.: Procoagulant and anticoagulant factor abnormalities following the Fontan procedure: increased factor VIII may predispose to thrombosis. *J Thorac Cardiovasc Surg* 125:1260–1267, 2003.

Ohdan H, Yang YG, Shimizu A, et al.: Mixed chimerism induced without lethal conditioning prevents cell and anti-Gal, alpha (1,3) Gal mediated graft rejection. *J Clin Invest* 104:281–290, 1999.

Okada A, Takagi Y, Fukuzawa M, et al.: [Intestinal failure—Its concept, physiopathology and treatment]. *Nippon Geka Gakkai Zasshi* 95:1–6, 1994.

Opolon P, Rapin JR, Huguet C, et al.: Hepatic failure coma (HFC) treated by polyacrylonitrile membrane (PAN) hemodialysis (HD). *Trans Am Soc Artif Intern Organs* 22:701–710, 1976.

OPTN/UNOS: Database. 2005. Available at: from http://www.optn.org/latestData/rptData.asp

OPTN/UNOS: Pediatric transplantation. 2002 Annual Report. Available at: http://www.optn.org/data/ar2002/ar02_chapter_five.htm

OPTN/UNOS: Transplants by donor type. Transplants by donor type from January 1988 to October 2004. Available at: http://www.unos.org

Organization for Economic Cooperation and Development: Advances in transplantation biotechnology: Animal to human organ transplants (xenotransplantation). Paris, 1996.

Otte JB, de Ville de Goyet J, et al.: Size reduction of the donor liver is a safe way to alleviate the shortage of size-matched organs in pediatric liver transplantation. *Ann Surg* 211:146–157, 1990.

Outwater KM, Rockoff MA: Diabetes insipidus accompanying brain death in children. *Neurology* 34:1243, 1984.

Ozcay F, Tokel K, Varan B, et al.: Cardiac evaluation of pediatric liver transplantation candidates. *Transplant Proc* 34:2150–2152, 2002.

Ozier YM, Le Cam B, Chatellier G, et al.: Intraoperative blood loss in pediatric liver transplantation: Analysis of preoperative risk factors. *Anesth Analg* 81:1142–1147, 1995.

Pagel PS, Hettrick DA, Kersten JR, et al.: Etomidate adversely alters determinants of left ventricular afterload in dogs with dilated cardiomyopathy. *Anesth Analg* 86:932–938, 1998.

Pahl E, Crawford SE, Swenson JM et al.: Dobutamine stress echocardiography: Experience in pediatric heart transplant recipients. *J Heart Lung Transplant* 18:725–732, 1999.

Pahl E, Naftel DC, Canter CE, et al.: Death after rejection with severe hemodynamic compromise in pediatric heart transplant recipients: A multi-institutional study. *J Heart Lung Transplant* 20:279–287, 2001.

Papadakis MA, Arieff AI: Unpredictability of clinical evaluation of renal function in cirrhosis. Prospective study *Am J Med* 82:945–952, 1987.

Papalois VE, Najarian JS: Pediatric kidney transplantation: Historic hallmarks and a personal perspective. *Pediatr Transplant* 5:239, 2001.

Paradis K, Langford G, Zhifeng L, et al.: The Xen 111 Study Group. Search for cross–species transmission of porcine endogenous retrovirus in patients treated with living pig tissue. *Science* 21:975–982, 1999.

Pasque MK, Cooper JD, Kaiser LR, et al.: Improved technique for bilateral lung transplantation: rationale and initial clinical experience. *Ann Thorac Surg* 49:785–791, 1990.

Patel R, Snydman DR, Rubin RH, et al.: Cytomegalovirus prophylaxis in solid organ transplant recipients. *Transplantation* 61:1279–1289, 1996.

Patience C, Takeuchi Y, Weiss RA: Infection of human cells by an endogenous retrovirus of pigs. *Nat Med* 3:282, 1997.

Paty B, Lanz K, Kendall D, et al.: Restored hypoglycemic counterregulation is stable in successful pancreas transplant recipients for up to 19 years after transplantation. *Transplantation* 72:1103–1107, 2001.

Peabody JL, Emery JR, Ashwal S: Experience with anencephalic infants as prospective organ donors. *N Engl J Med* 321:344–350, 1989.

Peck–Radosavljevic M: Thrombocytopenia in liver disease. *Can J Gastroenterol* 14(Suppl D):60D–66D, 2000.

Pennington DG, Swartz MT: Circulatory support in infants and children. *Ann Thorac Surg* 55:233–237, 1993.

Pienne J, Nakhleh RE, Dunn DL, et al.: Graft-versus-host disease after multiorgan transplantation. *J Surg Res* 50:622, 1991.

Pigott JD, Murphy JD, Barber G, Norwood WI: Palliative reconstructive surgery for hypoplastic left heart syndrome. *Ann Thorac Surg* 45:122–128, 1988.

Pinsker KL, Koerner SK, Kamholz SL, et al.:. Effect of donor bronchial length on healing: a canine model to evaluate bronchial anastomotic problems in lung transplantation. *J Thorac Cardiovasc Surg* 77:669–673, 1979.

Pinson CW, Chapman WC, Wright JK, et al.: Experience with Neoral versus Sandimmune in primary liver transplant recipients. *Transpl Int* 11(suppl 1): 278–283, 1998.

Pirenne J, Gruessner AC, Benedetti E, et al.: Donor-specific unmodified bone marrow transfusion does not facilitate intestinal engraftment after bowel transplantation in a porcine model. *Surgery* 121:79–88, 1997.

Planinsic RM, Nicolau-Raducu R, Eghtesad B, et al.: Diagnosis and treatment of intracardiac thrombosis during orthotopic liver transplantation. *Anesth Analg* 99:353–356, 2004.

Polson RJ, Park GR, Lindop MJ, et al.: The prevention of renal impairment in patients undergoing orthotopic liver grafting by infusion of low dose dopamine. *Anaesthesia* 42:15–19, 1987.

Poon M, Marx SO, Gallo R, et al.: Rapamycin inhibits vascular smooth muscle cell migration. *J Clin Invest* 98:2277–2283, 1996.

Porte RJ, Molenaar IQ, Begliomini B, et al.: Aprotinin and transfusion requirements in orthotopic liver transplantation: A multicentre randomised double-blind study. EMSALT Study Group. *Lancet* 355:1303–1309, 2000.

Porte RJ: Antifibrinolytics in liver transplantation: They are effective, but what about the risk-benefit ratio? *Liver Transpl* 10:285–288, 2004.

Portela D, Patel R, Larson-Keller J, et al.: CV OKT3 treatment for allograft rejection is a risk factor for cytomegalovirus disease in liver transplantation. *J Infect Dis* 71:1014–1018, 1995.

Poston RS, Billingham M, Hoyt EG et al.: Rapamycin reverses chronic graft vascular disease in a novel cardiac allograft model. *Circulation* 100:67–74, 1999.

Powers AC: Diabetes mellitus. In Brawnwald E, Fauci AS, Kasper DL, et al., editors. *Harrison's principles of internal medicine.* New York:, 2001, McGraw-Hill; 2001–2002, pp. 2109–2138.

Psacharopoulos HT, Mowat AP, Cook PJ, et al.: Outcome of liver disease associated with alpha 1 antitrypsin deficiency (PiZ): Implications for genetic counseling and antenatal diagnosis. *Arch Dis Child* 58:882–887, 1983.

Qvist E, Krogerus L, Rönnholm K, et al.: Course of renal transplantation in early childhood. *Transplantation* 70:480, 2000.

Qvist E, Pihko H, Fagerudd P, et al.: Neurodevelopmental outcome in high-risk patients after renal transplantation in early childhood. *Pediatr Transplantation* 6:53, 2002.

Rabbat C, Treleaven D, Russell D, et al.: Prognostic value of myocardial perfusion studies in patients with end-stage renal disease assessed for kidney or kidney-pancreas transplantation: a meta-analysis. *J Am Soc Nephrol* 14:431–439, 2003.

Rahman TM, Hodgson HJ: Review article: Liver support systems in acute hepatic failure. *Aliment Pharmacol Ther* 13:1255–1272, 1999.

Ramamoorthy C, Tabbutt S, Kurth CD, et al.: Effects of inspired hypoxic and hypercapnic gas mixtures on cerebral oxygen saturation in neonates with univentricular heart defects. *Anesthesiology* 96:283–288, 2002.

Randhawa PS, Shapiro R, Jordan ML, et al.: The histopathological changes associated with allograft rejection and drug toxicity in renal transplant recipients maintained on FK506. Clinical significance and comparison with cyclosporine. *Am J Surg Pathol* 17:60–68, 1993.

Randhawa PS, Starzl T, Ramos HC, et al.: Allografts surviving for 26 to 29 years following living-related kidney transplantation: analysis by light microscopy, in situ hybridization for the Y chromosome, and anti-HLA antibodies. *Am J Kidney Dis* 24:72–77, 1994.

Reding R, Tri T, Bourdeaux C, et al.: Pediatric liver transplantation with living-related donors provides significantly better graft survival than LT with post-mortem donors: A comparative study in 236 children. *Am J Transplant* 3(Suppl 5):306, 2003.

Reemtsma K, McCracken BH, Schlegel JU, et al.: Renal heterotransplantation in man. *Ann Surg* 160:384–410, 1964.

Reemtsma K: Clinical urgency and media scrutiny. *Hastings Cent Rep* 15:10–11, 1985.

Reemtsma K: Xenotransplantation–A brief history of clinical experiences: 1900–1965. In Cooper DKC, Kemp E, Reemtsma K, White D, editors: New York, 1991, Springer-Verlag, pp 10–12.

Reinhartz O, Keith FM, El-Banayosy A, et al.: Multicenter experience with the Thoratec ventricular assist device in children and adolescents. *J Heart Lung Transplant* 20:439–448, 2001.

Renz JF, Emond JC, Yersiz H, et al.: Split-liver transplantation in the United States: Outcomes of a national survey. *Ann Surg* 239:172–181, 2004.

Report of Special Task Force: Guidelines for the determination of brain death in children. *Pediatrics* 80:298, 1988.

Reuler JB: Hypothermia: Pathophysiology, clinical settings and management. *Ann Intern Med* 89:519, 1978.

Reyes J, Fishbein T, Bueno J, et al.: Reduced-size orthotopic composite liver-intestinal allograft. *Transplantation* 66:489–492, 1998.

Ricordi C: Human islet cell transplantation: new perspectives for an old challenge. *Diabetes Rev* 4:356–369, 1996.

Ricordi C, Karatzas T, Nery J, et al.: High-dose donor bone marrow infusions to enhance allograft survival: the effect of timing. *Transplantation* 63:7–11, 1997.

Ricordi C, Lacy PE, Finke EH, et al.: Automated method for isolation of human pancreatic islets. *Diabetes* 37:413–420, 1988.

Ricordi C, Murase N, Rastellini C, et al.: Indefinite survival of rat islet allografts following infusion of donor bone marrow without cytoablation. *Cell Transplant* 5:53–55, 1996.

Ricordi C, Tzakis AG, Carroll PB, et al.: Human islet isolation and allotransplantation in 22 consecutive cases. *Transplantation* 53:407–414, 1992.

Rimola A, Gavaler JS, Schade RR, et al.: Effects of renal impairment on liver transplantation. *Gastroenterology* 93:148–156, 1987.

Roberts J, Hulbert-Shearon T, Merion R, et al.: Outcomes of whole deceased, split deceased, and living donor transplant in pediatric recipients. *Am J Transplant* 3(Suppl 5):305, 2003.

Robertson K: Transplantation. In Gambling D, Douglas M, editors: *Obstetric anesthesia and uncommon disorders.* Philadelphia, 1998, WB Saunders, pp 145–170.

Robertson KM, Hramiak IM, Gelb AW: Thyroid function and haemodynamic stability after brain death. *Can J Anaesth* 35:102, 1988.

Rogel-Gilliard C, Bouirgeaux N, Billault A, et al.: Construction of swine BAC library: Application to the characterization and mapping porcine type C endoviral elements. *Cytogenet Cell Genet* 85:205–211, 1999.

Rogers AJ, Trento A, Siewers RD, et al.: Extracorporeal membrane oxygenation for postcardiotomy cardiogenic shock in children. *Ann Thorac Surg* 47:903–906, 1989.

Rosen DA, Rosen KR, Silvasi DL: In vitro variability in fentanyl absorption by different membrane oxygenators. *J Cardiothorac Anesth* 4:332–335, 1990.

Rosendale JD, Chabalewski FL, McBride MS, et al.: Increased transplanted organs from the use of a standardized donor management protocol. *Am J Transplant* 2:761–768, 2002.

Rosendale JD, Kauffman HM, McBride MA, et al.: Aggressive pharmacologic donor management results in more transplanted organs. *Transplantation* 75:482–487, 2003.

Rosengard B, Feng S, Alfrey E, et al.: Report of the Crystal City meeting to maximize the use of organs recovered from the cadaver donor. *Am J Transplant* 2:701–711, 2002.

Rosenzweig EB, Kerstein D, Barst RJ: Long-term prostacyclin for pulmonary hypertension with associated congenital heart defects. *Circulation* 99: 1858–65, 1999.

Rozenbaum JL, Kramer MS, Raja R, et al.: Resin hemoperfusion: A new treatment for acute drug intoxication. *N Engl J Med* 284:874–883, 1971.

Rubin RH, Tolkoff-Rubin NE: The impact of infection on the outcome of transplantation. *Transplant Proc* 23:2068–2074, 1991.

Sadamori H, Yagi T, Inagaki M, et al.: High-flow-rate haemodiafiltration as a brain-support therapy proceeding to liver transplantation for hyperacute fulminant hepatic failure. *Eur J Gastroenterol Hepatol* 14:435–439, 2002.

Salomon DR: Invited comment. *J Heart Transplant* 11:396–397, 1992.

Sandrin MS, Mckenzie IFC: Recent advances in xenotransplantation. *Curr Opin Immunol* 11:527–531, 1999.

Sauer IM, Obermeyer N, Kardassis D, et al.: Development of a hybrid liver support system. *Ann N Y Acad Sci* 944:308–319, 2001.

Sauer IM, Zeilinger K, Obermayer N, et al.: Primary human liver cells as source for modular extracorporeal liver support: A preliminary report. *Int J Artif Organs* 25:1001–1005, 2002.

Scheule AM, Zimmerman GJ, Johnston JK, et al.: Duration of graft cold ischemia does not affect outcomes in pediatric heart transplant recipients. *Circulation* 106(12 Suppl I):I163–I167, 2002.

Schlechter DC, Nealon TF, Gibbon JH: A simple extracorporeal device for reducing elevated blood ammonia levels. *Surgery* 44:892–897, 1958.

Schindler E, Muller M, Kwapisz M, et al.: Ventricular cardiac-assist devices in infants and children: anesthetic considerations. *J Cardiothorac Vasc Anesth* 17:617–621, 2003.

Schmid C, Heemann U, Azuma H, et al.: Rapamycin inhibits transplant vasculopathy in long-surviving rat heart allografts. *Transplantation* 60:729–73, 1995.

Schmidt LE, Sorensen VR, Svendsen LB, et al.: Hemodynamic changes during a single treatment with the molecular adsorbents recirculating system in patients with acute on chronic liver failure. *Liver Transpl* 7:1034–1039, 2001.

Schnuelle P, Lorenz D, Mueller A et al.: Donor catecholamine use reduces acute allograft rejection and improves graft survival after cadaveric renal transplantation. *Kidney Int* 56:738–746, 1999.

Schott R, Chaouat A, Launoy A, et al.: Improvement of pulmonary hypertension after liver transplantation. *Chest* 115:1748–1749, 1999.

Schowengerdt KO, Naftel DC, Seib PM, et al.: Infection after pediatric heart transplantation: results of a multiinstitutional study. The Pediatric Heart Transplant Study Group. *J Heart Lung Transplant* 16:1207–12, 1997.

Schratz LM, Meyer RA, Schwartz DC: Serial intracoronary ultrasound in children: Feasibility, reproducibility, limitations, and safety. *J Am Soc Echocardiogr* 15:782–790, 2002.

Schreiber SL, Crabtree GR: The mechanism of action of cyclosporin A and FK506. *Immunol Today* 13:136–142, 1992.

Schreier MH, Baumann G, Zenke G: Inhibition of T-cell signaling pathways by immunophilin drug complexes: Ae side effects inherent to immunosuppressive properties? *Transplant Proc* 25(1 pt 1):502–50, 1993.

Schulte-Sasse U, Hess W, Tarnow J: Pulmonary vascular responses to nitrous oxide in patients with normal and high pulmonary vascular resistance. *Anesthesiology* 57:9–13, 1982.

Schumann R: Intraoperative resource utilization in anesthesia for liver transplantation in the United States: A survey. *Anesth Analg* 97:21–28, 2003.

Schure AY, Holzman RS: Anesthesia in a child with severe restrictive pulmonary dysfunction caused by chronic graft-versus-host disease. *J Clin Anesth* 12:482, 2000.

Schwarz B, Pomaroli A, Hoermann C, et al.: Liver transplantation without venovenous bypass: morbidity and mortality in patients with greater than 50% reduction in cardiac output after vena cava clamping. *J Cardiothorac Vasc Anesth* 15:460–462, 2001.

Schwarzenberg SJ, Sharp HL: Pathogenesis of alpha 1-antitrypsin deficiency-associated liver disease, 1990. *J Pediatr Gastroenterol Nutr* 10:5–12, 1990.

Scott VL, De Wolf AM, Kang Y, et al.: Ionized hypomagnesemia in patients undergoing orthotopic liver transplantation: A complication of citrate intoxication. *Liver Transpl Surg* 2:343–347, 1996.

Seikaly M, Ho PL, Emmett L, et al.: The 12th Annual Report of the North American Pediatric Renal Transplant Cooperative Study: Renal transplantation from 1987 through 1998. *Pediatr Transplant* 5:215–231, 2001.

Shapiro H, editor: *Experience with human heart transplantation.* Durban, South Africa, 1969, Butterworths, pp 227–228.

Shapiro AM, Gallant H, Hao E, et al.: Portal vein immunosuppressant levels and islet graft toxicity. *Transplant Proc* 30:641, 1998.

Shapiro R, Rao AS, Fontes P, et al.: Combined kidney/bone marrow transplantation. *Arch Dialysis Transplant* 5: 282–285, 1996.

Sharples LD, Tamm M, McNeil K, et al.: Development of bronchiolitis obliterans syndrome in recipients of heart-lung transplantation—Early risk factors. *Transplantation* 61:560–566, 1996.

Shaw BW Jr, Martin DJ, Marquez JM, et al.: Advantages of venous bypass during orthotopic transplantation of the liver. *Semin Liver Dis* 5:344–348, 1985.

Shaw BW Jr, Martin DJ, Marquez JM, et al.: Venous bypass in clinical liver transplantation. *Ann Surg* 200:524–534, 1984.

Shaw LM, Bonner HS, Schuchter L, et al.: Pharmacokinetics of amifostine: Effects of dose and method of administration. *Semin Oncol* 26(2 Suppl 7): 34, 1999.

Shekerdemian L: Nonpharmacologic treatment of acute heart failure. *Curr Opin Pediatr* 13:240, 2001.

Sigal NH, Dumont FJ: Cyclosporin A, FK506, and rapamycin: Pharmacologic probes of lymphocyte signal transduction. *Annu Rev Immunol* 10:519–50, 1992.

Singh A, Stablein D, Tejani A: Risk factors for vascular thrombosis in pediatric renal transplantation: A special report of the North American Pediatric Renal Transplantation Cooperative Study. *Transplantation* 63:1263, 1997.

Singh N, Yu VL, Gayowski T: Central nervous system lesions in adult liver transplant recipients: Clinical review with implications for management. *Medicine (Baltimore)* 73:110–118, 1994.

Sklarin NT, Dutcher JP, Wiernik PH: Lymphomas following cardiac transplantation. Case report and review of the literature. *Am J Hematol* 37:105–111, 1991.

Smiley RM, Navedo AT, Kirby T, et al.: Postoperative independent lung ventilation in a single-lung transplant recipient. *Anesthesiology* 74:1144–1148, 1991.

Smith JM, Ho PL, McDonald RA: Renal transplant outcomes in adolescents: A report of the North American Pediatric Renal Transplant Cooperative Study. *Pediatr Transplant* 6:493, 2002.

So SK, Chang PN, Najarian JS, et al.: Growth and development in infants after renal transplantation. *J Pediatr* 110:343, 1987.

Sollinger HW, Odorico JS, Knechtle SJ, et al.: Experience with 500 simultaneous pancreas-kidney transplants. *Ann Surg* 228:284–296, 1998.

Sondheimer JM, Asturias E, Cadnapaphornchai M: Infection and cholestasis in neonates with intestinal resection and long-term parenteral nutrition. *J Pediatr Gastroenterol Nutr* 27:131–137, 1998.

Soon-Shiong P, Heintz RE, Merideth N, et al.: Insulin independence in a type 1 diabetic patient after encapsulated islet transplantation. *Lancet* 343:950–951, 1994.

Sorrentino F: Prime ricerche per la realizzazione di un fegato artificiale. *Chir Patol Sperim* 4:1401–1404, 1956.

Sosef MN, Abrahamse LS, van de Kerkhove MP, et al.: Assessment of the AMC-bioartificial liver in the anhepatic pig. *Transplantation* 73:204–209, 2002.

Stange J, Hassanein TI, Mehta R, et al.: The molecular adsorbents recycling system as a liver support system based on albumin dialysis: A summary of preclinical investigations, prospective, randomized, controlled clinical trial, and clinical experience from 19 centers. *Artif Organs* 26:103–110, 2002.

Starnes VA, Woo MS, MacLaughlin EF, et al.: Comparison of outcomes between living donor and cadaveric lung transplantation in children. *Ann Thorac Surg* 68:2279–2283, 1999.

Starr NJ, Sethna DH, Estafanous FG: Bradycardia and asystole following the rapid administration of sufentanil with vecuronium. *Anesthesiology* 64:521–523, 1986.

Starzl TE: Chimerism and tolerance in transplantation. *Proc Natl Acad Sci U S A* 101(Suppl 2):14607–14614, 2004.

Starzl TE, Demetris AJ, Murase N, et al.: Cell migration, chimerism, and graft acceptance. *Lancet* 339:1579–1582, 1992.

Starzl TE, Demetris AJ, Murase N, et al.: Donor cell chimerism permitted by immunosuppressive drugs: a new view of organ transplantation. *Trends Pharmacol Sci* 14:217–223, 1993.

Starzl TE, Demetris AJ, Trucco M, et al.: Systemic chimerism in human female recipients of male livers. *Lancet* 340:876–877, 1992.

Starzl TE, Demetris AJ, Trucco M, et al.: Cell migration and chimerism after whole-organ transplantation: the basis of graft acceptance. *Hepatology* 17:1127–1152, 1993.

Starzl TE, Fung J, Todo S, et al.: Notes on FK 506. *Transplant Proc* 23:2178–2179, 1991a.

Starzl TE, Fung JJ, Tzakis A, et al.: Baboon-to-human liver transplantation. *Lancet* 341:65–71, 1993.

Starzl TE, Groth CG, Brettschneider L, et al.: Orthotopic homotransplantation of the human liver. *Ann Surg* 168:392–415, 1968.

Starzl TE, Hakala TR, Shaw BW Jr, et al.: A flexible procedure for multiple cadaveric organ procurement. *Surg Gynecol Obstet* 158:223–230, 1984.

Starzl TE, Iwatsuki S, Van Thiel DH, et al.: Evolution of liver transplantation. *Hepatology* 2:614–636, 1982.

Starzl TE, Iwatsuki S: Transplantation of the liver. In Schiff L, Schiff ER, editors: *Diseases of the liver,* 6th ed. Philadelphia, 1987, JB Lippincott, p 255.

Starzl TE, Kaupp HA: Mass homotransplantation of abdominal organs in dogs. *Surg Forum* 11:28, 1960.

Starzl TE, Rowe MI, Todo S, et al.: Transplantation of multiple abdominal viscera. *JAMA* 261:1449–1457, 1989.

Starzl TE, Todo S, Fung J, et al.: FK 506 for liver, kidney, and pancreas transplantation. *Lancet* 2:1000–1004, 1989.

Starzl TE, Todo S, Tzakis A, et al.: The many faces of multivisceral transplantation. *Surg Gynecol Obstet* 172:335–344, 1991b.

Starzl TE: Medawar Prize Lecture. Liver allo- and xenotransplantation. *Transplant Proc* 25(1 pt 1):15–17, 1993.

Stegall MD, Wachs ME, Everson G, et al.: Prednisone withdrawal 14 days after liver transplantation with mycophenolate: A prospective trial of cyclosporine and tacrolimus. *Transplantation* 64:1755–1760, 1997.

Steib A, Gohard R, Beller JP, et al.: Mixed venous oxygen saturation monitoring during liver transplantation. *Eur J Anaesthesiol* 10:267–271, 1993.

Stein RA, Messino MJ, Hessel EA: Anaesthetic implications for bone marrow transplant recipients. *Can J Anaesth* 37:571, 1990.

Steiner C, Mitzner S: Experiences with MARS liver support therapy in liver failure: Analysis of 176 patients of the International MARS Registry. *Liver* 22(suppl 2):20–25, 2002.

Stieber AO, Boillot O, Scotti-Foglieni C, et al.: The surgical implications of the posttransplant lymphoproliferative disorders. *Transplant Proc* 23(1 pt 2): 1477–1479, 1991.

Stiller B, Hetzer R, Weng Y, et al.: Heart transplantation in children after mechanical circulatory support with pulsatile pneumatic assist device. *J Heart Lung Transplant* 2003; 22:1201–1208, 2003.

Stockmann HB, Hiemstra CA, Marquet RL, et al.: Extracorporeal perfusion for the treatment of acute liver failure. *Ann Surg* 231:460–470, 2000.

Stoye JP: Xenotransplantation: Proviruses pose potential problems. *Nature* 386:126, 1997.

Strom S, Fisher R: Hepatocyte transplantation: New possibilities for therapy. *Gastroenterology* 124:568–571, 2003.

Studies of Pediatric Liver Transplantation (SPLIT): Year 2000 outcomes. *Transplantation* 72:463–476, 2001.

Sudan DL, Kaufman SS, Shaw BW Jr, et al.: Isolated intestinal transplantation for intestinal failure. *Am J Gastroenterol* 95:1506–1515, 2000.

Sudan D, Sudan R, Stratta R: Long-term outcome of simultaneous kidney-pancreas transplantation: analysis of 61 patients with more than 5 years follow-up. *Transplantation* 69:550–555, 2000.

Suh KS, Lilja H, Kamohara Y, et al.: Bioartificial liver treatment in rats with fulminant hepatic failure: Effect on DNA-binding activity of liver-enriched and growth-associated transcription factors. *J Surg Res* 85:243–250, 1999.

Suriani RJ, Cutrone A, Feierman D, et al.: Intraoperative transesophageal echocardiography during liver transplantation. *J Cardiothorac Vasc Anesth* 10:699–707, 1996.

Sutherland DE, Goetz FC, Najarian JS: Intraperitoneal transplantation of immediately vascularized segmental pancreatic grafts without duct ligation. A clinical trial. *Transplantation* 28:485–491, 1979.

Sutherland D, Gruessner R, Dunn D, Matas A, et al.: Lessons learned from more than 1,000 pancreas transplants at a single institution. *Ann Surg* 233: 463–501, 2001.

Sutherland DE, Goetz FC, Sibley RK: Recurrence of disease in pancreas transplants. *Diabetes* 38(Suppl 1):85–87, 1989.

Svensson KL, Sonander HG, Henriksson BA, et al.: Whole-body oxygen consumption during liver transplantation. *Transplant Proc* 19(4 Suppl 3):56–58, 1987.

Sweet SC, Spray TL, Huddleston CB, et al.: Pediatric lung transplantation at St. Louis Children's Hospital, 1990–1995. *Am J Respir Crit Care Med* 155:1027–1035, 1997.

Sweet SC: Pediatric lung transplantation: Update 2003. *Pediatr Clin North Am* 50.1393–1417, 2003.

Swygert TH, Roberts LC, Valek TR, et al.: Effect of intraoperative low-dose dopamine on renal function in liver transplant recipients. *Anesthesiology* 75:571–576, 1991.

Sykes MK, Hurtig JB, Tait AR, et al.: Reduction of hypoxic pulmonary vasoconstriction in the dog during administration of nitrous oxide. *Br J Anaesth* 49:301–307, 1977.

Tabbutt S, Ramamoorthy C, Montenegro LM, et al.: Impact of inspired gas mixtures on preoperative infants with hypoplastic left heart syndrome during controlled ventilation. *Circulation* 104:I159–164, 2001.

Tackle SJ, Kurth K, Denner J: Porcine endogenous retroviruses inhibit human immune cell function: Risk for xenotransplantation. *Virology* 268:87–93, 2000.

Takeyoshi I, Zhang S, Nomoto M, et al.: Mucosal damage and recovery of the intestine after prolonged preservation and transplantation in dogs. *Transplantation* 71:1–7, 2001.

Tanaka K, Uemoto S, Tokunaga Y, et al.: Liver transplantation in children from living-related donors. *Transplant Proc* 25(1 pt 2):1084–1086, 1993.

Tanner GE, Angers DG, Barash PG, et al.: Effect of left-to-right, mixed left-to-right, and right-to-left shunts on inhalational anesthetic induction in children: a computer model. *Anesth Analg* 64:101–107, 1985.

Tejani AH, Sullivan EK, Alexander SR, et al.: Predictive factors for delayed graft function (DFG) and its impact on renal graft survival in children: A report of the North American Pediatric Renal Transplant Cooperative Study (NAPRTCS). *Pediatr Transplant* 3:293, 1999.

Teramoto S, Ishii T, Ouchi Y: The mechanism of hypoxemia in liver disease with pulmonary hypertension. *Chest* 117:614–615, 2000.

Terasaki PI, Cecka JM, Cho Y, et al.: A report from the UNOS Scientific Renal Transplant Registry. *Transplant Proc* 23:53–54, 1991.

The Diabetes Control and Complications Trial/Epidemiology of Diabetes Intervention and Complications Research Group. Retinopathy and nephropathy in patients with type 1 diabetes four years after a trial of intensive therapy. *N Engl J Med* 342:381–389, 2000.

The Diabetes Control and Complications Trial Research Group: The effect of intensive treatment of diabetes on the development and progression of long-term complications in insulin-dependent diabetes mellitus. *N Engl J Med* 329:977–986, 1993.

The U.S. Multicenter FK506 Liver Study Group: A comparison of tacrolimus (FK506) and cyclosporine for immunosuppression in liver transplantation. *N Engl J Med* 331:1110–1115, 1994.

Thistlethwaite JR Jr, Stuart JK, Mayes JT, et al.: Complications and monitoring of OKT3 therapy. *Am J Kidney Dis* 11:112–119, 1988.

Thistlethwaite JR Jr, Emond JC, Heffron TG, et al.: Innovative use of organs for liver transplantation. *Transplant Proc* 23:2147–2151, 1991.

Tisone G, Gunson BK, Buckels JA, et al.: Raised hematocrit—A contributing factor to hepatic artery thrombosis following liver transplantation. *Transplantation* 46:162–163, 1988.

Todd TR: Early postoperative management following lung transplantation. *Clin Chest Med* 11:259–267, 1990.

Todo S, Reyes J, Furukawa H, et al.: Outcome analysis of 71 clinical intestinal transplantations. *Ann Surg* 222:270–280; discussion 280–282, 1995.

Todo S, Tzakis A, Abu-Elmagd K, et al.: Current status of intestinal transplantation. *Adv Surg* 27:295–316, 1994a.

Todo S, Tzakis A, Reyes J, et al.: Small intestinal transplantation in humans with or without the colon. *Transplantation* 57:840–848, 1994b.

Toledo-Pereyra HL: Xenotransplantation: the promise of transplanting animal organs into humans. *JAMA* 285, 2001.

Toledo-Pereyra LH, Hau T, Simmons RL, Najarian JS: Lung preservation techniques. *Ann Thorac Surg* 23:487–494, 1977.

Toledo-Pereyra LH, Lopez-Neblina F: Xenotransplantation: a view to the past and an unrealized promise to the future. *Exp Clin Transplant* 1:1–7, 2003.

Tomichek RC, Rosow CE, Philbin DM, et al.: Diazepam-fentanyl interaction – hemodynamic and hormonal effects in coronary artery surgery. *Anesth Analg* 62:881–884, 1983.

Triantafillou AN, Heerdt PM: Lung transplantation. *Int Anesthesiol Clin* 29:87–109, 1991.

Trotter JF, Wachs M, Bak T, et al.: Liver transplantation using sirolimus and minimal corticosteroids (3 day taper). *Liver Transplant* 7:343–351, 2001.

Trotter JF, Wachs M, Everson GT, et al.: Adult-to-adult transplantation of the right hepatic lobe from a living donor. *N Engl J Med* 346:1074–1082, 2002.

Turenne MN, Port FK, Strawderman RL, et al.: Growth rates in pediatric dialysis patients and renal transplant recipients. *Am J Kid Dis* 30:93, 1997.

Tzakis A, Todo S, Starzl TE: Orthotopic liver transplantation with preservation of the inferior vena cava. *Ann Surg* 210:649–652, 1989.

US Department of Health and Human Services, Public Health Service: Draft guidelines on infectious disease issues in xenotransplantation. *Fed Register* 61:49920, 1996.

UK Advisory Group on the Ethics of Xenotransplantation (Kennedy Report): *Animal tissues into humans.* Norwich, UK, 1997, Her Majesty's Stationery Office.

UK Department of Health: *The government response to animal tissues into humans.* (UK Xenotransplantation Interim Regulatory Authority set up. Interim until National Standing Committee on Xenotransplantation is formed.) London, 1997, Her Majesty's Stationery Office.

UNOS/OPTN: Annual Report of the U.S. Scientific Registry of Transplant Recipients and the Organ Procurement and Transplantation Network, 2005

Valeriano V, Funaro S, Lionetti R, et al.: Modification of cardiac function in cirrhotic patients with and without ascites. *Am J Gastroenterol* 95:3200–3205, 2000.

Velidedeoglu E, Mange KC, Frank A, et al.: Factors differentially correlated with the outcome of liver transplantation in HCV+ and HCV– recipients. *Transplantation* 77:1834–1842, 2004.

Vichinsky E: New therapies in sickle cell disease. *Lancet* 360:629–631, 2002.

Vincenti, F, Kirkman, R, Light, S, et al.: Interleukin-2-receptor blockade with daclizumab to prevent acute rejection in renal transplantation. Daclizumab Triple Therapy Study Group. *N Engl J Med* 338:161–165, 1998.

Wagner K, Oliver MC, Boyle GJ et al.: Endomyocardial biopsy in pediatric heart transplant recipients: A useful exercise? (Analysis of 1,169 biopsies.) *Pediatr Transplant* 4:186–192, 2000.

Wah TM, Moss HA, Robertson RJ, Barnard DL: Pulmonary complications following bone marrow transplantation. *Br J Radiol* 76:373, 2003.

Wall WJ, Adams PC: Liver transplantation for fulminant hepatic failure: North American experience. *Liver Transpl Surg* 1:178–182, 1995.

Wallace KB: Doxorubicin–induced cardiac mitochondrionopathy. *Pharmacol Toxicol* 93:105–115, 2003.

Walsh CK, Krongrad E: Terminal cardiac electrical activity in pediatric patients. *Am J Cardiol* 51:557, 1983.

Wang CS, Wang ST, Chang TT, et al.: Smoking and alanine aminotransferase levels in hepatitis C virus infection: Implications for prevention of hepatitis C virus progression. *Arch Intern Med* 162:811–815, 2002.

Wasa M, Takagi Y, Sando K, et al.: Long-term outcome of short bowel syndrome in adult and pediatric patients. *JPEN J Parenter Enteral Nutr* 23(5 Suppl):S110–S112, 1999.

Watson CJ, Friend PJ, Jamieson NV, et al.: Sirolimus: A potent new immunosuppressant for liver transplantation. *Transplantation* 67:505–509, 1999.

Webber SA: The current state of, and future prospects for, cardiac transplantation in children. *Cardiol Young* 13:64–83, 2003.

Weinberg PM, Peyser K, Hackney JR: Fetal hydrops in a newborn with hypoplastic left heart syndrome: tricuspid valve "stopper". *J Am Coll Cardiol* 6:1365–1369, 1985.

Weinhaus L, Canter C, Noetzel M, et al.: Extracorporeal membrane oxygenation for circulatory support after repair of congenital heart defects. *Ann Thorac Surg* 48:206–212, 1989.

Weiss RA: Transgenic pigs and virus adaptation. *Nature* 391:327–328, 1998.

West JB: Blood flow to the lung and gas exchange. *Anesthesiology* 41:124–138, 1974.

Wetzel RC, Setzer N, Stiff JL, et al.: Hemodynamic responses in brain dead organ donor patients. *Anesth Analg* 64:125–128, 1985.

Wheeldon DR, Potter CD, Oduro A, et al.: Transforming the "unacceptable" donor: Outcomes from the adoption of a standardized donor management technique. *J Heart Lung Transplant* 14:734–742, 1995.

Wiesner RH: A long-term comparison of tacrolimus (FK506) versus cyclosporine in liver transplantation: A report of the United States FK506 Study Group. *Transplantation* 66:493–499, 1998.

Wigle ED, Sasson Z, Henderson MA, et al.: Hypertrophic cardiomyopathy. The importance of the site and the extent of hypertrophy. A review. *Prog Cardiovasc Dis* 28:1–83, 1985.

Wijdicks EFM: *Brain death.* Philadelphia, 2001, Lippincott Williams & Wilkins.

Wilmut I, Schnieke AE, McWhir J, et al.: Viable offspring derived from fetal and adult mammalian cells. *Nature* 385:281–290, 1997.

World Health Organization draft recommendations on xenotransplantation and infectious disease prevention and management. Prepared by the Division of Emerging and Other Communicable Disease Surveillance and Control, Geneva, Switzerland, 1997, World Health Organization.

Wszolek ZK, McComb RD, Pfeiffer RF, et al.: Pontine and extrapontine myelinolysis following liver transplantation: Relationship to serum sodium. *Transplantation* 48:1006–1012, 1989.

Wynands JE, Townsend GE, Wong P, et al.: Blood pressure response and plasma fentanyl concentrations during high- and very high-dose fentanyl anesthesia for coronary artery surgery. *Anesth Analg* 62:661–665, 1983.

Yankaskas JR, Mallory GB, Jr: Lung transplantation in cystic fibrosis: consensus conference statement. *Chest* 113:217–226, 1998.

Yarmush ML, Dunn JC, Tompkins RG: Assessment of artificial liver support technology. *Cell Transplant* 1:323–341, 1992.

Yamazaki K, Kamai F, Ieszuki Y, et al.: Extracorporeal methods of liver failure treatment. *Biomater Artif Cells Artif Organs* 15:667–675, 1987.

Yu J, Zheng SS, Liang TB, et al.: Possible causes of central pontine myelinolysis after liver transplantation. *World J Gastroenterol* 10:2540–2543, 2004.

Yuan HC, Wu TC, Huang IF, et al.: Hepatopulmonary syndrome in a child. *J Chin Med Assoc* 66:127–130, 2003.

Zapol WM, Snider MT, Hill JD, et al.: Extracorporeal membrane oxygenation in severe acute respiratory failure. A randomized prospective study. *JAMA* 242:2193–2196, 1979.

Zaroff JG, Rosengard BR, Armstrong WF, et al.: Consensus conference report: maximizing use of organs recovered from the cadaver donor: cardiac recommendations. *Circulation* 106:836–841, 2002.

Zuckerman L, Cohen E, Vagher JP, et al.: Comparison of thromboelastography with common coagulation tests. *Thromb Haemost* 46:752–756, 1981.

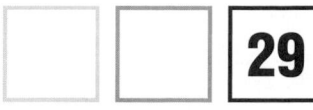

29 Anesthesia for Children with Burns

John E. McCall • Carl G. Fischer

Children are often the victims of burns and scalds. Burns are the leading cause of accidental in-home deaths for children less than 15 years of age, with the peak incidence occurring in children aged 1 to 5 years, mostly due to scalds. In the United States, there is a 1:70 lifetime chance of being hospitalized for a burn injury, and an average of 12,000 burn fatalities are reported in the United States each year (Lloyd, 1977). Only motor vehicle trauma causes more accidental deaths than burns (Feck and Baptiste, 1979).

Burns can be inflicted by various modalities including radiation, electrical, thermal, and caustic chemicals. The causes of thermal burns are scald, contact, and/or flame (Parks et al., 1977).

Burns are classified as follows (Table 29–1):

- A first-degree burn involves only the epithelial layer of the skin; these burns are erythematous and may be quite painful but heal with no scarring. These injuries are typical of sunburn (Fig. 29–1A).
- A second-degree burn involves the epithelial layer and to a varying degree the underlying dermis. These burns are characterized by the formation of blisters or a pink, moist appearance. Pain is an important component. Reepithelialization occurs because of sparing of the dermal appendages. The amount of pain and scarring produced depends on the depth of the dermal injury. Healing, if it occurs, should be complete in 7 to 14 days (Fig. 29–1B).
- A deep dermal or deep second-degree burn involves most of the dermis, resulting in survival of few dermal appendages. Blister formation is seldom seen due to the thickness of the dead tissue. These burns are characterized by red or white, depending on depth of injury, colorless skin. These burns may be indistinguishable from third-degree burns. This may be unimportant as excision and grafting almost certainly are needed (Fig. 29–1C).
- A third-degree or full-thickness burn involves the entire skin thickness, epidermis as well as dermis. It has the waxy white appearance of avascular tissue. Excision and grafting are mandated, or scarring will be severe (Fig. 29–1D).
- Fourth-degree burns are full-thickness burns that extend into the supporting structures under the fascia.

■ **TABLE 29–1.** Burn wound classification

First degree	• Involves epithelial layer of skin only • Erythematous in appearance—typical of sunburn • Pain (+) • Heals without scarring
Second degree	• Involves epithelial layer plus varying degree of underlying dermis • **Superficial** ○ Uniformly pink, moist ○ Pain (+/+) ○ Heals within 2 weeks without scarring or functional impairment • **Deep** ○ White or mottled red, fairly dry. May be difficult to differentiate from third degree ○ Pain (+/–) ○ Most often will need excision and grafting or will have scarring
Third degree	• Involves epithelial as well as full dermal layer • White, cherry red, or black ○ Elasticity of skin missing ○ Dry, hard, leathery appearance • Pain (+/–) • Need excision and grafting or will have major scarring
Fourth degree	• Full-thickness extending into the supporting structures under the fascia

Modified from De Campo T, Aldrete JA: The anesthetic management of the severely burned patient. *Intensive Care Med* 7:55, 1981.

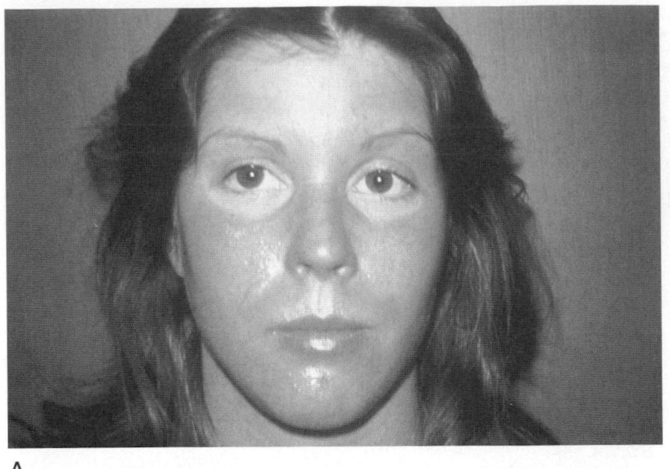

A

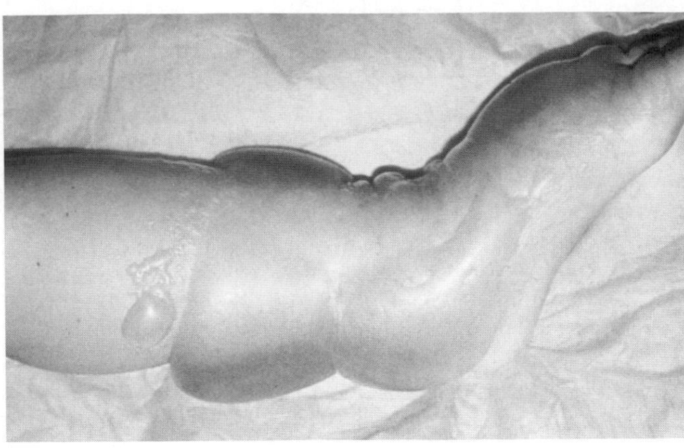

B

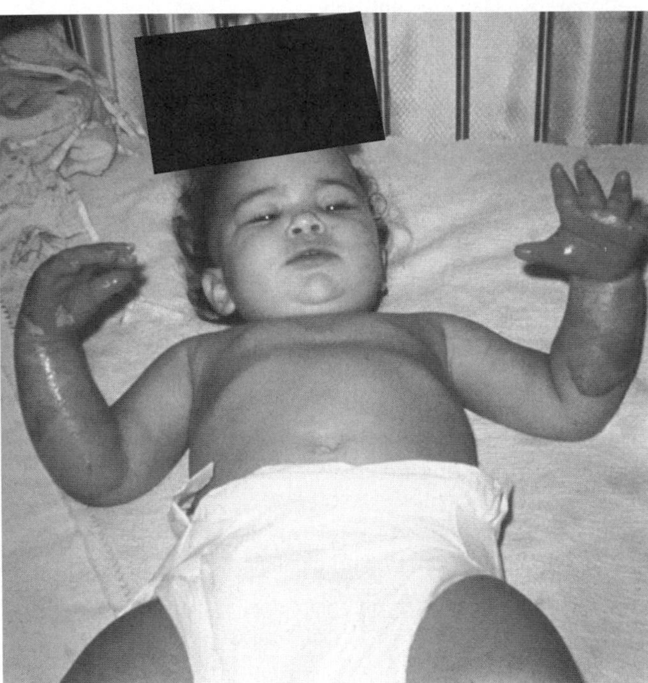

C

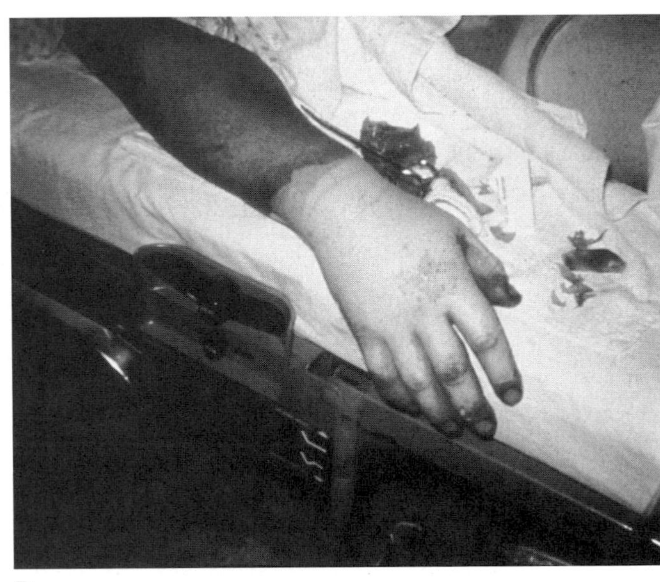

D

■ **FIGURE 29–1.** Degrees of burn severity. *A*, Patient with a first-degree burn. *B*, Patient with a second-degree burn. *C*, Patient with a deep second-degree burn. *D*, Patient with a third-degree burn.

To assess the total surface area of burn involvement, various tools and diagrams have been used. The diagram and chart in Figure 29–2 are of great use and require little learning curve.

The exact classification of burn injury may not be defined on the first examination; this is especially true of scald injuries. Watchful waiting eventually gives a true picture of the severity and extent of the injury and clarifies the extent of surgery that might be required. The amount of physiologic derangement, morbidity, and even mortality associated with a burn depends on the size and depth of injury. An inhalation injury adds to this derangement. Burn severity can be classified as minor, moderate, and major as originally determined by the American Burn Association and the American College of Surgeons Committee on Trauma (Table 29–2).

Abnormalities seen in burn patients include metabolic derangements, neurohumoral responses, massive fluid shifts, possible sepsis, and systemic effects of massive tissue destruction (Szyfelbein et al., 1993). Even minor burns may be associated with some systemic effects. The anesthesiologist who cares for these patients must be well versed in the treatment of these potentially altered pathophysiologic, pharmacologic, and anatomic derangements seen in burn patients.

Burn care has improved with resulting increase in survival rates even with extremely large burns. Now patients with burns of 80% have a survival rate of over 50%, and in adolescents and young adults this estimate probably is too low (Saffle, 1998). In this chapter we hope to convey the information that has made many of these advances possible.

■ PATHOPHYSIOLOGY OF THE BURN PATIENT

■ RESPIRATORY DERANGEMENTS

Airway Injury

The air temperature in a room containing a fire may exceed 1000°F (Trunkey, 1978). Due to the combination of efficient

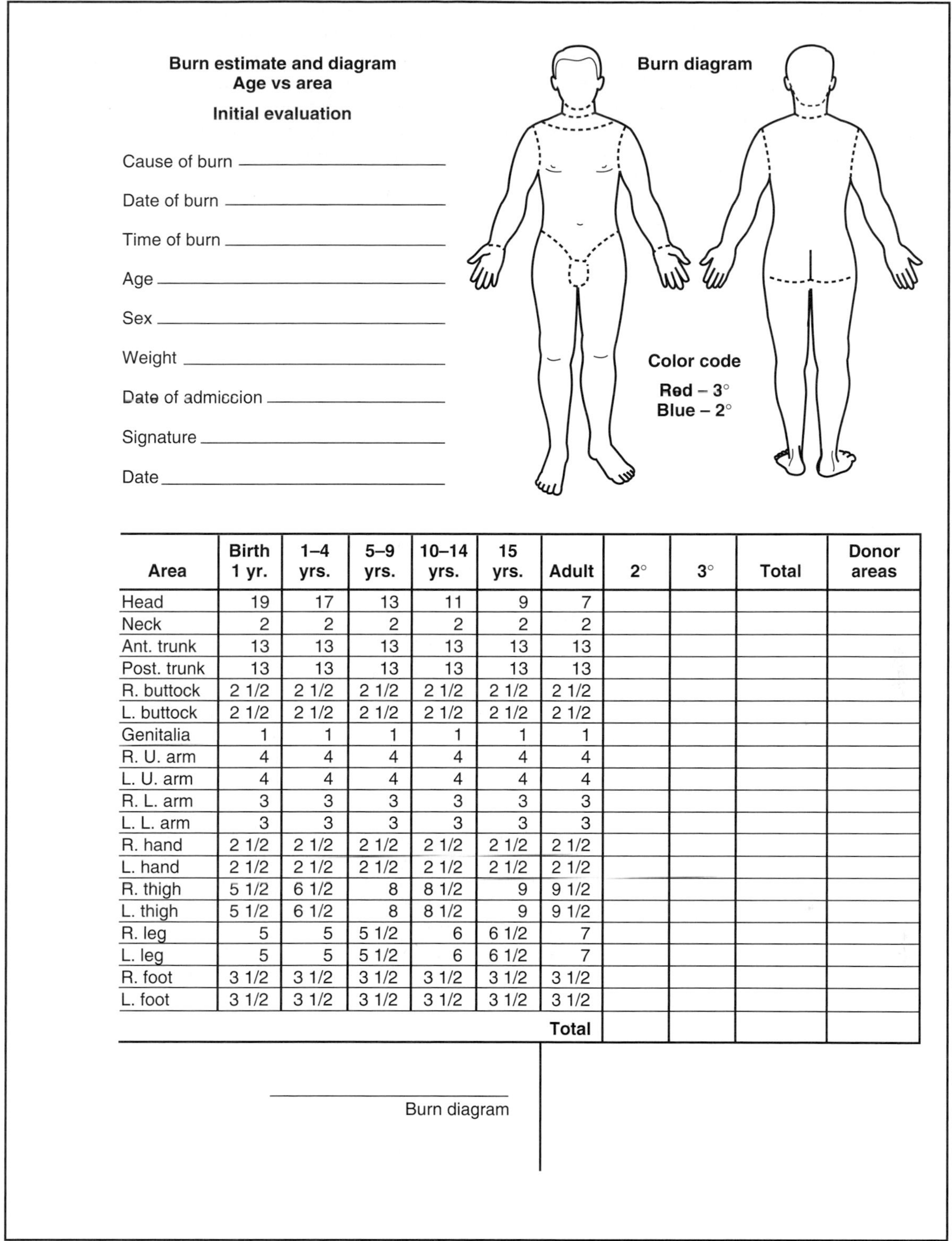

Burn estimate and diagram
Age vs area

Initial evaluation

Cause of burn ______

Date of burn ______

Time of burn ______

Age ______

Sex ______

Weight ______

Date of admiccion ______

Signature ______

Date ______

Area	Birth 1 yr.	1–4 yrs.	5–9 yrs.	10–14 yrs.	15 yrs.	Adult	2°	3°	Total	Donor areas
Head	19	17	13	11	9	7				
Neck	2	2	2	2	2	2				
Ant. trunk	13	13	13	13	13	13				
Post. trunk	13	13	13	13	13	13				
R. buttock	2 1/2	2 1/2	2 1/2	2 1/2	2 1/2	2 1/2				
L. buttock	2 1/2	2 1/2	2 1/2	2 1/2	2 1/2	2 1/2				
Genitalia	1	1	1	1	1	1				
R. U. arm	4	4	4	4	4	4				
L. U. arm	4	4	4	4	4	4				
R. L. arm	3	3	3	3	3	3				
L. L. arm	3	3	3	3	3	3				
R. hand	2 1/2	2 1/2	2 1/2	2 1/2	2 1/2	2 1/2				
L. hand	2 1/2	2 1/2	2 1/2	2 1/2	2 1/2	2 1/2				
R. thigh	5 1/2	6 1/2	8	8 1/2	9	9 1/2				
L. thigh	5 1/2	6 1/2	8	8 1/2	9	9 1/2				
R. leg	5	5	5 1/2	6	6 1/2	7				
L. leg	5	5	5 1/2	6	6 1/2	7				
R. foot	3 1/2	3 1/2	3 1/2	3 1/2	3 1/2	3 1/2				
L. foot	3 1/2	3 1/2	3 1/2	3 1/2	3 1/2	3 1/2				
						Total				

______
Burn diagram

■ **FIGURE 29–2.** Burn size estimate diagram, age versus area. (Redrawn from Lund CC, Browder NC: The estimation of areas of burns. *Surg Gynecol Obstet* 79:352–357, 1994; now *J Am Coll Surg.*)

heat dissipation in the upper airway, low heat capacity of air, and reflex closure of the larynx, superheated air usually causes thermal injury only to airway structures above the carina (Pruitt et al., 1979). Thermal injury to these airway structures may result in massive swelling of the tongue, epiglottis, or aryepiglottic folds with the resultant airway obstruction. These injuries are poorly tolerated, especially by infants and young children who have small airway size in absolute terms, high minute ventilation, and poorly developed respiratory muscles that fatigue easily (Keens et al., 1978). This scenario is further complicated by the possibility that the anatomic distortion caused by the massive swelling makes intubation very difficult. Because airway swelling develops over a matter of hours as fluid resuscitation is ongoing, the initial evaluation of the child might not provide a good indication of the severity of obstruction that may occur later. A high index of suspicion must be maintained and the child's respiratory

TABLE 29–2. Burn definitions

	Burn Classification
Minor	Superficial burns of less than 15% TBSA (total body surface area)
Moderate	• Superficial burns of 15–25% TBSA in adults • Superficial burns of 10–20% TBSA in children • Full-thickness burns of less than 10% TBSA and burns not involving the eyes, ears, face, hands, feet, or perineum
Major	• A second-degree burn greater than 25% TBSA • A third-degree burn greater than 10% TBSA • Any size burn with accompanying inhalation injury • Electrical burns • Any complicated burn injury, ie., patients with underlying disease, patients with burns to the eyes, ears, face, hands, feet, or perineum

As adapted from criteria of the American Burn Association and the American College of Surgeons Committee on Trauma.

Modified from De Campo T, Aldrete JA: The anesthetic management of the severely burned patient. *Intensive Care Med* 7:55, 1981.

status must be continuously monitored to assess the need for airway control and ventilator support. If the history and initial examination lead one to suspect significant thermal injury to the upper airway, intubation or tracheostomy for airway protection and possible ventilatory support should be considered early rather than later.

Inhalation Injury

In addition to the upper airway injury mentioned, the child with a burn may also have an inhalation injury. Inhalation injury is produced by the exposure of the lower respiratory tract to smoke, carbon monoxide, hydrogen cyanide, or, more commonly, a combination of these elements. A history of exposure to a closed space fire, loss of consciousness, and the presence of chemical irritants, along with a physical examination revealing carbonaceous sputum and singed nasal or facial hair, are all suggestive of inhalation injury. The presence of inhalation injury increases fluid requirements for resuscitation from burn shock by approximately 50% (Navar et al., 1985) and is a major source of mortality in burn patients (Thompson et al., 1986).

Smoke Inhalation

The chemical injury due to smoke inhalation occurs when toxic particles or gases are inhaled and damage small airways and alveoli. The combustion of most substances generates materials that are toxic to the respiratory tract. For example, burning rubber and plastic products produce sulfur dioxide, nitrogen dioxide, ammonia, and chlorine, which form strong acids or alkali when combined with water in the airways and alveoli. Glues in laminated furniture and wall paneling may release cyanide gas, which is rapidly absorbed. Burning cotton or wool produces aldehydes that precipitate pulmonary edema (Fein et al., 1980).

Almost all smoke-related toxins damage both airway epithelial and capillary endothelial cells. Histologic changes resemble those seen with tracheobronchitis. Mucociliary transport is destroyed, inhibiting the clearance of secretions, debris, and bacteria. The early inflammatory changes that occur in the airway are followed by a period of diffuse exudate formation (Herndon et al., 1986). Alveolar macrophages are damaged and produce chemotaxins, further enhancing the inflammatory response (Loke et al., 1984). Bronchiolar edema may become quite severe. The combination of the resulting necrotizing bronchitis, bronchial swelling, and bronchospasm results in obstruction of both large and small airways. Wheezing occurs as a result of bronchial swelling and irritant receptor stimulation. Alveolar collapse and atelectasis occur due to surfactant loss (Herndon et al., 1985). A generalized increase in capillary permeability aggravates airway and pulmonary edema.

The end result of smoke inhalation is pulmonary failure occurring 12 to 48 hours after the smoke exposure and is due to a decrease in lung compliance, an increase in airway and tissue resistance, an increase in ventilation/perfusion mismatch, and an increase in dead space ventilation. In several days, the injury may progress to sloughing of airway mucosa and intrapulmonary hemorrhage, which may result in mechanical obstruction of the lower airways and flooding of the alveoli. Air trapping, occurring distal to airway obstruction, may result in volutrauma and ventilator-induced lung injury. Due to ulceration and extensive necrosis of the respiratory epithelium, children with an inhalation injury may be predisposed to secondary bacterial invasion and subsequent development of a superimposed bacterial pneumonia several days after injury (Pruitt et al., 1975; Boutros and Hoyt, 1976; Rue et al., 1993). Although treatment is mainly supportive with mechanical ventilation, inhaled bronchodilators and mechanical methods of enhancing clearance of debris from the lower airways may be beneficial. If the child survives, pulmonary function may not return to normal for several months (Madden et al., 1986).

Carbon Monoxide/Cyanide Poisoning

Carbon monoxide is an odorless, tasteless, nonirritating gas that is a product of incomplete combustion. Children exposed to a closed-space fire have a high likelihood of carbon monoxide poisoning even if they have no thermal burns. Carbon monoxide levels may exceed 10% in a closed space with a fire; significant injury may occur in a short period of time with exposure to as little as 1% (Fig. 29–3). Carbon monoxide poisoning is a major source of early morbidity in the burned child, with many fatalities occurring at the scene of the fire (Trunkey, 1978). With an affinity for hemoglobin 200 times greater than that for oxygen, carbon monoxide effectively competes with oxygen for hemoglobin binding. This not only shifts the oxyhemoglobin dissociation curve to the left but also alters its shape. Oxygen delivery to tissues is severely compromised due to both the reduced oxygen-carrying capacity of blood and the less efficient dissociation of oxygen from hemoglobin at the tissue level (Fig. 29–4). In addition, carbon monoxide competitively inhibits intracellular cytochrome oxidase enzyme systems, most notably cytochrome P-450, resulting in an inability of cellular systems to utilize oxygen (Goldbaum et al., 1976). Inhaled hydrogen cyanide, which is produced during the combustion of numerous household materials, also affects the cytochrome oxidase system and thus may have a synergistic effect with carbon monoxide, producing an increase in tissue hypoxia and acidosis as well as a decrease in cerebral oxygen consumption and metabolism (Moore et al., 1991).

Carbon monoxide poisoning may be difficult to detect. The absorbance spectra of carboxyhemoglobin and oxyhemoglobin are very similar. Pulse oximeters cannot distinguish between the two forms of hemoglobin, and oximeter readings are normal even when lethal amounts of carboxyhemoglobin are present. A PaO_2 obtained from an arterial blood gas measures the amount of oxygen dissolved in the plasma but does not quantitate

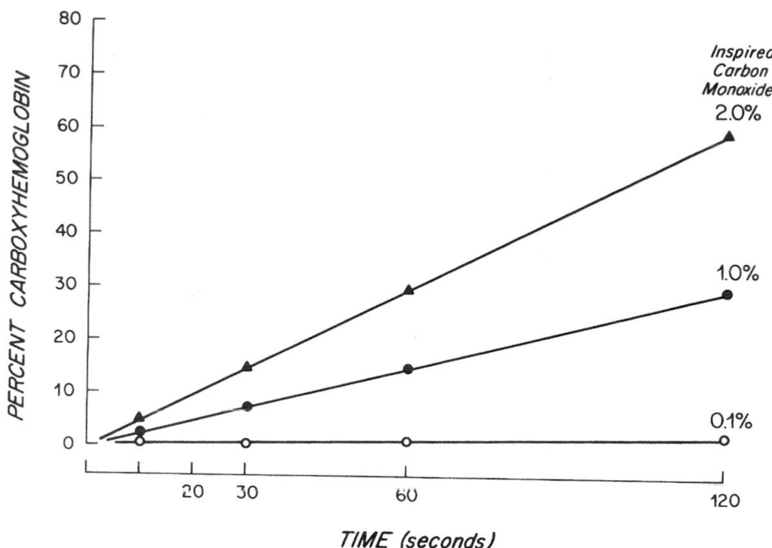

■ **FIGURE 29–3.** Hemoglobin is rapidly converted to carboxyhemoglobin in the presence of carbon monoxide. (Modified from Stewart RD, Stewart RS, Stamm W, et al.: Rapid estimation of carboxyhemoglobin level in fire fighters. *JAMA* 235:390, 1976.)

hemoglobin saturation, which is the true measure of the oxygen-carrying capacity of the blood. Carboxyhemoglobin levels may be measured directly, but this test is rarely available at the scene. Due to the inevitable time delay between exposure and testing, levels measured on arrival at a health care facility do not reflect the true extent of poisoning, especially when the child has been breathing high concentrations of oxygen.

The half-life of carboxyhemoglobin is 250 minutes for the victim breathing room air; this is reduced to 40 to 60 minutes with the inhalation of 100% oxygen (Crapo, 1981). Any child suspected of carbon monoxide exposure should receive high levels of oxygen until carbon monoxide poisoning has been ruled out. If the patient is unconscious or cyanotic, intubation for the administration of high oxygen concentrations is indicated.

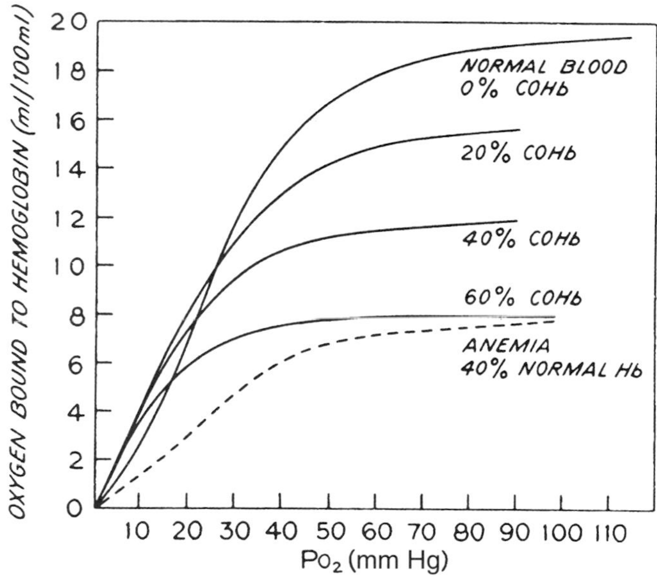

■ **FIGURE 29–4.** Carboxyhemoglobin-induced changes in the oxygen-hemoglobin dissociation curve. (From Fein A, Leff A, Hopewell PC: Pathophysiology and management of the complications resulting from fire and the inhaled products of combustion: review of the literature. *Crit Care Med* 8:94, 1980.)

While hyperbaric oxygenation further reduces the half-life of carboxyhemoglobin, the hyperbaric chamber is a difficult environment in which to monitor the patient and to perform fluid resuscitation and early burn care such as escharotomies and dressing changes. It is the opinion of most burn experts that hyperbaric oxygen treatment should be reserved for the child with minimal to no cutaneous burns or other injuries (Grube et al., 1988).

Additional External Factors

Circumferential burns of the chest may cause a mechanical restrictive effect and further compromise ventilation. Escharotomies in the anterior axillary lines, in conjunction with appropriately placed transverse escharotomies, may allow some patients to avoid mechanical ventilation.

BURN SHOCK AND HEMODYNAMIC DERANGEMENTS

Proper fluid management is critical to the survival of the child with a major burn. Although we have a better understanding of the massive fluid shifts and vascular changes that occur during burn shock than in the past, inadequate fluid resuscitation remains one of the most common causes of death within the first 10 days after burn injury (Artz and Moncrief, 1969). Further complicating the alterations in fluid homeostasis, children with major burns commonly exhibit systemic inflammatory response syndrome (SIRS), which ranges in severity from the presence of tachycardia, tachypnea, fever, and leukocytosis to refractory hypotension and, in its most severe form, shock and multiple organ dysfunction syndrome (MODS). Table 29–3 summarizes the systemic effects of burn injury (Szyfelbein et al., 1993).

Proinflammatory cytokines, chemokines, and noncytokine inflammatory mediators all play a role in the pathophysiology of SIRS and MODS. Tumor necrosis factor-α (TNFα), which is released from macrophages in response to local or systemic injury, is a classic mediator of systemic inflammation, and modulates a variety of immunologic and metabolic events (Spooner et al., 1992). The release of TNFα activates antimicrobial defense mechanisms and tissue repair, but paradoxically it may begin a sequence of events leading to tissue injury, organ dysfunction, and even apoptosis in a variety of cell types (Voss and Cotton, 1998).

■ **TABLE 29–3.** Systemic effects of burn injury

System	Early	Late
Cardiovascular	↓ CO due to decreased circulating blood volume, myocardial depressant factor	↑ CO due to sepsis ↑ CO 2 to 3 times > baseline for months (hypermetabolism) Hypertension
Pulmonary	Upper airway obstruction due to edema Lower airway obstruction due to edema, bronchospasm, particulate matter ↓ FRC ↓ Pulmonary compliance ↓ Chest wall compliance	Bronchopneumonia Tracheal stenosis ↓ Chest wall compliance
Renal	↓ GFR (a) Secondary to ↓ circulating blood volume (b) Myoglobinuria (c) Hemoglobinuria Tubular dysfunction	↑ GFR secondary to ↑ CO Tubular dysfunction
Hepatic	↓ Function due to ↓ circulating blood volume, hypoxia, hepatotoxins	Hepatitis ↑ Function due to hypermetabolism, enzyme induction, ↑ CO ↓ Function due to sepsis, drug interaction
Hematopoietic	↓ Red blood cell mass ↓ Platelets ↑ Fibrin split products, consumptive coagulopathy, anemia	↑ Platelets ↑ Clotting factors Possible AIDS, hepatitis
Neurologic	Encephalopathy Seizures ↑ ICP	Encephalopathy Seizures ICU psychosis
Skin	↑ Heat, fluid, electrolyte loss	Contractures, scar formation
Metabolic	↓ Ionized calcium	↑ Oxygen consumption ↑ Carbon dioxide production ↓ Ionized calcium
Pharmacokinetics	Altered volume of distribution Altered protein binding Altered pharmacokinetics Altered pharmacodynamics	↑ Tolerance to narcotics, sedatives Enzyme induction, altered receptors Drug interaction

↓, Decrease in; ↑, increase in; AIDS, acquired immunodeficiency syndrome; CO, cardiac output; FRC, functional residual capacity; GFR, glomerular filtration rate; ICP, intracranial pressure; ICU, intensive care unit.

Reproduced with permission from Szyfelbein SK, Martyn JA, Coté CJ: Burn injuries. In Coté CJ, Ryan JF, Todre ID, Goudsouzian NG, editors: *A practice of anesthesia for infants and children,* 2nd ed. Philadelphia, 1993, WB Saunders Co.

In addition, TNFα leads to the release of other mediators such as interleukins (IL-1, IL-6, and others) and interferon γ (IFNγ). Interleukins potentiate the destructive effects of TNFα and elevated levels may be predictive of a poor outcome (Van der Poll and van Deventer, 1999). IFNγ stimulates cytokine secretion, phagocytosis, and the respiratory burst activity of macrophages, thus amplifying the inflammatory response (Tominaga et al., 2000). Chemokines, such as IL-8, function as chemoattractants for leukocytes and play a role in tissue destruction (Laffon et al., 1999). Nuclear factor-κB (NFκB) is a transcription factor that may regulate many of the previously mentioned factors through transcription of a number of cytokine, chemokine, adhesion molecule, and enzyme genes leading to the clinical manifestation of SIRS. NFκB may be associated with poor outcome in patients with sepsis (Bohrer et al., 1997). It has been demonstrated that NFκB plays a key role in the molecular and cellular events leading to acid-induced lung injury (Madjdpour et al., 2003); a similar role in SIRS can be hypothesized. Noncytokine factors, such as platelet activation factor, eicosanoids, leukotrienes, and thromboxane A_2, also play a role in SIRS and MODS. Additionally, complement activation causes leukocyte attraction and activation, leading to cellular destruction through the release of reactive oxygen intermediates and proteases (Czermak et al., 1999). This hyperactive inflammatory response, with its numerous and complex interacting mediators, results in alterations of cardiovascular, metabolic, gastrointestinal, and coagulation systems. (A more detailed discussion of the subject is beyond the scope of this text.)

Burn shock is a combination of hypovolemic and cellular shock and is characterized by changes that include decreases in cardiac output and plasma volume resulting in decreased blood flow to major organs. In burn shock, resuscitation is complicated by massive transvascular fluid shifts that are unique to thermal trauma (Warden, 2002). Fluid requirements are initially increased due to a marked increase in vascular permeability in the area of the burn; however, this increased permeability becomes generalized in a patient with burns of greater than 30% of the body surface area (Moncrief, 1973). Edema occurs due to local thermally induced changes in the microcirculation and an increase in total body capillary permeability. The failure of semipermeable membranes leads to tremendous loss of fluids, electrolytes, and plasma proteins from the intravascular space. Maximum edema formation occurs from 8 to 24 hours after the burn, and the progression of edema is dependent on the adequacy of resuscitation. As in other types of shock, the primary goal is to restore and preserve tissue perfusion in order to avoid ischemia. Inadequate resuscitation results in severe depletion of plasma volume, which in turn increases morbidity and mortality due to adverse effects on cardiac output, renal function, and perfusion of burn wounds.

Children who are inadequately resuscitated from burn shock may not be able to increase their cardiac output to the extent needed to maintain arterial pressure in the face of excessive vasodilation and therefore exhibit signs of hypotension and shock. These patients may demonstrate a reduced vascular responsiveness to vasoconstrictors. It has been hypothesized that the presence of endotoxin or bacteria in the blood plays a role in this clinical picture (Traber et al., 1988). Proinflammatory cytokines, chemokines, noncytokine inflammatory mediators, and vasoactive substances with potentially deleterious effects are released from burned tissue, including vasoconstricting and vasodilating prostaglandins, kinins, serotonin, histamine, oxygen radicals, and lipid peroxidases (Demling, 1985). Administration of adequate volumes of fluid, during resuscitation as well as in the operating room, is of paramount importance.

Once adequate fluid resuscitation has been completed, the clinical picture of the burned child is that of a patient with a hyperdynamic circulation characterized by low systemic vascular resistance and high cardiac output. Blood flow to all major organs is increased (Wilmore et al., 1980). The degree of increase in cardiac output is a function of wound size. As the child stabilizes in the early postburn shock period, sustained hypertension is frequently present, probably mediated by renin, antidiuretic hormone (ADH), or catecholamines (Falkner et al., 1978).

HEMATOLOGIC DERANGEMENTS

A major burn also causes significant hematologic derangements in a characteristic biphasic response. Initial anemia is due to erythrocyte loss, the degree of which is proportional to the burn size. The loss occurs due to a number of etiologies. Red blood cell destruction occurs as a direct result of the burn injury and due to loss into capillary thrombi, which are produced through burn activation of the complement and coagulation cascades. Burn injury also induces alterations in the erythrocytes, via release of oxygen free radicals and proteases, which lead to their destruction (Heatherill et al., 1986). Red cell loss may approach 20% in the first 24 hours after a major burn and may continue at a rate of 1% to 2% per day until the wounds are grafted (Deitch and Sittig, 1993). If an increase in hemoglobin is observed during burn resuscitation, this is due to hemoconcentration and is an indication for an increase in fluid administration. During recovery from burn injury, anemia is due to a decrease in production of red cells. Erythropoietin levels are elevated, but the bone marrow remains hyporesponsive, possibly due to high circulating levels of various cytokines and other inflammatory mediators (Jelkmann et al., 1990).

Thrombocytopenia occurs early after burn injury due to increased platelet aggregation, consumption during the formation of microemboli, and dilution during fluid resuscitation (Lawrence and Atac, 1992). At 10 to 14 days postinjury, an increase in platelet count occurs, which may last several months (Heideman, 1979).

Burn patients experience activation of both the thrombotic and fibrinolytic pathways. This may increase the likelihood of disseminated intravascular coagulation (DIC) early in the course of patients with major burns (Kowal-Vern et al., 1992). As the child recovers from burn injury, factors V, VII, and VIII and fibrinogen may be elevated for several months; however, the child does not become hypercoagulable (Simon et al., 1977).

METABOLIC AND NUTRITIONAL DERANGEMENTS

The metabolic consequences of major burn injury in a child are profound and constitute a major challenge to effective treatment. Metabolic rates of children with burns can be twice normal and three to four times that of an unburned adult. Catabolic activity and nitrogen losses are greater than are seen with any other catastrophic illness (Wilmore and Aulick, 1978). Elevated levels of epinephrine and norepinephrine are present for a prolonged period after burn injury. Derangements in other hormones such as glucagon, glucocorticoids, growth hormone, and thyroid hormone are also present (Wilmore et al., 1974). Manifestations of hypermetabolism include persistent hyperpyrexia, tachycardia, hyperpnea, body wasting, increased oxygen consumption, and increased carbon dioxide production. The degree of hypermetabolism correlates with burn size. Protein catabolism, ureagenesis, lipolysis, accelerated gluconeogenesis, skeletal muscle proteolysis, elevated free fatty acids, glycogen mobilization, insulin resistance, and glucose intolerance are all indicators of the hypermetabolic state (De Campo and Aldrete, 1981).

RENAL DERANGEMENTS

The renal function of a child with a major burn may be impaired due to hypovolemia, hypotension, hypoxemia, myoglobinuria, hemoglobinuria, or a combination. Oliguria during burn resuscitation is due to a decrease in renal blood flow (Aikawa et al., 1990). Inadequate resuscitation early in burn shock exacerbates renal damage; fluid therapy should be directed toward the maintenance of 0.5 to 1.0 mL/kg per hr of urine output. Stress-induced elevation of serum glucose levels may cause an osmotic diuresis even in the face of hypovolemia; adequate urine output may give the false impression that renal blood flow is adequate as well. Children with burns of greater than 40% of the total body surface area (TBSA) may have tubular dysfunction as evidenced by an inadequate renal response to ADH and aldosterone (Moncrief and Teplitz, 1964).

The renal system may be further compromised by other factors. High levels of stress hormones and impairment of atrial natriuretic polypeptide secretion may contribute to reduced renal function (Aikawa et al., 1990). The kidneys may be exposed to nephrotoxic antibiotics as well as other nephrotoxins such as free hemoglobin (Sawada et al., 1984). Most cases of renal failure occur 5 days or more after burn injury; four fifths of these patients have inhalation injury as well (Holm et al., 1999). Even after the completion of resuscitation from burn shock, the pharmacology of drugs excreted by the kidney may be altered in an unpredictable fashion (Loirat et al., 1978).

HEPATIC DERANGEMENTS

Like the kidneys, the liver of the child with a major burn may experience insults due to hypovolemia, hypotension, hypoxemia, inflammation, or a combination. Other potential insults include drug toxicity, sepsis, and infection due to exposure to multiple blood products. Liver damage may be manifest by hepatic edema and release of hepatic enzymes (Jeschke et al., 2001). Liver injury may be due to hypoperfusion as well as insult from inflammatory cytokines such as IL-1 and TNFα (Jeschke et al., 1999).

In the early stages of burn resuscitation hepatic blood flow is decreased; once burn shock has resolved, the child enters the hypermetabolic phase and liver blood flow increases along with an increase in the metabolism of glucose and fats. The increased hepatic flow increases drug delivery to the liver (Martyn, 1986); protein binding may be altered, so pharmacokinetics of various drugs may be altered in an unpredictable fashion (Wilmore et al., 1980). Hepatic protein synthesis shifts from constitutive proteins such as albumin, prealbumin, and transferrin to acute phase proteins (Jeschke et al., 2001); albumin falls to critically low levels during the acute phase. In most cases, liver function returns to normal within 1 week of burn injury unless further insults occur.

PHARMACOLOGIC CONSIDERATIONS IN THE BURN PATIENT

Burns involving more than 10% to 15% of the TBSA in patients give rise to a cascade of systemic and localized physiologic responses (Demling, 1984, 1985). These responses include alterations in metabolic rate and cardiac output, alterations in fluid compartments, glomerular filtration, hepatic perfusion, reduction in serum albumin levels, and increases in α_1-acid glycoproteins. The greater the magnitude of the burn, the more profound are these changes. The response to medication in any patient may be unpredictable, but this is especially true in major burn patients and thus it is necessary to titrate to effect any and all medications given. This subject has been well reviewed (Martyn, 1986).

There are multiple other factors that may interact to alter pharmacokinetics. These may include sepsis, other drugs that may induce or inhibit metabolic pathways, drugs that are hepatotoxic or nephrotoxic, malnutrition, and parenteral nutrition. In addition, there may be burn-induced hepatic, renal, and pulmonary dysfunction.

In the early or acute stage of burn injury, known as the resuscitative phase, blood flow is decreased to organs and tissue for several reasons, including increased blood viscosity, hypovolemia, and decreased cardiac function secondary to circulating proinflammatory and vasoactive substances. Especially in this phase, only the intravenous route of medication administration should be used, titrating the desired effect of the medication with small repetitive doses. Subcutaneous and intramuscular routes of administration should be avoided due to variable uptake.

In the second stage of burn injury, known as the hypermetabolic phase, hypermetabolism and increased blood flow to all major organs are predominant (Wilmore et al., 1980). In this phase, it is not clear if drug metabolism is increased (Martyn, 1986). Many drugs are bound to plasma proteins, albumin for acidic drugs, and α_1-acid glycoproteins for basic drugs; binding to other proteins occurs to a much smaller extent. This binding is usually reversible and drugs compete with one another for binding sites. Examples of drugs bound to proteins include benzodiazepines and antiepileptics, which are acidic and when bound to albumin have an increased free component in the acute stages, and basic drugs such as tricyclic antidepressants and neuromuscular relaxants, which bind to α_1-acid glycoprotein and have a decreased free component in this phase (Martyn et al., 1984). In most instances, increased protein-binding leads to a decreased volume of distribution for any given drug (Stanski and Watkins, 1982).

MUSCLE RELAXANTS

Because of the well-known response of hyperkalemia with the use of succinylcholine in the burn patient (Gronert and Theye, 1975; Tolmie et al., 1967) and the controversy over when this response becomes manifest (MacLennan et al., 1998; Gronert, 1999; Martyn, 1999) this drug should not be stocked in any operating room in which a burn patient is to have surgery. The onset of hyperkalemia is as early as 24 to 48 hours after injury and may continue for up to 2 years after the burn injury

TABLE 29–4. Emergency department values of vecuronium in burn patients and control patients

Study Group (% TBSA burn)	ED_{50} (mcg/kg)	ED_{95} (mcg/kg)
Controls	17.6 (15.4–19.9)	35.3 (30.6–42.3)
<40	34.0* (29.3–38.7)	68.2* (59.8–79.9)
40–60	55.4* (48.1–62.1)	111.1* (99.8–126.2)
>60	64.5* (57.4–71.9)	129.4* (113.0–154.0)

Numbers in parentheses represent lower and upper 95% confidence limits.
TBSA, total body surface area.
*Significantly different from controls, $P<0.01$.
The effective doses for 50% and 95% twitch suppression (ED_{50} and ED_{95}) for vecuronium are significantly increased in burned children compared with controls. The shift in the dose response curve is related to the magnitude of burn.
From Mills AK, Martyn JA: Neuromuscular blockade with vecuronium in paediatric patients with burn injury. *Br J Clin Pharm* 28:155, 1989.

(Martyn et al., 1982). Although the duration of the hyperkalemic response is controversial, it can easily be avoided with the use of fairly rapid-onset nondepolarizing agents.

As noted, the increased levels of α_1-acid glycoprotein leads to lower free fractions of muscle relaxants in the plasma. Resistance to atracurium (Dwersteg et al., 1986), vecuronium (Mills and Martyn, 1989), curare (Martyn et al., 1980), and pancuronium (Martyn et al., 1983) has been demonstrated. Table 29–4 demonstrates this very well using vecuronium as an example (Mills and Martyn, 1989). A major reason may also be the increased number of receptors on the muscle membranes (Martyn et al., 1980). Most experts believe that altered pharmacokinetics and increased plasma protein binding contribute little to the phenomenon (Leibel et al., 1981; Martyn et al., 1982). The larger the burn, the more this effect is noted. The effect is noted beginning about the sixth day, peaks at days 15 to 40, and has decreased by day 70 after the burn; however, some resistance may be seen at 500 days after the burn (Dwersteg et al., 1986; Martyn et al., 1982). As an example, patients with burns of 50% to 60% may require doses 2.5 to 5 times that in nonburned patients. Interestingly, despite the large doses used, the serum half-life is unchanged and the reversal of nondepolarizing muscle relaxants using the usual drugs is accomplished without a problem.

ANALGESICS

Pain control in burn patients is a major issue that in the past has received little attention in the literature. In many instances, pain control has been woefully neglected, especially in children who are too young to speak or are intubated and cannot speak. Concerns with possible addiction or the impaired drug elimination in these patients are some of the reasons given for this and leads to severe undermedication. In a survey of multiple burn centers, no cases of such addiction have been discovered (Perry and Heidrich, 1982).

It is a well-known phenomenon with practitioners who routinely work with burn patients that the opioid requirements for pain relief are often increased. This may be due to changes in pharmacokinetic and pharmacodynamic factors. Tolerance to opioids develops quickly, but addiction develops very rarely in patients treated with opioids for pain relief (Porter and Hick, 1980). Withdrawal is usually not a problem in that opioids are gradually tapered as the healing takes place and the number of procedures is reduced.

The main drugs in the armamentarium for pain management remain morphine and fentanyl. A continuous infusion of morphine for pain control is preferred when necessary, and fentanyl is usually used only intraoperatively. Although remifentanil is an excellent agent with fast awakening, the painful procedures that many burn patients undergo make this agent less than ideal.

ANXIOLYTICS

Sedatives and anxiolytics are often administered to burn patients, especially those on ventilators. In burn patients given a single dose of diazepam, there is a rapid fall in drug concentration in the plasma and the therapeutic effect is short lived. This is due to the rapid uptake of the drug by the tissue and the high lipid solubility of the medication (Greenblatt et al., 1983). In those patients on diazepam for prolonged periods, high levels of parent drug have been found in the plasma for up to 2 weeks after the last dose. Active metabolites were found after an even longer period (Martyn et al., 1983). Lorazepam may be better used in burn patients due to its alternate metabolic pathway and due to the fact that the clearance is unimpaired even in the face of altered volume of distribution (Greenblatt et al., 1983).

ANESTHETICS

Inhaled Anesthetics

Halothane is and has been used extensively in many pediatric burn centers. It is often switched to isoflurane for the maintenance phase, especially in older children and adolescents. The newer anesthetics, including sevoflurane, have not played a major role, other than being used for a "smoother and faster" induction. In the same way that inductions are faster, awakening is equally as rapid. In many burn cases a slower emergence is preferred. The same can be said about the use of remifentanil. Both of these agents are excellent when one wants a rapid onset and an early awakening. However, due to the residual pain involved in acute burn surgery, the residual effects of the older inhalation agents and the lingering effects of morphine and even fentanyl are of some benefit. Although sevoflurane and remifentanil certainly may have a place during the reconstructive phase of burn anesthesia and surgery, they have not become important agents in the burn unit. There is little in the literature that promotes these agents or techniques for use in the acute phase of burn anesthesia.

Multiple administrations of halothane have not led to profound liver dysfunction (Gronert et al., 1967) or to an increased risk of halothane hepatitis in this population (Martyn, 1986). If indeed halothane hepatitis is due to an allergic phenomenon, the anergic state of the burn patient may in part be responsible for its absence.

Most inhalation agents have been clinically studied in the burn patient, but there are little data concerning uptake, distribution, and elimination (Martyn, 1986). Further discussion of these agents is given in the anesthetic management section.

Ketamine

There is a large body of literature documenting the use of ketamine in burn patients as both an induction agent and one used for the maintenance of anesthesia. Ketamine is well known for its cardiovascular stimulating properties, its analgesic effects, and its versatility (Slogoff et al., 1974). Tolerance may be exhibited (White et al., 1982), and high doses may prolong awakening in some patients. Dosing, as stated for all drugs in the burn patient, must be individualized. Side effects may be the same as in nonburned patients and, when used, may cause hallucinations and other untoward effects. These effects may be minimized by a small dose of benzodiazepine preceding the ketamine. It should also be mentioned that ketamine in the volume-depleted patient may cause hypotension.

RESUSCITATION AND INITIAL MANAGEMENT OF THE BURN PATIENT

AIRWAY AND VENTILATORY MANAGEMENT

As with any severely injured child, airway management is of utmost importance in the child with a major burn. Initial assessment should include a brief but directed history and physical examination. The history should focus on the mechanism of injury and underlying risk factors. Salient points include exposure to smoke in a closed space (i.e., car, house, or trailer fire), loss of consciousness at the scene with the resultant loss of protective airway reflexes, and a history of reactive airway disease, bronchitis, or other chronic diseases of the airways.

Physical examination of the child with an acute burn should focus on assessment of the risk of airway obstruction, respiratory failure, or both and the need for early establishment of an artificial airway. A child with an inhalation injury may develop massive swelling of the airway within a matter of hours after the injury as fluid resuscitation contributes to edema formation in thermally injured tissues of the upper airway. The extent of airway edema correlates with the body surface area burned. Not only does edema have the potential to cause mechanical obstruction of the supraglottic airway (see section on pathophysiology), it also makes endotracheal intubation extraordinarily difficult. Clinical suspicion of inhalation injury should be aroused by the above-mentioned risk factors in the history, as well as clinical features such as burns of the face and neck, singed nasal hairs, carbonaceous sputum, and hoarseness. Fiberoptic bronchoscopy may contribute to the diagnosis (Hunt et al., 1975) but should not take the place of clinical judgment. Blood gases may be normal for the first few hours after injury and thus may not be helpful, especially before fluid resuscitation is complete. Intubation and mechanical ventilation may also be indicated in a child with carbon monoxide poisoning and depressed airway reflexes, even without thermal injury.

Some authors believe that intubation of an inflamed airway increases the risk of damage to the larynx (Colice et al., 1986). Not every child with a face burn requires intubation; as mentioned, a delay in establishing an airway may result in a much more difficult scenario several hours later. The risk of losing an airway is much greater in attempting intubation after airway edema has resulted in severe distortion of airway structures, as in a child with acute epiglottitis. Although fiberoptic intubation figures prominently in the American Society of Anesthesiologists' difficult airway algorithm, if intubation of the burned child is delayed to the point where airway edema has developed to any significant degree, use of a fiberoptic technique is not helpful, as airway edema and secretions immediately obscure the endoscopic view.

Direct laryngoscopy with a rigid blade allows for mechanical displacement of edematous tissues and affords the best possible view of the airway. These children should not be given muscle relaxants as their use is likely to lead to a "cannot intubate, cannot ventilate" situation. Awake intubation is not a viable option in most children, including those with burns.

Judicious administration of intravenous ketamine (1 to 1.5 mg/kg) allows one to sedate the child while maintaining spontaneous ventilation. Whether airway reflexes are maintained with ketamine is subject to debate; however, aspiration has not been reported as a problem during early airway management of burned children. Because the airway obstruction is the result of supraglottic edema, the laryngeal mask airway (LMA) may in theory provide a useful temporary airway until intubation or a surgical airway is accomplished. The use of the LMA in this situation has not been reported in the literature.

If intubation is predicted to be or proves to be impossible, a tracheostomy may be considered. In the past, authors have stated that a tracheostomy in a child with a burned airway was associated with a mortality of close to 100% (Eckhauser et al., 1974). Later studies have refuted this statement (Palmieri et al., 2002; Saffle et al., 2002) and proved that tracheostomy is safe and may actually improve patient comfort. A tracheostomy is the airway of choice for a child with deep burns of the lower face, where an endotracheal tube would complicate skin grafting, and for patients who are anticipated to require greater than 2 to 3 weeks of mechanical ventilation.

FLUIDS

Many have debated the most appropriate type of fluid for resuscitation of the patient in burn shock; however, the adequacy of volume of fluid and replacement of extracellular salt lost into the burned tissue are the most reliable predictors of successful resuscitation (Neely et al., 1988). Crystalloid, in particular lactated Ringer's solution and Normosol, are the most popular resuscitation fluids currently used (Warden, 2002). The modified Parkland formula recommends 4 mL/kg per percent burn in the first 24 hours with one half administered in the first 8 hours. To this amount is added to 1500 mL/m^2 to account for normal maintenance (Merrell et al., 1986). Studies indicate that hypertonic saline may be beneficial in modulating the inflammatory cascade and restoring hemodynamic parameters and microcirculatory flow (Junger et al., 1997).

It is important to realize that regardless of the resuscitation formula and fluid that are used, these formulas are only guidelines and provide a starting point. Rates of fluid administration should be titrated to maintain a urine output of 1 mL/kg per hr. Central venous pressures may also be useful in guiding fluid therapy, providing the tip of the catheter is properly placed in the central circulation. Femoral catheters are usually too short to reach the level of the diaphragm and therefore do not adequately reflect true right heart filling pressures. Once resuscitation is complete, fluids can be decreased to a maintenance rate that takes into account the burn size and extra evaporative losses that are expected (Warden, 2002). Using the following formula, daily maintenance fluids (in milliliters per 24 hours) can be calculated:

$$[(\%\ \text{TBSA burned} + 35) \times \text{body surface area } (\text{m}^2) \times 24] + 1500\ \text{mL/m}^2$$

As with resuscitation fluids, it must be remembered that formulas only provide a starting point; the actual rate of fluid administration must be dictated by patient response (i.e., urine output). The importance of maintaining a normal circulating blood volume cannot be overemphasized.

EARLY NUTRITION AND METABOLIC NEEDS

The child with a major burn, even if he or she is able to eat, rarely is able to consume an adequate number of calories. Despite the ileus, which is almost universally present in the first few days after a major burn, it has been demonstrated that enteral feedings can be started safely within hours of burn injury. Early enteral feeding improves nitrogen balance and overall nutrition (McDonald et al., 1991) and reduces the incidence of stress ulceration (Demling, 1985). Tube feedings administered through nasal jejunal tubes do not need to be stopped before surgery but can be continued throughout the perioperative period without increased risk of aspiration or other complications (Jenkins et al., 1994). This reduces interruptions in feedings and therefore ensures adequate nutrition for patients undergoing multiple procedures and may also reduce infectious complications.

Failure to recognize and satisfy these exaggerated metabolic needs results in impaired wound healing, cellular dysfunction, and decreased resistance to infection. Environmental stress adds significantly to metabolic rate. Maintaining a high ambient temperature and humidity may reduce caloric requirements by up to 20% (Wilmore et al., 1974) and should be a standard of care in all burn centers as well as in the operating room. In addition, whether inside or outside the hospital, meticulous attention must be paid to the maintenance of normothermia during transport of the burned child. Metabolic needs do not return to normal until all burn wounds are covered and healed.

ESCHAROTOMIES

Burned tissue becomes inelastic. If a patient has a circumferential burn, the inelastic eschar will not expand to accommodate the inevitable tissue swelling occurring beneath it and tissue pressures increase. If the circumferential burn involves a limb, a compartment syndrome may develop. If the chest is involved, a restrictive pattern of ventilatory failure may develop. If the abdomen is involved, elevated intra-abdominal pressures may result in an intra-abdominal compartment syndrome, leading to a decrease in venous return, a decrease in urine output, and respiratory failure. With any of these scenarios, urgent escharotomies are required (Figs. 29–5 and 29–6). This can be accomplished in the operating room, or often more readily at the bedside using ketamine for sedation and analgesia. If electrocautery is used to perform the procedure, blood loss is usually minimal.

ASSOCIATED INJURIES

When caring for the child with a major burn, associated injuries are easily overlooked. Although management of the child's airway and volume status is a top priority, other injuries should be sought if a history of trauma is elicited, such as burns associated with a motor vehicle accident or a fall from a burning building. Long bone fractures, closed head injury, skull fracture, and intra-abdominal hemorrhage may complicate burn injury. In the older child and teenager, the presence of alcohol or illicit drugs may complicate management. A rapid yet thorough physical examination accompanied by a focused history should help to elucidate any additional injuries.

SPECIAL CONSIDERATIONS FOR ELECTRICAL BURNS

Electrical burns are truly a unique form of thermal injury. They may be classified into low voltage (≤400 V) and high voltage (>1000 V) injuries. Low voltage injuries are commonly seen in home settings, and high voltage injuries in industrial settings (Warden, 2003).

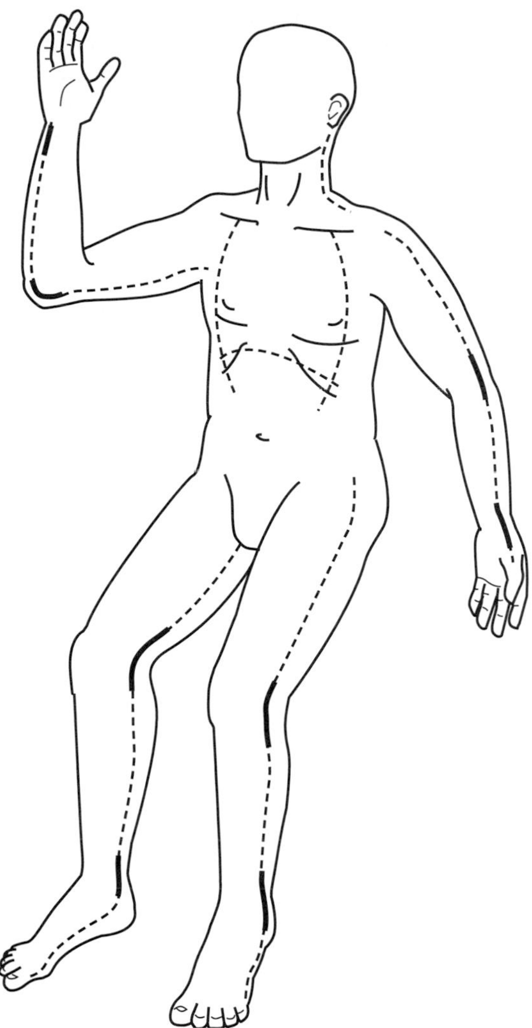

■ **FIGURE 29–5.** Escharotomy sites. (Redrawn from Pruitt BA, Dowling JA, Moncrief JA: Escharotomy in early burn care. *Arch Surg* 96:502, 1968.)

One type of injury is a purely contact burn in which there is no true entrance or exit wound. They are usually full-thickness burns due to prolonged contact with the element. They are treated as a true thermal burn, are usually caused by low voltage contact, and are of a limited extent. Of these, the most devastating are probably those in small children who bite an electric cord, causing injury to either one or both of the commissures of the mouth.

Another type is the electrical flash. These are not truly burns but rather injury due to an electrical discharge. They also may be treated as though a thermal burn.

The most devastating type of electrical burn is caused by high-voltage injuries. These injuries result from true electrical damage to a vast area of tissues and organs, including the heart, respiratory system, circulatory system, central nervous system, peripheral nervous tissue, eyes, kidney, and the integument and bones. The visible injury may be only the tip of the iceberg, with the major injury being to the underlying structures.

Lightning strikes remain a significant problem to the population, causing approximately 1320 deaths from 1980 through 1995; of these deaths, 85% occurred in males. The greatest number of deaths occurred in the 15- to 19-year-old group (Morbidity Mortality Weekly Report, 1998). Almost 30% of the people struck by lightening die, especially those with cranial and/or burns of the feet. As in electrical burns, the observed peripheral injury may be only the tip of the iceberg as many underlying structures may be involved.

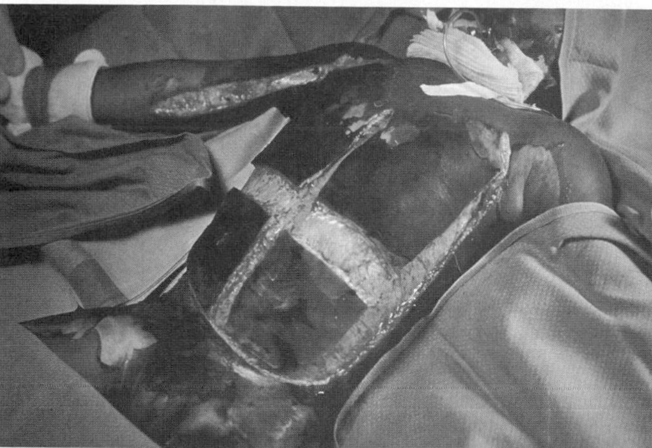

■ **FIGURE 29–6.** Extensive escharotomies required in a child with a major burn.

In patients with low-voltage injuries, the deep burn usually corresponds to the area of superficial involvement. This is usually not the case with high-voltage injuries. In the latter injuries, the current often passes up the center of the limb as if it were a conducting cable causing extensive damage to vessels, muscles, and nerves. Nevertheless, vascular damage may be present in any of these injuries, causing problems to structures distal to the involved site.

Early major problems in patients with major electrical/lightening burns may be cardiac arrhythmias and/or damage to muscle with release of free hemoglobin and myoglobin with subsequent hemoglobinuria and myoglobinuria. The latter is manifest by red to red-black urine and must be treated by maintaining high urine output. A urine output of 1 to 2 mL/kg per hr must be maintained until the pigment load is decreased, or there may be serious tubular damage to the kidneys resulting in oliguric renal failure. Mannitol is often added to the resuscitation fluids, in these cases, in order to increase urine output. Some clinicians also add sodium bicarbonate to the intravenous solutions to alkalinize the urine (Warden, 2003). This is one of the few burn problems that may be taken to the operating room within the first 24 hours of injury before stabilization is complete. The usual reason is for decompression of the extremity or extremities to maintain circulation. The decompression is necessary due to tissue swelling as well as injury to the blood vessels (the path of least resistance) from the current. Often, these patients need to return to the operating room at frequent intervals, even in the first 24 to 48 hours, to have the nonviable tissue débrided. This nonviable tissue may underlie normal skin (Warden, 2003).

This section is not meant to be a complete guide to treatment of severe electrical burns and thus a textbook of burn surgery should be referenced for a more thorough treatment of severe electrical injuries. Suffice it to say that on a percent burn injury, major electrical burns may be more devastating than a pure thermal burn.

■ PERIOPERATIVE MANAGEMENT

Once initial resuscitation and stabilization are complete, patients with full-thickness or deep partial-thickness burns begin a series of trips to the operating room for wound excision and coverage, either with autograft or with a temporary covering such as cadaver skin. Early excision of burn tissue may result in fewer complications, especially those due to infection (Demling, 1985). The child presenting to the operating room for excision, grafting of burn wounds, or both almost always require general anesthesia.

PERIOPERATIVE EVALUATION

During the preanesthetic evaluation of a child with a major burn, special attention should be focused on areas most likely to be adversely affected by the burn injury. These include the airway, respiratory system, cardiovascular system, and volume status. The physical examination should include an assessment of sites for monitoring blood pressure, electrocardiography, pulse oximetry, and temperature. A review of the past anesthetic records is always helpful, especially if the child has undergone prior anesthetics during the current admission. Ventilator settings should be noted and a determination made as to whether the intensive care unit ventilator should be brought into the operating room. Intravenous access must be adequate in view of the blood and fluid requirements likely to be encountered. Laboratory values should be checked, with special attention to the acid-base balance, hematocrit, calcium, and electrolytes. If a large blood loss is anticipated, consider initiating transfusion in advance of the procedure. A recent chest radiograph should be reviewed.

Most important, the time should be taken to discuss the proposed anesthetic management with the child and his or her family. The risks and benefits should be discussed along with a nontechnical explanation of anesthetic and operating room procedures. The child and family should be reassured that the child's safety and comfort are of utmost importance and will be maintained intraoperatively and postoperatively to the greatest degree possible.

INDUCTION AND AIRWAY MANAGEMENT

Transport to the operating room should be well planned and efficient. Preoperative sedation and analgesia should be provided if tolerated by the patient, as the trip to the operating room may be anxiety provoking and painful. Measures to prevent heat loss should be instituted prior to transport, as children with burns are especially susceptible to hypothermia and do not tolerate caloric stress well. If the patient is dependent on mechanical ventilation, current settings, including peak end-expiratory pressure (PEEP), should be duplicated during transport.

The child with burns should have standard monitors placed before induction. Sites for monitors may be problematic. Blood pressure cuffs usually continue to function adequately even when placed over dressings. Because extensive burns often involve the hands and feet, sites for an oximeter probe are often scarce. Probes may be placed on the tongue, lip, or any other novel site that produces an adequate signal. Additional monitors, such as invasive arterial and/or venous pressure monitoring or bladder catheterization, may be considered but possibly delayed until after induction. Alligator clips attached to wet dressings usually provide adequate electrocardiographic tracings; these may be changed to needle electrodes once the child is anesthetized.

If possible, induction of anesthesia prior to transfer to the operating table is more comfortable for the child. If volume status is adequate, any induction agent may be used with careful titration to effect. If the patient has any evidence of myocardial depression or decreased intravascular volume, ketamine may be the preferred induction agent due to its sympathomimetic effects. High concentrations of volatile agents should be used with caution while monitoring for myocardial depression. In any case, induction agents should be carefully titrated to effect.

A poor mask fit due to facial edema, burns, or bulky dressings may complicate management of an already difficult airway. Due to airway edema, intubation may be difficult for the first 5 to 7 days after acute burn injury, especially if the patient has sustained an inhalation injury (see sections on pathophysiology and airway management). Inelastic eschar around the mouth of a child with facial burns may limit mouth opening and jaw mobility. If difficult airway maintenance or intubation is anticipated, spontaneous ventilation should be maintained until the airway is secured. Judicious use of ketamine or a controlled inhalation induction may be useful in this regard.

Staged early excision and grafting require numerous trips to the operating room, possibly four or five times in a week. While data are sparse, there is concern that the repetitive intubation/extubation sequence has the potential to cause laryngeal injury, especially to the already inflamed airway (Colice et al., 1986). With this in mind, McCall and others (1999) advocate the use of the LMA for intraoperative airway management of these patients whenever possible. In their study, using the LMA in 88 pediatric burn patients for 141 general anesthetics, 20% of the patients required a minor intraoperative airway intervention (most commonly reseating or repositioning of the LMA after intraoperative patient position changes), but only 2% required LMA removal and intubation (McCall et al., 1999). Of note, no patient sustained airway injury or aspirated, despite the fact that many patients were placed in the lateral or prone position.

Whether airway maintenance is performed with an endotracheal tube or an LMA, it is often difficult to secure the device due to facial burns and/or dressings. Twill tape may be tied around the child's neck, or cloth tape may be stapled to the face. Staples leave very little in the way of scarring, especially when used in an area that is to be excised in the future. During the course of burn surgery, the child may be repositioned on the operating table numerous times; the airway must be well secured. If long-term intubation is anticipated, a nasal endotracheal tube may be preferable for patient comfort, stability, mouth care, and potential ability to communicate by lip reading.

The child with a major burn has a high cardiac output and increased levels of oxygen consumption and CO_2 production requiring the minute ventilation at least twice normal. Failure to adjust intraoperative ventilation accordingly leads to hypercapnia and hypoxemia. The child with an inhalation injury or acute respiratory distress syndrome may have noncompliant lungs; the child with an extensive burn of the trunk may have a noncompliant chest wall. Both conditions require higher-than-usual airway pressures and PEEP to maintain acceptable ventilation and gas exchange. End-tidal P_{CO_2} monitoring may underestimate arterial P_{CO_2} due to an increase in physiologic dead space and shunt. If the anesthesia machine ventilator is not capable of delivering the required pressures, an intensive care unit ventilator may be used. In the burned child with respiratory failure, it may be necessary to use a noncompliant anesthesia circuit and a cuffed endotracheal tube to allow delivery of adequate ventilator pressures.

MAINTENANCE OF ANESTHESIA

Maintenance of anesthesia may be accomplished by a number of techniques, including nitrous oxide/opioid, ketamine, propofol, volatile anesthetic agent, or a combination dictated by the child's overall clinical condition. If opioids, benzodiazepines, vasopressors, or inotropic agents are infused preoperatively, they most likely should be continued into the intraoperative and postoperative periods. When dosing analgesics and muscle relaxants, it must be remembered that the child with a burn may have increased requirements due to altered metabolism, pharmacokinetics, and pharmacodynamics. If ketamine is used for maintenance during long procedures, it may result in prolonged emergence. Hallucinations and other unpleasant emergence phenomena may occur, especially in the older child and teenager who receive ketamine; the incidence of these side effects may be reduced by the addition of a benzodiazepine or propofol.

The metabolic demands of the child must be met even while in the operating room. The child must be kept warm, as each calorie lost to the environment is a calorie lost to wound healing. The operating room must often be kept uncomfortably warm; fluids and blood must also be warmed. Consideration should also be given to using warming blankets and warmed and humidified inspired gases and covering the child with plastic or thermal blankets (especially the head). Forced warm air devices are difficult to use in this environment due to the large amount of body surface exposed.

Nutrition must be maintained as well as possible to minimize protein catabolism and promote wound healing. Children with extensive burns require enteral feedings. Nutrition is usually supplied through a nasoduodenal tube. In this setting, because this tube exits distal to the pylorus, feedings can be continued throughout the perioperative period including the intraoperative period as long as the nasogastric tube aspirate does not contain tube-fed material. This practice is essential to maintain caloric balance in these hypermetabolic children and has not led to an increase in aspiration or other complications. Adequate pain control, a warm environment, and early wound closure all help reduce the catabolic state of these children.

INTRAOPERATIVE BLOOD LOSS

Blood loss during burn excision is likely to be rapid and extensive. Quantity of loss is difficult to estimate because much of the hemorrhage ends up on the table, in the drapes, or on the floor. One may calculate appropriate preoperative blood ordering by estimating that 3% of the child's blood volume is lost for every 1% of the body surface excised (Housinger et al., 1993). Thus, an excision of a 20% TBSA burn results in a loss of 60% of the child's blood volume. Burns of the face, head, and neck produce even greater blood loss when excised. During skin grafting, which typically occurs 1 day after excision, one should expect the blood loss to be two thirds the amount that occurred during the prior excision (i.e., 2% of blood volume lost for every 1% of the body grafted). As blood loss occurs quickly, transfusion should begin before the patient arrives in the operating room and additional units of blood should be immediately available and checked. Needless to say, blood and blood products should be warmed due to the rapidity of transfusion. Adequacy of transfusion may be assessed by clinical signs such as blood pressure, heart rate, peripheral perfusion, urine output, and arterial or central venous pressure monitoring.

If transfusion exceeds one blood volume, one must consider the alterations in coagulation and metabolism that may occur. Administration of calcium may be required due to the quantity of citrate preservative in the banked blood. Platelets, fibrinogen, and other clotting factors may require replacement. The complications of major transfusion are discussed in detail elsewhere (see Chapter 12, Blood Conservation). Intraoperative laboratory determination of hemoglobin level may be helpful but should be repeated several hours postoperatively, as blood loss and other major fluid shifts may continue during this time. Although attempts are made to limit transfusion as much as possible, a hematocrit of at least 30% is recommended in children with large burns to maintain adequate oxygen-carrying capacity.

Adequate venous access is mandatory. Catheters must be as large as possible. Peripheral venous access is acceptable, but sites are limited in children with major burns. Central venous catheters are preferable and lead to few complications provided they are moved to a new site on a regular basis. Central venous catheters may be inserted through burned tissue if necessary.

The surgeon may be able to decrease blood loss to some extent by the subcutaneous infusion of an isotonic crystalloid solution into the burn wound to be excised. This solution is infused by roller pump and contains 1 to 2 mg of epinephrine/L, thus decreasing blood flow to the area via a hydrostatic and a vasoconstrictor mechanism. The amount of this solution infused may exceed the patient's blood volume, but despite the massive amount of volume and epinephrine delivered, few adverse effects are noted clinically, probably due to the loss from the surgical site and the slow uptake of the solution. This same solution is also used to prepare intact skin for harvest of split-thickness skin grafts.

In summary, the key to maintaining adequate circulating blood volume during a major burn excision is to anticipate the need for rapid transfusion. Beginning transfusion before surgery may be justified, even if the preoperative hematocrit is above 30%. Published studies have demonstrated complications related to blood loss may be reduced by limiting the length of the procedure to less than 2 hours, the area excised to less than 15% of the body surface area, and the blood loss to less than 50% of the patient's blood volume (Engrav et al., 1983). These are practical suggestions, but they are often difficult to carry out in practice.

POSTOPERATIVE PAIN CONTROL

High levels of postoperative pain must be anticipated. Preoperative infusions of opioids, anxiolytics, and other sedatives should be continued throughout the perioperative period. Additional opioids and sedatives should be titrated intraoperatively according to patient response, keeping in mind the increased dosing requirements and altered pharmacokinetics of the child with a major burn.

It is well recognized that donor site pain is the most intense that the burned child experiences. As mentioned, an isotonic crystalloid solution is infused into donor site tissues prior to skin harvesting. In order to decrease postoperative pain from these donor sites, an addition of 2 to 2.5 mg/kg of bupivacaine to the solution to be infused is recommended. The safety and efficacy of this practice have been confirmed through assays of bupivacaine blood levels and effective postoperative pain control (unpublished observations). Even very dilute solutions of subcutaneous bupivacaine are found to be very effective in reducing donor site pain.

SURGICAL RECONSTRUCTIVE PHASE OF BURN CARE

As one can well imagine, major burns, especially in children, in some respects may present a lifetime of care due to the need for

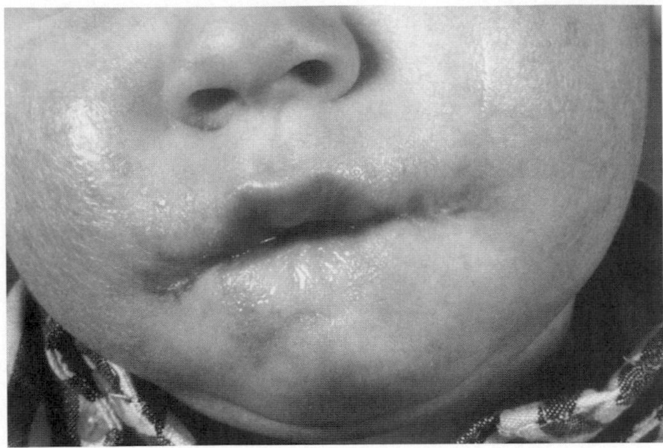

■ **FIGURE 29–7.** Marked scarring of the oropharynx after lye ingestion. Oral opening 6 mm by 10 mm. The child could only eat "one half of an M and M" according to the mother.

scar revisions, psychological support, and in many cases cosmetic surgery to help make the patient more comfortable in the acts of daily living.

These patients with burns continue to present the anesthesiologist/anesthetist with potentially serious problems in the operating room; especially those who have had major burns of the face and head come readily to mind. There may be contractures of the mouth, making access for the airway extremely difficult. Neck contractures can significantly impede visualization of the glottis and intubation. One must plan ahead in preparing for a procedure that includes various means and instruments to aid in securing a safe, effective airway.

In cases of microstomia with scarred nares or marked scarring in the oropharynx (Fig. 29–7), a technique of anesthetic care might be needed in which the mouth opening is enlarged prior to endotracheal intubation. One approach is a technique of intravenous sedation, including ketamine, and then injections of local anesthetic with epinephrine into the oral commissures and cheek. The surgeon then makes surgical incisions in order to enlarge the mouth opening, making oral intubation possible. This technique, although not presented in the literature, has worked well at the institution where surgeons and anesthesiologists have worked together for many years. One must be aware in using this technique, however, that if the condition has persisted for a long time, the temporomandibular joint may be involved and there may still be limitations in the mouth opening.

Many of these children have undergone numerous surgical procedures in the past, including those during the acute phase of treatment. Many are, therefore, very anxious preoperatively and need reassurance as well as satisfactory preoperative medications. Intravenous access can also be a challenge in these patients, due to the burns and grafting procedures that obliterate peripheral sites. As in many children, these individuals often are afraid of needles and a mask induction may be preferred.

In the reconstructive phase of burn treatment, anesthetic choices are those preferred by the anesthesiologist and the patient and those that are compatible with the procedure being performed. These choices include any and all that would be used in the everyday anesthetic management of the child.

The incidence of nausea and vomiting is extremely high in the postoperative period in this patient population. In the scalp-expander group, prior to instituting a rigorous regimen of antiemetic drugs, the incidence was nearly 100% (Stubbs, 1999). However, this problem is seen in many pediatric hospitals where the incidence of nausea and vomiting is reported to be high, especially with certain procedures such as tonsillectomy/adenoidectomies (40% to 88%) (Carithers et al., 1987; Sukhani et al., 2002) and strabismus surgery (50% to 80%) (Watcha et al., 1991; Gurkan et al., 1999). The propofol-based anesthetic technique has markedly decreased postoperative nausea and vomiting, even with a background infusion of 10 to 20 mcg/kg per min.

■ SUMMARY

Care of the burn patient, especially those children with major burns, demands a meticulous approach by a multidisciplinary team of physicians, nurses, pharmacists, physical therapists, blood bank and laboratory technicians, and social workers. These children and their families require multiple hours of attention for not only their medical care but also for the psychologic support of both the patient and his or her family. This is important during the acute phases of burn care but also may stretch into many years of contact during the physical maturing of the burn scars, with the attendant releases mandated not only by dense scar tissue but also the psychologic maturing of both the patient and his or her family. Although these patients may be readily accepted in the hospital setting, returning to community living presents its own problems for both the patient and the family. The anesthetic management must be geared to the constantly changing physical condition of the patient. Even the burn patient who returns after the acute phase of treatment for reconstructive procedures may well challenge the anesthesiologist in safely securing the airway and certainly in being able to secure vascular access. Although most anesthesiologists have limited contact and experience with burn patients, it must be kept in mind that they might be called on, at any time, to help in the initial resuscitation of a burn victim as well as in securing the airway.

Acknowledgments

We offer special thanks to Ms. Linda Holbrook for her excellent administrative support.

REFERENCES

Aikawa N, Wakabayashi G, Ueda M, et al.: Regulation of renal function in thermal injury. *J Trauma* 30:S174, 1990.

Artz CP, Moncrief JA: The burn problem. In Artz CP, Moncrief JA, editors: *The treatment of burns.* Philadelphia, 1969, WB Saunders, pp 1–22.

Bohrer H, Qui F, Zimmerman T, et al.: Role of NFκB in the mortality of sepsis. *J Clin Invest* 100:972, 1997.

Boutros AR, Hoyt JR: Management of carbon monoxide poisoning in the absence of hyperbaric oxygen chamber. *Crit Care Med* 4:144, 1976.

Carithers JS, Gebhart DE, Williams JA: Postoperative risks of pediatric tonsilloadenoidectomy. *Laryngoscope* 97:422, 1987.

Colice GL, Munster AM, Haponik EF: Tracheal stenosis complicating cutaneous burns: An underestimated problem. *Am Rev Respir Dis* 134:1315, 1986.

Crapo RO: Smoke inhalation injuries. *JAMA* 246:1694–1696, 1981.

Czermak BJ, Sarma V, Pierson CL, et al.: Protective effects of C5a blockade in sepsis. *Nature Med* 5:788, 1999.

de Campo T, Aldrete JA: The anesthetic management of the severely burned patient. *Intensive Care Med* 7:55–62, 1981.

Deitch EA, Sittig KM: A serial study of the erythropoietic response to thermal injury. *Ann Surg* [illegible]

Demling RH: Effect of early burn excision and grafting on pulmonary function. *J Trauma* 24:830, 1984.

Demling RH: Burns. *N Engl J Med* 313:1389, 1985.

Dwersteg JF, Pavlin EG, Heimbach DM: Patients with burns are resistant to atracurium. *Anesthesiology* 65:517, 1986.

Eckhauser FE, Billote J, Burke JF, et al.: Tracheostomy complicating massive burn injury. A plea for conservatism. *Am J Surg* 127:418, 1974.

Engrav LH, Heimbach DM, Reus JL, et al.: Early excision and grafting vs. nonoperative treatment of burns of indeterminate depth: A randomized prospective study. *J Trauma* 23:1001, 1983.

Falkner B, Roven S, DeClement FA, et al.: Hypertension in children with burns. *J Trauma* 18:213, 1978.

Feck G, Baptiste MS: The epidemiology of burn injury in New York. *Public Health Rep* 94:312, 1979.

Fein A, Leff A, Hopewell PC: Pathophysiology and management of the complications resulting from fire and the inhaled products of combustion: review of the literature. *Crit Care Med* 8:94, 1980.

Goldbaum LR, OrellanoT, Dergal E: Mechanism of the toxic action of carbon monoxide. *Ann Clin Lab Sci* 6:372, 1976.

Greenblatt DJ, Shader RI, Abernethy DR: Current Status of benzodiazepines. *N Engl J Med* 309:354, 1983.

Gronert GA: Succinylcholine hyperkalemia after burns. *Anesthesiology* 91:320, 1999.

Gronert GA, Schaner PJ, Gunther RD: Multiple halothane anesthesia. *Pacif Med Surg* 75:28, 1967

Gronert GA, Theye RA: Pathophysiology of hyperkalemia induced by succinylcholine. *Anesthesiology* 43:89, 1975.

Grube BJ, Marvin JA, Heimbach DM: Therapeutic hyperbaric oxygen: Help or hindrance in burn patients with carbon monoxide poisoning? *J Burn Care Rehabil* 9:249, 1988.

Gurkan Y, Kilickan L, Toker K: Propofol-nitrous oxide versus sevoflurane-nitrous oxide for strabismus surgery in children. *Paediatr Anaesth* 9:495, 1999.

Heatherill RJ, Till GO, Burner LH, et al.: Thermal injury, intravascular hemolysis, and toxic oxygen products. *J Clin Invest* 78:629, 1986.

Heideman M: The effect of thermal injury on hemodynamic, respiratory and hematologic variables in relationship to complement activation. *J Trauma* 19:239, 1979.

Herndon DN, Thompson RB, Traber DL: Pulmonary injury in burned patients. *Crit Care Clin* 1:79, 1985.

Herndon DN, Traber LD, Linares H, et al.: Etiology of the pulmonary pathophysiology associated with inhalation injury. *Resuscitation* 14:43, 1986.

Holm C, Horbrand E, von Donnersmarch GH, et al.: Acute renal failure in severely burned patients. *Burns* 25:171, 1999.

Housinger TA, Lang D, Warden GD: A prospective study of blood loss with excisional therapy in pediatric burn patients. *J Trauma* 34:262, 1993.

Hunt JL, Agee RN, Pruitt BA: Fiberoptic bronchoscopy in acute inhalation injury. *J Trauma* 15:641, 1975.

Jelkmann W, Wolff M, Fandrey J: Modulation of the production of erythropoietin by cytokines: in vitro studies and their clinical implications. *Contrib Nephrol* 87:68, 1990.

Jenkins M, Gottschlich AM, Mayes T, et al.: Enteral feeding during operative procedures. *J Burn Care Rehabil* 15:199, 1994.

Jeschke MG, Herndon DN, Wolf SE, et al.: Recombinant human growth hormone alters acute phase reactant proteins, cytokine expression and liver morphology in burn rats. *J Surg Res* 83:22, 1999.

Jeschke MG, Low JFA, Spies M, et al.: Cell proliferation, apoptosis, NF-kappaB expression, enzyme, protein, and weight changes in livers of burned rats. *Am J Physiol Gastrointest Liver Physiol* 280:G1314, 2001.

Junger WG, Coimbra R, Liu FC, et al.: Hypertonic saline resuscitation: A tool to modulate immune function in trauma patients? *Shock* 8:235, 1997.

Keens TG, Bryan AC, Levison H, et al.: Developmental pattern of muscle fiber types in human ventilatory muscles. *J Appl Physiol* 44:909, 1978.

Kowal-Vern A, Gamelli RL, Walenga JM, et al.: The effect of burn wound size on hemostasis: A correlation of the hemostatic changes to the clinical state. *J Trauma* 33:50, 1992.

Laffon M, Pittet J, Modelska K, et al.: Interleukin-8 mediates injury from smoke inhalation to both the lung endothelial and alveolar epithelial barriers in rabbits. *Am J Respir Crit Care Med* 160:1443, 1999.

Lawrence C, Atac B: Hematologic changes in massive burn injury. *Crit Care Med* 20:1284, 1992.

Leibel WS, Martyn JA, Szyfelbein SK, et al.: Elevated plasma binding cannot account for the burn related d-tubocurarine hyposensitivity. *Anesthesiology* 54:378, 1981.

Lightning-associated deaths–United States, 1980-1995. *Morb Mortal Wkly Rep* 47:391–394, 1998.

Lloyd JR: Thermal trauma: Therapeutic achievements and investigative horizons. *Surg Clin North Am* 57:121, 1977.

Loirat P, Rohan J, Baillet A, et al.: Increased glomerular filtration rate in patients with major burns and its effect on the pharmacokinetics of tobramycin. *N Engl J Med* 299:915, 1978.

Loke J, Paul E, Virgulto JA, et al.: Rabbit lung after acute smoke inhalation. *Arch Surg* 119:956, 1984.

MacLennan N, Heimbach DM, Cullen BF: Anesthesia for major thermal injury. *Anesthesiology* 89:749, 1998.

Madden MR, Finkelstein JL, Goodwin CW: Respiratory care of the burn patient. *Clin Plast Surg* 13(1):29, 1986.

Madjdpour L, Kneller S, Booy C, et al.: Acid induced lung injury. *Anesthesiology* 99:1323, 2003.

Martyn JA: Clinical pharmacology and drug therapy in the burned patient. *Anesthesiology* 65:67, 1986.

Martyn JA: Succinylcholine hyperkalemia after burns. *Anesthesiology* 91:321, 1999.

Martyn JA, Abernethy DR, Greenblatt DJ: Plasma protein binding of drugs after severe burn injury. *Clin Pharmacol Ther* 35:534, 1984.

Martyn JA, Greenblatt DJ, Quinby WC: Diazepam kinetics following burns. *Anesth Analg* 51:293, 1983.

Martyn JA, Liu LM, Szyfelbein SK, et al.: The neuromuscular effects of pancuronium in burned children. *Anesthesiology* 59:561, 1983.

Martyn JA, Matteo RS, Lebowitz PW, et al.: Pharmacokinetics of d-tubocurarine in patients with thermal injury. *Anesth Analg* 61:241, 1982.

Martyn JA, Matteo RS, Szyfelbein SK, et al.: Unprecedented resistance to neuromuscular blocking effects of metocurine with persistence after complete recovery in a burned patient. *Anesth Analg* 61:614, 1982.

Martyn JA, Szyfelbein SK, Ali HH, et al.: Tubocurarine requirement following major thermal injury. *Anesthesiology* 52:352, 1980.

McCall JE, Fischer CG, Schomaker E, et al.: Laryngeal mask airway use in children with acute burns: intraoperative airway management. *Paediatr Anaesth* 9:515, 1999.

McDonald W, Sharp D, Deitch E: Immediate enteral feeding in burn patients is safe and effective. *Ann Surg* 213:177, 1991.

Merrell SW, Saffle JR, Sullivan JJ, et al.: Fluid resuscitation in thermally injured children. *Am J Surg* 152:664, 1986.

Mills AK, Martyn JA: Neuromuscular blockade with vecuronium in paediatric patients with burn injury. *Br J Clin Pharm* 28:155, 1989.

Moncrief JA: Burns. *N Engl J Med* 288:444, 1973.

Moncrief JA, Teplitz C: Changing concepts in burn sepsis. *J Trauma* 4:233, 1964.

Moore SJ, Ho IK, Hume AS: Severe hypoxia produce by concomitant intoxication with sublethal doses of carbon monoxide and cyanide. *Toxicol Appl Pharmacol* 109:412, 1991.

Navar PD, Saffle JR, Warden GD: Effect of inhalation injury on fluid resuscitation requirements after thermal injury. *Am J Surg* 150:716, 1985.

Neely A, Nathen P, Highsmith R: Plasma proteolytic activity following burns. *J Trauma* 28:362, 1988.

Palmieri TL, Jackson W, Greenhalgh DG: Benefits of early tracheostomy in severely burned children. *Crit Care Med* 4:922, 2002.

Parks DH, Carvajal HF, Larson DL: Management of burns. *Surg Clin North Am* 57:875, 1977.

Perry S, Heidrich G: Management of pain during débridement: A survey of U.S. burn units. *Pain* 13:267, 1982.

Porter J, Hick H: Addiction rare in patients treated with narcotics. *N Engl J Med* 302:123, 1980.

Pruitt BA, Erickson DR, Morris A: Progressive pulmonary insufficiency and other pulmonary complications of thermal injury. *J Trauma* 15:369, 1975.

Pruitt BA, Flemma RJ, Divincenti, et al.: Complications in burn patients. *J Thorac Cardiovasc Surg* 59:7, 1979.

Roughton FJW, Darling RC: The effect of carbon monoxide on the oxyhemoglobin dissociation curve. *Am J Physiol* 141:17, 1944.

Rue LW III, Cioffi WG Jr, Mason AD Jr, et al.: Improved survival of burned patients with inhalation injury. *Arch Surg* 128:772, 1993.

Saffle JR, Morris SE, Edelman L: Early tracheostomy does not improve outcome in burn patients. *J Burn Care Rehabil* 23:431, 2002.

Saffle JR: Predicting outcomes of burns. *N Engl J Med* 338:387, 1998.

Sawada Y, Momma S, Takamizawa A, et al.: Survival from acute renal failure after severe burns. *Burns* 11:143, 1984.

Simon TL, Curreri PW, Harder LA: Kinetic characterization of hemostasis in thermal injury. *J Lab Clin Med* 89:702, 1977.

Slogoff S, Allen GW, Wessels JV, et al.: Clinical experience with subanesthetic ketamine. *Anesth Analg* 53:356, 1974.

Spooner C, Markowitz N, Saravolatz L: The role of tumor necrosis factor in sepsis. *Clin Immunol Immunopathol* 62:S11, 1992.

Stanski DR, Watkins DW: *Drug disposition in anesthesia.* New York, 1982, Grune & Stratton.

Stewart RD, Stewart RS, Stamm W, et al.: Rapid estimation of carboxyhemoglobin level in fire fighters. *JAMA* 235:390, 1976.

Stubbs TK, Saylors S, Jenkins M, et al.: Pediatric patients experiencing postoperative nausea and vomiting after burn reconstruction surgery: an analysis. *J Burn Care Rehabil* 20:236, 1999.

Sukhani R, Pappas AL, Lurie J, et al.: Ondansetron and dolasetron provides equivalent postoperative vomiting control after ambulatory tonsillectomy in dexamethasone pretreated children. *Anesth Analg* 95:1230, 2002.

Szyfelbein SK, Martyn JA, Coté CJ: Burn injuries. In Coté C, Ryan J, Todres I, et al., editors: *A practice of anesthesia for infants and children.* Philadelphia, 1993, WB Saunders, pp 357–376.

Thompson PB, Herdon DN, Traber DL, et al.: Effect on mortality of inhalation injury. *J Trauma* 26:163, 1986.

Tolmie JD, Joyce TH, Mitchell GD: Succinylcholine danger in the burned patient. *Anesthesiology* 28:467, 1967.

Tominaga K, Yoshimoto T, Torigoe K, et al.: IL-1 synergizes with IL-8 or IL-1β for IFN-γ production from human T cells. *Int Immunol* 12:151, 2000.

Traber DL, Redl H, Schlag G, et al.: Cardiopulmonary responses to continuous administration of endotoxin. *Am J Physiol* 254:H833, 1988.

Trunkey DD: Inhalation injury. *Surg Clin North Am* 58:1133, 1978.

Van der Poll T, van Deventer S: Cytokines and anticytokines in the pathogenesis of sepsis. *Infect Dis Clin North Am* 13:403, 1999.

Voss M, Cotton M: Mechanisms and clinical implications of apoptosis. *Hosp Med* 59:924, 1998.

Warden G: Fluid resuscitation and early management. In Herndon D, editor: *Total burn care,* 2n ed. London, 2002, WB Saunders, pp 88–90.

Warden GD, Stratta RJ, Laffle JR, et al.: Plasma exchange therapy in patients failing to resuscitate from burn shock. *J Trauma* 23:9456, 1983.

Warden GD: *Words of wisdom,* 8th ed. Shriners Hospital for Children, 2003.

Watcha MF, Simeon RM, White PF, et al.: Effect of propofol on the incidence of postoperative vomiting after strabismus surgery in pediatric outpatients. *Anesthesiology* 75:204, 1991.

White PF, Way WL, Trevor AJ: Ketamine: Its pharmacology and therapeutic uses. *Anesthesiology* 56:119, 1982.

Wilmore D, Long J, Mason A, et al.: Catecholamines: Mediators of the hypermetabolic response to thermal injury. *Ann Surg* 180:653, 1974.

Wilmore DW, Aulick LH: Metabolic changes in burned patients. *Surg Clin North Am* 58:1173, 1978.

Wilmore DW, Goodwin CW, Aulick LH, et al.: Effect of injury and infection on visceral metabolism and circulation. *Ann Surg* 192:491, 1980.

30 Perioperative Management of the Pediatric Trauma Patient

Paul I. Reynolds • Oliver Soldes • Shobha Malviya • Peter J. Davis

Childhood injuries are a major public health problem. Trauma is the number one killer of Americans aged 1 to 19 years, causing more than 16,000 deaths in 1999 in the United States. More than 60% of the deaths in this age group are related to injuries (Anderson, 2001), with traumatic brain injury (TBI) being the leading cause of death (70%) and long-term disability. Thoracic and abdominal injuries are the cause of death in 20% and 10% of trauma fatalities, respectively (Cooper et al., 1994).

Pediatric trauma remains a surgical disease, despite the large numbers of minor childhood injuries and successes in the nonoperative management of many solid organ injuries. Nonoperative management is more widely used in the pediatric trauma population than in adults. Operative management of solid organ injuries is required when hemodynamic instability or severe physiologic compromise develops. Data from an analysis of the National Pediatric Trauma Registry (NPTR) demonstrate that more than half of injured children have a diagnosis that requires evaluation by a surgeon and 11% require an operative procedure. Tepas and others (2003) reported that 32% of children in their study sample were considered at potential risk of death from their injuries. Of these, 86% had injuries requiring surgical evaluation, 21% required an operative procedure, and 12% died.

With careful assessment and continuing reassessment, many blunt head, chest, and abdominal injuries can be managed nonoperatively. The decision to pursue nonoperative therapy should be made by the surgical specialist caring for the patient. The periodic failure of nonoperative management requires rapid recognition and a decision to perform an urgent operation.

Trauma injuries can be broadly divided into (1) blunt and penetrating trauma and (2) burns. Blunt trauma is considerably more difficult to evaluate than penetrating trauma and relies more heavily on imaging studies. Nonburn traumatic injuries in children are approximately 90% blunt and 10% penetrating (Potola et al., 2000); urban centers may have a higher proportion of penetrating trauma. Thermal and chemical burn injuries are discussed in Chapter 29, Anesthesia for Children with Burns.

TRAUMA CENTERS AND CLASSIFICATION

Death from pediatric trauma occurs at three periods: (1) within seconds of the traumatic event due to overwhelming injuries; (2) within minutes to hours of the event (the "golden hour"), when aggressive intervention with attention to the ABCs (airway, breathing, and circulation) can make a difference in survival (Roback, 2000); and (3) days to weeks after the initial event when complications such as organ failure, sepsis, or brain death arise. An effective way to minimize morbidity and mortality due to trauma arose from lessons learned in the management of injured men and women during the Korean Conflict and Vietnam War (Morrison, 2002). During the past several decades, the American College of Surgeons and other organizations developed a three-tiered system for trauma center designation and verification (Table 30–1). Level I centers offer the widest range of services for the most severely injured patient, whereas level III centers allow for stabilization and triage. Because 25% of all trauma occurs in children, specific systems of pediatric trauma care developed within the adult systems. The first pediatric-specific trauma centers were developed in the early 1970s in Boston, Ann Arbor, Baltimore, Washington, DC, Toronto, and Brooklyn (Morrison et al., 2002). Since that time, more than 15 level I and level II pediatric trauma centers have been certified by the American College of Surgeons.

TRAUMA RESUSCITATION, DIAGNOSIS, AND PRIORITIZATION

The initial phase of the acute care of the trauma patient is resuscitation. This dynamic and crucial period involves continuous

TABLE 30–1. American College of Surgeons trauma center levels and descriptions

Level I
Provides comprehensive trauma care, serves as a regional resource, and provides leadership in education, research, and system planning. A level I center is required to have immediate availability of trauma surgeons, anesthesiologists, physician specialists, nurses, and resuscitation equipment. American College of Surgeons' volume performance criteria further stipulate that level I centers treat 1200 admissions a year or 240 major trauma patients per year or an average of 35 major trauma patients per surgeon.
Level II
Provides comprehensive trauma care either as a supplement to a level I trauma center in a large urban area or as the lead hospital in a less population-dense area. Level II centers must meet essentially the same criteria as level I but volume performance standards are not required and may depend on the geographic area served. Centers are not expected to provide leadership in teaching and research.
Level III
Provides prompt assessment, resuscitation, emergency surgery, and stabilization with transfer to a level I or II as indicated. Level III facilities typically serve communities that do not have immediate access to a level I or II trauma center.

From MacKenzie EJ, et al.: National inventory of hospital trauma centers. *JAMA* 289:1516, 2003. © 2003 American Medical Association.

TABLE 30–2. University of Michigan pediatric trauma classification

Level 1
Pediatric Patients with Single or Multisystem Injuries and Unstable Vital Signs with One or More of the Following 1. Respiratory distress as evidenced by a. Intubation prior to arrival b. Compromised airway c. Absent/significantly diminished breath sounds d. Significant retractions/nasal flaring e. Significantly increased or decreased respiratory rate for age 2. Shock a. Transfer patients from other hospitals receiving blood to maintain vital signs b. Confirmed age-specific hypotension at any time c. Delayed capillary refill >3 seconds thought to be due to hypovolemia 3. Neurologic injury a. Glasgow Coma Scale (GCS) score of <8 and/or focal neurologic finding with mechanism attributed to trauma b. Deteriorating level of consciousness (an acute change of >2 points from initial evaluation) c. Acute traumatic paralysis/paraplegia or quadriplegia 4. Specific traumatic injuries a. Gunshot wounds to the abdomen, chest, head, or neck b. Any burns with unstable vital signs
Level 2
Pediatric Patients with Multisystem Injuries and Stable Vital Signs 1. Neurologic status: GCS score of <9, no change in GCS score from the initial evaluation, and no focal neurologic findings 2. Children with open fractures 3. All patients with partial- or full-thickness burns >20% total burn surface area (TBSA), electrical or lightning injuries, full-thickness circumferential burns, or inhalation injury with threat of airway compromise, with stable vital signs
Level 3 ("trauma consult")
Pediatric Patients who are Conscious with an Apparent Isolated Injury and Stable Vital Signs with a Mechanism of Injury with a Low Potential for Multisystem Injuries 1. All pediatric patients with a mechanism of injury that has the potential for suspected child abuse 2. All patients with partial-thickness burns >5% TBSA, full-thickness burns >2% TBSA, or any burn with serious threat of functional or cosmetic impairment that involves the face, hands, feet, genitalia, perineum, or major joints

assessment with concurrent diagnostic and therapeutic procedures to preserve life and prevent morbidity (Rhodes, 1998). The Advanced Trauma Life Support (ATLS) course of the American College of Surgeons provides the basis of a systematic protocol to guide initial resuscitation and evaluation of the trauma patient and is summarized later (American College of Surgeons Committee on Trauma, 1997). The care of a trauma patient is divided into several phases: primary survey with concurrent resuscitation, secondary survey, and definitive care. Trauma patients require continuous reassessment for missed injuries and changes in known injuries.

PRIMARY SURVEY WITH CONCURRENT RESUSCITATION

According to basic and advanced pediatric life support guidelines, the primary survey is a rapid evaluation and treatment phase focusing on the "ABCDEs":

Airway: Ensure a patent airway.
Breathing: Assess and provide adequate respiration.
Circulation: Assess and assist the circulation with intravenous fluids and cardiopulmonary resuscitation (CPR) as needed.
Disability: Assess the neurologic injury.
Expose: Remove clothing to assess and evaluate for further injury and then take appropriate steps to prevent hypothermia.

The secondary survey is composed of a complete physical examination, patient history, laboratory tests, and radiologic imaging. This phase may be delayed or completed in the operating room in patients who require urgent interventions. Definitive care occurs in the intensive care unit and/or operating room and often involves care by pediatric surgical subspecialists (neurosurgeons, orthopedic surgeons). Patients may also require transfer to comprehensive trauma centers during this phase (Krantz, 1996).

During the primary and secondary stage of evaluation, patients may be categorized using a grading system based on acuity and severity of their trauma. A pediatric trauma classification system is outlined in Table 30–2. In addition, Figure 30–1 illustrates guidelines for airway and cardiovascular assessment in the traumatized pediatric patient.

AIRWAY AND BREATHING

The first step in trauma resuscitation is securing an airway and ensuring adequate respirations. Indications for endotracheal intubation include oxygenation and ventilation, and protection of the airway against aspiration. Appropriate management of the airway may be challenging or difficult without proper preparation and familiarity with the unique characteristics of the pediatric airway. In a young child or infant, the tongue is relatively large and the larynx and glottic opening are more anterior. The most obvious differences are that the child's airway has a smaller diameter and a shorter length. Airway edema occurring in an already

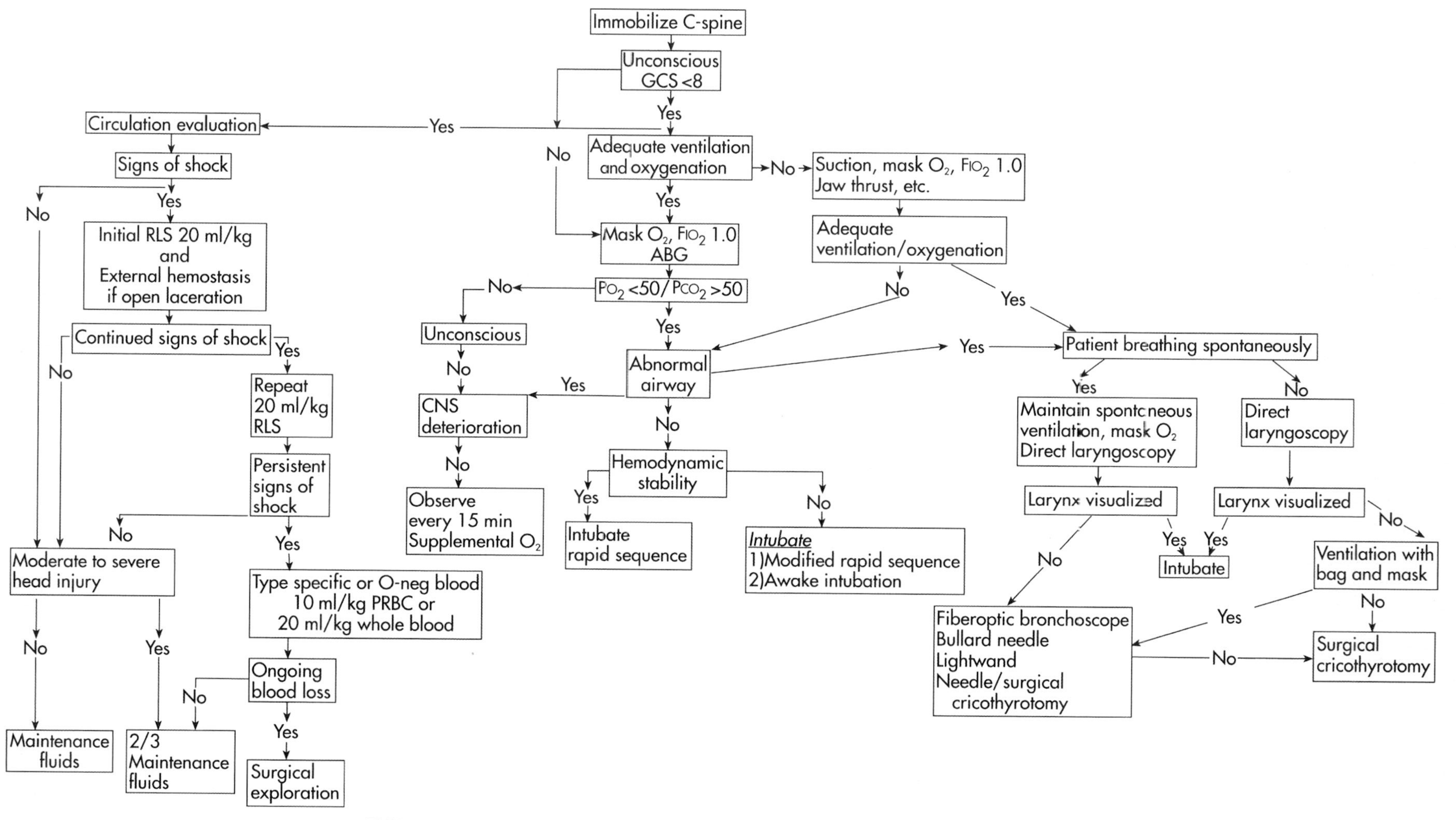

■ **FIGURE 30–1.** Guidelines for airway and cardiovascular assessment in the traumatized pediatric patient.

small airway results in significant changes in the internal diameter of the airway and in increased resistance to airflow. The short length of the trachea makes right mainstem intubations more likely and increases the likelihood of extubation from small positional changes of the endotracheal tube. The narrowest anatomic portion of the pediatric airway is at the cricoid cartilage throughout childhood, unless the glottis is partially or completely closed.

The initial management of the pediatric airway involves bag-valve-mask ventilation with a jaw-thrust maneuver and an Ambu bag. Intubation is indicated in patients with respiratory or cardiac compromise or an altered level of consciousness. Endotracheal intubation is the preferred definitive airway. Nasotracheal intubation may be suboptimal and difficult because of the small size and acute angle of the nasopharynx and the more anterior and cephalad position of the glottic opening. A laryngeal mask airway (LMA) may be used temporarily by persons familiar with their use but less skilled in intubation. However, it must be recognized that the LMA does not protect the airway from aspiration and must be replaced by an endotracheal tube as soon as skilled personnel become available. Endotracheal intubation of pediatric trauma patients in emergency situations is associated with a 25% rate of complications, such as bronchial intubation (Nakayama et al., 1990).

The head and neck must be protected from unnecessary movement. The physician managing the airway (positioned at the head of the patient) must maintain the head and neck in anatomic alignment with the body. Forceful axial traction may cause further disruption of an unstable spine and must be avoided. In an unconscious, head-injured child, endotracheal intubation will protect the airway and provide ventilatory support. When endotracheal intubation is required before a radiograph of the cervical spine (C-spine) has been obtained, a spinal injury should always be assumed (American College of Surgeons Committee on Trauma, 1997). Children are more likely—because of their neck musculature, their disproportionately large head size, and the elasticity of their supporting structures—to sustain cervical neck injuries above C3. It is frequently difficult to rule out a spinal cord injury because 50% of these injuries exist in the absence of radiographic findings.

Intubation of the child with a cervical neck injury requires keeping the patient supine and the neck in a neutral position and avoiding any head-tilt and or chin-lift maneuvers. While intubating patients with actual or presumed C-spine injuries, an assistant must apply manual inline axial stabilization—that is, the assistant holds a hand over each ear while keeping the patient's shoulders and occiput firmly on a rigid backboard (Fig. 30–2). Intubation techniques involving rapid sequence, the use of the Bullard laryngoscope, flexible fiberoptic bronchoscopy, and techniques involving the use of fluoroscopy have all been described for patients with presumed C-spine injuries (Watts et al., 1997; Criswell et al., 1994; Morell et al., 1997; Zanette et al., 1997) (see Chapter 10, Induction of Anesthesia). Hastings and Wood (1994) have shown that in patients without head or neck stabilization, exposure of the arytenoid cartilage and best view of the glottis were achieved with 10 and 15 degrees of head extension, respectively. Head immobilization reduces the extension angles to 4 degrees for arytenoid exposure and 5 degrees for the best view of the glottis.

Short-acting sedatives to facilitate intubation are preferred in head-injured patients to allow reexamination. A quick and focused neurologic assessment should be performed before administering sedatives or paralytics, when medically safe.

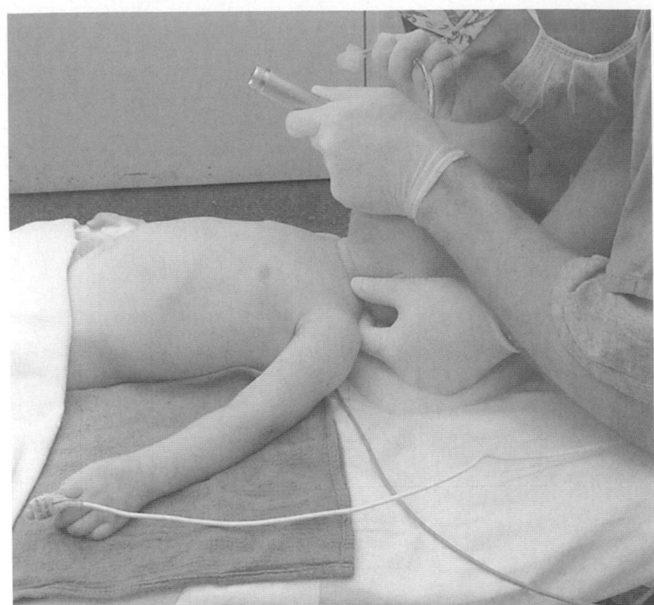

■ **FIGURE 30–2.** Manual axial inline stabilization during direct laryngoscopy.

Children commonly develop gastric distention because of crying or bag-and-mask positive-pressure ventilation. A distended stomach may compromise ventilation and increase the risk of aspiration (Fig. 30–3). The stomach should be decompressed with a nasogastric or an orogastric tube after intubation and a chest radiograph obtained to verify endotracheal tube position.

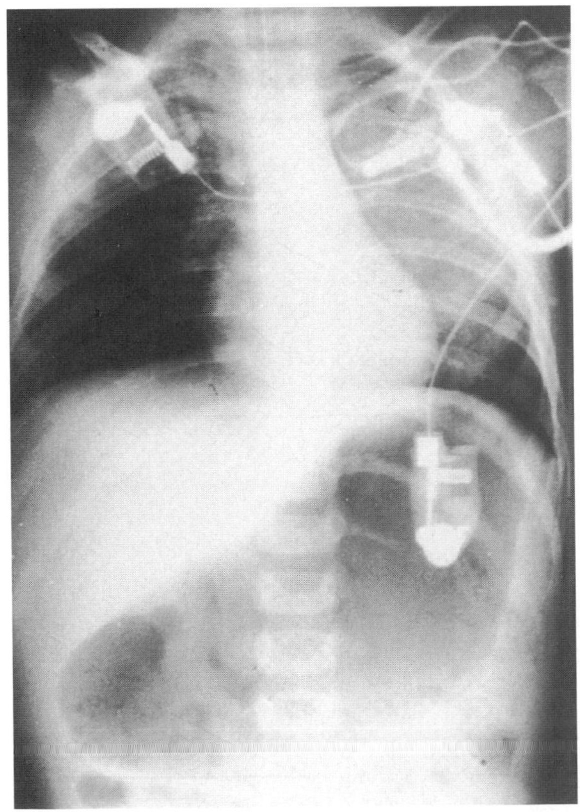

■ **FIGURE 30–3.** Gastric dilation frequently occurs after crying or positive-pressure ventilation by gas and mask.

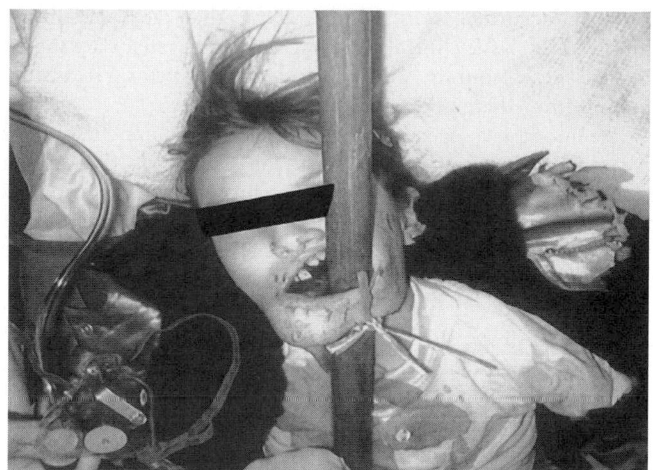

■ **FIGURE 30–4.** An 11-year-old girl fell 10 to 15 feet while sliding down the school banisters onto a plant supported by a thick wooden pole. She eventually was intubated orally with direct laryngoscopy. (From Melillo EP, Hawkins DJ, Lynch L, MacNamara A: Difficult airway management of a child impaled through the neck. *Paediatr Anaesth* 11:615–617, 2001.)

Depending on the nature of the underlying injury, securing the airway in a patient who has sustained multiple injuries or even isolated facial injuries can be extremely complicated (Melillo et al., 2001) (Fig. 30–4). The management of such cases calls upon the resourcefulness and skills of the anesthesiologist and requires careful consideration of damage to surrounding structures such as major blood vessels and the airway structures themselves, the ability to maintain a patent airway via facemask, and the potential for an expanding hematoma that may subsequently compromise an airway that may be patent at the current time. Additional considerations include the risks of increased intracranial pressure (ICP) in the case of concomitant head trauma, of exacerbating an existing C-spine injury, and of aspiration during airway manipulation. The presence of rhinorrhea, otorrhea, or ecchymoses around the eyes should raise suspicion about a possible basilar skull fracture, and any instrumentation of the nasal passages, including passage of an endotracheal tube or a nasogastric tube, should be avoided. Similarly, crepitus at the neck may herald the presence of a tracheal or bronchial disruption, and intubation under direct vision using a flexible fiberoptic scope in a spontaneously breathing patient should be considered to avoid false passage of the endotracheal tube.

In cases where airway difficulty is anticipated, it may be prudent to transport the child to the operating room with an anesthesiologist and otolaryngologist in attendance once the child has been stabilized hemodynamically and additional injuries have been ruled out. The airway may then be secured with preparations to perform an emergent tracheostomy in case of failure to intubate the trachea via direct laryngoscopy. A careful induction of anesthesia via the inhaled route may be tolerated by the patient who has received adequate volume resuscitation and permits direct laryngoscopy while the patient is breathing spontaneously. The use of muscle relaxants is best avoided until the airway is secured. If intravenous agents are required to induce anesthesia, it is preferable to use short-acting agents such as propofol and remifentanil. These agents effectively blunt ICP responses to direct laryngoscopy and allow for spontaneous respiration to occur in case of a failed intubation. The use of a combined propofol and remifentanil technique provides an alternative to a traditional rapid sequence induction (Haughton et al., 1999).

Ensuring adequate ventilation is the next task after securing the airway. Breathing is best assessed by auscultation and observation of chest motion. Young children in respiratory distress may exhibit subcostal and intercostal retractions. Nasal flaring and grunting also signal breathing difficulty. Assessment of tracheal position and jugular venous distention (for possible pneumothorax and cardiac tamponade) may be difficult because of the child's short, fat neck. Pallor, cyanosis, and an altered level of consciousness are late signs of respiratory insufficiency and demand immediate intervention. End-tidal CO_2 monitoring, pulse oximetry, and blood gas determinations are useful adjuncts. Many injuries that impair respiration include simple tension and open pneumothorax, massive hemothorax, flail chest, and pulmonary contusion.

CIRCULATION

Children who sustain multiple injuries frequently present in hypovolemic or hemorrhagic shock that must be promptly recognized and treated. Unlike adults, children maintain an almost normal blood pressure until 25% to 35% of their circulating blood volume is lost (Fig. 30–5). This is likely due to their high sympathetic tone that causes peripheral vasoconstriction in an effort to maintain blood pressure in the face of a diminished blood volume. Tachycardia is an earlier sign of impending shock than is hypotension. Tachycardia generally indicates a loss of at least 10% of the patient's blood volume. In addition, signs of poor peripheral perfusion such as delayed capillary refill (>2 seconds), weak or thready pulses, mottling or cyanosis of the skin, and impaired consciousness are earlier indicators of shock than low blood pressure. The presence of hypotension as a result of hypovolemia should be considered an ominous sign that usually heralds impending cardiovascular collapse. In children, hypotension as a result of hemorrhage corresponds to a loss of

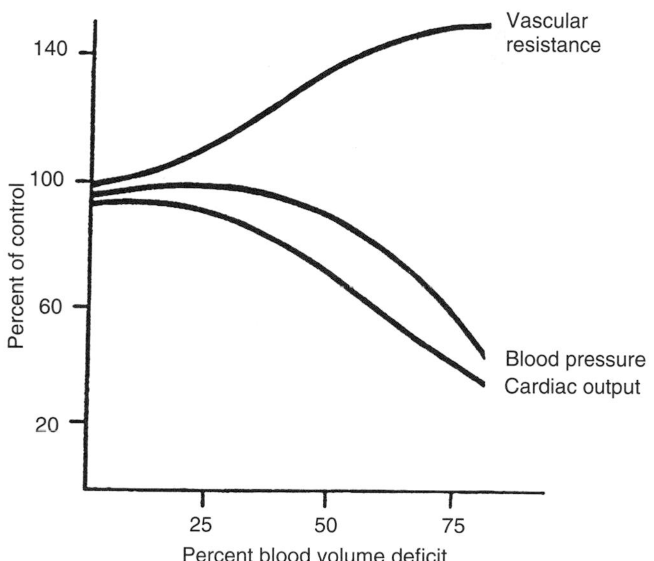

■ **FIGURE 30–5.** Increase in systemic vascular resistance in response to hypovolemia preserves blood pressure until 25% of blood volume is lost. Hypotension is a late sign of hypovolemia. (From Rasmussen GE, Grandes CM: Blood, fluids, and electrolytes in the pediatric trauma patient. *Int Anesthesiol Clin* 32:79–101, 1994.)

■ TABLE 30–3. Stages of pediatric blood volume loss (shock) and associated clinical signs

Blood Volume Loss	Clinical Signs	
<20%	CV:	Tachycardia; weak, thready pulses
	Skin:	Cool to touch, capillary refill 2 to 3 seconds
	Renal:	Slight decrease in urine output, increase in specific gravity
	CNS:	Irritable, may be combative
25%	CV:	Tachycardia; weak, thready distal pulses
	Skin:	Cold extremities, cyanosis and mottling
	Renal:	Decrease in urine output
	CNS:	Confusion, lethargy
40%	CV:	Frank hypotension; tachycardia may progress to bradycardia
	Skin:	Pale, cold
	Renal:	No urine output
	CNS:	Comatose

CV, cardiovascular; CNS, central nervous system.
From Rasmussen GE, Grandes CM: Blood, fluids, and electrolytes in the pediatric trauma patient. *Int Anesthesiol Clin* 32:79–101, 1994.

approximately 25% of the blood volume, or 20 mL/kg (American College of Surgeons Committee on Trauma, 1997). Bradycardia is a dangerous sign that indicates hypoxemia, impending arrest, or increased ICP. Table 30–3 describes the stages of pediatric shock and clinical signs seen at these stages.

It is imperative to rapidly assess the pediatric trauma patient for signs of shock on arrival at the emergency department and at frequent intervals thereafter. The initial fluid bolus administered in the trauma setting should be warmed isotonic crystalloid (lactated Ringer's or normal saline) in an intravenous bolus of 20 mL/kg. The pulse, capillary refill, and blood pressure should then be reassessed. A second bolus of 20 mL/kg should be administered if there is no significant response or only a transient improvement in these parameters. A third crystalloid bolus may be given, if necessary, to maintain appropriate vital signs and circulation. Then 10 mL/kg of blood should be administered next if additional fluid resuscitation is required. The need for blood transfusion initially is uncommon and usually signals "surgical bleeding" that may require operation.

If shock persists and fails to respond to fluid therapy, other causes should be sought. Such causes may include long bone or pelvic fractures. Pericardial effusion and tamponade are less common occurrences in blunt trauma than are penetrating injuries. The classic clinical signs of cardiac tamponade are shock, muffled heart sounds, and distended neck veins. Treatment requires immediate pericardiocentesis.

Pneumothorax is a common complication of blunt chest injury in children, with nearly one fourth under tension (Nakayama et al., 1989). Unilateral or bilateral tension pneumothoraces may produce hypotension and hypoxemia. The classic signs of tension pneumothorax are ipsilateral tympany, shift of the trachea to the contralateral side, and distended neck veins.

Significant occult blood loss may be overlooked on the initial examination of the small child and infant. Because the absolute blood volume of a child is small, the significance of external blood loss may be underestimated. In addition, blood accumulation in the infant's large, expandable head, and open fontanels can produce shock. Careful assessment of the abdomen is central to evaluation of the injured patient in shock.

VASCULAR ACCESS

Adequate large-bore intravenous access must be established as early as possible in the course of the resuscitation. Although peripheral routes offer the most rapidly accessible sites, such access may be difficult or impossible to obtain in the child with depleted intravascular volume or shock and resultant peripheral vasoconstriction. In such cases, a central venous catheter may be placed in the femoral vein if personnel with the necessary skills are available. Central venous catheters (specifically of the internal jugular or subclavian vein) are not recommended as a primary intravascular route during initial resuscitation because of the risk of pneumothorax or hemothorax during their insertion. Placement of these catheters is difficult in small children and infants under the best of circumstances, and C-spine immobilization precludes the appropriate neck position required for safe technique. Delays in establishing vascular access may be life threatening. Therefore, if these routes fail, intraosseous access should be rapidly initiated to expedite the administration of volume expanders and necessary pharmacologic agents. Once the child has been resuscitated, additional catheters should be placed.

Intraosseous access is placed in the medial surface of the proximal tibia 1 to 3 cm below the tibial tuberosity or the distal femoral metaphysis and has been used as a life-saving measure to establish short-term vascular access in critically ill or injured children (Figs. 30–6 and 33–2). In a review of the use of intraosseous access in pediatric trauma patients under 10 years of age, Guy and others

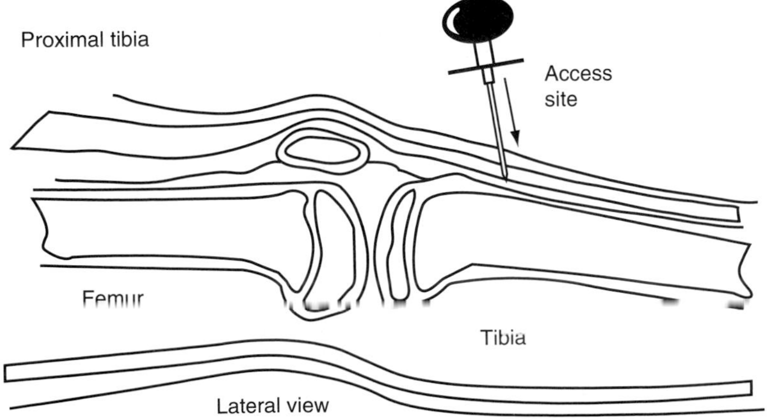

■ FIGURE 30–6. Appropriate placement of the intraosseous infusion needle on the medial surface, distal to tibial tuberosity. (From Ellemunter H: *Arch Dis Child Fetal Neonatal Ed* 80:74F, 1999.)

(1993) reported successful placement in 28 of 32 attempts. In this study, intraosseous access was established successfully by paramedics, nurses, and physicians. There were no long-term complications in the survivors, and there was one minor incident involving extravasation of fluid. The most common complication of intraosseous access is subperiosteal infiltration, which generally resolves spontaneously without further problems. Intraosseous access has a low complication rate; osteomyelitis and cellulitis occur in 0.6% and 0.7%, respectively (Rosetti et al., 1985; Fiser, 1990). Other rare complications include fractures and emboli. Although very few complications have been reported with this technique, it must be recognized that the high mortality in patients who require intraosseous access prevents assessment of long term complications.

DISABILITY AND DIAGNOSTIC EVALUATION

The diagnostic evaluation of the injured child involves clinical examination supplemented by radiologic examinations and laboratory testing. Imaging plays a major role in the evaluation of the injured child (Vane, 2002). Improvements in imaging techniques have allowed progress in nonoperative management of abdominal and thoracic trauma, supplanting exploratory laparotomy and diagnostic peritoneal lavage (DPL) in many hemodynamically stable patients.

Initial plain film screening examinations in injured children who have mechanisms of injury compatible with serious injuries are generally limited to chest, pelvis, and lateral C-spine radiographs obtained in the emergency department trauma bay. Further radiographs are directed by physical findings (e.g., extremity deformity, spine tenderness). Spine films are obtained when spine tenderness, deformity, neurologic deficits, or inadequate examination in a patient prevents clinical spine clearance (Fig. 30–7).

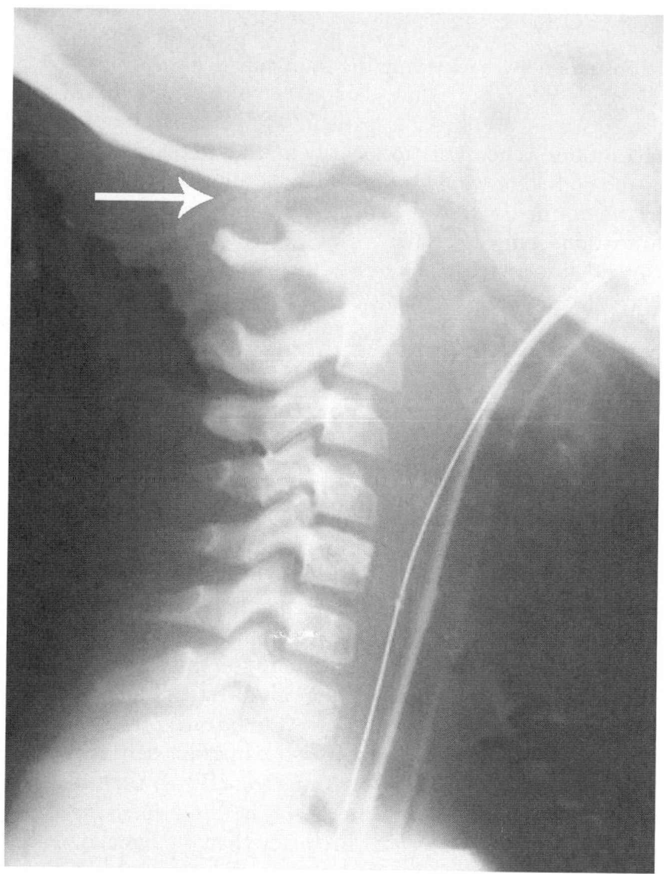

FIGURE 30–7. Lateral cervical spine radiograph of a 9-year-old involved in an automobile accident. *Arrow* points to an occipitoatloid (C1) dislocation. The patient died.

Computed tomography (CT) is widely used in the evaluation of pediatric trauma. Head CT scans are routinely obtained in children with a history of loss of consciousness, altered mental status, and focal neurologic deficits. Neck CT is obtained to supplement cervical radiographic studies or when a C-spine injury may exist on the basis of clinical signs and symptoms. Whenever C-spine injuries may exist based on clinical judgment or the mechanism of injury, C-spine precautions and immobilization should be maintained. C-spine clearance in the brain-injured patient may not be possible until the patient's mental status has improved.

CT of the abdomen and pelvis is routinely used in the evaluation of abdominal injuries and tenderness or as a screening tool in obtunded patients (Haftel et al., 1988; Vane et al., 2002). CT scans are invaluable for the evaluation of injuries to solid organs or retroperitoneum. They are useful but less sensitive and specific for evaluation of hollow viscous injuries or intestinal perforation (Bulas et al., 1989). CT scanning has largely replaced DPL in the initial evaluation of blunt pediatric abdominal trauma, although DPL may be a useful adjunct in selected patients. Focused abdominal sonogram for trauma (FAST) is of more limited value in the pediatric trauma population because many solid organ injuries produce minimal free fluid (lesser grades of spleen, liver, and kidney injuries) such that it may not be detected (Coley et al., 2000).

As most pediatric trauma patients are generally healthy before their injury and take few or no medications, screening laboratory examinations are limited and focused. Children with minor injuries (e.g., upper extremity fractures) may undergo no or very limited laboratory testing. In more seriously injured patients, laboratory testing may generally be safely limited to specific clinical indications, rather than a generalized routine "trauma panel" (Chu et al., 1996). A complete blood count, blood gas, blood typing and screening, and urinalysis are suggested for initial testing in seriously injured patients. Routine testing of liver functions, pancreatic enzymes, and coagulation parameters is of limited value and should be obtained only when clinically indicated.

DISABILITY (NEUROLOGIC ASSESSMENT)

A brief rapid neurologic evaluation is performed as part of the primary survey. It should include assessment of the patient's level of consciousness and pupillary function. The AVPU method (*A*lert, responds to *V*oice, responds only to *P*ain, *U*nresponsive to stimuli) or the more detailed Glasgow Coma Scale (GCS) should be used. If AVPU is selected, the GCS calculation is performed during the secondary survey with a detailed neurologic examination. Periodic reassessment of the level of consciousness is necessary to detect neurologic deterioration due to progression of TBI, hypoxemia, or hypovolemia. Changes in mental status require prompt reevaluation of the ABCs. If the ABCs are adequately managed, then deterioration in mental status should be considered as due to TBI, prompting further brain imaging and consultation with a neurosurgeon.

EXPOSURE

Exposure involves removing the trauma patient's garments, usually with shears, to allow detailed physical examination and detect injuries. Rolling the patient, while maintaining C-spine precautions, is necessary to identify injuries to the dorsal surface of the body that would otherwise be occult. Padding should be placed on the backboard at this time to prevent decubitus ulcer formation. This assessment should be rapid and the patient covered in warmed blankets and/or with a warming device to prevent hypothermia. In addition, intravenous fluids should be warmed and the room temperature raised. This is especially important in small children who are more prone to hypothermia due to their larger ratio of surface area to volume.

SPECIFIC INJURIES

FACIAL TRAUMA

Although severe facial trauma in children is a relatively uncommon event (Zerfowski and Bremerich, 1998), when it does occur, it can make endotracheal intubation challenging, if not impossible (Fig. 30–8; also see Fig. 30–4). Blood, secretions, hematomas, damaged tissues, and dentition may all obstruct the airway during respiration, ventilation, direct laryngoscopy, and fiberoptic intubation. Facial injuries can be categorized (in order of decreasing frequency) as soft tissue injuries, dental injuries, and facial fractures. As depicted in Figure 30–9, the frequency of these injuries varies with the age of the child. In all instances, injuries are more common in males than in females. Facial trauma in children under 5 years of age is less severe because of the protective environment under parental supervision (Kaban, 1993). However, Shaikh and Worrall (2002) found that 42% of the pediatric population they sampled with facial injuries were younger than 5 years, with soft tissue injuries more common. The vast majority of these injuries were caused by falls, due to insecurities in motion and lack of coordination preventing victims from shielding their face or turning their head. The injury is then focused on a relatively small area of the face, from the nose to the mentum, referred to as "the falling zone" (Zerfowski and Bremerich, 1998). Rates of soft tissue injuries rise again in adolescence, possibly explained by more aggressive, risky behavior, which may be related to alcohol consumption or sporting activities.

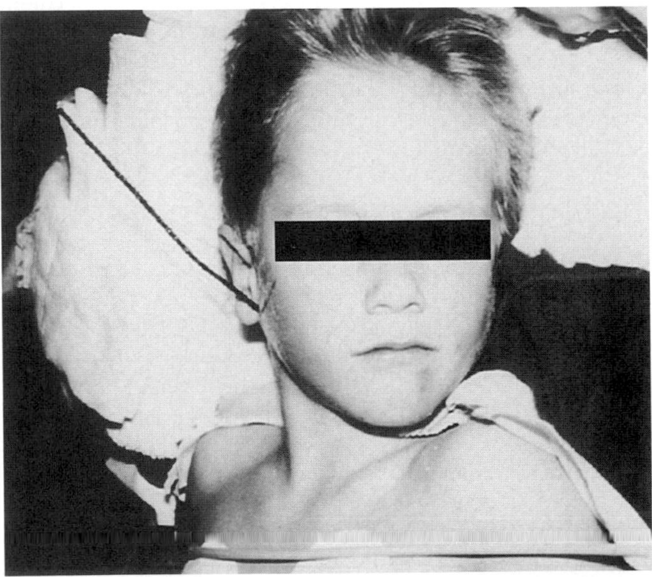

FIGURE 30–8. Protruding objects in the neck should never be pulled out because major vascular structures may be involved. In addition, hypertension during intubation must be avoided, as well as "awake" intubation.

Dental injuries occur at a lesser rate throughout childhood (compared with soft tissue injuries). Accidental aspiration of teeth before or during resuscitation can complicate care and necessitate removal via bronchoscopy. The least common form of pediatric facial trauma, accounting for only 8% of patients in the study by Zerfowski and Bremerich (1998), was facial fractures. Nasal fractures are the most common facial fractures in children, accounting for more than 50% of all facial fractures in one study, followed by mandibular fractures and, last, maxillary fractures.

Another form of pediatric facial injury that can pose a challenge to anesthesiologists is oropharyngeal lacerations or impalement. It is not uncommon for children to fall with foreign objects in their mouths (e.g., pencil, toothbrush, etc.), sometimes sustaining abrasions or lacerations to the soft palate or oropharynx. Most are mild and spontaneously heal without intervention (Hellmann et al., 1993). However, children require surgical extraction of the foreign body (Fig. 30–10). In these instances, before extraction of a foreign body, an angiogram should be performed to determine if any vascular structures are involved. Moriarty and others (1997) have reported carotid artery thrombosis and stroke in a 2-year-old following blunt pharyngeal trauma from a fall with a toothbrush.

Dog bites are another common cause of facial injury in children. In a study by Mcheik and others in 2000, the majority of children (68%) were less than 5 years of age. The goals of immediate surgical repair are to diminish scarring and decrease the rate of wound infection.

Last, extrusion of eye contents through a full-thickness penetrating ocular laceration may result in permanent loss of vision (Fig. 30–11). Intraoperative anesthetic management of open globe injuries is discussed further in Chapter 22, Anesthesia for Ophthalmic Surgery.

As with other trauma, facial injuries in children should be evaluated in the field or the emergency department during the primary survey. If there is any evidence of airway obstruction or respiratory insufficiency, the airway should be secured immediately with direct laryngoscopy, with LMA, or surgically. As mentioned previously, special attention to C-spine stability during direct laryngoscopy should be accomplished with inline stabilization of the neck. Once the airway is secured, a secondary survey can be performed to ascertain the extent of the facial injury and the need for surgical intervention.

CHEST INJURIES

Chest injuries may be immediately life threatening due to impairment of breathing or circulation or as a result of exsanguinating hemorrhage. Life-threatening injuries that impair breathing include open or tension pneumothorax, flail chest, and injuries to the trachea or bronchi. Fortunately, most pediatric chest injuries (78%) can be managed safely with observation or tube thoracostomy (Rielly et al., 1993).

Tension pneumothorax is an urgent yet manageable complication of chest injury that produces diminished breath sounds, tracheal deviation, hypotension, and increasing airway pressure to ventilate (i.e., decreased lung compliance). Tension pneumothorax

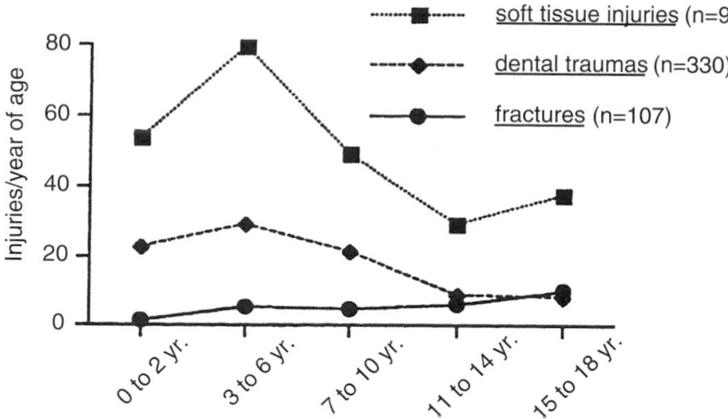

■ **FIGURE 30–9.** Type of injuries per year of age, demonstrated separately for soft tissue injuries, dental trauma, and fractures. (From Ferfowski M, Bremerich A: Facial trauma in children and adolescents. *Clin Oral Invest* 2:120–124, 1998.)

occurs due to accumulation of air in the pleural space under pressure. Air from the injured lung is trapped in the pleural space by an air leak, which acts as a one-way valve such that each subsequent breath introduces air under progressively increasing pressure. This impairs breathing and venous return to the heart. It should be treated immediately with needle catheter decompression by inserting a large-bore intravenous catheter in the second intercostal space, followed by chest tube placement. Simple pneumothorax also causes lung collapse and impaired breathing but to a lesser degree than tension pneumothorax.

Open pneumothorax occurs when injury has produced a chest wall defect. This equalizes the pressure between the pleural space and the environment, causing collapse of the ipsilateral lung and to-and-fro movements of air with breathing through the chest wall defect rather than the airway. It is managed by covering the defect with an occlusive dressing taped on three sides. This allows the patient to breathe and prevents the accumulation of a tension pneumothorax.

The pediatric chest wall is more compliant than that of the adult. The chest wall has a significant cartilaginous component and the ribs are not completely ossified. Consequently, rib fractures and flail chest are less common in children than in adults.

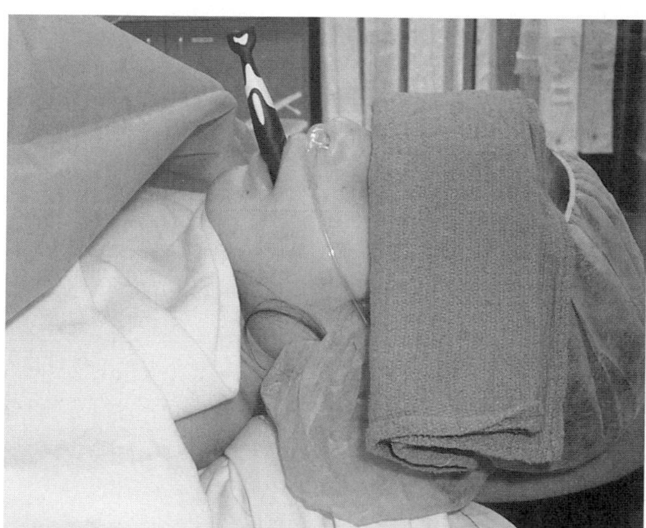

■ **FIGURE 30–10.** The left tonsillar bed of a 6-year-old girl was impaled after she fell with a toothbrush in her mouth. She was intubated orally with direct laryngoscopy.

However, significant intrathoracic injury, such as pulmonary contusion, may occur in the absence of a rib fracture. Flail chest occurs when four or more ribs are each fractured in two places by blunt trauma. The floating fracture segments produce paradoxical movement of the chest wall and reduce ventilation of the lung. An underlying pulmonary contusion impairs gas exchange or ventilation.

Injury to the airway may result in severe impairment of breathing, airway obstruction or hemorrhage, or tension pneumothorax. This may be immediately or rapidly lethal. Establishing adequate ventilation may require placement of a double-lumen endotracheal tube or selective intubation of the main bronchus.

The mediastinum is highly mobile in children. Aortic tears are rare in children (Eddy et al., 1990). When they occur, free rupture results in rapid demise of the patient. With contained rupture, the patients are frequently stable. Contained aortic injuries are managed operatively after life-threatening abdominal and head injuries are initially managed. A widened mediastinum, fractures of the first rib, or presence of an apical pleural "cap" on the left side each raises the possibility of an aortic disruption. An angiogram is essential for further evaluation (Akins et al., 1981) (Fig. 30–12). Significant cardiac injuries are uncommon in children (Langer et al., 1989). Injuries to the heart, great vessels, or lung hilus may result in massive hemorrhage and impaired circulation. Penetrating chest injuries that usually occur as a result of violent acts are fortunately rare in children. In most cases, pneumothorax and hemothorax respond rapidly to the placement of chest tubes. Thoracotomy is required only in the infrequent cases of massive air leak, persistent bleeding with shock, or transfusion requirements exceeding 10 mL/kg per hour.

ABDOMINAL INJURIES

Abdominal injuries are the cause of death in approximately 10% of trauma fatalities (Cooper et al., 1994). Blunt trauma as a result of motor vehicle accidents (as passengers or pedestrians) and falls are the most common mechanisms of injury in children. The vast majority of children with solid visceral injuries and bleeding do not require a laparotomy (Haller et al., 1994; Mehall et al., 2001; Mooney, 2002). The bleeding usually stops without surgical intervention. Nonoperative management of blunt trauma requires careful physical examination and imaging (usually CT scanning) for detection of injuries followed by observation and serial examination.

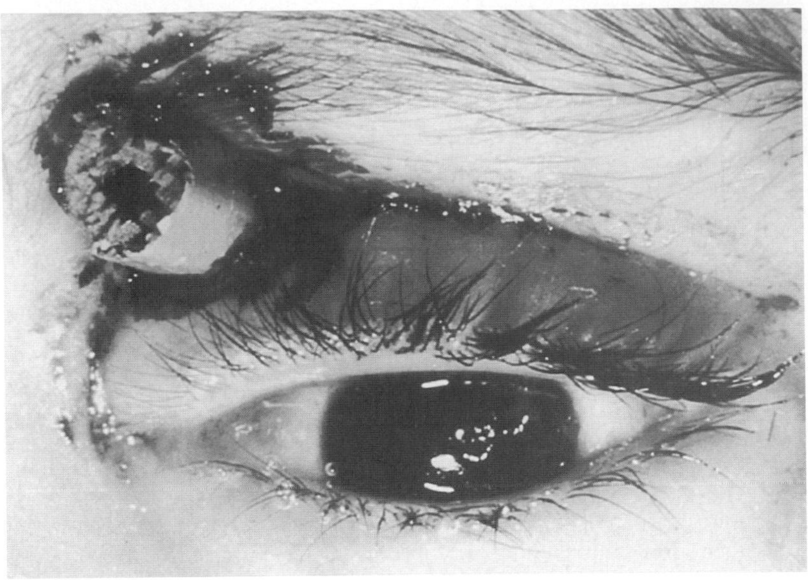

■ **FIGURE 30–11.** Open-eye injury in children is often caused by a projectile object.

Trauma laparotomy is infrequently performed in pediatric trauma centers, occurring in 0.3% of trauma admissions (Green and Rothrock, 2002). Laparotomies are performed when signs of bowel perforation (pneumoperitoneum, peritonitis) or hemodynamic instability occur due to suspected intra-abdominal injury. Gunshot wounds to the abdomen and lower chest, evisceration, and symptomatic stab wounds are also indications for laparotomy (Furnival, 2001; Stafford et al., 2002). Patients with asymptomatic anterior stab wounds are evaluated by local wound exploration and serial examinations. Asymptomatic flank and back stab wounds are evaluated by local exploration, serial examination, or contrast CT (American College of Surgeons Committee on Trauma, 1997). The introduction of laparoscopy may reduce the number of laparotomies or replace DPL in cases when physical examination is unreliable and there is a concern for possible intra-abdominal injuries (e.g., head-injured multitrauma patients, seat belt injuries, and abdominal tenderness). Indications for operative management of specific severe injuries (e.g., pancreatic head or ductal injuries, bile leak) and complications are beyond the scope of this chapter.

Most renal injuries and lacerations do not require immediate surgery (Cass, 1983; Bergren et al., 1987). Injury to the blood supply of the kidney that results in devascularization requires an operation. Devascularizing injuries can be diagnosed by the kidney failing to opacify with contrast material (Karp et al., 1986; Kisa and Schenk, 1986). Blood at the urethral meatus suggests trauma to the lower urinary tract (McAninch and Carroll, 1988). Retrograde urethrography and voiding cystourethrography are required studies. Transsection of the bladder neck can occur with major pelvic trauma and is suggested by the inability to feel the prostate on rectal examination.

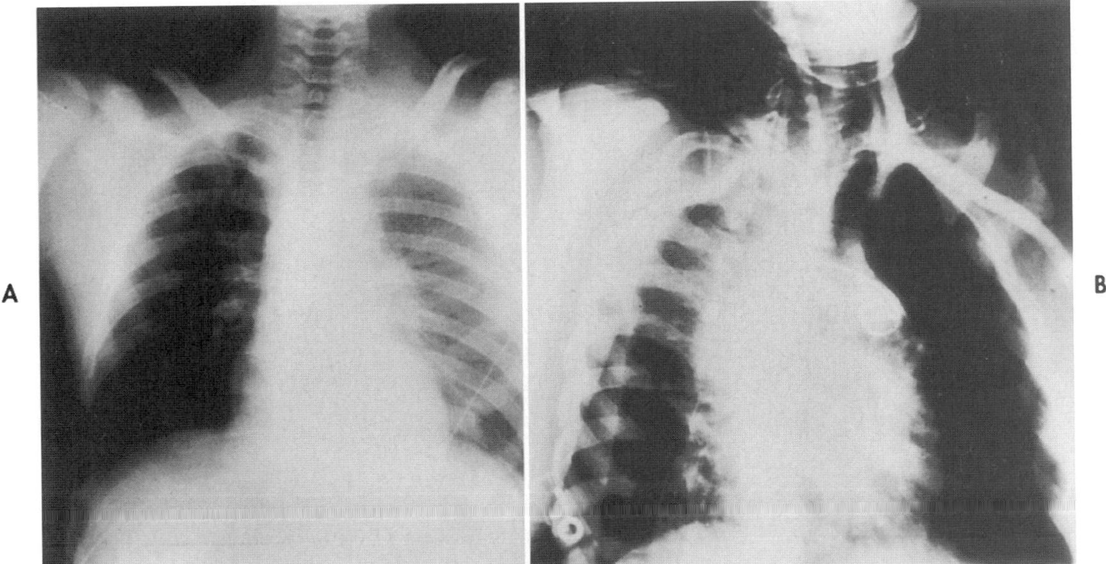

■ **FIGURE 30–12.** (*A*) This child presented with a widened mediastinum following blunt chest trauma. (*B*) An immediate arteriogram revealed a disrupted aortic arch.

TABLE 30–4. Glasgow Coma Scale (GCS) and Pediatric Glasgow Coma Scale

Best Response	Adult GCS	Pediatric GCS	Score
Eye	No eye opening	No eye opening	1
	Eye opening to pain	Eye opening to pain	2
	Eye opening to verbal command	Eye opening to speech	3
	Eyes open spontaneously	Eyes open spontaneously	4
Verbal	No verbal response	No vocal response	1
	Incomprehensible sounds	Inconsolable, agitated	2
	Inappropriate words	Inconsistently consolable, moaning	3
	Confused conversation	Cries, but is consolable, inappropriate interactions	4
	Oriented	Smiles, oriented to sounds, follows objects, interacts	5
Motor	No motor response	No motor response	1
	Extension to pain	Extension to pain	2
	Flexion to pain	Flexion to pain	3
	Withdrawal from pain	Withdrawal from pain	4
	Localizing pain	Localizing pain	5
	Obeys commands	Obeys commands	6

GCS ≥13, mild brain injury; GCS 9 to 12, moderate brain injury; GCS <8, severe brain injury.
From Marcin JP, Pollack MM: Triage scoring systems, severity of illness measures, and mortality prediction models in pediatric trauma. *Crit Care Med* 30:S457–S467, 2002.

TRAUMATIC BRAIN INJURY

TBI is the leading cause of mortality in the pediatric trauma patient (Tepas et al., 1990), accounting for over 70% of the deaths. Although motor vehicle accidents are the most common mechanism of head injury, 30% to 50% of TBI cases in children under 4 years of age are attributed to falls or abuse (Dashti et al., 1999). Multisystem injury due to trauma is almost always associated with head injury in children. The disproportionately large head and relatively weak neck musculature, with a high center of gravity in children less than 3 years, puts them at risk for coup-countercoup brain injuries even at low velocities (Dykes, 1999). Other factors contributing to the increased risk of TBI in children include thinner cranial bones and less myelinated nerve tissue, making them more vulnerable to damage.

Diffuse brain injury, the most common type of TBI in children, can range from a mild concussion to diffuse axonal injury resulting in permanent disability (Bruce, 1981). Focal cerebral contusions may be located in the area of impact (coup) or on the opposite side of the brain (countercoup), or both. Intracranial hemorrhage can present in the epidural, subdural, subarachnoid, or intracerebral spaces. Epidural hematomas occur as a result of a tear in the middle meningeal artery, but subdural hematomas usually result from a tear in the bridging veins. In case of an epidural hematoma, rapid decompression is usually required due to the arterial nature of the bleeding, to avoid death or permanent disability. In addition, children may sustain concomitant skull fractures, which if open may require early surgical intervention.

The three phases of TBI are (1) the primary injury, (2) the secondary injury due to cerebral response to trauma, and (3) the secondary injury due to the systemic response to trauma (Vavilala and Lam, 2002). The goal of the clinician caring for a child with TBI is to minimize neurologic effects of secondary injury, because this contributes largely to eventual morbidity and mortality. TBI should be considered in all children after trauma regardless of the absence of neurologic signs and symptoms. Initial assessment of the pediatric patient should include the GCS (Table 30–4), the most widely used and best known of all trauma scores (Teasale and Jennett, 1974). This scale has been validated in many studies as a reliable measure of neurologic outcome and is an excellent tool for following the neurologic status of a patient with TBI. The GCS has been modified for pediatric patients (Marcin and Pollack, 2002) but can also be used for the cognitively impaired child. A GCS score of 13 or greater is associated with mild brain injury; 9 to 12, moderate brain injury; and less than 8, severe. In all children with head injuries, a pediatric GCS should be assigned on arrival and at each reexamination. Significant or progressive intracranial injury, as suggested by localizing neurologic signs, a GCS less than 13, or a decrease in the GCS of 2 points from the initial level, is an indication for a CT scan of the head (Dykes, 1999). Seizures are not uncommon in children after even minor TBI (Bruce et al., 1979). Loss of consciousness and/or seizure activity may increase the risk of vomiting and subsequent aspiration.

There should be a low threshold for intubation in the child with TBI, for airway protection and hyperventilation. Waxing and waning mental status, or a GCS score of less than 8, is an indication for intubation and hyperventilation (to prevent increased arterial carbon dioxide and the resultant cerebral vasodilatation and brain swelling). It must be remembered that the presence or suspicion of a basilar skull fracture is a contraindication for a nasal intubation. Although little can be done to minimize the cerebral damage due to the primary injury, every effort should be made to minimize subsequent brain injury due to hypoxic or ischemic insult. Systemic abnormalities such as shock, hypotension, hypoxemia, and hypercarbia as a result of coexisting injuries may lead to further brain injury and should be promptly managed as discussed previously.

The reaction of the brain to the initial trauma develops over a 3- to 5-day period with potential for loss of autoregulation, cellular edema, and breakdown of the blood–brain barrier (Vavilala and Lam, 2002). Cerebral blood flow (CBF), ICP, cerebral metabolic rate ($CMRO_2$), mean arterial pressure (MAP), cerebral perfusion pressure (CPP), and acid-base status all may be affected by diffuse cerebral swelling, which may occur in TBI.

Also, reperfusion following ischemic brain injury may be accompanied by activation of the inflammatory cascade (Jean et al., 1998). The resultant influx of calcium, free radicals, cytokines, and other harmful inflammatory mediators has been implicated in the exacerbation of existing neuronal damage. Animal studies have demonstrated some benefits in terms of neurologic improvement by administration of anti-inflammatory antibodies, but human studies have not adequately addressed their use. Indeed, corticosteroids have a limited role in the routine management of the child with head trauma because they do not improve neurologic outcome and may predispose the child to infection (Bracco and Bissonnette, 2002).

Children with cerebral edema or intracranial hypertension may require an ICP monitor or ventriculostomy to be placed. Figure 30–13 depicts an algorithm for maintaining normal ICP/CPP in the pediatric patient. Figure 30–14 demonstrates changes in MAP, ICP, and CPP with age. By manipulating MAP and CBF with vasopressors and hyperventilation, draining cerebrospinal fluid, and decreasing $CMRO_2$ with sedatives or barbiturates, the goals of maintaining a normal ICP/CPP may be met. Refractory intracranial hypertension may require barbiturate coma, aggressive hyperventilation with CBF and/or jugular venous monitoring, or even decompressive craniectomy. Therapeutic hypothermia (to a temperature of 32° to 33°C for 24 hours) has been shown to improve long-term neurologic outcomes in a controlled randomized study involving 82 adults with TBI (Marion et al., 1997). However, hypothermia should be used only in selected patients with TBI because it did not improve outcomes in patients in whom ICP could be controlled by conventional measures (Shiozaki et al., 1999).

The mortality rate for children with severe head injuries (GCS score <8) is as high as 32% (Ward, 1995). Despite this

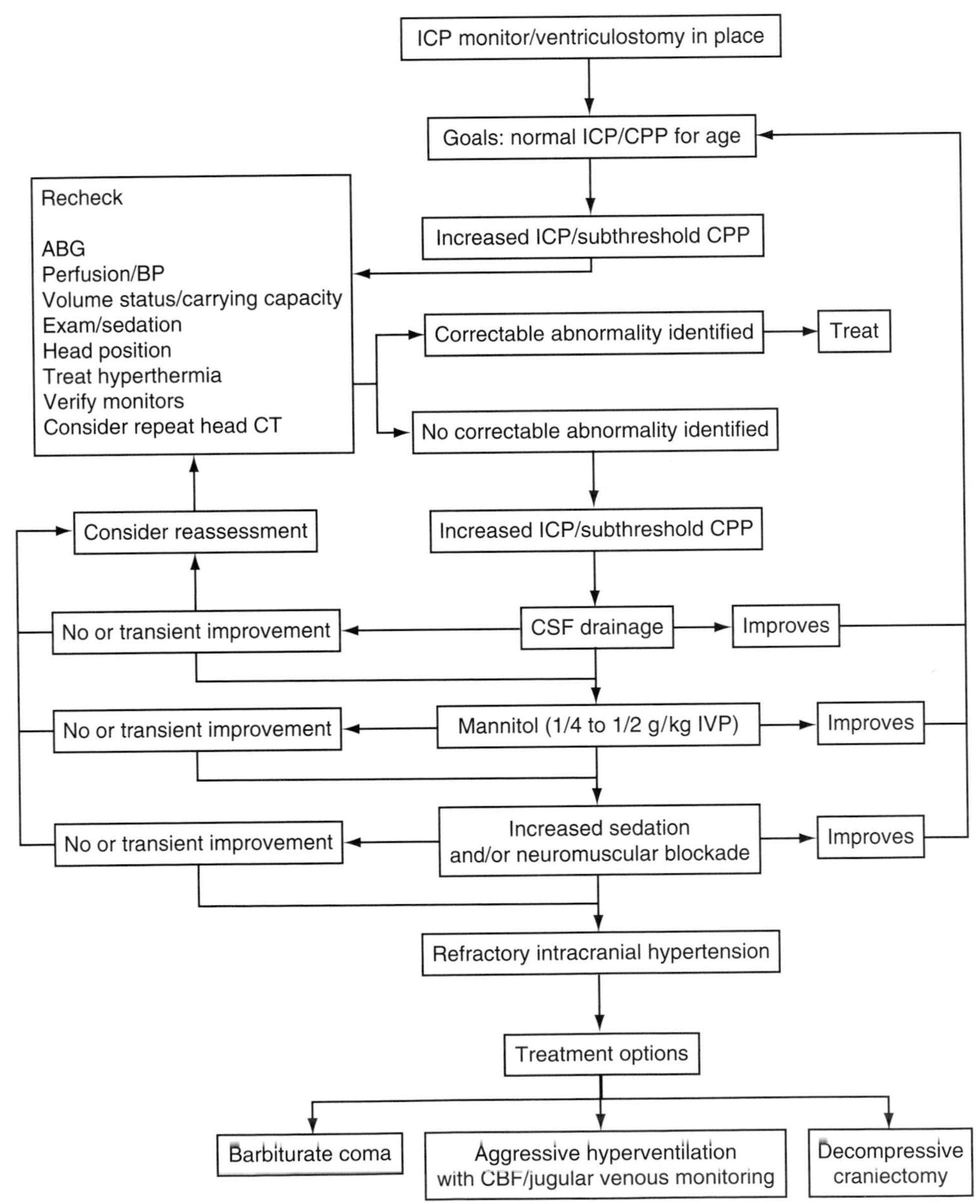

■ **FIGURE 30–13.** The University of Michigan C. S. Mott Children's Hospital algorithm for the treatment of intracranial hypertension in children. (Courtesy of C. S. Mott Children's Hospital, Ann Arbor, MI.)

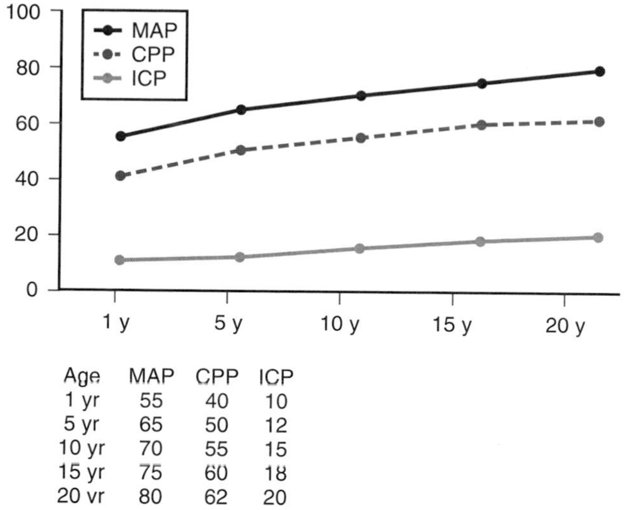

Age	MAP	CPP	ICP
1 yr	55	40	10
5 yr	65	50	12
10 yr	70	55	15
15 yr	75	60	18
20 yr	80	62	20

■ **FIGURE 30–14.** Age-related increases in mean arterial pressure (MAP), cerebral perfusion pressure (CPP), and intracranial pressure (ICP).

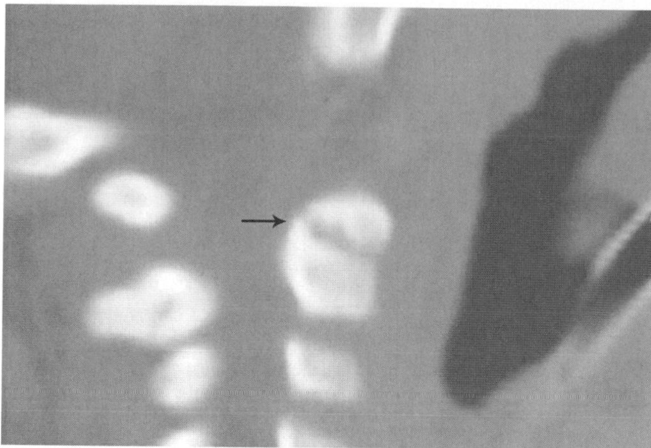

■ **FIGURE 30–15.** Magnetic resonance image of a 22 month old boy who fell off of a grocery cart onto his head. *Arrow* points to a nondisplaced fracture of the ondontoid process in C2.

high mortality rate, the functional outcome in children is thought to be better than that in adults. It is therefore imperative that the clinician manage children with TBI by rapidly alleviating the effects of the primary insult and aggressively treating the secondary injuries. TBI is discussed further in Chapter 18, Anesthesia for Neurosurgery.

■ SPINAL INJURIES

Although vertebral fractures in children are less common than in adults, it may be prudent to assume that any pediatric patient with a major traumatic injury has a spinal injury until proven otherwise. Cervical spine fractures occur in 7% to 10% of children with TBI, with 20% of these patients presenting with a second noncontiguous spinal injury. There are several anatomic differences between the adult and pediatric C-spine that account for the differences in the type of injuries incurred by each group. The fulcrum of cervical mobility in an infant or a young child is at the level of C2-3, compared with C5-6 or C6-7 in an adult. For this reason, 60% to 70% of pediatric fractures occur in the C1 or C2 vertebrae compared with only 16% in the adult population (Hasue et al., 1974). C-spine fractures are less common in children because of ligamental laxity, but this does not prevent spinal cord damage in this population. By the time the child has reached 8 years of age, the C-spine has fully matured (Eichelberger, 1993).

Fracture of the ondontoid process (dens) of the C2 vertebra is one of the most common vertebral injuries in children (Figs. 30–15 and 30–16). This is due to the inherent weakness of the growth plate at the base of the dens. These are usually flexion injuries that rarely cause initial neurologic impairment. Spinal cord damage is associated with hyperextension of the neck and posterior displacement of the dens into the cord. It is imperative, therefore, that any spinal injury is not exacerbated by manipulation of the neck during interventions such as endotracheal intubation. The presence of neck or back pain, altered mental status, or abnormal peripheral neurologic findings (e.g., priapism, paresthesia, and/or dysesthesia) should necessitate C-spine immobilization and a radiographic examination of the spine. A pediatric C-spine evaluation protocol is presented in Figure 30–17.

Radiographic evaluation of the C-spine should not take precedence over the ABCs, but studies should be performed in a timely fashion. In the absence of a fracture, the diagnosis of spinal cord injury in children is confounded by ligamental laxity, larger acceptable predental spaces, and C2-3 override (Swischuk, 1986) (Table 30–5). If intubation is required, the neck should be maintained in a neutral position with a cervical collar. Older children may tolerate awake, fiberoptic intubation with or without sedation. The very young or uncooperative child or any patient with bloody secretions in the airway may not be suitable for this technique and requires a rapid sequence induction with inline stabilization of the neck.

■ LAWNMOWER-RELATED INJURIES

Lawnmowers cause more than 9400 injuries in children less than 18 years of age annually in the United States, with almost a fourth of these injuries occurring in children less than 5 years of age (US Consumer Product Safety Commission, 1990–1999) (Fig. 30–18). The age distribution is bimodal, with peaks at

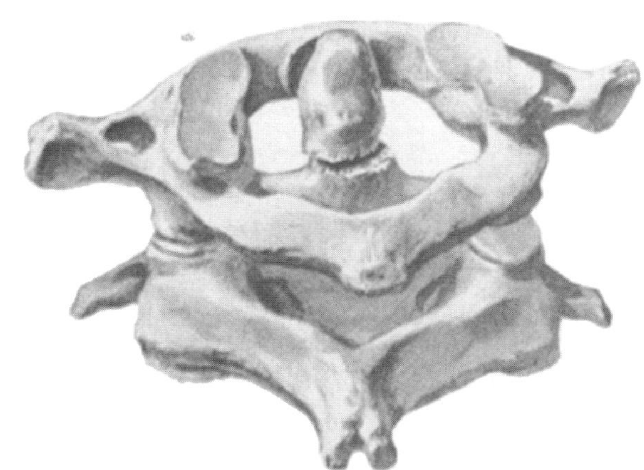

■ **FIGURE 30–16.** Posterior view of C2 ondontoid (dens) fracture. (From Netter F, editor: *The Ciba collection of medical illustrations, vol 1; nervous system.* Summit, NJ, 1953, p 83.)

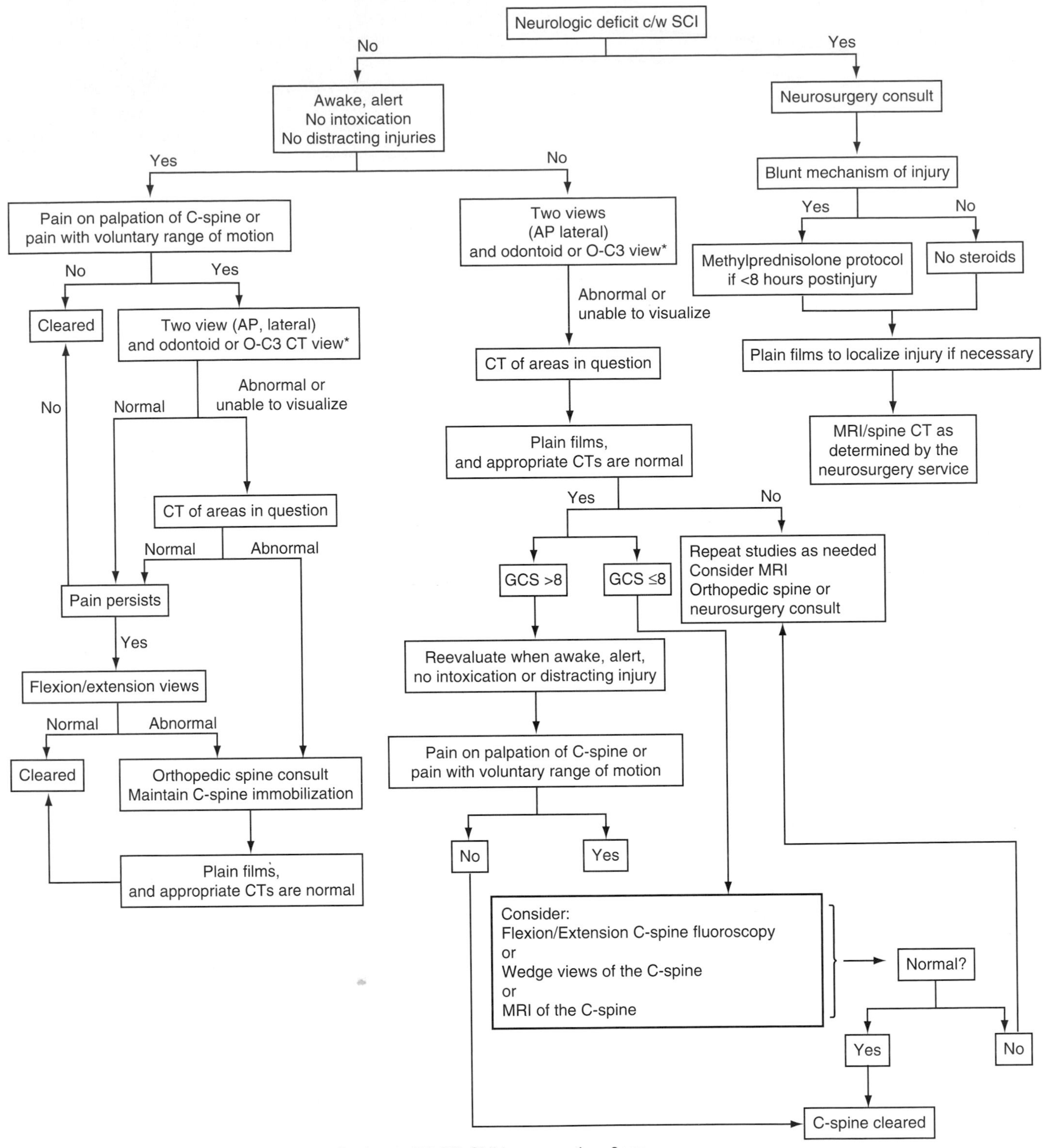

*Children less than 8 should always undergo Occiput to C3 CT, Children more than 8 yrs can undergo either CT or odontoid view. Children undergoing a head CT should have occiput to C3 CT rather than odontoid view

■ **FIGURE 30–17.** The University of Michigan C. S. Mott Children's Hospital algorithm for cervical spine evaluation in a pediatric trauma patient. (Courtesy of C. S. Mott Children's Hospital, Ann Arbor, MI.)

■ TABLE 30–5. Upper normal limits of cervical spine measurements in adults and children

	Adults	Children
Predental space	2.5 mm	4 to 5 mm
C2-3 override (flexion)	3 mm	4 to 5 mm
Prevertebral space (extension)	7 mm	$^1/_2$ to $^2/_3$ AP distance vertebral body

From Eichelberger MR: *Pediatric trauma prevention, acute care, rehabilitation.* St. Louis, 1993, Mosby–Year Book, p 45.

2 and 15 years, probably representing injuries to bystanders versus injuries to operators. More than 7% of children who incur mower-related injuries require hospitalization, about twice the rate for consumer product–related injuries. Riding lawnmowers, commonly used for lawn and field maintenance in this country, are more powerful and complex to operate than are walk-behind mowers. With an injury rate of more than three times that of walk-behind mowers, they carry a higher risk of injury and possible death than walk-behind mowers (Adler, 1994). In 1993, a U.S. Consumer Product Safety Commission report identified four mechanisms of injury due to riding lawnmowers: loss of mower stability, blade contact, layout and function of the mower controls, and running over or backing over young children (Adler, 1993). Backover injuries occurred approximately twice as often as did runover injuries, with about 85% of these injuries occurring in children between 15 months and 10 years of age. Typically, this occurs when the child is playing in the area, is following the mower, or falls off the back of the mower (Deppa, 1994).

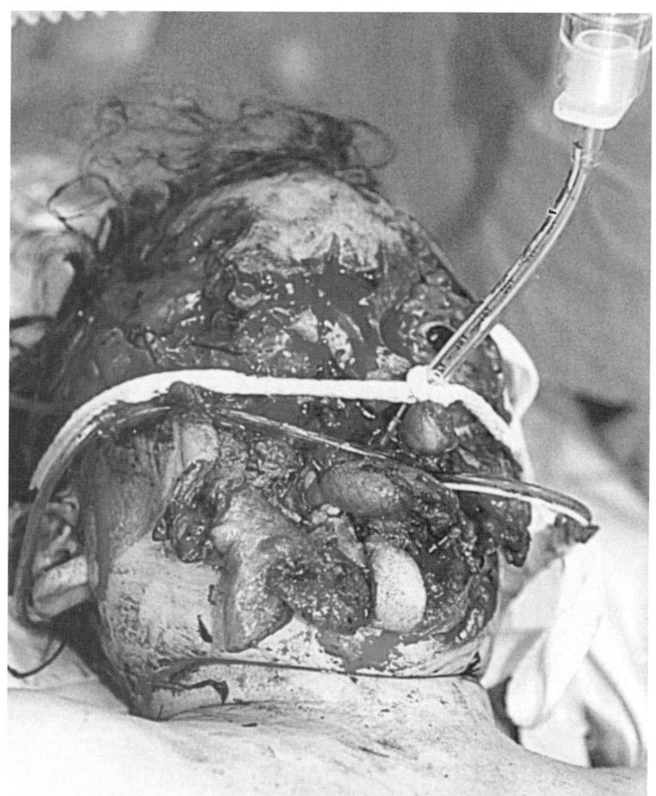

■ FIGURE 30–18. Photograph of a 3-year-old child who was backed over by a riding lawnmower and sustained massive facial trauma and amputation of the left foot.

The types of injuries incurred by children range from lacerations (41%) to amputations and avulsions (7%) (US Consumer Product Safety Commission, 1990–1999). Aside from initial stabilization and treatment, children with these injuries may require repeated anesthetics for wound debridement, reductions of bony fractures, skin grafts, or reconstructive surgery. A child presenting with a lower extremity injury may benefit from combined epidural and general anesthesia, with continued epidural analgesia in the postoperative period. The following are some of the recommendations of the American Academy of Pediatrics Committee on Injury and Poison Prevention (Smith and *Prevention*, 2001).

1. Manufacturers of riding lawnmowers should sell only tractors that will not mow in reverse without a manual override.
2. Children younger than 6 years of age should be kept indoors when lawnmowers are being operated.
3. Children must not be allowed to ride on mowers as passengers.
4. Children should not operate lawnmowers until they have displayed the necessary levels of judgment, strength, skill, and maturity. Most children will not be ready to operate a walk-behind mower until 12 years of age, and a riding mower until at least 16 years.

■ SKELETAL INJURIES

Musculoskeletal injuries are rarely life threatening except when they are associated with ongoing severe hemorrhage, yet they are a leading cause of morbidity and long-term disability, and if not managed appropriately and in a timely manner, long-term sequelae including limb deformities, permanent neurologic and joint dysfunction, and loss of limb viability may result. Additional considerations in children include premature growth arrest and potential for growth plate injuries. In the multiply injured child, it is important to identify the priorities of treatment. Control of bleeding as a result of skeletal injuries should occur as part of the primary survey. Once life-threatening injuries such as head and chest injuries are addressed and initially stabilized, the extent of skeletal injuries should be carefully assessed based on symptoms, physical examination, and radiography. Appropriate initial measures include functional bracing or splinting to alleviate pain and immobilization of bone fragments to prevent further injury of adjacent neurovascular structures, allow safe transport of the patient, and minimize impairment of limb function. In patients with adequate alignment of fracture segments, this may be the only necessary treatment. Other interventions that may be needed in case of displaced fractures include external traction, external fixation, and internal fixation.

Urgent or emergent surgical interventions are usually indicated in the case of complex or displaced fractures associated with vascular damage and potential for limb ischemia or neurologic dysfunction, open fractures, joint dislocations that cannot be reduced, and compartment syndromes (Musgrave and Mendelson, 2002). Vascular injuries in conjunction with limb fractures are, fortunately, rare in children. Although the majority of vascular injuries are associated with supracondylar distal humerus fractures, they may also occur in conjunction with fractures of the distal femur, proximal tibia, displaced pelvic fractures, and knee dislocations. Children with suspected vascular injuries may require an angiogram to delineate the extent of the injury and to determine the need for revascularization. In the case of open fractures, wound irrigation and debridement with extensive removal of contaminated and necrotic tissue are required. Children with open fractures frequently require repeated debridement under general anesthesia every 48 to 72 hours until all of the devitalized tissue has been removed. Pain out of proportion to the extent of the injury should raise concern about compartment syndrome. In these cases, emergent fasciotomies of all involved compartments is indicated because significant muscle necrosis can occur if intracompartment pressures exceed 30 mm Hg for longer than 8 hours (Musgrave and Mendelson, 2002).

Fractures of the femur in children most commonly involve the femoral shaft or the distal femoral physis. Femoral shaft fractures can result in significant blood loss from the fracture segments, and such blood loss may not be readily recognized because the blood accumulates in the large thigh compartments. Serial hematocrits should be obtained in children with femur fractures, and they should be adequately volume resuscitated before the induction of anesthesia to avoid cardiovascular collapse on induction. A high index of suspicion for compartment syndrome should be maintained, particularly in the patient with concomitant head trauma who may be difficult to evaluate. Children with distal femur fractures are at risk of arterial injury and compartment syndrome; attention should be focused on the neurovascular status of the limb (Musgrave and Mendelson, 2002).

The issue of early versus delayed stabilization of femur fractures in children with closed head injuries remains contentious. Interpretation of the existing literature is confounded by variability in study design, small sample size of patients studied, differences in severity of head injury in the early versus late treatment groups, and variable definitions of early versus late treatment. Previous studies in adults have found that early fixation significantly reduced the incidence of severe pulmonary complications, including respiratory distress syndrome, pneumonia, and pulmonary emboli (Bone et al., 1989; Behrman et al., 1990). Pediatric studies found that early stabilization did not lessen the risk of pulmonary complications in the multiply injured child. A retrospective study by Hedequist and others (1999) identified 25 children with femur fractures and central nervous system injury (GCS score, 8). Seven of these children underwent early stabilization, of whom 4 (57%) experienced a respiratory complication compared with 8 complications in 18 (44%) who underwent delayed fixation. In another retrospective study in children, Mendelson and others (2001) reported twice the number of respiratory complications in the late treatment group (4 of 13 versus 2 of 12, P = NS). This difference may be clinically significant, but the groups were dissimilar in that children in the late treatment group had a higher incidence of increased intracranial pressure. Other purported benefits of early fixation include early patient mobilization, shorter hospital and intensive care unit stays, improved predictability of fracture outcome, and decreased costs.

Proponents of late stabilization argue that minor hemodynamic changes, including shifts in blood pressure and volume status, may potentiate secondary brain injury and lead to adverse neurologic outcomes. Previous investigators have reported a greater frequency of intraoperative hypotension and hypoxemia and lower mean GCS scores in patients undergoing early fracture stabilization (Jaicks et al., 1997; Townsend et al., 1998). Yet, other studies have found no relationship between timing of fracture fixation and head trauma outcome (McKee et al., 1997; Kalb et al., 1998; Mendelson et al., 2001). The Committee on Trauma of the American College of Surgeons has recommended that femoral fractures be treated early provided hemodynamic stability has been achieved (Burgess and Cates, 1993). The appropriate timing of femur fracture fixation in a head-injured child remains open to further investigation. Until more definitive data become available, it may be prudent to delay operative fixation of femur fractures until stabilization of hemodynamic and neurologic status are achieved. Also, adequate volume resuscitation and careful monitoring of end-organ perfusion and pressure, including blood pressure and ICP monitoring, should be strongly considered to guide intraoperative interventions that reduce the risk of secondary brain injury.

PERIOPERATIVE MANAGEMENT

Children with multiple injuries frequently present with an unusual combination of anesthetic problems that present a challenge to the anesthesiologist. It must be emphasized that the likelihood of a successful outcome is greatly enhanced by the initial stabilization efforts that must include early initiation of critical care management in the emergency department based on appropriate and rapid physical examination and diagnostic studies rather than an urgent rush to the operating room for emergency surgical interventions (Meyer, 1999). Respiratory stabilization and suitable hemodynamic support including volume resuscitation prevent further decompensation and the development of secondary injuries. This in turn requires a well-coordinated effort by all members of the health care team, including the anesthesiologist, the emergency physician, surgeons of the relevant specialties, respiratory therapists, and critical care physicians and nurses. Only in rare instances is there too little time for the initial stabilization such that a child must undergo surgery emergently to ensure a favorable outcome. In such instances, there must be clear communication between the anesthesiologist and surgeon regarding the time available for resuscitation, securing vascular access, and invasive monitoring capabilities.

Ideally, the role of anesthesiologists in the care of the child who has sustained significant trauma should begin with securing the airway in the emergency department. However, if this cannot be accomplished, it is imperative that they become familiar with the immediate and ongoing resuscitative efforts, as well as the extent and nature of the injuries and the pertinent details regarding the patient's past medical history. The following addresses the anesthetic management of the child who presents for emergent surgery following multiple trauma. The major concerns include (1) NPO status, (2) airway management, (3) anesthetic agents, (4) patient monitoring, and (5) fluid and blood resuscitation.

NPO STATUS

It is common practice to consider all trauma patients at risk for aspiration regardless of the time of last oral intake. The rationale for this approach is that major injury, the presence of pain and anxiety, and/or the administration of opioid analgesics delay gastric emptying. Additionally, bag and mask ventilation at the scene of the accident or in the ED leading to gastric distention, and the use of oral contrast solutions for diagnostic imaging studies may further increase the risk for aspiration. Indeed, previous investigators have demonstrated that patients who present for emergency surgery are at five times the risk for aspiration compared with those who undergo elective surgery (Olsson et al., 1986). Other investigators reported a 17% incidence of vomiting and 3% incidence of aspiration in 60 children less than 19 years of age who required emergency endotracheal intubation after they sustained a severe traumatic injury (Nakayama et al., 1992). Interestingly, residual gastric volume has been previously found to have a greater correlation with the interval from oral intake to injury than with actual fasting interval (Bricker et al., 1989).

These data raise two questions regarding the management of anesthetic induction for the trauma patient: Can we predict the safe interval between oral intake, injury, and induction of anesthesia? Does imposing a fasting duration once the trauma has already occurred offer any benefit in terms of reduction in aspiration risk? Goodwin and Robinson (2000) surveyed 167 practicing anesthesiologists in the United Kingdom regarding their practice in three different scenarios following a forearm fracture in a child. Approximately one third of the respondents did not believe there was any benefit in delaying the procedure and would perform a rapid sequence induction and endotracheal intubation regardless of the fasting duration, whereas almost two thirds of the respondents would delay the procedure if it were not emergent and then use an LMA or facemask as they would for elective cases. Such variability in clinical practice related to the management of the trauma patient is likely due to the difficulty in predicting a safe interval between oral intake, injury, and induction of anesthesia with regard to aspiration risk. All trauma patients should have full stomach precautions and be considered at risk for aspiration.

ANESTHETIC AGENTS

Induction of Anesthesia

Anesthetic induction techniques should be individualized depending on the nature of the injuries, whether the airway has been secured before arrival in the operating suite, anticipated airway difficulty, hemodynamic status of the patient, and the presence of ongoing hemorrhage. The child with head trauma merits special consideration due to the risk of increased ICP during induction of anesthesia. Selection of an induction technique in these patients must be made with the goal of avoiding secondary brain injury. Intravenous induction agents such as thiopental, propofol, or etomidate may be preferred due to their beneficial effects on ICP and $CMRO_2$. On the other hand, a child with an anticipated difficult airway may be more easily managed with an inhaled route of induction so that spontaneous breathing is ensured. Induction of anesthesia in a patient with dehydration or hypovolemia may lead to cardiovascular collapse. It is therefore imperative to have adequate intravenous access and to rehydrate these patients before the induction of anesthesia. A brief description of commonly used induction agents and pitfalls with the use of each in a child with trauma follows (see Chapter 6, Pharmacology of Pediatric Anesthesia, and Chapter 11, Intraoperative and Postoperative Management).

Thiopental. The barbiturates have a long history of use as neuroprotectants. Thiopental has been extensively used as an induction agent in head-injured patients because it is a cerebral vasoconstrictor and decreases CBF, $CMRO_2$, and ICP in a dose-dependent manner. Another beneficial central nervous system effect is reduction in epileptiform activity. Furthermore, thiopental reliably attenuates the increase in ICP caused by noxious interventions such as direct laryngoscopy and endotracheal tube placement. Thiopental should be used with caution in a child with multiple trauma because it is a direct myocardial depressant and may produce a decrease in cardiac output and systemic blood pressure with a resultant decrease in CPP. These effects are more pronounced in patients who have been inadequately volume resuscitated, and the use of alternative induction agents such as etomidate should be strongly considered in patients with a questionable volume status or with uncontrolled, ongoing hemorrhage.

Propofol. Induction of anesthesia with propofol even in healthy children is frequently associated with a significant (10% to 20%) decrease in MAP due to its direct relaxant effects on vascular smooth muscle, causing a reduction in systemic vascular resistance and preload. It should, therefore, be used with caution, if at all, in patients with depleted intravascular volume. Its beneficial effects of cerebral vasoconstriction, reduced CBF, and $CMRO_2$ in patients with head trauma are offset to an extent by a reduction in CPP due to a decrease in systemic blood pressure. It has been further hypothesized that the decrease in CPP may lead to reflex cerebral vasodilation to maintain CBF, thereby also negating its beneficial effects in reducing ICP (Spitzfaden et al., 1999).

The adult literature evaluating the use of propofol in neurosurgical patients has yielded conflicting results. Previous studies have demonstrated that while propofol effectively lowered ICP in patients with elevated ICP following TBI and during cerebral aneurysm surgery, there was a reduction in CPP because of the greater decrease in MAP than in ICP caused by propofol (Herregods et al., 1988; Ravussin et al., 1988; Pinaud et al., 1990). Other investigators reported no reduction in ICP with propofol sedation in adults with head trauma (Stewart et al., 1994). Finally, in adult closed head injury patients administered propofol along with other measures to lower ICP (e.g., mannitol and hyperventilation), these combined measures provided significant reductions in ICP without affecting MAP. Consequently, CPP improved (Farling et al., 1989).

Data are limited with regard to the neurologic effects of propofol in children. Spitzfaden and others (1999) reported that propofol sedation produced significant reductions in ICP in two children with elevated ICP that had been previously refractory to other measures such as hyperventilation, mannitol, and sedation with midazolam and morphine. However, the effects of propofol on MAP were not reported in one child, and the other child required dopamine to maintain MAP so that CPP was not compromised. Taken together, the results of these studies suggest that further data are required to evaluate the use of propofol in the patient with reduced intracranial compliance.

Etomidate. Etomidate provides both hemodynamic stability and cerebral protection, making it the ideal anesthetic induction agent for emergency surgery in a child with multiple trauma. Although it does cause a direct myocardial depressant effect, it does so to a significantly lesser extent than equipotent doses of other induction agents, including thiopental, propofol, and ketamine (Stowe et al., 1992). Etomidate, however, maintains sympathetic outflow and produces no significant changes in blood pressure making it the agent of choice in the hemodynamically unstable patient. Similar to thiopental and propofol, it is a cerebral vasoconstrictor and causes a reduction in ICP, CBF, and $CMRO_2$. However, because MAP is maintained with etomidate, CPP is also maintained. Perhaps the only concern with its use has been adrenal suppression; however, this is believed to have questionable clinical significance with brief use (Crozier et al., 1987). A recent retrospective review reported successful fracture reduction in 52 of 53 patients who received etomidate alone or in combination with midazolam and/or opioids (Dickinson et al., 2001). This study found a low incidence of minor side effects, including nausea and vomiting, mild hypotension, and prolonged sedation in one patient each.

Ketamine. Ketamine is a dissociative anesthetic that is frequently selected for induction in hypovolemic children because its sympathomimetic actions result in an increase in blood pressure and heart rate. However, like the other induction agents described earlier, ketamine has direct myocardial depressant effects and direct vasodilatory effects. In fact, significant hypotension has been reported following ketamine administration in critically ill patients, likely due to its direct myocardial-depressant effects, which occur in the presence of depleted catecholamine stores (Waxman et al., 1980).

Ketamine, however, is a potent cerebral vasodilator causing a marked increase in CBF. While $CMRO_2$ usually remains unchanged following ketamine administration, ICP may increase, especially in patients with intracranial pathology. However, data regarding the effects of ketamine on ICP remain inconclusive, with some studies demonstrating modest decreases in ICP following ketamine administration, particularly when administered concomitantly with other sedatives (Mayberg et al., 1995; Albanese et al., 1997). A controlled, randomized, double-blind trial found no differences in mean daily values of ICP, CPP, and number of episodes of ICP elevations in patients with severe TBI sedated with ketamine and midazolam compared with those sedated with sufentanil and midazolam (Bourgoin et al., 2003). Yet, its cerebral vasodilatory effects preclude the use of ketamine as an induction agent in patients with head trauma.

Maintenance of Anesthesia

Selection of agents for maintenance of anesthesia should be based on the nature and duration of the proposed procedure; the extent of injuries; the child's ventilatory, hemodynamic, and neurologic status; and whether postoperative mechanical ventilation is anticipated. In hemodynamically stable patients, a standard general anesthetic may be used, including volatile agents, opioids for postoperative pain relief, and muscle relaxants as needed to provide good operating conditions. A technique using an opioid, hypnotic, muscle relaxant and oxygen may be more suitable in a child with unacceptably low blood pressure who may not tolerate the negative inotropic effects of potent volatile anesthetics. In such cases, fentanyl or sufentanil would be the preferred opioid because these do not significantly alter hemodynamic parameters, especially blood pressure. In children with uncertain injuries, nitrous oxide is best avoided because it may diffuse into closed air spaces such as the pleural cavity. In such cases, the use of amnestic agents such as benzodiazepines is useful in reducing the likelihood of awareness.

In a child with severe head trauma, efforts must be directed at preventing secondary brain injury and protecting the injured brain from further ischemia by selecting anesthetic techniques that maintain cardiovascular stability while reducing ICP. All volatile anesthetics cause cerebral vasodilation that is dose (minimum alveolar concentration [MAC]) related (Vavilal and Lam, 2002). Isoflurane affects CBF and cerebral autoregulation to a lesser extent than does halothane. Sevoflurane offers greater advantages in that CBF velocities do not increase significantly with less than 1 MAC (Monkhoff et al., 2001), and cerebral pressure autoregulation is maintained up to 1.5 MAC sevoflurane. For these reasons, sevoflurane may be the preferred volatile anesthetic for the child with TBI and it would be prudent to limit its use to 1 MAC.

Opioids (fentanyl, sufentanil, or remifentanil) are frequently administered as intermittent bolus doses or continuous infusions to supplement volatile anesthetics, for postoperative analgesia, and as additional measures to lower ICP. Increased ICP has been reported in an 11-year-old with closed head injury following fentanyl administration that responded to hyperventilation and barbiturates (Tobias, 1994). In addition, studies in adults have reported a transient but very significant increase in ICP accompanied by a decrease in MAP and CPP following bolus doses of morphine, fentanyl, sufentanil, and alfentanil (Albanese et al., 1999; de Nadal et al., 2000). The exact mechanism of these changes remains unknown, but impaired cerebrovascular autoregulation and direct cerebral vasodilatory effects of opioids have been implicated. Such effects may have important implications in the management of the child with head trauma. Until additional data become available, the judicious use of opioid infusions with careful monitoring of hemodynamic parameters is recommended.

PATIENT MONITORING

In addition to routine monitors, placement of invasive monitors, including arterial and central venous catheters, and a urinary catheter must be considered in the child with extensive injuries and those with head trauma. Placement of such catheters should be efficient, and in some cases when the surgery must be performed expeditiously, invasive monitors may need to be placed while the procedure is already under way. An arterial catheter is invaluable in cases of head, chest, and extensive abdominal trauma. Invasive catheters allow for continuous blood pressure management and frequent arterial blood gas, electrolyte, and serial hematocrit determination. Central venous pressure monitoring is useful in patients in whom large fluid shifts are expected and when rapid ongoing blood loss is anticipated. Central venous access also allows for mixed venous blood gas determination. Urine output is an important measure of fluid status. The need for additional monitors such as ICP and somatosensory evoked potential monitors must be individualized. In some cases of chest trauma, echocardiography may be useful in diagnosing injuries such as cardiac contusion causing ventricular wall motion abnormalities, aortic aneurysm, and cardiac tamponade.

Temperature monitoring and preventing hypothermia are an important aspect of trauma resuscitation but one that is frequently overlooked due to other priorities such as resuscitation. In the traumatized child, several factors contribute to ongoing heat loss and subsequent hypothermia. These factors include exposure to a cold environment at the scene of the accident, large open wounds, rapid infusion of cold intravenous fluids and blood products, and exposure of body cavities with consequent evaporative heat loss during operative procedures. Hypothermia has significant deleterious effects that may hinder resuscitative efforts. Such effects include myocardial dysfunction, cardiac irritability, and dysrhythmias. Other effects of hypothermia include acid-base disturbances, unpredictable dose-response curves of the anesthetic agents, a leftward shift of the oxyhemoglobin dissociation curve, and coagulopathies. Continuous temperature monitoring in all pediatric trauma patients is therefore essential. Every effort should be made to maintain temperature, including use of warm intravenous fluids, keeping the child covered once initial evaluation is completed, maintaining a warm environment, use of radiant warmers for infants, and the use of forced air warming devices. If possible, the head should be wrapped in plastic, and if the intestines are exposed, they should be placed in a plastic bag to help reduce heat loss by radiation and evaporation.

FLUID AND BLOOD RESUSCITATION

Shock is defined as a metabolic demand that exceeds either oxygen supply or oxygen delivery (Rasmussen and Grande, 1994). When a child who has sustained multiple injuries presents for surgical intervention, the fluid status must be quickly assessed before induction of anesthesia based on a physical examination and on fluid resuscitation administered before arrival in the operating suite. The anesthesiologist must be prepared to continue the fluid resuscitation in case of ongoing blood loss or third space fluid losses. The goals of fluid resuscitation should be to maintain normovolemia and osmolar and oncotic pressures in the intravascular space. Crystalloid solutions such as lactated Ringer's solution or normal saline are most commonly used in the initial stages of resuscitation. Hypertonic saline solutions (3%) have also been used in this setting based on the premise that they increase serum osmolality and thereby maintain intravascular volume for longer periods and with smaller volumes administered than isotonic solutions (Rasmussen and Grande, 1994). However, the data that support these arguments are inconclusive and further research in this area is needed. The decision to administer glucose-containing solutions must be based on serial blood glucose values. The issue of glucose administration is of greatest importance in the presence of head trauma because elevated blood glucose levels have been found to correlate significantly with indicators of the severity of brain injury and poor neurologic outcomes in children with severe brain injuries (Michaud et al., 1991) (see Chapter 18, Anesthesia for Neurosurgery).

Colloid solutions such as 5% albumin and hydroxyethyl starch have also been used for fluid resuscitation. Hydroxyethyl starch may exacerbate existing coagulopathy by interfering with platelet function, decreasing fibrinogen activity, and interfering with factor VIII (Niemi and Kuitunen, 1998; Deusch et al., 2003). It is therefore unsuitable for the pediatric trauma patient. The purported benefits of colloid solutions include their ability to increase colloid oncotic pressure, prolonged maintenance of intravascular volume, and smaller volumes required compared with crystalloid solutions (Niemi and Kuitunen, 1998). For these reasons, colloids may also be beneficial in children with head trauma because the smaller volume of fluids administered may reduce the likelihood of cerebral edema. One of the major concerns with the use of colloids has been the cost. In most patients who require massive fluid resuscitation, the cost of using colloids to supplement crystalloids may be justified. The discussion of the crystalloid versus colloid controversy has been reviewed elsewhere (Imm and Carlson, 1993; Rizoli, 2003).

Blood Administration

The primary purposes for transfusion of blood products in a pediatric trauma patient are to maintain oxygen delivery and to ensure hemostasis. Packed red blood cells (PRBCs) are required when oxygen-carrying capacity is inadequate to meet tissue demands and metabolic rate. Losses of up to 40% of blood volume can usually be replaced with isotonic crystalloid solutions or colloids without physiologic signs of inadequate oxygen delivery (Solheim and Wesenberg, 2001). When estimated blood volume losses exceed 40%, the decision to transfuse blood should be based on an overall assessment of the patient that includes the hemodynamic status, extent of ongoing blood loss, and underlying comorbidity. Some children may require blood transfusion with blood volume losses less than 40% if the blood loss has been rapid or if they have a significant underlying medical condition such as congenital cyanotic heart disease or blood dyscrasias. Although there can be no fixed numerical transfusion trigger in all trauma patients, Table 30–6 presents formulas that may be used as general guidelines to calculate allowable blood losses (Rasmussen and Grande, 1994). In most centers, blood banks supply blood components rather than whole blood. The primary advantage of component therapy is more efficient and cost-effective use of resources by eliminating the transfusion of unnecessary components and making components from a single blood donation available to several patients. It also permits improved preservation of individual components.

TABLE 30–6. Formulas to use as a general guideline to calculate allowable blood loss

Calculation 1*	ABL = EBV × (HCT initial − HCT target) HCT initial
Calculation 2	ERCM = EBV × HCT starting
	ERCM target = EBV × HCT target
	ARCL = ERCM − ERCM target
	ABL = ARCL × 3

ABL, allowable blood loss; EBV, estimated blood volume; HCT, hematocrit; ERCM, estimated red cell mass; ARCL, allowable red cell loss.

*The ABL, in milliliters, must be multiplied by 3 if replacement is by crystalloid and replaced, 1:1 if blood is to be used.

Calculations for allowable blood volume from Rasmussen GE, Grandes CM: Blood, fluids, and electrolytes in the pediatric trauma patient. *Int Anesthesiol Clin* 32:79–101, 1994.

The unstable patient in hemorrhagic shock may need blood before cross-matching procedures can be completed. The possibility of encountering a clinically significant, non-ABO antibody is rare in children. Type O Rh-negative non–cross-matched blood is preferred for emergency transfusions (Schwab et al., 1986).

Packed Red Blood Cells

The indication to transfuse PRBCs is to increase oxygen-carrying capacity. PRBCs are supplied in units of approximately 250 mL with hematocrits ranging from 60% to 80%. The units are preserved either in CPD (citrate, phosphate, and dextrose) with a shelf-life of 21 days or in CPD-A (citrate, phosphate, dextrose, and adenine) with a shelf-life of 35 days. The citrate in the preservative chelates calcium; therefore intravenous calcium supplement (calcium gluconate or chloride) must be readily available when transfusing PRBCs, especially at a rapid rate. The usual starting dose of PRBCs is 10 to 20 mL/kg depending on rapidity of blood loss. Banked red blood cells have a number of features with significant clinical effects, as summarized in Table 30–7.

Fresh Frozen Plasma

Fresh frozen plasma (FFP) must be separated from whole blood within 6 to 8 hours of collection. It generally takes approximately

TABLE 30–7. Differences in composition of major blood products

	Normal Whole Blood (in vivo)	Citrated Whole Blood (2 Weeks Old) CPD	Citrated Packed Red Blood Cells*	Frozen Packed Red Blood Cells	FFP
pH	7.4	6.6–6.9	6.6–6.9	6.6–7.2	6.6–6.9
P_{CO_2}	35–45	180–210	180–210	0–10	180–210
Base deficit (mmol/L)	0	9–15	9–15	?	9–15
Potassium (mmol/L)	3.5–5.0	18–26	18–26 (mmol/L)	1–2 mmol/L	4–8
Citrate	None	++++	++	None	++++
Factors V and VIII	Normal	20%–50%	20%–50%	None	85%–100%
Fibrinogen	Normal	Normal	Normal	None	Normal
Platelets	240,000–400,000	None	None	None	None
2,3-DPG	Normal	3% of normal	3% of normal	Nearly normal	—
Hematocrit	35–45	35–45	60–70	50–95	—
Temperature	37°C	4°–6°C	4°–6°C	4°–6°C	Cold

CPD: Citrate-phosphate-dextrose; FFP: fresh frozen plasma

*Citrated whole blood and citrated packed red blood cells have the same chemical composition, but citrated red blood cells have considerably less plasma volume.

(From Coté CJ, Ryan JF, Todres DD, et al.: *A practice of anesthesia for infants and children*, 2nd edition, New York, 1993, Grune & Stratton, p 186. Modified from Miller RD: *Refresher Courses in Anesthesiology* 1:101, 1973.)

45 minutes to thaw because it is stored at −18°C, and it must be used within 24 hours once thawed. FFP provides factors II, V, VIII, IX, X, and XI and antithrombin III. Most clotting factors are stable in banked CPD blood, but levels of factors V and VIII fall, reaching 15% and 50% of normal levels, respectively, at 21 days after collection. Only 20% of factor V and 30% of factor VIII are required to support adequate coagulation, so clotting tests should guide the replacement of clotting factors with FFP. In general, FFP should be transfused when clotting studies become abnormal, including a prolonged prothrombin time (PT) or activated partial thromboplastin time (aPTT). Nonsurgical bleeding in children who receive more than 1 blood volume of PRBCs frequently require FFP due to factor V and VIII deficiency. The recommended initial dose of FFP is 10 to 15 mL/kg. Constituents of FFP are listed in Table 30–7.

Platelets

Platelets are prepared through centrifugation and recentrifugation of fresh whole blood. Dilutional thrombocytopenia is the most likely cause of nonsurgical or microvascular bleeding following massive blood transfusion, and usually platelets are required before FFP for this condition. Transfusion of 0.1 unit/kg will raise the platelet count by approximately 20,000. Because platelet counts of 50,000 are adequate to achieve surgical hemostasis, doses in excess of 0.2 unit/kg are rarely required.

Cryoprecipitate

Cryoprecipitate that is produced by refreezing the insoluble portion of plasma is rich in factor VIII and fibrinogen. The insoluble portion from 1 unit of FFP yields 100 units of cryoprecipitate. The primary indications for cryoprecipitate in the trauma patient are bleeding abnormalities following massive transfusion, disseminated intravascular coagulation (DIC), and decreased fibrinogen levels. The recommended initial dose of cryoprecipitate is 0.1 unit/kg.

Massive Blood Replacement

Massive blood replacement is defined as the administration of 1 blood volume or more within a 24-hour period. It causes a number of physiologic derangements that can be detrimental in the child with multiple injuries, including coagulation defects, electrolyte and acid-base abnormalities, and hypothermia. Dilutional thrombocytopenia and clotting factor deficiencies have been primarily implicated in the etiology of nonsurgical bleeding following massive blood transfusion. However, mathematical models have demonstrated that a third of the patient's own blood remains after a single blood volume exchange, thereby retaining sufficient platelets and clotting factors to permit hemostasis (Marsaglia and Thomas, 1971). Other factors such as incompatibility of transfused blood and DIC have also been implicated in the etiology of nonsurgical bleeding in the trauma patient.

SUMMARY

Pediatric trauma accounts for 25% of all trauma cases in the United States. ATLS should be thought of as a continuum, beginning with the traumatic event; continuing through resuscitation and stabilization in the emergency department, diagnostic areas, and the operating room; and ending at discharge of a stable patient in the recovery room or intensive care unit. Careful evaluation with good teamwork and meticulous attention to detail can contribute to a positive outcome.

REFERENCES

Adler P: *Ride-on mower hazard analysis (1987-1990)*. Washington, DC, 1993, Directorate for Epidemiology, US Consumer Product Safety Commission.

Adler P: *Ride-on mower hazard analysis (1991-1993)*. Washington, DC, 1994, Directorate for Epidemiology, US Consumer Product Safety Commission.

Akins CW, Buckley MJ, Daggett W, et al.: Acute traumatic disruption of the thoracic aorta: A ten-year experience. *Am Coll Surg* 31:305, 1981.

Albanese J, Arnaud S, Rey M, et al.: Ketamine decreases intracranial pressure and electroencephalographic activity in traumatic brain injury patients during propofol sedation. *Anesthesiology* 87:1328–1334, 1997.

Albanese J, Viviand X, Potie F, et al.: Sufentanil, fentanyl, and alfentanil in head trauma patients: A study on cerebral hemodynamics. *Crit Care Med* 27:262–263, 1999.

American College of Surgeons Committee on Trauma: *Advanced trauma life support for doctors*. Chicago, 1997, American College of Surgeons.

Anderson PJ: Fractures of the facial skeleton in children. *Injury* 26:47–50, 1995.

Anderson RN: Deaths: Leading causes for 1999. *Natl Vital Stat Rep* 49:1–87, 2001.

Aun CS, Sung RY, O'Meara ME, et al.: Cardiovascular effects of I.V. induction in children: Comparison between propofol and thiopentone. *Br J Anaesth* 70:647–653, 1993.

Behrman SW, Fabian TC, Kudsk KA, et al.: Improved outcome with femur fractures: Early vs. Delayed fixation. *J Trauma* 30:792–797, 1990.

Bergren CT, Chan FN, Bodzin JH: Intravenous pyelogram results in association with renal pathology and therapy in trauma patients. *J Trauma* 27:515–518, 1987.

Bone LB, Johnston KD, Weigelt J, Scheinberg R: Early versus delayed stabilization of femoral fractures. A prospective randomized study. *J Bone Joint Surg Br* 71:336–340, 1989.

Bourgoin A, Albanese J, Wereszczynski N, et al.: Safety of sedation with ketamine in severe head injury patients: Comparison with sufentanil. *Crit Care Med* 31:711–717, 2003.

Bracco D, Bissonnette B: *Neurosurgery and neurotraumatology: Anesthetic considerations and postoperative management.* New York, 2002, McGraw-Hill.

Bricker SR, McLuckie A, Nightingale DA: Gastric aspirates after trauma in children. *Anaesthesia* 44:721–724, 1989.

Bruce DA, Raphaely RC, Goldberg AI, et al.: Pathophysiology, treatment and outcome following severe head injury in children. *Childs Brain* 5:174–191, 1979.

Bruce DA: Diffuse cerebral swelling following head injuries. *J Neurosurg* 54:170–178, 1981.

Bulas DI, Taylor GA, Eichelberger MR: The value of CT in detecting bowel perforation in children after blunt abdominal trauma. *AJR Am J Roentgenol* 153:561–564, 1989.

Burgess RC, Cates H: Deformities of the forearm in patients who have multiple cartilaginous exostosis. *J Bone Joint Surg Am* 75:13–18, 1993.

Cass AS: Blunt renal trauma in children. *J Trauma* 23:123–127, 1983.

Chu UB, Clevenger FW, Imami ER, et al.: The impact of selective laboratory evaluation on utilization of laboratory resources and patient care in a level-I trauma center. *Am J Surg* 172:558–562; discussion 562–553, 1996.

Coley BD, Mutabagani KH, Martin LC, et al.: Focused abdominal sonography for trauma (FAST) in children with blunt abdominal trauma. *J Trauma* 48:902–906, 2000.

Cooper A, Barlow B, DiScala C, String D: Mortality and truncal injury: The pediatric perspective. *J Pediatr Surg* 29:33–38, 1994.

Criswell JC, Parr MJ, Nolan JP: Emergency airway management in patients with cervical spine injuries. *Anaesthesia* 49:900–903, 1994.

Crozier TA, Beck D, Schlaeger M, et al.: Endocrinological changes following etomidate, midazolam, or methohexital for minor surgery. *Anesthesiology* 66:628–635, 1987.

Dashti SR, Decker DD, Razzaq A, Cohen AR: Current patterns of inflicted head injury in children. *Pediatr Neurosurg* 31:302–306, 1999.

de Nadal M, Munar F, Poca MA, et al.: Cerebral hemodynamic effects of morphine and fentanyl in patients with severe head injury: Absence of correlation to cerebral autoregulation. *Anesthesiology* 92:11–19, 2000.

Deppa RW: *Options package for riding mowers.* Washington, DC, 1994, Directorate for Engineering Sciences, US Consumer Product Safety Commission.

Deusch E, Gamsjager T, Kress HG, Kozek-Langenecker SA: Binding of hydroxyethyl starch molecules to the platelet surface. *Anesth Analg* 97:680–683, 2003.

Dickinson R, Singer AJ, Carrion W: Etomidate for pediatric sedation prior to fracture reduction. *Acad Emerg Med* 8:74–77, 2001.

Dykes EH: Paediatric trauma. *Br J Anaesth* 83:130–138, 1999.

Eddy AC, Rusch VW, Fligner CL, et al.: The epidemiology of traumatic rupture of the thoracic aorta in children: A 13-year review. *J Trauma* 30:989–991; discussion 991–982, 1990.

Eichelberger MR: *Pediatric trauma: Prevention, acute care, rehabilitation.* St. Louis, 1993, Mosby–Year Book, Inc.

Farling PA, Johnston JR, Coppel DL: Propofol infusion for sedation of patients with head injury in intensive care. A preliminary report. *Anaesthesia* 44:222–226, 1989.

Fiser DH: Intraosseous infusion. *N Engl J Med* 322:1579–1581, 1990.

Furnival RA: Controversies in pediatric thoracic and abdominal trauma. *Clin Pediatr Emerg Med* 2:48–62, 2001.

Goodwin MW, Robinson KN: A pragmatic approach to fasting in paediatric trauma? *Paediatr Anaesth* 10:452–453, 2000.

Green SM, Rothrock SG: Is pediatric trauma really a surgical disease? *Ann Emerg Med* 39:537–540, 2002.

Gupta S, Heath K, Matta BF: Effect of incremental doses of sevoflurane on cerebral pressure autoregulation in humans. *Br J Anaesth* 79:469–472, 1997.

Guy J, Haley K, Zuspan SJ: Use of intraosseous infusion in the pediatric trauma patient. *J Pediatr Surg* 28:158–161, 1993.

Haftel AJ, Lev R, Mahour GH, et al.: Abdominal CT scanning in pediatric blunt trauma. *Ann Emerg Med* 17:684–689, 1988.

Haller JA Jr, Papa P, Drugas G, Colombani P: Nonoperative management of solid organ injuries in children. Is it safe? *Ann Surg* 219:625–628; discussion 628–631, 1994.

Hastings RH, Wood PR: Head extension and laryngeal view during laryngoscopy with cervical spine stabilization maneuvers. *Anesthesiology* 80:825–831, 1994.

Hasue M, Hoshino R, Omata S, et al.: Cervical spine injuries in children. *Fukushima J Med Sci* 20:115–123, 1974.

Haughton A, Turley A, Pollock N: Remifentanil for rapid sequence induction. *Anaesth Intensive Care* 27:319–320, 1999.

Hedequist D, Starr AJ, Wilson P, Walker J: Early versus delayed stabilization of pediatric femur fractures: Analysis of 387 patients. *J Orthop Trauma* 13:490–493, 1999.

Hellmann JR, Shott SR, Gootee MJ: Impalement injuries on the palate in children: Review of 131 cases. *Int J Pediatr Otorhinolaryngol* 26:157–163, 1993.

Herregods L, Verbeke J, Rolly G, Colardyn F: Effect of propofol on elevated intracranial pressure. Preliminary results. *Anaesthesia* 43:107–109, 1988.

Imm A, Carlson RW: Fluid resuscitation in circulatory short. *Crit Care Clin* 9:313–333, 1993.

Jaicks RR, Cohn SM, Moller BA: Early fracture fixation may be deleterious after head injury. *J Trauma* 42:1–5; discussion 5–6, 1997.

Jean WC, Spellman SR, Nussbaum ES, Low WC: Reperfusion injury after focal cerebral ischemia: The role of inflammation and the therapeutic horizon. *Neurosurgery* 43:1382–1396, 1998.

Kaban LB: Diagnosis and treatment of fractures of the facial bones in children. *J Oral Maxillofac Surg* 51:722–729, 1993.

Kalb DC, Ney AL, Rodriguez JL, et al.: Assessment of the relationship between timing of fixation of the fracture and secondary brain injury in patients with multiple trauma. *Surgery* 124:739–744; discussion 744–735, 1998.

Karp MP, Jewett TC Jr, Kuhn JP, et al.: The impact of computed tomography scanning on the child with renal trauma. *J Pediatr Surg* 21:617–623, 1986.

Kisa E, Schenk WG 3rd: Indications for emergency intravenous pyelography (IVP) in blunt abdominal trauma: A reappraisal. *J Trauma* 26:1086–1089, 1986.

Krantz B: Initial assessment. In Feliciano DV, Mattox KL, editors: *Trauma,* 5th ed. Stamford, 1996, Appleton & Lang, pp 123–129.

Kruskall MS, Mintz PD, Bergin JJ, et al.: Transfusion therapy in emergency medicine. *Ann Emerg Med* 17:327–335, 1988.

Langer JC, Winthrop AL, Wesson DE, et al.: Diagnosis and incidence of cardiac injury in children with blunt thoracic trauma. *J Pediatr Surg* 24:1091–1094, 1989.

Marcin JP, Pollack MM: Triage scoring systems, severity of illness measures, mortality prediction models in pediatric trauma. *Crit Care Med* 30:S457–467, 2002.

Marion DW, Penrod LE, Keley SF, et al.: Treatment of traumatic brain injury with moderate hyperthermia. *N Engl J Med* 336:540–546, 1997.

Marsaglia A, Thomas ED: Mathematical consideration of cross circulation and exchange transfusion. *Transfusion* 11:216–219, 1971.

Mayberg TS, Lam AM, Matta BF, et al.: Ketamine does not increase cerebral blood flow velocity or intracranial pressure during isoflurane/nitrous oxide anesthesia in patients undergoing craniotomy. *Anesth Analg* 81:84–89, 1995.

McAninch JW, Carroll PR: Genitourinary trauma. In Mattox KL, Moore EE, Feliciano DV, editors: *Trauma.* Norwalk, 1988, Appleton & Lange, pp 537–552.

Mcheik JN, Vergnes P, Bondonny JM: Treatment of facial dog bite injuries in children: A retrospective study. *J Pediatr Surg* 35:580–583, 2000.

McKee MD, Schemitsch EH, Vincent LO, et al.: The effect of a femoral fracture on concomitant closed head injury in patients with multiple injuries. *J Trauma* 42:1041–1045, 1997.

Mehall JR, Ennis JS, Saltzman DA, et al.: Prospective results of a standardized algorithm based on hemodynamic status for managing pediatric solid organ injury. *J Am Coll Surg* 193:347–353, 2001.

Melillo EP, Hawkins DJ, Lynch L, Macnamara A: Difficult airway management of a child impaled through the neck. *Paediatr Anaesth* 11:615–617, 2001.

Mendelson SA, Dominick TS, Tyler-Kabara E, et al.: Early versus late femoral fracture stabilization in multiply injured pediatric patients with closed head injury. *J Pediatr Orthop* 21:594–599, 2001.

Meyer PG: Critical care management of severe paediatric trauma: A challenge for anaesthesiologists. *Paediatr Anaesth* 9:373–376, 1999.

Michaud LJ, Rivara FP, Longstreth WT Jr, Grady MS: Elevated initial blood glucose levels and poor outcome following severe brain injuries in children. *J Trauma* 31:1356–1362, 1991.

Monkhoff M, Schwarz U, Gerber A, et al.: The effects of sevoflurane and halothane anesthesia on cerebral blood flow velocity in children. *Anesth Analg* 92:891–896, 2001.

Mooney DP: Multiple trauma: Liver and spleen injury. *Curr Opin Pediatr* 14:482–485, 2002.

Morell RC, Colonna DM, Mathes DD, Wilson JA: Fluoroscopy-assisted intubation of a child with an unstable subluxation of c1/c2. *Neurosurg Anesthesiol* 9:25–28, 1997.

Moriarty KP, Harris BH, Benitez-Marchand K: Carotid artery thrombosis and stroke after blunt pharyngeal injury. *J Trauma Injury Infect Crit Care* 42:541–543, 1997.

Morrison W, Wright JL, Paidas CN: Pediatric trauma systems. *Crit Care Med* 30:S448–456, 2002.
Musgrave DS, Mendelson SA: Pediatric orthopedic trauma: Principles in management. *Crit Care Med* 30:S431–443, 2002.
Nakayama DK, Gardner MJ, Rowe MI: Emergency endotracheal intubation in pediatric trauma. *Ann Surg* 211:218–223, 1990.
Nakayama DK, Ramenofsky ML, Rowe MI: Chest injuries in childhood. *Ann Surg* 210:770–775, 1989.
Nakayama DK, Waggoner T, Venkataraman ST, et al.: The use of drugs in emergency airway management in pediatric trauma. *Ann Surg* 216:205–211, 1992.
Niemi TT, Kuitunen AH: Hydroxyethyl starch impairs in vitro coagulation. *Acta Anaesthesiol Scand* 42:1104–1109, 1998.
Olsson GL, Hallen B, Hambraeus-Jonzon K: Aspiration during anaesthesia: A computer-aided study of 185,358 anaesthetics. *Acta Anaesthesiol Scand* 30:84–92, 1986.
Pinaud M, Lelausque JN, Chetanneau A, et al.: Effects of propofol on cerebral hemodynamics and metabolism in patients with brain trauma. *Anesthesiology* 73:404–409, 1990.
Potoka DA, Schall LC, Gardner MJ, et al.: Impact of pediatric trauma centers on mortality in a statewide system. *J Trauma* 49:237–245, 2000.
Rasmussen GE, Grande CM: Blood, fluids, and electrolytes in the pediatric trauma patient. *Int Anesthesiol Clin* 32:79–101, 1994.
Ravussin P, Guinard JP, Ralley F, Thorin D: Effect of propofol on cerebrospinal fluid pressure and cerebral perfusion pressure in patients undergoing craniotomy. *Anaesthesia* 43:37–41, 1988.
Rhodes M: Trauma resuscitation. In Peitzman AB, Rhodes M, Schwab CW, Yealy DM, editors: *The trauma manual.* Philadelphia, 1998, Lippincott-Raven, pp 82–90.
Rielly JP, Brandt ML, Mattox KL, Pokorny WJ: Thoracic trauma in children. *J Trauma* 34:329–331, 1993.
Rizoli SB: Crystalloids and colloids in trauma resuscitation: A brief overview of the current debate. *J Trauma* 54:S82–S88, 2003.
Roback MG: America's tragedy: Pediatric trauma. *Emerg Med Serv* 29:61–65, 2000.
Rosetti VA, Thompson BM, Miller J, et al.: Intraosseous infusion: An alternative route of pediatric intravascular access. *Ann Emerg Med* 14:885–888, 1985.
Schwab CW, Shayne JP, Turner J: Immediate trauma resuscitation with type O uncrossmatched blood: A two-year prospective experience. *J Trauma* 26:897–902, 1986.
Shaikh ZS, Worrall SF: Epidemiology of facial trauma in a sample of patients aged 1-18 years. *Injury* 33:669–671, 2002.
Shiozaki T, Kato A, Taneda M, et al.: Little benefit from mild hypothermia therapy for severely head injured patients with low intracranial pressure. *J Neurosurg* 91:185–191, 1999.
Smith GA and Committee on Injury and Poison Prevention: Technical report: lawnmower-related injuries to children. *Pediatrics* 107:E106, 2001.
Solheim BG, Wesenberg F: Rational use of blood products. *Eur J Cancer* 37:2421–2425; discussion 2425–2427, 2001.
Spitzfaden AC, Jimenez DF, Tobias JD: Propofol for sedation and control of intracranial pressure in children. *Pediatr Neurosurg* 31:194–200, 1999.
Stafford PW, Blinman TA, Nance ML: Practical points in evaluation and resuscitation of the injured child. *Surg Clin North Am* 82:273–301, 2002.
Stewart L, Bullock R, Rafferty C, et al.: Propofol sedation in severe head injury fails to control high ICP, but reduces brain metabolism. *Acta Neurochir Suppl* 60:544–546, 1994.
Stowe DF, Bosnjak ZJ, Kampine JP: Comparison of etomidate, ketamine, midazolam, propofol, and thiopental on function and metabolism of isolated hearts. *Anesth Analg* 74:547–558, 1992.
Swischuk LE: *The spine and spinal cord: Emergency radiology of the acutely ill or injured child.* Baltimore, 1986, Williams & Wilkins.
Teasdale G, Jennett B: Assessment of coma and impaired consciousness: A practical scale. *Lancet* 2:81–84, 1974.
Tepas JJ 3rd, DiScala C, Ramenofsky ML, Barlow B: Mortality and head injury: The pediatric perspective. *J Pediatr Surg* 25:92–95; discussion 96, 1990.
Tepas JJ 3rd, Frykberg ER, Schinco MA, et al.: Pediatric trauma is very much a surgical disease. *Ann Surg* 237:775–780, 2003.
Tobias JD: Increased intracranial pressure after fentanyl administration in a child with closed head trauma. *Pediatr Emerg Care* 10:89–90, 1994.
Townsend RN, Lheureau T, Protech J, et al.: Timing fracture repair in patients with severe brain injury (Glasgow Coma Scale score <9). *J Trauma* 44:977–982, 1998.
US Consumer Product Safety Commission. *National Electronic Injury Surveillance System (Database):* Bethesda, MD: US Consumer Product Safety Commission; 1990–1999.
Vane DW: Imaging of the injured child: Important questions answered quickly and correctly. *Surg Clin North Am* 82:315–323, 2002.
Vavilala MS, Lam AM: Perioperative considerations in pediatric traumatic brain injury. *Int Anesthesiol Clin* 40:69–87, 2002.
Ward JD: Craniocerebral injuries. *Management of pediatric trauma.* Buntain WL, editor: Philadelphia, 1995, WB Saunders, pp 177–188.
Watts AD, Gelb AW, Bach DB, Pelz DM: Comparison of the Bullard and Macintosh laryngoscopes for endotracheal intubation of patients with a potential cervical spine injury. *Anesthesiology* Dec; 87(6):1335–1342, 1997.
Waxman K, Shoemaker WC, Lippmann M: Cardiovascular effects of anesthetic induction with ketamine. *Anesth Analg* 59:355–358, 1980.
Zanette G, Ori C, Zadra N, et al.: Hangman's fracture in a paediatric patient: Considerations for anaesthesia. *Paediatr Anaesth* 7:473–475, 1997.
Zerfowski M, Bremerich A: Facial trauma in children and adolescents. *Clin Oral Invest* 2:120–124, 1998.

Associated Problems

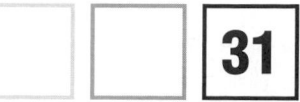

31 Malignant Hyperthermia

Barbara W. Brandom

Deaths during anesthesia associated with high fever and tachycardia were described repeatedly in the first half of the 20th century (Moschcowitz, 1916; Burford, 1940). These deaths were sometimes ascribed to heatstroke and dehydration, factors that were likely to occur in a time when intravenous hydration and air conditioning were unknown. In 1915 and 1919, two deaths occurred during chloroform anesthesia in one family. In these cases, severe muscle spasm was observed before cardiac arrest. In 1987, a young child from this family died during anesthesia for dental surgery. Subsequent in vitro contracture testing demonstrated susceptibility to malignant hyperthermia (MH) in several relatives (Harrison and Isaacs, 1992).

Denborough and others were the first to describe MH as a clinical entity (Denborough and Lovell, 1960; Denborough et al., 1962). They reported the case of a young Australian patient with a broken bone who was afraid to undergo general anesthesia because many of his relatives had died during ether anesthesia. The patient received halothane (a new drug at the time) as his anesthetic agent. Although the patient became febrile, tachycardic, cyanotic, and hypotensive, he survived the event. Extensive laboratory investigations of this patient were unrevealing. Further investigation of his family's medical history, however, showed a pattern of anesthetic deaths consistent with an autosomal dominant trait. Since then, MH has been recognized as a pharmacogenetic disorder of calcium regulation in muscle cells.

Several genetic differences may result in similar syndromes of increased metabolism and muscle cell injury (Gillard et al., 1991; Deufel et al., 1992; Levitt et al., 1992; Olckers et al., 1992). However, in the majority of families in whom linkage to MH has been studied, mutations have been found (MacLennan et al., 1992) in the gene encoding the skeletal muscle calcium release channel, the ryanodine receptor *(RYR1)*. The ryanodine receptor is located at 19q13.1.

An episode of MH is identified by documenting an increased metabolic rate after exposure to a triggering agent. Rhabdomyolysis may also be observed. Susceptibility to MH is rarely associated with clinically evident hypermetabolism in the absence of drugs used during anesthesia (Gronert et al., 1980; Tobin et al., 2001). Halothane and succinylcholine, two drugs formerly used frequently in pediatric anesthesia, are two of the most potent triggers of MH. A review of 25 years of halothane anesthetics in one pediatric hospital (Warner et al., 1984) found the incidence of acute MH episodes to range from 1:20,000 to 1:40,000 anesthetic procedures. Because choice of anesthetic and neuromuscular blocker are likely to influence the development of this potentially lethal syndrome, MH is a disease of particular concern to the pediatric anesthesiologist who chooses to administer inhalation anesthetics and succinylcholine. The purpose of this chapter is to review the clinical manifestations, management, and underlying pathophysiology of MH.

The broad clinical spectrum of MH contributes to difficulty defining its incidence. In the past, some clinicians based the diagnosis of MH on the occurrence of masseter spasm alone, whereas others required total body rigidity, signs of hypermetabolism, and a positive contracture test for a definitive diagnosis. The contracture test is difficult to apply to large populations because of technical and financial reasons. In vitro examination of muscle for contracture threshold in the presence of halothane alone and caffeine alone remains the most reliable method to assess the potential for MH to develop in a particular North American patient (Larach, 1993). Although there is a difference between the details of contracture testing in North America and Europe (European Malignant Hyperpyrexia Group, 1984; Ording et al., 1984, 1997; Larach, 1989), the diagnostic results are very similar with either method (Fletcher et al., 1999). Intensive evaluation of anesthetic records and contracture test results in large genealogies from limited populations may reduce the number of individuals who are treated as MH susceptible (MHS) (Bachand et al., 1997). This type of careful review is needed to determine the prevalence of MH susceptibility, as opposed to the incidence of acute MH episodes.

A countrywide study was undertaken in Denmark (Ording, 1985) to define the risk of MH and its relation to type of anesthetic. The Danish figures are based on 386,250 anesthetic experiences in 87 hospitals in patients of all ages during a 6½-year period starting with January 1978. They report that fulminant MH, defined as a rapid increase in temperature with potentially life-threatening metabolic changes, arrhythmias, and elevated creatine kinase (CK), occurred in 1:250,000 cases of general anesthesia. No fulminant MH occurred during regional or intravenous anesthesia. These findings are similar to reports in the United Kingdom, where fulminant MH occurs once in 200,000 anesthetic procedures (Ellis and Halsall, 1980). The Danish study further reported that masseter spasm occurred in 1:12,000 cases in which succinylcholine was used, along with both potent inhaled and intravenous anesthetics. Overall, suspicion of MH was raised in 1:16,000 anesthetic procedures and in 1:4,200 anesthetic procedures in which potent inhalation agents were combined with succinylcholine. The mortality rate for fulminant MH reported in this study was 10% (Ording, 1985). Britt and Kalow (1970) noted a mortality rate of 64% in the era before dantrolene.

In 1997, a code specific for MH was added to the *International Classification of Diseases, Ninth Revision*. The Healthcare Cost and Utilization Project reports about 400 cases per year using the *ICD-9-CM* code specific for hyperthermia related to anesthesia. Only a few of these cases are called into the MH Hotline Consultation Service. Unfortunately, overlap between these two independent sources of suspected cases of MH is small; the incidence of acute MH episodes may be greater than 500 per year in the United States.

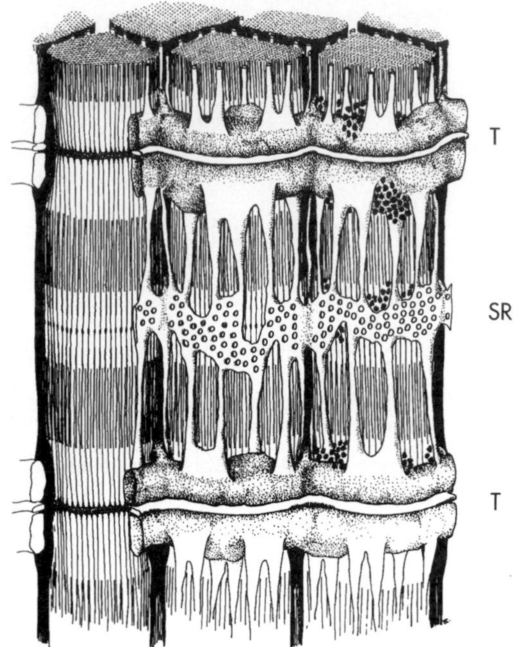

FIGURE 31–1. This three-dimensional reconstruction of the sarcoplasmic reticulum (SR) illustrates the continuity of the transverse tubules (T) surrounding the myofibrils and the fenestrations of the collar of the sarcoplasmic reticulum overlying the center of the A band of the myofibril. (From Engel AG, Banker BQ, editors: *Myology basic and clinical.* New York, 1986, McGraw-Hill Book Co. Modified from Peachey LD: *J Cell Biol* 25:209, 1965, by copyright permission of The Rockefeller University Press.)

MUSCLE PHYSIOLOGY

NORMAL MUSCLE PHYSIOLOGY

The propagation of an action potential down a motor nerve fiber produces depolarization of that fiber and release of acetylcholine at the neuromuscular junction. Acetylcholine combines with its receptors at the neuromuscular junction, initiating a wave of depolarization along the muscle cell membrane or sarcolemma. The propagated depolarization wave spreads internally via transverse tubules that abut the sarcoplasmic reticulum (Fig. 31–1). The wall of the transverse tubule contains the dihydropyridine receptor, a voltage-dependent calcium channel that in turn triggers the calcium-sensitive ryanodine receptor (RYR), to release large amounts of calcium from the sarcoplasmic reticulum (Melzer and Dietze, 2001).

The RYR forms the footplate between the transverse tubule and the sarcoplasmic reticulum. The RYR is the largest known receptor in the body, four times the size of the acetylcholine receptor (Wagenknecht et al., 1989). RYR reacts with several other proteins. Type 1 ryanodine receptors are found in all skeletal muscle, in smooth muscle, in neurons, and in B lymphocytes. Type 2 ryanodine receptors are found in cardiac muscle, brain, and some hemopoietic cells. Type 3 ryanodine receptors are found in skeletal and smooth muscle and, to a lesser extent, in brain. Abnormalities in the type I ryanodine receptor *(RYR1)* cause MH (Franzini-Armstrong and Protasi, 1997).

The sarcoplasmic reticulum is an internal cellular structure that forms a major storage site for calcium ions. When the muscle cell is depolarized, the sarcoplasmic reticulum releases calcium ions, which combine with troponin affixed to actin filaments. When troponin is bound to calcium ions, cross-bridges can form between actin and myosin filaments, and lead to muscle contraction. When the wave of depolarization ceases, calcium ions dissociate from troponin and are removed by adenosine triphosphate (ATP), requiring calcium pumps sequestered in the sarcoplasmic reticulum and other organelles. In short, calcium release leads to muscle contraction, and when calcium reuptake occurs, muscle fibers relax. Coupling of the excitation of the muscle membrane and contraction of the muscle cell entails changes in intracellular calcium concentration. Calcium release also initiates the breakdown of ATP and metabolic processes that support the energy needed for muscle contraction (e.g., glycolysis).

PATHOPHYSIOLOGY OF MALIGNANT HYPERTHERMIA

MH in humans is a result of failure of the muscle cell to maintain intracellular calcium homeostasis during excitation–contraction coupling. This can be due to malfunction of the *RYR1* (Censier et al., 1998). In porcine MH, there is a specific single-point mutation in the *RYR1* in all major susceptible breeds (Fuji et al., 1991). However, this point mutation is seen in a minority of human MHS families. Initial studies showed that only a third of patients (Sambuughin, 2001) who have had positive contracture tests and therefore carry the diagnosis of MHS have a mutation in *RYR1*. However, as a larger proportion of the *RYR1* is studied, the percentage of MHS patients with *RYR1* mutations has increased. MH causative mutations have been located in three regions of this large receptor. The heterogeneous nature of human MH may be due to one of a number of mutations in *RYR1* or to abnormalities in other entities such as the dihydropyridine (Gallant and Lentz, 1992) receptor, hormone-sensitive lipase, other aspects of fatty acid metabolism, increased sensitivity to catecholamines, or inositol triphosphate. All of these entities affect calcium release mechanisms.

The metabolic dysfunction of MH is caused by increased intracellular free ionized calcium (Mickelson and Louis, 1996). The direct result of increased intracellular calcium is to increase the need for intracellular ATP to drive calcium pumps that transfer calcium into the sarcoplasmic reticulum, across the sarcolemma into the extracellular fluid, or into mitochondria. Increased demands for ATP lead to the clinically detectable manifestations of MH (e.g., an increase in metabolism). The elevation of intracellular calcium observed in MH muscle is decreased by dantrolene (Lopez et al., 1985; Mickelson and Louis, 1996). There are other conditions, such as mitochondrial myopathies and some enzyme deficiencies, in which generation of ATP in muscle is compromised. In such situations, the patient may have increased metabolism, but it is not clear how useful dantrolene would be. Dantrolene can produce weakness and decrease metabolism in normal muscle and in MHS muscle (Flewellen et al., 1983).

Motor nerve activity and neuromuscular transmission are normal in MHS patients (Gronert, 1980). However, susceptible porcine muscle has a lower mechanical threshold than does normal muscle (Moulds and Denborough, 1974; Okumura et al., 1979), and less depolarization is required compared with normal muscle (Gronert, 1980). Calcium release from the sarcoplasmic reticulum occurs at more negative potentials in the presence of *RYR1* mutations seen with MH, and calcium-induced calcium release from the sarcoplasmic reticulum is abnormal in susceptible subjects. The abnormal *RYR1* is resistant to the inhibitory effects of both calcium and magnesium (Mickelson and Louis, 1996).

During an episode of MH, lactate release from muscle increases before mixed venous oxygen tension decreases (Gronert and Theye, 1976a). This sequence is consistent with intracellular ATP depletion (Gronert, 1986). Using magnetic resonance imaging (MRI) techniques, Olgin and others (1988) noted an increased ratio of inorganic phosphate to phosphocreatine in vivo in human muscle susceptible to MH. This ratio is an indicator of the energy state of the muscle (Chance et al., 1985a, 1985b). An increased ratio suggests either impaired synthesis of ATP or increased breakdown of ATP. During an episode of MH, the use of high-energy phosphates exceeds their production, resulting in an increased ratio of inorganic phosphorus to phosphocreatine. A more subtle abnormality exists in the "unchallenged" metabolism of MHS muscle (Allsop et al., 1991; Olgin et al., 1991; Bendahan et al., 2002).

MECHANISM OF ACTION OF DANTROLENE

Since dantrolene was introduced in the 1970s, its use has remarkably improved the treatment and survival of patients with MH. Dantrolene inhibits the release of calcium from the sarcoplasmic reticulum (Fruen et al., 1997) by limiting the activation of the calcium-dependent ryanodine receptor. Dantrolene does not act at the neuromuscular junction and has no effect on the passive or active electrical properties of the surface and tubular membranes of skeletal muscle fibers. Patients administered dantrolene have normal electromyographic results and depressed force of muscle contraction. Some situations where weakness is induced by dantrolene could be clinically significant. The protective effects of dantrolene against MH require significant depression of the force of contraction (Flewellen et al., 1983).

CLINICAL PRESENTATION

The initial clinical signs of an impending episode of MH are nonspecific; they may include tachycardia, arrhythmias, and tachypnea (Box 31–1). Rigidity of the extremities and the jaw may be present. When MH is fulminant, there is severe metabolic acidosis (base deficit often greater than −8 mEq/L), respiratory acidosis ($Pa{CO_2}$ > 60 mm Hg) (Gronert, 1980), tachycardia with arrhythmias, a rapid increase in body temperature to 39.5°C or greater, hyperkalemia, myoglobinuria, and a marked increase in serum CK. However, because of modern comprehensive monitoring and increased awareness of MH, fulminant MH is rarely observed. The clinical diagnosis of MH is often considered before metabolism and temperature reach these extremes (Karan et al., 1994). The patient's medical history and clinical course usually, but not

BOX 31–1 Steps in Identifying and Treating Malignant Hyperthermia (MH)

Clinical Events During MH

Total body rigidity
Masseter spasm
Increased oxygen consumption
Inappropriate increase in temperature; rapidly rising temperature (>1.5°C over 5 min) or temperature >38.8°C
Rapid respiratory rate and/or respiratory acidosis, P_{ETCO_2} >55 mm Hg with appropriately controlled ventilation
Inappropriate sinus tachycardia
Ventricular tachycardia or ventricular fibrillation
Profuse sweating
Mottled, cyanotic skin
Cola-colored urine

- If any two or more of these events occur, determine venous blood $P{CO_2}$, $P{O_2}$, base excess, lactate, potassium ion, creatine phosphokinase, and myoglobin to rule out MH and consider discontinuing trigger agents.
- If total body rigidity is present, send blood for laboratory evaluation, discontinue trigger agents, and begin treatment for acute MH episode.

Laboratory Evaluation: Positive Findings Consistent with MH

Venous $P{CO_2}$ >65 mm Hg
Arterial $P{CO_2}$ >60 mm Hg or 65 mm Hg with spontaneous ventilation
Arterial base excess more negative than −8 mEq/L
Arterial pH <7.25
Potassium ion >6 mEq/L
Creatine kinase >10,000 IU/L after anesthetic without succinylcholine
Myoglobin in serum >170 mcg/L
Myoglobin in urine >60 mcg/L

always (Allen and Rosenberg, 1990), help to differentiate fulminant MH from other metabolic or endocrine crises such as porphyria, thyroid storm, and untreated pheochromocytoma. Some other conditions that produce signs similar to MH are sepsis, drug reactions, intracranial trauma, and hypoxic encephalitis.

MH may also occur in an abortive (Ording, 1985) or insidious form. There may be only mild symptoms or signs suggestive of MH (e.g., moderate increases in heart rate, blood pressure, and temperature along with a slight metabolic or respiratory acidosis). Masseter spasm may or may not occur (Ellis et al., 1990). There may be a moderate increase in CK and serum myoglobin. Myoglobin appears in the plasma within minutes of muscle injury. However, CK will continue to increase for 8 to 20 hours after a transient injury (Florence et al., 1985) even in normal patients. According to Ording (1985), the incidence of abortive MH is as high as 1:4,200 anesthetic procedures when succinylcholine is used in combination with potent inhalation anesthetics. There is disagreement about when and whether to terminate anesthetic administration in cases of "abortive MH."

"Abortive MH" may also be confused with sudden fulminant rhabdomyolysis, which has occurred in pediatric patients after the administration of succinylcholine. In this condition, the sudden severe increase in plasma potassium can be fatal, but metabolic abnormalities are secondary to cardiac failure, not skeletal muscle pathophysiology, as in MH (Delphin et al., 1987; Rosenberg and Gronert, 1992; Tang et al., 1992; Larach et al., 1997, 2001).

In a group of 48 children, 17 of whom later proved to be MHS by muscle biopsy, two or more adverse signs or abnormal laboratory findings were present in all patients with positive in vitro contracture tests (Larach et al., 1987). Yet similar adverse events occurred in 83% of the children who had negative muscle biopsy findings. Generalized muscle rigidity was the single factor significantly associated with positive biopsy findings for MH. However, generalized muscle rigidity was not an absolute predictor of MH susceptibility. Three of 24 patients who were referred for biopsy and who had negative contracture test results had experienced generalized muscle rigidity during induction of anesthesia. Signs consistent with abortive MH, such as tachycardia, premature ventricular contractions, elevated end-tidal carbon dioxide (Lanier et al., 1990), and increase in tension of the masseter muscle (Van der Spek et al., 1987, 1988), may be observed in the normal pediatric patient administered halothane or sevoflurane and succinylcholine. Larach and others (1987; Hackl et al., 1990) could not identify the MHS patient on the basis of these signs.

It has been recommended that to most effectively treat or prevent the crisis of MH, the anesthesiologist must presume an episode of MH is occurring before the patient's temperature increases. If events during the induction of anesthesia require explanation beyond light anesthesia or hypoventilation, further investigation to rule out the diagnosis of MH must be undertaken immediately, before surgery begins.

To confirm the diagnosis of MH, the anesthesiologist must document the presence of increased metabolic rate, rather than the decreased metabolic rate that usually follows induction of anesthesia. Evidence of an increase in oxygen consumption would be a simple confirmation that MH was occurring. Because oxygen consumption may be difficult to document, however, other diagnostic steps must be taken. Venous or arterial blood should be obtained for measurement of P_{CO_2}, lactate, potassium, myoglobin, and CK. Mixed venous blood, which is most likely to show significant alterations in P_{CO_2} (Gronert and Theye, 1976a, 1976b), often is not readily available. During anesthesia there is increased arterial-to-venous shunting through the skin. Despite this fact, blood from a large peripheral vein, femoral or antecubital, may demonstrate increasing carbon dioxide tension and worsening base deficit before these changes are found in arterial blood. Increasing end-tidal carbon dioxide concentrations, particularly with increased minute ventilation, suggest that an episode of MH is occurring. Evidence of muscle injury, such as the presence of myoglobin in the serum and urine, and elevated CK and other enzymes in the blood, may not be observed if MH is treated very quickly. Once a hypermetabolic state is recognized, appropriate actions must be taken without delay, as described later.

MASSETER SPASM

Masseter spasm (also termed masseter muscle rigidity or trismus) is a marked increase in tension of the masseter that prevents opening of the mouth when succinylcholine has produced neuromuscular blockade. Masseter spasm may be an early sign of MH. However, succinylcholine can produce increased tension in normal muscle at the same time that it produces block of neuromuscular transmission (van der Spek, 1987, 1988). Many anesthesiologists believe that only if the jaw cannot be forced open should this phenomenon be called masseter spasm. Hannallah and Kaplan (1994) distinguish between masseter rigidity and trismus. In masseter rigidity, the mouth cannot be fully opened even with firm pressure on the incisors, but intubation of the trachea is possible. In trismus, the mouth cannot be fully opened and intubation of the trachea is not possible. Using this definition of masseter rigidity, Hannallah and Kaplan noted muscle rigidity to occur in 0.2% of 500 children anesthetized with halothane and administered succinylcholine. None of these 500 patients experienced trismus (Hannallah and Kaplan, 1994). It may be that the severalfold greater incidence of masseter spasm noted in the 1980s included some cases of incomplete jaw relaxation (i.e., the mouth opens fully with firm manual separation of the teeth), which was observed in 4.4% of these 500 pediatric patients. The 22 patients with incomplete jaw relaxation in this study continued to receive halothane anesthesia with no apparent complications. It seems likely that most of the cases in which the term "masseter spasm" was applied in the past were not trismus according to the definition of Hannallah and Kaplan.

Masseter spasm has been touted as a specific early warning sign of MH. Undoubtedly, deaths from MH have occurred during anesthetic procedures in which masseter spasm was observed. It may be that when masseter spasm is accompanied by rigidity of the entire body, MH is very likely to occur. However, transient increase in jaw stiffness, or resting tension of jaw muscles, is a normal response to succinylcholine (van der Spek et al., 1987, 1988; Plumley et al., 1990). Increased tension of the masseter muscle after administration of succinylcholine is most easily appreciated by the clinician after induction of anesthesia with potent inhalation anesthetics. Increase in masseter muscle tension occurs in normal mammals after the administration of succinylcholine following prior administration of epinephrine (Pryn and van der Spek, 1990). There is a greater increase in jaw tension after administration of succinylcholine during halothane anesthesia than in the presence of barbiturates.

Jaw tension is also increased in animals that are febrile as opposed to those that are normothermic (Storella et al., 1993). Temporomandibular joint abnormalities may confuse the diagnosis of masseter spasm by interfering with jaw opening.

Although masseter spasm usually occurs after anesthesia induction with halothane and the administration of succinylcholine, it may occur with other anesthetic agents (Larach et al., 1987; Marohn and Nagia, 1992). Masseter spasm may be transient (Rosenberg, 1987) or persistent. It occurs despite abolition of evoked muscle function in the extremities. Tachycardia or other nonspecific arrhythmias may accompany masseter spasm. MH may follow masseter spasm immediately; in the continued presence of anesthetic trigger agents, however, a period of 10 or more minutes often intervenes between masseter spasm and the clinical presentation of MH (Rosenberg, 1987; O'Flynn et al., 1994). In the O'Flynn and others study, clinical presentation of MH was defined as arterial PCO_2 greater than or equal to 50 mm Hg, pH less than 7.25, and base deficit more negative than −8 mEq/L.

Anesthesia with halothane has been continued after isolated masseter spasm, with no increased metabolism or cardiovascular instability. Littleford and others (1991) reported on 57 such children, of whom 33% experienced transient arrhythmias intraoperatively. Most of these children also had some degree of hypercarbia and/or metabolic acidosis. CK levels measured 18 to 24 hours postoperatively were elevated in all but one of these children, and CK levels greater than 20,000 U/L were observed in many. However, there were 11 children who experienced generalized rigidity in combination with masseter muscle spasm (MMS). Anesthesia was aborted for four of these children and continued without inhalation agents in three. None of these children developed fulminant MH in the perioperative period. The remaining four patients who developed generalized rigidity received dantrolene.

Kaplan and Rushing (1992) documented a case of masseter spasm in which clinical abnormalities prompted administration of dantrolene, and postoperative creatine kinase was 40,000 IU. Nine years later this healthy adolescent underwent extensive evaluation for neuromuscular disorders, including in vitro testing for MH caffeine-halothane contracture test (CHCT). The patient and family remain well without signs, symptoms, or diagnosis of any myopathy. If this patient had been labeled MHS, it would have been a misdiagnosis.

Children exhibiting a normal response to succinylcholine (slight or no increase in jaw tension, transient arrhythmias, transient increase in exhaled carbon dioxide) are not at increased risk for the development of MH. How can the clinician know which child with increased resistance to mouth opening after succinylcholine administration is responding in a slightly exaggerated fashion to succinylcholine and which child may develop MH? This is often impossible to determine, especially within the few minutes during induction in which a decision must be made.

One could argue that true masseter spasm is a relatively infrequent event and that associated MH susceptibility (Ording et al., 1984; Rosenberg and Fletcher, 1986; O'Flynn et al., 1994) has been overemphasized. In vitro contracture tests have documented an interaction between halothane and succinylcholine. In a study by Fletcher and Rosenberg (1985), the combination of halothane and succinylcholine produced greater contractures in muscle from patients who had a history of masseter spasm compared with those who did not, regardless of whether the muscle had produced a degree of contracture diagnostic of MH susceptibility. Contracture also occurred in normal muscle when it was exposed to halothane before succinylcholine was administered. Masseter spasm certainly has physiologic significance, but its clinical significance remains uncertain. Perhaps the incidence of masseter spasm will decrease further when halothane is completely replaced by sevoflurane, desflurane, or other anesthetics.

After an episode of masseter spasm, myalgia and occasionally weakness may be present for several days or longer. Elevation of CK levels characteristically follows masseter spasm within 24 hours (Rosenberg, 1987). In normal patients undergoing ophthalmic surgery with halothane anesthesia who received succinylcholine intraoperatively, an increase in CK level was noted 24 hours after surgery. The highest postanesthetic CK level in these otherwise normal patients was 40 times normal (Inness and Stromme, 1973). Myoglobin appears quickly in the plasma after halothane anesthesia and succinylcholine administration even in children who had no masseter spasm (Plotz and Braun, 1982). If radioimmunoassay is used to measure serum myoglobin concentrations, increases in myoglobin can be measured within the first hour after succinylcholine administration in normal children anesthetized with isoflurane or halothane. Myoglobinemia was greater during halothane than during isoflurane anesthesia in these children (Harrington and Ford, 1986). Inhalation anesthesia without succinylcholine was associated with fewer episodes of both fulminant (2 versus 8) and abortive (17 versus 110) MH than was succinylcholine with potent inhalation anesthetics in a Danish population (Ording, 1985). Thus, avoiding succinylcholine administration to pediatric patients anesthetized with halothane, or other inhalation anesthetics, not only avoids the diagnostic uncertainties associated with masseter spasm but also produces fewer episodes of MH and other adverse events (Delphin et al., 1987; Rosenberg and Gronert, 1992). Pediatric anesthesiologists may choose to administer succinylcholine only when definite indications for this drug have been identified.

MANAGEMENT OF MASSETER SPASM

There is no agreement among experienced clinicians concerning the preferred management of patients with incomplete relaxation of the masseter after the administration of succinylcholine (Kaplan et al., 1993). If jaw stiffness was mild, so that the mouth could be opened with increased effort, there was no rigidity in the rest of the body, and cardiovascular function was stable, anesthesia may be continued with careful documentation of capnography and core temperature. Fluid deficits should be replaced completely so that urine output is greater than 3 mL/kg per hour. Urine should be obtained in the early postoperative period to check for the presence of myoglobin. Blood should be obtained for measurement of electrolytes and CK. It is not necessary to terminate anesthetic administration unless signs of increasing metabolic rate occur. If jaw stiffness is so great that the mouth cannot be opened, there are several reasons to terminate elective anesthetic administration, not the least of which may be the need to clear the upper airway. If the jaw is tight, signs of MH should be sought. Venous blood should be obtained for gas analysis and measurement of electrolytes, myoglobin, and CK. If surgery must continue, anesthesia can be changed to nontriggering drugs. Intra-arterial, central venous, and bladder catheters are useful if evidence of increased metabolism is found and dantrolene is administered. Muscle tension of the rest of the body should be noted. Total body rigidity accompanying masseter muscle rigidity does not absolutely guarantee that the patient has MH (Larach et al., 1987). Anesthetic depth may have been misjudged. Alternatively, the patient may have occult myotonia.

Postoperative renal failure has occurred in patients who had myoglobinuria after administration of succinylcholine during anesthesia. In any situation in which injury to muscle may occur, it is important to document that myoglobinuria is *not* present. If any increased muscle stiffness was noted after administration of succinylcholine or the child complains of muscle pain postoperatively, urine should be obtained. If there is no blood in the urine as assessed by orthotolidin (Hematest), then there is no myoglobin present. If the response to blood is positive on the dipstick, urine should be examined for the presence of red blood cells, and free hemoglobin and myoglobin measured. If myoglobin is present, the patient should remain in the hospital. The patient should be observed for signs of MH, evaluated for the presence of occult muscle disease, and hydrated. Alkaline urine reduces the risk of renal tubular injury from myoglobin.

TREATMENT OF AN ACUTE EPISODE OF MALIGNANT HYPERTHERMIA

When the diagnosis of MH is made or strongly suspected, the most important step to take is to administer dantrolene. The other steps in management are to discontinue the triggering anesthetic agents immediately, increase minute ventilation severalfold with 100% oxygen, and alert the surgeon that the procedure must be concluded promptly. Other anesthesiologists or paramedical personnel or both should be called in at once for assistance.

As noted earlier, dantrolene is a calcium channel antagonist, specific for the ryanodine receptor. Dantrolene must be diluted with sterile, preservative-free, distilled water, which should be stored in large quantities with the drug (see Table 31-1). It is important to store sterile water in clearly labeled containers of a different size from those used for routine intravenous solutions and to keep a mixing system nearby. Dantrolene will dissolve faster as temperature increases from 20° to 40°C (Mitchell, 2003). When the dantrolene preparation is dissolved, the initial intravenous dose should be 2.5 mg/kg, although much higher doses may be needed to control the episode. Repeated dosing of dantrolene should be guided by clinical and laboratory signs.

TABLE 31–1. Drugs and dosages used to treat an acute episode of malignant hyperthermia

Dantrolene*	2.5 to 10.0 mg/kg or more (sterile water must be available to dilute dantrolene)
Sodium bicarbonate	2 mmol/kg PRN
Iced normal saline solution	PRN (10 to 12 L for 50-kg patient)
Mannitol	300 mg/kg (note there is 150 mg of mannitol per milligram of dantrolene in the vial)
Furosemide	0.5 to 1.0 mg/kg
Insulin (regular)	10 U regular insulin in 50 ml of 50% dextrose titrated to produce normokalemia
Lidocaine	1 mg/kg

*Dantrolene administration should be repeated until physical and chemical signs have returned to normal. When this degree of physiologic stability has been obtained, dantrolene [1 mg/kg or more] should be repeated approximately every 6 hours until creatine kinase has decreased consistently.

A flow sheet including minute ventilation, end-tidal carbon dioxide concentration, heart rate and rhythm, arterial blood pressure, central venous pressure, core temperature, and urine output, along with arterial and venous blood gas tensions, serum electrolytes, and glucose and total fluid intake, provides a useful guide for continued therapeutic interventions. Dantrolene must be administered until respiratory and metabolic acidosis has resolved. The usual upper limit of 10 mg/kg may be exceeded as necessary. The most frequent side effects of dantrolene administration are muscle weakness and phlebitis.

The anesthesia machine need not be switched to a standby unit that has been kept free of inhalation anesthetics. After 10 minutes of 10 L/min fresh gas flow, the isoflurane concentration at the gas outlet of the Datex-Ohmeda anesthesia workstation is less than 2 ppm (Schonell et al., 2003). Gas flow of 12 L/min or more will remove residual volatile agent from an anesthesia machine within 6 to 12 minutes (McGraw and Keon, 1989). When practical, the carbon dioxide absorber and circuit tubing should be changed. If this is not done, 30 minutes is needed to reach 2 ppm isoflurane with an anesthesia workstation (Schonell et al., 2003). If a vaporizer, which could continue to deliver anesthetic vapor despite being turned off, is present in the circuit, such as the Fluotec Mk.3 or Mini Boyle machine with cage-mounted vaporizer, it should be drained (Ritchie et al., 1988).

Procedures to cool the body should be instituted quickly. The goal is to reduce muscle metabolism and avoid exposure to a critical core temperature of greater than 40°C (Bouchama and Knochel, 2002). A core temperature of less than 36°C may not be beneficial. Drapes should be removed, heated humidifiers turned off, and water mattresses turned to cooling temperatures. Cold normal saline solution can be given intravenously to maintain normal central venous pressure. The stomach can be irrigated with iced saline solution through an orogastric tube. Open body cavities can also be lavaged with iced saline solution, and ice packs can be placed in the groin and axillae where large vessels come close to the skin surface. Wet cloths and a fan to facilitate surface evaporation can be useful. Even extracorporeal bypass with a heat exchanger was used successfully to cool patients with MH in the era before dantrolene was available. Now that dantrolene is readily available, extracorporeal bypass is not likely to be necessary to treat an episode of MH. An arterial catheter should be inserted to observe the patient's hemodynamic status and acid-base balance. A central venous catheter is useful for obtaining cardiac filling pressures and blood gas tensions, as well as for administering intravenous fluids. A pulmonary artery catheter will allow measurement of mixed venous blood gases and lactate and adjustment of cardiac filling pressures in the patient with pulmonary edema. Mixed venous blood is a more sensitive indicator than arterial blood of the patient's acid-base status. A blood sample should be taken to determine the blood gases and pH, potassium, glucose, CK, myoglobin, creatinine, and clotting profile as soon as feasible.

Arrhythmias usually stop when the episode is controlled with dantrolene. Lidocaine is recommended for treatment of arrhythmias in MH, because concern about amide-type local anesthetics such as lidocaine triggering or worsening an episode of MH has decreased.

Both metabolic acidosis and respiratory acidosis occur in MH. Increased metabolic rate leads to marked increases in carbon dioxide production, which can exceed the capability of breathing circuits to eliminate it. In addition, lactate production results when the body tries to maintain energy supplies through anaerobic metabolism. Treatment of the acidosis should include bicarbonate and hyperventilation. If a Mapleson system is used, very high flows are required for effective hyperventilation. High fresh gas flows also remove carbon dioxide adequately from a circle system.

Hyperkalemia results when cell membranes are disrupted. This is recognized on the electrocardiogram as increased T-wave amplitude in the early stages and later by widening QRS complexes, interventricular conduction delays and blocks, and finally no organized rhythm at all. Glucose and insulin (10 U regular insulin in 50 mL of 50% glucose titrated to effect) can be administered to lower serum potassium temporarily. β-Agonists can also be useful to move potassium intracellularly. Intravenous calcium is appropriate emergency treatment of the hyperkalemia associated with MH (Gronert et al., 1986).

Large losses of intravascular volume should be anticipated. Evaporative loss of fluid may be great, and edema formation may occur in muscle and in other tissues during fulminant MH. Intravenous fluids should be given to maintain normal cardiac filling pressures, as evidenced by adequate perfusion pressure, urine output, and capillary refill. Although an osmotic diuresis may be induced to protect renal tubule function in the presence of myoglobinuria, it will promote acute intravascular volume loss. The management of the acute MH episode is summarized in Box 31–2.

Because calcium channel blockers might interfere with excitation-contraction coupling (Lynch et al., 1986) and conserve energy reserves, it is reasonable to ask whether they might be useful in the treatment of MH or prophylaxis for MH susceptibility. Not all calcium channel–blocking drugs have the same effects in MHS subjects. Diltiazem inhibits halothane-induced contracture in MHS pig muscle (Illias et al., 1985), thus confirming a single similar observation in human muscle. Verapamil, however, is not a therapeutic agent in porcine MH (Gallant et al., 1985). Furthermore, verapamil and dantrolene interact to produce severe hyperkalemia and myocardial depression (Lynch et al., 1986; Rubin and Zablocki, 1987). Nifedipine administration has been associated with the development of MH in a child with underlying neuromuscular disease (Cook and Henderson-Tilton, 1985). At this time it seems prudent to administer calcium channel–blocking drugs to patients with a history of MH or neuromuscular disease only with extreme caution. Calcium channel blockers are not recommended in the management of acute MH. If dantrolene must be administered to a patient who is also receiving calcium channel–blocking drugs, invasive hemodynamic monitoring and frequent measurement of serum potassium levels are recommended (Lynch et al., 1986; Rubin and Zablocki, 1987).

BOX 31–2 Management of the Acute Malignant Hyperthermia (MH) Episode

- Stop inhalation anesthetics immediately.
- Cancel or conclude surgery as soon as possible.
- Hyperventilate with high flow of 100% oxygen.
- Administer dantrolene (2.5 mg/kg) IV over 5 min and repeat as needed. Give more dantrolene if signs of MH reappear.
- Initiate cooling with hypothermia blanket; intravenous cold saline solution (15 mL/kg over 10 min), ice packs in the axillae and groin, and lavage of body cavities with cold saline solution if the core temperature is greater than 39°C. Stop cooling when the core temperature falls to 38°C.
- Correct metabolic acidosis with 1 to 2 mEq/kg of sodium bicarbonate as an initial dose.
- Administer calcium (10 mg/kg of calcium chloride) or insulin (0.2 mcg/kg) in 50% dextrose in water (1mL/kg) to treat the effects of hyperkalemia.
- Administer lidocaine (1 mg/kg) to treat ventricular arrhythmias.
- Maintain urine output of 2 mL/kg per hour with furosemide (1 mg/kg) and additional mannitol if needed.
- Insert arterial and central venous catheters.
- Repeat venous blood gas and electrolyte analysis every 15 min until these and vital signs normalize.

POSTANESTHETIC CONSIDERATIONS

A patient in whom MH has been successfully treated in the operating room requires intensive care to continue treatment and to monitor for late manifestations of the disease.

Continuation of treatment is necessary because recrudescence of MH can occur after an apparently successfully treated episode. This usually happens in the first few hours after the initial event. As much as 12 mg/kg of dantrolene has been required to treat recurrences over one 12-hour period (Pollock et al., 1992). Continuous monitoring of vital signs and frequent measurement of venous lactate, blood gases, and electrolytes should detect metabolic changes. Dantrolene should be administered intravenously as necessary, not only until no evidence of metabolic acidosis remains but also until serum myoglobin levels decrease toward normal. The half-life of myoglobin in the blood is normally 1 to 3 hours. In contrast, CK peaks 24 to 36 hours after injury and usually decreases about 40% per day thereafter (Salluzzo, 1992). The CK may be measured repeatedly to demonstrate that it is decreasing and therefore that the process that produced rhabdomyolysis has abated.

After an acute episode, the patient with MH may die of a recrudescence, disseminated intravascular coagulopathy, or other nonspecific systemic injury. Disseminated intravascular coagulopathy is a frequent finding in fatal MH. The administration of dantrolene should be continued to stop the disruption of muscle, the presumed underlying cause of disseminated intravascular coagulopathy. Supportive care should be given as indicated, and coagulation function carefully monitored during and after an episode of MH.

Late manifestations of an episode of MH range from mild muscle pain to multiorgan system failure. Cerebral edema may occur. Fulminant cases of MH may have permanent neurologic sequelae (coma, paralysis) for no apparent reason. Even satisfactory care during anesthesia may not prevent these neurologic complications (Gronert, 1980). Rehabilitation can take months after an episode of fulminant MH.

Pulmonary edema may occur owing to marked shifts in intravascular volume and to myocardial dysfunction. Its presence requires more careful assessment of the circulatory status to improve cardiac filling pressures and inotropic state. Areas of myocardium may have abnormal conduction, decreased contractility, or both. It is important to maintain adequate renal perfusion because massive myoglobinuria produced by fulminant MH can cause acute renal failure. Mannitol, which is part of the dantrolene formulation (150 mg of mannitol/mg of dantrolene), induces an alkaline osmotic diuresis and therefore helps to prevent precipitation of myoglobin in the renal tubules. Sufficient muscle damage to produce myoglobinuria and acute renal failure can occur in the absence of pigmenturia or dramatic elevation of CK (Grossman et al., 1974). If myoglobin (or hemoglobin) is present, urine gives a positive reaction with orthotolidin (Hematest). In the presence of myoglobinuria, normal saline solution should be given to force a diuresis of at least 3 mL/kg per hour. If urine output is less than this, then mannitol (1 mL of 25% solution) and bicarbonate (1 mEq) in D_5W (8 mL) should be given at twice the maintenance fluid rate. Rapidly increasing serum creatinine signals the onset of renal failure.

All cases of MH, anesthetic-related episodes of increased metabolism or rhabdomyolysis, isolated masseter spasm, and anesthetics administered to patients who have undergone a CHCT should be reported to the Malignant Hyperthermia Registry, so that the epidemiologic study of MH may have as broad a scope and as complete a collection of data as possible. Report forms may be obtained by telephone (412-692-5464).

PROPHYLACTIC MANAGEMENT

INDICATIONS FOR MUSCLE BIOPSY AND GENETIC EVALUATION OF TYPE I RYANODINE RECEPTOR

Indications may vary depending on the particular goals being addressed. Individuals, both patients and physicians, concerned with improving the diagnostic tests for MH may urge all patients with any symptoms consistent with MH and those with a clear history of fulminant MH to undergo muscle biopsy. Others prefer to advise that this invasive test be performed only when the predictive value of the test may be helpful for patient management.

A new benefit of undergoing muscle biopsy and contracture testing is that patients with contracture tests indicating MH susceptibility are candidates for genetic study. Between 30% and 70% of such individuals have been found to have mutations in the ryanodine receptor gene that causes MH (Sambuughin et al., 2001; Robinson et al., 2003; Sambuughin et al., 2005). The process of evaluating MH susceptibility in relatives can begin with genetic evaluation in search of the familial mutation (Urwyler et al., 2001; Girard et al., 2004). A panel of *RYR1* mutations has been selected to be the initial genetic test of MH susceptibility in North America (Sei et al., 2004). Currently, genetic testing of MH susceptibility will be less sensitive (Nelson et al., 2004) but less invasive and less costly than muscle biopsy and contracture testing. The genetics of MH susceptibility is not completely known. In large families, there has been discordance between contracture test results and genetic results (Brown et al., 2000; Robinson et al., 2003). Continued evaluation of MH susceptibility by more than one type of test is needed to explain discordance. Genetic testing is of value for determining affected family members in a family in which an *RYR1* mutation has been associated with MH in an affected individual. However, the value of genetic testing for *RYR1* mutations as an initial screening for MH susceptibility has not been determined.

The sensitivity and specificity of the CHCT have been determined (Larach et al., 1992, 1993; Ording et al., 1997; Allen et al., 1998). General statements about the predictive value of this test can be made. *Sensitivity* is the probability that a test result will indicate the disease is present, when in fact the individual tested has the disease in question. *Specificity* is the probability that a test result will indicate disease is not present, when in fact the individual tested does not have the disease in question. The clinician is interested in the predictive value of a test because the clinician does not know whether the patient has the disease of interest but can obtain the results of the diagnostic test.

The *positive predictive value (PPV)* of a test is the probability that an individual whose test result indicates that the disease is present does indeed have the disease of interest. The *negative predictive value (NPV)* of a test is the probability that an individual whose test result indicates that disease is absent does not have the disease in question. By definition, the predictive value depends on the probability that the individual has the disease in question before the test results are obtained, as well as the sensitivity and specificity of the test (Rosner, 1990). This probability may be thought of as the prior probability of the individual having the disease of interest or, if a population rather than an individual is considered, the incidence of the disease in the population (Box 31–3).

Rather than speculate on what a group of clinical findings suggests about the probability of MH susceptibility in an individual, one may use the test characteristics (sensitivity and

BOX 31–3 Interpretation of a Test

Sensitivity = Pr (T^+/D^+) = Probability (Pr) the test (T) is positive given that the disease (D) is present
Sensitivity = Pr (T^-/D^-) = Probability the test is *not* positive given that the disease is *not* present
Predictive value of a positive test = Pr (D^+/T^-)

$$\text{PPV} = \frac{\text{Prevalence} \times \text{Sensitivity}}{\text{Prevalence} \times \text{Sensitivity} + (1-\text{Prevalence}) \times (1-\text{Specificity})}$$

Predictive value of a negative test = Pr (D^-/T^+)

$$\text{NPV} = \frac{(1-\text{Prevalence}) \times \text{Specificity}}{(1-\text{Prevalence}) \times \text{Specificity} + \text{Prevalence} \times (1-\text{Sensitivity})}$$

Prior probability and prevalence may be used interchangeably in these equations.

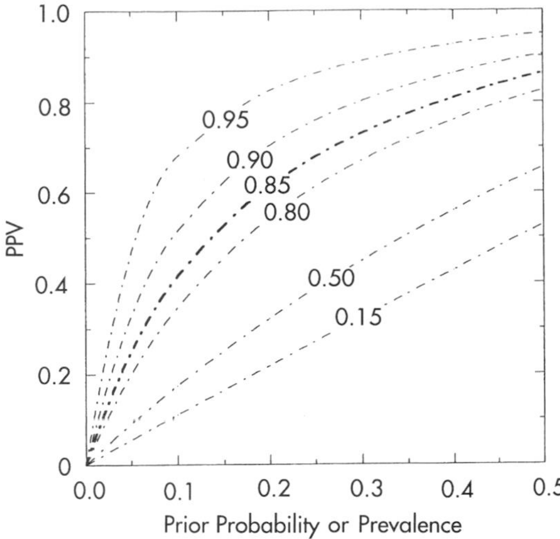

■ **FIGURE 31–2.** The y-axis is the positive predictive value (PPV) of the caffeine-halothane contracture test (CHCT). This figure illustrates the fact that when the sensitivity is 95% and the specificity is 85%, the positive predictive value is less than 50% when the prior probability is less than 15%.

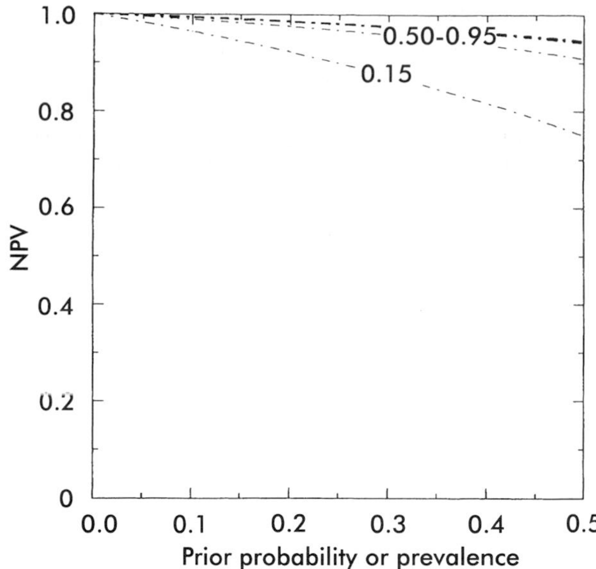

■ **FIGURE 31–3.** The y-axis is the negative predictive value (NPV) of the caffeine-halothane contracture test (CHCT). NPV is less altered by specificity than is positive predictive value (PPV) when prior probability is less than 50%. Thus the NPVs coincide for specificities from 85% to 95%.

specificity) to calculate the predictive value of the CHCT over a wide range of prior probabilities (Figs. 31–2 and 31–3). For example, if a patient with a history of isolated masseter spasm is thought to have a less than 25% chance of having MH, then, if the sensitivity of the CHCT is 99% and the specificity is 85%, the positive predictive value of the CHCT in that individual is less than 69% and the negative predictive value is greater than 99%. In other words, the chance of that individual having a false-positive result of CHCT is at least 30% and the chance of a false-negative result is less than 1%. In contrast, if a patient with a strong family history of MH has many of the clinical signs of MH, it might be judged that the probability of that individual having MH, before obtaining the result of the CHCT, would be 80%. The positive and negative predictive value of the CHCT would be 96% and 99%, respectively, for such a patient. These statements are oversimplifications in that these calculations assume that the disease being tested for has similar manifestations in all affected individuals. Certainly this is not the case for MH. Nevertheless, appreciation of the concept of the predictive value of a test is important when questions arise regarding the meaning of clinical events and test results. These concepts have been used to argue that the index case should be the first person to undergo contracture testing, followed by first-degree relatives (Loke and MacLennan, 1998; Larach and MacLennan, 1999).

Currently, muscle biopsy for CHCT is the only way to evaluate the diagnosis of MH susceptibility in the absence of an episode of fulminant MH. For satisfactory in vitro testing, 1 g of muscle must be removed from the thigh. A child weighing less than 20 kg may be too small to undergo a muscle biopsy. In general, children younger than 10 years are too young to undergo CHCT.

Parents of an affected child may wish to have a muscle biopsy performed. The relatives of the parent whose findings are negative (assuming autosomal dominant inheritance) can then be reassured, without biopsy, that they have no increased risk of MH. Ideally, siblings and first cousins on the affected side should be informed and offered biopsy testing. Financial and geographic considerations often discourage families in these endeavors. At the very least, relatives of an MHS patient should be informed about the presence of MH susceptibility in their family and its implications.

__Figures 31–2 and 31–3__ illustrate the relationship between the sensitivity and specificity of a test, the prior probability of the disease, and the predictive value of that test (see definitions in Box 31–3). The probabilities on the graphs are shown as decimals between 0 and 1. In both figures, the x-axis is prior probability of MH susceptibility in the individual under consideration. This may be thought of as the probability that the individual under examination is MH susceptible before the results of the CHCT are considered. This probability ranges from 0 to 0.5, or 50%, in these figures. In both figures, the sensitivity of the test is 0.95 or 95%. In both figures, the specificity of the CHCT varies between 0.95 (95%) and 0.15 (15%), as labeled on the dotted lines. The heavy line is the predictive value of the CHCT when sensitivity is 95% and specificity is 85%.

A valuable self-help resource is the Malignant Hyperthermia Association of the United States (MHAUS, P.O. Box 1069, 11 East State St., Sherburne, NY 13460 (Fax 1-607-674-7910). This organization offers information, expert consultation, and referral and provides family counseling. Their newsletter contains up-to-date information and reviews of the recent professional literature on topics related to MH. MHAUS maintains a 24-hour, professionally staffed telephone line to provide information on diagnosis, treatment, and referral of patients with MH (telephone: 1-800-644-9737).

CARE OF PATIENTS WITH A HISTORY OF MALIGNANT HYPERTHERMIA

When a patient is referred preoperatively because of "possible MH," one should determine how the diagnosis was made. At times, patients are erroneously told they "must have had an episode of MH" because a slight increase in temperature or transient ventricular arrhythmias occurred and no diligent effort was made to clarify the causes or to obtain biochemical evidence of hypermetabolism or rhabdomyolysis. Many cases of increased jaw tension, arrhythmia, or mild elevation of myoglobin or CK following the administration of succinylcholine occur in the absence of MH susceptibility. When the issue of MH susceptibility has been raised, the personal and family history should be examined for previous adverse sequelae to anesthetics, sudden cardiovascular collapse suggestive of arrhythmias or heatstroke, and any evidence of musculoskeletal disorders including cramping with exercise. A positive finding suggests that consultation with a neurologist, a muscle biopsy, and in vitro contracture testing may be warranted.

CK levels, at rest, are of no predictive value in the general population (Britt et al., 1976; Paasuke and Brownell, 1986). If a relative of a patient known to be susceptible to MH has an elevated CK level, that individual has an increased likelihood of also being susceptible. This will not hold for patients with other problems producing CK elevations (e.g., Duchenne's muscular dystrophy). In some populations (Ellis et al., 1975), more than 25% of the patients with elevated CK levels were not susceptible to MH on in vitro testing.

PREOPERATIVE CARE OF MALIGNANT HYPERTHERMIA–SUSCEPTIBLE PATIENTS

When it is clear that the suspected episode was MH and especially when contracture testing has already been done and shows a typical MH pattern, several decisions must be made. If it is at all possible, regional or local anesthesia should be chosen. Although some theoretic objections to amide-type local anesthetics exist, data in animals and humans have not shown any local anesthetic to trigger MH. Review of anesthesia during biopsy suggests that nerve blocks with small volumes of amide local anesthetics do not provoke an episode of MH (Berkowitz and Rosenberg, 1985). Regional anesthesia with lidocaine, bupivacaine, ropivacaine, or another local anesthetic is an acceptable choice for the MHS patient.

One must decide whether the risks of preoperative prophylactic dantrolene (muscle weakness, disequilibrium, and nausea) (Flewellen et al., 1983) justify its potential benefits. Because many muscle biopsies and other operations have been performed in patients with positive CHCT, without preoperative administration of dantrolene or postoperative complications (Ording et al., 1991), it is considered acceptable to withhold preoperative dantrolene. These patients must be closely monitored during anesthesia with nontriggering agents. If there are no signs of increased metabolism or rhabdomyolysis and if no dantrolene was administered, then MHS patients may be safely discharged on the day of surgery (Yentis et al., 1992).

When a very strong family or personal history of MH suggests that the risks of dantrolene may be acceptable, dantrolene can be given orally over several days or intravenously immediately before surgery. Treatment with what was expected to be adequate doses of oral dantrolene has not always prevented the development of hypermetabolism during anesthesia with nontriggering agents (Fitzgibbons, 1980). It appears most appropriate to administer prophylactic dantrolene intravenously while monitoring muscle strength.

The dose-response relationship of dantrolene in children has not been reported. Available data suggest that the half-life of dantrolene in children is somewhat shorter than that in adults: 7.3 to 9.8 hours (Lietman et al., 1974; Lerman et al., 1989) (Fig. 31–4) and 12.1 hours (Flewellen et al., 1983), respectively. In adults, a cumulative dose of 2.2 to 2.5 mg/kg of dantrolene administered intravenously over 125 minutes produced a steady plasma concentration of dantrolene for longer than 5 hours

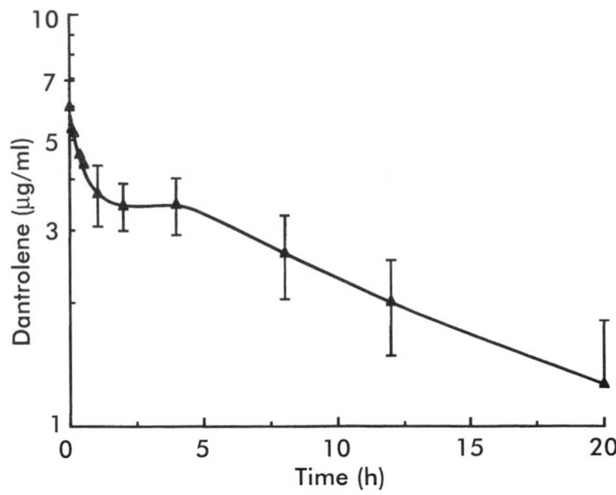

FIGURE 31–4. Dantrolene plasma concentration versus time in 10 children after intravenous administration of 2.4 mg/kg over 10 to 12 min. (From Lerman J, McLeod ME, Strong HA: Pharmacokinetics of intravenous dantrolene in children. *Anesthesiology* 70:625, 1989.)

(Flewellen et al., 1983). Orally administered dantrolene, a total of 5 mg/kg in three or four divided doses administered every 6 hours to MHS adults, has also been shown to produce protective plasma concentrations of dantrolene for at least 6 hours after induction of anesthesia (Allen et al., 1988). In children, intravenous administration of 2.4 mg/kg of dantrolene infused over 10 minutes produced stable blood levels of about 3.5 mcg/mL for 4 hours, after which a slow decline in plasma concentration occurred (Lerman et al., 1989). Hence, it may be reasonable to repeat doses of dantrolene in the range of 1 to 2 mg/kg every 5 to 7 hours for prophylaxis. The dose and timing are not rigid because they should be titrated to effect. It is likely that when plasma concentrations of dantrolene are sufficient to inhibit an episode of MH, the patient experiences weakness and possibly disequilibrium.

A dynamometer could be used to assess grip strength objectively, but this requires the patient's cooperation. In a study of adults, the dose of dantrolene that produced maximal depression of grip strength and evoked force of thumb contraction had no significant effect on vital capacity (Flewellen et al., 1983). Similar studies have not been performed in children. Clinical experience (Brandom and Carroll, unpublished observations) suggests that less than 2 mg/kg of dantrolene administered intravenously to a child preoperatively can be associated with significant hypotonia in the postoperative period. If the patient is unable to maintain grasp, it is wise to stop dantrolene administration. Weakness induced by dantrolene could compromise the ability to swallow (Flewellen et al., 1983) and even necessitate artificial protection of the airway and mechanical ventilation, although this has never been reported in the literature. Intravenous dantrolene should be administered in settings where support of airway and ventilation can be easily provided.

PERIOPERATIVE CARE OF PATIENTS WITH SUSPECTED MALIGNANT HYPERTHERMIA SUSCEPTIBILITY

One may encounter patients who have had an anesthetic course or who have a family history that suggests MH susceptibility but who have not had that possibility evaluated by means of muscle biopsy and in vitro contracture testing. A reasonable approach to providing anesthesia for such patients is to administer a "nontriggering" anesthetic and monitor carefully for signs of MH. Dantrolene must be available but need not be administered prophylactically. It would be inappropriate to label an individual as MHS and administer dantrolene without obtaining some evidence of a hypermetabolic response to anesthesia in that individual or a similarly convincing history in a first-degree relative. There are many causes of perioperative muscle injury. It may not be possible to diagnose the underlying muscle disorder, but it is easy to demonstrate that there is no myoglobin in the urine. Urine should be examined prior to discharge if a diagnosis of MH or other occult muscle disease is suspected. If there is no myoglobin in the urine, the patient has little risk of renal injury.

ANESTHETIC TECHNIQUES

Physiologic responses to stress may play a part in the initiation of an episode of MH in humans, as well as in pigs (Gronert et al., 1980; Gronert and Theye, 1976a, 1976b). Anesthesia for the MHS patient should be designed to be as "stress-free" as possible, so that any tachycardia and arrhythmias that may occur are more likely to be associated with impending MH than with the stress of anesthetic, induction, or surgery.

There are many "nontriggering" techniques for general anesthesia (Table 31–2). Local anesthetic cream can produce topical analgesia of the skin, which may facilitate intravenous catheter placement. Preoperative medication with midazolam 0.3 to 0.7 mg/kg orally or 0.2 to 0.3 mg/kg nasally often produces sedation adequate to facilitate the placement of an intravenous catheter in a child. Preoperative sedation is an important part of the anesthetic management for MHS patients in the opinion of some anesthesiologists. After placement of an intravenous catheter, anesthesia may be induced with barbiturates or propofol (Raff and Harrison, 1989; Harrison, 1991) and narcotics as indicated by the planned surgery and other characteristics of the patient. Prior administration of benzodiazepine can reduce chest and truncal rigidity commonly observed after the administration of a synthetic narcotic. A nondepolarizing neuromuscular blocking agent may be administered if necessary. It is helpful to use a peripheral nerve stimulator when a neuromuscular blocker is administered so that the dose of drug can be titrated to the desired effect. Similarly, an anticholinesterase should be administered as indicated by the results of peripheral nerve stimulation.

TABLE 31–2. Malignant hyperthermia and drugs used during anesthesia

Drugs Likely to Trigger MH	Drugs that Do Not Trigger MH
Potent inhalation anesthetics: Halothane, isoflurane, enflurane, desflurane, sevoflurane, ether	Narcotics
Depolarizing neuromuscular blockers: Succinylcholine	Benzodiazepines
	Barbiturates
	Propofol
	Ketamine
	Nondepolarizing (competitive) neuromuscular blockers
	Anticholinesterases and anticholinergics
	Local anesthetics
	Nonsteroidal anti-inflammatory drugs
	Calcium

There are rare reports of changes compatible with MH occurring after the use of such "safe" general anesthetic drugs (Fitzgibbons, 1980; Pollock et al., 1992). For susceptible patients, there is no "safe" general anesthetic technique, merely drugs that are less likely to trigger MH. It is advisable to avoid drugs that may affect temperature regulation and sympathetic tone to such an extent that it might be difficult to detect early signs of insidious MH. Furthermore, serotonergic agonists and some psychotropic drugs (MDMA [Ecstasy]) have produced MH episodes in susceptible pigs (Wappler et al., 1997; Fiege et al., 2003). Large doses of phenothiazines and anticholinergics are not drugs of choice for the MHS patient. Atropine is administered only when there is significant risk of bradycardia. However, some anesthesiologists have found ketamine to be a useful anesthetic in patients susceptible to MH.

Monitoring and preparedness to treat acute MH are of the utmost importance. In addition to precordial heart tones, electrocardiogram, blood pressure, and oxygen saturation, end-tidal carbon dioxide concentrations should be monitored. Core temperature should be measured. Arterial and urinary bladder catheters are not needed for all surgery in MHS patients, but they are convenient for repeated blood sampling and close monitoring of hemodynamic stability and urine myoglobin. The anesthesia machine can be sufficiently flushed of potent inhalation agents by 12 minutes of 10 L/min oxygen flow (McGraw and Keon, 1989). Anesthesia workstations require 20 minutes of flushing if carbon dioxide absorbers and the respiratory circuit are not removed (Schonell et al., 2003).

It is helpful to keep drugs (see Table 31–1) and supplies to treat MH in a portable container, such as a carryall or rolling cart that is immediately accessible in the operating room and recovery room and can easily be transported to other areas in the hospital. The necessary supplies include at least 5 to 10 mg/kg of dantrolene and liter quantities of sterile, preservative-free, distilled water in which to dissolve the dantrolene. Ice or cold packs should be ready, and large volumes of normal saline solution should be available in a nearby refrigerator. Water mattresses that can both cool and warm the patient should be placed under the MHS patient from the start of the anesthetic procedure.

ANESTHETIC MANAGEMENT FOR MUSCLE BIOPSY

The preceding recommendations for anesthetic care of patients with MH susceptibility apply to the patient undergoing diagnostic muscle biopsy except that prophylactic dantrolene is never given. Dantrolene may prevent the in vitro response to halothane and caffeine, causing a false-negative result. Biopsy for CHCT can be done only in one of the specialized centers that support the performance of this in vitro test. The list of currently active centers may be obtained from the Malignant Hyperthermia Association of the United States (www.mhaus.org).

The child scheduled for a biopsy usually weighs more than 20 kg. Some biopsy center directors will test only children who are at least 10 years old. The patient may be mature enough to have regional anesthesia. In a cooperative child, the use of lateral femoral-cutaneous nerve block and intravenous sedation is often successful (Berkowitz and Rosenberg, 1985). If the child cannot cooperate, general anesthesia may be induced and maintained with various agents, including benzodiazepines, narcotics, propofol or barbiturates, nondepolarizing relaxants, and nitrous oxide.

POSTOPERATIVE CARE OF THE MALIGNANT HYPERTHERMIA–SUSCEPTIBLE PATIENT

If anesthesia has proceeded uneventfully and prophylactic dantrolene has not been administered, the patient should be transported to the recovery room for the usual monitoring of vital signs, electrocardiogram, mental status, and urine output and color. A dipstick should be used to check urine for blood. The reaction of heme with orthotolidine will occur if myoglobin, free hemoglobin, or red blood cells are present. If no sign of MH appears, the patient may be transferred to the floor after an ordinary length of stay in the recovery room. After observing such patients for 4 hours and finding no abnormalities, they may be discharged from the hospital. In this way, it is possible for a child who is susceptible to MH to be treated successfully as an outpatient (Yentis et al., 1992; Pollock et al., 2004).

If there is any evidence of hypermetabolism or if continued treatment with intravenous dantrolene is contemplated, the patient should be cared for in an intensive care area. When preoperative prophylactic dantrolene has been administered but continuing treatment is not necessary and the patient is metabolically and hemodynamically stable, discharge from the recovery room is based on the same clinical criteria as for other patients who have been given muscle relaxants. Guidelines for heart rate, temperature, and other monitoring should be included in the postoperative orders. In a postoperative MH patient, the anesthesiologist should be called to evaluate fever or tachycardia. The causes are usually related to pain, mild dehydration, atelectasis, or bacteremia. Nevertheless, MH has been reported to occur several hours postoperatively. The patient must be examined carefully for signs of MH or altered mental status, venous blood gas tension and lactate should be measured, and urine should be tested for myoglobin. If signs of hypermetabolism or rhabdomyolysis are present, the patient should be treated with intravenous dantrolene and transferred to an intensive care unit.

DISORDERS ASSOCIATED WITH MALIGNANT HYPERTHERMIA

A number of disorders have been thought to be related to the MH syndrome because their presence appears to increase the risk of MH during anesthesia. A complete understanding of these syndromes could contribute to understanding the pathophysiology of MH.

The earliest large study of MH epidemiology (Britt and Kalow, 1970) provided a review of the case histories of 89 MHS patients. Thirty-two of these patients had preexisting musculoskeletal abnormalities; most frequent were ptosis, strabismus, idiopathic kyphoscoliosis, and hernias—congenital inguinal hernia, umbilical hernia, and diaphragmatic hernia. A few patients also reported a tendency to have severe muscle cramps in the extremities unrelated to either cold or exercise. Other abnormalities noted included recurrent spontaneous dislocations of the hip, clubfoot, and pes excavatum.

Although not all myopathic patients are MHS, the presence of a known or suspected myopathy should alert the anesthesiologist that there may be increased potential for MH susceptibility and/or anesthetic complications that may mimic MH (Heytens et al., 1992). It has been claimed that Duchenne's muscular dystrophy (DMD) coexists with MH susceptibility (Heiman-Patterson et al., 1986). However, the genetic defect that produces DMD is distinct from genetic loci that have been associated with MH susceptibility. DMD is caused by a lack of dystrophin. The gene responsible for the production of normal dystrophin is located at chromosomal position Xp21. One genetic locus associated with MH is on chromosome 19q13.1. This gene codes the ryanodine receptor (Thompson, 1994). There may be another genetic locus associated with MH on chromosome 17q (Levitt et al., 1992).

Many patients with DMD have received potent inhalation anesthetics without MH occurring (Peluso and Bianchini, 1992), but dystrophic muscle is fragile. Even mild exercise in DMD patients results in a marked egress of sarcoplasmic components into the plasma, most notably myoglobin, CK, and potassium (Florence et al., 1985). These patients can have rhabdomyolysis during anesthesia with potent inhalation anesthetics even without the administration of succinylcholine (Rubiano et al., 1987). It is not surprising that anesthetic complications with many of the qualities of MH occur in patients with abnormal dystrophin (Kleopa et al., 2000) (see Chapter 32, Systemic Disorders). Nevertheless, at least one patient with dystrophinopathy had a negative contracture test, ruling out MH susceptibility (Gronert et al., 1992).

Several extensive family studies of central core disease (Shy and Magee, 1956; Byrne et al., 1982) have documented morphologically abnormal muscle, that is, central cores of oddly aligned fibers, in some patients with MH. The histologic abnormality of central core disease (CCD) is not a marker for MH. However, CCD is the only myopathy for which a definite genetic link to MH has been shown (Kausch et al., 1990). Several mutations in *RYR1* cause CCD and/or MH susceptibility (Loke and MacLennan, 1998; Tilgen et al., 2001). It is advisable to treat a patient with central core disease as MHS.

Another familial myopathy, the King-Denborough syndrome (King and Denborough, 1973), is associated with MH susceptibility. Affected individuals have proximal muscle weakness, postural imbalances, cryptorchidism, webbed neck, pectus deformities, delayed development, and elevated levels of CK (Jurkatt-Rott et al., 2000).

In the past, other disorders in which patients appeared to have MH susceptibility included myotonia congenita, osteogenesis imperfecta (Rampton et al., 1984), Schwartz-Jampel syndrome (dwarfism, craniofacial and skeletal abnormalities, blepharophimosis, and muscle stiffness), and possibly arthrogryposis (Fowler et al., 1974; Baines et al., 1986). These syndromes may be associated with many of the symptoms of MH, but these symptoms are not specific for MH. Many patients with these and other muscular disorders have received inhalation anesthetics without complications. For example, a pyloromyotomy was performed in an infant with paramyotonia congenita during sevoflurane anesthesia (Ay et al., 2004). Sometimes evaluation of suspect cases has found CHCT to be negative (Hopkins et al., 1991).

The neurolept malignant syndrome (NMS) (Guzé, 1985; Cohen et al., 1985; Mann et al., 2003) is a disorder recognized by psychiatrists that may clinically resemble MH. It occurs in one of 200 patients taking neuroleptic drugs that produce dopaminergic blockade. Most of the patients are young men with schizophrenia or mania treated with the potent piperazine phenothiazines or haloperidol, but more than 25 drugs have been implicated (Heiman-Patterson, 1993). NMS may also occur when the administration of antiparkinsonian drugs is stopped. NMS may be fatal. Its manifestations are hypermetabolism with fever, tachycardia, muscle rigidity, and myoglobinuria. NMS has all the clinical features of MH, including acute renal failure and multiorgan failure, but it progresses over hours to days rather than minutes.

The inciting events of NMS are not the same as those for MH. There are several reasons that blockade of dopamine receptors can produce hyperthermia and rigidity (Heiman-Patterson, 1993). Dantrolene has been used successfully for treatment of this syndrome (Granati et al., 1983), as has bromocriptine, a dopamine agonist (Caroff, 1980). The results of CHCT in patients with a history of NMS have been inconsistent (Caroff et al., 1987; Adnet et al., 1989). Drugs that are known triggers of MH have been well tolerated in patients who have had NMS. However, repeated exposure of MHS pigs to a serotonin-2 receptor agonist can induce typical MH symptoms, without causing the same syndrome in normal animals (Gerbershagen et al., 2003). This suggests that serotonin syndrome (tremor, diaphoresis, shivering, and myoclonus in the presence of serotoninergic medication) could be elicited more easily in MHS individuals (Mann et al., 2003). Dantrolene can delay serotonin-induced contractures (Wappler et al., 1997).

■ CONTRACTURE TEST

The CHCT is the best laboratory test available to investigate susceptibility to MH. The methods for performance of the test have been standardized in North America (Larach et al., 1989). However, the European protocol differs from that in North America. Both tests provide consistent normal population values for comparison with diagnostic biopsies. In both North America and Europe, the CHCT is a concentration-response curve to caffeine alone, halothane alone, or their combination. Unlike usual concentration-response phenomena, differences between MHS and normal persons do not appear as altered ED_{50} or as a change in slope, but as a change in threshold. That is, when does a contracture begin to develop? At least three muscle strips are examined under each test condition (Larach, 1989). These must be about the same weight, length, and thickness and start with equivalent baseline tension. Shorter muscle bundles deteriorate more rapidly due to the current of injury from the cut muscle end, and thicker bundles yield greater contractures. The upper limit of a normal contracture response is somewhat arbitrary. A muscle strip must respond with an active twitch to electrical stimulation; that is, it must be viable. The test should be completed within 5 hours of the excision of muscle from the patient's thigh. There are slight differences in European and North American protocols, which account for differences in threshold (Ording and Bendixen, 1992).

The European protocol defines a positive caffeine contracture test as tension greater than 0.2*g* in the presence of 2 mmol/L caffeine or less. In this test, caffeine is added incrementally to concentrations of 0.5, 1, 1.5, 2, 3, 4, and 32 mmol/L to the bath surrounding the muscle strip. A positive halothane contracture test is the development of greater than 0.2*g* tension in the presence of 0.5%, 1.0%, or 2.0% halothane. In this test, muscle that has not been exposed to caffeine is bathed with Krebs' medium in which halothane concentrations have been verified. The combination of caffeine and halothane is not part of the European protocol. If one of the several strips tested has a positive response to caffeine and another strip has a positive response to halothane, the patient is considered MHS. If one muscle strip reacts to only one agent, the patient is MH equivocal by European standards.

The North American protocol includes exposure of muscle strips to 0.5, 1, 2, 4, 8, and 32 mmol/L caffeine. A positive caffeine contracture test is often defined as an increase in tension of 0.2*g* in the presence of 2 mmol/L caffeine or less. However, a cutoff of 0.3*g* or 0.4*g* may be preferred to increase the specificity of the test (Larach, 1989). The caffeine-specific concentration (CSC) is the mmol/L concentration of caffeine at which a 1*g* increase in tension occurs. A CSC of less than 4 mmol/L is considered a positive response. A positive halothane contracture test is the development of more than 0.2*g* to 0.7*g* tension (depending on the controls in that laboratory) in the presence of 3% halothane (Larach et al., 1989). In the United States, if one muscle strip produces a positive reaction in either caffeine or halothane, the patient is said to be MHS.

The joint halothane-caffeine assay is an optional test that is not performed by all laboratories. To perform this test, muscle strips are exposed to 1% halothane for 10 to 15 minutes; then caffeine is added incrementally to the bath to a maximum concentration of 32 mmol/L. Normal muscle is expected to produce 1*g* of tension at greater than 1 mmol/L caffeine. The results of this test may be reported in terms of the halothane-caffeine specific concentration, or the concentration of caffeine, in the presence of halothane, at which greater than 1*g* of tension is produced.

Some patients whose muscle reacts normally to both caffeine and halothane alone may have an abnormally low halothane-caffeine specific concentration. This reaction is referred to as a type K response, using the initial of Kalow, who proposed that this response may indicate an intermediate genotype (Kalow et al., 1979).

The significance of the type K response is controversial. About 20% of normal subjects exhibit a type K response; such individuals may respond normally to the clinical use of halothane and succinylcholine. There are some reports of MHS patients who had relatives whose muscle tested as type K. A similar phenomenon has been noted in the porcine model of MH.

Other laboratory tests have been evaluated for their diagnostic usefulness in MH; these include calcium uptake into frozen muscle, skinned fiber testing, platelet nucleotide depletion measurement, and the measurement of abnormal proteins in MH muscle. None of these is generally accepted, because none has been shown to reproduce the results of the in vitro muscle contracture tests (Lee et al., 1985; Britt and Scott, 1986; Whistler et al., 1986; Nagarjan et al., 1987). Several of the proposed tests produced inconsistent results (Ording et al., 1990; Quinlan et al., 1990).

Attempts have been made to develop relatively less invasive tests of MH susceptibility. The ryanodine receptor expressed on B-lymphocytes responds abnormally to agonists in the presence of mutations causative of MH (Girard et al., 2001; Sei et al., 2002; Kraev et al., 2003; Loke et al., 2003). Cultured human muscle from MHS patients also has greater increases in intracellular calcium with exposure to halothane than does normal muscle (Girard et al., 2002). Microdialysis of caffeine or halothane into muscle in vivo is being examined (Anetseder et al., 2002; Bina et al., 2003; Textor et al., 2002). Abnormal force of contracture and abnormal rate of increase of force have been demonstrated in MHS pigs (Quinlan et al., 1986). Studies of mechanical and electrical responses to repetitive nerve stimulation have been performed (Balog et al., 2000; Hoyer et al., 2001, 2002). A noninvasive in vivo test for MH susceptibility has been developed using phosphorus magnetic resonance spectroscopy (^{31}P NMR) (Olgin et al., 1988). This test is not specific for MH; it will yield a positive result, an elevated ratio of inorganic phosphate to phosphocreatine, in patients with mitochondrial myopathies (Argov et al., 1987a), muscular and myotonic dystrophies (Younkin et al., 1987), metabolic myopathies associated with secondary atrophy (Argov et al., 1987b), polymyositis, hypothyroid myopathy (Argov et al., 1987c), advanced denervating muscle disorders (Zochodne et al., 1986), and muscle injury (McCully et al., 1987). Although ^{31}P NMR is unlikely to be specific for MH, it could be useful as a screening test. An individual with a questionable clinical history could be evaluated by ^{31}P NMR. If abnormal results were obtained, muscle biopsy and follow-up with a neurologist would definitely be indicated.

MH is a disorder of muscle that is subclinical until the muscle is stressed. Tests discern MH susceptibility only if they impose a stress on the intact tissue or organism or detect a genetic difference that has been demonstrated to be causative (Urwyler et al., 2003). MH muscle testing is generally designed to avoid false-negative diagnoses; hence, there may be false-positive results of the CHCT. Findings suggest that, as with all tests, there are some rare false-negative contracture test results (Larach, 1993). However, overall, MH contracture testing appears accurate, and patients with negative findings on CHCT can receive safe anesthetics with drugs that could trigger MH (Ording et al., 1991). Failure to detect an *RYR1* mutation does *not* imply that the patient is *not* MHS. If a patient undergoes genetic evaluation prior to contracture testing and no MH causative mutation is found, the patient must undergo contracture testing in order to support the diagnosis of *not* MHS. All patients should be monitored for signs of MH responses during anesthesia. It is possible that under certain conditions, an MH response to anesthesia may be acquired. Furthermore, MH can occur without the use of triggering drugs such as succinylcholine and potent inhalation anesthetics (Fitzgibbons, 1980; Pollock et al., 1992).

■ ANESTHESIOLOGISTS' RESPONSIBILITY TO OTHER PHYSICIANS

MH has been known for more than 40 years, yet many primary care physicians, dentists, and surgeons still are unaware of its life-and-death significance. Malignant Hyperthermia Association of the United States published a letter from a parent:

> Your information will be most helpful for my married out-of-state, pregnant daughter—who tried to explain that MH existed in our family… . They told her nobody could be allergic to anesthetics, which was the same thing I was told 22 years ago when my son's tonsils were removed. We had lost many relatives to ether for minor surgery over the years. Trying to explain MH in places that don't have large amounts of it is difficult. Some won't listen … .—Anonymous, 1986

Physicians who are aware of the potential seriousness of MH may ask what the implications of the diagnosis of MH susceptibility are for the patient's daily life. MH susceptibility has been associated with fourfold increases in plasma catecholamines with graded exercise (Wappler et al., 2000) and rapid exhaustion after intense exercise (Rueffert et al., 2004). However, MHS individuals have performed farm labor in the hot sun without precipitating an MH attack. Early studies of metabolic responses during noncompetitive, low-intensity, steady-state exercise found no difference between control and MHS patients (Green et al., 1987). Slower recovery of muscle pH and phosphocreatine/inorganic phosphate ratios have been observed in MHS patients (Allsop et al., 1991, Olgin et al., 1991). MHS patients should be encouraged to refrain from strenuous exercise if they experience cramps or fever under such circumstances (Davis et al., 2002). Some patients with exertional heat stroke are MHS (Bendahan et al., 2001; Tobin, et al., 2001; Wappler et al., 2001). The psychoactive drug MDMA has been shown to trigger MH in susceptible swine (Fiege et al., 2003). Dantrolene may be therapeutic when these symptoms occur (Gronert, 1980).

Sudden death from undetermined cause may be part of the history of MHS families. In adults these sudden deaths may be due to arrhythmias. As of yet there are no published data regarding possible changes in muscle function with age in MHS patients, but it is noteworthy that in some MHS families the young adults are muscular and strong, whereas older adults may fatigue easily.

The North American Malignant Hyperthermia Registry, now at the University of Pittsburgh Medical Center in Pittsburgh, Pennsylvania (Dr. Barbara W. Brandom, Director), collects data from practitioners and testing centers in Canada and the United States. This registry provides a database by which to define clinical MH and to study aspects of its presentation, treatment, and diagnostic methods. Because MH is a rare event, it is necessary to collect clinical reports from a large geographic area over an extended period of time to improve understanding of the clinical problem. Because MH is rare, all practitioners should have a responsibility to report such cases or suspected cases to the registry.

■ SUMMARY

MH is a potentially lethal pharmacogenetic syndrome. It has been of particular concern to pediatric anesthesiologists because succinylcholine and halothane are potent triggers of MH and have been popular drugs in the practice of pediatric anesthesia. With the advent of improved monitoring techniques and universal availability of intravenous dantrolene, mortality from MH has plummeted. However, the definitive diagnosis of MH is still not simple or easy. It falls to anesthesiologists to choose anesthetic agents and adjuvants that maximize the safety of the patient, to identify as potentially MHS those individuals who experience adverse reactions consistent with MH, and to counsel and refer those individuals and families to appropriate diagnostic centers. Anesthesiologists must also make fellow physicians and other health care providers aware of the existence and the seriousness of MH and of its effective treatment and prevention. When capnography, blood gas analysis, temperature monitoring, and dantrolene are available, patients with a history of MH susceptibility may safely receive routine anesthetic care with nontriggering anesthetics.

Acknowledgments

We would like to acknowledge the extensive contributions of Joan Carroll, Henry Rosenberg, and Gerald Gronert to previous editions of this chapter and the editorial contribution of Philip Morgan to the current chapter.

REFERENCES

Adnet PJ, Krivosic-Horber RM, Adamantidis MM, et al.: The association between neuroleptic malignant syndrome and malignant hyperthermia. *Acta Anaesth Scand* 33:676, 1989.

Allen GC, Cattran CB, Peterson RG, et al.: Plasma levels of dantrolene following oral administration in malignant hyperthermia-susceptible patients. *Anesthesiology* 69:900, 1988.

Allen GC, Larach MG, Kunselman AR: The sensitivity and specificity of the caffeine-halothane contracture test: A report from the North American Malignant Hyperthermia Registry. *Anesthesiology* 88:579, 1998.

Allen GC, Rosenberg H: Phaeochromocytoma presenting as acute malignant hyperthermia—A diagnostic challenge. *Can J Anaesth* 37:593, 1990.

Allsop P, Jorfeldt L, Rutberg H, et al.: Delayed recovery of muscle pH after short duration, high intensity exercise in malignant hyperthermia susceptible subjects. *Br J Anaesth* 66:541, 1991.

Anetseder M, Hager M, Muller CR, et al.: Diagnosis of susceptibility to malignant hyperthermia by use of a metabolic test. *Lancet* 359:1579, 2002.

Argov Z, Bank WJ, Maris J, et al.: Bioenergetic heterogeneity of human mitochondrial myopathies as demonstrated by in vivo phosphorus magnetic resonance spectroscopy. *Neurology* 37:257, 1987a.

Argov Z, Bank WJ, Maris J, et al.: Muscle energy metabolism in McArdle's syndrome by in vivo phosphorus magnetic resonance spectroscopy (31P NMR). *Neurology* 37:1720, 1987b.

Argov Z, Renshaw P, Bank WJ: Abnormal oxidative metabolism of hypothyroid muscle: In vivo 31P NMR of humans and rats. *Neurology* 36(suppl 1): 138, 1987c.

Ay B, Gercek A, Dogan VI, et al.: Pyloromyotomy in a patient with paramyotonia congenital. *Anesth Analg* 98:68, 2004.

Bachand M, Vachon N, Boisvert M, et al.: Clinical reassessment of malignant hyperthermia in Abitibi-Temiscamingue. *Can J Anaesth* 44:685, 1997.

Baines DB, Douglas ID, Overton JH: Anaesthesia for patients with arthrogryposis multiplex congenita: What is the risk of malignant hyperthermia? *Anaesth Intensive Care* 14:370, 1986.

Balog EM, Enzmann NR, Gallant EM: Malignant hyperthermia: Fatigue characteristics of skeletal muscle. *Muscle Nerve* 23:223, 2000.

Bendahan D, Kozak-Ribbens G, Confort-Gouny S, et al.: A noninvasive investigation of muscle energetics supports similarities between exertional heat stroke and malignant hyperthermia. *Anesth Analg* 93:683, 2001.

Bendahan D, Mattei JP, Kozak-Ribbens G, et al.: Non invasive investigation of muscle diseases using 31P magnetic resonance spectroscopy: Potential in clinical applications. *Rev Neurol (Paris)* 158:527, 2002.

Berkowitz A, Rosenberg H: Femoral block with mepivacaine for muscle biopsy in malignant hyperthermia patients. *Anesthesiology* 62:651, 1985.

Bina S, Cowan G, Muldoon S, et al.: Diagnosis of susceptibility to malignant hyperthermia using microdialysis technique. *Anesthesiology* 99:A97, 2003.

Bouchama A, Knochel JP: Heat stroke. *N Engl J Med* 346; 1978, 2002.

Britt BA, Endrenyi L, Peters PL, et al.: Screening of malignant hyperthermia susceptible families by creatine phosphokinase measurement and other clinical investigations. *Can Anaesth Soc J* 23:263, 1976.

Britt BA, Kalow W: Malignant hyperthermia: A statistical review. *Can Anaesth Soc J* 17:293, 1970.

Britt BA, Scott EA: Failure of the platelet-halothane nucleotide depletion test as a diagnostic or screening test for malignant hyperthermia. *Anesth Analg* 65:171, 1986.

Brown RL, Pollock AN, Couchman KG, et al.: A novel ryanodine receptor mutation and genotype-phenotype correlation in a large malignant hyperthermia New Zealand Maori pedigree. *Hum Mol Genet* 9:1515, 2000.

Burford GE: Hyperthermia following anesthesia: Consideration of control of body temperature during anesthesia. *Anesthesiology* 1:208, 1940.

Byrne E, Blumbergs PC, Hallpike JF: Central core disease: Study of a family with five affected generations. *J Neurol Sci* 53:77, 1982.

Caroff SN: The neuroleptic malignant syndrome. *J Clin Psychiatry* 41: 79, 1980.

Caroff SN, Rosenberg H, Fletcher JE, et al.: Malignant hyperthermia susceptibility in neuroleptic malignant syndrome. *Anesthesiology* 67:20, 1987.

Censier K, Urwyler A, Zorzato F, et al.: Intracellular calcium homeostasis in human primary muscle cells from malignant hyperthermia susceptible and normal individuals. Effect of overexpression of recombinant wild-type and Arg163Cys mutated ryanodine receptors. *J Clin Invest* 101:1233, 1998.

Chance B, Clark BJ, Nioka S, et al.: Phosphorus nuclear magnetic resonance spectroscopy in vivo. *Circulation* 72:103, 1985a.

Chance B, Leigh JS, Clark BJ, et al.: Control of oxidative metabolism and oxygen delivery in human skeletal muscle: a steady-state analysis of the work/energy cost transfer function. *Proc Natl Acad Sci USA* 82:8384, 1985b.

Cohen BM, Baldessamini RJ, Pope HG, et al.: Neuroleptic malignant syndrome. *N Engl J Med* 313:1293, 1985.

Cook JD, Henderson-Tilton AC: Malignant hyperthermic reaction to nifedipine in a child with Schwartz-Jampel syndrome. *Ann Neurol* 18:402, 1985.

Davis M, Brown R, Dickson A, et al.: Malignant hyperthermia associated with exercise-induced rhabdomyolysis or congenital abnormalities and a novel RYR1 mutation in New Zealand and Australian pedigrees. *Br J Anaesth* 88:508, 2002.

Delphin E, Jackson D, Rothstein P: Use of succinylcholine during elective pediatric anesthesia should be re-evaluated. *Anesth Analg* 66:1190, 1987.

Denborough MA, Forster FA, Lovell RRH, et al.: Anaesthetic deaths in a family. *Br J Anaesth* 34:395, 1962.

Denborough MA, Lovell RRH: Anaesthetic deaths in a family. *Lancet* 2: 45, 1960.

Deufel T, Golla A, Iles D, et al.: Evidence for genetic heterogeneity of malignant hyperthermia susceptibility. *Am J Hum Genet* 50:1151, 1992.

Ellis FR, Clarke MC, Modgill M, et al.: Evaluation of creatine phosphokinase in screening patients for malignant hyperthermia. *Br Med J* 3:511, 1975.

Ellis FR, Halsall PJ: Malignant hyperpyrexia. *Br J Hosp Med* 24:318–321, 323, 325 327, 1980.

Ellis FR, Halsall PJ, Christian AS: Clinical presentation of suspected malignant hyperthermia during anesthesia in 402 probands. *Anaesthesia* 45:838, 1990.

European Malignant Hyperpyrexia Group: A protocol for the investigation of malignant hyperpyrexia group. *Br J Anaesth* 56:1267, 1984.

Fiege M, Wappler M, Weisshorn R, et al.: Induction of malignant hyperthermia in susceptible swine by 3,4-methylenedioxymethamphetamine ("ecstasy"). *Anesthesiology* 99:1132, 2003.

Fitzgibbons DC: Malignant hyperthermia following preoperative oral administration of dantrolene. *Anesthesiology* 54:73, 1980.

Fletcher JE, Rosenberg H: In vitro interaction between halothane and succinylcholine in human skeletal muscle: Implications for malignant hyperthermia and masseter muscle rigidity. *Anesthesiology* 63:190, 1985.

Fletcher JE, Rosenberg H, Aggarwal M: Comparison of European and North American malignant hyperthermia diagnostic protocol outcomes for use in genetic studies. *Anesthesiology* 90:654, 1999.

Flewellen EH, Nelson TE, Jones WP, et al.: Dantrolene dose response in awake man: Implications for management of malignant hyperthermia. *Anesthesiology* 59:275, 1983.

Florence JM, Fox PT, Planer J, and Brooke MH: Activity, creatine kinase, and myoglobin in Duchenne muscular dystrophy: A clue to etiology? *Neurology* 35:758, 1985.

Fowler WM, Fayzer RB, Taylor RG, et al.: The Schwartz-Jampel syndrome: Its clinical, physiological and histologic expressions. *J Neurol Sci* 22:127, 1974.

Franzini-Armstrong C, Protasi F: Ryanodine receptors of striated muscles: A complex channel capable of multiple interactions. *Physiol Rev* 77:699, 1997.

Fruen BR, Mickelson JR, Louis CF: Dantrolene inhibition of sarcoplasmic reticulum Ca^{2+} release by direct and specific action at skeletal muscle ryanodine receptors. *J Biol Chem* 272:26965, 1997.

Fuji J, Otsu K, Zorzato F, et al.: Identification of a point mutation in porcine ryanodine receptor associated with malignant hyperthermia. *Science* 253:448, 1991.

Gallant EM, Foldes FF, Rempel WE, et al.: Verapamil is not a therapeutic adjunct to dantrolene in porcine MH. *Anesth Analg* 64:601, 1985.

Gallant EM, Lentz LR: Excitation-contraction coupling in pigs heterozygous for malignant hyperthermia. *Am J Physiol* 262:C422, 1992.

Gerbershagen MU, Wappler F, Fiege M, et al.: Effects of a 5HT(2) receptor agonist on anesthetized pigs susceptible to malignant hyperthermia. *Br J Anaesth* 91:281, 2003.

Gillard EF, Otsu K, Fujii J, et al.: A substitution of cysteine for arginine 614 in the ryanodine receptor is potentially causative of human malignant hyperthermia. *Genomics* 11:751, 1991.

Girard T, Cavagna D, Padovan E, et al.: B-lymphocytes from malignant hyperthermia-susceptible patients have an increased sensitivity to skeletal muscle ryanodine receptor activators. *J Biol Chem* 21:276, 2001.

Girard T, Treves S, Censier K, et al.: Phenotyping malignant hyperthermia susceptibility by measuring halothane induced changes in myoplasmic calcium concentration in cultured human skeletal muscle cells. *Br J Anaesth* 89:571, 2002.

Girard T, Treves S, Voronkov E, et al.: Molecular genetic testing for malignant hyperthermia susceptibility. *Anesthesiology* 100:1076, 2004.

Granati JE, Stern BJ, Ringel A: Neuroleptic malignant syndrome: successful treatment with dantrolene and bromocriptine. *Ann Neurol* 14:89, 1983.

Green JH, Ellis FR, Halsall PJ, et al.: Thermoregulation, plasma catecholamine and metabolite levels during submaximal work in individuals susceptible to malignant hyperthermia. *Acta Anaesthesiol Scand* 31:122, 1987.

Gronert GA: Malignant hyperthermia. *Anesthesiology* 53:395, 1980.

Gronert GA: Malignant hyperthermia. Treatment of acute episodes. In Banker BQ, Engel AG, editors: *Myology: Basic and clinical,* vol 2. New York, 1986, McGraw-Hill Book Co., p 1775.

Gronert GA, Ahern CP, Milde JH, et al.: Effect of CO_2, calcium, digoxin, and potassium on cardiac and skeletal muscle metabolism in malignant hyperthermia susceptible swine. *Anesthesiology* 64:24, 1986.

Gronert GA, Fowler W, Cardinet GH, et al.: Absence of malignant hyperthermia contractures in Becker-Duchenne dystrophy at age 2. *Muscle Nerve* 15:52, 1992.

Gronert GA, Theye RA: Halothane-induced porcine malignant hyperthermia: Metabolic and hemodynamic changes. *Anesthesiology* 44:36, 1976a.

Gronert GA, Theye RA: Suxamethonium-induced porcine malignant hyperthermia. *Br J Anaesth* 48:513, 1976b.

Gronert GA, Thompson RL, Onofrio BM: Human malignant hyperthermia: Awake episodes and correction by dantrolene. *Anesth Analg* 59:377, 1980.

Grossman RA, Hamilton RW, Morse BM, et al.: Nontraumatic rhabdomyolysis and acute renal failure. *N Engl J Med* 291:807, 1974.

Guzé BH, Baxter LR: Neuroleptic malignant syndrome. *N Engl J Med* 313: 163, 1985.

Hackl W, Mauritz W, Schemper M, et al.: Prediction of malignant hyperthermia susceptibility: statistical evaluation of clinical signs. *Br J Anaesth* 64: 425, 1990.

Hannallah RS, Kaplan RF: Jaw relaxation after a halothane/succinylcholine sequence in children. *Anesthesiology* 81:99, 1994.

Harrington JF, Ford DJ: Myoglobinemia after succinylcholine in children undergoing isoflurane anesthesia. *Anesth Analg* 65:569, 1986.

Harrison GG: Propofol in malignant hyperthermia. *Lancet* 337:503, 1991.

Harrison GG, Isaacs H: Malignant hyperthermia: an historical vignette. *Anaesthesia* 47:54, 1992.

Heiman-Patterson TD: Neuroleptic malignant syndrome and malignant hyperthermia. *Med Clin North Am* 77:477, 1993.

Heiman-Patterson TD, Natter HM, Rosenberg HR, et al.: Malignant hyperthermia susceptibility in X-linked muscle dystrophies. *Pediatr Neurosci* 2:356, 1986.

Heytens L, Martin JJ, Van de Kleft E, et al.: In vitro contracture tests in patients with various neuromuscular diseases. *Br J Anaesth* 68:72, 1992.

Hopkins PM, Ellis FR, Halsall PJ: Hypermetabolism in arthrogryposis multiplex congenital. *Anaesthesia* 46:374, 1991.

Hoyer A, Veeser M, Albrecht Y, et al.: Relaxation times of malignant hyperthermia-susceptible human muscles (MHS) and non-susceptible human muscles (MHN) differ distinctly under the influence of repetitive stimulation in vivo. *Anesthesiology* A-1025, 2001.

Hoyer A, Veeser M, Schaupp F, et al.: The initially higher contraction velocity of malignant hyperthermia (MH)-susceptible human muscles (MHS) decreases earlier and more distinctly under the influence of repetitive stimulation (RS) than in non-susceptibles (MHN). *Anesthesiology* A-1014, 2002.

Illias WK, Williams CH, Fulfer RT, et al.: Diltiazem inhibits halothane-induced contractions in malignant hyperthermia-susceptible muscles in vitro. *Br J Anaesth* 57:994, 1985.

Inness RKR, Stromme JH: Rise in serum creatine phosphokinase associated with agents used in anaesthesia. *Br J Anaesth* 45:185, 1973.

Jurkat-Rott K, McCarthy T, Lehmann-Horn F: Genetics and pathogenesis of malignant hyperthermia. *Muscle Nerve* 23:4, 2000.

Kalow W, Britt BA, Chan FY: Epidemiology and inheritance of malignant hyperthermia. In Britt BA, editor: Malignant hyperthermia. *Int Anesthesiol Clin* 17:119, 1979.

Kaplan RF, Iaizzo P, Van der Spek AFL, et al.: Management of incomplete jaw relaxation after succinylcholine-responses from MH hotline consultants (abstract). *Anesthesiology* 79:A919, 1993.

Kaplan RF, Rushing E: Isolated masseter muscle spasm and increased creatine kinase without malignant hyperthermia susceptibility or other myopathies. *Anesthesiology* 77:820, 1992.

Karan SM, Crowl F, and Muldoon SM: Malignant hyperthermia masked by capnographic monitoring. *Anesth Analg* 78:590, 1994.

Kausch K, Grimm T, Janka M, et al.: Evidence for linkage of the central core disease locus to chromosome 19q. *J Neurol Sci* 98(suppl):549, 1990.

Kleopa KA, Rosenberg H, Heiman-Patterson T: Malignant hyperthermia-like episode in Becker Muscular Dystrophy. *Anesthesiology* 93:1535, 2000.

King JO, Denborough MA: Anesthetic-induced malignant hyperthermia in children. *J Pediatr* 83:37, 1973.

Kraev N, Loke JC, Kraev A, MacLennan DH: Protocol for the sequence analysis of ryanodine receptor subtype 1 gene transcripts from human leukocytes. *Anesthesiology* 99:289, 2003.

Lanier WL, Iaizzo PA, Milde JH: The effects of intravenous succinylcholine on cerebral function and muscle afferent activity following complete ischemia in halothane-anesthetized dogs. *Anesthesiology* 73:465, 1990.

Larach MG: Should we use muscle biopsy to diagnose malignant hyperthermia susceptibility? *Anesthesiology* 79:1, 1993.

Larach MG, for the North American Malignant Hyperthermia Group: Standardization of the caffeine halothane muscle contracture test. *Anesth Analg* 69:511, 1989.

Larach MG, Landis JR, Bunn JS, et al.: The North American Malignant Hyperthermia Registry: prediction of malignant hyperthermia susceptibility in low-risk subjects. *Anesthesiology* 76:16, 1992.

Larach MG, Localio AR, Allen GC, et al.: A clinical grading scale to predict malignant hyperthermia susceptibility. *Anesthesiology* 80:771, 1994.

Larach MG, MacLennan DH: How carefully can we phenotype patients suspected of malignant hyperthermia susceptibility? *Anesthesiology* 90: 645, 1999.

Larach MG, Rosenberg H, Gronert GA, et al.: Did anesthetics trigger cardiac arrests in patients with occult myopathy? *Anesthesiology* 94:933, 2001.

Larach MG, Rosenberg H, Gronert GA, et al.: Hyperkalemic cardiac arrest during anesthesia in infants and children with occult myopathies. *Clin Pediatr* 36:9, 1997.

Larach MG, Rosenberg H, Larach DR, et al.: Prediction of malignant hyperthermia susceptibility by clinical signs. *Anesthesiology* 66:547, 1987.

Lee MB, Adragna MG, Edwards L: Use of a platelet nucleotide assay as a possible diagnostic test for malignant hyperthermia. *Anesthesiology* 63: 311, 1985.

Lerman J, McLeod ME, Strong HA: Pharmacokinetics of intravenous dantrolene in children. *Anesthesiology* 70:625, 1989.

Levitt RC, Olckers A, Meyers S, et al.: Evidence for the localization of a malignant hyperthermia susceptibility locus (MHS2) to the human chromosome 17q. *Genomics* 14:562, 1992.

Lietman PS, Haslam RHA, Walcher JR: Pharmacology of dantrolene sodium in children. *Arch Phys Med Rehabil* 55:388, 1974.

Littleford JA, Patel LR, Bose D, et al.: Masseter muscle spasm in children: Implications of continuing the triggering anesthetic. *Anesth Analg* 72:151, 1991.

Loke J, MacLennan DH: Bayesian modeling of muscle biopsy contracture testing for malignant hyperthermia susceptibility. *Anesthesiology* 88:589, 1998.

Loke J, MacLennan DH: Malignant hyperthermia and central core disease: Disorders of Ca^{2+} release channels. *Am J Med* 104:470, 1998.

Loke JC, Kraev N, Sharma P, et al.: Detection of a novel ryanodine receptor subtype 1 mutation (R328W) in a malignant hyperthermia family by sequencing of a leukocyte transcript. *Anesthesiology* 99:297, 2003.

Lopez JR, Alamo L, Caputo C, et al.: Intracellular ionized calcium concentrations in muscles from humans with malignant hyperthermia. *Muscle Nerve* 8:355, 1985.

Lynch C, Durbin CG, Fisher NA, et al.: Effects of dantrolene and verapamil on atrioventricular conduction and cardiovascular performance in dogs. *Anesth Analg* 65:252, 1986.

MacLennan DH, Otsu K, Fujii J, et al.: The role of the skeletal muscle ryanodine receptor gene in malignant hyperthermia. *Symp Soc Exp Biol* 46: 189, 1992.

Mann SC, Caroff SN, Keck PE, et al.: *Neuroleptic malignant syndrome and related conditions.* 2nd ed. Washington, DC, 2003, American Psychiatric Publishing, Inc.

Marohn ML, Nagia AH: Masseter muscle rigidity after rapid-sequence induction of anesthesia. *Anesthesiology* 77:205, 1992.

McCully KK, Argov Z, Boden B, et al.: Detection of muscle injury in humans with 31P magnetic resonance spectroscopy. *Muscle Nerve* 1:62, 1987.

McGraw TT, Keon TP: Malignant hyperthermia and the clean machine. *Can Anaesth J* 36:530, 1989.

Melzer W, Dietze B: Malignant hyperthermia and excitation-contraction coupling. *Acta Physiol Scand* 171:367, 2001.

Mickelson JR, Louis CF: Malignant hyperthermia: excitation-contraction coupling, Ca^{2+} release channel, and cell Ca^{2+} regulation defects. *Physiol Rev* 76:537, 1996.

Mitchell LW, Leighton BL: Warmed diluent speeds dantrolene reconstitution. *Can J Anaesth* 50:127, 2003.

Moschcowitz AV: Postoperative heat stroke. *Surg Gynecol Obstet* 28:443, 1916.

Moulds RFW, Denborough MA: Biochemical basis of malignant hyperpyrexia. *Br Med J* 2:241, 1974.

Nagarjan K, Fishbein WN, Muldoon SM, et al.: Calcium uptake in frozen muscle biopsy sections compared with other predictors of malignant hyperthermia susceptibility. *Anesthesiology* 66:680, 1987.

Nelson TE, Rosenberg H, Muldoon S: Genetic testing for malignant hyperthermia in North America. *Anesthesiology* 100:212, 2004.

Nigrovic V, McCullough LS, Wajskol A, et al.: Succinylcholine-induced increases in plasma catecholamine levels in humans. *Anesth Analg* 62: 627, 1983.

O'Flynn R, Shutack J, Rosenberg H, et al.: Masseter muscle rigidity and malignant hyperthermia susceptibility in pediatric patients: An update on management and diagnosis. *Anesthesiology* 80:1228, 1994.
Okumura F, Cracker BD, Denborough MA: Identification of susceptibility to malignant hyperthermia in swine. *Br J Anaesth* 51:171, 1979.
Olckers A, Meyers DA, Meyers S, et al.: Adult muscle sodium channel a-subunit is a gene candidate for malignant hyperthermia susceptibility. *Genomics* 14:829, 1992.
Olgin J, Argov Z, Rosenberg H, et al.: Non-invasive evaluation of malignant hyperthermia susceptibility with phosphorus nuclear magnetic resonance spectroscopy. *Anesthesiology* 68:507, 1988.
Olgin J, Rosenberg H, Gregory A, et al.: A blinded comparison of non-invasive, in vivo phosphorus nuclear magnetic resonance spectroscopy and the in vitro halothane/caffeine contracture test in the evaluation of malignant hyperthermia susceptibility. *Anesthesiology* 72:36, 1991.
Ording H: Incidence of malignant hyperthermia in Denmark. *Anesth Analg* 64:700, 1985.
Ording H, Bendixen D: Sources of variability in halothane and caffeine contracture tests for susceptibility to malignant hyperthermia. *Eur J Anaesthesiol* 9:367, 1992.
Ording H, Brancadoro V, Cozzolino S, et al.: In vitro contracture test for diagnosis of malignant hyperthermia following the protocol of the European MH Group: Results of testing patients surviving fulminant MH and unrelated low-risk subjects. *Acta Anaesthesiol Scand* 41:955, 1997.
Ording H, Foder B, Scharff O: Cytosolic free calcium concentrations in lymphocytes from malignant hyperthermia susceptible patients. *Br J Anaesth* 64:341, 1990.
Ording H, Hedegran AM, Skovgaard LT: Evaluation of 119 anaesthetics received after investigation for susceptibility to malignant hyperthermia. *Acta Anaesthesiol Scand* 35:711, 1991.
Ording H, Ranklev E, Fletcher R: Investigation of malignant hyperthermia in Denmark and Sweden. *Br J Anaesth* 56:1183, 1984.
Paasuke RT, Brownell AKW: Serum creatine kinase level as a screening test for susceptibility to malignant hyperthermia. *JAMA* 255:769, 1986.
Peluso A, Bianchini A: Malignant hyperthermia susceptibility in patients with Duchenne's muscular dystrophy. *Can J Anaesth* 39:1117, 1992.
Plotz J, Braun J: Failure of "self-taming" doses of succinylcholine to inhibit increases in post-operative serum creatine kinase activity in children. *Anesthesiology* 56:207, 1982.
Plumley MH, Bevan JC, Saddler JM, et al.: Dose-related effects of succinylcholine on the adductor pollicis and masseter muscles in children. *Can J Anaesth* 37:15, 1990.
Pollock N, Hodges M, Sendall J: Prolonged malignant hyperthermia in the absence of triggering agents. *Anaesth Intensive Care* 20:520, 1992.
Pollock N, Langtont E, Stowell K, et al.: Safe duration of postoperative monitoring for malignant hyperthermia susceptible patients. *Ansesth Intensive Care* 32:502, 2004.
Pryn SJ, van der Spek AF: Comparative pharmacology of succinylcholine on jaw, eye, and tibialis muscle (abstract). *Anesthesiology* 73:A859, 1990.
Quinlan JG, Iaizzo PA, Gronert GA, et al.: Use of dantrolene plus multiple pulses to detect stress-susceptible porcine muscles. *J Appl Physiol* 60:1313, 1986.
Quinlan JG, Wedel DJ, Iaizzo PA: Multiple-pulse stimulation and dantrolene in malignant hyperthermia. *Muscle Nerve* 13:904, 1990.
Raff M, Harrison GG: The screening of propofol in MHS swine. *Anesth Analg* 68:750, 1989.
Rampton AJ, Kelly DA, Shanahan EC, et al.: Occurrence of malignant hyperpyrexia in a patient with osteogenesis imperfecta. *Br J Anaesth* 56:1443, 1984.
Ritchie PA, Cheshire MA, Pearce NH: Decontamination of halothane from anaesthesia machines achieved by continuous flushing with oxygen. *Br J Anaesth* 60:859, 1988.
Robinson RL, Anetseder MJ, Brancadoro V, et al.: Recent advances in the diagnosis of malignant hyperthermia susceptibility: How confident can we be of genetic testing? *Eur J Hum Genet* 11:342, 2003.
Rosenberg H: Trismus is not trivial (editorial). *Anesthesiology* 67:453, 1987.
Rosenberg H, Fletcher JE: Masseter muscle rigidity and malignant hyperthermia susceptibility. *Anesth Analg* 65:161, 1986.
Rosenberg H, Gronert GA: Intractable cardiac arrest in children given succinylcholine. *Anesthesiology* 77:1054, 1992.
Rosner B: *Fundamentals of biostatistics*. 3rd ed. Boston, 1990, PWS Kent Publishing Co.
Rubiano R, Chang JL, Carroll J, et al.: Acute rhabdomyolysis following halothane anesthesia without succinylcholine. *Anesthesiology* 67:856, 1987.
Rubin AS, Zablocki AD: Hyperkalemia, verapamil, and dantrolene. *Anesthesiology* 66:246, 1987.
Rueffert H, Olthoff D, Deutrich C: Spontaneous occurrence of the disposition to malignant hyperthermia. *Anesthesiology* 100:731–3, 2004.
Salluzzo RF: Rhabdomyolysis. In Rosen P, Barkin RM, editors: *Emergency medicine—Concepts and clinical practice*, vol 3. St. Louis, 1992, Mosby–Year Book, p 2237.
Sambuughin N, Holley H, Muldoon S, et al.: Screening of the entire ryanodine receptor type 1 coding region for sequence variants associated with malignant hyperthermia susceptibility in the North American population. *Anethesiology* 102:515, 2005.
Sambuughin N, Sei Y, Gallagher KL, et al.: North American malignant hyperthermia population screening of the ryanodine receptor gene and identification of novel mutations. *Anesthesiology* 95:594, 2001.
Schonell LH, Sims C, Bulsara M: Preparing a new generation of anaesthetic machine for patients susceptible to malignant hyperthermia. *Anaesth Intensive Care* 31:58, 2003.
Sei Y, Brandom BW, Bina S, et al.: Patients with malignant hyperthermia demonstrate an altered calcium control mechanism in B lymphocytes. *Anesthesiology* 97:1052, 2002.
Sei Y, Sambuughin N, Muldoon S: Malignant hyperthermia genetic testing in North America Working Group Meeting. *Anesthesiology* 100:464, 2004.
Shy GM, Magee KR: A new congenital non-progressive myopathy. *Brain* 79:610, 1956.
Storella RJ, Keykhah MM, Rosenberg H: Halothane and temperature interact to increase succinylcholine-induced jaw contracture in the rat. *Anesthesiology* 79:1261, 1993.
Tang TT, Oechler HW, Siker D, et al.: Anesthesia-induced rhabdomyolysis in infants with unsuspected Duchenne dystrophy. *Acta Paediatr* 81:716, 1992.
Textor Z, Beer M, Anetseder M, et al.: Caffeine impairs intramuscular energy balance in patients susceptible to malignant hyperthermia. *Muscle Nerve* 28:353, 2002.
Thompson MW: The genetic transmission of muscle diseases. In Engel AG, Franzini-Armstrong C, editors: *Myology, basic and clinical*, vol 1. New York, 1994, McGraw-Hill, p 1074.
Tilgen N, Zorzato F, Halliger-Keller B, et al.: Identification of four novel mutations in the C-terminal membrane spanning region of the ryanodine receptor 1: association with central core disease and alteration of calcium homeostasis. *Hum Mol Genet* 10:2879, 2001.
Tobin JR, Jason DR, Challa VR, et al.: Malignant hyperthermia and apparent heat stroke. *JAMA* 286:168, 2001.
Urwyler A, Duefel T, McCarthy T, West S: European Malignant Hyperthermia Group: Guidelines for molecular genetic detection of susceptibility to malignant hyperthermia. *Br J Anaesth* 86:283, 2001.
Urwyler A, Halsall PJ, Mueller C, Robinson R: Ryanodine receptor gene (RYR1) mutations for diagnosing susceptibility to malignant hyperthermia. *Acta Anaesth Scand* 47:492, 2003.
van der Spek AFL, Fang WB, Ashton-Miller JA, et al.: The effects of succinylcholine on mouth opening. *Anesthesiology* 67:459, 1987.
van der Spek AFL, Fang WB, Ashton-Miller JA, et al.: Increased masticatory muscle stiffness during limb muscle flaccidity associated with succinylcholine administration. *Anesthesiology* 69:11, 1988.
Wagenknecht T, Grassucci R, Frank J, et al.: Three-dimensional architecture of the calcium channel/foot structure of sarcoplasmic reticulum. *Nature* 338:167, 1989.
Wappler F, Fiege M, Antz M, et al.: Hemodynamic and metabolic alterations in response to graded exercise in a patient susceptible to malignant hyperthermia. *Anesthesiology* 92:268, 2000.
Wappler F, Fiege M, Steinfath M, et al.: Evidence for susceptibility to malignant hyperthermia in patients with exercise-induced rhabdomyolysis. *Anesthesiology* 94:95, 2001.
Wappler F, Scholz J, von Richthofen V, et al.: Attenuation of serotonin-induced contractures in skeletal muscle from malignant hyperthermia-susceptible patients with dantrolene. *Acta Anaesth Scand* 41:1312, 1997.
Warner LO, Beach TP, Garvin JP, et al.: Halothane and children: the first quarter century. *Anesth Analg* 63:838, 1984.
Whistler T, Isaacs H, Badenhorst M: No abnormal low molecular weight proteins identified in human malignant hyperthermic muscle. *Anesthesiology* 64: 795, 1986.
Yentis SM, Levine MF, Hartley EJ: Should all children with suspected or confirmed malignant hyperthermia susceptibility be admitted after surgery? A 10-year review. *Anesth Analg* 75:345, 1992.
Younkin DP, Berman P, Sladky J, et al.: ^{31}P NMR studies in Duchenne muscular dystrophy: age related metabolic changes. *Neurology* 37:165, 1987.
Zochodne DW, Thompson RT, Driedger AA, et al.: Topical ^{31}P NMR spectroscopy in human forearm denervation. *Neurology* 36(suppl 1):138, 1986.

Systemic Disorders in Infants and Children

Lynne Maxwell • Salvatore R. Goodwin • Thomas J. Mancuso • Victor C. Baum • Aaron L. Zuckerberg • Philip G. Morgan • Etsuro K. Motoyama • Peter J. Davis

Among patients presenting special problems for pediatric anesthesiologists are children whose underlying conditions complicate anesthetic management and may be associated with an increased risk of morbidity. The number of rare diseases that may be encountered in infants and children is great, although only a few are mentioned here. Chosen for discussion are the diseases seen with some frequency, those carrying an increased risk related to anesthetic management, and a few of unusual interest. Modifications to the understanding of mechanisms of coagulation are included along with consideration of coagulopathic states. Katz and Steward (1993) have provided a complete review of the anesthetic implications of uncommon pediatric diseases. A list of syndromes with possible anesthetic implications is included in Appendix D.

ENDOCRINE DISORDERS

DIABETES MELLITUS

The endocrine problem most frequently dealt with in the perioperative period is the management of glucose homeostasis in children with diabetes mellitus. The prevalence of type 1 (insulin-dependent) diabetes in the United States has remained stable for the past 15 years at 1 in 500 school-aged children (CDC, 2003), whereas the incidence of type 2 diabetes is increasing, especially among American Indian, African American, and Hispanic children and adolescents. Diabetes mellitus is the result of an absolute or functional deficiency of insulin production by the pancreas. In type 1 diabetes, this deficiency is caused by an autoimmune pathophysiologic process. Insulin deficiency results in abnormalities of glucose transport and storage and in lipid and protein synthesis. These metabolic derangements result in vascular pathology over time, which leads to the end-stage complications of renal, cardiac, and eye disease, which rarely occur before adulthood. The anesthetic implications of type 1 diabetes in childhood differ from those seen in adults with the same disease, for whom the primary concern is about the type and severity of end-organ disease.

Children with insulin-dependent diabetes may be treated with different kinds of insulin on a daily basis to maintain tight glucose control, with the aid of frequent blood glucose monitoring. Since 1982, most newly approved insulin preparations have been produced using recombinant DNA technology with laboratory-cultivated bacteria or yeast. This process allows the bacteria or yeast cells to produce complete human insulin. Recombinant human insulin has mostly replaced animal-derived insulin, such as pork and beef insulin, in diabetes

■ **TABLE 32–1.** Kinetics of commonly used insulins

Insulin Products	Route	Onset (hr)	Peak (hr)	Effective Duration (hr)
Human				
Lispro (Humalog)	SC	0.25	0.5 to 1.5	3 to 5
Regular	IV, SC	0.5 to 1.0	2 to 3	5 to 8
NPH	SC	1 to 3	4 to 10	12 to 20
Glargine (Lantus)	SC	2 to 4	No peak	>30
Animal				
Regular	IV, SC	0.5 to 1.0	2 to 5	4 to 6

IV, intravenous; SC, subcutaneous.

management (Plotnick, 1998). Insulin products called *insulin analogs* are produced so that the structure differs slightly from human insulin (by one or two amino acids) to change onset and peak of action. An example of an analog is human lispro (Humalog, NovoLog), an ultra-short-acting insulin, which is given only 15 minutes before a meal and whose peak and duration of action parallel the glucose rise resulting from carbohydrate ingestion.

Another new insulin is glargine (Lantus), which almost mimics an insulin pump, providing a 24-hour, continuous low background level of insulin. Table 32–1 lists some of the insulin preparations most commonly used in children. Some children may be managed with an external insulin pump, which provides a low background infusion of insulin and the ability to give small boluses before meals. Most diabetic children administer insulin at least three times and check blood sugar at least four times each day. Type 2 diabetes in children and adolescents may be controlled with diet and exercise, but they also may be taking metformin (Glucophage).

Insulin-dependent diabetic children are at risk for significant perioperative difficulties even when their preoperative glucose control is good because of the effects of surgical stress on glucose homeostasis. Brittle or noncompliant diabetic patients have additional problems, including an increased risk of perioperative hypoglycemia or hyperglycemia, osmotic diuresis with resultant hypovolemia, and altered mental status. The physician must document the child's current insulin regimen, degree of compliance, preoperative glucose control, and risk of hypoglycemia from preoperative fast. Much of this information can be obtained from the patient's endocrinologist or by examination of the child's blood glucose monitoring log. A recent growth history can indicate how well controlled the child's diabetes may be. Coordination and cooperation among the patient, parents, pediatrician, endocrinologist, and anesthesiologist are essential if the goal of optimal perioperative glucose homeostasis is to be achieved. The anesthesiologist must particularly heed the advice and counsel of the diabetic child's primary physician.

Insulin is an anabolic hormone that promotes glycogen and triglyceride storage and protein synthesis. It decreases glycogenolysis, gluconeogenesis, and lipolysis, with resultant ketogenesis and protein breakdown. It is present in small amounts even in the fasting state. Its complete absence at the time of surgery puts the patient in a state of starvation in which caloric intake is greatly restricted and substrate demands (e.g., for healing) are at their highest. The risk of a catabolic state is increased by the release of stress hormones, including catecholamines, cortisol, and glucagon. Perioperative insulin administration is essential for glucose control and to promote an anabolic state, which is most conducive to speedy healing and metabolic homeostasis.

Preoperative Evaluation

The preoperative evaluation should include measurements of the hematocrit, electrolyte levels, and glucose levels. A hemoglobin A_{1C} level (i.e., glycosylated hemoglobin assay), although a useful index of long-term glucose control (Nathan et al., 1984), is unlikely to affect the anesthetic plan and is not a necessary preoperative test. If glycohemoglobin results are available, one must realize that different laboratories have different ranges for hemoglobin A_{1C} in normal subjects. The normal range may change from time to time even in the same laboratory. It is therefore important to know the laboratory's normal range to interpret results in diabetic patients. The normal range of hemoglobin A_{1C} is 4.5% to 6.1% (Siberry and Iannone, 2000).

Several systemic abnormalities may be present in the child with diabetes mellitus. Nineteen percent of diabetic children have a vital capacity two standard deviations below the predicted mean value, suggesting the presence of restrictive lung disease (Buckingham et al., 1986). No apparent association exists between decreased vital capacity and duration of diabetes or presence of other diabetic complications. Abnormal lung elasticity (Schuyler et al., 1976) and thickening of the alveolar basal laminae (Vracko et al., 1980) have been reported in children with diabetes. Routine preoperative pulmonary function tests are not indicated in the asymptomatic diabetic child.

Decreased atlantooccipital joint mobility, resulting in difficult intubation, may be present in a subset of adolescents with a syndrome of diabetes mellitus, short stature, and tightness of small joints of the fingers, wrists, ankles, and elbows (Salzarulo and Taylor, 1986). Abnormal cross-linking of collagen by nonenzymatic glycosylation is the postulated cause of this syndrome (Chang et al., 1980).

Perioperative Management

Various regimens for managing insulin therapy perioperatively have been proposed, three of which are discussed here (Table 32–2). Essential to optimal management, no matter which regimen is chosen, is the scheduling of elective surgery for the diabetic child as early as possible in the day (first case) to minimize the time the patient is fasting. Fasting interval should be the same as that recommended for nondiabetic patients: no solid food or milk for 8 hours, and clear liquids permissible until 2 hours before the scheduled time of surgery (Schreiner et al., 1990). Children with diabetes should be encouraged to continue taking clear liquids until 2 hours before. If this is not possible, an intravenous infusion should be started (described later). As recommended in adult patients with type 1 diabetes, Glucophage should be stopped 48 hours before surgery, because of reports of lactic acidosis in patients who remain on the drug and are in a fasting state perioperatively.

Although some investigators have recommended the withholding of preoperative sedation from diabetic patients to better monitor for signs of hypoglycemia, premedication is recommended in children. The use of agents such as benzodiazepines, opioids, or barbiturates does not alter glucose metabolism, and the failure to use such agents may elevate the blood sugar level due to anxiety, which causes a stress response with catecholamine release.

TABLE 32–2. Protocols for perioperative insulin therapy

Regimen	Morning of surgery procedure
Classic regimen	Start intravenous infusion of 5% dextrose in 0.45% saline or Ringer's lactate solution at 1500 mL/m² per day. Administer one half of usual morning insulin dose as regular insulin. Check blood glucose before induction and during and after anesthesia.
Continuous insulin infusion	Start intravenous infusion of 5% dextrose in 0.45% saline or Ringer's lactate solution at 1500 mL/m² per day. Add 1 to 2 units of insulin per 100 mL of 5% dextrose. Starting insulin dose is 0.02 units/kg per hour. Check blood glucose before induction and during and after anesthesia.
Insulin- and glucose-free regimen (for operative procedures of short duration)	Withhold morning insulin dose. If indicated for procedure, give glucose-free solution (e.g., Ringer's lactate) at maintenance rate. Check blood glucose before induction and during and after anesthesia.

From Maxwell LG, Deshpande JK, Wetzel RC: Preoperative evaluation of children. *Pediatr Clin North Am* 41:93, 1994.

Classic Regimen

On the morning of surgery, one half of the usual dose of NPH insulin is administered subcutaneously after establishing an intravenous infusion of 5% glucose-containing solution at a rate of 100 mg/kg of glucose per hour (see Table 32–2). Plasma glucose concentrations should be maintained between 100 and 180 mg/dL. This target range is chosen because mild to moderate hyperglycemia (without ketosis) usually does not present a serious problem to the child, whereas hypoglycemia has devastating consequences. Hyperglycemia greater than 250 mg/dL should be avoided because of associated mental status changes, diuresis, and subsequent dehydration, which can occur because of the hyperosmolar state. Hyperglycemia has been associated with poorer outcomes in patients at risk for central nervous system (CNS) ischemia, including those undergoing cardiopulmonary bypass (Lanier et al., 1987; Lanier, 1991). Postoperatively, supplemental subcutaneous doses of short-acting insulin can be given on a sliding scale to maintain the desired plasma glucose level. This regimen should be restricted to patients who are scheduled for short surgical procedures after which they are expected to resume eating promptly.

Insulin Infusion

If a long procedure or a prolonged period of postoperative fasting is anticipated, the continuous intravenous infusion of glucose and insulin may provide the best control. On the morning of surgery, a glucose infusion is begun at a maintenance rate of 100 mg/kg per hour, with the insulin infusion of 0.02 to 0.05 U/kg per hour "piggy-backed" into the glucose infusion. The glucose infusion can be D_5 or D_{10} in half-normal saline with 10 to 20 mEq/L of potassium chloride. These infusions should be begun 2 hours before surgery to minimize the fasting interval and decrease the risk of the development of a catabolic state. Insulin is absorbed by intravenous bags and tubing. When the insulin solution is prepared, the first portion of the solution should be run through the tubing and discarded to saturate the sites in the tubing that bind insulin (Kaufman et al., 1996). Blood glucose levels should be checked hourly for the first few hours, and adjustments of +0.01 U/kg per hour in the insulin rate should be made to keep the blood sugar in the acceptable range of 80 to 180 mg/dL. The glucose and insulin should be infused through a dedicated intravenous cannula to enable it to be well regulated apart from non–glucose-containing crystalloid solutions administered to replace blood or fluid losses. Most investigators believe that lactated Ringer's solution should not be used for blood and fluid replacement, as lactate is a glycogenic precursor and may result in higher blood glucose levels. This continuous infusion regimen has been shown to yield better control of glucose concentrations than the regimen in which intermittent subcutaneous insulin is administered (Kaufman et al., 1996). There is no role for the administration of intermittent large intravenous insulin doses. This can result in big swings in glucose concentration (high and low) and a greater chance of lipolysis and ketogenesis. Patients with insulin pumps should have them turned off in the perioperative period and replaced by the continuous infusion regimen, as most anesthesiologists are not familiar with the details of operation of such pumps. Fifty percent dextrose solution should be available for administration in case of the development of hypoglycemia; 0.1 g/kg of dextrose raises the blood glucose level by approximately 30 mg/dL.

Alternative Procedure

For *extremely brief* procedures after which prompt resumption of oral intake is expected, the third protocol involves the administration of no insulin or glucose before or during surgery. When oral intake is established postoperatively, 40% to 60% of the usual daily insulin dose is given (Stevens and Roizen, 1987). Myringotomy with tube placement is an example of a procedure for which this regimen would be appropriate. The surgical procedure should be performed as the first case on the morning schedule to avoid prolonged fasting and excessive delay in insulin administration.

The most serious perioperative complication that can occur in the diabetic child is hypoglycemia. Common signs of low blood glucose levels include tachycardia, tearing, diaphoresis, and hypertension. In the anesthetized patient, these signs may be misinterpreted as caused by inadequate anesthesia. Because the clinical signs of hypoglycemia are masked by sedation or anesthesia, frequent measurement of the serum glucose level (every hour) is critical for the prevention of hypoglycemia, independent of the glucose-insulin regimen chosen. Glucose test strips (ChemStrip bG, Roche Diagnostics Corp., Indianapolis, IN), with or without the use of a reflectance photometer, provide quick, convenient, and reliable bedside blood sugar measurements to guide therapy. Blood glucose determinations performed with reflectance photometers (Accu-Chek, Roche Diagnostics Corp., Indianapolis, IN) provide results that are generally within 10% of clinical laboratory glucose determinations done on the same specimen (Chen et al., 2003). Visual evaluation of blood glucose strips is less accurate (Arslanian et al., 1994). Postoperative insulin administration is determined by the time the patient's oral or enteral feeding resumes and the postoperative blood glucose concentration. The endocrinologist and surgeon should be active partners in the choice of an appropriate insulin regimen because they will be responsible for monitoring glucose homeostasis after the patient leaves the recovery room.

For day-surgery patients, contingency planning for insulin management and mechanism for follow-up and consultation should be clearly defined for members of the care team and family.

Regional or general anesthesia is appropriate for the child with diabetes mellitus. If tolerated with minimal sedation, regional anesthesia might be argued to offer the advantage of allowing for observation of the level of consciousness as a monitor of hypoglycemia. Practically speaking, most children require general anesthesia, even when regional techniques are employed. The ease and availability of point-of-care glucose determination from venous or fingerstick specimens obviate the need for monitoring cerebral function.

Occasionally, diabetics require surgery for trauma or infection while in a state of ketoacidosis. Diabetic ketoacidosis occurs when there is hyperglycemia (plasma glucose concentration > 300 mg/dL) with glucosuria, ketonemia (ketones strongly positive at greater than 1:2 dilution of serum), ketonuria, and acidemia (pH < 7.30 or serum bicarbonate < 15 mEq/L, or both). It is common for intraabdominal catastrophes with infection to precipitate ketoacidosis. Foster and McGarry (1983) have succinctly summarized the pathophysiology of diabetic ketoacidosis. The initiating event is usually cessation of insulin therapy or onset of stress that renders the usual dose of insulin inadequate. Glucagon, catecholamines, cortisol, and growth hormone levels rise. A catabolic state is produced as substrates are mobilized, resulting in hepatic production of glucose and ketone bodies, which causes hyperglycemia and ketoacidosis. Subclinical brain swelling nearly always occurs during diabetic ketoacidosis therapy, although most patients remain asymptomatic (Krane et al., 1985). Fatalities from cerebral edema do occur, and some studies suggest that high rates of fluid administration early in treatment (>50 mL/kg in the first 4 hours) greatly increase the risk of herniation (Mahoney et al., 1999). Studies using 4 L/m^2 for the first 24 hours followed by 1 to 1.5 times maintenance resulted in clearance of ketoacidosis equal to that in patients given more fluid, but there remained a low but persistent incidence of symptomatic cerebral edema (0.35% to 0.5%) (Felner and White, 2001). Administration of isotonic fluid only and frequent monitoring of serum osmolality by direct measurement or calculation to ensure that elevated osmolality is reduced gradually are the best methods to prevent the development of this devastating complication. Insulin therapy should be tailored to decrease the blood glucose concentration at a rate no greater than 100 mg/dL per hour. To prevent a more rapid decrease in blood glucose concentration, 5% dextrose, and, if necessary, 10% dextrose should be added to the rehydration solution to slow the rate of fall, rather than decreasing the rate of insulin infusion (Arslanian et al., 1994). Fortunately, the anesthesiologist is rarely called on to administer anesthesia during this severe metabolic derangement. If an anesthetic is required during diabetic ketoacidosis, preoperative attention should be directed toward the correction of hypovolemia and hypokalemia along with beginning an insulin infusion. Invasive hemodynamic monitoring may be indicated preoperatively to optimize the patient's fluid and electrolyte balance and to monitor the patient's hemodynamic status accurately. Surgery should not be delayed inordinately because correction of the metabolic derangements may be impossible before the underlying source of infection or organ dysfunction is corrected. For patients with signs of cerebral edema, intracranial pressure monitoring may be necessary.

DIABETES INSIPIDUS

Diabetes insipidus is a clinical syndrome of hypotonic polyuria in the face of elevated plasma osmolality that results from inadequate production of, or inadequate response to, antidiuretic hormone (ADH). Central diabetes insipidus results from inadequate production or release of ADH from the posterior pituitary gland. ADH is synonymous with arginine vasopressin. Nephrogenic diabetes insipidus is characterized by partial or complete renal tubular unresponsiveness to endogenous ADH or exogenously administered arginine vasopressin.

The causes of diabetes insipidus are outlined in Box 32–1. This discussion will focus on central diabetes insipidus. Nephrogenic diabetes insipidus has been reviewed by Cramolini (1993) and Malhotra and Roizen (1987). The clinical manifestations of diabetes insipidus are polyuria and polydipsia. The urine is hypotonic relative to the plasma. The urine osmolality is usually less than 200 mOsm/L, and urine specific gravity is less than 1.005 (Weigle, 1987). When there has been inadequate access to water, severe dehydration and hypernatremia ensue because a large volume of dilute urine is continually produced.

Patients with preexisting diabetes insipidus may come for incidental surgery. These patients are usually taking maintenance doses of vasopressin, which for relatively short, uncomplicated, elective procedures, should be continued through the perioperative period. Desmopressin (1-desamino-8-D-arginine vasopressin [DDAVP]),

BOX 32–1 Causes of Diabetes Insipidus

Vasopressin Deficiency (Neurogenic Diabetes Insipidus)

Acquired
- Idiopathic
- Traumatic (accidental, surgical)
- Neoplastic (craniopharyngioma, metastasis, lymphoma)
- Granulomatous (sarcoid, histiocytosis)
- Infectious (meningitis, encephalitis)
- Vascular (Sheehan's syndrome, aneurysm)

Familial (autosomal dominant)

Excessive Water Intake (Primary Polydipsia)

Acquired
- Idiopathic (resetting of the osmostat)
- Psychogenic

Vasopressin Insensitivity (Nephrogenic Diabetes Insipidus)

Acquired
- Infectious (pyelonephritis)
- Postobstructive (urethral, ureteral)
- Vascular (sickle cell disease or trait)
- Infiltrative (amyloid)
- Cystic (polycystic disease)
- Metabolic (hypokalemia, hypercalcemia)
- Granulomatous (sarcoid)
- Toxic (lithium, demeclocycline)
- Solute overload (glucosuria, postobstructive)

Familial (X-linked recessive)

Adapted from Malhotra N, Roizen MF: Patients with abnormalities of vasopressin secretion and responsiveness. *Anesthesiol Clin North Am* 5:400, 1987.

a longer-acting (8 to 20 hours) vasopressin analog, has a decreased vasopressor effect relative to its antidiuretic effect (Hays, 1990). DDAVP is usually given intranasally (2.5 to 10 mcg once or twice daily) to prevent diuresis (Lee et al., 1976), but also may be given subcutaneously or intravenously (1 to 2 mcg twice daily). The most common situation encountered by the anesthesiologist, however, is the development of diabetes insipidus intraoperatively or postoperatively in patients having surgery for pituitary or hypothalamic tumors, most commonly craniopharyngiomas. Perioperative diabetes insipidus may present in one of four ways:

1. Transient polyuria probably is related to the onset and resolution of transient cerebral edema rather than to injury to the pituitary stalk. It usually resolves in 24 to 36 hours.
2. A triphasic pattern with an interlude of normal urine output reflects the release of stored vasopressin from the posterior lobe or median eminence of the pituitary. This is followed by resumption of polyuria when the stored supply of vasopressin is exhausted.
3. Mild polyuria reflects partial diabetes insipidus, which is exaggerated by local edema and corticosteroid administration.
4. Permanent diabetes insipidus is caused by destruction or removal of all cells capable of producing and storing vasopressin.

If any degree of diabetes insipidus is going to occur, the onset is most commonly within 18 hours after operation. A review of craniopharyngioma resection in children found a very high incidence of the development of diabetes insipidus (30 of 32 patients). Recommendations for therapy are reviewed by Lehrnbecher and others (1998).

The goal of perioperative management of diabetes insipidus is to maintain normal fluid and electrolyte balance, urine output, and hemodynamic stability. Urine output may be prodigious (10 to 20 mL/kg per hour). Care must be taken to differentiate polyuria caused by diabetes insipidus (urine specific gravity < 1.005) from diuresis caused by mannitol administration or hyperglycemia (urine specific gravity usually > 1.015), or simple excessive administration of crystalloid (urine specific gravity > 1.005). Patients with partial ADH deficiency usually do not require supplemental aqueous vasopressin perioperatively because large quantities of ADH are produced in response to surgical stress (Malhotra and Roizen, 1987). Serum osmolality should be measured frequently, however, and aqueous vasopressin should be given if the plasma osmolality exceeds 290 mOsm/L (Malhotra and Roizen, 1987).

If central diabetes insipidus is present preoperatively and the planned surgery is prolonged, an infusion of aqueous vasopressin is begun preoperatively and continued intraoperatively. The recommendations for adults include a bolus of 100 mU of aqueous vasopressin followed by a continuous infusion of 100 to 200 mU/hour, accompanied by the intraoperative administration of isotonic fluids (Malhotra and Roizen, 1987). For the pediatric population, an infusion is begun at 0.5 mU/kg per hour and increased until a urine osmolality twice that of plasma and a urine output of less than 2 mL/kg per hour are achieved. It is rarely necessary to use more than 10 mU/kg per hour (Weigle, 1987). Side effects from vasopressin administration are minimal at doses used for antidiuresis; at larger doses, generalized vasoconstriction can occur and has resulted in tissue ischemia and myocardial infarction.

DDAVP, rather than aqueous vasopressin, is the drug of choice for treatment of perioperative diabetes insipidus because of its potent antidiuretic effect with minimal pressor activity or other side effects. In the perioperative period, it may be given intravenously until intranasal administration can be started or resumed. The suggested intravenous dose is 0.5 to 4.0 mcg, with a single dose having a duration of action of 4 to 23 hours (Harris, 1989; Lehrnbecher et al., 1998). The ease of intermittent dosing with DDAVP with low incidence of side effects must be balanced against the ability to titrate the continuous vasopressin infusion cited earlier. In either case, careful monitoring of fluid balance is essential.

The anesthesiologist rarely may encounter children who are receiving nightly nasal DDAVP for the treatment of enuresis. A review of its use reveals a negligible incidence of water intoxication (and no permanent effect on enuresis when treatment is stopped) (van Kerrebroeck, 2002). Given the known duration of action, DDAVP given the night before outpatient surgery should not affect the urine output on the day of surgery.

SYNDROME OF INAPPROPRIATE ANTIDIURETIC HORMONE SECRETION

Just as central diabetes insipidus is caused by ADH deficiency, syndrome of inappropriate ADH secretion (SIADH) is caused by an excess production of ADH, which is inappropriate with respect to the state of the intravascular volume. The most common causes of SIADH are listed in Box 32–2. The hallmark of SIADH is hyponatremia in the face of high urine osmolality and sodium levels. A comparison of the urine and serum electrolyte status seen in diabetes insipidus and SIADH is presented in Table 32–3. The treatment for mild cases of SIADH is fluid

BOX 32–2 **Causes of Syndrome of Inappropriate Secretion of Antidiuretic Hormone**

Central Nervous System

Infection
Meningitis
Encephalitis
Abscess
Guillain-Barré syndrome

Neoplastic Process

Tumor

Trauma

Subarachnoid hemorrhage

Infectious Process

Pneumonia
Tuberculosis
Shigellosis
Infant botulism

Positive Pressure Ventilation

Drugs

Vincristine
Vinblastine

■ **TABLE 32–3.** Comparison of diabetes insipidus and syndrome of inappropriate antidiuretic hormone secretion

Laboratory Test	Results for Diabetes Insipidus	Results for SIADH
Urine specific gravity	≤1.005	≥1.005
Urine osmolality	50 to 200 mOsm/L	>200 mOsm/L
Serum osmolality	>280 mOsm/L	<280 mOsm/L
Serum sodium	High (usually >148 mEq/L)	Low (usually <132 mEq/L)
Urine sodium	<20 mmol/L	>20 mmol/L

restriction (50% to 60% of maintenance fluid requirement) or insensible loss (400 mL/m^2 per day, plus one half to three fourths of the urine output). If hyponatremia is severe enough to cause coma or seizures, treatment with hypertonic saline (3%) solution may be indicated, but caution should be employed because the administration of hypertonic saline may cause circulatory overload, because the intravascular volume is already increased. A too-rapid rise of osmolarity (>20 mOsm/kg or >10 mmol/L of sodium in 24 hours) carries a risk of central pontine myelinolysis, a condition that can result in death (Laureno, 1983). This syndrome is thought to be caused by the sudden shrinkage of brain cells in response to rapidly increasing extracellular osmolality.

ADRENAL INSUFFICIENCY

Adrenal Insufficiency because of Primary Abnormalities of the Hypothalamic-Pituitary-Adrenal Axis

Adrenal insufficiency is an uncommon disease in childhood, but when it occurs, there are significant implications for the anesthesiologist. The causes of adrenal insufficiency are listed in Box 32–3. Adrenal insufficiency may include glucocorticoid deficiency with or without mineralocorticoid deficiency. Isolated hypoaldosteronism is rare. The signs and symptoms of glucocorticoid and mineralocorticoid deficiency are presented in Box 32–4. In the perioperative period, children with congenital adrenal insufficiency require glucocorticoid and mineralocorticoid replacement.

Chronic deficits in adrenal function result in the classic findings of Addison's disease, including hyperpigmentation, weakness, and hyponatremia. The hyperpigmentation results from high levels of adrenocorticotropic hormone (ACTH) and unopposed melanophore-stimulating hormone caused by cortisol insufficiency. The additional presence of aldosterone insufficiency may produce hyponatremia, hyperkalemia, hypotension, and a small cardiac silhouette resulting from hypovolemia (Keon and Templeton, 1993).

Perioperative Steroid Management

The preoperative recognition of adrenal insufficiency and appropriate preoperative therapy minimize the likelihood of significant perioperative complications. Ninety percent of patients with congenital adrenal hyperplasia with adrenal insufficiency have 21-hydroxylase deficiency (Migeon and Donohoue, 1994). Virilization of the external genitalia occurs in female patients, and they frequently require surgical revision of their external genitalia. An abnormal genital pigmentation occurs in male patients, but this finding may be subtle. Infants with undiagnosed congenital

BOX 32–3 Causes of Adrenal Insufficiency

Primary Adrenocortical Insufficiency

Congenital form

Enzyme Deficiency

Adrenal aplasia
Adrenocortical unresponsiveness to adrenocorticotropic hormone (ACTH)
Adrenoleukodystrophy or adrenomyeloneuropathy

Trauma or Septic Origin

Adrenal hemorrhage of newborn
Adrenal hemorrhage of acute infection
Chronic hypoadrenocorticism (Addison's disease)

Related to Deficient ACTH Secretion

Hypopituitarism
Cessation of glucocorticoid therapy
Resection of unilateral cortisol-producing tumor
Infants born to steroid-treated mothers
Respiratory distress syndrome
Anencephaly
Inanition, anorexia nervosa

Related to End-Organ Unresponsiveness

Pseudohypoaldosteronism
Cortisol resistance

adrenal hyperplasia may undergo exploratory laparotomy for acute abdomen because of nausea and vomiting. It is important to be attuned to the signs and symptoms in the history, physical, and laboratory evaluation that point to this diagnosis to prevent or treat shock, which may occur because of failure to administer steroid replacement.

Mineralocorticoid deficiency can be managed by administering saline solution and avoiding potassium in intravenous fluids. Mineralocorticoid secretion rates in children are similar to those in adults, and the replacement dose is independent of age and weight. Desoxycorticosterone acetate is administered intramuscularly in a dose of 1 mg/day. The intramuscular injection may be replaced by a single daily oral dose of 9-α-fluorocortisol acetate (Florinef, 0.05 to 0.10 mg) when it is clear that an oral medication can be tolerated and absorbed.

Glucocorticoid deficiency is treated with cortisol (hydrocortisone) replacement. The importance of cortisol replacement for patients with known adrenal insufficiency should not be underestimated, although vastly excessive doses are unwarranted. In the normal individual the adrenal gland secretes 12 ± 2 mg of cortisol per square meter of body surface area every 24 hours (Kenny and Preeyasombat, 1966). The normal replacement dose prescribed for unstressed children is 25 mg/m^2 per day; the dose is double the normal production because of factors of bioavailability and half-life (Migeon and Donohoue, 1994). In response to stress (fever, acute illness, surgery, and anesthesia), the normal adrenal gland secretes 3 to 15 times this amount. Consequently, in the past, the recommendations for "stress" steroid coverage in the perioperative period ranged from 36 to 180 mg/m^2 per day.

More important than just the dose of steroid to be given, consideration should be devoted to the type of glucocorticoid administered, its half-life, the route of administration, and the

BOX 32–4 Signs and Symptoms of Adrenal Insufficiency

Glucocorticoid Deficiency

Fasting hypoglycemia
Increasing insulin sensitivity
Decreased gastric acidity
Gastrointestinal symptoms (nausea, vomiting)
Fatigue

Mineralocorticoid Deficiency

Muscle weakness
Weight loss
Fatigue
Nausea, vomiting, anorexia

Salt Craving

Hypotension
Electrolyte disturbance
Hypokalemia
Hyponatremia
Acidosis

Adrenal Androgen Deficiency

Decreased pubic and axillary hair
Decreased libido
Increased β-lipoprotein levels
Hyperpigmentation

timing of doses. The equivalencies for different steroid preparations in terms of their relative glucocorticoid and mineralocorticoid effects are presented in Table 32–4. The most frequently cited recommendation for perioperative steroid coverage is hydrocortisone hemisuccinate (Solu-Cortef), given intravenously as 2 mg/kg immediately preoperatively and every 6 hours on the day of surgery, with reductions in the postoperative period depending on the degree of stress. Some practitioners feel that the half-life of hydrocortisone is so short that a 6-hour dosing interval may lead to periods of inadequate "coverage." These practitioners recommend a preinduction dose of 25 mg/m^2 of hydrocortisone given intravenously, followed by a continuous infusion of 50 mg/m^2 administered during the estimated period of anesthesia. Postoperatively, 50 mg/m^2 by continuous infusion is administered over the remainder of the first 24 hours. The total dose for the first 24 hours is 125 mg/m^2, or 10 times normal physiologic production (Migeon and Donohoue, 1994). The first bolus dose must be administered before induction of anesthesia rather than waiting for an intravenous cannula to be placed after inhalational induction because of the stress associated with anesthetic induction itself. In the postoperative period, the steroid dose is tapered to a level commensurate with the residual stress. It is replaced with the child's usual oral preparation when he or she clearly can tolerate and absorb oral medication.

Hypothalamic-Pituitary-Adrenal Axis Suppression Caused by Exogenous Steroid Therapy

In addition to the diseases discussed previously, suppression of the hypothalamic-pituitary-adrenal (HPA) axis can also occur after exogenous steroid usage, such as that administered for the treatment of inflammatory (e.g., Crohn's disease, asthma) or autoimmune (e.g., lupus, juvenile rheumatoid arthritis) disease. Fifty years ago, two patients were reported (Fraser et al., 1952; Lewis et al., 1953) who developed irreversible shock perioperatively after glucocorticoid administration was stopped preoperatively. Both patients were found to have adrenal atrophy and hemorrhage at autopsy. These two cases led to suggestions for "stress" steroid coverage in the perioperative period. HPA suppression places the steroid-dependent child at increased risk for complications in the perioperative period because these patients may be unable to respond to stress with an appropriate increase in the adrenal secretion of glucocorticoid. Dosages of cortisol or its equivalent that exceed 15 mg/m^2 per day for more than 2 to 4 weeks invariably produce HPA suppression. A study in children with relatively short-term exposure to prednisolone or dexamethasone (5 and 3 weeks, respectively) for treatment of acute lymphoblastic leukemia showed that recovery of normal adrenal function (in response to ACTH stimulation) had a very

TABLE 32–4. Potency of commonly used steroid preparations

Generic Name	Trade Name	Glucocorticoid Effect Equal to 100 mg of Cortisol	Sodium Retention Effect Equal to 0.1 mg of Florinef	Duration of Action
Hydrocortisone	Hydrocortisone Solu-Cortef	100	20	S
Cortisone	Cortone	125	20	S
Prednisolone	Delta-Cortef	20	50	I
Prednisone	Deltasone Meticorten	25	50	I
Methylprednisolone	Medrol Solu-Medrol	15	No effect	I
Triamcinolone	Aristocort Kenacort	10	No effect	I
Dexamethasone	Decadron Hexadrol	1.5	No effect	L
Betamethasone	Celestone	3	No effect or salt loss	L
Aldosterone	NCA	300	0.1 to 0.04	—
9α-Fludrocortisone acetate	Florinef	6.5	0.1	I
Desoxycorticosterone acetate	NCA	0	1.0 (intramuscularly)	I

I, intermediate (12- to 36-hour biologic half-life); L, long (36- to 72-hour biologic half-life); NCA, not commercially available; S, short (8- to 12-hour biologic half-life).

Adapted from Migeon C, Donohoue PA: Adrenal disorders. In Kappy MS, Blizzard RM, Migeon CJ, editors: *The diagnosis and treatment of endocrine disorders in childhood and adolescence*. Springfield, IL, 1994, Charles C Thomas.

wide range, occurring between 2 weeks and 8 months (Petersen et al., 2003).

Although high dosages, prolonged therapy, and short duration between discontinuance of therapy and the surgical procedure increase the likelihood of HPA suppression, no practical test is available that unequivocally identifies patients who will need intraoperative steroids. Metyrapone (Metopirone) depresses the production of cortisol by the adrenal glands and can be used to test the capacity of the pituitary gland to respond to decreased plasma cortisol concentrations by increasing ACTH secretion (Haynes, 1990). This test, however, takes 3 days, is expensive, and has the risk of inducing adrenal insufficiency. Similarly, an ACTH stimulation test can be performed at great expense to test adrenal responsiveness. However, even if cost and time were not issues, a study has shown a poor correlation between tests indicating normal HPA function and dose or duration of glucocorticoid therapy or basal cortisol levels (Schlaghecke et al., 1992). Clinically significant events rarely occur during the perioperative period in unsupplemented patients who were receiving steroid medications for diseases other than adrenal insufficiency. Nevertheless, the potential for symptomatic adrenal insufficiency, although rare, coupled with the low risk of steroid-induced complications for short-term administration, suggests that steroids should be given in uncertain cases. If steroid therapy has been discontinued within the previous year, Migeon and Donohoue (1994) make the following recommendations:

1. If the dose of the glucocorticoid administered was less than replacement levels, independent of the duration of administration, there will be no major HPA suppression and therefore no need for supplementation.
2. If the dose of glucocorticoid administered was greater than replacement levels, HPA suppression will occur. If treatment lasted less than 2 weeks, suppression is transient, with prompt recovery (<2 weeks). If treatment lasted more than 2 weeks, HPA suppression may persist for 1 week to 6 months, with 50% of patients recovering function within 6 weeks. This is the case even if the glucocorticoid was administered on an every-other-day basis.

HPA suppression also can result from modes of steroid administration other than oral, including topical, nasal spray, and inhalers. Although adrenal suppression is rarely symptomatic with these modes of administration, some drugs, especially fluticasone propionate (Flovent), in high doses have been associated with growth failure and adrenal suppression (Duplantier et al., 1998). With surgical stress, patients with adrenal suppression may become symptomatic, as has been reported for other kinds of stress. The patients reported by Drake and others (2002) all had been taking fluticasone and presented with hypoglycemia at times of stress from intercurrent illness. Anesthesiologists should have a high index of suspicion of adrenal suppression if an asthmatic child on inhaled steroids develops hypotension or hypoglycemia in the perioperative period.

For children who have been on prolonged courses of high-dose steroids (e.g., for asthma, treatment of ALL), the glucocorticoid regimen should follow that described earlier for patients with adrenal insufficiency. The dose given should be commensurate with the normal physiologic corticosteroid production in response to stress (as described), and does not need to be a multiple of the pharmacologic dose being administered for the underlying medical illness.

The dose administered should also be proportional to the perceived degree of surgical stress. For brief procedures, such as upper endoscopy, a single preoperative dose of steroids is suggested (50 mg/m^2 of hydrocortisone); for more complicated cases, such as appendectomy or major intraabdominal operations, 100 mg/m^2 is administered as a continuous infusion or divided into four doses per day. This dose is usually continued for 1 to 3 days after more complex surgical procedures (Krasner, 1999). The dose is tapered postoperatively and replaced with the patient's usual oral steroid preparation and dose when he or she is able to tolerate oral medications. The dose these patients frequently take for the underlying disease often exceeds even maximum "stress" doses described for congenitally adrenal insufficient patients, and treatment required for the underlying disease may limit further tapering of the steroid dose. A small study of adults comparing "stress steroids" with saline showed no adverse effects in patients who continued their usual steroid dose for their underlying disease (Glowniak and Loriaux, 1997).

THYROID DISORDERS

Hypothyroidism

Hypothyroidism occurs because of abnormally low production of thyroid hormone. It may be caused by primary thyroid dysfunction or result from pituitary failure with decreased production of thyroid-stimulating hormone (TSH). Normal values for routinely performed thyroid function tests are presented in Table 32–5. The interpretation of these test results with regard to diagnosis is presented in Table 32–6.

Primary thyroid dysfunction may be congenital or acquired. Congenital hypothyroidism usually appears in infancy. Classic features in the infant include large fontanelles, wide sutures, large tongue, umbilical hernia, and decreased deep tendon reflexes. In the older child, manifestations include slow heart rate, narrow pulse pressure, growth failure, hypothermia, and cold intolerance. Severe hypothyroidism is rare but may be associated with coma, cardiovascular collapse, hyponatremia, hypothermia, and respiratory failure. Keon and Templeton (1993) reviewed the anesthetic management of patients with hypothyroidism and stressed the importance of correcting hypothyroidism gradually over a 2-week period. Sudden death has been reported in children with myxedematous heart disease 2 to 3 weeks into therapy (LaFranchi, 1979). It is suggested that these children receive one fourth of the maintenance dose of thyroid hormone (6 to 8 mcg/kg per day for an infant) (Siberry and Iannone, 2000), with gradual incremental increases over a period of 2 to 4 weeks until a maintenance dose is reached. Patients who are adequately replaced will have normal thyroid hormone and TSH levels. Patients with incompletely restored thyroid hormone levels may require hemodynamic monitoring and support to maintain hemodynamic stability. Patients with severe hypothyroidism may have associated adrenal insufficiency and, if so, should receive stress steroid coverage as outlined earlier.

The anesthetic care of the symptomatic patient with hypothyroidism can be problematic and requires caution when any depressant medications are given. Prolonged effects may result from decreased drug metabolism. Table 32–7 outlines important considerations in the management of hypothyroidism as described by Keon and Templeton (1993). Invasive monitoring may be indicated when significant blood loss or

TABLE 32–5. Thyroid function tests

Test	Age	Normal Values
T_4 RIA (µg/dL)	1 to 3 days	11.0 to 21.5
	1 to 4 weeks	8.2 to 16.6
	1 to 12 months	7.2 to 15.6
	1 to 5 years	7.3 to 15.0
	6 to 10 years	6.4 to 13.3
	11 to 15 years	5.6 to 11.7
	16 to 20 years	4.2 to 11.8
T_3 resin RU		25% to 35%*
T index		1.25 to 4.20†
Free T_4 (ng/dL)	1 to 10 days	0.6 to 2.0
	>10 days	0.7 to 1.7
T_3 RIA (ng/dL)	1 to 3 days	100 to 380
	1 to 4 weeks	99 to 310
	1 to 12 months	102 to 264
	1 to 5 years	105 to 269
	6 to 10 years	94 to 241
	11 to 15 years	83 to 213
	16 to 20 years	80 to 210
TSH RIA (mIU/mL)	1 to 3 days	<2.5 to 13.3
	1 to 4 weeks	0.6 to 10.0
	1 month to 15 years	0.6 to 6.3
	16 to 20 years	0.2 to 7.6
TBG (mg/dL)	1 to 3 days	—
	1 to 4 weeks	0.5 to 4.5
	1 to 12 months	1.6 to 3.6
	1 to 5 years	1.3 to 2.8
	6 to 20 years	1.4 to 2.6
Reverse T_3‡ (mg/dL)	Newborns	90 to 250
	Adults	10 to 50

*Measures thyroid hormone binding, not T_3.
†T_4 RIA × T_3 RU.
‡Reverse T_3.
RIA, radioimmunoassay; RU, reuptake; T_3, triiodothyronine; T_4, thyroxine; TBG, thyroid-binding globulin; TSH, thyroid-stimulating hormone.
Adapted from Johnson KB, editor: *The Harriet Lane handbook*. St Louis, 1993, Mosby–Year Book.

fluid shifts occur. Care should be taken to minimize heat loss intraoperatively. Postoperative care should include monitoring of oxygen saturation, blood pressure, heart rate, and respiratory rate; postoperative ventilation may be necessary in the patient with delayed emergence from anesthesia.

Hyperthyroidism

Hyperthyroidism is a syndrome produced by excess levels of circulating thyroid hormone. The most common causes are congenital hyperthyroidism and Graves' disease (i.e., toxic goiter). Less commonly, acute suppurative thyroiditis, hyperfunctioning thyroid carcinoma, thyrotoxicosis factitia (i.e., exogenous administration of thyroid hormone), and toxic uninodular goiter (i.e., Plummer's disease) may produce this syndrome. The McCune-Albright syndrome (i.e., precocious puberty with polyostotic fibrous dysplasia) is also frequently associated with hyperthyroidism (Jones, 1988).

TABLE 32–6. Interpretation of thyroid function tests

Finding	T_4 RIA	T_3 RU	T index	Free T_4	TSH
Primary hypothyroidism	L	L	L	L	H
Secondary hypothyroidism	L	L	L	L	L, N, or H
TBG deficiency	L	H	N	N	N
Hyperthyroidism	H	H	H	H	L

L, low; H, high; N, normal; RIA, radioimmunoassay; RU, reuptake; T_3, triiodothyronine; T_4, thyroxine; TBG, thyroid-binding globulin; TSH, thyroid-stimulating hormone
Adapted from Johnson KB, editor: *The Harriet Lane handbook*. St Louis, 1993, Mosby–Year Book.

TABLE 32–7. Anesthetic implications of hypothyroidism

Anesthetic Considerations	Comments
Pharmacologic	Possible lower minimum alveolar concentration (MAC) value, prolonged recovery from opioid anesthesia.
Cardiovascular	Decreased cardiac output, heart rate, and stroke volume; increased peripheral vascular resistance and decreased intravascular volume; myocardial depression resulting from impaired cellular metabolism or myxedematous infiltration; baroreceptor dysfunction
Respiratory	Abnormal response to hypercapnia and hypoxia
Temperature	Hypothermia resulting from reduced basal metabolic rate and reduced ability to increase core temperature
Endocrine	Increased incidence of adrenal insufficiency; consideration for stress steroid coverage
Metabolic	Syndrome of inappropriate secretion of antidiuretic hormone; hypoglycemia with prolonged fasting
Gastrointestinal	Delayed gastric emptying; consideration for full-stomach precautions

Congenital Hyperthyroidism

Congenital hyperthyroidism is a transient phenomenon seen in newborns that results from the transplacental transfer of thyroid-stimulating antibody from mothers who commonly have a history of Graves' disease. Most of these infants have a goiter and typically appear anxious and restless or irritable. Signs of hypermetabolism, including tachycardia, tachypnea, and elevated temperature, may be present. In the severely affected infant, symptoms may progress to weight loss, severe hypertension, and high output cardiac failure with hepatomegaly (Smith et al., 2001). Appropriate medical therapy (propylthiouracil) should be instituted early. Because maternal immunoglobulins have a short half-life in the infants, the hyperthyroid state resolves in a few weeks to a few months, and it sometimes may be followed by a period of hypothyroidism (Higuchi et al., 2001).

Graves' Disease

Diffuse toxic goiter (Graves' disease) is the most common cause of hyperthyroidism in children. Its peak incidence occurs during adolescence, and it is five times more common in girls than in boys. The clinical course is generally gradual, with symptoms developing over a period of 6 to 12 months. Early signs include motor hyperactivity, emotional disturbances, and nervousness. Affected children are progressively more irritable and restless, and may have increased sweating, increased appetite, palpitations, and tremors of their fingers. Most children have obvious exophthalmos and an enlarged palpable thyroid. The cardiopulmonary symptoms of hyperthyroidism include systolic hypertension, tachycardia, palpitations, dyspnea, and cardiac enlargement, which may progress to frank cardiac decompensation. On rare occasions, atrial fibrillation or mitral regurgitation may also be present.

Thyroid Storm

An acute onset of hyperthermia, severe tachycardia, and restlessness comprises the syndrome of acute uncompensated thyrotoxicosis, or "thyroid storm." Without appropriate and timely therapy, the patient's condition may deteriorate to delirium, coma, and death. Therapy includes treatment of hyperthermia by cooling; maintenance of intravascular volume with balanced salt solutions; and β-adrenergic blockers, such as propranolol, titrated to ameliorate the cardiovascular response. Specific thyroid suppression therapy with propylthiouracil should be instituted. The clinical presentation of thyroid storm may occur intraoperatively, and this hypermetabolic state may be mistaken for malignant hyperthermia (Peters et al., 1981). It is well known that perioperative surgical stress can trigger the development of thyroid storm in a patient with previously unrecognized thyrotoxicosis (Stevens, 1983). For this reason, patients with signs and symptoms that may indicate the presence of hyperthyroidism should be carefully evaluated. Patients should be rendered euthyroid before any elective surgery, even if it is minor. The use of dantrolene mitigated the clinical signs in a patient who turned out to have thyroid storm (Bennett and Wainwright, 1989).

Laboratory Evaluation

Serum levels of thyroxine (T_4) and triiodothyronine (T_3) are usually elevated in hyperthyroidism. TSH secretion is suppressed and may be unmeasurable. T_3 toxicosis (elevated T_3 level with normal amounts of T_4) is more common in adult patients and rarely seen in children. For borderline cases, thyrotropin-releasing hormone (TRH) stimulation tests may be needed. Many patients with Graves' disease of recent onset may have elevated levels of thyroid-stimulating immunoglobulin. Radionuclide scans can also be helpful in making a diagnosis. If a large goiter is present, neck radiographs, computed tomography (CT), or magnetic resonance imaging may be used to evaluate the degree of tracheal compression and deviation.

Treatment

The management of hyperthyroidism is aimed at controlling the cardiovascular effects. β-Adrenergic receptor blockade, usually with propranolol (1 to 2 mg/kg per day), is titrated to effect. Antithyroid medications include propylthiouracil and methimazole, both of which inhibit the incorporation of inorganic iodide into organic compounds. Propylthiouracil inhibits the conversion of T_4 to T_3. Although early studies suggested that these agents might inhibit the formation of thyroid antibodies, later studies that included careful histopathologic analysis have shown this to be false (Paschke et al., 1995). Saturated solutions of potassium iodide may be administered orally (one drop every 8 hours) to suppress thyroid hormone secretion. The clinical response to therapy is evident in 1 to 3 weeks, and the patient may require up to 3 months for adequate control to be achieved. Patients must have appropriate, regular surveillance to ensure that the T_3 and T_4 levels are in the normal range and TSH concentrations are normal. Clinically, the patient demonstrates a euthyroid state by return of the heart rate, blood pressure, and reflexes to normal.

Radioactive iodine is frequently used to treat hyperthyroidism in adults. Such therapy is avoided in children, however, because of side effects such as thyroid cancer, genetic damage to germ cells, and a higher incidence of hypothyroidism than occurs with pharmacologic therapy.

Anesthetic Management

Preoperatively, patients should be pharmacologically euthyroid. Any residual cardiovascular signs and symptoms should be well controlled through the use of a β-adrenergic receptor blocker. Esmolol is an excellent choice for intraoperative use. A large goiter may produce tracheal deviation or compression, and the possibility of airway compromise should be evaluated preoperatively with radiographic studies. Any commonly used sedative may be given for premedication. Atropine and other anticholinergics should be avoided or used with extreme caution because they decrease sweating and may interfere with thermoregulation. Medications, including antithyroid drugs and β-adrenergic blockers, should be administered through the morning of surgery.

Intraoperative Management of Patients for Thyroidectomy

In children with large goiters who have a compromised airway, anesthesia should be managed with caution, as in any other child with upper airway obstruction. A sedated fiberoptic intubation may be chosen or an inhalational induction performed with maintenance of spontaneous ventilation until the airway is secured. If a large goiter has caused prolonged tracheal compression, there may be a segment of tracheomalacia, and an armored endotracheal tube may be indicated.

For patients without issues of tracheal compression, anesthesia may be induced with thiopental or propofol. If the patient remains hyperthyroid, ketamine should be avoided, however, because of its effect on catecholamine release. Mask inductions may be prolonged in these patients because of an increased cardiac output, resulting in a slower rise in the alveolar concentration of the anesthetic if the ventilation is kept constant. Minute ventilation may be reduced if significant airway obstruction resulting from goiter or tracheomalacia is present. Care should be taken to lubricate, pad, and appropriately protect the eyes, especially if they are protuberant because of Graves' disease.

With respect to choice of drugs, muscle relaxants with few cardiovascular side effects, such as *cis*-atracurium, vecuronium, or rocuronium, provide a potential benefit by minimizing the occurrence of tachycardia. Similarly, for the maintenance of general anesthesia, anesthetics that have sympathomimetic effects should be avoided. If the child is in a hypermetabolic state, drug biotransformation may be accelerated; therefore, agents such as halothane, which has toxic metabolic products, are potentially more hazardous. Another reason to avoid halothane is its sensitization of the myocardium to catecholamines. If the patient is in a hypermetabolic state, controlled ventilation should be employed during the surgical procedure to minimize the development of hypercapnia, which can contribute to further sympathetic stimulation.

Anesthetic management at the conclusion of surgery may include deep extubation with direct or fiberoptic laryngoscopy performed to evaluate the presence or absence of vocal cord paralysis, which may result from surgical trauma to the recurrent laryngeal nerve (traction or section). Care should be taken after extubation to observe for signs of airway obstruction due to residual tracheomalacia. The decision to evaluate the airway prospectively at the time of extubation should be made jointly by the anesthesiologist and surgeon and is based on the likelihood of residual tracheal obstruction caused by tracheomalacia or of vocal cord paralysis because the surgeon thinks surgical trauma likely.

Postoperative Care

Children who have undergone thyroidectomy require close observation in the postoperative period (Fewins et al., 2003). They may develop postextubation croup or upper airway obstruction as a result of paralysis of the vocal cords, tetany, residual tracheomalacia, or tracheal compression resulting from a hematoma. Patients with postextubation croup may respond to supportive measures, including humidified supplemental oxygen, nebulized racemic epinephrine, and possibly continuous positive airway pressure (or BIPAP). Occasionally, these patients require brief reintubation before they can be successfully extubated. Unilateral vocal cord paralysis may go unnoticed or be associated with only mild stridor. Bilateral vocal cord paralysis, on the other hand, may manifest as severe stridor and upper airway obstruction. The child with bilateral vocal cord paralysis requires reintubation for airway support. A muscle relaxant such as rocuronium should be used to facilitate reintubation to avoid damage to the abducted cords. If the paralysis is prolonged, the child may subsequently require tracheostomy. Compression of the trachea by a hematoma may occur immediately after the operation or over the course of several hours. The child requires reintubation and surgical evacuation of the hematoma to relieve tracheal compression. Opening the wound in the recovery room may be necessary and lifesaving. After the extrinsic obstruction has been relieved and the incision closed again (if necessary), the child may be safely extubated.

Inadvertent resection of the parathyroid glands during thyroidectomy may result in acute hypoparathyroidism after surgery. Clinical signs of hypocalcemia may become manifest within the first postoperative day or take as long as 72 hours to develop. A low serum ionized calcium level and a low concentration of parathyroid hormone are diagnostic. Clinical hypocalcemia, including tetany, is treated with intravenous calcium therapy. Surgical manipulation of the trachea and neck tissues can also lead to subcutaneous emphysema and the more serious possibility of pneumomediastinum or pneumothorax. Postoperative evaluation should include radiologic examination of the chest if respiratory distress occurs.

PHEOCHROMOCYTOMA

Pheochromocytoma is a catecholamine-secreting tumor of chromaffin cells that most commonly arises in the adrenal medulla (DiGeorge, 1987). It may be found anywhere along the abdominal sympathetic chain, however, particularly near the aorta at the inferior mesenteric artery or the aortic bifurcation. Other sites include the neck, the mediastinum, and the walls of the bladder or ureters. Pheochromocytoma is a rare neoplasm in the pediatric population. Less than 5% of the reported cases occur in children. The tumors may occur bilaterally or in multiple sites. It can be inherited as an autosomal dominant trait (most frequently in association with von Hippel-Lindau syndrome) or as part of a multiple endocrine neoplasia syndrome (MEN type II or III) (Table 32–8).

The abnormally high plasma levels of epinephrine and norepinephrine produce a clinical syndrome with signs and symptoms related directly to the level of each hormone present in the patient. Hypertension is common and frequently leads to hypertensive encephalopathy and seizures. In particular, paroxysmal hypertension is most suggestive of pheochromocytoma. The patient may also complain of associated headaches and palpitation, pallor, sweating, and vomiting. In severe cases, patients

TABLE 32–8. Multiple endocrine neoplasia syndromes

MEN Syndrome	Affected Organs	Disorder Features
Werner's syndrome (MEN type I, familial)	Parathyroid gland; pancreas; pituitary gland	Hypercalcemia; hypoglycemia; peptic ulcer
Sipple's syndrome (MEN type II, autosomal dominant)	Thyroid and parathyroid glands; adrenal medulla	Medullary carcinoma; hypercalcemia; pheochromocytoma
MEN type III	Nervous system; thyroid gland; adrenal medulla	Multiple neuromas; medullary carcinoma; pheochromocytoma

MEN, multiple endocrine neoplasia.

develop chest pain that radiates to the arms, pulmonary edema, and cardiac decompensation. The catecholamine-induced hypermetabolism also can cause patients to have a voracious appetite but still lose weight and become cachectic. Polyuria, polydipsia, and abdominal pain may occur and be confused with diabetes mellitus.

Diagnosis

It is extremely important to establish the diagnosis of pheochromocytoma before induction of anesthesia and start of surgery. The significant cardiovascular effects of excess catecholamines can pose difficulties for the anesthesiologist and endanger the patient during the perioperative period if an appropriate diagnosis is not made preoperatively. These tumors can produce paroxysms of hypertension and other symptoms. Between paroxysms, the patient may be totally asymptomatic, making diagnosis extremely difficult. The demonstration of increased levels of catecholamines is the most specific diagnostic test. Although pheochromocytomas can produce norepinephrine and epinephrine, the predominant catecholamine produced in children is norepinephrine, which leads to chronic hypertension. Urine catecholamine concentrations are directly proportional to circulating levels, and determination of 24-hour urinary excretion of the primary catecholamines and their metabolites (i.e., 3-methoxy-4-hydroxy vanillyl-mandelic acid [VMA] and metanephrine) used to be the primary means of establishing the diagnosis. The plasma-free metanephrine determination has better sensitivity (100%) and specificity (94%). Because normal values differ with age, it is important to use age-specific norms when interpreting results (Weise et al., 2002).

The differential diagnosis includes renal vascular disease, hyperthyroidism, Cushing's syndrome, coarctation of the aorta, adrenal cortical tumors, and essential hypertension. Cerebral disorders, diabetes mellitus, and diabetes insipidus may produce similar symptoms. Neoplasms of neural origin (e.g., neuroblastoma, ganglioneuroma) may also secrete catecholamines.

Before any contemplated anesthesia and surgery, the patient must undergo a complete evaluation to localize the tumor. Urinary catecholamine levels should be measured and a CT scan performed to localize the tumor. Differential venous catheterization may be needed to obtain blood from various sites for catecholamine levels. A radionuclide (I 131 meta-iodobenzylguanidine [MIBG]) scan may also help to localize the tumor. Sedation or anesthesia may be required to perform these studies in infants and children. Before sedation for these diagnostic studies, hemodynamic abnormalities must be normalized. Drugs that induce catecholamine secretion or histamine release should be avoided. General anesthesia for the diagnostic procedures must be conducted with the same extreme caution one would exercise for resection of the tumor itself.

Preoperative Preparation and Evaluation

Preoperative evaluation should include the measurement of serum electrolytes, determination of renal function, and a glucose tolerance test or test for fasting blood glucose level. Excessive serum epinephrine levels may be associated with hyperglycemia and hypokalemia. An electrocardiogram and echocardiogram are important to evaluate cardiac rhythm, size, and function. Some patients with pheochromocytoma have a catecholamine-induced cardiomyopathy with decreased left ventricular contractility. The patient should be evaluated for associated endocrinopathies that may be present as part of MEN II or III.

Symptomatic treatment includes the administration of phenoxybenzamine over a period of several days to weeks before surgery. Phenoxybenzamine is a long-acting, orally administered α-adrenergic blocking agent that attenuates the effects of catecholamines on the peripheral circulation by blocking excessive vasoconstriction (Hoffman and Lefkowitz, 1990). There are no established starting doses of phenoxybenzamine for pediatric patients, although 0.2 mg/kg once daily is suggested (adult starting dose is 10 mg). The dose is then increased gradually until a clinical effect is obtained, that is, the patient's hematocrit decreases (because of vasodilation and increased blood volume), and the patient develops orthostatic changes in vital signs. Long-standing vasoconstriction produced by chronically high catecholamine levels causes decreased intravascular volume. Although the use of phenoxybenzamine will restore vascular capacity to normal, increased oral fluid intake should accompany administration of phenoxybenzamine to avoid severe orthostatic changes. In some children, β-adrenergic blocking drugs such as propranolol may be needed to control heart rate and blood pressure. However, β-blocking agents should **never** be used without concurrent α-blockade therapy because of the deleterious effects of unopposed α-agonism, which may result in cardiac failure due to increased afterload. Labetalol may have a role in the management of pheochromocytoma (Blom et al., 1987), because it has α- and β-adrenergic blocking properties. It can be useful in minimizing the cardiovascular effects of excess catecholamines during the perioperative period, but it is not as potent an α-blocker as phenoxybenzamine for preoperative treatment.

In addition to the pharmacologic preparation, children with pheochromocytoma benefit from preoperative sedation to reduce the release of catecholamines caused by anxiety. Oral or intravenous midazolam alone or in combination with an opioid provides a good level of sedation.

Anesthetic Induction

Induction of anesthesia is accomplished with intravenous anesthetics. Ketamine is specifically contraindicated because it induces catecholamine release. Halothane should be avoided because it may sensitize the myocardium to catecholamines and produce dysrhythmias. Mask induction with sevoflurane is well tolerated if hemodynamic parameters are well controlled, and intravenous cannula placement can be deferred until after induction. Intubation may proceed in the usual fashion, facilitated by a hemodynamically neutral nondepolarizing muscle relaxant such as vecuronium. Pancuronium, which causes muscarinic blockade and tachycardia, should be avoided. Despite the fact that atracurium causes histamine release and vasodilation, it has been used safely in adult patients with pheochromocytoma (Prys-Roberts, 2000). Before intubation, intravenous lidocaine (1 mg/kg) or fentanyl (2 to 5 mcg/kg), or both, are effective in minimizing the hemodynamic response to intubation.

Intraoperative Management

After induction of anesthesia, an intraarterial catheter is placed to monitor the blood pressure continuously. Before induction, a reliable automated blood pressure device can provide frequent, accurate blood pressure measurements. A central venous catheter provides direct and reliable access for the assessment of intravascular volume and for infusions of fluids and emergency medications.

Anesthesia may be maintained with isoflurane or sevoflurane, air, and oxygen. Both anesthetic agents have been used without exacerbation of hypertension, despite the fact that they do not blunt the production of norepinephrine in response to surgical stimulation (Suzukawa, et al., 1983). Desflurane should be avoided because of its tendency to cause tachycardia and hypertension. The addition of moderately large doses of fentanyl (10 mcg/kg) or remifentanil (0.3 to1 mcg/kg per minute) will minimize the stress response and provide stable hemodynamics. If remifentanil is chosen, it is important to give a longer-acting opioid before the end of surgery to avoid hypertension due to pain on awakening. Adjunctive use of epidural anesthesia (i.e., local anesthetic with or without a small dose of fentanyl) is an excellent method of reducing the stress response and catecholamine release caused by usual surgical stimulation. None of these anesthetic strategies, however, blocks catecholamine release resulting from direct surgical manipulation of tumor tissue.

Blood pressure control during the induction and maintenance of anesthesia is best accomplished by an infusion of sodium nitroprusside or phentolamine. In addition to using propranolol preoperatively, esmolol has been effective as a continuous infusion titrated to the level of surgical stimulation (Nicholas et al., 1988). Infusions of only short-acting vasodilators are recommended for control of hypertension before tumor resection, because with removal of the tumor, vasodilation due to persistent α-blockade and loss of excess catecholamines may lead to precipitous hypotension. Because phenoxybenzamine has a long half-life, some physicians recommend discontinuing it 24 hours before surgery to decrease the likelihood that persistent vasodilation due to α-blockade will cause severe hypotension after the tumor is removed because of withdrawal of the catecholamines of tumor origin (Prys-Roberts, 2000). Hypotension is best treated with discontinuation of vasodilator infusions, titration of anesthetic agents, and administration of crystalloid or colloid and blood products if indicated by the magnitude of blood loss. If these measures are ineffective, vasopressors may be necessary, but the patient may be relatively resistant to α-agonists due to persistent α-blockade. If this occurs, judicious use of small doses of more potent, direct-acting vasoconstrictors (e.g., norepinephrine, epinephrine) may be necessary.

During surgery, arterial blood gases, serum glucose, urine output, and body temperature should be closely monitored. Hyperglycemia may occur in response to high catecholamine levels. Hypoglycemia may occur when the tumor is removed and catecholamine levels decrease. Because of the potential for dysrhythmias, the electrocardiogram should also be continuously monitored.

At the end of surgery, the muscle paralysis is reversed. Extubation can be accomplished when the patient meets all normal extubation criteria. Despite the recent increase in laparoscopic adrenalectomies for pheochromocytoma in adults, an open approach continues to be the norm in children. No alteration in hemodynamic parameters has been seen with the laparoscopic approach in adults; there have been no adverse effects on hemodynamics from insufflation of carbon dioxide. If laparoscopic surgery is proposed, anesthetic management is as outlined previously.

Postoperative Care

Postoperatively, the patient should be observed in an intensive care unit, with continuous monitoring of the arterial blood pressure and electrocardiogram. Hypertension usually resolves within 24 to 48 hours after surgery. If symptoms persist beyond this period, further investigation for residual pheochromocytoma is warranted. Good postoperative analgesia is provided with epidural infusion or intravenous patient (parent or nurse) controlled analgesia.

RESPIRATORY DISORDERS

UPPER RESPIRATORY TRACT INFECTION

Viral upper respiratory tract infections (URIs) are mild processes that do not preclude school attendance and other routine activities. However, URIs hold much greater significance for anesthesiologists. For many anesthesiologists, it is standard practice to avoid general anesthesia for elective surgery in children with a URI because of the respiratory complications during and after anesthesia reported in multiple small case series (McGill et al., 1979; Cohen and Cameron, 1991; Konarzewski et al., 1992; Williams et al., 1992). Unfortunately, the vexing problem of runny noses in children is accentuated by the difficulty of differentiating URI from other causes of runny nose, such as allergic rhinitis, which does not increase the risk of complications.

Pathophysiology of Upper Tract Respiratory Infection

Many investigators suggest that complications, including bronchospasm (Olsson, 1987), intraoperative hypoxemia with an increased alveolar-arterial oxygen gradient (McGill et al., 1979), and postoperative hypoxemia (DeSoto et al., 1988), occur more frequently in children who undergo anesthesia while they have a URI. The proclivity for these complications may be related to peripheral airway abnormalities, which have been demonstrated experimentally in adult humans (Johanson et al., 1969; Fridy et al., 1974) and animals (Dueck et al., 1991) infected with viral respiratory pathogens. These abnormalities include decreased diffusing capacity and increased closing volume, factors that can predispose patients to intrapulmonary shunting and hypoxemia, especially when combined with the effect of general anesthesia on lung volumes (decreased functional residual capacity) (Murat et al., 1985) (see Chapter 2, Respiratory Physiology). These studies were done in adults who had infections involving their entire respiratory tracts, rather than isolated URIs. These results may support separation of treatment of patients with truly isolated upper airway infections from those with any symptoms of more global airway or pulmonary parenchymal involvement. Although the mechanisms by which viral respiratory infections lead to alterations in airway function are unclear, these experimental studies support the clinical impression that increased risk of perioperative hypoxemia occurs in patients with a recent viral respiratory infection. Empey and others (1976) demonstrated in adult patients that acute viral respiratory tract infection (influenza) produced marked bronchial reactivity to experimental bronchoconstrictor challenge that may last for 6 weeks. Mechanisms by which viral infections lead to increased airway reactivity include the release of immunologic and inflammatory mediators such as leukotrienes, bradykinin, and histamine, which cause bronchoconstriction. Vagal-mediated mechanisms may be involved because viral infections have been associated with changes in muscarinic receptors on airway smooth muscle (Fryer et al., 1990). Tissue concentrations of important enzymes such as neutral endopeptidase, which break down the neuropeptides that cause bronchoconstriction, are also decreased in viral infections (Jacoby et al., 1988; Dusser et al., 1989). These patients and animals, however, cannot be said to have only URIs because the airways below the larynx are clearly affected as well. Patients whose infections are truly uncomplicated URI or those with noninfectious causes of runny nose should be differentiated from those who have evidence of lower respiratory involvement.

Perioperative Risk

Many case reports in the literature document respiratory complications in the perioperative period in children with URIs, including bronchospasm, stridor caused by subglottic edema, hypoxia, and atelectasis (McGill et al., 1979; Konarzewski et al., 1992; Williams et al., 1992). Three prospective studies have shown that patients with an active or recent URI had a 2- to 10-fold higher risk of bronchospasm or laryngospasm (Olsson and Hallen, 1984; Olsson, 1987; Cohen and Cameron, 1991). The incidence was higher among younger children, especially those younger than 2 years, and in those whose tracheas were intubated (Cohen and Cameron, 1991). Tait and others (1987b, 2001) have contributed retrospective studies of much larger numbers of patients. These studies show that there may actually be a higher risk of respiratory complications in asymptomatic children with history of a URI within the 2 to 4 weeks preceding surgery than in those with an acute URI. Tait and others (2000, 2001) found that the factors increasing the risk of adverse events were intubation, history of prematurity or reactive airways disease (RAD), parental smoking, airway surgery, copious secretions, and nasal congestion. Despite this increased risk of adverse events, complications usually were easily treated and were not associated with any significant prolonged morbidity (Rolf and Cote, 1992; Tait et al., 2000, 2001). However, some patients in one study developed atelectasis severe enough to require bronchoscopy and prolonged postoperative mechanical ventilation. Although most of these studies evaluated children having relatively minor elective surgery, Malviya and others (2003) reported that children with URI symptoms at the time of cardiac surgery also had increased risks for respiratory and other complications, including nonrespiratory infection. Despite these findings, patients' hospital stays were not prolonged, and the incidence of long-term sequelae was not increased.

One study found that children with URIs who undergo mask halothane–nitrous oxide–oxygen anesthesia for myringotomy surgery had reduced severity and duration of the URI symptoms in the postoperative period (Tait and Knight, 1987a). However, this reduction in symptoms may have resulted from the drainage and removal of infectious foci rather than from the beneficial effects of general anesthetics. Other investigators have reported no significant respiratory complications when children with URI were anesthetized (Hinkle, 1989; Jacoby and Hirschman, 1991). It is extraordinarily difficult to integrate the contradictory conclusions of these various series of patients to develop a logical algorithm for dealing with the child with a URI.

Anesthetic Decision-Making

It is apparent that no consensus has been reached in the literature or in the general anesthesia community with regard to the wisdom and safety of anesthetizing children with active or recent URI. The bulk of the literature, clinical and experimental, suggests that recent viral infection increases the perioperative risk for respiratory complications, albeit mild and treatable, when the surgical and anesthetic plans require intubation. In children with underlying RAD, the risk for pulmonary complications immediately after an acute URI is much greater than in the normal patient population, making intraoperative bronchospasm much more likely. The threshold for postponing surgery in the asthmatic child with a recent URI who requires intubation is much lower. These risks must be weighed against the physiologic, psychologic, and financial implications of delaying surgery.

The most conservative approach to the child with a URI or recent URI is to postpone elective procedures for 1 to 2 weeks for uncomplicated rhinorrhea, congestion, and nonproductive cough and for 4 to 6 weeks for patients with lower airway involvement (e.g., wheezing, productive cough). However, this may be an overly cautious and somewhat unrealistic recommendation. Normal children have an average of three to eight colds per year, and children whose mothers smoke, who live in crowded conditions, and who attend day care centers have a 61% incidence of URIs over a 2-week period (Fig. 32–1) (Fleming et al., 1987). It may be nearly impossible to find a period when the child does not have a URI or is not recovering from one. The needs of the family must be considered. Often, parents have traveled significant distances, have taken time off from work, and have made alternative child care arrangements for their other children. Because the available data do not clearly indicate a single best approach to these patients, each anesthesiologist should develop a consistent approach appropriate to the individual practice.

The following is a summary of an approach to the child with symptoms of a URI. First, many children undergo operations directed at ameliorating their chronic upper respiratory tract symptoms. In cases such as myringotomy with tube placement, tonsillectomy, adenoidectomy, and cleft palate repair, the procedures are not automatically canceled or postponed unless the child's signs and symptoms are clearly "different from baseline" or clearly involve more than the upper respiratory tract. Children who undergo the procedures just listed have a high incidence of upper respiratory tract symptoms and may always have manifestations consistent with URI. Most parents will honestly state whether their child is more congested than usual.

Elective surgeries other than those cited previously are postponed if any of the following are present: "croupy" cough; rectal temperature greater than 38°C associated with any URI sign or symptom; malaise or decreased appetite; any evidence or recent history of lower respiratory tract involvement such as rales, wheezes, productive cough, or abnormal chest radiograph (Box 32–5). Laboratory and radiographic tests are usually not helpful in the decision-making process, although some investigators recommend obtaining a chest radiograph and a white blood cell count to evaluate the child with a URI. The white blood cell count is neither sensitive nor specific in identifying URI, and chest radiography associated with a normal auscultative examination is unlikely to identify abnormalities (Brill et al., 1973). The presence of rales or wheezes should lead to a postponement of elective surgery, regardless of the findings on the chest radiograph. A suggested algorithm for making decisions about proceeding with surgery is presented in Figure 32–2.

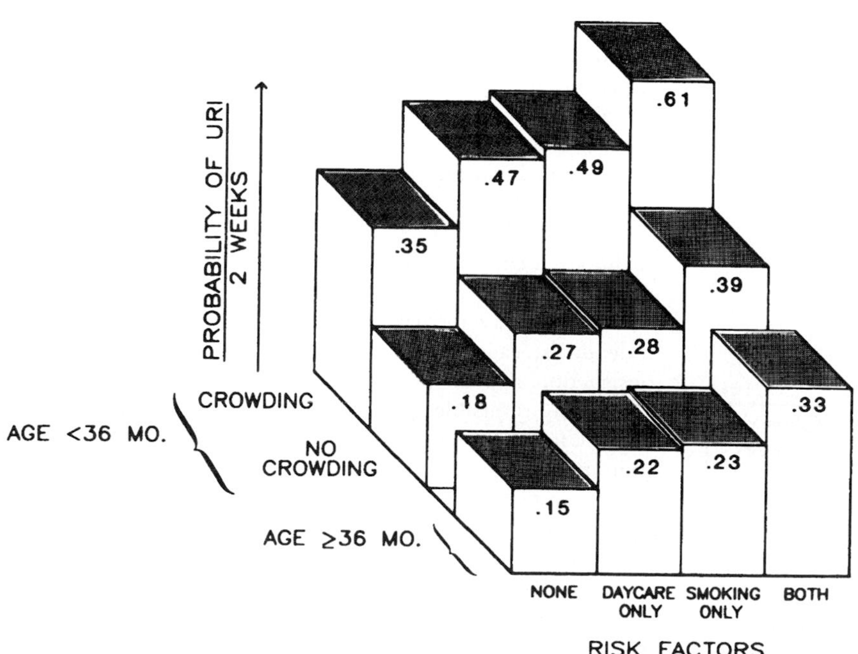

■ **FIGURE 32–1.** Probability of upper respiratory tract infection according to age, crowding, maternal smoking, and day care status. (From Fleming DW, Cochi SL, Hightower AW, et al.: Childhood upper respiratory tract infections: To what degree is incidence affected by day-care attendance? *Pediatrics* 79:55, 1987.)

BOX 32–5 Signs and Symptoms of Upper Respiratory Tract Infections

1. Mild sore or scratchy throat*
2. Mild malaise
3. Sneezing
4. Rhinorrhea
5. Nasal congestion or stuffiness
6. Nonproductive cough
7. Fever greater than 101°F (38°C)
8. Laryngitis

*To diagnose an upper respiratory tract infection, two of any of the signs or symptoms are required. If 1 and 2, 3 and 4, or 5 and 6 are combined, one additional sign or symptom is required.

Adapted from Tait AR, Knight PR: The effects of general anesthesia on upper respiratory tract infections in children. *Anesthesiology* 67:930, 1987a.

Anesthetic Management

Several major principles of anesthetic management can be suggested in dealing with children with an acute or recent URI (Tait and Malviya, 2005). These are especially important in anesthetizing children when surgery is urgent and cannot be delayed. In elective situations, it is best to avoid intubation if possible (if the surgical procedure allows), instead using regional anesthesia or general anesthesia by mask or laryngeal mask airway (LMA). A randomized, prospective study demonstrated a much lower incidence of bronchospasm in children with URI managed with LMA rather than ETT (0% versus 12.2%) (Tait et al., 1998). The incidence of all respiratory complications was reduced by 50% for the LMA group (19% versus 35%). LMA may be an excellent alternative for airway management for patients with URI if the planned surgical procedure and NPO status are compatible with its use. If intubation is indicated, it should be accomplished when the patient is at a deep plane of anesthesia using an endotracheal tube at least one size (0.5 cm) smaller than age would determine. Any intravenous induction agent is acceptable, with the most important guiding principle being that enough should be given to achieve a deep level of anesthesia. An alternative is mask induction of inhalation anesthesia with sevoflurane, nitrous oxide, and oxygen. If the procedure is expected to be prolonged, heated humidification should be used, because use of dry gas may lead to inspissation of secretions. Adjunctive agents such as intravenous lidocaine (1 mg/kg) or opioid, or both, decrease airway reflexes (Hirshman, 1983). The preoperative use of anticholinergic agents (i.e., atropine and glycopyrrolate) theoretically may block muscarinic receptors, thereby interrupting the airway reflex arc (Jacoby and Hirshman, 1991). Their properties as antisialagogues may be helpful. These agents have not been shown to be beneficial in prospective studies. The use of glucocorticoids experimentally has decreased viral associated tachykinin-induced airway edema formation (Piedimonte et al., 1990), although glucocorticoids are not routinely prescribed in this clinical situation, in contrast to their use in the patient with RAD. If intubation is necessary, tracheal suction of URI-associated secretions after intubation and before extubation may decrease the chance of atelectasis and mucus plugging, although this has not been studied.

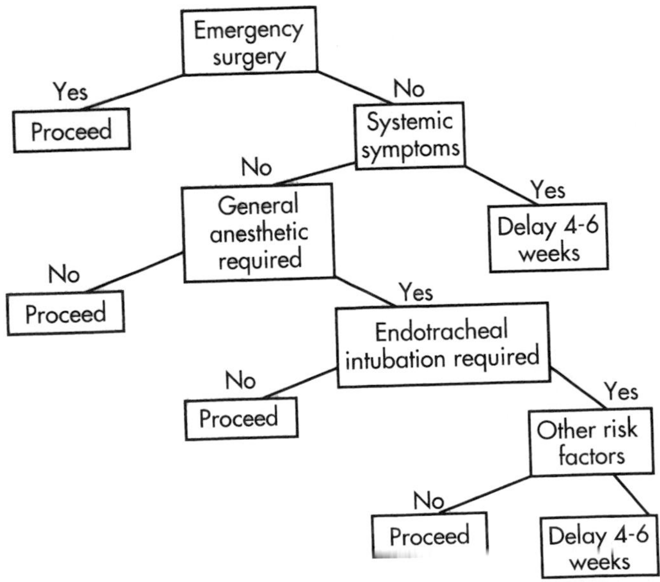

FIGURE 32–2. Algorithm for clinical decision-making for patients with upper respiratory tract infection. (From Martin LD: Anesthetic implications of an upper respiratory tract infection in children. *Pediatr Clin North Am* 41:121, 1994.)

Management of children with URI requires a logical approach. When this issue arises in the preoperative period, the patient, parents, surgeon, and anesthesiologist must participate in an informed fashion in the decision-making process. However, "in the final analysis, the name of the game is clinical judgment and a degree of good fortune" (Berry, 1990).

REACTIVE AIRWAYS DISEASE

Reactive Airway Disease (RAD), or asthma, is the most common chronic disease of childhood in industrialized countries. It has received wide public attention in recent years because of increases in morbidity and mortality. Asthma is the major cause of restricted activity, absence from school, and hospital admission in children, and it is responsible for significant health care costs in the United States (Newacheck and Halfon, 2000). The prevalence of asthma among children is greater than among adults, and it has increased by an average of 4.3% each year between 1980 and 1996 (Akinbami and Schoendorf, 2002). Beginning in 1997, the survey questions used to determine the prevalence of asthma were changed, which resulted in a slightly lower prevalence than in previous years, but the increasing trend has remained constant (Measuring childhood asthma, 2000).

Etiologic Factors and Pathophysiology

Asthma is a chronic inflammatory disorder of airways in which many cell types play a role, including mast cells and eosinophils. These cells release mediators of inflammation that, in susceptible individuals, cause symptoms associated with variable airway obstruction and airway hyperreactivity, which is partially or completely reversible spontaneously or with appropriate treatment. Understanding the important role of inflammation in the immunopathogenesis of asthma in recent years has changed the focus to a newer therapeutic approach using antiinflammatory agents. Among the immune regulatory pathways involved in the pathogenesis of asthma, two cytokines, interleukin-4 and interferon-γ, appear to be important in controlling IgE production. In asthmatic individuals, mast cells and eosinophils are attracted to airways and release cytokines and lipid mediators

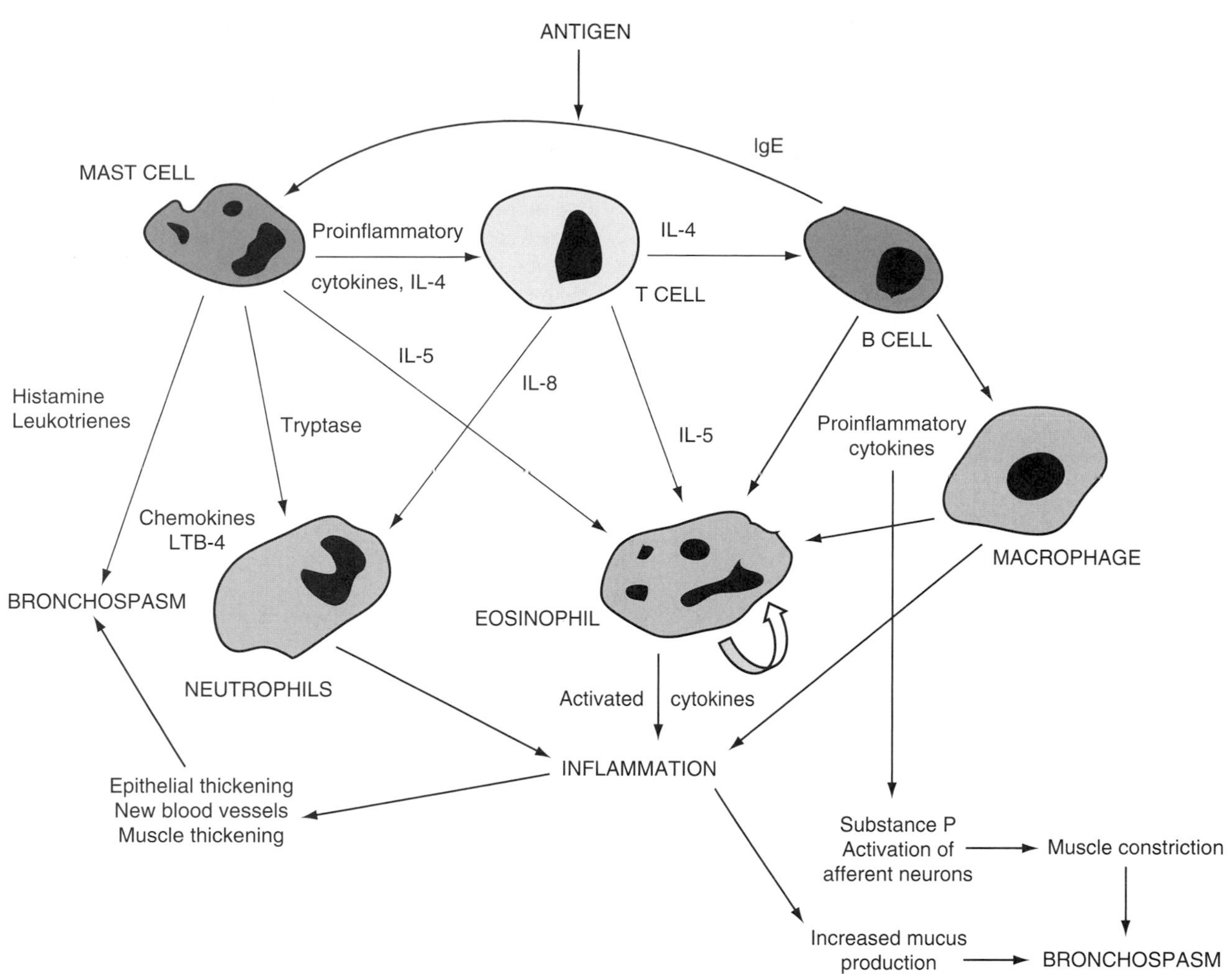

FIGURE 32–3. Pathophysiology of asthma.

that cause inflammation (Goldstein et al., 1994). The interplay of allergen/irritant, mast cells, eosinophils and their mediators, and the end effects on pulmonary vessels and airways is depicted in Figure 32–3. Airway obstruction in asthma results from a combination of several factors, including airway smooth muscle spasm, airway mucosal edema, hypersecretion, and mucus plugging of small bronchi and bronchioles (Djukanovic et al., 1990). These changes result in airway obstruction, increased work of breathing, uneven distribution of ventilation, and, in severe disease, air trapping, hyperinflation, and ventilation-perfusion imbalance, which leads to hypoxemia, diaphragmatic fatigue, hypercapnia, and respiratory failure.

There is a strong association between asthma and allergy. Up to 90% of children with frequent wheezing respond positively to bronchoconstrictor challenge, especially when associated with atopy (Clough et al., 1991). There is an increased prevalence of asthma among first-degree relatives of asthmatic subjects; over two thirds of children with asthma appear to have a familial predisposition (Clifford et al., 1989). Various environmental factors precipitate airway hyperreactivity and trigger asthma.

The onset of asthmatic symptoms is often associated with viral lower respiratory tract infection, particularly respiratory syncytial virus (RSV) infection in infants and children (Rooney and Williams, 1971). Severe viral bronchiolitis in infancy is significantly associated with the subsequent development of airway hyperreactivity and asthma, although familial factors cannot be ruled out (Rooney and Williams, 1971; Gurwitz et al., 1981). The development of IgE antibody to the RSV may play an important role in inducing an allergic response to the virus (Welliver et al., 1989). Children who experience respiratory failure and mechanical ventilation during infancy and early childhood, such as those with bronchopulmonary dysplasia (BPD), neonatal repair of congenital diaphragmatic hernia, or severe viral bronchiolitis, develop and sustain airway hyperreactivity even without a family history of asthma (Mallory et al., 1989; Nakayama et al., 1991). Prematurity alone may be associated with a higher incidence of asthma in preadolescent children (von Mutius et al., 1993). The primary site of airway obstruction and hyperreactivity in children with a history of neonatal respiratory failure appears to be in relatively small airways. This is in contrast to relatively large central airway obstruction and hyperreactivity in those with typical allergic (i.e., IgE antibody–mediated) asthma (Mallory et al., 1991).

In children with RAD, parental smoking (passive smoking) increases the incidence of severity of symptoms and exacerbates airway hyperreactivity (Soussan et al., 2003). Intrauterine exposure to maternal smoking also increases the incidence of airway hyperresponsiveness in infants (Singh et al., 2003). Infants with gastroesophageal reflux and chronic esophagitis often develop

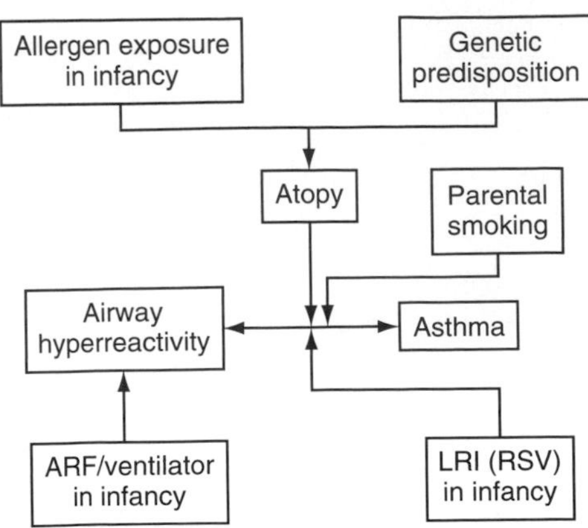

■ **FIGURE 32–4.** Contributing factors to the development of reactive airways disease. ARF, acute renal failure; LRI, lower respiratory tract infection; RSV, respiratory syncytial virus.

airway hyperresponsiveness with or without chronic aspiration and resultant tracheobronchial inflammation (Sheikh et al., 1999). Causative factors responsible for the development of airway hyperreactivity and asthma are listed in Figure 32–4.

Precipitating Factors for Reactive Airways Disease

Viral lower respiratory infections, particularly those due to RSV and influenza, sensitize airways and provoke airway hyperreactivity even in nonasthmatic, nonallergic individuals for as long as 6 weeks (Empey et al., 1976). Exposure to dry, cold air can precipitate tracheobronchial constriction in asthmatic subjects, presumably in response to reduced tracheal temperature caused by evaporative heat loss (Gilbert et al., 1988). The same mechanism appears to be responsible for exercise-induced bronchospasm and precipitation of asthma with excitement, anxiety, and hyperventilation (McFadden and Gilbert, 1994).

The period before and during the induction of anesthesia is uniquely suited to trigger bronchospasm in susceptible individuals because of the patient's emotional stress, fear, and excitement. There is resultant hyperventilation with mouth breathing of dry anesthetic gas mixtures, airway irritation by volatile anesthetics, and mechanical stimulation of the pharyngeal and laryngeal mucosa by laryngoscopy and endotracheal tube (Box 32–6).

> BOX 32–6 **Precipitating Factors for Bronchospasm**
>
> Lower respiratory tract infection (adenovirus, respiratory syncytial virus)
> Irritants (cigarette smoke, inhaled anesthetics)
> Allergens (inhaled)
> Emotional stress; fear and excitement
> Exercise, hyperventilation
> Cold or dry gas (anesthetic gases without humidification)
> Manipulation or mechanical stimulation of pharynx and larynx
> Gastroesophageal reflux

Pharmacologic Agents for Asthma

The pharmacologic management of asthma consists of bronchodilators and antiinflammatory drugs and includes six different classes of drugs: β-adrenergic agonists, leukotriene inhibitors, methylxanthines, anticholinergics, cromolyn (or nedocromil), and corticosteroids. Initial treatment for asthma most commonly consists of inhaled corticosteroids and β-adrenergic agonists, with inhaled corticosteroids often being the first line drugs. Other first, line alternatives are cromolyn (or nedocromil) or, increasingly, leukotriene receptor antagonists (zafirlukast, montelukast) and leukotriene synthesis (5-lipoxygenase) inhibitors (zileuton). Montelukast (Singulair) has been used widely in children. Drugs in common use in children are listed in Table 32–9. Theophylline has reentered the treatment algorithm if patients have exacerbations despite inhaled corticosteroids and β-adrenergic agonists. Oral corticosteroids in brief high-dose pulses are reserved for patients with moderate to severe asthma unresponsive to combinations of the other drugs (Stempel, 2003).

β_2-Adrenergic Agonists

β_2-Adrenergic agonists initiate their action on the receptor sites of airway smooth muscle cells and increase adenylate cyclase activity, which produces cyclic adenosine monophosphate (cAMP) from adenosine triphosphate (ATP) and results in smooth muscle relaxation and bronchodilation.

β_2-agonists are the most potent bronchodilators available and are the drugs of choice for the treatment of acute exacerbation in mild asthmatics, for maintenance therapy in more severe RAD, and for the prevention of exercise-induced bronchoconstriction. The recommended doses of commonly used β_2-agonists are listed in Table 32–9.

Methylxanthines

Methylxanthines (e.g., theophylline) produce bronchodilation by inhibiting adenosine-induced bronchoconstriction in asthmatic patients rather than, as was formerly thought, competitively inhibiting phosphodiesterase, which metabolizes cAMP (Holgate et al., 1984). Although theophylline was the mainstay of pediatric asthma therapy in the 1970s and 1980s, it is no longer used for therapy in acute exacerbations of RAD (Rooklin, 1989). Theophylline still has a role in decreasing the severity of persistent bronchospasm, especially that which occurs at night. Theophylline has a narrow therapeutic index with greatest efficacy at serum levels of from 5 to 15 mcg/mL. Levels greater than 20 mcg/mL are associated with symptoms of toxicity, such as nausea, irritability, learning difficulties in children, and headache (Creer and Gustafson, 1989). Vomiting, tachyarrhythmias, and seizures can occur at higher levels. The great variability of drug metabolism and the necessity for monitoring of blood levels is one reason the use of theophylline has declined (Drugs for asthma, 2002).

Anticholinergics

Ipratropium bromide is an atropine derivative and is available as a metered-dose inhaler and as a nebulizable solution. Ipratropium has a slower onset of action than β_2-agonists, but the duration of action is longer (up to 8 hours). Side effects are uncommon.

Cromolyn Sodium and Nedocromil Sodium

Cromolyn sodium does not have a bronchodilator effect and, therefore, is exclusively a prophylactic agent and has no bearing on anesthetic practice. It attenuates bronchoconstriction caused

■ **TABLE 32–9.** Drugs for asthma

Drug	Formulation	Dosage
Antiinflammatory Drugs		
Inhaled Corticosteroids		
Beclomethasone dipropionate (Vanceril)	MDI, 42 mcg/puff	2 to 4 puffs bid
Budesonide (Pulmicort)	DPI, 200 mcg/inhalation	1 to 2 inhalations bid
Flunisolide (AeroBid)	MDI, 250 mcg/puff	2 puffs bid
Fluticasone propionate (Flovent)	MDI, 44, 110, or 220 mcg/puff	1 to 2 puffs bid (max, 440 mcg/day)
(Flovent Rotadisk)	DPI, 50 mcg/inhalation	1 inhalation bid
Triamcinolone acetonide	MDI, 100 mcg/puff; DPI, 50 mcg/inhalation	2 to 4 puffs or inhalations bid
Oral Corticosteroids		
Prednisone or prednisolone (Prelone, Pediapred)	Oral tablets, 1, 2.5, 5, 10, or 20 mg Oral liquid, 1 mg/mL	Acute: 1 mg/kg qd or bid × 5 to 14d Chronic: 0.25 to 2 mg/kg qod Preoperative: 1 mg/kg/day × 3 days Max 60 mg/day
Leukotriene Modifiers		
Montelukast (Singulair)	Oral granules/chewable tablets, 4 or 5 mg	12 mo to 5 yr: 4 mg qd 6 to 14 yr: 5 mg qd
Zafirlukast (Accolate)	Tablets, 20 mg	10 mg bid
Cromolyn (Intal)	Spinhaler (DPI), 20 mg/capsule	1 capsule tid
Nedocromil (Tilade)	MDI, 1.75 mg/puff	2 to 4 puffs bid
Bronchodilators		
β_2-Agonists (inhaled or enteral)	MDI, 90 mcg/puff	2 puffs q 4 to 6 hr prn
Albuterol (Proventil, Ventolin)	Rotacaps (DPI), 200 mcg/capsule	
	Nebulized solution, 0.83 mg/mL; 0.63 or	1 to 2 inhalations prn
	1.25 mg/3 mL; 5 mg/mL	0.1 to 0.15 mg/kg prn
Levalbuterol (Xopenex)	Nebulized solution, 0.31 or 0.63 mg/mL	0.31 to 0.63 mg prn
Pirbuterol (Maxair)	MDI, 200 mcg/puff	2 puffs prn
Terbutaline (Bricanyl, Turbuhaler)	DPI, 50 mcg/inhalation	1 puff q 4 to 6 hr prn
Metaproterenol (Alupent)	MDI, 200 mcg/puff	1 puff prn
Salmeterol (Serevent)	MDI, 21 mcg/puff	1 to 2 puffs bid
Methylxanthines		
Theophylline	Oral solution, 90mg/5 mL Tablet (immediate release), 100 mg Capsule (sustained release), 125, 200, or 300 mg	10 mg/kg/day Max 16 mg/kg/day (>1 yr) Max 5 mg/kg/day + 0.2 (age in weeks) (<1 yr)
Anticholinergics		
Ipratropium bromide (Atrovent)	MDI, 20 mcg/puff	1 to 2 puffs qid (3 to 14 yr) 2 puffs qid (>14 yr)

DPI, dry powder inhaler; MDI, metered-dose inhaler.
Adapted from Drugs for asthma. *Treat Guidel Med Lett* 1:7, 2002.

by allergen, exercise, and bronchial challenge (Stempel, 2003). Nedocromil sodium has similar chemical and biologic properties to cromolyn, which became available in the early 1990s (Van Bever and Stevens, 1992). Cromolyn and nedocromil are thought to act on pulmonary mast cells and stabilize cell membranes. They reduce IgE antibody-induced release of inflammatory mediators, including histamine and leukotrienes, from activated mast cells (Douglas, 1985). Maintenance therapy with cromolyn or nedocromil is recommended in children with moderate to severe asthma.

Leukotriene-Modifying Drugs

Leukotriene-receptor antagonists and leukotriene synthesis inhibitors are a class of drugs recently developed for the prevention and treatment of bronchial asthma. The formation of leukotrienes through the 5-lipoxygenase pathway depends on lipoxygenation of arachidonic acid, a major constituent of cell membrane phospholipids, detached by phospholipase A_2 activity. Leukotrienes (LTs) are potent bronchial smooth muscle constrictors; on the molecular basis, LTC_4 and LTD_4 are approximately 1000 times more potent than histamine (Undem and Lichtenstein, 2001). Bronchial smooth muscle constriction by leukotrienes is considered a major cause of asthmatic symptoms. Leukotriene-receptor antagonists (e.g., zafirlukast, montelukast) are selective high-affinity LT1 receptor antagonists (Jones et al., 1995). Leukotriene synthesis inhibitors, such as zileuton, inhibit the formation of LTC_4, LTD_4, and LTB_4, a potent chemotactic autocoid, and other eicosanoids that depend on LTA_4 synthesis (Undem and Lichtenstein, 2001). Montelukast has been reported to be effective as maintenance therapy in children with moderate to severe asthma with or without concomitant steroid therapy with minimal side effects (Knorr et al., 2001; Phipatanakul et al., 2003).

Corticosteroids

Inhaled corticosteroids have become popular for the treatment of asthma because of their potent antiinflammatory effect on the airways with limited systemic effects compared with oral steroids. Regular use of an inhaled corticosteroid allows effective control of symptoms and improvement in lung function, reduces airway inflammation, and results in a gradual reduction in airway hyperreactivity (Konig, 1988; Juniper et al., 1991). Recommended doses of inhaled corticosteroids generally have minimal effects on the HPA axis (Barnes and Pedersen, 1993); however, high doses, especially of fluticasone (Flovent), have resulted in reduction of cortisol levels and symptomatic adrenal insufficiency in children (Drake et al., 2002; Eid et al., 2002). Oral or parenteral corticosteroids are most effective for acute exacerbations of asthma unresponsive to maximal bronchodilator therapy (Chapman et al., 1991).

Preanesthetic Considerations

The goal of the preoperative assessment of children with asthma is to ensure that each patient receives optimal treatment before reaching the operating room. The patient's history, physical examination, and laboratory tests are all helpful to determine if the patient's condition is adequately managed. Children with RAD rarely require preoperative pulmonary function testing, but they are commonly monitored by pulmonology or allergy and immunology services with frequent assessment of pulmonary function testing (i.e., spirometry with flow-volume curves). Some families use the peak expiratory flow rate (PEFR) for home assessment. If this is so, the family should be queried to ensure that PEFR is maximized.

Careful history taking is the single most important element of the preoperative evaluation of asthmatic children. The profile of a typical acute episode, precipitating factors, and time of the most recent episode of asthma should be obtained. Previous and current drug therapy, dosage, effectiveness, and side effects, if any, should also be documented. Specific points of importance in the history include the following:

1. Determine if the child has had episodes of bronchospasm and bronchodilator treatment in the previous 4 to 6 weeks. Ideally, elective surgery should be postponed for at least 4 to 6 weeks after an episode of symptomatic asthma because airway hyperreactivity may be worsened after acute exacerbations, and pulmonary gas exchange may still be impaired because of bronchoconstriction, mucosal edema, and mucus plugs.
2. Determine if there is a recent history of a URI or if the symptoms of URI still exist. A URI in children with RAD is frequently associated with the exacerbation of bronchospasm and requires a more conservative approach than in nonasthmatic children. Optimally the child with a history of RAD should be free of URI symptoms for 4 to 6 weeks before an elective procedure, unless the URI symptoms recur so frequently that an asymptomatic period is difficult to attain. If the child has had a lower respiratory infection, such as influenza, within the past 6 weeks, the postponement of scheduled surgery should be seriously considered because airway hyperreactivity would be exaggerated as long as 6 weeks even in nonasthmatic patients.
3. Ascertain the child's steroid requirements over the past year and the possible need for perioperative stress-dose steroid coverage (see preceding discussion). Children who often have bronchospasm that is poorly controlled with maximal therapy and require frequent courses of oral steroids may benefit from a short preoperative course of prednisone (1 mg/kg/day to a maximum of 60 mg once daily for 3 days, including the day of surgery), especially if endotracheal intubation is planned.

Physical examination should be focused on careful auscultation of the chest for clinical evidence of bronchoconstriction: expiratory wheezing; use of the accessory muscles of respiration; and a prolonged expiratory phase. During severe episodes of bronchospasm, air movement may become so limited that wheezing may be barely audible. Patients with a history of BPD and asthma are most likely to have lower airway obstruction and small airway hyperreactivity; wheezing and rhonchi may not be present.

Anesthetic Management

The anesthesiologist must get to know the asthmatic child and his or her parents and gain their confidence to minimize the child's anxiety before anesthesia induction. The child should be well sedated to avoid struggle and hyperventilation, which can provoke "exercise-induced" asthma. Midazolam, which may be administered transmucosally (oral, nasal, rectal) in infants and young children and orally or intravenously (if intravenous access present) in older children, works well for sedation. A β_2-adrenergic agonist may be given prophylactically using a metered-dose inhaler or nebulizer before induction (see Table 32–9). Otherwise, the drug can be given after the induction of anesthesia through the endotracheal tube using the metered-dose inhaler and an aerosol chamber inserted in between the ET tube adapter and the anesthesia circuit.

The preanesthetic level of oxygen saturation should be obtained with a pulse oximeter while the child is breathing room air to determine the baseline oxygen saturation and to look for any preexisting hypoxemia. This information is exceptionally valuable for the postoperative assessment of lung function and gas exchange.

The anesthetic approach is similar to that for children with a URI. After applying standard monitors (a minimum of a pulse oximeter and precordial stethoscope if the child resists), the inhalation induction should be smooth and progress swiftly with sevoflurane and nitrous oxide (see Chapter 9, Pediatric Anesthesia Equipment and Monitoring). For infants and young children, heated humidification should be used; the dry gas mixture from the anesthesia machine is a perfect environment for provocation of bronchospasm in an asthmatic child as a result of irritation and reduced tracheal temperature from evaporative heat loss of the tracheal mucosa (McFadden and Gilbert, 1994).

For intravenous induction, propofol may be a better agent of choice than thiopental because it suppresses airway reflexes compared with barbiturates (Brown et al., 1992), although thiopental, despite risk of histamine release, is not necessarily contraindicated in patients with asthma (Gal, 1994). Propofol may also produce bronchodilation in patients with other types of airway disease (Conti et al., 1993). Regardless of the drug chosen, it is important to give sufficiently large intravenous doses to blunt the response and to start adding sevoflurane before the peak effect of the intravenous agent is lost.

Whenever possible, endotracheal intubation should be avoided in asthmatic patients because the endotracheal tube stimulates large airway irritant receptors and can trigger bronchospasm (Hirshman, 1983). When no contraindications exist, a laryngeal mask airway is a good choice for patients with RAD, as its use avoids the laryngeal and tracheal stimulation of intubation (Groudine et al., 1995). It may also be prudent to avoid anesthetic agents that might release histamine (e.g., atracurium, morphine), although there is little clinical evidence that such drugs actually cause intraoperative bronchospasm.

An anesthetic technique using a volatile anesthetic may be preferable to a balanced technique (i.e., nitrous oxide, opioid, and a muscle relaxant) for asthmatic patients because of the salutary bronchodilating properties of volatile agents. Regional anesthesia can be combined with inhalation anesthesia with sevoflurane, halothane, or isoflurane.

Intraoperative Wheezing

The differential diagnosis of intraoperative wheezing includes "light anesthesia," kinked endotracheal tube, mainstem bronchial intubation, increased airway secretions, airway foreign body, pulmonary edema, embolus, and aspiration. In the child with RAD, wheezing can result from exacerbation of airway hyperreactivity and requires immediate attention. The treatment of intraoperative bronchospasm is detailed in Box 32–7. Treatment should begin after chest auscultation to confirm that there are bilateral breath sounds, and therefore no mainstem intubation. The first step includes increasing the inhaled concentration of oxygen and deepening the level of anesthesia with volatile anesthetics, or administering intravenous ketamine (0.5 to 2.0 mg/kg), a known bronchodilator (Corssen et al., 1972; Hirshman et al., 1979). Lidocaine (1 mg/kg) may also be given intravenously to reduce airway reactivity at the earliest sign of bronchospasm. Administration of muscle relaxant and suctioning of the ETT may be performed if the patient is intubated. The second step consists of the administration of β_2 agonists given by a metered-dose inhaler and a nebulizer chamber through the endotracheal tube followed by squeezing the anesthesia bag manually to provide a vital capacity maneuver to distribute the bronchodilator mist to the tracheobronchial tree. This maneuver should be repeated two to three times. If the nebulization chamber is not readily available, 4 to 8 puffs of a β_2 -agonist may be administered through the endotracheal tube, because only 5% to 10% of the administered dose may reach the end of the endotracheal tube and contact the airway. Parasympatholytic agents (atropine, 0.02 to 0.03 mg/kg) or antihistamines (Benadryl, 0.5 mg/kg) are indicated when wheezing is associated with increased vagal tone or histamine release, respectively. The development of hypotension and urticaria or flushing should lead to the consideration of anaphylaxis. Corticosteroids (e.g., 2 mg/kg of intravenous hydrocortisone) should be given and circulation supported with appropriate vasoactive agents (see Chapter 18, Anesthesia for Pediatric Neurosurgery).

BOX 32–7 Treatment of Intraoperative Bronchospasm

- Confirm the diagnosis (exclude main stem bronchus intubation, mucus plug, pneumothorax, anaphylaxis, congestive heart failure).
- Deepen anesthesia with a volatile agent.
- Administer inhaled β-agonists and ipratropium.
- Consider propofol or ketamine to further deepen anesthesia.
- Consider intravenous lidocaine or atropine, or both.
- Administer an intravenous corticosteroid.
- Modify ventilation to avoid stacking breaths, gas trapping, and barotrauma.

Techniques of Extubation

At the conclusion of surgery and anesthesia, the asthmatic patient can be extubated "deep" or "awake" to avoid laryngospasm. Upper airway obstruction caused by soft tissue collapse in the pharynx is the major disadvantage of deep extubation. Deep extubation can be accomplished safely provided the maintenance of upper airway patency was satisfactory during the induction of anesthesia before intubation and there are no excessive secretions or blood in the airway. If maintaining airway patency was difficult during induction, the patient may become obstructed during the time of emergence from anesthesia. If this was the case, airway patency may be facilitated by prophylactic placement of an oropharyngeal or nasopharyngeal airway, well lubricated with lidocaine jelly when the patient is still deeply anesthetized. Successful deep extubation is facilitated by the achievement of spontaneous breathing before attempted extubation.

For a successful "awake" extubation, prophylactic treatment with the inhalation of a β_2-agonist must be given even if a dose was previously given during or after the induction of anesthesia. Tracheal suction of any secretions before emergence may decrease coughing due to migration of mucus plugs. Lidocaine (1 mg/kg) given intravenously on emergence is helpful in minimizing tracheal stimulation as the patient awakens. The use of intravenous atropine (0.02 mg/kg), given for its vagolytic and bronchodilator effects, may be an additional safety precaution before extubation.

BRONCHOPULMONARY DYSPLASIA

BPD is a chronic disease of lung parenchyma and small airways with chronic respiratory insufficiency in prematurely born infants (see Chapter 16, Anesthesia for Neonates and Premature Infants). As originally described by Northway and others (1967), BPD developed after a period of acute and subacute ventilator-induced lung injury and oxygen toxicity, in prematurely born infants with severe respiratory distress syndrome (Hazinski, 1990). Although Northway's original series involved infants born at a mean gestational age of 34 weeks, all of whom had received excessive concentrations of oxygen during mechanical ventilation with a primitive ventilator by modern standards, over time, BPD has been seen in infants who had prolonged barotrauma (or volutrauma) in the absence of "excessive" oxygen. Early series were characterized by a high incidence of mortality with persistent respiratory symptoms and oxygen requirement beyond 4 weeks of age. Chest radiographs were abnormal and characterized by hyperinflation of the lungs with focal areas of increased density. They called this condition *bronchopulmonary dysplasia* to "emphasize the involvement of all the tissues of the lungs in the pathologic process" (Northway et al., 1967; Northway, 2001). The incidence of BPD has not decreased over the past 2 decades despite improved neonatal intensive care, probably because of the survival of more infants who are premature. However, the clinical picture has changed with the advent of antenatal steroids, the use of surfactant therapy, and advances in ventilatory strategies for reducing volutrauma and ventilator-induced lung injury, including noninvasive techniques. Most infants who develop BPD are born at 24 to 28 weeks' gestation and rarely are older than 32 weeks' gestation (Hazinski, 1990), whereas the mean gestational age of Northway's original series was 34 weeks. Due to these changes in neonatal intensive care and affected patient population, many aspects of BPD have changed, including the definition, theories of pathogenesis, pathology, and clinical picture (Jobe and Ikegami, 2000; Jobe and Bancalari, 2001).

Infants with BPD today are likely to have a minimal respiratory distress syndrome that does not progress after surfactant administration. The reason for prolonged ventilation in these very premature infants is more frequently apnea or poor respiratory effort, which may be related to immaturity of central respiratory control mechanisms. These infants rarely require the high airway pressures and high oxygen concentration that led to the "old" BPD. This newer clinical picture had been referred to as chronic lung disease or new BPD, but it is now simply called BPD. The current definition of BPD is oxygen dependence at 36 weeks postconceptual age (with a total duration of oxygen therapy of more than 28 days) in infants with birth weights between 500 and 1500 g. Prevalence varies between 67% in the smallest weight group to 1% in the largest (Bancalari et al., 2003).

Pathogenesis

In the past, the development of BPD was associated with a condition that caused respiratory failure in the neonatal period (e.g., prematurity with respiratory distress syndrome, meconium aspiration syndrome, congenital diaphragmatic hernia). Mechanical ventilation with high concentrations of oxygen (i.e., an acute insult to immature lungs) was employed, usually lasting more than 1 week. Oxygen free radicals, which are not well handled by an immature antioxidant host-defense system in the neonatal lungs, can cause direct cellular injury (Ackerman, 1994). Although much lower concentrations of oxygen are now used than in the past, even room air (21% oxygen) is relatively hyperoxic for a premature infant whose in utero Po_2 is less than 30 mm Hg (Hazinski, 1990). Excessive hydration and patent ductus arteriosus with increased pulmonary fluid have been recognized as additional important factors contributing to the development of BPD (Gerhardt and Bancalari, 1980; Van Marter et al., 1992). The current theory of the mechanism of injury in BPD also emphasizes the role of infection and inflammation (Gonzalez et al., 1996; Sadeghi et al., 1998). Recurrent bacterial or viral infections in these infants may cause persistent alveolitis, which worsens alveolar and airway damage (Rojas et al., 1995; Hannaford et al., 1999). Multiple markers of inflammation (e.g., lipid mediators, proteases, oxygen free radicals, cytokines) are elevated (Groneck et al., 1994; Pierce and Bancalari, 1995). Nutritional deficiencies may also play a role (Sosenko et al., 2000).

Immature, inflamed lungs with decreased compliance are most susceptible to high-volume trauma (i.e., volutrauma) and low-volume trauma (i.e., shear stress trauma) with marked distortion and distension of terminal bronchioles at high positive pressures (Hazinski, 1990). In earlier pathologic examination in lungs of infants dying with BPD, peribronchiolar fibrosis and smooth muscle thickening were seen. This has also been found in animal models exposed to prolonged positive pressure ventilation and hyperdistention (Coalson et al., 1999). The pathology now seen in extremely premature infants reflects the very immature state of their pulmonary parenchyma, with enlarged and simplified alveolar structure and a reduced number of capillaries, which are dysmorphic in appearance. Fibroproliferation may still occur but is more variable. Changes in larger blood vessels are less prominent with less indication of pulmonary hypertension than seen in "old BPD." Airway smooth muscle hyperplasia may still occur but is more variable (Coalson, 2000). After this damage has occurred to immature lungs, infants may require prolonged mechanical ventilation and high oxygen concentration for weeks or months, despite having not required high oxygen concentrations in the first few weeks of life. Although less common than with "old BPD," progressive respiratory failure with associated pulmonary hypertension with or without *cor pulmonale* may follow.

Even after the perinatal period, RAD persists in infants with BPD. Mallory and others (1991) studied lung function in infants with moderate to severe BPD longitudinally during the first 4 years of life with the forced deflation technique and found that airway hyperresponsiveness or hyperreactivity continued to be present in all children studied. They postulated that airway hyperreactivity is an important etiologic factor for the pathogenesis of lower airway obstruction in BPD.

Preanesthetic Considerations

Most infants with moderate to severe BPD remain oxygen dependent, with or without continuous positive airway pressure, or ventilator dependent beyond 4 weeks of age. They have persistent lower airway obstruction and airway hyperreactivity (Mallory et al., 1991). Tachypnea and dyspnea may be intermittently or chronically present. Growth failure because of chronic hypoxia despite oxygen therapy and *cor pulmonale* associated with pulmonary hypertension may occur (Hazinski, 1990). Wheezing may or may not be present on auscultation because the site of airway hyperreactivity is primarily in the periphery of the lungs. The chest wall may appear hyperinflated or flat (Edwards and Hilston, 1987). In addition to lower airway obstruction primarily involving small airways, infants who were intubated for prolonged periods sometimes develop large airway disease such as subglottic stenosis (which may or may not be recognized), tracheomalacia, and bronchomalacia (Miller et al., 1987; McCubbin et al., 1989). A later study also found a greater degree of upper airway obstruction in children with a history of BPD compared with age-matched children with asthma (Sadeghi et al., 1998).

Infants with mild forms of BPD improve with age and may become asymptomatic, but airway hyperreactivity may persist. Parents of the infant may not be aware of the history of BPD even when their child received prolonged mechanical ventilation as a neonate. It is appropriate, therefore, to assume that a child has or had BPD and has RAD if he or she was born prematurely and was mechanically ventilated for more than 1 week during the neonatal period. Inguinal hernia is often present in infants with BPD, probably as the result of prematurity and continually increased abdominal pressure resulting from airway obstruction and increased inspiratory effort. Prematurely born infants may require postoperative admission for monitoring because they have an increased risk of postoperative apnea, as discussed in Chapters 2 (Respiratory Physiology) and 16 (Anesthesia for Neonates and Premature Infants).

As with asthmatic patients, careful history taking is of utmost importance before anesthetizing an infant with BPD or a history of BPD. These patients may have failure to thrive (a sign of chronic hypoxia), worsening of symptoms, or even respiratory failure with lower respiratory tract infection. The patient may be taking β_2-agonists or other treatments for asthma. Other medications may include diuretics. A family history of allergy and asthma is significant because premature birth may be linked to smooth muscle hyperresponsiveness and asthma (Bertland et al., 1985).

Relatively common surgical conditions in infants and children with BPD or a history of BPD include inguinal hernia, direct laryngoscopy and bronchoscopy for subglottic stenosis, and surgical procedures of the larynx for the complications of prolonged intubation or tracheostomy (e.g., excision of granuloma, laryngotracheoplasty).

Anesthetic Management

Anesthetic management of infants and children with BPD or a history of BPD is similar to those with asthma. Before anesthetizing the child with a history of BPD, it is imperative to obtain a baseline oxygen saturation measurement with a pulse oximeter (SpO_2), although a normal oxygen saturation level does not necessarily guarantee the absence of lung dysfunction. Many infants and young children with a history of BPD maintain remarkably good SpO_2 values, presumably because of hypoxic pulmonary vasoconstriction (HPV). The infant with BPD with near normal SpO_2 in room air may develop marked desaturation after induction with halothane or sevoflurane, presumably due to a loss of HPV under general anesthesia, although HPV in healthy human volunteers may be insignificant (Benumof, 1994). If this occurs, oxygen saturation may be maintained better with intravenous techniques using opioids and propofol. Prophylactic treatment with a β_2-adrenergic agonist by a metered-dose inhaler may be beneficial for patients with possible airway hyperreactivity to prevent perioperative bronchoconstriction. For intubating a child with a history of mechanical ventilation, it is prudent to start with an endotracheal tube one size (0.5 mm inner diameter) smaller than the appropriate size for the age for subglottic narrowing, which may be the result of prolonged intubation. If rapid sequence intubation is required due to fasting violation or intestinal obstruction, desaturation may be rapid when apnea occurs, and gentle ventilation by mask with maintenance of cricoid pressure may be necessary to maintain saturation if intubation is not rapidly accomplished.

CYSTIC FIBROSIS

Cystic fibrosis (CF), an autosomal recessive disorder, is the most common lethal inherited disorder among whites (Wood et al., 1976). In the United States, the gene frequency (heterozygotes) in whites is about 1 in 25; it is uncommon among Hispanics (1 in 46) and African Americans (1 in 65) and lowest among Asians and Native Americans (1 in 90). The disease incidence among whites is approximately 1 in 2500 live births. With early diagnosis and aggressive treatment over the past 40 years, the mean survival of a CF patient has increased to 31 years by 2000.

In 1985, Tsui and others localized the gene responsible for the manifestation of CF to 250 kilobases on the long arm of chromosome 7 (Kerem et al., 1989). The deletion of three base pairs removing a phenylalanine residue at position 508 (d508) from a 1480–amino acid protein called *cystic fibrosis transmembrane conductance regulator*, a cAMP-dependent chloride ion channel, accounts for approximately 70% of CF chromosome abnormalities (Cystic Fibrosis Genetic Analysis Consortium, 1990). The remaining cases are accounted for by more than 700 mutations (Mickle and Cutting, 1998), of which 20 account for most of the remaining 30% of cases.

Pathogenesis

The disease is characterized by exocrine gland dysfunction resulting in chronic pulmonary disease, pancreatic dysfunction, and abnormalities in electrolyte reabsorption in the sweat duct with increases in sweat sodium and chloride concentrations and electrolyte imbalance. CF patients have sweat chloride levels in excess of 60 mEq/L (normal < 40 mEq/L) as measured by pilocarpine iontophoresis. In addition to pulmonary disease, other significant clinical manifestations of CF include those listed in Table 32–10.

TABLE 32–10. Organ system involvement in cystic fibrosis

Organ System	Incidence (%)
Pulmonary	
Pneumothorax due to bleb rupture	5 to 8
Obstructive lung disease	>90%
Ear, nose, and throat	
Pansinusitis	90 to100
Nasal polyps	20
Gastrointestinal	
Pancreatic enzyme deficiency	85 to 90
Diabetes, second-degree pancreatic failure	15
Intestinal	
Meconium ileus (newborn)	7 to 20
Distal intestinal obstruction syndrome (includes intussusception)	10 to 30
Rectal prolapse	20
Gastroesophageal reflux disease	50
Hepatic	
Liver failure	5 to 20
Coagulopathy due to vitamin K deficiency	100 if untreated

Pulmonary disease is the most common cause of death. Enhanced absorption of sodium across the airway epithelium and failure to secrete chloride and fluid toward the airway lumen is thought to lead to dehydration and thickening of airway mucus and abnormal mucociliary clearance. The patients are initially colonized with Haemophilus influenzae and then by *Staphylococcus aureus*, and eventually by the mucoid variant of *Pseudomonas aeruginosa*. Colonization with Aspergillus and atypical mycobacteria may occur. The chronic infection in the periphery of the tracheobronchial tree results in bronchiolitis, which may lead to airway hyperresponsiveness, bronchiectasis, lobar or segmental atelectasis, and pneumothorax. Hemoptysis, and eventually *cor pulmonale* and respiratory failure, ensues (Aitken and Fiel, 1993).

Small airways obstruction, hyperinflation, and ventilation-perfusion imbalance are the most common and important pulmonary changes in children with moderate to severe CF. The early signs of lung dysfunction include a reduction in maximum expiratory flow rates at low lung volumes (e.g., FEF_{25-75}, FEF_{50}, FEF_{75}) and an increase in residual volume to total lung capacity (RV/TLC) ratio (see Chapter 2, Respiratory Physiology in Infants and Children). Airway hyperreactivity is often present, probably in response to airway inflammation. Some patients have good response to bronchodilators but others have inconsistent or even paradoxical responses, sometimes worsening airway function because of the relaxation of airway smooth muscles and resultant increases in airway collapsibility (Pattishall, 1990).

Treatment

Patients with CF take multiple medications, including pancreatic enzyme replacement. Patients with a prominent bronchospastic component will be on β_2-agonist therapy. They frequently take inhaled or oral antibiotics for prophylaxis or treatment of pulmonary infection. Patients infected with *Pseudomonas aeruginosa* frequently take aerosolized tobramycin, which, when administered on an every-other-month basis, has been shown to preserve pulmonary function and reduce hospitalization (Ramsey et al., 1999). Patients with infectious exacerbations are treated with intravenous antibiotics in hospital or at home. Chest physiotherapy several times a day is a mainstay of CF treatment. Inhaled mucolytics (*N*-acetylcysteine-Mucomyst) have long been used to decrease the viscosity of pulmonary secretions, but there is little in the literature documenting its efficacy (Duijvestijn and Brand, 1999). Pulmozyme (i.e., human recombinant DNase), which dissolves DNA released from neutrophils, has improved pulmonary function and reduced the frequency of infection (Fuchs et al., 1994).

Preanesthetic Considerations

Common surgical indications in infants and children with CF are listed in Table 32–11. Management of children with CF is a challenge to the anesthesiologist. These patients are often frail and malnourished. Decreased plasma albumin levels may affect anesthetic potency. Intravascular volume may be diminished because of chronic diarrhea, poor oral intake, and diuretic therapy. Electrolyte imbalance may result from excessive chloride and sodium losses. Pulmonary function ranges from near normal without airway obstruction to severe obstruction, air trapping, hypoxemia, and hypercapnia. Copious secretions and resultant ventilation-perfusion imbalance may prolong mask induction with volatile anesthetics. Nasal polyps may block the nasal airway completely during mask induction. Secretions may irritate the larynx and precipitate laryngospasm. Pathophysiologic considerations in patients with CF that may affect anesthetic management are listed in Table 32–12.

The preoperative evaluation should include the assessment of pulmonary function by history, physical examination, and pulmonary function testing. The pulmonary function testing should include lung volume measurements and response to bronchodilators. An increase in TLC and the RV/TLC ratio with decreased vital capacity indicates the presence of hyperinflation and air trapping. Lower airway obstruction with small airway involvement is demonstrated when FEF_{25-75}, FEF_{50}, and especially FEF_{75} are markedly decreased from predicted values. A preoperative chest radiograph is needed in patients with moderate to severe pulmonary disease. Preoperative oxygen saturation should be obtained by means of pulse oximetry in room air for postoperative comparison. Recent tracheal culture results should be reviewed as a guide to choice of perioperative antibiotic therapy. In patients with significant lower airway obstruction and air trapping, preoperative arterial blood gas measurement is recommended to assess the degree of hypoxemia more accurately and to evaluate acid-base status and the presence of hypercapnia. In those with long-standing hypoxemia, pulmonary hypertension and *cor pulmonale* should be suspected. These patients should have preoperative electrocardiography and echocardiography to evaluate myocardial function and reserve. Blood sugar, liver function tests, and coagulation studies may be indicated.

The child with CF and his or her family are exceedingly knowledgeable regarding the pathogenesis and treatment of the disease. A lack of knowledge of CF in general and of the patient's past history and present conditions in particular at the time of the preoperative visit could quickly undermine the confidence of the family in the anesthesiologist. More importantly, the CF patient is often petrified by the thought of death under anesthesia. It is therefore prudent for the anesthesiologist to gain the patient's and his or her parents' confidence and administer preoperative sedation, such as oral benzodiazepine (Lamberty and Rubin, 1985). Opioid premedication should be avoided in severe cases because of possible respiratory depression and hypoxemia.

TABLE 32–11. Surgical indications for patients with cystic fibrosis

Conditions	Typical Age Range
Meconium ileus or equivalent	1 day to 3 years
Nasal polyps or sinusitis	10 to 18 years
Other procedures	10 to 18 years
Bronchoscopy	
Feeding gastrostomy; port-A-Cath or	
PICC venous access	
Lobectomy; thoracoplasty or thoracoscopy	
Organ transplantation (double lungs; heart-lungs)	

PICC, peripherally inserted central catheter.

TABLE 32–12. Pathophysiology of cystic fibrosis: Effect on anesthetic management

Pathophysiology	Possible Outcome
Pulmonary dysfunction	
Airway obstruction	Prolonged mask induction
V/Q imbalance	Prolonged mask induction
Copious secretions	Laryngospasm, bronchospasm
Airway hyperreactivity	Laryngospasm, bronchospasm
Nasal polyps	Upper airway obstruction
Gastrointestinal and hepatobiliary disorders	Upper airway obstruction
Decreased serum albumin levels	Increased drug potency
Coagulopathies	Increased bleeding
Diabetes or glucose intolerance	Hyperglycemia, acidosis
Abnormal sweat gland function	Electrolyte imbalance
Cor pulmonale	Hemodynamic instability; arrhythmia

Anesthetic Management

Because of copious secretions in affected patients, it is preferable to schedule surgery later in the day to allow enough time for ambulation and chest physiotherapy in the morning to facilitate expectoration of secretions retained overnight. The baseline oxygen saturation in room air is measured with a pulse oximeter before administering oxygen and anesthetics.

In patients with significant pulmonary involvement, intravenous access should be established before the induction of anesthesia because of prolonged mask induction and possible nasal obstruction from nasal polyps. An anticholinergic may be given during induction. Concern about excessive drying of secretions is unfounded because atropine decreases secretions without changes in viscosity and has not been a significant problem in clinical practice (Lamberty and Rubin, 1985). Intravenous propofol may be preferred to thiopental because it is less irritating to the upper airways and actually causes bronchodilation. Ketamine, despite its bronchodilating properties, is relatively contraindicated because it tends to increase secretions and may cause laryngospasm. Fifty percent of children with CF have gastroesophageal reflux disease (GERD) and may require rapid sequence intubation. Inhalation induction is usually satisfactory in young children with mild lung disease. Anesthetic gases should be heated and humidified to prevent irritation of the upper airways and laryngospasm, and to avoid drying and inspissation of secretions. Nitrous oxide should be avoided in patients with suspected or pulmonary function test-proven trapped gas volume to prevent its expansion and the potential danger of bleb rupture.

Endotracheal intubation with muscle relaxation is mandatory in patients with severe respiratory involvement, although the anesthesiologist should be exceedingly careful not to hyperdistend already air-trapped lungs. When a nondepolarizing muscle relaxant is chosen, the effect of aminoglycoside antibiotics to prolong the duration of action of such drugs must be kept in mind and monitoring of train-of-four used to guide relaxant administration. It is also mandatory to carefully monitor end-tidal pCO_2 to prevent hyperventilation and maintain preoperative arterial pCO_2 levels, which may be elevated. Sudden hypocapnia in a chronic hypercapnic patient can be disruptive of the patient's ventilatory control mechanisms, increasing the chance that the patient might require postoperative ventilation. After intubation, tracheobronchial suction should be performed and repeated at intervals throughout surgery and before extubation to improve pulmonary gas exchange. Although the use of an LMA might be an option for short cases, disadvantages include inability to suction secretions, obstruction of the LMA "grate" by thick secretions, risk of laryngospasm, and risk of aspiration in patients with GERD. Intraoperatively, glucose should be monitored in patients with glucose intolerance. Care should be taken to conserve heat in these patients with reduced body fat.

Regional anesthesia should be considered whenever applicable. Although regional anesthetic techniques without general anesthesia might be useful in some situations, these techniques should be carefully considered in children with severe pulmonary disease. Depression of abdominal and intercostal muscle function by thoracic levels of spinal or epidural anesthesia may not be tolerated. Pediatricians and pulmonologists often request regional anesthesia instead of general anesthesia because of fear that severely afflicted CF patients will not tolerate general anesthesia or may become ventilator dependent after endotracheal intubation. However, most of these sick CF patients, dyspneic or orthopneic with hypercapnia and oxygen dependence, may not tolerate even a short surgical intervention, such as central venous catheter or MediPort insertion, with local anesthesia and sedation. Instead, general endotracheal anesthesia with an inhaled agent, supplemented by caudal, lumbar, or thoracic epidural anesthesia for abdominal or thoracic procedures, is much better tolerated, safer, and provides good operative conditions, rapid emergence, and a pain-free postoperative state (Dalens et al., 1986). If epidural anesthesia is to be used, coagulopathy should be ruled out, and the appropriate concentration of local anesthetic drugs chosen to minimize motor block. Continuous caudal or epidural anesthesia with local anesthetic with or without carefully chosen doses of an opioid provides prolonged postoperative pain relief and facilitates coughing and deep breathing after upper abdominal or thoracic procedures. If regional anesthesia is not appropriate, judicious use of inhalation agents and short-acting opioids and wound infiltration with local anesthetic by the surgeon should facilitate early extubation, which is desirable in most cases. After surgeries without a high risk of postoperative bleeding, the use of NSAIDs may be effective in reducing the amount of opioid needed for analgesia.

Cystic Fibrosis and Lung Transplantation

For patients with end-stage pulmonary disease, lung transplantation may be the final surgical option. In general, CF patients with an FEV_1 less than 30%, PaO_2 less than 55 mg Hg, or $PaCO_2$ more than 50 mm Hg have a 50% 2-year survival (Kerem et al., 1992) and may be candidates for lung transplantation (i.e., double-lung or heart-lung procedure). The 3-year survival rate is 60%, which is similar to that seen in non-CF patients (Sweet et al., 1997). Twenty-seven percent of lung transplant patients develop bronchiolitis obliterans, which is responsible for 64% of the late deaths. Among the survivors of lung transplantation, there has been no recurrence of CF in the transplanted lungs measured by the transepithelial potential differences (Alton et al., 1991). The management of end-stage CF patients for lung transplantation is described in Chapter 2 (Respiratory Physiology) and Chapter 28 (Anesthesia for Organ Transplantation).

CARDIOVASCULAR DISORDERS

Cardiovascular disorders are commonly encountered in the pediatric population. The baseline incidence of congenital heart disease is approximately 0.8 in 100 births, on which is superimposed an incidence of acquired heart disease. Congenital and acquired diseases have the ability to affect myocardial function, valve function, and conduction tissue, all of which can be affected by anesthetics. Anesthetic effects on vascular tone can also have a positive or negative impact on myocardial function and shunting of blood through intracardiac defects.

Patients with cardiac disease should be identified preoperatively. Although children with congenital heart disease having noncardiac surgery should generally do well with appropriate anesthetic and perioperative care, there is preliminary information that, in the aggregate, congenital cardiac disease of even a moderate degree can negatively impact mortality after noncardiac surgery (Baum et al., 2000). Certainly even hemodynamically insignificant lesions can alter perioperative management as children with such abnormalities can require perioperative antibiotics for endocarditis prophylaxis; however, not all surgical procedures or all children with cardiac disease require endocarditis prophylaxis. Recommendations are outlined in Tables 32–13 and 32–14, in Boxes 32–8 and 32–9, and on the Internet (http://www.americanheart.org/presenter.jhtml?identifier=1745).

ANESTHETIC MANAGEMENT

Although the specifics of the anesthetic management of individual cardiac problems are discussed in Chapter 17 (Anesthesia for Cardiovascular Surgery), the following general areas should be emphasized.

Preoperative Period

Prolonged preoperative fasting should be avoided in cyanotic children with significant erythrocytosis to avoid dehydration and further exaggeration of the elevated hematocrit and blood viscosity. Small infants with clinically significant heart failure and failure to thrive can have inadequate glycogen reserves and are at risk for hypoglycemia if fasted for many hours. Otherwise appropriate preoperative sedation is in no way contraindicated in children with cyanotic or acyanotic heart disease unless the child has profound heart failure. DeBock and others (1990) demonstrated that SpO_2 frequently increases with preanesthetic medication in children with cyanotic and acyanotic heart defects.

■ **TABLE 32–13.** Endocarditis prophylaxis regimens for dental, oral, respiratory tract, or esophageal procedures

Situation	Agent	Regimen
Standard general prophylaxis	Amoxicillin	50 mg/kg PO 1 hr before procedure (adults, 2 g)
Unable to take orally	Ampicillin	50 mg/kg IM or IV within 30 min of procedure (adults, 2 g)*
Allergic to penicillin	Clindamycin	20 mg/kg PO 1 hr before procedure (adults, 600 mg)
	or Cephalexin or cefadroxil	50 mg/kg PO 1 hr before procedure (adults, 2 g)
	or Azithromycin or clarithromycin	15 mg/kg PO 1 hr before procedure (adults, 500 mg)
Allergic to penicillin and unable to take orally	Clindamycin	20 mg/kg IV within 30 min of procedure (adults, 600 mg)*
	or Cefazolin	25 mg/kg IM or IV within 30 min of procedure (adults, 1 g)*

*The pediatric dose should not exceed the adult dose. It is appreciated that many children do not have intravenous access before surgery. Intravenous antibiotics should be given as soon as possible after induction and intravenous catheter placement and before the surgical incision is made.

IM, intramuscularly; IV, intravenously; PO, orally.

Adapted from Dajani AS, Taubert KA, Wilson W, et al.: Prevention of bacterial endocarditis. Recommendations by the American Heart Association. *JAMA* 277:1794, 1997.

Intraoperative Period

Although much discussion is appropriately given to the specifics of cardiac pathophysiology, most children with congenital heart disease who develop problems during anesthesia do so for primarily noncardiac reasons, particularly airway compromise. Cyanotic infants, in particular, begin with decreased oxygen saturation, and can rapidly desaturate with transient interruption in breathing, whether due to apnea or airway obstruction with failure to establish effective ventilation. Children with severe congestive failure or cyanosis will have a decreased margin of safety and will tolerate failures of respiratory or hemodynamic management poorly.

Much time is often spent discussing the effects of left to right and right to left shunts on the onset time of intravenous and volatile anesthetics. Although there are differences, they usually are so small as to be clinically irrelevant. In the absence of a complication such as loss of the airway or the development of a hypercyanotic "tet" spell in children with tetralogy of Fallot or variants, oxygen saturation in cyanotic children almost invariably increases with the induction of anesthesia (Greeley et al., 1986; Laishley et al., 1986). There are several possible reasons for this, one of the most likely being a decrease in oxygen consumption causing an increase in mixed venous oxygen saturation, and subsequently higher arterial oxygen saturation when some of this blood is shunted right to left.

Minimization of right-to-left shunting at the atrial level is primarily addressed by increasing intravascular volume. Minimizing shunt at the ventricular and great vessel levels is primarily modulated by changes in pulmonary and systemic vascular resistance. Increasing systemic resistance or decreasing pulmonary resistance will increase left to right shunting (or decrease right to left shunting) and vice versa.

Nitrous oxide is a mild myocardial depressant. In adult patients, it can increase pulmonary vascular resistance (PVR), particularly in patients in whom PVR is already elevated (Schulte-Sasse et al., 1982). In children, however, no significant increase in PVR has been observed with 50% nitrous oxide regardless of the preexisting PVR (Hickey et al., 1986).

Cyanotic patients and patients with elevated central venous pressure, in particular, are at risk for increased perioperative blood loss and require adequate intravenous access. Not only do all cyanotic patients require that intravenous catheters be kept clear of air bubbles to avoid systemic air emboli, but there can also be small amounts of right-to-left shunting during the cardiac cycle even with lesions thought of as left-to-right shunting lesions. Therefore, all intravenous catheters and tubings need to be cleared of air for all patients with shunt lesions, regardless of predominant direction of shunt flow. Stopcocks are common sites for air to be introduced inadvertently.

■ **TABLE 32–14.** Endocarditis prophylaxis regimens for genitourinary and gastrointestinal (excluding esophageal) procedures

Situation	Agents	Regimen
High-risk patients*	Ampicillin + gentamicin	Ampicillin, 50 mg/kg IM or IV, plus gentamicin, 1.5 mg/kg within 30 min of starting the procedure;† 6 hr later: ampicillin, 25 mg/kg IM or IV, or amoxicillin, 25 mg/kg PO Adults: ampicillin, 2 g, and gentamicin, 1.5 mg/kg (up to 120 mg); 6 hr later: ampicillin, 1g IM or IV, or amoxicillin, 1 g PO
High-risk patients* allergic to penicillin	Vancomycin + gentamicin	Vancomycin, 20 mg/kg by slow IV infusion, plus gentamicin, 1.5 mg/kg IM or IV, to be completed within 30 min of starting the procedure† Adults: vancomycin, 1 g, and gentamicin, 1.5 mg/kg (up to 120 mg)
Moderate-risk patients*	Amoxicillin or ampicillin	Amoxicillin, 50 mg/kg PO 1 hr before the procedure, or ampicillin, 50 mg/kg IM or IV within 30 minutes of starting the procedure† Adults: amoxicillin, 2 g, or ampicillin, 2 g
Moderate-risk patients* allergic to ampicillin or amoxicillin	Vancomycin	Vancomycin, 20 mg/kg by slow IV infusion, completed within 30 min of starting the procedure† Adults: 1 g

*See Box 32–8 for definitions of medium-risk and high-risk groups.

†The pediatric dose should not exceed the adult dose. It is appreciated that many children do not have intravenous access before surgery. Intravenous antibiotics should be given as soon as possible and before the surgical incision is made.

IM, intramuscularly; IV, intravenously; PO, orally.

Adapted from Dajani AS, Taubert KA, Wilson W, et al.: Prevention of bacterial endocarditis. Recommendations by the American Heart Association. *JAMA* 277:1794, 1997.

BOX 32–8 Cardiac Conditions Requiring Antibiotic Endocarditis Prophylaxis

Prophylaxis Recommended

Prosthetic valves (i.e., bioprosthetic and homograft)*
Previous bacterial endocarditis*
Complex cyanotic heart disease*
Systemic-pulmonary shunts (e.g., Blalock-Taussig)*
Most cardiac structural abnormalities not delineated above or below†
Acquired valve dysfunction (e.g., rheumatic)†
Hypertrophic cardiomyopathy†
Mitral valve prolapse with insufficiency†

Prophylaxis Not Required‡

Isolated secundum atrial septal defect
Surgical repair beyond 6 months without residua
- Secundum atrial septal defect
- Ventricular defect
- Patent ductus arteriosus

Mitral valve prolapse without insufficiency
Cardiac pacemaker (i.e., intravenous and epicardial)
Functional murmur

*High risk.
†Moderate risk.
‡Endocarditis risk no higher than for the general population.
(Adapted from Djinni AS, Aubert KA, Wilson W, et al.: Prevention of bacterial endocarditis. Recommendations by the American Heart Association. *JAMA* 277:1794, 1997.)

End-tidal P_{CO_2} correlates with arterial P_{CO_2} in acyanotic patients. However, in children and adults with cyanotic congenital heart disease end-tidal P_{CO_2} tends to underestimate arterial P_{CO_2} in patients with normal, decreased, or increased total pulmonary blood flow (Burrows, 1989).

BOX 32–9 Procedures for Which Endocarditis Prophylaxis Is Not Recommended

Orotracheal intubation
Injection of intraoral anesthetics
Tympanostomy tube placement
Flexible bronchoscopy with or without biopsy*
Cardiac catheterization
Endoscopy with or without biopsy* (includes transesophageal echocardiography)
Cesarean section
In the absence of infection: urethral catheterization, dilatation and curettage, uncomplicated vaginal delivery,* therapeutic abortion, sterilization procedures, insertion or removal of intrauterine devices
Cardiac catheterization
Implanted pacemakers
Incision or biopsy of surgically scrubbed skin
Circumcision

*Prophylaxis is optional in the high-risk group (see Box 32–8 for delineation of high-risk patients).
(Adapted from Djinni AS, Aubert KA, Wilson W, et al.: Prevention of bacterial endocarditis. Recommendations by the American Heart Association. *JAMA* 277:1794, 1997.)

Postoperative Period

The specific length of observation in a postanesthesia care unit depends on the patient and the surgical procedure and cannot be generalized. Patients with good hemodynamic function may undergo relatively minor noncardiac surgery on an ambulatory basis and are not automatically excluded because of their cardiac disease.

When not under anesthesia, patients with cyanotic heart disease have little increase in systemic oxygen saturation in response to supplemental oxygen. Similarly, oxygen saturation will not be markedly decreased by removing supplemental oxygen (other causes for postoperative hypoxemia being absent). Knowledge of the patient's normal preoperative range of oxygen saturation will avoid unnecessary prolongation of the PACU stay because of a fear of removing supplemental oxygen.

Hypovolemia from continued surgical blood or fluid loss postoperatively can worsen right-to-left shunting in cyanotic patients, and it should be rapidly corrected. The onset of hypovolemia can be insidious if caused by gradual oozing from surgical drains. Cyanotic patients should have hematocrit levels measured serially after surgery, especially after significant blood loss. They may require a higher than normal hematocrit level to ensure adequate oxygen delivery. In general, a level similar to the preoperative hematocrit should be maintained.

Patients with labile pulmonary arterial hypertension would particularly benefit from good postoperative analgesia. Even cyanotic patients have a normal ventilatory response to hypercarbia and respond in a normal fashion to appropriate doses of parenteral, intrathecal, or epidural opiates, and age- and weight-appropriate doses of analgesic drugs should be given. Patients who have had a Glenn or Fontan procedure (i.e., single-ventricle physiology) depend on low pulmonary vascular resistance for maintenance of adequate pulmonary blood flow. If these patients require postoperative ventilatory support, pulmonary vascular resistance should be minimized by limiting positive inspiratory pressure and by using low levels of PEEP to optimize functional residual capacity, which minimizes pulmonary vascular resistance.

THE CHILD WITH A MURMUR AND POSSIBLE HEART DISEASE

Cardiac murmurs are exceedingly common in normal children with an overall incidence of about 80%. Most of these are the somewhat inappropriately called *functional murmurs* (also called *innocent*). The incidence of functional murmurs is highest at about 3 to 4 years of age. Functional murmurs represent the sound of blood flowing through a structurally normal heart (Fig. 32–5). There is no anesthetic concern about these murmurs, other than reassurance to the family. There are several commonly recognized functional murmurs. Almost all are short, soft, and louder when supine. Most functional murmurs will become louder with increased cardiac output, as would occur with anemia, fever, exercise, or anxiety. The most common is Still's murmur. This has a very typical musical or vibratory quality and is a mid-systolic murmur heard between the mid-left sternal border and the apex. Soft pulmonary flow murmurs at the upper left sternal border are commonly heard in thin-chested older children and adolescents. The murmur is softer than true pulmonic stenosis and is unaccompanied by a systolic ejection click. Peripheral pulmonic stenosis generates an ejection murmur from the left upper sternal border to the axillae and back in neonates. It is generated by turbulent flow when blood passes

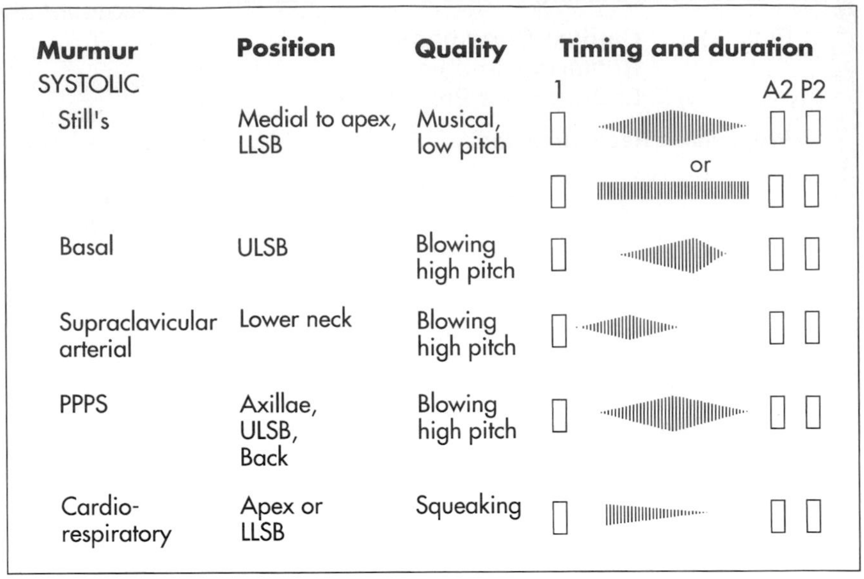

■ **FIGURE 32–5.** Description of innocent murmurs. A, aortic; LLSB, lower left sternal border; P, pulmonic; PPPS, physiologic peripheral pulmonic stenosis; ULSB, upper left sternal border; 1 and 2, first and second heart sounds. (From Hoffam JE: Cardiovascular examination. In Rudolph AM: *Rudolph's pediatrics,* 19th ed. Norwalk, CT, 1991, Appleton and Lange.)

Murmur	**Position**	**Quality**	**Timing and duration**
SYSTOLIC			1 A2 P2
Still's	Medial to apex, LLSB	Musical, low pitch	or
Basal	ULSB	Blowing high pitch	
Supraclavicular arterial	Lower neck	Blowing high pitch	
PPPS	Axillae, ULSB, Back	Blowing high pitch	
Cardio-respiratory	Apex or LLSB	Squeaking	

from the main to the branch pulmonary arteries. In the neonate, the branch pulmonary arteries, unaccustomed to accommodating large amounts of pulmonary blood flow in utero, form an acute angle with the main pulmonary artery. By about 6 months of age, the vessels remodel and the murmur disappears.

Less common innocent murmurs are the venous hum and the mammary souffle. Both of these are continuous murmurs and are exceptions to the rule that diastolic murmurs are always pathologic. The venous hum represents blood draining down the jugular into the subclavian veins. It is heard over the left or right upper chest with the patient upright. It disappears when the patient lies down, with gentle compression of the jugular vein, or with a Valsalva maneuver. The mammary souffle can be heard over the breasts of lactating women. Unlike functional murmurs, pathologic murmurs are generated by a normal amount of blood across an abnormal valve or opening, or an abnormal amount of blood passing through normal valves.

Occasionally, children arrive for a preanesthetic evaluation, and a murmur is identified for the first time. The exact method of evaluation remains somewhat controversial (Yu et al., 2002). Isolated chest radiographs and electrocardiograms are generally a poor investment (Yu et al., 2002). In any event, electrocardiograms interpreted by computer or an adult cardiologist may need to be reinterpreted using age-corrected normal values.

In general, children who are acyanotic and growing well, with a soft systolic murmur and good exercise tolerance, will tolerate anesthesia well. Signs of heart disease in infants differ somewhat from adults and older children. Perioral cyanosis can be a normal finding in neonates, especially with crying, and needs to be differentiated from central cyanosis (confirmed by pulse oximetry). Heart failure often manifests in young infants by tachypnea, diaphoresis with eating (in excess of the normal sweating of the head many infants have), and hepatomegaly. Increased pulmonary blood flow can impinge on small bronchioles, causing airway obstruction and expiratory wheezing ("cardiac asthma"). Peripheral edema due to congestive heart failure is distinctly uncommon in children. Blood pressure measurements in both arms and a leg can confirm or exclude coarctation of the aorta. When caring for children with known heart disease or a history of cardiac surgery, the child's pediatrician or cardiologist should be contacted and a copy of the most recent evaluation obtained.

■ NONCARDIAC MANIFESTATIONS OF CONGENITAL HEART DISEASE

Long-standing cyanotic and acyanotic congenital disease can have effects on the function of a variety of other organ systems. Some of these may not become clinically apparent until years after surgical correction of the underlying cardiac defect. These are summarized in Table 32–15.

■ KAWASAKI DISEASE

Originally named *mucocutaneous lymph node syndrome* after its major manifestations, Kawasaki disease is the most common cause of acquired heart disease in children in the United States. The cause has yet to be determined. In the United States, the peak incidence is between 13 and 24 months of age. Current diagnosis and therapy have been reviewed in detail (Mason and Takahashi, 1999). The acute illness is associated with fever, intense conjunctival injection, red cracked lips, lymphadenitis of the neck, and erythema of the palms and soles followed weeks later by desquamation of the fingers and toes. The most concerning feature of the disease is that it causes an infantile periarteritis nodosa-like vasculitis of medium and large arteries in 10% to 15% of children. Of particular concern is involvement of coronary arteries (Fig. 32–6) with the risk of subsequent thrombosis or, less commonly, rupture. The risk of coronary artery aneurysms is higher in infants. The acute phase of the illness can also be associated with myocarditis, usually mild, but sometimes associated with heart failure. Myocarditis is usually transient, lasting several weeks. Laboratory findings during the acute phase include elevated sedimentation rate, C-reactive protein, and thrombocytosis to more than 800,000/mm^3.

Coronary artery aneurysms will become apparent within the first two weeks of disease in about 5% of children who have been treated with intravenous injection of gamma globulin (IVIG),

■ **TABLE 32–15.** Potential noncardiac manifestations of congenital heart disease

Organ System and Manifestations	Comments
Pulmonary or Thoracic	
Decreased dynamic lung compliance	Occurs in lesions with increased pulmonary blood flow (i.e., left-to-right shunting)
	Pulmonary venous obstruction
	Can require higher airway pressure for ventilation
	Can impinge on small airways, resulting in air trapping, wheezing
Scoliosis	More common with cyanotic lesions
	Can manifest in adolescence, years after corrective cardiac surgery
Hemoptysis	Can occur in end-stage Eisenmenger syndrome (i.e., pulmonary hypertension due to prolonged excessive pulmonary blood flow)
Phrenic nerve injury	From prior surgery
	Particularly after surgery at the apices of the thorax (e.g., patent ductus arteriosus ligation, coarctation, pulmonary artery banding, Blalock-Taussig shunt)
Recurrent laryngeal nerve injury	From prior surgery or from an enlarged hypertensive pulmonary artery
Blunted ventilatory response to hypoxemia	In cyanotic patients
	Normalizes after surgical repair
	Normal ventilatory response to hypercarbia
Hematologic	
Symptomatic hyperviscosity	Occurs with hematocrit higher than about 65% (or lower if iron deficient)
	May cause neurologic symptoms
Bleeding diathesis	Abnormalities of many factors have been described in cyanotic patients, with no consistent pattern
	Elevated central venous pressure can cause increased operative bleeding, as can increased tissue vascularity with cyanotic disease (collateral blood vessel formation)
	Increased risk of bleeding with prior thoracic surgery during repeat thoracic procedures
Gallstones	Calcium bilirubinate stones from increased heme turnover in cyanotic disease
	Symptomatic years after corrective cardiac surgery
Neurologic	
Paradoxical emboli to central nervous system	Occur with right-to-left intracardiac shunts
	Occur even with a predominantly left-to-right shunt lesion
Brain abscess in patients with right-to-left shunts	Can present with seizure focus years later
Cerebral thrombosis	Polycythemia in children
Vascular	
Femoral vein complications	Thrombosis or ligation from prior cardiac catheterization
Reduced lower extremity blood pressure	Coarctation of the aorta; left arm involvement is variable
Reduced upper extremity blood pressure	With classic Blalock-Taussig anastomosis
	Stenosis of the subclavian artery after modified Blalock-Taussig anastomosis
Artifactually elevated right arm blood pressure	Supravalvar aortic stenosis (i.e., Coanda effect)

and in 20% to 25% of children who have not. Early aneurysms can resolve spontaneously or progress.

Treatment in the acute phase includes IVIG and aspirin (acetylsalicylic acid) for 4 days, followed by aspirin for 6 to 8 weeks. If IVIG therapy fails, children are at high risk for the development of coronary artery complications, which may be treatable with corticosteroids.

If coronary artery aneurysms do develop, about one half regress within 1 to 2 years, and about one fifth develop coronary stenoses. Smaller aneurysms (<8 mm in diameter) and fusiform aneurysms are more likely to regress than larger or saccular aneurysms. Larger aneurysms can develop thromboses or stenosis with subsequent ischemia, or can rupture. Rupture is rare and usually occurs within the first month or two of disease. Ischemia can develop years after the acute illness. Even if aneurysms regress, intimal proliferation can result in endothelial dysfunction (Furuyama et al., 2003). Warfarin has been used in some centers to treat children with giant aneurysms. Angioplasty has been attempted in several centers with mixed results, and surgical bypass grafting has been done on occasion for high-grade obstruction of the left main coronary artery or at least two of the major coronary arteries. Due to the young age of the patients, grafting is done with arterial rather than venous grafts (Kitamura et al., 1994).

TAKAYASU'S ARTERITIS

This vasculitis of the aorta and its major branches, sometimes known by its catchy synonym "pulseless disease," is an uncommon disease of children. However, 75% of patients begin to develop symptoms during their teenage years, and it is an important cause of hypertension in adolescents in Asia, where it is more common. It occurs eight times more often in females. Narrowing of major arteries results in limb claudication or end-organ disease. Limb blood pressures can be artifactually low or unobtainable. Early vessel inflammation is followed by fibrosis. Headaches are a common symptom. The subclavian artery is involved in 90% of cases, and two thirds involve the supradiaphragmatic and infradiaphragmatic aorta. The carotid artery, usually the left, is involved in one half of the cases. Stenoses are more common than occlusion, and occlusion is more common than aneurysm formation. There is mural inflammation and thickening. Both coronary arteries and pulmonary arteries are uncommonly affected. Initial treatment is with corticosteroids.

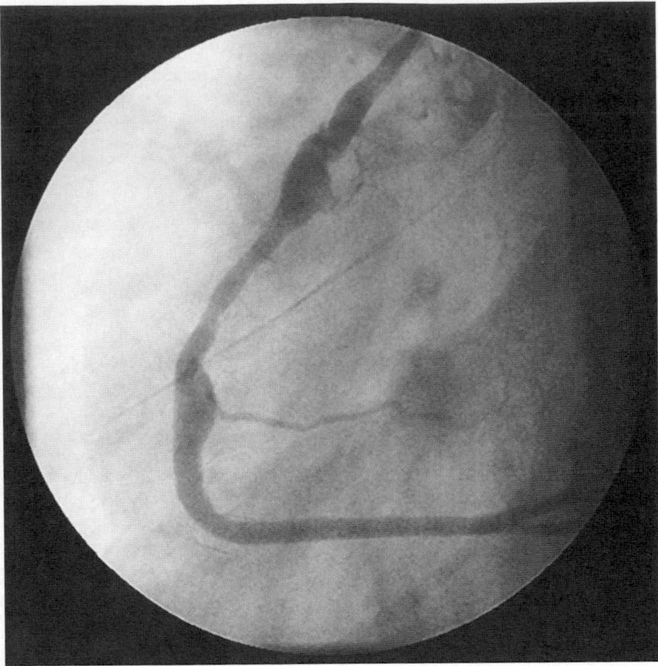

■ **FIGURE 32–6.** Large aneurysms of the left main coronary artery in a child with Kawasaki syndrome. (Courtesy of Jonathan Rome, M.D.)

Long-term therapy is often required, and cytotoxic drugs are sometimes added. After fibrosis has occurred, the treatment is stenting or surgery (Rigby et al., 2002).

■ HEMATOLOGIC-ONCOLOGIC DISORDERS

■ HEMOGLOBINOPATHIES

Hemoglobin Structure, Development, and Function

Hemoglobin (Hb) is composed of two pairs of subunits containing protoheme and globin (Box 32–10). The globin imparts the spatial structure responsible for many characteristics of hemoglobin, including oxygen affinity. The various globin chains differ in the number and sequence of amino acids and are designated by α, β, γ, δ, ε, ζ, and θ. Normal adult red blood cells (RBCs) have three types of hemoglobin: HbA ($\alpha_2\beta_2$), approximately 95%; HbA_2 ($\alpha_2\delta_2$), approximately 2.5%; and HbF ($\alpha_2\gamma_2$) (Table 32–16) (Lane, 1996). The intricate spatial relationship of the four subunits determines oxygen affinity and changes in affinity during oxygen loading and unloading, as well as physical properties such as hemoglobin solubility.

At birth, RBCs contain 70% to 90% HbF, which is predominant until 2 to 4 months of age in normal patients. β-Chain production begins before birth, and γ-chain production wanes, resulting in a normal adult profile by age 4 months. Disorders of the β chain do not manifest in the first few months and are not identified by precipitation screening tests. HbF persists in many conditions and offers a protective effect when present in many hemoglobinopathies. Some experimental interventions to treat sickle cell patients attempt to stimulate HbF production.

Hemoglobinopathies can result from production of an abnormal hemoglobin molecule or by underproduction of a given chain. The most common mechanism of the former type is the result of a single substitution of one amino acid for another on the protein chain. Underproduction of a given chain results in thalassemia.

BOX 32–10 Hemoglobinopathies: Glossary of Terms

CVA:	cerebrovascular accident
HBE:	hemoglobin A
HbA_2:	hemoglobin A_2
HBF:	hemoglobin F
HbS:	hemoglobin S
HbAS:	sickle cell trait
HBSS:	sickle cell C disease
ISC:	irreversibly sickled cell
SCD:	sickle cell disease

Sickle Cell Disease

Sickle cell disease (SCD) is an autosomal recessive inherited disease. Eight percent of the African American population of the United States are carriers (HbSA, sickle trait), and 1 in 625 has the disease (HbSS, SCD).

Sickle cell disease results from a single amino acid substitution on position 6 of the β chain (Glu → Val). The SCD patient has two normal α chains and two abnormal β chains in the S hemoglobin, which makes up roughly 90% of the hemoglobin. The remainder is HbF and HbA_2. The substituted amino acid (valine) increases the rate of polymerization (gel formation). This decreases the hemoglobin solubility. Polymerization is *increased* by increases in temperature and H^+ concentration and is *decreased* by oxygen and other non-S hemoglobin. As oxygen is unloaded, polymerization increases in a single direction, and subsequent alignment of multiple polymers results in sickling. Some sickled cells can regain normal conformation and some do not (i.e., irreversibly sickled cells). The irreversibly sickled cells are rigid, viscous, and more adherent to endothelium and result in arteriolar and capillary vaso-occlusion. This pathology results in acute crisis and in long-term chronic problems, which the anesthesiologist must consider. Table 32–16 provides information on diagnostic findings and relative severity of the spectrum various sickle variants (Lane, 1996).

Acute Crisis

Although the most important crises to consider during the perioperative period are the *vaso-occlusive* crises in the form of *acute chest syndrome* and *stroke*, the physician should also be aware of the other crises. *Acute splenic sequestration* may occur from 5 months to 2 years of age. Acute pooling of large amounts of blood results in profound anemia and shock. *Aplastic crisis* manifests as an acute decrease in RBC production, usually as a result of infection (e.g., parvovirus B19). *Hyperhemolytic crises* may result from infection or G6PD deficiency.

The *vaso-occlusive crises* are episodes of ischemia, pain, and infarctions of various organs. Those commonly seen are painful crisis (hand-foot syndrome in infancy), cerebrovascular accident (infarctive in infants and hemorrhagic in older patients), acute chest syndrome, and priapism. *Vaso-occlusive crises* occur with greater frequency during the perioperative period and prevention of these episodes is the primary goal when deciding the best transfusion and anesthetic approach.

■ **TABLE 32–16.** Common sickle cell syndromes: diagnostic testing and clinical severity

	RELATIVE CLINICAL SEVERITY				HEMOGLOBIN ELECTROPHORESIS IN OLDER CHILDREN					
Syndrome	**Genotype**	**Hemolysis**	**Vasoocclusion**	**Neonatal Screen***	**HbA (%)**	**HbS (%)**	**HbF (%)**	**HbA_2 (%)**	**HbC (%)**	**Solubility Test†**
Sickle cell anemia (HbSS)	SS	++++	++++	FS	0	80 to 95	2 to 20	<3.5	0	Positive
Sickle β^0 thalassemia‡	Sβ^0	+++	+++	FS	0	80 to 92	2 to 15	3.5 to 7	0	Positive
Sickle Hb C disease (HbSC)	SC	+	++	FSC	0	45 to 50	1 to 5	NA§	45 to 50	Positive
Sickle β^+ thalassemia‡	Sβ^+	+	+	FSA or FS‖	5 to 30	65 to 90	2 to 10	3.5 to 6	0	Positive
Sickle trait	AS	0	0	FAS	50 to 60	35 to 45	<2	<3.5	0	Positive
Normal	AA	0	0	FA	95 to 98	0	<2	<3.5	0	Negative

*Hemoglobin reported in order of quantity (e.g., FSA=F>S>A); F, fetal hemoglobin; S, sickle hemoglobin; C, hemoglobin C; A, hemoglobin A.
†False-negative results occur during infancy in all sickle syndromes.
‡β^0 Indicates thalassemia mutation with absent production of β-globin; β^+ indicates thalassemia mutation with reduced (but not absent) production of β-globin.
§Quantity of HbA_2 cannot be measured in presence of HbC.
‖Quantity of HbA at birth is sometimes insufficient for detection.
From Lane PA: Sickle cell disease. *Pediatr Clin North Am* 43:639, 1996.

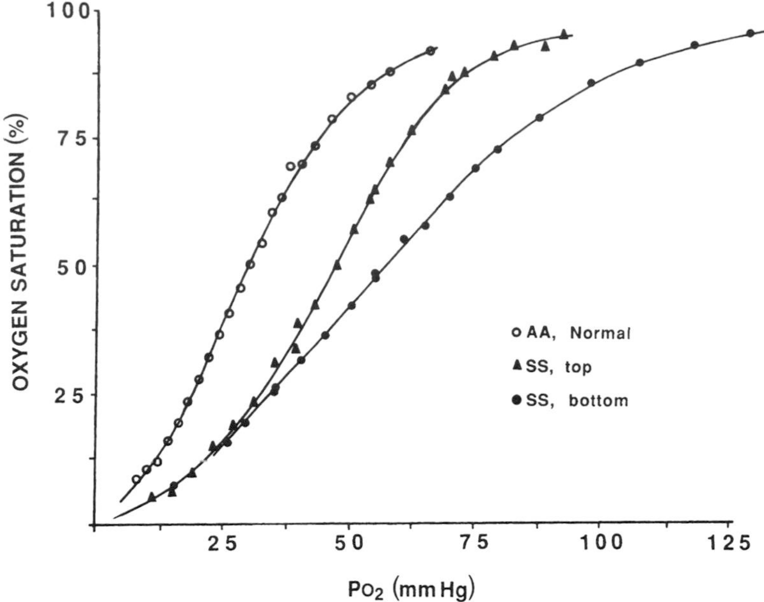

■ **FIGURE 32–7.** Oxygen hemoglobin dissociation curves from top and bottom layers of HbS red blood cells. Notice the heterogeneous nature of the P_{50} values. (From Seakins M, Gibbs WN, Milner PF, et al.: Erythrocyte Hb-S concentration. An important factor in the low oxygen affinity of blood in sickle cell anemia. *J Clin Invest* 52:422, 1973.)

Acute chest syndrome is a common and important perioperative complication of complex pathophysiology likely resulting at least in part from pulmonary vaso-occlusion due to sequestration of sickled cells in small pulmonary vessels. Symptoms of fever, tachypnea, pleuritic pain, and cough are difficult to distinguish from pneumonia and may begin as pneumonia. Infection or fat emboli may lead to vaso-occlusion and sequestration. Chest radiograph can range from normal to complete opacification but usually demonstrates a new lobar infiltrate. The mortality rate of patients with acute chest syndrome is from 2% to 12% depending on the series (Vichinsky et al., 1994, 1997). It is the second most common cause of hospitalization and accounts for 25% of deaths in sickle cell patients. Patients may rapidly develop respiratory failure and should be treated with hydration, oxygen, antibiotics, and in many cases exchange transfusion. There may be a role for inhaled nitric oxide in treating severe cases (Sullivan et al., 1999).

Chronic Problems

A lifetime of intermittent vaso-occlusion and endothelial damage results in a host of chronic problems in many patients. These include decreased growth and maturation, increased nutritional requirements, retinopathy, hearing loss, stroke, high output cardiac failure, pulmonary insufficiency, loss of renal concentrating ability, jaundice, bone and joint destruction, leg ulceration and splenic infarction (infection risk). Cardiomegaly and high output failure from anemia are common. Increased left ventricular end-diastolic volume and increased cardiac index have been reported in symptomatic children (Rees et al., 1978).

Survival of sickle cells in vivo is 5 to 15 days, compared with 120 days for RBCs containing hemoglobin A. The oxygen-dissociation curve in SCA is shifted to the right (i.e., the hemoglobin molecules' affinity for oxygen is less), and theoretically, the cells are predisposed to sickling (Bromberg et al., 1967; Milner, 1974). The cause of this rightward shift is unknown, but it is probably related to increased 2,3-diphosphoglycerate levels and to increased mean corpuscular hemoglobin concentration. Of interest is the heterogeneous nature of the P_{50} value among the cells with HbS, which varies from 27 to 42 mm Hg (Fig. 32–7).

Renal dysfunction is frequent in patients with sickle cell disease. Hematuria and hyposthenuria are hallmark findings in patients with SCA. Because sickle cell patients are unable to concentrate their urine, intravenous hydration should be started the night before surgery (Buckalew and Someren, 1974).

Neurologic impairment can be a devastating consequence of this disease. Cerebrovascular disease occurs in approximately 8% of children with sickle cell disease. Transfusion programs aimed at maintaining HbS levels at less than 30% reduce the risk of recurrent stroke from 60% to 70% to less than 10% (Lane, 1996). Evidence of a stroke or residual hemiparesis should be documented, and neuromuscular monitoring on the affected extremities should be avoided, because increased twitch responses may falsely minimize the degree of neuromuscular blockade. This can be considered to be as much an endothelial disease as an RBC disease. Every vascular bed is affected.

Anesthetic Management

Preoperative Transfusion. Surgical morbidity and mortality rates are increased for sickle cell patients. Early reviews reported mortality rates as high as 10% and complication rates as high as 50% (Holzmann et al., 1969). In later reviews, Platt and others (1994) reported some interesting statistics on mortality of patients with sickle cell disease. The perioperative mortality rate for sickle cell patients was 1.1%, clearly above that of the general population, and 7% of the deaths reviewed were surgically related. The mean age of death for sickle cell patients was 42 years.

Griffin and Buchanan (1993) reported their experience with nontransfused children with sickle cell disease having elective surgery. Although there were no intraoperative complications or perioperative deaths among 54 children undergoing 66 procedures, 26% experienced postoperative complications. They concluded that preoperative transfusion could be avoided in patients having low-risk procedures and that those having high-risk procedures (i.e., thoracotomy, laparotomy, or tonsillectomy and adenoidectomy) should receive preoperative transfusion.

The Cooperative Study of Sickle Cell Disease group observed nearly 4000 patients over a 10-year period and reported a 1.1% mortality rate when 717 patients underwent 1079 procedures (Koshy et al., 1995). This was a descriptive report without randomized comparisons, and it provided little insight about how differences in practice affect outcomes.

Because of these concerns, most anesthesiologists adopted some form of aggressive transfusion therapy for certain subgroups of patients or procedures when they thought the patients were at high risk for complications. This aggressive therapy often included a hypertransfusion protocol or acute exchange transfusion to a predetermined Hb and HbS level. Frequently, the goal of transfusion was to attain an Hb level of 9 to 10, with HbS accounting for less than 30%. Until recently, the value and consequence of such aggressive therapy was unknown.

In 1995, the results of the Preoperative Transfusion in Sickle Cell Disease Study Group were published (Vichinsky et al., 1995). This group, consisting of 36 centers, randomized 604 cases into a "simple transfusion arm" and an "aggressive transfusion arm." The former group received a simple transfusion to a hemoglobin level of 10 g/dL, and the later group received transfusions sufficient to attain an HbS level of less than or equal to 30% and a hemoglobin level of 10 g/dL (Table 32–17). Only higher-risk surgery and the existence of pulmonary disease were associated with serious complications. Most complications were in the postoperative period.

Since this study, anesthesiologists and hematologists have meaningful data on which to base transfusion guidelines. However, if a physician were to adopt a simple transfusion practice as described in this study, it would be prudent to adopt similar preoperative, intraoperative, and postoperative practice guidelines for the nontransfusional care of these patients. Each center should review the literature and adopt guidelines with guidance from the hematologists and transfusion medicine specialists in their own institution.

Sickle cell patients come to the operating room most often for cholecystectomy. Haberkern and others (1997) described the 364-patient subset of the Preoperative Transfusion in Sickle Cell Disease Study Group that was undergoing this procedure. As in the parent study, complications were similar in the aggressive versus simple transfusion. However, the nonrandomized, nontransfused group had the highest incidence of sickle cell-related complications, including a 19% incidence of acute chest syndrome. This rate was twice that of the transfused groups. This perhaps provides the most compelling data that some form of transfusion practice is prudent in patients with sickle cell disease undergoing surgery.

TABLE 32–17. Aggressive versus simple transfusion protocols for sickle cell patients

Characteristic	Aggressive Arm	Simple Arm
Hemoglobin S (HbS)	31%	59%
Hemoglobin (Hb)	11.1 g/dL	10.6 g/dL
Units transfused	5	2.5
Hospital days (for transfusion)	4	2.5
Complications	31%	35%
Transfusion-related	14%	7%
Acute chest syndrome	10%	10%
Death	1%	0

Data from Vichinsky EP, Haberkern CM, Neumayr L, et al.: The preoperative transfusion in sickle cell disease study group: A comparison of conservative and aggressive transfusion regimens in the perioperative management of sickle cell disease. *N Engl J Med* 333:206, 1995.

Recommendations for preoperative preparation for most patients include hydration and simple transfusion for correction of anemia. Very-high-risk patients, such as those with stroke or recent or frequent acute chest syndrome, will likely require a more aggressive transfusion regimen. Communication between the hematologist, anesthesiologist, and surgeon is essential to prepare these children for surgery. For patients who require transfusion, it is extremely important to keep the hemoglobin level less than 12 mg/dL to avoid potentially devastating problems, such as stroke, which may be associated with hyperviscosity.

Intraoperative Management. No particular anesthetic or technique has proved to be more or less advantageous for sickle cell disease patients. Arguments can be made for and against regional techniques for sickle cell patients. In the Cooperative Study of Sickle Cell Disease series, the non–sickle cell disease–related outcomes of fever and infection were higher in the regional group (Koshy et al., 1995). However, this group contained a large portion of obstetric patients receiving epidural anesthesia. This subpopulation is known to have a higher complication rate than other surgical groups. Some physicians suggest that the compensatory vasoconstriction in nonblocked areas, lack of control of ventilation, and potential for stasis during regional anesthesia create an environment in which sickling can occur (Scott-Conner and Brunson, 1994). Others feel that regional techniques do not create this milieu. In one series, epidural anesthesia and analgesia was successfully used to treat painful vaso-occlusive crisis (Yaster et al., 1994). Suffice it to say that the technique of anesthetic is likely much less important than the meticulous attention to detail in the areas of perioperative hydration, perfusion, oxygenation, and temperature control.

The advisability of tourniquet use in patients with sickle cell disease has been debated. Although no prospective studies have been performed to address this issue, there are several small retrospective reports touting its safety (Adu-Gyamfi et al., 1993). If one chooses to use a tourniquet, the extremity should be carefully exsanguinated before inflation. The value of administering sodium bicarbonate or creating mild respiratory alkalosis before deflation has not been critically evaluated.

Postoperative Management. Most of the serious sickle cell disease-related complications occur in the postoperative period (Holzmann et al., 1969; Goodwin, 1998), the most common of which are vaso-occlusive crises (painful crisis, acute chest syndrome, and stroke). For these reasons, it is important to comply with the regimen used by the Preoperative Transfusion in Sickle Cell Disease Study Group (Vichinsky, et al., 1995), which includes postoperative oxygen supplementation, hydration, and pulse oximeter monitoring. This has obvious implications with respect to advisability of outpatient surgery for these patients.

Myringotomy. In a later report, the Study Group compared perioperative morbidity in children having tonsillectomy, adenoidectomy, or myringotomy (Waldron et al., 1999). Most of the children having myringotomy received the same preoperative and postoperative care as described previously. There were no differences in the aggressive versus simple transfusion regimens. Four of 11 randomized, transfused patients had complications (recurrent cerebrovascular accident, 1; airway obstruction, 2; URI, 1). Of 18 nonrandomized children, 14 were not transfused. In this group, one child had a vaso-occlusive event on postoperative day 10, and one had an aplastic event on day 23. In the transfused group, a single patient had a complication of a period of bradycardia in the recovery room. Eight of 29 patients having myringotomy had at least one serious perioperative complication. Realizing that this was not specifically studied, the Study Group speculated that transfusion before myringotomy may not improve outcome. They emphasize, however, that the physician should give attention to hydration, oxygenation, and temperature control during the preoperative and postoperative period.

Sickle Trait

By definition, patients with sickle trait (HbSA) have at least 50% HbA. Under physiologic conditions, problems are rare. Intracellular polymerization begins below oxygen saturations of 85% in HbSS, but this does not occur in HbSA until saturations are below 40%. It is generally accepted that children with sickle trait do not require transfusions. However, attention to hydration, perfusion, ventilation, and temperature control is prudent.

Sickle Hemoglobin C Disease

In general, patients with HbS and HbC (HbSC or S-C disease) have less frequent and usually milder vaso-occlusive episodes. In the Preoperative Transfusion in Sickle Cell Disease Study Group, there were 92 patients with HbSC disease. This group was reported separately (Neumayr et al., 1998). Nontransfused patients undergoing intraabdominal procedures had a higher incidence of sickle cell–related complications (35%) compared with those who were transfused (0%). There were two deaths in the nontransfused group and none in the transfused group. The investigators concluded that transfusion appears to be beneficial in HbSC disease patients undergoing abdominal procedures but is not necessary in minor procedures. Because these patients are usually only mildly anemic, partial exchange transfusions may be required to keep hemoglobin levels to less than 12 mg/dL.

Thalassemia

Characteristics

Underproduction of a given chain results in thalassemia. *α-Thalassemia* represents defective α-chain production of which there are four types. The severity of the syndrome depends on how many of the four α-globulin genes are absent (one had the trait, two had mild anemia, three had thalassemia intermedia-like syndrome [HbH disease], and four were stillborn).

β-Thalassemia results from an underproduction of β chains and has 60 forms. The gene is commonly seen in countries bordering the Mediterranean Sea. Homozygotes (β^0) have a profound, transfusion-dependent anemia known as *thalassemia major, Cooley's anemia, or β-thalassemia.* However, a patient can be homozygous for a milder form (β^-) and have mild to moderate anemia (i.e., thalassemia intermedia). These patients do produce β chains but in lower amounts. Heterozygotes for β^- or β^0 (i.e., thalassemia minor) demonstrate a mild hypochromic microcytic anemia.

Anemia and problems associated with chronic anemia and frequent transfusions are the issues facing the anesthesiologist. These patients will not recover from blood loss during surgery as would otherwise be expected. Patients can be heterozygous for two disorders such as sickle cell disease and β-thalassemia. Those with sickle β^0-thalassemia have no normal HbA, and those with sickle β^--thalassemia have some normal HbA (see Table 32–16).

Screening

Many U.S. states include hemoglobin testing as part of the newborn screening blood tests. The degree to which parents are aware and understand the results is variable. Because the postoperative mortality and morbidity of SCD patients are significantly greater, many centers choose to screen patients at risk for sickle cell disease. This can be done with the newborn screen or with rapid prep tests with follow-up electrophoresis on positive prep tests to distinguish trait from disease. Ninety percent of SCD patients have some clinical manifestation by their 10th birthday.

With the completion of the Preoperative Transfusion of Sickle Cell Disease Study Group data, there are now reasonable guidelines to approach most surgical situations. It seems prudent to adopt the standard practices of preoperative hydration, intraoperative vigilance, and postoperative oxygen supplementation and oximetry monitoring, employed by the Study Group. Special circumstances of high-risk procedures and high-risk patients will continue to require careful consideration and consultation. Only through effective communication between surgery, anesthesiology, and hematology specialists will the individual unique patient considerations be appropriately managed.

ONCOLOGIC ISSUES

Epidemiology

Each year in the United States, 1 in 7000 children younger than age 20 years is diagnosed with a new cancer. Childhood cancer remains the leading cause of disease-related mortality in children 1 to 14 years old. Acute lymphoblastic leukemia and CNS tumors are the two most common types of neoplasm in children. They comprise 23.5% and 22.1%, respectively, of cancer diagnosis (Fig. 32–8). Five-year survival rates have improved dramatically over the past several decades (Fig. 32–9).

From the time a child is first diagnosed with a malignancy to the end of a successful treatment course, the anesthesiologist assumes a very important role in his or her care. Historically painful procedures such as lumbar punctures and bone marrow aspirations were performed under local anesthesia with or without sedation. This was only minimally effective in reducing pain and anxiety. Parents had to deal with the anguish and uncertainty of the cancer diagnosis and the horror of watching their children suffer through multiple painful procedures. In many centers, an anesthesiologist is present when diagnostic procedures are performed, when central venous access devices are implanted, when a tumor is removed, when the radiation treatments are performed, through all of the surveillance procedures, and when the central venous devices are removed after a cure is effected. Anesthesiologists individually and entire departments often develop close relationships with these children and their families. The anesthetic management in off-site venues and for specific malignancies is discussed in Chapter 25 (Anesthesia for Procedures Outside the Operating Room). In the following section, we review the anesthetic implications of cancer chemotherapy.

Anesthetic Implications of Cancer Chemotherapy

General Toxicity

Acute toxicities common to most agents include myelosuppression, alopecia, nausea, vomiting, mucositis, and liver dysfunction. Myelosuppression produces pancytopenia. Profoundly neutropenic

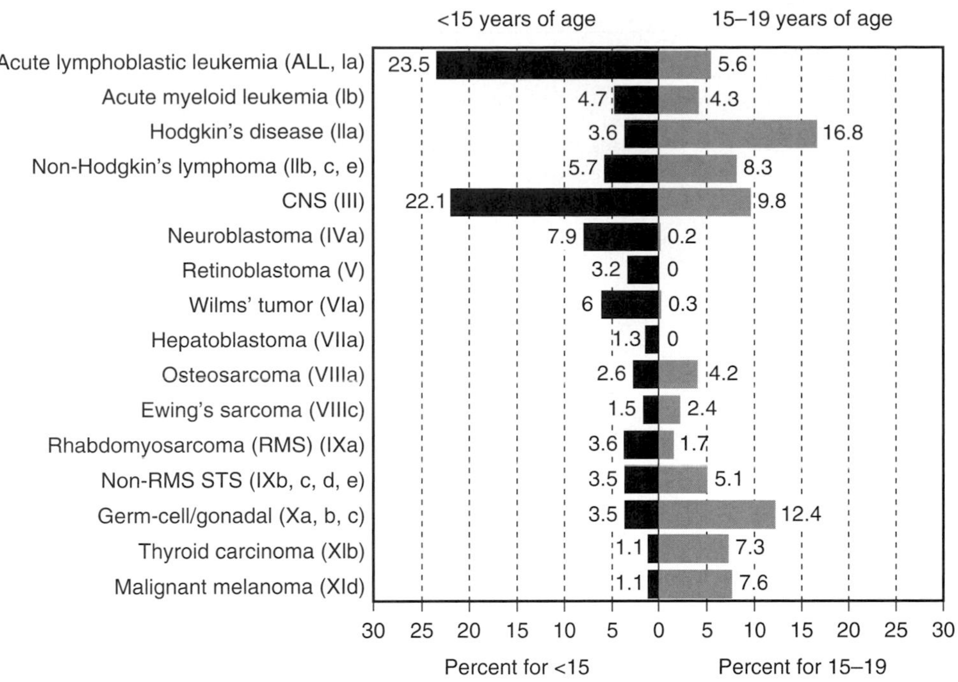

■ **FIGURE 32–8.** Distribution of specific cancer diagnosis for children (0 to 14 years) and adolescents (15 to 19 years) for 1990 to 1997. Percent distribution is given by international classification of childhood cancer diagnostic groups and subgroups for those younger than 15 to 19 years old (all races and both sexes). CNS, central nervous system; RMS, rhabdomyosarcoma; STS, soft tissue sarcoma. (Incidence data are from the Surveillance, Epidemiology and End Results program, National Cancer Institute; redrawn from Smith MA, Rloeckler Ries LA: Childhood cancer: Incidence, survival and mortality. In Pizzo PA, Poplack DG, editors: *Pediatric oncology*, 4th ed. Philadelphia, 2002, Lippincott, Williams & Wilkins, p 2.)

patients may require protective isolation. These children may be better served by avoiding the preoperative holding area and being recovered in a separate area. Rectal temperatures and medications should be avoided in neutropenic children. The need for platelet transfusion in thrombocytopenic children depends on the type of procedure and the function of the existing platelets. Neuraxial anesthesia may be contraindicated in patients with platelet counts of less than 80,000. These issues should be decided with consultation from, and in partnership with, the hematologist-oncologist before the procedure. The decision as to when and how to transfuse RBCs should also be discussed with the hematologist. RBCs may require irradiation to prevent graft-versus-host disease and should be screened for cytomegalovirus and other known viruses. Individual drugs produce unique toxicities (Table 32–18). Those that produce cardiac and pulmonary injury are of special interest to the anesthesiologist and warrant discussion.

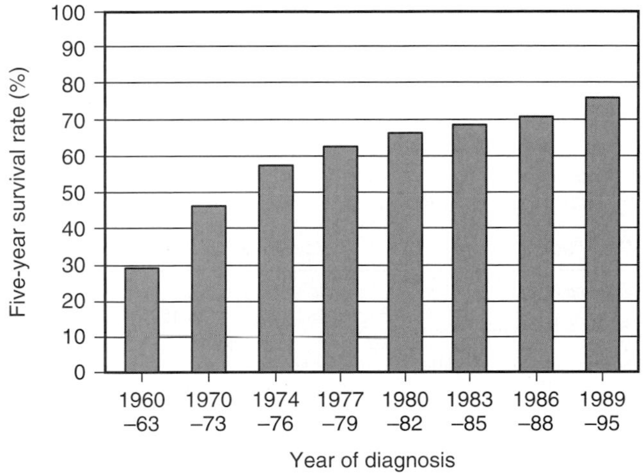

■ **FIGURE 32–9.** Five-year survival rate for all childhood cancers diagnosed between 1960 and 1995. (Data from Greenlee RT, Murray T, Bolden S, Wingo PA: Cancer statistics, 2000. *CA Cancer J Clin* 2000;50:7; redrawn from Balis FM, Holcenberg JS, Blaney SM: In Pizzo PA, Poplack DG, editors: *Pediatric oncology*, 4th ed. Philadelphia, 2002, Lippincott, Williams & Wilkins, p 238.)

Cardiac Toxicity

Several chemotherapeutic agents have cardiac toxicities that may be acute, chronic, or both. The most notorious agents for cardiac toxicity are the anthracycline agents: doxorubicin (Adriamycin), daunorubicin (Cerubidine), and idarubicin (Giantris et al., 1998; Singal and Iliskovic, 1998; Balis et al., 2002). These agents can cause acute alterations in the electrocardiogram (e.g., decreased QRS amplitude, nonspecific ST and T wave changes) and rhythm disturbances (e.g., supraventricular tachycardia, premature ventricular contraction). Another acute complication in children is a reduction in ventricular function reaching a nadir at 24 hours after administration. A rare form of this is the myocarditis-pericarditis syndrome. This can occur after one to three doses of doxorubicin and results in CHF with a variable course from complete recovery to cardiogenic shock.

Chronic toxicity may occur weeks, months (early form), and years (late form) after administration. The early form causes histopathologic changes within the myocyte, including cytoplasmic vacuolization and myofibrillary lysis, with degeneration of nuclei and mitochondria. Oxygen free radicals generated by metabolism of the drug are thought to be responsible for these changes. Myocardial dysfunction may cause congestive heart failure that is poorly responsive to inotropic medications. Its incidence correlates with cumulative dose. The incidence of congestive heart failure increases when doses exceed 450 mg/m^2 for doxorubicin and 700 mg/m^2 for daunorubicin. However, cardiac toxicity has occurred with doxorubicin doses as low as 220 mg/m^2. The cumulative toxic dose of idarubicin is not

TABLE 32–18. Toxicity of chemotherapeutic agents

Organ or System Effect	Drug Examples	Comments and Anesthetic Implications
Bone marrow suppression	All cytotoxics	Anemia, leukopenia, and thrombocytopenia occur to a variable degree
Nonthrombocytopenic bleeding	Mithramycin	Hemorrhagic pancreatitis
Lungs: fibrosis or pneumonitis	Bleomycin Mitomycin C Carmustine (BCNU) Procarbazine	Oxygen toxicity particularly associated with high doses; postoperative adult respiratory distress syndrome reported with high inspired oxygen concentrations and excessive intravenous fluids; synergistic with radiotherapy
Heart: cardiomyopathy, electrocardiographic, and echocardiographic changes	Cyclophosphamide Adriamycin Daunorubicin Epirubicin	Acute cardiomyopathy; cardiomyopathy months after therapy; echocardiographic changes may occur
	Cisplatin Mitoxantrone	Rarely cardiotoxic
Central nervous system	Ifosfamide	Corneal effects
	Fluorouracil	Cerebellar ataxia
	Vincristine Vinblastine L-Asparaginase Cisplatin Procarbazine	Encephalopathy, impaired sensorium, lethargy, convulsions, stroke, syndrome of inappropriate secretion of antidiuretic hormone (SIADH)
Peripheral nervous system: neuropathy	Vincristine, vinblastine Cisplatin, procarbazine	
Autonomic nervous system	Vincristine Vinblastine	Can lead to surgical abdominal crisis
Liver	6-Mecaptopurine Methotrexate	Common
	Streptozocin Dacarbazine	Uncommon
Kidneys	All drugs	Uric acid nephropathy at start of treatment. Prophylactic allopurinol and fluid therapy necessary
	Ifosfamide	Tubular and glomerular damage
	Vincristine Vinblastine Mithramycin	SIADH
	BCNU and CCNU	Glomerular damage, dose related
	Cisplatin	Glomerular and tubular damage, dose related; low calcium and magnesium blood levels possible
Gastrointestinal epithelium	Methotrexate Fluorouracil Bleomycin	Stomatitis, diarrhea, cachexia, mucous membrane ulceration
Skin	Bleomycin	Eruption may parallel pulmonary toxicity
	Procarbazine	Rash
Immunosuppression	Antimetabolites	Possible increased requirement for nondepolarizing relaxants
Endocrine	Alkylating agents	Inhibition of plasma cholinesterase
	Mithramycin	Possible increased apnea from suxamethonium
	Streptozocin	Electrolyte disturbances Hypoinsulinism
General	Procarbazine	MAO inhibitor effects; care with vasopressors, sedatives, narcotics; influenza symptoms can manifest

Adapted from Hain WR, Jones SEF: Diseases of blood. In Katz J, Steward DJ, editors: *Anesthesia and uncommon pediatric diseases,* 2nd ed. Philadelphia, 1993, WB Saunders, p 665.

known, but a dose of 150 mg/m² appears to be well tolerated. The risk is also increased with mediastinal irradiation (Table 32–19) (Allen, 1992). Late cardiotoxicity is more common in children and may be related to the inability of the heart to grow with the child. Although this complication was thought to occur primarily with doses of doxorubicin greater than 300 mg/m², some children suffer this complication at lower doses. Cardiac dysfunction may occur from 7 to 14 years after therapy. Children seem to have a higher incidence at lower doses than adults. Children treated with these medications should receive pretreatment echocardiograms and serial follow-up monitoring studies for many years after treatment.

Cyclophosphamide, especially in high doses (excess of 100 to 200 mg/kg) can cause severe CHF from hemorrhagic myocarditis. Cardiac tamponade from pericardial effusions has been reported with cardiotoxicity from this agent. Toxicity may occur at lower doses in children who have also received anthracyclines.

TABLE 32–19. Risk factors and effects of anthracycline cardiac toxicity

Risk Factor	Incidence and Effects
Cumulative dose	<1%: <300 mg/m² 5% to 10%: 350 to 450 mg/m² 30%: >550 mg/m²
Schedule of administration	Risk greatest with bolus administration Less risk with continuous infusion Less risk with dexrazoxane
Mediastinal irradiation	Strong association with increasing risk
Cardiac disease	Preexisting coronary artery disease, valvular heart disease, hypertension
Age	Young children Adults >70 yr

From Swafflor J, Gibbs HR: Cardiac complications of cancer treatment. *Anesthesiol Clin North Am* 16:598, 1998.

Radiation applied to thoracic tumors can result in cardiac toxicity. Early toxicity may cause pericarditis with effusion and possible tamponade. Most long-term effects occur with cumulative doses exceeding 4000 cGy, and they may not manifest for up to 10 years after treatment (Applefield et al., 1982). The dose of radiation absorbed is defined as energy expressed in units of joules deposited per kilogram (J/kg), which is denoted as gray (Gy) units. One Gy is equal to 100 rad in the old system, and 1 rad is equal to 1 cGy.

Preoperative assessment of many of these patients will include a cardiology consultation and echocardiogram in high-risk patients. Selection of induction and maintenance agents will obviously be influenced if ventricular dysfunction is present or suspected. Intraoperative fatalities have occurred in children with chemotherapy-induced cardiomyopathy in the presence of potent inhaled anesthetics (McQuillan et al., 1988). This has been most marked with halothane, because of its myocardial depressant effects on an already compromised myocardium.

Pulmonary Toxicity

Many, if not most, cancer chemotherapeutic agents cause some degree of pulmonary toxicity. Because immunosuppressed children are predisposed to lung infections, it is often difficult to sort out toxicity from infectious and toxic inflammatory processes. Because multimodal chemotherapy and radiation therapy are used to treat many forms of cancer, it is often difficult to pinpoint the specific causative agent.

Alkylating agents such as *busulfan, cyclophosphamide, melphalan,* and *chlorambucil* are associated with cytotoxic lung injury. Busulfan may cause lung injury when given as a single agent; the others do so only when given in high doses or as part of multidrug therapy. Busulfan lung injury occurs 6 weeks to 10 years after therapy with an average time interval from treatment to symptoms of 3 years. Dyspnea, fatigue, nonproductive cough, weight loss, unexplained fever, and bi-basilar reticular infiltrates are hallmarks of this complication. This pulmonary fibrosis carries a poor prognosis. Toxicity appears to be idiosyncratic and is not dose dependent.

Cytotoxic antibiotics such as *bleomycin* and its analogs, peplomycin and talisomycin S_{10}b, as well as mitomycin, an alkylating agent, have pulmonary toxicities. Bleomycin lung injury has become the prototype for interstitial pneumonitis and pulmonary fibrosis. A synergistic relationship exists between high inspired oxygen concentration and bleomycin toxicity. Although the exact mechanism is unclear, oxygen concentrations above 30% can rapidly precipitate acute lung injury and acute respiratory distress syndrome (Mathes, 1995; Maher and Daley, 1993). Mortality from this injury ranges from 13% to 83% in various studies. High dose corticosteroids may have a beneficial effect in this lung injury (Maher and Daley, 1993).

Antimetabolites such as *cytosine arabinoside (ara-C), fludarabine, methotrexate, and 6-mercaptopurine* also cause various degrees of lung injury. In general, these are dose-related toxicities and usually carry a better long-term prognosis.

Thoracic radiation causes clinically significant lung injury in 5% to 15% of patients who receive this treatment. Several phases of lung injury are described. The latent or early phase occurs within 1 to 2 months of exposure. The exudative or intermediate phase is 4 to 6 months after this; symptoms of pneumonitis develop. The late phase brings the development of pulmonary fibrosis and occurs from 6 to 12 months after exposure. Factors that influence the risks of this complication include the total dose of irradiation, volume of lung treated, and fraction size. Pulmonary toxicity has decreased significantly over the past decade because of refined techniques in radiotherapy (Hassink et al., 1993). Toxicity does not usually occur until more than 3000 cGy is delivered to more than 50% of the lung when radiation therapy alone is used in adult patients. The mechanism of injury appears to be different in children younger than 3 years, in whom interference with growth of the lung and chest wall may occur (Miller et al., 1986). In these children, restrictive lung disease has occurred with doses of 1100 to 1400 cGy.

Children who have received multimodal chemotherapy with and without thoracic radiation may be at risk for pulmonary toxicity. Preoperative assessment may include chest roentgenograms in selected patients. Determination of oxygen saturation with the patient breathing room air will identify those with intrapulmonary shunting and diffusion abnormalities. Children at risk for pulmonary toxicity should receive the minimum inspired oxygen concentration required to provide acceptable oxygen saturation values (Klein and Wilds, 1983). This vigilance should be observed in the postoperative period as well.

■ COAGULATION AND HEMOSTASIS: DEVELOPMENTAL ASPECTS, DISORDERS, AND PERIOPERATIVE MANAGEMENT

Coagulation abnormalities provide many challenges for the pediatric anesthesiologist. Children with known coagulation disorders require disease-specific perioperative management. Often the child in the operating room is to be treated for the complications of a bleeding diathesis. More challenging is the intraoperative investigation and management of children who develop coagulopathy in the operating room from preexisting but undiagnosed diseases or from acquired disorders. The following sections focus on the endogenous control of hemostasis, developmental changes in coagulation, and commonly inherited coagulopathies and their management (Box 32–11).

■ OVERVIEW OF HEMOSTASIS

The hemostatic system is designed to maintain blood in a fluid state until vessel injury occurs, at which point a rapid cascade of events is activated to terminate blood loss by sealing off the vascular defect. Hemorrhage occurs if the response is inadequate; thrombosis occurs if the response is dysregulated. The vascular endothelial cell is at the fulcrum of this delicate balance. The normal endothelial cell maintains blood in its fluid state by inhibiting platelet aggregation and blood coagulation through the production of prostacyclin, nitric oxide, and antithrombin III and by promoting fibrinolysis through the conversion of plasminogen to plasmin. Physically, the endothelial cell is a barrier between the platelets and procoagulant proteins derived from reactive components present in the deeper layers of the vessel wall. These components include collagen, fibronectin, von Willebrand factor (vWF), and tissue factor (TF), all of which stimulate platelet adhesion and aggregation and trigger the coagulation cascade.

Primary Phase of Hemostasis

The platelet is central to the primary phase of hemostasis. A graphic representation of the hemostatic mechanism is shown in Figure 32–10. The normal circulating platelet count ranges from 150,000 to 400,000/mL. An additional 33% of all platelets are sequestered within the spleen. After *vascular injury*, the

BOX 32–11 Coagulation: Glossary of Terms

ACT: activated clotting time
APC: activated protein C
aPTT: activated partial thromboplastin time
AT_{III}: antithrombin III
EACA: ε-aminocaproic acid
GPIIb/IIIa: platelet surface glycoprotein receptor IIb/IIIa
INR: international normalized ratio
PAI: plasminogen activator inhibitor
PIVKA: proteins induced in vitamin K's absence
PT: prothrombin time
rFVIIa: recombinant factor VIIa
SCIDS: severe combined immune deficiencies syndrome
TAFI: thrombin-activatable fibrinolysis inhibitor
TA-GVHD: transfusion-associated graft-versus-host disease
TEG: thromboelastography
TF: tissue factor
TFPI: tissue factor pathway inhibitor
TPA: tissue plasminogen activator
TRALI: transfusion-related acute lung injury
TXA_2: thromboxane A_2
vWF: von Willebrand factor

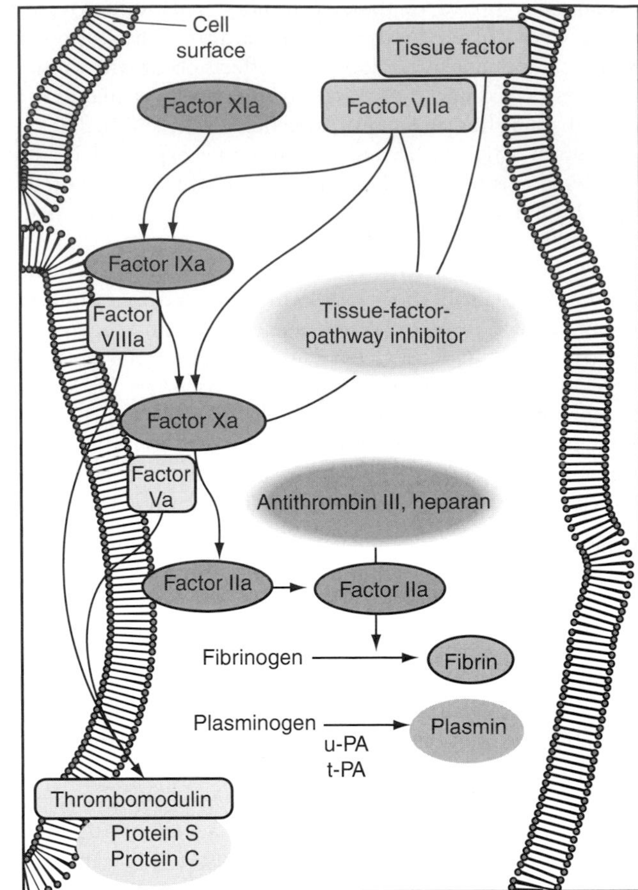

■ **FIGURE 32–10.** Regulation of coagulation. The coagulation cascade is regulated by a number of plasma proteins. The tissue-factor-pathway inhibitor forms a quaternary structure with tissue factor, factor VIIa, and factor Xa. The thrombomodulin–protein C–protein S pathway inactivates factors Va and VIIIa. Antithrombin III inactivates factors XIa, IXa, Xa, and IIa in a reaction that is accelerated by the presence of heparan sulfate. In the fibrinolytic pathway, tissue-type plasminogen activator (t-PA) and urokinase-type plasminogen activator (u-PA) convert plasminogen to plasmin. Once generated, plasmin proteolytically degrades fibrin. (Redrawn from Rosenberg RD, Aird WC: Vascular bed specific hemostasis and hypercoagulable states. *N Engl J Med* 340:1555, 1999.)

affected *vessel constricts* proximally, diverting blood flow away from the site of endothelial disruption. *Extravasated blood* is exposed to subendothelial structures and the platelets are stimulated by their exposure to collagen. The *platelets become adherent* to the subendothelial infrastructure, anchored through the binding of vWF to the platelet surface glycoprotein Ib. Once the platelet adhesion occurs, *platelet activation* results in (1) the release of platelet agonists, such as epinephrine and serotonin from the dense granules; (2) the synthesis of thromboxane A_2 by cyclooxygenase (COX) from the conversion of arachidonic acid, released from the platelet lipid membrane; and (3) a 50% increase in the number of platelets and a conformational change in the platelet surface glycoprotein receptor IIb/IIIa (GPIIb/IIIa), which binds to fibrinogen, vWF, and fibronectin (Shattil et al., 1998).

Platelet activation increases fibrinogen's affinity for the GPIIb/IIIa receptor and results in clustering of receptors on the platelet surface. *Platelet aggregation*, through the linkage of GPIIb/IIIa to the GPIIb/IIIa on other platelets by bridging fibrinogen or vWF, increases the size of the initial platelet plug, creating a mass of aggregated platelets at the site of injury. Thromboxane A_2 (TXA_2) binds to a G protein–coupled receptor on the platelet surface leading to an increase in intracellular calcium and activation of protein kinase C. TXA_2 induces aggregation of other platelets and promotes vascular smooth muscle constriction, producing local *vasoconstriction*, which limits blood loss and increases the effectiveness of the platelet plug by decreasing the effective surface area the platelet plug needs to cover. TXA_2 amplifies the platelet's responses to weak agonists such as ADP and epinephrine (Funk, 2001). The initial platelet plug is friable. It is stabilized by an increase in platelet cytosolic calcium that is mediated through platelet agonist exposure, which initiates actin filament turnover that modulates the cytoskeletal changes. These changes enable GPIIb/IIIa clustering and binding of fibrinogen and vWF. The conformational change of GPIIb/IIIa, induced by ligand binding, exposes new ligand binding sites and additional merging of receptors on the platelet surface, resulting in clot retraction (Wartlier et al., 2002).

Secondary Phase of Hemostasis

The exposure of subendothelial structures to circulating blood simultaneously activates the coagulation cascade (the secondary phase of hemostasis) to produce a cross-linked fibrin clot. Of the coagulation proteins, prothrombin (II), protein C, protein S and factors VII, IX, and X are synthesized as prozymogens and activated to serine proteases through a vitamin K–dependent hepatic enzyme (Furie and Furie, 1990). This modification is required for calcium binding, serving as a bridge for binding the factors to the phospholipid surface.

New Model of Cell-Based Coagulation

In earlier schemes, the coagulation cascade had been divided into intrinsic (e.g., XII, XI, IX, VIII) and extrinsic pathways (e.g., TF, factor VII). This traditional scheme is depicted in Figure 32–11.

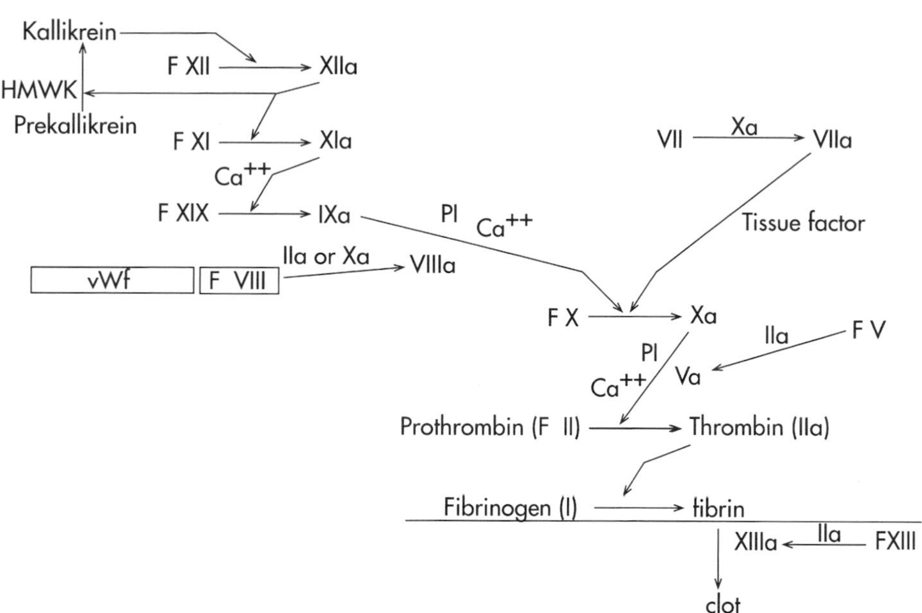

■ **FIGURE 32–11.** Mechanism of hemostasis. HMWK, high-molecular-weight kininogen; vWF, von Willebrand factor.

This model is primarily useful for the interpretation of in vitro laboratory tests, the activated partial thromboplastin time (aPTT), and the prothrombin time (PT). The common pathway of the clotting cascade is the production of factor Xa (FXa) that, in concert with FVa, cleaves prothrombin to thrombin resulting in fibrin production. It became apparent that deficiencies in the intrinsic pathway did not produce bleeding conditions, and that the concept was not clinically relevant.

In vivo, the critical component in the initiation of coagulation is TF, a membrane receptor for factor VII. TF is expressed constitutively on cells that are not in direct contact with blood, such as vascular smooth muscle, fibroblasts, and macrophages, forming a hemostatic envelope around the vascular endothelium (Mann et al., 1998). In response to cytokine exposure, mononuclear cells and vascular endothelial cells can be induced to express TF (Camerer et al., 1996; Levi et al., 2002). TF complexes with factor VII and activates it to factor VIIa. The TF/factor VIIa complex then activates factors X and IX. The TF/factor VIIa complex converts factor X to factor Xa directly. Factor Xa combines with its cofactor (factor Va) on the TF-bearing cell and generates small amounts of thrombin. This limited amount of thrombin is sufficient to activate platelets in the local area, as well as activating factor V, factor VIII, and factor XI, but it is insufficient to cleave fibrinogen. Factor VIII is cleaved off vWF and is then activated to factor VIIIa. Factor Xa produced in this manner cannot easily diffuse to the platelet surface because its two potent inhibitors, antithrombin III and TF pathway inhibitor, are present in sufficient concentrations. Therefore, its lifetime is limited to seconds.

Once activated by this small amount of thrombin, the platelet surface becomes coated with negatively charged phospholipid, an ideal catalytic surface for binding factor Va and factor VIIIa. Circulating platelets and adherent platelets can be activated in this manner. TF/FVIIa binds to factor IXa and then moves to the platelet surface as a complex. Factor IXa, in concert with factor VIIIa, produces factor Xa. This platelet, localized factor Xa, binds to factor Va on the platelet surface and catalyzes the conversion of prothrombin to thrombin at the rapid rate necessary for adequate hemostasis. The site at which factor Xa is produced is critical in this process (Hoffman et al., 1998). Thrombin formation is accelerated, fibrinogen is cleaved, and the coagulation complex is further activated, further augmenting thrombin formation. The fibrin monomers undergo spontaneous polymerization to form the fibrin clot, which is then stabilized by cross-linking, mediated by factor XIIIa. The net result is a firm, platelet-fibrin clot that, over the course of time, decreases in size, mediated by platelets. The graphic representation of this new model of cell-based coagulation, which replaces the former intrinsic pathway, is shown in Figure 32–12 (Gailani, 1991).

Modulators of Coagulation

Coagulation is modulated by a number of other plasma proteins, the most important of which are antithrombin III, thrombomodulin, TF pathway inhibitor, protein C, protein S, and factor V. Antithrombin III is a potent inhibitor of thrombin, factors IXa and Xa, and XIIIa. Inhibition of thrombin by antithrombin III is potentiated by heparin. Tissue factor pathway inhibitor (TFPI) limits factor Xa production to the IXa/VIIIa complex pathway. Activated protein C (APC), activated by the presence of thrombin, proteolytically inactivates FVIII/FVIIIa and FV/FVa, thereby downregulating production of factor Xa and thrombin. Protein S alone has little cofactor activity, but in the presence of factor V, its activity is dramatically increased. Factor V uniquely has procoagulant and anticoagulant activities. Genetic alterations in factor V (i.e., factor V Leiden) or deficiencies of protein C may result in excessive procoagulant activity, which may result in venous thromboembolism (Tormene et al., 2002). When factor V is cleaved by thrombin, a number of intermediates are formed in addition to factor Va, the essential cofactor to factor Xa. These intermediates are cofactors for APC and act as anticoagulants. APC can cleave factor V directly, producing an anticoagulant and precluding factor V's transformation to factor Va (Thorelli, 1999).

Fibrinolysis

Fibrinolysis occurs simultaneously with the initiation of clot formation. Fibrinolysis limits thrombosis to the local area of injury and begins the process of clot revision, vascular damage repair,

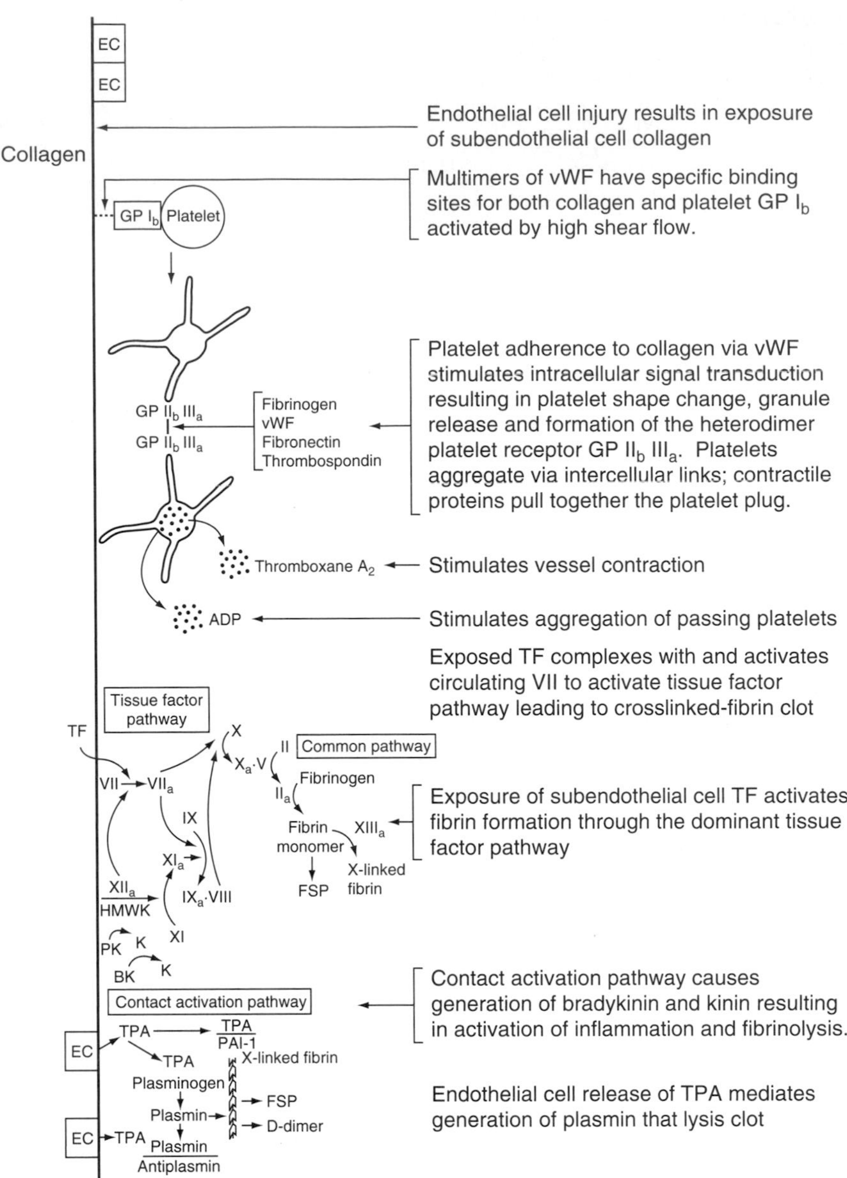

■ **FIGURE 32–12.** Hemostatic mechanism: cell-based coagulation model. BK, bradykinin; EC, endothelial cell; FSP, fibrin split products; GP, glycoprotein; K, kallikrein; PAI, plasminogen activator inhibitor; PK, prekallikrein; TF, tissue factor; TPA, tissue plasminogen activator; vWF, von Willebrand factor. (Redrawn from Manco-Johnson M, Nuss R: Hemostasis in the neonate. *Neoreviews* 1:191, 2000.)

and ultimately vessel recanalization. During the initial phase of hemostasis, endothelial cells and platelets release plasminogen activator inhibitors (PAIs), which facilitate fibrin formation. In response to thrombin, endothelial cells begin to release tissue-type plasminogen activator (TPA), which along with prourokinase, converts plasminogen to plasmin. The plasminogen, which is bound to fibrin in the hemostatic plug is much more reactive to TPA than is circulating plasmin. After plasmin is produced locally at the site of the hemostatic plug, fibrinolysis or fibrin degradation can occur. Fibrinolysis at the hemostatic plug is opposed by ongoing coagulation and by antifibrinolysis mediated by α_2-plasmin inhibitor, which also binds to fibrin.

The spectrum of endothelial cell and platelet interactions in the setting of clotting factors, adhesive proteins, fibrinolytic proteins, and the myriad inhibitors promotes an equilibrium which promotes fluidity of circulating blood and localization of hemostasis, and injury repair. Derangements in any portion of this precariously balanced mechanism can lead to a hemorrhagic or thrombotic complication. A defect in clot formation in the setting of physiologic fibrinolysis will lead to bleeding, as will normal clot formation in the setting of premature fibrinolysis. Thrombosis can occur in the setting of endothelial cell expression of TF, reduction in antithrombin function, and in excessive platelet aggregation and activation.

Laboratory Evaluation of Coagulation

The panel of tests routinely used to evaluate coagulation includes the platelet count, PT, aPTT, and the bleeding time.

The *normal platelet count* is between 150,000 and 500,000/mL, but increased bleeding due to thrombocytopenia rarely occurs at counts above 50,000/mL. Bleeding may also occur when platelets are relatively normal in number, but dysfunctional with regard to their role in coagulation.

The *normal PT,* which ranges from 11.5 to 14 seconds, reflects normal amounts of factors II, V, VII, and X, which are the vitamin K–dependent factors. Defects in the vitamin K–dependent clotting factors may be due to a deficiency of the vitamin, poor responsiveness to the vitamin because of liver disease, or to exposure to warfarin agents that impair vitamin K's transition to the reduced form. The international normalized ratio (INR) can be used to estimate the degree of factor deficiency. An INR in the range of 2 to 3 correlates with factor concentrations of 10%, between 3 and 4 correlates with concentrations of 5%, and more than 4 correlates with concentrations of 1% (Boulis et al., 1999).

The *normal aPTT* is between 25 and 40 seconds. It requires normal levels of vWF and factors XII, XI, IX, and VIII.

The *bleeding time* assesses the integrity of the vascular and platelet aspects of coagulation. It is prolonged in patients with reduced numbers of platelets (<100,000/mL), in patients with defective platelet function (e.g., after aspirin, NSAID, or valproic acid administration), and in patients with von Willebrand's disease. The bleeding time is performed using a standardized template device to guide the incision with a tourniquet placed on the arm at 40 mm Hg for children, 30 mm Hg for newborns at term, and 20 mm Hg for premature infants. The bleeding time has suffered from a reputation of being difficult to perform and poorly reproducible, especially in newborns and infants. Results may be affected by skin thickness and device used to puncture the skin (surgical blade, manufactured bleeding time device), location of incision, and body temperature. A bleeding time device (Surgicutt, ITC, Edison, NJ) has been developed. It comes in three sizes for adults, children (5 months to 15 years), and newborns (up to 5 months). The blades are different lengths (and depth for newborns) and afford a standardized incision, rather than a puncture. This standardization should decrease the variability in bleeding times that result from different incision techniques and skin thickness related to age, but this has not been studied in a controlled fashion. The blood is blotted with filter paper every 30 seconds. Normal bleeding time is between 4 and 8 minutes in adults and may be as low as 2 minutes in newborns. The bleeding time in very-low-birth-weight infants is decreased after transfusion to a hematocrit of greater than 28% (Sola et al., 2001). It is unknown whether the longer bleeding times at lower hematocrits are associated with an increased risk of clinical bleeding.

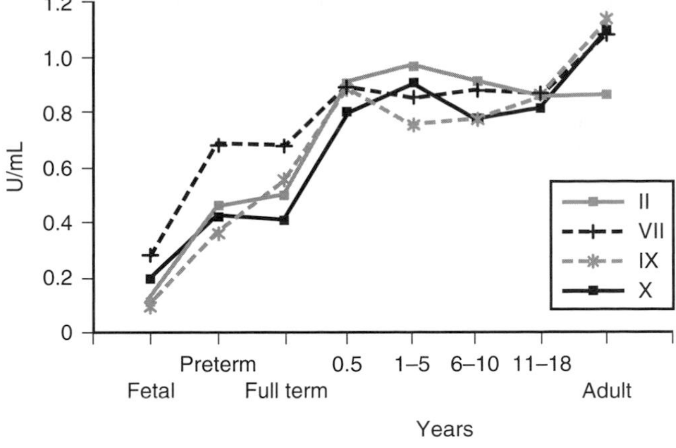

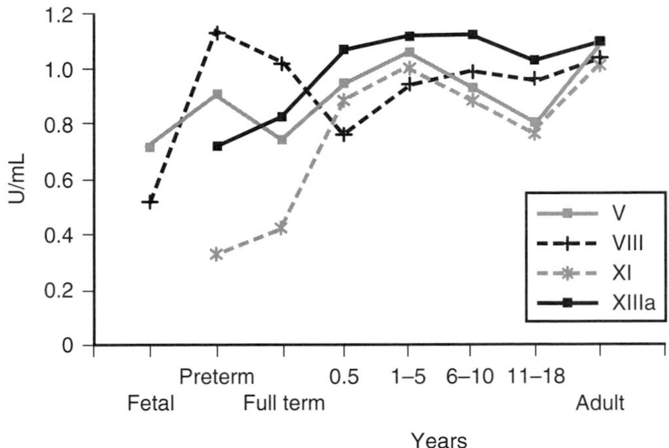

FIGURE 32–13. Developmental hemostasis: changes in plasma concentration of coagulation proteins over the course of development. (Redrawn from Andrew M: Developmental hemostasis: Relevance to thromboembolic complications in pediatric patients. *Thromb Haemost* 74(Suppl):415, 1995.)

DEVELOPMENTAL HEMOSTASIS

The hemostatic system in the newborn and young child is significantly different from that of the adult. Although considered immature, the hemostatic system is functional in that the young child is successfully protected from hemorrhagic and thrombotic complications. These differences are most exaggerated in the hemostatic mechanism of the newborn. As the coagulation and fibrinolytic factors do not cross the placenta, the proposed causes for the differences in the newborn's hemostatic system include decreased factor synthesis, enhanced clearance, general activation of the coagulation system with resulting factor consumption, and the synthesis of less active fetal forms of some proteins.

One of the most notable features of the coagulation system of the infant is that plasma clotting factors are inconsistently different from adult levels, as shown in Figure 32–13. The most well known ontogenetic differences in the hemostatic system involve the vitamin K–dependent factors. These proteins are present at low levels at birth and coagulation is severely impaired in the absence of vitamin K supplementation, called *hemorrhagic disease of the newborn*. The levels of the four vitamin K–dependent coagulation factors (i.e., II, VII, IX, and X) and the contact factors (i.e., XI, XII, prekallikrein, and kininogen) are all less than 50% of adult values and slowly rise to within 20% of adult levels by 6 months of age (Andrew et al., 1990a). Factor VII levels increase rapidly after birth in premature and full-term infants. Factors II and VII remain less than adult values for most of childhood (Andrew et al., 1992; Andrew, 1995). Factor IX activity can be as low as 15% of adult levels, and reach adult levels at 9 months of age. On the other hand, the levels of fibrinogen and factors V, VIII, and XIII are normal at birth; fibrinogen and factor VIII levels are at the high end of the normal range (Andrew et al., 1987). VWF levels are increased during the first weeks of life and return to adult levels between 2 to 6 months of life (Thomas et al., 1995). The net effect of these differences in the newborn's hemostatic system is delayed thrombin generation, similar to that seen in adults receiving anticoagulant medications, such as Coumadin or subcutaneous heparin (Andrew et al., 1990b). Thrombin generation in newborn plasma critically depends on the concentration of prothrombin, whereas the rate of thrombin production is proportional to the levels of the coagulation proteins. The plasma of children has a delayed and decreased (80% adult) capacity to generate thrombin. This has minimal hemostatic significance, but may contribute to a lower risk of thromboembolic phenomena (Andrew et al., 1994).

In addition to these changes in thrombin, newborn concentrations of plasminogen are markedly reduced, and levels of TPA

■ **TABLE 32–20.** Concentration of coagulation factors in the term and preterm newborn

Factor	Level at Term (% of Adult)	Level at Preterm (% of Adult)
Thrombin	50	40
Factor VII	66	66
Factor IX	50	35
Factor X	40	40
Fibrinogen	100	100
Factor V	75	88
Factor VIII	100	110
Factor X	40	40
Factor XI	40	40
Factor XII	50	30
Factor XIII	75	80
Heparin cofactor II	25	33
Antithrombin	50	40
α_2-Macroglobulin	150 to 200	150 to 200
Protein C	25	10
Protein S	40	25
Plasminogen	50	55
α_2-Antiplasmin	100	130
Tissue plasminogen activator (TPA)	200	200
Plasminogen activator inhibitor	180	180

and PAI-1 are increased. Suppressed fibrinolysis appears to be associated with the development of intraventricular hemorrhages in preterm neonates (Chen and Lorch, 1996). The concentration of coagulation factors in term and preterm infants relative to adult values is summarized in Table 32–20.

Laboratory Evaluation of Coagulation in the Newborn

Newborns with suspected coagulopathies are evaluated with PT, aPTT, platelet count, and levels of fibrinogen and fibrin degradation products. Patients suspected of having vitamin K deficiency should have evaluation of the proteins produced in vitamin K's absence. In newborns, as a result of the developmental differences in the coagulation protein levels, the PT and aPTT are prolonged compared with adult values. Because of the low plasma concentrations of many of the clotting factors in the newborn, the aPTT is markedly elevated. The developmental progression of the PT and aPTT in term and preterm infants is summarized in Table 32–21.

Developmental Changes beyond the Neonatal Period

Many of the proteins that regulate coagulation and thrombin generation are also decreased in early infancy. Antithrombin III and heparin cofactor II are markedly decreased to levels that might predispose to spontaneous thromboembolic events. The α_2-macroglobulin levels at birth are greater than those of adults and remain so until the third decade of life. By 6 months of life, antithrombin III levels exceed levels seen in adults. Protein C and protein S concentrations at birth are also substantially less than those seen in adults, and they remain low throughout childhood (Andrew et al., 1992). Fibrinolysis is also suppressed throughout childhood. During childhood, plasminogen levels increase to adult levels, but the TPA/PAI-1 ratio is significantly lower than in adults, which explains the decrease in fibrinolysis in children (Siegbahn and Ruusuvaara, 1988).

Developmental Aspects of Platelet Number and Function

Although normal in number, neonatal platelets are hyporeactive. This hyporeactivity is attributed to a defect in the signal transduction pathway (Rao et al., 1993). Neonatal platelet aggregation is diminished in response to certain physiologic agonists, such as ADP, thromboxane, and epinephrine. Intracellular calcium transport is decreased as well, resulting in diminished granule release and slowed conformational change (Kuhne and Imbach, 1998; Gelman et al., 1996). Increased vWF levels in the newborn period contribute to decreased bleeding times (Andrew et al., 1997). Platelet function in the neonate is aided by a relatively high hematocrit. This causes an increased concentration of platelets directed to the wall by the dynamics of laminar flow. Platelet function improves over the first 48 hours of life (Rajasekhar et al., 1994, 1997).

The most serious manifestation of thrombocytopenia in the newborn period is intraparenchymal brain hemorrhage. Of neonates with spontaneous intraparenchymal hemorrhage, one third will have an associated coagulopathy, such as vitamin K deficiency, hemophilia, or thrombocytopenia. Three studies in neonates with intraparenchymal hemorrhage identified a platelet count of less than 50,000 as a significant risk factor for hemorrhage, even in full term neonates (Nanigan et al., 1995; Sandberg et al., 2001; Jhawar et al., 2003).

■ INHERITED COAGULOPATHIES

Hemostasis usually requires activity levels of coagulation factors at least 30% of normal. The aPTT may be normal with a factor level as low as 15% to 18% of normal. Past medical history and family history are invaluable tools in the evaluation of a bleeding patient. Substantial hemorrhage after oral cavity manipulation (whether by dentist or toothbrush) is frequently a sign of an underlying bleeding disorder, reflecting an imbalance between

■ **TABLE 32–21.** Developmental changes in the prothrombin time and activated partial thromboplastin time

Age of Infant	Day 1	Day 5	Day 30	Day 90	Adult
Term					
PT	13 ± 1.4	12.4 ± 1.5	11.8 ± 1.3	11.9 ± 1.2	12.4 ± 0.8
aPTT	42.9 ± 5.8	42.6 ± 8.6	40.4 ± 7.4	37.1 ± 6.5	33.5 ± 3.4
Preterm (30 to 36 Weeks)					
PT	13.0 ± 1.5	12.5 ± 1.3	11.8 ± 0.9	12.3 ± 1.2	12.4 ± 0.8
aPTT	53.6 ± 13	50.5 ± 12	44.7 ± 9	50.5 ± 12	33.5 ± 3.4

aPTT, activated partial thromboplastin time; PT, prothrombin time.
Adapted from Andrew M and others, 1987; 1988.

abnormal clot formation and normal salivary fibrinolysis. Patients with mild bleeding disorders who have never had trauma or surgery may present rather late in life and may have normal screening tests. Prenatal diagnosis of most congenital factor deficiencies can now be made from fetal DNA (Andrew and Brooker, 1995).

Hemophilia

Of the inherited deficiencies of coagulation factors, the most common are the X-linked recessive hemophilias; hemophilia A is factor VIII deficiency, and hemophilia B (i.e., Christmas disease) is factor IX deficiency. Thirty percent of cases arise from spontaneous mutation. Approximately 50% of mutations of factor VIII result from inversions of the DNA sequence within intron 22 (Lakich et al., 1993). The incidence of hemophilia A is 1 in 5000 male live births, and that of hemophilia B is 1 in 30,000 (Tuddenham and Cooper, 1994). Hemophilia B can result from spontaneous mutations, which cause decreased rates of activation of factor IX, altered binding of factor IX to phospholipid membranes, or reduced circulation times. Patients with factor IX Leyden, a single nucleotide substitution in the transcriptional promoter, have severe hemophilia until puberty, at which point factor IX spontaneously increases to 50% (Briet et al., 1982; Stowell et al., 1993). This suggests that the transcription of factor IX gene is in part hormonally mediated. Factor IX is a smaller molecule than factor VIII and has a greater volume of distribution.

The clinical severity of hemophilia is usually dictated by the degree of clotting factor deficiency. Patients with severe hemophilia, less than 1% of normal plasma levels, have an annual average of 20 to 30 bleeds, bleeding events which may be spontaneous or marked by excessive bleeding after minor trauma, characteristically into joints or muscle. These patients are usually diagnosed within the first 2 years of life. Bleeding is less common in the newborn period than in later months, but when it occurs, it is most common after circumcision. Of newborns presenting with hemophilia, 30% bled from circumcision sites, 27% had intracranial hemorrhage, 16% had persistent bleeding from puncture sites, and 1% had subgaleal or cephalohematomas (Girolami et al., 1985; Kulkarni and Lusher, 2001). Infants with severe hemophilia A or B have a 2% to 8% risk of spontaneous intracranial hemorrhage (Bray and Luban, 1987). Patients with mild and moderate disease, corresponding to 6% to 30% and 1% to 5% of normal factor levels, respectively, usually bleed excessively only after trauma or surgery, and they are managed with on-demand factor replacement. These patients are often diagnosed later in life (White et al., 2001).

Hemophilia A and hemophilia B are characterized by a prolonged aPTT with a normal PT. Because the neonate's aPTT is physiologically prolonged, it cannot be used to diagnose hemophilia in this age group. Instead, the factor VIII level must be directly measured. Factor IX levels are physiologically low at birth and do not reach adult levels until 6 months of age, making confirmation of the diagnosis of hemophilia B uncertain until later infancy, except in severe cases. The treatment of hemophilia has changed dramatically over the past 3 decades from the availability of plasma derived replacement factors in the 1970s to the engineering of recombinant factors in the 1990s to the recently begun trials of gene replacement therapy (Mannucci and Tuddenham, 2001).

Preoperative Preparation of the Child with Hemophilia

Preparation of the child with hemophilia for surgery depends on the severity of the patient's disease and the proposed procedure. Patients with mild hemophilia A who have demonstrated an adequate response to DDAVP in the past can undergo minor procedures after intravenous DDAVP administration (0.3 mcg/kg) 30 minutes before surgery (Mannucci, 1997).

Factor Replacement

Hemophilia A. The type, timing, and dose of factor to be administered should be decided in advance in consultation with the patient's hematologist. In general, children with hemophilia A who require major procedures should have their factor VIII level maintained close to 100% of normal from 30 minutes before surgery through the first 2 to 7 days of the postoperative period. Factor VIII levels can then be weaned to 30% to 50% of normal for the next 3 to 7 days. Children undergoing minor procedures can be adequately covered with factor VIII levels of 50% after the second postoperative day (Martlew, 2000; Kapural and Sprung, 1999). In determining factor replacement, it should be remembered that the plasma volume is 45 to 50 mL/kg. Because 1 mL of plasma contains one unit of factor VIII, 50 units per kg of factor VIII will increase the patient's level to 100% (rise of 2% per unit of factor VIII/kg). In the absence of inhibitors, the half-life of factor VIII in vivo is 8 to 12 hours; subsequent doses are timed to maintain the desired level of activity. The first dose has a somewhat shorter half-life than subsequent doses. Therefore, the second dose should be given after a somewhat shorter interval (6 hours).

Factor VIII may be administered as cryoprecipitate (0.2 bags/kg should raise factor VIII level to 50%), but the factor VIII level in cryoprecipitate is variable and plasma levels should be followed if bleeding is not well controlled. The use of heat- or detergent-treated factor concentrates (Monoclate, Hemofil-M) has been replaced with recombinant factor VIII preparations (Humate P). Although the treated factor concentrates had a lower risk of transmission of viruses (e.g., human immunodeficiency virus [HIV]; hepatitis A, B, or C) compared with cryoprecipitate, recombinant factor VIII carries no risk of viral transmission, but it is unknown whether the albumin in the recombinant preparations may have a risk of prion and parvovirus B19 transmission.

Hemophilia B. Children with hemophilia B should be given factor IX concentrate, maintaining similar levels to hemophilia A patients. The factor IX level is raised 1% for each unit of factor IX concentrate/kg. Only plasma-derived factor IX is available; there is currently no recombinant factor IX. Because the half-life of factor IX is 12 to 24 hours, it requires less frequent dosing to maintain adequate levels (Shopnick and Brettler, 1996). As with factor VIII, the second dose should be give at a somewhat shorter interval than subsequent doses (6 to 8 hours).

Hemophilia C. Hemophilia C is factor XI deficiency (i.e., Rosenthal's syndrome), an autosomally recessive disease that is most commonly reported in Ashkenazi Jews. The incidence in the Ashkenazic population is 3 in 1000, compared with a rate of 1 in 1,000,000 in the general population (Weinstock and Schwartz, 1995). There is an increased incidence of hemophilia C among people with Noonan's syndrome (Singer et al., 1997). Factor XI deficiency presents with a prolongation of the aPTT, with a normal PT. There is an incomplete correlation between the severity of factor deficiency and hemorrhagic symptoms, in that some patients with very low factor levels have no history of bleeding. Bleeding typically occurs after trauma or surgery, and it is commonly seen in sites that have a high fibrinolytic rate, such as the genitourinary tract, and after circumcision (Andrew, 1997).

Because factor XI levels are physiologically low in the neonatal period, the diagnosis is confirmed through levels obtained in later infancy. The perioperative management of these patients is dictated by their bleeding risk. Patients with factor XI levels of >15% without a previous history of bleeding, or patients with levels of 5% to 14% who have had previous surgery without significant bleeding without fresh frozen plasma (FFP) administration can be considered low risk. Patients with factor levels of less than 15%, a history of spontaneous bleeding, bleeding during previous surgeries, or those with a family history of such bleeding complications can be considered high risk. Depending on the surgical procedure, patients who are considered low risk can be managed with FFP immediately available. High-risk patients should receive FFP 2 hours before surgery (Borud et al., 1999).

Von Willebrand's Disease

Characteristics

Von Willebrand's disease, the most common congenital bleeding disorder, is a deficiency or dysfunction of the adhesive glycoprotein vWF, which is produced in endothelial cells and megakaryocytes and is stored in Weibel-Palade bodies in endothelial cells and platelets. VWF is fundamental in platelet binding to damaged endothelial surfaces, promotes the secretion of factor VIII, and binds, carries, and protects factor VIII in plasma. von Willebrand's disease affects 1 in 1000 individuals and is inherited in an autosomal fashion (usually dominant), with males and females affected equally. It is characterized by impaired platelet adhesion to exposed subendothelium in high shear vessels. Because of the reduced or defective vWF, factor VIII is reduced to a mild and variable degree because of decreased secretion and enhanced clearance. Because von Willebrand's disease is a disorder of the protein responsible for the adherence of platelets to damaged endothelial surfaces, the clinical manifestations in affected individuals resemble those seen in patients with platelet disorders (i.e., mucocutaneous bleeding [nose, gingiva], menorrhagia, and increased bleeding with trauma or surgery).

There are three variants of von Willebrand's disease. Patients with the type 1 variant, the most common (80%), have a heterozygous quantitative deficiency of vWF (20% to 40% of normal) associated with diminished factor VIII levels. Type 1 patients frequently present with menorrhagia or mild to moderate bleeding from mucocutaneous sites. Medications that affect platelet function (e.g., NSAIDs) can cause hemorrhage in a previously asymptomatic patient with type 1 von Willebrand's disease. Type 2 von Willebrand's disease (17%) is characterized by the production of qualitatively abnormal vWF. Some of these patients have an associated thrombocytopenia, whereas others have a factor VIII deficiency that is out of proportion to the level of vWF. Type 3 von Willebrand's disease (3%) is marked by profound deficiencies of vWF and factor VIII. Homozygous patients may experience severe bleeding and spontaneous hemarthrosis. Because vWF levels are higher at birth and the proportion of the most functional high-molecular-weight multimeric units is increased, the incidence of bleeding in newborns is very low. When newborns with von Willebrand's disease bleed, it is the result of concomitantly low factor VIII levels. Acquired von Willebrand's disease has been associated with Wilms' tumor, systemic lupus erythematosus, congenital heart defects, and hemoglobin E-Thalassemia (Jakway, 1992).

The laboratory diagnosis of von Willebrand's disease is based on a prolonged bleeding time and on decreased levels of vWF antigen and factor VIII in the face of normal PT, fibrinogen, and platelet count. The aPTT may be normal or mildly prolonged. Ristocetin cofactor assay, which measures vWF induced platelet agglutination, is used to identify type 2 von Willebrand's disease. It is recommended that screening be performed on three separate occasions before ruling out von Willebrand's disease because functional and antigenic vWF levels may overlap that of normal patients and vWF levels can fluctuate in unpredictable ways. The vWF levels rise during pregnancy. There is a significant linkage between ABO locus and the vWF antigen, such that patients with A and B blood types have marked higher levels (100% to 115%) of factor than those with type O (75%) (Souto et al., 2000).

Preoperative Preparation

Most patients with type 1 disease respond to the intravenous administration of 0.3 mcg/kg of DDAVP 30 minutes before surgery. DDAVP induces the release of vWF from endothelial storage granules (Weibel-Palade bodies) into the circulation (Mannucci, 1997) and results in a twofold to threefold increase in plasma von Willebrand antigen levels within 30 to 60 minutes, with the effect lasting more than 6 hours (Mannucci, 1997). DDAVP may be administered two to three times each day, although tachyphylaxis may develop (Mannucci et al., 1992). Because 10% of patients with type 1 von Willebrand's disease fail to respond to DDAVP (Nolan et al., 2000), the response (increased factor VIII levels and normalization of bleeding time) should be documented before surgery to make sure it is adequate to prevent excessive perioperative bleeding. If it is effective, it may be used as the sole agent for the treatment of minor bleeding (e.g., epistaxis) or perioperatively for minor surgery, such as dental extraction.

Patients with type 2 and type 3 diseases usually require replacement of factor VIII and vWF to control bleeding. DDAVP is contraindicated in type 2b disease because it may exacerbate thrombocytopenia. Those who do respond to DDAVP may also need factor replacement before major surgical procedures or for major trauma. Plasma-derived, human factor VIII concentrate, which has a high concentration of vWF (Humate-P), is effective and is approved for replacement therapy in von Willebrand's disease (Federici et al., 2002).

If the patient's response to DDAVP is adequate and bleeding is not a problem, liberal DDAVP administration may be substituted for factor concentrate in the postoperative period. Close monitoring of bleeding and communication with the hematologist should guide postoperative management of these patients.

Factor XIII Deficiency

The role of factor XIII in hemostasis is in stabilizing newly formed clot by cross-linking fibrin monomers. Plasma levels as low as 1% to 2% are usually adequate for hemostasis. Patients with factor XIII deficiency have bleeding despite a normal PT, aPTT, and platelet count. Factor XIII deficiency is a rare bleeding disorder that is inherited in an autosomal recessive manner and has an estimated incidence of 1 in 2 million (Board et al., 1993). Typical symptoms are delayed hemorrhages after mild trauma. The most common manifestation is prolonged bleeding from the newborn's umbilical stump, which is virtually pathognomonic for this deficiency, or after circumcision. The major morbidity in factor XIII deficient children is a marked propensity for intracranial hemorrhages, up to 30% in some series

(Anwar and Miloszewski, 1999). Seriously affected patients are treated with cryoprecipitate or purified factor concentrate. All traumatic brain or closed-head injuries are treated prophylactically.

Factor VII Deficiency

Factor VII has the shortest half-life of all the clotting factors, estimated to be 6 hours. Factor VII deficiency is a rare autosomal recessive disorder. The severity of the hemorrhagic diathesis does not correlate with factor VII levels. Many individuals have mutations of factor VII but are asymptomatic, and they come to medical attention as a result of an isolated PT prolongation. Much more common than an inherited factor VII deficiency is an acquired factor VII deficiency. Because the exquisitely short half-life of factor VII, liver failure, vitamin K deprivation, or oral anticoagulant toxicity first manifests as factor VII deficiency with an isolated increased PT value.

Platelet Abnormalities

Congenital Coagulopathies due to Platelet Abnormalities

Inherited coagulopathies include diseases associated with quantitative and qualitative platelet dysfunction. Wiskott-Aldrich syndrome is an X-linked disorder characterized by thrombocytopenia, immunodeficiency, and eczema. Newborns typically present with thrombocytopenia, due to underproduction. These platelets are abnormally small. The disease results from the mutation of the Wiskott-Aldrich syndrome Protein (WASP), a cytoskeletal regulatory protein found in megakaryocytes and lymphocytes (Caron, 2002). Symptomatic bleeding is treated with platelet transfusions. Congenital bone marrow failure syndromes that result in congential thrombocytopenia include Diamond Blackfan syndrome anemia, Schwachman Diamond syndrome, and Fanconi anemia. These infants present with severe mucocutaneous bleeding or intracranial hemorrhage as a result of profound thrombocytopenia. These patients depend on platelet transfusions. Thrombocytopenia with absent radii (TAR) is another cause of neonatal thrombocytopenia that is associated with skeletal anomalies. The thrombocytopenia is most pronounced in the first year of life, when mucocutaneous bleeding commonly occurs, and platelet transfusions are required.

Thrombocytopenia of Immune Origin

Immune-mediated thrombocytopenias occur in the setting of isoimmunization, with transplacental transfer of maternal alloantibodies directed against paternally inherited antigens present on fetal platelets, or of maternal autoimmune diseases such as idiopathic thrombocytopenic purpura (ITP) and systemic lupus erythematosus (SLE). Thrombocytopenia is most severe in isoimmune disease. Isoimmune thrombocytopenia occurs in 1 of 1000 deliveries. The distinguishing characteristic is the maternal platelet count, which is normal in isoimmune disease and decreased in autoimmune disease. Infants are usually asymptomatic unless the platelet count is less than 10,000. Mucocutaneous, spinal cord, and intracranial hemorrhages are seen prenatally and postnatally in isoimmune disease (Blanchette, 1988; Abel et al., 2003). The bleeding in autoimmune thrombocytopenia is usually not as severe, but the risk of intracranial hemorrhage increases when the platelet count is less than 40,000 in the newborn. Both diseases are treated with platelet transfusions, intravenous gamma globulin, and corticosteroids. The established treatment of alloimmune neonatal thrombocytopenia is the administration of washed, irradiated maternal platelets (10 mL/kg) (Rothenberger, 2002), but donor platelets screened for the absence of human platelet antigen 1a (HPA-1a) have been shown to be effective (Rayment et al., 2003).

Thrombocytopathies

Inherited qualitative platelet defects are uncommon conditions. They present with bleeding in the newborn period as well. Glanzmann thrombasthenia is an autosomal recessive deficiency of GPIIb/IIIa, impairing fibrinogen binding on platelets. Patients present with mucocutaneous bleeding in the neonatal period and have a life-long risk of bleeding. Platelet count and morphology are normal, but bleeding time, clot retraction, and platelet aggregation tests are all abnormal, and flow cytometry is required to confirm the GPIIb/IIIa deficiency. Bleeding is managed with platelet transfusions. Bernard Soulier syndrome is an autosomal recessive deficiency of the platelet vWF receptor. These patients have mild to moderate bleeding and have unusually large platelets. The diagnosis is confirmed by failure of agglutination in the presence of ristocetin.

Bleeding Diathesis Associated with Blood Vessel Abnormalities

Hereditary blood vessel disorders associated with a bleeding diathesis include uncommon connective tissue diseases such as Ehlers-Danlos and Marfan syndromes.

ACQUIRED COAGULOPATHIES

Vitamin K Deficiency

Hemorrhagic disease of the newborn is a bleeding disorder that is caused by a deficiency of vitamin K. Clinical bleeding occurs in 1 in 1000 to 1 in 10,000 babies who do not receive vitamin K supplementation. Vitamin K is poorly transferred across the placenta and is present in very low concentration in breast milk. Hemorrhagic disease of the newborn can be temporally divided into three types: early, classic, and late-onset. Bleeding within the first 24 hours of life is defined as *early disease* and is generally seen in infants born to mothers receiving oral anticoagulants or antiepileptic drugs. These infants often have serious bleeding, including intracranial hemorrhage. Bleeding within the first week of life is *classic disease* and usually involves cutaneous, gastrointestinal, or circumcision bleeding in infants who did not receive vitamin K supplementation at birth and who are usually breast-fed. Bleeding in the first 3 months of life is referred to as *late-onset disease*, and it is seen in exclusively breast-fed infants and in infants with disorders of fat absorption such as CF, biliary atresia, and celiac disease (Lane and Hathaway, 1985; Sutor et al., 1999). The diagnosis is confirmed with a prolonged PT, increased levels of proteins produced in the absence of vitamin K, and a low vitamin K level. Administration of vitamin K subcutaneously or intravenously increases coagulation factors within 2 hours, with complete correction within 24 hours. Serious bleeding may be treated with FFP (10 to 20 mL/kg) or with a purified factor IX product.

Hepatic Dysfunction–Related Coagulopathy

Liver disease resulting in synthetic dysfunction has a major impact on hemostasis, because many of the coagulation factors are synthesized in the liver. Levels of these proteins are the first to decline with worsening liver disease, especially the very short-lived factor VII. Measurement of factor V, a hepatically synthesized, non–vitamin K–dependent protein, which is present in similar amounts in the newborn and the adult, is useful in differentiating vitamin K deficiency from hepatic dysfunction. Fibrin degradation products are increased as a result of their decreased clearance in the setting of hepatic dysfunction. The development of ascites results in further loss of coagulation proteins.

Perioperative management of these patients includes determination of the patient's exact deficiencies and correcting them with targeted management. Prolongation of the PT, resulting from depletion of vitamin K–dependent factors, can be treated with vitamin K or FFP. Vitamin K should normalize the PT in 6 to 8 hours. Hypofibrinogenemia should be treated with cryoprecipitate. Recombinant FVIIa has been successfully used to correct the coagulopathy associated with liver failure (Bernstein et al., 1997). FVIIa has been used in very small numbers of patients to decrease transfusion requirements during liver transplantation, despite the fact that bleeding in that setting is multifactorial in nature (Kalicinski et al., 1999; Hendriks et al., 2001).

Anticoagulant-Related Coagulopathy

Patients receiving therapeutic anticoagulation are at risk for devastating hemorrhagic complications. They have a 1% incidence of intracranial hemorrhage, either intracerebral or subdural, both associated with very high morbidity and mortality rates (Wintzen et al., 1984). If surgery is contemplated or when procedural heparinization must be reversed, anticoagulation is reversed with protamine administered intravenously over 10 minutes. The dosage of protamine is based on the interval since the last dose of heparin, and it can be calculated using the following formula:

$$\left.\begin{matrix}\text{Protamine dose}\\ \text{(mg/100 U heparin)}\end{matrix}\right\} = 1 - ([\text{time since last heparin (min)} \div 30] \cdot 0.25)$$

Low-molecular-weight heparin anticoagulation is also reversed with protamine, in a dose of 1 mg of protamine per 1 mg (100 Units) of low-molecular-weight heparin administered within the previous 3 to 4 hours (Monagle et al., 2001). Protamine is given slowly, as rapid administration may cause profound hypotension.

Children receiving oral anticoagulation may be difficult to maintain in a therapeutic range because of variations in diet, concurrent medications, and underlying disease processes. Breast-fed infants are very sensitive to oral anticoagulants because of low concentrations of vitamin K in breast milk. Many of the common medications that are prescribed for children, including prednisone, amoxicillin, trimethoprim-sulfamethoxazole, and ranitidine, increase the INR of children on oral anticoagulants (Michelson et al., 1995).

Acquired Thrombocytopathy

Aspirin and nonsteroidal antiinflammatory drugs (NSAIDs) are the most commonly used medications that affect the coagulation system. These medications inhibit platelet COX, blocking thromboxane synthesis and leading to a partial impairment of platelet function (Clarke et al., 1991). Aspirin ingestion prolongs the bleeding time by 2 to 3 minutes. Two COX isoenzymes have been characterized: COX-1, which is always present on platelets and the gastric mucosa, and COX-2, which is upregulated during inflammation (Cryer and Feldman, 1998). Nonspecific COX inhibitors increase perioperative bleeding complications after adenoidectomy. Preoperative administration of NSAIDs, such as ketorolac, increased blood loss by 70% to 80% in children undergoing tonsillectomy. In a meta-analysis of seven studies comprising 262 patients who received NSAIDs after tonsillectomy and 243 control patients, postoperative administration of NSAIDs resulted in a doubling of the number of children experiencing postoperative bleeding and a fivefold increase in reoperation for bleeding (Marret et al., 2003).

Many anesthetic agents have been implicated in platelet dysfunction, as measured by platelet aggregometry; among them are inhaled anesthetics, such as propofol and ketamine (Nakagawa et al., 2002). However, there are no data that demonstrate that these agents increase perioperative bleeding or transfusion requirements in the clinical setting (Faraday, 2002).

Another class of drugs that may interfere with platelet function is the anticonvulsants, such as sodium valproate. Valproate has caused mild thrombocytopenia, neutropenia, and even red cell aplasia, and patients taking valproate should be evaluated before surgery with a complete blood count with platelet count. Bone marrow suppression usually occurs with levels higher than 100 mcg/mL and usually responds to a decrease in dose (Acharya and Bussel, 2000). Bleeding time may be prolonged in patients taking valproic acid, but usually not to a clinically significant extent. Twenty percent of a small series of patients taking valproic acid were shown to have acquired von Willebrand's disease, with low ristocetin cofactor activity, although only two of six affected children were symptomatic (epistaxis) (Serdaroglu et al., 2002). One case report documented severe factor XIII deficiency resulting in severe intracranial bleeding after craniotomy for epilepsy surgery (Pohlmann-Eden et al., 2003). This deficiency was reversible with cessation of valproic acid therapy. An extensive evaluation of the procoagulant and anticoagulant effects of valproate showed that the procoagulant effects might balance the anticoagulant effects and thereby reduce the risk of bleeding (Banerjea et al., 2002). The blood loss during and after spinal surgery was evaluated in a small series of children with cerebral palsy, some of whom were taking valproic acid (Chambers et al., 1999). There was a 30% increase in mean blood loss in the children taking valproic acid (38.6 versus 30 mL/kg), and increased postoperative blood product administration. These children also had a greater likelihood of having longer bleeding times. Therefore, the anesthesiologist should have a heightened awareness of the possibility of excessive surgical bleeding, especially during and after craniotomy, in patients taking valproic acid. Routinely performing a bleeding time in all children taking valproic acid is likely to have an extremely low yield and bleeding times are more difficult to perform, especially in young children. Nevertheless, some hematologists recommend a bleeding time for children scheduled for craniotomy, with further investigation including vWF and ristocetin cofactor and possible preoperative administration of DDAVP if indicated (Acharya and Bussel, 2000).

Other Acquired Coagulopathies

Disseminated Intravascular Coagulation

Disseminated intravascular coagulation (DIC) is the unregulated activation of the hemostatic system characterized by generation of activated clotting factors, fibrin, and accelerated fibrinolysis. Conditions associated with DIC are listed in Box 32–12. Patients can present with bleeding, thrombosis, or only laboratory evidence

BOX 32–12 Conditions Associated with Disseminated Intravascular Coagulation

Sepsis
Shock
Heat stroke
Acidosis
Hypoxia*
Trauma
  Head injury
  Fat embolism
  Crush injury
  Burn injury
Toxin exposure†
Severe allergic reaction
Intravascular hemolysis
Liver disease
Cancer
  Myeloproliferative disease
Vascular anomalies
  Kasabach-Merritt syndrome
Extracorporeal circulation
Obstetric complications
  Amniotic fluid embolism
  Placental abruption
  Preeclampsia

*Antenatal hypoxia (Hannam et al., 2003).
†Snake bite (Gold et al., 2003).

of DIC. DIC is the result of the significant exposure of circulating blood to TF, commonly from endothelial disruption or from hypoxia, acidosis, and sepsis.

No single laboratory test can establish or exclude the diagnosis of DIC. The most common laboratory abnormalities include thrombocytopenia or a rapidly falling platelet count and elevated D-dimer levels. Less commonly, microangiopathic hemolytic anemia, hypofibrinogenemia, PT and aPTT prolongation are seen (Bick and Baker, 1986). D-dimers may be present in premature infants without DIC. Antithrombin III levels can be markedly depressed as well. *The treatment of DIC is principally focused on eradicating the precipitating process; treating the consequences without treating the underlying cause is certain to fail.* There is no evidence that prophylactic administration of platelets or plasma will improve the outcome of a nonbleeding patient. FFP, cryoprecipitate, and platelet transfusions are used only to treat bleeding symptoms in the older child. In the neonatal period, however, because of the risk of intracerebral hemorrhage, many aim to correct a platelet count of less than 50,000, fibrinogen level of less than 100 mg/dL, and an INR of more than 1.5. Sequential thromboelastograms (TEGs) are useful in monitoring the correction of DIC in the perioperative period (Stammers et al., 2000). Activated protein C (i.e., drotrecogin alfa), a specific inhibitor of the TF/factor VIIa/factor Xa complex, is in clinical trials for the treatment of DIC (Levi and ten Cate, 1999).

Acquired Hemophilia

Antibodies to coagulation factors develop in hemophiliacs treated with factor replacement and in nonhemophiliacs who have no prior exposure to hemostatic therapy. These acquired inhibitors to coagulation factors occur most commonly against factor VIII. Although many patients with acquired hemophilia are elderly, children can be affected in a devastating manner (Stein and Ratnoff, 1993). Patients who develop inhibitors commonly have coexisting diseases, such as lupus or rheumatoid arthritis, or they have been recently treated for rheumatic fever (Moraca and Ragni, 2002). Transplacental transfer of acquired inhibitors has been reported, resulting in hemorrhagic complications in the newborn period (Ries et al., 1995). Patients with acquired inhibitors most frequently have bleeding into fascial planes and mucous membranes, rather than joints. The diagnosis is elusive due to inconsistent test results. There is no correlation between inhibitor titers and the severity or pattern of bleeding (Yee et al., 2000).

In patients with inhibitors, even large amounts of cryoprecipitate or FFP may not promote satisfactory hemostasis. FFP administration leads to an anamnestic response. Factor VIII autoantibodies in acquired hemophilia are usually incompletely inhibitory so that factor VIII levels are usually detectable and may be as high as 10% to 20% of normal values. DDAVP is effective in many cases of inhibitor-associated hemorrhage (Mudad and Kane, 1993). Porcine factor VIII is a viable therapeutic alternative in acquired hemophilia patients, because most autoantibodies are usually species specific, and therefore these patients have low or undetectable titers of anti-porcine factor VIII (Kobrinksy et al., 2002). Treatment is initiated with a dose of 50 to 100 IU/kg and titrated to maintain therapeutic levels. The development of neutralizing antibodies to the porcine factor takes 7 to 10 days to develop. Rarely, transfusion reactions and thrombocytopenia can develop. There are no reports of the transmission of a porcine virus to a human recipient (Rubinger et al., 1997). Another therapeutic alternative is one of the commercially available activated prothrombin complex concentrates that, by bypassing factor VIII, stimulate fibrin clot formation in the presence of factor inhibitors. These agents are effective hemostatic agents in most bleeding patients with inhibitors (Negrier et al., 1997). The risk of adverse effects such as thrombotic complications and disseminated intravascular coagulation are small but are increased in the settings of patients with extensive crush injuries, marked hepatic dysfunction, or with prolonged administration (Teitel, 1999).

Recombinant Factor VIIa

In the presence of inhibitory antibodies, recombinant factor VIIa administered at a starting dose of 90 mcg/kg is effective at normalizing bleeding in more than 90% of surgical procedures, and in achieving adequate hemostasis in 78% of patients with life- or limb-threatening bleeding (Scharrer, 1999; Arkin et al., 2000). The clinical response did not correlate with the degree of decrease of the PT after the recombinant factor VIIa infusion (Hay et al., 1997). Immunomodulation therapy should be instituted concomitantly with hemostatic therapy. As there is no consensus on the optimal regimen, many have used multiple agents of demonstrable efficacy, such as intravenous immune globulin, corticosteroids and alkylating agents to reduce inhibitor levels.

INTRAOPERATIVE COAGULOPATHIES

Patients with no preoperative disorders of coagulation who have surgery may develop coagulopathy due to a combination of blood loss, fluid replacement, and other intraoperative circumstances. Conditions associated with the development of intraoperative coagulopathy are listed in Box 32–13.

BOX 32–13 Conditions Associated with Development of Intraoperative Coagulopathy

Neurologic conditions
- Intracranial surgery
- Traumatic brain injury

Cardiovascular conditions
- Congenital heart disease
- Shock
- Kasabach-Merritt syndrome

Trauma

Orthopedic conditions
- Fat embolism
- Scoliosis surgery
- Osteogenesis imperfecta
- Intramedullary nailing of long bone fractures

Miscellaneous conditions
- Citrate-induced hypocalcemia
- Factor V inhibition from exposure to bovine topical thrombin

Data from Iberrti et al., 1994; Hymel et al., 1997; Byrick RJ, 2001; Robinson et al., 2001; Vavilala et al., 2001; Keegan et al., 2002; Murshid et al., 2002; Neschis et al., 2002.

Colloid-Induced von Willebrand's Syndrome

The administration of some synthetic colloids as volume expanders may be associated with the development of acquired von Willebrand's disease. Large amounts of dextran decrease vWF and factor VIII levels and enhance fibrinolysis (Batlle et al., 1985). The increase in bleeding times after dextran infusion can be completely normalized by the administration of DDAVP. Dextran's anticoagulant properties have been used to prevent postoperative thromboembolic complications (Clagett et al., 1998). Patients receiving dextran intraoperatively required more blood transfusions than did those receiving heparin prophylaxis (De Jonge and Levi, 2001). Dextran also changes the structure of the thrombus formation and increases the clot's susceptibility to fibrinolysis.

High-molecular-weight hydroxyethyl starch (HES) is the only starch approved for use in the United States for plasma expansion, and is associated with decreases in plasma vWF and factor VIII levels, as well as increases in fibrinolysis and platelet dysfunction (Egli et al., 1997). The aPTT is prolonged, the bleeding time is increased, and TEGs demonstrate prolonged clot formation and increased clot lysis (Mortier et al., 1997). Changing the molecular weight of the starch and modifying its in vivo degradation rate do not seem to decrease the risk of development of an induced von Willebrand syndrome (De Jonge et al., 2001). Smaller volumes of HES seem to cause less hemostatic perturbation (Treib et al., 1996).

Children are rarely given HES. They more commonly receive human serum albumin for volume expansion. Human serum albumin administration causes minimal changes in plasma factor VIII and vWT levels. However, albumin does prolong the bleeding time based on impairment of platelet aggregation (Kim et al., 1999). In adult studies, when albumin is compared with dextran and high-molecular-weight HES, it is associated with less postoperative blood loss. Preliminary studies with middle-molecular-weight HES and albumin suggest that there is a minimal difference in postoperative blood loss. In patients with even mild forms of von Willebrand's disease, the administration of artificial colloid in patients can be associated with significant hemorrhagic complications; albumin or crystalloid should be used preferentially (De Jonge and Levi, 2001).

Hypothermia

There is substantial data that suggest that hypothermia is an independent and dramatic contributor to coagulopathy. Mild hypothermia of 35°C significantly prolongs the PT, aPTT, and bleeding time (Valeri et al., 1987). A decrease of 1.6°C in a randomized study of normothermia compared with mild hypothermia in hip procedures resulted in a 30% increase in blood loss and transfusion requirements (Schmied et al., 1996). At a core temperature of 34°C, coagulation and platelet function are severely altered, despite normal fibrinolytic function (Watts et al., 1998). The degree of hypothermia during cardiopulmonary bypass in infants undergoing correction of congenital heart disease has a high correlation with blood loss and transfusion requirements (Williams et al., 1999a). The transfusion of platelets and clotting factors does not correct the hypothermic coagulopathy completely in the absence of rewarming.

Both components of the hemostatic mechanism appear to be deleteriously affected by hypothermia. Platelet function is seriously impaired by mild hypothermia, due to a reduction in thromboxane A_2 release (Michelson et al., 1994). The clotting cascade involves a series of enzymatic reactions, all of which are slowed by hypothermia. The laboratory detection of hypothermic coagulopathy is often missed because most laboratories perform clotting tests at 37°C (Eddy et al., 2000). The PT and aPTT performed at the patient's actual core temperature will be prolonged (Rohrer and Natale, 1992). Some studies suggest that fibrinolysis is accelerated during hypothermia (Yoshihara, 1985); TEG data suggest that hypothermia impairs clot formation rather than enhancing fibrinolysis (Kettner et al., 1998). Thromboelastography can be adjusted to a patient's core body temperature to adequately evaluate the contribution hypothermia plays in a hypothermic coagulopathy.

Hemodilution

Acute normovolemic hemodilution to minimize red cell transfusion requirements often results in alterations of hemostasis. Quantitative modeling of acute normovolemic hemodilution demonstrates that patients often attain inadequate fibrinogen levels (<100 mg/dL) before they would reach the hematocrit threshold for red cell transfusion, or the threshold for platelet transfusions (Singbartl et al., 2003).

Massive Transfusion

Massive blood loss is defined as the loss of over one blood volume in a 24-hour period, the normal blood volume being 7% of ideal body weight in an adult and 8% to 9% in an infant. In the operating room, early recognition of major blood loss can be appreciated using the definitions of massive blood loss as occurring at the rate of 2 to 3 mL/kg per minute or 50% of blood volume in a 3-hour period (Fakhry and Sheldon, 1994).

The progression from dilutional coagulopathy to dilutional thrombocytopenia is seen in massive transfusion and in extreme hemodilution. During the era of whole blood administration, thrombocytopenia was the initial coagulopathic event (Counts et al., 1979). Currently, blood loss is most often replaced with plasma-poor RBC products, which are devoid of most coagulation factors. Under these conditions, dilution of coagulation factors is the initial coagulopathic event (marked by prolongation of the PT), and hypofibrinogenemia is the first factor deficiency that occurs, even while the platelet count is greater than 150,000/μL (Hiippala et al., 1995; Murray et al., 1995). The PT becomes prolonged when less than one blood volume is lost, but a clinical coagulopathy does not occur until the PT and PTT exceed 1.5 to 1.8 times the control values (Cote, 1991; Hirshberg et al., 2003). Fibrinogen concentrations fall below the hemostatically critical level of 100 mg/dL when blood loss is in excess of 150% of the patient's blood volume, and the remaining coagulation factors fall below 25%, after 200% blood loss. A platelet count of less than 50,000 should be anticipated when more than two blood volumes have been lost (Hiippala et al., 1995; Stainsby et al., 2000).

Because patients with severe traumatic injury often lose almost 70% of their blood volume before transfusion therapy and operative intervention, FFP administration should be given early to patients with exsanguinating injuries (Hirshberg et al., 2003). Simple dilution is the cause of these early coagulation abnormalities observed in patients with massive blood loss. Consumption, as a result of TF elaboration or excessive fibrinolysis, with production of fibrin degradation products, prolonged shock, or acidosis results in hemostatic failure at a much lower volume loss (Drummond and Petrovich, 2001).

Treatment should be anticipated when blood loss approaches 150% of blood volume. In this setting, if rapid laboratory corroboration is possible, a complete coagulation profile should be obtained to determine the patient's specific replacement needs. In the absence of timely data or with continuing hemorrhage, empirical therapy with FFP is justified. FFP at a dose of 20 mL/kg will increase fibrinogen by about 60 mg/dL and increase clotting factors by 20%.

Traumatic Coagulopathy Independent of Blood Loss or Replacement

Traumatic coagulopathy manifests as a hypocoagulable state associated with hypothermia, acidosis, clotting factor dilution, and tissue destruction, which is directly proportional to the severity of the traumatic injury (Kaufmann, 1997). Four risk factors have been identified as increasing the likelihood of the development of traumatic coagulopathy: pH less than 7.10, temperature less than 34°C, systolic blood pressure less than 70 mm Hg, and an injury severity score higher than 25 (Cosgriff et al., 1997). Extensive tissue destruction releases tissue thromboplastins, which activate the clotting process and result in a consumptive coagulopathy. TPA and PAI-1 are released from the extensively damaged tissue bed. In the first few hours after traumatic injury, TPA increases out of proportion to PAI-1 and produces a systemic activation of fibrinolysis (Enderson et al., 1991). This coagulopathy resembles that of DIC, but the diffuse microthrombi that are classically seen in DIC are not seen in traumatic coagulopathy.

The aggressive fluid management required by these patients produces a concomitant dilutional coagulopathy as well. Vigorous fluid resuscitation can result in a confluence of circumstances that in and of itself contributes to the traumatic coagulopathy. By increasing intravascular volume, blood pressure, and vasodilation, hemorrhage is further potentiated. These hemodynamic and rheologic perturbations increase the likelihood that hemostatic plug formation will not occur, and that blood will continue to leak around and through the hemostatic plug (Riddez et al., 1998; Orlinsky et al., 2001).

Traumatic coagulopathy is diagnosed clinically by pathologic oozing from tissue. Early ACT values can be used to predict which traumatically injured patients are at risk for developing traumatic coagulopathy. However, because the ACT test is performed at 37°C, the contribution of hypothermia to the development of this coagulopathy will be underappreciated (Aucar et al., 2003).

Intraoperative Evaluation of the Bleeding Patient

Activated clotting time (ACT) is a modification of a whole blood clotting test that uses kaolin or celite to accelerate coagulation by activating the contact pathway (Box 32–14). A fixed volume of blood is placed into a tube with activator at 37°C for 60 seconds, after which the contents are stirred until a clot

BOX 32–14 Evaluation of the Bleeding Child

Platelet Assessments

Abnormal number: thrombocytopenias, hemangiomas
Abnormal morphology: inherited platelet defects
Abnormal function: inherited or acquired

Prothrombin Time (PT) and Activated Partial Thromboplastin Time (aPTT) Assessments

Abnormal PT, normal aPTT
- Factor VII deficiency
- Vitamin K deficiency, liver disease
- Factor deficiencies: II, V, VII, X
- Drug related: Coumadin

Normal PT, abnormal aPTT
- Factor deficiencies: VIII, IX, XI, XII, kallikrein, prekallikrein, high-molecular-weight kininogen, von Willebrand's disease
- Drug related: heparin

Abnormal PT, abnormal aPTT
- Vitamin K deficiency, liver disease
- Factor deficiencies: II, V, X
- Dysfibrinogenemia
- Drug related: heparin and Coumadin

Abnormal PT, abnormal aPTT, thrombocytopenia
- Disseminated intravascular coagulation
- Liver disease
- Dysfibrinogenemia

Normal PT, normal aPTT, normal platelets
- Factor XIII deficiency
- α_2-Antiplasmin deficiency

Thrombin Time*

Normal
- Liver disease, vitamin K deficiency
- Factor deficiencies: II, V, and X
- Drug related: Coumadin

Abnormal
- Liver disease
- Disseminated intravascular coagulation
- Dysfibrinogenemia
- Drug related: heparin

*Useful in cases of abnormal PT and abnormal aPTT.

is formed. The normal ACT range is 80 to 120 seconds. This test can be performed easily at the bedside using commercially available equipment. ACT levels correlate well with anti-factor Xa heparin levels in the pre-cardiopulmonary bypass period, and are commonly used to monitor the adequacy of heparin anticoagulation levels during extracorporeal circulation (Despotis et al., 1999). The relationship of ACT with heparin dosing is linear in the setting of normal antithrombin III concentrations and factor XII activity, normothermia, a platelet count of more than 50,000, intact platelet function, and a fibrinogen level greater than 100 mg/mL (Spiess, 1998). However, in the absence of extracorporeal circulation, ACT has a much poorer correlation with plasma heparin concentrations than does the aPTT (Koerber et al., 1999). ACT is insensitive to many coagulation abnormalities, such that clotting deficiencies and platelet abnormalities can be present with a normal ACT (Girardi et al., 2000). Nevertheless, in the setting of major trauma, intraoperative ACT measurements were able to discriminate between patients who became coagulopathic and those who did not (Aucar et al., 2003). ACT levels do not correlate well with low-molecular-weight heparin anti-Xa levels (Henry et al., 2001).

The thromboelastograph is a point-of-care evaluation of a patient's hemostatic balance, from initial clot formation to clot retraction or dissolution. Coagulation of blood has been compared with building a house: TEG profiling does not end when the foundation stone is laid, as do the other clinically employed clotting studies. The TEG also reflects the speed of the building process, whether the building will be sturdy, and whether it is likely to be damaged soon after it is built. Initially described in 1948, the TEG examines the elastic properties of blood as it clots. Placed into a rotating cup with an immersed pin, liquid blood begins to clot by forming fibers between the cup and the pin, transmitting motion to the pin. The TEG measures the elastic shear modulus of the clot, providing information about the rate of clot formation, clot strength, platelet function, and fibrinolytic activity, reflected in the characteristics of the tracing produced (Samana, 2001; Srinivasa et al., 2001). The maximal elastic sheer modulus depends on platelet count, function, and the amount of fibrin deposited on the pin. The TEG is a global measure of hemostasis, useful when there are multiple hemostatic defects. The weakness of TEG is its inability to identify specific clotting abnormalities. The TEG is a sensitive indicator of hypocoagulable and hypercoagulable perturbations. The typical hypercoagulable TEG profile has the appearance of a cognac glass (Fig. 32–14) (Traverso et al., 1995).

The TEG parameters are illustrated in Figure 32–15:

R (i.e., reaction time): latency to initial clot formation; from onset of the tracing until a 2-mm amplitude on the tracing. This is similar to whole blood clotting time; it depends on an intact intrinsic pathway and an adequate generation of thrombin.
Prolonged: clotting deficiencies, heparin, thrombocytopenia
Correlated: aPTT
K (i.e., coagulation rate): rate of fibrin buildup and cross-linking, occurring from 2 to 20 mm
Prolonged: clotting deficiencies, platelet dysfunction, thrombocytopenia, hypofibrinogenemia
α angle: rate of increase in elastic shear modulus; the rate of fibrin buildup and cross-linking; slope of divergence of tracing from R
MA: maximal elastic shear modulus. Measured at maximal divergence of the graph, after the clot is entirely formed,

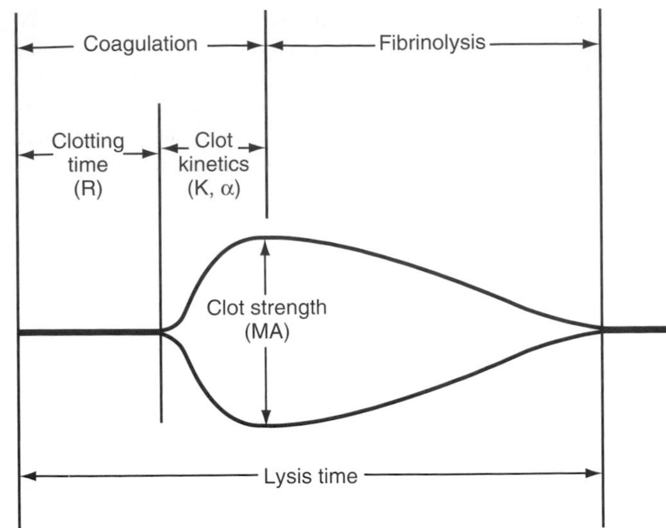

■ **FIGURE 32–14.** Parameters of the thromboelastograph.

this is the maximal clot strength. A typical clot has an MA of 50 mm, which is equivalent to 5000 dynes/cm^2. MA is the best description of the competency of the clot. MA depends on platelet count and function and on the fibrinogen level, as defined by the equation (Chandler, 1995):

$$\text{MA (mm)} = 0.12\ (\text{platelet count } [1000/\mu\text{L}]) + 0.081\ (\text{fibrinogen } [\text{mg/dL}]) + 15.2$$

Decreased: thrombocytopenia, platelet dysfunction hypofibrinogenemia, deficiencies of factor VIII and factor XIII
Increased: prothrombotic state
A_{30}, A_{60}: represents the percentage of fibrinolysis or clot retraction at 30 and 60 minutes; percent relative to MA

A typical tracing and the parameters of the TEG are illustrated in Figure 32–14. Figure 32–15 shows the tracings seen on the TEG for common disorders of hemostasis.

The R of patients receiving Coumadin increases with INR, but it may remain within a normal range (Hepner et al., 2002). Patients with decreased clotting factors have decreased R and K values and a prolonged PT, or they have a decreased angle and a prolonged aPTT. Hypofibrinogenemia is associated with

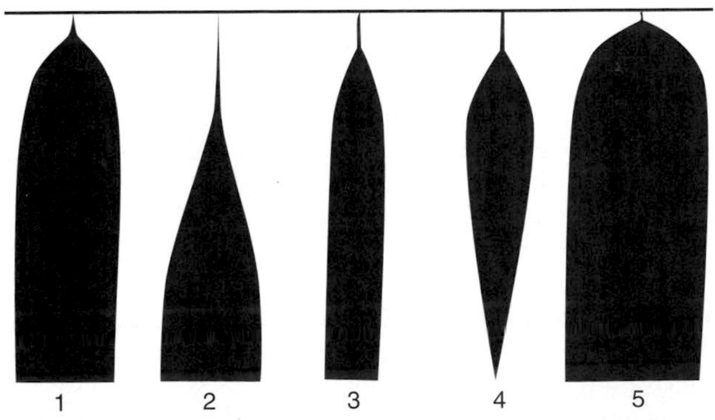

■ **FIGURE 32–15.** Thromboelastographic tracings of common hemostatic abnormalities. 1, normal; 2, hemophilia; 3, thrombocytopenia; 4, fibrinolysis; 5, hypercoagulation.

decreased R and K times, decreased angle, and decreased MA. Hyperfibrinolysis is characterized by reduced amplitude at 30 and 60 minutes.

The conditions under which a TEG is performed can be optimized to best define the clinical scenario. A TEG can be performed at the patient's core temperature to identify hemostatic perturbations due to modulation of body temperature. Additives have been employed to activate the coagulation process for TEG analysis, which shortens the study and reduces sample variability (Yamakage et al., 1998).

The TEG has been used in the pediatric population. Miller looked at the effects of age on TEG variables in children younger than 24 months of age undergoing elective noncardiac procedures. He found that all of the TEG variables in children less than 1 year of age were different from that of an adult control group. The rates of clot initiation and clot buildup, as well as clot strength, were all greater in the infant groups. Despite ontogenetic differences in clotting factor concentrations, the investigators concluded that the hemostatic mechanism of the infant is balanced. The coagulation indices were not reported in his original paper. Using the reported data, all children had a coagulation index of more than 2.0, suggesting a hypercoagulable state (Miller et al., 1997). The trend toward a hypercoagulable state in children was confirmed in a celite-activated TEG study as well (Pivalizza et al., 2001). TEG has also been used to document the intraoperative development of a hypercoagulable state in children undergoing craniotomy and resection of brain tissue (Goobie et al., 2001).

TREATMENT OF THE BLEEDING PATIENT

SAFETY OF TRANSFUSION AND FACTOR REPLACEMENT

Complications of life-threatening blood-borne virus transmission have been markedly reduced by the institution of multiple screening steps in the procurement of donor-derived plasma products. However, the risks of transfusion-associated transmission of thermostable viruses, such as hepatitis A and parvovirus B19, remain. Reports of transfusion associated-transmission of West Nile virus highlight the continued risks of using the blood supply as the principle source for hemostatic agents. Two nucleic acid–based tests for West Nile virus are in clinical trials and appear to be effective in detecting virus in asymptomatic donors. The list of potential blood-borne pathogens is long and continues to grow, although not all blood-borne viruses have been demonstrated to be pathogenic to humans (Quirolo, 2002). Unfortunately, these concerns are not completely alleviated by the use of recombinant factor concentrates. With the outbreak of new-variant Creutzfeldt-Jakob disease in the United Kingdom, there is concern that prion proteins may be contained in and transmitted by the human albumin used in the manufacture and formulation of some recombinant factors (Ludlam, 1997). Recombinant factor IX is unique because no human or animal protein is used in its preparation or formulation (White et al., 1998).

TREATMENT TRIGGERS

The ASA Task Force on Blood Component therapy recommended that the triggers for treatment of the patient who is at risk for bleeding be multiple and not depend on a single factor. Often, the critically ill child may require an emergent invasive procedure before a complete hemostatic profile has been determined. In these circumstances, bleeding from puncture sites or general oozing in the surgical field may necessitate empirical treatment with FFP (American Society of Anesthesiologists, 1996). Generally accepted treatment triggers for component therapy are listed in Box 32–15.

BOX 32–15 Recommendations for Blood Component Therapy

Platelets:	<50k for acute bleeding <100k for intracranial, subarachnoid, or extracorporeal circulation procedures
FFP:	aPTT > 1.5 times normal PT > 1.5 times normal
Fibrinogen:	<100 mg/dL

aPTT, activated partial thromboplastin time; FFP, fresh frozen plasma; PT, prothrombin time.

ANTICOAGULANT-INDUCED COAGULOPATHY

Patients who are experiencing severe bleeding should receive FFP in a dose of 20 mL/kg until vitamin K administration increases endogenous synthesis. Factor IX levels may be low in FFP (Makris et al., 1997). Infusion of factor IX complex concentrate, which contains high concentrations of the activated vitamin K–dependent factors (II, VII, IX, X) can correct anticoagulation rapidly without the excessive fluid volume exposure of FFP. Factor IX complex, at a dose of 40 IU/kg in addition to an FFP infusion successfully corrected the INR in patients with intracranial hemorrhage in one third of the time with 9% of total fluid volume administered as compared with FFP alone (Boulis et al., 1999). Recombinant factor VIIa is also able to correct oral anticoagulant-induced coagulopathy.

DDAVP is an analog of vasopressin that recruits factor VIII from storage sites within endothelial cells and may raise baseline factor VIII levels by 2-fold to 20-fold in normal patients and patients with mild hemophilia (Mannucci, 1997). This increase in factor level is often sufficient to prevent or limit minor bleeding. DDAVP also increases the release of high-molecular-weight vWF multimers from the endothelium. DDAVP is the treatment of choice for children with type 1 von Willebrand's disease, mild hemophilia, or platelet dysfunction, including uremia and drug-induced bleeding diatheses. In one study, preoperative administration of DDAVP was efficacious in controlling perioperative bleeding in more than 94% of children with von Willebrand's disease undergoing adenotonsillectomy. Complications of DDAVP included hyponatremia and seizure, which occurred in three patients and one patient, respectively (Allen et al., 1999). DDAVP is also effective in treating hemorrhage in patients with acquired inhibitors to factor VIII or factor IX (McFarland, 1999). DDAVP has also been reported to improve the bleeding diathesis in osteogenesis imperfecta, which is due to abnormal collagen-induced platelet aggregation dysfunction (Keegan et al., 2002).

DDAVP has been employed in a variety of procedures associated with risk of large volume blood loss in an attempt to decrease perioperative blood loss and transfusion requirements.

Despite early studies to suggest that DDAVP reduced blood loss in cardiac surgery patients, most studies suggest that DDAVP is not efficacious in uncomplicated cardiac surgery (Hedderich et al., 1990). Children undergoing complex congenital heart repair did not have any reduction in bleeding or transfusion requirements with the prophylactic use of DDAVP (Oliver et al., 2000). Similarly, DDAVP does not appear to reduce blood loss in spinal fusion for patients with idiopathic scoliosis or for those with cerebral palsy–associated neuromuscular scoliosis (Theroux et al., 1997; Alanay et al., 1999).

A test dose of DDAVP should be given in patients with von Willebrand's disease to predict the hemostatic effect before relying solely on this drug for treatment. The response can be measured by shortening of the bleeding time and the aPTT. Side effects include facial flushing, transient headache, tachycardia, and mild, transient decreases in systolic blood pressure. A dose of 0.3 mcg/kg administered intravenously over 20 to 30 minutes or intranasally (150 mcg for children weighing less than 50 kg and 300 mcg for those weighing more than 50 kg) increases factor VIII levels by 62%, and this dose may be repeated every 8 to 12 hours to control bleeding. Peak effects occur within 30 to 60 minutes after intravenous infusion and 60 to 90 minutes after intranasal administration (Lethagen et al., 1987). Tachyphylaxis may occur after three or four doses (Mannucci et al., 1992). Because severe hyponatremia-associated seizures have been reported with the use of DDAVP, close observation of fluid status and electrolyte balance is mandated (Sutor, 1998; Allen et al., 1999; Francis et al., 1999). Arterial thrombosis has occurred in some patients treated with DDAVP (Desmopressin and arterial thrombosis, 1989).

AGENTS USED TO CONTROL BLEEDING

Factor VIII

One unit of factor VIII per kilogram will increase the plasma factor VIII concentration by 2%. The half-life of infused factor VIII is shorter in hemophiliac patients with blood group O than in those with blood group A in the presence of active bleeding or after recent surgery. The half-life is increased with age and plasma concentration of vWF (Bjorkman et al., 1994; Vlot et al., 2000). The goal is a peak post infusion factor VIII level of about 0.3 to 1 U/mL (30% to 100% of normal), depending on the severity of bleeding. This can be achieved with the administration of 15 to 50 U/kg of factor VIII concentrate. For perioperative prophylaxis, plasma concentrations should be followed. Most mild bleeding episodes respond to a single dose of factor VIII, but additional follow-up treatments at 12 and 24 hours may be needed. For severe bleeding or after major surgery or trauma, therapeutic factor VIII concentrations with a nadir of more than 0.5 U/mL should be maintained for 5 to 14 days. A continuous infusion of factor VIII at a rate of 1 to 4 U/kg per hour or administered by intermittent injection (6 to 24 U/kg every 6 to 12 hours), guided by close monitoring of the aPTT, should maintain therapeutic levels.

Von Willebrand Factor Concentrate

Patients with von Willebrand's disease who are unresponsive to DDAVP administration have been treated in the past with multiple units of cryoprecipitate, resulting in exposure to a large number of allogeneic donors, each with a finite infectious risk. Virally inactivated, pooled factor VIII concentrates with a high vWF content have become available; Humate P is one of these products that has been approved for use in treating von Willebrand's disease. The ristocetin cofactor assay of Humate P, a measure of vWF activity, is twice that of its factor VIII content (Bolan et al., 2001).

Factor IX

The biologic half-life of factor IX is 24 hours, which is twice that of factor VIII. For severe bleeding in hemophilia B patients, an initial dose of 75 to 100 U/kg of factor can achieve the desired plasma level of greater than 0.75 U/mL, after which a continuous infusion or intermittent injections may be given. The levels of factor achieved after administration of recombinant factor IX are often markedly lower than with equivalent dosages of plasma-derived factor IX, mandating that serum levels be followed (Roth et al., 2001).

Antifibrinolytics

Two classes of antifibrinolytics have been employed to optimize hemostasis in the setting of a bleeding diathesis and to reduce blood loss and transfusion requirements during major procedures: the synthetic lysine analogs, e-aminocaproic acid (EACA) and tranexamic acid, and the serine protease inhibitor, aprotinin. Antifibrinolytic drugs are commonly employed when bleeding occurs in sites that are rich in plasminogen activator and other fibrinolytic enzymes, such as the endometrium, the gastrointestinal tract, and the urinary tract (Mannucci, 1998).

EACA binds to the lysine site on plasminogen and plasmin preventing plasmin binding to fibrin. Fibrinolysis is inhibited and clot stabilization is allowed to continue. EACA has been shown to be effective in decreasing blood loss in children undergoing cardiac surgery (Williams et al., 1999b). Children undergoing posterior lumbar fusion who received 100 mg/kg of EACA followed by an infusion of 10 mg/kg per hour had less blood loss and required less red cell transfusions than did a randomized control group (Florentino-Pineda et al., 2001).

Aprotinin is a naturally occurring serine protease inhibitor that affects hemostasis through several mechanisms; it is an antifibrinolytic, inhibits kallikrein, plasmin, trypsin, and inhibits activated protein C. Aprotinin inhibits the initiation of fibrinolysis and the contact phase of coagulation. Aprotinin has no effects on platelet function. Aprotinin is inactive when given orally. Aprotinin was first shown to be effective in reducing blood loss in coronary artery bypass graft operations (Lemmer et al., 1996). Aprotinin has been shown to be effective in reducing perioperative bleeding and transfusion requirements in cardiac surgery, liver transplantation, hip replacements, and in posterior spine fusion (Urban et al., 2001; Samama et al., 2002).

Mouth bleeding is common in hemophilia patients, resulting in part from the potent fibrinolytic activity of saliva. For oral or gastrointestinal bleeding in hemophiliacs, EACA is often very effective and may dramatically reduce the need for additional coagulation factor infusions when given at a dose of 100 mg/kg orally every 6 hours for 5 to 10 days after a hemorrhagic episode. Antifibrinolytic mouthwashes allow for the performance of dental extractions on patients receiving long-term oral anticoagulant treatment without lowering the degree of anticoagulation (Sindet-Pedersen et al., 1989).

Recombinant Factor VIIa

Recombinant factor VIIa (rFVIIa) is a synthetic clotting factor that was originally developed for use in patients with hemophilia who have developed inhibitors to factor VIII or factor IX. The rationale behind the development and clinical success of rFVIIa underscores the new paradigm of cell-based hemostasis presented earlier. Hemophiliacs are unable to generate the platelet-localized factor Xa necessary for explosive thrombin production because of deficiencies in factor VIII or factor IX. Hedner and Kisiel (1983) demonstrated that plasma-derived factor VIIa was effective in hemophilia A. Factor VIIa complexes with TF exposed at areas of vascular injury, acting as a local catalyst for coagulation. In sufficient quantities, factor VIIa binds to activated platelets and restores platelet-surface thrombin generation (Monroe et al., 1997). Augmented thrombin production increases platelet activation and thrombin-activatable fibrinolysis inhibitor (TAFI), which decreases fibrinolysis. The FVIIa/TF/Xa complex can overcome a deficiency of factor VIII or factor IX, the foundation for rFVIIa's sole evidence-based indication. For hemophiliacs with high inhibitor titers, rFVIIa has been effective in randomized, controlled trials in adults and children to prevent or minimize spontaneous bleeding and to decrease intraoperative blood loss, and it has been approved for use in patients with inhibitors (Leach et al., 1999; O'Connell et al., 2002).

The successful use of rFVIIa in mitigating uncontrollable bleeding in nonhemophiliac pediatric patients in a variety of clinical situations has been reported in numerous anecdotal accounts (Tobias et al., 2003a, 2003b). Because factor VII is the first of the clotting factors to become deficient in liver failure, rFVIIa has been used in the setting of hepatic dysfunction and vitamin K antagonism. The enhanced platelet activation that results from increased thrombin production has led to the use of rFVIIa in treating quantitative and qualitative platelet dysfunction (D'Oiron et al., 2000; Patel et al., 2001). In thrombocytopenia patients rFVIIa resulted in a reduction in bleeding time in 50% of patients. The clot formed with rFVIIa use has a denser mesh of fibrin fibers, which is more resistant to plasmin degradation (Hedner, 1998). Recombinant factor VIIa has been used in the massively transfused patient whose coagulopathy has been recalcitrant to conventional plasma component therapy.

The use of rFVIIa has many advantages. It is completely synthetic, decreasing the risks of infectious complications. The drug can be quickly reconstituted from powder, eliminating the time needed for thawing and procurement of products from the blood bank, and it is dissolved in a small volume, minimizing excessive volume load, electrolyte perturbations, and the latency between institution of treatment and correction of the hemostatic defect.

Recombinant factor VIIa has limitations as well. The efficacy of rFVIIa depends on the presence of the other clotting factors. In the setting of the massive transfusion, factor VIIa is not the only clotting factor that is deficient. Most of the anecdotal reports about the use of rFVIIa in massive transfusion-associated bleeding are in the context of earlier administration of FFP. RFVIIa has a short half-life, necessitating frequent dosing. In the context of liver failure or dilutional coagulopathy, dosing was required every 12 hours. In the presence of inhibitors to factor VIII or factor IX, doses must be given every 2 to 4 hours until hemostasis is maintained. Although no thrombotic complications have been reported in the limited anecdotal reports of the use of rFVIIa in the setting of noninhibitor coagulopathies, thrombotic events have been reported in patients with circulating inhibitors who have received rFVIIa. In an initial safety report, two episodes of DIC have been reported in a registry of 1947 uses of rFVIIa, an incidence of 0.1% (Roberts, 1998). In another report of adverse events, there were four fatal thromboembolic events in more than 5500 patients treated with factor VIIa from 1996 to 2000 (Martinowitz et al., 2001). Whether the difference in thrombotic complications is because of the limited experience with rFVIIa or is demonstrative of the differential prothrombotic tendency of rFVIIa under a variety of hemostatic conditions is unknown.

There is evidence that the interaction of TF and factor VIIa may have deleterious effects on the pulmonary vascular bed, with reports of the development of acute respiratory distress syndrome (ARDS) at the time of rFVIIa administration. TF-factor VIIa increases the expression of vascular endothelial growth factor, which is a key factor in the development of the capillary leak syndrome found in ARDS. Blockade of TF with site-inactivated factor VIIa, a competitive TF inhibitor, appeared to prevent the development of ARDS, renal insufficiency, and the systemic release of interleukin-6 and interluekin-8 in a baboon model of sepsis-induced organ dysfunction (Welty-Wolf et al., 2001; Carraway et al., 2003). TF blockade appears to protect the lung from *Escherichia coli* lipopolysaccharide–induced lung injury as well (Miller et al., 2002).

The recommended dose of rFVIIa is 90 mcg/kg administered over 2 to 5 minutes. Because of its short half-life, additional doses must be given every 2 to 4 hours until hemostasis is achieved. The dose for factor VII–deficient patients is 25 mcg/kg. In a series of 67 treatments of bleeding in patients with inhibitors to coagulation factors, there were three episodes of thrombophlebitis, and there was no evidence of disseminated intravascular coagulation or organ dysfunction caused by thrombotic complications (Scharrer, 1999). No laboratory parameter is available to determine an adequate dose or whether a hemostatically relevant endpoint has been reached.

Although potentially promising, at this point, the role of rFVIIa in the treatment of the perioperative bleeding should be relegated to that of rescue therapy for the intractably bleeding patient in whom conventional transfusion treatment has been unsuccessful. Specifically, the use of rFVIIa in patients at risk for catastrophic thrombotic complications, such as children with small vessel anastomoses or palliative cardiac shunts should be approached with caution until further experience is garnered. After randomized, controlled trials have been completed to better define the thrombotic and pulmonary risks, rFVIIa may become a first-line agent for many of the coagulopathies that plague patients in the perioperative period.

Hemostatic Formulary

Table 32–22 summarizes the blood-based components available for treatment of the bleeding patient, including their constituents and indications for their use.

Platelets

Each unit of platelets contains 5.5 to 7.5 × 10^{10} platelets diluted in 50 mL of plasma. An apheresis platelet unit contains more than 3 × 10^{11} platelets in 250 to 300 mL of plasma. One third of all transfused platelets undergo splenic sequestration. In nonsurgical patients, spontaneous bleeding with a platelet count higher than 20,000 is uncommon. The ASA Task Force suggests that patients receive transfusions for platelet counts below 50,000/μL and that platelet transfusions be considered for patients with platelet counts between 50,000 and 100,000/μL, taking into consideration the risks and consequences of postoperative bleeding from the surgical site. If concurrent platelet dysfunction exists, the threshold for platelet transfusion should be raised. The ideal platelet dose is between 0.07 and 0.15 × 10^{11} platelets/kg, which is approximately 10 mL/kg. A dose of 5 to 10 mL/kg or 1 unit/10 kg can increase the platelet count to 50,000.

TABLE 32–22. Hemostatic formulary

Component	Contents	Indications	Adult Dose	Outcome
Whole blood	Hematocrit: 30% to 40% Most clotting factors ↓ Factor V, factor VIII No platelets	Neonatal surgery Massive transfusion		
Fresh frozen plasma, 225 mL	All clotting factors 2 mg/mL of fibrinogen	Hemodilution Liver failure Factor XI deficiency Disseminated intravascular coagulation Warfarin toxicity	10 to 15 mL/kg (2 units) 5 to 8 mL/kg	↑ 15% in factors ↑ 40 mg/dL of fibrinogen
Platelets, 50 mL	$>5.5 \times 10^{10}$ 50 mL of plasma	Thrombocytopenia Platelet dysfunction	5 to 10 mL/kg 1 unit/10 kg (10 units)	↑ 50,000
Cryoprecipitate, 25 mL*	Fibrinogen >150 mg Factor VIII >80 units von Willebrand factor >80 units Factor XIII >80 units	↓ Fibrinogen Hemophilia A von Willebrand's disease	1 to 2 units/10 kg (10 units)	↑ 60 to 100 mg/dL of fibrinogen

*Cryo units = (desired fibrinogen–initial fibrinogen) × Plasma Volume ÷ 100 mL/dL
150 mg fibrinogen/unit
†Factor VIII dosing: desired FVIII – initial FVIII × plasma volume; about 1 unit/kg produces an increase of 2% factor activity.

Platelets are much more likely than RBCs to cause bacterial sepsis, because they are stored at room temperature for up to 5 days and potentially have a higher bacterial load. The reported incidence of bacterial contamination of platelet products is one case per 2000 units (Snyder and Rinder, 2003). Storing the platelets in galactose-containing solution has been found to preserve platelet function despite chilling, and this approach may reduce the risk of bacterial contamination (Hoffmeister et al., 2003). Platelet concentrates are more frequently contaminated but are diluted before administration. Single-donor platelets have a greater volume with higher numbers of bacteria per unit administered and are more frequently implicated in sepsis (Busch, 2001). Platelet transfusions can also be associated with the development of pulmonary microvascular injury called transfusion-related acute lung injury (TRALI). TRALI is clinically similar to ARDS (discussed later). Within 6 hours of receiving a plasma-containing product, fever, tachypnea, dyspnea, progressive hypoxemia, radiographic evidence of pulmonary edema, and hypotension occur. The prevalence of TRALI in patients with platelet transfusions is estimated to be 3 per 1000 units of concentrate (Silliman, 1999).

Fresh Frozen Plasma

FFP contains 250 mL of plasma and 500 mg of fibrinogen in a citrate anticoagulant. One unit of FFP has a concentration of coagulation factors similar to that of 4 to 5 units of platelet concentrates, 1 apheresis unit of platelets, and 1 unit of fresh whole blood; 1 mL/kg of FFP raises most factor levels by approximately 1%. After a dose of 10 to 15 mL/kg of FFP, plasma clotting factors rise about 15%, and the fibrinogen level rises by 40 mg/dL. However, FFP contains only 0.6% of factor VIII.

FFP use is indicated for treatment of microvascular bleeding in massively transfused patients, for documented coagulopathy (PT > 1.5 times) in the massively transfused patient, for urgent reversal of anticoagulant therapy, and for active bleeding with a history or course suggesting an inherited or acquired coagulopathy, for which specific factor concentrates are not available.

Cryoprecipitate

Cryoprecipitate is the most practical source for fibrinogen replacement. Each unit contains approximately 200 mg of fibrinogen and more than 80 units of factor VIII, vWF, fibronectin, and factor XIII. Achieving fibrinogen plasma levels of 80 to 100 mg/dL and maintaining this level above 50 to 60 mg/dL usually controls hemorrhagic symptoms. To raise the fibrinogen level 100 mg/dL, 0.17 unit of cryoprecipitate per 1 kg of body weight should be infused. Fibrinogen has a long half-life, and replacement therapy, therefore, can be given at intervals of 3 to 4 days.

Cryoprecipitate is indicated for several uses:

1. Prophylactic use in patients with congenital fibrinogen deficiencies, von Willebrand's disease unresponsive to DDAVP, and factor VIII deficiency when factor VIII concentrate is not available
2. Bleeding patients with von Willebrand's disease or factor VIII deficiency when factor VIII concentrate is not available
3. Consumptive coagulopathies when the fibrinogen level is less than 80 to 100 mg/dL
4. Microvascular bleeding in the massively transfused patient when hypofibrinogenemia cannot be immediately documented

Factors V, X, XI, and XIII

The only source of *factor V* is FFP. Normal hemostasis is achieved with levels above 25 U/dL. This can be achieved with a loading dose of 20 mL/kg of FFP, followed by infusions of 6 mL/kg every 12 hours. Factor V is very labile in FFP, and recently donated FFP should be used. FFP (1 mL/kg) increases the plasma level of factor X by 1 U/dL. FFP (1 mL/kg) increases circulating factor XI by 1.5 U/dL. Hemostatic levels of factor XIII are 2 to 3 U/dL. FFP (5 to 10 mL/kg) is adequate to achieve therapeutic levels. Cryoprecipitate may also be used. One bag of cryoprecipitate contains 75 U of factor XIII.

COMPLICATIONS OF THE TREATMENT OF THE BLEEDING PATIENT

Citrate Intoxication

Citrate, when infused rapidly as the storage solution of blood products, can cause a temporary reduction in ionized calcium levels. FFP has considerably more citrate than does packed

RBCs in CPDA-1. The signs of citrate intoxication include hypotension, narrow pulse pressure, flattening of the instantaneous slope of the arterial catheter tracing, elevated end diastolic pressures, prolongation of the QT interval, widening of the QRS complexes, and flattening of the T waves. Hypocalcemia is directly related to the rate of citrate administration, and it is unlikely to occur unless transfusions exceed 1 mL/kg per minute. Impaired perfusion or liver dysfunction lowers this threshold for potential hypocalcemia. Slow calcium administration during rapid blood product administration can avert this induced hypocalcemia (Cote et al., 1988).

Transfusion-Related Acute Lung Injury

TRALI usually manifests as bilateral pulmonary infiltrates within 4 hours of transfusion. The clinical picture is that of ARDS. There are two proposed mechanisms for TRALI. Granulocytes from transfused blood products interact with antibodies in the pulmonary microvasculature leading to endothelial injury and alveolar exudation. Anti-leukocyte antibodies are found in this group of patients. The other proposed mechanism involves clinical settings such as trauma, sepsis, or massive transfusion, in which cytokine production partially activates endogenous neutrophils. These neutrophils become adherent to the pulmonary microvascular endothelium. On exposure to the lipids contained in transfused blood products, neutrophil activation becomes complete and endothelial damage results in the clinical picture of TRALI (Silliman et al., 1998; Silliman, 1999).

Transfusion-Associated Graft-versus-Host Disease

Transfusion associated graft-versus-host disease (TA-GVHD) results when immunocompetent lymphocytes are transfused into a patient who is unable to reject allogeneic cells. The pathogenesis of TA-GVHD appears to require recipient secretion of tumor necrosis factor and interleukin-1 in response to preexisting injury or infection to enhance antigen recognition by donor T cells (Ferrara and Krenger, 1998). These transfused lymphocytes react with host antigens producing fever, skin rash, pancytopenia, diarrhea, and abnormal liver function test results. TA-GVHD can occur 10 to 28 days after transfusion. The pancytopenia is profound and mortality approaches 100%. Median survival is only 21 days after transfusion. Patients who are at high risk for developing TA-GVHD include neonates, patients with congenital immunodeficiency, leukemia, or lymphoma and those who have received intensive chemotherapy and bone marrow or solid organ transplants. Infants and children with severe combined immunodeficiency syndrome (SCIDS) are of most concern, in part because SCIDS is often unrecognized at birth or in early infancy. Although many children with SCIDS are diagnosed by 6 months of age, children have been diagnosed with SCIDS up until 2 years of age. Children with the DiGeorge anomaly and those with conotruncal defects or Tetralogy of Fallot in whom immunodeficiency has not been excluded should be considered at risk for TA-GVHD as well (Neill and Zuckerberg, 1995). Patients with HIV do not appear to be at increased risk for TA-GVHD, as only one case has been reported despite significant transfusion support (Kruskall et al., 2001). The lack of TA-GVHD in HIV patients may underscore the key role the recipient's CD4 cells, which are depleted early in the course of HIV infection, plays in the pathogenesis of TA-GVHD (Ammann, 1993).

TA-GVHD can occur in patients without an immunodeficiency. Patients who receive products from a donor who is homozygous for a shared haplotype are also at risk for TA-GVHD. The chance of receiving haplotype homozygous blood from an unrelated donor varies in different countries, ranging from 1 in 874 in Japan, 1 in 7147 whites in the United States, and 1 in 16,835 in France. Trauma patients with no known risk factors for TA-GVHD had evidence of microchimerism for as long as 1.5 years after transfusion (Lee et al., 1999). The spectrum of patients who are at potential risk for TA-GVHD is likely to increase with the use of immunosuppressive regimens in the treatment of autoimmune and inflammatory bowel diseases.

The prevention of TA-GVHD lies in attenuation of donor lymphocyte reactivity. The only method approved by the U.S. Food and Drug Administration (FDA) is irradiation (Williamson et al., 1995). Irradiation damages the DNA in donated T cells, which precludes their proliferation and prevents TA-GVHD development (Shlomchik, 1999). Most blood centers rely on a nominal dose of 25Gy. Patients at risk for TA-GVHD should receive only irradiated RBCs, platelets, and granulocytes. A summary of situations in which irradiated blood products should be administered is presented in Box 32–16.

BOX 32–16 Indications for Irradiated Blood Products

- Intrauterine transfusions
- Patients < 2 years old
- Transplantation
  - Bone marrow transplantation
  - Organ transplantation
- Oncologic conditions
  - Lymphoma
  - Neuroblastoma
  - Glioblastoma
  - Rhabdomyosarcoma
- Immunodeficiency
  - Congenital immunodeficiency
    - Wiskott-Aldrich syndrome
    - Conotruncal abnormalities
  - Acquired immunodeficiency
    - Human immunodeficiency virus infection
    - Patients receiving immunosuppressive drugs
- Recipients of blood products from first-degree relatives

To avoid the risk of TA-GVHD in patients with late-presenting severe combined immunodeficiency syndrome (SCIDS), all children younger than 2 years should receive only irradiated products. Blood components donated from first- or second-degree relatives should be irradiated, because there is usually homozygosity for an HLA haplotype (Kanter, 1992). FFP and cryoprecipitate do not need to be irradiated, because most authorities feel that the freezing and thawing process destroys any donor T cells (Luban, 2002). Nevertheless, there are reports of some progenitor cells that have survived the freezing and thawing process, suggesting that even FFP and cryoprecipitate be irradiated as well (Anderson, 1995; Wieding et al., 1994).

Hyperkalemia

Acute hemodynamic decompensation after red cell transfusions should be considered hyperkalemia, until proved otherwise. Large volumes (>25 mL/kg) of stored red cells given rapidly to infants have been associated with hyperkalemic arrests (Hall et al., 1993). The combination of perturbations of calcium and potassium concentrations in the context of central venous blood administration may be sufficient to produce a hyperkalemic dysrhythmia (Eder, 2002).

■ MISCELLANEOUS PROBLEMS

■ ACQUIRED IMMUNODEFICIENCY SYNDROME

Clinical Presentation

The acquired immunodeficiency syndrome (AIDS) epidemic has had an enormous deleterious impact on worldwide health and this effect has not spared children. In 1997, the World Health Organization (WHO) estimated that there were more than 30 million people worldwide who were infected with HIV (Kahn and Walker, 1998). Of this number, 1.1 million were younger than 15 years. Most people infected with HIV live outside the United States. HIV/AIDS incidence varies by both ethnicity and geography. In the United States, AIDS is seen more frequently in Hispanic and African-American children than in Caucasians. In 1996, the CDC National HIV/AIDS surveillance system reported that 58% of the children with AIDS in the United States were African American, 23% were Hispanic, and 18% were white. Most U.S. cases have been reported in the Northeast (44%) and the South (36%), primarily in larger metropolitan areas. Although adolescents comprise a small percentage of cases of HIV/AIDS, the number of adolescents with HIV/AIDS is growing rapidly.

Transmission of HIV can occur through parenteral exposure to blood, sexual contact, or through vertical transmission from mother to child. In the United States, most HIV infections in children younger than 13 years have resulted from vertical transmission. Approximately 6000 to 7000 children are born to HIV-positive mothers annually in the United States. Women of childbearing are one of the fastest growing groups of individuals with AIDS in the United States, accounting for greater than 20% of adult AIDS cases reported (CDC, 1996). Transmission of HIV from mother to child can occur before, during, or after delivery. The highest percentage of HIV-infected children acquire the virus during delivery, most likely through exposure to infected blood and secretion during delivery. Chance of transmission is increased with preterm births, low birth weight, low maternal CD4 counts, and intravenous drug use during pregnancy. Transmission has been decreased by cesarean section and with prenatal, intrapartum, and postnatal zidovudine (AZT) treatment (CDC, 1997).

In the United States, postpartum transmission by breast-feeding is the least common mode of perinatal transmission; however, it is quite important in developing countries. Transmission of HIV through contaminated blood or blood products accounts for approximately 3% of AIDS cases in the United States. Blood product screening for HIV began in the United States in 1985, and since then, the risk of transmission has decreased dramatically. Sexual transmission of HIV is rare in pediatric patients, but a small number of cases have been reported (American Academy of Pediatrics, 2001a). The age at which AIDS is diagnosed in children varies with the mode of transmission. Children who were infected by transfusion of contaminated blood or blood products, primarily between the years of 1978 and 1985, are now teens or young adults. Children who acquired the disease during birth can be diagnosed as infants with detection of virus as early as 1 week of age. The viral load increases with time, and by 4 months of age, almost all infected infants have virus detectable in the peripheral blood (American Academy of Pediatrics, 1997). There are three patterns of progression of HIV in infected infants and children. Some newborns, those who were infected during gestation, develop symptoms within the first few months of life. Without treatment, these infants often die before their first birthday. These infants have detectable virus very early in life. Most newborns acquire the infection during birth, and these infants have a much slower progression of disease. The viral load increases in the first few months of life then declines over the subsequent 2 years. A small percentage of infants with perinatal infection survive for extended periods with minimal progression of the disease.

Children infected with HIV have generally the same immunologic effects as adults. Because infants and children have a lymphocytosis, true lymphopenia is relatively rare. However, there is progressive depletion of CD4 lymphocytes with development of opportunistic infections. The CDC classification system for HIV in young children includes the presence of signs and symptoms, the state of immunodeficiency, and the immunologic category of the disease (CDC, 1994). The recommendations for initiation of antiretroviral therapy in infants, children, and adolescents are summarized in Tables 32–23 and 32–24 (CDC, 1998). In the perioperative environment, caring for children with HIV/AIDS centers on two major considerations: the effects of this systemic infection and its treatment on the child's readiness for anesthesia and surgery and the protection of health care workers from infection from these children. Infants and children with HIV/AIDS have many opportunistic infections, which may involve all organ systems. The most common serious infections

■ TABLE 32–23. Indications for initiation of antiretroviral therapy in children younger than 12 months with human immunodeficiency virus infection

Clinical Category*		$CD4^+$ Cell Percentage	Plasma HIV RNA Copy Number†	Recommendation
Symptomatic (clinical category A, B, or C)	*OR*	<25% (immune category 2 or 3)*	Any value	Treat*
Asymptomatic (clinical category N)	*AND*	≥25% (immune category 1)	Any value	Consider treatment‡

*Clinical and immune category parameters and specific treatment guidelines with recommended drugs can be found at http://aidsinfo.nih.gov/guidelines.

†Plasma human immunodeficiency virus (HIV) RNA levels are higher in HIV-infected infants than in older infected children and adults, and they may be difficult to interpret in infants younger than 12 months because overall HIV RNA levels are high, and there is an overlap in HIV RNA levels between infants who have and those who do not have rapid disease progression.

‡Because HIV infection progresses more rapidly in infants than on older children or adults, some experts treat all HIV-infected infants younger than 6 months or younger than 12 months, regardless of clinical, immunologic, or virologic parameters.

Adapted from http://aidsinfo.nih.gov/guidelines.

■ TABLE 32–24. Indications for initiation of antiretroviral therapy in children 1 year old or older with human immunodeficiency virus infection

Clinical Category*		CD4⁺ Percentage		Plasma HIV RNA Copy Number	Recommendation
Acquired immunodeficiency syndrome (AIDS) (clinical category C)	*OR*	<15% (immune category 3)		Any value	Treat
Mild to moderate symptoms (clinical category A or B)	*OR*	15% to 25%† (immune category 2)	*OR*	≥100,000 copies/mL‡	Consider treatment
Asymptomatic (clinical category N)	*AND*	>25% (immune category 1)	*AND*	<100,000 copies/mL‡	Many experts defer therapy and closely monitor clinical and viral parameters

*Clinical and immune category parameters and specific treatment guidelines with recommended drugs can be found at http://aidsinfo.nih.gov/guidelines.
†Many experts initiate therapy if the CD4⁺ cell percentage is between 15% and 20%, and they defer therapy and increase monitoring frequency for children with CD4⁺ cell percentages between 21% and 25%.
‡There is controversy among pediatric human immunodeficiency virus (HIV) experts regarding the plasma HIV RNA threshold warranting consideration of therapy in children in the absence of clinical or immune abnormalities; some experts consider initiation of therapy in asymptomatic children if the plasma HIV RNA levels are between 50,000 and 100,000 copies/mL.
Adapted from http://aidsinfo.nih.gov/guidelines

are pneumonia, bacteremia, and sepsis; nearly every organ system may be affected by opportunistic infections.

Anesthetic Considerations

As many as 80% of children with HIV develop lung disease (McSherry, 1996). Pulmonary function is compromised by bacterial and viral infections, but many children with AIDS also develop lipoid interstitial pneumonia (LIP) (Rubinstein et al., 1986). The incidence of LIP in HIV-infected children is approximately 20% to 30%. Clinical characteristics of this condition include tachypnea, wheezing, cough, hypoxemia, and even clubbing. This condition presents with bilateral infiltrates. Severely affected children may have bronchiectasis and lung cysts. The most common opportunistic infection in children with AIDS is probably *Pneumocystis carinii* pneumonia. Most people are infected with this very common organism in childhood, but disease is caused only in immunocompromised individuals. The peak incidence of this infection is in children younger than 1 year. *Pneumocystis carinii* pneumonia is often characterized by the acute onset of fever, hypoxemia, and respiratory distress, but a more slowly progressing disease also occurs (Simonds and Orejas, 1999). Infection with respiratory viruses in children with HIV are common and often more severe in these patients. In children with AIDS, infections with RSV, parainfluenza viruses, and influenza viruses are more likely to be symptomatic, and infections with adenovirus or measles may lead to serious morbidity (Englund and King, 1998).

Children with LIP and/or infectious pneumonia may present to the operating room for bronchoscopy with bronchoalveolar lavage for diagnosis. These children are often hypoxemic and in respiratory distress before the procedure. These cases are often quite challenging because establishing a diagnosis is important in prescribing therapy; the procedure cannot be delayed until the child's condition improves. Children who are infected in the perinatal period with HIV often have involvement of the CNS, although opportunistic infections of the CNS are uncommon. In toddlers, the presentation is that of a progressive encephalopathy with loss of developmental milestones or arrest of development. CNS pathology includes low brain weight, acquired microcephaly, inflammatory infiltrates, and calcific vasculopathy of the basal ganglia vessels. As the encephalopathy progresses, there may be loss of fine and gross motor skills, loss of language skills, and development of behavioral problems. In older children, the clinical picture often becomes one of a static encephalopathy (Browers et al., 1998). Seizures and focal neurologic signs are unusual, and their presence should prompt a search for other causes such as infection, stroke, or a tumor.

Approximately 10% to 20% of children with HIV infections have clinically significant cardiovascular involvement. Careful echocardiographic and electrocardiographic evaluations of children with AIDS may uncover subtle abnormalities in a much higher percentage of patients (Lipshultz et al., 1989). Common abnormalities include resting sinus tachycardia, sinus arrhythmias, and ventricular hypertrophy. Echocardiographic studies of children with HIV infection have demonstrated both LV diastolic and systolic dysfunction. One center reported that 10% of children with HIV required temporary treatment for congestive heart failure, generally during an intercurrent illness (Luginbuhl et al., 1993).

Hepatosplenomegaly and a gallop are indications of congestive heart failure in these patients. Medical therapy has been generally effective in reversing the symptoms of congestive heart failure. In children with advanced AIDS, hemodynamic instability may occur (Evenhouse et al., 1987; Stewart et al., 1989).

Children with AIDS often have lowered counts of all the formed elements of the blood. Poor bone marrow function in these patients may be due to the disease itself, poor nutrition, or the side effect of the medications used to treat the disease. As with many chronic conditions, the anemia seen in AIDS patients is often normochromic or normocytic, with low reticulocyte counts. In the preoperative evaluation of these children, other causes for anemia, such as occult bleeding, should be ruled out (Morse, 2002). Treatment of anemia in HIV-infected children should address the cause but also often includes administration of erythropoietin (rh-EPO). Perioperative transfusion of RBCs should be undertaken only to provide a minimally acceptable level of oxygen delivery and after careful consideration of the possible deleterious effects in patients with HIV/AIDS (Hillyer et al., 1999; Jacobson et al., 1990). Only cytomegalovirus-negative, leukocyte-depleted RBCs should be used. Thrombocytopenia has a high prevalence in patents with HIV. The cause is sometimes difficult to determine, but both impaired production and increased destruction have been found in AIDS patients. Complicating thrombocytopenia, a lupus-type anticoagulant was found in 20% of AIDS patients undergoing routine coagulation testing (Cohen et al., 1986).

Gastrointestinal and nutritional problems can be very common and very difficult to treat in children with AIDS. Infections of the gastrointestinal tract cause major morbidity and can be quite severe in these patients (Doyle and Pickering, 1990). Oral infections with candida or ulcerative gingivitis are seen in HIV-infected children. Bacterial, viral, or fungal infections may cause diarrhea. With recurrent or chronic diarrhea, children develop malnutrition and failure to thrive. Although linear growth may correlate with the severity of viremia, growth failure in these children can result from malabsorption, poor nutrient intake, and altered energy use. Hepatosplenomegaly is seen in up to 80% to 90% of children infected with HIV, and it is associated elevated levels of serum aminotransferase. Coinfection with hepatitis B or C virus is common in HIV-infected children. Pancreatitis can occur, usually as a complication of the drug therapy for HIV or one of the opportunistic infections. Other clinical manifestations of HIV infection include various rashes such as eczema or seborrhea and manifestation of renal dysfunction such as proteinuria, hematuria, hypoalbuminemia, and edema.

Anesthesia and Procedures

The procedures that children with HIV/AIDS commonly undergo are diagnostic bronchoscopies with bronchoalveolar lavage, diagnostic upper and lower endoscopies, placement of gastrostomy tubes for nutritional support, and placement of central venous catheters. In addition to procedures specific to this systemic infection, these children can require anesthesia for any other surgical or diagnostic procedure such as myringotomy, herniorrhaphy, and others. In the evaluation of these children before anesthesia, the effects of the infection on the organ systems should be evaluated as outlined previously. The anesthesiologist should be aware of medications taken and of their effects and side effects. In addition to medications specific for the treatment of AIDS, these children are often being treated with antibiotics and with corticosteroids. Pulmonary insufficiency is often seen in patients with AIDS, and despite meticulous care during the procedure, clinical deterioration commonly occurs after the procedure. During the preanesthetic visit, the anesthesiologist should, when indicated, discuss the possibility of postoperative intubation and ventilation. In advanced cases for which there is a do not resuscitate (DNR) or other advance directive in place, the anesthesiologist should discuss these plans thoroughly with the child and family (Truog et al., 1999). It may be that the person caring for the child is not a biologic parent, necessitating additional administrative steps in the informed consent process.

Although the specific agents and techniques chosen for a case will depend on the particular child and situation, there are several points to keep in mind when making those choices. CNS involvement is relatively common, and CNS depressants such as barbiturates, benzodiazepines, and opioids should be carefully titrated. If liver or renal dysfunction occurs, drug metabolism and elimination will be impaired. Attention to sterile technique, often not a priority among anesthesiologists, is important in these children who have severe immunocompromise.

Pain Management

There are many causes for pain and suffering in infected children in addition to postoperative pain. The anesthesiologist/pediatric pain specialist should be prepared to participate in management of both the acute and chronic pain that afflicts these children. The clinical presentations of pain and suffering in children with AIDS are varied and the pharmacologic and nonpharmacologic treatments that may be employed are very broad. Assessment is often very difficult because of the nature of the discomfort and to the difficulty of communication with children afflicted with encephalopathy.

Health Care Providers and Exposure to Human Immunodeficiency Virus

Those caring for a child with AIDS must take prudent steps to prevent transmission. Although HIV has been isolated from saliva, the titer is generally low. Studies of hundreds of household contacts have confirmed that the risk of transmission from casual contact is nearly zero. It is, therefore, very unlikely that operating room personnel would contract AIDS from passive contact with an HIV-positive child. By far the greatest risk of contracting AIDS for health care workers is by a needlestick with a contaminated needle. Seroconversion is not a common occurrence after accidental needlestick in health care workers. An earlier report found that seroconversion occurred in 0.4% of all health care workers and that all the conversions occurred after needlesticks or lacerations.

Hollow-bore needles, those used to administer medications, give a much larger inoculum of blood and infectious agent than solid needles. After parenteral exposure to HIV, three steps should be taken: postexposure prophylaxis, postexposure treatment, and follow-up. A health care worker who has a parenteral exposure to blood or body fluids from a child known or suspected to have AIDS should have the wound thoroughly washed and then irrigated with saline. Exposed mucous membranes should be thoroughly irrigated with saline. The exposure should be immediately reported to the institutional employee health service or the "stick team." As prophylaxis is begun, the employee should be tested to document HIV status. Subsequent testing should occur at 6 and 12 weeks. Postexposure prophylaxis should be undertaken immediately after the parenteral exposure to the blood or body fluid from a child suspected or known to have HIV infection.

A retrospective study done by the CDC was undertaken to determine the rate of seroconversion of health care workers. The study involved health care workers in England, France, and the United States. There were three conclusions: exposure to a large quantity of blood was associated with a higher rate of seroconversion; seroconversion was more likely when the exposure was from a patient in the terminal stages of AIDS; and there was a 79% decrease in seroconversion when zidovudine was begun after exposure. Guidelines for treatment of exposed health care workers recommend initiation of zidovudine with the possible addition of lamivudine or indinavir. Anesthesiologists should be familiar with the needlestick policy of their institution and be prepared to follow it and advise others of the policy in the event of an exposure. Following universal precautions, as recommended by the CDC (Michna and Mason, 2002), should be the practice for all health care workers who have direct patient contact or exposure to patients' bodily fluids.

LATEX ALLERGY

The first published report in an American medical journal of allergy to rubber gloves appeared in 1933 (Downing, 1933). Subsequently, there were sporadic reports until the late 1980s and early 1990s, after which there was a sharp increase in the reporting of allergic reactions to latex. This increase is thought to reflect the increased exposure of health care workers and patients after the CDC's publication of the Universal Precautions Guidelines (CDC, 1987). The annual use of surgical gloves in the United States increased by a factor of 25, from 800 million to 20 billion. Allergic reactions to latex were first reported by pediatric anesthesiologists in 1991, before the Medical Alert circulated in 1991 by the FDA warning health care workers of this emerging problem (Holzman et al., 1990).

Latex allergy is a significant problem in health care. As of 1997, the FDA had received through its mandatory reporting database reports of more than 2300 allergic reactions involving latex-containing medical products, with 225 cases of anaphylaxis, 53 cardiac arrests, and 17 deaths. Patient populations at increased risk for latex allergy have been identified (Hochleitner et al., 2001; Randolph, 2001; Hourihane et al., 2002):

Patients who have undergone multiple surgical procedures
Patients with spina bifida (Myelomeningocele)
Patients with bladder exstrophy
Health care personnel
Individuals with a history of atopy
Individuals with a history of allergy to tropical fruits

Many children who have experienced allergic reactions to latex in the operating room have had spina bifida or urinary tract anomalies. These two groups undergo multiple surgical procedures, making it difficult to ascertain whether the high prevalence of latex allergy is caused by frequent exposure or an immunologic response associated with specific conditions. Reactions to latex have been divided into three types: irritant contact dermatitis; type IV hypersensitivity (i.e., skin reactions similar to poison ivy); and type I, or IgE-mediated, hypersensitivity. Type I hypersensitivity is by far the more severe reaction. All the deaths reported to the FDA were caused by type I hypersensitivity. This type of response to latex has been reported in many clinical settings, including intraabdominal surgery, genitourinary surgery, dental procedures, and even while putting on latex-containing gloves. Manifestations of type I, IgE-mediated hypersensitivity include the following:

1. Hives, urticaria, red eyes, angioedema of the eyelids
2. Nasal congestion
3. Gastrointestinal cramping, nausea, diarrhea
4. Headache, anxiety
5. Shortness of breath, tachycardia, hypotension, anaphylaxis

Intraoperative type I hypersensitivity generally does not occur immediately at the beginning of the surgical procedure but after exposure of the peritoneum or other mucous membrane to latex. The presentation includes bronchospasm, hypoxemia, hypotension, and tachycardia. There may also be skin manifestations such as urticaria or flushing. The bronchospasm and hypotension are difficult to treat, even with IV epinephrine, and the syndrome persists until the exposure is stopped. In a series of patients reported by Holzman, the mean Spo_2 fell from 100% to 92% (Holzman, 1993).

Treatment of Intraoperative Anaphylaxis

As more and more medical equipment is manufactured free of latex, it is important to maintain vigilance to the possibility of inadvertent exposure of an at-risk patient with resultant reaction. Delay in diagnosis of an episode of latex anaphylaxis will only make treatment more difficult due to continued exposure to the offending allergen. The mainstays of treatment are *stopping the latex exposure* and *resuscitation.*

All latex must be removed from the surgical field and the procedure ended as rapidly as possible. Materials whose latex content is unknown should also be removed. If blood and/or antibiotics are being administered, this administration should be stopped. Consideration should be given to evaluating the patient for a transfusion reaction if the symptoms and signs of anaphylaxis began during blood administration. Resuscitation efforts are directed toward stabilization of the vital signs and reversal of the pathophysiology of anaphylaxis. Because these reactions often occur during intraabdominal surgery, the patients are usually already intubated when the reaction occurs. If the patient is not intubated, strong consideration should be given to intubation. Based on the progress of the surgery and the patient's vital signs, administration of anesthetic agents should be stopped. Intravenous fluid and epinephrine doses should be given to maintain blood pressure, a Foley catheter placed, invasive hemodynamic monitoring should be instituted, and inhaled bronchodilators should be given through the endotracheal tube. If repeated doses of epinephrine are needed, as often occurs, an infusion of 0.05 to 0.1 mcg/kg per minute should be started. The patient may require treatment as outlined previously for several hours and intensive care admission should be arranged. A *Latex Alert* sign should be placed outside the patient's operating room and in the intensive care unit, and the condition should be noted prominently in the medical record. After the vital signs are stable, secondary treatments can begin. These include administration of diphenhydramine, ranitidine, and hydrocortisone. Further therapy depends on the patient's condition as the resuscitation progresses.

Diagnosis of Latex Anaphylaxis

After the patient is stabilized, tests to document the diagnosis of latex allergy can be performed. Although there are many tests available to confirm the diagnosis, there is not a universally accepted serum test for the diagnosis of a type I hypersensitivity reaction. An elevated level of serum tryptase occurs in the first four hours in patients who have experienced anaphylaxis with mast-cell degranulation, regardless of the cause. The latex radioallergosorbent (RAST) or enzyme allergosorbent (EAST) tests are available for specific proteins. Blood should be sent for testing, even if an individual may or may not be reacting to that particular protein. Nevertheless, a skin prick test using antigen extracted from latex similar to that used in medical products is used to determine type I hypersensitivity to latex. However, testing materials and methods have only recently begun to be standardized (Hamilton et al., 2002). The patient should be referred to a specialist in allergy and immunology for complete evaluation. The performance of skin testing should be delayed until 4 to 6 weeks after the anaphylactic event to allow time for cellular inflammatory mediators released as a consequence of the reaction to be reconstituted (Dakin and Yentis, 1998). Performance of testing before allowing time for reconstitution increases the risk of false-negative results. This testing must be done carefully and in the proper setting because severe reactions have been seen in sensitive individuals even with the exposure due to this test (Kelly et al., 1993). After the diagnosis is confirmed, the patients should be offered the opportunity to wear a MedicAlert bracelet.

Recommendations

Avoidance of latex exposure is by far the best approach to this problem (Holzman, 1997). Many operating rooms are working toward becoming completely latex free, but this goal has not yet been achieved. Avoidance, therefore, depends on recognizing those at risk for latex sensitivity. Specific at-risk groups are known, such as children with spina bifida and urinary tract anomalies. The preanesthetic assessment should include questions about atopy and allergy to foods, especially tropical fruits. Children thought to be at risk based on the history simply should not be exposed to latex. If a child is thought to be at risk for latex sensitivity but, when questioned, denies (or the parents deny) facial redness after touching balloons or after dental care and has not undergone latex-sensitivity testing, it seems prudent to avoid latex-containing products, especially because more and more products are manufactured to be latex free. The operating room should have *Latex Alert* warning signs that can be placed outside the door for these patients to help avoid inadvertent exposure to latex. Clinicians must keep themselves informed about the progress in this area. Products formerly unsafe may become safe with a change in manufacturing, but given the high morbidity of an anaphylactic reaction, it is essential that caregivers be certain of the safety of the medical products used in children at risk for latex sensitivity. All equipment used by anesthesiologists is available free of latex. Intravenous sets and tubing, breathing circuits and breathing bags, and sterile and nonsterile gloves are available latex free. Most multidose vials are made with latex-free stoppers. Unfortunately, not all medical equipment and products are latex free, and it is important to check each new product for possible latex content.

Prophylaxis and Desensitization

Although it is difficult to create a completely latex-free environment, the consensus opinion seems to be that prophylaxis of patients with known or suspected latex sensitivity need not be undertaken. There are case reports of patients who developed anaphylaxis after exposure to latex despite preoperative administration of the recommended prophylactic medication (Kwittken et al., 1992; Setlock et al., 1993). Those who endorse prophylaxis propose administration of diphenhydramine, ranitidine, and corticosteroids from the preoperative through the postoperative period. There have been interesting reports of efforts to desensitize latex-sensitive patients. Children with spina bifida or urologic anomalies, or both, were not included in the reports. Many of the participants in these efforts were actually health care workers, and none of them had suffered anaphylaxis after exposure to latex. Although most patients were adults, one report included subjects as young as 8 years of age. The techniques used were cutaneous exposure over a 12-month period and rush, 4-day, desensitization by means of sublingual exposure (Patriarca et al., 2002a, 200b). At this point, however, desensitization does not appear to be an option for children with type I hypersensitivity to latex.

Occupational Latex Allergy

In 1998, a report of latex sensitivity among the staff of the anesthesiology department at the Johns Hopkins Department of Anesthesiology (Brown et al., 1998) documented a 24% incidence of irritant or contact dermatitis and nearly13% incidence of latex-specific IgE positivity, although pediatric anesthesiologists may have a somewhat lower incidence (Ben-David and Gaitini, 1997; Greenberg et al., 1999). A large meta-analysis of all health care workers showed a 0% to 30% prevalence of type I latex allergy in the group. The investigators did not have data that elucidated the reasons for the large variation in prevalence (Garabrant and Schweitzer, 2002). In other reports, there has been a suggestion that avoidance of latex reverses the sensitivity, at least in health care workers (Zeldin et al., 1996). The creation of a latex-free operating room environment will benefit the patients and those who care for them.

EPIDERMOLYSIS BULLOSA

The term *epidermolysis bullosa* encompasses a heterogeneous group of congenital, hereditary blistering disorders. The disease is subdivided into three major subtypes: epidermolysis bullosa simplex, junctional epidermolysis bullosa, and dystrophic epidermolysis bullosa. These types differ in histology, clinical severity, and mode of inheritance, but all are characterized by the easy development of blisters after minor trauma or friction. The review by Smith (1993) remains an important source of information regarding the anesthetic management of children with one of these rare conditions. Junctional epidermolysis bullosa is often clinically apparent early in life and heal with scarring. A discriminating feature of this variant is the relative sparing of the hands and feet. Involvement of the mucous membranes may be severe, however, and ulceration of the respiratory epithelium has been documented. The recessive variant of dystrophic epidermolysis bullosa may be the most severe form of the condition. Mucous membranes lesions are common in this variant. Treatment of children with this condition is supportive. Infections are frequent and should be promptly treated. Adequate nutrition is paramount but often difficult to provide in cases with esophageal blisters. Children with the more severe forms may come to the operating room for a variety of procedures, such as scar revisions, corrections of digital fusions, placement of gastrostomy tubes, and colonic interpositions.

Anesthetic Management

The preanesthetic evaluation of a child with epidermolysis bullosa should involve the dermatologist and pediatrician who care for the patient. These physicians can advise the anesthesiologist about the child's general course with regard to blistering, skin infections, and nutritional status, as well as the possible utility of additional steroid administration. In addition to assessing the child's general condition and health, the physical examination should focus on the airway, which may be compromised by scarring around the mouth, intravenous access sites, and the location and condition of existing and recent blisters.

Friction and secondary pressure must be avoided in caring for children with this condition in the perioperative period. Monitoring must adhere to the ASA standards but the application of the monitors should be modified. The precordial stethoscope is placed onto the chest, the temperature is monitored with an axillary probe, and soft padding is placed between the skin and blood pressure cuffs. Electrocardiographic leads should be nonadhesive, and intravenous and arterial catheters are sutured and covered with a gauze bandage that is lightly applied. The eyes should be lubricated but not held closed with adhesive tape. Endotracheal tubes are secured with umbilical tape lubricated with steroid cream rather than taped to facial skin.

A variety of anesthetic techniques have been used for procedures performed on these challenging patients (Holzman et al., 1987; Smith, 1993). An oral premedication may be useful in children with epidermolysis bullosa coming to the operating room because a struggling child who is restrained may develop blisters where he or she is held by the operating room team. Alternatively, intramuscular ketamine has been used to induce and maintain anesthesia in these patients (Idvall, 1987; LoVerme and Oropollo, 1977). The induction technique chosen depends on the preoperative assessment and the planned procedure. Induction of general anesthesia can be achieved with an inhalational technique, but contact with the child's face must be very gentle. Oropharyngeal airways should be avoided. Laryngoscopy with a straight blade without contact with the epiglottis is preferred, and intubation with a smaller than predicted, lubricated endotracheal tube after muscle relaxation can minimize trauma to the tracheal mucosa. If there are no contraindications, a deep extubation will decrease tracheal trauma due to coughing. Cases of postoperative bullae in the pharynx, some of which caused airway obstruction, have been reported but predisposing factors are difficult to identify (James and Wark, 1982). Laryngeal mask airways should not be used due to the large area of contact/pressure of the "cuff" with the pharyngeal wall. The decision to admit these children after the procedure must be made on an individual basis. However, these patients warrant careful observation in a well-monitored environment after surgery and anesthesia. Although general anesthesia is used very frequently in these patients, reports of successful regional techniques have been published (Kaplan and Strauch, 1987).

DOWN SYNDROME

The incidence of trisomy 21 is 1 in 600 to 800 live births. More than one half of trisomy conceptions spontaneously abort early in pregnancy. The syndrome has many clinical manifestations, some of which are of particular note to the anesthesiologist.

Approximately 40% of children with trisomy 21 have anomalies of the cardiovascular system. The three most common anomalies seen in these children are complete atrioventricular canal (comprising approximately 40% of the total), ventricular septal defect (25%), and atrial septal defect (10% to 15%). Children with Down syndrome who undergo repair of complete atrioventricular canal have significantly higher perioperative mortality than those without trisomy 21. The outcome after surgery is not different for other cardiac anomalies, however. These defects have in common the propensity for increased pulmonary blood flow, which the anesthetic plan should attempt to minimize. Repair or palliation of a cardiac defect does not eliminate the need for particular attention to the cardiovascular system in the evaluation of these patients preoperatively.

Children with Down syndrome have various degrees of mental retardation, and it is important to be aware of the degree of intellectual impairment when meeting and talking with these patients. Hypotonia is one the most common clinical features seen in these children, and it may affect the adequacy of the upper airway. Partial airway obstruction while awake and during sleep is often seen in children with trisomy 21. This situation is exacerbated by the administration of sedatives and during inhalation inductions. The incidence of hearing loss and of hypothyroidism is increased in these children (Tuysuz and Beker, 2001). There is an increased incidence of subglottic stenosis in trisomy 21 children, and often, the proper-sized endotracheal tube for a given child is smaller than would have been predicted. The relatively large tongue, short neck, and crowded midface and laryngomalacia contribute to the upper airway obstruction (Clark et al., 1980; Kanamori et al., 2000; Mitchell et al., 2003). The orthopedic anomaly of great concern in these children is ligamentous laxity of the atlantoaxial joint that may predispose affected individuals to C1-C2 subluxation and possible spinal cord damage. The incidence of this anomaly is 12% to 32%, depending on the ages of the children studied and the exact definition of laxity used. Other associated findings in patients with Down syndrome are included in Box 32–17.

Perioperative Management

The preoperative evaluation of a child with Down syndrome should focus particular attention on the organ systems commonly affected in this condition. The history of prior surgeries should be reviewed. These children often have undergone cardiac procedures, removal of the tonsils and adenoids, myringotomy and tube placement, and other common pediatric procedures. Records from other doctors may have helpful information about associated conditions such as obstructive sleep apnea syndrome, atlantoaxial laxity, or subluxation. Management of these children regarding possible C1-C2 subluxation is a difficult matter. The American Academy of Pediatrics (AAP) has published statements by the committee on Genetics and the Committee on Sports Medicine and Fitness that include discussion of this clinical problem. The Committee on Genetics policy statement on health care supervision of children with Down syndrome recommends radiographs looking for evidence of

BOX 32–17 Associated Findings in Patients with Down Syndrome

General findings
- Low birth weight
- Short stature

Cardiovascular findings
- Congenital heart disease
- Increased susceptibility to pulmonary hypertension
- Atropine sensitivity

Respiratory findings
- High-arched, narrow palate
- Macroglossia
- Micrognathia
- Increased susceptibility to respiratory infections
- Subglottic stenosis
- Postextubation stridor
- Upper airway obstruction, sleep apnea

Gastrointestinal findings
- Dental abnormalities
- Duodenal obstruction
- Gastroesophageal reflux
- Hirschsprung's syndrome

Nervous system findings
- Mental retardation
- Epilepsy
- Strabismus

Musculoskeletal findings
- Hypotonia
- Hyperextensibility or flexibility
- Dysplastic pelvis
- Atlantoaxial subluxation

Immune system findings
- Immunosuppression
- Leukemia (acute lymphoblastic, acute myeloid forms)

Hematologic findings
- Neonatal polycythemia

Endocrine findings
- Low circulating level of catecholamine
- Hypothyroidism

atlantoaxial instability or subluxation be performed between 3 and 5 years of age (American Academy of Pediatrics, 2001b). The Committee on Sports Medicine and Fitness reviewed the topic of atlantoaxial instability in Down Syndrome in a 1995 publication and tentatively concluded that lateral plain films are of potential but unproved value in detecting patients at risk for developing spinal cord injury during participation in sports (1995). The Special Olympics does not plan to remove its requirement that all athletes with Down syndrome receive lateral spine radiographs (Special Olympics Bulletin, 1983). In 1984, the Committee on Sports Medicine and Fitness published a paper recommending that all children with Down syndrome have cervical spine radiographs, a much stronger endorsement of the practice (American Academy of Pediatrics, 1984). Some conclusions can be drawn for the published case reports summarized in the AAP Committee on Sports Medicine Subject Review and the recommendations cited earlier (American Academy of Pediatrics, 1995).

The preoperative history and physical examination should include a careful search for evidence of cervical instability. The parent should be questioned about past cervical radiographs, if they were taken. The family and patient should be questioned about the occurrence of any type of neck pain, limitation of neck mobility, torticollis, head tilt, abnormalities of gait, bowel or bladder dysfunction, or other signs of upper motor neuron dysfunction. The examination similarly should look for spasticity, hyperreflexia, extensor-plantar reflex, or clonus. If the history and physical examination reveal problems or the cervical radiographs show an atlantodens interval of more than 5 mm, the child's elective surgery is delayed, and neurosurgical consultation is sought. If previous radiographs were negative and the history and physical examination findings did not suggest a problem, it is not certain whether the x-ray films should be repeated. Although there is a very low incidence of worsening of the atlantodens interval over time (Pueschel et al., 1992; Pueschel, 1998), some patients did show progression. Even in asymptomatic patients, there is the possibility that a postoperative neurologic disability may occur (Williams et al., 1987). Whatever the result of the evaluations, if surgery and anesthesia are undertaken, there is general agreement that these patients should be kept in the neutral position throughout the perioperative period. A reassuring study of children with Down syndrome with cervical radiographs who underwent tonsillectomy and adenoidectomy in the usual position showed no changes in the latency or amplitude of the somatosensory potentials (Abramson et al., 1995). It should be noted that atlantoaxial instability occurs in conditions other than Down syndrome and at much higher frequency (Box 32–18).

BOX 32–18 Conditions Associated with Atlantoaxial Dislocation

Congenital abnormalities
- Trisomy 21
- Klippel-Feil syndrome
- Larsen's syndrome
- Mucopolysaccharidoses
- Spondyloepiphyseal dysplasia
- Metatropic dwarfism
- Kniest syndrome
- Chondrodysplasia punctata
- Chondrodystrophia calcificans congenita
- 22q-syndrome

Infection
- Pharyngeal

Tumors

Trauma (especially in young children)

Postoperative complication (especially after airway surgery)

Arthritis
- Rheumatoid
- Ankylosing spondylitis

GENETIC MUSCLE DISORDERS

Characteristics and Classification

Genetic studies during the past several years have led to a clearer understanding of the molecular causes of genetic-based muscle diseases. In most cases, the identification of the proteins altered in the disease states has added to our understanding of the function of muscle and the neuromuscular junction. However, the anesthetic management suggested for these diseases and syndromes has not changed as a result of the knowledge. The purpose of this section will be to review what is presently known concerning the generation of muscle contraction in a normal cell (Fig. 32–16), molecular nature of diseases of the neuromuscular system, the clinical presentations of these diseases and their anesthetic implications.

The genetic muscle diseases can be divided into four broad categories: muscular dystrophies, myotonic syndromes, mitochondrial myopathies, and myasthenic syndromes. Though there is some overlap between malignant hyperthermia and the other genetic muscle diseases, malignant hyperthermia is included in this section where overlap exists between malignant hyperthermia and other muscle diseases. For further discussion of malignant hyperthermia, see Chapter 32 (Malignant Hyperthermia). The general location in the muscle cell of the molecular changes leading to these classes of genetic muscle diseases are shown in Figure 32–17. Generally, the syndromes are caused by the following changes:

1. *Myasthenic syndromes* affect transmission of the action potential from the motor neuron to the muscle cell. This generally involves a disruption of the signal carried by the neurotransmitter, acetylcholine, across the synaptic cleft (see Fig. 32–17*A*). The molecular changes may affect release of the neurotransmitter, acetylcholine, or its action at the postsynaptic receptor.
2. *Myotonic syndromes* affect transmission of the action potential along the muscle membrane and are generally caused by abnormalities in sodium, chloride, or potassium channels (see Fig. 32–17*B*). These changes cause a prolonged depolarization of the muscle membrane, which leads to prolonged contraction of the muscle. A subgroup of these syndromes causes muscle degeneration and is called *myotonic dystrophy*.
3. *Mitochondrial myopathies* are caused by abnormalities in mitochondrial function. Because mitochondria are important for supplying ATP in most tissues (most importantly nerve and muscle), the symptoms of mitochondrial myopathies often involve the nervous system and muscle (see Fig. 32–17*C*). The lack of ATP in muscle leads primarily to weakness and

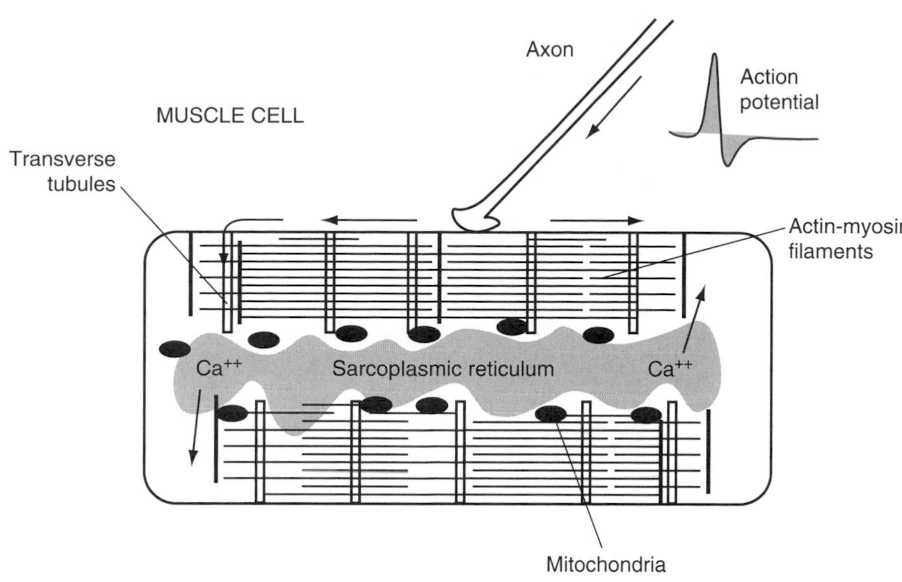

■ **FIGURE 32–16.** A schematic diagram of the muscle cell and motor neuron. An action potential travels down the motor neuron causing the release of acetylcholine and the neuromuscular junction (NMJ). An action potential is generated in the muscle, travels down the transverse tubules, and causes the influx of calcium at the base of the tubules. The small calcium currents trigger release of larger amounts of calcium from the calcium stores in the sarcoplasmic reticulum into the matrix of the muscle cell. This activates the actin-myosin filaments to contract. The filaments attach (not shown) to the surface of the cell and the extracellular matrix to cause effective mechanical contraction.

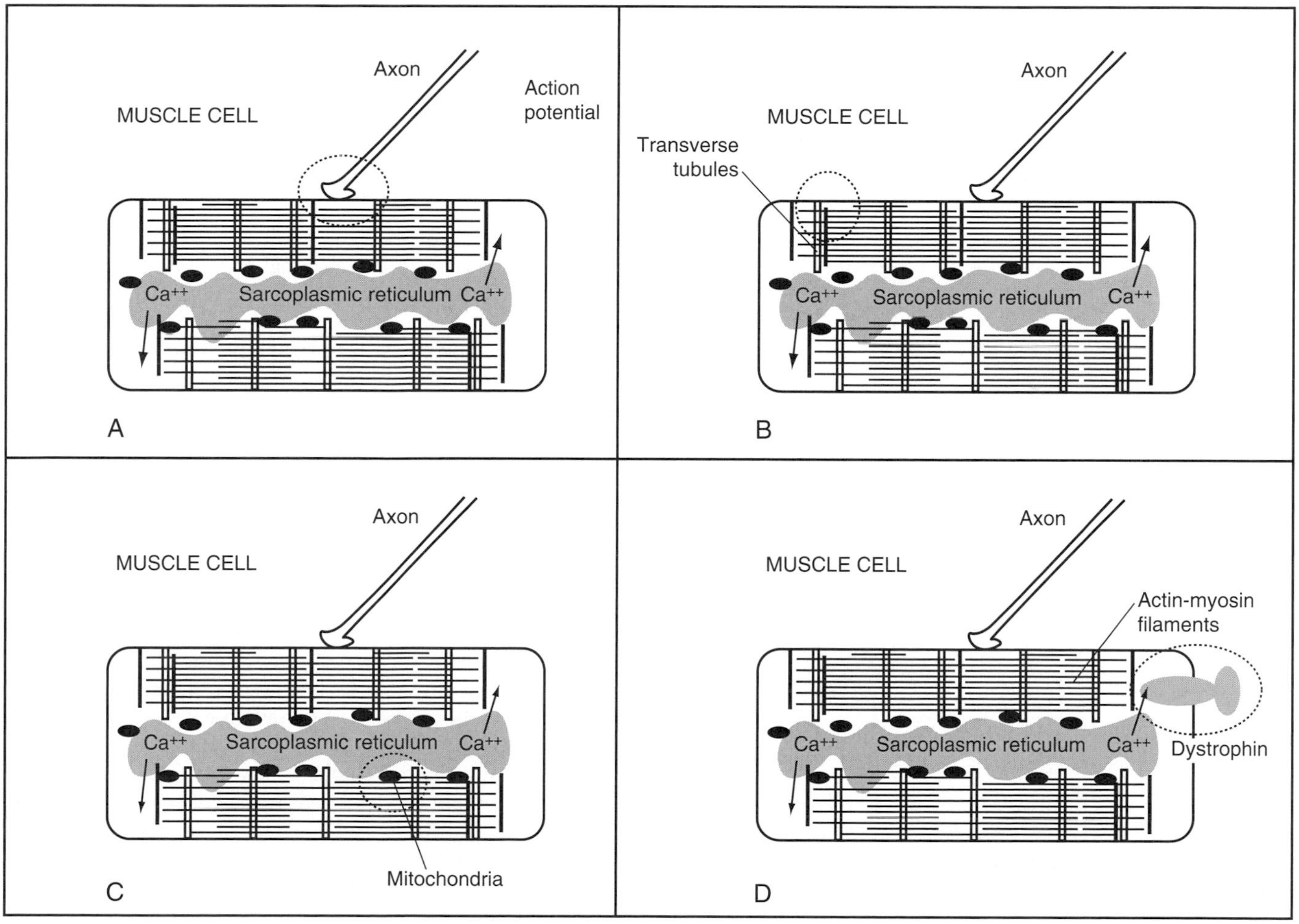

■ **FIGURE 32–17.** The diagram in Figure 32–16 is expanded to show the main areas of defects leading to muscular disease. *A,* Disruption of the signal across the neuromuscular junction (NMJ) leads to myasthenic syndromes. *B,* Defects in the calcium, potassium, and sodium channels in the muscle cell membrane give rise to myotonias. The membranes remain depolarized too long, causing the inability to relax. *C,* Mitochondrial dysfunction leads to decreased intracellular levels of ATP. The decreased ATP concentration is responsible for the inability to contract strongly and defects in the reuptake of calcium into the sarcoplasmic reticulum. *D,* Defects in the attachment of the actin-myosin filaments to the cell surface and extracellular matrix produce muscular dystrophies. These attachments are important for mechanical force and for organizing and stabilizing the membrane.

wasting of muscle. Mitochondrial myopathies are a complex and diverse group of diseases with a wide range of clinical implications.

4. *Muscular dystrophies* result from the dissociation of contractile force from the muscle to the surrounding connective tissue. The actin-myosin filaments in the muscle cell contract but they are no longer adequately connected to the cell membrane or the surrounding tissue. As a result, there is the equivalent of electromechanical dissociation (see Fig. 32–17*D*), which is the electrical signal from the muscle cell membrane that is not translated into effective mechanical force.

Skeletal muscle contraction is accomplished by the generation of a neuronal action potential that terminates at the neuromuscular synapse (see Fig. 32–16). The neuronal action potential (AP) stimulates sodium channels in the neuronal axon that propagates the signal along the axon. As the AP reaches the end of the axon, voltage-gated calcium channels are activated, allowing the influx of calcium into the neuron. This influx of calcium stimulates the release of a neurotransmitter, acetylcholine, from the nerve terminal into the synapse. Acetylcholine binds to acetylcholine receptors on the cell surface of the postsynaptic cell, in this case the muscle. Binding of acetylcholine to its receptors allows influx of sodium into the muscle, generating a new AP, which propagates a transmembrane signal that spreads along the membrane of the muscle cell.

The AP is carried from the cell surface into the interior of the cell by a series of invaginations of the cell membrane known as transverse-tubules. These structures allow transmembrane electrical depolarizations to be carried deeply within the cell, where they would otherwise not be generated. At the ends of the T-tubules the sodium currents are replaced by calcium currents, resulting from the activation of a voltage-gated calcium channel known as the *dihydropyridine receptor* (Fig. 32–18). These calcium currents stimulate a greater release of calcium from the large stores of calcium in the sarcoplasmic reticulum through a calcium-sensitive calcium channel, the ryanodine receptor. These larger fluxes of calcium stimulate movement of the actin-myosin filaments, an ATP-requiring step (and therefore dependent on functioning mitochondria). The filaments are attached to the surface of the muscle and the surrounding matrix through a variety of proteins, most notably dystrophin. Movement of the filaments is transduced into shortening of the cell (i.e., muscle contraction) by the connection to the cell surface and surrounding matrix. Relaxation is accomplished by reuptake of the intracellular calcium primarily back into the sarcoplasmic reticulum. This reuptake is energy requiring ATP-dependent calcium pumps. Because reuptake of calcium requires energy, it also depends on mitochondrial function and ATP generation.

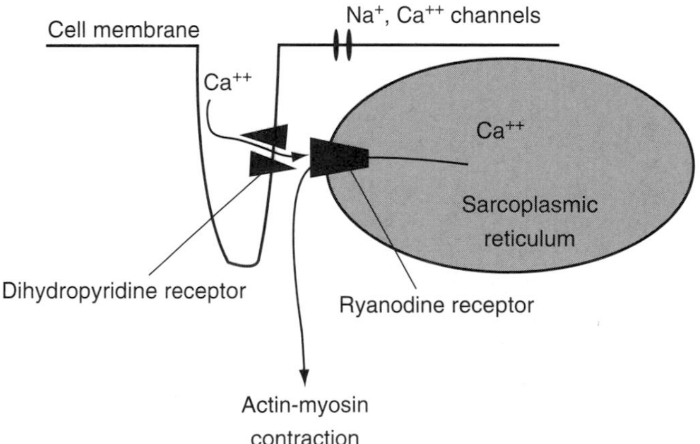

■ **FIGURE 32–18.** An expansion of the region of the transverse tubules (T-tubules). Sodium, potassium, and calcium channels on the cell surface are responsible for propagation of the action potential (AP) along the cell membrane and into the T-tubules. When the AP reaches the terminus of the T-tubule, the sodium currents are replaced by calcium currents through the voltage-gated dihydropyridine receptor. These calcium currents trigger release of calcium through the ryanodine receptor from the large calcium stores in the sarcoplasmic reticulum.

This normal flow of electrical signal transduced to mechanical force can be disrupted at many places. As anesthesiologists, we often inhibit the transmission of the signal across the neuromuscular junction with the use of neuromuscular blockers such as vecuronium. Such an effect is similar to a myasthenic syndrome. The use of local anesthetics directly on muscle blocks voltage-gated sodium channels in the muscle membrane and acts oppositely to the changes seen in myotonic syndromes. Volatile anesthetics are also inhibitors of the voltage-gated membrane channels (sodium, potassium, and calcium) and act oppositely of myotonia. However, these drugs also inhibit mitochondria, and are capable of causing a relaxation effect in a manner similar to a mitochondrial myopathy. These examples are given only to further acquaint the anesthetist with the underlying causes of the myopathies; the drugs certainly do not cause these diseases. However, these similar effects largely predict the interactions of the drugs with the disease states.

Myasthenic Syndromes

Myasthenic syndromes are the result of the failure of transmission of the signal from the terminal of a motor neuron to the muscle innervated by the neuron. Most myasthenic syndromes are the result of immune responses against components of the neuromuscular junction (primarily the post-synaptic acetylcholine receptors) and are not truly genetic diseases. The symptoms result from decreased neurotransmission across the neuromuscular junction, and task-specific fatigue is the hallmark of these diseases (see Fig. 32–17*A*).

The classic disease of myasthenia gravis is an example of such a disorder, though it is primarily a disease of adulthood. Myasthenia gravis can occur neonatally due to placental transfer of maternal antibodies. Rarely, inherited disorders of neuromuscular transmission, known as *congenital myasthenic syndromes*, can result from acetylcholine receptor mutations or other mutations involving the release of acetylcholine. Included in this group are familial infantile myasthenia, familial limb-girdle myasthenia, end-plate acetylcholinesterase deficiency, and syndromes with altered or deficient acetylcholine receptors (Vincent et al., 1997; Menold et al., 1998). As an example, Maselli and others describe a form of congenital myasthenia gravis that results from a deficiency in the calcium-induced release of neurotransmitter or impaired recycling of synaptic vesicles (Maselli et al., 2001). These genetic diseases can mimic myasthenia gravis in their presentation and implications for anesthesia and can manifest in children (Dalal et al., 1972). Juvenile-onset myasthenia gravis is also associated with thymoma (Kiran et al., 2000). Because these syndromes are not well described, their management is determined by analogy to that for adult-onset myasthenia gravis.

Anesthetic Considerations

The primary concern during the perioperative period for patients with myasthenic syndromes is to avoid respiratory compromise from weakened respiratory muscles or upper airway muscles (Abel and Eisenkraft, 2002; Brown et al., 1990). For this reason nondepolarizing muscle relaxants are used sparingly, if at all, in these patients. Patients with myasthenia gravis or myasthenic syndromes are often resistant to succinylcholine (Baraka, 2001). It is important to remember that patients can appear strong on awakening only to become fatigued later in the recovery period. Itoh and others (2002) showed that seronegativity for the anti-acetylcholine receptor antibody (seen in myasthenia gravis) did not predict a normal response to muscle relaxants. Myasthenia gravis patients "cured" by thymectomy may also retain a high sensitivity to muscle relaxants (Itoh et al., 2002). The conclusion of these reports is that the anesthesiologist must presume a high sensitivity to muscle relaxants in all patients with myasthenic syndromes, even if they are functioning well after medical or surgical treatment. When muscle relaxants are needed, short-acting agents are favored.

Techniques using short-acting anesthetics without the addition of muscle relaxants have been very successful (McBeth and Watkins, 1996; Della Rocca et al., 2003). It should be remembered that the volatile anesthetics are also muscle relaxants and may accentuate the compromised strength in myasthenic patients. Short-acting inhaled anesthetics (sevoflurane or desflurane) would seem to have a useful role with these patients. Opioids must also be used sparingly, when possible, to avoid adding to inhibition of respiratory effort. It is advisable to monitor the ventilatory status of myasthenic patients for a longer time than that done normally.

Myotonias

Myotonia is a temporary, involuntary contraction of muscle fibers due to transient hyperexcitability of the surface membrane (Miller, 1989). In general, the myotonias may be thought of as a family of channelopathies mostly affecting muscle (Jurkat-Rott et al., 2002; Rosenbaum and Miller, 2002). The abnormalities in the channels leads to prolonged depolarization in the membrane once an action potential is generated (see Fig. 32–18) and leads to prolonged or increased release of calcium into the cell. This leads to prolonged stimulation of the actin-myosin contractile apparatus of the muscle cell (Fig. 32–19). The persistent contracture of the skeletal muscle generally occurs after muscle stimulation but may be triggered by other stimuli such as cold, pain, or stress. A classic finding in patients with myotonia is the inability to easily relax after a firm handshake.

Two forms of myotonia (myotonia congenita and Becker's disease) result from defects in the *same* skeletal muscle chloride channel (ClC-1) (Pusch, 2002; Renner and Ptacek, 2002; Jurkat-Rott et al., 2002). Myotonia congenita (i.e., Thomsen's disease) is an autosomal dominant disease, presenting in childhood associated with a normal life expectancy and minimal symptoms (Grunnet et al., 2003). Becker's disease, not to be confused with Becker muscular dystrophy, is an autosomal recessive form of this channelopathy, appearing in childhood also (Pusch, 2002). Some mutations in this chloride channel cause a variant of dominant myotonia with a milder phenotype, myotonia levior (Ryan et al., 2002; Farbu et al., 2003). These myotonic diseases are nonprogressive and do not have a dystrophic component (i.e., there is no deterioration of the muscle over time). Other, milder myotonias result from abnormalities in sodium or potassium channels on the muscle cell membrane. These include paramyotonia congenital (sodium channel), hyperkalemic periodic paralysis (sodium channel) and hypokalemic periodic paralysis (calcium, sodium, or potassium channels) (Jurkat-Rott et al., 2002).

Anesthetic Considerations

Myotonic contractions may be precipitated by stress, cold, and pain. These triggering factors must be carefully avoided during the perioperative period for these patients. Regional anesthesia and neuromuscular blockade *do not* reverse the contractions because they act upstream from the molecular causes of the syndrome (compare Figs. 32–17*A* and 32–17*B*). Succinylcholine has been noted to precipitate contractions, as have neuromuscular blocking reversal agents. These contractions have been most notable in the occurrence of masseter spasm after the use of succinylcholine, but they can also involve other muscles and lead to extreme difficulty with positive pressure ventilation and intubation (Farbu et al., 2003). For these reasons, the use of succinylcholine is discouraged in patients with myotonia. If an episode of myotonia occurs during anesthesia, volatile anesthetics, quinine, or procainamide can be used for relaxation. Because the myotonias occur as the result of abnormal ion channels, great care must be taken to keep electrolytes normal at all times. Although myotonic syndromes may have symptoms in common with malignant hyperthermia (especially muscle contracture after the administration of succinylcholine), they are not associated with true malignant hyperthermia.

Myotonic Dystrophy

Myotonic dystrophy (i.e., Steinert muscular dystrophy) is the most common form of myotonia (Anderson and Brown, 1989). This disease is a form of muscular dystrophy and includes congenital

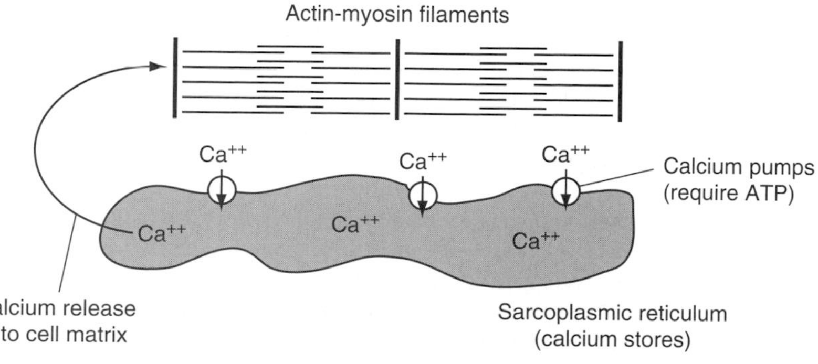

■ **FIGURE 32–19.** Calcium is released from the sarcoplasmic reticulum and causes contraction of the actin-myosin filaments. Calcium reuptake is achieved by ATP-dependent calcium pumps. Contraction and reuptake depend on the function of mitochondria.

myotonic dystrophy. Myotonic dystrophy is discussed here instead of with other muscular dystrophies because its presentation is different, more resembling the myotonias than the dystrophies.

It has been shown that myotonic dystrophy actually includes two different molecular diseases (Ranum and Day, 2002). Myotonic dystrophy type 1 results from alterations in the human dystrophica myotonica-protein kinase gene *(DMPK)* (Amack and Mahadevan, 2004). The precise mechanism by which this mutation causes the disease is not clear but the dystrophy results from abnormal development of the muscle cells (Wansink and Wieringa, 2003; Martorell et al., 2004). However, the myotonia probably is the result of abnormal phosphorylation of sodium channels resulting in delayed inactivation after channel opening (Lee et al., 2003). The prolonged channel activation causes prolonged muscle contraction. The changes in the protein kinase gene are in the promoter or starting region of the gene and are the result of duplications in short repetitive sequences (i.e., CTG triplets). The number of repetitive sequences is often increased in the offspring compared with an affected parent. As a result, each successive generation tends to exhibit a more severe form of the disease. Myotonic dystrophy type 2 has a clinically diverse presentation, including myotonia, proximal muscle wasting, and endocrine, cardiac, and cerebral abnormalities. Myotonic dystrophy 2 also results from expansion of a sequence in the promotor of a gene, but the gene is separate from that causing myotonic dystrophy type 1 and codes for a probable transcription factor, ZNF9 (Finsterer, 2002; Liquori et al., 2003). The precise physiologic changes leading to myotonic or dystrophic changes are not known. In both disease states, the abnormalities result from abnormal RNA species that disrupt normal development of the cells (Mankodi and Thornton, 2002).

Anesthetic Considerations. Production of muscle relaxation can be very difficult in these patients. As with the other forms of myotonia, cold, stress, pain, and succinylcholine can precipitate myotonia. Because this is a dystrophy with muscle wasting, succinylcholine can elicit a hyperkalemic response and should be avoided. Unlike the other myotonias, myotonic dystrophy leads to deterioration of the muscle fibers, affects tissue other than skeletal muscle, and is associated with weakness and hypotonia in infants and children. Paradoxically, however, the patients can trigger a myotonic episode as well. These patients can have profound respiratory depression, severe cardiac conduction abnormalities, cardiomyopathy, developmental delay, dysphagia, and decreased gastric motility. Muscle relaxants must be used with great care, if at all, in these patients. Smaller doses are probably necessary and a neuromuscular blockade monitor is advised. As with other myotonias, reversal agents may induce myotonia. Because respiratory depression is notable in these patients, the respiratory status is potentially fragile when any narcotic or general anesthetic is used. Their care presents challenges involving several physiologic systems. Myotonic dystrophy and their anesthetic implications have been reported (White and Bass, 2003). Although myotonic dystrophy is also commonly thought to be associated with malignant hyperthermia and shares similar features with malignant hyperthermia, nonetheless, myotonic dystrophy is not associated with true malignant hyperthermia.

Mitochondrial Myopathies

An increasingly large list of disease syndromes is associated with mitochondrial dysfunction. The more commonly seen mitochondrial syndromes are Leigh disease, Kearns-Sayre syndrome, and Leber hereditary optic neuropathy. However, mitochondrial dysfunction is also associated with unnamed myopathies and encephalopathies and with symptoms of failure to thrive. Mitochondrial abnormalities have been involved in some forms of autism and Parkinson's disease. The presentation of mitochondrial disease may be quite varied.

Mitochondria are the principal source of energy metabolism within cells, especially those of nerve and muscle (see Fig. 32–17*C*). Within mitochondria reside the enzymes responsible for the Krebs cycle, fatty acid β-oxidation, and, most importantly, oxidative phosphorylation (Fig. 32–20). Mitochondria contain the enzymes that metabolize glucose, fatty acids, and amino acids to generate NADH and succinate, which are used as electron donors for the electron transport chain. By passing electrons down the electron transport chain (complexes I to IV), a proton gradient is generated across the mitochondrial inner membrane, and electrons are donated to oxygen to generate water. The proton gradient is then used to drive an ATP synthase (complex V). The coupling of electron transfer to phosphorylation is known as *oxidative phosphorylation,* and it is overwhelmingly the major source of ATP and other high-energy phosphate bonds supplying energy to the cell. ATP is necessary for actin-myosin filament contraction and for reuptake of calcium by ATP-dependent calcium pumps into the sarcoplasmic reticulum (see Fig. 32–19).

Mitochondrial complexes are composed of groups of proteins ranging from just a few (complex II) to over 40 (complex I). The dehydrogenases, membrane transporters, and structural proteins raise the number of functional proteins in the mitochondria into the hundreds. Some of the proteins are encoded for by genes in the cell's chromosomes, whereas some are encoded by the mitochondria's own DNA. The genetics of mitochondrial disease is complicated by the fact that mitochondria are inherited from the mother. However, different populations of mitochondria may be passed to different offspring, so that the inheritance pattern can be quite varied. Mitochondrial dysfunction has effects other than energy depletion. Increased free radical damage to other cellular components and alterations in protein phosphorylation may be seen with mitochondrial disease. Each of these effects can give rise to mixed, but wide-ranging, functional changes in affected individuals.

It is a common mistake to group all mitochondrial diseases together as similar entities. Because a mutation can occur in any of the mitochondrial proteins, the resulting functional protein changes can manifest differently. Mitochondria in different tissues can be quite varied in their activity. The differences among tissues with regard to mitochondrial function, coupled with the varied inheritance pattern discussed previously, give rise to different clinical symptoms even among members of a family carrying identical mutations. It is dangerous to assume that, because an anesthetic technique was successful in a few patients with mitochondrial disease, the same technique would be safe for all patients with mitochondrial dysfunction.

Muscle and nerve cells uniquely depend on the energy delivered by these mitochondria. Mutations in mitochondrial proteins are responsible for the clinical features, including myopathy, cardiomyopathy, encephalopathy, seizures, and cerebellar ataxia. Because motor neurons may be affected, a hyperkalemic response to succinylcholine may occur. Malignant hyperthermia is thought to be associated with some forms of mitochondrial myopathies, but the nature of this relationship is unclear (Fricker et al., 2002; Keyes et al., 1996).

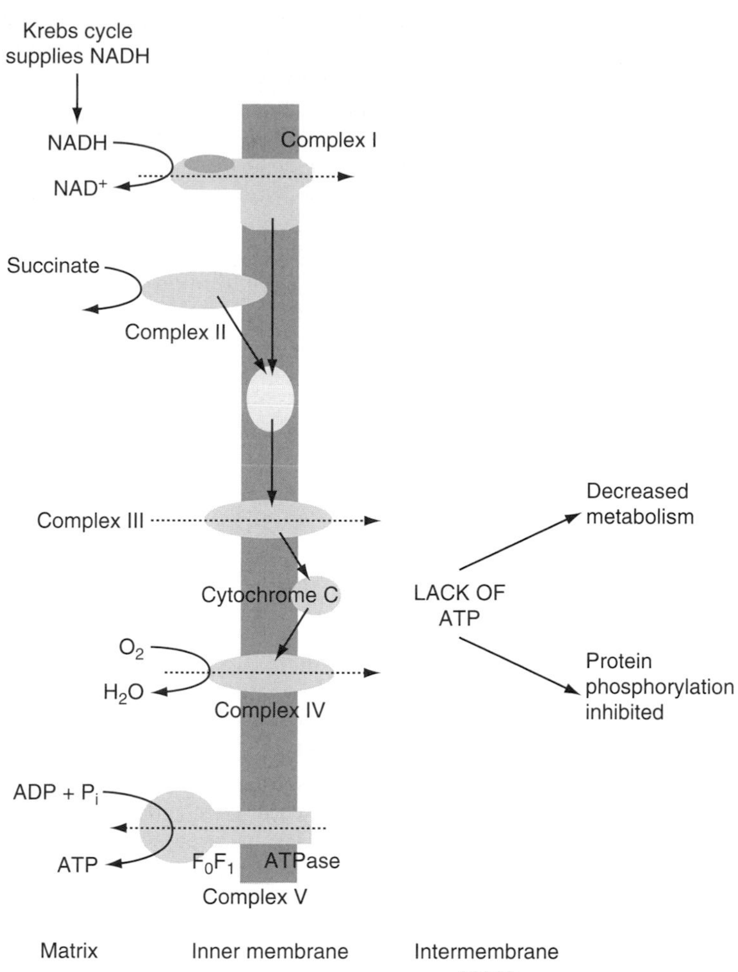

■ **FIGURE 32–20.** A representation of the electron transport chain (ETC) of mitochondria. Substrates for the ETC are generated from the Krebs cycle and enter the ETC at complex I or complex II. Protons are pumped into the intermembrane space *(arrows)* and return through complex V to drive the production of ATP. The figure demonstrates the complexity of the ETC and surrounding matrix.

Anesthetic Considerations

The perioperative period is a time during which a patient may be exposed to periods of stress. Conditions of stress may lead to inadequate ATP levels relative to energy demands. Shivering due to hypothermia probably represents the greatest threat to these patients. However, hyperthermia and stress from untreated pain also represent serious risks. The failure for ATP production to meet metabolic demands inevitably leads to a lactic acidosis, often of profound significance. To avoid such problems great care must be taken to keep patients normothermic during surgical procedures and to adequately treat postoperative pain. Postoperative pain represents a particularly troublesome problem because narcotics can further compromise the patient's respiratory status.

Patients with mitochondrial disorders may become acidemic due to high levels of lactate as a result of hypovolemia. Prolonged preoperative fasting should be avoided in these patients. If fasting is necessary, intravenous fluids containing glucose must be administered to avoid anaerobic metabolism. As cyanide inhibits the respiratory chain, sodium nitroprusside should be avoided. For similar reasons, tourniquets should be avoided if possible. It is not clear what hematocrit is adequate in these patients, but it is probably prudent to maintain a near normal level. Although mild levels of hypotension are commonly used in many patients to avoid blood loss, such an approach is less desirable in patients with mitochondrial disease. These patients are probably less able to compensate for decreased oxygen delivery.

Unfortunately, essentially every general anesthetic studied has been shown to depress mitochondrial function. The most notable of these are the inhaled anesthetics and propofol. It is reported that these agents significantly depress mitochondrial function at doses higher than their clinical concentrations. However, studies have also shown that even at doses commonly used in the operating room, anesthetics cause a significant depression of mitochondrial function from normal patients (Miro et al., 1999). Studies in animals have shown that when complex I is abnormal, sensitivity to volatile anesthetics is markedly increased (Kayser et al., 1999). Case reports have also indicated that some children exhibit an increased sensitivity to sevoflurane (Morgan et al., 2002). Wolf and others (2001) have shown that the propofol infusion syndrome probably occurs by means of mitochondrial inhibition. This has been interpreted to indicate that propofol also should be used with caution and increased monitoring in patients with mitochondrial disease. Because propofol and inhaled anesthetics primarily inhibit complex I function (see Fig. 32–20), patients with complex I-specific defects may have increased susceptibility to these drugs.

There is a strong clinical impression that children with mitochondrial myopathies have an increased risk during surgery (Bolton et al., 2003; Morgan et al., 2002). Because metabolism is altered in patients with mitochondrial disease, the abilities of the cell to generate ATP and to effectively use oxygen are diminished; consequently, exposure to anesthetics probably represents an increased risk compared with other patients (Bolton et al., 2003). The use of regional anesthetics should be considered if appropriate for the patient. However, it has also been noted that mitochondria are the probable target for the cardiac complications of bupivacaine (Weinberg et al., 2000); patients with mitochondrial myopathies may be at increased risk with this drug as well. Lastly, these patients (as with all patients with myopathies) must not be stressed with respect to their respiratory status. Caution must be used in weaning them from mechanical ventilation to ensure adequate spontaneous ventilation with minimal increases in the work of breathing.

The primary complications of mitochondrial myopathies include respiratory failure, cardiac depression, cardiac conduction defects, and dysphagia. Each of the volatile anesthetics depresses respiration, although to different degrees. However, because volatile anesthetics do not require metabolism for excretion, this route of elimination may present an advantage over intravenous anesthetics, which depend on energy-requiring mechanisms for their metabolism.

During the past decade, the intravenous anesthetic propofol has become increasingly popular as a maintenance anesthetic. However, it has many of the same side effects as volatile anesthetics. One notable exception is that it is not known to cause much muscle relaxation. Although propofol is viewed as a very-short-acting drug, its ultimate excretion is metabolism dependent, and patients with mitochondrial myopathy may have an increased risk for developing propofol infusion syndrome during prolonged exposure (Wolf et al., 2001).

Although all of the general anesthetic agents are known to directly inhibit mitochondrial function, all of these agents have been successfully used in patients with mitochondrial disease. It may be that as the different types of mitochondrial disease are better defined, preferences for an anesthetic in certain cases may become clear. It is imperative that patients with mitochondrial diseases are monitored closely, and the effects of the anesthetics have dissipated before assuming that the patient can ventilate adequately.

Patients with mitochondrial myopathies respond well to the nondepolarizing relaxants, though they probably have an increased sensitivity. These drugs should be titrated to the desired effect, monitored by nerve stimulation, and reversed fully before discontinuing ventilatory support. Because motor neurons may be affected, a hyperkalemic response to succinylcholine may be seen. Succinylcholine should be used only when absolutely necessary in these patients. Succinylcholine and volatile anesthetics are also known as triggers for malignant hyperthermia. Malignant hyperthermia is thought to be associated with some forms of mitochondrial myopathies, but the nature of this relationship is unclear. It may be that a group of mitochondrial myopathies mimics malignant hyperthermia by having inadequate ATP for reuptake of calcium from the cytoplasm of muscle cells into the sarcoplasmic reticulum. Such a failure could cause prolonged muscle contraction and lead to increased metabolism, and this represents a complicated problem in these patients. Whether they will increase their temperature or become acidemic will depend on the quality and severity of their disease.

There is no perfect anesthetic for patients with mitochondrial myopathies. When possible, consideration should be given to the use of local anesthetics in small amounts. When a general anesthetic is necessary, probably each of the general anesthetics in use has its place. At present it is not possible to eliminate one group as less safe than others. What is clear is that these patients must be monitored closely.

Muscular Dystrophy

At least five forms of muscular dystrophy are clinically relevant for anesthesiologists (Farrell, 1994). These include Becker's, Duchenne's, facioscapulohumeral, Emery-Dreifuss, and limb-girdle muscular dystrophies. These entities vary greatly in severity of presentation (Kerr et al., 2001; Schmidt et al., 2003). Duchenne's muscular dystrophy is an X-linked disorder resulting from deletion mutations in the dystrophin gene resulting in a complete lack of dystrophin in skeletal muscles (see Fig. 32–17*D*). The defect is present in about 1/3500 live births with the onset of disease often before school age and progressing to wheelchair dependence by the second decade of life. Dystrophin is a large protein which helps anchor the contractile components (the actin-myosin filaments) to the cell membrane and indirectly to the surrounding extracellular matrix (Fig. 32–21). Loss of this protein leads to profound muscle weakness and eventual respiratory insufficiency (Muntoni et al., 2003; Finsterer and Stollberger, 2003). Other, less global changes in this same gene

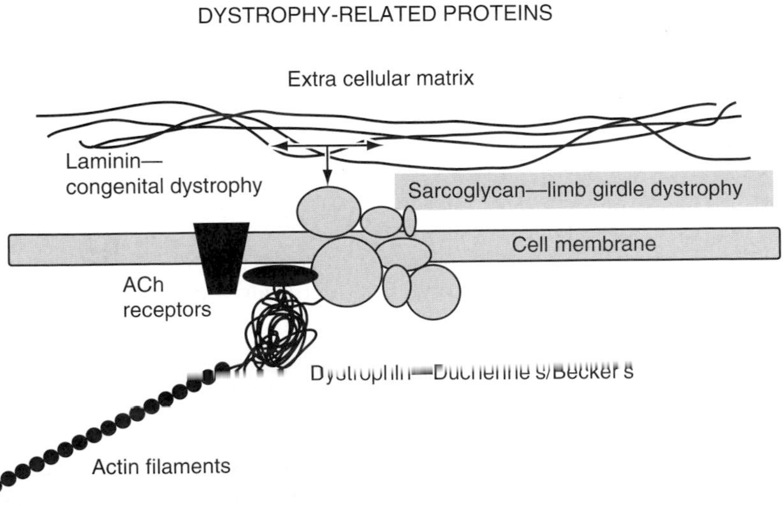

DYSTROPHY-RELATED PROTEINS

Extra cellular matrix

Laminin—congenital dystrophy

Sarcoglycan—limb girdle dystrophy

Cell membrane

ACh receptors

Dystrophin—Duchenne's/Becker's

Actin filaments

■ **FIGURE 32–21.** Representation of attachments of the actin filaments to the cell membrane and extracellular matrix. Disruption of these attachments alters protein distribution in the membrane and membrane stability. Some of the specific proteins that cause dystrophies are listed.

cause Becker's muscular dystrophy and the related disease, X-linked dilated cardiomyopathy. Cardiomyopathy is occasionally seen in female heterozygote carriers of the mutation.

Dystrophin is also found in cells other than skeletal muscle and has an apparent role in organizing protein complexes in the membrane and stabilizing the membrane. Absence of the protein leads to membrane instability which causes eventual muscle cell deterioration. Associated defects seen in patients with Duchenne's muscular dystrophy and Becker's muscular dystrophy include cardiomyopathy, cardiac conduction defects, and occasionally, mild mental retardation. The presence of the protein in other cell types provides an explanation for the involvement of the nervous system in affected patients.

Dystrophin also is important in organizing the postsynaptic acetylcholine receptors (Muntoni et al., 2003). In its absence, abnormalities occur both in the types of receptors and in their number and location. In the absence of dystrophin, there is an increase in expression of acetylcholine receptor subunits and changes in interacting proteins (Chen et al., 2000). The membrane instability coupled with changes in acetylcholine receptors may explain the sensitivity of the muscle to succinylcholine and volatile anesthetics.

Anesthetic Considerations

The main anesthetic implications of Duchenne's muscular dystrophy and Becker's muscular dystrophy are related to the profound myopathies. As would be expected in patients with muscle weakness, significant postoperative respiratory insufficiency can result from either disease. Cardiac muscle and conduction are also involved and drugs that further depress cardiac function, or which increase the likelihood of arrhythmias, should be avoided. All patients with Duchenne's muscular dystrophy or Becker's muscular dystrophy should receive a full cardiology evaluation and pulmonary function tests before any surgery. Dysphagia is common and gastric motility may be decreased requiring expedient control of the airway. The association of malignant hyperthermia with Duchenne's muscular dystrophy and Becker's muscular dystrophy appears to be coincidental only.

Both Duchenne's muscular dystrophy and Becker's muscular dystrophy patients can have rhabdomyolysis and hyperkalemia in response to succinylcholine; succinylcholine, therefore, is contraindicated in these patients. It is unclear whether volatile anesthetics alone can cause rhabdomyolysis in these patients.

Other Dystropies

Other forms of congenital muscular dystrophy exist that also involve other proteins necessary for attaching the contractile machinery to the extracellular matrix (see Fig. 32–21). Although this is a heterogeneous group of mutations, it is probably best to treat these patients as if they had Duchenne Muscular Dystrophy.

More than 30 different forms of congenital muscular dystrophy are now known, and are caused by defects in a wide array of components of the basement cell membrane and extracellular matrix (Engvall and Wewer, 2003). These are not discussed in detail as their clinical implications are similar to each other. Examples are the absence of laminin, or a related protein merosin, which give rise to similar forms of congenital dystrophies. These often have profound effects both on skeletal muscle and the nervous system.

The most common remaining dystrophies—facioscapulohumeral, Emery-Dreifuss, and limb-girdle muscular dystrophy—are much milder in their presentations (Emery, 2002). Facioscapulohumeral is one of the most common muscular dystrophies, but the molecular basis of facioscapulohumeral is unknown. Facioscapulohumeral is the most benign muscular dystrophy usually with little respiratory involvement (Fitzsimons, 1999). However, the neck, face, and scapular stabilizing muscles are often weak, and the ability to raise the head (at the end of anesthesia) may be of little use in determining respiratory muscle strength. Of clinical importance is that these patients may lose the ability to swallow well and therefore be unable to protect their airway during emergence from anesthesia.

Emery-Dreifuss dystrophy may result from multiple causes. The most common form has its onset in the teenage years and results from mutations in emerin, an inner nuclear membrane protein that interacts with laminin (part of the nuclear matrix) and transcription regulators (see Fig. 32–21). These patients have cardiac conduction defects, cardiomyopathy, contractures (positioning problems) and often a fusion of C3-C5, resulting in a less mobile neck (difficulty during intubation) (Aldwinckle and Carr, 2002; Shende and Agarwal, 2002).

Limb-girdle dystrophy results from mutations in several proteins (at least 11 are known), such as α-sarcoglycan, which associate with dystrophin. Limb-girdle disease is associated with some respiratory muscle weakness and significant cardiac conduction abnormalities. At least some cases of Limb-girdle disease result from a defect in a protein which interacts with muscle cell membrane and is implicated in membrane repair (Capanni et al., 2003).

Anesthetic Considerations

There is little experience in the literature on the interaction of anesthetics with LG dystrophy (Pash et al., 1996). In all three forms of muscular dystrophy, succinylcholine should be avoided because hyperkalemia can result. Malignant hyperthermia is not reported in these three milder forms of muscular dystrophy. Although not universal, the recurring themes with muscular dystrophy are to avoid succinylcholine, to watch for respiratory depression, and to avoid cardiac depressants and arrhythmogenic drugs. Anesthetic complications have been reported for most of these forms of muscular dystrophy (Farrell, 1994). These episodes most commonly result from a hyperkalemic episode and sudden cardiac arrest may occur. Such events can occur in patients who are still in a subclinical stage of their disease and in whom the crisis may be the first manifestation. For this reason, many clinicians limit their use of succinylcholine in children.

METABOLIC DISEASES

Several other genetic diseases of muscle exist which are of interest to anesthesiologists. These include primary diseases of metabolism which lead to chronically weak muscles or muscles that are prone to damage when exposed to high metabolic stress. *McArdle disease,* an inherited disorder of muscle phosphorylase activity which downregulates a Na^+-K^+ membrane pump, is a prototypic disorder of this type (Clausen, 2003). Muscle from patients with McArdle disease can function normally until stressed by exercise or ischemia, at which time severely painful electrically silent contracture develops, which can be followed by rhabdomyolysis, myoglobinuria, renal failure, and death. This sequence is similar to anesthesia-induced malignant hyperthermia. Several patients with anesthesia complications suggestive of malignant hyperthermia have had features of metabolic dysfunction on muscle biopsy, raising the possibility that disorders of intracellular energy production may underlie the malignant hyperthermia phenotype in some patients (Isaacs et al., 1989).

Patients with other less common diseases, such as Schwartz-Jampel syndrome, King-Denborough syndrome, and Lambert-Brody disease, are also prone to anesthetic complications. In each case, malignant hyperthermia–like responses have been reported, but their exact relationship to malignant hyperthermia is not clear. *King-Denborough syndrome* is a progressive myopathy, and affected patients have short stature, severe scoliosis, pectus deformities, ptosis, low-set ears, and cryptorchism (Heiman-Patterson et al., 1986). Anesthesia-related deaths, fulminant episodes of malignant hyperthermia, and positive in vitro contracture test results have been commonly associated with this disorder (Isaacs and Badenhorst, 1992). Because this disease is rare, genetic information about it is still lacking.

Patients with *Brody's disease* (i.e., Lambert-Brody disease) elicit a decreased ability to relax on repeated activation of their muscle that results from an identified defect of the sarcoplasmic reticulum Ca^{2+}-ATPase (Odermatt et al., 2000). An in vitro contracture test performed on muscle from such a patient was abnormal, which may indicate that such patients may be at risk for malignant hyperthermia-like syndrome (Froemming and Ohlendieck, 2001). Severe myotonia or neuromyotonia is a common feature of Schwartz-Jampel syndrome, in which hyperexcitability can be exacerbated by anesthetic agents and muscle relaxants considered as triggering agents for malignant hyperthermia (Seay and Ziter, 1978; Ray and Rubin, 1994). It is unclear whether true malignant hyperthermia is associated with this syndrome. Abnormal neck and laryngeal structure leading to difficulty with intubation has been reported (Stephen and Beighton, 2002).

Unfortunately, the molecular and genetic studies of these diseases raise nearly as many questions as they answer. Recommendations for the anesthetic care of these patients remain rather general. Physicians probably should avoid the use of succinylcholine and volatile anesthetics. The use of nontriggering anesthetics seems to be safe for these patients, although any muscle relaxant must be used with the utmost caution.

Most myopathies have been shown to be unrelated to malignant hyperthermia, though some overlap in their response to drugs may exist. However, the use of succinylcholine should be avoided. Other muscle relaxants can be used as necessary, but the anesthesiologist must carefully monitor their effects. Volatile anesthetics alone may present a risk of rhabdomyolysis in some muscular dystrophies. Mitochondrial disease represents a wide array of molecular changes and clinical presentations. The response of patients with mitochondrial disorders to anesthetic agents does not appear to be consistent.

SUMMARY

The anesthetic care of the pediatric patient with a systemic disorder provides myriad challenges for the anesthesiologist. A thorough understanding of the patient's disease and the effect that the anesthetic will have on the disease process are the two most important issues the anesthesiologist must address. For some of these patients, appropriate consultation with the surgeon, pediatrician, and pediatric subspecialist is essential to the proper management of these potentially difficult and challenging anesthetics.

REFERENCES

Abel M, Bona M, Zawodniak L: Cervical spinal cord hemorrhage secondary to neonatal alloimmune thrombocytopenia. *J Pediatr Hematol Oncol* 25:340, 2003.

Abel M, Eisenkraft JB: Anesthetic implications of myasthenia gravis. *Mt Sinai J Med* 69:31, 2002.

Abramson PJ, Todd NW, Holt PJ, et al.: Neck flexion and extension in children with Down syndrome: A somatosensory study. *Laryngoscope* 105:1209, 1995.

Acharya S, Bussel JB: Hematologic toxicity of sodium valproate. *J Pediatr Hematol Oncol* 22:62, 2000.

Ackerman VL: Bronchopulmonary dysplasia. In Loughlin GM, Eigen H, editors: *Respiratory disease in children, diagnosis and management.* Baltimore, 1994, Williams & Wilkins, p 383.

Adu-Gyamfi Y, Sankarakutty M, Marwa S: Use of a tourniquet in patients with sickle cell disease. *Can J Anaesth* 40:24, 1993.

Aitken ML, Fiel SB: Cystic fibrosis. Dis Mon 39:1, 1993.

Akinbami LJ, Schoendorf KC: Trends in childhood asthma: Prevalence, health care utilization and mortality. *Pediatrics* 110:315, 2002.

Alanay A, Acaroglu E, Ozdemir O, et al.: Effects of deamino-8-D-arginin vasopressin on blood loss and coagulation factors in scoliosis surgery. A double-blind randomized clinical trial. *Spine* 24:877, 1999.

Aldwinckle RJ, Carr AS: The anesthetic management of a patient with Emery-Dreifuss muscular dystrophy for orthopedic surgery. *Can J Anaesth* 49:467, 2002.

Allen A: The cardiotoxicity of chemotherapeutic drugs. *Semin Oncol* 19:529, 1992.

Allen GC, Armfield DR, Bontempo FA, et al.: Adenotonsillectomy in children with von Willebrand disease. *Arch Otlaryngol Head Neck Surg* 125:547, 1999.

Almeida AM, Khair K, Hann I, et al.: The use of recombinant factor VIIa in children with inherited platelet function disorders. *Br J Haematol* 121:477, 2003.

Alton E, Khagani A, Taylor RF, et al.: Effect of heart-lung transplantation on airway potential difference in patients with and without cystic fibrosis. *Eur Respir J* 4:5, 1991.

Amack JD, Mahadevan MS: Myogenic defects in myotonic dystrophy. *Dev Biol* 265:294, 2004.

American Academy of Pediatrics: Adolescents and human immunodeficiency infection: The role of the pediatrician in prevention and intervention. American Academy of Pediatrics, Committee on Pediatric AIDS and Committee on Adolescence. *Pediatrics* 107:188, 2001a.

American Academy of Pediatrics: Atlantoaxial instability in Down syndrome. American Academy of Pediatrics, Committee on Sports Medicine. *Pediatrics* 74:152, 1984.

American Academy of Pediatrics: Atlantoaxial instability in Down syndrome: Subject review. American Academy of Pediatrics, Committee on Sports Medicine and Fitness. *Pediatrics* 96:151, 1995.

American Academy of Pediatrics: Evaluation and medical treatment of the HIV-exposed infant. American Academy of Pediatrics, Committee on Pediatric AIDS. *Pediatrics* 99:909, 1997.

American Academy of Pediatrics: Health supervision for children with Down syndrome: *Pediatrics* 107:442, 2001b.

American Society of Anesthesiologists: Practice guidelines for blood component therapy. A report by the American Society of Anesthesiologists Task Force on Blood Component Therapy. *Anesthesiology* 84:732, 1996 (updated on ASA web site, 2003: www.asahq.org/publicationsAndServices/blood_component.html).

Ammann AJ: Hypothesis: Absence of graft-versus-host disease in AIDS is a consequence of HIV-1 infection of CD4+ T cells. *J Acquir Immune Defic Syndr* 6:1224, 1993.

Amrein PC, Ellman L, Harris WH: Aspirin induced prolongation of bleeding time and perioperative blood loss. *JAMA* 245:1825, 1981.

Anderson BJ, Brown TC: Congenital myotonic dystrophy in children—a review of ten years' experience. *Anaesth Intensive Care* 17:320, 1989.

Anderson KC: Current trends: Evolving concepts in transfusion medicine. Leukodepleted cellular blood components for prevention of transfusion-associated graft-versus-host disease. *Transfus Sci* 16:265, 1995.

Andrew M: Developmental hemostasis: relevance to hemostatic problems during childhood. *Semin Thromb Hemost* 21:341, 1995.

Andrew M: The relevance of developmental hemostasis to hemorrhagic disorders of the newborn. *Semin Perinatol* 21:70, 1997.

Andrew M, Brooker LA: Blood component therapy in neonatal hemostatic disorders. *Transfus Med Rev* 9:231, 1995.

Andrew M, Mitchell L, Vegh P, et al.: Thrombin regulation in children differs from adults in the absence and presence of heparin. *Thromb Haemost* 72:836, 1994.

Andrew M, Paes B, Johnston M: Development of the hemostatic system in the neonate and young infant. *Am J Pediatr Hematol Oncol* 12:95, 1990a.

Andrew M, Paes B, Milner R, et al.: Development of the human coagulation system in the full-term infant. *Blood* 70:165, 1987.

Andrew M, Paes B, Milner R, et al.: Development of the human coagulation system in the healthy premature infant. *Blood* 72:1651, 1988.

Andrew M, Schmidt B, Mitchell L, et al.: Thrombin generation in newborn plasma is critically dependent on the concentration of prothrombin. *Thromb Haemost* 63:27, 1990b.

Andrew M, Vegh P, Johnston M, et al.: Maturation of the hemostatic system during childhood. *Blood* 80:1998, 1992.

Anwar R, Miloszewski KJA: Factor XIII deficiency. *Br J Haematol* 107:468, 1999.

Applefield MM, Slawson RG, Spicer KM, et al.: Long term cardiovascular evaluation of patients with Hodgkin's disease treated by thoracic mantle radiation therapy. *Cancer Treat Rep* 66:1003, 1982.

Arkin S, Blei F, Fetten J, et al.: Human coagulation factor FVIIa (recombinant) in the management of limb-threatening bleeds unresponsive to alternative therapies: Results from the NovoSeven emergency use programme in patients with severe hemophilia or with acquired inhibitors. *Blood Coagul Fibrinolysis* 11:255, 2000.

Arslanian S, Becker D, Drash A: Diabetes mellitus in the child and adolescent. In Kappy MS, Blizzard RM, Migeon CJ, editors: *The diagnosis and treatment of endocrine disorders in childhood and adolescence*. Springfield, IL, 1994, Charles C Thomas.

Aucar JA, Norman P, Whitten E, et al.: Intraoperative detection of traumatic coagulopathy using the activated coagulation time. *Shock* 19:404, 2003.

Balis FM, Holcenberg JS, Blaney SM: General principles of chemotherapy. In Pizzo PA, Poplack DDG, editors: *Pediatric oncology*, 4th ed. Philadelphia, 2002, Lippincott Williams & Wilkins, p 272.

Bancalari E, Claure N, Sosenko IR: Bronchopulmonary dysplasia: Changes in pathogenesis, epidemiology and definition. *Semin Neonatol* 8:63, 2003.

Banerjea MC, Diener W, Kutschke G, et al.: Pro- and anticoagulatory factors under sodium valproate therapy in children. *Neuropediatrics* 33:215, 2002.

Baraka A: Anesthesia and critical care of thymectomy for myasthenia gravis. *Chest Surg Clin N Am* 11:337, 2001.

Barnes PJ, Pedersen S: Efficacy and safety of inhaled corticosteroids in asthma. Report of a workshop held in Eze, France, October 1992. *Am Rev Respir Dis* 148:S1, 1993.

Batlle J, del Rio F, Lopez F, et al.: Effect of dextran on factor VIII/von Willebrand factor structure and function. *Thromb Haemost* 54:697, 1985.

Baum VC, Barton DM, Gutgesell HP: Influence of congenital heart disease on mortality following noncardiac surgery in hospitalized children. *Pediatrics* 105:332, 2000.

Ben-David B, Gaitini L: Compliance with gloving in anesthesia: An observational study of gloving practice at induction of general anesthesia. *J Clin Anesth* 9:527, 1997.

Bennett MH, Wainwright AP: Acute thyroid crisis on induction of anaesthesia. *Anaesthesia* 44:28–30, 1989.

Benumof JL: *Anesthesia for thoracic surgery*. Philadelphia, 1995, WB Saunders.

Benumof JL: Respiratory physiology and respiratory function during anesthesia. In Miller RD, editor: *Anesthesia,* 5th ed. New York, 1994, Churchill-Livingstone, p 557.

Bernstein DE, Jeffers L, Erhardtsen E, et al.: Recombinant factor VIIa corrects prothrombin time in cirrhotic patients: A preliminary study. *Gastroenterology* 114:1930, 1997.

Berry FA: The child with the runny nose. In Berry FA, editor: *Anesthetic management of difficult and routine pediatric patients*, ed 2, New York, 1990, churchill Livingstone.

Bertland JM, Riley SP, Popkin J, et al.: The long term pulmonary sequelae of prematurity: The role of familial airway hyperreactivity and the respiratory distress syndrome. *N Engl J Med* 312:742, 1985.

Bick RL, Baker W: Diagnostic efficacy of the D-dimer assay in DIC and related disorders. *Blood* 68:329, 1986.

Bjorkman S, Carlsson M, Berntorp E: Pharmacokinetics of factor IX in patients with haemophilia B. Methodologic aspects and physiological interpretation. *Eur J Pharmacol* 46:325, 1994.

Blanchette VS: Neonatal alloimmune thrombocytopenia: A clinical perspective. *Curr Stud Hematol Blood Transfus* 54:112, 1988.

Blom HJ, Karsdorp V, Birnie R, et al.: Phaeochromocytoma as a cause of pulmonary edema. *Anaesthesia* 42:646, 1987.

Board PG, Losowsky MS, Miloszewski KJ: Factor XIII: Inherited and acquired deficiency. *Blood Rev* 7:229, 1993.

Bolan CD, Rick ME, Polly DW Jr: Transfusion medicine management for reconstructive spinal repair in a patient with von Willebrand's disease and a history of heavy surgical bleeding. *Spine* 26:E552, 2001.

Bolton P, Peutrell J, Zuberi S, et al.: Anaesthesia for an adolescent with mitochondrial encephalomyopathy-lactic acidosis-stroke-like episodes syndrome. *Paediatr Anaesth* 13:453, 2003.

Borud LJ, Matarasso A, Spaccavento CM, et al.: Factor XI deficiency: Implications for management of patients undergoing aesthetic surgery. *Plast Reconstr Surg* 104:1907, 1999.

Boulis NM, Bobek M, Schmaier A: Use of factor IX complex in warfarin-related intracranial hemorrhage. *Neurosurgery* 45:1113, 1999.

Bray GL, Luban NL: Hemophilia presenting with intracranial hemorrhage. An approach to the infant with intracranial bleeding and coagulopathy. *Am J Dis Child* 141:1215, 1987.

Briet E, Bertina RM, Van Tilburg NA, et al.: Hemophilia B Leyden: A sex linked hereditary disorder that improves after puberty. *N Engl J Med* 306:782, 1982.

Brill PW, Ewing ML, Dunn AA: The value of routine chest radiography in children and adolescents. *Pediatrics* 52:125, 1973.

Bromberg PA, Jensen WN: Blood oxygen dissociation curves in sickle cell disease. *J Lab Clin Meb* 70:480, 1967.

Browers P, Wolters P, Civitello L: Central nervous system assesment and management. In Pizzo PA, Wilfert CM, editors: *Pediatric AIDS*: New York, 1998, Lippincott Williams & Wilkins, p 297.

Brown RH, Pizov R, Mennes M, et al.: The incidence and relative risk of wheezing during induction of anesthesia in asthmatics. *Anesthesiology* 77:A1209, 1992.

Brown RH, Schauble JF, Hamilton RG: Prevalence of latex allergy among anesthesiologists: Identification of sensitized but asymptomatic individuals. *Anesthesiology* 89:292, 1998.

Brown TC, Gebert R, Meretoja OA, et al.: Myasthenia gravis in children and its anaesthetic implications. *Anaesth Intensive Care* 18:466, 1990.

Buckalew VM Jr, Someren A: Renal manifestations of sickle cell disease. *Arch Intern Med* 133:660, 1974.

Buckingham B, Perejda AJ, Sandborg C, et al.: Skin, joint and pulmonary changes in type I diabetes mellitus. *Am J Dis Child* 140:420, 1986.

Burrows FA: Physiologic dead space, venous admixture, and the arterial to end-tidal carbon dioxide difference in infants and children undergoing cardiac surgery. *Anesthesiology* 70:219, 1989.

Busch MP: Closing the windows on viral transmission by blood transfusion. In Stramer SL, editor: *Blood safety in the new millennium*. Bethesda, MD, 2001, American Association of Blood Banks, p 233.

Camerer E, Kolsto AB, Prydz H: Cell biology of tissue factor, the principal initiator of blood coagulation. *Thromb Res* 81:1, 1996.

Capanni C, Sabatelli P, Mattioli E, et al.: Dysferlin in a hyperCKaemic patient with caveolin 3 mutation and in C2C12 cells after p38 MAP kinase inhibition. *Exp Mol Med* 35:538, 2003.

Caron E: Regulation of Wiskott-Aldrich syndrome protein and related molecules. *Curr Opin Cell Biol* 14:82, 2002.

Carraway MS, Welty-Wolf KE, Miller DL, et al.: Blockade of tissue factor: Treatment for organ injury in established sepsis. *Am J Respir Crit Care Med* 167:1200, 2003.

Centers for Disease Control and Prevention (CDC): Recommendations for prevention of HIV transmission in health-care settings. *MMWR Morb Mortal Wkly Rep* 36(Suppl 2):1S, 1987.

Centers for Disease Control and Prevention (CDC): 1994 Revised classification system for human immunodeficiency virus infection in children less than 13 years of age. *MMWR Morb Mortal Wkly Rep* 43:RR-12, 1994.

Centers for Disease Control and Prevention (CDC): Guidelines for the use of antiretroviral agents in pediatric HIV infection. *MMWR Mor Mortal Wkly Rep* 47:RR-4, 1998.

Centers for Disease Control and Prevention (CDC): HIV/AIDS surveillance report. *MMWR Morb Mortal Wkly Rep* 8:2, 1996.

Centers for Disease Control and Prevention (CDC): Update: Perinatally acquired HIV-1/AIDS—United States. *MMWR Morb Mortal Wkly Rep* 46:1086, 1997.

Centers for Disease Control and Prevention (CDC): Public health dispatch: Investigations of West Nile virus infections in recipients of blood transfusions. *MMWR Morb Mortal Wkly Rep* 51:973, 2002.

Centers for Disease Control and Prevention (CDC). www.cdc.gov/diabetes/pubs/factsheet.htm

Chambers HG, Weinstein CH, Mubarak SJ, et al.: The effect of valproic acid on blood loss in patients with cerebral palsy. *J Pediatr Orthop* 19:792, 1999.

Chandler WL: The thromboelastograph and the thromboelastograph technique. *Semin Thromb Hemost* 21:S1, 1995.

Chang K, Uitto J, Rowold EA, et al.: Increased collagen cross linkages in experimental diabetes: Reversal by beta-amino propionitrile and D-penicillamine *Diabetes* 29:778, 1980.

Chapman KR, Verbeck PR, White JG, et al.: Effects of a short course of prednisone in the prevention of early relapse after the emergency room treatment of acute asthma. *N Engl J Med* 324:788, 1991.

Chen ET, Nichols JH, Duh SH, et al.: Performance evaluation of blood glucose monitoring devices. *Diabetes Technol Ther* 5:749, 2003.

Chen JP, Lorch V: Intraventricular hemorrhage in preterm infants: Evidence of suppressed fibrinolysis. *Blood Coagul Fibrinolysis* 7:289, 1996.

Chen YW, Zhao P, Borup R, et al.: Expression profiling in the muscular dystrophies: Identification of novel aspects of molecular pathophysiology. *J Cell Biol* 151:1321, 2000.

Chuansumrit A, Chantarojanasiri T, Isarangkura P, et al.: Recombinant activated factor VII in children with acute bleeding resulting from liver failure and disseminated intravascular coagulation. *Blood Coagul Fibrinolysis* 11:S101, 2000.

Clagett GP, Anderson FAJ, Geerts W, et al.: Prevention of venous thromboembolism. *Chest* 114:531S, 1998.

Clark RW, Schmidt HS, Schuller DE: Sleep-induced ventilatory dysfunction in Down syndrome. *Arch Intern Med* 140:45, 1980.

Clarke RJ, Mayo G, Price P, et al.: Suppression of thromboxane A_2 but not of systemic prostacyclin by controlled release aspirin. *N Engl J Med* 325:1137, 1991.

Clausen T: Na^+-K^+ pump regulation and skeletal muscle contractility. *Physiol Rev* 83:1269, 2003.

Clifford RD, Radford M, Howell JB, et al.: Prevalence of respiratory symptoms among 7 and 11 year old school children and association with asthma. *Arch Dis Child* 64:1118, 1989.

Clough JB, Williams JD, Holgate ST: Effect of atopy on the natural history of symptoms, peak expiratory flow, and bronchial responsiveness in 7 and 8 year old children with cough and wheeze. *Am Rev Respir Dis* 143:755, 1991.

Coalson J: Pathology of chronic lung disease of early infancy. In Bland RJ, Coalson JJ, editors: *Chronic lung disease in early infancy*. New York, 1999, Marcel Dekker, p 85.

Cohen AJ, Philips TM, Kessler CM: Circulating coagulation inhibitors in the acquired immunodeficiency syndrome. *Ann Intern Med* 104:175, 1986.

Cohen MM, Cameron CB: Should you cancel the operation when a child has an upper respiratory tract infection? *Anesth Analg* 72:282, 1991.

Conti G, Dellutri D, Viraldi V, et al.: Propofol induces bronchodilation in mechanically ventilated chronic obstructive pulmonary disease (COPD) patients. *Acta Anaesthesiol Scand* 37:105, 1993.

Corssen G, Gutierrez J, Reves JG, et al.: Ketamine in the anesthetic management of asthmatic patients. *Anesth Analg* 51:588, 1972.

Cosgriff N, Moore EE, Sauaia A, et al.: Predicting life-threatening coagulopathy in the massively transfused trauma patient: Hypothermia and acidoses revisited. *J Trauma* 42:857, 1997.

Cote CJ: Blood colloid and crystalloid therapy. *Anesthesiol Clin North Am* 9:865, 1991.

Cote CJ, Drop LJ, Hoaglin DC, et al.: Ionized hypocalcemia after fresh frozen plasma administration to thermally injured children: Effects of infusion rate, duration and treatment with calcium chloride. *Anesth Analg* 67:152, 1988.

Counts RB, Haisch C, Simon TL, et al.: Hemostasis in massively transfused trauma patients. *Ann Surg* 190:91, 1979.

Cramolini GM: Diseases of the renal system. In Katz J, Steward DJ, editors: *Anesthesia and uncommon pediatric diseases*. Philadelphia, 1993, WB Saunders.

Creer TL, Gustafson KE: Psychological problem associated with drug therapy in childhood asthma. *J Pediatr* 115:850, 1989.

Cryer B, Feldman M: Cyclooxgenase-1 and cyclooxygenase-2 selectivity of widely used nonsteroidal anti-inflammatory drugs. *Am J Med* 104:413, 1998.

Cystic Fibrosis Genetic Analysis Consortium: Worldwide survey of the d508 mutation Report from the Cystic Fibrosis Genetic Analysis Consortium. *Am J Hum Genet* 47:354, 1990.

Dajani AS, Taubert KA, Wilson W, et al.: Prevention of bacterial endocarditis. Recommendations by the American Heart Association. *JAMA* 277:1794, 1997.

Dakin MJ, Yentis: Latex allergy: A strategy for management. *Anaesthesia* 53:774, 1998.

Dalal FY, Bennett EJ, Gegg WS: Congenital myasthenia gravis and minor surgical procedures. A review with two case reports. *Anaesthesia* 27:61, 1972.

Dalens B, Tanguy A, Haberer JP: Lumbar epidural anesthesia for operative and postoperative pain in infants and young children. *Anesth Analg* 65:1069, 1986.

DeBock TL, Davis PJ, Tome J, et al.: Effect of premedication on arterial oxygen saturation in children with congenital heart disease. *J Cardiothorac Anesth* 4:425, 1990.

De Jonge E, Levi M: Effects of different plasma substitutes on blood coagulation: A comparative review. *Crit Care Med* 29:1261, 2001.

De Jonge E, Levi M, Buller HR, et al.: Decreased circulating levels of von Willebrand factor after intravenous administration of a rapidly degradable hydroxyethyl starch (HES 200/0.5/6) in healthy human subjects. *Intensive Care Med* 27:1825, 2001.

Della Rocca G, Coccia C, Diana L, et al.: Propofol or sevoflurane anesthesia without muscle relaxants allow the early extubation of myasthenic patients. *Can J Anaesth* 50:547, 2003.

Desmopressin and arterial thrombosis [editorial]. *Lancet* 1:938, 1989.

DeSoto H, Patel RI, Soliman IE, et al.: Changes in oxygen saturation following general anesthesia in children with upper respiratory infection and symptoms undergoing otolaryngological procedures. *Anesthesiology* 68:276, 1988.

Despotis GJ, Gravlee G, Filos K, et al.: Anticoagulation monitoring during cardiac surgery: A review of current and emerging techniques. *Anesthesiology* 91:1121, 1999.

DiGeorge AM: Excessive secretion of catecholamines. In Behrman RE, Vaughan VC III, editors: *Nelson's textbook of pediatrics*. Philadelphia, 1987, WB Saunders.

Djukanovic R, Roche WR, Wilson JW, et al.: Mucosal inflammation in asthma. *Am Rev Respir Dis* 142:434, 1990.

D'Oiron R, Menart C, Trzeciak MC, et al.: Use of recombinant factor VIIa in three patients with inherited type I Glanzmann's thrombasthenia undergoing invasive procedures. *Thromb Haemost* 83:644, 2000.

Douglas WW: Histamine and 5-hydroxytrptamine (serotonin) and their antagonists. In Gilman AG, Goodman LS, Rall TW, et al., editors: *Goodman and Gilman's the pharmacological basis of therapeutics*, 7th ed. New York, 1985, Macmillan.

Downing J: Dermatitis from rubber gloves. *N Engl J Med* 208:196, 1933.

Doyle MG, Pickering LK: Gastrointestinal tract infections in children with AIDS. *Semin Pediatr Infect Dis* 1:64, 1990.

Drake AJ, Howells RJ, Shield JP, et al.: Symptomatic adrenal insufficiency presenting with hypoglycaemia in children with asthma receiving high dose inhaled fluticasone proprionate. *BMJ* 324:1081, 2002.

Dresner DL, Ali HH: Anaesthetic management of a patient with facioscapulohumeral muscular dystrophy. *Br J Anaesth* 62:331, 1989.

Drugs for asthma. *Treat Guidel Med Lett* 1:7, 2002.

Drummond JC, Petrovich CT: The massively bleeding patient. *Anesthesiol Clin North Am* 19:633, 2001.

Dueck R, Prutow R, Richman D: Effect of parainfluenza infection on gas exchange and PRC response to anesthesia in sheep. *Anesthesiology* 74:1044, 1991.

Duijvestijn YC, Brand PL: Systemic review of *N*-acetylcysteine in cystic fibrosis. *Acta Pediatr* 88:38, 1999.

Duplantier JE, Nelson RP Jr, Morelli AR, et al.: Hypothalamic-pituitary-adrenal axis suppression associated with the use of inhaled fluticasone proprionate. *J Allergy Clin Immunol* 102:699, 1998.

Dusser DJ, Jacoby DB, Djokic TD, et al.: Virus induces airway hyperresponsiveness to tachykinins: Role of neutral endopeptidase. *J Appl Physiol* 67:1504, 1989.

Eddy VA, Morris JA Jr, Cullinane DC: Hypothermia, coagulopathy and acidosis. *Surg Clin North Am* 80:845, 2000.

Eder AF: Donor limitation of neonatal and pediatric transfusion. In Herman JH, Manno CS, editors: *Pediatric transfusion therapy*, Bethesda, MD, 2002, AABB Press, p 193.

Edwards DK, Hilston SVW: Flat chest in chronic bronchopulmonary dysplasia. *Am J Radiol* 149:1213, 1987.

Egli GA, Zollinger A, Seifert B, et al.: Effect of progressive haemodilution with hydroxyethyl starch, gelatin and albumin on blood coagulation. *Br J Anaesth* 78:684, 1997.

Eid N, Morton R, Olds B, et al.: Decreased morning serum cortisol levels in children with asthma treated with inhaled fluticasone propionate. *Pediatrics* 109:217, 2002.

Emery AE: The muscular dystrophies. *Lancet* 359:687, 2002.

Empey DW, Laitinen LA, Jacobs L, et al.: Mechanisms of bronchial hyperreactivity in normal subjects after upper respiratory tract infection. *Am Rev Respir Dis* 113:131, 1976.

Enderson BL, Chen JP, Robinson R, et al.: Fibrinolysis in multisystem trauma patients. *J Trauma* 31:1240, 1991.

Englund JA, King JC Jr: Respiratory viral infections in children infected with HIV. In Pizzo P, Wilfert C, editors: *Pediatric AIDS*. New York, 1998, Lippincott Williams & Wilkins, p 227.

Engvall E, Wewer UM: The new frontier in muscular dystrophy research: Booster genes. *FASEB J* 17:1579, 2003.

Evenhouse M, Haas E, Snell E, et al.: Hypotension in infection with the human immunodeficiency virus. *Ann Intern Med* 107:590, 1987.

Fakhry SM, Sheldon GF: Massive transfusion in the surgical patient. In Jeffries LC, Brecher ME, editors: *Massive transfusion*. Bethesda, MD, American Association of Blood Banks, 1994.

Faraday N: Platelets, perioperative hemostasis and anesthesia. *Anesthesiology* 96:1042, 2002.

Farbu E, Softeland E, Bindoff LA: Anaesthetic complications associated with myotonia congenita: Case study and comparison with other myotonic disorders. *Acta Anaesthesiol Scand* 47:630, 2003.

Farrell PT: Anaesthesia-induced rhabdomyolysis causing cardiac arrest: Case report and review of anaesthesia and the dystrophinopathies. *Anaesth Intensive Care* 22:597, 1994.

Federici AB, Baudo F, Caracciolo C, et al.: Clinical efficacy of highly purified doubly virus-inactivated factor VIII/von Willebrand factor concentrate (Fanhdi) in the treatment of von Willebrand disease: A retrospective clinical study. *Haemophilia* 8:761, 2002.

Felner EI, White PC: Improving management of diabetic ketoacidosis in children. *Pediatrics* 108:735, 2001.

Ferrara JL, Krenger W: Graft-versus-host disease: The influence of type 1 and type 2 T cell cytokines. *Transfus Med Rev* 12:1, 1998.

Fewins J, Simpson CB, Miller FR: Complications of thyroid and parathyroid surgery. *Otolaryngol Clin North Am* 36:189, 2003.

Finsterer J. Myotonic dystrophy type 2. *Eur J Neurol* 9:441, 2002

Finsterer J, Stollberger C: The heart in human dystrophinopathies. *Cardiology* 99:1, 2003.

Fitzsimons RB: Facioscapulohumeral muscular dystrophy. *Curr Opin Neurol* 12:501, 1999.

Fleming DW, Cochi SL, Hightower AW, et al.: Childhood upper respiratory infections: To what degree is incidence affected by day care attendance. *Pediatrics* 79:55, 1987.

Florentino-Pineda I, Blakemore L, Thompson GH, et al.: The effect of (epsilon) aminocaproic acid on perioperative blood loss in patients with idiopathic scoliosis undergoing posterior spinal fusion: A preliminary prospective study. *Spine* 26:1147, 2001.

Foster DW, McGarry JD: The metabolic derangements and treatment of diabetic ketoacidosis. *N Engl J Med* 309:159, 1983.

Francis JD, Leary T, Niblett DJ: Convulsions and respiratory arrest in association with desmopressin administration for the treatment of a bleeding tonsil in a child with borderline hemophilia. *Acta Anesthesiol Scand* 43:870, 1999.

Fraser CG, Preuss FS, Bigford WD: Adrenal atrophy and irreversible shock associated with cortisone therapy. *JAMA* 149:1542, 1952.

Fricker RM, Raffelsberger T, Rauch-Shorny S, et al.: Positive malignant hyperthermia susceptibility in vitro test in a patient with mitochondrial myopathy and myoadenylate deaminase deficiency. *Anesthesiology* 97:1635, 2002.

Fridy WW Jr, Ingram RH Jr, Hierholzer JC, et al.: Airway function during mild viral respiratory illnesses. *Ann Intern Med* 80:150, 1974.

Friederich PW, Wever PC, Briet C, et al.: Successful treatment with recombinant factor VIIa of therapy-resistant severe bleeding in a patient with acquired von Willebrand disease. *Am J Hematol* 66:292, 2001.

Froemming GR, Ohlendieck K: The role of ion-regulatory membrane proteins of excitation-contraction coupling and relaxation in inherited muscle diseases. *Front Biosci* 6:D65, 2001.

Fuchs HJ, Borowitz DS, Christiansen DH, et al.: Effect of aerosolized recombinant human DNase on exacerbations of respiratory symptoms and on pulmonary function in patients with cystic fibrosis. The Pulmozyme Study Group. *N Engl J Med* 331:637, 1994.

Funk CD: Platelet eicosanoids. In Colman RW, Jirsh J, Marder VJ, et al., editors: *Hemostasis and thrombosis: Basic principles and clinical practice.*, 4th ed. Baltimore, MD, 2001, Lippincott Williams & Wilkins, pp 533–539.

Furie B, Furie BC: Molecular basis of vitamin K–dependent gamma carboxylation. *Blood* 75:1753, 1990.

Furuyama H, Odagawa Y, Katoh C, et al.: Altered myocardial flow reserve and endothelial function late after Kawasaki disease. *J Pediatr* 142:149, 2003.

Gailani D: Factor XI activation in a revised model of blood coagulation. *Science* 9912:909, 1991.

Gal TJ: Bronchial hyperresponsiveness and anesthesia: Physiologic and therapeutic perspectives. *Anesth Analg* 78:559, 1994.

Garabrant DH, Schweitzer S: Epidemiology of latex sensitization and allergies in health care workers. *J Allergy Clin Immunol* 110:S82, 2002.

Gelman B, Setty Y, Chen D, et al.: Impaired mobilization of intracellular calcium in neonatal platelets. *Pediatr Res* 39:692, 1996.

Gerhardt T, Bancalari E: Lung compliance in newborns with patent ductus arteriosus before and after surgical ligation. *Biol Neonate* 38:96, 1980.

Giantris A, Abdurrahman L, Hinkle A, et al.: Anthracycline-induced cardiotoxicity in children and young adults. *Crit Rev Oncol Hematol* 61:53, 1998.

Gilbert IA, Fouke JM, McFadden ER Jr: Intra-airway thermodynamics during exercise and hyperventilation in asthmatics. *J Appl Physiol* 64:2167, 1988.

Girardi L, Sudi K, Muntean W: Effect of heparin, platelets, activated platelets, platelet fragments and hematocrit on activated clotting time. *Artif Organs* 24:507, 2000.

Girolami A, DeMarco L, Dal Bo Zanon R, et al.: Rarer, quantitative and qualitative abnormalities of coagulation. *Clin Haemotol* 14:385, 1985.

Glowniak JV, Loriaux DL: A double-blind study of perioperative steroid requirements in secondary adrenal insufficiency. *Surgery* 121:123, 1997.

Gold BS, Dart RC, Barish RA: Bites of venomous snakes. *N Engl J Med* 83:177, 2003.

Goldstein RA, Paul WE, Metcalfe DD, et al.: NIH conference. Asthma. *Ann Intern Med* 121:698, 1994.

Gonzalez A, Sosenko IR, Chandar J, et al.: Influence of infection on patent ductus arteriosus and chronic lung disease in premature infants weighing 1000 grams or less. *J Pediatr* 128:470, 1996.

Goobie SM, Soriano SG, Zurakowski D, et al.: Hemostatic changes in pediatric neurosurgical patients as evaluated by thromboelastograph. *Anesth Analg* 93:887, 2001.

Goodwin SR: Perioperative implications of hemoglobinopathies. *Anesth Analg* 86(Suppl):39, 1998.

Greeley WJ, Bushman GA, Davis DP, et al.: Comparative effects of halothane and ketamine on systemic arterial oxygen saturation in children with cyanotic heart disease. *Anesthesiology* 65:666, 1986.

Greenberg RS, Hamilton RG, Brown RH: Differential latex allergy prevalence in anesthesiology subspecialties. *Anesthesiology* 90:1238, 1999.

Griffin TX, Buchanan GR: Elective surgery in children with sickle cell disease without preoperative blood transfusion. *J Pediatr* Surg 28:681, 1993.

Groneck P, Gotze-Speer B, Oppermann M, et al.: Association of pulmonary inflammation and increased microvascular permeability during the development of bronchopulmonary dysplasia: A sequential analysis of inflammatory mediators in respiratory fluids of high risk preterm neonates. *Pediatrics* 93:712, 1994.

Groudine SB, Lumb PD, Sandison MR: Pressure support ventilation with the laryngeal mask airway: A method to manage severe reactive airway disease postoperatively. *Can J Anaesth* 42:341, 1995.

Grunnet M, Jespersen T, Colding-Jorgensen E, et al.: Characterization of two new dominant ClC-1 channel mutations associated with myotonia. *Muscle Nerve* 28:722, 2003.

Gurwitz D, Mirdorff C, Levison H: Increased incidence of bronchial reactivity in children with a history of bronchiolitis. *J Pediatr* 98:551, 1981.

Haberkern CM, Neumayr LD, Orringer EP, et al.: Cholecystectomy in sickle cell anemia patients: Perioperative outcome of 364 cases from the National Preoperative Transfusion Study. *Blood* 89:1533, 1997.

Hall TL, Barnes A, Miller JR, et al.: Neonatal mortality following transfusion of red cells with high plasma potassium levels. *Transfusion* 33:606, 1993.

Hamilton RG, Peterson EL, Ownby DR: Clinical and laboratory-based methods in the diagnosis of natural rubber latex allergy. *J Allergy Clin Immunol* 110:S47, 2002.

Hannaford K, Todd DA, Jeffrey H, et al.: Role of *Ureaplasma urealyticum* in lung disease of prematurity. *Arch Dis Child Fetal Neonatal Ed* 81:F162, 1999.

Hannam S, Lees C, Edwards RJ, et al.: Neonatal coagulopathy in preterm, small-for-gestational-age infants. *Biol Neonate* 83:177, 2003.

Harris AS: Clinical experience with desmopressin: Efficacy and safety in central diabetes insipidus and other conditions. *J Pediatr* 114:711, 1989.

Hassink EA, Souren TS, Boersma LJ, et al.: Pulmonary morbidity 10-18 years after irradiation for Hodgkin's disease. *Eur J Cancer* 29A:343, 1993.

Hay CR, Negrier C, Ludlam CA: The treatment of bleeding in acquired hemophilia with recombinant factor VIIa: A multicenter study. *Thromb Haemost* 78:1463, 1997.

Haynes RC Jr: Adrenocorticotropic hormone: Adrenocortical steroids and their synthetic analogs: Inhibitors of adrenocortical steroid biosynthesis. In Goodman AG, Rall TW, Nies AS, et al., editors: *Goodman and Gilman's the pharmacological basis of therapeutics,* 8th ed. New York, 1990, Macmillan.

Hays RM: Agents affecting the renal conservation of water. In Goodman AG, Rall TW, Nies AS, et al., editors: *Goodman and Gilman's the pharmacological basis of therapeutics,* 8th ed. New York, 1990, Macmillan.

Hazinski TA: Bronchopulmonary dysplasia. In Chernick V, editor: *Kendig's disorders of the respiratory tract in children*, 5th ed. Philadelphia, 1990, WB Saunders, p 300.

Hedderich GS, Petsikas DJ, Cooper BA, et al.: Desmopressin acetate in uncomplicated coronary artery bypass surgery: A prospective randomized clinical trial. *Can J Surg* 33:33, 1990.

Hedner U: Recombinant activated factor VII as a universal haemostatic agent. *Blood Coagul Fibrinolysis* 9:S147, 1998.

Hedner U, Kisiel W: Use of human factor VIIa in the treatment of two hemophilia A patient with high titer inhibitors. *J Clin Invest* 71:1836, 1983.

Heiman-Patterson TD, Rosenberg HR, et al.: King-Denborough syndrome: Contracture testing and literature review. *Pediatr Neurol* 2:175, 1986.

Hendriks HG, Meijer K, deWolf JT, et al.: Reduced transfusion requirements by recombinant factor VIIa in orthotopic liver transplantation: A pilot study. *Transplantation* 71:402, 2001.

Henry TD, Satran D, Knox LL: Are activated clotting times helpful in the management of anticoagulation with subcutaneous low molecular weight heparin? *Am Heart J* 142:590, 2001.

Hepner DL, Concepcion M, Bhavani-Shankar K: Coagulation status using thromboelastography in patients receiving warfarin prophylaxis and epidural analgesia. *J Clin Anesth* 14:405, 2002.

Hickey PR, Hansen DD, Strafford M, et al.: Pulmonary and systemic hemodynamic effects of nitrous oxide in infants with normal and elevated pulmonary vascular resistance. *Anesthesiology* 65:374, 1986.

Higuchi R, Kumagai T, Kobayashi M, et al.: Short-term hyperthyroidism followed by transient pituitary hypothyroidism in a very low birth weight infant born to a mother with uncontrolled Graves' disease. *Pediatrics* 107:E57, 2001.

Hillyer CD, Lankford KV, Roback JD, et al.: Transfusion of the HIV-seropositive patient: Immunomodulation, viral reactivation, and limiting exposure to EBV (HHV-4), CMV (HHV-5), and HHV-6, 7, and 8. *Transfus Med Rev* 13:1, 1999.

Hinkle AJ: What wisdom is there in administering elective general anesthesia to children with active upper respiratory tract infection? *Anesth Analg* 68:413, 1989.

Hiippala S: Replacement of massive blood loss. *Vox Sang* 74:399, 1998.

Hiippala ST, Myllyla GJ, Vahtera EM: Hemostatic factors and replacement of major blood loss with plasma poor red cell concentrates. *Anesth Analg* 81:360, 1995.

Hirshberg A, Dugas M, Banez EI, et al.: Minimizing dilutional coagulopathy in exsanguinating hemorrhage: A computer simulation. *J Trauma* 54:454, 2003.

Hirshman CA: Airway reactivity in humans: Anesthetic implications. *Anesthesiology* 68:170, 1983.

Hirshman CA, Downes H, Farbood A, et al.: Ketamine block of bronchospasm in experimental canine asthma. *Br J Anesth* 51:713, 1979.

Hochleitner BW, Menardi G, Haussler B, et al.: Spina bifida as an independent risk factor for sensitization to latex. *J Urol* 166:2370, 2001.

Hoffman BB, Lefkowitz RJ: Adrenergic receptor antagonists. In Goodman AG, Rall TW, Nies AS, et al., editors: *Goodman and Gilman's the pharmacological basis of therapeutics*, 8th ed. New York, 1990, Macmillan.

Hoffman M, Monroe DM III, Roberts HR: Activated factor VII activates factors IX and X on the surface of activated platelets: Thoughts on the mechanism of action of high-dose activated factor VII. *Blood Coagul Fibrinolysis* 9:S61, 1998.

Hoffmeister KM, Josefsson EC, Isaac NA, et al.: Glycosylation restores survival of chilled blood platelets. *Science* 301:1531, 2003.

Holgate ST: Pharmacological modulation of airway caliber and mediator release in human models of bronchial asthma. In Austen KF, Lichenstein LM, Kay AB, editors: *Asthma: Physiology, immunopharmacology and treatment.* London, 1984, Academic Press.

Holzmann L, Finn H, Lichtman HC, et al.: Anesthesia in patients with sickle cell disease: A review of 112 cases. *Anesth Analg* 48:566, 1969.

Holzman RS: Clinical management of latex-allergic children. *Anesth Analg* 85:529, 1997.

Holzman RS: Latex allergy: An emerging operating room problem. *Anesth Analg* 76:635, 1993.

Holzman RS, Pascucci R, Sethna N: Hypotension, flushing and bronchospasm in myelodysplasia patients undergoing surgery: Section on Anesthesiology [abstract]. American Academy of Pediatrics, 1990.

Holzman RS, Worthen HM, Johnson KL: Anesthesia for children with junctional epidermolysis bullosa (letalis): *Can J Anesth* 34:395, 1987.

Hourihane JO, Allard JM, Wade AM, et al.: Impact of repeated surgical procedures on the incidence and prevalence of latex allergy: A prospective study of 1263 children. *J Pediatr* 140:479, 2002.

Hymel KP, Abshire TC, Luckey DW, et al.: Coagulopathy in pediatric abusive head injury patients. *Pediatrics* 99:371, 1997.

Iberrti TJ, Miller M, Abalos A: Abnormal coagulation profile in brain tumor patients during surgery. *Neurosurgery* 34:389, 1994.

Idvall J: Ketamine monoanesthesia for major surgery in epidermolysis bullosa. Case report. *Acta Anaesthesiol Scand* 31:658, 1987.

Isaacs H, Badenhorst ME: Dominantly inherited malignant hyperthermia (MH) in the King-Denborough syndrome. *Muscle Nerve* 15:740, 1992.

Isaacs H, Badenhorst ME, Du Sautoy C: Myophosphorylase B deficiency and malignant hyperthermia. *Muscle Nerve* 12:203, 1989.

Itoh H, Shibata K, Nitta S: Sensitivity to vecuronium in seropositive and seronegative patients with myasthenia gravis. *Anesth Analg* 95:109, 2002.

Iwamoto M, Jernigan DB, Guasch A, et al.: Transmission of West Nile virus from organ donor to four transplant recipients. *N Engl J Med* 348:2196, 2003.

Jobe AH, Ikegami M: Lung development and function in pattern infants in the surfactant treatment era. *Ann Rev Physiol* 62:825, 2000.

Jobe AH, Bancalari E: Bronchopulmonary dysplasia. *Am J Respir Crit Care Med* 163:1723–1729, 2001.

Jacobson MA, Peiperl L, Volberding PA, et al.: Red cell transfusion therapy for anemia in patients with AIDS and ARC: Incidence, associated factors, and outcome. *Transfusion* 30:133, 1990.

Jacoby DB, Hirshman CA: General anesthesia in patients with viral respiratory infections: An unsound sleep? *Anesthesiology* 74:969, 1991.

Jacoby DB, Tamaoki J, Borson DB, et al.: Influenza infection causes airway hyperresponsiveness by decreasing enkephalinase. *J Appl Physiol* 64:2653, 1988.

Jakway JL: Acquired von Willebrand's disease. *Hematol Oncol Clin North Am* 6:1409, 1992.

James I, Wark H: Airway management during anesthesia in patients with epidermolysis bullosa dystrophica. *Anesthesiology* 56:323, 1982.

Jhawar BS, Ranger A, Steven D, et al.: Risk factors for intracranial hemorrhage among full-term infants: A case-control study. *Neurosurgery* 52:581, 2003.

Jobe AH, Ikegami M: Lung development and function in preterm infants in the surfactant treatment era. *Ann Rev Physiol* 62:825–846, 2000.

Johanson WG Jr, Pierce AK, Sanford JP: Pulmonary function in uncomplicated influenza. *Am Rev Respir Dis* 100:141, 1969.

Jones KL: *Smith's recognizable patterns of human malformation*, 4th ed. Philadelphia, 1988, WB Saunders.

Jones TR, Labelle M, Belley M, et al.: Pharmacology of montelukast sodium (Singulair), a potent and selective liukotriene D4 receptor antagonist. *Can J Physiol Pharmacol* 73:191, 1995.

Juniper EF, Kline PA, Vanzieleghem MA, et al.: Reduction of budesonide after a year of increased use: A randomized controlled trial to evaluate whether improvements of airway responsiveness and clinical asthma are maintained. *J Allergy Clin Immunol* 87:473, 1991.

Jurkat-Rott K, Lerche H, Lehmann-Horn F: Skeletal muscle channelopathies. *J Neurol* 249:1493, 2002.

Kahn JO, Walker BD: Acute human immunodeficiency virus type 1 infection. *N Engl J Med* 339:33, 1998.

Kalicinski P, Kaminski A, Drewniak H, et al.: Quick correction of hemostasis in two patients with fulminant liver failure undergoing liver transplantation by recombinant activated factor VII. *Transplant Proc* 21:378, 1999.

Kanamori G, Witter M, Brown J, et al.: Otolaryngologic manifestations of Down syndrome. *Otolaryngol Clin North Am* 33:1285, 2000.

Kanter MH: Transfusion associated graft-versus-host disease: Do transfusions from second-degree relatives post a greater risk than those from first-degree relatives? *Transfusion* 32:323, 1992.

Kaplan R, Strauch B: Regional anesthesia in a child with epidermolysis bullosa. *Anesthesiology* 67:262, 1987.

Kapural L, Sprung J: Perioperative anticoagulation and thrombolysis in congenital and acquired coagulopathies. *Anesthesiol Clin North Am* 17:923, 1999.

Katz, J, Steward DJ, editors: *Anesthesia and uncommon pediatric diseases*, 2nd ed. Philadelphia, 1993, WB Saunders.

Kaufmann CR: Usefulness of thromboelastography in assessment of trauma patient coagulation. *J Trauma* 43:716, 1997.

Kaufman FR, Devgan S, Roe TF, et al.: Perioperative management with prolonged intravenous insulin infusion versus subcutaneous insulin in children with type I diabetes mellitus. *J Diabetes Complications* 10:6, 1996.

Kayser EB, Morgan PG, Sedensky MM: GAS-1: A mitochondrial protein controls sensitivity to volatile anesthetics in the nematode *Caenorhabditis elegans. Anesthesiology* 90:545, 1999.

Keegan MT, Whatcott BD, Harrison BA: Osteogenesis imperfecta perioperative bleeding and desmopressin. *Anesthesiology* 97:1011, 2002.

Kelly KJ, Kurup V, Zacharisen M, et al.: Skin and serologic testing in the diagnosis of latex allergy. *J Allergy Clin Immunol* 91:1140, 1993.

Kenny FM, Preeyasombat C: Cortisone production rate. II. Normal infants, children and adults. *Pediatrics* 37:34, 1966.

Keon TP, Templeton JJ: Diseases of the endocrine system. In Katz J, Steward DJ, editors: *Anesthesia and uncommon pediatric diseases.* Philadelphia, 1993, WB Saunders.

Kerem B, Rommens JM, Buchanan JA, et al.: Identification of cystic fibrosis gene: Genetic analysis. *Science* 245:1073, 1989.

Kerem E, Reisman J, Corey M, et al.: Prediction of mortality in patients with cystic fibrosis. *N Engl J Med* 326:1187, 1992.

Kerr TP, Duward A, Hodgson SV, et al.: Hyperkalaemic cardiac arrest in a manifesting carrier of Duchenne muscular dystrophy following general anaesthesia. *Eur J Pediatr* 160:579, 2001.

Kettner SC, Kozek SA, Groetzner JP, et al.: Effects of hypothermia on thrombelastography in patients undergoing cardiopulmonary bypass. *Br J Anaesth* 80:313, 1998.

Keyes MA, Van de Wiele BV, Stead SW: Mitochondrial myopathies: An unusual cause of hypotonia in infants and children. *Paediatr Anaesth* 6:329, 1996.

Kim SB, Chi HS, Park JS, et al.: Effect of increasing serum albumin on plasma D-dimer, von Willebrand factor, and platelet aggregation in CAPD patients. *Am J Kidney Dis* 33:312, 1999.

Kiran U, Choudhury M, Saxena N, et al.: Sevoflurane as a sole anaesthetic for thymectomy in myasthenia gravis. *Acta Anaesthesiol Scand* 44:351, 2000.

Kitamura S, Kameda Y, Seki T, et al.: Long-term outcome of myocardial revascularization in patients with Kawasaki coronary artery disease. A multicenter cooperative study. *J Thorac Cardiovasc Surg* 107:663, 1994.

Klein DS, Wilds PR: Pulmonary toxicity of antineoplastic agents. Anesthetic and postoperative implication. *Can Anaesth Soc J* 30:399, 1983.

Knorr B, Franchi LM, Bisgaard H, et al.: Montelukast, a leukotriene receptor antagonist, for the treatment of persistent asthma in children aged 2 to 5 years. *Pediatrics* 108:E748, 2001.

Kobrinsky NL, Stegman D, Sjolander D: Management of spontaneous inhibitors in children with porcine factor VIII. *Haemophilia* 8(Suppl 1):1, 2002.

Koerber JM, Smythe MA, Begle RL, et al.: Correlation of activated clotting time and activated partial thromboplastin time to plasma heparin concentration. *Pharmacotherapy* 19:922, 1999.

Konarzewski WH, Ravindran N, Findlow D, et al.: Anesthetic death of a child with a cold. *Anaesthesia* 47:624, 1992.

Konig P: Inhaled corticosteroids—their present and future role in the management of asthma. *J Allergy Clin Immunol* 82:297, 1988.

Koshy M, Weiner J, Miller S, et al.: The Cooperative Study of Sickle Cell Disease: Surgery and anesthesia in sickle cell disease. *Blood* 86:3676, 1995.

Krane EJ, Rockoff MA, Wallman JK, et al.: Subclinical brain swelling in children during treatment of diabetic ketoacidosis. *N Engl J Med* 312:1147, 1985.

Krasner AS: Glucocorticoid-induced adrenal insufficiency. *JAMA* 282:671, 1999.

Kruskall MS, Lee TH, Assmann SF, et al.: Survival of transfused donor white blood cells in HIV-infected recipients. *Blood* 98:272, 2001.

Kuhne T, Imbach P: Neonatal platelet physiology and pathophysiology. *Eur J Pediatr* 157:87, 1998.

Kulkarni R, Lusher J: Perinatal management of newborns with haemophilia. *Br J Haematol* 112:264, 2001.

Kwittken PL, Becker J, Oyefara B, et al.: Latex hypersensitivity reactions despite prophylaxis. *Allergy Proc* 13:123, 1992.

LaFranchi SH: Hypothyroidism. *Pediatr Clin North Am* 26:33, 1979.

Laishley RS, Burrows FA, Lerman J, et al.: Effect of anesthetic induction regimens on oxygen saturation in cyanotic congenital heart disease. *Anesthesiology* 65:673, 1986.

Lakich D, Kazazian HH Jr, Antonarakis SE, et al.: Inversions disrupting the factor VIII gene are a common cause of severe haemophilia A. *Nat Genet* 5:236, 1993.

Lamberty JM, Rubin BK: The management of anesthesia for patients with cystic fibrosis. *Anaesthesia* 40:448, 1985.

Lane PA, Hathaway WE: Vitamin K in infancy. *J Pediatr* 106:351, 1985.

Lane PA: Sickle cell disease. *Pediatr Clin North Am* 43:639, 1996.

Lanier WL: Glucose management during cardiopulmonary bypass: Cardiovascular and neurologic implications. *Anesth Analg* 72:423, 1991.

Lanier WL, Stangland KJ, Scheithauer BW, et al.: The effects of dextrose infusion and head position on neurologic outcome after complete cerebral ischemia in primates: Examination of a model. *Anesthesiology* 66:39, 1987.

Laureno R: Central pontine myelinolysis following rapid correction of hyponatremia. *Ann Neurol* 13:232, 1983.

Leach M, Makris M, Hampton KK, et al.: Spinal epidural haematoma in haemophilia A with inhibitors—efficacy of recombinant factor VIIa concentrate. *Haemophilia* 5:209, 1999.

Lee HC, Patel MK, Mistry DJ, et al.: Abnormal Na channel gating in murine cardiac myocytes deficient in myotonic dystrophy protein kinase. *Physiol Genomics* 12:147, 2003.

Lee TH, Paglieroni T, Ohto H, et al.: Survival of donor leukocyte subpopulations in immunocompetent transfusion recipients: Frequent long-term microchimerism in severe trauma patients. *Blood* 93:3127, 1999.

Lee WP, Lippe B, LaFranchi M, et al.: Vasopressin analog DDAVP in the treatment of diabetes insipidus. *Am J Dis Child* 130:166, 1976.

Lehrnbecher T, Muller-Scholden J, Danhauser-Leistner I, et al.: Perioperative fluid and electrolyte management in children undergoing surgery for craniopharyngioma. A 10-year experience in a single institution. *Childs Nerv Syst* 14:276, 1998.

Lemmer JH, Dilling EW, Morton JR, et al.: Aprotinin for primary coronary artery bypass grafting: A multicenter trial of three dose regimens. *Ann Thorac Surg* 62:1659, 1996.

Lethagen S, Harris AS, Sjorin E, et al.: Intranasal and intravenous administration of desmopressin: Effect on FVIII/vWF, pharmacokinetics and reproducibility. *Thromb Haemost* 58:1033, 1987.

Levi M, ten Cate H: Disseminated intravascular coagulation. *N Engl J Med* 341:586, 1999.

Levi M, ten Cate H, van der Poll T: Endothelium: Interface between coagulation and inflammation. *Crit Care Med* 30:S220, 2002.

Lewis L, Robinson RF, Yee J, et al.: Fatal adrenal cortical insufficiency precipitated by surgery during prolong continuous cortisone infusion. *Ann Intern Med* 39:116, 1953.

Lipshultz, SE, Chanock S, Sanders SP, et al.: Cardiovascular manifestations of human immunodeficiency virus infection in infants and children. *Am J Cardiol* 63:1489, 1989.

Liquori CL, Ikeda Y, Weatherspoon M, et al.: Myotonic dystrophy type 2: Human founder haplotype and evolutionary conservation of the repeat tract. *Am J Hum Genet* 73:849, 2003.

LoVerme SR, Oropollo AT: Ketamine anesthesia in dermolytic bullous dermatosis (epidermolysis bullosa). *Anesth Analg* 56:398, 1977.

Luban NC: Irradiation for neonatal and pediatric tranfusions. In Herman JH, Manno CS, editors: *Pediatric transfusion therapy*. Bethesda, MD, 2002, AABB Press, p 147.

Ludlam CA: New-variant Creutzfeldt-Jakob disease and treatment of haemophilia. *Lancet* 350:1704, 1997.

Luginbuhl LM, Orav EJ, McIntosh K, et al.: Cardiac morbidity and related mortality in children with HIV infection. *JAMA* 269:2869, 1993.

Maher J, Daley DA: Severe bleomycin lung toxicity: Reversal with high dose corticosteroids. *Thorax* 48:92, 1993.

Makris M, Greaves M, Phillips WS, et al.: Emergency oral anticoagulant reversal: The relative efficacy of infusions of fresh frozen plasma and clotting factor concentrate on correction of the coagulopathy. *Thromb Haemost* 77:477, 1997.

Malhotra N, Roizen MF: Patients with abnormalities of vasopressin secretion and responsiveness. *Anesthesiol Clin North Am* 5:395, 1987.

Mallory GB Jr, Motoyama EK, Koumbourlis AC, et al.: Bronchial reactivity in infants in acute respiratory failure with viral bronchiolitis. *Pediatr Pulmonol* 6:253, 1989.

Mallory GB Jr, Chaney H, Mutich RL, et al.: Longitudinal changes in lung function during the first three years in prematurely born infants with moderate to severe bronchopulmonary dysplasia. *Pediatr Pulmonol* 11:8, 1991.

Malviya S, Voepel-Lewis T, Siewert M, et al.: Risk factors for adverse postoperative outcomes in children presenting for cardiac surgery with upper respiratory tract infections. *Anesthesiology* 98:628, 2003.

Mankodi A, Thornton CA: Myotonic syndromes. *Curr Opin Neurol* 15:545, 2002.

Mann KG, van't Veer C, Cawthern K, et al.: The role of the tissue factor pathway in initiation of coagulation. *Blood Coagul Fibrinolysis* 9(Suppl 1):S3, 1998.

Mannucci PM: Desmopressin (DDAVP) in the treatment of bleeding disorders. The first 20 years. *Blood* 90:2515, 1997.

Mannucci PM: Hemostatic drugs *N Engl J Med* 339:245, 1998.

Mannucci PM, Bettega D, Cattaneo M: Patterns of development of tachyphylaxis in patients with hemophilia and von Willebrand disease after repeated doses of desmopressin (DDAVP). *Br J Haematol* 82:87, 1992.

Mannucci PM, Tuddenham EGD: The hemophilias—from royal genes to gene therapy. *N Engl J Med* 344:1773, 2001.

Marret E, Flahault A, Samama CM, et al.: Effects of postoperative, nonsteroidal anti-inflammatory drugs on bleeding risk after tonsillectomy: Meta-analysis of randomized, controlled trials. *Anesthesiology* 98:1497, 2003.

Martinowitz U, Kenet G, Segal E, et al.: Recombinant activated factor VII for adjunctive hemorrhage control in trauma. *J Trauma* 51:431, 2001.

Martlew VJ: Perioperative management of patients with coagulation disorders. *Br J Anaesth* 85:446, 2000.

Martorell L, Gamez J, Cayuela ML, et al.: Germline mutational dynamics in myotonic dystrophy type 1 males: Allele length and age effects. *Neurology* 62:269, 2004.

Maselli RA, Kong DZ, Bowe CM, et al.: Presynaptic congenital myasthenic syndrome due to quantal release deficiency. *Neurology* 24;57:279, 2001.

Mason WS, Takahaski M: Kawasaki syndrome. *Clin Infect Dis* 28:169, 1999.

Mathes DD: Bleomycin and hyperoxia exposure in the operating room. *Anesth Analg* 81:624, 1995.

Maxwell LG, Deshpande JK, Wetzel RC: Preoperative evaluation of children. *Pediatr Clin North Am* 41:93, 1994.

McBeth C, Watkins TG: Isoflurane for sedation in a case of congenital myasthenia gravis. *Br J Anaesth* 77:672, 1996.

McCubbin M, Frey EE, Wagner JS, et al.: Large airway collapse in bronchopulmonary dysplasia. *J Pediatr* 114:304, 1989.

McFadden ER Jr, Gilbert IA: Exercise-induced asthma. *N Engl J Med* 330:1362, 1994.

McFarland JG: Perioperative blood transfusions: Indications and options. *Chest* 115:113S, 1999.

McGill WA, Coveler LA, Epstein BS: Subacute upper respiratory infection in small children. *Anesth Analg* 58:331, 1979.

McQuillan PJ, Morgan BA, Ramwell J: Adriamycin cardiomyopathy. Fatal outcome of general anesthesia in a child with adriamycin cardiomyopathy. *Anesthesia* 432:301, 1988.

McSherry GD: Human immunodeficiency virus-related pulmonary infections in children. *Semin Respir Infect* 11:173, 1996.

Measuring childhood asthma prevalence before and after the 1997 redesign of the National Health Interview Survey. *MMWR Morb Mortal Wkly Rep* 49:908, 2000.

Menold MM, Sadeh M, Lennon F, et al.: Evidence for genetic heterogeneity supports clinical differences in congenital myasthenic syndromes. *Hum Hered* 48:325, 1998.

Michelson AD, Bovill E, Andrew M: Antithrombotic therapy in children. *Chest* 108:506S, 1995.

Michelson AD, MacGregor H, Barnard MR, et al.: Reversible inhibition of human platelet activation by hypothermia in vivo and in vitro. *Thromb Haemost* 71:633, 1994.

Michna E, Mason KP: AIDS and the Health Care worker. In Nedeljkovic SS, editor: *Pain management, anesthesia and HIV/AIDS*. Boston, 2002, Butterworth-Heinemann, p 187.

Mickle JE, Cutting GR: Clinical implications of cystic fibrosis transmembrane conductance regulator mutations. *Clin Chest Med* 19:443, 1998.

Migeon C, Donohoue PA: Adrenal disorders. In Kappy MS, Blizzard RM, Migeon CJ, editors: *The diagnosis and treatment of endocrine disorders in childhood and adolescence*. Springfield, IL, 1994, Charles C Thomas.

Miller BE, Bailey JM, Mancuso TJ, et al.: Functional maturity of the coagulation system in children: An evaluation using thrombelastography. *Anesth Analg* 84:745, 1997.

Miller DL, Welty-Wolf KE, Carraway MS, et al.: Extrinsic coagulation blockade attenuates lung injury and proinflammatory cytokine release after intratracheal lipopolysaccharide. *Am J Respir Cell Mol Biol* 26:650, 2002.

Miller G: Myopathies of infancy and childhood. *Pediatr Ann* 18:439, 1989.

Miller RW, Fusner JE, Fink RJ, et al.: Pulmonary function abnormalities in long-term survivors of childhood cancer. *Med Pediatr Oncol* 14:202, 1986.

Miller RW, Woo P, Kellman RK, et al.: Tracheobronchial abnormalities in infants with bronchopulmonary dysplasia. *J Pediatr* 111:779, 1987.

Milner PF: Oxygen transport in sickle cell anemia. *Arch Intern Med* 133:565, 1974.

Miro O, Barrientos A, Alonso JR, et al.: Effects of general anaesthetic procedures on mitochondrial function of human skeletal muscle. Eur *J Clin Pharmacol* 55:41, 1999.

Mitchell RB, Call E, Kelly J: Ear, nose, and throat disorders in children with Down syndrome. *Laryngoscope* 113:259, 2003.

Monagle P, Michelson AD, Bovill E, et al.: Antithrombotic therapy in children. *Chest* 119(Suppl 1):344S, 2001.

Monroe DM, Hoffman M, Oliver JA, et al.: Platelet activity of high-dose factor VIIa is independent of tissue factor *Br J Haematol* 99:542, 1997.

Moraca RJ, Ragni MV: Acquired anti-FVIII inhibitors in children. *Haemophilia* 8:28, 2002.

Morgan PG, Hoppel CL, Sedensky MM: Mitochondrial defects and anesthetic sensitivity. *Anesthesiology* 96:1268, 2002.

Morse DS: HIV infection and transfusion. In Nedeljkovic SS, editor: *Pain management, anesthesia, and HIV/AIDS*. Boston, 2002, Butterworth-Heinemann, p 231.

Mortier E, Ongenae M, De Baerdemaeker L, et al.: In vitro evaluation of the effect of profound hemodilution with hydroxyethyl starch 6%, modified fluid gelatin 4% and dextran 40 10% on coagulation profile measured by thromboelastography. *Anaesthesia* 52:1061, 1997.

Mudad R, Kane WH: DDAVP in acquired hemophilia A: Case report and review of the literature. *Am J Hematol* 43:295, 1993.

Muntoni F, Torelli S, Ferlini A: Dystrophin and mutations: One gene, several proteins, multiple phenotypes. *Lancet Neurol* 2:731, 2003.

Murat I, Deleur MM, Macgee K, et al.: Changes in ventilatory patterns during halothane anesthesia in children. *Br J Anaesth* 57:569, 1985.

Murray DJ, Pennel BJ, Weinstein SL, et al.: Packed red cells in acute blood loss: Dilutional coagulopathy as a cause of surgical bleeding. *Anesth Analg* 80:336, 1995.

Murshid WR, Gader AG: The coagulopathy in acute head injury: Comparison of cerebral versus peripheral measurements of haemostatic activation markers. *Br J Neurosurg* 16:362, 2002.

Nakagawa T, Hirakata H, Sato M, et al.: Ketamine suppresses platelet aggregation possibly by suppressed inositol triphosphate formation and subsequent suppression of cytosolic calcium increase. *Anesthesiology* 96:1147, 2002.

Nakayama DK, Motoyama EK, Mutich RI, et al.: Pulmonary dysfunction in newborns after repair of congenital diaphragmatic hernia. *Pediatr Pulmonol* 11:49, 1991.

Nanigan WC, Powell FC, Miller TC, et al.: Symptomatic intracranial hemorrhage in full-term infants. *Childs Nerv Syst* 11:698, 1995.

Nathan DM, Singer DE, Hurxthal K, et al.: The clinical information value of the glycosylated hemoglobin assay. *N Engl J Med* 310:341, 1984.

Negrier C, Goudemand J, Sultan Y, et al.: Multicenter retrospective study on the utilization of FEIBA in France in patients with factor VIII and factor IX inhibitors. French FEIBA Study Group. Factor eight bypassing activity. *Thromb Haemost* 77:1113, 1997.

Neill CA, Zuckerberg AL: Syndromes and congential heart defects. In Nichols DG, Cameron DE, Greeley WJ, et al., editors: *Critical heart disease in infants and children*. Baltimore, 1995, Mosby, p 987.

Neschis DG, Heyman MR, Cheanvechai V, et al.: Coagulopathy as a result of factor V inhibitor after exposure to bovine topical thrombin. *J Vasc Surg* 35:400, 2002.

Neumayr L, Koshy M, Haberkern C, et al.: Surgery in patients with hemoglobin SC disease. *Am J Hematol* 57:101, 1998.

Newacheck PW, Halfon N: Prevalence, impact and trends in childhood disability due to asthma. *Arch Pediatr Adolesc Med* 154:287, 2000.

Nicholas E, Deutschman CS, Allo M, et al.: Use of esmolol in the intraoperative management of pheochromocytoma. *Anesth Analg* 67:1114, 1988.

Nolan B, White B, Smith J, et al.: Desmopressin: Therapeutic limitations in children and adults with inherited coagulation disorders. *Br J Haematol* 109:865, 2000.

Northway WH: Bronchopulmonary dysplasia: thirty-three years later. *Pediatr Pulmonol* Suppl 23:5, 2001.

Northway WH, Rosan RC, Porter DI: Pulmonary disease following respiratory therapy of hyaline membrane disease. *N Engl J Med* 276:357, 1967.

O'Connell N, McMahon C, Smith J, et al.: Recombinant factor VIIa in the management of surgery and acute bleeding episodes in children with haemophilia and high responding inhibitors. *Br J Haematol* 116:632, 2002.

Odermatt A, Barton K, Khanna VK, et al.: The mutation of Pro789 to Leu reduces the activity of the fast-twitch skeletal muscle sarco(endo)plasmic reticulum Ca^{2+} ATPase (SERCA1) and is associated with Brody disease. *Hum Genet* 106:482, 2000.

Oliver WC, Santrach PJ, Danielson GK, et al.: Desmopressin does not reduce bleeding and transfusion requirements in congenital heart disease operations. *Ann Thorac Surg* 70:1923, 2000.

Olomu N, Kulkarni R, Manco-Johnson M: Treatment of severe pulmonary hemorrhage with activated recombinant factor VII (rFVIIa) in very low birth weight infants. *J Perinatol* 22:672, 2002.

Olsson GL: Bronchospasm during anesthesia. A computer aided incidence study of 136,929 patients. *Acta Anaesthesiol Scand* 31:244, 1987.

Olsson GL, Hallen B: Laryngospasm during anaesthesia. A computer-aided incidence study in 136, 929 patients. *Acta Anaesthesiol Scand* 28:567, 1984.

Orenstein DM: Cystic fibrosis. *Semin Respir Med* 6:252, 1985.

Orlinsky M, Shoemaker W, Reis ED, et al.: Current controversies in shock and resuscitation. *Surg Clin North Am* 81:1217, 2001.

Paschke R, Vogg M, Kristoferitsch R, et al.: Methimazole has no dose-related effect on the intensity of the intrathyroidal autoimmune process in relapsing Graves' disease. *J Clin Endocrinol Metab* 80:2470, 1995.

Pash MP, Balaton J, Eagle C: Anaesthetic management of a parturient with severe muscular dystrophy, lumbar lordosis and a difficult airway. *Can J Anaesth* 43:959, 1996.

Patel RK, Savidge GF, Rangarajan S: Use of recombinant factor VIIa for postoperative hemorrhage in a patient with Glanzmann's thrombasthenia and human leukocyte antigen antibodies. *Br J Haematol* 114:245, 2001.

Patriarca G, Nucera A, Buonomo M, et al.: Latex allergy desensitization by exposure protocol: Five case reports. *Anesth Analg* 94:754, 2002a.

Patriarca G, Nucera E, Pollastrini E, et al.: Sublingual desensitization: A new approach to latex allergy problem. *Anesth Analg* 95:956, 2002b.

Pattishall EN: Longitudinal response of pulmonary function to bronchodilators in cystic fibrosis. *Pediatr Pulmonol* 9:80, 1990.

Peters KR, Nance P, Wingard DW: Malignant hyperthyroidism or malignant hyperthermia? *Anesth Analg* 60:613, 1981.

Petersen KB, Mueler J, Rosmussen M, et al: Impaired adrenal function after glucocorticoid therapy in children with acute lymphoblastic leukemia. *Med Pediatr Oncol* 41:110–114, 2003.

Phipatanakul W, Greene C, Downes SJ, et al.: Montelukast improves asthma control in asthmatic children maintained on inhaled corticosteroids. *Ann Allergy Asthma Immunol* 91:49, 2003.

Piedimonte G, McDonald DM, Nadel JA: Glucocorticoids inhibit neurogenic plasma extravasation and prevent virus-potentiated extravasation in the rat trachea. *J Clin Invest* 86:1409, 1990.

Pierce MR, Bancalari E: The role of inflammation in the pathogenesis of bronchopulmonary dysplasia. *Pediatr Pulmonol* 19:371, 1995.

Pivalizza EG, Pivalizza PJ, Gottschalk LI, et al.: Celite-activated thrombelastography in children. *J Clin Anesth* 13:20, 2001.

Platt OS, Brambiller DJ, Rosse WF, et al.: Mortality in sickle cell disease: Life expectancy and risk factors for early death. *N Engl J Med* 303:1639, 1994.
Plotnick L, Henderson R: *Clinical management of the child and teenager with diabetes*. Baltimore, MD, 1998, The Johns Hopkins University Press, pp 77–96.
Pohlmann-Eden B, Peters CN, Wennberg R, et al.: Valproate induces reversible factor XIII deficiency with risk of perioperative bleeding. *Acta Neurol Scand* 108:104, 2003.
Poon MC, D'Oiron R: Recombinant activated factor VII treatment of platelet related bleeding disorders. International registry on recombinant factor VIIa and congential platelet disorders. *Blood Coagul Fibrinolysis* 11(Suppl 1):S55, 2000.
Prys-Roberts C: Phaeochromocytoma—recent progress in its management. *Br J Anaesth* 85:44, 2000.
Pueschel SM: Should children with Down syndrome be screened for atlantoaxial instability? *Arch Pediatr Adolesc Med* 152:123, 1998.
Pueschel SM, Scola FH, Pezzullo JC: A longitudinal study of atlanto-dens relationships in asymptomatic individuals with Down syndrome. *Pediatrics* 89:1194, 1992.
Pusch M: Myotonia caused by mutations in the muscle chloride channel gene CLCN1. *Hum Mutat* 19:423, 2002.
Quirolo KC: Transfusion medicine for the pediatrician. *Pediatr Clin North Am* 49:1211, 2002.
Rajasekhar D, Barnard MR, Bednarek FJ, et al.: Platelet hyporeactivity in very low birth weight neonates. *Thromb Haemost* 77:1002. 1997.
Rajasekhar D, Kestin AS, Bednarek FJ, et al.: Neonatal platelets are less reactive than adult platelets to physiological agonists in whole blood. *Thromb Haemost* 72:957, 1994.
Ramsey BW, Pepe MS, Quan JM, et al.: Intermittent administration of inhaled tobramycin in patients with cystic fibrosis. *N Engl J Med* 340:23, 1999.
Randolph C: Latex allergy in pediatrics. *Curr Probl Pediatr* 31:131, 2001.
Ranum LP, Day JW: Myotonic dystrophy: Clinical and molecular parallels between myotonic dystrophy type 1 and type 2. *Curr Neurol Neurosci Rep* 2:465, 2002.
Rao GH: Signal transduction, second messengers, and platelet function *J Lab Clin Med* 121:18, 1993.
Ray S, Rubin AP: Anaesthesia in a child with Schwartz-Jampel syndrome. *Anaesthesia* 49:600, 1994.
Rayment R, Birchall J, Yarranton H, et al.: Neonatal alloimmune thrombocytopenia *Br Med J* 327:33, 2003.
Rees AH, Stefadouros MA, Strong WB, et al.: Left ventricular performance in children with homozygous sickle cell anaemia. *Br Heart J* 40:690, 1978.
Renner DR, Ptacek LJ: Periodic paralyses and nondystrophic myotonias. *Adv Neurol* 88:235, 2002.
Riddez L, Johnson L, Hahn RG: Central and regional hemodynamics during crystalloid fluid therapy after uncontrolled intra-abdominal bleeding. *J Trauma* 44:433, 1998.
Ries M, Wolfel D, Maier-Brandt B: Severe intracranial hemorrhage in a newborn infant with transplacental transfer of an acquired factor VII:C inhibitor *J Pediatr* 127:649, 1995.
Rigby WFC, Fan CM, Mark EJ: A 35-year-old man with headache, deviation of the tongue, and unusual radiographic abnormalities. *N Engl J Med* 347:2061, 2002.
Rigby WFC, Fan CM, Mark EJ: Case records of the Massachusetts General Hospital. *N Engl J Med* 347:2061, 2002.
Roberts HR: Clinical experience with activated factor VII: Focus on safety aspects. *Blood Coagul Fibrinolysis* 9:S115, 1998.
Robinson CM, Ludlam CA, Ray DC, et al.: The coagulative and cardiorespiratory responses to reamed intramedullary nailing of isolated fractures. *J Bone Joint Surg Br* 83:963, 2001.
Rohrer M, Natale A: Effect of hypothermia on the coagulation cascade. *Crit Care Med* 20:1402, 1992.
Rojas MA, Gonzalez A, Bancalari E, et al.: Changing trends in the epidemiology and pathogenesis of neonatal chronic lung disease. *J Pediatr* 126:605, 1995.
Rolf N, Cote CJ: Frequency and severity of desaturation events during general anesthesia in children with and without upper respiratory infection. *J Clin Anesth* 4:200, 1992.
Rooklin A: Theophylline: Is it obsolete for asthma? *J Pediatr* 115:841, 1989.
Rooney JC, Williams H: The relationship between proved viral bronchiolitis and subsequent wheezing. *J Pediatr* 79:744, 1971.
Rosenbaum HK, Miller JD: Malignant hyperthermia and myotonic disorders. *Anesthesiol Clin North Am* 20:623, 2002.
Roth DA, Kessler CM, Pasi KJ, et al.: Human recombinant factor IX: Safety and efficacy studies in hemophilia B patients previously treated with plasma-derived factor IX concentrate. *Blood* 98:3600, 2001.
Rothenberger S: Neonatal alloimmune thrombocytopenia. *Ther Apher* 6:32, 2002.
Rubinger M, Houston DS, Schwetz N, et al.: Continuous infusion of porcine factor VIII in the management of patients with factor VIII inhibitors. *Am J Hematol* 56:112, 1997.
Rubinstein A, Morecki R, Silverman B, et al.: Pulmonary disease in children with acquired immune deficiency syndrome and AIDS-related complex. *J Pediatr* 108:498, 1986.
Ryan A, Rudel R, Kuchenbecker M, et al.: A novel alteration of muscle chloride channel gating in myotonia levior. *J Physiol* 545(Pt 2):345, 2002.
Sadeghi H, Lowenthal DB, Dozor AJ: Inspiratory flow limitation in children with bronchopulmonary dysplasia. *Pediatr Pulmonol* 26:167, 1998.
Salzarulo HH, Taylor LA: Diabetic "stiff joint syndrome" as a cause of difficult endotracheal intubation. *Anesthesiology* 64:366, 1986.
Samama CM, Langeron O, Rosencher N, et al.: Aprotinin versus placebo in major orthopedic surgery: A randomized double-blinded, dose ranging study. *Anesth Analg* 95:287, 2002.
Samana CM: Thromboelastography: The next step. *Anesth Analg* 92:563, 2001.
Sandberg DI, Lamerti-Pasculli M, Drake JM, et al.: Spontaneous intraparenchymal hemorrhage in full-term neonates. *Neurosurgery* 48:1042, 2001.
Scharrer I: Recombinant factor VIIa for patients with inhibitors to factor VIII or IX or factor VII deficiency. *Haemophilia* 5:253, 1999.
Schlaghecke R, Komely E, Santen RT, et al.: The effect of long term glucocorticoid therapy on pituitary-adrenal responses to exogenous corticotropin-releasing hormone. *N Engl J Med* 326:226, 1992.
Schmidt GN, Burmeister MA, Lilje C, et al.: Acute heart failure during spinal surgery in a boy with Duchenne muscular dystrophy. *Br J Anaesth* 90:800, 2003.
Schmied H, Kurz A, Sessler DI, et al.: Mild intraoperative hypothermia increases blood loss and allogeneic transfusion requirements during total hip arthroplasty. *Lancet* 347:289, 1996.
Schreiner M, Triebwasser A, Keon T: Ingestion of liquids compared with preoperative fasting in pediatric patients. *Anesthesiology* 72:593, 1990.
Schulte-Sasse U, Hess W, Tarnow J: Pulmonary vascular responses to nitrous oxide in patients with normal and high pulmonary vascular resistance. *Anesthesiology* 57:9, 1982.
Schuyler MR, Niewoehner DE, Inkley SR, et al.: Abnormal lung elasticity in juvenile diabetes mellitus. *Am Rev Respir Dis* 113:37, 1976.
Scott-Conner CE, Brunson CD: The pathophysiology of the sickle hemoglobinopathies and implications of perioperative management. *Am J Surg* 168:268, 1994.
Seakins M, Gibbs WN, Milner PF, et al.: Erythrocyte Hb-S concentration. An important factor in the low oxygen affinity of blood in sickle cell anemia. *J Clin Invest* 52:422, 1973.
Seay AR, Ziter FA: Malignant hyperpyrexia in a patient with Schwartz-Jampel syndrome. *J Pediatr* 93:83, 1978.
Serdaroglu G, Tutuncuoglu S, Kavakli K, et al.: Coagulation abnormalities and acquired von Willebrand's disease type 1 in children receiving valproic acid. *J Child Neurol* 17:41, 2002.
Setlock MA, Cotter TP, Rosner D: Latex allergy: Failure of prophylaxis to prevent severe reaction. *Anesth Analg* 76:650, 1993.
Shattil SJ, Kashiwagi H, Pampori N: Integrin signaling: The platelet paradigm. *Blood* 91:2645, 1998.
Sheikh S, Stephen T, Howell L, et al.: Gastroesophageal reflux in infants with wheezing. *Pediatr Pulmonol* 28:181, 1999.
Shende D, Agarwal R: Anaesthetic management of a patient with Emery-Dreifuss muscular dystrophy. *Anaesth Intensive Care* 30:372, 2002.
Shlomchik WD, Couzens MS, Tang CB, et al.: Prevention of graft versus host disease by inactivation of host antigen present cells. *Science* 285:412, 1999.
Shopnick RI, Brettler DB: Hemostasis: A practical review of conservative and operative care. *Clin Orthop* 328:34, 1996.
Siberry GK, Iannone R, editors: *The Harriet Lane handbook*. St. Louis, 2000, Mosby.
Siegbahn A, Ruusuvaara L: Age dependence of blood fibrinolytic components and the effects of low dose oral contraceptive on coagulation and fibrinolysis in teenagers. *Thromb Haemost* 60:361, 1988.
Silliman CC: Transfusion-related acute lung injury. *Transfus Med Rev* 13:177, 1999.
Silliman CC, Voelkel NF, Allard JD, et al.: Plasma and lipids from stored packed red blood cells cause acute lung injury in an animal model. *J Clin Invest* 101:1458, 1998.
Simonds RJ, Orejas G: *Pneumocystis carinii* pneumonia and toxoplasmosis. In Pizzo PA, Wilfert CM, editors: *Pediatric AIDS*. New York, 1999, Lippincott Williams & Wilkins, p 251.
Sindet-Pedersen S, Ramstrom G, Bernvil S, et al.: Hemostatic effect of tranexamic acid mouthwash in anticoagulant-treated patients undergoing oral surgery. *N Engl J Med* 320:840, 1989.
Singal PK, Iliskovic N: Doxorubicin-induced cardiomyopathy. *N Engl J Med* 339:900, 1998.

Singbartl K, Innerhofer P, Radvan J, et al.: Hemostasis and hemodilution: A quantitative mathematical guide for clinical practice. *Anesth Analg* 96:929, 2003.

Singer ST, Hurst D, Addiego JE Jr: Bleeding disorders in Noonan syndrome: Three case reports and review of the literature. *J Pediatr Hematol Oncol* 19:130, 1997.

Singh SP, Barrett EG, Kalra R, et al.: Prenatal cigarette smoke decreases lung cAMP and increases airway hyperresponsiveness. *Am J Respir Crit Care Med* 168:342, 2003.

Smith C,Thomsett M, Choong C, et al.: Congenital thyrotoxicosis in premature infants. *Clin Endocrinol* 54:371–376, 2001.

Smith MF: Skin and connective tissue diseases. In Katz JD, Steward DJ, editors: *Anesthesia and Uncommon Pediatric Diseases*. Philadelphia, 1993, WB Saunders.

Snyder EL, Rinder HM: Platelet storage—time to come in from the cold? *N Engl J Med* 348:2032, 2003.

Sola MC, del Vecchio A, Edwards TJ, et al.: The relationship between hematocrit and bleeding time in very low birth weight infants during the first week of life. *J Perinatol* 21:368, 2001.

Sosenko IR, Kinter MT, Roberts RJ: Nutritional issues in chronic lung disease of premature infants. In Bland RJ, Coalson JJ, editors: *Chronic lung disease in early infancy*. New York, 2000, Marcel Dekker, p 285.

Soussan D, Liard R, Zureik M, et al.: Treatment compliance, passive smoking, and asthma control: A three year cohort study. *Arch Dis Child* 88:229, 2003.

Souto JC, Almasy L, Muinz-Diaz E, et al.: Functional effects of the ABO locus polymorphism on plasma levels on von Willebrand factor, factor VIII, and activated partial thromboplastin time. *Arterioscler Thromb Vasc Biol* 20:2024, 2000.

Spiess B: Perioperative coagulation monitoring. In Bruce B, Counts R, Gould S, editors: *Perioperative transfusion medicine*. Baltimore, 1998, Williams & Wilkins, p 239.

Srinivasa V, Gilbertson LI, Bhavani-Shankar K: Thromboelastography: Where is it heading? *Int Anesthesiol Clin* 39:35, 2001.

Stainsby DL, MacLennan S, Hamilton PJ: Management of massive blood loss: A template guideline. *Br J Anaesth* 85:487, 2000.

Stammers AH, Rauch ED, Willett LD, et al.: Preoperative coagulopathy management of a neonate with complex congential heart disease: A case study. *Perfusion* 15:161, 2000.

Stein J, Ratnoff OD: An inhibitor of antihemophiliac factor (factor VIII) in an 18-month old nonhemophilic child. *Am J Pediatr Hematol Oncol* 15:346, 1993.

Stempel DA: The pharmacologic management of childhood asthma. *Pediatr Clin North Am* 50:609, 2003.

Stephen LX, Beighton PH: Oro-dental manifestations of the Schwartz-Jampel syndrome. *J Clin Pediatr Dent* 27:67, 2002.

Stevens JJ: A case of thyrotoxic crisis that mimicked malignant hyperthermia. *Anesthesiology* 59:263, 1983.

Stevens A, Roizen MF: Patients with diabetes mellitus and disorders of glucose metabolism. *Anesthesiol Clin North Am* 5:339, 1987.

Stewart JM, Kaul A, Gromisch DS, et al.: Symptomatic cardiac dysfunction in children with human immunodeficiency virus infection. *Am Heart J* 117:140, 1989.

Stowell KM, Figueiredo MS, Brownlee GG, et al.: Haemophilia B Liverpool: A new British family with mild haemophilia B associated with a –6 G to A mutation in the factor IX promoter. *Br J Haematol* 85:188, 1993.

Strauss RG, Stansfield C, Henriksen RA, et al.: Pentastarch may cause fewer effects on coagulation than hetastarch. *Transfusion* 28:257, 1988.

Sullivan KJ, Goodwin SR, Evangelist J, et al.: Nitric oxide successfully used to treat acute chest syndrome of sickle cell disease in a young adolescent. *Crit Care Med* 27:2563, 1999.

Sutor AH: Desmopressin (DDAVP) in bleeding disorders of childhood. *Semin Thromb Hemost* 24:555, 1998.

Sutor AH, von Kries R, Cornelissen EA, et al.: Vitamin K deficiency bleeding (VKDB) in infancy. ISTH pediatric/perinatal subcommittee. International society on thrombosis and haemostasis. *Thromb Haemost* 81:456, 1999.

Suzukawa M, Michaels IA, Ruzbarsky J, et al.: Use of isoflurane during resection of pheochromocytoma. *Anesth Analg* 62:100, 1983.

Swafflor J, Gibbs HR: Cardiac complications of cancer treatment. *Anesthesiol Clin North Am* 16:598, 1998.

Sweet SC, Spray TL, Huddleston CB, et al.: Pediatric lung transplantation at St Louis Children's Hospital, 1990-1995, *Am J Respir Crit Care Med* 155:1027, 1997.

Tait AR, Knight PR: The effects of general anesthesia on upper respiratory tract infections in children. *Anesthesiology* 67:930, 1987a.

Tait AR, Knight PR: Intraoperative respiratory complications in patients with upper respiratory tract infections. *Can J Anesth* 34:300, 1987b.

Tait AR, Malviya S: Anesthesia for the child with an upper respiratory tract infection: still a dilemma? Review *Anesth Analg* 100:59–65, 2005.

Tait AR, Malviya S, Voepel-Lewis T, et al.: Risk factors for perioperative adverse respiratory events in children with upper respiratory tract infections. *Anesthesiology* 95:299, 2001.

Tait AR, Pandit UA, Voepel-Lewis T, et al.: Use of the laryngeal mask airway in children with upper respiratory tract infections: A comparison with endotracheal infection. *Anesth Analg* 86:706, 1998.

Tait AR, Voepel-Lewis T, Malviya S: Perioperative considerations for the child with an upper respiratory tract infection. *J Perianesth Nurs* 15:392, 2000.

Teitel JM: Recombinant factor VIIa versus aPCCs in hemophiliacs with inhibitors; treatment and cost considerations. *Haemophilia* 5(Suppl 3):43, 1999.

Theroux MC, Corddry DH, Tietz AE, et al.: A study of desmopressin and blood loss during spinal fusion for neuromuscular scoliosis: A randomized, controlled, double-blinded study. *Anesthesiology* 87:260, 1997.

Thomas KB, Sutor AH, Altinkaya N, et al.: Von Willebrand factor-collagen binding activity is increased in newborns and infants. *Acta Paediatr* 84:697, 1995.

Thorelli E: Mechanisms that regulate the anticoagulant function of coagulation factor V. *Scand J Clin Lab Invest Suppl* 229:19, 1999.

Tobias JD: Synthetic factor VIIa to treat dilutional coagulopathy during posterior spinal fusion in two children. *Anesthesiology* 96:1522, 2002.

Tobias JD, Berkenbosch JW, Russo P: Recombinant factor VIIa to treat bleeding after cardiac surgery in an infant. *Pediatr Crit Care* 5:49, 2003a.

Tobias JD, Groeper K, Berkenbosch JW: Preliminary experience with the use of recombinant factor VIIA to treat coagulation disturbances in pediatric patients. *South Med J* 96:12, 2003b.

Tormene D, Simioni P, Prandoni P, et al.: The incidence of venous thromboembolism in thrombophilic children: A prospective cohort study. *Blood* 100:2403, 2002.

Traverso CL, Caprini JA, Arcelus JI: The normal thromboelastogram and its interpretation. *Semin Thromb Hemost* 21:S7, 1995.

Treib J, Haass A, Pindur G, et al.: All medium starches are not the same: Influence of the degree of hydroxyethyl substitution of hydroxyethyl starch on plasma volume, hemorheologic conditions, and coagulation. *Transfusion* 36:450, 1996.

Truog RD, Waisel DB, Burns JP: DNR in the OR: A goal-directed approach: *Anesthesiology* 90:289, 1999.

Tsui LC, Buchwald M, Barker D, et al.: Cystic fibrosis locus difined by a genetically linked polymorphic DNA marker. *Science* 230:1054, 1985.

Tuddenham EGD, Cooper DN: *The molecular genetics of haemostasis and its inherited disorders*. Oxford monographs in medical genetics No. 25. Oxford, England, 1994, Oxford University Press.

Tuysuz B, Beker DB: Thyroid dysfunction in children with Down's syndrome. *Acta Paediatr* 90:1389, 2001.

Undem BJ, Lichtenstein LM: Drugs used in the treatment of asthma. In Hardman JG, Limbird LE, Gilman AG, editors: Goodman and Gilman's The pharmacological basis of therapeutics, 10th edition. 2001, The McGraw-Hill Companies, p 733.

Urban MK, Beckman J, Gordon M, et al.: The efficacy of antifibrinolytics in the reduction of blood loss during complex adult reconstructive spine surgery. *Spine* 26:152, 2001.

Valeri CR, Cassidy G, Khuri S, et al.: Hypothermia induced reversible platelet dysfunction. *Ann Surg* 205:175, 1987.

Van Bever HP, Stevens WJ: Pharmacotherapy of childhood asthma. An inflammatory disease. *Drugs* 44:36, 1992.

Van Kerrebroeck PE: Experience with the long-term use of desmopressin for nocturnal enuresis in children and adolescents. *BJU Int* 89:420, 2002.

Van Marter LJ, Pagano M, Allred EN, et al.: Rate of bronchopulmonary dysplasia as a function of neonatal intensive care practices. *J Pediatr* 120:938, 1992.

Vavilala MS, Dunbar PJ, Rivara FP, et al.: Coagulopathy predicts poor outcome following head injury in children less than 16 years of age. *J Neurosurg Anesthesiol* 13:18, 2001.

Vichinsky E, Williams R, Das M, et al.: Pulmonary fat embolism: A distinct cause of severe acute chest syndrome in sickle cell anemia. *Blood* 83:3107, 1994.

Vichinsky EP, Haberkern CM, Neumayr L, et al.: The preoperative transfusion in sickle cell disease study group: A comparison of conservative and aggressive transfusion regimens in the perioperative management of sickle cell disease. *N Engl J Med* 333:206, 1995.

Vichinsky EP, Styles LA, Colangelo LH, et al.: Acute chest syndrome in sickle cell disease clinical presentation and course. *Blood* 89:1787, 1997.

Vincent A, Newland C, Croxen R, et al.: Genes at the junction—candidates for congenital myasthenic syndromes. *Trends Neurosci* 20:15, 1997.

Vlot AJ, Mauser-Bunschoten EP, Zarkova AG, et al.: The half-life of infused factor VIII is shorter in hemophiliac patients with blood group O than in those with blood group A. *Thromb Haemost* 83:65, 2000.

Von Mutius E, Nicolai T, Martinez FD: Prematurity as a risk factor for asthma in preadolescent children. *J Pediatr* 123:223, 1993.

Vracko R, Pecoraro RE, Carter WB: Overview article: Basal lamina of epidermis, muscle fibers, muscle capillaries, and renal tubules: Changes with aging and in diabetes mellitus. *Ultrastruct Pathol* 1:559, 1980.

Waldron P, Pegelow C, Neumayr L, et al.: Tonsillectomy, adenoidectomy, and myringotomy in sickle cell disease: Perioperative morbidity. Preoperative Transfusion in Sickle Cell Disease Study Group. *J Pediatr Hemotol Oncol* 21:129, 1999.

Wansink DG, Wieringa B: Transgenic mouse models for myotonic dystrophy type 1 (DM1). *Cytogenet Genome Res* 100:230, 2003.

Wartlier DC, Kam PC, Egan MK: Platelet glycoprotein IIb/IIIa antagonists: Pharmacology and clinical developments. *Anesthesiology* 96:1237, 2002.

Watts DD, Trask A, Soeken K, et al.: Hypothermic coagulopathy in trauma: Effect of varying levels of hypothermia on enzyme speed, platelet function, and fibrinolytic activity. *J Trauma* 44:846, 1998.

Weigle CGM: Metabolic and endocrine disease in pediatric intensive care. In Rogers MC, editor: *Textbook of pediatric intensive care*. Baltimore, 1987, Williams & Wilkins.

Weinberg GL, Palmer JW, VadeBoncouer TR, et al.: Bupivacaine inhibits acyl-carnitine exchange in cardiac mitochondria. *Anesthesiology* 92:523, 2000.

Weinstock DJ, Schwartz AD: Factor XI deficiency in an Ashkenazi Jewish child, causing severe postoperative hemorrhage. *J Pediatr Surg* 30:1746, 1995.

Wiese M, Merke DP, Pacak K, et al.: Utility of plasma free metanephrines for detecting childhood pheochromocytoma. *J Clin Endocrinol Metab* 87:1955–1960, 2002.

Welliver RC, Kaul TN, Ogra P: The appearance of cell bound IgE in respiratory tract epithelium after respiratory-syncytial-virus infection. *N Engl J Med* 303:166, 1989.

Welty-Wolf KE, Carraway MS, Miller DL, et al.: Coagulation blockade prevents sepsis-induced respiratory and renal failure in baboons. *Am J Respir Crit Care Med* 15:1988, 2001.

White G, Shapiro A, Ragni M, et al.: Clinical evaluation of recombinant factor IX. *Semin Hematol* 35(Suppl 2):33, 1998.

White GC 2nd, Rosendaal FR, Aledort LM, et al.: Definitions in hemophilia. *Thromb Haemost* 85:560, 2001.

White RJ, Bass SP: Myotonic dystrophy and paediatric anaesthesia. *Paediatr Anaesth* 13:94, 2003.

Wieding JU, Vehmeyer K, Dittman J, et al.: Contamination of fresh frozen plasma with viable white cells and proliferable stem cells. *Transfusion* 34:185, 1994.

Williams GD, Bratton SL, Ramamoorthy C: Factors associated with blood loss and blood product transfusions: A multivariate analysis in children after open heart surgery. *Anesth Analg* 89:57, 1999a.

Williams GD, Bratton SL, Riley EC, et al.: Efficacy of epsilon-aminocaproic acid in children undergoing cardiac surgery. *J Cardiothorac Vasc Anesth* 13:304, 1999b.

Williams JP, Somerville GM, Miner ME, et al.: Atlanto-axial subluxation and trisomy-21: Another perioperative complication. *Anesthesiology* 67:253, 1987.

Williams OA, Hills R, Goddard JM: Pulmonary collapse during anesthesia in children with respiratory tract symptoms. *Anaesthesia* 47:411, 1992.

Williamson LM, Warwick RM: Transfusion-associated graft-versus-host disease and its prevention. *Blood Rev* 9:251, 1995.

Wintzen AR, de Jonge H, Loeliger EA, et al.: The risk of intracerebral hemorrhage during oral anticoagulant treatment: A population study. *Ann Neurol* 16:553, 1984.

Wolf A, Weir P, Segar P, et al.: Impaired fatty acid oxidation in propofol infusion syndrome. *Lancet* 357:606, 2001.

Wood RE, Boat TF, Doershuk CF: Cystic fibrosis, state of the art. *Am Rev Respir Dis* 113:833, 1976.

Yamakage M, Tsujiguchi N, Kohro S, et al.: The usefulness of celite-activated thromboelastography for evaluation of fibrinolysis. *Can J Anaesth* 45:993, 1998.

Yaster M, Tobin JR, Billett C, et al.: Epidural analgesia in the management of severe vaso-occlusive sickle cell crisis. *Pediatrics* 93:310, 1994.

Yee TT, Taher A, Pasi KR, et al.: A survey of patients with acquired haemophilia in a haemophilia center over a 28-year period. *Clin Lab Haematol* 22:275, 2000.

Yoshihara H, Yamamoto T, Mihara H: Changes in coagulation and fibrinolysis occurring in dogs during hypothermia. *Thromb Res* 37:503, 1985.

Yu MS, Kimball TR, Tsevat J, et al.: Evaluation of heart murmurs in children: Cost-effectiveness and practical implications. *Pediatrics* 141:504, 2002.

Zeldin RR, Hamilton G, Adkinson N: The effects of avoidance on natural history of latex rubber allergy. *J Allergy Clin Immunol* 97:429A, 1996.

33 Pediatric Cardiopulmonary Resuscitation

R. Blaine Easley • Charles L. Schleien • Donald H. Shaffner

In the late 1950s, children with cardiac arrest during anesthesia received 1.5 minutes of knee-to-chest "artificial respiration" (Rainer, 1957), followed by a thoracotomy for internal cardiac massage. In 1958, closed-chest compressions were successfully performed on a 2-year-old child (Sladen, 1984). The resuscitation of this child, along with several successful resuscitations of subsequent patients (many undergoing anesthesia), led to the reporting of closed-chest compressions (Kouwenhoven et al., 1960). The high rate of successful resuscitation after cardiac arrest in the operating room (42%) (Jude et al., 1961) helped establish closed-chest compression as the standard for cardiopulmonary resuscitation (CPR).

Despite the success rate of resuscitation during anesthesia, the potential for disaster and the increased likelihood of arrests in young children require that pediatric anesthesiologists have a complete understanding of the physiology and pharmacology of CPR. "No more depressing shadow can darken an operating room than that occasioned by the death of a child" (Leigh and Belton, 1949).

■ INCIDENCE OF CARDIAC ARREST DURING ANESTHESIA

Anesthesia-related cardiac arrest and *anesthesia-related mortality* are the commonly used terms that suggest a general association between the delivery of anesthesia and the most devastating events that can result from the care of a child by an anesthesiologist in the operating room or in the perioperative period. To better understand and, it is hoped, prevent these events, it is necessary to know both the likelihood of their occurrence and their associated risk factors. The likelihood (or frequency) of a cardiac arrest is usually described as either a percentage of occurrence within a subgroup (children) compared with the main group (all patients) or an incidence of occurrence expressed as a ratio of a total number of anesthetic procedures for a group. The presentation of the likelihood of cardiac arrest as a percentage can be misleading because the groups being compared often do not have the same denominator of anesthetics performed. For example, the impact of a 20% anesthesia-related cardiac arrest rate for children depends upon the percentage of the anesthetics at an institution that were performed in children. Incidence data are more informative but less available than percentage-based data because most data sets collect events and are unlikely to have the denominators that include the number of uneventful anesthetics for each group. A compilation of data regarding the incidence of cardiac arrest and mortality from the anesthesia literature is available in Table 33-1.

Multiple risk factors for "anesthesia-related" cardiac arrest have been suggested and include the patient's age, their condition or "physical status," and the emergency nature of the procedure. Age is a risk factor for an increased incidence of both cardiac arrest

TABLE 33–1. Incidence of cardiac arrests and mortality by age (per 10,000 anesthetic procedures)*

	Anesthesia Related						All Causes					
	CARDIAC ARREST			MORTALITY			CARDIAC ARREST			MORTALITY		
Age	*Incidence*	*Range*	*No. of Studies*	*Incidence*	*Range*	*No. of Studies*	*Incidence*	*Range*	*No. of Studies*	*Incidence*	*Range*	*No. of Studies*
Neonates							83	83	1	83	83	1
Infants	15	9.2 to 19	4	4.2	0 to 9.3	4	19	16 to 24	2	62	12 to 165	3
Children	3.3	0 to 4.3	4	0.9	0 to 3.2	4	5.2	4.4 to 6.0	2	22	1.8 to 59	3
All pediatric groups	1.8	0.4 to 5.5	9	0.5	0 to 4.7	7	3.1	2.7 to 14	5	18	3.8 to 88	3
All ages	1.6	0.1 to 7.8	12	0.8	0.1 to 7.9	13	7.5	1.5 to 27	10	12	0.9 to 189	10

*The incidence of cardiac arrest and mortality for all ages includes studies that combine pediatric and adult patients.

and mortality (see Table 33–1). The data in the table for neonates are incomplete because incidence data were not available for "anesthesia-related" events, but one study was available for "all causes" of intraoperative events in neonates. Neonates and infants appear to be at the greatest risk for both cardiac arrest and mortality. Children have the lowest incidence compared with neonates and infants. The table indicates that the group "All pediatric groups" has a lower incidence than the group "Children" because "All pediatric groups" includes two studies with very large denominators and low incidence rates that did not break down all pediatric cases into children and infant age subgroups. Pediatric and adult studies often have similar incidences of anesthesia-related cardiac arrest because both have high-risk groups at the extremes of age. The incidence of cardiac arrest is low for both older children and young adults, but the risk of cardiac arrest increases for the youngest children and the eldest adults (see Table 33–1).

Review of the effect of the physical condition of the patient shows that the American Society of Anesthesiologists (ASA) physical status correlates with the incidence of cardiac arrest and mortality (Table 33–2). ASA physical status as an indicator of the patient's physical condition represents another risk for both cardiac arrest and mortality. Unfortunately, there is a lack of incidence data for pediatrics, with only one cardiac arrest study and no mortality studies; the table represents the effect of ASA physical status for patients of all ages. "ASA physical status V" patients are not included in most reports of "anesthesia-related" events because by definition they have a low likelihood of survival, making it difficult to determine if events are a result of their condition or related to anesthesia. ASA physical status IV and V patients have a 30 to 300 times greater risk of cardiac arrest than ASA I or II patients (Rackow et al., 1961; Newland et al., 2002). Prematurity, congenital heart disease, and congenital defects are common pediatric comorbidities that increase the risk for children (Morray, 2000).

The designation of an emergency status to patient's procedure is a third risk factor for both cardiac arrest and mortality. Emergency surgery is associated with a six times increased incidence of anesthetic cardiac arrest (6.5 versus 1.1 per 10,000, $P = 0.0001$) (Keenan and Boyan, 1985). In addition to a higher incidence of arrests during an emergent procedure, a poorer outcome is also likely (Vacanti et al., 1970; Marx et al., 1973; Olsson and Hallen, 1988; Morray, 2000; Biboulet et al., 2001; Newland et al., 2002; Sprung et al., 2003). It is not clear that the emergent procedures have increased risk because of the patient's condition, the lack of optimal personnel, or both. The extremes of age, ASA physical status, and emergency status are the three most commonly reported risk factors for cardiac arrest and mortality in the operating room.

■ ETIOLOGY OF CARDIAC ARREST DURING ANESTHESIA

The etiologies of cardiac arrest during anesthesia are typically grouped by either the organ systems involved or the interventions applied. The Pediatric Perioperative Cardiac Arrests (POCA) Registry uses a classification system that involves both interventions and organ systems, thus grouping arrests as being either "medication," "cardiovascular," "respiratory," or "equipment" related (Morray, 2000). Some etiologies may be difficult to classify because they could fit into several grouping schemes. For example, a succinylcholine-induced dysrhythmia may be classified as either a "medication" or a "cardiovascular" cause of cardiac arrest. A set of guidelines for reporting cardiac arrest data in children, known as the pediatric Utstein guidelines, suggests an organ system-based classification for etiologies (Zaritsky et al., 1995). The Utstein guidelines use three groups, consisting of cardiac, pulmonary, and cardiopulmonary, for the comparison of etiologies of cardiac arrest in children. The Utstein guidelines have not yet been incorporated into much of the anesthesia cardiac arrest literature. A summary from the anesthesia literature of etiologies of cardiac arrest is listed in Box 33–1 (grouped as commonly reported in the anesthesia literature).

"Medication-related" causes are some of the most frequent causes of cardiac arrest related to anesthesia in children and adults, representing approximately 35% (range, 4% to 54%) of the arrests (Rackow et al., 1961; Salem et al., 1975; Keenan and Boyan, 1985; Olsson and Hallen, 1988; Morgan et al., 1993; Morray, 2000; Biboulet et al., 2001; Newland et al., 2002; Kawashima et al., 2003; Sprung et al., 2003). For general anesthetics, the frequently reported causes of cardiac arrest are inhalational agent overdose, intravenous agent overdose, succinylcholine-induced dysrhythmia, neostigmine-induced dysrhythmia, and medication "swaps." The intravenous administration of local anesthetic intended for the caudal space, high spinal anesthesia, and local anesthesia toxicity is a commonly reported cause of arrest during regional anesthesia. The inadequate reversal of a paralytic agent and opioid-induced respiratory depression are medication-related causes of cardiac arrest that present in the postoperative period.

"Cardiovascular-related" causes of cardiac arrest represent approximately 20% (range, 0% to 45%) of cardiac arrest related to anesthesia in children and adults (Rackow et al., 1961; Salem et al., 1975; Keenan and Boyan, 1985; Olsson and Hallen, 1988; Morgan et al., 1993; Morray, 2000; Biboulet et al., 2001; Newland et al., 2002; Kawashima et al., 2003; Sprung et al., 2003). Arrests due to intravascular volume are the most frequently reported in this group and may include inadequate volume administration, excessive hemorrhage, or inappropriate volume/transfusion administration. The other causes of cardiovascular collapse in this group may or may not involve dysrhythmias. Dysrhythmias may be caused by hyperkalemia seen with succinylcholine, transfusion, reperfusion, myopathy, or renal insufficiency. Dysrhythmia or cardiovascular collapse (asystole) may have a vagal etiology due to traction, pressure, or insufflation involving the abdomen, eye, neck, or heart. Cardiovascular collapse can occur with anaphylaxis from exposure to latex, contrast, drugs, or dextran. Venous air embolism is another important cause of cardiovascular collapse and cardiac arrest under anesthesia. Malignant hyperthermia is an infrequently reported cause of cardiac arrest in this group.

"Respiratory-related" causes involve approximately 31% (range, 11% to 51%) of cardiac arrests related to anesthesia in children and adults (Rackow et al., 1961; Salem et al., 1975; Keenan and Boyan, 1985; Olsson and Hallen, 1988; Morgan et al., 1993; Morray, 2000; Biboulet et al., 2001; Newland et al., 2002; Kawashima et al., 2003; Sprung et al., 2003). Inadequate ventilation and oxygenation are broad categories often expressed in this group of causes of cardiac arrest. "Loss of the airway" may involve laryngospasm/bronchospasm, a difficult-to-manage anatomy, or a misplaced, kinked, plugged, or inadvertently removed endotracheal tube. Aspiration remains a cause of respiratory-related cardiac arrest but appears to be decreasing in occurrence.

"Equipment-related" causes involve approximately 4% (range, 0% to 20%) of cardiac arrest related to anesthesia in children and adults (Rackow et al., 1961; Salem et al., 1975;

TABLE 33–2. Incidence of cardiac arrests or mortality by American Society of Anesthesiology physical status for all ages (per 10,000 anesthetic procedures)

	Anesthesia Related						All Causes					
	CARDIAC ARREST			MORTALITY			CARDIAC ARREST*			MORTALITY		
ASA Class	*Incidence*	*Range*	*No. of Studies*	*Incidence*	*Range*	*No. of Studies*	*Incidence*	*Range*	*No. of Studies*	*Incidence*	*Range*	*No. of Studies*
I	0.7	0.2 to 0.9	2	0.3	0 to 1.1	2				6.0	6.0	1
II	5.3	0.7 to 7.1	2	0.5	0.4 to 0.9	2				47	47	1
III	11	6.5 to 13	2	11	3.3 to 29	2				440	440	1
IV	24	19 to 25	2	47	19 to 75	2				2349	2349	1
V										5077	5077	1

*No data available.

BOX 33–1 Etiologies of Cardiac Arrest During Anesthesia

Medication-Related Causes

Anesthetic overdose (including relative overdose)
 Inhalational agent, intravenous agent
Succinylcholine-induced dysrhythmia
Neostigmine-induced dysrhythmia
Medication "swaps"

Drug Reactions

Intravenous administration of local anesthetic intended for the caudal space
High spinal anesthesia*
Local anesthesia toxicity
Inadequate reversal of a paralytic (PACU)
Opioid-induced respiratory depression (PACU)

Cardiovascular-Related Causes

Intravascular volume/hemorrhage (inadequate or inappropriate volume administration*)
Hyperkalemia (succinylcholine, transfusion, reperfusion, myopathy, or renal insufficiency)
Hypocalcemia (citrate intoxication from rapid blood administration)
Hypoglycemia
Vagal episodes (traction, pressures, or insufflation involving the abdomen, eye, neck, or heart)
Central catheter (dysrhythmia, hemorrhage/tamponade)
Anaphylaxis (latex, contrast, drugs, or dextran)
Embolism (air, clot, or fat)
Temperature (malignant hyperthermia, hypothermia)
Myocardial ischemia
Sepsis
Adrenal insufficiency

Respiratory-Related Causes

Inadequate ventilation and oxygenation*
"Loss of the airway" (laryngospasm/bronchospasm, a difficult-to-manage anatomy, or a misplaced, kinked, plugged, or inadvertently removed endotracheal tube)
Residual neuromuscular weakness
Aspiration
Pneumothorax

PACU, postanesthesia care unit.
*Causes of cardiac arrest that have low resuscitation and high mortality rates.

Keenan and Boyan, 1985; Olsson and Hallen, 1988; Morgan et al., 1993; Morray, 2000; Biboulet et al., 2001; Newland et al., 2002; Kawashima et al., 2003; Sprung et al., 2003). The categories of equipment-related cardiac arrest that are most frequently described involve central line-induced bleeding or dysrhythmias and breathing circuit disconnection. Other groups of cardiac arrest are reported in some studies and include multiple events (3%) (Morray, 2000), inadequate vigilance (6%) (Kawashima et al., 2003), or an unclear etiology (9%; range, 1% to 18%) (Olsson and Hallen, 1988; Morray, 2000; Biboulet et al., 2001).

THE RELATIONSHIP OF THE ETIOLOGY OF A CARDIAC ARREST TO THE ANESTHESIA CARE

The determination that a cardiac arrest is "anesthesia related" is subjective, as is the extent to which a cardiac arrest is related to the anesthesia care. Patient-related factors, procedure-related factors, and anesthesia care-related factors are the three most important determinants of the etiology of cardiac arrest in the operating room. Trying to determine the extent of the contribution by anesthesia care has evolved terms such as *anesthesia-associated cardiac arrest* and *anesthesia-attributable cardiac arrest.* The determination of anesthesia contribution is complicated by the contribution of the patient and procedure factors. As an example, to what extent is the anesthesia care involved in an arrest related to surgical bleeding in a coagulopathic patient? Is failing to keep up with major hemorrhage or to correct a coagulopathy related to the procedure or patient compared with the anesthesia care? To avoid some of these subjective determinations, many studies use the term *anesthesia related* to describe a cardiac arrest after an anesthesiologist has been involved in the care of the patient.

Non-anesthesia-related cardiac arrest is most often due to the patient's underlying condition or the procedure being performed. Trauma, exsanguination, and failure to wean from cardiopulmonary bypass are three of the most often reported causes of non-anesthesia-related cardiac arrest. Myocardial infarction, pulmonary embolus, sepsis, and ruptured aneurysm are other, less frequently observed, patient-related causes of cardiac arrest. Procedure-related causes include technical problems, caval compression, vagal asystole related to traction or insufflation, and complications related to transplantation.

OUTCOME FROM CARDIAC ARREST DURING ANESTHESIA

The terminology used to describe outcome from cardiac arrest can be confusing as many different end points are reported. The term *survival* is commonly used to describe a positive outcome for a patient who sustains a cardiac arrest. The term *survival* is imprecise as to the duration or quality of the patient's outcome. A patient may "survive" initial resuscitation attempts but subsequently die in the intensive care unit from persistent hemodynamic instability or devastating neurologic injury. The term *return of spontaneous circulation* (ROSC) describes the immediate success of the resuscitation effort (initial survival). ROSC means that the native heartbeat and blood pressure are adequate for a period of at least 20 minutes. Although ROSC indicates a successful reversal of cardiac arrest, it may not be a meaningful indicator if many patients subsequently die in the intensive care unit. The number of patients with ROSC after cardiac arrest is usually much greater than the number of patients who have a longer, more meaningful, period of survival such as survival to discharge from the hospital. Although "survival to discharge from the hospital" indicates a longer survival period than ROSC, surviving a longer time period does not address the quality of that outcome. An assessment of the quality of survival should acknowledge the presence either of a new neurologic deficit or of the patient's return to baseline neurologic status. These terms are found in some of the descriptions in the anesthesia literature of the outcome of children who sustain cardiac arrest (Table 33–3).

It is presumed that the duration and quality of survival from arrest in the operating room should be good because the personnel who witness the arrests and provide the resuscitation are trained and prepared. A review of the anesthesia literature reveals that cardiac arrest can be reversed in approximately 90% of the anesthesia-related episodes. The likelihood of ROSC drops from about 90% to 50% to 60% if the causes of the arrest include those that are not related to anesthesia. The patient's

TABLE 33–3. Outcome from cardiac arrest

	Anesthesia Related						All Causes					
	PEDIATRICS			COMBINED			PEDIATRICS			COMBINED		
Outcome	*%*	*Range*	*No. of Studies*	*%*	*Range*	*No. of Studies*	*%*	*Range*	*No. of Studies*	*%*	*Range*	*No. of Studies*
Return of spontaneous circulation	92	83 to 100	2	87	78 to 95	4	51	32 to 70	2	58	47 to 65	5
Died	32	0 to 100	10	34	8 to 55	7	72	60 to 88	3	59	35 to 72	7
Survival to discharge	68	0 to 100	9	65	45 to 92	7	28	12 to 40	3	36	28 to 41	6
New neurologic deficits	5	0 to 16	5	5	4 to 7	3	14	12 to 15	2	4	2 to 7	3
Return to baseline neurologic status	57	21 to 92	5	69	44 to 85	3	22	20 to 25	2	33	30 to 35	3

survival to hospital discharge after an anesthetic-related cardiac arrest appears to be approximately 65% to 68% (the range for pediatric studies of this variable is very large). This survival to discharge falls to 30% if nonanesthesia causes of cardiac arrest are included. Comparing these data with descriptions from the nonanesthesia literature reveals that studies of "in-hospital" cardiac arrests in children show a survival to discharge percentage of 23% (range, 8% to 42%) (Gillis et al., 1986; Von Seggern et al., 1986; Davies et al., 1987; Carpenter and Stenmark, 1997; Para et al., 2000; Suominen et al., 2000; Reis et al., 2002). In-hospital cardiac arrests are comparable to perioperative arrests because both include the presence of trained witnesses. This 23% survival to discharge rate is comparable to the 30% rate for "all causes" and much lower than the 65% rate for "anesthesia-related" causes of cardiac arrest in the operating room. The vigilance and training of the witnesses are expected to be higher when anesthesiologists are involved. The presence of anesthesiologists may account, in part, for the better survival outcomes in anesthesia-related cardiac arrests.

Outcome studies should include a determination of the presence of new neurologic injuries due to the hypoperfusion of the brain during the period of cardiac arrest. Pediatric studies from the nonanesthesia literature of "in-hospital" cardiac arrests show a 71% favorable neurologic outcome for the survivors (range, 45% to 90%) (Gillis et al., 1986; Davies et al., 1987; Carpenter and Stenmark, 1997; Para et al., 2000; Suominen et al., 2000; Reis et al., 2002). The anesthesia literature shows that 57% of the children survive and return to their baseline neurologic status, whereas 5% survive with a new neurologic deficit (see Table 33–3). This frequency of 57% at baseline of the 62% total for survivors gives a rate of 92% with a favorable neurologic outcome in survivors of an "anesthesia-related" cardiac arrest. This percentage for pediatric survivors falls to 22% with return to baseline of 36% total survivors or a 61% favorable neurologic outcome when "all causes" of cardiac arrest are included. The 71% favorable neurologic outcome for in-hospital cardiac arrests is comparable to the 61% rate for "all causes" and lower than the 92% rate for "anesthesia-related" causes of cardiac arrest in the operating room. Note that the number of studies and patients for these estimates are small and the ranges are large. These data indicate that both the duration and quality of survival are favorable for children who arrest from anesthesia-related causes.

There are many potential explanations for the increased resuscitation rate (ROSC, approximately 92% versus 51%) from "anesthesia-related" cardiac arrest. Factors such as the resuscitation skills of the anesthesiologist, the preparation by the anesthesiologist for emergencies, the reversibility of the causes of cardiac arrest in the operating room, and the increased monitoring during anesthesia to provide early recognition of problems may contribute to improved resuscitation rates during anesthesia care. The survival rate after cardiac arrest is affected by many factors, some of which are the same that predispose a patient to cardiac arrest. The risk factors for cardiac arrest, consisting of the patient's age, his or her ASA physical status, and emergency procedures, are also determinants of mortality (see Tables 33–1 and 33–2). The etiology of the cardiac arrest also impacts the likelihood of both resuscitation and survival. The mortality is increased if the etiology of the cardiac arrest is hemorrhage or is associated with protracted hypotension (both $P < 0.001$) (Girardi and Barie, 1995; Newland et al., 2002; Sprung et al., 2003).

Resuscitation-related factors also have an effect on outcome. The rhythm during resuscitation and the duration of the resuscitation attempts have been related to the outcome of the patient. "No-flow" and "low-flow" states occur during the arrest and resuscitation process. A no-flow state occurs when a patient is in cardiac arrest before receiving resuscitation efforts. A low-flow state occurs when a patient is arrested and receiving resuscitation that is unable to provide adequate circulation. The longer the patient is in a "no-flow" state or a "low-flow" state, the worse the outcome is likely to be.

Asystole is a rhythm that, if present during resuscitation, has been associated with a decreased incidence of both ROSC and survival to discharge for children with cardiac arrest outside of the operating room. Usually, asystole is due to a prolonged period of hypoxia or ischemia of the myocardium and represents a terminal rhythm. The prolonged hypoxia causes the myocardium to be more resistant to resuscitation efforts. The prolonged global hypoxia leading to asystole usually also causes severe neurologic injury. If the heart can be resuscitated, there is still the likelihood of a poor outcome. Asystole in the operating room is much more likely to be associated with a good outcome. In the operating room, the continuous monitoring of the patient decreases the risk of prolonged periods of hypoxia or ischemia. Instead of a terminal rhythm, asystole in the operating room is often an initial rhythm caused by a vagal stimulation. As an initial rhythm, asystole is much more likely to be reversed. Usually, discontinuation of the vagal stimulus and support of the heart rate chemically are effective resuscitation measures. Unlike non-operating room arrests, asystole is a commonly reported rhythm with anesthesia-related cardiac arrest and is associated with a good prognosis (Sprung et al., 2003).

The duration of the resuscitative efforts also has an effect on the patient's outcome. Prolonged duration of CPR increases the possibility of low-flow intervals resulting in myocardial and cerebral injury. The need for CPR for longer than 15 minutes has been determined to be a predictor of mortality in anesthesia-related cardiac arrests ($P < 0.001$) (Girardi and Barie, 1995). The interpretation of these data is complicated by the possibility of successful outcomes even after very prolonged periods of resuscitation efforts. Up to 3 hours of CPR has been reported in anesthetic-related cardiac arrests with eventual resuscitation and a good outcome (Cleveland et al., 1971; Lee et al., 1994). The rapid initiation of resuscitative efforts by the anesthesia team can result in effective, even if prolonged, CPR. In summary, the etiology of the arrest, the rhythm disturbance, and the duration of CPR have an impact on the outcome from cardiac arrest in the operating room.

PREVENTION OF CARDIAC ARREST DURING ANESTHESIA

"Anesthesia-related" cardiac arrest is preventable 53% of the time, and "anesthesia-related" mortality is preventable 22% of the time (Kawashima et al., 2003). Human error may be the most important factor in deaths attributable to anesthesia and manifests not as a fundamental ignorance but as a failure in the application of existing knowledge (Olsson and Hallen, 1988). Poor preoperative preparation and inadequate vigilance are frequently reported errors that could be avoided. Examples of poor preoperative preparation relevant to the pediatric anesthesiologist include failure to identify patients with unrecognized skeletal myopathy, coronary involvement with Williams syndrome, prolonged QT syndrome, and undiagnosed cardiomyopathy. Another category of preventable causes is inadequate vigilance such as failure to recognize progressive bradycardia and failure to respond to persistent hypotension. In addition to improving preparation and vigilance, the use of test dosing and divided dosing when administering medications (especially to unstable patients) is suggested to minimize medication errors. Other important and preventable etiologies of "anesthesia-related" cardiac arrest include transfusion-related hyperkalemia, local anesthetic toxicity, and inhalational anesthetic overdose (Morray, 2000).

PHYSIOLOGY OF CARDIOPULMONARY RESUSCITATION

Successful resuscitation of a victim of cardiopulmonary arrest requires that the anesthesiologist: (1) recognizes inadequate ventilation or circulation and the need for CPR and (2) reestablishes and maintains both ventilation and circulation until the underlying pathology can be corrected. These steps are the same for all resuscitations whether they occur on the street or in the operating room. The more rapidly these steps are achieved, the better is the outcome.

RECOGNITION OF THE NEED FOR CARDIOPULMONARY RESUSCITATION

The decision to begin CPR for a child in the operating room requires the recognition that the patient's vital signs are inadequate. An understanding of the cerebral and cardiac perfusion requirements in children is necessary to determine the adequacy of the vital parameters. Exact data are lacking to address these requirements for the wide range of patients who come under the pediatric anesthesiologist's care. Specific pediatric experience and training provide the background necessary to make decisions about these perfusion requirements. A lower rate of CPR in children receiving anesthetics by anesthesiologists trained in pediatric anesthesiology suggests that the knowledge of the appropriate hemodynamic variables in children may reduce the need for resuscitation (Keenan et al., 1991).

CPR should be started immediately when the circulation is inadequate to deliver oxygen, substrates, or resuscitative drugs to the heart or brain. The presence of inadequate ventilation or circulation should be evident in the patient undergoing extensive monitoring in the operating room. In the absence of extensive monitoring, health care workers should use palpation of the umbilical artery for the newly born, of the brachial artery for an infant, and of the carotid artery for a child to detect a heart rate abnormality (Cavallaro and Melker, 1983; Lee and Bullock, 1991; American Heart Association, 2000). The presence of either a heart rate or a blood pressure alone should not result in an assumption that the circulation is sufficient as both an adequate heart rate (>60 beats per minute) and signs of good perfusion are necessary (adequate blood pressure values in Table 33–4).

REESTABLISHMENT OF VENTILATION

The finding that exhaled air from the rescuer (16% oxygen) may provide adequate oxygenation of the victim (SaO_2 of ≥90%) (Elam et al., 1954) is the basis for bystander CPR when supplemental oxygen is not available. The administration of 100% oxygen via tracheal intubation during CPR helps to maximize oxygen delivery to the vital organs. The need to optimize oxygen delivery outweighs the risk of oxygen toxicity during resuscitation, and 100% oxygen should be used when available. The rare exception is the child with a circulatory condition such as a hypoplastic left heart whose poor systemic perfusion may be the result of pulmonary overcirculation. In such a case, the anesthesiologist needs to decide whether high levels of oxygen administration contribute to the poor systemic circulation.

TABLE 33–4. Adequate vital signs for children

	Heart Rate (bpm)*			Blood Pressure (mm Hg)
Age	*Bradycardia*	*Normal*	*Tachycardia*	*Hypotension*
Neonates	<80	100 to 170	>220	SBP <60
Infants	<60	65 to 140	>190	SBP <70
Children	<60	65 to 140	>180	SBP <70 + (2 × age in years)
>10 Years	<50	60 to 120	>180	SBP <90

SBP, systolic blood pressure.

*Note: Significant bradycardia is typically defined as 2 SDs below the low end of normal.

Modified from American Heart Association in collaboration with the International Liaison Committee on Resuscitation: Guidelines 2000 for cardiopulmonary resuscitation and emergency cardiovascular care. Part 10: Pediatric advanced life support. *Circulation* 102:I291, 2000.

Initially, researchers believed that closed-chest compression alone provided adequate ventilation to the victim requiring CPR (Kouwenhoven et al., 1960). The possibility that compressions alone may provide ventilation for adult victims has resulted in over-the-telephone instruction for compressions-alone CPR to untrained bystanders or those unwilling to provide mouth-to-mouth ventilation. Unfortunately, soft tissue obstruction may prevent adequate ventilation in humans without intubation and positive-pressure ventilation (Safar et al., 1961). An unprotected airway puts patients at greater risk for aspiration during CPR. Unlike fibrillatory arrests, a model of asphyxial arrest shows the greatest benefit with the combination of compressions and ventilations compared with compression or ventilation alone (Berg et al., 2000). Tracheal intubation is the optimal means to ensure ventilation during CPR for pediatric anesthesiologists because they maintain the training to do so.

The laryngeal mask airway (LMA) is an airway adjunct that the anesthesiologist may be using when a child experiences a cardiac arrest. The LMA compares favorably to mouth-to mouth, mask ventilation, and other airway adjuncts during CPR (Rumball and MacDonald, 1997; Stone et al., 1998). There are limited data available for a comparison of LMA to tracheal intubation during CPR (Samarkandi et al., 1994). Tracheal intubation is considered a more stable and protective airway than the LMA during resuscitation. Airway adjuncts remain not recommended as a replacement for tracheal intubation during CPR in children, especially when an anesthesiologist is available (Grayling et al., 2002). The tracheal tube (TT) remains the airway of choice for patients requiring CPR, and appropriate placement can be verified by the presence of end-tidal CO_2 ($ETCO_2$).

The incidence of accidentally placing a TT in the esophagus of a child is greater during an arrest than during a nonarrest intubation (19% to 26% esophageal intubation rate during arrest versus 3% for nonarrest situations) (Bhende et al., 1992; Bhende and Thompson, 1995). The demonstration of persistent (after six ventilations) $ETCO_2$ after intubation is extremely

TABLE 33–5. Vascular access during cardiopulmonary resuscitation

Route	Characteristics
Peripheral venous access (IV)	Route of first choice if vascular access not present. Rapidly and easily placed. Any drug or fluid may be administered by this route. Need to flush each drug with 0.25 mL/kg normal saline to ensure central delivery (20 mL in adults).
Intraosseous access (IO)	Easier to obtain in <6 years old; can use for any age. Any drug or fluid may be administered by this route. Use flush as with peripheral venous access.
Intratracheal route (TT)	Use only if no IV or IO access. Only administer lidocaine, atropine, naloxone, and epinephrine (LEAN drugs) by TT. Note: TT drug delivery requires 2 to 10 times IV dose. Use 1 to 2 mL of normal saline in TT to increase distribution into distal bronchial tree (10 mL in adults).
Central venous catheter	Central access is first choice if already in place. Place if no IV or IO access is obtained. Requires flush if catheter tip is below diaphragm.
Cutdown saphenous	Use when other options have failed. Requires special skill; high complication rate.

PACU, causes of arrest likely to occur in the postanesthesia care unit.
*Causes of cardiac arrest that have low resuscitation and high mortality rates.

reliable to confirm correct placement of the TT in children with spontaneous circulation (Bhende et al., 1992). The lack of presence of $ETCO_2$ in the TT implies esophageal intubation but can be misleading during cardiac arrest. After cardiac arrest, the decreased pulmonary blood flow produced during CPR causes $ETCO_2$ to be falsely low or absent in correctly placed TTs (14% to 15% of TTs had no $ETCO_2$ in arrested children receiving CPR) (Bhende et al., 1992; Bhende and Thompson, 1995). Continually detectable $ETCO_2$ is proof of tracheal intubation even during arrest. In the absence of $ETCO_2$ and unless pulmonary circulation is restored, the TT placement should be visually inspected to discriminate esophageal intubation. The TT also provides access to the circulation for drug administration (Table 33–5).

A comparison of different patterns of ventilation during chest compression revealed differences in oxygenation, ventilation, and hemodynamics (Wilder et al., 1963). Both oxygen administration without pressure and continuous positive airway pressure produce adequate oxygenation but not ventilation or hemodynamic effects. Ventilation independent of compression, ventilation interposed between compressions, and ventilation synchronized with compression allow both adequate oxygenation and ventilation, but their effects on hemodynamic pressures vary. Delivery of positive-pressure ventilation has an impact on the hemodynamic variables due to the changes in intrathoracic pressure. Simultaneous compression and ventilation yield improvement in blood flow and survival in this canine model but has not shown the same benefit in humans and remains an experimental mode of CPR. The current recommendations are that in unintubated patients, ventilations should be interposed between compressions to maximize effectiveness of the ventilation, at least until the airway is secured (American Heart Association et al., 2000). The recommendations for the ratio of chest compressions to ventilation during CPR vary with the age of the child, whether the airway is secured, and the number of rescuers. The younger the child, the greater the need for an increase in the number of ventilations during CPR. The neonate and newly born require a 3:1 ratio or about 90 compressions and 30 breaths per minute whether one or two rescuers are used and whether or not the child is intubated. The infant and child aged 1 to 8 years require a 5:1 ratio or about 100 compressions and 20 breaths per minute whether one or two rescuers are used and whether or not the child is intubated. The older child and adult should receive a 15:2 ratio or about 90 compressions and 12 breaths per minute for both one and two rescuers if not intubated; the older child or adult should receive a 5:1 ratio for two rescuers once intubated.

The decreased compression-to-ventilation ratios used for the youngest victims allow more ventilation and may be more effective in the age groups at highest risk of respiratory etiology of arrest. The decreased compression ratio in the older victim allows the delivery of more uninterrupted compressions. Data in animals suggest that longer periods of uninterrupted compressions result in increased coronary perfusion (Kern et al., 1992, 1998). Interposed ventilation interrupts chest compression and, if prolonged, causes a reduction in CPR-generated perfusion pressure and recovery time to regain perfusion pressure when compressions are restarted (Berg et al., 2001).

Other significant interruptions to chest compressions include patient assessment for return or spontaneous circulation, intubation, central line placement, and placement of adhesive pads for defibrillation. These interruptions should be minimized or compressions continued when possible. The accomplishment of 80 chest compressions per minute has been correlated with successful resuscitation (Yu et al., 2002). Once the patient is intubated, the pauses for ventilations can be minimized and the need to interrupt compressions decreased. In the operating room, the airway should be secured as soon as possible and the compressions performed without interruption. The anesthesiologist can use the age-specific ratios of compressions to ventilations or adjust them as appropriate for the etiology of the arrest (Table 33–6).

TABLE 33–6. Basic life support procedures

	Newly Born (<12 hr old)	Infant (<1 yr old)	Child (1 to 8 yr old)	Adult (>8 yr old)
Ventilation rate, breaths/min	30	20	20	12
Pulse check	Umbilical cord	Brachial/femoral	Carotid	Carotid
Compression area	Below nipples	Lower 1/2 of sternum	Lower 1/2 of sternum	Lower 1/2 of sternum
Compress with	Two fingers/encircle	Two fingers/encircle	One hand	Two hands
Compression depth	1/3 AP diameter	1/3 to 1/2 AP diameter	1/3 to 1/2 AP diameter	1/3 to 1/2 AP diameter
Compression rate, /min	90	100 minimum	100	100
Compression-to-ventilation ratio	3:1	5:1	5:1	15:2 (5:1 if intubated)

Data from American Heart Association in collaboration with the International Liaison Committee on Resuscitation: Guidelines 2000 for cardiopulmonary resuscitation and emergency cardiovascular care. Part 10: Pediatric advanced life support. *Circulation* 102:I291, 2000.

REESTABLISHMENT OF CIRCULATION

Mechanisms of Blood Flow During Cardiopulmonary Resuscitation

Kouwenhoven and others (1960) proposed that external chest compressions squeeze the heart between the sternum and the vertebral column, forcing blood to be ejected. This assumption of direct cardiac compression during external CPR became known as the *cardiac pump mechanism* of blood flow. The cardiac pump mechanism proposes that the atrioventricular (AV) valves close during ventricular compression and that ventricular volume decreases during ejection of blood. During chest relaxation, ventricular pressures fall below atrial pressures, enabling the AV valves to open and the ventricles to fill. This sequence of events resembles the normal cardiac cycle and occurs with the direct cardiac compression during open-chest CPR.

Several observations of the hemodynamics during external CPR are inconsistent with the cardiac pump mechanism for blood flow (Table 33–7). First, similar elevations in the arterial and venous intrathoracic pressures during closed-chest CPR suggest a generalized increase in intrathoracic pressure (Weale and Rothwell-Jackson, 1962). Second, reconstructing the integrity of the thorax of patients with flail sternums improves the blood pressure during CPR (unexpected, because a flail sternum should allow direct cardiac compression during closed-chest CPR) (Rudikoff et al., 1980). Third, patients who develop ventricular fibrillation (VF) produce sufficient blood flow to maintain consciousness by repetitive coughing or deep breathing (MacKenzie et al., 1964; Criley et al., 1976; Niemann et al., 1980; Harada et al., 1991). These observations suggest a generalized increase in intrathoracic pressure may contribute to the production of blood flow during CPR. The finding that changes in intrathoracic pressure without direct cardiac compression (i.e., a cough) produce blood flow epitomizes the *thoracic pump mechanism* of blood flow during CPR. Extensive research has addressed the involvement of the cardiac and thoracic pump mechanisms in blood flow during CPR.

Thoracic Pump Mechanism

Chest compressions during CPR generate almost equal pressures in the left ventricle, aorta, right atrium, pulmonary artery, airway, and esophagus (MacKenzie et al., 1964; Criley et al., 1976; Chandra et al., 1981a; Niemann et al., 1981a; Cohen et al., 1982; Raessler et al., 1988; Swenson et al., 1988; Paradis et al., 1989). Because all intrathoracic vascular pressures are equal, the suprathoracic arterial pressures must be greater than the suprathoracic venous pressures for a cerebral perfusion gradient to exist. Venous valves, either functional or anatomic, prevent the direct transmission of the elevation in intrathoracic pressure to the suprathoracic veins. These jugular venous valves are present in animals (Rudikoff et al., 1980; Chandra et al., 1980, 1981a; Niemann et al., 1981b; Fisher et al., 1982; Guerci et al., 1985; Criley et al., 1986; Gudipati et al., 1986) and humans (Niemann et al., 1981b; Swenson et al., 1988; Paradis et al., 1989; Chandra et al., 1990; Goetting and Paradis, 1991a, 1991b). This unequal transmission of the intrathoracic pressure to the suprathoracic vasculature establishes the gradient necessary for cerebral blood flow during closed-chest CPR.

During normal cardiac activity, the lowest pressure occurs on the atrial side of the AV valves, providing a downstream effect that allows venous return to the pump. The extrathoracic

TABLE 33–7. Comparison of mechanisms of blood flow during closed-chest compressions

	Cardiac Pump	Thoracic Pump
Proposed Mechanism		
	Sternum and spine compress heart	General increase in intrathoracic pressure
Findings During Compression		
Atrioventricular valves	Close	Stay open
Aortic diameter	Increases	Decreases
Blood movement	Left ventricle to aorta	Pulmonary veins to aorta
Ventricular volume	Decreases	Little change
Compression rate	Dependent	Little effect
Duty cycle	Little effect	Dependent
Compression force	Increases role	Decreases role
Clinical Situations		
	Small chest High compliance	Large chest Low compliance

shift of this low-pressure area to the cephalic side of the jugular venous valves during the thoracic pump mechanism of blood flow implies that the heart is merely a conduit during this mechanism. Angiographic studies show blood passing from the vena cavae, through the right heart, to the pulmonary artery and from the pulmonary veins, through the left heart, to the aorta during a single chest compression (Niemann et al., 1981b; Cohen et al., 1982). Unlike normal cardiac activity and open-chest CPR, echocardiographic studies during closed-chest CPR in both dogs (Niemann et al., 1981b; Cohen et al., 1982) and humans (Rich et al., 1981; Werner et al., 1981; Clements et al., 1986) have shown that the AV valves are open during blood ejection. In addition, unlike native cardiac activity and open-chest CPR, aortic diameter decreases instead of increasing during blood ejection (Niemann et al., 1981b; Werner et al., 1981). These findings during closed-chest CPR support the thoracic pump theory and suggest that the heart becomes a passive conduit for blood flow.

Cardiac Pump Mechanism

Despite evidence for the importance of the thoracic pump mechanism of blood flow during external chest compressions, there are specific situations in which the cardiac pump mechanism predominates during closed-chest CPR. First, applying more force during chest compressions (as in High Impulse Cardiopulmonary Resuscitation, see later) increases the likelihood of direct cardiac compression. Increasing the force of chest compressions in animals undergoing CPR increases the closure of the AV valves, implying more direct cardiac compression (Feneley et al., 1987; Hackl et al., 1990). Second, a smaller chest size seems to allow more direct cardiac compression. Adult dogs with small chests have better hemodynamics during closed-chest CPR than do dogs with large chests (Babbs et al., 1982a). Third, the very compliant infant chest should permit more direct cardiac compression. During closed-chest CPR in an infant swine model, excellent blood flows are produced compared with most adult models (Schleien et al., 1986). Unlike the adult model, the addition of simultaneous ventilation with compression (SCV) does not augment the flow produced during piglet CPR (Berkowitz et al., 1989).

SCV-CPR fails to augment the already high flows that occur in small dogs with conventional chest compression (Babbs et al., 1982a). The lack of contribution of SCV-CPR in the infant or small adult animal models implies that excellent compression (probably direct cardiac) occurs and that the additional intrathoracic pressure is of no benefit.

Transesophageal echocardiography studies demonstrate the closing of the AV valves during the compression phase of CPR in humans (Higano et al., 1990; Kuhn et al., 1991) and during thoracic pump models of CPR in animals (Beattie et al., 1991). These findings support the occurrence of cardiac compression during conventional CPR, suggesting both mechanisms of blood flow may occur during CPR. As seen later, varying the CPR technique may alter the contribution of each mechanism.

Distribution of Blood Flow During Cardiopulmonary Resuscitation

The overall blood flow to the tissues is decreased during CPR compared with the normal physiologic state. A redistribution of the blood flow during CPR optimizes perfusion to the heart and brain. This redistribution toward the vital organs should enhance outcome. Maintenance of myocardial blood flow during CPR is necessary for the ROSC, and maintenance of cerebral blood flow determines the quality of the eventual neurologic outcome. The distribution of blood flow to both the heart and brain during CPR is influenced by the development of regional gradients.

The distribution of blood flow to the brain depends on the development of three regional gradients: intrathoracic-suprathoracic, intracranial-extracranial, and caudal-rostral gradients. The first gradient, intrathoracic-suprathoracic, provides the flow of oxygenated blood from the chest to the upper extremities and head. Either venous collapse, secondary to the elevated intrathoracic pressure, or closure of anatomic valves in the jugular system prevents the transmission of intrathoracic pressure to the suprathoracic venous system (Rudikoff et al., 1980; Niemann et al., 1981b; Fisher et al., 1982). When CPR is effective, arterial collapse does not occur and elevated intrathoracic pressure results in a gradient that promotes suprathoracic blood flow.

The second gradient, intracranial-extracranial, directs blood to the brain away from the extracranial suprathoracic vessels and toward the intracranial vessels. The α-adrenergic agonist vasoconstrictors constrict the extracranial vessels but have little effect on the intracranial vessels, resulting in increased intracranial blood flow. Use of the a-agonist vasoconstrictor epinephrine increases intracranial blood flow while decreasing flow in the cephalic skin, muscle, and tongue (Schleien et al., 1986).

The third gradient, caudal-rostral, occurs within the intracranial vessels. CPR alone seems to increase the distribution of flow to caudal areas of the brain, and ischemia preceding CPR significantly increases the distribution of flow to these areas (Michael et al., 1984; Shaffner et al., 1998, 1999). This pattern of caudal redistribution of flow also occurs in other models of global ischemia and may provide relative sparing of the brainstem (Jackson et al., 1981).

Myocardial blood flow does not have the advantage of the large extrathoracic pressure gradient that augments cerebral flow. The thoracic pump generates equal increases in all intrathoracic structures. This lack of a gradient causes poor myocardial blood flow during external chest compressions. Several studies have shown much lower blood flow to the myocardium compared with the cerebrum during closed-chest CPR (Ditchey et al., 1982; Michael et al., 1984; Schleien et al., 1986).

The type of CPR influences the production of myocardial blood flow. Methods that are more likely to cause direct cardiac compression, such as high-impulse CPR, result in increased myocardial blood flow (Ditchey et al., 1982; Maier et al., 1984). Myocardial blood flow may be present only during relaxation of chest compression (Maier et al., 1984), correlating with a "diastolic" pressure (Cohen et al., 1982) or, in other methods, during compression, correlating with a "systolic" pressure (Michael et al., 1984; Schleien et al., 1986). Regional flow within the heart also changes during CPR, with a shift in the ratio of subendocardial-subepicardial blood flow from the normal 1.5:1 to 0.8:1 (Schleien et al., 1986). This ratio reverts to normal with epinephrine administration.

Blood flow to organs other than the heart or brain falls dramatically during CPR. The lack of valves in the infrathoracic veins causes retrograde transmission of venous pressure and decreases the gradient for blood flow below the diaphragm in animals (Brown et al., 1987b). Regional blood flows for infrathoracic organs (small intestine, pancreas, liver, kidney, and spleen) during CPR are usually less than 20% of prearrest rates and often close to zero (Koehler and Michael, 1985a, 1985b; Voorhees et al., 1983; Michael et al., 1984; Sharff et al., 1984). The addition of abdominal compressions does not alter the infrathoracic organ blood flow (Koehler and Michael, 1985a, 1985b; Voorhees et al., 1983). Administration of epinephrine during closed-chest CPR almost eliminates flow to the subdiaphragmatic organs, with the exception of the adrenal glands (Ralston et al., 1984).

Few data are available regarding pulmonary blood flow during CPR. Pulmonary blood flow occurs primarily at times of low intrathoracic pressure during closed-chest CPR (Cohen et al., 1982). High extrathoracic venous pressure builds up during compression and results in pulmonary filling during relaxation as intrathoracic pressure falls. Resuscitation methods that lower intrathoracic pressure may augment pulmonary vascular filling.

Rate and Duty Cycle

In 1986, the American Heart Association *Guidelines for CPR and Emergency Cardiac Care* recommended increasing the rate of chest compressions from 60 to 100 per minute. This change represented a compromise between advocates of the thoracic pump mechanism and those of the cardiac pump mechanism (Feneley et al., 1988). The mechanics of these two theories of blood flow differ, but a faster compression rate could augment both. It is necessary to understand the concepts of *compression rate*, *duty cycle*, and *compression force* to understand the mechanics of CPR.

Compression rate is the number of cycles per minute. *Duty cycle* is the ratio of the duration of the compression phase to the entire compression-relaxation cycle expressed as a percentage. For example, a rate of 60 compressions per minute (total cycle, 1 second), a 0.6-second compression time, produces a 60% duty cycle (0.6 second/1.0 second = 60%). The impact of duty cycle differs between the two mechanisms of blood flow (see Table 33–7). *Compression force* is the pressure and the acceleration applied to the chest.

If direct cardiac compression generates blood flow (cardiac pump mechanism), then the force of the compression determines the stroke volume. Prolonging the compression (increasing the duty cycle) beyond the time necessary for full ventricular ejection fails to produce any additional increase in stroke volume in this model. In contrast, increasing the rate of compressions increases cardiac output since a fixed ventricular blood volume ejects with each cardiac compression. Therefore, in the cardiac pump mechanism, blood flow is rate sensitive but duty cycle insensitive.

If the thoracic pump mechanism is producing blood flow, the reservoir of blood to be ejected is the large capacitance of the intrathoracic vasculature. With the thoracic pump mechanism, increasing either the force of compression or the duty cycle enhances flow by emptying more of the large intrathoracic capacity. Changes in the compression rate have less effect on flow over a wide range of rates (Halperin et al., 1986a). Blood flow in the thoracic pump mechanism is duty cycle sensitive but rate insensitive.

Mathematical models of the cardiovascular system confirm that both the applied force and the duration of compression determine blood flow with the thoracic pump mechanism (Beyar et al., 1984; Halperin et al., 1987). Animal data suggest that either the thoracic pump or the cardiac pump mechanism can effectively generate blood flow during closed-chest CPR. Discrepancies among the results of various studies can be attributed to differences in CPR models and in compression techniques. These differences may involve issues of chest compliance and geometry, maturity of different animal species, or chest compression techniques. For example, either mechanism may come into play in an infant with a very compliant chest wall. Differences in techniques may include the magnitude of sternal displacement, compression force, compression rate, and duty cycle.

Several studies in dogs show a benefit of a fast compression rate (120 per minute) over slower rates during conventional CPR (Maier et al., 1984; Feneley et al., 1988; Sanders et al., 1990). Studies in piglets (Dean et al., 1990), puppies (Fleisher et al., 1987), and humans (Taylor et al., 1977; Ornato et al., 1988; Chandra et al., 1990) find no difference in the effectiveness of conventional CPR at various rates. A piglet CPR study found that the duty cycle was the major determinant of cerebral perfusion pressure (Chandra et al., 1981a). The duty cycle at which venous return becomes limited varies with age. Increasing the duty cycle is more effective in younger piglets and more likely to limit venous return in the adult models.

The discrepancy between the importance of rate and duty cycle in various models by different investigators generates confusion. Increasing the rate of compressions during conventional CPR to 100 per minute satisfies both those who prefer the faster rates and those who support a longer duty cycle. This is true because it is physically easier for a rescuer to produce a 50% duty cycle at a rate of 100 than at 60 compressions per minute (holding compression is physically difficult at slow rates). This is the reason behind the rate change in the 1986 American Heart Association guidelines for CPR. This increased rate continues to be recommended (American Heart Association et al., 2000).

Chest Geometry

Chest geometry plays an important role in the ability of chest compressions to generate intrathoracic pressures. *Shape, compliance,* and *deformability* are chest characteristics with a significant impact during CPR. The age of the patient affects each of these characteristics, which may explain some differences in CPR between the pediatric and adult models.

Chest Shape

During anterior-to-posterior-delivered compressions, the change in cross-sectional area of the chest relates to its shape (Fleisher et al., 1987). The thoracic index refers to the ratio of the anteroposterior diameter to the lateral diameter. A keel-shaped chest, as in an adult dog, has a greater anteroposterior diameter and thus a thoracic index greater than 1. A flat chest, as in a thin human, has a greater lateral diameter and thus a thoracic index of less than 1. A circular chest would have a thoracic index of 1. A circular chest with the same perimeter would also have a larger cross-sectional area than either elliptical chest shape. As an anteroposterior compression flattens a circle, it decreases the cross-sectional area and compresses the contents. In contrast, as a keel-shaped chest approaches a circular shape, the cross-sectional area increases during the application of anteroposterior compression. The cross-sectional area of the keel-shaped chest does not decrease until the compression continues past the circular shape to flatten the chest. This implies a threshold distance past which the compression must proceed before the intrathoracic contents are compressed (Dean et al., 1987). The rounded, flatter chests of small dogs and pigs may require less displacement than the keel-shaped chests of adult dogs to generate thoracic ejection of blood. The rounded chests of small dogs improve the efficacy of external thoracic compression compared with the keel-shaped chests of adult dogs (Babbs et al., 1982a).

Chest Compliance

With increasing age, the cartilage in the chest becomes calcified and the compliance changes. The stiffer or less compliant, older chest may require greater compression force to generate the same anteroposterior displacement. Three-month-old swine require a much greater pressure for anteroposterior displacement than do their 1-month-old counterparts (Dean et al., 1987). The compliance of the chest affects not only the amount of displacement but also the structures compressed. Direct cardiac compression is more likely to occur in the more compliant chests of younger animals. Cerebral blood flow production in a piglet model of external CPR was much greater than expected compared with the usual findings in adult animals (Schleien et al., 1986). The more compliant infant chest may allow more direct cardiac compression, accounting for the high flows that resemble those produced by open-chest cardiac massage.

Chest Deformation

Chest deformation occurs as CPR becomes prolonged. The chest assumes a flatter shape as compressions continue, producing larger decreases in cross-sectional area at the same displacement. Progressive deformation may be beneficial if it leads to more direct cardiac compression. Unfortunately, too much deformation may decrease the recoil of the chest wall during release of compression. Decreased chest recoil with progressing deformation limits the displacement and produces less effective compression. A pediatric model of conventional CPR shows a progressive decrease over time in the effectiveness of chest compressions to produce blood flow (Schleien et al., 1986; Dean et al., 1991). The permanent deformation of the chest in this model approaches 30% of the original anteroposterior diameter. Attempting to limit the deformation by increasing intrathoracic pressure from within during compression with SCV-CPR was ineffective (Berkowitz et al., 1989). Neither the amount of deformation nor the time to deterioration of flow was different.

In an attempt to limit the production of deformation, investigators used a third mode of infant animal CPR with a vest to deliver compressions. The vest distributes compression force diffusely around the thorax and greatly decreases permanent deformation (3% versus 30%) (Fisher et al., 1982; Shaffner et al., 1990). Unfortunately, the deterioration of blood flows with time still occurs and appears to be unrelated to the amount of deformation in this model.

The relevance to humans of chest geometry characteristics found in animal studies is unclear. Body weight, surface area, chest circumference, and chest diameter did not correlate with the aortic pressure produced during CPR in a study of nine adults already declared dead (Swenson et al., 1988). There has not been a direct comparison of adult and pediatric human CPR. The increased compliance and deformability of the infant chest make it likely that CPR would be more effective in children than in adults (as seen in animal models).

MAINTENANCE OF CIRCULATION

Efficacy of Blood Flow During Cardiopulmonary Resuscitation

The level of blood flow to the vital organs produced by conventional closed-chest CPR without pharmacologic support is disappointingly low. The range of cerebral blood flow in dogs is 3% to 14% of prearrest levels (Bircher and Safar, 1981; Koehler and Michael, 1985a; Koehler et al., 1983; Jackson et al., 1984; Luce et al., 1984). Cerebral perfusion pressures are also low, 4% to 24% of prearrest levels in animals (Bircher and Safar, 1981; Koehler and Michael, 1983a, 1983b; Luce et al., 1984) and only 21 mm Hg in humans (Goetting and Paradis, 1991b). Myocardial blood flows in this basic CPR mode are also discouragingly low at 1% to 15% of prearrest levels in dogs (Chandra et al., 1981a; Voorhees et al., 1983; Koehler and Michael, 1985a; Halperin et al., 1986a; Shaffner et al., 1990). Myocardial perfusion pressures (MPPs) correlate with myocardial blood flow. Plotting myocardial blood flow in milliliters per minute per gram versus MPP in mm Hg gives a slope of 0.01 to 0.015 (Voorhees et al., 1983; Ralston et al., 1984). These data imply a one-to-one relationship between myocardial blood flow (when measured in mL/min per 100 g) and MPP (mm Hg).

In addition to pharmacologic support, several other factors affect cerebral and myocardial blood flow during CPR. These factors include the victim's age, intracranial pressure, duration of CPR, and duration of preresuscitation ischemia.

Age affects cerebral blood flow during closed-chest CPR. Two-week-old piglets have substantially higher cerebral blood flows (50% of prearrest) and slightly higher myocardial flows (17% of prearrest) than those reported for adult models (Schleien et al., 1986). Two studies on slightly older pigs yielded opposing results. Cerebral blood flows in these two studies were 26% to 95% and 1% to 4% of prearrest values, with corresponding myocardial values of 2% to 8% and 1% to 6% (Sharff et al., 1984; Brown et al., 1987b). The cerebral blood flow in the first of these two studies was markedly higher than in adult models during closed-chest CPR, and neither of the myocardial flows was different from that in adult models. No human data exist with blood flows at different ages during CPR.

Intracranial pressure can represent the downstream pressure for cerebral blood flow and, if elevated, can inhibit cerebral perfusion. Increasing intrathoracic pressure with closed-chest CPR causes intracranial pressure to increase (Rogers et al., 1979). This relationship is linear; one third of the increase in intrathoracic pressure is transmitted to the intracranial pressure (Guerci et al., 1985). The carotid arteries and jugular veins do not appear to be involved in the transmission of intrathoracic pressure to the intracranial contents. The transmission can be partially blocked by occluding the cerebrospinal fluid or vertebral vein flow (Guerci et al., 1985). The rise in intracranial pressure with chest compressions becomes more significant in the setting of baseline increased intracranial pressure (two thirds of the intrathoracic pressure is transmitted to the intracranial pressure). Clinicians need to be aware that the efficacy of CPR to perfuse the brain deteriorates markedly in the face of elevated intracranial pressure. When possible, the intracranial pressure should be lowered early in the resuscitation (i.e., shunt tapped, hematoma drained) to increase the effectiveness of resuscitative efforts.

Increased duration of CPR has a negative effect on cerebral blood flow and seems to be most detrimental in the infant preparation (Sharff et al., 1984; Schleien et al., 1986). The length of the ischemic period before CPR begins also has a negative effect on cerebral blood flow (Lee et al., 1984; Shaffner et al., 1999). Forebrain blood flow during subsequent CPR is reduced more than brainstem as the preceding ischemic interval is increased (Shaffner et al., 1998, 1999). Hypothermia has some protective effect and prevents this reduction in the ischemic intervals tested in dogs (Shaffner et al., 1998). The cause of these detrimental effects on cerebral blood flow is unclear. It remains obvious that a short ischemic period and quick resuscitation improve eventual outcome.

There appear to be thresholds for minimal vital organ blood flow during CPR. The inability to maintain blood flow above these thresholds during CPR results in organ malfunction. A myocardial blood flow of 20 mL/min per 100 g or greater is necessary for successful defibrillation in dogs (Guerci et al., 1985; Sanders et al., 1985a). A cerebral blood flow of greater than 15 to 20 mL/min per 100 g is necessary to maintain normal electrical activity during CPR (Michael et al., 1984).

Monitoring the Effectiveness of Cardiopulmonary Resuscitation

Monitoring the effectiveness of CPR can be difficult. An adequate MPP is necessary to allow the ROSC during CPR. The above data suggest that a myocardial blood flow of 20 mL/min per 100 g is necessary for the resumption of myocardial activity. This flow would correlate with an MPP of 20 mm Hg (aortic relaxation pressure minus right atrial relaxation pressure). Data from CPR in humans show that an MPP of 15 mm Hg was necessary for, but did not guarantee, ROSC (Paradis et al., 1990). Often right atrial relaxation pressure is low and the aortic "diastolic" pressure represents the MPP. In clinical practice, detection of this "diastolic" pressure is difficult without an arterial catheter. With the use of an arterial catheter during CPR, the anesthesiologist can observe the effects of interventions on the "diastolic" pressure as a guide to optimizing the impact of the resuscitative efforts on myocardial perfusion.

Measurement of venous oxygen saturation has been described as a method to monitor the effectiveness of CPR. In humans, the level of venous oxygen saturation correlated with the ROSC (Snyder et al., 1991; Rivers et al., 1992). This observation may be of use during CPR in victims with central venous access. Patients with a mixed venous oxygen saturation of less than 30% are receiving inadequate CPR and are unlikely to have an ROSC

(Rivers et al., 1992). If the patient has a central catheter in place during CPR, this method can be useful in determining the effectiveness of resuscitative efforts.

Another method to monitor the effectiveness of myocardial perfusion during CPR is to follow the production of $ETCO_2$. $ETCO_2$ monitoring is particularly useful to determine the effectiveness of CPR as the patient is more likely to have a TT than an arterial catheter or a central catheter in place. The amount of CO_2 exhaled and measured in the TT depends on the amount of pulmonary blood flow. In general, $ETCO_2$ levels decrease as pulmonary blood flow falls during CPR. As blood flow to the heart and lungs improves during CPR, $ETCO_2$ should return toward arterial CO_2 levels.

An $ETCO_2$ measured during CPR of less than 10 mm Hg predicts an inability to restore spontaneous circulation (Callaham and Barton, 1990; Wayne et al., 1995; Levine et al., 1997). Alternatively, an $ETCO_2$ greater than 15 mm Hg during CPR predicts resuscitation (Sanders et al., 1989; Barton and Callaham, 1991; Bhende and Thompson, 1995). These studies imply that $ETCO_2$ monitoring is useful in determining the effectiveness of CPR and that the production of $ETCO_2$ of less than 10 to 15 mm Hg suggests a need to modify CPR to improve blood flow. $ETCO_2$ may also detect cardiac output during electromechanical dissociation (Barton and Callaham, 1991), the ROSC during CPR (Garnett et al., 1987), and the presence of spontaneous circulation during cardiopulmonary bypass (Gazmuri et al., 1991).

The measurement of $ETCO_2$ for patients receiving CPR without tracheal intubation appears useful to determine the effectiveness of cardiac compressions at producing blood flow (Nakatani et al., 1999). In nonintubated patients receiving CPR with a facemask or an LMA, the level of $ETCO_2$ correlated with the rate of ROSC. The correlation was not as close as reports from studies of intubated patients. More patients with a low $ETCO_2$ had ROSC and fewer with higher $ETCO_2$ had ROSC than in studies with intubated patients.

There are pitfalls in the monitoring of $ETCO_2$ during CPR. Administration of bicarbonate increases CO_2 production and may elevate $ETCO_2$ without a corresponding increase in pulmonary blood flow. Administration of epinephrine may decrease $ETCO_2$ despite an increase in the myocardial perfusion, causing a misinterpretation that CPR has become less effective (Martin et al., 1990). Contamination of disposable $ETCO_2$ detectors by resuscitation medications (epinephrine, atropine, or lidocaine) or gastric acid may decrease their accuracy in the assessment of CPR effectiveness or the detection of esophageal intubation (Muir et al., 1990). The cause of the arrest may also have an impact on the interpretation of quantitative $ETCO_2$ analysis during CPR. The initial $ETCO_2$ measurements are higher following asphyxial arrest than fibrillatory arrest, and the ability to predict ROSC from initial $ETCO_2$ levels was better with fibrillatory arrest (Grmec et al., 2003).

An additional monitoring tool during CPR is the electrocardiogram (ECG) when the arrest is ventricular fibrillation. Fibrillation with large amplitude and long latency (coarse fibrillation) represents less cellular ischemia and a more resuscitatable situation. As myocardial perfusion continues to deteriorate, the fibrillation becomes finer and the myocardium less responsive to resuscitation. Effective CPR can reverse a fine fibrillation to a coarser pattern. Analyzing fibrillation waveforms may allow the rescuer to deliver defibrillation attempts when optimal (Hayes et al., 2003).

METHODS OF CARDIOPULMONARY RESUSCITATION

CONVENTIONAL CARDIOPULMONARY RESUSCITATION

Conventional CPR includes closed-chest compressions delivered manually with ventilations interposed after every 5th or 15th compression (see Table 33–6 for basic life support procedures). This method of CPR can be delivered in any setting without additional equipment and with a minimum of training. No large randomized study exists to demonstrate the superiority of any alternative method of CPR over conventional CPR.

Rescuer fatigue is a major problem with manual CPR in the field. Individual variation among rescuers performing manual CPR is another problem both in the field and in the laboratory. Mechanical devices are available to deliver chest compressions to prevent fatigue and to standardize compression delivery. Mechanical devices are presently limited to adult CPR and are not recommended for children (American Heart Association, 2000). The overall low efficacy of conventional CPR has led to investigations of multiple CPR modalities. These methods usually reflect attempts to enhance the contribution of the thoracic pump or cardiac pump to blood flow during CPR (Table 33–8). For example, the use of both hands to encircle the chest of an infant while using the thumbs to apply sternal compression attempts to both raise intrathoracic pressure and compress the heart (Todres and Rogers, 1975; David, 1988). This two-thumb encircling technique of CPR generates higher blood pressures and is recommended over the two-finger technique for infants (Dorfsman et al., 2000).

CONVENTIONAL CARDIOPULMONARY RESUSCITATION IN THE PRONE POSITION

Conventional CPR is usually performed with sternal compressions applied to a supine patient. Patients who are prone and undergoing posterior cranial or spine surgery when they sustain a cardiac arrest may not be able to be quickly repositioned to supine. An unstable spine, protruding stabilizers, and ongoing blood loss are factors that may delay turning the patient and necessitate starting CPR in the prone position. Two methods for posterior chest compression in the prone position have been suggested. The first uses two hands, one spread over each scapula (Tobias et al., 1994), and the second uses the heel of one hand on the spine (second hand on top of the first, similar to sternal

TABLE 33–8. Contribution of cardiac or thoracic pump to various methods of cardiopulmonary resuscitation

Cardiopulmonary Resuscitation Method	Cardiac Pump	Thoracic Pump
Open chest	++	0
High impulse	++	+
Conventional	0/+	+
Abdominal binding	0/+	++
Interposed abdominal compression*	0/+	++
Simultaneous compression		
Ventilation	0/+	++
Vest	0	++
Cough	0	++

*Also moves blood by abdominal compression alone.

■ **TABLE 33–9.** Risk factors for cardiac arrest in the prone position

Cardiac anomalies in patients undergoing major spinal surgery
Hypovolemia
Air embolism
Wound irrigation with H_2O_2
Poor positioning
Occluded venous return

From Brown J, Rogers J, Soar J: Cardiac arrest during surgery and ventilation in the prone position: A case report and systematic review. *Resuscitation* 50:233, 2001.

compression) (Sun et al., 1992; Dequin et al., 1996). Counterpressure under the sternum with another rescuer's hand or fist or a sandbag has also been suggested (Sun et al., 1992; Dequin et al., 1996; Mazer et al., 2003). When possible, patients should be turned supine for CPR.

In addition to chest compressions, defibrillation may be necessary in a prone patient. Prior placement of self-adhesive defibrillation pads is advised as intraoperative placement of paddles may be difficult and requires time. The placement of gel pads on the back on either side of the surgical incision in left mid-axillary lines and inferior to right scapula has been successful for defibrillating a prone patient (Miranda and Newton, 2001). Prone defibrillation may be attempted if the defibrillator is available and the patient cannot be turned immediately. Risk factors for cardiac arrest in the prone position are listed in Table 33–9.

■ SIMULTANEOUS COMPRESSION-VENTILATION CARDIOPULMONARY RESUSCITATION

Simultaneous compression-ventilation CPR (SCV-CPR) represents an attempt to augment conventional CPR by increasing the contribution of the thoracic pump mechanism to blood flow. Delivering ventilation simultaneously with every compression (instead of interposed after every fifth compression) adds to the intrathoracic pressure and should augment blood flow produced by conventional closed-chest CPR. Several studies suggest that SCV-CPR increases the carotid blood flow compared with conventional CPR (Harris et al., 1967; Chandra et al., 1980, 1981a; Bircher and Safar, 1981; Babbs et al., 1982a). Studies show an advantage of SCV-CPR in large canine models (Koehler and Michael, 1985a, 1985b; Luce et al., 1983) but no advantage over conventional CPR in infant pigs (Berkowitz et al., 1989) and small dogs (Babbs et al., 1982a, 1982b; Sanders et al., 1982). In small animals, the compliance of the chest may allow more direct cardiac compression and higher intravascular pressure than with conventional CPR (Schleien et al., 1986; Dean et al., 1987, 1990). Human studies comparing SCV to conventional CPR show minimal improvement (Harris et al., 1967) or detrimental effect (Martin et al., 1986) on the coronary perfusion pressure. Survival is worse in both animals (Sanders et al., 1982) and humans (Krischer et al., 1989) when SCV-CPR is compared with conventional CPR. No study has shown an increased survival with this CPR technique.

■ ABDOMINAL BINDING

Researchers have used abdominal binders and military antishock trousers (MAST) to augment closed-chest CPR. Both methods apply continuous compression circumferentially below the diaphragm. Abdominal binding augments CPR by (1) decreasing the compliance of the diaphragm, which results in increased intrathoracic pressure; (2) forcing blood out of the subthoracic structures, which increases the circulating blood volume (an autotransfusion effect); and (3) increasing the resistance in the subdiaphragmatic vasculature, which increases suprathoracic blood flow. The increases in intrathoracic pressure and blood volume lead to increased aortic pressure and carotid blood flow in both animals (Lee et al., 1981; Koehler and Michael, 1985a, 1985b; Niemann et al., 1984) and humans (Chandra et al., 1981b; Lilja et al., 1981).

Unfortunately, as the aortic pressure increases, the right atrial "diastolic" pressure increases to a greater extent, resulting in a decrease in the coronary perfusion pressure (Sanders et al., 1982; Niemann et al., 1984). This deterioration of coronary perfusion pressure is coincidental with a decreased myocardial blood flow (Niemann et al., 1984). This technique also decreases the cerebral perfusion pressure via transmission of the intrathoracic pressure to the intracranial vault, raising the intracranial pressure (Guerci et al., 1985). The use of abdominal binders or MAST to augment CPR does not increase survival in clinical studies (Sanders et al., 1982; Mahoney and Mirick, 1983; Niemann et al., 1990). Liver laceration from abdominal binder CPR has been reported (Harris et al., 1967) but is no more frequent than with conventional CPR (Redding, 1971; Rudikoff et al., 1980; Mahoney and Mirick, 1983; Niemann et al., 1984). There are no data to support the use of these techniques clinically during CPR, and the potential for complications should discourage their application.

■ ABDOMINAL COMPRESSION

Interposed abdominal compression CPR (IAC-CPR) is the delivery of an abdominal compression during the relaxation phase of chest compression. IAC-CPR may augment conventional CPR (1) by increasing venous return to the chest during the abdominal compression/chest relaxation phase and "priming the pump" (Ralston et al., 1982; Voorhees et al., 1983), (2) through abdominal compression during IAC-CPR, increasing intrathoracic pressure and adding to the duty cycle of the chest compression (Einagle et al., 1988), and (3) via the effect of abdominal compression on the aorta, which may send blood retrograde to the carotids or coronaries (Ralston et al., 1982). Several studies have shown hemodynamic improvements secondary to IAC-CPR. In animals, cardiac output and cerebral and coronary blood flow improved when IAC-CPR was compared with conventional CPR in adult models (Ralston et al., 1982; Voorhees et al., 1983; Walker et al., 1984; Einagle et al., 1988) but not in an infant swine model (Eberle et al., 1990). Human studies have also shown an increase in aortic pressure and coronary perfusion pressure during IAC-CPR compared with conventional CPR (Berryman and Phillips, 1984; Howard et al., 1984, 1987; Ward et al., 1989; Barranco et al., 1990; Chandra et al., 1990).

Although one study reports a 10% aspiration rate (Walker et al., 1984), most report no aspiration or liver lacerations (Voorhees et al., 1983; Berryman and Phillips, 1984; Mateer et al., 1985; Einagle et al., 1988; Ward et al., 1989; Barranco et al., 1990; Sack et al., 1992). Clinically, IAC-CPR requires extra manpower or equipment and remains experimental. Outcome studies have mixed results, showing no increase in survival with prehospital arrests but increased survival with in-hospital arrests (Mateer et al., 1985; Sack et al., 1992). Although an alternative technique for in-hospital CPR in adults, a lack of data prevents a recommendation for the use of IAC-CPR in children.

VEST CARDIOPULMONARY RESUSCITATION

Vest CPR uses an inflatable bladder that is wrapped circumferentially around the chest and is cyclically inflated. This method of delivering chest compressions by diffuse application of pressure has two unique characteristics. First, the increase in intrathoracic pressure occurs with only minimal change in chest dimensions, making direct cardiac compression unlikely (an almost purely thoracic pump technique). Second, the diffuse distribution of pressure decreases the likelihood of trauma. Vest CPR in dogs improves cerebral and myocardial blood flows and survival compared with conventional CPR (Luce et al., 1983; Criley et al., 1986; Halperin et al., 1986a, 1986b). In a pediatric model of vest CPR, only a 3% permanent chest deformation occurred after 50 minutes of vest CPR (Shaffner et al., 1990) compared with almost 30% deformation produced by an equivalent period of conventional CPR (Schleien et al., 1986). In humans, vest CPR increases aortic systolic pressure but does not significantly increase diastolic pressure compared with conventional CPR (Swenson et al., 1988). In a preliminary study of vest CPR in victims of out-of-hospital arrest, increased aortic and coronary perfusion pressures were demonstrated, and there was a trend toward a greater ROSC compared with standard CPR (Halperin et al., 1993). A large clinical trial is under way to determine if these benefits improve outcome.

The lack of metallic parts has allowed vest CPR to be used experimentally during nuclear magnetic resonance spectroscopy to study brain intracellular pH (Eleff et al., 1992). In addition, the vest has been used as an external cardiac assist device in nonarrested dogs with heart failure (Beyar et al., 1989; Chandra et al., 1991). Clinically, the use of vest CPR depends on sophisticated equipment and the technique remains experimental at this time.

HIGH-IMPULSE CARDIOPULMONARY RESUSCITATION

High-impulse CPR involves the application of greater than usual force during chest compression. This increase in force can be in the form of greater mass, greater velocity, or both. It is hypothesized that the larger impulses result in greater chest deflection, causing more contact with the heart (Kernstine et al., 1982). Direct cardiac compression is more likely with this form of closed-chest CPR. High-impulse CPR can generate myocardial blood flows as high as 60% to 75% of prearrest values (Maier et al., 1984). In humans, high-impulse CPR generates increased aortic pressures (Swenson et al., 1988). An outcome study in dogs compared high-impulse CPR with conventional closed-chest CPR and found no significant improvement in resuscitation, survival, or neurologic outcome (Kern et al., 1986).

ACTIVE COMPRESSION–DECOMPRESSION CARDIOPULMONARY RESUSCITATION

Active compression-decompression (ACD) CPR requires a device that attaches to the chest and allows the rescuer to pull up on the sternum and decompress the thorax between compressions. The theoretical advantages of decompressing the chest between compressions include restoring chest wall shape and creating a negative intrathoracic pressure that pulls gas into the lungs and pulls blood into the intrathoracic vessels. These characteristics allow for more effect from the subsequent compression as more intrathoracic pressure can be generated and more blood ejected. Preliminary studies in humans have shown that after advanced cardiac life support failed, ACD-CPR was more effective than standard CPR at improving hemodynamic variables (Cohen et al., 1992). Following a witnessed in-hospital arrest, more patients had ROSC and survival at 24 hours and had a better Glasgow Coma Scale score when they received ACD-CPR than when standard CPR was applied (Cohen et al., 1993).

A larger study of in-hospital cardiac arrest victims failed to show any difference in the resuscitation or outcomes between patients receiving ACD-CPR or standard CPR (Stiell et al., 1996). Several large studies of patients who sustained an out-of-hospital cardiac arrest did not find a difference in the effectiveness of ACD-CPR or standard CPR for improving the incidence of ROSC, hospital admission, hospital discharge, or short-term neurologic outcome (Lurie et al., 1994; Schwab et al., 1995; Mauer et al., 1996; Stiell et al., 1996; Nolan et al., 1998).

Complication rates following CPR were not different following ACD-CPR or standard CPR in most studies (Lurie et al., 1994; Schwab et al., 1995; Mauer et al., 1996). It is interesting that the same study that showed that ACD had more complications than standard CPR (hemoptysis and sternal dislodgment) was also one of the few large studies that found ACD-CPR more effective than standard CPR for out-of-hospital arrests (Plaisance et al., 1997). ACD-CPR is considered an optional technique for adults, but the absence of clinical data prevents a recommendation for children.

Impedance threshold valve (ITV) describes the use of a device on the TT or facemask that impedes the inflow of inspiratory gas during reexpansion of the chest between CPR compressions when not actively ventilating the patient. The impedence of gas inflow promotes negative intrathoracic pressure development during chest reexpansion. This increase in the negative intrathoracic pressure facilitates blood return to the thorax with chest recoil prior to the next chest compression (Lurie et al., 2002). The use of an ITV has been shown to improve coronary perfusion pressure and vital organ blood flow with both standard and ACD-CPR in adult and pediatric animal models (Langhelle et al., 2002; Voelckel et al., 2002). Improved levels of $ETco_2$, diastolic and coronary perfusion pressure occurred in a prospective, randomized controlled trial in adults with ACD-CPR with ITV compared with ACD-CPR without ITV. A decrease in the time to achieve an ROSC was also seen with ACD-CPR with ITV (Plaisance et al., 2000). A prospective controlled trial comparing standard CPR and ACD-CPR with ITV found significantly improved short term survival (24 hours) in adult patients (Wolcke et al., 2003). Further studies are needed to determine the effectiveness of the use of an ITV for pediatric resuscitation.

PHASED CHEST ABDOMINAL COMPRESSION–DECOMPRESSION CARDIOPULMONARY RESUSCITATION

Another manual method of CPR known as phased chest and abdominal compression-decompression (PCACD) cardiopulmonary resuscitation is being investigated (Tang et al., 1997). PCACD CPR resembles a combination of active compression-decompression CPR and interposed abdominal compression CPR. It requires a device that attaches to both the abdomen and chest and is used to alternately compress and reexpand both structures. It offers the theoretical advantages of both methods because chest shape is restored and blood and gas are pulled into the thorax during active decompression of the chest and blood flow is augmented due to the compression, and active decompression, of the abdomen. Coronary perfusion pressure, ROSC, short-term survival, and neurologic outcome were improved in a porcine model of fibrillatory cardiac arrest resuscitated using PCACD CPR (Tang et al., 1997).

OPEN-CHEST CARDIOPULMONARY RESUSCITATION

Open-chest CPR involves a thoracotomy and the application of direct compression of the heart to generate blood flow. The use of this technique requires a high level of preparation and training as well as special equipment and facilities. These requirements limit open-chest CPR to certain hospital settings.

Open-chest CPR represents a model of the cardiac pump mechanism for generation of blood flow. In theory, this model eliminates the production of intrathoracic pressure, which, if transmitted, could reduce the gradients for blood flow. This enhanced gradient combined with directly applied compression can result in near-normal blood flows. In experimental models, open-chest CPR produces cardiac outputs of 25% to 61% of prearrest values (Weiser et al., 1962; Bircher and Safar, 1981; Bartlett et al., 1984). These studies and others demonstrate cardiac outputs two to three times larger than those with conventional closed-chest CPR (Weiser et al., 1962; Del Guercio et al., 1965; Bircher et al., 1980; Bircher and Safar, 1981; Bartlett et al., 1984). Increases in cerebral perfusion pressure have been significant in some studies (Bircher et al., 1980) but not in others (Del Guercio et al., 1965; Bircher and Safar, 1981). MPPs are significantly increased compared with closed-chest CPR (Bircher et al., 1980; Sanders et al., 1984b). Cerebral blood flow in dogs of 150% of prearrest values can be produced with open-chest CPR (Jackson et al., 1984). Cross-clamping the descending aorta during open-chest CPR further increases carotid blood flow.

Survival in dogs can be improved by use of open-chest CPR after inadequate closed-chest CPR (Sanders et al., 1984a). Dogs with MPP of less than 30 mm Hg after 15 minutes of closed-chest external CPR received 2 to 4 minutes of either open-chest or closed-chest external CPR before defibrillation was attempted. The dogs that received open-chest CPR had significantly greater MPPs and survival rates.

The length of time of closed-chest CPR affects the success of subsequent open-chest CPR (Sanders et al., 1985b). After 20 and 25 minutes of closed-chest CPR, the success rate of open-chest CPR decreased to 38% and 0%, respectively. This implies that the benefits from open-chest CPR are time limited and that early application is crucial. There are no data to recommend the routine use of open-chest CPR in the pediatric patient. Postoperative cardiac patients with a recent sternotomy may benefit from open-chest CPR. They have easier access and can be inspected for tamponade, and suture lines can be inspected and avoided.

CARDIOPULMONARY BYPASS

Cardiopulmonary bypass (CPB) is a very effective way to restore circulation after cardiac arrest. Animal studies show that CPB increases 72-hour survival and recovery of consciousness and preserves myocardium better than conventional CPR (Levine et al., 1987; Pretto et al., 1987). In dogs, CPB results in better neurologic outcome than continued conventional CPR after a 4-minute ischemic period (neurologic outcome was dismal in both groups when the ischemic period lasted for 12 minutes) (Levine et al., 1987; Pretto et al., 1987). Twenty-four-hour survival is possible for at least 90% of dogs after 15 or 20 minutes of cardiac arrest but for only 10% of dogs after 30 minutes of arrest with CPB stabilization during defibrillation (Reich et al., 1990). CPB decreases myocardial infarct size in a model involving coronary artery occlusion, compared with conventional CPR (Angelos et al., 1990). In most animal models, CPB facilitates resuscitation and improves success compared with conventional CPR.

There is increasing experience with CPB for cardiac arrest in humans outside the cardiac operating room. Timely application of percutaneous femoral artery and vein bypass has been successful in resuscitating patients with "refractory" cardiac arrest. Unfortunately, many patients who are stabilized on CPB after standard CPR fails cannot be weaned off CPB or have a low likelihood of long-term survival or of good neurologic outcome (Mattox and Beall, 1976; Phillips et al., 1983; Hartz et al., 1990; Reichman et al., 1990; Martin et al., 1998). There are reports of patients with cardiac arrest in the operating room or catheterization suite who have cardiac arrest under anesthesia and fail to respond to conventional CPR but benefit from the institution of CPB. These patients are reported to have good neurologic outcomes despite over 30 minutes (even over 2 hours and transfer to another facility) of failed conventional resuscitation efforts (Lee et al., 1994; Cochran et al., 1999).

CPB rescue for cardiac arrest requires considerable technical support and experience. It is remarkable that the procedure can be fully operational in less than 10 minutes after it is requested (Mattox and Beall, 1976; Phillips et al., 1983). Despite rapid availability and restoration of circulation, the lack of effective resuscitation before institution of CPB reduces the ability to preserve neurologic or cardiac function. Because of these limitations, CPB may have limited value for patients who sustain out-of-hospital cardiac arrest or require more than 30 minutes of conventional CPR (Hartz et al., 1990; Tisherman et al., 1991; Martin et al., 1998). The patient who arrests in the operating room may be the ideal candidate for CPB rescue because intervention and application of CPR are usually immediate. For many patients, extracorporeal membrane oxygenation (ECMO) can extend the CPR duration to 50 to 60 minutes with an acceptable survival and neurologic outcome rates (del Nido et al., 1992; Dalton et al., 1993; Duncan et al., 1998; Chen et al., 2003).

The anesthesiologist can make a decision about attempting CPB rescue of cardiac arrest that is based on the reversibility of the cause of arrest and the effectiveness of the ongoing CPR. A patient with a cardiac arrest from a very reversible cause, with immediate and effective CPR, may be helped by CPB rescue even if the CPR has been longer than 60 minutes.

VASCULAR ACCESS FOR DRUG AND FLUID ADMINISTRATION

PERIPHERAL AND CENTRAL VASCULAR ACCESS

Emergency situations require prioritization of events and escalation to invasive measures (Fig. 33–1). Vascular access is crucial to

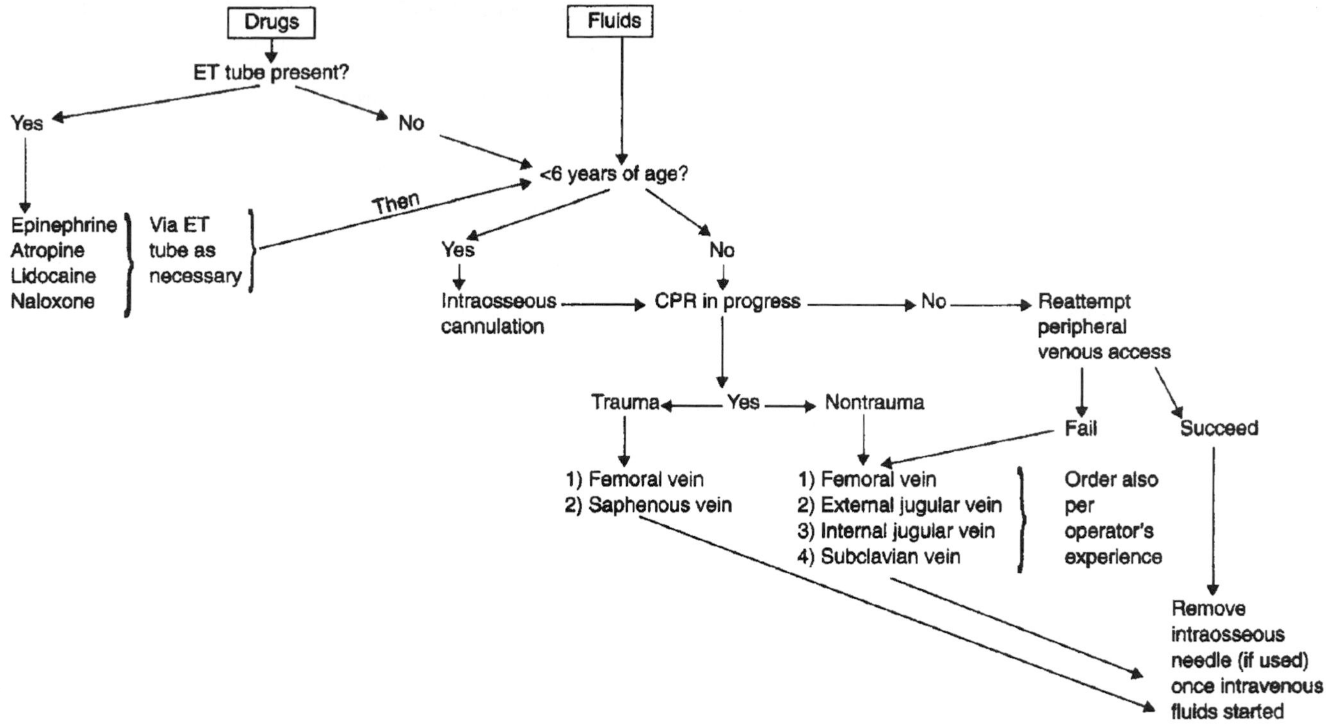

■ **FIGURE 33–1.** Algorithm for peripheral vascular access during emergencies in pediatric patients. (From Chameides L, Hazinski MF, editors: Vascular access. In *Pediatric advanced life support.* Dallas, TX, 1997, American Heart Association.)

the effective administration of drugs and fluids for resuscitation but may be difficult to achieve in pediatric victims. During cardiac arrest, attempts to obtain peripheral venous access in infants and children should be limited to 90 seconds. After 90 seconds, an intraosseous catheter should be placed, percutaneous central venous access attempted, or the administration of drugs in the TT started.

During CPR, the optimal location of intravascular catheterization provides ready access to the anesthesiologist and minimizes the interruption of resuscitation efforts. Peripheral venous access, femoral central access, and intraosseous access can usually be accomplished without interruption of airway management or chest compressions. The use of a saline flush for medications administered in peripheral access, intraosseous access, and central lines with the catheter tip below the diaphragm improves drug delivery to the heart in the low-flow state of CPR. A flush with 5 to 20 mL of normal saline administered into the catheter should drive the medication up the vein into the central circulation (0.25 mL/kg was effective in an animal model). For most CPR events, peripheral vascular access should be adequate for resuscitation medication if obtainable (see Table 33–5).

INTRAOSSEOUS ACCESS

Intraosseous cannulation provides a rapid, safe, and reliable route to vascular access via the marrow venous plexus. Intraosseous access can be accomplished within 30 to 60 seconds (American Heart Association, 2000). All drugs, crystalloids, colloids, and blood can be administered via this route. The preferred site of placement is the anterior tibia, but other sites include the distal femur, medial malleolus, iliac crest, and, in older children and adults, the distal radius, distal ulna, proximal tibia, and sternum (risk of cardiac laceration) (Glaeser et al., 1993; Guy et al., 1993; Waisman and Waisman, 1997; Calkins et al., 2000) (Fig. 33–2). Specially designed intraosseous needles should be readily available in the operating room for such emergencies. Complications from intraosseous placement are rare (<1% of patients) but include bone fracture, compartment

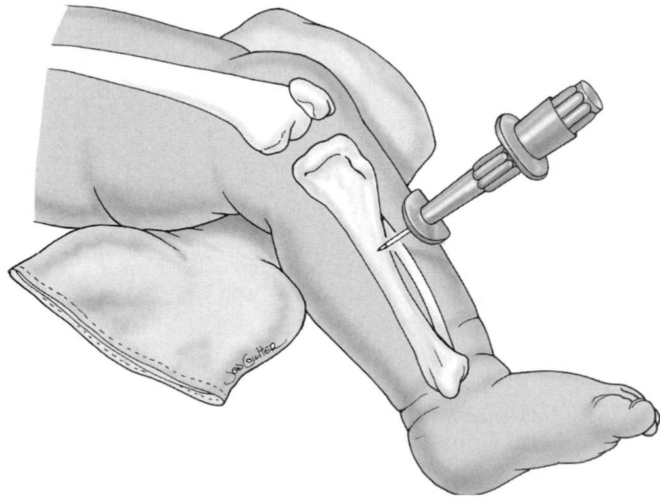

■ **FIGURE 33–2.** Intraosseous needle insertion into the proximal tibia.

syndrome, fluid extravasation, osteomyelitis, and fat embolism (Orlowski et al., 1989).

INTRATRACHEAL ACCESS

Intratracheal administration of drugs may be used for lipid-soluble resuscitation drugs. As most anesthetized children have this route available, it must be considered early, especially if vascular access is a problem. Drugs that can be administered via the trachea are **l**idocaine, **e**pinephrine, **a**tropine, and **n**aloxone (remember the pneumonic "LEAN"). Animal studies suggest that standard intravenous doses given via the trachea achieve serum concentrations approximately 10% of that of intravenously administered drugs (Kleinman et al., 1999); the recommended intratracheal dose of epinephrine is 10 times the intravascular dose. The technique for administration is to flush the drug with 2 to 5 mL of normal saline into the endotracheal tube and provide five manual ventilation breaths to deliver the medication into the distal airways and alveoli. This technique is favored over catheter or feeding tube delivery because of ease and practicality (Jasani et al., 1994).

FLUID RESUSCITATION

Based on the initial findings of the POCA Registry (Morray, 2000), hemorrhage and inadequate fluid therapy accounted for 41% of arrests and contributed to 18% of reported pediatric deaths from cardiac arrest. Postarrest fluid status can often be difficult to evaluate, necessitating the need for more invasive monitoring (such as an arterial and central venous catheters) and secure large-bore vascular access for continued resuscitation. In the setting of hemorrhage or surgical bleeding, for every 1.5 mL/kg lost, 5 mL/kg of isotonic fluid or 1:1 mL/kg of red blood cells should be administered (Barcelona and Coté, 2001). Such bleeding, if anticipated, often necessitates a large-bore catheter to permit such rapid fluid and blood product administration. Complications of any fluid resuscitation, whether colloid or crystalloid, are electrolyte abnormalities, hypothermia, metabolic abnormalities, coagulopathies, and hemoglobin abnormalities (both high and low).

Isotonic crystalloid solutions are preferred for volume expansion. Normal saline or Ringer's lactate should be used. Early volume expansion has been shown to prevent progression of patients to shock and cardiac arrest (Carcillo et al., 1991). Dextrose-containing fluids should not be used for the initial fluid resuscitation because of the complications of hyperglycemia and secondary osmotic diuresis. Further, hyperglycemia prior to cerebral ischemia may worsen neurologic outcome (Cherian et al., 1997). Dextrose-containing fluids should be used to treat documented or suspected hypoglycemia (see section on glucose). The use of colloid fluids (e.g., albumin, dextran, hetastarch, etc.) has the theoretic benefit of improving oncotic pressure as well as volume expansion, although studies have failed to prove a clear benefit over crystalloid (Schierhout and Roberts, 1998). Caution should be taken in aggressively fluid-resuscitating a postarrest patient with poor urine output as acute tubular necrosis or other forms of renal insufficiency often occur. If low blood pressure and poor perfusion persist after adequate pharmacologic and fluid resuscitation, other causes should be sought and consideration given to evaluation of cardiac function (pulmonary artery catheter placement, echocardiogram, or both).

ELECTRICAL INTERVENTIONS IN ARREST

PACING

Physiology of Bradycardia

Bradyarrhythmias are frequent complications in children in the perioperative period. Bradycardia is the rhythm seen most often before cardiac arrest in pediatric patients. Most bradycardic events are precipitated by hypoxemia, vagal stimuli, or the side effects of medications. In the operating room, hypoxia and the depressant effects of anesthetic agents were identified as the probable causes of intraoperative arrest (Morray, 2000). Sinus bradycardia results from slowed or suppressed sinoatrial node depolarization. However, other pathologic causes can occur and should be considered in the settings of trauma, cardiac surgery, and structural heart disease. A sufficiently slow heart rate in an infant or a child that results in hemodynamic instability and fails to respond to ventilation, oxygenation, epinephrine, atropine, and chest compressions is an indication for electrical pacing. The probability of successfully pacing after cardiac arrest decreases with increasing duration of CPR (Quan et al., 1992; Beland et al., 1988). If a bradyarrhythmia persists despite resuscitative and electrical support, other forms of cardiovascular support should be sought, such as cardiopulmonary bypass or extracorporeal membrane oxygenation therapies. These therapies, although not curative, can provide the time needed to diagnose the cause and allow time for recovery (Fig. 33–3).

Sinus Bradycardia

Great variability exists in infant and pediatric heart rates (see Table 33–4). Lower limits of heart rates serve as guidelines but may not be indicative of pathology. Diagnosis of sinus bradycardia implies a normal p wave is present on 12-lead ECG evaluation. Hemodynamic instability may or may not be present and is not essential for the diagnosis. Underlying etiologies should be sought, such as increased vagal tone (from suctioning), elevated intracranial pressure, hypoxia, metabolic abnormalities (hypokalemia or hypercalcemia), and drug effects.

Sinus and Atrioventricular Block

Sinus block or sinus node arrest is characterized by absence of p waves from the ECG and are usually related to a toxic ingestion or underlying cardiac disease. This can also present as asystole. Often suppression of the sinus node results in activation of extranodal pacing with variable electrical activity. Recognition and prompt initiation of transcutaneous pacing are crucial and can be lifesaving (Beland et al., 1998).

Various degrees of heart block will appear as a bradyarrhythmia (Fig. 33–4*A*). Often, 12-lead ECG is needed to diagnose properly the changes in the PR interval and potential conduction delays. First-degree heart block is the prolongation of the PR interval beyond normal. Normal PR interval can vary with age and is usually less than 0.16 second. Such prolongation can be normal or a sign of underlying disease or medication effects. Most patients with first-degree heart block are hemodynamically stable and require monitoring for progression to other forms of heart block. No emergent intervention is required.

Second degree AV block is characterized by the frequent occurrence of a p wave without a QRS complex. Progressive lengthening of the PR interval until this occurs is called a Wenkebach (Mobitz type 1) rhythm (Fig. 33–4*B*). If the QRS complex is repeatedly absent without a change in the PR interval, it is a Mobitz type 2 rhythm (Fig. 33–4*C*). Both are forms of second-degree heart block caused by delayed or absent conduction through the AV node. Some medications, hypoxia, myocarditis, and other conditions can create this problem. As long as the ventricular rate maintains adequate perfusion, no immediate treatment is necessary and diagnosis with elimination of the causative factor can be curative. However, if the patient is not stable hemodynamically, attempts to increase conduction by increasing heart rate with atropine or epinephrine may be useful and a pediatric cardiologist should be consulted.

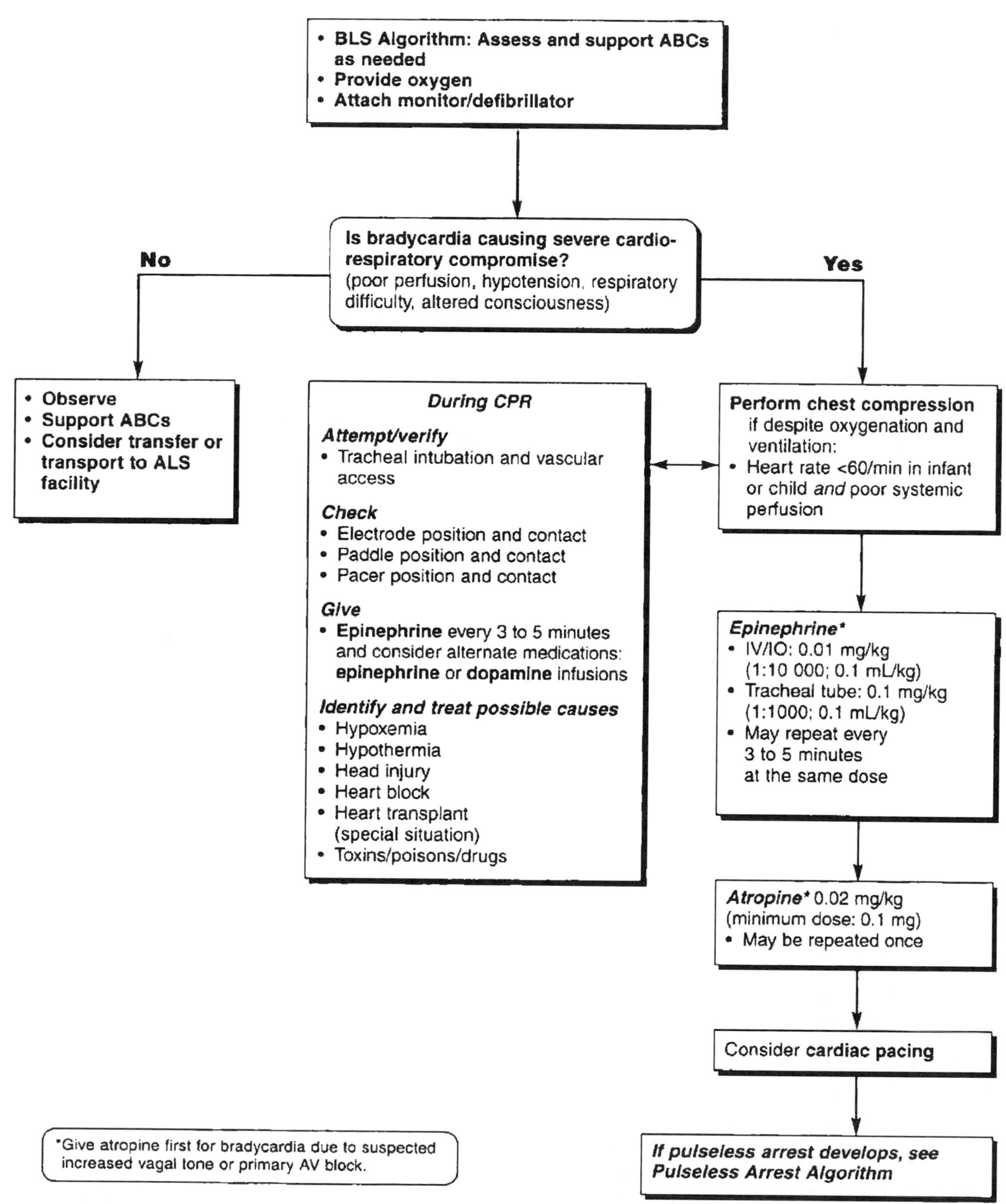

■ **FIGURE 33–3.** PALS bradycardia algorithm.

■ **FIGURE 33–4.** Arrhythmias from delayed atrioventricular node conduction.

A) First degree heart block.

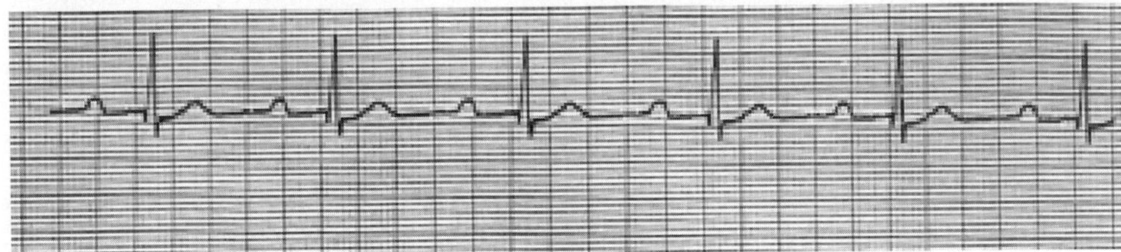

B) Second Degree Heart Block, Type 1: Wenckebach/Mobitz 1

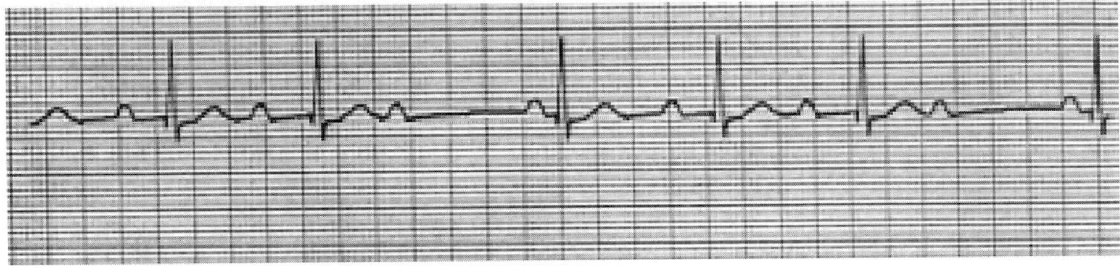

C) Second Degree Heart Block, Type 2/ Mobitz 2

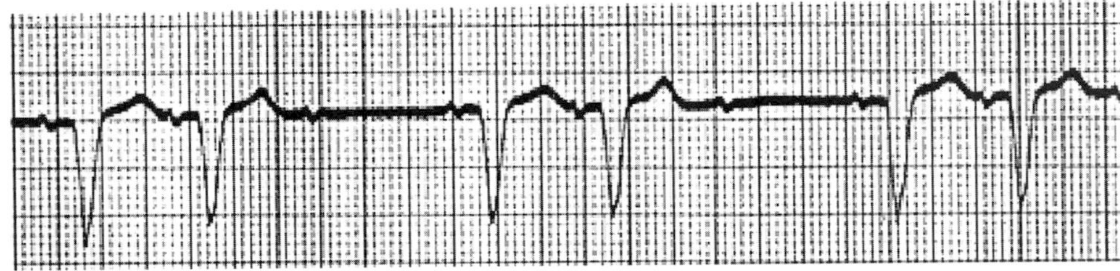

D) Third degree – complete heart block.

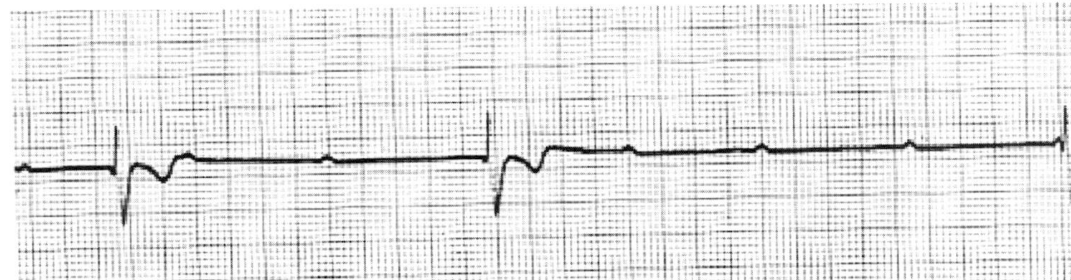

Third-degree AV block, or complete heart block, is characterized by electrical and mechanical dissociation between the atrial and ventricular rates (see Fig. 33–4*D*). ECG analysis demonstrates p waves at one rate and QRS complexes at a separate rate. As with other forms of heart block, finding and eliminating the causative agent is curative. If the patient is hemodynamically stable, observation is often suitable. However, if the rhythm becomes unstable, some form of supportive pacing is required. If the third-degree block is congenital in origin or is persistent from surgical correction of a congenital heart lesion, a permanent pacemaker is often required.

Treatment of Bradycardia

The treatment of all causes of bradycardia should focus on the underlying causes. If the patient is hemodynamically unstable, immediate measures should be taken to improve the heart rate. The first line of therapy is administration of a vagolytic agent and stopping all sedatives/medications that may be aggravating the bradycardia. The POCA Registry demonstrated epinephrine with or without atropine was most successful in returning stable heart rate and circulation (Morray, 2002). If the patient is hypoxic, improved oxygenation and oxygen delivery often result in improvement in heart rate. Bradycardia secondary to vagal stimulus can be treated by the removal of the stimulus and the administration of a vagolytic agent. Further treatment with adrenergic agents, such as epinephrine, is reasonable and effective. Epinephrine may be the first-choice treatment for bradycardia if severe hypotension is present. Severe hypotension refers to inadequate cerebral or myocardial perfusion. Prior recommendations had included use of isoproterenol, a potent β-selective adrenergic agent, to provide "chemical" pacing. However, because of its tendency to vasodilate resulting in inadequate coronary perfusion, it is no longer recommended and the next line of therapy is electrical pacing (see Fig. 33–3).

Transcutaneous/Transesophageal Pacing

Most modern defibrillator/cardioversion units have the capability for cardiac pacing. For transcutaneous pacing, the external pacing electrodes should be positioned anteriorly on the left sternal border and posteriorly between the scapulae. For most resuscitative efforts, the demand mode (not sensing) is selected for overdrive pacing. Initial settings should be set at the desired age appropriate rate, and the output set at zero. The output should then be increased rapidly until capture or pacing occurs. Note that the required output is usually "relative" and not in a defined milliamperage (mA) like epicardial or transvenous pacer units. Once electrical capture is seen on the monitor, mechanical association should be assessed by palpation of a pulse (Beland et al., 1988).

Transesophageal pacing is another minimally invasive technique. Lead positioning is technically more challenging and can be uncomfortable depending on the level of consciousness of the infant or child. Positioning can be confirmed by ECG monitoring with an arm lead attached to the esophageal electrode, by chest radiograph, by clinical response of electrical capture, or by a combination. Because of the higher electrical output required, ventricular capture rarely occurs with a conventional epicardial pacer unit. A defibrillator/cardioversion unit should be used for transesophageal pacing as described for transcutaneous pacing to obtain electrical capture. Although both transcutaneous and transesophageal methods can be used to overdrive pace complex supraventricular tachycardia (SVT), the transesophageal electrode also has diagnostic use. Diagnostic and therapeutic consultation with a cardiologist is usually warranted.

Transvenous Pacing

When transcutaneous pacing fails to provide results, transvenous pacing is often attempted in adults. Experience with transvenous pacing techniques in children has primarily occurred in the catheterization laboratory. Limited data are available using this technique in children during CPR. One study retrospectively reviewed experience with five children with various etiologies for cardiac arrest. Four of the patients had restoration of cardiac output and stability for 10 to 60 minutes with subsequent arrest and death (Greismann et al., 1995). The pacing wire can be placed via a vascular introducer into the right atrium or right ventricle. The techniques for setting the output and sensitivity are then the same as for the epicardial pacing leads. Although there is limited published experience, many anesthesiologists and intensivists attempt such interventions as a bridge to more definitive or supportive therapy.

Epicardial Pacing

Many infants and children undergoing cardiac surgery have atrial and ventricular epicardial pacing wires placed during the procedure for postoperative management. During resuscitation, if both atrial and ventricular leads are available, the ventricular leads should be used to maintain cardiac output. Note that most pacemaker generators can sense as well as pace depending on the mode. It may be necessary to adjust the sensitivity and output to produce ventricular depolarization with every paced beat. Pacing in asynchronous ventricular fixed-rate or ventricle-inhibited pacing ensures the most consistent cardiac output. Again, electrical activity should be monitored for electrical association and pulses or arterial waveform monitored to evaluate the mechanical results.

For routine use in the postoperative period, the pacer is often attached with the output at 0 mA and sensitivity at 0 mA. For initial testing of the pacemaker, the rate of the pacer should be set 20 beats per minute higher than the monitored rate. The sensitivity can then be increased until the pacing unit indicates adequate sensing with every stimulus. Then the pacer output can be adjusted up until electrical capture is seen on the monitor. The pacer rate can be adjusted down to an age appropriate backup rate, and the output turned up (by several mA) to provide a margin of safety if emergent pacing is required.

CARDIOVERSION

Physiology of Tachycardia

The analysis of a tachyarrhythmia must discriminate between a supraventricular, junctional, or ventricular etiology. The source of the reentrant or excitable focus creates variations of wide or narrow QRS complexes. Those tachycardias with narrow complexes (<0.08 second) are often atrial or high junctional (between the atria). Sinus tachycardia is the most common tachycardia seen in the pediatric patient during anesthesia. This may be brought on by pain, hyperthermia, light anesthesia, hypercarbia, hypoxia, and hypoglycemia. Most often, these events are limited. It is not uncommon to have a child with a heart rate 20% to 30% above baseline in the postoperative period because of these various factors. However, many common pathologic tachycardias present in the perioperative period that must be recognized and distinguished from sinus tachycardia. Often, a 12-lead ECG is required along with evaluation and elimination of the possible causes. SVT, atrial fibrillation, atrial flutter, and junctional ectopic tachycardia (JET) present with narrow QRS complex. Ventricular tachycardia, often surprisingly well tolerated by pediatric patients, usually presents with widened QRS complex.

Supraventricular Tachycardia

SVT is the most common tachyarrhythmia and nonarrest arrhythmia in children and is the most common arrest arrhythmia in infancy (Fig. 33–5). The cause is often a reentrant mechanism producing a rapid and narrow QRS complex (<0.08 second) on ECG. Rates are greater than 220 beats per minute in infancy and greater than 180 beats per minute in childhood. Ability of

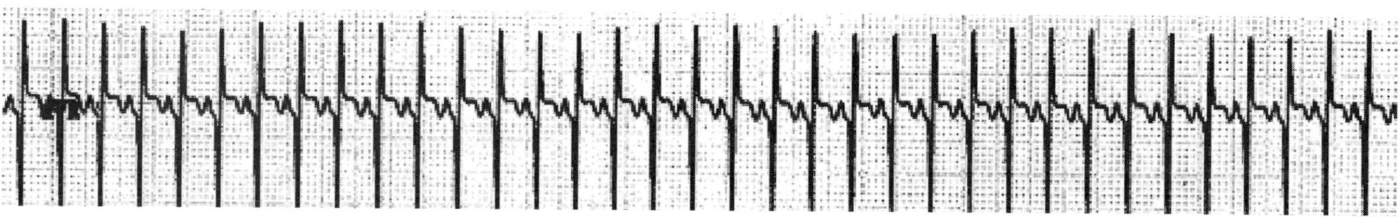

■ **FIGURE 33–5.** Supraventricular tachycardia.

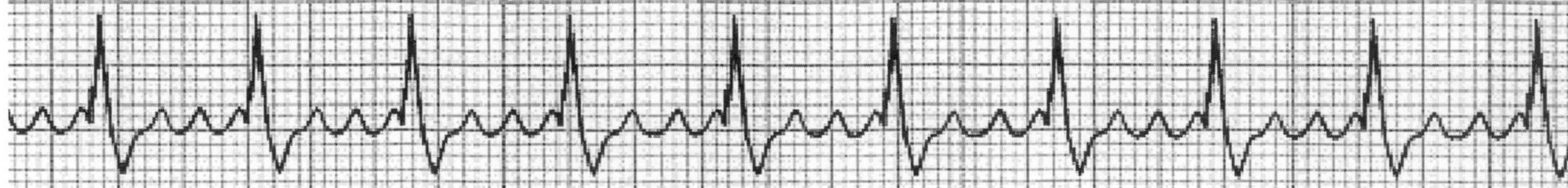

■ **FIGURE 33–6.** Atrial flutter.

a pediatric patient to tolerate the arrhythmia depends on prior diseases, possible initiating factors, and duration of the SVT event. In infants, the presenting signs are irritability and poor feeding. Older children often complain of lightheadedness, fatigue, and sometimes chest discomfort. In anesthetized patients, the difficulty often is in differentiating the rhythm from sinus tachycardia. In this situation, it is important to rule out possible causes of sinus tachycardia such as fever, pain, hypovolemia, hypoxia, hypercarbia, and myocardial failure. If the patient becomes hemodynamically unstable, synchronized cardioversion is the treatment of choice. The initial dose is 0.5 to 1 J/kg. If SVT persists or recurs after countershock, additional synchronized cardioversion can occur with the dose increased to 2 J/kg. If vascular access is available, adenosine (see Adenosine) can be attempted but no delays for vascular access should occur.

In a stable pediatric patient with SVT, vagal maneuvers can be the first line of therapy. Gag and diving reflex can be attempted. Ocular rubs are no longer recommended because of the risk for ocular trauma. Intraoperatively, some of these maneuvers are unavailable. Ice applied to the face, Valsalva maneuvers, and carotid sinus massage have potential benefit and may be attempted until adenosine dosing is prepared (see Adenosine). An electrical intervention can be overdrive pacing with an esophageal or epicardial lead. Failure of these methods may indicate a more complex arrhythmia and necessitate consultation with a pediatric cardiologist.

Atrial Fibrillation/Atrial Flutter

Atrial flutter and fibrillation are extremely rare in children (Figs. 33–6 and 33–7). Atrial flutter is often a rapid and regular rhythm, and in children, it is often associated with structural heart disease. The underlying physiology is a macroreentry phenomenon creating a rapid, regular tachycardia. Atrial rates of 200 to 500 beats per minute are usually present, and "sawtoothed" waves or f waves are present on the ECG.

Atrial fibrillation is a rapid, irregular tachycardia. Atrial rates can be as high as 600 beats per minute. The rhythm occurs because of multiple microreentrant circuits in the atria creating the variable ventricular response and irregular atrial rate. Treatment options are variable and depend on the underlying structural etiology. If the rhythm is sustained and stable, consultation with a pediatric cardiologist should be sought. If unstable, synchronized cardioversion with 0.5 to 2 J/kg is treatment of choice.

Anesthesiologists are often consulted to provide sedation or anesthesia during elective cardioversion. Of importance are the duration and level of anticoagulation that should be present in these patients to help decrease the risk of atrial thrombus formation. Heparin or coumadin or both are often used and should be considered if the atrial fibrillation/flutter has been present for longer than 2 days. Presence of clot can often be excluded by transthoracic or transesophageal echocardiography but is not absolute. Chemical conversion with amiodarone and/or ibutilide may be an alternative consideration in those patients with clot or stable atrial fibrillation or flutter (Bernard et al., 2003).

Junctional Ectopic Tachycardia

JET is seen in the days following cardiac surgery for congenital heart disease. It is narrow and rapid with complete AV dissociation resulting in a ventricular rate that is more rapid than the atrial rate. Many describe the arrhythmia as a narrow-complex SVT brought on by increased automaticity of the AV node or in the bundle of His. Occasional atrial beats are conducted through to the ventricles depending on the timing of the electrical pulse. Hemodynamic instability depends on the heart rate and degree of AV dissociation. If there is no instability, there is no need for treatment. However, as cardiac output becomes diminished, more aggressive treatment is warranted. Current treatment involves elimination of painful stimuli, metabolic acidosis, electrolyte abnormalities, and fever. Further interventions involve cooling the child, intravenous amiodarone (see Amiodarone) and pacing the atria at an increased rate to provide improved atrial synchrony and forward blood flow. These efforts are supportive until the JET rhythm resolves over 2 to 4 days (Hoffman et al., 2002).

Ventricular Tachycardia

Ventricular tachycardia (VT) is defined as a rapid, wide-complex QRS tachycardia (Fig. 33–8). The etiology of the tachycardia is below the bifurcation of the bundle of His. This can result from either a reentrant phenomena or increased automaticity. At a minimum, there are three wide QRS complexes in series with no evident p wave. When there are more wide-complex beats that

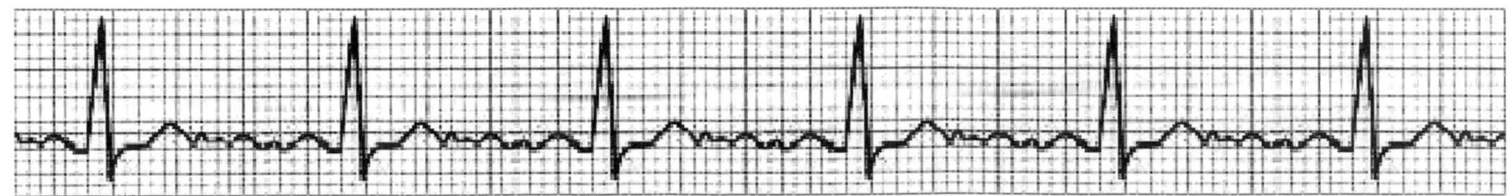

■ **FIGURE 33–7.** Atrial fibrillation.

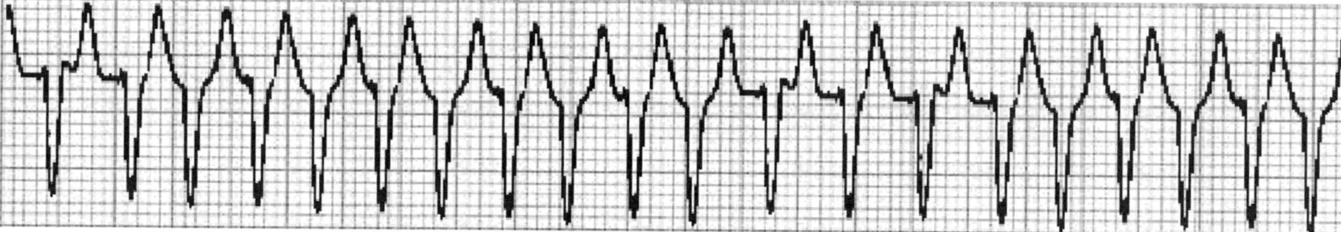

■ **FIGURE 33–8.** Ventricular tachycardia.

persist in runs of 30 seconds or greater, sustained VT is present. If there are unstable vital signs, VT should be treated emergently with synchronized cardioversion. Countershock should start with 0.5 to 1 J/kg and increase to 2 J/kg with subsequent countershocks (Fig. 33–9, Pediatric Advanced Life Support [PALS] algorithm for VT without pulse). If the patient is stable, then medical intervention with intravenous amiodarone can be attempted (Fig. 33–10, PALS algorithm for VT with pulse). After initial stabilization, electrolytes should be measured, medications reviewed for possible toxic/adverse effects, and potential structural or conductive abnormalities explored. Myocarditis and myocardial ischemia, although rare in pediatrics, should always be in the differential diagnosis.

Technique for Synchronized Cardioversion

Correct paddle size and position are important to the success of defibrillation. Three paddle sizes are available for external defibrillation: 13 cm in diameter for adults, 8 cm for older children, and 4.5 cm for infants. The largest paddle size that can be used without causing the paddles to touch should be used. The large surface area reduces the density of current flow, which reduces myocardial damage. However, if the entire paddle does not rest firmly on the chest wall, a high-density current is delivered to a small contact point on the skin. The paddles should be positioned on the chest wall with most of the myocardium included between them. If for some reason two paddles cannot be placed on the anterior chest, an alternate approach is to place one paddle anteriorly over the left precordium and the other paddle posteriorly between the scapulae.

The interface between the paddle and chest wall can be electrode cream, saline, paste, soap, or moist gauze pads. The cream produces lower impedance than does the paste. Care should be taken not to allow the substance from one paddle to touch that from the other paddle, as electrical current follows the path of least resistance. This is especially important in infants, in whom the distance between electrodes is very small.

The defibrillator/cardioversion unit should be set with "sensing" on. This mode permits coordination of the countershock with the electrical activity of the heart. Once the patient is adequately sedated (if necessary) and the paddles are positioned for optimal contact, the monitor should be indicating adequate sensing and charge set to deliver 0.5 to 1 J/kg. Once cardioversion occurs, a follow-up ECG should be obtained and the rhythm strip reviewed to identify the resulting rhythm. Repeat dosing with up to 2 J/kg is sometimes required with the same technique. Often other antiarrhythmic therapy can be initiated if the rhythm is transiently responsive to the cardioversion. For resistant tachycardias, hypoxemia, acidosis, hypoglycemia, and electrolyte abnormalities should be sought and corrected if present as they can interfere with the success of cardioversion.

■ DEFIBRILLATION

Physiology of Ventricular Fibrillation

Ventricular fibrillation (VF) is a sustained burst of multiple, uncoordinated regional ventricular depolarizations and contractions, resulting in an ineffective cardiac output and cessation of myocardial blood flow. Reentrant impulses, generated within the ventricles with multiple, shifting circuits, maintain VF. Several physiologic conditions lower the threshold for fibrillation, including hypoxia, hypercapnia, myocardial ischemia, hypothermia, metabolic acidosis, and electrolyte disturbances, including those of potassium, calcium, sodium, and magnesium. VF is a relatively uncommon rhythm during cardiac arrest in children. Typically, an initial ECG finding of a bradyarrhythmia, which progresses to asystole, is found. One study showed VF to be the initial rhythm in 19% of children presenting with cardiac arrest (Mogayzel et al., 1995). The etiologies of VF in that study were medical illness, toxic overdose, drowning, trauma, and congenital heart defect.

When either VT or VF with significant hypotension or absent pulses is present, electrical countershock is the treatment of choice (Fig. 33–11). Drug treatment by itself cannot be relied on to terminate VF. High-voltage electrical countershock, when correctly applied, sends more than 2 amps through the heart and can terminate VF by simultaneously depolarizing and causing a sustained contraction of the myocardium. This allows spontaneous cardiac contractions to commence if the myocardium is in a well-oxygenated environment with a normal acid-base status. The amount of myocardial damage produced by the countershock relates proportionally to the amount of energy delivered (Dahl et al., 1974; DiCola et al., 1976). In addition, the incidence of postdefibrillation arrhythmias increases as the energy dose increases (Peleska, 1963). Frequent, concentrated, high-density electrical current can damage the myocardium, decrease the likelihood of successful defibrillation, and lead to postdefibrillation arrhythmias (Weaver et al., 1982). These arrhythmias are thought to be associated with prolonged depolarization of the myocardial cell membrane, which increases with the intensity of the stimulus (Jones et al., 1978; Anderson et al., 1980) and provides an ideal setting for reentrant arrhythmias (Anderson et al., 1980).

Technique for Defibrillation

When the onset of VF is observed, defibrillation should be attempted as soon as possible. If three rapidly administered shocks of 2, 4, and 4 J/kg are unsuccessful, basic life support should be continued, epinephrine administered, and sodium bicarbonate given (if metabolic acidosis is documented or if the duration of cardiac arrest warrants its administration). If subsequent defibrillation attempts are necessary, 360 J of delivered energy to adults or 4 J/kg in children should be used. If VF is

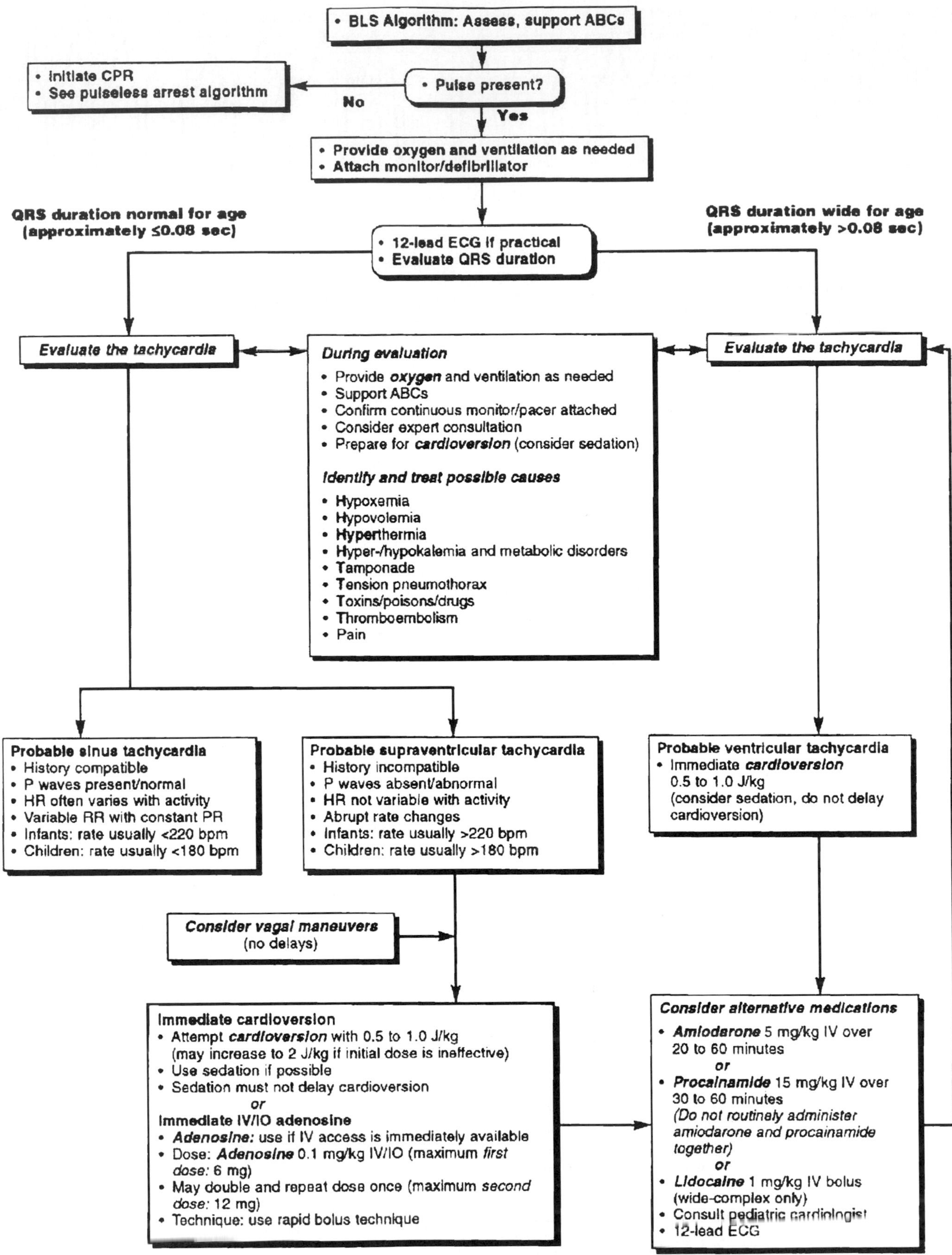

■ **FIGURE 33–9.** PALS tachycardia algorithm for infants and children with rapid rhythm and evidence of poor perfusion.

recurrent, an antiarrhythmic can be used (see later). It is not necessary to increase the energy dose for successive defibrillation attempts. On the contrary, the potential for successful defibrillation often increases after CPR and the administration of resuscitation medications improves the metabolic environment in the myocardium.

Open-chest internal defibrillation should be performed when the chest is already open during surgery or is reopened following surgery. Paddles made specifically for this purpose are applied directly to the heart. Internal paddles have a diameter of 6 cm for adults, 4 cm for children, and 2 cm for infants. The handles should be insulated. The paddles are applied with saline-soaked pads. One electrode is placed behind the left ventricle and the other over the right ventricle on the anterior surface of the heart. To perform open-chest defibrillation, a dose of 5 to 20 J of delivered energy should be used, beginning with the lowest energy level.

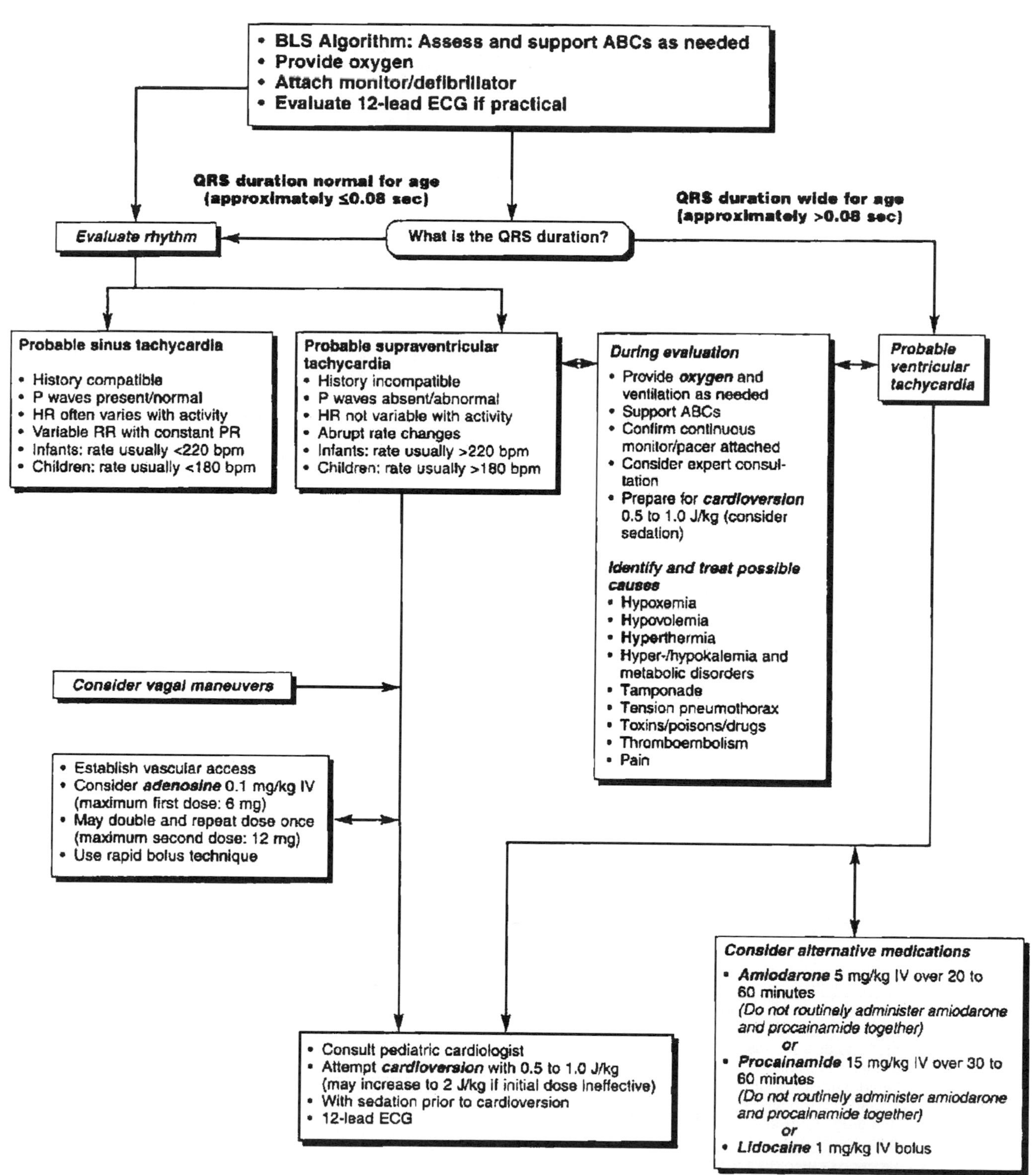

■ FIGURE 33–10. PALS tachycardia algorithm for infants and children with rapid rhythm and adequate perfusion.

The optimal dose of electrical energy required to defibrillate the heart of an infant or a child is not conclusively established. The available data suggest an initial dose of 2 J/kg for external defibrillation (no data exist for internal defibrillation doses in children) (Gutgesell et al., 1976). If the initial dose is unsuccessful, then a dose of 4 J/kg should be used on the second and subsequent attempts at defibrillation. The initial three defibrillation doses should be given in succession, followed by medication administration. This pattern can be maintained as either cycles of "CPR-drug-shock, CPR-drug-shock" or as "CPR-drug-shock-shock-shock." The technique for lead/paddle placement/paddle size is similar to synchronized cardioversion (see Technique for

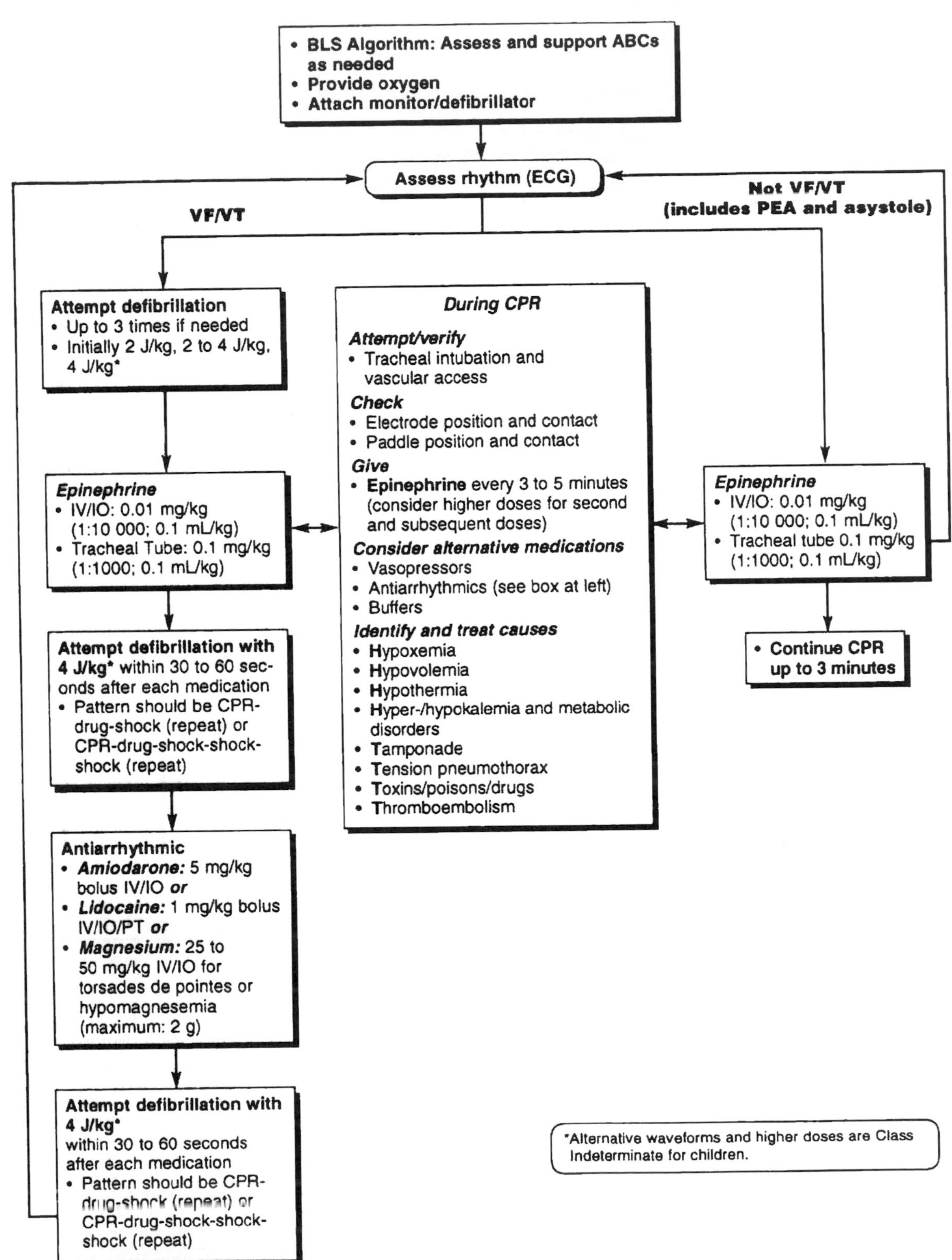

■ **FIGURE 33–11.** PALS pulseless arrest algorithm.

Synchronized Cardioversion). The major difference is that no sensing of the intrinsic rhythm is performed, and countershock is administered immediately on discharge of the device.

Defibrillators are available that use a biphasic waveform. This waveform variant appears to be more effective at producing defibrillation/cardioversion at lower dosages (Tang et al., 2002). The advantage of lower dose and potentially less risk of injury have made biphasic defibrillators appealing. Data are not available for lower dosages of shocks for defibrillation in pediatric patients.

Several clinical factors affect the success rate of ventricular defibrillation in humans. Success decreases with an increased duration of VF. Short fibrillation time is the most accurate predictor for successful defibrillation (Kerber and Sarnat, 1979; Pionkowski et al., 1983). Defibrillation attempts were successful in patients shocked within 8 minutes of fibrillation, whereas attempts were unsuccessful in patients shocked at an average of 17 minutes after the onset of VF (Kerber and Sarnat, 1979). A brief period of myocardial perfusion in dogs before electrical countershock improves cardiac resuscitation outcome after prolonged VF (Niemann et al., 1992). Acidosis and hypoxia also decrease the success of defibrillation (Kerber and Sarnat, 1979). The temperature of the patient does not alter the energy dose required for successful defibrillation (Tacker et al., 1981). Patients with terminal illness are more resistant to successful defibrillation (Gascho et al., 1979), as are those who fibrillate later in the course of a myocardial infarction.

■ AUTOMATED EXTERNAL DEFIBRILLATION

Automated external defibrillators (AEDs) are becoming the standard therapy for VF in the out-of-hospital environment because early defibrillation is the key to successful resuscitation for adult patients (Weaver et al., 1988). Current recommendations support the use of AEDs in early rhythm identification in children as young as 1 year. A retrospective review of 18 adolescents and children aged 5 to 15 years receiving AED treatment by emergency medical services crews showed accurate rhythm detection and shock delivery (Atkins et al., 1998). The use of AEDs has generally been limited to adults because of the lower incidence of VF in children. However, with the increasing recognition of VF as a cause of cardiac arrest in children, the use of AED for children may be more beneficial, resulting in the alteration of AED use from older than 8 years to older than 1 year (Atkins et al., 1998). The dosage delivered by most AED devices (150 to 200 J) exceeds recommended dosages for children younger than 8 years of age or weighing less than 25 kg. The risk of delivering a shock that may cause myocardial injury needs to be considered against the possibility of diagnosis and early treatment of VF. Low-energy (150-J) impedance-adjusted shocks for adults appear to be clinically safe and effective (Cummins et al., 1987). Studies have demonstrated biphasic waveform transthoracic defibrillation to be effective with lower energy levels in both adults and children (Samson et al., 2003). Triphasic waveform defibrillation is under investigation (Tang et al., 2002). These AED units continue to improve with the implementation of lower energy delivery and pediatric rhythm recognition software (Niskanen, 1997).

Pulseless Electrical Activity

Pulseless electrical activity (PEA) is a clinical state characterized by monitored electrical activity in the absence of detectable cardiac output. This is a preterminal condition that often leads to asystole. Typically, it is characterized by a slow wide-complex rhythm in a child without pulses who has experienced a prolonged period of hypoxia, ischemia, and/or hypercarbia. If the condition occurs rapidly, it may result from a reversible cause. This subcategory of cardiac arrest was previously described as electromechanical dissociation (EMD). Recognition and treatment of one of the four H's (**h**ypovolemia, **h**ypoxemia, **h**ypothermia, and **h**yperkalemia) or the four T's (**t**ension pneumothorax, pericardial **t**amponade, **t**hromboembolism to the lungs, and **t**oxins) often result in rapid relief of PEA.

Treatment

PEA should be managed according to the pulseless arrest algorithm (see Fig. 33–11). In the setting of the operating room, many episodes of PEA in children are fortunately related to treatable causes that, if promptly recognized and treated, result in survival.

■ PHARMACOLOGY OF RESUSCITATION

■ ANTIARRHYTHMIC AGENTS

Atropine

Clinical Effects

Atropine is a parasympatholytic agent that acts by reducing vagal tone to the heart. This results in the increased discharge rate of the sinus node, enhanced AV conduction, and activated latent ectopic pacemakers (Gillette and Garson, 1981). Atropine has minimal effects on systemic vascular resistance, myocardial perfusion, and myocardial contractility (Gilman et al., 1990).

Indications

Atropine is indicated for treatment of asystole, pulseless electrical activity, bradycardia associated with hypotension (Goldberg, 1974), ventricular ectopy, second- and third-degree heart block, and slow idioventricular rhythms (Scheinman et al., 1975). Atropine is a useful drug in clinical states associated with excessive parasympathetic tone. Acute myocardial infarction may augment parasympathetic tone and lead to arrhythmias (including asystole) that are responsive to atropine. In pediatric patients who present in cardiac arrest, bradycardia or asystole is commonly the initial rhythm and atropine is therefore a first-line drug for such patients. In infants, during the perioperative period, any type of stress (e.g., laryngoscopy) may result in severe bradycardia or even asystole secondary to enhanced parasympathetic tone. These conditions should be treated with atropine.

Dosage

The recommended adult dose of atropine is 0.5 mg IV given every 5 minutes until a desired heart rate is obtained or to a maximal dose of 2 mg. Full vagal blockade occurs in adults who receive a dose of 2 mg. For asystole, 1 mg IV should be given and repeated every 5 minutes if asystole persists. The pediatric dose for atropine is 0.02 mg/kg, with a minimal dose of 0.15 mg and a maximal dose of 2 mg. A minimal dose is necessary because of the possible occurrence of paradoxical bradycardia resulting from a central stimulating effect on the medullary vagal nuclei (Kottmeier and Gravenstein, 1968). Atropine may be given via any route: intravenous, endotracheal, intraosseous, intramuscular, or subcutaneous (intramuscular and subcutaneous routes may not have adequate perfusion and absorption during cardiac arrest or CPR). Onset of action occurs within 30 seconds and the peak effect occurs 1 to 2 minutes after an IV dose.

TABLE 33–10. First-line antiarrhythmic administration during cardiopulmonary resuscitation

Atropine	
Indications	Symptomatic bradycardia with AV node block Vagal bradycardia during intubation attempts After epinephrine for bradycardia with poor perfusion
Dose	0.02 mg/kg intravenous or intraosseous after ensuring oxygenation (2.5 times dose if given via TT) Repeat every 3 to 5 min at the same dose Maximum single dose 0.5 mg in a child and 1 mg in an adolescent Maximum total dose 1 mg in a child and 2 mg in an adolescent
Adenosine	
Indications	First line after vagal maneuvers fail for supraventricular tachycardia (SVT)
Dose	First dose 0.1 mg/kg rapid IV bolus, second dose increase to 0.2 mg/kg rapid IV bolus (maximum single dose, 12 mg) Note: Must be followed with 0.5 to 1 mL/kg normal saline flush over 1 to 2 seconds to have effect
Amiodarone	
Indication	Supraventricular and ventricular tachyarrhythmia
Dose	5 mg/kg IV over 20 to 60 minutes

Data from American Heart Association in collaboration with the International Liaison Committee on Resuscitation: Guidelines 2000 for cardiopulmonary resuscitation and emergency cardiovascular care. Part 10: Pediatric advanced life support. *Circulation* 102:I291, 2000.

Adverse Effects

Atropine should not be used in patients in whom tachycardia is undesirable. Following myocardial infarction or ischemia with persistent bradycardia, atropine should be administered in the lowest dose possible that increases heart rate. Tachycardia, which increases myocardial oxygen consumption and can lead to VF, is common after large doses of atropine in patients with myocardial ischemia. Caution should also be used when administering atropine to patients with pulmonary or systemic outflow tract obstruction or idiopathic hypertrophic subaortic stenosis as tachycardia can decrease ventricular filling and lower cardiac output (Table 33–10). Electrical pacing may be a safer means of maintaining a desired heart rate in these patients.

Adenosine

Clinical Effects

Adenosine is a purine nucleoside that is first-line treatment for SVT for children and adults. It is an endogenous molecule involved in the various precursors of adenosine triphosphate (ATP). Adenosine acts by binding directly to adenosine receptors in the myocardium and peripheral vasculature. Binding to the receptor initiates intracellular signaling via G proteins and results in a prolonged refractory period of the AV node and slowed conduction. This breaks the reentrant circuit responsible for most SVT (Crosson et al., 1994).

Clinical Indications

Treatment of narrow-complex QRS tachyarrhythmia (<0.08 second) with adenosine results in conversion to sinus rhythm in 75% of patients with few side effects. Adenosine can be used diagnostically to differentiate between VT and SVT. The half-life is <10 seconds because of rapid uptake by red blood cells and endothelial cells and metabolism by adenosine deaminase on the red cell surface. Adenosine is then completely cleared from the plasma in less than 30 seconds, giving it the rapid onset and short duration of action (Losek et al., 1999).

Dosage

A rapid primary bolus of 100 mcg/kg (maximum, 6 mg) is given. If SVT resumes or no electrical response is seen, another higher bolus of 200 mcg/kg (maximum, 12 mg) is given and may be repeated if no response is seen or there is a limited duration of effect. The technique of administration is critical for the success of the therapy. Central administration is preferable when available. A stopcock should be used with 10 mL of saline flush and the adenosine dosages drawn up. Thus, three saline doses and the progressively larger dosages of adenosine should be prepared and ready for administration. Each dose should be followed by a rapid injection of the 10-mL flush to drive the medicine centrally.

Adverse Effects

Reported complications are rare considering adenosine's frequency of use. Hypotension, bradycardia, and brief AV block have been reported. Less likely complications are bronchospasm, facial flushing, headache, dyspnea, chest pain, nausea, lightheadedness, complete AV block, and ventricular standstill. If complications do occur, they are often brief secondary to the short duration of action of adenosine. Note that doses may need to be increased in patients receiving methylxanthines (e.g., theophylline) because these agents are adenosine antagonists (see Table 33–10).

Amiodarone

Clinical and Pharmacologic Effects

Amiodarone hydrochloride is a diiodinated benzofuran derivative containing a diethylated tertiary amine chain. It is strongly lipophilic and has extensive tissue distribution. The drug is metabolized in the liver with mainly bile elimination. There is little renal elimination. Amiodarone has a long elimination half-life ranging from 20 to 47 days (Chow, 1996).

Amiodarone has a broad range of pharmacologic effects, including all four antiarrhythmic classes (Singh et al., 1989). It has potassium channel-blocking action, blocks the inward sodium current, is a noncompetitive b-blocker, and has calcium channel-blocking properties. Interestingly, its major electrophysiologic effect is dependent on the route (and duration) of administration (Bauman, 1997). With long-term treatment, its predominant activity is in its ability to increase the action potential duration in most cardiac tissue, a class III effect. When used acutely via the intravenous route, the drug increases AV node refractoriness and intranodal conduction interval time, class II antiadrenergic effect, or calcium channel blocker effect (Nattel, 1993). Additionally, amiodarone causes both coronary and systemic vasodilation (Coté et al., 1979). It does have phosphodiesterase inhibition (Harris et al., 1993) and is a selective inhibitor of thyroid hormone metabolism (Singh et al., 1989).

Clinical Indications

Amiodarone has been studied as both a prophylactic long-term medication for patients with high arrhythmogenic potential due to organic heart disease and for the use of acute life-threatening arrhythmias. It has been shown to be effective when lidocaine or bretylium was not for VT or VF in over

15 studies (Bauman et al., 1987; Helmy et al., 1988; Roberts et al., 1994; Podrid, 1995; Chow, 1996). When intravenous amiodarone was compared with placebo in a randomized trial (ARREST trial), there was significant improvement in the number of patients surviving to the emergency department following an out-of-hospital arrest (Gonzales et al., 1998). Amiodarone was shown to improve survival to admission when given to adults with out-of-hospital arrest and shock-resistant VF (Kudenchuk et al., 1999). A study comparing the efficacy of lidocaine with that of amiodarone for shock-resistant VF in out-of-hospital arrest demonstrated 15% versus 27% survival of adult patients to admission (Dorian et al., 2002). These adult studies further support the superior performance of amiodarone for ventricular arrhythmias.

Amiodarone has been studied in children with generally favorable outcome. Perry and others (1993) showed arrhythmia resolution in 6 of 10 children (mean age, 6.8 years) for whom multiple other antiarrhythmic agents had failed. Figa and others (1994) studied 30 infants and children with life-threatening arrhythmias, including SVT and VT. Arrhythmias were eliminated in 71% of patients, and an additional 23% experienced a significant improvement in clinical status and rhythm (Figa et al., 1994). Burri and others (2003) demonstrated safety and efficacy of treatment in infants. They treated 23 infants with hemodynamically unstable tachycardias. Of the infants treated, only one was unresponsive. Dosages ranged from 5 to 26 mcg/kg per min (mean, 15 mcg/kg per min). Adverse effects were seen in only four infants.

Dosage

There are limited data of amiodarone pharmacokinetics in children. Intravenous administration for active arrhythmias is common practice, followed by a continuous infusion and/or transition to oral medication if ongoing treatment is indicated. An initial intravenous dose of 5 mg/kg can be followed by additional doses or a continuous infusion of 5 mcg/kg per min. Increases in the infusion can occur up to a maximum of 10 mcg/kg per min or 20 mg/kg per 24 hr (Perry et al., 1996).

Adverse Effects

All of the adverse effects of amiodarone appear to be less frequent at lower dosages (Singh, 1996). Cardiovascular effects appear to be the most common and include hypotension due to the acute vasodilation and negative inotropic effects of the drug. Bradyarrhythmias, congestive heart failure, cardiac arrest, and VT have all been reported. Proarrhythmias, although possible, are seen less frequently than with other class III antiarrhythmic agents with an incidence of approximately 2%. Torsades de pointes occurs in one third of these cases (Perry et al., 1993). The most common noncardiovascular toxicities are pulmonary complications. Interstitial pneumonitis is the most frequent, usually associated with oral long-term treatment. A hypersensitivity pneumonitis can occur early in the course of treatment. Symptoms include cough, low-grade fever, dyspnea, weight loss, respiratory associated chest pain, and bilateral interstitial infiltrates. These symptoms are usually reversible upon cessation of the drug (Jessurun et al., 1998). Hepatotoxicity can occur and is more common with oral use. Thyroid dysfunction may occur in as many as 10% of patients resulting in either hypo- or hyperthyroidism. Optic neuritis or neuropathy resulting in decreased acuity or blurred vision can progress to permanent blindness. Neurologic symptoms include ataxia, tremor, peripheral neuropathy, malaise or fatigue, sleep disturbance, dizziness, and headache. Dermatologic reactions include allergic rash, photosensitivity, and blue-gray skin discoloration (Hilleman et al., 1998) (see Table 33–10).

Lidocaine

Chemistry

Lidocaine, a class 1B antiarrhythmic, depresses the fast inward sodium channel, which results in an increased refractory period and shortening of the total action potential. The drug is metabolized primarily in the liver by the microsomal enzyme system (Collinsworth et al., 1974). Up to 10% of the drug is excreted unchanged in the urine. The amount excreted unchanged increases in acidic urine. There is no biliary excretion or intestinal absorption in humans.

Electrophysiology

Lidocaine causes a decrease in automaticity and in spontaneous phase 4 depolarization of pacemaker tissue. The drug increases the VF threshold while having essentially no effect on the ventricular diastolic threshold for depolarization. It decreases the duration of the action potential of Purkinje fibers and ventricular muscle while increasing the effective refractory period of these fibers. Lidocaine does not affect conduction time through the AV node or intraventricular conduction time. By decreasing automaticity, lidocaine prevents or terminates ventricular arrhythmias caused by accelerated ectopic foci. Lidocaine abolishes reentrant ventricular arrhythmias by decreasing action potential duration and conduction time of Purkinje fibers, thus reducing the nonuniformity of action. The effect on ischemic tissues in which lidocaine delivery may be limited is unknown (Collinsworth et al., 1974).

Hemodynamic Effects

In animal models, rapid intravenous delivery of lidocaine causes a decrease in stroke work, blood pressure, systemic vascular resistance (Constantino et al., 1967), and left ventricular contractility (Austen and Moran, 1965) and a slight increase in heart rate. In healthy adults, the drug does not appear to cause any change in heart rate or blood pressure (Jewitt et al., 1968; Schumacher et al., 1968) but patients with cardiac disease have a slight decrease in ventricular function (Schumacher et al., 1969). In most patients, even in those who have sustained a recent myocardial infarction, a 1- to 2-mg/kg bolus of lidocaine does not alter cardiac output, heart rate, or blood pressure (Jewitt et al., 1968). Excessive doses of lidocaine given via rapid infusion may decrease cardiac function in patients with cardiac disease, especially in those with an acute myocardial infarction. Slow intravenous administration at no greater than 50 to 100 mg/min in adults is recommended (Collinsworth et al., 1974). When given to a patient with a normal heart, lidocaine usually causes few, if any, hemodynamic changes.

Antiarrhythmic Effects

Lidocaine is effective in terminating ventricular premature beats (VPBs) and VT in humans during the perioperative period of general or cardiac surgery, after an acute myocardial infarction, and in patients with digitalis intoxication. Treatment of VPBs after myocardial infarction is indicated if they are of unifocal origin occurring at a rate of more than five per minute, they occur on a normal T wave, they are multifocal, or if runs of VPBs occur (VT). Lidocaine is also effective in preventing and treating ventricular arrhythmias during cardiac catheterization. The drug is second-line therapy for VF, especially when VF or tachycardia recurs. Lidocaine is not effective in the treatment of atrial or AV junctional arrhythmias.

Pharmacokinetics

To achieve and maintain therapeutic levels of lidocaine, a bolus dose should be given at the initiation of a constant infusion. If an infusion is begun without an initial bolus, approximately five half-lives are required to approach a plateau serum concentration (half-life of 108 minutes) (Collinsworth et al., 1974). When a bolus administration is used alone, ventricular arrhythmias often return within 15 to 20 minutes because of its rapid clearance (Bartlett et al., 1984). Lidocaine toxicity with serum concentration greater than 7 to 8 mcg/mL occurs most commonly in patients with severe hepatic disease or severe congestive heart failure. Decreased cardiac output results in decreased hepatic blood flow, which leads to decreased lidocaine clearance. During CPR, lidocaine clearance is decreased because of the inherent decrease in cardiac output and very low hepatic blood flow. In dogs, with the use of conventional CPR to obtain a blood pressure of 20% of control values, an intravenous lidocaine bolus of 2 mg/kg resulted in very elevated blood and tissue concentrations. During CPR, distribution of the drug, which is usually complete in 20 minutes, was still not complete after 1 hour. In addition, lidocaine clearance and distribution may be altered owing to changes in protein binding and metabolism during CPR (Chow et al., 1983). In humans, high peak blood and tissue concentrations of lidocaine occur during CPR, with a delay in the time to peak concentration. Comparison of the peripheral, central, and intraosseous routes of administration of lidocaine during open-chest CPR in dogs revealed no difference in time to peak serum concentration (Chow et al., 1981).

Dosage

In patients with normal cardiac and hepatic function, an initial intravenous bolus of lidocaine 1 mg/kg is given, followed by a constant intravenous infusion at a rate of 20 to 50 mcg/kg per min (Table 33–11). If the arrhythmia recurs, a second intravenous bolus of the same dose can be given (Greenblatt et al., 1976). In patients with severe diminution of cardiac output, a bolus no greater than 0.75 mg/kg should be administered, followed by an infusion at a rate of 10 to 20 mcg/kg per min. In patients with hepatic disease, dosages should be decreased by 50% of normal. Patients with chronic renal disease on hemodialysis have normal lidocaine pharmacokinetics. Drug interactions with lidocaine are common. Phenobarbital increases lidocaine metabolism, requiring increased doses. Isoniazid and chloramphenicol decrease lidocaine metabolism, so a decreased dosage should be used. Any drug that decreases cardiac output (e.g., β-blockers) increases the serum concentration of lidocaine, whereas drugs (e.g., isoproterenol) that increase cardiac output and hepatic blood flow cause the serum concentration to be lower than predicted.

Adverse Effects

The toxic effects of lidocaine generally involve the central nervous system and include seizures, psychosis, drowsiness paresthesias, disorientation, muscle twitching, agitation, and respiratory arrest. Treatment for seizures and psychosis consists of a benzodiazepine or a barbiturate. True allergic reactions to lidocaine are extremely rare. Cardiovascular side effects (discussed earlier) are usually observed in patients whose myocardial function is already decreased. Conversion of second-degree to complete heart block has been described (Lichstein et al., 1973). Further slowing of sinus bradycardia has also been observed. These effects are infrequent and occur with large-dose administration. These potential side effects do not prohibit the use of lidocaine in these patients (see Table 33–11).

■ **TABLE 33–11.** Second-line antiarrhythmic administration during cardiopulmonary resuscitation

Lidocaine	
Indications	Ventricular arrhythmias (not ventricular escape rhythm) Suppress ventricular ectopy Raise threshold for fibrillation
Dose	1 mg/kg intravenous or intraosseous bolus (2.5 times dose if given via TT) 20 to 50 mcg/kg per min intravenous or intraosseous infusion Reduce infusion rate if low cardiac output or liver failure
Procainamide	
Indications	Refractory ventricular arrhythmias Possibly junctional ectopic tachycardia
Dose	5 to 15 mg/kg load intravenously or intraosseously over 30 to 60 minutes 20 to 80 mcg/kg per min intravenous or intraosseous infusion
Magnesium	
Indications	Torsades de pointes Hypomagnesemia
Dose	25 to 50 mg/kg intravenous or intraosseous (maximum, 2 g/dose)

TT, intratracheal route

Data from American Heart Association in collaboration with the International Liaison Committee on Resuscitation: Guidelines 2000 for cardiopulmonary resuscitation and emergency cardiovascular care. Part 10: Pediatric advanced life support. *Circulation* 102:I291, 2000.

Procainamide

Clinical Effects

Procainamide is a class IA antiarrhythmic agent and is metabolized to *N*-acetyl procainamide (NAPA), which has class III antiarrhythmic properties. Procainamide is a sodium channel-blocking agent that prolongs the refractory period of both atria and ventricles and slows the conduction velocity of the conducting system. This results in prolonged QT and PR intervals. Approximately 50% of the dose is excreted as unchanged drug and the other half is metabolized by *N*-acetylation in the liver (Elson et al., 1975). The efficacy and toxicity of procainamide has been linked to the activity of the *N*-acetyl transferase enzyme. Rapid acetylators have a significantly higher NAPA/procainamide ratio than do slow acetylators (Reidenberg et al., 1975). Reports in children have demonstrated potential benefit in the treatment of atrial fibrillation, flutter, and SVT, as well as the treatment of postoperative JET (Luedtke et al., 1997; Walsh et al., 1997). Despite its long history of use in children, there are little data to compare its effectiveness with that of other antiarrhythmic agents. In PALS recommendations, procainamide serves as a second- or third-line treatment for perfusing VT.

Dosage

An initial intravenous load of 5 to 15 mg/kg over 30 to 60 minutes is followed by an infusion of 20 to 80 mcg/kg per min. The infusion should be stopped if the QRS complex increases to greater than 50% of baseline, hypotension occurs, or both occur. Because the use of procainamide increases the likelihood of torsades de pointes, it should not be used in combination with other agents that prolong the QT interval, such as amiodarone. Both Walsh and others (1997) and Mandapati and others (2000) reported infusion rates of greater than 40 mcg/kg per min were necessary to cause decreases in heart rates greater than180 beats per minute. Therapeutic serum levels of procainamide are 4 to 10 mcg/mL, and procainamide plus NAPA is 10 to 30 mcg/mL. The medication can also be given intramuscularly and orally.

Adverse Effects

Reported complications of procainamide use in children are hypotension, arrhythmia (both bradyarrhythmias and tachyarrhythmias), and hepatotoxicity. Prolongation of the QT interval is a real and demonstrated complication of coadministration with other agents such as amiodarone. However, careful monitoring during administration and halting of infusion represents the treatment for most of the adverse effects. Patients on therapy should have blood levels monitored, with rising levels thought to be associated with a greater number of side effects (see Table 33–11).

Magnesium

Clinical Effects and Indications

Only two clinical scenarios are indications for emergent magnesium therapy in children: hypomagnesemia and polymorphic VT (torsades de pointes). Magnesium is an intracellular cation with less than 1% of the body's store available in the serum. The ionized fraction is physiologically active, much like calcium, and serves as a cofactor in enzymatic reactions. Low serum magnesium levels often develop in critically ill patients and patients post cardiopulmonary bypass. Whether the decline is caused by stress or creates any physiologic problems in many clinical scenarios is unknown.

Other situations have been studied, but the benefits of magnesium administration are controversial, such as myocardial ischemia, premature ventricular contractions and atrial arrhythmias, and asthma. Dorman and others (2000) and Dittrich and others (2003), in a randomized, double-blind prospective study, demonstrated that treatment with magnesium (whether via bolus or infusion) prevented falls in magnesium levels and resulted in a lower incidence of hemodynamically unstable arrhythmias than in the placebo groups. However, another study showed other interventions (such as amiodarone treatment) to be more efficacious in dealing with these same postoperative arrhythmias (Hoffman et al., 2002). The exact mechanism of magnesium on the conduction pathways of the heart is not known. Studies have demonstrated antagonism of calcium channels. Such "antagonism of calcium" has been shown to block the rise of intracellular calcium during periods of hypoxia.

Dosage

Treatment with magnesium sulfate starts with 25 to 50 mg/kg per dose (maximum, 2 g/dose) given intravenously over 20 to 30 minutes. Serum levels should be monitored, with some controversy regarding the usefulness of monitoring ionized levels. Note that 1 g of magnesium sulfate is equivalent to 4 mmol, 8 mEq, or 98 mg of elemental magnesium. Magnesium sulfate can be administered via the intravenous, intraosseous, and oral route.

Adverse Effects

A rapid rate of administration can cause a fall in systemic vascular resistance by as much as 30%. This hypotension can be treated by either slowing or stopping the dose. Apnea and weakness are possible complications but are not routinely seen until toxic levels of greater than 4 mmol/L. Potentiation of neuromuscular blockade and neuromuscular weakness has been reported at lower serum levels (see Table 33–11).

Bretylium

Bretylium is no longer part of the American Heart Association protocols for treatment of ventricular arrhythmias. Its removal is based primarily on the lack of supporting evidence for its continued use in the face of more effective treatments. Bretylium is included here in the discussion of CPR medications because of its historical and controversial significance.

Chemistry

Bretylium, a class III antiarrhythmic (prolongs phase 3 repolarization, prolonging the refractory period), is a bromobenzyl quaternary ammonia compound not structurally related to lidocaine. Its half-life gradually increases over time, with a mean elimination half-life of 9.8 hours (Romhilt et al., 1972). The drug is 80% excreted unchanged in the urine over the first 24 hours. An additional 10% of the drug is excreted in the urine during the next 72 hours (Kuntzman et al., 1970).

Mechanism of Action

The mechanism of action of bretylium is still controversial, but it appears to act by adrenergic stimulation. There is an initial release of norepinephrine from adrenergic nerve endings, with subsequent inhibition of norepinephrine release (Markis and Koch-Weser, 1971). There is also blockade of the reuptake of norepinephrine and epinephrine by adrenergic nerve endings, thereby potentiating the action of these agonists on adrenal receptors. Bretylium increases the action potential duration of cardiac muscle and increases the effective refractory period of Purkinje and ventricular muscle fibers. In dogs, bretylium decreases the disparity in action potential duration between normal and infarcted areas of the heart, probably the major physiologic explanation for its antiarrhythmic actions (Chatterjee et al., 1973). Bretylium also increases the VF threshold in normal and infarcted myocardium. It has been known to defibrillate a heart without electrical countershock (Bacaner, 1966).

Clinical Effects

Bretylium has been shown to be effective in suppressing ventricular arrhythmias when other antiarrhythmics are not, including VF resistant to electrical countershock (Zipes et al., 1975). There was no difference in out-of-hospital resuscitation of VF when the number of patients achieving a stable rhythm, the time needed to achieve that rhythm, the number of defibrillation shocks required, and the numbers of patients discharged from the hospital were compared. In that study, none of the patients were defibrillated with electrocardioversion (Bacaner, 1966).

Dosage

The dose of bretylium used to treat VF or VT is 5 to 10 mg/kg given via rapid intravenous bolus. If the drug can be given less urgently, 500 mg should be diluted in not less than 50 mL of fluid given over 10 minutes. The slower regimen decreases the incidence of nausea in the awake patient. Close monitoring, including an ECG and blood pressure, is critical during bretylium administration. Its onset of action in suppressing VF and facilitating electrocardioversion is within minutes, although it can be delayed by up to 10 to 15 minutes. After an intramuscular injection, the drug is effective in 20 to 60 minutes. Its duration of action is 6 to 12 hours (Haynes et al., 1981). After an intravenous dose of bretylium is given, an electrical countershock should be administered. If the arrhythmia then persists, the drug can be repeated every 15 to 30 minutes, up to a total dose of 30 mg/kg. If the arrhythmia is abolished, a maintenance dose, the same as the initial dose, can be given every 6 to 8 hours. In treating VT, the second dose should be repeated in 1 to 2 hours and then for maintenance every 6 to 8 hours. The drug can also be given by constant infusion at 1 to 2 mg/min in adults.

Adverse Effects

Hypertension due to norepinephrine release is the most commonly seen side effect due to bretylium (Bernstein and Koch-Weser, 1972). In addition, bretylium appears to have an inotropic effect (Markis and Kock-Weser, 1971). After the initial hypertensive response, more than half of the patients subsequently show a mild decrease in blood pressure including orthostatic changes (Koch-Weser, 1979) due to the adrenergic-blocking effects of bretylium (Markis and Koch-Weser, 1971). After receiving bretylium, a patient may have an exaggerated response to dopamine, norepinephrine, and epinephrine because of the impaired uptake of those drugs. With rapid infusions of the drug, nausea and vomiting are common. Parotid swelling and pain are complications of oral use of bretylium (Koch-Weser, 1979).

VASOACTIVE DRUGS

Adrenergic Agonists

Redding and Pearson (1963) first described the use of adrenergic agonists during CPR and demonstrated that early administration of epinephrine during cardiac arrest improved the success rate for resuscitation. They also demonstrated that the increase in diastolic pressure produced by administration of adrenergic agonist drugs was responsible for the success of resuscitation (Pearson and Redding, 1965). They theorized that vasopressors such as epinephrine were of value because they increase systemic vascular resistance. Since that time, epinephrine has been the drug of choice during CPR, without compelling evidence for a change in that role.

Yakaitis and others (1979) investigated the relative importance of α- and β-adrenergic agonist actions during resuscitation. Also using a canine model of arrest, they found only one in four animals receiving both the pure β-adrenergic agonist isoproterenol and an α-adrenergic antagonist was successfully resuscitated. In contrast, all the dogs treated with both an α-adrenergic agonist drug and a β-adrenergic antagonist were successfully resuscitated. These data suggest that the α-adrenergic agonist action of epinephrine is responsible for successful resuscitation after cardiac arrest. Further studies have confirmed this notion. Michael and others (1984) demonstrated that the effects of epinephrine during CPR are mediated by selective vasoconstriction of peripheral vessels, excluding those supplying the brain and heart. Epinephrine infusions maintain a higher aortic pressure and result in a higher perfusion pressure to both the heart and the brain (Michael et al., 1984). Even with the increase in both mean and diastolic aortic pressure, the flow to other "nonvital" organs, such as the kidneys and small intestine, becomes compromised because of intense vasoconstriction of their blood supply (Michael et al., 1984; Koehler and Michael, 1985b; Schleien et al., 1986).

Effects on Coronary Blood Flow

The increase and maintenance of aortic diastolic pressure associated with the administration of α-adrenergic agonists during CPR are critical for coronary blood flow and ultimately the rate of successful resuscitation. In the beating heart, the contractile state of the myocardium is increased by β-adrenergic receptor agonist action. During CPR, these drugs may stimulate spontaneous myocardial contractions and increase the intensity of VF. In the fibrillating heart, the inotropic effect of β-adrenergic agonists might be deleterious by increasing intramyocardial wall pressure (Livesay et al., 1978). This increased wall pressure contributes to decreased coronary perfusion pressure and diminished myocardial blood flow. In addition, β-adrenergic stimulation increases myocardial oxygen demand by increasing cellular metabolism and oxygen consumption. The superimposition of an increased oxygen demand on the low myocardial blood flow available during CPR probably contributes to ischemia.

Other α-adrenergic agonist drugs (such as methoxamine and phenylephrine) have been used successfully during CPR. As with epinephrine, the increase in aortic diastolic pressure results in an increased coronary blood flow. However, the absence of direct β-adrenergic stimulation avoids an increase in oxygen uptake by the myocardium, resulting in a more favorable oxygen demand-to-supply ratio in the ischemic heart. These nonepinephrine, α-adrenergic agonists have contributed to successful resuscitation (Redding and Pearson, 1963; Pearson and Redding, 1965; Yakaitis et al., 1979; Schleien et al., 1989) and maintain myocardial blood flow during CPR as effectively as epinephrine (Yakaitis et al., 1979). Schleien and others (1989) found that high aortic pressures can be sustained in a canine model of CPR with phenylephrine, a pure α-adrenergic agonist. The debate continues about the merits of pure α-adrenergic agonist drugs for resuscitation because of the confusion regarding the benefit versus detriment of the β-adrenergic effects of epinephrine (Brown et al., 1987a, 1987c; Holmes et al., 1980).

Effects on Cerebral Blood Flow

During CPR, the generation of cerebral blood flow, like coronary blood flow, depends on the vasoconstriction of peripheral vessels. This vasoconstriction is enhanced by administration of α-adrenergic agonists. Epinephrine and other α-agonist drugs produce selective vasoconstriction of noncerebral peripheral vessels to areas of the head and scalp (e.g., tongue, facial muscle, and skin) without causing cerebral vasoconstriction in adult (Koehler and Michael, 1985a, 1985b, Beattie et al., 1991) and infant models of CPR (Schleien et al., 1986). Infusion of either epinephrine or phenylephrine maintained cerebral blood flow and oxygen uptake at prearrest levels for 20 minutes in a canine model of CPR. This implies that blood flow was higher than that needed to maintain adequate cerebral metabolism (Schleien et al., 1989). There were no differences in neurologic outcome 24 hours after resuscitation when either epinephrine or phenylephrine was administered 9 minutes after VF (Brillman et al., 1985). Other investigators found epinephrine to be more beneficial in generating vital organ blood flow (Brown et al., 1986b, 1987, 1987c). This may have been due to the use of drug dosages that were not equipotent in generating vascular pressure and subsequent blood flow.

Cerebral oxygen uptake may be increased by a central β-adrenergic receptor effect if sufficient amounts of epinephrine cross the blood-brain barrier during or after resuscitation (MacKenzie et al., 1976; Carlsson et al., 1977). In addition, epinephrine may have either a vasoconstriction or vasodilation effect on cerebral vessels, depending on the balance between α- and β-adrenergic actions (Winquist et al., 1982). When cerebral ischemia is brief and the blood-brain barrier remains intact, epinephrine and phenylephrine have similar effects on cerebral blood flow and metabolism (Schleien et al., 1989). Catecholamines may cross the blood-brain barrier when mechanical disruption occurs or when enzymatic barriers to vasopressors (e.g., monoamine oxidase inhibitors) are overwhelmed during tissue hypoxia (Edvinsson et al., 1978; Lasbennes et al., 1983). During CPR, the blood-brain barrier may be disrupted owing to the generation of large fluctuations in cerebral venous and arterial pressures during chest compressions. In addition, the permeability of the barrier may increase because of the arterial pressure surge that occurs in a maximally dilated vascular bed after resuscitation (Arai et al., 1981). An increase in cerebral oxygen demand when cerebral blood flow is limited could affect cerebral recovery adversely. In an infant model of CPR producing 8 minutes of cardiac arrest, disruption of the blood-brain barrier was present 4 hours after defibrillation (Schleien et al., 1991). In similar protocols involving 8 minutes of cardiac arrest, endothelial vacuolization has been shown, with extravasation of protein through the blood-brain barrier (Schleien et al., 1992a). These theoretical effects of catecholamines on the cerebral circulation need to be further clarified and do not represent a contraindication to the administration of epinephrine during cardiac arrest.

Dosage

The administration of high-dose epinephrine is no longer recommended. Studies have examined the physiologic response of animals and humans to higher doses of epinephrine. Cerebral blood flow increases further in response to administration of larger doses of epinephrine (Brillman et al., 1985; Brown et al., 1986a; Berkowitz et al., 1991). Although myocardial and endocardial blood flow increases, animal models suggest that there is a disproportionate rise in myocardial oxygen consumption with high-dose epinephrine (Jackson et al., 1984; Maier et al., 1984; Brown et al., 1988a, 1988b; Ditchey and Lindenfeld, 1988). In a swine model, high-dose epinephrine failed to increase myocardial blood flow to levels achieved with a lower dose (Berkowitz et al., 1991). Studies in humans have been contradictory regarding survival of patients who were given high-dose epinephrine after cardiac arrest. In earlier studies, investigators were optimistic that higher doses of epinephrine would increase aortic diastolic pressure and therefore improve the return to spontaneous circulation compared with standard epinephrine doses. Gonzalez and others (1988, 1989) demonstrated a dose-dependent increase in aortic blood pressure for patients who failed to respond to prolonged resuscitation efforts.

Paradis and others (1990) showed increased aortic diastolic pressure and successful resuscitation for patients for whom advanced cardiac life support (ACLS) protocols failed. They also reported on seven pediatric patients treated successfully with 0.2 mg/kg of epinephrine (Goetting and Paradis, 1989). Other investigators have also reported higher aortic diastolic pressures and an improvement in ROSC (Martin et al., 1990; Paradis et al., 1990; Cipolotti et al., 1991). In these nonrandomized, unblinded studies, there were few survivors, although three patients survived in the pediatric study. Subsequently, three large multicenter studies were published that dampened the enthusiasm for the use of high-dose epinephrine.

Stiell and others (1992) reported on 650 adult patients who sustained cardiac arrest. These patients were randomly assigned to either a standard or a high-dose (7 mg) epinephrine protocol. High-dose epinephrine did not improve survival (18% versus 23% 1-hour survival; 3% versus 5% hospital discharge) or alter neurologic outcome. In a multicenter prospective study, Brown and others (1992) reported on 1280 adult patients who received either standard (0.02 mg/kg) or high-dose (0.2 mg/kg) epinephrine after cardiac arrest. Again, no differences were seen between groups in ROSC, short-term survival, survival to hospital discharge, or neurologic outcome between patients treated with a standard dose of epinephrine and those treated with a high dose. Callaham and others (1992), in a study of 816 adults, reported a higher rate of ROSC in the high-dose epinephrine group. However, there were no differences in the rate of hospital discharge or survival of these patients.

There is concern that high-dose epinephrine may account for some of the adverse effects that occur after resuscitation. High doses may worsen myocardial ischemia and result in arrhythmias, hypertensive crisis, pulmonary edema, digitalis toxicity, hypoxemia, and cardiac arrest (Brown et al., 1992; Schleien et al., 1992b). Tang and others (1991) showed that epinephrine induced a decrease in Pa_{O_2} and an increase in alveolar dead space ventilation, thought to be due to a redistribution of pulmonary blood flow, compared with an α-agonist.

In children, the dosing scheme is explicit. Higher doses are preferred when epinephrine is given through the endotracheal tube because of its decreased bioavailability. All endotracheal tube doses are 0.1 mg/kg (1:1000). To treat a pulseless arrest in children, the first and all intravenous or intraosseous doses are 0.01 mg/kg (1:10,000) repeated every 3 to 5 minutes (Table 33–12).

Other Adrenergic Agents

Dopamine and dobutamine are additional agents used for vasopressor support postarrest in infants and children. Guidelines for postresuscitation support advocate their use as they cause less tachycardia, myocardial ectopy, and hypertension in the postarrest patient. Dopamine hydrochloride is often used as an infusion of 2 to 20 mcg/kg per min. At higher doses (>10 mcg/kg per min rates), α-adrenergic activity is dominant and increases in blood pressure are observed. Dobutamine hydrochloride is another adrenergic agent used for inotropic support. Dobutamine infusions are maintained between 2 and 20 mcg/kg per min. Decreases in systemic vascular resistance can be observed with its predominant β-adrenergic effects (Table 33–13).

Phosphodiesterase Inhibitors

Amrinone and milrinone are increasingly used to support inotropic myocardial function during the perioperative period

■ TABLE 33–12. Epinephrine administration during cardiopulmonary resuscitation

Actions	Decreases perfusion to nonvital organs (α-adrenergic effect) Improves coronary perfusion (aortic diastolic pressure) (α-adrenergic effect) Increases intensity of ventricular fibrillation (β-adrenergic effect) Stimulates cardiac contractions (β-adrenergic effect) Intensifies cardiac contractions (β-adrenergic effect)
Indications	Bradyarrhythmia with hemodynamic compromise Asystole or pulseless arrest
Dosage	Bradycardia 0.01 mg/kg intravenous or intraosseous or 0.1 mg/kg TT Repeat every 3 to 5 min at the same dose Pulseless First dose 0.01 mg/kg intravenous or intraosseous or 0.1 mg/kg TT Repeat every 3 to 5 min.

TT, intratracheal route

Data from American Heart Association in collaboration with the International Liaison Committee on Resuscitation: Guidelines 2000 for cardiopulmonary resuscitation and emergency cardiovascular care. Part 10: Pediatric advanced life support. *Circulation* 102:I291, 2000.

in children undergoing congenital heart surgery. The benefits of these agents are multiple: increased inotropy (force of left ventricular contraction), increased dromotropy (speed and efficiency of myocardial conductive pathways), and increased lusitropy (left ventricular diastolic relaxation). There is no effect on chronotropy (rate of contraction). All of these effects are accomplished through nonadrenergic mechanisms; the impact on myocardial oxygen consumption is minimal. In addition, the risk of arrhythmias is lower. The side effects of these agents are predominantly on platelet function and decreases in systemic vascular resistance.

Because of the increased incidence of thrombocytopenia seen with amrinone, milrinone has become the drug of choice. Milrinone is usually administered with a loading dose of 50 mcg/kg over 30 minutes followed by an infusion of 0.5 to 1 mcg/kg per min. The benefits in the postoperative cardiac period at preventing low cardiac output states has been supported by a single double-blind randomized prospective study (Hoffman et al., 2003). In an animal model of CPR with fibrillatory arrest, the treatment with a loading dose and maintenance infusion of milrinone improved stroke volume and sustained rhythm after arrest (Niemann et al., 2003). There are no studies of this category of drug in adults or children in the postarrest period.

■ TABLE 33–13. Vasopressor infusions in the postarrest period

Agent	Dose	Comments
Epinephrine:	0.05 to 1.0 mcg/kg per min	Inotrope
Dopamine:	2 to 20 mcg/kg per min	Inotrope, chronotrope; dilates the splanchnic vasculature at lower doses, pressor effect at higher doses
Dobutamine:	2 to 20 mcg/kg per min	Inotrope, decreased SVR
Milrinone:	Load: 50 to 75 mcg/kg Infusion: 0.5 to 1 mcg/kg per min	Inotrope, improve diastolic relaxation, decreased SVR

Vasopressin

Clinical Effects. Renewed interest for the vasoconstrictor vasopressin has brought it into the CPR literature. Vasopressin is a pituitary hormone that binds to specific receptors located throughout the vasculature (V_1 receptors, vasoconstriction) and in the renal tubules (V_2 receptors, facilitate water reabsorption). L-Arginine vasopressin is the exogenously administered compound used to treat diabetes insipidus, gastric hemorrhage, and adult cardiac arrest. Both endogenous and administered vasopressin are cleared and inactivated from plasma during passage through the liver and kidneys. This results in an elimination half-life of about 10 to 20 minutes. Studies in both animals and humans show its efficacy in restoring a life-sustaining rhythm for cardiac arrest with VF (Lindner et al., 1993, 1995; Prengel et al., 1996b; Strohmenger et al., 1996) but not with pulseless electrical activity (Morris et al., 1997).

Mechanism of Action. For the treatment of VF, vasopressin has a theoretical advantage compared with epinephrine because it is a vasoconstrictor without adrenergic activity, so it does not increase oxygen demand at a time when oxygen delivery is limited. In addition, vasopressin should result in less ventricular ectopy and tachycardia in the postresuscitation period. These advantages may be offset by intense vasoconstriction following ROSC, potentially worsening myocardial ischemia (Prengel et al., 1996a, 1998; Wenzel and Lindner, 2002).

Dosage. No controlled study has shown improved survival in humans with vasopressin compared with epinephrine. One study showed improved ROSC with vasopressin. In an uncontrolled trial, vasopressin (40 units IV) was administered to eight adults with in-hospital VF in whom conventional resuscitation, including epinephrine, had failed. All eight patients recovered spontaneous circulation, and three were eventually discharged with intact neurologic function (Lindner et al., 1996). In an out-of-hospital randomized controlled trial comparing epinephrine with vasopressin (40 units IV) after an initial unsuccessful defibrillation attempt, there was a trend (14 of 20 versus 7 of 20, $P = 0.06$) toward more successful resuscitation with vasopressin. However, survival to hospital discharge was not different ($P = 0.16$) between the groups (Lindner et al., 1997).

In a prospective double-blind randomized study, the efficacy of 1 mg of epinephrine was compared against two injections of 40 U of vasopressin in adults with out-of-hospital arrest. Vasopressin and epinephrine were comparable in ROSC and hospital admission in those patients with VF and PEA. However, vasopressin was superior to epinephrine for patients with asystole (29.0% versus 20.3% in the epinephrine group, $P = 0.02$ for hospital admission; 4.7% versus 1.5%, $P = 0.04$ for hospital discharge). Further, a subgroup of 732 adults who failed to have return of circulation after vasopressin dosing were treated with epinephrine with significant improvement in rates of admission. This may suggest that refractory arrest patients are more responsive to epinephrine after treatment with vasopressin (Wenzel et al., 2004).

Adult dosing recommendations are the administration of vasopressin 40 U intravenously times two dosages for refractory VT. Currently, there are no recommendations for the use of vasopressin in pediatric patients. However, there has been some limited experience to suggest that it may be of similar benefit in children. Two studies have evaluated the effects of vasopressin therapy in children with cardiac compromise. A retrospective review showed that four of six children experiencing cardiac arrest had ROSC after dosage with vasopressin (0.4 U/kg) (Mann et al., 2002). In two of the patients, a second dose of vasopressin of 0.4 U/kg was given. In a non-cardiac arrest study of 11 children undergoing cardiac surgery, vasopressin infusion improved blood pressure and myocardial function for 9 of 11 patients (Cipolotti et al., 1991). Vasopressin was administered by continuous infusion of 0.0003 to 0.002 U/kg per min. During the first hour of treatment, systolic blood pressure rose from 65 to 87 mm Hg ($P < 0.0001$; n = 11), and epinephrine administration was decreased in a majority of children. Ultimately, the role of vasopressin in the treatment of children is to be determined.

Adverse Effects. The most common side effects seen with vasopressin treatment in children receiving treatment for diabetes insipidus and gastric hemorrhage are nausea, vomiting, and abdominal pain. This may be related to vasoconstriction of the splanchnic vasculature. Rare adult reports of bowel ischemia, skin necrosis, and myocardial ischemia have been made that may be related to the vasoconstrictive effects of vasopressin. Anaphylactic and other allergic reactions have also been reported but are rare (Wenzel et al., 2002).

OTHER RESUSCITATION MEDICATIONS

Sodium Bicarbonate

Clinical Effects. Sodium bicarbonate use during CPR is one of the most controversial issues in the cardiac arrest literature. This stems from its potential side effects and the lack of evidence in animals and humans of any benefit from receiving bicarbonate during CPR. Administration of sodium bicarbonate results in an acid-base reaction in which bicarbonate combines with hydrogen ions to form water and carbon dioxide, resulting in an elevated blood pH:

$$HCO_3^- + H^+ \rightarrow H_2CO_3 \rightarrow H_2O + CO_2$$

Because bicarbonate generates carbon dioxide, adequate alveolar ventilation must be present before its administration. Sodium bicarbonate administration transiently elevates CO_2 levels in the blood so that administration during cardiac arrest may worsen preexisting respiratory acidosis if ventilation is not adequate to remove the elevated CO_2. This may be more of an issue for children because a major cause of cardiac arrest is respiratory failure.

Indications. Sodium bicarbonate is indicated for correction of significant metabolic acidosis. Acidosis depresses myocardial function by decreasing spontaneous cardiac activity, the electrical threshold for VF, the inotropic state of the myocardium, and the cardiac responsiveness to catecholamines and by prolonging diastolic depolarization (Pannier and Leusen, 1968; Cingolani et al., 1970; Orlowski, 1980; Steinhart et al., 1983). Acidosis also decreases systemic vascular resistance and blunts the vasoconstrictive response of peripheral vessels to catecholamines (Wood et al., 1963). In addition, pulmonary vascular resistance increases with acidosis in patients with a reactive pulmonary vascular bed (Rudolph and Yuan, 1966). Therefore, correction of acidosis may be of help in resuscitating patients who have the potential for right-to-left shunting. Sodium bicarbonate is also indicated in hyperkalemic arrest because the increase in pH drives potassium intracellularly, resulting in a lowered serum potassium concentration. Hypermagnesemia, tricyclic antidepressant overdose, and overdose from sodium channel-blocking medications including cocaine, β-blockers, and diphenhydramine are other indications for bicarbonate (Kilecki and Curry, 1997; Donovan et al., 1999; Mullins et al., 1999; American Heart Association, 2000).

Dosage. When the $PaCO_2$ and pH are known, the dose of bicarbonate needed to correct the pH to 7.40 can be calculated from the formula (0.3 × weight [kg] × base deficit) = mEq bicarbonate. Because of the possible side effects of bicarbonate and the large arterial-to-venous carbon dioxide gradient that develops during CPR, giving half the dose based on a volume of distribution of 0.6 is recommended. If blood gases are not available, the initial dose is 1 mEq/kg, followed by 0.5 mEq/kg every 10 minutes of ongoing arrest (Martinez et al., 1979). The importance of alveolar ventilation cannot be overemphasized, as well as the need for repeated arterial blood gas analyses.

Adverse Effects. The multiple side effects that are seen with bicarbonate administration include metabolic alkalosis, hypernatremia (Worthley, 1976), hypercapnia, and hyperosmolarity (Mattar et al., 1974), all of which are associated with an increased mortality rate. Metabolic alkalosis causes a leftward shift of the oxyhemoglobin dissociation curve that impairs the release of oxygen from hemoglobin to tissues at a time of low cardiac output and low oxygen delivery (Bishop and Weisfeldt, 1976). Hypernatremia and hyperosmolarity may decrease organ perfusion by increasing interstitial edema in microvascular beds.

There are various theoretical adverse effects created by bicarbonate administration. A marked hvpercapnic acidosis in both systemic venous and coronary sinus blood develops during cardiac arrest and may be worsened by administration of bicarbonate (Grundler et al., 1986; Weil et al., 1986). Hypercapnic acidosis in the coronary sinus may cause decreased myocardial contractility (Pannier and Leusen, 1968; Cingolani et al., 1970; Deshmukh et al., 1986). Falk and others (1988) measured the mean venoarterial difference of $PaCO_2$ as 23.8 ± 15.1 mm Hg in five patients during CPR. In one patient, the difference increased from 16 mm Hg to 69 mm Hg after administration of sodium bicarbonate. In another study of 16 patients during CPR, the venoarterial gradient for carbon dioxide was 42 mm Hg (Weil et al., 1986).

In the central nervous system, intracellular acidosis probably does not occur unless overcorrection of the pH occurs. After administration of two doses of bicarbonate of 5 mEq/kg to neonatal rabbits recovering from hypoxic acidosis, the arterial pH increased to 7.41 and the intracellular brain pH increased to prehypoxic levels (Sessler et al., 1987). A paradoxical intracellular acidosis did not develop. In a study in rats, the intracellular brain ATP concentration did not change during 70 minutes of extreme hypercarbia, despite a decrease in the intracellular brain pH to 6.5 (Cohen et al., 1990). After hypercarbia, these animals could not be distinguished from normal controls and their brains were not morphologically different from those of control animals. Eleff and others (1992), using nuclear magnetic resonance spectroscopy to measure brain pH in dogs during CPR, showed that brain pH decreased to 6.29 after 6 minutes of VF, with total depletion of brain ATP. After 6 minutes of effective CPR, the ATP level returned to 86% of prearrest levels, and after 35 minutes of CPR, brain pH had returned to normal despite ongoing peripheral arterial acidosis (Eleff et al., 1992) (Table 33–14).

TABLE 33–14. Sodium bicarbonate administration during cardiopulmonary resuscitation

Indications	Hyperkalemia Preexisting metabolic acidosis Long cardiopulmonary resuscitation time without blood gas availability Pulmonary hypertensive crisis
Dose	1 mEq/kg intravenous or intraosseous empirically, or calculated from base deficit Ensure adequate ventilation when administering bicarbonate
Complications	Metabolic alkalosis Impairs O_2 delivery by shift of oxyhemoglobin dissociation Decreases cardiac contractility Increases possibility for fibrillation Decreases plasma K^+ and Ca^{2+} by intracellular shift Hypernatremia Hyperosmolarity Hypercapnia Paradoxical intracellular acidosis

Several other alkalinizing agents have been used experimentally in animals and humans to avoid the real and theoretical side effects of sodium bicarbonate. Unfortunately, none have demonstrated real advantages over sodium bicarbonate. Carbicarb (International Medication Systems, Ltd.), a solution of equimolar amounts of sodium bicarbonate and sodium carbonate, works by consuming carbon dioxide and water to generate bicarbonate ion and sodium:

$$Na_2CO_3 + CO_2 + H_2O \rightarrow 2HCO_3^- + 2Na^+$$

In animal models, Carbicarb administration resulted in a higher elevation of pH and a lesser increase in $PaCO_2$, lactate, and serum osmolarity compared with sodium bicarbonate (Sun et al., 1987; Bersin and Arieff, 1988; Gazmuri et al., 1990).

Dichloroacetate (DCA), another alkalinizing agent, works by stimulating the activity of pyruvate dehydrogenase, which facilitates the conversion of lactate to pyruvate (Stacpoole, 1989). Initial studies have shown that DCA decreased lactate concentration by half and increased bicarbonate concentration and pH when administered to humans (Stacpoole et al., 1988). It was also shown to improve cardiac output, possibly by enhancing myocardial metabolism of lactate and carbohydrate (Wargovich et al., 1988; Stacpoole et al., 1987). Unfortunately, in a multicenter trial that studied patients with lactic acidosis, DCA did not improve outcome or survival compared with standard alkalinizing agents (Stacpoole et al., 1992).

Tromethamine (THAM), or tris-[hydroxymethyl] aminomethane, is an organic amine that attracts and combines with hydrogen ions. It is available as a 0.3 mol/L solution adjusted to pH 8.6. A dose of 3 mL/kg should raise the bicarbonate concentration by 3 mEq/L. Side effects of this drug include hyperkalemia, hypoglycemia, acute hypocarbia, and apnea. Most important, it also acts as a peripheral vasodilator when administered during CPR, which may worsen myocardial perfusion. THAM is contraindicated for patients with renal failure.

Calcium

Clinical Effects

Indications for the administration of calcium during CPR are now limited to a few specific problems. This is primarily due to the possibility that in the setting of ischemia-reperfusion injury, calcium administration may worsen postischemic hypoperfusion and hasten the development of intracellular cytotoxic events that lead to cell death. Intracellular calcium overload occurs in many pathologic conditions, including ischemia, and may be a part of the common pathway of cell death (Katz and Reuter, 1979; White et al., 1983). Nevertheless, no study has shown that transient elevation of plasma calcium concentration worsens the outcome after cardiac arrest.

The calcium ion is essential in myocardial excitation-contraction coupling and myocardial contractility, and it enhances ventricular automaticity during asystole (Greenblatt et al., 1976). Therefore, calcium should be useful in the setting of asystole or EMD. Ionized hypocalcemia leads to decreased ventricular performance, peripheral vasodilatation, and blunting of the hemodynamic response to catecholamines (Bristow et al., 1977; Scheidegger et al., 1977; Drop and Scheidegger, 1980; Marquez et al., 1986; Urban et al., 1986). Severe ionized hypocalcemia (mean, 0.67 mmol/L) was present in adult patients who experienced out-of-hospital cardiac arrest (Urban et al., 1988). Evidence for beneficial clinical effects of calcium during these clinical situations is lacking (Dembo, 1981; Stueven et al., 1985a, 1985b).

Calcium channel blockers improve blood flow and function after ischemia to the heart (Clark et al., 1979), kidney (Burke et al., 1984), and brain (Holthoff et al., 1990). Calcium channel blockers also raise the threshold of the ischemic heart to VF (Resnekov, 1981). The use of calcium in these settings seems contraindicated.

Indications

The few firm indications for calcium use during CPR include cardiac arrest secondary to total or ionized hypocalcemia, hyperkalemia, hypermagnesemia, or an overdose of a calcium channel blocker. Hypocalcemia occurs with a vast array of conditions that predispose to low total body calcium stores, including the long-term use of loop diuretics. Ionized hypocalcemia may coexist with a normal total plasma calcium concentration. This occurs in the presence of severe alkalosis, which may be seen in the operating room secondary to iatrogenic hyperventilation. Ionized hypocalcemia also follows massive or rapid transfusion of citrated blood products into patients during surgery. The degree of hypocalcemia caused by citrated products depends on the rate of administration, the total dose, and the hepatic and renal function of the patient. Administration of 2 mL/kg per min of citrated whole blood causes a significant but transient decrease in the ionized calcium in anesthetized patients (Denlinger et al., 1976). Because calcium administration is not a first-line treatment during CPR, hypocalcemia must be considered as a cause of cardiac arrest, particularly in the operating room, and, if present, must be treated aggressively.

Dosage

The pediatric dose is 20 mg/kg or 0.2 mL/kg of the 10% calcium chloride solution. Calcium gluconate is as effective as calcium chloride in raising ionized calcium concentration during CPR (Heining et al., 1984). However, calcium chloride was more effective than calcium gluconate in supporting blood pressure in the hypotensive child (Broner et al., 1990). Calcium gluconate can be given as a dose of 30 to 100 mg/kg, with a maximal dose of 2 g in pediatric patients. Note that calcium preparations can be administered via the intraosseous route.

TABLE 33–15. Calcium chloride administration during cardiopulmonary resuscitation

Indications	Hyperkalemia Hypocalcemia Hypermagnesemia Calcium channel blocker overdose
Dose	20 mg/kg IV or IO

Adverse Effects

Calcium should be given slowly through a large-bore, free flowing intravenous line, preferably a central venous line. Severe tissue necrosis can occur when calcium infiltrates subcutaneous tissue. When administered too rapidly, calcium may cause severe bradycardia, heart block, or ventricular standstill (Table 33–15).

Glucose

Glucose administration during CPR should be restricted to documented hypoglycemia because of the possible detrimental effects of hyperglycemia during brain ischemia. Myers and others (1979) first hypothesized that hyperglycemia worsens the neurologic outcome after cardiac arrest. Siemkowicz and Hansen (1978) confirmed this finding when they found that after 10 minutes of global brain ischemia the neurologic recovery of hyperglycemic rats was worse than in normoglycemic control animals. Hyperglycemia exaggerates ischemic neurologic injury by increasing the production of lactic acid in the brain by anaerobic metabolism. During ischemia under normoglycemic conditions, brain lactate concentration reaches a plateau. However, when hyperglycemia is present, the brain lactate concentration continues to rise for the duration of the ischemic period (Siesjo, 1984). The severity of intracellular acidosis during brain ischemia is directly proportional to the preischemic plasma glucose concentration. These negative effects of hyperglycemia during brain ischemia are based on the existence of at least a small amount of blood flow to brain tissue. In one study, collaterally perfused but not end-arterial brain tissue had greater neuronal damage during hyperglycemic focal ischemia (Prado et al., 1988).

Clinical studies have shown a direct correlation between the initial glucose concentration and a poor neurologic outcome (Pulsinelli et al., 1983; Longstreth and Inui, 1984; Woo et al., 1988; Ashwal et al., 1990). Longstreth and others (1986) suggested that a higher admission plasma glucose concentration may be an endogenous response to severe stress and not the cause of more severe brain injury. Given the likelihood of additional ischemic events during the postresuscitation period, it may be wise to maintain serum glucose in the normal range. Voll and Auer (1988) showed that administration of insulin to hyperglycemic rats after global brain ischemia improved the neurologic outcome. It is not known if active treatment of hyperglycemia enhances the clinical outcome after an ischemic episode. This effect of insulin may be independent of its glucose-lowering properties, because normoglycemic treated rats had a better outcome than did placebo-treated controls (Voll and Auer, 1991). Before any surgical procedure, when the possibility of brain ischemia exists, tight preoperative and intraoperative control of the serum glucose level is desirable (Sieber and Traystman, 1992).

Infants, patients with hepatic disease, and debilitated patients with low endogenous glycogen stores are prone to hypoglycemia when stressed, as may occur during surgery. In these patients, bedside monitoring of the serum glucose level is critical during the perioperative period. In cardiac arrest, glucose is administered to the hypoglycemic patient to maintain normal substrate delivery to vital organs. To treat hypoglycemia, an intravenous dose of 1 mL/kg of 50% dextrose for adults, 2 mL/kg of 25% dextrose in children, or 3 to 5 mL/kg of 10% dextrose for infants can be administered.

POSTRESUSCITATION CARE

Vital organ perfusion remains a priority in the postresuscitation period. Maintaining adequate metabolic supply requires attention to blood pressure, ventilation, and glucose levels. Avoiding increased metabolic demand involves prevention of hyperthermia and seizures. In the postresuscitation period, blood pressure should be maintained adequate for vital organ perfusion and may require the administration of fluids, vasoactive medication, or pacing. Ventilation should be normocapnic, avoiding hyperventilation and hypoventilation. Blood glucose levels should also be normalized, avoiding hyperglycemia and hypoglycemia. Postresuscitation hyperthermia is common as patients are often excessively rewarmed. This overwarming can increase metabolic demands, thus worsening outcome, and should be avoided. In fact, hypothermia may be neuroprotective and was recommended for adult victims of cardiac arrest.

The International Liaison Committee on Resuscitation recommends that unconscious adult patients with spontaneous circulation after out-of-hospital cardiac arrest be cooled to 32° to 34°C for 12 to 24 hours when the initial rhythm was VF (Nolan et al., 2003). Consideration should also be given to cooling for other rhythms or in-hospital cardiac arrest. These recommendations are based on the results from two prospective randomized clinical studies that compared hypothermia to normothermia in comatose survivors of cardiac arrest (Bernard et al., 2002; Hypothermia after Cardiac Arrest Study Group, 2002). These European and Australian studies excluded children and cardiac arrests of noncardiac etiology. Animal models of asphyxial arrest are reporting protective effects of hypothermia in rats (Xiao et al., 1998; Hickey et al., 2000; Hicks et al., 2000; Hachim-Idrissi et al., 2001) and piglets (Agnew et al., 2003). There is insufficient evidence to make a recommendation on the use of therapeutic cooling for children resuscitated from cardiac arrest.

SUMMARY

CPR is not a definitive treatment for cardiac arrest but rather a means of maintaining respiration and circulation until the underlying pathology can be corrected. In children, the inciting event is often related to the airway, and restoring the airway by initiating CPR can be therapeutic. Because of the limited efficacy of CPR, it is important to identify the underlying pathology as early as possible and correct it so that spontaneous circulation can be restored. During anesthesia, this often means restoring the airway, reducing the anesthetic level, or correcting vascular volume deficits. If EMD is present, hypovolemia, tension pneumothorax, and pericardial tamponade must be considered if no improvement occurs with restoration of the airway. If VF is present, then electrolyte disorders, hypoglycemia, hypothermia, and digitalis or tricyclic antidepressant overdose must be considered.

Preparation for CPR during anesthetic management begins with knowledge of the most current recommendations for treating children during cardiopulmonary arrest. However, the anesthesiologist must have at his or her disposal the appropriate medications and devices necessary to treat these emergencies.

REFERENCES

Agnew DM, Koehler RC, Guerguerian AM, et al.: Hypothermia for 24 hours after asphyxic cardiac arrest in piglets provides striatal neuroprotection that is sustained 10 days after rewarming. *Pediatr Res* 54:253, 2003.

American Heart Association in collaboration with the International Liaison Committee on Resuscitation: Guidelines 2000 for cardiopulmonary resuscitation and emergency cardiovascular care. Part 10: Pediatric advanced life support. *Circulation* 102:I291, 2000.

Anderson GJ, Reiser J, McAllister H, et al.: Electro-physiological characterization of myocardial injury induced by defibrillation shocks. *Med Instrum* 14:54, 1980.

Angelos MG, Gaddis ML, Gaddis GM, et al.: Improved survival and reduced myocardial necrosis with cardiopulmonary bypass reperfusion in a canine model of coronary occlusion and cardiac arrest. *Ann Emerg Med* 19:1122, 1990.

Arai T, Watanabe T, Nagaro T, et al.: Blood-brain barrier impairment after cardiac resuscitation. *Crit Care Med* 9:444, 1981.

Ashwal S, Schneider S, Tomasi L, et al.: Prognostic implications of hyperglycemia and reduced cerebral blood flow in childhood near-drowning. *Neurology* 40:820, 1990.

Atkins DL, Hartley LL, York DK: Accurate recognition and effective treatment of ventricular fibrillation by automated external defibrillators in adolescents. *Pediatrics* 101:393, 1998.

Austen WG, Moran JM: Cardiac and peripheral vascular effects of lidocaine and procainalol. *Am J Cardiol* 16:701, 1965.

Babbs CF, Fitzgerald KR, Voorhees WD, et al.: High-pressure ventilation during CPR with 95% O_2:5% CO_2. *Crit Care Med* 10:505, 1982b.

Babbs CF, Tacker WA, Paris RL, et al.: CPR with simultaneous compression and ventilation at high airway pressure in 4 animal models. *Crit Care Med* 10:501, 1982a.

Bacaner MB: Bretylium tosylate for suppression of induced ventricular fibrillation. *Am J Cardiol* 17:528, 1966.

Barcelona SL, Coté CJ: Pediatric resuscitation in the operating room. *Anesthesiol Clin North Am* 19:339, 2001.

Barranco F, Lesmes A, Irles JA, et al.: Cardiopulmonary resuscitation with simultaneous chest and abdominal compression: Comparative study in humans. *Resuscitation* 20:67, 1990.

Bartlett RL, Stewart NJ, Taymond J, et al.: Comparative study of three methods of resuscitation: Closed-chest, open chest manual, and direct mechanical ventricular assistance. *Ann Emerg Med* 13:773, 1984.

Barton C, Callaham M: Lack of correlation between end-tidal carbon dioxide concentrations and $PaCO_2$ in cardiac arrest. *Crit Care Med* 19:108, 1991.

Bauman JL, Berk SI, Hariman RJ, et al.: Amiodarone for sustained ventricular tachycardia: Efficacy, safety, and factors influencing long-term outcome. *Am Heart J* 114:1436, 1987.

Bauman JL: Class III antiarrhythmic agents: The next wave. *Pharmacotherapy* 17:76S, 1997.

Beattie C, Guerci AD, Hall T, et al.: Mechanisms of blood flow during pneumatic vest cardiopulmonary resuscitation. *J Appl Physiol* 70:454, 1991.

Beland MJ, Hesslein PS, Rowe RD: Ventricular tachycardia related to transcutaneous pacing. *Ann Emerg Med* 17:279, 1988.

Berg RA, Hilwig RW, Kern KB, et al.: "Bystander" chest compressions and assisted ventilation independently improve outcome from piglet asphyxial pulseless "cardiac arrest." *Circulation* 101:1743, 2000.

Berg RA, Sanders AB, Kern KB, et al.: Adverse hemodynamic effects of interrupting chest compressions for rescue breathing during cardiopulmonary resuscitation for ventricular fibrillation cardiac arrest. *Circulation* 104:2465, 2001.

Berkowitz ID, Chantarojanasiri T, Koehler RC, et al.: Blood flow during cardiopulmonary resuscitation with simultaneous compression and ventilation in infant pigs. *Pediatr Res* 26:558, 1989.

Berkowitz ID, Gervais H, Schleien CL, et al.: Epinephrine dosage effects on cerebral and myocardial blood flow in an infant swine model of cardiopulmonary resuscitation. *Anesthesiology* 75:1041, 1991.

Bernard EO, Schmid ER, Schmidlin D, et al.: Ibutilide versus amiodarone in atrial fibrillation: A double-blinded, randomized study. *Crit Care Med* 31:1031, 2003.

Bernard SA, Gray TW, Buist MD, et al.: Treatment of comatose survivors of out-of-hospital cardiac arrest with induced hypothermia. *N Engl J Med* 346:557, 2002.

Bernstein JG, Koch-Weser J: Effectiveness of bretylium tosylate against refractive ventricular arrhythmias. *Circulation* 45:1024, 1972.

Berryman CR, Phillips GM: Interposed abdominal compression-CPR in human subjects. *Ann Emerg Med* 13:226, 1984.

Bersin RM, Arieff AI: Improved hemodynamic function during hypoxia with Carbicarb, a new agent for the management of acidosis. *Circulation* 77:227, 1988.

Beyar R, Halperin HR, Tsitlik JE, et al.: Circulatory assistance by intrathoracic pressure variations: optimization and mechanisms studied by a mathematical model in relation to experimental data. *Circ Res* 64:703, 1989.

Beyar R, Kishon Y, Sideman S, et al.: Computer studies of systemic and regional blood flow mechanisms during cardiopulmonary resuscitation. *Med Biol Eng Comput* 22:499, 1984.

Bhende MS, Thompson AE, Cook DR, et al.: Validity of a disposable end-tidal CO_2 detector in verifying endotracheal tube placement in infants and children. *Ann Emerg Med* 21:142, 1992.

Bhende MS, Thompson AE: Evaluation of an end-tidal CO_2 detector during pediatric cardiopulmonary resuscitation. *Pediatrics* 95:395, 1995.

Biboulet P, Aubas P, Dubourdieu J, et al.: Fatal and nonfatal cardiac arrests related to anesthesia. *Can J Anaesth* 48:326, 2001.

Bircher N, Safar P, Stewart R: A comparison of standard, "MAST"-augmented, and open-chest CPR in dogs: A preliminary investigation. *Crit Care Med* 8:147, 1980.

Bircher N, Safar P: Comparison of standard and "new" closed-chest CPR and open-chest CPR in dogs. *Crit Care Med* 9:384, 1981.

Bishop RL, Weisfeldt ML: Sodium bicarbonate administration during cardiac arrest: Effect on arterial pH, PCO_2, and osmolality. *JAMA* 235:506, 1976.

Brillman JA, Sanders AB, Otto CW, et al.: Outcome of resuscitation from fibrillatory arrest using epinephrine and phenylephrine in dogs. *Crit Care Med* 13:912, 1985.

Bristow MR, Schwartz HD, Binetti G, et al.: Ionized calcium and the heart. Elucidation of in vivo concentration-response relationships in the open chest dog. *Circ Res* 41:565, 1977.

Broner CW, Stidham GL, Westenkirchner DF, et al.: A prospective, randomized, double-blind comparison of calcium chloride and calcium gluconate therapies for hypocalcemia in critically ill children. *J Pediatr* 115:988, 1990.

Brown CG, Birinyi F, Werman HA, et al.: The comparative effects of epinephrine versus phenylephrine on regional cerebral blood flow during cardiopulmonary resuscitation. *Resuscitation* 14:171, 1986b.

Brown CG, Davis EA, Werman RL: Methoxamine versus epinephrine on regional cerebral blood flow during cardiopulmonary resuscitation. *Crit Care Med* 15:682, 1987c.

Brown CG, Martin DR, Pepe PE, et al.: A comparison of standard-dose and high-dose epinephrine in cardiac arrest outside the hospital. *N Engl J Med* 327:1051, 1992.

Brown CG, Taylor RB, Werman HA, et al.: Effect of standard doses of epinephrine on myocardial oxygen delivery and utilization during cardiopulmonary resuscitation. *Crit Care Med* 16:536, 1988b.

Brown CG, Taylor RB, Werman HA, et al.: Myocardial oxygen delivery/consumption during cardiopulmonary resuscitation: A comparison of epinephrine and phenylephrine. *Ann Emerg Med* 17:302, 1988a.

Brown CG, Werman HA, Davis EA, et al.: Comparative effects of graded doses of epinephrine on regional brain blood flow during CPR in a swine model. *Ann Emerg Med* 15:1138, 1986a.

Brown CG, Werman HA, Davis EA, et al.: The effect of high-dose phenylephrine versus epinephrine on regional cerebral flow during CPR. *Ann Emerg Med* 16:743, 1987a.

Brown CG, Werman HA, Davis EA, et al.: The effects of graded doses of epinephrine on regional myocardial blood flow during cardiopulmonary resuscitation in swine. *Circulation* 75:491, 1987b.

Brown J, Rogers J, Soar J: Cardiac arrest during surgery and ventilation in the prone position: A case report and systematic review. *Resuscitation* 50:233, 2001.

Burke TJ, Arnold PE, Gordon JA, et al.: Protective effect of intrarenal calcium membrane blockers before or after renal ischemia: Functional, morphological, and mitochondrial studies. *J Clin Invest* 74:1830, 1984.

Burri S, Hug MI, Bauersfeld U: Efficacy and safety of intravenous amiodarone for incessant tachycardias in infants. *Eur J Pediatr* 162:880, 2003.

Calkins MD, Fitzgerald G, Bentley TB, et al.: Intraosseous infusion devices: A comparison for potential use in special operations. *J Trauma* 48:1068, 2000.

Callaham M, Barton C: Prediction of outcome of cardiopulmonary resuscitation from end-tidal carbon dioxide concentration. *Crit Care Med* 19:358, 1990.

Callaham M, Madsen CD, Barton CW, et al.: A randomized clinical trial of high-dose epinephrine and norepinephrine versus standard-dose epinephrine in prehospital cardiac arrest. *JAMA* 268:2667, 1992.

Carcillo JA, Davis AL, Zaritsky A: Role of early fluid resuscitation in pediatric septic shock. *JAMA* 266:1242, 1991.

Carlsson C, Hagerdal M, Kaasid AE, et al.: A catecholamine-mediated increase in cerebral oxygen uptake during immobilization stress in rats. *Brain Res* 119:223, 1977.

Carpenter TC, Stenmark KR: High-dose epinephrine is not superior to standard-dose epinephrine in pediatric in-hospital cardiopulmonary arrest. *Pediatrics* 99:403, 1997.

Cavallaro DL, Melker RJ: Comparison of two techniques for detecting cardiac activity in infants. *Crit Care Med* 11:189, 1983.

Chandra N, Rudikoff M, Weisfeldt ML: Simultaneous chest compression and ventilation at high airway pressure during cardiopulmonary resuscitation. *Lancet* 1:175, 1980.

Chandra N, Snyder LD, Weisfeldt ML: Abdominal binding during cardiopulmonary resuscitation in man. *JAMA* 246:351, 1981b.

Chandra N, Tsitlik J, Halperin HR, et al.: Observations of hemodynamics during human cardiopulmonary resuscitation. *Crit Care Med* 18:929, 1990.

Chandra N, Weisfeldt ML, Tsitlik J, et al.: Augmentation of carotid flow during cardiopulmonary resuscitation by ventilation at high airway pressure simultaneous with chest compression. *Am J Cardiol* 48:1053, 1981a.

Chandra NC, Beyar R, Halperin HR, et al.: Vital organ perfusion during assisted circulation by manipulation of intrathoracic pressure. *Circulation* 84:279, 1991.

Chatterjee K, Mandel WJ, Vyden JK, et al.: Cardiovascular effects of bretylium tosylate in acute myocardial infarction. *JAMA* 223:757, 1973.

Chen YS, Chao A, Yu HY, et al.: Analysis and results of prolonged resuscitation in cardiac arrest patients rescued by extracorporeal membrane oxygenation. *J Am Coll Cardiol* 41:197, 2003.

Cherian L, Goodman JC, Robertson CS: Hyperglycemia increases brain injury caused by secondary ischemia after cortical impact injury in rats. *Crit Care Med* 25:1378,1997.

Chow MS: Intravenous amiodarone: Pharmacology, pharmacokinetics, and clinical use. *Ann Pharmacother* 30:637, 1996.

Chow MSS, Ronfeld RA, Hamilton RA, et al.: Effect of external cardiopulmonary resuscitation on lidocaine pharmacokinetics in dogs. *J Pharmacol Exp Ther* 224:531, 1983.

Chow MSS, Ronfeld RA, Ruffett D, et al.: Lidocaine pharmacokinetics during cardiac arrest and external cardiopulmonary resuscitation. *Am Heart J* 102:799, 1981.

Cingolani HE, Mattiazi AR, Blesa ES: Contractility in isolated mammalian heart muscle after acid-base changes. *Circ Res* 26:269, 1970.

Cipolotti G, Paccagnella A, Simini G: Successful cardiopulmonary resuscitation using high doses of epinephrine. *Int J Cardiol* 33:430, 1991.

Clark RE, Kristlieb IY, Henry PD: Nifedipine: A myocardial protective agent. *Am J Cardiol* 44:825, 1979.

Clements FM, De Bruijn NP, Kisslo JA: Transesophageal echocardiographic observations in a patient undergoing closed-chest massage. *Anesthesiology* 64:826, 1986.

Cleveland JC: Complete recovery after cardiac arrest for three hours. *N Engl J Med* 284:334, 1971.

Cochran JB, Tecklenburg FW, Lau YR, et al.: Emergency cardiopulmonary bypass for cardiac arrest refractory to pediatric advanced life support. *Pediatr Emerg Care* 15:30, 1999.

Cohen JM, Chandra M, Alderson PO, et al.: Timing of pulmonary and systemic blood flow during intermittent high intrathoracic pressure cardiopulmonary resuscitation in the dog. *Am J Cardiol* 49:1883, 1982.

Cohen TJ, Goldner BG, Maccaro PC, et al.: A comparison of active compression-decompression cardiopulmonary resuscitation with standard cardiopulmonary resuscitation for cardiac arrests occurring in the hospital. *N Engl J Med* 329:1918, 1993.

Cohen TJ, Tucker KJ, Lurie KG, et al.: Active compression-decompression. A new method of cardiopulmonary resuscitation. Cardiopulmonary Resuscitation Working Group. *JAMA* 267:2916, 1992.

Cohen Y, Chang LH, Litt L, et al.: Stability of brain intracellular pH during prolonged hypercapnia in rats. *J Cereb Blood Flow Metab* 10:277, 1990.

Collingsworth KA, Kalman SM, Harrison DC: The clinical pharmacology of lidocaine as an antiarrhythmic drug. *Circulation* 50:1217, 1974.

Constantino RT, Crockett SE, Vasko JS: Cardiovascular effects and dose response relationships of lidocaine. *Circulation* 36:89, 1967.

Coté P, Bourassa MG, Delaye J, et al.: Effects of amiodarone on cardiac and coronary hemodynamics and on myocardial metabolism in patients with coronary artery disease. *Circulation* 59:1165, 1979.

Criley JM, Blaufuss AH, Kissel GL: Cough-induced cardiac compression: self-administered form of cardiopulmonary resuscitation. *JAMA* 236:1246, 1976.

Criley JM, Niemann JT, Rosborough JP, et al.: Modification of cardiopulmonary resuscitation based on the cough. *Circulation* 74(suppl IV):IV-42, 1986.

Crosson JE, Etheridge SP, Milstein S, et al.: Therapeutic and diagnostic utility of adenosine during tachycardia evaluation in children. *Am J Cardiol* 74:155, 1994.

Cummins RO, Eisenberg MS, Litwin PE, et al.: Automatic external defibrillators used by emergency medical technicians. A controlled clinical trial. *JAMA* 257:1605, 1987.

Dahl CF, Ewy GA, Warner ED, et al.: Myocardial necrosis from direct current countershock: effect of paddle electrode size and time interval between discharges. *Circulation* 50:956, 1974.

Dalton HJ, Siewers RD, Fuhrman BP, et al.: Extracorporeal membrane oxygenation for cardiac rescue in children with severe myocardial dysfunction. *Crit Care Med* 21:1020, 1993.

David R: Closed chest cardiac massage in the newborn infant. *Pediatrics* 81:552, 1988.

Davies CR, Carrigan T, Wright JA, et al.: Neurologic outcome following pediatric resuscitation. *J Neurosci Nurs* 19:205, 1987.

Dean JM, Koehler RC, Schleien CL, et al.: Age-related changes in chest geometry during cardiopulmonary resuscitation. *J Appl Physiol* 62:2212, 1987.

Dean JM, Koehler RC, Schleien CL, et al.: Age-related effects of compression rate and duration in cardiopulmonary resuscitation. *J Appl Physiol* 68:554, 1990.

Dean JM, Koehler RC, Schleien CL, et al.: Improved blood flow during prolonged cardiopulmonary resuscitation with 30% duty cycle in infant pigs. *Circulation* 84:896, 1991.

Del Guercio LR, Feins NR, Cohn JD, et al.: Comparison of blood flow during external and internal cardiac massage in man. *Circulation* 32(suppl I):I-171, 1965.

del Nido PJ, Dalton HJ, Thompson AE, et al.: Extracorporeal membrane oxygenator rescue in children during cardiac arrest after cardiac surgery. *Circulation* 86(suppl II):II-300-II-304, 1992.

Dembo DH: Calcium in advanced life support. *Crit Care Med* 9:358, 1981.

Denlinger JK, Nahrwold MLL, Gibbs PS, et al.: Hypocalcemia during rapid blood transfusion in anaesthetized man. *Br J Anaesth* 48:995, 1976.

Dequin PF, Hazouard E, Legras A, et al.: Cardiopulmonary resuscitation in the prone position: Kouwenhoven revisited. *Intensive Care Med* 22:1272, 1996.

Deshmukh HG, Gudipati CV, Weil MH, et al.: Myocardial respiratory acidosis during CPR. *Crit Care Med* 14:433, 1986.

DiCola VC, Freedman GS, Downing SE, et al.: Myocardial uptake of technetium-99m stannous pyrophosphate following direct current transthoracic countershock. *Circulation* 54:980, 1976.

Ditchey RV, Lindenfeld J: Failure of epinephrine to improve the balance between myocardial oxygen supply and demand during closed chest resuscitation in dogs. *Circulation* 78:382, 1988.

Ditchey RV, Winkler JV, Rhodes CA: Relative lack of blood flow during closed-chest resuscitation in dogs. *Circulation* 66:297, 1982.

Dittrich S, Gemanakis J, Dahnert I, et al.: Randomized trial on the influence of continuous magnesium infusion on arrhythmias following cardiopulmonary bypass surgery for congenital heart disease. *Intensive Care Med* 29;1141, 2003.

Donovan KD, Gerace RV, Dreyer RF: Acebutolol-induced ventricular tachycardia reversed with sodium bicarbonate. *J Toxicol Clin Toxicol* 37:481-4, 1999.

Dorfsman ML, Menegazzi JJ, Wadas RJ, et al.: Two-thumb versus two-finger chest compression in an infant model of prolonged cardiopulmonary resuscitation. *Acad Emerg Med* 7:1077-82, 2000.

Dorian P, Cass D, Schwartz B, et al.: Amiodarone as compared with lidocaine for shock-resistant ventricular fibrillation. *N Engl J Med* 346:884, 2002.

Dorman BH, Sade RM, Burnette JS, et al.: Magnesium supplementation in the prevention of arrhythmias in pediatric patients undergoing surgery for congenital heart defects. *Am Heart J* 139:522, 2000.

Drop LJ, Scheidegger D: Plasma ionized calcium concentration: Important determinant of the hemodynamic response to calcium infusion. *J Thorac Cardiovasc Surg* 79:425, 1980.

Duncan BW, Ibrahim AE, Hraska V, et al.: Use of rapid-deployment extracorporeal membrane oxygenation for the resuscitation of pediatric patients with heart disease after cardiac arrest. *J Thorac Cardiovasc Surg* 116:305, 1998.

Eberle B, Schleien CL, Shaffner DH, et al.: Effects of three modes of abdominal compression on vital organ blood flow in a piglet CPR model. *Anesthesiology* 73:A300, 1990.

Edvinsson L, Hardebo JE, MacKenzie ET, et al.: Effect of endogenous noradrenaline on local cerebral blood flow after osmotic opening of the blood-brain barrier in the rat. *J Physiol (Lond)* 274:149, 1978.

Einagle V, Bertrand F, Wise RA, et al.: Interposed abdominal compressions and carotid blood flow during cardiopulmonary resuscitation. *Chest* 93:1206, 1988.

Elam JO, Brown ES, Elder JD: Artificial respiration by mouth-to-mask method. *N Engl J Med* 250:749, 1954.

Eleff SM, Schleien CL, Koehler RC, et al.: Brain bioenergetics during cardiopulmonary resuscitation in dogs. *Anesthesiology* 76:77, 1992.

Elson J, Strong JM, Lee WK, et al.: Antiarrhythmic potency of N-acetylprocainamide. *Clin Pharmacol Ther* 17:134, 1975.

Falk JL, Rackow EC, Weil MH: End-tidal carbon dioxide concentration during cardiopulmonary resuscitation. *N Engl J Med* 318:607, 1988.

Feneley MP, Maier GW, Gaynor JW, et al.: Sequence of mitral valve motion and transmitral blood flow during manual cardiopulmonary resuscitation in dogs. *Circulation* 76:363, 1987.

Feneley MP, Maier GW, Kern KB, et al.: Influence of compression rate on initial success of resuscitation and 24 hour survival after prolonged manual cardiopulmonary resuscitation in dogs. *Circulation* 77:240, 1988.

Figa FH, Gow RM, Hamilton RM, et al.: Clinical efficacy and safety of intravenous Amiodarone in infants and children. *Am J Cardiol* 74:573, 1994.

Fisher J, Vaghaiwall F, Tsitlik J, et al.: Determinants and clinical significance of jugular venous valve competence. *Circulation* 65:188, 1982.

Fleisher G, Delgado-Paredes C, Heyman S: Slow versus rapid closed-chest cardiac compression during cardiopulmonary resuscitation in puppies. *Crit Care Med* 15:939, 1987.

Garnett AR, Ornato JP, Gonzales ER, et al.: End-tidal carbon dioxide monitoring during cardiopulmonary resuscitation. *JAMA* 257:512, 1987.

Gascho JA, Crampton RS, Cherwek ML, et al.: Determinants of ventricular defibrillation in adults. *Circulation* 60:231, 1979.

Gazmuri RJ, Planta M, Weil MH, et al.: Cardiac effects of carbon dioxide-consuming and carbon dioxide-generating buffers during cardiopulmonary resuscitation. *JAMA* 15:482, 1990.

Gazmuri RJ, Weil MH, Bisera J, et al.: End-tidal carbon dioxide tension as a monitor of native blood flow during resuscitation by extracorporeal circulation. *J Thorac Cardiovasc Surg* 101:984, 1991.

Gillette PC, Garson A: *Pediatric cardiac dysrhythmias.* New York, 1981, Grune & Stratton.

Gillis J, Dickson D, Rieder M, et al.: Results of inpatient pediatric resuscitation. *Crit Care Med* 14:469, 1986.

Gilman AG, Rall TW, Nies AS, et al.: *Goodman and Gilman's the pharmacological basis of therapeutics,* 8th ed. Elmsford, NY, 1990, Pergamon Press.

Girardi LN, Barie PS: Improved survival after intraoperative cardiac arrest in noncardiac surgical patients. *Arch Surg* 130:15, 1995.

Glaeser PW, Hellmich TR, Szewczuga D, et al.: Five-year experience in prehospital intraosseous infusions in children and adults. *Ann Emerg Med* 22:1119, 1993.

Goetting MG, Paradis MA: Right atrial-jugular venous pressure gradients during CPR in children. *Ann Emerg Med* 20:27, 1991a.

Goetting MG, Paradis NA, Appleton TJ, et al.: Aortic-carotid artery pressure differences and cephalic perfusion pressure during cardiopulmonary resuscitation in humans. *Crit Care Med* 19:1012, 1991b.

Goetting MG, Paradis NA: High dose epinephrine in refractor pediatric cardiac arrest. *Crit Care Med* 17:1258, 1989.

Goldberg AH: Cardiopulmonary arrest. *N Engl J Med* 290:381, 1974.

Gonzalez ER, Kannewurf BS, Ornato JP: Intravenous amiodarone for ventricular arrhythmias: Overview and clinical use. *Resuscitation* 39:33, 1998.

Gonzalez ER, Ornato JP, Garnett AR, et al.: Dose-dependent vasopressor response to epinephrine during CPR in human beings. *Ann Emerg Med* 18:920, 1989.

Gonzalez ER, Ornato JP, Levine RL: Vasopressor effect of epinephrine with and without dopamine during cardiopulmonary resuscitation. *Drug Intell Clin Pharm* 22:868, 1988.

Grayling M, Wilson IH, Thomas B: The use of the laryngeal mask airway and Combitube in cardiopulmonary resuscitation; a national survey. *Resuscitation* 52:183, 2002.

Greenblatt DJ, Gross PL, Bolognini V: Pharmacotherapy of cardiopulmonary arrest. *Am J Hosp Pharm* 33:379, 1976.

Greissman A, Silver P, Nimkoff L, et al.: Transvenous right ventricular pacing during cardiopulmonary resuscitation of pediatric patients with acute cardiomyopathy. *Pediatr Emerg Care* 11:17, 1995.

Grmec S, Lah K, Tusek-Bunc K: Difference in end-tidal CO_2 between asphyxia cardiac arrest and ventricular fibrillation/pulseless ventricular tachycardia cardiac arrest in the prehospital setting. *Crit Care* 7:R139, 2003.

Grundler W, Weil MH, Rackow EC: Arteriovenous carbon dioxide and pH gradients during cardiac arrest. *Circulation* 77:234, 1986.

Gudipati CV, Weil MH, Deshmukh HG, et al.: Right atrial-jugular venous pressure gradients during experimental CPR. *Chest* 89:443s, 1986.

Guerci AD, Shi A, Levin H, et al.: Transmission of intrathoracic pressure to the intracranial space during cardiopulmonary resuscitation in dogs. *Circ Res* 56:20, 1985.

Gutgesell HP, Tacker WA, Geddes LA, et al.: Energy dose for ventricular defibrillation of children. *Pediatrics* 58:898, 1976.

Guy J, Haley K, Zuspan SJ: Use of intraosseous infusion in the pediatric trauma patient. *J Pediatr Surg* 28:158, 1993.

Hachimi-Idrissi S, Corne L, Huyghens L: The effect of mild hypothermia and induced hypertension on long term survival rate and neurological outcome after asphyxial cardiac arrest in rats. *Resuscitation* 49:73, 2001.

Hackl W, Simon P, Mauritz W, et al.: Echocardiographic assessment of mitral valve function during mechanical cardiopulmonary resuscitation in pigs. *Anesth Analg* 70:350, 1990.

Halperin HR, Guerci AD, Chandra N, et al.: Vest inflation without simultaneous ventilation during cardiac arrest in dogs: Improved survival from prolonged cardiopulmonary resuscitation. *Circulation* 74:1407, 1986b.

Halperin HR, Tsitlik JE, Beyar R, et al.: Intrathoracic pressure fluctuations move blood during CPR: Comparison of hemodynamic data with predictions from a mathematical model. *Ann Biomed Eng* 15:385, 1987.

Halperin HR, Tsitlik JE, Gelfand M, et al.: A preliminary study of cardiopulmonary resuscitation by circumferential compression of the chest with use of a pneumatic vest. *N Engl J Med* 329:762, 1993.

Halperin HR, Tsitlik JE, Guerci AD, et al.: Determinants of blood flow to vital organs during cardiopulmonary resuscitation in dogs. *Circulation* 73:539, 1986a.

Harada Y, Fuseno H, Ohtomo T, et al.: Self-administered hyperventilation cardiopulmonary resuscitation for 100 s of cardiac arrest during Holter monitoring. *Chest* 99:1310, 1991.

Harris L, Kimura Y, Shaikh NA: Phospholipase inhibition and the electrophysiology of acute ischemia: Studies with amiodarone. *J Mol Cell Cardiol* 25:1075, 1993.

Harris LC, Kirimli B, Safar P: Ventilation-cardiac compression rates and ratios in cardiopulmonary resuscitation. *Anesthesiology* 28:806, 1967.

Hartz R, LoCicero J, Sanders JH, et al.: Clinical experience with portable cardiopulmonary bypass in cardiac arrest patients. *Ann Thorac Surg* 50:437, 1990.

Hayes MM, Berg RA, Otto CW: Monitoring during cardiac arrest: Are we there yet? *Curr Opin Crit Care* 9:211, 2003.

Haynes RE, Chinn TL, Copass MK, et al.: Comparison of bretylium tosylate and lidocaine in management of out-of-hospital ventricular fibrillation: A randomized clinical trial. *Am J Cardiol* 48:353, 1981.

Heining MPD, Band DM, Linton RAF: Choice of calcium salt: A comparison of the effects of calcium chloride and gluconate on plasma ionized calcium. *Anaesthesia* 39:1079, 1984.

Helmy I, Herre JM, Gee G, et al.: Use of intravenous amiodarone for emergency treatment of life-threatening ventricular arrhythmias. *J Am Coll Cardiol* 12:1015, 1988.

Hickey RW, Ferimer H, Alexander HL, et al.: Delayed, spontaneous hypothermia reduces neuronal damage after asphyxial cardiac arrest in rats. *Crit Care Med* 28:3511, 2000.

Hicks SD, DeFranco DB, Callaway CW: Hypothermia during reperfusion after asphyxial cardiac arrest improves functional recovery and selectively alters stress-induced protein expression. *J Cereb Blood Flow Metab* 20:520, 2000.

Higano ST, Oh JK, Ewy GA, et al.: The mechanism of blood flow during closed chest cardiac massage in humans: Transesophageal echocardiographic observations. *Mayo Clin Proc* 65:2, 1990.

Hilleman D, Miller MA, Parker R, et al.: Optimal management of amiodarone therapy: Efficacy and side effects. *Pharmacotherapy* 18:138S, 1998.

Hoffman TM, Bush DM, Wernovsky G, et al.: Postoperative junctional ectopic tachycardia in children: Incidence, risk factors, and treatment. *Ann Thorac Surg* 74:1607, 2002.

Hoffman TM, Wernovsky G, Atz AM, et al.: Efficacy and safety of milrinone in preventing low cardiac output syndrome in infants and children after corrective surgery for congenital heart disease. *Circulation* 107:996, 2003.

Holmes HR, Babbs CF, Voorhees WD, et al.: Influence of adrenergic drugs upon vital organ perfusion during CPR. *Crit Care Med* 8:137, 1980.

Holthoff V, Beil C, Hartmann-Klosterklotter U, et al.: Effect of nimodipine on glucose metabolism in stroke patients. *Stroke* 21(suppl IV):IV-95, 1990.

Howard M, Carruba C, Foss F, et al.: Interposed abdominal compression-CPR: Its effects on parameters of coronary perfusion in human subjects. *Ann Emerg Med* 16:253, 1987.

Howard M, Carruba C, Guiness M, et al.: Interposed abdominal compression CPR: Its effects on coronary perfusion pressure in human subjects. *Ann Emerg Med* 13:989, 1984.

Hypothermia after Cardiac Arrest Study Group: Mild therapeutic hypothermia to improve the neurologic outcome after cardiac arrest. *N Engl J Med* 346:549, 2002.

Jackson DL, Dole WP, McGloin J, et al.: Total cerebral ischemia: Application of a new model system to studies of cerebral microcirculation. *Stroke* 12:66, 1981.

Jackson RE, Joyce K, Danosi SF, et al.: Blood flow in the cerebral cortex during cardiac resuscitation in dogs. *Ann Emerg Med* 13:657, 1984.

Jasani MS, Nadkarni VM, Finkelstein MS, et al.: Effects of different techniques of endotracheal epinephrine administration in pediatric porcine hypoxic-hypercarbic cardiopulmonary arrest. *Crit Care Med* 22:1174, 1994.

Jessurun GA, Boersma WG, Crijns HJ: Amiodarone-induced pulmonary toxicity. Predisposing factors, clinical symptoms and treatment. *Drug Saf* 18:339, 1998.

Jewitt DE, Kishow Y, Thomas M: Lidocaine in the management of arrhythmias after myocardial infarction. *Circulation* 37:965, 1968.

Jones JL, Lepeschkin E, Jones RE, et al.: Response of cultured myocardial cells to countershock-type electrical field stimulation. *Am J Physiol* 235:H214, 1978.
Jude JR, Kouwenhoven WB, Knickerbocker GG: Cardiac arrest: Report of application of external cardiac massage on 118 patients. *JAMA* 178:1063, 1961.
Katz AM, Reuter M: Cellular calcium and cardiac cell death. *Am J Cardiol* 44:188, 1979.
Kawashima Y, Takahashi S, Suzuki M, et al.: Anesthesia-related mortality and morbidity over a 5-year period in 2,363,038 patients in Japan. *Acta Anaesthesiol Scand* 47:809, 2003.
Keenan RL, Boyan CP: Cardiac arrest due to anesthesia: A study of incidence and causes. *JAMA* 253:2373, 1985.
Keenan RL, Shapiro JH, Dawson KD: Frequency of anesthetic cardiac arrests in infants: Effect of pediatric anesthesiologists. *J Clin Anesth* 3:433, 1991.
Kerber RE, Sarnat W: Factors influencing the success of ventricular defibrillation in man. *Circulation* 60:226, 1979.
Kern KB, Carter AB, Showen RL, et al.: Twenty-four hour survival in a canine model of cardiac arrest comparing three methods of manual cardiopulmonary resuscitation. *J Am Coll Cardiol* 7:859, 1986.
Kern KB, Hilwig RW, Berg RA, et al.: Efficacy of chest compression-only BLS CPR in the presence of an occluded airway. *Resuscitation* 39:179, 1998.
Kern KB, Sanders AB, Raife J, et al.: A study of chest compression rates during cardiopulmonary resuscitation in humans. The importance of rate-directed chest compressions. *Arch Intern Med* 152:145, 1992.
Kernstine KH, Tyson GS, Maier GW, et al.: Determinants of direct cardiac compression during external cardiac massage in intact dogs. *Crit Care Med* 10:231, 1982.
Kilecki PF, Curry SC: Poisoning by sodium channel blocking agents. *Crit Care Clin* 13:829-48, 1997.
Kleinman MF, Oh W, Stonestreet BS: Comparison of intravenous and endotracheal epinephrine during cardiopulmonary resuscitation in newborn piglets. *Crit Care Med* 27:2748, 1999.
Koch-Weser J: Drug therapy, bretylium. *N Engl J Med* 300:473, 1979.
Koehler RC, Chandra N, Guerci AD, et al.: Augmentation of cerebral perfusion by simultaneous chest compression and lung inflation with abdominal binding after cardiac arrest in dogs. *Circulation* 67:266, 1983.
Koehler RC, Michael JR, Guerci AD, et al.: Beneficial effect of epinephrine infusion on cerebral and myocardial blood flow during CPR. *Ann Emerg Med* 14:744, 1985a.
Koehler RC, Michael JR: Cardiopulmonary resuscitation, brain blood flow, and neurologic recovery. *Crit Care Clin* 1:205, 1985b.
Kottmeier CA, Gravenstein JS: The parasympathomimetic activity of atropine and atropine methylbromide. *Anesthesiology* 29:1125, 1968.
Kouwenhoven WB, Jude JR, Knickerbocker GG: Closed-chest cardiac massage. *JAMA* 173:1064, 1960.
Krischer JP, Fine EF, Weisfeldt ML, et al.: Comparison of prehospital conventional and simultaneous compression-ventilation cardiopulmonary resuscitation. *Crit Care Med* 17:1263, 1989.
Kudenchuk PJ, Cobb LA, Copass MK, et al.: Amiodarone for resuscitation after out-of-hospital cardiac arrest due to ventricular fibrillation. *N Engl J Med* 341:871, 1999.
Kuhn C, Juchems R, Frese W: Evidence for the "cardiac pump theory" in cardiopulmonary resuscitation in man by transesophageal echocardiography. *Resuscitation* 22:275, 1991.
Kuntzman R, Tsai I, Chang R: Disposition of bretylium in man and rat: A sensitive chemical method for its estimation in plasma and urine. *Clin Pharmacol Ther* 11:829, 1970.
Langhelle A, Stromme T, Sunde K, et al.: Inspiratory impedance threshold valve during CPR. *Resuscitation* 52:39, 2002.
Lasbennes F, Sercombe R, Seylaz J: Monoamine oxidase activity in brain microvessels determined using natural and artificial substances: Relevance to the blood-brain barrier. *J Cereb Blood Flow Metab* 3:521, 1983.
Lee CJ, Bullock LJ: Determining the pulse for infant CPR: Time for a change? *Milit Med* 156:190, 1991.
Lee G, Antognini JF, Gronert GA: Complete recovery after prolonged resuscitation and cardiopulmonary bypass for hyperkalemic cardiac arrest. *Anesth Analg* 79:172, 1994.
Lee HR, Wilder RJ, Downs P, et al.: MAST augmentation of external cardiac compression: Role of changing intrapleural pressure. *Ann Emerg Med* 10:560, 1981.
Lee SK, Vaagenes P, Safar P, et al.: Effect of cardiac arrest time on cortical cerebral blood flow generated by subsequent standard external cardiopulmonary resuscitation in rabbits. *Ann Emerg Med* 13:385, 1984.
Leigh MD, Belton MK: Anesthetic deaths in infants and children. *J Mich Med Soc* 48:871, 1949.
Levine R, Gorayeb M, Safar P, et al.: Cardiopulmonary bypass after cardiac arrest and prolonged closed-chest CPR in dogs. *Ann Emerg Med* 16:620, 1987.
Levine RL, Wayne MA, Miller CC: End-tidal carbon dioxide and outcome of out-of-hospital cardiac arrest. *N Engl J Med* 337:301, 1997.
Lichstein E, Chadda KD, Gupta PK: Atrioventricular block with lidocaine therapy. *Am J Cardiol* 31:277, 1973.
Lilja GP, Long RS, Ruiz E: Augmentation of systolic blood pressure during external cardiac compression by use of the MAST suit. *Ann Emerg Med* 10:182, 1981.
Lindner KH, Brinkmann A, Pfenninger EG, et al.: Effect of vasopressin on hemodynamic variables, organ blood flow, and acid-base status in a pig model of cardiopulmonary resuscitation. *Anesth Analg* 77:427, 1993.
Lindner KH, Dirks B, Strohmenger HU, et al.: Randomized comparison of epinephrine and vasopressin in patients with out-of-hospital ventricular fibrillation. *Lancet* 349:535, 1997.
Lindner KH, Prengel AW, Brinkmann A, et al.: Vasopressin administration in refractory cardiac arrest. *Ann Intern Med* 124:1061, 1996.
Lindner KH, Prengel AW, Pfenninger EG, et al.: Vasopressin improves vital organ blood flow during closed-chest cardiopulmonary resuscitation in pigs. *Circulation* 91:215, 1995.
Livesay JJ, Follette DM, Fey KH, et al.: Optimizing myocardial supply/demand balance with alpha-adrenergic drugs during cardiopulmonary resuscitation. *J Thorac Cardiovasc Surg* 76:244, 1978.
Longstreth WT, Diehr P, Cobb LA, et al.: Neurologic outcome and blood glucose levels during out-of-hospital cardiopulmonary resuscitation. *Neurology* 36:1186, 1986.
Longstreth WT, Inui TS: High blood glucose level on hospital admission and poor neurological recovery after cardiac arrest. *Ann Neurol* 15:59, 1984.
Losek JD, Endom E, Dietrich A, et al.: Adenosine and pediatric supraventricular tachycardia in the emergency department: Multicenter study and review. *Ann Emerg Med* 33:185, 1999.
Luce JM, Rizk NA, Niskanen RA: Regional blood flow during cardiopulmonary resuscitation in dogs. *Crit Care Med* 12:874, 1984.
Luce JM, Ross BK, O'Quin RJ, et al.: Regional blood flow during cardiopulmonary resuscitation in dogs using simultaneous and nonsimultaneous compression and ventilation. *Circulation* 67:258, 1983.
Luedtke SA, Kuhn RJ, McCaffrey FM: Pharmacologic management of supraventricular tachycardias in children. Part 2: Atrial flutter, atrial fibrillation, and junctional and atrial ectopic tachycardia. *Ann Pharmacother* 31:1347, 1997.
Lurie KG, Shultz JJ, Callaham ML, et al.: Evaluation of active compression-decompression CPR in victims of out-of-hospital cardiac arrest. *JAMA* 271:1405, 1994.
Lurie KG, Zielinski T, Voelckel W, et al.: Augmentation of ventricular preload during treatment of cardiovascular collapse and cardiac arrest. *Crit Care Med* 30:S162-5, 2002.
MacKenzie ET, McCulloch J, O'Keane M, et al.: Cerebral circulation and norepinephrine: Relevance of the blood-brain barrier. *Am J Physiol* 231:483, 1976.
MacKenzie GJ, Taylor SH, McDonald AH, et al.: Haemodynamic effects of external cardiac compression. *Lancet* 1:1342, 1964.
Mahoney BD, Mirick MJ: Efficacy of pneumatic trousers in refractory prehospital cardiopulmonary arrest. *Ann Emerg Med* 12:8, 1983.
Maier GW, Tyson GS, Olsen CO, et al.: The physiology of external cardiac massage: High-impulse cardiopulmonary resuscitation. *Circulation* 70:86, 1984.
Mandapati R, Byrum CJ, Kavey RE, et al.: Procainamide for rate control of postsurgical junctional tachycardia. *Pediatr Cardiol* 21:123, 2000.
Mann K, Berg RA, Nadkarni V: Beneficial effects of vasopressin in prolonged pediatric cardiac arrest: A case series. *Resuscitation* 52:149, 2002.
Markis JE, Koch-Weser J: Characterizations and mechanisms of inotropic and chronotropic actions of bretylium tosylate. *J Pharmacol Exp Ther* 178:94, 1971.
Marquez J, Martin D, Virja MA, et al.: Cardiovascular depression secondary to ionic hypocalcemia during hepatic transplantation in humans. *Anesthesiology* 65:457, 1986.
Martin D, Werman HA, Brown CG: Four case studies: high dose epinephrine in cardiac arrest. *Ann Emerg Med* 19:322, 1990.
Martin GB, Carden DL, Nowak RM, et al.: Aortic and right atrial pressures during standard and simultaneous compression and ventilation CPR in human beings. *Ann Emerg Med* 15:125, 1986.
Martin GB, Gentile NT, Paradis NA, et al.: Effect of epinephrine on end-tidal carbon dioxide monitoring during CPR. *Ann Emerg Med* 19:396, 1990.
Martin GB, Rivers EP, Paradis NA, et al.: Emergency department cardiopulmonary bypass in the treatment of human cardiac arrest. *Chest* 113:743, 1998.
Martinez LR, Holland S, Fitzgerald J, et al.: pH homeostasis during cardiopulmonary resuscitation in critically ill patients. *Resuscitation* 7:109, 1979.
Marx GF, Mateo CV, Orkin LR: Computer analysis of postanesthetic deaths. *Anesthesiology* 39:54, 1973.
Mateer JR, Stueben HA, Thompson BM, et al.: Pre-hospital IAC-CPR versus standard CPR: Paramedic resuscitation of cardiac arrests. *Am J Emerg Med* 3:143, 1985.

Mattar JA, Weil MH, Shubin H, et al.: Cardiac arrest in the critically ill: II. Hyperosmolal states following cardiac arrest. *Am J Med* 56:162, 1974.

Mattox KL, Beall AC: Resuscitation of the moribund patient using portable cardiopulmonary bypass. *Ann Thorac Surg* 22:436, 1976.

Mauer D, Schneider T, Dick W, et al.: Active compression-decompression resuscitation: A prospective, randomized study in a two-tiered EMS system with physicians in the field. *Resuscitation* 33:125, 1996.

Mazer SP, Weisfeldt M, Bai D, et al.: Reverse CPR: A pilot study of CPR in the prone position. *Resuscitation* 57:279, 2003.

Michael JR, Guerci AD, Koehler RC, et al.: Mechanisms by which epinephrine augments cerebral and myocardial blood perfusion during cardiopulmonary resuscitation in dogs. *Circulation* 69:822, 1984.

Miranda CC, Newton MC: Successful defibrillation in the prone position. *Br J Anaesth* 87:937, 2001.

Mogayzel C, Quan L, Graves JR, et al.: Out-of-hospital ventricular fibrillation in children and adolescents: Causes and outcomes. *Ann Emerg Med* 25:484,1995.

Morgan CA, Webb RK, Cockings J, et al.: The Australian Incident Monitoring Study. Cardiac arrest—an analysis of 2000 incident reports. *Anaesth Intensive Care* 21:626, 1993.

Morray JP, Geiduschek JM, Ramamoorthy C, et al.: Anesthesia-related cardiac arrest in children: initial findings of the Pediatric Perioperative Cardiac Arrest (POCA) Registry. *Anesthesiology* 93:6, 2000.

Morray JP: Anesthesia-related cardiac arrest in children. An update. *Anesthesiol Clin North Am* 20:1, 2002.

Morris DC, Dereczyk BE, Grzybowski M, et al.: Vasopressin can increase coronary perfusion pressure during human cardiopulmonary resuscitation. *Acad Emerg Med* 4:878, 1997.

Muir JD, Randalls PR, Smith GB: End tidal carbon dioxide detector for monitoring cardiopulmonary resuscitation. *Br Med J* 301:41, 1990.

Mullins ME, Pinnick RV, Terhes JM: Life threatening diphenhydramine overdose treated with charcoal hemoperfusion and hemodialysis. *Ann Emerg Med* 33:104-7, 1999.

Myers R: Lactic acid accumulation as a cause of brain edema and cerebral necrosis resulting from oxygen deprivation. In Korbin R, Gilleminault C, editors: *Advances in perinatal neurology*. New York, 1979, Spectrum, p 84.

Nakatani K, Yukioka H, Fujimori M, et al.: Utility of colorimetric end-tidal carbon dioxide detector for monitoring during prehospital cardiopulmonary resuscitation. *Am J Emerg Med* 17:203, 1999.

Nattel S: Comparative mechanisms of action of antiarrhythmic drugs. *Am J Cardiol* 72:13F, 1993.

Newland MC, Ellis SJ, Lydiatt CA, et al.: Anesthetic-related cardiac arrest and its mortality: A report covering 72,959 anesthetics over 10 years from a US teaching hospital. *Anesthesiology* 97:108, 2002.

Niemann JT, Cairns CB, Sharma J, et al.: Treatment of prolonged ventricular fibrillation: immediate countershock versus high-dose epinephrine and CPR preceding countershock. *Circulation* 85:281, 1992.

Niemann JT, Garner D, Khaleeli E, et al.: Milrinone facilitates resuscitation from cardiac arrest and attenuates post-resuscitation myocardial dysfunction. *Circulation* 108:3031, 2003.

Niemann JT, Rosborough JP, Hausknecht M, et al.: Blood flow without cardiac compression during closed chest CPR. *Crit Care Med* 9:380, 1981a.

Niemann JT, Rosborough JP, Hausknecht M, et al.: Cough-CPR: documentation of systemic perfusion in man and in an experimental model: A "window" to the mechanism of blood flow in external CPR. *Crit Care Med* 8:141, 1980.

Niemann JT, Rosborough JP, Hausknecht M, et al.: Pressure-synchronized cineangiography during experimental cardiopulmonary resuscitation. *Circulation* 64:985, 1981b.

Niemann JT, Rosborough JP, Pelikin PCD: Hemodynamic determinants of subdiaphragmatic venous return during closed-chest CPR in a canine cardiac arrest model. *Ann Emerg Med* 19:1232, 1990.

Niemann JT, Rosborough JP, Ung S, et al.: Hemodynamic effects of continuous abdominal binding during cardiac arrest and resuscitation. *Am J Cardiol* 53:269, 1984.

Niskanen RA: Automated external defibrillators: Experiences with their use and options for their further development. *New Horiz* 5:137, 1997.

Nolan J, Smith G, Evans R, et al.: The United Kingdom pre-hospital study of active compression-decompression resuscitation. *Resuscitation* 37:119, 1998.

Nolan JP, Morley PT, Vanden Hoek TL, et al.: Therapeutic hypothermia after cardiac arrest. An advisory statement by the Advanced Life Support Task Force of the International Liaison Committee on Resuscitation. *Circulation* 108:118-121, 2003.

Olsson GL, Hallen B: Cardiac arrest during anaesthesia. A computer-aided study in 250,543 anaesthetics. *Acta Anaesthesiol Scand* 32:653, 1988.

Orlowski JP, Julius CJ, Petras RE, et al.: The safety of intraosseous infusions: Risks of fat and bone marrow emboli to the lungs. *Ann Emerg Med* 18:1062, 1989.

Orlowski JP: Cardiopulmonary resuscitation in children. *Pediatr Clin North Am* 27:495, 1980.

Ornato JP, Gonzalez ER, Garnett AR, et al.: Effect of cardiopulmonary resuscitation compression rate on end-tidal carbon dioxide concentration and arterial pressure in man. *Crit Care Med* 16:241, 1988.

Pannier JL, Leusen I: Contraction characteristics of papillary muscle during changes in acid-base composition of the bathing fluid. *Arch Int Physiol Biochem* 76:624, 1968.

Paradis NA, Martin GB, Goetting MG, et al.: Simultaneous aortic, jugular bulb, and right atrial pressures during cardiopulmonary resuscitation in humans: Insights into mechanisms. *Circulation* 80:361, 1989.

Paradis NA, Martin GB, Rivers EP, et al.: Coronary perfusion pressure and the return of spontaneous circulation in human cardiopulmonary resuscitation. *JAMA* 263:1106, 1990.

Parra DA, Totapally BR, Zahn E, et al.: Outcome of cardiopulmonary resuscitation in a pediatric cardiac intensive care unit. *Crit Care Med* 28:3296-300, 2000.

Pearson JW, Redding JS: Influence of peripheral vascular tone on resuscitation. *Anesth Analg* 44:746, 1965.

Peleska B: Cardiac arrhythmias following condenser discharges and their dependence upon strength of current and phase of cardiac cycle. *Circ Res* 13:21, 1963.

Perry JC, Fenrich AL, Hulse JE, et al.: Pediatric use of intravenous amiodarone: efficacy and safety in critically ill patients from a multicenter protocol. *J Am Coll Cardiol* 27:1246-1250, 1996.

Perry JC, Knilans TK, Marlow D, et al.: Intravenous amiodarone for life-threatening tachyarrhythmias in children and young adults. *J Am Coll Cardiol* 22:95, 1993.

Phillips SJ, Ballentine B, Slonine D, et al.: Percutaneous initiation of cardiopulmonary bypass. *Ann Thorac Surg* 36:223, 1983.

Pionkowski RS, Thompson BM, Gruchow HW, et al.: Resuscitation time in ventricular fibrillation: A prognostic indicator. *Ann Emerg Med* 12:733, 1983.

Plaisance P, Adnet F, Vicaut E, et al.: Benefit of active compression-decompression cardiopulmonary resuscitation as a prehospital advanced cardiac life support. A randomized multicenter study. *Circulation* 95:955, 1997.

Plaisance P, Lurie KG, Payen D: Inspiratory impedance during active compression-decompression cardiopulmonary resuscitation—A randomized evaluation in patients in cardiac arrest. *Circulation* 101:989-94, 2000.

Podrid PJ: Amiodarone: Reevaluation of an old drug. *Ann Intern Med* 122:689, 1995.

Prado R, Ginsberg MD, Dietrich WD, et al.: Hyperglycemia increases infarct size in collaterally perfused but not end-arterial vascular territories. *J Cereb Blood Flow Metab* 8:186, 1988.

Prengel AW, Lindner KH, Keller A, et al.: Cardiovascular function during the post-resuscitation phase after cardiac arrest in pigs: A comparison of epinephrine versus vasopressin. *Crit Care Med* 24:2014, 1996a.

Prengel AW, Lindner KH, Keller A: Cerebral oxygenation during cardiopulmonary resuscitation with epinephrine and vasopressin in pigs. *Stroke* 27:1241, 1996b.

Prengel AW, Lindner KH, Wenzel V, et al.: Splanchnic and renal blood flow after cardiopulmonary resuscitation with epinephrine and vasopressin in pigs. *Resuscitation* 38:19, 1998.

Pretto E, Safar P, Saito R, et al.: Cardiopulmonary bypass after prolonged cardiac arrest in dogs. *Ann Emerg Med* 16:611, 1987.

Pulsinelli WA, Levy DE, Sigsbee B, et al.: Increased damage after ischemic stroke in patients with hyperglycemia with or without established diabetes mellitus. *Am J Med* 74:540, 1983.

Quan L, Graves JR, Kinder DR, et al.: Transcutaneous cardiac pacing in the treatment of out-of-hospital pediatric cardiac arrests. *Ann Emerg Med* 21:905, 1992.

Rackow H, Salanitre E, Green LT: Frequency of cardiac arrest associated with anesthesia in infants and children. *Pediatrics* 28:697, 1961.

Raessler KL, Kern KB, Sanders AB, et al.: Aortic and right atrial systolic pressures during cardiopulmonary resuscitation: A potential indicator of the mechanism of blood flow. *Am Heart J* 115:1021, 1988.

Rainer EH: Respiratory and cardiac arrest during anaesthesia in children. *Br Med J* 2:1024, 1957.

Ralston SH, Babbs CF, Niebauer MJ: Cardiopulmonary resuscitation with interposed abdominal compression in dogs. *Anesth Analg* 61:645, 1982.

Ralston SH, Voorhees WD, Babbs CF: Intrapulmonary epinephrine during prolonged cardiopulmonary resuscitation: Improved regional blood flow and resuscitation in dogs. *Ann Emerg Med* 13:79, 1984.

Redding JS, Pearson JW: Evaluation for drugs for cardiac resuscitation. *Anesthesiology* 24:203, 1963.

Redding JS: Abdominal compression in cardiopulmonary resuscitation. *Anesth Analg* 50:668, 1971.

Reich H, Angelos M, Safar P, et al.: Cardiac resuscitability with cardiopulmonary bypass after increasing ventricular fibrillation times in dogs. *Ann Emerg Med* 19:887, 1990.

Reichman RT, Joyo CI, Dembitsky WP, et al.: Improved patient survival after cardiac arrest using a cardiopulmonary support system. *Ann Thorac Surg* 49:101, 1990.

Reidenberg MM, Drayer DE, Levy M, et al.: Polymorphic acetylation procainamide in man. *Clin Pharmacol Ther* 17:722, 1975.

Reis AG, Nadkarni V, Perondi MB, et al.: A prospective investigation into the epidemiology of in-hospital pediatric cardiopulmonary resuscitation using the international Utstein reporting style. *Pediatrics* 109:200, 2002.

Resnekov L: Calcium antagonist drugs: Myocardial preservation and reduced vulnerability to ventricular fibrillation during CPR. *Crit Care Med* 9:360, 1981.

Rich S, Wix HL, Shapiro EP: Clinical assessment of heart size and valve motion during cardiopulmonary resuscitation by two-dimensional echocardiography. *Am Heart J* 102:368, 1981.

Rivers EP, Martin GB, Smithine H, et al.: The clinical implications of continuous central venous oxygen saturation during human CPR. *Ann Emerg Med* 21:1094, 1992.

Roberts SA, Viana MA, Nazari J, et al.: Invasive and noninvasive methods to predict the long-term efficacy of amiodarone: A compilation of clinical observations using meta-analysis. *PACE Pacing Clin Electrophysiol* 17:1590, 1994.

Rogers MC, Nugent SK, Stidham GL: Effects of closed-chest cardiac massage on intracranial pressure. *Crit Care Med* 7:454, 1979.

Romhilt DW, Bloodfield SS, Lipicky RJ: Evaluation of bretylium tosylate for the treatment of premature ventricular contractions. *Circulation* 45:800, 1972.

Rudikoff MT, Maughan WL, Effron M, et al.: Mechanism of blood flow during cardiopulmonary resuscitation. *Circulation* 61:345, 1980.

Rudolph AM, Yuan S: Response of the pulmonary vasculature to hypoxia and hydrogen ion concentration changes. *J Clin Invest* 45:399, 1966.

Rumball CJ, MacDonald D: The PTL, Combitube, laryngeal mask, and oral airway: A randomized prehospital comparative study of ventilatory device effectiveness and cost-effectiveness in 470 cases of cardiorespiratory arrest. *Prehosp Emerg Care* 1:1, 1997.

Sack JB, Kesselbrenner MB, Bregman D: Survival from in-hospital cardiac arrest with interposed abdominal counterpulsation during cardiopulmonary resuscitation. *JAMA* 267:379, 1992.

Safar P, Brown TC, Holtey WJ, et al.: Ventilation and circulation with closed-chest cardiac massage in man. *JAMA* 176:92, 1961.

Salem MR, Bennett EJ, Schweiss JF, et al.: Cardiac arrest related to anesthesia. Contributing factors in infants and children. *JAMA* 233:238, 1975.

Samarkandi AH, Seraj MA, el Dawlatly A, et al.: The role of laryngeal mask airway in cardiopulmonary resuscitation. *Resuscitation* 28:103, 1994.

Samson RA, Berg RA, Bingham R, et al.: Pediatric Advanced Life Support Task Force, International Liaison Committee on Resuscitation: Use of automated external defibrillators for children: An update: An advisory statement from the Pediatric Advanced Life Support Task Force, International Liaison Committee on Resuscitation. *Circulation* 107:3250, 2003.

Sanders AB, Atlas M, Ewy GA, et al.: Expired PCO_2 as an index of coronary perfusion pressure. *Am J Emerg Med* 3:147, 1985a.

Sanders AB, Ewy GA, Alferness CA, et al.: Failure of one method of simultaneous chest compression, ventilation, and abdominal binding during CPR. *Crit Care Med* 10:50913, 1982.

Sanders AB, Ewy GA, Taft TV: Prognostic and therapeutic importance of the aortic diastolic pressure in resuscitation from cardiac arrest. *Crit Care Med* 12:871, 1984b.

Sanders AB, Kern KB, Ewy GA, et al.: Improved outcome from cardiac arrest with open-chest massage. *Ann Emerg Med* 13:672, 1984a.

Sanders AB, Kern KB, Ewy GA: Time limitations for open-chest cardiopulmonary resuscitation from cardiac arrest. *Crit Care Med* 13:897, 1985b.

Sanders AB, Kern KB, Fonken S, et al.: The role of bicarbonate and fluid loading in improving resuscitation from prolonged cardiac arrest with rapid manual chest compression CPR. *Ann Emerg Med* 19:1, 1990.

Sanders AB, Kern KB, Otto CW, et al.: End-tidal carbon dioxide monitoring during cardiopulmonary resuscitation: A prognostic indicator for survival. *JAMA* 262:1347, 1989.

Scheidegger D, Drop LJ, Laver MB: Interaction between vasoactive drugs and plasma ionized calcium. *Intensive Care Med* 3:200, 1977.

Scheinman MM, Thorburn D, Abbott JA: Use of atropine in patients with acute myocardial infarction and sinus bradycardia. *Circulation* 52:627, 1975.

Schierhout G, Roberts I: Fluid resuscitation with colloid or crystalloid solutions in critically ill patients: A systematic review of randomized trials. *BMJ* 316:961, 1998.

Schleien CL, Caceres MJ, Kuluz JW, et al.: Light and electron microscopic blood-brain barrier (BBB) changes following cardiopulmonary resuscitation in young piglets. *Anesthesiology* 77(suppl IIIA):712, 1992.

Schleien CL, Dean JM, Koehler RC, et al.: Effect of epinephrine on cerebral and myocardial perfusion in an infant animal preparation of cardiopulmonary resuscitation. *Circulation* 73:809, 1986.

Schleien CL, Koehler RC, Gervais H, et al.: Organ blood flow and somatosensory evoked potentials before and after cardiopulmonary resuscitation with epinephrine and phenylephrine. *Circulation* 79:1332, 1989.

Schleien CL, Koehler RC, Shaffner DH, et al.: Blood-brain barrier disruption after cardiopulmonary resuscitation in immature swine. *Stroke* 22:477, 1991.

Schleien CL, Kuluz JW, Shaffner DH, et al.: Cardiopulmonary resuscitation. In Rogers MC, editor: *Textbook of pediatric intensive care,* 2nd ed. Baltimore, 1992, Williams & Wilkins, p 52.

Schumacher RR, Lieberson AD, Childress RH, et al.: Hemodynamic effects of lidocaine in patients with heart disease. *Am J Cardiol* 24:191, 1968.

Schwab TM, Callaham ML, Madsen CD, et al.: A randomized clinical trial of active compression-decompression CPR versus standard CPR in out-of-hospital cardiac arrest in two cities. *JAMA* 273:1261, 1995.

Sessler D, Mills P, Gregory G, et al.: Effects of bicarbonate on arterial and brain intracellular pH in neonatal rabbits recovering from hypoxic lactic acidosis. *J Pediatr* 111:817, 1987.

Shaffner DH, Eleff SM, Brambrink AM, et al.: Effect of arrest time and cerebral perfusion pressure during cardiopulmonary resuscitation on cerebral blood flow, metabolism, ATP recovery, and pH in dogs. *Crit Care Med* 27:1335, 1999.

Shaffner DH, Eleff SM, Koehler RC, et al.: Effect of the no-flow interval and hypothermia on cerebral blood flow and metabolism during cardiopulmonary resuscitation in dogs. *Stroke* 29:2607, 1998.

Shaffner DH, Schleien CL, Koehler RC, et al.: Cerebral and coronary perfusion with vest cardiopulmonary resuscitation in piglets. *Crit Care Med* 18:S243, 1990.

Sharff JA, Pantley G, Noel E: Effect of time on regional organ perfusion during two methods of cardiopulmonary resuscitation. *Ann Emerg Med* 13:649, 1984.

Sieber FE, Traystman RJ: Special issues: Glucose and the brain. *Crit Care Med* 20:104, 1992.

Siemkowicz E, Hansen AJ: Clinical restitution following cerebral ischemia in hypo-, normo- and hyperglycemic rats. *Acta Neurol Scand* 58:1, 1978.

Siesjo BK: Cerebral circulation and metabolism. *Neurosurgery* 60:883, 1984.

Singh BN, Venkatesh N, Nademanee K, et al.: The historical development, cellular electrophysiology and pharmacology of amiodarone. *Prog Cardiovasc Dis* 31:249, 1989.

Singh BN: Antiarrhythmic actions of amiodarone: A profile of a paradoxical agent. *Am J Cardiol* 78:41, 1996.

Sladen A: Closed-chest massage. *JAMA* 251:3137, 1984.

Snyder AV, Salloum LJ, Barone JE, et al.: Predicting short-term outcome of cardiopulmonary resuscitation using central venous oxygen tension measurements. *Crit Care Med* 19:111, 1991.

Sprung J, Warner ME, Contreras MG, et al.: Predictors of survival following cardiac arrest in patients undergoing noncardiac surgery: A study of 518,294 patients at a tertiary referral center. *Anesthesiology* 99:259, 2003.

Stacpoole PAW, Gonzalez MG, Vlasak J, et al.: Dichloroacetate derivatives. Metabolic effects and pharmacodynamics in normal rats. *Life Sci* 41:2167, 1987.

Stacpoole PAW, Lorenz AC, Thomas RG, et al.: Dichloroacetate in the treatment of lactic acidosis. *Ann Intern Med* 108:58, 1988.

Stacpoole PAW, Wright EC, Baumgartner TG: A controlled clinical trial of dichloroacetate for treatment of lactic acidosis in adults. *N Engl J Med* 327:1564, 1992.

Stacpoole PAW: The pharmacology of dichloroacetate. *Metab Clin Exp* 38:1124, 1989.

Steinhart CR, Permutt S, Gurtner GH, et al.: Beta-adrenergic activity and cardiovascular response to severe respiratory acidosis. *Am J Physiol* 244:H46, 1983.

Stiell IG, Hebert PC, Weitzman BN, et al.: High-dose epinephrine in adult cardiac arrest. *N Engl J Med* 327:1045, 1992.

Stiell IG, Hebert PC, Wells GA, et al.: The Ontario trial of active compression-decompression cardiopulmonary resuscitation for in-hospital and prehospital cardiac arrest. *JAMA* 275:1417, 1996.

Stone BJ, Chantler PJ, Baskett PJ: The incidence of regurgitation during cardiopulmonary resuscitation: A comparison between the bag valve mask and laryngeal mask airway. *Resuscitation* 38:3, 1998.

Strohmenger HU, Lindner KH, Keller A, et al.: Effects of graded doses of vasopressin on median fibrillation frequency in a porcine model of cardiopulmonary resuscitation: Results of a prospective, randomized, controlled trial. *Crit Care Med* 24:1360, 1996.

Stueven HA, Aprahamian C, Tonsfeldt DJ, et al.: Lack of effectiveness of calcium chloride in refractory asystole. *Ann Emerg Med* 14:630, 1985.

Stueven HA, Thompson BM, Aprahamian C, et al.: The effectiveness of calcium chloride in refractory electromechanical dissociation. *Ann Emerg Med* 14:626, 1985.

Sun JH, Filley GF, Hord K, et al.: Carbicarb: an effective substitute for $NaHCO_3$ for the treatment of acidosis. *Surgery* 102:835-839, 1987.

Sun W, Huang F, Kung K, et al.: Successful cardiopulmonary resuscitation of two patients in the prone position reversed precordial compression. *Anesthesiology* 77:202, 1992.

Suominen P, Olkkola KT, Voipio V, et al.: Utstein style reporting of in-hospital paediatric cardiopulmonary resuscitation. *Resuscitation* 45:17-25, 2000.

Swenson RD, Weaver WD, Niskanen RA, et al.: Hemodynamics in humans during conventional and experimental methods of cardiopulmonary resuscitation. *Circulation* 78:630, 1988.

Tacker WA Jr, Babbs CF, Abendschein DR, et al.: Transchest defibrillation under conditions of hypothermia. *Crit Care Med* 9:390, 1981.

Tang W, Weil MH, Gazmuri RJ, et al.: Pulmonary ventilation/perfusion defects induced by epinephrine during cardiopulmonary resuscitation. *Circulation* 84:2101, 1991.

Tang W, Weil MH, Jorgenson D, et al.: Fixed-energy biphasic waveform defibrillation in a pediatric model of cardiac arrest and resuscitation. *Crit Care Med* 30:2736-41, 2002.

Tang W, Weil MH, Schock RB: Phased chest and abdominal compression-decompression. A new option for cardiopulmonary resuscitation. *Circulation* 95:1335, 1997.

Taylor GJ, Tucker WM, Greene HL, et al.: Importance of prolonged compression during cardiopulmonary resuscitation in man. *N Engl J Med* 296:1515, 1977.

Tisherman SA, Safar P, Abramson NS, et al.: Feasibility of emergency cardiopulmonary bypass for resuscitation from CPR-resistant cardiac arrest: A preliminary report. *Ann Emerg Med* 20:491, 1991.

Tobias JD, Mencio GA, Atwood R, et al.: Intraoperative cardiopulmonary resuscitation in the prone position. *J Pediatr Surg* 29:1537, 1994.

Todres ID, Rogers MC: Methods of external cardiac massage in the newborn infant. *J Pediatr* 86:781, 1975.

Urban P, Scheidegger D, Buchmann B, et al.: Cardiac arrest and blood ionized calcium levels. *Ann Intern Med* 109:110, 1988.

Urban P, Scheidegger D, Buchmann B, et al.: The hemodynamic effects of heparin and their relation to ionized calcium levels. *J Thorac Cardiovasc Surg* 91:303, 1986.

Vacanti CJ, VanHouten RJ, Hill RC: A statistic analysis of the relationship of physical status to postoperative mortality in 68,388 cases. *Anesth Analg* 49:564, 1970.

Voelckel WG, Lurie KG, McKnite S, et al.: Effects of epinephrine and vasopressin in a piglet model of prolonged ventricular fibrillation and cardiopulmonary resuscitation. *Crit Care Med* 30:957-62, 2002.

Voll CL, Auer RN: Insulin attenuates ischemic brain damage independent of its hypoglycemic effect. *J Cereb Blood Flow Metab* 11:1006, 1991.

Voll CL, Auer RN: The effect of postischemic blood glucose levels on ischemic brain damage in the rat. *Ann Neurol* 24:638, 1988.

Von Seggern K, Egar M, Fuhrman BP: Cardiopulmonary resuscitation in a pediatric ICU. *Crit Care Med* 14:275-277, 1986.

Voorhees WD, Niebauer MJ, Babbs CF: Improved oxygen delivery during cardiopulmonary resuscitation with interposed abdominal compressions. *Ann Emerg Med* 12:128, 1983.

Waisman M, Waisman D: Bone marrow infusion in adults. *J Trauma* 42:288, 1997.

Walker JW, Bruestle JC, White BC, et al.: Perfusion of the cerebral cortex by use of abdominal counterpulsation during cardiopulmonary resuscitation. *Am J Emerg Med* 2:391, 1984.

Walsh EP, Saul JP, Sholler GF, et al.: Evaluation of a staged treatment protocol for rapid automatic junctional tachycardia after operation for congenital heart disease. *J Am Coll Cardiol* 29:1046, 1997.

Ward KR, Sullivan RJ, Zelenak RR, et al.: A comparison of interposed abdominal compression CPR and standard CPR by monitoring end-tidal PCO_2. *Ann Emerg Med* 18:831, 1989.

Wargovich TJ, MacDonald RG, Hill JA, et al.: Myocardial metabolic and hemodynamic effects of dichloroacetate in coronary artery disease. *Am J Cardiol* 61:65, 1988.

Wayne MA, Levine RL, Miller CC: Use of end-tidal carbon dioxide to predict outcome in prehospital cardiac arrest. *Ann Emerg Med* 25:762, 1995.

Weale FE, Rothwell-Jackson RL: The efficiency of cardiac massage. *Lancet* 1:990, 1962.

Weaver WD, Cobb LA, Copass MK, et al.: Ventricular defibrillation: A comparative trial using 175-J and 320-J shocks. *N Engl J Med* 307:1101, 1982.

Weaver WD, Hill D, Fahrenbruch CE, et al.: Use of the automatic external defibrillator in the management of out-of-hospital cardiac arrest. *N Engl J Med* 319:661, 1988.

Weil MH, Rackow EC, Trevino R, et al.: Differences in acid-base state between venous and arterial blood during cardiopulmonary resuscitation. *N Engl J Med* 315:153, 1986.

Weiser FM, Adler LN, Kuhn LA: Hemodynamic effects of closed and open chest cardiac resuscitation in normal dogs and those with acute myocardial infarction. *Am J Cardiol* 10:555, 1962.

Wenzel V, Krismer AC, Arntz HR, et al.: European Resuscitation Council Vasopressor during Cardiopulmonary Resuscitation Study Group: A comparison of vasopressin and epinephrine for out-of-hospital cardiopulmonary resuscitation. *N Engl J Med* 350:105, 2004.

Wenzel V, Lindner KH: Arginine vasopressin during cardiopulmonary resuscitation: Laboratory evidence, clinical experience and recommendations, and a view to the future. *Crit Care Med* 30:S157, 2002.

Werner JA, Greene HL, Janko CL, et al.: Visualization of cardiac valve motion in man during external chest compression using two-dimensional echocardiography: Implications regarding the mechanism of blood flow. *Circulation* 63:1417, 1981.

White BC, Winegar CD, Wilson RF, et al.: Possible role of calcium blockers in cerebral resuscitation: A review of the literature and synthesis for future studies. *Crit Care Med* 11:202, 1983.

Wilder RJ, Weir D, Rush BF, et al.: Methods of coordinating ventilation and closed chest cardiac massage in the dog. *Surgery* 53:186, 1963.

Winquist RJ, Webb RC, Bohr OF: Relaxation to transmural nerve stimulation and exogenously added norepinephrine in porcine vessels. A study utilizing cerebrovascular intrinsic tone. *Circ Res* 51:769, 1982.

Wolcke BB, Mauer DK, Schoefmann MF, et al.: Comparison of standard cardiopulmonary resuscitation versus the combination of active compression-decompression cardiopulmonary resuscitation and an inspiratory impedance threshold device for out-of-hospital cardiac arrest. *Circulation* 108:2201, 2003.

Woo E, Chan YW, Yu YL, et al.: Admission glucose level in relation to mortality and morbidity outcome in 252 stroke patients. *Stroke* 19:185, 1988.

Wood WB, Manley ES Jr, Woodbury RA: The effects of CO_2 induced respiratory acidosis on the depressor and pressor components of the dog's blood pressure to epinephrine. *J Pharmacol Exp Ther* 139:238, 1963.

Worthley LS: Sodium bicarbonate in cardiac arrest. *Lancet* 2:903, 1976.

Xiao F, Safar P, Radovsky A: Mild protective and resuscitative hypothermia for asphyxial cardiac arrest in rats. *Am J Emerg Med* 16:17, 1998.

Yakaitis RW, Otto CW, Blitt CD: Relative importance of alpha and beta adrenergic receptors during resuscitation. *Crit Care Med* 7:293, 1979.

Yu T, Weil MH, Tang W, et al.: Adverse outcomes of interrupted precordial compression during automated defibrillation. *Circulation* 106:368, 2002.

Zaritsky A, Nadkarni V, Hazinski MF, et al.: Recommended guidelines for uniform reporting of pediatric advanced life support: The pediatric Utstein Style. A statement for healthcare professionals from a task force of the American Academy of Pediatrics, the American Heart Association, and the European Resuscitation Council Writing Group. *Circulation* 92:2006, 1995.

Zipes DP, Fischer J, King RM, et al.: Termination of ventricular fibrillation in dogs by depolarizing a critical amount of myocardium. *Am J Cardiol* 36:37, 1975.

34 Safety and Outcome in Pediatric Anesthesia

Etsuro K. Motoyama

The safety of infants and children undergoing general anesthesia has improved considerably since the 1970s, as evidenced by significant decreases in anesthesia mortality despite the fact that more complicated surgical procedures have been performed on sicker children and more premature infants.

Since the 1980s, anesthesiologists' awareness of and interest in the subject of patient safety have reached a new peak (Smith and Norman, 1987; Runciman, 1988a; Runciman et al., 1988b), and a number of new steps have been taken to ensure perioperative patient safety (Keats and Siker, 1985). In addition to advanced technology for patient monitoring, standards for basic patient monitoring have been implemented (American Society of Anesthesiologists, 1986; Eichhorn et al., 1986). Documentation of the quality assurance (QA) process has been emphasized as an integral and essential component for hospital accreditation by the Joint Commission on Accreditation of Healthcare Organizations (JCAHO) in the United States. To further improve the quality of patient care, a number of national and international organizations have been created, including the International Committee on Prevention of Anesthesia Mortality and Morbidity (Cooper, 1988), the Anesthesia Patient Safety Foundation (Cooper and Pierce, 1986), and the Australian Patient Safety Foundation (Pierce, 1988; Runciman, 1988b).

Nevertheless, anesthesia-related morbidity and mortality still do occur during the administration of anesthesia, and can happen with any anesthesiologist under various situations. An analysis of anesthetic mishaps from U.S. closed anesthesia malpractice claims, before the new patient monitoring standards with pulse oximetry and capnography were instituted, indicated that at least 80% of the claims consist of preventable hypoxic damage caused by human errors rather than mechanical failures (Davis, 1984).

Allnutt (1987), a member of the British Army Personnel Research Establishment, examined human factors in anesthesia-related mishaps in comparison with those in military aviation accidents. He stresses that "both pilots and doctors make many errors" (that is, performance that deviates from the ideal). "Usually there is sufficient slack in the system for the error to be... noticed and corrected, but some apparently innocuous errors are not noticed and some systems are not so forgiving as others" (such as a high performance aircraft in flight). "Thus recovery from a control error when flying at high speed, low level may not be possible, whereas the same error in the cruise [at high altitude] might barely occasion comment." A basic tenet of Allnutt's theory is that "all human beings, without any exception whatsoever, make errors and that such errors are a completely normal and necessary part of human cognitive function." He goes on to state that "to claim exemption on the grounds of being a senior professor [or a] test pilot ... or of having 30 years' experience or 3000 accident-free hours, is the first step on the road to disaster." The first step toward the prevention of catastrophe is for the pilot or the anesthetist to accept that he or she is as likely as anyone else to make an error (Pierce, 1988).

In this chapter, some of the important aspects of patient safety—the incidence and causes of mortality and morbidity and measures for the prevention of anesthesia-related mishaps—are discussed.

ANESTHESIA-RELATED MORTALITY

OVERALL ANESTHESIA-RELATED MORTALITY

The number of deaths associated with general anesthesia has declined steadily over the past several decades as the standard of anesthesia practice has improved and as advances have been made in instrumentation, anesthetic and adjuvant drugs, and safety monitors and standards. The extensive survey of 10 university hospitals by Beecher and Todd (1954) involving nearly 600,000 anesthetic cases between 1948 and 1952 suggested that mortality primarily attributable to anesthesia occurred in 1:2680 anesthetic cases (3.7:10,000), whereas the overall anesthesia-associated mortality was 1:1580 (6.3:10,000) anesthetics (Graff et al., 1964).

A survey by Dornette and Orth (1956) showed similar mortality rates. The data from the Baltimore Anesthesia Study Committee (1953 to 1963) showed an anesthesia-related death rate of 2.7:10,000 cases. During the 1970s and 1980s, statistics on anesthesia-related mortality in the United States were scarce, apparently because of medicolegal concerns. The anesthesia-related mortality from Canadian, British, and European sources during this period ranged from 0.7 to 2.2:10,000 anesthetic procedures (Bodlander, 1975; Harrison, 1978; Hovi-Viander, 1980; Turnbull et al., 1980; Lunn and Mushin, 1982; Hatton et al., 1983; Vickers and Lunn, 1983).

In the 1980s, European and Australian studies had shown much lower rates of operative mortality that were directly attributed to anesthesia. The report from the British Confidential Enquiry into Perioperative Deaths (CEPOD), a survey that was jointly organized by the Associations of Anaesthetists and Surgeons of Great Britain and Ireland during 1985 to 1986 and included more than 480,000 general anesthetic procedures, indicated the mortality attributable to anesthesia alone was 1:185,000 (0.054:10,000) anesthetics (Buck et al., 1987). However, anesthesia, along with other causes, was thought to be a contributory factor in the death of between 1.4 (surgeons' estimate) and 9.8 (anesthetists' estimate) per 10,000 cases. A prospective survey of anesthesia outcome by the French Health Ministry during the 1978-1982 period, in which nearly 200,000 general anesthetic cases were documented, revealed an intraoperative and early postoperative death rate solely attributable to anesthesia to be 0.76:10,000 anesthetics, and an intraoperative death rate of 0.44:10,000 anesthetics (Tiret et al., 1986, 1988) (Table 34–1).

Clearly, it is difficult to compare the incidence of anesthesia-related death among reports from different parts of the world because the definition and inclusion criteria (all inclusive versus American Society of Anesthesiologists [ASA] physical status [PS] 1 and 2), duration (perioperative, 48 hours versus 30 days), and the definition of anesthetic contributions (anesthesia contributory versus primary cause) to mortality may differ markedly.

A longitudinal comprehensive anesthesia-related mortality study from New South Wales, Australia, which has been continuous by the same author using the same criteria since 1960 (interrupted between 1980 and 1983 because of the temporary loss of legal confidentiality), has indeed shown a steady decline in anesthetic mortality from 1.8:10,000 cases in 1960 to 0.38:10,000 cases by 1984 (Holland, 1984, 1987). Similarly, a longitudinal study from South Africa has also shown the trend of decreases in anesthesia-related mortality from 3.3:10,000 in 1956-1965 to 0.7:10,000 in 1983-1987 (Harrison, 1978, 1990) (Table 34–2).

In the United States, Eichhorn (1989) analyzed the data from nine Harvard University-affiliated hospitals between 1976 and 1988. He reported 11 major anesthesia-related intraoperative accidents, including five deaths based on more than 1 million anesthetic procedures in relatively healthy patients (ASA PS 1 and 2); the anesthetic mortality was 0.05:10,000 cases; postoperative mortality, including two deaths from halothane hepatitis, was excluded from these statistics. After implementation of the patient monitoring standards in 1985 (Eichhorn et al., 1986), there was only one serious accident (no mortality) in 319,000 general anesthetic procedures. Of the 11 major accidents, eight cases were considered preventable with proper monitoring, especially with capnography. Unrecognized hypoventilation was the most common cause (seven cases) of major mishaps. Inadequate supervision of residents and nurse anesthetists was also contributory. Although Eichhorn's statistics were based on a malpractice insurance database and are likely different and considerably lower than the data based on a peer review process, anesthetic safety appears to have improved significantly.

Anesthesiology was the first medical specialty to consider patient safety as an independent problem and has institutionalized patient safety in its scientific and governing bodies (such as the ASA Anesthesia Patient Safety Foundation and similar organizations in other countries) (Cooper and Gaba, 2002). In 1999, the Committee on Quality of Health Care in America for the Institute of Medicine published a report entitled *To Err Is Human: Building a Safer Health Care System* (Kohn et al., 1999). The report stated: "Anesthesia is an area in which very impressive improvements in safety have been made." This statement was based on the statistics that anesthesia-related mortality rates have decreased from two deaths per 10,000 anesthetic procedures in the 1980s to about one death per 200,000 to 300,000 anesthetic procedures administered today (probably quoting the report by Eichhorn et al. [1989]). Such dramatic decreases in anesthetic mortality have been attributed to a variety of mechanisms, including the wide acceptance of new monitoring guidelines, the improvement in monitoring techniques, safer anesthetic drugs, and the adoption of QA mechanisms and other systematic approaches for reducing human and systemic errors (Gaba, 2000; Stoelting, 2000; Lagasse, 2002).

TABLE 34–1. Historical changes in anesthesia-related mortality (all ages)

Authors (Country)	Study Years	Incidence per 10,000
Beecher and Todd (United States)	1948 to 1952	3.7
Graff et al. (United States)	1953 to 1963	2.7
Hovi-Viander (Finland)	1975	2.0
Lunn and Mushin (United Kingdom)	1978 to 1979	1.0
Tikkanen (Finland)	1986	0.6
Tiret and others (France)	1978 to 1982	0.76*
Buck and others, CEPOD (United Kingdom)	1985 to 1986	0.05*
Eichhorn (United States)	1976 to 1988 (ASA PS 1 or 2)	0.05*
Lagasse (United States)	1995 to 1999	0.75
Fasting and Gisvold (Canada)	1996 to 2000	0.12

ASA PS, American Society of Anesthesiologists physical status; CEPOD, Confidential Enquiry into Perioperative Death.
*Anesthesia primarily responsible only.

TABLE 34–2. Anesthesia-related mortality: Longitudinal study at the same institution

Authors (Country)	Study Years	Incidence per 10,000
Holland (Australia)	1960 to 1969	1.8
	1970 to 1980	0.97
	1983 to 1985	0.38
Harrison (South Africa)	1956 to 1965	3.3
	1967 to 1976	2.2
	1983 to 1985	0.7

Based on the extensive analyses of 23 publications by 21 different investigators on anesthesia-related deaths between 1955 and 1999, Lagasse (2002) challenged the assertion of "impressive" gains in anesthesia patient safety published by the Institute of Medicine (Kohn et al., 1999). Lagasse's analyses demonstrated that the anesthesia-related mortality rate ranged between 1:1388 (7.2:10,000) and 1:85,708 (0.12:10,000) (mean, 2.17:10,000), a majority of which could have been preventable. The mortality in which anesthesia was considered solely responsible ranged between 1:6795 and 1:200,200 (1.47 to 0.05:10,000). However, he found no statistically significant decrease in mortality rates since the 1970s (Lagasse, 2002).

Furthermore, Lagasse (2002) pointed out the inaccuracy of estimating the anesthesia-related mortality rates based on malpractice insurance claim statistics. Data from two (urban and suburban) university hospitals between 1992 and 1999 revealed 17 anesthesia-related deaths (N = 184,472). Most of these deaths occurred in sick patients (ASA PS 5) and there was no trend of improved mortality with time (Lagasse, 2002). Four out of these 17 patients (0.22:10,000) died as the result of major anesthetic mishaps and three of these four cases resulted in legal action; only one (0.08:10,000) occurred in a patient whose ASA PS was in the 1 or 2 category (Lagasse, 2002). Thus, the mortality rate reported by Einhorn and others (1989) could have been underestimated.

One major drawback of Lagasse's assertion challenging the commonly held belief of marked improvement in anesthesia safety in recent years (2002) may be that his data base included disproportionately few reports after the 1990s when, in part as the result of the new perioperative monitoring guidelines (including pulse oximeter and capnography), the anesthesia-related morbidity and mortality rates have declined considerably.

In the editorial accompanying the article by Lagasse (2002), Cooper and Gaba (2002) refuted Lagasse's conclusion by quoting more recent studies demonstrating that anesthesia has indeed become much safer in recent years. "Has anesthesia safety reached a plateau? Lagasse's data from hospitals in the 1990s contain too few patients for a definite conclusion but such a plateau is possible" (Cooper and Gaba, 2002). On the other hand, if the low probability of anesthetic mortality in healthy patients is taken for granted, the goal of anesthesia patient safety may compete inappropriately against the economical pressure of efficiency and cost containment (Cooper and Gaba, 2002).

MORTALITY IN INFANTS AND CHILDREN

Among the pediatric age group, the anesthesia-related mortality has been reported to be disproportionately high in the literature. In the 1950s, Beecher and Todd (1954) and Stevenson and others (1953) found that accidental deaths resulting from anesthesia were disproportionately high during the first decade of life. Between 1947 and 1956 at the Babies Hospital/Columbia-Presbyterian Medical Center, Rackow, Salanitre, and Green (1961) found that the frequency of cardiac arrest associated with anesthesia in infants less than 1 year of age (1 in 617 cases, or 16.2:10,000) was higher than in children aged 1 to 12 years (1 in 1678, or 6.0:10,000) and in adults (1 in 2580, or 3.9:10,000) (Beecher and Todd, 1954). Hypoventilation and hypoxia from ether overdosage were among the common causes of death. Smith (1956) emphasized the importance of certain factors contributing to the high anesthetic mortality in pediatric anesthesia. These factors included lack of proper equipment, improper preoperative rehydration and stabilization, inadequate intraoperative monitoring,

TABLE 34–3. Anesthesia-related mortality in children (N > 10,000)

Authors (City)	Study Years	Age (yr)	Incidence per 10,000
Rackow (New York City)	1947 to 1956	<1.0	16.2
		1 to 12	6.0
Graff and others (Baltimore)	1957 to 1964	<15 15 to 24	3.3 0.6
Smith (Boston)	1957 to 1966	<10	1.9
	1969 to 1978	<10	0.64
Elwyn (Salt Lake City)	1970 to 1975	<11	0.34
Morray and others (POCA Registry)	1994 to 1997	<18	0.34*
Tay and others (Singapore)	1997 to 1999	<18	0
Murat and others (Paris)	2000 to 2002	<16	0

POCA, Pediatric Perioperative Cardiac Arrest.
*Estimated

error in fluid replacement, and aspiration of vomitus. Today, half a century later, some of these factors are still applicable.

In the report by the Baltimore Anesthesia Study Committee (Phillips and Frazier, 1957; Graff et al., 1964), anesthesia-related mortality for children less than 15 years of age was found to be 3.3:10,000 cases (versus 0.6:10,000 for the 15- to 24-year-old group). These authors also found that the ratio of anesthesia deaths to total surgical deaths was higher in the neonatal period than in any other age group. Furthermore, 57% of the deaths related to anesthesia occurred in healthy children (ASA PS 1 and 2). Respiratory problems were implicated in 83% of the anesthesia-related deaths (Graff et al., 1964) (Table 34–3).

In contrast, in a review of 73 anesthesia-related cardiac arrests in children between 1960 and 1972 (33% resulted in death), Salem and others (1975) found that both respiratory (airway obstruction) and cardiovascular causes (blood loss, preoperative anemia, inappropriate injection of succinylcholine and potassium) were equally responsible. In retrospect, most of these accidents were preventable.

In an attempt to improve anesthesia patient safety in infants and children, a number of important innovations and improvements in perioperative management and monitoring had been made by the pioneering pediatric anesthesiologists in the 1950s and 1960s. These innovations included homemade pediatric blood pressure cuffs and precordial stethoscopes (by Robert Smith in Boston) and endotracheal intubation (by Margo Demming in Philadelphia). Fellowship training in pediatric anesthesia also began in several cities in North America and in the United Kingdom in the 1950s and spread across the continent by the early 1970s (see Chapter 35, History of Pediatric Anesthesia).

By the mid-1970s, anesthesia-related morbidity and mortality decreased considerably. Management of known hazards, such as the full stomach, preoperative fever, and hypovolemia, was greatly improved by increased experience and knowledge (Smith, 1975). Smith (1980) reported the anesthesia-related mortality rate of 2.0:10,000 general anesthetic cases in children (0 to 10 years old) during the decade ending in 1966 at the Children's Hospital in Boston; the mortality rate decreased to 0.6:10,000 anesthetic cases in the decade ending in 1978. Furthermore, there was a series of 35,710 consecutive tonsillectomies and adenoidectomies, mostly in children, without a single death at the Eye and Ear Hospital of Pittsburgh (Petruscak et al., 1974).

There were 7500 consecutive anesthetics for cleft lip and cleft palate repairs without a death at the Children's Hospital in Boston (Smith, 1975). Elwyn, in his 5-year study between 1970 and 1975 at the Primary Children's Hospital in Salt Lake City, reported one anesthetic death in 29,101 anesthetic procedures (0.34:10,000) in children under 11 years of age (Smith, 1980). Downes and Raphaelly (1979) reported an anesthetic mortality of 0.2:10,000 cases (from a total of 50,000 patients) at Children's Hospital of Philadelphia. Most fatalities occur during the first year of life, beyond which the risk of mortality is no higher than that in teenagers and young adults (Smith, 1975) (see Table 34–3).

Despite advances in pediatric anesthesia, statistics in the 1980s still show anesthesia-related mortality rates in children that are three to four times higher than in the general patient population, although the mortality rates in children have decreased considerably and appeared to have reached a plateau (Keenan and Boyan, 1985; Gibbs, 1986; Olsson and Hallen, 1988).

As part of a closed anesthesia malpractice claims study by the Committee on Professional Liability of ASA, Morray and others (1993) compared pediatric and adult closed claims and found a different distribution of serious outcomes in children compared with those in adults. Of 2400 closed malpractice claims, 238 (10%) were in the pediatric age group (≤15 years old). A majority of cases involved children less than 3 years of age, and 28% of all pediatric cases involved infants less than 1 year of age. Respiratory events (mostly inadequate ventilation) were more common than among adult claims (43% versus 30%) and mortality was higher (50% versus 35%), mostly attributable to inadequate ventilation. Anesthesia care was judged inadequate more often. The authors concluded that 89% of the pediatric claims that were related to inadequate ventilation could have been prevented with proper monitoring using pulse oximetry and capnography (Morray et al., 1993).

Analysis of anesthesia-related incidents reported to the Australian Incident Monitoring Study (AIMS) showed almost identical characteristics among pediatric age groups (van der Walt et al., 1993). Of the first 2000 cases reported, 10% involved infants and children. Incidents involving respiratory and breathing circuit systems accounted for nearly half of the adverse incidents. As with the ASA closed claims study, the Australian reviewers estimated that 89% of all applicable problems in AIMS could have been detected and potentially prevented by the combination of pulse oximetry and capnography (van der Walt et al., 1993).

Has anesthesia-related mortality in pediatric patients decreased over the past decade, or has it reached the plateau as Lagasse's (2002) controversial analysis concluded? A study from Singapore based on the QA database reports no fatalities among 10,000 consecutive general pediatric anesthetic procedures from 1997 to 1999 (Tay et al., 2001). A 2004 QA database study from Hopital d'Enfants Armand Trousseau in Paris also reports zero mortality among 24,165 general anesthetic procedures in children between 2000 and 2002 (Murat et al., 2004). On the other hand, from the Pediatric Perioperative Cardiac Arrest (POCA) Registry in the United States (see later) between 1994 and 1997, the anesthesia-related mortality rate was estimated to be 0.36:10,000 (Morray et al., 2000). Obviously, a large-scale prospective and longitudinal study is needed to determine the overall pediatric anesthesia-related mortality in the early 21st century.

ANESTHESIA-RELATED MORBIDITY IN INFANTS AND CHILDREN

PERIOPERATIVE CARDIAC ARRESTS

Incidences of perioperative cardiac arrests have been reported from North America, Europe, and Australia. Estimated incidence of cardiac arrests ranged 17 to 24:10,000, and, as with the mortality rates, the rates are 3 to 10 times higher in infants than in older children (Olsson and Hallen, 1988; Tiret et al., 1988; Cohen et al., 1990). Studies by Keenan and Boyan (1985) and by Morgan and others (1993) also showed higher incidences of cardiac arrest in younger (<10 to 12 years) than in older children. Most frequent causes leading to cardiac arrest involved respiratory and cardiovascular systems and included relative drug overdosage, vagal stimulation, hypoventilation, and succinylcholine-induced asystole.

Keenan and others (1991) reported the effect of specialty training in pediatric anesthesia on the safety of children, especially in infants. In a single university hospital setting, the incidence of perioperative cardiac arrest in infants less than 1 year of age was 19:10,000 with mortality, when residents were supervised by nonpediatric attending anesthesiologists, whereas no arrest occurred when pediatric anesthesiologists were in charge.

Pediatric Perioperative Cardiac Arrest (Poca) Registry

In order to accurately estimate the incidence of cardiac arrests and adverse outcomes, the POCA Registry was formed in 1994 under the combined auspices of the ASA Committee on Professional Liability, the Quality Assurance Committee of the Section on Anesthesiology of the American Academy of Pediatrics (Morray, 2004). The registry included 63 institutions, of which 75% were university hospitals and 40% were children's hospitals. All cardiac arrests requiring cardiopulmonary resuscitation during the immediate perioperative period are eligible for inclusion. During the first 4 years of the registry (1994-1997), participating institutions administered an estimated total of 1,089,200 cases of anesthesia in children younger than 18 years (Morray et al., 2000). A total of 289 cardiac arrests were registered, of which 150 cases were considered as anesthesia contributory. The mean overall incidence of anesthesia-related cardiac arrest was 1.4:10,000 with a mortality rate of 26% (0.36:10,000). Of the total anesthesia-related cardiac arrests, 55% occurred in infants less than 11 months of age (Morray et al., 2000).

Of the major causes of anesthesia-related cardiac arrests, medication-related (37%) and cardiovascular causes (32%) were most common, together accounting for 69% (Table 34–4). In contrast, the respiratory causes represented only 20%, a marked reduction from the incidence of 43% reported by the ASA closed malpractice claim study (Morray et al., 2000). Equipment-related causes comprised 7% of the total (Morray et al., 2000). Of the patients' physical status, 33% were those with ASA PS 1 and 2, a significant decrease from earlier studies of pediatric mortality (57% of deaths) (Graff et al., 1964), a significant improvement, and a move in the right direction, although it is still too high. Of medication-related cardiac arrests, cardiovascular depression with halothane alone, or in combination with other drugs (mostly opioids), accounted for 66% of all medication-related arrests. In healthy children with ASA PS 1 and 2, 64% of arrests were medication related in comparison with 23% in those with ASA PS 3 to 5 (Morray et al., 2000; Mason, 2004) (Fig. 34–1).

■ **TABLE 34–4.** Mechanism of cardiac arrest

Mechanism	No. of Arrests
Medication Related Inhalation Agents	**55 (37%)**
Halothane alone	26 (46%)
Halothane plus an intravenous medication	11 (20%)
Sevoflurane alone	2 (4%)
Intravenous Medications	
Single	5 (9%)
Combination	5 (9%)
Intravenous injection of local anesthetic	5 (9%)
Succinylcholine-induced hyperkalemia	1 (2%)
Cardiovascular	**48 (32%)**
Presumed cardiovascular, unclear etiology	18 (38%)
Hemorrhage, transfusion related	8 (17%)
Inadequate/inappropriate fluid therapy	6 (13%)
Arrhythmia	5 (10%)
Hyperkalemia	4 (8%)
Air embolism	2 (4%)
Pacemaker related	2 (4%)
Vagal response	1 (2%)
Pulmonary hypertension	1 (2%)
Tetralogy hypercyanotic spell	1 (2%)
Respiratory	**30 (20%)**
Laryngospasm	9 (30%)
Airway obstruction	8 (27%)
Difficult intubation	4 (13%)
Inadequate oxygenation	3 (10%)
Inadvertent extubation	2 (7%)
Presumed respiratory, unclear etiology	2 (7%)
Inadequate ventilation	1 (3%)
Bronchospasm	1 (3%)
Equipment Related	**10 (7%)**
Central line	4 (40%)
Breathing circuit	2 (20%)
Peripheral intravenous catheter	1 (10%)
Other	**3 (30%)**
Multiple Events	**5 (3%)**
Hypothermia	**1 (<1%)**
Unclear Etiology	**1 (<1%)**

Modified from Morray JP, Geiduscheck JM, Ramamoorthy C, et al.: Anesthesia-related cardiac arrest in children: Initial findings of the Pediatric Perioperative Cardiac Arrest (POCA) Registry. *Anesthesiology* 93:6–14, 2000, Table 2, p. 9.

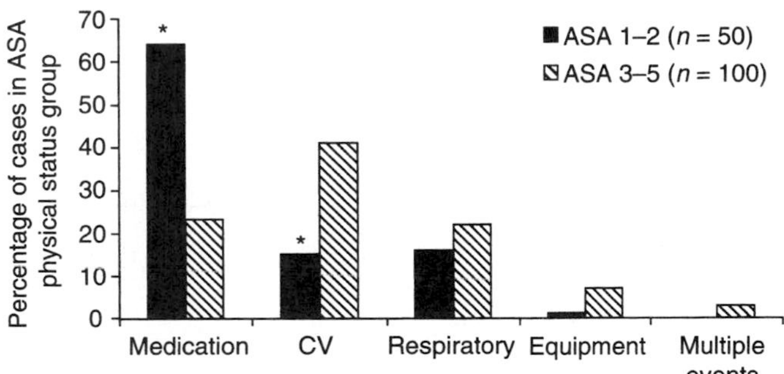

■ **FIGURE 34–1.** Primary cause of anesthesia-related cardiac arrest in American Society of Anesthesiologists (ASA) physical status 1 to 2 and 3 to 5 patients compared with ASA physical status 3 to 5 patients. $*P < 0.01$. [From Morray JP, Geiduschek JM, Ramamoorthy C, et al.: Anesthesia-related cardiac arrest in children: Initial findings of the Pediatric Perioperative Cardiac Arrest (POCA) Registry. *Anesthesiology* 93:6–14, 2000, Fig. 1, p. 10, reproduced with permission.]

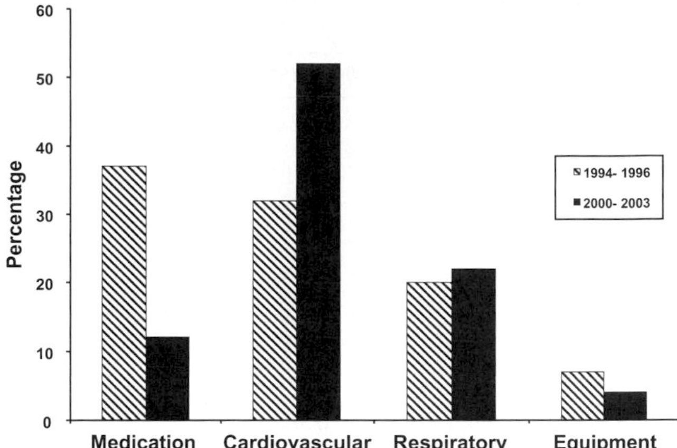

■ **FIGURE 34–2.** Causes of anesthesia-related cardiac arrest in children in two time periods: 1994 to 1996 versus 2000 to 2003. (From Morray JP: Unexpected cardiac arrest in the anesthetized child. Presented at Society of Pediatric Anesthesia spring meeting, March 4–7, 2004, figure reproduced with permission.)

Among the patients who sustained anesthesia-related cardiac arrest in the POCA Registry, death was associated most strongly with ASA PS 3 to 4 and emergency surgery (Morray et al., 2000). Similar correlations between cardiac arrest or death and ASA PS 3 to 4 were found in the earlier study by Keenan and Boyan (1985).

Since the last publication of the POCA Registry, based on data between 1994 and 1997, more than 200 POCA cases have been added to the registry (2000-2003); about one half of these arrests were found to be anesthesia contributory (Morray, 2004). In this new series of cardiac arrests in a recent preliminary report, the cause profile has changed considerably from 1994 through 1997 (Morray, 2004) (Fig. 34–2). Medication-related arrests have decreased markedly from 37% to 12% of the total causes, due primarily to the near disappearance of cardiovascular depression by inhaled anesthetics causing cardiac arrest (Morray, 2004). These welcome changes appear to coincide with the replacement of halothane with sevoflurane as an anesthetic of choice for induction, with its far less myocardial depression and bradycardia. As the consequence of reductions in cardiac arrests with medication (primarily halothane), cardiovascular causes of arrests increased relatively, from 32% to 52%. Hypovolemia from hemorrhage and a metabolic consequence of massive transfusion and resultant hyperkalemia were the frequent causes of arrests under this category (Morray, 2004). Also, with a reduction in medication-related arrests in healthy infants, the incidence of arrests in patients with ASA PS 1-2 has declined considerably from 33% to 19%, one of the most remarkable differences between the 1994-1997 and 2000-2003 databases (Table 34–5).

OTHER PERIOPERATIVE ADVERSE EVENTS

Computerized data acquisition on nonfatal adverse outcome has become commonplace in most hospitals for the QA or quality improvement (QI) survey; such information in pediatric anesthesia has started to appear in the literature. Excellent reviews on this subject have been published (Holzman, 1994; Duncan, 1995).

■ TABLE 34–5. Comparison of demographic data from Pediatric Perioperative Cardiac Arrest Registry cases 1994 to 1997 Versus 2000 to 2003

	1994 to 1997	2000 to 2003
ASA PS		
1	15%	4%
2	18%	15%
3	37%	46%
4	27%	22%
5	2%	13%
Age		
<1 mo	15%	13%
1 to 5 mo	28%	25%
6 to 11 mo	13%	10%
12 mo to 5 yr	31%	25%
6 to 18 yr	13%	27%
Emergency surgery	**21%**	**30%**
Mortality	**26%**	**27%**

ASA PS, American Society of Anesthesiologists physical status.
Modified from Morray JP: Unexpected cardiac arrest in the anesthetized child. Presented at Society of Pediatric Anesthesia spring meeting, March 4–7, 2004.

Cohen and others (1990) reviewed perioperative adverse events in over 29,000 children between 1982 and 1987 at Winnipeg's Children's Hospital. Unlike the adult surgical population, a majority (70%) of children were healthy and had no preoperative medical problems. Infants under 1 year of age, particularly those under 1 month of age (61% of whom underwent intra-abdominal, intrathoracic, or major cardiovascular surgery), had a significantly increased incidence of airway obstruction and other adverse respiratory events (9.4%) and hypotension (3.9%) intraoperatively. Among children 1 to 10 years of age, the most frequent problem was arrhythmias (3.9% to 9.3%). In the recovery room, infants less than 1 month of age had frequent hypotension (13.9%), respiratory events (11.6%), and abnormal temperature (4.7%). In older children, the most common adverse event in the recovery period was vomiting (5.9%), followed by airway obstruction (3.2%). This study was performed during the presevoflurane era when essentially all inhalation inductions were performed with halothane, with potent myocardial depression and bradycardia (Table 34–6).

A report from Hopital d'Enfants Armand Trousseau in Paris was based on the Quality Assurance database involving over 24,000 pediatric anesthesia cases for a 30-month period between 2000 and 2002, when halothane had been completely eliminated from clinical use (Murat et al., 2004). Although this database did not include open heart and neurosurgical cases, the nature of adverse events and their frequency have changed considerably. As a whole, respiratory events were most frequent, representing 53% of all intraoperative events (Table 34–7). As with other reports, respiratory events were more frequent among infants (3.6:10,000 versus <1.5:10,000 in older children), in ears, nose, and throat (ENT) surgery than in other surgery, in children who were intubated versus not intubated, and in those with ASA PS 3 to 5 versus 1 or 2 (Murat et al., 2004). Cardiac events represented 12.5% of all intraoperative events and were mostly observed in sick children (ASA PS 3 to 5).

■ TABLE 34–6. Perioperative events by age of child, 1982 to 1987 (rate per 10,000 anesthetic cases)

	Age					
	<1 mo (n = 361)	*1 to 12 mo (n = 2544)*	*1 to 5 yr (n = 12,484)*	*6 to 10 yr (n = 7184)*	*11+ yr (n = 5647)*	*Total (N = 29,220)*
Intraoperative						
Vomiting	28	47	56*	99	136*	81
Cardiac arrest	28	12	3	4	5	5
Arrhythmia	166	86	391	933	561	528†
Blood pressure	388*	55	22*	19	46	34
Temperature	83	24	13	8	16	14
Airway obstruction	222	200*	99	86	90	105
Other respiratory problems	720*	318*	118	82*	99	130
Drug incident	—	20	20	28	35	25
Surgical problems	28	31	39	43	39	39
Death	83*	8	3	1	2	4
Recovery Room						
Laryngospasm	28	43	187	177	165	166†
Vomiting	—	83	410	855	935	587†
Cardiac arrest	55*	4	2	1	—	2
Arrhythmia	—	12	8	15	9	10
Blood pressure	1385*	12	10*	15*	32	17
Temperature	471*	138	57*	86	159*	96
Airway obstruction	28	161	444	260	184	319†
Other respiratory problems	1163*	248*	105	78*	103	126
Drug incident	—	20	19	19	30	21
Surgical problems	28	63	131	167	76	122

*$P < 0.01$, exact tail probability calculation based on Poisson distribution.
†$P < 0.01$ χ^2 test for association.
Modified from Cohen MM, et al.: *Anesth Analg* 70:160, 1990.

■ **TABLE 34–7.** Details of respiratory and cardiac adverse events observed during anesthesia and in postanesthesia care unit (PACU) in different age groups

				PACU		
Intraoperative	*0 to 1 yr*	*1 to 7 yr*	*8 to 16 yr*	*0 to 1 yr*	*1 to 7 yr*	*8 to 16 yr*
Respiratory Event						
No. of anesthetics	3681	12,495	6867	3681	12,495	6867
Bronchospasm	19	25	4	4	11	5
Hypercarbia	8	10	1	5	5	8
Hypoxemia	56	90	24	21	34	15
Aspiration	2	4	4	1	5	3
Unanticipated difficult intubation	9	7	6	—	—	—
Esophageal intubation	3	2	1	—	—	—
Endobronchial intubation	6	3	1	3	5	7
Laryngospasm	17	31	9	1	6	4
Pulmonary edema	0	0	2	1	9	7
Pneumothorax	0	2	0	1	7	6
Reintubation	13	17	7	5	11	9
Dental trauma	—	—	—	0	3	1
Respiratory depression	—	—	—	12	17	10
Total	133	191	59	54	113	75
Rate per 1000 anesthetics	36.1	15.3	8.6	14.7	9.0	10.9
Cardiac Event						
No. of anesthetics	3681	12,495	6867	3681	12,495	6867
Cardiac arrest	4	2	2	0	0	0
Bradycardia	12	9	10	0	1	0
Hypertension	0	0	0	1	0	0
Hypotension	4	6	11	0	0	0
Hypovolemia	8	6	3	0	0	1
Circulatory insufficiency	3	2	1	1	0	0
Tachycardia	0	0	1	0	0	0
Arrhythmia	0	2	5	0	0	0
Total	31	27	33	2	1	1
Rate per 1000 anesthetics	8.4	2.2	4.8	0.5	0.1	0.2

Modified from Murat I, Constant I, Maud'huy H: Perioperative anaesthetic morbidity in children: A database of 24,165 anaesthetics over a 30-month period. *Pediatr Anesth* 14:161, 2004.

In contrast to earlier reports, the incidence of bradycardia was greatly decreased (13:10,000) and arrhythmias essentially disappeared. There were eight cardiac arrests (3.3:10,000), of which five children were in the ASA PS 3 to 5 category and four were infants 6 months old or younger (see Table 34–7). There were no anesthesia-related deaths (Murat et al., 2004). Vomiting was the commonest adverse event postoperatively, with an overall incidence of 6%. As with previous studies, vomiting was more frequent in older children than in infants and occurred more often after ENT surgery compared with other surgery and in children who were intubated versus those who were not (Murat et al., 2004). Similarly, based on QA data of 10,000 surgical cases, Tay and others (2001) in Singapore found critical perioperative incidents four times higher in infants less than 1 year of age than older children (8.6% versus 2.1%). Respiratory events were most common (77.4%) with laryngospasm, accounting for 35.7%. There were no anesthesia-related deaths (Tay et al., 2001).

Bradycardia

An outcome study from the Medical College of Virginia examined the incidence of bradycardia in nearly 8000 children less than 4 years of age (Keenan et al., 1994). Bradycardia (<100 beats per minute) was more frequent in infants (1.27%) and decreased with age. The incidence in the 4-year-old group was only 0.16%. Causes of bradycardia included disease or surgery (35%), inhalation anesthesia (35%), and hypoxemia (22%). Of these children, hypotension occurred in 30%, asystole or ventricular fibrillation in 10%, and death in 8%. Significant associated factors predisposing children to bradycardic events, based on multiple logistic regression analysis, were ASA PS, emergency surgery, duration of surgery (> 4 hours), and the absence of a trained pediatric anesthesiologist supervising the anesthetic management (Keenan et al., 1994).

Laryngospasm and Bronchospasm

The incidence of laryngospasm and bronchospasm has been studied in a series of large population studies in Stockholm by Olsson and others (1984, 1987). The incidence of laryngospasm in children less than 9 years of age was 1.7%. The presence of respiratory infection raises the incidence to 9.6%. The incidence of laryngospasm was also increased in patients with obstructive lung disease (6.4%) and in those with a history of previous anesthetic complications (5.5%). The incidence of bronchospasm in the same age group increased from 0.4% to 4.1% in those with respiratory infection. The incidence of bronchospasm was also elevated (2.4%) in patients at high risk (ASA PS 3 or higher) (Olsson, 1987).

Possible effects of recent or current upper respiratory tract infection (URI) and incidence of respiratory events have been studied by a number of investigators using parental interview or written questionnaires. Of more than 1500 children, Schreiner and others (1996) from Children's Hospital of Philadelphia found that patients who developed laryngospasm were more than twice as likely to have an active URI than were patients in the control group without URI. A survey of more than 2000 children by Parnis and others (2001) from Adelaide, Australia, did not find statistically significant differences in the long-term outcome of children with a recent history of URI. They did, however, find that orotracheal intubation was associated with an increased probability of respiratory complications compared with facemask or laryngeal mask airway. Similarly, in more than 1000 children, Tait and others (2001) found no difference between children with active or recent URI versus asymptomatic children, with respect to the incidence of laryngospasm, bronchospasm, or long-term respiratory sequelae. However, children with current or recent URI had significantly more overall adverse respiratory events, including breath holding and major desaturation ($Spo_2 < 90\%$). Independent risk factors for adverse respiratory outcome in children with active URI included tracheal intubation (<5 years of age), history of prematurity, reactive airway disease, parental smoking, surgery involving the airway, and the presence of copious secretions and nasal congestion (Tait et al., 2001).

Aspiration

Studies before the 1970s reported high morbidity and mortality from pulmonary aspiration of gastric contents (Mendelson, 1946). The Baltimore Anesthesia Study Committee reported a mortality rate of 39% in children associated with pulmonary aspiration (Graff et al., 1964) (see Chapter 10, Induction of Anesthesia and Maintenance of the Airway). Studies reported since the 1980s, however, indicate marked improvements in outcome.

From a computer database between 1967 and 1985, Olsson and others (1986) identified 83 cases of pulmonary aspiration of gastric content of more than 185,000 anesthetic cases in all ages (4.7:10,000 cases). The rate of gastric aspiration in children less than 9 years of age (8.6:10,000) was nearly three times higher than that in young adults (20 to 49 years old). In 47% of patients with aspiration, pneumonia or atelectasis developed, as confirmed by chest radiograph. The mortality rate in children was relatively low (0.2:10,000) (Olsen et al., 1986). Risk factors associated with aspiration included the skill and experience of anesthetists, a number of coexisting diseases, ASA PS 3-5, emergency surgery, nighttime operation, history indicating an increased risk of regurgitation (esophageal disease, pregnancy), and difficult intubation. Other high-risk categories included children with intestinal obstruction, increased intracranial pressure, increased abdominal pressure, and obesity. Incidence of gastric aspiration was even lower in studies from the French-speaking countries (1.0:10,000) (Tiret et al., 1988) and from Norway (2.9:10,000) (Mellin-Olsen, Fasting and Gisvold, 1996) in the 1980s. No fatalities were reported.

Borland and others (1998) studied the incidence and outcome of perioperative aspiration during the 5-year period between 1988 and 1993 involving over 50,000 general anesthetic cases at Children's Hospital of Pittsburgh. They identified 52 cases of aspiration (10.2:10,000 cases), of which 25 patients aspirated gastric content (4.9:10,000) (and the rest were blood or pharyngeal secretions). Approximately 80% of aspirations occurred during induction. Most patients were treated aggressively with fiberoptic bronchoscopy through the endotracheal tube, removal of solid particles, and continuous positive pressure ventilation. Most patients had radiographic evidence of aspiration (infiltration, pneumonia, atelectasis, or pulmonary edema), but fulminant chemical pneumonitis secondary to aspiration, as reported in early publications (Mendelson, 1946), was absent. No death was attributable to aspiration. Among the different pediatric age groups, the incidence of aspiration was highest among children 6 to 11 years of age (0.22%). Several risk factors for intraoperative aspiration were identified: ASA PS 3 or higher, a history of previous esophageal surgery, and patients with previous chemotherapy undergoing central venous catheter (Broviac) placement. Twenty-nine percent of these children were kept intubated in the postanesthetic care unit (PACU) for several hours or longer, but only 23% of these patients stayed overnight. None of these children developed clinically significant pneumonia, and there were no deaths (Borland et al., 1998).

Similarly, a study from the Mayo Clinic reported a low incidence of aspiration (3.8:10,000). In this report, however, the incidence of aspiration was similar to that of adults (3.1:10,000). There was no serious respiratory morbidity and no associated deaths (Warner et al., 1999). These epidemiologic studies suggest that the incidence of gastric aspiration and associated morbidity and mortality, especially in children, has declined considerably. The risk of aspiration in general, with the exception of the Mayo Clinic report (Warner et al., 1999), remained higher in infants and children than in adults (Olsson et al., 1986; Tiret et al., 1988; Flick et al., 2002).

POSTOPERATIVE COMPLICATIONS

Postoperative Hypoxemia

During general anesthesia, static tension of the thoracic inspiratory muscle is abolished and the balance between the outward recoil of the thorax and the inward recoil of the lungs is altered. This change in balance results in the reduction of resting lung volume (functional residual capacity [FRC]), airway closure, collapse of alveoli (microatelectasis), and increased venous admixture, particularly in infants and young children (see Chapter 2, Respiratory Physiology in Infants and Children). By means of pulse oximetry, Motoyama and Glazener (1986) were the first to demonstrate that a large proportion (42%) of healthy infants and children undergoing simple elective surgical procedures become hypoxemic in the postoperative recovery room (PACU). Patients sleeping in the PACU tend to be more hypoxemic and for a longer duration than those who are awake and sitting up (Motoyama and Glazener, 1986), but the presence of hypoxemia is not clinically obvious and does not correlate with the recovery score (Soliman et al., 1988). In a study involving a large number (N = 1152) of healthy infants, children, and adults (ASA PS 1) undergoing plastic surgical procedures, postoperative oxygen saturation (Spo_2) was followed frequently for two hours. The incidences of both moderate (Spo_2, 86% to 90%) and severe (Spo_2 < 86%) hypoxemia were the highest among infants (36.6% and 16.7%, respectively), followed by toddlers (20% and 10% in 1- to 3-year-olds), children (14% and 3.3%), and adults (8% and 0.6%). The duration of hypoxemia was also significantly longer in infants than in older age groups (Xue et al., 1996) (Fig. 34–3).

Patients also become hypoxemic as often during the short transport from the operating room to the PACU (Pullerits et al., 1987) because the benefit of oxygen breathing to maintain oxygenation lasts only a few minutes. Children with upper respiratory infection (DeSoto et al., 1988) and infants younger than 6 months of age are at increasing risk of developing hypoxemia

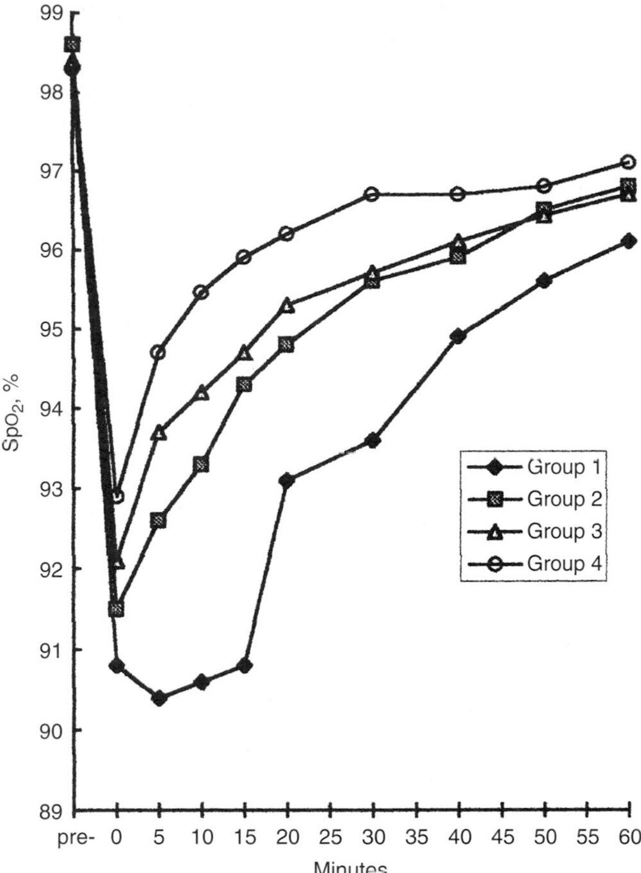

■ **FIGURE 34–3.** The recovery tendencies of arterial oxygen saturation (SpO_2) within the first hour after operation in four age groups. Group 1: infants <1 year; group 2: toddlers 1 to 3 years; group 3: children 3 to 14 years; group 4: teenagers and adults 14 to 58 years. (From Xue FS, Huang YG, Tong SY, et al.: A comparative study of early postoperative hypoxemia in infants, children, and adults undergoing elective plastic surgery. *Anesth Analg* 83:709–715, 1996, Fig. 1, p. 712, reproduced with permission.)

(Kataria et al., 1988; Xue et al., 1996). Most pediatric anesthesiologists, therefore, recommend routine oxygen administration during the transport of children to and in the PACU (Duncan, 1995).

Postoperative Apnea

Postoperative apnea in prematurely born infants has become a major clinical concern since the early 1980s, when the number of premature infants surviving neonatal intensive care started to increase. Apnea is usually defined as the cessation of breathing lasting longer than 15 to 20 seconds or lasting for a lesser duration associated with bradycardia, cyanosis, or pallor (Thach, 1985). Apneic spells in these infants after simple surgical procedures are mostly central in origin (cessation of respiratory effort), although some infants have mixed (central and obstructive) apneas (Kurth et al., 1991). Postoperative apnea occurs more commonly in infants with a previous history of apnea (Liu et al., 1983) and those younger than 42 to 44 weeks' postconception. Apnea is infrequent after 44 weeks' postconception (Malviya et al., 1993), although apnea in older ex-premature infants (up to 55 weeks' postconception) has been reported after more extensive surgical procedures (Kurth et al., 1987). Malviya and others (1993) recommend that all former premature infants of less than 44 weeks' postconception be monitored for at least 12 hours postoperatively. Another important risk factor for postoperative apnea appears to be the presence of anemia (Welborn et al., 1991).

In 1995, Coté and others published the results of meta analysis of the data from eight published reports of postoperative apnea between 1987 and 1993 involving 384 ex-premature infants following inguinal hernia repair. They concluded that (1) apnea was strongly and inversely correlated both with gestational age and postconceptual age; (2) an associated risk factor was continuing episodes of apnea at home; (3) small-for-gestational-age infants seemed to be somewhat protected from apnea compared with those with normal or large-for-gestational-age infants; (4) anemia (hematocrit < 30) was a significant risk factor even beyond 43 weeks postconceptual age; and (5) relationships of postoperative apnea with history of necrotizing enterocolitis, neonatal apnea, respiratory distress syndrome, bronchopulmonary dysplasia, or operative use of opioids and/or muscle relaxants could not be determined (Coté et al., 1995). The probability of apnea in nonanemic infants, free of apnea in the recovery room, decreases with postconceptual and postnatal ages but is not less than 5% (with 95% confidence limits) until postconceptual age of 48 weeks (with gestational age, 35 weeks) and not less than 1% until postconceptual age of 56 weeks (gestational age, 32 weeks) or postconceptual age of 54 weeks (gestational age, 35 weeks) (Coté et al., 1995) (Fig. 34–4).

Based on these findings, it is generally recommended that ex-premature infants less than 44 to 46 weeks' postconception be admitted overnight for monitoring following general anesthesia in the United States. Whether the infant with postconceptual age between 46 and 48 weeks or even 52 weeks is admitted overnight depends on the decision made case by case between the anesthesiologist and the surgeon, based on a number of factors. These factors include the general health of the infant and his or her home environment (parents, passive smoking, distance from the hospital, etc.). However, the decision often depends on the general policies of the hospital administration and insurance providers, and these policies do not necessarily represent the best interest of the patient or the health care providers. In countries like France and Japan, where economic pressure on health care resources is less stringent than in the United States, most infants less than 60 weeks' postconception are admitted overnight for monitoring (Murat, 2002).

Incidence of postoperative apnea was reported to be lower after spinal anesthesia alone than after general (halothane) anesthesia, but spinal anesthesia combined with ketamine increases

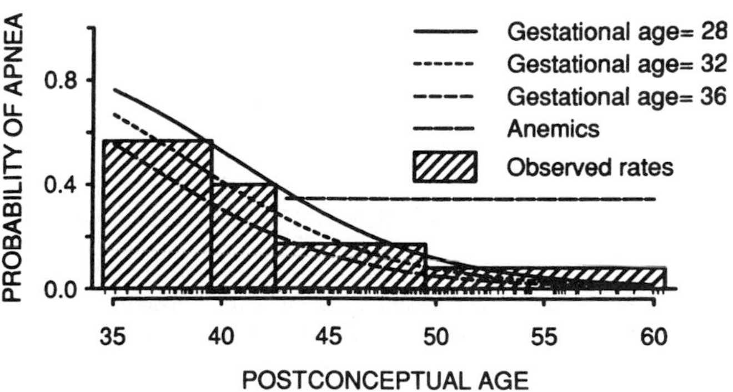

■ **FIGURE 34–4.** Probability of postoperative apnea versus postconceptual and gestational ages of former preterm infants. (From Coté CJ, Zaslavsky A, Downes JJ, et al.: Postoperative apnea in former preterm infants after inguinal herniorrhaphy. A combined analysis. *Anesthesiology* 82:809–822, 1995, Fig. 2, p. 813, reproduced with permission.)

the incidence of apnea more than that with general anesthesia (Welborn et al., 1990). Caffeine seems to be helpful in preventing postoperative apnea (Welborn et al., 1988).

Postintubation Croup

The major cause of postintubation croup is subglottic injury and edema associated with traumatic intubation, especially with an oversized endotracheal tube. Koka and others (1977) made an important observation that the incidence of postintubation croup increases markedly when there is no air leak around the endotracheal tube with the airway pressure exceeding 40 cm H_2O. Consequently, it has become a standard practice in pediatric anesthesia to choose an endotracheal tube that produces air leak around the tube with a pressure lower than 30 cm H_2O. With this preventive measure in clinical practice, the incidence of postintubation croup has decreased dramatically from 1% to less than 0.1%, along with reductions in the severity of croup (Litman and Keon, 1991). With the presence of URI, however, the incidence of airway complications and the tendency for oxygen desaturation increase (Cohen and Cameron, 1992; Rolf and Coté, 1992).

Postoperative Nausea and Vomiting

Although rarely life-threatening, postoperative nausea and vomiting (PONV) remains the single most common complication resulting in unscheduled overnight admissions in same-day surgery settings (Cohen et al., 1990; Patel and Rice, 1991). The average incidence of PONV in children over 3 years of age was reported to be over 40%. The incidence of PONV has decreased considerably with newer anesthetics and techniques as well as with more effective medications (Murat et al., 2004). The incidence of PONV is higher after certain types of surgery including adenotonsillectomy, eye muscle surgery for strabismus, and orchiopexy. Other factors affecting the incidence of PONV include the gender and age of the child (infrequent in infants), PONV after previous surgery or history of motion sickness, anesthetic techniques (inhaled anesthetics and nitrous oxide versus intravenous anesthesia with propofol), intraoperative opioids, inadequate pain control, gastric distention, and the skill of the anesthesiologist (Patel and Rice, 1991; Martin et al., 1993; Weir et al., 1993; Weinstein et al., 1994; Duncan, 1995). A mandatory requirement for oral fluid intake and early ambulation before discharge from the short stay unit was also associated with increased incidence of vomiting (Schreiner et al., 1992; Weinstein et al., 1994). Serotonin (5-HT_3) receptor antagonists (such as ondansetron and granisetron) have shown to be highly effective in preventing or treating PONV (Patel et al., 1996; Fujii et al., 1996). Prophylactic use of dexamethasone was also found to be effective (Aouad et al., 2001) (see Chapter 11, Intraoperative and Postoperative Management).

COMPLICATIONS OF REGIONAL ANESTHESIA

A survey by the ASA Closed Claims Study on the complication of regional anesthesia revealed that of 2400 closed anesthesia malpractice claims cases, 29 adult patients and 1 pediatric patient were identified who developed cardiac arrest during regional anesthesia, resulting in death or severe brain damage (Morray et al., 1993). From the analysis of these data, it can be concluded that (1) cardiac arrest resulting in death or other major outcomes can occur during apparently well-managed spinal or epidural anesthesia in young, healthy patients undergoing relatively minor procedures, because respiratory insufficiency from sedation is not recognized, and (2) pulse oximetry would have given an early warning of respiratory insufficiency (Caplan et al., 1988; Cheney, 1988; Keats, 1988).

Valley and Bailey (1991), in a retrospective survey involving 138 pediatric patients who received caudal morphine, reported 11 patients (8%) with postoperative respiratory depression. All but one incident occurred in infants less than 12 months of age and within 12 hours of caudal morphine administration (70 mcg/kg). Krane (1988) reported a life-threatening delayed respiratory depression in a 2.5-year-old boy 3.5 hours after the administration of caudal morphine (100 mcg/kg, a much higher dose than today's standards of 30 to 50 mcg/kg) for postoperative analgesia. Intravenous naloxone was continued until 16.5 hours after caudal morphine to maintain adequate breathing. Jones and others (1984) used intrathecal morphine in 56 children undergoing open-heart surgery. Respiratory depression occurred (most frequently, 3.5 to 4.5 hours after morphine administration) in 6 of 27 patients (22%) who received 30 mcg/kg of morphine and 3 of 29 children (10%) who received 20 mcg/kg. Patients receiving epidural or intrathecal morphine should therefore be admitted overnight and their respiration continuously monitored.

Giaufré, Dalens, and Gombert (1996) reported a 1-year prospective study (1993-1994) of morbidity/mortality associated with regional anesthesia by the French Language Society of Pediatric Anesthesia involving over 24,000 regional blocks of about 85,000 pediatric anesthesia cases of which central blocks (approximately 15,000 cases [62%]) were the most common, followed by peripheral nerve blocks (17%) and others (22%). Of the central block, caudal block was most common (12,000, or 80% of central block or 50% of the total), followed by lumbar epidural (1700) and spinal anesthesia (500). A total of only 23 incidents was reported, including 0% for peripheral blocks, 11% (0.7:1000) for caudal blocks, 9% (3.7:1000) for lumbar epidural blocks, 2% (6.8:1000) for sacral epidural blocks, and 1% (2:1000) for spinal anesthesia (Giaufré, et al., 1996). Complications included eight dural punctures (resulting in total spinal block in four), six intravascular injections (resulting in seizures or arrhythmias), two overdosage with arrhythmias, and one opioid-related apnea. No fatalities were reported.

COMPLICATIONS ARISING FROM SEDATION

According to the data compiled by the U.S. Department of Health and Human Services, more than 80 deaths attributable to midazolam occurred within 3 years after its introduction for clinical use in 1986. Midazolam was used, often in combination with fentanyl, for the sedation of patients undergoing various procedures without the supervision of anesthesiologists (Bailey et al., 1990). Of these deaths associated with midazolam, 78% were respiratory events, with opioids being used in 57% of these cases (Bailey et al., 1990).

A collaborative study by the American Society of Gastrointestinal Endoscopy and the U.S. Food and Drug Administration, involving over 21,000 endoscopic procedures under sedation, revealed the incidence of serious cardiorespiratory outcome to be 54:10,000 cases with a mortality rate of 3:10,000 (Arrowsmith et al., 1991); that is 10 to 50 times higher than the reported deaths associated with general anesthesia (Tiret et al., 1986, 1988; Buck et al., 1987; Holland, 1987; Eichhorn, 1989). These extremely high morbidity and mortality rates of conscious and deep sedations (apparently including inadvertent general anesthesia and deaths) performed by nonanesthesiologists without adequate skills, proper monitoring, or supervision have led the way to the establishment and modifications of the new sedation guidelines by the Section of Anesthesiology, American Academy of Pediatrics (Committee on Drugs, Section on Anesthesiology, American Academy of Pediatrics, 1985, 1992). Although the terminology adopted ("conscious" sedation in particular) were misnomers (if not oxymorons), in hindsight the guidelines included the approach similar to that commonly practiced by anesthesiologists, that is, proper fasting, preprocedural history and physical examinations with a special attention to airways, informed consent, monitoring including pulse oximetry, documentation of drugs used and vital signs during and after the procedure, and discharge criteria (Coté, 2004).

The Joint Commission on the Accreditation of Healthcare Organizations in the United States (JCAHO, 1992) modified its regulations and published rules to develop new guidelines in each health care institution it accredits (available at www.jcaho.org). To further improve patient safety for sedation in accordance with the new JCAHO regulations, a task force by the ASA developed new guidelines for sedation by nonanesthesiologists (Gross et al., 2002). The sedation guidelines were again updated in 2002 (American Society of Anesthesiologists Task Force on Sedation and Analgesia by Non-Anesthesiologists, 2002) with the new terminology (available at ASA Web site: www.asahq.org/standards) and were later incorporated by JCAHO and by the AAP (Committee on Drugs, Section on Anesthesiology, American Academy of Pediatrics, 2002). The term "conscious sedation" has been eliminated, and instead, three stages of procedural sedation are described: minimal, moderate, and deep stages (plus general anesthesia) (Coté, 2004).

Under the new JCAHO regulations, the director of anesthesia service in each institution has a responsibility for developing new "within-institution" sedation guidelines by nonanesthesiology services to further improve patient safety. General guidelines include onsite availability of oxygen and positive pressure oxygen delivery system (which can provide the minimum of 90% oxygen for 60 minutes), availability of a resuscitation kit (including drugs, laryngoscope, and endotracheal tubes), a suction apparatus, and monitors (pulse oximeter, electrocardiography, and blood pressure apparatus). Documentation for sedation should include evaluation of health status before sedation, informed consent, record of drugs given (the time and doses), and vital signs (oxygen saturation, heart and respiratory rates). For deep sedation, there must be a dedicated person (registered nurse, respiratory therapist, etc.) in addition to the practitioner, whose responsibility is only monitoring and who is trained to perform resuscitation.

Using the QA database created specifically for procedural sedation, Malviya and others (1997) identified 239 adverse outcomes (20% of 1140 children), mostly after receiving recommended doses of chloral hydrate. Oxygen desaturation (5.5%) was the most common adverse outcome including laryngospasm and apnea in five children. Inadequate sedation occurred in 150 (13.2%) children. These findings appear to indicate that the establishment and enforcement of safety guidelines for procedural sedation have considerably reduced the incidence of adverse outcomes.

Analysis of adverse sedation events reported to the U.S. Food and Drug Administration between 1969 and 1996 by Coté and others (2000) revealed that of 95 incidents reported, 60 ended up in death (51) or permanent neurologic injury (9). Although the incidence of respiratory events (about 80% of all events, mostly hypoxia, laryngospasm, and/or apnea) was similar between hospital and nonhospital settings, inadequate resuscitation (57.1% versus 2.3%) and death or permanent neurologic injury (92.8% versus 37.2%) occurred more frequently in nonhospital versus in hospital environments. Death or severe outcome occurred disproportionately more often (32 of 95 cases) involving sedation for dental procedures (mostly at nonhospital settings). Ten children sustained death or permanent neurologic injury in the car or at home after being discharged from medical supervision despite deep levels of residual sedation. Unsupervised sedative medication by a parent at home (or by a technician at a facility) caused an additional two arrests in the car on the way to the hospital or clinic (Coté et al., 2000). The results of this report imply the inadequacy of existing (or the nonexistence of) discharge criteria and their practice. Two reports have further addressed these issues.

Motas and others (2004) studied the efficacy and safety of procedural (light or deep grade) sedation in 86 children under 12 years of age undergoing sedation by nonanesthesia services (for computed tomography scans, cardiac catheterizations, gastrointestinal endoscopy, and dental procedures). A variety of medications were used by different services, including intravenous pentobarbital, intravenous midazolam with fentanyl or meperidine, oral chloral hydrate with meperidine and hydroxyzine, and intramuscular or intravenous ketamine (Motas et al., 2004). An independent observer applied the Bispectral Index (BIS) monitor (40 to 60, general anesthesia; 61 to 70, deep sedation; 71 to 90, minimum, and >90, awake) and the University of Michigan Sedation Scale (UMSS) (0 to 4 observational scale: 0, awake; 1, minimal sedation [tired, sleepy]; 2, moderately sedated [easily arousable]; 3, deeply sedated [deep sleep, arousable only with strong stimulus]; and 4, unarousable or general anesthesia) at 10-minute intervals for 1 hour. The goal of either light or deep sedation was attained in 53% (BIS) and 72% (UMSS). Depth consistent with general anesthesia was observed in 35% (BIS) and 0% (UMSS) of patients, and those consistent with awake state (failure) was observed in 12% (BIS) and 28% (UMSS). About 8% of patients experienced desaturation and airway events. The patients were often sedated either too deeply or not enough, and the goal of either light or deep procedural sedation was not achieved in large numbers of children.

Malviya and others (2004) assessed the readiness of discharge in 29 children following the procedural sedation for echocardiographic examinations with either chloral hydrate (93%) or midazolam with diphenhydramine (7%). A trained observer used BIS monitor, UMSS scores every 10 to 15 minutes, a Modified Maintenance of Wakefulness Test (MMWT), and the visual observation of the time the child was able to stay awake for 20 minutes, until revised discharge criteria were met (BIS > 90, UMSS of 0 or 1, MMWT > 20 minutes). There were moderate correlations among BIS, UMSS, and MMWT ($P < 0.01$). Revised criteria correctly identified wakefulness (BIS value > 90) in 88% of patients. However, when discharged by the nurse, only 55% of patients returned to the baseline BIS value (>90); it took longer to meet the revised criteria (more appropriate and safer) compared with standard criteria (nursing judgment) (75 minutes versus 13 minutes, $P = 0.001$).

Thus, Melviya and others (2004) clearly demonstrated that sedation with chloral hydrate can result in prolonged sedation even after the children reached currently used (but unsatisfactory) discharge criteria by nurses, with a potential for airway obstruction and adverse outcome (Coté et al., 2000). The results of this study have several important implications. First, the currently practiced guidelines are inadequate and need changes, using more reliable criteria, such as UMSS, MMWT, BIS monitor, or their combinations, to further improve patient safety associated with procedural sedations. Second, the duration of postsedation monitoring should be increased beyond what is currently practiced, and the hospital must respond to increase staffing needs for nurses in the recovery area and to provide additional space for adequate patient observation (quiet space for MMWT) and recovery, changes that have associated cost increases. Third, anesthesia service should provide additional guidelines to nonanesthesiologists for the proper selection of sedative and hypnotic drugs, with shorter elimination half-life to shorten the recovery time (Coté, 2004). In addition, office-based procedures under sedation should either be performed under the care of anesthesiologists within the office setting or moved to hospital-based facilities to further decrease untoward events (see Chapter 26, Office-Based Anesthesia).

COMMON CAUSES OF ANESTHESIA-RELATED MISHAPS

JUDGMENT ERRORS

If one accepts the theory that "to err is human" (Kohn et al., 1999) and recognizes that "all human beings, without any exception whatsoever, make errors and [errors]... are a completely normal and necessary part of human cognitive function" (Allnut, 1987), then it is not surprising to realize that most anesthetic mishaps involve human errors and are preventable (Salem et al., 1975; Cooper et al., 1978; Holland, 1987). Cooper and others (1978), with the use of a carefully structured interview technique with a group of anesthesiologists, collected incidents in which human error or equipment failure occurred. These investigators found that 82% of incidents were caused by preventable human error; the remaining incidents were mostly caused by equipment failure. Analysis of 238 closed anesthesia malpractice claims involving pediatric patients revealed that 43% of these claims were related to inadequate ventilation and resulted in death or severe permanent neurologic damage (Morray et al., 1993). Morray and others concluded that 89% of these cases could have been prevented if they were monitored with pulse oximetry or capnography.

Holland (1987) compared incidences of various categories of mishaps during his three decades of investigation involving anesthesia-related mortality in patients of all ages (Table 34–8). In the 1960s, anesthetic overdose, wrong choice of anesthetics, inadequate preoperative preparation, and inadequate crisis management dominated as frequent causes of adverse outcomes, indicating inadequacy (according to today's standard) of equipment and physician experience administering anesthesia. The total incidence of management errors involving fatality was 2.7:10,000 anesthetics. There has been a dramatic decrease in the incidence of management errors with time as well as changes in the dominant categories of error in management over the decades. In the 1980s, inadequate preparation and inadequate postoperative management ranked high among the categories of errors causing anesthesia-related fatalities. Incidence of management errors decreased to 0.55:10,000 anesthetics, about one fifth that in the 1960s. Factors frequently associated with preventable adverse outcomes (both fatal and nonfatal) include a failure to perform proper review of patients and anesthesia apparatus, distraction (inattention, haste, fatigue, and boredom), lack of experience, and lack of a skilled assistant (Craig and Wilson, 1981; Derrington and Smith, 1987).

EMERGENCY OR URGENT CASES

Inadequate preanesthetic preparation occurs most frequently with emergency or "urgent" cases and most commonly represents failure to appreciate the degree of dehydration and electrolyte imbalance (Holland, 1987). In the British CEPOD study cited previously, more than 20% of anesthesia-related deaths occurred after surgery performed as emergencies and an additional 40% occurred in operations classified as urgent (Buck et al., 1987). In the New South Wales study, the risk of anesthesia-attributable death in patients undergoing emergency anesthesia is 10 times that of the overall incidence (Holland, 1987). In the CEPOD study, anesthetists were dissatisfied with preoperative preparations in 14% of cases that ended with anesthesia-related deaths, but they presumably were pressured or persuaded by surgeons into administering anesthesia. On the basis of these findings, Lunn and Devlin (1987) emphasize the importance of proper preanesthetic preparation as an important deterrent of tragic outcome. In children the incidence of bradycardic episodes, both fatal and

TABLE 34–8. Errors of management: Numbers and rank order of frequency

	1960 to 1969		1970 to 1980		1983 to 1985		Whole Series	
Error	*No.*	*Rank*	*No.*	*Rank*	*No.*	*Rank*	*No.*	*Rank*
Inadequate preparation	102	3	93	1	23	1	218	1
Wrong choice	120	2	65	3	13	4	198	4
Overdose	127	1	34	7	14	3	175	4
Aspiration	41	9	18	11	1	9	60	10
Inadequate resuscitation	63	7	49	4	6	5	118	6
Hypoxic mixture	14	12	0	—	0	—	14	12
Inadequate ventilation	68	5	21	9	1	9	90	7
Inadequate monitoring	22	11	19	10	6	5	47	11
Technical mishap	25	10	40	6	1	9	66	9
Inadequate crisis management	102	3	80	2	4	8	186	3
Inadequate reversal	52	8	22	8	5	7	79	8
Inadequate postoperative management	68	5	43	5	16	2	127	5
Total errors	804		484		90		1378	
Errors per patient	2.4		2.0		1.8		2.2	

Modified from Holland R: *Br J Anaesth* 59:834, 1987.

nonfatal, during anesthesia was reported to be significantly higher among emergency surgical procedures (2.7%) than in elective procedures (1.1%) (Keenan et al., 1994).

TIMING OF OCCURRENCE

Keenan and Boyan (1985), in a 15-year study of cardiac arrest resulting from anesthesia in a university hospital setting, found 18 of 27 cases occurred during the induction of anesthesia, whereas the remaining 9 occurred intraoperatively. However, in five of six patients in the pediatric age group who sustained cardiac arrest (1 day to 6 years), the arrest occurred during the maintenance of anesthesia. In most other reports, critical incidents or mishaps have occurred most frequently during the maintenance period of anesthesia (Cooper et al., 1978; Craig and Wilson, 1981; Gibbs, 1986). The maintenance period is not the quiet interlude between often stormy induction and emergence that many anesthesiologists had for a long time supposed (Epstein, 1978). In the survey involving 112,000 general anesthetic cases in a teaching hospital between 1975 and 1983 (Cohen, Duncan, and Tait, 1988), the incidence of intraoperative adverse events among adults was lower than events in the PACU. In contrast, the incidence of adverse events in children tended to be higher in the PACU (12.9% to 13.2%) than during surgery (8.6% to 9.5%) (Tiret et al., 1988). Machine-patient disconnection was a frequent occurrence in the 1970s (Cooper et al., 1978) before the disconnect alarm became a standard feature of anesthesia machines, mandated by the American National Standard Institute Z79 Committee on Anesthesia Equipment.

ANESTHETIC OVERDOSAGE

Drug overdose as the cause of anesthetic death occurs, although the incidence has decreased since the 1980s (Holland, 1984, 1987), and it accounted for only 5.4% of anesthetic deaths reported to the Medical Defense Union of the United Kingdom between 1970 and 1979 (Utting, Gray, and Shelley, 1979). In a 15-year study between 1969 and 1983 by Keenan and Boyan (1985), an "absolute" overdosage (a dose well in excess of the usual clinical range) caused one third of all cardiac arrests resulting from anesthesia. Of six incidents of cardiac arrest in children in this series, absolute overdosage with halothane was responsible in five cases; the other resulted from airway obstruction during nitrous oxide–curare anesthesia.

As described earlier, the POCA Registry database revealed that between 1994 and 1997, cardiovascular depression with halothane accounted for 66% of all medication-related cardiac arrests. In healthy children with ASA PS 1 or 2, 64% of all arrests were medication related in comparison with 23% in those with ASA PS 3 to 5 (Morray et al., 2000). The database between 2000 and 2003, when halothane had been replaced by sevoflurane as the primary inhalation induction agent, showed a dramatic decrease in medication-related cardiac arrest, from 37% to 12% of the total arrests (Morray, 2004), indicating the importance of safer anesthetic drugs for reducing medication-related complications (see Fig. 34–2).

RISK FACTORS IN PEDIATRIC ANESTHESIA

A number of perioperative risk factors specific to infants and children have been identified.

Age

Infants less than 1 year of age are at higher risk of developing complications (Tiret et al., 1988; Cohen et al., 1990). A prospective survey in France between 1978 and 1982 involving 440 institutions and a total of 40,240 anesthetic procedures found 27 major complications, of which 9 occurred in infants (0.43:10,000 cases), an incidence significantly higher than that in children (0.05:10,000) (Tiret et al., 1988). Infants less than 1 year of age also showed a significantly higher incidence of airway obstruction and other respiratory problems than did older children (Cohen et al., 1990). Cohen and others (1990) reported that the intraoperative incidence of complications in children was about the same as that in adults, but postoperative complications (35%) were twice as frequent as in adults (17%). The POCA Registry database (1994-1997) revealed 83 of 150, or 55%, anesthesia-related cardiac arrests occurred in infants less than 12 months of age (Morray et al., 2000) (see Table 34–5).

Physical Status

Correlation between perioperative cardiac arrest and ASA PS has been reported in adults (Keenan and Boyan, 1985). In a large-scale prospective survey in France involving infants and children, Tiret and others (1988) showed a highly significant correlation between the ASA PS classification and the incidence of major perianesthetic complications in children (Table 34–9). They also found a highly significant correlation between the perioperative adverse outcomes and the number of coexisting diseases. The POCA Registry database between 1994 and 1997 showed 100 of 150 (66.7%) of all anesthesia-related cardiac arrests occurred among children with ASA PS 3 to 5 (Morray et al., 2000) (see Table 34–5).

TABLE 34–9. Risks of pediatric anesthesia

	No. of Anesthetics	Rate of Complications (per 1000)	Significance
ASA PS			
1	36,903	0.4	
2	1461	3.4	$P < 0.001$
3	518	11.6	
4, 5	122	16.4	
No. of Coexisting Diseases			
0	36,544	0.5	
1	3064	1.3	$P < 0.001$
2	490	4.1	
≥3	142	21.1	
Previous Anesthetic			
No	25,517	0.5	
Yes	11,343	1.1	$P < 0.05$
Duration of Preoperative Fasting (hours)			
<8	5189	1.5	
>8	34,067	0.6	$P < 0.05$
Emergency			
No	33,391	0.5	
Yes	5918	1.5	$P < 0.05$

ASA PS, American Society of Anesthesiologists physical status.
Modified from Tiret L, et al.: *Br J Anaesth* 61:263, 1988.

Emergency Surgery

The French study (Tiret et al., 1988) showed a three-fold increase in perioperative complications in pediatric emergency cases compared with the scheduled cases (see Table 34–9). Similarly, Keenan and others (1994) found a highly significant increase of bradycardic episodes in children during emergency surgery compared with those with elective procedures (2.7% versus 1.1%).

Training

Proper training or experience is particularly important in pediatric anesthesia for minimizing the incidence of adverse outcome. In a retrospective study in a large university hospital over a span of 7 years, Keenan and others (1991) reviewed the incidence of cardiac arrests occurring in infants less than 1 year of age. No anesthesia-related cardiac arrests occurred when trained pediatric anesthesiologists were in charge of pediatric cases. In contrast, when nonpediatric anesthesiologists were supervising, cardiac arrests occurred at a frequency of 19.7:10,000 pediatric anesthetics, including deaths. In a subsequent prospective study from the same institution for the period of 9 years ending in 1992, the incidence of bradycardic episodes was significantly higher when pediatric anesthesiologists were not supervising the trainees administering anesthetics to infants (2.1%) compared with when pediatric anesthesiologists supervised the trainees (0.8%) (Keenan et al., 1994).

PREVENTION OF ANESTHESIA-RELATED MISHAPS

The first important step toward patient safety is prevention of critical events. As is clear from the foregoing discussion, a number of steps should be taken to achieve this goal.

PREANESTHETIC PREPARATION

Preoperatively, the patient's past medical history, especially anesthetic history, if any, should be reviewed thoroughly, and the patient should be examined carefully. The anesthesia machine, accessories, and drugs should also be checked carefully, because failure to perform these steps properly has been identified as a major cause of anesthesia-related mishaps, including death (Holland, 1984, 1987; Derrington and Smith, 1987). In an emergency or urgent situation (perhaps with the exception of exsanguination, cardiac tamponade, or acute upper airway obstruction), one should try to take at least minimal necessary steps (e.g., fluid resuscitation, transfusion, correction of electrolytes, acid-base imbalance, and fever) to stabilize the patient for anesthesia and surgery in a coordinated effort with the surgeon. One should not yield to unreasonable pressures to start the case before the patient is best prepared under these circumstances. Indeed, hypovolemia and anemia are reported to be the major causes of anesthesia-related cardiac arrest in infants and children (Salem et al., 1975).

If the anesthesiologist is unfamiliar or uncomfortable with uncommon pathophysiology (for instance, an infant with cyanotic heart disease coming for noncardiac surgery or a child with craniopharyngioma and diabetes insipidus), the anesthesiologist should not hesitate to ask for consultation with a senior anesthesiologist or other specialists. In addition, especially in an emergency situation (such as post-tonsillectomy bleeding or acute epiglottitis), an experienced assistant, preferably an attending pediatric anesthesiologist, should be standing by for the induction. Keenan and others (1994) found a significantly lower incidence of bradycardic events with the presence of a pediatric anesthesiologist during induction. In teaching institutions, resident trainees should always be supervised by a pediatric attending anesthesiologist for a pediatric patient. Lack of an experienced assistant has been associated with anesthesia-related mortality and major morbidity (Craig and Wilson, 1981; Derrington and Smith, 1987; Eichhorn et al., 1989; Keenan et al., 1994). A reluctance to ask for help, whether out of insecurity, pride, or ill-conceived heroism (or machismo), has no place in a pediatric anesthesia emergency and is the first step toward disaster.

VIGILANCE

A timely recovery from impending failure is the key to patient safety. It is, therefore, extremely important to recognize without delay that something is going wrong. Sustained attention or vigilance is essential for patient safety during the maintenance of anesthesia, when critical events most frequently occur (Cooper et al., 1978; Craig and Wilson, 1981; Gibbs, 1986) at the time of presumably reduced mental and physical workload (Gaba et al., 1987). One should develop the habit of scanning all of the monitors regularly in an orderly fashion, as a pilot in flight scans the instrument panel at regular intervals, to keep up with minute deviations in the patient's cardiorespiratory stability. A survey by Cooper and others (1984), however, suggests that at least 33% of critical incidents occurring during the maintenance of anesthesia resulted from errors in judgment rather than from inattentiveness. Vigilance is an important deterrent but by itself is not sufficient for prevention of critical incidents. However, the notion that all human beings, including all anesthesiologists, make mistakes (Allnutt, 1987) should not be used as an excuse to discount the importance of vigilance, especially in pediatric anesthesia. One should aim for near perfection by minimizing factors that adversely affect vigilance, such as fatigue, distraction, and boredom. A better understanding and application of ergonomic principles may improve vigilance and help reduce anesthesia-related mishaps in the future (Gravenstein and Weinger, 1986).

MONITORS AND MONITORING STANDARDS

The fact that most anesthesia-related fatalities involve human error clearly supports the concept that monitoring devices are essential for patient safety even for the experienced, conscientious, and vigilant anesthesiologist. The ASA Closed Malpractice Claims Study indicated that in 28% of these cases, proper monitoring already available commercially could have averted the mishaps (Cheney, 1988). Of particular interest to anesthesiologists is that the median cost of legal settlement in cases in which improved monitoring would probably have prevented the complication or death was more than 10 times higher than in cases in which better monitoring would have had no effect on occurrence or outcome (Cheney, 1988). In a similar review involving 238 (10% of 2400 total claims) closed anesthesia malpractice claims concerning children, a vast majority (estimate, 89%) of pediatric claims that were related to inadequate ventilation (43% of total) could have been prevented with pulse oximetry, capnography, or both (Morray et al., 1993).

In 1985, minimum standards for patient monitoring during anesthesia at Harvard University teaching hospitals were adopted and later published (Eichhorn et al., 1986). Similar but slightly more specific standards for basic intraoperative monitoring, proposed by the ASA, were approved by the House of Delegates in 1986. Both of these standards specifically mandate that oxygenation, ventilation, circulation, and body temperature be evaluated continually (at frequent intervals) or continuously (without interruption). For each of the components, the clear objective to ensure adequacy, followed by specific methods, is stated (see Chapters 9 and 11, Anesthetic Equipment and Monitoring and Intraoperative and Postoperative Management). There is a strong emphasis on combining clinical evaluation and technologic methods. Although no specific methodology or instrumentation is mandated for monitoring cardiopulmonary and other indices, the ASA standards strongly encourage quantitative methods, such as pulse oximetry and capnography, over qualitative clinical assessment, with inspection and auscultation for cardiopulmonary monitoring. In addition, the New York State Hospital Code (1988) dictates that pulse oximetry and capnography be used to monitor all patients undergoing general anesthesia to reduce anesthesia-related morbidity and mortality. Eventually, most other states have followed with similar laws mandating intraoperative monitoring with pulse oximetry and capnography. Accordingly, most malpractice liability insurers in the United States have required that anesthesiologists follow these standards whenever possible (Orkin, 1989).

Similar standards for basic patient monitoring have also been proposed in the United Kingdom (Sykes, 1987), Australia (Cass, Crosby, and Holland, 1988; Runciman, 1988b), and other industrialized countries. They are similar to the ASA standards in terms of machine monitoring (oxygen analyzer, low-flow alarm, and ventilator disconnect alarm). The standards for minimum patient monitoring, however, differ considerably, depending in part on the patient's physical status and the degree of surgical involvement (minor, standard, or major operation) (Sykes, 1987).

With the advent of pulse oximetry in the late 1980s, the anesthesiologist's ability to detect hypoxemia has improved markedly (see Chapter 9, Anesthesia Equipment and Monitoring). Coté and others (1988, 1991) have demonstrated that major hypoxemic events ($SaO_2 \leq 80\%$ lasting more than 30 seconds) can occur without visible cyanosis or obvious changes in the cardiorespiratory patterns in children and that pulse oximetry detects such events more quickly than other means of monitoring. Cooper and others (1987), as part of perianesthetic QA activity, found a significant reduction in undesirable anesthesia-related incidents that require intervention after the introduction of pulse oximetry in the operating room.

SELECTION OF SAFER ANESTHETICS AND ADJUVANT DRUGS

The POCA Registry data analyses have clearly demonstrated the safety of sevoflurane over halothane as the agent of choice for inhalation induction of anesthesia (Morray, 2004). During the period between 1994 and 1997, cardiac arrest associated with medication accounted for 37% of all arrests, of which halothane with or without other drugs accounted for 66% (Morray et al., 2000). During the period from 2000 to 2003, when sevoflurane had replaced halothane as the inhalation induction agent of choice, medication-related cause of cardiac arrests decreased drastically, from 37% to 12%. Concomitantly, the incidence of arrests among healthy children (ASA PS 1 or 2) decreased from 33% to 19% of all arrests (Morray, 2004). Although halothane may still be useful and could even be superior (and definitely far less expensive) than sevoflurane for anesthetic maintenance in certain situations (such as bronchoscopy) in experienced hands, there is no question that halothane should be avoided as an induction agent, especially for inexperienced trainees without close supervision. There is a strong indication that the clinical availability of halothane may end in the near future in the United States. A similar comparison can also be made with bupivacaine versus less toxic ropivacaine and levobupivacaine for conduction anesthesia in children (Ala-Kokko et al., 2002; Bosenberg et al., 2002; Mazoit and Dalens, 2004) (see Chapter 14, Pediatric Regional Anesthesia).

BETTER EDUCATION AND TRAINING

The steady decline in anesthesia-related mortality and morbidity over the past several decades has been attributed to increases in better-trained and better-qualified physicians administering anesthesia (Holland, 1987). In a survey of potentially harmful anesthesia-related events, Cooper and others (1978) found that 25% of these events were associated with inadequate training or unfamiliarity with equipment or devices; further training of these anesthetists (presumably trainees) would have prevented some of these events. In addition, an anesthesia-related mortality study from Harvard University (Eichhorn, 1989) has shown that in 8 of 11 cases of fatalities attributed primarily to anesthesia, inadequate supervision of residents, medical students, and nurse anesthetists was considered contributory.

As mentioned previously, Keenan and others (1991) reported the importance of specialty training in pediatric anesthesia for the reduction of cardiac arrests in infants. No anesthesia-related cardiac arrests occurred when trained pediatric anesthesiologists were in charge of pediatric cases, whereas arrests occurred at a frequency of 19.7:10,000 when nonpediatric anesthesiologists were supervising trainees. The same investigators also reported in a subsequent prospective study that the incidence of bradycardic episodes was significantly higher when pediatric anesthesiologists were not supervising the trainees anesthetizing infants (2.1%) than when trained pediatric anesthesiologists were in charge (0.8%) (Keenan et al., 1994). These results emphasize the importance of training and experience for a better anesthetic outcome.

QUALITY ASSURANCE

Documentation of the QA or QI process, especially that of fatal and morbid events, has been mandated in an effort to reduce the risk to and improve the outcome of patients undergoing anesthesia. In a pilot prospective study, Currie and others (1988) found the QA survey helpful in identifying nonfatal, nonmorbid, often transient events for peer review soon after such events took place. The survey demonstrated disproportionately high incidences of nonfatal events occurring with pediatric and emergency or out-of-hours cases. Induction and maintenance periods seem to be equally hazardous, up to four times more so than the emergence and recovery periods. As noted in other studies (Cooper et al., 1978, 1984; Craig and Wilson, 1981), airway events were most frequent (53%). The authors concluded that the advantage of their method lies for the most part in its inherent lack of inertia—rapid evaluation, response, and feedback—in a confidential and nonjudgmental atmosphere, resulting in the improvement of patient care in a unique manner (Cooper et al., 1978; Currie et al., 1988). QA or QI programs should be continued to prevent adverse events due to human factors or errors (active failure) by learning from events and "near-misses" as a group. Equally important, the QA program is the process of continually evaluating the environment, in which anesthesia is practiced, and identifying systemic problems (environmental factors or latent failures) responsible for or potentially causing adverse events, which have not been obvious, so as to implement strategies or new guidelines to improve the structure or environment and prevent future occurrence of adverse events.

Environmental factors (latent failures) may play a major role and may be responsible for adverse outcomes impeding the safety and quality of patient care. These factors may include inadequate safety mechanisms (organizational, clear drug labeling, etc.), inadequate or nonfunctional monitoring systems, and poor communication among the surgeons, anesthesiologists, and operating room personnel. Indeed, in an analysis of 110 adverse events from more than 13,000 anesthetic procedures, Lagasse and others (1995) identified only 8% caused by human errors, whereas 92% of adverse events were attributable to system errors.

Critical events related to anesthesia occur frequently during the practice of anesthesia. A well-trained, motivated, vigilant anesthesiologist normally detects these events in time and takes proper measures to prevent disaster. Anesthesia-related accidents causing catastrophic injury or death, therefore, are very rare, especially in relation to the frequency of such potentially harmful events. Because humans are imperfect and make mistakes as part of normal human cognitive behavior, catastrophic accidents can occur almost at random to any anesthesiologist (Allnutt, 1987). The availability of both machine and patient monitors and adherence to monitoring standards are indispensable.

From the foregoing presentation, it is apparent that young children, especially infants, are more vulnerable to anesthesia-related mishaps, whereas such a risk in older, healthy children is relatively low. Because of the small size and physiologic differences in cardiopulmonary and other organ systems in young infants, as outlined earlier in this book, safety in pediatric anesthesia demands additional clinical training and vigilance. Anesthetic complications in infants and children and their management, when applicable, have been discussed in appropriate chapters elsewhere in this book.

For the safety of infants and young children, a high-risk group in terms of anesthesia-related morbidity and mortality, more clinical training, adequate preoperative preparation, more vigilance, and adherence to monitoring standards (especially the use of a pulse oximeter and precordial stethoscope continuously) are all important and indispensable. When in doubt, one should not hesitate to transfer the young and unstable patient to a specialized center for pediatric anesthesia and surgery to provide a better opportunity for survival.

■ SUMMARY

Anesthesia-related mortality has declined steadily over the past several decades as the percentage of general anesthetics administered by trained anesthesiologists has increased and as newer and safer anesthetics and adjuvant drugs, anesthetic equipment, monitoring, and safety standards in the industrialized nations have improved. Yet, anesthesia-related adverse events remain relatively higher in infants less than 1 year of age than in older children and adults. As in adults, anesthetic catastrophe is still caused predominantly by judgment errors and environmental factors that are potentially preventable. Critical incidents occur more frequently during the induction and maintenance of anesthesia than during emergence and recovery. Emergency surgery and "urgent" surgery are associated with a disproportionately high incidence of anesthesia-related adverse events, in part because of inadequate preanesthetic patient preparation.

Analyses of closed malpractice insurance claims as well as the POCA Registry sponsored by the ASA have been informative in developing a future strategy for preventing anesthesia-related mishaps. Emphasis on strict monitoring standards and QA surveillance, developed and sustained since the late 1980s, seem valuable both in preventing "near-misses" and in heightening anesthesiologists' awareness of such events. For patient safety in pediatric anesthesia, better clinical training, adequate preanesthetic preparations, vigilance, and adherence to monitoring standards are all important and essential.

REFERENCES

Ala-Kokko TI, Karinen J, Reiha E, et al.: Pharmacokinetics of 0.75% ropivacaine and 0.5% bupivacaine after ilioinguinal-iliohypogastric nerve block in children. *Br J Anaesth* 89:438–441, 2002.

Allnutt MF: Human factors in accidents. *Br J Anaesth* 59:856–864, 1987.

American Society of Anesthesiologists: *Standards for basic intraoperative monitoring.* Oct 1986. http://www.asahq.org/publicationsAndServices/standards/02.pdf#2

American Society of Anesthesiologists Task Force on Sedation and Analgesia by Non-Anesthesiologists: Pediatric guidelines for sedation and analgesia by non-anesthesiologists. *Anesthesiology* 96:1004–1017, 2002.

Arrowsmith JB, Gerstman BB, Fleischer DE, Benjamin SB: Results from the American Society for Gastrointestinal Endoscopy/U.S. Food and Drug Administration collaborative study on complication rates and drug use during gastrointestinal endoscopy. *Gastrointest Endosc* 37:421, 1991.

Aouad MT, Siddik SS, Rizk LB, et al.: The effect of dexamethasone on postoperative vomiting after tonsillectomy. *Anesth Analg* 92:636–640, 2001.

Bailey PL, Pace NL, Ashburn MA, et al.: Frequent hypoxemia and apnea after sedation with midazolam and fentanyl. *Anesthesiology* 73:826–830, 1990.

Beecher HK, Todd DP: A study of the deaths associated with anesthesia and surgery based on a study of 599,548 anesthesias in ten institutions 1948-1952, inclusive. *Ann Surg* 140:2, 1954.

Bodlander FMS: Deaths associated with anesthesia. *Br J Anaesth* 47:36, 1975.

Borland LM, Sereika SM, Woelfel SK, et al.: Pulmonary aspiration in pediatric patients during general anesthesia: Incidence and outcome. *J Clin Anesth* 10:95–102, 1998.

Bosenberg A, Thomas J, Lopez T, et al.: The efficacy of caudal ropivacaine 1, 2 and 3 mg x (-1) for postoperative analgesia in children. *Paediatr Anaesth* 12:53–58, 2002.

Buck N, Devlin HB, Lunn JN: *The report of the confidential inquiry into perioperative deaths.* London, 1987, Nuffield Provincial Hospitals Trust/King's Fund.

Caplan RA, Ward RJ, Posner K, Cheney FW: Unexpected cardiac arrest during spinal anesthesia: A closed claims analysis of predisposing factors. *Anesthesiology* 68:5–11, 1988.

Cass NM, Crosby WM, Holland RB: Minimal monitoring standards. *Anaesth Intensive Care* 16:110, 1988.

Cheney FW: Anesthesia: Potential risks and causes of incidents. In Gravenstein JS, Holzer JF, editors: *Safety and cost containment in anesthesia.* Boston, 1988, Butterworths.

Cohen MM, Cameron CB: Should you cancel the operation when a child has an upper respiratory tract infection? *Anesth Analg* 72:282–288, 1991.

Cohen MM, Cameron CB, Duncan PG: Pediatric anesthesia morbidity and mortality in the perioperative period. *Anesth Analg* 70:160–167, 1990.

Cohen MM, Duncan PG, Tate RB: Does anesthesia contribute to operative mortality? *JAMA* 260:2859–2863, 1988.

Committee on Drugs, Section on Anesthesiology, American Academy of Pediatrics: Guidelines for the elective use of conscious sedation, deep sedation and general anesthesia in pediatric patients. *Pediatrics* 76:317–321, 1985.

Committee on Drugs, Section on Anesthesiology, American Academy of Pediatrics: Guidelines for monitoring and management of pediatric patients during and after sedation for diagnostic and therapeutic procedures. *Pediatrics* 89:1110–1115, 1992.

Committee on Drugs, Section on Anesthesiology, American Academy of Pediatrics: Guidelines for monitoring and management of pediatric patients during and after sedation for diagnostic and therapeutic procedures: Addendum. *Pediatrics* 110:836–838, 2002.

Cooper JB: Conference report: 1986 Meeting of the International Committee for Prevention of Anesthesia Mortality and Morbidity. *Can J Anaesth* 35: 287, 1988.

Cooper JB, Cullen DJ, Nemeskal R, et al.: Effects of information feedback and pulse oximetry on the incidence of anesthesia complications. *Anesthesiology* 67:686–694, 1987.

Cooper JB, Gaba D: No myth: Anesthesia is a model for addressing patient safety (editorial). *Anesthesiology* 97:1335–1337, 2002.

Cooper JB, Newbower RS, Kitz RJ: An analysis of major errors and equipment failures in anesthesia management: Considerations for prevention and detection. *Anesthesiology* 60:34–92, 1984.

Cooper JB, Newbower RS, Long CD, McPeek B: Preventable anesthesia mishaps: A study of human factors. *Anesthesiology* 49:399–406, 1978.

Cooper JB, Pierce EC Jr: Safety foundation organized: Statement of purpose. *Anesthesia Patient Safety Foundation Newsletter* 1:1, 1986.

Coté CJ: Discharge criteria for children sedated by nonanesthesiologists. *Anesthesiology* 100:207–209, 2004.

Coté CJ, Goldstein EA, Coté MA, et al.: A single-blind study of pulse oximetry in children. *Anesthesiology* 68:184–188, 1988.

Coté CJ, Nottermann DA, Karl HW, et al.: Adverse sedation events in pediatrics: A critical incident analysis of contributing factors. *Pediatrics* 105:805–814, 2000.

Coté CJ, Rolf N, Liu LMP, Goudsouzian NG: A single-blind study of pulse oximetry and capnography in children. *Anesthesiology* 74:980–987, 1991.

Coté CJ, Zaslevsky A, Downes JJ, et al.: Postoperative apnea in former preterm infants after inguinal herniorrhaphy. A combined analysis. *Anesthesiology* 82:809–822, 1995.

Craig J, Wilson ME: A survey of anaesthetic misadventures. *Anaesthesia* 36:933–936, 1981.

Currie M, Pybus DA, Torda TA: A prospective survey of anaesthetic critical events. A report on a pilot study of 88 cases. *Anaesth Intensive Care* 16:103–107, 1988.

Davis DA: An analysis of anesthetic mishaps from medical liability claims. *Int Anesthesiol Clin* 22:31–42, 1984.

Derrington MC, Smith G: A review of studies of anaesthetic risk, morbidity and mortality. *Br J Anaesth* 59:815–833, 1987.

DeSoto H, Patel RI, Soliman IE, Hannallah RS: Changes in oxygen saturation following general anesthesia in children with upper respiratory infection signs and symptoms undergoing otolaryngological procedures. *Anesthesiology* 68:276–279, 1988.

Diaz JH: Halothane anesthesia in infancy: Identification and correlation of preoperative risk factors with intraoperative arterial hypotension and postoperative recovery. *J Pediatr Surg* 20:502–507, 1985.

Dornette WHL, Orth OS: Death in the operating room. *Anesth Analg* 35:545, 1956.

Downes JJ, Raphaely RC: Anesthesia and intensive care. In Ravitch MM, Welch KJ, Benson CD, et al., editors: *Pediatric surgery,* 3rd ed. Chicago, 1979, Year Book Medical Publishers.

Duncan PG: Clinical pearls-pediatric anesthesia. IARS Review Course Lectures. *Anesth Analg* (Suppl) March:9, 1995.

Eichhorn JH: Prevention of intraoperative anesthesia accidents and related severe injury through safety monitoring. *Anesthesiology* 70:572–577, 1989.

Eichhorn JH, Cooper JB, Cullen DJ, et al.: Standards for patient monitoring at Harvard Medical School. *JAMA* 256:1017–1020, 1986.

Epstein RM: Morbidity and mortality from anesthesia: A continuing problem. *Anesthesiology* 49:388–389, 1978.

Fasting S, Gisvold SE: Data recording of problems during anaesthesia: presentation of a well-functioning and simple system. *Acta Anaesthesiol Scand* 40:1173–1183, 1996.

Flick RP, Schears GJ, Warner MA: Aspiration in pediatric anesthesia: Is there a higher incidence compared with adults? *Curr Opin Anesthesiol* 15:323–327, 2002.

Fujii Y, Toyooka H, Tanaka H: Antiemetic efficacy of granisetron and metoclopramide in children undergoing ophthalmic or ENT surgery. *Can J Anaesth* 43:1095–1099, 1996.

Gaba DM: Anesthesiology as a model for safety in health care. *Br Med J* 320:785–788, 2000.

Gaba DM, Maxwell M, DeAnda A: Anesthetic mishaps: Breaking the chain of accident evolution. *Anesthesiology* 66:670–676, 1987.

Giaufré E, Dalens B, Gombert A: Epidermiology and morbidity of regional anesthesia in children: a one-year prospective survey of the French-Language Society of Pediatric Anesthesiologists. *Anesth Analg* 83:904–912, 1996.

Gibbs JM: The Anaesthetic Mortality Assessment Committee 1979-1984. *N Z Med J* 99:55–59, 1986.

Graff TD, Phillips OC, Benson DW, Kelley E, Baltimore Anesthesia Study Committee: Factors in pediatric anesthesia mortality. *Anesth Analg* 43:407, 1964.

Gravenstein JS, Weinger MB: Why investigate vigilance? *J Clin Monit* 2:145–147, 1986.

Gross JB, Bailey PL, Caplan RA, et al.: Practice guidelines for sedation and analgesia by non-anesthesiologists: A report by the American Society of Anesthesiologists Task Force on Sedation and Analgesia by Non-Anesthesiologists. *Anesthesiology* 96:1004–1017, 2002.

Harrison GG: Death attributable to anaesthesia. *Br J Anaesth* 50:1041, 1978.

Harrison GG: Death due to anesthesia at Groote Schuur Hospital, Cape Town—1956–1987. Part II. Causes and changes in aetiological pattern of anesthetic-contributory death. *S Afr Med J* 77:416–421, 1990.

Hatton F, Tiret L, Vourc'h G, et al.: Morbidity and mortality associated with anaesthesia—French survey: Preliminary results. In Vickers MD, Lunn JN, editors: *Mortality in anaesthesia.* Berlin, 1983, Springer-Verlag, p. 25.

Holland R: Anaesthesia-related mortality in Australia. *Int Anesthesiol Clin* 22:61, 1984.

Holland R: Anaesthetic mortality in New South Wales. *Br J Anaesth* 59:834–841, 1987.

Holzman RS: Morbidity and mortality in pediatric anesthesia. *Pediatr Clin North Am* 41:239–256, 1994.

Hovi-Viander M: Death associated with anesthesia in Finland. *Br J Anaesth* 52:483–489, 1980.

Joint Commission on Accreditation of Healthcare Organizations: *Joint Commission Accreditation Manual on Hospitals, Vol 3.* Oak Brook Terrace, IL, 1992, JCAHO.

Jones SEF, Beasley JM, MacFarlane WR, et al.: Intrathecal morphine for post-operative pain relief in children. *Br J Anaesth* 56:137–140, 1984.

Kataria BK, Harmik EV, Michard R, et al.: Postoperative arterial oxygen saturation in the pediatric population during transportation. *Anesth Analg* 67:280–282, 1988.

Keats AS: Anesthesia mortality: A new mechanism. *Anesthesiology* 68:2–4, 1988.

Keats AS, Siker ES: International Symposium on Preventable Anesthetic Morbidity and Mortality, Boston, Oct. 8-10, 1984. *Anesthesiology* 63:349, 1985.

Keenan RL: Anesthetic disasters: Incidence, causes and preventability. *ASA Refresher Course* 16:125, 1988.

Keenan RL, Boyan CP: Cardiac arrest due to anesthesia. A study of incidence and causes. *JAMA* 253:2373–2377, 1985.

Keenan RL, Shapiro JH, Dawson K: Frequency of anesthetic cardiac arrest in infants: Effect of pediatric anesthesiologists. *J Clin Anesth* 3:433–437, 1991.

Keenan RL, Shapiro JH, Kane FR, Simpson PM: Bradycardia during anesthesia in infants. An epidemiologic study. *Anesthesiology* 80:976–982, 1994.

Kohn L, Corrigan J, Donaldson M, editors: *Committee on Quality of Health Care in America: To err is human: Building a safer health care system in America.* Institute of Medicine, 1999, National Academy Press, p. 241.

Koka BV, Jeon IS, Andre JM, et al.: Postintubation croup in children. *Anesth Analg* 56:501–505, 1977.

Krane EJ: Delayed respiratory depression in a child after caudal epidural morphine. *Anesth Analg* 67:79–82, 1988.

Kurth CD, LeBard SE: Association of postoperative apnea, airway obstruction, and hypoxemia in former premature infants. *Anesthesiology* 75:22–26, 1991.

Kurth CD, Spitzer AR, Broennle AM, Downes JJ: Post-operative apnea in preterm infants. *Anesthesiology* 66:483–488, 1987.

Lagasse RS: Anesthesia safety: Model or myth? *Anesthesiology* 97:1609–1617, 2002.

Lagasse RS, Steinberg ES, Katz RI, Saubermann AJ: Defining quality of perioperative care by statistical process control of adverse outcomes. *Anesthesiology* 82:1181–1188, 1995.

Litman RS, Keon TP: Postintubation croup in children. *Anesthesiology* 75:1122–1123, 1991.

Liu LM, Coté CJ, Goudsouzian NG, et al.: Life-threatening apnea in infants recovering from anesthesia. *Anesthesiology* 59:506–510, 1983.

Lunn JN, Devlin HB: Lessons from the confidential enquiry into perioperative deaths in three NHS regions. *Lancet* 2:1384–1386, 1987.

Lunn JN, Mushin WW: *Mortality associated with anaesthesia.* London, 1982, Nuffield Provincial Hospitals Trust.

Malviya S, Swartz J, Lerman J: Are all preterm infants younger than 60 weeks postconceptual age at risk for postanesthetic apnea? *Anesthesiology* 78:1076–1081, 1993.

Malviya S, Voepel-Lewis T, Ludomirsky A, et al.: Can we improve the assessment of discharge readiness? *Anesthesiology* 100: 218–224, 2004.

Malviya S, Voepel-Lewis T, Tait AR: Adverse events and risk factors associated with the sedation of children by nonanesthesiologists. *Anesth Analg* 85: 1207–1213, 1997.

Martin TM, Nicolson SC, Bargas MS: Propofol anesthesia reduces emesis and airway obstruction in pediatric outpatients. *Anesth Analg* 76:144–148, 1993.

Mason LJ: An update on the etiology and prevention of anesthesia-related cardiac arrest in children. *Pediatr Anesth* 14:412–416, 2004.

Mazoit JX, Dalens BJ: Pharmacokinetics of local anesthesia in infants and children. *Clin Pharmacokinet* 43:17–32, 2004.

Mellin-Olsen J, Fasting S, Gisvold SE: Routine preoperative gastric emptying is seldom indicated. A study of 85,594 anaesthetics with special focus on aspiration pneumonia. *Acta Anaesthesiol Scand* 40:1184–1188, 1996.

Mendelson CL: Aspiration of stomach contents into lungs during obstetric anesthesia. *Am J Obstet Gynecol* 51:889–892, 1996.

Morgan CA, Webb RK, Cockings J, et al.: The Australian Incident Monitoring Study. Cardiac arrest-an analysis of 2000 incident reports. *Anaesth Intensive Care* 21:626–637, 1993.

Morray JP: Unexpected cardiac arrest in the anesthetized child. Presented at Society of Pediatric anesthesia spring meeting. March 4–7, 2004.

Morray JP, Geiduschek JM, Caplan RA, et al.: A comparison of pediatric and adult anesthesia closed malpractice claims. *Anesthesiology* 78:461–467, 1993.

Morray JP, Geiduscheck JM, Ramamoorthy C, et al.: Anesthesia-related cardiac arrest in children: Initial findings of the Pediatric Perioperative Cardiac Arrest (POCA) registry. *Anesthesiology* 93:6–14, 2000.

Motas D, McDermott NB, Vansickle T, Friesen RH: Depth of consciousness and deep sedation attained in children as administered by nonanesthesiologists in a children's hospital. *Pediatr Anesth* 14:256–260, 2004.

Motoyama EK, Glazener CH: Hypoxemia after general anesthesia in children. *Anesth Analg* 65:267–272, 1986.

Murat I: Mortality, morbidity and outcome. In Bissonette B, Dalens B, editors: *Pediatric anesthesia: Principle and practice.* New York, 2002, McGraw-Hill, Chapter 79, pp. 1465–1478.

Murat I, Constant I, Maud'Huy H: Perioperative anaesthetic morbidity in children: A database of 24,165 anaesthetics over a 30 month period. *Pediatr Anesth* 14:158–166, 2004.

New York State Hospital Code, Section 405.13, endorsed by the New York State Hospital Review and Planning Council, June 9, 1988; approved by the Commissioner of the New York State Department of Health for Jan. 1, 1989, implementation.

Olsson GL: Bronchospasm during anesthesia. A computer-aided incidence study of 136,929 patients. *Acta Anesthesiol Scand* 31:244–252, 1987.

Olsson GL, Hallen B: Cardiac arrest during anaesthesia: A computer-aided study in 250,543 anaesthetics. *Acta Anaesthesiol Scand* 32:653–654, 1988.

Olsson GL, Hallen B: Laryngospasm during anesthesia: A computer-aided incidence study in 136,929 patients. *Acta Anaesthesiol Scand* 28:567–575, 1984.

Olsson GL, Hallen B, Hambraeus-Jonzon K: Aspiration during anaesthesia: A computer-aided study of 185,358 anaesthetics. *Acta Anaesthesiol Scand* 30: 84–92, 1986.

Orkin FK: Practice standards: The Midas touch or the emperor's new clothes? *Anesthesiology* 70:567–571, 1989.

Parnis SJ, Barker DS, van der Walt JH: Clinical predictors of anaesthetic complications in children with respiratory tract infections. *Paediatr Anaesth* 11:29–40, 2001.

Patel RI, Rice LJ: Special considerations in the recovery room of children from anesthesia. *Int Anesthesiol Clin* 29:55–68, 1991.

Patel RI, Verghese ST, Hannallah RS, et al.: Fast-tracking children after ambulatory surgery. *Anesth Analg* 92:918–922, 2001.

Petruscak J, Smith RN, Breslin P: Mortality related to ophthalmological surgery. *Surv Anesthesiol* 18:87, 1974.

Phillips OC, Frazier TM: Baltimore Anesthesia Study Committee: Organization and preliminary report. *Anesthesiology* 18:33, 1957.

Pierce EC Jr: Analysis of anesthetic mishaps. Historical perspectives. *Int Anesthesiol Clin* 22:116, 1984.

Pierce EC Jr: Safety in anesthesia. *Curr Opin Anaesth* 1:532, 1988.

Practice guidelines for sedation and analgesia by non-anesthesiologists. A report by the American Society of Anesthesiologists Task Force on Sedation and Analgesia by Non-Anesthesiologists. *Anesthesiology* 84:459, 1996.

Pullerits J, Burrows FA, Roy WL: Arterial desaturation in healthy children during transfer to the recovery room. *Can J Anaesth* 34:470–473, 1987.

Rackow H, Salanitre E, Green LT: Frequency of cardiac arrest associated with anesthesia in infants and children. *Pediatrics* 28:697, 1961.

Rolf N, Coté CJ: Frequency and severity of desaturation events during general anesthesia in children with and without upper respiratory infection. *J Clin Anesth* 4:200–203, 1992.

Runciman WB: Monitoring and patient safety: An overview. *Anaesth Intensive Care* 16:11–13, 1988a.

Runciman WB: The Australian Patient Safety Foundation. *Anaesth Intensive Care* 16:114, 1988b.

Runciman WB, Ilsley AH, Holland RB, Russell WJ: Symposium issue: Monitoring and patient safety. *Anaesth Intensive Care* 16:1–116, 1988.

Salem MR, Bennett EJ, Schweiss JF, et al.: Cardiac arrest related to anesthesia. Contributing factors in infants and children. *JAMA* 233:238–241, 1975.

Schreiner MS, Nicholson SC, Martin T, Whitney L: Should children drink before discharge from day surgery? *Anesthesiology* 76:528–533, 1992.

Schreiner MS, O'Hara I, Markakis DA, Politis GD: Do children who experience laryngospasm have an increased risk of upper respiratory tract infection? *Anesthesiology* 85:475–480, 1996.

Smith G, Norman J, editors: Symposium on complications and medico-legal aspects of anesthesia. *Br J Anaesth* 59:813, 1987.

Smith RM: Some reasons for the high mortality in pediatric anesthesia. *N Y State J Med* 56:2212, 1956.

Smith RM: The pediatric anesthetist, 1950-1975. *Anesthesiology* 43:144, 1975.

Smith RM, editor: *Anesthesia for infants and children,* ed 4. St. Louis, 1980, CV Mosby.

Soliman IE, Patel RI, Ehrenpreis MB, Hannallah RS: Recovery scores do not correlate with postoperative hypoxemia in children. *Anesth Analg* 67:53–56, 1988.

Stevenson HE, Reid LC, Hinton JW: Some common denominators in 1200 cases of cardiac arrest. *Ann Surg* 137:731, 1953.

Stoelting R: APSF response to IOM medical error report. *Anesthesia Patient Safety Foundation Newsletter* 15:1, 2000.

Sykes MK: Essential monitoring. *Br J Anaesth* 59:901–912, 1987.

Tait AR, Malviya S, Voepel-Lewis T, et al.: Risk factors for perioperative adverse respiratory events in children with upper respiratory tract infections. *Anesthesiology* 95:299–306, 2001.

Tay CLM, Tan GM, Ng SBA: Critical incidents in paediatric anaesthesia: An audit of 10 000 anaesthetics in Singapore. *Paediatr Anaesth* 11:711–718, 2001.

Thach BT: Sleep apnea in infancy and childhood. *Med Clin North Am* 69:1289–1315, 1985.

Tiret L, Desmonts JM, Hatton F, et al.: Complications associated with anaesthesia: A prospective survey in France. *Can Anaesth South J* 33:336, 1986.

Tiret L, Nivoche Y, Hatton F, et al.: Complications related to anaesthesia in infants and children: A prospective survey of 40240 anaesthetics. *Br J Anaesth* 61:263–269, 1988.

Turnbull KW, Fancourt-Smith PF, Banting GC: Death within 48 hours of anaesthesia at the Vancouver General Hospital. *Can Anaesth Soc J* 27:159–163, 1980.

Utting JE, Gray TC, Shelley FC: Human misadventure in anaesthesia. *Can Anaesth Soc J* 26:472–478, 1979.

Valley RD, Bailey AG: Caudal morphine for postoperative analgesia in infants and children: a report of 138 cases. *Anesth Analg* 72:120–124, 1991.

van der Walt JH, Sweeney DB, Runciman WB, Webb RK: Pediatric incidents in anaesthesia: An analysis of 2000 incidents reports. *Anaesth Intensive Care* 21:655–658, 1993.

Vickers MD, Lunn JN: *Mortality in anaesthesia.* Berlin, 1983, Springer-Verlag, p. 19.

Warner MA, Warner ME: Warner DO, et al.: Perioperative pulmonary aspiration in infants and children. *Anesthesiology* 90:66–71, 1999.

Weinstein MS, Nicholson SC, Schreiner MSS: A single dose of morphine sulfate increases the incidence of vomiting after outpatient inguinal surgery in children. *Anesthesiology* 81:572–577, 1994.

Weir PM, Munro HM, Reynolds PI: Propofol infusion and the incidence of emesis in pediatric outpatient strabismus surgery. *Anesth Analg* 76:760–764, 1993.

Welborn LG, deSoto H, Hannallah RS, et al.: The use of caffeine in the control of post-anesthetic apnea in former premature infants. *Anesthesiology* 68:796–798, 1988.

Welborn LG, Hannallah RS, Luban NLC, et al.: Anemia and postoperative apnea in former premature infants. *Anesthesiology* 74:1003–1006, 1991.

Welborn LG, Rice LJ, Hannallah RS, et al.: Postoperative apnea in former preterm infants: Prospective comparison of spinal and general anesthesia. *Anesthesiology* 72:838–842, 1990.

Xue FS, Huang YG, Tong SY, et al.: A comparative study of early postoperative hypoxemia in infants, children, and adults undergoing elective plastic surgery. *Anesth Analg* 83:709–715, 1996.

35 History of Pediatric Anesthesia

Robert M. Smith • Mark A. Rockoff

The goal of the individual pediatric anesthesiologist is generally neither to diagnose nor to cure but rather to guide and support each young patient through the operative experience with the least possible mental and physical stress. The history of pediatric anesthesia is best told by tracing the steps toward increasing precision in the regulation (maintaining within normal limits) or controlling (carrying beyond normal limits) of neurologic, respiratory, cardiovascular, and other body systems to serve both surgeon and child (Smith, 1991).

The goals of pediatric anesthesiology as a specialty include the reduction of perioperative morbidity and mortality and the promotion of ancillary resuscitative and supportive fields through teaching, research, and organizational activity throughout the world.

PHASE I: PEDIATRIC ANESTHESIA BEFORE 1940

PRIMITIVE PERIOD

Before the introduction of ether in 1846, not only circumcisions but amputations, excisions of tumors, and correction of gross deformities were performed on infants and children without any relief of pain. Struggling could be controlled by use of force, but pain was accepted as an unavoidable part of life. Crude attempts occasionally made with alcoholic "spirits," nerve compression, or even brief strangling, coupled with headlong surgical speed, resulted in predictably poor outcome for both operation and patient. Harelip repair had been attempted without pain relief measures in many parts of the world for hundreds of years. In Japan, general anesthesia with the herb mixture *tsu san sen* was used successfully for breast cancer operations in 1804 by Seishu Hanaoka. In 1837, Gancho Homma reported a series of general anesthesia with the use of the same herb mixture for children over 5 years of age for harelip repair but withheld it from use in younger patients because of its toxicity (Iwai and Satoyoshi, 1992). The conviction that small infants did not need anesthesia was not effectively suppressed until recently (Anand and Hickey, 1987). For many years, the "whiskey nipple" had been used widely as a sedative supplement to local anesthesia in infants undergoing abdominal procedures; wine has been given for ritual circumcisions for millennia.

EARLY CONTROL OF PAIN: ETHER AND CHLOROFORM

The introduction of ether was the first giant step in the history of anesthesia. Although Crawford Long used ether in his rural practice in Georgia beginning in 1842 and his third ether anesthetic procedure was for a toe amputation in a 7-year-old boy (Long, 1849), it was not until the famous public demonstration of ether anesthesia at the Massachusetts General Hospital in Boston in 1846 that ether was widely accepted for use during surgery (Morton, 1847). The discovery that sensation, or pain, could be abolished temporarily by ether, and along with it consciousness and motion, was widely acclaimed, but little was known about its actions, how to use it, or what its dangers might be. Ether was accepted only gradually over several years, with many surgeons retaining the belief that ordinary men (the wealthy excluded) should be able to tolerate surgery without anesthesia! However, for children and ladies, who were considered to be "more sensitive," anesthesia was considered appropriate (Warren, 1847; Pernick, 1975), although Morton himself was reluctant to administer it to very young subjects because of the high incidence of nausea and vomiting in this population (Bigelow, 1846).

It was soon found that pouring ether onto a handkerchief or small cloth was a practical method of administration with small children. One simply pressed the cloth to the patient's face until the child was quiet and limp. Then it was withdrawn, and the surgeon was granted 3 or 4 minutes to operate as the child regained consciousness. The use of continuous administration of ether caught on slowly with gradual familiarization with the new agent. The early impression that ether was easy to administer, effective, and safe led to the belief that it was a trivial service that any inexperienced person, often an orderly or a parent, could perform. The unfortunate result of this in the United States was that throughout the rest of the century, the administration of anesthesia continued to be held in poor repute as a medical activity, rarely attracting physicians with special interest or ability in the field. Nurses eventually began to assume increasing responsibilities for providing anesthesia care. As late as 1940, a physician, in the lead article published in the first edition of the new journal *Anesthesiology,* noted, "During my internship I was trained by a nurse. I was given a cone, a can of ether and a few empirical tricks" (Haggard, 1940).

In England, chloroform was accepted more readily because of its smoother and more rapid action. Soon, however, the incidence of deaths became so alarming that the British established a dictum that only physicians should be allowed to administer anesthesia (Eckenhoff, 1966). The fortunate result was that throughout the British Empire anesthesia flourished as a medical specialty, its workers gaining equal status with other physicians, and establishing early leadership in this field for several decades, particularly in the development of pediatric anesthesia.

Another great advantage for the British in the early development of anesthesia was the presence of the astounding John Snow (1813–1858), whose contributions included epidemiologic advances of national importance and an active medical practice while keeping notes on hundreds of anesthetic experiences and research experiments, mostly between 1846 and his death a decade later (Griffith, 1934). Snow formulated the first description of signs by which one could monitor and control the depth of anesthesia in patients of all ages (Snow, 1847). His five stages of anesthesia, based on excitement, loss of consciousness, relaxation, eye movement, and depth of respiration, served as guidelines throughout the remainder of the century and formed the basis of Guedel's important guide *Inhalation Anesthesia,* published in 1937. Snow explored both ether and chloroform, preferring the latter, which he found well suited to infants and children. However, he warned of its danger with excessive depth (Snow, 1858). His record of successfully anesthetizing 147 infants for harelip repair is hardly conceivable in view of the mortality that this operation continued to bear well into the next century!

Following the remarkable beginning made by Snow, anesthesia in England progressed at a slower pace. For nearly 20 years, chloroform and ether remained the only anesthetic agents available, and progress consisted chiefly of developing methods of their administration, comparing their advantages and dangers, and simply trying to find out how to keep children asleep and still for longer periods of time. Despite its recognized danger, chloroform remained the principal agent in England and throughout Europe. Efforts to reduce the complications associated with chloroform included many warnings as well as more effective steps, such as diluting it with ether (CE) and with alcohol and ether (ACE). The introductions of nitrous oxide into general use by 1870 and ethyl chloride shortly after 1900 were important advances, reducing or replacing the use of chloroform in many operations not requiring relaxation. The fact that both of these agents were nonirritating and relatively acceptable made them particularly adaptable for induction and initiated early interest in special methods of handling this troublesome stage of anesthesia.

British physician anesthetists began to publish articles and texts in increasing numbers. Buxton alone producing five editions of his *Anaesthetics: Their Uses and Administration* between 1888 and 1912. Many adult texts contained advice on pediatric problems, among which that of harelip continued to attract the most attention. Numerous references to pediatric anesthesia could be found in *The Lancet,* Britain's premier medical journal, and in 1923 C. Langton Hewer wrote *Anaesthesia for Children,* the first text on pediatric anesthesia to be written in English.

In the United States, the special needs of children were given slight consideration for many years. The child was treated as "a little man," surgeons operated with large instruments, and all equipment was adult sized. Ether remained the principal agent. Although criticism of chloroform became more vehement (Kopetsky, 1903), its use was advocated in the United States as recently as 1957 (Schwartz, 1957). Progress was made by trial and error, with little communication among those using anesthesia. Most literature in the United States concerning anesthesia for children was written by surgeons before 1900.

Interest grew slowly in widely separated areas where adept nurses and occasionally unsuccessful surgeons developed skills sufficient to carry children through longer and more difficult procedures. Tonsillectomy, practiced since 1887, was being performed by the thousands in 1900, and appendectomy became an accepted, although often dangerous, procedure. Orthopedic surgery was definitely the most active type of pediatric surgery at the turn of the century, and most procedures were easily managed by simple ether techniques. One of the first signs of concern for the child's anxiety when undergoing anesthesia was voiced by James Gwathmey in 1907, when he recommended that one should "add a few drops of the mother's cologne to the ether mask and induce the child in the mother's arms." Another step toward easing induction came in 1928 with the entry of tribromoethanol, the German Avertin, which was used widely as a rectal agent. It provided almost certain sleep in 7 to 8 minutes and was of special value prior to ether induction because, unlike the barbiturates used later, it had a bronchodilating effect and facilitated rather than retarded induction. Unfortunately, the drug required preparation immediately before use and that, plus the frequent occurrence of fecal incontinence, led to its abandonment.

Between 1925 and 1940, activity in both pediatric surgery and anesthesia began to accelerate. William Ladd, whose interest stemmed from his experience in caring for children injured in a massive explosion in Halifax, Nova Scotia in 1917, led the development of pediatric surgery in North America (Goldbloom, 1917; Steward, 1983). His work at Children's Hospital Boston was particularly devoted to the correction of neonatal defects including, of course, harelip. He performed harelip repair seated, with the infant held facing him in the lap of a nurse, while the anesthetist stood behind the nurse, directing ether from a vaporizing bottle into the infant's mouth via a metal mouth hook.*

The introduction of cyclopropane in 1930 proved particularly helpful for pediatric anesthetists in the management of infants, although it required assembly of a closed-system apparatus. Lamont and Harmel developed a miniaturization of the

*An accurate description of the first anesthetic agents given by one of the writers (R.M.S.) for Dr. Ladd at Children's Hospital Boston in 1946.

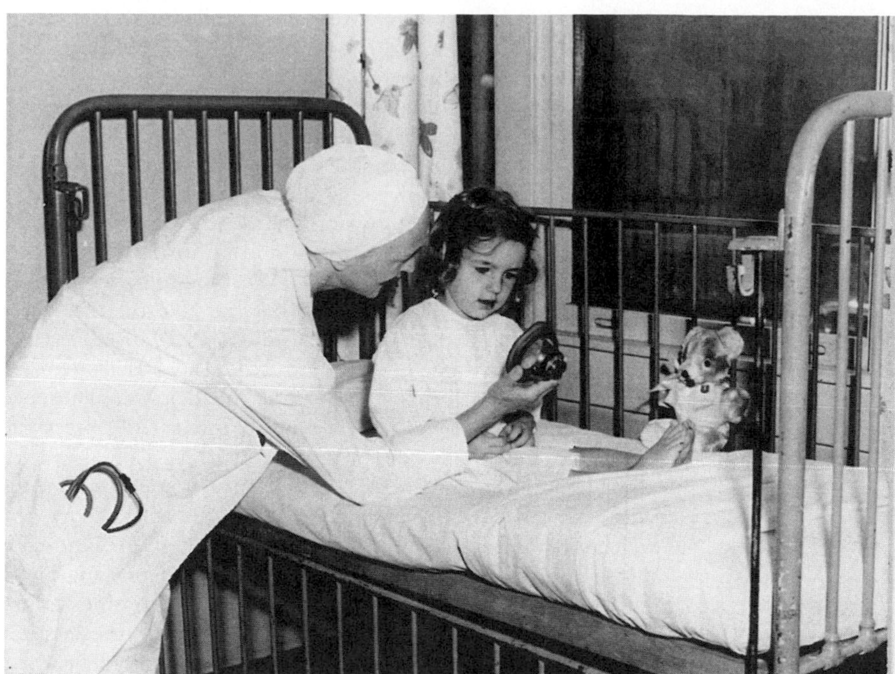

■ **FIGURE 35–1.** Ms. Betty Lank served as chief nurse anesthetist at Children's Hospital Boston from 1935 to 1969 (see text).

to-and-fro canisters Waters described in Wisconsin and used this technique for Blalock's "blue baby" (tetralogy of Fallot) operations at Johns Hopkins Hospital. In Boston, Betty Lank (Fig. 35–1),* an enterprising nurse anesthetist, further redesigned the miniature to-and-fro apparatus with less dead space and shrank adult celluloid masks to infant size, enabling her to provide anesthesia, relaxation, and controlled respiration for Ladd's infants as well as for Robert Gross' widely heralded division of a patent ductus arteriosus in 1938—without endotracheal intubation.

By 1940, considerable progress had been made in the ability of minimally trained anesthetists to provide quite satisfactory operating conditions for the surgeons of that time. Ladd strenuously corrected the previous concept by establishing the dictum "the child is *not* a little man." Supportive warming, preoperative correction of electrolyte balance, and intraoperative charting became standardized. Clinical signs of anesthetic depth, described by Guedel in 1937, served well. This might be termed the height of the art of pediatric anesthesia in the United States, where simple expedients still prevailed.

In England, there had been more progress in airway control. Following World War I, Magill and Rowbotham popularized tracheal intubation for adult procedures, and in 1937, Philip Ayre of Newcastle-Upon-Tyne reported his classic method of endotracheal intubation with a T-tube device for harelip repair in neonates (Ayre, 1937). Although Robson of Toronto had described intubation of children using digital guidance rather than a laryngoscope (Robson, 1936), it had received little attention.

*Ms. Lank, who served as chief nurse anesthetist at Children's Hospital Boston from 1935 to 1969, was one of several remarkable nurses who provided much of the anesthesia care for children at major pediatric centers in the United States until physician anesthesiologists trained and experienced during World War II returned home and began developing interest and expertise in pediatric care.

■ PHASE II: EMERGENCE OF PEDIATRIC ANESTHESIA (1940–1960)

■ FACTORS IN THE RAPID DEVELOPMENT OF INTEREST

Before and during this period, activity accelerated in related fields and much information became available defining normal and abnormal infants in such texts as Clement Smith's *The Physiology of the Newborn Infant* (1945), Taussig's *Congenital Malformations of the Heart* (1947), and *Nelson's Textbook of Pediatrics* (Nelson, 1950). The practice of adult anesthesia had become established, providing fresh information on new agents and techniques easily adaptable to children. As yet, the only established pediatric anesthesiologist in North America was Charles Robson, in Toronto, and in England, Robert Cope, at London's Hospital for Sick Children. Among those who became interested in pediatric anesthesia, M. Digby Leigh made himself well known (Fig. 35–2). Trained by Waters in Wisconsin, he was appointed head of anaesthesia at Montreal Children's Hospital, where he taught and innovated and, with his invaluable associate Kathleen Belton, authored *Paediatric Anaesthesia* (1948), the first North American text on this subject. Here, they described the use of spinal anesthesia for intrathoracic procedures, an original pediatric circle absorption apparatus, and a nonrebreathing valve. Leigh moved to Vancouver, British Columbia in 1947 and to Los Angeles in 1954, where he started the first annual pediatric anesthesia teaching conference in America. He was a brilliant technician and a stern teacher, and he delighted his audiences with his stinging repartee. His foresighted attempts to monitor exhaled carbon dioxide in 1952, however, were rebuffed by incredulous scoffers (Conn, 1992).

In the meantime, in Liverpool, G. Jackson Rees (Fig. 35–3) had been named anaesthetist at the Alder Hey Children's Hospital by his mentor and teacher Cecil Grey. Together, they conceived the idea that practically all surgery could be performed under the simple and nonexplosive combination of nitrous oxide

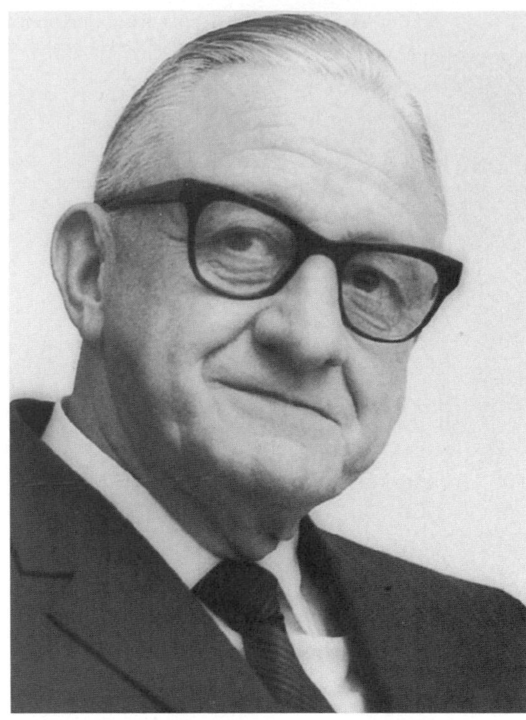

■ **FIGURE 35–2.** Dr. M. Digby Leigh.

and curare. Rees, adapting the Ayre T-tube system by adding an expiratory limb and breathing bag (the well-known Jackson Rees system), proceeded to carry out this concept with astounding success. With minor alterations this technique was to survive through years of short-lived, complicated types of apparatus.

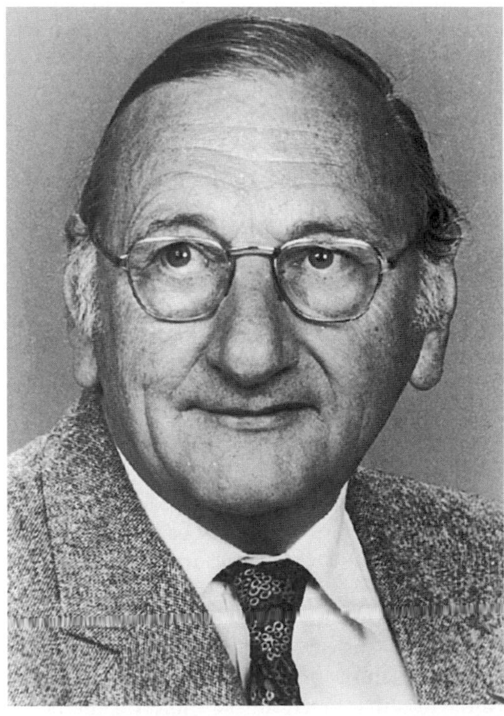

■ **FIGURE 35–3.** Dr. G. Jackson Rees.

Rees' conviction that respiration be controlled in infants with reduced tidal volumes and rates of 60 to 80 times per minute also met criticism but proved to be rational when increased tidal volumes were found to cause surfactant washout and barotrauma.

The new field of pediatric surgery, spearheaded by Gross, was calling for more skilled anesthetists, and at the end of World War II, large numbers of young physicians were released from military service, many of whom chose the uncharted field of pediatric anesthesia. McQuiston and Smith found posts at children's hospitals in Chicago and Boston, respectively, and Rackow worked at Columbia Presbyterian Hospital in New York, each to participate in early advances. In 1946, C. Everett Koop recruited Margo Deming to head the Department of Anesthesia at the Children's Hospital of Philadelphia as a teacher and investigator. Dr. Koop is currently Professor of Surgery at Dartmouth Medical School.

Little had happened in anesthesia on the home front during World War II. After the war, numerous problems, many not even envisioned at the outset, were resolved by the exceptionally harmonious cooperation between pediatric surgeons and anesthesiologists. While the success of individual operations is the natural goal of the surgeon, and improved supportive measures are the steps noted by anesthesiologists, all are interdependent and are considered together.

■ FOUNDATIONS OF CLINICAL CONTROL AND SUPPORT

Neonatal Surgery and Anesthesia

Chief among the surgical challenges at the beginning of this period were three congenital defects: tracheoesophageal fistula (TEF), omphalocele, and congenital diaphragmatic hernia (CDH). Both Leven and Ladd performed secondary multiprocedure repair of TEF in 1939. Primary repair, first accomplished by Haight in 1941, then became the most important challenge in pediatric surgery, each case demanding all-out day and night efforts of all participants. In Boston, the operation was carried out under cyclopropane by mask with a to-and-fro apparatus, endotracheal intubation then being reserved for emergency use during operation. Control of the exposed pleura during esophageal anastomosis required complete immobility, and the operation, in the words of Ladd, was "like stitching the wing of a butterfly." Supportive management played a large part in the survival of these infants, both during and after the operation. Warmth was maintained by heating and humidifying the operating room, wrapping limbs in sheet-wadding, and using a semiclosed to-and-fro absorption technique. Blood pressure was measured by a locally introduced cuff with a latex bladder encircling the arm (Fig. 35–4). Fluids and blood were administered via a open-top burette with rubber tubing and "cut down" metal cannula in the saphenous vein. Postoperative survival depended largely on the remarkably able service of one or two very special nurses.

Repair of omphalocele posed different problems. Here the forceful closure of the abdomen over the extruded viscera often caused severe compression of the lungs and abdominal blood vessels. The challenge to the anesthetist was that of providing adequate relaxation while preserving ventilation and circulation. Skin closure was possible only rarely, leaving the alternative of delayed closure, which frequently failed. The use of muscle relaxants facilitated closure but increased the risk of postoperative hypoventilation. Mortality was appreciable.

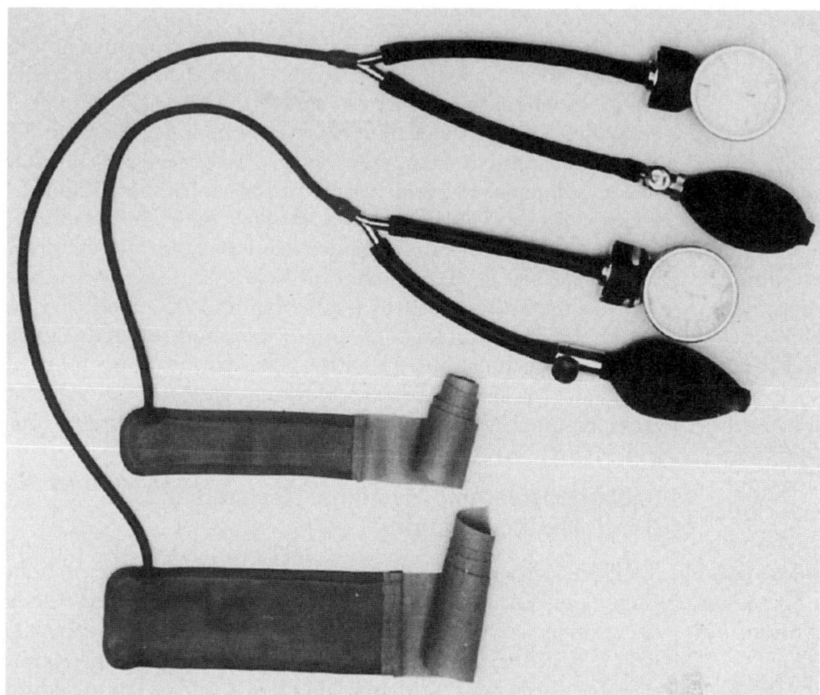

■ **FIGURE 35–4.** Smith's latex blood pressure cuffs: newborn and infant sizes.

Of the three defects, CDH at first appeared to be the easiest to correct, and anesthesia frequently was managed with open-drop ether without mortality. By 1950, however, postoperative deaths became an obvious but unsolved problem until it became evident that they were caused by earlier recognition of the defect in sicker infants who previously would have died before repair could be attempted. The management of CDH subsequently became, and still is, one of the most engrossing problems of neonatal surgery.

Herniorrhaphy and Pyloromyotomy

Herniorrhaphy and pyloromyotomy could be performed under local anesthesia by the average surgeon, but open-drop divinyl ether (Vinethene)-ether was definitely preferable. The problem most often encountered in infants with inguinal hernia was whether to cancel the operation when the infant's hemoglobin was 9.8 g/dL instead of the "required" 10 g/dL or to transfuse. Transfusion frequently was chosen. Before 1912, attempts to correct pyloric stenosis by gastroenterostomy had resulted in a 50% mortality rate. The Ramstedt pyloromyotomy effected one of the great achievements of pediatric surgery in creating a simple procedure for this commonly occurring lesion, thereby saving the life of an otherwise normal child. Anesthetic management after early diagnosis centered on the prevention of aspiration of the accumulated stomach contents, best accomplished by drainage via a large-bore urethral catheter immediately before operation. In Boston, trachea intubation was not considered necessary unless contrast medium had been used for diagnosis, whereas intubation was routinely used in other centers. In cases of delayed diagnosis, operation was postponed for rehydration and correction of electrolyte disorders or anemia.

Early Attempts to Control Fear

It soon became evident that for the small child, the fear of needles and the horrors of anesthetic induction were deeply upsetting and of long duration. Concern about this most unfortunate anesthetic byproduct was voiced by psychologists (Levy, 1945), pediatricians (Jackson, 1951), anesthesiologists (Eckenhoff, 1953), and others, as well as numerous mothers reporting prolonged night terrors, bed-wetting, and dependence.

Some attention had been paid to premedication shortly before this time. French Armand-Delille (1932) recommended morphine and Waters (1938) promoted the combination of morphine and scopolamine, but the response to the outburst of concern came in a flood of reports on a variety of ineffective agents. The basic error in most studies was, and still is, the use of age and/or weight for estimation of drug dosage, when neither reflects the child's state of mind. General use of intramuscular barbiturates plus morphine mixed with either atropine or scopolamine resulted in severe horror of needles, an uncomfortably dry mouth, and an unpredictable degree of sedation, seldom better than 65% successful. Attempts to improve this record continued to play a large part in the activities and literature of pediatric anesthesiologists with only slight improvement with regard to the effectiveness of sedative drugs. However, the concentration of attention of numerous investigators on this problem did result in the development of close personal interest in each child studied, quite possibly responsible for much of the benefit credited to the drug being promoted.

Methods of induction showed somewhat more success than those of sedation. Thiopental replaced rectal Avertin, providing greater ease of administration via either the intravenous or the rectal route (Weinstein, 1939), whereas induction with nitrous oxide, cyclopropane, or divinyl ether eliminated much use of the dreaded ether. With the repeated failure of sedative agents, greater skills were developed by caring anesthetists to gain the confidence of children in preoperative visits and then to divert their attention at induction by telling them stories or by simply lulling them to sleep. Hypnosis was used for induction by Betcher (1958), Marmer (1959), and a few others for the total operation in short procedures. It was particularly valuable for the repair of facial lacerations in small children who had recently eaten. Unfortunately, this potentially useful and harmless method gained only limited acceptance.

Control of the Airway

The importance of airway management became evident with the first anesthetics, and after years of progress it still presents formidable difficulties. For patients of all ages, hypoxia resulting from laryngospasm, oral secretions or blood, abscesses or tumors, aspiration of vomitus, or simply blockage by the tongue has been an ever-present danger. Many deaths from early harelip procedures resulted primarily from hemorrhage, as were later deaths from tonsillectomy.

By 1940, two simple but extremely fundamental aids had been introduced. To prevent obstruction by the tongue, metal and rubber oral airways, often fitted with a metal nipple for insufflation of vaporized ether, had been used successfully for a decade. Suction apparatus was first available in the form of bulb syringes used alone or fitted with rubber catheters and then later as portable motorized pumps situated at the head of the operating table (ether and cyclopropane notwithstanding) or by means of a centrally operated pipeline.

Endotracheal Intubation

The outstanding advance in pediatric anesthesia between 1940 and 1960 was in control of the airway by tracheal intubation. Early use in England and Canada met with little resistance. In the United States, however, opposition by surgeons raised the first major obstacle to progress in the new specialty. (One must admit that reasonable concern had been aroused in those who had witnessed the traumatic attempts of inexperienced individuals to perform unnecessary intubations.) It was the efforts of Rees in England, Leigh, then in Canada, the British-American Gillespie (1939), and Americans Deming (1952), Pender (1954), and others, and their supportive younger surgeons, that brought forth grudging acceptance of tracheal intubation of infants and children in the United States in the 1940s and 1950s.

The ongoing development of this technique led to (1) an increased understanding of laryngeal anatomy (Eckenhoff, 1951); (2) replacement of the "classic" hyperextension of the head by use of the "sniffing" position for intubation; (3) a succession of different types of tracheal tubes, including the tapered tube of Cole (1945) that enjoyed more than a decade of popularity; (4) a variety of tube materials progressing from coarse rubber to nonreactive plastic; and (5) laryngoscopes of several types and sizes.

As with ether and other major advances, the advent of tracheal intubation brought a host of disadvantages and a few real dangers that, in turn, led to a glut of literature concerning complications (Flagg, 1951), including subglottic stenosis (Colgan and Keats, 1957), laryngeal irritation from large tubes (Baron and Kohlmoos, 1951), and tracheitis caused by contamination (Smith, 1953a). This proved to be just the beginning.

"Total Control" of Respiration: The Muscle Relaxants

Following the first clinical use of *d*-tubocurarine by Griffith and Mitchell in Canada in 1942, Canadians and British accepted it readily and began extensive use in both children and adults (Anderson, 1951; Stead, 1955; Leigh et al., 1957; Rees, 1958), to be followed by much investigation in later years. Again, in the United States there was much opposition, this time by anesthesiologists (Beecher and Todd, 1954) as well as surgeons (Gross, 1953), to whom the concept of total "takeover" of an essential body function, termed *controlled respiration*, appeared to be a dangerous and unacceptable "physiologic trespass." Beecher threatened one of these writers (R.M.S.) that "heads would roll" if he and others persisted in support of its use. In the meantime, Cullen (1943) had found it quite safe for adults and children, using it as a sole agent for infant surgery. This practice was abandoned after Scott Smith of Utah (Smith, 1947; Smith et al., 1947) was tested under total curarization and suffered acutely on painful stimulation. As with tracheal intubation, the total acceptance of neuromuscular blocking agents in the United States required many years. By 1960, however, the terms "controlled" and "assisted" respiration had gained widespread use.

Pediatric Breathing Systems: Assisted and Controlled Respiration

With the stimulating effect of ether on respiration in light surgical planes, assisted respiration was seldom needed. Open chest surgery, cyclopropane, and particularly muscle relaxants definitely changed this picture and led to a succession of considerably diverse devices (Dorsch and Dorsch, 1975). The to-and-fro absorption method, using soda lime canisters of graduated sizes, was particularly adaptable to infants but caused heat retention and the aspiration of lime dust. For larger children, the canisters were bulky and heat retention was even more troublesome.

Special interest was taken in infant circle absorption systems. The Leigh (Leigh and Belton, 1948), Ohio, and Bloomquist models were not only difficult to handle but also introduced the problems of valve resistance and dead space.

To eliminate problems of carbon dioxide accumulation, several nonrebreathing valves were designed by Leigh (1948), Stephen and Slater (1948), and others. Although compact in design, they were not easy to manage and were definitely ill suited for use with explosive agents.

The saga of apparatus variously called rebreathing (British), nonrebreathing (United States), and partial rebreathing (general) is complicated and involved numerous studies and modifications of the basic Ayre T-system (Ayre, 1937) (Fig. 35–5) over a period of 30 years. Following the Rees elongation of the expiratory limb with an attached breathing bag, the addition of exhaust valves placed either proximal (Mapleson A) or distal (Mapleson D) to the face brought intensive examination, as did the estimation of proper flow rates of incoming gases. Evaluation by Mapleson (1954) and Inkster (1956) did much to clarify these issues at the time, but more problems lay ahead.

Cardiovascular and Thermal Control

Between 1940 and 1960, revolutionary advances were made in several areas involving the combined efforts of anesthesiologists and surgeons. The intentional reduction of arterial blood pressure, extensively explored by Enderby (1950) and others in England, was cautiously extended to pediatric use by Sheila Anderson (1955) with trimethaphan camphorsulfonate (Arfonad). This served as a reasonably safe agent. It was the initial step in induced hypotension to reduce surgical blood loss in major pediatric surgery and to prevent excessive blood pressure elevation during correction of coarctation of the aorta. However, the agent was unpredictable and soon was replaced by more controllable agents and techniques.

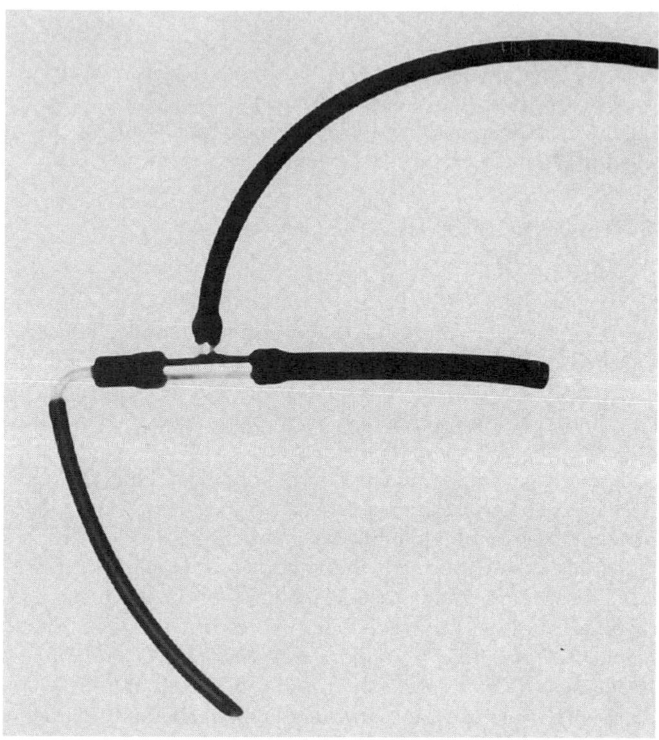

■ **FIGURE 35–5.** Original Ayre T-tube nonrebreathing system.

Controlled Reduction of Body Temperature and Cardiopulmonary Arrest

Following Gross' ligation of a patent ductus arteriosus in 1938, correction of coarctation of the aorta, repair of vascular rings, and shunt procedures for tetralogy of Fallot were successfully performed under closed or semiclosed inhalation anesthesia, usually with cyclopropane (Harmel and Lamont, 1948; Harris, 1950; Smith, 1952). McQuiston, endeavoring to reduce the oxygen requirement of Dr. Potts' cyanotic infants, cooled them 3° to 4°C on a simple ice-water mattress, thereby introducing the practice of hypothermic control of body metabolism into pediatric anesthesia (McQuiston, 1949). Efforts to reduce oxygen demand by further lowering temperatures to 30°C with immersion in ice water provided surgeons time for simple intracardiac aortic or pulmonary valvotomy (Lewis and Taufic, 1953; Virtue, 1955).

The drive to bypass both heart and lungs initiated by Gibbon in 1937 became exciting in the early 1950s, with competing surgeons Lillihei, Kirklin, and Kay and their respective anesthesiologists Matthews, Buckley, and Van Bergen (1957), Patrick, Theye, and Moffit (1957), and Mendelsohn, Mackrell, Machlan, and others (1957) all contributing toward the first practical use of the pump oxygenator in 1955, 2 years before publication of the articles cited.

The supplementation to bypass perfusion by moderate hypothermia (30°C) and different methods of induced cardiac arrest produced the greatest "takeover" of body function to date and the means of performing intracardiac surgery on all but small infants.

Mild and moderate hypothermia techniques were also used in this period for neurosurgery, orthopedic surgery, and harelip repair (Kilduff et al., 1956).

Control During Maintenance of Anesthesia

As more extensive procedures were developed and surgeons began to prefer accuracy to speed, 4-hour operations became more frequent and the methods of maintenance and support more demanding. Experience, skill, and constant observation were still primary factors, assisted by a few simple devices (Fig. 35–6). During this time the precordial stethoscope became essential for use with every infant or child throughout anesthesia (Smith, 1953b). A precordial or esophageal stethoscope (Smith, 1991) served, first, to keep the anesthetist in direct contact with the child at all times, providing unaltered information as to the clarity and strength of breath sounds and the rate, rhythm, and strength of heart sounds. Strength of heart sounds was an important guide to the degree of blood loss at that time. Arterial blood pressure could be obtainable with standard apparatus for larger children and with a specially constructed latex cuff with an inflatable bladder for infants (Smith cuff). During this phase, the electrocardiograph was occasionally brought into operating rooms, encased in antiexplosive shielding (shaped like a torpedo), and served relatively little purpose. Body temperature was measured intermittently at oral, nasal, or rectal sites, the standard glass thermometer giving way to the safer but less accurate thermostat devices. The anesthesia chart was considered a necessary item, gaining in importance as procedures grew increasingly complex and legal suits more frequent.

Control of Blood Loss

Methods of estimating blood loss at the time consisted of assessing blanching of conjunctivae, evaluating the strength of heart sounds, measuring arterial blood pressure, and weighing bloodied sponges, purposely used without moistening. While speed was

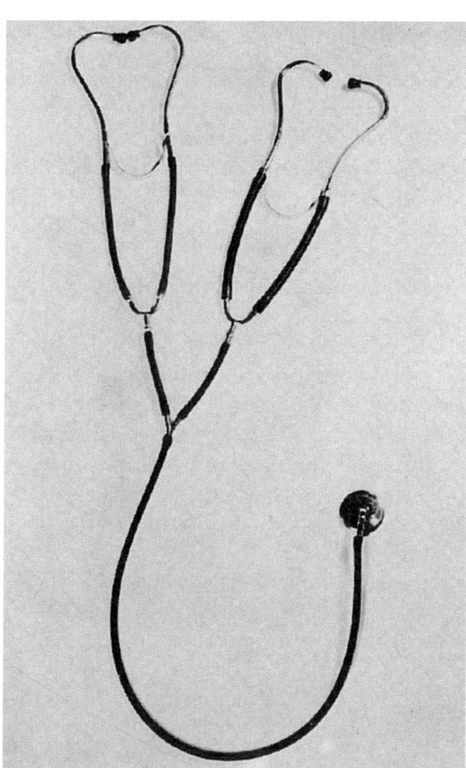

■ **FIGURE 35–6.** Smith's teaching precordial stethoscope with a single chest piece and two headpieces.

still considered essential in pediatric surgery during the excision of Wilms' and other large tumors, massive hemorrhage might exsanguinate small infants before replacement was possible. Attempts to restore the loss with cold, acidified blood brought failing hearts to irreversible arrest. A major advance to control these situations occurred when surgeons were persuaded to time their work by the advice of the anesthesiologist rather than by the clock. Although the cautery soon reduced blood loss drastically when used, it was not adopted immediately by all.

Progress in Local Anesthesia

Ladd had used local infiltration for abdominal procedures in premature infants in the late 1930s, and Leigh wrote of spinal anesthesia for open chest work in the 1940s, but improved inhalation methods outmoded both. Except for brachial plexus block (Small, 1951; Eather, 1958), little attention was paid to these methods in the United States. In many other countries, however, where inhalation anesthesia was less advanced, there was considerable dependence on regional and spinal anesthesia for both infants and children.

Halothane Opens a New Era

Although anesthesia with relaxants and nitrous oxide permitted the use of electrical instruments in the operating room, explosive gases were still popular until the introduction of halothane. Following its first use in England by Johnstone in 1956 (in 10% concentration), this nonflammable, nonirritating, and potent agent was promptly introduced in Canada by Junkin, Smith, and Conn (1957) and in the United States by Stephen, Lawrence, Fabian, and others (1958). Subsequently flammable anesthetic agents were totally abolished in the United States, thus opening the way to revolutionary changes, first in the control of blood loss by cautery and then in the development of electronic devices for monitoring and physiologic control.

Supportive Care and Oxygen Therapy

Related fields brought important aid to pediatric anesthesiologists during this period. The time-honored rule developed by Holliday and Segar (1957) for pediatric fluid administration based on metabolic requirements serves to this day. Also of great importance, particularly in reducing the morbidity and mortality of small surgical infants, was the control of infection by the use of antibiotic agents.

The interest of pediatricians caring for neonates led to the development of enclosed incubators with regulated oxygen, warmth, and humidification for infants with respiratory distress syndrome. Improved oxygen tents were developed for older children including those with cystic fibrosis. The poliomyelitis epidemics of the 1950s in Europe and North America initiated a succession of ventilating devices to replace the enclosed "iron lung" in use since 1929. Pediatric anesthesiologists and pediatricians shared responsibility for this work, which opened a new field for anesthesiologists.

In related areas, Virginia Apgar introduced her scoring system for neonatal assessment (Apgar, 1953), Peter Safar launched his crusade for mouth-to-mouth ventilation and further work in cardiopulmonary resuscitation, and the first multidisciplinary adult intensive care unit in North America was developed (Safar, 1950).

The first pediatric intensive care unit was established in Goteburg, Sweden, in 1955. Similar units were established in Stockholm (Hans Feychtung), Liverpool (Rees), and Melbourne (MacDonald and Stocks) between 1960 and 1964. In North America, the first pediatric intensive care unit was established by John J. Downes at the Children's Hospital of Philadelphia in 1967, followed by Children's Hospital of Pittsburgh (Kampschulte), Yale-New Haven Hospital (Gilman), Massachusetts General Hospital (Todres and Shannon), and the Hospital for Sick Children in Toronto (Conn) within the following 4 years (Downes, 1992).

TEACHING AND RESEARCH

Throughout Europe and North America, communication among anesthesiologists began to accelerate. The Great Ormand Street Hospital for Sick Children in London and the Alder Hey Hospital in Liverpool became teaching centers in England; the Hospital for Sick Children in Toronto in Canada and the Children's Hospitals of Boston and Los Angeles in the United States became centers to which various novice and experienced anesthetists came from all parts of the world for clinical training. Residents on affiliation from teaching hospitals were rotated through brief training periods for instruction in basic, safe, and practical methods of anesthetic control of children undergoing standard operations and in special methods for those at higher risk.

On the heels of Leigh and Belton's *Pediatric Anesthesia* (1948), Stephen's *Elements of Pediatric Anesthesia* (1954) and Smith's *Anesthesia for Infants and Children* (1959) were published, with details of advances to date. Articles on new agents and techniques steadily increased in the anesthetic literature. While some reported personal early experiences based on limited numbers, many were of lasting value, including those involving tracheal abnormalities by Eckenhoff (1951) and Colgan and Keats (1957), tracheoesophageal repair by Zindler and Deming (1953), and the important warning of Leigh, McCoy, Belton, and others (1957) concerning bradycardia after the intravenous administration of succinylcholine.

Research, on the other hand, was still in its infancy, there being little space, time, or funds for sophisticated investigation. As previously mentioned, many clinical studies offered practical current value concerning new agents and techniques. While those concerning preoperative sedation outnumbered others, many reports covered airway resistance, valves, and dead space (Macon and Bruner, 1950; Mapleson, 1954; Orkin et al., 1954; Hunt, 1955; Inkster, 1956). The introduction of muscle relaxants initiated other studies, including those of Stead (1955), Hodges (1955), Telford and Keats (1957), and Bush and Stead (1962). The addition of halothane late in this period led to a more critical analysis of this agent than had been done for previous anesthetics.

This period established such fundamental techniques and basic concepts that Rees subsequently (1991) stated, "Paediatric anaesthesia in Great Britain and Ireland shows that by 1950 it had reached a point at which current practice is recognizable… . Future pediatric anesthetists are therefore unlikely to experience the great excitement their predecessors enjoyed between 1930 and 1950, but will derive satisfaction from changes less dramatic as the curve of improvement approaches perfection."

PHASE III: ERA OF NONFLAMMABLE ANESTHETICS (1960–1980)

With sound fundamental approaches defined and restrictions resulting from flammable agents eliminated, the way was cleared for rapid and extensive advances in all areas of pediatric anesthesia. Clinical control would drive ahead and research would become more productive, but this period saw the greatest progress in the development of organized teaching and communication.

Unfortunately, progress was not marked in the control of fear. Despite continued efforts to address this problem by many skilled workers (Poe and Karp, 1946; Rackow and Salanitre, 1962; Root, 1962), sedatives were still unpredictable and intramuscular needles were still in general use. The introduction of ketamine (Ketalar) by Domino, Chodoff, and Corsson (1965) created mixed feelings based on its early postoperative psychologic reactions, but the agent found a place in pediatric use for uncontrollable patients and to accomplish minor but painful procedures.

A major change in the methods for controlling fear was in giving permission to parents, first, for free admission to the child's bedside at all times, including "sleep-in" privileges, and later, to preinduction and induction areas. While many parents were assuaged by these moves, statistics failed to show great help for the children (Schulman et al., 1967).

INCREASING CLINICAL PRECISION

Modification of the partial rebreathing systems by Bain and Spoerel (1972), by which the exhalation tube passes inside the inhalation arm, provided a means of scavenging expired gases, thereby greatly enhancing the use of this popular pediatric method. This marked a major evolution of airway systems for pediatric anesthesia.

Steps toward greater precision in monitoring were taken in the measurement of infant blood pressure by Doppler sonography and by oscillotonometry (Dinamap) (Marcy and Cook, 1988). In the determination of arterial oxygen saturation, the transcutaneous electrode (ear oximetry) was used with limited success (Saunders et al., 1976). It was during this period that "control by the numbers" gained predominance over the unreliable art of anesthesia. Led by Downes of Philadelphia and others, arterial blood gas determinations, blood sugar, hemoglobin, electrolytes, and other measurements were serially evaluated intraoperatively in adjacent laboratories. Insertion of arterial and central venous catheters became commonplace, and urinary catheterization became an important guide to fluid and electrolyte replacement.

Progress in controlling fluid balance included the recognition of the importance of electrolytes in all intravenous solutions (Bennett et al., 1970; Herbert et al., 1971). New concepts concerning blood replacement included Davenport's practical recommendation to give blood when loss reached 10% of blood volume (Davenport and Barr, 1963), followed later by Furman's more precise suggestion to maintain the hematocrit level above 28% to 30% in children and 40% in the newborn (Furman et al., 1975). At this time, the concept of replacement of preoperative fluid deficit was widely adopted.

Airway problems presented ongoing challenges, and their management continued to register improved methods of control. Great emphasis was placed on the prevention of food aspiration and the damaging effects of hypoxia. The Sellick maneuver (1961) and Salem's many warnings about "the full stomach" (1970) were forever fixed in the mind of each new resident.

The treatment of acute epiglottitis by nasotracheal intubation instead of the former mandatory use of tracheostomy was a major change and clear advance, speeding recovery and significantly reducing serious complications (Oh and Motoyama, 1977).

Management of "the difficult airway" began to assume a larger role in both adult and pediatric anesthesia as more complicated procedures were undertaken on more deformed patients. By this time, some 120 different types of laryngoscope blades had been invented, each with some minor modifications to suit the designer, usually with no major advantage. It was the introduction of the fiberoptic laryngoscope (Taylor and Towley, 1972; Stiles, 1974) that enabled anesthesiologists to intubate infants and children for whom this had been virtually impossible.

The startling appearance of what became known as malignant hyperthermia caused great concern, but widespread warnings about "triggering agents" and the discovery of a specific counteragent, dantrolene, usually brought it under reasonable control at least when recognized early (Denborough et al., 1960; Britt, 1979; Gronert, 1980).

SURGICAL PROGRESS

Interesting progress occurred in the evolution of infant surgery. Tracheoesophageal fistula repair became a standardized procedure, and mortality was generally limited to infants with serious cardiac defects. Problems related to omphalocele repair were largely overcome by the introduction of Schuster's staged mesh sac closure (1967). Congenital diaphragmatic hernia, however, brought increasing difficulties as smaller and more premature infants were encountered. Acidosis, shunting (Raphaely and Downes, 1973), and pulmonary hypertension (Dibbins, 1976) posed problems yet to be solved. Attempts to use extracorporeal membrane oxygenation (ECMO) predicted later value (Bartlett et al., 1979).

Following the breakthrough in cardiac surgery accomplished by the establishment of extracorporeal circulation in larger children, the next step was to find a means of operating within the hearts of neonates, without obstruction by intracardiac catheters. In 1965 the use of hyperbaric oxygenation served as a temporary answer, providing surgeons 3 to 5 minutes of inflow occlusion for the performance of aortic valvotomy and other brief procedures (Bernhard et al., 1966). The use of oxygen at 3 to 4 atmospheres of pressure substantially increased plasma oxygen-carrying capacity, while presenting increased potency of nitrous oxide and increased flammability (Smith et al., 1964).

The final hurdle in the approach to infant cardiac surgery was passed by the successful combination of deep hypothermia (Horiuchi et al., 1963) and extracorporeal circulation (Hikasa et al., 1967), providing time for the most complicated reconstruction of neonatal cardiac defects. Rendering an infant virtually dead by complete cessation of respiration and circulation, at a body temperature of 15°C, appeared to be the ultimate in physiologic control. Agents and techniques have undergone several changes in subsequent years but remain fundamentally similar.

Somewhat less dramatic, but also of great importance, was the initiation of renal transplantation in 1950, which saved the lives of thousands of children and adults with end-stage renal disease.

Among many well-known tenets established, two of particular interest to anesthesiologists were the danger of succinylcholine in patients with elevated serum potassium levels (Powell and Miller, 1975) and the evident tolerance to anesthesia in patients with hemoglobin levels as low as 6 g/dL.

The craniofacial repair devised by Tessier and others (1967) for correction of the disfiguring deformities of Apert's and Crouzon's diseases was a bold undertaking. It was equally challenging for the anesthesiologists involved, with difficult airway management, prolonged maintenance, marked fluid and blood loss, and a particularly precarious period of recovery while the child's head was so completely swathed in tight bandaging that only the endotracheal tube was visible.

Anesthetic management to separate conjoined twins at birth was of such unique interest that any report of a single case was welcomed for publication. A separate team of surgeons and anesthesiologists was assigned to each twin, and multiple problems of shared organ systems, hemorrhage, and airway obstruction were noted (Furman et al., 1971; Winston et al., 1987).

POSTOPERATIVE PATIENT MANAGEMENT: VENTILATION, RESUSCITATION, AND INTENSIVE CARE

For many years, much attention had been directed toward controlling the responses of children during the introductory phases of anesthesia. Postoperative care, however, often consisted of little more than a prompt return to the child's room with orders for checks every 4 hours and nothing by mouth. The advent of various new and extensive operations made it evident that the survival of patients depended to a large extent on their supportive control during recovery—a third dimension of anesthesia.

One of the first needs to be met was the ability to provide prolonged tracheal intubation, fostered by Brandstater (1962), MacDonald and Stocks (1965), and Hatch (1968). The continuation of earlier efforts to devise ventilation machines for infants and children with cardiopulmonary pathology brought a succession of models, some as adaptations of those made for adults and others designed specifically for younger patients.

So-called recovery rooms or postanesthesia care units (PACUs) for routine postoperative care had been established in many hospitals over previous decades, but areas staffed by highly trained personnel and fully equipped for high-risk patient care became mandatory. The earliest units of this type, termed critical care or intensive care units, appeared in Goteburg, Sweden, in 1955*; others were established in France in 1962, England in 1964, Australia in 1963, and America by those in Philadelphia in 1967, Pittsburgh and Boston in 1969, and Toronto in 1971, where Conn established a prototype of the modern multidisciplinary unit for infants and children, including near-drowning survivors (Downes and Raphaely, 1975; Conn et al., 1980).

Important new approaches to resuscitation replaced such outmoded maneuvers as anal dilatation, drugs promoted as respiratory stimulants, and the prone pressure method. During the trial-and-error development of pediatric cardiac surgery and the poliomyelitis epidemics, apparent death became an indication for immediate slashing into the chest and manual cardiac compression. When it became evident that the patients occasionally survived both the original insult and the therapeutic assault, the term "cardiac arrest" was coined (Singer, 1977). Because the exact cause of these mishaps frequently was uncertain, each was considered "an act of God" and successful resuscitation was considered a feather in the cap of any anesthesiologist who had been associated with one. Intelligent procedures of ventilation and closed-chest cardiac compression, combined with electric and pharmacologic stimulation, brought far greater reason, order, and success.

*The excellent first-hand report of Downes (1992) on the development of pediatric critical care is recommended.

ORGANIZED TEACHING

This period marked the definite establishment of teaching facilities for the specialized training of pediatric anesthesiologists. With markedly enlarged departmental staffs, didactic and clinical instruction became available in numerous institutions. Residents became capable of managing most types of cases and also received instruction in ancillary services. Accreditation for residency training in pediatric centers was established in Boston in 1970, to be followed by several others by 1980.

Teaching clinics were established for residents and others throughout the United States, Canada, and England. Edward Eger stood out as teacher par excellence over three decades. Annual symposia on pediatric anesthesia initiated by Leigh in 1962 were followed by those organized by Conn in Toronto, Downes in Philadelphia, Salem in Chicago, Ryan in Boston, and others. Literature became increasingly available in periodicals, including both new editions of previously published texts and added texts such as those by Davenport (1967) of Canada and an excellent Australian text by Brown and Fisk (1979). Early exponents of the specialty became popular at local and national meetings, and an international exchange of speakers grew rapidly, stimulating interest and exchanging information on the rapidly developing scene.

International Progress

At this time, it became evident that considerable progress was being made in many parts of the world. In France, M. Delegue pioneered the modern stage, her text *Memento a l'Uusage de l'Anesthesiologiste-Reanimateur Pediatrique* passing through several editions. Rapid advances have taken place in France in many aspects of pediatric anesthesia. A marked difference in their approach appeared with their use of combinations of intravenous phenothiazines, antihistamines, and barbiturates in place of inhalation agents, with remarkable success (G. Durand-Gurry, personal communication, 1993). Their work in regional anesthesia and pharmacology has also been outstanding (Saint Maurice et al., 1986; Murat et al., 1988).

Other early leaders in Europe include Suuterinen of Finland, Swensson, Feyting, and Ekstrom-Jodal of Sweden, and Rondio and Wezyk of Poland. South African and Australian workers, adopting British methods, also kept abreast or ahead of other areas. Douglas Wilson has been called the real pioneer of pediatric anesthesia in Western Australia, and Margaret McLellan, John Stocks, Ian McDonald, M. A. Denborough, and others have contributed on local and international levels. Japanese interest in pediatric anesthesia began later but proceeded vigorously beginning in 1958 (Iwai and Satoyoshi, 1992); the publication of *Pediatric Anesthesia* in 1958 by Onchi and Fujita served as a valuable guide. Throughout Latin America, Brazilian physicians (Fortuna, 1967) and others followed North American methods to some extent, but in these countries, and especially in Mexico, local and regional anesthetic techniques were depended on and consequently more highly developed than inhalation anesthesia (Melman et al., 1975). The great number of students who studied in North America and Europe from India, the Philippine Islands, and other Asiatic areas resulted in growth of this organized activity and clinical excellence in their respective nations.

Research Stimulated by Clinical Advances

The introduction of various breathing devices, new muscle relaxants, and the halogenated agents alone provided material for extensive investigation, and other problems still lay unanswered. The demonstration of the more rapid uptake of anesthetic gases by infants than by adults (Salanitre and Rackow, 1969) became a classic study, as did Motoyama's measurements of pulmonary mechanics (Motoyama, 1977; Motoyama and Cook, 1980), with some of his many contributions elaborating the pulmonary physiology of infants and children. Bush and Stead (1962), Cook (1974), Goudsouzian and others (1975), and other researchers did much to establish the comparable actions of successive neuromuscular blocking agents in the search for safer, shorter-acting, and reversible types—hence, greater control. The advent of new halogenated agents aroused the pharmacologic investigation of metabolism, toxicity, cardiovascular depression, and seizures, and the increased potency demanded vaporizers of greater accuracy (Brennan, 1957; Fabian et al., 1958; Lomaz, 1965). Other notable achievements included the establishment of minimum effective doses (ED_{50}) of halothane by Nicodemus, Nassiri-Rahimi, Bachman, and others (1969) and the minimum alveolar concentration (MAC) as a standard measure of potency (Eger et al., 1965), followed by the application of MAC to demonstrate the higher halothane requirement for infants than for adults (Gregory et al., 1969).

PHASE IV: PROGRESS AND SOPHISTICATION (1980–PRESENT)

This latest phase consists of many events now in progress that are described in this book. The entire scenario in the operating room has evolved enormously with anesthesiologists setting their multicomputerized monitors and infusion pumps, with numerous syringes loaded and coded, and a large cabinet within reach, holding drugs and other equipment for all possible occasions. The patient is brought in, and anesthesia is induced with minimal resistance. The next variable time is consumed while surgeons await the fixation of monitors, endotracheal tubes, and numerous catheters. Multiple medications are delivered by the intravenous route, frequently measured now by micrograms or "mics" per kilogram. The ventilator is set at a prescribed rate and tidal volume, and surgeons are allowed to approach and drape the patient, erecting a high sterile shield between themselves and the anesthesiologist. Charting is frequently automated. Chatting occurs with other anesthesiologists and the surgeons and nurses. Boredom in long simple cases can be a major hazard, as is a tendency to watch the monitors rather than the patient.

Fortunately, this is only one part of the picture. In the next room, a premature infant may be receiving spinal anesthesia for herniorrhaphy, and in a third, a liver transplantation may have been in progress for the past 8 hours. In the remaining 20 operating rooms, various procedures go on, more than half of which are outpatient cases.

RECOGNITION OF RISK

During this period, there has been a widespread appreciation that infants and very small children are at increased risk of complications from anesthesia and surgery. Previous reports (Salem, 1975) had shown that these were frequently related to cardiovascular factors (including hypovolemia, anemia), respiratory difficulties (airway obstruction, hypoxia, inadequate ventilation), or electrolyte imbalance (hyperkalemia, hyponatremia, hypoglycemia). Additional reports from the United States (Morray et al., 1993; Keenan et al., 1994; Holzman, 1994) described some of the problems in greater detail, as did others from France (Tiret et al., 1988), Scandinavia (Olsson and Hallen, 1988), Canada (Cohen et al., 1990), and England (Lunn, 1992). In particular, postoperative apnea, especially in very premature infants, was noted by several investigators (Steward, 1982; Gregory and Steward, 1983; Liu et al., 1983), and overnight hospitalization in these situations was widely adopted. Furthermore, there were indications that risk in small children could be decreased if individuals specially trained and experienced in pediatric anesthesia provided the anesthesia care (Keenan et al., 1991; Morray, 1994; Berry, 1995; Downes, 1995). Although this concept remains controversial, surgeons, pediatricians, and parents increasingly began to appreciate the important role of pediatric anesthesiologists.

GROWTH IN PEDIATRIC FACILITIES

In part because the post-World War II "baby boomers" were now having their own children, pediatric facilities exhibited enormous growth. Freestanding children's hospitals, which had existed for more than a century, expanded and new pediatric hospitals were established. Some of these evolved as pediatric "hospitals within a hospital," whereby large general hospitals developed specific buildings, wings, or floors to provide specialized care for children. Currently, several large children's hospitals in the United States are performing more than 20,000 surgical procedures per year. Some children's hospitals perform more operations and have more operating rooms and staff than major hospitals caring for adult patients. Reports are being published indicating that the outcome, at least for some conditions in small children, is better if surgery is performed by pediatric specialists in large pediatric centers (Bratton et al., 2001; Kososka et al., 2001). The American Academy of Pediatrics (2002, 2003) has disseminated several policy statements emphasizing the need to have proper personnel and facilities available whenever children require surgery and/or anesthesia.

CHANGING PATTERNS OF CARE

There has also been a great impetus to perform surgical procedures in younger and younger patients. While this was not possible or was fraught with danger in earlier eras, better equipment and surgeons well trained in pediatric subspecialties have made this not only feasible, but also ultimately desirable for children. Outcome studies in several areas have shown that corrective procedures performed in infancy, rather than palliative procedures done initially followed by full repair later in life, lead to improved long-term results. For example, the American Academy of Pediatrics in 1975 advocated surgical repair of elective urologic defects in children after the age of 4 years, but by 1996 was recommending these repairs occur in infancy. Likewise, repair of congenital cardiac anomalies shifted from early palliative procedures (largely shunts) to corrective repairs in the neonatal period (Jenkins et al., 1995). This tendency to perform more complex surgical procedures in younger patients undoubtedly contributed to the growth of major pediatric centers.

At the opposite end of the age spectrum, pediatric institutions were also seeing an increasing population of older patients who had survived diseases generally considered pediatric in nature. For example, patients treated for cystic fibrosis, meningomyelocele and hydrocephalus, congenital heart disease, leukemias, and many "syndromes" were now routinely surviving into adulthood and presenting well past childhood for surgical procedures. Hospitals and/or their physicians catering to adults often exhibited a reluctance to manage these patients. This has led to the interesting paradox of pediatric subspecialists and pediatric hospitals being involved in the ongoing management of patients who clearly are no longer children. Compounding this has been the growth of surgical specialties where the care of children and adults is frequently undertaken simultaneously, such as fetal surgery or transplantation from living related donors. Thus, pediatric hospitals are now caring for patients well into their 20s, 30s, and beyond.

It is not simply the age of patients requiring surgery that has been changing but also the setting of much of the surgery itself. The vast majority of pediatric surgical procedures currently occurs in ambulatory patients who never remain overnight in the hospital. Patients frequently arrive for their procedure in the morning and go home later the same day. This creates additional challenges to anesthesiologists who must rely on surgeons to screen patients for significant coexisting medical problems, because patients are usually not seen in advance of the procedure by their anesthesiologist. Even when hospitalization following surgery is required, elective patients are rarely admitted prior to the day of the procedure. This is the case even when the surgical procedure will be quite complex, such as scoliosis repair, craniofacial reconstruction, repair of congenital cardiac lesions, etc. For these situations, anesthesiologists developed preoperative clinics where patients can be evaluated by an anesthesiologist along with any necessary consultants and have laboratory and radiologic studies obtained and blood cross-matched when necessary. This also provides an opportunity to answer questions about anesthesia and/or the perioperative experience and attempt to manage patient and parental anxiety.

Finally, pediatric anesthesiologists have become increasingly involved in caring for children outside the operating rooms when immobility and/or analgesia is required for nonsurgical procedures. This has largely occurred in the radiology departments, where increasingly sophisticated equipment and techniques have led to major advances in diagnosis (computed tomography, magnetic resonance imaging, positron emission tomography, etc.) and new, less-invasive treatment options (in the catheterization laboratory, radiation therapy suite, etc.). Anesthesiologists are being requested to provide care for patients in several other areas of the hospital as well, including the gastrointestinal suite for endoscopy, oncology unit for lumbar punctures and bone marrow aspirations, and so on. While children clearly benefit from relief of pain and anxiety in these situations, this has greatly increased demands for anesthesia services.

When anesthesiologists are unable or unwilling to assist in these areas, physicians from other specialties (including pediatricians, intensivists, hospitalists) or nurses have stepped in (Malviya et al., 1997; Lowrie et al., 1998). Whether this affords a comparable degree of safety to administration of anesthesia by anesthesiologists in these situations remains to be seen. In any case, the large number of children requiring sedation/immobilization for nonoperative procedures has led to the development of "sedation guidelines" by several organizations representing anesthesiologists, pediatricians, emergency physicians, dentists, and others, with some variability among them (American Academy of Pediatrics, 1992; American Society of Anesthesiologists, 1996; American College of Emergency Physicians, 1997; American Academy of Pediatric Dentistry, 1997). A group of pediatric anesthesiologists at Dartmouth Hitchcock Medical Center convened a conference in 2000 to try to develop consensus among physicians from varied disciplines in this regard, and they continue to disseminate a bulletin via email to individuals interested in this ongoing issue (Dartmouth, 2000).

NEW DEVELOPMENTS IN ANESTHESIA

Although the scope of new developments in anesthesia is the subject of much of the remainder of this book, there are several major changes worth noting. The age-old, frequently used restriction of preoperative intake ultimately underwent scrutiny with resulting changes in concept and reduction of fasting time (Coté, 1990; Ferrari et al., 1999).

New, potent, inhalational anesthetic agents have been developed, virtually replacing halothane as the "standard" for the previous generation. To induce anesthesia via mask, sevoflurane is used almost exclusively because it acts faster and results in less bradycardia and hypotension (Sarner et al., 1995; Holzman et al., 1996). This has been especially important in infants. Isoflurane is frequently used for maintenance of anesthesia, in part because it is currently less expensive; desflurane may be used when particularly rapid awaking is desired, although the need for special, temperature-regulated vaporizers has limited its popularity. None of these newer agents, however, have the smooth induction properties of sevoflurane. Concerns have been raised about breakdown products that may develop when sevoflurane interacts with some carbon dioxide absorbents, especially when dessicated, leading to overheating of the absorbent system, carbon monoxide production, or both (Holak et al., 2003). The clinical significance of this remains to be determined.

A new, major feature in airway management has been the promotion of the laryngeal mask airway to eliminate tracheal intubation for many simple procedures, as well as provide airway access in emergency situations when intubation is difficult (Brain, 1983; Mason and Bingham, 1990; Pennant and White, 1993). Endoscopes have also been developed that permit fiberoptic intubation even in small children.

Several "descendents" of fentanyl have been developed, with remifentanil capable of providing very potent and transient analgesia when administered via constant intravenous infusion (Davis et al., 2001; Galinkin et al., 2001; Ross et al., 2001). Fentanyl transcutaneous "patches" have also been developed, largely to provide analgesia for chronic pain, and fentanyl is sometimes administered transnasally or transorally (Friesen et al., 1995; Viscusi et al., 2004). Potent opioids have been particularly useful for cardiac procedures when inhaled anesthetic agents are not well tolerated (Hickey and Hansen, 1984). Perhaps more significant, the prolonged debate over the need for anesthesia at all during surgery on small infants was finally terminated when Anand and Hickey (1987) produced evidence of physiologic stress in infants under light anesthesia. This brought general agreement that all infants should receive anesthesia during surgery, although the best method for doing this, especially when the patient is a fetus, remains to be fully elucidated.

Propofol has become the most common intravenous induction agent for adults but has not completely replaced thiopental in children because propofol causes some discomfort when injected into small peripheral veins. Midazolam has replaced diazepam as the intravenous benzodiazepine of choice for sedation in children; midazolam is also the most popular oral sedative in the preoperative setting (Kain et al., 2000). Midazolam can also be administered via several other routes (including intranasal) and is sometimes used rectally because production of methohexital, often used for this purpose, has ceased for economic reasons. The use of lidocaine-prilocaine (EMLA) or other creams

(Freeman et al., 1993) for skin desensitization eases the discomfort of venipuncture for intravenous induction but requires adequate time to become effective. Intramuscular injections are rarely necessary now in pediatric anesthesia practice.

Several new, nondepolarizing muscle relaxants have replaced curare. Although pancuronium is commonly used for lengthy procedures, several shorter-acting agents (especially cisatracurium and vecuronium) are frequently administered for brief procedures and have fewer side effects. Rocuronium is often used to facilitate emergency endotracheal intubation, and succinylcholine is no longer administered without good cause, because masseter spasm, malignant hyperthermia, or both occasionally develop after its administration, especially in the presence of potent inhaled anesthetic agents (Schwartz et al., 1984). In addition, the Food and Drug Administration (1997) issued a "black box" warning due to serious complications (including cardiac arrest resulting from acute hyperkalemia) associated with its use, particularly in young boys with unrecognized muscular dystrophy.

Although there had been some use of local and regional anesthesia for children before 1940, the development of improved inhalation methods soon largely displaced other forms of anesthesia. Regional anesthesia has become more commonplace in children, beginning in Europe, with "single-shot" techniques (spinal, caudal, peripheral nerve block) reducing the requirements for general anesthesia and providing postoperative analgesia (Abajian et al., 1984; Yaster and Maxwell, 1989). In addition, continuous infusions of local anesthetics with or without fentanyl are often delivered intraoperatively and postoperatively via catheters placed during surgery, especially via the epidural route. This is a reflection of the much greater emphasis being devoted to the needs of the pediatric patient in the postoperative period. Pain control following surgery has been a major focus of pediatric anesthesiologists with patient-, parent-, or nurse-controlled analgesia available via computer-controlled infusion pumps for delivery of medications by the intravenous or epidural route. Pain treatment services have become more important aspects of the mission of most departments of pediatric anesthesia; they provide care for children with medical, as well as surgical, pain (Zeltzer et al., 1989; Schecter et al., 2002).

In addition, outpatient pain treatment clinics evaluate and treat many chronic pain conditions in childhood; although largely directed by anesthesiologists, these are best multidisciplinary in nature and use many different techniques (including nerve blocks, oral medications, acupuncture, hypnosis, behavioral modification) and involve the participation of neurologists, neurosurgeons, physiatrists, physical therapists, psychologists, and many other ancillary medical and nursing personnel. Greater attention has also been directed toward assessing and allaying preoperative fears and anxiety of patients and their families. Preoperative clinics are used to evaluate many patients in advance of their procedures, and significant attention has been devoted to methods of easing induction of anesthesia, especially the use of oral premedicants and parental presence during mask induction (Kain et al., 1998, 2003). In all instances, kindness remains the essential feature in preoperative management.

PROGRESS IN MONITORING

Technical advances have also greatly enhanced patient monitoring. Smaller equipment is now readily available so that very young patients can be monitored as carefully as critically ill adults. Percutaneous catheters can be inserted directly into virtually any peripheral vein or artery; the Seldinger technique (if necessary with ultrasound guidance) can be used to insert central catheters. Echocardiography can be performed transthoracically or transesophageally in small children as well as in adults. Its use has greatly facilitated the ability of cardiac surgeons to assess the repair of congenital heart lesions intraoperatively (Ungerleider et al., 1990). "Standard" monitoring is now quite extensive and sophisticated as promulgated by the American Society of Anesthesiologists in 1986 and includes continuous pulse oximetry and capnography. It appears that the average anesthesiologist is frequently able to manage a procedure with little or no direct observation of the patient, although a precordial or an esophageal stethoscope is still considered valuable by many pediatric anesthesiologists.

Advances in the intensive care unit also have been significant during this time and extended into the operating rooms. Patients with severe lung injury are now managed with several new forms of respiratory support, including advanced mechanical ventilators, inhaled nitric oxide, and ECMO (Neonatal Inhaled Nitric Oxide Study Group, 1997; Bartlett et al., 2000; Aharon et al., 2001; Campbell et al., 2003). This latter technique can be used for weeks at a time and as an emergency method of resuscitation from cardiac arrest when a reversible condition is suspected (Laussen, 2002).

ADVANCES IN SURGERY

Numerous developments have occurred in surgical techniques that have greatly influenced anesthesia practice and are discussed elsewhere in this text. However, it is worthwhile noting that laparoscopic techniques, robotics, and intraoperative imaging have progressed so extensively and so rapidly into pediatric practice that anesthesiologists have had to accommodate the special problems and challenges presented by these situations. Perhaps nowhere is this more apparent than the field of fetal surgery, where surgeons, obstetricians, anesthesiologists, and neonatologists must collaborate to care for two patients simultaneously as techniques for surgical repair of prenatal anomalies are developed and assessed (Harrison et al., 1982, 1993; Rosen, 1992).

Organ transplantation has extended beyond kidneys, and transplantation of the liver (Starzl et al., 1963) became a major challenge for pediatric surgeons and anesthesiologists. To support a young patient who has hepatic failure through a repeat liver transplant requiring replacement of multiple blood volumes while monitoring and maintaining cardiac function, temperature, and many components of blood chemistry during an 8- to 12-hour operation is one of the most demanding anesthetic tasks known. The record of 1000 liver transplantations performed at the Children's Hospital of Pittsburgh between 1980 and 1990 with a nearly 70% survival rate stands as a remarkable accomplishment of both surgeons and anesthesiologists (Robertson and Borland, 1990). Transplantation of the heart, lungs, or both appears similarly impressive, although it is not associated with the same degree of blood loss (Jamieson et al., 1984). In any case, a shortage of available organs, especially those of a small size, greatly limits pediatric transplantation, and attempts to grow organs in cell culture has evolved into the new and fascinating field of tissue engineering (Lanza et al., 2000).

RESEARCH EFFORTS

Activity in research is reaching a new level of excellence and productivity, while demands for clinical service and limitations of funding make this an ongoing challenge and old problems persist. As noted by Berry (1993), failure in the endless search for better preoperative sedation lies in controversies regarding basic ground rules for investigation, especially in children. In many fields, understanding of the problems has been gradually extended, with resultant improvement in the practical management of patients. Physiologic studies of cerebral circulation in the neonate by Rogers, Nugent, and Trystman (1980), gas exchange in cardiac patients (Lindahl, 1989; Fletcher, 1993), pharmacologic biotransformation of sedatives (Saint-Maurice et al., 1986), the infant and the myoneural junction (Goudsouzian and Standaert, 1986), and hypoxia in children following anesthesia (Motoyama and Glazener, 1986) are but a few of the important initial studies. The report by Lerman and others (1986) concerning postanesthetic vomiting after strabismus surgery is another illustration of one of the problems of the conscious child that remains particularly difficult to control. Advances in molecular biology, mapping the human genome, and genomic pharmacology offer great hope that it will be possible to "customize" care for individual patients in a continuing attempt to drive the curve of improvement mentioned by Rees (1991) "closer to perfection."

DEVELOPMENT OF THE SUBSPECIALTY

Pediatric anesthesia organizations have advanced greatly over the recent generation. Although a small group of anesthesiologists from the United States and Canada have had a section within the American Academy of Pediatrics since 1966 (now called the Section on Anesthesiology and Pain Medicine), it was not until 1973 that pediatric activities formally became a part of the American Society of Anesthesiologists. At this same time, a separate organization devoted to pediatric anesthesiology was established in the United Kingdom, but it was not until 1986 that the Society for Pediatric Anesthesia (SPA) was created in the United States. This is now the largest organization in the world devoted to pediatric anesthesiology, with more than 4000 members largely from the United States. The SPA has held annual meetings since 1987 in association with the annual meeting of the American Society of Anesthesiologists; for several years, it has also organized an additional winter educational meeting. The goals of the SPA are listed in Box 35–1; the society's presidents are listed in Table 35–1.

The SPA collaborated with other groups interested in pediatric anesthesiology in developing a proposal to have fellowship training formally accredited by the Accreditation Council for Graduate Medical Education (Rockoff and Hall, 1997). This was successful in 1997; there are 43 programs in the United States that offer 1 year of training in pediatric anesthesiology to individuals who have completed a basic residency in anesthesiology (American Medical Association, 2003). Furthermore, subspecialization within pediatric anesthesiology continues to advance informally with individuals developing additional experience in areas such as pediatric pain medicine, pediatric intensive care, pediatric cardiac anesthesiology, and others.

Finally, many additional textbooks directed to pediatric anesthesia have been published and several have been updated into multiple editions; these include texts by Gregory (2002); Coté, Todres, Goudsouzian, and Ryan (2001); Smith (now edited by Motoyama and Davis, 2005); Berry (1990); Brown and Fisk (1992); Sumner and Hatch (1999); Steward and Lerman (2001); Bisonnette and Dalens (2002); and others. The further development of pediatric anesthesiology into subspecialties became evident in texts on topics such as uncommon diseases (Katz and Steward, 1993), neonatal anesthesia (Hatch, Sumner, and Hellmann, 1995), pediatric pain (Bush and Harkins, 1991; Tobias, 1996; Schechter, Berde and Yaster, 2002), regional anesthesia (Saint-Maurice and Steinberg, 1990), cardiac anesthesia (Lake, 1998), and intensive care (Rogers, 1996; Todres, 1996; and others). The journal *Paediatric Anaesthesia*, originally edited by Bush in Liverpool and Saint-Maurice in Paris, became the first independent monthly publication devoted to this field; with its international editorial board members, it has led to enhanced worldwide relationships among pediatric anesthesiologists. *Anesthesia & Analgesia*, one of the largest anesthesia journals in the world, has also developed a separate section devoted to pediatric anesthesia. Furthermore, pediatric anesthesiologists are members of the editorial boards of *Anesthesiology* and several other well-respected international anesthesia journals.

Table 35–1. Presidents of the Society for Pediatric Anesthesia

Year	President	Location
1986 to 1988	Myron Yaster, M.D.	Baltimore, MD
1988 to 1990	Robert Crone, M.D.	Seattle, WA
1990 to 1992	Aubrey Maze, M.D.	Phoenix, AZ
1992 to 1994	Charles Lockhart, M.D.	Denver, CO
1994 to 1996	William Greeley, M.D.	Durham, NC
1996 to 1998	Mark Rockoff, M.D.	Boston, MA
1998 to 2000	Steven Hall, M.D.	Chicago, IL
2000 to 2002	Peter Davis, M.D.	Pittsburgh, PA
2002 to 2004	Anne Lynn, M.D.	Seattle, WA
2004 to 2006	Francis McGowan, M.D.	Boston, MA

BOX 35–1 Goals of the Society for Pediatric Anesthesia

1. To advance the practice of pediatric anesthesia through new knowledge
2. To provide educational programs on clinical, scientific, and political issues that are important to pediatric anesthesia practice
3. To promote scientific research in pediatric anesthesia and related disciplines
4. To provide a forum for exchange of ideas and knowledge among practitioners of pediatric anesthesia
5. To support the goals of the American Society of Anesthesiologists and the American Academy of Pediatrics

SUMMARY

Pediatric anesthesia has advanced enormously from the days when anesthesiologists and surgeons adapted adult techniques and equipment to small children. It is clear that pediatric anesthesiology is a well-established and well-recognized subspecialty in its own right. It is one of the most popular fields to pursue by individuals who desire further training after completing basic anesthesia residency, and its practitioners are desired by surgeons, pediatricians, and parents alike.

Challenges are ongoing as more complex surgical and diagnostic techniques are performed on younger and younger patients. In addition, society will always have limited resources, and ensuring adequate allocation of funding, personnel, and research priorities is an increasing problem for those who care for children as the "baby-boomer" population ages, adults live longer with ever more complicated medical conditions, and geriatric problems demand society's greater attention.

Nevertheless, history has shown that talented and dedicated individuals can and will meet the challenges ahead, and there are few who doubt that things are better now for pediatric anesthesiologists—and most important, for their patients—than ever before.

REFERENCES

Abajian JC, Mellish RW, Browne AF, et al.: Spinal anesthesia for the high-risk infant. *Anesth Analg* 63:359, 1984.

Aharon AS, Drinkwater DC, Churchwell KB, et al.: Extracorporeal membrane oxygenation after repair of congenital cardiac lesions. *Ann Thorac Surg* 72:2095, 2001.

American Academy of Pediatric Dentistry: Guidelines for the elective use of pharmacologic conscious sedation and deep sedation in pediatric dental patients. *Pediatr Dent* 19:48, 1997.

American Academy of Pediatrics, Clinical Report: Facilities and equipment for the care of pediatric patients in a community hospital. *Pediatrics* 111:1120, 2003.

American Academy of Pediatrics, Committee on Drugs, Section on Anesthesiology: Guidelines for monitoring and management of pediatric patients during and after sedation for diagnostic and therapeutic procedures. *Pediatrics* 89:1110, 1992.

American Academy of Pediatrics, Section on Urology: Timing of elective surgery on the genitalia of male children with particular reference to the risks, benefits, and psychologic effects of surgery and anesthesia. *Pediatrics* 97:590, 1996.

American Academy of Pediatrics, Surgical Advisory Panel: Guidelines for referral to pediatric surgical specialists. *Pediatrics* 110:187, 2002.

American College of Emergency Physicians: The use of pediatric sedation and analgesia. *Ann Emerg Med* 29:834, 1997.

American Medical Association: *Graduate Medical Education Directory*. Chicago, 2003, AMA.

American Society of Anesthesiologists Task Force on Sedation and Analgesia by Non-Anesthesiologists: Practice guidelines for sedation and analgesia by non-anesthesiologists. *Anesthesiology* 84:459, 1996.

Anand KJS, Hickey PR: Pain and its effects in the human neonate and fetus. *N Engl J Med* 317:1321, 1987.

Anderson SM: Controlled hypotension with Arfonad in pediatric surgery. *Br Med* 72:103, 1955.

Anderson SM: Use of depressant and relaxant drugs in infants and children. *Lancet* 2:965, 1951.

Apgar V: Proposal for new method of evaluation of newborn infants. *Anesth Analg* 32:260, 1953.

Armand-Delille PF: Morphine injection before induction of general anesthesia in children. *Bull Acad Natl Med* 107:890, 1932.

Ayre P: Endotracheal anesthesia for babies with special reference to harelip and cleft lip operations. *Anesth Analg* 16:330, 1937.

Bain JA, Spoerel WE: A streamlined anaesthetic system. *Can Anaesth Soc J* 19:426, 1972.

Baron SH, Kohlmoos HW: Laryngeal sequelae of endotracheal anesthesia. *Ann Otol Rhinol Laryngol* 60:67, 1951.

Bartlett RH, Gazzaniga AB, Huxtable RH: Extracorporeal membrane oxygenation (ECMO) in newborn respiratory failure: Technical consideration. *Trans Am Soc Artif Organs* 25:473, 1979.

Bartlett RH, Roloff DW, Custer JR, et al.: Extracorporeal life support: The University of Michigan experience. *JAMA* 283:904, 2000.

Beecher HK, Todd DP: A study of the deaths associated with anesthesia and surgery. *Ann Surg* 140:2, 1954.

Bennett EJ, Bowyer DE: *Principles of pediatric anesthesia*. Springfield, IL, 1982, Charles C Thomas.

Bennett EJ, Dougherty MJ, Jenkins MT: Fluid requirements for neonatal anesthesia and operation. *Anesthesiology* 32:343, 1970.

Bernhard WF, Navarro RV, Yagi H, et al.: Cardiovascular surgery in infants performed under hyperbaric conditions. *Vasc Dis* 3:33, 1966.

Berry FA: Anesthesia for the child with a difficult airway. In Berry FA: *Anesthetic management of difficult and routine pediatric patients*. New York, 1986, Churchill Livingstone.

Berry FA: *Anesthetic management of difficult and routine pediatric patients*, 2nd ed. New York, 1990, Churchill Livingstone.

Berry FA: Editorial: When is a control group not a control? *Paediatr Anaesth* 3:63, 1993.

Berry FA: The winds of change. *Paediatr Anaesth* 5:279, 1995.

Betcher AM: Hypno-induction techniques in pediatric anesthesia. *Anesthesiology* 19:279, 1958.

Bigelow HJ: Insensibility during surgical operations produced by inhalation. *Boston Med Surg J* 35:16, 1846.

Bissonnette B, Dalens BJ: *Pediatric anesthesia: Principles and practice*. New York, 2002, McGraw-Hill, Medical Pub. Division.

Black TCK, Fisk GC: *Anaesthesia for children including aspects of intensive care*. London, 1979, Blackwell Scientific Publications.

Brain AIJ: The laryngeal mask: A new concept in airway management. *Br J Anaesth* 55:801, 1983.

Brandstater BM: Prolonged intubation: An alternative to tracheostomy in infants. In Proceedings of the European Congress of Anaesthesia, 1962.

Bratton SL, Haberkern CM, Waldhausen JHT, et al.: Intussusception: Hospital size and risk of surgery. *Pediatrics* 107:299, 2001.

Brennan HJ: Vaporizer for fluothane. *Br J Anaesth* 29:332, 1957.

Britt BA: Etiology and patho-physiology of malignant hypothermia. *Fed Proc* 38:44, 1979.

Brown TCK, Fisk GC: *Anaesthesia for children*. Oxford, 1979, Blackwell Publishing.

Brown TCK, Fisk GC: *Anaesthesia for children*, 2nd ed. Oxford, 1992, Blackwell.

Bush GH, Stead AL: The use of d-tubocurarine in neonatal anaesthesia. *Br J Anaesth* 34:721, 1962.

Bush JP, Harkins SW: *Children in pain: Clinical and research issues from a developmental perspective*. New York, 1991, Springer-Verlag.

Buxton DW: *Anaesthetics: Their use and administration*. London, 1888, HK Lewis Co Ltd.

Campbell BT, Braun T, Schumacher R, et al.: Impact of ECMO on neonatal mortality in Michigan (1980-1999). *J Pediatr Surg* 38:290, 2003.

Cohen MM, Cameron CB, Duncan PG: Pediatric anesthesia morbidity and mortality in the perioperative period. *Anesth Analg* 70:160, 1990.

Cole F: A new endotracheal tube for infants. *Anesthesiology* 6:87, 1945.

Colgan FC, Keats AS: Subglottic stenosis, a cause of difficult intubation. *Anesthesiology* 18:265, 1957.

Conn AW, Montes JE, Barker GA, et al.: Cerebral salvage in near-drowning following neurological classification by triage. *Can Anaesth Soc J* 27:201, 1980.

Conn AW: Origins of paediatric anaesthesia in Canada. *Paediatr Anaesth* 2:179, 1992.

Cook DR: Neonatal anesthetic pharmacology: A review. *Anesth Analg* 53:544, 1974.

Cook DR, Marcy JH: *Neonatal anesthesia*. Pasadena, CA, 1988, Appleton Davies.

Coté CJ: NPO after midnight for children: A reappraisal. *Anesthesiology* 72:589, 1990.

Coté CJ, Todres ID, Goudsouzian N, Ryan JF: *A practice of anesthesia for infants and children*, 3rd ed. Philadelphia, 2001, WB Saunders.

Crasilneck HB, Hally JA: *Clinical hypnosis: Principles and application*, 2nd ed. New York, 1985, Grune & Stratton, p. 262.

Cullen SC: The use of curare for the improvement of abdominal muscle relaxation during inhalation anesthesia. *Surgery* 14:261, 1943.

Dartmouth Pediatric Sedation Project Site: Available at http://an.hitchcock.org/PediSedation.

Davenport HT: *Paediatric anaesthesia*. Philadelphia, 1967, Lea & Febiger.

Davenport HT, Barr MN: Blood loss during pediatric operations. *Can Med Assoc* 789:1309, 1963.

Davis PJ, Galinkin J, McGowan FX, et al.: A randomized multicenter study of remifentanil compared with halothane in neonates and infants undergoing pyloromyotomy. *Anesth Analg* 93: 1380, 1387, 2001.

Deming MV: Agents and techniques for induction of infants and young children. *Anesth Analg* 31:113, 1952.

Denborough MA, Forster FA, Lovell RRH, et al.: Anaesthetic deaths in a family. *Lancet* 2:45, 1960.

Dibbins AW: Neonatal diaphragmatic hernia: A physiologic challenge. *Am J Surg* 131:408, 1976.

Domino EF, Chodoff P, Corssen G: Pharmacologic effects of CI-581, a new dissociative anesthetic in man. *Clin Pharm Ther* 6:279, 1965.

Dorsch JA, Dorsch SE: *Understanding anesthetic equipment*. Baltimore, 1975, Williams & Wilkins.

Downes JJ, Raphaely RC: Pediatric intensive care. *Anesthesiology* 43:238, 1975.

Downes JJ: The historical evolution, current status, and prospective development of pediatric critical care. *Crit Care Clin* 8:1, 1992.

Downes JJ: What is a paediatric anaesthesiologist? The American perspective. *Paediatr Anaesth* 5:277, 1995.

Eather KE: Axillary brachial plexus block. *Anesthesiology* 19:683, 1958.

Eckenhoff JE: *Anesthesia from Colonial times.* Philadelphia, 1966, JB Lippincott, p. 27.

Eckenhoff JE: Relationship of anesthesia to postoperative personality changes in children. *Am J Dis Child* 86:587, 1953.

Eckenhoff JE: Some anatomic considerations of the infant larynx influencing endotracheal intubation. *Anesthesiology* 12:401, 1951.

Eger EI, Saidman LJ, Branstater B: Minimum alveolar concentration: A standard of anesthetic potency. *Anesthesiology* 26:756, 1965.

Enderby GEH: Controlled circulation with hypotensive drugs and posture to reduce bleeding in surgery. *Lancet* 1:1145, 1950.

Fabian LW, Newton GW, Stephen CR: Simple and accurate Fluothane vaporizer. *Anesthesiology* 19:284, 1958.

Ferrari LR, Rooney FM, Rockoff MA: Preoperative fasting practices in pediatrics. *Anesthesiology* 90:978, 1999.

Finch E, Jamleson S: Anesthesia for combined heart and lung transplantation. In Brown BR Jr, editor: *Anesthesia and transplantation surgery: Contemporary anesthesia practice.* Philadelphia, 1987, FA Davis.

Flagg PJ: Endotracheal inhalation anesthesia: Special reference to postoperative reaction and suggestions for their elimination. *Laryngoscope* 61:1, 1951.

Fletcher R: Gas exchange during anaesthesia and controlled ventilation in children with congenital heart disease. *Paediatr Anaesth* 3:5, 1993.

Food and Drug Administration: Cardiac arrest in children and adolescent patients receiving succinylcholine: Succinylcholine-induced hyperkalemia. Available at http://www.fda.gov/medwatch/safety/1997/succin.htm.

Fortuna A: Caudal analgesia: A simple and safe technique in paediatric surgery. *Br J Anaesth* 39:165, 1967.

Freeman JA, Doyle E, Im NG, et al.: Topical anaesthesia of the skin. *Paediatr Anaesth* 3:129, 1993.

Friesen RH, et al.: Oral transmucosal fentanyl citrate for preanaesthetic medication for pediatric cardiac surgery patients. *Paediatr Anaesth* 5:29, 1995.

Furman EB, Roman DG, Hairabet J, et al.: Management for surgical separation of newborn conjoined twins. *Anesthesiology* 34:95, 1971.

Furman EB, Roman DG, Hemmer E, et al.: Specific therapy in water, electrolyte and blood volume replacement during pediatric surgery. *Anesthesiology* 42:187, 1975.

Galinkin JL, Davis PJ, McGowan FX, et al.: A randomized multicenter study of remifentanil compared with halothane in neonates and infants undergoing pyloromyotomy. *Anesth Analg* 93:1387, 2001.

Gibbon JH: Artificial maintenance of circulation during experimental occlusion of pulmonary artery. *Arch Surg* 34:1105, 1937.

Gillespie NA: Endotracheal anaesthesia in infants. *Br J Anaesth* 17:2, 1939.

Goldbloom RB: Halifax and the precipitate birth of pediatric surgery. *Pediatrics* 11:164, 1917.

Goudsouzian NG, Donlon JN, Savarese JJ: Re-evaluation of dosage and duration of action of d-tubocurarine in the pediatric age group. *Anesthesiology* 43:416, 1975.

Goudsouzian NG, Standaert FG: The infant and the myoneural junction. *Anesth Analg* 65:1208, 1986.

Graff TD, Benson DW, Holzman RS, et al.: Acid-base balance in infants during halothane anesthesia with the use of an adult circle absorption system. *Anesth Analg* 43:583, 1964.

Gregory GA: *Pediatric anesthesia,* 4th ed. Philadelphia, 2002, Churchill Livingstone.

Gregory GA, Eger EI, Munson ES: The relationship between age and halothane requirement. *Anesthesiology* 31:344, 1969.

Gregory GA, Steward DJ: Life-threatening perioperative apnea in the ex-premie. *Anesthesiology* 59:495, 1983.

Griffith HR: John Snow, pioneer specialist in anesthesia. *Anesth Analg* 13:45, 1934.

Gronert GA: Malignant hyperthermia. *Anesthesiology* 53:395, 1980.

Gross RE: *The surgery of infancy and childhood.* Philadelphia, 1953, WB Saunders.

Guedel A: *Inhalation anesthesia.* New York, 1937, The Macmillan Co.

Gwathmey JT: Anesthesiology in infants and children. *Pediatrics* 19:734, 1907.

Haggard HW: The place of the anesthetist in American medicine. *Anesthesiology* 1:1, 1940.

Harmel HH, Lamont A: Anesthesia in the surgical treatment of congenital pulmonary stenosis. *Anesthesiology* 7:477, 1948.

Harris AJ: Management of anesthesia for congenital heart operation in children. *Anesthesiology* 11:328, 1950.

Harris JS: Special pediatric problems in fluid and electrolyte therapy in surgery. *Ann N Y Acad Sci* 66:966, 1957.

Harrison MR, Adzick NS, Flake AW, et al.: Correction of congenital diaphragmatic hernia in utero: VI. Hard lessons learned. *J Pediatr Surg* 28:1411, 1993.

Harrison MR, Adzick NS, Longaker MT, et al.: Successful repair in utero of a fetal diaphragmatic hernia after removal of herniated viscera from the left thorax. *N Engl J Med* 322:1582, 1990.

Harrison MR, Golbus MS, Filly RA, et al.: Open fetal surgery was performed at UCSF. *N Engl J Med* 308:591, 1982.

Hatch D, Sumner E, Hellmann J: *Surgical neonate: Anaesthesia and intensive care,* 3rd ed. New York, 1995, Oxford University Press.

Hatch DJ: *Neonatal anaesthesia.* London, 1984, Churchill Davidson.

Hatch DJ: Prolonged nasotracheal intubation in infants and children. *Lancet* 1:1272, 1968.

Herbert WI, Scott EB, Lewis GB: Fluid management of pediatric patients. *Anesth Analg* 50:376, 1971.

Hewer CL: *Anaesthesia in children.* London, 1923, HK Lewis Co. Ltd.

Hickey PR, Hansen DD: Fentanyl- and sufentanil-oxygen-pancuronium anesthesia for cardiac surgery in infants. *Anesth Analg* 63:117, 1984.

Hikasa Y, Shirocani H, Satomura K, et al.: Open-heart surgery in infants with an aid of hypothermic anesthesia. *Arch Jpn Chir* 36:495, 1967.

Hodges RJH: *Suxamethonium tolerance and pseudocholinesterase levels in children.* Proceedings of World Conference of Anaesthetists, Sheveningen, the Netherlands, September 5–10, 1955, pp. 247–251.

Holak EJ, Mei DA, Dunning MB, et al.: Carbon monoxide production from sevoflurane breakdown: Modeling of exposures under clinical conditions. *Anesth Analg* 96:757, 2003.

Holliday MA, Segar WE: The maintenance need for water in parenteral fluid therapy. *Pediatrics* 19:823, 1957.

Holzman RS: Morbidity and mortality in pediatric anesthesia. *Pediatr Clin North Am* 41:239, 1994.

Holzman RS, van der Velde ME, Kaus SJ, et al.: Sevoflurane depresses myocardial contractility less than halothane during induction of anesthesia in children. *Anesthesiology* 85:1260, 1996.

Horiuchi T, Koyamada K, Matano I, et al.: Radical operation for ventricular septal defect in infancy. *J Thorac Cardiovasc Surg* 46:180, 1963.

Hunt KH: Resistance in respiratory valves and canisters. *Anesthesiology* 16:190, 1955.

Inkster JS: The T-piece technique in anaesthesia. *Br J Anaesth* 28:512, 1956.

Iwai S, Satoyoshi M: History of paediatric anaesthesia in Japan. *Paediatr Anaesth* 2:275, 1992.

Jackson K: Psychological preparation as a method of reducing the emotional trauma of anesthesia in children. *Anesthesiology* 12:293, 1951.

Jamieson SW, Stinson EB, Baldwin JC, Shumway NE: Operative technique for heart-lung transplantation. *J Thorac Cardiovasc Surg* 87:930, 1984.

Jenkins KJ, Newburger JW, Lock JE, et al.: In-hospital mortality for surgical repair of congenital heart defects: Preliminary observations of variation in caseload. *Pediatrics* 95:323, 1995.

Johnstone M: The human cardiovascular response to Fluothane anesthesia. *Br J Anaesth* 28:392, 1956.

Junkin CL, Smith C, Conn AW: Fluothane for pediatric anesthesia. *Can Anaesth Soc J* 4:259, 1957.

Kain ZN, Caldwell-Andrews AA, Wang SM, et al.: Parental intervention choices for children undergoing repeated surgeries. *Anesth Analg* 96:970, 2003.

Kain ZN, Hofstadter MB, Mayes LC, et al.: Midazolam: effects on amnesia and anxiety in children. *Anesthesiology* 93:676, 2000.

Kain ZN, Mayes LC, Wang SM, et al.: Parental presence during induction of anesthesia versus sedative medication: Which intervention is more effective? *Anesthesiology* 89:1147, 1998.

Kass E: Timing of elective surgery on the genitalia of male children with particular reference to the risks, benefits, and psychological effects of surgery and anesthesia. *Pediatrics* 97:590, 1996.

Katz J, Steward DJ: *Anesthesia and uncommon pediatric diseases,* 2nd ed. Philadelphia, 1993, WB Saunders.

Keenan RL, Boyan CP: Cardiac arrest due to anesthesia. *JAMA* 253:2373, 1985.

Keenan RL, Shapiro JH, Dawson K: Frequency of anesthetic cardiac arrests in infants: Effect of pediatric anesthesiologists. *J Clin Anesth* 3:433, 1991.

Keenan RL, Shapiro JH, Kane FR, Simpson PM: Bradycardia during anesthesia in infants: an epidemiologic study. *Anesthesiology* 80:976, 1994.

Kilduff CJ, Wyant GM, Dale RH: Anaesthesia for repair of cleft lip and palate in infants using moderate hypothermia. *Can Anaesth Soc J* 3:102, 1956.

Kopetsky SJ: The selection of anesthesia in children. *Med Rec* 14:534, 1903.

Kososka ER, Minkes RK, Silen ML, et al.: Effect of pediatric surgical practice on the treatment of children with appendicitis. *Pediatrics* 107:1298, 2001.

Lake CL: *Pediatric cardiac anesthesia,* 3rd ed. Stamford, CT, 1998, Appleton & Lange.

Lanza RP, Langer R, Vacanti JP: *Principles of tissue engineering,* 2nd ed. New York, 2000, Academic Press.

Laussen PC: Mechanical support of the circulation: The ABC&E of pediatric resuscitation. Available at http://web1.tch.harvard.edu/heartmurmurs/fall2002/art1.html. Accessed March 24, 2005.

Leigh MD, Belton MK: *Pediatric anesthesia.* New York, 1948, The Macmillan Co.

Leigh MD, McCoy DD, Belton MK, et al.: Bradycardia following intravenous administration of succinylcholine chloride to infants and children. *Anesthesiology* 18:698, 1957.

Lerman J, Eustis S, Smith DR: Effect of droperidol pretreatment on postanesthetic vomiting in children undergoing strabismus surgery. *Anesthesiology* 65:322, 1986.

Levy DM: Psychic trauma of operation in children. *Am J Dis Child* 69:75, 1945.

Lewis FJ, Taufic M: Closure of atrial septal defect with the aid of hypothermia: Experimental accomplishments and report of one successful case. *Surgery* 33:52, 1953.

Lindahl SGE: Oxygen consumption and carbon dioxide elimination in infants and children during anaesthesia and surgery. *Br J Anaesth* 62:70, 1989.

Liu LMP, Coté CJ, Goudsouzian NG, et al.: Life-threatening apnea in infants recovering from anesthesia. *Anesthesiology* 59:506, 1983.

Lomaz JG: Halothane and jaundice in paediatric anesthesia. *Anaesthesia* 20:70, 1965.

Long CW: An account of the first use of sulphuric ether by inhalation as an anaesthetic in surgical operations. *S Med Surg J* 5:45, 1849.

Lowrie L, Weiss AH, Lacombe C: The pediatric sedation unit: A mechanism for pediatric sedation. *Pediatrics* 102:E30, 1998.

Lunn JN: Implications of the national confidential enquiry into perioperative deaths for paediatric anaesthesia. *Paediatr Anaesth* 2:69, 1992.

MacDonald IH, Stocks JG: Prolonged nasotracheal intubation: A review of its development in a paediatric hospital. *Br J Anaesth* 37:161, 1965.

Macon EB, Bruner HD: The scientific aspect of endotracheal tubes. *Anesthesiology* 11:313, 1950.

Malviya S, Voepel-Lewis T, Tait AR: Adverse events and risk factors associated with the sedation of children by non-anesthesiologists. *Anesth Analg* 85:1207, 1997.

Mapleson WW: The elimination of rebreathing in various semi-closed anesthetic systems. *Br J Anaesth* 26:323, 1954.

Marcy JH, Cook DR: Basic neonatal anesthesia and monitoring. In March JH, Cook DR, editors: *Neonatal anesthesia.* Pasadena, CA, 1988, Appleton Davies.

Marmer MJ: Hypnosis as an adjunct to anesthesia in children. *Am J Dis Child* 97:314, 1959.

Mason DG, Bingham RM: The laryngeal mask airway in children. *Anaesthesia* 45:760, 1990.

Matthews JH, Buckley JJ, Van Bergen FH: Acute effect of low-flow extracorporeal circulation on cerebral circulation. *Anesthesiology* 18:169, 1957.

McQuiston WO: Anesthetic problems in cardiac surgery in children. *Anesthesiology* 10:590, 1949.

Melman E, Pennelas J, Maruffo J: Regional anesthesia in children. *Anaesth Analg* 54:387, 1975.

Mendelsohn D Jr, Mackrell TN, Machlan MA, et al.: Experiences using the pump-oxygenator for open heart surgery in man. *Anesthesiology* 18:223, 1957.

Morray JP: Implications for subspecialty care of anesthetized children. *Anesthesiology* 80:969, 1994.

Morray JP, et al.: A comparison of pediatric and adult anesthesia closed malpractice claims. *Anesthesiology* 78:461, 1993.

Morray JP, Geiduschek JM, Ramamoorthy C, et al.: Anesthesia-related cardiac arrest in children: Initial findings of the Pediatric Perioperative Cardiac Arrest (POCA) Registry. *Anesthesiology* 93:6, 2000.

Morton WTG: *Remarks on the proper mode of administering the sulphuric ether by inhalation.* Boston, 1847, Dutton & Wentworth, Printers.

Motoyama EK: Pulmonary mechanics during early postnatal years. *Pediatr Res* 11:220, 1977.

Motoyama EK, Cook CD: Respiratory physiology. In Smith RM, editor: *Anesthesia for infants and children,* 4th ed. St. Louis, 1980, CV Mosby, pp. 38–87.

Motoyama EK, Davis PJ: *Smith's anesthesia for infants and children,* 7th ed. Philadelphia, 2005, Elsevier.

Motoyama EK, Glazener CH: Hypoxemia after general anesthesia in children. *Anesth Analg* 65:267, 1986.

Murat I, Montay G, Delleur MM, et al.: Bupivacaine pharmacokinetics during epidural anaesthesia in children. *Eur J Anaesthesiol* 5:113, 1988.

Nelson WE: *Nelson's textbook of pediatrics.* Philadelphia, 1950, WB Saunders.

Neonatal Inhaled Nitric Oxide Study Group: Inhaled nitric oxide and hypoxic respiratory failure in infants with congenital diaphragmatic hernia. *Pediatrics* 99:838, 1997.

Nicodemus HF, Nassiri-Rahimi C, Bachman L, et al.: Median effective doses (ED50) of halothane in adults and children. *Anesthesiology* 31:344, 1969.

Oh TH, Motoyama EK: Comparison of nasotracheal intubation and tracheostomy in management of epiglottitis. *Anesthesiology* 46:214, 1977.

Olsson GL, Hallen B: Cardiac arrest during anesthesia: A computerized study. *Acta Anaesthesiol Scand* 32:653, 1988.

Onchi O, Fujita M: *Pediatric anesthesia.* Tokyo, 1958, Nankodo & Co Ltd.

Onchi Y, Hayashi T, Veyama H: Studies on the Ayre T piece technique. *Far East J Anaesth* 1:30, 1947.

Orkin LK, Siegel M, Rovenstine EA: I. Resistance to breathing by apparatus used in anesthesia. *Anesth Analg* 33:217, 1954.

Patrick RT, Theye RA, Moffitt EA: Studies in extracorporeal circulation. V. Anesthesia and supportive care during intracardiac surgery with the Gibbon-type pump-oxygenator. *Anesthesiology* 18:673, 1957.

Pender JW: Endotracheal anesthesia in children. *Anesthesiology* 15:495, 1954.

Pennant JH, White PF: Review article: The laryngeal mask airway. Its uses in anesthesiology. *Anesthesiology* 79:144, 1993.

Pernick MS: *A calculus of suffering.* New York, 1975, Columbia University Press.

Poe MF, Karp M: Seconal as a basal anesthetic in children: A preliminary report. *Anesth Analg* 25:88, 1946.

Powell DR, Miller RD: The effect of repeated doses of succinylcholine on serum potassium in patients with renal failure. *Anesth Analg* 54:746, 1975.

Rackow H, Salanitre E: A dose effect study of preoperative medication in children. *Anesthesiology* 23:747, 1962.

Raphaely RC, Downes JJ Jr: Congenital diaphragmatic hernia: Prediction of survival. *J Pediatr Surg* 8:815, 1973.

Rees GJ: An early history of paediatric anaesthesia. *Paediatr Anaesth* 1:3, 1991.

Rees GJ: Paediatric anaesthesia. *Br J Anaesth* 32:132, 1960.

Rees GJ: The child as a subject for anaesthesia. In Evans FT, Gray TC, editors: *Modern trends in anaesthesia.* New York, 1958, Harper & Row, Publishers.

Rice LJ, Baker SB: Review article: Congenital diaphragmatic hernia. Does extracorporeal membrane oxygenation (ECMO) improve survival? *Paediatr Anaesth* 3:205, 1993.

Robertson K, Borland LM: Anesthesia for organ transplantation. In Motoyama EK, Davis PJ: *Smith's anesthesia for infants and children.* St. Louis, 1990, CV Mosby.

Robson CH: Anesthesia in children. *Am J Surg* 34:468, 1936.

Rockoff MA, Hall SC: Subspecialty training in pediatric anesthesiology: What does it mean? *Anesth Analg* 85:1185, 1997.

Rogers MC: *Textbook of pediatric intensive care,* 3rd ed. Baltimore, 1996, Williams & Wilkins.

Rogers MC, Nugent S, Traystman RJ: Control of cerebral circulation in the neonate and infant. *Crit Care Med* 8:570, 1980.

Root B: Problems in evaluating effects of premedication in children. *Anesth Analg* 41:180, 1962.

Rosen MA: Anesthesia for fetal procedures and surgery. In Snider SM, Levinson G, editors: *Anesthesia for obstetrics,* 3rd ed. Baltimore, 1992, Williams & Wilkins, pp. 281–285.

Ross AK, Davis PJ, Dear G, et al.: Pharmacokinetics of remifentanil in anesthetized pediatric patients undergoing elective surgery or diagnostic procedures. *Anesth Analg* 93:1393, 2001.

Rowe MI, Oribe FL: Hypoxia and the newborn infant: Blood gas and pH considerations. *Surgery* 70:758, 1971.

Safar P: Ventilatory efficiency of mouth-to-mouth artificial respiration. *JAMA* 167:335, 1958.

Saint-Maurice C, Meistelman C, Rey E, et al.: The pharmacokinetics of rectal midazolam for premedication in children. *Anesthesiology* 65:536, 1986.

Saint-Maurice C, Steinberg OS: *Regional anaesthesia in children.* Fribourg, Switzerland, 1990, Mediglobe.

Salanitre E, Rackow H: The pulmonary exchange of nitrous oxide and halothane in infants and children. *Anesthesiology* 30:388, 1969.

Salem MR: Anesthetic management of patients with a "full stomach." A critical review. *Anesth Analg* 49:47, 1970.

Salem MR, Bennett EJ, Schweiss JF, et al.: Cardiac arrest related to anesthesia. Contributing factors in infants and children. *JAMA* 233:238–241, 1975.

Sarner JB, Levine M, Davis PJ, et al.: Clinical characteristics of sevoflurane in children: A comparison with halothane. *Anesthesiology* 82:38, 1995.

Saunders NA, Powles ACP, Rebuck AS: Ear oximetry accuracy practicability in the assessment of arterial oxygenation. *Am Rev Respir Dis* 113:745, 1976.

Schechter NL, Berde CB, Yaster M: *Pain in infants, children, and adolescents,* 2nd ed. Baltimore, 2002, Williams & Wilkins.

Schulman JL, Foley JM, Vernon DTA, et al.: A study of the effect of the mother's presence during anesthesia induction. *Pediatrics* 39:111, 1967.

Schuster SR: A new method for the staged repair of large omphaloceles. *Surg Gynecol Obstet* 125:837, 1967.

Schwartz H: Chloroform anesthesia for ophthalmic examination. *Am J Ophthalmol* 43:27, 1957.
Schwartz L, Rockoff MA, Koka BV: Masseter spasm with anesthesia: incidence and implications. *Anesthesiology* 61:772, 1984.
Sellick BA: Cricoid pressure to control the regurgitation of stomach contents during induction of anaesthesia. *Lancet* 2:204, 1961.
Singer JJ: Cardiac arrest in children. *J Am Coll Emerg Physicians* 6:198, 1977.
Small GA: Brachial plexus block anesthesia in children. *JAMA* 147:1648, 1951.
Smith AOC: An endo-oesophageal stethoscope. *Anesthesiology* 15:566, 1954.
Smith CA: *The physiology of the newborn infant.* Springfield, IL, 1945, Charles C Thomas.
Smith RM: *Anesthesia for infants and children.* St. Louis, 1959, CV Mosby.
Smith RM: Anesthesia for pediatric surgery. In Gross DE, editor: *Surgery of infants and children.* Philadelphia, 1953b, WB Saunders.
Smith RM: Circulatory factors affecting anesthesia in surgery for congenital heart disease. *Anesthesiology* 13:38, 1952.
Smith RM: Progress in paediatric anaesthesia in the United States. *Paediatr Anaesth* 1:63, 1991.
Smith RM: The prevention of tracheitis in children following endotracheal anesthesia. *Anesth Analg* 32:102, 1953a.
Smith RM, Crocker DC, Adams JG: Anesthetic management of patient under hyperbaric oxygenation. *Anesth Analg* 43:766, 1964.
Smith SM: The use of curare in infants and children. *Anesthesiology* 8:176, 1947.
Smith SM, Brown H, Toman J, et al.: The lack of cerebral effects of d-tubocurarine. *Anesthesiology* 8:1, 1947.
Snow J: *On chloroform and other anesthetics.* London, 1858, John Churchill.
Snow J: *On the inhalation of the vapour of ether.* London, 1847, John Churchill.
Stanley CJ, Hirschl RB, Schumacher RE, et al.: Extracorporeal life support for neonatal respiratory failure: 20 Year experience. *Ann Surg* 220:269, 1994.
Starzl TE, Marchioro TL, von Kaulla KN, et al.: Homo-transplantation of the liver in human. *Surg Gynecol Obstet* 117:659, 1963.
Stead AL: The response of the newborn infant to muscle relaxants. *Br J Anaesth* 27:124, 1955.
Stehling L: *Common problems in pediatric anesthesia,* 2nd ed. St. Louis, 1992, Mosby-Year Book.
Stephen CR: *Elements of paediatric anaesthesia.* Springfield, IL, 1954, Charles C Thomas.
Stephen CR, Lawrence JH, Fabian LW, et al.: Clinical experience with fluothane—1,400 cases. *Anesthesiology* 19:197, 1958.
Stephen CR, Slater HM: A non-rebreathing, non-resisting valve. *Anesthesiology* 9:550, 1948.
Steward DJ: History of pediatric anesthesia. In Gregory GA, editor: *Pediatric anesthesia.* New York, 1983, Churchill Davidson.
Steward DJ: Preterm infants are more prone to complications following minor surgery than are term infants. *Anesthesiology* 56:304, 1982.
Steward DJ, Lerman J: *Manual of pediatric anesthesia,* 5th ed. New York, 2001, Churchill Livingstone.
Stiles CM: A flexible fiberoptic bronchoscope for endotracheal intubation of infants. *Anesth Analg* 53:1017, 1974.
Sumner E, Hatch D: *Paediatric anaesthesia,* 2nd ed. New York, 1999, Oxford University Press.
Task Force on Sedation by Non-Anesthesiologists: Practice guidelines for sedation and analgesia by non-anesthesiologists. *Anesthesiology* 84:459, 1996.
Taussig HB: *Congenital malformations of the heart.* New York, 1947, The Commonwealth Fund.
Taylor PA, Towley RM: The broncho-fiberscope as an aid to endotracheal intubation. *Br J Anaesth* 46:611, 1972.
Telford J, Keats AS: Succinylcholine in cardiovascular surgery in infants and children. *Anesthesiology* 18:841, 1957.
Tessier P, Guiot G, Delbet JP, et al.: Osteotomies cranio-naso-orbito-faciales hypertelorisme. *Ann Chir Plast Esthet* 12:103, 1967.
Tiret L, Nivoche Y, Hatton F, Desmonts JM, Vourc'h G: Complications related to anaesthesia in infants and children. *Br J Anaesth* 61:263, 1988.
Tobias JD, Deshpande JK: *The pediatric pain handbook.* St. Louis, 1996, Mosby.
Todres ID, Fugate JH: *Critical care of infants and children.* Boston, 1996, Little, Brown.
Ungerleider RM, Greeley WJ, Sheikh KH, et al.: Routine use of intraoperative epicardial echocardiography and Doppler color flow imaging to guide and evaluate repair of congenital heart lesions: A prospective study. *J Thorac Cardiovasc Surg* 100: 297, 1990.
Virtue RW: *Hypothermic anesthesia.* Springfield, IL, 1955, Charles C Thomas.
Viscusi ER, Reynolds L, Chung F, et al.: Patient-controlled transdermal fentanyl hydrochloride vs intravenous morphine pump for postoperative pain: A randomized controlled trial. *JAMA* 291:1333, 2004.
Warren JM: Inhalation of ether. *Boston Med Surg J* 36:160, 1847.
Waters RM: Pain relief for children. *Am J Surg* 39:470, 1938.
Weinstein ML: Rectal pentothal sodium: A new pre- and basal anesthetic drug in the practice of surgery. *Anesth Analg* 18:221, 1939.
Winston KR, Rockoff MA, Mullikan JB, et al.: Surgical division of craniopagi. *Neurosurgery* 21:782, 1987.
Yaster M, Aranoff D, Kornhauser DM, et al.: Pharmacokinetics of lidocaine during caudal anesthesia in children. *Anesthesiology* 63:A465, 1985.
Yaster M, Maxwell LG: Pediatric regional anesthesia. *Anesthesiology* 70:324, 1989.
Zeltzer LK, Jay SM, Fisher DM: The management of pain associated with pediatric procedures. *Pediatr Clin North Am* 36:941, 1989.
Zindler M, Deming MV: The anesthetic management of infants for repair of congenital atresia of the esophagus with tracheo-esophageal fistula. *Anesth Analg* 32:180, 1953.

36 Medicolegal and Ethical Aspects

Eva Vogeley • Jodi Innocent

The topic of the ethics and medicolegal aspects of pediatric anesthesia is very broad and could fill volumes. Although the law may differ from state to state and from country to country, bioethical issues are generally applicable to all people. This chapter of necessity emphasizes some topics while neglecting others. Because medical malpractice and risk management are emphasized in most writings on the law and anesthesia, this topic is only summarized here. The emphasis of this chapter includes the intention torts, the doctrine of informed consent, and issues related to research involving children as subjects. A glossary of terms and abbreviations is provided in Box 36–1.

BOX 36–1 Glossary of Terms and Abbreviations

Assault: Causing apprehension of battery
Battery: Harmful or offensive touching
Capacity: Attribute of having legal competency to act
Consortium: Inability of family members of the plaintiff to have normal relations with him or her
Defendant: Party sued in a legal action
Duty: Legal obligation, the breach of which can lead to liability
EMTALA: Emergency Medical Treatment and Active Labor Act
FDA: Food and Drug Administration
HIPAA: Health Insurance Portability and Accountability Act of 1996
OHRP: Office for Human Research Protections
Plaintiff: Party who initiates a lawsuit by filing a complaint
Res ipsa loquitur: Literally, "the thing speaks for itself"; an exception to the rule that a plaintiff must show defendant's actions caused injury
Standard of care: Level of skill and learning commonly possessed by members of a profession who are in good standing
Tort: Civil wrong that results in an injury to another

ETHICAL CONCEPTS

The traditional ethical principles of beneficence, respect for persons, and justice* must guide physicians in all aspects of their professional lives, including the treatment of patients, the education of health care personnel, and research involving human subjects. As with overarching principles in general, it is difficult at times to apply these broad rules in individual instances. This is especially true in dealing with children, who do not have the capacity to consent on their own behalf.

The term "justice" encompasses the concept of fairness of distribution. The principle is often stated as requiring that people similarly situated should be treated similarly. Although pediatric anesthesiologists share the concerns of the greater medical community about issues of access to health care by families who are uninsured or underinsured, the principle of justice becomes more intense when there is inequality of treatment of pain based on age, gender, or both. There is a substantial body of literature dealing with the physiologic and autonomic concomitants of pain that makes it clear that even the smallest of preemies experiences distress when subjected to noxious stimuli. Because pain management often falls within the purview of departments of anesthesiology, there is the opportunity to ensure the compassionate and just treatment of all.

The Hippocratic oath reminds all physicians of the ethical mandate to do no harm. The principle of beneficence goes beyond this in that it requires the making of efforts to secure the well-being of patients. This, in turn, requires maximizing benefit and minimizing risk. It is important to remember that risks to patients involve more than physical risks. Especially in the area of anesthesiology, it is essential that physicians be mindful of psychological issues implicit in being rendered entirely dependent on a stranger, as occurs during general anesthesia. Sensitive and age-appropriate discussion can minimize these potential psychological harms to children and adolescents.

*These principles are those that were enunciated in the Belmont Report, which continues to serve as the guiding document for research in human subjects.

For example, the expression "put to sleep" may have one meaning for an anesthesiologist but quite another for a child whose pet was recently euthanized.

The principle of respect for persons requires acknowledgement of autonomy. This means that people who have decisional capacity should be given sufficient information to make informed choices. In turn, such informed choices should be honored. As a corollary, however, respect for persons also requires protection of those with diminished capacity to make decisions. By legal definition, most minors are held to lack full decisional capacity. However, it is also clear that decisional capacity does not develop at a single age, legislatively defined. To the contrary, decisional capacity develops over the lifetime of an individual with considerable variation from person to person. For practitioners of pediatric anesthesia, the principle of respect for persons requires not only that the parents of children are given sufficient information to make choices about treatment but also that information is given to children in a manner that they can understand so that their assent to treatment can be obtained. Problematic are those situations in which a parental decision conflicts with that of a minor child. For example, what happens if a parent consents for anesthesia for a debulking operation for metastatic cancer when the child wants no further therapy? What if a teenager wants a cosmetic operation but the parent is opposed and refuses to consent for the operation? One of the unique features of pediatric anesthesiology is that the person consenting to anesthesia is not the patient but rather a legally authorized representative, usually a parent who can consent on the child's behalf. If consent is not obtained or the obtained consent is in some way defective, the treating physician runs the risk of committing medical negligence or an intentional tort, both of which are discussed in more detail later.

MEDICAL MALPRACTICE

The mere utterance of the word "lawsuit" strikes terror in the hearts of most physicians. Although there is no doubt that some frivolous lawsuits are won not on the merits of the case but rather on the basis of emotional issues, it should be reassuring to pediatric anesthesiologists that in most instances a plaintiff must fulfill some clearly defined elements in order to prevail. These requirements are as follows.

DUTY

In the law, a duty arises when there is a relationship that requires that a person conduct himself or herself according to a certain standard. If a physician is walking across a bridge and notices a person who is threatening to jump, it may be morally reprehensible for the physician simply to continue to walk across the bridge. It is not, however, an act of negligence because there is no relationship between the physician and the potential jumper that creates a duty for the physician to act in a certain way. In contrast, when a physician agrees to perform a medical service for a patient, then that physician has a duty to conduct himself or herself according to professional standards. In general, for a duty to arise, the physician and a patient must have entered into a physician-patient relationship. In some situations, however, a duty may be inferred even though no formal physician-patient relationship has been established. For example, it is not unusual for a pediatric anesthesiologist to be called to the emergency department or onto one of the wards in a hospital when a patient, previously unknown to the anesthesiologist, develops airway difficulties or otherwise requires intubation. If an anesthesiologist has agreed to be available for such an emergency situation, then he or she has a duty to such a patient, even though a formal relationship has not been previously established.

BREACH OF THE DUTY OF DUE CARE

This element of a medical malpractice suit prevents a bad outcome alone from being sufficient to prevail against the treating pediatric anesthesiologist. The patient alleging malpractice must, in addition to showing that there was a bad outcome, establish that (1) there is a standard, a level of skill and learning, commonly possessed by members of the profession in good standing and (2) that the physician's action fell short of this standard.

Historically, the standard to which a physician's conduct was held was determined locally. This approach was based on the belief that the standard for a practitioner in a small rural community understandably differed from that of a specialist in a large metropolitan medical center. With the development of medical boards and specialty boards, the concept of a local standard was supplanted by a national standard related to one's specialty, rather than to one's location. To the extent that professional societies have promulgated practice guidelines, these can be used as evidence of a national standard. In the absence of such accepted guidelines, the standard of care is less clear and must be established through expert testimony. In cases in which competent members of the profession differ on what the standard should be (subscribe to different schools of thought), the adherence to one or the other approach does not constitute negligence.

An illustration may be helpful. Pediatric anesthesiologists may differ in whether a straight or curved blade is preferable when performing an intubation. The choice of one type over another does not constitute negligence. In contrast, there is a standard for ensuring that an esophageal intubation has not occurred. If a pediatric anesthesiologist has intubated a child's esophagus and continues on without confirming endotracheal tube placement, this would constitute a breach of the duty of due care.

The absence of Food and Drug Administration (FDA) approval for a drug or device has also been used by plaintiffs to establish a standard of care. Although physicians have the legal right to prescribe any FDA-approved medication for any condition or age group, it may be problematic when such a use results in an unfortunate or unforeseen outcome. If, for example, a medical device has been approved for ablation of varicose veins and an ophthalmologist uses it to treat blood vessels in an eye, the lack of FDA approval for this use might be persuasive evidence that there was a breach of the standard of care. In the area of pediatric anesthesia, however, the lack of FDA approval for the use of an agent in children does not in and of itself constitute evidence of breech of a national standard. Until very recently, there was little incentive for pharmaceutical companies to sponsor trials of drugs to permit FDA approval for children. Often, drugs used in adults were tried in children, were found to be successful, and became widely used without ever having undergone the stringent testing required for FDA approval. For example, the drug albuterol that is widely used by pediatricians and pediatric anesthesiologists to treat bronchospasm has never received FDA approval for young children. The lack of FDA approval for a drug that is widely used and adequately studied in children is unlikely to be held to be a breach of the standard of care. However, an off-label use of a drug in children that has not been widely studied may give rise to such a finding. Fortunately, legislation has been enacted that promises extension of exclusivity rights to pharmaceutical companies that are willing to undertake pediatric trials. It is hoped that this will give rise to more FDA approval of drugs used in children.

CAUSATION

In order for a plaintiff to prevail in a malpractice action against an anesthesiologist, it is not sufficient to show that the physician had a duty and breached the standard of care. The plaintiff must also show that the act or omission of the anesthesiologist was what caused harm. Two different tests are used to determine if a physician's actions were the cause of a patient's harm. The first is the "but for" test. This test asks if "but for" the actions (or inactions) of the physician, would the patient have had the same untoward outcome? On the one hand, this test makes sense. If the patient's injuries would have occurred regardless of whether the physician did or did not act in a certain way, then it does not seem reasonable to hold the physician liable. Unfortunately, the "but for" test can give rise to unintended results that offend common sense. For example, an infant with congenital heart disease may not have had operative complications "but for" the fact that anesthesiologist had been willing to cover the heart cases on that day. This does not, however, prove that the anesthesiologist's decision to cover the heart cases was responsible for the harm. To avoid results that offend basic logic, courts may also apply the "significant factor" test in order to determine whether an anesthesiologist's action was an important cause of the operative injuries. If both these tests are met, then it is likely that the plaintiff has met the burden of proving causation.

In general, plaintiffs must specifically prove the element of causation. In a relatively few instances, the plaintiff does not have this burden because of the doctrine of *res ipsa loquitur*, which literally means, "The thing speaks for itself." When his or her doctrine is invoked, the plaintiff no longer has the burden of proof; instead, the physician must prove that his or her actions were not the cause of the patient's harm. In order to invoke the doctrine of *res ipsa loquitur*, the plaintiff must demonstrate the following:

1. The injury is of a type that does not ordinarily occur without negligence.
2. The instrumentality of the injury was under the exclusive control of the defendant(s).
3. The plaintiff did not contribute to the injury

Some courts add a fourth requirement—that the actual explanation for the injury is more accessible to the defendant than the plaintiff. In the case of pediatric anesthesiologists, this fourth requirement is easily met, because their patients are often minors who are either unconscious or have been given sedatives in combination with agents that produce amnesia.

One of the most famous cases to invoke the doctrine of *res ipsa loquitur* is the case of *Ybarra v. Spanard* [154 P.2d 687 (Cal. 1944)]. In this case, the plaintiff underwent an appendectomy. After the operation, he had pain in his shoulder due to an injury sustained during the operation. He sued the surgeon, the hospital, and the anesthesiologist, alleging that at least one of them had to have been negligent for his injury to have occurred. The court found in favor of the plaintiff on the basis of *res ipsa loquitur*, holding that it was unreasonable to require the plaintiff to identify the party that had been negligent as he was anesthetized, that each of the plaintiffs owed him a duty of care, and that a shoulder injury was unlikely to result from appendectomy surgery absent negligence.

DAMAGES

Even if a plaintiff shows that a pediatric anesthesiologist owed him a duty and there was a breach of the standard of care, he must also show that the resultant harm resulted in damages. Most jurisdictions require an actual physical harm before damages for nonphysical harms such as emotional distress may be awarded. Damage awards consist of what the fact finder (jury or judge) believes to be the actual harm (medical bills and actual economic losses, which in the case of children are mostly future loss of wages) and compensation of less tangible harms such as pain, suffering, and loss of consortium.

Negligence is not the only cause of action that can be brought against a pediatric anesthesiologist. Suits based on intentional torts have also been successfully brought against physicians.

INTENTIONAL TORTS

The term "tort" refers to civil as opposed to criminal wrong-doing. As discussed earlier, most cases of medical malpractice come under the tort of negligence. The intentional torts present an area of special concern for health care professionals because many malpractice policies exclude coverage for these actions. Another important consequence of the distinction between intentional torts and negligence is that in an action for negligence, the physician is generally held liable only for the consequences that were foreseeable; the physician who commits an intentional tort is liable for every result stemming from his conduct regardless of its predictability or ability to be foreseen. The following illustration shows this distinction:

D intentionally hits P on the head, intending merely to annoy him. P is slightly injured and taken to the hospital. There, by gross and completely unforeseeable error, a nurse gives him a poison instead of medication and P dies. D will be liable for P's death, not just the minor injury. But if D had merely negligently given P the same minor injury, he would not be liable for the unanticipated death (Rest.2d,§435B, Illustration 1).

The intentional torts of most interest to physicians are those of battery and assault. *Battery* is the intentional infliction of a harmful or offensive bodily contact. *Assault* is the intentional causing of an apprehension of harmful or offensive bodily contact. It is important to note that the bodily contact need not be harmful but need only be offensive or to offend one's sense of dignity. A troubling example is illustrated by the case of *Mohr v. Williams* [104 N.W. 12 (Minn. 1905)]. In this case, a patient consulted an otolaryngologist about her right ear and consented to an operation on that ear. During the operation, the physician discovered that it was actually the left ear that was diseased and operated on it. The court held that the surgery on the left ear was an offensive contact that constituted battery even though there was no harm to the patient. The amount of damages awarded to the plaintiff in this case was $39.00. Nearly everything that pediatric anesthesiologists do to patients would constitute a battery were it not for obtaining consent. Even if obtained, if the informed consent process is incomplete or in some other fashion defective, then the action of the physician may constitute a battery or, more likely, medical negligence.

Although the intentional torts of assault and battery are those of which physicians are accused if valid consent is not obtained, several other intentional torts merit mention.

Claims for invasion of privacy can arise from unauthorized release of information concerning patients. With the implementation of the privacy rule of the Health Insurance Portability and

Accountability Act of 1996 (HIPAA), most hospitals have reevaluated and refined their privacy policies. However, the temptation to discuss interesting cases with students on an elevator can still lead to inadvertent disclosures of private health information. Additionally, the increasing use by physicians of email to communicate with their patients carries the risk of protected health information being made available to persons who should not have such access. Finally, the convenience of the cellular phone must be balanced against the potential for a conversation being overheard by others. Prudence dictates that patients are informed if a cellular phone is being used so that they can decide whether to continue the cellular conversation or to call at another time.

Intentional infliction of emotional distress is another intentional tort that includes outrageous conduct that results in emotional trauma. This is the tort that perhaps may easily be avoided if the physician remembers to treat patients and families with respect at all times. Because the health care context is one that lends itself to at times challenging one's most strongly held beliefs, it is at times possible to get caught up in the emotionality of the moment and engage in conduct that could be construed as sufficiently outrageous to constitute intentional infliction of emotional distress. For example, a family who sought to discontinue life support alleged that hospital personnel accused them in a nonprivate area of the hospital of trying to murder the patient. The appeals court held that such conduct could be considered sufficiently outrageous as to permit a finding of intentional infliction of emotional distress [Gregg v. Calandra, 297 Ill.App.3d 639 (1998)].

False imprisonment is the unlawful restriction of a person's freedom, usually through physical restraint, although threats of harm can constitute false imprisonment in certain circumstances. During outpatient surgical procedures, most hospitals encourage a parent to remain in the waiting room. If a parent told the anesthesiologist that she planned to go out to a restaurant during her son's tonsillectomy and the anesthesiologist stated that if she left he would notify Child Protective Services and have her child placed in foster care, this might be held to constitute false imprisonment.

■ INFORMED CONSENT

Depending on the state in which a physician practices, the courts may distinguish between lack of consent and lack of informed consent. As described, lack of consent to touch or treat a patient can result in a claim for battery. There is no need for physical injury, but only some contact; the matter of permission goes to the quality of the contact, and consent to being so touched is a defense [Chandler v. Cook, 438 Pa. 447, 265 A.2d 794 (1970)]. In contrast, in an informed consent claim grounded in negligence, the matter of permission goes to the scope of the contract between physician and patient, and the primary inquiry is whether the injury suffered was within the known risks of which the patient was informed, or whether the information, such as to alternative procedures, was complete [*Grabowski v. Quigley,* 454 Pa. Super. 27, 684 A2d 610, 616 (Pa, Super. 1996)]. For various procedural and evidentiary reasons, many attorneys will plead both battery and medical negligence when asserting a claim of lack of informed consent.

A claim of lack of informed consent also may be supported by state law. Moreover, a claim of lack of informed consent may be limited by applicable state law or case law to only those procedures that are considered invasive. For example, Pennsylvania requires that informed consent be obtained, except in emergencies, prior to conducting the following procedures (40 P.S. 1301.811-A):

1. Surgery, including the related administration of anesthesia
2. Administration of radiation or chemotherapy
3. Administration of a blood transfusion
4. Inserting a surgical device or appliance
5. Administration of an experimental medication, use of an experimental device, or use of an approved medication or device in an experimental manner

Valid informed consent discussion, of necessity, requires that the person obtaining consent have detailed knowledge of the procedure. It is unlikely that a surgeon can discuss anesthesia with as much depth as an anesthesiologist. Similarly, physicians in training may lack sufficient knowledge and experience to conduct a consent interveiw.

■ IMPLIED CONSENT AND DECISIONAL CAPACITY

In some instances, consent to medical treatment can be implied by a patient's behavior. In the case of *O'Brien v. Cunard SS Co* [28 N.E. 266 (Mass. 1891)], decided in 1891, a passenger on a ship bound for the United States was told that she could not enter unless she had a certificate to show that she had been vaccinated. The patient stood in line and held up her arm. She then sued for battery, claiming that she had not consented to the vaccination. The court said that the behavior of the patient was such that it was reasonable for the physician to conclude that she had consented. The finding of implied consent in the modern medical setting, however, would be very unusual, and in some states that by regulation mandate the obtaining of written consent for certain procedures, the doctrine of implied consent cannot be used as a defense. The better practice is to adhere to the frequently quoted maxim, "If it isn't evidenced in a writing, it didn't happen."

In order for consent to be valid, the person giving consent must have the capacity to do so. In general (with some exceptions listed here), children do not have the capacity to consent for medical treatment. In addition, persons who are premedicated, unconscious, or severely intoxicated do not have the capacity to consent. Commentators on decisional impairment have pointed out that in many cases there is a continuum of decisional capacity so that persons who are mildly intoxicated or persons with some degree of mental retardation can in some circumstances give legally effective consent, whereas in other circumstances they cannot. It is the obligation of the physician obtaining consent to determine the decisional capacity, either alone or in consultation with a colleague, and to present materials in a way that can be understood by the patient in light of their innate abilities, education, and other circumstances.

When treating minors, the issue of decisional capacity also goes to the authority of the person who is acting as the representative of the minor. In some states when children are placed in foster homes, parental rights are not terminated, and therefore the consent of the parent, rather than that of the foster parent, is required for almost all medical procedures. Even routine health care may not be the province of the foster parent but rather reside with the county agency.

There are some situations in which the patient's consent will be implied "as a matter of law" if certain conditions are met, including the following:

1. The patient or person from whom consent must be obtained is incapacitated because of unconsciousness or a similar condition.
2. Failure to act would result in death or other serious harm.
3. There is no reason to believe that the patient would not consent.
4. A reasonable person would consent under the circumstances (Rest.2d, § 62).

EMANCIPATED MINOR AND THE MATURE MINOR DOCTRINE

The use of the term "emancipated minor" is dependent on the context in which the term is used. A minor may be emancipated for some things, such as receiving public assistance, and not considered emancipated for others, such as signing a contract or entering into a lease for an apartment. A minor may be emancipated due to certain circumstances defined by statute or as a result of being legally granted such status by a court of law. In many states, minors are considered "emancipated" for purposes of consenting to health care if they have met certain conditions. The definition of "emancipated minor" for purposes of health care consent may vary in detail from state to state, but the law in Pennsylvania is quite typical. It states

> Any minor who is eighteen years of age or older, or has graduated from high school, or has married, or has been pregnant, may give effective consent to medical, dental, and health services for himself or herself, and the consent of no other person shall be necessary (Act of Feb. 13, 1970, pl 19, No. 10 §1, 35 P.S. § 10101).

It should be noted that statutes such as this, while giving minors the ability to consent to medical care, do not necessarily give such persons the right to consent to participate in research.

Some jurisdictions, mostly through case law as opposed to legislation, have adopted the "Mature Minor Doctrine" as an exception to the usual rule requiring parental consent to medical treatment for the minor. A typical example comes from the case of *Cardwell v. Bechtol* [724 S.W.2d 739 (Tenn. 1987)], in which an adolescent sought care for back pain. The physician did not inquire about parental consent but rendered manipulative treatment because he believed that the adolescent was old enough to consent to the treatment on her own behalf. The parents of the adolescent brought suit when complications developed. The Supreme Court of Tennessee held that the adolescent was a mature minor and that the defendant could not be held to have committed a battery when he failed to obtain parental consent prior to treatment. An interesting extension of the concept of the "mature minor" was made in the case of *Larry D. Belcher, Sr., Administrator of the Estate of Larry D. Belcher, Jr., Deceased, Plaintiff Below, Appellant v. Charleston Area Medical Center, a Corporation, Charleston Pediatric Group, a West Virginia Corporation, and M.B. Ayoubi, MD, Defendant Below, Appellees* [422 S.E.2d 827 (West Va. 1992)] in which the parents told the treating physician that they did not want their 17-year-old son, who had muscular dystrophy, to be intubated unless their son desired it. The son died and was not resuscitated. The executors of the son's estate brought an action for wrongful death based on the theory that, as a mature minor, the son should have been consulted prior to the issuance of a do not resuscitate (DNR) order. The court held that if the son was a mature minor, he was entitled to consent to his medical treatment decisions. The case was remanded to the lower court to try the issue of whether the son in this case was a mature minor. Under the mature minor doctrine, whether a child has the capacity to consent depends upon the age, ability, experience, education, training, and degree of maturity or judgment obtained by the child. According to the court, in situations in which there is a conflict between the intentions of one or both parents and the minor, the physician's good faith assessment of the minor's maturity level would immunize him or her from liability for the failure to obtain parental consent.

EMERGENCY MEDICAL TREATMENT AND ACTIVE LABOR ACT

When working in a health care facility, the physician has additional obligations to act even in the absence of written informed consent. The Emergency Medical Treatment and Active Labor Act (EMTALA) was included in the Consolidated Omnibus Budget Reconciliation Act of 1986 (COBRA) in response to some hospitals' refusal to treat indigent patients. EMTALA imposes the following requirements on all hospitals that participate in Medicare:

1. An appropriate screening examination must be provided to anyone who comes to the health care facility seeking medical care.
2. If the health care facility determines that the individual has an emergency medical condition, the facility must treat and stabilize the patient.

It should be noted that the EMTALA requirements apply for all patients, not just those who are covered by Medicare. The penalties for violation of EMTALA are quite draconian and include fines as well as exclusion from Medicare, and giving rise to private causes of action. In practical terms, this means that an anesthesiologist summoned to the emergency department has an obligation to intubate and otherwise stabilize a child, even if the parents have not yet consented to treatment.

RISK MANAGEMENT

It goes without saying that the best way to avoid legal liability is to always get complete and informed consent from the person authorized to give consent and to practice impeccably so as to avoid all possible harm to patients. It is also common wisdom that if a physician has an excellent relationship with a patient and the patient's family, the likelihood of a lawsuit is lessened. In most cases, the avoidance of litigation based on interpersonal relationship is not available to pediatric anesthesiologists. In most instances, the interaction of a pediatric anesthesiologist is brief and takes place at a stressful time when there is an anticipation of surgery or another frightening procedure. This may be part of the reason why pediatric anesthesiologists may be sued, even if they are always mindful of the requirements for informed consent and scrupulously follow the standards of practice for their profession.

There are, however, other strategies that may help to minimize the risk. With the realization that untoward events occur despite flawless medical care, the pediatric anesthesiologist must be prepared to deal with unexpected outcomes. The best defense in any malpractice case is a careful, legible medical record with detailed preoperative assessments, anesthetic record, and postoperative notes. It is also prudent to discuss adverse events directly with the patient or the patient's family. It is tempting to defer these discussions to the surgeon, but an honest, caring, and open discussion between the anesthesiologist and patients and their families may prevent the filing of a suit. A careful note in the chart describing the adverse event, the factors that led to the event, and a description of actions that were undertaken to minimize harm is also essential when it is realized that it may be years between the adverse event and any resultant lawsuit. Because the statute of limitations for negligence suits only begins when a child reaches the age of majority, a lawsuit may be brought against a pediatric anesthesiologist as late as 20 years after the event. It goes without saying that any urge to revise the chart should be assiduously avoided. Erasures and marginal notes may be used by the plaintiff's attorneys to great advantage to cast doubt on one's integrity.

Finally, once a physician receives notice that a lawsuit has been filed, he or she should immediately contact the malpractice carrier and the legal department of the institution in which the activity giving rise to the claim occurred. To be a defendant in a malpractice suit can be emotionally devastating, and there is a tendency to want to solicit support and advice from friends and colleagues. As understandable as it is to try to gain solace, it is prudent to discuss the matter only with one's attorney, who cannot testify as to those conversations because of attorney-client privilege.

RESEARCH IN CHILDREN

Any institution that receives federal monies for research, including grants from the National Institutes of Health (NIH), must have a federalwide assurance from the Office for Human Research Protections (OHRP) in order to conduct any research involving human subjects. As a part of this assurance, the institution must pledge to follow the Belmont Report in all research activities regardless of the source of funding. The overarching principles of the Belmont Report have been codified at 45 CFR 46 with similar regulations covering Food and Drug Administration-controlled test articles found at 21 CFR 50. Subpart D of both of these statutes contains the additional protections afforded children when they become research subjects. In addition to requiring written permission from parents, the regulations require that the institutional review board (IRB) responsible for the conduct of the research ensures that there are adequate provisions for soliciting the assent of children who are developmentally capable of giving consent. Although many IRBs and researchers use 7 years as the age when most children are capable of giving assent, this is not the position taken by the regulations. To the contrary, the regulations provide that this determination should be made on the basis of the age, maturity, and psychological state of the involved child.

Apart from the requirement of assent, the most important statutory difference between the statutory requirements for conducting research with children and that with adults is that research involving children falls into one of four permissible categories. Once a given risk-benefit category is assigned, additional protections must be met.

The categories of permissible research in children and their attendant requirements are as follows.

1. Research Not Involving Greater Than Minimal Risk (45 CFR 46.404, 21 CFR 50.51)*

Under the federal regulations, "minimal risk" is defined as the probability and magnitude of harm encountered by healthy children in their ordinary life experiences including routine physical examinations and educational/psychometric testing. Under this definition, studies that involve the sampling of a small amount of blood or a urine test are considered minimal risks because such activities might be encountered during a routine physical examination. When research with children falls into this category, the only additional requirement is permission from parents and the assent of the child subjects.

2. Research Involving Greater Than Minimal Risk but Presenting the Prospect of Direct Benefit to the Individual Subjects (45 CFR 46.405, 21 CFR 50.52)

Under this category, the research intervention must hold the possibility of contributing to the subjects' well-being. In addition to the requirements for permission from parents and assent from children, research under this category must be such that the risk is justified by the anticipated benefit to the subjects and that the relation of the anticipated benefit to the risk is at least as favorable to the subject as that presented by available alternative approaches.

Whether a placebo-controlled study can be approved under this category depends, in part, on whether the determination is made before or after randomization. The regulations are silent as to when the determination should be made, so there is variation among IRBs in interpretation. In general, however, placebo-controlled studies can be approved under this category if (1) there is no standard treatment for the condition under study or (2) the standard treatment carries significant risk or toxicity.

3. Research Involving Greater Than Minimal Risk and No Prospect of Direct Benefit to the Individual Subjects but Likely to Yield Generalizable Knowledge About the Subject's Disorder or Condition (45 CFR 46.406, 21 CFR 50.53)

It is important to note that research cannot be conducted on healthy control subjects under this category because they do not have a disorder or condition. In advice from the OHRP, however, a genetic propensity to a disease may be construed as a condition. It might, then, be possible to conduct research on a child at risk of malignant hyperthermia under this category, even if the diagnosis had not yet been firmly established.

An additional requirement for research in this category is that the intervention or procedure presents experiences to the subject that are reasonably commensurate with those inherent in his or her actual or expected medical, dental, psychological, social, or educational situations. Thus, a child with leukemia might be able to undergo bone marrow aspiration as part of a research study as this is consistent with the child's actual medical experiences; a liver biopsy, on the other hand, probably could not be justified.

For an IRB to approve research under this category, two additional findings must be made. The risk must represent only a minor increase over minimal risk, and the IRB must find that the research is likely to yield generalizable knowledge about the subject's disorder or condition that is of vital importance for the understanding or amelioration of that condition. Many IRBs have difficulty applying these statutory requirements because there

*CFR is the abbreviation for the Code of Federal Regulations.

is little guidance to help with the interpretation of "minor increase over minimal risk" and "vital importance." Further guidance from the OHRP is anticipated.

Finally, as an added protection for children in whom research is being conducted under this category, the written permission of both parents is required if they are reasonably available.

4. Research Not Otherwise Approvable That Presents an Opportunity to Understand, Prevent, or Alleviate a Serious Problem Affecting the Health or Welfare of Children (45 CFR 46.407 and 21 CFR 50.54)

Research in this category cannot be approved by local IRBs but must be referred to OHRP or the FDA for consideration by a panel of experts, as well as an opportunity for public review and comment.

There has not been extensive case law interpreting these regulations governing research in children, but an important case was decided by the Maryland Supreme Court. In *Grimes v. Kennedy Krieger Institute* (366 Md 29, 782 A2d 807, 2001), the plaintiffs were children enrolled in a study to evaluate different methods of lead abatement in the Baltimore area. The plaintiffs alleged that they were encouraged to remain in the study houses so that their lead levels could be monitored over time even when there was knowledge that lead had not been completely removed. In addition, one child was found to have a significant elevation in his blood lead level, and the parents were never informed of this finding. The trial court found in favor of Kennedy Krieger Institute on the basis that the researchers had no duty to warn the subjects about the presence of lead dust. The court of appeals reversed and held that the federal regulations governing research may create an affirmative duty for researchers that are enforceable in state negligence actions. More important, the trial court stated the following:

In our view, otherwise healthy children should not be subjects of non-therapeutic research that has the potential to be harmful to the child. It is first and foremost the responsibility of the researcher and the research entity to see to the harmlessness of such non-therapeutic research. Consent of parents can never relieve the researchers of this duty (366 Md 29, 782 A2d 807, 2001).

The court further stated:

We hold that in Maryland a parent, appropriate relative, or other appropriate surrogate cannot consent to the participation of a child or other person under legal disability in non-therapeutic research or studies in which there is any risk of injury or damage to the health of the subject (366 Md 29, 782 A2d 807, 2001).

This latter holding has engendered considerable concern in the pediatric research community. There are many currently approved studies in institutions across the United States in which children are enrolled in nontherapeutic studies. Measurements of certain physiologic functions (e.g., nerve conduction studies or electromyograms) that do not lengthen the duration of anesthesia have been seen by many IRBs as constituting minimal risk. Under the Maryland holding, such studies are not approvable because they are nontherapeutic. At the time of this writing, the Maryland standard has not been adopted in any other jurisdictions.

■ DEATH AND ORGAN DONATION

For centuries, the definition of *death* was based on the cessation of respiration and heartbeat. With the advent of the modern intensive care unit with respirators and extracorporeal membrane oxygenation devices, this definition was no longer useful. In 1974, the House of Delegates of the American Medical Association recognized a definition of *death* based on the irreversible cessation of all brain functions.

When death is declared, there is no longer a patient but only a dead body. This is so even if heartbeat and respirations and other functions are preserved while awaiting the harvesting of organs for transplantation. Insurance companies cease to pay for any medical or surgical treatments once death has been declared. If there is any payment for the services rendered to a dead body to preserve organs for transplantation, it is from the insurance company of the recipients.

An ethical dilemma that occurred at the Children's Hospital of Pittsburgh, which is likely to occur elsewhere (if it has not already), is when the parent of a child who has been declared dead but whose heartbeat and respirations are being maintained for transplantation wants to be present when the organs are harvested. Despite the medical acceptance of brain criteria for death, it is difficult for some parents to fully grasp this concept when their child's body remains warm and pink and has a pulse. At this institution, this dilemma was handled through counseling of the family and the nursing and support staff so that a solution was found that was acceptable to all. This situation may well illustrate the increasingly complicated and fascinating legal and ethical dilemmas that pediatric anesthesiologists will face over the next decade.

■ SUMMARY

The practice of pediatric anesthesiology not only requires an extensive knowledge of pediatrics and the principles of anesthesia but also demands an understanding of basic legal and ethical concepts. Although it is unpleasant to contemplate the possibility of a lawsuit, a basic understanding of the elements that must be proved by a malpractice plaintiff may provide some reassurance that merely having been named does not mean that the plaintiff will prevail. Pediatric anesthesiology is an exciting, fluid, and developing field, and an understanding of regulations governing research with children provides a foundation for contributing to the knowledge of an interesting and essential field that delivers excellent health care to children.

Appendix A Pediatric Drug Dosages

Franklyn P. Cladis

Generic Name (Trade Name)	Route	Dose	Indication	Side Effects
Acetaminophen (Tylenol)	PO PR	10 to 15 mg/kg q 4 to 6 hr 20 to 40 mg/kg initial dose, then 20 mg/kg q 6 hr	Pain/fever	
Adenosine	IV	0.1 mg/kg bolus; if not effective, 0.2 mg/kg (12 mg maximum single dose)	SVT	Flushing, chest pain, bronchospasm
Albuterol	Nebulized	0.15 mg/kg in 2 mL normal saline solution	Bronchospasm	Tachycardia
Alfentanil	IV	10 to 150 mcg/kg bolus 0.5 to 3 mcg/kg per min	Anesthesia Adjunct for anesthesia maintenance	Apnea, bradycardia
Alprostadil	IV	0.05 to 0.1 mcg/kg per min	Patency of ductus arteriosus	Fever, apnea, arrhythmias
Aminocaproic acid (Amicar)	IV	100 mg/kg bolus, infusion 30 mg/kg per hr	Excessive bleeding from fibrinolysis	Hypotension, bradycardia, arrhythmias
Aminophylline	PO, IV	100 mg/kg load: 100 mg/kg dose every 6 hr 5 mg/kg load, infusion 1 mg/kg per hr	Bronchospasm	Arrhythmias
Amiodarone	IV	5 mg/kg bolus slowly, infusion 5 to 10 mcg/kg per min	Ventricular arrhythmias	Hypotension, arrhythmias (torsades de pointes)
Ampicillin	IV	50 mg/kg	Endocarditis prophylaxis	
Aprotinin (Trasylol)	IV load Load IV infusion	10,000 units test done, 30,000 units/kg over 30 min 30,000 units/kg in the pump prime 10,000 to 30,000 units/kg per hr (turn off during cardiopulmonary bypass and at end of surgery)	To decrease bleeding, used mostly in cardiac surgery	Anaphylaxis, celite ACT prolonged by aprotinin
Atracurium (Tracrium)	IV	0.5 mg/kg intubation 5 to 15 mcg/kg per min infusion	Neuromuscular blocker	Histamine release
Atropine	IV	0.01 to 0.02 mg/kg	Bradycardia	
Bretylium	IV	5 to 10 mg/kg load, q 10 to 20 min for a total of 30 mg/kg 1 to 2 mg/min infusion (≥12 yr old)	Refractory ventricular tachycardia and fibrillation	Hypotension
Bupivacaine (Marcaine)	Neuraxial, peripheral	2.5 mg/kg	Epidural, caudal, peripheral nerve blockade	Seizures, arrhythmias
Butorphanol	IV	10 mcg/kg	Pain/fever	CNS depression, respiratory depression
Caffeine	PO, IV	5 to 10 mg/kg as caffeine base (10 to 20 mg/kg as caffeine citrate)	Apnea of prematurity	Tachyarrhythmias
Calcium chloride	IV	10 to 20 mg/kg (via central venous line)	Hypocalcemia, hypotension	Tissue necrosis
Calcium gluconate	IV	30 to 45 mg/kg	Hypocalcemia, hypotension	Tissue necrosis
Cefazolin (Ancef)	IV	25 mg/kg	Wound prophylaxis	
Chloral hydrate	PO/PR	50 to 75 mg/kg	Sedation	Arrhythmias
Cimetidine (Tagamet)	IV/PO	5 to 15 mg/kg q 6 to 12 hr	Gastric pH control	Confusion, headache
Cisatracurium (Nimbex)	IV	0.1 to 0.2 mg/kg bolus, infusion 1 to 5 mcg/kg per min	Neuromuscular blockade	
Clindamycin (Cleocin)	IV	5 to 10 mg/kg (slowly) q 6 to 8 hr 20 mg/kg (slowly) for SBE prophylaxis	Wound prophylaxis (penicillin [PCN] allergic)	Thrombophlebitis, hypotension
Clonidine	Neuraxial	1 to 3 mcg/kg	Enhance neuraxial blockade	Hypotension, sedation
Codeine	PO	0.5 to 1 mg/kg	Pain	Sedation, nausea, vomiting, respiratory depression
Dantrolene	IV	2.5 mg/kg to maximum 10 mg/kg	Malignant hyperthermia	Slow to solubilize, drowsiness, muscle weakness

Continued

Generic Name (Trade Name)	Route	Dose	Indication	Side Effects
Desmopressin (DDAVP)	IV	0.3 mcg/kg (over 15 min)	Platelet dysfunction, von Willebrand disease	Hyponatremia, hypertension, flushing
	IV	2 to 4 mcg/day in 2 doses (≥12 years old)	Diabetes insipidus	Hyponatremia, hypertension, flushing
Dexamethasone (Decadron)	IV	0.5 to 1 mg/kg (maximum 16 to 20 mg)	Croup, airway edema, cerebral edema	Hypertension, headache, hyperglycemia
Diazepam (Valium)	PO	0.2 to 0.3 mg/kg 45 to 60 minutes preprocedure	Preoperative sedation	Hypotension, bradycardia
	IV	0.05 to 0.3 mg/kg		
Digoxin	IV	0.03 mg/kg <2 years old 0.01 to 0.04 mg/kg >2 years old (digitalizing dose; $^1/_2$ dose initially then $^1/_4$ q 6 hr × 2)	SVT, CHF	Arrhythmias, atrioventricular block
	IV maintenance	2 to 10 mcg/kg per day (IV dose = 75% oral dose)		
Diphenylhydantoin (Dilantin)	IV	12 to 20 mg/kg (over 30 min to avoid hypotension; limit infusion rate to 50 mg/min)	Seizure, digoxin toxicity	Hypotension, skin necrosis at IV site, ataxia, gingival hyperplasia
Diphenhydramine (Benadryl)	IV	0.5 to 2 mg/kg (maximum single dose 50 mg) (maximum 150 mg/day if <12 years old, 300 mg if >12 years old)	Sedation, pruritus, acute dystonic reactions	Paradoxical excitement
Dobutamine	IV	2 to 15 mcg/kg per min (maximum dose 40 mcg/kg/min)	Heart failure	Increased heart rate, ectopy, hypotension
Dopamine	IV	2.5 to 20 mcg/kg per min	Heart failure, increased renal blood flow—low dose	Increased heart rate, ectopy
Doxacurium	IV	0.05 to 0.1 mg/kg intubation	Neuromuscular blocker	
Droperidol	IV	10 to 75 mcg/kg (maximum dose 1.25 mg)	Antiemetic	Hypotension, arrhythmias (FDA warning)
d-Tubocurarine	IV	0.3 to 0.6 mg/kg	Neuromuscular blocker	Histamine release
Edrophonium (Enlon, Tensilon)	IV	0.5 to 1.0 mg/kg	Neuromuscular blocking reversal agent	Bradycardia
EMLA cream	Topical	0 to 3 mo maximum 1 g (10 cm^2), 3 to 12 mo maximum 2 g (20 cm^2), 1 to 6 years old maximum 10 g (100 cm^2), 7 to 12 years old maximum 20 g (200 cm^2)	Dermal anesthesia for venipuncture	Methemoglobinemia, blanching of skin
Ephedrine	IV	0.02 to 0.2 mg/kg	Hypotension	Bradycardia, hypotension, confusion
Epinephrine (Adrenalin)	IV	10 mcg/kg q 3 to 5 min, infusion 0.01 to 1 mcg/kg per min	Cardiac arrest, hypotension, heart failure	Tachycardia
	Endotracheal	100 mcg/kg		
Epinephrine, racemic	Nebulized	<2 years old 0.25 mL, >2 years old 0.5 mL of 2.25% solution in 3 mL normal saline solution	Upper airway edema	Tachycardia
Esmolol	IV	500 mcg/kg per min loading dose for one minute, 50 to 300 mcg/kg per min infusion	Hypertension, tachycardia	Bradycardia
Etomidate	IV	0.3 mg/kg (0.2 to 0.6 mg/kg)	Anesthetic induction	Myoclonus, pain on injection, adrenal suppression
Fentanyl	IV	0.5 to 3 mcg/kg (may repeat q 30 min)	Analgesia and sedation	Apnea, cough, laryngospasm, chest wall rigidity, bradycardia
		2 to 10 mcg/kg bolus, infusion 1 to 4 mcg/kg per hr	Adjunct for induction and maintenance of anesthesia	
Fentanyl (Oralet, Actiq)	PO	5 to 15 mcg/kg (200 mcg is smallest dose)	Sedation preoperatively	Sedation, pruritis, oxygen desaturation
Flumazenil	IV	0.01 mg/kg (maximum dose 0.2 mg) q 1 min up to 1 mg (maximum cumulative dose)	Benzodiazepine antagonist	Altered blood pressure, arrhythmias
Furosemide (Lasix)	IV	1 to 2 mg/kg q 6 hr (6 mg/kg per day maximum dose)	Diuretic	Hypokalemia, hyponatremia, potential ototoxicity
Gentamicin	IV	1.5 to 2.5 mg/kg	Endocarditis prophylaxis	Nephrotoxicity, ototoxicity, potentiate neuromuscular blockade
Glucagon	IM, IV	<20 kg 0.5 mg, >20 kg 1 mg	Antihypoglycemic, relaxant for gastrointestinal tract	Tachycardia
Glucose	IV	200 mg/kg, 4 mg/kg per min	Hypoglycemia	
Glycopyrrolate (Robinul)	IV	0.005 to 0.01 mg/kg	Antisialagogue, bradycardia	Tachycardia, flushing
Hydralazine	IV	0.05 to 0.3 mg/kg (15 min onset)	Hypertension	Tachycardia, flushing
Hydrocortisone (Solu-Cortef)	IV	1 to 2 mg/kg q 6 hr	Adrenal suppression, asthma	Hypertension, hyperglycemia
Hydromorphone (Dilaudid)	IV	0.01 to 0.015 mg/kg	Analgesia	Sedation, nausea, vomiting, respiratory depression

Generic Name (Trade Name)	Route	Dose	Indication	Side Effects
Hydroxyzine (Atarax, Vistaril)	IM	0.5 to 1 mg/kg q 4 to 6 hr	Sedation	Drowsiness
Ibuprofen	PO	10 mg/kg q 6 hr	Analgesic/ antiinflammatory	Inhibition of platelet aggregation, renal failure
Inamrinone	IV	Load 3 to 4.5 mg/kg over 30 min, then 3 to 10 mcg/kg per min infusion	Heart failure	Arrhythmias, thrombocytopenia
Insulin, regular	IV	Load 0.01 to 0.1 unit/kg, infuse 0.1 unit/kg per hr	Hyperglycemia, DKA	Hypoglycemia
Isoproterenol (Isuprel)	IV	0.05 to 1 mcg/kg per min	Bradycardia	Tachycardia, ventricular arrhythmias, hypotension
Ketamine	IV	0.5 to 1 mg/kg	Sedation	
	IV	1 to 2 mg/kg	Anesthesia	Hallucinations, tachycardia, may increase intracranial and intraocular hypersalivation, pressure, apnea, vomiting
	IM	3 to 5 mg/kg	Sedation	
	IM	5 to 10 mg/kg	Anesthesia	
	PO	5 to 10 mg/kg	Sedation	
Ketorolac (Toradol)	IV	0.5 to 1 mg/kg	Analgesia	Inhibition of platelet aggregation, renal failure
Labetalol	IV	0.2 to 0.5 mg/kg (q 5 min)	Tachycardia, hypertension	Hypotension, bradycardia
Lidocaine	IV	1 mg/kg	Ventricular arrhythmias	Seizures
	IV	20 to 50 mcg/kg per min infusion		
Lidocaine	Intratracheal	3 to 4 mg/kg	Topical anesthesia	Arrhythmias, seizures
Lorazepam	IV	0.05 to 0.1 mg/kg (maximum 4 mg)	Sedation, anxiolysis	Neurotoxicity in neonates (preservative)
Mannitol	IV	0.25 to 1 g/kg (over 20 min)	Increased intracranial pressure, diuresis	
Meperidine (Demerol)	IV	1 to 2 mg/kg	Analgesia, preoperative sedation	Accumulation of normeperidine in renal dysfunction
	IM	1 to 2 mg/kg		
Methadone	IV	0.1 mg/kg	Analgesia	Sedation, nausea, vomiting, respiratory depression
Methohexital (Brevital)	IV	1 to 2 mg/kg	Anesthesia	Apnea
	PR	25 to 35 mg/kg (10% solution)	Sedation/anesthesia	
Methylene blue	IV	1 to 2 mg/kg may repeat in 1 hr	Antidote for drug-induced methemoglobinemia	Stains skin
Methylprednisolone (Solu-Medrol)	IV	2 mg/kg load, 0.5 to 1 mg/kg q 6 hr	Asthma exacerbation	Hypertension, psychosis, glucose intolerance
	IV	30 mg/kg over 15 min, infusion 5.4 mg/kg per hr for 23 hr	Acute spinal cord injury	
Metoclopramide (Reglan)	IV	0.1 to 0.2 mg/kg	Antiemetic	Extrapyramidal reactions
Midazolam (Versed)	IV	0.05 to 0.1 mg/kg	Sedation	Hypotension in neonates, hiccups
	IN	0.2 to 0.3 mg/kg (5 to 10 min onset)	Sedation	Nasal irritation
	PO	0.5 to 1 mg/kg (20 to 30 min onset)	Sedation	Bad taste
Milrinone	IV	50 mcg/kg load, infusion 0.25 to 0.75 mcg/kg per min	Heart failure	Hypotension
Mivacurium	IV	0.2 to 0.3 mg/kg intubation; 10 to 15 mcg/kg per min infusion	Neuromuscular blocker	Histamine release
Morphine	IV/IM	0.05 to 0.1 mg/kg	Analgesia	Histamine release, apnea, sedation, nausea, vomiting
Naloxone (Narcan)	IV/IM	1 to 10 mcg/kg titrated	Apnea/sedation after opioids	Hypertension
Naproxen (Naprosyn)	PO	5 to 10 mg/kg q 12 hr	Analgesia, anti-inflammatory	Inhibition of platelet aggregation, renal failure
Neostigmine	IV	0.05 to 0.07 mg/kg	Neuromuscular blockade reversal	Bradycardia, secretions
Nicardipine	IV	0.5 to 5 mcg/kg per min	Induced hypotension, hypertension	Hypotension
Nitroglycerin	IV	0.5 to 3 mcg/kg per min	Venodilation, myocardial ischemia	Hypotension
Nitroprusside	IV	0.5 to 10 mcg/kg per min	Induced hypotension, hypertension	Cyanide toxicity
Norepinephrine (Levophed)	IV	0.1 to 1 mcg/kg per min	Hypotension	Arrhythmias
Ondansetron (Zofran)	IV	0.05 to 0.1 mg/kg (maximum 4 mg)	Antiemetic	Headache
Oxycodone	PO	0.05 to 0.15 mg/kg q 4 to 6 hr	Analgesia	Sedation, nausea, vomiting, respiratory depression
Pancuronium (Pavulon)	IV	0.08 to 0.15 mg/kg	Neuromuscular blocker	Tachycardia
Pentobarbital (Nembutal)	IV	1 to 3 mg/kg (maximum 100 mg)	Sedation	Respiratory depression, apnea

Continued

Generic Name (Trade Name)	Route	Dose	Indication	Side Effects
Phenylephrine (Neo-Synephrine)	IV	1 to 10 mcg/kg	Hypotension	Hypertension
	IV	0.1 to 0.5 mcg/kg/min infusion		
Potassium chloride	IV	0.5 mEq/kg (via CVP over 30 to 45 min)	Hypokalemia	Arrhythmias with rapid infusion
Procainamide	IV	3 to 6 mg/kg per dose over 5 min q 5 to 10 min (maximum 15 mg/kg), infusion 20 mcg/kg per min	Ventricular and atrial arrhythmias	Hypotension, QT prolongation
Prochlorperazine (Compazine)	IV/IM	0.1 to 0.15 mg/kg q 6 hr (IV not recommended)	Antiemetic	High incidence of extrapyramidal reactions, sedation, hypotension
	PO/PR	0.4 mg/kg per day divided q 6 to 8 hr		
Promethazine (Phenergan)	IV/IM	0.25 to 0.5 mg/kg q 4 to 6 hr	Antiemetic	Sedation
Propofol	IV	2 to 3 mg/kg; 100 to 200 mcg/kg per min infusion	Anesthesia	Apnea, hypotension
Propranolol (Inderal)	IV	0.01 to 0.1 mg/kg (over 10 min)	Tachycardia, hypertension	Hypotension, bradycardia
Prostaglandin E_1	IV	0.05 to 0.1 mcg/kg per min	Maintain patent ductus arteriosus	Fever, apnea
Protamine	IV	1 mg for every 100 U of heparin to be neutralized	Heparin neutralization	Hypotension, bradycardia, pulmonary hypertension
Ranitidine (Zantac)	IV	1 to 1.5 mg/kg per day divided q 8 hr	Gastric pH control	
	PO	2 to 3 mg/kg per day divided q 12 hr		
Remifentanil	IV	1 to 4 mcg/kg bolus, infusion 0.1 to 0.5 mcg/kg per min	Analgesia, adjunct to anesthesia	Apnea, bradycardia
Rocuronium (Zemuron)	IV	0.6 to 1.2 mg/kg	Neuromuscular blocker	
Scopolamine	IV/IM	6 to 10 mcg/kg (maximum 0.3 mg/dose)	Antisialagogue, amnestic	Tachycardia, confusion
Sodium bicarbonate	IV	0.5 to 1 mEq/kg	Metabolic acidosis	
Succinylcholine	IV	1.5 to 2 mg/kg (fast onset)	Neuromuscular blocker (depolarizing)	Hyperkalemia, malignant hyperthermia trigger
	IM	5 mg/kg	Neuromuscular blocker	
Sufentanil	IV	0.25 to 1 mcg/kg bolus	Anesthesia	Apnea, chest wall rigidity
	IV	0.1 to 1 mcg/kg per hr infusion	Adjunct for maintenance of anesthesia	
Thiopental	IV	3 to 7 mg/kg	Anesthesia	Apnea
Vancomycin	IV	10 mg/kg (over 30 min)	Wound prophylaxis	Hypotension, histamine release, red man syndrome
Vasopressin	IV	0.0005 to 0.005 unit/kg per min	Vasopressor, diabetes insipidus	Hypertension
Vecuronium (Norcuron)	IV	0.07 to 0.2 mg/kg	Neuromuscular blocker	
		0.8 to 1 mcg/kg per min infusion		
Verapamil	IV	0.1 to 0.3 mg/kg (1 to 15 years old)	SVT, CHF	Bradycardia hypotension

IM, intramuscular; IN, intranasal; IV, intravenous; CHF, congestive heart failure; PR, per rectum; SVT, supraventricular tachycardia; DKA, diabetic ketoacidosis; PO, orally; ACT, activated clotting time.

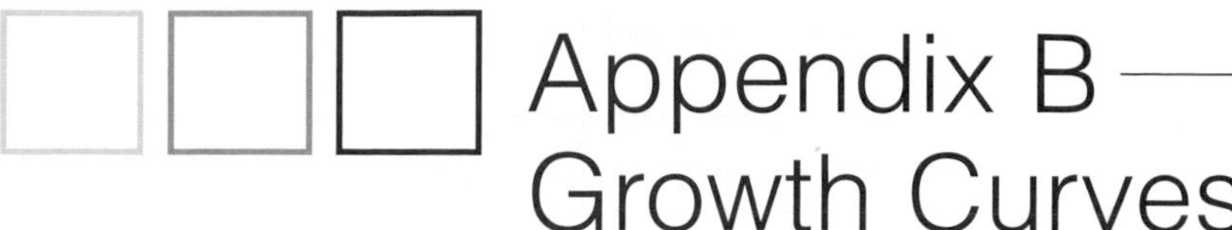

Appendix B
Growth Curves

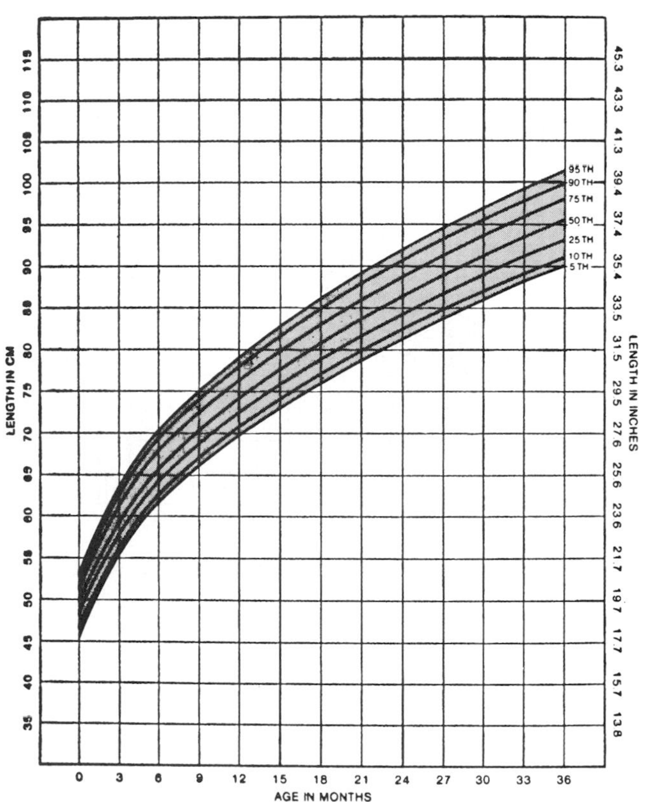

■ **FIGURE B–1.** Girls from birth to 36 months: Length by age.

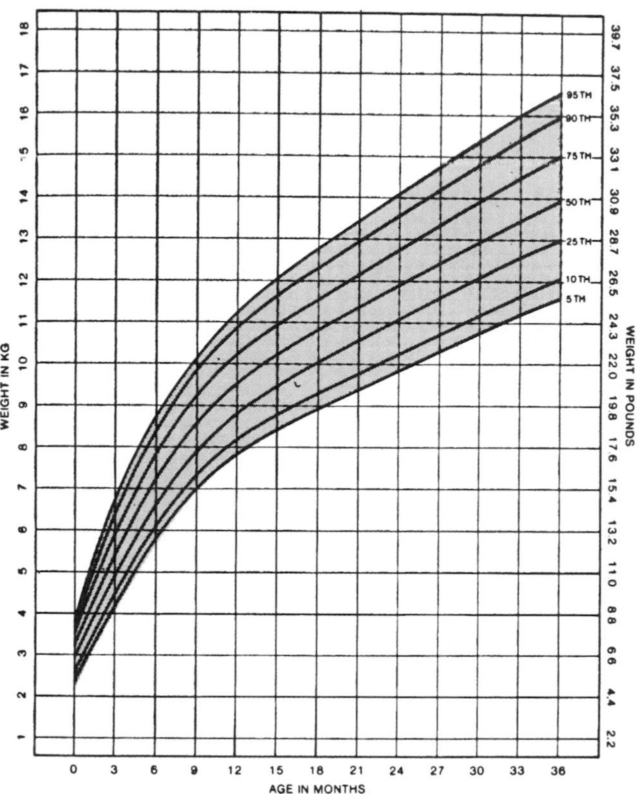

■ **FIGURE B–2.** Girls from birth to 36 months: Weight by age.

GIRLS STATURE BY AGE PERCENTILES
AGES 2-18 YEARS

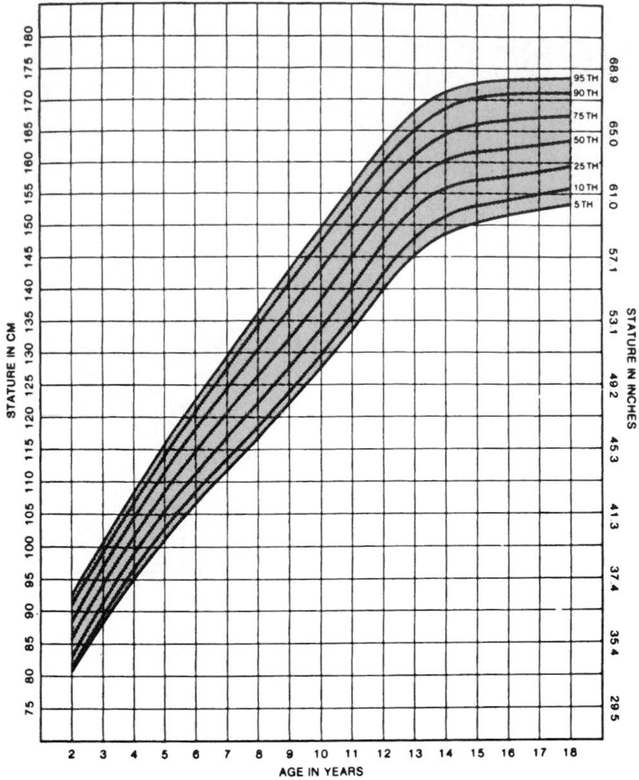

■ **FIGURE B–3.** Girls from 2 to 18 years: Stature by age.

GIRLS WEIGHT BY AGE PERCENTILES
AGES 2-18 YEARS

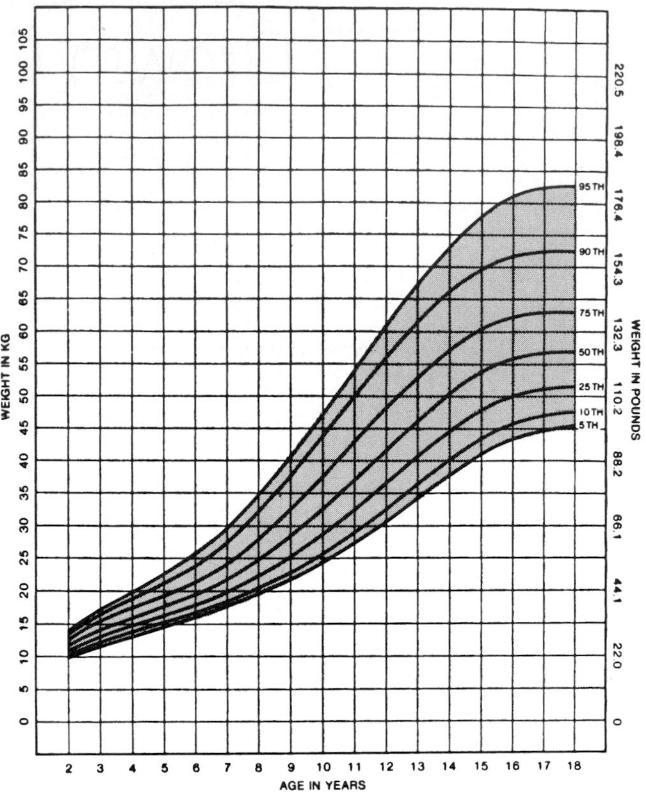

■ **FIGURE B–4.** Girls from 2 to 18 years: Weight by age.

BOYS LENGTH BY AGE PERCENTILES
AGES BIRTH-36 MONTHS

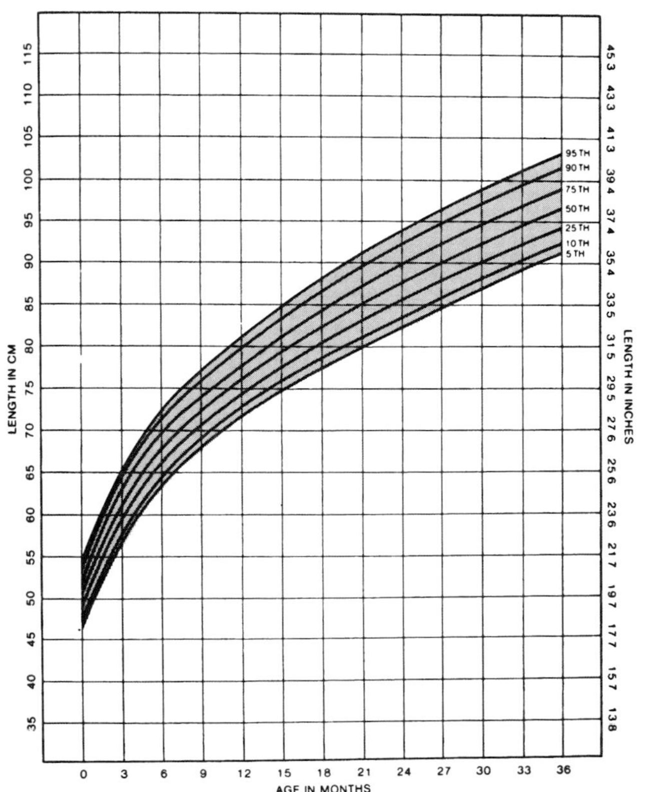

■ **FIGURE B–5.** Boys from birth to 36 months: Length by age.

BOYS WEIGHT BY AGE PERCENTILES
AGES BIRTH-36 MONTHS

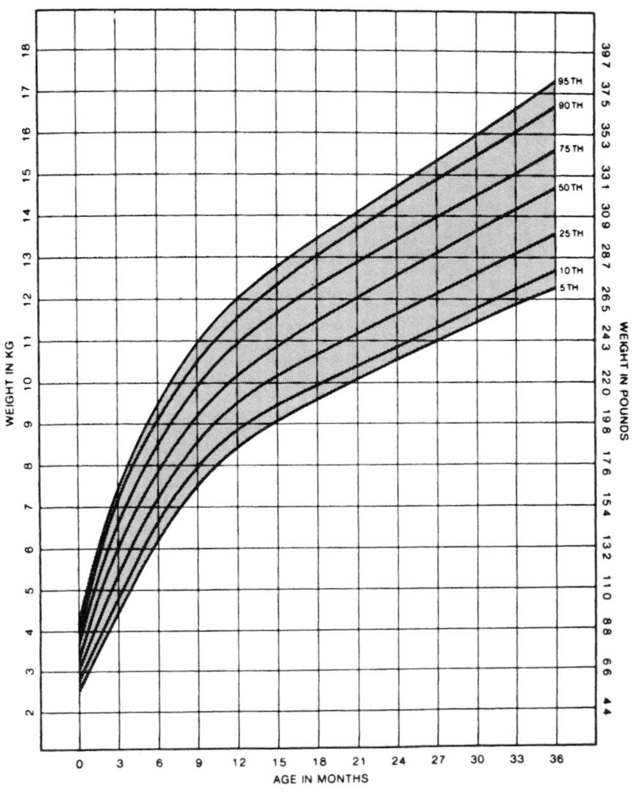

■ **FIGURE B–6.** Boys from birth to 36 months: Weight by age.

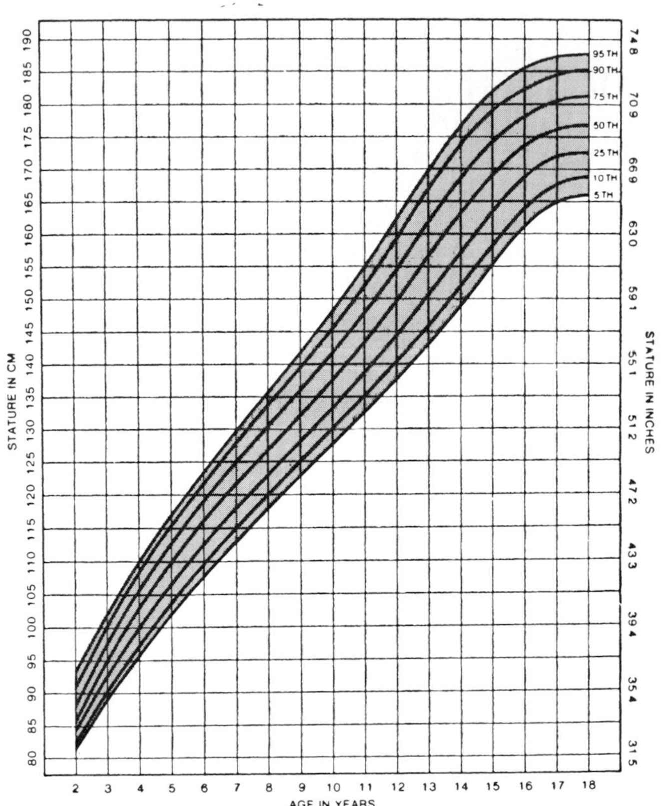

■ **FIGURE B–7.** Boys from 2 to 18 years: Stature by age.

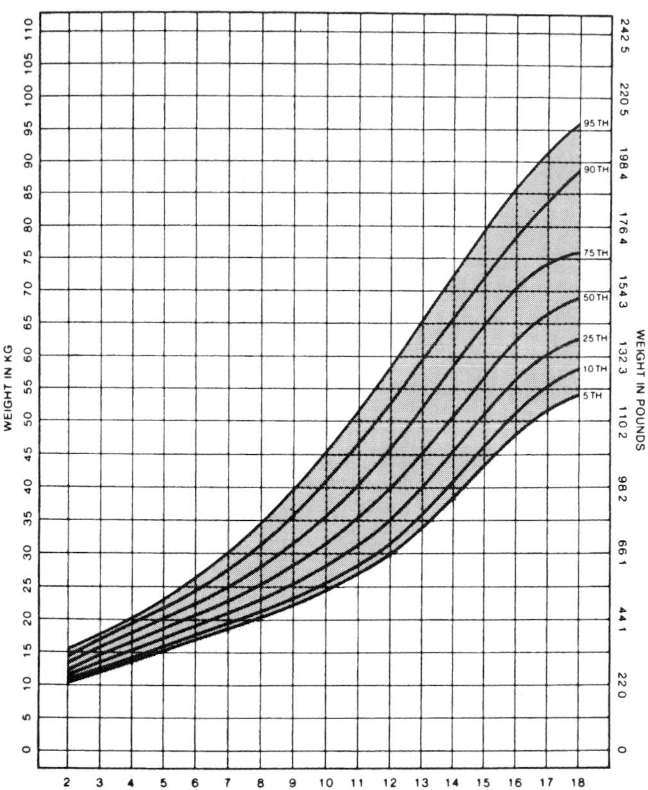

■ **FIGURE B–8.** Boys from 2 to 18 years: Weight by age.

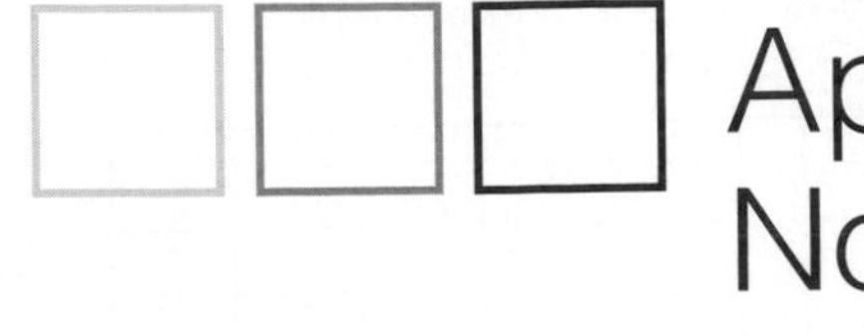

Appendix C Normal Pulmonary Function Values

■ **TABLE C–1.** Vital capacity (VC) in relation to body height in boys

Height (cm)	VC (mL)		
	Mean	*Lower Limits*	*Upper Limits*
115	1,418	1,238	1,623
116	1,452	1,269	1,662
118	1,523	1,330	1,743
120	1,596	1,394	1,827
122	1,671	1,460	1,912
124	1,748	1,527	2,001
126	1,828	1,597	2,092
128	1,909	1,668	2,186
130	1,994	1,742	2,282
132	2,080	1,817	2,381
134	2,169	1,895	2,482
136	2,260	1,974	2,587
138	2,354	1,056	2,694
140	2,450	2,140	2,804
142	2,548	2,226	2,917
144	2,649	2,315	3,032
146	2,753	2,405	3,151
148	2,859	2,498	3,273
150	2,968	2,593	3,397
152	3,079	2,690	3,524
154	3,193	2,790	3,655
156	3,310	2,892	3,788
158	3,429	2,996	3,925
160	3,551	3,102	4,065
162	3,676	3,211	4,207
164	3,803	3,323	4,353
166	3,934	3,437	4,503
168	4,067	3,553	4,655
170	4,203	3,672	4,811
172	4,342	3,793	4,970
174	4,484	3,917	5,132
176	4,629	4,044	5,298
178	4,776	4,173	5,467
180	4,927	4,304	5,639

Formula: $\log y = a + b \cdot \log x$;
y = VC (mL); x = Body height (cm);
$\log VC (mL) = -2.5768 + 2.7799 \cdot \log height (cm)$;
$SD \log y \cdot x = \pm 0.0294$; $n = 86$; $r = +0.96$.

■ **TABLE C–2.** Vital capacity (VC) in relation to body height in girls

Height (cm)	VC (mL)		
	Mean	*Lower Limits*	*Upper Limits*
115	1,365	1,128	1,651
116	1,396	1,154	1,689
118	1,461	1,207	1,767
120	1,527	1,262	1,847
122	1,595	1,318	1,930
124	1,665	1,376	2,014
126	1,736	1,435	2,101
128	1,810	1,496	2,190
130	1,886	1,559	2,281
132	1,963	1,623	2,375
134	2,043	1,688	2,471
136	2,124	1,756	2,569
138	2,207	1,824	2,670
140	2,293	1,895	2,774
142	2,380	1,967	2,879
144	2,469	2,041	2,987
146	2,561	2,117	3,098
148	2,654	2,194	3,211
150	2,750	2,273	3,327
152	2,848	2,354	3,445
154	2,948	2,436	3,566
156	3,050	2,521	3,689
158	3,154	2,607	3,815
160	3,260	2,695	3,944
162	3,369	2,784	4,075
164	3,479	2,876	4,209
166	3,592	2,969	4,346
168	3,708	3,065	4,485
170	3,825	3,162	4,628
172	3,945	3,261	4,772
174	4,067	3,362	4,920
176	4,191	3,465	5,071
178	4,318	3,569	5,224
180	4,447	3,676	5,380

Formula: $\log y = a + b \cdot \log x$;
y = VC (mL); x = Body height (cm);
$\log VC (mL) = -2.2970 + 2.6361 \cdot \log x$;
$SD \log y \cdot x = \pm 0.0415$; $n = 87$; $r = +0.94$.

From Zapletal A, Sambanek M, Paul T: *Lung function in children and adolescents. Progress in respiration research*, vol 22. New York, 1987, S Karger.

TABLE C–3. Total lung capacity measured in a body plethysmograph (TLC_{box}) in relation to body height in boys

Height (cm)	TLC_{box} (mL)		
	Mean	*Lower Limits*	*Upper Limits*
115	1,966	1,732	2,232
116	2,011	1,771	2,283
118	2,101	1,851	2,385
120	2,194	1,932	2,490
122	2,289	2,016	2,599
124	2,387	2,102	2,709
126	2,487	2,109	2,823
128	2,589	2,281	2,940
130	2,695	2,374	3,059
132	2,803	2,469	3,182
134	2,913	2,566	3,307
136	3,026	2,666	3,436
138	3,142	2,767	3,567
140	3,260	2,872	3,701
142	3,381	2,978	3,839
144	3,505	3,087	3,979
146	3,631	3,199	4,123
148	3,761	3,313	4,269
150	3,893	3,429	4,419
152	4,028	3,548	4,572
154	4,165	3,669	4,729
156	4,306	3,793	4,888
158	4,449	3,919	5,051
160	4,595	4,048	5,217
162	4,744	4,179	5,386
164	4,896	4,313	5,558
166	5,051	4,449	5,734
168	5,209	4,587	5,914
170	5,370	4,730	6,096
172	5,534	4,874	6,282
174	5,701	5,021	6,472
176	5,870	5,171	6,665
178	6,043	5,323	6,861
180	6,220	5,468	7,061

Formula: $\log y = a + b \cdot \log x$;
$y = TLC_{box}$ (mL); x = Body height (cm);
$\log TLC_{box}$ (mL) $= -2.0018 + 2.5698 \cdot \log$ height (cm);
SD $\log y \cdot x = \pm 0.0276$; $n = 82$; $r = +0.96$.

TABLE C–4. Total lung capacity measured in a body plethysmograph (TLC_{box}) in relation to body height in girls

Height (cm)	TLC_{box} (mL)		
	Mean	*Lower Limits*	*Upper Limits*
115	1,860	1,575	2,196
116	1,902	1,611	2,245
118	1,987	1,683	2,346
120	2,075	1,758	2,450
122	2,166	1,834	2,556
124	2,258	1,913	2,666
126	2,353	1,993	2,778
128	2,451	2,076	2,893
130	2,551	2,161	3,011
132	2,653	2,247	3,132
134	2,758	2,336	3,255
136	2,865	2,427	3,382
138	2,975	2,520	3,512
140	3,087	2,615	3,644
142	3,202	2,712	3,780
144	3,319	2,812	3,918
146	3,439	2,914	4,060
148	3,562	3,017	4,205
150	3,687	3,124	4,353
152	3,815	3,232	4,504
154	3,946	3,343	4,658
156	4,079	3,456	4,816
158	4,216	3,571	4,976
160	4,354	3,689	5,140
162	4,496	3,809	5,307
164	4,640	3,931	5,478
166	4,787	4,055	5,651
168	4,937	4,183	5,828
170	5,090	4,312	6,009
172	5,247	4,444	6,193
174	5,405	4,578	6,380
176	5,566	4,715	6,570
178	5,730	4,854	6,765
180	5,898	4,996	6,962

Formula: $\log y = a + b \cdot \log x$;
$y = TLC_{box}$ (mL); x = Body height (cm);
$\log TLC_{box}$ (mL) $= -2.0377 + 2.5755 \cdot \log$ height (cm);
SD $\log y \cdot x = \pm 0.0361$; $n = 72$; $r = +0.96$.

■ TABLE C–5. Functional residual capacity measured in a body plethysmograph (FRC_{box}) in relation to body height in boys

Height (cm)	FRC_{box} (mL)		
	Mean	*Lower Limits*	*Upper Limits*
115	941	790	1,121
116	963	809	1,148
118	1,008	846	1,201
120	1,054	885	1,256
122	1,101	925	1,312
124	1,150	965	1,370
126	1,200	1,007	1,429
128	1,251	1,050	1,490
130	1,303	1,094	1,553
132	1,357	1,140	1,617
134	1,413	1,186	1,683
136	1,469	1,233	1,750
138	1,527	1,282	1,819
140	1,587	1,332	1,890
142	1,648	1,383	1,962
144	1,710	1,435	2,037
146	1,774	1,489	2,113
148	1,839	1,544	2,190
150	1,905	1,600	2,270
152	1,974	1,657	2,351
154	2,043	1,715	2,434
156	2,114	1,775	2,518
158	2,187	1,836	2,605
160	2,261	1,898	2,693
162	2,337	1,962	2,784
164	2,414	2,027	2,876
166	2,493	2,093	2,970
168	2,574	2,161	3,066
170	2,656	2,230	3,163
172	2,739	2,300	3,263
174	2,825	2,372	3,365
176	2,912	2,445	3,468
178	3,000	2,519	3,574
180	3,091	2,595	3,681

Formula: $\log y = a + b \cdot \log x$;
$y = FRC_{box}$ (mL); x = Body height (cm);
$\log FRC_{box}$ (mL) $= -2.4915 + 2.6523 \cdot \log$ height (cm);
SD $\log y \cdot x = \pm 0.0381$; $n = 82$; $r = +0.94$.

■ TABLE C–6. Functional residual capacity measured in a body plethysmograph (FRC_{box}) in relation to body height in girls

Height (cm)	FRC_{box} (mL)		
	Mean	*Lower Limits*	*Upper Limits*
115	906	707	1,160
116	926	723	1,186
118	969	756	1,241
120	1,012	790	1,296
122	1,057	825	1,354
124	1,103	861	1,412
126	1,150	898	1,473
128	1,198	936	1,535
130	1,248	974	1,598
132	1,299	1,014	1,663
134	1,351	1,055	1,730
136	1,404	1,097	1,799
138	1,459	1,139	1,869
140	1,515	1,183	1,940
142	1,572	1,228	2,014
144	1,631	1,273	2,089
146	1,691	1,320	2,165
148	1,752	1,368	2,244
150	1,815	1,417	2,324
152	1,879	1,467	2,406
154	1,944	1,518	2,489
156	2,011	1,570	2,575
158	2,079	1,623	2,662
160	2,148	1,677	2,751
162	2,219	1,733	2,842
164	2,292	1,789	2,935
166	2,365	1,847	3,029
168	2,441	1,906	3,126
170	2,517	1,966	3,224
172	2,596	2,027	3,324
174	2,675	2,089	3,426
176	2,756	2,152	3,530
178	2,839	2,217	3,636
180	2,923	2,283	3,744

Formula: $\log y = a + b \cdot \log x$;
$y = FRC_{box}$ (mL); x = Body height (cm);
$\log FRC_{box}$ (mL) $= -2.4314 + 2.6149 \cdot \log$ height (cm);
SD $\log y \cdot x = \pm 0.0538$; $n = 72$; $r = +0.91$.

■ TABLE C–7. Forced expiratory volume in the first second (FEV_1) in relation to body height in boys

	FEV_1 (mL)		
Height (cm)	*Mean*	*Lower Limits*	*Upper Limits*
115	1,135	952	1,352
116	1,163	976	1,386
118	1,222	1,025	1,456
120	1,282	1,076	1,528
122	1,345	1,128	1,602
124	1,409	1,182	1,679
126	1,475	1,238	1,758
128	1,544	1,295	1,839
130	1,614	1,354	1,923
132	1,686	1,415	2,009
134	1,761	1,478	2,098
136	1,837	1,542	2,189
138	1,916	1,608	2,283
140	1,997	1,676	2,380
142	2,080	1,746	2,479
144	2,165	1,817	2,580
146	2,253	1,891	2,685
148	2,343	1,966	2,792
150	2,435	2,043	2,901
152	2,529	2,123	3,014
154	2,626	2,204	3,129
156	2,725	2,287	3,248
158	2,827	2,372	3,369
160	2,931	2,460	3,493
162	3,038	2,549	3,620
164	3,147	2,641	3,749
166	3,258	2,734	3,882
168	3,372	2,830	4,018
170	3,489	2,928	4,157
172	3,608	3,028	4,299
174	3,730	3,130	4,445
176	3,854	3,235	4,593
178	3,982	3,342	4,744
180	4,112	3,451	4,899

Formula: $\log y = a + b \cdot \log x$;
$y = FEV_1$ (mL); x = Body height (cm);
$\log FEV_1$ (mL) = −2.8652 + 2.8729 · log height (cm);
SD $\log y \cdot x = \pm 0.0380$; n = 60; $r = +0.94$.

■ TABLE C–8. Forced expiratory volume in the first second (FEV_1) in relation to body height in girls

	FEV_1 (mL)		
Height (cm)	*Mean*	*Lower Limits*	*Upper Limits*
115	1,105	883	1,382
116	1,131	905	1,415
118	1,186	948	1,483
120	1,242	993	1,553
122	1,299	1,039	1,625
124	1,358	1,086	1,699
126	1,419	1,135	1,775
128	1,482	1,185	1,853
130	1,546	1,236	1,934
132	1,612	1,289	2,016
134	1,680	1,344	2,101
136	1,750	1,399	2,188
138	1,821	1,457	2,278
140	1,895	1,515	2,369
142	1,970	1,575	2,463
144	2,047	1,637	2,560
146	2,126	1,700	2,658
148	2,207	1,765	2,759
150	2,289	1,831	2,863
152	2,374	1,898	2,969
154	2,461	1,968	3,077
156	2,549	2,039	3,188
158	2,640	2,111	3,301
160	2,732	2,185	3,417
162	2,827	2,261	3,535
164	2,924	2,338	3,656
166	3,023	2,417	3,780
168	3,124	2,498	3,906
170	3,227	2,580	4,035
172	3,332	2,664	4,166
174	3,439	2,750	4,300
176	3,549	2,838	4,437
178	3,660	2,927	4,577
180	3,774	3,018	4,719

Formula: $\log y = a + b \cdot \log x$;
$y = FEV_1$ (mL); x = Body height (cm);
$\log FEV_1$ (mL) = −2.6056 + 2.7413 · log height (cm);
SD $\log y \cdot x = \pm 0.0483$; n = 51; $r = +0.93$.

■ TABLE C–9. Peak expiratory flow rate (PEFR) in relation to body height in boys and girls

Height (cm)	PEFR (L/sec)		
	Mean	*Lower Limits*	*Upper Limits*
115	2.85	2.05	3.96
116	2.91	2.09	4.04
118	3.03	2.18	4.21
120	3.15	2.26	4.38
122	3.27	2.35	4.55
124	3.40	2.44	4.73
126	3.53	2.54	4.91
128	3.66	2.63	5.09
130	3.80	2.73	5.28
132	3.94	2.83	5.47
134	4.08	2.93	5.67
136	4.22	3.04	5.87
138	4.37	3.14	6.08
140	4.52	3.25	6.28
142	4.67	3.36	6.50
144	4.83	3.47	6.71
146	4.99	3.59	6.93
148	5.15	3.70	7.16
150	5.31	3.82	7.39
152	5.48	3.94	7.62
154	5.65	4.07	7.86
156	5.83	4.19	8.10
158	6.00	4.32	8.34
160	6.18	4.45	8.59
162	6.36	4.58	8.85
164	6.55	4.71	9.11
166	6.74	4.85	9.37
168	6.93	4.99	9.64
170	7.13	5.13	9.91
172	7.32	5.27	10.18
174	7.53	5.41	10.46
176	7.73	5.56	10.75
178	7.94	5.71	11.03
180	8.15	5.86	11.33

Formula: $\log y = a + b \cdot \log x$;
y = PEFR (L/sec); x = Body height (cm);
log PEFR (L/sec) = −4.3722 + 2.3422 · log height (cm);
SD $\log y \cdot x = \pm 0.0717$; n = 76; $r = +0.83$.

■ TABLE C–10. Maximum mid-expiratory flow ($MMEF_{25\text{-}75\%\ VC}$) in relation to body height in boys and girls

Height (cm)	$MMEF_{25\text{-}75\%\ VC}$ (L/sec)		
	Mean	*Lower Limits*	*Upper Limits*
115	1.57	1.11	2.20
116	1.60	1.13	2.25
118	1.66	1.18	2.34
120	1.73	1.23	2.43
122	1.80	1.28	2.53
124	1.87	1.33	2.63
126	1.94	1.38	2.73
128	2.02	1.43	2.84
130	2.09	1.49	2.94
132	2.17	1.54	3.05
134	2.25	1.60	3.16
136	2.33	1.65	3.27
138	2.41	1.71	3.39
140	2.49	1.77	3.50
142	2.58	1.83	3.62
144	2.66	1.89	3.75
146	2.75	1.95	3.87
148	2.84	2.02	4.00
150	2.93	2.08	4.12
152	3.02	2.15	4.26
154	3.12	2.22	4.39
156	3.22	2.29	4.52
158	3.31	2.36	4.66
160	3.41	2.43	4.80
162	3.52	2.50	4.95
164	3.62	2.57	5.09
166	3.72	2.65	5.24
168	3.83	2.72	5.39
170	3.94	2.80	5.54
172	4.05	2.88	5.70
174	4.16	2.96	5.86
176	4.28	3.04	6.02
178	4.39	3.12	6.18
180	4.51	3.21	6.34

Formula: $\log y = a + b \cdot \log x$;
y = ($MMEF_{25\text{-}75\%\ VC}$) (L/sec); x = Body height (cm);
log ($MMEF_{25\text{-}75\%\ VC}$) (L/sec) = −4.6651 + 2.3588 · log height (cm);
SD $\log y \cdot x = \pm 0.0746$; n = 108; $r = +0.78$.

■ TABLE C–11. Maximum expiratory flow rate at 50% of vital capacity($\dot{V}max_{50\% VC}$, $MEF_{50\% VC}$) in relation to body height in boys and girls

Height (cm)	$\dot{V}max_{50\% VC}$ (L/sec)		
	Mean	*Lower Limits*	*Upper Limits*
115	1.86	1.35	2.55
116	1.89	1.38	2.59
118	1.96	1.43	2.69
120	2.04	1.48	2.79
122	2.11	1.54	2.90
124	2.19	1.59	3.00
126	2.27	1.65	3.11
128	2.34	1.71	3.21
130	2.43	1.77	3.33
132	2.51	1.83	3.44
134	2.59	1.89	3.55
136	2.68	1.95	3.67
138	2.76	2.01	3.79
140	2.85	2.08	3.91
142	2.94	2.14	4.03
144	3.03	2.21	4.16
146	3.12	2.28	4.28
148	3.22	2.35	4.41
150	3.31	2.42	4.54
152	3.41	2.49	4.68
154	3.51	2.56	4.81
156	3.61	2.63	4.95
158	3.71	2.71	5.09
160	3.81	2.78	5.23
162	3.92	2.86	5.37
164	4.02	2.94	5.52
166	4.13	3.01	5.67
168	4.24	3.09	5.82
170	4.35	3.17	5.97
172	4.47	3.26	6.12
174	4.58	3.34	6.28
176	4.69	3.42	6.44
178	4.81	3.51	6.60
180	4.93	3.60	6.76

Formula: $\log y = a + b \cdot \log x$;
$y = \dot{V}max_{50\% VC}$ (L/sec); x = Body height (cm);
$\log \dot{V}max_{50\% VC}$ (L/sec) $= -4.2168 + 2.1771 \cdot \log$ height (cm);
SD $\log y \cdot x = \pm 0.0689$; n = 101; $r = +0.79$.

■ TABLE C–12. Maximum expiratory flow rate at 25% of vital capacity ($\dot{V}max_{25\% VC}$, $MEF_{25\% VC}$) in relation to body height in boys and girls

Height (cm)	$\dot{V}max_{25\% VC}$, liters/s		
	Mean	*Lower Limits*	*Upper Limits*
115	0.94	0.63	1.41
116	0.96	0.64	1.44
118	1.00	0.67	1.49
120	1.04	0.69	1.55
122	1.08	0.72	1.61
124	1.11	0.75	1.66
126	1.16	0.77	1.73
128	1.20	0.80	1.79
130	1.24	0.83	1.85
132	1.28	0.86	1.91
134	1.32	0.89	1.98
136	1.37	0.92	2.04
138	1.41	0.95	2.11
140	1.46	0.98	2.18
142	1.51	1.01	2.25
144	1.55	1.04	2.32
146	1.60	1.07	2.39
148	1.65	1.11	2.46
150	1.70	1.14	2.54
152	1.75	1.17	2.61
154	1.80	1.21	2.69
156	1.86	1.24	2.77
158	1.91	1.28	2.85
160	1.96	1.31	2.93
162	2.02	1.35	3.01
164	2.07	1.39	3.09
166	2.13	1.43	3.18
168	2.19	1.47	3.26
170	2.25	1.50	3.35
172	2.30	1.54	3.44
174	2.36	1.58	3.53
176	2.42	1.62	3.62
178	2.49	1.67	3.71
180	2.55	1.71	3.80

Formula: $\log y = a + b \cdot \log x$;
$y = \dot{V}max_{25\% VC}$ (L/sec); x = Body height (cm);
$\log \dot{V}max_{25\% VC}$ (L/sec) $= -4.5808 + 2.2116 \cdot \log$ height (cm);
SD $\log y \cdot x = \pm 0.0874$; n = 101; $r = +0.76$.

■ TABLE C–13. Tidal volume (VT) in relation to body height in boys and girls

Height (cm)	VT (mL)		
	Mean	Lower Limits	Upper Limits
115	279	185	421
116	283	188	428
118	293	194	442
120	302	200	456
122	311	206	470
124	321	213	484
126	331	219	499
128	341	226	514
130	351	232	529
132	361	239	544
134	371	246	560
136	381	253	575
138	392	260	591
140	403	267	607
142	413	274	624
144	424	281	640
146	435	289	657
148	447	296	674
150	458	303	691
152	469	311	708
154	481	319	726
156	493	327	743
158	505	334	761
160	517	342	779
162	529	350	798
164	541	358	816
166	553	367	835
168	566	375	854
170	578	383	873
172	591	392	892
174	604	400	911
176	617	409	931
178	630	418	951
180	643	426	971

Formula: $\log y = a + b \cdot \log x$;
$y = V_T$ (mL); x = Body height (cm);
$\log V_T \text{ (mL)} = -1.3956 + 1.8643 \cdot \log \text{height (cm)}$;
SD $\log y \cdot x = \pm 0.0903$; $n = 170$; $r = +0.65$.

■ TABLE C–14. Tidal volume (VT) in relation to age in boys and girls

Age (yr)	VT (mL)		
	Mean	Lower Limits	Upper Limits
6	278	178	432
7	313	201	486
8	347	223	539
9	380	244	590
10	412	265	640
11	443	285	689
12	474	305	737
13	504	324	784
14	534	343	830
15	563	362	875
16	592	381	920
17	620	399	964

Formula: $\log y = a + b \cdot \log x$;
$y = V_T$ (mL); x = Age (yr);
$\log V_T \text{ (mL)} = 1.8438 + 0.7713 \cdot \log \text{age (yr)}$;
SD $\log y \cdot x = \pm 0.0969$; $n = 170$; $r = +0.57$.

■ TABLE C–15. Minute ventilation (MV) in relation to body height in boys and girls

	MV (mL/min)		
Height (cm)	*Mean*	*Lower Limits*	*Upper Limits*
115	5,872	4,454	7,741
116	5,958	4,520	7,855
118	6,132	4,652	8,084
120	6,308	4,785	8,316
122	6,486	4,920	8,550
124	6,666	5,056	8,787
126	6,847	5,194	9,027
128	7,031	5,333	9,269
130	7,217	5,474	9,514
132	7,405	5,617	9,761
134	7,594	5,761	10,011
136	7,786	5,906	10,264
138	7,979	6,053	10,519
140	8,175	6,201	10,777
142	8,372	6,351	11,037
144	8,571	6,502	11,300
146	8,772	6,654	11,565
148	8,976	6,808	11,832
150	9,180	6,964	12,103
152	9,387	7,121	12,375
154	9,596	7,279	12,650
156	9,806	7,439	12,928
158	10,019	7,600	13,208
160	10,233	7,762	13,490
162	10,449	7,926	13,775
164	10,667	8,091	14,062
166	10,886	8,258	14,352
168	11,108	8,426	14,643
170	11,331	8,595	14,938
172	11,556	8,766	15,235
174	11,783	8,938	15,534
176	12,012	9,112	15,835
178	12,242	9,286	16,139
180	12,474	9,463	16,445

Formula: $\log y = a + b \cdot \log x$;
y = MV (mL/min); x = Body height (cm);
log MV (mL/min) = −0.3035 + 1.6815 · log height (cm);
SD $\log y \cdot x = \pm 0.0607$; n = 170; $r = +0.75$.

■ TABLE C–16. Minute ventilation (MV) in relation to age in boys and girls

	MV (mL/min)		
Age (yr)	*Mean*	*Lower Limits*	*Upper Limits*
6	5,864	4,287	8,022
7	6,524	4,769	8,924
8	7,154	5,230	9,787
9	7,761	5,674	10,616
10	8,347	6,102	11,418
11	8,916	6,518	12,196
12	9,468	6,922	12,951
13	10,007	7,315	13,688
14	10,532	7,700	14,407
15	11,047	8,076	15,111
16	11,551	8,444	15,800
17	12,045	8,805	16,476

Formula: $\log y = a + b \cdot \log x$;
y = MV (mL/min); x = Age (yr);
log MV (mL/min) = 3.2305 + 0.6910 · log age (yr);
SD $\log y \cdot x = \pm 0.0689$; n = 170; $r = +0.66$.

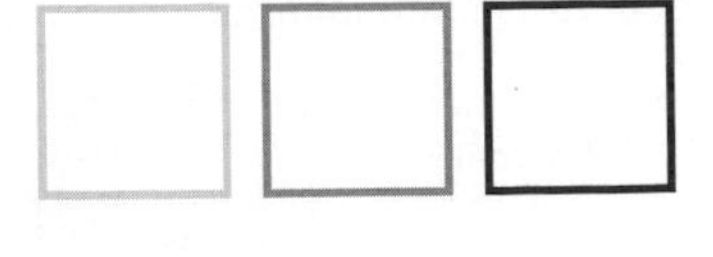

Appendix D Index of Syndromes and Their Pediatric Anesthetic Implications

Franklyn P. Cladis

DVD, Section 6

Name	Description	Anesthetic Implications	References
A			
Aarskog syndrome	Mutation in faciodigitogenital gene, growth retardation, rare congenital heart disease, mental retardation, hypermobility of cervical spine with possible hypoplasia, cryptorchidism	Care with neck manipulation	Baum and O'Flaherty, 1999; Butler and others, 2000
Aase syndrome	May be variant of Diamond Blackfan syndrome, anemia, radial hypoplasia	Check preoperative hematocrit, radial anomalies make arterial catheter insertion more difficult	Baum and O'Flaherty, 1999
Abetalipoproteinemia	Absence of apolipoprotein B, neuropathy with sensory and motor loss, malabsorption of lipids	May be deficient in fat-soluble vitamins with elevation in prothrombin time, succinylcholine is contraindicated with demyelination	Baum and O'Flaherty, 1999
Achondrogenesis	Types 1 and 2 result in severe defect in the development of bone and cartilage, micrognathia, very short stature, large cranium, micromelia, usually lethal	May be difficult airway, difficult intravenous access, care with positioning	Baum and O'Flaherty, 1999; Butler and others, 2000
Achondroplasia	Premature fusion of the bones, macrocephaly, sleep apnea, chest wall deformities—scoliosis and small rib cage, brainstem compression, spine stenosis and fusion, small stature, obesity, normal intelligence	May be difficult airway, may have cervical spine compression with positioning, altered lung mechanics secondary to chest wall deformity, regional anesthesia has been performed	Kalla and others, 1986; Berkowitz and others, 1990; Baum and O'Flaherty, 1999
Adrenoleukodystrophy	Adrenal cortical deficiency and CNS demyelination, secondary to accumulation of very long chain fatty acids, visual changes, retinopathy, hypotonia, ataxia, apraxia, neuropathy, spastic paraparesis, seizures, GERD	Concern regarding succinylcholine with demyelination and muscle atrophy, risk of aspiration, inhibitors of dopamine may exacerbate movement disorder, may require stress-dose steroids	Tobias, 1992; Nishina and others, 1993; Baum and O'Flaherty, 1999
Aicardia syndrome	Seen only in females, agenesis of corpus callosum, hypotonia, infantile spasm and seizures, kyphoscoliosis	Risk for aspiration, chronic antiseizure medication	Baum and O'Flaherty, 1999; Butler and others, 2000
Alagille syndrome	Congestive heart disease, biliary hypoplasia or atresia, HTN, vitamin K deficiency, renal dysplasia or stenosis	May have cirrhosis and portal HTN, increased prothrombin time, preoperative cardiac evaluation, check renal function	Choudry and others, 1998; Baum and O'Flaherty, 1999
Albright osteodystrophy	See Pseudohypoparathyroidism		
Alport syndrome	Sensorineural hearing loss, renal failure, can have myopathy or peripheral neuropathy	Check renal function preoperatively, possible hyperkalemia with myopathy or neuropathy and succinylcholine	Baum and O'Flaherty, 1999
Alström syndrome	Vision and hearing loss, cardiomyopathy uncommon, progressive renal dysfunction, obesity	Check renal function preoperatively, may need cardiac evaluation preoperatively	Baum and O'Flaherty, 1999
Angelman syndrome	Severe mental retardation, laughing, ataxia, seizures, "happy puppet syndrome"	Chronic antiseizure medications	Baum and O'Flaherty, 1999; Butler and others, 2000
Antley-Bixler syndrome	Craniosynostosis, frontal bossing, choanal stenosis or atresia with severe upper airway obstruction, proptosis	Choanal atresia may require early airway intervention (tracheostomy), may preclude the use of nasal tubes, eye protection for proptosis	LeBard and Thiemann, 1998; Baum and O'Flaherty, 1999

Name	Description	Anesthetic Implications	References
Apert syndrome	Craniosynostosis, midface hypoplasia, may have tracheal stenosis, congenital heart disease, mental retardation, increased ICP, syndactyly, renal anomalies, fusion of cervical vertebrae	May be difficult intubation due to midface hypoplasia, cervical fusion and tracheal stenosis, preoperative cardiac evaluation, caution with premedication if ICP elevated, intravenous access may be difficult	Baum and O'Flaherty, 1999; Butler and others, 2000
Argininosuccinic acid lyase and argininosuccinic acid synthetase deficiency	Urea cycle defect with hyperammonemia, mental retardation, seizures	Need high carbohydrate intake perioperatively with low protein intake, protein load (blood) may cause acute metabolic encephalopathy	Baum and O'Flaherty, 1999
Arthrogryposis multiplex	Multiple congenital contractures, small mandible, short neck, may be associated myopathy or neuropathy	May be difficult intubation, difficult intravenous access, no known association with malignant hyperthermia	Baum and O'Flaherty, 1999
Asplenia	Duplication of right-sided structures, two right lungs, two right atria, usually a form of anomalous venous return, two sinoatrial nodes, absent spleen, may have malrotation	Preoperative cardiac evaluation, risk of infection from encapsulated organisms	Baum and O'Flaherty, 1999
Ataxia-telangiectasia syndrome	Oculocutaneous telangiectalas, cerebellar ataxia, peripheral nerve degeneration, immunodeficiency, recurrent lung infections, predisposition to malignancies	Aseptic technique with invasive procedures, potential hyperkalemia with succinycholine in setting of neuropathy, may have glucose intolerance	Baum and O'Flaherty, 1999
B			
Baller-Gerold syndrome	Craniosynostosis, micrognathia, radial aplasia, congenital heart disease common, mental retardation, renal anomalies	Micrognathia may make intubation difficult, preoperative cardiac evaluation, check renal function, radial artery catheterization may be difficult	Baum and O'Flaherty, 1999; Butler and others, 2000
Bartter syndrome	Abnormalities in Na^+, K^+, and Cl^- transport with hypokalemia, hypochloremia, metabolic alkalosis, mental retardation, muscle weakness	Check electrolytes (Na^+, K^+, and Cl^-) preoperatively, may have ileus secondary to hypokalemia, may have decreased muscle tone	Higa and others, 1993; Kannan and others, 1995; Baum and O'Flaherty, 1999
Becker muscular dystrophy	Abnormality in size or amount of dystrophin, later age of onset and milder course, respiratory muscle weakness, cardiomyopathy	Hyperkalemia with succinylcholine, possible risk of malignant hyperthermia, risk of aspiration, preoperative cardiac evaluation	Baum and O'Flaherty, 1999; Russell and Hirsch, 1994
Beckwith-Wiedemann syndrome	Macroglossia, macrosomia, visceromegaly, increased risk of intra-abdominal tumors, hypoglycemia, neonatal polycythemia, omphalocele, may have congenital heart disease	May have significant upper airway obstruction, preoperative cardiac evaluation, monitor blood glucose	Gurkowski and Rasch, 1989; Suan and others, 1996; Baum and O'Flaherty, 1999; Butler and others, 2000
Bernard-Soulier syndrome	Disorder of platelet function	May require platelet transfusion	Baum and O'Flaherty, 1999
Blackfan-Diamond syndrome	Congenital red cell hypoplasia, steroid therapy common	Check preoperative hemoglobin, may require transfusions, may need stress-dose steroids	Baum and O'Flaherty, 1999
Branchio-oculofacial syndrome	Defects of the branchial arch involving the eye and face, pseudocleft lip, renal anomalies	No reports of difficult airway, check renal function preoperatively	Baum and O'Flaherty, 1999
C			
Camptomelic dysplasia	Short stature, micrognathia, short neck, kyphoscoliosis	May be difficult intubation, may have unstable cervical spine	Baum and O'Flaherty, 1999; Butler and others, 2000
Carpenter syndrome	Craniosynostosis, hypoplastic mandible, congenital heart disease common, may have increased ICP, mental retardation, obesity	May be difficult intubation, preoperative cardiac evaluation, may need to manage elevated ICP	Baum and O'Flaherty, 1999; Butler and others, 2000
Cat-eye syndrome	Colobomas of iris, may have choanal atresia, congenital heart disease, anal atresia, renal abnormalities, radial anomalies	Check renal function, preoperative cardiac evaluation, radial artery catheter may be difficult	Baum and O'Flaherty, 1999; Butler and others, 2000
Catch-22 syndrome	See DiGeorge syndrome		
Catel-Manzke syndrome	Severe micrognathia, short neck, congenital heart disease common,	May have significant upper airway obstruction, ventilation and intubation may be very difficult, preoperative cardiac evaluation	Baum and O'Flaherty, 1999; Butler and others, 2000
Central core disease	Congenital myopathy with defect in ryanidine receptor	Risk of malignant hyperthermia	Baum and O'Flaherty, 1999; Frank and others, 1980
Cerebrocostomandibular syndrome	Severe micrognathia, gap in ribs with small thoracic cage, congenital heart disease	Intubation may be very difficult, severe restrictive lung disease, preoperative cardiac evaluation	Baum and O'Flaherty, 1999
Cerebrooculofacioskeletal syndrome	Degeneration of brain and spinal cord, hypotonia, hyporeflexia, micrognathia	May have hyperkalemia with succinylcholine	Baum and O'Flaherty, 1999; Butler and others, 2000
Charcot-Marie-Tooth syndrome	Hereditary peripheral neuropathy, respiratory insufficiency later in life, muscle atrophy	May have hyperkalemia with succinylcholine, may have perioperative respiratory complications	Anotgnini, 1992; Greenberg and Parker, 1992; Baraka, 1997; Baum and O'Flaherty, 1999

Continued

Name	Description	Anesthetic Implications	References
CHARGE association	**C**olobomas of the eye, **h**eart disease (tetralogy of Fallot), **a**tresia of choanae, **r**etarded growth, **g**enital anomalies (hypogonadism), **e**ar anomalies (deafness)	May be difficult intubation secondary to micrognathia, preoperative cardiac evaluation, respiratory distress from choanal atresia	Stack and Wyse, 1991; Baum and O'Flaherty, 1999; Butler and others, 2000
Chédiak-Higashi syndrome	Defect in granular cells (neutrophils, monocytes, lymphocytes), immunodeficient, partial albinism, peripheral neuropathy, may have platelet abnormalities, steroid therapy	Risk for bacterial infections, use aseptic technique, may have hyperkalemia with succinylcholine, may require platelet transfusion, consider stress-dose steroids	Baum and O'Flaherty, 1999
CHILD syndrome	**C**ongenital **h**emidysplasia, **i**chthyosiform erythroderma, **l**imb **d**efects, congenital heart disease, hypomelia, renal agenesis	Intravenous access may be difficult, preoperative cardiac evaluation, check renal function preoperatively	Baum and O'Flaherty, 1999
Chotzen syndrome	See Saethre-Chotzen syndrome		
Cockayne syndrome	UV light–induced DNA damage, small mandible, small trachea, precocious coronary artery disease and HTN, ataxia, muscle atrophy, vertebral abnormalities, kyphoscoliosis	Difficult intubation has been reported, may need smaller endotracheal tube, preoperative cardiac evaluation for ischemia, may need to treat HTN, check renal function preoperatively, succinylcholine may cause hyperkalemia with muscle atrophy	Cook, 1982; Woolridge and others, 1996; Sasaki and others, 1997; Baum and O'Flaherty, 1999
Coffin-Siris syndrome	Microcephaly, congenital heart disease, mental retardation, hypoplastic digits, renal anomalies, aggressive behavior	Preoperative cardiac evaluation, check renal function preoperatively	Baum and O'Flaherty, 1999; Butler and others, 2000
Cohen syndrome	Micrognathia, mitral valve prolapse, mental retardation, hypotonia, muscle weakness, obesity	May be difficult intubation, may be difficult ventilation secondary to obesity, subacute bacterial, endocarditis prophylaxis, perioperative complications secondary to obesity and muscle weakness	Baum and O'Flaherty, 1999; Butler and others, 2000
Congenital adrenal hyperplasia	Defect in the synthesis of cortisol with overproduction of an androgen cortisol precursor, virilization, clinical features depend on enzyme deficiency, may have salt wasting, may have hypoglycemia, may have hypokalemia and HTN, defect in aldosterone synthesis common	Check Na^+, K^+, and glucose preoperatively, stress-dose steroids, salt losing can be treated with salt-containing intravenous fluids and mineralocorticoid	White and others, 1987; Baum and O'Flaherty, 1999
Cornelia de Lange syndrome	Micrognathia and short neck, occasional congenital heart disease, severe mental retardation, seizures, apnea, GERD, micromelia	May be difficult intubation, risk of perioperative respiratory complications from GERD and apnea, may be difficult intravenous access	Munoz Corsini and others, 1998; Baum and O'Flaherty, 1999
Costello syndrome	Short neck, oral and nasal papillomas, hypertrophic cardiomyopathy, arrhythmias, congenital heart disease, mental retardation, swallowing difficulty and GERD	Airway papillomas may make intubation difficult, preoperative cardiac evaluation, perioperative respiratory complications secondary to swallowing difficulty and GERD	Dearlove and Harper, 1997; Baum and O'Flaherty, 1999; Butler and others, 2000
Cri du chat syndrome	Partial deletion of chromosome 5p, high pitched cry, may have micrognathia and short neck, long epiglottis, laryngeal deformity, severe mental retardation, recurrent aspiration, congenital heart disease common	Difficult intubation described, preoperative cardiac evaluation, risk of aspiration at baseline, airway obstruction secondary to hypotonia	Yamashita and others, 1985; Brislin and others, 1995; Baum and O'Flaherty, 1999; Butler and others, 2000
Crouzon's syndrome	Craniosynostosis, proptosis, hypoplastic maxilla, rarely elevated ICP	Possible difficult intubation, eye care with proptosis	Payne and Cranston, 1995; Baum and O'Flaherty, 1999
Cutis laxa	Disorder of elastin synthesis, emphysema, aortic dilation, coronary artery disease, pulmonary HTN, pendulous skin	Preoperative cardiac evaluation, intravenous access may be difficult	Baum and O'Flaherty, 1999
Cystic fibrosis	See Chapter 32		
D			
Dejerine-Sottas syndrome	Motor and sensory neuropathy, distal muscle atrophy and weakness, may have autonomic abnormalities	May develop hyperkalemia with succinylcholine, autonomic dysfunction may cause thermal lability, no known association with malignant hyperthermia	Baum and O'Flaherty, 1999
Diastrophic dysplasia	Short stature, can have subluxation of C2-3, micrognathia, laryngotracheal stenosis, limited joint mobility	May be difficult intubation, may require smaller-than-expected endotracheal tube, cervical subluxation possible, care with positioning	Baum and O'Flaherty, 1999; Butler and others, 2000
DiGeorge syndrome (CATCH-22 syndrome)	Microdeletion on chromosome 22, abnormalities of thymus, parathyroids, and great vessels, choanal atresia, may have micrognathia and short trachea, congenital heart disease, hypocalcemia and seizures in neonates, cellular immunodeficiency	May be difficult intubation, endobronchial intubation more likely with short trachea, preoperative cardiac evaluation, avoid nasal tubes with choanal atresia, monitor calcium, irradiate blood products	Flashburg and others, 1983; Wells and others, 1989; Baum and O'Flaherty, 1999; Butler and others, 2000

Name	Description	Anesthetic Implications	References
Down syndrome (trisomy 21 syndrome)	Trisomy 21, macroglossia, pharyngeal hypotonia, smaller trachea, obstructive sleep apnea, recurrent lung infections, congenital heart disease common, atlantoaxial instability, duodenal atresia, congenital hypothyroidism	Airway obstruction may occur intraoperatively and postoperatively, reports of subluxation after intubation, may require neck films if symptomatic, may need smaller endotracheal tube, preoperative cardiac evaluation, bradycardia common after inhalation induction	Williams and others, 1987; Baum and O'Flaherty, 1999; Butler and others, 2000; Williams and others, 1987
Dubowitz syndrome	Small facies, mental deficiency, growth deficiency, rare congenital heart disease, micrognathia	May be difficult airway, preoperative cardiac evaluation, may have behavioral disturbance	Baum and O'Flaherty, 1999; Butler and others, 2000
Duchenne muscular dystrophy	X-linked muscular dystrophy, lack of dystrophin in muscle, respiratory muscle weakness, restrictive lung disease, cardiomyopathy, heart block or arrhythmias, scoliosis, delayed gastric emptying, obesity in second decade	Preoperative cardiac evaluation, postoperative mechanical ventilation possible, hyperkalemia with succinylcholine, unclear association with malignant hyperthermia, possible increased risk of aspiration secondary to respiratory muscle weakness and delayed gastric emptying	Baum and O'Flaherty, 1999; Butler and others, 2000
Dutch-Kentucky syndrome (Hecht Beals syndrome)	Limited mouth opening, mitral valve prolapse, flexion deformities	Difficult intubation reported requiring fiberoptic technique, preoperative cardiac evaluation	Browder and others, 1986; Geva and others, 1997; Baum and O'Flaherty, 1999
E			
Eagle-Barrett syndrome	See prune belly syndrome		
Edwards syndrome	See Trisomy 18		
Ehlers-Danlos syndrome	Defect in gene encoding collagen, 10 types, possible tracheal dilation, lung cysts, mitral valve prolapse, aortic root dilation, congenital heart disease, coronary disease, joint laxity, poor wound healing, vascular abnormalities (aneurysm) with poor integrity, platelet abnormalities	May bleed significantly from vascular aneurysm and bleeding diathesis, preoperative cardiac evaluation for congenital defects, premature ischemic heart disease, and conduction abnormalities, risk for pneumothorax, may be difficult intravenous access	Baum and O'Flaherty, 1999; Butler and others, 2000
Ellis-van Creveld syndrome	Dwarfism, micrognathia, may have short trachea, congenital heart disease, restrictive lung disease	May be difficult intubation, endobronchial intubation more likely with short trachea, preoperative cardiac evaluation	Wells and others, 1989; Baum and O'Flaherty, 1999
Epidermolysis bullosa	Abnormality of dermis and mucous membranes, degree of skin separation, bullae formation and scarring depends on type, may limit mouth opening, airway bleeding and obstruction possible	Any adhesive may cause skin sloughing and bullae formation; use nonadhesive technique to secure endotracheal tube, monitors, and intravenous catheters; protect skin from blood pressure cuff; pad pressure points; cover facemask with Xeroform or lubricate, may be difficult intubation; eye protection with lubricant; may be at risk for aspiration from esophageal disease	Baum and O'Flaherty, 1999
Escobar syndrome	See multiple pterygium syndrome		
F			
Fabry disease	Deficiency in lysosomal alphagalactosidase A, may have temporomandibular joint involvement, may have ischemic heart disease, HTN, valvular disease, cerebrovascular disease, extremity pain, lymphedema, renal failure, hypohidrosis, angiokeratomas	May be difficult intubation from limited mouth opening, preoperative cardiac evaluation for ischemic heart disease and HTN, check renal function preoperatively, consider avoiding anticholinergics with hyperhidrosis	Baum and O'Flaherty, 1999
Facioauriculovertebral syndrome	See Goldenhar syndrome		
Fascioscapulohumeral muscular dystrophy	Weakness of facial and ocular muscles, no cardiac involvement, neck and shoulder muscle weakness	Hyperkalemia with succinylcholine, no reports of malignant hyperthermia	Dresner and Ali, 1989; Baum and O'Flaherty, 1999
Familial dysautonomia	See Riley-Day syndrome		
Familial periodic paralysis	See Chapter 32		
Fanconi syndrome	Proximal renal tubular dysfunction (renal tubular acidosis), renal loss of amino acids, phosphate, glucose, bicarbonate, and potassium, may have muscle weakness from hypokalemia, may develop chronic renal failure	Check electrolytes preoperatively (potassium, phosphate, chloride, and bicarbonate), check renal function preoperatively, check acid-base status preoperatively	Joel and Rosales, 1981; Baum and O'Flaherty, 1999

Continued

Name	Description	Anesthetic Implications	References
Farber disease	Deficiency of lysosomal enzyme ceramidase, ceramide deposition and granuloma formation may be disseminated, oral and laryngeal granulomas, pulmonary and cardiac granulomas, mental retardation, peripheral neuropathy with muscle atrophy	May be difficult airway secondary to oral granulomas, preoperative cardiac evaluation for valvular granulomas, succinylcholine can cause hyperkalemia	Baum and O'Flaherty, 1999
Femoral hypoplasia-unusual facies syndrome	Craniosynostosis, cleft palate, micrognathia, may have congenital heart disease, femoral hypoplasia, may have renal anomalies	May be difficult intubation from micrognathia, preoperative cardiac evaluation, check renal function preoperatively	Baum and O'Flaherty, 1999; Butler and others, 2000
Fetal alcohol syndrome	Secondary to in-utero exposure to alcohol, micrognathia, short neck, congenital heart disease, mental retardation, growth deficiency	May be difficult intubation, preoperative cardiac evaluation	Baum and O'Flaherty, 1999
Fetal hydantoin (Dilantin) syndrome	Secondary to in-utero exposure to Dilantin, microcephaly, midface hypoplasia, webbed neck, congenital heart disease, may have mental retardation, growth delay, hirsutism	May be a difficult intubation, preoperative cardiac evaluation	Baum and O'Flaherty, 1999; Butler and others, 2000
Fetal rubella syndrome	Secondary to maternal rubella infection during first trimester, microcephaly, hearing loss, congenital heart disease, mental retardation, anemia and thrombocytopenia in the neonate, cataracts and glaucoma	Preoperative cardiac evaluation, check preoperative hemoglobin and platelet count during neonatal period	Baum and O'Flaherty, 1999
Fetal valproate syndrome	Secondary to in utero exposure to valproic acid, congenital heart disease, meningomyelocele, radial anomalies	Preoperative cardiac evaluation	Baum and O'Flaherty, 1999; Butler and others, 2000
Fetal warfarin syndrome	Secondary to in utero exposure to warfarin, microcephaly, congenital heart disease, severe mental retardation, seizures	May have upper airway obstruction, preoperative cardiac evaluation, chronic antiseizure medication	Baum and O'Flaherty, 1999
Fibrodysplasia ossificans progressiva syndrome	Progressive ossification of muscles, joints, and subcutaneous tissue, affects neck, spine, shoulders, and jaw, may develop restrictive lung disease, cardiac conduction abnormalities, steroid therapy	May be very difficult intubation due to limited cervical motion and mouth opening, preoperative cardiac evaluation for conduction defects and supraventricular tachycardia, may need stress-dose steroids	Lininger and others, 1989; Newton and others, 1990; Baum and O'Flaherty, 1999; Butler and others, 2000
Fragile X syndrome	Defect in X chromosome, acromegalic facies, large ears, prognathism, mitral valve prolapse, mental retardation, behavioral issues, seizures	Preoperative cardiac evaluation for mitral valve prolapse, may have behavioral difficulties, chronic antiseizure medication	Baum and O'Flaherty, 1999; Butler and others, 2000
Fraser syndrome	Absent palpebral fissures with skin overlying the eyes (cryptophthalomas), choanal atresia, tracheal stenosis, micrognathia, congenital cardiac defects, syndactyly, renal anomalies	May be difficult intubation from laryngeal or tracheal stenosis, avoid nasal tubes if choanal atresia, preoperative cardiac evaluation, check renal function preoperatively	Jagtap and others, 1995; Baum and O'Flaherty, 1999
Freeman-Sheldon syndrome (also Sheldon-Freeman syndrome and whistling face syndrome)	Slowly progressive myopathy, increased muscle tone of face with microstomia, micrognathia, upper airway obstruction from increased tone of pharynx, dysphagia, joint contractures	May be very difficult intubation from microstomia and micrognathia, fiberoptic intubation through an LMA has been described, aspiration risk with vomiting, hyperkalemia possible with myopathy, unclear association with malignant hyperthermia	Jones and Dolcourt, 1992; Vas and Naregal, 1998; Baum and O'Flaherty, 1999; Butler and others, 2000
Friedreich ataxia	Degeneration of corticospinal, spinocerebellar, and pyramidal tracts, ataxia, cardiomyopathy is common	Preoperative cardiac evaluation, hyperkalemia reported with succinylcholine	Baum and O'Flaherty, 1999
Fryn's syndrome	Micrognathia, congenital diaphragmatic hernia, congenital heart disease, mental retardation, may have renal anomalies	Difficult intubation, may have significant respiratory distress or death from congenital diaphragmatic hernia, preoperative cardiac evaluation, check renal function preoperatively	Baum and O'Flaherty, 1999; Butler and others, 2000
G			
Gaucher disease	Lysosomal storage disease, trismus in infants, pulmonary HTN, seizures and apnea in infants, cranial nerve involvement, splenomegaly with thrombocytopenia and anemia	May be difficult intubation from trismus, may be at risk for aspiration, check hematocrit and platelet count preoperatively	Tobias and others, 1993; Baum and O'Flaherty, 1999
Goldenhar syndrome	A subset of hemifacial microsomia. hemifacial microsomia, epibulbar dermoid, and rib, vertebral, scapular anomalies. Microtia with hearing loss, congenital heart disease, renal anomalies, may have hydrocephalus, radial anomalies	May be very difficult intubation and mask ventilation, may have increased ICP, preoperative cardiac evaluation, check renal function preoperatively	Scholtes and others, 1987; Madan and others, 1990; Baum and O'Flaherty, 1999; Butler and others, 2000

Name	Description	Anesthetic Implications	References
Gorlin syndrome	Pigmented and atrophic skin changes, may have oral papillomas, congenital heart disease, GERD, renal dysplasia	May be difficult ventilation and intubation from papillomas, care with positioning with joint hypermobility, preoperative cardiac evaluation	Baum and O'Flaherty, 1999; Butler and others, 2000
H			
Hajdu-Cheney syndrome	Abnormality in skeletal tissue development, failure of cranial suture ossification, hypoplastic mandible, dental loss, cervical instability, short stature, cystic renal disease	May be difficult intubation from hypoplastic mandible and cervical instability, check renal function preoperatively	Baum and O'Flaherty, 1999; Butler and others, 2000
Hallerman-Streiff syndrome	Birdlike facies, mandibular hypoplasia, tracheomalacia, chronic upper airway obstruction, may have cor pulmonale, joint hyperextensibility	May be difficult intubation, can have significant airway obstruction, care with positioning	Ravindran and Stoops, 1979; Baum and O'Flaherty, 1999; Butler and others, 2000
Hallervorden-Spatz disease	Iron deposition in CNS, oromandibular rigidity, dystonia, rigidity, dementia, spasticity	Succinylcholine is contraindicated secondary to bedridden condition, oromandibular rigidity resolves under anesthesia, neuroleptic malignant syndrome has been reported	Roy and others, 1983; Hayashi and others, 1993; Baum and O'Flaherty, 1999
Henoch-Schönlein purpura	Usually postinfectious small vessel vasculitis, edema, renal dysfunction, lower extremity, and abdominal pain	Check renal function preoperatively	Baum and O'Flaherty, 1999
Holt-Oram syndrome	Upper limb defects and congenital heart disease	Preoperative cardiac evaluation	Baum and O'Flaherty, 1999
Hunter syndrome	Mucopolysaccharidosis II from lack of iduronate sulfatase, coarse facial features, soft tissue stiffness of lips and mouth, joint stiffness, coronary artery narrowing, hydrocephalus	Can be extremely difficult intubation, fiberoptic scope and LMA have been used, preoperative cardiac evaluation for ischemia, care with positioning	Baum and O'Flaherty, 1999; Butler and others, 2000
Hurler syndrome	Mucopolysaccharidosis IH from abnormality in α-L-iduronidase (clinically similar to Hunter syndrome but more severe and rapid clinical course), coarse facial features, soft tissue stiffness of lips and mouth, joint stiffness, coronary artery narrowing, hydrocephalus, mental retardation	Extremely difficult intubation, fiberoptic scope and LMA have been used, preoperative cardiac evaluation for ischemia, care with positioning	Baum and O'Flaherty, 1999; Butler and others, 2000
J			
Jarcho-Levin syndrome	Dwarfism, limited cervical motion, short thoracic cage, rib anomalies, congenital heart disease	May be difficult intubation, preoperative cardiac evaluation, may have restrictive lung disease	Baum and O'Flaherty, 1999; Butler and others, 2000
Jervell and Lange-Nielsen syndrome	See Prolonged QT syndrome		
Jeune syndrome	Asphyxiating thoracic dystrophy, thoracic cage deformity, lung hypoplasia, may have pulmonary HTN, chronic renal failure	Severe respiratory insufficiency, preoperative cardiac evaluation for pulmonary HTN and cor pulmonale, check renal function preoperatively	Borland, 1987; Baum and O'Flaherty, 1999; Butler and others, 2000
K			
Kabuki syndrome	Similarity in facial appearance with Japanese Kabuki actors, congenital heart disease, may have pectus excavatum, mental retardation, renal anomalies	Preoperative cardiac evaluation, check renal function preoperatively	Baum and O'Flaherty, 1999; Butler and others, 2000
Kartagener syndrome	Marked by situs inversus and immotile cilia, chronic sinusitis, chronic respiratory tract infection, bronchiectasis, dextrocardia, may be asplenic, immotile sperm	Thick secretions may complicate airway management, nasal intubation relatively contraindicated in chronic sinusitis, situs inversus reverses many procedures: mainstem intubation occurs on left, reverse placement of electrocardiographic and defibrillator pads	Baum and O'Flaherty, 1999; Ho and Friedland, 1992
Kasabach-Merritt syndrome	Hemangioma and thrombocytopenia, high output cardiac failure, microangiopathic hemolytic anemia, may develop disseminated intravascular coagulation	May need transfusion therapy with red cells, platelets, and fresh frozen plasma	Baum and O'Flaherty, 1999
Kearns-Sayre syndrome	Mitochondrial myopathy, external ophthalmoplegia, heart block, cardiomyopathy, proximal muscle weakness, ataxia, may have elevated lactate with exercise	May develop lactic acidosis, consider avoiding lactated Ringer's, preoperative cardiac evaluation for heart block and myopathy, possible hyperkalemia with succinylcholine and mitochondrial myopathy, may be sensitive to non-depolarizing muscle relaxants, no clear association between mitochondrial myopathy and malignant hyperthermia	Baum and O'Flaherty, 1999

Continued

Name	Description	Anesthetic Implications	References
Klinefelter syndrome (XXY syndrome)	47, XXY karyotype, developmental delay, behavioral problems, hypogonadism, infertility	Behavioral problems may complicate the perioperative period	Baum and O'Flaherty, 1999
Klippel-Feil sequence	Short neck and limited cervical spine immobility, micrognathia, congenital heart disease, may have renal anomalies	Intubation may be extremely difficult, neurologic injury may occur with neck hyperextension, preoperative cardiac evaluation	Baum and O'Flaherty, 1999; Butler and others, 2000
Klippel-Trénaunay-Weber syndrome	Unilateral extremity hypertrophy with arteriovenous fistulas and hemangiomas, may have high output failure, may have facial, intracranial, and epidural hematomas	May have significant bleeding from arteriovenous fistulae, may have thrombocytopenia, preoperative cardiac evaluation for high output failure, neuraxial hemangiomas may complicate epidural and spinal anesthesia	Baum and O'Flaherty, 1999; Ezri and others, 1996
L			
Langer-Giedion syndrome	Micrognathia, may have congenital heart disease, may have seizures, may have anemia, vertebral and rib anomalies	May be difficult intubation, preoperative cardiac evaluation, check hematocrit preoperatively	Baum and O'Flaherty, 1999; Butler and others, 2000
Larsen syndrome	Flat face, subglottic stenosis, tracheomalacia, congenital heart disease, cervical spine instability, multiple joint dislocations	Care with intubation with neck extension, smaller endotracheal tube with subglottic stenosis, preoperative cardiac evaluation, care with positioning with joint dislocations	Stevenson and others, 1991; Baum and Tobias, 1996; Baum and O'Flaherty, 1999; Butler and others, 2000
LEOPARD syndrome	**L**entigines, **e**lectrocardiographic conduction abnormalities, **o**cular hypertelorism, **p**ulmonic stenosis, **a**bnormal genitalia **r**etarded growth, **d**eafness	May be deaf, preoperative cardiac evaluation for conduction defects and pulmonic stenosis	Rodrigo and others, 1990; Baum and O'Flaherty, 1999
Leprechaunism	Mutation of insulin receptor gene, hyperglycemia and hypoglycemia, precocious puberty	Check perioperative glucose	Baum and O'Flaherty, 1999
Lesch-Nyhan syndrome	Developmental delay, hypertonia, spasticity, self-mutilation, hyperuricemia and renal stones, megaloblastic anemia	Check hematocrit preoperatively, check renal function preoperatively	Williams and others, 1997; Baum and O'Flaherty, 1999
Liddle syndrome	Defect in sodium channel, HTN, hypokalemic metabolic alkalosis, may have renal failure	Check preoperative electrolytes (K^+, HCO_3^-), check renal function, check blood pressure preoperatively	Baum and O'Flaherty, 1999
Limb-girdle muscular dystrophy	Respiratory tract infections, conduction disorder, muscle weakness of pelvis and legs	Preoperative cardiac evaluation for conduction disorders, succinylcholine may cause hyperkalemia, no known association with malignant hyperthermia	Baum and O'Flaherty, 1999
Lowe syndrome	Cataracts, mental retardation, renal failure, rickets	Check renal function preoperatively, check electrolytes (Ca^{2+}) preoperatively	Baum and O'Flaherty, 1999
Lown-Ganong-Levine syndrome	Accessory pathway that bypasses atrioventricular node, atrial tachyarrhythmias	Reentrant tachycardia can be treated with adenosine or β-blockade	Baum and O'Flaherty, 1999
M			
Marfan syndrome	Connective tissue disorder, defect in fibrillin, lens dislocations, pectus excavatum, pulmonary blebs, pneumothorax, dilation of aorta and pulmonary artery, aortic insufficiency and mitral valve prolapse, recurrent joint dislocations	Preoperative cardiac evaluation for aortic and valvular pathology, aortic dissection possible, pneumothorax possible with positive pressure ventilation, care with positioning	Wells and Podolakin, 1987; Baum and O'Flaherty, 1999; Butler and others, 2000
Maroteaux-Lamy syndrome	Mucopolysaccharidosis, heart failure common in second and third decade, recurrent respiratory infections, obstructive sleep apnea, short stature, decreased joint mobility, anemia and thrombocytopenia	May be very difficult intubation, preoperative cardiac evaluation, care with positioning, check preoperative hematocrit and platelet count	Baum and O'Flaherty, 1999
McArdle syndrome	Glycogen storage disease (V) with subsequent myopathy, muscle pain, no cardiac involvement	May develop hyperkalemia with succinylcholine	Baum and O'Flaherty, 1999
McCune-Albright syndrome	Fibrous dysplasia of bones, café-au-lait spots, precocious puberty, may have thyrotoxicosis and hyperadrenalism	Care with positioning secondary to pathologic fractures, cushingoid patients may have difficult intravenous access	Baum and O'Flaherty, 1999
Meckel-Gruber syndrome (Meckel syndrome)	Microcephaly, short neck, micrognathia, congenital heart disease, may have occipital encephalocele, hydrocephalus, seizures, renal dysplasia	May be difficult intubation, preoperative cardiac evaluation, check preoperative renal function, anticonvulsant medications may affect neuromuscular blockade and opioid metabolism	Baum and O'Flaherty, 1999; Butler and others, 2000
MELAS syndrome	**M**itochondrial myopathy, **e**ncephalopathy, **l**actic **a**cidosis, **s**troke. Blindness and hearing loss, cardiomyopathy, diffuse CNS degeneration with strokelike infarcts	Preoperative cardiac evaluation, possible hyperkalemia with succinylcholine, no clear association with malignant hyperthermia	Baum and O'Flaherty, 1999

Name	Description	Anesthetic Implications	References
Melnick-Needles syndrome	Small face, micrognathia, glaucoma, respiratory track infections, may have pulmonary HTN, hypotonia	May be difficult intubation	Baum and O'Flaherty, 1999; Butler and others, 2000
Menkes kinky hair syndrome (Menkes syndrome)	Abnormal copper transport, microcephaly, cerebral degeneration, seizures, characteristic kinky hair, gastroesophageal reflux	Difficult ventilation and intubation is described, anticonvulsant medications may affect neuromuscular blockade and opioid metabolism	Baum and O'Flaherty, 1999; Butler and others, 2000
MERRF syndrome	**M**yoclonus, **e**pilepsy, **r**agged **r**ed **f**ibers Defect in mitochondrial DNA, hearing loss, epilepsy, myopathy, CNS degeneration	May be acidemic, avoid lactated Ringer's in those with lactic acidosis, possible hyperkalemia with succinylcholine, no clear association with malignant hyperthermia	Baum and O'Flaherty, 1999
Miller syndrome (postaxial acrofacial dysostosis syndrome)	Craniofacial syndrome, malar hypoplasia, eyelid colobomas, micrognathia, congenital heart disease, postaxial limb deficiency, renal anomalies	May be very difficult ventilation and intubation, preoperative cardiac evaluation, check preoperative renal function, may be difficult intravenous access, eye care essential	Baum and O'Flaherty, 1999; Butler and others, 2000
Möbius sequence	Congenital sixth and seventh cranial nerve palsy, micrognathia, feeding difficulties and aspiration, congenital cardiac defects possible, limb defects	May be difficult to intubate, decreased ability to manage secretions, eye care essential, preoperative cardiac evaluation, may develop perioperative apnea or hypoventilation	Baum and O'Flaherty, 1999; Butler and others, 2000
Morquio syndrome	Mucopolysaccharidosis (IV), short neck with decreased mobility, spine and thoracic deformities with respiratory insufficiency, aortic valve pathology, atlantoaxial instability, short stature	Preoperative cervical spine evaluation, may be difficult intubation, preoperative cardiac evaluation for aortic valve, care with positioning	Baum and O'Flaherty, 1999
Multiple pterygium syndrome	Multiple pterygia, micrognathia, decreased range of motion of neck, rare congenital heart defects	Difficult intubation described, LMA has been used, care with positioning, malignant hyperthermia has been reported—association with malignant hyperthermia not clear	Baum and O'Flaherty, 1999; Butler and others, 2000
Multiple synostosis syndrome	Multiple synostosis of digits with decreased joint mobility, developmental delay	Care with positioning	Baum and O'Flaherty, 1999; Butler and others, 2000
Myotonia congenita	See Chapter 32		
Myotonic dystrophy	See Chapter 32		
N			
Nager syndrome (mandibulofacial dysostosis syndrome)	Absent zygomatic arches, downsloping palpebral fissures, colobomas, hearing loss, micrognathia, congenital heart disease, radioulnar synostosis, similar to Treacher Collins	Difficult or impossible intubation described, intravenous access may be difficult due to limb anomalies, preoperative cardiac evaluation	Baum and O'Flaherty, 1999; Butler and others, 2000
Neu-Laxova syndrome	Microcephaly, micrognathia, short neck, canine facies, congenital heart disease, renal anomalies, usually lethal	May be difficult intubation, preoperative cardiac evaluation, check preoperative renal function	Baum and O'Flaherty, 1999; Butler and others, 2000
Neurofibromatosis (von Recklinghausen disease)	Neurofibromas of central and peripheral nervous system, café-au-lait spots and bone lesions, association with pheochromocytoma	Neurofibromas may involve airway, increased sensitivity to succinylcholine and nondepolarizing muscle relaxants described, neurofibromas may involve neuraxial space	Yamashita and others, 1977; Baum and O'Flaherty, 1999; Butler and others, 2000
Noonan syndrome	Webbed neck, low-set ears, micrognathia, pectus excavatum, congenital heart disease especially pulmonic stenosis, chylothorax, lymphedema, mental retardation, platelet and coagulation disorders, renal dysfunction	May be difficult intubation, may have bleeding diathesis, preoperative cardiac evaluation, check preoperative renal function, intravenous access may be difficult with lymphedema	Campbell and Bousfield, 1992; Schwartz and Eisenkraft, 1992; Baum and O'Flaherty, 1999; Butler and others, 2000
O			
Oculodentodigital syndrome (oculodento-osseous dysplasia)	Micro-ophthalmia, cleft lip or palate, micrognathia or mandibular overgrowth, small nose, syndactyly	May be difficult intubation	Baum and O'Flaherty, 1999; Butler and others, 2000
Oral-facial-digital-syndrome (Type I)	Cleft lip and palate, micrognathia, choanal atresia, mental retardation, hydrocephalus, syndactyly, digital asymmetry, polycystic kidney disease, affects females, Types II-IX clinically similar to Type I	Upper airway obstruction possible, check renal function preoperatively	Baum and O'Flaherty, 1999; Butler and others, 2000
Oromandibular-limb hypogenesis	Small mouth, cleft palate, moebius, micrognathia, limb deficiency	May be difficult intubation	Baum and O'Flaherty, 1999; Butler and others, 2000
Osler-Weber-Rendu syndrome (hereditary	Vasculopathy with multiple telagiectases, pulmonary arteriovenous fistula with right-to-left shunting, paradoxical emboli,	Patients can have life-threatening bleeding from nose, lung, brain, and gastrointestinal tract, check hematocrit	Waring and others, 1990; Radu and others, 1992; Baum and O'Flaherty, 1999

Continued

Name	Description	Anesthetic Implications	References
hemorrhagic telangiectasia)	and bleeding, CNS arteriovenous fistulas and aneurysms, gastrointestinal bleeding	preoperatively, avoid nasal instrumentation, care with laryngoscopy to avoid bleeding, paradoxical emboli can occur, consider avoiding neuraxial blocks	
Osteogenesis imperfecta	Mutation in a gene for collagen, four types, blue sclera in type I, hearing loss, kyphoscoliosis, restrictive hearing loss, extremely fragile bones, multiple fractures, hyperextensibility, short stature	Fractures may occur with any manipulation, care with intubation, care with positioning, consider radiologic evaluation for fractures, type I may have platelet dysfunction, malignant hyperthermia not clearly associated	Barros, 1995; Porsborg and others, 1996; Baum and O'Flaherty, 1999; Butler and others, 2000
P			
Pallister Hall syndrome	Hypothalamic hamartoblastoma, panhypopituitarism, imperforate anus, cleft lip and/or palate, micrognathia, dysplastic tracheal cartilage, hypoplastic lung, congenital heart disease, thyroid hypoplasia	May be difficult intubation, abnormal tracheal cartilage may alter tracheal tube size, preoperative cardiac evaluation, preoperative evaluation of hypothalamic pituitary axis, may require stress-dose steroids	Baum and O'Flaherty, 1999; Butler and others, 2000
Pearson syndrome	Sideroblastic anemia, exocrine pancreatic dysfunction (may have Fanconi syndrome)	Preoperative hematocrit, preoperative electrolytes (K^+, Cl^-, HCO_3^-, PO_4^-)	Baum and O'Flaherty, 1999; Butler and others, 2000
Pendred syndrome	Deafness, hypothyroid, goiter	Preoperative thyroid studies	Baum and O'Flaherty, 1999
Pentalogy of Cantrell	Defect in ventral midline development, cystic hygroma, cleft lip and/or palate, congenital diaphragmatic hernia, pulmonary hypoplasia, omphalocele, renal anomalies, congenital heart disease	Preoperative cardiac evaluation, may have significant pulmonary hypoplasia and pulmonary HTN	Laloyaux and others, 1998; Baum and O'Flaherty, 1999
Peter's plus syndrome	Ophthalmologic anomalies (glaucoma, decreased vision), micrognathia, congenital heart disease, dwarfism, developmental delay, seizures	May be difficult intubation (rare), preoperative cardiac evaluation, anticonvulsant medication may affect neuromuscular blockade and opioid metabolism	Baum and O'Flaherty, 1999; Butler and others, 2000
Pfeiffer syndrome	Acrocephalosyndactyly, coronal and/or sagittal synostosis, midface hypoplasia, proptosis, obstructive sleep apnea, congenital heart defects, broad thumbs and broad great toes, may have fused elbows, usually normal intelligence	May be difficult intubation (rare), may have increased ICP, preoperative cardiac evaluation, may have airway obstruction	Tobias and others, 1998; Baum and O'Flaherty, 1999
Pierre Robin sequence	Micrognathia, glossoptosis, airway obstruction, may also have cleft palate (not necessary for diagnosis)	May be very difficult to intubate, successful intubation described with fiberoptic scopes, LMA, and Bullard, prone positioning, and tongue suture to displace tongue forward	Populaire and others, 1985; Schelle and Schulman, 1991; Baraka, 1996; Perkins and others, 1997; Baum and O'Flaherty, 1999; Butler and others, 2000
Poland syndrome	Hypoplasia of chest muscles and ribs on one side, rare dextrocardia, unilateral syndactyly	Respiratory complications	Sethuraman and others, 1998; Baum and O'Flaherty, 1999
Pompe disease	Glycogen storage disease, macroglossia, respiratory and swallowing muscle weakness, cardiomegaly, hypotonia	May be difficult to ventilate and intubate, increased risk for perioperative respiratory complications, preoperative cardiac evaluation	McFarlane and Soni, 1986; Rosen and Broadman, 1986; Baum and O'Flaherty, 1999
Porphyria	Defect in heme synthesis with overproduction of heme precursors, precipitating factors include infection, starvation, drugs, and pregnancy, acute attacks cause abdominal pain, autonomic instability with HTN, neuropathy, neuropsychiatric abnormalities, electrolyte abnormalities. May also have hemolytic anemia, hepatic failure, and cirrhosis.	Preoperative fasting should be minimized, can administer glucose-containing solution, premedication may decrease stress, avoid barbiturates, etomidate pentazocine. Ketamine may be safe, safe anesthetics include opioids, propofol, nitrous oxide, isoflurane, sevoflurane, desflurane, and muscle relaxants, neuropathy may cause respiratory muscle weakness and aspiration	Jensen and others, 1995; Kanbak, 1997; Baum and O'Flaherty, 1999
Potter syndrome	Secondary to oligohydramnios, low-set ears, beaked nose, micrognathia, lung hypoplasia, renal agenesis	May be difficult intubation, respiratory failure secondary to pulmonary hypoplasia, check preoperative renal function	Baum and O'Flaherty, 1999
Prader-Willi syndrome	Secondary to partial deletion of chromosome 15, obesity, hypotonia, developmental delay, hypogonadism, obstructive sleep apnea, may have pulmonary HTN, hypotonia, developmental delay, hypogonadism, diabetes mellitus	Anesthetic concerns related to obesity, difficult mask ventilation, potential difficult airway, decreased functional residual capacity, perioperative respiratory complications, monitor perioperative glucose	McKenzie, 1991; Dearlove and others, 1998; Baum and O'Flaherty, 1999; Butler and others, 2000
Progeria	Premature aging, micrognathia, beaked nose, premature coronary artery disease, cerebrovascular disease, HTN, diabetes mellitus	Perioperative cardiac evaluation for ischemic heart disease, may be difficult intubation secondary to micrognathia and stiff joints	Chapin and Kahre, 1979; Baum and O'Flaherty, 1999; Butler and others, 2000
Prolonged QT interval syndrome (Jervell-Lange-Nielson	Prolonged QT interval on electrocardiogram, congenital deafness with Jervell-Lange Nielson syndrome	Tachydysrhythmias and sudden death, torsades de pointes, prevention by avoiding drugs that prolong QT interval,	Dunn and others, 1991; Richardson and others, 1992; Holland, 1993; Michaloudis and others, 1996

Name	Description	Anesthetic Implications	References
syndrome; Romano-Ward syndrome)		volatile anesthetics prolong QT interval, avoid epinephrine, treat torsades with defibrillation, magnesium, correcting electrolytes, β-blocker	
Proteus syndrome	Hemihypertrophy, hypertrophic cardiomyopathy, emphysematous lung disease, renal anomalies, cervical spine abnormalities	Perioperative cardiac evaluation, may have abnormal lung function, check preoperative renal function	Pennant and Harris, 1991; Baum and O'Flaherty, 1999
Prune-belly syndrome (Eagle-Barrett syndrome)	Absence of abdominal wall musculature, urinary tract dilation, cryptorchidism, lung hypoplasia secondary to in-utero urinary tract obstruction with oligohydramnios, may have congenital heart disease	Increased risk of perioperative respiratory complications secondary to decreased ability to cough, check preoperative renal function, preoperative cardiac evaluation	Henderson and others, 1987; Baum and O'Flaherty, 1999
R			
Rett syndrome	Only in females, progressive encephalopathy beginning at 6 to 18 months, seizures, spasticity, behavioral problems	Anticonvulsant medication may affect neuromuscular blockade and opioid metabolism	Dearlove and Walker, 1996; Baum and O'Flaherty, 1999
Riley-Day syndrome (familial dysautonomia)	Deficiency of dopamine hydroxylase, blood pressure instability, abnormal sweating, hypersensitivity to catecholamine, emotional lability, decreased respiratory drive to hypercarbia and hypoxia, decreased or lack of tear formation, decreased peripheral pain sensation	Increased risk of aspiration, may have exaggerated response to inotropes, may have exaggerated depression of respiratory drive with narcotics, perioperative eye care, decreased postoperative pain requirements	Stenquist and Sigurdsson, 1982; Axelrod and others, 1988; Baum and O'Flaherty, 1999
Riley-Smith syndrome	Macrocephaly, mild developmental delay, lipid storage myopathy, seizures	Anticonvulsant medication may affect neuromuscular blockade and opioid metabolism, may develop hyperkalemia with succinylcholine	Baum and O'Flaherty, 1999
Robinow syndrome (fetal face syndrome)	Frontal bossing, micrognathia, may have congenital heart disease, genitourinary and renal anomalies	May be difficult intubation, check preoperative renal function, preoperative cardiac evaluation	Baum and O'Flaherty, 1999; Butler and others, 2000
Rubinstein-Taybi syndrome	Defect in cAMP-mediated induction of protein synthesis, microcephaly, micrognathia, obstructive sleep apnea, congenital heart disease in 30%, developmental delay, seizures, broad thumbs and toes	May be difficult to intubate, preoperative cardiac evaluation, anticonvulsant medication may affect neuromuscular blockade and opioid metabolism, may have delayed recovery from anesthesia	Stirt, 1981; Dunkley and Dearlove, 1996; Baum and O'Flaherty, 1999; Butler and others, 2000
Russell-Silver syndrome	Short stature, micrognathia, café-au-lait spots, normal intelligence hypoglycemia with fasting	May be difficult to intubate, monitor perioperative glucose and use glucose-containing solutions	Diner and others, 1994; Baum and O'Flaherty, 1999; Butler and others, 2000
S			
Saethre-Chotzen syndrome	Acrocephalosyndactyly, craniosynostosis, maxillary hypoplasia, normal intelligence, syndactyly	No reports of difficult intubation, may have increased ICP	Baum and O'Flaherty, 1999
Sanfilippo syndrome	Mucopolysaccharidosis III, coarse facies, rare cardiac involvement, severe developmental delay, behavioral disturbances, seizures	May be difficult intubation, anticonvulsant medication may affect neuromuscular blockade and opioid metabolism, may have behavioral problems	Kempthorne and Brown, 1983; Myles and Westhorpe, 1989; Baum and O'Flaherty, 1999
Schinzel-Giedion syndrome	Growth and mental deficiencies, congenital heart disease, seizures, renal anomalies, choanal atresia	Preoperative cardiac evaluation, anticonvulsant medication may affect neuromuscular blockade and opioid metabolism, check preoperative renal function	Baum and O'Flaherty, 1999; Butler and others, 2000
Schwartz-Jampel syndrome	Myotonia secondary to sodium channel defect, micrognathia, joint contractures	May be difficult intubation, myotonic contractures can occur during anesthetic or surgical manipulation, muscle relaxation does not relax contractions, hyperkalemia with succinylcholine, myotonic contractures can be precipitated by reversal of muscle relaxant, may be associated with malignant hyperthermia	Ray and Rubin, 1994; Theroux and others, 1995; Baum and O'Flaherty, 1999; Butler and others, 2000
Scimitar syndrome	Partial anomalous pulmonary venous return, hypoplastic right lower lobe, recurrent pulmonary infections, pulmonary HTN	Preoperative cardiac evaluation	Baum and O'Flaherty, 1999
Shprintzen syndrome	See Velocardiofacial syndrome		
Shwachman syndrome	Metaphyseal chondrodysplasia, recurrent pneumonia, hypotonia, short stature, exocrine pancreatic insufficiency, pancytopenia, immunologic abnormalities	Preoperative hematocrit and platelet count	Baum and O'Flaherty, 1999

Continued

Name	Description	Anesthetic Implications	References
Smith-Lemli-Opitz syndrome	Abnormality in cholesterol synthesis, microcephaly, micrognathia, lung hypoplasia, congenital heart disease, mental retardation, seizures, renal anomalies, thymic hypoplasia	May be difficult intubation, preoperative cardiac evaluation, anticonvulsant medication may affect neuromuscular blockade and opioid metabolism, blood should be irradiated if thymic hypoplasia, no clear association with malignant hyperthermia	Peterson and Crouch, 1995; Haji-Michael and Hatch, 1996; Baum and O'Flaherty, 1999; Butler and others, 2000
Sotos syndrome	Cerebral gigantism, excessive head growth, congenital heart disease, mental retardation, behavioral problems	No reports of difficult airway, preoperative cardiac evaluation	Jones and others, 1991; Baum and O'Flaherty, 1999
Stevens-Johnson syndrome	Secondary to hypersensitivity to exogenous agents (drugs), erythema multiforme, urticarial lesions	Placement of monitors may be difficult secondary to skin lesions, care with positioning	
Stickler syndrome	Flat facies, hearing loss, cleft palate, pectus excavatum, hyperextensible joints, may be associated with Pierre Robin sequence	May be difficult intubation, may have hearing loss	Baum and O'Flaherty, 1999
Sturge-Weber syndrome	Capillary hemangiomas in distribution of cranial nerve V, port wine stain, congenital glaucoma, may have mental retardation and seizures	Hemangiomas of the mouth and upper airway may make intubation difficult, may have increased intraocular pressure, anticonvulsant medication may affect neuromuscular blockade and opioid metabolism	Batra and others, 1994; Baum and O'Flaherty, 1999; Butler and others, 2000
T			
Tangier disease	Low high-density lipoprotein and serum cholesterol, orange tonsils, neuropathic abnormalities with cranial, sensory, or motor findings, muscle wasting, splenomegaly, hemolytic anemia, platelet dysfunction	Succinylcholine may cause hyperkalemia, check preoperative hematocrit and platelet count, possible premature ischemic heart disease	Mentis, 1996; Baum and O'Flaherty, 1999
Thrombocytopenia-absent radius syndrome (TAR syndrome)	Thrombocytopenia precipitated by stress, infection, surgery, congenital heart disease, bilateral absence of radii (thrombocytopenia worst during infancy)	Preoperative cardiac evaluation, check preoperative platelet count	Baum and O'Flaherty, 1999
Tourette syndrome	Involuntary motor and vocal tics, behavioral abnormalities	No specific anesthetic concerns	Morrison and Lockhart, 1986
Treacher Collins syndrome	Mandibulofacial dysostosis, malar hypoplasia, downsloping palbebral fissures, micro-ophthalmia, low-set ears, small mouth, micrognathia, obstructive sleep apnea, congenital heart disease	May be extremely difficult airway, fiberoptic endoscopy, LMA, and Bullard laryngoscope have all been used, preoperative cardiac evaluation	Rasch and others, 1986; Brown and others, 1993; Inada and others, 1995; Baum and O'Flaherty, 1999; Butler and others, 2000
Trisomy 8 syndrome	Strabismus, micrognathia, webbed neck, congenital heart disease, mental retardation, seizures	May be difficult intubation, anticonvulsant medication may affect neuromuscular blockade and opioid metabolism, preoperative cardiac evaluation	Baum and O'Flaherty, 1999
Trisomy 9 syndrome	May have microcephaly, cleft lip and palate, micrognathia, congenital heart disease, profound mental retardation	May be difficult intubation, anticonvulsant medication may affect neuromuscular blockade and opioid metabolism, preoperative cardiac evaluation	Baum and O'Flaherty, 1999
Trisomy 13 syndrome (Patau syndrome)	Occipital scalp defect, low-set ears, cleft lip and palate, micrognathia, congenital heart disease common, severe mental retardation, seizures, renal anomalies, capillary hemangiomas, most die within 6 months, radial anomalies	May be difficult intubation, preoperative cardiac evaluation, check preoperative renal function, placement of radial catheter may be difficult, anticonvulsant medication may effect neuromuscular blockade and opioids	Pollard and Beasley, 1996; Baum and O'Flaherty, 1999; Butler and others, 2000
Trisomy 18 syndrome (Edwards syndrome)	Prominent occiput, microcephaly, micrognathia, short sternum, congenital heart disease, clenched hands, rocker bottom feet, renal anomalies	May be difficult intubation, preoperative cardiac evaluation, check preoperative renal function	Baum and O'Flaherty, 1999; Butler and others, 2000
Trisomy 21 syndrome	See Down syndrome		
Tuberous sclerosis	Triad of mental retardation, seizures, and adenoma sebaceum on face, hamartomas of the lung, cardiac rhabdomyomas, may develop endocrinopathies	Oral adenomas may make intubation difficult, preoperative cardiac evaluation, spontaneous pneumothorax may occur, anticonvulsant medication may affect neuromuscular blockade and opioid metabolism	Lee and others, 1994; Schweiger and others, 1994; Baum and O'Flaherty, 1999; Butler and others, 2000
Turner syndrome	Caused by single X chromosome, micrognathia and short webbed neck, broad chest, congenital heart disease (coarctation), HTN, short stature, lymphedema of hands and feet, renal anomalies, may be hypothyroid	May be difficult intubation, preoperative cardiac evaluation, intravenous access may be difficult secondary to lymphedema, check preoperative renal function	Divekar and others, 1983; Baum and O'Flaherty, 1999; Butler and others, 2000

Name	Description	Anesthetic Implications	References
V			
VATER association	**V**ertebral anomalies, **a**nal atresia, **t**racheoesophageal fistula, **e**sophageal atresia, **r**adial and renal anomalies. Increased incidence in tracheoesophageal fistula, diabetic mothers, and trisomy 18	Preoperative cardiac evaluation, check radiographs of vertebrae and radii, check preoperative renal function	Baum and O'Flaherty, 1999; Butler and others, 2000
Velocardiofacial syndrome (Shprintzen syndrome)	Deletion of chromosome 22, microcephaly, micrognathia, congenital heart disease, developmental delay, may have T-cell immunodeficiency, neonatal hypocalcemia	May be difficult intubation, preoperative cardiac evaluation, blood should be irradiated if T-cell immunodeficiency, check preoperative calcium in neonates	Baum and O'Flaherty, 1999
von Hippel Lindau syndrome	Retinal, CNS, and visceral hemangioblastomas, may be associated with pheochromocytoma, may have renal, pancreatic, or hepatic cysts, may develop cerebellar tumors	Epidural analgesia has been described despite descriptions of spinal cord involvement, may have increased ICP, preoperative evaluation for pheochromocytoma	Matthews and Halshaw, 1986; Mugawar and others, 1998; Baum and O'Flaherty, 1999
W			
Walker-Warburg syndrome (HARD syndrome)	Retinal defects, microtia, cleft lip and palate, CNS anomalies, hydrocephalus, seizures, mental retardation, muscular dystrophy	May have increased intraocular pressure and ICP, anticonvulsant medication may affect neuromuscular blockade and opioid metabolism, succinylcholine may cause hyperkalemia	Baum and O'Flaherty, 1999
Watson syndrome	Valvular pulmonary stenosis, slightly decreased intelligence, may have neurofibromas and café-au-lait spots	Preoperative cardiac evaluation	Baum and O'Flaherty, 1999; Butler and others, 2000
Weaver syndrome	Macrocephaly, large tongue, short neck, developmental delay, seizures, behavioral problems	May be very difficult intubation, anticonvulsant medication may affect neuromuscular blockade and opioid metabolism	Turner and Downing, 1985; Baum and O'Flaherty, 1999
Weber-Christian disease	Fevers and panniculitis, necrosis of fat involving the retroperitoneal, pericardial, and meningeal areas, may have heart failure, involvement of retroperitoneal tissue may cause adrenal insufficiency, may develop restrictive pericarditis and seizures	Preoperative cardiac evaluation for cardiac failure, avoid trauma to fat, anticonvulsant medication may affect neuromuscular blockade and opioid metabolism	Baum and O'Flaherty, 1999
Weill-Marchesani syndrome	Glaucoma, blindness, subvalvular aortic stenosis	Preoperative cardiac evaluation	Baum and O'Flaherty, 1999
Werdnig-Hoffman disease	Spinal muscular atrophy, anterior horn cell degeneration, decreased ability to swallow, respiratory tract infections, may have respiratory failure spine deformities, normal intelligence	Increased risk of perioperative aspiration, may be chronically ventilated, succinylcholine may cause hyperkalemia	Baum and O'Flaherty, 1999; Butler and others, 2000
Whistling face syndrome	See Freeman-Sheldon syndrome		
Williams syndrome (Williams-Beuren syndrome)	Deletion of elastin gene on chromosome 7, elfin facies, severe congenital heart disease, high incidence of sudden death, mild developmental delay, may be very gifted musically, precocious social skills, "cocktail party personality," rarely has behavioral problems, may be hypercalcemic	Preoperative cardiac evaluation	Baum and O'Flaherty, 1999; Butler and others, 2000; Kececioglu and others, 1993
Wiskott-Aldrich syndrome	Recurrent pulmonary infections, vasculitis may affect coronary and cerebral arteries, renal insufficiency, thrombocytopenia, eczema, immune deficiency	Check preoperative platelet count and hematocrit, irradiate blood products, consider preoperative cardiac evaluation of coronary arteries, check preoperative renal function, consider stress-dose steroids if taking steroids on a chronic basis	Baum and O'Flaherty, 1999
Wolff-Parkinson-White syndrome	Accessory pathway bypasses atrioventricular node, reentrant tachycardia, may have structural heart disease	Adenosine and β-blockade terminate the tachycardia	Lavoie and others, 1995
Z			
Zellweger syndrome	Dysfunction and absence of peroxisomes, micrognathia, congenital heart disease, hypotonia with respiratory insufficiency, adrenal atrophy, contractures	Preoperative cardiac evaluation, care with positioning, may require stress-dose steroids	Baum and O'Flaherty, 1999

CNS, central nervous system; GERD, gastrointestinal reflux disease; HTN, hypertension; ICP, intracranial pressure; LMA, laryngeal mask airway.

REFERENCES

Antognini JF: Anaesthesia for Charcot-Marie-Tooth disease: A review of 86 cases. *Can J Anaesth* 39:398–400, 1992.

Axelrod FB, Donenfelf RF, Danziger RF, et al.: Anesthesia in familial dysautonomia. *Anesthesiology* 68:631–635, 1988.

Baraka A: Laryngeal mask airway for resuscitation of a newborn with Pierre Robin syndrome. *Anesthesiology* 83:645–646, 1996.

Baraka AS: Vecuronium neuromuscular blockade in a patient with Charcot-Marie-Tooth syndrome. *Anesth Analg* 84:927–928, 1997.

Barros F: Caudal block in a child with osteogenesis imperfecta, type II [letter]. *Paediatr Anaesth* 5:398–399, 1995.

Batra RK, Gulaya V, Madan R, et al.: Anaesthesia and the Sturge-Weber syndrome. *Can J Anaesth* 41:133–136, 1994.

Baum VC, O'Flaherty JE: *Anesthesia for genetic, metabolic, and dysmorphic syndromes of childhood.* Lippincott Williams and Wilkins, 1999, Philadelphia.

Berkowitz I, Raja S, Bender K, et al.: Dwarfs: Pathophysiology and anesthetic implications. *Anesthesiology* 73:39–59, 1990.

Borland LM: Anesthesia for children with Jeune's syndrome. *Anesthesiology* 66:86–88, 1987.

Brislin RP, Stayer SA, Schwartz RE: Anaesthetic considerations for the patient with cri du chat syndrome. *Paediatr Anaesth* 5:139–141, 1995.

Browder FH, Lew D, Shahbazian TS: Anesthetic management of a patient with Dutch-Kentucky syndrome. *Anesthesiology* 65:218–219, 1986.

Brown RE, Vollers JM, Rader GR, et al.: Nasotracheal intubation in a child with Treacher Collins syndrome using the Bullard intubating laryngoscope. *J Clin Anesth* 5:492–493, 1993.

Butler MG, Hayes BG, Hathaway MH, Begleiter ML: Specific genetic diseases at risk for sedation/anesthesia complications. *Anesth Analg* 91:837–855, 2000.

Campbell AM, Bousfield JD: Anaesthesia in a patient with Noonan's syndrome and cardiomyopathy. *Anaesthesia* 47:131–133, 1992.

Chapin JW, Kahre J: Progeria and anesthesia. *Anesth Analg* 58:424–425, 1979.

Choudry DK, Rehman MA, Schwartz RE, et al.: The Alagille syndrome and its anaesthetic considerations. *Paediatr Anaesth* 8:79–82, 1998.

Cook S: Cockayne syndrome: Another cause of difficult intubation. *Anaesthesia* 37:1104–1107, 1982.

Dearlove O, Dobson A, Super M: Anaesthesia and Prader-Willi syndrome. *Pediatr Anaesth* 8:267–271, 1998.

Dearlove O, Harper N: Costello syndrome. *Paediatr Anaesth* 7:476–477, 1997.

Dearlove OR, Walker RWM: Anaesthesia for Rett syndrome. *Paediatr Anaesth* 6:155–158, 1996.

Diner M, Goldin EZ, Ward R, et al.: Russell-Silver syndrome: Anesthetic implications. *Anesth Analg* 78:1197–1199, 1994.

Divekar VM, Kothari MD, Kamdar BM: Anaesthesia in Turner's syndrome. *Can Anaesth Soc J* 30:417–418, 1983.

Dresner DL, Ali HH: Anaesthetic management of a patient with fascioscapulohumeral muscular dystrophy. *Br J Anaesth* 62:331–334, 1989.

Dunkley CJA, Dearlove OR: Delayed recovery from anaesthesia in Rubinstein-Taybi syndrome. *Paediatr Anaesth* 6:245–246, 1996.

Dunn CM, Gunter JB, Quattromani A, et al.: Esmolol in the anaesthetic management of a boy with Romano-Ward syndrome. *Paediatr Anaesth* 1:129–132, 1991.

Ezri T, Szmuk P, Pansky A: Anaesthetic management for Klippel-Trenauney-Weber syndrome. *Paediatr Anaesth* 6:81, 1996.

Flashburg MH, Dunbar DS, August G, et al.: Anaesthesia for surgery on an infant with DiGeorge syndrome. *Anesthesiology* 58:479–480, 1983.

Frank JP, Harati Y, Butler IJ, et al.: Central cord disease and malignant hyperthermia. *Ann Neurol* 7:11–17, 1980.

Geva D, Ezri T, Szmuk P, et al.: Anaesthesia for Hecht Beals syndrome. *Paediatr Anaesth* 7:178–179, 1997.

Greenberg RS, Parker SD: Anesthetic management for the child with Charcot-Marie-Tooth disease. *Anesth Analg* 74:305–307, 1992.

Gurkowski MA, Rasch DK: Anesthetic considerations for Beckwith-Wiedemann syndrome. *Anesthesiology* 70:711–712, 1989.

Haji-Michael PG, Hatch DL: Smith-Lemli-Opitz syndrome and malignant hyperthermia. *Anesth Analg* 83:200, 1996.

Hayashi K, Chihara E, Sawa T, et al.: Clinical features of neuroleptic malignant syndrome: Spontaneous presentation in a patient with Hallervorden-Spatz syndrome in the absence of neuroleptic drugs. *Anaesthesia* 48:499–502, 1993.

Henderson AM, Vallis CJ, Sumner E: Anaesthesia and the prune-belly syndrome. *Anaesthesia* 42:54–60, 1987.

Higa K, Ishino H, Sato S, et al.: Anesthetic management of a patient with Bartter's syndrome. *J Clin Anesth* 5:321–324, 1993.

Ho AM, Friedland MJ: Kartagener's syndrome: Anesthetic considerations. *Anesthesiology* 77:386–388, 1992.

Holland JJ: Cardiac arrest under anaesthesia in a child with previously undiagnosed Jervell and Lange-Neilson syndrome. *Anaesthesia* 48:149–151, 1993.

Inada T, Fujise K, Kazuya T, et al.: Orotracheal intubation through the LMA in paediatric patients with Treacher Collins syndrome. *Paediatr Anaesth* 5:129–132, 1995.

Jagtap SR, Malde AD, Pantvaidya SH: Anaesthetic considerations in a patient with Fraser syndrome. *Anaesthesia* 50:39–41, 1995.

Jensen NF, Fiddler DS, Striepe V: Anesthetic considerations in porphyrias. *Anesth Analg* 80:591–599, 1995.

Joel M, Rosales JK: Fanconi syndrome and anesthesia. *Anesthesiology* 55:455–456, 1981.

Jones D, Doughty L, Brown K: Anaesthesia for a patient with Soto's syndrome. *Anaesth Intensive Care* 19:298–299, 1991.

Jones R, Dolcourt JL: Muscle rigidity following halothane anesthesia in two patients with Freeman-Sheldon syndrome. *Anesthesiology* 77:599–600, 1992.

Kalla GN, Fening E, Obiaya MO: Anaesthetic management of achondroplasia. *Br J Anaesth* 58:117–119, 1986.

Kanbak M: Ketamine and porphyria (letter). *Anesth Analg* 84:1395, 1997.

Kannan S, Delph Y, Moseley HSL: Anaesthetic management of a child with Bartter's. *Can J Anaesth* 42:808–812, 1995.

Kececioglu D, Kotthoff S, Vogt J: Williams-Beuren syndrome: A 30 year follow up of natural and postoperative course. *Eur Heart J* 14:1458–1464, 1993.

Kempthorne PM, Brown TCK: Anaesthesia and mucopolysaccharidosis: A survey of techniques and problems. *Anaesth Intensive Care* 11:203–207, 1983.

Laloyaux P, Veyckemans F, Van Dyck M: Anaesthetic management of a prematurely born infant with Cantrell's pentalogy. *Paediatr Anaesth* 8:163–166, 1998.

Lavoie J, Walsh EP, Burrows FA, et al.: Effects of propofol and isoflurane anesthesia on cardiac conduction in children undergoing radiofrequency catheter ablation for tachydysrhythmias. *Anesthesiology* 82:884–887, 1995.

LeBard SE, Thiemann LJ: Antley-Bixler syndrome: A case report and discussion. *Paediatr Anaesth* 8:89–91, 1998.

Lee JJ, Imrie M, Taylor V: Anaesthesia and tuberous sclerosis. *Br J Anaesth* 73:421–425, 1994.

Lininger TE, Brown EM, Brown M: General anesthesia and fibrodysplasia ossificans progressiva. *Anesth Analg* 68:175–176, 1989.

Madan R, Trikha, Venkataraman RK, et al.: Goldenhar's syndrome: An analysis of anaesthetic management. *Anaesthesia* 45:49–52, 1990.

Matthews AJ, Halshaw J: Epidural anesthesia in von Hippel Lindau disease: Management of childbirth and anaesthesia for cesarean section. *Anaesthesia* 41:853–855, 1986.

McFarlane HJ, Soni M: Pompe's disease and anaesthesia. *Anaesthesia* 41: 1219–1224, 1986.

McKenzie JW: Anaesthesia and the Prader-Willi syndrome. *J R Soc Med* 84:239, 1991.

Mentis SW: Tangier disease. *Anesth Analg* 83:427–429, 1996.

Michaloudis D, Fraisakis O, Lefaki I, et al.: Anaesthesia and the QT interval in humans: The effects of isoflurane and halothane. *Anaesthesia* 51:219–224, 1996.

Morrison JE, Lockhart CH: Tourette syndrome: Anesthetic complications. *Anesth Analg* 65:200–202, 1986.

Mugawar M, Rajender Y, Purohit AK, et al.: Anesthetic management of von Hippel-Lidau syndrome for excision of cerebellar hemangioblastoma and pheochromocytoma surgery. *Anesth Analg* 86:673–674, 1998.

Munoz Corsini L, Stefano G, Porras MC, et al.: Anaesthetic implications of Cornelia de Lange syndrome. *Paediatr Anaesth* 8:159–161, 1998.

Myles PS, Westhorpe RN: A patient with Sanfilippo syndrome and pseudocholinesterase deficiency, further complicated by post-tonsillectomy haemorrhage. *Anaesth Intensive Care* 17:86–88, 1989.

Newton MC, Allen PW, Ryan DC: Fibrodysplasia ossificans progressiva. *Br J Anaesth* 64:246–250, 1990.

Nishina K, Mikawa K, Maekawa N, et al.: Anaesthetic considerations in a child with leukodystrophy. *Paediatr Anaesth* 3:313–316, 1993.

Payne JF, Cranston AJ: Postoperative airway problems in a child with Crouzon's disease. *Paediatr Anaesth* 5:331–333, 1995.

Pennant JH, Harris MF: Anaesthesia for Proteus syndrome. *Anaesthesia* 46: 126–128, 1991.

Perkins JA, Sie KC, Milczuk H, et al.: Airway management in children with craniofacial anomalies. *Cleft Palate Craniofac J* 34:135–140, 1997.

Peterson WC, Crouch ER: Anesthesia induced rigidity, unrelated to succinylcholine, associated with Smith-Lemli-Opitz syndrome and malignant hyperthermia. *Anesth Analg* 80:606–608, 1995.

Pollard RC, Beasley JM: Anaesthesia for patients with trisomy 13 (Patau's syndrome). *Paediatr Anaesth* 6:151–153, 1996.

Populaire C, et al.: Elective tracheal intubation in the prone position for a neonate with Pierre Robin syndrome (letter). *Anesthesiology* 62:214, 1985.

Porsborg P, Astrup G, Bendixen D, et al.: Osteogenesis imperfecta and malignant hyperthermia: Is there a relationship? *Anaesthesia* 51:863–865, 1996.

Radu C, Reich DL, Tamman R: Anesthetic consideration in a cardiac surgical patient with Osler-Weber-Rendu disease. *J Cardiothorac Vasc Anesth* 6:461–464, 1992.

Rasch DK, Browder F, Barr M, et al.: Anaesthesia for Treacher Collins and Pierre Robin syndromes: A report of three cases. *Can Anaesthet Soc J* 33: 363–370, 1986.

Ravindran R, Stoops CM: Anaesthetic management of a patient with Hallerman-Streiff syndrome. *Anesth Analg* 58:254–255, 1979.

Ray S, Rubin AP: Anaesthesia in a child with Schwartz-Jampel syndrome. *Anaesthesia* 49:600–602, 1994.

Richardson MG, Roark GL, Helfaer MA: Intraoperative epinephrine induced torsades de pointes in a child with prolonged QT syndrome. *Anesthesiology* 76:647–649, 1992.

Rodrigo MRC, Cheng CH, Tai YT, et al.: "Leopard" syndrome. *Anaesthesia* 45:30–33, 1990.

Rosen KR, Broadman LM: Anaesthesia for diagnostic muscle biopsy in an infant with Pompe's disease. *Can Anaesth Soc J* 33:790–794, 1986.

Roy RC, McLain S, Wise A, et al.: Anesthetic management of a patient with Hallervorden-Spatz syndrome. *Anesthesiology* 58:382–384, 1983.

Russell SH, Hirsch NP: Anaesthesia and myotonia. *Br J Anaesth* 72:210–216, 1994.

Sasaki R, Hirota K, Masuda A: Nifedipine-induced transient cerebral ischaemia in a child with Cockayne syndrome. *Anaesthesia* 52:1236, 1997.

Schelle JG, Schulman SR: Fiberoptic bronchoscopic guidance for intubation of a neonate with Pierre Robin syndrome. *J Clin Anesth* 3:45–47, 1991.

Scholtes JL, Veyckemans F, Van Obbergh L, et al.: Neonatal anaesthetic management of a patient with Goldenhar's with hydrocephalus. *Anaesth Intensive Care* 15:338–340, 1987.

Schwartz N, Eisenkraft JB: Anesthetic management of a child with Noonan's syndrome and idiopathic subaortic stenosis. *Anesth Analg* 74:464–466, 1992.

Schweiger JW, Schwartz RE, Stayer SA: Anaesthetic management of the patient with tuberous sclerosis complex. *Paediatr Anaesth* 4:339–342, 1994.

Sethuraman R, Kannan S, Bala I, et al.: Anaesthesia and Poland syndrome. *Can J Anaesth* 45:277–279, 1998.

Stack CG, Wyse RK: Incidence and management of airway problems in CHARGE association. *Anaesthesia* 46:582–585, 1991.

Stenquist O, Sigurdsson J: The anaesthetic management of a patient with familial dysautonomia. *Anaesthesia* 37:929–932, 1982.

Stevenson GW, Hall SC, Palmieri J: Anesthetic considerations for patients with Larsen's syndrome. *Anesthesiology* 75:142–144, 1991.

Stirt JA: Anesthetic problems in Rubinstein-Taybi syndrome. *Anesth Analg* 60:534–536, 1981.

Suan C, Ojeda R, Garcia-Perla JL, et al.: Anaesthesia and the Beckwith-Wiedemann syndrome. *Paediatr Anaesth* 6:231–233, 1996.

Theroux MC, Kettrick RG, Khine HH: Laryngeal mask airway and fiberoptic endoscopy in an infant with Schwartz-Jampel syndrome. *Anesthesiology* 82:605, 1995.

Tobias J, Jones B, Jimenez DF, et al.: Anesthetic implications of Pfieffer syndrome. *Am J Anesth* 25:79–83, 1998.

Tobias JD: Anesthetic considerations for the child with leukodystrophy. *Can J Anaesth* 39:394–397, 1992.

Tobias JD: Anesthetic implications of Larsen's syndrome. *J Clin Anesth* 8:255–257, 1996;

Tobias JD, Atwood RA, Lowe S, et al.: Anesthetic considerations in the child with Gaucher disease. *J Clin Anesth* 5:150–153, 1993.

Turner DR, Downing JW: Anaesthetic problems associated with Weaver syndrome. *Br J Anaesth* 57:1260–1263, 1985.

Vas L, Naregal P: Anaesthetic management of a patient with Freeman Sheldon syndrome. *Paediatr Anaesth* 8:175–177, 1998.

Waring PH, Shaw DB, Brumfield CG: Anesthetic management of a parturient with Osler-Weber-Rendu syndrome and rheumatic heart disease. *Anesth Analg* 71:96–99, 1990.

Wells AL, Wells TR, Landing BH, et al.: Short trachea: A hazard in tracheal intubation of neonates and infants. *Anesthesiology* 71:367–373, 1989.

Wells DG, Podolakin W: Anaesthesia and Marfan's syndrome: Case report. *Can J Anaesth* 34:311–314, 1987.

White PC, New MI, Dupont B: Congenital adrenal hyperplasia. *N Engl J Med* 316:1580, 1987.

Williams JP, Someville GM, Miner ME, et al.: Atlanto-axial subluxation and trisemy-21: another preoperative complication. *Anesthesiology* 67:233–254, 1987.

Williams KS, Hankerson JG, Ernst M, et al.: Use of propofol anesthesia during outpatient radiographic imaging studies in patients with Lesch-Nyhan syndrome. *J Clin Anesth* 9:61–65, 1997.

Woolridge WJ, Dearlove OR, Khan AA: Anaesthesia for Cockayne syndrome: Three case reports. *Anaesthesia* 51:478–481, 1996.

Yamashita M, Matsuki A, Oyama T: Anaesthetic considerations in von Recklinghausen's disease: abnormal response to muscle relaxants. *Anaesthetist* 26: 317–318, 1977.

Yamashita M, Tanioka F, Taniguchi K, et al.: Anesthetic considerations in cri du chat syndrome: A report of three cases. *Anesthesiology* 63:201–202, 1985.

Index

Note: Page numbers followed by b indicate boxed material; those followed by f indicate figures; those followed by p indicate plates, and those followed by t indicate tables.

A

B

D

E

F

G

H

I

M

O

P

Q

R

S

T

U

V

W

X

Z